CORNEA

ELSEVIER DVD-ROM LICENSE AGREEMENT

PLEASE READ THE FOLLOWING AGREEMENT CAREFULLY BEFORE USING THIS DVD-ROM PRODUCT. THIS DVD-ROM PRODUCT IS LICENSED UNDER THE TERMS CONTAINED IN THIS DVD-ROM LICENSE AGREEMENT ('Agreement'). BY USING THIS DVD-ROM PRODUCT, YOU, AN INDIVIDUAL OR ENTITY INCLUDING EMPLOYEES, AGENTS AND REPRESENTATIVES ('You' or 'Your'), ACKNOWLEDGE THAT YOU HAVE READ THIS AGREEMENT, THAT YOU UNDERSTAND IT, AND THAT YOU AGREE TO BE BOUND BY THE TERMS AND CONDITIONS OF THIS AGREEMENT. ELSEVIER INC. ('Elsevier') EXPRESSLY DOES NOT AGREE TO LICENSE THIS DVD-ROM PRODUCT TO YOU UNLESS YOU ASSENT TO THIS AGREEMENT. IF YOU DO NOT AGREE WITH ANY OF THE FOLLOWING TERMS, YOU MAY, WITHIN THIRTY (30) DAYS AFTER YOUR RECEIPT OF THIS DVD-ROM PRODUCT RETURN THE UNUSED, PIN NUMBER PROTECTED, DVD-ROM PRODUCT, ALL ACCOMPANYING DOCUMENTATION TO ELSEVIER FOR A FULL REFUND.

DEFINITIONS

As used in this Agreement, these terms shall have the following meanings:

'Proprietary Material' means the valuable and proprietary information content of this DVD-ROM Product including all indexes and graphic materials and software used to access, index, search and retrieve the information content from this DVD-ROM Product developed or licensed by Elsevier and/or its affiliates, suppliers and licensors.

'DVD-ROM Product' means the copy of the Proprietary Material and any other material delivered on DVD-ROM and any other human-readable or machine-readable materials enclosed with this Agreement, including without limitation documentation relating to the same.

OWNERSHIP

This DVD-ROM Product has been supplied by and is proprietary to Elsevier and/or its affiliates, suppliers and licensors. The copyright in the DVD-ROM Product belongs to Elsevier and/or its affiliates, suppliers and licensors and is protected by the national and state copyright, trademark, trade secret and other intellectual property laws of the United States and international treaty provisions, including without limitation the Universal Copyright Convention and the Berne Copyright Convention. You have no ownership rights in this DVD-ROM Product. Except as expressly set forth herein, no part of this DVD-ROM Product, including without limitation the Proprietary Material, may be modified, copied or distributed in hardcopy or machine-readable form without prior written consent from Elsevier. All rights not expressly granted to You herein are expressly reserved. Any other use of this DVD-ROM Product by any person or entity is strictly prohibited and a violation of this Agreement.

SCOPE OF RIGHTS LICENSED (PERMITTED USES)

Elsevier is granting to You a limited, non-exclusive, non-transferable license to use this DVD-ROM Product in accordance with the terms of this Agreement. You may use or provide access to this DVD-ROM Product on a single computer or terminal physically located at Your premises and in a secure network or move this DVD-ROM Product to and use it on another single computer or terminal at the same location for personal use only, but under no circumstances may You use or provide access to any part or parts of this DVD-ROM Product on more than one computer or terminal simultaneously.

You shall not (a) copy, download, or otherwise reproduce the DVD-ROM Product in any medium, including, without limitation, online transmissions, local area networks, wide area networks, intranets, extranets and the Internet, or in any way, in whole or in part, except for printing out or downloading nonsubstantial portions of the text and images in the DVD-ROM Product for Your own personal use; (b) alter, modify, or adapt the DVD-ROM Product, including but not limited to decompiling, disassembling, reverse engineering, or creating derivative works, without the prior written approval of Elsevier; (c) sell, license or otherwise distribute to third parties the DVD-ROM Product or any part or parts thereof; or (d) alter, remove, obscure or obstruct the display of any copyright, trademark or other proprietary notice on or in the DVD-ROM Product or on any printout or download of portions of the Proprietary Materials.

RESTRICTIONS ON TRANSFER

This License is personal to You, and neither Your rights hereunder nor the tangible embodiments of this DVD-ROM Product, including without limitation the Proprietary Material, may be sold, assigned, transferred or sublicensed to any other person, including without limitation by operation of law, without the prior written consent of Elsevier. Any purported sale, assignment, transfer or sublicense without the prior written consent of Elsevier will be void and will automatically terminate the License granted hereunder.

TERM

This Agreement will remain in effect until terminated pursuant to the terms of this Agreement. You may terminate this Agreement at any time by removing from Your system and destroying the DVD-ROM Product. Unauthorized copying of the DVD-ROM Product, including without limitation, the Proprietary Material and documentation, or otherwise failing to comply with the terms and conditions of this Agreement shall result in automatic termination of this license and will make available to Elsevier legal remedies. Upon termination of this Agreement, the license granted herein will terminate and You must immediately destroy the DVD-ROM Product and accompanying documentation. All provisions relating to proprietary rights shall survive termination of this Agreement.

LIMITED WARRANTY AND LIMITATION OF LIABILITY

NEITHER ELSEVIER NOR ITS LICENSORS REPRESENT OR WARRANT THAT THE DVD-ROM PRODUCT WILL MEET YOUR REQUIREMENTS OR THAT ITS OPERATION WILL BE UNINTERRUPTED OR ERROR-FREE. WE EXCLUDE AND EXPRESSLY DISCLAIM ALL EXPRESS AND IMPLIED WARRANTIES NOT STATED HEREIN, INCLUDING THE IMPLIED WARRANTIES OF MERCHANTABILITY AND FITNESS FOR A PARTICULAR PURPOSE. IN ADDITION, NEITHER ELSEVIER NOR ITS LICENSORS MAKE ANY REPRESENTATIONS OR WARRANTIES, EITHER EXPRESS OR IMPLIED, REGARDING THE PERFORMANCE OF YOUR NETWORK OR COMPUTER SYSTEM WHEN USED IN CONJUNCTION WITH THE DVD-ROM PRODUCT. WE SHALL NOT BE LIABLE FOR ANY DAMAGE OR LOSS OF ANY KIND ARISING OUT OF OR RESULTING FROM YOUR POSSESSION OR USE OF THE SOFTWARE PRODUCT CAUSED BY ERRORS OR OMISSIONS, DATA LOSS OR CORRUPTION, ERRORS OR OMISSIONS IN THE PROPRIETARY MATERIAL, REGARDLESS OF WHETHER SUCH LIABILITY IS BASED IN TORT, CONTRACT OR OTHERWISE AND INCLUDING, BUT NOT LIMITED TO, ACTUAL, SPECIAL, INDIRECT, INCIDENTAL OR CONSEQUENTIAL DAMAGES. IF THE FOREGOING LIMITATION IS HELD TO BE UNENFORCEABLE, OUR MAXIMUM LIABILITY TO YOU SHALL NOT EXCEED THE AMOUNT OF THE LICENSE FEE PAID BY YOU FOR THE SOFTWARE PRODUCT. THE REMEDIES AVAILABLE TO YOU AGAINST US AND THE LICENSORS OF MATERIALS INCLUDED IN THE SOFTWARE PRODUCT ARE EXCLUSIVE.

If this DVD-ROM Product is defective, Elsevier will replace it at no charge if the defective DVD-ROM Product is returned to Elsevier within sixty (60) days (or the greatest period allowable by applicable law) from the date of shipment.

Elsevier warrants that the software embodied in this DVD-ROM Product will perform in substantial compliance with the documentation supplied in this DVD-ROM Product. If You report a significant defect in performance in writing to Elsevier, and Elsevier is not able to correct same within sixty (60) days after its receipt of Your notification, You may return this DVD-ROM Product, including all copies and documentation, to Elsevier and Elsevier will refund Your money.

YOU UNDERSTAND THAT, EXCEPT FOR THE 60-DAY LIMITED WARRANTY RECITED ABOVE, ELSEVIER, ITS AFFILIATES, LICENSORS, SUPPLIERS AND AGENTS, MAKE NO WARRANTIES, EXPRESSED OR IMPLIED, WITH RESPECT TO THE DVD-ROM PRODUCT, INCLUDING, WITHOUT LIMITATION THE PROPRIETARY MATERIAL, AND SPECIFICALLY DISCLAIM ANY WARRANTY OF MERCHANTABILITY OR FITNESS FOR A PARTICULAR PURPOSE.

If the information provided on this DVD-ROM Product contains medical or health sciences information, it is intended for professional use within the medical field. Information about medical treatment or drug dosages is intended strictly for professional use, and because of rapid advances in the medical sciences, independent verification of diagnosis and drug dosages should be made.

IN NO EVENT WILL ELSEVIER, ITS AFFILIATES, LICENSORS, SUPPLIERS OR AGENTS, BE LIABLE TO YOU FOR ANY DAMAGES, INCLUDING, WITHOUT LIMITATION, ANY LOST PROFITS, LOST SAVINGS OR OTHER INCIDENTAL OR CONSEQUENTIAL DAMAGES, ARISING OUT OF YOUR USE OR INABILITY TO USE THE DVD-ROM PRODUCT REGARDLESS OF WHETHER SUCH DAMAGES ARE FORESEEABLE OR WHETHER SUCH DAMAGES ARE DEEMED TO RESULT FROM THE FAILURE OR INADEQUACY OF ANY EXCLUSIVE OR OTHER REMEDY.

U.S. GOVERNMENT RESTRICTED RIGHTS

The DVD-ROM Product and documentation are provided with restricted rights. Use, duplication or disclosure by the U.S. Government is subject to restrictions as set forth in subparagraphs (a) through (d) of the Commercial Computer Restricted Rights clause at FAR 52.22719 or in subparagraph (c)(1)(ii) of the Rights in Technical Data and Computer Software clause at DFARS 252.2277013, or at 252.2117015, as applicable. Contractor/Manufacturer is Elsevier Inc., 360 Park Avenue South, New York, NY 10010 USA.

GOVERNING LAW

This Agreement shall be governed by the laws of the State of New York, USA. In any dispute arising out of this Agreement, You and Elsevier each consent to the exclusive personal jurisdiction and venue in the state and federal courts within New York County, New York, USA.

CORNEA

THIRD EDITION

Jay H Krachmer MD

Professor and Chair
Department of Ophthalmology
University of Minnesota Medical School
Minneapolis MN
USA

Mark J Mannis MD FACS

Professor and Chair
Department of Ophthalmology & Vision Science
UC Davis Health System Eye Center
University of California, Davis
Sacramento CA
USA

Edward J Holland MD

Professor of Ophthalmology
University of Cincinnati
Director, Cornea Services
Cincinnati Eye Institute
Cincinnati OH
USA

MOSBY
ELSEVIER

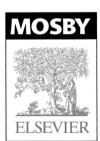

MOSBY
ELSEVIER

MOSBY is an imprint of Elsevier Inc.

First edition 1997
Second edition 2005

Notices

Knowledge and best practice in this field are constantly changing. As new research and experience broaden our understanding, changes in research methods, professional practices, or medical treatment may become necessary. Practitioners and researchers must always rely on their own experience and knowledge in evaluating and using any information, methods, compounds, or experiments described herein. In using such information or methods they should be mindful of their own safety and the safety of others, including parties for whom they have a professional responsibility. With respect to any drug or pharmaceutical products identified, readers are advised to check the most current information provided (i) on procedures featured or (ii) by the manufacturer of each product to be administered, to verify the recommended dose or formula, the method and duration of administration, and contraindications. It is the responsibility of practitioners, relying on their own experience and knowledge of their patients, to make diagnoses, to determine dosages and the best treatment for each individual patient, and to take all appropriate safety precautions.

To the fullest extent of the law, neither the Publisher nor the authors, contributors, or editors, assume any liability for any injury and/or damage to persons or property as a matter of products liability, negligence or otherwise, or from any use or operation of any methods, products, instructions, or ideas contained in the material herein.

ISBN 978 0 323 06387 6

Mosby
British Library Cataloguing in Publication Data
Cornea. – 3rd ed.
1. Cornea – Diseases.
I. Krachmer, Jay H. II. Mannis, Mark J. III. Holland, Edward J.
617.7′19 – dc22

Library of Congress Cataloging in Publication Data

The publisher's policy is to use paper manufactured from sustainable forests

A catalog record for this book is available from the Library of Congress
Printed in China
Last digit is the print number: 9 8 7 6 5 4 3 2 1

Commissioning Editor: Russell Gabbedy
Development Editor: Sharon Nash
Editorial Assistant: Kirsten Lowson
Project Manager: Alan Nicholson
Design: Charles Gray
Illustration Manager: Gillian Richards
Illustrator: Marion Tasker
Multimedia Producer: Fraser Johnston

Contents

Part VII: Diseases of the Cornea

Section 1: Developmental Abnormalities of Cornea

Section 2: Corneal Manifestations of Systemic Disease and Therapies

Section 3: Corneal Dystrophies, Ectatic Disorders, and Degenerations

Section 4: Corneal Infections

Section 5: Interstitial Keratitis

Section 6: Noninfectious Keratopathy

Section 7: Immunologic Disorders of the Cornea

DVD Contents

Clip	Clip title	Video contributor/s	Length
114.1	Penetrating Keratoplasty	David D. Verdier	00:02:51
114.2	Combined Penetrating Keratoplasty and Cataract Extraction	David D. Verdier	00:05:28
114.3	Penetrating Keratoplasty and Intraocular Lens Exchange	Michael L. Nordlund, Edward J. Holland	00:03:22
115.1	Femtosecond Assisted Penetrating Keratoplasty: Donor Preparation	Marjan Farid, Sumit Garg, Roger F. Steinert	00:01:26
115.2	Femtosecond Assisted Penetrating Keratoplasty: Dissection of Recipient Button and Donor Suturing	Marjan Farid, Sumit Garg, Roger F. Steinert	00:00:52
115.3	Femtosecond Assisted Penetrating Keratoplasty: Laser Incision	Marjan Farid, Sumit Garg, Roger F. Steinert	00:00:19
115.4	Femtosecond Assisted DALK (Zigzag Pattern)	Marjan Farid, Sumit Garg, Roger F. Steinert	00:03:00
130.1	Techniques of Anterior Lamellar Keratoplasty: Stromal Delamination	Luigi Fontana	00:01:02
130.2	Techniques of Anterior Lamellar Keratoplasty: ALTK 1	Luigi Fontana	00:08:47
130.3	Techniques of Anterior Lamellar Keratoplasty: ALTK 2	Luigi Fontana	00:06:12
130.4	Techniques of Anterior Lamellar Keratoplasty: Big Bubble	Luigi Fontana	00:04:26
130.5	Techniques of Anterior Lamellar Keratoplasty: Donor Preparation	Luigi Fontana	00:01:03
131.1	Intra-Operative and Post-Operative Complications of Anterior Lamellar Keratoplasty: Rupture of Descemet's Membrane (DM)	Shigeto Shimmura	00:05:07
134.1	Manual Dissection of the Donor for DSEK	Kenneth M. Goins	00:04:38
134.2	Microkeratome Dissection of the Donor for DSAEK	Kenneth M. Goins	00:02:37
134.3	Femtosecond Laser Donor Preparation for DSAEK	Greg Schmidt, Kenneth M. Goins	00:02:36
134.4	DMEK Donor Preparation	Greg Schmidt, Kenneth M. Goins	00:01:36
135.1	DSAEK Precut Tissue	W. Barry Lee	00:02:45
136.1	The New Triple Procedure	Michael L. Nordlund, Kristiana D. Neff, Edward J. Holland	00:09:50
139.1	Management of Corneal Perforations: Corneal Gluing	Andrew J.W. Huang	00:02:31
140.1	Therapeutic Lamellar Keratoplasty	Richard A. Eiferman, Sonya Yoo	00:01:12
142.1	Surgical Management of Superficial Corneal and Conjunctival Disease	Joseph M. Biber, Edward J. Holland	00:02:16
144.1	Harvesting the Conjunctival Autograft: Superficial Dissection Technique	Donald Tan, Cordelia Chan	00:00:34
144.2	Suturing the Conjunctival Autograft	Donald Tan, Cordelia Chan	00:00:56
144.3	Primary Pterygium Excision	Donald Tan, Cordelia Chan	00:02:15
144.4	Pterygium Excision with Conjunctival Autografting with Fibrin Glue	Donald Tan, Cordelia Chan	00:01:19
146.1	Orientation of the Amniotic Membrane	Jose L. Güell, Oscar Gris, Felicidad Manero, Marta Calatayud, Marta Torrabadella, Merce Morral	00:00:44
146.2	Amniotic Membrane Transplantation	Jose L. Güell, Oscar Gris, Felicidad Manero, Marta Calatayud, Marta Torrabadella, Merce Morral	00:03:27
148.1	Iris Reconstruction Surgery: ICE-IPS	Michael E. Snyder, Jason H. Bell	00:05:22
148.2	Iris Reconstruction Surgery: Humanoptics Iris for ICE	Michael E. Snyder, Jason H. Bell	00:00:27
148.3	Iris Reconstruction Surgery: Humanoptics Iris Injected	Michael E. Snyder, Jason H. Bell	00:03:00
148.4	Iris Reconstruction Surgery: Morcher 50-F	Michael E. Snyder, Jason H. Bell	00:01:55
148.5	Iris Reconstruction Surgery: Toric Disco 50-F	Michael E. Snyder, Jason H. Bell	00:03:32
151.1	Types and Techniques of Keratoprosthesis: OOKP Stage 1	Masahiko Fukuda, Oliver Comyn, Christopher Liu	00:02:03
151.2	Types and Techniques of Keratoprosthesis: OOKP Stage 2	Masahiko Fukuda, Oliver Comyn, Christopher Liu	00:02:55
155.1	Surgical Techniques for Ocular Surface Reconstruction: Clip 1	Edward J. Holland, Gary S. Schwartz, Sheraz M. Daya, Ali Djalilian	00:01:14
155.2	Surgical Techniques for Ocular Surface Reconstruction: Clip 2	Edward J. Holland, Gary S. Schwartz, Sheraz M. Daya, Ali Djalilian	00:01:15
155.3	Surgical Techniques for Ocular Surface Reconstruction: Clip 3	Edward J. Holland, Gary S. Schwartz, Sheraz M. Daya, Ali Djalilian	00:00:48
155.4	Surgical Techniques for Ocular Surface Reconstruction: Clip 4	Michael L. Nordlund, Edward J. Holland	00:03:50
157.1	Corneal Transplantation in Ocular Surface Disease	Joseph M. Biber, Kristiana D. Neff, Edward J. Holland, Mark J. Mannis	00:02:57
162.1	Keratome ILASIK	Stephen S. Lane, Deval R. Paranjpe, David H. Park	00:05:36
163.1	Femtosecond Laser LASIK	David R. Hardten	00:02:23
170.1	Peripheral Corneal Relaxing Incisions	Leela V. Raju, Douglas D. Koch	00:01:13
171.1	Alcon Acrysof Phakic IOL	David Park, Stephen Lane	00:05:01
	Total time of DVD:		**02:06:42**

Preface

In the age of instantaneous electronic information, a bound textbook may seem to some, perhaps, anachronistic. We, and even more so, our residents and fellows are accustomed to finding quick facts and lengthy lists of citations with but a few key strokes at the computer. The time spent rifling through the pages of journals in a library or working one's way through a hard copy text is, for better or worse, diminishing in favor of the agility of the computer – ever faster, ever smaller, and ever more convenient. Indeed, there are some advantages to modern day electronic texts – universal access in spite of time of day or location, portability, rapidity of information access, and the ability to do complex Boolean searches in moments. Such features save hours of time. For these very reasons, this edition is made available in an electronic format as well as the print version.

At the same time, a multi-authored text which has been forged through the process of gathering the best minds in the field, written and rewritten through a laborious and meticulous editing process, and presented as a comprehensive and authoritative source that can be turned to repeatedly is highly desirable as a bound document – codifying the current state of our knowledge in one place.

The practice of our subspecialty in ophthalmology is more diversified than ever before. The proliferation of new surgical procedures targeted to specific corneal abnormalities, a variety of new diagnostic testing capabilities, and a dramatic broadening of our understanding of the pathophysiology of the cornea and ocular surface have revolutionized what we know about the remarkable structure through which we view the world. We hope that this book will continue to serve as a useful tool to all students and practitioners in our field, both in print and electronic forms.

Jay H Krachmer
Mark J Mannis
Edward J Holland

Acknowledgments

These volumes are the result of the very hard work and thoughtful contributions of many people. First and foremost, we thank the contributing authors who provided extensive updates of previous work and a wealth of new material in this edition and who were so responsive to the demands of the editorial process. In addition, we cannot adequately thank Sharon Nash and Russell Gabbedy at Elsevier for their guidance, efficiency, responsiveness, resilience and good humor in the process of birthing this text. And as always, we thank our families who gave up so much time with us so that this book could be written.

To

my wife, Kathryn
our children, Edward, Kara, and Jill
our parents, Paul and Rebecca Krachmer
and Louis and Gertrude Maraist
with great love and appreciation

Jay H Krachmer

To

my sister, Libby, and in memory of my brother, Norman

Mark J Mannis

To

my wife, Lynette who is a great partner and always supportive
and our children, Colson, Kelsey and Natalie who keep me entertained,
challenged and grounded

Edward J Holland

Contributors

Richard L Abbott MD
Thomas W. Boyden, Endowed Chair
Health Science Clinical Professor of Ophthalmology
Research Associate, Francis I. Proctor Foundation
UCSF Department of Ophthalmology
San Francisco CA, USA
Chapter 122

Sean D Adrean MD
Vitreoretinal Fellow
Department of Ophthalmology
University of California Davis
Sacramento CA, USA
Chapter 38

Abdulrahman Al-Muammar MBBS FRCSC
Cornea, External Diseases and Uveitis Fellow
University of Ottawa Eye Institute
Ottawa ON, Canada
Chapter 161

Jihan Akhtar MD
Research Fellow
Department of Ophthalmology and Visual Sciences
College of Medicine, University of Illinois at Chicago
Chicago, IL, USA
Chapter 128

Eduardo C Alfonso MD
Medical Director, Ocular Microbiology Laboratory
Professor, Edward W D Norton Chair in Ophthalmology
Bascom Palmer Eye Institute
University of Miami
Miami FL, USA
Chapter 82

Richard C Allen MD PhD
Private Practice
Eye Associates of New Mexico
Albuquerque NM, USA
Chapter 31

M Camille Almond MD
Fellow
Department of Ophthalmology
University of Minnesota Medical School
Minneapolis MN, USA
Chapter 107

Lênio Alvarenga MD
Cornea and External Disease Fellow
External Eye Disease and Cornea Section
University of California, Davis
Federal University of São Paulo – UNIFESP
São Paulo SP
Brazil
Chapter 44

Wallace LM Alward MD
Professor of Ophthalmology
Director of Glaucoma Service
Department of Ophthalmology
University of Iowa Carver College of Medicine
Iowa City IA, USA
Chapter 58

Renato Ambrósio Jr MD
Medical Director
Visare Personal Laser and Refracta-RIO
Instituto de Olhos Renato Ambrósio
Rio de Janeiro RJ
Brazil
Chapter 164

Mohammad Anwar FRCS Edin FRCOphth
Senior Consultant Ophthalmic Surgeon
Cornea and External Diseases
Magrabi Eye Hospital
Dubai UAE
Chapter 129

Dimitri T Azar MD
B.A. Field Chair of Ophthalmologic Research
Professor and Head
Department of Ophthalmology and Visual Science
Illinois Eye and Ear Infirmary
Chicago IL, USA
Chapters 161 and 165

James L Ball MA FRCOphth
Consultant Ophthalmologist
Private Practice
Yorkshire Eye Hospital
Apperley Bridge
Bradford, UK
Chapter 132

Neal P Barney MD
Associate Professor of Ophthalmology
Department of Ophthalmology and Visual Sciences
University of Wisconsin School of Medicine
Madison WI, USA
Chapter 49

Rebecca M Bartow MD
Physician
Private Practice
Marshfield Clinic
Department of Ophthalmology
Marshfield WI, USA
Chapter 64

Jules Baum MD
Research Professor
Department of Ophthalmology
Tufts University School of Medicine
Boston MA, USA
Chapter 43

Michael W Belin MD FACS
Adjunct Professor of Ophthalmology and former Director of Cornea and Refractive Surgery
Department of Ophthalmology
Albany Medical College
Albany NY, USA
Chapters 151 and 160

Jason H Bell MD
Senior Resident
University of Cincinnati
University of Cincinnati Medical Center
Cincinnati OH, USA
Chapter 148

Beth Ann Benetz CRA FOPS
Associate Professor
Case Western Reserve University
University Hospitals Case Medical Center
Cleveland OH, USA
Chapter 14

Zachary Berbos MD
Medical Resident
Ophthalmology Department
Mayo Medical Center
Minneapolis MN, USA
Chapter 66

Roger W Beuerman PhD
Professor of Ophthalmology
Louisiana State University Health Sciences Center
School of Medicine
New Orleans LA, USA
Chapter 3

Arpita Kadakia Bhasin MD PhD
University of Illinois at Chicago
College of Medicine
Flossmoor IL, USA
Chapter 156

Pooja V Bhat MD
Clinical Research Fellow
David D Cogan Ophthalmic Pathology Lab
Massachusetts Eye and Ear Infirmary
Boston MA, USA
Chapter 41

Joseph M Biber MD
Resident
Horizon Eye Care
Charlotte NC, USA
Chapter 104

Maria Bidros MD MS
Resident of Ophthalmology
Department of Ophthalmology
University Hospitals Case Medical Center
Cleveland OH, USA
Chapter 14

Andrea D Birnbaum MD
Resident
University of Illinois at Chicago
Chicago IL, USA
Chapters 105 and 110

Charles S Bouchard MD
Professor and Chairman
Department of Ophthalmology
Loyola University Medical Center
Maywood IL, USA
Chapter 5

Jay C Bradley MD
Assistant Professor of Cornea and External Disease and Refractive Surgery
Department of Ophthalmology and Visual Sciences
Texas Tech University, HSC
Lubbock TX, USA
Chapters 119 and 152

James D Brandt MD
Professor and Director, Glaucoma Service
Department of Ophthalmology and Vision Science
University of California, Davis
Sacramento CA, USA
Chapter 124

Richard D Brasington MD FACP
Associate Professor of Medicine
Division of Rheumatology
Washington University School of Medicine
St. Louis MO, USA
Chapter 92

Harilaos S Brilakis MD MPH
Ophthalmic Surgeon
UltraLase Visual Correction
Athens
Greece
Chapter 52

Cat N Burkat MD
Assistant Professor
Department of Ophthalmology and Visual Sciences
University of Wisconsin Hospital and Clinics
Madison WI, USA
Chapter 29

Marta Calatayud MD
Department of Ophthalmology
Cornea and Ocular Surface Unit
Vall d'Hebron Hospitals
Barcelona, Spain
Chapter 146

J Douglas Cameron MD
Professor of Ophthalmology
Department of Ophthalmology
Mayo Clinic
Rochester MN, USA
Chapters 2 and 40

Mauro Campos MD
Professor of Ophthalmology
Department of Ophthalmology
Federal University of São Paulo
Vision Institute IPEPO
São Paulo-SP
Brazil
Chapter 169

Emmett F Carpel MD
Clinical Professor
Department of Ophthalmology
University of Minnesota
Hennepin County Medical Center
Minneapolis MN, USA
Chapter 75

H Dwight Cavanagh MD PhD
Vice Chairman of Ophthalmology and Associate Dean for Clinical Services
University of Texas Southwestern Medical Center
Dallas TX, USA
Chapters 15 and 101

Cordelia Chan MBBS FRCSEd MMed(Ophth) FAMS
Senior Consultant Ophthalmologist
Cornea and External Eye Disease Service
Singapore National Eye Centre
Singapore
Chapter 144

Richard I Chang MD
Medical Director
North Carolina Eye Bank
Graystone Eye Surgery Center
Hickory NC, USA
Chapter 76

Bernard H Chang MD
Private Practice
Cornea Consultants of Nashville
Nashville TN, USA
Chapter 90

Kenneth C Chern MD MBA
Clinical Professor of Ophthalmology
University of California San Francisco
Peninsula Ophthalmology Group
Burlingame CA, USA
Chapter 81

Steven Ching MD
Professor of Ophthalmology
University of Rochester Eye Institute
Rochester NY, USA
Chapter 76

James Chodosh MD
Professor of Opthalmology
University of Oklahoma Health Sciences Center
Oklahoma City OK, USA
Chapter 150

Phillip H Choo MD
Assistant Professor of Clinical Ophthalmology
Department of Ophthalmology
University of California Davis
Sacramento CA, USA
Chapter 38

Gary Chung MD
Private Practice
Evergreen Eye Center
Auburn WA, USA
Chapter 94

Joseph B Ciolino MD
Cornea Fellow
Massachusetts Eye and Ear Infirmary
Boston MA, USA
Chapter 151

Janine A Clayton (formerly Smith) MD
Deputy Clinical Director
Office of the Clinical Director
National Eye Institute
Bethesda MD, USA
Chapter 86

Elisabeth J Cohen MD
Director Cornea Service, Attending Surgeon
Cornea Service
Wills Eye Hospital
Philadelphia PA, USA
Chapters 18; 23 and 102

Oliver Comyn MA MRCOphth
Specialty Registrar in Ophthalmology
Sussex Eye Hospital
Brighton, UK
Chapter 151

M Soledad Cortina MD
Cornea and Refractive Surgery Fellow
Department of Ophthalmology
University of Illinois at Chicago Eye and Ear Infirmary
Chicago IL, USA
Chapter 93

John W Cowden MD
Professor of Ophthalmology
Department of Ophthalmology
Mason Eye Institute
Columbia MO, USA
Chapter 126

Christopher R Croasdale MD
Assistant Clinical Professor and Assistant Director of the Corneal Transplant and Refractive Surgery Fellowship program
Department of Ophthalmology
Cornea, External Disease and Refractive Surgery
University of Wisconsin
Davis Duehr Dean
Madison WI, USA
Chapter 24

Richard S Davidson MD
Assistant Professor
Rocky Mountain Lions Eye Institute
University of Colorado School of Medicine
Aurora CO, USA
Chapter 88

Elizabeth A Davis MD FACS
Adjunct Clinical Assistant Professor
Minnesota Eye Consultants
Minneapolis MN, USA
Chapter 163

Sheraz M Daya MD FACP FACS FRCS(Ed) FRCOphth
Medical Director
Centre for Sight
Director and Consultant
Corneo Plastic Unit and Eye Bank
Queen Victoria Hospital
East Grinstead, UK
Chapter 155

Denise de Freitas MD
Department of Ophthalmology
Federal University of São Paulo
São Paulo SP, Brazil
Chapter 127

David L DeMill BA
Medical Student
The University of Utah School of Medicine
Salt Lake City, Utah, USA
Chapter 118

Lauro Augusto de Oliveira MD
Keratoprosthesis Sector Coordinator
Vision Institute
Federal University of São Paulo – Brasil
São Paulo SP, Brazil
Chapter 153

Marc D de Smet MDCM PhD FRCSC FRCOphth
Professor and Head
Department of Ophthalmology
Academic Medical Center
Amsterdam, The Netherlands
Chapter 107

Luciene B de Sousa MD
Affiliated Professor
Federal University of São Paulo
Head of Cornea and External Diseases Section
UNIFESP
Medical Director
Sorocaba Eye Banking
President
APABO
São Paulo, Brazil
Chapter 72

Ali R Djalilian MD
Assistant Professor
Department of Ophthalmology and Visual Sciences
University of Illinois at Chicago
Chicago IL, USA
Chapters 36; 128; 155 and 156

Claes H Dohlman MD PhD
Professor of Ophthalmology
Harvard Medical School
Chief Emeritus
Massachusetts Eye and Ear Infirmary
Boston MA, USA
Chapter 150

Eric D Donnenfeld MD FACS
Clinical Professor of Ophthalmology, NYU
Trustee, Dartmouth Medical School
Founding Partner
Ophthalmic Consultants of Long Island
Rockville Centre NY, USA
Chapter 141

Richard K Dortzbach MD
Professor Emeritus
Department of Ophthalmology and Visual Sciences
University of Wisconsin – Madison
Madison WI, USA
Chapter 29

William T Driebe Jr MD
Professor of Ophthalmology/Cornea and External Disease
Department of Ophthalmology
University of Florida
Gainesville FL,USA
Chapter 54

Steven P Dunn MD
Director, Cornea Services
Department of Ophthalmology
William Beaumont Hospital
Royal Oak MI, USA
Chapter 50

Ralph C Eagle Jr MD
Director, Department of Pathology
Wills Eye Institute
Philadelphia PA, USA
Chapter 18

Sean L Edelstein MD
Instructor: Cornea, External Disease, and Refractive Surgery
Saint Louis University Department of Ophthalmology
Saint Louis MO, USA
Chapter 77

Richard A Eiferman MD FACS
Ophthalmologist, Surgeon
Corneal Surgery and External Eye Disease
Springs Medical Center
Louisville KY, USA
Chapter 140

Joseph A Eliason MD
Clinical Professor of Ophthalmology
Chair, Division of Ophthalmology
Santa Clara Valley Medical Center
San Jose CA, USA
Chapter 33

Marjan Farid MD
Assistant Professor
Department of Ophthalmology
University of California Irvine
Irvine CA, USA
Chapter 115

William J Faulkner MD
Cornea Specialist
Cincinnati Eye Institute
Cincinnati OH, USA
Chapter 10

Robert S Feder MD MBA
Associate Professor
Director, Cornea and External Disease Service
Department of Ophthalmology
Feinberg School of Medicine
Northwestern University
Chicago IL, USA
Chapter 74

Vahid Feiz MD
Assistant Professor of Ophthalmology
Department of Ophthalmology
University of California
Sacramento CA, USA
Chapter 21

Matthew T Feng MD
Research Fellow
Department of Ophthalmology and Vision Science
University of Arizona
Tucson AZ, USA
Chapter 86

John H Fingert MD PhD
Resident
Department of Ophthalmology and Visual Sciences
University of Iowa Hospitals and Clinics
Iowa City IA, USA
Chapter 12

George J Florakis MD
Associate Professor of Clinical Ophthalmology
Columbia University
New York NY, USA
Chapter 61

Luigi Fontana MD PhD
Cornea Service
Ospedale Maggiore
Director, Emilia-Romagna Eye Bank
Bologna, Italy
Chapter 130

Richard K Forster MD
Professor
The Richard K. Forster Chair in Corneal and External Ocular Diseases
Bascom Palmer Eye Institute
Miami FL, USA
Chapter 20

C Stephen Foster MD
Professor of Ophthalmology
The Massachusetts Eye and Ear Infirmary
Cambridge MA, USA
Chapter
Chapter 51

F Stuart Foster PhD
Professor
University of Toronto
Sunnybrook Health Sciences Centre
Toronto ON
Canada
Chapter 16

Gary N Foulks MD FACS
Arthur and Virginia Keeney Professor of Ophthalmology
University of Louisville School of Medicine
Louisville KY
USA
Chapters 34 and 121

Mitchell H Friedlander MD
Division Head
Ophthalmology
Scripps Clinic CA, USA
Chapter 48

Masahiko Fukuda MD DSc
Assistant Professor
Department of Ophthalmology
Kinki University School of Medicine
Osaka, Japan
Chapter 151

Anat Galor MD
Associate Professor of Clinical Ophthalmology
Department of Ophthalmology
Bascom Palmer Eye Institute
Miami FL, USA
Chapter 82

Theresa J Gan MD
Resident in Ophthalmology
Northwestern University
Chicago IL, USA
Chapter 74

Prashant Garg MD
Distinguished Chair of Education
Consultant, Cornea and Anterior Segment Services
Medical Director, Ramayamma International Eye Bank
L V Prasad Eye Institute
L V Prasad Marg
Banjara Hills
Hyderabad
Andhra Pradesh, India
Chapters 84 and 95

Sumit Garg MD
Clinical Instructor in Ophthalmology
The Gavin Herbert Eye Institute
Department of Ophthalmology
University of California, Irvine
Irvine CA, USA
Chapter 115

David B Glasser MD
Assistant Professor of Ophthalmology
Johns Hopkins University School of Medicine
Columbia MD, USA
Chapter 28

Kenneth M Goins MD
Professor of Clinical Ophthalmology
Corneal and External Diseases
University of Iowa Hospitals and Clinics
Iowa City IA, USA
Chapter 134

Debra A Goldstein MD FRCS(C)
Associate Professor of Ophthalmology
Director, Uveitis Service
Department of Ophthalmology and Visual Sciences
University of Illinois at Chicago
Chicago IL, USA
Chapter 110

Chloe Gottlieb MD FRCSC
Clinical Fellow, Uveitis and Ocular Immunology
National Eye Institute
National Institutes of Health
Bethesda, MD, USA
Chapter 105

Michael R Grimmett MD FACP FACS
Assistant Professor of Ophthalmology
Bascom Palmer Eye Institute
University of Miami School of Medicine
Miami FL, USA
Chapter 63

Oscar Gris MD
Instituto de Microcirugia Ocular (IMO)
Barcelona, Spain
Chapter 146

Erich B Groos Jr MD
Partner
Cornea Consultants of Nashville
Nashville TN, USA
Chapter 90

William D Gruzensky MD
Corneal Consultant and Anterior Segment Surgeon
Pacific Cataract and Laser Institute
Tacoma WA, USA
Chapter 47

Jose L Güell MD APO
Associate Professor of Ophthalmology
Autonoma University of Barcelona
Director of Cornea and Refractive Surgery Unit
Instituto Microcirugia Ocular de Barcelona
Barcelona, Spain
Chapter 146

Preeya K Gupta MD
Resident
Department of Ophthalmology
Duke University School of Medicine
Duke University Eye Center
Durham NC, USA
Chapter 57

M Bowes Hamill MD
Associate Professor
Department of Ophthalmology
Baylor College of Medicine
Houston TX, USA
Chapters 97 and 149

Kristin M Hammersmith MD
Assistant Surgeon
Cornea Service
Wills Eye Hospital
Instructor, Thomas Jefferson Medical College
Philadelphia PA, USA
Chapters 18 and 123

Pedram Hamrah MD
Assistant Professor, Department of Ophthalmology
Director, Ocular Surface Imaging Center
Attending Physician, Cornea and Refractive Surgery
Massachusetts Eye and Ear Infirmary
Harvard Medical School
Boston, MA, USA
Chapters 36 and 128

Sadeer B Hannush MD
Assistant Professor of Ophthalmology
Jefferson Medical College
Attending Surgeon
Cornea Service
Wills Eye Institute
Philadelphia PA
USA
Chapters 113 and 152

David R Hardten MD FACS
Director of Refractive Surgery
Adjunct Associate Professor of Ophthalmology
University of Minnesota
Minnesota Eye Consultants
Minneapolis MN, USA
Chapter 163

Andrew Harrison MD
Associate Professor
Director, Oculoplastic and Orbital Surgery
Departments of Ophthalmology and Otolaryngology
University of Minnesota
Minneapolis MN, USA
Chapter 4

Ellen L Heck MT MA
Director
Transplant Services Center
University of Texas Southwestern Medical Center
Dallas TX, USA
Chapter 27

David G Heidemann MD
Private Practice
Michigan Cornea Consultants
Southfield MI, USA
Chapter 50

David C Herman MD MSMM
Associate Professor of Ophthalmology
Mayo Clinic College of Medicine
Rochester MN, USA
Chapter 109

J Martin Heur MD PhD
Clinical Instructor of Ophthalmology
Doheny Eye Insitute
Los Angeles CA, USA
Chapter 17

William G Hodge MD MPH PhD FRCSC
Associate Professor of Ophthalmology
Cornea and External Disease
The University of Ottawa Eye Instiure
The Ottawa Hospital
Ottawa ON, Canada
Chapter 106

Carol J Hoffman MD
Medical Director
Eye Surgeons
Kremer Laser Eye Center
Wilmington DE, USA
Chapter 69

Edward J Holland MD
Professor of Ophthalmology
University of Cincinnati
Director, Cornea Services
Cincinnati Eye Institute
Cincinnati OH, USA
Chapters 52; 55; 79; 112; 136; 154; 155; 156 and 157

Gary N Holland MD
Vernon O Underwood Family Professor of Ophthalmology
Chief, Cornea-External Ocular Disease and Uveitis Division
University of California, Los Angeles
Los Angeles CA, USA
Chapter 67

Marc A Honig MD
Attending Surgeon
Private Practice
Brull and Honig
Owings Mills MD
USA
Chapter 139

Christopher T Hood MD
Resident in Ophthalmology
The Cleveland Clinic Foundation
Cleveland OH
USA
Chapter 67

Eliza N Hoskins MD
Proctor Fellow
Francis I Proctor Foundation for Research in Ophthalmology
University of California, San Francisco
San Francisco, CA, USA
Chapter 122

Andrew J W Huang MD MPH
Professor, Ophthalmology and Visual Sciences
Department of Ophthalmology
Washington University School of Medicine
St Louis MO, USA
Chapter 77

David Huang MD PhD
Associate Professor of Ophthalmology
Department of Ophthalmology
Doheny Eye Institute
University of Southern California
Los Angeles CA, USA
Chapter 17

Jennifer I Hui MD
Professor of Clinical Ophthalmology
Bascom Palmer Eye Institute
University of Miami Miller School of Medicine
Miami FL
USA
Chapter 32

Joseph D Iuorno MD
Clinical Instructor
Department of Ophthalmology
University of Minnesota
Minneapolis MN, USA
Chapter 26

W Bruce Jackson MD FRCS
Professor and Chairman
Department of Ophthalmology
University of Ottawa
Director General
University of Ottawa Eye Institute
Ottawa ON, Canada
Chapter 161

Frederick A Jakobiec MD DSc(Med)
Professor Emeritus of Ophthalmology and Pathology
Massachusetts Eye and Ear Infirmary
David G Cogan Ophthalmic Pathology Laboratory
Boston MA, USA
Chapters 39 and 41

Bennie H Jeng MD
Associate Professor of Clinical Ophthalmology
Director, Ocular Surface and Keratoprosthesis Program
Chief, Department of Ophthalmology
San Francisco General Hospital
University of California, San Francisco
San Francisco CA, USA
Chapters 67 and 122

James V Jester PhD
Professor of Ophthalmology
The Eye Institute
University of California, Irvine
Orange CA, USA
Chapter 15

David R Jordan MD FRCSC
Professor of Ophthalmology
Department of Ophthalmology
University of Ottawa Eye Institute
Ottawa ON, Canada
Chapter 37

Terry L Kaiura MD FACS
Assistant Professor of Ophthalmology
New York Eye and Ear Infirmary
Mineola NY, USA
Chapter 61

Carol L Karp MD
Associate Professor of Clinical Ophthalmology
Department of Ophthalmology
Bascom Palmer Eye Insititute
Miami FL, USA
Chapter 20

Douglas G Katz MD
Assistant Professor
Cornea, External Disease and Refractive Surgery
Department of Ophthalmology
University of Kentucky
Lexington KY, USA
Chapter 116

Stephen C Kaufman MD PhD
Professor and Lyon Endowed Chair of Ophthalmology
Director of Cornea and Refractive Surgery
Department of Ophthalmology
University of Minnesota
Minneapolis MN, USA
Chapter 19

Robert C Kersten MD
Associate Professor of Ophthalmology
University of Cincinnati Medical School
Cincinnati Eye Institute
Cincinnati OH, USA
Chapter 30

Stephen S Khachikian MD
Cornea Fellow
Department of Ophthalmology
Albany Medical College
Albany NY, USA
Chapter 160

Jennifer H Kim MD
Resident
Wills Eye Hospital
Philadelphia PA, USA
Chapter 23

Joung Y Kim MD
Assistant Professor
Department of Ophthalmology
Emory University School of Medicine
Atlanta GA, USA
Chapter 78

Stella K Kim MD
Assistant Professor
Section of Ophthalmology
MD Anderson Cancer Center
Houston TX, USA
Chapter 68

Terry Kim MD
Professor of Ophthalmology
Duke University School of Medicine
Associate Director
Cornea and Refractive Surgery
Duke University Eye Center
Durham NC, USA
Chapter 57

Colin M Kirkness
Tennent Professor of Ophthalmology
Department of Ophthalmology
Faculty of Medicine
University of Glasgow
Glasgow UK
Chapter 62

Stephen D Klyce PhD
Adjunct Professor of Ophthalmology
Mount Sinai School of Medicine
New York NY, USA
Chapter 13

Douglas D Koch MD
Professor of Ophthalmology
Department of Ophthalmology
Baylor College of Medicine
Houston TX, USA
Chapter 170

Regis P Kowalski MS (M)ASCP
Associate Professor of Ophthalmology
Associate Director of the Charles T. Campbell Ophthalmic Microbiology Laboratory
Ophthalmic Microbiology
The Eye and Ear Institute
University of Pittsburgh
Pittsburgh PA, USA
Chapter 11

Jay H Krachmer MD
Professor and Chair
Department of Ophthalmology
University of Minnesota Medical School
Minneapolis MN, USA
Chapters 9 and 66

Peter R Laibson MD
Professor of Ophthalmology
Thomas Jefferson University School of Medicine
Director Emeritus
Cornea Service
Wills Eye Institute
Philadelphia PA, USA
Chapters 69 and 71

Stephen S Lane MD
Adjunct Clinical Professor
Department of Ophthalmology
University of Minnesota
Associated Eye Care
Stillwater MN, USA
Chapters 162 and 171

Jonathan H Lass MD
Charles I Thomas Professor and Chairman
Department of Ophthalmology and Visual Sciences
University Hospitals Case Medical Center
Cleveland OH, USA
Chapter 14

W Barry Lee MD
Cornea, External Disease, and Refractive Surgery
Eye Consultants of Atlanta
Atlanta GA, USA
Chapters 80 and 135

Olivia A Lee MD
Cornea, External Disease and Refractive Surgery Fellow
Associate Faculty
Department of Ophthalmology
Emory University School of Medicine
Atlanta GA, USA
Chapters 125

Michael A Lemp MD
Clinical Professor of Ophthalmology
Department of Ophthalmology
Georgetown and George Washington Universities
Washington DC, USA
Chapters 3; 8 and 34

Phoebe D Lenhart MD
Assistant Professor of Ophthalmology
Emory Eye Center
Emory University School of Medicine
Atlanta GA, USA
Chapter 125

Yan Li PhD
Senior Research Associate
Department of Ophthalmology
University of Southern California
Doheny Eye Institute
Los Angeles CA, USA
Chapter 17

Thomas J Liesegang MD
Professor of Ophthalmology
Mayo Clinic College of Medicine
Jacksonville FL, USA
Chapter 80

Michele C Lim MD
Medical Director
University of California Davis Health Service
Department of Ophthalmology and Vision Science
Sacramento CA, USA
Chapter 124

Lily Koo Lin MD
Assistant Professor
Department of Ophthalmology
University of California Davis Eye Center
Sacramento CA, USA
Chapter 38

Michael P Lin MD MS
Resident Physician
Aesthetic and Plastic Surgery Institute
University of California, Irvine
Orange CA, USA
Chapter 4

Thomas D Lindquist MD PhD
Director, Corneal and External Disease Service
Group Health Cooperative
Medical Director, SightLife
Group Health Eastside Speciality Center
Redmond WA, USA
Chapters 42 and 46

Richard L Lindstrom MD
Adjunct Professor of Ophthalmology
University of Minnesota Medical School
Minnesota Eye Consultants, PA
Minneapolis MN, USA
Chapter 163

David Litoff MD
Chief of Ophthalmology
Kaiser Permanente
Clinical Institute at University of Colorado
Boulder CO, USA
Chapter 25

Christopher Liu FRCOphth
Honorary Clinical Senior Lecturer
Consultant Ophthalmic Surgeon
Sussex Eye Hospital
Brighton
Sussex, UK
Chapter 151

Careen Y Lowder MD PhD
Staff Physician
Division of Ophthalmology
Cole Eye Institute
Cleveland Clinic Foundation
Cleveland OH, USA
Chapter 67

Anthony J Lubniewski MD
Associate Professor
Cornea, External Disease and Refractive Surgery
Washington University
St Louis MO, USA
Chapter 92

Hall T McGee MD
Specialist in Medical and Surgical Treatment of the Cornea
Everett and Hurite Ophthalmic Association
Pittsburgh PA, USA
Chapter 6

Ian W McLean MD
Formerly
Chief
Division of Ophthalmic Pathology
Armed Forces Institute of Pathology
Washington DC, USA
Chapter 40

Marian S Macsai MD
Chief, Division of Ophthalmology
Evanston Northwestern Healthcare
Professor and Vice Chair
Department of Ophthalmology
Northwestern University Feinberg School of Medicine
Glenview IL, USA
Chapter 147

Felicidad Manero MD
Instituto de Microcirugia Ocular (IMO)
Barcelona, Spain
Chapter 146

Mark J Mannis MD FACS
Professor and Chair
Department of Ophthalmology & Vision Science
UC Davis Health System Eye Center
University of California, Davis
Sacramento, CA, USA
Chapters 9; 44; 53; 72; 88; 112; 145; 153 and 157

Dimosthenis Mantopoulos MD
Clinical Fellow
Harvard Medical School
Boston MA, USA
Chapter 128

Carlos E Martinez MD MS
Assistant Clinical Professor of Ophthalmology
University of California Irvine, Irvine CA
Director, Eye Physicians of Long Beach
Long Beach CA, USA
Chapter 13

Csaba L Mártonyi CRA FOPS
Emeritus Associate Professor
Department of Ophthalmology and Visual Sciences
University of Michigan Medical School
Ann Arbor MI, USA
Chapter 7

Raneen S Mashor MD
Ophthalmologist, Corneal Fellow
Toronto Western Hospital
University of Toronto
Toronto, Canada
Chapter 59

William D Mathers MD
Professor of Ophthalmology
Oregon Health and Science University
Casey Eye Institute
Portland OR, USA
Chapter 6

Manisha N Mehta MD
Pathology Fellow,
Massachusetts Eye and Ear Infirmary
Boston MA, USA
Chapter 39

David M Meisler MD FACS
Professor of Ophthalmology
Cleveland Clinic Lerner College of Medicine
Cole Eye Institute
Cleveland OH, USA
Chapters 67 and 81

Shahzad I Mian MD
Assistant Professor
Ophthalmology and Visual Sciences Department
Kellogg Eye Institute
University of Michigan
Ann Arbour MI, USA
Chapter 96

Darlene Miller MPH MA SM
Technical Director – Ocular Microbiology
Laboratory Director
University of Miami Miller School of Medicine
Miami FL, USA
Chapter 82

Corey A Miller MD
Clinical Associate Professor
Department of Ophthalmology
University of Utah
Salt Lake City UT, USA
Chapter 118

Monty Montoya BS MBA
President and CEO
Sightlife
Seattle WA, USA
Chapter 27

Merce Morral MD PhD
Specialist in Cornea and Refractive Surgery
Instituto de Microcirugia Ocular (IMO)
Institut Clínic d'Oftalmologia (ICOF)
Hospital Clinic i Provincial de Barcelona
Barcelona, Spain
Chapter 146

Andrew L Moyes MD
Clinical Assistant Professor
University of Kansas
Moyes Eye Center
Kansas City MO, USA
Chapter 35

Michael L Murphy MD FACS
Ophthalmic Plastic and Reconstructive Specialty General Ophthalmology Surgeon
Private Practice
Medical Eye Associates
Moreland Medical Center
Waukesha WI, USA
Chapter 31

Nariman Nassiri MD
Research Fellow
Department of Ophthalmology and Visual Sciences
University of Illinois at Chicago
Chicago IL, USA
Chapter 36

Kristiana D Neff MD
Assistant Professor of Clinical Ophthalmology
Department of Ophthalmology
University of South Carolina
Columbia SC, USA
Chapters 55; 79; 136; 157 and 166

J Daniel Nelson MD FACS
Professor of Ophthalmology
University of Minnesota
Associate Medical Director
HealthPartners Medical Group
Minneapolis MN, USA
Chapter 2

Jeffrey A Nerad MD FACS
Professor of Ophthalmology and Otolaryngology
Director, Oculoplastic, Orbital and Oncology Service
Department of Ophthalmology
University of Iowa Hospitals and Clinics
Iowa City IA, USA
Chapter 31

Marcelo V Netto MD
Cornea and Refractive Surgery Staff
Department of Ophthalmology
University of São Paulo
São Paulo, Brazil
Chapter 164

Christopher J Newton MD
Cornea Fellow
Department of Ophthalmology
University of Minnesota Medical School
Minneapolis MN, USA
Chapter 62

Lisa M Nijm MD JD
Senior Fellow
Department of Ophthalmology and Vision Science
University of California Davis
Sacramento CA, USA
Chapters 91 and 112

Teruo Nishida MD DSc
Dean, Professor and Chairman
Department of Ophthalmology
Yamaguchi University Graduate School of Medicine
Ube
Yamaguchi, Japan
Chapter 1

Bruce A Noble BSc FRCS FRCOphth
Consultant Ophthalmologist
BUPA Hospital
Leeds, UK
Chapter 132

Michael L Nordlund MD PhD
Assistant Professor of Ophthalmology
University of Cincinnati and Cincinnati Eye Institute
Cincinnati OH, USA
Chapter 136 Phacoemulsification and Endothelial Keratoplasty: the New Triple Procedure
Chapter 155

Robert B Nussenblatt MD MPH
Chief, Laboratory of Immunology
National Eye Institute
Bethesda MD, USA
Chapter 105

David G O'Day MD
Ophthalmic Surgeon
Charleston Cornea and Refractive Surgery, PA
Mount Pleasant SC, USA
Chapter 124

Jenny V Ongkosuwito MD
Assistant Professor
Department of Ophthalmology
Academic Medical Center
University of Amsterdam
Amsterdam, The Netherlands
Chapter 107

Karen W Oxford MD
Director of Corneal and External Diseases
Pacific Eye Associates
San Francisco CA, USA
Chapter 122

David A Palay MD
Associate Clinical Professor
Department of Ophthalmology
Emory University School of Medicine
Atlanta GA, USA
Chapter 22

Florentino E Palmon MD
Medical Director
Southwest Florida Eye Care
Fort Myers FL, USA
Chapter 52

Deval R Paranjpe MD ScB
Assistant Professor of Ophthalmology
Drexel University College of Medicine
Pittsburgh PA, USA
Chapters 62 and 162

Mansi Parikh MD
Assistant Professor
Casey Eye Institute
Oregon Health & Science University
Portland OR, USA
Chapter 58

David H Park MD
Adjunct Assistant Professor
Department of Ophthalmology
University of Minnesota
Stillwater MN, USA
Chapters 162 and 171

D J John Park MD
Resident
Aesthetic and Plastic Surgery Institute
University of California, Irvine
Orange CA, USA
Chapter 4

Matthew R Parsons MD
Chief
Corneal Service
Excel Eye Center
Provo UT, USA
Chapter 91

Charles J Pavlin MD FRCS(Can)
Professor, University of Toronto
Department of Ophthalmology
Mount Sinai Hospital
Toronto ON, Canada
Chapter 16

Eric S Pearlstein MD
Assistant Attending
Ophthalmology Associates of Bay Ridge
Brooklyn NY, USA
Chapter 103

Alicia Perry BA
Ophthalmic Consultants of Long Island
New York, NY USA
Chapter 141

W Matthew Petroll MD
Professor of Ophthalmology
Department of Ophthalmology
University of Texas Southwestern Medical Center
Dallas TX, USA
Chapter 15

Daryl R Pfister MD
Private Practice
Chandler AZ, USA
Chapters 98 and 99

Roswell R Pfister MD
Professor of Ophthalmology
University of Alabama
Birmingham AL, USA
Chapters 98 and 99

Stephen C Pflugfelder MD
Professor of Ophthalmology
Department of Ophthalmology
The Cullen Eye Institute
Baylor College of Medicine
Houston TX, USA
Chapter 36

Francis W Price Jr MD
President
Price Vision Group
Indianapolis IN, USA
Chapter 133

Marianne O Price PhD
Director of Research and Education
Cornea Research Foundation of America
Indianapolis IN, USA
Chapter 133

Louis E Probst MD
Medical Director
TLC Vision
Ann Arbor MI, USA
Chapter 166

John J Purcell Jr MD FACS
Clinical Professor of Ophthalmology
Department of Ophthalmology
St Louis University School of Medicine
St Louis MO, USA
Chapter 117

Andrew A E Pyott MBChB BSc FRCs(Glas) FRCOphth
Consultant Ophthalmologist
Head of Service, Department of Ophthalmology
Raigmore Hospital
Inverness, UK
Chapter 62

Michael B Raizman MD
Private Practice
Ophthalmic Consultants of Boston
Boston MA, USA
Chapters 48 and 104

Leela V Raju MD
Clinical Fellow – Cornea, Cataract, Refractive, and External Disease
Cullen Eye Institute
Baylor College of Medicine
Houston TX, USA
Chapter 170

J Bradley Randleman MD
Associate Professor
Emory Eye Institute
Atlanta GA, USA
Chapters 167 and 168

Gullapalli N Rao MD
Distinguished Chair of Eye Health
L V Prasad Eye Institute
L V Prasad Marg
Banjara Hills
Hyderabad
Andhra Pradesh, India
Chapter 84

Christopher J Rapuano MD
Co-Director, Cornea Service
Professor of Ophthalmology
Jefferson Medical College
Wills Eye Hospital
Philadelphia PA, USA
Chapters 18; 23; 123; 139; 142 and 143

Charles D Reilly MD Maj USAF MC FS
Fellow, Cornea and External Disease
University of California Davis Medical Center
Sacramento CA, USA
Chapter 53

Adimara de Candelaria Renesto MD
Fellow of Refractive Surgery
Department of Ophthalmology
Federal University of São Paulo
Vision Institute IPEPO
São Paulo-SP, Brazil
Chapter 169

Renata A Rezende MD
Assistant Professor of Ophthalmology
Pontificia University of Rio de Janeiro
Cornea Specialist
Hospital Sao Vicente de Paulo
São Paulo-SP, Brazil
Chapter 18

Danielle M Robertson OD PhD FAAO
Assistant Professor
Department of Ophthalmology
University of Texas Southwestern Medical Center
Dallas TX, USA
Chapter 101

David S Rootman MD FRCSC
Associate Professor
Toronto Western Hospital
Toronto ON, Canada
Chapter 45

Jason S Rothman MD
Private Practice
Ophthalmic Consultants of Boston
Beverly Hospital
Beverly MA, USA
Chapter 48

Roy Scott Rubinfeld MD
Clinical Associate Professor of Ophthalmology
Georgetown University
Washington Hospital Center
Washington Eye Physicians and Surgeons
Chevy Chase MD, USA
Chapter 87

Alan E Sadowsky MD
Adjunct Assistant Professor
Division of Ophthalmology
University of Minnesota
Fridley MN, USA
Chapter 65

Shizuya Saika MD PhD
Professor and Chairman
Department of Ophthalmology
Wakayama Medical University School of Medicine
Wakayama, Japan
Chapter 1

Monali V Sakhalkar MD
Assistant Professor of Ophthalmology
Department of Ophthalmology
University of Florida, Gainesville
Gainesville FL, USA
Chapter 54

James J Salz MD
Clinical Professor of Ophthalmology
Cornea Genetic Eye Institute
Cedars-Sinai Medical Center
Los Angeles CA, USA
Chapter 159

Virender S Sangwan MD
Associate Director
L V Prasad Eye Institute
L V Prasad Marg
Banjara Hills
Hyderabad
Andhra Pradesh, India
Chapter 95

Marinho Scarpi MD
Professor of Ophthalmology
Federal University of Sao Paulo (UNIFESP/EPM)
Sao Paulo SP, Brazil
Chapter 44

Bradley H Scharf MD
Private Practice
Eye Specialists of Westchester
New Rochelle NY, USA
Chapter 119

Greg Schmidt BS CEBT
Laboratory/EK Manager
Iowa Lions Eye Bank
Iowa City, IA, USA
Chapter 134

Artur Schmitt MD
Bascom Palmer Eye Institute
Cornea, Cataract and Refractive Surgery Research Fellow
Miller School of Medicine
University of Miami
Miami FL, USA
Chapter 137

Fernanda Piccoli Schmitt MD
Cornea, Cataract and Refractive Surgery Research Fellow
Bascom Palmer Eye Institute
Miller School of Medicine
University of Miami
Miami FL, USA
Chapter 137

Miriam T Schteingart MD
Assistant Clinical Professor
Department of Ophthalmology
Michigan State University
Saginaw MI, USA
Chapter 108

Ivan R Schwab MD FACS
Professor of Ophthalmology
Department of Ophthalmology
University of California at Davis
Sacramento CA, USA
Chapter 89

Brian L Schwam MD
Director, Medical Affairs and Ocular Sciences
Johnson and Johnson Vision Care
Jacksonville FL, USA
Chapter 104

Gary S Schwartz MD
Adjunct Associate Professor
Department of Ophthalmology
University of Minnesota
Stillwater MN, USA
Chapters 55; 79; 154 and 155

H Nida Sen MD MHSc
Staff Clinician
Director, Uveitis and Ocular Immunology Fellowship Program
National Eye Institute
National Institutes of Health
Bethesda, MD, USA
Chapter 105

Michael B Shapiro MD MS ACPE
Chief in Ophthalmology
St Joseph Hospital
Hillsboro WI
Anderson & Shapiro Eye Care
Madison WI, USA
Chapter 24

Shigeto Shimmura MD
Associate Professor
Department of Ophthalmology
Keio University School of Medicine
Shinjuku-ku
Tokyo, Japan
Chapter 131

Neera Singal MD FRCSC
Cataract Surgeon
Toronto Eye Surgery Centre
Toronto ON, Canada
Chapter 45

Heather M Skeens MD
Assistant Professor
Department of Ophthalmology
Medical University of South Carolina
Charleston SC, USA
Chapter 120

Craig A Skolnick MD
Assistant Professor of Clinical Ophthalmology
Bascom Palmer Eye Institute
Palm Beach Gardens FL, USA
Chapter 100

Allan R Slomovic MA MD FRCS(C)
Associate Professor of Ophthalmology
University of Toronto
Toronto Western Hospital
Toronto ON, Canada
Chapter 59

Janine A Smith MD
Senior Staff Fellow
Clinical Immunology Section
Laboratory of Immunology
National Eye Institute
National Institutes for Health
Bethesda MD, USA
Chapter 86

Michael E Snyder MD
Ophthalmologist
Cincinnati Eye Institute
Blue Ash OH, USA
Chapter 148

Renée Solomon MD
Private Practice
New York NY, USA
Chapter 141

Sarkis H Soukiasian MD
Assistant Clinical Professor
Tufts University School of Medicine
Lahey Clinic
Peabody MA, USA
Chapter 43

Sathish Srinivasan MBBS FRCSEd FRCOphth
Consultant Ophthalmic and Corneal Surgeon
Department of Ophthalmology
Ayr Hospital
Ayr UK
Chapter 59

John F Stamler MD PhD
Clinical Instructor
Department of Ophthalmology
University of Iowa
Iowa City IA, USA
Chapter 12

Roger F Steinert MD
Professor of Ophthalmology
Professor of Biomedical Engineering
Director of Cornea, Refractive and Cataract Surgery
Vice Chair of Clinical Ophthalmology
Irvine CA, USA
Chapter 115

Glenn L Stoller MD
Assistant Clinical Professor of Ophthalmology
Ophthalmic Consultants of Long Island
Rockville Centre NY, USA
Chapter 61

Barbara W Streeten MD
Professor of Ophthalmology and Pathology
Upstate Medical Center
State University of New York at Syracuse
Syracuse NY, USA
Chapter 73

R Doyle Stulting MD PhD
Professor of Ophthalmology
Emory Eye Center
Atlanta GA, USA
Chapter 125

Alan Sugar MD
Professor of Ophthalmology and Visual Sciences
University of Michigan
Ann Arbor MI, USA
Chapter 96

Joel Sugar MD
Professor of Ophthalmology
Eye and Ear Institute
University of Illinois at Chicago
Chicago IL, USA
Chapter 93

Donald Tan MBBS FRCS(G) FRCS(Ed) FRCOphth FAMS
Deputy Director
Singapore National Eye Centre
Singapore
Chapter 144

Joseph Tauber MD
Clinical Professor of Ophthalmology
Kansas University School of Medicine
Tauber Eye Center
Kansas City MO, USA
Chapter 111

Mark A Terry MD
Director, Corneal Services
Clinical Professor,
Department of Ophthalmology
Devers Eye Institute
Oregon Health Sciences University
Portland OR, USA
Chapter 138

Howard H Tessler MD
Professor of Ophthalmology
Department of Ophthalmology
University of Illinois at Chicago
Chicago IL, USA
Chapters 108 and 110

Marta Torrabadella MD
Department of Ophthalmology
Cornea and Ocular Surface Unit
Vall d'Hebron Hospitals
Barcelona, Spain
Chapter 146

Elias I Traboulsi MD
Professor of Ophthalmology
The Cole Eye Institute
Cleveland Clinic Foundation
Cleveland OH, USA
Chapter 60

William B Trattler MD
Cornea Specialist, Center for Excellence in Eye Care
Volunteer Assistant Professor of Ophthalmology
Bascom Palmer Eye Institute
Miami FL, USA
Chapter 159

Julie H Tsai MD
Assistant Professor
Department of Opthalmology
University of South Carolina
Columbia SC, USA
Chapter 56

David T Tse MD FACS
Professor of Ophthalmology
Dr Nasser Ibrahim Al-Rashid Chair in Ophthalmic Plastic Orbital Surgery and Oncology
Bascom Palmer Eye Institute
Miami FL, USA
Chapter 32

Elmer Y Tu MD
Associate Professor of Clinical Ophthalmology
Director of the Cornea and External Disease Service
University of Illinois at Chicago
Chicago IL, USA
Chapter 83

Roxana Ursea MD
Assistant Professor of Ophthalmology
Director, Cornea and Refractive Surgery Division
Department of Ophthalmology
University of Arizona
Tucson AZ, USA
Chapter 86

Pravin K Vaddavalli MD
Consultant, Cornea and Anterior Segment Service
Contact Lens and Refractive Surgery Service
L V Prasad Eye Institute
Hyderabad, India
Chapter 84

Woodford S Van Meter MD
Associate Clinical Professor
Department of Ophthalmology
University of Kentucky School of Medicine
Lexington KY, USA
Chapter 116

Gary A Varley MD
Ophthalmologist
Cincinnati Eye Institute
Cincinnati OH, USA
Chapter 10

Roshni Vasaiwala MD
Resident
University of Illinois Eye and Ear Infirmary
Department of Ophthalmology and Visual Sciences
Chicago IL, USA
Chapter 161

Anthony J Verachtert OD
Clinical Director
Moyes Eye Center
Kansas City MO, USA
Chapter 35

David D Verdier MD
Clinical Professor
Department of Surgery,
Ophthalmology Division
Michigan State University College of Human Medicine
Verdier Eye Center
Grand Rapids MI, USA
Chapter 114

Ana Carolina Vieira MD
Fellow in Cornea and External Diseases
Post-graduation Student
Federal University of Sao Paulo
Post-doctoral Research Fellow
University of California, Davis
Sacramento CA, USA
Chapters 89 and 145

Vanee V Virasch MD
Cornea Fellow
Department of Ophthalmology
Washington University in St Louis
St. Louis MO, USA
Chapter 92

Li Wang MD PhD
Assistant Professor
Department of Ophthalmology
Baylor College of Medicine
Houston TX, USA
Chapter 170

George O Waring III MD FACS FRCOphth
Founding Surgeon
InView
Atlanta GA, USA
Chapters 5 and 158

George O Waring IV MD
Clinical Assistant Professor of Ophthalmology
Emory University School of Medicine
Refractive and Intraocular Lens Surgeon
Private Practice
Atlanta GA, USA
Chapter 158

Michael A Warner MD PC
Private Practice
Inland Eye and Cosmetic Surgery Institute
Hermiston OR, USA
Chapters 39 and 41

Kevin J Warrian BA (Hons) BSc (Med) MD MA
Ophthalmic Surgical Resident
Ivey Eye Institute
London ON, Canada
Chapter 106

Guy F Webster MD PhD FAAD
Private Practice
Webster Dermatology PA
Hockessin DE, USA
Chapter 52

Mitchell P Weikert MD MS
Department of Ophthalmology
Laser Eye Surgeon
Baylor College of Medicine
Houston TX, USA
Chapter 170

Robert W Weisenthal MD FACS
Clinical Professor of Ophthalmology
Upstate Medical Center
State University of New York at Syracuse
DeWitt NY, USA
Chapter 73

Jayne S Weiss MD
Professor of Ophthalmology and Pathology
Kresge Eye Institute
Detroit MI, USA
Chapter 70

Pongmas Wichiensin MD
Attending Surgeon
Department of Ophthalmology
Rajavithi Hospital
Bangkok, Thailand
Chapter 77

Kirk R Wilhelmus MD PhD
Professor of Ophthalmology
Department of Ophthalmology
Cullen Eye Institute
Baylor College of Medicine
Houston TX, USA
Chapter 85

Steven E Wilson MD
Professor of Ophthalmology
Staff Cornea and Refractive Surgeon
Director of Corneal Research
The Cole Eye Institute
The Cleveland Clinic
Cleveland OH, USA
Chapter 164

Maria A Woodward MD
Corneal Fellow
Emory Eye Center
Atlanta GA, USA
Chapter 168

Richard W Yee MD
Clinical Professor
Department of Ophthalmology and Visual Science
University of Texas Science Center,
Director of Corneal and External Diseases and Refractive Surgery
Hermann Eye Center
Memorial Hermann Hospital
Houston TX, USA
Chapter 14

Sonya Yoo MD
Associate Professor of Clinical Ophthalmology
Bascom Palmer Eye Institute
University of Miami Miller School of Medicine
Miami FL, USA
Chapter 137

PART I

BASIC SCIENCE: CORNEA, SCLERA, OCULAR ADNEXA ANATOMY, PHYSIOLOGY AND PATHOPHYSIOLOGIC RESPONSES

Chapter 1

Cornea and Sclera: Anatomy and Physiology

Teruo Nishida, Shizuya Saika

Introduction

The avascular cornea is not an isolated tissue. It forms, together with the sclera, the outer shell of the eyeball, occupying one-third of the ocular tunic. Although most of both the cornea and sclera consist of dense connective tissue, the physiological roles of these two components of the eye shell differ. The cornea serves as the transparent 'window' of the eye that allows the entry of light, whereas the sclera provides a 'darkbox' that allows the formation of an image on the retina. The cornea is exposed to the outer environment, whereas the opaque sclera is covered with the semitransparent conjunctiva and has no direct exposure to the outside. The differences in the functions of the cornea and sclera reflect those in their microscopic structures and biochemical components.

Interwoven fibrous collagen is responsible for the mechanical strength of both the cornea and sclera, protecting the inner components of the eye from physical injury and maintaining the ocular contour.[1] The corneal epithelium forms an effective mechanical barrier as a result of interdigitation of cell membranes and the formation of junctional complexes such as tight junctions and desmosomes between adjacent cells. Together with the cellular and chemical components of the conjunctiva and tear film, the corneal surface protects against potential pathological agents and microorganisms.

The smooth surface of the cornea contributes to visual clarity. The regular arrangement of collagen fibers in the corneal stroma accounts for the transparency of this tissue.[2] Maintenance of corneal shape and transparency is critical for light refraction, with the cornea accounting for more than two-thirds of the total refractive power of the eye. A functionally intact corneal endothelium is important for maintenance of stromal transparency as a result of regulation by the endothelium of corneal hydration.

Anatomy and Physiology

Structure of the cornea and sclera

The anterior corneal surface is covered by the tear film, whereas the posterior surface is bathed directly by the aqueous humor. The highly vascularized limbus, which is thought to contain a reservoir of pluripotent stem cells, constitutes the transition zone between the cornea and sclera. The anterior corneal surface is convex and aspheric (Fig. 1.1), and it is transversely oval as a result of scleralization superiorly and inferiorly.

The adult human cornea measures 11 to 12 mm horizontally and 9 to 11 mm vertically. It is approximately 0.5 mm thick at the center, with the thickness increasing gradually toward the periphery, where it is about 0.7 mm thick.[3] The curvature of the corneal surface is not constant, being greatest at the center and smallest at the periphery. The radius of curvature is between 7.5 and 8.0 mm at the 3-mm central optical zone of the cornea, where the surface is almost spherical. The refractive power of the cornea is 40 to 44 diopters, constituting about two-thirds of the total refractive power of the eye.

The sclera, a tough and nontransparent tissue, shapes the eye shell, which is approximately 24 mm in diameter in the emmetropic eye. The anterior part of the sclera is covered with the bulbar conjunctiva and Tenon's capsule, which consists of loose connective tissue and is located beneath the conjunctiva (Fig. 1.2). The nontransparency of the sclera prevents light from reaching the retina other than through the cornea, and, together with the pigmentation of the choroid and retinal pigment epithelium, the sclera provides a dark box for image formation. The scleral spur is a projection of the anterior scleral stroma toward the angle of the anterior chamber and is the site of insertion for the anterior ciliary muscle. Contraction of this muscle thus opens the trabecular meshwork. At the posterior pole of the eyeball, where the optic nerve fibers enter the eye, the scleral stroma is separated into outer and inner layers. The outer layer fuses with the sheath of the optic nerve, dura, and arachnoid, whereas the inner layer contains the sievelike structure of the lamina cribrosa. The rigidity of the lamina cribrosa accounts for the susceptibility of retinal nerve fibers to damage during the development of chronic open-angle glaucoma. The sclera contains six insertion sites of the extraocular muscles as well as the inputs of arteries (anterior and posterior ciliary arteries) and outputs of veins (vortex veins) that circulate blood through the uveal tissues.

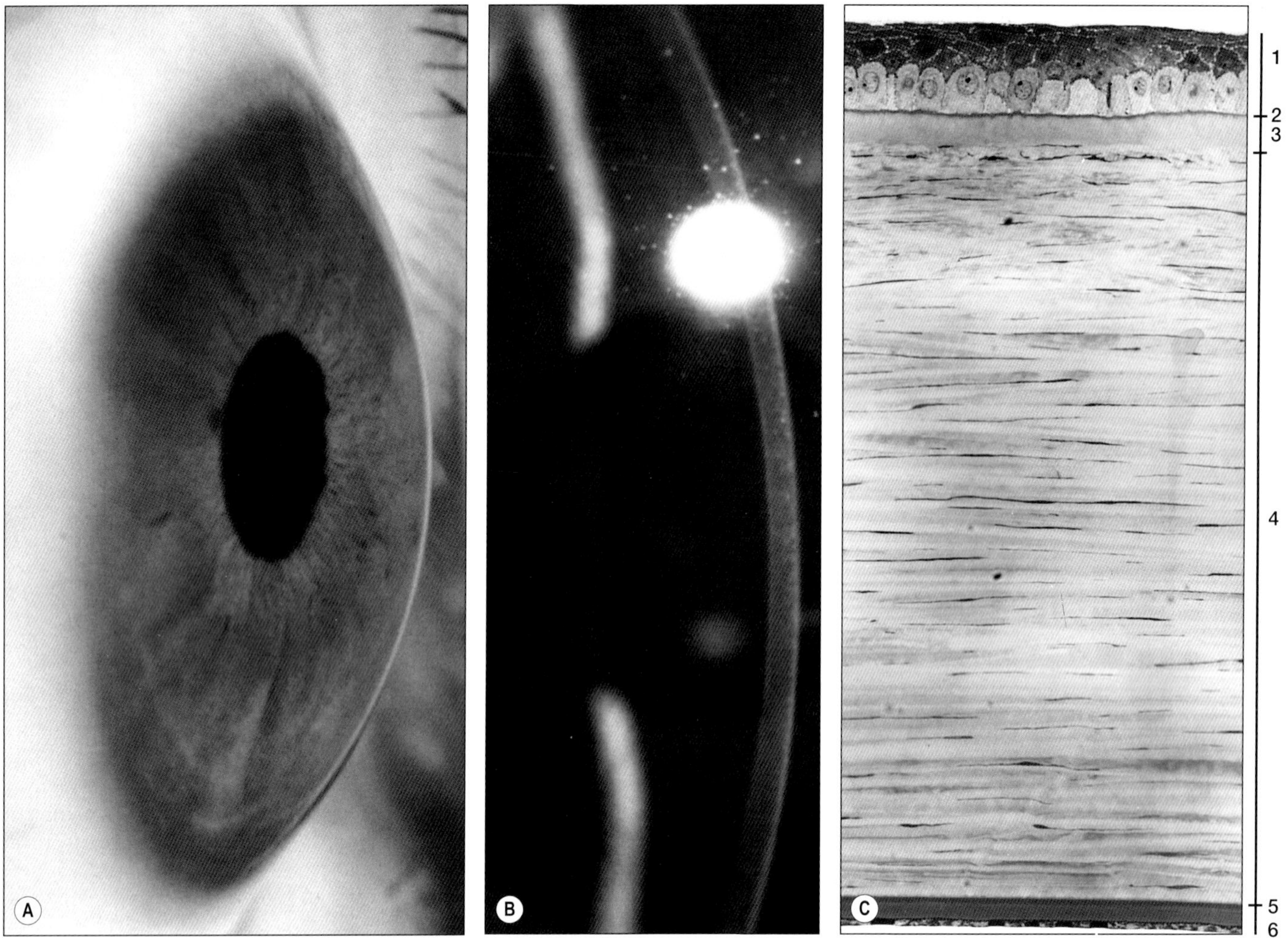

Fig. 1.1 Anatomy of the human cornea. (**A**) Lateral view of the cornea. (**B**) Higher-magnification view of the cornea provided by a slit lamp microscope. (**C**) Histology of the cornea showing the epithelium (*1*), epithelial basement membrane (*2*), Bowman's layer (*3*), stroma (*4*), Descemet's membrane (*5*), and endothelium (*6*).

Optical properties of the cornea

The optical properties of the cornea are determined by its transparency, surface smoothness, contour, and refractive index of the tissue.[4] If the diameter of (or the distance between) collagen fibers in the corneal stroma becomes heterogeneous (as occurs in fibrosis or edema), incident light rays are scattered randomly and the cornea loses its transparency. Given that the spherocylindrical surface of the cornea has both minor and major axes, changes in corneal contour caused either by pathological conditions such as scarring, thinning, or keratoconus or by refractive surgery render the surface regularly or irregularly astigmatic.

The total refractive index of the cornea is determined by the sum of refraction at the anterior and posterior interfaces as well as by the transmission properties of the tissue. The refractive indexes of air, tear fluid, corneal tissue, and aqueous humor are 1.000, 1.336, 1.376, and 1.336, respectively. The refractive power of a curved surface is determined by the refractive index and the radius of curvature. The refractive power at the central cornea is about +43 diopters, being the sum of that at the air–tear fluid (+44 diopters), tear fluid–cornea (+5 diopters), and cornea–aqueous humor (–6 diopters) interfaces. Most keratometry and topography measurements assume a standard refractive index of 1.3375.

Innervation

Innervation of the cornea is required for pain sensation as well as for tissue repair. In addition, autonomic innervation of the scleral spur and of blood vessels in the episclera, the surface of the sclera immediately beneath the subconjunctival connective tissue, plays an important role in the regulation of intraocular pressure.

The cornea is one of the most heavily innervated and most sensitive tissues in the body. The density of nerve endings in the cornea is thus about 300 to 400 times greater than that in the skin.[5,6] Most of the sensory nerves in the cornea are derived from the ciliary nerves of the ophthalmic branch of the trigeminal nerve. The long ciliary nerves provide the perilimbal nerve ring. Nerve fibers penetrate the cornea in the deep peripheral stroma radially and then

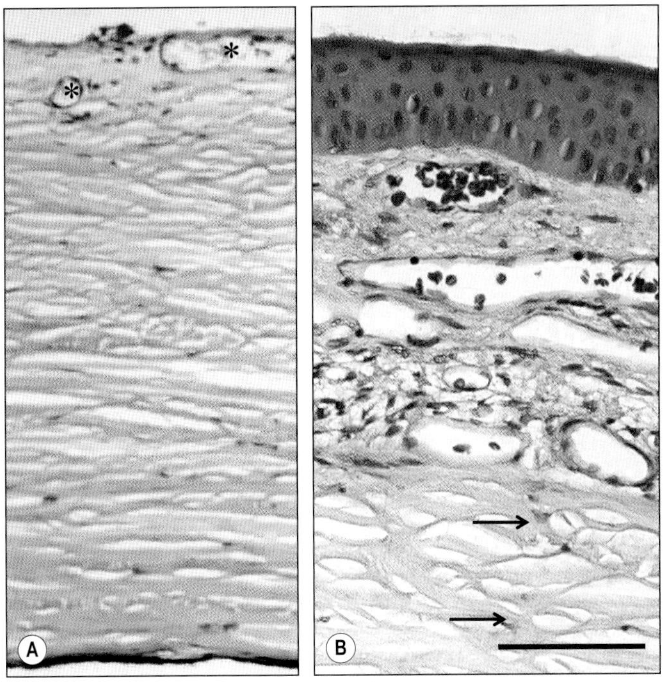

Fig. 1.2 Histology of the human sclera. (**A**) Hematoxylin & eosin staining of a cross-section of the sclera. Blood vessels (*asterisks*) are largely restricted to the episclera (upper region of section). (**B**) Higher-magnification view of the conjunctiva and episclera as well as of stromal fibroblasts (*arrows*) in the sclera. Bars, 100 μm.

course anteriorly, forming a terminal subepithelial plexus.[7] The nerve fibers lose their myelination within a short distance of their point of entry into the cornea, penetrate Bowman's layer, and terminate at the wing cell level of the epithelium. Loss of the superficial corneal epithelium results in exposure of the nerve endings and consequent severe ocular pain.

Slit lamp microscopy allows observation of nerve fibers in the corneal stroma. The fibers are especially prominent at the corneal periphery, where their diameter is relatively large. Laser-scanning confocal biomicroscopy has revealed networks of fine nerve fibers (subepithelial nerve plexuses) in or below the basal cell layer of the corneal epithelium.[6,8,9] The diameter of these nerve fibers increases with distance from the anterior corneal surface (Fig. 1.3).

Histochemical studies have revealed the presence of various neurotransmitters, including substance P, calcitonin gene-related peptide, neuropeptide Y, vasoactive intestinal peptide, galanin, methionine-enkephalin, catecholamines, and acetylcholine, in the cornea.[6,10–21] The cornea thus contains peptidergic, sympathetic, and parasympathetic nerve fibers. Degeneration or dysfunction of sensory nerves (trigeminal nerve branches) in the cornea can result in delayed healing of corneal injuries and the development of neurotrophic ulcer.

The short and long posterior ciliary nerves, which are branches of the trigeminal nerve, penetrate the sclera and provide fine sensory branches to the scleral stroma. In addition, nerve fibers are also present in the episclera. These fibers include those of vasodilative and vasoconstrictive nerves and are thought to regulate blood flow and volume in the episcleral vessels for modulation of episcleral venous pressure and outflow facility.[22] Cells in the scleral spur are also thought to contribute to the regulation of intraocular pressure. Axons of presumably parasympathetic origin are present in the scleral spur of humans. On the other hand, cholinergic innervation of scleral spur cells appears to be rare or absent.[23]

Vascular system

The cornea is one of the few avascular tissues in the body. Although the normal cornea does not contain blood vessels, factors derived from the blood play important roles in corneal metabolism and wound healing. The anterior ciliary artery, which is derived from the ophthalmic artery, forms a vascular arcade in the limbal region that anastomoses with vessels derived from the facial branch of the external carotid artery. The cornea is thus supplied with blood components by both internal and external carotid arteries. In certain pathological conditions, new vessels enter the transparent corneal stroma from the limbus and result in a loss of corneal transparency.

In contrast to the cornea, the episclera is highly vascularized. The episcleral vasculature shows a specialized morphology characterized by the absence of capillaries, numerous arteriovenous anastomoses, and a muscle-rich venous network, which is thought to play an important role in the regulation of intraocular pressure. Such vascularization is also apparent in the loose connective tissue of Tenon's capsule. The scleral stroma contains few blood vessels with the exception of the input and output of the vessels of the choroidal circulation.

Oxygen and nutrient supply

Corneal epithelial and endothelial cells are metabolically active. Cellular activities require adenosine triphosphate (ATP) as an energy source, with catabolism of glucose by glycolysis and the citric acid cycle generating ATP under aerobic conditions. A supply of glucose and oxygen is thus essential to maintain the normal metabolic functions of the cornea.[24–27] The cornea is supplied with glucose by diffusion from the aqueous humor. In contrast, oxygen is supplied to the cornea primarily by diffusion from tear fluid, which absorbs oxygen from the air. Direct exposure of tear fluid to the atmosphere is thus essential for oxygenation of the cornea. Disruption of the oxygen supply to the cornea, such as that resulting from the wearing of contact lenses with less gas permeability, can lead to corneal hypoxia and consequent stromal edema.[28–31] Closure of the eyelids during sleep also reduces the amount of oxygen that reaches the cornea. Corneal metabolism therefore changes from aerobic to anaerobic (with consequent accumulation of lactate) during sleep.[32,33]

Tear fluid

The corneal surface is covered by tear fluid, which protects the cornea from dehydration and helps to maintain the smooth epithelial surface. The thickness and volume of the

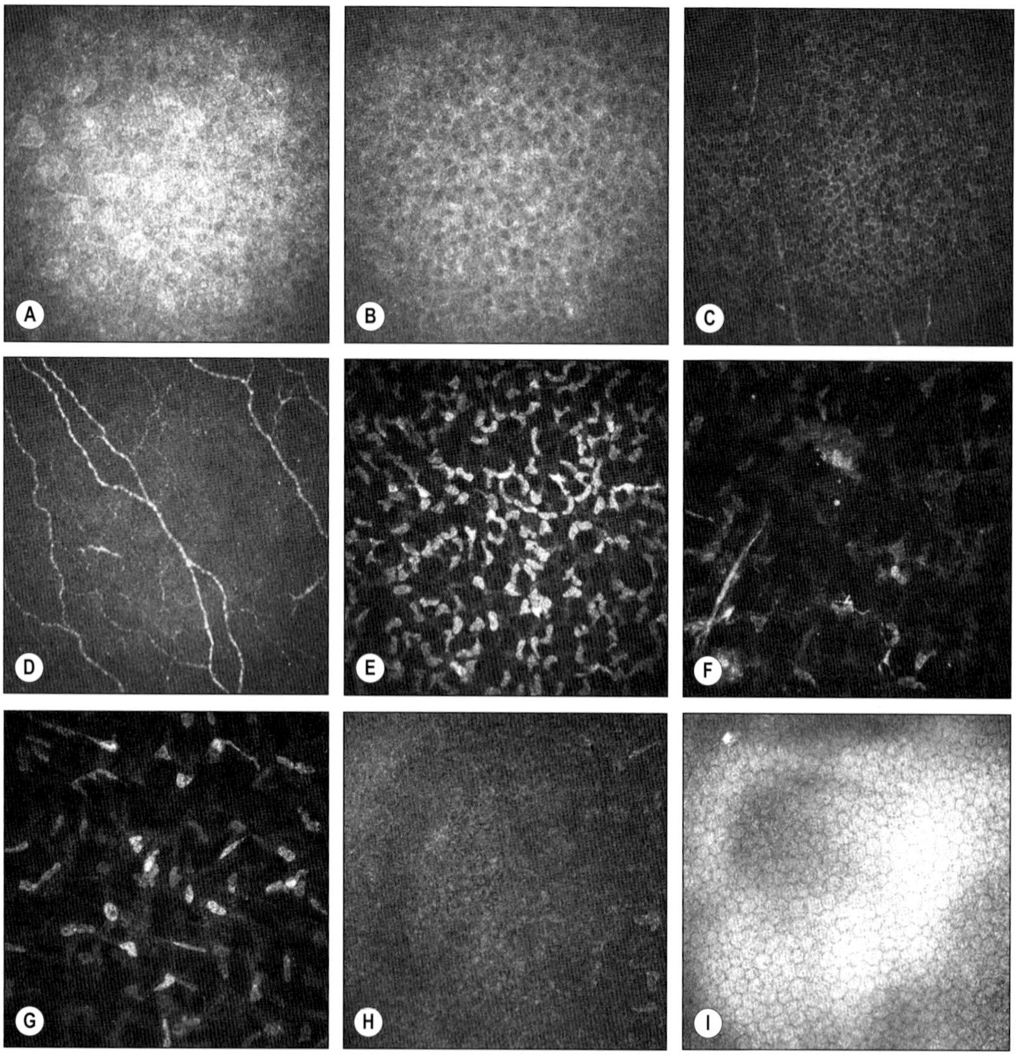

Fig. 1.3 Confocal biomicroscopy of the human cornea. (**A–C**) Superficial, wing, and basal cell layers of the corneal epithelium. (**D**) Subepithelial nerve plexus. (**E**) Shallow layer of the stroma, containing a high density of polygonal keratocytes. (**F**) Mid layer of the stroma, containing thick nonbranching nerve fibers. (**G**) Deep layer of the stroma, containing keratocytes. (**H**) Amorphous appearance of Descemet's membrane. (**I**) Endothelium, comprising hexagonal endothelial cells of uniform size.

tear film are about 7 μm and 6.5 μL, respectively.[34,35] The tear film consists of three layers: a superficial lipid layer (≈0.1 μm), an aqueous layer (≈7 μm), and a mucinous layer (0.02–0.05 μm).[36] More than 98% of the total volume of the tear film is water. However, tear fluid also contains many biologically important ions and molecules, including electrolytes, glucose, immunoglobulins, lactoferrin, lysozyme, albumin, and oxygen. Moreover, it contains a wide range of biologically active substances such as histamine, prostaglandins, growth factors, and cytokines (Table 1.1). The tear film thus serves not only as a lubricant and source of nutrients for the corneal epithelium but also as a source of regulatory factors required for epithelial maintenance and repair.[37–54]

The components of the superficial lipid layer of the tear film are supplied by meibomian glands and other secretory glands of the eyelid. The aqueous layer is derived from the lacrimal gland and accessory lacrimal glands, and the mucinous layer is produced largely by goblet cells in the conjunctival epithelium. Hypolacrimation (dry eye syndrome) can thus be classified basically into three categories attributable to lipid, aqueous, or mucin deficiency.

Histology and Biochemistry

The cornea consists of three different cellular layers and two interfaces: the epithelium, Bowman's layer, the stroma, Descemet's membrane, and the endothelium (see Fig. 1.1).[55] The cell types that constitute the cornea thus include epithelial cells, keratocytes (corneal fibroblasts), and endothelial cells. Components of the cornea interact with each other to maintain the integrity and function of the tissue, with the precise arrangement of the various components contributing to its transparency and strength.

Table 1.1 Components of tear fluid

Tear layer	Origin	Components	Physiological functions
Lipid layer	Meibomian glands, accessory lacrimal glands	Wax, cholesterol, fatty acid esters	Lubrication, prevention of evaporation, stabilization
Aqueous layer	Lacrimal gland, accessory lacrimal glands	Water, electrolytes (Na^+, K^+ Cl^-, HCO_3^-, Mg^{2+}), proteins (albumin, lysozyme, lactoferrin,transferrin, ceruloplasmin), immunoglobulins (IgA, IgG, IgE, IgM), cytokines, growth factors (EGF, TGF-α, TGF-β1, TGF-β2, bFGF, HGF, VEGF, substance P), others (glucose, vitamins)	Lubrication, antimicrobial, bacteriostasis, supply of oxygen and nutrients, mechanical clearance, regulation of cellular functions
Mucinous layer	Conjunctival goblet cells, conjunctival epithelial cells, corneal epithelial cells	Sulfomucin, cyalomucin, MUC1, MUC4, MUC5AC	Lowering of surface tension, stabilization of aqueous layer

Corneal epithelium

The corneal and conjunctival epithelia are continuous and together form the ocular surface. They are both composed of nonkeratinized, stratified, squamous epithelial cells. Although their characteristics differ, both corneal and conjunctival epithelia cooperate to provide the biodefense system of the anterior surface of the eye.[56,57] The thickness of the corneal epithelium is approximately 50 µm, which is about 10% of the total thickness of the cornea (see Fig. 1.1), and it is constant over the entire corneal surface.

The corneal epithelium consists of five or six layers of three different types of epithelial cells: superficial cells, wing cells, and columnar basal cells, the latter of which adhere to the basement membrane adjacent to Bowman's layer (Fig 1.4). Only the basal cells of the corneal epithelium proliferate. The daughter cells differentiate into wing cells and subsequently into superficial cells, gradually emerging at the corneal surface. The differentiation process requires about 7 to 14 days, after which the superficial cells are desquamated into the tear film.[58] Ultraviolet radiation, hypoxia, or mechanical stress induces apoptosis (programmed cell death) and desquamation of corneal epithelial cells.[59–62]

An important physiological role of the corneal epithelium is to provide a barrier to external stimuli. The presence of junctional complexes between adjacent corneal epithelial cells prevents the passage of such agents into the deeper layers of the cornea. Both cell–cell and cell–matrix interactions are important for maintenance of the normal stratified structure and physiological functions of the corneal epithelium. The characteristics of the different types of intercellular junctional complexes present in the corneal epithelium are summarized in Table 1.2 and in Figures 1.4, 1.5, and 1.6. Tight junctions (zonula occludens) are present mostly between cells of the superficial cell layers and provide a highly effective barrier to prevent the penetration of tear fluid and its chemical constituents. Hemidesmosomes (zonula adherens) and desmosomes are present in all layers of the corneal epithelium, whereas gap junctions, which allow the passage of small molecules between cells, are present in the wing cells and basal cells. After damage to the corneal epithelium, actively migrating epithelial cells no longer manifest gap junctions or desmosomes in the wounded region lacking a basement membrane. Reestablishment of the continuity of the corneal epithelium is accompanied by the synthesis and deposition of basement membrane proteins and by the reassembly of the various types of junctional apparatus, suggesting that the presence of the basement membrane may be required for re-formation of cell–cell junctions in the corneal epithelium (Fig. 1.6).[63]

In corneal epithelial cells, intermediate filaments of the cytoskeleton are formed by specific types of acidic (type I) and basic (type II) keratin molecules. Basal cells of the corneal epithelium express keratin 5/14, like basal epidermal cells of the skin. However, keratin 3/12 (64-kDa keratin) is specifically expressed in the epithelium of the cornea, not being found in that of the conjunctiva or in the epidermis.[64,65] Genetic mutation of the keratin 12 gene is responsible for Meesmann's dystrophy of the corneal epithelium.[66]

Replacement of most organs or tissues by transplantation from a genetically nonidentical individual is associated with an immune response that may lead to rejection. In contrast, the cornea is 'immune privileged,' a characteristic that is critical for the success of corneal transplantation. Dendritic Langerhans cells, specialized macrophages derived from the bone marrow that are implicated in antigen processing, are abundant at the periphery of the corneal epithelium but are not present in the central region of the normal cornea.[67,68] These cells express human leukocyte antigen (HLA) class II molecules and are thought to function in the afferent arm of the ocular immune response by presenting antigens to T lymphocytes.[69,70] Injury to the central cornea results in the rapid migration of peripheral Langerhans cells to the damaged area.

Superficial cells

The surface of the corneal epithelium contains two to three layers of terminally differentiated superficial cells. In contrast to the epidermis of the skin, the corneal epithelium is not normally keratinized, although it may become so under pathological conditions such as vitamin A deficiency. These cells are flat and polygonal with a diameter of 40–60 µm and a thickness of 2–6 µm (see Table 1.2). Their surface is covered

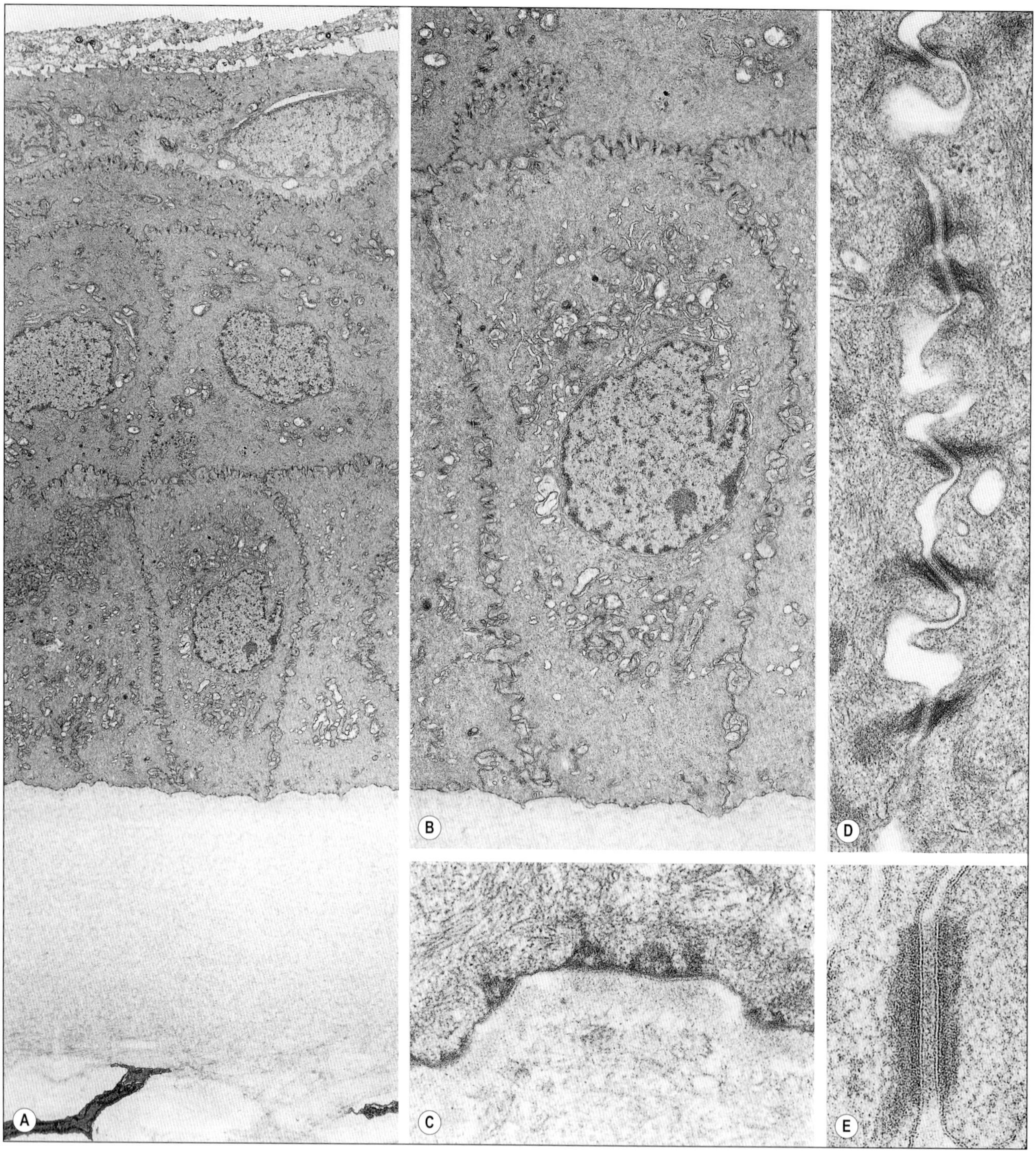

Fig. 1.4 Transmission electron microscopy of the human corneal epithelium. (**A**) The epithelium comprises five or six layers of epithelial cells. The electron-dense cell is about to undergo desquamation. (**B**) Basal cells. Note the numerous junctional complexes. (**C**) Basement membrane and anterior portion of Bowman's layer. Note hemidesmosomes at the basal surface of the epithelial cells. (**D**) Interdigitation and junctional complexes at the lateral surface of basal epithelial cells. (**E**) Gap junction at the lateral surface of basal cells.

Table 1.2 Characteristics of the various types of corneal epithelial cells

	Shape	Layers	Size	Mitotic activity	Interdigitation	Junctional complexes	Cytoplasmic organelles	Keratin	Microfilaments (actin)	Microtubules
Superficial cells	Flat Microvilli Microplicae	2–4	40–60 μm in diameter 4–6 μm thick at the nucleus 2 μm thick at the periphery	–	Entire surface	Desmosomes Tight junctional complexes (zonula occludens)	Sparse	+	+	?
Wing cells	Winglike processes	2–3		–	Entire surface	Desmosomes Gap junctions	Sparse	+++	+	+/–
Basal cells	Columnar	Mono layer	18–20 μm high 8–10 μm in diameter Flat at posterior surface	+	Apical surface	Desmosomes Gap junctions Hemidesmosomes	More than superficial cells Large numbers of glycogen granules Prominent mitochondria and Golgi apparatus	+++	+	+

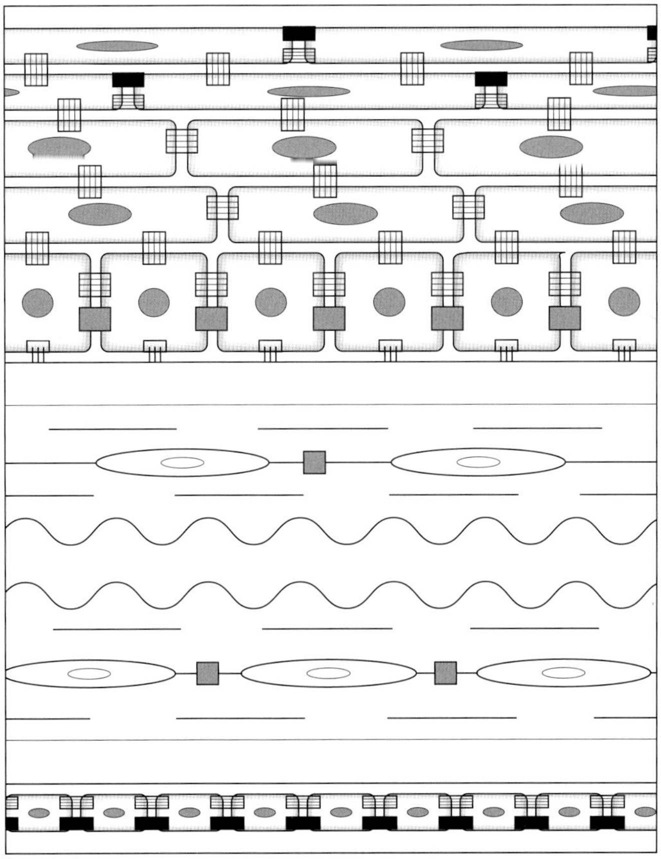

Fig. 1.5 Schematic representation of the localization of tight junctions (*dark boxes*), desmosomes or hemidesmosomes (*hatched boxes*), and gap junctions (*dotted boxes*) in the cornea.

with microvilli.[71] Given that superficial cells are well differentiated, they do not proliferate.

Numerous glycoprotein and glycolipid molecules are embedded in the cell membrane of epithelial cells. These oligosaccharide-containing molecules form floating particles in the membrane that are collectively termed the glycocalyx and which confer hydrophilic properties on the anterior surface of the superficial epithelial cells. The glycocalyx interacts with the mucinous layer of the tear film and helps to maintain the trilayered structure of the latter.[72,73] Loss either of the glycocalyx of corneal epithelial cells or of goblet cells in the conjunctival epithelium results in tear film instability and the mucin-deficiency form of dry eye.

The superficial cells of the corneal epithelium are joined by desmosomes, adherens junctions, and tight junctions (see Figs 1.4, 1.5, and 1.6), which prevent the passage of substances through the intercellular space. Examination of fluorescein penetration into the corneal stroma with a fluorophotometer provides a measure of the barrier function of the corneal epithelium.[74]

Wing cells

Beneath the superficial cells lie two to three layers of wing cells, so called because of their characteristic winglike shape. Wing cells are in an intermediate state of differentiation between basal and superficial cells and are rich in intracellular tonofilaments composed of keratin (see Table 1.2). The cell membranes of adjacent wing cells are interdigitate. Numerous desmosomes, adherens junctions, and gap junctions are present between wing cells (see Figs 1.4, 1.5, and 1.6).

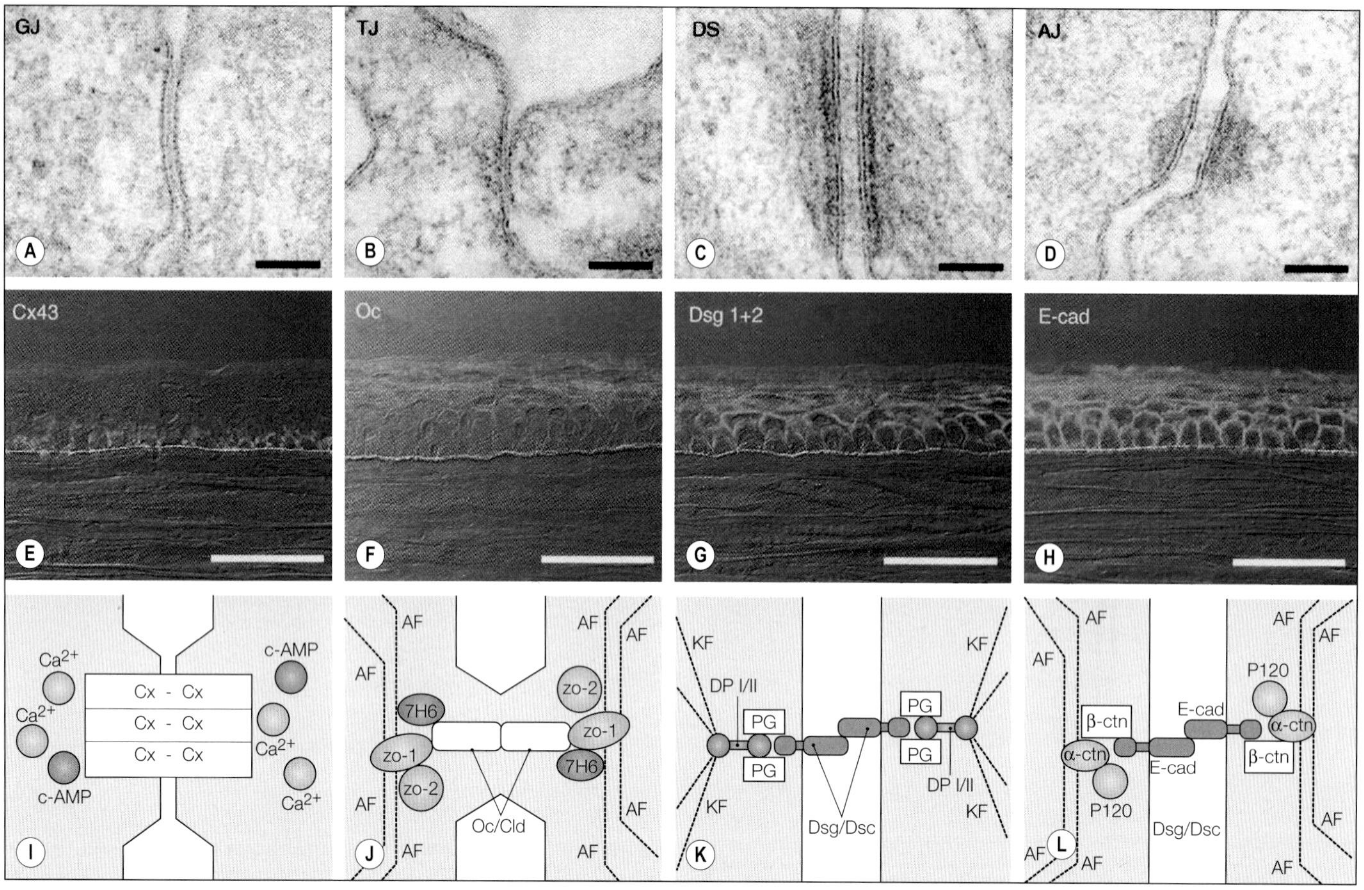

Fig. 1.6 Intercellular junctions in the corneal epithelium. Upper panels: **(A–D)** Transmission electron micrographs of the human corneal epithelium. Scale bars, 50 nm. Middle panels: (**E–H**) Immunofluorescence micrographs of the rat corneal epithelium stained with antibodies to the indicated proteins. Scale bars, 50 μm. Lower panels: (**I–L**) Schematic representation of intercellular junctions in the corneal epithelium. GJ, gap junction; TJ, tight junction; DS, desmosome; AJ, adherens junction; Cx43, connexin 43; Oc, occludin; Dsg 1+2, desmogleins 1 and 2; E-cad, E-cadherin; c-AMP, cyclic adenosine monophosphate; Cld, claudin; zo-1 and -2, zonula occludens-1 and -2; 7H6, 7H6 antigen; AF, actin filament; Dsc, desmocollin; DP I/II, desmoplakin I or II; PG, plakoglobin; KF, keratin filament; α- and β-ctn, α- and β-catenin; P120, P120 catenin. (From Suzuki K et al. Cell–matrix and cell–cell interactions during corneal epithelial wound healing. *Prog Retin Eye Res* 22:113-133, 2003 Copyright Elsevier.)

Basal cells

The single layer of columnar basal cells of the corneal epithelium rests on the basement membrane. Basal cells, unlike superficial and wing cells, possess mitotic activity, and they differentiate consecutively into wing and superficial cells (see Table 1.2). Neighboring basal cells interdigitate laterally and are joined by desmosomes, gap junctions, and adherens junctions. The posterior surface of basal cells is flat and abuts the basement membrane.

Basal cells adhere to the basement membrane via hemidesmosomes that are linked to anchoring fibrils of type VII collagen secreted by themselves (see Fig. 1.4).[75,76] The anchoring fibrils penetrate the basement membrane and course into the stroma, where they form anchoring plaques together with type I collagen, a major component of the stroma. The adherens junctions are present at the lateral surface of the basal cells of the corneal epithelium and are thought to mediate cell–cell interaction.[77]

Members of the integrin family of cell surface receptors for extracellular matrix components (ECM) proteins exist as heterodimers of α and β subunits.[78] The integrin α5β1 heterodimer, which is the major receptor for fibronectin, is present at the surface of basal cells in the normal corneal epithelium.[79–83] All epithelial cells undergoing active migration after debridement of the corneal epithelium express integrin α5β1.[83,84]

Basement membrane

As in epithelia in other parts of the body, basal cells of the corneal epithelium are anchored to a basement membrane. The presence of the basement membrane between the basal epithelium and the underlying stroma fixes the polarity of epithelial cells. Ultrastructurally, the basement membrane, which is 40–60 nm thick, is composed of a pale layer (the lamina lucida) immediately posterior to the cell membrane of the basal epithelial cells as well as an electron-dense layer (the lamina densa) (see Fig. 1.4). Type IV collagen and laminin are major components of the basement membrane (Fig. 1.7).

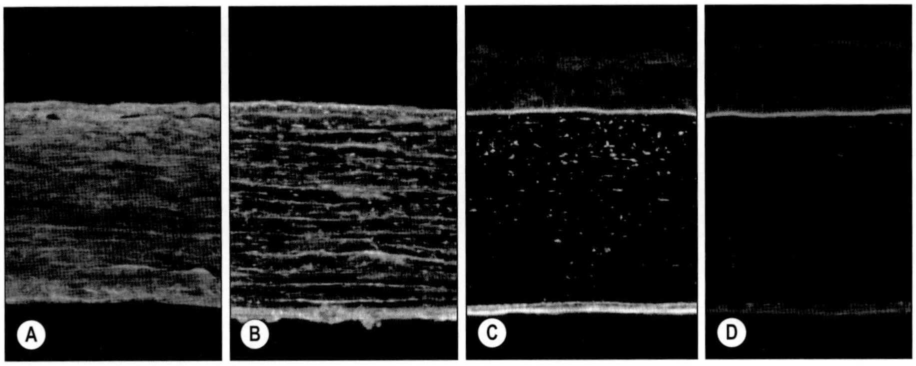

Fig. 1.7 Immunofluorescence analysis of the expression of matrix proteins in the rat corneal epithelium. (**A**) Fibronectin. (**B**) Type I collagen. (**C**) Type IV collagen. (**D**) Laminin.

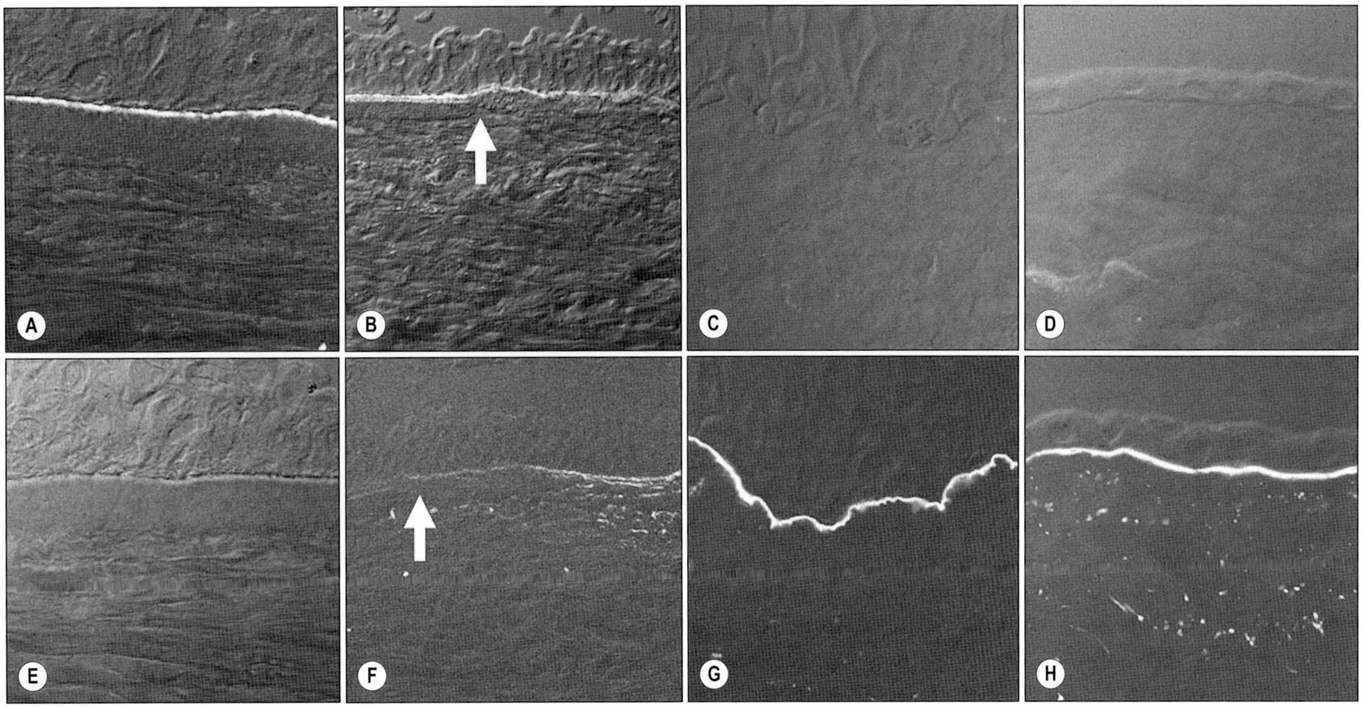

Fig. 1.8 Differential expression of α2(IV) and α5(IV) isoforms of type IV collagen in the human cornea, conjunctiva, and amniotic membrane. The arrow shows the termination of Bowman's layer. (Reprinted with permission from: Fukuda K et al. Differential distribution of subchains of the basement membrane components type IV collagen and laminin among the amniotic membrane, cornea, and conjunctiva. *Cornea* 18:73-79, 1999.)

The basement membranes of the corneal and conjunctival epithelia contain different type IV collagen chains, although the functional relevance of this difference is unknown. Whereas collagen α5(IV) is present in the corneal basement membrane, collagen α2(IV) is present in the conjunctival basement membrane (as well as in the amniotic membrane) (Fig. 1.8).

Bowman's layer

An acellular, membrane-like zone known as Bowman's layer, or Bowman's membrane, is detectable by light microscopy at the interface between the corneal epithelium and stroma in humans and certain other mammals (but not in rodents). Given that this structure, which is 12 μm thick, is not a membrane but rather a random arrangement of collagen fibers and proteoglycans, the term Bowman's layer is preferable. The collagen fibers in Bowman's layer are primarily collagen types I and III. The diameter of these fibers is 20–30 nm, which is smaller than that of the collagen fibers present in the corneal stroma (22.5–35 nm) (see Fig. 1.4).

Bowman's layer is considered to be the anterior portion of the corneal stroma. The anterior surface of this layer, which faces the basement membrane, is smooth. Given that the collagen fibers in Bowman's layer are synthesized and secreted by stromal keratocytes, they appear continuous with those in the stroma.

Biological functions originally attributed to Bowman's layer are now thought to be mediated by the basement membrane. Bowman's layer does not regenerate after injury. Recent clinical experience with excimer laser photoablation demonstrates that a normal epithelium is formed and maintained even in the absence of Bowman's layer. Furthermore, many mammals do not have a Bowman's layer but still exhibit a well-organized epithelial structure. The physiological role of Bowman's layer therefore remains unclear.

Stroma of the cornea and sclera

Overview

The stroma constitutes the largest portion, more than 90%, of the thickness of the cornea. The peripheral portion of the cornea connects to the anterior sclera at the limbus, where the tissue loses its transparency. Many characteristics of the cornea, including its physical strength, stability of shape, and transparency, are largely attributable to the anatomic and biochemical properties of the stroma. The uniform arrangement and continuous slow turnover (production and degradation) of collagen fibers in the stroma are essential for corneal transparency.

The sclera is also composed mostly of collagen fibers and other matrix macromolecules, but nonuniformity in the arrangement of these fibers accounts for its lack of transparency.[85] The thickness of the scleral stroma ranges from approximately 0.5 nm to 1.0 mm depending on the area, with the exception of the sites of insertion for the rectus muscle, where the sclera is thinnest. The toughness of the scleral stroma is essential for its role as a container of the intraocular tissues. Scleral fibroblasts are embedded within the collagen lamellae.

Cells

Keratocytes are the predominant cellular components of the corneal stroma and are thought to turn over about every 2 to 3 years. The spindle-shaped keratocytes are scattered among the lamellae of the stroma (Fig. 1.9). These cells extend long processes, and the processes of neighboring cells are connected at their tips by gap junctions (Fig. 1.10).[86] The three-dimensional network structure of keratocytes can be observed by light microscopy in flat preparations of the corneal stroma by confocal biomicroscopy, and, after digestion of stromal collagen, by scanning electron microscopy (Fig. 1.10).[87]

Keratocytes are similar to fibroblasts and possess an extensive intracellular cytoskeleton, including prominent actin filaments. Keratocytes are thus quiescent in the normal cornea but are readily activated and undergo transformation into myofibroblasts, that express α-smooth muscle actin, in response to various types of insult to the stroma.[88] Myofibroblasts produce ECM, collagen-degrading enzymes, matrix metalloproteinases (MMPs), and cytokines for stromal tissue repair, and their ability to contract contributes to wound closure.

Although scleral fibroblasts are not as well characterized as keratocytes, they are thought to be similar to fibroblasts in other parts of the body. As in the corneal stroma, a slow turnover of collagen fibers by scleral fibroblasts is required for connective tissue homeostasis. Matrix degradation by scleral fibroblasts is promoted by prostaglandin derivatives, which accounts in part for the increase in uveoscleral outflow of aqueous humor and the reduction in intraocular pressure induced by such drugs.[89] Activation of scleral fibroblasts by external stimuli, such as injury or surgery, also results in their transdifferentiation into myofibroblasts and consequent tissue fibrosis.

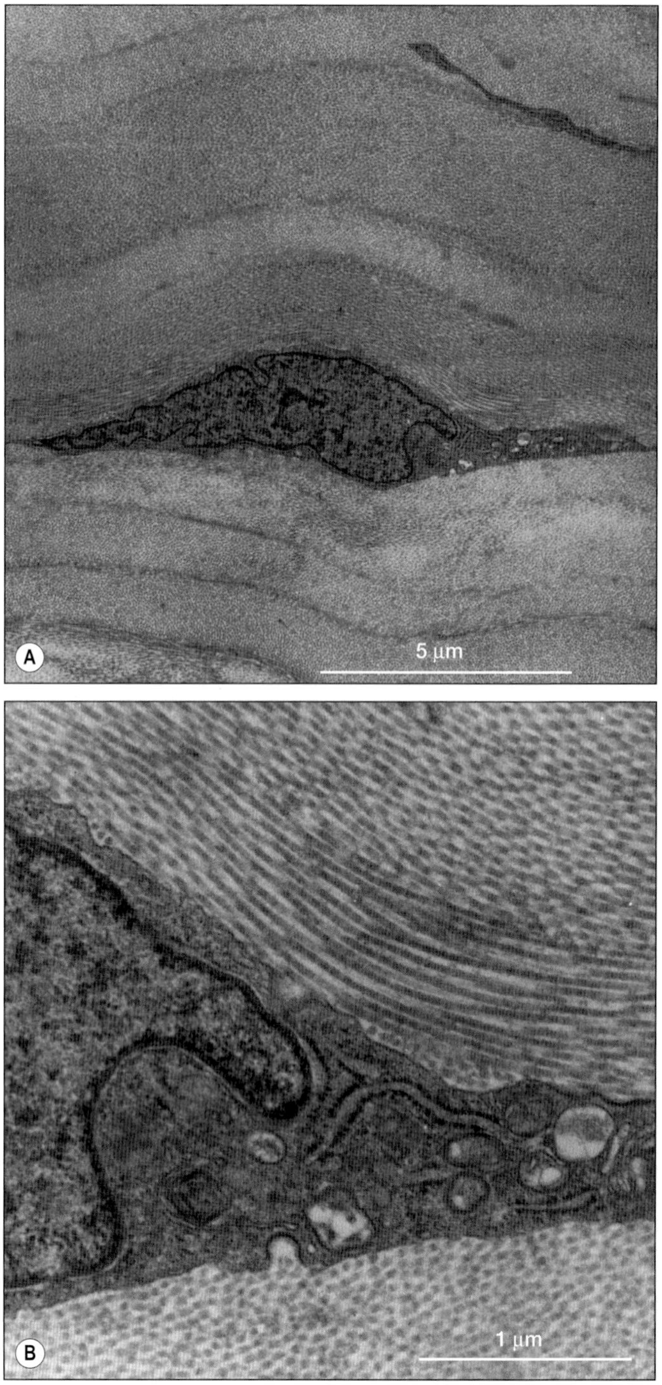

Fig. 1.9 Transmission electron microscopy of the human corneal stroma. (**A**) A keratocyte localized between stromal lamellae. (**B**) A higher-magnification view showing a keratocyte in relation to collagen fibers coursing in various directions.

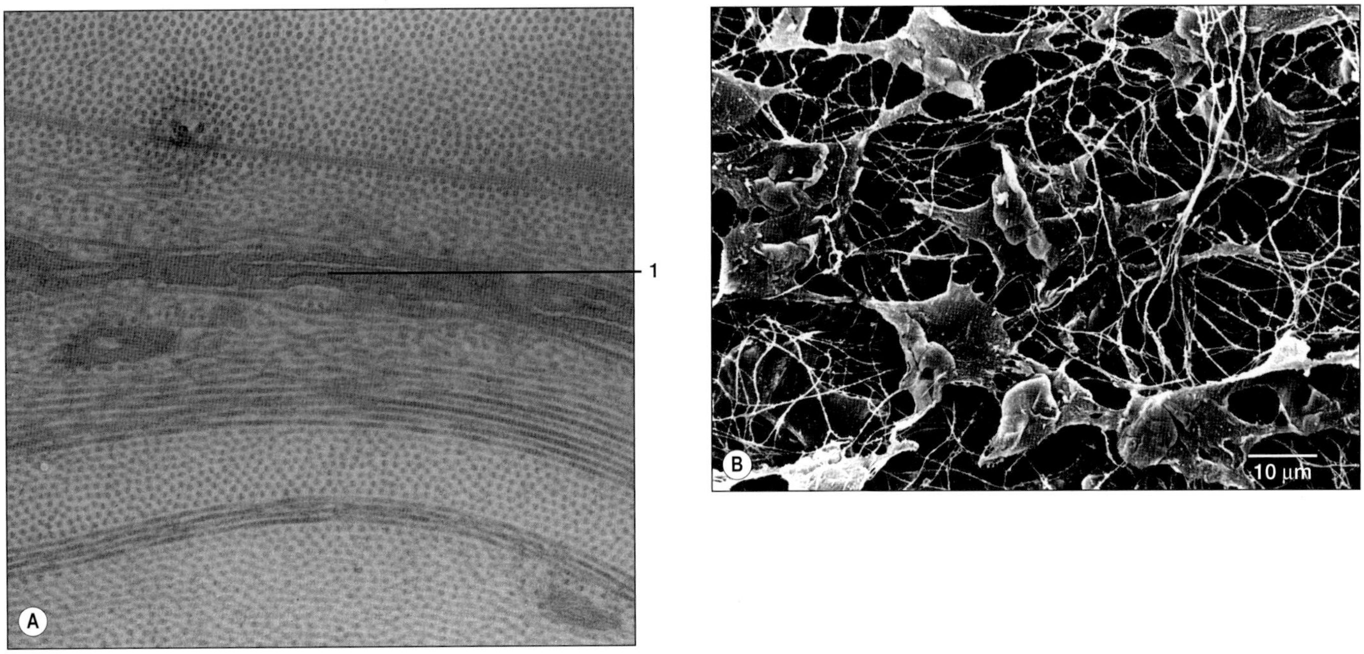

Fig. 1.10 Electron microscopy of the corneal stroma. (**A**) Lamellar structure of collagen fibers and electron-dense gap junctions (*1*) between the cellular processes of keratocytes in the human cornea. (**B**) Three-dimensional view of keratocytes in the rat cornea after digestion of collagen. Note the cellular network formed by keratocytes.

Collagen

The cellular components (mainly keratocytes) occupy only 2–3% of the total volume of the corneal stroma,[90] with the remaining portion comprising mostly the ECM components collagen and proteoglycans. Collagen constitutes more than 70% of the dry weight of the cornea. Collagen in the corneal stroma is mostly type I, with smaller amounts of types III, V, and VI also present.[91–100] Proteoglycans are distributed among the major collagen fibers.

Both the mean diameter of collagen fibers and the mean distance between such fibers in the corneal stroma are relatively homogeneous and are less than half of the wavelength of visible light (400–700 nm). This anatomic arrangement is thought to be responsible for the fact that scattering of an incident ray of light by each collagen fiber is canceled by interference from other scattered rays,[4] allowing light to pass through the cornea. If the diameter of or the distance between collagen fibers becomes heterogeneous (as occurs in fibrosis or edema), incident rays are scattered randomly and the cornea loses its transparency.

Procollagen molecules are secreted by keratocytes into the extracellular space, after which the propeptides at both ends are cleaved to yield the mature collagen molecules. The collagen molecules self-assemble into fibrils with a diameter of 10–300 nm, and these fibrils subsequently further assemble into collagen fibers. Individual collagen fibers in the corneal stroma can be observed by transmission electron microscopy (see Fig. 1.9). As mentioned above, both the diameter of (22.5–35 nm)[99,101] and distance between (41.4 ± 0.5 nm)[102] collagen fibers in the corneal stroma are highly uniform, with this regular arrangement being a major determinant of corneal transparency. At high magnification, each collagen fiber exhibits a characteristic cross-striation pattern with a periodicity of 67 nm (see Fig. 1.9). In the corneal stroma, the collagen fibers form about 300 lamellae.[103] Each lamella courses parallel to the surface of the cornea from limbus to limbus. The turnover of collagen molecules in the cornea is slow, requiring 2 to 3 years.

The histological features of the scleral stroma are similar to those of the corneal stroma, with the scleral stroma also being composed largely of major collagen fibers and proteoglycans.[104] The collagen types detected in the scleral stroma are also similar to those in the corneal stroma. In contrast, the matrix components present in the spaces between the major collagen fibers in the scleral stroma differ from those in the corneal stroma. This difference in the noncollagenous matrix largely accounts for the difference in ultrastructure between the cornea and sclera. Whereas the collagen fibers in the corneal stroma are highly uniform in diameter, those in the scleral stroma range in diameter from 25 to 250 nm. Furthermore, whereas collagen fibers are arranged regularly with a relatively uniform interfiber distance in the corneal stroma, the distance between collagen fibers in the scleral stroma varies. The ECM of the scleral stroma, including both collagen and noncollagenous components, is produced by the stromal fibroblasts.

Proteoglycans

Proteoglycans, the major matrix components located in the spaces among major collagen fibers in the stroma of the cornea and sclera, are composed of a core protein and glycosaminoglycan chains and are thought to modulate collagen fibrillogenesis.[105] Glycosaminoglycans themselves also play important roles regardless of the core protein to which they are attached. The functions of proteoglycans can thus be considered from the points of view of both the core protein and glycosaminoglycans.

With the exception of hyaluronan (hyaluronic acid), the glycosaminoglycans of the corneal stroma are present in the form of proteoglycans. The most abundant glycosaminoglycan in the cornea is keratan sulfate,[106] constituting about 65% of the total glycosaminoglycan content. The remaining glycosaminoglycans include chondroitin sulfate and dermatan sulfate. Glycosaminoglycans have the ability to absorb and retain large amounts of water. Although corneal hydration is regulated predominantly by an endothelial pump, it is also influenced by the epithelial barrier, surface evaporation, intraocular pressure, and stromal swelling pressure. The tendency of the stroma to swell results from interfibrillary imbibition of fluid and repulsion between the fixed negative charges on keratan sulfate and chondroitin sulfate. This swelling tendency has been termed the swelling pressure (SP) and is approximately 50 mmHg in the excised cornea. The negative pressure that draws fluid into the cornea is termed the imbibition pressure (IP), which, in the excised cornea, is equal to the swelling pressure. In vivo, however, the imbibition pressure is lower than the swelling pressure because of the compressive effect of intraocular pressure (IOP). The relationship between these three parameters is described by the equation:

$$\mathrm{IP} = \mathrm{IOP} - \mathrm{SP}$$

An appreciation of the dynamics of corneal edema therefore requires an understanding of the role of the stromal ground substance (glycosaminoglycan chains of proteoglycans) in the hydration state (and hence the clarity) of the cornea. If the pump function of the corneal endothelium is lost, the corneal stroma swells, leading to a disturbance in the regular spacing between collagen fibers. The irregularity of the interfiber distance results in scattering of incident light and renders the cornea hazy.

In terms of core proteins, the corneal stroma contains lumican, keratocan, and mimecan (osteoglycin) as keratan sulfate proteoglycans as well as decorin and biglycan as chondroitin sulfate or dermatan sulfate proteoglycans (Table 1.3).[107,108] These core proteins are members of the family of small leucine-rich proteoglycans (SLRPs), which contain a common central domain consisting of about 10 leucine-rich repeats.[109] They first accumulate as low-sulfate glycoproteins in the embryonic stroma and subsequently bind glycosaminoglycans to form proteoglycans typical of the adult cornea. Although the roles of specific proteoglycans in the maintenance of corneal transparency or shape under physiological conditions or in the development of corneal haziness under pathological conditions remain unclear, spontaneous mutation of a core protein gene has provided some insight. Mutation of the keratocan gene was recently shown to result in cornea plana, an anomaly characterized by abnormal corneal curvature, but it did not affect the transparency of the corneal stroma.[110,111]

Recent studies with transgenic or knockout mice have also provided insight into the roles of proteoglycan core proteins. Lumican-deficient mice have been shown to undergo age-dependent opacification of the corneal stroma.[112,113] Transmission electron microscopy revealed an irregular arrangement of collagen fibers in the posterior stroma of these animals. Humans with a mutated lumican gene have not yet been described, however. Keratocan-deficient mice show a change in the shape of the eye shell, but the transparency of the corneal stroma is not affected.[110] Mice lacking decorin exhibit abnormal collagen fibrillogenesis in the tail tendon but not in the corneal stroma,[114] indicating that decorin may not play an important role in maintenance of corneal stromal transparency, despite its abundance in the stroma. Such genetically modified mice not only shed light on the functions of specific molecules but also provide models of human genetic disorders of the cornea.

Table 1.3 Glycosaminoglycans and proteoglycan core proteins in the cornea

Glycosaminoglycan	Size (kDa)	Constituent disaccharide
Heparan sulfate	5–12	*N*-acetylgalactosamine, glucuronic acid
Heparin	6–25	*N*-acetylgalactosamine, glucuronic acid
Dermatan sulfate	15–49	*N*-acetylgalactosamine, iduronic acid
Chondroitin 4,6-sulfate	5–50	*N*-acetylgalactosamine, glucuronic acid
Keratan sulfate	4–19	*N*-acetylgalactosamine, galactose
Hyaluronan	4–8000	*N*-acetylgalactosamine, glucuronic acid

Core protein	Glycosaminoglycan	Function
Lumican	Keratan sulfate	Interaction with corneal epithelial cells
Keratocan	Keratan sulfate	Mutation causes cornea plana
Mimecan	Keratan sulfate	Unknown
Decorin	Chondroitin sulfate or dermatan sulfate	Wound healing

In the normal cornea, proteoglycans are synthesized by stromal keratocytes. They are transiently synthesized by corneal epithelial cells during the early phase of wound healing.

The main difference between the proteoglycan composition of the sclera and that of the cornea is the absence of keratocan, a specific marker of keratocyte differentiation,[108] in the sclera. However, this difference alone does not explain the lack of uniformity in the size and arrangement of collagen fibers in the sclera. The relative amounts of proteoglycan components in the sclera are changed in an animal model of myopia.[115] Recent studies suggest that matrix components of the cornea or sclera play specific roles in regulation of the shape or size of the eye shell. The eyeball of lumican-deficient mice is larger than that of wild-type animals, whereas that of keratocan-deficient mice is smaller.[110,112,113]

Descemet's membrane

Descemet's membrane, the basement membrane of the corneal endothelium, gradually increases in thickness from birth (3 μm) to adulthood (8–10 μm) in humans. Histological analysis reveals it to be stratified into a thin (0.3 μm) nonbanded layer adjacent to the stroma, an anterior banded zone (2–4 μm), and a posterior amorphous, nonbanded zone (>4 μm), the latter of which can represent up to two-thirds of the thickness of the membrane and is laid down over time.[116]

Descemet's membrane is composed primarily of collagen types IV and VIII and laminin[117] but also contains fibronectin.[118,119] Type VIII collagen, which is produced by the corneal endothelium, forms a hexagonal lattice that is substantially different from the structure of type IV collagen in the basement membrane. Collagen fibrils in the stroma are continuous with those in Bowman's layer but not with those in Descemet's membrane. Descemet's membrane adheres tightly to the posterior surface of the corneal stroma and reflects any change in the shape of the stroma. Rupture of Descemet's membrane by physical stress, such as compression birth injury, results in the penetration of aqueous humor into the corneal stroma and consequent stromal edema. Descemet's membrane does not regenerate after endothelial cells re-cover the ruptured area. Diseases such as Fuchs' dystrophy are associated with an atypical striated pattern of collagen deposition in Descemet's membrane.[120] A patient with early-onset Fuchs' dystrophy was found to harbor a mutation in *COL8A2*,[121] which encodes the α2 chain of type VIII collagen.

Endothelium

A single layer of corneal endothelial cells covers the posterior surface of Descemet's membrane in a well-arranged mosaic pattern (Fig. 1.11). These cells are uniformly 5 μm in thickness and 20 μm in width and are polygonal (mostly hexagonal) in shape. The uniformity of endothelial cell size has been evaluated by statistical analysis based on photographs taken by a wide-field specular microscope. In young adults, the cell density is about 3500 cells/mm^2. The coefficient of variation of mean cell area (standard deviation of mean cell area/mean cell area) is a clinically valuable marker and is about 0.25 in the normal cornea. An increase in the variability of cell area is termed polymegathism. Another

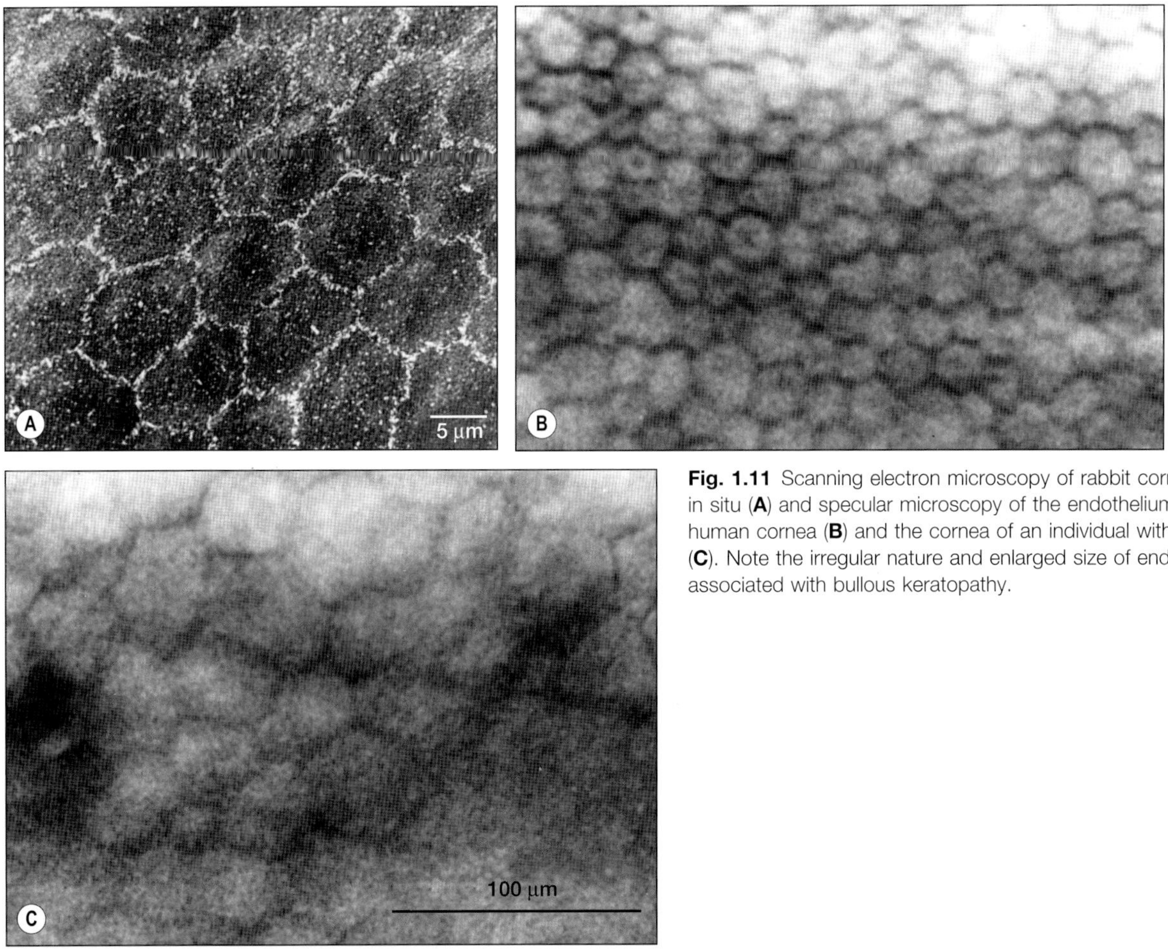

Fig. 1.11 Scanning electron microscopy of rabbit corneal endothelial cells in situ (**A**) and specular microscopy of the endothelium in both a normal human cornea (**B**) and the cornea of an individual with bullous keratopathy (**C**). Note the irregular nature and enlarged size of endothelial cells associated with bullous keratopathy.

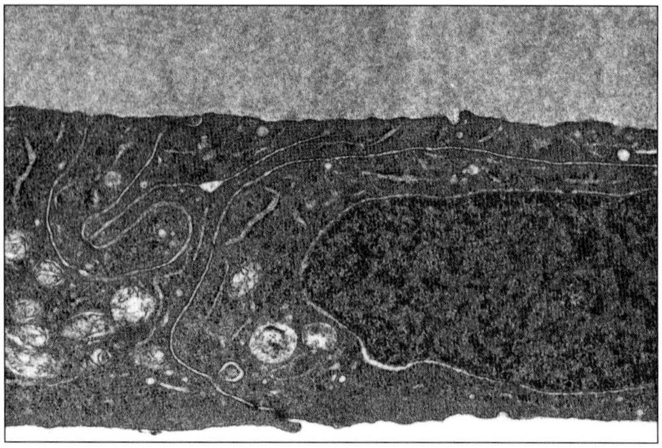

Fig. 1.12 Transmission electron microscopy of the human corneal endothelium.

morphometric parameter of the state of the endothelium is hexagonality. In the normal healthy cornea, about 70–80% of endothelial cells are hexagonal. However, endothelial damage can result in a decrease in the hexagonality value and an increase in the variability of cell area (Fig. 1.11). Deviation from hexagonality is referred to as pleomorphism.

Endothelial cells contain a large nucleus and abundant cytoplasmic organelles, including mitochondria, endoplasmic reticulum, free ribosomes, and Golgi apparatus (Fig. 1.12), suggesting that they are metabolically active. The endothelial cells interdigitate and contain various junctional complexes, including zonula occludens, macula occludens, and macula adherens. In addition, gap junctions allow the transfer of small molecules and electrolytes between the endothelial cells. The interconnected endothelial cell layer provides a leaky barrier to aqueous humor.

Loss of or damage to corneal endothelial cells results in increased imbibition of water by the corneal stroma. The endothelial cells contain ion transport systems that counteract the imbibition of water into the stroma. An osmotic gradient of Na^+ is present between the aqueous humor (143 mEq/L) and the stroma (134 mEq/L). This gradient results in the flow of Na^+ from the aqueous humor to the stroma and in a flux of K^+ in the opposite direction. The Na^+- and K^+-dependent ATPase and the Na^+/H^+ exchanger are expressed in the basolateral membrane of corneal endothelial cells. Carbon dioxide also diffuses into the cytoplasm of these cells and, together with water, generates bicarbonate ions (HCO_3^-) in a reaction catalyzed by carbonic anhydrase. The HCO_3^- then diffuses or is transported into the aqueous humor. Coupled with this movement of HCO_3^- is a flux of water across endothelial cells into the aqueous humor. Given that this ion transport system is partially dependent on cellular energy, cooling of the cornea results in its thickening and in it becoming opaque. The return of the cornea to normal body temperature, however, results in restoration of its normal thickness and clarity in a phenomenon known as temperature reversal.

Corneal endothelial cells essentially do not proliferate in humans, monkeys, and cats, but they do divide in rabbits. Endothelial cell density in the normal healthy cornea decreases with age.[122] It is important that corneal endothelial cells are protected during surgery. The loss of endothelial cells for any reason results in enlargement of the remaining neighboring cells and their spreading to cover the defective area, without an increase in cell number. The indices based on specular microscopy fluctuate as endothelial damage is resurfaced by the migration and enlargement of the remaining endothelial cells. The coefficient of variation of mean cell area is the most sensitive index of corneal endothelial dysfunction, whereas hexagonality is a good index of the progress of endothelial wound healing.

Maintenance of Normal Corneal Integrity

Overview

Maintenance of corneal structure is crucial for the physiological roles of this tissue in refraction and biodefense. A smooth epithelium, a transparent stroma, and a functioning endothelium are all essential for clear vision. The cornea is vulnerable to various chemical or biological agents as well as physical events in the outside world. It is, therefore, equipped with an active maintenance system responsible for renewal of the corneal epithelium and wound healing.

The widespread application of corneal surgery, including keratoplasty and refractive surgery, has necessitated a more detailed understanding of recent advances in cellular and molecular biology of corneal wound healing. In most parts of the body, wound healing is initiated by the extravasation of blood constituents that accompanies disruption of blood vessels. The cornea, however, is an avascular tissue. The mechanism of wound healing in the cornea thus differs from that elsewhere in the body.

Epithelial maintenance

Role of limbal stem cells

Corneal epithelial cells renew continuously to maintain the normal layered structure of the epithelium. The centripetal movement of corneal epithelial cells has been well demonstrated, as has the fact that only the basal epithelial cells are capable of proliferation. Thoft and Friend proposed that an equilibrium exists between the centripetal movement of epithelial cells, the differentiation of basal cells into superficial cells, and the desquamation of epithelial cells from the corneal surface (X, Y, Z hypothesis).[123] The existence of corneal epithelial stem cells at the limbus has also been postulated.[124] Indeed, the limbal epithelium exhibits a higher proliferative activity and a lower differentiation capability than those of the corneal epithelium, and basal limbal epithelial cells are thought to be a type of undifferentiated stem cell because they do not express corneal epithelium-specific keratin (keratin 3/12).[125]

Basal epithelial cells of the human limbus express various possible stem cell markers.[126] The expression of p63, a-enolase, keratin 5/14, and the hepatocyte growth factor (HGF) receptor has also been shown to be higher in the limbal epithelium than in the corneal epithelium. Although no direct evidence for the existence of limbal stem cells has been obtained to date, ABCG2 appears to be the most promising surface marker for the identification of such cells. Deficiency of limbal stem cells has been suggested to result in impairment of corneal epithelial homeostasis in individuals with aniridia, inflammatory disorders of the ocular surface such as Stevens–Johnson syndrome, or severe alkali burn of the ocular surface.[127]

Epithelial movement

Injury to the corneal surface is not uncommon and results in an epithelial defect, the rapid resurfacing of which is required for restoration of the continuity of the corneal epithelium. Repair of epithelial defects occurs in three distinct phases characterized by epithelial cell migration, proliferation, and differentiation, resulting in restoration of the stratified structure of the epithelium.

Epithelial migration is thus the initial step in the resurfacing of epithelial defects.[128] Trauma to the corneal epithelium induces the sliding and migration of the remaining epithelial cells adjacent to the injury site toward the defective area.[129–132] Dynamic changes in cell–cell and cell–matrix (fibronectin–integrin system) interactions, up-regulation of hyaluronan, and modulation of the ECM by newly expressed proteolytic enzymes play important roles in these two types of epithelial cell movement in response to injury. Such changes are under the overall control of growth factors and cytokines.

Fibronectin–integrin system

Fibronectin provides a provisional matrix during the first phase of epithelial wound healing in many tissues.[133] Fibronectin appears at the newly exposed corneal surface soon after epithelial or stromal injury,[118,119] and epithelial cells then attach to and spread over the fibronectin matrix.[79,134,135]

Adhesion of migrating corneal epithelial cells to a fibronectin matrix is mediated by integrins, which constitute a family of cell surface receptor proteins. To date, this family has been shown to include 24 different α subunits and nine different β subunits, with the selective combination of these α and β subunits determining the specificity of binding to ECM proteins. The integrin subunits α2, α3, α5, α6, αv, β1, β4, and β5 have been detected in the human cornea.[136] The binding of integrins α5β1, αvβl, and αIIβ3 to fibronectin is mediated by the RGD sequence. The appearance and disappearance of the integrin β1 chain and fibronectin during corneal epithelial wound healing are well coordinated (Fig. 1.13).[83] Immediately after an incision to

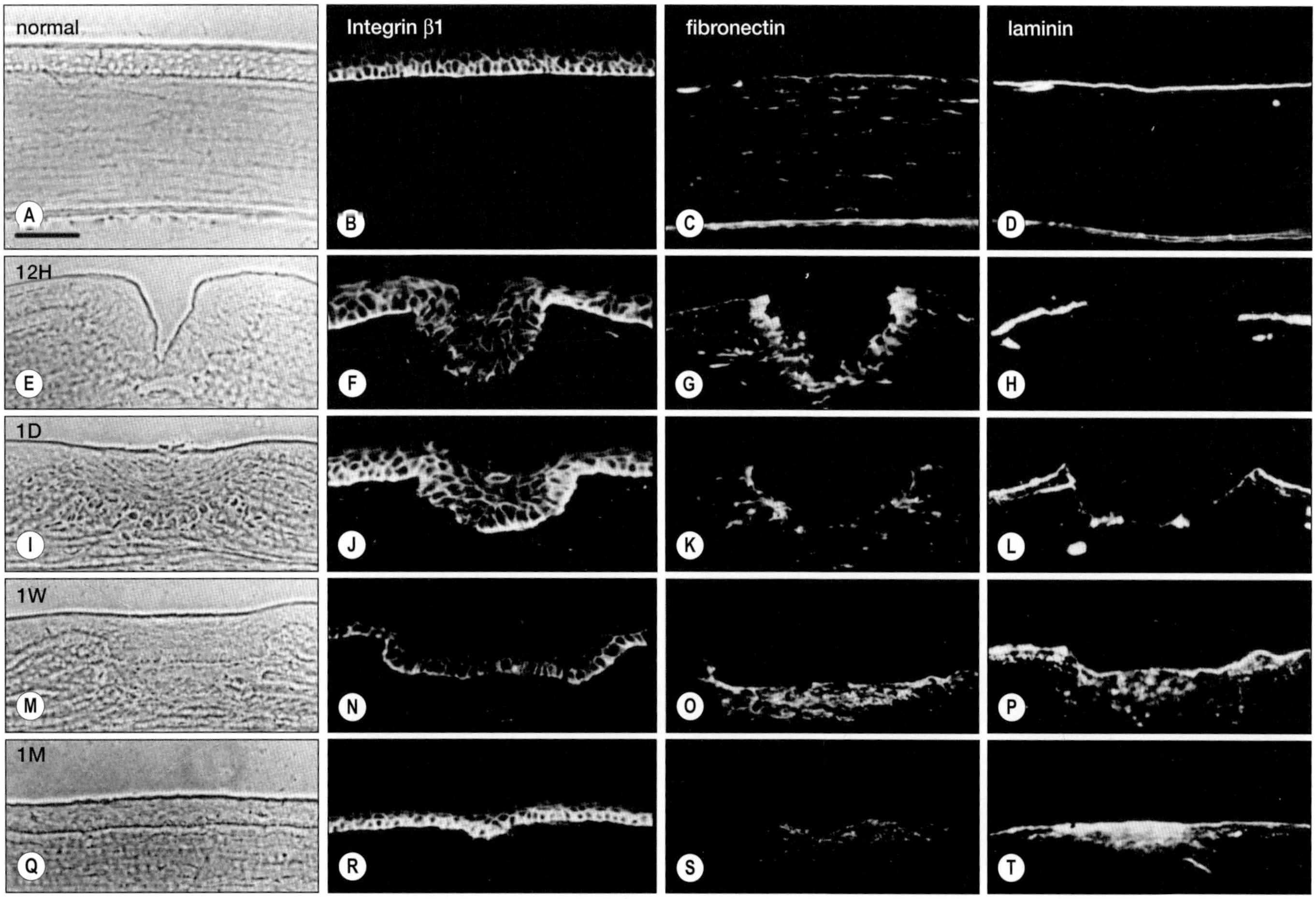

Fig. 1.13 Changes in the localization of the integrin β1 chain, fibronectin, and laminin after a nonpenetrating incision in the rat cornea.

the rat cornea, fibronectin was detected on the surface of the V-shaped defect in the stroma. Epithelial cells expressing the integrin β1 subunit then began to migrate over and to fill in the defect. With the exception of that in basal cells, expression of the integrin β1 chain in epithelial cells was down-regulated coincident with the completion of wound healing. The abundance of fibronectin at the interface between the new epithelium and the stroma also markedly decreased at this time.

The integrin α6β4 heterodimer is a component of hemidesmosomes and is not related to fibronectin-mediated cell adhesion and migration. In response to wounding of the corneal epithelium, hemidesmosomes in the basal cell layer are disassembled. They eventually reappear after migration of the remaining epithelium has resulted in a recovering of the denuded area.[137]

Hyaluronan

Hyaluronan is also recognized as a biological signaling molecule and, like fibronectin, plays an important role in inflammation and wound healing.[138] Hyaluronan is not present in the normal cornea. Unlike other glycosaminoglycans, a core protein for hyaluronan binding has not yet been identified. Hyaluronan is transiently expressed in the rabbit cornea during wound healing.[139,140] These observations suggest that hyaluronan plays a key role in the late stages of corneal wound healing.

Exogenous hyaluronan also increases the rate of corneal epithelial wound healing. The administration of hyaluronan eyedrops thus promotes corneal epithelial wound closure after epithelial debridement in rabbits[141] and in diabetic rats.[142,143]

Proteolytic enzymes

Proteolytic enzymes also play an important role in wound healing. Cellular motility depends not only on the interaction of cells with the underlying ECM but also on the termination of such interaction by degradation of matrix proteins. Proteases, including plasminogen activator, have been detected in tear fluid.[143–146] MMPs are also up-regulated in the migrating corneal epithelium.[147]

Cytokines and growth factors

Epidermal growth factor

The roles of various cytokines and growth factors in the regulation of corneal epithelial migration have also been investigated.[148] In general, these molecules modulate corneal epithelial wound healing by regulating the various healing-related systems described above.

Epidermal growth factor (EGF) was first isolated from the mouse submaxillary gland as a factor that stimulates eye opening and incisory tooth eruption in newborn mice.[149] This 53-amino acid polypeptide is a potent stimulator of proliferation in a variety of cell types, including corneal epithelial cells.[150,151] It was also found to promote corneal epithelial wound closure in animals.[152,153]

The continuous exposure of the corneal epithelium to EGF present in tear fluid suggests that the stimulatory effect of this growth factor on epithelial cell proliferation must be counteracted if the normal thickness and function of the epithelium are to be maintained. In addition to its stimulatory effect on cell proliferation, EGF exerts a variety of other actions in corneal epithelial cells, including promotion of cell adhesion to a fibronectin matrix.[154,155]

Transforming growth factor-β

Corneal epithelial cells express transforming growth factor (TGF)-β1.[156] The stimulatory effects of EGF on corneal epithelial cell proliferation, attachment to fibronectin, and migration are modulated by TGF-β.[157,158] Although TGF-β alone inhibits corneal epithelial cell proliferation, it has no effect on cell attachment to a fibronectin matrix in the absence of EGF. Endogenous TGF-β also promotes corneal epithelial cell migration.

Basic fibroblast growth factor and platelet-derived growth factor

Basic fibroblast growth factor (bFGF) is another polypeptide growth factor that stimulates the proliferation of various cell types of mesodermal or neuroectodermal origin.[159] The application of recombinant human bFGF (200–500 ng, twice a day) was shown to accelerate corneal epithelial wound closure in rabbits.[160] Rabbit corneal epithelial cells also express both the β and α type of receptors for platelet-derived growth factor (PDGF) at a density of 4.3×10^4 and 2.8×10^3/cell, respectively.[161] Consistent with this observation, the BB and AB isoforms of PDGF increased the cytosolic concentration of free Ca^{2+} in these cells. Although Ca^{2+} is implicated as a second messenger in regulation of a variety of functions in many cell types, a role for this ion in corneal epithelial wound healing remains to be determined.

Interleukins

Interleukins are cytokines that regulate the function of the immune system, inflammation, and other reactions of tissue to external stimuli.[162] They modulate the activities of immune or inflammatory cells both locally in tissue as well as systemically in the circulation and in bone marrow. Although 35 members of the interleukin family (IL-1 to IL-35) have been identified to date, the roles of many of these proteins in corneal wound healing remain to be investigated. For example, the corneal epithelium expresses IL-1, and exogenous IL-1 promotes the healing of corneal epithelial wounds.[163] Corneal epithelial cells also express IL-6.[164] Exposure of rabbit corneal epithelial cells in culture to IL-6 resulted in a marked increase in the number of cells that attached to a fibronectin matrix. IL-6 stimulates the expression of integrin α5β1 in corneal epithelial cells, suggesting that this cytokine may regulate corneal epithelial migration through modulation of the fibronectin–integrin system.[53,165,166]

Neural regulation

The physiological role of corneal innervation in corneal epithelial wound healing remains to be fully clarified. The loss of corneal sensation, however, often results in breakdown of the normal integrity of the cornea. Persistent corneal epithelial defects or delayed epithelial wound healing are frequently observed in individuals with a reduced corneal sensation, such as those infected with herpes simplex or herpes zoster virus as well as those with diabetes mellitus. Abuse of topical anesthetics also impairs corneal epithelial migration in an organ culture system.[167] Furthermore, frank corneal ulceration has been shown to develop in anesthetized eyes. These various observations thus implicate neural regulation in maintenance and repair of the corneal epithelium.

As discussed earlier, the cornea is densely innervated by sensory nerve fibers of trigeminal nerve origin which contain the sensory neurotransmitter substance P. Substance P is thought to regulate various physiological processes, including plasma extravasation, vasodilatation, and the release of histamine from mast cells.[168–171] Exposure of rabbit corneal epithelial cells in culture to the combination of substance P and insulin-like growth factor-1 (IGF-1) resulted in a marked increase in the number of cells that attached to a fibronectin matrix.[154] Substance P has also been implicated in neuronal responses to various stimuli in the eye as well as in other tissues.[20,172,173]

Trigeminal denervation correlates with a reduction in the abundance of substance P in the cornea.[174] Sectioning of the trigeminal nerve results in trophic or degenerative changes in the cornea as well as in the depletion of substance P.[175] Substance P may thus contribute to maintenance of the normal integrity of the corneal epithelium. The combination of substance P and IGF-1 synergistically promotes corneal epithelial migration, with neither agent alone having an effect on this process. Furthermore, the administration of eyedrops containing IGF-1 and either substance P or a tetrapeptide derived from its carboxyl terminus has been shown to be an effective treatment for persistent corneal epithelial defects in individuals with neurotrophic keratopathy or diabetic neuropathy.[176–178]

Nerve growth factor (NGF), first discovered by Levi-Montalcini in the early 1950s,[179] is a polypeptide that stimulates the regeneration of peripheral nerve fibers.[180] Furthermore, eyedrops containing NGF promote resurfacing of persistent corneal epithelial defects in animals and humans.[181–185]

Stromal maintenance

Extracellular matrix and stromal repair

Structural and biochemical homeostasis of the ECM in the corneal stroma is thus maintained by a balance in the keratocyte regulation of the synthesis and degradation of ECM components. In response to corneal injury, keratocytes transdifferentiate into myofibroblasts and actively produce matrix components for healing of the injured stroma, with each newly expressed macromolecule appearing to play an important role in the repair process.

During infectious ulceration of the corneal stroma, enzymes that degrade the ECM of the stroma are released by both host cells and the infecting bacteria. Furthermore, pseudomonal elastase degrades collagen directly as well as promotes collagen degradation by keratocytes, in part, via activation of pro-MMPs.[186] Thus, there appear to be at least three different pathways for the degradation of stromal collagen fibers in individuals with infectious corneal ulceration: (1) direct degradation by bacterial collagenase, (2) degradation by MMPs released from keratocytes (or myofibroblasts) activated by bacterial factors such as elastase, or (3) activation by infiltrated inflammatory cells.

Cytokines and growth factors

Both keratocytes and infiltrated cells, such as lymphocytes, neutrophils, and macrophages, secrete cytokines or growth factors and modulate behaviors of cells in the healing corneal stroma. Each cytokine or growth factor activates signal transduction pathways that regulate the expression of specific genes that contribute to the inflammatory response. Targeting of such regulation at the ligand or signaling level may provide new strategies for treatment of wound-related pathology. TGF-β is thought to play a key role in healing of the corneal stroma.[187,188] It is expressed by both epithelial cells and stromal cells (keratocytes or scleral fibroblasts) as well as by inflammatory cells that activate stromal cells and promote their transdifferentiation into myofibroblasts. Myofibroblasts contribute not only to wound repair but also to post-injury stromal scarring in the cornea and sclera as a result of the overproduction of matrix components. Blockade of TGF-β signaling effectively reduces the fibrogenic reaction and consequent scarring and opacification in a mouse model of corneal alkali burn.[187,188]

The proinflammatory cytokine tumor necrosis factor (TNF)-α is also up-regulated in response to injury.[189] TNF-α induces various effects in the cornea under pathological conditions such as injury, allergy, and infection.[190–193] However, the complete loss of TNF-α in the cornea of knockout mice results in enhancement of post-alkali burn inflammation, suggesting that the role of TNF-α in the cornea might depend on the specific condition.[194]

Neovascularization in the corneal stroma

The cornea is an avascular tissue and must remain transparent in order to refract light properly. Neovascularization in the cornea resulting from inflammation associated with various conditions such as trauma, microbial infection, or alkali burn or from limbal stem cell deficiency can thus impair vision. Cytokines and growth factors orchestrate cell behavior associated with the development of corneal neovascularization. Vascular endothelial growth factor (VEGF) and TGF-β thus contribute to injury-induced neovascularization, with ECM components supporting the growth of new vessels. These factors are up-regulated in the corneal stroma (in both inflammatory cells and resident cells) during wound healing or inflammatory disorders.[195]

Development of the Anterior Eye Segment

Characterization of the development of ocular tissues during embryogenesis is important for understanding the pathogenesis of congenital anomalies of the cornea and

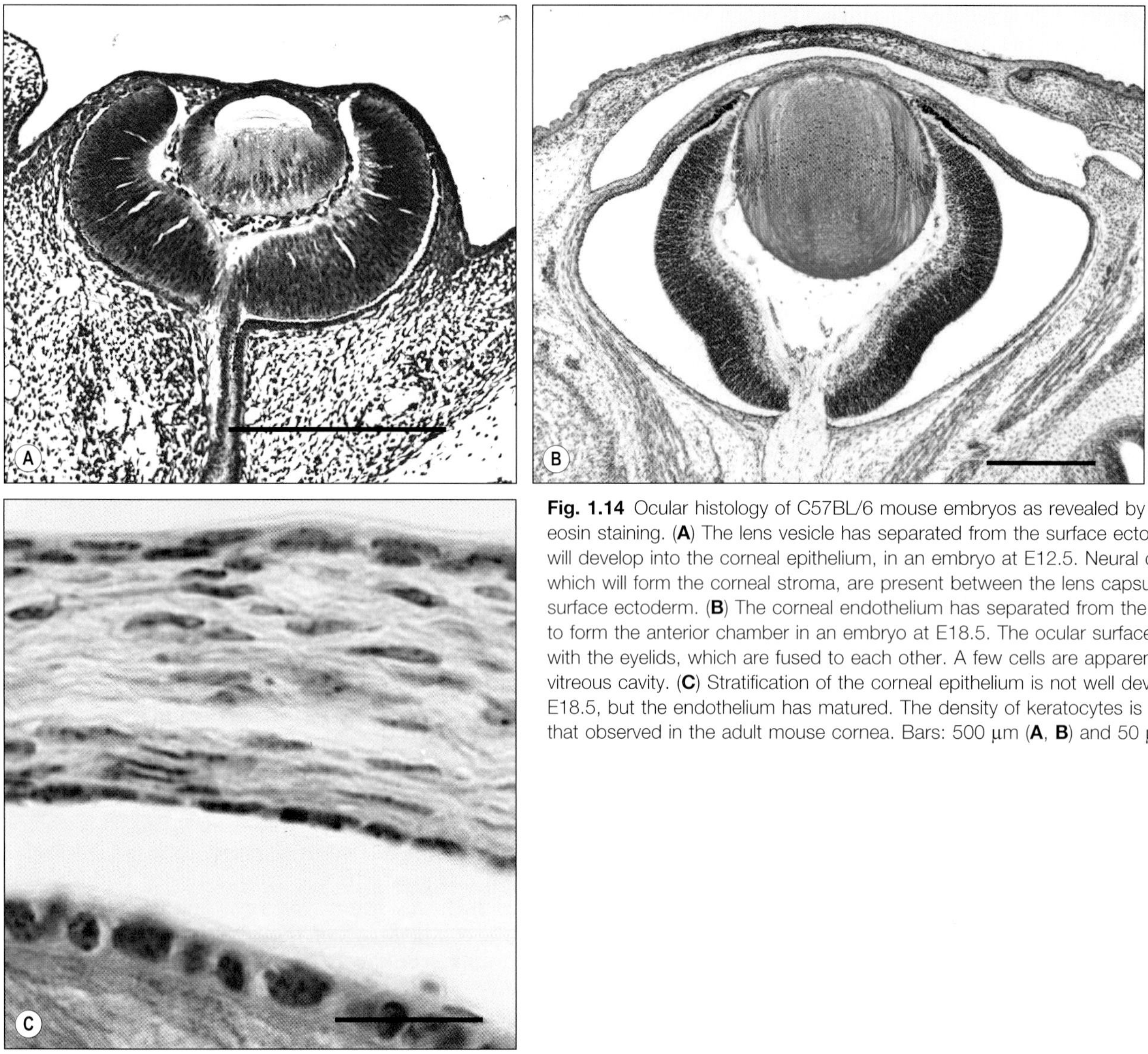

Fig. 1.14 Ocular histology of C57BL/6 mouse embryos as revealed by hematoxylin & eosin staining. (**A**) The lens vesicle has separated from the surface ectoderm, which will develop into the corneal epithelium, in an embryo at E12.5. Neural crest cells, which will form the corneal stroma, are present between the lens capsule and surface ectoderm. (**B**) The corneal endothelium has separated from the lens capsule to form the anterior chamber in an embryo at E18.5. The ocular surface is covered with the eyelids, which are fused to each other. A few cells are apparent in the vitreous cavity. (**C**) Stratification of the corneal epithelium is not well developed at E18.5, but the endothelium has matured. The density of keratocytes is higher than that observed in the adult mouse cornea. Bars: 500 μm (**A**, **B**) and 50 μm (**C**).

anterior eye segment (Fig. 1.14).[196,197] Morphogenesis of the eye is achieved by cell lineages of various origins including the surface and neural ectoderm during embryonic development. Epithelial cells of the cornea are derived from the epidermal ectoderm, whereas keratocytes, scleral fibroblasts, and endothelial cells are of neural crest (neuroectodermal) origin. The surface ectoderm above the neuronal optic cup invaginates to form the crystalline lens. After the lens vesicle has separated from the surface ectoderm, the epithelium on the immature lens differentiates into the corneal epithelium. Neural crest-derived mesenchymal cells migrate in the space between the lens and primitive corneal epithelium and develop into the corneal stroma, endothelium, iris, and trabecular meshwork. Many anomalies of the anterior eye segment result from impaired differentiation of these neural crest-derived tissues.

The surface ectoderm above the optic cup invaginates during the fifth week of gestation in humans, and the primitive corneal epithelium develops junctional complexes by the sixth week. Most scleral fibroblasts differentiate from neural crest cells that surround the optic cup during the sixth week. Mesodermal cells also contribute to development of the sclera and the extraocular muscles. The neural crest cell-derived mesenchyme migrates into the space between the primitive corneal epithelium and lens vesicle in three waves during the seventhh week. The first wave of migration results in formation of the corneal endothelium and trabecular endothelium; the second wave of cells differentiates into keratocytes; and the third wave gives rise to the iris. During the eighth week, the keratocytes form five to eight layers of collagen lamellae and the corneal endothelium starts to form Descemet's membrane. Defects in the migration of neural crest-derived mesenchymal cells are responsible for anomalies of the cornea and anterior eye segment including Peters' anomaly. Several genes, including those encoding TGF-β2 and the transcription factor FOXC, have been implicated in the differentiation of neural crest cells into the primitive corneal stroma in mice.[198]

The spaces among collagen fibers become occupied by proteoglycans that are formed as a result of the binding of glycosaminoglycan chains to previously accumulated core proteins. Even by the sixth month of gestation, the cornea is still not fully mature. The epithelium has only three or four layers of cells, and keratan sulfate proteoglycans continue to accumulate. During the seventh month, however, the cornea is well developed, with the epithelium consisting of four or five layers with readily recognizable basal, wing, and superficial cells. The stroma is also almost fully developed at this time, with the accumulation of keratan sulfate proteoglycans among collagen fibers being virtually complete. Hyaluronan is a major glycosaminoglycan in the corneal stroma during the early stages of embryonic development, but its abundance declines concomitantly with the increase in that of keratan sulfate, chondroitin sulfate, and dermatan sulfate, giving rise to a glycosaminoglycan composition similar to that of the adult stroma.[199]

Recent advances in transgenic and gene knockout technologies in mice have provided important insight into the role of specific genes in the development and homeostasis of corneal tissue as well as into congenital anomalies in humans.[199,200] Interpretation of such studies also depends on an understanding of the normal process of eye development in the mouse (see Fig. 1.14). The surface ectoderm invaginates into the optic cup at embryonic day (E) 10.5 in mice. At E12.5, the primitive lens has already separated from the surface ectoderm, which will become the corneal epithelium, and the neural crest-derived mesenchyme has begun to migrate into the space between the primitive corneal epithelium and lens. In contrast to the human embryo, the neural crest-derived cells migrate into this space in a single wave. At E14.5, the embryo has already developed the epithelium, stroma, and endothelium of the cornea, and at E18.5 the corneal stroma has increased in thickness as a result of the synthesis of matrix macromolecules. The upper and lower eyelids fuse to each other between E14.5 and E16.5; the eyelids separate and the eyes reopen after birth, and the corneal epithelium then undergoes final maturation.

References

1. Birk DE, Trelstad RL. Extracellular compartments in matrix morphogenesis: collagen fibril, bundle, and lamellar formation by corneal fibroblasts. *J Cell Biol.* 1984;99:2024–2033.
2. Freegard TJ. The physical basis of transparency of the normal cornea. *Eye.* 1997;11:465–471.
3. Mishima S. Corneal thickness. *Surv Ophthalmol.* 1968;13:57–96.
4. Maurice DM.The cornea and sclera. In: Davson H, ed. *The eye.* Orlando, FL: Academic Press; 1984:1–158.
5. Rozsa AJ, Beuerman RW. Density and organization of free nerve endings in the corneal epithelium of the rabbit. *Pain.* 1982;14:105–120,
6. Muller LJ, Marfurt CF, Kruse F, et al. Corneal nerves: structure, contents and function. *Exp Eye Res.* 2003;76:521–542.
7. Hogan MJ, Alvarado JA, Weddell JE. *Histology of the human eye.* Philadelphia, PA: WB Saunders; 1971.
8. Grupcheva CN, Wong T, Riley AF, et al. Assessing the sub-basal nerve plexus of the living healthy human cornea by in vivo confocal microscopy. *Clin Exp Ophthalmol.* 2002;30:187–190.
9. Oliveira-Soto L, Efron N. Morphology of corneal nerves using confocal microscopy. *Cornea.* 2001;20:374–384.
10. Jones MA, Marfurt CF. Peptidergic innervation of the rat cornea. *Exp Eye Res.* 1998;66:421–435.
11. Tervo K, Tervo T, Eranko L, et al. Substance P-immunoreactive nerves in the human cornea and iris. *Invest Ophthalmol Vis Sci.* 1982;23:671–674.
12. Lehtosalo JI. Substance P-like immunoreactive trigeminal ganglion cells supplying the cornea. *Histochemistry.* 1984;80:273–276.
13. Beckers HJ, Klooster J, Vrensen GF, et al. Substance P in rat corneal and iridal nerves: an ultrastructural immunohistochemical study. *Ophthalmic Res.* 1993;25:192–200.
14. Marfurt CF, Murphy CJ, Florczak JL. Morphology and neurochemistry of canine corneal innervation. *Invest Ophthalmol Vis Sci.* 2001;42:2242–2251.
15. Stone RA, Kuwayama Y, Terenghi G, et al. Calcitonin gene-related peptide: occurrence in corneal sensory nerves. *Exp Eye Res.* 1986;43:279–283.
16. Uusitalo H, Krootila K, Palkama A. Calcitonin gene-related peptide (CGRP) immunoreactive sensory nerves in the human and guinea pig uvea and cornea. *Exp Eye Res.* 1989;48:467–475.
17. Stone RA. Neuropeptide Y and the innervation of the human eye. *Exp Eye Res.* 1986;42:349–355.
18. Ueda S, del Cerro M, LoCascio JA, et al. Peptidergic and catecholaminergic fibers in the human corneal epithelium. An immunohistochemical and electron microscopic study. *Acta Ophthalmol Suppl.* 1989;192:80–90.
19. Stone RA, Tervo T, Tervo K, et al. Vasoactive intestinal polypeptide-like immunoreactive nerves to the human eye. *Acta Ophthalmol (Copenh).* 1986;64:12–18.
20. Unger WG, Butler JM, Cole DF, et al. Substance P, vasoactive intestinal polypeptide (VIP) and somatostatin levels in ocular tissue of normal and sensorily denervated rabbit eyes. *Exp Eye Res.* 1981;32:797–801.
21. Terenghi G, Zhang SQ, Unger WG, et al. Morphological changes of sensory CGRP-immunoreactive and sympathetic nerves in peripheral tissues following chronic denervation. *Histochemistry.* 1986;86:89–95.
22. Selbach JM, Rohen JW, Steuhl KP, et al. Angioarchitecture and innervation of the primate anterior episclera. *Curr Eye Res.* 2005;30:337–344.
23. Tamm ER, Koch TA, Mayer B, et al. Innervation of myofibroblast-like scleral spur cells in human monkey eyes. *Invest Ophthalmol Vis Sci.* 1995;36:1633–1644.
24. Aguayo JB, McLennan IJ, Graham C Jr, et al. Dynamic monitoring of corneal carbohydrate metabolism using high-resolution deuterium NMR spectroscopy. *Exp Eye Res.* 1988;47:337–343.
25. Gottsch JD, Chen CH, Aguayo JB, et al. Glycolytic activity in the human cornea monitored with nuclear magnetic resonance spectroscopy. *Arch Ophthalmol.* 1986;104:886–889.
26. Riley MV. Glucose and oxygen utilization by the rabbit cornea. *Exp Eye Res.* 1969;8:193–200.
27. Weissman BA, Fatt I, Rasson J. Diffusion of oxygen in human corneas in vivo. *Invest Ophthalmol Vis Sci.* 1981;20:123–125.
28. Holden BA, Sweeney DF, Vannas A, et al. Effects of long-term extended contact lens wear on the human cornea. *Invest Ophthalmol Vis Sci.* 1985;26:1489–1501.
29. Ichijima H, Ohashi J, Cavanagh HD. Effect of contact-lens-induced hypoxia on lactate dehydrogenase activity and isozyme in rabbit cornea. *Cornea.* 1992;11:108–113.
30. Polse KA, Decker M. Oxygen tension under a contact lens. *Invest Ophthalmol Vis Sci.* 1979;18:188–193.
31. Thoft RA, Friend J. Biochemical aspects of contact lens wear. *Am J Ophthalmol.* 1975;80:139–145.
32. Sack RA, Tan KO, Tan A. Diurnal tear cycle: evidence for a nocturnal inflammatory constitutive tear fluid. *Invest Ophthalmol Vis Sci.* 1992;33:626–640.
33. Sack RA, Beaton A, Sathe S, et al. Towards a closed eye model of the pre-ocular tear layer. *Prog Retin Eye Res.* 2000;19:649–668.
34. Mishima S, Gasset A, Klyce SD Jr, et al. Determination of tear volume and tear flow. *Invest Ophthalmol.* 1966;5:264–276.
35. Scherz W, Doane MG, Dohlman CH. Tear volume in normal eyes and keratoconjunctivitis sicca. *Graefe's Arch Clin Exp Ophthalmol.* 1974;192:141–150.
36. Holly FJ, Lemp MA. Tear physiology and dry eyes. *Surv Ophthalmol.* 1977;22:69–87.
37. van Setten GB, Viinikka L, Tervo T, et al. Epidermal growth factor is a constant component of normal human tear fluid. *Graefe's Arch Clin Exp Ophthalmol.* 1989;227:184–187.
38. Ohashi Y, Motokura M, Kinoshita Y, et al. Presence of epidermal growth factor in human tears. *Invest Ophthalmol Vis Sci.* 1989;30:1879–1882.
39. Gupta A, Monroy D, Ji Z, et al. Transforming growth factor β-1 and β-2 in human tear fluid. *Curr Eye Res.* 1996;15:605–614.
40. van Setten GB. Basic fibroblast growth factor in human tear fluid: detection of another growth factor. *Graefe's Arch Clin Exp Ophthalmol.* 1996;234:275–277.

41. van Setten GB, Macauley S, Humphreys-Beher M, et al. Detection of transforming growth factor-a mRNA and protein in rat lacrimal glands and characterization of transforming growth factor-α in human tears. *Invest Ophthalmol Vis Sci.* 1996;37:166–173.
42. Li Q, Weng J, Mohan RR, et al. Hepatocyte growth factor and hepatocyte growth factor receptor in the lacrimal gland, tears, and cornea. *Invest Ophthalmol Vis Sci.* 1996;37:727–739.
43. Barton K, Monroy DC, Nava A, et al. Inflammatory cytokines in the tears of patients with ocular rosacea. *Ophthalmology.* 1997;104: 1868–1874.
44. Vesaluoma M, Teppo AM, Gronhagen-Riska C, et al. Platelet-derived growth factor-BB (PDGF-BB) in tear fluid: a potential modulator of corneal wound healing following photorefractive keratectomy. *Curr Eye Res.* 1997;16:825–831.
45. Goren MB. Neural stimulation of lactoferrin and epidermal growth factor secretion by the lacrimal gland. *Cornea.* 1997;16:501–502.
46. Schechter J, Warren DW, Wood RL. The distribution of FGF-2 and TGF-β within the lacrimal gland of rabbits. *Adv Exp Med Biol.* 1998; 438:511–514.
47. Wilson SE, Liang Q, Kim WJ. Lacrimal gland HGF, KGF, and EGF mRNA levels increase after corneal epithelial wounding. *Invest Ophthalmol Vis Sci.* 1999;40:2185–2190.
48. Kurpakus MA, Wheater M, Kernacki KA, Hazlett LD. Corneal cell proteins and ocular surface pathology. *Biotech Histochem.* 1999;74: 146–159.
49. Pflugfelder SC, Jones D, Ji Z, et al. Altered cytokine balance in the tear fluid and conjunctiva of patients with Sjögren's syndrome keratoconjunctivitis sicca. *Curr Eye Res.* 1999;19:201–211.
50. Nishida T, Nakagawa S, Awata T, et al. Fibronectin promotes epithelial migration of cultured rabbit cornea in situ. *J Cell Biol.* 1983;97: 1653–1657.
51. Watanabe K, Nakagawa S, Nishida T. Stimulatory effects of fibronectin and EGF on migration of corneal epithelial cells. *Invest Ophthalmol Vis Sci.* 1987;28:205–211.
52. Tsutsumi O, Tsutsumi A, Oka T. Epidermal growth factor-like, corneal wound healing substance in mouse tears. *J Clin Invest.* 1988;81: 1067–1071.
53. Nishida T, Nakamura M, Mishima H, et al. Interleukin 6 promotes epithelial migration by a fibronectin-dependent mechanism. *J Cell Physiol.* 1992;153:1–5.
54. Nishida T, Tanaka T. Extracellular matrix and growth factors in corneal wound healing. *Curr Opin Ophthalmol.* 1996;7:2–11.
55. Beuerman RW, Pedroza L. Ultrastructure of the human cornea. *Microsc Res Tech.* 1996;33:320–335.
56. Sack RA, Nunes I, Beaton A, et al. Host-defense mechanism of the ocular surfaces. *Biosci Rep.* 2001;21:463–480.
57. Thoft RA, Friend J, Kenyon KR. Ocular surface response to trauma. *Int Ophthalmol Clin.* 1979;19:111–131.
58. Hanna C, Bicknell DS, O'Brien JE. Cell turnover in the adult human eye. *Arch Ophthalmol.* 1961;65:695–698.
59. Esco MA, Wang Z, McDermott ML, et al. Potential role for laminin 5 in hypoxia-mediated apoptosis of human corneal epithelial cells. *J Cell Sci.* 2001;114:4033–4040.
60. Ma X, Bazan HE. Platelet-activating factor (PAF) enhances apoptosis induced by ultraviolet radiation in corneal epithelial cells through cytochrome c-caspase activation. *Curr Eye Res.* 2001;23:326–335.
61. Li L, Ren DH, Ladage PM, et al. Annexin V binding to rabbit corneal epithelial cells following overnight contact lens wear or eyelid closure. *CLAO J.* 2002;28:48–54.
62. Estil S, Primo EJ, Wilson G. Apoptosis in shed human corneal cells. *Invest Ophthalmol Vis Sci.* 2000;41:3360–3364.
63. Suzuki K, Tanaka T, Enoki M, et al. Coordinated reassembly of the basement membrane and junctional proteins. *Invest Ophthalmol Vis Sci.* 2000;41:2495–2500.
64. Schermer A, Galvin S, Sun TT. Differentiation-related expression of a major 64K corneal keratin in vivo and in culture suggests limbal location of corneal epithelial stem cells. *J Cell Biol.* 1986;103:49–62.
65. Kurpakus MA, Stock EL, Jones JC. Expression of the 55-kD/64-kD corneal keratins in ocular surface epithelium. *Invest Ophthalmol Vis Sci.* 1990;31:448–456.
66. Nishida K, Honma Y, Dota A, et al. Isolation and chromosomal localization of a cornea-specific human keratin 12 gene and detection of four mutations in Meesmann corneal epithelial dystrophy. *Am J Hum Genet.* 1997;61:1268–1275.
67. Hacket DJ, Bakos I. Langerhans cells in the normal conjunctiva and peripheral cornea of selected species. *Invest Ophthalmol Vis Sci.* 1981;21:759–765.
68. Gillette TE, Chandler JW, Greiner JV. Langerhans cells of the ocular surface. *Ophthalmology.* 1982;89:700–710.
69. Rubsamen PE, McCulley J, Bergstresser PR, et al. On the Ia immunogenicity of mouse corneal allografts infiltrated with Langerhans cells. *Invest Ophthalmol Vis Sci.* 1984;25:513–518.
70. Whitsett CF, Stulting RD. The distribution of HLA antigens on human corneal tissue. *Invest Ophthalmol Vis Sci.* 1984;25:519–524.
71. Pfister RR. The normal surface of corneal epithelium: a scanning electron microscopic study. *Invest Ophthalmol.* 1973;12:654–668.
72. Argueso P, Gipson IK. Epithelial mucins of the ocular surface: structure, biosynthesis and function. *Exp Eye Res.* 2001;73:281–289.
73. Pflugfelder SC, Liu Z, Monroy D, et al. Detection of sialomucin complex (MUC4) in human ocular surface epithelium and tear fluid. *Invest Ophthalmol Vis Sci.* 2000;41:1316–1326.
74. Yokoi N, Kinoshita S. Clinical evaluation of corneal epithelial barrier function with the slit-lamp fluorophotometer. *Cornea.* 1995;14: 485–489.
75. Gipson IK, Spurr-Michaud SJ, Tisdale AS. Anchoring fibrils form a complex network in human and rabbit cornea. *Invest Ophthalmol Vis Sci.* 1987;28:212–220.
76. Bentz H, Morris NP, Murray LW, et al. Isolation and partial characterization of a new human collagen with an extended triple-helical structural domain. *Proc Natl Acad Sci USA.* 1983;80:3166–3172.
77. Takahashi M, Fujimoto T, Honda Y, et al. Immunoelectron microscopy of E-cadherin in the intact and wounded mouse corneal epithelium. *Acta Histochem Cytochem.* 1991;24:619–623.
78. Hynes RO. Integrins: bidirectional, allosteric signaling machines. *Cell.* 2002;110:673–687.
79. Nishida T, Nakagawa S, Watanabe K, et al. A peptide from fibronectin cell-binding domain inhibits attachment of epithelial cells. *Invest Ophthalmol Vis Sci.* 1988;29:1820–1825.
80. Paallysaho T, Williams DS. Epithelial cell-substrate adhesion in the cornea of actin, talin, integrin and fibronectin. *Exp Eye Res.* 1991;52:261–267.
81. Tervo K, Tervo T, van Setten G-B, et al. Integrins in human corneal epithelium. *Cornea.* 1991;10:461–465.
82. Lauweryns B, van den Oord JJ, Volpes R, et al. Distribution of very late activation integrins in the human cornea. An immunohistochemical study using monoclonal antibodies. *Invest Ophthalmol Vis Sci.* 1991;32:2079–2085.
83. Murakami J, Nishida T, Otori T. Coordinated appearance of β1 integrins and fibronectin during corneal wound healing. *J Lab Clin Med.* 1992;120:86–93.
84. Nishida T, Nakagawa S. Expression of fibronectin receptors in corneal epithelial cells. In: Beuerman RW, Crosson CE, Kaufman HE, eds. *Healing processes in the cornea.* The Woodlands, TX: Portfolio Publishing Co.; 1989:127–135.
85. Watson PG, Young RD. Scleral structure, organisation and disease. A review. *Exp Eye Res.* 2004;78:609–623.
86. Ueda A, Nishida T, Otori T, et al. Electron-microscopic studies on the presence of gap junctions between corneal fibroblasts in rabbits. *Cell Tissue Res.* 1987;249:473–475.
87. Nishida T, Yasumoto K, Otori T, et al. The network structure of corneal fibroblasts in the rat as revealed by scanning electron microscopy. *Invest Ophthalmol Vis Sci.* 1988;29:1887–1890.
88. Tomasek JJ, Gabbiani G, Hinz B, et al. Myofibroblasts and mechanoregulation of connective tissue remodelling. *Nat Rev Mol Cell Biol.* 2002;3:349–363.
89. Toris CB, Gabelt BT, Kaufman PL. Update on the mechanism of action of topical prostaglandins for intraocular pressure reduction. *Surv Ophthalmol.* 2008;53(suppl 1):S107-S120.
90. Otori T. Electrolyte content of rabbit corneal stroma. *Exp Eye Res.* 1967;6:356–367.
91. Dodson JW, Hay ED. Secretion of collagen by corneal epithelium. II. Effect of the underlying substratum on secretion and polymerization of epithelial products. *J Exp Zool.* 1974;189:51–72.
92. Linsenmayer TF, Fitch JM, Mayne R. Extracellular matrices in the developing avian eye: type V collagen in corneal and noncorneal tissues. *Invest Ophthalmol Vis Sci.* 1984;25:41–47.
93. Fitch JM, Gross J, Mayne R, et al. Organization of collagen type I and V in the embryonic chicken cornea: monoclonal antibody studies. *Proc Natl Acad Sci USA.* 1984;81:2791–2795.
94. Konomi H, Hayashi T, Nakayasu K, et al. Localization of type V collagen and type IV collagen in human cornea, lung, and skin. Immunohistochemical evidence by anti-collagen antibodies characterized by immunoelectroblotting. *Am J Pathol.* 1984;116:417–426.
95. Birk DE, Fitch JM, Linsenmayer TF. Organization of collagen type I and V in the embryonic chicken cornea. *Invest Ophthalmol Vis Sci.* 1986;27:1470–1477.
96. Yue BYJT, Sugar J, Schrode K. Collagen staining in corneal tissues. *Curr Eye Res.* 1986;5:559–564.

97. McLaughlin JS, Linsenmayer TF, Birk DE. Type V collagen synthesis and deposition by chicken embryo corneal fibroblasts in vitro. *J Cell Sci.* 1989;94:371–379.
98. Kern P, Menasche M, Robert L. Relative rates of biosynthesis of collagen type I, type V and type VI in calf cornea. *Biochem J.* 1991;274:615–617.
99. Komai Y, Ushiki T. The three-dimensional organization of collagen fibrils in the human cornea and sclera. *Invest Ophthalmol Vis Sci.* 1991;32:2244–2258.
100. Doane KJ, Yang G, Birk DE. Corneal cell-matrix interactions: Type VI collagen promotes adhesion and spreading of corneal fibroblasts. *Exp Cell Res.* 1992;200:490–499.
101. Giraud JP, Pouliquen Y, Offret G, et al. Statistical morphometric studies in normal human and rabbit corneal stroma. *Exp Eye Res.* 1975;21:221–229.
102. Hamada R, Pouliquen Y, Giranud JP, et al. Quantitative analysis on the ultrastructure of human fetal cornea. In: Yamada E, Mishima S, eds. *The structure of the eye III.* Tokyo: *Jpn J Ophthalmol.* 1976:49–62.
103. Hamada R, Giraud JP, Graf B, et al. Etude analytique et statistique des lamelles, des keratocytes, des fibrilles de collagene de la region centrale de la cornee humaine normale. [Analytical and statistical study of the lamellae, keratocytes and collagen fibrils of the central region of the normal human cornea (light and electron microscopy).] *Arch Ophtalmol Rev Gen Ophtalmol.* 1972;32:563–570.
104. Ihanamaki T, Pelliniemi LJ, Vuorio E. Collagens and collagen-related matrix components in the human and mouse eye. *Prog Retin Eye Res.* 2004;23:403–434.
105. Iozzo RV. Matrix proteoglycans: from molecular design to cellular function. *Annu Rev Biochem.* 1998;67:609–652.
106. Funderburgh JL. Keratan sulfate: structure, biosynthesis, and function. *Glycobiology.* 2000;10:951–958.
107. Funderburgh JL, Corpuz LM, Roth MR, et al. Mimecan, the 25-kDa corneal keratan sulfate proteoglycan, is a product of the gene producing osteoglycin. *J Biol Chem.* 1997;272:28089–28095.
108. Liu CY, Shiraishi A, Kao CW, et al. The cloning of mouse keratocan cDNA and genomic DNA and the characterization of its expression during eye development. *J Biol Chem.* 1998;273:22584–22588.
109. Kao WW, Liu CY. Roles of lumican and keratocan on corneal transparency. *Glycoconj J.* 2002;19:275–285.
110. Liu CY, Birk DE, Hassell JR, et al. Keratocan-deficient mice display alterations in corneal structure. *J Biol Chem.* 2003;278:21672–21677.
111. Pellegata NS, Dieguez-Lucena JL, Joensuu T, et al. Mutations in KERA, encoding keratocan, cause cornea plana. *Nat Genet.* 2000;25:91–95.
112. Chakravarti S, Magnuson T, Lass JH, et al. Lumican regulates collagen fibril assembly: skin fragility and corneal opacity in the absence of lumican. *J Cell Biol.* 1998;141:1277–1286.
113. Saika S, Shiraishi A, Liu CY, et al. Role of lumican in the corneal epithelium during wound healing. *J Biol Chem.* 2000;275:2607–2612.
114. Danielson KG, Baribault H, Holmes DF, et al. Targeted disruption of decorin leads to abnormal collagen fibril morphology and skin fragility. *J Cell Biol.* 1997;136:729–743.
115. Paluru PC, Scavello GS, Ganter WR, et al. Exclusion of lumican and fibromodulin as candidate genes in MYP3 linked high grade myopia. *Mol Vis.* 2004;30:917–922.
116. Johnson DH, Bourne WM, Campbell RJ. The ultrastructure of Descemet's membrane. I. Changes with age in normal corneas. *Arch Ophthalmol.* 1982;100:1942–1947.
117. Fitch JM, Birk DE, Linsenmayer C, et al. The spatial organization of Descemet's membrane-associated type IV collagen in the avian cornea. *J Cell Biol.* 1990;110:1457–1468.
118. Suda T, Nishida T, Ohashi Y, et al. Fibronectin appears at the site of corneal stromal wound in rabbits. *Curr Eye Res.* 1981;1:553–556.
119. Fujikawa LS, Foster CS, Harrist TJ, et al. Fibronectin in healing rabbit corneal wounds. *Lab Invest.* 1981;45:120–129.
120. Bourne WM, Johnson DH, Campbell RJ. The ultrastructure of Descemet's membrane. III. Fuchs' dystrophy. *Arch Ophthalmol.* 1982;100:1952–1955.
121. Biswas S, Munier FL, Yardley J, et al. Missense mutations in COL8A2, the gene encoding the alpha2 chain of type VIII collagen, cause two forms of corneal endothelial dystrophy. *Hum Mol Genet.* 2001;10:2415–2423.
122. Laule A, Cable MK, Hoffman CE, et al. Endothelial cell population changes of human cornea during life. *Arch Ophthalmol.* 1978;96:2031–2035.
123. Thoft RA, Friend J. The X, Y, Z, hypothesis of corneal epithelial maintenance. *Invest Ophthalmol Vis Sci.* 1983;24:1442–1443.
124. Cotsareils G, Cheng S-Z, Dong G, et al. Existence of slow-cycling limbal epithelial basal cells that can be preferentially stimulated to proliferate: implications on epithelial stem cells. *Cell.* 1989;57:201–209.
125. Daniels JT, Harris AR, Mason C. Corneal epithelial stem cells in health and disease. *Stem Cell Rev.* 2006;2:247–254.
126. O'Sullivan F, Clynes M. Limbal stem cells, a review of their identification and culture for clinical use. *Cytotechnology.* 2007;53:101–106.
127. Secker GA, Daniels JT. Corneal epithelial stem cells: deficiency and regulation. *Stem Cell Rev.* 2008;4:159–168.
128. Binder PS, Wickham MG, Zavala EY, et al. Corneal anatomy and wound healing. In: Barraque JI, Binder PS, Buxton JN, et al, eds. *Symposium on medical and surgical diseases of the cornea.* St. Louis, MO: Mosby; 1980:1–35.
129. Kuwabara T, Perkins DG, Cogan DG. Sliding of the epithelium in experimental corneal wounds. *Invest Ophthalmol Vis Sci.* 1976;15:4–14.
130. Buck RC. Cell migration in repair of mouse corneal epithelium. *Invest Ophthalmol Vis Sci.* 1979;18:767–784.
131. Hanna C. Proliferation and migration of epithelial cells. *Am J Ophthalmol.* 1966;61:55–63.
132. Matsuda H, Smelser GK. Electron microscopy of corneal wound healing. *Exp Eye Res.* 1973;16:427–442.
133. Proctor RA. Fibronectin: a brief overview of its structure, function, and physiology. *Rev Infect Dis.* 1987;9(suppl 4):S317-S321.
134. Cameron JD, Hagen ST, Waterfield RR, et al. Effects of matrix proteins on rabbit corneal epithelial cell adhesion and migration. *Curr Eye Res.* 1988;7:293–301.
135. Nakagawa S, Nishida T, Kodama Y, et al. Spreading of cultured corneal epithelial cells on fibronectin and other extracellular matrices. *Cornea.* 1990;9:125–130.
136. Stepp MA, Spurr-Michaud S, Gipson IK. Integrins in the wounded and unwounded stratified squamous epithelium of the cornea. *Invest Ophthalmol Vis Sci.* 1993;34:1829–1844.
137. Latvala T, Tervo K, Tervo T. Reassembly of the $\alpha 6\beta 4$ integrin and laminin in rabbit corneal basement membrane after excimer laser surgery: a 12-month follow-up. *CLAO J.* 1995;21:125–129.
138. Itano N. Simple primary structure, complex turnover regulation and multiple roles of hyaluronan. *J Biochem.* 2008;144:131–137.
139. Fitzsimmons TD, Fagerholm P, Harfstrand A, et al. Hyaluronic acid in the rabbit cornea after excimer laser superficial keratectomy. *Invest Ophthalmol Vis Sci.* 1992;33:3011–3016.
140. Fagerholm P, Fitzsimmons T, Harfstrand A, et al. Reactive formation of hyaluronic acid in the rabbit corneal alkali burn. *Acta Ophthalmol Suppl (Copenh).* 1992;202:67–72.
141. Nakamura M, Hikida M, Nakano T. Concentration and molecular weight dependency of rabbit corneal epithelial wound healing on hyaluronan. *Curr Eye Res.* 1992;11:981–986.
142. Nakamura M, Sato N, Chikama TI, et al. Hyaluronan facilitates corneal epithelial wound healing in diabetic rats. *Exp Eye Res.* 1997;64:1043–1050.
143. Nakamura M, Nishida T. Recent developments in the use of hyaluronan in wound healing. *Exp Opin Invest Drugs.* 1995;4:175–188.
144. Nishida T, Nakamura M, Mishima H, et al. Hyaluronan stimulates corneal epithelial migration. *Exp Eye Res.* 1991;53:753–758.
145. Salonen E-M, Tervo T, Torma E, et al. Plasmin in tear fluid of patients with corneal ulcers: basis for new therapy. *Acta Ophthalmol.* 1987;65:3–12.
146. Hayashi K, Sueishi K. Fibrinolytic activity and species of plasminogen activator in human tears. *Exp Eye Res.* 1988;46:131–137.
147. Sivak JM, Fini ME. MMPs in the eye: emerging roles for matrix metalloproteinases in ocular physiology. *Prog Retin Eye Res.* 2002;21:1–14.
148. Barrientos S, Stojadinovic O, Golinko MS, et al. Growth factors and cytokines in wound healing. *Wound Repair Regen.* 2008;16:585–601.
149. Cohen S. Isolation of a mouse submaxillary gland protein accelerating incisor eruption and eyelid opening in the new-born animal. *J Biol Chem.* 1962;237:1555–1562.
150. Frati L, Daniele S, Delogu A, et al. Selective binding of the epidermal growth factor and its specific effects on the epithelial cells of the cornea. *Exp Eye Res.* 1972;14:135–141.
151. Savage CRJ, Cohen S. Proliferation of corneal epithelium induced by epidermal growth factor. *Exp Eye Res.* 1973;15:361–366.
152. Ho PC, Davis WH, Elliott JH, et al. Kinetics of corneal epithelial regeneration and epidermal growth factor. *Invest Ophthalmol Vis Sci.* 1974;13:804–809.
153. Gonul B, Koz M, Ersoz G, et al. Effect of EGF on the corneal wound healing of alloxan diabetic mice. *Exp Eye Res.* 1992;54:519–524.
154. Nishida T, Nakamura M, Murakami J, et al. Epidermal growth factor stimulates corneal epithelial cell attachment to fibronectin through a fibronectin receptor system. *Invest Ophthalmol Vis Sci.* 1992;33:2464–2469.
155. Nishida T, Nakamura M, Mishima H, et al. Differential modes of action of fibronectin and epidermal growth factor on rabbit corneal epithelial migration. *J Cell Physiol.* 1990;145:549–554.

156. Wilson SE, Lloyd SA, He YG. EGF, basic FGF, and TGFβ-1 messenger RNA production in rabbit corneal epithelial cells. *Invest Ophthalmol Vis Sci.* 1992;33:1987–1995.
157. Roberts AB, Russo A, Felici A, et al. Smad3: a key player in pathogenetic mechanisms dependent on TGF-β. *Ann NY Acad Sci.* 2003;995:1–10.
158. Mishima H, Nakamura M, Murakami J, et al. Transforming growth factor-β modulates effects of epidermal growth factor on corneal epithelial cells. *Curr Eye Res.* 1992;11:691–696.
159. Steiling H, Werner S. Fibroblast growth factors: key players in epithelial morphogenesis, repair and cytoprotection. *Curr Opin Biotechnol.* 2003;14:533–537.
160. Rieck P, Assouline M, Savoldelli M, et al. Recombinant human basic fibroblast growth factor (Rh-bFGF) in three different wound models in rabbits: corneal wound healing effect and pharmacology. *Exp Eye Res.* 1992;54:987–998.
161. Knorr M, Steuhl K, Tatje D, et al. A rabbit corneal epithelial cell line expresses functional platelet-derived growth factor β-type receptors. *Invest Ophthalmol Vis Sci.* 1992;33:2207–2211.
162. Steinke JW, Borish L. 3. Cytokines and chemokines. *J Allergy Clin Immunol.* 2006;117:S441-S445.
163. Wilson SE, Liu JJ, Mohan RR. Stromal-epithelial interactions in the cornea. *Prog Retin Eye Res.* 1999;18:293–309.
164. Sakamoto S, Inada K, Chiba K, et al. Production of IL-6 and IL-1a by human corneal epithelial cells. *Acta Soc Ophthalmol Jpn.* 1991;95: 728–732.
165. Nishida T, Nakamura M, Mishima H, et al. Interleukin 6 facilitates corneal epithelial wound closure in vivo. *Arch Ophthalmol.* 1992;110: 1292–1294.
166. Ohashi H, Maeda T, Mishima H, et al. Up-regulation of integrin α5β1 expression by interleukin-6 in rabbit corneal epithelial cells. *Exp Cell Res.* 1995;218:418–423.
167. Bisla K, Tanelian DL. Concentration-dependent effects of lidocaine on corneal epithelial wound healing. *Invest Ophthalmol Vis Sci.* 1992;33: 3029–3033.
168. Pernow B. Substance P. *Pharmacol Rev.* 1983;35:85–141.
169. McGillis JP, Organist ML, Payan DG. Substance P and immunoregulation. *Fed Proc.* 1987;46:196–199.
170. Payan DG. Neuropeptides and inflammation: the role of substance P. *Annu Rev Med.* 1989;40:341–352.
171. Wallengren J, Hakanson R. Effects of substance P, neurokinin A and calcitonin gene-related peptide in human skin and their involvement in sensory nerve-mediated responeses. *Eur J Pharmacol.* 1987; 143:267–273.
172. Shimizu Y. Localization of neuropeptides in the cornea and uvea of the rat: an immunohistochemical study. *Cell Mol Biol.* 1982;28:103–110.
173. Nishiyama A, Masuda K, Mochizuki M. Ocular effects of substance P. *Jpn J Ophthalmol.* 1981;25:362–369.
174. Cook GA, Elliott D, Metwali A, et al. Molecular evidence that granuloma T lymphocytes in murine *Schistosomiasis mansoni* express an authentic substance P (NK-1) receptor. *J Immunol.* 1994;152:1830–1835.
175. Kaplan JE. Plasma fibronectin and resistance to thrombosis during sepsis. *Adv Shock Res.* 1982;7:159–172.
176. Brown SM, Lamberts DW, Reid TW, et al. Neurotrophic and anhidrotic keratopathy treated with substance P and insulinlike growth factor 1. *Arch Ophthalmol.* 1997;115:926–927.
177. Chikama T, Fukuda K, Morishige N, et al. Treatment of neurotrophic keratopathy with substance-P-derived peptide (FGLM) and insulin-like growth factor I. *Lancet.* 1998;351:1783–1784.
178. Morishige N, Komatsubara T, Chikama T, et al. Direct observation of corneal nerve fibres in neurotrophic keratopathy by confocal biomicroscopy. *Lancet.* 1999;354:1613–1614.
179. Levi-Montalcini R. The nerve growth factor 35 years later. *Science.* 1987;237:1154–1162.
180. Rask CA. Biological actions of nerve growth factor in the peripheral nervous system. *Eur Neurol.* 1999;41(suppl 1):14–19.
181. Levi-Montalcini R, Hamburger V. A diffusible agent of mouse sarcoma producing hyperplasia of sympathic ganglia and hyperneurotization of the chick embryo. *J Exp Zool.* 1953;123:233–388.
182. Lambiase A, Rama P, Bonini S, et al. Topical treatment with nerve growth factor for corneal neurotrophic ulcers. *N Engl J Med.* 1998;338:1174–1180.
183. Lambiase A, Pagani L, Di Fausto V, et al. Nerve growth factor eye drop administrated on the ocular surface of rodents affects the nucleus basalis and septum: biochemical and structural evidence. *Brain Res.* 2007;1127:45–51.
184. Lambiase A, Manni L, Bonini S, et al. Nerve growth factor promotes corneal healing: structural, biochemical, and molecular analyses of rat and human corneas. *Invest Ophthalmol Vis Sci.* 2000;41:1063–1069.
185. Bonini S, Lambiase A, Rama P, et al. Topical treatment with nerve growth factor for neurotrophic keratitis. *Ophthalmology.* 2000;107:1347–1351. discussion 1351–1342.
186. Nagano T, Hao JL, Nakamura M, et al. Stimulatory effect of pseudomonal elastase on collagen degradation by cultured keratocytes. *Invest Ophthalmol Vis Sci.* 2001;42:1247–1253.
187. Saika S. TGF-β signal transduction in corneal wound healing as a therapeutic target. *Cornea.* 2004;23:S25-S30.
188. Saika S, Yamanaka O, Sumioka T, et al. Fibrotic disorders in the eye: targets of gene therapy. *Prog Retin Eye Res.* 2008;27:177–196.
189. Brenner MK. Tumour necrosis factor. *Br J Haematol.* 1988;69:149–152.
190. Hong J-W, Liu JJ, Lee J-S, et al. Proinflammatory chemokine induction in keratocytes and inflammatory cell infiltration into the cornea. *Invest Ophthalmol Vis Sci.* 2001;42:2795–2803.
191. Keadle TL, Usui N, Laycock KA, et al. IL-1 and TNF-α are important factors in the pathogenesis of murine recurrent herpetic stromal keratitis. *Invest Ophthalmol Vis Sci.* 2000;41:96–102.
192. Dekaris I, Zhu SN, Dana MR. TNF-α regulates corneal Langerhans cell migration. *J Immunol.* 1999;162:4235–4239.
193. Planck SR, Rich LF, Ansel JC, et al. Trauma and alkali burns induce distinct patterns of cytokine gene expression in the rat cornea. *Ocul Immunol Inflamm.* 1997;5:95–100.
194. Saika S, Ikeda K, Yamanaka O, et al. Loss of tumor necrosis factor α potentiates transforming growth factor β-mediated pathogenic tissue response during wound healing. *Am J Pathol.* 2006;168:1848–1860.
195. Ma DH, Chen JK, Zhang F, et al. Regulation of corneal angiogenesis in limbal stem cell deficiency. *Prog Retin Eye Res.* 2006;25:563–590.
196. Graw J. Genetic aspects of embryonic eye development in vertebrates. *Dev Genet.* 1996;18:181–197.
197. Sevel D, Isaacs R. A re-evaluation of corneal development. *Trans Am Ophthalmol Soc.* 1988;86:178–207.
198. Kim JE, Han MS, Bae YC, et al. Anterior segment dysgenesis after overexpression of transforming growth factor-beta-induced gene, beta igh3, in the mouse eye. *Mol Vis.* 2007;13:1942–1952.
199. Saika S, Liu CY, Azhar M, et al. TGFβ2 in corneal morphogenesis during mouse embryonic development. *Dev Biol.* 2001;240:419–432.
200. Kao WW, Xia Y, Liu CY, et al. Signaling pathways in morphogenesis of cornea and eyelid. *Ocul Surf.* 2008;6:9–23.

Chapter 2

The Conjunctiva: Anatomy and Physiology

J. Daniel Nelson, J. Douglas Cameron

Critical to maintaining the integrity of the eye, the conjunctiva is a mucous membrane that protects the soft tissues of the eyelid and orbit, allows extensive movement of the eye and is the main site for the production of the aqueous and mucous components of tears. The sebaceous glands of the eyelid produce the third component of the tear film. The conjunctiva also provides a source of immune tissue and antimicrobial agents to protect the ocular surface. Abnormalities of the conjunctiva may lead to restriction of ocular movement, deficiency of the tear film, and decreased host resistance to infection. In addition, the cornea may ultimately be adversely affected because of conjunctival disease.

Embryology

The conjunctiva arises from surface ectoderm and neural crest tissues in the region of the optic vesicle.[1] At 8 weeks (32- to 37-mm stage) the eyelids form from folds of the surface ectoderm and fuse together. The conjunctiva develops within the lid folds from surface ectodermal and neural crest tissue along the posterior surface of the lids and from similar tissues around the developing cornea. The conjunctival epithelium differentiates from the cutaneous epithelium and corneal epithelium as early as the tenth week and definitely by the twelfth (60- to 70-mm stage). Budding of the epithelium in the conjunctival fornices forms the lacrimal gland superotemporally and accessory lacrimal glands of Wolfring and Krause in the inferior and superior fornices (12 weeks, 50- to 55-mm stage). The caruncle arises as a sequestration of the medial lower eyelid to accommodate the development of the nasolacrimal duct. The caruncle is composed of tissues found both in the conjunctiva and skin; however, the surface epithelium is nonkeratinized. The plica semilunaris (semilunar fold) lies between the caruncle and globe. It is similar to the nicatating membrane of certain mammals but does not contain cartilage.

Anatomy

The conjunctiva extends from the corneoscleral limbus to the mucocutaneous junction on the eyelids. The conjunctiva reflects to form a fornix on three sides and an extendible plica medially. The redundant conjunctiva in this region allows for independent movement of the eye and eyelids. Conjunctival surface folds increase the surface area of the conjunctiva, decrease the area of contact, and reduce friction between the bulbar and tarsal conjunctiva (Fig. 2.1).

The larger superior fornix is maintained by fine smooth muscle slips passing from the deep surface of the levator palpebrae muscle to insert into the conjunctiva. These effectively prevent the superior forniceal conjunctiva from falling down and blocking vision during upward gaze. The temporal conjunctiva is attached by fine fibrous slips to the lateral rectus tendon, which maintains the position of the conjunctiva during horizontal gaze. A true fornix does not exist medially except in adduction. Fine fibrous strips from the medial rectus tendon insert deep into the plica and caruncle. With contraction of the medial rectus, these slips tighten and form a cul-de-sac medially as the eye adducts. The total surface area for the adult conjunctival sac including the cornea averages 16 cm^2 for one eye.

The plica semilunaris is a crescent-shaped fold of conjunctiva with its free lateral border lying 3–6 mm lateral to the caruncle. On adduction, a cul-de-sac of approximately 2–3 mm in depth is formed that mostly disappears on abduction. The epithelium contains goblet cells, Langerhans cells, and dendritic melanocytes. The substantia propria, or conjunctival stroma, is highly vascularized and may contain nonstriated muscle, sympathetic nerves, cartilage, and fatty tissue. The caruncle measures 4–5 mm horizontally and 3–4 mm vertically and is located at the most medial aspect of the interpalpebral fissure. The caruncle is attached to the medial rectus and moves with the plica semilunaris during movement of the globe. The caruncle is composed of pilosebaceous units, accessory lacrimal gland tissue, fibrofatty tissue, occasional smooth muscle fibers, and eccrine glands. Deep to the caruncle there may be several large sebaceous glands without cilia, similar to meibomian glands, which open onto the surface. At the mucocutaneous junction of the eyelid margin, there is an abrupt transition from the keratinized, stratified squamous epithelium to the nonkeratinized stratified squamous epithelium of the palpebral conjunctiva. Meibomian glands of the eyelid are seen easily through the transparent palpebral conjunctiva as yellow lobulated structures separated by vascular arcades in the tarsus of the upper and lower eyelids running perpendicular to the eyelid margin. Overlying the mucocutaneous junction is a hydrophobic strip of lipid secreted by the meibomian glands, which separates the dry anterior keratinized portion

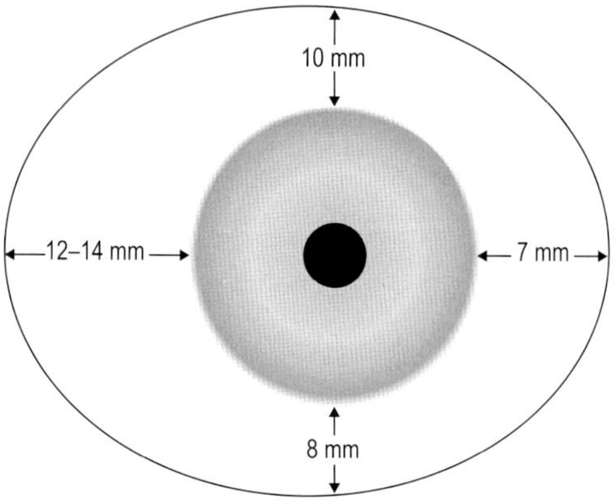

Fig. 2.1 Geography of the fornices. Distance from the corneoscleral limbus to the fornix.

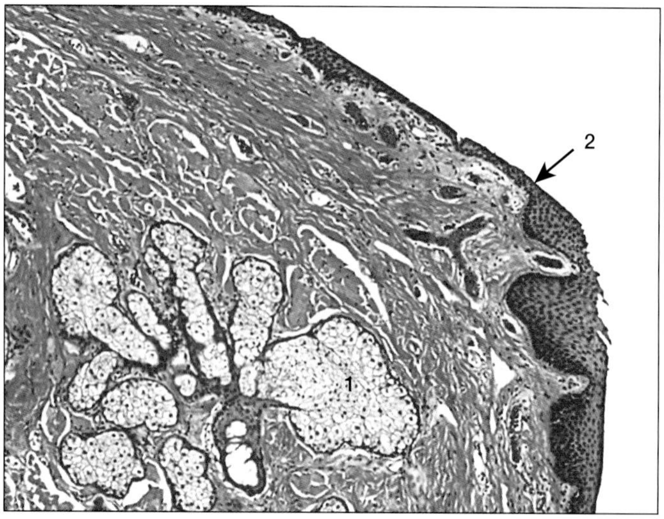

Fig. 2.2 Histologic section through the upper eyelid. Meibomian glands (1) and the mucocutaneous junction (2) can be seen.

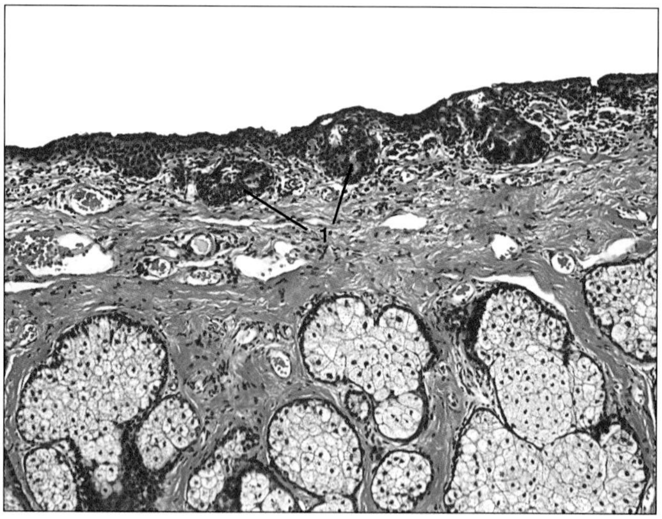

Fig. 2.3 Histologic section of tarsal conjunctiva showing the pseudocrypts of Henle (1).

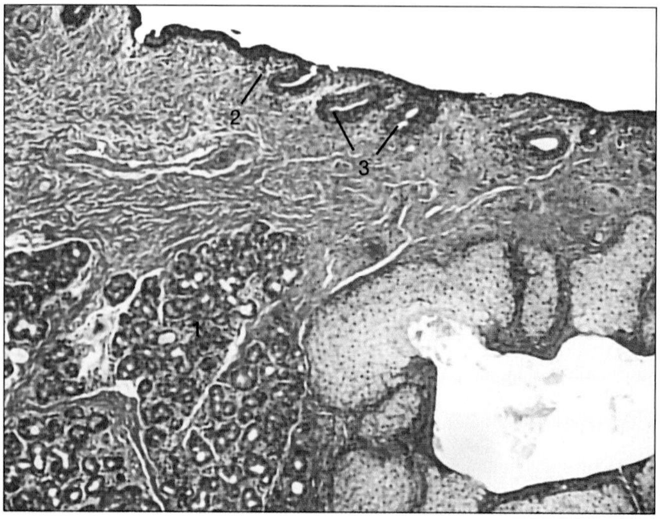

Fig. 2.4 Histologic section through the superior tarsus demonstrating the glands of Wolfring (1), lymphocytes in the adenoid layer (2), and pseudocrypts of Henle (3).

of the eyelid from the wet posterior, nonkeratinized part. The exact position of the mucocutaneous junction is determined by the air–fluid interface of the tear film meniscus. Ectropion will cause the mucocutaneous junction to move posteriorly, while entropion will cause the mucocutaneous junction to move anteriorly.

The tarsal conjunctiva is tightly adherent to the substance of the tarsus to present a smooth surface to interface the anterior corneal surface. Consequently, there is no accessible subconjunctival tissue plane for dissection of the tarsal conjunctiva. Along the tarsal surface, 2 mm posterior to the lid margin, lies a shallow subtarsal groove less than 1-mm deep. The subtarsal groove is situated parallel to the eyelid margin for most of the length of the tarsus. In this region there is transition from the nonkeratinizing stratified epithelium of the lid margin to the more cuboidal epithelium of the tarsal conjunctiva (Fig. 2.2). Between the eyelid margin and the tarsal groove are multiple ridges and grooves that communicate with goblet cell-lined invaginations of the conjunctival epithelium (the pseudocrypts of Henle) (Fig. 2.3). Few crypts are present at birth; most develop at puberty. After age 50 years the crypts are found in about one-third of specimens.[2] The crypts are more numerous in the nasal conjunctiva and around the plica. Accessory lacrimal glands are located in the forniceal conjunctiva (glands of Krause) and in the palpebral conjunctiva above or within the tarsus (glands of Wolfring) (Fig. 2.4).

The bulbar conjunctiva is smoother and more loosely adherent to underlying tissues than the tarsal conjunctiva. At the corneoscleral limbus there is a series of fibrovascular ridges perpendicular to the corneal margin (palisades of Vogt). These arcades are formed by the epithelial rete ridges and the stromal condensations beneath them and may become accentuated to form peripheral corneal neovascularization (corneal pannus).

Histology

The conjunctival surface is composed of stratified nonkeratinizing epithelium and varies in thickness and appearance from the eyelid margin to the limbus. Unlike any other stratified squamous epithelium, goblet cells are dispersed among and attached to neighboring epithelial cells. There is some controversy as to the location of the conjunctival stem cells. They may be uniformly distributed throughout the bulbar and forniceal conjunctiva,[3] located at the mucocutaneous junction on the eyelid,[4] or at the corneal–scleral limbus and the mucocutaneous junction.[5] Recent work further supports the uniform distribution of conjunctival epithelial stem cells in the bulbar conjunctiva.[6] Ectopically, corneal epithelial cells may reside in the conjunctival epithelium and participate in corneal re-epithelialization in cases where the corneal stem cells are compromised.[7]

Palpebral and forniceal conjunctiva

The forniceal conjunctival epithelium is two to three cell layers thick over the superior tarsus and four to five cell layers thick over the inferior tarsus. The forniceal conjunctival epithelium tends to be more columnar in nature, whereas the palpebral conjunctival epithelium is more cuboidal. Subepithelial cysts often arise from invaginated areas of surface palpebral conjunctival epithelium or crypts that have closed off (pseudocrypts of Henle). These cysts are lined by surface epithelial cells and contain mucin secreted from goblet cells. Near the eyelid margin, the stratified columnar epithelium of the conjunctiva contains more tonofilaments and merges imperceptibly with the keratinized, stratified squamous epithelium of the eyelid skin (see Fig. 2.2). The surface epithelium beyond the eyelid margin becomes keratinized where the surface is not covered by fluid and is continuously exposed to air.

Bulbar conjunctiva

The bulbar conjunctival epithelium consists of six to nine layers of stratified nonkeratinizing squamous epithelial cells arranged in an irregular fashion in contrast to the more regularly arranged corneal epithelium. Cytoplasmic organelles are similar to those of the cornea but more abundant. The basal and intermediate epithelial cells contain more and larger mitochondria than the corneal epithelium, suggesting a higher level of oxidative metabolism. Cytoplasmic tonofilaments are present and form dense bundles, some closely associated with desmosomes. Fewer desmosomes are present than in the corneal epithelium. The epithelial cellular membranes show marked infoldings, with incomplete interdigitation with adjacent cells. This configuration produces wide intracellular spaces in which antibodies and other plasma constituents and inflammatory cells from underlying vessels can accumulate. In addition, infectious and topically applied substances can gain access to the intracellular spaces and then to the subconjunctival capillaries and systemic circulation. Apically, a glycocalyx is secreted from mucin-containing intraepithelial vesicles[8] (Fig. 2.5). The vesicles release their contents by fusing with the apical membrane forming the glycocalyx, consisting of transmembrane mucins (MUC1, MUC4, MUC16). The long-chain glycoprotein molecules maintain tear film stability by anchoring the mucin produced by the goblet cells (MUC5AC) to the conjunctival surface and also bind immunoglobulins. The bulbar conjunctival epithelium is attached to a thin basement membrane, which is discontinuous in some places, by relatively few hemidesmosomes. This configuration allows wandering cells access to the conjunctival stroma. Lymphocytes, dendritic melanocytes, and Langerhans cells may be seen in the suprabasal region of the epithelium.

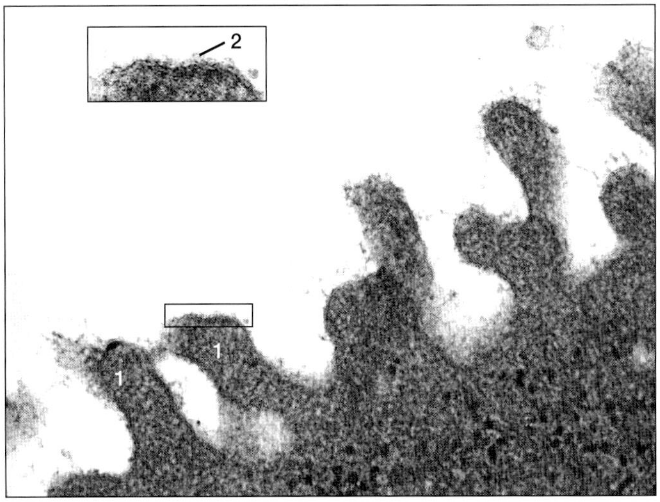

Fig. 2.5 Electron micrograph of the conjunctiva showing the microvilli (1) and glycocalyx (2, inset).

The conjunctival basement membrane zone (BMZ) does not normally show immunochemical reactivity to any immunoglobulins, complement components, or albumin. The superficial cells in normal subjects do show variable amounts of IgA and IgG reactivity. BMZ immunoreactivity to IgM, IgD, and IgE may be seen in patients with ocular cicatricial pemphigoid but is not found in normal conjunctiva. Fibrinogen is normally found at the BMZ and can serve as a positive control when processing conjunctival specimens for immunoreactivity.[9]

The corneoscleral limbus

Similar to the palpebral eyelid margin, there is a gradual transition at the limbus from the stratified, nonkeratinized columnar epithelium of the conjunctiva to the stratified, nonkeratinized squamous epithelium of the cornea (Fig. 2.6). There are seven to ten layers of cells at the limbus, which have cell-to-cell and cell-to-substrate attachments similar to those of the cornea. The areas of stratified nonkeratinizing squamous epithelium at the eyelid margin and limbus correspond to the areas of most common contact and greatest pressure between the palpebral and bulbar surfaces maintained by the muscle of Riolan of the eyelid margin. This mechanical appositional pressure, along with eyelid movement, has been suggested as the greatest stimulus for the formation of stratified squamous epithelium at the eyelid margins and limbus.[10] The stem cells for corneal epithelium reside at the limbus in the basal layer. The limbus may also be a source of conjunctival stem cells.[5]

Conjunctival goblet cells

Goblet cells are unicellular, mucin-secreting glands that account for approximately 5% to 10% of basal cells.[11] They

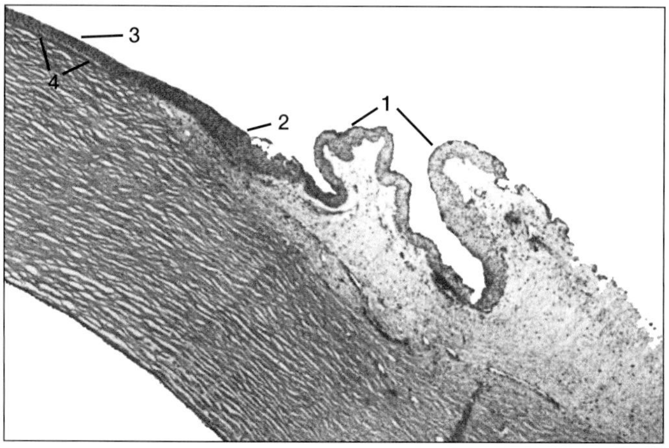

Fig. 2.6 Histologic section demonstrating the conjunctival (1), limbal (2), and corneal (3) epithelium, and Bowman's membrane (4).

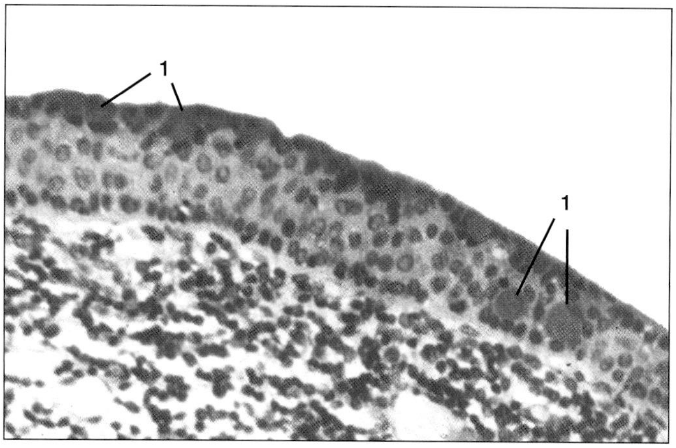

Fig. 2.7 Photomicrograph of conjunctival epithelium with periodic acid–Schiff-positive staining goblet cells (1).

are likely apocrine in nature, with all the secretory granules secreted once the cell has been activated.[12] They are the primary source of the large soluble mucins in the tear film. Goblet cells release their secretory granules in response to activation of the parasympathetic nerves that surround them. The neurotransmitters acetylcholine and vasoactive intestinal peptide (VIP) are know neurotransmitters that stimulate goblet cell mucin secretion.[13] Sympathetic nerves also surround the goblet cells.[14,15] While sensory nerves surround conjunctival squamous epithelial cells, they do not appear to surround the goblet cells.[12] The mucin synthesized by goblet cells of normal human conjunctiva is identified as MUC5AC. The cysteine-rich domains at the N and C termini lead to a viscous mucus (gel-forming) that provides a scaffolding for the mucin layer of the tear film.[16] Goblet cells may also secrete other proteins. Transmembrane mucins MUC1, MUC4, and MUC16 are expressed at the ocular surface.[16–18] These mucins function to protect, hydrate, and lubricate the ocular surface. They are also involved in cell signaling and may be abnormally released from the ocular surface in conditions associated with inflammation (e.g. dry eye).[19]

Goblet cells likely arise from common bipotential progenitor cells distributed in the bulbar and palpebral conjunctiva.[3] The nucleus and cytoplasmic organelles are displaced toward the basal aspect of the cells with mucin packets located apically, accounting for its goblet-like appearance (Fig. 2.7). Although tonofilaments are present, they are not highly differentiated. Tight junctions attach goblet cells with adjacent epithelial cells. The density of conjunctival goblet cells is between 1000 and 56 000 cells/mm^2. They are not distributed uniformally, may occur singly or in random groups, and are more numerous over the tarsal and inferonasal bulbar conjunctiva[20,21] and less dense temporally and at the limbus. The density of goblet cells peaks in young adults and then decreases until age 30 years, remaining constant thereafter.[21] The density of goblet cells is influenced by local ocular disease such as keratoconjunctivitis sicca, ocular pemphigoid, Stevens–Johnson syndrome, and chemical injuries,[22,23] and by factors in the external environment such as humidity, temperature, and pollution.[24]

In ocular cicatricial pemphigoid,[25] vitamin A deficiency,[26] and atopic keratoconjunctivitis,[27] there is an increase in the conjunctival epithelial mitotic rates. Although conjunctival goblet cell density is decreased in ocular cicatricial pemphigoid, it is increased in atopic keratoconjunctivitis. Recent evidence suggests that goblet cells are innervated by cholinergic and sympathetic nerves.[14,15] The hormonal control of goblet cells is not known. In vitamin A deficiency, goblet cells are lost and epithelium becomes keratinized (squamous metaplasia). This suggests that vitamin A may play an important role in conjunctival differentiation and in the pathogenesis of some ocular surface diseases. The loss of goblet cells is an early sign of squamous metaplasia.[28]

Substantia propria

The conjunctiva rests on fibrovascular connective tissue, which varies in thickness and density (substantia propria). In the tarsal conjunctiva, the substantia propria is thin and compact and is attached to the tarsus more firmly superiorly than inferiorly. In the fornices, it is thick and loosely attached to the globe and orbital septum. The substantia propria extends temporally behind the canthus and nasally to the semilunar fold. At the limbus it is thin and compact, and merges with Tenon's fascia and episcleral tissues.

The substantia propria can be divided into superficial and deep layers. The superficial layer of the substantia propria consists of loose, interconnected connective tissue. This layer is not present at birth and begins to form at 8 to 12 weeks of age. In adults there is a 50- to 70-mm thick layer of lymphocytes (adenoid layer), which is more prominent inferiorly. In normal, noninflamed conjunctiva, there are no true follicles with germinal centers; however, lymphocytes can be stimulated by viral or chlamydial infections or by a toxic reaction to certain topical medications to form follicles with reactive germinal centers. Follicles tend to elevate the conjunctival epithelium, producing a round, fish-egg-like mound. Similar to other lymphoid organs, sensory nerves have been found in association with the conjunctival mucosa-associated lymphoid tissue in monkeys.[29] Papillae form from a reactive, histamine-mediated vascular reaction.

Papillae are characterized by chronic inflammatory cells (lymphocytes and plasma cells) and the presence of a central vascular core.[2]

The deeper, fibrous layer contains vessels, lymphatics, and nerves. Capillaries arise from the anterior ciliary arteries, which are branches of the ophthalmic artery, and drain into the episcleral venous plexus. Lymphatics drain into the episcleral plexus, which joins the drainage system of the eyelids, draining into the submandibular and preauricular lymph node systems. There is no lymphoid drainage posterior to the orbital septum. Sensory nerves arise from the ophthalmic division of the trigeminal nerve (V_1).

Vascular Supply

The palpebral conjunctiva and lids share a common arterial blood supply that arises from terminal branches of the ophthalmic artery: the dorsal, nasal, frontal, supraorbital, and lacrimal arteries. The facial, superficial, temporal, and infraorbital branches from the facial artery provide supplemental blood supply. In the bulbar conjunctiva, branches from the anterior ciliary arteries, which are a continuation of the muscular branches supplying the rectus muscles, form a superficial marginal plexus at the limbus, giving rise to the terminal vessels of the peripheral arcades and the palisades of Vogt. Branches of the bulbar anterior ciliary arterial system anastomose in the fornices with recurrent vessels from the palpebral conjunctiva. Conjunctival vessels maintain their superficial position, and a deeper circulation furnishes blood supply to the peripheral corneal arcades, iris, and ciliary body. Inflammatory processes of the conjunctiva result in prominence of the superficial vessels, which increases away from the limbus. Inflammatory processes of the cornea, iris, or ciliary body result in prominence of the deep vessels, which increases toward the limbus. Clinically, this process is manifest as coronal or ciliary flush.

Conjunctival capillaries are fenestrated. Fenestrae are specialized plasma membrane microdomains in endothelial cells that are involved in vascular permeability. They appear as circular discontinuities of $\approx$60 nm in diameter and usually occur in clusters in the most attenuated regions of the endothelial cell.[30] Each fenestration is covered by the plasma membrane of the underlying endothelial cell. Some of the deeper vessels are not fenestrated. Fenestration allows more rapid passage of luminal contents in inflammation. After intravenous injection of fluorescein, conjunctival vessels can be seen to leak in a time and concentration sequence similar to that of the choroidal capillaries. The vessels at the palisades of Vogt may be more competent and leak less than conjunctival vessels elsewhere.[31] Conjunctival inflammation, infections, irritation, or severe intraorbital inflammation cause the conjunctival capillaries to leak plasma proteins faster than the fluid can pass between the epithelial cells. This process causes thickening of the epithelium and chemosis of the conjunctiva.[32] Vessel engorgement varies during the menstrual cycle.[33]

Venous drainage from the palpebral conjunctiva joins the post-tarsal veins of the eyelids and the deep facial branches of the anterior facial vein and pterygoid plexus. The bulbar conjunctival veins drain into the episcleral venous plexus, which drains into the intrascleral plexus. Wind, cold, heat, and endocrine changes associated with menstruation and early pregnancy dilate the venous side of circulation.[33]

Lymphatic Drainage

The conjunctiva contains a rich anastomotic network of lymphatic channels that drain into the episcleral lymphatic plexus. Many small, irregular lymphatic channels arise 1 mm peripheral to the limbus and anastomose to form larger collecting channels in the deep layer of the substantia propria. Occasionally, these can be seen as irregular, dilated, sausage-shaped channels (lymphangiectasia). Lymphatics of the conjunctiva join the lymphatics of the eyelids and drain medially to the submandibular lymph node and laterally to the preauricular (intraparotid) lymph node system.

Nerve Supply

Proper sensory innervation of the conjunctiva is essential to maintain its health and ultimately the health of the eye. The conjunctiva is richly supplied with free nerve endings that arise from the lacrimal, supraorbital, supratrochlear, and infraorbital branches of the ophthalmic branch of the trigeminal nerve (V_1). The threshold for tactile conjunctival sensitivity is 100 times greater than that of the center of the cornea. This is likely due to lower innervation density and that the nerve endings innervating the conjunctival epithelium are further away from the surface and less exposed to stimuli compared to the cornea. It is least sensitive in the perilimbal area and most sensitive along the marginal palpebral conjunctiva. Pain can occur with inflammation, an epithelial defect, hypoxia, and osmotic shock, all of which cause deformation of the nerve endings. Small peptides produced by inflammation may stimulate free nerve endings and increase pain. Inflammation can also lower the threshold to pain (primary hyperalgesia). When the pain threshold is exceeded, pain may become more intense and severe (secondary hyperalgesia). The most common sensations are foreign body sensation, burning, and itching. The conjunctiva is also capable of low-threshold temperature sensitivity.[34]

In the rat, conjunctival nerve fibers contain neuropeptide Y, vasoactive intestinal peptide (VIP), histidine, isoleucine, helospectin, substance P, and calcitonin gene-related peptide. The superior cervical ganglion (sympathetic) contributes the most to innervation via neuropeptide Y-containing fibers. VIP-containing fibers (parasympathetic) arise from the sphenopalatine ganglion. Substance P-containing fibers (sensory) travel to the trigeminal ganglion.[35] In humans, the accessory lacrimal glands of Zeiss and Wolfring, the glands of Moll, and goblet cells are innervated by VIP-containing nerve fibers.[36] Parasympathetic nerves and M(1), M(2), and M(3) muscarinic receptors as well as sympathetic nerves are present on mouse and human goblet cells.[15] Adrenergic receptors are also present on mouse and human goblet cells.[15]

Normal Flora

The conjunctiva is well protected from infectious disease. The mechanical sweeping of the lids and the presence of tear lysozyme and lactoferrin, as well as other antimicrobial factors in the tears, are available defense mechanisms. In addition, the migration of antibodies and inflammatory cells, which are supplied across the conjunctival epithelium from the indigenous lymphocytic population and from the systemic circulation, participate in this defense. There is also a delicate balance between host tolerance and parasitic invasiveness. Any alteration of this delicate balance can lead to tissue destruction. The normal conjunctival flora is relatively consistent worldwide. If an organism is present in one eye, it is usually cultured from the other eye. Organisms cultured from the conjunctival sac are almost always found on the eyelids. When organisms are found on the eyelids, however, only about one-half are cultured from the conjunctival sac.[37]

The ocular surface of healthy individuals supports a relatively small population of bacteria, typically coagulase negative staphylococci, of which *Staphylococcus epidermidis* is the most common isolate. Bacteria are more frequently isolated from individuals with dry eye compared to normals.[38] A greater diversity of conjunctival bacteria are isolated from normals by using molecular cloning and DNA sequencing, including *Corynebacterium*, *Propionibacterium*, *Rhodococcus erythropolis*, *Klebsiella* spp., *Erwinia* spp.[38] Ten percent of adults', 5% of children's, and 1% of infants' eyes are culture positive for fungi.[39] Conjunctival cultures of adults have shown a greater number of aerobic and anaerobic bacterial species than those from children, while *Streptococcus* spp. were more commonly isolated from children.[40]

Physiology of the Conjunctiva

The conjunctiva provides a barrier to exogenous infectious agents and foreign bodies and allows rotation of the globe. The human conjunctiva occupies 17 times more surface area than the cornea, is more permeable than the cornea, and likely exerts more effect on the tear film than the cornea.[41] The conjunctival epithelium has sufficient water permeability and the transporters necessary to contribute significantly to tear film volume that may represent basal tear secretion.[42,43] The conjunctiva not only secretes electrolytes, water, and mucin into the tear film but also is capable of absorbing electrolytes, water, and other compounds from the tear film. It plays an important role in the absorption of ophthalmic drugs applied to the ocular surface.[44] Under pathological conditions such as inflammation or the application of substances that increase vascular permeability, there is leak of plasma, electrolytes, water, and proteins, which can alter the composition of the tear film. Under normal conditions there is fluid transport across the epithelium. This secretion is regulated by nerves, growth factors, and other types of agonists such as the $P2Y_2$ agonists UTP and ATP. Mucin secretion by goblet cells and fluid secretion by stratified squamous cells is likely controlled by different nerves.[44]

Nutrition to the conjunctiva comes from underlying blood vessels and the tear film. Conjunctival epithelium differs from corneal epithelium in gross and histologic appearance and in its biochemical functions. The cornea is a clear, regular, refracting and reflecting surface without blood vessels. The conjunctiva, in contrast, is translucent, irregular, and vascularized. The cornea is devoid of goblet cells; the conjunctiva has numerous goblet cells. The corneal epithelium is five to six layers thick with an orderly progression from basal to wing to superficial cells on an avascularized stroma, whereas the conjunctiva consists of six to nine layers of cells arranged in an irregular fashion on a vascularized stromal bed. Nutrition for the cornea must diffuse across a great distance through the corneal epithelium, endothelium, and stroma. Conjunctival nutrition comes directly from nearby blood vessels. The corneal epithelial cells maintain and require large stores of glycogen for epithelial wound healing; the conjunctiva does not (Table 2.1).

Table 2.1 Comparison of conjunctiva and corneal anatomy, histology, and physiology

Characteristic	Conjunctiva	Cornea
Clarity	Translucent	Clear
Epithelium	6–9 less orderly layers	5–6 orderly layers
Goblet cells	Present	Absent
Stromal bed	Vascular	Avascular
Source of nutrition	Conjunctival vessels, tear film	Anterior chamber, tear film
Glycogen content	Low	High
Dependence on glycogen	Low	High

The conjunctiva is an important source of tear mucin, which arises from the goblet cells (MUC5AC) and conjunctival epithelium (MUC1, MUC2, MUC4). Goblet cells account for 5% to 10% of all ocular surface cells.[11] Carbohydrates, amino acids, and other nutrients are readily available from nearby conjunctival vessels. Small amounts of glycogen are present, since less stored glycogen is needed to meet metabolic needs in case of a crisis. The conjunctiva depends much less on oxidative pathways than does the cornea.[45] There are high levels of glycolic, tricarboxyacetic acid, and respiratory chain enzymes, and low hexose monophosphate shunt activity.[46]

Limbal corneal epithelium with its stems cells act as a barrier that prevents migration of conjunctival epithelial cells on to the cornea.[47] With corneal abrasions that involve the limbus or in ocular surface conditions that result in loss of corneal limbal stem cells (e.g. ocular cicatricial pemphigoid, Stevens–Johnson syndrome, and alkali burns), conjunctival epithelium can migrate onto the cornea. 'Conjunctivialization' of the cornea is usually accompanied by blood vessels and is characterized cytologically by the presence of goblet cells.[48] Conjunctival epithelium on the cornea is not stable, does not tolerate trauma well, and is prone to epithelial defects. It has been thought that conjunctival epithelium on the denuded corneal surface eventually undergoes transdifferentiation from conjunctival to corneal epithelium. Recent work suggests that transdifferentiation does not occur in humans and that conjunctival epithelium is instead replaced by normal corneal epithelium from remaining limbal stem cells[49] or from ectopic corneal epithelial cells in the conjunctival epithelium.[7]

References

1. Spencer W, Zimmerman L, eds. *Conjunctiva*. Philadelphia: WB Saunders; 1985.
2. Kessing S. On the conjunctiva papillae and follicles. *Acta Ophthalmol (Copenh)*. 1966;44:846–851.
3. Pellegrini G, Golisano O, Paterna P, Lambiase A. Location and clonal analysis of stem cells and their differentiated progeny in the human ocular surface. *J Cell Biol*. 1999;145:769–782.
4. Wirtschafter J, Ketcham J, Weinstock R, Tabesh T, McCloon L. Mucocutaneous junction as the major source of replacement palpebral conjunctival epithelial cells. *Invest Ophthalmol Vis Sci*. 1999;40:3138–3146.
5. Peer J, Zajicek G, Greifner H, Kogan M. Streaming conjunctiva. *Anat Rec*. 1996;245:36–40.
6. Nagasaki T, Zhao J. Uniform distribution of epithelial stem cells in the bilbar conjunctiva. *Invest Ophthalmol Vis Sci*. 2005;46:126–132.
7. Kawasaki S, Tanioka H, Yamasaki K, Norihiko Y, Komuro A, Kinoshita S. Clusters of corneal epithelial cells reside ectopically in human conjunctival epithelium. *Invest Ophthalmol Vis Sci*. 2006;47:1359–1367.
8. Dilly P, Makie I. Surface changes in the anesthetic conjunctiva in man with special reference to the production of mucin from non-goblet cell source. *Br J Ophthalmol*. 1981;65:833–842.
9. Foster C, Dutt J, Rice B, Kupferman A, Lane L. Conjunctival epithelial basement membrane zone immunohistology: normal and inflamed conjunctiva. *Int Ophthalmol Clin*. 1994;34:209–214.
10. Podhorany G, Sallai V, Feher J. A kotohartyaham qualitativ adaptatios keszsege. *Szemeszet*. 1967;104:276–281.
11. Thoft R, Friend J. Ocular surface evaluation. In: Francois J, Brown S, Itoi M, eds. *Proceedings of the symposium of the International Society for Corneal Research (Doc Ophthalmol Proc Series 20)*. The Hague: Junk, The Netherlands; 1980.
12. Dartt D. Regulation of mucin and fluid secretion by conjunctival epithelial cells. *Prog Ret Eye Res*. 2002;21:555–576.
13. Rios J, Ghinelli J, Hodges R, Dartt D. Role of neurotrophins and neurotrophin receptors in rat conjunctival goblet cell secretion and proliferation. *Invest Ophthalmol Vis Sci*. 2007;48:1543–1551.
14. Dartt D, McCarthy D, Mercer H, Kessler T, Chung E, Zieske J. Localization of nerves adjacent to goblet cells in rat conjunctiva. *Curr Eye Res*. 1995;14:993–1000.
15. Diebold Y, Rios J, Hodges R, Rawe I, Dartt D. Presence of nerves and their receptors in mouse and human conjunctival goblet cells. *Invest Ophthalmol Vis Sci*. 2001;42:2270–2282.
16. Jumblatt M, McKenzie R, Jumblatt J. MUC5AC is a component of the human precorneal tear film. *Invest Ophthalmol Vis Sci*. 1999;40:43–49.
17. Berry M, Ellingham R, Corfield A. Membrane-associated mucins in normal human conjunctiva. *Invest Ophthalmol Vis Sci*. 2000;41:398–403.
18. Argueso P, Spurr-Michaud S, Russo C, Tisdale A, Gipson I. MUC16 mucin is expressed by the human ocular surface epithelial and carries the H185 carbohydrate epitope. *Invest Ophthalmol Vis Sci*. 2003;44:2487–2495.
19. Blalock T, Spurr-Michaud S, Tisdale A, Gipson I. Release of membrane-associated mucins from ocular surface epithelia. *Invest Ophthalmol Vis Sci*. 2008;49:1864–1871.
20. Allansmith M, Baird G, Greiner G. Density of goblet cells in vernal conjunctivitis and contact lens associated giant papillary conjunctivitis. *Arch Ophthalmol*. 1981;99:884–885.
21. Kessing S. Mucous gland system of the conjunctiva. *Acta Ophthalmol (Copenh)*. 1968;95(suppl):1–133.
22. Nelson J, Wright J. Conjunctival goblet cell densities in ocular surface disease. *Arch Ophthalmol*. 1984;102:1049–1051.
23. Ralph R. Conjunctival goblet cell density in normal subjects and in dry eye syndromes. *Invest Ophthalmol Vis Sci*. 1975;14:299–302.
24. Waheed M, Basu M. The effect of air pollutants on the eye. I. The effects of an organic extract on the conjunctival goblet cells. *Can J Ophthalmol*. 1970;5:226–230.
25. Thoft R, Friend J, Kinoshita S, Nikolic S, Foster C. Ocular cicatricial pemphigoid associated with hyperproliferation of the conjunctival epithelium. *Am J Ophthalmol*. 1984;98:37–42.
26. Rao V, Friend J, Thoft R, Underwood B, Reddy P. Conjunctival goblet cells and mitotic rate in children with retinol deficiency and measles. *Arch Ophthalmol*. 1987;105:378–380.
27. Roat M, Ohji M, Hunt L, Thoft R. Conjunctival epithelial cell hypermitosis and goblet cell hyperplasia in atopic keratoconjunctivitis. *Am J Ophthalmol*. 1993;116:456–463.
28. Tseng S, Hirst L, Maumenee A, Kenyon K, Sun T, Green W. Possible mechanisms for the loss of goblet cells in mucin-deficient disorders. *Ophthalmology*. 1984;91:545–552.
29. Ruskell G, VanderWerf F. Sensory innervation of conjunctival lymph follicles in cynomolgus monkeys. *Invest Ophthalmol Vis Sci*. 1997;38:884–892.
30. Palade G, Simionescu M, Simionescu N. Structural aspects of the permeability of the microvascular endothelium. *Acta Physiol Scand Suppl*. 1979;463:11–32.
31. Goldberg M, Bron A. Anatomy and angiography of the palisades of Vogt. *Trans Am Ophthalmol Soc*. 1982;80:201–206.
32. Lockard I, Debacker H. Conjunctival circulation in relation to circulatory disorders. *JSC Med Assoc*. 1967;63:201–206.
33. Landsman R, et al. The vascular bed of the bulbar conjunctiva in the normal menstrual cycle. *Am J Obstet Gynecol*. 1953;66:988–998.
34. Burton H, ed. *Somatosensory features of the eye*. 9th ed. St Louis: Mosby; 1987:71–100.
35. Elsas T, Edvinsson L, Sundler F, Uddman R. Neuronal pathways to the rat conjunctiva revealed by retrograde tracing and immunochemistry. *Exp Eye Res*. 1994;58:117–126.
36. Seifert P, Spitznas M. Vasoactive intestinal peptide (VIP) innervation of the human eyelid glands. *Exp Eye Res*. 1999;68:685–692.
37. Allansmith M, Osler H, Butterwoth M. Concomitance of bacteria in various areas of the eye. *Arch Ophthalmol*. 1969;82:37–42.
38. Graham J, Moore J, Jiru X, et al. Ocular pathogen or commensal: A PCR-based study of surface bacterial flora in normal and dry eyes. *Invest Ophthalmol Vis Sci*. 2007;48:5616–5623.
39. Hammeke J, Ellis P. Mycotic flora of the conjunctiva. *Am J Ophthalmol*. 1960;49:1174–1178.
40. Singer T, Isenberg S, Apt L. Conjunctival anaerobic and aerobic bacterial flora in paediatric versus adult subjects. *Br J Ophthalmol*. 1988;72:448–451.
41. Watsky M, Jablonski M, Edelhauser H. Comparision of conjunctival and corneal surface areas in rabbit and human. *Curr Eye Res*. 1988;7:519–531.
42. Li Y, Kuang K, Yerxa B, Wen Q, Rosskothen H, Fischbarg J. Rabbit conjunctival epithelium transports fluid, and P2Y2(2) receptor agonists stimulate Cl^- and fluid secretion. *Am J Physiol Cell Physiol*. 2001;281:C595–602.
43. Shiue M, Kulkarni A, Gukasyan H, Swisher J, Kim K, Lee V. Pharmacological modulation of fluid secretion in the pigmented rabbit conjunctiva. *Life Sci*. 2000;66:PL105–111.
44. Yang J, Ueda H, Kim K, Lee V. Meeting future challenges in topical ocular drug delivery: development of an air-interfaced primary culture of rabbit conjunctival epithelial cells on a permeable support for drug transport studies. *J Controlled Rel*. 2000;65:1.
45. Thoft R, Friend J. Biochemical transformation of regenerating ocular surface epithelium. *Invest Ophthalmol Vis Sci*. 1977;16:14–20.
46. Baum B. A histochemical study of corneal respiratory enzyme. *Arch Ophthalmol*. 1963;70:59.
47. Tseng S. Concept and application of limbal stem cells. *Eye*. 1989;3:141–157.
48. Thoft R, Friend J, Murphy H. Ocular surface epithelium and corneal vascularization. *Invest Ophthalmol Vis Sci*. 1979;18:85–92.
49. Dua H. The conjunctiva in corneal epithelial wound healing. *Br J Ophthalmol*. 1998;82:1407–1411.

Chapter 3

Tear Film

Michael A. Lemp, Roger W. Beuerman

Overview and Function

The tear film is a complex composite whose components have multiple sources, which include the lacrimal gland, meibomian glands, goblet cells, and accessory lacrimal glands of the ocular surface. Additional secretory contributions from the ocular surface, which contains several types of embedded tissues, such as the glands of Krause, Moll, and Wolfring, have a structure very similar to that of the main lacrimal gland.[1,2] The base of the tear film is the outer surface membrane of the corneal or conjunctival epithelial cells. The membrane of the corneal cells is striking in appearance. The membrane is thrown into folds called microplicae or microvilli and the membrane leaflet touching the tear film is very osmophilic. It is usually assumed that the reason for the elaborate folds and filaments extending into the tear film is to aid adherence of the tear film. However, the tear film extends over the conjunctiva as well, and the outer surface of those cells do not show the same elaborations to the extent seen for the corneal cells (Fig. 3.1), but both structures serve to increase the surface area, presumably aiding in tear–epithelial adhesion. The tears have been reviewed often and there are classic texts that detail the well-accepted concepts of the tears; in the present work the emphasis will be on the evolving concepts of the tears.[3,4]

The function of the tear film includes lubrication, protection from disease, nutrition of the cornea, and a critical role in the optical properties of the eye.[5] In fact, the crisp optical (corneal) reflex commonly seen in clinical or casual photographs of the eye provides evidence of the mirror-like quality of the optical function of this surface and an indication that the tear film is intact. Normal tear volume is around 6 μL and production is about 1.2 μL/minute with a turnover rate of about 16% per minute.[6] The precorneal tear film is a metastable structure between blinks allowing for clear vision; this limited stability is compromised in dry eye disease, leading to optical image degradation between blinks.[7]

Although early studies separated the tear film into three discernable layers, that structural rigidity has changed with time, and the tear layers are considered to be more of a continuum with the lipid layer most anterior to the aqueous and mucin components. The aqueous component of the tear film contains proteins, and electrolytes of lacrimal gland origin, and other ocular surface sources. Normal tears contain 6–10 mg/mL total proteins[8] and almost 500 proteins have been reported.[9] Major tear proteins include lysozyme, lactoferrin, secretory immunoglobulin A (sIgA), serum albumin, lipocalin[10] (previously called tear-specific prealbumin), and lipophilin.[11] Tears are a dilute protein solution and both the electrolyte and protein content of the tears varies from that of the serum. Chloride and potassium are higher in the tears (tears, 120 mEq/L and 20 mEq/L; serum, 102 mEq/L and 5 mEq/L, respectively) and glucose concentration is lower in the tears (about 2.5 mg/100 mL) compared to plasma (85 mg/L). The osmotic pressure of the tears in normals ranges between 280 and 305 mOsm/L, whereas in plasma the value is about 6 atm.[3,4]

Tear proteins vary with the state of health of the ocular surface. Measured levels of proteins such as β2-microglobulin (Mw = 11.8 kDa[12]), cystatins (Mw = 14 kDa[13,14]), substance P,[15] epidermal growth factor (EGF),[16] transforming growth factor β1 (TGF-β1) and β2 (TGF β2),[17] plasmin,[18] tryptase,[19] and α1-antitrypsin[20] change depending on conditions, although how these change is not always clear. Examination of the levels of IgE and IgA antibodies to grass and tree allergens in serum and tears in a series of patients showed the same specificity for many allergans.[21] Elevated tear plasmin concentrations were observed after anterior keratectomy,[18] and tryptase levels were elevated in tears of patients with active ocular allergy.[22] Growth factors, EGF, TGF-β1, and TGF-β2, are present in normal tear fluids and have been associated with corneal wound healing.[23] In addition to these components of the tear proteome, genetic markers for both ocular and systemic diseases have been reported to be present in tears.[24] Rapid, reliable analysis of tear properties such as tear osmolarity and individual components such as proteins may be useful in the clinical diagnosis of eye diseases such as dry eye disease[25,26] and conjunctivitis.[27] Sampling of tears, however, presents certain challenges and almost certainly affects results (vide infra).

Control of Tear Secretion

Control of the tears and hence the activity of the tears has recently been suggested to be under constant neural regulation: a somewhat different concept from the more traditional one that thought only reflex tears are a result of neural participation and that normal tears were the results of

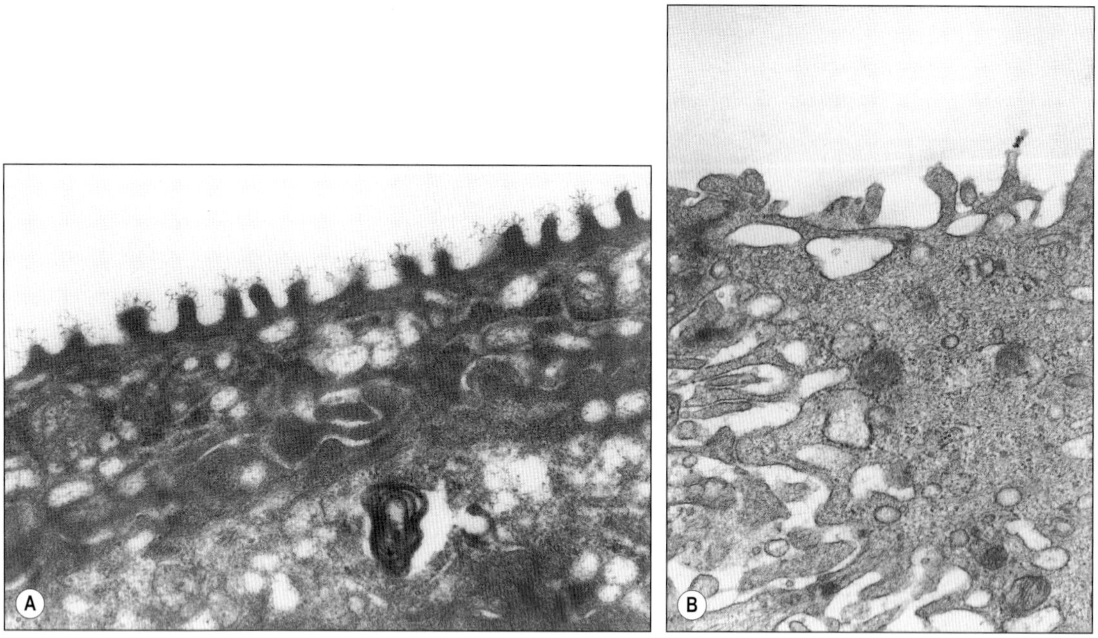

Fig. 3.1 As shown in the transmission electron micrographs of the surface cell layer of the cornea (**A**) and conjunctiva (**B**), the outer membrane of these epithelial cells is thrown into folds that will increase the total surface area in contact with the tears. However, the membrane of the corneal epithelial cells shows the additional specializations of the very dense osmium staining, and the very fine filaments that radiate into the tear layer. This difference in surface articulations between cornea and conjunctiva is similar for humans, nonhuman primates, and rabbits. Both tissues are from human material fixed at 2–3 hours postmortem. The cornea (**A**, × 51 587) is from a 66-year-old individual, and the bulbar conjunctiva (**B**, × 50 000) from an 86-year-old.

intrinsic lacrimal gland activity. Obviously, either too little or too much aqueous secretion will present a problem with visual function. Thus, there is a means for the ongoing homeostatic regulation of the ocular surface, which is under a control mechanism whose components include afferent nerves from the cornea and other ocular surface tissues, central nervous system relay nuclei, and efferent nerves which comprise the autonomic innervation to secretory tissues whose products contribute to the tear film (Fig. 3.2).[28–30] This mechanism is suggested to supply a relatively constant level of neural signals that precisely meter the amount of tears secreted by the main lacrimal gland, but also may mediate lipid production by the meibomian glands and mucin secretion from the goblet cells. The accessory lacrimal glands have been shown to have local innervation, but it is not known if these nerves are included in the homeostatic mechanism or if secretion from the accessory lacrimal glands can be stimulated by transmitter release as part of the lacrimal reflex (Fig. 3.3). Interruption of the neural pathway by different means such as LASIK or anesthesia of the cornea decreases tear flow.[31,32]

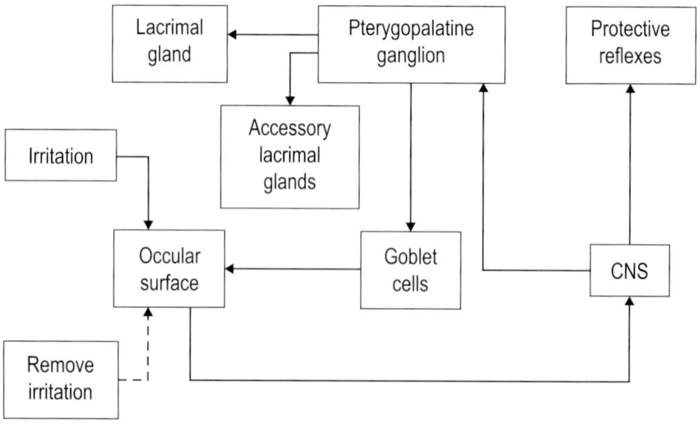

Fig. 3.2 The small sensory nerve endings located just below the epithelial surface of the cornea, lid margin, and conjunctiva constantly respond to drying and temperature change as well as contact and chemical changes, by sending intensity-coded neural signals to the spinal trigeminal nucleus located in the brain stem. A multisynaptic pathway to the preganglionic parasympathetic nuclei in the superior salivatory nucleus forms the output to the secretory tissue. An irritation to the ocular surface gives rise to a large neural input, which provides the neural signal for reflex tearing. The loop is reset when the irritation is removed by copious tearing. For simplicity, some of the components of the neural pathways such as the trigeminal ganglion, sympathetic nerves, and meibomian glands, have been omitted.

Tear Layer Thickness

Although its importance may not be immediately apparent, the thickness of the tear layer has received a great deal of attention. It is of interest to know the volume of the tears over the surface of the eye, particularly the cornea, as it is a reservoir for drugs that have been delivered by either topical or systemic routes for penetration into the eye. As a major risk to vision, the lack of a sufficient amount of tears is the primary problem in aqueous-deficient dry eye. The contact lens industry has been interested in the thickness of the tear layer as contact lenses need the support of the tear layer for both optical placement and comfort. From

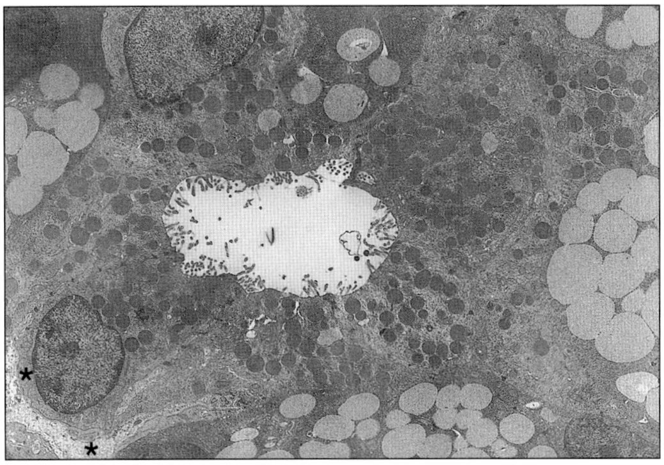

Fig. 3.3 Transmission electron micrograph of the accessory lacrimal gland of the tarsal conjunctiva of the upper eyelid from a nonhuman primate (× 6000). The basic secretory morphology is very similar to that of the orbital lacrimal gland. Small unmyelinated axons (*asterisks*) are seen adjacent to the basal aspect of the acinar cells.

earlier studies, the thickness of the tear layer was found to be about 7–8 μm.[33] Studies by Prydal using confocal microscopy and interferometry, however, estimated tear film thickness to be over 40 μm.[34] The use of lipid interference patterns to monitor the lipid component of tears have produced interesting new insights and it has been found that several orders of interference patterns could be used to detect changes in the lipid layer and that a dry eye patient was deficient in this regard.[35] Recent studies have reported that the lipid layer of the tears is thinner in many patients with dry eye disease.[36]

However, the controversy has continued. Making use of innovative methods, additional thickness values are still being offered. Using reflection spectra of the human tear film, it was found that there were no oscillations that compared to Prydal's measurements or of earlier estimates. Rather, the results of this study suggested a tear film of about 3 μm.[37] A study of the mouse tear film using a microelectrode technique found the tear film to be about 7 μm.[38] In infants, the lipid layer was found to be thicker than in adults, which may be a response to a thinner aqueous layer.[39]

Analytical Methods

The tears are an attractive source for sampling due to their accessibility, rich content, and largely acellular structure. This latter quality means that unlike the processing of blood samples necessary to separate the cells from serum, direct measurements of tear samples are possible. As mentioned above, tears have an extensive proteome and genomic markers have been reported. There are, however, challenges to sampling tears. Most tear samples are collected using a glass capillary tube applied to the inferior marginal tear strip. Since the entire volume of minimally stimulated tears (ordinary environmental stimulation) is around 7 μL and only about 2–3 μL are in the inferior marginal tear strip, and there is minimal exchange between the marginal tear strip and other compartments of tears, collection of more than 2 μL samples at a single sampling implies reflex tearing. The lacrimal functional unit is composed of the cornea, conjunctiva, tears, lids, and drainage pathways. As outlined above, this neurally controlled unit responds to perturbations in an attempt to maintain a homeostatic environment for cells of the ocular surface. Both changes in volume and composition are induced. Increased secretion from the lacrimal glands and increased passage of transconjunctival fluid result in reflex tearing. Tear composition changes with an increase in some tear proteins and a decrease in others. This leads to great variability in many components of tears, creating clinical variances depending on the degree of induced reflex tearing. Attempts to measure glucose, for example, have been plagued by large differences which are thought to be due to influx of glucose from serum across the conjunctiva induced by sampling stimulation.[40]

Despite the sampling problems described above, a number of analytical methods that couple microliter sample sizes with high sensitivity and resolution have prompted more detailed studies of event-related changes in tear composition. Qualitative and quantitative techniques include one- and two-dimensional polyacrylamide gel electrophoresis (PAGE),[11,41–43] isoelectric focusing (IEF),[11,41] crossed immunoelectrophoresis, enzyme-linked immunosorbent assay (ELISA), and high-pressure liquid chromatography (HPLC) techniques such as size-exclusion HPLC,[44–46] reversed-phase HPLC,[12] and ion-exchange HPLC.[12] Matrix-assisted laser desorption/ionization (MALDI) mass spectrometry has also been applied to study changes in tear proteins before and after corneal wound healing,[47] and proteomic methods have been used to map tear protein profiles.[48,49]

Electrophoresis and 2D-PAGE have been used extensively for tear protein analysis. However, these methods are limited due to the large volume of tears required and the time required to perform the analysis. Furthermore, 2D-PAGE is limited in its ability to analyze small proteins, extremely acidic or basic proteins, or hydrophobic proteins. MALDI provides mass information, but using this technique for quantification can be difficult, although progress is being made in this area.[49]

Surface-enhanced laser desorption-time of flight (SELDI-TOF) ProteinChip technology has recently been introduced as an alternative to 2D-PAGE.[50–52] This technology utilizes affinity surfaces to retain adherent proteins based on their physical or chemical characteristics, which is then followed by direct analysis using TOF-MS. It is a rapid and reproducible technique used to generate protein expression profiles known as 'phenomic fingerprints.' SELDI-TOF is more sensitive and requires smaller amounts of tear samples (2–3 μL) than 2D-PAGE (Fig. 3.4). This system has enabled detection of critical proteins directly from crude mixtures without time- and labor-intensive preprocessing and has been proven to be a very useful tool to identify biomarkers in various cancers and biomarkers of disease and trauma.[53,54] This method is promising for a rapid scan of tear proteins; however, it requires some additional precision to accurately determine mass and, hence, exact protein information.

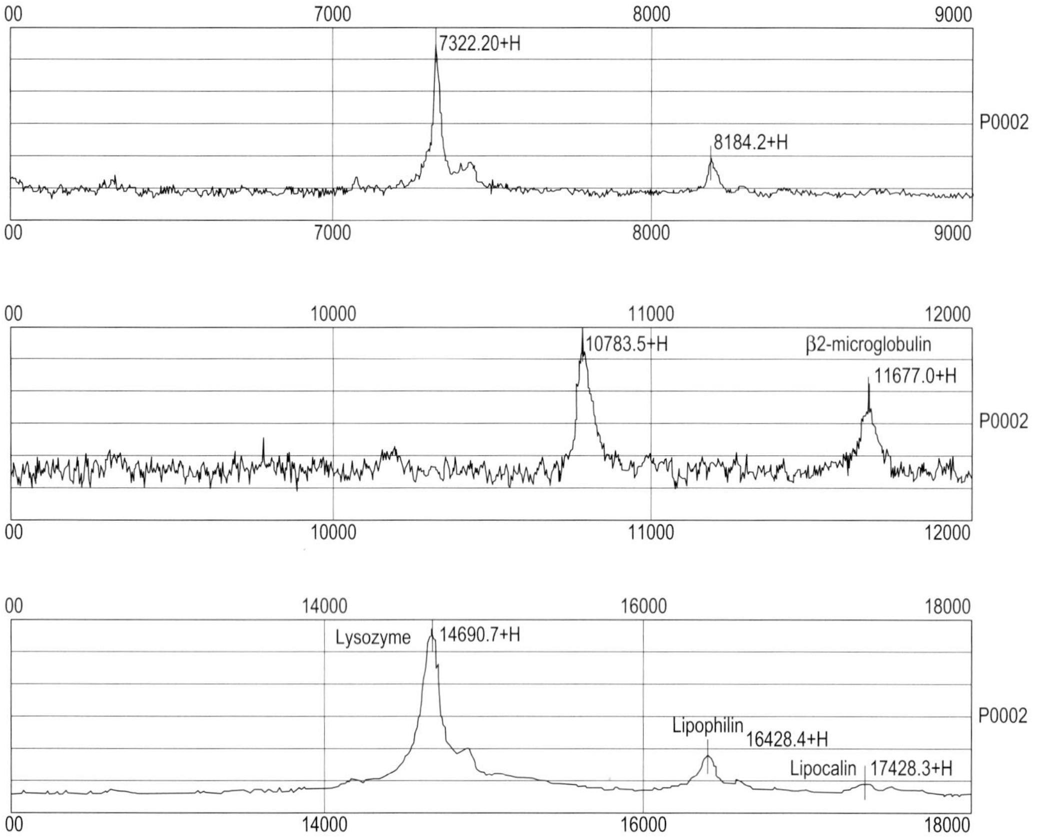

Fig. 3.4 Tear mass spectrogram from a 3 μL sample of human tears of a normal eye from a SELDI chip. Some of the common tear components are noted as part of identified peaks. The SELDI chip is a rapid method for obtaining a composite spectrogram of many peptide peaks that can undergo further analysis of specific peptide components.

Peptide Components of Tears

As seen in Table 3.1, peptides in the tear film include a heterogeneous variety of bioactive molecules, including a wide range of growth factors with multicellular targets and neuropeptides. There has been a longstanding interest in molecules which augment corneal wound healing, as well as understanding how some of these growth factors (shown in Table 3.1) may complicate wound healing by stimulating scar formation. Epidermal growth factor (EGF) has been shown to stimulate migration of corneal epithelial cells in tissue culture. However, it was found that EGF is a naturally occurring component of the tears.[55,56] Uncovering antimicrobial peptides in tears was an early initiative due to the vulnerability and devastating effect of infectious disease on the cornea, and continues with additional vigor today, augmented by more sensitive instrumentation. In fact, activity in this area has increased as it has become clear that these peptides have a number of properties in addition to their antimicrobial properties and may in fact be active in the wound response. The cornea and ocular surface, although small in area, are critical for vision and extremely vulnerable to airborne and contact-transmitted pathogens. Accordingly, there has been a great deal of work to determine the presence and activity of the members of these molecular species. Antimicrobial peptides form the system of innate immunity of the ocular surface and are evolutionarily old. These naturally occurring antibiotics act against a wide range of viruses, bacteria, and fungi; however, recently these have been suggested to directly participate in wound healing. The tears have been shown to have lysozyme, lactoferrin, and both α- and β-defensins. [57–89] PMNs which contribute to some of the tear peptides are not found in great numbers in normal tears, but following stress of the ocular surface these are abundant in tears and clearly contribute to the protein milieu. These references represent a good survey of the reports of protein substances within tears thought to play a role in mediating responses to environmental, infectious challenges and disease states.

The defensin family of peptides has received a great deal of attention as there is considerable evidence for multifunctionality of antimicrobial and wound healing effects. Defensins are a family of small, cationic antimicrobial peptides containing an average of 35 amino acids with molecular weights around 3–4 kDa.[90,91] They possess six cysteine residues that form three intramolecular disulfide bonds and have broad-spectrum antimicrobial action against Gram-positive and Gram-negative bacteria, fungi, and some viruses.[92,93] More recently, human α-defensins (HNP-1, HNP-2, and HNP-3) have been shown to possess anti-HIV activity for human CD8+ T lymphocytes.[94,95] In humans, six α-defensins (HNP-1–4, HD-5, and HD-6) and three β-defensins

Table 3.1 Functional peptides of tears

	References	Association
Growth factors		
Epidermal growth factor (EGF)	55, 56, 57, 58, 59	Epithelial wound healing Tear concentration higher than saliva or serum
Transforming growth factor alpha (TGF-α)	60, 61	Wound response
Transforming growth factor beta-1 (TGF-β1)	62, 63	Wound response
Transforming growth factor beta-2 (TGF-β2)	62, 64, 65	Found in normal tears, increases after wounding
Hepatocyte growth factor (HGF)	66, 67	Wound response
Basic fibroblast growth factor (FGF-2)	68	Wound response
Vascular endothelial growth factor (VEGF)	64, 69	Wound response, increases after wounding
Platelet derived growth factor-BB	69, 70	Did not change after PRK
Neuropeptides		
Substance P	15, 71, 72	Wound healing, neurogenic inflammation
Calcitonin gene related peptide	64, 73	Wound healing, neurogenic inflammation
Interleukins		
IL-4	76	Increases in vernal conjunctivitis
IL-1α, IL-1β	77, 78	Elevation of IL-1 in dry eye patients
IL-2, IL-4, IL-6, IL-8, IL-10	79, 80, 81	Increases with contact lens wear, ocular allergy
Immunoglobulins		
IgA, IgE, IgG(1–4) and complement	21, 82	Ocular allergy
Proteases		
MMP-1, MMP-3, MMP-9, TIMP-1, capthepsin, alpha2-macroglobulin	83, 84, 85, 86	Role in pterygium migration and vernal keratoconjunctivitis, protection of the ocular surface
Antimicrobial peptides		
Lysozyme, lactoferrin, α and β defensins, phospholipase A2	87, 88, 89, 90, 91, 92	Increases in infections, wound healing, may decrease in dry eye

(hBD-1-3) have been identified. The α-defensins are most probably released into the tear fluids by resident or passing neutrophils and secretion from lacrimal ductular epithelia. However, other biological functions of defensins have been reported or suggested, such as accelerating epithelial wound healing and mediating inflammatory process.[96,97] Tumor necrosis factor has already been found to be a tear component in vernal conjunctivitis, but the interactions between these many indicators of immune disease are not yet clear.[98]

Tear research should continue the present resurgence of interest over the next several years and, with the ability to measure a wide range of peptides in a single small volume sample, the diagnostic value of tears may become a reality for diseases such as KCS, immune disease, and for a wide range of corneal infections. Certainly, working out the tear proteome would be a much-needed early step to understand how these peptides affect the health of the ocular surface and vision and to develop the research background for targeted therapies. At this time, however, the clinical utility of tear levels of individual proteins and peptides is limited by the volume of tears necessary for most analyses requiring reflex tear samples. Progress in this field may depend on the development of new methods of sampling which collect small samples without inducing reflex tearing and nanoassay techniques for quantitative analysis. Identification of proteins which are not normally present in tears, e.g. IgE in ocular allergy, presents a binary approach which may not be as dependent on quantitative assays.

Another approach is to measure properties of the whole of the tear film rather than individual components, e.g. tear stability and tear concentration of electrolytes or its surrogate, tear osmolarity. Tear film break-up time is a measure of the stability of the tear film; a recently reported new technology for sampling nanoliter quantities of tear atraumatically and measurement of tear osmolarity on samples of 40 nL size may represent a new platform on which to develop diagnostic tests without prior sample processing and suitable for use in the clinical setting.[99]

Acknowledgments

Supported by the following grants: NEI EY 12416 and EY 02377, Research to Prevent Blindness (US National Institutes of Health) and NMRC proto-PG002, NMRC-IBG (Singapore). (RB) We would like to extend our appreciation to our colleague, Dr. Zhou Lei, for the mass spectrogram.

References

1. Maitchouk DY, Beuerman RW, Ohta T, et al. Tear production after unilateral removal of the main lacrimal gland in squirrel monkeys. *Arch Ophthalmol.* 2000;118:246–252.
2. Seifert P, Spitznas M. Vasoactive intestinal polypeptide (VIP) innervation of the human eyelid glands. *Exp Eye Res.* 1999;68:685–692.
3. Van Haeringen NJ. Clinical biochemistry of tears. *Surv Ophthalmol.* 1981;26:84–96.
4. Farris RL. Abnormalities of the tears and treatment of dry eyes. Chapter 6. In: Kaufman HE, Barron BA, McDonald MB, Waltman SR, eds. *The cornea.* New York: Churchill Livingstone; 1988:139–155.
5. Klyce SD, Beuerman RW. Structure and function of the cornea. Chapter 1. In: Kaufman HE, Barron BA, McDonald MB, Waltman SR, eds. *The cornea.* New York: Churchill Livingstone; 1988:3–54.
6. Mishima S, Gassett A, Klyce SD, et al. Determination of tear volume and tear flow. *Invest Ophthalmol Vis Sci.* 1966;5:264–269.
7. Goto E, Ishida R, Kaido M, et al. Optical aberrations and visual disturbances with dry eye. *Ocul Surf.* 2006;4(4):207–213.
8. Berta A. *Enzymology of the tears.* Boca Raton: CRC Press; 1992.
9. De Souza GA, Godov LM, Mann M. Identification of 491 proteins in the tear proteome reveals a large number of proteases and protease inhibitors. *Genome Biol.* 2006;7(8):R72.
10. Redl B. Human tear lipocalin. *Biochim Biophys Acta.* 2000;1482: 241–248.
11. Lehrer RI, Xu GR, Abduragimov A, et al. Lipophilin, a novel heterodimeric protein of human tears. *FEBS Letters.* 1998;432:163–167.
12. Baier G, Wollensak G, Mur E, et al. Analysis of human tear proteins by different high performance liquid chromatographic techniques. *J Chromatogr.* 1990;525:319–328.
13. Barka T, Asbell PA, van der Noen H, et al. Cystatins in human tear fluid. *Curr Eye Res.* 1991;10:25–34.
14. Reitz C, Breipohl W, Augustin A. Analysis of tear proteins by one- and two-dimensional thin-layer iosoelectric focusing, sodium dodecyl sulfate electrophoresis and lectin blotting. Detection of a new component: cystatin C. *Graefe's Arch Clin Exp Ophthalmol.* 1998;236:894–899.
15. Varnell RJ, Freeman JY, Maitchouk D, et al. Detection of substance P in human tears by laser desorption mass spectrometry and immunoassay. *Curr Eye Res.* 1997;16:960–963.
16. Van Setten GB, Viinikka L, Tervo T, et al. Epidermal growth factor is a constant component of normal human tear fluid. *Graefe's Arch Clin Exp Ophthalmol.* 1989;227:82–87.
17. Gupta A, Monroy D, Ji Z, et al. Transforming growth factor beta-1 and beta-2 in human tear fluid. *Curr Eye Res.* 1996;15:605–614.
18. Van Setten GB, Salonen EM, Vaheri A, et al. Plasmin and plasminogen activator activities in tear fluid during corneal wound healing after anterior keratectomy. *Curr Eye Res.* 1989;8:1293–1298.
19. Butrus SI, Ochsner KI, Abelson MB, et al. The level of tryptase in human tears. An indicator of activation of conjunctival mast cells. *Ophthalmology.* 1990;97:1678–1683.
20. Sen DK, Sarin GS. In: Holly FJ, ed. *The preocular tear ?lm in health, disease, and contact lens wear.* Lubbock TX: Dry Eye Institute; 1986:192–199.
21. Aghayan-Ugurluoglu R, Ball T, Vrtala S, et al. Dissociation of allergen-specific IgE and IgA responses in sera and tears of pollen-allergic patients: a study performed with purified recombinant pollen allergens. *J Allergy Clin Immunol.* 2000;105:803–813.
22. Schultz G, Khaw PT, Oxford K, et al. Growth factors and ocular wound healing. *Eye.* 1994;8:184–187.
23. Grus FH, Sabuncuo P, Augustin AJ. Analysis of tear protein patterns of dry-eye patients using fluorescent staining dyes and two-dimensional quantification algorithms. *Electrophoresis.* 2001;22:1845–1850.
24. Fukuda M, Deai T, Higaki S, Hayashi K, Shimomura Y. Presence of a large amount of herpes simplex virus genome in tear fluid of herpetic stromal keratitis and persistent epithelial defects. *Semin Ophthalmol.* 2008; 23(4):217–220.
25. Grus FH, Augustin AJ, Evangelou NG, et al. Analysis of tear-protein patterns as a diagnostic tool for the detection of dry eyes. *Eur J Ophthalmol.* 1998;8:90–97.
26. Boukes RJ, Boonstra A, Breebaart AC, et al. Analysis of human tear protein profiles using high performance liquid chromatography (HPLC). *Doc Ophthalmol.* 1987;67:105–113.
27. Rapacz P, Tedesco J, Donshik PC, et al. Tear lysozyme and lactoferrin levels in giant papillary conjunctivitis and vernal conjunctivitis. *CLAO J.* 1988;14:207–209.
28. Stern ME, Beuerman RW, Fox RI, et al. The pathology of dry eye: the interaction between the ocular surface and lacrimal glands. *Cornea.* 1998;17:584–589.
29. Stern ME, Beuerman RW, Fox RI, et al. A unified theory of the role of the ocular surface in dry eye. In: Sullivan DA, Dartt DA, Meneray MA, eds. *Lacrimal gland, tear film, and dry eye syndromes 2: basic science and clinical relevance,* New York: Plenum Press; 1998:643–651; *Adv Exp Med Biol.* 1998;438:643–651.
30. Beuerman RW, Maitchouk DY, Varnell RJ, Pedroza-Schmidt L. Interactions between lacrimal function and the ocular surface. In: Kinoshita S, Ohashi Y, eds. *Proceedings of the 2nd annual meeting of the Kyoto Cornea Club, The Hague.* The Netherlands: Kugler Publications; 1998:1–10.
31. Wilson SE, Ambrosio R. Laser in situ keratomileusis-induced neurotrophic epitheliopathy. *Am J Ophthalmol.* 2001;132:405–406.
32. Sugar A, Rapuano CJ, Culbertson WW, et al. Laser in situ keratomileusis for myopia and astigmatism: safety and efficacy: a report by the American Academy of Ophthalmology. *Ophthalmology.* 2002;109:175–187.
33. Mishima S. Some physiological aspects of the precorneal tear film. *Arch Ophthalmol* 1965;73:233–241.
34. Prydal JI, Artal P, Woon H, et al. Study of human tear film thickness and structure using laser interferometry. *Invest Ophthalmol Vis Sci.* 1992;33:2006.
35. Goto E, Dogru M, Kojima T, et al. Computer-synthesis of an interference color chart of human tear lipid layer, by a colorimetric approach. *Invest Ophthalmol Vis Sci.* 2003;44:4693–4697.
36. Foulks GN The correlation between the tear film lipid layer and dry eye disease. *Surv Ophthalmol.* 2007;52(4):369–374.
37. King-Smith PE, Fink BA, Fogt N, et al. The thickness of the human precorneal tear film: evidence from reflection spectra. *Invest Ophthalmol Vis Sci.* 2000;41:3348–3359.
38. Tran CH, Routledge C, Miller J, et al. Examination of the murine tear film. *Invest Ophthalmol Vis Sci.* 2003;44:3520–3525.
39. Isenberg SJ, DelSignore M, Chen A, et al. The lipid layer and stability of the preocular tear film in newborns and infants. *Ophthalmology.* 2003;110:1408–1411.
40. Baca JT, Finegold DN, Asher SA. Tear glucose analysis for the non-invasive detection and monitoring of diabetes mellitus. *Ocul Surf.* 2007;5(4):280–293.
41. Wollensak G, Mur E, Mayr A, et al. Effective methods for the investigation of human tear film proteins and lipids. *Graefe's Arch Clin Exp Ophthalmol.* 1990;228:78–82.
42. Molloy MP, Bolis S, Herbert BR, et al. Establishment of the human reflex tear two-dimensional polyacrylamide gel electrophoresis reference map: New proteins of potential diagnostic value. *Electrophoresis.* 1997;18: 2811–2815.
43. Mii S, Nakamura K, Takeo K, et al. Analysis of human tear proteins by two-dimensional electrophoresis. *Electrophoresis.* 1992;13:379–382.
44. Fullard RJ. Identification of proteins in small tear volumes with and without size exclusion HPLC fractionation. *Curr Eye Res.* 1988;7: 163–179.
45. Fullard RJ, Snyder C. Protein levels in nonstimulated and stimulated tears of normal human subjects. *Invest Ophthalmol Vis Sci.* 1990;31: 1119–1126.
46. Fullard RJ, Tucker DL. Changes in human tear protein levels with progressively increasing stimulus. *Invest Ophthalmol Vis Sci.* 1991;32: 2290–2301.
47. Varnell RJ, Maitchouk DY, Beuerman RW, et al. Small-volume analysis of rabbit tears and effects of a corneal wound on tear protein spectra. *Adv Exp Med Biol.* 1998;438:659–664.

48. Evans VE, Cordwell S, Vockler C, et al. Ten isoforms of human tear lipocalin demonstrated with 2D-PAGE and MALDI-TOF analysis. *Invest Ophthalmol Vis Sci.* 2000;41:S69.
49. Bucknall M, Fung KY, Duncan MW. Practical quantitative biomedical applications of MALDI-TOF mass spectrometry. *J Am Soc Mass Spectrom.* 2002;13:1015–1027.
50. Hutchens TW, Yip T-T. New desorption strategies for the mass spectrometric analysis of macromolecules. *Rapid Commun Mass Spectrom.* 1993;7:576–580.
51. Jain KK. Recent advances in oncoproteomics. *Curr Opin Mol Ther.* 2002;4:203–209.
52. Issaq HJ, Veenstra TD, Conrads TP, et al. The SELDI-TOF MS approach to proteomics: protein profiling and biomarker identification. *Biochem Biophys Res Commun.* 2002;292:587–592.
53. Zhou L, Beuerman RW, Barathi A, Tan D. Analysis of rabbit tear proteins by high-pressure liquid chromatography/electrospray ionization mass spectrometry. *Rapid Commun Mass Spectrom.* 2003;17(5):401–412.
54. Wang S, Diamond DL, Hass GM, et al. Identification of prostate specific membrane antigen (PSMA) as the target of monoclonal antibody 107-1A4 by proteinchip; array, surface-enhanced laser desorption/ionization (SELDI) technology. *Int J Cancer.* 2001;92:871–876.
55. Hayashi T, Sakamoto S. Radioimmunoassay of human epidermal growth factor-hEGF levels in human body fluids. *J Pharmacobiodyn.* 1988;11: 146–151.
56. Ohashi Y, Motokura M, Kinoshita Y, et al. Presence of epidermal growth factor in human tears. *Invest Ophthalmol Vis Sci.* 1989;30:1879–1882.
57. van Setten GB, Viinikka L, Tervo T, et al. Epidermal growth factor is a constant component of normal human tear fluid. *Graefe's Arch Clin Exp Ophthalmol.* 1989;227:184–187.
58. van Setten GB, Tervo T, Tevo K, et al. Epidermal growth factor (EGF) in ocular fluids: presence, origin, and therapeutical considerations. *Acta Ophthalmol Suppl.* 1992;202:54–59.
59. Schuller S, Knorr M, Steuhl KP, et al. Lacrimal secretion of human epidermal growth factor in perforating keratoplasty. *Ger J Ophthalmol.* 1996;5:268–274.
60. van Setten GB, Schultz G. Transforming growth factor-alpha is a constant component of human tear fluid. *Graefe's Arch Clin Exp Ophthalmol.* 1994;232:523–526.
61. Schultz G, Rotatori DS, Clark W. EGF and TGF-alpha in wound healing and repair. *J Cell Biochem.* 1991;45:346–352.
62. Gupta A, Monroy D, Ji Z, et al. Transforming growth factor beta-1 and beta-2 in human tear fluid. *Curr Eye Res.* 1996;15:605–614.
63. Vesaluoma M, Teppo AM, Gronhagen-Riska C, et al. Release of TGF-beta 1 and VEGF in tears following photorefractive keratectomy. *Curr Eye Res.* 1997;16:19–25.
64. Vesaluoma MH, Tervo T. Tenascin and cytokines in tear fluid after photorefractive keratectomy. *J Refract Surg.* 1998;14:447–454.
65. Kokawa N, Sotozono C, Nishida K, Kinoshita S. High total TGF-beta 2 levels in normal tears. *Curr Eye Res.* 1996;15:341–343.
66. Wilson SE, Li Q, Mohan RR, Tervo T, et al. Lacrimal gland growth factors and receptors: lacrimal fibroblastic cells are a source of tear HGF. *Adv Exp Med Biol.* 1998;438:625–628.
67. Grierson I, Heathcote L, Hiscott P, et al. Hepatocyte growth factor/scatter factor in the eye. *Prog Retin Eye Res.* 2000;19:779–802.
68. van Setten GB. Basic fibroblast growth factor in human tear fluid: detection of another growth factor. *Graefe's Arch Clin Exp Ophthalmol.* 1996;234:275–277.
69. Vesaluoma M, Teppo AM, Gronhagen-Riska C, Tervo T. Platelet-derived growth-BB (PDGF-BB) in tear fluid: a potential modulator of corneal healing following photorefractive keratectomy. *Curr Eye Res.* 1997;16: 825–831.
70. Tuominen IS, Tervo T, Teppo AM, et al. Human tear fluid PDGF-BB, TNF-alpha, and TGF-beta 1 vs corneal haze and regeneration of corneal epithelium and subbasal nerve plexus after PRK. *Exp Eye Res.* 2001;72: 631–641.
71. Fujishima H, Takeyama M, Takeuchi T, et al. Elevated levels of substance P in tears of patients with allergic conjunctivitis and vernal conjunctivitis. *Clin Exp Allergy.* 1997;27:372–378.
72. Yamada, M, Ogata M, Kawai M, Mashima Y. Decreased substance P concentrations in tears from patients with corneal hypesthesia. *Am J Ophthalmol.* 2000;129:671–672.
73. Merrtaniemi P, Ylatupa S, Partanen P, Tervo T. Increased release of immunoreactive calcitonin gene-related peptide (CGRP) in tears after excimer laser keratectomy. *Exp Eye Res.* 1995;60:659–665.
74. Vesluoma M, Tervo T. Tear fluid changes after photorefractive keratectomy. *Adv Exp Med Biol.* 1998;438:515–521.
75. Leonardi A, DeFranchis G, Zancanaro F, et al. Identification of local Th2 and Th0 lymphocytes in vernal conjunctivitis by cytokine flow cytometry. *Invest Ophthalmol Vis Sci.* 1999;40:3036–3040.
76. Uchio E, Ono SY, Ikezawa Z, Ohno S. Tear levels of interferon-gamma, interleukin (IL)-2, IL-4 and IL-5 in patients with vernal keratoconjunctivitis, atopic keratoconjunctivitis and allergic conjunctivitis. *Clin Exp Allergy.* 2000;30:103–109.
77. Thakur A, Willcox MD. Contact lens wear alters the production of certain inflammatory mediators in tears. *Exp Eye Res.* 2000;70:255–259.
78. Solomon A, Dursun D, Liu Z, et al. Pro-and anti-inflammatory forms of interleukin-1 in the tear fluid and conjunctiva of patients with dry-eye disease. *Invest Ophthalmol Vis Sci.* 2001;42:2283–2292.
79. Malecaze F, Simorre V, Chollet P, et al. Interleukin-6 in tear fluid after photorefractive keratectomy and its effects on keratocytes in culture. *Cornea.* 1997;16:580–587.
80. Schultz CL, Kunert KS. Interleukin-6 levels in tears of contact lens wearers. *J Interferon Cytokine Res.* 2000;20:309–310.
81. Cook EB, Stahl JL, Lowe L, et al. Simultaneous measurement of six cytokines in a single sample of human tears using particle-based flow cytometry: allergics vs. non-allergics. *J Immunol Methods.* 2001;254: 109–118.
82. Baudoin C, Bourcier T, Brignole F, et al. Correlation between tear IgE levels and HLA-DR expression by conjunctival cells in allergic and nonallergic chronic conjunctivitis. *Graefe's Arch Clin Exp Ophthalmol.* 2000;238:900–914.
83. Leonadi A, Brun P, Abatangelo G, et al. Tear levels and activity of matrix metalloproteinase (MMP)-1 and MMP-9 in vernal keratoconjunctivitis. *Invest Ophthalmol Vis Sci.* 2003;44:3052–3058.
84. Sack RA, Beaton A, Sathe S, et al. Towards a closed eye model of the preocular tear layer. *Prog Retin Eye Res.* 2000;19:649–668.
85. Di Girolamo N, Wakefield D, Coroneo MT. Differential expression of matrix metalloproteinases and their tissue inhibitors at the advancing pterygium head. *Invest Ophthalmol Vis Sci.* 2000;41:4142–4149.
86. Sobrin L, Liu Z, Monroy DC, et al. Regulation of MMP-9 activity in human tear fluid and corneal culture supernatant. *Invest Ophthalmol Vis Sci.* 2000;41:1703–1709.
87. Nevalainen TJ, Aho HJ, Peuravuori H. Secretion of group 2 phospholipase A2 by lacrimal glands. *Invest Ophthalmol Vis Sci.* 1994;35:417–421.
88. Qu XD, Lehrer RI. Secretory phospholipase A2 is the principal bactericide for staphylococci and other Gram-positive bacteria in human tears. *Infect Immun.* 1998;66:2791–2797.
89. Gasymov OK, Adburagimov AR, Yusifov TN, et al. Interaction of tear lipocalin with lysozyme and lactoferrin. *Biochem Biophys Res Commun.* 1999;265:322–325.
90. Haynes RJ, Tighe PJ, Dua HS. Antimicrobial defensin peptides of the human ocular surface. *Br J Ophthalmol.* 1999;83:737–741.
91. Paulsen FP, Pufe T, Schaudig U, et al. Detection of natural peptide antibiotics in human nasolacrimal ducts. *Adv Exp Med Biol.* 2001;42: 2157–2163.
92. Caccavo D, Pelligrino NM, Altamura M, et al. Antimicrobial and immunoregulatory functions of lactoferrin and its potential therapeutic application. *J Endotoxin Res.* 2002;8:403–417.
93. Goebel C, Mackay LG, Vickers ER, et al. Determination of defensin HNP-1, HNP-2, and HNP-3 in human saliva by using LC/MS. *Peptides.* 2000;21:757–765.
94. Lehrer RI, Ganz T. Defensins of vertebrate animals. *Curr Opin Immunol.* 2002;14:96–102.
95. Zhang L, Yu W, He T, et al. Contribution of human alpha-defensin 1, 2, and 3 to the anti-HIV-1 activity of CD8 antiviral factor. *Science.* 2000;298:995–1000.
96. Murphy CJ, Foster BA, Mannis MJ, et al. Defensins are mitogenic for epithelial cells and fibroblasts. *J Cell Physiol.* 1993;155:408–413.
97. Chaly YV, Paleolog EM, Kolesnikova TS, et al. Neutrophil alpha-defensin human neutrophil peptide modulates cytokine production in human monocytes and adhesion molecule expression in endothelial cells. *Eur Cytokine Netw.* 2000;11:257–266.
98. Leonardi A, Brun P, Tavolato M, et al. Tumor necrosis factor-alpha (TNF-alpha) in seasonal allergic conjunctivitis and vernal conjunctivitis. *Eur J Ophthalmol.* 2003;13:606–610.
99. Sullivan B. Fourth International Conference on the Lacrimal Gland, Tear Film & Ocular Surface and Dry Eye Syndromes. *Adv Exp Med Biol.* 2004.

Chapter 4

The Eyelids

Michael P. Lin, D.J. John Park, Andrew R. Harrison

Introduction

The eyelids are a thin, complex, and dynamic structure, whose primary function is to protect the ocular surface of the eye. They cleanse and lubricate the eye, protecting it from desiccation as well as damage from foreign bodies and, in doing so, maintain optical visual clarity of the cornea. They serve as both a physical and immunological barrier providing a crucial means of defense against infection. In addition, the eyelids also serve as an important facial aesthetic subunit, and play an essential part of facial expression and cultural identification. It is for these reasons that the eyelids are not only critical for human survival but also for maintenance of quality of life.

The eyelid can be conceptualized as a trilamellar structure. The anterior layer is composed of the eyelid skin and orbicularis oculi and is contiguous with the skin and superficial muscular aponeurotic system of the face and the galea aponeurosis of the scalp. The posterior layer consists of the palpebral conjunctiva and underlying smooth muscle fibers and is contiguous with bulbar conjunctiva by way of the fornix. The anterior and posterior lamellae are separated by a middle tarsofascial layer, which is composed of the orbital septum anteriorly and the retractors of the eyelid posteriorly. The septum and retractors are separated by orbital fat, bound near the eyelid margin by the tarsus. Near the eyelid margin, the orbital fat is attenuated and the septum and eyelid retractors are fused. In the upper lid, the lid retracting structures are the levator palpebrae and its aponeurosis, while in the lower lid they are the inferior retractors and capsulopalpebral fascia.[1,2]

Embryology

The formation of the eyelid starts the first week of gestation and continues until birth. During the first nine weeks of gestation, the primitive optic vesicle is covered with a layer of surface ectoderm that is destined to eventually form the future eyelids, conjunctiva, and cornea. Despite their close proximity, the presence of an eye is not required for lid formation.[3] During the second month of gestation, the surface ectoderm further proliferates and divides to form a multilayered epithelium. A rudimentary fold forms above and below the eye, which is the primitive 'bud' of eyelid formation.[4,5] The fold destined to become the upper eyelid appears slightly before that of the lower eyelid. As these folds continue to grow and lengthen, the outer layer of epithelium forms the skin, while the inner layer becomes the conjunctiva.

Within the primitive eyelid is a layer of mesoderm. The upper lid mesoderm is derived from paraxial mesoderm, while the lower lid develops from visceral mesoderm. Shortly following ectodermal development, the mesoderm begins to thicken and form the basement membrane under the epithelium. Blood vessels then invade the basal portion of each eyelid. The mesoderm will ultimately become the muscles, connective tissues, and tarsus of the eyelids.[5,6]

Around the eighth and ninth week of gestation, the lacrimal glands are formed, and glandular secretion begins. At week nine, the eyelids have elongated enough to abut each other. Lid fusion then occurs, starting from the medial and lateral canthal regions and moving centrally, progressing from the inner eyelid outward. This is thought to be a true epithelial junction as electron microscopic studies have demonstrated evidence of desmosome formation.[7] After fusion of the eyelids is complete, the closed conjunctival sac becomes filled with lacrimal secretion, and is separated from the amniotic sac.[5]

Upon complete fusion of the eyelids, glandular formation begins. Epithelial invaginations from the fused lid margins form the primitive cilia hair bulbs. This formation begins anteriorly on the lid margin and proceeds posteriorly. Also around the tenth week of gestation, primitive muscle is developing underneath the skin, and the tarsus is beginning to form.[5,8] Major glandular formation occurs at the fourth month of gestation. The meibomian glands develop as epithelial cell invaginations into the tarsus along the posterior region of the fused lid margins. Lateral outgrowths of epithelial cells from hair follicles initiate the formation of the glands of Zeis and Moll. The glands of Zeis are holocrine glands with sebaceous secretion, while the glands of Moll are modified apocrine sweat glands whose secretions efflux at the base of eyelashes and appear to have immunoprotective properties.[6,7] Further differentiation of meibomian glands and the glands of Zeis and Moll occurs later in gestation, including acinar formation and maturation into functional, secreting glands.[5,6]

Around twenty weeks' gestation, the eyelids begin to separate. This is preceded by the production of lipid in the glands of Zeis and Moll at the lid margin and keratinization of the walls of the glandular ducts.[5] Eyelid disjunction begins anteriorly and progresses in a posterior direction, requiring three weeks for full separation. By this time, the major elements of the lid are present. Glandular differentiation and maturation continues after lid separation, to produce the developed eyelid.[4–6,8]

Anatomy

Epithelium

The skin of the eyelid is the thinnest and most pliable on the human body, ranging from 500 to 1000 μm in thickness. It is thinnest near the lid margin and thickest near the orbital rims, where it is contiguous with infrabrow skin superiorly and malar skin inferiorly. Because of its physical characteristics, the eyelid skin contains more wrinkles than infrabrow or cheek skin, and replacement of eyelid skin may pose a challenge in finding donor sites with comparably thin skin.

Histologically, the skin of the eyelid closely resembles other facial skin, composed of keratinized stratified squamous epithelium. At the mucocutaneous junction of the eyelid (Marx's line), which is located on the eyelid margin just posterior to the orifices of the meibomian glands, the stratified squamous epithelium becomes nonkeratinized (Fig. 4.1).[9]

The dermis of the eyelid is also very thin when compared to skin on the rest of the face and body, and nearly nonexistent. It is composed of loose collagenous fibers interspersed with a rich elastic fiber network. Sparse glands and hair follicles, when present, are contained in the dermis.

The eyelids are relatively hairless, except for laterally where nonpigmented vellus hairs may be found. These vellus hairs may convert into pigmented hairs on hirsute people. Eyelashes are a relatively sparse, specialized type of hair, which may serve as sensory structures causing a reflex eyelid closure when dust or foreign bodies hit them. There are approximately 100 eyelashes in the upper eyelid and 50 in the lower eyelid.[10] In addition, eyelashes serve an important role for eyelid aesthetics. Their limited length, increased shaft diameter, and unique curvature set them apart from any other hair on the body.

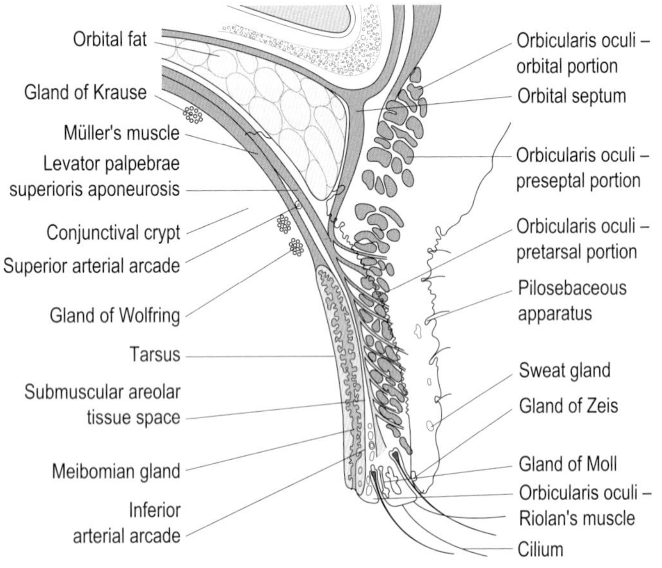

Fig 4.1 Magnified view of the upper eyelid and margin.

Glandular structures contained within eyelid skin include sebaceous glands and sweat glands, which are present at higher density at the peripheral portions of the eyelid, away from the eyelid margin. The lash line also contains two types of glandular structures. The glands of Zeis are holocrine sebaceous glands which secrete their contents into the eyelash duct, which is lined by epithelium continuous with the eyelash follicle. Clinically, these glands are significant due to their potential for malignant transformation into sebaceous cell carcinoma.[11] The glands of Moll are apocrine sweat glands, which empty into the follicle of the eyelash or directly onto the surface of the lid margin. These glands are less numerous than the glands of Zeis and have the potential of forming cystic tumors (sudoriferous cysts).[12]

The subcutaneous space of the eyelid is essentially devoid of fat. The eyelid skin is directly attached to the underlying orbicularis muscle by way of loose connective tissue. At the upper eyelid crease, the canthal angles, and the eyelid margin, the skin is more firmly adherent to the orbicularis.[1,9,13]

Orbicularis oculi

The orbicularis oculi is a sphincter-like muscle that lies directly beneath the skin of the eyelids and extends from the lid margin and eyelash follicles to beyond the superior and inferior orbital rims. The muscle originates from and inserts into medial and lateral canthal tendons. It is densely adherent to the lower tarsal plate and the superior tarsal plate.

The muscle is divided into three concentric portions, named anatomically according to the underlying structures of the eyelids: pretarsal, preseptal, and orbital orbicularis muscle. The orbital and preseptal orbicularis are under voluntary control, whereas the pretarsal muscle is almost exclusively responsible for the involuntary corneal blink reflex, which plays an important role in lubricating the cornea. The orbicularis is a striated muscle with diffuse innervation by multiple branches of the facial nerve, including frontal, zygomatic, and buccal branches. This muscle is the first of the facial nerve-innervated muscles to begin contracting in utero, which is observed between the eighth and ninth weeks of gestation.[9,14]

The orbicularis muscle is crucially important for eyelid closure, protection of the globe, and maintenance of corneal moisture. Horner's muscle is a branch of the orbicularis oculi muscle that passes posterior to the lacrimal sac. It divides the lacrimal sac into upper and lower compartments, and covers the lateral component of the lacrimal canaliculus, and contributes to the lacrimal pump.[15] The muscle of Riolan consists of marginal fibers of the palpebral portion of the orbicularis muscle, and is believed to form the 'gray line' at the margin of the eyelid. It functions to hold the lacrimal punctum against the sclera for proper drainage of tears.[16]

Orbital septum

The orbital septum is a thin membranous structure that originates from the arcus marginalis of the orbital rim and fuses with the lid-retracting structures (levator palpebrae superioris aponeurosis superiorly and capsulopalpebral fascia inferiorly). It serves as a demarcation point, separating the preseptal space anteriorly and the orbit posteriorly. Anteriorly, the orbital septum lies subjacent to the thin, areolar connective tissue known as the postorbicularis fascia. Retro-orbicularis fat may be found within this space. Deep to the orbital septum lie the upper and lower orbital fat pads. In the lateral superior orbit, the orbital septum abuts the orbital lobe of the lacrimal gland. The orbital septum does not contribute to movement of the eyelid, but rather acts as a retinacular membrane that prevents prolapse of orbital contents. Indeed, its attenuation with age is associated with steatochalasis of the upper and lower eyelids.

Retractors

Levator palpebrae superioris

The upper orbit has two distinct muscles for supraduction of the globe (superior rectus) and for retraction of the eyelid (levator palpebrae superioris). The inferior orbit has a solitary muscle (inferior rectus) that subserves movement of both the globe and eyelid. Consequently, the upper eyelid is capable of 10–14 mm of excursion, but the lower eyelid is capable of only 4–5 mm.[17]

The levator palpebrae superioris arises from the annulus of Zinn above the superior rectus muscle. It is innervated on its undersurface by the third cranial nerve. The levator muscle passes along with the superior rectus muscle through the posterior orbit, loosely attached to the rectus muscle by intermuscular septa. Where the superior rectus attaches to the globe, the levator muscle transitions to a fascial sheet known as the levator aponeurosis. The levator aponeurosis is a fan-like structure that securely inserts at multiple points on the anterior surface of the tarsus, and to the canthal tendons via more loose attachments. Moreover, extensions of the levator aponeurosis attach to the orbital septum, orbicularis muscle, and pretarsal skin near the upper tarsal border, forming the upper eyelid crease.

Müller's muscle

Just deep to the levator aponeurosis lies the Müller's muscle. The Müller's muscle is composed of smooth muscle fibers and is innervated by sympathetic input. It inserts upon the superior tarsal border and is densely adherent to the underlying conjunctiva. At resting tone, it is responsible for approximately 1–2 mm of vertical elevation of the upper eyelid, whereas at times of stress, its contraction is responsible for creating a look of surprise or shock.[18]

Capsulopalpebral fascia and inferior retractors

In the inferior orbit, the inferior rectus muscle is responsible for inferior displacement of the globe and lower eyelid. A fibrous tissue expansion known as capsulopalpebral fascia extends from the inferior rectus muscle to the anterior surface of the lower tarsus, transmitting pull from the inferior rectus muscle. This fascia is analogous to the levator aponeurosis, and is capable of moving the lower eyelid approximately 4–5 mm from extreme upward gaze to extreme downward gaze. This is under control by cranial nerve III and its action is yoked to the action of the inferior rectus. The inferior orbital septum fuses to the capsulopalpebral fascia 3–4 mm inferior to the tarsus. In addition, a narrow strip of nonstriated muscle known as the inferior tarsal muscle, analogous to Müller's muscle, attaches to the inferior tarsal border. The inferior tarsal muscle is innervated by sympathetic fibers.[18]

Tarsal plates

The tarsal plates are composed of a firm, densely packed collection of collagen fibers. They provide structural stability to the eyelids and also serve as a platform upon which the orbicularis muscle and levator muscle insert. The tarsal plates are tethered medially and laterally by their respective canthal tendons, forming a tarsoligamentous sling upon which the forces of the protractors and the retractors act. The tarsal plates measure approximately 25–30 mm in horizontal length and 0.75 mm in thickness. The vertical length of the tarsal plates is generally 10 mm centrally in the upper eyelid and 4–5 mm in the lower eyelid (Fig. 4.2).

Contained within tarsal plates are the meibomian glands. These glands contribute the oily portion of the tear film, which is important for stabilizing the tear film, and preventing rapid evaporation. The meibomian glands are found in greater numbers in the upper eyelid compared to the lower eyelid (approximately 40 versus 25).[9] Also, the glands are longer in the upper eyelid. Both of these factors may explain the increased production of lipid material by glands of the upper eyelid relative to the lower eyelid. The meibomian glands are a frequent site of chronic granulomatous inflammation of the lids, and rarely may undergo malignant transformation into sebaceous cell carcinomas.[19]

Conjunctiva

The conjunctiva is the mucous membrane that lines the inner surface of the eyelids and the anterior surface of the globe. Histologically, it is composed of a nonkeratinized stratified epithelium with goblet cells. The underlying substantia propria, or stroma, is richly vascularized and contains numerous immune defense cells. The histology of the epithelium varies depending on location, from squamous epithelium near the lid margin to columnar epithelium in the tarsal area. In the fornix, the conjunctiva transitions to a prismatic cell type, and to a cuboidal cell type in the bulbar area. Finally it transitions back to squamous epithelium near the limbus. The conjunctiva is continuous with the eyelid skin through the mucocutaneous junction at the lid margin (Marx's line), with the corneal epithelium at the corneoscleral limbus, and with the respiratory mucosa through the lacrimal puncta. The marginal mucosa of the conjunctiva is responsible for spreading the tear film.[20]

At the superior and inferior fornices, the conjunctiva is adherent to underlying structures through the attachment

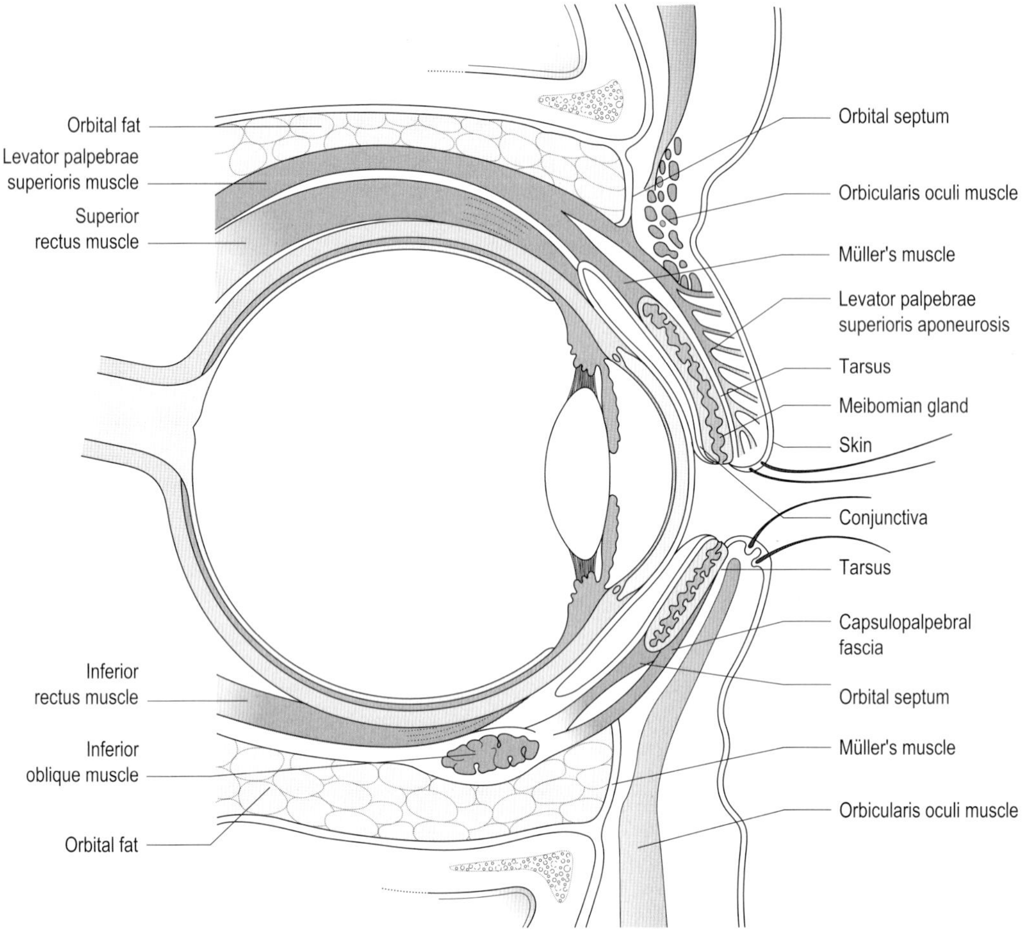

Fig 4.2 Sagittal section of the upper and lower eyelid.

of fibrous extensions from the superior and inferior rectus muscles, respectively. These attachments maintain the shape and integrity of the fornices and prevent prolapse of the conjunctival tissue into the lid aperture. The fornices also contain numerous accessory lacrimal glands of Wolfring and Krause within its submucosal tissue. These lacrimal structures are more numerous in the superior fornix than inferior fornix.

Eyelid margin

The lid margin is a short 2-mm wide segment that contains the mucocutaneous junction that demarcates keratinized epithelium anteriorly and conjunctival nonkeratinized epithelium posteriorly, and is composed of pseudostratified squamous mucosa. There are three clinically apparent lines on the eyelid margin. At the posterior eyelid margin, where the horizontal component of the eyelid ends and the vertical component begins, the mucosa makes an abrupt transition into stratified columnar epithelium. Anterior to this lies the gray line which represents an optical reflection of the marginal portion of the orbicularis (muscle of Riolan), and which lies coincident with meibomian gland orifices. The mucocutaneous junction itself lies just posterior to the gray line and is not clinically apparent. At the anterior eyelid margin is the lash line. Chronic inflammation, as in the case of blepharitis, can lead to disruption of these distinct transitions as well as effacement and anterior migration of the mucocutaneous junction.[9,16]

The suspensory system of the eyelids

The medial and lateral commissures are located at either corner of the eye where the upper and lower eyelids meet. These important structures are supported by the medial and lateral canthal tendons, which create a sling-like structure to support the lid margin and maintain apposition against the globe.

The medial canthal tendon has two limbs, an anterior and a posterior limb. The anterior limb is a broader band arising from the superficial head of the pretarsal orbicularis muscle and inserting onto the anterior lacrimal crest. The posterior limb of the medial canthal tendon arises from the deep head of the pretarsal and preseptal orbicularis muscles and inserts onto the posterior lacrimal crest.

The lateral canthal tendon has a superior crus arising from the superior tarsus and an inferior crus arising from the inferior tarsus. The superior and inferior crura fuse at the lateral border of the tarsal plates to join the lateral retinaculum which attaches to Whitnall's tubercle, located 2–4 mm posterior to the lateral orbital rim, and 9–12 mm below the zygomaticofrontal suture.[21]

When observed straight on, the lateral canthus appears about 2 mm higher than the medial canthus, subtending a 15-degree inclination from the medial canthus to the lateral canthus.[9]

Whitnall's ligament is a superior transverse ligament that acts as the main suspensory ligament of the upper eyelid, as a support ligament for the conjunctival fornix, and also as a check ligament for the levator complex. It extends from the periorbita of the trochlea medially to the frontozygomatic suture laterally. It is located 15–20 mm superior to the superior border of the tarsus.

Lockwood's ligament acts as a suspensory sling or 'hammock' for the globe. It also anchors the inferior conjunctival fornix. It is composed of a fibrous condensation of the capsulopalpebral fascia, Tenon's capsule, intramuscular septa, check ligaments, and fibers from the inferior rectus sheath. It attaches medially to the medial canthal tendon and laterally to the lateral canthal tendon.[21]

Orbital fat compartments

Superior orbital fat contains two separate compartments, the preaponeurotic and the medial fat pads, separated by the trochlea. The medial fat pad is firmer and pale white in color, and is associated with the medial palpebral artery and infratrochlear nerve. The preaponeurotic fat pad is more yellow in color due to increased carotenoid content[22] and extends laterally over the lacrimal gland. Due to their close proximity to the trochlea, superior oblique palsy and Brown syndrome have been reported following excision of fat during upper eyelid blepharoplasty.[23] The superior orbital fat compartments are bordered posteroinferiorly by the levator aponeurosis, anteriorly by the orbital septum, and inferiorly by the fusion of both.

The inferior orbital fat contains three distinct compartments. The medial and central fat compartments are separated by the inferior oblique muscle. The central and lateral fat compartments are separated by the arcuate expansion of the inferior oblique muscle. The inferior orbital fat compartments are bordered posterosuperiorly by the capsulopalpebral fascia and anteriorly by the orbital septum.[24]

Vascular supply

The eyelids are encircled by superior and inferior palpebral vascular arcades with extensive contributions from both the internal and external carotid artery systems. The lower eyelid has a single arcade that lies between the inferior tarsal muscle and the confluence of the orbital septum and capsulopalpebral fascia, just below the inferior limit of the tarsus. The upper eyelid contains two discrete arcades: the marginal, which lies 2 mm from the eyelid, margin and peripheral arcade, which lies between the levator aponeurosis and the Müller's muscle just above the superior limit of the tarsus.

At the medial canthus, the superior and inferior palpebral arcades receive contributions from the medial palpebral arteries, arising from the ophthalmic branch of the internal carotid artery. The superomedial portion receives contributions from the supratrochlear and supraorbital arteries, which are also derived from the ophthalmic artery. At the superolateral aspect of the orbit, the superior palpebral arcade anastomoses with the zygomatico-orbital branch of the superficial temporal artery. Near the lateral canthal area, the superior and inferior palpebral arcades anastomose with the two lateral palpebral branches from the lacrimal artery, a branch of the ophthalmic artery. The inferolateral lower eyelid receives most of its contributions from the transverse facial artery, whereas the inferomedial lower eyelid receives major contributions from the angular artery, a terminal branch of the facial artery. The superficial temporal artery, transverse facial artery, and facial artery are derived from the external carotid system. The ophthalmic artery is the first branch of the internal carotid artery.

Venous drainage of the eyelids is through the anterior facial and superior temporal veins into the external jugular system and through the ophthalmic vein into the cavernous sinus and internal jugular system.[25,26]

Lymphatic drainage

The lateral aspect of the upper and lower eyelids drains into the preauricular nodes and to a lesser extent into the parotid gland nodes. The medial aspect of the upper and lower eyelids drains into the submandibular nodes and to a lesser extent into the submental nodes.[1]

Sensory innervation

The sensory innervation of the upper lid is derived from the ophthalmic division of the trigeminal nerve (CN V) and its branches: supraorbital, supratrochlear, lacrimal, and infratrochlear. Sensation to the lower lid is supplied by the maxillary division of the trigeminal nerve via the infraorbital branch. The medial and lateral canthi are supplied by overlapping branches of the ophthalmic and maxillary divisions of the trigeminal nerve

Blink reflex

Closure of the eyelids can be under voluntary or involuntary control. The eyelids serve the critical role of distributing the tear film over the anterior surface of the globe to maintain moisture. Continuous spreading of the tear film depends on the subconscious blink reflex, which occurs every 6 to 10 seconds. The afferent pathway of this reflex is dependent on the trigeminal nerve, while the facial nerve controls the efferent pathway through the pretarsal portion of the orbicularis muscle.[27]

References

1. Kikkawa DO, Vasani SN. Ophthalmic facial anatomy. In: Chen WP, ed. *Oculoplastic surgery: the essentials*. New York: Thieme; 2001.
2. Newman MI, Spinelli HM. Reconstruction of the eyelids, correction of ptosis, and canthoplasty. In: Thorne CH, Beasley RW, Aston SJ, et al., eds. *Grabb & smith's plastic surgery*. 6th ed. Philadelphia: Lippincott Williams & Wilkins; 2007.
3. Eayrs JT. The factors governing the opening of the eyes in the albino rat. *J Anat*. 1951;85:330–337.
4. Pearson AA. The development of the eyelids Part 1: external features. *J Anat*. 1980;130:33–42.
5. Hamming N. Anatomy and embryology of the eyelids: a review with special reference to the development of divided nevi. *Ped Dermatol*. 1983;1(1):51–58.
6. Andersen H, Ehler N, Matthiessen ME. Histochemistry and development of the human eyelids. *Acta Ophthalmol*. 1965;43:642–668.

7. Stoeckelhuber M, Stoeckelhuber B, Welsch U. Human glands of Moll: histochemical and ultrastructural characterization of the glands of Moll in the human eyelid. *J Invest Dermatol.* 2003;121:28–36.
8. Candy R. *Development of the visual system. Visual development, diagnosis, and treatment of the pediatric patient.* Philadelphia: Lippincott Williams & Wilkins; 2006.
9. Wolfley DE. Eyelids. In: Krachmer JH, Mannis MJ, Holland EJ, eds. *Cornea.* 2nd ed. Philadelphia: Elsevier; 2005.
10. Nerad JA, Chang A. Trichiasis. In: Chen WP ed. *Oculoplastic surgery: the essentials.* New York: Thieme; 2001.
11. Honavar SG, Shields CL, Maus M, et al. Primary intraepithelial sebaceous gland carcinoma of the palpebral conjunctiva. *Arch Ophthalmol.* 2001;119:764–767.
12. Jordan DR. Common eyelid lumps and bumps. *Insight: A Quarterly Report For Health Care Professionals Delivering Eye Care.* 1997;3(4):1–2.
13. Wobig JL, Dailey RA. Anatomy and physiology of the eyelids. In: Wobig JL, Dailey RA, eds. *Oculofacial plastic surgery.* New York: Thieme; 2004.
14. Humphrey T. Some correlations between the appearance of human fetal reflexes and the development of the nervous system. *Prog Brain Res.* 1964;4:93–135.
15. Kakizaki H, Zako M, Miyaishi O, et al. The lacrimal canaliculus and sac bordered by the Horner's muscle form the functional lacrimal drainage system. *Ophthalmology.* 2005;112(4):710–716.
16. Lipham WJ, Tawfik HA, Dutton JJ. A histologic analysis and three-dimensional reconstruction of the muscle of Riolan. *Ophthal Plast Reconstr Surg* 2002;18(2):93–98.
17. Dresner S. Ptosis management a practical approach. In: Chen WP, ed. *Oculoplastic surgery: the essentials.* New York: Thieme; 2001.
18. Felt DP, Frueh BR. A pharmacologic study of the sympathetic eyelid tarsal muscles. *Ophthal Plast Reconstr Surg.* 1988;4(1):15–24.
19. Khan JA, Doane JF, Grove AS Jr. Sebaceous and meibomian carcinomas of the eyelid. Recognition, diagnosis, and management. *Ophthal Plast Reconstr Surg.* 1991;7(1):61–66.
20. Mastrota KM. The conjunctiva and dry eye. *Contact Lens Spectrum.* Feb 2009 <http://www.clspectrum.com/article.aspx?article=102543>.
21. Bedrossian EH Jr. Surgical anatomy of the eyelids. In: Della Rocca RC, Bedrossian EH, Arthurs BP, eds. *Ophthalmic plastic surgery: decision making and techniques.* New York: McGraw-Hill Professional; 2002.
22. Sires BS, Saari JC, Garwin GG, et al. The color difference in orbital fat. *Arch Ophthalmol.* 2001;119:868–871.
23. Wilhelmi BJ, Mowlavi A, Neumeister MW, Codner MA. Upper blepharoplasty with bony anatomical landmarks to avoid injury to trochlea and superior oblique muscle tendon with fat resection. *Plast Reconstr Surg.* 2001;108(7):2137–2140.
24. Hwang K, Kim DJ, Chung RS. Pretarsal fat compartment in the lower eyelid. *Clin Anat.* 2001;14(3):179–183.
25. Snell RS, Lemp MA. The orbital blood vessels. In: Snell RS, Lemp MA, eds. *Clinical Anatomy of the Eye.* Hoboken, NJ: Wiley-Blackwell; 1997.
26. Hayreh SS. Orbital vascular anatomy. *Eye.* 2006;20(10):1130–1144.
27. Pearce JM. Observations on the blink reflex. *Eur Neurol.* 2008;59(3–4): 221–223.

Chapter 5

A Matrix of Pathologic Responses in the Cornea

George O. Waring III, Charles S. Bouchard

Anatomical Regions of the Cornea

Anatomically, the cornea consists of two cellular layers, the epithelium and the endothelium. Each rests on a basement membrane: the epithelial basement membrane and Descemet membrane, respectively. These two cellular layers sandwich a thin layer of acellular connective tissue (Bowman's layer) and a thicker, cellular layer of connective tissue (stroma). For the purpose of discussing pathologic responses in the cornea, we can divide the cornea into four regions (Fig. 5.1):

1. Epithelium
2. Subepithelial zone
   a. Epithelial basement membrane
   b. Bowman's layer
   c. Superficial stroma
3. Stroma
4. Endothelium and Descemet's membrane

A whole spectrum of pathologic processes can disrupt the structure of these four zones and interfere with corneal function. However, the cornea can generate only a limited number of responses to these insults. Although there is some overlap among them, these responses can be grouped conveniently into six categories (see Fig. 5.1):

1. Defects (and their repair)
2. Fibrosis and vascularization
3. Edema and cysts
4. Inflammation and immune responses
5. Deposits
6. Proliferation

To provide the ophthalmology resident, the corneal fellow, and the practicing clinician with a useful perspective, the authors describe concisely the patterns of tissue response that characterize each zone, and provide representative clinicopathologic examples, as originally presented by Waring and Rodrigues[1] and elaborated by Freddo and Waring[2] (Fig. 5.2).

Clinical details and the pathophysiology – including the molecular biology – of the disorders and the pathologic processes discussed here are found in relevant chapters throughout this textbook.

General Pathologic Responses of the Cornea

1. Defects and their repair

Defects are a partial or complete absence of a portion of corneal tissue. A defect is acute if it appears suddenly and heals (e.g. corneal abrasion and breaks in Descemet's membrane and the endothelium in acute hydrops of keratoconus). It is recurrent if it appears repeatedly (e.g. recurrent epithelial erosion). A defect is chronic or persistent if healing stops and the defect remains (e.g. sterile, indolent epithelial ulcer associated with herpes simplex keratitis).

2. Fibrosis and vascularization

Fibrosis and vascularization are part of the normal repair process in connective tissues. In most tissues, these processes have a beneficial effect; in the cornea, however, fibrosis and vascularization lead to stromal scarring with opacification and disruption of optical function. Because the normal cornea is avascular, the appearance of blood vessels in the cornea is always abnormal.

3. Edema and cysts

Edema and cysts are grouped together for simplicity and because they often resemble each other clinically. When edema (i.e. excess fluid in or between cells) occurs, the normal architecture is disrupted, leading to opacification. The edema can be diffuse (stromal edema) or focal (epithelial bullae). Corneal cystic areas are focal collections of fluid or solid material without an epithelial lining.

4. Inflammation and immune responses

Inflammation and immune reactions result from a variety of insults which can lead to reversible or irreversible changes. In general, three basic steps are involved: (1) an inciting pathologic event, either exogenous (e.g. infection) or endogenous (e.g. autoimmune), acute or chronic; (2) a host cellular and humoral inflammatory and/or immune response; and (3) a repair process. These three steps are beneficial when they contain and control the pathologic process (e.g. eliminate an epithelial viral infection); however, they can be harmful if they concurrently damage the cornea. Details are presented in the latter part of this chapter.

5. Deposits

Abnormal types or amounts of material can be deposited in the cornea. Exogenous sources include drugs (more than 50); endogenous sources include excess material from metabolic diseases (e.g. Wilson's disease with deposits of copper in Descemet's membrane), and corneal dystrophies and degenerations (e.g. excess glycosaminoglycans in the stroma and endothelium in macular dystrophy), and autologous breakdown products (e.g. iron deposits which occur as iron lines in the basal epithelium).

6. Proliferation

There are three basic types of abnormal proliferative responses: (1) abnormalities of growth and maturation (e.g. hypertrophy, hyperplasia, metaplasia, and dysplasia/neoplasia – such as corneal intraepithelial neoplasia [CIN]); (2) ectopic migration such as epithelial ingrowth; and (3) corneal stem cell deficiency, leading to conjunctivalization of the ocular surface.

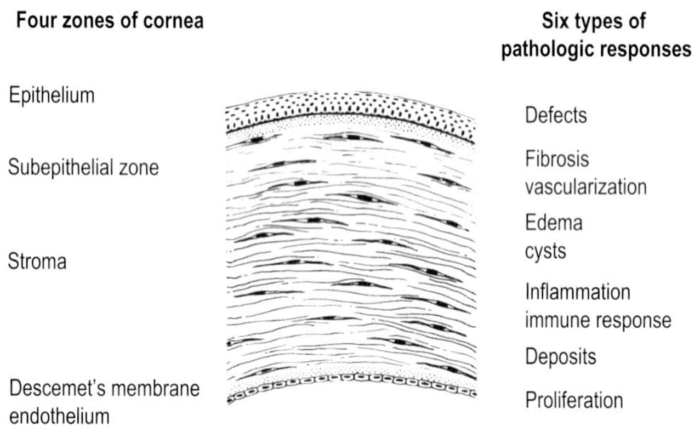

Fig. 5.1 To simplify the discussion of pathologic responses of the cornea, we artificially divide the cornea into four zones. Each zone can manifest six types of responses. (Modified from Waring GO 3rd, Rodrigues MM. Patterns of pathologic response in the cornea. *Surv Ophthalmol* 1987; 31:262. Copyright Elsevier 1987.)

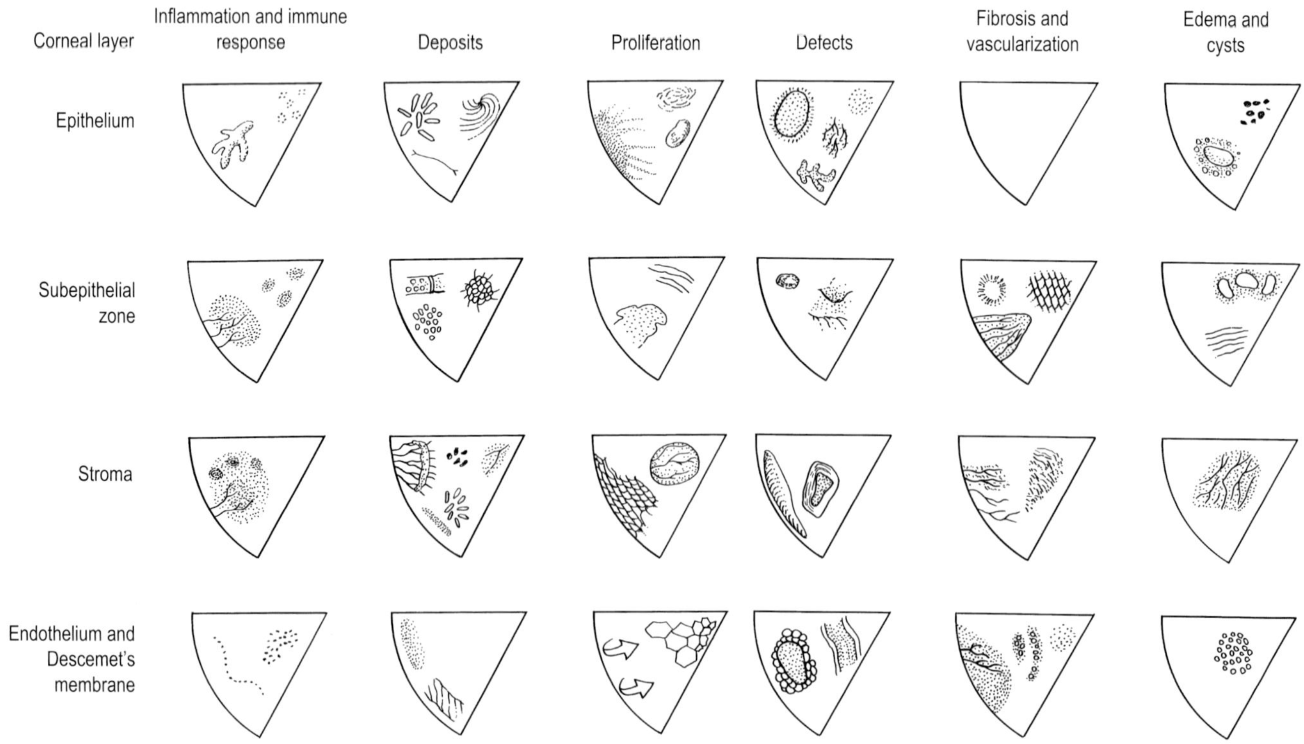

Fig. 5.2 This matrix of the four corneal zones and six types of pathologic responses can include almost all corneal diseases, as demonstrated by the listed examples. (Modified from Waring GO 3rd, Rodrigues MM. Patterns of pathologic response in the cornea. *Surv Ophthalmol* 1987; 31:262. Copyright Elsevier 1987.)

PATHOLOGIC RESPONSES OF THE CORNEA
Examples of Each Represented by Drawings

Corneal Layer	Defects	Fibrosis and Vascularization	Edema and Cysts
Epithelium	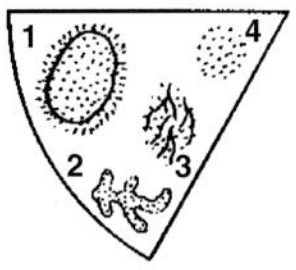 1. Neurotrophic keratopathy 2. Herpes simplex dendrite 3. Recurrent erosion 4. Punctate epithelial keratopathy	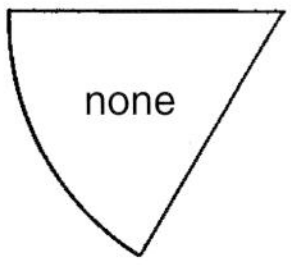 None	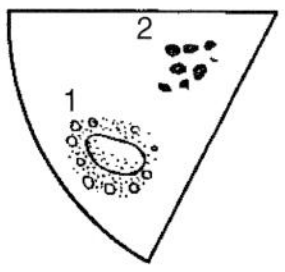 1. Microcystic edema, bulla 2. Cysts in epithelial basement membrane dystrophy
Subepithelial zone	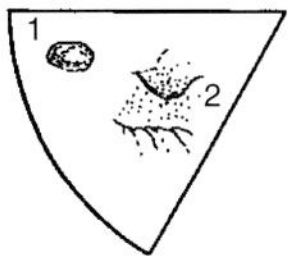 1. Foreign body 2. Keratoconus	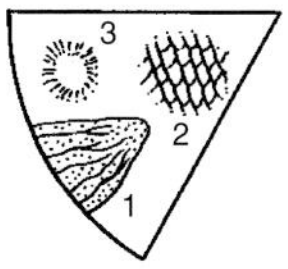 1. Pterygium 2. Salzmann's nodular degeneration 3. Pannus	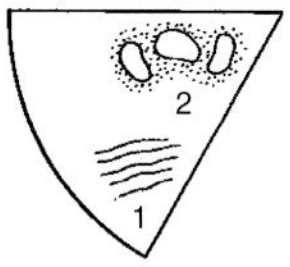 1. Basement membrane folds 2. Subepithelial bulla
Stroma	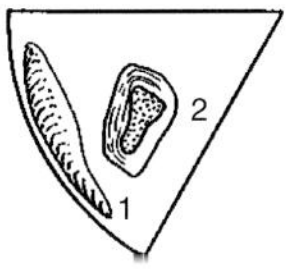 1. Terrien's degeneration 2. Sterile stromal ulcer	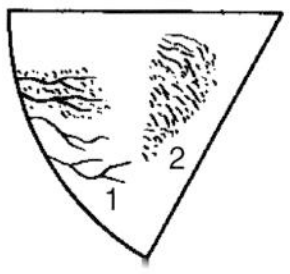 1. Vascularization and scarring 2. Avascular scar	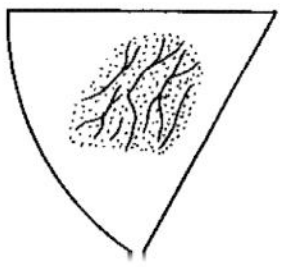 Stromal edema
Endothelium and Descemet's Membrane	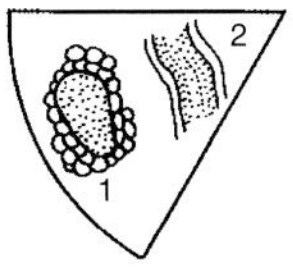 1. Focal damage during surgery 2. Birth trauma	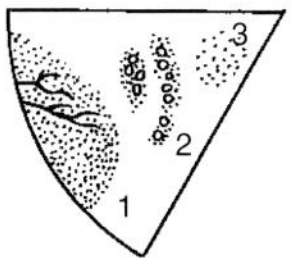 1. Posterior collagenous layer 2. Posterior polymorphous dystrophy 3. Cornea guttata	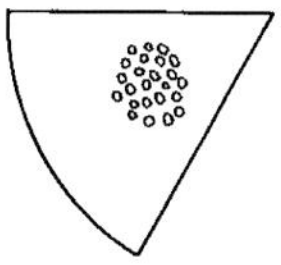 Endothelial edema

Fig. 5.2, cont'd

PATHOLOGIC RESPONSES OF THE CORNEA
Examples of Each Represented by Drawings

Corneal Layer	Inflammation and Immune Responses	Deposits	Proliferation
Epithelium	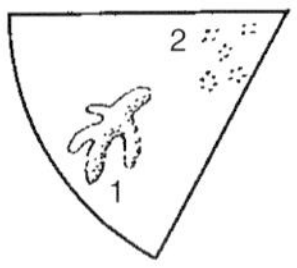 1. Zoster dendrite 2. Thygeson's superficial punctate keratitis	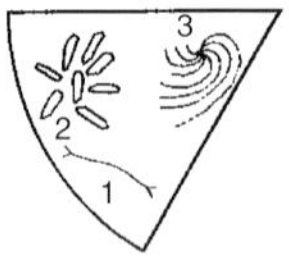 1. Hudson-Stähli line 2. Crystals 3. Amiodarone or chloroquine	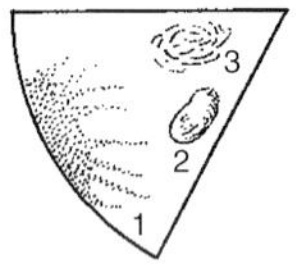 1. Corneal intraepithelial neoplasia 2. Facet 3. Keratinization
Subepithelial zone	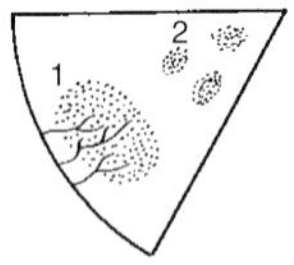 1. Phlyctenulosis 2. Adenovirus punctate keratitis	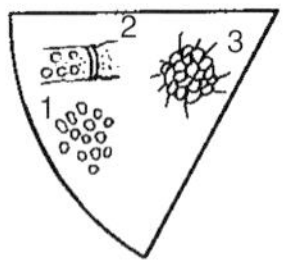 1. Spheroidal degeneration 2. Calcific band keratopathy 3. Reis-Bücklers' dystrophy	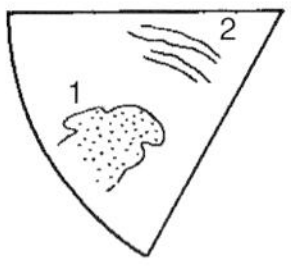 1. Maps and 2. Fingerprints in epithelial basement membrane dystrophy Bowman's layer does not proliferate
Stroma	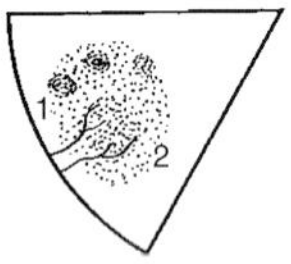 1. Suppuration in herpes simplex keratitis 2. Immune ring	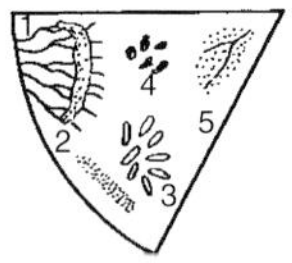 1. Vessels with lipid leakage 2. Corneal arcus 3. Crystals in gammopathy 4. Granular dystrophy 5. Lattice dystrophy	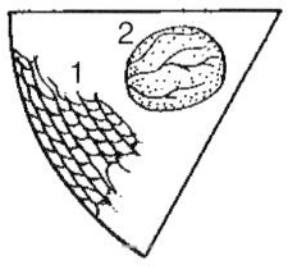 1. Fibrous ingrowth 2. Dermoid
Endothelium and Descemet's Membrane	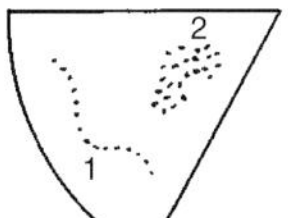 1. Allograft rejection line 2. Keratic precipitates	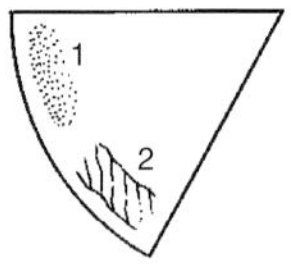 1. Corneal arcus 2. Wilson's disease	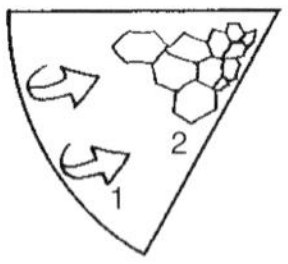 1. Spread in ICE syndrome 2. Hypertrophic cells

Fig. 5.2, cont'd

Specific Pathologic Responses of the Cornea

A summary of the six pathologic responses as each relates to the four corneal zones is presented in Figure 5.2. Representative disorders occupy each box of this pathophysiologic matrix. The amount of functional deficit inflicted by a disease process depends on:

- The type of insult
- The duration of the insult
- The severity of the insult

- The portion of the cornea affected
- The cornea's ability to repair and restore normal structure and function

In managing corneal disease, the clinician seeks to inhibit repair responses in some cases and to encourage them in others. For example, in the management of herpes simplex disciform keratitis, the goal is to prevent scarring and vascularization of the stroma in order to protect the refractive and image transmission functions of the cornea. In contrast, in the management of an alkali burn of the cornea, the goal often is to encourage scarring and vascularization in order to maintain the structural and protective functions of the cornea.

Pathologic Responses of the Corneal Epithelium

1. Defects (and their repair)

The normal corneal epithelium is replaced continuously every 4 to 7 days, involving three processes: (1) differentiation of the basal cells toward the surface; pathologic example: epidermalization and keratinization in vitamin A deficiency; (2) centripetal movement of limbal and peripheral cells; pathologic example: chemical damage of the limbal epithelium; (3) desquamation of epithelial cells from the surface; pathologic example: extended-wear soft contact lenses interfering with normal desquamation. Among the causes of epithelial defects are acute corneal abrasions (including excimer laser photorefractive keratotomy), focal foreign bodies, viral invasion by herpes simplex and herpes zoster, and sloughing of cells in recurrent epithelial erosion, neurotrophic keratopathy (Fig. 5.3). Healing of a defect in the corneal epithelium involves four major stages: sliding of cells to cover the defect, mitosis of cells to restore normal thickness, attachment of cells to the basement membrane, and remodeling to establish normal architecture.[3,4]

Four factors are required to reestablish normal epithelial integrity: a normal basement membrane, vitamin A, normal tear film, and intact sensory innervation. The edges of sliding, healing epithelium often abut to form a dendriform figure that can be confused with a herpes simplex dendrite.

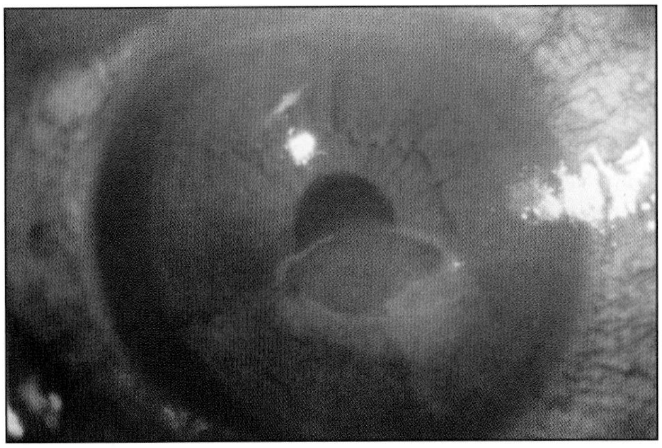

Fig. 5.3 Neurotrophic keratopathy can create a central epithelial defect, here stained with rose Bengal. (From Leibowitz HM, Waring GO, III. Corneal Disorders. Clinical Diagnosis and Management 2nd edn. Philadelphia, W.B. Saunders Company, 1998. Copyright Elsevier 1998.)

2. Fibrosis and vascularization

The corneal epithelium contains no connective tissue and therefore is not subject to fibrosis or vascularization. However, either process can occur subepithelially and may adversely affect epithelial repair, particularly after complete epithelial debridement, following which either limbal stem cell differentiation or conjunctival transdifferentiation is required to resurface the cornea.[5]

3. Edema and cysts

The epithelium takes on a cystic appearance when edema develops within or between the cells (e.g. endothelial dysfunction) and when changes in epithelial maturation create small, debris-filled cystic spaces (e.g. Cogan's microcysts in epithelial basement membrane degeneration). These changes reduce visual acuity if they create an irregular surface or if they diffract and scatter light. If they cause a break in the epithelial surface or loosen the epithelium so that it shifts during blinking, pain can result from sensory nerve stimulation.

Epithelial edema

There are two common causes of epithelial edema: endothelial dysfunction and epithelial hypoxia and trauma. When fluid lifts cells from the basement membrane, blister-like bullae appear. At this stage, the epithelial sheet is held together by desmosomal connections (Fig. 5.4).

Epithelial hypoxia and trauma

Contact lens-induced edema is caused by epithelial hypoxia, hypercapnia, trauma due to improper fitting or overwear, or a combination of these. Hypoxia causes depletion of glycogen stores and an increase in lactate accumulation, indicative of a conversion to anaerobic metabolism. Intracellular edema results when the compensatory abilities of the epithelium are exceeded. Chronicity can stimulate angiogenesis.

Changes in epithelial maturation

Cysts can result from accumulation of rapidly multiplying (e.g. Meesmann's dystrophy) or degenerating (e.g. epithelial basement membrane degeneration) epithelial cells.

In recurrent epithelial erosions, chronically regenerating epithelium often manifests clusters of clear, pinpoint microcysts in the area of a previous erosion. Many disorders produce a punctate epithelial keratopathy (PEK; sometimes called superficial punctate keratopathy [SPK]) that often takes on a cystic appearance, especially in retroillumination, as a result of focal accumulation of dead or dying epithelial cells.

4. Inflammation and immune response

In corneal allograft rejection, the donor epithelium may be attacked by sensitized cytotoxic T lymphocytes. This is a specific response to foreign antigens (e.g. the human leukocyte antigens [HLAs] in the epithelial cells or in Langerhans cells) and appears clinically as a serpentine line that spreads from the graft–host margin toward the center of the transplant.

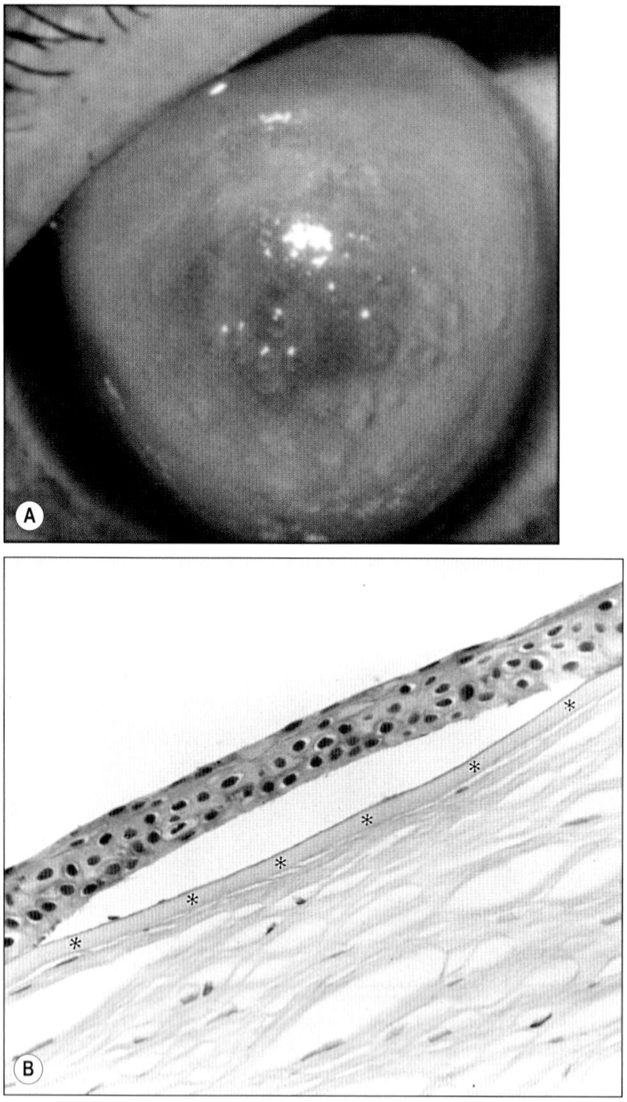

Fig. 5.4 Corneal edema. (**A**) Diffuse corneal edema with epithelial bullous elevations from a spontaneous break in Descemet's membrane and endothelium in keratoconus (corneal hydrops). (**B**) Histopathology shows an epithelial bulla with fluid separation of corneal epithelium from Bowman's layer (*asterisks*). (From Leibowitz HM, Waring GO, III. Corneal Disorders. Clinical Diagnosis and Management 2nd edn, Philadelphia, W.B. Saunders Company, 1998. Copyright Elsevier 1998.)

Fortunately, epithelial healing often keeps pace with cell death; in this instance, the epithelial rejection lines are a passing, asymptomatic phenomenon and no surface defect occurs. In contrast, Thygeson's superficial punctate keratitis is a recurrent disorder characterized by focal, intraepithelial white infiltrates that appear clinically as fine spots of crushed chalk.

Herpes simplex epithelial dendriform keratitis is a combination of epithelial defect and infection-inflammation (Fig. 5.5).

5. Deposits

Epithelial deposits can be divided into four categories based on their origin: (1) elements (iron, copper), (2) drugs (topical and systemic), (3) systemic diseases and (4) corneal dystrophies and degenerations.

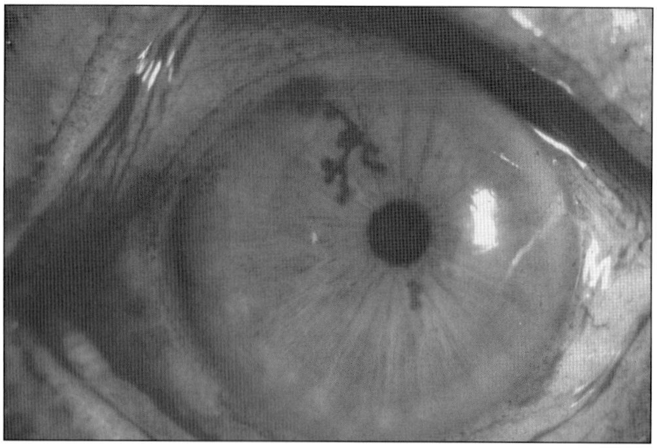

Fig. 5.5 Herpes simplex viral keratitis shows a dendriform epithelial lesion, here stained with rose Bengal. (From Leibowitz HM, Waring GO, III. Corneal Disorders. Clinical Diagnosis and Management 2nd edn, Philadelphia, W.B. Saunders Company, 1998. Copyright Elsevier 1998.)

Elements: iron deposits

The most common intraepithelial deposit is an iron line where hemosiderin pigment is deposited in lysosomes of the basal epithelial cells. Iron lines also commonly appear adjacent to elevated areas of the cornea (Fig. 5.6).[6]

Drugs: topical and systemic[7]

Numerous systemically administered drugs accumulate in the epithelium, including the antiarrhythmic drug amiodarone with its whorl-hurricane pattern (90% incidence in patients on long-term therapy) the psychotropic drug chlorpromazine, the antiinflammatory drug indometacin (rarely), the antimetabolite tilorone, and the numerous antimalarials including chloroquine; other drugs include naproxen, perhexiline, suramin, the thioxanthines, and tamoxifen. These drugs probably gain access to the cornea through the tears. The severity of the deposits is directly proportional to the total drug dose. Generally, when the drug is withdrawn, the corneal deposits disappear gradually. These drugs enter the cytoplasmic lysosomes where they become trapped, combine with bipolar lipids, and produce lipid–drug lamellar complexes refractory to enzymatic digestion.

Systemic diseases

Epithelial deposits from systemic diseases seldom reduce visual acuity. Exceptions include certain of the inherited metabolic disorders (e.g. mucopolysaccharidosis type VI-A, Maroteaux-Lamy, and the sphingolipidosis of Fabry's disease with its whorl pattern (vortex or cornea verticillata).

Multiple myeloma and other dysproteinemias may deposit fine, grayish crystals of immunoglobulins in the cytoplasm. Intraepithelial crystals of cystine are found in cystinosis.

The limbal conjunctival melanocytes of non-Caucasians frequently migrate into the epithelium, especially in eyes with a chronic superficial keratopathy, forming a streaming whorl called striate melanosis.

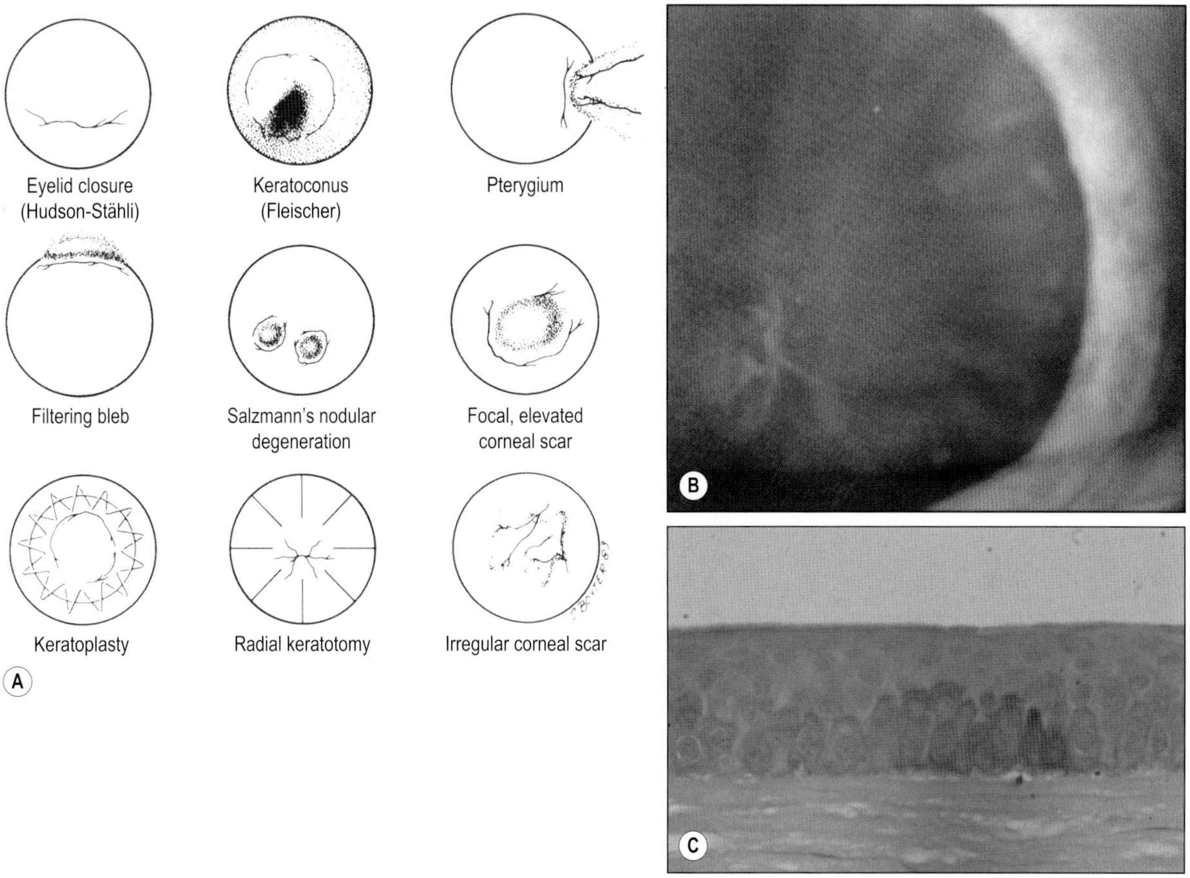

Fig. 5.6 (**A**) Nine types of iron lines in the corneal epithelium. (From Steinberg EB, Wilson LA, Waring GO 3rd, et al. Stellate iron lines in the corneal epithelium after radial keratotomy. *Am J Ophthalmol* 1984; 98:416.) (**B**) Irregular epithelial iron line with whorl-shaped brownish deposits in Fuchs' dystrophy with chronic corneal edema and an irregular epithelial surface. (**C**) Histopathology demonstrates dark stain of iron deposits in the basal layer of corneal epithelium. (**B** and **C**) From Leibowitz HM, Waring GO, III. Corneal Disorders. Clinical Diagnosis and Management. 2nd edn. Philadelphia, W.B. Saunders Company, 1998. Copyright Elsevier 1998.

Corneal dystrophies and degenerations

Few of the corneal dystrophies produce deposits within the epithelium. Exceptions include Meesmann's epithelial dystrophy (see Edema and cysts above).

6. Proliferation

The epithelium manifests a full spectrum of disorders of growth and maturation, including hyperplasia, metaplasia, and dysplasia-neoplasia. Because the epithelium conforms to the contour of the underlying basement membrane and stroma, its thickness varies. Areas of atrophy or thinning occur over elevations (e.g. over Salzmann's nodules) whereas areas of hyperplasia or thickening occur when the epithelium fills in focal defects (e.g. a facet) or in a broader defect (e.g. that caused by excimer laser photorefractive keratectomy). These adjustments in epithelial thickness appear to be efforts to preserve a smooth corneal surface in order to maintain optimal optical function, but the mechanisms through which this adjustment is accomplished are unknown.

Epithelial filaments are caused by the attachment of strands of mucus to punctate epithelial defects, followed by abnormal proliferation of epithelium and basement membrane around the strands. After an accidental or surgical perforating trauma, proliferating corneal epithelium can invade the anterior chamber through a fistula and form a cyst or a sheet. Epithelium can proliferate as ingrowth under a laser in situ keratomileusis (LASIK) flap.

Metaplasia from a normal to a keratin-forming abnormal epithelium can occur in severe ocular inflammation such as ocular cicatricial pemphigoid and Stevens-Johnson syndrome.

The epithelium is the only layer of the cornea that can become neoplastic, giving rise to squamous cell carcinoma, predominantly at the limbus.[8] Because the epithelia of the cornea, conjunctiva, and limbus are contiguous, benign and malignant neoplastic disorders commonly affect all three epithelia simultaneously. The full spectrum of changes, from mild dysplasia through carcinoma in situ, is grouped under the term 'intraepithelial neoplasia.'[9,10] It appears as a gray intraepithelial sheet advancing onto clear cornea as a sharply demarcated margin with finger-shaped extensions and clusters of islands (Fig. 5.7) Invasive squamous cell carcinoma of the cornea/conjunctiva is amenable to resection under frozen section control.

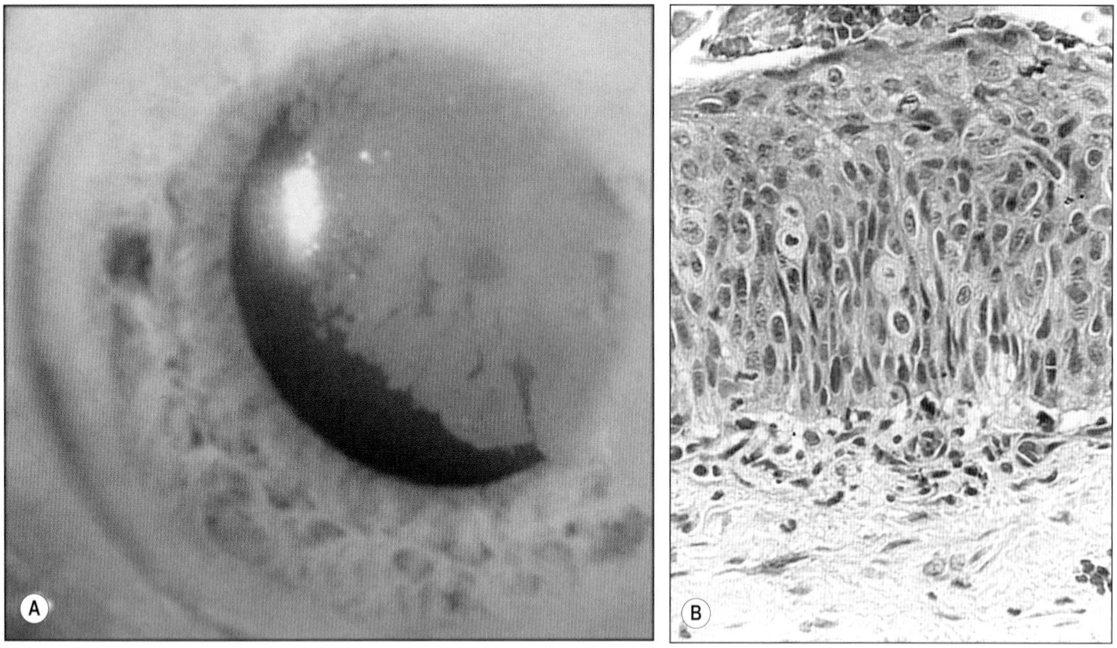

Fig. 5.7 (**A**) Corneal intraepithelial neoplasia. A flat limbal mass extends onto the cornea as a gray, opaque sheet with a sharply marginated, fimbriated leading edge. (From Leibowitz HM, Waring GO, III. Corneal Disorders. Clinical Diagnosis and Management. 2nd edn, Philadelphia, W.B. Saunders Company, 1998. Copyright Elsevier 1998.) (**B**) Histopathology demonstrates thickened epithelium with loss of normal maturation and basilar neoplastic cells. (From Waring GO 3rd, Roth AM, Ekins MB. Clinical and pathological description of 17 cases of clinical intraepithelial neoplasia. *Am J Ophthalmol* 1984; 97:547.)

The Pathologic Responses of the Subepithelial Zone

1. Defects (and their repair)

The epithelial basement membrane and Bowman's layer are both acellular, but their healing responses differ. The basement membrane is secreted by the basal epithelial cells and, therefore, can be regenerated or produced in excess or altered form. Bowman's layer, once damaged or destroyed, does not regenerate. A defect in Bowman's layer fills with fibroblasts and connective tissue, creating a permanent scar (e.g. keratoconus).

2. Fibrosis and vascularization

Neither the epithelial basement membrane nor Bowman's layer can become fibrotic or vascularized; however, fibrous or vascular tissues can spread between the basement membrane and Bowman's layer and replace the latter or grow into the anterior stroma immediately posterior to Bowman's layer as a pannus (Latin: carpet), either as avascular fibrosis or vascular fibrosis.

Subepithelial avascular fibrosis

Patches of avascular fibrous tissue appear beneath the epithelium as a nonspecific response. Examples include (1) corneal edema after cataract surgery, (2) advanced Fuchs' endothelial dystrophy, (3) granular and lattice corneal dystrophies, and (4) chronic superficial keratitis (e.g. phlyctenulosis). Another example is the subepithelial opacity from excimer laser photorefractive keratectomy, At 4 to 8 weeks after photorefractive keratectomy, a subepithelial haze may occur, which corresponds to a layer of subepithelial collagen and proteoglycans[11] that gradually is remodeled so that the subepithelial zone becomes clearer, although permanent scars can occur (Fig. 5.8).

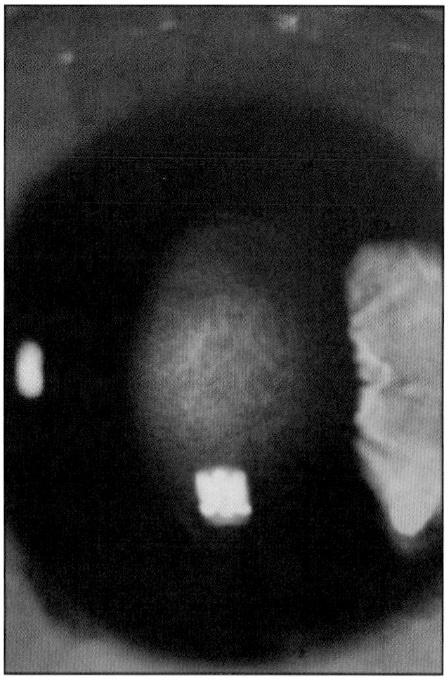

Fig. 5.8 Subepithelial central scar from excimer laser photorefractive keratectomy. (From Leibowitz HM, Waring GO, III. Corneal Disorders. Clinical Diagnosis and Management. 2nd edn, Philadelphia, W.B. Saunders, 1998. Copyright Elsevier 1998.)

Salzmann's nodular degeneration is a distinctive type of nonspecific avascular subepithelial fibrosis. The bluish-gray nodules usually appear in corneas afflicted by chronic, superficial inflammation that began in childhood, such as vernal keratoconjunctivitis. The nodules of hyaline and basement membrane material accumulate between Bowman's layer and the thinned but continuous epithelium and can be scraped off readily, with minimal chance of recurrence.

Subepithelial vascular fibrosis

Subepithelial vascular fibrosis involves three basic cells: leukocytes, proliferating vascular endothelial cells, and active fibroblasts that secrete an extracellular connective tissue matrix. This process occurs (1) after mild insults (e.g. hypoxia beneath an extended-wear soft contact lens), in which a very fine sheet of fibrovascular tissue slowly migrates in from the limbus, (2) during chronic long-lasting insult such as trachomatous eyelid scarring and entropion where a progressive dense pannus spreads centrally, as well as (3) after devastating insults (e.g. alkali burns) in which a thick layer of exuberant fibrovascular tissue can progress across the entire cornea (Fig. 5.9).

3. Edema and cysts

Subepithelial edema arises from endothelial dysfunction, as described above. Diffuse stromal edema can throw the epithelial basement membrane into folds, referred to as shift lines.

4. Inflammation and immune responses

Damage to the subepithelial zone from inflammation and innate immune response accompanies severe bacterial or fungal infection or trauma and usually is characterized by an epithelial defect and focal white superficial infiltrate that damages Bowman's layer and the superficial stroma. Subepithelial infiltrates can also be caused by antigens and toxins that pass through the intact epithelium into Bowman's layer and the superficial stroma, where they elicit immune and inflammatory responses that cause focal areas of infiltration and edema, generally in the absence of concurrent epithelial defects or ulcers.

There are two general locations of subepithelial infiltrates: the first is central and paracentral, where chronic, focal, ground-glass spots accumulate following acute adenoviral keratoconjunctivitis[12] and protein-coated, extended-wear soft contact lenses or dendriform or geographic pattern infiltrates occur after herpes simplex epithelial keratitis, and herpes zoster keratitis. Following penetrating keratoplasty, chronic 0.5-mm subepithelial infiltrates, confined to the donor button, reflect a mild form of allograft rejection. The second location of subepithelial infiltrates is paralimbal. These acute focal, dense, flat marginal 'staphyloccal catarrhal' corneal infiltrates are separated from the limbus by a clear zone, and those of phlyctenular keratoconjunctivitis have no intervening clear zone, becoming vascularized.

5. Deposits

Deposits in the epithelial basement membrane, such as silver granules from topical medications, are seldom visible clinically. Topical and systemic drugs rarely accumulate subepithelially. One exception is epinephrine, which deposits within and below the epithelium as adrenochrome pigment.

Systemic diseases rarely leave deposits selectively in Bowman's layer. Superficial, iron-containing foreign bodies embedded in the cornea can deposit a rust ring in Bowman's layer and the superficial stroma.

Reis-Bücklers and related corneal dystrophies produce deposition of fine, curled filaments 10 nm in diameter that replace Bowman's layer. These filaments give the cornea a central fish-net appearance and disrupt the epithelial basement membrane, causing painful erosions.

In Avellino corneal dystrophy, the granular dystrophy-like deposits are most dense in the anterior stroma.

A form of amyloid is deposited subepithelially in primary, gelatinous, droplike dystrophy, in which milky white, nodular opacities create mulberry-like lesions.

Calcium deposited in Bowman's layer as band-shaped keratopathy represents a degeneration that usually begins as a turbid haziness and gradually progresses within the palpebral fissure as a chalk-white plaque. Peripheral, arcuate calcific anterior stromal deposits may result from hypercalcemia.

Spheroidal degeneration of the cornea with its yellowish, round deposits in Bowman's layer and the anterior stroma within the palpebral fissure is also known as climatic droplet keratopathy and occurs in people who work in climatic. Focal spherules of a proteinaceous, autofluorescent material accumulate in Bowman's layer consisting of some constituent of plasma or tears in addition to elastotic fibrillar degeneration of collagen.[13]

6. Proliferation of the epithelial basement membrane

The basal corneal epithelial cells can secrete exuberant amounts of basement membrane, both subepithelially and within the epithelium. This excess tissue appears in primary epithelial disorders (e.g. epithelial basement membrane degeneration/dystrophy[14] with its patterns of maps, gray lines, refractile parallel lines (fingerprint lines), and gray putty-like intraepithelial cysts) (Fig. 5.10), as a nonspecific response (e.g. chronic corneal edema, Salzmann's degeneration), and as a manifestation of systemic diseases (e.g. diabetes mellitus).

Pathologic Responses of the Corneal Stroma

The structural integrity, tensile strength, and contour of the cornea are derived primarily from stromal collagen, predominantly type 1.

1. Defects (and their repair)

Stromal defects often occur acutely after accidental or surgical trauma and are repaired according to the principles of normal corneal wound healing. Acute stromal defects also result from ulceration due to microbial invasion; their repair requires elimination of the microorganism and control of the inflammation. Chronic defects often are progressive and

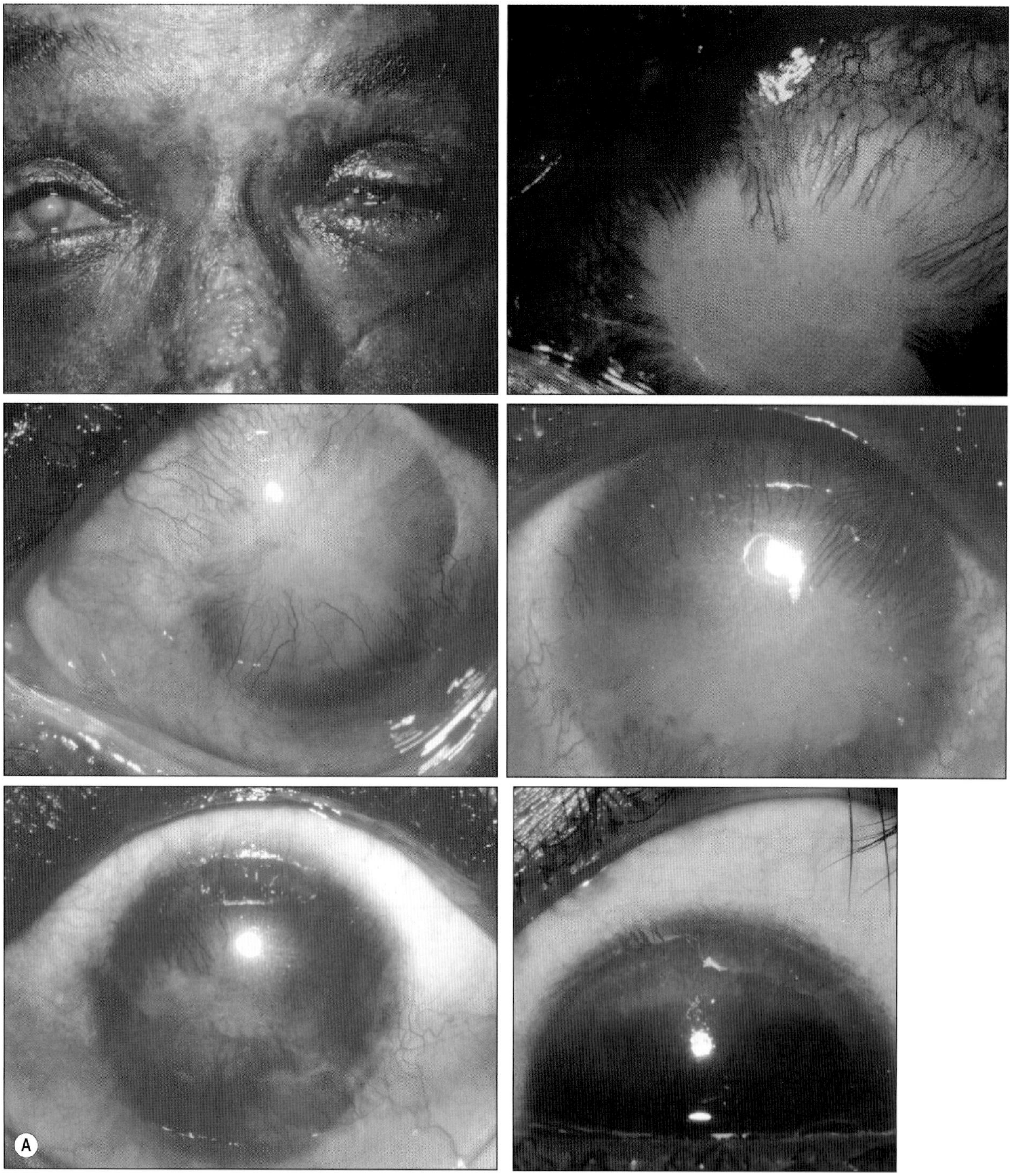

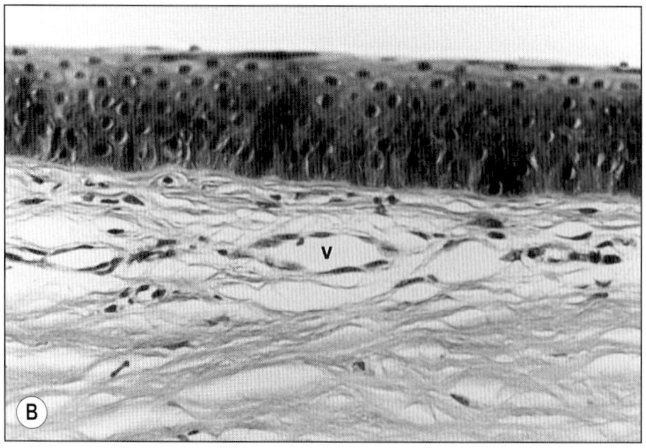

Fig. 5.9 (**A**) Set of images showing subepithelial vascular fibrosis in an alkali burn of the cornea. (**B**) Histopathology of subepithelial vascular fibrosis demonstrates thickened epithelium, diffuse fibrosis, and vessels (*v*). (From Leibowitz HM, Waring GO, III. Corneal Disorders. Clinical Diagnosis and Management, 2nd edn. Philadelphia, W.B. Saunders Company, 1998. Copyright Elsevier 1998).

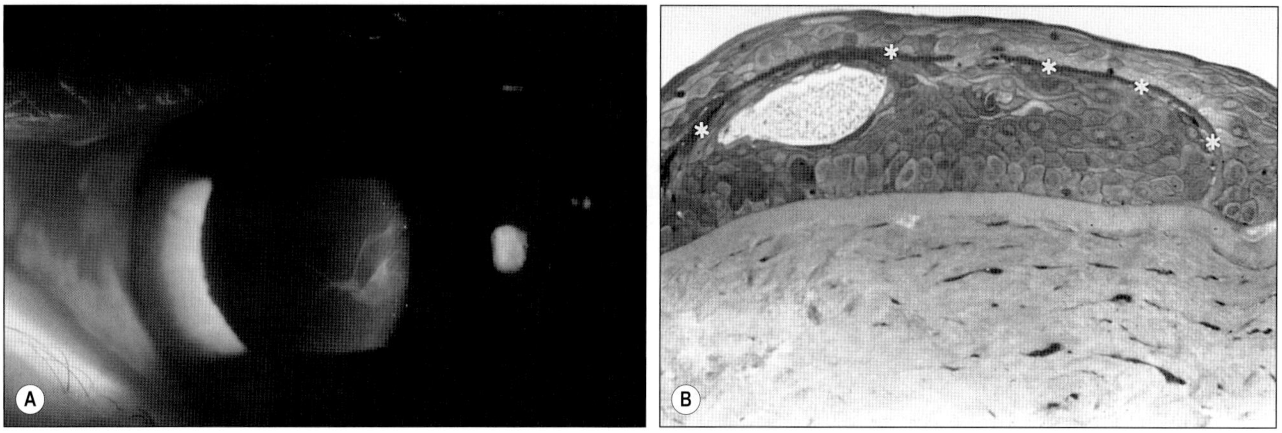

Fig. 5.10 Epithelial basement membrane degeneration. (**A**) An irregular, gray maplike pattern of epithelial basement membrane. (**B**) Histopathology demonstrates basement membrane duplication (*asterisks*) within the epithelium, trapping epithelial cells that show thickening and degeneration (the basis of the map figure, clinically) and focal cyst-like formation (*white area*) which create 'Cogan's microcysts.' (From Leibowitz HM, Waring GO, III. Corneal Disorders. Clinical Diagnosis and Management. 2nd edn. Philadelphia, W.B. Saunders Company, 1998. Copyright Elsevier, 1998.)

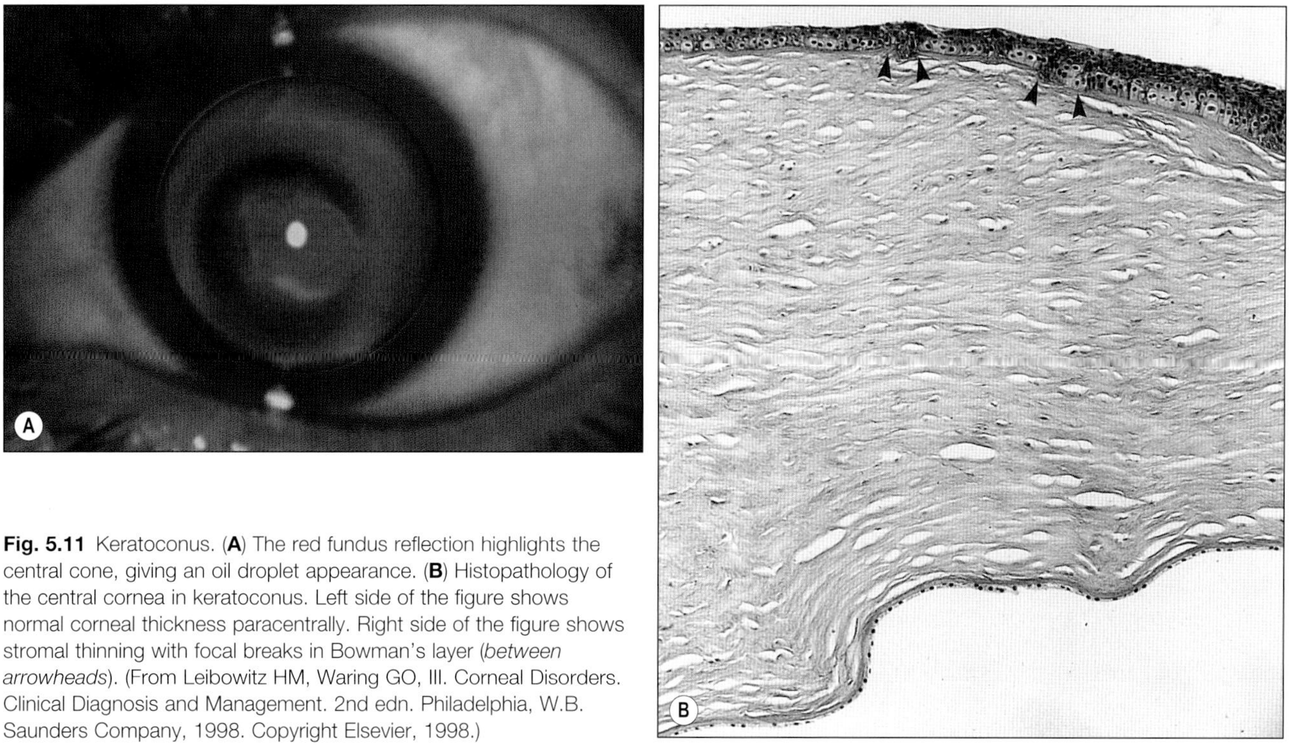

Fig. 5.11 Keratoconus. (**A**) The red fundus reflection highlights the central cone, giving an oil droplet appearance. (**B**) Histopathology of the central cornea in keratoconus. Left side of the figure shows normal corneal thickness paracentrally. Right side of the figure shows stromal thinning with focal breaks in Bowman's layer (*between arrowheads*). (From Leibowitz HM, Waring GO, III. Corneal Disorders. Clinical Diagnosis and Management. 2nd edn. Philadelphia, W.B. Saunders Company, 1998. Copyright Elsevier, 1998.)

fall into three categories: (1) stromal thinning without ulceration, (2) sterile stromal ulceration, and (3) congenital posterior corneal defects (see Endothelium).

Stable or progressive thinning of the stroma without epithelial ulceration or stromal inflammation occurs in keratoconus (Fig. 5.11),[15] keratoglobus, pellucid marginal degeneration, Terrien's marginal degeneration, and LASIK – especially with postoperative corneal ectasia. Stromal thinning alters corneal curvature and may create irregular astigmatism. The thinner the cornea, the less protection it affords the intraocular contents, the less stable it is, and the less it is amenable to optical or surgical vision correction. In general, a thickness of 250–300 μm is required to preserve corneal integrity and normal contour.

Keratoconus[15] is a variably progressive disorder of central corneal thinning and ectasia with a decrease in the number of stromal collagen lamellae, from about 350 to about 150 (see Fig. 5.11). Despite thinning, corneas with this disorder rarely perforate, even after a rupture of Descemet's membrane and the endothelium in acute hydrops. The term keratoglobus is applied colloquially to advanced keratoconus with total corneal thinning. The most extreme corneal

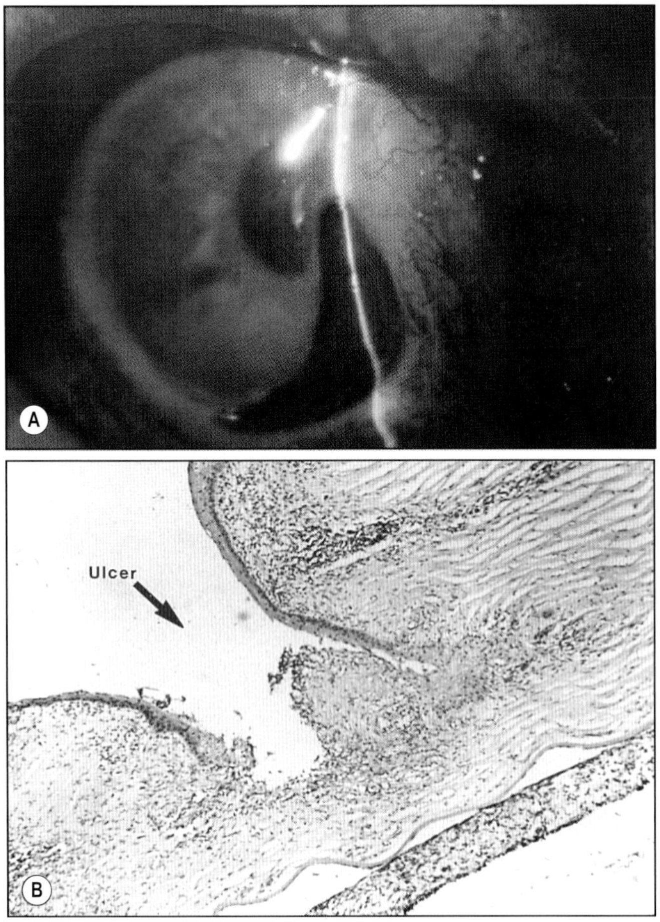

Fig. 5.12 Sterile stromal defect. (**A**) Marginal corneal ulcer in rheumatoid arthritis is stained with rose Bengal. (**B**) Histopathology demonstrates epithelial and stromal defects (*arrow*) with inflammatory cell infiltration. (From Leibowitz HM, Waring GO, III. Corneal Disorders. Clinical Diagnosis and Management, 2nd edn. Philadelphia, W.B. Saunders Company, 1998. Copyright Elsevier, 1998.)

thinning occurs in keratoglobus as part of the autosomal recessive connective tissue disease Ehlers-Danlos type VI A; minor trauma can rupture these corneas.

A variety of corneal diseases – including herpes simplex keratitis, alkali burns, systemic connective tissue disease such as rheumatoid arthritis (Fig. 5.12), bacterial and fungal keratitis, neurotrophic keratitis, and drug toxicity[16] – may set off a chain of destructive inflammatory and enzymatic events[16] that result in a persistent, sterile, sharply demarcated stromal defect, sometimes progressing to a descemetocele and corneal perforation.

2. Fibrosis and vascularization

Two of the most common and nonspecific pathologic processes that opacify the stroma are fibrosis (scarring) and vascularization.

Wound healing in the corneal stroma occurs slowly, presumably because the tissue is avascular and its rate decreases with age. The resultant scar tissue is weaker than the normal stroma, as evidenced by traumatic dehiscence of penetrating keratoplasty wounds many years after surgery, a circumstance obviated by lamellar corneal transplant techniques such as deep anterior lamellar keratoplasty (DALK) and endothelial keratoplasty techniques.

There are three basic phases in the healing of stromal wounds: (1) the destructive phase involves removal of abnormal tissues by polymorphonuclear (PMN) leukocytes and macrophages, aided by collagenases and proteoglycanases from epithelial cells, fibroblasts, and inflammatory cells; (2) the synthetic phase involves closure of the wound through synthesis of new collagens and proteoglycans by stromal fibroblasts, aided by epithelial cells; and (3) in the remodeling phase, the newly synthesized materials are initially assembled into a fine scar that is slowly remodeled into a clearer structure that more closely resembles normal cornea but never achieves total transparency or normal strength.

If the destructive phase is not constrained, melting of the corneal stroma can lead to corneal perforation. If the synthetic phase is inhibited by drugs (e.g. corticosteroids) or disease (e.g. rheumatoid arthritis), healing is delayed and wound strength may be decreased. In contrast, if the synthetic phase proceeds uncontrolledly, optically destructive scars can result. If the remodeling phase is incomplete, a larger scar persists.

Within hours of anterior stromal wounding, a fibrin clot fills the defect, fluid from the tears and aqueous humor produces swelling of the adjacent stroma, PMNs migrate into the wound from the tears, keratocytes at the edge of the wound die, and the epithelium migrates toward the wound. Epithelial–stromal interaction is important in corneal wound healing. The healing epithelium elaborates cytokines (e.g. interleukin [IL]-1, tissue growth factor [TGF]-β), which stimulate stromal keratocytes to transform into fibroblasts and myofibroblasts and to secrete extracellular matrix. This response is seen after excimer laser photorefractive keratectomy,[17] where the healing epithelium is in direct contact with the underlying stroma (without Bowman's layer) (see Fig. 5.8). However, the same excimer laser photoablation done under a flap of anterior cornea (LASIK) does not elicit a diffuse haze,[18] presumably because of an absence of epithelial–stromal interaction so that minimal activation of keratocytes occurs, except at the edge of the flap, where a linear scar results (Fig. 5.13).[19] The same mechanism keeps the stroma clear with the creation of intrastromal pockets for the implantation of ring segments and refractive lenticules. Similarly, intrastromal femtosecond laser wounds do not stimulate the profibrotic cytokine TGF-β1, which helps explain the lack of scarring in procedures such as Intracor circular intrastromal spots to treat presbyopia/hyperopia,[20] and the femtosecond laser creation of an intrastromal lenticule that is removed for refractive effect.

Stromal fibrosis

Alterations in the regular alignment of collagen fibrils greater than a 20-nm distance (i.e. one-half the wavelength of visible light) cause scattering of light. The observer sees this as a stromal opacity (back scatter), and the patient experiences glare (forward scatter). The opacity can take the form of a nebula (a mild, diffuse cloudiness), a macula (a moderately dense spot), or a leukoma (a markedly white opacity).

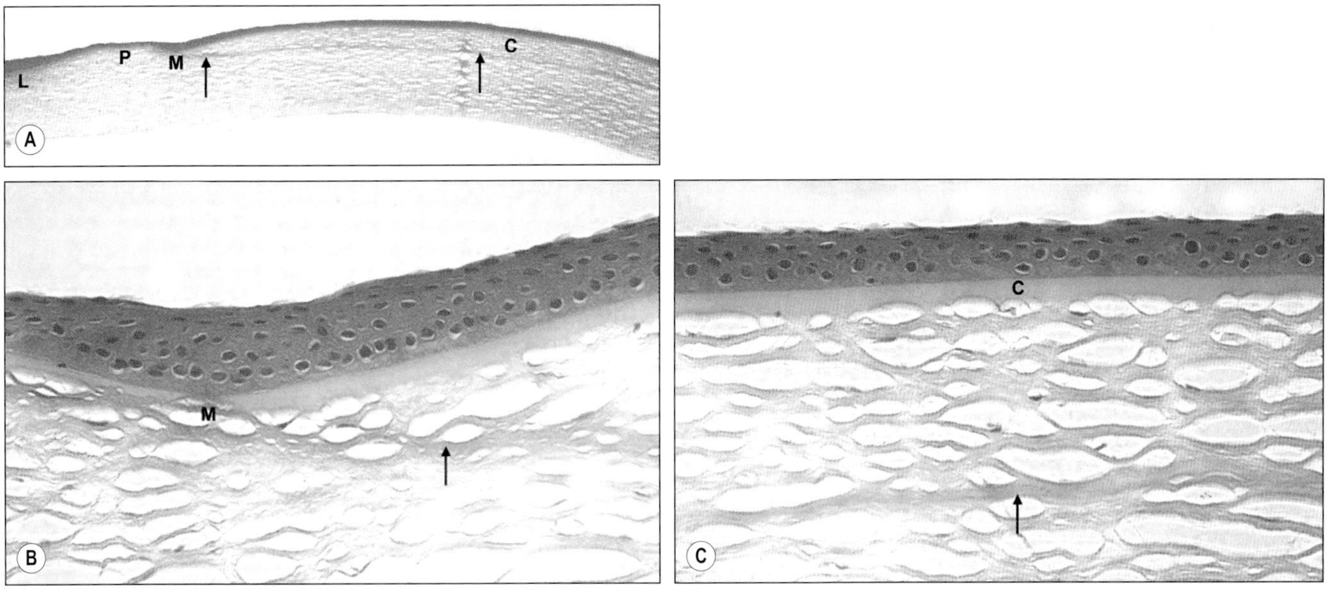

Fig. 5.13 Histopathlogy of human laser in situ keratomileusis (LASIK) demonstrates two types of avascular stromal wound healing: (**A**) a fibrocellular scar that is around the edge of the LASIK flap where the epithelium is in contact with the healing stroma, and (**B**) an acellular scar in the stromal interface that is separated from the epithelium and consists mainly of proteoglycans with negligible fibrosis. (**A**) L, limbus; P, peripheral cornea outside flap; M, margin of flap; C, central corneal flap; *arrows* indicate the stromal interface between flap and bed. (**B**) M, margin of flap showing slight epithelial thickening over the break in Bowman's layer and fibrocellular wound healing (*arrow*). (**C**) corneal flap with intact Bowman's layer (*C*) and hypocellular healing in the stromal interface (*arrow*). (Courtesy Daniel Dawson, MD.)

In general, it is not the specific disease but rather its severity and duration and the extent of healing that determine the degree of corneal scarring.

The pattern of a corneal scar usually is not diagnostic, but some processes leave characteristic scars. Bacterial and fungal keratitis usually create a focal, sharply demarcated scar whose depth reflects the degree of penetration of the stromal abscess. Vernal keratitis creates a discrete, shield-shaped anterior opacity, generally in the superior half of the cornea. Alkali burns leave diffuse, opaque, marbleized scars. Syphilitic interstitial keratitis is characterized by deep stromal scarring with ghost vessels and lipid deposits. Surgical scars, such as those produced by radial keratotomy, clear cornea cataract surgery, and penetrating keratoplasty also are characteristic.

Stromal vascularization

Vascularization of the corneal stroma is a nonspecific pathologic response; the location and number of vessels reflect the location and severity of the inflammatory response.[21,22] Stromal vessels can reduce vision in three ways: (1) they disrupt the normal stromal architecture, (2) they allow leakage of lipid into the stroma, and (3) they increase the potential for allograft rejection corneal transplantation. In most instances, the clinician tries to prevent stromal vascularization to preserve vision. At times, however (e.g. stromal melting), ingrowth of blood vessels is desirable because it helps prevent corneal perforation by facilitating the transport of nutrients, immunoprotective factors, antimicrobial factors, antiproteases, and fibroblasts to the stroma.

Stromal vessels characteristically grow at three levels: (1) subepithelial and superficial stromal vessels appear in response to superficial corneal disease (e.g. chronic blepharitis, phlyctenulosis, contact lens wear, recurrent epithelial defects; see Subepithelial Zone); (2) vessels appear in the middle layers of the stroma in response to chronic inflammation (e.g. necrotizing stromal herpes simplex keratitis, bacterial or fungal abscesses, chemical burns); and (3) vessels appear in the deep stroma, anterior to Descemet's membrane, and in eyes with keratouveitis (e.g. syphilitic interstitial keratitis).

Blood vessels that invade the stroma arise from superficial conjunctival vessels, deep scleral vessels, or iris vessels when the iris is in contact with the cornea. The vessels spread along the natural collagen lamellar planes but do not grow in an anterior–posterior direction unless a scar is present along which they can migrate.

In inflammatory conditions, the pattern of the vessels often follows that of the leukocytic infiltrate. Triangular tufts grow toward focal inflammation (e.g. infiltrates in rosacea keratoconjunctivitis). In contrast, a ring of vessels surrounds the cornea in limbal vernal conjunctivitis and the host–graft junction in penetrating keratoplasty. Generally, no single pattern characterizes a particular disease; exceptions include the superior limbal pannus of trachoma and superior limbic keratoconjunctivitis and the 360-degree limbal tufts from excessive soft contract wear. During active inflammation, stromal vessels dilate; when inflammation subsides, the vessels gradually shrink to endothelium-lined tubes without blood flow (i.e. ghost vessels), which refill with blood if inflammation recurs or if ischemia develops (e.g. contact lens wear). Large single stromal vessels can be treated by occlusion with argon laser photocoagulation (preferably yellow dye)[23] or with photodynamic therapy,[24] but this cannot be done effectively for diffuse fans of vessels.

Topical or subconjunctival bevacizumab – and possibly other vascular endothelial growth factor (VEGF) inhibitors – can inhibit stromal vascularization.[25]

3. Edema and cysts

Edema of the stroma is a common clinical sign;[26] epithelial-lined cysts of the corneal stroma occur rarely.

Edema of the corneal stroma occurs when its water content rises above the normal 78%. In most cases, corneal stromal edema results from disruption of endothelial or epithelial functions and manifests itself as an increase in corneal thickness. Fluid accumulates in the glycosaminoglycans (not in the collagen fibrils) of the stroma, altering the regular arrangement of collagen fibrils Clinically, stromal edema appears as a gray, ground-glass haze that varies from a fine, diffuse granularity to a dense, gray opacity, with clear, cyst-like lakes of fluid sometimes present. As the stroma swells, the anterior curvature of the cornea, as established by Bowman's layer, remains fixed, whereas the more elastic Descemet's membrane is displaced posteriorly toward the anterior chamber, developing folds, clinically termed corneal striae. As the glycosaminoglycans expand and the collagen fibrils separate, the cornea thickens from its normal central value of approximately 530 μm to as much as 1500 μm, as measured by optical or ultrasonic pachymetry or optical coherence tomography.

Disruption of the endothelium is the most common cause of stromal edema. It occurs frequently (1) after the trauma of intraocular surgery, (2) as part of Fuchs' endothelial dystrophy or the ICE syndrome, (3) in cases of severe iridocyclitis, herpes simplex disciform keratitis, and acute angle-closure glaucoma, and (4) in the most extreme circumstance, when there is a defect in Descemet's membrane and the endothelium is absent in that location either acutely (e.g. hydrops in keratoconus, forceps injury during birth) or congenitally (e.g. Peters' anomaly).

Stromal edema usually remains confined to the area in which the endothelial or epithelial damage has occurred, presumably because the functioning endothelium in the other areas continues to pump fluid from the stroma. For example, edema often remains central in Fuchs' endothelial dystrophy, superior or temporal adjacent to a cataract incision, and inferior in association with a retained anterior chamber foreign body.

With corneal edema, so-called 'cystic' spaces are fluid-filled lacunae caused by extreme stromal edema, and do not have an epithelial lining. An extreme example is the fluid interface syndrome after LASIK, in which high intraocular pressure and/or a dysfunctional endothelium allow fluid accumulation between the corneal flap and the stromal bed (Fig. 5.14).[27]

Epithelium-lined intrastromal cysts occur rarely after penetrating corneal trauma.[28] Sometimes they contain cloudy material, probably accumulated epithelial cells and debris.

4. Inflammation and immune responses

Numerous infections, immunologic diseases, and traumatic disorders have as their common denominator the aggregation of leukocytes in the corneal stroma. Details of corneal inflammation are presented in a later section of this chapter. On clinical inspection, leukocytes migrating through the corneal stroma have a faint, gray-brown, granular appearance. When leukocytes congregate at the site of attack, they create foci of yellow-white suppuration. If corneal damage secondary to leukocytic infiltration is severe, the stroma thickens with edema and pus, becomes gelatinous, and begins to melt. The destructive activity of leukocytes usually is repaired by fibrosis with or without vascularization, and the resulting scar causes decreased vision if it is central or paracentral.

Histopathologically, leukocytes migrate along stromal lamellae and congregate with varying density. Bacteria, particularly Gram-negative bacteria, cause severe stromal suppuration and destruction. An extreme example is *Pseudomonas aeruginosa* keratitis, in which both the PMNs and the bacteria secrete proteolytic enzymes that can lead to corneal perforation in a short time.

Immune-based stromal inflammation is more complicated and stems from deposition of antigen–antibody complexes and complement-mediated hypersensitivity as well as from alteration of stromal cell surface antigenicity through previous exposure to an infectious agent, such as herpes simplex virus (HSV).

As one example, the peripheral corneal stromal melting associated with adult rheumatoid arthritis (see Fig. 5.12) likely results from deposition of immune complexes that activate the complement cascade, which results in chemotaxis of PMNs, leading to lysosomal enzyme release and stromal melting.

Herpes simplex stromal keratitis probably is mediated not by active viral replication but by deposition of viral antigens into the stroma and subsequent immune complex hypersensitivity with the migration of PMNs and lymphocytes to form a centripetally migrating immune ring (Wessley ring). In contrast, herpes simplex disciform keratitis more likely represents a delayed-type hypersensitivity response prompted by HSV-induced modification of membrane surface expression in corneal stromal cells or by damage to the underlying endothelium.

5. Deposits

Deposits of substances in the stroma disrupt image formation in proportion to their central location and density.

Topical and systemic drugs

Few drugs accumulate in the stroma. One example: the compounds of gold sometimes used in the treatment of rheumatoid arthritis can accumulate in the cytoplasm of keratocytes, appearing as myriad, fine, distinct, round, ashlike particles varying in color from gold to violet (ocular chrysiasis).[29]

Ocular diseases

A foreign body that is retained in the corneal stroma, such as a fragment of wood or dirt, if not removed surgically, is expelled as part of the inflammatory response. Other less reactive foreign bodies are encased in subsequent scarring: glass, sand, pencil lead, and nylon or polypropylene sutures. These need little attention unless they lie in the central cornea and interfere with light transmission.

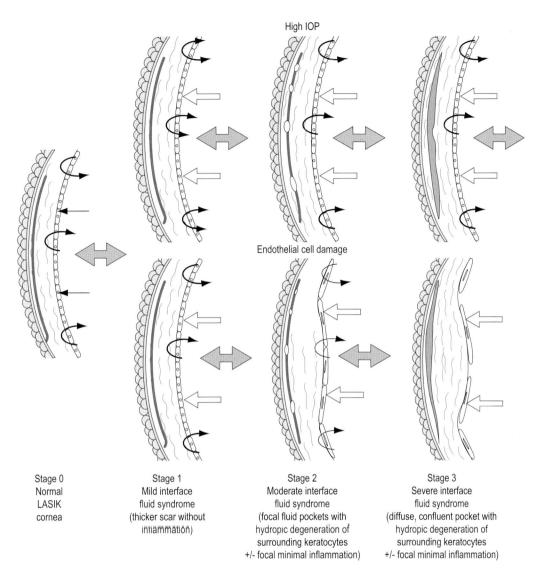

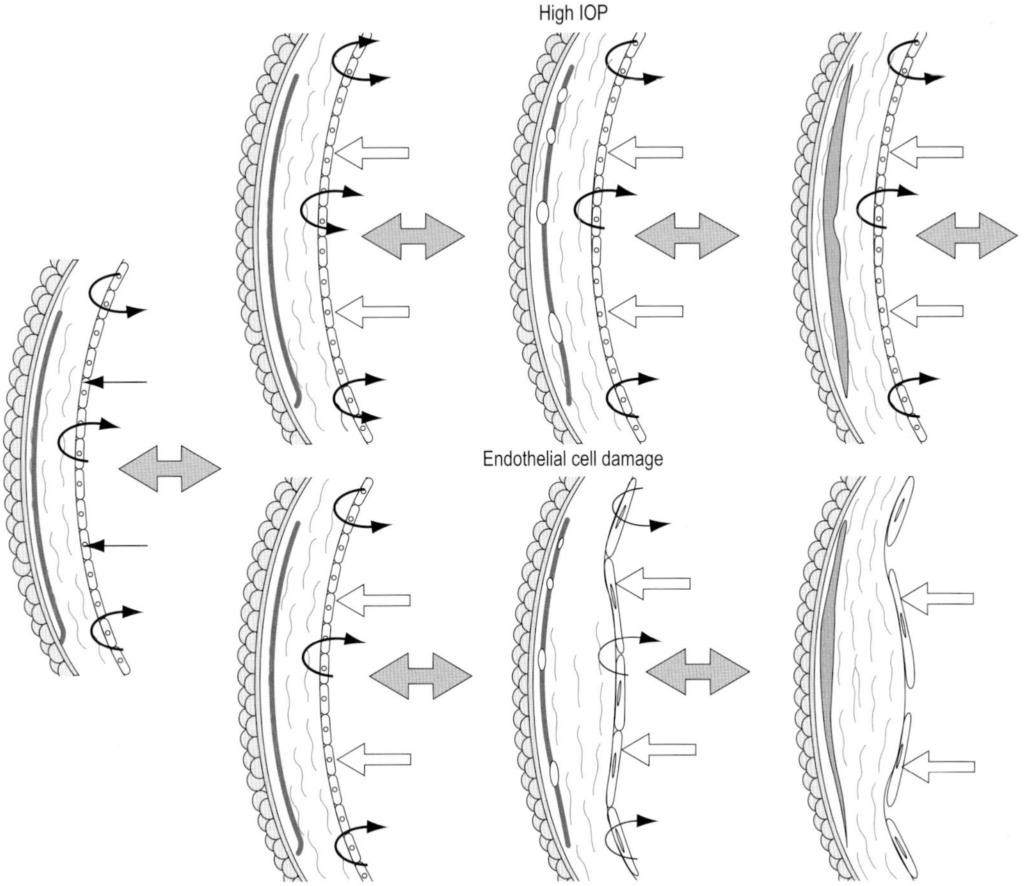

Fig. 5.14 Stromal edema in the interface fluid syndrome (IFS) after LASIK. A summary of the typical clinical slit lamp characteristics seen in each stage of the LASIK interface fluid syndrome, whether caused by elevated intraocular pressure (IOP) or by endothelial cell damage. Normal corneas after LASIK have a clear flap, interface, and residual stromal bed (RSB), with variable haze at the flap wound margin. LASIK corneas with normal endothelium and high IOP can have: (1) asymptomatic thickening of the central stromal LASIK interface, (2) symptomatic smudgy interface haze and thickening of the interface tissue, or (3) a clear fluid cleft and a clear and compressed flap and RSB. LASIK corneas with damaged endothelium (with or without high IOP) have similar findings in the interface but also have a clear to mildly hazy flap and a hazy, thickened, edematous RSB. (From Dawson DG, Schmack I, Holley GP, et al. Interface fluid syndrome in human eye bank corneas after LASIK: causes and pathogenesis. *Ophthalmology* 2007; 114:1857. Copyright Elsevier, 2007.)

Lipid deposits in the cornea are common,[30,31] not only in humans but also in dogs.[32] Lipids can leak from stromal blood vessels. These deposits vary from refractile crystals at the tip of a vessel to a full-thickness stromal mass that pushes Descemet's membrane posteriorly. Laser photocoagulation sometimes can occlude feeder vessels, allowing the lipids to regress. Only a small percentage of vascularized corneas manifest lipid deposits. Stromal keratocytes are capable of synthesizing lipids, which suggests that lipid precursors can leak from vessels and may be absorbed by the keratocytes, which synthesize and secrete cholesterol and fatty acids. Lipids can deposit around a corneal inlay, such as ring segments for myopia and keratoconus[33] but not all inlays manifest these deposits. Corneal arcus is the most common lipid deposition in the cornea and is considered a normal change of aging unless it appears before the mid-30s, when it is suggestive of hyperlipoproteinemia.[34,35]

Blood staining of the cornea occurs after anterior chamber hemorrhage (hyphema), particularly if there is a persistent increase in the intraocular pressure (IOP) or damage to the corneal endothelium (Fig. 5.15).

Systemic diseases

In certain systemic diseases, nonimmune deposits can appear in the corneal stroma, either because the keratocytes are

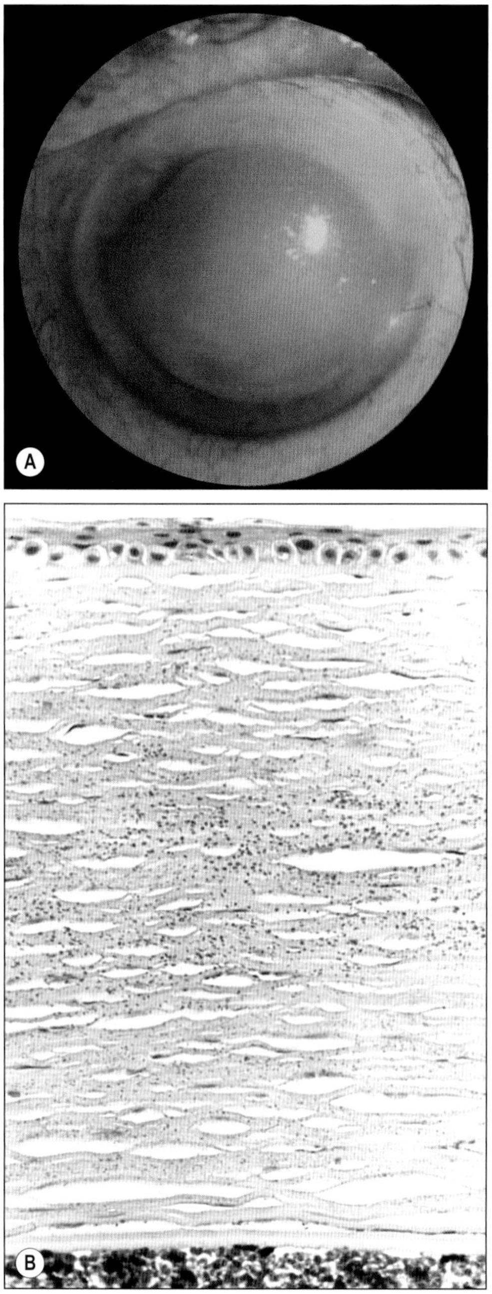

Fig. 5.15 Blood-stain deposit in corneal stroma. (**A**) Brownish, well-circumscribed blood staining in an eye with a chronic hyphema. (**B**) Histopathology demonstrates particulate hemosiderin pigment throughout the corneal stroma. Intact erythrocytes fill the anterior chamber (*bottom of figure*). (From Leibowitz HM, Waring GO, III. Corneal Disorders. Clinical Diagnosis and Management. 2nd edn. Philadelphia, W.B. Saunders Company, 1998. Copyright Elsevier, 1998.)

involved in an inherited metabolic disorder (e.g. disorders of lipid metabolism, the mucopolysaccharidoses, cystinosis) or because the corneal stroma is a repository for abnormal, circulating substances (e.g. globulin crystals in multiple myeloma,[36] benign monoclonal gammopathy).

Central corneal lipid deposits are found as part of rarer genetic disorders of high-density lipoprotein (HDL) metabolism such as lecithin-cholesterol acyltransferase (LCAT) deficiency.

In the mucopolysaccharidoses, corneal deposits of excess dermatan sulfate and keratan sulfate create a diffuse, ground-glass appearance in the stroma.

Deposits from dystrophies and degenerations of the stroma

Deposits of abnormal substances or abnormal amounts of normal substances can create opacities in corneal stromal dystrophies,[37,38] such as a form of amyloid in lattice and Avellino dystrophies, phospholipids in granular and Avellino dystrophies, glycosaminoglycans in fleck and macular dystrophies, and lipid in Schnyder's central crystalline dystrophy.

6. Proliferation

Stromal proliferation usually occurs in the peripheral cornea and can be congenital or acquired. The congenital type includes dermoid choristomas, which are histologically normal tissues in an abnormal location, appear most commonly at the limbus, either as an isolated finding or as part of a systemic syndrome (e.g. Goldenhar's syndrome, organoid nevus syndrome),[39] vary from small white spots to large masses, occupy the anterior one-third to one-half of the stroma, and do not enlarge after birth.

The acquired type includes connective tissue elements of the stroma that proliferate at a surgical or accidental wound without vascularization. This can occur anteriorly any time after trauma, because the defect in Bowman's layer persists indefinitely, allowing stromal outgrowth that appears as a flat, gray plaque with a feathered leading edge, spreading centripetally in between the epithelium and Bowman's layer (e.g. after penetrating keratoplasty). If the tissue interferes with vision, it can be peeled easily from Bowman's layer. Proliferation of the corneal stroma posteriorly through a penetrating keratoplasty, or a posterior lamellar graft[40] wound or along a keratoprosthesis[41] across the posterior surface of the cornea, possibly with the assistance of fibroblast-transformed corneal endothelial cells, can form a thick gray layer, a retrocorneal membrane. The potential for posterior stromal proliferation ceases if the endothelium secretes a new basement membrane over the posterior surface of the wound.

Pathologic Responses of the Corneal Endothelium and Descemet's Membrane

1. Defects (and their repair)

Normal adult endothelial cell density is approximately 2500 cells/mm^3 and normal cell size is approximately 250 μm. Defects in the endothelium can occur alone or in combination with defects in Descemet's membrane. In either case, aqueous humor rushes through the defect into the corneal stroma, producing stromal and epithelial edema that persists until a functioning endothelial monolayer reestablishes itself.

Defects in the endothelium

Defects in the endothelium may occur acutely (after accidental or surgical trauma by a phacoemulsification tip or an intraocular lens [IOL]) or chronically (in diseases that cause gradual attrition of endothelial cells with 'micro-defects' between the sick cells – as in Fuchs' dystophy). The endothelial defect is difficult to visualize with the slit lamp or specular microscope if there is overlying corneal edema.[42]

The wounded corneal endothelium repairs itself primarily through limited migration and hypertrophy and minimally through cell division.[43] The corneal endothelium does not divide under normal circumstances but can be stimulated by injury to divide. The regenerative potential of the endothelium in children is substantial and can produce excess Descemet membrane, but it decreases with age. After an injury, only cells adjacent to the defect participate directly in wound healing; those farther from the site retain their normal configuration, although the limbal endothelium may be a source of regenerative cells. Stromal edema resolves when the endothelial monolayer and barrier and pump functions are reestablished.

Alterations in individual endothelial cell area and shape occur during healing. Enlarged cells represent those that spread out to cover the defect, while smaller cells represent those that result from mitotic division or are still in the process of desquamating. In normal corneas, 48–90% of endothelial cells are hexagonal; as the cells spread and heal, the number of hexagonal cells decreases. Thus, variation in cell size and shape reflects the severity of the damage. There is a poor correlation between the size of an endothelial cell and its function. Presumably, enlarging endothelial cells develop more pump sites in their lateral plasma membranes, and barrier and pump functions remain at a normal level. Corneas with cell densities as low as 500 cells/mm^3, a figure that corresponds to an average cell size of approximately 2000–3000 µm^2, can remain clear.

Acute damage to the endothelium is most commonly surgically induced during cataract extraction[44] or corneal transplantation – especially posterior lamellar endothelial keratoplasty techniques that involve the folding and manipulation of the posterior stromal/endothelial donor disc.[45]

Chronic diseases of the endothelium, such as Fuchs' endothelial dystrophy[46] and chronic touch by an anterior chamber IOL (pseudophakic corneal edema)[47] cause a progressive loss of endothelial cells. As cells are lost, the remaining cells progressively enlarge and flatten to maintain a continuous covering over Descemet's membrane. If cell loss continues, however, the capacity of the remaining cells to maintain corneal deturgescence is exceeded and corneal decompensation results, with stromal and epithelial edema. After penetrating keratoplasty, endothelial cell density drops for about 5 years and then becomes relatively stable.[48]

Defects in Descemet's membrane

Descemet's membrane has less tensile strength than full-thickness stroma; therefore, conditions in which the cornea is stretched may produce breaks in this membrane. The size of these defects is enlarged by retraction and coiling of Descemet's membrane along the edge of the break. For example, birth forceps injury compresses the globe vertically, stretching Descemet's membrane horizontally and creating vertical or oblique breaks; elevated IOP in infantile glaucoma stretches the cornea, creating serpentine or circular breaks in Descemet's membrane; and the thin, ecstatic keratoconic cornea can stretch sufficiently to produce a focal spontaneous, elliptical rupture in the endothelium and Descemet's membrane (acute corneal hydrops) (see Fig. 5.4).

In all of these disorders, Descemet's membrane can separate from the overlying stroma to form a ledge or strand in the anterior chamber. Because most of these disorders occur in children and young adults, the corneal endothelium can repair and cover the defect, usually with production of a thick subendothelial fibrillar matrix (posterior collagenous layer). The retracted, coiled ends of the ruptured Descemet's membrane do not reapproximate, even when endothelial continuity is reestablished.[49]

Congenital, focal defects in Descemet's membrane and the endothelium are present in most cases of Peters' anomaly and its variants. These range from a slight indentation (posterior localized keratoconus) to an excavation that reaches Bowman's layer and is accompanied by focal stromal defects and scarring.

2. Fibrosis and vascularization posterior to Descemet's membrane

Like stromal keratocytes, with which the healing corneal endothelium has a common mesenchymal origin in the neural crest, endothelial cells also can transdifferentiate into epithelium-like cells (e.g. posterior polymorphous dystrophy).

The endothelium and Descemet's membrane contain no connective tissue and do not respond to adverse stimuli with classical fibrosis or vascularization. However, when the endothelium is damaged or diseased, it secretes a layer of abnormal fibrillar tissue on the posterior surface of the original Descemet's membrane (Fig. 5.16).

Posterior collagenous layer

Clinically, this tissue appears as a gray sheet at the level of Descemet's membrane and has been called a 'thickened' or 'multilaminar' Descemet's membrane or retrocorneal membrane. The term 'posterior collagenous layer' (PCL) is preferable because: (1) it designates the tissue as a distinct abnormality; (2) it locates the tissue in the posterior cornea rather than mislabeling it 'behind' the cornea, since endothelial cells are often present on its posterior surface; (3) it describes the layered architecture; and (4) it indicates that collagen is a major component.[50]

A posterior collagenous layer has been described by various names in more than 30 different corneal disorders. Examples include cornea guttata and Fuchs' endothelial dystrophy, the refractile ridges in syphilitic interstitial keratitis, and the gray 'thickened Descemet's membrane' apparent in pseudophakic corneal edema. Clinically, the posterior collagenous layer is best seen in a broad slit beam that sweeps tangentially across the posterior surface of the cornea to reveal the plaques or sheets of gray, swirling, crinkled tissue.

With light microscopy, the periodic acid-Schiff (PAS) stain demonstrates the original uniform Descemet's membrane

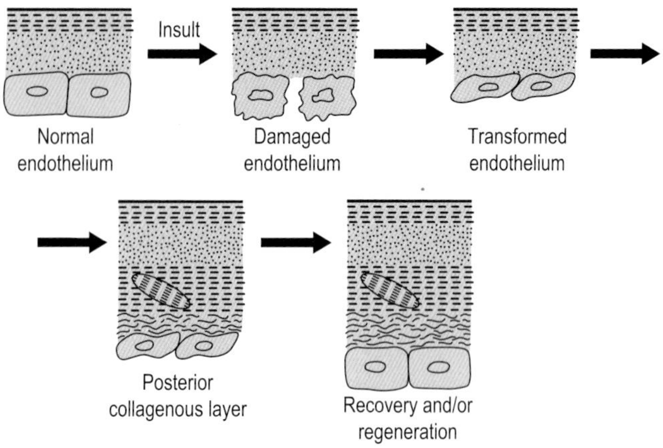

Fig. 5.16 A variety of endothelial insults transform corneal endothelial cells to fibroblast-like cells that secrete extracellular matrix on the posterior surface of the original Descemet's membrane, forming a posterior collagenous layer. Normal endothelial morphology can recover, depending on the severity and duration of the insult. (From Leibowitz HM, Waring GO, III. Corneal Disorders. Clinical Diagnosis and Management, 2nd edn. Philadelphia. W.B. Saunders, 1998. Copyright Elsevier, 1998.)

adjacent to the stroma, with the posterior collagenous layer behind it, consisting of multiple lamellae of varying thickness and staining. Immunohistochemistry indentifies five different collagen types and proteoglycans in the abnormal layers.[51]

Using the posterior collagenous layer to date the onset of endothelial or Descemet's membrane disease with transmission electron microscopy

Under normal conditions, Descemet's membrane thickens throughout life, increasing from approximately 3 μm at birth to approximately 18 μm by age 90 years. When viewed by transmission electron microscopy, the anterior banded portion of Descemet's membrane is present at birth. The posterior, homogeneous, nonbanded layer is produced and thickens throughout life.

The multiple lamellae of the posterior collagenous layer that result from disease in or trauma to the endothelium accumulate as a historical record, like geologic strata or tree rings.[50] By noting whether abnormalities exist in the anterior banded or posterior nonbanded portion of Descemet's membrane, one can reasonably infer whether a corneal disease process is congenital or acquired. For example, in corneas affected by the iridocorneal endothelial (ICE) syndrome, the layers of normal banded and nonbanded Descemet's membrane are present, bounded posteriorly by abnormal posterior collagenous layers, indicating an acute onset of the endothelial disorder in adulthood.[52] A contrasting example is Fuchs' dystrophy, where abnormal wide-spacing collagen bundles are present throughout the nonbanded layer, indicating the disorder began early in life, although it is not manifested clinically until the fifth or sixth decade.[53] Similarly, posterior polymorphous dystrophy demonstrates abnormalities in the anterior portion of the nonbanded layer, indicating it is onset congenitally.

Vascularization does not occur in Descemet's membrane or in the posterior collagenous layer. Certain thick, fibrocellular membranes that are truly retrocorneal can become vascularized, but most of these are connected to the stroma through a wound, often with adherent iris.

3. Edema and cysts

Edema of the endothelium is usually associated with decreased endothelial function and overlying stromal edema. True cysts do not occur in these layers. Accumulated fluid within and between endothelial cells forms dilated spaces, creating a dewdrop, beaten-metal appearance sometimes called 'pseudo-guttata.' Specular photomicrographs show the swollen endothelial cells as a patchy array of dark spots that do not have the central white reflection characteristic of cornea guttata.[54]

Inflammation affecting the endothelium is the most common cause of endothelial edema; herpetic disciform edema is believed to result from an endotheliitis.

Because Descemet's membrane is a compact tissue that is readily permeable to water and contains only small amounts of glycosaminoglycans, it does not become edematous. However, Descemet's membrane can be displaced from the posterior stroma by edema, focal hemorrhage or a pocket of pus to form a posterior bulge, folds, or ledges. Posterior polymorphous dystrophy is characterized by focal, round, small lesions that resemble a group of vesicles or blisters. However, these are not true vesicles but are small pits in the posterior stroma lined by a thin Descemet's membrane.[55]

4. Inflammation and immune responses

The endothelium indirectly becomes involved in inflammatory processes in disorders such as microbial keratitis and iridocyclitis, in which vasodilatory and chemotactic factors bring it into contact with leukocytes, forming various patterns of keratic precipitates. Keratic precipitates form a variety of patterns, including (1) a nonspecific spattering on the posterior cornea (e.g. ankylosing spondylitis), (2) a focal aggregation (e.g. disciform herpes simplex keratitis), and (3) a central, inferior, elliptical or triangular pattern (e.g. sarcoid uveitis). The endothelium also becomes directly involved in inflammatory processes in disorders such as herpetic disciform keratitis and allograft reactions, in which antigens on the endothelial cell surface stimulate the inflammatory process, for example an endothelial rejection line on the donor.[56,57]

PMNs and mononuclear leukocytes adhere to the endothelial cell surface, penetrate between the cells, and intersperse themselves between Descemet's membrane and the endothelium. If the inflammatory process is mild to moderate or is appropriately treated, the leukocytes migrate back into the anterior chamber, and the endothelial monolayer recovers functional viability. If the inflammatory process is more severe and prolonged or is inadequately treated, endothelial cells show increasing vacuolization, separation from Descemet's membrane, desquamation into the anterior chamber, and death.

Descemet's membrane is remarkably resistant to the proteolytic enzymes elaborated by microorganisms, leukocytes, and epithelial cells. It resists destruction in the presence of severe keratitis, iridocyclitis, and endophthalmitis, and acts as a barrier that prevents the passage of leukocytes and most microorganisms between the anterior chamber and the stroma.[58] Fungi are an exception; many elaborate enzymes that enable them to penetrate Descemet's membrane. After severe stromal melting, Descemet's membrane, bulging anteriorly as a descemetocele, may persist as the only intact structure in the cornea.

Inflammation directed specifically at Descemet's membrane is rare. A granulomatous reaction can occur around a fragmented Descemet's membrane, most commonly in chronic ulcerative herpes simplex keratitis, although it also is encountered in other inflammatory disorders.[59]

5. Deposits

Topical and systemic drugs

Drugs and metals deposit in Descemet's membrane, whereas melanin pigment selectively deposits in or on the endothelium. Although they are seldom used today, prolonged topical administration of silver-containing medications (e.g. Argyrol) historically was the most common source of deposits in Descemet's membrane.

Ocular and systemic diseases

The most common deposit in Descemet's membrane resulting from a systemic disease is copper, which appears as the Kayser-Fleischer ring in Wilson's disease (hepatolenticular degeneration).[60] Clinically, the copper accumulates in the peripheral part of Descemet's membrane, initially in superior and inferior arcs that eventually become confluent and form a 360-degree greenish brown deposit).

Certain ocular diseases result in deposition of melanin pigment in or on the endothelium. This occurs from four different sources within the eye, each with distinctive clinical and histopathologic features.

1. Endothelial cells phagocytose pigment in disorders such as pigment dispersion syndrome and Fuchs' endothelial dystrophy, creating the clinical appearance of fine dusting of the posterior surface of the cornea, often in the form of a vertical, central Krukenberg's spindle The vertical pattern of distribution comes about as the result of aqueous humor rising posteriorly in proximity to the warm iris and falling anteriorly on contact with the cooler cornea.
2. Iris stromal melanocytes can migrate over the posterior cornea, particularly in areas where there has been endothelial damage or where iris adhesions are present, forming a faint, brownish membrane that often consists of individual dendriform-shaped cells.
3. Iris pigment epithelial cells migrate onto the posterior surface of the cornea, especially in areas where the endothelium is damaged or absent or where iris adhesions are present, and create sharply marginated, rounded patches of dense, round, dark-brown pigment.
4. Pigmented macrophages also may be found in the endothelium but generally are not visible clinically.

Other types of material deposit on the endothelial surface: lymphocytes and keratic precipitates in inflammation, clumps or sheets of red blood cells in anterior chamber hemorrhage, tumor cells in lymphoproliferative disorders, white flakes in the exfoliation syndrome, and pieces of lens cortex or capsule after extracapsular cataract extraction.

Corneal dystrophies and degenerations

Among corneal dystrophies, only macular dystrophy produces deposits in the endothelium and Descemet's membrane.[61]

The most common material deposited in Descemet's membrane is lipid as part of a corneal arcus. Because Descemet's membrane ends abruptly at Schwalbe's line, the lipid material appears with a sharp outer margin and a diffuse inner margin.

6. Proliferation

The production of excess basement membrane and collagenous tissue by the endothelium (posterior collagenous layer) is discussed in the section on fibrosis. There are no neoplastic or dysplastic disorders of the endothelium, as might be expected in a tissue with minimal regenerative capacity.

Endothelial cells are capable of transforming into both fibroblast-like and epithelium-like cells. In fibroblastic metaplasia, endothelial cells secrete extracellular collagenous tissue (the posterior collagenous layer). Patches of keratin-containing, epithelium-like cells occupy the posterior cornea in posterior polymorphous dystrophy,[62] the ICE syndrome, congenital hereditary endothelial dystrophy, and Fuchs' endothelial dystrophy.[63]

Despite minimal regenerative capacity, the endothelium can proliferate over the surface of the trabecular meshwork, iris, and vitreous under specific circumstances, especially in children. When this occurs, the endothelium itself is not visible but the basement membrane it produces (ectopic Descemet's membrane) is visible and is often described as a glass, cuticular, or hyaline membrane. The process is sometimes referred to as endothelialization or descemetization of the anterior chamber and can result in glaucoma and distortion of the iris and pupil.[50]

The ICE syndrome has been called 'primary proliferative endothelial degeneration.' Its common feature is an ectopic proliferation of the endothelium across the trabecular meshwork and onto the iris, where it secretes an ectopic basement membrane that contracts, forming unilateral peripheral anterior synechiae, distorting the pupil and creating iris stromal tufts or nodules.[64]

The Immune Response: Components and Reactions in the Eye

Overview

The ocular immune response involves a complex set of interactions between local and systemic immunocompetent and parenchymal cells that communicate through specialized cell surface receptors and soluble mediators to protect the delicate functional and structural integrity of the eye. Immunocompetent cells include those of the lymphoid system (lymphocytes) and those of the myeloid system (macrophages, polymorphonuclear leukocytes, eosinophils, basophils, and antigen presenting cells [APCs]). Antigen presenting cells include macrophages, Langerhans cells, and B lymphocytes. Soluble components of the immune system include immunoglobulins, cytokines (peptide/glycopeptide intercellular mediators), chemokines (molecules with chemoattractant and cytokine properties), and complement.[65]

The immune system has primary and secondary tissue components. Primary lymphoid tissue includes the thymus, spleen, and bone marrow. Lymph nodes and the mucosa-associated lymphoid tissue (MALT) comprise the secondary tissue. The eye has its own MALT and is composed of the conjunctival lymphoid elements and lacrimal gland.

Adhesion molecules are a family of cell-surface glycoproteins located on a variety of circulating and fixed cells that mediate cell communication and migration. Special receptors on the surface of some lymphocytes (homing receptors) regulate the traffic of sensitized cells across the vascular endothelium into local lymphoid tissues of the MALT.[65] During the immune response, several families of adhesion receptors participate in a cascade of binding events that control cell migration out of the vascular compartment and also within the tissues themselves. Expressed at low levels under normal conditions, adhesion molecules can be dramatically up-regulated during an immune or inflammatory response.

There are two broad types of immune response to antigens: the innate or natural immune response and the adaptive or acquired immune response.[65] The innate response is the first line of defense against foreign agents. It is rapid in onset (minutes), lacks memory, and does not have the capacity for a more aggressive immune response following subsequent exposure to a specific agent (anamnestic response). Elimination of antigen occurs through cellular elements such as macrophages, polymorphonuclear leukocytes, and certain lymphocytes (natural killer [NK] cells). Soluble factors also participate, and in the eye they include complement, lysozyme, and some inflammatory mediators.

The more complex adaptive immune response has both humoral (antibody) and cell-mediated immune (CMI) pathways and occurs over a longer time frame (hours, days). Both cells (B and T lymphocytes) and soluble components such as antibodies and cytokines also participate in this specific response to antigen. In humans, the major histocompatibility complex (MHC) gene codes for MHC surface proteins whose primary function is to distinguish between self and nonself.[65] These MHC molecules play an integral role in antigen recognition and presentation.

The adaptive immune response has three phases. First, the afferent arm involves an initial antigen recognition process followed by antigen presentation to host T lymphocytes. Antigen presentation involves the interaction between an APC and a helper T lymphocyte. The second phase involves antigen processing and activation of lymphocytes (B cells and T cells), as well as differentiation and proliferation of specific effector lymphocytes. Finally, mature specialized cells interact with their specific target antigens. Subsequent exposure to antigen generates a more aggressive (anamnestic) response through the activation of memory cells that have been sensitized to that specific antigen.[65]

Regulation of the immune response is complex and involves both soluble and cellular factors. Many immunoregulatory phenomena occur in the anterior segment, including tissue transplantation (corneal, stem cell), immune privilege, immune tolerance, and autoimmunity.[66]

Although the immune response is usually protective, tissue injury may occur subsequent to an exuberant immune reaction. Four well-characterized hypersensitivity reactions account for a variety of immunopathologic mechanisms in the anterior segment, although a single pure hypersensitivity reaction in the eye is uncommon.[65]

Finally, the ocular immune response, in particular, occurs through a complex and integrated system involving many cellular and tissue structures of the eye. This chapter discusses basic principles of the immune response in general and focuses particular attention on special features of immune privilege and the ocular immune response.[66–68] The cascade of events is illustrated in Figure 5.17 for acute inflammation and Figure 5.18 for chronic inflammation.

Cells of inflammation and the immune response

The major types of immunocompetent cells include lymphocytes (B cells, T cells, and non-B, non-T cells), cells of the mononuclear phagocytic system (monocytes and macrophages), cells of the myeloid system (polymorphonuclear leukocytes), and auxiliary cells. The latter group includes a variety of constitutive and facultative antigen presenting cells, dendritic cells, platelets, and endothelial cells.[65]

Lymphocytes, which cannot be distinguished morphologically, are defined on the basis of their development, cellular products, and characteristic cell membrane receptors.[66] These surface receptors are characteristic of different cell lines, stages in development of a specific cell line, or activation levels of a specific cell type. The identification of a growing number of specific lymphocyte subsets has been facilitated by the use of monoclonal antibodies that bind to specific cell surface glycoproteins. The current nomenclature utilizes a universal system based on 'clusters of differentiation' (CD) designations.[65] Table 5.1 lists the major soluble mediators and receptors of inflammation.

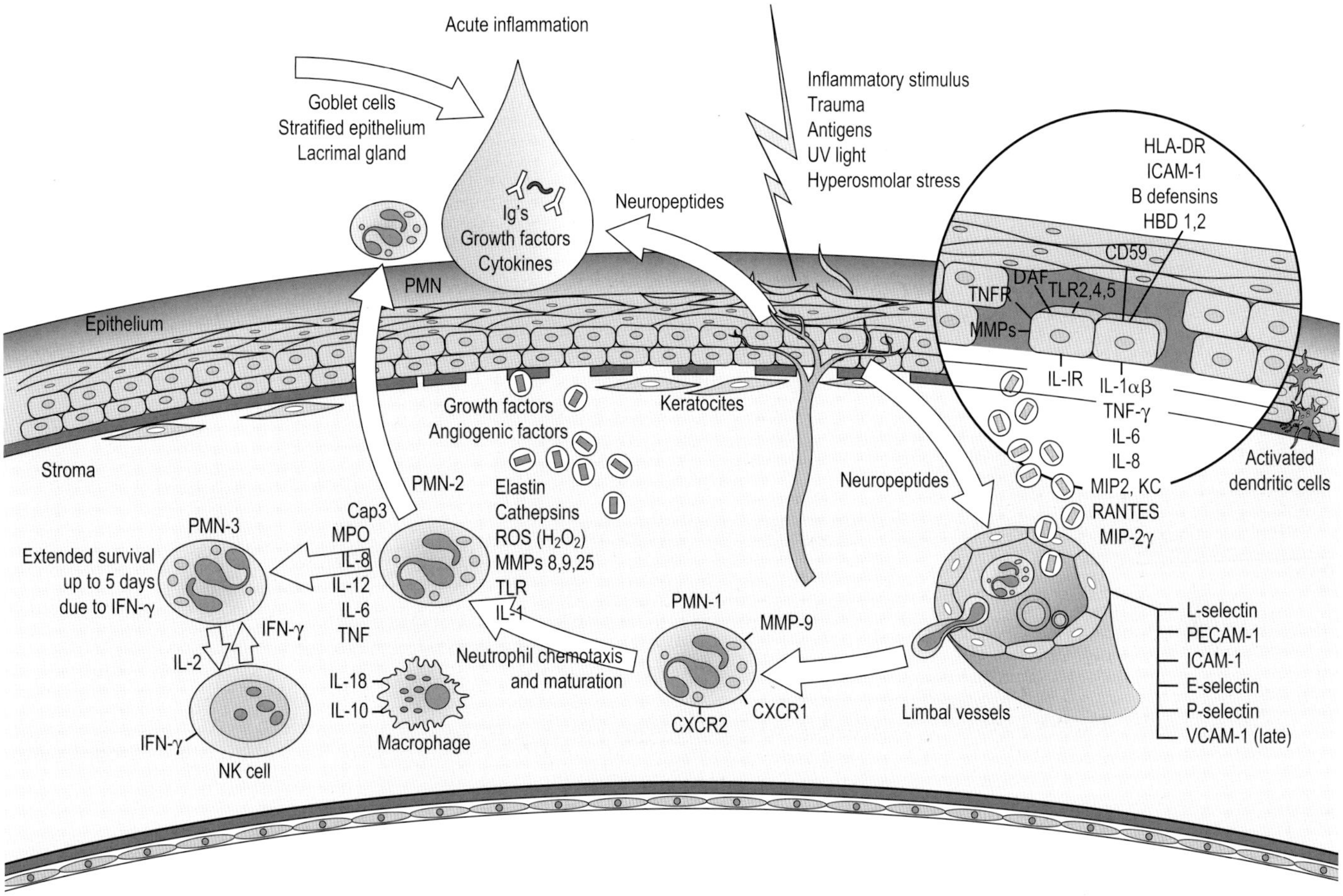

Fig. 5.17 Acute inflammation. Following an acute stimulus, cells release IL-1, IL-6, IL-8, and TNF α, which stimulates the migration of limbal Langerhans cell into the central cornea. These cytokines also upregulate ICAM-1, E-selectin, L-selectin, PECAM-1 on the vascular endothelium of the limbus, and facilitate PMN (PMN-1) infiltration. Complement becomes activated and local receptors regulate the complement response. Specific growth factors and angiogenic factors are also released. Keratomalacia may result from IL-1-stimulated IL-8 release and activation of PMNs (PMN-2), which release metalloproteinase (MMP) and other lysozomal enzymes that cause corneal ulceration. IFN-γ and IL-2 release may exend PMN (PMN-3) and recruitment of NK cells.

Cells of the lymphoid system

B lymphocytes

B lymphocytes constitute 5–15% of the circulating lymphocytes and are primarily responsible for the humoral (antibody) arm of the adaptive immune response. B cells manufacture a large number (20000 to 200000) of specific immunoglobulins, which are expressed on their cell surface. There are five subclasses of B lymphocytes: IgG, IgA, IgM, IgE, IgD.

There are many surface markers on B cells. Most human B cells in the peripheral blood express IgM and IgD. The receptor for the Fc portion of IgG (FcγRII, CD32) is also expressed on B cells. Major histocompatibility class (MHC) II antigens are also located on most B cells and provide the 'antigen-presenting' capacity of these cells. B cells can endocytose and present antigen to helper T lymphocytes in the context of their surface MHC class II molecules.

T lymphocytes

T lymphocytes make up 65–85% of peripheral blood lymphocytes and direct the cell-mediated arm of the adaptive immune response.[65] T cells develop from cell precursors within the thymus where 90% of cells are T lymphocytes. During intrathymic differentiation, the repertoire of T-cell antigen receptor (TCR) specificities is generated. The T-cell antigen receptor is the definitive marker for T lymphocytes. Each T-cell antigen receptor is also associated with the CD3 or T-cell differentiation antigen, which is made up of five polypeptides. T cells have MHC class II HLA-DR surface antigens.

Three major functional subsets of helper T cells have been characterized: Th1, Th2 and Th17. The differences between the three major subtypes are defined primarily by their unique patterns of cytokine secretion. Regulation of the immune responses through these three subsets of T helper cells is depicted in Figure 5.19. Th1 cells manufacture IFN-γ and TNF-β. IFN-γ increases the production of IL-12 by

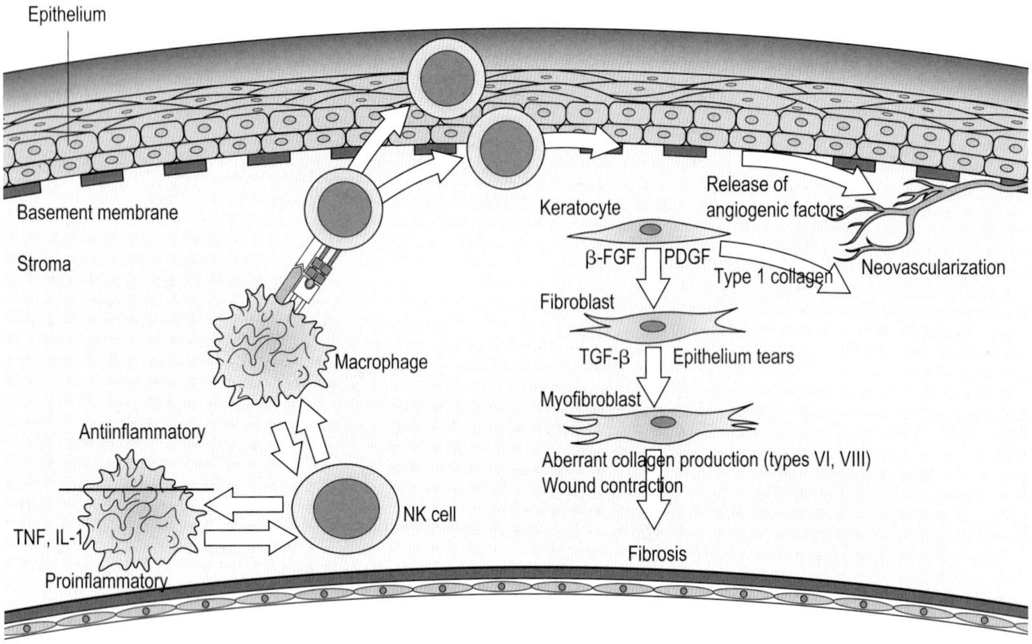

Fig. 5.18 Chronic immune/inflammatory response. In the chronic phases of immune/inflammatory responses, infiltrating lymphocytes (NK cells) release IFN-γ, which stimulates an upregulation of ICAM-1 and HLA-DR coexpression on the corneal stroma/endothelium, thereby providing the mechanism for HLA-DR-dependent cell-mediated cytotoxicity. Macrophages may play either a proinflammatory or antiinflammatory role depending on the cytokines released. Specific immune responses through antigen processing (between the macrophage and T lymphocyte) result in the production of Th1 or Th2 lymphocytes. The Th1 responses result in release of IL-2, IFN-γ associated with viral infections, graft rejection, and dry eye. Th2 responses result in the release of IL-4, IL-5, and IL-13. These are associated with allergic and parasitic reactions. In addition, keratocytes through the action of bFGF and PDGF transform into fibroblasts and through TGF-β become myofibroblasts producing aberrant collagen (types V, VIII) leading to stromal scarring. Angiogenic factors also result in abnormal stromal vascularization.

Table 5.1 Soluble mediators and receptors of inflammation (important examples)

Group	Example	Source/cell	Target/ligand/action
Adhesion molecule	Intercellular adhesion molecule 1 (ICAM-1)	Endothelial cells (EC)	Lymphocyte function associated antigen 1 (LFA-1) Promote leukocyte recruitment
	Very late antigen 1 (VLA-1)	T cells	Collagen, fibronectin, laminin
	Vascular cell adhesion molecule (VCAM)	Endothelial cells (EC) Macrophage (MΦ)	Very late antigen 4 (VLA4)
	Platelet endothelial cell adhesion molecule (PECAM)	T cells	Endothelial cells (EC) Platelets
	Fas ligand (Fas L)	Many cells	Fas ligand receptor (FasR) Apoptosis Cytotoxic T-cell activity Corneal immune privilege
	Tumor necrosis factor (TNF)-related apoptosis inducing ligand (TRAIL)	T cells	Apoptosis Death receptors DR4 (TRAIL-RI) and DR5 (TRAIL-RII).
	Mucosal adressin cell adhesion molecule 1 (MAdCAM-1)	T lymphocytes (T)	Lymphocyte Peyer's patch HEV adhesion molecule 1 (LPAM-1 or integrin α4β7)
	P-selectin	Endothelial cells (EC)	White blood cells (WBC)

Table 5.1 Soluble mediators and receptors of inflammation (important examples) – cont'd

Group	Example	Source/cell	Target/ligand/action
	E-selectin	Endothelial cells (EC)	White blood cells (WBC)
	L-selectin	White blood cells (WBC)	Endothelial cells (EC)
Chemokines	Chemokine ligand 5 (CCL5), Regulated in activation of normal T cells expressed and secreted (RANTES)	T cells Basophils (BΦ) Eosinophils (EΦ)	Chemotactic for T cells, eosinophils, basophils Activation of natural killer (NK) cells
	CXCR1,2	Natural killer (NK) cells, basophils (BΦ)	IL-8
	Interleukin 8 (IL-8)	Fibroblasts Corneal epithelial cells (EpC)	Corneal neovascularization Attract neutrophils
Chemotactic factors	Eosinophil chemotactic factor	Mast cells (MC)	Attract eosinophils
	Neutrophil chemotactic factor	Mast cells (MC)	Attract neutrophils
	Eotaxin	Eosinophils (EΦ)	Attract eosinophils
	Macrophage migration inhibiting factor (MIF)	T cells	Cell-mediated immunity (CMI) Immunoregulation Inflammation
	Platelet activating factor (PAF)	Mast cell (MC)	Vasodilatation Increase permeability
Clotting and fibrinolytic factors	Fibrin (factor Ia)	Fibrinogen	Clotting Inflammation
	Thrombin (factor XIII)	Endothelial cells	Converts fibrinogen to fibrin
	Fibrinogen (factor I)	Liver	Fibrin precursor
	Laminin	Basal epithelial cells	Integrins
	Fibronectin	Macrophages (MΦ)	
Complement	Complement factor C5a	Hepatocytes, APC	Anaphylatoxin Histamine release from mast cells Neutrophil chemotaxis
	Complement factor C3a	Macrophages	Chemotaxis Anaphylatoxin
	Complement factor C3b (opsonin)		Opsonize bacteria by macrophage (MΦ)
	Decay accelerating factor (DAF)	Corneal epithelial cells (EpC)	Complement regulation prevents the assembly of the C3bBb complex
Colony stimulating factors	Granulocyte-macrophage colony-stimulating factor (GM-CSF)	Macrophages (MΦ), fibroblasts (FB)	Macrophage activation
Cytokines	Interleukin 1 (IL-1α, β)	Corneal epithelial cells (EpC) Macrophages (MΦ), Langerhans cells (LC)	T-cell stimulation, metalloproteinase induction, Adhesion molecule expression
	Interleukin 1 receptor (IL-1R)		
	Interleukin 2 (IL-2)	T helper 1 cells (Th1) Natural killer (NK) cells Keratocytes	T: proliferation and lymphokine secretion Th2: induces interferon gamma (IFN-γ) secretion

Table 5.1 Soluble mediators and receptors of inflammation (important examples) – cont'd

Group	Example	Source/cell	Target/ligand/action
	Interleukin 4 (IL-4)	T helper 2 cells (Th2) Natural killer (NK) cells Mast cells (MC)	Increase IgE Decrease proinflammatory cytokines Suppress T helper 1 (Th1)
	Interleukin 6 (IL-6) (IFN-β2)	T helper 2 cells (Th2) Macrophages (MΦ) Dendritic cells (DC) Mast cells (MC)	T-cell activation B-cell Ig secretion Macrophages (MΦ) differentiation
	Interleukin 10 (IL-10)	T helper 2 cells (Th2) Macrophages (MΦ) Mast cells (MC)	Th1: inhibit IL-2, IL-3, interferon gamma (IFN-γ) synthesis Th1: inhibit DTH Macrophage (MΦ): inhibit TNF, IL-1, IL-12 production
	Interleukin 12 (IL-12)	Macrophages (MΦ) Dendritic cells (DC)	T helper 1 (Th1) differentiation Interferon gamma (IFN-γ) production
	Interleukin 18 (IL-18)	Macrophages (MΦ)	Cell-mediated immunity (CMI) Inflammation
	Tumor necrosis factor alpha (TNF-α)	T cells Macrophages (MΦ) Mast cells (MC)	T-cell stimulation Matrix metalloproteinase (MMP) induction Adhesion molecule expression
	Interferon gamma (IFN-γ)	T cells Natural killer (NK) cells	HLA-DR expression Activation of: T cells, natural killer (NK) cells, macrophages (MΦ)
	Interferon alpha (IFN-α) (14 subtypes)	Macrophages (MΦ) Leukocytes	Innate immune response (virus) IFN-α receptor (IFNAR)
Eicosanoids	Leukotriene B4	Mast cells (MC)	Promotes inflammation and breakdown blood–ocular barriers
	Leukotriene C4	Eosinophils (EΦ)	Increase capillary permeability
	Prostaglandin D2 (PGD2)	Mast cells (MC)	Vasodilatation
Growth factors	Vascular endothelial factor (VEGF-A, B, C, D)	RPE and neurosensory retinal cells	Angiogenesis Lymphangiogenesis Macrophage chemotaxis Vasodilation
	TGF-β	Many cells	Fibroblast proliferation Collagen synthesis Decrease matrix metalloproteinases Decrease T-cell proliferation Decrease proinflammatory cytokines
	TGF-α	Macrophages (MΦ)	Epithelial growth Neural cell development
	Nerve growth factor (NGF)	B cells T cells Fibroblasts	Nerve proliferation and development
	Basic fibroblast growth factor (bFGF)	Basement membrane Vascular subendothelial matrix	Angiogenesis
	Epidermal growth factor (EGF)	Macrophages Platelets	Epidermal growth factor receptor (EGFR) Epithelial migration
	Platelet derived growth factor (PDGF)	Platelets	Angiogenesis

Table 5.1 Soluble mediators and receptors of inflammation (important examples) – cont'd

Group	Example	Source/cell	Target/ligand/action
Immunoglobulins	Immunoglobulin A (IgA)	B lymphocytes	Mucosal immunity
	Immunoglobulin D (IgD)	Immature B cells	B-cell activation
	Immunoglobulin E (IgE)	B lymphocytes	Allergy, type I reactions Binds to Fc receptors on mast cells (MC)
	Immunoglobulin G (IgG)	B lymphocytes	Ig2a fixes complement
	Immunoglobulin M (IgM)	B lymphocytes	Complement activation
Kinin forming system	Bradykinin	Vascular endothelial cells	Increase vascular permeability Vasodilator
Leukocyte oxidants	Hydrogen peroxide	Polymorphonuclear cells	Oxidizes free radicals
Neuropeptides	Substance P	Neural cells	Inflammation and pain neurokinin 1 receptor (NK1-receptor, NK1R)
	Alpha melanocyte stimulating hormone (α-MSH)	Pituitary cells	Suppresses inflammation and T-cell responses
Proteases/enzymes	Collagenase (MMP-1,8,13,18)	Keratocytes (K) Corneal epithelial cells (EpC) Polymorphonuclear cells	Degrade collagen and stromal matrix
	Membrane type matrix metalloproteinases (MMP, 14–17)	Keratocytes (K)	Activate progelatinase A
	Gelatinases (matrix metalloproteinases [MMP] 2,9)	Keratocytes (K)	Native type IV, V, VII collagens Fibronectin
	Matrilysins (matrix metalloproteinases [MMP] 7,12,19,20)	Keratocytes (K)	Gelatins Fibronectin Elastin
	Stromelysins (matrix metalloproteinases [MMP] 3,10,11)	Keratocytes (K)	Proteoglycans, fibronectin, serine proteinase inhibitors
	Cathepsins (A and B)	Lysosomes	Protease activity
	Tryptase	Mast cell (MC)	Complement activation
	Peroxidase	Eosinophil (EΦ)	Epithelial cytotoxicity
	Lysozyme	Macrophages (MΦ) Lacrimal acinar cells (AC)	Degrade bacterial cell walls
Vasoactive amines	Histamine	Mast cell (MC)	Dilate blood vessels
Other	MBP	Eosinophil (EΦ)	Mast cell degranulation
	Heparin	Mast cell (MC)	Anticoagulation
	Cationic protein	Eosinophil (EΦ)	Epithelial cytotoxicity
	Lactoferrin	Lacrimal acinar cells	Monocytes, macrophages, PMN Antimicrobial activity Binds divalent cations

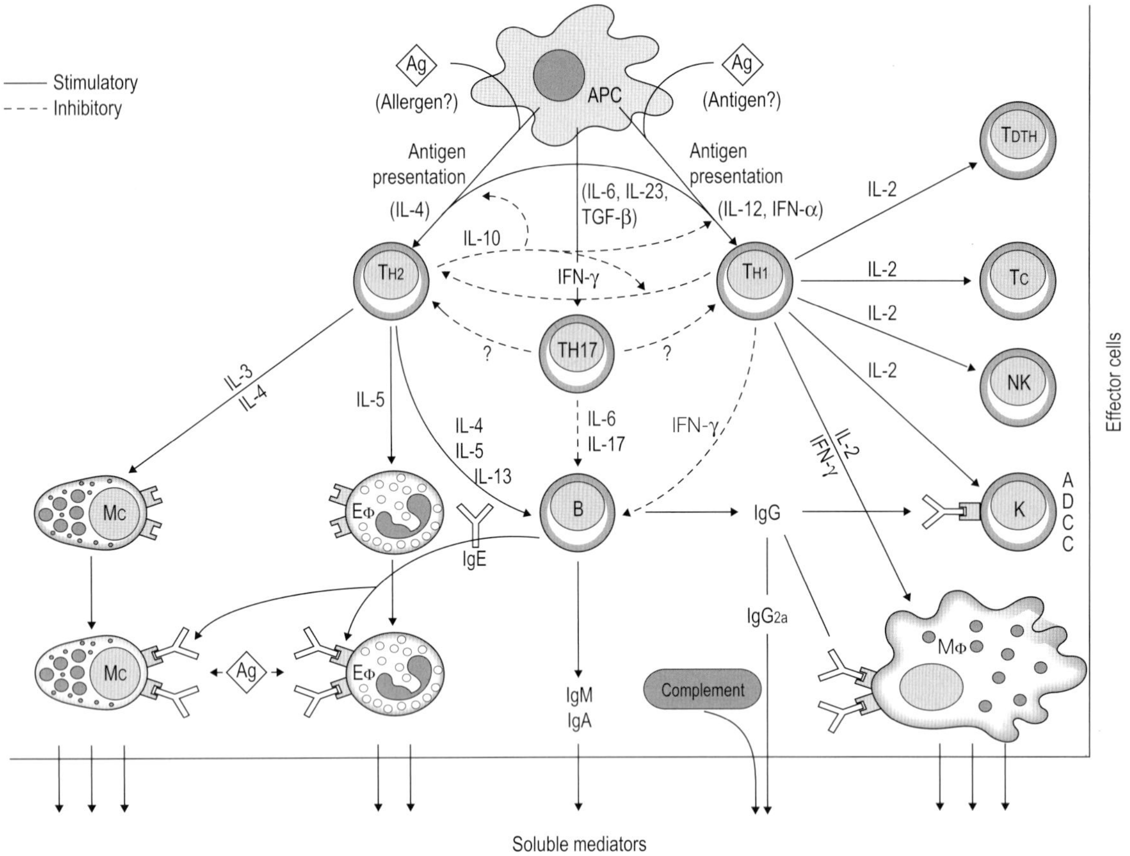

Fig. 5.19 Cytokine regulation of the acquired immune response. Hypothetical activation pathways of proposed Th1, Th2 and Th17 cells leading to effector cell stimulation are depicted. Hypothetical stimulatory pathways (*solid arrows*) and inhibitory effects (*dashed arrows*) are shown. Th1 cells release IFN-γ, which inhibits Th2 cells. Th2 cells release IL-10, which may inhibit IFN-γ production and APC activation of Th1 cells. Th17 cells produce IL-17, IL-6 and G-CSF. Allergens seem to preferentially activate Th2 cells, which stimulate IgE-mediated allergic responses (including IgE F_{ce} receptors). IL-3 and IL-4 release would also activate mucosal mast cells, and IL-5 stimulates eosinophil proliferation. Activation of Th1 cells would also be inhibited. On the other hand, APCs seem to present antigens more to the Th1 side of the immune response. These cells release IL-2 and IFN-γ, mediating CTL and macrophage activation and IgG_{2a} production. Antibody-dependent, cell-mediated cytotoxicity (ADCC) and delayed-type hypersensitivity (DTH) responses are also mediated by this pathway. This response is characteristic for responses to intracellular (viral, parasitic) antigens. (Adapted from Roitt IM, Brostoff J, Male DK, eds. *Immunology*, London, 1993, Mosby; Niederkorn JY, Li XY. *Invest Ophthalmol Vis Sci* 1995; 35:S817.)

dendritic cells and macrophages, and via positive feedback, IL-12 stimulates the production of IFN-γ in helper T cells, thereby promoting the Th1 profile. Th2 cells secrete IL-4, IL-5, IL-6, IL-10, and IL-13. The Type 2 response promotes its own profile using two different cytokines. IL-4 acts on helper T cells to promote the production of Th2 cytokines , while IL-10 inhibits a variety of cytokines including IL-2 and IFN-γ in helper T cells and IL-12 in dendritic cells and macrophages. T helper 17 cells (Th17) are a newly discovered subset of T helper cells producing IL-17, IL-6, IL-22, and G-CSF. They are considered developmentally distinct from Th1 and Th2 cells and excessive amounts of the cell are thought to play a key role in inflammation and autoimmune disease such as autoimmune uveitis, juvenile diabetes, rheumatoid arthritis. IL-22 may play an important role in mucosal immunity.

Cytotoxic T cells (Tc) are CD8+ positive and carry the TCR-2 receptor. They participate in reactions related to cell destruction. They are MHC class I restricted and destroy viral infected cells and foreign allogeneic cells.

Null lymphocytes

Natural killer (NK) cells are a heterogeneous population of granular, nonadherent, nonphagocytic lymphocytes found in the peripheral blood, spleen, and lymph nodes. They represent 10–15% of circulating lymphocytes or 5% of all white cells. There are more NK cells in circulation than B cells.

NK cells function in immune surveillance. They destroy cells without prior sensitization or interaction with antigen presenting cells. NK cells participate in the innate arm of the immune response and kill tumor cells, viral infected cells, and xenogeneic cells. NK cells release IFN-γ, TNF-α, and IL-1 as well as other soluble cytotoxic factors, including NK cytotoxic factor. The cytolytic activity of NK cells may be enhanced by several lymphokines including IFN-α, IFN-β, IL-2, and IL-4.[65]

Cells of the myeloid system

Macrophages and the mononuclear phagocytic system

The mononuclear phagocyte system consists of a single population of cells called macrophages (MΦ). Macrophages are located throughout the body and provide a number of important functions in host defense. These bone marrow-derived cells develop from a myeloid progenitor cell, enter the bloodstream as monocytes, and migrate into various tissues as macrophages.

Macrophages are the preeminent APC. They serve as a link between the innate and adaptive immune responses, actively participating in innate immune responses through phagocytosis of foreign material. Macrophages mediate the initiation and effector phases of immune responses. They also influence lymphocyte responses to antigen and can stimulate T lymphocytes directly.

Macrophages produce a variety of important secretory factors including proteases, collagenases, angiotensin-converting enzyme, lysozyme, fibronectin, platelet activating factor, arachidonic acid derivatives, prostaglandins, leukotrienes, and oxygen metabolites. Macrophages also release soluble products called monokines, which include IFN-α, IL-1, IL-6, and TNF-α.[65]

Dendritic cells

Dendritic cells (DC) make up a system of specialized APCs within the mononuclear phagocytic system. This network of highly motile cells initiates a variety of immune responses, particularly antigen recognition and processing. Dendritic cells migrate between tissues and home to specific T-cell-dependent areas of lymph nodes and other lymphoid structures. Dendritic cells contain specialized cell surface adhesion molecules (β2 integrins), which are associated with their homing function. Dendritic cells are found in a variety of nonlymphoid tissues including the epithelium of the skin, the ocular surface, iris, ciliary body, and other mucosal epithelia.[67–69]

Langerhans cells

Langerhans cells (LC) are bone marrow-derived DC that are also part of the monocyte/macrophage family. Langerhans cells are found in the thymus, lymph nodes, and epithelial layers of the skin, oral cavity, esophagus, nasopharynx, cervix, conjunctiva, and cornea.[67–70] They are important immunocompetent cells of the ocular surface and mucosal immune system. Langerhans cells have been extensively studied for their capacity to present antigen to T lymphocytes and trigger T-cell proliferative responses.

Other cells of the myeloid system

Polymorphonuclear leukocytes

The myeloid system is made up of erythrocytes, platelets, monocytes, and granulocytes. Polymorphonuclear (PMN) leukocytes (also called granulocytes) are divided into three categories: neutrophils, basophils, and eosinophils. Granulocytes represent 60–70% of circulating white cells and are relatively short lived. They participate in the innate immune response by migrating into tissues at sites of inflammation and releasing mediators.[65]

The neutrophil is the first cell type to appear at sites of inflammation and infection. It possesses two types of cytoplasmic granules: primary (azurophilic or lysosomal) and secondary (specific) granules. These granules contain a variety of enzymes including myeloperoxidase, acid and alkaline phosphatases, and lysozyme. They phagocytose organisms and degrade them through their lysosomal enzymes. The cell surface of neutrophils contains many types of adhesion molecules that regulate their migration out of the vascular compartment and into the tissues.

Eosinophils

Eosinophilic granulocytes (eosinophils) represent about 2–5% of peripheral leukocytes. They possess intracellular granules rich in acid phosphatase and peroxidase and have the capacity to activate a wide variety of other cells including basophils, neutrophils, and platelets. Eosinophil major basic protein (MBP) is released by these cells and induces the production of IL-8 by other eosinophils, macrophages, and T cells.[65] Eosinophils are phagocytic and participate in the ingestion of antigen as well as antibody complexes. They can present antigen through their cell surface MHC class II antigen.

Basophils

Basophilic granulocytes (basophils) make up less than 0.5% of all circulating leukocytes. Mast cells have characteristics similar to basophils, including receptors for Ig. However, basophils release different cytokines (IL-4, IL-13) and have different cell surface receptors for cytokines (IL-1 to IL-5).[65] Basophils circulate in the peripheral blood, and have life spans of several days, like other granulocytes. They migrate to sites of inflammation, particularly during the late phase of allergic reactions and possess a wide variety of cell surface receptors for adhesion molecules.[71]

Mast cells

Mast cells play active roles in both innate and adaptive immune responses.[65,66] Mast cells have receptors for IL-4, IL-6 and release TNF-α, IL-3 to -6, -10, -13, -16, VEGF, and GM-CSF (see Table 5.1). Mast cells are present only in mucosal epithelia and connective tissue and have life spans of months. They participate in all four types of hypersensitivity responses.

Two functionally and structurally distinct types of mast cells are characterized by their surface receptors, tissue distribution, and cell products. Mucosal mast cells (MMC) are located primarily in the gut, lung, and eye.[71,72] The connective tissue mast cells (CTMC) are found in the skin and peritoneum. MMCs are regulated in part through IL-3 released by Th2 lymphocytes. CTMC, however, are not T cell/IL-3 dependent. MMC contain IgE both on their surface and within the cell, whereas CTMC contain IgE only on the surface. MMC release tryptase and chrondroitan sulfate, whereas CTMC release tryptase and chymase as specific proteases.

Soluble Mediators/Receptors of Inflammation

Adhesion molecules

Adhesion molecules are cell-surface proteins that regulate cell–cell interactions, as well as cellular contact with intercellular matrix proteins such as collagen and fibronectin. Adhesion molecules participate in a variety of processes including antigen presentation, migration of leukocytes to inflammatory sites, lymphocyte homing to specific tissues, and adherence of immunocompetent cells to resident (target) cells. Adhesion molecules are selected to perform distinct effector functions based on their cell background and factors present in the local environment.

A multistep process occurs for neutrophil and monocyte migration out of the vascular system into sites of inflammation. This combination of steps and multiplicity of ligand pairs provides the diversity for regulating the multitude of leukocyte functions in vivo. This cascade of overlapping but successive phases is similar to the multistep process involved in blood clotting and complement-mediated killing.

Adhesion molecules are classified into several groups of similar structures: selectins, integrins, and immunoglobulins.[65] The selectins regulate the first phase of 'tethering and rolling' of leukocytes along the margin of the vascular endothelium. The slowing down of cells ends with the more firm adhesion of the cell to the endothelium. The second 'activation' phase results from chemoattractants, or chemokines, released from the vessel wall, which activate the second group of adhesion molecules, the integrins, on the leukocyte to mediate 'firm adhesion' to their immunoglobulin superfamily ligands on the vascular wall. The final phase of 'transendothelial migration' of leukocyte entry into inflamed tissue is also mediated by integrin molecules. Certain endothelial adhesion molecules also demonstrate organ- and tissue-specific expression and specific leukocytes also have specific homing molecules with differential expression. Blocking the expression of these molecules may inhibit inflammatory processes.

Cytokines

The term cytokine refers to any intercellular peptides or glycopeptides secreted by immune and nonimmune cells.[65,66] Cytokines act on other hematopoietic cells to modulate immune and inflammatory responses. They differ from hormones and growth factors, which act on nonhematopoietic cells. The group of cytokines includes the interleukins, TNF, chemokines, colony-stimulating factors, interferons, and growth factors (see Table 5.1).

Different cytokines can act on the same cell type to mediate similar effects (redundancy). Cytokine receptors generally consist of two polypeptide chains: a ligand binding receptor, and a nonbinding signal transducer. Different ligand binding molecules may share the same signal transducer, which may explain in part the redundancy in cytokine effects. The effects of each cytokine also depend on the specific target cell (pleiotropism). Many cytokines function as part of a complex cascade of cytokine responses between cells and can act synergistically as well.

Because cytokines depend on a variety of factors, including the specific combination and concentration of each cytokine, the effects of the cytokine network is determined to a large extent by the local environment. Because of their role in inflammation, synthesis of most cytokines is highly regulated, especially in the cornea where unchecked inflammation could lead to significant functional loss.[65,66,68]

Chemokines

Chemokines are small secreted molecules which have both chemoattractant and cytokine properties.[65,66,73] They have four families, comprising: CXC (α), CC (β), XC (γ), and CX3C (δ) (see Table 5.1). Chemokines can be divided into constitutive (SDF-1, TARC, SLC, etc.) and inducible (RANTES, MIP1s, IL-8, and MCP). Constitutive chemokines are expressed in primary and secondary lymphoid organs and regulate lymphocyte traffic in physiologic conditions while the inducible chemokines play roles in response to inflammatory conditions. One of the important features of chemokines is their redundancy: most receptors interact with multiple chemokines and most chemokines bind to most receptors.[65,74]

Complement

The complement system is a potent mechanism for initiating and amplifying the inflammatory host response against bacteria and foreign antigens. The complement system involves a set of proteins numbered C1 to C9, which interact in a cascade-like fashion determined by a series of enzymatic steps. It is an integral component of the humoral immune response and participates in types II and III hypersensitivity responses.[65] It also participates in discrimination between self and nonself. Both recognition and effector pathways promote the inflammatory response, assist in immune complex formation, and alter the plasma membrane of cells leading to cell death. Three major functions of complement are opsonization of bacteria/immune complexes, target cell lysis, and activation of phagocytosis.

Two pathways can activate the complement cascade. The classic pathway is activated by IgG or IgM bound to a specific target. C1 has three components: C1q, C1r, and C1s. C1q binds with the Fc receptor on the Ig molecule and becomes activated. Activated C1 then initiates the cascade of proteolytic events.

The alternative pathway (also called the properdin system) directly activates the complement system without the participation of antibody. This process occurs through stimulation by several factors including the Fab (in contrast to the Fc of the classic pathway) area of immunoglobulin complexes (IgA, IgE, IgG), zymosan, endotoxin, and bacterial cell walls.

Formation of C3 convertase is a critical step in both classic and alternative pathways. This enzyme stimulates the formation of C3b (the opsonin component) and C4b, which bind to cell membranes. The final common pathway of the complement system is cell destruction by osmotic lysis, which is mediated by the formation of membrane attack complex (MAC) (factors C5–C9). C5a, the chemoattractant component, serves to recruit other inflammatory cells.

In the eye, activation of the complement cascade must be controlled to focus on foreign targets and not on host cells, and mechanisms are in place to regulate this process (see Fig. 5.17). C1–7 and factors B and P have all been identified in the cornea.

There are three principal locations of complement regulatory proteins: fluid phase (C1-INH, Factors I and H, S protein-40 [SP-40]); cell membranes (decay accelerating factor (DAF, CD55), membrane cofactor protein (MCP, CD46), and CD59, and membrane C3 proteinases; and matrix (decorin).[65] All cell membrane regulatory proteins (DAF, MCP, CD59, and decorin) are expressed differentially in the normal human cornea (see Fig. 5.17). CD59 blocks the interaction of C9 and C8, preventing the formation of membrane attack complexes and subsequent polymerization of C9. DAF, MCP, and CD59 are strongly expressed in the corneal epithelium and limbus, whereas CD59 is expressed more than DAF or MCP on the keratocytes, suggesting that a complement regulatory system in the eye inhibits destruction of normal tissue. Decorin, a dermatan sulfate proteoglycan, binds C1q with high affinity.

Tissue Components of the Ocular Immune System

Mucosa-associated immune system (MALT)

Granulocytes and monocytes are eliminated during inflammation. Lymphocytes, APCs (macrophages), and DC, however, recirculate from the spleen and lymph nodes through the blood and lymphatic system to sites where specific antigen was first encountered. More than 1% of the total lymphocyte pool circulates every hour. Lymphocyte migration from the blood vessels into specific tissues is controlled by the expression of complementary pairs of homing receptors (HR) on lymphocytes and vascular addressins (VA) on endothelial cells. Addressins are tissue- and organ-specific endothelial cell glycoproteins that bind to specific adhesion molecules on specific lymphocytes. The vascular addressins are constitutively expressed on various tissue components of the mucosa-associated lymphoid tissue (MALT).

MALT is a distinct network of diffuse aggregates of lymphoid tissue located in a variety of mucosal surfaces including the gut (GALT), bronchus (BALT), conjunctiva (CALT), nasal mucosa (NALT), and mammary gland.[75] Because mucosa-associated lymphocytes actually recirculate throughout the many sites, the various components actually compose a distinct lymphoid structure. Antigenic access is augmented through specialized epithelial cells which work with other APCs in the conjunctiva, particularly Langerhans cells.[67,68] The processess of antigen presentation, Ig production and T-cell activation then take place. T-suppressor cells predominate over Th cells in the conjunctiva.

The lacrimal functional unit (LFU)

The lacrimal gland, tear film, ocular surface epithelium (cornea and conjunctiva, and the meibomian glands), eyelids, and the interconnecting sensory and motor nerves comprise a complex functional unit which modulates the homeostasis of the ocular surface.[73,75,76] The local immune pathways are determined by a wide variety of factors including the products of the lacrimal gland. In the normal lacrimal gland, the predominant lymphocytic cell type in the lymphocytic aggregates of the interstitium is the plasma cell (IgA and IgD), important vehicles of the adaptive immune response. Tc cells constitute the predominant cell type in the interstitium away from the lymphoid aggregates. With age, the acinar elements undergo degenerative changes, atrophy, and decrease in number. The IgA secretory piece, which binds two IgA molecules, is produced by the acinar epithelial cells.

The Cell-Mediated Immune (CMI) Response

Major histocompatibility complex[65]

The major histocompatibility complex (MHC) is a region on human chromosome 6p21.31 which is the most gene-dense region of the human genome. The MHC is divided into three regions: class I, class II, and class III. These genes code for cell membrane glycoproteins important in immune regulation. Class I antigens consist of a single glycoprotein chain that is noncovalently associated with a smaller protein, α2 microglobulin. These antigens code for the HLA-A, HLA-B, and HLA-C antigens found on all nucleated cells. Class I molecules present peptides from endogenous antigens to CD8+ T cells. Class II antigens consist of two noncovalently linked glycoprotein chains, α and β. These code for HLA-DP, HLA-DQ, and HLA-DR antigens, which are present on several important immunocompetent cells including monocytes, macrophages, dendritic cells (including Langerhans cells), and B lymphocytes. These molecules present peptides from exogenous antigens to CD4+ T cells. Cells not normally expressing class II antigens may be stimulated to express them by certain cytokines such as IFN-γ (from Th1, NK cells). Class II antigens function in regulating the immune response primarily through interactions between lymphocytes and macrophages or antigen presenting cells. The class III region contains genes which code for molecules of the complement system, inflammation, and other system functions.

Antigen presentation and T-cell activation[65]

Antigen processing is a complex sequence of events between a T lymphocyte and an antigen processing cell. This involves a complex process of antigen recognition, antigen uptake, intracellular processing, and finally presentation to resting Th lymphocytes. Activated Th cells then interact with and sensitize other cells to bring about immune responses. Although macrophages, monocytes, and DC are the most important antigen processing cells, other parenchymal cells may be stimulated by IFN-γ to acquire antigen-presenting capacity. The activated Th cell then stimulates the differentiation and clonal expansion of a variety of committed antigen-specific effector cells through the secretion of a variety of cytokines including IL-2 to IL-6, IFN-γ, and TNF-β. IL-2 stimulates antigen-responding cytotoxic T cells (Tc) to mediate the direct tissue destruction and cells of delayed-type hypersensitivity to mediate DTH responses. IL-2, IL-4, and IL-5 also stimulate B cells to produce memory cells and antibody-producing plasma cells.

Cell-mediated immune response

A variety of cell-mediated immune (CMI) responses can be T-cell dependent or T-cell independent.[65] T-cell-independent responses constitute the innate immune response and include phagocytosis by PMNs, complement-mediated cell destruction, and cytotoxic activity of NK cells and macrophages. Th-cell-dependent responses are more complex, and the mechanism by which specific pathways are selected is unknown. There is some evidence that allergens may preferentially activate Th2 cells, whereas antigens mediate their effects through Th1 activation (see Fig. 5.19). Th cells contribute to the differentiation and proliferation of effector cells and the final mechanism of target cell/antigen destruction/elimination. The main effector cell pathways take place via cytotoxic lymphocytes (Tc, NK, K), but also through mast cells and eosinophils through antigen-specific IgE. In antibody-dependent cell-mediated cytotoxicity (ADCC), cytotoxic cells that possess the Fc receptor for IgG on their cell membrane mediate cell destruction through the release of cytotoxic cytokines (TNF-α, TNF-β, IFN-γ). Complement also may play a role in this mechanism. Finally, lymphokine-mediated macrophage activation also occurs through T_{DTH} cells. If the CMI response fails to effectively eliminate the antigen, tumor cells, or transplant antigen, then the localization of T cells, immune complexes, macrophages, and PMN may lead to chronic inflammation and granuloma formation.

The Humoral (Antibody-Mediated) Immune Response

Binding of antigen to antibodies located on the plasma membrane leads to B-cell activation. After contact with antigen, Ig actively migrates within the cell membrane to form a 'cap,' which is then either internalized or shed. B cells respond to specific antigenic stimulation, with help from T-helper cells (Th cells), by blastogenic transformation. This transformation is associated with increased protein and DNA synthesis, antibody synthesis, and finally differentiation into plasma and memory cells. Plasma cells are immunoglobulin 'factories' that manufacture a specific antibody. Memory cells are previously sensitized cells that manufacture a specific antibody. They account for the more rapid and effective immune response following reexposure to antigen.

Immunoglobulins

Characteristics of immunoglobulins[65]

Antibodies are immunoglobulins (Ig) produced by B lymphocytes in response to antigenic stimulation. They play a key role together with the T-cell antigen receptors in providing the characteristic specificity of the adaptive immune response. Immunoglobulins are composed of four polypeptide chains linked together by disulfide bonds. Two of the chains are longer than the others and are termed heavy (H) chains; the two shorter chains are termed light (L) chains. Similar amino acid sequences are termed constant (C) regions, while other sequences are variable (V). A small sequence that is quite variable is termed hypervariable. This region is associated with the antigen-binding portion of the immunoglobulin. Antibody-mediated immunity requires noncovalent contact between the antigen and antibody. Antigenicity is the physicochemical binding of an antigen to an antibody while immunogenicity is the ability to induce the biosynthesis of antibody in a physiological property.

There are five classes of immunoglobulins in humans: IgG, IgA, IgM, IgE, and IgD. IgG accounts for about 75% of the serum Ig and it is the principal antibody of the secondary immune response. It fixes complement (IgG2a) and plays an important role in mediating inflammation and fighting infection through types II, III, and IV hypersensitivity reactions. By binding to Fc receptors on macrophages, NK cells, mast cells, and basophils, it also functions in the cytotoxic arm of the immune response through ADCC.

IgA is the next most common serum Ig and makes up about 15–20% of circulating Ig molecules. IgA functions primarily in opsonization, neutralization of toxins, and agglutination. IgA is a dimer with a secretory form containing a stabilizing secretory component that is synthesized by glandular epithelial cells (lacrimal). The secretory component protects the Ig from proteolysis by enzymes usually found on the mucosal (ocular) surface. IgA, and more specifically secretory IgA (sIgA), is the predominant Ig found in external secretions such as tears, saliva, milk, and the mucosa of the respiratory and digestive tracts. Therefore, it participates in the peripheral surveillance system of the mucosa-associated lymphoid tissue (MALT) where there is frequent exposure to a wide variety of foreign antigens.

IgM is the largest Ig and is composed of five Ig molecules. It constitutes only 5–10% of the total serum Ig. IgM is the predominant Ig formed after initial exposure to antigen and plays a dominant role in agglutination, complement fixation, and cytolysis. Because of its size and structure, IgM has a high antigen-combining capacity and does not migrate across the placenta.

IgE is an important mediator of anaphylactic responses and ocular allergy. The IgE molecule is fixed to mast cells and basophils through the Fc receptor. There are several types of Fc receptors with variable affinities. In an immune response to allergen, Th2 cells respond by releasing IL-4, which promotes an isotype switching to IgE production (see Fig. 5.19). After binding with antigen, IgE mediates the type I hypersensitivity immune response characterized by histamine and vasoactive mediator release.

Anterior Chamber Associated Immune Deviation (ACAID)

There are many physiological and regulatory phenomena which provide 'immune privilege' to the anterior segment.

These include anterior chamber associated immune deviation (ACAID), and soluble and cell membrane-bound immunosuppressive factors in the anterior segment.[66]

ACAID is an unusual systemic immune response, whereby, following foreign antigen injection into the anterior chamber of the eye, a signal is produced that communicates with the immune system through the spleen. A series of events occurs that has several important features: (1) an inhibition of systemic DTH; (2) an inhibition of a complement-fixing antibody response; (3) the maintenance of a normal cytotoxic T-cell and humoral immune response; and (4) the capacity to adoptively transfer ACAID through antigen-specific splenic suppressor T cells, both CD4+ and CD8+, to immunologically naive recipients. As DTH and complement fixing antibodies would generate intense local immunogenic inflammation, the eye has developed a mechanism to reduce this type of immune response.

Niederkorn and Kaplan describe three phases of ACAID.[66] The first 'ocular phase' involves an antigen-specific signal which is generated in the eye and delivered to the systemic immune system. F4/80+ APC in the anterior chamber constitute this signal. These cells are exposed to a variety of immunosuppressive agents which lead to: (1) a reduced capacity to produce Th1 inducing IL-12; (2) enhanced production of the Th2 cytokine IL-10; (3) reduced expression of CD40 costimulatory molecule; and (4) autocrine production of TGF-β. The presence of Fas ligand (CD95L) in the eye is also essential for the generation of these cells. In the second 'thymic' phase, F4/80+ APC migrate to the thymus where they generate NK1.1+, CD8+CD4- efferent cells which suppress DTH. Finally, the 'splenic' phase requires the spleen for at least 7 days. F4/80+ APC also migrate to the spleen where they generate CD8+ regulatory suppressor cells. B cells, T cells bearing the γd T-cell receptor, and B cells are also required for ACAID.

Two cell populations are responsible for ACAID. The first are CD4+ cells which produce increased amounts of IL-10 and decreased amounts of IFN-γ. These Th1-type cells are termed 'afferent suppressor cells.' These cells are required to generate a second population of CD8+ cells which inhibit the expression of DTH responses and are termed 'efferent suppressor cells.'

In addition to ACAID, there are many immunoregulatory phenomena in the anterior segment which contribute to ocular inmmune privilege. The blood–ocular barrier, located at the tight junctions of the ciliary epithelium of the ciliary body, physically provides a barrier to cellular infiltration. Soluble factors also inhibit a variety of immunological processes including: (1) T cell proliferation; (2) IFN-γ production by Th1 cells; (3) proinflammatory factors secreted by macrophages; (4) NK cell activity; (5) DTH response; and (6) infiltrating cells by FasL.

Immune Hypersensitivity Reactions

When the adaptive ocular immune response occurs in an excessive or inappropriate form and results in damage to ocular tissue, it is termed a hypersensitivity response. In 1968, Gell and Coombs described four classic types of hypersensitivity responses.[77] Types I through III are antibody mediated, and type IV is cell mediated (T cells and macrophages). Many clinical entities probably result from a combination of mechanisms.

Type I hypersensitivity response (atopic, allergic reactions)

After exposure to antigen, an antigen presenting cell (APC) presents antigen to a helper 2 T lymphocyte (Th2), causing the release of cytokines interleukins 4 and 5, which stimulate the (excessive) antigen-specific synthesis of IgE antibodies by B lymphocytes. IL-3 and IL-4 also stimulate the proliferation of $Fc_{\epsilon}RI$ + mucosal mast cells. After secondary exposure to antigen, eosinophils and mast cells with antigen-specific IgE respond to antigen by bridging two immunoglobulin molecules. An aggregation of receptors in the membrane then causes a rapid membrane-coupled activation of adenylate cyclase, which leads to the increase in cyclic adenosine monophosphate (cAMP). This leads to the degranulation of preformed mediators of inflammation and allergy from storage granules. Newly synthesized mediators are also generated.

Mast cells and basophils release a variety of mediators. Some are preformed, and others must be synthesized. Preformed mediators include an amine (histamine or serotonin), proteoglycans (heparin or chondroitin sulfate), and many different neutral proteases, including aryl sulfatase. Newly formed mediators are usually produced following an IgE-mediated activation. Different profiles of newly formed mediators are probably produced by different populations of mast cells. The newly formed mediators include arachidonic acid metabolites, prostaglandins (PGD_2), products of the cyclooxygenase (thromboxanes) and lipooxygenase pathways (leukotriene C_4, D_4, B_4), and cytokines including TNF-α, IL-3 to IL-6, IL-10, IL-13, and VEGF. The release of vasoactive mediators results in the familiar clinical signs of chemosis, vascular injection, itching, and increases in local (tear) IgE levels.

Type II (cytotoxic) hypersensitivity response

A type II hypersensitivity response results from complement-fixing antibodies (IgG_1, IgG_3, or IgM), which bind to endogenous (acetylcholine receptor in myasthenia gravis, basement membrane zone in ocular cicatricial pemphigoid) or exogenous (microbes, transplanted cells) membrane antigens.

Cell damage is mediated by several mechanisms. Through one mechanism, a variety of phagocytic effector cells (macrophages, neutrophils, eosinophils, NK cells) can bring about cell destruction through binding via their Fc receptor and release proteolytic and collagenolytic enzymes. Significant 'bystander' damage may result when the target tissue (basement membrane) is too large to be engulfed by the phagocyte. Neutrophils play an important role in this reaction.

Through antibody-dependent cell cytoxicity (ADCC), rather than through enzymatic membrane destruction, NK cells cause direct cell damage through nonspecific binding of antibody to their Fc receptor. These cells release proteolytic enzymes, resulting in target cell destruction.

Finally, antibodies also may activate complement through the classic and lytic pathways, resulting in the deposition of the C5b-9 membrane attack complex. C3b can also bind to target cells and mediate membrane damage via the C3b receptor on phagocytic cells. C3a and C5a are also powerful chemoattractants of inflammatory cells including mast cells, macrophages, and T lymphocytes. These cells also release their own inflammatory mediators. Mast cells release IL-8, ECF, LTB_4, and vasoactive amines. Macrophages release LTB_4, IL-1, and TNF-α, and T cells release IFN-γ, IL-8, and TNF-α/β (see Table 5.1). These mediators further attract inflammatory cells.

Type III hypersensitivity response (immune complex)

In the type III hypersensitivity response, soluble antigen–antibody complexes bind complement and either it becomes deposited into blood vessels throughout the body or the antigen combines with the antibody in the extracellular space. PMNs and phagocytes are attracted into the tissue and directly or indirectly destroy it. The same complement-fixing antibodies in the type II response (IgG and IgM) participate.

Antigen–antibody complexes are normally eliminated through the reticuloendothelial system (larger complexes). This system may become overloaded, resulting in the deposition of complexes into tissues. The outcome usually depends on the size of the complexes, with smaller complexes not deposited in the tissues and larger ones being cleared by the reticuloendothelial system. The intermediate-sized complexes are the most likely to lead to deposition.

Persistent antigen exposure to specific body sites may generate a systemic circulating antibody response with local deposition. Increases in vascular permeability through vasoactive amine release or previous damage to the endothelium is necessary for the complexes to exit the circulatory system and deposit into the tissues. Potential inciting antigens include microbes, drugs, or autoantigens.

Type IV (delayed-type hypersensitivity [DTH]) response

Type IV reactions are mediated by macrophages and antigen-specific T lymphocytes rather than antibodies. They are different from the other hypersensitivity reactions in that they are reactions to fixed, rather than soluble, antigens. These include infectious agents, tumors, and foreign grafts. Antigen is presented to T cells by an antigen presenting cell (APC), which then migrates to lymphoid tissue where it presents to resting T lymphocytes. Once activated, these antigen-specific sensitized cells respond by direct cytotoxic attack or through the release of cytokines that have secondary effects including macrophage chemotaxis and activation. It requires about 48 hours to elicit a maximum response through antigen-specific T cells. Tc and T_{DTH} cells directly attack the target cell. Macrophages are also recruited through cytokine release by these lymphocytes and participate in the elimination of the fixed tissue antigen or organism. Three types of type IV hypersensitivity responses are currently recognized: contact hypersensitivity, tuberculin-type hypersensitivity, and granulomatous hypersensitivity. Corneal allograft rejection results from this process.

References

1. Waring GO 3rd, Rodrigues MM. Patterns of pathologic response in the cornea. *Surv Ophthalmol.* 1987;31:262–266.
2. Leibowitz HM, Waring III GO. *Corneal disorders. Clinical diagnosis and management.* 2nd ed. Philadelphia, WB: Saunders Company; 1998: 154–200.
3. Ambrósio Jr R, Kara-José N, Wilson SE. Early keratocyte apoptosis after epithelial scrape injury in the human cornea. *Exp Eye Res.* 2009;89:597–599.
4. Lagali NS, Germundsson J, Fagerholm P. The role of Bowman's layer in anterior corneal regeneration after phototherapeutic keratectomy: a prospective, morphological study using in-vivo confocal microscopy. *Invest Ophthalmol Vis Sci.* 2009;50:4192–4198.
5. Dua HS, Miri A, Alomar T, Yeung AM, Said DG. The role of limbal stem cells in corneal epithelial maintenance: testing the dogma. *Ophthalmology.* 2009;116:856–863.
6. Steinberg EB, Wilson LA, Waring GO 3rd, Lynn MJ, Coles WH. Stellate iron lines in the corneal epithelium after radial keratotomy. *Am J Ophthalmol.* 1984;98:416–421.
7. Fraunfelder FW. Corneal toxicity from topical ocular and systemic medications. *Cornea.* 2006;5:1133–1138.
8. Hamam R, Bhat P, Foster CS. Conjunctival/corneal intraepithelial neoplasia. *Int Ophthalmol Clin.* 2009;49:63–70.
9. Waring GO 3rd, Roth AM, Ekin MB. Clinical and pathologic description of 17 cases of corneal intraepithalial neoplasia. *Am J Ophthalmol.* 1984;97:547–559.
10. Ballalai PL, Erwenne CM, Martins MC, Lowen MS, Barros JN. Long-term results of topical mitomycin C 0.02% for primary and recurrent conjunctival-corneal intraepithelial neoplasia. *Ophthal Plast Reconstr Surg.* 2009;25:296–299.
11. Dawson DG, Grossniklaus HE, McCarey BE, Edelhauser HF. Biomechanical and wound healing characteristics of corneas after excimer laser keratorefractive surgery: is there a difference between advanced surface ablation and sub-Bowman's keratomileusis? *J Refract Surg.* 2008;24: S90–S96.
12. Randleman JB, Hewitt SM, Stulting RD. Delayed reactivation of presumed adenoviral subepithelial infiltrates after laser in situ keratomileusis. *Cornea.* 2004;23:217–219.
13. Waring GO 3rd, Malaty A, Grossniklaus H, Kaj H. Climatic proteoglycan stromal keratopathy, a new corneal degeneration. *Am J Ophthalmol.* 1995;20:330–341.
14. Itty S, Hamilton SS, Baratz KH, Diehl NN, Maguire LJ. Outcomes of epithelial debridement for anterior basement membrane dystrophy. *Am J Ophthalmol.* 2007;144:217–221.
15. Kenney MC, Brown DJ, Rajeev B. Everett Kinsey lecture. The elusive causes of keratoconus: a working hypothesis. *CLAO J.* 2000;26:10–13.
16. Hsu JK, Johnston WT, Read RW, et al. Histopathology of corneal melting associated with diclofenac use after refractive surgery. *J Cataract Refract Surg.* 2003;29:250–256.
17. Kremer I, Kaplan A, Novikov I, Blumenthal M. Patterns of late corneal scarring after photorefractive keratectomy in high and severe myopia. *Ophthalmology.* 1999;106:467–473.
18. Dawson DG, Edelhauser HF, Grossniklaus HE. Long-term histopathologic findings in human corneal wounds after refractive surgical procedures. *Am J Ophthalmol.* 2005;139:168–178.
19. Meltendorf C, Burbach GJ, Ohrloff C, Ghebremedhin E, Deller T. Intrastromal keratotomy with femtosecond laser avoids profibrotic TGF-β1 induction. *Invest Ophthalmol Vis Sci.* 2009;50:3688–3695.
20. Ruiz LA, Cepeda LM, Fuentes VC. Intrastromal correction of presbyopia using a femtosecond laser system. *J Refract Surg.* 2009;25:847–854.
21. Montezuma SR, Vavvas D, Miller JW. Review of the ocular angiogenesis animal models. *Semin Ophthalmol.* 2009;24:52–61.
22. Lee P, Wang CC, Adamis AP. Ocular neovascularization: an epidemiologic review. *Surv Ophthalmol.* 1998;43:245–269.
23. Baer JC, Foster CS. Corneal laser photocoagulation for treatment of neovascularization. Efficacy of 577 nm yellow dye laser. *Ophthalmology.* 1992;99:173–179.
24. Sheppard JD Jr, Epstein RJ, Lattanzio Jr FA, Marcantonio D, Williams PB. Argon laser photodynamic therapy of human corneal neovascularization after intravenous administration of dihematoporphyrin ether. *Am J Ophthalmol.* 2006;141:524–529.
25. Dastjerdi MH, Al-Arfaj KM, Nallasamy N, et al. Topical bevacizumab in the treatment of corneal neovascularization: results of a prospective, open-label, noncomparative study. *Arch Ophthalmol.* 2009;127:381–389.
26. Levenson JE. Corneal edema: cause and treatment. *Surv Ophthalmol.* 1975;20:190–204.

27. Dawson DG, Schmack I, Holley GP, et al. Interface fluid syndrome in human eye bank corneas after LASIK: causes and pathogenesis. *Ophthalmology*. 2007;114:1848–1859.
28. Reed JW, Dohlman CH. Cornea cysts: a report of eight cases. *Arch Ophthalmol*. 1971;86:648–652.
29. Singh AD, Puri P, Amos RS. Deposition of gold in ocular structures, although known, is rare. A case of ocular chrysiasis in a patient of rheumatoid arthritis on gold treatment is presented. *Eye*. 2004;18:443–444.
30. Barchiesi BJ, Eckel RH, Ellis PP. The cornea and disorders of lipid metabolism. *Surv Ophthalmol*. 1991;36:1–22.
31. Loeffler KU, Seifert P. Unusual idiopathic lipid keratopathy: a newly recognized entity? *Arch Ophthalmol*. 2005;123:1435–1438.
32. Waring GO, MacMillan AD, Roth AM, Spangler WL, Elkins MB. Lipid corneal opacities in beagles and Siberian huskies. *Proc Am Coll Vet Ophthalmol*. 1979;10:1–27.
33. Twa MD, Ruckhofer J, Kash RL, Costello M, Schanzlin DJ. Histologic evaluation of corneal stroma in rabbits after intrastromal corneal ring implantation. *Cornea*. 2003;22:146–152.
34. Fernandez AB, Keyes MJ, Pencina M, et al. Relation of corneal arcus to cardiovascular disease (from the Framingham Heart Study data set). *Am J Cardiol*. 2008;103:64–66.
35. Crispin S. Ocular lipid deposition and hyperlipoproteinaemia. *Prog Retin Eye Res*. 2002;21:169–224.
36. Nakatsukasa M, Sotozono C, Tanioka H, Shimazaki C, Kinoshita S. Diagnosis of multiple myeloma in a patient with atypical corneal findings. *Cornea*. 2008;27:249–251.
37. Waring GO 3rd, Rodrigues MM, Laibson PR. Corneal dystrophies: I. Dystrophies of the epithelium, Bowman's layer and stroma. *Surv Ophthalmol*. 1978;23:71–122.
38. Weiss JS, Møller HU, Lisch W, et al. The IC3D classification of the corneal dystrophies. *Cornea*. 2008;27(Suppl 2):S1–S83.
39. Kaufman A, Medow N, Phillips R, Zaidman G. Treatment of epibulbar limbal dermoids. *J Pediatr Ophthalmol Strabismus*. 1999;36:136–140.
40. Sbarbaro JA, Eagle RC, Thumma P, Raber IM. Histopathology of posterior lamellar endothelial keratoplasty graft failure. *Cornea*. 2008;27:900–904.
41. Hicks CR, Hamilton S. Retroprosthetic membranes in AlphaCor patients: risk factors and prevention. *Cornea*. 2005;24:692–698.
42. Edelhauser HF. The resiliency of the corneal endothelium to refractive and intraocular surgery. *Cornea*. 2000;19:263–273.
43. Waring GO 3rd, Bourne WM, Edelhauser HF, Kenyon KR. The corneal endothellium. Normal and pathologic structure and function. *Ophthalmology*. 1982;89:531–590.
44. Claesson M, Armitage WJ, Stenevi U. Corneal oedema after cataract surgery: predisposing factors and corneal graft outcome. *Acta Ophthalmol*. 2008;87:154–159.
45. Mehta JS, Por YM, Poh R, Beuerman RW, Tan D. Comparison of donor insertion techniques for Descemet stripping automated endothelial keratoplasty. *Arch Ophthalmol*. 2008;126:1383–1388.
46. Afshari NA, Pittard AB, Siddiqui A, Klintworth GK. Clinical study of Fuchs' corneal endothelial dystrophy leading to penetrating keratoplasty: a 30-year experience. *Arch Ophthalmol*. 2006;124:777–780.
47. Waring GO 3rd. The 50-year epidemic of pseudophakic corneal edema. *Arch Ophthalmol*. 1989;107:657–659.
48. Patel SV, Hodge DO, Bourne WM. Corneal endothelium and postoperative outcomes 15 years after penetrating keratoplasty. *Trans Am Ophthalmol Soc*. 2004;102:57–65; discussion 65–66.
49. Waring GO, Laibson PR, Rodrigues MM. Clinical and pathologic alterations of Descemet's membrane: with emphasis on endothelial metaplasia. *Surv Ophthalmol*. 1974;18:325–368.
50. Waring GO. Posterior collagenous layer of the cornea: ultrastructural classification of abnormal collagenous tissue posterior to Descemet's membrane in 30 cases. *Arch Ophthalmol*. 1982;100:122–134.
51. Dogru M, Kato N, Matsumoto Y, et al. Immunohistochemistry and electron microscopy of retrocorneal scrolls in syphilitic interstitial keratitis. *Curr Eye Res*. 2007;32:863–870.
52. Alvarado JA, Murphy CG, Maglia M, Hetherlington J. Pathogenesis of Chandler's syndrome, essential iris atrophy and the Cogan-Reese syndrome. II: Estimated age at disease onset. *Invest Ophthalmol Vis Sci*. 1986;27:873–882.
53. Bourne WM, Johnson DH, Campbell RJ. The ultrastructure of Descemet's membrane: III. Fuchs' dystrophy. *Arch Ophthalmol*. 1982;100:1948–1951.
54. Krachmer JH, Schnitzer JI, Fratkin J. Cornea pseudogutta: a clinical and histopathologic description of endothelial cell edema. *Arch Ophthalmol*. 1981;99:1377–1381.
55. Mazzotta C, Baiocchi S, Caporossi O, et al. Confocal microscopy identification of keratoconus associated with posterior polymorphous corneal dystrophy. *J Cataract Refract Surg*. 2008;34:318–321.
56. Olsen TW, Hardten DR, Meiusi RS, Holland EJ. Linear endotheliitis. *Am J Ophthalmol*. 1994;117:468–474.
57. Suzuki T, Ohashi Y. Corneal endotheliitis. *Semin Ophthalmol*. 2008;23:235–240.
58. Vemuganti GK, Garg P, Gopinathan U, et al. Evaluation of agent and host factors in progression of mycotic keratitis: a histologic and microbiologic study of 167 corneal buttons. *Ophthalmology*. 2002;109:1538–1546.
59. Weiner JM, Carroll N, Robertson IF. The granulomatous reaction in herpetic stromal keratitis: immunohistological and ultrastructural findings. *Aust N Z J Ophthalmol*. 1985;13:365–372.
60. Liu M, Cohen EJ, Brewer GJ, Laibson PR. Kayser-Fleischer ring as the presenting sign of Wilson disease. *Am J Ophthalmol*. 2002;133:832–834.
61. Santos LN, Fernandes BF, de Moura LR, et al. Histopathologic study of corneal stromal dystrophies: a 10-year experience. *Cornea*. 2007;26:1027–1031.
62. Jirsova K, Merjava S, Martincova R, et al. Immunohistochemical characterization of cytokeratins in the abnormal corneal endothelium of posterior polymorphous corneal dystrophy patients. *Exp Eye Res*. 2007;84:680–686.
63. Hidayat AA, Cockerham GC. Epithelial metaplasia of the corneal endothelium in Fuchs endothelial dystrophy. *Cornea*. 2006;25:956–959.
64. Doe EA, Budenz DL, Gedde SJ, Imami NR. Long-term surgical outcomes of patients with glaucoma secondary to the iridocorneal endothelial syndrome. *Ophthalmology*. 2001;108:1789–1795.
65. Delves PJ, Martin SJ, Burton DR, Roitt IM, eds. *Roitt's essential immunology*. 11th ed. New York: Wiley-Blackwell; 2006.
66. Niederkorn JY, Kaplan HJ, eds. *Immune response and the eye*. 2nd, revised edition. Basel: Karger AG; 2007.
67. Zierhut M, Rammensee H-G, Streilein JW, eds. *Antigen-presenting cells and the eye*. New York: Informa Health Care; 2007.
68. Hendricks R. Interaction of angiogenic and immune mechanisms in the eye. *Semin Ophthalmol*. 2006;21:37–40.
69. Shen L, Barabino S, Taylor AW, Dana MR. Effect of the ocular microenvironment in regulating corneal dendritic cell maturation. *Arch Ophthalmol*. 2007;125(7):908–915.
70. Chan JH, Amankwah R, Robins RA, Gray T, Dua HS. Kinetics of immune cell migration at the human ocular surface. *Br J Ophthalmol*. 2008;92:970–975.
71. Ono S, Abelson M. Allergic conjunctivitis: update on pathophysiology and prospects for future treatment. *J All Clin Immunol*. 2005;115:118–122.
72. Pawankar R, Holgate ST, Rosenwasser, LJ, eds. *Allergy frontiers: clinical manifestations*, Philadelphia: Springer; 2009.
73. Pflugfelder SC, Beuerman RW, Stern ME, eds. *Dry eye and ocular surface disorders*. New York: Informa Health Care; 2004.
74. Xue ML, Thakur A, Cole N, et al. A critical role for CCL2 and CCL3 chemokines in the regulation of polymorphonuclear neutrophils recruitment during corneal infection in mice. *Immunol Cell Biol*. 2007;85:525–531.
75. Steven P, Gebert A. Conjunctiva-associated lymphoid tissue – current knowledge, animal models and experimental prospects. *Ophthalmol Res*. 2009;42:2–8.
76. Zierhut M, Stern ME, Sullivan DA, eds. *Immunology of the lacrimal gland, tear film and ocular surface*. New York: Informa Health Care; 2005.
77. Gell PGH, Coombs RRA, eds. *Clinical aspects of immunology*. Oxford: Blackwell; 1968.

PART II

EXAMINING AND IMAGING THE CORNEA AND EXTERNAL EYE

Chapter **6**

Examination of the Lids

Hall T. McGee, William D. Mathers

General Principles

As with all other aspects of ophthalmic examination, having a routine aids in ensuring that the examination has been both complete and expeditious. One example routine is provided in Box 6.1, and although it covers the major aspects of the examination it should be modified as necessary.

History of Patient

Symptoms from eyelid disease are frequently quite vague and non-specific; nevertheless, the customary questions about onset, severity, duration, exacerbation, localization, and history of previous treatments are still appropriate.

Of course, the examination begins during the history taking. As patients are often distracted, this is an excellent time to observe such behaviors as eye rubbing, scratching itchy skin, or wiping away excess tears. One should also observe the manner and rate of blinking, particularly noting whether blinks are forced or incomplete. Patients taking psychotropic drugs and those with central nervous system disease, for example, may blink much less frequently.

Dermatologic Examination

A general examination of the lids begins with the skin around the orbit and face. This is aided by examining the patient in fairly bright, diffuse lighting as close in color to daylight as possible; darkened rooms and artificial light will distort the true color and translucency of tissues. Many patients have dermatologic conditions of which they are unaware.

Contact dermatitis involving the eyelids is quite common and is associated with other ocular allergies.[1] In this condition the skin slightly away from the lid margin is usually more involved. The skin may be quite erythematous, edematous, and display considerable scaling. A recent history of use of lotions, creams, or any topical application to the area should be diligently sought. Atopic dermatitis, or eczema, can be associated with severe keratoconjunctivitis. The periorbital skin may be thickened, scaly, erythematous, and even fissured. Patients may also be aware of lesions elsewhere on their skin, but may not have associated their dermatitis with their eye condition.

Rosacea is a common dermatologic condition of unknown etiology that affects up to 10% of the population and is most commonly found in those of northern European origin. Rosacea dermatitis is characterized by malar flushing, telangiectasias, papules, pustules, and sebaceous gland hypertrophy.

Bacterial infections can also occur, causing preseptal cellulitis, or even progressing to orbital cellulitis. Xanthelasma can also provide evidence of lipid abnormalities.

Eyelid Position

It is important to pay close attention to the position of the eyelids, since many patients with exposure keratopathy do not complain of their condition.[2] The distance between the upper and lower eyelids in the center of the cornea should be evaluated for symmetry. Eyes with large interpalpebral fissures have a much greater surface area. Because evaporation is a direct function of surface area, patients with larger interpalpebral apertures and somewhat compromised tear production are more likely to experience dry eye from increased exposure. One should also observe the position of the eyes when the lids are closed, and look for the presence of corneal and conjunctival exposure. It is important not to allow the patient to force lid closure. Thus, it is best to wait at least 1 minute with the lids closed to allow time for the patient to relax and reveal the true position of the lids.

The examination for ectropion and entropion is important because symptoms are often non-specific.[3] Ectropion often produces abnormalities in the tear film and dryness even to cause keratinization of the conjunctiva. Entropion produces irritation and vascularization of the conjunctiva and corneal surface, both of which also increase evaporation and make any dry eye condition worse. Sometimes 'spastic' entropion, which occurs after a forced blink, can be observed following ophthalmic surgery. It is also important to note the position of the lashes with attention to trichiasis and distichiasis.

Eyelid laxity is relatively common, and is easily evaluated by manipulating the lids themselves. Gently pulling the lid straight away from the eye surface tests how much it can be displaced, while pulling a lower lid downward toward the cheek and releasing tests the ability of the lid to snap back to its original location. Excessive laxity may precede

Box 6.1 A recommended order for examination of the eyelids

- Take history and observe patient's behavior and habits
  - Note eye rubbing, blink rate, blotting of tears
- Examine face and eyelids in ambient lighting
  - Note signs of atopic or contact dermatitis, rosacea, tumors, infection, entropion, ectropion, scarring or other signs of trauma
- Examine tear meniscus and puncta with slit lamp (before administering drops or dyes of any kind)
  - Note the height of the meniscus, the presence of debris or bubbles, and any punctal ectropion or stenosis
- Examine anterior eyelid
  - Note any eyelash changes and crusting, tumors, nodules
- Examine posterior eyelid
  - Note erythema, telangiectasis, pouting of meibomian gland orifices, distichiasis, rounding of posterior eyelid border
- Express the meibomian glands
  - Note the quantity and character of the fluid expressed
- Step back again and examine the mechanical properties of the lids
  - Note eyelid laxity, and measure the interpalpebral fissure
- Instill dye into the eye (fluorescein, lissamine green or rose Bengal)
  - Use slit lamp again to note the presence and location of the Marx line (mucocutaneous junction) relative to the meibomian orifices
- Consider imaging studies as appropriate (generally for research applications)

ectropion and is often associated with corneal exposure and dryness. Occasionally the lids are relatively tight for the given eye, and this can be associated with problems with diseases such as superior limbic keratoconjunctivitis and exopthalmos.

Floppy eyelid syndrome (Fig. 6.1) results from excessive eyelid elasticity and usually presents with conjunctival injection, mucous discharge, and irritation that is often worse in the morning and not associated in the patient's mind with eyelid disease.[4–7] These patients are usually obese and frequently report snoring and sleeping face-down. Examination involves first having the patient look down. The examiner then places both thumbs on the superotemporal orbital rims and draws the upper eyelid up and temporally. Floppy eyelids are diagnosed when the upper lid stretches excessively, often to the superior orbital rim, and the tarsal plate everts exposing the palpebral conjunctiva. The syndrome involves not only the presence of floppy eyelids but also signs and symptoms of chronic irritation, including conjunctival injection, thickening, and a papillary response. The cornea also may show mild to moderate vascularization, particularly in the inferior and temporal limbal area.

Tear Meniscus and Puncta

When performing biomicroscopy, the tear lake should be examined first. The tear meniscus should be examined with

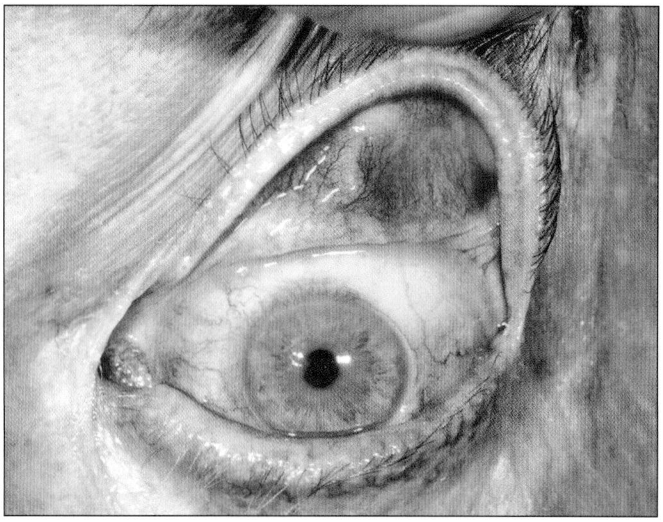

Fig. 6.1 Floppy eyelid syndrome depicting eversion of the upper lid with exposure of the conjunctiva.

a slit lamp, but with the light turned off and the ambient light just sufficient to reveal the size of the meniscus. It is also best to refrain from manipulating the eyelids before examining the tear lake. Once the tear meniscus has been carefully examined, slit lamp illumination can be turned on and the degree of reflex tearing noted. The intersection between the lid margin and the ocular surface contains the tear meniscus. The height and volume can reveal the relative severity of dry eye and the amount of debris in the tear film.[8–10] Foamy tears generally indicate meibomian gland dysfunction.

Patients with a very small tear meniscus who are unable to generate a response to the slit lamp light are much more likely to have difficulty with dry eye than a person who is still capable of a significant reflex tearing.[10–12]

The positions of the upper and lower puncta are important for normal function. The lower punctum may be everted even if the position of the central part of the eyelid is relatively normal. Punctal ectropion will reduce its ability to drain the tear lake, leading to epiphora. A punctum that is rotated inward rarely causes a problem. Puncta may be scarred closed from a variety of conjunctival diseases or as a treatment for dry eye, although patients may be unaware of previous occlusions. Pemphigoid and alkali burns frequently lead to occlusion of the punctum.[13,14]

Anterior Eyelid

Although it is best to examine the patient first in ambient lighting with attention to color, transparency, induration, and other general characteristics, any nodules or other suspicious lesions should be examined with the biomicroscope as well. Eyelid scaling, separation, scarring, and atrophic changes are also more easily seen with magnification.

Examination of the lashes is most readily performed with the biomicroscope. The length of the lashes and the number of white, broken and missing lashes should be noted. Particular attention should be paid to the presence of very small

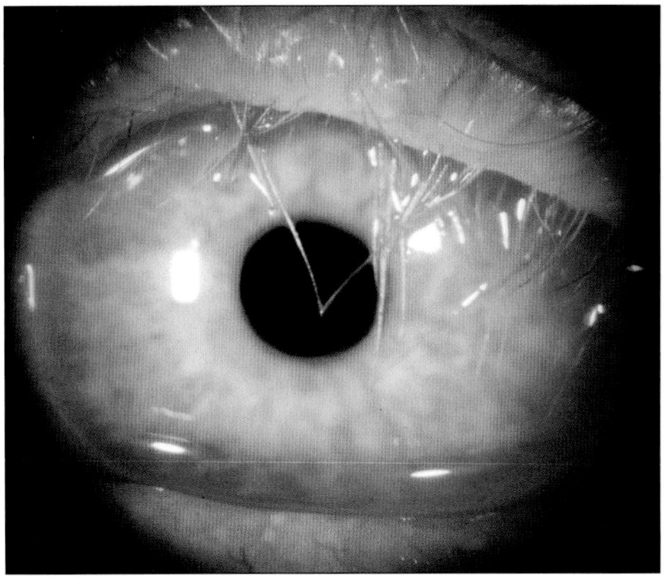

Fig. 6.2 Trichiasis from lid margin scarring can be seen in blepharitis as well as in Stevens–Johnson syndrome and other scarring diseases of the conjunctiva.

lashes that may be directed posteriorly (Fig. 6.2). In some patients, particularly those with Stevens–Johnson syndrome and related diseases, trichiasis of very small lashes is a very difficult problem and may lead to severe symptoms, inflammation, and scarring of the corneal surface.[15]

A collarette, which forms in areas of inflammation or hyperkeratinization, is simply mucous debris that adheres to the lash and becomes visible as the lash grows. Collarettes are a relatively non-specific sign of inflammation. The lashes also should be examined for signs of infestation. Lice are relatively easy to see on the lashes, whereas Demodex organisms are much smaller and more difficult to identify.[16–19] Infectious processes may occur at the lashes and are usually evident by swelling and pus noted at the base. Such hordeola of the hair follicles are often associated with a more generalized bacterial infection of other lid structures.[20,21]

Posterior Eyelid

Inflammatory stimuli or infections of the eyelid may induce rounding of the posterior lid margin, which normally has a squared edge in profile.[22] In normal, noninflamed lids very small capillaries can be identified, but large vessels are not seen. Atrophy and inflammation of the entire lid margin will also cause the appearance of hypervascularity, in part because atrophy causes an increased transparency of the lid margin which makes the deeper vessels more visible. These vascular changes are relatively nonspecific but are often associated with obstructive meibomian gland dysfunction, rosacea, or infections, but not with seborrheic meibomian gland dysfunction (Fig. 6.3).

Besides trauma, chalazia are the most common cause of lid scarring, and may leave notches that distort the smooth contour of the lid. These notches are also associated with

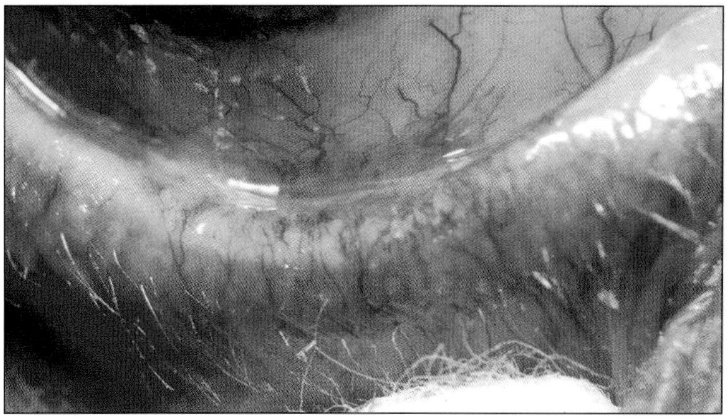

Fig. 6.3 Vascularization and hypertrophy along the lid margin which alters the normal contours and obscures landmarks.

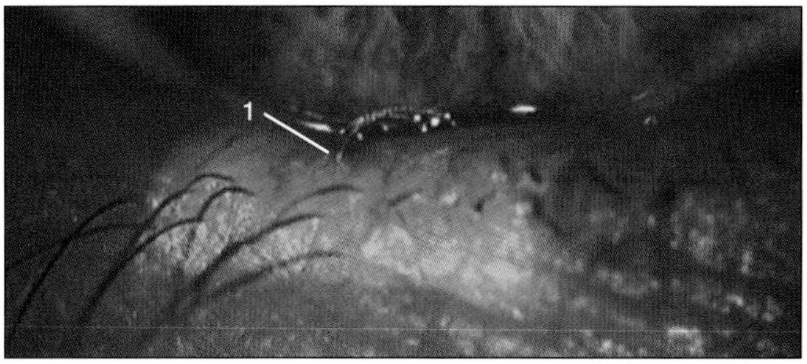

Fig. 6.4 Scarring line on the lid margin from chalazia formation may produce a loss of tissue, which appears as a notch on the lid margin. Lashes are often found within the notch (1).

trichiasis and are indicative of obstructive meibomian gland dysfunction (Fig. 6.4).

Allergic processes cause thickening of the conjunctiva and may also cause chronic changes to the lid margin. In severe disease, deep furrows in the skin and conjunctival surface of the lid margin develop which may become secondarily infected and lead to frank ulceration.[23] The openings of the meibomian glands should be inspected carefully for signs of chronic disease. Periglandular atrophy renders the ducts more evident as the lid margin recedes around the keratinized duct.[24] Hyperkeratinization of the ductal epithelium also may occlude the meibomian orifice entirely.[25–27] In some instances, partial occlusion from keratinization will add to obstruction from dry and hardened inflammatory debris and further obstruct the meibomian gland. Chronic changes also occur simply from aging, and are exacerbated by the effects of long-term obstructive meibomian gland dysfunction and dry eye.[28]

Meibomian Gland Expression

Meibomian gland expression is an essential part of the lid examination.[28,29] Digital pressure is applied to the meibomian gland through the skin just distal to the opening of the gland duct with the patient in upward gaze. A cotton swab may be used to press on the lid. Firm pressure sufficient to indent the contour of the globe is usually required to express meibomian gland excreta. The pressure may need to

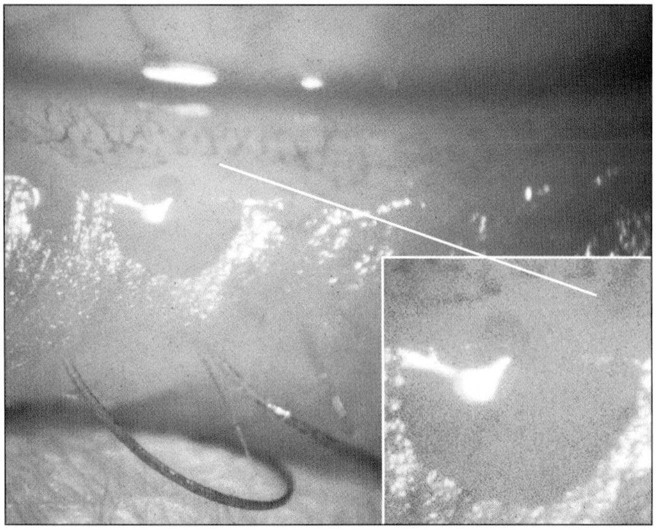

Fig. 6.5 Lipid expressed with digital pressure on an eyelid with seborrheic meibomian gland dysfunction reveals semi-transparent liquid of increased volume.

be maintained for several seconds to evaluate adequately the appearance of the expressible lipid. Usually 20–25 meibomian glands are present in the lower lid; two or three can be compressed at one time. The entire lid margin should be examined and the volume and viscosity of the excreta noted. Particular attention should be directed at those glands with abnormal findings, as normal glands are commonly found next to glands with severe disease.

The volume of the meibomian excreta can be recorded as the diameter of the lipid dome that forms after several seconds of pressure. The normal diameter of each dome is 0.5–0.7 mm. The volume of lipid is increased if any of the lipid domes are 0.8 mm or larger; this finding is sufficient to diagnose seborrheic meibomian gland dysfunction (Fig. 6.5). Meibomian gland lipid production may also be measured by evaluating the area of increased transparency of a paper strip placed against the meibomian orifices.[30,31] Smaller lipid volumes or totally obstructed glands that cannot be expressed with digital pressure are associated with obstructive meibomian gland dysfunction.

The viscosity and opacity of the expressed lipid are important signs of eyelid disease. Normal meibomian lipid is liquid at body temperature, flows easily, and is completely transparent. Seborrheic meibomian gland dysfunction is associated with a more opaque lipid that remains liquid. In obstructive meibomian gland dysfunction the viscosity increases, the transparency of the liquid declines, and the volume usually declines as well. At the highest level of viscosity lipid will emerge slowly like toothpaste, will not flow except under pressure, and will be totally opaque, with a white or light yellow color (Fig. 6.6).[28] Although such increased viscosity is usually associated with obstructive meibomian gland dysfunction, it is also found in some subjects with rosacea.[29] The differences in consistency of meibomian excreta have been found to be due to changes in lipid composition.[32]

Meibomian glands may also become infected, whereupon expression will often produce pus from an orifice and will

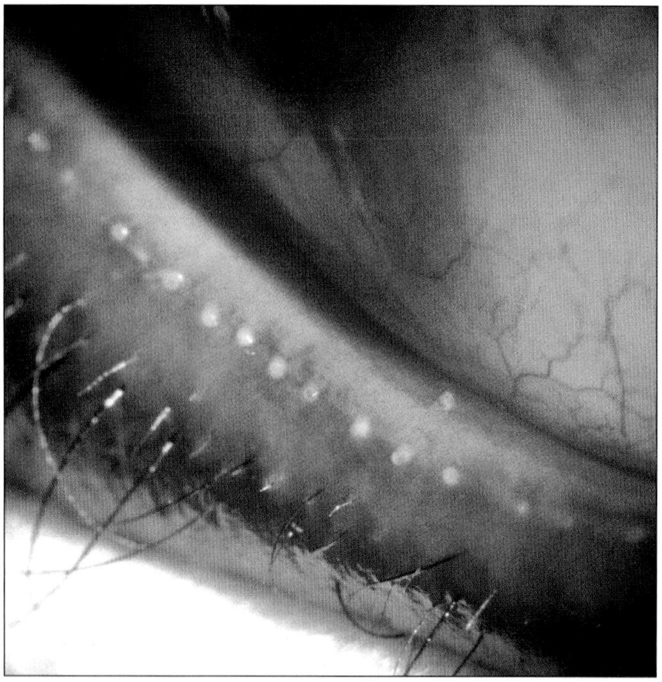

Fig. 6.6 Meibomian gland expression from a lid with obstructive meibomian dysfunction showing thickened and opaque lipid (toothpaste).

be quite tender. This condition should not be confused with staphylococcal blepharitis, which is usually the result of an immune response to heavy staphylococcal overgrowth on the eyelids.[33] *Staphylococcus* and *Streptococcus* organisms are usually responsible, and culturing the organism for antibiotic sensitivity may be helpful.[34–36] Because nearly all eyelids harbor such organisms, it may be difficult to determine the significance of the bacteria found with eyelid cultures. There is some evidence that different strains of bacteria are involved in different forms of blepharitis.[34] Blepharitis patients may also have heavier growth of bacteria on their lids.[33] The relative contribution of bacterial overgrowth, infection, bacterial toxins, and abnormal immune responses towards the development of blepharitis and meibomian gland dysfunction is a subject of continuing controversy and investigation.

In clinical practice, although much is often made of examination techniques to distinguish between infectious and inflammatory blepharitis, such distinctions may not be critical as the use of topical antibiotics, steroids, and systemic tetracyclines reduces the bacterial load and alters the immune response for most patients.[37] It is important, however, to recognize the presence of meibomian gland disease to enable appropriate treatment.

Mucocutaneous Junction

The mucocutaneous junction is where the keratinized squamous epithelium of the skin meets the moist, nonkeratinized squamous epithelium of the conjunctiva, and it normally lies just posterior to the opening of the meibomian orifices.[22,38] After instilling lissamine green, rose Bengal or

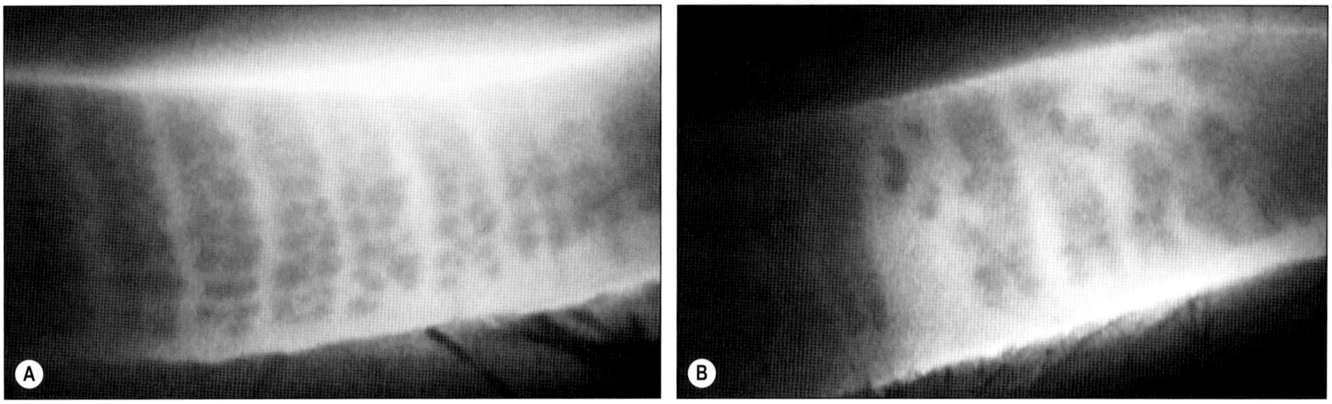

Fig. 6.7 Meibomian gland imagery. **A,** Transillumination of a normal eyelid showing evenly spaced glands. **B,** An infrared image with transillumination of the lower lid showing loss of glands.

fluorescein onto the ocular surface, a visible line of demarcation, called the Marx line, is often apparent on the lid margin. This line is thought to represent the mucocutaneous junction, and anterior displacement relative to the meibomian gland orifices may correlate with gland dysfunction.[38] Other authors have disagreed, finding that, although meibomian secretion declines with age, no age-related changes occur with the position of the mucocutaneous junction.[22]

Meibomian Gland Imagery

Albeit often reserved for research settings, transillumination of the lids can clearly image the morphology of individual glands. Either lid can be transilluminated, but the lower is considerably easier to evert. Digital infrared images of the entire lid can now be obtained with resolution approximately equal to that of infrared film.[39–41]

In humans, one can see evidence of gland loss, ductal dilation, chalazion formation, microcyst formation, and aberrant gland development (Fig. 6.7). Animal investigations demonstrate similar pathophysiologic processes.[25,27] The most obvious change seen with transillumination is gland dropout. Dropout is associated with obstructive meibomian gland dysfunction and is not associated with infectious blepharitis, allergic phenomenon, or seborrheic meibomian gland dysfunction. Seborrheic meibomian gland dysfunction shows no abnormalities of gland morphology. Patients with rosacea often reveal a mixed picture. Some areas of the lid will reveal gland dropout and increased lipid viscosity, whereas other areas will have increased lipid volume without gland dropout. This is consistent with the report that chalazia are more common in patients with rosacea than in normals.[42] Active chalazia often induce such thickening and induration of the lid that the details of meibomian glands cannot be seen with transillumination. Following resolution of the acute inflammation, a scarred area that may contain small cystic structures is usually evident.

Patients receiving isotretinoin (Accutane) therapy will have diminished lipid density in their meibomian glands, and the images will be much fainter, especially when the dosage has been relatively high. In such cases the meibomian glands seem almost to disappear, but will return to a normal appearance several weeks to months after cessation of therapy.[43,44]

Radiation to the orbit also damages meibomian glands, which are quite radiosensitive; in such cases transillumination shows that the number of glands is reduced, as is the volume of lipid secretion, and the viscosity is often increased.

In vivo confocal microscopy has also been used to image living meibomian glands in great detail both in normal patients and in cases of inflammatory meibomian gland obstruction. The obstruction causes a reduction in the number of acini and dilation of the ones that remain, as well as glandular atrophy and surrounding fibrosis in advanced cases.[45] This provides useful insight into the sequence of events that leads to gland dropout, and may become more clinically useful in predicting those patients who are most likely to benefit from lid margin treatment. To that end, the same technique can also be used to monitor the meibomian glands for treatment effects.[46]

References

1. Fonacier L, Luchs J, Udell I. Ocular allergies. *Curr Allergy Asthma Rep.* 2001;1(4):389–396.
2. Cosar CB, Cohen EJ, Rapuano CJ, et al. Tarsorrhaphy: clinical experience from a cornea practice. *Cornea.* 2001;20(8):787–791.
3. Vallabhanath P, Carter SR. Ectropion and entropion. *Curr Opin Ophthalmol.* 2000;11(5):345–351.
4. Madjlessi F, Kluppel M, Sundmacher R. [Operation of the floppy eyelid. Symptomatic cases require surgical eyelid stabilization]. *Klin Monatsblatt Augenheilkde.* 2000;216(3):148–151.
5. Culbertson WW, Tseng SC. Corneal disorders in floppy eyelid syndrome. *Cornea.* 1994;13(1):33–42.
6. van den Bosch WA, Lemij HG. The lax eyelid syndrome. *Br J Ophthalmol.* 1994;78(9):666–670.
7. Boulton JE, Sullivan TJ. Floppy eyelid syndrome and mental retardation. *Ophthalmology.* 2000;107(11):1989–1991.
8. Doughty MJ, Laiquzzaman M, Button NF. Video-assessment of tear meniscus height in elderly Caucasians and its relationship to the exposed ocular surface. *Curr Eye Res.* 2001;22(6):420–426.
9. Yaylali V, Ozyurt C. Comparison of tear function tests and impression cytology with the ocular findings in acne rosacea. *Eur J Ophthalmol.* 2002;12(1):11–17.
10. Tomlinson A, Blades KJ, Pearce EI. What does the phenol red thread test actually measure? *Optom Vis Sci.* 2001;78(3):142–146.
11. Tsubota K, Kaido M, Yagi Y, et al. Diseases associated with ocular surface abnormalities: the importance of reflex tearing. *Br J Ophthalmol.* 1999;83(1):89–91.

12. Yokoi N, Kinoshita S, Bron AJ, et al. Tear meniscus changes during cotton thread and Schirmer testing. *Invest Ophthalmol Vis Sci.* 2000;41(12):3748–3753.
13. McNab AA. Lacrimal canalicular obstruction associated with topical ocular medication. *Aust NZ J Ophthalmol.* 1998;26(3):219–223.
14. Sakol PJ. Tearing: lacrimal obstructions [Review]. *Pa Med.* 1996; 99(Suppl):99–104.
15. Lehman SS. Long-term ocular complication of Stevens–Johnson syndrome. *Clin Pediatr.* 1999;38(7):425–427.
16. Key JE. A comparative study of eyelid cleaning regimens in chronic blepharitis. *CLAO J.* 1996;22(3):209–212.
17. Demmler M, de Kaspar HM, Mohring C, Klauss V. [Blepharitis. *Demodex folliculorum*-associated pathogen spectrum and specific therapy]. *Ophthalmologe.* 1997;94(3):191–196.
18. Junk AK, Lukacs A, Kampik A. [Topical administration of metronidazole gel as an effective therapy alternative in chronic Demodex blepharitis – a case report]. *Klin Monatsblatt Augenheilkd.* 1998;213(1):48–50.
19. Burkhart CN, Burkhart CG. Oral ivermectin therapy for phthiriasis palpebrum. *Arch Ophthalmol.* 2000;118(1):134–135.
20. Kiratli HK, Akar Y. Multiple recurrent hordeola associated with selective IgM deficiency. *J AAPOS.* 2001;5(1):60–61.
21. Lederman C, Miller M. Hordeola and chalazia. *Pediatr Rev.* 1999;20(8):283–284.
22. Hykin PG, Bron AJ. Age-related morphological changes in lid margin and meibomian gland anatomy. *Cornea.* 1992;11(4):334–342.
23. Inoue Y. Ocular infections in patients with atopic dermatitis. *Int Ophthalmol Clin.* 2002;42(1):55–69.
24. Bron AJ, Benjamin L, Snibson GR. Meibomian gland disease. Classification and grading of lid changes. *Eye.* 1991;5(Pt 4):395–411.
25. Jester JV, Rife L, Nii D, et al. In vivo biomicroscopy and photography of meibomian glands in a rabbit model of meibomian gland dysfunction. *Invest Ophthalmol Vis Sci.* 1982;22(5):660–667.
26. Robin JB, Jester JV, Nobe J, et al. In vivo transillumination biomicroscopy and photography of meibomian gland dysfunction. A clinical study. *Ophthalmology.* 1985;92(10):1423–1426.
27. Jester JV, Rajagopalan S, Rodrigues M. Meibomian gland changes in the rhino (hrrhhrrh) mouse. *Invest Ophthalmol Vis Sci.* 1988;29(7):1190–1194.
28. Mathers WD, Shields WJ, Sachdev MS, et al. Meibomian gland dysfunction in chronic blepharitis. *Cornea.* 1991;10(4):277–285.
29. Mathers WD, Lane JA, Sutphin JE, Zimmerman MB. Model for ocular tear film function. *Cornea.* 1996;15(2):110–119.
30. Chew CK, Jansweijer C, Tiffany JM, Dikstein S, Bron AJ. An instrument for quantifying meibomian lipid on the lid margin: the Meibometer. *Curr Eye Res.* 1993;12(3):247–254.
31. Chew CK, Hykin PG, Jansweijer C, et al. The casual level of meibomian lipids in humans. *Curr Eye Res.* 1993;12(3):255–259.
32. Shine WE, McCulley JP. Association of meibum oleic acid with meibomian seborrhea. *Cornea.* 2000;19(1):72–74.
33. Groden LR, Murphy B, Rodnite J, Genvert GI. Lid flora in blepharitis. *Cornea.* 1991;10(1):50–53.
34. Dougherty JM, McCulley JP. Bacterial lipases and chronic blepharitis. *Invest Ophthalmol Vis Sci.* 1986;27(4):486–491.
35. Dougherty JM, McCulley JP. Comparative bacteriology of chronic blepharitis. *Br J Ophthalmol.* 1984;68(8):524–528.
36. McCulley JP, Dougherty JM, Deneau DG. Classification of chronic blepharitis. *Ophthalmology.* 1982;89(10):1173–1180.
37. Dougherty JM, McCulley JP, Silvany RE, Meyer DR. The role of tetracycline in chronic blepharitis. Inhibition of lipase production in staphylococci. *Invest Ophthalmol Vis Sci.* 1991;32(11):2970–2975.
38. Yamaguchi M, Kutsuna M, Uno T, et al. Marx line: fluorescein staining line on the inner lid as indicator of meibomian gland function. *Am J Ophthalmol.* 2006;141(4):669–675.
39. Shimazaki J, Goto E, Ono M, et al. Meibomian gland dysfunction in patients with Sjögren syndrome. *Ophthalmology.* 1998;105(8):1485–1488.
40. Lee SH, Tseng SC. Rose Bengal staining and cytologic characteristics associated with lipid tear deficiency. *Am J Ophthalmol.* 1997;124(6):736–750.
41. Mathers WD, Daley T, Verdick R. Video imaging of the meibomian gland [letter]. *Arch Ophthalmol.* 1994;112(4):448–449.
42. Lempert SL, Jenkins MS, Brown SI. Chalazia and rosacea. *Arch Ophthalmol.* 1979;97(9):1652–1653.
43. Mathers WD, Shields WJ, Sachdev MS, et al. Meibomian gland morphology and tear osmolarity: changes with Accutane therapy. *Cornea.* 1991;10(4):286–290.
44. Lambert RW, Smith RE. Pathogenesis of blepharoconjunctivitis complicating 13-*cis*-retinoic acid (isotretinoin) therapy in a laboratory model. *Invest Ophthalmol Vis Sci.* 1988;29(10):1559–1564.
45. Matsumoto Y, Sato E, Ibrahim O, et al. The application of in vivo laser confocal microscopy to the diagnosis and evaluation of meibomian gland dysfunction. *Mol Vis.* 2008;14:1263–1271.
46. Matsumoto Y, Shigeno Y, Sato EA, et al. The evaluation of the treatment response in obstructive meibomian gland disease by in vivo laser confocal microscopy. *Graefe's Arch Clin Exp Ophthalmol.* 2008 Dec. 20 (Epub ahead of print).

Chapter 7

Slit Lamp Examination and Photography

Csaba L. Mártonyi

'On August 3, 1911, Alvar Gullstrand presented his first rudimentary model of the slit lamp ... and explained its optics and applications.'*

An occasion of tremendous significance to ophthalmology had taken place. Gullstrand had introduced a device with the potential to advance the understanding of the eye and its problems as profoundly as did the direct ophthalmoscope 50 years earlier.

This chapter will deal primarily with techniques of examination (all applicable to the photographic process) and will address special considerations required for photodocumentation under the heading Photography, below.

At present, only an appropriately equipped photo slit lamp biomicroscope (PSL) is able to reproduce the information seen at the clinical slit lamp.

The Instrument: Examination and Photography

The principle underlying the slit lamp biomicroscope is isolation. This instrument provides precise and modifiable illumination plus magnification with which to isolate, and thereby make visible, fine detail (Fig. 7.1).

Composed of two primary components, the biomicroscope and the slit illuminator, today's slit lamp is both highly efficient and accommodating. The addition of available accessories provides for an impressive array of functions.

Most biomicroscopes consist of a parallel, Galilean telescope design. Utilizing optical changers, interchangeable oculars, or both, these instruments produce an effective range of magnification with excellent resolution. Many offer optional beam splitters to accommodate one-to-one teaching or to accept a video camera for real-time display or recording for later use.

The slit beam delivery system is basically a projector, with the slit aperture as the actual 'object' focused on a plane corresponding to the focal length of the biomicroscope. The foremost prowess of the slit lamp is its ability to create a focused, well-delineated, narrow slit beam that forms an optic section in transparent and translucent tissue. Not restricted to a single configuration, however, this beam is highly malleable through the use of simple controls that dictate its size and shape. It finds many additional applications in its various forms.

The biomicroscope and the illuminator are mounted on a common axis in a copivotal arrangement. This arrangement facilitates the parfocal (biomicroscope and slit beam are focused on the same plane) and isocentric (the slit beam is centered in the field of view) relationships essential for practical function. A departure from these relationships can be purposely created for certain techniques of examination; otherwise, the absence of isocentricity or parfocality indicates a faulty condition requiring adjustment or repair.

The Instrument: Photography

Good photographic results require the use of a PSL equipped with the following additional elements:

Beam splitter: A beam splitter provides the necessary coaxial view shared by the examiner and the camera back. That is the only arrangement whereby complete control over the image can be exercised before it is recorded. Beam splitters will divert from 50% to 85% of the light to the camera to ensure satisfactory exposures with most forms of illumination. As more light is diverted to the camera back, less remains for the examiner. A suitable compromise must be established for practical use, especially when the same instrument serves both examination and photography.

Electronic flash: Electronic flash produces light of high intensity at an effective duration of exposure of approximately 1 ms, the speed required to arrest the motion of the eye at high magnifications. The flash delivery system must be coaxial with the ambient light from the slit beam illuminator to reproduce the effect of lighting established by the examiner.

Fill light: The fill light is an accessory source of diffuse illumination unique to the PSL. It provides partial compensation for the loss of the dynamic, three-dimensional character of an examination by contributing the important element of perspective in situations that call for limited direct focal illumination. The addition of diffused, overall light places isolated elements into context. In a single image, the fill light provides overall, general information about the eye, and the slit beam is used to highlight specific changes in the cornea (Fig. 7.2). The fill light also must be equipped

* From Berliner ML. *Biomicroscopy of the eye*. Vol 1. New York: Paul B. Hoeber; 1949.

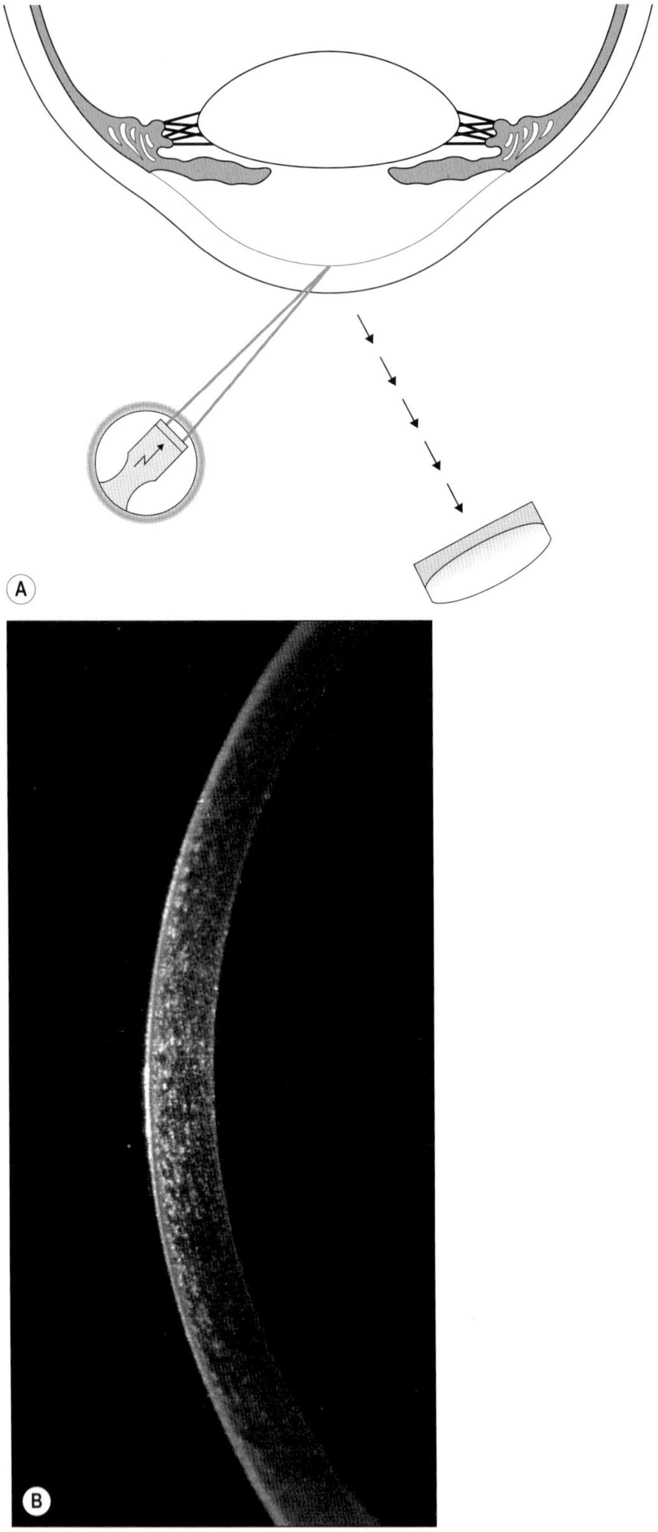

Fig. 7.1 (**A**) Slit illuminator and biomicroscope. (Redrawn from Mártonyi CL, Bahn CF, Meyer RF. *Clinical slit lamp biomicroscopy and photo slit lamp biomicrography*. Ann Arbor: Time One Ink, Ltd; 1985.) (**B**) The magnified optic section is the most important capability of the slit lamp biomicroscope. (From Mártonyi CL, Bahn CF, Meyer RF. *Slit lamp: examination and photography.* Sedona: Time One Ink, Ltd; 2007.)

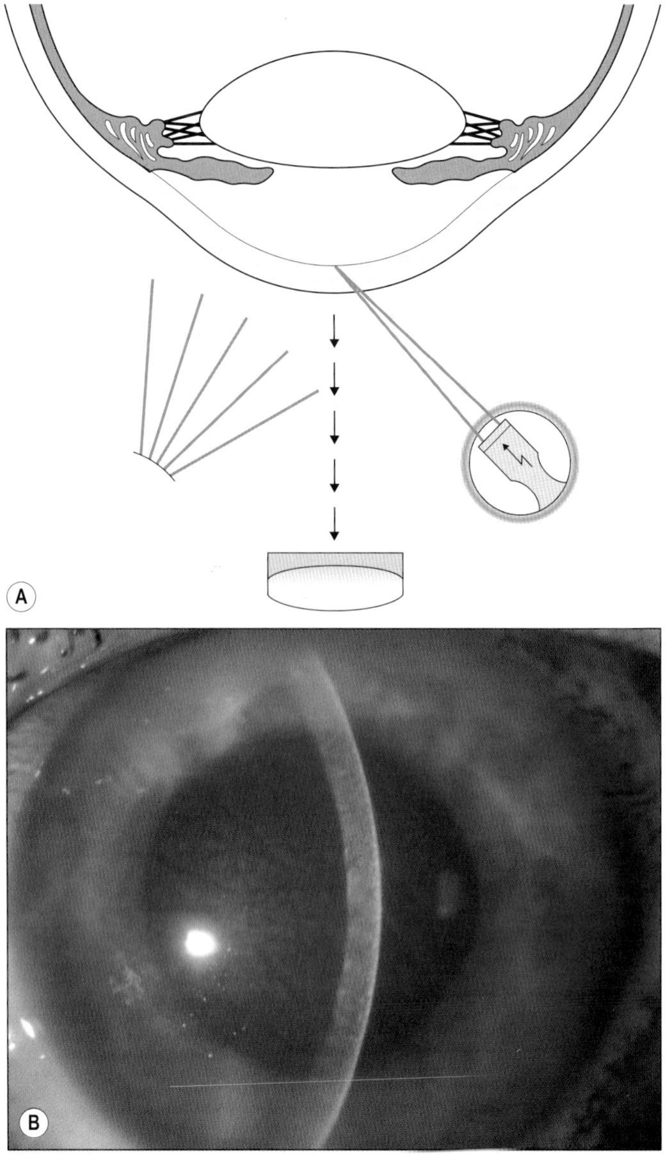

Fig. 7.2 (**A**) Diagrammatic representation of the slit lamp illuminator, biomicroscope objective lens, and fill light. (**B**) Chemical injury to the cornea seen in optic section combined with diffuse illumination from the fill light. (**A**, Redrawn from Mártonyi CL. et al. *Clinical slit lamp biomicroscopy and photo slit lamp biomicrography.* Ann Arbor: Time One Ink, Ltd; 1985. **B**, Mártonyi CL. *Landscapes of the eye: images from ophthalmology.* A Photographic Exhibit, 1993.)

with electronic flash proportioned to an output of approximately two stops lower than that of the slit illuminator. This relationship provides the necessary contrast between the diffusely illuminated background and the bright, narrow slit beam.

Preparing for Photography

The basic protocol for photodocumentation is essentially the same as for slit lamp biomicroscopy. One begins with an overview and proceeds to isolate further with illumination and magnification the salient features of the condition under consideration. Techniques of illumination that produce specific information over a wide area of distribution should be considered whenever applicable. The most utilized images are those that present findings in recognizable context.

Essential detail, however, should not be compromised in an attempt to include everything in a single view, and the fill light should not be used in conjunction with indirect forms of illumination. While such photographs are often used to obviate the need for multiple images, the results will always be compromised.

Although the fundamental principles of clinical slit lamp biomicroscopy and photo slit lamp biomicrography are essentially the same, additional considerations are necessary for successful photodocumentation. Chief among these considerations is the conscious awareness that slit lamp illumination, by its very nature, is a compromise. The larger the area of simultaneous illumination, the less fine detail is seen. Conversely, the more detail elicited by selective illumination, the more out of context that information will be. During a dynamic, three-dimensional examination of the eye, these limitations have little effect on the process of gathering information. The result of a thorough examination is a complete mental image of the condition of the eye. By comparison, a static, two-dimensional photograph is not only deprived of the elements of motion and the third dimension, but is also limited to a single moment of such an examination. As such, it is amazing how effective a single photograph can be.

Several components have been discussed as essential to the PSL. Additional factors must be considered to produce consistently accurate and pleasing photographs. Correct mechanical focus, format, magnification, centration, control of artifacts, and optimum exposure are elements that combine to reproduce visual impressions most accurately.

Focus

The maintenance of a sharp image in the biomicroscope is a continuous element of a dynamic slit lamp examination. Focus is a perpetual, flowing transition as the slit beam is played over the gently curving surfaces of the eye. In a practical sense, there are no specifically individual images, but rather a compendium of infinite, transitional views that produce an aggregate impression. Each photograph, however, is but a single slice of that examination. Therefore, preparations for photo documentation must include the selection of the most informative single view (or the first in a series of views) and the perception of its appearance as a static, two-dimensional image. To ensure a sharp image, precise mechanical focus of the biomicroscope at the time of exposure is critical.

The view seen in the biomicroscope is an aerial image. An aerial image is suspended in space rather than projected onto a flat, immovable plane (as the focusing screen of a single lens reflex camera). Because the view through the biomicroscope would be unacceptably diffused by such a focusing screen, it is not used. The aerial image system, therefore, is the most practical in such an application, but not without limitation. With the image literally floating in air, the mechanical position of the biomicroscope (and the camera back) can be unwittingly altered from its correct focal distance through simple accommodation. Although seen as a sharp image by the examiner, the resultant photograph may be so unsharp as to be unusable. To produce a sharp image on film, a specific protocol is followed.

To facilitate the correct focus of the biomicroscope, a 'cross-hair' reticle is used in one ocular for reference. To use the reticle correctly, the ocular must be adjusted for the user's refractive error. That is best achieved by first turning the eyepiece adjustment to its maximum plus setting. Then, while the user looks through the eyepiece, with accommodation completely relaxed, the setting is adjusted toward the minus side while observing the reticle. This rotation toward the minus should be relatively brisk and should result in a sharp impression of the reticle at or near the user's refractive error, or at zero for an emmetrope. This exercise should be repeated until consistent results are achieved. The image in the biomicroscope should be treated as an object at infinity and viewed with the accommodation completely relaxed. The reticle is always used in the ocular that shares the image with the camera back.

The 35-mm format

The circular field seen in the biomicroscope must be reduced to a corresponding rectangle within that circle. The areas beyond the rectangle, which had been used for examining the eye, must now be disregarded and the intended picture area confined to the photographic format. As a guide, a reticle eyepiece including the rectangular outline is an ideal solution.

Magnification

Many PSLs demonstrate an apparent difference between the image size seen in the microscope and the recorded image. Although the actual magnification is the same, the resultant photographic image appears disappointingly small. This discrepancy results from the larger physical area of the film or sensor as compared with the area within the oculars. To obtain a photograph that matches more closely the image seen in the oculars, the photograph must be taken at one magnification setting higher. On some PSLs, this can be accomplished by placing a 2× optical magnifier between the microscope and the camera back. When a 2× magnifier is not used, the image of the eye to be photographed is viewed at the magnification desired; then, just before taking the photograph, the magnification changer is advanced to the next higher setting. Once the image is recorded, the magnification can be returned to the setting that best delineates visually the next field under consideration.

Centration

The need to ensure that the principal subject is in the center of the photographic field seems obvious. Nevertheless, this element is frequently compromised. The most common cause may be a momentary disregard of the rectangular format in favor of the full, circular field seen in the oculars. Additionally, when the isocentric relationship between the slit illuminator and the biomicroscope is left intact when using indirect forms of illumination, the subject area becomes decentered in favor of the isocentric incident beam. The beam must always be decentered to allow centration of the principal subject area when indirect forms of illumination are used.

Control of artifacts

To be effective, a photograph must first include the principal subject area. Of equal importance is the elimination of unwanted elements that either obscure the desired detail or distract attention from the principal subject.

The most distracting artifacts of illumination are the ubiquitous specular reflections seen during the course of an examination. They are of little concern as they come and go, because their effect is nullified by their momentary presentation during the dynamic examination. In a static photograph, however, such artifacts can considerably compromise an otherwise excellent image. When final adjustments are made preparatory to making an exposure, it is important to view the image only through the ocular that shares that image with the camera back. On most photo slit lamps, the camera back is mounted to share the view seen with the right eye. By closing the left eye, the monocular image on the right, as seen by the camera, will be much more manageable in terms of minimizing artifacts and maximizing desirable elements before its capture.

Exposure

A good exposure results from correct white balance, media sensitivity, intensity of illumination, subject reflectivity, and duration of exposure.

Color balance and sensitivity

Unlike film, digital cameras provide for easy adjustment to match the color temperature of various light sources. This process is called 'white balance' and should be set following the instructions for the camera back used. It will ensure accurate color reproduction in captured images. For electronic flash, the setting is approximately 5400K (degrees Kelvin).

Sensitivity refers to the responsiveness of film and digital media to light, stated in ISO numbers. Low ISO settings will provide better image quality when there is sufficient light for a good exposure. When the captured image is too dark and the flash intensity is already set to maximum, the ISO should be increased sufficiently to obtain good results.

Intensity of illumination

The light output, or flash intensity, of the PSL, while seemingly very bright, is the limiting factor in the use of low ISO values for certain forms of illumination. Flash intensity should be set to maximum for demanding situations before increasing ISO settings for better image quality.

Subject reflectivity

Subject reflectivity is an element of great influence. In recording conditions by direct illumination, levels of subject reflectivity may dictate an adjustment of one to two f-stops for a good exposure at either extreme. In certain applications of indirect illumination, however, a range of four to five f-stops may have to be considered.

Duration of exposure

Duration of exposure is dictated by the electronic flash source, as mentioned earlier. Of very short duration, it makes the effective 'shutter speed' approximately 1/1000th of a second, an ideal speed to arrest motion. This flash duration is not variable. The shutter speed setting on the camera back must be set to the speed prescribed by the manufacturer for electronic flash synchronization – the maximum speed at which both shutter curtains are simultaneously clear of the full frame to permit the short-duration flash to expose the entire image area. Using higher shutter speeds results in the loss of all or part of the frame.

Exposure is everything! The most skilled and experienced clinician will fail to produce good slit lamp images if exposure is miscalculated or neglected. The ability of our eyes to adapt over a wide range of light intensity is not even remotely shared by the camera. Elements of interest that are easily appreciated visually may be completely off the scale from the standpoint of exposure. The development of a thorough exposure guide is an excellent investment, as it provides predictable exposures for most situations. The successful photographer will also have cultivated an intuitive sense for differences beyond the obvious—differences that are subtle visually but require exposure compensation for best results.

Forms of Illumination: Examination and Photography

While there are only a few basic forms of illumination, most have variable uses and are highly effective in specific applications. This chapter concentrates on those forms of illumination and techniques of examination and photography that specifically address the eyelids, conjunctiva, cornea, sclera, and iris. Other structures are mentioned as their examination may be helpful in establishing a diagnosis of conditions involving the principal structure under consideration.

Techniques of illumination are broadly divided into direct and indirect forms. Direct illumination, as the term implies, describes any situation where the beam of light is directed to strike the principal subject area. Direct illumination may be diffused or focal. Indirect illumination techniques use a secondary surface that reflects light onto the principal subject area or light transmitted through tissue from an area of adjacent illumination.

Direct Illumination

Diffuse illumination: examination

Diffuse illumination facilitates simultaneous observation of large areas at low magnification. The area surrounding the eyes, the eyelids, conjunctiva, sclera, cornea, and iris can be quickly reviewed for gross abnormalities. Initiating the slit lamp examination in this manner generates an early, overall

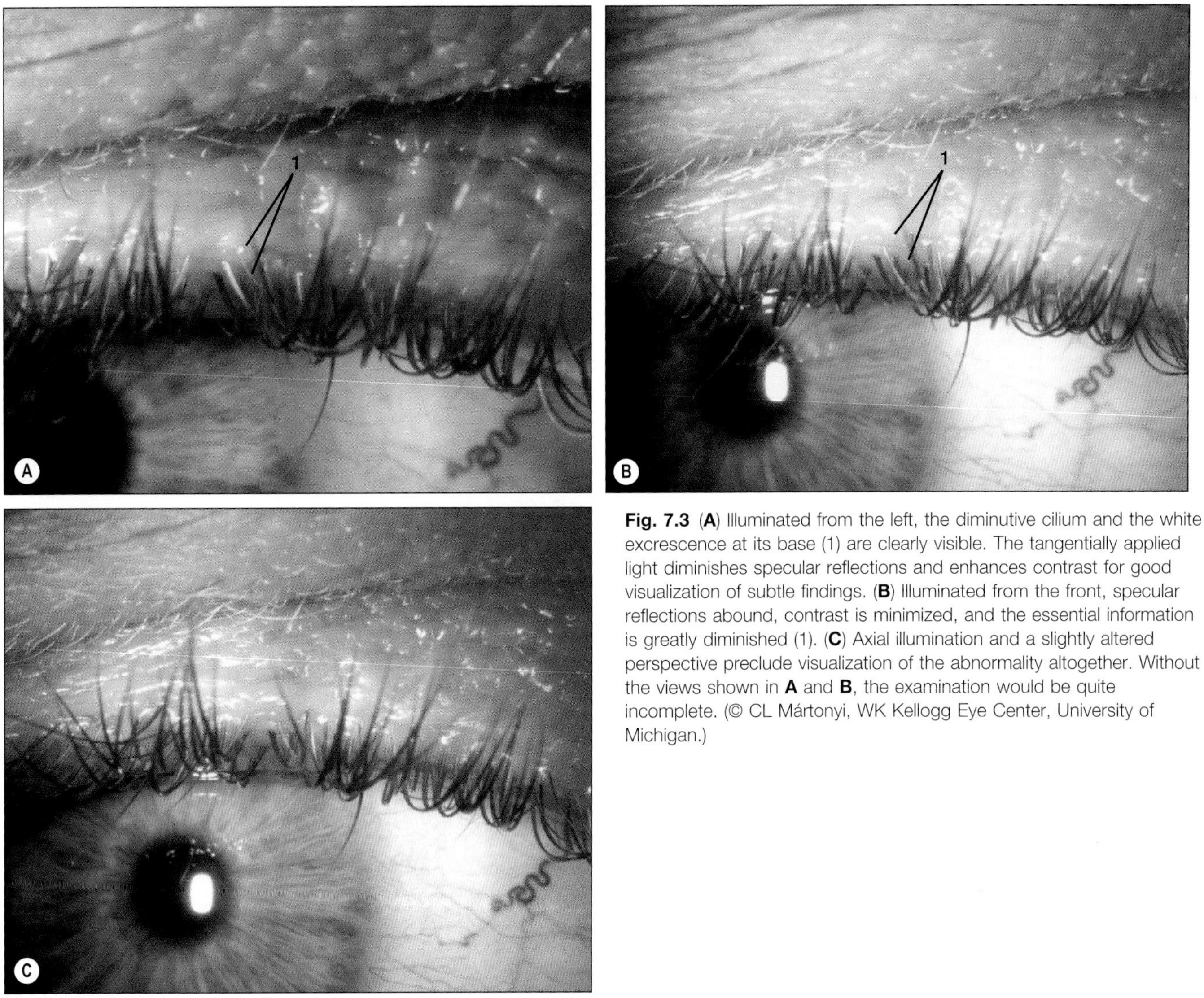

Fig. 7.3 (**A**) Illuminated from the left, the diminutive cilium and the white excrescence at its base (1) are clearly visible. The tangentially applied light diminishes specular reflections and enhances contrast for good visualization of subtle findings. (**B**) Illuminated from the front, specular reflections abound, contrast is minimized, and the essential information is greatly diminished (1). (**C**) Axial illumination and a slightly altered perspective preclude visualization of the abnormality altogether. Without the views shown in **A** and **B**, the examination would be quite incomplete. (© CL Mártonyi, WK Kellogg Eye Center, University of Michigan.)

impression and provides a unifying matrix for the more isolating magnifications and forms of illumination to follow. With the slit illuminator set at its largest aperture and the diffuser in place, the illuminator is rotated through its arc of travel from side to side. The effect is to create alternating axial and tangential illumination. Tangentially applied light, even when diffused, produces highlights and shadows and enhances the visibility of many changes. As shadows and highlights wax and wane with the oscillating illumination, alterations from normal topography become exaggerated and more readily apparent. A subtle presentation of molluscum contagiosum, for example, possibly hidden by cilia, may elude detection in static light, but may become quite obvious through the motion of the illuminator and the biomicroscope. Abnormalities of the lashes, such as collarettes, scales, and broken or missing lashes, are well enhanced with this approach. Because of shadows cast by cilia and foreign matter and the generally translucent nature of such deposits, static light may not provide adequate discrimination. The dynamic travel of light, however, animates shadows and cascades highlights to fully dimensionalize and identify even mild expressions of various conditions (Fig. 7.3).

Focal alterations in skin color (e.g. hyperemia, hyperpigmentation, or hypopigmentation) also present more readily under diffused and dynamically altered light. Focal illumination tends to isolate an area with a proportionate loss of perspective. Additionally, the brightness of focal illumination, with its inherent contrast, makes slight differences in color difficult to appreciate. Another factor to limit the usefulness of focal illumination in this application is the possibly enhanced reflectivity of the skin of the eyelids. Secretions from resident sebaceous glands can engender considerable specular reflections, greatly limiting a view beyond the episurface.

As stated earlier, the initial survey of the conjunctiva, sclera, cornea, and iris in diffuse illumination provides a

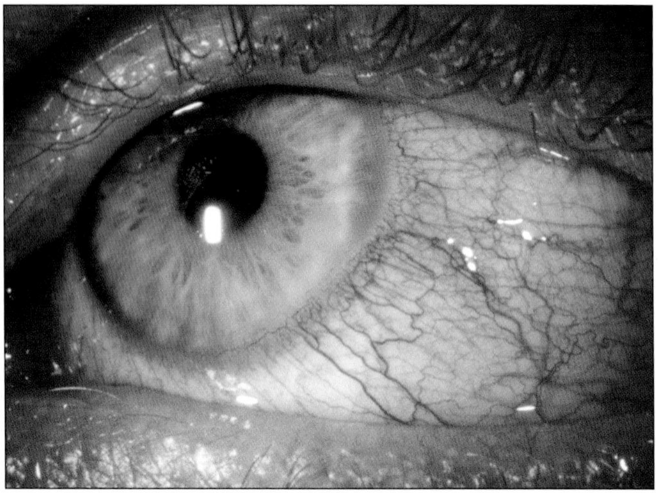

Fig. 7.4 Staphylococcal keratoconjunctivitis and blepharitis are presented in diffuse illumination. (From Mártonyi CL et al. *Slit lamp: examination and photography.* Sedona: Time One Ink, Ltd; 2007.)

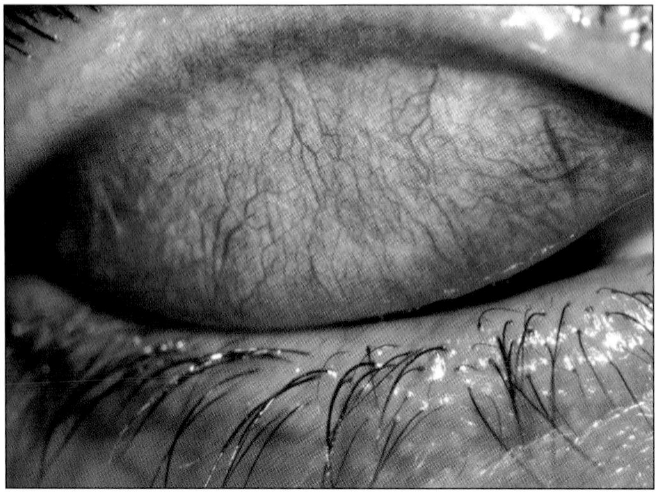

Fig. 7.5 Trachoma with linear scarring seen in diffuse Illumination. (From Mártonyi CL et al. *Slit lamp: examination and photography.* Sedona: Time One Ink, Ltd; 2007.)

useful introduction to overall condition (Fig. 7.4). Many abnormalities are easily visualized with this technique. Findings such as conjunctival injection, follicles, papillae, chemosis, membranes/pseudomembranes, and scarring are recognizable in diffused light and should prompt examination with additional forms of illumination. The inferior and superior palpebral conjunctivae and much of the fornices can be given a preliminary review in the same manner. Tangentially applied diffuse illumination, with increased magnification, is an excellent technique for initial examination of these surfaces (Fig. 7.5).

Inspection in diffuse light often provides the first indication of abnormalities present in the cornea (Box 7.1). Gross opacification or changes that affect its topography present with little coaxing. After such an overview, further investigation can continue with more selective illumination and magnification.

Box 7.1 Examples of conditions seen in diffuse illumination

Sclerocornea	Pterygium
Band keratopathy	Follicles
Trichiasis	Hypopion
Distichiasis	Ectropion
Pinguecula	Corneal pannus
Papillae	Blepharitis
Hordeolum	Arcus senilis
Entropion	Xanthelasma
Megalocornea	Chalazion
Lagophthalmos	Hyphema
Poliosis	

Diffuse illumination: photography

Diffuse illumination is required to show large areas simultaneously at low magnification. By diffusing the light from the slit illuminator, along with the fill light, two sources of diffuse light are available to produce even illumination of the external eye (Fig. 7.6). Such overviews are useful for demonstrating the general condition of the eye and serve as introductions for more isolated views.

Focal illumination

Broad-beam illumination: examination

The term broad-beam illumination is variably used and highly subject to interpretation. It can vary from a beam width of 1 mm to its full size of approximately 11 mm. In this discussion a flexible width is assumed. As with the recommended oscillation of the slit illuminator, a dynamically altered beam width is also beneficial. In this application, the beam is intended only as a source of bright, focal illumination, with the width adjusted to maximize information within the area under study. As the light strikes tissue interfaces, it is reflected, refracted, transmitted, scattered, and absorbed in a highly variable fashion. Thus, a given width of beam, with its corresponding overall intensity, may provide good information to confirm a particular entity, but may overpower findings associated with another. A beam width of 2–3 mm can provide a good starting point (Fig. 7.7). Although width is an important factor in the beam's efficiency in specific applications, its intensity also affects its usefulness. A beam that is too bright will produce scatter, reducing the examiner's ability to discriminate. Conversely, a beam intensity that is too 'gentle' (in deference to patient comfort, for example) may preclude detection of mild departures from the normal.

As various tissues are examined, suspected alterations from the normal will either be confirmed or will prompt the examiner to use more or less light in their continued pursuit. As a general rule, forms of illumination should be exaggerated in both directions beyond the ideal setting, especially

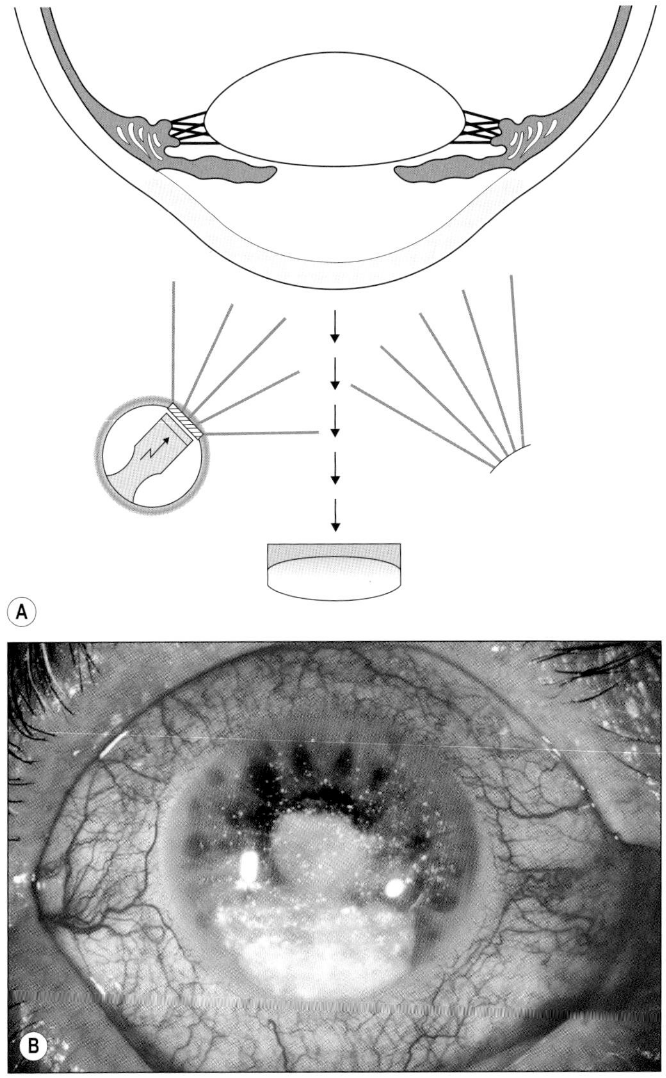

Fig. 7.6 (**A**) Two sources of diffuse illumination. (**B**) A case of phakolytic glaucoma is seen in dual, diffuse illumination. (**A**, From Mártonyi CL et al. *Slit lamp: examination and photography.* Sedona: Time One Ink, Ltd; 2007. **B**, © CL Mártonyi, WK Kellogg Eye Center, University of Michigan.)

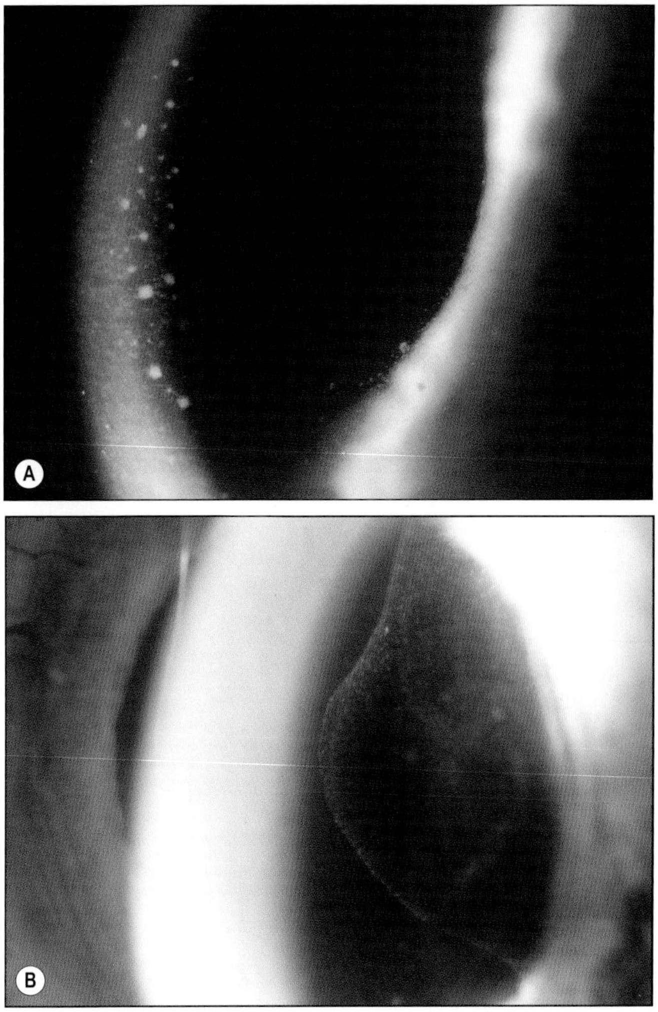

Fig. 7.7 (**A**) Keratic precipitates are well visualized with a moderate, direct beam. (**B**) Vitreous presenting in the anterior chamber is illuminated with a broad beam of a much higher intensity than would be used for tissue of greater reflectivity. (**A**, © CL Mártonyi, WK Kellogg Eye Center, University of Michigan, **B**, From Mártonyi CL et al. *Slit lamp: examination and photography.* Sedona: Time One Ink, Ltd; 2007.)

with the use of broad-beam illumination. The beam should be narrowed to the point of diminished width and then increased in width beyond the ideal setting to the point at which information loss occurs once again. Only by testing these limits will optimum size and intensity become apparent.

Many conditions are seen best using broad-beam illumination (Box 7.2). All changes that are fairly opaque and reflect or absorb considerable amounts of light can be visualized easily. The light should be applied tangentially for maximum effectiveness. Topographic changes will become dramatically sculpted by the raking light. Additionally, oblique illumination will obviate the dazzling specular reflections resulting from axial lighting (Fig. 7.8). Tangentially applied broad-beam illumination is one of the most effective forms for examining the iris surface (Fig. 7.9).

Box 7.2 Examples of conditions seen in broad-beam illumination

Corneal vascularization	Corneal scars
Basement membrane dystrophy	Lisch nodules
Reis-Bücklers' dystrophy	Keratic precipitates
Schnyder's crystalline dystrophy	Granular dystrophy
Terrien's marginal dystrophy	Iris atrophy
Amiodarone vortex dystrophy	Pterygium
Prominent corneal nerves	Band keratopathy
Salzmann's nodular degeneration	Macular dystrophy
Posterior embryotoxon	Arcus senilis

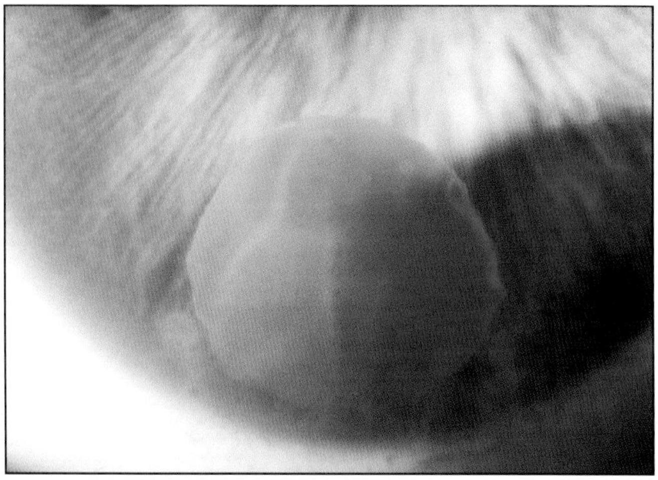

Fig. 7.8 Broad-beam illumination demonstrating a luxated, mature lens nucleus. The tangentially applied light dramatizes dimension and minimizes reflections from overlying surfaces. (From Mártonyi CL et al. *Slit lamp: examination and photography.* Sedona: Time One Ink, Ltd; 2007.)

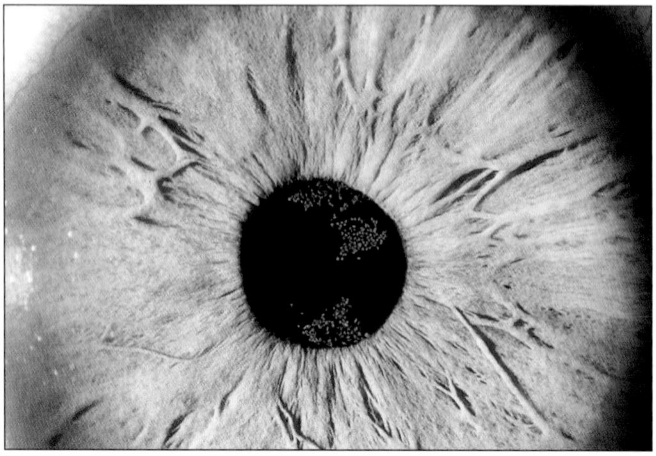

Fig. 7.9 Broad-beam illumination of the iris and anterior lens surface in Rieger's syndrome. (From Mártonyi CL et al. *Slit lamp: examination and photography.* Sedona: Time One Ink, Ltd; 2007.)

When no abnormalities are seen with this technique, more selective forms of illumination are indicated. The absence of findings under broad-beam illumination should never encourage the conclusion that abnormalities are not present. However useful in the applications described above, broad-beam illumination can be quite counterproductive to the detection of many alterations of subtle expression.

Broad-beam illumination: photography

When diffused light causes too much scatter or when a specific element of a condition must be emphasized, a broad beam, without fill light, can be used. Beam size is important to the outcome. Although desirable from the standpoint of an all-inclusive photograph, when beam size is enlarged to include too much, the results are often compromised. The effect of illumination must be observed carefully while dynamically altering beam width to determine the optimum setting (see Figs 7.7–7.9). Exposure is not a problem because this form of illumination returns the largest percentage of the light available. Magnification should be increased to make best use of the photographic format.

The presentation of the beam should be as oblique as possible. Axial light is reflected axially from surfaces overlying the condition or object to be photographed and further reduces dimensional information within the subject area (Fig. 7.10). The tangential presentation of light, however, facilitates illumination of the subject without overlying reflections to diffuse information and simultaneously enhances its topography (Fig. 7.11). This form can also be used to isolate abnormalities of high reflectance in transparent tissue. When photographing an object within the lens or the anterior vitreous, a well-dilated pupil is necessary to accommodate a sufficiently tangential presentation of light to obviate reflections from overlying surfaces (Fig. 7.12).

Optic section: examination

This narrowest slit beam is, in effect, a fine blade of light that makes possible the virtual serial sectioning of transparent tissues in the living eye. The tangential presentation of these 'light slices' facilitates an essentially cross-sectional view of the cornea and lens, even though these structures are largely parallel with the plane of observation. The sharply focused light is completely confined to the optic section, reducing scatter and maximizing contrast between the illuminated section and the dark, unilluminated surround. The result is a clear, basically uncompromised view of the tissue within the beam. As the slit beam is projected from an increasingly lateral position (away from the axis of the biomicroscope), the greater angular presentation has the effect of increasing the distance between the anterior and posterior surfaces of the structure under study. This increase serves to clarify intrastructural relationships and localization of abnormalities within.

This capability represents the most selective and most isolating manner in which such tissue may be illuminated and observed (Box 7.3). For maximum effectiveness, the light intensity is set to maximum, and the slit beam is diminished in width to a point just before the optic section loses structural integrity. The thinner the beam, the more selective the optic section, thus producing finer delineation of information within that section. Beam width, however, should never be reduced to the point at which information is compromised because of light loss.

The transparency of the cornea, coupled with its propensity for both primary and secondary expressions of numerous diseases, makes it the most important component of the eye to section with light. Although remarkably transparent, normal corneal tissue is sufficiently relucent to reflect the narrow slit beam and articulate the optic section.

A high-magnification view of the optic section will produce excellent discrimination of the substantial corneal layers. Beginning with the tear film, each layer may be selectively examined for departures from the normal (Fig. 7.13). The normal tear film will 'flow' dynamically within the slit beam following each blink of the eyelids. Its reflectivity will alter with the amount of refreshed, protective lipid on its

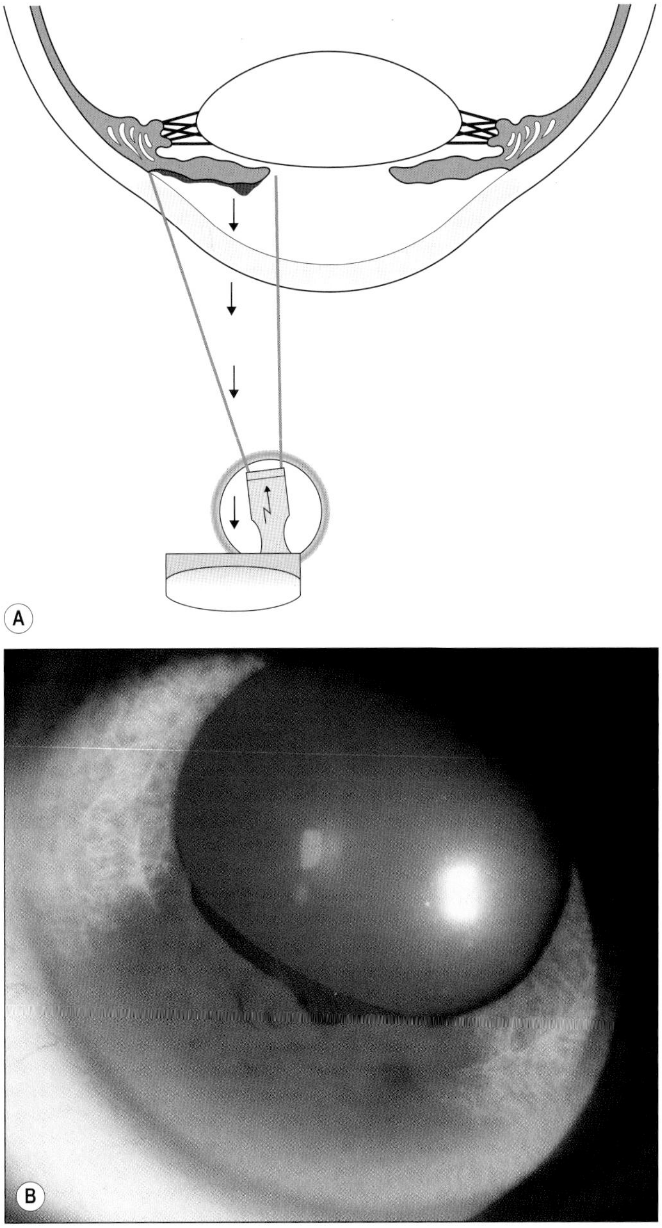

Fig. 7.10 (**A**) and (**B**) This iris lesion is de-emphasized by the diffusing axial reflection of light and the lack of highlights and shadows to demonstrate its dimensional nature. (From Mártonyi CL et al. *Slit lamp: examination and photography.* Sedona: Time One Ink, Ltd; 2007.)

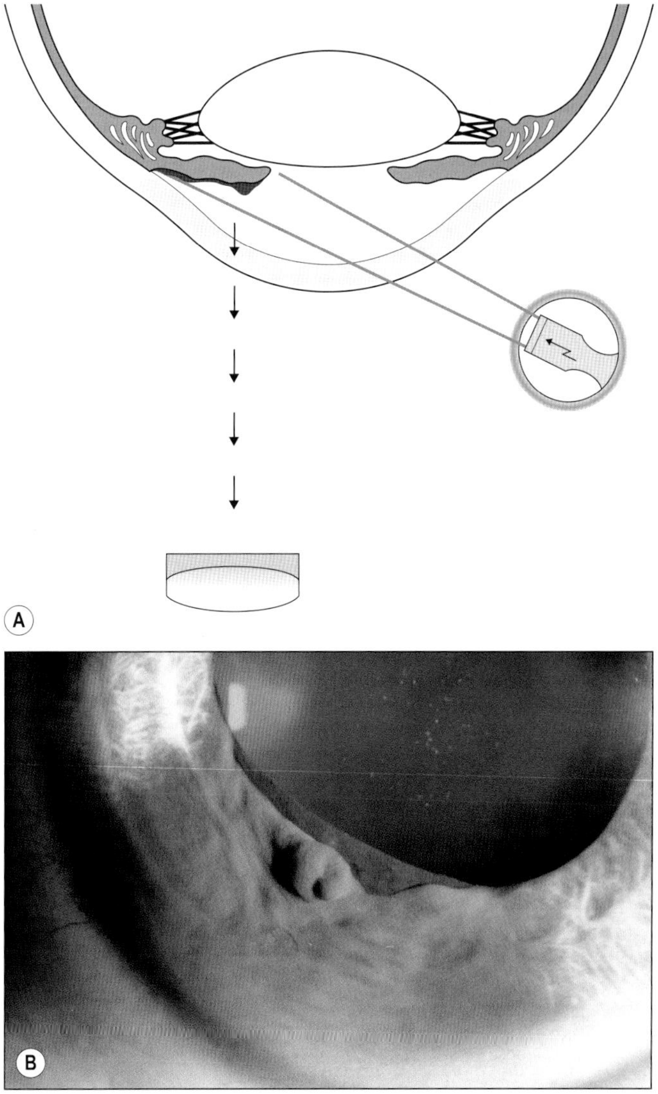

Fig. 7.11 (**A**) and (**B**) A tangentially applied beam will obviate the reflections inherent in axial illumination and will dimensionalize the subject with the highlights and shadows it creates. (From Mártonyi CL et al. *Slit lamp: examination and photography.* Sedona: Time One Ink, Ltd; 2007.)

surface, but will maintain a constant thickness and a smooth anterior face. The epithelium is seen as a line of nonreflectance or greatly diminished reflectance between reflections from the tear film and Bowman's layer, which is contiguous with (and largely indistinguishable from) the anterior-most reflection from the stroma. The stroma itself is quite transparent. By encroaching on the zone of specular reflection, however, its reflectance can be enhanced considerably for better visualization of its structure. The optic section will terminate with the heightened reflection from the endothelium.

As corneal transparency is lost to disease or injury, an increased amount of light is reflected. (The condition of a

Box 7.3 Examples of conditions seen in optic section

Edema	Lens opacities
Stromal opacities	Dellen
Marginal dystrophy	Microcysts
Kayser-Fleisher ring	Bullae
Fuchs' dystrophy	Ectatic changes
Corneal pannus	Anterior chamber depth
Epithelial defect	Tear film deficiency
Corneal infiltrates	Corneal thinning
Furrow dystrophy	

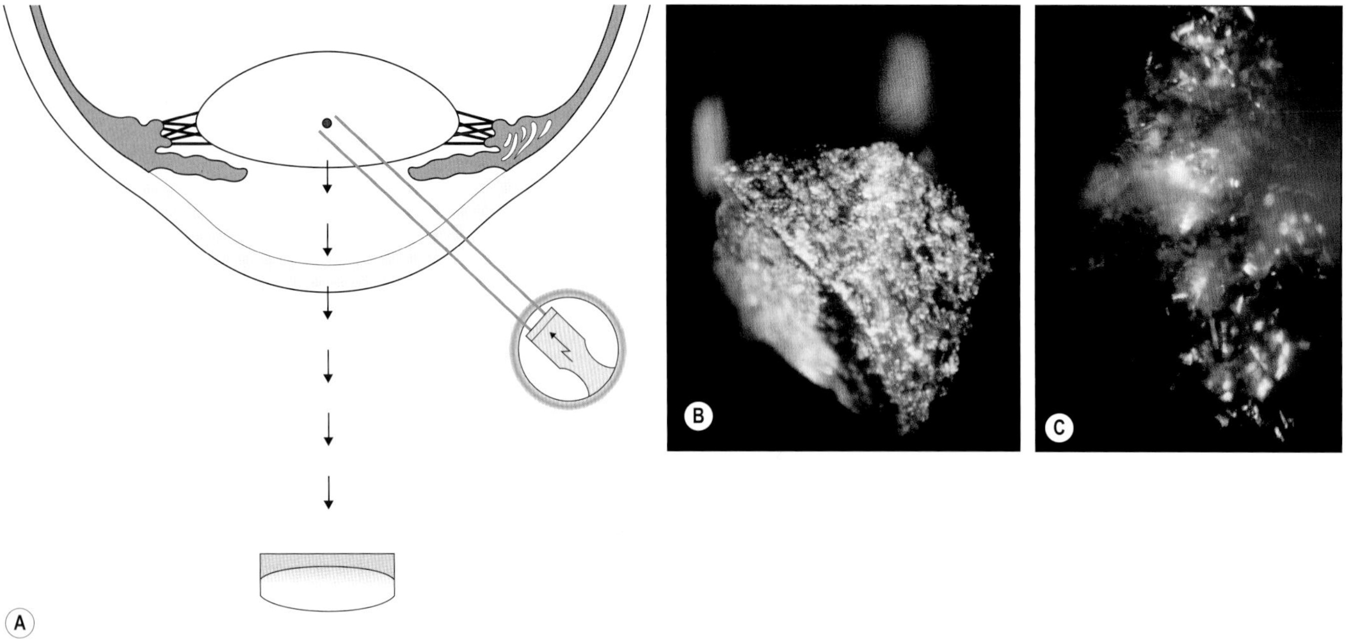

Fig. 7.12 (**A**) and (**B**) Metallic foreign body in a clear lens, isolated with a moderate, tangentially applied beam. (**C**) 'Christmas tree' cataract shown in great clarity due to the unilluminated surfaces in front and behind the subject, facilitated by tangential illumination. (From Mártonyi CL et al. *Slit lamp: examination and photography.* Sedona: Time One Ink, Ltd; 2007.)

sclerotic, totally opaque cornea represents the extreme, or terminal, end of this transmission spectrum. In this condition, much of the light is reflected by the surface, limiting visual access to deeper layers. In such cases, moderate amounts of illumination will be considerably more informative, and a thorough examination will necessitate the use of indirect techniques, as discussed later in this chapter.)

An inadequate tear film will present as a compromise to the normally smooth, unbroken reflection of the beam (Fig. 7.14). An edematous epithelium will become dimensional in the optic section and reflect increasing amounts of light (Fig. 7.15). Focal density changes will be isolated to the anterior, mid, or posterior cornea (Figs 7.16 and 7.17). Descemet's membrane will become visible when abnormal mechanical forces alter its normal topography (Fig. 7.18). The endothelium will reflect increased amounts of light when affected by changes such as Fuchs' dystrophy (Fig. 7.19). Within the visual axis, relatively mild expressions of tissue compromise can cause notable symptoms. Determining exact location and distribution is significant for arriving at a diagnosis.

As the cornea is scanned in optic section, the relationship of the anterior to the posterior surface is also observed for changes in normal thickness and curvature. Ectatic changes, such as keratoconus or keratoglobus, will become readily apparent (Fig. 7.20). Focal elevations or depressions also become obvious as the slit beam deviates toward or away from the light source (Fig. 7.21).

The narrow slit beam is important to apply to all ocular surfaces. A thorough scan of the lid margins, the bulbar and palpebral conjunctiva, the plica, caruncle, and corneal limbus will provide confirmatory information or add to what was gleaned using the modalities described earlier. The narrow slit beam is most effective in detecting topographic changes in these structures (Fig. 7.22). Follicles, papillae, or other dimensional alterations are well stated in this manner. All tissue will demonstrate some penetration by the beam. The degree of penetrativeness is variably limited by the optical density of the tissue under study. Although actual penetration may be minimal, the information produced can be valuable. Of equal or greater importance is the indirect, proximal illumination simultaneously achieved (see section entitled Indirect Illumination).

The relationship between the cornea and iris is also evaluated with a narrow slit beam. By projecting the light from a moderate angle and observing the distance between the reflections from the cornea and the iris, a good estimate of anterior chamber depth can be obtained. Observing this relationship at the limbus provides information regarding the grade of the angle.[1] A completely closed segment of the angle is indicated by a contiguous presentation of corneal and iris reflections (Fig. 7.23). In a similar fashion, anterior synechiae may present as focal areas of contact between the reflected beams at the posterior corneal surface. This condition is confirmed by observing the slit beam coursing up the side of the tented iris tissue to make contact with the reflection from the posterior corneal surface (Fig. 7.24).

Optic section: photography

Easily applied at the clinical slit lamp, the optic section remains a challenge to reproduce photographically. The primary problem is insufficient light. Most PSLs do not generate sufficient flash power to adequately expose a thin slit beam in relatively clear cornea. As a result, the most refined sectioning capabilities of the slit beam may have to be sacrificed in the interest of exposure. A wider than optimum beam may have to be used as the standard; however, the beam should not be widened to the point at which the optic sectioning capability is lost. Rather than settling for a beam too wide, one should consider increasing the ISO setting.

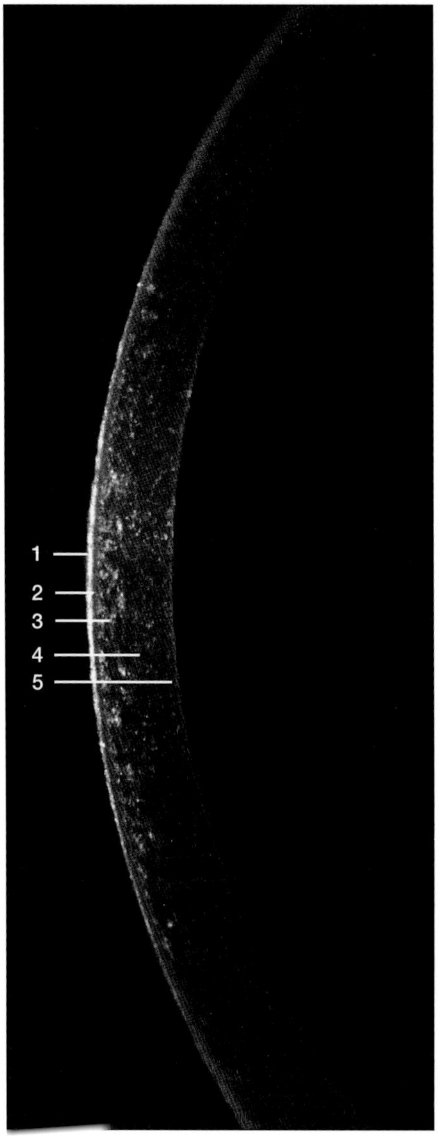

Fig. 7.13 Optic section through a normal cornea demonstrating its principal layers. (1) Tear film, (2) epithelium, (3) anterior stroma with high density of keratocytes, (4) posterior stroma with lower density of keratocytes, (5) posterior layer (Descemet's membrane and endothelium). (From Mártonyi CL et al. *Slit lamp: examination and photography.* Sedona: Time One Ink, Ltd; 2007.)

Once the best compromise between beam width and exposure is achieved, the instrument should be calibrated to reproduce that same width whenever the situation calls for an optic section. The use of maximum flash power is assumed.

Photographs of the optic section can convey precise information regarding the condition of the cornea and other structures (see Figs 7.13 through 7.24).

Combined direct focal and diffused illumination: photography

This type of illumination produces one of the most informative single images of the eye. It combines the narrow slit

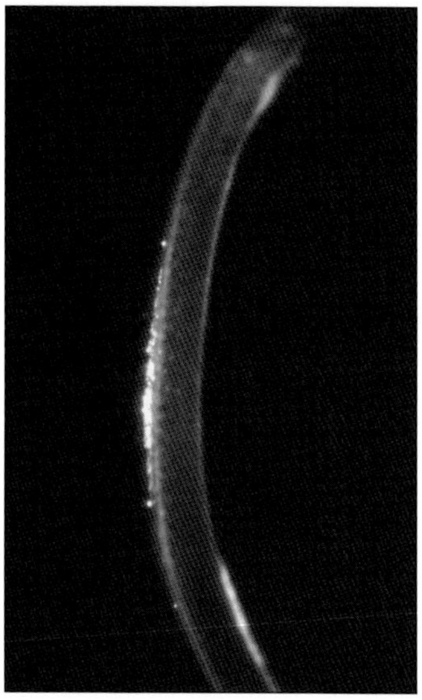

Fig. 7.14 The fragmented reflection from the corneal surface indicates an inadequate tear film, an uneven epithelial surface, or both. (From Mártonyi CL et al. *Slit lamp: examination and photography.* Sedona: Time One Ink, Ltd; 2007.)

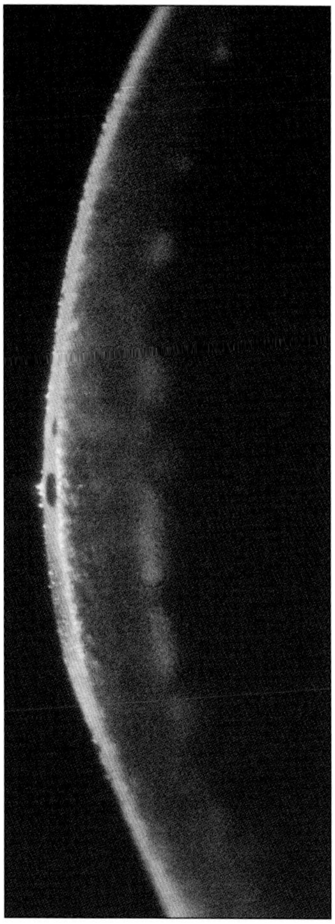

Fig. 7.15 The normally nonreflective epithelium is visible when edematous. The reflection is contiguous with the reflections from the tear film and the stroma. Two small edema clefts are seen in optic section. (From Mártonyi CL et al. *Slit lamp: examination and photography.* Sedona: Time One Ink, Ltd; 2007.)

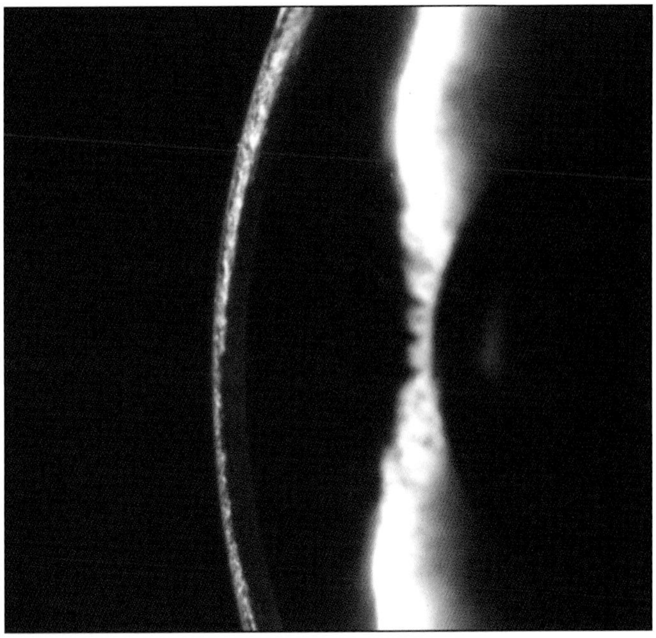

Fig. 7.16 Anterior to mid-stromal deposits are seen in a patient with dystonia. (Copyright Mártonyi CL, WK Kellogg Eye Center, University of Michigan.)

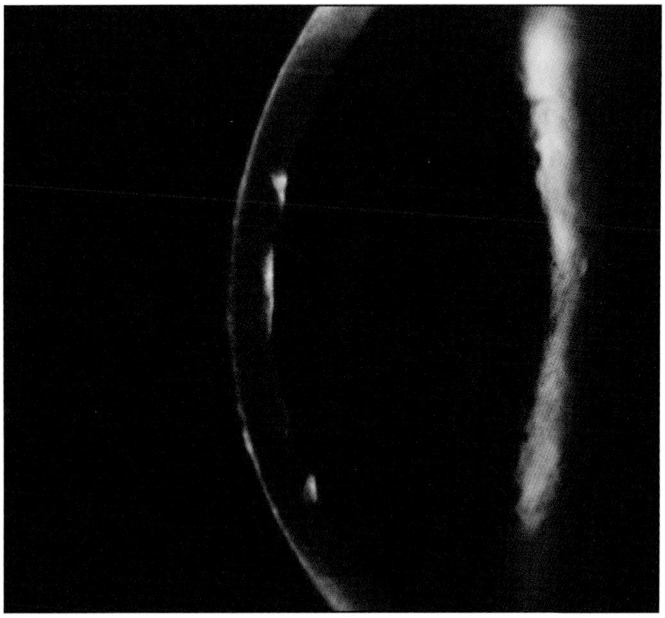

Fig. 7.18 The normally nonreflective Descemet's membrane layer is made visible by the reflection of light from its disturbed architecture in pseudophakic bullous keratopathy. (From Mártonyi CL et al. *Slit lamp: examination and photography*. Sedona: Time One Ink, Ltd; 2007.)

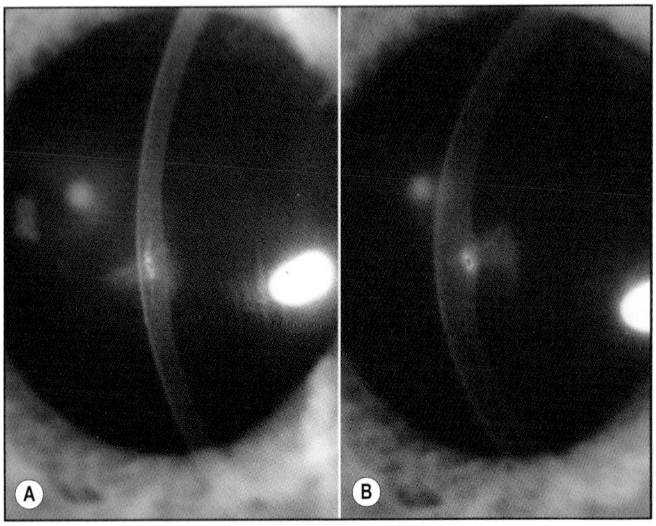

Fig. 7.17 (**A**) and (**B**) Two images demonstrating the right-to-left, anterior-to-posterior track of a penetrating foreign body. (From Mártonyi CL et al. *Slit lamp: examination and photography*. Sedona: Time One Ink, Ltd; 2007.)

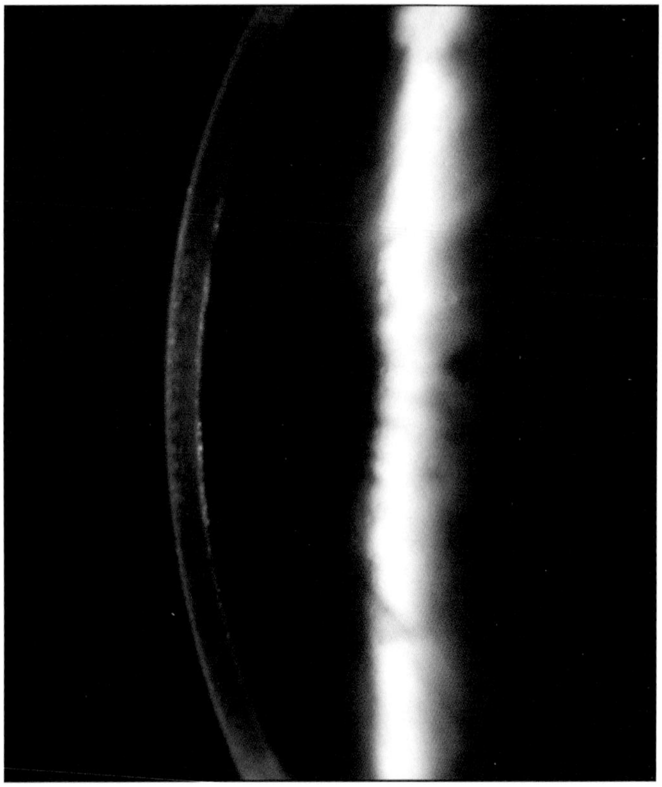

Fig. 7.19 Abnormal amounts of light are seen reflected from the endothelial layer in Fuchs' dystrophy. (From Mártonyi CL et al. *Slit lamp: examination and photography*. Sedona: Time One Ink, Ltd; 2007.)

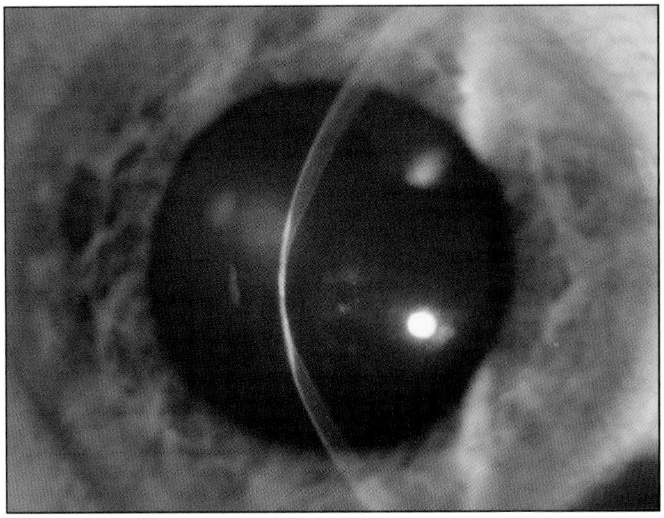

Fig. 7.20 Central thinning is obvious in this optic section of keratoconus. (From Mártonyi CL et al. *Slit lamp: examination and photography.* Sedona: Time One Ink, Ltd; 2007.)

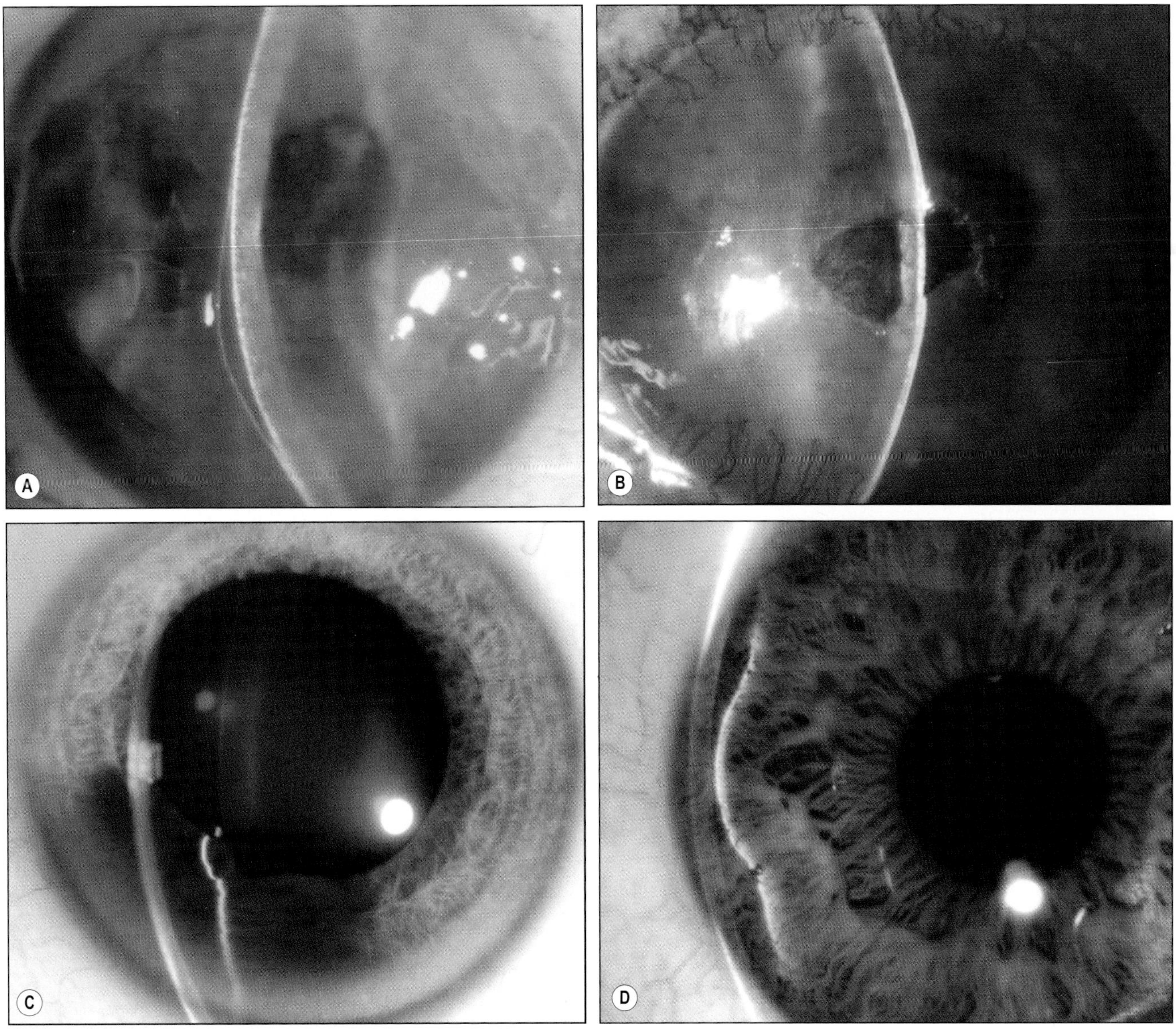

Fig. 7.21 (**A**) Aphakic bullous keratopathy with the large bulla well described by the slit beam. (**B**) Chemical injury with central loss of epithelium and limbal vascularization. (**C**) An iris lesion, clearly seen as elevated by the contour of the slit beam. (**D**) The deviating slit beam indicates a focal elevation of the iris by a ciliary body cyst. (From Mártonyi CL et al. *Slit lamp: examination and photography.* Sedona: Time One Ink, Ltd; 2007.)

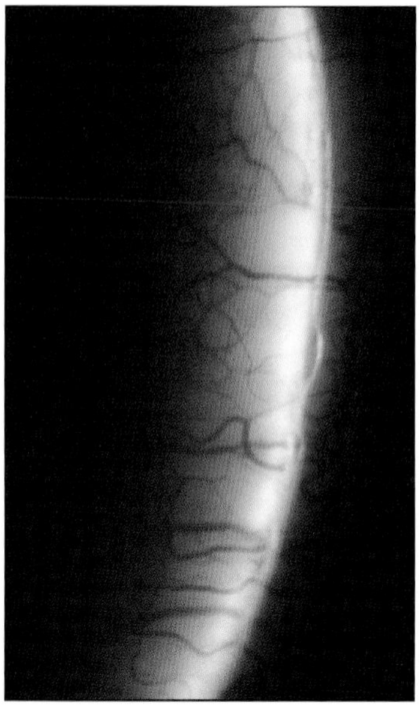

Fig. 7.22 The slit beam deviates toward the source, confirming elevations in the bulbar conjunctiva. (From Mártonyi CL et al. *Slit lamp: examination and photography.* Sedona: Time One Ink, Ltd; 2007.)

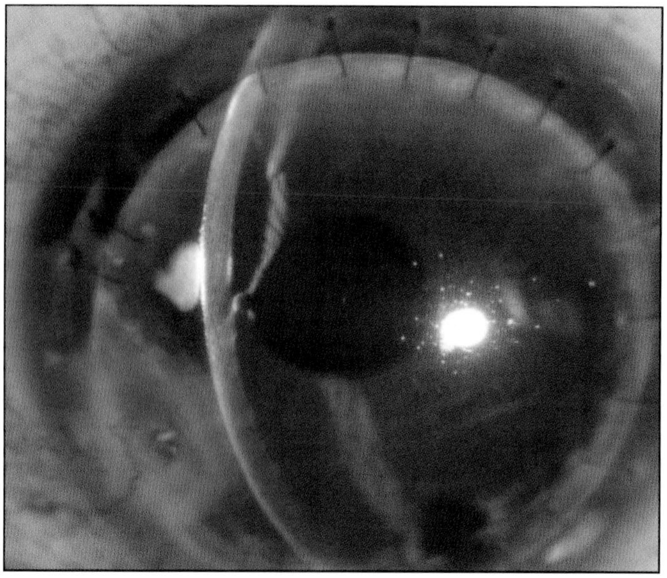

Fig. 7.24 Iris tissue adherent to the posterior corneal surface in an eye that, following successful penetrating corneal transplantation, suffered a penetrating foreign body injury. (From Mártonyi CL et al. *Slit lamp: examination and photography.* Sedona: Time One Ink, Ltd; 2007.)

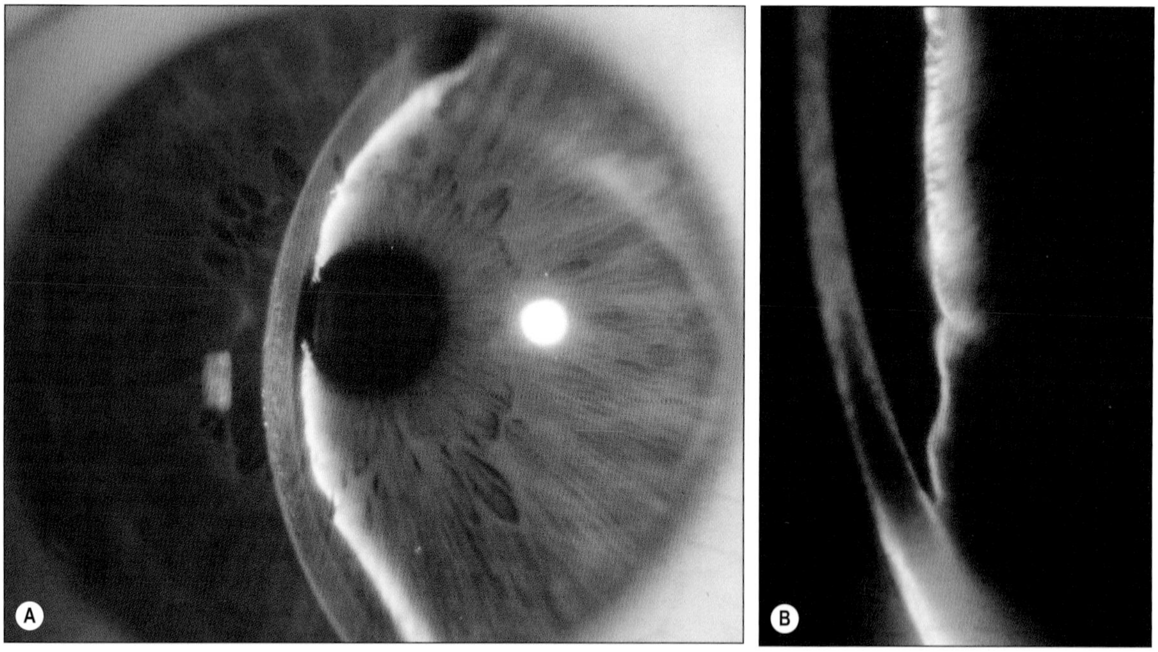

Fig. 7.23 (**A**) A very shallow anterior chamber is evidenced by the proximity of reflections from the iris and the corneal endothelium. Superiorly, contiguous reflections indicate an area of closed angle. (**B**) An area of the angle closed by an iris lesion. (**A**, From Mártonyi CL et al. *Slit lamp: examination and photography.* Sedona: Time One Ink, Ltd; 2007. **B**, © CL Mártonyi, WK Kellogg Eye Center, University of Michigan.)

beam discussed above with diffuse illumination from the fill light. The fill light is responsible for mean exposure and, therefore, the slit beam is used at an intensity that technically constitutes an overexposure. This relationship is necessary to demonstrate adequate background information and a sufficiently brilliant slit beam to highlight information within the section. Numerically, the slit beam is approximately two f-stops (four times) brighter than the fill light. This combination is excellent for portraying conditions of the cornea and also applicable to numerous other situations (see Figs 7.20 through 7.24).

Tyndall's light/anterior chamber cells and flare: examination

Based on Tyndall's phenomenon, pinpoint illumination is maximally effective at isolating aqueous cells and flare. The anterior chamber is considered optically empty, as its contents do not reflect sufficient light to express the beam in the normal state. The cells and protein that present in response to local inflammation, therefore, can be seen readily when isolated within the well-defined, narrow tunnel of light produced by pinpoint illumination.

A small, round beam of high intensity is directed tangentially through the anterior chamber, and the focal point of the light (and the biomicroscope) is swept through the aqueous to determine the presence and density of cells and flare. For maximum contrast, when conditions permit, cells and flare should be observed against the dark background of a dilated pupil, while minimizing the light striking the iris.

Although the 'pinpoint' or 'pencil of light' configuration represents the most discriminating technique,[2] the standard grading system used to describe the concentration of cells and flare assumes the use of a beam approximately 1 × 3 mm in size. The number of actual cells seen simultaneously within that beam is the stated degree of the condition. The amount of abnormal protein is determined by the examiner's impression of the reflectivity (or Tyndall effect) of the aqueous. The degree of expression of these two conditions is stated in terms of one to four-plus cells and/or flare (Fig. 7.25).

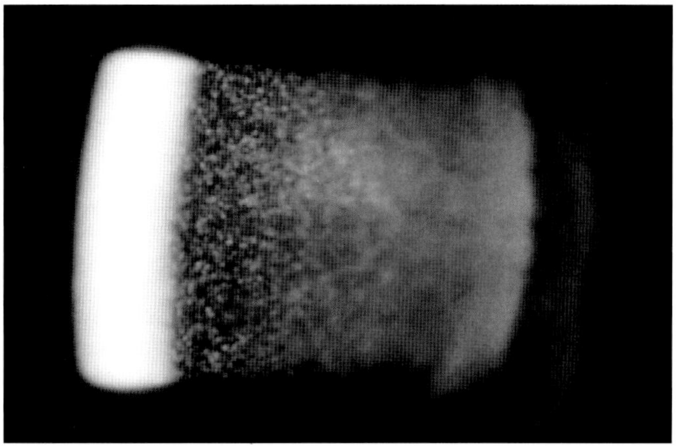

Fig. 7.25 A dramatic expression of four-plus aqueous cells in a case of endophthalmitis. (From Mártonyi CL et al. *Slit lamp: examination and photography.* Sedona: Time One Ink, Ltd; 2007.)

Tyndall's light/anterior chamber cells and flare: photography

Documentation of this condition is clearly the most challenging task in slit lamp photography. Although cells and flare are easily visualized, their low reflectivity makes it difficult to obtain an adequate exposure. Even 'four-plus' expressions will be marginally exposed at a sensitivity below 3200 ISO.[2]

The beam should be configured into a small spot or 'pencil of light' to produce maximum isolation.[3] With a fairly tangential presentation of the beam at moderate magnification, useful images can be achieved. For maximum contrast and best results, the focal point of the beam should be placed over the dark, unilluminated pupil (Fig. 7.26).

Specular reflection: examination

The bright, mirrored reflections of light sources are considered regular, or specular, reflections, as opposed to the more common, irregular reflections whereby most objects are seen.[3] Specular reflections are subject to Snell's law of optics,

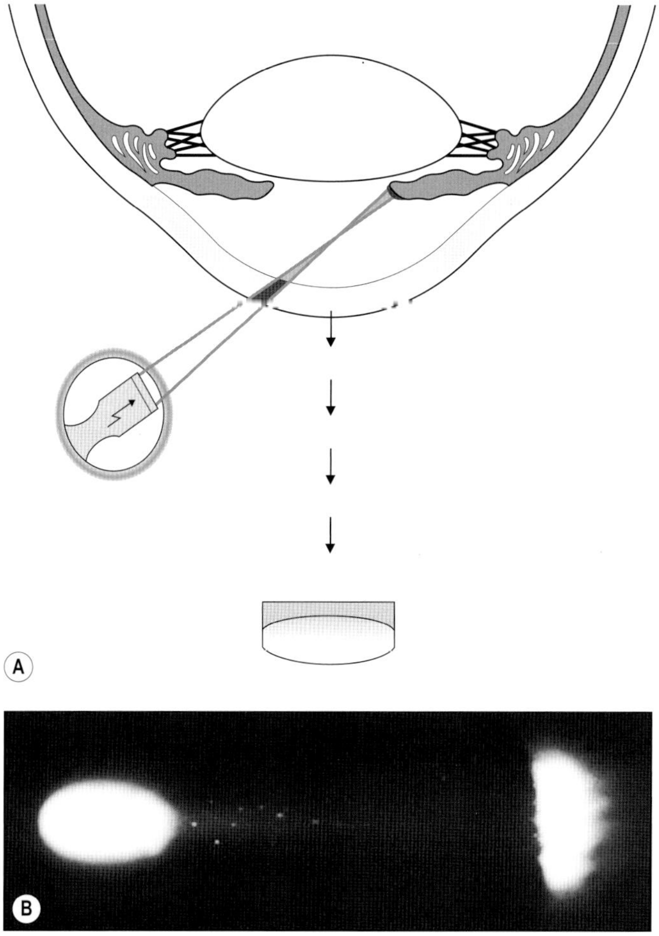

Fig. 7.26 (**A**) and (**B**) Pinpoint illumination of cells and flare, recorded on 400 ISO film push-processed to 1000 ISO. (From Mártonyi CL et al. *Slit lamp: examination and photography.* Sedona: Time One Ink, Ltd; 2007.)

which states that the angle of reflection equals the angle of incidence. That suggests a level of difficulty associated with the location of such a reflection that is simply not present when examining the eye. On the curved ocular surfaces, specular reflections are easily elicited. The convex cornea and the high reflectivity of its anterior-most layer, the tear film, combine to make such reflections more or less ever-present companions during the course of an examination. While at times annoying, these reflections are, in fact, of great value for gathering information about the condition of the eye.

As the eye is viewed in direct illumination, the zone of specular reflection is studied as an expression of surface integrity. This evaluation should be performed under a fairly low light level, so as to diminish scatter and make visible detail within the zone of specular reflection. The area of specular reflection is not only a mirror image of the source but also faithfully mirrors the topographic condition of the surface on which it rests. Therefore, a compromised corneal surface will produce an abnormal reflection of the light source. Broken or granular reflections may indicate an inadequate tear film, the presence of foreign material, or a compromise to underlying tissue expressed as an alteration from normal topography. A greatly diminished or irregular reflection is always a clear sign of abnormality (Fig. 7.27).

The most important application of the specular reflection is in the evaluation of the corneal endothelium. While not expressly difficult, this technique may prove initially challenging. The reflectivity of the endothelial surface is so much lower than that of the tear film layer that the specular reflection may not be appreciated even when present. An angular difference of 30 to 40 degrees between the slit illuminator and the biomicroscope will make the task easier by producing greater separation between the two reflections. Moving the incident beam laterally across the face of the cornea will elicit the bright specular reflection from the tear film layer. By observing the adjacent area on the side away from the light source, the more demure endothelial reflection is seen. Moving the biomicroscope forward approximately 0.5 mm will bring into focus the endothelial layer and cellular detail should become apparent. To obtain a clear view of endothelial cells, especially those that populate the uncompromised, young cornea, a magnification of 25× to 40× is required (Fig. 7.28). When such levels of magnification are not available, the endothelium can still be evaluated with this technique. The reflection is observed for continuity and uniform intensity as the light is played across the endothelium. When conditions such as guttae are present, the homogeneity of the reflection is interrupted (Fig. 7.29).

In severe expressions of disease-related endothelial compromise, such as advanced Fuchs' dystrophy, the reflection may become totally altered from the normal. Coalesced guttae may cause it to appear patchy or quite dark overall and, even when viewed at high magnification, information about individual cell borders may not be present (Fig. 7.30). In such conditions, even specular micrography may fail to produce satisfactory information regarding cell morphology or density.

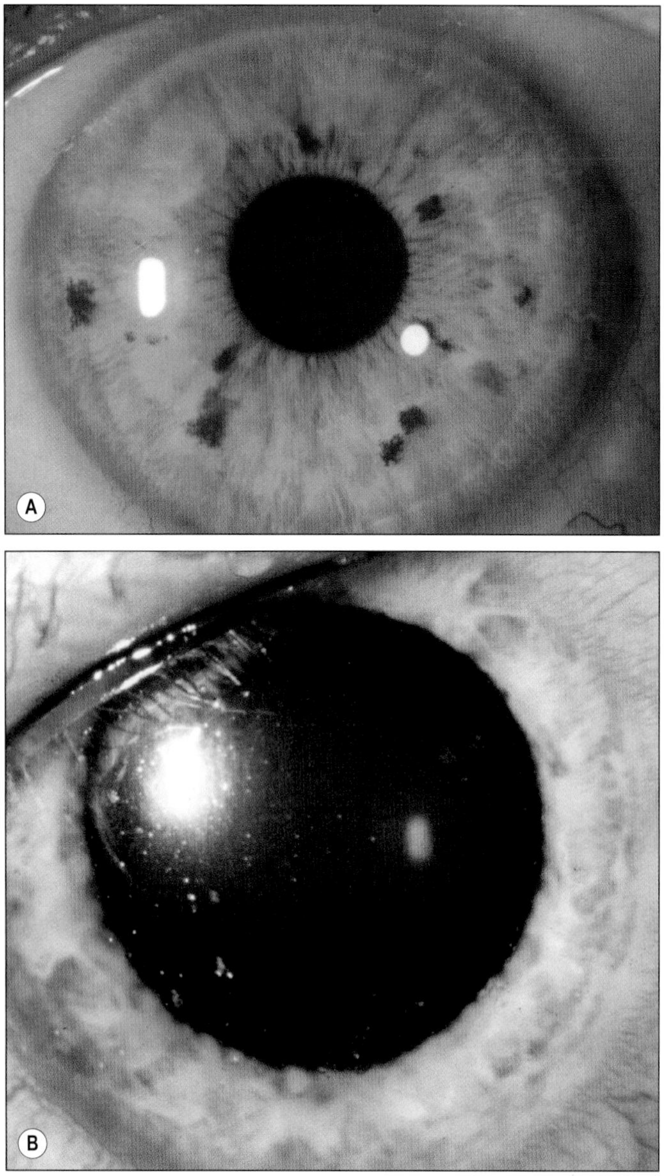

Fig. 7.27 (**A**) Specular reflections faithfully reproduce the shapes of light sources on the surface of a normal tear film layer. (**B**) The specular reflections are altered from normal by the condition of interstitial keratitis. (**A**, From Mártonyi CL et al. *Slit lamp: examination and photography.* Sedona: Time One Ink, Ltd; 2007.)

The specular reflection can also be used to examine the surface of the conjunctiva and the anterior and posterior surfaces of the lens.

Specular reflection: photography

Although the reflection from the endothelium is much less intense when compared to the reflection from the epithelium (or more accurately, the tear film layer), there is more than adequate light with which to obtain a good exposure. Photographs should be taken at high magnifications (25× to 40×) to show cellular detail. Critical focus is essential (see Fig. 7.28).

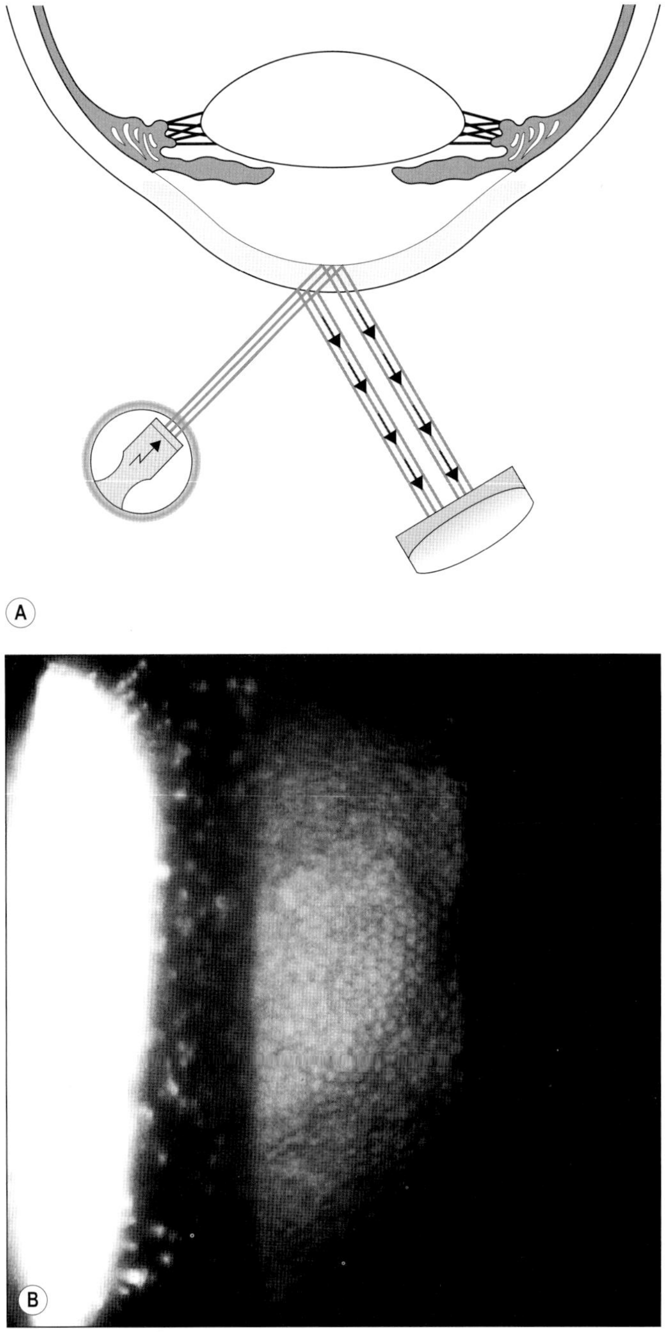

Fig. 7.28 (**A**) The bright specular reflection from the tear film layer is easily seen. The reflection from the endothelium is found just adjacent on the side opposite the light source. (**B**) At 40× magnification, even the small cells of this young, healthy endothelium are appreciable. (From Mártonyi CL et al. *Slit lamp: examination and photography.* Sedona: Time One Ink, Ltd; 2007.)

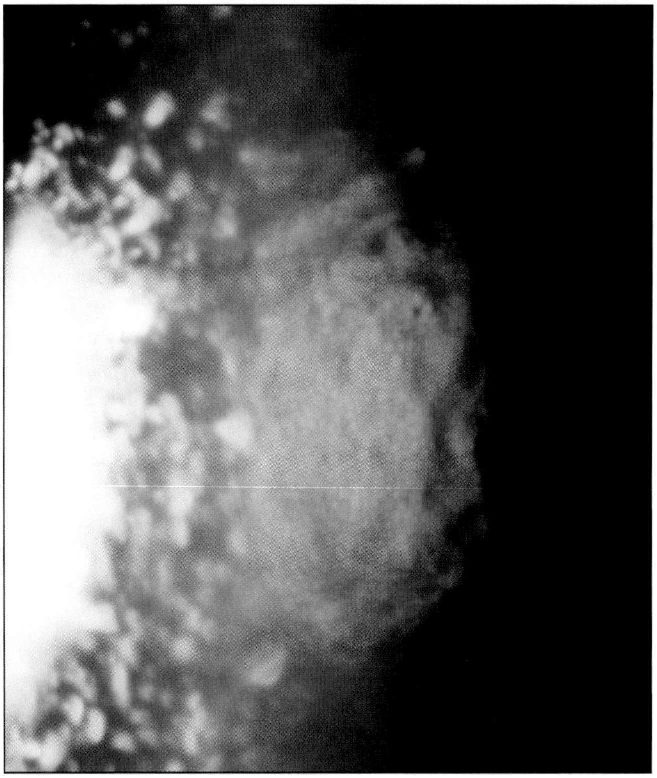

Fig. 7.29 The normally smooth specular reflection is altered by low- or off-axis reflections. (From Mártonyi CL et al. *Slit lamp: examination and photography.* Sedona: Time One Ink, Ltd; 2007.)

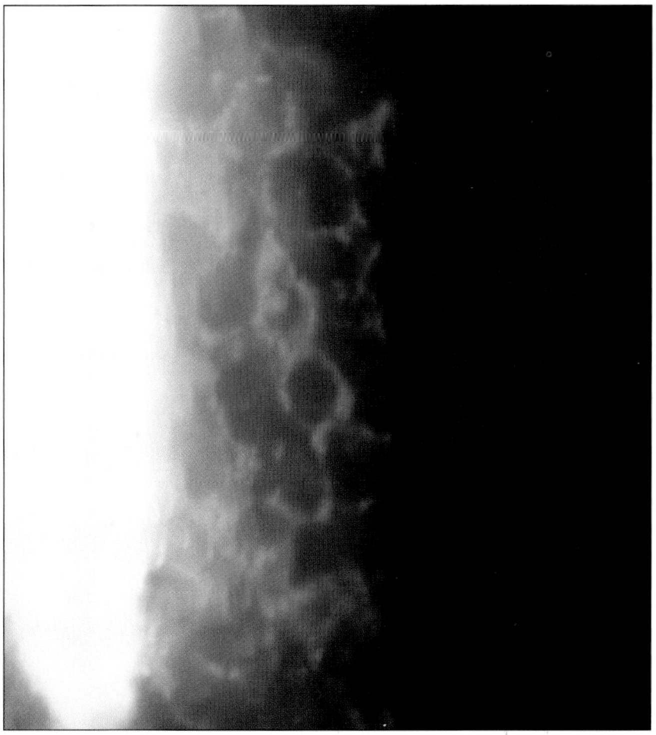

Fig. 7.30 Severe Fuchs' dystrophy preventing a view of endothelial cells. (From Mártonyi CL et al. *Slit lamp: examination and photography.* Sedona: Time One Ink, Ltd; 2007.)

Indirect Illumination

Proximal illumination: examination

In proximal illumination, the light is directed to strike an area just adjacent to the area to be examined. The principal subject, therefore, is illuminated by light transmitted through tissue. The effect is one of retroillumination from deeper layers. It is remarkably effective for observing subsurface changes in tissue of sufficient opacity to prevent light penetration to the desired level with direct illumination (Fig. 7.31). Similarly, proximal illumination can facilitate location and determination of size and shape of an imbedded foreign body or one obscured by soft tissue reaction. It also can be helpful in gathering additional information about abnormalities that are apparent in direct focal illumination. By observing conjunctival or skin alterations with this modality, the specular reflections produced by direct illumination are eliminated, and another, valuable perspective is obtained in what becomes a form of retroillumination (Fig. 7.32).

The benefits of proximal illumination are probably exploited more frequently than may be realized. A scan of

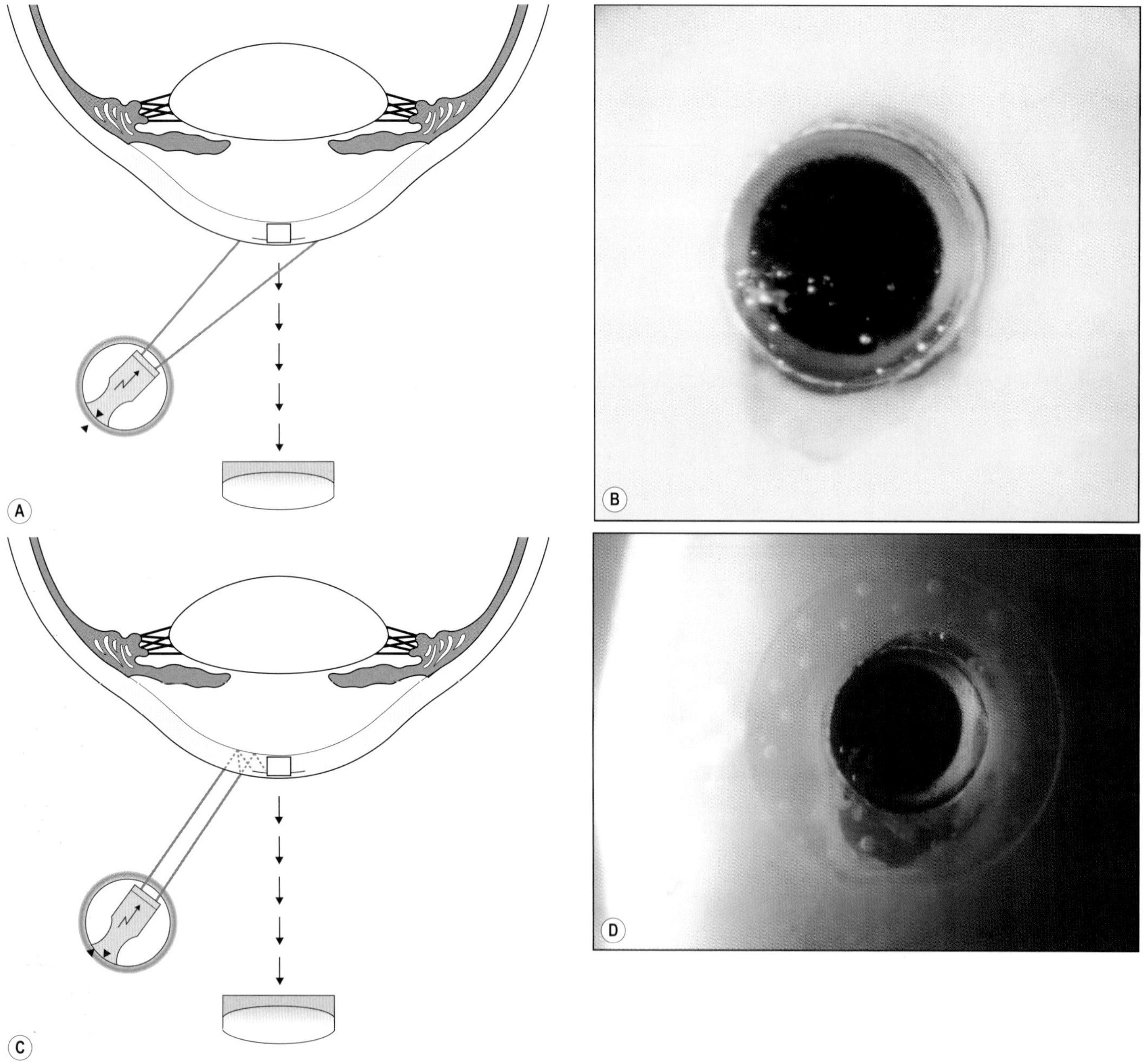

Fig. 7.31 (**A**) and (**B**) Direct, broad-beam illumination of a Cardona keratoprosthesis is ineffective in demonstrating the flange of the device by light reflected by the sclerotic corneal tissue. (**C**) and (**D**) Proximal illumination transmits light behind the flange, creating a light background against which the flange is easily seen. Additionally, the material of the flange 'pipes' the light to make its contours quite visible. (From Mártonyi CL et al. *Slit lamp: examination and photography.* Sedona: Time One Ink, Ltd; 2007.)

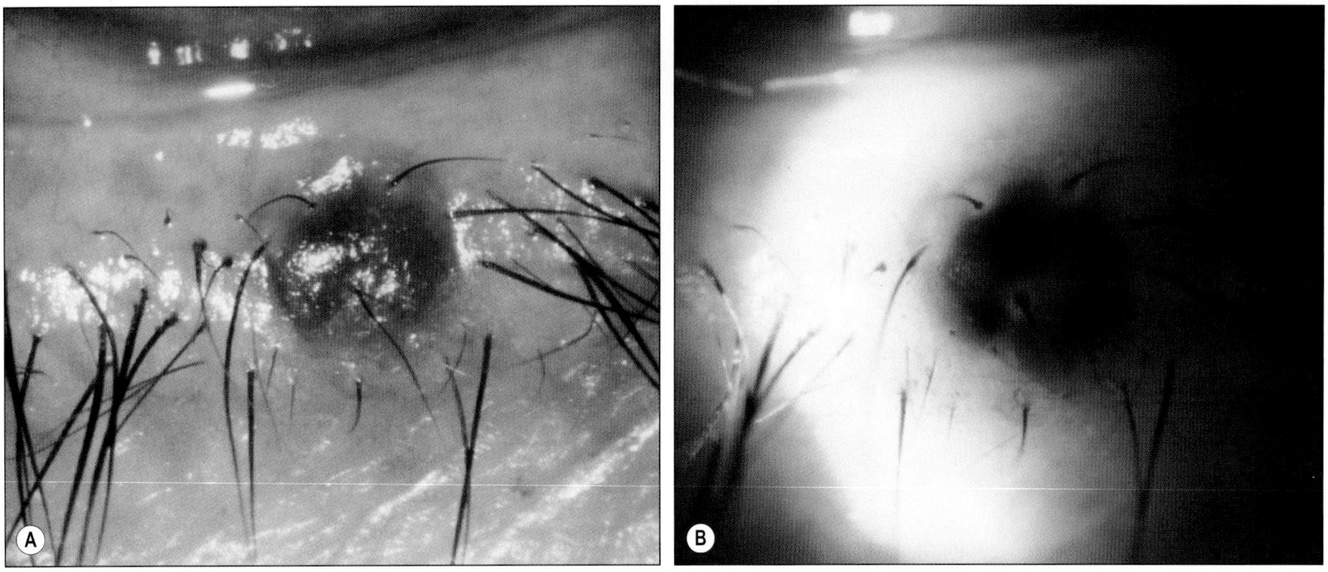

Fig. 7.32 The size, shape, and density of an eyelid nevus are better appreciated when viewed in both direct (**A**) and proximal (**B**) illumination. (From Mártonyi CL et al. *Slit lamp: examination and photography.* Sedona: Time One Ink, Ltd; 2007.)

the conjunctiva in direct focal illumination (e.g. with a narrow slit beam) includes making use of the information seen in the adjacent area of proximal illumination. Proximal illumination may not be the conscious goal of the examiner, but information from this zone is nonetheless gleaned. In fact, without it, the examination would be incomplete.

When high magnification is used in observations by proximal illumination, the subject area may become sufficiently decentered to make viewing cumbersome. In such cases, the slit illuminator must be decentered from its normal isocentric position to permit centration of the principal subject area within the field of view.

Proximal illumination: photography

All indirect forms of illumination require decentration of the slit beam for the maintenance of a centered principal subject area. Although it may be unnecessary for most of a slit lamp examination, decentration of the incident beam is essential to the success of each slit lamp photograph.

Proximal illumination poses quite a challenge in achieving good exposure. The amount of light by which such changes are visible represents a small percentage of the light used to directly illuminate the adjacent area. For this reason, the exposure is frequently underestimated. The area of direct illumination must be dramatically overexposed as compared with the area of indirect illumination. This is an unavoidable by-product of this technique, which the photographic process exaggerates beyond the visual impression. In some cases, the distraction factor of this zone of overexposure may be tempered by increasing magnification to the exclusion of the directly illuminated area. The important goal, however, is to use sufficient incident light to adequately expose the principal subject area. Although somewhat variable because of differences in tissue reflectivity and absorption, an increase of approximately three f-stops of light is required (see Figs 7.31 and 7.32).[2]

Sclerotic scatter: examination

Specifically applicable to the cornea, sclerotic scatter permits the illumination of the entire cornea against a largely unilluminated background. An intense beam of moderate size is directed at the corneoscleral junction. The light travels the breath and width of the cornea by total internal reflection. In the normal cornea, this light passes through the stroma undisturbed and is visible only as a ring of light at the limbus, where it intersects, and is reflected by, the sclera. The brightest portion of this ring of light is located directly opposite the source. The normal cornea itself will appear unilluminated. Because of the extreme degree to which the cornea must be decentered to accommodate illumination of the limbus, the slit illuminator must be disengaged from its normal, isocentric relationship with the biomicroscope to allow centration of the cornea within the field of view (Fig. 7.33). In the abnormal cornea, the light that is axially reflected or refracted makes the abnormality visible. The degree to which this light is visible depends on the optical density and other characteristics of the abnormality and the size and intensity of the incident light beam (Fig. 7.34).

Sclerotic scatter is quite remarkable for its sensitivity to subtle change while yielding information over a large area of distribution (Box 7.4). That combination is not possible with most forms of illumination. The ever-present compromise of 'area versus detail' limits each application.[2] Generally, the larger the area of simultaneous illumination, the more light that will be scattered, producing a corresponding loss of fine detail. However, in sclerotic scatter, as the cornea is illuminated by a source that is comparatively small (the size of the beam directed at the limbus), this technique is not strictly subject to this limitation. In reality, sclerotic scatter provides a simultaneous view of a large expanse of cornea, making it useful in identifying certain disease entities through recognition of a characteristic, overall pattern.

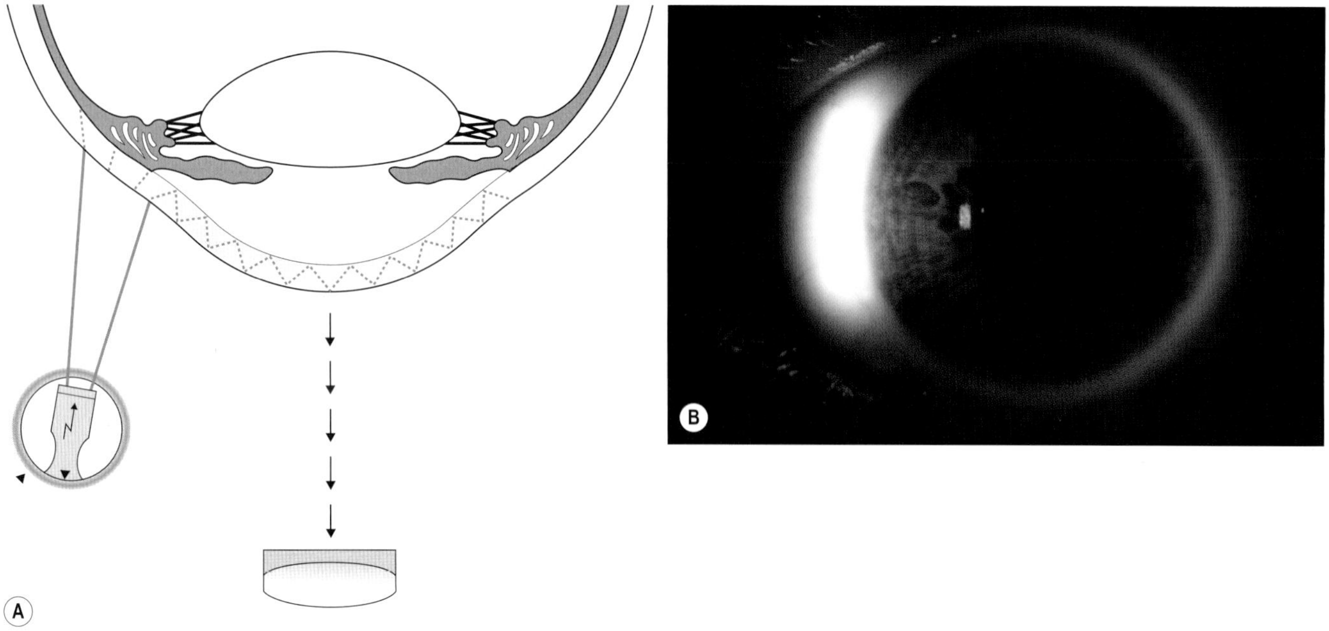

Fig. 7.33 **A**, The beam is decentered to facilitate centration of the cornea in the biomicroscope. (**B**) The light at the corneoscleral junction illuminates the cornea by total internal reflection. The normal cornea will not reflect the light along the viewing axis and remains dark against an essentially dark background. (From Mártonyi CL et al. *Slit lamp: examination and photography.* Sedona: Time One Ink, Ltd; 2007.)

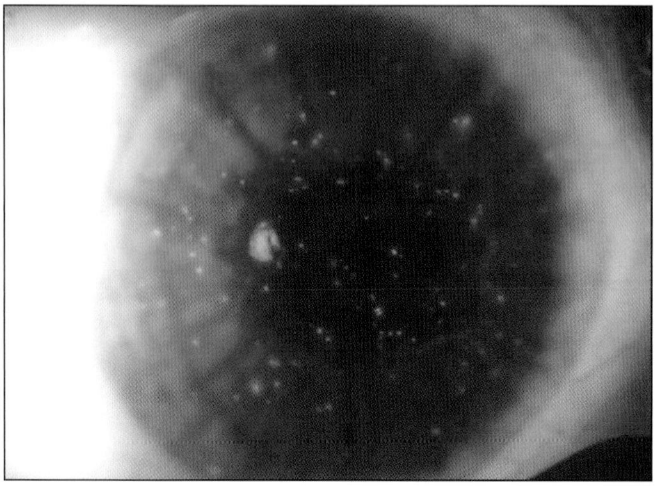

Fig. 7.34 Multiple fiberglass foreign bodies are seen over a wide distribution with the technique of sclerotic scatter. The light color (low optical density) of these particles makes them excellent candidates for viewing in what becomes, in effect, darkfield illumination. (From Mártonyi CL et al. *Slit lamp: examination and photography.* Sedona: Time One Ink, Ltd; 2007.)

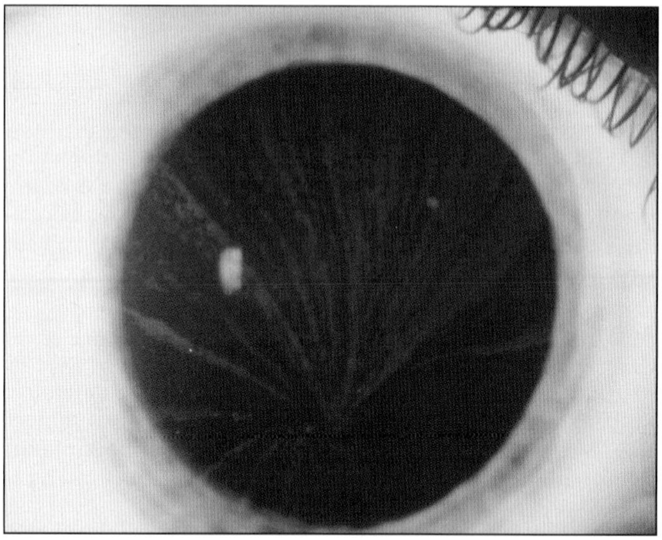

Fig. 7.35 The subtle cornea verticillata in Fabry's disease is best seen in sclerotic scatter against the dark background of a well-dilated pupil. (From Mártonyi CL et al. *Slit lamp: examination and photography.* Sedona: Time One Ink, Ltd; 2007.)

In certain instances, the incidental light that falls on the iris, especially one of light pigmentation, may become a significant negative factor. Thus, a condition of subtle expression (e.g. cornea verticillata in Fabry's disease) can be best appreciated against the dark background of a dilated pupil (Fig. 7.35).[2]

Sclerotic scatter: photography

Sclerotic scatter can produce information over a wide expanse of cornea in a single photograph. It is best used to

Box 7.4 Examples of conditions seen in sclerotic scatter

Corneal foreign bodies	Interstitial keratitis
Corneal edema	Granular dystrophy
Keratic precipitates	Radial keratotomy scars
Verticillata	Hydrops

delineate alterations that are of low optical density. This technique requires a complete decentration of the slit beam to permit centration of the cornea in the final image (see Fig. 7.33). It also requires the maximum light output from the power supply. Obvious conditions, such as the bright foreign bodies seen in Figure 7.34, are easily exposed. More subtle entities, such as the verticillate pattern in Fabry's disease may require a setting of 400–800 ISO. Dilating the pupil ensures a sufficiently dark background to provide the contrast necessary for good visualization (see Fig. 7.35).

Direct and indirect retroillumination from the iris: examination

Representing two distinct forms from the standpoint of how they function, direct and indirect retroillumination from the iris are most informative when used together. This combined technique is the most important to the thorough examination of the cornea. It actually produces three types of illumination with corresponding zones of information. With the beam applied tangentially, the area of the cornea observed against the directly illuminated iris (direct retroillumination from the iris) demonstrates alterations that are chiefly opaque. The zone of cornea that falls on either side of the illuminated background, i.e. cornea that lies in front of unilluminated iris or pupil (the zone of indirect retroillumination from the iris), demonstrates primarily refractile changes and changes of low optical density. Of greatest importance is the interface between light and dark backgrounds, where the most subtle changes may be seen. Abnormalities that both refract and reflect light become most dimensional in this zone between light and dark backgrounds.

Technically, this juncture is an interface rather than a true zone. Because the biomicroscope (and therefore the slit beam) is focused at the level of the cornea, however, the interface is formed by divergent rays, resulting in an unsharp image at the level of the iris. Because this unsharp image of an unsharp interface appears to occupy space by virtue of its broader appearance, it becomes a zone in the practical sense (Fig. 7.36). The entire cornea can thus be examined for both subtle and obvious alterations. The beam of light is applied tangentially and moved across the cornea while observing the three zones simultaneously, with particular attention paid to the interface of light and dark backgrounds.[2] To ensure that all information about the cornea has been gathered with this modality, the scan should be repeated, with the light applied from both the temporal and nasal sides.

Many entities are easily visualized and identified in this manner (Box 7.5). Lattice dystrophy, with its characteristic signature, is seen in all three zones of illumination (see Fig. 7.36). Folds in Descemet's membrane are best seen in indirect retroillumination from the iris, but close to the interface

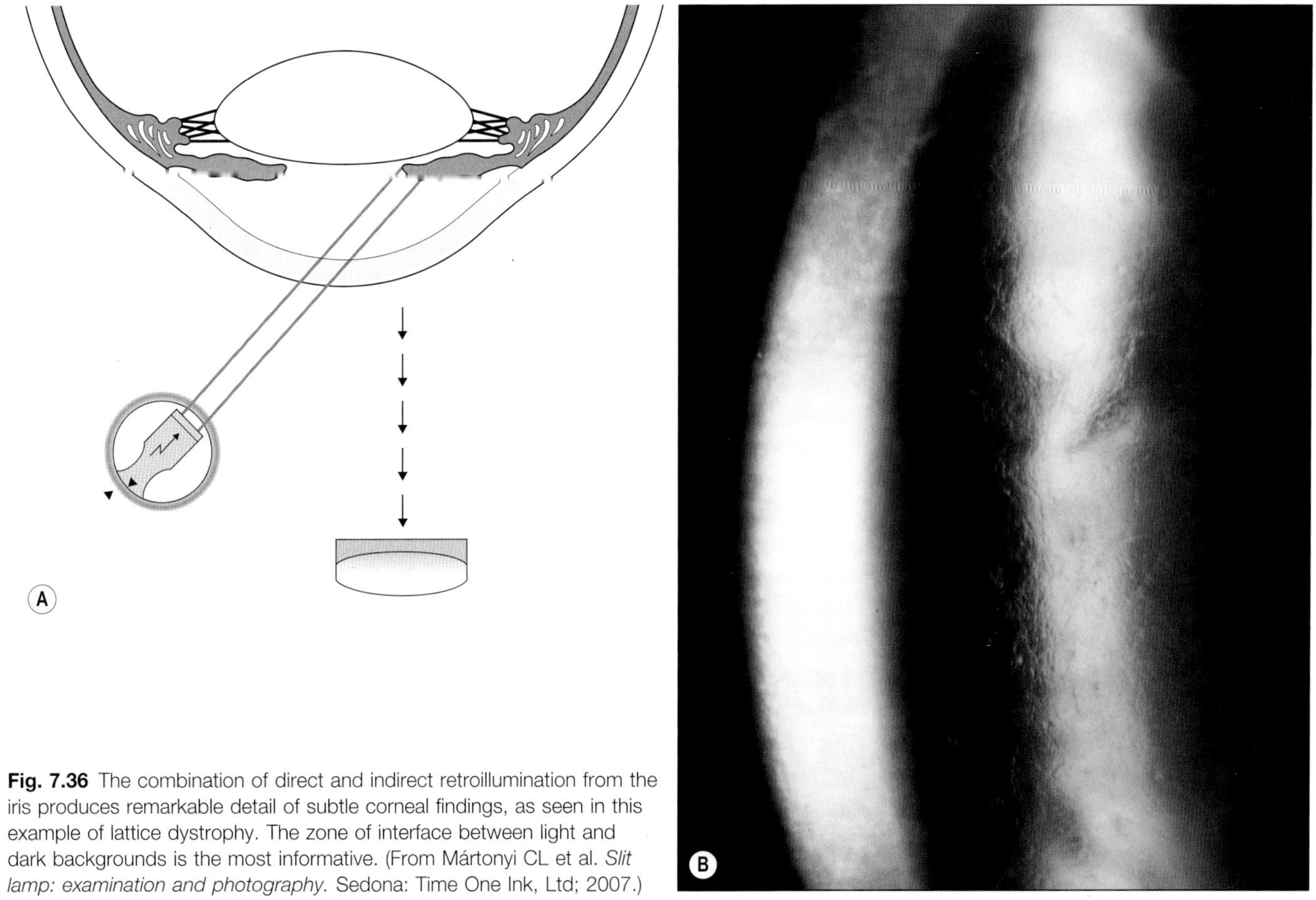

Fig. 7.36 The combination of direct and indirect retroillumination from the iris produces remarkable detail of subtle corneal findings, as seen in this example of lattice dystrophy. The zone of interface between light and dark backgrounds is the most informative. (From Mártonyi CL et al. *Slit lamp: examination and photography.* Sedona: Time One Ink, Ltd; 2007.)

of light and dark backgrounds (Fig. 7.37). The classic, bubble-like microcysts characterizing Meesmann's dystrophy are most dimensionally described within the interface zone (Fig. 7.38).

Direct retroillumination from the iris: photography

A beam of moderate width is projected onto the iris to create a light background against which opaque changes are visible. When the condition presents in an eye with a light iris, the exposure appropriate to the documentation of that iris in direct illumination is sufficient. When the condition presents against a dark iris, an increase in exposure is required. The

Box 7.5 Examples of conditions seen in direct and indirect retroillumination from the iris

Lattice dystrophy	Corneal infiltrates
Corneal foreign bodies	Early edema
Meesmann's dystrophy	Filaments
Map-dot-fingerprint	Microcysts
Cornea farinata	Fuchs' dystrophy
Descemet's folds	Corneal scars
Keratic precipitates	
Thygeson's superficial punctate keratitis	

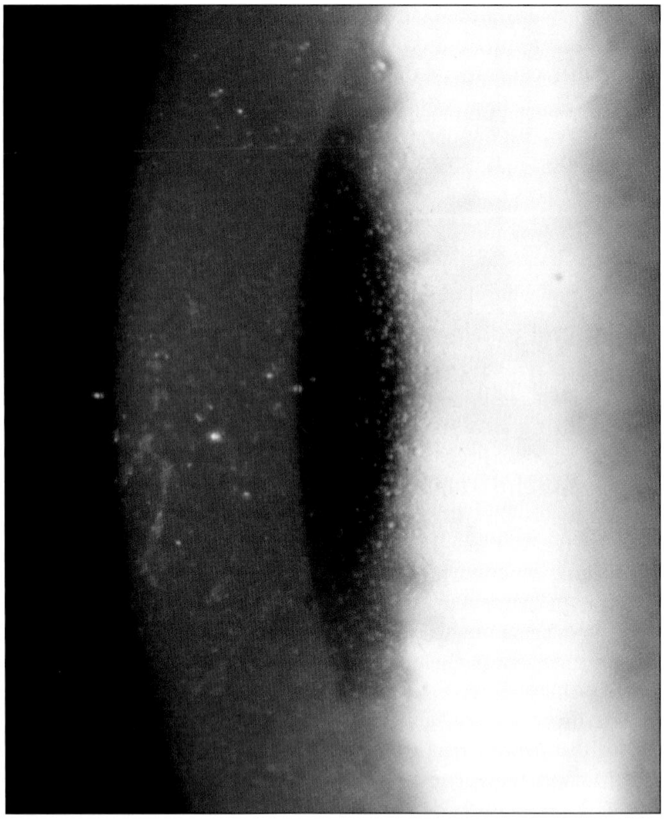

Fig. 7.38 Meesmann's dystrophy is effectively demonstrated in indirect retroillumination from the iris. (From Mártonyi CL et al. *Slit lamp: examination and photography.* Sedona: Time One Ink, Ltd; 2007.)

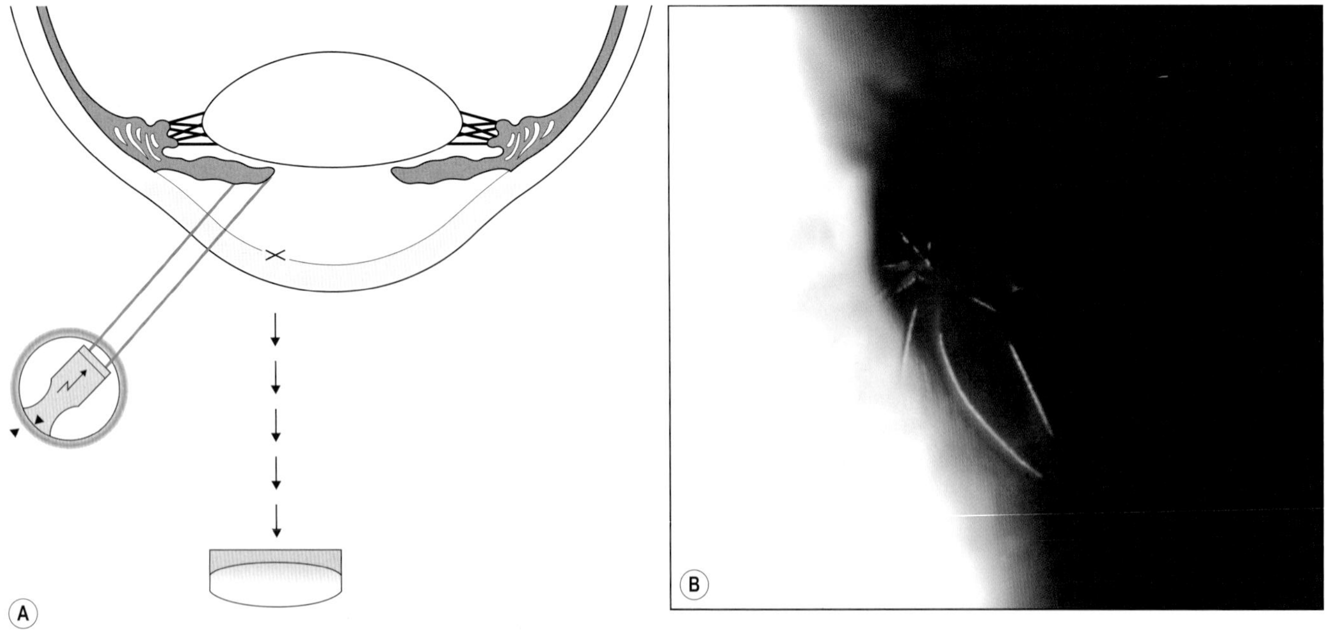

Fig. 7.37 (**A**) and (**B**) Wrinkles in Descemet's membrane are primarily refractile and are best seen against a dark background directly adjacent to the illuminated background. (From Mártonyi CL et al. *Slit lamp: examination and photography.* Sedona: Time One Ink, Ltd; 2007.)

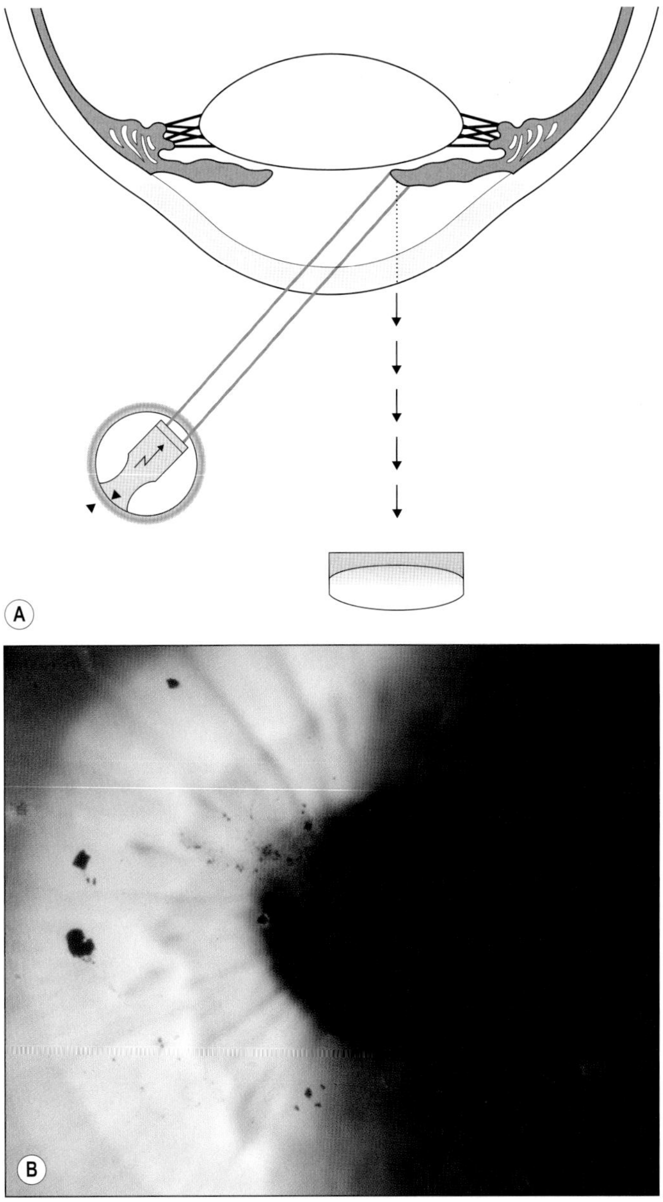

Fig. 7.39 (**A**) Direct retroillumination from the iris. (**B**) Opaque corneal foreign bodies silhouetted against an illuminated, lightly pigmented iris. (From Mártonyi CL et al. *Slit lamp: examination and photography.* Sedona: Time One Ink, Ltd; 2007.)

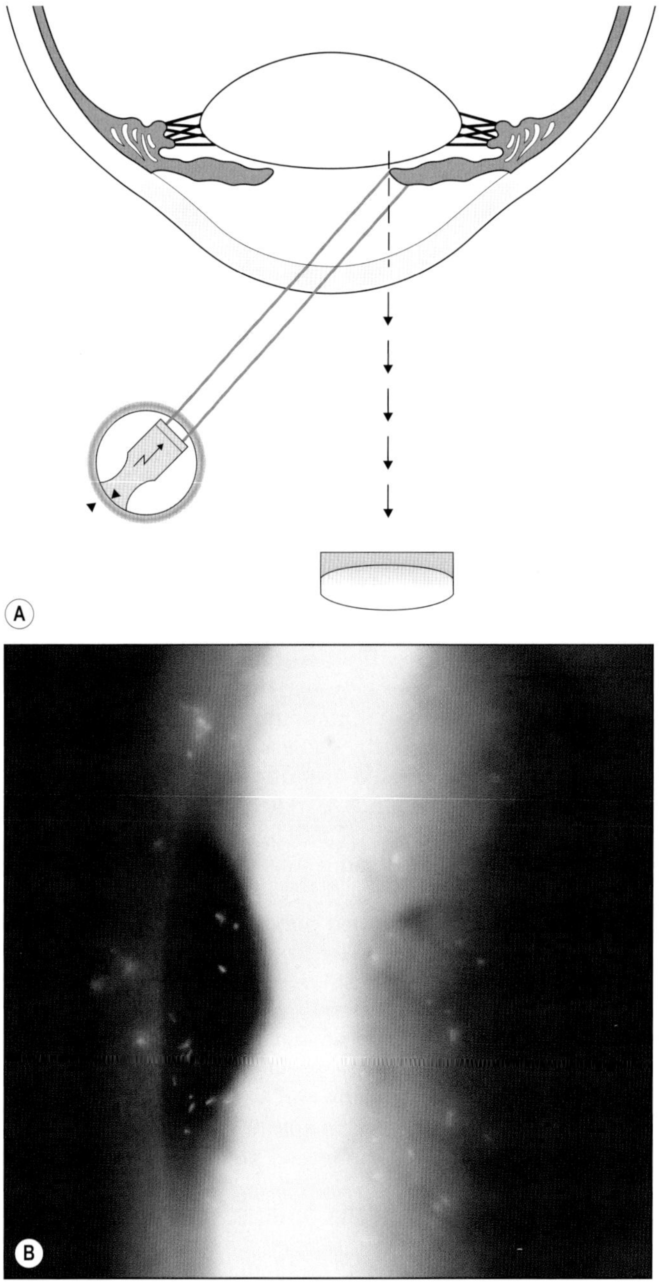

Fig. 7.40 (**A**) Indirect retroillumination from the iris. (**B**) Fiberglass particles in the cornea seen in indirect retroillumination from the iris. The light particles are nicely contrasted against the dark pupil. A two f-stop overexposure of the iris was required. (From Mártonyi CL et al. *Slit lamp: examination and photography.* Sedona: Time One Ink, Ltd; 2007.)

beam should be wide enough to create an adequate background, without directly illuminating the corneal condition (Fig. 7.39).

Indirect retroillumination from the iris: photography

The photography involved in this technique is somewhat more challenging because the light available to illuminate the abnormal condition is but a small portion of the light striking the iris (Fig. 7.40). With increased pigmentation of the iris, light loss also increases, requiring a greater adjustment in exposure. Many changes are visible in this form of illumination. Alterations that are primarily refractile are especially well described in this manner. Such changes are the most striking at the interface of light and dark backgrounds, demanding careful attention to exposure (see Figs 7.36 through 7.38). As a general rule, the exposure used for direct illumination of the iris should be increased by one f-stop to provide good exposure of refractile changes at the interface generated by a light iris, and up to three f-stops when the condition is being photographed at the interface created by the surface of a darkly pigmented iris.

Retroillumination from the fundus: examination

Using the light reflected by the retinal pigment epithelium, the anterior vitreous, lens, and cornea may be examined in retroillumination. The slit lamp illuminator is placed into an axial position with the biomicroscope and the light is introduced through a dilated pupil to illuminate the fundus. With modest excursions of the illuminator to either side of center, the optimum position is established when the greatest retroillumination effect is achieved. A large pupil is required for maximum effectiveness. After configuring a moderately sized beam, the entire instrument can be moved from side to side to facilitate examination of most of the cornea. Decentering the slit to one side of the available pupil and then to the other facilitates a serial, uncompromised view of both sides of the subject stratum, and the area under study remains centered in the biomicroscope. Leaving the iris unilluminated ensures maximum visibility of the abnormality. Light striking the iris causes scatter and reduces the effectiveness of this valuable form of illumination.

One major advantage of this modality is that it produces excellent delineation of subtle changes over a wide area of distribution. In that regard, it is similar to sclerotic scatter. The principal difference between the two is that sclerotic scatter produces darkfield illumination (objects illuminated against a dark background), whereas retroillumination from the fundus is a brightfield technique (objects silhouetted against a bright background). Darkfield excels at demonstrating changes that primarily reflect light, and brightfield produces best contrast for opaque changes and those that are refractile (Box 7.6). Much of the cornea or lens may be visualized simultaneously, limited only by the size of the pupil and shallow depth of field. The classic findings in fingerprint dystrophy are beautifully displayed in this form of illumination (Fig. 7.41). Similarly, many lens changes are most easily identified in this manner. Cataract formation and subluxation of the lens are dramatically demonstrated (Fig. 7.42). The essentially colorless lens and cornea are transformed into structures that are seen in additional contrast by virtue of the color reflected by the retinal pigment epithelium.

Retroillumination from the fundus: photography

Exposure is generally not a problem. With a well-dilated pupil and clear media, excellent images of corneal or lenticular changes can be captured.

The slit beam is configured into a short rectangle or, when possible, into a half-moon shape to permit maximum illumination of the background (the retinal pigment epithelium) without allowing the light to strike the iris. The light beam is then displaced to the side of the pupil that causes the least compromise to the information to be recorded. A considerable decentration of the beam is necessary to maintain centration of the pupillary area (see Fig. 7.42). When necessitated by the presentation of the condition, the beam is moved to the other side of the pupil for additional photographs to provide complete documentation.

Box 7.6 Examples of abnormalities seen in retroillumination from the fundus

Lattice dystrophy	Map-dot-fingerprint dystrophy
Pseudoexfoliation	Lens vacuoles
Keratic precipitates	Cataract
Corneal scars	Corneal rejection lines
Meesmann's dystrophy	

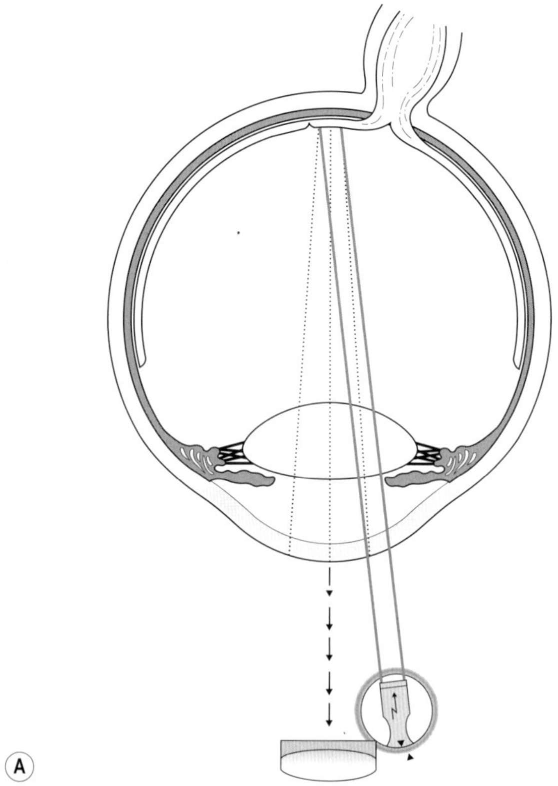

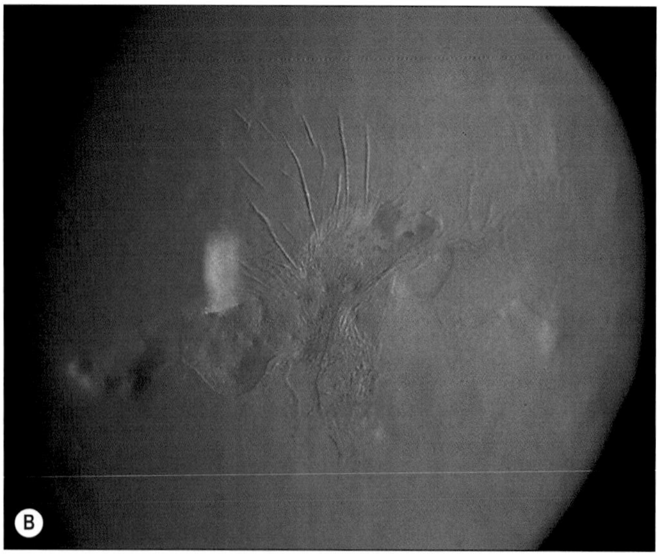

Fig. 7.41 (**A**) and (**B**) Epithelial fingerprint dystrophy is best visualized in retroillumination from the fundus. (From Mártonyi CL et al. *Slit lamp: examination and photography.* Sedona: Time One Ink, Ltd; 2007.)

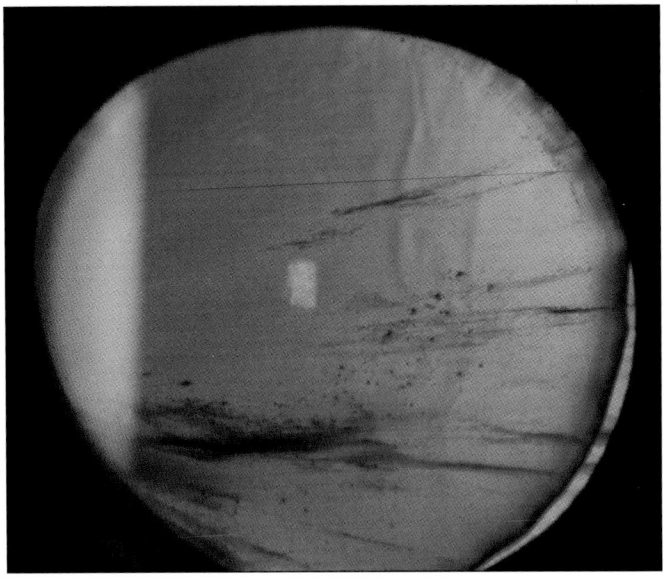

Fig. 7.42 A traumatically subluxated lens is seen with blood on its posterior surface, well demonstrated in retroillumination from the fundus. (From Mártonyi CL et al. *Slit lamp: examination and photography.* Sedona: Time One Ink, Ltd; 2007.)

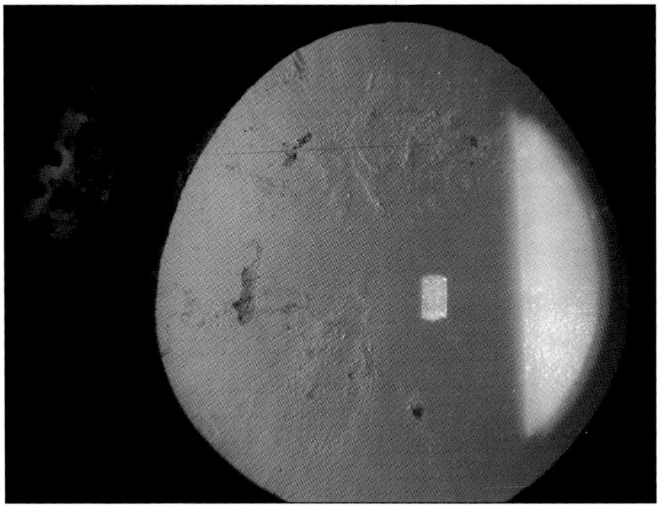

Fig. 7.43 Cataract formation and iris atrophy, resulting from a contusion injury, are simultaneously observed in retroillumination from the fundus and transillumination of the iris. (From Mártonyi CL et al. *Slit lamp: examination and photography.* Sedona: Time One Ink, Ltd; 2007.)

In the absence of optimum conditions, coupled with a heavily pigmented retinal pigment epithelium, exposure may need to be increased considerably. When maximum retroillumination is required, the eye is rotated to cause the incident beam to strike the optic nerve head, producing more intense retroillumination from that highly reflective surface.

Transillumination of the iris: examination

Iris transillumination is a simple extension of the technique just described (Fig. 7.43). An important difference is the optimum pupil size. A completely dilated pupil is counterproductive to iris transillumination; a pupil size of 2–3 mm is ideal. Through such an opening, a moderate beam of high intensity can be introduced to illuminate the fundus. In that presentation, the iris is still sufficiently attenuated to demonstrate even subtle expressions of transillumination (Fig. 7.44).[2]

Transillumination of the iris: photography

Figure 7.43 required midrange intensity of illumination, whereas Figure 7.44 required the maximum light output of the PSL.

The peripheral cornea (gonioscopy): examination

The peripheral cornea cannot be examined without the use of a gonioscope. Indirect lenses provide the ideal view with a choice of mirror angles and reduced light scatter. Once the lens is placed, the optic section can provide information regarding the posterior surface of the cornea and the condition of the angle. A wider beam, which is conformed to the area under study, is useful for the simultaneous view of a larger area to assess structural relationships further. Confining the beam to the zone of immediate attention minimizes distracting reflections that inevitably reduce contrast and detail (Fig. 7.45). The anterior chamber angle is extremely reflective in most eyes, and moderate amounts of light are suggested for its examination.

The peripheral cornea: photography

Photography of the peripheral cornea requires the same basic techniques as photography of the filtration angle. Both areas are imaged simultaneously, and the delineation of the principal subject area is largely a matter of focus. The best access to this area is provided with the most oblique mirror in the Goldmann three-mirror lens, set at an angle of 59 degrees. In this application, the more oblique view provides better access to this zone of the anterior chamber. For some conditions, the 67-degree mirror produces a better overview, providing an enhanced perspective (Fig. 7.46). Because of the highly reflective nature of this area, the danger of overexposure is much greater than underexposure. Because findings in this zone are frequently subtle, it is doubly important to avoid overexposing the image. In some instances, a moderate underexposure produces a more saturated image containing more detailed information (see Fig. 7.45). Previewing the image with only the eye that shares the image with the camera back will help in managing unwanted reflections from the flat surface of the contact lens.

Vital dyes: examination

Vital dyes provide information important to a complete ocular examination. Their application is essential to determine the condition of the corneal and conjunctival epithelium. Because these dyes can cause irritation (rose Bengal, in particular) and because their presence may interfere with the

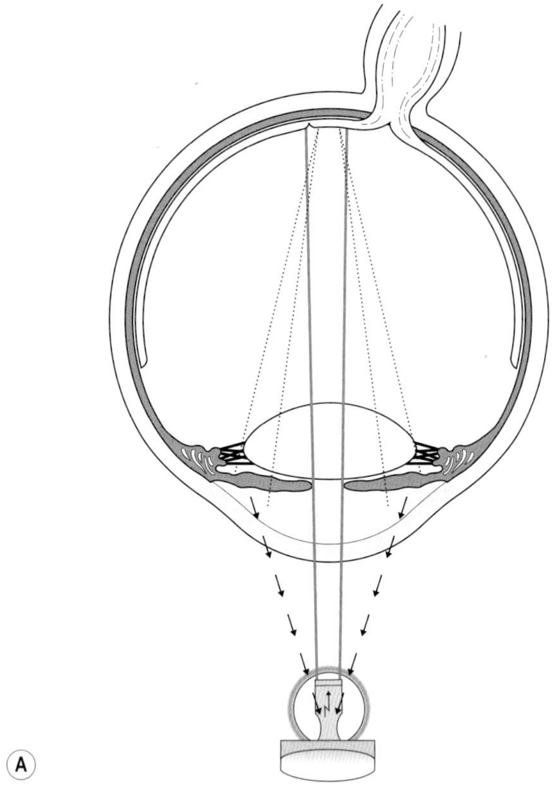

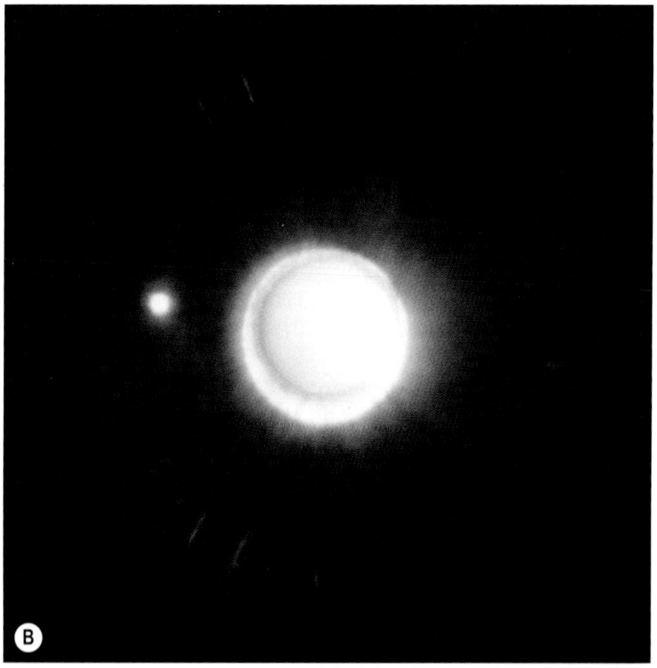

Fig. 7.44 (**A**) and (**B**) Information regarding transmission defects of the iris in pigment dispersion syndrome is maximized by projecting a small, round beam through a partially dilated pupil. (From Mártonyi CL et al. *Slit lamp: examination and photography.* Sedona: Time One Ink, Ltd; 2007. **B**, Copyright Mártonyi CL: WK Kellogg Eye Center, University of Michigan.)

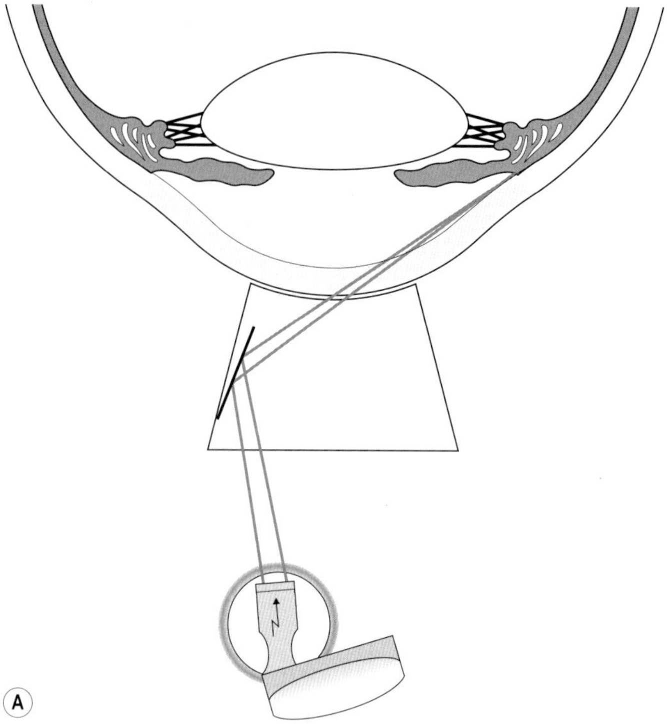

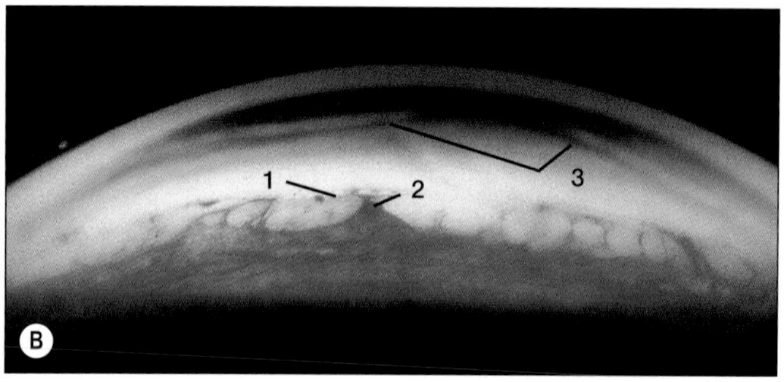

Fig. 7.45 (**A**) View of the peripheral cornea through a three-mirror lens. (**B**) A prominent Schwalbe's line (1) is seen, with adherent iris strands (2). Haab's striae (3) of the cornea prevent an optimum view in this case of Axenfeld's syndrome. (From Mártonyi CL et al. *Slit lamp: examination and photography.* Sedona: Time One Ink, Ltd; 2007.)

assessment of deeper layers of the cornea, they may be best used toward the end of the examination.

Fluorescein is a good indicator of contact lens fit. With the blue exciter filter in place and the light intensity sufficiently increased, such information is easily obtained (Fig. 7.47). Similarly, tear film break-up time can be ascertained (Fig. 7.48). Conditions that disturb the normal tear film also can be confirmed (or detected[4]) with this same technique (Fig. 7.49).

To determine the presence of epithelial compromise, the dyes can be used individually or mixed and applied in combination. The irritation caused by rose Bengal may warrant the use of a topical anesthetic before instillation. The cornea and conjunctiva should be examined for signs of staining with both white and blue light (Fig. 7.50). Because

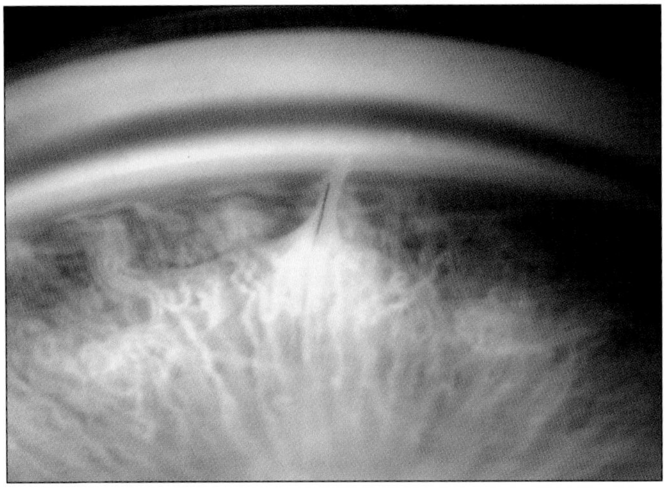

Fig. 7.46 The 67-degree mirror produces a view that provides better perspective for this presumed (by history) caterpillar hair in the angle. (From Mártonyi CL et al. *Slit lamp: examination and photography.* Sedona: Time One Ink, Ltd; 2007.)

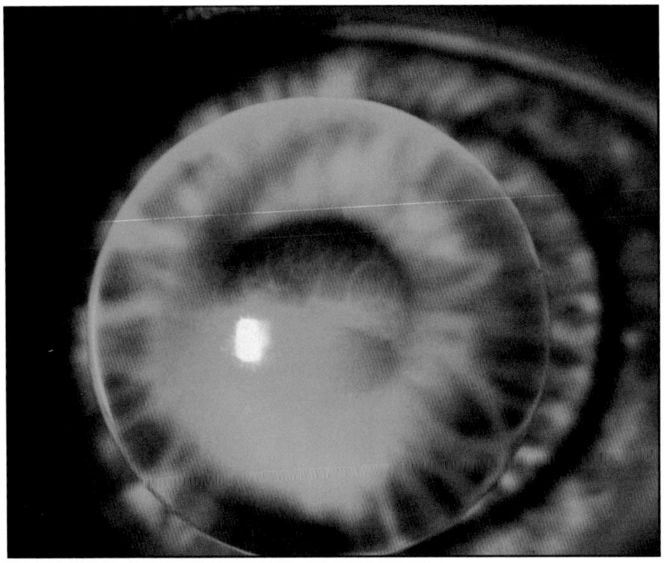

Fig. 7.47 Fluorescein pooled under a poorly fitting contact lens. (From Mártonyi CL et al. *Slit lamp: examination and photography.* Sedona: Time One Ink, Ltd; 2007.)

devitalized epithelium stains with rose Bengal and areas that are de-epithelialized stain with both rose Bengal and fluorescein, the subtle areas of rose Bengal staining may be better appreciated when viewed in a matrix of fluorescein. Since rose Bengal absorbs much of the incident blue light, its consequently dark appearance contrasts well with a brightly fluorescing background (Fig. 7.51).

The patient should blink repeatedly to help differentiate pooling from staining. Areas of staining become apparent as they move with the eye. Pooled dye appears somewhat static by comparison. A definitive differentiation can be made only by rinsing the pooled dye. A particularly dry eye will certainly require rinsing before an accurate assessment can be made regarding actual staining.

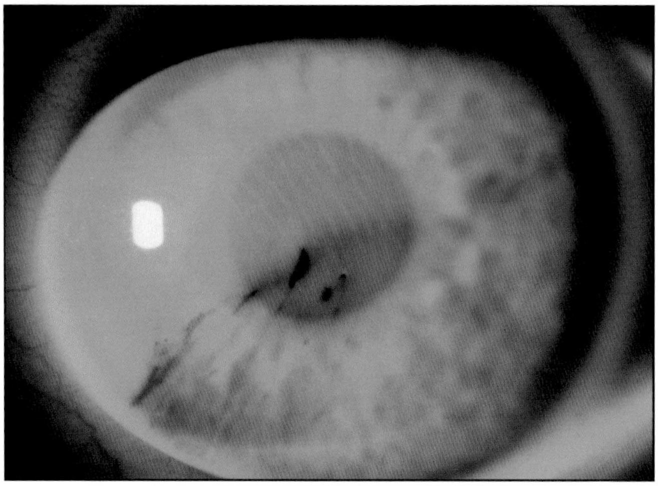

Fig. 7.48 Tear film break-up in a normal eye. (From Mártonyi CL et al. *Slit lamp: examination and photography.* Sedona: Time One Ink, Ltd; 2007.)

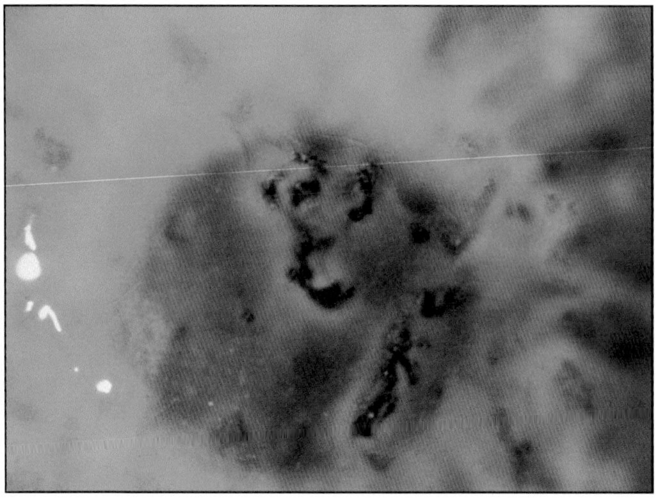

Fig. 7.49 Tear film interrupted by changes in lattice dystrophy. (From Mártonyi CL et al. *Slit lamp: examination and photography.* Sedona: Time One Ink, Ltd; 2007.)

The Seidel test: examination

The Seidel test is used to determine corneal or conjunctival patency. When the escape of aqueous is suspected, fluorescein dye is applied directly to the site of suspected leakage. When present, escaping aqueous dilutes the fluorescein as it flows down the surface of the eye. The rate of dilution is the indicator of the dynamic of the positive test. The application of concentrated fluorescein results in a dark, nonfluorescing background, against which the diluted and now brightly fluorescing dye is highly visible, even in the presence of a modest flow (Fig. 7.52).[5]

Vital dyes: photography

Vital dyes are best photographed in direct, broad-beam illumination. Of great importance is the removal of excess dye

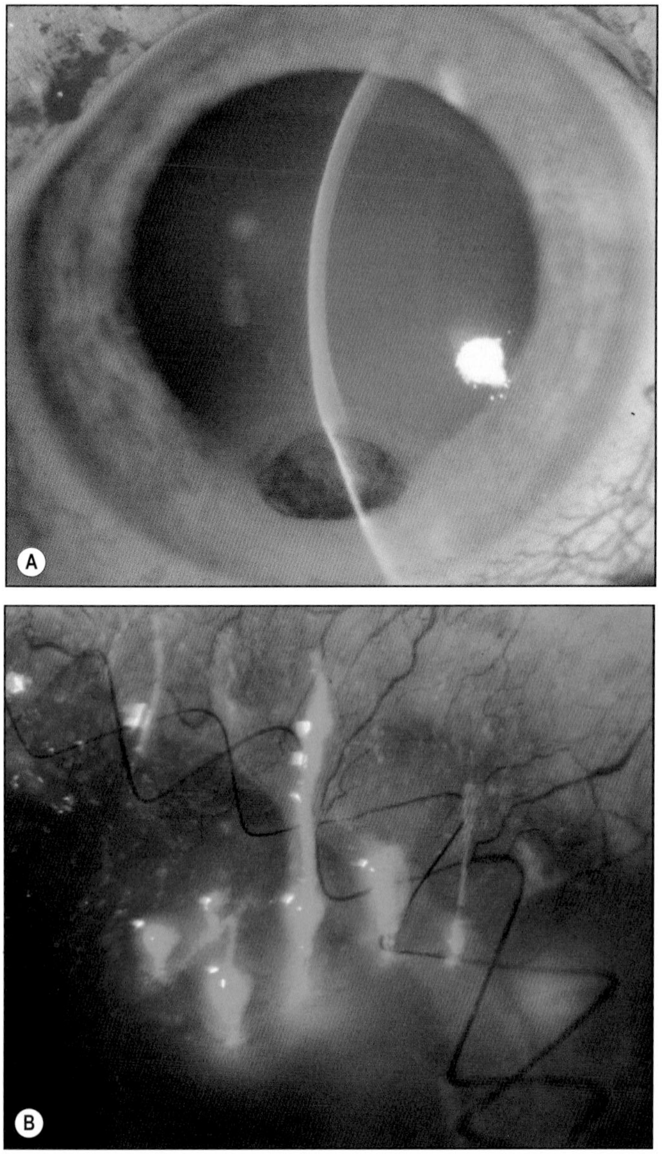

Fig. 7.50 (**A**) An obviously compromised cornea stained with rose Bengal and fluorescein, seen in white light. (**B**) Corneal filaments stained with fluorescein seen in a recently transplanted cornea. (**A**, From Mártonyi CL et al. *Slit lamp: examination and photography.* Sedona: Time One Ink, Ltd; 2007. **B**, Copyright Mártonyi CL, WK Kellogg Eye Center, University of Michigan.)

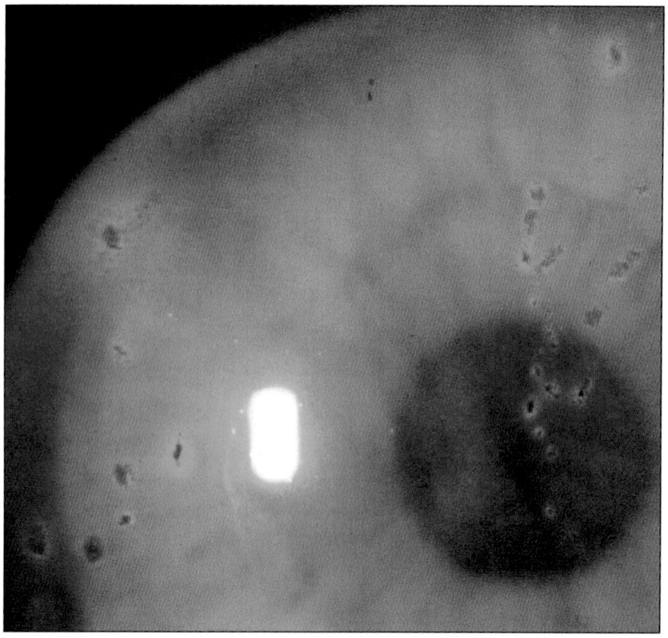

Fig. 7.51 A case of dendritic keratitis, stained with rose Bengal and fluorescein. Rose Bengal absorbs the blue light, resulting in a dark signature against the fluorescing surround. (From Mártonyi CL et al. *Slit lamp: examination and photography.* Sedona: Time One Ink, Ltd; 2007.)

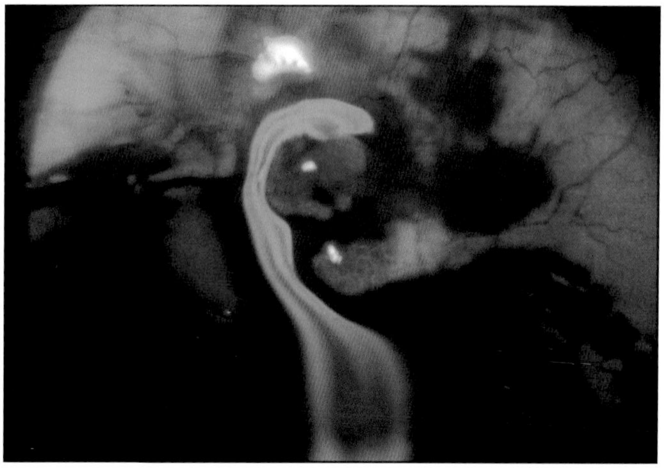

Fig. 7.52 A Seidel-positive filtering bleb. (From Mártonyi CL et al. *Slit lamp: examination and photography.* Sedona: Time One Ink, Ltd; 2007.)

before photodocumentation. Thus, only actual staining is recorded. This is important to the accurate recording of both rose Bengal and fluorescein staining.

Rose Bengal staining is easily photographed, requiring only minor adjustments from the normal exposure used for broad-beam illumination. Since rose Bengal delineates subtle areas of epithelial compromise, care must be taken to preserve the subtle nature of the information. The light beam is applied tangentially to avoid obscuring information with overlying specular reflections. In most cases, a slight underexposure will better express subtle focal staining (Fig. 7.53).

Fluorescein is best viewed and photographed under blue light (approximately 480 nm) used to excite the dye to fluorescence. Because the blue filter diminishes overall light intensity, adjustment in exposure is required. About two f-stops of additional light are needed, depending on the actual filter used. For most applications, only an excitation filter is required (see Figs 7.47–7.49). For photographs that demonstrate extremely subtle staining, a barrier filter (approximately 520 nm) is added to provide adequate discrimination.[6] An additional increase in exposure may be necessary.

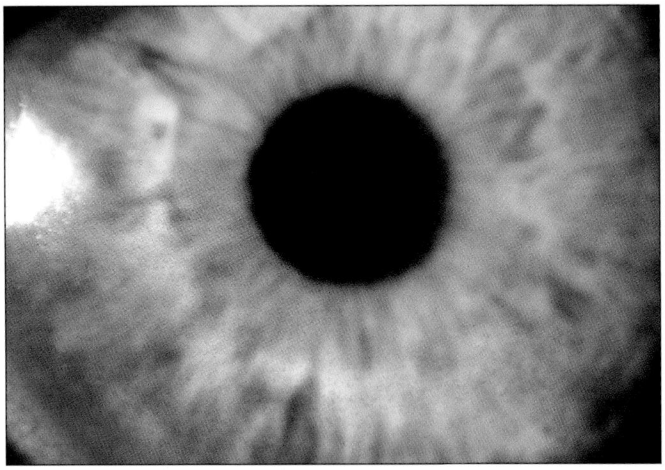

Fig. 7.53 A punctate pattern of rose Bengal staining of the inferior cornea in a case of toxic keratitis (polyurethane foam vapors). From Mártonyi CL et al. *Slit lamp: examination and photography.* Sedona: Time One Ink, Ltd; 2007.)

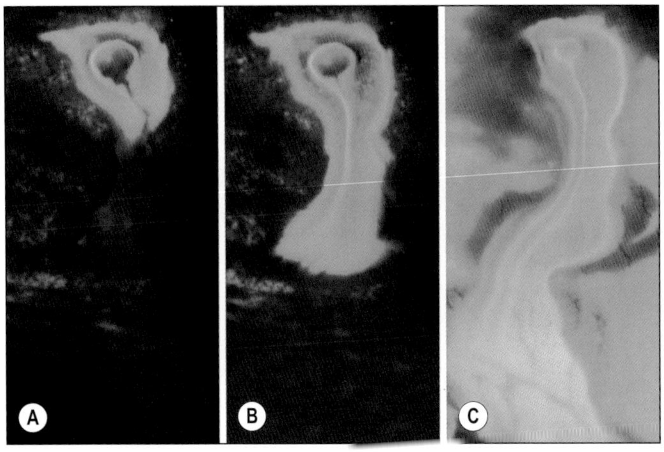

Fig. 7.54 (**A**) The Seidel test. The fluorescein is applied directly to the site of suspected compromise to demonstrate leakage of aqueous through a perforated cornea. (**B**) and (**C**) Moments later, the pattern progresses to demonstrate the highly dynamic flow of aqueous. (From Mártonyi CL et al. *Slit lamp: examination and photography.* Sedona: Time One Ink, Ltd; 2007.)

Combining rose Bengal and fluorescein can add a further dimension to such coverage, as discussed above under 'Examination' (see Fig. 7.51).

The Seidel test: photography

To produce photographs of this technique, the blue filter is placed over the light source, which is set to produce full, broad-beam illumination, and the exposure is set for routine fluorescein photographs. The fluorescein is applied directly to the suspected site of leakage and the image captured as the diluted fluorescein cascades down the surface of the eye (Fig. 7.54).[5]

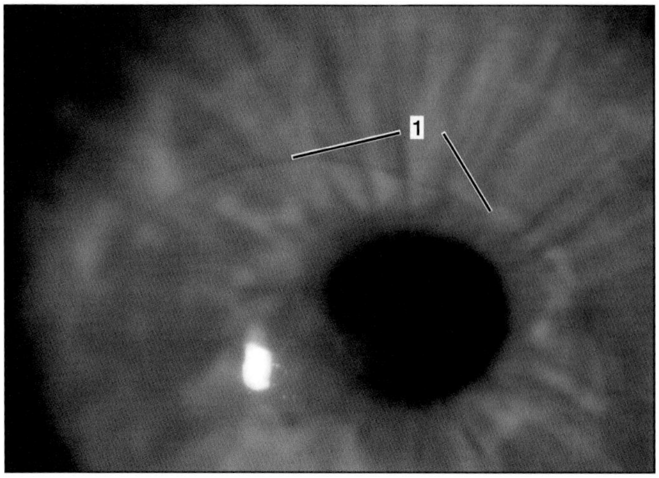

Fig. 7.55 The iron line (1), or Fleischer ring, seen in keratoconus can be enhanced with blue light. Because the basis for greater visibility is rendering the ring darker through its absorption of the incident blue light, this technique is effective only in eyes with lightly pigmented irides. (From Mártonyi CL et al. *Slit lamp: examination and photography.* Sedona: Time One Ink, Ltd; 2007.)

Techniques specific to keratoconus: photography

Documenting the Fleischer ring

The Fleischer ring may be documented by using the blue filter described earlier for exciting fluorescein. In this case, the blue light is absorbed by the iron line, delineating the conus and causing it to appear dark in the resultant photograph. It is only effective, however, when the iron line is seen against a light iris (Fig. 7.55).

Munson's sign

Munson's sign is a simple and graphic means of demonstrating the abnormal corneal outline. By asking the patient to look down, the lid margin conforms to the cornea's horizontal profile, boldly revealing the condition (Fig. 7.56).

A vertical profile can be documented by turning the patient's head in the chin rest assembly sufficiently to obtain a temporal view. By directing a moderate beam of light to strike the nasal bridge behind the cornea, a light background is produced, against which the condition is presented in a dramatic and pleasing manner (Fig. 7.57).

The Examination

'The examination of the eyes is begun after establishing the history of the case. In making this examination, too much stress can not be laid upon the necessity of proceeding systematically, since otherwise important matters can very readily be overlooked. We first examine the patient with regard to his general physical condition as well as with regard to the expression of his countenance, and then, in observing the eyes themselves, proceed gradually from the

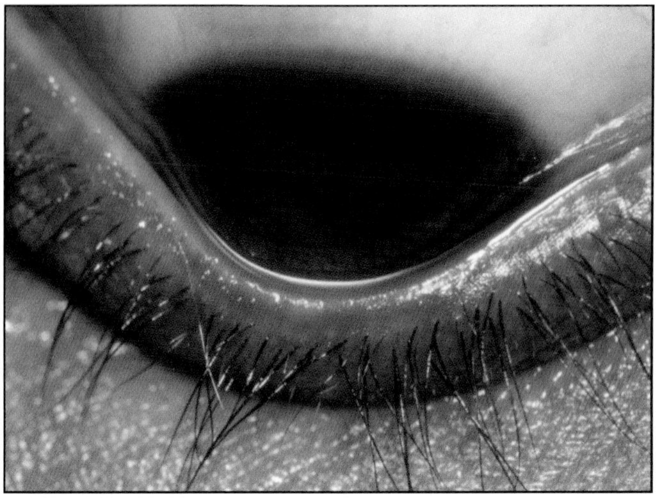

Fig. 7.56 Munson's sign in keratoconus. (From Mártonyi CL et al. *Slit lamp: examination and photography.* Sedona: Time One Ink, Ltd; 2007.)

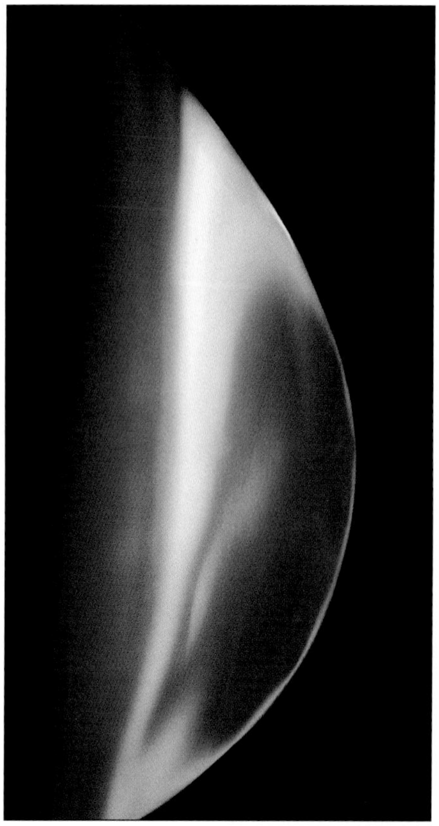

Fig. 7.57 A corneal profile of mild keratoconus seen against the illuminated nasal bridge. (From Mártonyi CL et al. *Slit lamp: examination and photography.* Sedona: Time One Ink, Ltd; 2007.)

superficial parts – lids, conjunctiva, and cornea – to the deeper portions.'**

The ideal examination includes a careful, highly dynamic analysis of all structures, using each applicable form of illumination. The result should be a fully detailed, three-dimensional mental image of the segments of the eye. Although many abnormalities are easily identified, some of subtle expressivity cannot be ruled out without having exercised fully the capabilities of the slit lamp. In the absence of clear clinical signs, with only vague symptomatology reported, the examiner must exhaust all possibilities. After the abnormality is identified, additional information about its severity, extent, or particular characteristics can be gleaned through observation under all forms of illumination.

The importance of a dynamic approach cannot be sufficiently stressed. Observing the eye in static light deprives the examiner of much of the available information. The process of examining the cornea in direct and indirect retroillumination from the iris, for instance, requires a scan of the cornea from one limbus to the other. This motion itself will reveal information that may otherwise go unnoted. It enhances the dimensional qualities of the information observed and results in a more accurate and complete impression of the extent and severity of the abnormality present. Similarly, observing the motion of the eye and the eyelids can provide important clues to normal or abnormal function.[7]

Establishing a routine protocol will minimize the time required to complete an examination and provides a fail-safe measure to ensure its completeness. As the examiner gathers experience, an individualized routine emerges. Type of practice and attendant patient population may be influencing factors in establishing a protocol. When circumstances permit, steps of an examination that may cause somewhat greater discomfort (e.g. eversion of the upper eyelid, application of vital dyes) may be best carried out toward the end of the routine to help ensure the patient's ability to cooperate throughout the examination.

** From Fuchs E. *Textbook of ophthalmology.* New York: D. Appleton & Co; 1892.

Further reading

For a more complete description of the slit lamp examination and photography techniques detailed in this chapter, refer to Mártonyi CL et al. *Slit lamp: examination and photography.* Sedona: Time One Ink, Ltd; 2007.

References

1. Van Herick W, Schaffer RN, Schwartz A. Estimation of width of angle of the anterior chamber. *Am J Ophthalmol.* 1969;68:626–629.
2. Mártonyi CL, Bahn CF, Meyer RF. *Clinical slit lamp biomicroscopy and photo slit lamp biomicrography.* Ann Arbor: Time One Ink, Ltd; 1985.
3. Berliner ML. *Biomicroscopy of the eye.* vol 1. New York: Paul B. Hoeber; 1949.
4. Shahinian L. Corneal valance: a tear film pattern in map-dot-fingerprint corneal dystrophy. *Ann Ophthalmol.* 1984;16:567–571.
5. Romanchuck KG. Seidel's test using 10% fluorescein. *Can J Ophthalmol.* 1979;14:253–256.
6. Justice J Jr, Soper JW. An improved method of viewing topical fluorescein. *Trans Am Acad Ophthalmol Otolaryngol.* 1976;81:927–928.
7. Arffa RC. *Grayson's diseases of the cornea.* 3rd ed. St Louis: Mosby; 1991.

Chapter 8

Tear Film Evaluation

Michael A. Lemp

The tear film is a critical component in maintaining the health of the ocular surface and as a pathway for repair. Oxygen captured from the atmosphere during the day and from the capillaries of the conjunctiva lining the upper lid during sleep supplies the cornea and conjunctiva, supporting the cellular turnover and maturation necessary to maintain a clear cornea for vision.[1] The tear film, moreover, provides an exit pathway for cellular debris, metabolic waste products, microbes, and other particulate matter in the tear film via drainage through the nasolacrimal ducts.[2] In addition, the ocular surface and the tear-producing structures (lacrimal glands, meibomian glands of the eyelid, and mucin-producing cells of the conjunctiva and the mucosal lining of the nasolacrimal ducts) are linked by a neural pathway forming an integrated functional unit that regulates epithelial cell turnover in health and epithelial repair processes in response to trauma or pathophysiological processes.[3,4] The tear film contains water, electrolytes, proteins (which form cytokines directing epithelial cell activities), mucins, sugars, and other water-soluble substances. Overlying this aqueous phase produced primarily by the main and accessory lacrimal glands (and to a lesser extent by the conjunctiva) is a thin lipid layer. The lipid is produced by the meibomian glands of the eyelids and serves to stabilize the tear film, retard evaporative tear loss, and prevent contamination of the ocular surface with skin lipids[5,6] The ocular surface is covered by a mucin layer consisting of two parts: a thin membrane-associated mucin produced by the epithelial cells and a thicker mucin blanket, the product of the goblet cells of the conjunctiva.[7] Mucin serves to render the epithelial cells wettable by aqueous tears and interacts with the overlying lipid layer to stabilize the tear film.

In dry eye disease there are qualitative and quantitative alterations in the volume, composition, and structure of the tear film. In this chapter we will consider examination techniques and clinical tests designed to aid in the diagnosis of dry eye disease.

General Inspection

Gross examination of the ocular adnexa can reveal significant structural changes important in the pathogenesis of dry eye disease. Alterations in the eyelid structure and function can be observed with bright natural or artificial light. The eyelids should approximate the ocular surface, and the upper lid travel over two-thirds of the cornea with each blink. Interpalpebral fissure widths vary greatly but an excessively wide interpalpebral fissure, e.g. in thyroid eye disease, is associated with increased evaporative tear loss.[8] Trichiasis, ectropion, or entropion can interfere with normal tear film dynamics, and incomplete closure of the lids can lead to localized areas of drying on the ocular surface. Bell's phenomenon in which the cornea rotates upward on lid closure ensures protection for the corneal surface. About 5% of the normal population will have an absent or deficient Bell's reflex. This can be estimated by asking the patient to close the eye while holding the lid and observing the cornea. A deficient Bell's reflex can lead to exposure keratopathy.

Slit Lamp Examination

Examination of the inferior marginal tear strip can yield information about the volume of tears present on the ocular surface. The tear strip is a line of tears just above the lower lid (Fig. 8.1). It is normally about 0.5 mm in width and has a concave upper aspect. When this strip is thin or discontinuous, it is evidence of deficient aqueous tear volume. The tear strip is better visualized by fluorescein staining but care must be taken not to flood the surface by overwetting the fluorescein strip; it should be just barely moistened. While thinning of the marginal tear strip is a relatively late sign of aqueous tear deficiency (ATD), attention to this area can yield valuable information.

Another feature frequently seen in dry eye is increased debris in the tear film. Bits of mucus, fragments of sheets of sloughed epithelial cells, and other foreign material trapped in the tear film are suggestive of delayed tear clearance seen in dry eye.[9] Examination of the ocular surface with the slit lamp can also reveal alterations in the morphology of the conjunctiva such as redundant folds in the bulbar conjunctival epithelium (conjunctivochalasis). This finding has been reported to be characteristic of dry eye.[10]

There are a variety of objective tests of tear film characteristics and function. Although most of these have some clinical utility, many have been relegated to a research setting or have not gained wide clinical acceptance. This chapter will confine itself to objective tests which are either in wide clinical use or are of such importance that they may become essential elements of routine clinical examination.

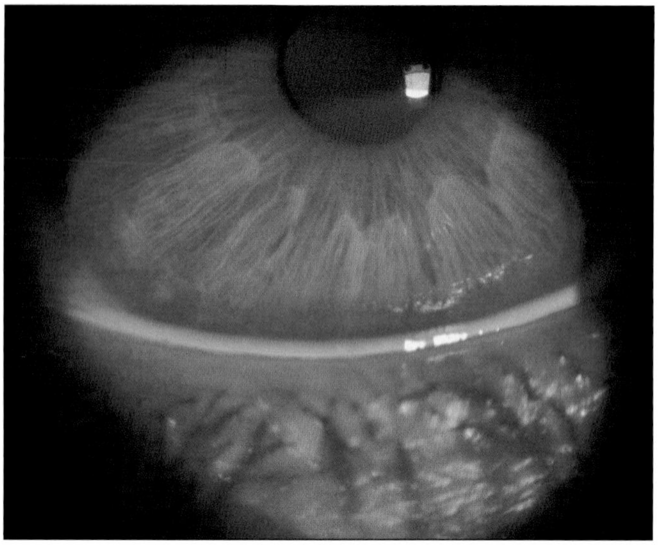

Fig. 8.1 Fluorescein-stained marginal tear strip.

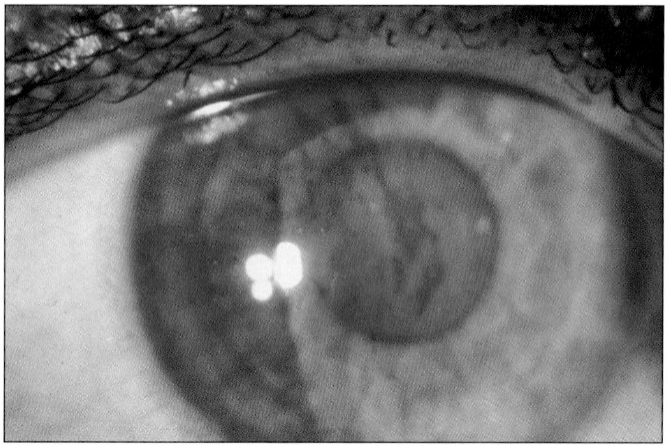

Fig. 8.2 Fluorescein-stained tear film break-up.

Tear Stability

In dry eye disease the tear film is unstable, resulting in an abnormally rapid break-up of the precorneal tear film between blinks.[11,12] After tears are surfaced by the action of the lids, a meta-stable tear film is established. Over time (usually 10–30 seconds) the tear film thins, leading to the development of randomly distributed dry spots in the precorneal tear film (Fig. 8.2). The interval between the last complete blink and the appearance of the first random dry spot is the break-up time (BUT). This is generally measured after a small amount of fluorescein has been instilled or a slightly moistened fluorescein strip has been applied to the superior aspect of the bulbar conjunctiva. A wide slit lamp beam with the cobalt blue filter is used to scan the cornea; the patient is instructed to blink several times and then not blink. A hand-held timer is used to measure the seconds until the appearance of the first randomly distributed dry spot in the fluorescein-stained precorneal tear film. This is repeated several times and averaged. Values of less than 10 seconds are considered abnormal.[13]

There are nonfluorescein (noninvasive) measurements[20] of BUT that employ reflective devices with a grid projected onto the corneal surface.[14] These values are slightly higher and require equipment not widely available.

BUT is a measure of the stability of the tear film; abnormally low values are seen in aqueous tear deficient and in evaporative dry eye. Abnormal BUT values are reflective of a tear film abnormality but do not specify the type of dry eye. The tear film will break up rapidly over an underlying epithelial irregularity such as superficial punctate keratopathy. The presence of corneal staining will result in a rapid BUT that is not necessarily evidence of an intrinsic tear abnormality but rather the epitheliopathy. BUT has been criticized as being quite variable in an individual.[15] This inter-test variability is probably due to the method with which the test is performed, variations in blink patterns, and the dynamics of tear production and flow. Consistent results below 10 seconds are, however, pathognomonic of a pathologically unstable tear film. More recently, a newer method of measuring and recording tear film break-up has been developed and is being used in clinical drug trials.[16] In this method a quantified amount of sodium fluorescein solution 1% is instilled into the conjunctival sac, blinking occurs and the appearance of the first randomly occurring corneal dry spot is video-recorded with a timer recording the time in 0.1 second increments. Three measurements are recorded and the timing measured by three independent observers. The authors have reported a new reference value for this technique. Values below 7 seconds are considered abnormal and reflective of the presence of dry eye disease.[16] The same authors have combined their BUT measurements with an assessment of the blink rate, which is calculated by dividing 60 by the number of observed blinks per second. The ratio of the tear film BUT over the interblink interval (IBI) is referred to as the Ocular Protection Index (OPI): OPI = BUT/IBI. Values below 1 are characteristic of tear film instability and dry eye disease.

Tear Production

The most widely used test to measure aqueous tear production is the Schirmer's test. In this test a standardized size strip of filter paper is inserted over the lower lid margin into the cul-de-sac, usually in the temporal one-third of the lid (Fig. 8.3). The patient is instructed to close the eyes and the strip is removed at 5 minutes; the extent of wetting of the strip is measured. Values below 5.5 mm of wetting are diagnostic of aqueous tear deficiency.[17] This test is performed both with and without the use of topical anesthesia. The so-called Schirmer's's II (with anesthesia) has been purported to measure 'basal' tear secretion, i.e. nonstimulated tears.[18] It has been demonstrated that, even with anesthesia of the cornea and conjunctiva, tear secretion is driven by sensory stimuli, e.g. the lids, lashes, air currents, and light.[19] The whole concept of 'basal' or unstimulated tears has been called into question. A Schirmer's's I (without anesthesia) has become the generally accepted method for assessing aqueous tear production.

This test has been criticized for its variability.[20] Differences in performance of the test will greatly influence the

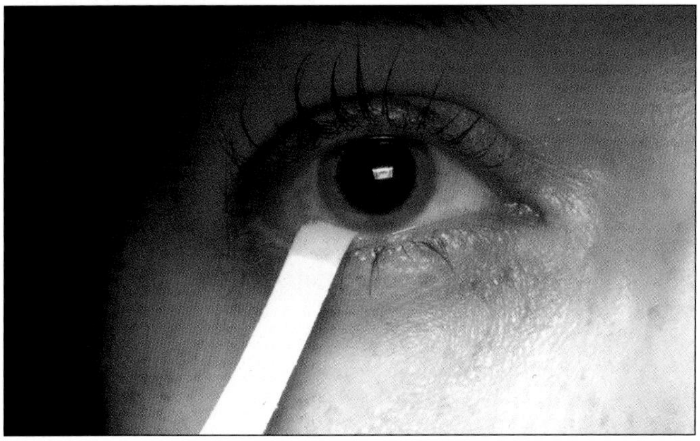

Fig. 8.3 Schirmer's strip in position on the temporal one-third of the lower lid.

sensory stimuli. The Schirmer's test, however, is a useful estimate of aqueous tear production because of its ease of performance, wide availability, and low cost. As aqueous tear-deficient dry eye disease progresses and the lacrimal glands lose their ability to respond to sensory stimuli or the sensory receptors on the ocular surface are compromised, results of the Schirmer's test become more consistent. Serially consistent Schirmer's I results below 5 mm of wetting at 5 minutes are highly suggestive of dry eye disease.

An alternative method of measuring aqueous tear production has been proposed – the phenol red test.[21] This involves the use of a special cotton thread that has been impregnated with a dye – phenol red. The thread is inserted over the inferior lid margin into the temporal conjunctival sac. At the end of 15 seconds, the dye, which is pH sensitive, turns color from yellow to orange, indicating the length of the thread wetted by tears. This test has been reported to be less uncomfortable and more specific in the diagnosis of aqueous tear-deficient dry eye disease.[22]

Tear Composition and Characteristics

Of the more than 200 proteins that have been identified in tears, several have been used as surrogate measures of aqueous tear production, i.e. lysozyme and lactoferrin. Lysozyme was first of interest because of its antibacterial activity. It has been demonstrated that tear lysozyme levels are decreased in aqueous tear-deficient dry eye disease.[23] Lysozyme is one of the principal protein components of tears. Its measurement is based on the enzyme's ability to lyse a suspension of the bacterium, *Micrococcus lysodeikticus*. When this suspension is placed in an agar gel, a tear sample is collected by micropipette and placed in a well in the suspension containing gel. The plate is incubated and the area of lysis noted. The larger the area of lysis, the greater the concentration of the enzyme. This method is not used very often because of lack of availability of the plates, cost, and the lack of specificity of the results. Decreased tear lysozyme levels are also seen in a number of inflammatory conditions.[24]

Of more recent interest is the tear protein lactoferrin, which also possess antibacterial activity.[25] In addition, it has a protective effect on the corneal and conjunctival epithelium.[26] Previously, an assay was based on a commercial solid-phase ELISA methodology but more recent reports of a colorimetric analysis of microvolumes of tears have shown good diagnostic utility.

In this method (Touch MicroAssay), a micropipette is used to collect a small volume of tears, which is then transferred to a cell where the tears are exposed to a reactive reagent that is colorimetrically tagged; the resultant sample is read in a commercially available colorimeter.[27] Clinical experience has, however, shown tear lactoferrin levels to be scattered over a broad area. Decreased lactoferrin secretion in aqueous tear-deficient dry eye disease would be expected to be counterbalanced by the tear-concentrating effects seen in both aqueous deficient and evaporative dry eye disease, yielding variable results. Ways to compensate for the increased tear concentration characteristic of dry eye disease might improve the diagnostic value of this marker for aqueous tear-deficiency dry eye disease.

Tear ferning

It has been observed that tear samples dried on a slide and examined under a microscope display a crystalline pattern of tear mucin. In aqueous tear deficiency, this pattern resembles ferns. A grading system has been developed and this test has been reported to have greater specificity and sensitivity than the Schirmer's test, particularly for more severe forms of dry eye disease.[28]

Tear osmolarity

It has been known that in dry eye disease the tear film is in a hyperosmolar state. This is true for both aqueous deficient and evaporative dry eye disease.[29] Tear film osmolarity has been measured using freezing point depression and vapor pressure measurement. Unfortunately, these methods have been limited primarily to a research setting, owing to their complexity, the high operator skill required and, most importantly, the need for relatively large volumes of tears, which necessitates stimulating tears for collection, and even this is insufficient in many dry eye subjects.[30] A large, recently published meta-analysis of the literature over the last 25 years identifies tear hyperosmolarity as the single diagnostic test with the highest accuracy in identifying patients with dry eye disease.[31] The advent of a new technology requiring tear samples of less than 50 nanoliters and measuring tear osmolarity easily and quickly in a clinical setting promises to provide a new practical diagnostic test suitable for clinical use. A recent report suggests very high sensitivity and specificity and positive predictive values for this TearLab technology, making this a new 'gold standard' in the diagnosis of dry eye disease.[32]

Meibomian Gland Structure and Excreta

The meibomian glands of the eyelid number between and 20 and 25 in each lid. They secrete a lipid mixture which is discharged onto the tear film: excretion of the lipid is effected primarily through the muscular contraction associated with blinking. Meibomian gland lipid forms the top layer of the tear film and both stabilizes the tear film and retards evaporative tear loss.[33] Evaluation of the functional status of these glands involves slit lamp inspection of the lid margin and an estimate of the quantity and quality of the excreted lipid (meibum). Evidence of altered meibomian gland structure includes increased vascularity of the lid margin, plugging of the orifices, and loss of orifices.[34] Increased vascularity of the lid margins occurs with advancing age and is not, by itself, a reliable indicator of meibomian gland disease.

Meibum can be evaluated by pressing against the lower lid with a finger about 1 mm below the lid margin. In the normal subject, it will be possible to express some lipid from about two-thirds of the glands at a given time. This excretion is normally fluid and clear. Lack of expression from the glands, and/or alteration in the character of the excretion, is critical in the diagnosis of meibomian gland dysfunction (MGD). As the disease process advances, the excretion will vary from turbid to coagulated (toothpaste-like). Such meibum is pathognomonic of MGD. A grading scale for assessing severity of meibomian gland dysfunction has been developed for use in clinical trails but is equally suitable for clinical practice.[35]

Another method of assessing meibomian gland dysfunction involves transillumination of the eyelid. Using an examining muscle light placed inside the lower eyelid (after topical anesthesia), it is possible to visualize the outline of the glandular structure. This visualization can be enhanced and recorded with the use of infrared film.[36] The normal pattern is that of branching ductules coming off a central vertical core. Obliteration of this structure is evidence of chronic inflammation and glandular dysfunction.

Tear Clearance Tests

Coincident with a decrease in aqueous tear production, there is a decrease in tear turnover, which is defined as the rate at which newly secreted tears reside within the tear film before they are lost either to evaporation or drainage through the lacrimal punctae and the nasolacrimal ducts. Tear volume and turnover are most accurately measured by dye dilution studies. In this methodology, a small amount of fluorescein dye is instilled into the tear film and the concentration of the dye is measured over time. Special fluorophotometers have been built to accurately measure dilution of the dye as new tears enter the tear film and old tears exit. Expense has limited the availability of this methodology. An alternative, inexpensive method of semiquantitatively grading fluorescein dilution has been proposed and is in use.[37] In this method (Fluorescein Clearance Test [FTC]), 5 μL of 1% fluorescein dye is instilled into the tear film. The patient is asked to blink to distribute the dye and serial 1-minute Schirmer's tests are performed every 10 minutes. Initially, the staining of the paper strip with the dye will be intense. Persistent staining (beyond 10 minutes) indicates delayed tear clearance (DTC).

A combined use of the Schirmer's II test with the FTC has been proposed.[38] This tear function index (TFI) is the ratio of the value of the Schirmer's test over the tear clearance rate. The use of the TFI in the diagnosis of dry eye disease is reported to demonstrate a specificity of 91% and a sensitivity of 79%.

Staining of the Ocular Surface

The normal ocular surface does not take up water-soluble dyes instilled into the tear film. With disruption of the mucin coating protecting the surface epithelial cells and/or damage to the epithelial cell walls, water-soluble dyes will diffuse into the surface cells. The three most commonly used dyes are fluorescein, rose Bengal (RB), and lissamine green (LG). Fluorescein, which stains damaged epithelial cells, is best visualized on the corneal surface. A 1% solution or a filter paper strip impregnated with fluorescein is used to introduce the dye into the tear film. The patient is instructed to blink to distribute the dye. The ocular surface is scanned using the broad beam of the slit lamp with the cobalt blue filter (or Wratten 47 blue filter). The extent and intensity of the stain are assessed. There are a number of grading scales, including the Van Bjisterveld, NEI/Industry Workshop, and Oxford systems.[39] The NEI/Industry Workshop grading system has the advantage of collecting data on five discrete subareas of the cornea separately, e.g the central cornea

Staining of the conjunctiva is seen when there are disruptions in the protective mucin coating; RB and LG are used. A 1% solution of either is instilled into the tear film, and the patient is asked to blink. The surface of the conjunctiva can be viewed within 10 seconds with RB but one should wait at least 2–3 minutes before viewing LG stain, and low light should be used. RB is more irritating to the patient and LG is gaining wider acceptance for this reason. Staining of the ocular surface is evidence of ocular surface damage and is characteristic of more severe dry eye.

Tests of visual function

Recently, attention has been directed to optical aberrations which have been identified in patients with dry eye disease. Although severe dry eye with significant staining of the central cornea has long been known to reduce visual acuity, recent studies have demonstrated that even in the absence of significant central corneal staining, the instability which is characteristic in all forms of dry eye disease results in rapid break-up of the tear film between blinks, compromising image quality. This effect on visual acuity is not captured during ordinary Snellen chart measurement of acuity because the patient can blink, momentarily improving vision. More rapid break-up occurs within 3 second of a blink in many dry eye patients, reducing their inter-blink acuity to levels of 20/60 or less.[40]

Recent work has developed two instruments to detect these changes. In one, the tear stability analysis system (TSAS), serial videokeratographic images are collected each second between blinks.[41] In another approach, a functional visual acuity (FVA) device has been developed which measures visual acuity by way of rapid presentation of optotypes. Both of these technologies promise to add to our armamentarium of diagnostic technologies in the near future.[42]

Conclusion

The various objective methods of examining the tear film can provide useful information, diagnosing, classifying, and grading the severity of dry eye.

References

1. Holly FJ, Lemp MA. Tear physiology and dry eyes: review. *Surv Ophthalmol.* 1977;22:69–87.
2. Doane EMG. Blinking and the mechanics of the lacrimal drainage system. *Ophthalmology.* 1981;88:844–851.
3. Stern ME, Beuerman RW, Fox RI, et al. The pathology of dry eye: the interaction between ocular surface and lacrimal glands. *Cornea.* 1998;17:584–589.
4. Paulsen FP, Schaudig U, Thale AB. Drainage of tears: impact on the ocular surface and lacrimal system. *Ocul Surf.* 2003;1(4):180–191.
5. Holly FJ. Formation and stability of the tear film. *Int Ophthalmol Clin.* 1973;13:73–96.
6. Lozato PA, Pisella PJ, Baudouin C. The lipid layer of the lacrimal tear film: physiology and pathology. *J Fr Ophtalmol.* 2001;24(6):643–658.
7. Watanabe H. Significance of mucin on the ocular surface. *Cornea.* 2002;21(2 Suppl 1):S17–S22.
8. Khurana AK, Sunder S, Ahluwalia BK, et al. Tear film profiles in Graves' ophthalmopathy. *Acta Ophthalmol (Copenh).* 1992;70:346–349.
9. Pflugfelder SC, Solomon A, Stern ME. The diagnosis and management of dry eye: a twenty-five year review. *Cornea.* 2000;19(5):644–649.
10. Meller D, Tseng SC. Conjunctivochalasis: literature review and possible pathophysiology. *Surv Ophthalmol.* 1998;43(3):225–232.
11. Norn MS. Desiccation of the precorneal tear film. I. Corneal wetting time. *Acta Ophthalmol (Copenh).* 1969;47:865–880.
12. Lemp MA, Holly FJ. Recent advances in ocular surface chemistry. *Am J Optom Arch Am Acad Optom.* 1970;47:669–672.
13. Lemp MA, Hamill JR. Factors affecting tear film breakup in normal eyes. *Arch Ophthalmol.* 1973;89:103–105.
14. Mengher LS, Bron AJ, Tonge SR, et al. A non-invasive instrument for clinical assessment of the pre-corneal tear film stability. *Curr Eye Res.* 1985;4:1–7.
15. Vanley GT, Leopold IH, Gregg TH. Interpretation of tear film breakup. *Arch Ophthalmol.* 1977;95:445–448.
16. Abelson M, Ousler G, Nally L. Alternate reference values for tear film break-up time in normal and dry eye populations. Lacrimal Gland, Tear Film, and Dry Eye Syndromes 3 Part B. *Adv Exp Med Biol.* 2002;506: 1121–1125
17. van Bijisterveld OP. Diagnostic tests in sicca syndrome. *Arch Ophthalmol.* 1969;82:10–14.
18. Jones LT. The lacrimal secretory system and its treatment. *Am J Ophthalmol.* 1966;62:47–60.
19. Jordan A, Baum J. Basic tear flow, does it exist? *Ophthalmology.* 1980;87:920–930.
20. Clinch TE, Benedetto DA, Felberg NT, et al. Schirmer's's test: a closer look. *Arch Ophthalmol.* 1983;101:1383–1386.
21. Hamano H, Hori M, Hamano T, et al. A new method for measuring tears. *CLAO J.* 1983;9:281–289.
22. Asbell PA, Chiang B, Li K. Phenol-red thread test compared to Schirmer's test in normal subjects. *Ophthalmology.* 1987;94(Suppl):128.
23. Regan E. The lysozyme content of tears. *Am J Ophthalmol.* 1950;33: 600–605.
24. Sapse AT, Bonavida B. Preliminary study of lysozyme levels in subjects with smog eye irritation. *Am J Ophthalmol.* 1968;66:79.
25. van Bijisterveld OP. The Sjogren syndrome and tear function profile. *Adv Exp Med Biol.* 1998;438:949–952.
26. Shimmura S, Shimoyama M, Hojo M, et al. Reoxygenation injury in a cultured corneal epithelial cell line protected by the uptake of lactoferrin. *Invest Ophthalmol Vis Sci.* 1998;39:1346–1351.
27. Foulks GN. Personal communication.
28. Albach KA, Lauer M, Stolze HH. Diagnosis of KCS in rheumatoid arthritis. *Ophthalmologe.* 1994;91(2):229–234.
29. Gilbard JP, Farris RL, Santamaria HJ. Osmolarity of tear film microvolumes in keratoconjunctivitis sicca. *Arch Ophthalmol.* 1978;96:677–681.
30. Nelson JD, Wright JC. Tear film osmolarity determination: an evaluation of potential errors in measurement. *Curr Eye Res.* 1986;5(9):677–681.
31. Tomlinson A, Khanal S, Ramesh K, Diaper C, McFayden A. Tear film osmolarity determination of a referent value for dry eye diagnosis. *Invest Ophthal Vis Sci.* 2006;47(10):4309–4315.
32. Tomlinson A, McCann L, Pearce I. Comparison of OcuSense and Clifton nanolitre osmometers. ARVO Abstract, 2009.
33. Driver PJ, Lemp MA. Meibomian gland dysfunction. *Surv Ophthalmol.* 1996;40:343–367.
34. Bron AJ, Benjamin L, Snibson GR. Meibomian gland disease. Classification and grading of lid changes. *Eye.* 1991;5:395–411.
35. Foulks GN, Bron AJ. Meibomian gland dysfunction: a clinical scheme for description, diagnosis, classification and grading. *Ocul Surf.* 2003;1(4): 107–126.
36. Mathers WD, Shields WJ, Sachdev MS, et al. Meibomian gland dysfunction in chronic blepharitis. *Cornea.* 1991;10:277–285.
37. Macri A, Rolando M, Pflugfelder S. A standardized visual scale for evaluation of tear fluorescein clearance. *Ophthalmology.* 2000;107:1338–1343.
38. Xu KP, Yagi Y, Toda I, et al. Tear function index: a new measure of dry eye. *Arch Ophthalmol.* 1995;113:84–88.
39. Foulks GN. Challenges and pitfalls in clinical trials of treatments for dry eye. *Ocul Surf.* 2003;1:20–30.
40. Goto E, Ishida R, Kaido M, et al. Optical aberrations and visual disturbance associated with dry eye. *Ocul Surf.* 2006;4(4):207–213.
41. Kojima T, Ishida R, Dogru M, et al. A new noninvasive tear stability analysis system for the assessment of dry eyes. *Invest Ophthalmol Vis Sci.* 2004;45:1369–1374.
42. Ishida R, Kojima T, Dogru M, et al. The application of a new continuous functional visual acuity measurement system in dry eye syndromes. *Am J Ophthalmol.* 2005;139:253–258.

Chapter **9**

Refraction of the Abnormal Cornea

Mark J. Mannis, Jay H. Krachmer

Refracting the abnormal cornea is as much art as it is science. The refractionist must often employ techniques not routinely used in the normal eye. If responsive, the patient can play a significant role in determining the final prescription, while patients with abnormal corneas who cannot provide subjective input, such as infants, present a greater challenge.

There are principles that, if understood, may enhance successful refraction of the abnormal cornea. The air–tear interface is the main refracting element of the eye. Tears assume the curvature of the underlying corneal tissue. There is a much greater change in the index of refraction between the air and tears than between tears and cornea, cornea and aqueous, aqueous and the crystalline or pseudophakic lens, lens and vitreous, or vitreous and retina. Therefore, pathology that causes even minor alterations in the surface curvature of the central cornea can result in significant degradation of vision.

Stromal opacities, on the other hand, that are not accompanied by irregularities of the corneal surface may be consistent with surprisingly good visual acuity. Even so, stromal opacities can reduce both visual acuity as well as contrast sensitivity, so that vision may be impaired both qualitatively and quantitatively.

Instrumentation

Four devices increase accuracy and reduce total time needed for refraction of the abnormal cornea. They are the retinoscope, the keratometer, computed topography, and the trial frame.

Retinoscopy

Retinoscopy is one of the most important tools in ophthalmology for determining refractive error and alterations in the corneal surface. A skillful retinoscopist understands what component the ocular media – cornea, anterior chamber, lens, and vitreous – play in vision. Opacities and irregularities in these structures degrade the image falling on the retina. Retinoscopy reveals critical and sometimes subtle anterior corneal abnormalities, axial corneal opacities, significant anterior chamber inflammation, opacities in and multiple refractive layers of the lens, as well as optically significant vitreous pathology. After years of experience, the skilled retinoscopist can predict best-corrected visual acuity assuming good neurologic (retina, optic nerve, visual pathway) health.

Subtle corneal anterior membrane pathology degrades the quality of the red reflex. Corneal curvature irregularities such as in keratoconus and pellucid marginal degeneration are recognized by characteristic scissoring of the retinoscopic streak. Indeed, the retinoscope is the instrument that is most sensitive to the early changes found in the noninflammatory ectatic diseases of the cornea.

Two refractive abnormalities in which retinoscopy is particularly useful are high astigmatism and high myopia or hyperopia. In the case of high astigmatism, retinoscopy can both determine, with remarkable precision, the *amount* of as well as the *axis* of the cylinder. Occasionally, moving closer to the patient with the retinoscope helps in this determination.

In high myopia, even in the presence of a relatively clear cornea, the red reflex is dull or dark. A high spherical error can be uncovered if the retinoscope sleeve is dropped; the red reflex will become brighter, and movement of the streak will be far more noticeable. Of course, in this circumstance the retinoscopist must remember to add corrective lenses in the opposite manner. For instance, with the sleeve dropped, minus lenses will be added if there is *with* motion rather than the usual *with* motion observed with plus lenses when the sleeve is in the up position.

There are times when the retinoscopic reflex is so poor, due to abnormal media, that retinoscopy can only be used as a diagnostic tool rather than a refracting device.

Keratometry

The Bausch & Lomb Keratometer™ is an extremely useful tool for quantification of corneal astigmatism and the diagnosis of curvature irregularities. It may help to predict the best-corrected visual acuity, assuming that the remainder of the eye is normal. Practitioners who examine a large number of patients with corneal abnormalities should consider including this instrument, in addition to a phoropter, in every examination room.

The keratometer can be used to evaluate the quality of the corneal surface as well as the dioptric curvature of the anterior cornea. It is important to remember that the

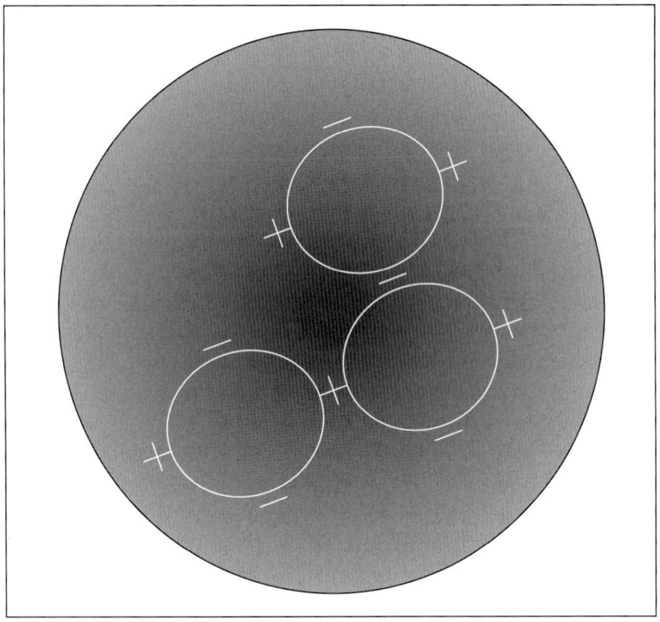

Fig. 9.1 Regular keratometry mires.

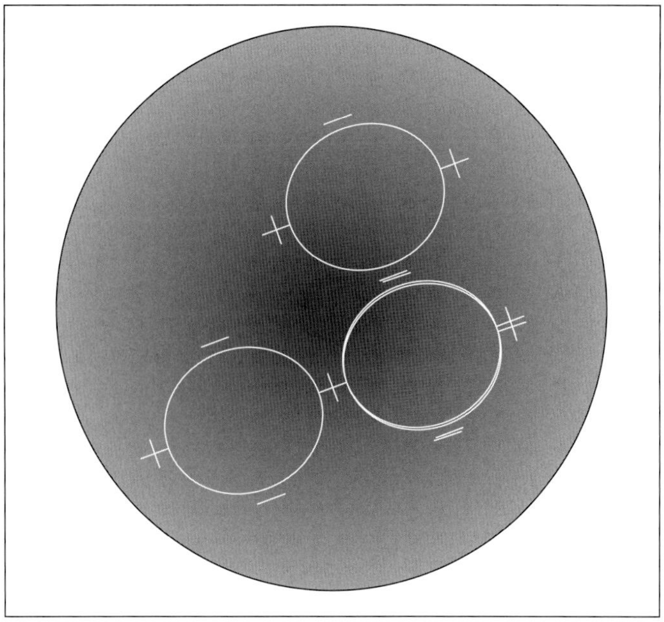

Fig. 9.2 Mildly irregular keratometry mires.

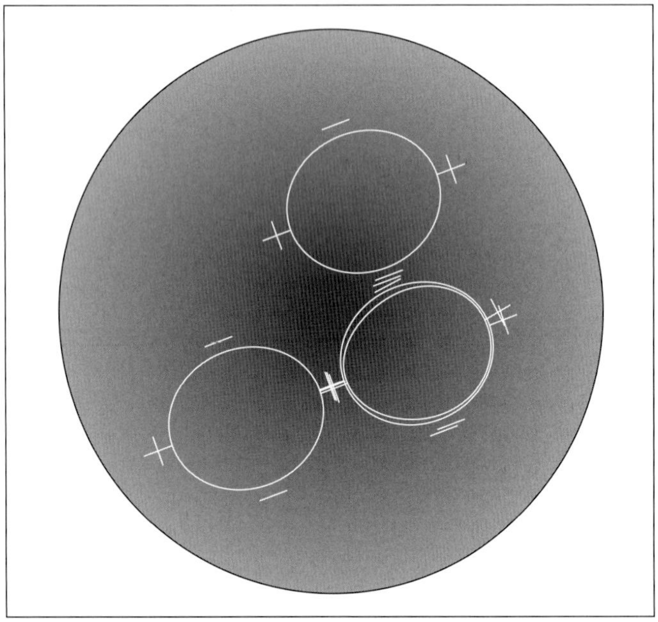

Fig. 9.3 Moderately irregular keratometry mires.

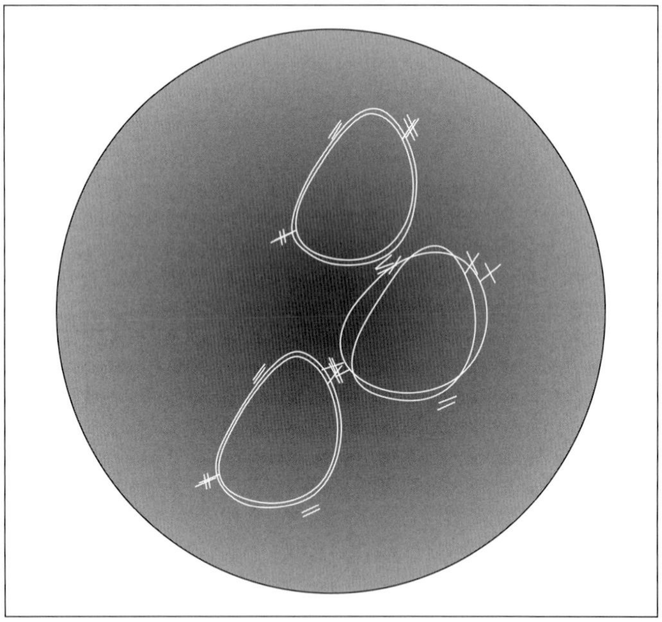

Fig. 9.4 Markedly irregular keratometry mires.

keratometric mires that reflect from the cornea fall on a very small area (3.0–3.5 mm) and do not represent the curvature of the entire cornea. For example, on a cornea of 45 spherical diopters, the diameter of the mire is 3.2 mm. If a 3.0 mm diameter drill were used to produce a hole through a steel ball having a 45-diopter curvature, and readings were taken with an axis through the center of the hole, the mires would be perfect. The mire would fall on the unaffected steel ball just outside the hole because its diameter on a 45 diopter curvature would be 3.2 mm. In the case of the human cornea with pathology in the central visual axis, the result is surface irregularity radiating from that pathology. In such a case, keratometric mires would be irregular. Therefore, even though the keratometer K measures a small, defined area, regularity of the mires is significantly affected by adjacent central pathology.

Every time K-readings are taken, the quality of the mires should be assessed and described. A useful convention is to describe them as regular (Fig. 9.1), mildly irregular (Fig. 9.2), moderately irregular (Fig. 9.3), or markedly irregular (Fig. 9.4). Mires are regular if they overlap perfectly. A patient can have 5 diopters of corneal astigmatism with perfectly overlapping mires. This would be described as 'regular' astigmatism. If keratoconus is present and the patient has 5 diopters of astigmatism, the mires will not overlap perfectly and can be described as mildly, moderately, or severely irregular. Other factors may contribute to irregularity of keratometric mires, including dry eye, eye drops used as part of the eye examination, and post-tonometry surface irregularities.

The skilled retinoscopist and examiner, adept in the use of the keratometer, can often predict best-corrected visual acuity and can judge from the anterior corneal surface abnormalities the visual potential. Perfect mires are compatible with 20/20 or better visual acuity. Mild irregularity may be compatible only with 20/25 to 20/40 visual acuity, moderate irregularity with 20/40 to 20/60 visual acuity, and severe irregularity with 20/60 to 20/200 visual acuity. These parameters are, of course, arbitrary, but with experience, each examiner develops his or her own empirical classification. Even with the advanced technologies of the current systems of topographic analysis (see Ch. 160), the keratometer can provide subtle visual information that is missed by the automated analyzers.

In the majority of cases of keratoconus, the earliest finding is steepening of the cornea below the visual axis. This inferior corneal steepening is easily observed by taking K-readings with the patient looking straight ahead and then asking the patient to look up slowly. The vertical mires slowly spread apart as they get smaller, indicating inferior steepening. At the point of maximum separation, a new reading can be taken, and the amount of dioptric steepening can be recorded.

When corneal steepening measures greater than 52 diopters, a +1.25 diopter trial lens can be taped over the opening on the front of the keratometer, and new readings are taken. One then adds 9 diopters to the reading for the final result. For example, if the curvature is greater than 52 diopters and a +1.25 diopter lens is taped over the front, a new drum reading of 49 diopters would be extrapolated to 58 diopters. When keratometer readings are less than 36 diopters, a −1.00 diopter lens can be taped to the keratometer and 6 diopters subtracted from the new reading. In this case, if the reading using a −1.00 diopter lens is 38 diopters, the reading would be extrapolated to 32 diopters. Standard nomograms for extension of the keratometer are available in tabular format from the manufacturer.

Computer-assisted topographic analysis

Of equal utility to the keratometer in facilitating the refraction of the abnormal cornea is computer-assisted topographic analysis. A standard topogram will often provide the refractionist with a clear cylinder axis, even when this is hard to determine with retinoscopy. Using the topogram, the refractionist can dial in both the axis of the cylinder as well as the approximate amount of astigmatism in diopters. As a general rule, the refractive cylinder is often roughly two-thirds of the topographically measured cylinder. Using this as a base, particularly in patients with high cylinder, one can often start the refraction with considerably less guesswork. Moreover, the topogram provides a reasonably accurate assessment of the degree of irregular astigmatism. This information can be gleaned by observing the color map or by using the numerical indices (e.g. surface regularity index) provided by some analyzers. While topographic analysis does not provide significantly greater refractive information than does a keratometer, the information is very easily accessible and is not subject to interpretation of the operator as is, to some extent, keratometry. Much in the same way in which topography aids in the determination of selective suture removal, it may be of use to the refractionist when the graft patient is ready for spectacle or contact lens prescription. Likewise, in the patient with an irregular cornea (e.g. keratoconus or scarring from trauma or infection), the topogram may explain why best-corrected acuity is not achieved even when retinoscopy provides distinct information about sphere and cylinder but acuity does not improve with spectacle refraction. (See Ch. 160 for a detailed analysis of contemporary computer-assisted topographic analysis systems.)

Trial frame

The patient with a high refractive error, significant corneal pathology, or inability to cooperate, is best refracted using a trial frame instead of a phoropter. A useful technique that may help define the axis of astigmatism preferred by the patient is to ask the patient to turn the dial on the trial frame that changes the axis (Fig. 9.5). The patient can accurately determine the axis by rotating the lens around the axis until the best vision is obtained. This technique is especially helpful in cases where the retinoscopic reflex is poor or when K-readings are moderately or severely irregular. It does, however, require a reasonably cooperative and observant patient. Moreover, vertex distance – especially important in high refractive errors – can be more accurately determined with the trial frame than with phoropter.

In patients with abnormal corneas, the manifest refraction found in the trial frame should always be used to test whether the expensive glasses to be purchased by the patient are likely to work. A 15-minute walk around the clinic while wearing the trial frames usually answers this question. If the

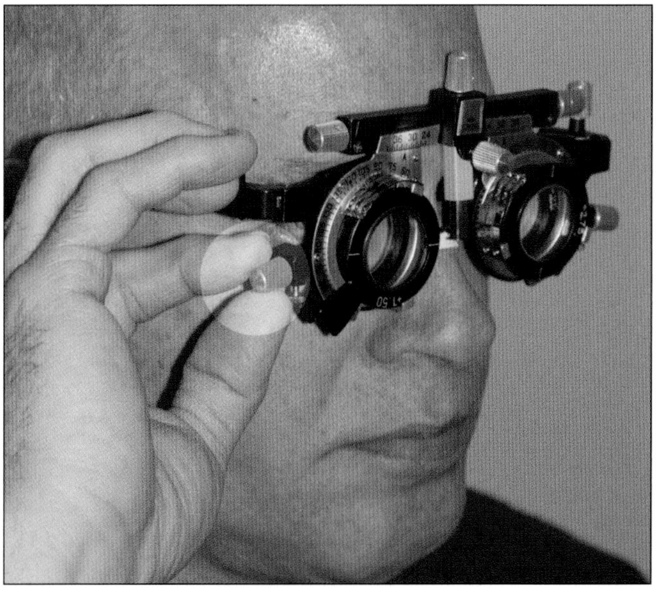

Fig. 9.5 Patient with high astigmatism helping with manifest refraction by turning cylinder screw of trial frame.

power in either eye or using both eyes together is not acceptable, changes in the sphere or cylinder may result in a better tolerated prescription, even if the visual acuity is not quite as good. Some patients, especially those with keratoconus, will accept a surprisingly high amount of anisometropia.

Refracting the Patient

How, then, are the retinoscope, keratometer, topography unit, and trial frame used together to refract the patient with an abnormal cornea? Although there is more than one strategy for use in the abnormal cornea, the approach here employes the procedural paradigm seen in Figure 9.6. Other strategies reflect the fact that there are different approaches which accomplish a successful result.[1,2]

One first uses the retinoscope to evaluate the quality of the red reflex and streak. At the same time, the refractionist can assess what the best-corrected visual acuity should be, assuming the remainder of the eye to be normal. If the retinoscopic reflex is reasonably good, one uses the trial frame to complete a manifest refraction. If the reflex is poor, one then uses the keratometer or topography unit to measure the curvature and evaluate the quality of the anterior surface, another predictor of best-corrected visual acuity. If there is minimal cylinder, one uses the measurement obtained along with retinoscopy and trial lenses to determine the refraction. The best-corrected visual acuity obtained with the manifest refraction should have been predicted with the retinoscope and keratometer or topography unit.

If the cylinder is moderate or high, one should start with three-quarters of the amount in a trial frame. For example, if there are 6 diopters of astigmatism by keratometry or topography, and the cylinder axis for the steeper reading is at 90 degrees, one can place a +4.5 diopter lens at 90 degrees in the trial frame. Retinoscopy is then used to determine the sphere. The examiner asks the patient to refine the axis by turning the screw on the trial frame. The manifest refraction can then be completed using cylindrical and spherical lenses. Once again, the best-corrected visual acuity should make sense from information gained by retinoscopy and keratometry. In the special case of the presence of a corneal graft, pre-refraction topography is often a great time saver for the refractionist. And in the case of a reasonably clear cornea with moderate to marked irregular astigmatism, as may be found in the post-keratoplasty patient, the use of a trial rigid contact lens with over-refraction can be very helpful in determining the role of irregular astigmatism in the decreased acuity.

An autorefracting device can sometimes be a useful piece of equipment but often provides erroneous readings due to the irregularity of the refracting surface.

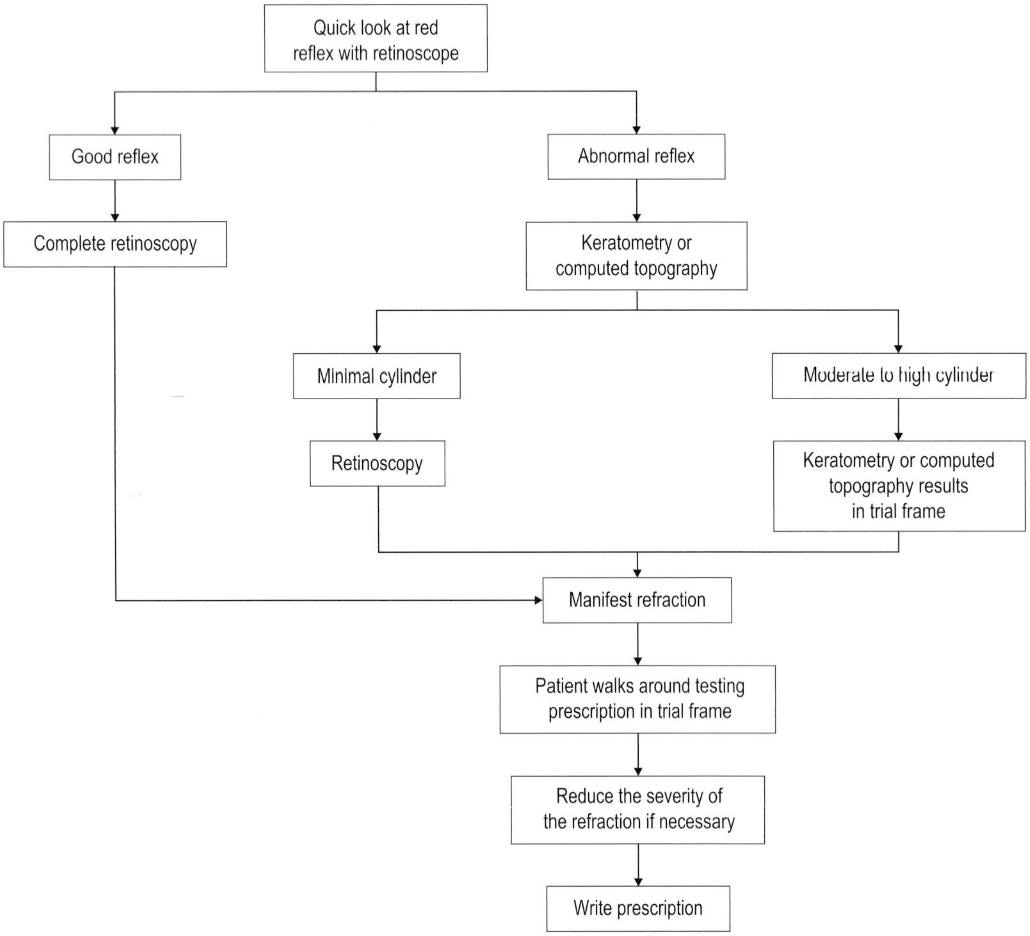

Fig. 9.6 Flowchart for refracting the patient with an abnormal cornea.

Conclusion

Refracting the patient with an abnormal cornea is a challenging, interesting, but most especially a rewarding experience for both patient and refractionist. Successful refraction of the abnormal cornea may require both the use of additional instrumentation as well as a change of the order in which the steps in refraction are employed.

References

1. Mannis MJ, Zadnik K. Refracting the corneal graft. *Surv Ophthalmol.* 1990;34:436–440.
2. Kielty DW. Refraction of the abnormal cornea. In: Krachmer JH, Mannis MJ, Holland EJ, eds. *Cornea*. St. Louis: Mosby; 1997.

Chapter **10**

Corneal Diagnostic Techniques

William J. Faulkner, Gary A. Varley

Corneal diagnostic techniques are specialized methods of examination that may involve simple or complex aids to yield valuable information for the diagnosis and treatment of ocular disease. These techniques are commonly but selectively used, depending on the patient's history and the goals of the examination. External examination of the lids, slit lamp biomicroscopy techniques, and tear film evaluation usually precede other diagnostic tests and have been discussed in previous chapters. Techniques discussed here are corneal staining, pachymetry, tests for corneal sensation, and osmolarity.

Corneal Staining

Corneal stains are diagnostic tools to assess the integrity of superficial cell layers of the cornea and the surface environment. These may be the most commonly performed tests in routine slit lamp biomicroscopy. Characteristic staining patterns aid in the diagnosis and management of corneal and external disease. Staining should be documented, noting depth and extent. Descriptions may specify micropunctuate (resembling small dots), macropunctuate (larger dots), or coalescent (a patch). Depth may be limited to the epithelium or include stroma.

Fluorescein and rose Bengal are the most common dyes used to evaluate the ocular surface. Both are halide derivatives of the hydroxyxanthene dye family. The addition of seven halogen atoms (three iodide and four chloride) to the hydroxyxanthene skeleton is responsible for the photophysical differences of rose Bengal. The spectroscopic absorption undergoes a red shift that contributes to the rose Bengal dye color.

Recently Feenstra and Tseng have demonstrated that the original concepts of fluorescein and rose Bengal staining have not been entirely correct.[1] While both dyes can stain living cells, rose Bengal does so more effectively and is intrinsically toxic. However, a healthy preocular tear film will block rose Bengal staining of healthy and damaged cells. The lack of a healthy precorneal tear film in keratoconjunctivitis sicca explains the clinical usefulness of rose Bengal staining in that disorder. Cell degeneration or death increases membrane permeability to both dyes, but rose Bengal diffusion into the stroma is limited. Its clinical usefulness is recognized in the evaluation of keratoconjunctivitis sicca, the interpretation of epithelial dendrites (Fig. 10.1), and dysplastic or neoplastic lesions.

Because of the fluorescence property of fluorescein, examination of a fluorescein-stained cornea is enhanced by the use of a cobalt (blue) filter along with a yellow (Wratten # 12) barrier filter. Conjunctival staining, otherwise often difficult to appreciate, becomes more visible. Fluorescein staining of healthy cells is limited, but fluorescein diffuses rapidly into the intercellular spaces or stroma when disruption of cell–cell junctions occurs. This diffusion property is responsible for the need to examine the cornea very soon after fluorescein is applied. Fine details of fluorescein staining may be lost after as little as 2–3 minutes (Fig. 10.2). One technique for visualizing staining (according to Korb) is as follows: instill a drop, have the patient blink three times, and wait 1–2 minutes. This is enough time for the stain to penetrate damaged epithelial cells but also leach out of the tear film.[2] Some pathologic conditions such as diabetes mellitus, as well as some medications, may increase epithelial permeability.[3] As noted earlier, cell degeneration or death increases membrane permeability to both dyes, and, given time, fluorescein will also stain dead cells.[1] These properties of fluorescein dye are responsible for its usefulness in the various forms of epithelial defect, in evaluating the status of precorneal tear film, in contact lens fitting, in detection of aqueous humor leakage, and to measure epithelial or endothelial permeability.

The technique of applying stain to the cornea can influence the information gathered for fluorescein. The clinician quickly learns 'less is more.' A very small amount of concentrated dye yields much better diagnostic information than a full drop. In fact, a full drop may overwhelm the cornea and mask subtle findings. Therefore, dye strips may be more useful, as well as more sanitary, than corresponding solution. Placing a small drop in the middle or proximal end of the strip and letting it run down to the end provides a small but highly concentrated volume of corneal stain.

Gross evidence of epithelial discontinuity can easily be seen after the instillation of dye but must be distinguished from 'pooling.' Pooling of the fluorescein tear film occurs in a depressed or irregular area of the cornea. The easiest method to distinguish pooling from staining uses a wisp of cotton from a cotton-tipped applicator. In an anesthetized cornea, without blinking, the cotton wisp is used to absorb the fluorescein tear film in the area of concern. If the

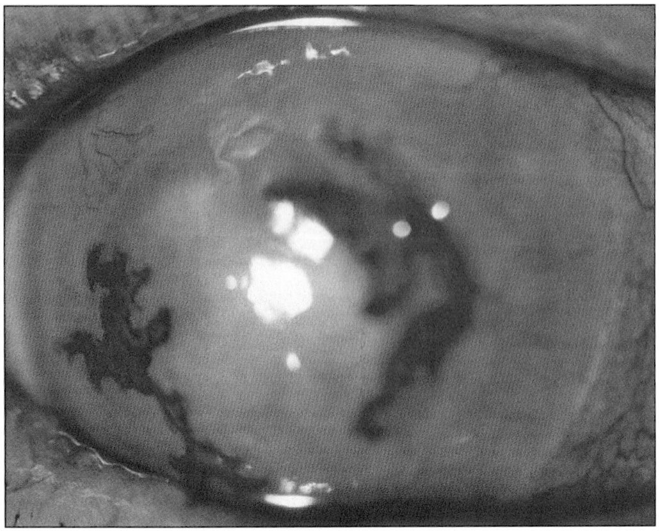

Fig. 10.1 Herpes simplex dendrites stained with rose Bengal.

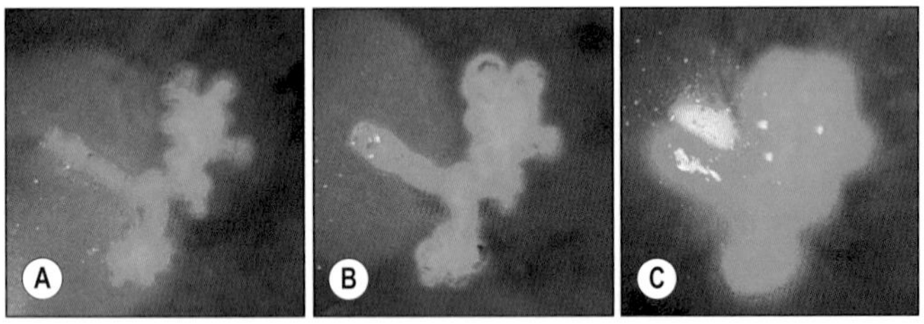

Fig. 10.2 Cornea stained with fluorescein strip demonstrating a herpes simplex dendrite. (**A**) Taken immediately after application of stain. (**B**) and (**C**) Taken 1 and 3 minutes later, respectively.

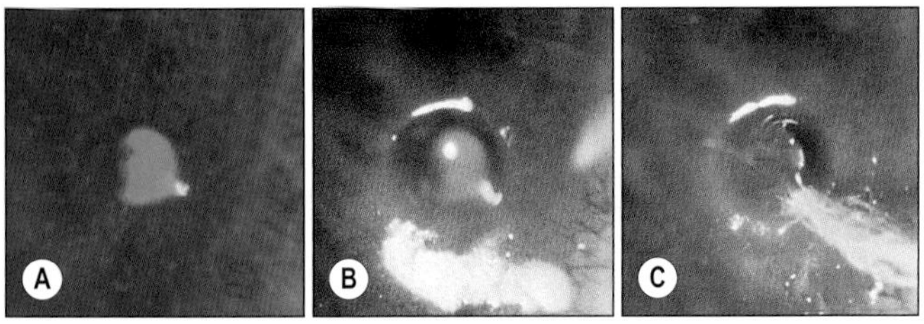

Fig. 10.3 Cornea with depressed area 2 weeks after removal of a foreign body. (**A**) demonstrates fluorescein in depressed area. After removal of fluorescein tear film with a wisp of cotton, (**B**) and (**C**), epithelium is found to be intact.

epithelium is intact, the pool of fluorescein will be removed and no staining in the base will be found (Fig. 10.3).

Ocular surface staining grading with fluorescein (yellow) filter is one of the four most common valuable examination techniques in assessing dry eye. Others include fluorescein break-up time (BUT), Schirmer's test, and meibomian examination. The monitoring and assessment of staining can be greatly enhanced by the use of a grading scale and standardized dye instillation and evaluation techniques. At least three grading systems (the Van Bijsterveld system, the Oxford system, and a standardized version of the NEI/

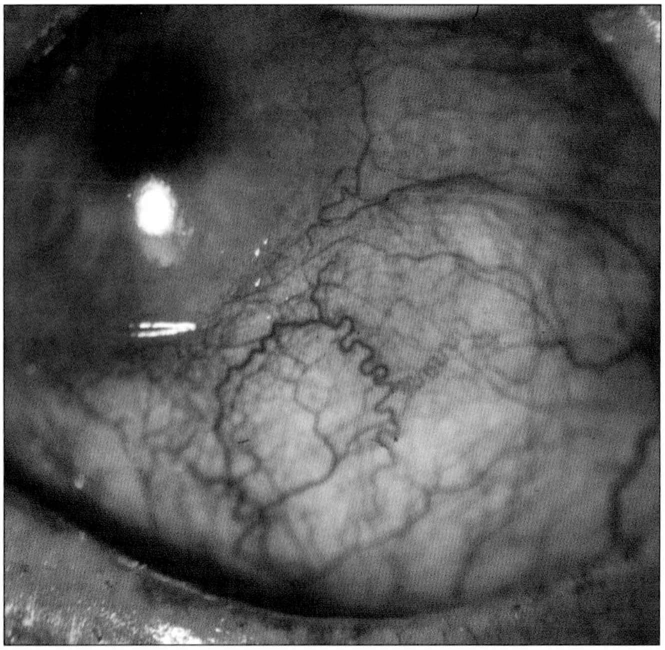

Fig. 10.4 Lissamine green staining in a 68-year-old female with Sjögren's syndrome and stem cell deficiency (secondary to long-term contact lens wear).

Industry Workshop system) are in current use or discussed in the International Dry Eye WorkShop (DEWS) report, 2007 (www.tearfilm.org).[4] Part of the difficulty in ocular surface disease diagnosis is the common scenario of a mismatch in the signs and symptoms. Indeed, the repeatability of both fluorescein and rose Bengal staining has been found to be poor.[5] In contrast, the repeatability of serial Schirmer's test was moderate, repeatability of tear break-up time was substantial, and repeatability of subjective symptoms (dryness and grittiness) was moderate to high. No single diagnostic test is a gold standard for diagnosis, but various combinations of tests have been recommended and shown to be more valid.

Another biological stain commonly used is lissamine green (Fig. 10.4). At least as effective in evaluating the ocular surface as rose Bengal, Manning et al. showed that it was better tolerated than rose Bengal by patients. Mean sensation score was significantly lower and duration of symptoms was shorter.[6] The effects of lissamine green and rose Bengal were compared on proliferating human corneal epithelial (HCE) cells in vitro. Rose Bengal stained normal proliferating HCE cells and adversely affected HCE cell viability, unlike lissamine green, which demonstrated neither of these characteristics.[7] When lissamine green is used, a relatively large volume (10–20 mL) is necessary to maximally view staining. Staining is enhanced by a red filter (Wratten # 25) as a barrier device on the slit lamp.

Characteristic corneal staining patterns may occur with corneal infections, inflammation, toxic changes, degenerative changes, and allergic conditions. Staining may be diffuse, regional, or focal depending on the underlying cause. Both the location and the pattern of corneal staining aid in diagnosis and management of corneal diseases (Fig.

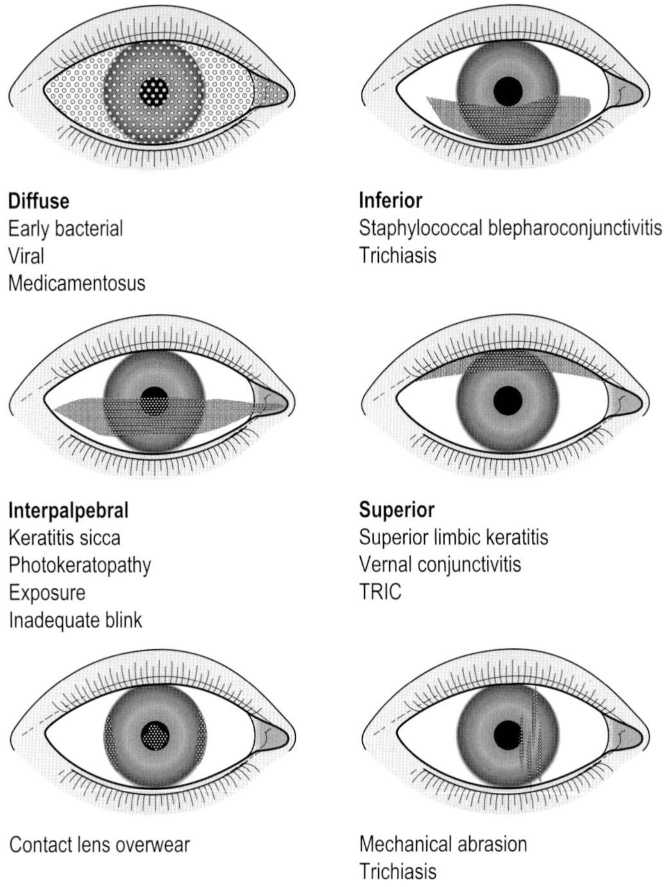

Fig. 10.5 Staining patterns of the cornea and conjunctiva in various disease states. TRIC, trachoma and inclusion conjunctivitis. (Reprinted with permission from Pavan-Langston D, ed. *Manual of ocular diagnosis and therapy.* Boston: Little Brown; 1991.)

10.5). For example, linear staining in the superior third of the cornea is typically found with a foreign body on the superior tarsal conjunctiva.[8] Linear staining in a contact lens wearer indicates a foreign body beneath the lens (Fig. 10.6). Superior bulbar conjunctival staining is characteristic of Theodore's superior limbic keratoconjunctivitis.

While some prefer to indicate any corneal staining as superficial punctate keratitis (SPK), it is more helpful to describe corneal staining precisely. Minute focal defects visualized at the slit lamp with fluorescein as small green dots are best described as punctate epithelial erosions (PEEs). While these are often the earliest stage of tear film instability or desiccation (Fig. 10.7), they are also found in some infectious disorders. Epithelial lesions with focal inflammatory infiltrates within the epithelium have punctate staining but also have areas of negative stain and are known as punctate epithelial keratitis (PEK). Finally, subepithelial infiltrates (SEIs) are deep to the epithelium and do not stain. Complete evolution of these staining patterns (PEE → PEK → SEI) occurs typically in some cases of adenoviral conjunctivitis and on occasion in herpes simplex, herpes zoster, chlamydia, and rosacea keratitis.

Negative staining patterns may provide as much information as positive staining of the cornea. Negative staining

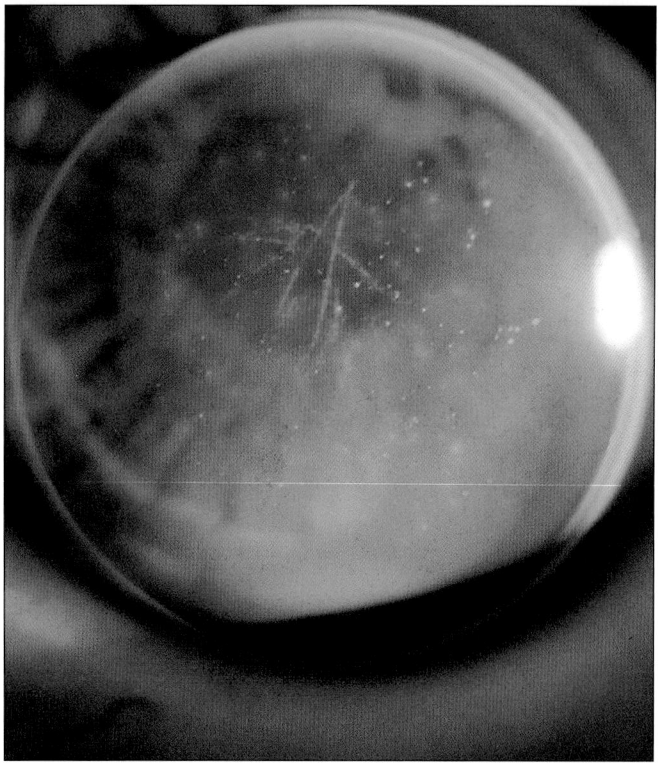

Fig. 10.6 Dust-trail linear abrasions from a rigid contact lens. These occur when a foreign body lodges between a contact lens and the patient's cornea.

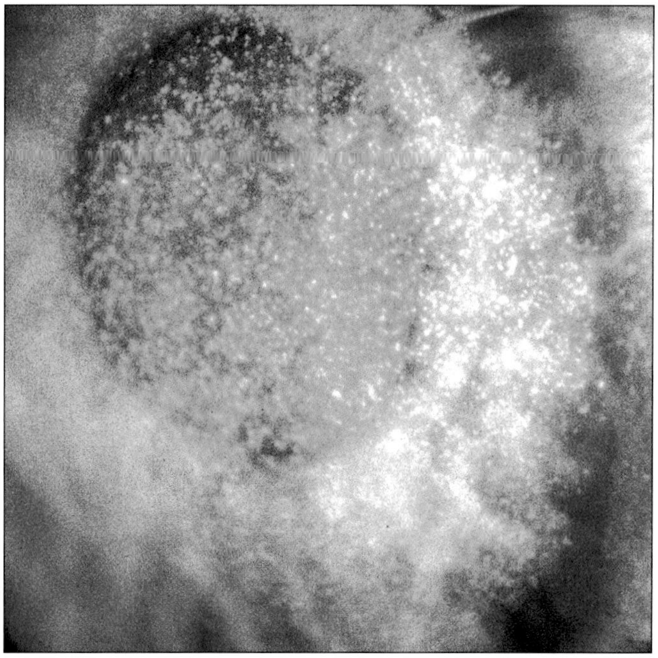

Fig. 10.7 Diffuse PEEs viewed with a cobalt light in a dry eye patient.

refers to an elevated or irregular area of the cornea with intact epithelium in which the normal fluorescein tear film quickly dissipates (Fig. 10.8). These patterns have both diagnostic and therapeutic implications in cases of recurrent corneal erosion. Negative staining may also demonstrate

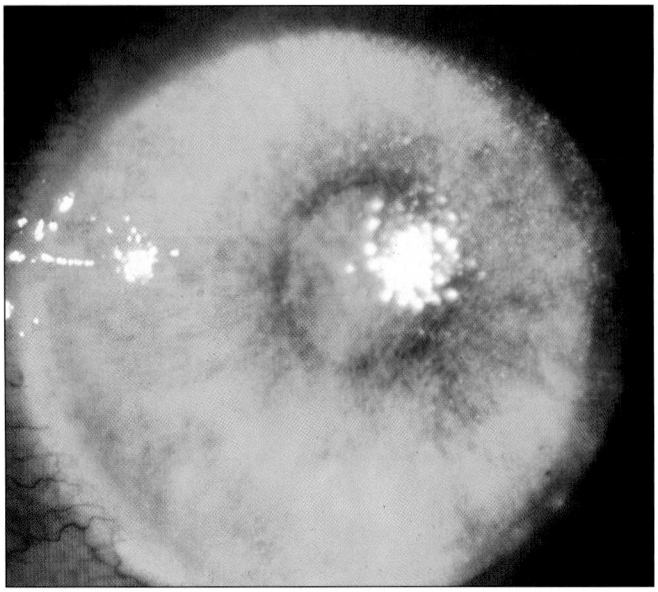

Fig. 10.8 Mixture of positive and negative staining in a patient with drug-induced epithelial toxicity.

elevated areas of the cornea that may be contributing to irregular astigmatism such as corneal scars, Salzmann's degeneration, or corneal striae after laser-assisted in situ keratomileusis (LASIK).

Pachymetry

Pachymetry, the measurement of cornea thickness, has become routine and is increasingly important in ophthalmic practice. Refractive surgeons invariably use central corneal thickness (CCT) in planning surgery,[9] as adequate thickness is key in avoiding postoperative ectasia. Glaucoma specialists have learned that cornea thinning is a cardinal risk factor for development of the disease,[10] and pachymetry is therefore performed as a standard in glaucoma consultation.

Pachymetry is an important indicator of corneal health but varies widely in 'normal' patients. The thinnest part of the cornea is usually located about 1.5 mm temporal to the center of the cornea.[11] Rapuano et al.[12] measured 303 normal corneas and found a range of 410 to 625 μm. Mean thickness was 515 μm in the central cornea. In the paracentral region, thickness varied from 522 μm inferiorly to 574 μm superiorly. In the peripheral zone, thickness was 633 μm inferiorly and 673 μm superiorly. No significant differences were noted in readings between right or left eyes, males or females, time of day, month of year, or systemic medication use.[12] Paracentral and peripheral, but not central, measurements tended to become thinner with age, but this trend was not statistically significant.[11] Since the absolute central value can vary significantly and still be 'normal,' the relationship of central, midperipheral, and peripheral corneal thickness is important and should remain constant. The central area (within a 4 mm optical zone) is typically thinner than the midperipheral cornea (4–9 mm optical zone), which is thinner than the peripheral cornea (outside a 9 mm optical zone). Therefore, a cornea with a central thickness greater than the thickness in the midperipheral should be considered suspicious for endothelial dysfunction centrally or thinning in the midperiphery, irrespective of the absolute values. In fact, a patient with early endothelial compromise may have a CCT equal to the midperipheral corneal thickness.

Corneal pachymetry abnormalities include both thinning disorders, such as keratoconus and pellucid marginal corneal degeneration, and thickened corneas with endothelial compromise, such as Fuchs' endothelial dystrophy and pseudophakic bullous keratopathy. While corneal thickness is an indirect measurement of the endothelial pump function, it is also affected to a lesser degree by the intraocular pressure.

One of the most common uses of corneal pachymetry is in assessing the extent of functional impairment of the endothelial pump in patients with Fuchs' endothelial dystrophy or previous intraocular surgery before a planned intraocular procedure. If the intraocular pressure is normal, epithelial edema develops when the stroma has swollen about 40%, to a corneal thickness greater than 700 μm. If, however, swelling is only 20% or pachymetry demonstrates corneal thickness greater than 620 μm, the risk of corneal decompensation after cataract surgery is significant.[13] Other uses of corneal pachymetry include determining the 'health' of a corneal transplant, evaluating a patient with keratoconus, and monitoring the degree of stromal edema in herpetic disciform keratitis. In contact lens wear, corneal edema and hypoxia can be assessed in daily wear, extended wear, or therapeutic lens patients. Corneal swelling averages 4% during eye closure, 9–10% with extended wear lenses, 11–14% during sleep, and up to 18% with contact lens wear. On slit lamp examination, corneal striae become visible at 4–8%, folds are seen at 11–12% swelling, and loss of transparency can occur at greater than 20% swelling.[14] High altitude causes a significant increase in CCT in healthy volunteers with normal corneas likely due to endothelial dysfunction.[15]

Techniques for measuring CCT include optical pachymetry, ultrasound pachymetry, confocal microscopy, ultrasound biomicroscopy, optical ray path analysis or scanning slit corneal topography, and optical coherence tomography.[16]

Optical methods of pachymetry were first described as early as 1951 by Maurice and Giardini.[17] Donaldson[18] and Mishima[19] also described manual slit lamp techniques to view the tear film or anterior corneal surface and the endothelial surface of the cornea. The Mishima-Hedbys fixation device for the Haag-Streit slit lamp reduced alignment problems. Various equations were used to calculate corneal thickness. Variables in these equations were the cornea's refractive index and the anterior radius of curvature. These variables, along with the subjective nature of optical pachymetry readings, led to imprecise measurements and further investigation.[12] Because of its subjective endpoints, the accuracy of optical pachymetry is partly dependent on the skill of the examiner. Advantages, however, include relatively low cost and noncontact technique.[20]

Some specular microscopes designed to evaluate the corneal endothelial cell count also measure corneal thickness using electromechanical devices. These were designed to measure central and apical readings only. The measurement derived is based on the distance from the posterior surface of the tear film to the posterior surface of Descemet's membrane, thus inducing an error of as much as 20 or 30 μm. In the contact mode, corneal touch is involved and compression may be another source of error.[20]

Another optical method of measuring corneal thickness utilizes the Orbscan II Anterior Segment Analysis System. While Orbscan central thickness measurements are statistically thinner than with ultrasound, there is a conversion factor to allow a surgeon to adjust the Orbscan value.[21] An advantage of the Orbscan data is the display of corneal thickness in a 'map' that facilitates evaluation of regional changes in corneal thickness.

Since its introduction in 1980, ultrasound technology has improved tremendously. Early units were more expensive, difficult to use, variable, and subject to alignment errors. Salz et al.[22] compared optical pachymetry with three ultrasonic pachymeters and concluded that optical pachymetry had more intersession variation, significant intraobserver variation, and significant right–left thickness differences.

Ultrasound pachymetry is not without disadvantages. Topical anesthesia is necessary due to direct contact with the cornea. Contact is undesirable in the early post-op period and the handheld nature of the probe limits measurement accuracy.[23] Ultrasound measurements generally read thicker than Orbscan II.[24] Recent studies reveal that optical methods of measurement (partial coherence interferometry) not only measure thinner than ultrasound but also have been quoted as 'more reproducible, more reliable',[25] and with the least intraobserver and interobserver variability.[26]

Sources of error in pachymetry may be 'systematic' or inherent in the methods used in the procedure. Stucchi et al.[27] studied several factors including repeated measurements, drying of the cornea, patient positioning, and marking. Repeated measurements of the same corneal point showed small variability (<1.5%) and were lower with blinking after each measurement (<1%). After lying down for 3 hours, thickness increased by 2.21%. Pachymetry performed after marking the cornea underestimated thickness in the marked area by an average of 2.7%.[27]

The evolution and growth of laser refractive surgery and the importance of preoperative knowledge of corneal thickness has supported significant improvements in pachymeters. OCT is capable of measuring flap thickness with great accuracy and can differentiate femtosecond laser-created planar flaps from microkeratome-created meniscus flaps.[28] Modern ultrasound pachymeters are far superior to their predecessors. Significant engineering improvements include the solid-tipped probe, defining the speed of sound in human cornea, continuous-read measurement, automatic gain and angle sensitivity within 5 degrees of axis, advanced electronics and microprocessor control, battery-powered operation, memory storage capability, and 50 MHz high-frequency transducer. Modern ultrasound pachymeters are as light as 3.6 ounces, have a reported accuracy of ±5 microns and resolution of 1 micron, and have an IOP correction factor available.[29] Intraoperative measurements of Intralase flaps are possible as well as an epithelium mode helpful in monitoring regression.[30]

Aesthesiometry

Corneal sensation is a function of the ophthalmic branch of the fifth cranial nerve (trigeminal). Abnormalities such as trauma, tumors, surgery, infection, and inflammation can affect normal corneal sensation. Both the corneal epithelium and, to a lesser extent, the endothelium depend on normal corneal innervation. Anesthetic corneas may develop a characteristic interpalpebral horizontal band of punctate epithelial staining. Untreated, this may progress to an epithelial defect and subsequent stromal loss (neurotrophic ulcer). Interestingly, the endothelium also depends on 'normal' corneal innervation for its functions. In some cases, abnormalities in corneal innervation have been associated with cold-induced corneal edema.[31] Therefore, defects in corneal sensation can adversely affect the cornea.

Tests for corneal sensitivity may be very simple or more complex. Obviously, topical anesthetics should be avoided before these tests. The easiest and most widely used technique employs a cotton-tipped swab. A wisp from the cotton tip may be used to assess corneal sensation grossly. Care should be taken to avoid frightening the patient by bringing the wisp from the side. The patient's response comparing the two corneas, as well as the examiner's observation of the blink reflex, contributes to this gross assessment of corneal sensation.

A more accurate measurement of corneal sensitivity is obtained with the Cochet-Bonnet aesthesiometer. This device has a 6.0 cm-long adjustable nylon monofilament. To measure sensation, the tip is moved onto the corneal surface perpendicularly. The pressure (from 11 to 200 mg/mm^2) exerted at the corneal surface directly relates to the length of the filament. Persons with normal corneal sensitivity sense touch at 6.0 cm length. If touch at 6.0 cm is not felt, the filament is reduced by 0.5 cm at a time until perceived. Measurements may be repeated and averaged.

Other methods of measuring corneal sensation primarily have research applications. Beuerman et al.[32] devised a technique based on warming the cornea with a jet of warm saline solution within a saline bath at ocular temperature. A 4.5°C increase in temperature elicited a response in a normal cornea.[33] Zaidman et al.[34] used a noncontact air puff technique to stimulate the cornea. Chemical stimulation of the cornea may be a reliable measure of sensation using the pungent substance capsaicin.[35] Brennan and Maurice stimulated the cornea thermally with a carbon dioxide laser, potentially a highly controllable technique.[36]

Ocular sensitivity is greatest in the central cornea[31] except in elderly patients, in whom the peripheral cornea is the most sensitive.[29] Sensitivity drops rapidly as distance from the limbus increases. The temporal limbus is significantly more sensitive than the inferior limbus. Short-term lens wear causes no significant loss of sensitivity; sensitivity falls with increasing age and is not affected by iris color.[37]

Corneal sensitivity may be the most reliable test of long-term corneal compromise. In contact lens wearers, Brennan and Bruce recorded six ocular parameters: visual function, microcysts, polymegathism, edema, oxygen flux, and sensitivity. They found a change in corneal sensitivity of up to 150% over 6 months of extended lens wear, the most dramatic and easily detected change of all parameters.[38] Long-term hypoxia is associated with loss of sensitivity. The mechanism in long-term contact lens wear includes altered acetylcholine levels with combined metabolic and respiratory acidosis and build-up of lactic acid and carbon dioxide.

After penetrating keratoplasty (PK), corneal sensitivity of the graft usually progressively improves with time. The peripheral cornea remains more sensitive than centrally, and some clear grafts remain completely anesthetic. Neither age, preoperative diagnosis, nor graft size was correlated with the recovery of sensitivity.[39] Rao et al.[40] found that the central graft never recovered normal sensitivity.

Topical medications may be associated with serious corneal problems in patients with decreased corneal sensation. Nonsteroidal antiinflammatory drugs (primarily generic diclofenac but also proprietary diclofenac and ketorolac) have been linked to punctate keratitis, erosions, sterile ulcers, and even perforations. The risk appears heightened in patients with compromised corneas from chronic ocular disease, decreased sensation, or severe dry eyes.

Corneal sensitivity may be reduced after radial keratotomy (RK). Shivitz and Arrowsmith observed this in 31% of RK patients after 6 months and 70% of astigmatic RK patients after 6 months, recovering to 9.5% and 47%, respectively, at 12 months.[41] This reduced sensitivity may help explain the ability of former contact lens-intolerant patients to wear lenses after RK. It may also be a factor in late infectious keratitis occurring months or years after RK.

Corneal sensitivity has been compared in laser refractive surgery patients. In a masked study, Kanellopoulos et al.[42] tested 40 consecutive patients 6 to 12 months following PRK and LASIK with the Cochet-Bonnet aesthesiometer. Patients undergoing LASIK had statistically better corneal sensation than those having PRK.[37] However, studies on patients undergoing LASIK have shown a decrease in corneal sensation following LASIK for 3 weeks to 9 months.[43,44] The location of the hinge in LASIK may be important in decreasing postoperative dry eye signs and symptoms. Donnenfeld et al.[45] showed that nasal hinge location preserved corneal sensation better than superior hinged flaps. This was felt to be due to sparing of one of two horizontal nerves entering the cornea at 3 and 9 o'clock positions.

Osmolarity

The etiology of a very common ocular surface disease, dry eye disease, has only recently been clarified. Indeed, from the 1997 first edition of this text, 'The mechanism for lacrimal gland dysfunction in this condition is unclear' (Vol. II, p. 647). Ten years later the DEWS report states, 'Tear osmolarity may reasonably be regarded as the signature feature that characterizes the condition of ocular surface dryness.'[4] The cutoff value of 316 mOsm/L is well validated. Although long used as a research tool, osmolarity measurement has until recently been only performed in a laboratory due to cost, lack of technology, and inconvenience. At least two separate methodologies are imminent, and one FDA application has been filed. Microscopic nanoliter tear volumes are required and readings are instantaneous.[46,47] This may become the gold standard for diagnosis.

Summary

The use of corneal dyes, pachymetry, and tests for corneal sensation may greatly enhance our ability to diagnose and manage corneal and external disease problems correctly. A thorough understanding of these techniques allows us to maximize the information obtained.

References

1. Feenstra RPG, Tseng SCG. Comparison of fluorescein and rose Bengal staining. *Ophthalmology.* 1992;99:605–617.
2. Korb DR. The tear film, its role today and in the future. *BCLA pubs Butterworth-Heinemann.* 2002:126–190.
3. Gobbels M, Spitznas M, Oldendoerp J. Impairment of corneal epithelial barrier function in diabetics. *Graefes Arch Clin Exp Ophthalmol.* 1989;227:142–144.
4. Bron Anthony J, et al. Methodologies to diagnose and monitor dry eye disease: Report of the Diagnostic Methodology Subcommittee of the International Dry Eye WorkShop (2007). *Ocul Surf.* 2007;5(2):108–152.
5. Nichols KK, Mitchell GL, Zadnik K. The repeatability of clinical measurements of dry eye. *Cornea.* 2004;23(3):272–285.
6. Manning FS, Wlehrly SR, Fopulks GN. Patient tolerance and ocular surface staining characteristics of lissamine green versus rose bengal. *Ophthalmology.* 1995;102:1953–1957.
7. Kim J, Foulks GN. Evaluation of the effect of lissamine green and rose bengal on human corneal epithelial cells. Presented at ARVO meeting. Ft. Lauderdale, FL, 1997.
8. Pavan-Langston D, Foulks GN. Cornea and external disease. In: Pavan-Langston D, ed. *Manual of ocular diagnosis and therapy.* Boston: Little Brown; 1991.
9. Marsich MM, Bullimore MA. The repeatability of cornea thickness measures. *Cornea.* 2000;19:792–795.
10. Kass MA, Heuer DK, Higginbotham EJ, et al. The Ocular Hypertension Treatment Study group: a randomized trial determines that topical ocular hypotensive medication delays or prevents the onset of primary open-angle glaucoma. *Arch Ophthalmol.* 2002;120:701–713.
11. Casebeer JC. *A system of precise, predictable keratorefractive surgery. A system for success, Chiron Ophthalmic Educational Series.* Irvine, CA: Chiron Corp; 1992.
12. Rapuano CJ, Fishbaugh JA, Strike DJ. Nine point corneal thickness measurements and keratometry readings in normal corneas using ultrasound pachymetry. *Insight.* 1993;18:16–22.
13. Reinstein DZ, Silverman RH, Rondeau MJ, et al. Epithelial and corneal thickness measurements by high frequency ultrasound digital signal processing. *Ophthalmology.* 1994;101:140–146.
14. Stiegemeier MJ. Pachometry: invaluable for specialty contact lens, refractive surgery arena. *Primary Care Optometry News.* 2000;5:10.
15. Morris D, Somner JEA, Scott K, et al. Corneal thickness at high altitude. *Cornea.* 2007;26:308–311.
16. Brugin E, Ghirlando A, Gambato C, Midena E. Central cornea thickness Z-ring corneal confocal microscopy versus ultrasound pachymetry. *Cornea.* 2007;26:303–307.
17. Maurice DM, Giardini AA. A simple optical apparatus for measuring the corneal thickness and the average thickness of the human cornea. *Br J Ophthalmol.* 1951;35:169–177.
18. Donaldson DD. A new instrument for the measurement of corneal thickness. *Arch Ophthalmol.* 1966;76:25–31.
19. Mishima S. Corneal thickness. *Surv Ophthalmol.* 1968;13:57–96.
20. Hoffman RF. Preoperative evaluation. In: Sanders DR, Hoffman RF, eds. *Refractive surgery: a text of radial keratotomy.* Thorofare, NJ: Slack; 1985.
21. Prisant O, Calderon N, Chastang P, et al. Reliability of pachymetric measurements using Orbscan after excimer refractive surgery. *Ophthalmology.* 2003;110:511–515.
22. Salz JJ, Azen AP, Berstein J, . Evaluation and comparison of sources of variability in the measurement of corneal thickness with ultrasonic and optical pachymeters. *Ophthalmic Surg.* 1983;14:750–754.
23. Much MM, Haigis W. Ultrasound and partial coherence interferometry with measurement of central corneal thickness. *J Refr Surg.* 2006;22: 665–670.
24. Kim SW, Byun YJ, Kim EK, Kim T. Central corneal thickness measurements in unoperated eyes after PRK for myopia using Pentacam, Orbscan II, and ultrasonic pachymetry. *J Refr Surg.* 2007;23:888–894.
25. Nemeth G, Tsorbatzoglou A, Kertesz K, et al. Comparison of central corneal thickness measurements with a new optical device and a standard ultrasonic pachymeter. *J Cataract Refract Surg.* 2006;32:460–463.

26. Ranier G, Findl O, Petternel V, et al. Central corneal thickness measurements with partial coherence interferometry, ultrasound, and the Orbscan system. *Ophthalmology.* 2004;111:875–879.
27. Stucchi CA, Genneri G, Aimino G, et al. Systematic error in computerized pachymetry. *Ophthalmologica.* 1993;207:208–214.
28. Rajecki R, Mauche EE. Accuracy of flap measurements during, after LASIK is examined in clinical trial. *Ophthalmol Times.* November, 2008:102.
29. DGH. pachymetry.com.
30. Sonogage. info@sonogage.com.
31. Thorgaard GL, Holland EJ, Krachmer JH. Corneal edema induced by cold in trigeminal nerve palsy. *Am J Ophthalmol.* 1987;103:641–646.
32. Beuerman RW, Maurice DM, Tanelian DL. Thermal stimulation of the cornea. In: Anderson D, Mathews B, eds. *Pain in the trigeminal region.* New York: North-Holland Biomedical; 1977.
33. Burman RW, Tanelian DL. Corneal pain evoked by thermal stimulation. *Pain.* 1979;7:1–4.
34. Zaidman G, Gould H, Weinstein C, et al. Corneal sensitivity mapping studies in post-surgical patients. *Invest Ophthalmol Vis Sci.* 1989;30(Suppl): 338.
35. Dupuy B, Thompson H, Beurman RW. Capsaicin: a psychophysical tool to explore corneal sensitivity. *Invest Ophthalmol Vis Sci.* 1988;29(Suppl):454.
36. Brennan NA, Maurice DM. Corneal esthesiometry with a carbon dioxide laser. *Invest Ophthalmol Vis Sci.* 1989;30(Suppl):148.
37. Lawrenson JG, Ruskell GL. Investigation of limbal touch sensitivity using a Cochet-Bonnet aesthesiometer. *Br J Ophthalmol.* 1993;77:339–343.
38. Brennan NA, Bruce AS. Esthesiometry as an indicator of corneal health. *Optom Vis Sci.* 1991;68:699–702.
39. Tutkum IT, et al. Corneal sensitivity after penetrating keratoplasty. *Eur J Ophthalmol.* 1993;3:66–70.
40. Rao GN, et al. Recovery of corneal sensitivity in grafts following penetrating keratoplasty. *Ophthalmology.* 1985;92:1408–1411.
41. Shivitz IA, Arrowsmith PN. Corneal sensitivity after radial keratotomy. *Ophthalmology.* 1988;95:827–832.
42. Kanellopoulos AJ, Pallikaris IG, Donnenfeld ED, et al. Comparison of corneal sensation following photorefractive keratectomy and laser in situ keratomileusis. *J Cataract Refract Surg.* 1997;23:34–38.
43. Chuck RS, Quiros PA, Perez AC, et al. Corneal sensation after laser in situ keratomileusis. *J Cataract Refract Surg.* 2000;26:337–339.
44. Nassaralla BA, McLeod SD, Nassaralla JJ. Effect of myopic LASIK on human corneal sensitivity. *Ophthalmology.* 2003;110:497–502.
45. Donnenfeld ED, Solomon K, Perry HD, et al. The effect of hinge position on corneal sensation and dry eye after LASIK. *Ophthalmology.* 2003;110: 1023–1030.
46. Ocusense. info@tearlab.com.
47. Lacripen, Lacri Sciences, LLC. tcappo@opticology.com.

Chapter **11**

Practical Ophthalmic Microbiology for the Detection of Corneal Pathogens

Regis P. Kowalski

Introduction

Practical laboratory tests for the detection of corneal pathogens provide pertinent information that impacts patient care. Practical tests are highly sensitive, 100% specific, involve easy specimen collection and transport to the testing center, and provide testing results within 24 to 72 hours, if not sooner. Clinical laboratory testing is a dynamic relationship between technology and managed care. Although technologic advances will provide newer sensitive tests, laboratories are limited within budgetary restraints to provide only essential testing. Managed care resulted in significant reduction of laboratory personnel because insurance reimbursement for testing has decreased, as in other fields of medicine. Laboratories operate under high regulatory standards that are mandated by Medicare and other insurance carriers. Laboratories must be certified for diagnostic testing by CLIA (Federal), JCAH (hospital), State, and CAP (independent) regulatory agencies. Most laboratories process specimens for routine and frequent repetitive testing because of cost-effectiveness and the ease to validate testing proficiency, which is necessary for reimbursement. Infrequent testing is not cost-effective due to overhead costs (waste of perishable media) and the necessity of dedicating valuable laboratory personnel for a few tests. Infrequent testing is generally handled with batch testing (waiting for an accumulation of similar testing) that delays laboratory results or by referring the specimens to a reference laboratory (a large hospital or government laboratory). It is very difficult for a laboratory to validate testing for an infrequent pathogen because of the lack of true positive specimens that may require an extended time to collect.

Many ophthalmologists will find it difficult to locate microbiology laboratories that cater to specific ocular infectious disease testing in a timely fashion. As this chapter will demonstrate, ophthalmic microbiology is unique but not necessarily so high-tech that diagnostic testing is not available. Ophthalmologists will have to investigate the availability of laboratory testing that is pertinent to their practice. This chapter will describe the best practical tests that are available for the detection of corneal pathogens. The ophthalmic microbiology tests presented in this chapter were established in a modern, fully certified, clinical laboratory that caters exclusively to detecting corneal and ocular pathogens.

Central Laboratory versus In-office Testing

Government regulations have made in-office testing an obsolete option for diagnosing ocular infections. All laboratory testing is regulated to assure that patient care is maximized, with qualified personnel who are certified or properly trained. Even if testing is provided free of charge, in-office testing must be regulated, which can be costly and invites a regulating agency to the office practice.

Communication: Ophthalmologist and Laboratory

Direct communication of the ophthalmologist with the diagnostic laboratory is essential. The laboratory must understand the specific needs of the ophthalmologist. The ophthalmologist must indicate the type of specimen, the possible pathogens involved in infection, and specific antibiotic susceptibilities that must be tested. Unusual pathogens (mycobacteria, *Acanthamoeba*, etc.) require planning and acquisition of media. Simply sending a single soft-tipped applicator to a laboratory and requesting isolation of all possible pathogens (bacteria – aerobic and anaerobic, virus, fungus, *Acanthamoeba*, etc.) is unreasonable, and valuable time is lost for the ophthalmologist, patient, and laboratory.

Corneal Specimen Collection

Corneal specimens can be collected with spatulas, jeweler's forceps, and surgical blades (Fig. 11.1). Cotton-tipped applicators can be used when less aggressive cultures need to be obtained or when less distinct areas of infection over a large area require culture. Sometimes, after an instrument is used, an additional specimen can be obtained with a soft-tipped applicator at the infected site. The instruments are used to collect specimens for planting media and placing on glass slides for cytologic examination. Each ophthalmologist should determine which collecting instrument is most

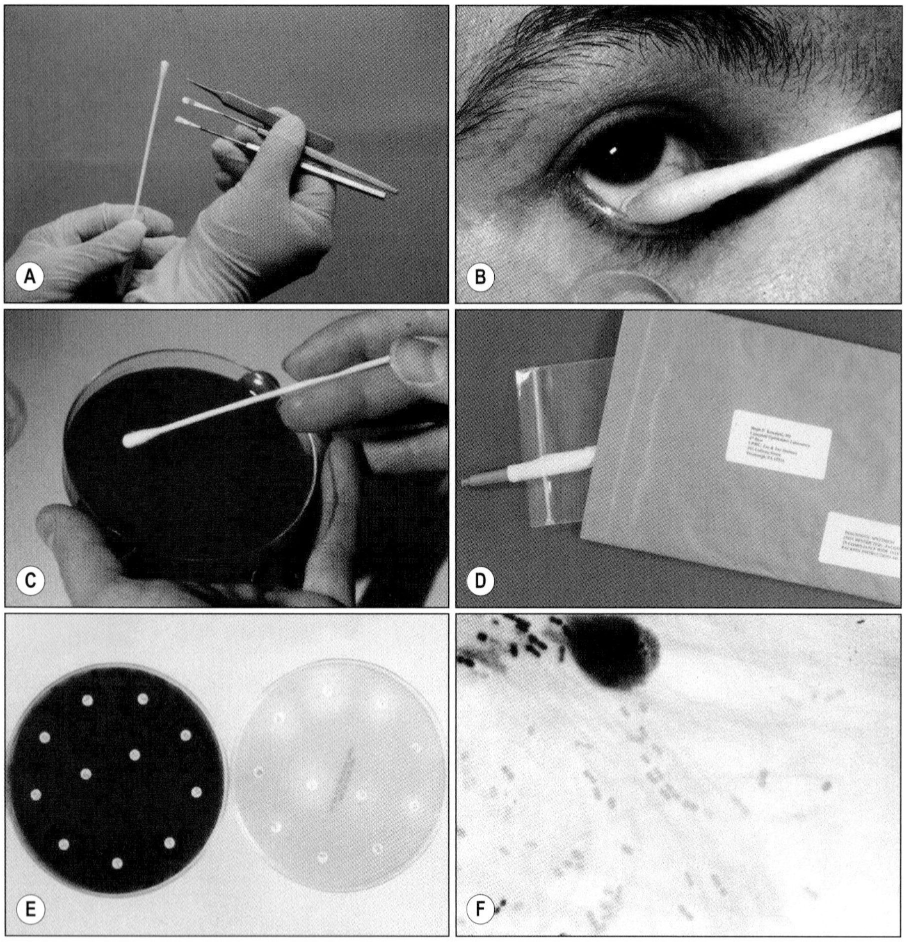

Fig. 11.1 Corneal specimen collection. (**A**) Corneal specimen collection instruments; (**B**) conjunctival culture; (**C**) specimen planting for bacterial isolation; (**D**) correct packing for transporting corneal specimen; (**E**) disk diffusion antibiotic susceptibility testing; (**F**) Gram stain of Gram-negative diplobacilli (*Moraxella*) from corneal tissue.

comfortable and provides the best specimen for laboratory diagnosis.

Conjunctival cultures can be diagnostic when corneal cultures are negative due to antibiotic pretreatment (Fig. 11.1). Conjunctival specimens are collected with soft-tipped applicators with plastic handles and heads composed of cotton, Dacron, or calcium alginate (Fig. 11.1). Calcium alginate swabs have been reported to produce a higher yield of bacterial organisms but these may not always be available; thus, cotton and Dacron are alternatives.[1]

Transport media

Direct inoculation of isolation media is best but this approach is not always possible. There are many transport systems for supporting bacteria, virus, and chlamydia prior to direct inoculation on proper isolation media. The ophthalmologist should ask advice from the laboratory on suggestions for transport media and reliable delivery of specimens to the laboratory.

Mailing of diagnostic specimens

Diagnostic specimens can be easily delivered through couriers and public mail with a few simple requirements as mandated by federal law. These samples must be double-sealed to prevent any leakage of sample. A proper amount of desiccant to absorb any leakage due to damage should also be packed within the double-sealed specimen. The sample should be marked to indicate that the package is a diagnostic specimen. For example, a corneal specimen collected on a soft-tipped applicator and placed in a plastic tube (transport sleeve, culturette™ (Becton Dickinson, Sparks, MD), wrapped in a paper towel, enclosed in a sealable vinyl zip-locked bag, placed in a bubble mailer addressed to the laboratory, and marked as 'Diagnostic Specimen (Not Restricted) – Packed in Compliance with IATA Packing Instructions 650' would be a properly sent diagnostic sample (Fig. 11.1).

Stains and Cytologic Specimens

The acquisition of tissue from infected corneas for cytologic examination is not only a rapid method for determining the presence of an infectious agent but also may be the only positive indication of a pathogen. Microscopic examination of cornea specimens is a function of an adequate specimen collected and the laboratory's expertise in interpreting the stained specimen. The ophthalmologist must be proficient in obtaining at least two corneal specimens for laboratory examination. One slide allows for the examination of microorganisms and the other for cytology. Additional samples

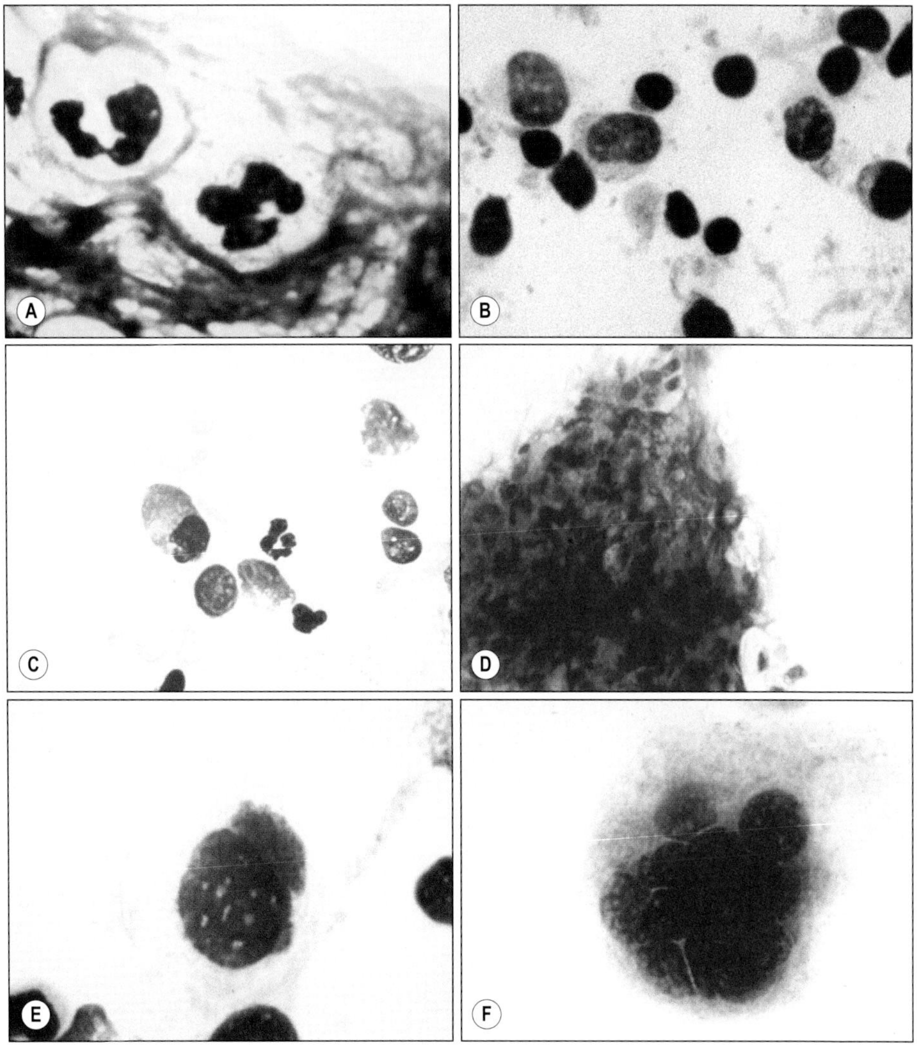

Fig. 11.2 Giemsa stain cytology. (**A**) Polymorphonuclear cells; (**B**) mononuclear and epithelial cells; (**C**) plasma cell in center; (**D**) *Acanthamoebae* cyst in middle; (**E**) dark purple chlamydial inclusion caps peripheral to nucleus of epithelial cell; (**F**) corneal multinucleated epithelial cell from HSV keratitis.

may be useful for additional staining procedures (i.e. acid-fast). Specimens should be collected with a spatula, forceps, or blade, placed in the middle of a glass microscopic slide, and circled with a wax pencil for location. No immediate fixation is necessary and the slides should be delivered to the diagnostic laboratory with directions indicating the differential diagnoses. Gram stain (Fig. 11.1) is the standard stain for determining the presence of Gram-positive (*Staphylococcus, Streptococcus*) and -negative (*Pseudomonas, Haemophilus*) bacteria, and other microbes (i.e. fungi, *Acanthamoeba*). Other stains for detecting microorganisms are acridine orange, calcofluor, and acid-fast.[2] The ophthalmologist must feel confident in the interpretation expertise of the laboratory. Confidence is gained with direct communication between ophthalmologist and microbiologist.

Historically, the Giemsa stain has been the standard for cytology examination and it may be necessary to use a pathology laboratory. Along with normal epithelial cells, inflammatory cells such as mononuclear, polymorphonuclear, eosinophils, basophils, plasma, leiber, etc., can be observed with smears stained by Giemsa (Fig. 11.2). In addition, abnormal epithelial cells from the upper tarsal conjunctiva can indicate malignancy, and multinucleated epithelial cells could indicate herpes simplex infection (Fig. 11.2). This powerful stain is excellent for depicting microorganisms, including chlamydia, which cannot easily be observed with other stains. Pathology laboratories may have other ideas for cytologic examination, with higher comfort levels using other stains and it may be advantageous to be receptive to other approaches.

Bacterial Laboratory Diagnosis

Laboratory studies for the isolation of bacterial pathogens from the cornea are widely available. Laboratories must be aware of the type (i.e. tissue, soft-tipped applicator) and location (i.e. cornea, conjunctiva, eyelid, vitreous, etc.) of submitted samples. The ophthalmologist must inform the laboratory of the possible pathogens that could be the etiologic agent in disease and provide enough time for the laboratory to acquire special media for infrequent pathogens (i.e. mycobacteria, *Acanthamoeba*). Ophthalmologists must inform laboratories that all bacteria isolated from the cornea

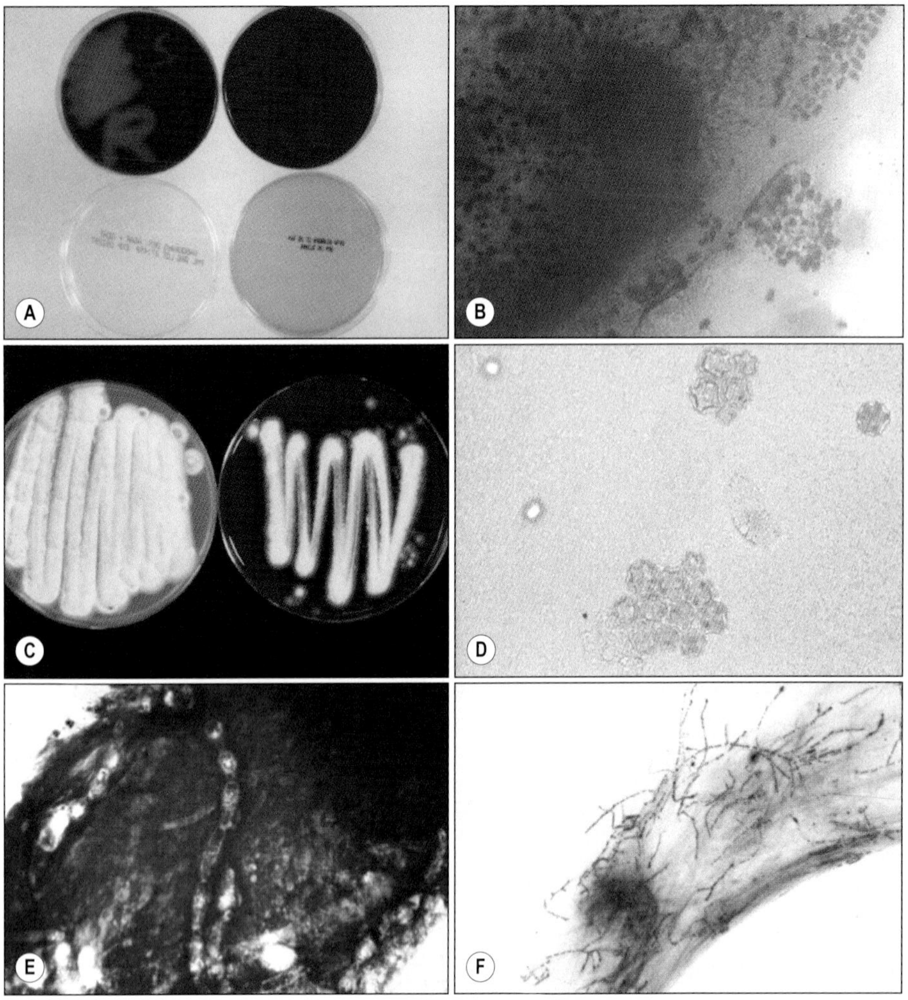

Fig. 11.3 Bacterial laboratory diagnosis. (**A**) Routine culture agar plates; (**B**) Microsporidia spores from stained corneal specimen (Courtesy of Darlene Miller, Bascom Palmer, Miami, FL); (**C**) mold growing on agar plates; (**D**) *Acanthamoebae* hexagonal cysts on non-nutrient agar with *Enterobacter aerogenes* overlay; (**E**) *Candida albicans* pseudohyphae on Giemsa-stained corneal specimen; (**F**) *Actinomyces* on Giemsa-stained corneal tissue.

should be considered pathogens and tested for antibiotic susceptibilities. It should be requested that inoculated culture media be held and examined for at least 5 days.

The routine media for isolating bacteria from the cornea, conjunctiva, and eyelids are broth-based agar with 5% sheep blood, chocolate agar, and mannitol salt agar (Fig. 11.3). The sheep blood agar will isolate most bacterial pathogens except *Haemophilus* species, *Neisseria gonorrhoeae,* and nutriently variant *Streptococcus* species that will grow on chocolate agar. Mannitol salt agar is an optional medium that is very helpful to the microbiologist for differentiating *Staphylococcus* species.[3] Enriched thioglycollate liquid medium will provide isolation for most bacteria, including anaerobes. Anaerobes are best isolated on special anaerobe media or a chocolate plate incubated under anaerobic conditions such as an oxygen-depleted jar or bag. Anaerobic cultures should be treated as special cultures, with preparation between physician and laboratory.

Mycobacteria

The detection of mycobacteria is a specialization within a large laboratory that is highly regulated and requires planning by the ophthalmologist. Mycobacteria can be quite fastidious and can require long incubation periods for isolation. The process of screening for all mycobacteria species is quite complex and probably unnecessary for ocular specimens. In general, mycobacteria keratitis is due to fast-growing species (growth within 7 days), *Mycobacterium chelonae* and *M. fortuitum,* which propagate on routine culture media (i.e. blood and chocolate agar).[4] Inoculating routine agar media plus a mycobacteria agar medium (i.e. Lowenstein-Jensen) and liquid medium (Middlebrook 7H9) should suffice. To culture for all species of mycobacteria, many laboratories prefer tissue for inoculating multiple media and for special stains (i.e. acid-fast). Submitting lone soft-tipped applicators for mycobacteria testing without previously notifying the laboratory will result in a delayed planted specimen that most likely will test negative or be designated as an insufficient specimen.

Nocardia and *Actinomyces*

Nocardia and *Actinomyces* are less frequent pathogens of the cornea. *Nocardia* are easily cultured on routine bacterial culture media and can be visualized on stained specimens as branching or partially branching filaments. *Actinomyces* are a more fastidious grower on culture media and require an extended growth period. Cytologic examination of corneal specimens by Giemsa and other stains is the best diagnostic test for detecting *Actinomyces*. *Actinomyces* appear as long, thin filaments with branching and sometimes as long thin rods (Fig. 11.3).

Antibiotic Susceptibility Testing

Antibiotic susceptibility testing is performed on fast-growing bacterial isolates to assess whether an antibiotic will be successful in therapy. Laboratories should be informed of the required antibiotics for which corneal bacterial isolates should be tested. Some laboratories may not provide antibiotic susceptibility testing on ocular bacterial isolates because no susceptibility standards exist for topical antibiotic therapy. The interpretation of antibiotic susceptibility for ocular isolates can be based on systemic standards if laboratories assume that the antibiotic levels in the ocular tissues are equal to or greater than the antibiotic levels reached in the blood serum. In vitro antibiotic susceptibility is determined using the disk diffusion and MIC methods.[5] Disk diffusion susceptibility is determined by placing paper disks impregnated with a set amount of antibiotics on a lawn of bacteria (see Fig. 11.1). After 24 hours of incubation, zones of inhibition are measured and compared to predetermined zone standards that represent susceptibility, intermediate susceptibility, and resistance. Methods of MIC determination include broth dilution, agar dilution, and E-tests. Using these methods, the minimum inhibitory concentration of antibiotic required to inhibit bacteria is determined and compared to predetermined concentrations that represent susceptibility. Bacterial corneal isolates should be tested for antibiotic susceptibility to ciprofloxacin, ofloxacin (levofloxacin), moxifloxacin, gatifloxacin, oxacillin (or cefoxitin for staphylococcal methicillin resistance),[5] cefazolin, vancomycin, gentamicin, tobramycin, sulfacetamide, polymyxin B, and bacitracin. There are no current systemic susceptibility standards for bacitracin, but an older manufacturer standard could be used to assess susceptibility with reservation.

Laboratory Diagnosis of Fungal Infection

As with mycobacteria, fungus isolation and identification is a specialized section in a microbiology laboratory, with special certification requirements. Many laboratories can isolate fungus from ocular cultures but must refer the identification to a reference laboratory. Most fungi that infect the cornea can be isolated on routine culture media (i.e. blood agar, chocolate agar, and Sabouraud's agar supplemented with gentamicin). In general, molds (hyphael elements extending over the agar medium that have a fuzzy appearance) (see Fig. 11.3) and yeasts (pasty bacteria-like colonies) are isolated within 3–7 days after inoculation. The most common molds isolated from fungal keratitis are *Aspergillus* and *Fusarium*, but other genera have been isolated.[6] *Candida albicans*, *C. parapsilosis*, and other *Candida* species are the most common yeast pathogens of the cornea, but other yeasts have been implicated.[7] Corneal specimens for microscopic examination by Giemsa or specialized mycology stain should be obtained and are highly recommended as a rapid detection test (see Fig. 11.3). Ophthalmologists should discuss with the laboratory the fungal possibilities and the range of fungal isolation and identification that is required. More invasive culturing may require a tissue specimen, which may necessitate a corneal biopsy.

Laboratory Detection of *Acanthamoeba* and Microsporidia

Acanthamoeba can be easily isolated in any laboratory, but stocking media for such an infrequent pathogen is not cost-effective for most laboratories. Corneal specimens, contact lenses, solutions, and water that possibly contain *Acanthamoeba* can easily be sent to laboratories that offer testing without loss of viability.[8] Routine corneal specimens are planted on non-nutrient agar plates that are overlaid with a heavy slurry of live *Enterobacter aerogenes* or *Escherichia coli*. After a few days of incubation, *Acanthamoeba* trophozoites can be microscopically observed with movement across the agar leaving tracks. Once the food source is exhausted, the trophozoites will form hexagonal cysts (see Fig. 11.3). Cultures using an axenic liquid medium and cell culture are also used to isolate *Acanthamoeba*.[9] Corneal specimens for microscopic examination by Giemsa, calcofluor, and acridine orange stain should be obtained and are highly recommended as a rapid detection test. Polymerase chain reaction (PCR) testing can also be used to detect *Acanthamoeba* DNA.[10]

The detection of Microsporidia from corneal specimens is determined through the examination of stained specimens. A modified trichrome staining of epithelial cells will reveal pinkish to red organisms.[11] Other stains such as Giemsa, Gram, periodic acid–Schiff, Grocott's methenamine silver, calcofluor, and acid-fast methods have been equally successful for visualizing Microsporidia (see Fig. 11.3).[12,13]

Laboratory Diagnosis of Adenovirus Infection

The laboratory diagnosis of adenovirus infection is a function of specimen collection after the onset of clinical presentation.[14] At the time of early clinical onset, the adenoviral titer is large in regards to live virus, capsid antigen, and viral DNA. This large titer decreases rapidly within days of clinical onset and dwindles to minute amounts within 1–2 weeks. Table 11.1 describes adenovirus laboratory testing as a function of the onset of clinical presentation. Adenovirus can be detected from ocular specimens using four methods: (1) cell culture isolation, (2) shell vial, (3) rapid antigen testing, and (4) PCR.

The isolation of adenovirus in cell culture is the 'gold standard' for detecting adenovirus from ocular samples. In general, cell culture isolation will not provide timely results for patient care. Clinical specimens are obtained from the cornea and/or conjunctiva using soft-tipped applicators and transported to a clinical virology laboratory in viral transport medium (Bartels Chlamydia transport medium, Wicklow, Ireland) or a viral culturette (see Fig. 11.1). Adenovirus is a very hardy virus and can be transported without loss of viability through mail carriers under normal conditions.[15,16] Most virology laboratories inoculate A549 monolayer cells

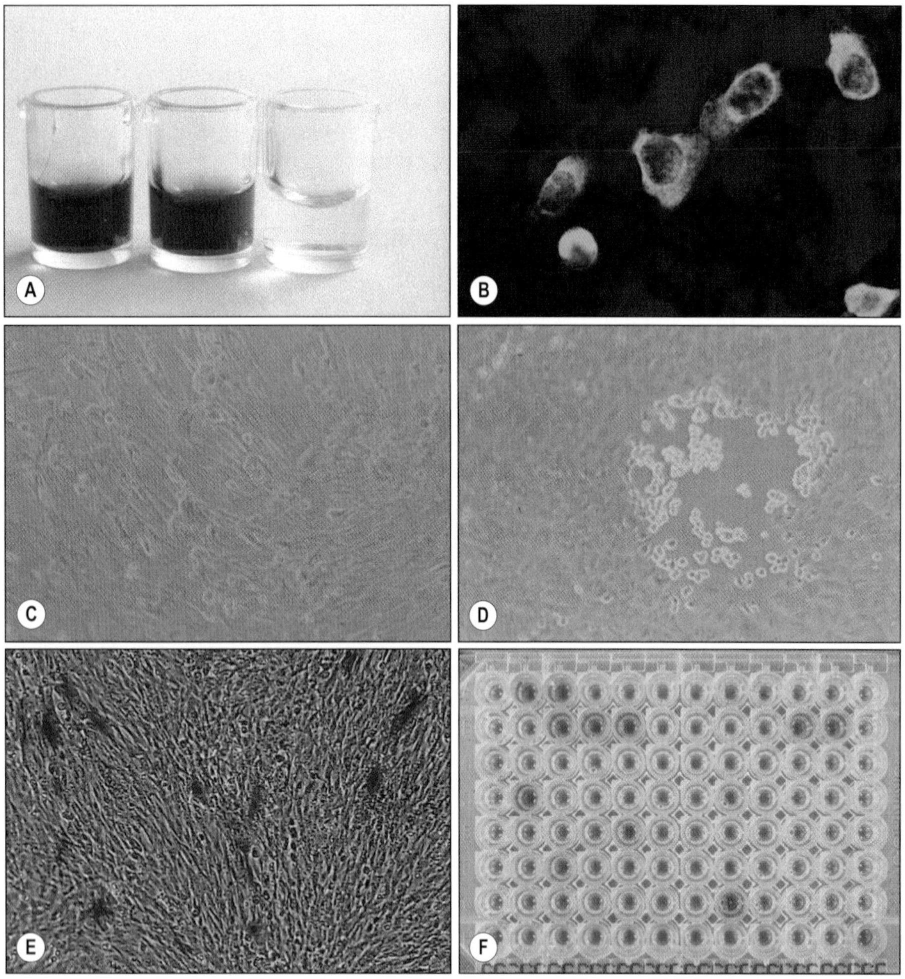

Fig. 11.4 Laboratory diagnosis of adenovirus infection. (**A**) Adenoclone® test; (**B**) positive adenovirus shell vial; (**C**) adenovirus CPE in cell culture; (**D**) herpes simplex virus CPE in cell culture; (**E**) positive ELVIS test for herpes simplex virus; (**F**) positive ELISA tests for chlamydial DNA after PCR amplification.

Table 11.1 Laboratory detection of adenovirus from ocular specimens as a function of clinical onset

	Clinical onset of infection		
Test	**3 days or less**	**3 to 7 days**	**Greater than 7 days**
Adenoclone™	Reliable only if positive	Rarely positive	Never positive
Cell culture isolation	Positive in 1 to 7 days	Positive in 3 to 10 days	Positive in 10 days to 3–4 weeks
Shell vial isolation	Positive in 3 days	Positive in 3 days	Positive in 3 days – less sensitive due to minute titer
Polymerase chain reaction	Positive in 1 to 3 days	Positive in 1 to 3 days	Positive in 1 to 3 days – less sensitive due to minute titer

(human lung carcinoma continuous cell line) for adenovirus isolation. Observance of characteristic cytopathic effect (cell rounding) is monitored for at least 3 weeks before finalizing cultures as negative with the immunoassay (Adenoclone®, Meridian, Cincinnati, OH) (Fig. 11.4). Ocular specimens obtained within the first 3 days of clinical onset will be positive in culture as early as 1 day (rare) but generally at 4–7 days with a few positive cultures at 8–10 days. Cultures obtained after 3 days of onset should include both eyes, since the fellow eye generally becomes involved at this time point. Specimens obtained at this later time of clinical onset generally require 10 days to 3 weeks or more for positive cell culture results.

The shell vial method is a cell culture technique that provides results in 3 days.[17] Viral specimens are inoculated on a glass cover-slip placed in a shell vial (small glass cylinder) layered with a monolayer of A549 cells. The inoculated shell vial is centrifuged and incubated for 3 days. Instead of waiting for the appearance of cell rounding, individual infected cells are stained with monoclonal antibodies conjugated with fluorescein isothiocyanate that appear apple-green using a fluorescent microscope (see Fig. 11.4). Shell vial detection is as sensitive as standard cell culture from patients cultured within 3 days of clinical onset of infection.[17]

The enzyme immunoassay, Adenoclone®, is a 90-minute antigen detection test that does not require the presence of live adenovirus. At its inception, Adenoclone® appeared to be a highly sensitive and specific test[18] but subsequent experience demonstrated a decrease in positive testing with a sensitivity of less than 50%.[19–21] Adenoclone® can provide rapid results when tests are positive, but all negative results require confirmation by cell culture isolation. Another rapid test, the RPS Adeno Detector™ was developed as a 'point of care' test to directly detect adenovirus antigen from the conjunctiva. The sensitivity of testing was 88%, the specificity was 91%, and it was demonstrated to be less reliable for testing samples from transport medium in the laboratory setting.[22,23]

An important advance in the detection of adenovirus is PCR technology. PCR tests for the presence of specific adenoviral DNA sequences by amplifying these sequences in a series of steps and then detecting the amplified product with DNA detection methods (i.e. gels, ELISA, real-time). Compared to cell culture isolation, the sensitivity of PCR is over 90% and equivalent to shell vial.[24] The lower sensitivity is probably due to the lower volume of sample tested. Only 5–10 μL of sample is tested for PCR, whereas 500 μL is used for cell culture isolation and 200 μL for shell vial. Advances in technology are making PCR more available but many molecular diagnostic laboratories may still be slow to offer adenoviral PCR testing due to validation testing. A dedicated molecular laboratory is capable of producing positive or negative results within 1–3 days of receipt of specimen. Real-time PCR for adenovirus DNA detection was determined to be 85% sensitive and 98% specific.[25]

Laboratory Testing for Herpes Simplex Virus

The laboratory diagnosis of active herpes simplex virus (HSV) from ocular specimens is widely available and positive results can be obtained within 24–72 hours of receipt at the testing center. In general, the diagnosis of HSV ocular disease is made at the initial slit lamp examination with characteristic epithelial presentations, but studies have reported that only 55–65% of patients with culture-positive proven infection are treated at this time.[26,27] This would indicate that HSV ocular infection is not always classical in appearance and that laboratory diagnosis may be crucial. Clinical specimens are obtained from the cornea and/or conjunctiva using soft-tipped applicators and transported to a clinical virology laboratory in viral transport medium (Bartels Chlamydia transport medium, Wicklow, Ireland) or a viral culturette. Care should be taken not to delay the delivery of the specimens, since HSV, an enveloped virus, is not as hardy as adenovirus.[28] The key laboratory methods for detecting HSV from ocular specimens are: (1) cell culture isolation, (2) ELVIS (enzyme linked virus induced system) one-day cell culture isolation, and (3) PCR.

The gold standard for the laboratory testing of HSV is cell culture isolation. This is a sensitive test that is processed by all virology laboratories and generally produces positive results within 2–3 days, but isolation can be delayed to 1 week or more in rare occasions. Clinical samples are inoculated to monolayers of A549, Vero, or other susceptible cell lines in glass test tubes. The monolayers are monitored every other day for 2–3 weeks for the observation of characteristic cytopathic effect (CPE – cell rounding) (see Fig. 11.4). Experienced laboratories can distinguish HSV from other viral CPE, while others can confirm the CPE with complementing tests (i.e. ELVIS, PCR).

A more rapid cell culture isolation method that can produce positive results within 24 hours is ELVIS.[29] In a similar fashion to the adenovirus shell vial test, 0.2 mL of clinical specimen is centrifuged on a specially engineered cell line that produces beta-galactosidase when HSV virus is introduced into the cell. After the clinical specimen is allowed to incubate on the cell line for 24 hours, the cell line is fixed and a substrate is added to react with the beta-galactosidase to produce a blue color within the cells, which are observed with a light microscope under 10–40× magnification (see Fig. 11.4). ELVIS is an uncomplicated test that provides 85% sensitivity.[29] The reduced sensitivity compared to standard cell culture is probably due to the reduction in inoculation volume and the decreased incubation period.

Most molecular diagnostic laboratories offer PCR testing for HSV DNA. This is an excellent alternative when central virology laboratories are unavailable and specimens must be sent through couriers to testing centers. Viable HSV is not necessary for PCR but negative tests should be confirmed with cell culture isolation because PCR may not be 100% sensitive.[illegible] Real-time PCR for HSV viral DNA detection was determined to be 98% sensitive and 100% specific.[25] In contrast, prospective studies indicated that PCR was more likely to detect the presence of HSV DNA with patients of suspected HSV ocular disease than cell culture isolation. Of 47 patients with positive PCR testing, only 28 tested for live virus in cell culture isolation.[30]

The laboratory diagnosis of HSV as an etiologic agent in pre-existing disease by submitting corneal buttons after keratoplasty for analysis is different than diagnosis for active infection. Corneal buttons from keratoplasty are generally negative for active infection but some success for detecting HSV from these samples has been had using PCR and immunohistochemistry methods.[31]

Laboratory Testing for Varicella-Zoster Virus and Epstein–Barr Virus

Varicella-zoster virus (VZV) is not a hardy virus that is readily isolated in cell culture. Cell culture isolation requires a vigorous collection of infected cells from the clinical ocular site and immediate inoculation on a susceptible cell line. Sometimes, the clinical sample is centrifuged to a cell monolayer contained in shell vials to provide better adsorption between infected cell and susceptible cell line.[32] The best method to detect VZV from ocular samples is PCR.[25] The method is available in many molecular diagnostic laboratories and testing results can be expected as soon as 48 hours after receipt of specimen. Real-time PCR for VZV DNA detection was determined to be 100% sensitive and 100% specific.[25]

Epstein–Barr virus (EBV) cannot be isolated from ocular samples. Studies have shown that the normal population without eye disease can be PCR positive for EBV.[33] The diagnosis of EBV can be supported with serology testing for different antigens that represent various times of EBV infection.[34]

Laboratory Testing for Chlamydia

Chlamydia from ocular samples can be detected using: (1) cell culture isolation, (2) Giemsa stain, and (3) PCR. Antigen and immunofluorescent tests are available but these are generally less sensitive and less than 100% specific for ocular samples.[35] Serology testing has been shown to support treatment when cell culture isolation was negative, but this method is not definitive and requires drawing blood.[36]

The fastidious nature of chlamydia weakens cell culture isolation as a reliable test for detecting chlamydia in ocular samples.[37] Clinical specimens are collected in a similar fashion to viral cultures. Many virology laboratories do offer this testing, but the specimens must be delivered immediately under low temperature requirements to obtain the best results. Observing chlamydial inclusion bodies on conjunctival specimens collected with a spatula, placed on glass slides, and stained with Giemsa is definitive when present, but this microscopic expertise is limited to a few laboratories. Giemsa-stained smears that present with slightly enlarged epithelial cells containing prominent nucleoli, polymorphonuclear cells, mononuclear cells, and plasma cells could support a chlamydial diagnosis but are not definitive.

PCR is the best diagnostic test for the laboratory diagnosis of ocular chlamydial infection.[38] PCR tests for chlamydial detection are commercially available as kits (COBAS Amplicor™ CT/NG Test, Roche Diagnostics Corp., Indianapolis, IN) and many central laboratories offer this as the sole technique. The PCR test is a 6-hour test that includes routine DNA amplification and amplified product detection with an ELISA (enzyme-linked immunosorbent assay) format (see Fig. 11.4). Transportation requirements are not a problem since live chlamydia is not essential, and results can be expected in 24–72 hours. Real-time PCR for chlamydial DNA detection was determined to be 94% sensitive and 100% specific.[25]

Laboratory Diagnosis: Unusual Requests

Any rare pathogen that cannot be easily cultured and has no commercial test for detection will need to be tested in special laboratories (i.e. Centers for Disease Control, State laboratories) or at facilities researching the particular disease. Sometimes, special in vitro antibiotic susceptibility testing for fungi and viruses may be requested. Laboratories in general should have reference laboratories to assist in these special cases, but final results may be delayed. Some infectious agents such as *Treponema pallidum* (syphilis) and *Borrelia burgdorferi* (Lyme disease) can be indirectly diagnosed with serology support.[39]

Summary

Modern practical microbiology tests are available to the ophthalmologist for detecting pathogens from the cornea. Ophthalmologists must become more involved in laboratory medicine in order to successfully manage corneal infections. Technology will develop more sensitive methods of detecting corneal pathogens, but new testing will need to be cost-effective in order to make an impact on patient care. Innovative methods to detect new pathogens and better techniques to detect existing pathogens will require a cooperative effort between the ophthalmologist and microbiology laboratory.

References

1. Benson WH, Lanier JD. Comparison of techniques for culturing corneal ulcers. *Ophthalmology.* 1992;99:800–804.
2. Matoba AY. Laboratory investigation: microbiologic and cytologic testing. In: Krachmer JH, Mannis MJ, Holland EJ, eds. *Cornea*. St. Louis, MO: Mosby; 1997:305–306.
3. Kowalski RP, Roat MI. Normal flora of the human conjunctiva and eyelid. In: Tasman W, Jaeger EA, eds. *Duane's foundations of clinical ophthalmology.* Philadelphia: Lippincott Williams and Wilkins; 1998 [Chapter 41].
4. Forbes BA, Sahm DF, Weissfeld AS. Mycobacteria. In: *Bailey and Scott's diagnostic microbiology.* 11th ed. St. Louis, MO: Mosby; 2002:240–271 [Chapter 48].
5. National Committee for Clinical Laboratory Standards. *Performance Standards for Antimicrobial Susceptibility Testing; Fourteenth Informational Supplement.* Villanova: PA National Committee for Clinical Laboratory Standards; January 2004. document M100-S14A5, vol. 20, No. 2.
6. Abad JC, Foster CS. Fungal keratitis. In: Albert DM, Jakobiec FA, eds. *Principles and practice of ophthalmology.* Philadelphia, PA: WB Saunders; 2000:906.
7. Tanure MA, Cohen EJ, Sudesh S, et al. Spectrum of fungal keratitis at Wills Eye Hospital, Philadelphia, PA. *Cornea.* 2000;19:307–312.
8. Kitay SE, Kowalski RP, Karenchak LM, Wiley L. Can acanthamoeba survive the U.S. Postal Service? *Invest Ophthalmol Vis Sci.* 1995;36(4 suppl):1524.
9. Visvesvara GS. Pathogenic and opportunistic free-living amebae. In: Murray PR, Baron EJ, Pfaller MA, et al, eds. *Manual of clinical microbiology.* 7th ed. Washington, DC: ASM Press; 1999:1386–1388.
10. Thompson PP, Shanks RMQ, Gordon YJ, Kowalski RP. Laboratory diagnosis of acanthamoeba keratitis using the Cepheid SmartCycler II in the presence of topical ophthalmic drugs. *J Clin Microbiol.* 2008;46;3232–3236.
11. Theng J, Chan C, Ling ML, Tan D. Microsporidial keratoconjunctivitis in a healthy contact lens wearer without human immunodeficiency virus infection. *Ophthalmology.* 2001;108:976–978.
12. Font RL, Samaha AN, Keener MJ, et al. Corneal microsporidiosis. Report of case, including electron microscopic observations. *Ophthalmology.* 2000;107(9):1769–1775.
13. Didier ES, Rogers LB, Brush AD, et al. Diagnosis of disseminated microsporidian Encephalitozoon hellem infection by PCR-Southern analysis and successful treatment with albendazole and fumagillin. *J Clin Microbiol.* 1996;34:947–952.
14. Kowalski RP, Gordon YJ. Comparison of direct rapid tests for the detection of adenovirus antigen in routine conjunctival specimens. *Ophthalmology.* 1989;96:1106–1109.
15. Nauheim RC, Romanowski EG, Cruz TA, et al. Prolonged recoverability of desiccated adenovirus type 19 from various surfaces. *Ophthalmology.* 1990;97:1450–1453.
16. Romanowski EG, Bartels SP, Vogel R, et al. Feasibility of an antiviral clinical trial requiring cross-country shipment of conjunctival adenovirus cultures and recovery of infectious virus. *Curr Eye Res.* 2004;29:195–199.
17. Kowalski RP, Karenchak LM, Gordon YJ. The evaluation of the shell vial technique for the detection of ocular adenovirus. *Ophthalmology.* 1999;106:1324–1327.
18. Wiley L, Springer D, Kowalski RP, et al. Rapid diagnostic testing for ocular adenovirus. *Ophthalmology.* 1988;95:431–433.

19. Roba LA, Kowalski RP, Gordon AT, et al. An analysis of clinical adenoviral ocular isolates by serotype, in vitro infectivity and clinical course. *Cornea.* 1995;14:388–393.
20. Wiley LA, Roba LA, Kowalski RP, et al. A 5-year evaluation of the adenoclone test for the rapid diagnosis of adenovirus from conjunctival swabs. *Cornea.* 1996;15:363–367.
21. Uchio E, Aoki K, Saitoh W, et al. Rapid diagnosis of adenoviral conjunctivitis swabs by 10-minute immunochromatography. *Ophthalmology.* 1997;104:1294–1299.
22. Sambursky R, Tauber S, Schirra F, et al. The RPS Adeno Detector for diagnosing adenoviral conjunctivitis. *Ophthalmology.* 2006;113:1758–1764.
23. Siamak NM, Kowalski RP, Thompson PP, et al. RPS Adeno Detector. *Ophthalmology.* 2009;116:591.
24. Kowalski RP, Suzow J, Karenchak LM, et al. Laboratory diagnosis of ocular adenovirus infection: Is there really one best test? *Invest Ophthalmol Vis Sci.* 2001;42(4 suppl):3106.
25. Kowalski RP, Thompson PP, Kinchington PR, Gordon YJ. Evaluation of the SmartCyclerII for real-time detection of viruses and chlamydia from ocular specimens. *Arch Ophthalmol.* 2006;124:1135–1139.
26. Kowalski RP, Gordon YJ. Evaluation of immunologic tests for the detection of ocular herpes simplex virus. *Ophthalmology.* 1989;96:1583–1586.
27. Kowalski RP, Gordon YJ, Romanowski EG, et al. A comparison of enzyme immunoassay and polymerase chain reaction with the clinical examination for diagnosing ocular herpetic disease. *Ophthalmology.* 1993;100:530–533.
28. Romanowski EG, Barnhorst DA, Kowalski RP, Gordon YJ. The survival of herpes simplex virus in multidose office ophthalmic solutions. *Am J Ophthalmol.* 1999;128:239–240.
29. Kowalski RP, Karenchak LM, Shah C, Gordon JS. ELVIS: a new 24-hour culture test for detecting herpes simplex virus from ocular samples. *Arch Ophthalmol.* 2002;120:960–962.
30. Cronin TH, Thompson PP, Kowalski RP. Clinical correlation of herpes simplex results: When PCR and standard viral culture results don't match. *Invest Ophthalmol Vis Sci.* 2007;(suppl):3798.
31. Kaye SB, Baker K, Bonshek R, et al. Human herpesviruses in the cornea. *Br J Ophthalmol.* 2000;84:563–571.
32. Schirm J, Meulenberg JJ, Pastoor GW, et al. Rapid detection of varicella-zoster in clinical specimens using monoclonal antibodies on shell vials and smears. *J Med Virol.* 1989;28:1–6.
33. Plugfelder SC, Crouse CA, Pereira I, Atherton S. Amplification of Epstein-Barr virus genomic sequences in blood cells, lacrimal glands, and tears from primary Sjögren's syndrome patients. *Ophthalmology.* 1990;97:976–984.
34. Matoba AY. Ocular disease associated with Epstein-Barr virus infection. *Surv Ophthalmol.* 1990;35:145–150.
35. Sheppard JD, Kowalski RP, Meyer MP, et al. Immunodiagnosis of adult chlamydial conjunctivitis. *Ophthalmology.* 1988;95:434–443.
36. Arffa RC, Kowalski RP, Springer PS. The value of serology in the diagnosis of adult chlamydial keratoconjunctivitis. *Ophthalmology.* 1988;95(9 Suppl):145.
37. Novak KD, Kowalski RP, Karenchak LM, Gordon YJ. The recovery of chlamydia from a non-porous surface. *Cornea.* 1995;14:523–526.
38. Kowalski RP, Uhrin M, Karenchak LM, et al. The evaluation of the Amplicor™ test for the detection of chlamydial DNA in adult chlamydial conjunctivitis. *Ophthalmology.* 1995;102:1016–1019.
39. Foulks GN, Gordon JS, Kowalski RP. Bacterial infections of the conjunctiva and cornea. In: Albert DM, Jakobiec FA, eds. *Principles and practice of ophthalmology.* Philadelphia: WB Saunders; 2000:901.

Chapter 12

Molecular Genetics of Corneal Disease

John F. Stamler, John H. Fingert

The Value of Molecular Genetics Study of Disease

The identification of disease-causing genes provides information about the pathogenesis of heritable corneal disorders at the most fundamental level. The function of disease-causing genes may suggest involvement of important biologic pathways in a particular disorder. In addition to clarifying mechanisms of disease, the discovery of disease genes will likely provide insights into the normal function of the cornea.

The discovery of the genes responsible for corneal disorders has important implications for patient care. As disease-causing genes are identified, DNA-based tests can be designed to aid with diagnosis and to help differentiate between clinically similar disorders. Such genetic tests have become available for many diseases on both a fee-for-service and a research basis (www.genetests.org). Identification of the specific mutation responsible for a patient's disease not only solidifies the diagnosis but also may often allow one to accurately predict the course of the disease. Mutation-specific phenotypes of many hereditary eye diseases including glaucoma,[1] retinitis pigmentosa,[2] and Von Hippel-Lindau[3] have been described and will be of increasing utility to clinicians in counseling patients about their prognosis in the coming years.

The identification of disease-causing genes is crucial to the development of therapies for heritable disorders. In some cases, the biologic function of a disease-causing gene may suggest the novel application of known medical and surgical therapies. In other cases, new interventions will be designed to mitigate or repair a gene defect once it has been discovered. Such interventions may include custom pharmaceuticals, gene replacement (replacing a defective gene using viral vectors) or other molecular genetic techniques such as suppressing expression of abnormal gene products using ribozymes.[4,5]

Understanding the molecular genetic basis of a disease not only suggests new avenues for medical and surgical interventions but also facilitates testing these therapeutics in animal models and human subjects. The most relevant animal models will be based upon genetic defects similar to those observed in human disease and will be used for testing the efficacy and safety of new interventions. While therapeutics are being tested in animal models, populations of human study patients with the same genetic basis of disease can be identified with diagnostic genetic tests and recruited for participation in future human studies. Clinically defined diseases, especially common ones like Fuchs' endothelial corneal dystrophy, are often really a group of similar-appearing diseases with different underlying mechanisms of disease. For this reason, it is unlikely that all subtypes of such a clinical disease will respond equally to a single therapy. The use of mechanistically homogeneous animal and patient populations will help to maximize the likelihood of identifying useful new therapies and targeting them to the right patients.

Review of Genetics and Human Disease

Genes are the most basic units of heredity. More specifically, genes are segments of deoxyribonucleic acid (DNA) molecules that specify the production of proteins, which in turn perform structural or enzymatic functions necessary for development and homeostasis. Other molecules necessary for life, such as carbohydrates and lipids, are produced as needed by proteins. In this fashion, information stored in the DNA of each cell in an organism is used to create and organize cellular building blocks and on a larger scale to determine recognizable qualities or traits. Heritable traits (and genetic diseases) are determined by variations in the DNA sequence of genes and the proteins they encode.

The DNA sequence of the human genome encodes approximately 30 000 genes divided among the 23 pairs of chromosomes (22 autosomes and the X and Y sex chromosomes). Each chromosome consists of a single, extremely long molecule of DNA that is complexed with proteins and extensively folded and packaged into a condensed element. Every cell of an organism contains a complete copy of all of its genes stored in chromosomes.

Although all of an organism's genes are present in each of its cells, only a fraction of these genes are active in a given cell. Some genes that perform basic functions necessary for survival, such as energy production, are active in every cell of the body, while others are tissue specific. Tissue-specific activation of genes occurs because proteins are not produced directly from DNA. The DNA sequence of a gene is first converted into ribonucleic acid (RNA) in a process known as

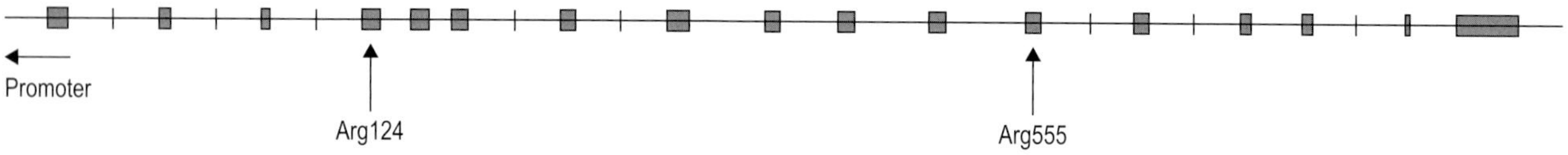

Fig. 12.1 The gene structure of the *BigH3* gene. The coding sequence of *BigH3* is divided into 17 exons (represented by the boxes) which are separated by 16 introns (represented by the space between the boxes). Upstream (to the left) of the coding sequences is the promoter region that regulates the transcription (expression) of the *BigH3* gene. The positions of the amino acids most commonly mutated in *BigH3*-associated corneal disease (Arg124 and Arg555) are shown with arrows. The drawing is to scale except that introns greater than 500 nucleotides long have been truncated (indicated with a vertical slash mark).

transcription. The nucleotide sequence of an RNA molecule specifies a series of amino acids that, when connected in succession, form a protein (translation). In a given cell of a complex organism, most genes lie dormant and are neither transcribed nor translated and the proteins which they encode are not produced. The subset of genes that are transcribed and subsequently translated into proteins give a cell specialized form and function, and is the basis of cellular differentiation and tissue formation.

The structure of a gene includes several domains necessary for the production of a particular protein in a coordinated fashion (Fig. 12.1). Only a portion of a gene's DNA sequence (the coding sequence) specifies the amino acids that compose the encoded protein. In eukaryotic cells, the coding sequence is usually divided into several segments called exons, which are separated by noncoding DNA segments called introns. 'Upstream' of the coding sequence is the promoter region of the gene which regulates transcription. The promoter contains DNA sequences that are binding sites for the enzyme (RNA polymerase) and cofactors that transcribe the gene from DNA into RNA. Tissue-specific activation of gene expression is primarily determined by differential binding of these cofactors to the promoter.

Techniques Used to Identify Disease-causing Genes

The general approaches that are used to identify genes responsible for heritable corneal diseases are population-based techniques (association studies or candidate gene screening) and family-based techniques (positional cloning). In the population-based approaches, the frequency of different types of genetic variations are compared between large numbers of patients with a disease and normal control subjects. Lately, there has been great success in studying populations of patients with eye disease using genome-wide association studies. In such studies, cohorts of patients and controls are typed with hundreds of thousands of genetic markers in search of a cluster of markers that are seen more frequently in patients than controls. These groups of disease-associated markers may define a region in the genome that contains a genetic risk factor for disease. Genome-wide association studies have been successful in mapping the location and identifying important genetic risk factors for common eye diseases such as age-related macular degeneration[6–8] and exfoliation syndrome.[9]

Another population-based technique for finding disease-causing genes is the candidate gene screening approach. With this method, a hypothesis about the mechanism of disease is used to select and prioritize candidate genes for mutation screening without regard to the chromosomal locations of the candidates. Genes are studied as possible causes of corneal disorders based upon their function or expression pattern. While it is true that some ocular diseases, such as gyrate atrophy[10] and Leber's hereditary optic neuropathy,[11] are caused by genes expressed ubiquitously, it is rarely true that ocular diseases are caused by genes that are not expressed in the eye. Therefore, genes expressed in the cornea would be given higher priority as candidate genes for corneal dystrophies than genes not expressed in the cornea. Genes with known functions that suggest an association with a corneal disorder would also be selected for further study. For example, the sulfotransferase gene *CHST6* was considered a good candidate for involvement in macular cornea dystrophy after biochemical studies identified a deficit of sulfated glycosaminoglycans in this disorder.[12,13] Finally, genes that cause corneal disease when disrupted in an animal model are excellent candidates for involvement in human corneal disease. For example, a keratin 12 'knock-out' mouse (i.e. a mouse genetically engineered to have a genome lacking the keratin 12 gene) has a fragile corneal epithelium and is predisposed to corneal abrasions and erosions.[14] This observation suggested that the keratin 12 gene was a good candidate for causing Meesmann corneal dystrophy. Candidate gene screening is a useful technique for identifying disease genes when only individuals or small families affected with a disease are available for study. Candidate genes are evaluated by screening large cohorts of patients for disease-causing mutations.

Family-based studies may also be used to identify disease-causing genes. Large families with many members affected with an eye disease may be studied using a positional cloning approach. With these studies, potential corneal disease genes are identified and evaluated, based on their chromosomal location. This method is dependent on the availability of large families transmitting disease in a mendelian fashion. The chromosomal location of the disease-causing gene in such pedigrees is determined by linkage analysis. Family members are typed with hundreds of genetic markers with known chromosomal locations in search of markers that are coinherited (or linked) with the disease more often than can be explained by chance. This coinheritance is related to their physical nearness on a chromosome because genetic markers in close proximity to the disease-causing gene are less likely to be separated by a meiotic crossover. The likelihood of a crossover occurring between a marker and a disease gene is proportional to the distance between them. The known position of a linked marker indicates the chromosomal location of the disease-causing gene. Positional cloning has some advantages over candidate gene screening. This approach requires no hypothesis regarding the pathogenesis of the disease studied or of the function of the disease-causing gene. This feature of linkage analysis is of great utility in studying disorders for which the disease pathways are only poorly understood.[15]

Disease-causing Mutations versus Nondisease-causing Sequence Variations

The human genome is composed of approximately three billion base-pairs of DNA and there are millions of DNA sequence differences between any two unrelated individuals. The vast majority of these differences are not associated with any detectable phenotype. Consequently, one of the challenges of studying the genetics of human disease is differentiating between disease-causing mutations and nondisease-causing sequence variations.

A variety of criteria have been used to judge which sequence variations are disease-causing and which are not. In general, even to be considered to be a disease-causing mutation, a variation must be present in patients more frequently than in control subjects and must either alter the expression level of a gene or alter the encoded protein sequence. Statistical methods, sequence analysis, and functional studies have been used to infer which of these variations are truly pathogenic.

One can use statistical approaches to demonstrate a significant association between a sequence variation and disease, but the statistical methods appropriate for studies of many unrelated patients are different from those used to study individual families with many members affected with disease. In population studies, the pathogenicity of gene variations may be strongly supported by demonstrating a significantly higher frequency of a certain variation among a large number of patients as compared to a large number of controls. A crucial aspect of this technique is that the subjects and controls are well matched. Some nondisease-causing variations are specific to certain ethnic groups and if the ethnicities of the subjects and controls are not well matched, such variations may incorrectly appear to be associated with disease. If a gene variation is found in affected members of a large family, one can use statistics to show that coinheritance of the variation and the disease occurs more likely than can be attributed to chance. Analysis of sequence homology can also lend support to the pathogenicity of a particular sequence variation. Alterations of portions of genes that are identical in disparate organisms are considered more likely to cause disease than those that occur in portions of genes not conserved during evolution. Similarly, variations within known functional domains of a gene are often considered more likely to cause disease than variations in other portions of a gene.

Perhaps the strongest support of the pathogenicity of a sequence variation is to show directly that the variation harms the function of the protein encoded by the gene. This can be done with in vitro assays as well as with various types of animal models. Using molecular genetic techniques, the pathogenicity of a specific gene variation can be evaluated by creating a cell line or an animal that has the gene defect of interest. If such a model expresses a phenotype similar to the human disease, it is likely that the particular gene variation does cause disease. The Meesmann corneal dystrophy-like phenotype of the keratin 12 knock-out mouse[14] is an excellent example of this type of evidence for disease causation.

The term 'dystrophy' has been used in the ophthalmic literature to refer to various types of disorders. However, it has become generally accepted that 'corneal dystrophy' is used to characterize 'a group of inherited corneal diseases that are typically bilateral, symmetric, slowly progressive, and without relationship to environmental or systemic factors' (IC3D classification). These are not absolute constraints, but rather general guidelines. Some dystrophies appear more sporadic than inherited, such as epithelial basement membrane dystrophy. Other disorders that are historically considered dystrophies are often asymmetric or unilateral, such as posterior polymorphous dystrophy. Still others, such as macular corneal dystrophy, may have systemic features.

Recently, the IC3D classification system for corneal dystrophies has been published.[16] This is the system that we have used here.

Epithelial and Subepithelial Corneal Dystrophies

Epithelial basement membrane dystrophy (EBMD, MIM #121820)

Poor adhesion of epithelium resulting in symptomatic recurrent erosions and the visual disturbances of glare and blur associated with irregular corneal epithelium is most often thought to be sporadic or of traumatic origin. However, familial cases have been reported.[17] Typically, there are no signs until adulthood, when irregular patches of epithelium are seen as hazy islands of epithelium with scalloped borders (maps) interspersed among pockets of round or oval gray inclusions (dots). Edges of overlapping epithelial layers can be seen as curvilinear lines (fingerprints). Episodic spontaneous erosions produce lacrimation, glare, and pain.

While most cases are sporadic or arise from superficial trauma, a subset of patients have been linked to mutations in the *TGFBI* gene on chromosome 5q31.[18]

Epithelial recurrent erosion dystrophy (ERED, MIM #122400)

The autosomal dominant ERED has an early onset in the first decade of life. Recurrent erosions occur spontaneously or after minimal trauma. A subepithelial haze may be present and, in the Smolandiensis variant, may be prominent enough to require corneal transplantation.[19] The genetic locus and genes are not known.

Subepithelial mucinous corneal dystrophy (SMCD)

A rare bilateral subepithelial haze involving the whole cornea, but most prominent in the center, has been described to occur in affected family members of this autosomal dominantly inherited dystrophy.[20] The opacities occur in the first decade of life and are accompanied by painful recurrent erosions. Only one family has been reported and the gene that causes corneal disease in this family has not been identified.

Meesmann corneal dystrophy (MCD, MIM #122100)

Multiple, tiny intraepithelial vesicles extend from limbus to limbus with intervening clear areas primarily in the intrapalpebral cornea in MCD. The lesions may appear as gray cysts or clear vacuoles on indirect illumination.[21] In the Stocker-Holt variant of MCD, the punctate epithelial opacities stain with fluorescein and fine linear whorls of opacities may be present.[22]

Mutations in the keratin genes, keratin 3 (*KRT3*) on chromosome 12q13 and keratin 12 (*KRT12*) on chromosome 17q12 have been implicated in MCD and MCD-Stocker-Holt variant.[23,24]

Lisch epithelial corneal dystrophy (LECD)

Localized gray punctate epithelial opacities radiate from the limbus to the center of the cornea in flame, band, or feather-like whorls in individuals affected with LECD. Patients are generally asymptomatic unless the opacities extend to the central cornea. The inheritance pattern is X-linked dominant with a locus at Xp22.3.[25] However, the disease-causing gene in this locus has not yet been identified.

Bowman Layer Dystrophies

Reis-Bücklers corneal dystrophy (RBCD, MIM #608470, *TGFBI* gene)

First described by Reis[26] and then by Bücklers,[27] RBCD presents as subepithelial reticular opacities that focally elevate the epithelium, appearing symmetrically in both corneas around 4–5 years of age. The opacities remain asymptomatic until they produce recurrent erosions. In the second and third decades of life the visual acuity is reduced as the corneal haze and irregular surface progresses. The inheritance is autosomal dominant and specific mutations in the *TGFBI* gene (Arg124Leu and Gly623Asp)[28,29] have been shown to cause disease.

Thiel-Behnke corneal dystrophy (TBCD, MIM #602082, *TGFBI* gene)

Thiel-Behnke corneal dystrophy is similar to RBCD in that it is characterized by subepithelial corneal opacities associated with symptomatic corneal erosions. However, the opacities can be differentiated by their honeycombed pattern and a clear zone near the corneoscleral limbus. Subepithelial fibrous tissue accumulates in wavelike patterns and is seen as the characteristic 'curly' fibers on transmission electron microscopy.[30]

TBCD can be caused by mutations in the *TGFBI* gene at locus 5q31.[28] However, another locus on chromosome 10 (10q23-q24)[31] has recently been identified, which suggests the existence of at least one additional gene that can cause TBCD.

The distinction between Reis-Bücklers and Thiel-Behnke corneal dystrophies has been a focus of controversy. In several early reports, descriptions of Reis-Bücklers dystrophy were based on patients that actually had Thiel-Behnke dystrophy.[30,32] Consequently, features of Thiel-Behnke corneal dystrophy (honeycomb opacities seen at the slit lamp and peculiar 'curly fibers' seen on electron microscopy) and those of Reis-Bücklers dystrophy (geographic opacities seen at the slit lamp and rodlike bodies on electron microscopy) were not precisely delineated. In an extensive review of the literature, Küchle et al. found that most American and British literature reports of Reis-Bücklers dystrophy (prior to 1995) were likely affected with Thiel-Behnke dystrophy.[30] More recently, several patients initially diagnosed with Reis-Bücklers corneal dystrophy were found to harbor an Arg555Gln *TGFBI* mutation[33] and later had their clinical diagnosis changed to Thiel-Behnke dystrophy (the dystrophy associated with this *TGFBI* mutation).[28] At present, histological confirmation may be necessary for a certain diagnosis.[30,34] However, as genotype–phenotype correlations are strengthened, the gold standard for diagnosing Reis-Bücklers or Thiel-Behnke may shift to *TGFBI* mutation screening.

Grayson-Wilbrandt (GWD)

One family has been described with variable patterns of subepithelial corneal opacities that range from diffuse mottling to scattered gray-white opacities. The inheritance appeared to be autosomal dominant, but no information about a chromosomal locus or causative gene is known.[35]

Stromal Dystrophies

TGFBI Dystrophies

Early in the molecular genetic investigation of corneal dystrophies it became evident that several different phenotypes can be caused by variations in a single gene. Linkage studies demonstrated that lattice, granular, and Avellino corneal dystrophies all mapped to the same chromosomal location at 5q31,[36] suggesting that they were caused by different variations in the same gene. Specific mutations in the beta-transforming growth factor induced gene (*TGFBI*, also known as *BIGH3*; MIM #601692) were later shown to be associated with each of these disorders. Later, *TGFBI* mutations were found to be associated with several additional corneal dystrophies (Fig. 12.2).

Classic lattice corneal dystrophy (LCD1), lattice variants, the two types of granular corneal dystrophy (GCD1 and GCD2), and the Bowman's layer dystrophies, Reis-Bücklers corneal dystrophy (RBCD) and Thiel-Behnke corneal dystrophy (TBCD), have all been associated with *TGFBI* mutations.[37] All of these dystrophies share the characteristics of being autosomal dominant and relatively sparing the peripheral 1–2 mm of cornea.

It was more than a little surprising to many clinicians to learn that the breadcrumb-like corneal deposits of granular dystrophy and the branching lines of lattice dystrophy were caused by mutations in the same gene. Specifically, alterations involving the arginine amino acids at positions 124 and 555 of the encoded protein were found to be responsible for these diseases.[38] Additional study has shown that alterations of these two amino acids are the most commonly detected mutations in patients with *TGFBI* corneal dystrophies.[28]

The protein encoded by *TGFBI* contains a host of protein-binding domains, suggesting that it may have a role in cell adhesion and has been shown to bind to type I, II, and IV collagens.[39]

Classic lattice corneal dystrophy (LCD1, MIM #122200, *TGFBI* gene)

Classic lattice corneal dystrophy (LCD1) typically is manifest during the first decade of life and is characterized by branching, linear, central corneal amyloid opacities within the stroma of both eyes. Corneal sensation is reduced and recurrent erosions are common. LCD1 is autosomal dominant and the majority of reported cases have been associated with mutations of C to T at nucleotide 417 in exon 4 of the *TGFBI* gene causing an Arg124Cys mutation; however, many other mutations in *TGFBI* have also been shown to cause forms of LCD1.[28,37]

Historically, several variants of lattice corneal dystrophy have been described, based on differences in phenotype, and are not included in the IC3D. These include types IIIA, I/IIIA, and IV. These subtypes are distinguished by the characteristics of the amyloid deposits, the age of onset, and the frequency of corneal erosions.

Lattice corneal dystrophy, gelosin type (LCD2, MIM #105120, *GSN* gene)

The gelosin type of lattice corneal dystrophy is not a true corneal dystrophy, but rather a systemic amyloidosis (also known as familial amyloid polyneuropathy type IV, Meretoja syndrome, MIM #105120).[40] In LCD2 the corneal opacities are short, radial, fine lines that are more peripheral with relative sparing of the central cornea and fewer in number than those seen in LCD1. Further differentiating features are a later onset in the third or fourth decade and infrequent erosions. Unlike LCD1, LCD2 has systemic features of cranial, autonomic, and peripheral neuropathies,

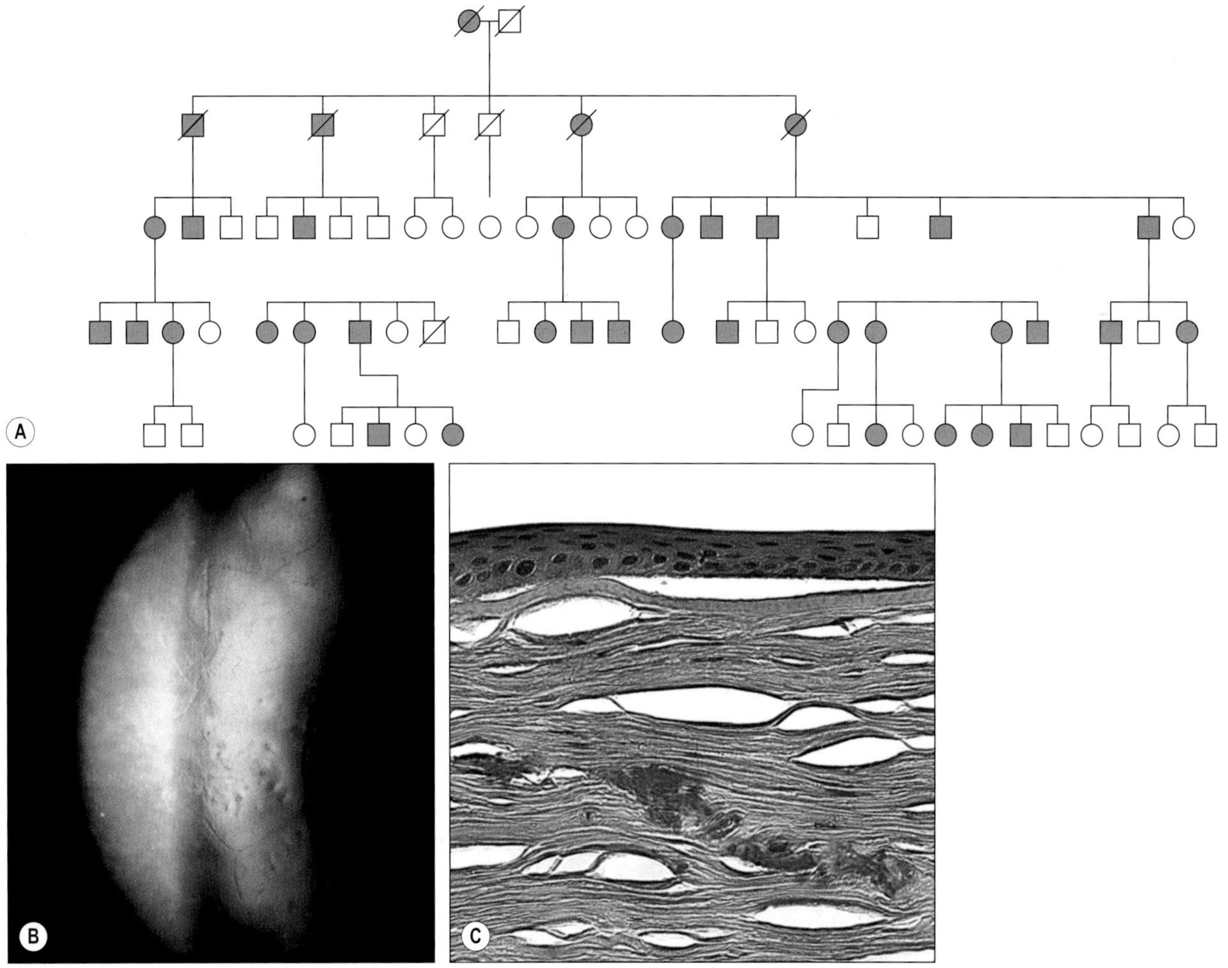

Fig. 12.2 Lattice dystrophy type I. (**A**) Pedigree of a large family. Affected members of this family were found to harbor an Arg124Cys *BigH3* mutation. (**B**) The slit lamp appearance of the cornea of a member of this family demonstrates the linear stromal opacities characteristic of this dystrophy. (**C**) Corneal tissue obtained from a member of this lattice dystrophy pedigree showed positive Congo red staining. Granular dystrophy type I.

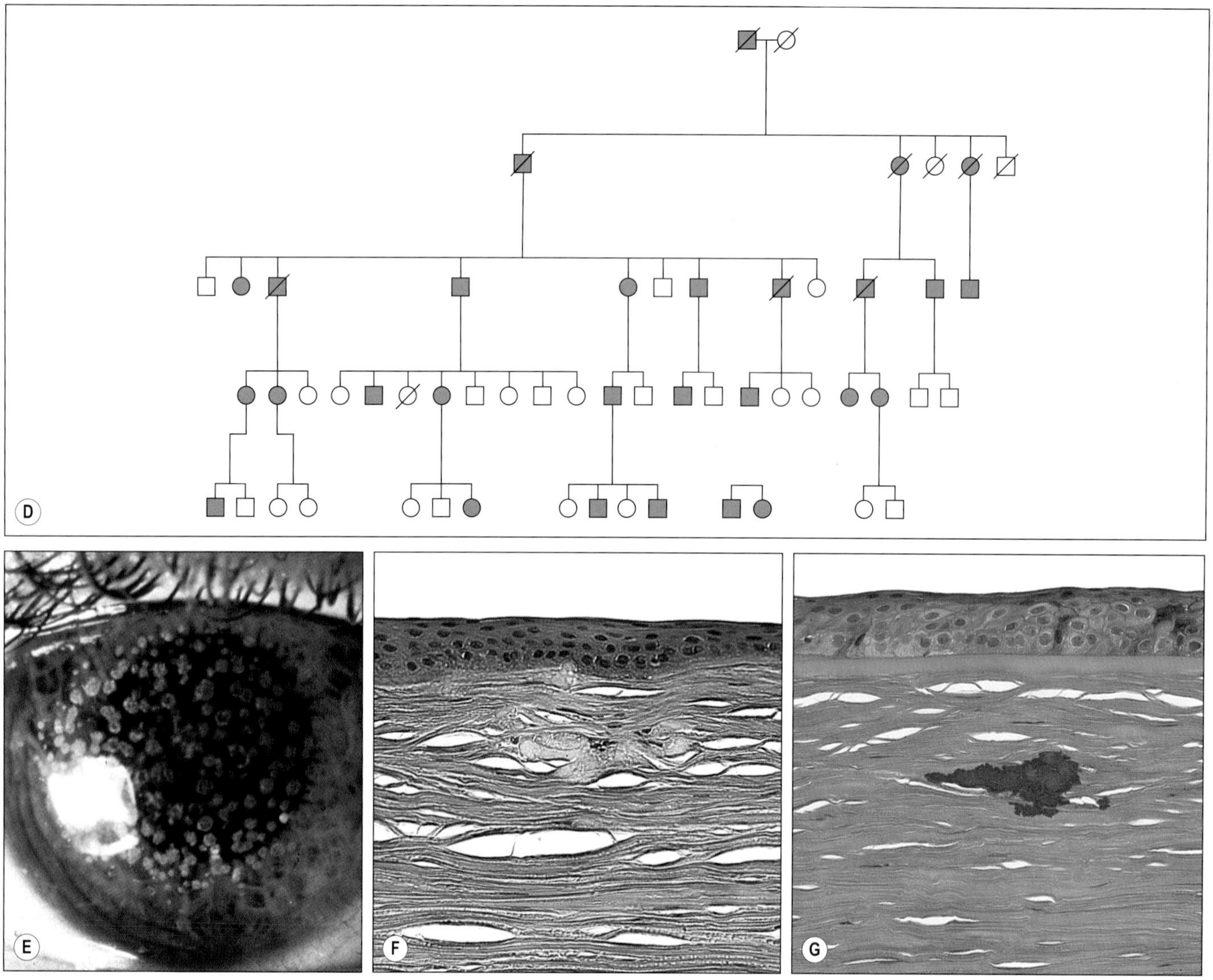

Fig. 12.2, cont'd (**D**) Pedigree of a large family with granular dystrophy in which an Arg555Trp *BigH3* mutation was detected. (**E**) The slit lamp appearance of the cornea of one of the affected members of this family demonstrates the breadcrumb-like stromal opacities characteristic of this disorder. (**F**) Corneal tissue obtained from a family member showed negative Congo red staining. (**G**) The same tissue showed positive Masson's trichrome staining. Granular dystrophy type II (Avellino).

and dry, lax skin. Also protruding lips, pendulous ears, and blepharochalasia are characteristic features.

The amyloid in LCD2 is a mutated form of gelosin that accumulates in the cornea between the epithelium and Bowman's layer. It is also found in heart, kidney, skin, nerves, vessel walls, and various other tissues.[41] The gelsolin gene (*GSN*), which is located on chromosome 9q34 and encodes an actin-modulating protein, is responsible for LCD2. Causative mutations in nucleotide 654 of G to A and G to T resulting in substitutions of asparagine or tyrosine for aspartic acid have been reported.[42]

Granular corneal dystrophy, type 1 (GCD1, MIM #121900, *TGFB1* gene)

The classic type of granular dystrophy, GCD1, generally presents in the first decade of life as discrete, bilateral, crumblike, corneal deposits in the anterior central stroma. Reduced visual acuity, increasing glare, photophobia, and recurrent erosions worsen as the corneal opacities gradually progress with age. Both Arg124Ser and Arg555Trp mutations in the TGFBI peptide have been identified to produce GCD1.[37]

Granular-lattice (Avellino) corneal dystrophy (GCD2, MIM #607541, *TGFB1* gene)

The second type of granular dystrophy, GCD2, contains features of both granular and lattice corneal dystrophies. This disorder has also been called Avellino corneal dystrophy because many of the families with GCD2 came from that region of Italy.[43] In GCD2, white, snowflake-like opacities appear in the central cornea in the first two decades of life. Then lattice lines and interstitial haze gradually develop.

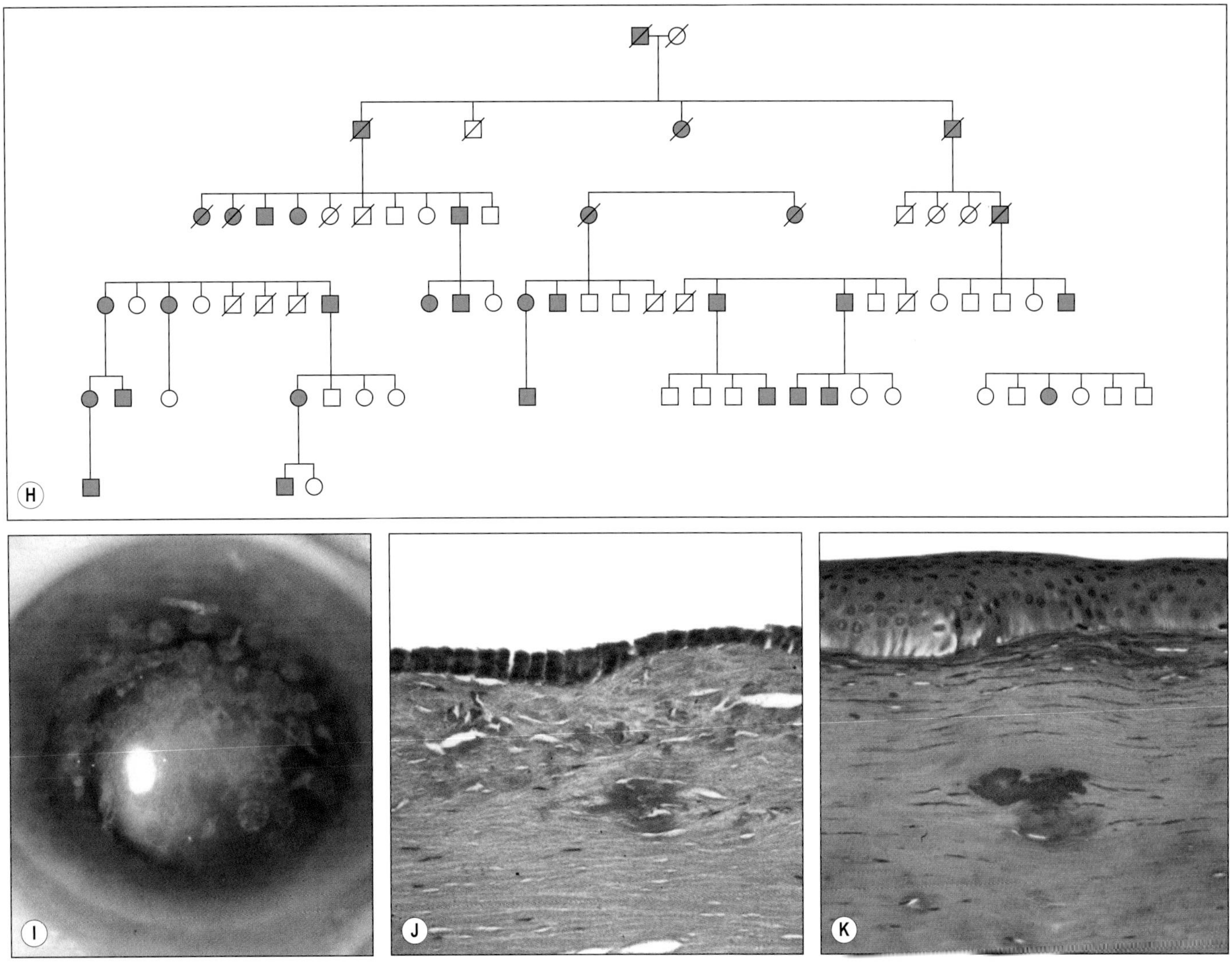

Fig 12.2, cont'd (**H**) Pedigree of a large family with Avellino dystrophy. (**I**) The slit lamp appearance of the cornea of a member of this family. (**J**) Tissue obtained during a corneal transplant operation on the photographed patient showed positive Congo red staining. (**K**) There was also positive Masson's trichrome staining.

Recurrent erosions are not common in GCD2 and the visual acuity is variably affected. GCD2 has been associated with the Arg124His mutation in *TGFB1*.[37]

Macular corneal dystrophy (MCD, OMIM #217800, *CHST6* gene)

The autosomal recessive macular corneal dystrophy (MCD) usually presents early in childhood as a diffuse stromal haze extending all the way to the limbus. As the patient ages, opacities gradually coalesce in the stroma to form irregular white patches or macules that give the dystrophy its name. However, in distinction with granular dystrophy, there are no clear areas between the opacities. MCD is not entirely a stromal condition. The deposits extend through the stroma to Descemet's membrane and the endothelium. Eventually, the endothelium decompensates and corneal edema develops, producing severe loss of vision in the second or third decades.[44]

MCD is characterized by intracellular accumulation of glycosaminoglycans (GAG) within the keratocytes and endothelium, but not the epithelial cells. Similarly, extracellular deposits of GAG are present throughout the stroma and Descemet's membrane.

Mutations in the carbohydrate sulfotransferase 6 gene (*CHST6*) on chromosome 16q22 produce most, but not all, cases of MCD. Well over a hundred different mutations have been identified and most are either missense or nonsense mutations that alter a single nucleotide of the *CHST6* gene. However, insertions and deletions in and around the coding regions of *CHST6* have also been detected.

There are three subtypes of MCD distinguished by the presence of keratan sulfate (KS). In type I, there is no detectable keratan sulfate in the cornea or serum. In type II, there are normal amounts of KS in both cornea and serum. The third type, IA, has KS in keratocytes, but not in serum. Although, these subtypes are not distinguishable clinically, specific classes of *CHST6* mutations are correlated with particular types of MCD. Patients with MCD type I have homozygous mutations in the coding sequence of *CHST6* that would be expected to inactivate the function of the sulfotransferase protein. The loss of *CHST6* function is thought to cause the formation of unsulfated keratan sulfate and accumulation of opaque deposits in the corneal stroma.[13] Alternatively, patients with MCD type II were found to harbor homozygous promoter sequence rearrangements in the *CHST6* gene. These promoter mutations appear to alter the tissue-specific expression of the gene, such that no CHST6 protein is produced in the corneal epithelium, while normal CHST6 is produced in the corneal stroma and in other tissues of the body. Without CHST6 activity in the corneal epithelium, unsulfated keratan sulfate is produced, leading to corneal opacification. The normal keratan sulfate levels observed in MCD type II are due to normal expression of *CHST6* in the corneal stroma and other tissues of the body.[13]

Schnyder corneal dystophy (SCD, MIM #121800, *UBIAD1* gene)

Although Schnyder crystalline corneal dystrophy has been a common name for SCD, the IC3D classification scheme recommends the term 'crystalline' not be used since only about half of involved patients have corneal crystals.[16] Early in life, central corneal haze or frank crystals become apparent in affected individuals. Often, a light yellow opacity forms a ring shape in the anterior stroma and Bowman's layer. The opacities increase with age, but remain primarily in the anterior cornea. Typically, SCD is bilateral, but often asymmetric.

The opacities correspond histological to both intra- and extracellular crystals of cholesterol and other lipids. While most cases of SCD lack any significant systemic abnormalities, many have hypercholesterolemia and its associated manifestations of arcus lipoides and xanthelasma.

Numerous mutations in UbiA prenyltransferase domain containing 1 (*UBIAD1*) gene on chromosome 1p36 have been found to produce autosomal dominant SCD.[44a–c]

Congenital stromal corneal dystrophy (CSCD, MIM #610048, *DCN* gene)

Only four families of this rare autosomal dystrophy have been reported. CSCD is characterized by the presence of diffuse, bilateral, tiny flakelike corneal opacities. The opacities are spread throughout the stroma. It is stable or slowly progressive. The epithelium and endothelium appear normal.

Defects in the decorin (*DCN*) gene on chromosome 12q21.33 have been associated with two families with CSCD.[45]

Fleck corneal dystrophy (FCD, MIM #121850, *PIP5K3* gene)

Fleck corneal dystrophy, an autosomal dominant corneal dystrophy, is characterized by multiple asymptomatic and nonprogressive tiny white opacities scattered throughout the cornea. The epithelium, Descemet's membrane, and endothelium appear normal. The flecks correspond to intracellular accumulations of glycosaminoglycans and lipids. Vision is not affected, with the possible exception of mild photophobia.[46]

Mutations in the phosphatidylinositol-3-phosphate/phosphatidylinositol-5-kinase type III (*PIP5K3*) gene on chromosome 2q35 cause FCD.[47]

Posterior amorphous corneal dystrophy (PACD)

The characteristic sheets of diffuse gray-white opacities of PACD are most prominent in the posterior stroma. The opacity may be noted in early life and may be congenital. The associated anterior abnormalities of prominent Schwalbe line, fine iris processes, iridocorneal adhesions, corectopia, and anterior stromal tags suggest that this may not be a true dystrophy, but more appropriately termed a mesodermal dysgenesis.[48]

PACD shows an autosomal dominant inheritance pattern, but no chromosomal locus or gene has been identified.

Central cloudy dystrophy of Francois (CCDF, MIM #217600)

The asymptomatic central polygonal or rounded stromal opacities that are surrounded by clear zones of CCDF are clinically indistinguishable from the corneal degeneration posterior crocodile shagreen. The opacities may be mucopolysaccharide and lipid.[49] Although apparent autosomal dominant patterns have been reported, the inheritance has not been clearly identified. No chromosomal locus or disease-causing gene has been identified.

Pre-Descemet's corneal dystrophy (PDCD)

The clinical and genetic features of PDCD have not been well defined. No definite inheritance pattern has been described and histopathologic studies have not been consistent. The corneal opacities have been described as fine, gray opacities in the deep stroma of various shapes along with more central, larger lesions. Typically, the vision is not affected and the patients are without symptoms.[50] No chromosomal locus or causative gene has been identified and there is debate as to whether PDCD is best described as a dystrophy or as a degeneration.

Descemet's Membrane and Endothelial Dystrophies

Fuchs' endothelial corneal dystrophy (FECD, MIM #1368000)

Classic FECD: Fuchs' endothelial corneal dystrophy (FECD) is characterized by progressive, bilateral accumulation of central, focal Descemet's membrane excrescences or guttae, loss of endothelial cells, leading to loss of vision from corneal edema. There are at least two clinical types of FECD. In the typical adult-onset or classic type, significant numbers of guttae usually do not become visible until the fourth or fifth decade of life. After the appearance of guttae, it usually takes one or two decades or more for significant compromise of endothelial function and corneal edema to develop.[51]

Late-onset FECD displays an autosomal dominant inheritance pattern with an unknown rate of incomplete penetrance.[52]

Recently, four different mutations in the *SLC4A11* gene were found in four of 89 FECD Chinese and Indian patients, but not in ethnically matched controls.[53] Because of this association and since the *SLC4A11* gene has been implicated in another endothelial cell dystrophy (CHED2), this gene is an appealing possible disease-causing candidate for FECD. In other studies, different FECD genetic loci (13pTel-13q12.13[54] and 18q21.2-q21.32[55]) have been identified with family-based research. Furthermore, a recent study of the candidate genes *COL8A1* and *COL8A2* detected no disease-causing mutations in late-onset FECD.[56] Consequently, it is likely that mutations in at least three different genes can cause the FECD phenotype.

Early-onset FECD: In contrast to the classic FECD presentation, a rare early-onset type of FECD has been described.[57] First signs appear as early as the first decade with significant edema and visual impairment by the third or fourth decade of life. In addition, the guttae differ in morphology between the two types. In the early-onset form they are small, rounded, and associated with the endothelial cell center. This is in distinction to the classic FECD guttae, which are larger, sharply peaked, and initially positioned at the edge of endothelial cells.

This early-onset form of FECD is also autosomal dominant in the reported families. Linkage analysis demonstrated a genetic locus of 1p34.3-p32.[58] The gene that codes for the alpha2 subunit of collagen VIII (*COL8A2*) is within this locus and is highly expressed in corneal endothelial cells. Two different mutations in separate families in the *COL8A2* gene segregate with the disease phenotype. In three families with early-onset FECD, a missense mutation of Gln455Lys was found to occur within the triple helical domain of the protein. In the original family described by Magovern et al.,[59] a mutation was identified that changes leucine to tryptophan at residue 450 of the protein.[57] This is convincing evidence for the disease-causing role of *COL8A2* mutations in the rare early-onset form of FECD.

Posterior polymorphous corneal dystrophy (PPCD, MIM #122000, #609140, #609141)

Posterior polymorphous corneal dystrophy (PPCD) is a rare disease of the corneal endothelium that has autosomal dominant inheritance.[60] PPCD is typically bilateral, with signs appearing in the first or second decade of life, and ranges from rapidly progressive and visually disabling to asymptomatic and stable. The endothelial cells in PPCD have epithelial characteristics such as multilaminar growth and the expression of cytokeratins that are not normally seen in endothelial cells but are typical of epithelial cells.[61,62] Additionally, Descemet's membrane is abnormal.[63]

Three distinct loci and two genes have been identified for PPCD. One large family was mapped to a 30-cM locus on 20q11.[64] Initial studies suggested that mutations in a candidate gene, *VSX1*, in this locus caused PPCD.[65] However subsequent studies have neither confirmed *VSX1* as a PPCD gene nor identified other disease-causing genes within the locus.[66–68]

An association of PPCD with a mutation in the collagen type VIII gene (*COL8A2*) located on the short arm of chromosome 1 has been reported.[58] However, other investigators have failed to find mutations in the *COL8A2* gene in PPCD families.[69–71]

A third PPCD 8.55-cM locus was found on chromosome 10.[72] A frameshift-causing 2-bp deletion (2916_2917delTG) in the last exon of the gene *TCF8* that codes for a transcription factor ZEB1 located within this locus was found to segregate with the disease in a large family.[71] Further analysis of 10 other families revealed mutations that frameshift or terminate this reading frame in four probands.[71] Subsequently, 10 more families (six Czech and four British) have been studied. Four novel pathogenic mutations were identified in the *TCF8* gene.[67]

In summary, there is compelling data that suggests mutations in the *TCF8* gene cause PPCD. However, the initial reports implicating the *VSX1* and *COL8A2* genes in PPCD have not been confirmed.

Congenital hereditary endothelial dystrophy (CHED)

Congenital hereditary endothelial dystrophy (CHED) is a disease of the corneal endothelium that is characterized by bilateral, symmetric stromal haze, which is apparent at or soon after birth. Diffuse opacification is secondary to edema caused by abnormal endothelial development.[73] CHED may be inherited in an autosomal dominant (CHED1) or autosomal recessive (CHED2) pattern.

Autosomal dominant congenital hereditary endothelial dystrophy (CHED1, MIM #121700)

The autosomal dominant form of CHED (CHED1) is slowly progressive and associated with significant vision loss usually requiring treatment with penetrating keratoplasty.[74] The gene that causes CHED1 has been mapped to a chromosome 20 locus. However, the disease-causing gene in this locus region has not been discovered.[75]

Autosomal recessive congenital hereditary endothelial dystrophy (CHED2, OMIM 217700)

Patients with CHED2 differ from those with CHED1 in that they have nystagmus and a nonprogressive course. Linkage analysis of an autosomal recessive pedigree mapped a gene that causes CHED2 locus to a chromosome 20p13 locus that is distinct from the nearby CHED1 locus.[76] Vithana et al. later showed that mutations in one of the genes in this locus, the sodium borate transporter (*SLC4A11*), are a likely cause of CHED2.[77] *SLC4A11* is expressed in human corneal endothelium and mutations in *SLC4A11* were identified in several CHED2 pedigrees.[77] Subsequent studies showed that mutations in *SLC4A11* are a common cause of CHED2.[78–83] However, no *SLC4A11* mutations were detected in some families with CHED2, which suggests that some cases may be caused by different genes.

X-linked endothelial corneal dystrophy (XECD)

Congenital bilateral diffuse hazelike ground glass or milky corneal clouding characterizes patients with XECD. The endothelium has indentations or 'moon craters' with missing endothelial cells. There are secondary epithelial changes of band keratopathy. The inheritance pattern is X-linked dominant and a gene that causes XECD has been mapped to chromosome Xq25;[25] however, no causative gene has been identified.

Keratoconus (OMIM 148300)

Keratoconus is a disorder of the corneal stroma in which progressive thinning of the central cornea induces myopia, irregular astigmatism, and conical surface contours.[84] The heritability of keratoconus has been suggested by twin studies[85–90] and by pedigrees demonstrating autosomal dominant transmission of the disease.[91–96] More recently, computerized corneal topographic methods have increased the sensitivity for detecting keratoconus and have provided additional evidence of mendelian inheritance of the disease.[94,95] The cause of keratoconus is unknown; however, it has been suggested that disturbances in protease regulation,[97,98] wound healing, or IL-1-mediated apoptosis might be involved.[99,100] Associations have also been reported between keratoconus and osteogenesis imperfecta,[101] mitral valve prolapse,[102–104] Down's syndrome,[105–108] Leber congenital amaurosis (LCA),[109,110] and eye rubbing.[106] Mutations in the *VSX1*[65] gene have been implicated in the pathogenesis of keratoconus; however, results from initial reports have not been replicated or confirmed.[111]

Recently, a locus for a putative disease-causing gene for keratoconus has been indentified on 13q32.[112]

X-linked megalocornea (MGC1, OMIM #309300)

Megalocornea is a heritable condition defined by bilateral enlargement of the corneas (greater than 12.5 mm in diameter). Most cases show X-linked inheritance, although there have been reports of autosomal dominant and autosomal recessive transmission. Arcus juvenilis and mosaic corneal dystrophy are frequently associated with megalocornea.[113] The gene causing megalocornea in one pedigree was mapped with linkage analysis to chromosome Xq12-q26.[114] The megalocornea disease gene at this locus is unknown.

Cornea plana (CNA2, OMIM #217300, gene *KERA*)

Cornea plana is a rare, heritable disorder in which the cornea has an abnormally flat curvature resulting in extreme hyperopia. Mutations in keratocan (*KERA*) which encodes a corneal proteoglycan, have been associated with autosomal recessive cornea plana (CNA2).[115] The gene or genes that cause autosomal dominant cornea plana (CNA1, OMIM #121400) have not yet been mapped to chromosomal loci and mutations associated with CNA1 have been excluded in CNA2.[116]

Conclusion

Recent molecular genetics research has provided startling insights into the pathogenesis of corneal disease showing that what were once thought to be disparate phenotypes are caused by mutations of the same gene and mutations in apparently unrelated genes could cause clinically indistinguishable disease. These molecular genetic discoveries have allowed for a reclassification of the corneal dystrophies and continue to provide greater understanding of corneal diseases and fertile soil for continued research.

References

1. Alward WL, Fingert JH, Coote MA, et al. Clinical features associated with mutations in the chromosome 1 open-angle glaucoma gene (GLC1A). *N Engl J Med.* 1998;338:1022–1027.
2. Berson EL, Rosner B, Sandberg MA, Dryja TP. Ocular findings in patients with autosomal dominant retinitis pigmentosa and a rhodopsin gene defect (Pro-23-His). *Arch Ophthalmol.* 1991;109:92–101.
3. Webster AR, Maher ER, Bird AC, Moore AT. Risk of multisystem disease in isolated ocular angioma (haemangioblastoma). *J Med Genet.* 2000;37:62–63.
4. Doudna JA, Cech TR. The chemical repertoire of natural ribozymes. *Nature.* 2002;418:222–228.
5. Sullenger BA, Gilboa E. Emerging clinical applications of RNA. *Nature.* 2002;418:252–258.
6. Klein R, Zeiss C, Chew E, et al. Complement factor H polymorphism in age-related macular degeneration. *Science.* 2005;308:385–389.
7. Edwards AO, Ritter R 3rd, Abel KJ, et al. Complement factor H polymorphism and age-related macular degeneration. *Science.* 2005;308:421–424.
8. Haines JL, Hauser MA, Schmidt S, et al. Complement factor H variant increases the risk of age-related macular degeneration. *Science.* 2005;308:419–421.
9. Thorleifsson G, Magnusson KP, Sulem P, et al. Common sequence variants in the LOXL1 gene confer susceptibility to exfoliation glaucoma. *Science.* 2007;317:1397–1400.
10. Valle D, Kaiser-Kupfer MI, Del Valle LA. Gyrate atrophy of the choroid and retina: deficiency of ornithine aminotransferase in transformed lymphocytes. *Proc Natl Acad Sci USA.* 1977;74:5159–5161.
11. Wallace C, Singh G, Lott MT, et al. Mitochondrial DNA mutation associated with Leber's hereditary optic neuropathy. *Science.* 1988;242:1427–1430.
12. Hassell JR, Newsome DA, Krachmer JH, Rodrigues MM. Macular corneal dystrophy: failure to synthesize a mature keratan sulfate proteoglycan. *Proc Natl Acad Sci USA.* 1980;77:3705–3709.
13. Akama TO, Nishida K, Nakayama J, et al. Macular corneal dystrophy type I and type II are caused by distinct mutations in a new sulphotransferase gene. *Nat Genet.* 2000;26:237–241.
14. Kao WW, Liu CY, Converse RL, et al. Keratin 12-deficient mice have fragile corneal epithelia. *Invest Ophthalmol Vis Sci.* 1996;37:2572–2584.
15. Ott J. *Analysis of human genetic linkage.* 3rd edn. Baltimore: Johns Hopkins University Press; 1999.
16. Weiss JS, Moller HU, Lisch W, et al. The IC3D classification of the corneal dystrophies. *Cornea.* 2008;27(Suppl 2):S1–S83.
17. Laibson PR, Krachmer JH. Familial occurrence of dot (microcystic), map, fingerprint dystrophy of the cornea. *Invest Ophthalmol.* 1975;14:397–399.
18. Boutboul S, Black GC, Moore JE, et al. A subset of patients with epithelial basement membrane corneal dystrophy have mutations in TGFBI/BIGH3. *Hum Mutat.* 2006;27:553–557.
19. Hammar B, Bjorck E, Lagerstedt K, Dellby A, Fagerholm P. A new corneal disease with recurrent erosive episodes and autosomal-dominant inheritance. *Acta Ophthalmol.* 2008;86:758–763.
20. Feder RS, Jay M, Yue BY, et al. Subepithelial mucinous corneal dystrophy. Clinical and pathological correlations. *Arch Ophthalmol.* 1993;111:1106–1114.
21. Fine BS, Yanoff M, Pitts E, Slaughter FD. Meesmann's epithelial dystrophy of the cornea. *Am J Ophthalmol.* 1977;83:633–642.
22. Stocker FW, Holt LB. A rare form of hereditary epithelial dystrophy of the cornea: a genetic, clinical, and pathologic study. *Trans Am Ophthalmol Soc.* 1954;52:133–144.
23. Irvine AD, Corden LD, Swensson O, et al. Mutations in cornea-specific keratin K3 or K12 genes cause Meesmann's corneal dystrophy. *Nat Genet.* 1997;16:184–187.
24. Klintworth GK, Sommer JR, Karolak LA, Reed JW. Identification of new keratin K12 mutations associated with Stocker-Holt corneal dystrophy that differs from mutations found in Meesmann corneal dystrophy. *Invest Ophthalmol Vis Sci.* 1999;40:S563.
25. Schmid E, Lisch W, Philipp W, et al. A new, X-linked endothelial corneal dystrophy. *Am J Ophthalmol.* 2006;141:478–487.
26. Reis W. Familiäre, fleckige hornhautentartung. *Dtsch Med Wochenschr.* 1917;43–575.

27. Bücklers M. Über eine weitere familiäre Hornhaut-dystrophie (Reis). *Klin Monasbl Augenkeilkd.* 1949;114:386–397.
28. Munier FL, Frueh BE, Othenin-Girard P, et al. BIGH3 mutation spectrum in corneal dystrophies. *Invest Ophthalmol Vis Sci.* 2002;43:949–954.
29. Afshari NA, Mullally JE, Afshari MA, et al. Survey of patients with granular, lattice, Avellino, and Reis-Bucklers corneal dystrophies for mutations in the BIGH3 and gelsolin genes. *Arch Ophthalmol.* 2001;119:16–22.
30. Küchle M, Green WR, Volcker HE, Barraquer J. Reevaluation of corneal dystrophies of Bowman's layer and the anterior stroma (Reis-Bucklers and Thiel-Behnke types): a light and electron microscopic study of eight corneas and a review of the literature. *Cornea.* 1995;14:333–354.
31. Yee RW, Sullivan LS, Lai HT, et al. Linkage mapping of Thiel-Behnke corneal dystrophy (CDB2) to chromosome 10q23-q24. *Genomics.* 1997;46:152–154.
32. Bron AJ. The corneal dystrophies. *Curr Opin Ophthalmol.* 1990;1:333–346.
33. Munier FL, Korvatska E, Djemai A, et al. Kerato-epithelin mutations in four 5q31-linked corneal dystrophies. *Nat Genet.* 1997;15:247–251.
34. Aldave AJ, McLeod SD. The molecular genetics of Bowman's layer dystrophies. *Cornea.* 2001;20:672–674.
35. Grayson M, Wilbrandt H. Dystrophy of the anterior limiting membrane of the cornea. (Reis-Buckler type). *Am J Ophthalmol.* 1966;61:345–349.
36. Stone EM, Mathers WD, Rosenwasser G, et al. Three autosomal dominant corneal dystrophies map to chromosome 5q. *Nat Genet.* 1994;6:47–51.
37. Munier FL, Korvatska E, Djemai A, et al. Kerato-epithelin mutations in four 5q31-linked corneal dystrophies. *Nat Genet.* 1997;15:247–251.
38. Korvatska E, Munier FL, Djemai A, et al. Mutation hot spots in 5q31-linked corneal dystrophies. *Am J Hum Genet.* 1998;62:320–324.
39. Skonier J, Neubauer M, Madisen L, et al. cDNA cloning and sequence analysis of beta ig-h3, a novel gene induced in a human adenocarcinoma cell line after treatment with transforming growth factor-beta. *DNA Cell Biol.* 1992;11(7):511–522.
40. de la Chapelle A, Tolvanen R, Boysen G, et al. Gelsolin-derived familial amyloidosis caused by asparagine or tyrosine substitution for aspartic acid at residue 187. *Nat Genet.* 1992;2:157–160.
41. Meretoja J. Comparative histopathological and clinical findings in eyes with lattice corneal dystrophy of two different types. *Ophthalmologica.* 1972;165:15–37.
42. Levy E, Haltia M, Fernandez-Madrid I, et al. Mutation in gelsolin gene in Finnish hereditary amyloidosis. *J Exp Med.* 1990;172:1865–1867.
43. Folberg R, Alfonso E, Croxatto JO, et al. Clinically atypical granular corneal dystrophy with pathologic features of lattice-like amyloid deposits. A study of these families. *Ophthalmology.* 1988;95:46–51.
44. Klintworth GK, Vogel FS. Macular corneal dystrophy. An inherited acid mucopolysaccharide storage disease of the corneal fibroblast. *Am J Pathol.* 1964;45:565–586.
44a. Orr A, et al. Mutations in the UBIAD1 gene, encoding a potential prenyltransferase, are causal for Schnyder crystalline corneal dystrophy. *PLoS ONE.* 2007;2:e685.
44b. Yellore VS, et al. Identification of mutations in UBIAD1 following exclusion of coding mutations in the chromosome 1p36 locus for Schnyder crystalline corneal dystrophy. *Mol Vis.* 2007;13:1777–1782.
44c. Weiss JS, et al. Mutations in the UBIAD1 gene on chromosome short arm 1, region 36, cause Schnyder crystalline corneal dystrophy. *Invest Ophthalmol Vis Sci.* 2007;48:5007–5002.
45. Bredrup C, Knappskog PM, Majewski J, Rodahl E, Boman H. Congenital stromal dystrophy of the cornea caused by a mutation in the decorin gene. *Invest Ophthalmol Vis Sci.* 2005;46:420–426.
46. Purcell JJ Jr, Krachmer JH, Weingeist TA. Fleck corneal dystrophy. *Arch Ophthalmol.* 1977;95:440–444.
47. Li S, Tiab L, Jiao X, et al. Mutations in PIP5K3 are associated with Francois-Neetens mouchetée fleck corneal dystrophy. *Am J Hum Genet.* 2005;77:54–63.
48. Johnson AT, Folberg R, Vrabec MP, et al. The pathology of posterior amorphous corneal dystrophy. *Ophthalmology.* 1990;97:104–109.
49. Karp CL, Scott IU, Green WR, Chang TS, Culbertson WW. Central cloudy corneal dystrophy of Francois. A clinicopathologic study. *Arch Ophthalmol.* 1997;115:1058–1062.
50. Curran RE, Kenyon KR, Green WR. Pre-Descemet's membrane corneal dystrophy. *Am J Ophthalmol.* 1974;77:711–716.
51. Adamis AP, Filatov V, Tripathi BJ, Tripathi RC. Fuchs' endothelial dystrophy of the cornea. *Surv Ophthalmol.* 1993;38:149–168.
52. Krachmer JH, Purcell JJ Jr, Young CW, Bucher KD. Corneal endothelial dystrophy. A study of 64 families. *Arch Ophthalmol.* 1978;96:2036–2039.
53. Vithana EN, Morgan PE, Ramprasad V, et al. SLC4A11 mutations in Fuchs endothelial corneal dystrophy. *Hum Mol Genet;* 2008;17:656–666.
54. Sundin OH, Jun AS, Broman KW, et al. Linkage of late-onset Fuchs' corneal dystrophy to a novel locus at 13pTel-13q12.13. *Invest Ophthalmol Vis Sci.* 2006;47:140–145.
55. Sundin OH, Broman KW, Chang HH, et al. A common locus for late-onset Fuchs' corneal dystrophy maps to 18q21.2-q21.32. *Invest Ophthalmol Vis Sci.* 2006;47:3919–3926.
56. Aldave AJ, Rayner SA, Salem AK, et al. No pathogenic mutations identified in the COL8A1 and COL8A2 genes in familial Fuchs' corneal dystrophy. *Invest Ophthalmol Vis Sci.* 2006;47:3787–3790.
57. Gottsch JD, Sundin OH, Liu SH, et al. Inheritance of a novel COL8A2 mutation defines a distinct early-onset subtype of Fuchs' corneal dystrophy. *Invest Ophthalmol Vis Sci.* 2005;46:1934–1939.
58. Biswas S, Munier FL, Yardley J, et al. Missense mutations in COL8A2, the gene encoding the alpha2 chain of type VIII collagen, cause two forms of corneal endothelial dystrophy. *Hum Mol Genet.* 2001;10:2415–2423.
59. Magovern M, Beauchamp GR, McTigue JW, Fine BS, Baumiller RC. Inheritance of Fuchs' combined dystrophy. *Ophthalmology.* 1979;86:1897–1923.
60. Cibis GW, Krachmer JA, Phelps CD, Weingeist TA. The clinical spectrum of posterior polymorphous dystrophy. *Arch Ophthalmol.* 1977;95:1529–1537.
61. Boruchoff SA, Kuwabara T. Electron microscopy of posterior polymorphous degeneration. *Am J Ophthalmol.* 1971;72:879–887.
62. Rodrigues MM, Sun TT, Krachmer J, Newsome D. Epithelialization of the corneal endothelium in posterior polymorphous dystrophy. *Invest Ophthalmol Vis Sci.* 1980;19:832–835.
63. Merjava S, Liskova P, Sado Y, et al. Changes in the localization of collagens IV and VIII in corneas obtained from patients with posterior polymorphous corneal dystrophy. *Exp Eye Res.* 2009;88:945–952.
64. Héon E, Mathers W, Alward W, et al. Linkage of posterior polymorphous corneal dystrophy to 20q11. *Hum Mol Genet.* 1995;4:485–488.
65. Héon E, Greenberg A, Kopp KK, et al. VSX1: a gene for posterior polymorphous dystrophy and keratoconus. *Hum Mol Genet.* 2002;11:1029–1036.
66. Aldave AJ, Yellore VS, Principe AH, et al. Candidate gene screening for posterior polymorphous dystrophy. *Cornea.* 2005;24:151–155.
67. Liskova P, Tuft SJ, Gwilliam R, et al. Novel mutations in the ZEB1 gene identified in Czech and British patients with posterior polymorphous corneal dystrophy. *Hum Mutat.* 2007;28:638.
68. Hosseini SM, Herd S, Vincent AL, Héon E. Genetic analysis of chromosome 20-related posterior polymorphous corneal dystrophy: genetic heterogeneity and exclusion of three candidate genes. *Mol Vis.* 2008;14:71–80.
69. Kobayashi A, Fujiki K, Murakami A, et al. Analysis of COL8A2 gene mutation in Japanese patients with Fuchs' endothelial dystrophy and posterior polymorphous dystrophy. *Jpn J Ophthalmol.* 2004;48:195–198.
70. Yellore VS, Papp JC, Sobel E, et al. Replication and refinement of linkage of posterior polymorphous corneal dystrophy to the posterior polymorphous corneal dystrophy 1 locus on chromosome 20. *Genet Med.* 2007;9:228–234.
71. Krafchak CM, Pawar H, Moroi SE, et al. Mutations in TCF8 cause posterior polymorphous corneal dystrophy and ectopic expression of COL4A3 by corneal endothelial cells. *Am J Hum Genet.* 2005;77:694–708.
72. Shimizu S, Krafchak C, Fuse N, et al. A locus for posterior polymorphous corneal dystrophy (PPCD3) maps to chromosome 10. *Am J Med Genet A.* 2004;130:372–377.
73. Maumenee AE. Congenital hereditary corneal dystrophy. *Am J Ophthalmol.* 1960;60:1114–1124.
74. Kirkness CM, McCartney A, Rice NS, Garner A, Steele AD. Congenital hereditary corneal oedema of Maumenee: its clinical features, management, and pathology. *Br J Ophthalmol.* 1987;71:130–144.
75. Toma NM, Ebenezer ND, Inglehearn CF, et al. Linkage of congenital hereditary endothelial dystrophy to chromosome 20. *Hum Mol Genet.* 1995;4:2395–2398.
76. Hand CK, Harmon DL, Kennedy SM, et al. Localization of the gene for autosomal recessive congenital hereditary endothelial dystrophy (CHED2) to chromosome 20 by homozygosity mapping. *Genomics.* 1999;61:1–4.
77. Vithana EN, Morgan P, Sundaresan P, et al. Mutations in sodium-borate cotransporter SLC4A11 cause recessive congenital hereditary endothelial dystrophy (CHED2). *Nat Genet.* 2006;38:755–757.
78. Jiao X, Sultana A, Garg P, et al. Autosomal recessive corneal endothelial dystrophy (CHED2) is associated with mutations in SLC4A11. *J Med Genet.* 2007;44:64–68.

79. Ramprasad VL, Ebenezer ND, Aung T, et al. Novel SLC4A11 mutations in patients with recessive congenital hereditary endothelial dystrophy (CHED2). Mutation in brief #958. Online. *Hum Mutat.* 2007;28: 522–523.
80. Sultana A, Garg P, Ramamurthy B, Vemuganti GK, Kannabiran C. Mutational spectrum of the SLC4A11 gene in autosomal recessive congenital hereditary endothelial dystrophy. *Mol Vis.* 2007;13:1327–1332.
81. Aldave AJ, Yellore VS, Bourla N, et al. Autosomal recessive CHED associated with novel compound heterozygous mutations in SLC4A11. *Cornea.* 2007;26:896–900.
82. Desir J, Abramowicz M. Congenital hereditary endothelial dystrophy with progressive sensorineural deafness (Harboyan syndrome). *Orphanet J Rare Dis.* 2008;3:28.
83. Shah SS, Al-Rajhi A, Brandt JD, et al. Mutation in the SLC4A11 gene associated with autosomal recessive congenital hereditary endothelial dystrophy in a large Saudi family. *Ophthalmic Genet.* 2008;29:41–45.
84. Rabinowitz YS. Keratoconus. *Surv Ophthalmol.* 1998;42:297–319.
85. Etzine S. Conical cornea in identical twins. *S Afr Med J.* 1954;28: 154–155.
86. Franceschetti A, Lisch K, Klein D. Two pairs of identical twins concordant for keratoconus. *Klin Monatsbl Augenheilkd.* 1958;133:15–30.
87. Krachmer JH, Feder RS, Belin MW. Keratoconus and related noninflammatory corneal thinning disorders. *Surv Ophthalmol.* 1984;28:293–322.
88. Woillez M, Razemon P, Constantinides G: [A recent case of keratoconus in univitelline twins]. *Bull Soc Ophtalmol Fr.* 1976;76:279–281.
89. Owens H, Watters GA. Keratoconus in monozygotic twins in New Zealand. *Clin Exp Optometry.* 1995;78:125–129.
90. Parker J, Ko WW, Pavlopoulos G, et al. Videokeratography of keratoconus in monozygotic twins. *J Refract Surg.* 1996;12:180–183.
91. Falls HF, Allen AW. Dominantly inherited keratoconus. *J Genet Hum.* 1969;17:317–324.
92. Hammerstein W: [Genetics of conical cornea (author's transl)]. *Graefe's Arch Klin Exp Ophthalmol.* 1974;190:293–308.
93. Ihalainen A. Clinical and epidemiological features of keratoconus genetic and external factors in the pathogenesis of the disease. *Acta Ophthalmol Suppl.* 1986;178:1–64.
94. Rabinowitz YS, Garbus J, McDonnell PJ. Computer-assisted corneal topography in family members of patients with keratoconus. *Arch Ophthalmol.* 1990;108:365–371.
95. Gonzalez V, McDonnell PJ. Computer-assisted corneal topography in parents of patients with keratoconus. *Arch Ophthalmol.* 1992;110: 1413–1414.
96. Rabinowitz YS, Nesburn AB, McDonnell PJ. Videokeratography of the fellow eye in unilateral keratoconus. *Ophthalmology.* 1993;100: 181–186.
97. Sawaguchi S, Yue BY, Sugar J, Gilboy JE. Lysosomal enzyme abnormalities in keratoconus. *Arch Ophthalmol.* 1989,107:1507–1510.
98. Sawaguchi S, Twining SS, Yue BY, et al. Alpha 2-macroglobulin levels in normal human and keratoconus corneas. *Invest Ophthalmol Vis Sci.* 1994;35:4008–4014.
99. Wilson SE, He YG, Weng J, et al. Epithelial injury induces keratocyte apoptosis: hypothesized role for the interleukin-1 system in the modulation of corneal tissue organization and wound healing. *Exp Eye Res.* 1996;62:325–327.
100. Bron AJ, Rabinowitz YS. Corneal dystrophies and keratoconus. *Curr Opin Ophthalmol.* 1996;7:71–82.
101. Beckh U, Schonherr U, Naumann GO. [Autosomal dominant keratoconus as the chief ocular symptom in Lobstein osteogenesis imperfecta tarda]. *Klin Monatsbl Augenheilkd.* 1995;206:268–272.
102. Beardsley TL, Foulks GN. An association of keratoconus and mitral valve prolapse. *Ophthalmology.* 1982;89:35–37.
103. Beauchamp G, Knepper P. Role of neural crest in the anterior segment development and disease. *J Pediatr Ophthalmol Strabismus.* 1984; 12:209–214.
104. Sharif KW, Casey TA, Coltart J. Prevalence of mitral valve prolapse in keratoconus patients. *J R Soc Med.* 1992;85:446–448.
105. Cullen JF, Butler HG. Mongolism (Down's syndrome) and keratoconus. *Br J Ophthalmol.* 1963;47:321–330.
106. Krachmer J, Feder RS, Belin MW. Keratoconus and related noninflammatory corneal thinning disorders. *Surv Ophthalmol.* 1984;28:293–322.
107. Shapiro MB, France TD. The ocular features of Down's syndrome. *Am J Ophthalmol.* 1985;99:659–663.
108. Cantor RM. Analysis of genetic data: methods and interpretation. In: King RA, Rotter JI, Motulsky AG, eds. *The genetic basis of common diseases.* New York: Oxford University Press; 1992:49–72.
109. Alstrom CH, Olson O. Heredo-retinopathia congenitalis. Monohybride recessiva autosomalis, *Hereditas Genttiskt.* 1957;43:672–676.
110. Elder MJ. Leber conetial amaurosis and its association with keratoconus and keratoglobus. *J Pediatr Ophthalmol Strabismus.* 1994;31:38–40.
111. Aldave AJ, Yellore VS, Salem AK, et al. No VSX1 gene mutations associated with keratoconus. *Invest Ophthalmol Vis Sci.* 2006;47:2820–2822.
112. Gajecka M, Radhakrishna U, Winters D, et al. Localization of a gene for keratoconus to a 5.6-Mb interval on 13q32. *Invest Ophthalmol Vis Sci.* 2009;50:1531–1539.
113. Mackey DA, Buttery RG, Wise GM, Denton MJ. Description of X-linked megalocornea with identification of the gene locus. *Arch Ophthalmol.* 1991;109:829–833.
114. Chen JD, Mackey DA, Fuller H, et al. X-linked megalocornea: close linkage to DXS87 and DXS94. *Hum Genet.* 1989;83:292–294.
115. Pellegata NS, Dieguez-Lucena JL, Joensuu T, et al. Mutations in KERA, encoding keratocan, cause cornea plana. *Nat Genet.* 2000;25:91–95.
116. Aldave AJ, Sonmez B, Bourla N, et al. Autosomal dominant cornea plana is not associated with pathogenic mutations in DCN, DSPG3, FOXC1, KERA, LUM, or PITX2. *Ophthalmic Genet.* 2007;28:57–67.

Chapter 13

Keratometry and Topography

Carlos E. Martinez, Stephen D. Klyce

Vision scientists have examined the shape of the cornea for over 300 years. The study of corneal curvature began in 1619 when Father Christoph Scheiner compared the reflections of window panes on marbles of known size to those reflections from the cornea to determine corneal curvature.[1] In 1839, Kohlraush introduced a telescope with adjustable mires to measure reflected images from the cornea.[2] In 1854, Helmholtz extended this work and constructed a complex instrument that he called an ophthalmometer,[3] which measured the curvatures of the cornea, the lens, and other dimensions of the eye. In 1881, Javal and Schiotz introduced a simplified ophthalmometer for clinical use.[4] This simplified the cumbersome Helmholtz instrument into a practical clinical tool to rapidly measure corneal astigmatism. The designation of the Javal instrument as an ophthalmometer was a misnomer since the adaptation of the Helmholtz instrument measured only the cornea and not the other parts of the eye.[5] Hence, the instrument was renamed the keratometer, which to this day is used to measure the curvature of the principal corneal meridians. In effect, many topographers currently used are based on the basic principles used by keratometers: the measurement of patterns reflected from the corneal surface. However, the real cornea is not well described by keratometry, which measures the curvature of the two principal meridians from only four locations on the cornea. Corneas are radially asymmetric, aspheric, and may be irregular.[6] This is particularly true for corneas of patients who have undergone keratorefractive surgery.

The rapid expansion of keratorefractive surgery over the last three decades has highlighted the need to measure corneal shape over a large area. Measuring corneal topography is now a fundamental part of evaluating patients preoperatively as well as understanding the basis for visual complaints after surgery. In this chapter, fundamentals of keratometry and corneal topography will be explored and their applications and limitations will be discussed. The discussion is illustrated with examples of corneal topography commonly seen in clinical practice.

Keratometry

Keratometry describes a method to measure the two principal meridional radii of curvature of the central cornea. The keratometer does this by measuring the size of mire reflections from the corneal surface. Each meridian of the central cornea is considered a section of a spherical convex reflecting mirror. From geometric optics, the magnification equation is:

$$\frac{h'}{h} = \frac{f}{x} \qquad (1)$$

where h' is the height of the virtual image of the mires, h is the physical height of the mire, f is the focal length of the mirror, and x is the distance from the mires to the principal focus.

The focal length (f) of a convex mirror is given by:

$$f = r/2 \qquad (2)$$

where r is the radius of curvature. Then

$$\frac{h'}{h} = \frac{r}{2x}$$

or

$$r = \frac{2xh'}{h} \qquad (3)$$

Since the distance (x) from the mires to the focal point of the mirror surface is not known, the distance from the mire to the surface is used (d).

$$r = \frac{2dh'}{h} \qquad (4)$$

This dimension, d, is generally called the working distance and is a reasonable approximation as long as the distance from the mire to the surface is large compared to the focal length of the surface. Since the distance (d) from the keratometer to the surface (the cornea) can be fixed and the height of the mire (h) is known, one can solve for the radius of curvature (r) by measuring the size of the virtual image (h'). The keratometer is calibrated with measurements on test balls. Since the central area of the *normal* cornea is nearly spherical, and the keratometer is designed to measure the curvature of the principal meridians at a 3–4-mm diameter, K readings can provide accurate measurements of curvature and cylinder within the pupil.

Although the radius of corneal curvature is useful for fitting contact lenses, corneal power is generally more useful for diagnostics and ontraocular lens (IOL) calculations.

Corneal power can be calculated from the radius of curvature:

$$P = \frac{(n' - n)}{r} \quad (5)$$

where P is the corneal power, n' is the corneal index of refraction and n is the index of refraction of air (1.000), and r is the corneal radius of curvature in meters. The index of refraction of the cornea is generally taken as 1.376. However, because the keratometer attempts to estimate the total refractive power of the cornea and not just the air–tear interface, a value of 1.3375 is generally used instead of the corneal index of refraction. This is called the keratometric index, an effective index of refraction, which accounts for the small negative power introduced by the endothelial surface. On average, the anterior cornea has a refractive power of +48 diopters (D) of convergence and the posterior cornea of −5 D of divergence. Thus, equation (5) becomes:

$$P = \frac{(1.3375 - 1.000)}{r} = \frac{0.3375}{r} \quad (6)$$

The keratometric index makes several approximations including the assumption of spherical radii of curvature for the anterior and posterior corneal surfaces. Corneal surgery or pathology that results in a significant alteration in corneal thickness or changes in the curvature of the anterior and/or posterior cornea will introduce errors in this power relationship. For this reason, K-values used in intraocular lens calculations should not be measured with keratometry in eyes that have undergone keratorefractive surgery or are irregular for any other reason;[7] average central corneal power indices are available on several corneal topographers for this purpose.

Corneal Topography

To extend measurement coverage of the corneal surface beyond the capabilities of the keratometer, the modern corneal topographer emerged via a series of instrument developments that began with the keratoscope, followed by the photokeratoscope, and finally the videokeratoscope. The videokeratoscope combines video capture of corneal images with computer processing to provide maps of the corneal surface power distribution. This is now called the corneal topographer. All of these use a more complete target to examine a wider area of the cornea than the keratometer. The most common target configuration used is still the circular mire pattern that characterized the Placido disk introduced by Antonio Placido in 1880.[8] The Placido disk consists of a target with concentric rings that alternate black and white mires with a central aperture through which the clinician could view the virtual image.

Photokeratoscopes that captured the Placido reflections from the corneal surface were useful for demonstrating irregular astigmatism in corneal grafts and the surface distortion in moderate keratoconus, but only qualitative information could be obtained, and the more modest corneal shape distortions that had a visual impact could not be detected by simple visual inspection of the mires (Fig. 13.1). Doss and associates published one of the first methods for calculating corneal power quantitatively from a photokeratoscope.[9] Klyce extended this approach and explored methods of representing the results to a clinical audience.[10] Further advances led to instrumentation that resulted in the video capture of Placido disk images, the automatic detection of the mires, and calculation of corneal shape and power distribution. These led to the development of the modern corneal topographer and the representation of corneal power with the color-coded contour map introduced by Maguire and associates.[11]

The development of widespread keratorefractive surgery in the 1980s was the impetus for this progress in corneal topography. The introduction of the personal computer (PC) helped make these systems available and useful in diagnosing pathology as well as understanding visual complaints with the early techniques of radial keratotomy and photorefractive keratectomy. Corneal topography has been essential to the development and evaluation of new techniques for refractive surgery. In the screening of refractive surgical can-

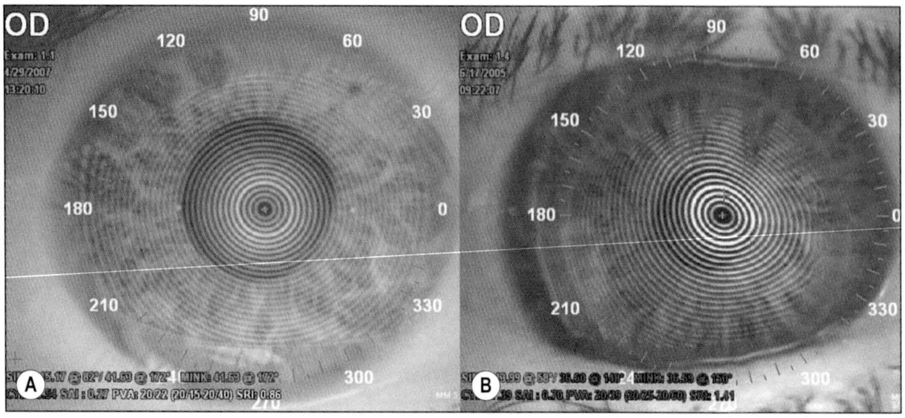

Fig. 13.1 Videokeratographs of astigmatic corneas. (**A**) This cornea has 3.54 D of keratometric cylinder, but this cannot be detected by visual inspection of the mires. (**B**) This cornea is status post-penetrating keratoplasty after suture removal with a residual of 7.39 D of keratometric cylinder. Note that the elliptical nature of the mires are notable in **B** with over 7 D of cylinder, but not in **A**. Computerized analysis is necessary since astigmatism less than about 4 D cannot be easily detected by observing the mires.

didates, corneal topography has become the standard of care.

Since the introduction of Placido-based topography, other methods to measure corneal shape have been explored. These technologies included scanning slit technology, raster stereography,[12] scanning high-frequency ultrasound,[13] holography, Fourier profilometry, and optical coherence tomography.[14] Two approaches are in general use currently: the Placido disk or reflection-based topographers, and the scanning slit-based tomographers.*

Placido disk-based topographers

Corneal topographers capture their images of the cornea with digital video cameras. The resolution of the different Placido disk-based topographers depends on the number and width of the mires. In general, the larger the spacing between the mires, the more interpolation between samples data points will be necessary. However, in clinical practice, 'fine' mire and 'wide' mire topographers can produce very similar topography displays (Fig. 13.2).

There are two different design types of Placido topographers: those with large-diameter targets and those with small, cone-type targets. The former have longer working distances and their respective larger targets help minimize issues related to alignment and focusing. Instruments with smaller targets and shorter working distances generally have sensitive focusing aids to achieve accuracy and repeatability. Images from the systems with larger targets are more likely to be affected by shadows from the nose and eyebrows that can produce inferonasal and superior areas that are be analyzed.

Placido disk reflection topographers are sensitive to disruptions in the tear film. Excessively increasing the amount of time between a blink and the time of capture can cause normal spherocylindrical corneas to exhibit irregularities.[15] The corneal topography examination should be done before drops are used or intraocular pressure is measured to maintain a regular, intact tear film. However, accommodation will not affect corneal topography in normal or keratoconic corneas,[16] while there may be a small effect of eyelid pressure on the corneal shape.[17] The eyelids cause a small amount of corneal distortion, primarily confined to the superior and inferior extrapupillary regions, and therefore have minimal effect on central corneal shape during the blink.

Slit scanning tomography

Corneal shape and thickness can be measured with the scanning slit beam. Placido topography utilizes the first Purkinje image reflected from the corneal surface. Under these conditions, the second Purkinje image from the endothelial surface of the cornea is not detectable with current instruments. With slit beam technology, light scatter from both corneal surfaces can be viewed, as is routinely done during a slit lamp examination. Because the elevation

*Strictly speaking, when slit data is used to calculate corneal power from shape measurements, this process is tomography.

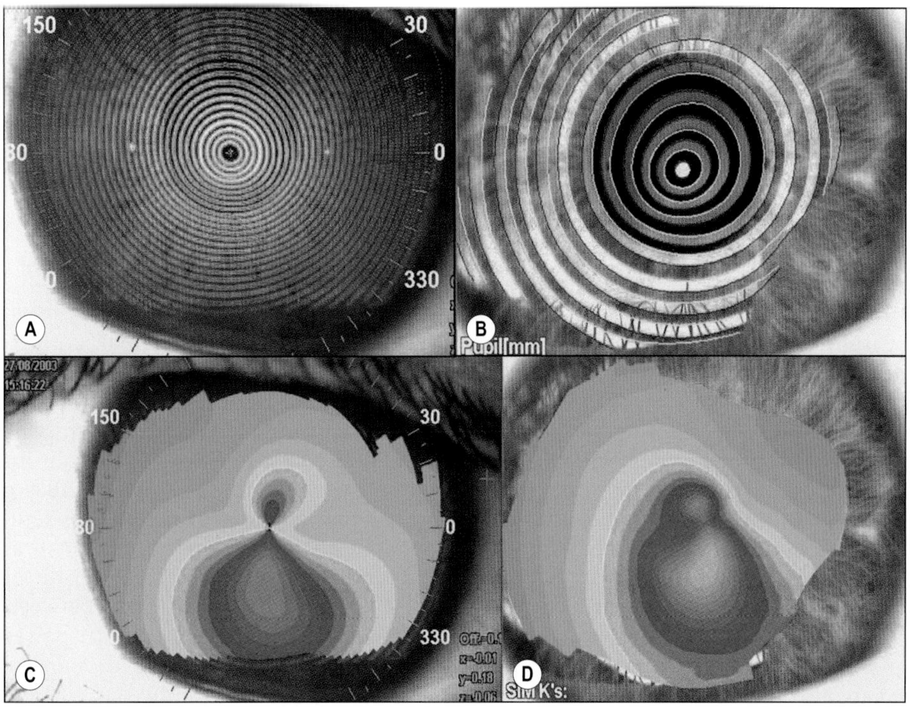

Fig. 13.2 Corneal topographers with different mire characteristics can produce similar results. (**A**) A fine mire topographer (NIDEK Magellan). The green dots show the found edges of each mire. (**B**) Color map of **A** shows a classic keratoconus pattern. (**C**) Wide mire topography (NIDEK OPD-Scan) of another keratoconus cornea. (Note the areas of missing mires caused by shadows from the brow and nose.) (**D**) Color map of **C** using the same color scale as in **B**.

of each surface can be measured directly with slit beam technology, no shape approximation errors should arise, as with some of the early Placido disk-based devices. Slit scanning tomographers project a series of slit beams at regular intervals. The successive images are captured with a digital camera over the course of 1–2 seconds. Image analysis is used to determine locations of points on the corneal surfaces. These data can then be processed to determine shape characteristics of both corneal surfaces as well as the thickness of the cornea. There are several instruments commercially available that use this method. The more widely distributed are the Orbscan (Model IIz, Bausch & Lomb, Rochester, NY) and the Pentacam (Model HR, Oculus, Inc., Wetzlar, Germany). The Orbscan is a hybrid system – both a topographer and a tomographer – that uses Placido disk technology to display conventional corneal topography, while the Pentacam derives corneal topography from the slit beam elevation data. Both instruments measure anterior and posterior surface elevations with scanning slits for the determination of corneal thickness. The Orbscan uses the projection of slit beams at 45-degree angles 20 times on each side of the video axis. This is done in two 0.75-second intervals. Note, however, that the cornea is in constant motion from microsaccadic movements and thus the entire image acquisition should ideally take less than 30 ms.

The Pentacam uses a scanning slit but with Scheimpflug optics, which increases the depth of focus. In doing so, simultaneous imaging of the cornea, lens, and iris is possible; this permits corneal, anterior chamber, and lens geometry to be imaged and analyzed. The Scheimpflug camera and a monochromatic slit light source rotate around the eye 180 degrees in 2 seconds, producing 25 images of the front and back surfaces of the cornea. Up to 25 000 elevation points are used to give a 3-D representation of the cornea. As with the Orbscan, the data must be translated and aligned to reduce errors due to eye movement during acquisition.

Calculations and Surface Reconstruction

Placido disk

Since curvature is generally calculated along meridians, the image of the Placido target is digitized and the radial positions of points along the mires are determined every 1 degree (see Fig. 13.2A,C). Computer algorithms are then used to calculate corneal curvatures that are consistent with the shapes of the mires. Again, close spacing of the mires will indicate a relatively steep portion of the cornea, while broadly spaced mires overlie regions of low power. This relationship is very clear in Figure 13.2 (compare the mires and curvature displays within the superior portion of the pupil to those within the lower portion of the pupil in C and D). The algorithms used to calculate corneal curvatures vary considerably among the different Placido-based topographers, but with proper consideration, good accuracy can be achieved.[18]

The keratometer suffers from the assumption that corneas are spherocylindrical. Corneal topographers are also usually calibrated using spherical test surfaces. However, modern calibration and the test surfaces used include shapes that are spherical, elliptical, and toric.[19] Using these can help evaluate the adequacy of certain corneal topographers in faithfully reproducing the topography of aberrated corneas. Obscure details of corneal topography that are important to understand certain aberrations that occur after corneal surgery need to be presented accurately in order to manage difficult cases. In particular, accurate portrayal of corneal shape is essential as excimer laser surgery adopts algorithms for corneal topography-guided ablations.

Slit scanning technology

The scanning slit systems capture light that is diffusely scattered from the two corneal surfaces and the obtained elevation data are used to calculate power in diopters from equation (5) above. For these topographers to calculate curvature with sufficient accuracy to differentiate between two curves that differ by 0.25 D, the resolution of this system needs to be less than 1 microns (μm).[20] However, this is difficult to achieve since the sensitivity of the slit scanning systems to changes in corneal power is some 20 times less than that of a Placido-based corneal topographer.

An additional challenge using slit-derived elevation data for calculation of curvature and power for the posterior corneal surface is that there is a lack of calibration surfaces. These must have dual surfaces from materials that mimic corneal scattering; this presents a problem.[21] The accuracy of slit-based posterior elevation maps and pachymetric maps has not yet been resolved because of this.

Presentation Methods

Color-coded maps

A graphic representation of the topographic distribution of local corneal dioptric power values can be achieved by presenting the results as a color-coded topographic map.[22] The 'warmer' colors represent higher dioptric powers (steeper curvatures), while the 'cooler' colors are used to represent the lower dioptric powers (flatter curvatures). Similar color-coded maps can be used to present changes in elevation.

The Normal Cornea

In 1989, Dingeldein and Klyce studied normal corneas with uncorrected vision of 20/20.[23] They found that the cornea does flatten towards the periphery and that the rate of peripheral flattening varies significantly amongst individuals. They also found that the color-coded contour maps of each individual have a unique pattern, like a fingerprint. Moreover, the topographies of fellow eyes tend to be mirror images of each other (enantiomorphs) as shown in Figures 13.3 and 13.4. A final characteristic of normal corneas is that even with these variations between individuals, normal corneas have relatively smooth power contours.

The scale used to display corneal topography is extremely important both for diagnostic purposes as well as to

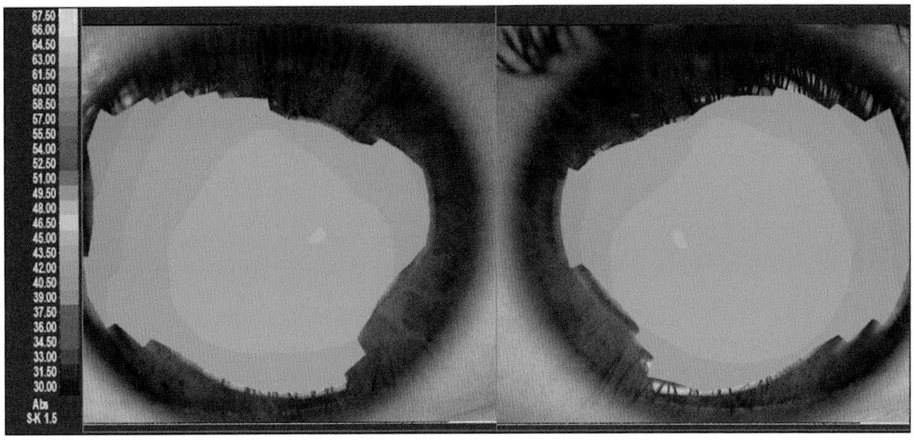

Fig. 13.3 Color-coded contour map from Placido-based topographies of an individual's normal corneas. Note the scale and color palette used are the universal standard scale from Smolek et al.[24] Note the nonsuperimposable mirror image symmetry. The underlying image of the eye is important to relate topographic features to the corneal surface.

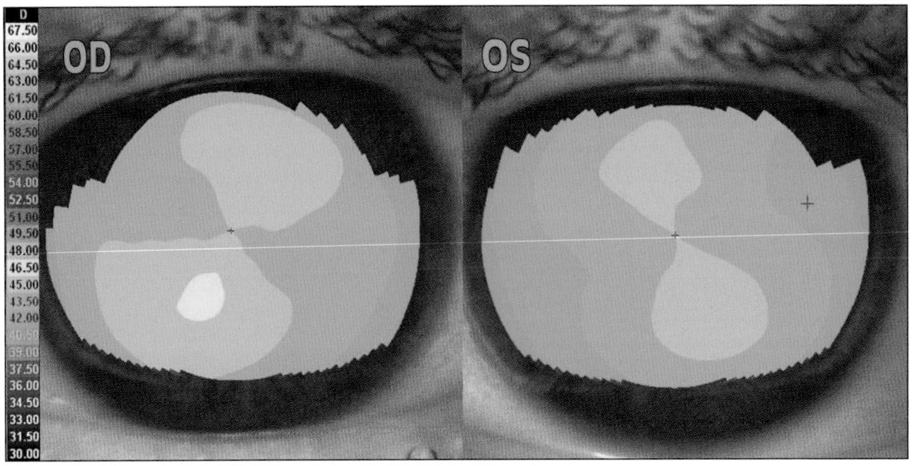

Fig. 13.4 Placido-based topography showing regular oblique astigmatism. Note how fellow eyes tend to be mirror images of each other.

appreciate features that might reduce vision. Most corneal topographers have implemented adjustable scales that allow the user to increase or decrease the sensitivity as well as the range of dioptric power. In addition, most corneal topographers allow the user to choose a self-adapting or normalized scale which will display every cornea with the same color range irrespective of its condition. The use of smaller dioptric intervals and a narrower range of powers may lead to a distracting amount of noise. On the opposite extreme, scales with broad dioptric intervals can lead to smoothing and masking of irregular astigmatism. The most effective color palette and dioptric interval has been evaluated in several studies (the Absolute Scale,[11] the Klyce/Wilson Scale,[22] and finally the Universal Standard Scale[24]). The Universal Standard Scale has been adopted by the ANSI standard on corneal topography.[19] With this scale, features such as regular corneal astigmatism can be visualized (Fig. 13.5) while masking corneal details irrelevant to interpretation. This scale is compared to other scales and different methods for corneal power calculation in Figure 13.6.

Axial Curvature Maps

The axial dioptric power map was the first standard method for presenting corneal topography. Axial power represents corneal curvature in a way similar to keratometry. The size of mires reflected from the corneal surface are determined and analyzed as if emanating from a sphere. Axial power is useful clinically because it relates corneal power to corneal shape. The cornea has a prolate shape, which means that it is steeper in the center than in the periphery; this helps compensate for spherical aberration. Axial power presents itself in the same manner: that is, higher in the center than in the periphery. For these reasons, axial power maps are the preferred clinical default for presenting corneal topography for routine diagnostic and screening purposes.

Refractive Power Map

Most clinicians are used to thinking of the cornea in terms of refractive power since that relates to corrective lenses as

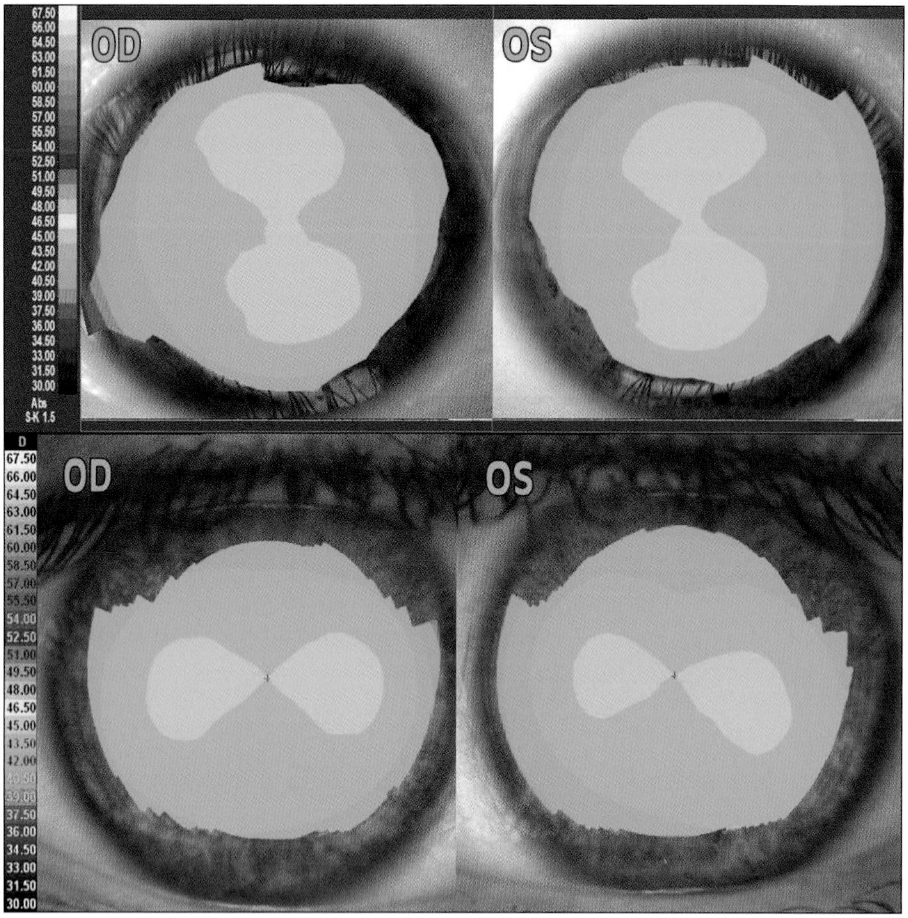

Fig. 13.5 Placido-based topography of astigmatism. *Top*: with-the-rule cylinder both eyes. *Bottom*: against-the-rule astigmatism. Note the classic bow tie shape of astigmatism on Placido-based topography which makes it easily recognizable.

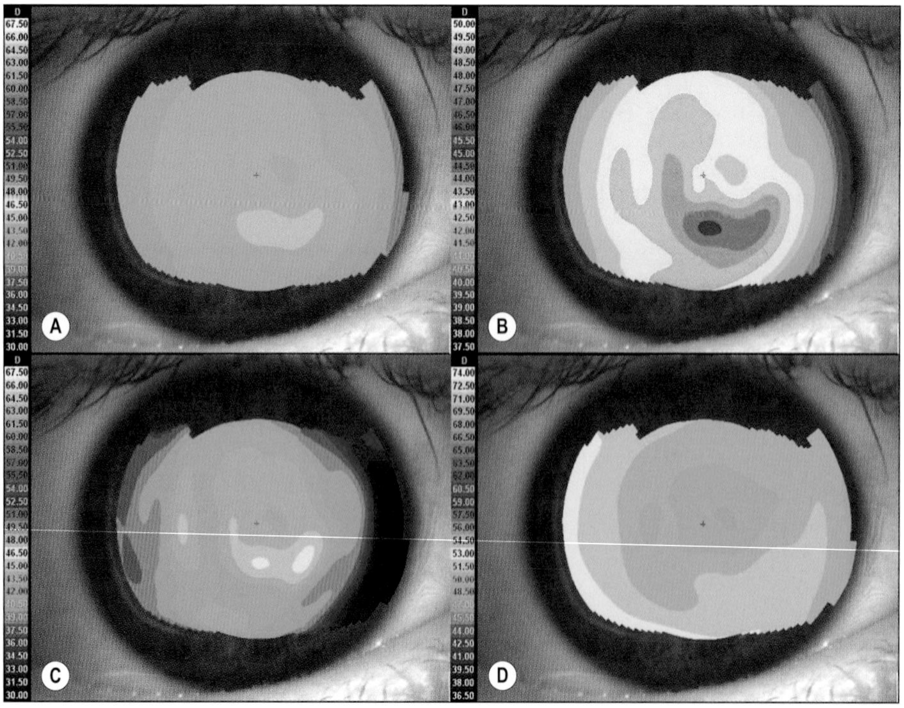

Fig. 13.6 Using different scales and different power calculations can confuse interpretation of corneal topography. The topographies in this figure are all presentations of the same data. (**A**) Normal corneal topography presented with axial power and the 1.5-D contour interval Universal Standard Scale.[41] (**B**) Axial power map with 0.5-D contour intervals. This gives the appearance of irregular astigmatism in this normal cornea. (**C**) Power map using tangential or instantaneous power calculation. Again, details are shown that confuse interpretation. (**D**) Power map using the calculation of refractive corneal power with Snell's Law. This true power calculation is useful for ray tracing, but obscures the relation of power to corneal shape: that the cornea flattens toward the periphery.

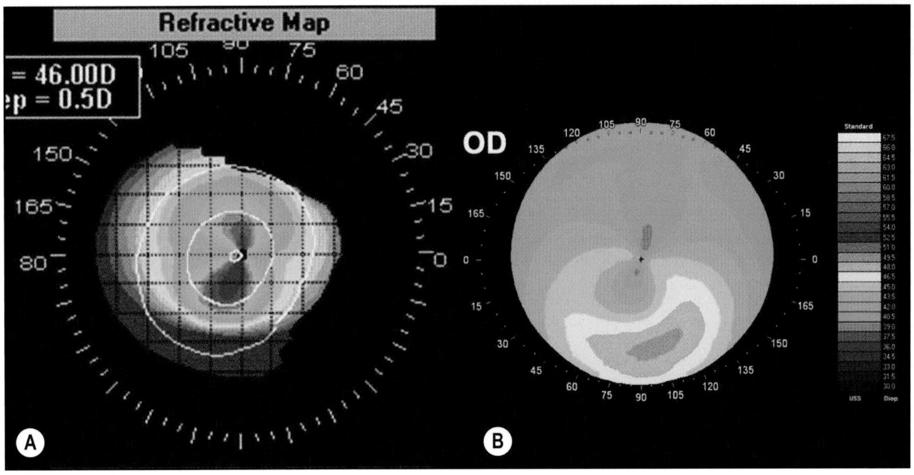

Fig. 13.7 The refractive power map can obscure the peripheral steepening characteristic of keratoconus and pellucid marginal degeneration. (**A**) Preoperative refractive power map of patient who developed ectasia subsequent to LASIK. The map can be interpreted as against-the-rule cylinder, but the inferior steepening is muted by the method. (**B**) Axial power map of a similar topography clearly showing the inferior steepening and 'C' shape in topography characteristic of pellucid marginal degeneration.

well as amounts of correction in refractive surgery. While axial power maps convey shape information, they are not a true representation of the refractive power of the cornea except centrally over the photopic pupil. Refractive power is calculated with Snell's Law; hence, as the angle of incidence of the incoming rays increases in the corneal periphery, the power increases. When this method is used to calculate corneal power, the normal cornea will have a higher calculated power peripherally than in the center (see Fig. 13.6D). This is due to the natural residual spherical aberration of the cornea. A spherical cornea would exhibit an even higher peripheral refractive power than the normal prolate cornea. The measurement of corneal spherical aberration is of importance in the choice of an aspheric intraocular lens.

Caveat: With the refractive power map, as noted above, there is an increased calculated power in the corneal periphery. Keratoconus and pellucid marginal degeneration are frequently expressed as inferior peripheral steepening; the use of the refractive power map can mask these pathologies. An example of such a case that resulted in ectasia following LASIK surgery is illustrated in Figure 13.7.

Instantaneous or Tangential Power Map

Another method for calculating corneal power is through the use of the instantaneous radius of curvature or tangential power map. The second derivative of the shape of the surface is used to calculate curvature in this method,[20] which can introduce mathematical noise or fluctuations in power values. The instantaneous power map is not recommended for routine clinical use because the measurement noise can obscure the true optical quality of a cornea. For example, the normal cornea shown in Figure 13.6C with this type of power calculation appears irregular even though the cornea has 20/15 visual potential. However, tangential power maps are extremely useful in the demonstration and measurement of the optical zone size in modern refractive surgery as they emphasize transition zone power changes (Fig. 13.8).

Difference Maps

Certain changes in corneal topography with time can be usefully explored by subtracting one map from another. For example, when following a keratoconus patient, it is of paramount importance, particularly with current corneal cross linking therapy, to make a prediction as to whether a cornea should be stabilized before functional vision is lost. Progression of keratoconus can be followed with difference maps and the consequences of refractive surgery evaluated (Fig. 13.9). When using differences maps, careful registration of the data may be necessary to reduce the positional errors due to microsaccades.

Elevation Maps

Except in the case of advanced disease such as keratoconus, distortions of corneal shape displayed with elevation data cannot be seen without amplification. Hence, elevation maps are generally displayed with reference to some standard shape. Commonly, the best-fitting sphere or toroidal surface is subtracted from the elevation data. However, there is no single known geometric shape that can approximate the cornea over its entirety.[25]

The Orbscan allows a choice of reference surface type, shape, size, and alignment as well as elevation direction. The Pentacam allows the user to use a best-fit sphere or an ellipsoid. Elevation maps generally use green to indicate zero difference from the reference surface. Warmer colors (red) represent areas higher than the reference surface and cooler

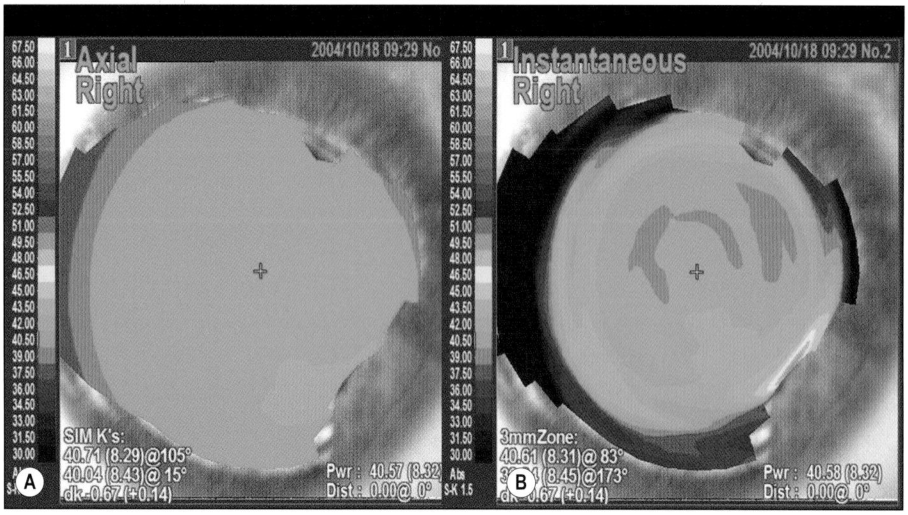

Fig. 13.8 Corneal topography of a −2.00 D LASIK treatment. (**A**) With the standard axial map, details of the treatment are obscure. (**B**) Using the tangential map, the transition zone between the treated area and the peripheral cornea is clearly demarcated.

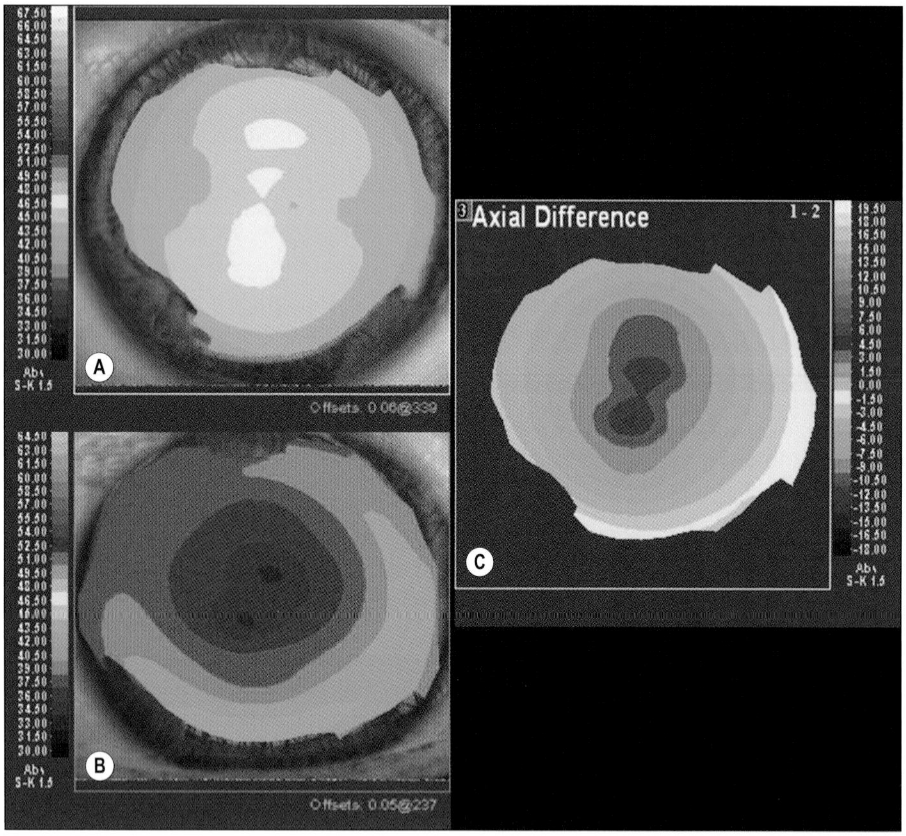

Fig. 13.9 The difference map can be used to confirm the power change induced by laser treatment. (**A**) Preoperative map of a cornea showing with-the-rule corneal cylinder. (**B**) Note the circular nature of the profile in the postoperative LASIK map. (**C**) The difference clearly shows the characteristics of the toric ablation used to reduce cylinder.

colors (blue) areas below the reference surface. For anterior and posterior elevation maps, Tanabe et al. addressed the issue of scale and suggested that 10-µm and 20-µm scales for the anterior and posterior elevation maps, respectively, appear most suitable.[26]

It has been suggested that changes in posterior corneal elevation might be the initial changes that can be detected in keratoconus.[27] Mean posterior corneal elevation has been studied in an effort to distinguish keratoconic corneas from normal corneas.[28] Posterior elevation values can be used to

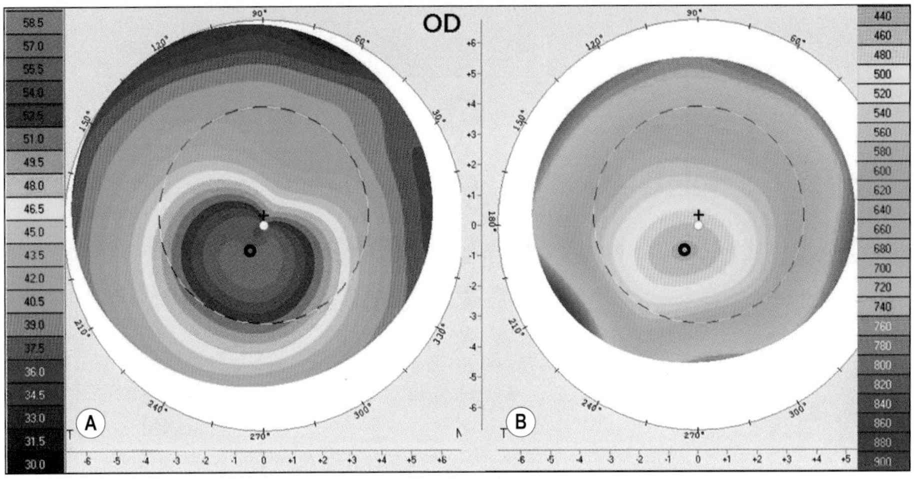

Fig. 13.10 Correlation of axial topography (**A**) and pachymetry (**B**) with the Pentacam. The dashed circle indicates the pupil margin and its center is marked with a cross. The filled white circle is the axis of the instrument while the empty black circle indicates the thinnest point.

distinguish normal and keratoconic corneas, but posterior elevations are not sensitive enough a measure to separately classify forme fruste keratoconus and normal corneas.

Pachymetric Maps

The slit-based tomographers have shown that the thinnest areas of the corneal stroma are generally inferotemporal to the fixation-reflex axis. Orbscan pachymetric central measurements tend to correlate with ultrasound measurements although they are consistently thicker by about 30 μm.[29,30] This offset may change for corneas after refractive surgery,[31,32] very thick corneas,[33] and for corneas in their periphery.[34] The Orbscan allows the user to shift all pachymetric measurements by a single acoustic factor in order to more closely match ultrasound measurements. However, the relationship between Orbscan pachymetry and ultrasound pachymetry may not be proportionate throughout the corneal thickness. Therefore, a single acoustic factor cannot be used on all measurements made by the Orbscan to equate the measurements made by the ultrasound pachymeter.[34,35] The factory-calibrated Pentacam may correlate better with ultrasound than the Orbscan after refractive surgery.[36] The important clinical advantage of slit scanning technology is that it provides a data-rich global map of corneal thickness which exceeds the normal capabilities of manual ultrasound measurements (Fig. 13.10).

Quantitative indices

Color-coded contour maps are very useful for diagnostics by recognition of patterns and by color association. Examples include the bowtie pattern that denotes corneal astigmatism and the red areas associated with moderate to advanced keratoconus cones. However, in order to derive quantitative measurements from corneal topography examinations, a number of statistical indices have been derived. The first of these was Simulated Keratometry or the SimKs SimK1 and SimK2.[37] To mimic keratometry, these indices report the power derived from the corneal topography principal meridians at the four points 3–4 mm apart, just where the keratometer mires would fall on a cornea. SimKs are important indices the clinician has been trained to use for numerous tasks from diagnostics to contact lens fitting.

Standard keratometry agrees with SimK values. Placido disk-based measurements of surfaces with marked and frequent curvature changes can provide repeatable measurements.[38] On the other hand, slit scanning systems can have artifacts of asymmetric topography which can confuse interpretation.

Keratometry by itself is not a good predictor of the visual potential of the eye as it does not evaluate the central cornea. Moreover, the simple visual inspection of irregularities in the power contours of a topography map cannot be used directly to predict their effect on visual acuity. The irregularity of the corneal topography over the pupil was developed with the Surface Regularity Index (SRI).[39] SRI is correlated to potential visual acuity and is a measure of local fluctuations in central corneal power. When the SRI is elevated, the corneal surface ahead of the entrance pupil will be irregular, leading to a reduction in best spectacle-corrected visual acuity. High SRI values are found with dry eyes, contact lens wear, trauma, and penetrating keratoplasty. Large amounts of corneal astigmatism that are induced with corneal grafts can be corrected to some extent with cylindrical lenses, but it is the irregular astigmatism (higher-order aberrations) that is often the major source of visual loss in these patients. SRI has been implemented on a number of corneal topography systems including models produced by Tomey Corp. (Nagoya, Japan) and by NIDEK, Inc. (Gamagori, Japan). Indices such as the Central Irregularity Measure, or CIM, displayed by the Humphrey Atlas (Carl Zeiss Meditec, Inc., Jena, Germany) corneal topographer have been developed as a similar means to understand the visual impact of irregularities in corneal topography. The Orbscan offers a surface irregularity index from its Placido data as well which is the statistical sum of the standard deviations of the curvatures in the mean and astigmatic power maps over a certain area.

Fourier transforms and Zernike polynomials are also quantitative descriptors of corneal surface and can be used

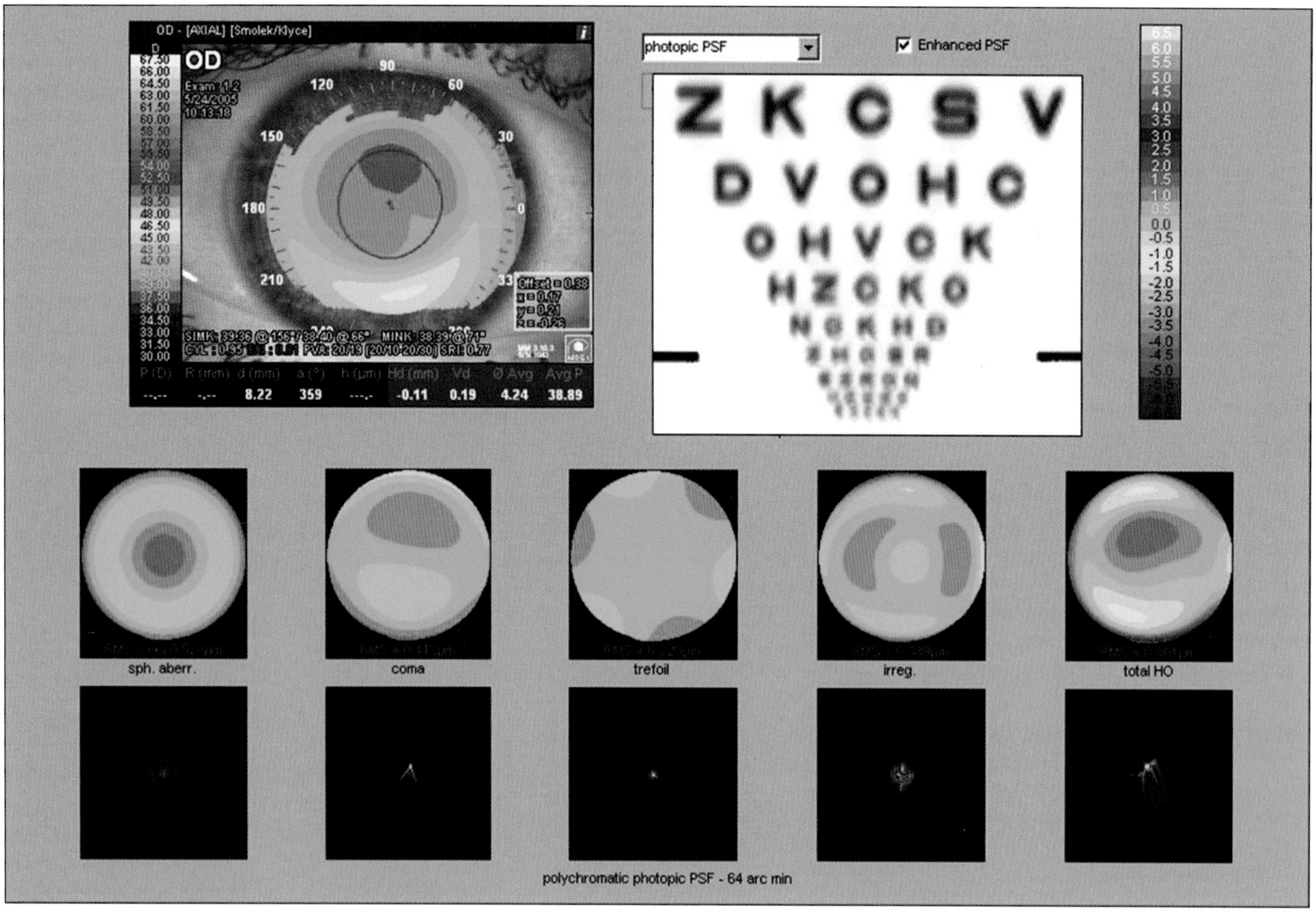

Fig. 13.11 Corneal wavefront analysis of a LASIK procedure with the NIDEK Magellan topographer. Using an aperture of 4.5 mm simulating the pupil of this eye under photopic conditions, vision is 20/20 (fourth line up from the bottom of the Snellen Chart segment). The blue circle outlines the pupil on the corneal topography map in the upper left. Zernike analysis allows display of (left to right) spherical aberration, coma, trefoil, residual higher-order aberrations, and total higher-order aberrations. The color scale in the upper right of the figure has a range of −6.5 to +6.5 mm of RMS wavefront error and corresponds to the wavefront displays. The lowest set of displays is a polychromatic representation of the point spread function for each of the individual aberration displays.

to calculate the aberrations of the cornea.[40–42] Point spread, optical transfer, and wave aberration functions have been used to measure optical quality of the eye, and these can be obtained from corneal measurements. Zernike coefficients can also be used to describe corneal aberrations. These are derived from conversion of corneal topography to corneal wavefront; the method is very useful for the presentation and evaluation of corneal optics (Figs 13.11, 13.12).

Corneal topography indices and screening methods

Topographic indices have been developed and used for corneal classification and screening. One of the first topographic indices developed for keratoconus detection is the I-S value introduced by Rabinowitz and McDonnell.[43] This index is helpful to recognize levels of corneal topographic asymmetry that are abnormal and are consistent with suspect keratoconus or clinical keratoconus. Additional sophistication was added with the recognition that central cones would not be detected with the I-S index, and that some keratoconus patterns involved skewing of the radial axes.[44] Since the topography of disorders characterized by corneal ectasia such as keratoconus and pellucid marginal degeneration can take several appearances (Figs 13.13–13.18), other indices were developed to detect specific patterns seen in keratoconus, and artificial intelligence techniques were used to recognize not only keratoconus but also several other abnormal corneal conditions (Fig. 13.19).[45–49]

As with most tests, patient history is of paramount importance. Contact lens warpage can mimic mild keratoconus and needs to be ruled out.[50] Patients who have with-the-rule corneal astigmatism are particularly at risk for the development of pseudo-keratoconus from contact lens wear, particularly from the wear of rigid lenses. To differentiate between contact lens-induced corneal asymmetry and true keratoconus, it is necessary for the patient to discontinue contact lens wear completely, and to be reexamined at intervals of 2–3 weeks until the corneal topography stabilizes. In general, if the asymmetry is due to contact lens wear, the cornea will

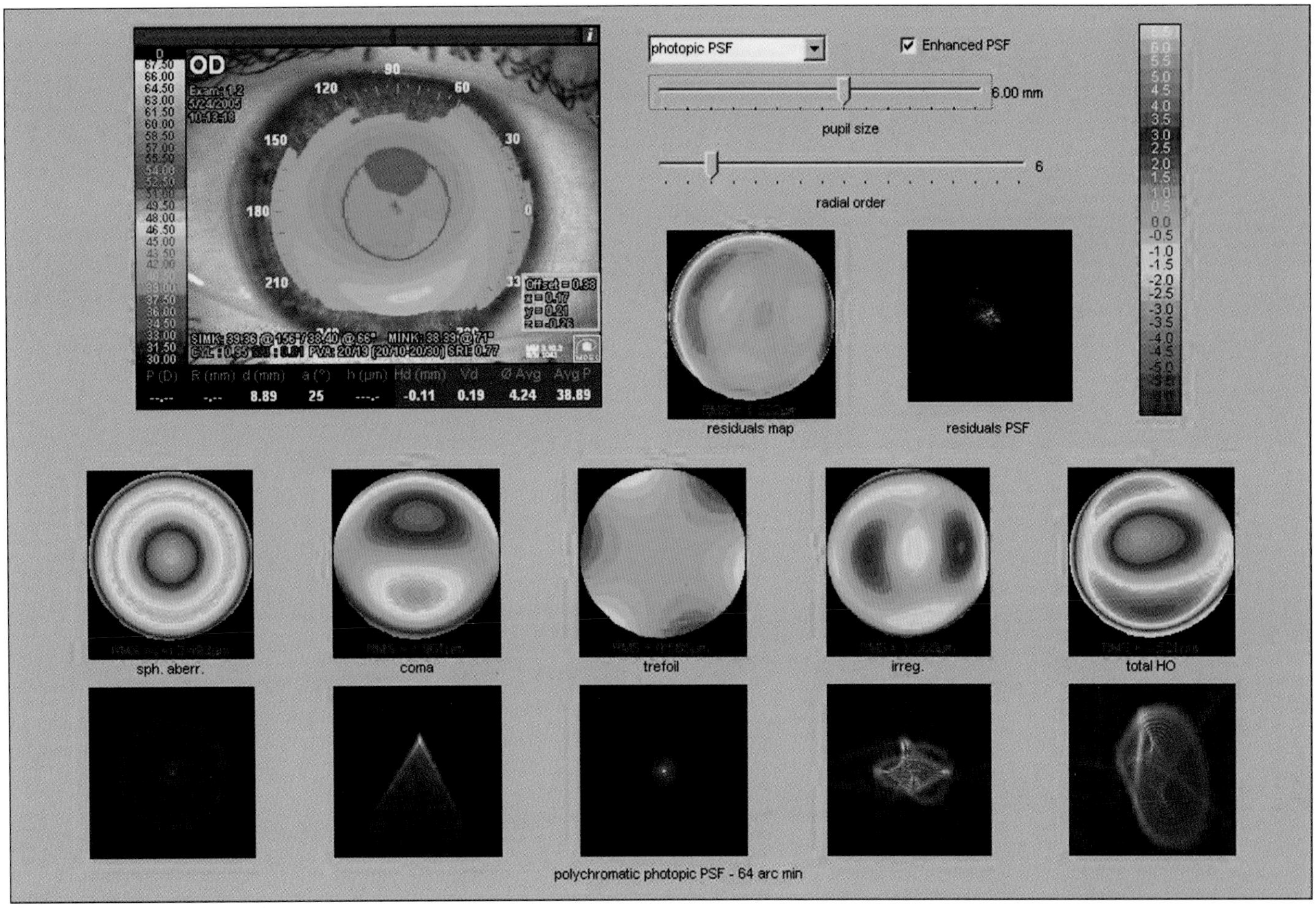

Fig. 13.12 Corneal wavefront analysis of the LASIK procedure shown in Figure 13.11. With a 7-mm pupil (black circle on topography map), mesopic vision is no better than 20/80 (top line on Snellen Chart segment). This is due to the 7-mm aperture encompassing regions of the cornea well beyond the optical zone. See Figure 13.11 for further details.

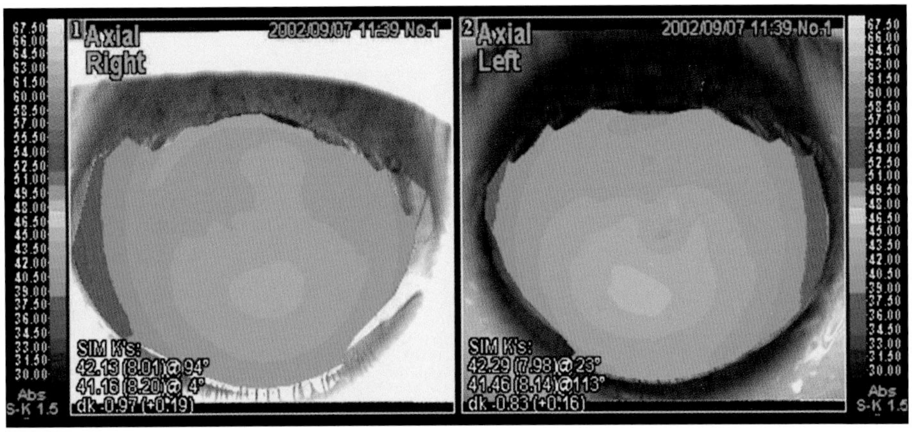

Fig. 13.13 The right eye of this patient is interpreted as keratoconus suspect while the left eye is advanced enough so that thinning or other clinical signs would confirm the diagnosis of clinical keratoconus.

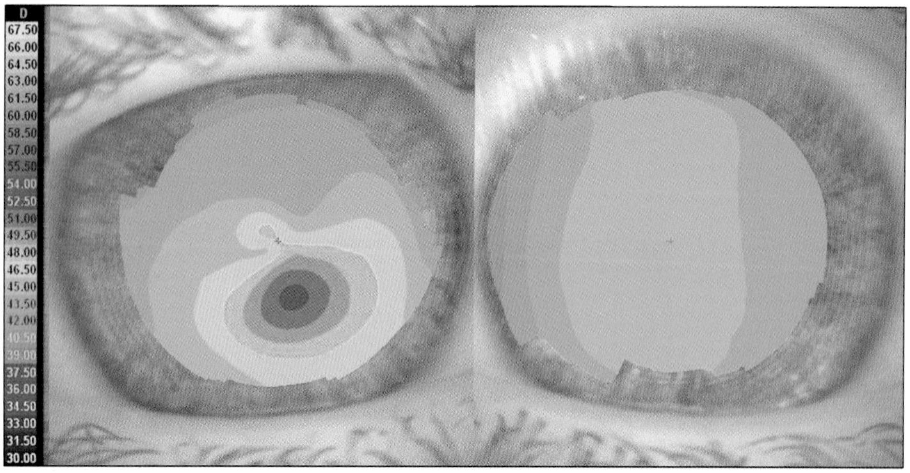

Fig. 13.14 'Unilateral' keratoconus. The right eye has a classic inferior cone, while there are no obvious signs of a cone in the left eye.

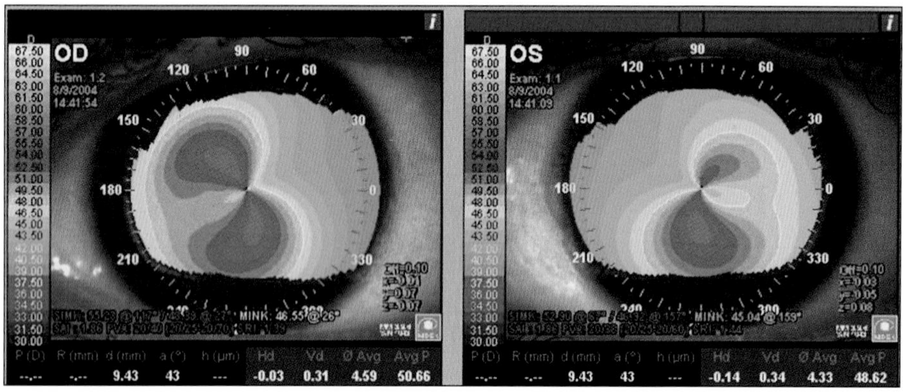

Fig. 13.15 Bilateral keratoconus in a patient who has marked skewing of the radial axes.

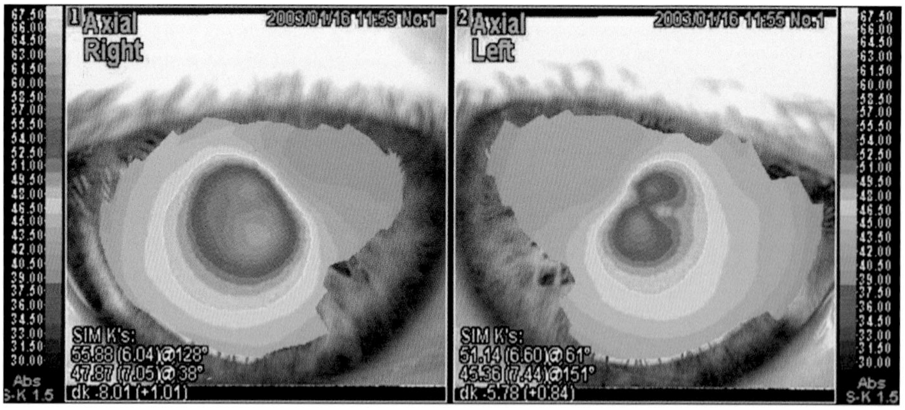

Fig. 13.16 Central keratoconus with a nearly circular pattern in the right cornea and a truncated bow tie in the left. Even if the bow tie were perfectly linear and symmetric, the truncated sign is important to recognize as one of the hallmarks of keratoconus.

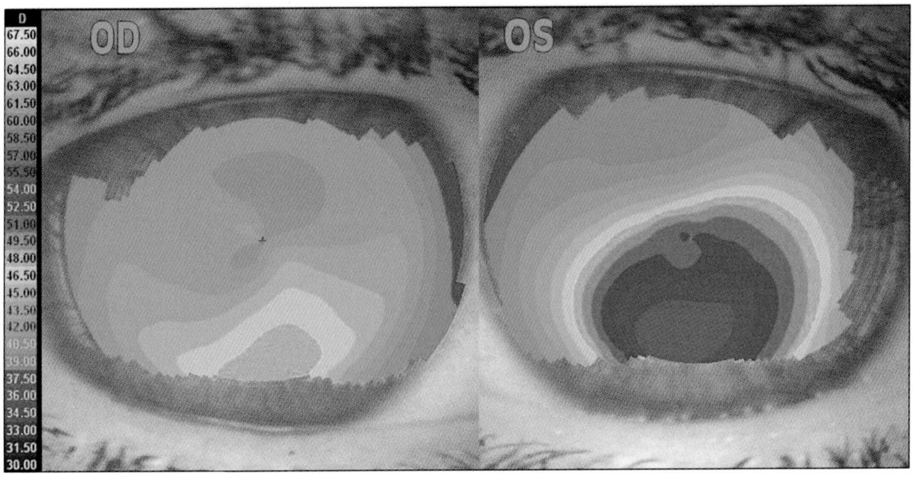

Fig. 13.17 This patient may be thought to have pellucid marginal degeneration in the right eye (note the abortive 'C' shape in the topography) and classic keratoconus in the left eye. However, the diagnosis of pellucid can only be made through careful examination of the thinning pattern: arcuate perilimbal thinning is pathognomonic for pellucid.

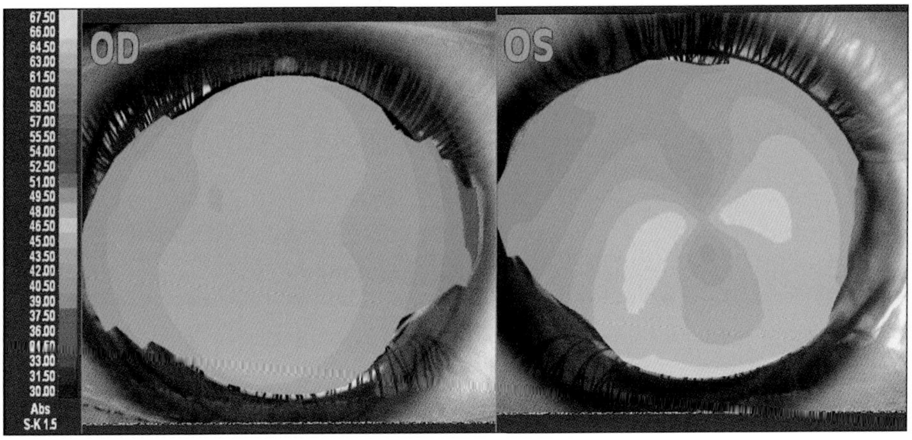

Fig. 13.18 Unilateral pellucid marginal corneal degeneration. Note the characteristic 'claw' or C-shaped pattern in the left eye.

become symmetrical; if the asymmetry is indeed owing to keratoconus, the corneal topography will become more asymmetric as contact lens wear tends to regularize an asymmetric cornea. Relaxation of the cornea from contact lens warpage can be a slow process taking weeks or months depending upon the degree of corneal distortion.[51] An example of this is shown in Figure 13.20.

Conclusion

Corneal topography now defines the standard of care in anterior segment surgery. Used wisely, it has guided the development of corneal surgery to reduce irregular astigmatism in corneal grafts, to minimize cataract incision size and to guide their placement, to understand the sources of night vision complaints after refractive surgery, to report the optical quality of the corneal surface in health, disease, and after surgery, and importantly in the early detection of corneal disease. Used well, corneal topography is a basic tool to prevent patients with signs of keratoconus or pellucid marginal degeneration from undergoing traditional laser refractive surgery.

In addition, describing corneal topography is essential to the understanding of its role in the optics of the eye. With over two-thirds of the total power of the eye, the corneal surface shape plays a major role in optical performance. The normal cornea is by no means a perfect optical component; yet some amount of astigmatism, residual spherical aberration, and even coma that are not compensated by the lens can be accommodated by neural adaptation. This becomes important when managing refractive corrective procedures, since eliminating all the measurable aberrations of the eye may not be acceptable to the patient, or even optically ideal even accounting for amelioration by neural readaptation. The new frontier in the management of refractive imperfections may be to discover what the optimal ocular wavefront should be for a given patient; most likely it will contain significant higher-order aberrations. The impressive feature is that the clinician now has the tools to produce the desired optical wavefront – once we discover what it is!

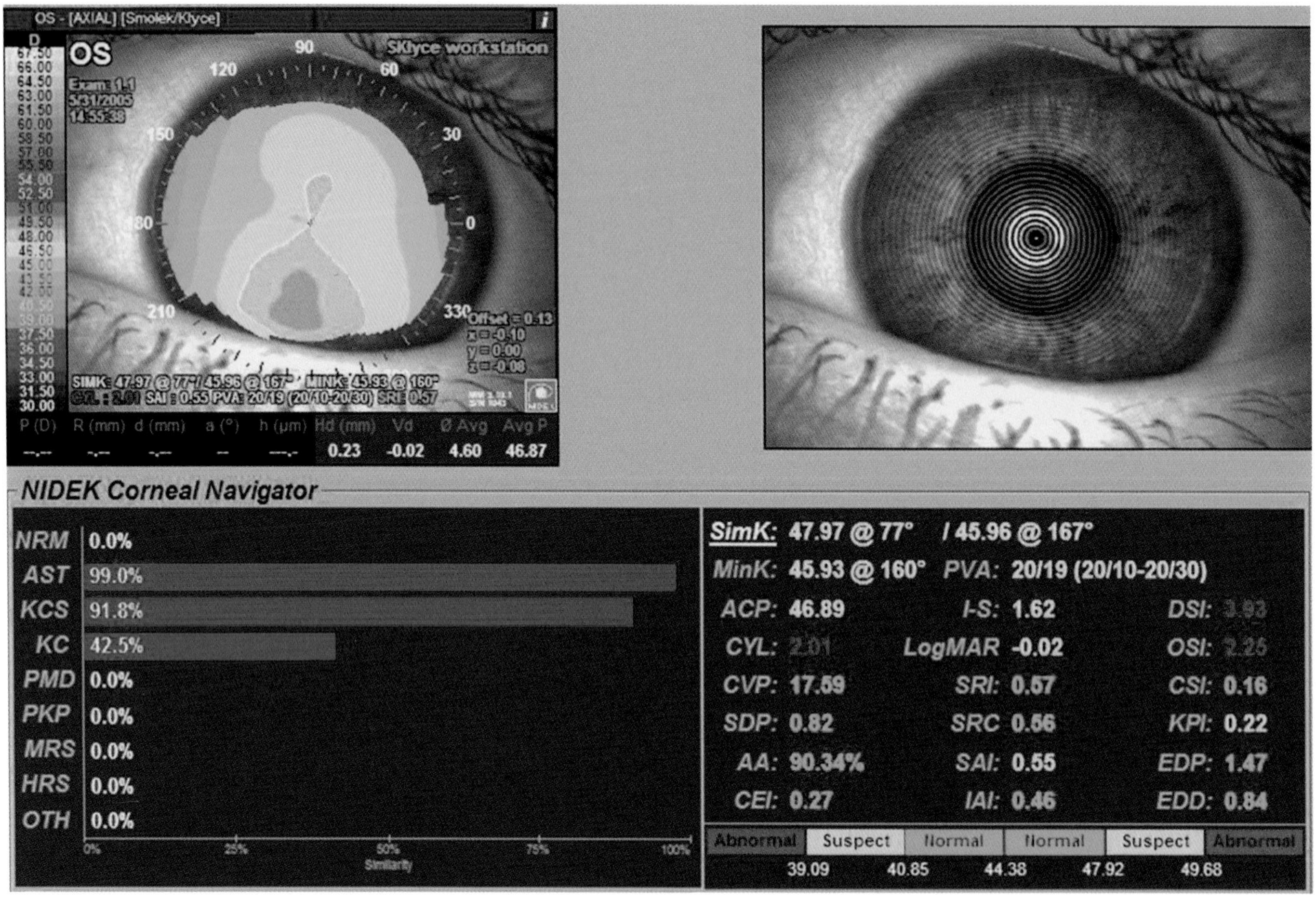

Fig. 13.19 This cornea has more asymmetry than would be found in the variations of normal corneal topography. It is recognized as having astigmatism, but also has characteristics associated with suspect keratoconus and clinical keratoconus. NIDEK Magellan topographer. This corneal topography has the characteristics associated with a cornea with 2.01 D of cylinder (AST = 99.0%). There are also features of this topography similar to keratoconus suspect (KCS = 91.8%). There are also features of this topography similar to clinical keratoconus (KC = 42.5%) with a severity index (KSI) of 2.7%.

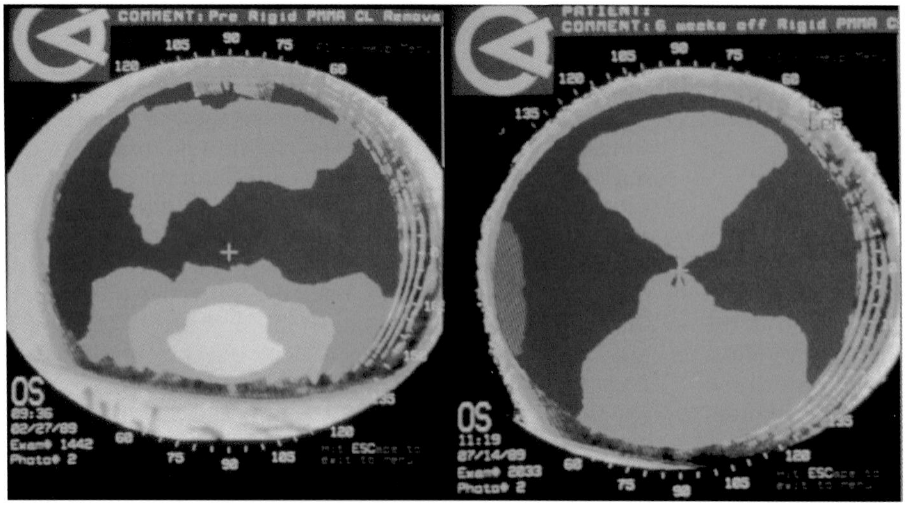

Fig. 13.20 Corneal warpage resembling a cone and cornea after removing lens for 6 weeks. (From Wilson SE, Lin DTC, Klyce SD, et al. Rigid contact lens decentration – a risk factor for corneal warpage. *CLAO J.* 1990;16:177–182.)

References

1. Scheiner C. *O Oculus, hoc est: fundamentum opticum*. Austria: Innsbruck; 1619.
2. Kohlraush J. Uber die messing des radius der vorderflache der hornhaut am libenden menschlichen Auge. *Okens Isis Jahrg*. 1840;5:886.
3. Helmholtz H. *Hanndbuch der Physiologieschen Optik*. Hamburg, Germany: Leopold Voss; 1909.
4. Javal L, Schiötz H. Un opthalmomètre pratique. *Annales d'Oculistique, Paris*. 1881;86:5–21.
5. Emsley H. Keratometry. In: *Visual optics*. London: Hatton Press Ltd; 1946:298–324.
6. Bogan SJ, Waring GO 3rd, Ibrahim O, Drews C, Curtis L. Classification of normal corneal topography based on computer-assisted videokeratography. *Arch Ophthalmol*. 1990;108:945–949.
7. Maeda N, Klyce SD, Smolek MK, McDonald MB. Disparity of keratometry readings and corneal power within the pupil after refractive surgery for myopia. *Cornea*. 1997;16:517–524.
8. Plácido A. Novo instrumento de exploracño da córnea. *Periodico d'Oftalmologia Pratica*. 1880;5:27–30.
9. Doss JD, Hutson RL, Rowsey JJ, Brown R. Method for calculation of corneal profile and power distribution. *Arch Ophthalmol*. 1981;99:1261–1265.
10. Klyce SD. Computer-assisted corneal topography. High-resolution graphical presentation and analysis of keratoscopy. *Invest Ophthalmol Vis Sci*. 1984;25:1426–1435.
11. Maguire LJ, Singer DE, Klyce SD. Graphic presentation of computer-analyzed keratoscope photographs. *Arch Ophthalmol*. 1987;105:223–230.
12. Warnicki JW, Rehkopf PG, Curtin DY, et al. Corneal topography using computer analyzed rastereography images. *Appl Optom*. 1988;27:1135–1140.
13. Reinstein DZ, Silverman RH, Trokel SJ, Coleman DJ. Corneal pachymetric topography. *Ophthalmology*. 1994;101:432.
14. Izatt JA, Hee MR, Swanson EA, et al. Micrometer-scale resolution imaging of the anterior eye in vivo with optical coherence tomography. *Arch Ophthalmol*. 1994;112:1584.
15. Buehren T, Collins MJ, Iskander DR, et al. The stability of corneal topography in the post-blink interval. *Cornea*. 2001;20:826–833.
16. Buehren T, Collins MJ, Loughridge J, Carney LG, Iskander DR. Corneal topography and accommodation. *Cornea*. 2003;22:311–316.
17. Lieberman DM, Grierson JW. The lids' influence on corneal shape. *Cornea*. 2000;19:336–342.
18. Wang J, Rice DA, Klyce SD. A new reconstruction algorithm for improvement of corneal topographical analysis. *Refract Corneal Surg*. 1989;5:379
19. American National Standard Ophthalmics-Corneal Topography Systems-Standard Terminology. Requirements. ANSI Z80.23–1999. Optical Laboratories Association, American National Standards Institute, Inc., 1999.
20. Roberts C. Corneal topography. In: Azar DT, Gatinel D, Hoang-Xuan T, eds. *Refractive surgery*. 2nd ed. Philadelphia: Elsevier/Mosby; 2007:103–116.
21. Cairns G, McGhee CJ. Orbscan computerized topography: attributes, applications, and limitations. *Cataract Refract Surg*. 2005;31:205–220.
22. Wilson SE, Klyce SD, Husseini ZM. Standardized color-coded maps for corneal topography. *Ophthalmology*. 1993;100:1723–1727.
23. Dingeldein SA, Klyce SD. The topography of normal corneas. *Arch Ophthalmol*. 1989;107:512.
24. Smolek MK, Klyce SD, Hovis JK. The Universal Standard Scale: proposed improvements to the American National Standards Institute (ANSI) scale for corneal topography. *Ophthalmology*. 2002;109:361–369.
25. Mandell RB. The enigma of corneal contour. *CLAO J*. 1992;18;267–273.
26. Tanabe T, Oshika T, Tomidokoro A, et al. Standardized color-coded scales for anterior and posterior elevation maps of scanning slit corneal topography. *Ophthalmology*. 2002;109:1298–1302.
27. Rao SN, Raviv T, Majmudar PA, Epstein RJ. Role of Orbscan II in screening keratoconus suspects before refractive corneal surgery. *Ophthalmology*. 2002;109:1642–1646.
28. De Sanctis U, Loiacono C, Richiardi L, et al. Sensitivity and specificity of posterior corneal elevation measured by Pentacam in discriminating keratoconus/subclinical keratoconus. *Ophtalmology*. 2009;116:816.
29. Yaylali V, Kaufman SC, Thompson HW. Corneal thickness measurements with the Orbscan Topography System and ultrasonic pachymetry. *J Cataract Refract Surg*. 1997;23:1345–1350.
30. Modis L Jr, Langenbucher A, Seitz B. Scanning slit and specular microscopic pachymetry in comparison with ultrasonic determination of corneal thickness. *Cornea*. 2001;20:711–714.
31. Cheng AC, Rao SK, Lau S, Leung CK, Lam DS. Central corneal thickness measurements by ultrasound, Orbscan II, and Visante OCT after LASIK for myopia. *J Refract Surg*. 2008;24:361–365.
32. Prisant O, Calderon N, Chastang P, Gatinel D, Hoang-Xuan T. Reliability of pachymetric measurements using Orbscan after excimer refractive surgery. *Ophthalmology*. 2003;110:511–515.
33. Cheng AC, Tang E, Mohamed S, Lam DS. Correction factor in Orbscan II in the assessment of corneal pachymetry. *Cornea*. 2006;25:1158–1161.
34. González-Méijome JM, Cerviño A, Yebra-Pimentel E, Parafita MA. Central and peripheral corneal thickness measurement with Orbscan II and topographical ultrasound pachymetry. *J Cataract Refract Surg*. 2003;29:125–132.
35. Jonuscheit S, Doughty MJ, Button NF. On the use of Orbscan II to assess the peripheral corneal thickness in humans: a comparison with ultrasound pachometry measures. *Ophthalmic Physiol Opt*. 2007;27:179–189.
36. Kim SW, Byun YJ, Kim EK, Kim TI. Central corneal thickness measurements in unoperated eyes and eyes after PRK for myopia using Pentacam, Orbscan II, and ultrasonic pachymetry. *J Refract Surg*. 2007;23:888–894.
37. Dingeldein SA, Klyce SD, Wilson SE. Quantitative descriptors of corneal shape derived from computer-assisted analysis of photokeratographs. *Refract Corn Surg*. 1989;5:372–378.
38. Tang W, Collins MJ, Carney L, Davis B. The accuracy and precision performance of four videokeratoscopes in measuring test surfaces. *Optom Vis Sci*. 2000;77:483–491.
39. Wilson SE, Klyce SD. Quantitative descriptors of corneal topography: a clinical study. *Arch Ophthalmol*. 1991;109:349–353.
40. Keeler P, van Saarloos P. Fourier transformation of corneal topography data. *Aust NZ J Ophthalmol*. 1997;25(Suppl 1):S53-S55.
41. Martínez CE, Applegate RA, Klyce SD, et al. Effect of pupillary dilation on corneal optical aberrations after photorefractive keratectomy. *Arch Ophthalmol*. 1998;116(8):1053–1062.
42. Endl MJ, Martínez CE, Klyce SD, et al. Effect of larger ablation zone and transition zone on corneal optical aberrations after photorefractive keratectomy. *Arch Ophthalmol*. 2001;119:1159–1164.
43. Rabinowitz YS, McDonnell PJ. Computer-assisted corneal topography in keratoconus. *Refract Corneal Surg*. 1989;5:400–408.
44. Rabinowitz YS. Videokeratographic indices to aid in screening for keratoconus. *J Refract Surg*. 1995;11:371–379.
45. Swartz T, Marten L, Wang M. Measuring the cornea: the latest developments in corneal topography. *Curr Opin Ophthalmol*. 2007;18:325–333.
46. Klyce SD, Karon MD, Smolek MD. Screening patients with the corneal navigator. *J Refract Surg*. 2005;21:S617–S622.
47. Maeda N, Klyce SD, Smolek MK, Thompson HW. Automated keratoconus screening with corneal topography analysis. *Invest Ophthalmol Vis Sci*. 1994;35:2749–2757.
48. Rabinowitz YS, Rasheed K. KISA% index: a quantitative videokeratography algorithm embodying minimal topographic criteria for diagnosing keratoconus. *J Cataract Refract Surg*. 1999;25:1327–1335.
49. Smolek MK, Klyce SD. Current detection methods compared with a neural network approach. *Invest Ophthalmol Vis Sci*. 1997;38:2290–2299.
50. Ruiz-Montenegro J, Mafra CH, Wilson SE, et al. Corneal topographic alterations in normal contact lens wearers. *Ophthalmology*. 1993;100:128–134.
51. Wilson SE, Lin DTC, Klyce SD, Reidy JJ, Insler MS. Rigid contact lens decentration – a risk factor for corneal warpage. *CLAO J*. 1990;16:177–182.

Chapter 14

Specular Microscopy

Beth Ann Benetz, Richard Yee, Maria Bidros, Jonathan Lass

The specular microscope is unlike most microscopes. Instead of imaging light transmitted through a substance, the specular microscope images light reflected from an optical interface. The optical interface giving the most interest is that between the corneal endothelium and the aqueous humor. The specular microscope, however, can also be used to image the corneal epithelium, stroma, and crystalline lens. Depending on the instrument used, the projected light can be in the form of a stationary slit, a moving slit, or a moving spot. The optical design can be either confocal or nonconfocal. The design of the equipment can be either contact or noncontact.

The young, normal corneal endothelium as seen by specular microscopy (Fig. 14.1) shows a quasi-regular array of hexagonal cells, all having nearly the same size. With aging, trauma, and corneal disease, this regularity is lost. In general, the more the endothelium differs from the normal appearance, the more difficult it is for the endothelium to maintain corneal clarity.

The first direct visualization of the endothelium was demonstrated by Vogt in 1918.[1] Using the slit lamp microscope, Vogt demonstrated that the endothelial mosaic could be visualized in the axis of the reflected light. In 1924, Graves used similar methods to describe Fuchs' endothelial corneal dystrophy in elderly patients.[2] It was not, however, until 1968 that David Maurice described the first laboratory specular microscope that could be used to study excised living corneas.[3,4] Modifications of this specular microscope were made by Laing et al.[5] and later by Bourne and Kaufman,[6] allowing routine clinical examination and photography of the corneal endothelium.

Specular microscopes have evolved from interest in wider field and higher-resolution contact microscopes[7,8] to narrower field, high-resolution noncontact microscopes equipped with software to obtain automated or semiautomated determination of endothelial cell density and morphology, including coefficient of variation and percentage of hexagonal cells.[9–13] Currently, specular microscopes are available for both clinical and eyebank use.

Optical Principles of Specular Microscopy

To properly interpret endothelial photomicrographs obtained clinically, it is helpful to understand the optical principles of the specular microscope. Light striking a surface can be reflected, transmitted, or absorbed. Generally, some combination of the three effects occurs. Of primary importance in clinical specular microscopy is the light that is reflected specularly (i.e. 'mirrorlike'), where the angle of reflection is equal to the angle of incidence. It is this light that is captured by the specular microscope and forms the image of interest.

For the normal transparent cornea, most visible light is transmitted through the cornea. Some light, however, can be absorbed by the tissue, and some can be reflected by various objects having a different index of refraction than the surrounding corneal tissue. Some of the reflected light is scattered (reflected at arbitrary angles) by cellular organelles. With an increase in corneal edema, the fraction of scattered light increases and can become the dominant element, giving rise to a 'hazy' cornea.

As light passes through the cornea, it encounters a series of interfaces between optically distinct regions. At each interface, some light is reflected back and some is transmitted deeper into the cornea. The greater the difference in index of refraction between the regions, the greater the intensity of reflected light. The more edematous the tissue, the more light is scattered. A portion of this reflected light

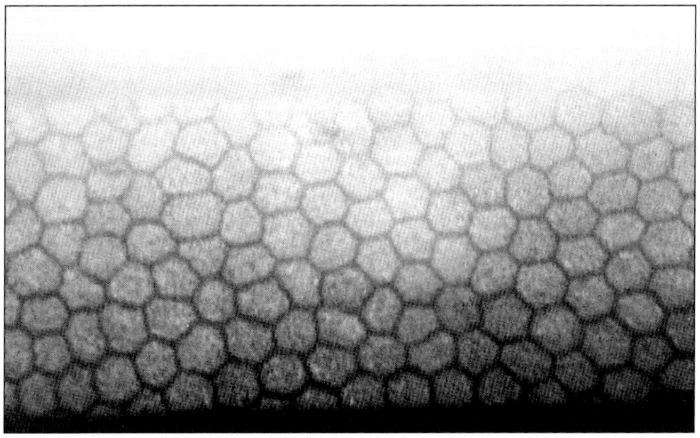

Fig. 14.1 Normal corneal endothelium as photographed by specular microscopy. A quasi-regular array of hexagonal cells, all having nearly the same area, is seen.

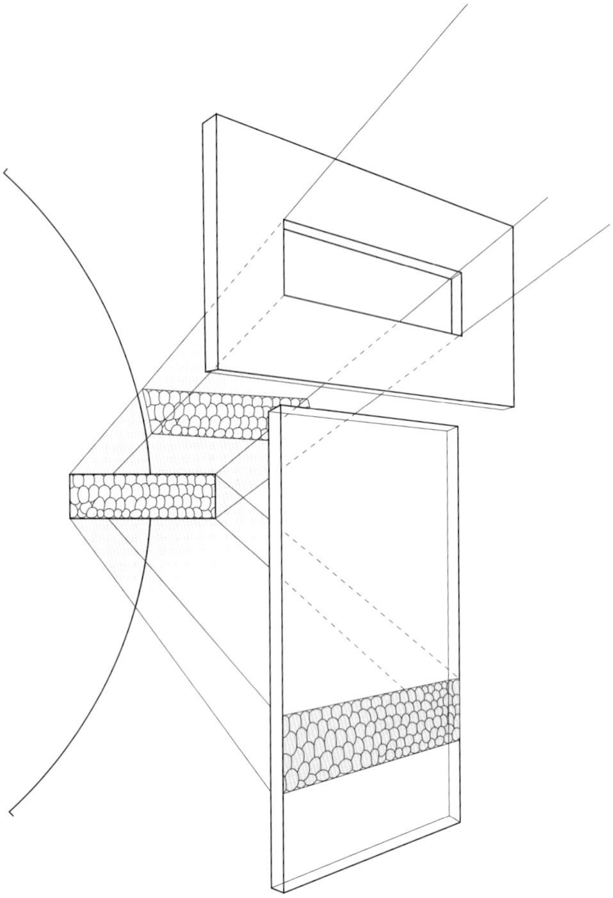

Fig. 14.2 Pathway of light from its source in the clinical specular microscope back to the film plane of the same instrument. Although both epithelium and endothelium are shown in focus on the film plane of the graphic representation, in practice only one layer is in focus at any one time because of the restricted depth of field of the specular microscope.

is collected by the objective lens of the specular microscope and forms, at the film plane of the microscope, an image of that part of the cornea on which the instrument is focused (Fig. 14.2).

Laing et al. have described the components of the images formed by reflected light from various interfaces in the cornea.[14] Figure 14.3A shows a narrow slit of light from a contact specular microscope that is focused on the posterior corneal surface. Most light is reflected at the major optical interfaces, labeled 1, 2, and 3. The greatest index of refraction exists between the objective lens and coupling fluid. Therefore, much more light is reflected from this interface (0.36%) than the interface formed by the coupling fluid and epithelium (0.025%) or, most importantly, the interface formed by the endothelium and aqueous humor (0.022%).

According to Laing, if the beam is narrowed sufficiently, four zones of reflection can be seen. Zone 1 is the brightest region and is formed by the interfaces formed by the lens, coupling fluid, and epithelium. Zone 2 is a larger region and represents light reflected from the stroma. Zone 3 is the endothelial region, and zone 4 represents light reflected from the aqueous humor. Unless considerable debris is present, little light is reflected from the aqueous. As a result, zone 4 is usually dark. The boundary, then, between the endothelial region (zone 3) and the aqueous (zone 4) is almost always dark and is termed the 'dark boundary.' In contrast, some light is scattered from the stroma (zone 2), making it brighter than the endothelial region (zone 3). The boundary, then, between the endothelial region (zone 3) and the stroma (zone 2) is usually bright and is termed the 'bright boundary.' When examining specular photomicrographs taken with a stationary slit of light, one can usually identify a brighter portion of the image (the bright boundary which, in the stationary slit images provided in this chapter, is the upper portion of the image) and a darker portion of the image (the dark boundary which, in the stationary slit images provided in this chapter, is the lower portion of the image).

If the angle of incidence of the illuminating source is increased, less overlap occurs and a wider slit can be used. As a result, a larger field of endothelial cells can be seen (Fig. 14.3B). The wider beam, however, illuminates more of the corneal stroma and epithelium, resulting in a greater amount of scattered light. The increase in scattered light from tissue overlying the endothelium results in a decrease in contrast, obscuring endothelial cell detail. A washed-out picture results with a decrease in contrast and loss of cellular definition. Furthermore, as the angle of incidence is increased, normal endothelial cells appear shortened in one direction. This distortion should be compensated for in morphometric analysis.

With widefield scanning slit or scanning spot confocal microscopes, the slit or spot is made very small to provide less interference and increased image quality. With the help of sensitive recording systems, the spot or slit can be scanned over the tissue and recorded to provide a high-quality image and a larger field of view. When using such equipment, dark and bright boundaries are generally no longer identifiable. These advancements have improved the ability to visualize the endothelium in edematous corneas and have allowed better visualization of stromal nerves and keratocytes. However, with the development of commercially available confocal microscopes, the limitations of the specular microscope to image with the thick cornea have been overcome by confocal technology (see Ch. 15).[15–17]

Patient Preparation

Commercially available contact and noncontact specular microscopes are easy to use with little, if any, patient discomfort. To obtain good patient cooperation and ultimately aquire quality images for analysis, it is important to first explain the procedure to the patient. The positioning of the head and establishing patient comfort are key to minimize movement and allow optimal images of the endothelium.

In noncontact specular microscopy, instructing the patient to blink to wet the cornea and then to hold still just

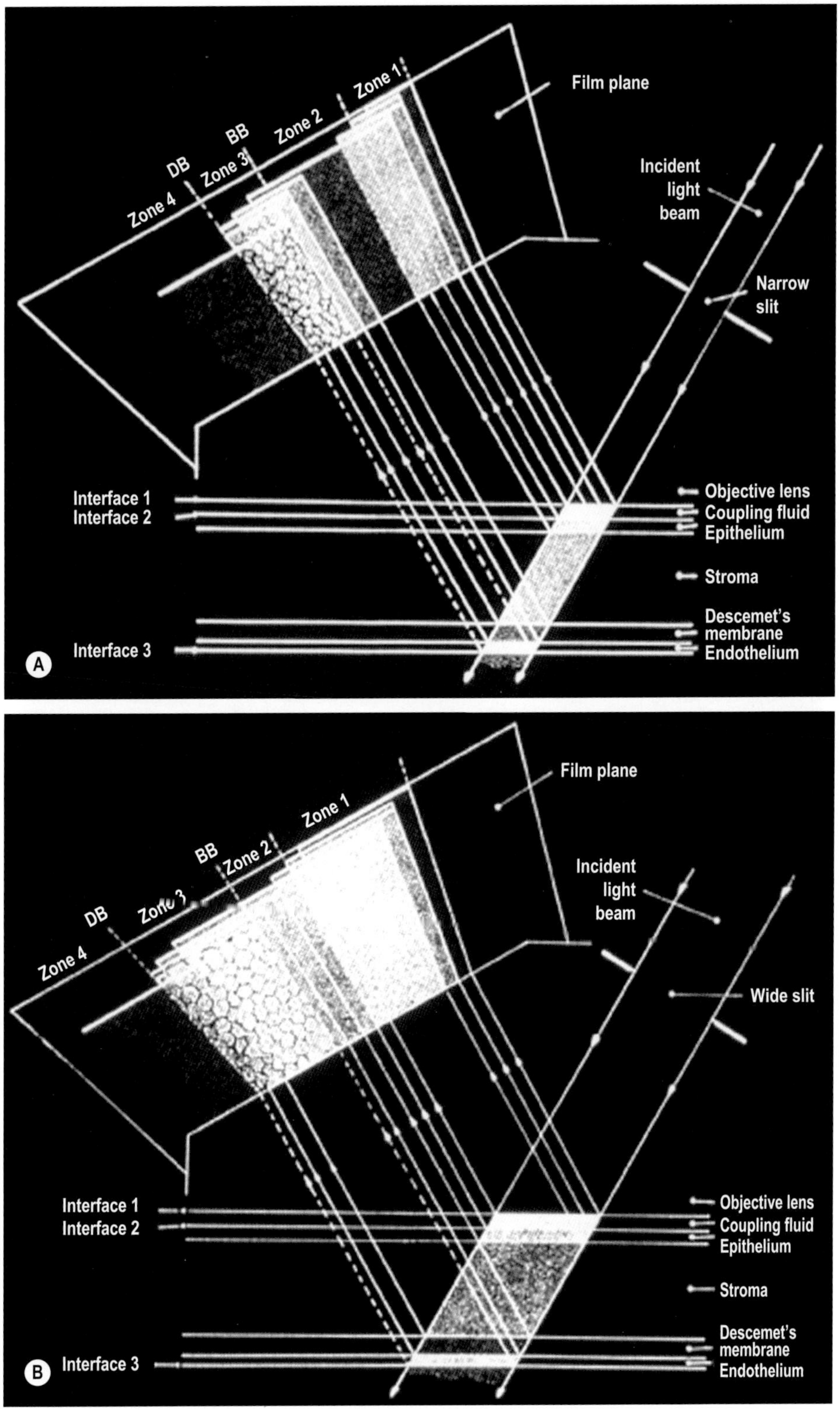

Fig. 14.3 Representation of an optical section when a narrow slit (**A**) or a wide slit (**B**) of light passes through various corneal layers and is focused on the posterior corneal surface. As drawn, the film plane is positioned at right angles to the plane of the paper. The zones are defined in the text. BB, bright boundary; DB, dark boundary.

prior to image capture improves image sharpness. Also of note with noncontact instruments is that imaging a thickened cornea will sometimes fail in the automated capture mode and may require the operator to use a manual mode. If using a contact specular microscope, one or two drops of proparacaine anesthetic should be used before the eye is contacted. Once the cornea is contacted, a few epithelial irregularities may be seen; however, these usually disappear within a few hours. Positioning the eye in a straight-ahead position is best achieved with an internal fixation point.

Optimal photographs are obtained when the cornea is relatively thin and clear, with minimal scarring or edema. Light reflexes from the iris can obscure the endothelial mosaic and are best eliminated by dilating the pupil.

Standardization of Imaging Techniques

A standard approach to examining the corneal endothelium is necessary for observing change over time. When using a contact specular microscope, the beam of light is directed through the pupil to ensure the placement of the cone on the most central portion of the cornea. Systematic scanning superiorly, inferiorly, nasally, and temporally will ensure a thorough evaluation of the endothelium. Noncontact specular microscopes use internal fixation points to provide a more standardized approach to consistently imaging the central endothelium, midperiphery, and periphery. With these systems, the patient view is shifted when the technician selects the desired region.

To best evaluate small changes over time in any region, including the central endothelium, the technician should image the region three times at the same sitting and record the average of the three images' analyses. This is particularly important with the higher-magnification microscopes as so few cells of the total corneal surface are captured in the final image. It is also important for the technician to use the same image analysis method from baseline and throughout the follow-up period. Most specular microscopic studies of the corneal endothelium determine solely the endothelial cell density of the central endothelium in order to attempt to consistently examine the same endothelial cell area over time. However, this may be misleading and does not necessarily reflect the impact of a surgical procedure that primarily damages the peripheral cornea. Changes in the central corneal endothelium in both density and morphology may take some time (months, years) to be reflected. In addition, the paracentral and peripheral endothelium, in particular superiorly, has a higher cell density than the central endothelium and may assist in maintaining central endothelial density and function.[18] Procedures in this area may therefore have an even greater impact on central endothelium over time.

Instrumentation

There are several specular microscopes commercially available, both contact and noncontact. In addition, confocal microscopes (see Ch. 15) are used clinically to capture and analyze endothelial cell density and morphology (Table 14.1). All the instruments have computer integration and semi- or fully-automated analyses. Some instruments allow manual analysis and/or adjustments to the automated analyses. The noncontact instruments use autotracking and focusing technology. Perhaps the most widely used clinical instrument in the United States is the Konan NonCon Robo Series (Torrance, CA). Using this instrument, tracking of the cornea and imaging of the endothelium are automated, requiring minimal intervention by the operator. Once the patient is aligned, the operator presses a button on the control box to start the imaging process. The optics of the instrument first objectively aligns themselves relative to the cornea by using the Purkinje images until the proper specular reflection mode is achieved. The instrument then objectively focuses back to the endothelial surface, the flash lamp is triggered, and the resulting endothelial photograph is displayed on the monitor. Other noncontact instruments image sequential images (Tomey, Inc., Phoenix, AZ) or provide a live view (HAI Labs, Inc., Lexington, MA), both automatically selecting the best images. As mentioned above, a limitation of the noncontact instruments is the difficulty of getting quality images when the cornea is thickened. HAI offers a contact specular microscope with a focal depth of 0–999 μm. Though less comfortable for the patient because it is a contact instrument, it obtains sharp, widefield images regardless of corneal thickness or disease.

Qualitative Specular Microscopy

Epithelium

Corneal epithelial cells do not normally present a flat surface suitable for specular microscopy. If a contact lens is pressed against the anterior surface of the eye, however, the epithelial cells can be flattened and can reflect light in a mirror-like fashion.[19] Tsubota and colleagues have described contact lens systems that enable photography of the superficial layer of epithelial cells using specular microscopy.[20–22] The reflection of the epithelium is reduced by the application of a soft contact lens with nearly the same index of refraction as the cornea, permitting the observation of individual epithelial cells. Combining these techniques with the higher resolution provided by modern widefield specular microscopes allows the study of even greater epithelial detail.

The normal corneal epithelium contains polygonal cells of varying brightness (Fig. 14.4). Most cells can be placed into one of three groups: dark, medium, and light. Hexagonal, pentagonal, and triangular cells may be present, but rounded, enlarged, or elongated cells are considered abnormal.

Elongated or enlarged corneal epithelial cells can be observed in wound healing processes such as penetrating keratoplasty (Fig. 14.5),[20,23,24] and epikeratophakia.[20,25,26] This is thought to be a result of the normal migration of cells during the wound healing response. Various other conditions can result in elongated or enlarged epithelial cells, including daily or extended soft contact lens wear,[27–29] dry eyes,[30] neurotrophic keratitis,[30] aphakia,[20] and diabetes.[20,28,31] Elongated cells are also seen in keratoconus patients, especially near the

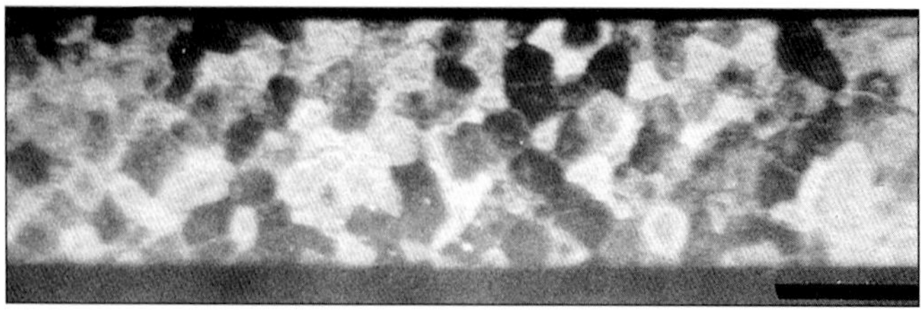

Fig. 14.4 Specular image of normal corneal epithelium. Note that there are three kinds of cell: dark cells, intermediate cells, and bright cells. No rounded or elongated cells are seen. The bar represents 100 μm.

cone's apex.[20,28,31,32] This has been shown to be a result of a keratoconic condition and not from the secondary changes due to contact lens wear.[33] Since the last edition of this text, there have been several updated methods to evaluate the corneal epithelium, such as the Pentacam comprehensive eye scanner and ultrasound pachymetry (Oculus, Inc., Lynnwood, WA).[34] Such techniques may be better in analyzing corneal thickness of keratoconic corneas with higher reliability than the current specular microscope systems.[35,36] Confocal microscopy has also provided new insights into appearance and changes in the basal epithelium, wing cells, and superficial cells in normals and in disease (Ch. 15).

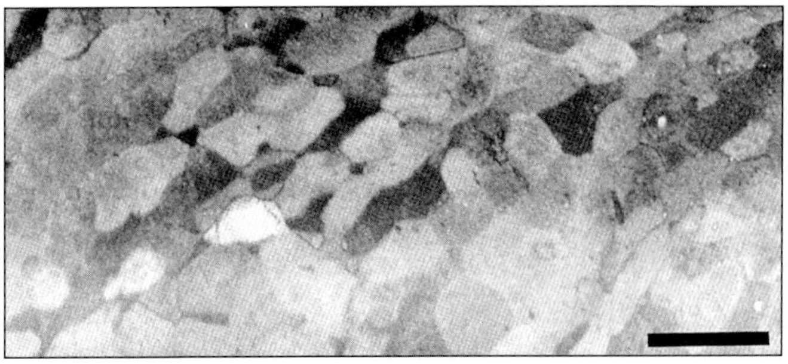

Fig. 14.5 Specular microscopic image of the corneal epithelium after penetrating keratoplasty. Note the enlargement and elongation of the cells. The bar represents 100 μm.

Table 14.1 Summary of currently available specular microscopes and the key advertised features of each instrument

Manufacturer	Type	Model	Analyses options	Advertised features	Sample image
HAI Labs, Inc. Lexington, MA	Contact	CL-1000xyz	Automated Fixed Frame Variable Frame Corners	– f.o.v. 250 μm × 400 μm – Focal depth of 0–999 μm – Pachymeter – Live sequence capture – HAI CAS/CL Cell Analysis System	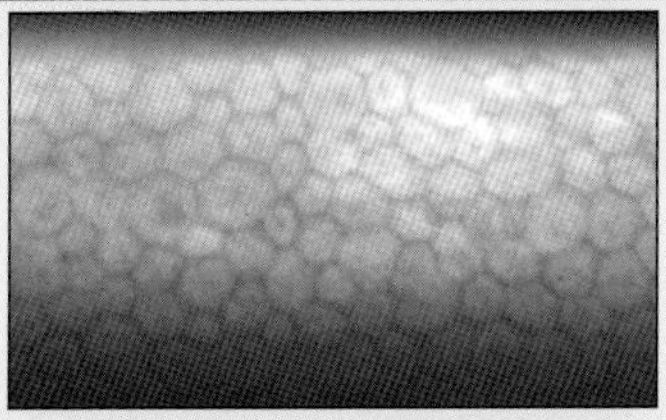
HAI Labs, Inc. Lexington, MA	Noncontact	CL-1000nc	Automated, Semiautomated	– Live view of endothelium – Automated selection of good images – Optical pachymetry – Central and peripheral points	
Heidelberg Engineering Vista, CA	Confocal Contact immersion	Corneal Module HRT	Semiautomated	– Layer by layer imaging – Uniform illumination, undistorted image – Movie capture – Manual pachymetry	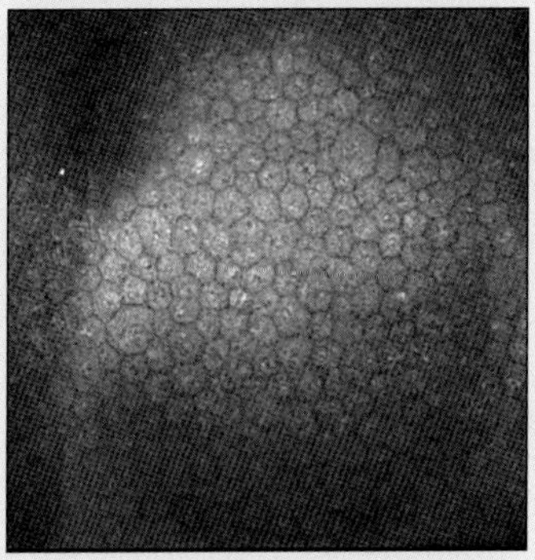

Continued

Table 14.1 Summary of currently available specular microscopes and the key advertised features of each instrument – cont'd

Manufacturer	Type	Model	Analyses options	Advertised features	Sample image
Konan Medical USA, Inc. Torrance, CA	Noncontact	CELLCHEK Series (CELLCHEK XL, SP, RU, SP-9000 PLUS)	Automated Semiautomated, Center, Center-Flex, Corner Method, Simple Grid, Screener	– Fully automated alignment and focus, easy to use – Five fixation points – Optical pachymetry at all five fixation points – Integrated computer system and analysis software	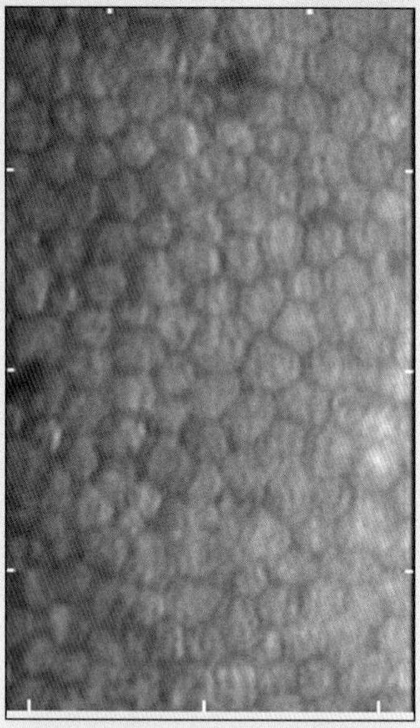
Nidek Fremont, CA	Confocal Noncontact (20×)	Confoscan 4	Automated	– Wide measurement area (up to 1000 cells/exam) – Fully noncontact (12-mm working distance) – Quality imaging through opacities and corneal haze	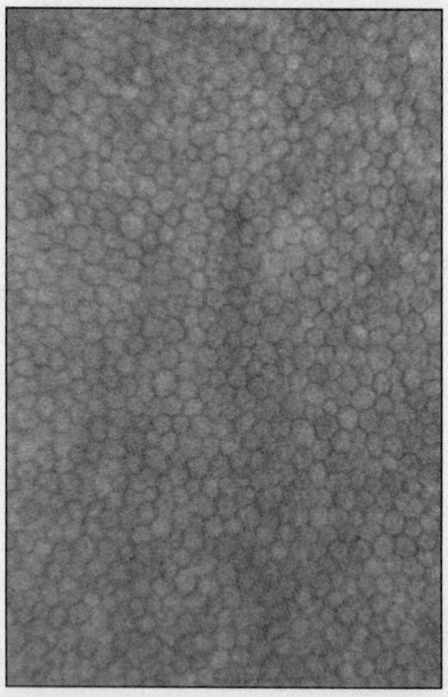
Nidek Fremont, CA	Confocal Contact immersion (40×)	Confoscan 4	Automated	– Combines live in-vivo confocal microscopy, endothelial microscopy, and pachymetry – Gel immersion exam – Automated alignment – Multiple internal fixation mires	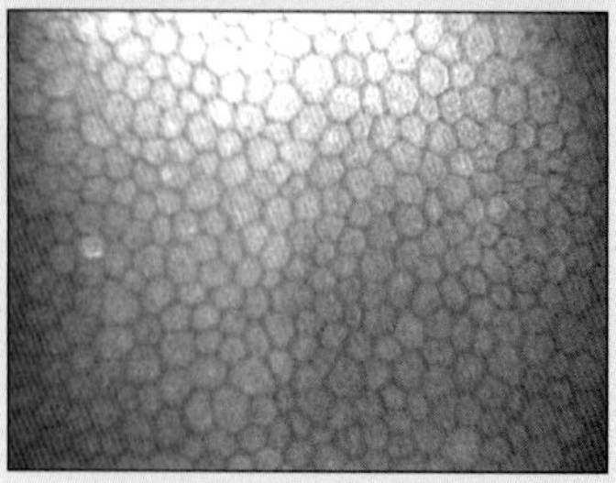

Table 14.1 Summary of currently available specular microscopes and the key advertised features of each instrument – cont'd

Manufacturer	Type	Model	Analyses options	Advertised features	Sample image
Tomey, Inc. Phoenix, AZ	Noncontact	EM-3000	Automated	– Easy 'touch alignment' – Serial photography (15 shots) – Wide field – f.o.v. 250 μm × 540 μm – Seven capture positions	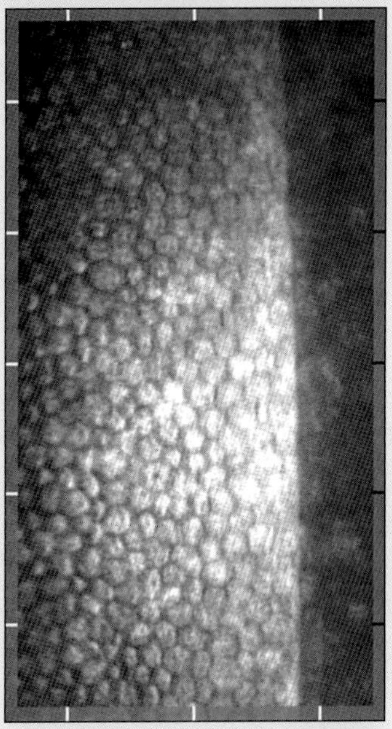
Topcon Medical, Inc. Tokyo, Japan*	Noncontact	SP-3000P	Automated	– Three modes for image capture (automated, semiautomated, manual) – Fast 3-D auto alignment and centering – Five fixation targets – Integrated color monitor and data analysis	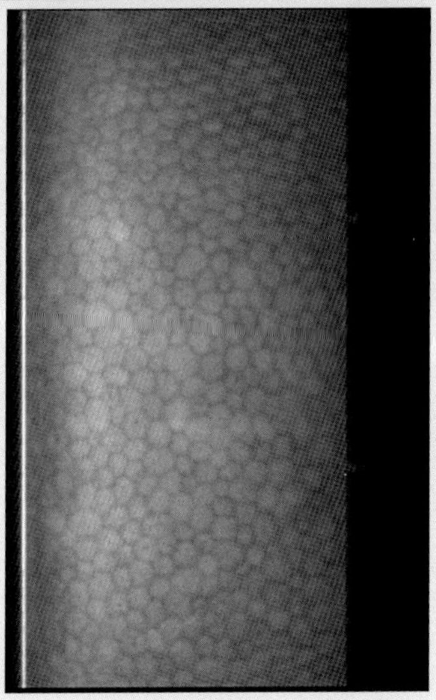

** Not available in the USA.*

Endothelium: miscellaneous bright and dark structures

A number of abnormal endothelial structures can be seen with specular microscopy.[37] One of the most notable is corneal guttae (Fig. 14.6A). Guttae are excrescences of Descemet's membrane. They can be seen with the specular microscope much earlier than with the slit lamp. They begin as small, dark structures, but, in time, these structures grow, often becoming larger than individual endothelial cells. The excrescences can be dome shaped, or they can assume the shape of a mushroom. If the excrescence assumes a mushroom shape with a flat top, light can be specularly reflected from the surface much like a mirror. When this occurs, a bright spot can be seen within the dark structure. In the case of Fuchs' endothelial corneal dystrophy, the surrounding

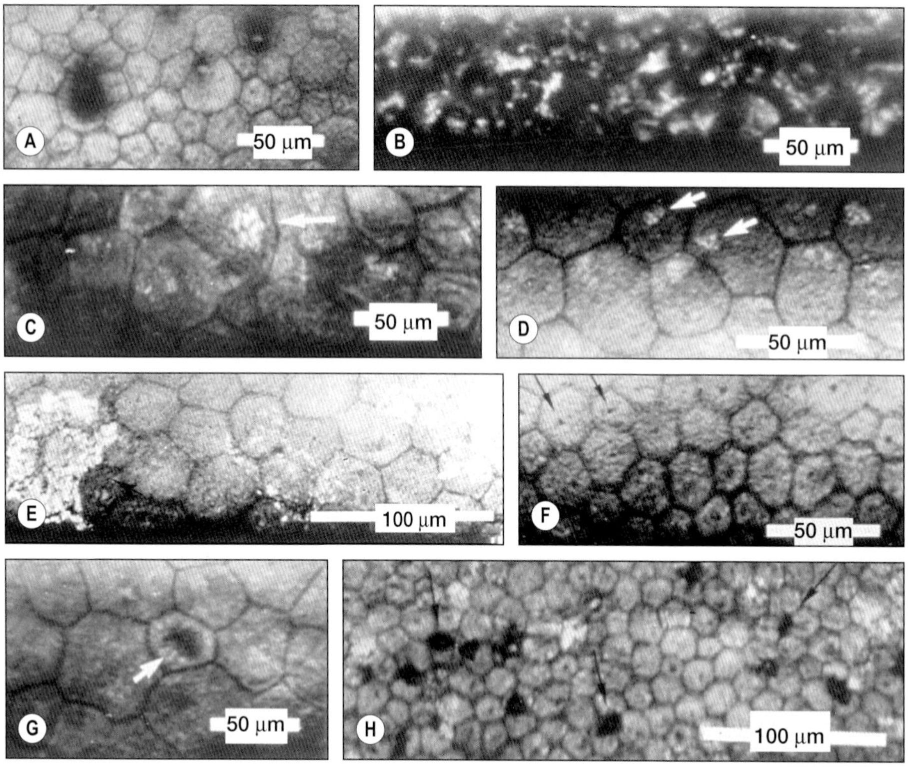

Fig. 14.6 Miscellaneous endothelial structures. Arrows indicate features mentioned. (**A**) Isolated smooth excrescences (corneal guttae). (**B**) Multiple coalesced excrescences. Only the bright reflection from the apex of each excrescence is clearly seen. (**C** and **D**) Intracellular bright structures possibly representing cell nuclei. (**E**) Pigmented endothelial deposits. (**F**) Dark structures possibly representing endothelial cilia. (**G**) Intracellular dark structures possibly representing intracellular vacuoles. (**H**) Intercellular dark structures believed to be invading inflammatory cells.

endothelial cells are often abnormally shaped. Guttae, however, can also be seen in the far periphery of young individuals. In this case, they are called Hassall-Henle warts. The excrescence is usually shaped more like a dome than a mushroom, and the surrounding endothelium does not appear as abnormal.

If the excrescences are very abundant, they may begin to touch each other and coalesce. It may become difficult to identify endothelial cells. This is often seen centrally in advanced stages of Fuchs' endothelial corneal dystrophy (Fig. 14.6B).

Intracellular bright structures can sometimes be seen (Fig. 14.6C,D).[37] They seem to be associated with stressed cells such as those seen after corneal transplantation. The size of the bright structure often corresponds to the size of the endothelial cell (the larger the cell, the larger the bright structure). This structure is felt to represent the cell nucleus.

Some bright structures span several endothelial cells and have sharp borders, indicating they are likely very near the endothelial–stromal interface (Fig. 14.6E). These structures are believed to represent pigment deposits on the endothelial surface.

Various dark structures can also be seen in specular micrographs. One such structure appears to be intracellular, is small, and has sharp borders. This structure is thought to represent endothelial cilia (Fig. 14.6F). Another intracellular dark structure is much larger and less distinct, suggesting that it is located within the cell (Fig. 14.6G). These are thought to represent intracellular vacuoles or blebs.

Specular microscopy of patients with anterior uveitis has revealed well-demarcated, dark structures usually located at endothelial cell intersections (Fig. 14.6H).[37] These structures are uniform in size and are thought to represent invading white blood cells.

Endothelium: morphometry

Analyzing specular micrographs can be done qualitatively by looking at the cellular morphology and giving an interpretation, or quantitatively by counting cell density and performing morphometric analysis. To properly recognize abnormal endothelium, however, requires knowledge of the appearance of normal endothelial (Fig. 14.7). Complete qualitative analysis requires knowledge of cell conformation, cell boundaries and their intersections, configuration of the dark boundary, and the presence of acellular structures.[14] Additionally, one must be able to recognize the presence of optical artifacts and eliminate them from consideration when performing both qualitative and quantitative analysis.

The normal specular micrograph of a young person should show a regular endothelial mosaic of hexagonal cells of approximately the same size. Cell boundaries should be well defined. With age, however, endothelial cells become larger and the cellular pattern becomes distinctly pleomorphic. Figure 14.8A–F demonstrates various examples of abnormal cell shapes. Laing has also described the appearance of abnormal cell boundaries, cell shapes, and other cell structures seen in specular microscopy.[38] It should be noted that, even though the cell pattern can be pleomorphic, the cell size is not always increased.

One of the simplest methods to determine cell area and cell density is comparison cell analysis. When using this method, the endothelial cell mosaic is compared to a cell pattern of known size.[39–41] The mean cell area and cell density can then be subjectively estimated.

Quantitative Specular Microscopy

There have been limited attempts to perform quantitative specular microscopy of corneal epithelial cell density and morphology impaired by the analysis of a multilayer structure, artifact induced by the higher resolution contact microscopes, and questionable value in the analysis of dynamic cell population undergoing constant turnover. Confocal microscopy has shown much greater value with its precise determination of depth of focus and the three-dimensional construction of images, including the epithelium (Ch. 15). The lens epithelium has also been studied in a limited manner by specular microscopy in a group of normal volunteers and cataract patients by using a noncontact specular microscope.[42] There was a statistically significant decrease in the cell density of the lens epithelium in a group of cataract patients over the age of 80 years. Cell area variation and the number of large black spots that were observed were not related to aging or cataract formation. Cell density of the lens epithelium decreased after the age of 80, but cataract formation did not affect the cell density or the variation in cell areas until the age of 80.

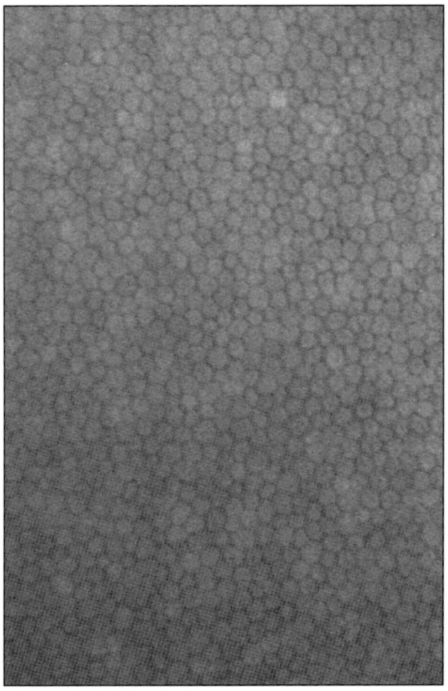

Fig. 14.7 Widefield confocal microscopic image of normal corneal endothelium (cell density 2933 cells/mm^2, mean cell area 341 mm^2, CV [coefficient of variation] 0.22, and hexagonal cells 80%).

There is an extensive literature on the quantitative analysis of the density and morphology of the corneal endothelium and this is where specular microscopy has played the greatest role in the clinical management of corneal conditions. Quantitative analysis of a specular photomicrograph is the objective description of the attributes of a selected cluster of individual endothelial cells from a specular photomicrograph. Examples include endothelial cell density (ECD) (measured as cells/mm^2), mean cell area (measured as μm^2/cell), coefficient of variation (CV) (standard deviation of cell areas/mean cell area), and pleomorphism (usually measured as a percentage of 6, <6 or >6-sided cells). Modern specular microscopes can calculate these values automatically or semiautomatically.

For quantitative analysis for the determination of ECD, at least one of the three methodologies are found in analysis software included with modern microscopes: fixed-frame, variable-frame or center methods (see Fig. 14.9A,B,D). In

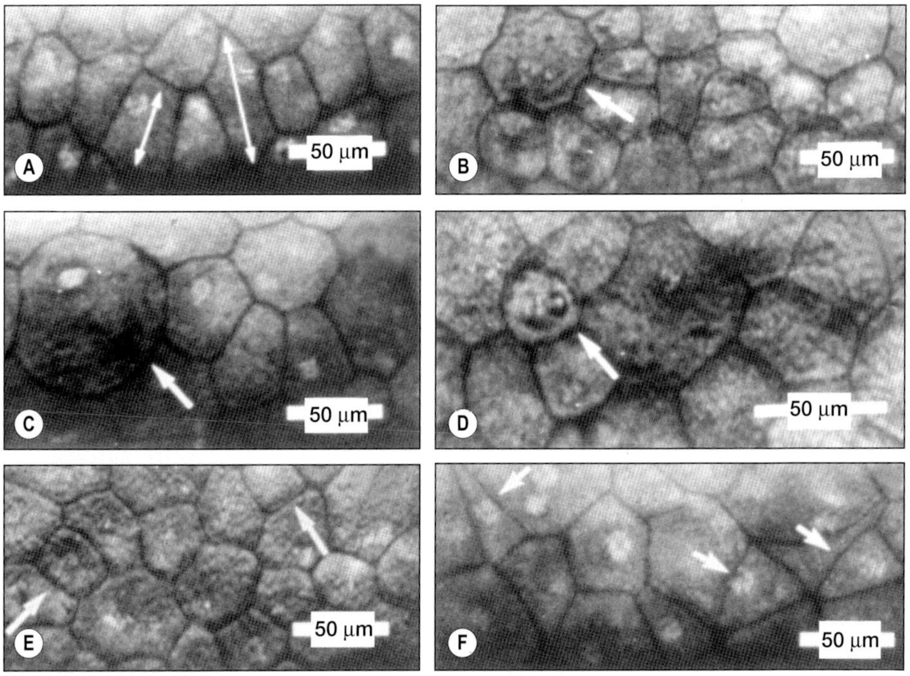

Fig. 14.8 Variations in the configuration of the corneal endothelium. (**A**) Enlarged and elongated cells. (**B**) Cells having scalloped edges. (**C** and **D**) Round cells. (**E**) Square cell. (**F**) Triangular cell. Arrows indicate the cell types mentioned.

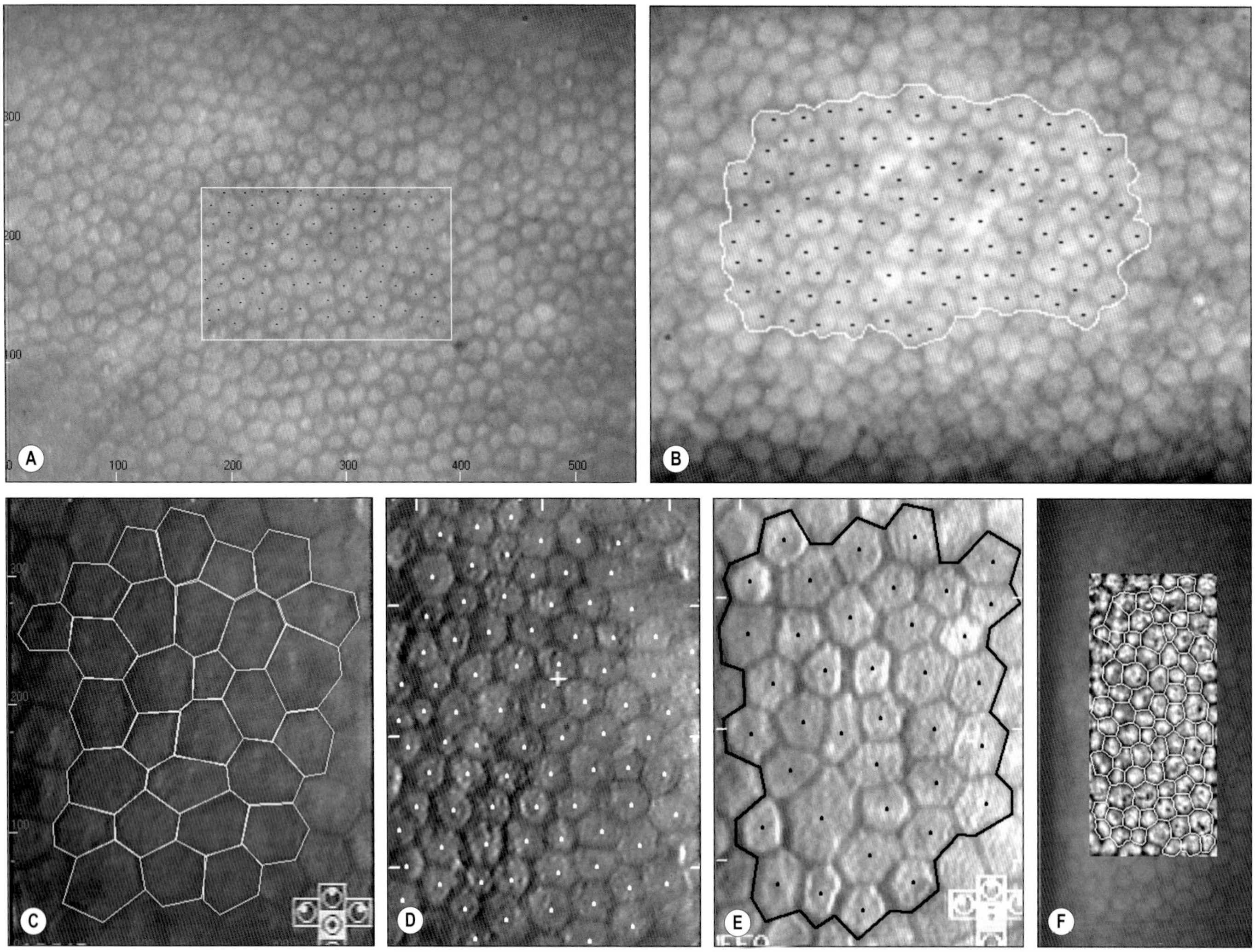

Fig. 14.9 Various analyses methods. (**A**) Fixed-frame analysis. Only the cells within the rectangle and those touching two adjacent borders are counted (dots). (**B**) Variable-frame analysis. The borders of a specific group of cells are outlined. The cells are then counted and the area calculated. (**C**) Corners analysis. The corner of each cell is marked. (**D**) Center analysis. The center of contiguous cells is marked. (**E**) Center-flex analysis. The center of cells are marked with an outlined area. (**F**) Automated. Instrument analyzes cells automatically.

addition, many modern instruments offer automated or semiautomated (manual adjustment by reader) analyses in the determination of both ECD and morphometric parameters. In fixed-frame analysis (Fig. 14.9A), the technician counts all the cells lying completely within a given area (in this case a square frame). To avoid overestimating the number of cells present, not all of the cells lying on the boundary of the frame are added. Usually the total number of cells lying on the boundary is divided by two, or only cells lying on two sides of the square are counted. The estimate of the total number of cells within this given area is then used to calculate cell density. In variable-frame analysis, (Fig. 14.9B) the technician traces the boundary of the largest possible known area of cells after calibration of the magnification of the image, preferably incorporating a minimum of 100 contiguous cells. The number of cells available for analysis is dependent on the magnification of the image and the size of the cells. The variable-frame analysis is more accurate than fixed-frame analysis because only whole cells are counted and it is not necessary to include portions of cells located on the frame boundary.

Cell density alone is not the most sensitive measure of endothelial health, as the endothelium functions even at low ECDs (under 500 cells/mm^2).[43] A number of authors have suggested that polymegathism (variation in cell area as determined by the CV) and pleomorphism (variation in cell shape as represented by the percentage of hexagonal cells) are a more sensitive measure of the endothelium under stress. As the CV goes up and the percentage of hexagonal cells goes down, this would indicate that the cell population has a less stable thermodynamic relationship between the individual cell and the adjoining neighbor cells, which correlates with declining endothelial function (loss of barrier function and pumping function). Yee et al.[44] have demonstrated the decreasing endothelial cell density and increasing pleomorphism seen with aging. These measurements, however, do not tend to vary greatly between paired human corneas.

The increased sensitivity of morphometric analysis can be illustrated in the following example. If only one cell is lost in a cluster of 100 cells, the mean cell area would increase maximally by 1%, a statistically nondetectable increase.[45] On the other hand, if a six-sided cell is lost in the cluster of 100 cells, at least two cells (2%) or possibly a maximum of six cells (6%) will show significant changes in cell pattern as adjacent cells stretch, slide, or even fuse together to repair the defect. It can, therefore, be seen how cell loss that is not detectable by cell density measurements alone may be detectable by quantification of cellular polymegathism and pleomorphism.

Most modern specular microscopes provide automated (Fig. 14.9F) or semiautomated morphometric analyses (Fig. 14.9A–E). For fully automated analyses, it is preferable to have the ability to make corrections (i.e. remove and redraw lines). The corners method (Fig. 14.9C) has been the standard method of morphometric analyses since the inception of specular microscopy more than 30 years ago.[6] With this method, the corner of each cell is denoted, and the software then connects these points to outline the cell borders, and then determines cell area. The Center method (Konan Medical USA) (Fig. 14.9D) was introduced in the late 1990s and incorporated a semiautomated method of generating morphometric data where the center of each cell and its adjoining cells are identified. This method requires the technician to accurately mark the center of an area of contiguous cells. All peripheral cells along the edge of the marked cells are discarded from analysis because there are no adjacent outer cells next to them, and adjacent cells are required to determine the distance from their centers. Thus, even if 50 cells are marked, only 25 cells may actually be analyzed. For this reason, when performing the center method, the technician should mark the center of a minimum of 100 cells. Konan has recently developed a new analysis, the center-flex method (Fig. 14.9E), which capitalizes on the advantages of both the variable-frame and center methods. With this method, the technician traces an area of cells with visible cell borders, boundaries, and centers and then marks the center of the cells within the traced area.

The accuracy of any quantitative analysis, both for ECD determination and for the determination of morphometric parameters, is dependent upon image quality, how closely the area sampled represents the entire population of endothelial cells, the technician's understanding of endothelial cell morphology, and the technician's understanding of and technique in performing the specific analysis method.[46] Image quality must be sufficient to enable the technician to identify the cell borders, boundaries, and centers. When using noncontact instruments, training is required to achieve optimal images, particularly on the thickened cornea. This typically requires the technician to take the instrument off automated into a manual capture mode. Sampling can be improved by capturing and analyzing three images taken at the same location (i.e. central corneal endothelium.) Technicians performing specular microscopy should be trained to recognize normal and abnormal corneal morphology. The most common errors seen in the clinical setting related to specular microscopy are related to improper application of the method of analysis or, in the case of automated analysis, not knowing it has failed. Examples of common errors (Fig. 14.10) are double counting or missing cells when performing the center method and failing to recognize when automated analysis has traced cell borders inaccurately.

Specular Microscopy in Clinical Trials and the Value of a Reading Center

Specular microscopy plays a significant role in safety and efficacy studies of anterior and even posterior segment procedures, devices, and pharmaceutical interventions. To minimize variability in FDA multicenter clinical trials, the following guidelines have been recommended for specular microsopy and endothelial analyses: (1) all participating sites should use the same specular microscope; (2) each individual site should use the same technician who is reading center certified in their ability to obtain good-quality images throughout the course of the study; (3) a centralized reading center should confirm calibration of each specular microscope used in the study; and (4) a single reader should analyze all the images.[46]

The Cornea Image Analysis Reading Center (CIARC), formerly the Specular Microscopy Reading Center (SMRC), at Case Western Reserve University and University Hospitals Case Medical Center in Cleveland, Ohio, has been one example that follows these guidelines. The CIARC has published its methodology for dual grading and adjudication for the determination of ECD in a multicenter clinical trial using a variety of specular microscopes.[47] The CIARC has developed these protocols to maximize the number of eligible sites, incorporate sites with noncontact microscopes that are dependent on a manufacturer's internal calibration of the image (e.g. Konan) to validate the calibration externally with a calibration tool developed jointly with the manufacturer and the CIARC, and minimize variability inherent in multicenter clinical trials. The CIARC provides the participating sites with detailed instructions for quality image capture techniques and microscope-specific quality standards. Multiple technicians can be certified for study participation based on their ability to consistently produce quality images, export the images, properly deidentify the images of all protected health information, label the images per protocol, and properly submit the images to the reading center.

The CIARC has developed standardized procedures to externally calibrate each commercially available specular microscope for the purposes of analysis at the reading center. The CIARC performs detailed training and certification procedures for each method of analysis employed by its readers so that the data are consistent over the course of a study regardless of staffing changes. The CIARC provides dual assessment of ECD[47] and morphometric parameters with adjudication to address interobserver variability and a retesting procedure to address intraobserver variability, assuring consistent standards over an extended period of time by the readers. In addition, the CIARC image quality criteria classification system[47] provides specific image quality criteria in order to evaluate factors that may influence image quality and affect endothelial analyses.

Through its work on the Specular Microscopy Ancillary Study (SMAS) and other multicenter studies, the CIARC has determined that, for multicenter clinical trials, a reproducible and reliable central reading center methodology for the

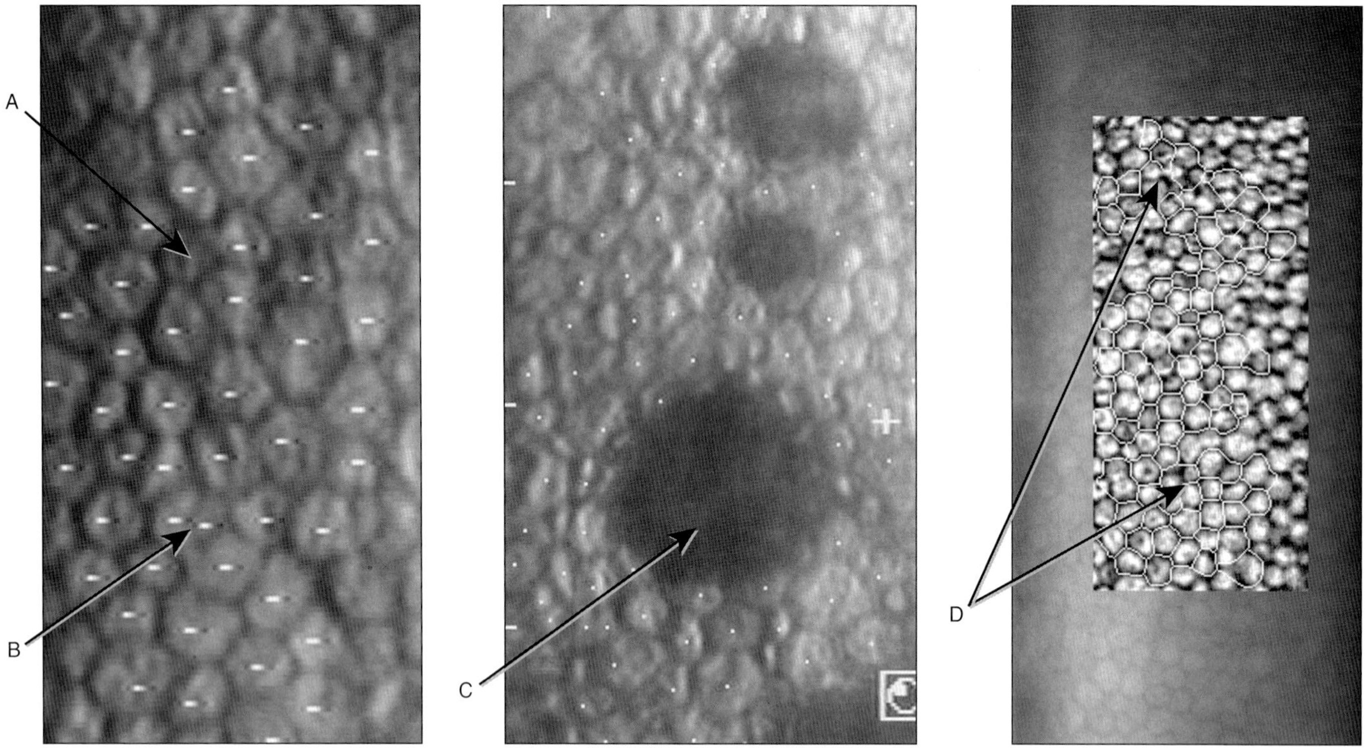

Fig. 14.10 Examples of common counting and analysis errors. (**A**) Missed cells. (**B**) Double counting. (**C**) Inclusion of unanalyzable areas in frame. (**D**) Automation failed to trace cell borders accurately.

assessment of endothelial image quality and ECD and morphometric analyses includes the use of certified readers, a defined image quality classification scheme, dual grading and adjudication, and masked quality control procedures are all critical for the conduct of large, multicenter, long-term studies.[47,48]

Clinical Applications for Specular Microscopy

Clinical specular microscopy is a practical tool not only for the cornea subspecialist in evaluating donor corneas and corneal dystrophies but also for the ophthalmic surgeon in identifying subtle as well as macroscopic changes in the cornea prior to surgery. A clear cornea with a normal pachymetry reading is no assurance of a normal endothelial morphology or cell density. The ECD at which corneal edema occurs is quite variable, but has been estimated to be between 300 and 700 cells per mm^2.[40,49,50] A recent study, however, has shown that at least in penetrating keratoplasty grafts, 14% of the clear grafts (40 of 277 participants) at 5 years had an ECD below 500 cells/mm^2.[43] Assuming a cell loss in the range of 0–30% for any given intraocular surgical event, a patient should have at least 1000 to 1200 cells per mm^2 to safely undergo most anterior segment surgery without an increased risk of permanent postoperative corneal edema. Moreover, when the ECD approaches this arbitrary cell count range, it behooves the surgeon to make certain that the patient understands the increased risk of postoperative corneal edema and subsequent corneal decompensation. Most patients, including those over the age of 70, should have an ECD of at least 2000 cells per mm^2; however, given the large variation of ECD among age groups, age alone cannot be used to predict ECD. Typically, there should be no significant difference in the ECD between eyes. With age, however, some people can develop a significant difference in the ECD. To be meaningful, this difference should be greater than 280 cells per mm^2.[51]

There is evidence that a polymegathic and pleomorphic corneal endothelium does not tolerate intraocular surgery as well as a more uniform endothelium. A cornea with a coefficient of variation greater than 0.40 or the presence of less than 50% hexagonal cells should be considered abnormal and at increased risk for postoperative edema. As in ECD measurements, there is a range of variation of polymegathism and pleomorphism in all age groups, and age alone cannot be used to predict the endothelial morphologic appearance.

When an endothelial abnormality is noted during the preoperative examination, specular microscopy can often provide valuable information that may affect management.[19] Such slit lamp abnormalities can include corneal guttae, keratic precipitates, pigmented and inflammatory cells, endothelial surface or Descemet's membrane irregularities, and increased corneal thickness. A history of possible endothelial abnormality, i.e. family history of corneal dystrophy,[52] trauma,[53] acute narrow-angle[54–56] or chronic open-angle glaucoma, uveitis,[57–60] keratitis, graft rejection,[61] previous ocular surgery,[62,63] secondary intraocular lens implantation,[64] or corneal transplantation,[65] can also affect the surgical outcome. When evaluating postoperative corneas, it is particularly important to utilize multiple images in the central, midperiphery, and even periphery, because a regional disparity in ECD and morphology in these postoperative corneas has been reported.[64,66,67]

Aging

In most individuals, ECD decreases (or mean cell area increases) throughout life.[68] Cell loss is most rapid from birth to the first few years of life.[69,70] Part of this decrease in ECD may be due to the normal enlargement of the globe during early childhood.[71] ECD is rather stable from age 20 through approximately age 50 years.[72] After the age of 60 years, ECD decreases significantly in most people, but there is a great degree of variability between individuals. On average, age-related cell loss is approximately 0.5% per year.[73] A higher variability in polymegathism and pleomorphism has also been shown to correlate with age.[74,75]

Corneal guttae

Corneal guttae is a common condition, the incidence of which increases significantly with age.[76,77] Corneal guttae are focal accumulations of collagen on the posterior surface of Descemet's membrane that are abnormal products formed by stressed or abnormal endothelial cells. Microscopically, they appear as mushroom-shaped excrescences of Descemet's membrane. These guttae can easily be seen by specular microscopy.[78–81]

Fuchs' endothelial corneal dystrophy

In 1910, Ernst Fuchs[82] initially described bilateral corneal stromal and epithelial edema in elderly patients without the benefit of slit lamp microscopy. With the advent of biomicroscopy, it became possible to diagnose early endothelial involvement by the presence of guttae, making it unclear whether the term Fuchs' endothelial corneal dystrophy (FECD) should be used for the early stage with endothelial changes or only for advanced disease associated with corneal edema.[83–85] It seems that most ophthalmologists, however, reserve the term FECD for guttae that are confluent by more than 1–2 mm centrally or paracentrally advancing to great confluence and corneal edema.[85]

FECD is usually bilateral and is more commonly seen in women in their thirties to sixties.[86] It is a progressive endothelial dystrophy that results in endothelial dysfunction, leading to progressive corneal stromal edema and eventually epithelial edema and subepithelial fibrosis (Fig. 14.11). Laing et al.[78] have described the progressive morphologic changes of corneal guttae in FECD. Five specific stages in the development of excrescences can be discerned during the early evolution of the disorder All five stages can occur in a cornea clinically free of edema. Several stages can be observed in the same cornea at a given time, although in most cases the majority of corneal guttae seem to have progressed to the same stage of development. More recently, there has been an early-onset form of FECD recognized, that has an equal representation in males and females, occurring below the age of 50, which notably has marked thickening of the anterior banded layer of the Descemet's membrane with a normal posterior nonbanded layer, unlike the more common late-onset disease in which this layer is predominantly affected.[87,88] This early-onset disease is noted to be due to a pathogenic mutation in *COL8A2* gene, which encodes the alpha2 subtype of collagen VIII, a major component of Descemet's membrane.

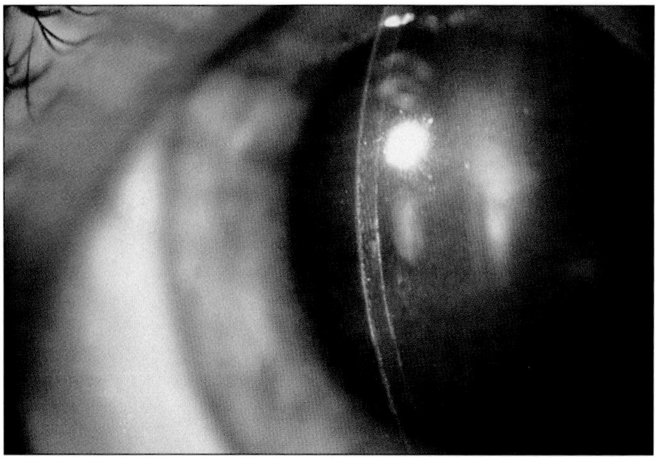

Fig. 14.11 Slit lamp photo of a patient with Fuchs' endothelial corneal dystrophy demonstrating guttae and subepithelial fibrosis.

Specular microscopy of the common late-onset form of FECD demonstrates that an individual excrescence begins as a very small structure, much smaller than an individual endothelial cell. Adjacent endothelial cells appear normal. In time, however, the excrescence grows and begins to distort overlying and adjacent endothelial cells, making the borders of these cells indistinct. The guttae themselves appear as dark spots, sometimes with bright central reflections. In the case of FECD, they are usually more numerous centrally. If the guttae are confluent, slit lamp microscopy can reveal a beaten-silver appearance of the posterior cornea, similar to that seen in the iridocorneal endothelial (ICE) syndrome. The images of the guttae and endothelium in the early-onset form of FECD have a distinctive difference from the late-onset form with every endothelial cell associated with a single, low-elevation gutta (Fig. 14.12), a pattern of high density that alternates with large areas devoid of guttae (early onset) compared to sharply raised guttae with higher elevation and areas of coalescence (late onset).[87]

Ultrastructural studies in late-onset FECD have revealed both smooth, rounded excrescences and excrescences with flat, broad posterior surfaces containing a central depression.[89,90] The latter umbilicated excrescences tend to be larger than the rounded excrescences, suggesting that the irregular posterior surface may represent a maturational change.

Many surgeons assess corneas with FECD before intraocular surgery to help predict the prognosis for postoperative corneal clarity. This specular evaluation, in addition to the clinical history of frequent fluctuating vision, abnormal pachymetry readings, and formation of microcystic bullae, and/or subepithelial fibrosis, can aid in deciding whether penetrating or endothelial keratoplasty is necessary at the time of intraocular surgery. If there are a significant number of peripheral endothelial cells and the guttae are primarily

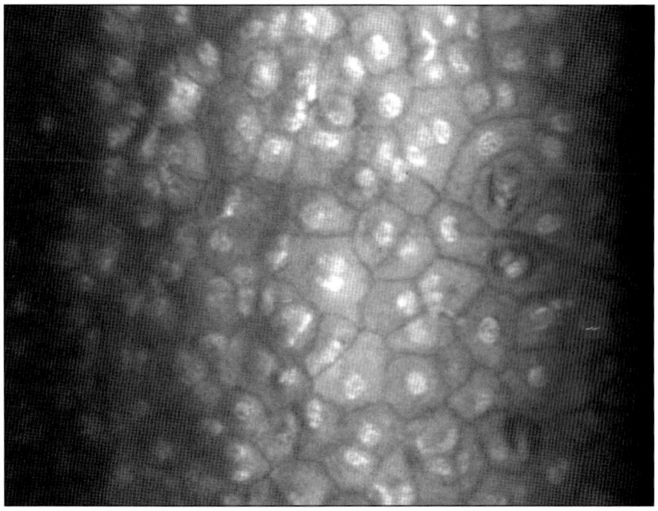

Fig. 14.12 Confocal microscopic image of a 32-year-old individual with early-onset FECD with the L450W-*COL8A2* mutation. (With permission, from *Invest Ophthalmol Vis Sci*, June 2005, Vol. 46, No. 6, page 1936, Fig. 3A.)

located centrally, there is a decreased likelihood that corneal transplantation will be necessary. On the other hand, if there is complete confluence of guttae even in the peripheral cornea associated with increased corneal thickness of over 0.68 microns (μm), one might consider a combined procedure.

Despite the advantages offered by specular microscopy, the likelihood of postoperative corneal clarity can be difficult to judge. For this reason, some surgeons do not consider keratoplasty combined with another intraocular procedure unless evidence of significant stromal edema is already present preoperatively.

Lattice corneal dystrophy

Lattice dystrophy is inherited in an autosomal dominant manner. Clinically, the dystrophy appears quite early – at the age of 2 to 7 years. As the disease progresses, the cornea becomes progressively cloudy, causing a marked reduction in acuity by age 20–30. The disease is caused by amyloid deposition throughout the stroma. Recurrent erosions sometimes result from the superficial nature of some of the deposits.

Specular microscopy of patients with lattice corneal dystrophy has revealed the presence of linear structures described as branching lines which crisscross the stroma. These lines are believed to be amyloid deposits or lesions caused by amyloid deposition.[91–93] A crater-form appearance has also been described.[91] Although abnormalities of both Bowman's layer and the epithelium have been documented histologically, no endothelial abnormalities have been found.[92]

Iridocorneal endothelial syndrome

The iridocorneal endothelial (ICE) syndrome is a progressive, nonfamilial group of disorders with female predominance. It consists of three variants, previously believed to be independent entities, but now grouped under the term ICE syndrome. These three variants are Chandler's syndrome, essential iris atrophy, and Cogan-Reese syndrome (the iris nevus syndrome).[94,95] All three are characterized by a fundamental abnormality of the corneal endothelium that is responsible for variable degrees of iris atrophy, secondary angle-closure glaucoma, and corneal edema.[96–98] The disease may be related to a herpes simplex virus (HSV) infection of the corneal endothelium.[99] This helps explain its unilateral clinical presentation; however, studies have demonstrated subclinical involvement of the contralateral eye, evidenced by a degree of endothelial cell pleomorphism and polymegathism that is inconsistent with the patient's age.[100–104]

Ultrastructural studies of the more involved eye reveal abnormal endothelium covering a thickened, multilayered Descemet's membrane which can extend over the inner surface of the trabecular meshwork and anterior iris surface.[95,105–108] Glaucoma may result from contraction of the membrane, which can also result in peripheral anterior synechiae with secondary glaucoma and various iris abnormalities.[98] The affected endothelial cells can also take on features of epithelial cells and can even become multilayered.[108]

The specular microscopic appearance of the endothelium is characterized as a rounding off of cell angles.[109,110] There is a loss of cellular definition and hexagonal shape, and many pentagonal cells are evident.[103,111] There can also be an increased granularity of the intracellular details, and small, centric dark areas in individual cells which can enlarge and become completely blacked-out areas within the cell.[110,112] Slit lamp examination will often reveal a characteristic hammered-silver appearance of the posterior cornea, which can involve the entire posterior corneal surface or only part of it.[97,108,110] As the disease progresses, the endothelial monolayer may no longer be recognizable as a mosaic of cells. A 'reversal appearance' may develop, with black central areas and white borders (Fig. 14.13).[103,108,110]

Posterior polymorphous corneal dystrophy

Posterior polymorphous corneal dystrophy (PPCD) is a disorder of the posterior, nonbanded layer of Descemet's membrane. It is usually bilateral and is usually inherited as an autosomal dominant trait with variable expressivity. The clinical manifestations of PPCD are similar to those of the ICE syndrome, which complicates the diagnosis. Unlike ICE syndrome, however, PPCD is generally bilateral, nonprogressive, and only occasionally associated with corneal decompensation, visual dysfunction, and glaucoma.[90]

A review of PPCD by Waring et al.[90] divides its appearance, as seen with the slit lamp, into three basic forms: vesicular, band, and diffuse. All forms demonstrate the classic posterior polymorphous vesicle, a small, round, blister-like lesion at the level of Descemet's membrane, surrounded by a ring of opacity (Fig. 14.14A).[113] Using specular microscopy, this vesicle can be used to differentiate PPCD from ICE syndrome. When examined with the specular microscope, the vesicle has a thick, dark border yielding a doughnut-like appearance (Fig. 14.14B). This structure appears to lie anterior to undistorted endothelial cells, which are generally more recognizable toward the center of the lesion.[113–115] A similar appearance can be seen when an

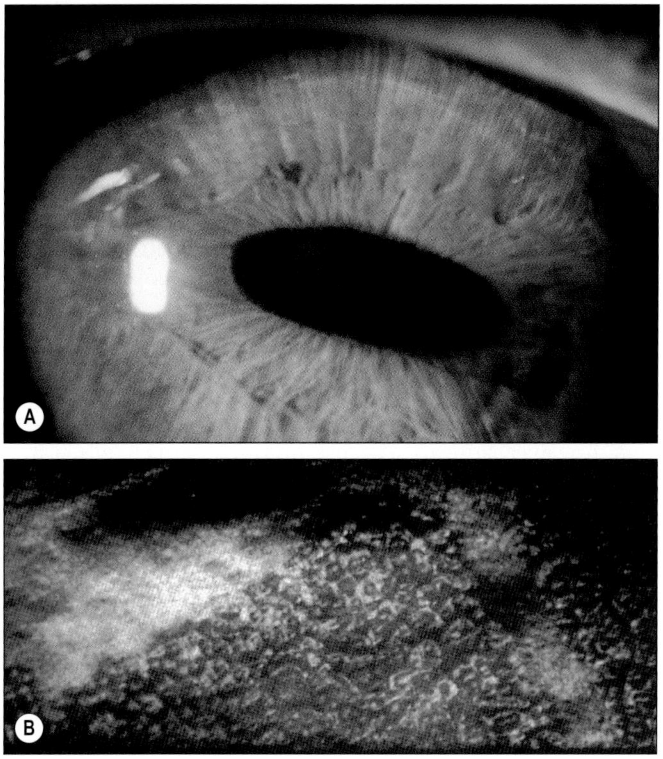

Fig. 14.13 Iridocorneal endothelial syndrome. (**A**) Slit lamp appearance of ICE (Chandler's) syndrome. (**B**) Specular micrograph showing more normal endothelium in the upper left quadrant and the adjacent characteristic 'reversal pattern' often seen in Chandler's syndrome.

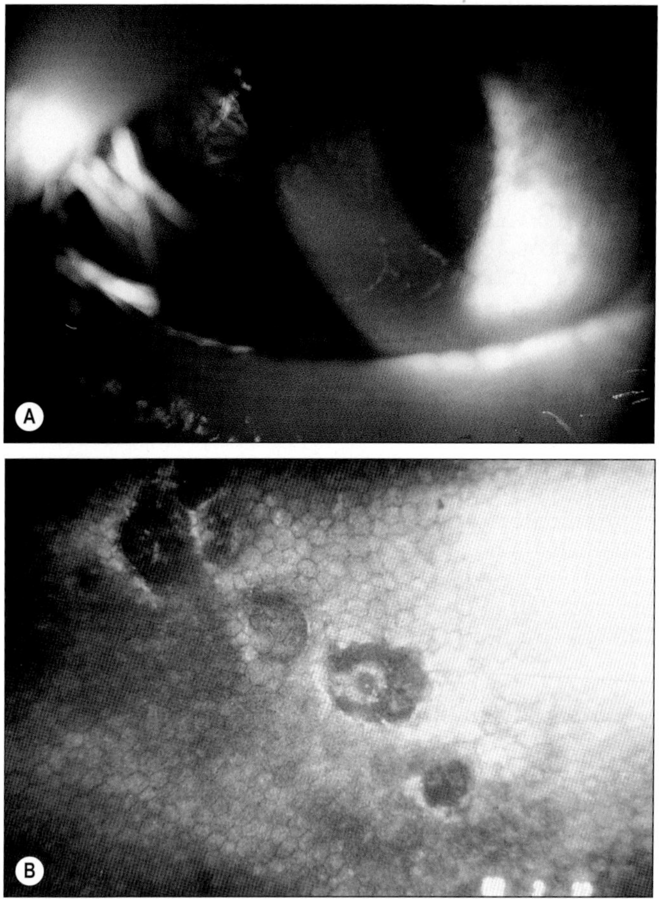

Fig. 14.14 Posterior polymorphous corneal dystrophy. (**A**) Slit lamp appearance of posterior corneal polymorphous dystrophy. (**B**) Specular micrograph demonstrates round vesicles circumscribed by elongated abnormal cells.

isolated patch of ICE cells (also known as an ICE-berg) is identified in a patient with ICE syndrome. In ICE syndrome, however, the lesion does not appear anterior to the endothelium as in PPCD, but appears to lie within the endothelium. Furthermore, the endothelial cells adjacent to the structure are not normal in appearance as in PPCD, but are distorted and commonly smaller than normal.[113,115]

Specular microscopy has also been useful in distinguishing PPCD from other problems causing corneal opacities. The parallel 'rail track' (straight) borders from old Descemet's tears, such as those from Haab's striae, can be distinguished from the 'snail tracks' (irregular) seen in the band presentation of PPCD.[115,116]

Keratoconus

Specular microscopy of keratoconic corneas has revealed two populations of endothelial cells, one larger and one considerably smaller than normal. The most striking abnormality in keratoconus, however, is elongation of endothelial cells.[117] The cells appear to have been stretched by the ectatic process with their long axis in the direction of the apex of the cone. This lends support to the concept that acute corneal hydrops is a result of stretching of the endothelium and Descemet's membrane. These structures are thought to be stretched to the point of rupture, allowing the passage of aqueous into the stroma. Dehydration of the cornea usually occurs, presumably a result of endothelial cell migration and enlargement to cover the defect. This concept is supported by the finding of localized areas of endothelial cells that are 7 to 10 times larger than normal near the site of rupture.[117,118] Away from the site of rupture, however, the endothelial cells are of a more normal size and morphologic appearance, suggesting that the area of enlarged cells represents the site of endothelial and Descemet's rupture and the subsequent changes necessary to repair the defect.

Other abnormal findings seen in keratoconus include the presence of dark bodies completely contained within an otherwise normal-appearing cell. These dark bodies occur less frequently in larger endothelial cells and are consistent in appearance with blebs or vacuoles seen with the electron microscope.[119] Their role in the pathogenesis of keratoconus is not presently understood.

Glaucoma

Persistently elevated intraocular pressure likely results in gradual loss of endothelial cells and progressive loss of endothelial function.[120] This is evidenced by the decreasing pressure at which the cornea becomes edematous in many glaucoma patients as their disease progresses.[120] In vitro experiments, however, revealed no morphologic changes despite elevated pressures, as long as normal aqueous flow was maintained.[121] These experiments suggest that endothelial cell loss is not a direct result of increased pressure, but rather some other disturbance such as prolonged low oxygen concentration in the aqueous humor. Furthermore, in patients with unilateral glaucoma or a history of unilateral attacks of glaucomatocyclitic crisis, specular microscopy reveals a decreased endothelial cell density in the eye affected with glaucoma.[122–124] If the pressure is medically controlled, cell loss is reduced.[122] Studies have shown varying cell loss connected with various glaucoma procedures, in particular trabeculomy and tube shunts.[125–128]

Intraocular inflammation

During an acute episode of anterior uveitis, mononuclear inflammatory cells penetrate apical junctional complexes and infiltrate both between endothelial cells and between endothelial cells and Descemet's membrane (see Fig. 14.6H). Endothelial cells, however, are not generally harmed by this process,[58] but in the most severe case can become dislodged and float free in the aqueous humor.[129]

Cataract extraction with intraocular lens implantation

Numerous investigators have reported findings on specular microscopy after cataract extraction.[63,130–159] Reports of endothelial cell loss after cataract surgery using a variety of surgical approaches have demonstrated variable cell loss ranging from no detectable cell loss to as much as 40% cell loss. Methods of cataract surgery, however, have changed dramatically through the years and are now much less damaging to the endothelium. Endothelial cell loss following uncomplicated phacoemulsification and posterior chamber intraocular lens implantation using viscoelastic and modern, small-incision techniques is quite low, ranging from no detectable cell loss to 20%.[131,133,135,136,141–144,159] There does not appear to be a statistical difference between endothelial cell loss resulting from phacoemulsification versus extracapsular cataract extraction.[135,138,140,159] Furthermore, suture fixation of a posterior chamber intraocular lens[160] or placement of an intraocular lens in the sulcus[132] appears to be no more traumatic and results in no more endothelial cell loss than a posterior chamber intraocular lens placed in the capsular bag. The implantation of an anterior chamber lens, however, has been shown to result in not only higher endothelial cell loss due to the procedure itself but also continued endothelial loss which is greater than that of posterior chamber intraocular lenses [64,148,161–163]

Endothelial damage during phacoemulsification has been attributed to mechanical injury caused by anterior chamber instrumentation and/or anterior chamber manipulation of a lens nucleus, heat generation, or prolonged intraocular irrigation.[164,165] Endothelial loss, however, also correlates with ultrasound time and power[140,142,143] and is greatest near the wound, which is also the area of maximal manipulation.[67,166–169] The endothelium suffering the least damage is the greatest distance away from the wound. Despite the ability of the endothelium to migrate during many forms of endothelial insult, this endothelial disparity may not correct with time.

In the past, significant endothelial damage could result from even momentary contact between the hydrophobic intraocular lens surface and the endothelium.[170–172] The development of viscoelastics significantly limited such injury. Additionally, modern intraocular lenses now have a hydrophilic surface that produces minimal endothelial damage, especially when used with viscoelastic. The choice, however, of a dispersive viscoelastic over a cohesive viscoelastic does not appear to result in any less endothelial cell loss,[133,139,149,150,173] even though one could reason that a dispersive viscoelastic might provide more endothelial protection.[170] Other surgical materials, such as stainless steel, also cause endothelial damage on contact. The natural crystalline lens, however, appears to cause minimal damage when it is in contact with the endothelium for short periods.

Refractive surgery

Numerous investigators have studied the effects of photorefractive keratectomy (PRK)[174–179] and laser-assisted in situ keratomileusis (LASIK)[174,180–184] on the corneal endothelium. Most studies have shown that neither LASIK nor PRK results in a decreased endothelial density.[180] Laser ablation of the stroma within 200 μm of the corneal endothelium, however, will result in endothelial structural changes and the formation of the amorphous substance deposited onto Descemet's membrane.[185] Only two clinical studies have reported endothelial cell loss after LASIK or PRK.[174,186] Each of these studies, however, was composed primarily of patients with high myopia requiring very deep ablations.

Interestingly, many investigators have described an increase in central endothelial cell density after PRK and LASIK.[179,180,184] This is felt to be a result of endothelial migration initiated by the discontinuation of contact lens wear[174] and not a result of refractive surgery.[179,180,184]

Several studies have been conducted on the effects of PRK, LASIK, and laser-assisted subepithelial keratectomy (LASEK) on ECD. Diakonis et al.[187] studied the effects of mitomycin-C (MMC), an intraoperative agent used to decrease haze and regression, on ECD after use during PRK. While there was a decrease in ECD at 1 month and 3 months postoperatively, the authors concluded this may be due to the issues encountered with the repeatablity of ECD determination.[187] Other studies on the effects of mitomycin-C during LASEK have also found no significant changes in the corneal endothelium.[188,189]

Azar et al.[190] studied the effects of uncomplicated intrastromal corneal ring segment placement on the corneal endothelium. ECD was determined preoperatively and at 6, 12, and 24 months. Significant endothelial cell loss was not present at the 6- and 12-month visits, but a decrease in ECD was found at the 24-month visit, which may or may not be related to surgery.

Previously, implantation of phakic intraocular lenses were thought to result in significant endothelial cell loss.[190–196] More recently, long-term studies on the FDA-approved Artisan/Verisyse phakic intraocular lens (IOL) have found acceptable mean cell loss rates of 1.8% per year after insertion to correct high myopia.[197] Hexagonality and coefficient of variation during a 4-year follow-up study were comparable to preoperative numbers.[188] Candidates who narrowly meet the minimal ECD of 2000 cells/mm^2,[198] are suggested to have greater anterior chamber depth due to greater cell loss.[199] Additionally, increased aqueous flare,[191] decreased crystalline lens transmittance,[191,195] pupillary ovalization,[192,193] and chronic inflammation[192,195] have been described after implantation of phakic intraocular lenses but these have been minimized with the use of iris-fixated IOLs, proper training, and strict exclusion criteria.[200]

Penetrating keratoplasty

Specular microscopy of successful penetrating keratoplasty (PKP) has revealed substantial but variable endothelial cell loss occurring during and shortly after surgery.[48,201–203] Furthermore, endothelial loss well above that found in normal eyes appears to continue throughout the life of the graft.[203–205] Ing et al.[204] have demonstrated that, 5 to 10 years after successful PKP for a variety of indications including keratoconus and endothelial dysfunction disorders, endothelial cell loss progresses at a rate seven times faster than normal. However, between 10 and 15 years, this rate substantially slows and approaches the rate of loss of endothelial cells in normal aging.[201] In the Specular Microscopy Ancillary Study (SMAS) of the multicenter Cornea Donor Study (CDS) examining the impact of donor age on graft survival and endothelial cell loss following PKP for endothelial dysfunction conditions only (FECD, pseudophakic/aphakic corneal edema), a substantial 70% median endothelial cell loss from baseline to 5 years postoperatively overall was noted (Fig. 14.15).[48] The younger age group (12–65 years old) experienced a substantial but slightly lower 69% median percentage cell loss, compared to the older group (66–75 years old) of 75% cell loss; however, graft clarity was equal in both groups at 5 years, at 86% of the 1090 grafts performed.[206] In part because of this difference between cell loss with comparable graft clarity, the study has now been extended to 10 years. Another longitudinal study following PKPs for a variety of conditions done by one surgeon has shown that of the 388 initial grafts used for analysis, the 67 cases available for analysis at year 15 had a 71% endothelial cell loss, which was unchanged from the 10-year analysis.[201]

Besides the contribution of the SMAS to our understanding of endothelial cell loss following PKP for at least the endothelial dysfunctions, the study also provided insight as to the importance of the quality of the specular image in achieving the most accurate cell count by the eye bank and also pointed out the variability of cell counting among eye banks and the importance of a reading center to provide the most accurate, standardized endothelial cell density (ECD) determination.[47,206a] Accuracy of counting by the eye bank correlated with image quality, while 35% of the cell counts determined by the eye banks were 10% higher or lower than the reading center.[206a] This study has prompted a need to develop new standards for cell counting among the eye banks in the United States.

It is fortunate that a surprisingly low endothelial cell density can maintain the cornea in a dehydrated, transparent state.[43,207] In the SMAS, 40 (14%) of 277 subjects with a clear graft after 5 years had an ECD below 500 cells/mm^2.[43] This had been previously shown in other studies.[207,208] Nonetheless, there is a critical endothelial cell density below which irreversible corneal edema occurs, explaining the sudden decompensation of some grafted corneas years after successful transplantation.[209]

Obata et al.[202] measured the endothelial cell density of 58 corneal grafts both before and after PKP. At the 2-week postoperative visit, endothelial cell density had decreased by only about 10%, indicating significant intraoperative endothelial loss had not occurred. Endothelial cell loss was most rapid during the early postoperative course but then gradually slowed. At the 3-month postoperative visit, endothelial cell loss averaged 33%. By 1 year, endothelial loss of all eyes averaged nearly 50%. Cell loss in the keratoconus subgroup, however, measured only 33% after 1 year. Langenbucher et al.[210] followed their patients beyond the initial postoperative period when cell loss is greatest and still noted a similar disparity among patients with keratoconus. They described an annual cell loss of only 2.9% in patients who underwent keratoplasty for keratoconus. On the other hand, patients who underwent PKP for FECD or bullous keratopathy had an annual cell loss of 11.2% and 19.3%, respectively. This was observed similarly in the SMAS.[48] Such findings have suggested that endothelial cells may migrate along a density gradient after penetrating keratoplasty.[211] This may explain the decreased endothelial cell loss seen in keratoconus, given the relatively normal peripheral host keratoconic endothelium. On the other hand, Ruusuvaara[212] has documented great endothelial disparities between the graft and the recipient, leading one to believe that migration may not occur in this fashion.

The presence or absence of a lens has also been shown to affect endothelial cell loss after PKP.[63,204] Ing et al.[204] have shown that patients who are aphakic have the least cell loss after PKP, and patients who are phakic or pseudophakic have the greatest cell loss. Some of this cell loss may, however, be attributable to increased cell loss during the actual surgical procedure. Bourne has demonstrated that phakic patients lose significantly more endothelial cells during PKP than do aphakic patients.[213] This finding was attributed to the deeper anterior chamber and the absence of endothelial trauma from the lens–iris diaphragm in the aphakic eye. The difference in endothelial cell loss between phakic and aphakic eyes, however, has not been confirmed by other studies[63,214] and needs further research.

Recent findings from the SMAS have shown that baseline donor ECD, at least following PKP for endothelial dysfunction disorders, does not predict graft failure 5 years postoperatively.[43] Interestingly, the 6-month ECD does predict failure. Among those that had not failed within the first 6 months, the 5-year cumulative incidence of failure was 13% in the 33 subjects with a 6-month ECD less than 1700 cells/mm^2 versus 2% in the 137 subjects with a 6-month ECD of 2500 cells/mm^2 or higher. These findings may not apply to endothelial keratoplasty (EK), which has an entirely different pattern of cell loss (see below) with usually twice as much loss in the first 6 months post EK, but a significantly lower rate of cell loss thereafter than PKP.

Although transplanted corneas recovered excellent deturgescence capabilities, Sato has demonstrated that, in comparison with normal corneas, a small but statistically

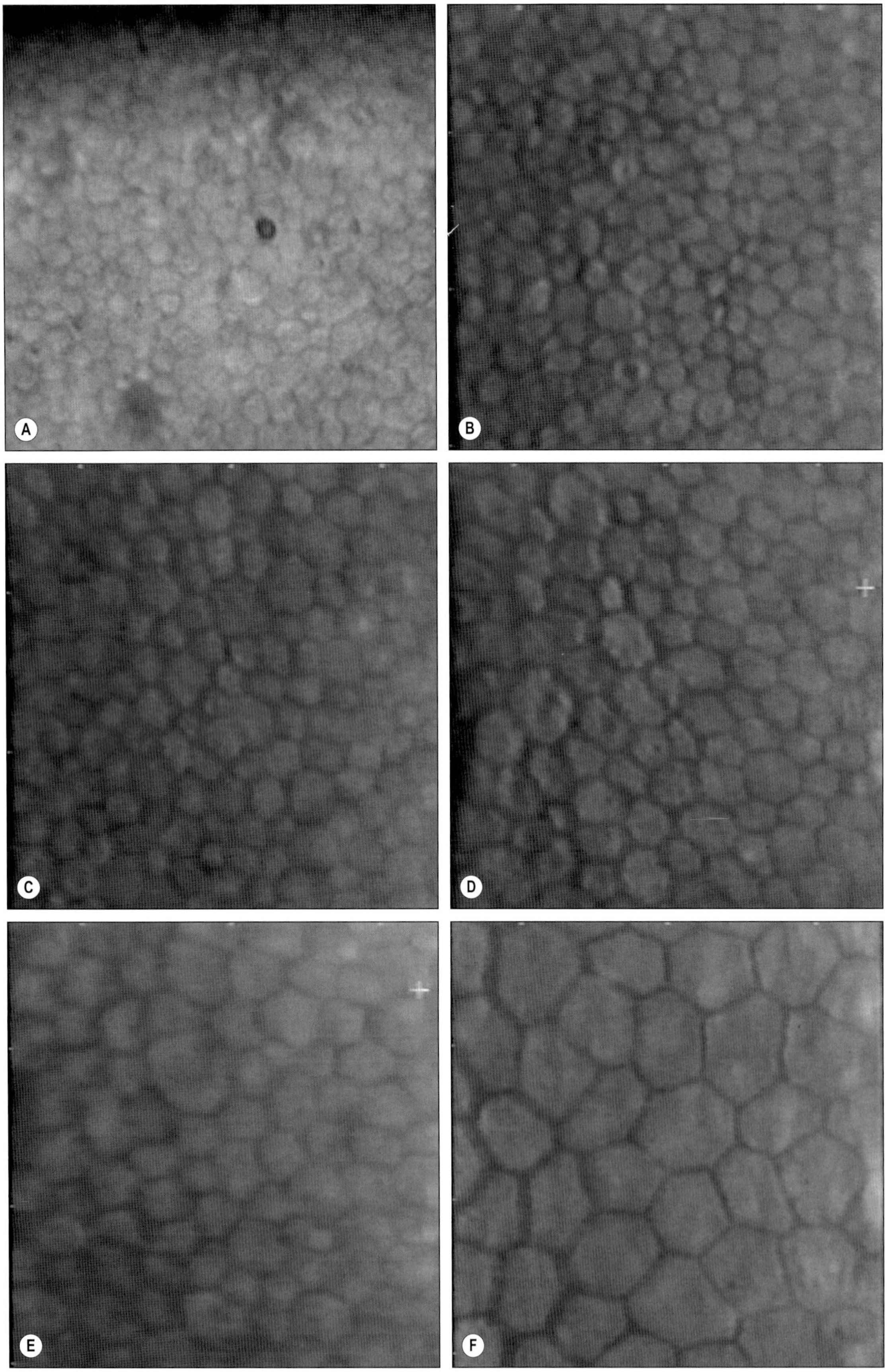

Fig. 14.15 Endothelial cell loss following PKP for endothelial dysfunction in the Specular Microscopy Ancillary Study with clear graft at 5 years. (**A**) baseline, (**B**) one year, (**C**) two years, (**D**) three years, (**E**) four years, and (**F**) five years.

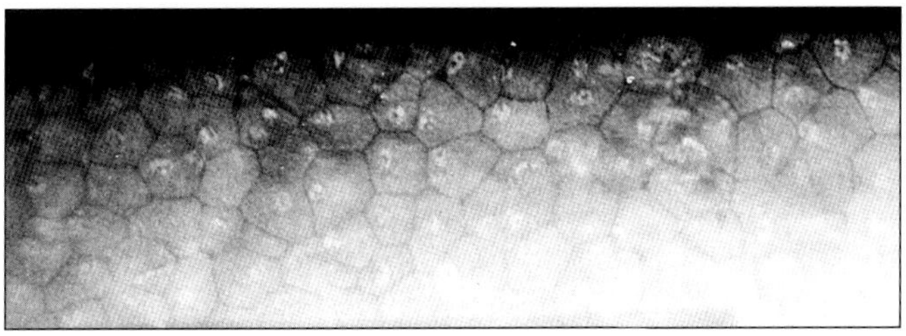

Fig. 14.16 Specular microscopic image of corneal endothelium during a corneal transplantation rejection reaction. Note the small particles adherent to the endothelium, presumably inflammatory cells.

significant increase in corneal thickness persisted.[215] The correlation between graft thickness and endothelial cell size or endothelial cell pleomorphism was not significant. The transfer coefficient of fluorescein from the aqueous humor to the cornea was, however, significantly greater in cases of uneventful PKP than in normal corneas, indicating a persistent increase in the endothelial permeability. Thus, endothelial function of the clear graft is not completely normal. The correlation between graft thickness and endothelial permeability (as measured by the transfer coefficient of fluorescein) is statistically significant,[213,215,216] suggesting that endothelial permeability, rather than the variation in cell size (polymegathism) or cell shape (pleomorphism) of endothelial cells, is the major factor that determines the thickness of a clear corneal graft. Additional longitudinal morphometric studies are needed to correlate changes in parameters such as the coefficient of variation (variation in cell size, polymegathism) and percentage of hexagonal cell (variation in cell shape, pleomorphism) with subsequent increase in corneal thickness and subsequent graft failure.

Besides quantitative determination of changes in cell density and morphometric parameters (CV, percentage hexagonal cells), qualitative specular microscopy can detect early evidence of graft rejection not detectable by clinical examination and can thus be of value in following certain high-risk patients. During graft rejection episodes, one sees intercellular bright bodies, black inflammatory cells, and generally recognizable keratic precipitates on the endothelial surface (Fig. 14.16).[217–219]

Endothelial keratoplasty

Endothelial keratoplasty (EK) has rapidly become the procedure of choice for endothelial dysfunction since 2006. According to the Eye Bank Association of America (EBAA) 2008 statistics, EK increased from 1429 to 18 221 of the total keratoplasty cases (3% to 30%), over the past 3 years in the United States.[220] The procedure has been applied to all endothelial failure conditions, including FECD, pseudophakic/aphakic corneal edema, the iridocorneal endothelial syndromes, posterior polymorphous corneal dystrophy, and failed graft.[221–235] The goal of EK is to remove only the diseased endothelial layer of the affected cornea. The first human cases were described by Melles[236,237] as posterior lamellar keratoplasty (PLK) in 1998, and refined by Terry using new instrumentation as deep lamellar endothelial keratoplasty (DLEK) in 2001.[238] Melles went on to develop a technique to excise Descemet's membrane from the recipient cornea (descemetorhexis).[239] Price performed the first procedure using stripping Descemet's membrane and named this form of EK, Descemet stripping endothelial keratoplasty (DSEK).[221] Gorovoy further refined the procedure utilizing a microkeratome to cut the donor, thus automated, and described the procedure as Descemet stripping automated endothelial keratoplasty (DSAEK).[222] Recently, Melles has developed a procedure solely transplanting Descemet's with endothelium, Descemet membrane endothelial keratoplasty (DMEK).[223,240,241]

EK has grown rapidly in popularity because of its many benefits over PKP, including smaller wound size, less astigmatism, less wound dehiscence, and faster visual recovery. These advantages are tempered by greater initial potential donor trauma, a higher primary donor failure rate, and common dislocation of the donor necessitating repositioning in the early postoperative period. Initial studies with experienced surgeons have shown comparable success to PKP in regards to graft clarity at 3 years postoperatively, but longer-term 5-year graft success remains to be determined.[227] There is limited endothelial cell loss data utilizing either specular microscopy or confocal microscopy for the most recent methods for EK, DSEK, and DSAEK. Most authors have reported significantly greater cell loss in the first 6 months after EK compared to PKP. For example, one EK study showed 34% cell loss after 6 months, and 38% at 1 year, comparable to other studies.[224,227,228,232,233] Interestingly, although there is greater loss at 1 year when compared to PKP, the rate of cell loss begins to level off around 6 months, unlike PKP, as observed by several authors.[224,227,228,232,242] After 1 year, there is minimal loss to the second and third years, 7% between 6 months and 2 years, and 8% between 6 months and 3 years, compared with 42% in the eyes that underwent PKP in the Specular Microscopy Ancillary Study (SMAS) of the Cornea Donor Study (CDS).[48,227] Only one group in a small series has reported greater cell loss at 1 year in the PKP group than the EK group.[235]

No significant differences in cell loss have been shown between donor posterior lenticule prepared by the surgeon versus the eye bank.[229–231] The influences of variations in technique related to EK, including wound size and insertion methods, have not been well studied. In regards to wound size, studies have shown that both in cadaver eyes and humans, a smaller-sized incision for EK surgery results in greater acute endothelial area damage than larger size (5 mm) incisions.[225,226]

There have been no randomized trials comparing EK to PKP, but Price et al. reported in a prospective series of EK cases performed by two experienced surgeons compared to a series of PKP cases from the SMAS that at 6 months cell loss was 34% versus 11% and 38% versus 20% at 1 year in the EK versus PKP group, respectively.[232] This multicenter study with cell counts determined in a masked fashion by the same specular microscopy reading center for both studies confirmed single-site studies that the endothelial damage at the time of EK is greater as reflected in the greater loss at 6 months, but that the rate of loss thereafter is significantly less than PKP. This difference may relate to the larger donor (9 mm) with 26% more endothelial cells transplanted than with PKP, less damage to the peripheral endothelium that may ultimately be reflected in less central cell loss where specular microscopy is performed, and perhaps a lower rejection rate.[18,227] Long-term studies are needed to see if this difference in the rate of loss after 6 months compared to PKP is reflected in improved long-term graft cell survival associated with a more stable endothelial cell population.

Donor corneas

Specular microscopy is a useful method of screening tissue for keratoplasty. Evaluation of corneal tissue can be performed on whole globes[243,244] as well as corneas stored in tissue culture media.[104,245,246] In addition to historical and slit lamp information, most eye banks provide the ECD and sometimes morphologic information to help decide if tissue is accepted or rejected. At the discretion of the local medical director of each eye bank, the minimum donor ECD is established for keratoplasty. Generally, this minimum has been established for most eye banks at 2000 cells/mm^2. There are no good scientific data why the minimum was established at this level, except for the success of keratoplasty over the past 20 years utilizing this minimum criteria.[247] The Specular Microscopy Ancillary Study has reported that baseline donor ECD does not predict graft failure 5 years after PKP; however, the 6-month ECD was predictive of subsequent failure, as previously described in the PKP section of this chapter.[43] Among those that had not failed within the first 6 months, the 5-year cumulative incidence of failure was 13% ± 12% in the 33 subjects with a 6-month ECD less than 1700 cells/mm^2 versus 2% ± 3% in the 137 subjects with a 6-month ECD of 2500 cells/mm^2 or higher.[43]

Intraocular irrigating solutions

Closed intraocular surgery (e.g. phacoemulsification, vitrectomy) requires the introduction into the eye of a large volume of an irrigating solution over a relatively prolonged time. Numerous studies describe the effects of intraocular irrigation solutions on the corneal endothelium.[165,248–262] Endothelial structure and function are best maintained when solutions resemble aqueous humor in composition. Irrigating solutions not satisfying the basal metabolic requirements of the corneal endothelium can rapidly produce adverse endothelial changes and corneal edema. In vitro perfusion experiments demonstrate that these endothelial changes and the resultant corneal swelling are caused by intraocular irrigating solutions that are deficient in certain essential components. As a result of these studies, intraocular irrigation solutions that more closely resemble aqueous humor are now commercially available.

Vitreocorneal contact

Persistent corneal edema, resulting from contact of formed vitreous humor with the corneal endothelium, can occur months to years after cataract extraction in which the posterior capsule is no longer intact, but the precise mechanism of corneal decompensation is not known.[263–266] Since corneal dehydration is controlled primarily by the endothelium, it is assumed that vitreous contact mechanically injures the endothelium and interferes with its physiologic function. Experimental evidence suggests that contact of solid, collagenous elements of the vitreous humor with the endothelium interferes with transport of fluid out of the cornea.[267] Contact between formed vitreous humor and the corneal endothelium, however, is not invariably followed by corneal edema. In those cases in which the phenomenon is encountered, the cornea may tolerate vitreous contact and remain clear and dehydrated for extended periods before edema is observed. Specular microscopic studies tend to support these concepts.[268,269] Several types of morphologic abnormalities are observed in the endothelium of corneas in the early stages of decompensation as a result of vitreous contact. Some endothelial cells are markedly enlarged and grossly abnormal in shape. Others contain abnormal bright or dark structures within their cell boundaries. Abnormal cell intersections and side length distribution are encountered, and the central guttate excrescences of FECD are often seen.

Removal of vitreous humor from the anterior chamber by closed vitrectomy, with the elimination of vitreous contact, may result in substantial improvement in the state of corneal hydration and in some cases in the elimination of clinically significant corneal edema.[268–272] Surprisingly, those endothelial changes seen in edematous corneas prior to vitrectomy appear to persist following vitrectomy and corneal deturgescence. Despite the seeming irreversibility of the endothelial changes, clinical reversal of corneal edema may occur on occasion in cases of moderately prolonged vitreous contact. Cases in which closed vitrectomy does not produce complete reversal of corneal edema are those with FECD and those with the most bizarre endothelium.

Epithelialization of the anterior chamber

The endothelial surface of the cornea has been photographed in vivo with the specular microscope during varying stages of epithelialization of the anterior chamber in an effort to define clinical signs that would permit a definite diagnosis to be made in the absence of histopathologic verification.[273–275] Evaluation of the corneal endothelium in this entity is laborious and demanding. Even in the most cooperative of patients, cellular structures may be difficult to detect, and often cannot be distinctly focused. A sharply defined border between normal corneal endothelial cells and the area of epithelial downgrowth is observed.[273] In contrast, in the region occupied by the clinically observed endothelial demarcation line, enlarged, abnormally shaped endothelial cells inferiorly blending into an acellular, structureless area superiorly have been noted.[274] By focusing more deeply in the seemingly structureless area superiorly, these investigators were able to visualize poorly defined structures that suggested multilayered epithelial cells. However, neither epithelial nor endothelial cells could be identified with certainty in the region above the demarcation line seen with the slit lamp biomicroscope; the diagnosis was later verified histopathologically. Improved resolution of the epithelial cells at the junction between epithelial downgrowth and the endothelial cells has been achieved.[276]

When the endothelium is successfully visualized with the specular microscope, it is usually abnormal even though the advancing demarcation line is far away from the cells being examined.[274] Considerable cell loss seems to occur, as evidenced by the large size of the remaining cells. Whether this cell loss results from a traumatic insult prior to surgery and contributes to the subsequent epithelial invasion of the anterior chamber or, alternatively, whether it is produced by the advancing layer of epithelium, is not clear. When epithelialization is moderately advanced, cellular structures are seen that do not have the morphologic appearance of endothelial cells. Presumably, these are epithelial cells, but this is not certain. In the most advanced cases, no distinct cell boundaries can be seen. Only a disorganized, amorphous, membranous layer containing some formed structures is visualized. This is believed to represent a thickened, multilayered epithelial membrane whose structure does not permit satisfactory resolution by the specular microscope. The inability to see endothelial structures distinctly with the specular microscope suggests either that the endothelium is disorganized or that more than a single layer of cells is present. The invading epithelium also produces an irregular layer of fibular material along the epithelium–Descemet's membrane interface[277] that may contribute to the gray appearance of the involved cornea and to the difficulty encountered in obtaining a clear image of the structures in the zone of specular reflection.

Blunt trauma

Blunt trauma to the cornea can damage the endothelium. Bourne and co-workers[278] have reported their findings on a 16-year-old boy who had suffered a pellet gun injury of the right eye 2 years previously. Clinically, both corneas were clear and free of edema. Evidence of prior endothelial damage was revealed only by clinical specular microscopy. The endothelial cells on the right were enlarged and the central endothelial cell density was only 47% of that of the opposite, normal, left eye. Although it is suspected that in such instances the residual endothelial cells might be more susceptible to subsequent trauma than normal cells, no additional cell loss was documented following cataract extraction by phacoemulsification in this particular case.

The impact of small, nonpenetrating foreign bodies on the cornea may give rise to posterior annular keratopathy, clinically apparent gray rings on the corneal endothelium.[279–281] Specular microscopic studies demonstrate that posterior annular keratopathy occurring after blunt corneal trauma in humans represents a contusion injury and consists of disrupted and swollen endothelial cells. Reproduction of these rings in experimental animals also reveals that they consist of swollen or disrupted endothelial cells.[281] The center of each ring corresponds to the epithelial impact site of the foreign body, with the least disruption of the endothelium occurring here. The damaged cells may still be evident many days after the clinically visible endothelial rings disappear and, indeed, permanent cell loss may occur. As might be expected, the degree of endothelial cell loss appears to be related to the severity of the injury; a measurable decrease in cell density occurs only in the more severely injured corneas.

Contact lens wear

Both acute and chronic endothelial changes are seen with the specular microscope following contact lens wear. Within minutes of application of a contact lens, small dark endothelial blebs occur that disappear quickly if the lens is removed.[275,282–284] These endothelial blebs reach a maximum size in 20–30 minutes from the time the contact lens is placed on the cornea and then gradually decrease in size. Similar blebs occur during prolonged lid closure, such as during sleep,[285] and may represent the effects of hypoxia or lactate accumulation.

Long-term wear of either hard or soft contact lenses results in an increased polymegathism[286–301] that is not reversed upon cessation of lens wear,[296,297] although some recovery towards normal might occur.[301,302] The degree of polymegathism increases as the period of time the lenses are worn increases.[288,290,291,293,297,298] The degree of polymegathism also depends upon the type of lens worn.

Diabetes

In type I diabetes the cell density significantly decreases with age.[303] However, no difference in corneal thickness or endothelial permeability to fluorescein has been described in two studies.[304,305] Whereas another study showed increased permeability in subjects with type 1 diabetes and exacerbated by cystic fibrosis.[306a] Diabetic corneas also exhibit increased polymegathism and pleomorphism and a decreased percentage of hexagonality.[294,303–309] However, Ohguro et al.[309] have demonstrated that topical administration of aldose reductase inhibitor can reverse these morphologic changes, suggesting that aldose reductase may be involved in the etiology of corneal endothelial variations in diabetic patients.

References

1. Vogt A. Die sichtbarkeit des lebenden hornhautendotheis. Ein beitrog zur methodik der spaltlampenmikroskopie. *Graefe's Arch Ophthalmol.* 1930;101:123–144
2. Graves B. A bilateral chronic affection of the endothelial face of the cornea of elderly persons, with an account of the technical and clinical principles of its slit-lamp observation. *Br J Ophthalmol.* 1924;8:502.
3. Maurice DM. Cellular membrane activity in the corneal endothelium of the intact eye. *Experientia.* 1968;24(11):1094–1095.
4. Maurice DM. A scanning slit optical microscope. *Invest Ophthalmol.* 1974;13(12):1033–1037.
5. Laing RA, Sandstrom MM, Leibowitz HM. In vivo photomicrography of the corneal endothelium. *Arch Ophthalmol.* 1975;93(2):143–145.
6. Bourne WM, Kaufman HE. Specular microscopy of human corneal endothelium in vivo. *Am J Ophthalmol.* 1976;81(3):319–323.
7. Lohman LE, Rao GN, Aquavella JA. Optics and clinical applications of wide-field specular microscopy. *Am J Ophthalmol.* 1981;92(1):43–48.
8. Sherrard ES, Buckley RJ. Visualisation of the corneal endothelium in the clinic. *Ophthalmologica.* 1983;187(2):118–128.
9. Doughty MJ, Aakre BM. Further analysis of assessments of the coefficient of variation of corneal endothelial cell areas from specular microscopic images. *Clin Exp Optom.* 2008;91(5):438–446.
10. Doughty MJ, Oblak E. A comparison of two methods for estimating polymegethism in cell areas of the human corneal endothelium. *Ophthalmic Physiol Opt.* 2008;28(1):47–56.
11. Sheng H, Parker EJ, Bullimore MA. An evaluation of the ConfoScan3 for corneal endothelial morphology analysis. *Optom Vis Sci.* 2007;84(9):888–895.
12. van Schaick W, van Dooren BT, Mulder PG, Volker-Dieben HJ. Validity of endothelial cell analysis methods and recommendations for calibration in Topcon SP-2000P specular microscopy. *Cornea.* 2005;24(5):538–544.
13. Oblak E, Doughty MJ, Oblak L. A semi-automated assessment of cell size and shape in monolayers, with optional adjustment for the cell–cell border width-application to human corneal endothelium. *Tissue Cell.* 2002;34:283–295.

14. Laing RA, Sandstrom MM, Leibowitz HM. Clinical specular microscopy. II. Qualitative evaluation of corneal endothelial photomicrographs. *Arch Ophthalmol.* 1979;97:1720–1725.
15. Cheung SW, Cho P. Endothelial cells analysis with the TOPCON specular microscope SP-2000P and IMAGEnet system. *Curr Eye Res.* 2000;21:788–798.
16. Kitzmann AS, Winter EJ, Nau CB, et al. Comparison of corneal endothelial cell images from a noncontact specular microscope and a scanning confocal microscope. *Cornea.* 2005;24(8):980–984.
17. Klais CM, Buhren J, Kohnen T. Comparison of endothelial cell count using confocal and contact specular microscopy. *Ophthalmologica.* 2003;217:99–103.
18. Amann J, Holley GP, Lee SB, Edelhauser HF. Increased endothelial cell density in the paracentral and peripheral regions of the human cornea. *Am J Ophthalmol.* 2003;135:584–590.
19. Mayer DJ. *Clinical wide-field specular microscopy.* London: Balliere Tindall; 1984.
20. Tsubota K, Yamada M, Naoi S. Specular microscopic observation of human corneal epithelial abnormalities. *Ophthalmology.* 1991;98(2): 184–191.
21. Tsubota K. A contact lens for specular microscopic observation. *Am J Ophthalmol.* 1988;106(5):627–628.
22. Tsubota K, Yamada M, Naoi S. Specular microscopic observation of normal human corneal epithelium. *Ophthalmology.* 1992;99(1):89–94.
23. Tsubota K, Mashima Y, Murata H, Yamada M, Sato N. Corneal epithelium following penetrating keratoplasty. *Br J Ophthalmol.* 1995;79(3): 257–260.
24. Lemp MA. The surface of the corneal graft: in vivo color specular microscopic study in the human. *Trans Am Ophthalmol Soc.* 1989;87: 619–657.
25. Tsubota K. Corneal epithelium following intraepikeratophakia. *J Cataract Refract Surg.* 1991;17(4):460–465.
26. Rao GN, Ganti S, Aquavella JV. Specular microscopy of corneal epithelium after epikeratophakia. *Am J Ophthalmol.* 1987;103(3 Pt 2):392–396.
27. Mathers WD, Sachdev MS, Petroll M, Lemp MA. Morphologic effects of contact lens wear on the corneal surface. *CLAO J.* 1992;18(1):49–52.
28. Tsubota K. In vivo observation of the corneal epithelium. *Scanning.* 1994;16(5):295–299.
29. Tseng SH, Yu CH, Wang ST. [Morphometric analysis of corneal epithelium in normal subjects and soft contact lens wearers]. *J Formos Med Assoc.* 1995;94(Suppl 1):S20–S25.
30. Lemp MA, Mathers WD. Corneal epithelial cell movement in humans. *Eye.* 1989;3(Pt 4):438–445.
31. Tsubota K, Chiba K, Shimazaki J. Corneal epithelium in diabetic patients. *Cornea.* 1991;10(2):156–160.
32. Pardos GJ, Krachmer JH. Comparison of endothelial cell density in diabetics and a control population. *Am J Ophthalmol.* 1980;90(2):172–174.
33. Tsubota K, Mashima Y, Murata H, Sato N, Ogata T. Corneal epithelium in keratoconus. *Cornea.* 1995;14(1):77–83.
34. Swartz ML, Wang M. Measuring the cornea: the latest developments in corneal topography. *Curr Opin Ophthalmol.* 2007;18:325–333.
35. Ucakhan OM, Kanpolat A. Corneal thickness measurements in normal and keratoconic eyes: Pentacam comprehensive eye scanner versus noncontact specular microscopy and ultrasound pachymetry. *J Cataract Refract Surg.* 2006;32:970–977.
36. Sanchis-Gimeno J HM, Lleo-Perez A, et al. Quantitative anatomical differences in central corneal thickness values determined with scanning-slit corneal topography and noncontact specular microscopy. *Cornea.* 2006;25:203–205.
37. Koester CJ. Comparison of optical sectioning methods. The scanning slit confocal microscope. In: Pawley J, ed. *The handbook of biological confocal microscopy.* Madison: IMR Press; 1989.
38. Laing RA. Specular microscopy of the cornea. *Curr Top Eye Res.* 1980;3:157–218.
39. Langston RH, Roisman TS. Comparison of endothelial evaluation techniques. *J Am Intraocul Implant Soc.* 1981;7(3):239–241.
40. Holladay JT, Bishop JE, Prager TC. Quantitative endothelial biomicroscopy. *Ophthalmic Surg.* 1983;14(1):33–40.
41. Yee RW, Matsuda M, Edelhauser HF. Wide-field endothelial counting panels. *Am Ophthalmol.* 1985;99:596–597.
42. Oharazawa H IN, Matsui H, Ohara K. Age-related changes of human lens epithelial cells in vivo. *Ophthalmic Res.* 2001;33:363–366.
43. Lass JH, Sugar A, Benetz BA, et al. Endothelial cell density to predict endothelial graft failure after penetrating keratoplasty. *Arch Ophthalmol.* 2010;128(1):63–69.
44. Yee RW, Matsuda M, Schultz RO, Edelhauser HF. Changes in the normal corneal endothelial cellular pattern as a function of age. *Curr Eye Res.* 1985;4:671–678.
45. Honda H, Ogita Y, Higuchi S, Kani K. Cell movements in a living mammalian tissue: long-term observation of individual cells in wounded corneal endothelia of cats. *J Morphol.* 1982;174(1):25–39.
46. McCarey BE, Edelhauser HF, Lynn MJ. Review of corneal endothelial specular microscopy for FDA clinical trials of refractive procedures, surgical devices, and new intraocular drugs and solutions. *Cornea.* 2008; 27(1):1–16.
47. Benetz BA, Gal RL, Rice C, et al. Dual grading methods by a central reading center for corneal endothelial image quality assessment and cell density determination in the Specular Microscopy Ancillary Study of the Cornea Donor Study. *Current Eye Res.* 2006;31:1–9.
48. Lass JH, Gal RL, Dontchev M, et al. Donor age and corneal endothelial cell loss 5 years after successful corneal transplantation. Specular microscopy ancillary study results. *Ophthalmology.* 2008;115(4):627–632.
49. Mishima S. Clinical investigations on the corneal endothelium. *Ophthalmology.* 1982;89(6):525–530.
50. Allansmith M. *The eye and immunology.* St. Louis: C.V. Mosby, 1982.
51. Bigar F. Specular microscopy of the corneal endothelium. Optical solutions and clinical results. *Dev Ophthalmol.* 1982;6:1–94.
52. Bigar F, Schimmelpfennig B, Hurzeler R. Cornea guttata in donor material. *Arch Ophthalmol.* 1978;96(4):653–655.
53. Roberson MC, Wicheta WE. Endothelial loss in corneal concussion injury. *Ann Ophthalmol.* 1985;17(8):457–458, 60.
54. Markowitz SN, Morin JD. The endothelium in primary angle-closure glaucoma. *Am J Ophthalmol.* 1984;98(1):103–104.
55. Setala K. Corneal endothelial cell density after an attack of acute glaucoma. *Acta Ophthalmol (Copenh).* 1979;57(6):1004–1013.
56. Olsen T. The endothelial cell damage in acute glaucoma. On the corneal thickness response to intraocular pressure. *Acta Ophthalmol (Copenh).* 1980;58(2):257–266.
57. Setala K. Corneal endothelial cell density in iridocyclitis. *Acta Ophthalmol (Copenh).* 1979;57(2):277–286.
58. Olsen T. Changes in the corneal endothelium after acute anterior uveitis as seen with the specular microscope. *Acta Ophthalmol (Copenh).* 1980;58(2):250–256.
59. Brooks AM, Gillies WE. Fluorescein angiography of the iris and specular microscopy of the corneal endothelium in some cases of glaucoma secondary to chronic cyclitis. *Ophthalmology.* 1988;95(12):1624–1630.
60. Brooks AM, Grant G, Gillies WE. Comparison of specular microscopy and examination of aspirate in phacolytic glaucoma. *Ophthalmology.* 1990;97(1):85–89.
61. Olsen T. The specular microscopic appearance of corneal graft endothelium during an acute rejection episode. A case report. *Acta Ophthalmol (Copenh).* 1979;57(5):882–890.
62. Olsen T. Variations in endothelial morphology of normal corneas and after cataract extraction. A specular microscopic study. *Acta Ophthalmol (Copenh).* 1979;57(6):1014–1019.
63. Abbott RL, Forster RK. Clinical specular microscopy and intraocular surgery. *Arch Ophthalmol.* 1979;97(8):1476–1479.
64. Glasser DB, Matsuda M, Gager WE, Edelhauser HF. Corneal endothelial morphology after anterior chamber lens implantation. *Arch Ophthalmol.* 1985;103(9):1347–1349.
65. Culbertson WW, Abbott RL, Forster RK. Endothelial cell loss in penetrating keratoplasty. *Ophthalmology.* 1982;89:600–604.
66. Matsuda M, Suda T, Manabe R. Serial alterations in endothelial cell shape and pattern after intraocular surgery. *Am J Ophthalmol.* 1984; 98(3):313–319.
67. Schultz RO, Glasser DB, Matsuda M, Yee RW, Edelhauser HF. Response of the corneal endothelium to cataract surgery. *Arch Ophthalmol.* 1986; 104(8):1164–1169.
68. Abib FC, Barreto J Jr. Behavior of corneal endothelial density over a lifetime. *J Cataract Refract Surg.* 2001;27:1574–1578.
69. Sherrard ES, Novakovic P, Speedwell L. Age-related changes of the corneal endothelium and stroma as seen in vivo by specular microscopy. *Eye.* 1987;1(Pt 2):197–203.
70. Nucci P, Brancato R, Mets MB, Shevell SK. Normal endothelial cell density range in childhood. *Arch Ophthalmol.* 1990;108(2):247–248.
71. Murphy C, Alvarado J, Juster R, Maglio M. Prenatal and postnatal cellularity of the human corneal endothelium. A quantitative histologic study. *Invest Ophthalmol Vis Sci.* 1984;25(3):312–322.
72. Sherrard ES, Buckley RJ. Relocation of specific endothelial features with the clinical specular microscope. *Br J Ophthalmol.* 1981;65(12):820–827.
73. Bourne WM, Hodge DO, Nelson LR. Corneal endothelium five years after transplantation. *Am J Ophthlamol.* 1994;118:185–196.

74. Ohara K, Tsuru T, Inoda S. [Morphometric parameters of the corneal endothelial cells]. *Nippon Ganka Gakkai Zasshi.* 1987;91(11):1073–1078.
75. Laing RA, Sandstrom MM, Berrospi AR, Leibowitz HM. Changes in the corneal endothelium as a function of age. *Exp Eye Res.* 1976;22:587–594.
76. Lorenzetti DW, Uotila MH, Parikh N, Kaufman HE. Central cornea guttata. Incidence in the general population. *Am J Ophthalmol.* 1967;64(6):1155–1158.
77. Goar EL. Dystrophy of the corneal endothelium (corneal guttae) with a report of a histological examination. *Am J Ophthalmol.* 1934;17:215–221.
78. Laing RA, Leibowitz HM, Oak SS, et al. Endothelial mosaic in Fuchs' dystrophy. A qualitative evaluation with the specular microscope. *Arch Ophthalmol.* 1981;99(1):80–83.
79. Jackson AJ, Robinson FO, Frazer DG, Archer DB. Corneal guttata: a comparative clinical and specular micrographic study. *Eye.* 1999;13 (Pt 6):737–743.
80. Chiou AG, Kaufman SC, Beuerman RW, et al. Confocal microscopy in cornea guttata and Fuchs' endothelial dystrophy. *Br J Ophthalmol.* 1999;83(2):185–189.
81. Mustonen RK, McDonald MB, Srivannaboon S, et al. In vivo confocal microscopy of Fuchs' endothelial dystrophy. *Cornea.* 1998;17(5):493–503.
82. Fuchs E. Dystrophia epithelialis corneae. *Graefe's Arch Klin Exp.* 1910;76:478–508.
83. Stocker FW. The endothelium of the cornea and its clinical implications. *Trans Am Ophthalmol Soc.* 1953;51:669–786.
84. Duke-Elder S, ed. *System of ophthalmology*. Volume III. St. Louis: Mosby; 1963.
85. Krachmer JH, Purcell JJ Jr, Young CW, Bucher KD. Corneal endothelial dystrophy. A study of 64 families. *Arch Ophthalmol.* 1978;96(11):2036–2039.
86. Gutti V, Bardenstein DS, Iyengar SI, Lass JH. Fuchs' Endothelial Corneal Dystrophy. In: Levin LA, Albert DM: *Ocular Disease: Mechanisms and Management.* London: Saunders; pp. 34–41.
87. Gottsch JD SO, Liu S, et al. Inheritance of a novel *COL8A2* mutation defines a distinct early-onset subtype of Fuchs' corneal dystrophy. *Invest Ophthalmol Vis Sci.* 2005;46:1934–1939.
88. Gottsch JD, Sundin O, et al. Fuchs' corneal dystrophy: aberrant collagen distribution in an L450W mutant of the *COL8A2* gene. *Invest Ophthalmol Vis Sci.* 2005;46:4504–4511.
89. Polack FM. The posterior corneal surface in Fuchs' dystrophy. Scanning electron microscope study. *Invest Ophthalmol.* 1974;13(12):913–922.
90. Waring GO 3rd, Rodrigues MM, Laibson PR. Corneal dystrophies. II. Endothelial dystrophies. *Surv Ophthalmol.* 1978;23(3):147–168.
91. Takahashi N, Sasaki K, Nakaizumi H, Konishi F. Specular microscopic findings of lattice corneal dystrophy. *Int Ophthalmol.* 1987;10(1):47–53.
92. Mayer DJ. *Lattice dystrophy in clinical wide-field specular microscopy.* London: Bailliere Tindall; 1984.
93. Smith ME, Zimmerman LE. Amyloid in corneal dystrophies. Differentiation of lattice from granular and macular dystrophies. *Arch Ophthalmol.* 1968;79(4):407–412.
94. Yanoff M. Iridocorneal endothelial syndrome: unification of a disease spectrum. *Surv Ophthalmol.* 1979;24(1):1–2.
95. Shields MB, McCracken JS, Klintworth GK, Campbell DG. Corneal edema in essential iris atrophy. *Ophthalmology.* 1979;86(8):1533–1550.
96. Halhal M, D'Hermies F, Morel X, Renard G. [Iridocorneal endothelial syndrome. Series of 7 cases]. *J Fr Ophtalmol.* 2001;24(6):628–634.
97. Shields MB. Progressive essential iris atrophy, Chandler's syndrome, and the iris nevus (Cogan-Reese) syndrome: a spectrum of disease. *Surv Ophthalmol.* 1979;24(1):3–20.
98. Campbell DG, Shields MB, Smith TR. The corneal endothelium and the spectrum of essential iris atrophy. *Am J Ophthalmol.* 1978;86(3):317–324.
99. Alvarado JA, Underwood JL, Green WR, et al. Detection of herpes simplex viral DNA in the iridocorneal endothelial syndrome. *Arch Ophthalmol.* 1994;112(12):1601–1609.
100. Liu Z, Zhang M, Chen J, et al. [The contralateral eye in patients with unilateral iridocorneal endothelial syndrome]. *Zhonghua Yan Ke Za Zhi.* 2002;38(1):16–20.
101. Lucas-Glass TC, Baratz KH, Nelson LR, Hodge DO, Bourne WM. The contralateral corneal endothelium in the iridocorneal endothelial syndrome. *Arch Ophthalmol.* 1997;115(1):40–44.
102. Kupfer C, Kaiser-Kupfer MI, Datiles M, McCain L. The contralateral eye in the iridocorneal endothelial (ICE) syndrome. *Ophthalmology.* 1983;90(11):1343–1350.
103. Hirst LW, Quigley HA, Stark WJ, Shields NB. Specular microscopy of iridocorneal endothelial syndrome. *Aust J Ophthalmol.* 1980;8(2):139–146.
104. Bourne WM. Examination and photography of donor corneal endothelium. *Arch Ophthalmol.* 1976;94(10):1799–1800.
105. Quigley HA, Forster RF. Histopathology of cornea and iris in Chandler's syndrome. *Arch Ophthalmol.* 1978;96(10):1878–1882.
106. Levy SG, McCartney AC, Sawada H, et al. Descemet's membrane in the iridocorneal-endothelial syndrome: morphology and composition. *Exp Eye Res.* 1995;61(3):323–333.
107. Patel A, Kenyon KR, Hirst LW, et al. Clinicopathologic features of Chandler's syndrome. *Surv Ophthalmol.* 1983;27(5):327–344.
108. Chiou AG, Kaufman SC, Beuerman RW, et al. Confocal microscopy in the iridocorneal endothelial syndrome. *Br J Ophthalmol.* 1999;83(6):697–702.
109. Ullern M, Massin M, Pozzo JM, Boureau C. [Specular microscopy in the diagnosis of the iridocorneal endothelial syndrome]. *J Fr Ophtalmol.* 1985;8(11):721–728.
110. Sherrard ES, Frangoulis MA, Muir MG. On the morphology of cells of posterior cornea in the iridocorneal endothelial syndrome. *Cornea.* 1991;10(3):233–243.
111. Setala K, Vannas A. Corneal endothelial cells in essential iris atrophy. A specular microscopic study. *Acta Ophthalmol (Copenh).* 1979;57(6):1020–1029.
112. Ullern M, Boureau C, Muzac MS, M'Rad A. [The value of specular microscopy in the diagnosis of endothelial iridocorneal syndrome]. *Bull Mem Soc Fr Ophtalmol.* 1982;94:339–342.
113. Laganowski HC, Sherrard ES, Muir MG. The posterior corneal surface in posterior polymorphous dystrophy: a specular microscopical study. *Cornea.* 1991;10(3):224–232.
114. Hirst LW, Waring GO 3rd. Clinical specular microscopy of posterior polymorphous endothelial dystrophy. *Am J Ophthalmol.* 1983;95(2):143–155.
115. Brooks AM, Grant G, Gillies WE. Differentiation of posterior polymorphous dystrophy from other posterior corneal opacities by specular microscopy. *Ophthalmology.* 1989;96(11):1639–1645.
116. Cibis GW, Tripathi RC. The differential diagnosis of Descemet's tears (Haab's striae) and posterior polymorpous dystrophy bands. A clinicopathologic study. *Ophthalmology.* 1982;89(6):614–620.
117. Laing RA, Sandstrom MM, Berrospi AR, Leibowitz HM. The human corneal endothelium in keratoconus: a specular microscopic study. *Arch Ophthalmol.* 1979;97(10):1867–1869.
118. Skuta GL, Sugar J, Ericson ES. Corneal endothelial cell measurements in megalocornea. *Arch Ophthalmol.* 1983;101(1):51–53.
119. Jakus MA. Further observations on the fine structure of the cornea. *Invest Ophthalmol.* 1962;1:202–225.
120. Irvine AR Jr. The role of the endothelium in bullous keratopathy. *AMA Arch Ophthalmol.* 1956;56(3):338–351.
121. Mortensen AC, Sperling S. Human corneal endothelial cell density after an in vitro imitation of elevated intraocular pressure. *Acta Ophthalmol (Copenh).* 1982;60(3):475–479.
122. Vannas A, Setala K, Ruusuvaara P. Endothelial cells in capsular glaucoma. *Acta Ophthalmol (Copenh).* 1977;55(6):951–958.
123. Setala K, Vannas A. Endothelial cells in the glaucomato-cyclitic crisis. *Adv Ophthalmol.* 1978;36:218–224.
124. Bigar F, Witmer R. Corneal endothelial changes in primary acute angle-closure glaucoma. *Ophthalmology.* 1982;89(6):596–599.
125. Lee EK, Yun YJ, Yim JH, Kim CS. Changes in corneal endothelial cells after Ahmed glaucoma valve implantation: 2-year follow-up. *Am J Ophthalmol.* 2009;148(3):361–367.
126. Storr-Paulsen NJ, Ahmed S, Storr-Paulsen A. Corneal endothelial cell loss after mitomycin C-augmented trabeculectomy. *J Glaucoma* 2008;17:654–657.
127. Nassiri NN, Rahnavardi M, Rahmani L. A comparison of corneal endothelial cell changes after 1-site and 2-site phacotrabeculectomy. *Cornea.* 2008;27:889–894.
128. Baratz KH, Nau CB, Winter EJ, et al. Effects of glaucoma medications on corneal endothelium, keratocytes, and subbasal nerves among participants in the ocular hypertension treatment study. *Cornea.* 2006;25(9):1046–1052.
129. Inomata H, Smelser GK. Fine structural alterations of corneal endothelim during experimental uveitis. *Invest Ophthalmol.* 1970;9(4):272–285.
130. Wirbelauer C, Anders N, Pham DT, Holschbach A, Wollensak J. [Early postoperative endothelial cell loss after corneoscleral tunnel incision and phacoemulsification in pseudoexfoliation syndrome]. *Ophthalmologe.* 1997;94(5):332–336.
131. Beltrame G, Salvetat ML, Driussi G, Chizzolini M. Effect of incision size and site on corneal endothelial changes in cataract surgery. *J Cataract Refract Surg.* 2002;28(1):118–125.

132. Amino K, Yamakawa R. Long-term results of out-of-the-bag intraocular lens implantation. *J Cataract Refract Surg.* 2000;26(2):266–270.
133. Maar N, Graebe A, Schild G, Stur M, Amon M. Influence of viscoelastic substances used in cataract surgery on corneal metabolism and endothelial morphology: comparison of Healon and Viscoat. *J Cataract Refract Surg.* 2001;27(11):1756–1761.
134. Basti S, Aasuri MK, Reddy S, Reddy S, Rao GN. Prospective evaluation of corneal endothelial cell loss after pediatric cataract surgery. *J Cataract Refract Surg.* 1998;24(11):1469–1473.
135. Diaz-Valle D, Benitez del Castillo Sanchez JM, Castillo A, Sayagues O, Moriche M. Endothelial damage with cataract surgery techniques. *J Cataract Refract Surg.* 1998;24(7):951–955.
136. Oshika T, Nagahara K, Yaguchi S, et al. Three year prospective, randomized evaluation of intraocular lens implantation through 3.2 and 5.5 mm incisions. *J Cataract Refract Surg.* 1998;24(4):509–514.
137. Wirbelauer C, Anders N, Pham DT, Wollensak J. Corneal endothelial cell changes in pseudoexfoliation syndrome after cataract surgery. *Arch Ophthalmol.* 1998;116(2):145–149.
138. Matheu A, Castilla M, Duch F, et al. Manual nucleofragmentation and endothelial cell loss. *J Cataract Refract Surg.* 1997;23(7):995–999.
139. Ravalico G, Tognetto D, Baccara F, Lovisato A. Corneal endothelial protection by different viscoelastics during phacoemulsification. *J Cataract Refract Surg.* 1997;23(3):433–439.
140. Diaz-Valle D, Benitez Del Castillo Sanchez JM, Toledano N, et al. Endothelial morphological and functional evaluation after cataract surgery. *Eur J Ophthalmol.* 1996;6(3):242–245.
141. Hayashi K, Hayashi H, Nakao F, Hayashi F. Corneal endothelial cell loss in phacoemulsification surgery with silicone intraocular lens implantation. *J Cataract Refract Surg.* 1996;22(6):743–747.
142. Dick HB, Kohnen T, Jacobi FK, Jacobi KW. Long-term endothelial cell loss following phacoemulsification through a temporal clear corneal incision. *J Cataract Refract Surg.* 1996;22(1):63–71.
143. Dick B, Kohnen T, Jacobi KW. [Endothelial cell loss after phacoemulsification and 3.5 vs. 5 mm corneal tunnel incision]. *Ophthalmologe.* 1995;92(4):476–483.
144. Oshika T, Tsuboi S, Yaguchi S, et al. Comparative study of intraocular lens implantation through 3.2- and 5.5-mm incisions. *Ophthalmology.* 1994;101(7):1183–1190.
145. Bourne WM, Nelson LR, Hodge DO. Continued endothelial cell loss ten years after lens implantation. *Ophthalmology.* 1994;101:1014–1022.
146. Hayashi K, Nakao F, Hayashi F. Corneal endothelial cell loss after phacoemulsification using nuclear cracking procedures. *J Cataract Refract Surg.* 1994;20(1):44–47.
147. Kim JY, Lee JH. The effect of extracapsular cataract extraction using nucleus dislocation into anterior chamber on the corneal endothelium. *Korean J Ophthalmol.* 1993;7(2):55–58.
148. Numa A, Nakamura J, Takashima M, Kani K. Long-term corneal endothelial changes after intraocular lens implantation. Anterior vs posterior chamber lenses. *Jpn J Ophthalmol.* 1993;37(1):78–87.
149. Cosemans I, Zeyen P, Zeyen T. Comparison of the effect of Healon vs. Viscoat on endothelial cell count after phacoemulsification and posterior chamber lens implantation. *Bull Soc Belge Ophtalmol.* 1999;274:87–92.
150. Colin J, Renard G, Ullern M, et al. [Comparative prospective study of effects of Biovisc and Healonid on endothelial cell loss and intraocular pressure in cataract surgery]. *J Fr Ophtalmol.* 1995;18(5):356–363.
151. Forstot SL, Blackwell WL, Jaffe NS, Kaufman HE. The effect of intraocular lens implantation on the corneal endothelium. *Trans Sect Ophthalmol Am Acad Ophthalmol Otolaryngol.* 1977;83(2):195–203.
152. Bourne WM, Kaufman HE. Cataract extraction and the corneal endothelium. *Am J Ophthalmol.* 1976;82(1):44–47.
153. Bourne WM, Kaufman HE. Endothelial damage associated with intraocular lenses. *Am J Ophthalmol.* 1976;81(4):482–485.
154. Hirst LW, Snip RC, Stark WJ, Maumenee AE. Quantitative corneal endothelial evaluation in intraocular lens implantation and cataract surgery. *Am J Ophthalmol.* 1977;84(6):775–780.
155. Cheng H, Sturrock GD, Rubinstein B, Bulpitt CJ. Endothelial cell loss and corneal thickness after intracapsular extraction and iris clip lens implantation: a randomised controlled trial (interim report). *Br J Ophthalmol.* 1977;61(12):785–790.
156. Sugar J, Mitchelson J, Kraff M. Endothelial trauma and cell loss from intraocular lens insertion. *Arch Ophthalmol.* 1978;96(3):449–450.
157. Drews RC, Waltman SR. Endothelial cell loss in intraocular lens placement. *J Am Intraocul Implant Soc.* 1978;4(2):14–16.
158. Kraff MC, Sanders DR, Lieberman HL. Specular microscopy in cataract and intraocular lens patients. A report of 564 cases. *Arch Ophthalmol.* 1980;98(10):1782–1784.
159. Ravalico G, Tognetto D, Palomba MA, Lovisato A, Baccara F. Corneal endothelial function after extracapsular cataract extraction and phacoemulsification. *J Cataract Refract Surg.* 1997;23(7):1000–1005.
160. Lee JH, Oh SY. Corneal endothelial cell loss from suture fixation of a posterior chamber intraocular lens. *J Cataract Refract Surg.* 1997;23(7):1020–1022.
161. Martin NF, Stark WJ, Maumenee AE. Continuing corneal endothelial loss in intracapsular surgery with and without Binkhorst four-loop lenses: a long-term specular microscopy study. *Ophthalmic Surg.* 1987;18(12):867–872.
162. Kraff MC, Sanders DR. Planned extracapsular extraction versus phacoemulsification with IOL implantation: a comparison of concurrent series. *J Am Intraocul Implant Soc.* 1982;8(1):38–41.
163. Team OCTaE. Long-term corneal endothelial cell loss after cataract surgery. Results of a randomized controlled trial. Oxford Cataract Treatment and Evaluation Team (OCTET). *Arch Ophthalmol.* 1986;104(8):1170–1175.
164. Binder PS, Sternberg H, Wickman MG, Worthen DM. Corneal endothelial damage associated with phacoemulsification. *Am J Ophthalmol.* 1976;82(1):48–54.
165. McCarey BE, Polack FM, Marshall W. The phacoemulsification procedure. I. The effect of intraocular irrigating solutions on the corneal endothelium. *Invest Ophthalmol.* 1976;15(6):449–457.
166. Hoffer KJ. Vertical endothelial cell disparity. *Am J Ophthalmol.* 1979;87(3):344–349.
167. Galin MA, Lin LL, Fetherolf E, Obstbaum SA, Sugar A. Time analysis of corneal endothelial cell density after cataract extraction. *Am J Ophthalmol.* 1979;88(1):93–96.
168. Inaba M, Matsuda M, Shiozaki Y, Kosaki H. Regional specular microscopy of endothelial cell loss after intracapsular cataract extraction: a preliminary report. *Acta Ophthalmol (Copenh).* 1985;63(2):232–235.
169. Azen SP, Burg KA, Smith RE, Maguen E. A study in the measurement of corneal endothelial cell density using the specular microscope. *Acta Ophthalmol (Copenh).* 1980;58(3):418–423.
170. Kaufman E, Katz JI. Endothelial damage from intraocular lens insertion. *Invest Ophthalmol.* 1976;15(12):996–1000.
171. Kaufman HE, Katz J, Valenti J, Sheets JW, Goldberg EP. Corneal endothelium damage with intraocular lenses: contact adhesion between surgical materials and tissue. *Science.* 1977;198(4316):525–527.
172. Kirk S, Burde RM, Waltman SR. Minimizing corneal endothelial damage due to intraocular lens contact. *Invest Ophthalmol Vis Sci.* 1977;16(11):1053–1056.
173. Lane SS, Naylor DW, Kullerstrand LJ, Knauth K, Lindstrom RL. Prospective comparison of the effects of Occucoat, Viscoat, and Healon on intraocular pressure and endothelial cell loss. *J Cataract Refract Surg.* 1991;17(1):21–26.
174. Pallikaris IG, Siganos DS. Excimer laser in situ keratomileusis and photorefractive keratectomy for correction of high myopia. *J Refract Corneal Surg.* 1994;10(5):498–510.
175. Spadea L, Dragani T, Blasi MA, Mastrofini MC, Balestrazzi E. Specular microscopy of the corneal endothelium after excimer laser photorefractive keratectomy. *J Cataract Refract Surg.* 1996;22(2):188–193.
176. Wojciechowska R, Bolek S, Gierek-Ciaciura S, Janiec S, Mrukwa E. [Corneal endothelium after photorefractive keratectomy procedures]. *Klin Oczna.* 1996;98(5):361–363.
177. Mardelli PG, Piebenga LW, Matta CS, Hyde LL, Gira J. Corneal endothelial status 12 to 55 months after excimer laser photorefractive keratectomy. *Ophthalmology.* 1995;102(4):544–549; discussion 8–9.
178. Nagy ZZ, Seitz B, Maldonado MJ, Simon M. Changes of the corneal endothelium after ultraviolet-B exposure in previously photokeratectomized eyes. *Acta Chir Hung.* 1995;35(3–4):325–332.
179. Perez-Santonja JJ, Meza J, Moreno E, Garcia-Hernandez MR, Zato MA. Short-term corneal endothelial changes after photorefractive keratectomy. *J Refract Corneal Surg.* 1994;10(2 Suppl):S194–S198.
180. Perez-Santonja JJ, Sahla HF, Alio JL. Evaluation of endothelial cell changes 1 year after excimer laser in situ keratomileusis. *Arch Ophthalmol.* 1997;115(7):841–846.
181. Chen J, Wang Z, Yang B, Li S. [Laser in situ keratomileusis for correction of myopia]. *Zhonghua Yan Ke Za Zhi.* 1998;34(2):141–145.
182. Kim T, Sorenson AL, Krishnasamy S, Carlson AN, Edelhauser HF. Acute corneal endothelial changes after laser in situ keratomileusis. *Cornea.* 2001;20(6):597–602.
183. Collins MJ, Carr JD, Stulting RD, et al. Effects of laser in situ keratomileusis (LASIK) on the corneal endothelium 3 years postoperatively. *Am J Ophthalmol.* 2001;131:1–6.
184. Perez-Santonja JJ, Sakla HF, Gobbi F, Alio JL. Corneal endothelial changes after laser in situ keratomileusis. *J Cataract Refract Surg.* 1997;23(2):177–183.

185. Edelhauser HF. The resiliency of the corneal endothelium to refractive and intraocular surgery. *Cornea.* 2000;19:263–273.
186. Pallikaris IG, Siganos DS. Laser in situ keratomileusis to treat myopia: early experience. *J Cataract Refract Surg.* 1997;23(1):39–49.
187. Diakonis PA, Kymionis G, Markomanolakis M. Alterations in endothelial cell density after photorefractive keratectomy with adjuvant mitomycin. *Am J Ophthalmol.* 2007;144:1009–1013.
188. de Benito-Llopis TM, Ortega M. Effect of intraoperative mitomycin-C on healthy corneal endothelium after laser-assisted subepithelial keratectomy. *J Cataract Refract Surg.* 2007;33:1009–1013.
189. Zhao LQ, Wei RL, Ma XY, Zhu H. Effect of intraoperative mitomycin-C on healthy corneal endothelium after laser-assisted subepithelial keratectomy. *J Cataract Refract Surg.* 2008;34(10):1715–1719.
190. Azar RG, Holdbrook MJ, Lemp M, Edelhauser HF. Two-year corneal endothelial cell assessment following INTACS implantation. *J Refract Surg.* 2001;17(5):542–548.
191. Jimenez-Alfaro I, Benitez del Castillo JM, Garcia-Feijoo J, Gil de Bernabe JG, Serrano de la Iglesia JM. Safety of posterior chamber phakic intraocular lenses for the correction of high myopia: anterior segment changes after posterior chamber phakic intraocular lens implantation. *Ophthalmology.* 2001;108(1):90–99.
192. Perez-Santonja JJ, Alio JL, Jimenez-Alfaro I, Zato MA. Surgical correction of severe myopia with an angle-supported phakic intraocular lens. *J Cataract Refract Surg.* 2000;26(9):1288–1302.
193. Leroux-Les-Jardins S, Ullern M, Werthel AL. [Myopic anterior chamber intraocular lens implantation: evaluation at 8 years]. *J Fr Ophtalmol.* 1999;22(3):323–327.
194. Fechner PU, Haubitz I, Wichmann W, Wulff K. Worst-Fechner biconcave minus power phakic iris-claw lens. *J Refract Surg.* 1999;15(2):93–105.
195. Perez-Santonja JJ, Bueno JL, Zato MA. Surgical correction of high myopia in phakic eyes with Worst-Fechner myopia intraocular lenses. *J Refract Surg.* 1997;13(3):268–281; discussion 81–84.
196. El Danasoury MA, El Maghraby A, Gamali TO. Comparison of iris-fixed Artisan lens implantation with excimer laser in situ keratomileusis in correcting myopia between −9.00 and −19.50 diopters: a randomized study. *Ophthalmology.* 2002;109(5):955–964.
197. Stulting R, et al. Three-year results of Artisan/Verisyse phakic intraocular lens implantation results of the United States Food and Drug Administration clinical trial. *Ophthalmology.* 2008;115:464–472.
198. Menezo J CA, Rodriguez-Salvador V. Endothelial study of iris claw phakic lens: four-year follow up. *J Cataract Refract Surg.* 1998;24:1039–1049.
199. Saxena R, Multer P, et al. Long term follow up of endothelial cell change after Artisan phakic intraocular lens implantation. *Ophthalmology.* 2008;115:608–613.
200. Budo C, Izak M, et al. Multicenter study of the Artisan phakic intraocular lens. *J Cataract Refract Surg.* 2000:1163–1171.
201. Patel SV, Hodge DO, Bourne WM. Corneal endothelium and postoperative outcomes 15 years after penetrating keratoplasty. *Am J Ophthalmol.* 2005;139(2):311–319.
202. Obata H, Ishida K, Murao M, Miyata K, Sawa M. Corneal endothelial cell damage in penetrating keratoplasty. *Jpn J Ophthalmol.* 1991;35(4):411–416.
203. Bourne WM. Cellular changes in transplanted human corneas. *Cornea.* 2001;20(6):560–569.
204. Ing JJ, Ing HH, Nelson LR, Hodge DO, Bourne WM. Ten-year postoperative results of penetrating keratoplasty. *Ophthalmology.* 1998;105(10):1855–1865.
205. Zacks CM, Abbott RL, Fine M. Long-term changes in corneal endothelium after keratoplasty. A follow-up study. *Cornea.* 1990;9:92–97.
206. Gal RL, Dontchev M, Beck RW, et al. The effect of donor age on corneal transplantation outcome results of the Cornea Donor Study. *Ophthalmology.* 2008;115(4):620–626.
206a. Lass JH, Gal RL, Ruedy KJ, Benetz BA, et al. An evaluation of image quality and accuracy of eye bank measurement of donor cornea endothelial cell density in the Specular Microscopy Ancillary Study. *Ophthalmology.* 2005;112:431–440.
207. Laing RA, Sandstrom M, Berrospi AR, Leibowitz HM. Morphological changes in corneal endothelial cells after penetrating keratoplasty. *Am J Ophthalmol.* 1976;82(3):459–464.
208. Bourne WM, He K. The endothelium of clear corneal transplants. *Arch Ophthalmol.* 1976;94:1730–1732.
209. Bell KD, Campbell RJ, Bourne WM. Pathology of late endothelial failure: late endothelial failure of penetrating keratoplasty: study with light and electron microscopy. *Cornea.* 2000;19(1):40–46.
210. Langenbucher A, Seitz B, Nguyen NX, Naumann GO. Corneal endothelial cell loss after nonmechanical penetrating keratoplasty depends on diagnosis: a regression analysis. *Graefe's Arch Clin Exp Ophthalmol.* 2002;240:387–392.
211. Ohguro N, Matsuda M, Shimomura Y, Inoue Y, Tano Y. Effects of penetrating keratoplasty rejection on the endothelium of the donor cornea and the recipient peripheral cornea. *Am J Ophthalmol.* 2000;129:468–471.
212. Ruusuvaara P. Endothelial cell densities in donor and recipient tissue after keratoplasty. *Acta Ophthalmol (Copenh).* 1980;58(2):267–277.
213. Bourne WM. Functional measurements on the enlarged endothelial cells of corneal transplants. *Trans Am Ophthalmol Soc.* 1995;93:65–79; discussion 82.
214. Rao GN, Stevens RE, Mandelberg AI, Aquavella JV. Morphologic variations in graft endothelium. *Arch Ophthalmol.* 1980;98(8):1403–1406.
215. Sato T. Studies on the endothelium of the corneal graft. *Jpn J Ophthalmol.* 1978;22:114–126.
216. Ota Y. Endothelial permeability of fluorescein in corneal grafts and bullous keratopathy. *Jpn J Ophthalmol.* 1975;19:286–295.
217. Khodadoust AA. The allograft rejection reaction. The leading cause of late failure of clinical corneal grafts. In: Jones B (ed). *Corneal graft failure. Ciba Foundation Symposium No 15.* Amsterdam: Associated Scientific Publishers; 1973.
218. Polack FM. Clinical and pathologic aspects of the corneal graft reaction. *Trans Am Acad Ophthalmol Otolaryngol.* 1973;77(4):OP418–32.
219. Hirst LW. *Specular microscopy of endothelial graft rejection. Symposium on endothelium.* Las Vegas: International Cornea Society; 1982.
220. Eye Bank Association of America. 2009 *Eye Banking Statistical Report.* 2009.
221. Price FW Jr, Price MO. Descemet's stripping with endothelial keratoplasty in 50 eyes: a refractive neutral corneal transplant. *J Refract Surg.* 2005;21(4):339–345.
222. Gorovoy MS. Descemet-stripping automated endothelial keratoplasty. *Cornea.* 2006;25(8):886–889.
223. Melles GR, Lander F, Rietveld FJ. Transplantation of Descemet's membrane carrying viable endothelium through a small scleral incision. *Cornea.* 2002;21(4):415–418.
224. Terry MA, Chen ES, Hoar KL, Phillips PM, Friend DJ. Endothelial keratoplasty: the influence of preoperative donor endothelial cell densities on dislocation, primary graft failure, and 1-year cell counts. *Cornea.* 2008;27:1131–1137.
225. Terry MA, Shamie N, et al. Endothelial keratoplasty: the influence of insertion techniques and incision size on endothelial survival. *Cornea.* 2009;28:24–31.
226. Price MO, Bidros M, Gorovoy M. Effect of incision width on graft survival and endothelial cell loss after DSAEK. *Cornea.* 2010;29:523–27.
227. Price FW Jr. Does endothelial survival differ between DSEK and standard PK? *Ophthalmology.* 2009;116:367–368
228. Price MO, Pricejr FW Jr. Endothelial cell loss after Descemet stripping with endothelial keratoplasty influencing factors and 2-year trend. *Ophthalmology.* 2008;115:857–865.
229. Price MO, Brubaker JW, Price FW Jr. Randomized, prospective comparison of precut vs surgeon-dissected grafts for Descemet stripping automated endothelial keratoplasty. *Am J Ophthalmol.* 2008;146:36–41.
230. Terry MA, Chen ES, Phillips PM, Hoar KL, Friend DJ. Precut tissue for Descemet's stripping automated endothelial keratoplasty: vision, astigmatism, and endothelial survival. *Ophthalmology.* 2009;116:248–256.
231. Chen ES, Terry MA, Shamie N, Hoar KL, Friend DJ. Precut tissue in Descemet's stripping automated endothelial keratoplasty donor characteristics and early postoperative complications. *Ophthalmology.* 2008;115(3):497–502
232. Price MO, Gorovoy M, Benetz BA, et al. Descemet's stripping automated endothelial keratoplasty outcomes compared with penetrating keratoplasty from the Cornea Donor Study. *Ophthalmology.* 2010;117:438–444.
233. Terry MA, Chen ES, Shamie N, Hoar KL, Friend DJ. Endothelial cell loss after Descemet's stripping endothelial keratoplasty in a large prospective series. *Ophthalmology.* 2008;115(3):488–496.
234. Price MO, Price FW Jr. Descemet stripping with endothelial keratoplasty for treatment of iridocorneal endothelial syndrome. *Cornea.* 2007;26(4):493–497.
235. Bahar I, McAllum P, Slomovic A, Rootman D. Comparison of posterior lamellar keratoplasty techniques to penetrating keratoplasty. *Ophthalmology.* 2008;115:1525–1533.
236. Melles GR, Eggink FA, Lander F, et al. A surgical technique for posterior lamellar keratoplasty. *Cornea.* 1998;17(6):618–626.
237. Melles GR, Lander F, Beekhuis WH, Remeijer L, Binder PS. Posterior lamellar keratoplasty for a case of pseudophakic bullous keratopathy. *Am J Ophthalmol.* 1999;127(3):340–341.

238. Terry MA, Ousley PJ. Deep lamellar endothelial keratoplasty in the first United States patients: early clinical results. *Cornea*. 2001;20(3):239–243.
239. Melles GR, Wijdh RH, Nieuwendaal CP. A technique to excise the Descemet membrane from a recipient cornea (descemetorhexis). *Cornea*. 2004;23(3):286–288.
240. Melles GR, Ong TS, Ververs B, van der Wees J. Descemet membrane endothelial keratoplasty (DMEK). *Cornea*. 2006;25(8):987–990.
241. Melles GR, Ong TS, Ververs B, van der Wees J. Preliminary clinical results of Descemet membrane endothelial keratoplasty. *Am J Ophthalmol*. 2008;145(2):222–227.
242. Terry MA, Chen ES, Shamie N, Hoar KL, Friend DJ. Endothelial cell loss after Descemet's stripping endothelial keratoplasty in a large prospective series. *Ophthalmology*. 2008;115(3):488–496.
243. Matsuda M, Yee RW, Glasser DB, Geroski DH, Edelhauser HF. Specular microscopic evaluation of donor corneal endothelium. *Arch Ophthalmol*. 1986;104:259–262.
244. Bigar F, Schimmelpfennig B, Gieseler R. Routine evaluation of endothelium in human donor corneas. *Graefe's Arch Klin Exp Ophthalmol*. 1976; 200(3):195–200.
245. Roberts CV, Rosskothen HD, Koester CJ. Wide field specular microscopy of excised donor corneas. *Arch Ophthalmol*. 1981;99(5):881–883.
246. Nesburn AB, Mandelbaum S, Willey DE, et al. A specular microscopic viewing system for donor corneas. *Ophthalmology*. 1983;90(6):686–691.
247. Eye Bank Association of America. *Medical Standards*. 2009.
248. Edelhauser HF, Van Horn DL, Hyndiuk RA, Schultz RO. Intraocular irrigating solutions. Their effect on the corneal endothelium. *Arch Ophthalmol*. 1975;93(8):648–657.
249. Edelhauser HF, Van Horn DL, Schultz RO, Hyndiuk RA. Comparative toxicity of intraocular irrigating solutions on the corneal endothelium. *Am J Ophthalmol*. 1976;81(4):473–481.
250. Joussen AM, Barth U, Cubuk H, Koch H. Effect of irrigating solution and irrigation temperature on the cornea and pupil during phacoemulsification. *J Cataract Refract Surg*. 2000;26(3):392–397.
251. Nuyts RM, Edelhauser HF, Holley GP. Intraocular irrigating solutions: a comparison of Hartmann's lactated Ringer's solution, BSS and BSS Plus. *Graefes Arch Clin Exp Ophthalmol*. 1995;233(10):655–661.
252. Puckett TR, Peele KA, Howard RS, Kramer KK. Intraocular irrigating solutions. A randomized clinical trial of balanced salt solution plus and dextrose bicarbonate lactated Ringer's solution. *Ophthalmology*. 1995;102(2):291–296.
253. Watsky MA, Edelhauser HF. Intraocular irrigating solutions: the importance of Ca++ and glass versus polypropylene bottles. *Int Ophthalmol Clin*. 1993;33(4):109–125.
254. Matsuda M, Kinoshita S, Ohashi Y, et al. Comparison of the effects of intraocular irrigating solutions on the corneal endothelium in intraocular lens implantation. *Br J Ophthalmol*. 1991;75(8):476–479.
255. Kramer KK, Thomassen T, Evaul J. Intraocular irrigating solutions: a clinical study of BSS plus and dextrose bicarbonate lactated Ringer's solution. *Ann Ophthalmol*. 1991;23(3):101–105.
256. Araie M. Barrier function of corneal endothelium and the intraocular irrigating solutions. *Arch Ophthalmol*. 1986;104(3):435–438.
257. Rosenfeld SI, Waltman SR, Olk RJ, Gordon M. Comparison of intraocular irrigating solutions in pars plana vitrectomy. *Ophthalmology*. 1986; 93(1):109–115.
258. Katz HR. Effects of intraocular irrigating solution on the corneal endothelium after in vivo anterior chamber irrigation. *Am J Ophthalmol*. 1985;100(4):622–623.
259. Adenis JP, Loubet A, Leboutet MJ, Loubet R. [Scanning electron microscopic study of the effect of some intraocular irrigating solutions on the corneal endothelium]. *Ophthalmologica*. 1980;180(6):344–349.
260. McEnerney JK, Peyman GA, Janevicius RV. A new irrigating solution for intraocular surgery: TC Earle Solution. *Ophthalmic Surg*. 1978;9(1): 66–72.
261. Peyman GA, Stainer GA, Asdourian G, Sicher S. Corneal thickness after vitrectomy and infusion with dextran solution. *Ann Ophthalmol*. 1977; 9(10):1241–1244.
262. Sanders DR, Peyman GA, McEnerney JK, Janevicius RV. In vitro evaluation of intraocular infusion fluids: effects on the lens and cornea. *Ophthalmic Surg*. 1977;8(5):63–67.
263. Leahy B. Bullous keratitis from vitreous contact. *Arch Ophthalmol*. 1951;46:22.
264. Chandler PA. Complications after cataract extraction: clinical aspects. *Trans Am Acad Ophthalmol Otolaryngol*. 1954;58(3):382–396.
265. Goar EL. Postoperative hyaloid adhesions to the cornea. *Am J Ophthalmol*. 1958;45(4 Part 2):99–102.
266. Jaffe NS. *Cataract surgery and its complications*. 2nd ed. St. Louis: Mosby; 1976.
267. Fischbarg J, Stuart J. The effect of vitreous humor on fluid transport by rabbit corneal endothelium. *Invest Ophthalmol*. 1975;14(7):497–506.
268. Leibowitz HM, Laing RA, Chang R, Theodore J, Oak SS. Corneal edema secondary to vitreocorneal contact. *Arch Ophthalmol*. 1981;99(3):417–421.
269. Homer PI, Peyman GA, Sugar J. Automated vitrectomy in eyes with vitreocorneal touch associated with corneal dysfunction. *Am J Ophthalmol*. 1980;89(4):500–506.
270. Snip RC, Kenyon KR, Green WR. Retrocorneal fibrous membrane in the vitreous touch syndrome. *Am J Ophthalmol*. 1975;79(2):233–244.
271. Wilkinson CP, Rowsey JJ. Closed vitrectomy for the vitreous touch syndrome. *Am J Ophthalmol*. 1980;90(3):304–308.
272. Schimek RA. Vitreous touch after phacoemulsification. *Ann Ophthalmol*. 1978;10(11):1591–1592.
273. Smith RE, Parrett C. Specular microscopy of epithelial downgrowth. *Arch Ophthalmol*. 1978;96(7):1222–1224.
274. Laing RA, Sandstrom MM, Leibowitz HM, Berrospi AR. Epithelialization of the anterior chamber: clinical investigation with the specular microscope. *Arch Ophthalmol*. 1979;97(10):1870–1874.
275. Zavala EY, Binder PS. The pathologic findings of epithelial ingrowth. *Arch Ophthalmol*. 1980;98(11):2007–2014.
276. Holliday JN, Buller CR, Bourne WM. Specular microscopy and fluorophotometry in the diagnosis of epithelial downgrowth after a sutureless cataract operation. *Am J Ophthalmol*. 1993;116(2):238–240.
277. Jensen P, Minckler DS, Chandler JW. Epithelial ingrowth. *Arch Ophthalmol*. 1977;95(5):837–842.
278. Bourne WM, McCarey BE, Kaufman HE. Clinical specular microscopy. *Trans Am Ophthalmol Soc*. 1976;81:743–752.
279. Maloney WF, Colvard M, Bourne WM, Gardon R. Specular microscopy of traumatic posterior annular keratopathy. *Arch Ophthalmol*. 1979; 97(9):1647–1650.
280. Forstot SL, Gasset AR. Transient traumatic posterior annular keratopathy of Payrau. *Arch Ophthalmol*. 1974;92(6):527–528.
281. Cibis GW, Weingeist TA, Krachmer JH. Traumatic corneal endothelial rings. *Arch Ophthalmol*. 1978;96(3):485–488.
282. Hamano H, Jacob JT, Senft CJ, et al. Differences in contact lens-induced responses in the corneas of Asian and non-Asian subjects. *CLAO J*. 2002; 28(2):101–104.
283. Barr JT, Schoessler JP. Corneal endothelial response to rigid contact lenses. *Am J Optom Physiol Opt*. 1980;57(5):267–274.
284. Ohya S, Nishimaki K, Nakayasu K, Kanai A. Non-contact specular microscopic observation for early response of corneal endothelium after contact lens wear. *CLAO J*. 1996;22(2):122–126.
285. Khodadoust AA, Hirst LW. Diurnal variation in corneal endothelial morphology. *Ophthalmology*. 1984;91(10):1125–1128.
286. Holden BA, Sweeney DF, Vannas A, Nilsson KT, Efron N. Effects of long-term extended contact lens wear on the human cornea. *Invest Ophthalmol Vis Sci*. 1985;26(11):1489–1501.
287. Holden BA. Contact lens-induced endothelial polymegathism. *Invest Ophthalmol Vis Sci*. 1985;26(Suppl):275.
288. Schoessler JP. Corneal endothelial polymegathism associated with extended wear. *Int Contact Lens Clin*. 1982;10:148–155.
289. Schoessler J. Corneal endothelium in veteran PMMA contact lens wearers. *Int Contact Lens Clin*. 1981;8:19–25.
290. Hirst LW, Auer C, Cohn J, Tseng SC, Khodadoust AA. Specular microscopy of hard contact lens wearers. *Ophthalmology*. 1984;91(10): 1147–1153.
291. Stocker EG, Schoessler JP. Corneal endothelial polymegathism induced by PMMA contact lens wear. *Invest Ophthalmol Vis Sci*. 1985;26(6): 857–863.
292. MacRae SM, Matsuda M, Yee R. The effect of long-term hard contact lens wear on the corneal endothelium. *CLAO J*. 1985;11(4):322–326.
293. MacRae SM. The effects of hard and soft contact lens wear on the corneal endothelium. *Am J Ophthalmol*. 1986;102:50–57.
294. Lass JH, Spurney RV, Dutt RM, et al. A morphologic and fluorophotometric analysis of the corneal endothelium in type I diabetes mellitus and cystic fibrosis. *Am J Ophthalmol*. 1985;100(6):783–788.
295. Carlson KH, Bourne WM, Brubaker RF. Effect of long-term contact lens wear on corneal endothelial cell morphology and function. *Invest Ophthalmol Vis Sci*. 1988;29(2):185–193.
296. MacRae SM, Matsuda M, Shellans S. Corneal endothelial changes associated with contact lens wear. *CLAO J*. 1989;15(1):82–87.
297. MacRae SM, Matsuda M, Phillips DS. The long-term effects of polymethylmethacrylate contact lens wear on the corneal endothelium. *Ophthalmology*. 1994;101(2):365–370.
298. Chang SW, Hu FR, Lin LL. Effects of contact lenses on corneal endothelium – a morphological and functional study. *Ophthalmologica*. 2001; 215(3):197–203.

299. McMahon TT, Polse KA, McNamara N, Viana MA. Recovery from induced corneal edema and endothelial morphology after long-term PMMA contact lens wear. *Optom Vis Sci.* 1996;73(3):184–188.
300. Gong XM, Shao MR, Tao XQ. [Effects of contact lens wear on the corneal endothelium and sensitivity]. *Zhonghua Yan Ke Za Zhi.* 1994; 30(3):207–209.
301. Sibug ME, Datiles MB 3rd, Kashima K, McCain L, Kracher G. Specular microscopy studies on the corneal endothelium after cessation of contact lens wear. *Cornea.* 1991;10(5):395–401.
302. Yamauchi K, Hirst LW, Enger C, Rosenfeld J, Vogelpohl W. Specular microscopy of hard contact lens wearers II. *Ophthalmology.* 1989;96(8): 1176–1179.
303. Schultz RO, Matsuda M, Yee RW, Edelhauser HF, Schultz KJ. Corneal endothelial changes in type I and type II diabetes mellitus. *Am J Ophthalmol.* 1984;98(4):401–410.
304. Keoleian GM, Pach JM, Hodge DO, Trocme SD, Bourne WM. Structural and functional studies of the corneal endothelium in diabetes mellitus. *Am J Ophthalmol.* 1992;113(1):64–70.
305. Watsky MA, McDermott ML, Edelhauser HF. In vitro corneal endothelial permeability in rabbit and human: the effects of age, cataract surgery and diabetes. *Exp Eye Res.* 1989;49(5):751–767.
306. Sieck E. Endothelial cell characteristics of diabetic donor corneas. *Invest Ophthalmol Vis Sci.* 1993;34(Suppl):772.
306a. Lass JH, Spurney RV, Dutt RM, et al. A morphologic and fluorophotometric analysis of the corneal endothelium in type 1 diabetes mellitus and cystic fibrosis. *Am J Ophthalmol.* 1985;100:783–788.
307. Aaberg TM. Correlation between corneal endothelial morphology and function. *Am J Ophthalmol.* 1984;98(4):510–512.
308. Dong XG, Xie LX. [Specular microscopy of the corneal endothelial cells in diabetes]. *Zhonghua Yan Ke Za Zhi.* 1994;30(1):14–15.
309. Ohguro N, Matsuda M, Ohashi Y, Fukuda M. Topical aldose reductase inhibitor for correcting corneal endothelial changes in diabetic patients. *Br J Ophthalmol.* 1995;79(12):1074–1077.

Chapter 15

Confocal Microscopy

W. Matthew Petroll, H. Dwight Cavanagh, James V. Jester

Background

It is well established that confocal microscopy provides higher-resolution images with better rejection of out-of-focus information than conventional light microscopy. The optical sectioning ability of confocal microscopy allows images to be obtained from different depths within a thick tissue specimen, thereby eliminating the need for processing and sectioning procedures. Thus, confocal microscopy is uniquely suited to the study of intact tissue in living subjects. In vivo confocal microscopy has been used in a variety of corneal research applications on experimental animals since its development over 20 years ago. However, in recent years, the use of the confocal microscope on human patients has also expanded dramatically. In this article we review the latest developments and most current applications of clinical confocal microscopy of the cornea. In addition, we discuss an emerging confocal imaging technique, multiphoton-second harmonic generation imaging, which allows noninvasive assessment of collagen matrix organization in intact corneal tissue.

Historical overview

The optical design of confocal microscopy is based on the principle of Lukosz, which states that resolution may be improved at the expense of field of view.[1] In 1955, Marvin Minsky developed the first confocal microscope for studying neural networks in the living brain.[2] The Minsky microscope condenser focused the light source within a small area of tissue, with concomitant focusing of the microscope objective lens on the same area. Because both condenser and objective lenses had the same focal point, the microscope was termed 'confocal.' Since the introduction of Minsky's original microscope, the optical theory of confocal microscopy has been more formally developed and improved. In modern confocal microscopy, a point (i.e. diffraction limited) light source is focused onto a small volume within the specimen, and a confocal point detector is used to collect the resulting signal. This technique results in a reduction of the amount of out-of-focus signal from above and below the focal plane which contributes to the detected image, and produces a marked increase in both lateral (x, y) and axial (z) resolution.[3–5]

The use of a point source/detector in the confocal optical design trades field of view for enhanced resolution; therefore, a full field of view must be built up by scanning. The first scanning confocal microscope, developed by Petran et al.,[6,7] used a modified Nipkow disk containing thousands of optically conjugate (source/detector) pinholes arranged in Archimedean spirals (Fig. 15.1A). Light from a broadband source passes through the pinholes on one side of the disk, and is focused into the specimen. Detector pinholes on the opposite side of the disk prevent light from outside the optical volume, determined by the objective lens and pinhole diameter, from reaching a camera or eyepiece. Rotation of the disk results in even scanning of the tissue in real time. Because the illumination and detection of light through conjugate pinholes occurs in tandem, this microscope was named the tandem scanning confocal microscope (TSCM).

Current confocal systems in clinical use

There are three main confocal imaging systems used clinically: the TSCM, the HRT III (a scanning laser system), and the Confoscan 4 (a scanning slit system). Much of the in vivo imaging to date has been accomplished with the TSCM design. The TSCM is well suited for in vivo applications because it generates images in real time, and uses a broadband light source which causes less tissue damage than laser sources. Egger and Petran obtained the first images of cells from uncut and unstained tissue blocks including the brain, retina, and other organs.[8,9] These initial observations were not repeated until 1985 when Boyde demonstrated the dramatic optical sectioning abilities of the TSCM by imaging osteocytes in intact bone without demineralization, grinding, or other destructive processing techniques.[10,11] In 1986, Lemp et al.[12] were the first to apply confocal imaging techniques to the study of the cornea ex vivo. This work led to the design of a TSCM with a horizontally oriented objective (Tandem Scanning Corp, Reston, VA), which was more suited to use in ophthalmology (Fig. 15.1B).[13] Most TSCM systems currently in use employ a specially designed surface contact objective (24×, 0.6 NA, 1.5-mm working distance). The position of the focal plane relative to the objective tip is varied by moving the lenses within the objective casing (Fig. 15.1C). Thus, the depth of the focal plane within the

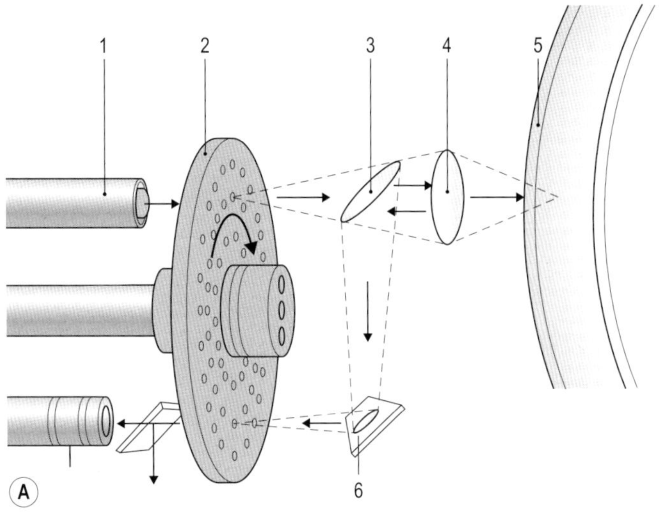

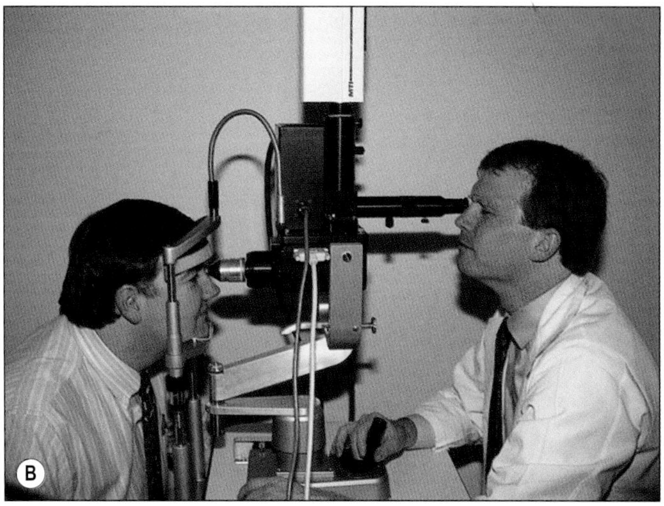

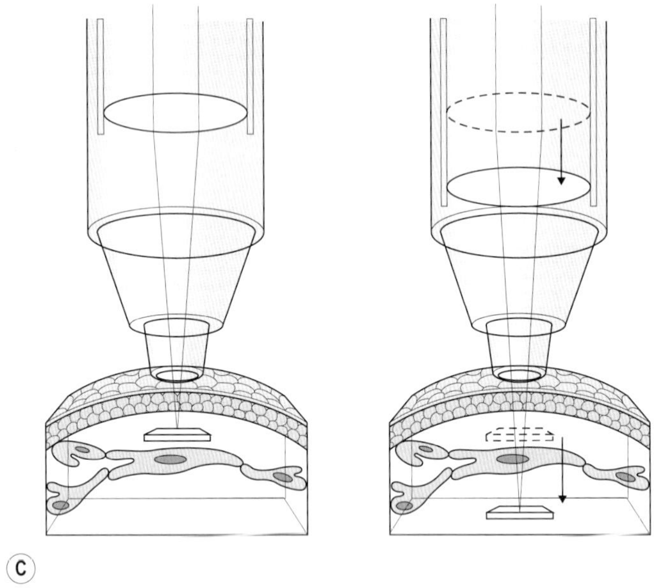

Fig. 15.1 The tandem scanning confocal microscope (TSCM). (**A**) An illustration of the optical pathway used in TSCM. Light from a broadband source (*1*) passes through the pinholes on one side of a Nipkow disk (*2*) and a beam splitter (*3*), and is focused by an objective lens (*4*) into the specimen (*5*). The reflected or emitted signal is then reflected by the beam splitter (*3*) and front surface mirror (*6*) to the conjugate pinholes on the opposite side of the disk, which prevent light from outside the optical volume from reaching a camera or eyepiece. Rotation of the disk results in even scanning of the tissue in real time. (From Cavanagh HD, Petroll WM, Alizadeh H, He Y-G, McCulley JP, Jester JV: Clinical and diagnostic use of in vivo confocal microscopy in patients with corneal disease, *Ophthalmology* 100:1444–1454, 1993.) (**B**) A TSCM adapted for use in ophthalmology (Tandem Scanning Corp., Reston, Virginia). (**C**) A simplified sketch of the TSCM objective, demonstrating how the depth or *z* position of the focal plane can be changed by moving the internal lenses. This allows acquisition of a series of optical sections through a single cell or other tissue structure. (From Petroll WM, Cavanagh HD, Jester JV: Three-dimensional reconstruction of corneal cells using in vivo confocal microscopy, *J Microsc* 170(3):213–219, 1993.)

tissue can be calibrated, and quantitative three-dimensional imaging is possible with this system.[14,15] With this objective, the TSCM has an axial (*z*-axis) resolution of approximately 9 μm.[14] The TSCM system is no longer commercially available.

The HRT III with Rostock Corneal Module (Heidelberg Engineering, GmBH, Dossenheim, Germany) is a laser scanning confocal microscope (Fig. 15.2). It operates by scanning a 670-nm laser beam (<1 μm diameter) in a raster pattern over the field of view. This is accomplished using horizontally and vertically oriented scanning mirrors. The reflected light from the cornea is descanned using the same two mirrors, and directed to a photodetector using a beam splitter. The system typically uses a 63× objective lens (0.9 NA), and provides images that are 400 μm × 400 μm in size. The microscope produces images with excellent resolution and contrast, and has better axial resolution than the TSCM, due to the higher NA objective.[15a,b]

The Confoscan 4 is a variable-slit, real-time scanning confocal microscope, available commercially from Nidek, Inc. (Fig. 15.3). This general design was originally described and applied to corneal imaging by Masters and Thaer.[16] Mounted on a slit lamp stand and using a 12 V halogen lamp for noncoherent illumination, the instrument can be used clinically in conjunction with a CCD video camera to examine the living eye. In this design, two independently adjustable slits are located in conjugate optical planes; a rapidly oscillating two-sided mirror is used to scan the image of the slit over the plane of the cornea to produce optical sectioning in real time.[17] The system uses a 40× objective lens (0.75 NA) and digitized images are 460 μm × 345 μm in size. This is a user-friendly instrument that incorporates automated alignment and scanning software. In addition, the scanning slit design allows better light throughput and provides images with a higher signal to noise ratio than the TSCM. However, this is achieved at

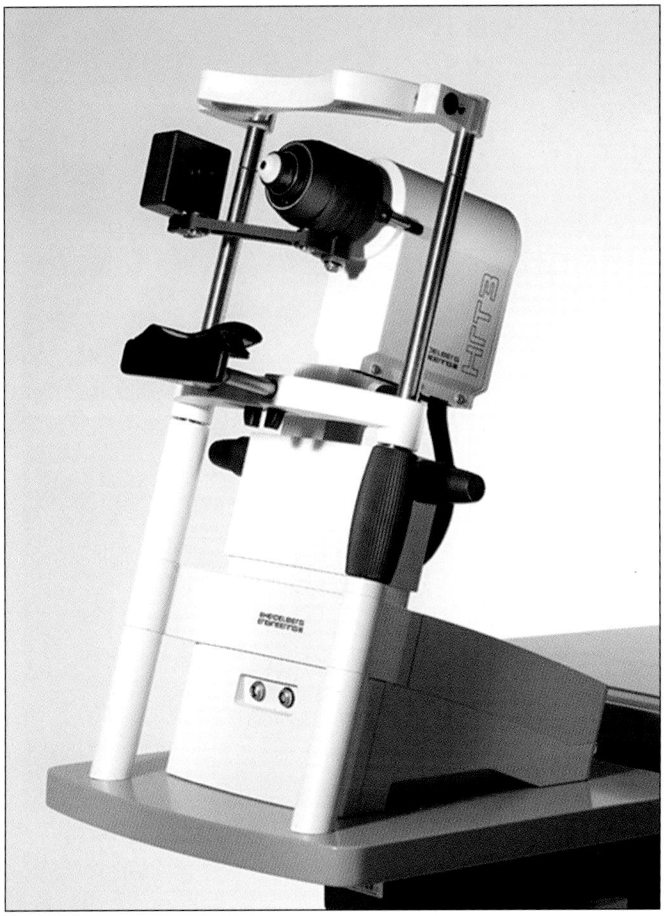

Fig. 15.2 The HRT III confocal scanning laser ophthalmoscope with the Rostock Cornea Module. (Provided by Heidelberg Instruments, Inc., with permission.)

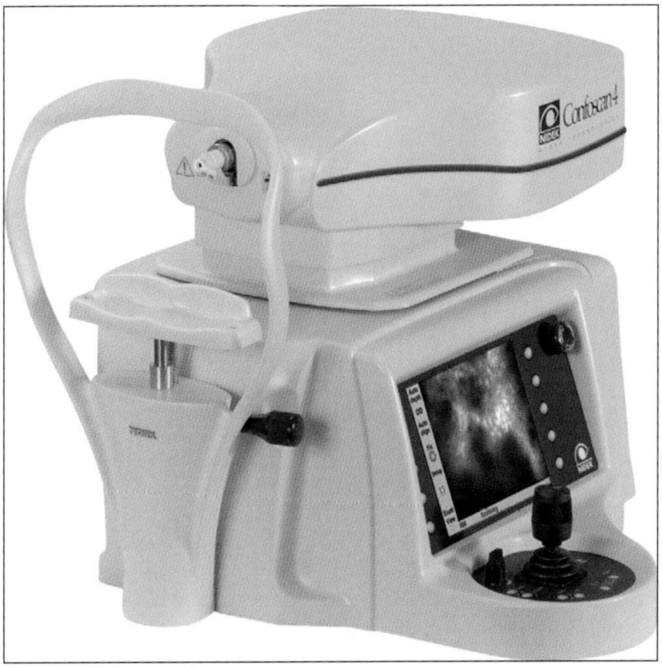

Fig. 15.3 The Confoscan 4 microscope (Courtesy of Nidek Technologies).

the expense of axial resolution, which has been measured at approximately 26 μm.[18]

In Vivo Confocal Imaging Techniques

Normal corneal structures

Many aspects of the clinical imaging procedure are similar for all three confocal instruments. Before observation, a drop of topical anesthetic is placed on the patient's eye. Next, a drop of methylcellulose or other viscous solution is applied to the tip of the objective lens in order to optically couple it to the cornea (i.e. as an immersion fluid). The objective is then aligned perpendicular to the surface of the cornea in a manner identical to specular microscopy. The x, y position of the image is controlled by moving the joystick on the microscope stand, and the z position of the focal plane is changed using the objective drive control. However, the objective drive and scanning software differ significantly between systems. More detailed descriptions of the individual scanning procedures used for each instrument can be found elsewhere.[19,20]

Normal corneal anatomy as observed with the TSCM is shown in Figure 15.4.[21] Confocal images are always taken en face: that is, the viewer sees thin slices of the cornea that are parallel to the epithelial surface. The borders of the surface epithelial cells are readily seen, as are the bright cell nuclei (Fig. 15.4A). Immediately beneath the basal epithelium, a fine nerve plexus can be detected (Fig. 15.4B).[22] In the corneal stroma, only cell nuclei are visible using TSCM under normal conditions, with a dark background in between (Fig. 15.4C, D). Interestingly, the interconnected cell processes of the keratocytes, which have been previously identified by Nishida et al.,[23] become visible under certain pathologic conditions, possibly due to tissue edema or cell activation. Large numbers of keratocytes are present in the anterior stroma as compared to the mid and deeper stroma, which show a lower cell density.[24] Prominent nerve fibers can be seen within the stroma, and tracked over long distances three-dimensionally. TSCM images of the normal endothelium appear similar to what is observed using specular microscopy (Fig. 15.4E).

HRT III images of a normal human cornea are shown in Figure 15.5. Due to its higher signal-to-noise ratio and improved axial and lateral resolution, intraepithelial sectioning can be achieved, and wing cells (15.5A) and basal cells (15.5B) can be easily distinguished. The sub-basal nerve plexus can be clearly imaged (15.5C), and dramatic montages can be generated in order to map temporal changes in the overall organization and nerve branching patterns over large areas of the cornea.[25] Langerhans cells can also be distinguished and their density quantified using the HRT III microscope.[26] Images of stromal cells (15.5D, E) and corneal endothelium (15.5F) are generally similar to that observed with the TSCM, albeit with higher contrast.

The Confoscan 4 can also provide images of the basal epithelial cells and the sub-basal nerve plexus, but with less resolution than the HRT III.[20] High-contrast images througout the corneal stroma can also be obtained. The Confoscan 4 is particularly well suited to imaging the corneal endothelial

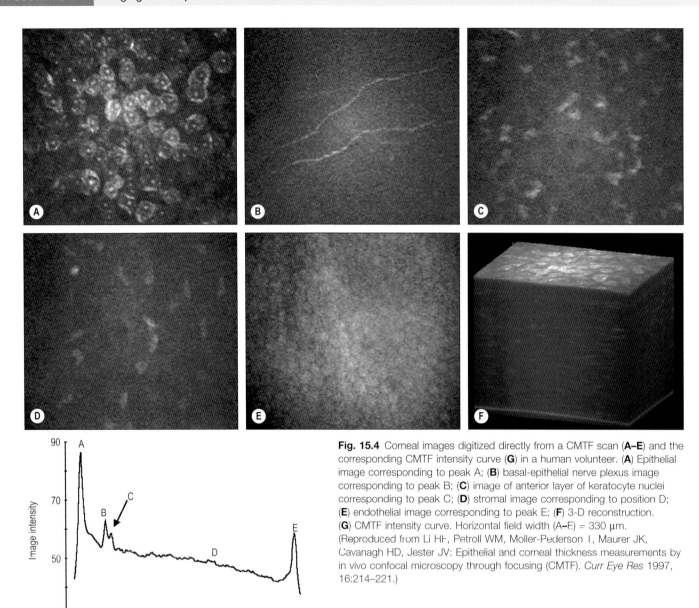

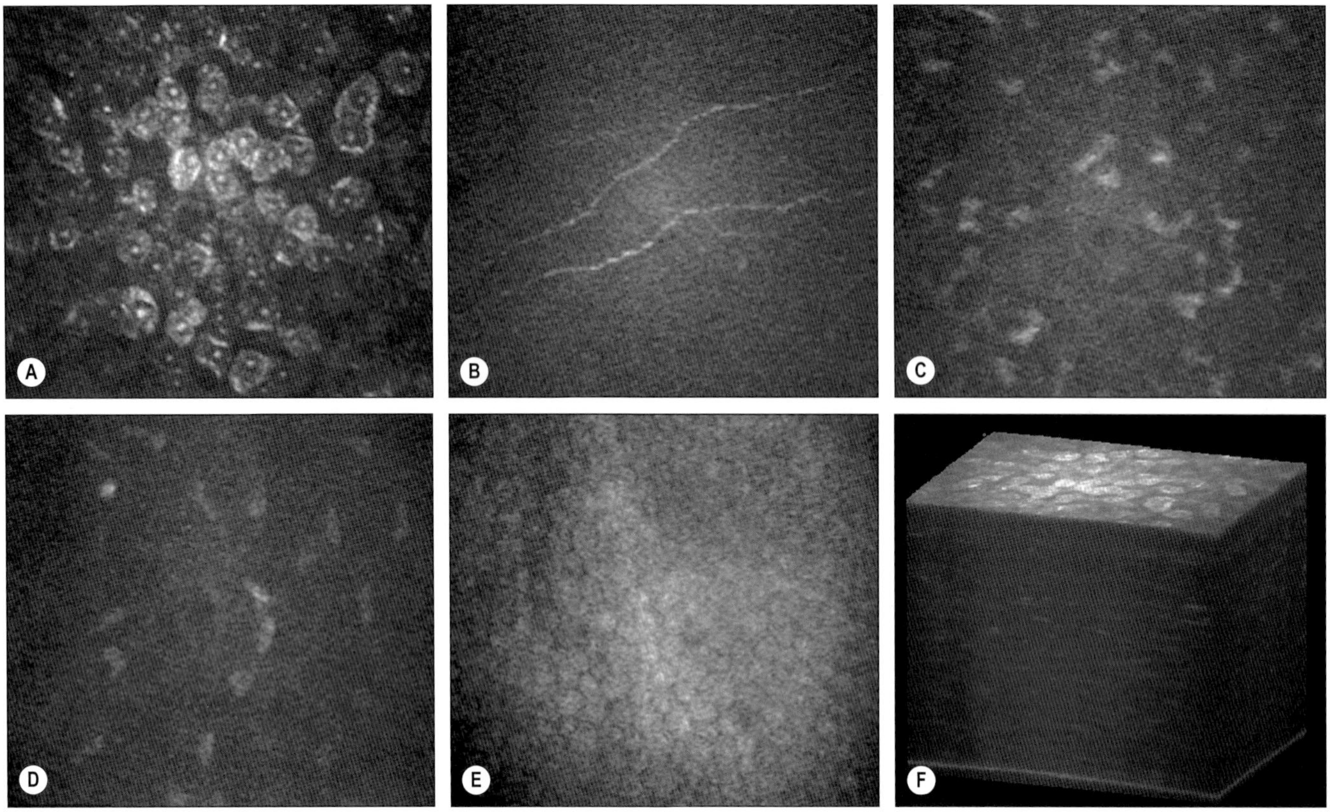

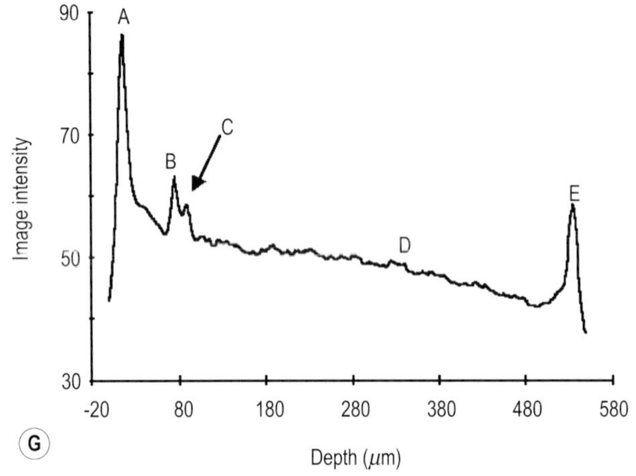

Fig. 15.4 Corneal images digitized directly from a CMTF scan (**A–E**) and the corresponding CMTF intensity curve (**G**) in a human volunteer. (**A**) Epithelial image corresponding to peak A; (**B**) basal-epithelial nerve plexus image corresponding to peak B; (**C**) image of anterior layer of keratocyte nuclei corresponding to peak C; (**D**) stromal image corresponding to position D; (**E**) endothelial image corresponding to peak E; (**F**) 3-D reconstruction. (**G**) CMTF intensity curve. Horizontal field width (A–E) = 330 μm. (Reproduced from Li HF, Petroll WM, Moller-Pederson T, Maurer JK, Cavanagh HD, Jester JV: Epithelial and corneal thickness measurements by in vivo confocal microscopy through focusing (CMTF). *Curr Eye Res* 1997, 16:214–221.)

cells. Due to its thicker optical volume and high light throughput, high contrast, full-field images are easily obtained. The thinner optical section thickness of the TSCM and HRT III make endothelial imaging somewhat more difficult. Unlike specular microscopy, the optical sectioning capability of confocal microscopy allows imaging through edematous corneas. Software for endothelial cell analysis is included with both the Confoscan 4 and HRT III instruments. The Confoscan 4 can also be used with a 20× nonimmersion (dry) objective lens for endothelium imaging.

Confocal microscopy through-focusing

To collect and quantify 3-D information from the cornea, a technique termed confocal microscopy through-focusing (CMTF) is typically used. Wiegand et al. originally demonstrated that by rapidly focusing through the cornea at high speed, a *z*-axis intensity profile of the tissue can be obtained.[27] This technique is based on the observation that different corneal sublayers generate different reflective intensities when imaged using confocal microscopy; thus, the intensity profile can provide information about the depth and thickness of corneal cell layers.

In the TSCM system, CMTF scans are obtained by scanning through the cornea from the epithelium to endothelium at a constant lens speed. Images are detected using a video camera and digitized into computer memory. The CMTF intensity curve is then generated by calculating the average pixel intensity in a central region of each image, and plotting versus *z* depth (Fig. 15.4G). After a *z* series of CMTF

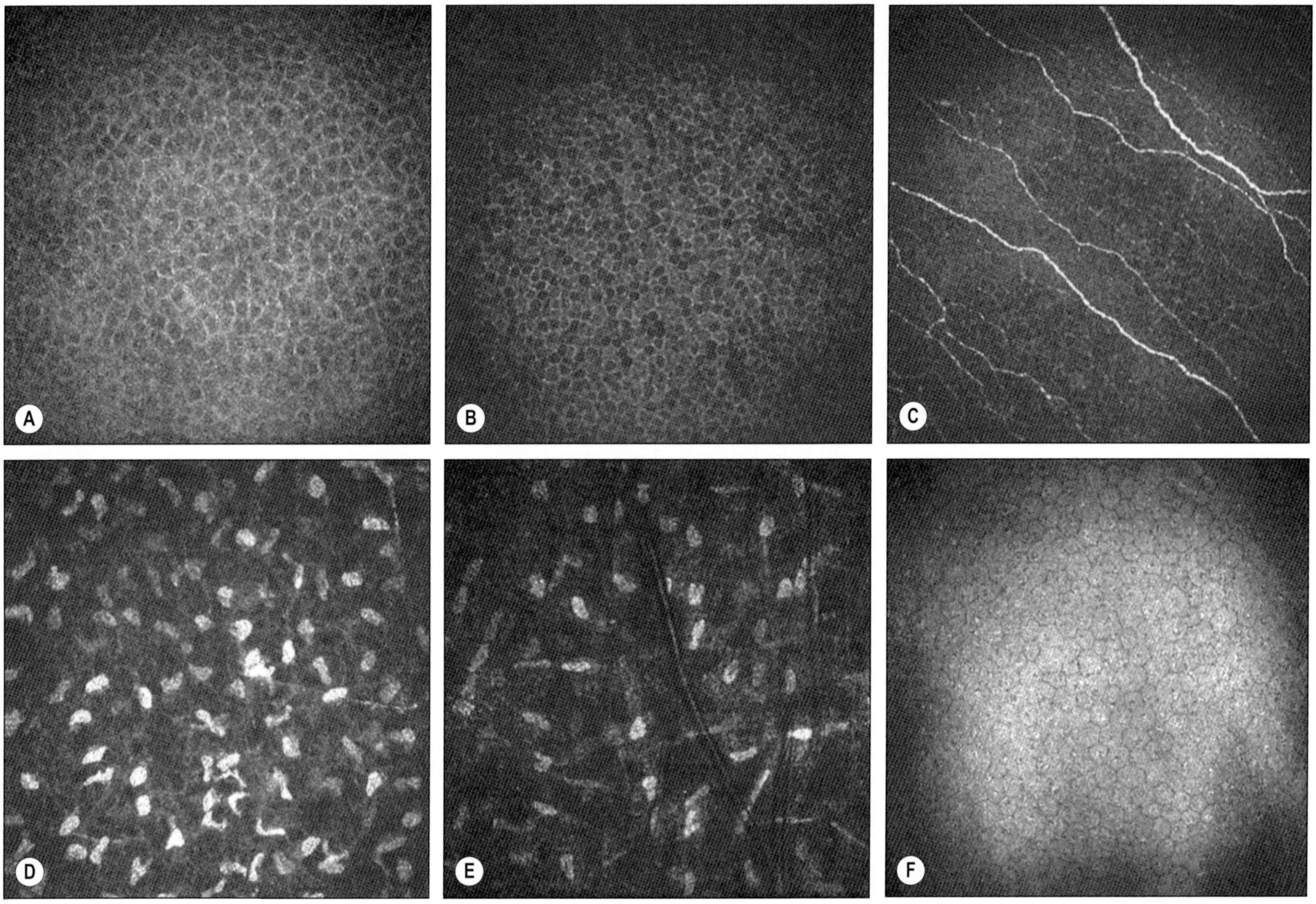

Fig. 15.5 Images of a normal cornea obtained using the HRT III. (**A**) Epithelial wing cells. (**B**) Basal epithelial cells. (**C**) Epithelial nerve plexus. (**D**) Anterior stroma just below Bowman's layer. (**E**) Mid stroma. Note decreased density of keratocyte nuclei as compared to (**D**). (**F**) Normal endothelium. Horizontal field width = 400 μm.

images have been digitized, a cursor can be moved along the intensity curve as corresponding images are displayed. In this way, the user can identify images of interest and record their exact *z* axis depth.[28,29] Two major peaks corresponding to the superficial epithelium anteriorly (Fig 15.4A) and the corneal endothelium posteriorly (Fig 15.4E) are present in normal CMTF curves. CMTF intensity profiles also showed smaller peaks corresponding to the basal corneal epithelial nerve plexus (Fig 15.4B) and the anterior layer of corneal keratocytes (Fig 15.4C). By measuring the distance between the various peaks, accurate and reproducible measurements of corneal, epithelial, and stromal thickness can be obtained.[28]

Unlike other more widely used methods for measuring corneal and epithelial thickness, confocal microscopy provides a series of high-resolution microscopic images which directly correspond to peaks in the intensive curve. Thus, the origin of the intensity peaks can be confirmed if necessary. CMTF scans can also be used to generate a 3-D image of the cornea by stacking the images and projecting them using surface or volume rendering (Fig 15.4F).

Cross-sections (*x-z* projection images) of CMTF scans from all three clinical confocal systems are shown in Figure 15.6. As mentioned previously, the TSCM uses an applanating objective which stabilizes the cornea, and the position of the focal plane within the tissue is changed by moving the lenses within the objective casing (Fig. 15.1C). A stack of evenly spaced images can thus be obtained and reconstructed (15.6A). The HRT III also uses an applanating tip to provide stability, and cross-sections with excellent resolution and contrast can be generated (Fig. 15.6B). Unfortunately, automated scans of only 60 μm can be generated at this time, and changing the focal plane over larger distances must be performed manually (by rotating the objective housing by hand). A modified prototype that overcomes this limitation has recently been described.[30] The Confoscan system uses a noncontact objective lens (for patient comfort), and movement of the entire objective lens is necessary to change the focal plane position within the cornea and generate CMTF scans. A trade-off with this design is that the cornea can move randomly with respect to the lens tip during a CMTF scan. A 'Z-Ring' which touches the corneal surface can be used to allow accurate calculation of *z*-axis position within the cornea during scanning,[31] but the distance between images in CMTF scans is generally not as uniform as that obtained using applanating objectives. As shown in Figure 15.6C, both the stability and axial resolution of the

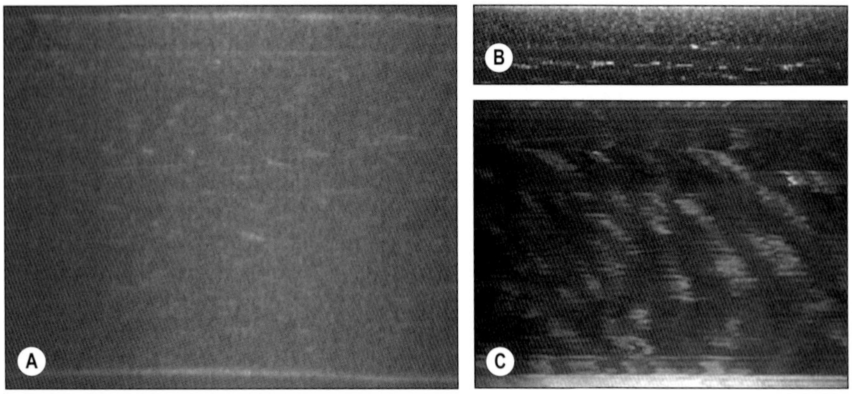

Fig. 15.6 Comparison of *x-z* reconstructions from CMTF scans through a human cornea in vivo using the TSCM (**A**), HRT III (**B**), and Confoscan 4 (**C**) microscopes.

Confoscan 4 are reduced as compared to the TSCM and HRT III. There are clearly trade-offs in all designs that must be considered when purchasing an instrument.

Clinical Applications

Although confocal microscopy has been used extensively in research applications on experimental animals, its noninvasive nature makes it ideally suited for clinical use in ophthalmology.[21] In recent years, the clinical application of in vivo confocal microscopy has expanded rapidly. Confocal microscopy has been used to monitor changes in keratocyte density during aging, in keratoconus patients, and following surgery.[24,32–35] In addition, temporal changes in the density and organization of subepithelial nerves in response to surgery or disease can be assessed.[36–40] The effects of contact lens wear on the morphology and thickness of the corneal epithelium has also been quantified, and such studies have provided important insight into how lens type and wear pattern influence bacterial binding and corneal epithelial homeostasis.[41–45] There are numerous other applications of this technology in the literature which cannot be covered here due to space limitations; many of these are discussed in several recent review articles.[19,46,47] Below, we discuss two of the most common applications of clinical confocal microscopy in more detail: (1) assessment of wound healing following refractive surgery, and (2) diagnosis of corneal infections.

Wound healing following refractive surgery

Because of its unique ability to image the cornea four-dimensionally at the cellular level (*x*, *y*, *z*, and *t*), confocal microscopy is ideally suited to monitoring the cellular events of epithelial and stromal wound healing, particularly following refractive surgical procedures (for reviews see references 48–50). For example, confocal microscopy allows measurement of wound gape, the depth of epithelial ingrowth, and the degree of corneal fibrosis in radial keratotomy wounds. Similar assessments can also be performed following penetrating keratoplasty (PK),[51,52] or lacerating injury. As detailed below, confocal microscopy is especially well suited to assessing the corneal response to photorefractive keratectomy (PRK) and laser assisted in situ keratomeliosis (LASIK). It has also been applied following related procedures such as LASEK[38,53] and epi-LASIK,[54] as well as emerging surgical techniques such as Descemet stripping with automated endothelial keratoplasty (DSAEK).[55]

PRK: CMTF has been used to assess multiple parameters associated with corneal wound healing following PRK.[56] Changes in corneal, epithelial, and stromal thickness following surgery can be made from the CMTF curves. In addition, confocal microscopy can be used to assess the degree of subepithelial haze induced by the procedure. Confocal microscopy following PRK has demonstrated that the development of corneal haze is correlated with the activation of corneal keratocytes and transformation to a fibroblast or myofibroblast phenotype.[57–60] These activated cells are more reflective than quiescent corneal keratocytes, and synthesize extracellular matrix components that also reduce corneal transparency. As shown in Figure 15.7, a 'haze peak' is observed in the CMTF curves after PRK, and the width and height of the haze peak indicate the thickness and reflectivity of the subepithelial tissue. An objective haze estimate can be obtained by calculating the area under the haze peak for each patient. Interestingly, increased subepithelial haze was been detected using CMTF in patients who were graded clinically clear using the slit lamp, demonstrating the higher sensitivity of confocal microscopy.[56] Nerve regeneration following PRK has also been assessed using confocal microscopy.[61,62] Interestingly, regenerating subepithelial nerve fibers have been detected as early as 7 days after PRK, but require at least 6–12 months for complete recovery, perhaps due to the persistence of the subepithelial scarring. Temporal changes in keratocyte density have also been documented following PRK.[32] Overall, in vivo confocal microscopy represents an important tool for quantitative assessment of initial photoablation depth, temporal changes in epithelial, stromal, and corneal thickness, cell loss and/or repopulation, and unbiased haze estimation after PRK.

LASIK: Confocal microscopy has also been used to assess numerous parameters following LASIK, such as epithelial thickness, flap thickness, interface particle density, keratocyte density, nerve damage and recovery, stromal cell activation, and interface haze.[33,38,62–74] Confocal microscopy has been used to assess the corneal response to both microkeratome-assisted LASIK, and LASIK with flap creation using IntraLase (IntraLASIK). Following traditional LASIK with a microkeratome, corneal haze is not generally observed

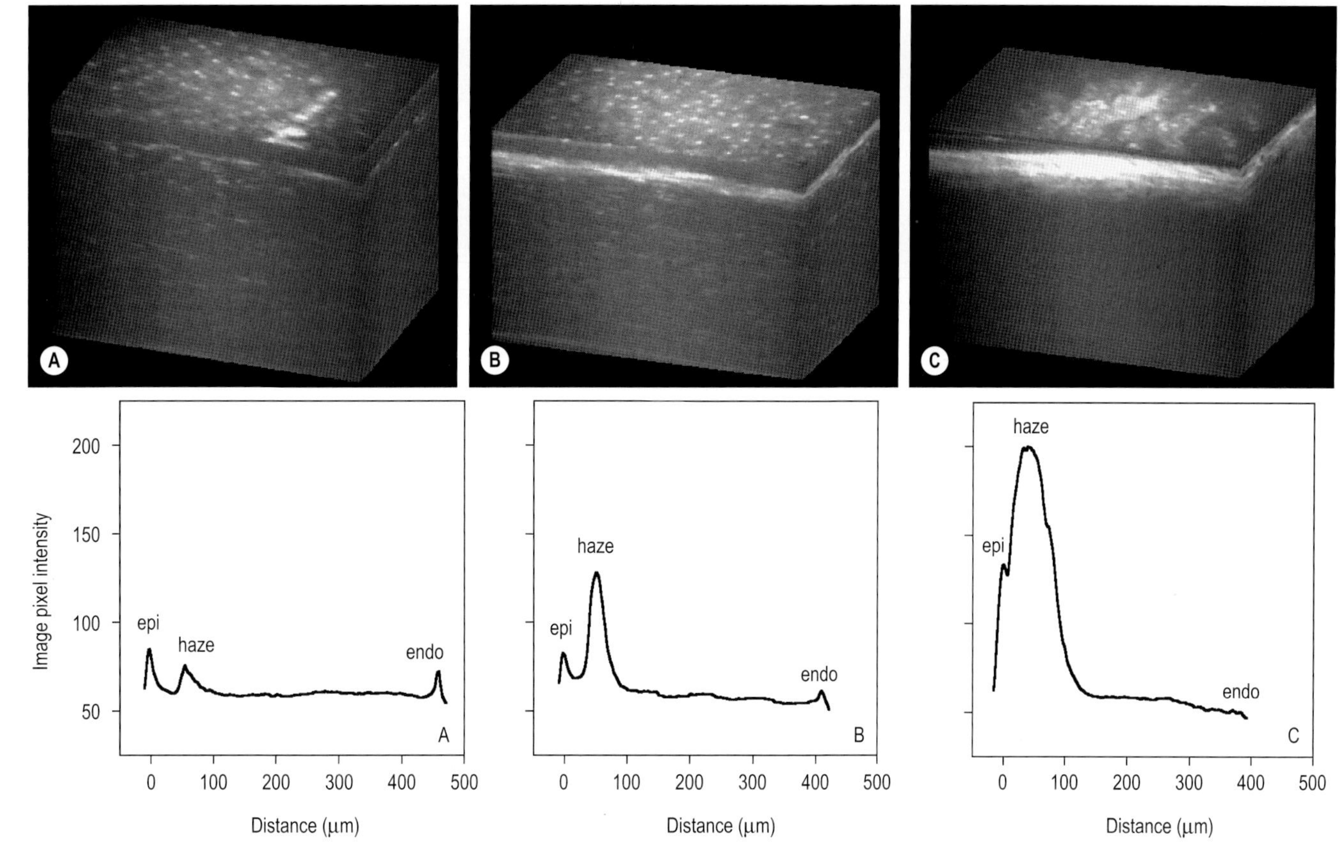

Fig. 15.7 Three-dimensional reconstructions and corresponding confocal microscopy through-focusing (CMTF) scans of three human corneas 1 month after photorefractive keratectomy. (**A**) A clinically clear cornea (grade 0 haze). (**B**) Cornea with clinical grade 2 haze. (**C**) Cornea with clinical grade 4 haze. Note the increased subepithelial reflectivity in all three corneas. In the corresponding CMTF scans, a profound increase in both haze thickness (haze peak width) and haze intensity (haze peak height) is seen with increasing clinical grades. (From Möller-Pederson T, Vogel M, Li HF, Petroll WM, Cavanagh HD, Jester JV. Quantification of stromal thinning, epithelial thickness, and corneal haze after photorefractive keratectomy using in vivo confocal microscopy. *Ophthalmology* 1997, 104:360–8.)

clinically. Although regions of keratocyte activation and changes in keratocyte density have been observed by confocal microscopy, the overall stromal wound healing response is much less pronounced than that of PRK.[33,63–66,75–78]

Previous clinical studies have shown that IntraLase® provides fewer complications than mechanical microkeratomes, and results in better visual outcomes in most patients.[79–84] Consistent with these results, studies using confocal microscopy have demonstrated that IntraLASIK provides more accurate and reproducible flap thickness, as well as a significant reduction in the number of interface particles detected.[70,85–89] One concern regarding IntraLase® is that the procedure for flap creation can induce more damage than a microkeratome, and therefore appears to stimulate a more pronounced wound healing response. To address this issue, IntraLase® has evolved in recent years with the development of new lasers with higher pulse frequencies, which allow for faster procedure time, tighter spot placement, and the use of lower raster energies than first-generation lasers.

Confocal microscopy has confirmed that IntraLase® can induce significant keratocyte activation, particularly at higher raster energies, and that this may underlie clinical observations of haze in some patients. An example of a cornea with keratocyte activation and ECM haze is shown in Figure 15.8. In this patient, a raster energy of 2.6 μJ was used. A CMTF stack is shown in Figure 15.8A. Note the areas of increased reflectivity near the flap interface (15.8A, *arrows*). Examination of individual images revealed keratocyte activation near the interface, as indicated by highly reflective nuclei (Fig 15.8B–D, *arrows*). An increase in ECM reflectivity (ECM haze) was also observed surrounding the cells in many cases (Fig. 15.8B–D). In addition, cell processes were sometimes visible, suggesting local stromal edema and/or fibroblast transformation of corneal keratocytes. Normal keratocytes are observed above and below (Fig. 15.8E, *arrowheads*) the region of activation.

In a recent paper, an analysis of confocal data from several studies was performed to determine the influence of different IntraLase® raster energies, pulse frequencies, and postoperative steroid treatments on the corneal response to IntraLASIK.[90] In this study, for patients with the same steroid dosing regimen, a decrease in the percentage of eyes with keratocyte activation as well as amount of interface reflectivity was found as the raster energy was reduced (from 2.8 μJ to 1.2 μJ). However, when the steroid treatment regimen was shortened, activation and reflectivity increased even if the

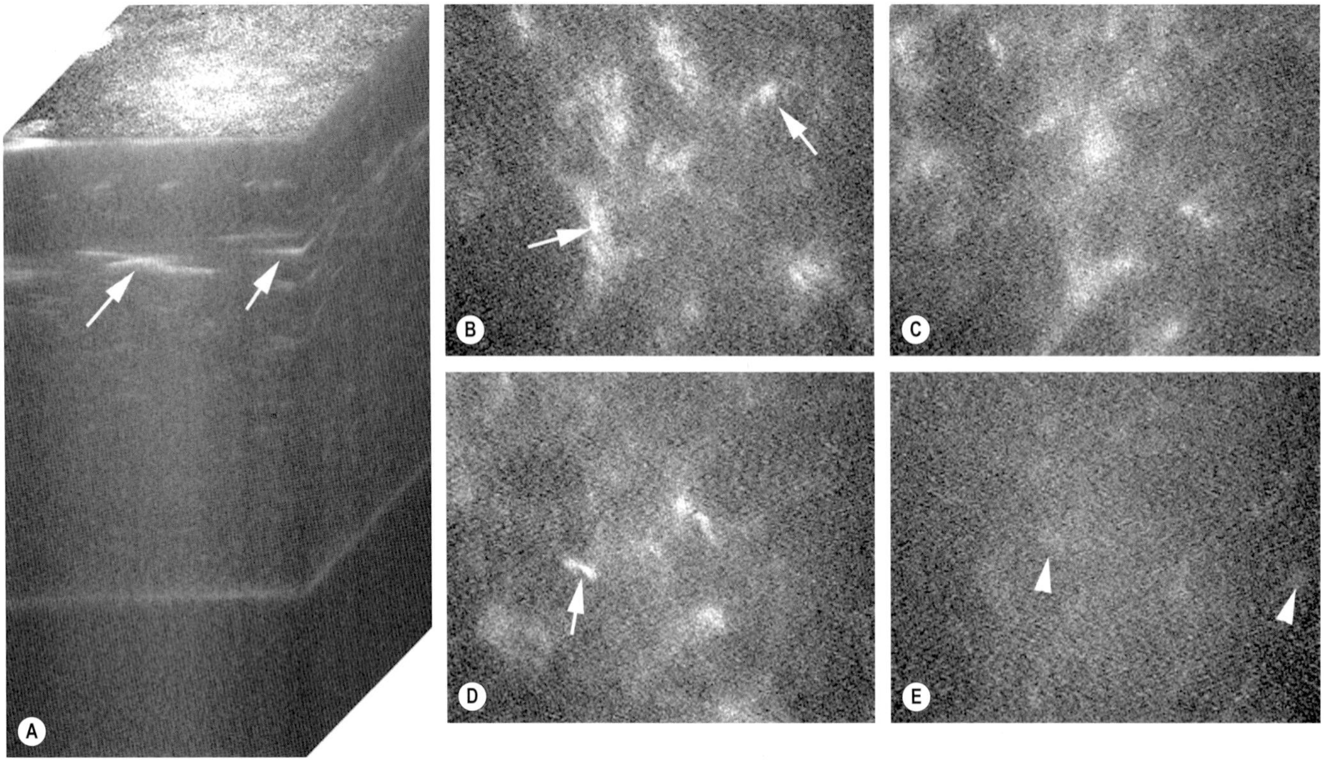

Fig. 15.8 (**A**) CMTF stack taken 3 months after LASIK with IntraLase®. Note the areas of increased reflectivity near the flap interface (*arrows*). (**B**) Single image taken from the CMTF stack in **A**, at the level of the flap interface. Note highly reflective keratocyte nuclei (*arrows*), indicating cell activation. An increase in ECM reflectivity (ECM haze) is also observed surrounding the cells (**C**) Single image from the CMTF stack taken 20 μm below the flap interface. Keratocyte activation and ECM haze is observed. (**D**) Single image from the CMTF stack taken 30 μm below the interface. A few activated keratocytes (*arrow*) and ECM haze is detected. (**E**) Single image taken 55 μm below the interface. Normal keratocytes are observed (*arrowheads*). Horizontal field width = 375 μm. (From Petroll WM, Goldberg D, Lindsey SS, et al. Confocal assessment of the corneal response to intracorneal lens insertion and LASIK with flap creation using IntraLase®. *J Cataract Refract Surg* 32:1119–1128, 2006, copyright Elsevier.)

raster energy was low. Most eyes with keratocyte activation had little or no haze detected by clinical examination. However, at the highest raster energy used, two eyes were found to have significant clinical haze by slit lamp examination. Overall, the confocal data suggests that IntraLase® can induce significant keratocyte activation, which may underlie clinical observations of haze in some patients. However, activation can be avoided by using lower raster energies and an extended steroid treatment regimen.

Infectious keratitis

Because it provides much higher magnification than a slit lamp biomicroscope, confocal microscopy is ideally suited for early detection and diagnosis of a number of infectious organisms (for review see references 19 and 47). One important clinical application of the TSCM is the localization of *Acanthamoeba* cysts and trophozoites in the living eye for diagnosis and assessment of the efficacy of ongoing medical treatment.[21,91–96] Figure 15.9A shows the appearance of a pig cornea infected with *Acanthamoeba castellanii* with active trophozoite forms of the infectious organism present just beneath the epithelium (*1*).[21] The cystic form is also seen (*2*); internal cyst detail can be noted with indentations suggestive of a double wall. The invading organism seems to 'hollow' the cornea in a series of internal tissue ridges, furrows, and cavities highly reminiscent of termites in solid wood. Figure 15.9B shows easily identifiable brightly reflective cysts (*1*) in a human patient who had a biopsy confirming *Acanthamoeba* infection. Figure 15.9C is from a patient who was being treated with Brolene™ (propamidine isetionate), and was showing symptoms of an active infection. Note the appearance of two types of highly reflective structures, presumably trophozoites (*1*) and cysts (*2*). The three-dimensional nature of this process can be assessed using confocal imaging; thus, the total spatial volume delineated by the infection can be quantitated, and response to antiamebal drug therapy monitored.

The detection of fungal keratitis has also become an important clinical application of confocal microscopy, due in part to the increased incidence of these infections in recent years.[97] Treatment of these infections is often slow and difficult, and early diagnosis is extremely important. Confocal microscopy has been shown to provide distinctive images of the filaments of *Fusarium solani* (Fig. 15.10)[98] and *Aspergillus* keratitis[64,99] in human patients, and may provide a unique means for early detection of these infections. Elongated particles resembling *Candida* pseudofilaments have

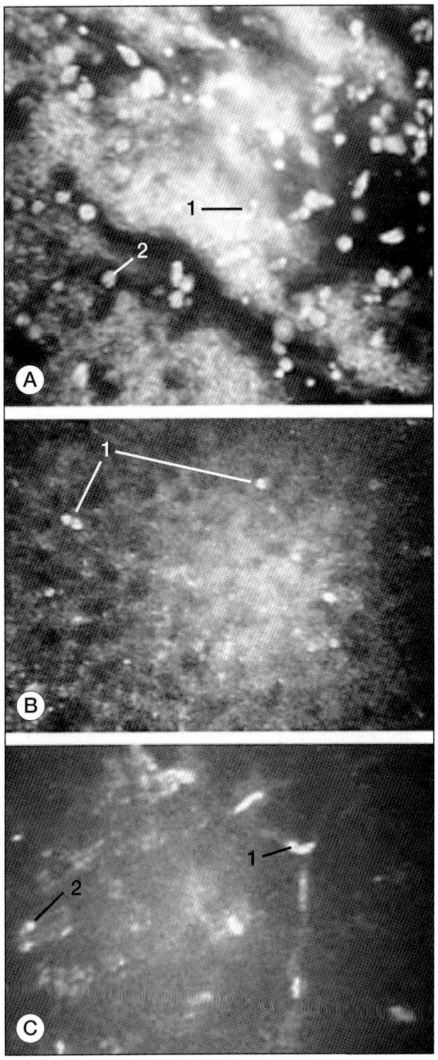

Fig. 15.9 *Acanthamoeba* keratitis. (**A**) 24 hours postinfection of a pig cornea, showing active trophozoites (*1*) and cysts (*2*) in the subepithelial region. Note the ridges and furrows (*dark areas*) within a markedly abnormal anterior corneal stroma. (From Cavanagh HD, Petroll WM, Alizadeh H, He Y-G, McCulley JP, Jester JV: Clinical and diagnostic use of in vivo confocal microscopy in patients with corneal disease, *Ophthalmology* 100:1444–1454, 1993.) (**B**) Easily identifiable brightly reflective cysts (*1*) in a human patient who had a biopsy confirming *Acanthamoeba* infection. (**C**) TSCM image from a patient who was being treated with Brolene™, and was showing symptoms of an active infection. Note the appearance of two types of highly reflective structures, presumably trophozoites (*1*) and cysts (*2*). Horizontal field width = 350 μm.

also been identified in infected corneas.[97] Other studies have demonstrated the potential usefulness of confocal microscopy in diagnosing bacterial contact lens-related keratitis,[100] microsporidial keratitis,[101,102] and *Borrelia* keratitis.[103] It should be noted that not all infectious agents can be detected and/or distinguished using confocal microscopy, and physical biopsy of the cornea is still often necessary to confirm diagnosis.[47,96,104] Bacterial and viral infections are difficult to image directly using current confocal systems, due to the small size of the infiltrates. Further studies are needed to

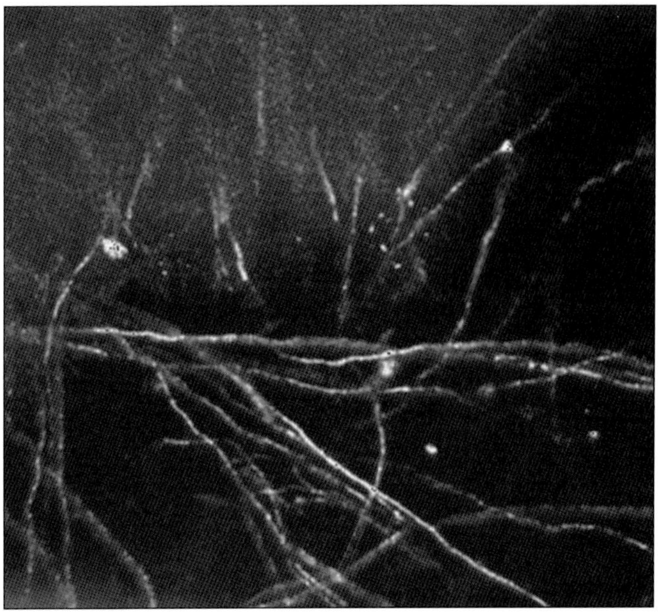

Fig. 15.10 Fungal keratitis. *Fusarium* imaged using the HRT III confocal microscope. Horizontal field width = 300 μm. (Courtesy of Dr Brasnu and Dr Baudouin, Paris, France, and courtesy of Heidelberg Engineering, Inc. All rights reserved.)

clarify which infectious organisms can be reliably detected and distinguished using confocal microscopy.

Imaging Corneal Collagen Using Second Harmonic Generated Signals

The application of lasers to biology and medicine, while not new, has been greatly expanded by the development of ultrafast, femtosecond lasers that enable the focusing of very high-intensity light within small optical volumes to generate nonlinear optical effects including two photon excited fluorescence (TPEF), second harmonic generated signals (SHG), and laser-induced optical break down (LIOB).[105] SHG has particular relevance to studying the structure of the cornea, since collagen fibrils generate strong SHG signals that can be imaged using optical microscopic techniques. To generate an SHG signal, a material is excited by the simultaneous absorption of two photons of light of the same frequency and then the material emits a single photon of light that is double the frequency or half the wavelength of the excitation light. The ability to generate SHG signals is limited to materials that are highly ordered and noncentrosymmetric, such as collagen.[106] Hochheimer, in 1982, was the first to show that SHG signals could be generated from the rabbit cornea.[107] Past studies have also shown that imaging of SHG signals can be used to establish collagen fibril orientation, as well as study the three-dimensional collagen organization.[108,109]

SHG imaging has more recently been used to study the supramolecular organization of collagen in the normal human and keratoconus cornea.[110,111] In these studies a Zeiss 510 Meta confocal microscope attached to a Coherent Chameleon tunable Ti:Sapphire femtosecond laser was used.

This system generated SHG signals from intact corneal tissue ex vivo using 800-nm infrared femtosecond pulses. Signals were then imaged using both the transmitted light detector and a 400-nm band pass filter (forward scattered signals) and the Meta detector collecting light in the 380–420-nm region (backscattered signals).[110]

Normal human corneal stromal collagen organization

Imaging of forwardscattered SHG signals from normal human cornea identifies distinct fiber-like structures, approximately 1 μm in diameter, that vary in length and orientation depending upon the depth within the cornea (Fig. 15.11A–C). Imaging of the backscattered signals, on the other hand, does not fully resolve individual collagen fibers as clearly as detected in the forwardscattered images taken from the same optical plane (Fig. 15.11D–F), although the general outline of the lamellar organization can still be detected. In the anterior cornea, small bands of five or fewer parallel fibers that run deeper into the cornea are seen as short segments aligned in random orientations (Fig. 15.11A). As in the forwardscattered image, backscattered images of the anterior cornea also show a highly interwoven lamellar organization in which narrow bands of collagen fibers run in random directions and cross over and under multiple lamellae (Fig. 15.11D). When both forward- and backscattered images are merged together, a more detailed view of the precise collagen organization can be detected (Fig. 15.12). Viewing of sequential images taken deeper within the cornea shows that these short collagen lamellae extend continuously deeper into the stroma, indicating that the short segments represented longer collagen fibers that run in and out of the plane of focus. This pattern indicates that the anterior collagen is organized into a highly interwoven lamellar structure with many lamellae running in a transverse, anterior–posterior direction and not parallel to the corneal surface. Deeper within the cornea, collagen bundles become wider, containing from five to ten fibers, but continue to pass through multiple optical planes, suggesting that lamellae continued to be highly interwoven (Fig. 15.11B). In the posterior cornea, large numbers of fibers can be detected that are grouped together into orthogonally arranged lamellae that run parallel to the corneal surface and show markedly less interweaving than observed in the other regions (Fig. 15.11C). Imaging of backscattered SHG signals

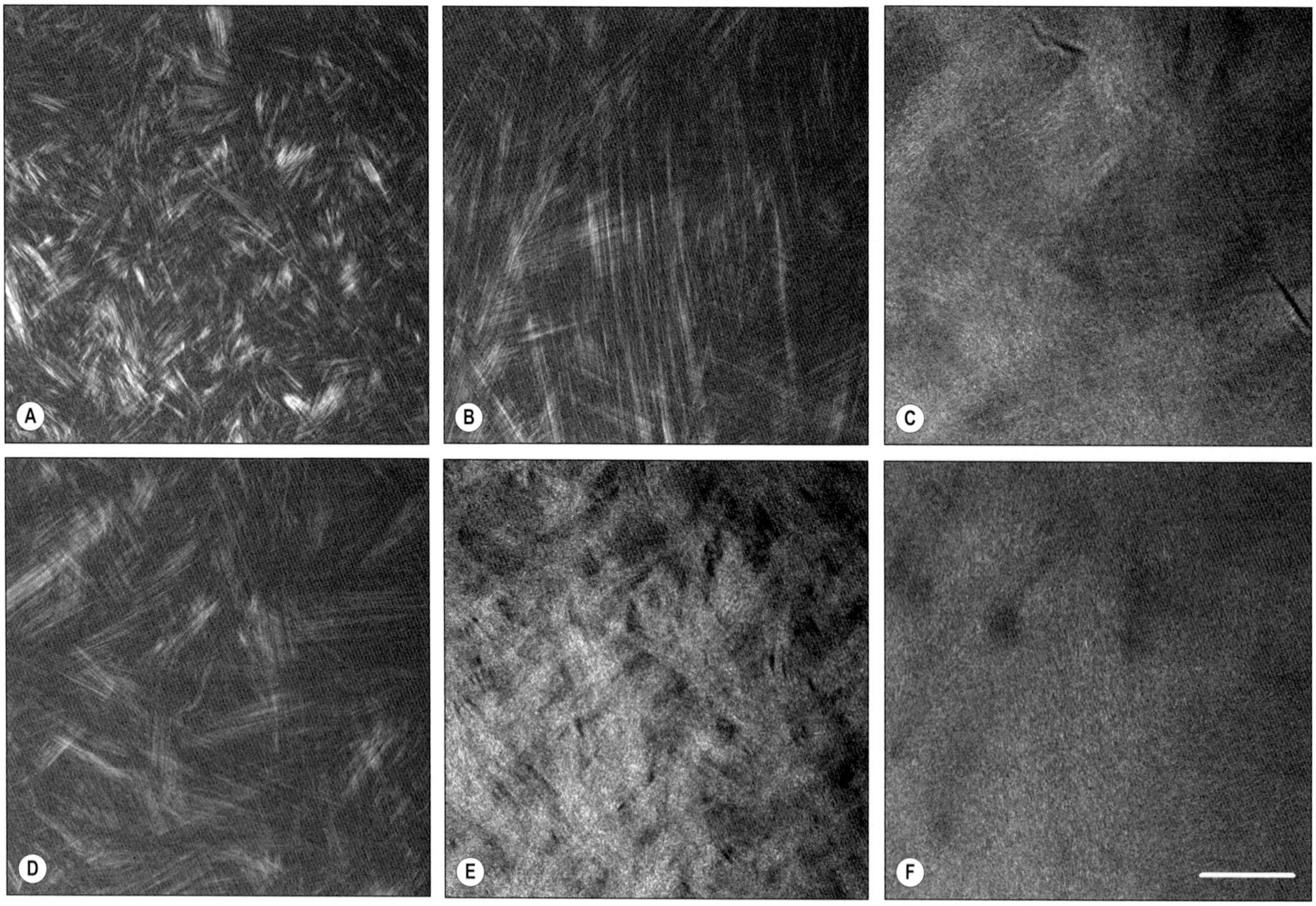

Fig. 15.11 Forwardscattered (**A–C**) and backscattered (**D–F**) SHG images of human corneal stroma taken in the anterior (**A** and **D**), middle (**B** and **E**), and posterior (**C** and **F**) cornea. Bar = 50 μm. (From Morishinge N, Petroll WM, Nishida T, et al. Non-invasive imaging of corneal stromal collagen using two photon generated second harmonic signals. *J Cataract Refract Surg.* 2006;32:1784.)

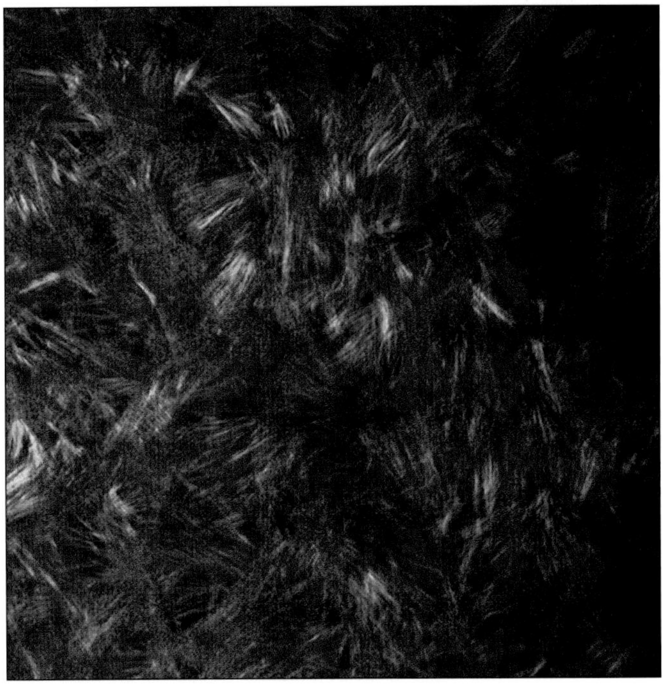

Fig. 15.12 Combined forwardscattered (*cyan*) and backscattered (*magenta*) image of SHG signal from the anterior human corneal stroma. Collagen fibril organization shows a highly interwoven pattern in the anterior cornea. (From Morishinge N, Wahlert AJ, Kenney MC, et al. Second harmonic imaging microscopy of normal human and keratoconus cornea. *Invest Ophthalmol Vis Sci.* 2007;48:1087–1094, Copyright, Association for Research in Vision and Ophthalmology.)

also detects interwoven yet broader lamellae within the middle layers of the stroma, similar to that detected in the forwardscattered image (Fig. 15.11E). In the posterior cornea the backscattered image is less distinct and does not show the same organizational pattern detected in the forwardscattered image (Fig. 15.11F).

Using digital image reconstruction, the anterior–posterior organizational pattern of collagen can also be evaluated using SHG imaging (Fig. 15.13). Such imaging shows that the anterior limiting lamina (ALL, Bowman's layer) generates a strong backscattered SHG signal that is detected between the corneal epithelium and the anterior stroma (*asterisk*). More strikingly, the transverse collagen lamellae detected in the anterior stroma can be seen inserting into the ALL (*double arrowheads*). The insertion of stromal collagen lamellae into the ALL has been previously detected by Komai and Ushiki using transmission electron microscopy.[112] Furthermore, as discussed by Bron, the anterior stromal collagen is known to have extensive anteroposterior interweaving with occasionally insertion into the ALL that may contribute to the anterior corneal mosaic.[113] The observations using SHG imaging complement these earlier observations and point to the extension of collagen lamellae from the ALL much deeper into the stroma than formerly appreciated. In this respect, studies by Muller et al.[113a] evaluating swollen human corneas have shown that the anterior 100–120 μm of stroma is resistant to swelling and maintains the corneal curvature. While it has been proposed that the

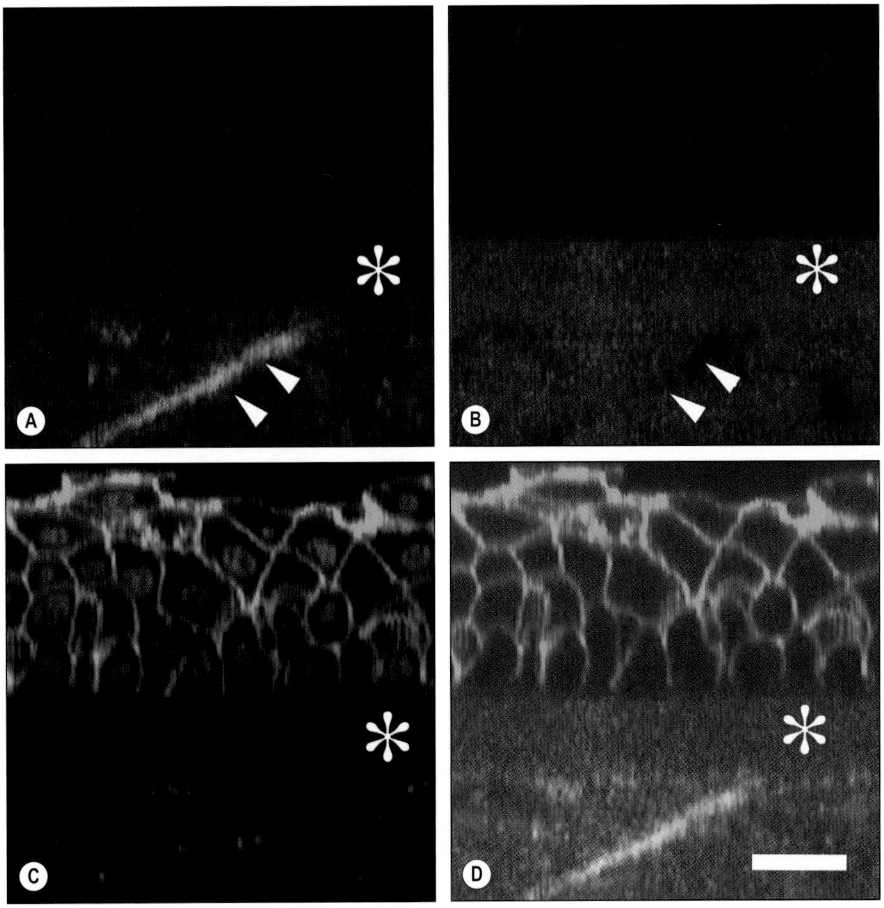

Fig. 15.13 Reconstructed cross-sectional images of human cornea showing forward (**A** *cyan*), backward (**B** *magenta*) SHG signal co-localized with Phalloidin to detect actin and Syto-59 to detect nuclei (**C** *green* and *red*, respectively). High-resolution images show that SHG imaging can detect the anterior limiting lamina (Bowman's layer, *asterisk*) and the insert of anterior collagen lamellae into the anterior limiting lamina (*double arrowheads*). Bar = 20 μm **D**. Four color overlay of A–C. (From Morishinge N, Petroll WM, Nishida T, et al. Non-invasive imaging of corneal stromal collagen using two photon generated second harmonic signals. *J Cataract Refract Surg.* 2006;32:1784.)

interwoven nature of the anterior cornea is responsible for this mechanical property, this region also corresponds to the region containing transverse lamellae that extends to a depth of approximately 130 μm. Therefore, it is likely that the presence of transverse lamellae that insert into the ALL explains the rigidity of the anterior corneal stroma, particularly if these lamellae extend out to the limbus as suggested by Bron.[113] In this respect, these transverse lamellae may represent a similar structural feature to that of 'sutural fibers' identified in the dogfish.[114,115] 'Sutural fibers' are thought to provide rigidity to the dogfish cornea and to play a role in the resistance to swelling following removal of the corneal endothelium, a similar function identified by Muller et al.[113a] for the anterior region of the human cornea.

Collagen organization in keratoconus corneas

Keratoconus is an acquired or genetic disorder that leads to thinning of the paracentral cornea, resulting in corneal steepening and cone formation. Histologic examination of end-stage keratoconus reveals disruption of the ALL and corneal scarring. These findings suggest that keratoconus involves a defect in the mechanical strength of the paracentral cornea that leads to progressive thinning. Since the biomechanical strength of the cornea is generally thought to be associated with the axial strength of the collagen fibrils, understanding the 3-D collagen organization of the keratoconus cornea compared to the normal cornea may provide insight into the pathogenesis of this disorder.

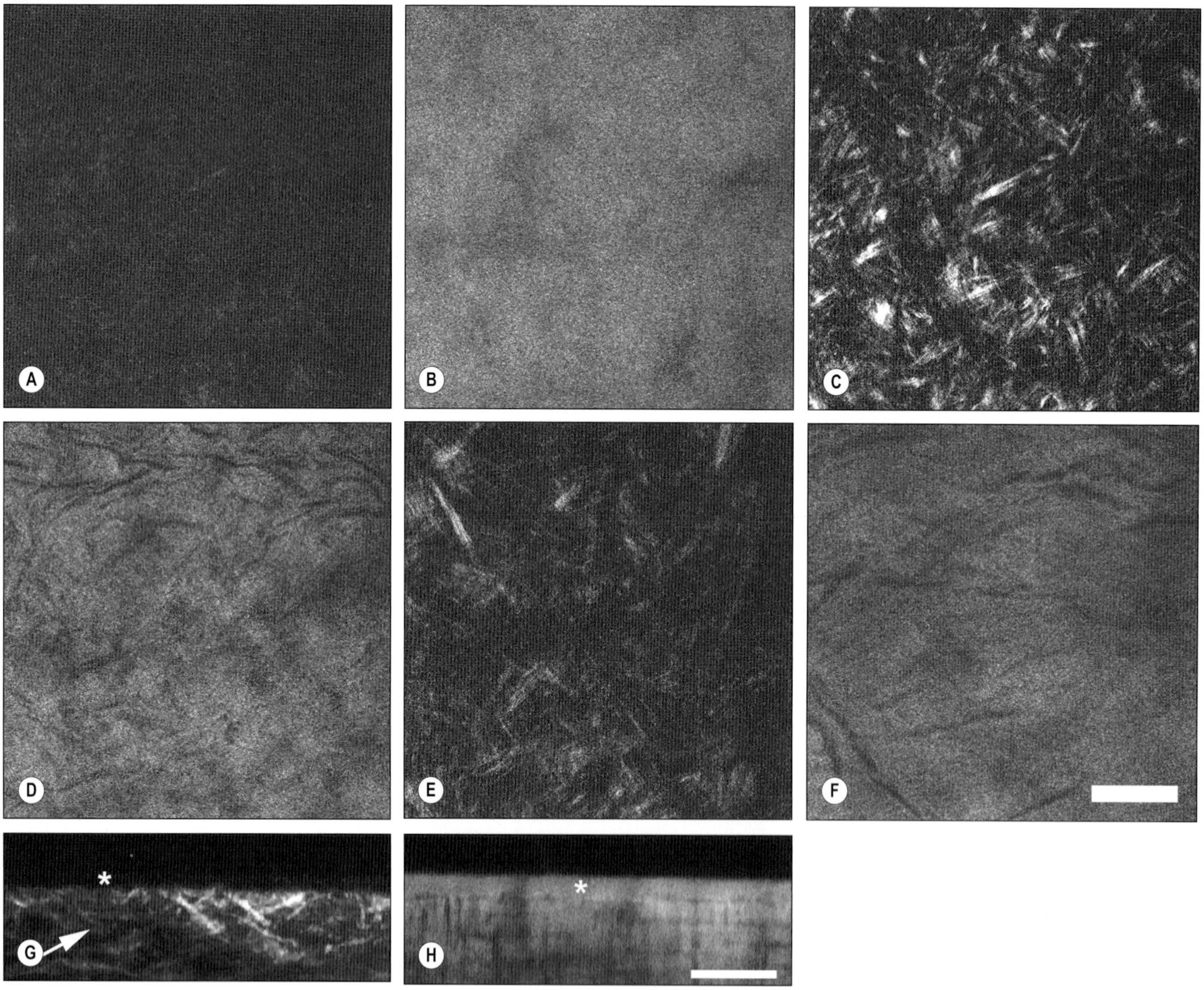

Fig. 15.14 Second harmonic signals from keratoconus corneas detected with the forward (**A**, **C**, **E**, **G**) and backward (**B**, **D**, **F**, **H**) detector. (**A**, **B**) Bowman's layer. (**C**, **D**) 10 μm below **A**. (**E**, **F**) 50 μm below **A**. (**G**) Three-dimensional reconstruction of the data set from forward detector showing a maximum intensity projection rotated 90° in the *y* axis through 230 μm of anterior stroma. Note that lamellae inserting into Bowman's layer are absent (*arrow*) or shortened. (**H**) Three-dimensional reconstruction of a 10 μm thick slice through the data set from the backward detector showing a maximum intensity projection rotated 90° in the *y* axis through 10 μm of anterior stroma. Asterisk = Bowman's layer. Bar = 50 μm. (From Morishinge N, Wahlert AJ, Kenney MC. Second-harmonic imaging microscopy of normal human and keratoconus cornea. *Int Ophthalmol Vis Sci.* 2007;48:1087.)

Using SHG imaging, a recent study evaluating 13 corneal buttons obtained following corneal transplant surgery for keratoconus noted a marked loss or decrease in the presence of transverse stromal lamellae that inserted into the ALL.[111] Images from a representative subject from that report are shown in Figure 15.14. In regions where the anterior limiting lamina was intact (Fig. 15.14A, B), a distinct decrease in the number of transverse lamellae was detected (Fig. 15.14C) along with less lamellar interweaving (Fig. 15.14D) compared to normal. Furthermore, deeper into the anterior stroma (50 µm), the loss of lamellae detected by the forward detector was more dramatic (Fig. 15.14E) and lamellar interweaving appeared completely absent in the backward detector image (Fig. 15.14F). Three-dimensional reconstructions and evaluation of the cross-sectional organization confirmed these findings and indicated that the number of lamellae inserting into the ALL (*asterisk*) was remarkably reduced in some regions (Fig. 15.14G, *arrow*) and, when present, only extended a short distance into the anterior cornea. Reconstruction of a 10 µm×230 µm slice through the three-dimensional data set taken from the backward detector also confirmed the marked lack of lamellar interweaving below the ALL (Fig. 15.14H), which was distinctly different from that of normal adult cornea.

Overall, based on SHG evaluation of 13 cases of keratoconus using maximum intensity projections to identify transversely oriented collagen lamellae, 12 of 13 showed marked abnormalities in the density and extent to which these 'sutural' lamellae extended deeper into the underlying corneal stroma.[111] These observations are in distinct contrast to SHG images obtained from similarly aged normal corneas which all show numerous transverse collagen lamellae that insert into the ALL. Overall, the findings based on SHG imaging suggest that there is an underlying defect in the organization of stromal collagen in keratoconus corneas that may explain the observed biomechanical differences between normal and keratoconus corneas.

Conclusions

This chapter has described the ability of confocal microscopy to resolve noninvasively structural and functional interrelationships, both temporally and spatially, in the corneas of human patients. Using confocal microscopy, the cellular details of fundamental biological processes such as inflammation, wound healing, toxicity, infection, and disease, which could previously be studied only under static or isolated conditions, can now be dynamically evaluated over time and the effectiveness of treatment modalities determined. The application of femtosecond laser-based nonlinear optical imaging of SHG signals from collagen is an important emerging technology which can be used to study noninvasively the structural organization of the human cornea with high spatial and lateral resolution. In the future, incorporation of multiphoton lasers into clincial confocal instruments may allow imaging of both cellular biology and interactions with extracellular matrix in human corneas, opening up a new world of potential applications.

References

1. Lukosz W. Optical systems with resolving powers exceeding the classical limit. *J Opt Soc Am.* 1966;57:1190.
2. Minsky M. Memoir on inventing the confocal scanning microscope. *Scanning J.* 1988;10:128–138.
3. Sheppard CJR. Axial resolution of confocal fluorescence microscopy. *J Microsc.* 1989;154:237–241.
4. Wilson T, Sheppard CJR. *Theory and practice of scanning optical microscopy.* London: Academic Press; 1984.
5. Wilson T. Confocal light microscopy. *Ann NY Acad Sci.* 1986;483:416–427.
6. Petran M, Hadravsky M, Egger MD, Galambos R. Tandem scanning reflected light microscope. *J Opt Soc Am.* 1968;58:661–664.
7. Petran M, Hadravsky M, Benes J, Kucera R, Boyde A. The tandem scanning reflected light microscope: Part I: the principle, and its design. *Proc R Microsc Soc.* 1985;20:125–129.
8. Egger MD, Petran M. New reflected light microscope for viewing unstained brain and ganglion cells. *Science.* 1967;157:305–307.
9. Petran M, Sallam ASM. Microscopical observation of the living (unprepared and unstained) retina. *Physiol Bohemoslov.* 1974;23:369.
10. Boyde A. The tandem scanning reflected light microscope. Part 2. Premicro '84 applications at UCL. *Proc R Microsc Soc.* 1985;20:130–139.
11. Petran M, Hadravsky M, Benes J, Boyde A. In vivo microscopy using the tandem scanning microscope. *Ann NY Acad Sci.* 1986;483:440–447.
12. Lemp MA, Dilly PN, Boyde A. Tandem scanning (confocal) microscopy of the full thickness cornea. *Cornea.* 1986;4:205–209.
13. Cavanagh HD, Shields W, Jester JV, Lemp MA, Essepian J. Confocal microscopy of the living eye. *CLAO J.* 1990;16:65–73.
14. Petroll WM, Cavanagh HD, Jester JV. Three-dimensional reconstruction of corneal cells using in vivo confocal microscopy. *J Microsc.* 1993;170:213–219.
15. Jester JV, Petroll WM, Feng W, Essepian J, Cavanagh HD. Radial keratotomy: I. The wound healing process and measurement of incisional gape in two animal models using in vivo confocal microscopy. *Invest Ophthalmol Vis Sci.* 1992;3:3255–3270.
15a. Guthoff RF, Baudouin C, Stave J. *Atlas of confocal laser scanning in vivo microscopy in ophthalmology.* Berlin: Heidelberg/Springer; 2006.
15b. Zhivov A, Stachs O, Stave J, et al. In vivo three-dimensional confocal laser scanning microscopy of corneal surface and epithelial. *Br J Ophthalmol.* 2009;93:667–672.
16. Masters BR, Thaer AA. Real-time scanning slit confocal microscopy of the in vivo human cornea. *Appl Optics.* 1994;33:695–701.
17. Brakenhoff GJ, Visscher K. Confocal imaging with bilateral scanning and array detectors. *J Microsc.* 1992;165:139–146.
18. Erie EA, McLaren JW, Kittleson KM, et al. Corneal subbasal nerve density: a comparison of two confocal microscopes. *Eye Contact Lens.* 2008;34:322–325.
19. Efron N. Contact lens-induced changes in the anterior eye as observed in vivo with the confocal microscope. *Prog Retin Eye Res.* 2007;26:398–436.
20. Szaflik JP. Comparison of in vivo confocal microscopy of human cornea by white light scanning slit and laser scanning systems. *Cornea.* 2007;26:438–445.
21. Cavanagh HD, et al. Clinical and diagnostic use of in vivo confocal microscopy in patients with corneal disease. *Ophthalmology.* 1993;100:1444–1454.
22. Vedas del Cerro M, LoCasio J, Aquavella JA. Peptidergic and catecholaminergic fibers in the human corneal epithelium. *Acta Ophthalmol.* 1989;67(suppl 192):80–90.
23. Nishida T, Yasumoto K, Otori T, Desaki J. The network structure of corneal fibroblasts in the rat as revealed by scanning electron microscopy. *Invest Ophthalmol Vis Sci.* 1988;29:1887–1890.
24. Patel SV, McLaren JW, Hodge DO, Bourne WM. Normal human keratocyte density and corneal thickness measurement by using confocal microscopy in vivo. *Invest Ophthalmol Vis Sci.* 2001;42:333–339.
25. Patel DV, McGhee CNJ. In vivo laser scanning confocal microscopy confirms that the human corneal sub-basal nerve plexus is a highly dynamic structure. *Invest Ophthalmol Vis Sci.* 2008;49.
26. Zhivov A, Stave J, Vollmar B, Guthoff R. In vivo confocal microscopic evaluation of Langerhans cell density and distribution in the corneal epithelium of healthy volunteers and contact lens wearers. *Cornea.* 2007;26:47–54.
27. Wiegand W, Thaer AA, Kroll P, Geyer OC, Garcia AJ. Optical sectioning of the cornea with a new confocal in vivo slit-scanning videomicroscope. *Ophthalmology.* 1993;100(9A):128.

28. Li HF, Petroll WM, Moller-Pedersen T, et al. Epithelial and corneal thickness measurements by in vivo confocal microscopy through focusing (CMTF). *Curr Eye Res*. 1997;16:214–221.
29. Li J, Jester JV, Cavanagh HD, Black TD, Petroll WM. On-line 3-dimensional confocal imaging in vivo. *Invest Ophthalmol Vis Sci*. 2000; 41:2945–2953.
30. Petroll WM, Cavanagh HD. Remote-controlled scanning and automated confocal microscopy through focusing using a modified HRT Rostock cornea module. *Eye Contact Lens*. 2009;35:302–308.
31. McLaren JW, Nau CB, Patel SV, Bourne WM. Measuring corneal thickness with the Confoscan 4 and Z-ring adapter. *Eye Contact Lens*. 2007;33:185–190.
32. Erie JC, Patel SV, McLaren JW, Hodge DO, Bourne WM. Corneal keratocyte deficits after photorefractive keratectomy and laser in situ keratomileusis. *Am J Ophthalmol*. 2006;141:799–809.
33. Erie JC, Nau CB, McLaren JW, Hodge DO, Bourne WM. Long-term keratocyte deficits in the corneal stroma after LASIK. *Ophthalmology*. 2004;111:1356–1361.
34. Ku JYF, Niederer RL, Patel DV, Sherwin T, McGhee CNJ. Laser scanning in vivo confocal analysis of keratocyte density in keratoconus. *Ophthalmology*. 2008;115:845–850.
35. Niederer RL, Perumal D, Sherwin T, McGhee CNJ. Laser scanning in vivo confocal microscopy reveals reduced innervation and reduction in cell density in all layers of the keratoconic cornea. *Invest Ophthalmol Vis Sci*. 2008;49:2964–2970.
36. Auran JD, Koester CJ, Kleiman NJ, et al. Scanning slit confocal microscopic obervation of cell morphology and movement within the normal human anterior cornea. *Ophthalmology*. 1995;102:33–41.
37. Masters BR, Thaer AA. In vivo human corneal confocal microscopy of identical fields of subepithelial nerve plexus, basal epithelial, and wing cells at different times. *Microsc Res Tech*. 1994;29:350–356.
38. Darwish T, Brahma A, O'Donnell C, Efron N. Subbasal nerve fiber regeneration after LASIK and LASEK assessed by noncontact esthesiometry and in vivo confocal microscopy: prospective study. *J Cataract Refract Surg*. 2007;33:1515–1521.
39. Benitez-del-Castillo JM, Acosta MC, Wassfi MA, et al. Relation between corneal innervation with confocal microscopy and corneal sensitivity with noncontact esthesiometry in patients with dry eye. *Invest Ophthalmol Vis Sci*. 2007;48:173–181.
40. Tuisku IS, Konttinen YT, Konttinen LM, Tervo TM. Alterations in corneal sensitivity and nerve morphology in patients with primary Sjögren's syndrome. *Exp Eye Res*. 2008;86:879–885.
41. Imayasu M, Petroll WM, Jester JV, Patel SK, Cavanagh HD. The relationship between contact lens oxygen transmissibility and binding of *Pseudomonas aeruginosa* to the cornea after overnight wear. *Ophthalmology*. 1994;101:371–386.
42. Ren DH, Yamamoto K, Ladage PM, et al. Adaptive effects of 30-night wear of hyper-O_2 transmissible contact lenses on bacterial binding and corneal epithelium: a 1-year clinical trial. *Ophthalmology*. 2002;109: 27–39.
43. Cavanagh HD, Ladage PM, Li SL, et al. Effects of daily and overnight wear of a novel hyper oxygen-transmissible soft contact lens on bacterial binding and corneal epithelium. *Ophthalmology*. 2002;109:1957–1969.
44. Ladage PM, Yamamoto K, Ren DH, et al. Effects of rigid and soft contact lens daily wear on corneal epithelium, tear lactate dehydrogenase, and bacterial binding to exfoliated cells. *Ophthalmology*. 2001;108:1279–1288.
45. Robertson DM, Petroll WM, Cavanagh HD. The effect of nonpreserved care solutions on 12 months of daily and extended silicone hydrogel contact lens wear. *Ophthalmology*. 2008;49:7–15.
46. Dhaliwal JS, Kaufman SC, Chiou AGY. Current applications of clinical confocal microscopy. *Curr Opin Ophthalmol*. 2007;18:300–307.
47. Labbe A, Khammari C, Dupas B, et al. Contribution of in vivo confocal microscopy to the diagnosis and management of infectious keratitis. *Ocul Surf*. 2009;7:41–52.
48. Petroll WM, Jester JV, Cavanagh HD. Clinical confocal microscopy. *Curr Opin Ophthalmol*. 1998;9:59–65.
49. Tervo T, Moilanen J. In vivo confocal microscopy for evaluation of wound healing following corneal refractive surgery. *Prog Retin Eye Res*. 2003;22:339–358.
50. Kaufman SC, Kaufman HE. How has confocal microscopy helped us in refractive surgery? *Curr Opin Ophthalmol*. 2006;17:380–388.
51. Richter A, Slowik C, Somodi S, Vick HP, Guthoff R. Corneal reinnervation following penetrating keratoplasty – correlation of esthesiometry and confocal microscopy. *German J Ophthalmol*. 1997;5:513–517.
52. Niederer RL, Patel DV, Sherwin T, McGhee CNJ. Corneal innervation and cellular changes after corneal transplantation: an in vivo confocal microscopy study. *Invest Ophthalmol Vis Sci*. 2007;48.
53. Darwish T, Brahma A, Efron N, O'Donnell C. Subbasal nerve regeneration after LASEK measured by confocal microscopy. *J Refract Surg*. 2007;23.
54. Chen WL, Chang HW, Hu FR. In vivo confocal microscopic evaluation of corneal wound healing after epi-LASIK. *Invest Ophthalmol Vis Sci*. 2008;49.
55. Kobayashi A, Mawatari Y, Yokogawa H, Sugiyama K. In vivo laser confocal microscopy after Descemet stripping with automated endothelial keratoplasty. *Am J Ophthalmol*. 2008;145.
56. Møller-Pedersen T, Vogel M, Li HF, Petroll WM, Cavanagh HD, Jester JV. Quantification of stromal thinning, epithelial thickness, and corneal haze after photorefractive keratectomy using in vivo confocal microscopy. *Ophthalmology*. 1997;104:360–368.
57. Møller-Pedersen T, Cavanagh HD, Petroll WM, Jester JV. Corneal haze development after PRK is regulated by volume of stromal tissue removal. *Cornea*. 1998;17:627–639.
58. Møller-Pederson T, Petroll WM, Cavanagh HD, Jester JV. Neutralizing antibody to TGFb modulates stromal fibrosis but not regression of photoablative effect following PRK. *Curr Eye Res*. 1998;17:736–747.
59. Møller-Pedersen T, Cavanagh HD, Petroll WM, Jester JV. Stromal wound healing explains refractive instability and haze development after photorefractive keratectomy. *Ophthalmology*. 2000;107:1235–1245.
60. Møller-Pedersen T, Li H, Petroll WM, Cavanagh HD, Jester JV. Confocal microscopic characterization of wound repair after photorefractive keratectomy using in vivo confocal microscopy. *Invest Ophthalmol Vis Sci*. 1998;39:487–501.
61. Linna T, Tervo T. Real-time confocal microscopic observations on human corneal nerves and wound healing after excimer laser photorefractive keratectomy. *Curr Eye Res*. 1997;16:640–649.
62. Erie JC, McLaren JW, Hodge DO, Bourne WM. Recovery of corneal subbasal nerve density after PRK and LASIK. *Am J Ophthalmol*. 2005;140: 1059–1064.
63. Buhren J, Kohnen, T. Stromal haze after laser in situ keratomileusis. Clinical and confocal microscopy findings. *J Cataract Refract Surg*. 2003;29:1718–1726.
64. Avunduk AM, Senft CJ, Emerah S, et al. Corneal healing after uncomplicated LASIK and its relationship to refractive changes: a six-month prospective confocal study. *Invest Ophthalmol Vis Sci*. 2004;45: 1334–1339.
65. Pisella P-J, Auzerie O, Bokobza Y, Debbasch C, Baudouin C. Evaluation of corneal stromal changes in vivo after laser in situ keratomileusis with confocal microscopy. *Ophthalmology*. 2001;108:1744–1750.
66. Vesaluoma M, Perez-Santonja J, Petroll WM, et al. Corneal stromal changes induced by myopic LASIK. *Invest Ophthalmol Vis Sci*. 2000; 41:369–376.
67. Gokmen F, Jester JV, Petroll WM, et al. In vivo confocal microscopy through focusing to measure corneal flap thickness after laser in situ keratomileusis. *J Cataract Refract Surg*. 2002;28:962–970.
68. Erie JC, Patel SV, McLaren JW, et al. Effect of myopic laser in situ keratomileusis on epithelial and stromal thickness. *Ophthalmology*. 2002;109:1447–1452.
69. Perez-Gomez I, Efron N. Confocal microscopic evaluation of particles at the corneal flap interface after myopic laser in situ keratomileusis. *J Cataract Refract Surg*. 2003;29:1373–1377.
70. Patel SV, Maguire LJ, McLaren JW, Hodge DO, Bourne WM. Femtosecond laser versus mechanical microkeratome for LASIK: a randomized controlled study. *Ophthalmology*. 2007;114:1482–1490.
71. Patel SV, Erie JC, McLaren JW, Bourne WM. Confocal microscopy changes in epithelial and stromal thickness up to 7 years after LASIK and photorefractive keratectomy for myopia. *J Refract Surg*. 2007;23.
72. Linna TU, Perez-Santonja JJ, Tervo KM, et al. Recovery of corneal nerve morphology following laser in situ keratomileusis. *Exp Eye Res*. 1998;66: 755–763.
73. Linna TU, Vesaluoma MH, Perez-Santonja JJ, et al. Effect of myopic LASIK on corneal sensitivity and morphology of subbasal nerves. *Invest Ophthalmol Vis Sci*. 2000;41:393–397.
74. Lee BH, McLaren JW, Erie JC, Hodge DO, Bourne WM. Reinnervation in the cornea after LASIK. *Invest Ophthalmol Vis Sci*. 2002;43:3660–3664.
75. Perez-Gomez I, Efron N. Change to corneal morphology after refractive surgery (myopic laser in situ keratomileusis) as viewed with a confocal microscope. *Optom Visi Sci*. 2003;80:690–697.
76. Mitooka K, Ramirez M, Maguire LJ, et al. Keratocyte density of central human cornea after laser in situ keratomileusis. *Am J Ophthalmol*. 2002; 133:307–314.
77. Ivarsen A, Thøgersen J, Keiding SR, Hjortdal JØ, Møller-Pedersen T. Plastic particles at the LASIK interface. *Ophthalmology*. 2004;111:18-23.
78. Dawson DG, Edelhauser HF, Grossniklaus HE. Long-term histopathologic findings in human corneal wounds after refractive surgical procedures. *Am J Ophthalmol*. 2005;139:168–178.

79. Binder PS. Flap dimensions created with the IntraLase FS laser. *J Cataract Refract Surg.* 2004;30:26–32.
80. Sugar A. Ultrafast (femtosecond) laser refractive surgery. *Curr Opin Ophthalmol.* 2002;13:4.
81. Durrie DS, Kezirian GM. Femtosecond laser versus mechanical keratome flaps in wavefront-guided laser in situ keratomileusis: prospective contralateral eye study. *J Cataract Refract Surg.* 2005;31:120–126.
82. Tran DB, Bor Z, Garufis C, et al. Randomized prospective clinical study comparing induced aberrations with IntraLase and Hansatome flap creation in fellow eyes. Potential impact on wavefront-guided laser in situ keratomileusis. *J Cataract Refract Surg.* 2005;31:97–105.
83. Kezirian GM, Stonecipher KG. Comparison of the IntraLase femtosecond laser and mechanical keratomes for laser in situ keratomileusis. *J Cataract Refract Surg.* 2004;30:804–811.
84. Nordan LT, Slade SG, Baker RN, et al. Femtosecond laser flap creation for laser in situ keratomileusis: six-month follow-up of initial U.S. clinical series. *J Refract Surg.* 2003;19:8–14.
85. Javaloy J, Vidal MT, Abdelrahman AM, Artola A, Alio JL. Confocal microscopy comparison of intralase femtosecond laser and Moria M2 microkeratome in LASIK. *J Refract Surg.* 2007;23:178–187.
86. Soniga B, Iordanidou V, Chong-Sit D, et al. In vivo corneal confocal microscopy comparison of Intralase femtosecond laser and mechanical microkeratome for laser in situ keratomileusis. *Invest Ophthalmol Vis Sci.* 2006;47:2803–2811.
87. Petroll WM, Goldberg D, Lindsey SS, et al. Confocal assessment of the corneal response to intracorneal lens insertion and LASIK with flap creation using Intralase. *J Cataract Refract Surg.* 2006;32:1119–1128.
88. Petroll WM, Bowman RW, Cavanagh HD, et al. Assessment of keratocyte activation following LASIK with flap creation using the IntraLase FS60 Laser. *J Refract Surg.* 2008;24:847–899.
89. Hu MY, McCulley JP, Cavanagh HD, et al. Comparison of the corneal response to laser in situ keratomileusis with flap creation using the FS15 and FS30 femtosecond lasers: clinical and confocal findings. *J Cataract Refract Surg.* 2007;33:673–681.
90. Petroll WM, McCulley JP. Quantitative assessment of corneal wound healing following IntraLASIK using in vivo confocal microscopy. Proceedings of the AOS. *Trans Am Ophthalmol Soc.* 2008;106:84–92.
91. Chew SJ, et al. Early diagnosis of infectious keratitis with in vivo real time confocal microscopy. *CLAO J.* 1992;18:197–201.
92. Auran JD, Starr MB, Koester CJ, La Bombardi VJ. In vivo scanning slit confocal microscopy of *Acanthamoeba* keratitis. *Cornea.* 1994;13: 183–185.
93. Silverman J, Ariyasu RG, Irvine JA. Observations with the tandem scanning confocal microscope in acute *Acanthamoeba* keratitis in the rabbit. *Invest Ophthalmol Vis Sci.* 1993;34(4):856.
94. Winchester K, Mathers WD, Sutphin JE, Daley TE. Diagnosis of *Acanthamoeba* keratitis in vivo with confocal microscopy. *Cornea.* 1995; 14:10–17.
95. Parmar DN, Awwad ST, Petroll WM, et al. Tandem scanning confocal corneal microscopy in the diagnosis of suspected *Acanthamoeba* keratitis. *Ophthalmology.* 2006;113:538–547.
96. Tu EY, Joslin CE, Sugar J, et al. The relative value of confocal microscopy and superficial corneal scrapings in the diagnosis of *Acanthamoeba* keratitis. *Cornea.* 2008;27:764–772.
97. Brasnu E, Bourcier T, Dupas B, et al. In vivo confocal microscopy in fungal keratitis. *Br J Ophthalmol.* 2007;91:588–591.
98. Florakis GJ, Moazami G, Schubert H, Koester CJ, Auran JD. Scanning slit confocal microscopy of fungal keratitis. *Arch Ophthalmol.* 1997;115: 1461–1463.
99. Winchester K, Mathers WD, Sutphin JE. Diagnosis of *Aspergillus* keratitis in vivo with confocal microscopy. *Cornea.* 1997;16:27–31.
100. Kaufman SC, Laird JA, Cooper R, Beuerman RW. Diagnosis of bacterial contact lens related keratitis with the white-light confocal microscope. *CLAO J.* 1996;22:274–277.
101. Shah GK, Pfister D, Probst LE, Ferrieri P, Holland E. Diagnosis of microsporidial keratitis by confocal microscopy and the chromatrope stain. *Am J Ophthalmol.* 1996;121:89–91.
102. Sagoo MS, Mehta JS, Hau S, et al. *Microsporidium* stromal keratitis: in vivo confocal findings. *Cornea.* 2007;26:870–873.
103. Linna T, Mikkila H, Karna A, et al. In vivo confocal microscopy: a new possibility to confirm the diagnosis of *Borrelia* keratitis? [letter]. *Cornea.* 1996;15:639–640.
104. Kanavi MR, Javadi M, Yazdani S, Mirdehghanm S. Sensitivity and specificity of confocal scan in the diagnosis of infectious keratitis. *Cornea.* 2007;26:782–786.
105. Masters BR, So PTC. *Biomedical nonlinear optical microscopy.* New York: Oxford University Press; 2008.
106. Mohler W, Millard AC, Campagnola PJ. Second harmonic generation imaging of endogenous structural proteins. *Methods.* 2003;29:97–109.
107. Hochheimer BF. Second harmonic light generation in the rabbit cornea. *Appl Opt.* 1982;1516–1518.
108. Stoller P, Kim BM, Rubenchik AM, Reiser KM, Da Silva LB. Polarization-dependent optical second-harmonic imaging of a rat-tail tendon. *J Biomed Opt.* 2002;7:205–214.
109. Yeh AT, Nassif N, Zoumi A, Tromberg BJ. Selective corneal imaging using combined second-harmonic generation and two-photon excited fluorescence. *Opt Lett.* 2002;27:2082–2084.
110. Morishige N, Petroll WM, Nishida T, Kenney MC, Jester JV. Noninvasive corneal stromal collagen imaging using two-photon-generated second-harmonic signals. *J Cataract Refract Surg.* 2006;32:1784–1791.
111. Morishige N, Wahlert AJ, Kenney MC, et al. Second-harmonic imaging microscopy of normal human and keratoconus cornea. *Invest Ophthalmol Vis Sci.* 2007;48:1087–1094.
112. Komai Y, Ushiki T. The three-dimensional organization of collagen fibrils in human cornea and sclera. *Invest Ophthalmol Vis Sci.* 1991;32: 2244–2258.
113. Bron AJ. The architectue of the normal corneal stroma. *Br J Ophthalmol.* 2001;85:379–381.
113a. Muller LJ, Pels E, Vrensen GFJM. The specific architecture of the anterior stroma accounts for maintenance of corneal curvature. *Br J Ophthalmol.* 2001;85:437–443.
114. Goldman JN, Benedek GB. The relationship between morphology and transparency in the nonswelling corneal stroma of the shark. *Invest Ophthalmol Vis Sci.* 1967;6:574–600.
115. Keller N, Pouliquen Y. Ultrastructural study of the posterior cornea of the dogfish *Scyliorhinus canicula*. *Cornea.* 1985;4:108–117.

Chapter 16

High-Resolution Ultrasound

Charles J. Pavlin, F. Stuart Foster

The use of high-frequency ultrasound as a diagnostic tool was pioneered at the University of Toronto.[1–7] We applied the term ultrasound biomicroscopy (UBM) to this method.[2] This method uses ultrasound in the frequency range of 25–100 MHz to produce cross-sectional subsurface images of the eye at an axial and lateral resolution ranging from 20 to 100 µm, depending on the choice of frequency. Ultrasound is increasingly attenuated at high frequencies, limiting penetration to the 4–15-mm range.

UBM has been used to examine a variety of pathologic conditions of the anterior segment and ocular adnexa including glaucoma,[8–10] anterior segment tumors,[11,12] intraocular lens-related problems,[13,14] trauma,[15] scleral disease,[16] and adnexal pathology. A non-specific imaging method, UBM can be used for any pathology that falls within its penetration limits. The superficial location of the cornea allows excellent penetration of this structure and the ability to image the majority of the underlying anterior segment. Ultrasound in the higher frequency ranges (60–80 MHz) can be used for corneal examination because of a lesser need for deep penetration and a greater need for high resolution. The cornea can usually be imaged by optical techniques, but in several conditions UBM can provide added information. Because sound is used instead of light, UBM provides a different type of information on internal structure and allows penetration of optical opacities. Accurate measurement of various corneal parameters can be performed.

This chapter reviews the use of UBM in corneal imaging and provides examples of clinical application.

Instrumentation

The instrumentation for UBM has been described extensively elsewhere.[1–3] A simplified block diagram of a UBM scanner is given in Figure 16.1. Signal processing in an ultrasound biomicroscope is identical to that in a conventional B-mode imaging system except that the operating frequency is approximately one order of magnitude higher. In this example, a 25–100-MHz transducer is moved linearly over the imaging field (typically 4–8 mm), collecting radiofrequency ultrasound data at each of 512 equally spaced lines (8 µm between lines for a 4-mm field of view). At each location, a 40–100-MHz ultrasound pulse is transmitted into the tissue, and the backscattered ultrasound is detected by the same transducer. The radiofrequency signal is received and amplified in proportion to the depth from which it originated, using time-gain compensation (TGC). By amplifying with the TGC signals from deeper structures more than superficial structures, it is possible to compensate for the attenuation of the ultrasound beam in the tissue. After the radiofrequency signal is processed nonlinearly to enhance the low-level signals, its envelope is 'detected' to produce the A-scan signal. This signal is then converted from analog to digital format and transferred to a special high-speed scan converter, stored, and displayed as B-scan data on a video monitor. The servo motion system and signal processing are controlled and synchronized by a computer. B-mode imaging is currently performed at 5–10 frames/second. This mode of ultrasonography has been shown to be safe for corneal use.[17] A variant of the instrumentation used is the arc scanner,[18] which moves the transducer in an arc that follows the curvature of the cornea. This instrument allows the transducer to remain relatively perpendicular to the corneal surface over the entire corneal curvature. This allows a complete corneal image in one pass and also allows construction of three-dimensional corneal maps by using multiple passes in various meridians.

Image resolution

Ultrasound biomicroscopy image quality is determined by the choice of transducer frequency and focusing characteristics. Because of the frequency-dependent nature of losses in tissue, the choice of these parameters is a trade-off between resolution and depth of penetration. For anterior segment imaging to a depth of approximately 5 mm, it is convenient to use frequencies in the 50 MHz range, where resolutions of the order of 35 µm in the axial direction and 60 µm in the lateral direction are achieved. In the cornea, however, where penetration of less than 1 mm is required, it is feasible to use higher frequencies and consequently achieve higher resolution. When possible, we try to scan the cornea using frequencies between 60 and 80 MHz.

An example of an echo (radiofrequency signal) obtained from a normal cornea made with a strongly focused 60-MHz transducer is shown in Figure 16.2. Note the three prominent specular echoes received from (1) the fluid couplant–epithelium interface, (2) the epithelium–Bowman's membrane interface, and (3) the endothelium/

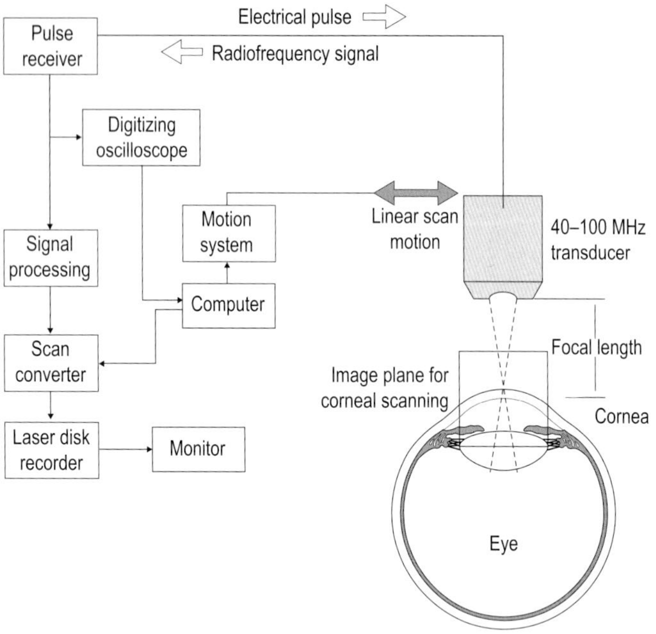

Fig. 16.1 Block diagram of ultrasound biomicroscopic system for corneal scanning.

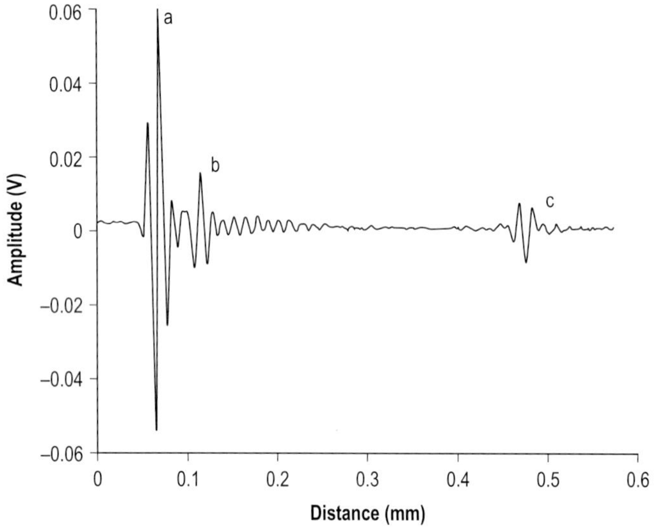

Fig. 16.2 Radiofrequency signal received from a normal cornea. Interfaces shown are (**a**) the fluid couplant–epithelium interface, (**b**) epithelium–Bowman's membrane interface, and (**c**) the endothelium–aqueous interface.

Descemet's membrane–aqueous interface. The axial resolution and separation between these surfaces is difficult to interpret from the radiofrequency signal. By envelope detecting the radiofrequency signal using a Hilbert transform to generate the A-scan, it is possible to make estimates of the axial resolution and layer thicknesses based on the equation:

$$z = ct/2$$

where z is the thickness of the layer or resolved structure, t is the time between echoes, and c is the speed of sound in the medium. There is currently debate over the speed of sound in corneal tissue in vivo. Measurements by Ye et al.,[19] made at 50 MHz, suggest that an appropriate value for c is 1575 m/s in this frequency range. Plots of radiofrequency and envelope amplitude versus z for the epithelial region of Figure 16.2 are given in Figure 16.3 A and B, respectively. The width of the signal from the fluid couplant–epithelium interface measured at one-half maximum is a measure of the axial resolution of the system. For this particular transducer, the axial resolution, z_{ax}, measures 20 μm. The epithelial thickness, z_{epi}, in this case measures 49.46 μm in thickness, with a precision (standard deviation) of 1.13 μm for eight independent measurements. Note that the precision for measuring the thickness of resolved parallel layers is many times greater than the axial resolution. Reinstein et al.[20] have shown that the precision of corneal epithelial measurements can be further improved using deconvolution approaches. The above techniques make measurement of corneal epithelial thickness practical.

The curvature of corneal surfaces can also be measured with reasonable accuracy. Various curve-fitting algorithms may be used. Three-dimensional reconstructions of corneal surfaces are also possible.

Examination Techniques

Ultrasound biomicroscopic examination with more commonly available commercial instrumentation is performed using an eye cup and a fluid couplant such as methylcellulose or saline. The viscosity of methylcellulose decreases fluid loss during examination. The moving transducer is inserted in the fluid couplant and scanning is begun (Fig. 16.4). The examination is performed with an unshielded moving transducer in close proximity to the eye, and care must be taken to prevent corneal contact. A membrane over the transducer can simplify the procedure at the expense of some sound attenuation, but this is more suitable for deep structures as the membrane echo interferes with corneal echoes.

The best image and most accurate measurement is achieved when the ultrasound beam is perpendicular to the structures being examined. Any obliquity will result in part of the backscattered signal not being detected. When the epithelial and endothelial reflections are maximized, one can be assured of reasonable perpendicularity to the cornea.

The Normal Cornea

The normal corneal surface on ultrasound biomicroscopy appears as a smooth, curved, specular reflection from the fluid couplant–epithelium interface (Fig. 16.5). Immediately below this interface is another smoothly reflective line that corresponds to the surface of Bowman's membrane. The distance between these two lines represents the epithelial thickness. The stroma has a uniform, low reflectivity. At the posterior aspect of the cornea is another highly reflective line that is the interface between Descemet's membrane/endothelium and the aqueous. Descemet's membrane and endothelium cannot usually be differentiated from each other.

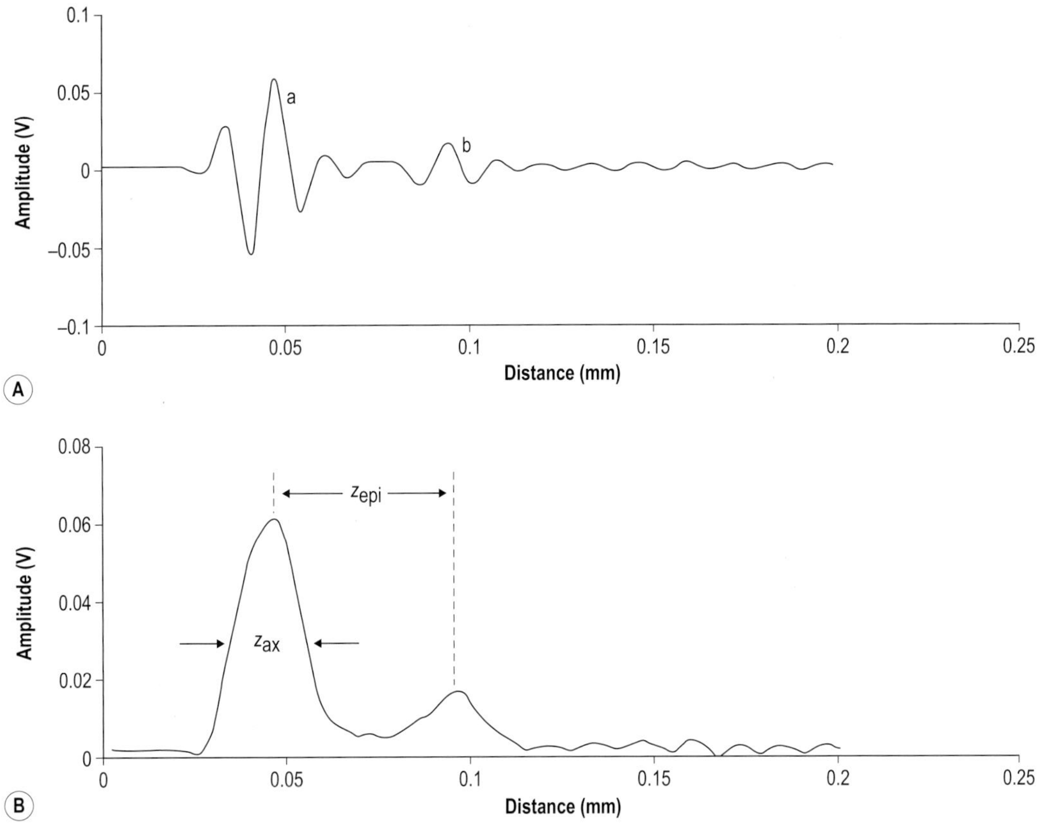

Fig. 16.3 Details of the radiofrequency signal (**A**) and envelope detected signal (**B**) received from the epithelial region of the cornea.

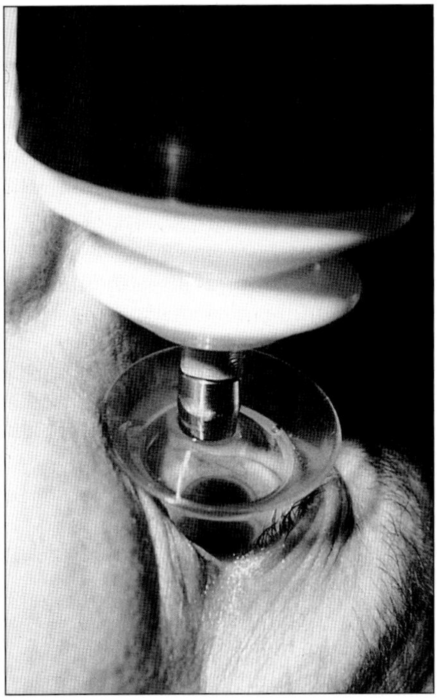

Fig. 16.4 An eye being examined using an eye cup with methylcellulose as a couplant. The moving transducer is placed in close proximity to the corneal surface. (From Pavlin CJ, Foster FS. *Ultrasound biomicroscopy of the eye.* New York: Springer Verlag; 1994. With kind permission of Springer Science & Business Media.)

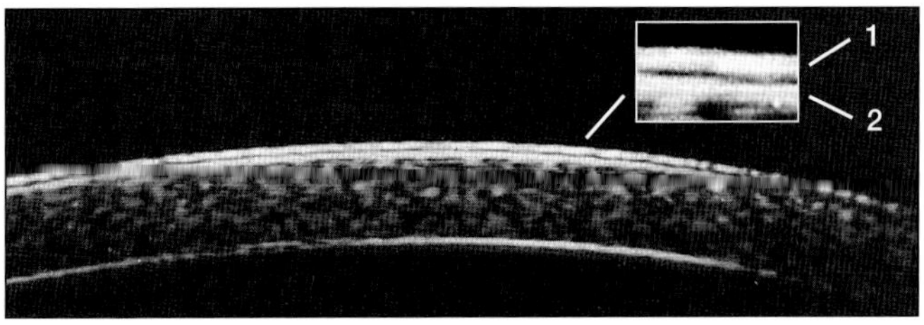

Fig. 16.5 Ultrasound biomicroscopic image of the normal cornea. The first smooth specular reflection (1) is from the epithelial surface. The second reflection (2) is from the interface between the epithelium and Bowman's membrane. The corneal stroma has a low regular internal reflectivity. The posterior aspect of the cornea is marked by a smooth, highly reflective line representing the endothelium/Descemet's membrane layer. (From Pavlin CJ et al. Ultrasound biomicroscopy in the assessment of anterior scleral disease. *Am J Ophthalmol.* 1993;116:628–635.

The corneoscleral junction is easily discerned (Fig. 16.6). The sclera is composed of irregular scleral collagen bundles which have a higher reflectivity than the regular corneal lamellae of the cornea. The junction shows a curved region of transition similar to that seen histologically. The scleral spur constitutes an easily identified landmark which is useful for measurements that require a fixed point of reference. The external limbus is about 1 mm medial to the scleral spur.

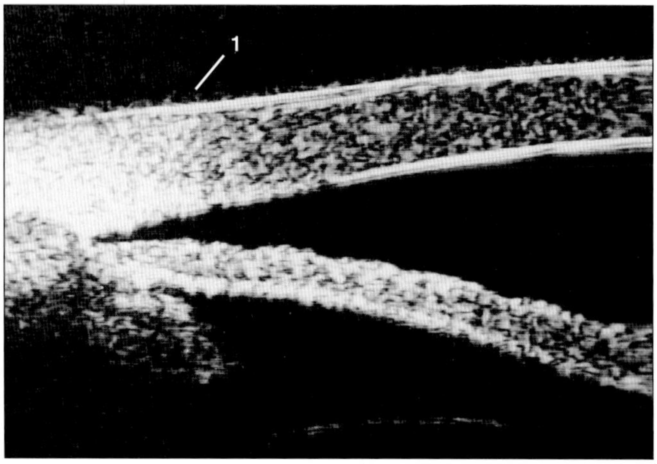

Fig. 16.6 Ultrasound biomicroscopic image through the corneoscleral junction (1). The sclera has a higher internal reflectivity than the cornea.

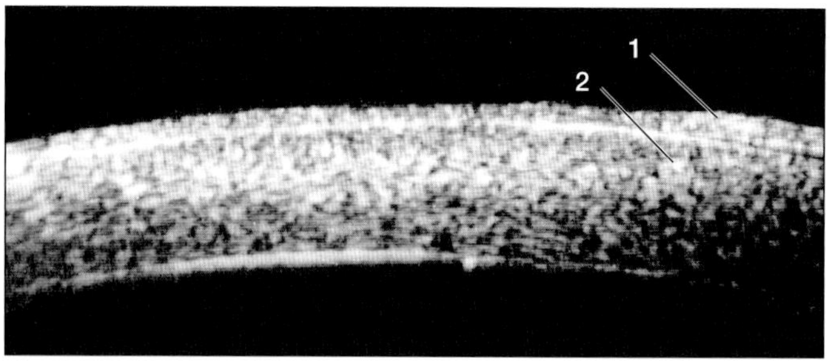

Fig. 16.7 Ultrasound biomicroscopic image of an edematous cornea. The epithelium (1) and corneal stroma (2) are both thickened. (From Pavlin CJ, Foster FS. *Ultrasound biomicroscopy of the eye.* New York: Springer Verlag; 1994. With kind permission of Springer Science & Business Media.)

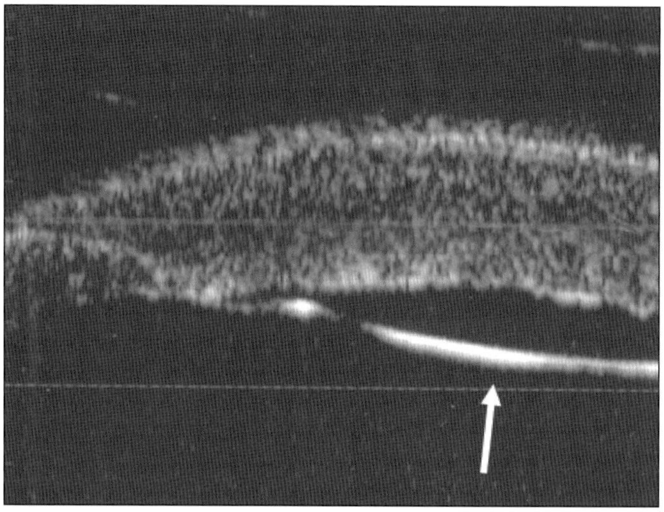

Fig. 16.8 Ultrasound biomicroscopic image in a case of Descemet's detachment following cataract surgery. The detached membrane is clearly imaged (*arrow*).

Corneal Disease

Corneal edema

Ultrasound biomicroscopy of an edematous cornea shows increased corneal thickness and higher reflectivity of the corneal stroma (Fig. 16.7). The epithelium is usually thickened, and the smooth, highly reflective surface line replaced by a more irregular, less reflective line. Epithelial bullae can be discerned as a slight separation of the corneal epithelium from the underlying Bowman's membrane. Ultrasound biomicroscopy provides an accurate quantitative method of measuring corneal thickness and of following progressive changes in corneal disease.

Descemet's membrane detachment

Descemet's membrane detachment can occur as a complication of intraocular surgery.[21] This generally results in corneal edema in the area involved and may result in the entire cornea becoming edematous, decreasing visibility. Ultrasound biomicroscopy images Descemet's membrane clearly (Fig. 16.8) when it is detached and can be used to map out the area of detachment prior to surgical repair.

Intraocular lens malposition

Intraocular lens displacement with corneal compromise can occur. This was more common with anterior chamber lenses, but can occur with posterior chamber lenses as well. The position of misplaced haptics is easily discernible by ultrasound biomicroscopy,

Imaging the anterior segment behind corneal opacities

Information on the status of the anterior segment behind corneal opacities can aid in planning pre-surgery.[4,22,23] Ultrasound biomicroscopy allows imaging of the entire anterior segment unless extensive corneal calcification produces shadowing. The depth of the anterior chamber and state of angle opening can be evaluated. The status of the lens and the presence of pupillary membranes can be determined. Descemet's membrane detachments and iris adhesions to the posterior corneal surface can be imaged (Fig. 16.9).

In pseudophakic corneal edema, the position of the intraocular lens can be determined. The position of haptics can be imaged and the amount of overlying tissue quantified if lens replacement is considered.[14]

Corneal dystrophies

Intrastromal corneal pathology can be imaged in corneal dystrophies, congenital abnormalities, and systemic diseases.[4,24–26] Abnormalities can be detected as either a disruption of the normal smooth corneal lamellae or a deposition of material of a different reflectivity from the normal cornea. Figure 16.10 shows a case of granular dystrophy.

Peripheral corneal degenerations

Peripheral corneal melting syndromes may be imaged by ultrasound biomicroscopy.[27] Areas of thinning can be

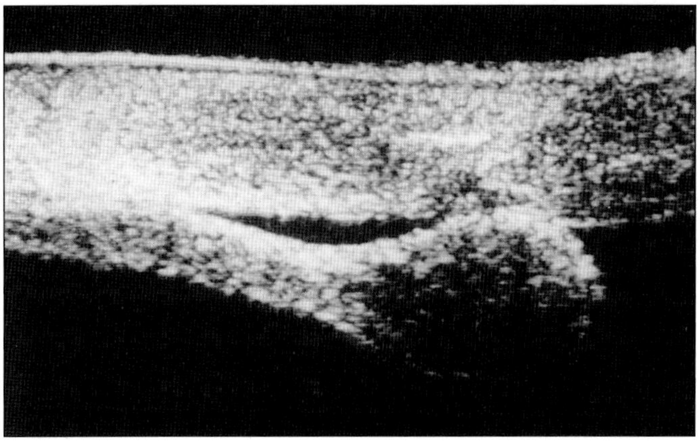

Fig. 16.9 Ultrasound biomicroscopic image through an opaque cornea shows a closed angle and adhesion of the iris tip to the inferior corneal surface. (From Pavlin CJ, Foster FS. *Ultrasound biomicroscopy of the eye.* New York: Springer Verlag; 1994. With kind permission of Springer Science & Business Media.)

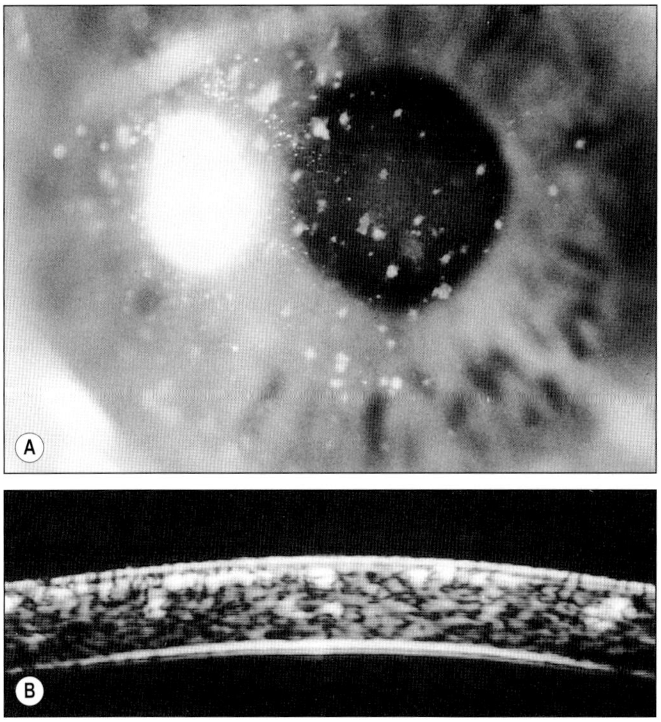

Fig. 16.10 Corneal dystrophies. (**A**) Clinical photograph of a patient with granular dystrophy. (**B**) Ultrasound biomicroscopic image shows the hyaline granules as highly reflective bodies in the superficial stroma, extending into Bowman's membrane. (From Pavlin CJ et al. Ultrasound biomicroscopic assessment of the cornea following excimer laser photokeratectomy. *J Cataract Refract Surg.* 1994;20:206–211.)

quantitatively assessed. Figure 16.11 shows the ultrasound biomicroscopic appearance of an area of peripheral corneal thinning in a case of Terrien's marginal degeneration. The affected area shows corneal thinning, with an hourglass shape indicating thinning from both sides.

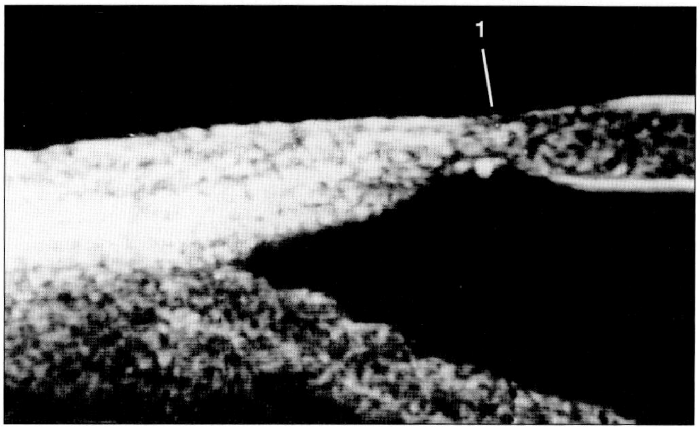

Fig. 16.11 Peripheral corneal thinning in a case of Terrien's marginal degeneration (1).

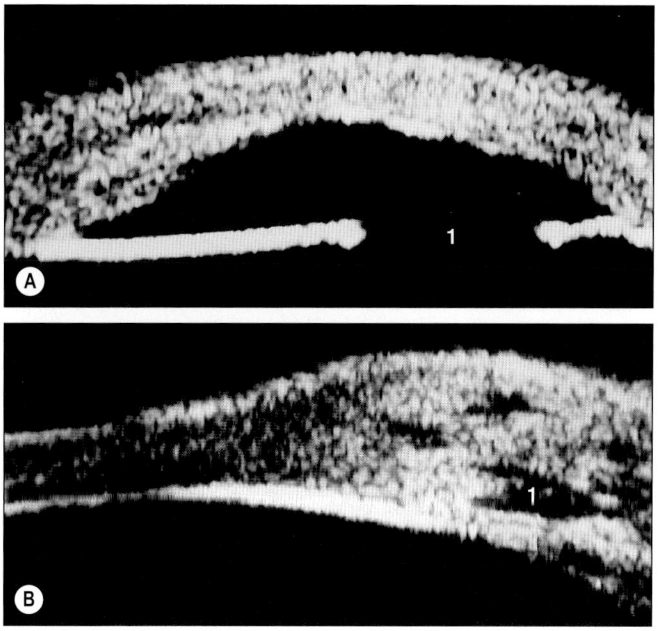

Fig. 16.12 Keratoconus. (**A**) Acute hydrops in a patient with keratoconus. Descemet's membrane and the endothelium have separated from the posterior corneal surface, showing a central defect (1). (**B**) Acute hydrops. The thickened cornea shows internal fluid spaces in the stroma (1). (Courtesy of N. Allemann, Sao Paulo.)

Keratoconus

Keratoconus can be assessed for variations in corneal curvature and corneal thickness.[28] Figure 16.12 shows the findings in a case of acute hydrops. The break in Descemet's membrane is clearly demonstrated.

Corneal Tumors

Various tumors can involve the cornea either directly or as part of involvement of adjacent structures. Congenital tumors such as dermoids can involve the cornea.[29–31] It

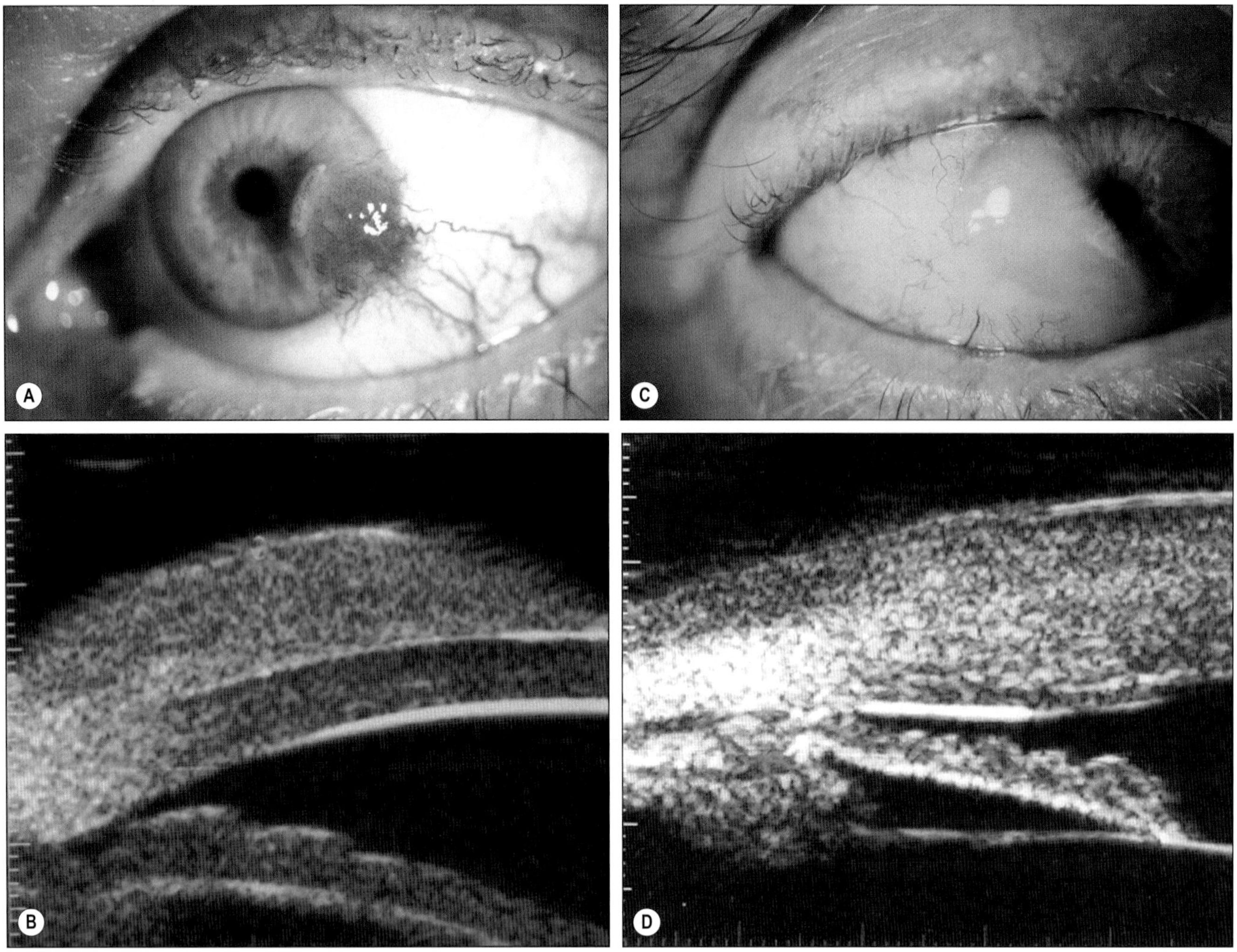

Fig. 16.13 Corneal tumors. (**A**) Clinical photograph of melanoma involving the cornea. (**B**) Ultrasound biomicroscopy shows the lesion is superficial to Bowman's membrane with normal-thickness underlying cornea. (**C**) Clinical photograph of a mucoepidermoid carcinoma involving the cornea. (**D**) Ultrasound biomicroscopy shows full-thickness corneal involvement.

is frequently uncertain as to whether these tumors are superficial, or whether they invade the cornea. This differentiation can be important in planning therapy. Ultrasound biomicroscopy can image these lesions at depth, and determine whether they are superficial to Bowman's membrane or involve the corneal stroma. In the illustrated cases, the first case was a melanoma (Fig. 16.13A). Ultrasound biomicroscopy indicated that the lesion was superficial to Bowman's membrane (Fig. 16.13B), and surgery was performed with removal of the tumor, leaving the cornea intact. The second case was diagnosed as a mucoepidermoid carcinoma (Fig. 16.13C). Ultrasound biomicroscopy revealed full-thickness corneal involvement (Fig. 16.13D). Local removal was not possible. This case was treated by plaque radiotherapy.

Corneal Surgery

Keratoplasty

Penetrating

The junction between the host cornea and the graft is imaged clearly by ultrasound biomicroscopy. Frequently, the host cornea has a higher internal reflectivity, depending on the initial pathology. The graft itself has a low internal stromal reflectivity if it is clear. Graft failure will result in the signs of corneal edema, as outlined previously. Graft thickness can be measured.

The image of the junction varies, depending on the particular features of the graft and the postoperative interval.

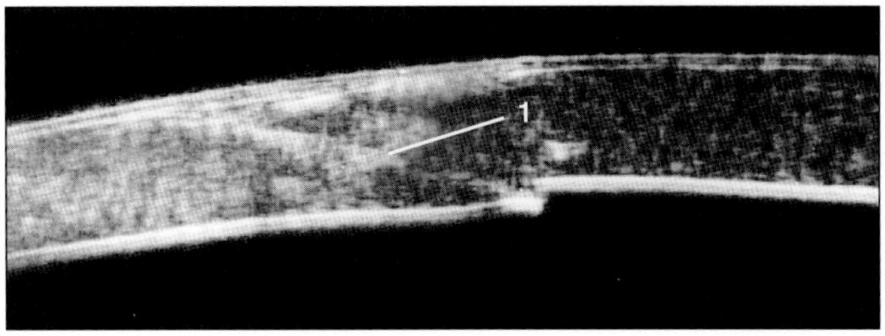

Fig. 16.14 Ultrasound biomicroscopic image of the margin of a penetrating corneal graft. The junction (1) is slanted. Epithelial and endothelial surfaces are reasonably well apposed.

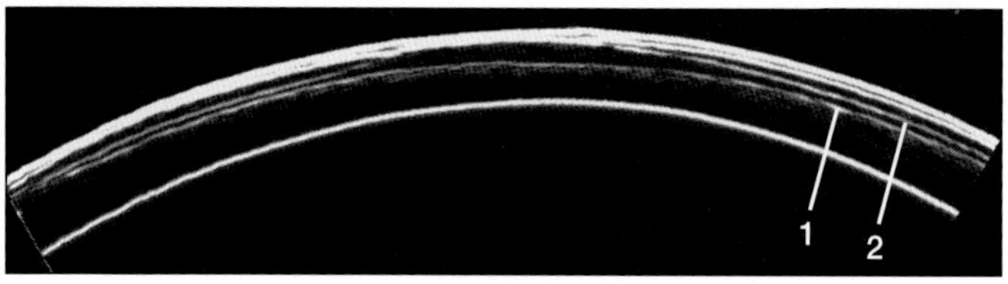

Fig. 16.16 Arc scan image of a cornea that has undergone LASIK with a buttonholed flap. Two separate flaps were created in this patient at different times. The first incision line is intact (1). The second more superficial incision line (2) extends to Bowman's membrane at the site where the flap was buttonholed. (Courtesy of D. Reinstein, New York.)

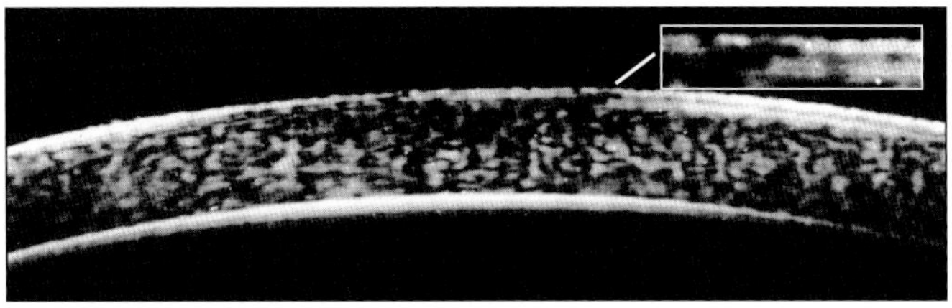

Fig. 16.15 Ultrasound biomicroscopic image of the junction between the treated and untreated region (*inset*) in a case of excimer laser photokeratoplasty. The double superficial echoes of the untreated region on the right give way to the single echo in the treated region where Bowman's membrane is missing. (From Pavlin CJ et al. Ultrasound biomicroscopic assessment of the cornea following excimer laser photokeratectomy. *J Cataract Refract Surg.* 1994;20:206–211.)

In the early postoperative period, a line indicating the junction can be discerned (Fig. 16.14). As healing takes place, the stromal junction becomes less clearly delineated. Discrepancy in thickness between the graft and host is frequently found, usually with a thicker host side, but occasionally, in a condition such as keratoconus, a thicker graft side can be noted. Irregularities of the inner wound can be discerned, with a step being present or an irregularity in Descemet's membrane being noted. Other features such as iris adhesions to the wound can be imaged.

Lamellar

The junction between the lamellar graft and the host graft bed can be imaged. Lamellar thickness and host cornea thickness can be measured independently. Irregularities such as elevated margins or epithelial ingrowth can be imaged.

Refractive surgery

Excimer laser keratectomy

Photorefractive and phototherapeutic keratectomy involve removing a thin layer of superficial cornea. The region of excimer laser photokeratectomy is imaged[32–34] as a loss of the double line found superficially in normal corneas (Fig. 16.15). The interface between the stroma and the regenerated epithelium is generally less reflective than the interface between the epithelium and Bowman's membrane. The junction between treated and untreated cornea can be detected by the transition from the double reflection to a single reflection. The fine superficial stromal haze is usually below the resolution level of ultrasound biomicroscopy. More extensive scarring, however, can be detected as more highly reflective regions in the superficial stroma. Ultrasound biomicroscopy can provide some indication of the depth of corneal pathology before considering phototherapeutic keratectomy.

Laser-associated in situ keratomileusis

In laser-associated in situ keratomileusis (LASIK) the keratome incision line can be imaged, allowing one to assess depth of the incision and irregularities such as epithelial ingrowth. Figure 16.16 shows an example of the ability to define the incision interface. This patient had two separate keratome flaps performed. The inferior incision line is intact, but the more superficial flap was buttonholed. Ultrasound biomicroscopy clearly shows the edges of the superficial flap extending to Bowman's membrane centrally. Use of the arc scanner has also allowed construction of three-dimensional maps of various layers.[35] Epithelial depth can be mapped using color coding (Fig. 16.17). This technique can shed light on the structural changes that are produced by this type of surgery, and follow variations such as epithelial and stromal thickness over time.

Summary

High-frequency ultrasound has provided a method of imaging ocular structural detail previously below the resolution of conventional ultrasound. The cornea is a good candidate for imaging with this technique because of its superficial location, which allows use of higher-frequency transducers with the highest possible resolution. Light-based techniques such as anterior segment optical coherence tomography can also produce high-resolution images of the cornea.[36] High-frequency ultrasound has superior penetration through opaque tissue and is preferable for determining the state of the underlying anterior segment.[37]

Acknowledgments

This chapter is supported in part by the National Cancer Institute of Canada.

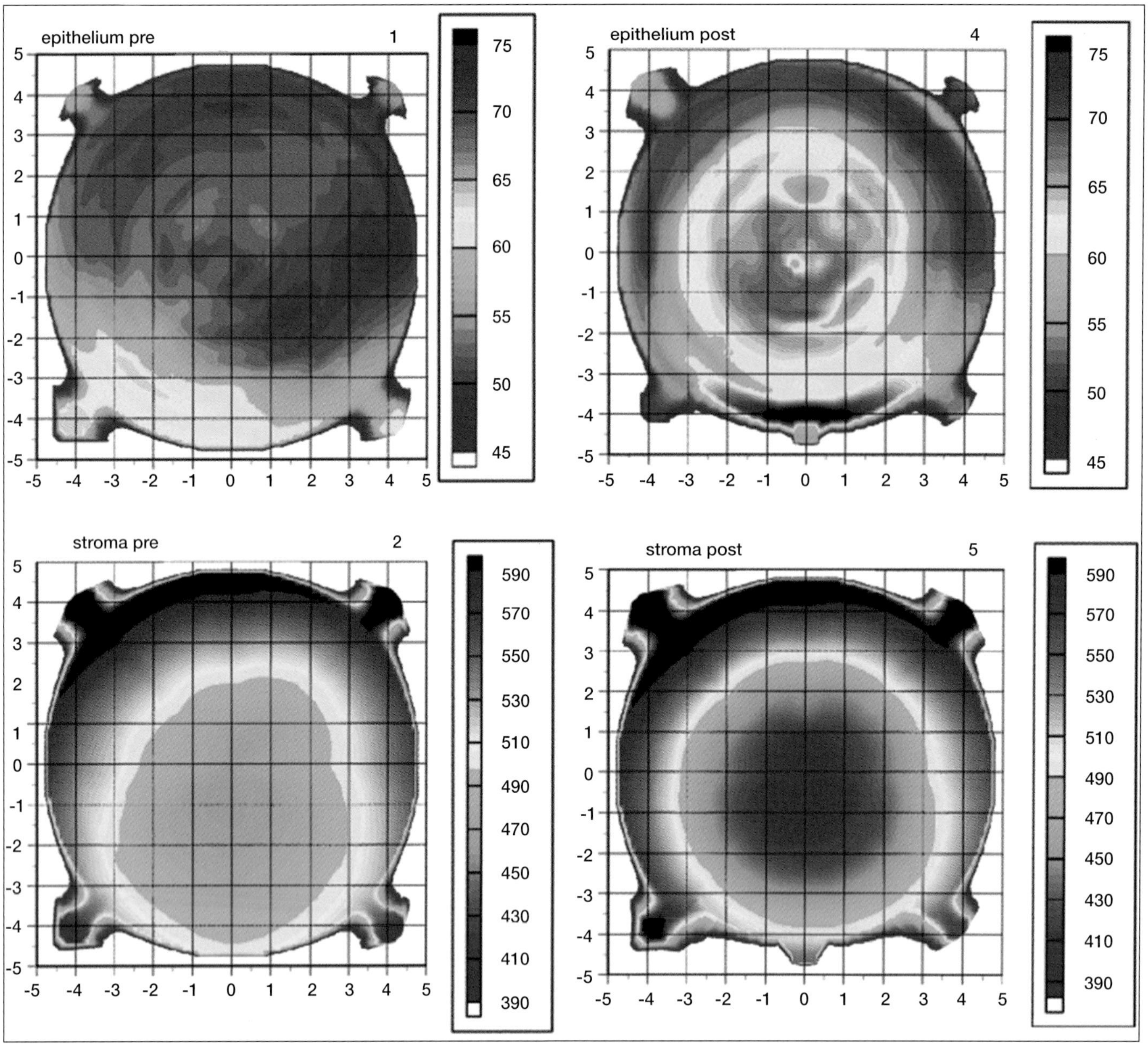

Fig. 16.17 Three-dimensional thickness maps of the corneal epithelium and stroma pre- and post-LASIK. The top two images show increased thickness and irregularity of the central epithelium. The bottom two images show decreased thickness of the central stroma. (Reproduced from Reinstein DZ et al. Arc-scanning very high-frequency digital ultrasound for 3D pachymetric mapping of the corneal epithelium and stroma in laser in situ keratomileusis *J Refract Surg.* 2000;16:414–430, by kind permission of Slack Inc.)

References

1. Pavlin CJ, Sherar MD, Foster FS. Subsurface ultrasound microscopic imaging of the intact eye. *Ophthalmology.* 1990;97:244–250.
2. Pavlin CJ, Sherar MD, Harasiewicz K, et al. Clinical use of ultrasound biomicroscopy. *Ophthalmology.* 1991;98:287–295.
3. Foster FS, Pavlin CJ, Lockwood GR, et al. Principles and applications of ultrasound backscatter microscopy. *Ultrasonics, Ferroelectrics and Frequency Control.* 1993;40:608–617.
4. Pavlin CJ, Foster FS. *Ultrasound biomicroscopy of the eye.* New York: Springer Verlag; 1994.
5. Pavlin CJ, Foster FS. Ultrasound biomicroscopy. High-frequency ultrasound imaging of the eye at microscopic resolution. *Radiol Clin North Am.* 1998;36:1047–1058.
6. Foster FS, Pavlin CJ, Harasiewicz KA, et al. Advances in ultrasound biomicroscopy. *Ultrasound Med Biol.* 2000;26(1):1–27.
7. Cavanagh HD, El-Agha MS, Petroll WM, et al. Specular microscopy, confocal microscopy, and ultrasound biomicroscopy: diagnostic tools of the past quarter century. *Cornea.* 2000;19:712–722.
8. Pavlin CJ, Harasiewicz K, Foster FS. Ultrasound biomicroscopy of anterior segment structures in normal and glaucomatous eyes. *Am J Ophthalmol.* 1992;113:381–389.
9. Pavlin CJ, Ritch R, Foster FS. Ultrasound biomicroscopy in plateau iris syndrome. *Am J Ophthalmol.* 1992;113:390–395.
10. Mandell MA, Pavlin CJ, Weisbrod DJ, Simpson ER. Anterior chamber depth in plateau iris syndrome and pupillary block as measured by ultrasound biomicroscopy. *Am J Ophthalmol.* 2003;136(5):900–903.
11. Pavlin CJ, McWhae J, McGowan H, et al. Ultrasound biomicroscopy of anterior segment ocular tumors. *Ophthalmology.* 1992;99:1220–1228.

12. Weisbrod DJ, Pavlin CJ, Emara K, et al. Small ciliary body tumors: ultrasound biomicroscopic assessment and follow-up of 42 patients. *Am J Ophthalmol.* 2006;141(4):622–628.
13. Pavlin CJ, Rootman D, Arshinoff S, et al. Determination of haptic position of transsclerally-fixated posterior chamber intraocular lenses by ultrasound biomicrocopy. *J Cataract Refract Surg.* 1993;19:573–577.
14. Rutnin S, Pavlin CJ, Slomovic A, et al. Using ultrasound biomicroscopy to determine the ease of removal of lens haptics prior to penetrating keratoplasty – IOL exchange surgery. *J Cataract Refract Surg.* 1997;23: 239–243.
15. Gentile RC, Pavlin CJ, Liebmann JM, et al. Diagnoses of traumatic cyclodialysis by ultrasound biomicroscopy. *Ophthalmic Surg Lasers.* 1996;27:97–105.
16. Pavlin CJ, Easterbrook M, Hurwitz JJ, et al. Ultrasound biomicroscopy in the assessment of anterior scleral disease. *Am J Ophthalmol.* 1993; 116:628–635.
17. Silverman RH, Lizzi FL, Ursea BG, et al. Safety levels for exposure of cornea and lens to very high-frequency ultrasound. *Ultrasound Med.* 2001;20:979–986.
18. Reinstein DZ, Silverman RH, Raevsky T, et al. Arc-scanning very high-frequency digital ultrasound for 3D pachymetric mapping of the corneal epithelium and stroma in laser in situ keratomileusis. *J Refract Surg.* 2000;16:414–430.
19. Ye SG, Harasiewicz KA, Pavlin CJ, et al. Ultrasound characterization of ocular tissue in the frequency range from 50 MHz to 100 MHz. *Ultrasonics, Ferroelectronics, and Frequency Control.* 1995;42:8–14.
20. Reinstein DZ, Silverman RH, Rondeau MJ, et al. Epithelial and corneal thickness measurements by high-frequency ultrasound digital signal processing. *Ophthalmology.* 1994;101:140–146.
21. Morinelli EN, Najac RD, Speaker MG, et al. Repair of Descemet's membrane detachment with the assistance of intraoperative ultrasound biomicroscopy. *Am J Ophthalmol.* 1996;121(6):718–720.
22. Milner MS, Liebmann JM, Tello C, et al. High resolution ultrasound biomicroscopy of the anterior segment in patients with dense corneal scars. *Ophthalmic Surg.* 1994;25:284–287.
23. Dada T, Aggarwal A, Vanathi M, et al. Ultrasound biomicroscopy in opaque grafts with post-penetrating keratoplasty glaucoma. *Cornea.* 2008;27(4):402–405.
24. Castelo Branco B, Chalita MR, Casanova FH, et al. Posterior amorphous corneal dystrophy: ultrasound biomicroscopy findings in two cases. *Cornea.* 2002;21:220–222.
25. Mungan N, Nischal KK, Heon E, et al. Ultrasound biomicroscopy of the eye in cystinosis. *Arch Ophthalmol.* 2000;118:1329–1333.
26. Kim T, Cohen EJ, Schnall BM, et al. Ultrasound biomicroscopy and histopathology of sclerocornea. *Cornea.* 1998;17:443–445.
27. Berrocal AM, Chen PC, Soukiasian SH. Ultrasound biomicroscopy of corneal hydrops in Terrien's marginal degeneration. *Ophthalmic Surg Lasers.* 2002;33:228–230.
28. Avitabile T, Marano F, Castiglione F, et al. Keratoconus staging with ultrasound biomicroscopy. *Ophthalmologica.* 1982;212(Suppl 1):10–12.
29. Haddad AM, Greenfield DS, Stegman Z, et al. Peter's anomaly: diagnosis by ultrasound biomicroscopy. *Ophthalmic Surg Lasers.* 1997;28:311–312.
30. Grant CA, Azar D. Ultrasound biomicroscopy in the diagnosis and management of limbal dermoid. *Am J Ophthalmol.* 1999;128:365–367.
31. Hoops JP, Ludwig K, Boergen KP, et al. Preoperative evaluation of limbal dermoids using high-resolution biomicroscopy. *Graefes Arch Clin Exp Ophthalmol.* 2001;239:459–461.
32. Pavlin CJ, Harasiewicz K, Foster FS. Use of ultrasound biomicroscopy in excimer laser photokeratectomy. *J Cataract Refract Surg.* 1994;20(Suppl): 206–211.
33. Reinstein DZ, Silverman RH, Trokel SL, et al. High frequency ultrasound digital signal processing for biometry of the cornea in planning phototherapeutic keratectomy (letter). *Arch Ophthalmol.* 1993;111:430–431.
34. Allemann N, Chamon W, Silverman RH, et al. High frequency ultrasound quantitative analysis of corneal scarring following excimer laser keratectomy. *Arch Ophthalmol.* 1993;111:968–973.
35. Reinstein DZ, Silverman RH, Sutton HF, et al. Very high-frequency ultrasound corneal analysis identifies anatomic correlates of optical complications of lamellar refractive surgery: anatomic diagnosis in lamellar surgery. *Ophthalmology.* 1999;106:474–482.
36. Lim LS, Aung HT, Aung T, Tan DT. Corneal imaging with anterior segment optical coherence tomography for lamellar keratoplasty procedures. *Am J Ophthalmol.* 2008;145(1):81–90.
37. Pavlin CJ, Vasquez L, Lee R, Simpson ER, Ahmed I. Anterior segment OCT and ultrasound biomicroscopy in the imaging of anterior segment tumors. *Am J Ophthalmol.* 2009;(2):214–219.

Chapter 17

Anterior Segment Optical Coherence Tomography

Martin Heur, Yan Li, David Huang

Introduction

Optical coherence tomography (OCT) was initially developed by Fujimoto, Huang, and colleagues as a way to obtain near-histological resolution images of tissue without biopsy.[1] In OCT, a beam of light, typically in the infrared wavelength range, is scanned across a sample such as the eye. The optical delay of the reflected light is determined by interferometry to generate a ranging measurement called the axial scan (A-scan). The axial resolution of the A-scan depends on the coherence length of the light used, and is typically several microns (μm). Transverse scanning of the beam yields information to build cross-sectional or three-dimensional images. The imaging principle of OCT is similar to ultrasound and radar, but the spatial resolution of OCT is much finer due to light's shorter wavelength. Izatt and colleagues reported the first application of OCT in imaging of the cornea and anterior segment in 1994.[2] Since then, anterior segment OCT has undergone several iterations of refinement.

Optical coherence tomography relies on interferometry to measure distance. In the interferometer, a broad-spectrum light, typically from an infrared superluminescent diode (SLD), is split into sample and reference beams through a beam splitter. The reflections from the sample and reference arms are recombined at the beam splitter and their interference pattern is detected by a photodetector and converted into a digital signal. A computer processes the digital data to generate a cross-sectional image. The original OCT technology is now classified as time-domain OCT (TD-OCT), in which the reference mirror is moved through a range of delay, and the resulting inference patterns between the sample and reference beams are processed into an axial image. The scanning speed in TD-OCT is limited by having to physically cycle the reference mirror through the delay range. In order to speed up image acquisition, a new technology called Fourier-domain OCT (FD-OCT) has been developed. In FD-OCT, the reference mirror is stationary and the A-scan is generated by Fourier transformation of spectral interference patterns between the sample and reference reflections. Advantages of FD-OCT include improvements in scanning speed and signal-to-noise ratio that are achieved through elimination of reference mirror movement and simultaneous detection of reflections from all layers of the target. The terms spectral OCT, spectral-domain OCT (SD-OCT), and frequency-domain OCT (FD-OCT) are synonymous with FD-OCT. Swept-source OCT (SS-OCT), also called optical frequency domain imaging (OFDI), is a subtype of FD-OCT. Table 17.1 lists the commercially available TD-OCT platforms for anterior segment imaging. An important consideration is the wavelength; longer wavelength light penetrates deeper into the sclera and iris, but has coarser resolution, and the best operating wavelength will depend on the intended application.

Keratoconus Screening

Keratoconus is an ectatic disorder of the cornea characterized by progressive stromal thinning and steepening of the cornea, leading to a loss of visual acuity. Moderate to advanced keratoconus is easily recognizable by several distinctive clinical features, but the diagnosis of forme fruste keratoconus can be challenging. Keratoconus evaluations, done through corneal topography-based algorithms, can sometimes be ambiguous. When a patient presents with normal vision and shows only a slight inferior steepening on topography, the clinician is left to wonder whether subclinical keratoconus is present. In such situations, OCT-generated pachymetry maps (Fig. 17.1) could help confirm the diagnosis by detecting the eccentric focal thinning characteristic of keratoconus. Studies of eyes of keratoconus and unaffected patients showed that presence of the following pachymetric parameters in the central 5-mm area of an unoperated cornea should raise concerns for keratoconus:

1. The difference in the minimum thickness and median thickness in the central 5-mm area is less than –63 μm (minimum – median < –63 μm).
2. The difference in average thickness of the inferior (I) octant and the superior (S) octant is less than –31 μm (I – S < –31 μm).
3. The difference in average thickness of the inferotemporal (IT) octant and the superonasal (SN) octant is less than –48 μm (IT – SN < –48 μm).
4. Minimum corneal thickness is less than 492 μm.
5. The thinnest region of the cornea is outside of the central 2-mm area.

The above parameters evaluate for the presence of asymmetry in corneal thickness and thinning. One abnormal param-

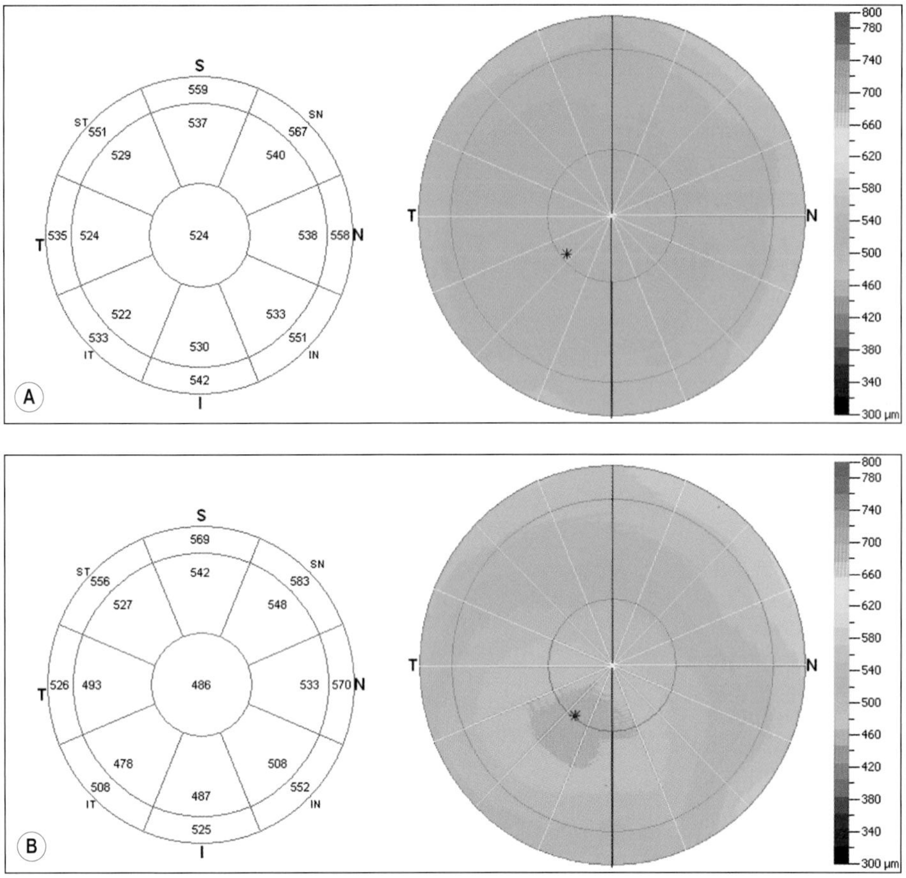

Fig. 17.1 RTVue-CAM OCT pachymetry maps. (**A**) Normal cornea. (**B**) Keratoconic cornea. Three pachymetry indices (I–S = –55µm, IT–SN = –69 µm, minimum = 462 µm) met diagnostic criteria for keratoconus.

Table 17.1 Commercially available TD-OCT platforms

Name	Manufacturer	Type	Wavelength	Resolution	Scan speed
Visante	Carl Zeiss Meditec, Inc.	TD-OCT	1310 nm	18 µm	2 kHz
Heidelberg SL-OCT	Heidelberg Engineering	TD-OCT	1310 nm	25 µm	0.2 kHz
RTVue	Optovue Inc.	FD-OCT	830 nm	5 µm	26 kHz
Bioptigen SD-OCT	Bioptigen, Inc.	FD-OCT	840 nm	3–5 µm	17 kHz
Casia SS-1000	Tomey USA	FD-OCT	1310 nm	10 µm	30 kHz

eter is suggestive while two or more abnormal parameters are diagnostic of keratoconus.[3]

Refractive Surgery Evaluation

LASIK flap evaluation

Optical coherence tomography allows for the visualization of the LASIK flap in the immediate postoperative period. Li and colleagues have shown that LASIK flaps were detectable in all patients at 1 day and 1 week after surgery.[4] Imaging of the flap in the immediate postoperative period allows for the evaluation of microkeratome and femtosecond laser performance (Fig. 17.2A). In addition to flap thickness evaluation, the flap morphology can also be analyzed. OCT analysis has shown that flaps created with the IntraLase femtosecond laser are more uniform in thickness, whereas those created with a microkeratome are thinner in the center.[5]

Refractive enhancement

Corneal ectasia occurring after laser vision correction is a well-documented complication, and an important risk factor is residual stromal bed thickness less than 250 µm.[6] The

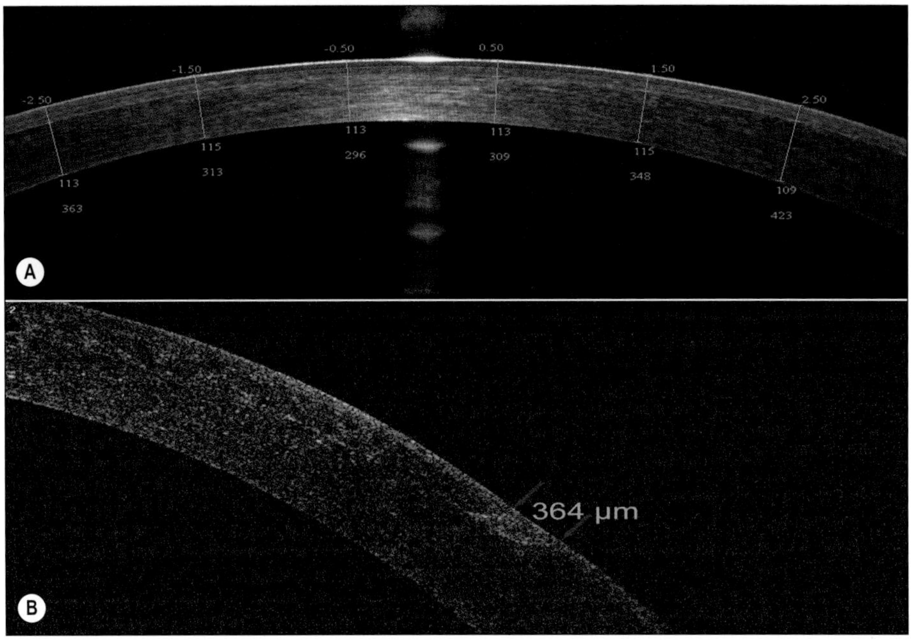

Fig. 17.2 (**A**) RTVue-CAM OCT image 1 week after LASIK with flap creation by a femtosecond laser (IntraLase®). The image's quality was enhanced by registering and averaging 16 consecutively acquired frames. The flap thickness was measured with computer calipers to be 109–115 µm. (**B**) RTVue-CAM OCT taken 2 weeks after LASIK. A gap filled with epithelium was visualized between the temporal edge of the flap and the stromal bed edge. The width of the gap was measured with computer calipers.

capability to analyze flaps several years after LASIK using OCT becomes useful in refractive enhancement evaluations. Accurate measurement of the residual stromal bed thickness can help determine whether a LASIK enhancement can be safely performed. An attractive feature of OCT is that, unlike an ultrasound pachymeter, it can measure the residual stromal bed thickness without the need for a flap lift.

LASIK complications

Optical coherence tomography can be valuable in the evaluation of LASIK cases with suboptimal outcomes. In a patient with decreased vision following LASIK, measuring the residual stromal bed thickness can aid in the evaluation for post-LASIK ectasia. The flap edge is usually well defined in OCT images, making it possible to visualize the position of the flap relative to the flap bed. In a case of decreased vision in the early post-LASIK period, flap striae were visualized at the slit lamp examination, but a gap between the flap and bed edges could not be appreciated. Optical coherence tomography was used to visualize the location of the gap and the direction of the flap shift (Fig. 17.2B). This was helpful for planning the flap lift and repositioning procedure.

Corneal Power Calculation

Fourier-domain optical coherence tomography is fast enough to calculate the central corneal power by averaging the measured instantaneous curvature of the central region. In post-refractive surgery patients, the usual relationship between anterior and posterior corneal curvatures no longer holds. Conventional keratometry can grossly overestimate the central corneal power after myopic LASIK and underestimate the central corneal power after hyperopic LASIK. A method that measures both anterior and posterior corneal curvatures is useful in calculating the true central corneal power in postrefractive surgery patients who are considering cataract surgery.

Corneal Opacities

Ultrasound has traditionally been used to provide imaging of and through an opacified cornea. In addition to higher resolution, OCT offers an additional advantage of being a non-contact modality. OCT can provide pachymetry mapping in opacified corneas more accurately than slit scanning devices.[7] OCT can also measure the depth of corneal opacity, thereby aiding in the preoperative planning (Fig. 17.3). Using the depth data, the surgeon can opt for an ablative approach such as phototherapeutic keratectomy if the superficial opacity can be removed while maintaining a residual stromal bed thickness of greater than 250 µm, or opt for anterior lamellar keratoplasty if replacement tissue is needed. If the opacity is too deep for ablation or anterior lamellar keratoplasty, then a penetrating keratoplasty can be considered. OCT can also be used to image anterior chamber structures such as the angle, iris and lens, iris and drainage tube through an opaque cornea, which can be helpful in assessing the mechanism of postoperative intraocular pressure elevation.[8]

Cornea Transplant

Posterior lamellar keratoplasty

Since the inception of modern posterior lamellar keratoplasty in the late 1990s by Melles, the technique has undergone several cycles of refinement to Descemet's stripping automated endothelial keratoplasty (DSAEK).[9] The primary advantages of DSAEK over penetrating keratoplasty (PK) are a smaller and more secure wound, lower postoperative

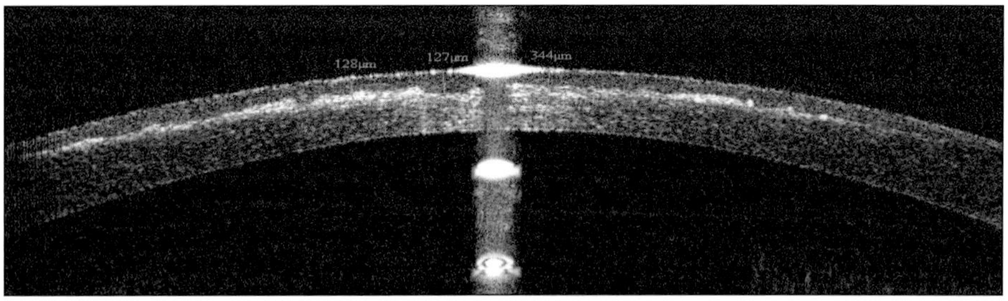

Fig. 17.3 RTVue-CAM OCT image of a cornea with severe haze and scarring after photorefractive keratectomy enhancement, limiting best spectacle-corrected visual acuity (BSCVA) to 20/50. The central corneal thickness was determined to be 344 μm while depth of the opacity was determined to be 127 μm, indicating that there was not sufficient stromal bed thickness for a phototherapeutic keratectomy to remove the haze. The BSCVA was improved to 20/20–3 with topical corticosteroid treatment.

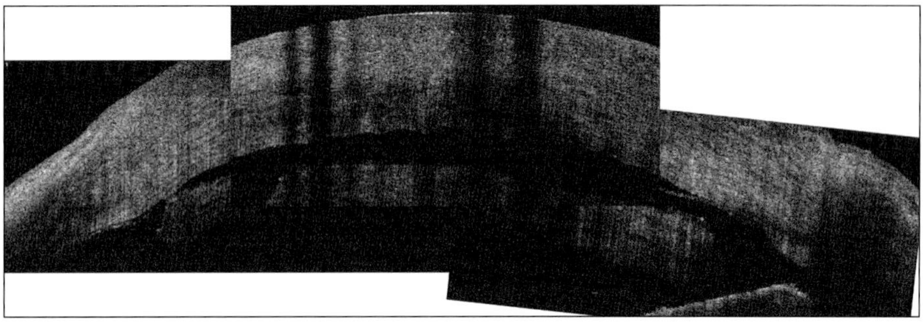

Fig. 17.4 Montage of RTVue-CAM OCT sections showing detachment of the endothelial graft 1 week following Descemet's stripping automated endothelial keratoplasty.

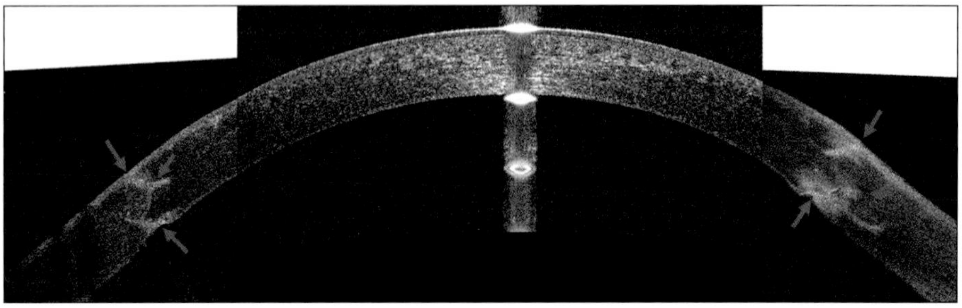

Fig. 17.5 Montage of RTVue-CAM OCT sections taken 4 months after IntraLase®-enabled penetrating keratoplasty. The sutures had been removed. The zigzag wound junctions (*red arrows*) were well apposed.

astigmatism, and faster visual rehabilitation.[10] Postoperative OCT scans can be used to monitor for lenticule detachment in patients with persistent postoperative corneal edema (Fig. 17.4).

Femtosecond-enabled keratoplasty

Penetrating keratoplasty (PK) is evolving due to the ability to make complex-shaped incisions using a femtosecond laser such as the IntraLase® (AMO, Inc., Santa Ana, CA). A concern of traditional PK performed using trephine blades is the slow wound healing and the weak host–donor junction. Shaped incision designs such as the zigzag, top hat, and mushroom configurations created using the femtosecond laser result in greater resistance to wound leakage when compared to traditional PK.[11] The wound may be stronger and heal faster due to the interlocking host–donor junction and greater wound contact area. Proper apposition of the interlocking wound can be visualized with OCT (Fig. 17.5). OCT can also be very helpful in confirming proper matching of laser cuts and developing the proper suturing technique to obtain good wound apposition, especially in the early phases of adopting a new wound architecture.

Refractive Implants

Corneal implants

Keratophakia involves implanting a lens within the corneal stroma, under a lamellar flap created using a microkeratome or femtosecond laser. Use of earlier synthetic material

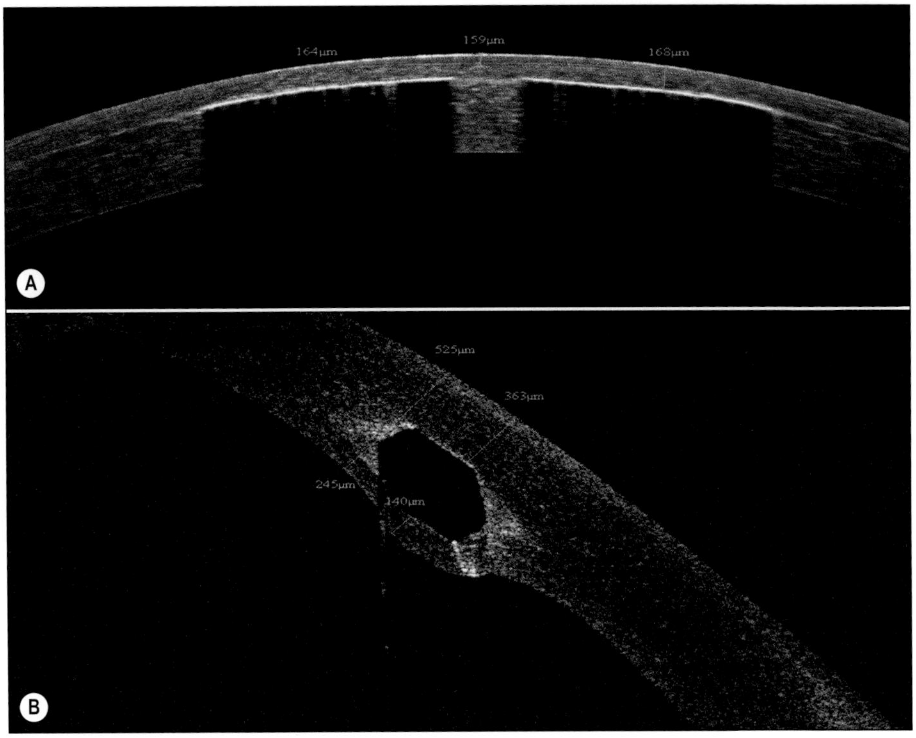

Fig. 17.6 (**A**) RTVue-CAM OCT horizontal section of an ACI 7000 corneal implant in a cornea. The device appears as a highly reflective band with shadowing of the underlying corneal stroma. Reprinted from Huang D (Ed). RTVue Fourier-Domain Optical Coherence Tomography Primer Series: Cornea and Anterior Segment. Optovue Inc. Fremont, CA, 2008, with permission from Optovue (**B**) RTVue-CAM OCT radial section showing an Intacs segment implanted in corneal stroma. The fractional depth of the implant at the inner edge was 68%, 525/(525+245), close to the target depth of 70%.

resulted in tissue necrosis and extrusion secondary to impermeability of the implanted material to nutrients within the corneal stroma.[12] A newer generation of synthetic material under development, such as silicone hydrogel, promises increased safety and refractive predictability. Keratophakic implants are optically clear on OCT and appear as dark spaces between the lamellar flap and stromal bed. OCT can be used to determine the position and depth of the implant within the cornea without the need of a flap lift.

The ACI 7000 (AcuFocus Inc., Irvine, CA and Bausch & Lomb, Rochester, NY) corneal implant is a ring made of an opaque biocompatible polymer that increases the depth of focus through the pinhole effect. It has shown promising results in an initial trial to treat presbyopia.[13] The ACI 7000 corneal implant is placed under a corneal flap cut by a microkeratome or femtosecond laser. OCT can be used to evaluate the implant depth and centration in situ (Fig. 17.6A).

Intacs intrastromal ring segments (Addition Technology Inc., Fremont, CA) were initially developed to treat low myopia. The 150-degree segments function as spacers between collagen fibers, shortening the arc length of the fibers and flattening of the central cornea.[14] The degree of flattening is proportional to the thickness of the ring segments. Intacs have been shown to improve the best-corrected visual acuity and decrease myopia and astigmatism in keratoconic eyes.[15] Proper implant depth is critical for ensuring good visual outcome. Intacs segments appear as dark spaces within the corneal stroma on OCT (Fig. 17.6B). The implant depth, ideally at 70%, should be measured at the inner edge of the segment to avoid compression and optical artifacts above and below the implant.

Phakic Intraocular Lenses

Phakic intraocular lenses (PIOL) are designed to treat myopia by providing additional refractive power. Two PIOL, Visian Implantable Collamer Lens (ICL) (STAAR Surgical Co., Monrovia, CA) and Verisyse PIOL (Ophtec USA Inc., Boca Raton, FL), have received FDA approval for treatment of myopia ranging from −3 diopters to −20 diopters with astigmatism less than 2.5 diopters. Potential advantages of PIOL over corneal refractive surgery include a larger range of treatable ametropia, faster visual recovery, and better quality of vision.[16,17] PIOL is also attractive for patients who are not candidates for corneal refractive surgery.

The refractive success and long-term safety of PIOL depend on preservation of the anterior segment structures such as the endothelium, trabecular meshwork, iris, and crystalline lens from mechanical trauma related to the PIOL. Currently used white-to-white angle measurement may not accurately reflect the internal anterior chamber width. OCT can provide accurate measurements such as anterior chamber widths, measured from angle recess to angle recess, along several meridians.[18] OCT can be used to determine the crystalline lens rise, the distance between the anterior pole of the lens and angle recess plane. Crystalline lens rise greater than 0.6 mm has been shown to be a risk factor for pigment dispersion in patients with Artisan PIOL.[19] OCT can also be used to simulate PIOL implantation to determine the virtual clearance of PIOL from the endothelium and crystalline lens.[20] OCT can provide the distances between the PIOL and the corneal endothelium, iris, and the crystalline lens postoperatively (Fig. 17.7). Long-term follow-up after PIOL

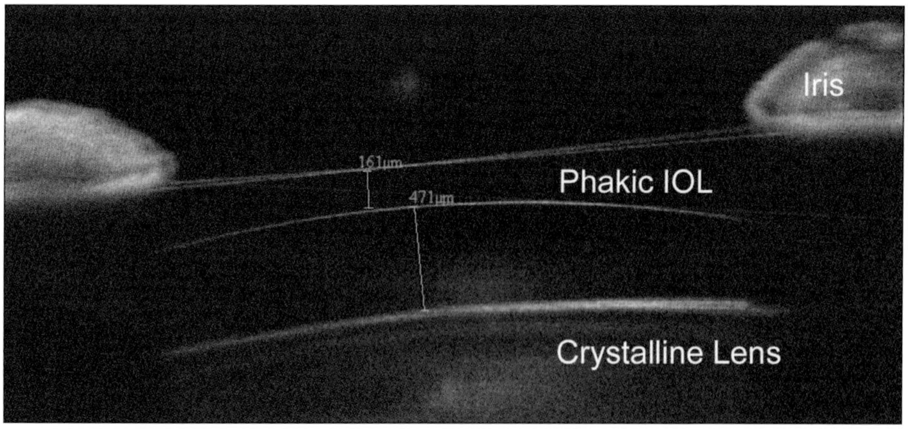

Fig. 17.7 RTVue-CAM OCT image showing a posterior phakic intraocular lens (Visian ICL) vaulting over the natural crystalline lens with good clearance of 471 μm as measured by computer calipers. Reprinted from Huang D (Ed). RTVue Fourier-Domain Optical Coherence Tomography Primer Series: Cornea and Anterior Segment. Optovue Inc. Fremont, CA, 2008, with permission from Optovue.

implantation using OCT can help to detect eyes at risk for complications such as corneal decompensation, pupillary block, and cataract formation from POIL-crystalline lens contact.

Financial interests

Yan Li and David Huang receive grant support and patent royalty from Optovue, Inc.; David Huang also received stock options and travel support from Optovue.

References

1. Huang D, Swanson EA, Lin CP, et al. Optical coherence tomography. *Science*. 1991;254(5035):1178–1181.
2. Izatt JA, Hee MR, Swanson EA, et al. Micrometer-scale resolution imaging of the anterior eye in vivo with optical coherence tomography. *Arch Ophthalmol*. 1994;112(12):1584–1589.
3. Li Y, Meisler DM, Tang M, et al. Keratoconus diagnosis with optical coherence tomography pachymetry mapping. *Ophthalmology*. 2008; 115(12):2159–2166.
4. Li Y, Netto MV, Shekhar R, et al. A longitudinal study of LASIK flap and stromal thickness with high-speed optical coherence tomography. *Ophthalmology*. 2007;114(6):1124–1132.
5. Ashrafzadeh A, Steinert RF. Evaluation of LASIK flaps. In: Steinert RF, Huang D, eds. *Anterior segment optical coherence tomography*. Thorofare, NJ: Slack; 2008.
6. Randleman JB, Russell B, Ward MA, et al. Risk factors and prognosis for corneal ectasia after LASIK. *Ophthalmology*. 2003;110(2):267–275.
7. Khurana RN, Li Y, Tang M, et al. High-speed optical coherence tomography of corneal opacities. *Ophthalmology*. 2007;114(7):1278–1285.
8. Memarzadeh F, Li Y, Francis BA, et al. Optical coherence tomography of the anterior segment in secondary glaucoma with corneal opacity after penetrating keratoplasty. *Br J Ophthalmol*. 2007;91(2):189–192.
9. Melles GR, Wijdh RH, Nieuwendaal CP. A technique to excise the descemet membrane from a recipient cornea (descemetorhexis). *Cornea*. 2004;23(3):286–288.
10. Price MO, Price FW. Descemet's stripping endothelial keratoplasty. *Curr Opin Ophthalmol*. 2007;18(4):290–294.
11. Farid M, Kim M, Steinert RF. Results of penetrating keratoplasty performed with a femtosecond laser zigzag incision initial report. *Ophthalmology*. 2007;114(12):2208–2212.
12. Horgan SE, Fraser SG, Choyce DP, Alexander WL. Twelve year follow-up of unfenestrated polysulfone intracorneal lenses in human sighted eyes. *J Cataract Refract Surg*. 1996;22(8):1045–1051.
13. Yilmaz OF, Bayraktar S, Agca A, et al. Intracorneal inlay for the surgical correction of presbyopia. *J Cataract Refract Surg*. 2008;34(11): 1921–1927.
14. Colin J, Cochener B, Savary G, Malet F. Correcting keratoconus with intracorneal rings. *J Cataract Refract Surg*. 2000;26(8):1117–1122.
15. Zare MA, Hashemi H, Salari MR. Intracorneal ring segment implantation for the management of keratoconus: safety and efficacy. *J Cataract Refract Surg*. 2007;33(11):1886–1891.
16. El Danasoury MA, El Maghraby A, Gamali TO. Comparison of iris-fixed Artisan lens implantation with excimer laser in situ keratomileusis in correcting myopia between −9.00 and −19.50 diopters: a randomized study. *Ophthalmology*. 2002;109(5):955–964.
17. Schallhorn S, Tanzer D, Sanders DR, Sanders ML. Randomized prospective comparison of visian toric implantable collamer lens and conventional photorefractive keratectomy for moderate to high myopic astigmatism. *J Refract Surg*. 2007;23(9):853–867.
18. Baikoff G, Jitsuo Jodai H, Bourgeon G. Measurement of the internal diameter and depth of the anterior chamber: IOLMaster versus anterior chamber optical coherence tomographer. *J Cataract Refract Surg*. 2005;31(9):1722–1728.
19. Baikoff G, Bourgeon G, Jodai HJ, et al. Pigment dispersion and Artisan phakic intraocular lenses: crystalline lens rise as a safety criterion. *J Cataract Refract Surg*. 2005;31(4):674–680.
20. Baikoff G, Lutun E, Wei J, Ferraz C. Contact between 3 phakic intraocular lens models and the crystalline lens: an anterior chamber optical coherence tomography study. *J Cataract Refract Surg*. 2004;30(9):2007–2012.

PART III

DIFFERENTIAL DIAGNOSIS OF SELECTED PROBLEMS IN CORNEAL AND EXTERNAL EYE DISEASE

Chapter 18

Congenital Corneal Opacities: Diagnosis and Management

Kristin M. Hammersmith, Renata A. Rezende, Elisabeth J. Cohen, Ralph C. Eagle Jr, Christopher J. Rapuano

Differential Diagnosis

The term congenital refers to conditions that are present in the newborn. Congenital corneal opacities may result from hereditary, developmental, or infectious causes. They can be bilateral, and can be seen in isolation or in association with other ocular or systemic abnormalities.

The prevalence of congenital corneal opacity is approximately 3:100000 newborns, and this figure increases to 6:100000 if congenital glaucoma is included.[1] Although congenital clouding of the cornea is rare, the ophthalmologist must make an accurate diagnosis to predict the natural history of the disorder, to look for associated ocular and systemic abnormalities, to provide genetic counseling, and to begin appropriate medical or surgical therapy promptly.[2]

Box 18.1 Congenital opacities of the cornea – STUMPED classification[2]

S	Sclerocornea
T	**Tears in Descemet's membrane** Congenital glaucoma Birth trauma
U	**Ulcer** Herpes simplex virus Bacterial Neurotropic
M	**Metabolic (rarely present at birth)** Mucopolysaccharidoses Mucolipidoses Tyrosinosis
P	**Posterior corneal defect** Peters' anomaly Posterior keratoconus Staphyloma
E	**Endothelial dystrophy** Congenital hereditary Posterior polymorphous corneal dystrophy Stromal: congenital stromal corneal dystrophy
D	Dermoid

From Waring GO, Rodrigues MM. Congenital and neonatal corneal abnormalities. In: Tasman, Jaeger eds. Duane's Ophthalmology, CD-Rom. *Philadelphia: Lippincott, Williams & Wilkins; 2002.*

This chapter will address the main features and differential diagnosis between the most common causes of corneal opacification seen at birth (Box 18.1).

History and Physical Examination

Diagnosing the condition causing congenital corneal clouding begins with the history and physical examination. A complete obstetric, maternal, paternal, and family history may be helpful in identifying many diseases. For example, the newborn's mother may have a history of a gestationally acquired rubella infection or previous vaginal or cervical herpes simplex infection. In addition there may be a relative with congenital hereditary endothelial dystrophy, making this diagnosis a strong possibility. After obtaining a detailed history, examination of the newborn is needed. This may be limited to a bedside or office evaluation. Often a careful slit lamp examination is possible using a handheld slit lamp. However, a complete examination is sometimes best accomplished under general anesthesia with the collaboration of a pediatric ophthalmologist, along with cornea and glaucoma specialists (Fig. 18.1). During the examination under anesthesia (EUA), A scan, B scan, and high-frequency ultrasound biomicroscopy (UBM) should be performed. UBM has been

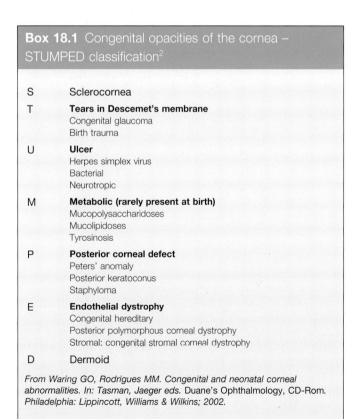

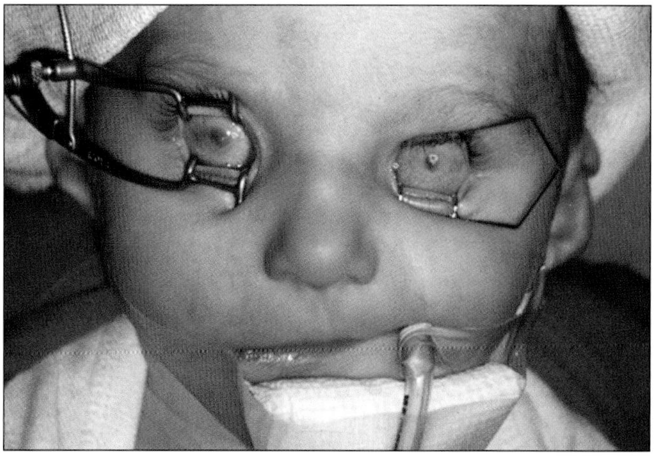

Fig. 18.1 An infant with sclerocornea being examined under general anesthesia.

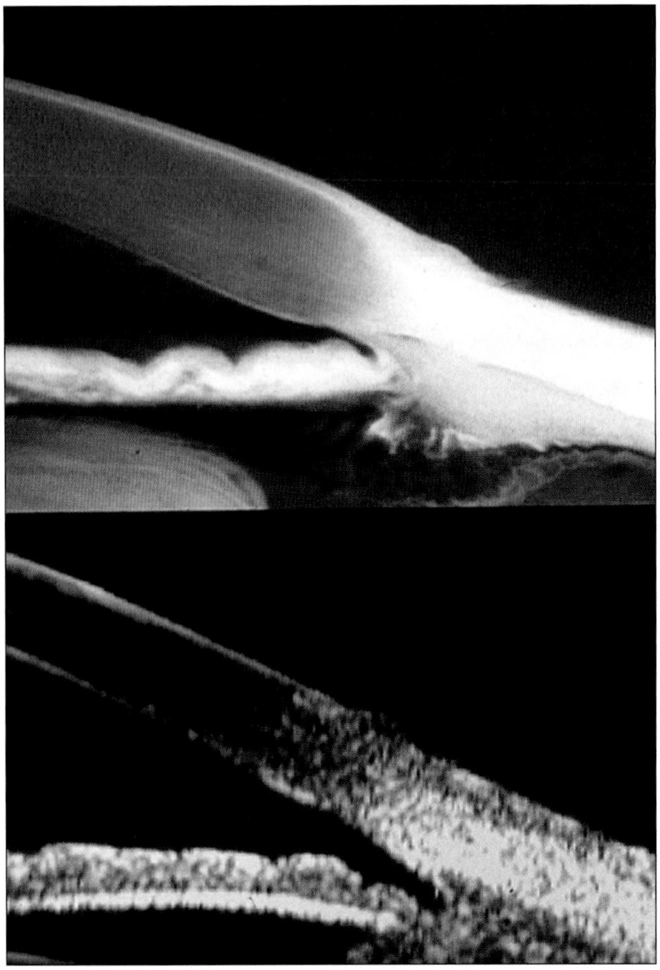

Fig. 18.2 Anatomical structures of the anterior segment shown in ultrasound biomicroscopy. (Courtesy of Elisabeth L. Affel, MS.)

widely used for imaging the anterior segment structures of the eye with exceptional resolution (Fig. 18.2). Some studies have demonstrated that UBM is capable of delineating the corneal layers, with the exception of distinguishing between Descemet's membrane and the endothelium.[3]

Biomicroscopic examination of the cornea and anterior segment can be performed with a handheld slit lamp at the bedside, in the office, or in the operating room. An infant lid speculum is sometimes used with topical anesthesia to provide exposure for a detailed examination, but it may be possible to examine the baby adequately by simply opening the lids. The portable slit lamp permits examination of the cornea with magnification and a slit beam. The slit beam makes this method superior to the operating microscope for corneal evaluation. Also, it is often easier to use than a regular slit lamp because the child can remain in the parent's lap during the examination and there is less movement of the patient's head.

When examining the corneal epithelium, a cobalt blue light with fluorescein can be used with the slit lamp or with a penlight to detect epithelial defects. Visualization through a cloudy cornea can be difficult, especially if the clouding is diffuse and dense. During an EUA, the view through the cornea may be improved by mechanically removing the epithelium. This can be accomplished with cellulose sponge debridement. If the baby is awake, a cotton fiber can be used to touch the cornea while movement of the other lid is used as an indicator of corneal sensation. This is especially important if herpes simplex keratitis or another disorder associated with decreased corneal sensitivity is suspected. If an infection is present and corneal cultures are needed, general anesthesia is required and the operating microscope is used for the procedure.

The diameter of the normal infant cornea is 10.0–10.5 mm. Corneal enlargement, especially if unilateral, can be a sign of congenital glaucoma. Although corneal enlargement can often be detected by gross inspection, a measurement should be obtained. Corneal diameters should be measured both vertically and horizontally with a caliper. A photograph of the child with a ruler on his or her forehead can also be used to assess corneal diameters.

Intraocular pressure measurement is part of the essential examination in a newborn with a congenital cloudy cornea. Several devices are available for intraocular pressure testing, including portable applanation (Perkins, Draeger), indentation (Schiotz), electronic (TonoPen), pneumatic or noncontact (air puff) tonometers, and finger tension measurement. One study showed the pneumatonometer to be the most accurate in children and the TonoPen the least.[4]

General anesthesia typically lowers intraocular pressures, which in premature infants has a mean of 10.11 ± 2.21 mmHg.[5] One study in Korea found an average IOP of 11.85 ± 1.35 mmHg in children under the age of 2. During EUA this measurement should be taken as soon as possible after induction. The finger tension technique helps to detect elevated intraocular pressure while the infant is asleep.

Gonioscopy in the neonate may be best accomplished using a Koeppe lens, and the operating microscope rotated to the correct angle for viewing. In the office, a Koeppe lens and the indirect ophthalmoscope with a 20 diopter lens gives an adequate view.[6]

Dilation of the pupil can sometimes expose the pupillary opening to areas of clear cornea, allowing a view of the posterior structures even in the presence of corneal opacities (Fig. 18.3). The direct ophthalmoscope can be used with a Koeppe lens to obtain a good view of the optic nerve and the macula. An indirect ophthalmoscope with a 14 diopter lens can also be used to examine the disk, and with a 20 or 28 diopter lens for the macula and peripheral retina. Retinoscopy should be done if possible, but can be difficult through a cloudy cornea.

When the corneal opacification is dense and visualization of ocular structures is impossible, there are other ways to evaluate the eye. A-scan ultrasonography can determine the position of the iris and the lens, as well as the length of the eye. For a better evaluation of the anterior segment, UBM should be performed. UBM examination is not only very useful in evaluating the clinical diagnosis in congenital corneal opacification but also it acts as a preoperative guide in cases undergoing penetrating keratoplasty by detecting keratolenticular and iridocorneal adhesions and other ocular abnormalities, such as aniridia and congenital aphakia.[1] Awareness of anterior segment abnormalities can help in

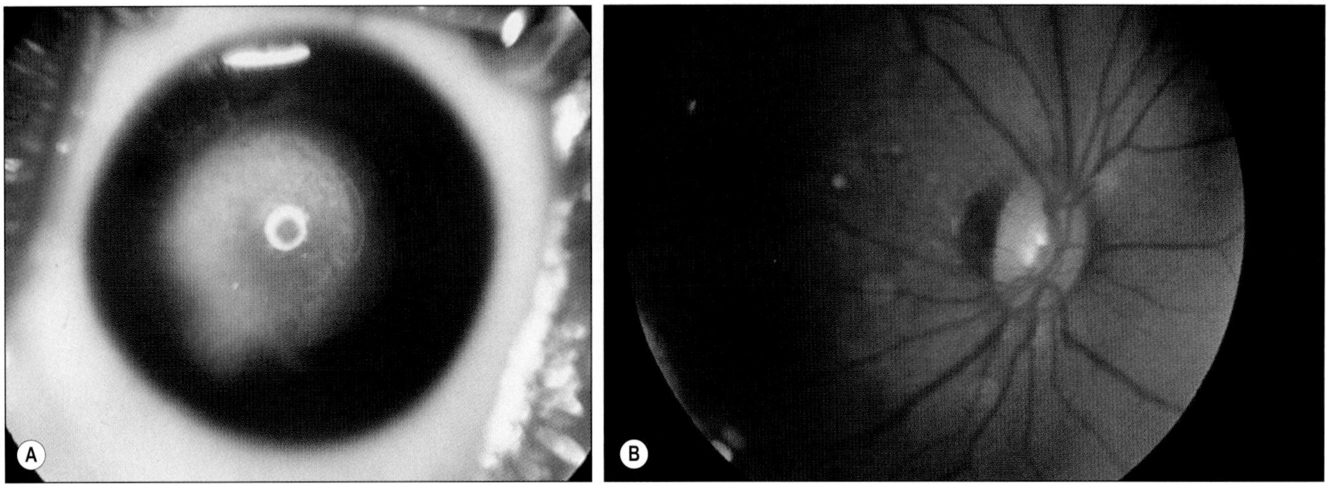

Fig. 18.3 A, Corneal opacity in a newborn with Peters' anomaly. **B**, Dilated fundus examination through the corneal opacity of the same patient.

planning surgery and preventing complications.[3] B-scan ultrasonography provides imaging of the vitreous and retina when there is no view due to anterior segment pathology.

Examination of the patient's parents may also be helpful in establishing the diagnosis of various inherited conditions. In unilateral conditions the healthy eye must be thoroughly examined to look for any abnormalities. This may also be helpful in making the diagnosis in the fellow eye.

When examining an infant with a cloudy cornea, it helps to remember the STUMPED mnemonic developed by Waring and colleagues.[2] This can be used as a guide to the differential diagnosis of the neonatal cloudy cornea (Box 18.1).

Sclerocornea (*S* TUMPED)

Sclerocornea is a primary anomaly in which scleralization of the peripheral part of the cornea, or of the entire tissue, occurs. It may occur alone or in association with other ocular defects. It generally appears sporadically, but can also be familial or autosomal dominant.[7] The embryogenesis and genetics are discussed in Chapter 57.

Sclerocornea is nonprogressive and is usually bilateral but commonly asymmetric (see Fig. 18.1).[8] The opacification of the cornea is smooth, white, and vascular; it appears to be an extension of the sclera without limbal landmarks, and is greater peripherally than centrally (Fig. 18.4). The vessels are fine continuations of conjunctival vessels, but deep vascularization can sometimes occur. Some patients have only the peripheral cornea involved (Fig. 18.4), whereas others have opacification of the entire cornea (Fig. 18.5).

Waring and Rodrigues have classified sclerocornea into four groups:[9,10]

- Isolated peripheral sclerocornea: abrupt change from scleral-like tissue to clear cornea with no other ocular abnormalities (Fig. 18.4).
- Sclerocornea plana: flat corneas with keratometry readings of less than 38 diopters, leading to high hyperopia. The anterior chamber is usually shallow, but glaucoma is

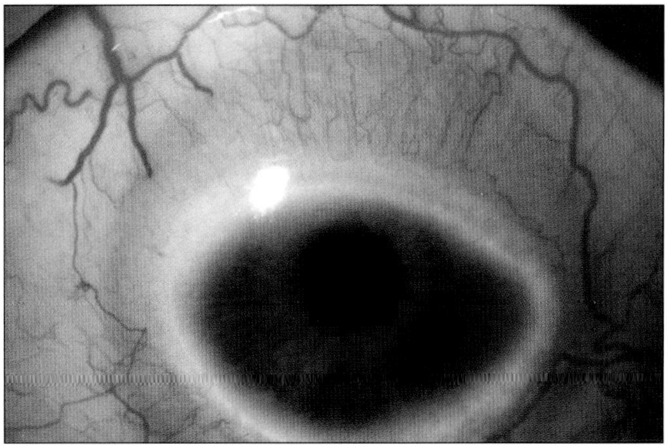

Fig. 18.4 Peripheral sclerocornea. Significant scleralization of the peripheral cornea sparing the central cornea.

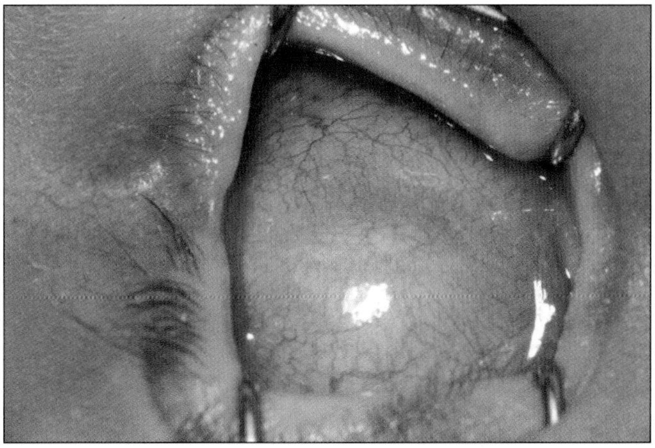

Fig. 18.5 Total sclerocornea: complete opacification of the entire cornea.

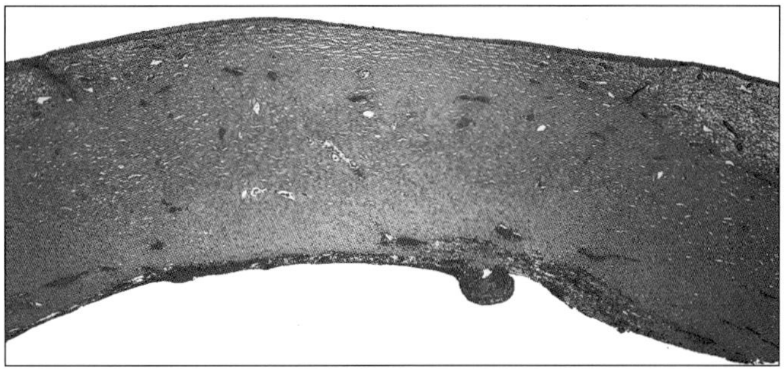

Fig. 18.6 Histopathology of sclerocornea (see also Box 18.2).

Box 18.2 Histopathology in sclerocornea

Corneal stroma resembles sclera morphologically
Precise arrangement of stromal lamellae absent
Irregular arrangement of collagen fibers; variable in diameter
Collagen fibrils thickened (up to 1500 Å in diameter); resemble scleral fibrils
Diameter of collagen fibrils decreases in posterior stroma
Changes in posterior cornea may resemble those seen in Peters' anomaly
(Descemet's membrane attenuated or absent)

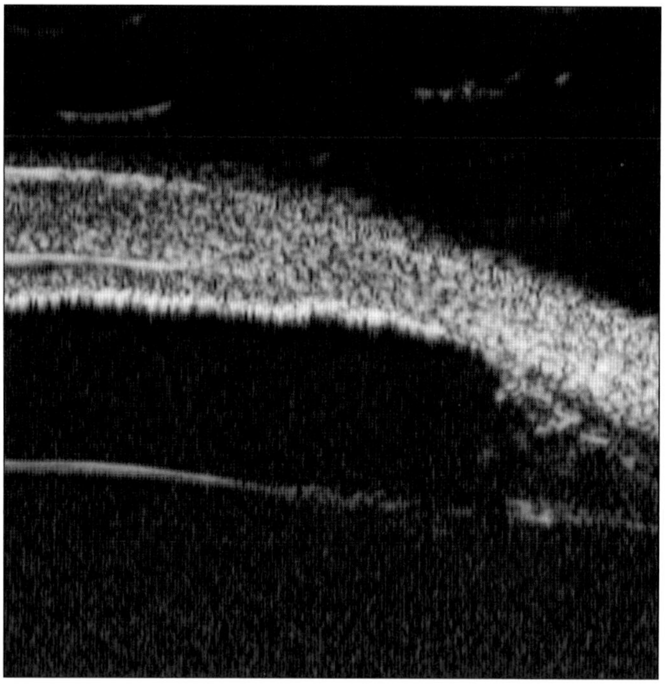

Fig. 18.7 Sclerocornea. Ultrasound biomicroscopy (UBM) demonstrates thickened cornea with collagenous tissue more dense than normal. (Courtesy of Elisabeth L. Affel, MS.)

apparently not frequent. Pseudoptosis can be seen because the flat cornea supports the upper lid poorly. Sharkey et al.[11] reported it in association with epidermolysis bullosa dystrophica. Reduced corneal sensitivity has also been reported in cornea plana.[12]

- Sclerocornea associated with anterior chamber cleavage anomalies: commonly associated with Peters' anomaly, characterized by paracentral corneal adhesions.
- Total sclerocornea: the most common form causing congenital corneal opacity (Fig. 18.5). The corneas are totally opaque and vascularized, but the central cornea is not as densely opaque as the peripheral cornea. The opacification generally affects the full thickness of the stroma, and visualization of the endothelium, pupil, and the anterior chamber structures may be difficult or impossible. Histopathologically, the corneal stroma in sclerocornea resembles sclera. Precisely arranged stromal lamellae are absent and stromal vascularization is often present (Fig. 18.6). Electron microscopy has shown that the collagen fibrils of the stroma are arranged irregularly and are variable in caliber. Most notably, their diameter often is markedly increased (up to 1500 Å), resembling the diameter of the scleral fibrils (Box 18.2). Furthermore, in contrast to the normal human cornea, the collagen fiber diameter in sclerocornea reduces gradually in magnitude from anterior to posterior.[10]

UBM has been reported to help the diagnosis of the sclerocornea itself (Fig. 18.7), to highlight potential associated structural abnormalities, and to facilitate surgical planning by identifying the pupil, which may or may not coincide with the clearest area of the cornea.[3] The usefulness of anterior segment OCT has also been described.[11] Patients with sclerocornea sometimes exhibit somatic abnormalities such as mental retardation, anomalies of the skin, facies, ears, cerebellum, and testes. A list of ocular and systemic abnormalities associated with sclerocornea is found in Chapter 57.

The differential diagnosis can be narrowed by history, clinical examination, ocular and systemic associations, and observations of the patient over time, and include arcus juvenilis, interstitial keratitis, Peters' anomaly, and microcornea (Table 18.1).

Management is similar to that of other congenital corneal opacities. If the disorder is unilateral and the other eye has good visual acuity, the decision to operate becomes more difficult, and surgery can be performed only if other ocular structures are relatively normal. If the condition affects the central corneas bilaterally, causing a significant reduction in visual acuity, penetrating keratoplasty should be performed in an attempt to obtain useful vision. Awareness of other ocular abnormalities can be made by the use of UBM or OCT prior to surgery, reducing the risk of complications.[14] However, the prognosis for a clear graft is still worse than in Peters' anomaly, but better in recent years with the use of topical ciclosporin.

Tears in the Endothelium and Descemet's Membrane (*S T* UMPED)

Congenital glaucoma

Congenital glaucoma is the most important disease in the differential diagnosis of congenital corneal clouding, because

Table 18.1 Differential diagnosis of sclerocornea

Sclerocornea	Arcus juvenilis	Interstitial keratitis	Peters' anomaly	Microcornea
Corneal opacification greater peripherally, smooth, white, and vascular extension of the sclera without limbal landmarks Fine vessel continuations of conjunctival vessels, but deep vascularization can sometimes occur. Some patients have opacification of the entire cornea Usually associated with other ocular abnormalities	Cornea is not vascularized Clear interval between the opacification and the limbus May be associated with lipid abnormalities	Later onset Associated with a red, inflamed eye	Central cornea more opaque than periphery	Steep corneal curvature Narrow angles Small anterior segments Different systemic associations

early diagnosis may allow adequate treatment and preservation of vision, and delayed diagnosis can result in irreversible visual loss. All infants with unilateral or bilateral cloudy corneas must be evaluated carefully for glaucoma. Primary congenital glaucoma is usually sporadic, but may be inherited as an autosomal recessive trait.

The first symptoms of primary congenital glaucoma are epiphora, photophobia, and blepharospasm. The first signs are elevated intraocular pressure, corneal enlargement and clouding, and optic nerve cupping.[15] The symptoms result from epithelial edema, caused by the elevated intraocular pressure. The cornea and sclera of infants and children are more elastic and distensible than those of adults. The infant's Descemet's membrane is also thinner (3–4 μm) than in the adult (10–12 μm). Therefore, the elevated intraocular pressure may lead to rapid enlargement of the eye (buphthalmos). As the eye enlarges, the cornea stretches, which causes Descemet's membrane to break. These ruptures disturb the endothelial barrier, and aqueous gains access to the corneal stroma and epithelium. The initial symptoms may worsen acutely with disruption of Descemet's membrane. In addition to the elevated intraocular pressure, breaks in Descemet's membrane contribute to diffuse corneal haziness. Early in the course of the disease, corneal clouding may be seen only intermittently and may precede breaks in Descemet's membrane.

Another corneal sign of congenital glaucoma is increased corneal diameter. The buphthalmic eye has a diameter greater than the normal infant corneal diameter of 10.0–10.5 mm. Parents sometimes bring these children after noticing slight haziness or enlargement of the corneas. The enlarged cornea and globe of buphthalmos generally are not present in the immediate postpartum period, but by 6 months of age approximately 75% of affected infants manifest corneal enlargement.[16]

The tears in Descemet's membrane can be single or multiple, and appear as elliptical, glassy, parallel ridges on the posterior cornea, either peripherally or across the visual axis. In congenital glaucoma these breaks have a random distribution, most commonly horizontal or concentric to the limbus, in contrast to the oblique and vertical orientation of the breaks in Descemet's membrane seen in birth trauma (Fig. 18.8).

The diagnosis of congenital glaucoma is not based on elevated intraocular pressure alone. Other signs, such as corneal haze, increased corneal diameter, increased cup to disk ratio, increased axial length, and gonioscopic abnormalities, support the diagnosis.

The management of congenital glaucoma is surgical. Procedures should be performed by a glaucoma specialist or a pediatric ophthalmologist, and initially include goniotomy and trabeculotomy. If these two procedures fail, trabeculectomy or aqueous shunt implantation are employed. Corneal clouding can complicate the treatment by making goniotomy and filtering trabeculotomy difficult owing to poor visualization of the anterior chamber angle.

Birth trauma

Injury to the cornea occurs from placement of the forceps blade across the globe and orbit during delivery, causing blunt trauma and rupture of Descemet's membrane.[17] Other soft tissue injuries such as unilateral periorbital edema and ecchymoses may accompany the trauma.[2] Left eyes seem to be affected more commonly than right eyes because neonates usually present in the left-occiput-anterior position.[18]

The elevation of intraocular pressure (IOP) is acute, distends the globe, exceeds the elasticity of Descemet's membrane, and produces tears that allow the cornea to imbibe aqueous with resultant stromal and epithelial edema.[2] The Descemet's tears in birth trauma are usually unilateral, central and, in contrast to congenital glaucoma, line up in a vertical or oblique pattern (Table 18.2; Fig. 18.9), presumably because the tip of the forceps has slipped over the rim of the orbit and compressed the globe vertically, stretching it horizontally to create the tears.[2]

Birth trauma produces diffuse stromal and epithelial edema in the immediate postpartum period (Table 18.2). If the damage is not too severe, the corneal edema usually clears within weeks to months.

The young endothelium resurfaces the posterior cornea, and it synthesizes a new thick basement membrane that

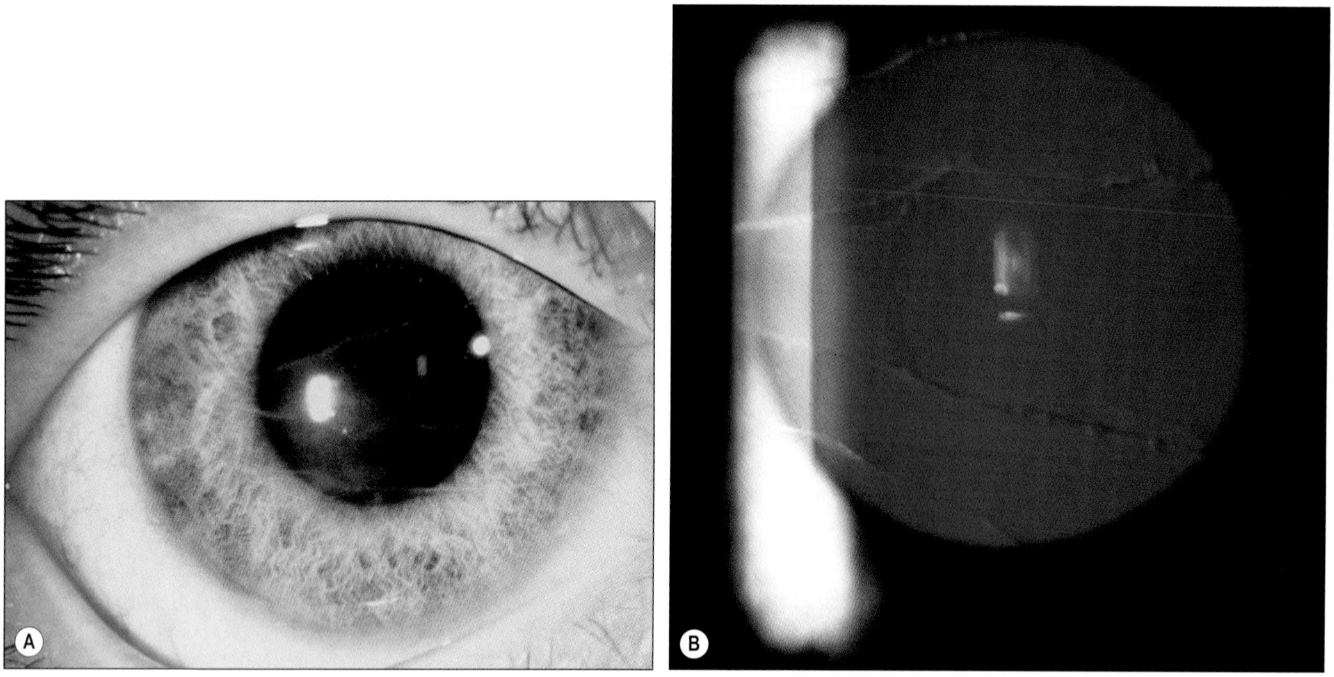

Fig. 18.8 Horizontal breaks in Descemet's membrane (Haab's striae) in an infant with congenital glaucoma. Striae are seen in (**A**) direct and (**B**) retroillumination.

Table 18.2 Differential diagnosis between birth trauma and congenital glaucoma

Birth trauma	Congenital glaucoma
Normal IOP	High IOP
Normal corneal diameter	Large corneal diameter with buphthalmos (may get back to normal with decrease in IOP)
Corneal edema in the immediate postpartum period	Corneal edema weeks or months after birth
Corneal edema clears after weeks to months	Corneal edema clears after lowering IOP
Tears in Descemet's membrane are vertical or oblique	Tears in Descemet's membrane are horizontal or concentric to the limbus
Left eyes seem to be more frequently affected and other soft tissue injuries may accompany the trauma	No preference for either eye
Usually no photophobia	Photophobia

accentuates the edges of the tear and fills in the dehiscence.[2] Once the corneal edema disappears, the edges of the break appear as rounded, glassy ridges that protrude from the posterior cornea and light up strikingly in retroillumination (Fig. 18.9B). Within the break, the new basement membrane has a beaten-metal, guttate appearance. Although the cornea remains clear, high residual corneal astigmatism, which may range from 4 to 9 diopters, requires urgent correction and amblyopia treatment. The steep meridian of the astigmatism parallels the Descemet's ruptures.[2] Rigid gas-permeable contact lenses (Fig. 18.10) and patching are the first choice of treatment. The diagnosis is based on the history and clinical findings.

Later in life, the previously stressed endothelium may decompensate, with resulting corneal edema that requires penetrating keratoplasty to restore vision.[18,19] The visual acuity may be limited by amblyopia from high astigmatism and anisometropia.

Refraction for glasses or contact lenses should be measured as soon as possible. Early fitting with rigid gas-permeable lenses has been reported in birth trauma (Fig. 18.10), showing excellent results in the prevention of amblyopia secondary to severe astigmatism.[20] Patching or atropine therapy is necessary to treat amblyopia. The corneal specialist should always try to work with a pediatric ophthalmologist in the treatment of amblyopia.

Another type of prenatal trauma that can produce a corneal opacity is an amniotic band that stretches across the face during development, often causing a cleft lip, sometimes associated with microphthalmia and a hazy cornea. The corneal haze probably represents direct trauma to the cornea and not tears in Descemet's membrane.[21]

Corneal Ulcers and Inflammation (ST *U* MPED)

Congenital opacities caused by corneal ulcers are rarely present at birth, but when a fluorescein-staining epithelial defect does occur in a neonate, the ophthalmologist should

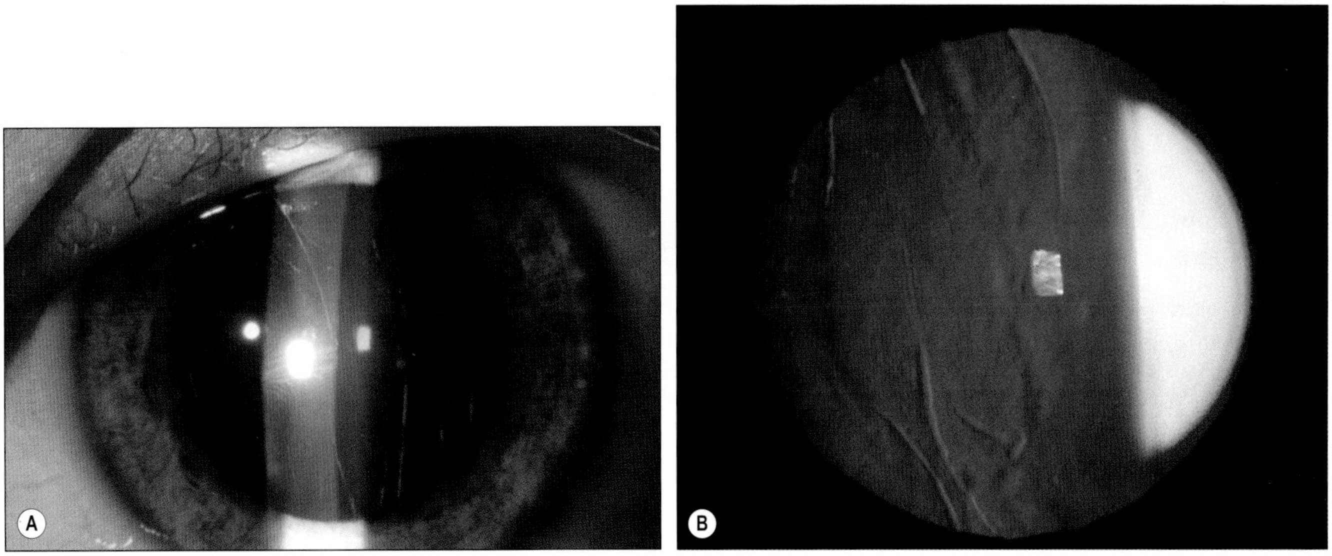

Fig. 18.9 Vertical and oblique distribution of Descemet's tears in birth trauma. The tears are seen in (**A**) direct but sometimes are better seen in (**B**) retroillumination.

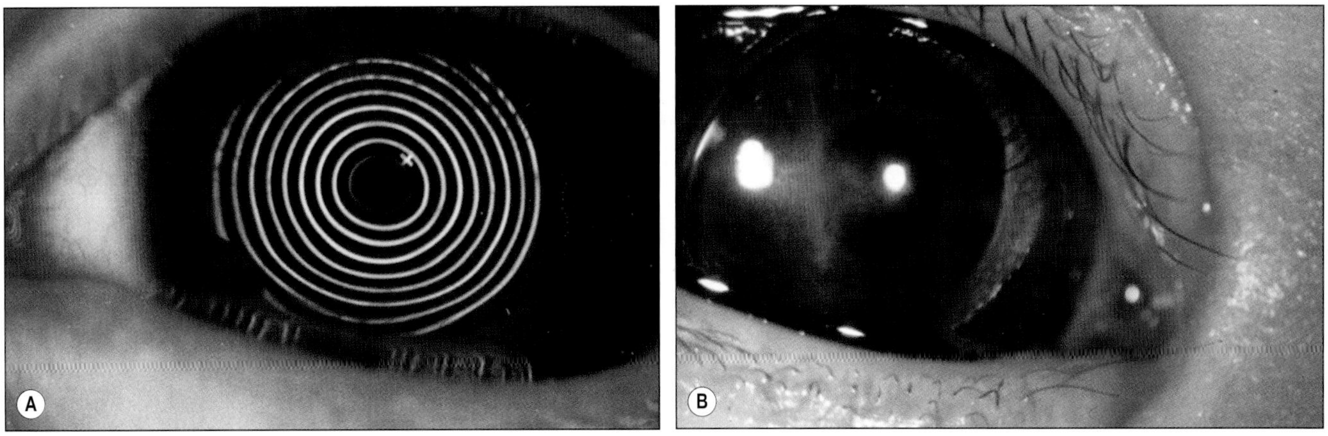

Fig. 18.10 Birth trauma. **A** and **B**, Rigid gas-permeable lenses fitting in a 2-month-old child with high with-the-rule astigmatism due to forceps injury.

consider herpes simplex keratitis, bacterial keratitis, and neurotrophic keratitis.

Viral diseases

Herpes simplex virus infection

Congenital herpes simplex virus (HSV) infection is generally contracted during delivery from an infected birth canal. Two cases of HSV infection acquired in utero have also been reported.[22,23] Neonatal herpes infection is secondary to pre- or perinatal viral contamination with HSV2 or HSV1 from the mother.[24] Approximately 80% of perinatal HSV infections are caused by HSV type 2 and 20% by type 1.

The infection represents a primary ocular infection that can later become recurrent despite the presence of neutralizing antibodies. Disseminated disease and central nervous system (CNS) involvement are common and are associated with significant mortality despite appropriate systemic antiviral therapy. Diagnosing HSV ocular infection is critical because it can be the first manifestation of perinatal systemic infection.

The diagnosis of neonatal ocular HSV infection must be considered in any newborn with conjunctivitis or keratitis. Ocular manifestations of the disease are usually apparent within 2 days to 2 weeks of life, but in two reported cases herpes simplex epithelial keratitis was present at birth.[22,23] Conjunctivitis is the most common finding and can be purulent or nonpurulent. Many forms of ulcerative keratitis are seen, including macrodendrites, geographic epithelial defects, and punctate keratopathy. The finding of a dendrite is indicative of HSV infection. Isolated stromal keratitis is unusual and may indicate the rarely reported intrauterine infection.[22] The eyelids are usually edematous and red, with or without skin vesicles. Many other ocular complications of HSV infection also occur, including necrotizing chorioretinitis, cataracts, optic neuritis, optic atrophy, strabismus, and phthisis.[23,24] A history of genital herpes in the mother strongly suggests herpetic eye disease. Use of a fetal scalp monitor is also associated with an increased risk of neonatal HSV infection.[24]

The diagnosis is made by history and clinical findings, but can be confirmed by additional laboratory evaluation. As more rapid and precise methods of viral diagnosis become available, scrapings from the cornea or conjunctiva may demonstrate the virus by fluorescein antibody or peroxidase antibody staining, and electron microscopy may be used to detect viral particles in tears. Immunologic testing using commercial kits is another available method of diagnosis. Acute and convalescent serum titers can also be used to confirm HSV primary infection.

The gravity of neonatal herpes warrants prophylactic measures, including cesarean section if the risk is high.[25] Cesarean section is mandatory in cases of genital primary infection or nonprimary maternal infection during the last month of pregnancy.[26] Antiviral treatment of the mother using aciclovir (ACV) is well tolerated and may be given to mothers at higher risk of transmission in the third trimester prior to delivery. An oral ACV–cesarean combination provides maximal protection for the neonate.[26]

The treatment for neonatal HSV keratitis or conjunctivitis is intravenous aciclovir. It is used in every case of HSV infection of the neonate because disseminated disease is common and can be fatal. Additionally, other vision-threatening ocular manifestations of the disease are best treated systemically.[27] The medication treats systemic disease, but therapeutic levels are also achieved in the aqueous and tears. Topical therapy is also used for ocular disease.

Trifluorothymidine (Viroptic) five to nine times daily is generally used first because of its superior effectiveness compared to the other commonly used antiviral agents. Vidarabine or aciclovir ointment or ganciclovir gel can also be used topically. Neither of the reported congenital cases responded to idoxuridine. The treatment for the skin lesions includes warm compresses followed by complete drying of the area and topical aciclovir ointment. Bacitracin, erythromycin, or other topical antibiotic ointments can be placed on the lesions to help prevent superinfection.[24] Consultation with pediatric or infectious disease specialists is imperative to help monitor the infant for CNS or disseminated disease.

Congenital rubella

Because rubella (German measles) vaccine is now routinely administered, conferring virtually lifelong immunity, the disorder rarely occurs in developed countries.

Rubella is usually accompanied by nondescript, catarrhal conjunctivitis. A mild form of follicular conjunctivitis may also occur and, more rarely, mild superficial punctate epithelial keratitis. Permanent corneal disease due to childhood rubella has not been described. Congenital rubella infection, however, causes microphthalmia, cataract, retinitis, iridocyclitis, corneal clouding, strabismus, nystagmus, nasolacrimal duct obstruction, and viral dacryoadenitis.[28,29]

Congenital rubella infection is acquired by the fetus transplacentally during the first trimester of gestation and represents an uncommon cause of congenital corneal opacity. Boniuk[29,30] has thoroughly described the congenital rubella syndrome, which includes ocular, otic, cardiac, and other visceral anomalies. Approximately 6% of infants of mothers who had rubella in the first trimester of pregnancy manifest three different types of corneal opacity at birth:[31]

1. Transient central stromal opacity that clears in the first weeks of life may result from viral infection of the endothelium.
2. Corneal edema may result from elevated intraocular pressure, but clears as the pressure spontaneously returns to normal.
3. Corneal edema and scarring may accompany severe microphthalmos with keratoiridial or corneal lenticular adhesions (Peters' anomaly).

Diagnosis of rubella-induced corneal opacification is based on history; typical visceral and radiographic anomalies; viral cultures of the throat, urine, or other secretions; and subsequent documentation of characteristic ocular fundus changes. Serologies of both infant and mother are obtained. The presence of rubella-specific IgM in the cord serum confirms the diagnosis, as IgM does not cross the placenta.

If the corneal clouding is related to glaucoma or lens–corneal touch, these two conditions must be treated appropriately. If the opacification is an isolated finding, it usually resolves spontaneously. If the opacification persists, penetrating keratoplasty can be performed[32] but is often very difficult because of inflammation in these eyes and the other associated ocular problems.

Bacterial diseases

Bacterial corneal ulcers do not appear at birth and are exceedingly rare in the neonate. Although in the late 19th and early 20th centuries bacterial conjunctivitis in the newborn commonly produced corneal ulceration and blindness, the advent of 1% silver nitrate prophylaxis and many effective topical antibiotics has virtually eliminated corneal ulceration in this age group.

The etiology of conjunctival infection is thought to be multifactorial. The neonate is exposed to many bacteria in the birth canal, and the duration of exposure, integrity of the ocular surface, and adequacy of antibiotic prophylaxis all factor into the development of ocular infection. Many Gram-positive and Gram-negative organisms have been implicated in these infections.

Neisseria gonorrhoeae can produce serious ocular and systemic complications if not treated appropriately. Gonorrheal ophthalmia neonatorum usually presents as a unilateral conjunctivitis with an incubation period of a few hours to 2–3 days. The disease is characterized by lid edema, severe bulbar conjunctival injection, and chemosis, with a watery or serosanguineous discharge. After 4 or 5 days the disease enters the purulent stage, with an increasingly copious purulent discharge and the formation of a pseudomembrane on the tarsal conjunctiva. Untreated, the conjunctival inflammation will slowly decrease, but conjunctival scarring may occur. The cornea can be involved, displaying peripheral corneal infiltrates that may ulcerate, or a central ulcer or a ring abscess. It can result in perforation if untreated, or if the infection occurs in utero. Systemic treatment is then necessary.

Prophylaxis using topical erythromycin is very effective in preventing many cases of neonatal conjunctivitis. Treatment for infections that do occur consists of broad-spectrum topical therapy replaced by a more specific agent when the offending microorganism is identified. Penicillin G systemic treatment is needed for *N. gonorrhoeae* infection. Saline irrigation of the fornices may also help in decreasing the bacterial load. For beta-lactamase-producing *N. gonorrhoeae*, intravenous cefotaxime is currently recommended by the Centers for Disease Control. Topical therapy can also be used. Infections caused by *Pseudomonas* species usually require fortified gentamicin or tobramycin drops.

Ophthalmia neonatorum caused by *Chlamydia*, albeit a common cause of ophthalmia neonatorum, rarely produces corneal ulceration or opacification. Erythromycin is given systemically to treat a possible associated systemic chlamydial infection.

Congenital syphilis is not a cause of congenital corneal opacification. Syphilitic interstitial keratitis occurs bilaterally in the first or second decade of life, and is probably immunologically mediated.

Neurotrophic keratitis

Familial dysautonomia (Riley–Day syndrome) is a condition associated with generalized dysfunction of the autonomic nervous system resulting in increased sweating, dermal discoloration, motor incoordination, cyclic vomiting, blood pressure lability, emotional difficulties, and frequent respiratory infections. It has been suggested that the corneal innervation may also be deficient. Therefore, decreased tearing, decreased corneal sensation, and sterile corneal ulceration are common, and may be present at birth or develop later. Most patients with this condition have a shortened lifespan, frequently dying from infection.

Metabolic diseases (STU *M* PED)

Even though corneal opacities due to metabolic diseases are rare, it is important for the clinician to be aware of them. Corneal opacification is usually not present at birth but develops later in the first year of life. Sometimes the corneal findings may be the first manifestation of the systemic disease.

Mucopolysaccharidoses and mucolipidoses are inherited lysosomal enzyme deficiencies. The enzyme deficiency leads to the accumulation of the mucopolysaccharides (now called glycosaminoglycans) or mucolipids that the deficient enzyme would normally metabolize. The enzyme deficiencies in these diseases are expressed at the level of the bone marrow stem cells, and so these disorders fall into the relatively small number of inborn errors of metabolism that are amenable to correction by allogeneic bone marrow transplantation.[33,34] They are all autosomally recessive, with the exception of mucopolysaccharidosis type II (Hunter's syndrome), which is X-linked recessive.

The prevalence of clinically apparent corneal opacification depends on the type of disease, the age of the patient, the method of examination, and the experience of the examining physician.

There are at least six types of mucopolysaccharidosis and 10 types of mucolipidosis, each with its own distinct clinical, biochemical, and genetic manifestations. These metabolic diseases are also discussed in Chapter 57.

Mucopolysaccharidosis

These diseases present differently, depending on the specific enzyme deficiency. Corneal clouding, pigmentary retinal abnormalities, and optic atrophy are the common ocular features of these diseases. Heparin and keratan sulfates are glycosaminoglycans that accumulate in the cells and extracellular matrix of the cornea.[17] Heparin sulfate also accumulates in the retina and CNS.[35] The syndromes most commonly involving the cornea are MPS I-H, I-S, IV A and B, and VI A and B.

Mild to severe corneal clouding within the first few years of life is typical of mucopolysaccharidosis type I-H (Hurler's syndrome) and type VI (Maroteaux–Lamy syndrome).

Hurler's syndrome (MPS I-H) or gargoylism is caused by a deficiency of alfa-l-iduronidase and the gene involved with this error is mapped to 4p16.3. Corneal clouding is a prominent feature of Hurler's syndrome (Table 18.3). Diffuse punctate stromal opacities are present without involvement of the epithelium and endothelium.[36] Corneal clouding is significant and helps differentiate this disease from Hunter's syndrome. The diagnosis can be confirmed by measuring the affected enzyme in peripheral leukocytes, cultured dermal fibroblasts, or amniotic cells.[37]

Maroteaux–Lamy syndrome (types VIA and VIB) is caused by arylsulfatase B deficiency and the causative gene was mapped to 5q13[38] (Fig. 18.11). Type A is the severe form of the disease and type B is the mild form (Table 18.4). Punctate corneal opacities are almost always present at birth, although sometimes they cannot be seen without a slit lamp biomicroscope. Narrow-angle glaucoma has also been reported.[39] Occasionally the corneal clouding is severe, necessitating penetrating keratoplasty (Fig. 18.11C).[40]

Scheie's syndrome (MPS I-S) is caused by a mutation in the gene encoding alfa-l-iduronidase, mapped to 4p16.3. Patients have normal intelligence, normal height, and a normal life expectancy[41] (Table 18.3). Corneal clouding results from the accumulation of acid mucopolysaccharides, occurs at birth or early in life, and slowly progresses to cause decreased vision by the second decade of life.[42] The cornea appears thickened or edematous.[42] Occasionally these corneal changes are more prominent in the corneal periphery. Glaucoma has also been reported.[43] Ultrastructural analysis of the cornea has found attenuated Bowman's layer and fibrous long-spacing collagen.[43] Penetrating keratoplasty can be performed if the opacification limits visual acuity.

Corneal opacification is found much less frequently in other mucopolysaccharidoses. Approximately 10% of patients with mucopolysaccharidosis type IV (Morquio's syndrome) develop corneal opacities after age 10, and corneal opacities are also seen in a small number of patients who have the milder phenotypes of mucopolysaccharidosis type II (Hunter's syndrome) and rarely mucopolysaccharidosis type III (Sanfilippo's syndrome).[44]

Table 18.3 Clinical features of mucopolysaccharidosis

I-H: Hurler	VI: Maroteaux–Lamy	I-S: Sheie	IV: Morquio	II: Hunter	III: Sanfilippo
Autosomal recessive Severe corneal clouding within the first few years	Autosomal recessive Severe corneal clouding within the first few years	Autosomal recessive Corneal opacification from birth and slowly progresses to cause decreased vision by the second decade of life[42]	Autosomal recessive Corneal opacities after[9] years old	X-linked recessive trait Does not present as a congenital corneal opacity	Autosomal recessive Rarely develops corneal opacity
Diffuse punctate stromal opacities are present without involvement of the epithelium and endothelium[36]	Narrow-angle glaucoma has been reported[39]	Cornea appears thickened or edematous[42] Corneal changes may be more prominent in the corneal periphery Glaucoma has also been reported[44]		Corneal opacity may occur later in life in milder phenotypes	
Syndrome: mental retardation, dwarfism, large head with abnormal-appearing face, enlarged abdomen, and contractures of the joints[37,45]	Mild facial abnormalities and multiple skeletal changes, dwarfism, kyphosis, protuberant sternum, and genu valgum[37]	Clawhand deformities, bony changes in the feet, and aortic valve abnormalities may be present	Dwarfism, aortic valvular disease, and laxity of the joints[44]	Clinically it appears similar to Hurler's syndrome	
Other abnormalities: hepatosplenomegaly; thickening of the skin, lips, and tongue; chest enlargement; hirsutism; deafness; neurologic defects; and cardiac defects[35]	Other abnormalities: optic neuropathy, hydrocephalus[53]			Deafness and heart defects are common	
Diagnosis confirmed by measuring the affected enzyme in peripheral leukocytes, cultured dermal fibroblasts, or amniotic cells[37]					

Table 18.4 Clinical features of mucolipidosis

Mucolipidoses	Systemic manifestations	Corneal manifestations	Other ocular manifestations
MLS I	Hepatosplenomegaly, hernias, moderate degree of mental retardation	Rare. Fine epithelial and stromal opacification	Cherry-red spot, spotlike cataracts, tortuous retinal and conjunctival vessels, and strabismus
MLS II (I-cell disease)	Severe mental retardation, skin and gingival thickening, skeletal deformities and hepatomegaly	Mild corneal haziness may appear at birth Megalocornea	Prominent eyes, retinal degeneration, cortical cataracts, glaucoma, and optic atrophy
MLS III (pseudo-Hurler)	Musculoskeletal abnormalities, small stature, moderate mental retardation, gargoyle-like facies	Fine corneal opacities that usually do not decrease visual acuity	Retinal and optic nerve abnormalities
MLS IV	More common in Ashkenazi Jews. Profound psychomotor retardation	Most severe corneal clouding of the MLSs At birth Epithelial irregularities and recurrent erosions	Cataract, retinal degeneration, optic atrophy

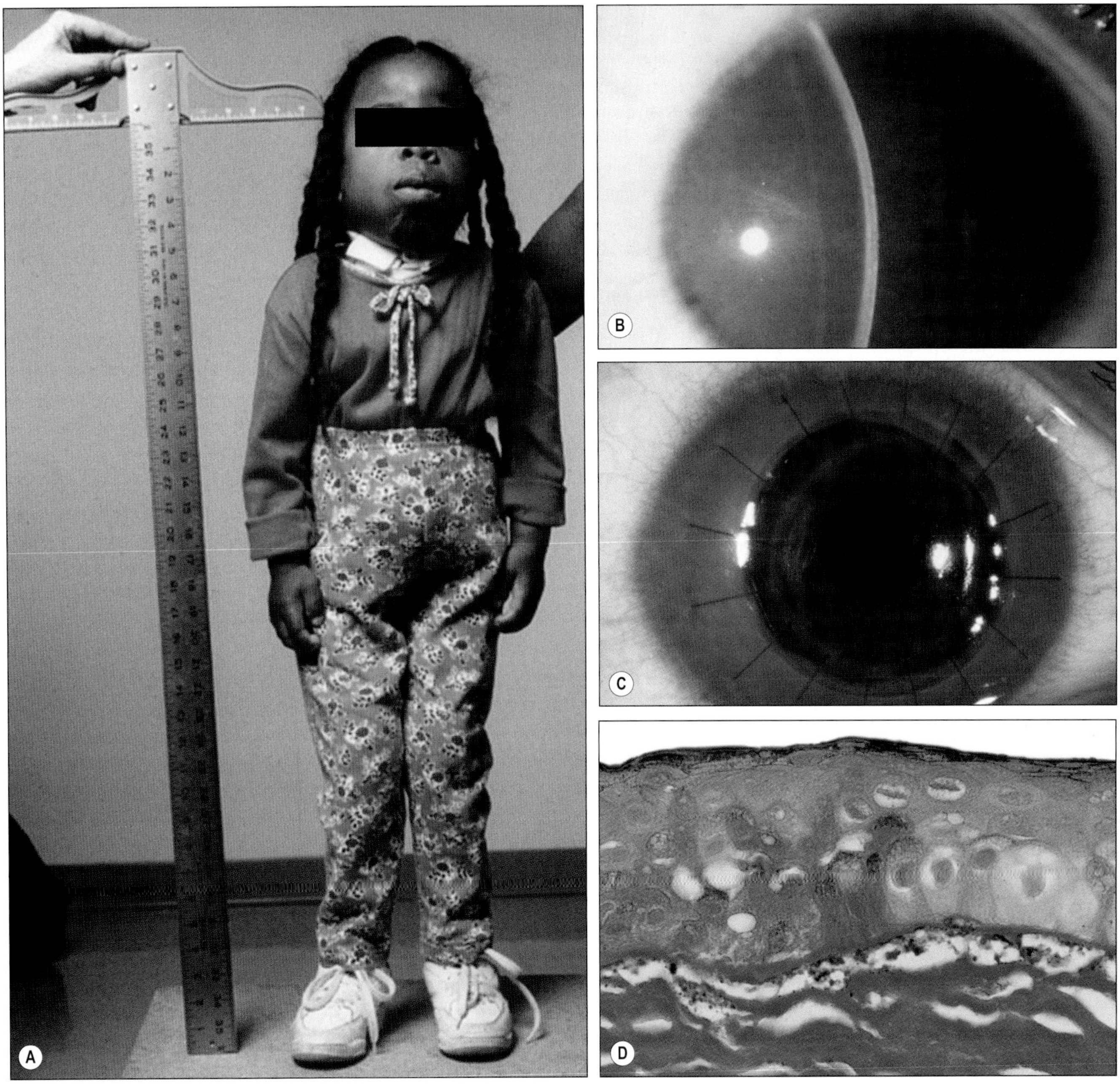

Fig. 18.11 A child with Maroteaux–Lamy syndrome with mild facial abnormality, dwarfism, and genu valgum (**A**) and a diffuse corneal haze (**B**). She underwent a penetrating keratoplasty (**C**). **D**, Colloidal iron stain shows deposition of acid mucopolysaccharide (blue staining) in apical cytoplasm of basal epithelial cells and subepithelial vacuoles. Bowman's membrane is absent. Hales colloidal iron, ×250.

Morquio's syndrome (MPS types IVA and IVB) has two subtypes, A and B, which result from a deficiency of galactosamine-6-sulfate sulfatase and beta-galactosidase, respectively. Variable haziness of the corneal stroma occurs and may not be evident for several years after birth (Table 18.3).

Hunter's syndrome (MPS II) is inherited as an X-linked recessive trait (gene mapped to Xq28) resulting in a deficiency of iduronate sulfatase and does not present as a congenital corneal opacity. Clinically it appears similar to Hurler's syndrome (Table 18.3). Corneal opacification may occur later in life in the mild form of the disease.[44]

Bilateral diffuse acid mucopolysaccharide accumulation in Bowman's membrane without evidence of systemic MPS has also been described as a cause of congenital cloudy corneas.[46]

Successful early bone marrow transplantation or allogenic stem cell transplantation for systemic mucopolysaccharidoses has been shown to lead to a reduction in the degree of corneal opacification in some patients.[47] Severe corneal opacities can be treated by penetrating keratoplasty, but retinal degeneration is a common concomitant and preoperative electroretinography (ERG) is mandatory to assess retinal function.[48] Other factors that limit the visual prognosis are glaucoma and optic nerve disease, as well as the risk of cataract and recurrence of opacification in the corneal graft. Both acute and chronic angle-closure glaucoma have been reported in types VI, I-H and I-S.[49–52] There is one case report of glaucoma in a patient with mucopolysaccharidosis type I-H, with a return of intraocular pressure to normal ranges after successful gene replacement by bone marrow transplantation.[52]

Mucolipidosis

Mucolipidoses (MLSs) are autosomal recessive metabolic diseases with neuraminidase deficiency that result in an abnormal accumulation of sphingolipids, glycolipids, and acid mucopolysaccharides. The mucolipidoses have phenotypic and biochemical features of both the mucopolysaccharidoses and the sphingolipidoses, without excessive urinary excretion of mucopolysaccharides.[2] Four diseases have been included in this category: MLS I to MLS IV. However, corneal opacities are commonly present at birth only in MLS II and MLS IV.[48] The latter is always accompanied by significant congenital corneal opacity. Mild congenital opacification is a feature in 40% of cases of type II mucolipidosis and in less than 20% of type I mucolipidosis and generalized gangliosidosis.[54–58] Mild clouding is found in all cases of type III mucolipidosis by age 10.[59]

Episodic ocular pain is an important symptom in mucolipidosis type IV. It is caused by corneal epithelial cytoplasmic accumulation of abnormal material with subsequent corneal surface irregularities.[60]

In mucopolysaccharidosis the urinary excretion of glycosaminoglycan is increased, but that is not a feature of the mucolipidoses. A definitive diagnosis of MLS is made by observing storage organelles on electron microscopy.[61] The main clinical features of this group of diseases are summarized in Table 18.4.

Usually, mucolipidoses types I, II, and III do not cause severe corneal disease and do not require ocular treatment. Management of MLS IV has centered on attempts to improve ocular comfort. The use of lubricants and therapeutic soft contact lenses helps to avoid painful erosive episodes.[62] Penetrating keratoplasty and lamellar keratoplasty have been reported to yield poor results because of the opacification of the transplanted tissue.[62] Mechanical debridement has also been attempted, with poor results. Conjunctival and limbal transplantation techniques have been suggested to provide a new population of corneal epithelial stem cells.[62–64]

Other metabolic diseases

Cystinosis

Cystinosis is a rare autosomal recessive metabolic disorder caused by a defect in cystine transport. It is characterized biochemically by an abnormally high intracellular content of free cystine; this in turn results in cystine crystal deposition in various tissues, including the eye, bone marrow, lymph nodes, leukocytes, and internal organs, including the kidneys.[65–67] The mutant gene for the infantile and juvenile forms has been mapped to chromosome 17p.[69,70]

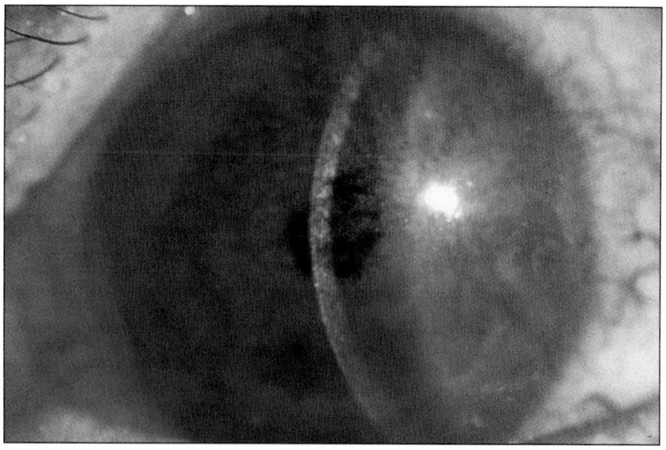

Fig. 18.12 Needle-like cystine crystal deposition in cystinosis.

Deposition of needle-like cystine crystals in the cornea and conjunctiva is usually seen by 1 year of age.[17] Deposits start centrally and progress until the entire cornea becomes involved (Fig. 18.12). Corneal irritation and erosions often occur, leading to photophobia and pain. The most severe form, which is infantile, is usually associated with death from renal failure in early childhood.[48,66] Other complications include hypothyroidism, pancreatic endocrine insufficiency, myopathy, and neurologic deficits.

Lubrication and therapeutic contact lenses can be employed in the treatment of corneal erosions caused by cystinosis. Cysteamine (beta-mercaptoethylamine) 0.5% topical solution has been used as a cystine-depleting therapy.[66,68] It has also been used after penetrating keratoplasty to prevent the redeposition of cystine crystals in the transplanted tissue. Additionally, cysteamine has also been used to reduce pain associated with corneal erosions. Trials with oral cysteamine have not proved beneficial.[67] If the corneal opacity becomes severe and does not respond to cysteamine, penetrating keratoplasty is indicated. Recurrence of crystalline deposits has been reported after penetrating keratoplasty.[65]

Fabry's disease

This is a sphingolipidosis caused by a lack of alfa-galactosidase A. It has X-linked recessive inheritance and it has been genetically mapped to chromosome Xq22. This is a multisystem disease characterized by angiokeratomatous skin lesions and may involve the genitourinary, nervous, musculoskeletal, and cardiovascular systems. It is not present at birth. Spaeth and Frost[71] have emphasized that the ophthalmologist is in an excellent position to diagnose Fabry's disease because the eye findings are conspicuous. Corneal opacities occur in 90% of cases, conjunctival vascular changes in 60%, retinal vessel tortuosity in 55%, and cataracts in only 50% of patients.[71] Corneal opacities are found in males and in many heterozygous females with the disease when other manifestations are very slight.[72] They occur as early as 6 months of age[71] and are due to the deposition of glycosphingolipid in the corneal epithelium, which coats the cornea with a diffuse, delicate haze. In more advanced cases the opacities are seen as fine, curving, creamy white lines radiating from a point below the center of the cornea, or as a fine whorl-like superficial corneal opacity, termed cornea verticillata.[72,73] Enzyme replacement therapy, using agalsidase alfa enzyme, may improve pain and stabilize renal and cardiac function, but is not yet approved for use in the United States.[74]

Tyrosinemia

There are five clinical syndromes in which elevated serum and urinary tyrosine levels and their metabolites can be detected, but only tyrosinemia type II is associated with corneal opacity.

Tyrosinemia type II (Richner–Hanhart syndrome) is a rare congenital error of metabolism characterized by a triad of dendriform keratitis, hyperkeratotic lesions of the palms and soles, and mental retardation.[75–77] Many of the early reported cases of this disease were in patients who were the product of consanguineous marriages, suggesting a possible autosomal recessive inheritance.[76,77] Ocular symptoms of photophobia and lacrimation in both eyes usually appear during the first few months of life. The affected patient has bilateral subepithelial central corneal ulcers with coarse dendritic branching, figures that may suggest herpes simplex and may develop with time into round whitish opacities with superficial new vessel formation.[77,78] The corneal ulceration probably results from the accumulation of intracellular crystals, presumably tyrosine. These crystals have been shown to enlarge, lacerate and rupture the cell, attract lysosomal enzymes, and trigger the inflammatory cycles.

The keratitis found in tyrosinemia type II can be distinguished from herpes simplex keratitis by its morphologic appearance, bilateral presentation, lack of response to antiviral therapy, and associated systemic findings.[75] Therefore, an infant or young child with bilateral dendritic keratitis should undergo serum and urinary evaluation for elevated levels of tyrosine and its metabolic byproducts. Ocular abnormalities can be reversed by restricting the intake of phenylalanine and tyrosine.[24]

The diagnosis of tyrosinemia type II may be confirmed by amino acid analysis of the blood and urine, which shows an increase of tyrosine and its metabolites only. The enzymatic basis of the syndrome is a defect in soluble hepatic cytosol tyrosine aminotransferase, whose gene has been mapped to chromosome 16 (16q22.1-q22.3).[76,79]

Gangliosidoses

The gangliosidoses are metabolic neurodegenerative diseases involving defects in ganglioside degradation. Gangliosides are glycosphingolipids that contain sialic acid in their oligosaccharide chain. These lipids are present in most cell types of the body. They are found in the greatest concentration in neurons and are of the highest content in the brain. Disorders of ganglioside degradation resulting in abnormal accumulation and storage of these glycolipids are of two major types: GM1 and GM2. GM1 is an autosomal recessive disorder that has been reported to cause mild congenital corneal opacity.[79]

Miscellaneous Syndromes

Fetal alcohol syndrome

Fetal alcohol syndrome occurs in the offspring of alcoholic mothers. Alcohol is thought to have a teratogenic effect on anterior segment structures during a critical period of their development.[80] The child may have cloudy corneas at birth, and pathologic studies have found malformations in Descemet's membrane and endothelium with secondary corneal edema.[81,82] Corneal abnormalities in infants with fetal alcohol syndrome (FAS) include Peters' anomaly with classic iridocorneal adhesions, Axenfeld–Rieger syndrome, and diffuse corneal clouding.[83]

The diagnosis of FAS is made historically and clinically. Facial abnormalities, mental retardation, lower weight and height, various cardiovascular and skeletal abnormalities, along with a history of maternal alcohol abuse, should alert the clinician to the possibility of FAS. The neonate's urine can be tested for the presence of alcohol. If positive, the diagnosis can be made with certainty.

If the corneal opacification is severe enough to warrant treatment, penetrating keratoplasty can be performed. If the corneal abnormality is Peters' anomaly, treatment and prognosis are similar to those that will be described in the discussion of Peters' anomaly.

Fryns syndrome

Fryns syndrome is a multiple congenital anomaly syndrome, with characteristic features including Dandy–Walker malformation, cleft lip and palate, diaphragmatic hernia, lung hypoplasia, cardiac defects, renal cysts, urinary tract malformations, distal limb anomalies, polydramnios, and neonatal death.[84,85] Congenital corneal opacity, irregularities of Bowman's layer, thickened posterior capsule, microphthalmia, and retinal dysplasia are associated with this autosomal recessive anomaly, which therefore must be considered in the differential diagnosis of congenital corneal opacity.

The corneal clouding may be caused by corneal endothelial dysfunction with abnormal composition of Descemet's membrane, as documented previously.[86]

Cerebro-oculofacio-skeletal syndrome

The cerebro-oculofacio-skeletal syndrome is associated with multiple ocular abnormalities, including congenital corneal clouding, microphthalmos, cataracts, and blepharophimosis.[87,88] Other findings in this disorder include microcephaly, hypotonia, micrognathia, widely set nipples, camptodactyly, flexure contractures at the elbows and knees, generalized osteoporosis, dysplastic acetabula, coxa valga, and vertical talus manifesting as rocker-bottom feet.[88] The diagnosis is made clinically in consultation with a pediatric genetics specialist. Corneal transplantation has been performed for the corneal clouding.[87]

Posterior Corneal Defect (STUM *P* ED)

The term anterior segment dysgenesis replaced the original classification of anterior chamber cleavage syndrome and

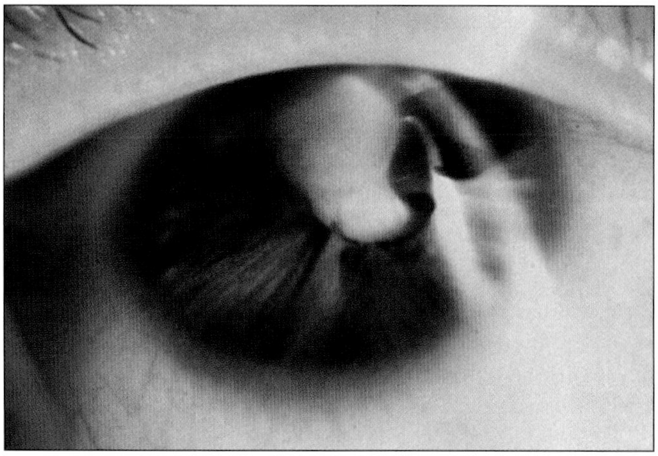

Fig. 18.13 Peters' anomaly patient with synechiae from the iris collarette to the edge of the posterior corneal defect.

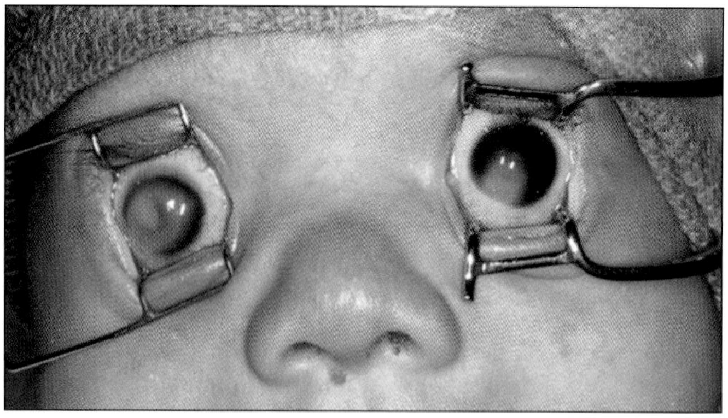

Fig. 18.14 Peters' anomaly infant with bilateral and asymmetric disease.

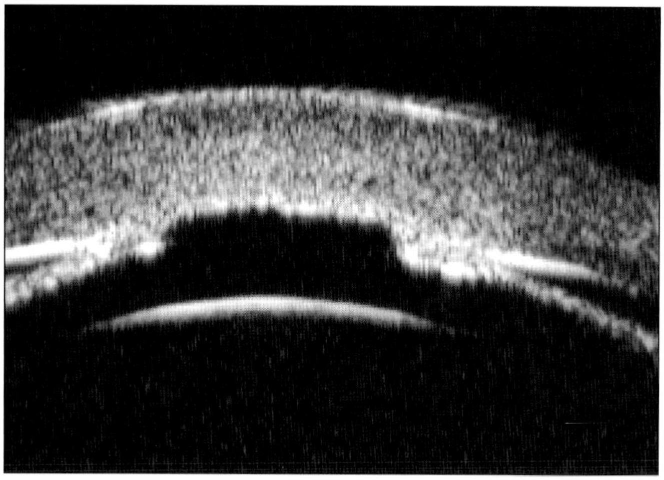

Fig. 18.15 UBM image of Peters' anomaly showing central posterior stromal defect with iridocorneal adhesions. (Courtesy of Elisabeth L. Affel, MS.)

refers to a spectrum of congenital eye conditions that are associated with posterior defects of the cornea. They can be peripheral or central. Peripheral abnormalities are not covered in this chapter because they are associated with insignificant congenital opacity of the cornea. Unlike the peripheral abnormalities, in which the abnormal anatomy is visible, the central anomalies are characterized by a focal absence of the corneal endothelium and Descemet's membrane, which results in an overlying corneal opacity.[9] This leukoma often obscures other anterior segment abnormalities.

The central abnormalities are often classified into three groups: Peters' anomaly, posterior keratoconus, and congenital anterior staphyloma.[9] Peters' anomaly is the most common congenital opacity presenting to the tertiary cornea specialist, followed in frequency by sclerocornea, corneal dermoids, congenital glaucoma, microphthalmia, birth trauma, and metabolic disease.[89]

Peters' anomaly (STUM *P* ED)

This congenital disorder is characterized by a central corneal opacity with corresponding defects in the posterior stroma, Descemet's membrane, and the endothelium.[9,90] The peripheral cornea is usually relatively clear.[91] Synechiae frequently extend from the iris collarette to the edge of the posterior corneal defect (Fig. 18.13). The iris strands can appear as filaments, thicker bands, or broad sheets which form an arcuate iridocorneal adhesion. Lens abnormalities, including cataract and central corneolenticular adhesion, as well as corneal staphyloma, are variably present.[92,93] The corneolenticular adhesion, when present, can be difficult to diagnose clinically because of the overlying leukoma. Incomplete development of the angle is common, helping to explain the high frequency of glaucoma (50–80%), which may present at birth or may develop later. The cornea is usually avascular.

Usually occurring bilaterally (80% of cases), but often asymmetrically (Fig. 18.14), Peters' anomaly may vary morphologically from its most simple presentation, described as Peters' anomaly type I (corneal opacity with iridocorneal adhesion),[94,95] to more severe cases, Peters' type II, with involvement of the lens and other ocular anomalies, in addition to the corneal opacity and iridocorneal synechiae (Table 18.5).[93] The corneal opacity (and the corresponding defect in Descemet's membrane and endothelium) coincides with the area of the corneolenticular contact.

Histopathologic findings used to be the only tool to help the diagnosis of Peters' anomaly in cases in which the leukoma was severe, but UBM has been demonstrated to be very useful, clearly detecting central corneal edema and absence of Descemet's membrane, as well as corneolenticular and iridocorneal adhesions when present (Fig. 18.15).[96] The histopathologic changes can be present in all layers of the central cornea (Fig. 18.16; Box 18.3).

Historically, the internal ulcer of Von Hippel has also been grouped with Peters' anomaly, but the former is

Table 18.5 Peters' anomaly types I and II

Type I	Type II
Corneal opacity + iridocorneal adhesions – unilateral involvement predominates – mild/dense central stromal nebular opacity bordered by iris strands that cross the anterior chamber from the iris collarette – peripheral cornea is usually clear, but peripheral edema or scleralization may be present – peripheral edema can regress (especially if associated with glaucoma successfully treated) – lens generally clear and in normal position – usually isolated – associated ocular anomalies may be present (microcornea, sclerocornea, and infantile glaucoma) – vitreoretinal abnormalities rare – good visual acuity potential – **systemic abnormalities** are uncommon	**Corneal opacity + iridocorneal adhesions + lens abnormality (position or transparency)** – denser corneal opacity – most frequently bilateral – thought to be secondary in nature, rarely demonstrating a primary hereditary pattern[94] – keratolenticular adherence varies **Most characteristic**: the lens directly adherent to the posterior corneal surface or firmly pressed against it Other cases: cortex or only lens fragments adhere to the corneal defect, the lens is in position but is cataractous – Severe ocular and systemic malformations – **Ocular abnormalities**: microphthalamic with vitreoretinal abnormalities (PHPV*), microcornea, cornea plana, glaucoma, sclerocornea, colobomas, aniridia, and optic atrophy – **Systemic conditions**: congenital cardiac defects, craniofacial dysplasia, skeletal abnormalities, and central nervous system and urogenital anomalies Other systemic conditions: external ear anomalies, pulmonary hypoplasia, syndactyly or polydactyly, camptodactyly, fetal transfusion syndrome, Wilms' tumor[91] Peters'-plus syndrome:[98] Peters' anomaly + short stature, brachymorphy, mental retardation, abnormal ears, and, in some patients, cleft lip and palate)[122] Krause-Kivlin syndrome:[99–100] Peters' anomaly + facial abnormalities, disproportionate short stature, retarded skeletal maturation and developmental delay (probably inherited in an autosomal recessive manner)

* *Persistent hyperplastic primary vitreous*

Box 18.3 Histopathology of Peters' anomaly

Central concave defect in the posterior corneal stroma (posterior ulcer)

Disorderly stromal lamellae in ulcer bed

Absence of corneal endothelium and Descemet's membrane in the posterior ulcer

Corresponding area of central corneal edema and opacification

Keratolenticular adhesions to posterior cornea in some cases

Iridocorneal adhesions to margin of ulcer in some cases

Bowman's layer thickened or absent

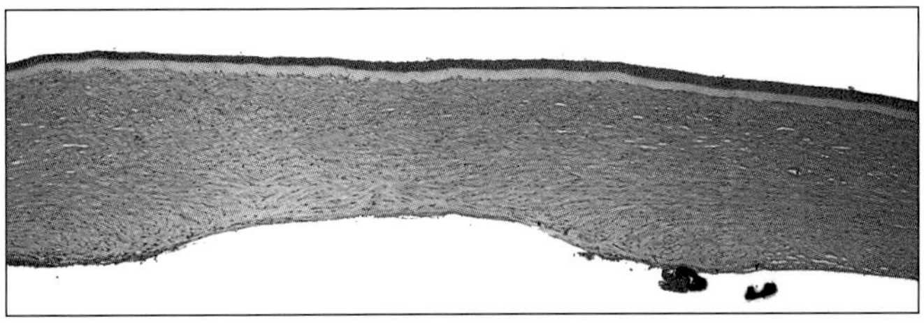

Fig. 18.16 Histopathology of Peters' anomaly (see also Box 18.3).

probably an intrauterine inflammatory condition rather than a true developmental defect, and it has been considered in the differential diagnosis of Peters' anomaly.[91] However, some authorities believe the posterior ulcer of Von Hippel to be identical to Peters' anomaly without lens abnormalities. Other conditions in the differential diagnosis of Peters' anomaly include sclerocornea, dermoid, congenital hereditary endothelial dystrophy (CHED), and posterior polymorphous corneal dystrophy (PPCD) (Table 18.6).

There are several proposed causes of Peters' anomaly (Box 18.4). The most often documented is the incomplete central migration of corneogenic mesenchyme (i.e., neural crest cells), accounting for posterior endothelial and stromal defects.[97] Goldenhar's syndrome is also due to the maldevelopment of neural crest cells and has been documented in association with Peters' anomaly.[97] Intrauterine infection, maternal alcoholism, and other teratogenic exposures can also be associated with Peters' anomaly (Box 18.4).[98]

Peters' anomaly occurs most often as a sporadic disorder; however, both recessive and dominant inheritance patterns have been observed. Hereditary syndromes featuring Peters' anomaly type II as the only anterior segment disturbance include Krause–Kivlin syndrome[99,100] and Peters'-plus syndrome (see Table 18.5). The diagnosis of Krause–Kivlin syndrome should be considered in any child with anterior segment anomaly who is small for gestational age or who develops short stature.[98] Mutations in the eye development genes *PAX6*, *PITX2*, *CYP1B1*, and *FOXC1* have been implicated in Peters' anomaly.[101]

The clinician dealing with an infant affected by Peters' anomaly should be aware of the possible associated malformations, obtain a thorough family history, and examine the eyes of the parents and the siblings. These patients should be screened for systemic malformations, especially those involving midline body structures such as the pituitary gland and the heart.[102] The management of these children should involve a multidisciplinary approach, including corneal and pediatric ophthalmologists, social workers, and – first and foremost – committed and informed parents.[103]

Table 18.6 Peters' anomaly – differential diagnosis

Peters' anomaly	Von Hippel's internal corneal ulcer	Sclerocornea	Dermoids	CHED	PPCD
Opacification central and localized	Inflammation characterizes von Hippel's internal corneal ulcer, differentiating it from Peters' anomaly	Diffuse full-thickness	Yellowish-white vascularized elevated nodules inferotemporal at the limbus junction may contain hair follicles, sebaceous and sweat glands, smooth and skeletal muscle, nerves, blood vessels, bone, cartilage, and teeth	Diffuse edema Absence of iris abnormalities 2 to 3 (up to 5) times normal thickness	Less edema than CHED but also diffuse; usually normal pachymetry
Iris strands attached to leukoma		More pronounced peripherally	Usually unilateral		Corneal changes in parents
Lens normal or abnormal			Can be central and often appear to have satellite lesions		
Normal peripheral endothelium and Descemet's membrane					

Box 18.4 Proposed causes of Peters' anomaly

Isolated Peters' anomaly
- Autosomal recessive defect
- Autosomal dominant defect
- Chromosomal defect
- Homeotic gene defect*

Peters' anomaly with other ocular malformations
- Monogenic defect
- Developmental field defect
- Homeolitic gene defect*

Peters' anomaly with systemic malformation
- Well-delineated single-gene disorders
- Developmental field defect
- Contiguous gene syndrome
- Homeolitic gene defect*

Teratogenic effects of alcohol, rubella virus, or retinoic acid

** Genes that control differentiation of primordial cells and the development of different body segments.*

Genetic counseling should take into consideration the fact that autosomal recessive inheritance is possible.

When glaucoma develops in infancy, it is treated surgically. In older children, medical therapy should be used initially. If the Peters' anomaly is bilateral and visually disabling, corneal transplantation is often required to provide a clear visual axis and to try to restore vision. If a cataract is also present and has to be removed, the prognosis is worse.[91] Glaucoma represents the most common complication after the surgery. Penetrating keratoplasty and combined placement of a Molteno implant has been described with success,[104] although it may be preferable to control the pressure first.

Theoretically, surgery at the youngest age possible would be best to minimize the risk of deprivation amblyopia, but the decision to operate at a young age should be made by considering the risks of undergoing general anesthesia (for the initial surgery and multiple EUAs for suture removal over 2 months postoperatively), as well as associated systemic abnormalities and the general health of the patient.

The management of Peters' and pediatric penetrating keratoplasty is discussed in detail in Chapter 57.

Posterior keratoconus (STUM *P* ED)

Posterior keratoconus is a very uncommon corneal abnormality characterized by a discrete local conical internal protrusion of the posterior corneal curvature with concomitant stromal thinning and variable haze. The lesion is usually circumscribed, crater-like, round or oval, and occurs centrally or eccentrically, singly or multiply. It may represent the mildest variant of Peters' anomaly.[9] It has no relationship to anterior keratoconus.

The defect in posterior keratoconus is usually central. Sometimes pigment surrounds the edges of the posterior depression, suggesting previous contact with the iris.[9] Posterior synechiae may rarely be seen in the affected area. The condition is usually focal, but can rarely occur in a generalized form, with the concavity involving the entire posterior surface of the cornea.

The condition is most commonly unilateral but may be bilateral.[9] It is nonprogressive and usually sporadic. Familial and posttraumatic cases have been reported. The pathogenesis and causes of this condition are unclear. Descemet's excrescences can also be present in or just outside of the area of involvement.[105] The corneal endothelium and Descemet's membrane are present. On histologic examination Descemet's membrane may be thinned, with a concomitant endothelial abnormality in the focally abnormal area.

Although the irregularity of the posterior cornea may affect vision to some extent, approximately 85% of the refractive power of the cornea is produced by the anterior surface, which is usually normal and uniform throughout the cornea. Keratometry and photokeratoscopy provide an incomplete picture of the surface geometry of posterior keratoconus, and more recent studies done with corneal topography evaluation detected changes on the anterior corneal curvature. Rao and Padmanabhan[106] demonstrated that posterior keratoconus manifests significant corneal surface alterations and that the changes in central and paracentral posterior keratoconus appear to progress with an increase in patient age. Mannis et al.[107] used topographic analysis to study the cornea of a patient with posterior keratoconus and demonstrated a central steepened 'cone' coincident with the area of circumscribed posterior keratoconus, as well as paracentral flattening.

Posterior keratoconus is commonly isolated but it can be associated with other ocular abnormalities, such as astigmatism, choroidal and/or retinal sclerosis, lens abnormalities, posterior polymorphous dystrophy, retinal coloboma, optic nerve hypoplasia, and ptosis. Systemic abnormalities can also be present, including mental retardation, hypertelorism, superiorly displaced lateral canthi, short stature, and genitourinary abnormalities.[108]

Visual acuity can be reduced due to amblyopia, refractive errors, or astigmatism, but vision is usually acceptable and keratoplasty is rarely indicated. Correction of refractive errors may be all that is needed to attain useful vision.

Congenital anterior staphyloma (STUM *P* ED)

Congenital anterior staphyloma (CAS) is characterized by a protuberant congenital corneal opacity.[109] The ectatic cornea often has a blue hue. It may extend beyond the plane of the eyelids, and secondary epithelial metaplasia into keratinized, stratified, squamous epithelium occurs. The anterior segment frequently is disproportionately enlarged and extremely disorganized. There is virtually no possibility of attaining useful vision. One or both eyes may be involved.

The lesion can be vascularized and can transilluminate easily.[9] The posterior portions of the thin cornea are usually lined by the remaining pigment epithelium of the atrophic iris.

As in Peters' anomaly, the lens may be adherent to the posterior cornea. The pathogenesis of CAS is unknown, but the condition is thought to be secondary to an intrauterine infection or related to a developmental abnormality such as a severe type of Peters' anomaly.[94] In several cases one eye showed a frank staphyloma while the other demonstrated a Peters' anomaly type II. In the CAS developmental abnormality there is failure of migration of mesenchymal tissues that ordinarily form the posterior corneal structures, iris, and angle. This maldevelopment, probably coupled with increased intraocular pressure caused by the angle abnormality, leads to corneal opacity and thinning, plus prominent buphthalmic enlargement of the entire anterior segment. Hereditary cases have been reported.

The diagnosis is made clinically and can be confirmed histopathologically if enucleation is performed. Descemet's membrane, Bowman's layer, and endothelium are typically absent.

The visual prognosis of CAS is very poor. Enucleation or evisceration may be considered in an attempt to improve cosmesis.

Endothelial Dystrophy (STUMP *E* D)

Three corneal dystrophies may exhibit diffuse corneal cloudiness at birth: congenital hereditary endothelial dystrophy, posterior polymorphous corneal dystrophy, and congenital stromal corneal dystrophy.

Congenital hereditary endothelial dystrophy

Congenital hereditary endothelial dystrophy (CHED), first documented in the English literature in 1960 by Maumenee, is a rare disease that that has two forms (see Box 18.5): CHED 1 and CHED 2.[110,111] The nomenclature for CHED and all corneal dystrophies has recently been standardized by the International Committee on the Classification of Corneal Dystrophies (IC3D).[111] CHED 1 is an autosomal dominant dystrophy, with its genetic locus at 20p11.2-q11. This has its onset in the first or second year of life, but is occasionally congenital. In these patients, corneal clouding ranges from a diffuse haze to a ground-glass, milky appearance. The corneal clouding is slowly progressive over 1–10 years. Patients usually present with photophobia and epiphora and the subsequent development of corneal clouding. The epiphora and photophobia resolve with the onset of clouding. Progressive diffuse corneal opacification develops, with an irregular edematous epithelial surface, scarring of Bowman's layer, and thickening of the stroma. The degree of clouding is usually symmetric, but occasionally one eye is more adversely affected.[112] The visual impairment in the dominant form is not initially as severe as in the recessive form, and patients therefore do not usually develop nystagmus.

CHED 2, previously referred to as Maumenee cornea dystrophy, is autsomal recessive and results from mutations in

Box 18.5 CHED 1 vs CHED 2

CHED 1
- Autosomal dominant
- Appears within the first 2 years of life
- Slowly progressive
- Pain, tearing, and photophobia
- Parents may have PPMD changes

CHED 2
- Autosomal recessive form
- Present at birth
- Nonprogressive nystagmus

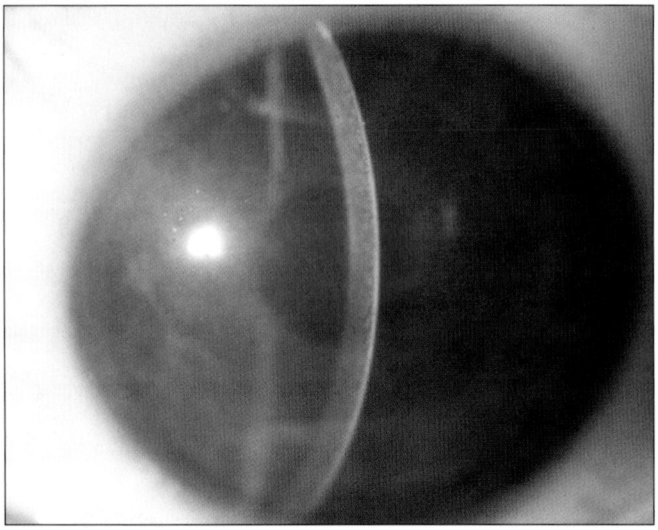

Fig. 18.17 Congenital hereditary endothelial dystrophy (CHED) with ground-glass diffuse stromal edema.

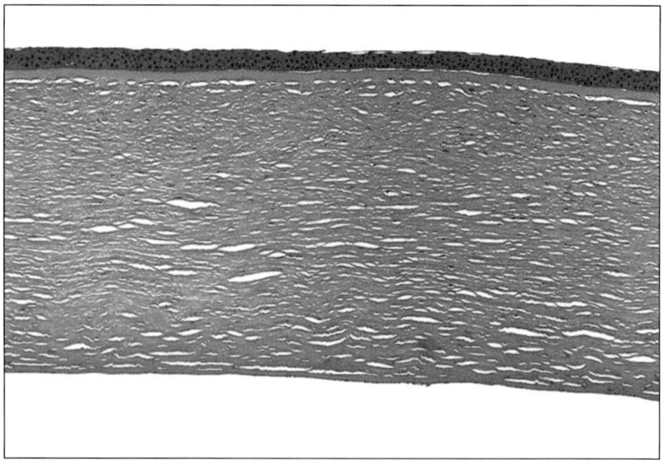

Fig. 18.18 Histopathology of CHED (see also Box 18.6).

the solute carrier family, located on chromosome 20p13.[111] This form of CHED generally presents as bilateral corneal clouding at birth or shortly thereafter.[113] The corneal changes are stable and do not progress or regress. There are no associated symptoms, such as epiphora or photophobia, but patients often develop nystagmus because of the severity of the early visual loss. Occasionally, visual acuity is retained despite considerable corneal clouding. On slit lamp examination the epithelium appears roughened secondary to nonbullous epithelial edema. The stroma is often two to three times normal thickness and has a diffuse blue-gray, ground-glass haze (Fig. 18.17). The endothelium is generally difficult to observe because of the stromal haze. If seen, the endothelium is atrophic, irregular, or absent, and Descemet's membrane is thickened without guttae (Box 18.6; Fig. 18.18).

The differential diagnosis of CHED includes congenital glaucoma, posterior polymorphous corneal dystrophy (PPCD), Peters' anomaly, and inborn errors of metabolism, especially the mucopolysaccharidoses (Table 18.7). Both CHED and congenital glaucoma originate from defects in the neural crest cell contribution to the development of the anterior segment of the eye. Bahn et al.[114] state that congenital glaucoma is a result of abnormal crest cell migration, whereas CHED results from abnormal crest cell differentiation. Differentiating CHED from congenital glaucoma can be particularly difficult because measurement of the intraocular pressure may give unreliable results in the presence of stromal edema, and if severe corneal opacity has developed the optic disks cannot be inspected.[114,115] These two entities may rarely coexist,[116] but inappropriate glaucoma surgery in CHED has been reported.[117]

It is important to distinguish between CHED and PPCD because the edema in posterior polymorphous corneal dystrophy may show slow clearing, so that penetrating keratoplasty may not be needed.[118]

Although the edema sometimes remains stationary, it usually progresses, and penetrating keratoplasty has been the recommended treatment of CHED to avoid amblyopia and restore vision.

Box 18.6 Histopathology of CHED[125,137]

The main characteristics are the severely degenerated corneal endothelial cells and abnormal thickening of Descemet's membrane

Changes in the epithelium, Bowman's layer, and the stroma are considered to be secondary to longstanding edema

Stromal lamellae irregular and separated by fluid pockets

Descemet's membrane: anterior banded zone normal; posterior nonbanded zone with aberrant collagen fibrils

Corneal endothelium atrophy with vacuolation, focal absence of cells and many multinucleated cells; melanin deposition can be present

Adapted from Witschel H et al. Congenital hereditary stromal dystrophy of the cornea. Arch Ophthalmol. *1978;96(6):1043–1051 and O'Grady RB, Kirk HQ: Corneal Keloids, Am J Ophthalmol 1972;73:206.*

Posterior polymorphous corneal dystrophy (PPCD)

Most reports on posterior polymorphous corneal dystrophy (PPCD) are based on adolescent or adult patients. PPCD is inherited as an autosomal dominant condition with variable expression in the vast majority of cases.[111]

Most patients with PPCD have bilateral, nonprogressive, asymptomatic disease that rarely requires penetrating keratoplasty. The pathogenesis of both CHED 1 and PPCD is considered to be due to a primary dysfunction of corneal endothelium.[110] These two entities also share clinical, histological, and embryological similarities, but significant differences between the phenotypic expression of these disorders exist (Table 18.7).

The severity and nature of the resulting endothelial dysfunction, which may be genetically controlled, ultimately determine the range of clinical signs that manifest in the form of CHED or PPCD.[110] PPCD is a milder disease

Table 18.7 Differential diagnosis of CHED

CHED	CSCD	PPCD	Congenital glaucoma	Birth trauma	Peters' anomaly	Mucopolysaccharidosis
Isolated disorder	Corneal opacity: central and flaky, feathery appearance	Less edema	Enlarged corneal diameter	Patchy corneal edema from rupture of Descemet's membrane	Central and localized opacity	Corneal clouding is not usually seen at birth
Cornea avascular	Normal pachymetry	Usually normal pachymetry	Increased ultrasonic axial length measurements		Normal peripheral endothelium and Descemet's membrane	Conjunctival biopsy may be helpful
Eye is not inflamed		More common than CHED	Elevated IOP			Raised levels of mucopolysaccharide in the urine
Absence of iris abnormalities		Corneal changes in parents	Haab's striae appear after the edema clears with the lowering of IOP			
Corneal edema: – diffuse – nonbullous – vary from a blue-gray ground-glass appearance to total corneal opacification						
Pachymetry: 2–3 times normal thickness						
Less common than PPCD but more likely to require surgery						

characterized clinically by the presence of grouped vesicles or bands, geographic-shaped discrete gray lesions, and broad bands with scalloped edges and vesicles on the endothelial surface of the cornea (Fig. 18.19). Descemet's membrane can be irregular and have a nodular or warty appearance.[119] These findings can be confirmed with specular microscopy.[119]

Although most patients with PPCD are asymptomatic, there is a form of PPCD characterized by congenital corneal edema which appears as a diffuse corneal haze at birth. In a review of eight families with PPCD, Cibis et al.[120] found great variation ranging from mild endothelial defects to severe stromal and epithelial edema (Fig. 18.20). The largest published series of PPCD is that of Krachmer,[121] who reported on clinical and pathological findings in 13 patients. Sometimes the cornea can be so opacified as to preclude detailed examination of the endothelium. The epithelium can be irregular, with a thickened stroma and deep feathery opacities (Fig. 18.20). If the endothelium is visible or the edema clears, findings are the same as those in adult PPCD described above. Nystagmus is present if the visual loss is significant.

It is important to differentiate PPCD from CHED, because the treatment is different. Some children with PPCD have experienced clearing of their corneal edema, eliminating the need for penetrating keratoplasty.[122] Examination of the child's parents may be helpful in making the diagnosis.[121] Despite the absence of significant symptoms, one of the parent's corneas will generally demonstrate the features of PPCD.

Several different loci have been identified in PPCD, including 20p11.2-q11.2, 1p34.3-p32.3, and 10p11.2. CHED 1 and PPCD share the 20p11.2-q11.2 locus. It has been proposed that CHED 1 may be allelic to PPCD.[123,124]

If the cornea does not clear spontaneously, penetrating keratoplasty should be performed. One review of corneal transplantation in children suggests that patients with congenital corneal opacities from PPCD have a better visual prognosis after surgery than patients with other causes of congenital corneal clouding.

The histopathology of PPCD demonstrates epithelialization of endothelial cells (Fig. 18.21),[120] with multilayered cells linked by desmosomes with surface microvilli and intracytoplasmic filaments.

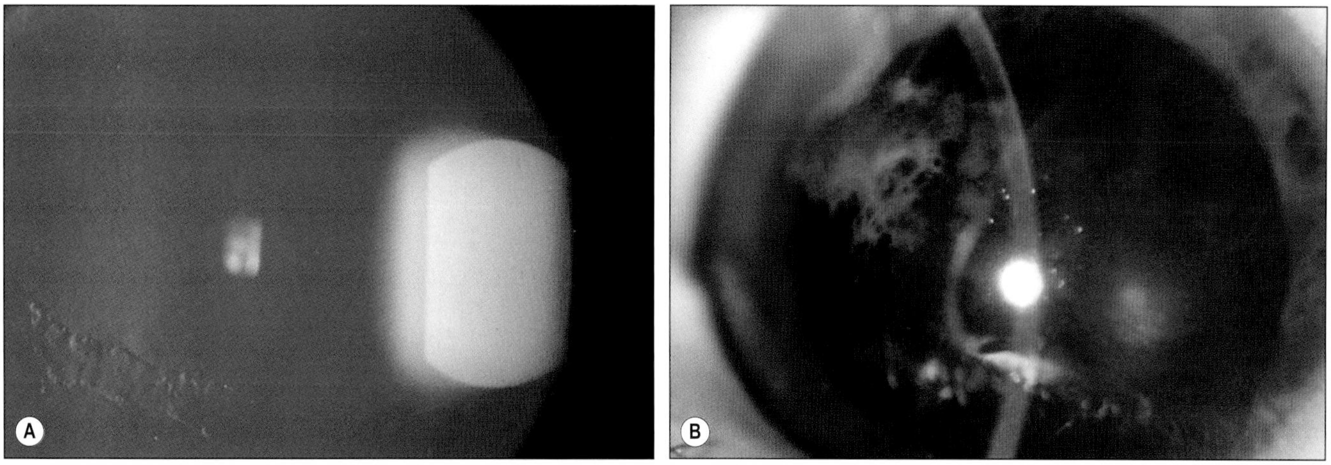

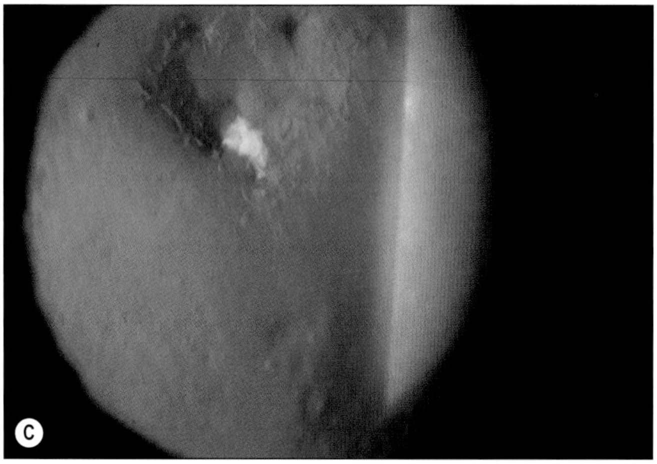

Fig. 18.19 PPCD. Geographic shape lesions and broad band vesicles: mild PPCD changes on retroillumination (**A**), and direct (**B**) and retroillumination (**C**) of moderate PPCD changes.

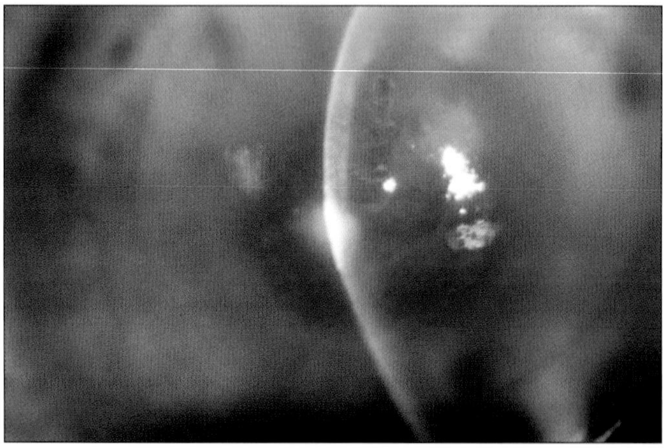

Fig. 18.20 Severe stromal and epithelial edema in a patient with advanced PPCD.

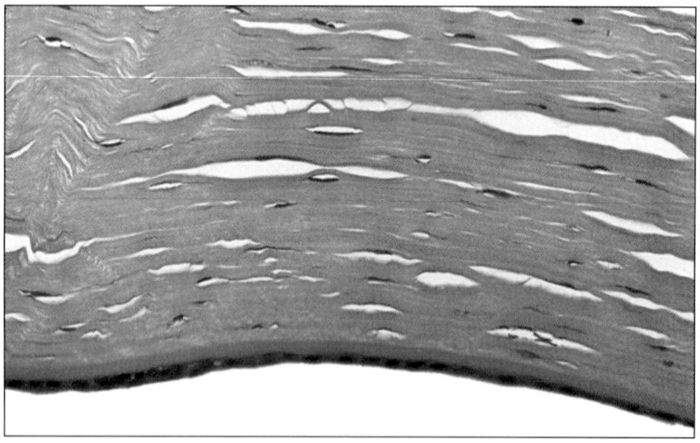

Fig. 18.21 Histopathology of PPCD showing epithelialization of endothelial cells.

Congenital stromal corneal dystrophy (CSCD)

Previously referred to as congenital hereditary stromal dystrophy, this is a rare dystrophy caused by a mutation on the decorin gene on chromosome 12.[111] It was thought that all hereditary congenital corneal dystrophies were caused by endothelial dysfunction until a report by Witschel et al.[125] demonstrated a true CSCD in a small number of dominant pedigrees.

The anterior stroma demonstrates a diffuse, flaky-feathery opacification caused by corneal lamellar irregularities that are denser centrally and anteriorly than peripherally and posteriorly. The changes are stationary from birth. Nystagmus and esotropia are often present secondary to the profound visual loss. The corneal thickness is normal, and the epithelium, Descemet's membrane, and endothelium appear normal. There are no associated systemic abnormalities.

If the clinical diagnosis of CSCD is in doubt, the histopathologic features of the corneal button are typical and usually result in accurate diagnosis. The histologic abnormalities are confined to the stroma. The anterior banded layer of Descemet's membrane is missing. This abnormality is questionably caused by early dysfunction of the endothelium that becomes normal later. The epithelium, basement membrane, Bowman's layer, endothelium, and posterior banded layer of Descemet's membrane are normal.

As with CHED, no medical therapy is available for CSCD. Penetrating keratoplasty can be performed if the corneal opacification is severe.

Other dystrophies

Posterior amorphous corneal dystrophy (PACD) is a rare autosomal dominant dystrophy characterized by bilateral sheet-like opacification of the posterior stroma in association with corneal flattening and thinning.[126,127] Other ocular findings include hyperopia, marked corneal astigmatism, and progressive ectasia of the cornea.[128] Dunn et al.[129] recognized other features, such as anterior iris surface and stromal abnormalities, fine iris processes extending to Schwalbe's line for 360°, and extension of the opacity to the limbus. No abnormalities of the endothelium were detected, and visual acuity was only mildly affected. The condition appears to be nonprogressive.

Two forms of the disease were documented by Moshegov: a centroperipheral and a peripheral form. The first is more severe and usually presents with keratometry readings below 41 diopters and central corneal thicknesses less than 0.5 mm, and the latter represents a less severe peripheral form with less hyperopia, some slight myopia, and keratometry readings above 41 diopters, but the central corneal thicknesses are similar to those with the centroperipheral form. Although the centroperipheral form of posterior amorphous corneal dystrophy is more likely to lead to presentation, most patients are asymptomatic. Castelo Branco et al.[130] recently reported two cases of PACD in the same family in which they studied the depth of stromal opacification using UBM.

This dystrophy can be very subtle in its appearance and easily overlooked. This led Moshegov et al.[127] to suspect that the prevalence of this condition is higher than the few reports in the ophthalmic literature suggest. Bowman's layer dysgenesis has been reported as a cause of congenital cloudy cornea.[131] It cannot be classified as a dystrophy because its inheritance is unknown. It presents as bilateral, noninflammatory, progressive corneal disease without associated systemic disease.[45]

Congenital Dermoids (STUMPE *D*)

Dermoids are solid benign congenital tumors that frequently arise at the inferotemporal corneoscleral junction. They are classified as choristomas[132] because they contain cellular elements not normally present in that location: ectodermal derivatives, such as hair follicles, as well as sebaceous and sweat glands embedded in connective tissue and covered by squamous epithelium. They can also contain smooth and skeletal muscle, nerves, blood vessels, bone, cartilage, and teeth. In the eye they most often present as yellowish-white, solid, vascularized, elevated nodules straddling the corneal limbus. They vary greatly in size ranging from 2 to 15 mm in diameter.[24] Corneal dermoids occur more commonly as single lesions but may be multiple, and they may be unilateral or bilateral, the former being the more common. Dermoids can be central and often appear to have satellite lesions.

These tumors usually occur in sporadic fashion, although their occurrence in cousins has been described.[133] Corneal dermoids have been genetically mapped to chromosome Xq24-qter. They usually exhibit little or no growth but can occasionally enlarge. They typically extend into the deeper stroma without affecting Descemet's membrane and the endothelium, but in some cases they replace all tissue anterior to the iris pigment epithelium.

Three different types of dermoid choristoma have been characterized according to the extent of involvement (Table 18.8).[134] The grade 1 dermoid is the most frequent type. It is small, usually measuring 5 mm in diameter or less, single, limbal or epibulbar (Fig. 18.22). Already present at birth, it may enlarge, especially at puberty. In general they are

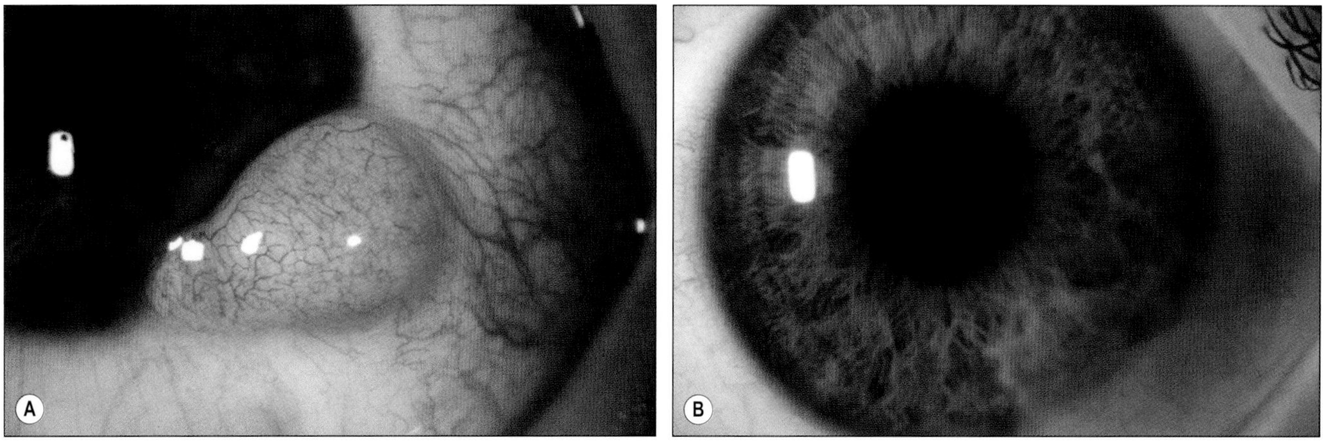

Fig. 18.22 Congenital dermoids. **A**, Limbal dermoid situated in the inferotemporal limbus. **B**, The same dermoid patient after lamellar keratectomy was successfully performed.

Table 18.8 Grading dermoids

Grade 1 (limbal or epibulbar)	Grade 2	Grade 3
– most frequent type	– much larger	– most severe type
– small (5 mm in diameter)	– covers part or entire central corneal surface	– very rare
– single	– varible depth of stromal extension[134]	– entire anterior segment is involved
– inferotemporal limbus	– does not involve Descemet's membrane or the corneal endothelium	– associated abnormalities: microphthalmos, posterior segment abnormalities
– it may enlarge (especially at puberty)		
– superficial		
– one-third of cases associated with Goldenhar's syndrome: nonfamilial; triad of epibulbar dermoids, preauricular appendages, and pretragal fistulas		
– other abnormalities: coloboma of the lids, aniridia, microphthalmos, anophthalmos, neuroparalytic keratitis, lacrimal stenosis, Duane's syndrome, cardiovascular abnormalities, facial hemiatrophy, atresia of the external auditory meatus, accessory auricles, nevus flammeus, and neurofibromatosis.[135]		

superficial, but can rarely involve deeper ocular structures such as the ciliary body or the anterior chamber angle. In approximately one-third of cases these dermoids are associated with a broader syndrome complex such as Goldenhar's syndrome. This syndrome is nonfamilial and consists of congenital abnormalities classically described by the triad of epibulbar dermoids, preauricular appendages, and pretragal fistulas. In one review of the literature, epibulbar dermoids were found in 76% of patients with Goldenhar's syndrome and were almost always located straddling the inferotemporal limbus (Fig. 18.22A).[135]

Other abnormalities associated with dermoids include coloboma of the lids, aniridia, all grades of microphthalmos, anophthalmos, neuroparalytic keratitis, lacrimal stenosis, Duane's syndrome, cardiovascular abnormalities, facial hemiatrophy, atresia of the external auditory meatus, accessory auricles, nevus flammeus, and neurofibromatosis.[135]

The second type, grade 2 dermoid, is much larger, covering part of (Fig. 18.23) or the entire corneal surface, with varible depth of stromal extension.[134] This type generally does not involve Descemet's membrane or the corneal endothelium. It is the most important type in the differential of congenital corneal opacities.

The third and most severe type, grade 3 dermoid, is fortunately the rarest. In this type, the entire anterior segment is involved. The tumor replaces the cornea, anterior chamber, and iris stroma, and is lined posteriorly by the pigment epithelium of the iris. Microphthalmos is common, and posterior segment abnormalities can also occur. Patients develop the different types of corneal dermoid depending on when during gestation the teratogenic effect took place. The earlier the onset, the more severe the malformation.

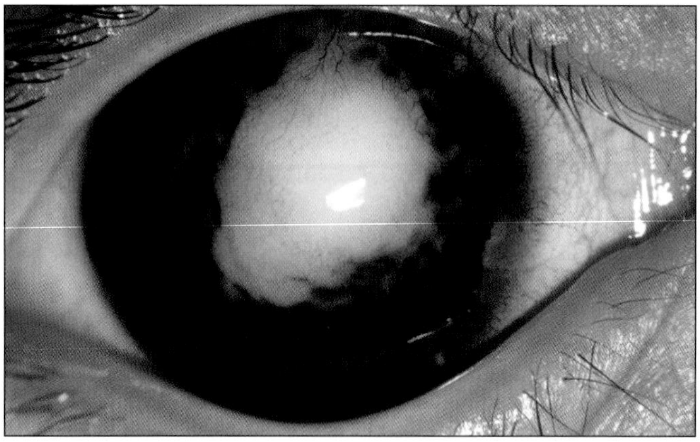

Fig. 18.23 Central dermoid.

Gonioscopic examination of the angle beneath the tumor and UBM (Fig. 18.24) can indicate the depth of extension.

The entities most likely to be confused diagnostically with corneal dermoids are corneal keloids, Peters' anomaly, CHED, and sclerocornea (Table 18.9).[136]

Limbal dermoids are usually a cosmetic rather than a visual problem; however, the vision may be impaired if there is encroachment into the pupillary area by either the tumor or the lipid infiltrate that is often present around the periphery. In some instances, irregular astigmatism appears. If astigmatism is the cause of visual loss in patients with corneal dermoid, correction of refractive errors can be attempted with spectacles, and patching may be necessary

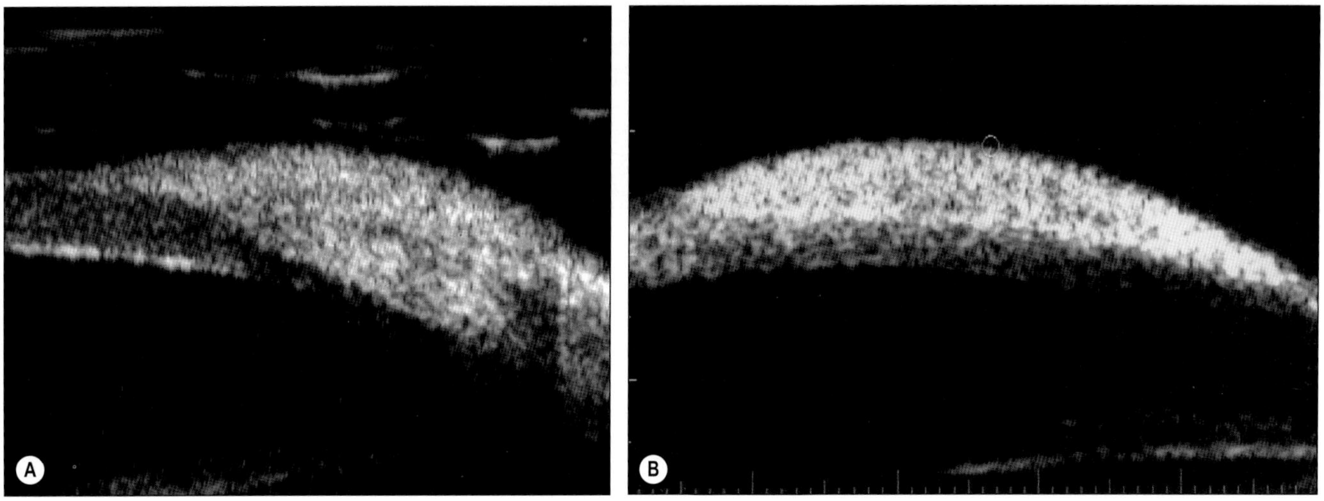

Fig. 18.24 Congenital dermoids. **A**, UBM shows a depth of a dermoid that reaches approximately 90% of the corneal stroma. Whenever excision is to be performed, a penetrating keratoplasty might be necessary. **B**, UBM image of another dermoid that leaves about 0.4 mm of cornea, indicating that in this case lamellar keratoplasty could be performed. (Courtesy of Elisabeth L. Affel, MS.)

Table 18.9 Differential diagnosis of dermoids

Dermoids	Corneal keloids	CHED	Peters' anomaly	Sclerocornea
Yellowish-white vascularized elevated nodules	Chalky white solid masses with glistening gelatinous texture	Diffuse corneal edema bilaterally; cornea is not vascularized; there are never hair follicles present	Corneal opacity + iridocorneal adhesions with or without lens abnormality (position or transparency)	Lost transition between cornea and sclera
– inferotemporal at the limbus junction		Inheritance may be recessive or dominant	– denser corneal opacity	Cornea plana commonly associated
– may contain hair follicles, sebaceous and sweat glands, smooth and skeletal muscle, nerves, blood vessels, bone, cartilage, and teeth			– most frequently bilateral	Peripheral cornea more opacified than central cornea
– usually unilateral				Surface vascularization
– can be central but do not involve the most peripheral cornea (leaving a definite sclerocorneal junction) and often appear to have satellite lesions				

to treat amblyopia. They can also cause irritation (due to a hair or mass effect), or produce drying of the surrounding cornea by lifting of the lid during blinking.

The tumor should be cut flush with the corneal surface (see Fig. 18.24B), but it may recur. If an effort is made to excise the entire tumor, perforation may occur. Therefore, it is advisable to have corneal tissue available. A good but not perfect cosmetic result can be achieved with a lamellar graft. The dermoid tissue is often not solid enough to retain sutures, so grafts must encompass the entire tumor. Dermoids that are incompletely excised can recur.

Dermoids that involve or distort the central cornea (Fig. 18.23) can reduce the quality of the visual image and create amblyopia. If the patient has bilateral visually disabling dermoids, treatment is indicated. If the central cornea is involved (Fig. 18.23), penetrating and lamellar keratoplasty are vision-restoring procedures.

Penetrating keratoplasty can be performed for central dermoids if they are 7 mm or less in diameter. Larger central dermoids require a two-stage procedure: first the tumor is excised and a large lamellar graft is placed in the bed; once that is healed, a smaller central penetrating keratoplasty is

Table 18.10 Differential diagnosis of corneal keloids

Keloid	Dermoid	Salzmann's nodules
White, sometimes protuberant, glistening and jellylike corneal masses	– yellowish-white solid	Not seen at birth
	– vascularized, elevated nodules	– multiple, bluish-white, superficial corneal nodules
	– corneal/scleral junction	– usually in the midperiphery
	May contain: hair follicles, sebaceous and sweat glands, smooth and skeletal muscle, nerves, blood vessels, bone, cartilage, and teeth	– may be related to previous inflammation (phlyctenular disease, vernal keratoconjunctivitis, trachoma, or lues and interstitial keratitis) or in patients with epithelial basement membrane dystrophy, contact lens wear, keratoconus, and after corneal surgery[142]

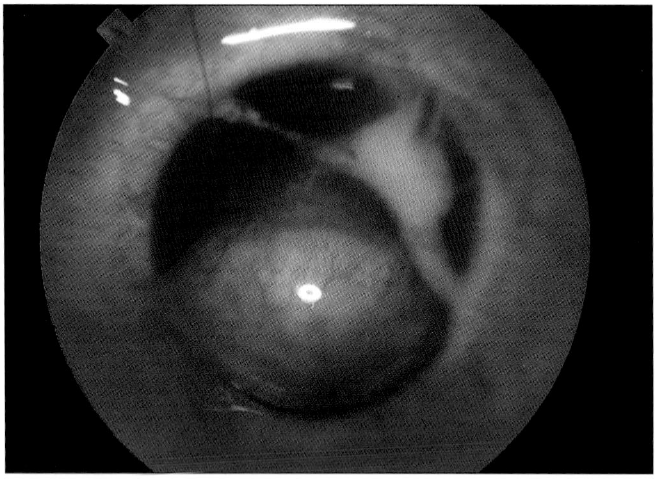

Fig. 18.25 Corneal keloid characterized by a protuberant, glistening corneal mass.

performed. An alternative method can utilize a corneoscleral rim. Operating for cosmetic reasons or mild irritation can be unsuccessful if unsightly scarring occurs.

Histologic examination confirms the diagnosis of the corneal dermoid.

Corneal Keloids

Keloids are reactive fibrous tissue proliferations that represent the exuberant response of embryonic connective tissue to injury.[137] They are thought to be secondary to a vigorous fibrocytic response to corneal perforation or injury.[137] Corneal keloids are seen as white, sometimes protuberant, glistening, masses (Fig. 18.25). They often assume tumoral proportions and bear a superficial resemblance to dermoids. They may be found in either the central or the peripheral cornea, and also resemble the nodules in Salzmann's degeneration (Table 18.10). Like dermoids, keloids show variable degrees of extension and may replace the cornea or the entire anterior segment, and can involve the entire corneal surface.[137] Subtle differences between corneal keloids and dermoids include the glistening and jellylike quality of the keloids. The definitive diagnosis can be made by performing a corneal biopsy.[137] Immunohistochemical and electron microscopic studies have demonstrated the presence of myofibroblasts in these lesions, differentiating them from Salzmann's nodules.[138]

Corneal keloids can be associated with Lowe's syndrome. However, the etiology of keloids in Lowe's syndrome remains obscure. Considerations include excessive local delivery of amino acids and unknown noxious substances through the leaking corneal vessels, seepage of similar substances across the defective blood–aqueous barrier and the decompensated endothelium, repeated external trauma with associated inflammation, phenytoin (Dilantin) therapy, and congenital predisposition. No data are available on the management of progressive corneal keloids. Possible empirical regimens include local excision, pressure therapy, topical corticosteroids, and cromolyn sodium.[139–141]

Study of enucleation specimens has revealed associated findings including cataract, anterior staphyloma, ruptured lens capsule with lens fragments in the wound, buphthalmos, chronic glaucoma, and angle-closure glaucoma.[142]

References

1. Nichal KK, Naor J, Jay V, et al. Clinicopathological correlation of congenital corneal opacification using ultrasound biomicroscopy. *Br J Ophthalmol.* 2002;86:62–69.
2. Waring GO, Rodrigues MM. Congenital and neonatal corneal abnormalities. In: Tasman W, Jaeger E, eds. *Duane's Ophthalmology, CD-Rom.* Philadelphia: Lippincott Williams & Wilkins; 2002.
3. Kim T, Cohen EJ, Schnall BM, et al. Ultrasound biomicroscopy and histopathology of sclerocornea. *Cornea.* 1998;17(4):443–445.
4. Eisenberg DL, Sherman BG, McKeown CA, et al. Tonometry in adults and children. A manometric evaluation of pneumatonometry, applanation, and TonoPen in vitro and in vivo. *Ophthalmology.* 1998;105:1173–1181.
5. Spierer A, Huna R, Hirsh A, et al. Normal intraocular pressure in premature infants. *Am J Ophthalmol.* 1994;117:801–803.
6. Dickens CJ, Hoskins KH Jr. Diagnosis and treatment of congenital glaucoma. In: Ritch R, Shields MB, eds. *The glaucomas.* Vol 2. St. Louis: Mosby; 1989.
7. Elliot JH, Feman SS, O'Day DM, et al. Hereditary sclerocornea. *Arch Ophthalmol.* 1985;103:676–679.
8. Kenyon KR. Mesenchymal dysgenesis in Peters' anomaly, sclerocornea and congenital endothelial dystrophy. *Exp Eye Res.* 1975;21:125–142.

9. Waring GO, Rodrigues MM, Laibson PR. Anterior chamber cleavage syndrome: a stepladder classification. *Surv Ophthalmol.* 1975;20:3–27.
10. Waring GO, Rodrigues MM. Ultrastructure and successful keratoplasty of sclerocornea in Mietens' syndrome. *Am J Ophthalmol.* 1980;90: 469–475.
11. Sharkey JA, et al. Cornea plana and sclerocornea in association with recessive epidermolysis bullosa dystrophica. *Cornea.* 1992;11(1):83–85.
12. Vesaluoma MH, Sankila EM, Gallar J, et al. Autosomal recessive cornea plana: in vivo corneal morphology and corneal sensitivity. *Invest Ophthalmol Vis Sci.* 2000;41(8):2120–2126.
13. Nischal KK. Congenital corneal opacities – a surgical approach to nomenclature and classification. *Eye.* 2007;21(10):1326–1337.
14. Kanai A, Wood TC, Polack FM, Kaufman HE. The fine structure of sclerocornea. *Invest Ophthalmol.* 1971;10(9):687–694.
15. Walton DS. Primary congenital open angle glaucoma. A study of the anterior segment abnormalities. *Trans Am Ophthalmol Soc.* 1979;77: 746–768.
16. Costenbader FD, Kwitko ML. Congenital glaucoma: an analysis of seventy-seven consecutive eyes. *J Pediatr Ophthalmol.* 1967;4:9.
17. Cotran PR, Bajart AM. Congenital corneal opacities. *Int Ophthalmol Clin.* 1992;32(1):93–105.
18. Wilson FM. Congenital anomalies. In: Smolin G, Thoft RA, eds. *The cornea.* ed 2. Boston: Little, Brown; 1987.
19. Spencer WH, Ferguson WJ Jr, Shaffer RN, Fine M. Late degenerative changes in the cornea following breaks in Descemet's membrane. *Trans Am Acad Ophthalmol Otolaryngol.* 1966;70(6):973–983.
20. Stein RM, Cohen EJ, Calhoun JH, et al. Corneal birth trauma managed with a contact lens. *Am J Ophthalmol.* 1987;103(4):596–598.
21. Kumar P, Tiwari VK. An unusual cleft lip secondary to amniotic bands. *Br J Plast Surg.* 1990;43(4):492–493.
22. Hutchison DS, Smith RE, Haughton PB. Congenital herpetic keratitis. *Arch Ophthalmol.* 1975;93:70–73.
23. Nahmias AJ, Visintine AM, Caldwell DR, et al. Eye infections with herpes simplex viruses in neonates. *Surv Ophthalmol.* 1976;21(2): 100–105.
24. Aujard Y. Modalities of treatment local and general, medicamentous or not, controlling neonate suspected to be infected/contaminated by HSV1 or HSV2. *Ann Dermatol Venereol.* 2002;129(4 Pt 2):655–661.
25. Sibony O. Antiviral and non-antiviral local and general treatments for herpes in the pregnant woman (including prevention of mother–infant transmission): alternative propositions. *Ann Dermatol Venereol.* 2002;129(4 Pt 2):652–654.
26. Henrot A. Mother–infant and indirect transmission of HSV infection: treatment and prevention. *Ann Dermatol Venereol.* 2002;129(4 Pt 2):533–549.
27. Azazi M, Malm G, Forsgren M. Late ophthalmologic manifestations of neonatal herpes simplex virus infection. *Am J Ophthalmol.* 1990; 109(1):1–7.
28. Wolff SM. The ocular manifestation of congenital rubella. *J Pediatr Ophthalmol.* 1973;10:101–141.
29. Boniuk V, Boniuk M. The congenital rubella syndrome. *Int Ophthalmol Clin.* 1968;8:487–514.
30. Boniuk V. Systemic and ocular manifestations of the rubella syndrome. *Int Ophthalmol Clin.* 1972;12(2):67–76.
31. Wolf SM. Ocular manifestations of congenital rubella: a prospective study of 328 cases of congenital rubella. *J Pediatr Ophthalmol.* 1973;10: 101.
32. Deluise VP, Cobo LM, Chandler D. Persistent corneal edema in the congenital rubella syndrome. *Ophthalmology.* 1983;90(7):835–839.
33. Whitley CB, Ramsay NCK, Kersey JH, Krivit W. Bone marrow transplantation for Hurler syndrome: assessment of metabolic correction. *Birth Defects.* 1986;22(1):7.
34. Schaison G, Bordigoni P, Leverger G. Bone marrow transplantation for genetic and metabolic disorders. *Nouv Rev Fr Hematol.* 1989;31(2): 119–123.
35. Friedlaender MH. Metabolic diseases. In: Smolin G, Thoft RA, eds. *The cornea.* ed 2. Boston: Little, Brown; 1987.
36. Goldberg MF, Maumenee AE, MuKusick VA. Corneal dystrophies associated with abnormalities of mucopolysaccharide metabolism. *Arch Ophthalmol.* 1965;74:516–520.
37. Frangieh GT, Traboulsi EI, Kenyon KR. Mucopolysaccharidoses. In: Gold DH, Weingeist TA, eds. *The eye in systemic disease.* Philadelphia: Lippincott; 1990.
38. Casanova FH, Adan CB, Allemann N, et al. Findings in the anterior segment on ultrasound biomicroscopy in Maroteaux–Lamy syndrome. *Cornea.* 2001;20(3):333–338.
39. Cantor LB, Disseler JA, Wilson FM 2nd. Glaucoma in the Maroteaux–Lamy syndrome. *Am J Ophthalmol.* 1989;15;108(4):426–430.
40. Varssano D, Cohen EJ, Nelson LB, et al. Corneal transplantation in Maroteaux–Lamy syndrome. *Arch Ophthalmol.* 1997;115(3):428–429.
41. Constantopoulos G, Dekaban AS, Scheie HG. Heterogeneity of disorders in patients with corneal clouding, normal intellect, and mucopolysaccharidosis. *Am J Ophthalmol.* 1971;72(6):1106–1116.
42. Scheie HG, Hambridk GW Jr, Barness LA. A newly recognized forme fruste of Hurler's disease (gargoylism). *Am J Ophthalmol.* 1962;53: 753.
43. Zabel RW, MacDonald IM, Mintsioulis G, et al. Scheie's syndrome. An ultrastructural analysis of the cornea. *Ophthalmology.* 1989;96(11): 1631–1638.
44. Kenyon KR. Ocular manifestations and pathology of systemic mucopolysaccharidoses. *Birth Defects.* 1976;12(3):133.
45. Gredrickson DS. Hereditary systemic diseases of metabolism that affect the eye. In: Mausolf FA, ed. *The eye and systemic disease.* St. Louis: Mosby; 1975.
46. Rodrigues MM, Calhoun J, Harley RD. Corneal clouding with increased acid mucopolysaccharide accumulation in Bowman's membrane. *Am J Ophthalmol.* 1975;79(6):916–924.
47. Summers CG, Purple RL, Krivit W, et al. Ocular changes in the mucopolysaccharidoses after bone marrow transplantation: a preliminary report. *Ophthalmology.* 1989;96(7):977–984.
48. Sugar J. Metabolic disorders of the cornea. In: Kaufman HE, Baron BA, McDonald MB, eds. *The cornea.* ed 2. on CD-Rom. Portland: Butterworth–Heinemann; 1999.
49. Cantor LB, Disseler JA, Wilson FM. Glaucoma in the Maroteaux–Lamy syndrome. *Am J Ophthalmol.* 1989;108(4):426–430.
50. Quigley HA, Maumenee AE, Stark WJ. Acute glaucoma in systemic mucopolysaccharidoses. *Am J Ophthalmol.* 1975;80(1):70–72.
51. Spellacy E, Bankes JL, Crow J, et al. Glaucoma in a case of Hurler's disease. *Br J Ophthalmol.* 1980;64(10):773–778.
52. Christiansen SP, Smith TJ, Henslee-Downey PJ. Normal intraocular pressure after a bone marrow transplant in glaucoma associated with mucopolysaccharidosis type I-H. *Am J Ophthalmol.* 1990;109(2):230–231.
53. Schwartz GP, Cohen EJ. Hydrocephalus in Maroteaux–Lamy syndrome. *Arch Ophthalmol.* 1998;116(3):400.
54. Cipolloni C, Boldrini A, Donti E, et al. Neonatal mucolipidosis II (I-cell disease): clinical, radiological and biochemical studies in a case. *Helv Paediatr Acta.* 1980;35:85.
55. Whelan D, Chang P, Cockshott P. Mucolipidosis II. The clinical, radiological and biochemical features in three cases. *Clin Genet.* 1983;24(2):90–96.
56. Sprigz R, Doughty R, Spackman T, et al. Neonatal presentation of I-cell disease. *J Pediatr.* 1978;93(6):954–958.
57. Libert J, Van Hoof F, Farriaux J, et al. Ocular findings in I-cell disease (mucolipidosis type II). *Am J Ophthalmol.* 1977;83(5):617–628.
58. Mueller O, Wasmuth J, Murray J, et al. Chromosomal assignment of *N*-acetylglucosaminylphosphotransferase, the lysosomal hydrolase targeting enzyme deficient in mucolipidosis II and III. *Cytogenet Cell Genet.* 1987;46:664.
59. Okada S, Owada M, Sakiyama T, et al. I-cell disease: clinical studies of 21 Japanese cases. *Clin Genet.* 1985;28(3):207–215.
60. Ben-Yoseph Y, Mitchell D, Yager R, et al. Mucolipidoses II and III variants with normal *N*-acetylglucosamine 1-phosphotransferase activity toward alpha-methylmannoside are due to nonallelic mutations. *Am J Hum Genet.* 1992;50(1):137–144.
61. Traboulsi E, Maumenee I. Ophthalmologic findings in mucolipidosis III. *Am J Ophthalmol.* 1986;102(5):592–597.
62. Newman NJ, et al. Corneal surface irregularities and episodic pain in a patient with mucolipidosis IV (clinical conference). *Arch Ophthalmol.* 1990;108(2):251–254.
63. Kenyon KR, Tseng SCG. Limbal autograft transplantation for ocular surface disorders. *Ophthalmology.* 1989;96:709–723.
64. Dangel ME, Bremer DL, Rogers GL. Treatment of corneal opacification in mucolipidosis IV with conjunctival transplantation. *Am J Ophthalmol.* 1985;99(2):137–141.
65. Katz B, Melles RB, Schneider JA. Crystal deposition following keratoplasty in nephropathic cystinosis. *Arch Ophthalmol.* 1989;107(12): 1727–1728.
66. Kaiser-Kupfer MI, et al. A randomized placebo-controlled trial of cysteamine eye drops in nephropathic cystinosis. *Arch Ophthalmol.* 1990;108(5):689–693.
67. Schneider JA, Schulman JD. Cystinosis. In: Stanbury JB, Wyngaarden JB, Fredrickson DS, eds. *The metabolic basis of inherited disease.* ed 5. New York: McGraw-Hill; 1983:1844.
68. Khan AO, Latimer B. Successful use of topical cysteamine formulated from the oral preparation in a child with keratopathy secondary to cystinosis. *Am J Ophthalmol.* 2004;138:674–675.

69. Gahl WA, et al. Lysosomal transport disorders: cystinosis and sialic acid storage disorders. In: Scriver CR, et al, *eds. The metabolic basis of inherited disease*. ed 7. New York: McGraw-Hill; 1995:3763.
70. Gahl WA, Thoene JG, Schneider JA. Cystinosis. *N Engl J Med.* 2002;347(2):111–121.
71. Spaeth GL, Frost P. Fabry's disease: its ocular manifestations. *Arch Ophthalmol.* 1965;74(6):760–769.
72. Hirano K, Murata K, Miyagawa A, et al. Histopathologic findings of cornea verticillata in a woman heterozygous for Fabry's disease. *Cornea.* 2001;20(2):233–236.
73. Massi D, Martinelli F, Battini ML, et al. Angiokeratoma corporis diffusum (Anderson–Fabry's disease): a case report. *J Eur Acad Dermatol Venereol.* 2000;14(2):127–130.
74. Morel CF, Clarke JT. The use of agalsidase alfa enzyme replacement therapy in the treatment of Fabry disease. *Exp Opin Biol Ther.* 2009;9(5): 631–639.
75. Charlton KH, Pinder PS, Wozniak L, et al. Pseudodendritic keratitis and systemic tyrosinemia. *Ophthalmology.* 1981;88(4):355–360.
76. Goldsmith LA, Kang E, Bienfang DC, et al. Tyrosinemia with plantar and palmar keratosis and keratitis. *J Pediatr.* 1973;83(5):798–805.
77. Sammartino A, de Crecchio G, Balato N, et al. Familial Richner–Hanhart syndrome: genetic, clinical, and metabolic studies. *Ann Ophthalmol.* 1984;16(11):1069–1074.
78. Macsai MS, Schwartz TL, Hinkle D, et al. Tyrosinemia type II: nine cases of ocular signs and symptoms. *Am J Ophthalmol.* 2001;132(4): 522–527.
79. Barton DE, Yang-Feng TL, Francke U. The human tyrosine aminotransferase gene mapped to the long arm of chromosome 16 (region 16q22–q24) by somatic cell hybrid analysis and in situ hybridization. *Hum Genet.* 1986;72(3):221–224.
80. Miller MT, et al. Anterior segment anomalies associated with the fetal alcohol syndrome. *J Pediatr Ophthalmol Strabismus.* 1984;21(1): 8–18.
81. Edward DP, Li J, Sawaguchi S, et al. Diffuse corneal clouding in siblings with fetal alcohol syndrome. *Am J Ophthalmol.* 1993;115(4):484–493.
82. Carones F, Brancato R, Venturi E, et al. Corneal endothelial anomalies in the fetal alcohol syndrome. *Arch Ophthalmol.* 1992;110(8):1128–1131.
83. Edward DP, et al. Diffuse corneal clouding in siblings with fetal alcohol syndrome. *Am J Ophthalmol.* 1993;115:484–493.
84. Pierson DM, Subtil A, Taboada E, et al. Newborn with anophthalmia and features of Fryns syndrome. *Pediatr Dev Pathol.* 2002;5(6): 592–596.
85. Ayme S, Julian C, Gambarelli D, et al. Fryns syndrome: report on 8 cases. *Clin Genet.* 1989;35(3):191–201.
86. Cursiefen C, Schlotzer-Schrehardt U, Holbach LM, et al. Ocular findings in Fryns syndrome. *Acta Ophthalmol Scand.* 2000;78(6):710–713.
87. Insler MS. Cerebro-oculo-facio-skeletal syndrome. *Ann Ophthalmol.* 1987;19(2):54–55.
88. Preus M, Fraser F. The cerebro-oculo-facio-skeletal syndrome. *Clin Genet.* 1974;5:294–302.
89. Rezende R, Uchoa UB, Uchoa R, et al. Congenital corneal opacities in a cornea referral practice. *Cornea.* 2004;23:565–570.
90. Dana MR, Schaumberg DA, Moyes AL, Gomes JAP. Corneal transplantation in children with Peters' anomaly. *Ophthalmology.* 1997;104:1580–1586.
91. Yang LLH, Lambert SR, Lynn MJ, Stulting RD. Long-term results of corneal graft survival in infants and children with Peters' anomaly. *Ophthalmology.* 1999;106:833–848.
92. Matsubara A, Ozeki H, Matsunaga N, et al. Histopathological examination of two cases of anterior staphyloma associated with Peters' anomaly and persistent primary vitreous. *Br J Ophthalmol.* 2001;85:1421–1425.
93. Zaidman GW, Juechter K. Peters' anomaly associated with protruding corneal pseudostaphyloma. *Cornea.* 1998;17(2):163–168.
94. Townsend WM. Congenital anomalies of the cornea. In: Kaufman HE, Baron BA, McDonald MB, eds. *The Cornea.* ed 2. on CD-Rom. Portland: Butterworth–Heinemann; 1999.
95. Townsend WM. Congenital corneal leukomas. *Am J Ophthalmol.* 1974;77:80–86.
96. Ozeki H, Shirai S, Nozaki M, et al. Ocular and systemic features of Peters' anomaly. *Graefes Arch Clin Exp Ophthalmol.* 2000;238:833–839.
97. Ghose S, Kishore K, Patil ND. Oculoauricular dysplasia syndrome of the Goldenhar and Peters' anomaly: a new association. *J Pediatr Ophthalmol Strabismus.* 1992;29:384–386.
98. Heon E, Barsoum-Homsy M, Cevrette L, et al. Peters' anomaly. The spectrum of ocular and associated malformations. *Ophthalmic Paediatr Genet.* 1992;13:137–143.
99. Kivlin J, Fineman RM, Crandall AS, Olson RA. Peters' anomaly as a consequence of genetic and nongenetic syndromes. *Arch Ophthalmol.* 1986;104(1):61–64.
100. Frydman M, Weinstock AL, Cohen HA, et al. Autosomal recessive Peters' anomaly, typical facies appearance, failure to thrive, hydrocephalus, and other anomalies: further delineation of the Krause–Kivlin syndrome. *Am J Med Genet.* 1991;40(1):34–40.
101. Ciralsky J, Colby K. Congenital corneal opacities: A review with a focus on genetics. *Semin Ophthalmol.* 2007;22:241–246.
102. Traboulsi EI, Maumenee IH. Peters' anomaly and associated congenital malformations. *Arch Ophthalmol.* 1992;110:1739–1741.
103. Gollamudi SR, Traboulsi EI, Chamon W, et al. Visual outcome after surgery for Peters' anomaly. *Ophthalmic Genet.* 1994;15(1):31–35.
104. Astle WF, Lin DTC, Douglas GR. Bilateral penetrating keratoplasty and placement of a Molteno implant in a newborn with Peters' anomaly. *Can J Ophthalmol.* 1993;28(6):276–282.
105. Krachmer JH, Rodriques MM. Posterior keratoconus. *Arch Ophthalmol.* 1978;96:1867–1873.
106. Rao SK, Padmanabhan P. Posterior keratoconus. An expanded classification scheme based on corneal topography. *Ophthalmology.* 1998;105(7): 1206–1212.
107. Mannis MJ, Lightman J, Plotnik RD. Corneal topography of posterior keratoconus. *Cornea.* 1992;11(4):351–354.
108. Rapuano CJ, Luchs JI, Kim T. *Anterior segment: the requisites in ophthalmology.* St. Louis: Mosby; 2000:46–61.
109. Zaidman GW, Juechter K. Peters' anomaly associated with protruding corneal pseudostaphyloma. *Cornea* 1998:17(2):163–168.
110. Toma NMG, Ebenezer ND, Inglehearn CF, et al. Linkage of congenital hereditary endothelial dystrophy to chromosome 20, *Hum Mol Genet.* 1995;4(12):2395–2398.
111. Weiss JS, Møller HU, Lisch W, et al. The IC3D classification of the corneal dystrophies. *Cornea.* 2008;27(Suppl 2):S1–S83.
112. Hirst LW. Congenital corneal problems. *Int Ophthalmol Clin.* 1984;24(1):55–71.
113. Levenson JE, Chandler JW, Kaufman HE. Affected asymptomatic relatives in congenital hereditary endothelial dystrophy. *Am J Ophthalmol.* 1973;76(6):967–971.
114. Bahn CF, Falls HF, Varley GA, et al. Classification of corneal endothelial disorders based on neural crest origin. *Ophthalmology.* 1984;91: 558–563.
115. Whitacre MM, Stein R. Sources of error with use of Goldmann-type tonometers. *Surv Ophthalmol.* 1993;38:1–30.
116. Mullaney PB, Risco JM, Teichmann K, et al. Congenital hereditary endothelial dystrophy associated with glaucoma. *Ophthalmology.* 1995;102:186–192.
117. Pedersen O, Rushood A, Olsen EG. Anterior mesenchymal dysgenesis of the eye. Congenital hereditary endothelial dystrophy and congenital glaucoma. *Acta Ophthalmol.* 1989;67:470–476.
118. Sekundo W, et al. An ultrastructural investigation of an early manifestation of the posterior polymorphous dystrophy of the cornea. *Ophthalmology.* 1994;101(8):1422–1431.
119. McCartney ACE, Kirkness CM. Comparison between posterior polymorphous dystrophy and congenital hereditary endothelial dystrophy of the cornea. *Eye.* 1988;2:63–70.
120. Cibis GW, Krachmer JA, Phelps CD, et al. The clinical spectrum of posterior polymorphous dystrophy. *Arch Ophthalmol.* 1977;95: 1529–1537.
121. Krachmer JH. Posterior polymorphous corneal dystrophy: a disease characterized by epithelial-like endothelial cells which influence management and prognosis. *Trans Am Ophthalmol Soc.* 1985;83:413–475.
122. Van Schooneveld MS, Dellerman JW, Beemer FE, et al. Peter's plus: a new syndrome. *Ophthalmol Pediatr Genet.* 1984;4(3):141–145.
123. Callaghan M, Hand CK, Kennedy SM, et al. Homozygosity mapping and linkage analysis demonstrate that autosomal recessive congenital hereditary endothelial dystrophy (CHED) and autosomal dominant CHED are genetically distinct. *Br J Ophthalmol.* 1999;83(1):115–119.
124. Kanis AB, Al-Rajhi AA, Taylor CM, et al. Exclusion of AR-CHED from the chromosome 20 region containing the PPMD and AD-CHED loci. *Ophthalmic Genet.* 1999;20(4):243–249.
125. Witschel H, et al. Congenital hereditary stromal dystrophy of the cornea. *Arch Ophthalmol.* 1978;96(6):1043–1051.
126. Roth SI, Mittelman D, Stock EL. Posterior amorphous corneal dystrophy. An ultrastructural study of a variant with histopathological features of an endothelial dystrophy. *Cornea.* 1992;11(2):165–172.
127. Moshegov CN, Hoe WK, Wiffen SJ, Daya SM. Posterior amorphous corneal dystrophy. A new pedigree with phenotypic variation. *Ophthalmology.* 1996;103(3):474–478.

128. Grimm BB, Waring GO 3rd, Grimm SB. Posterior amorphous corneal dysgenesis. *Am J Ophthalmol.* 1995;120(4):448–455.
129. Dunn SP, Krachmer JH, Ching SS. New findings in posterior amorphous corneal dystrophy. *Arch Ophthalmol.* 1984;102(2):236–239.
130. Castelo Branco B, Chalita MRC, Casanova FHC, et al. Posterior amorphous corneal dystrophy. Ultrasound biomicroscopy findings in two cases. *Cornea.* 2002;21(2):220–222.
131. Apple DJ, Olson RJ, Jones GR, et al. Congenital corneal opacification secondary to Bowman's layer dysgenesis. *Am J Ophthalmol.* 1984;98(3):320–328.
132. Hogan M, Zimmerman LE, eds. *Ophthalmic pathology.* ed 2. Philadelphia; WB Saunders: 1962.
133. Henkind P, Marinoff G, Manas A, et al. Bilateral corneal dermoids. *Am J Ophthalmol.* 1973;76(6):972–977.
134. Mann I. *Developmental anomalies of the eye.* London: Cambridge University Press; 1957.
135. Baum JL, Feingold M. Ocular aspects of Goldenhar's syndrome. *Am J Ophthalmol.* 1973;25(2):250–257.
136. Henkind P, et al. Bilateral corneal dermoids. *Am J Ophthalmol.* 1973; 76(6):972–977.
137. O'Grady RB, Kirk HQ. Corneal keloids. *Am J Ophthalmol.* 1972;73:206.
138. Holbach LM, Font RL, Shivitz IA, et al. Bilateral keloidlike myofibroblastic proliferations of the cornea in children. *Ophthalmology.* 1990;97:1198.
139. Cibis GW, Tripathi RC, Tripathi BJ, Harris DJ. Corneal keloid in Lowe's syndrome. *Arch Ophthalmol.* 1982;100(11):1795–1799.
140. Tripathi RC, Cibis GW, Tripathi BJ. Lowe's syndrome. *Trans Ophthalmol Soc UK.* 1980;100(Pt 1):132–139.
141. McElvanney AM, Adhikary HP. Corneal keloid: etiology and management in Lowe's syndrome. *Eye.* 1995;9(Pt 3):375–376.
142. Wood TO. Salzmann's nodular degeneration. *Cornea.* 1990;9(1):17–22.

Chapter 19

Peripheral Corneal Disease

Stephen C. Kaufman

The Peripheral Cornea: Its Susceptibility and Response to Disease

The peripheral cornea is generally considered to be that portion located between the central 50% of the cornea and the limbus. This is the thickest region of the cornea, which is directly adjacent to the corneal limbus and internal angle structures. Although the peripheral cornea manifests some of the same disorders as the central cornea, its proximity to the limbus and conjunctiva results in a unique collection of abnormalities. These frequently stem from the distinctive architecture of the limbus, which includes a highly vascular zone with associated lymphatic tissue, scleral collagen, corneal collagen, and limbal stem cells. Thus, vascular inflammatory disorders, limbal infections, collagen vascular disorders, neoplastic disease, and local degenerations may affect the peripheral cornea in a distinctive way.

This chapter discusses peripheral corneal diseases by categorizing the disorders into five groups: (1) congenital/developmental/inherited; (2) inflammatory/autoimmune; (3) neoplastic; (4) environmental exposure/degenerative/iatrogenic; and (5) infectious (Table 19.1). A number of these items could be classified under more than one heading; however, a single heading was chosen to reduce redundancy. To reduce further redundancy, this chapter includes an abbreviated discussion of each topic. If further information is desired, please refer to the specific chapter for that disorder.

Congenital/Developmental/Inherited Disorders of the Peripheral Cornea

Corneal dystrophies are rare, inherited, primary corneal disorders. There are no corneal dystrophies that exclusively affect the peripheral cornea, although *Lattice dystrophy* type II is associated with systemic amyloidosis and primarily involves the peripheral cornea.[1] A complete discussion of this disorder is found elsewhere in this book.

Certain congenital systemic disease manifest changes in the peripheral cornea. *Wilson's disease* is a genetic disorder which results in the accumulation of copper in a variety of tissues and affects the neurological system, liver and other organ systems. In the cornea Wilson's disease produces an orangey-brown ring in the periphery of the cornea. This *Kayser–Fleischer ring* consists of copper which is deposited in Descemet's membrane. *Iron deposition* can be seen in many situations and appears as a brown line or other shape. Intercellular deposits of iron have been seen in basal corneal epithelial cells as well as in Bowman's membrane. At first glance iron lines and rings can mimic the appearance of the copper deposits associated with Wilson's disease, but careful slit lamp examination will demonstrate that the brown iron deposits are located more superficially within the cornea, at the level of Bowman's membrane. The corneal copper deposition does not affect vision or require treatment. This autosomal recessive genetic disorder generally presents in the first two decades of life with liver dysfunction.[2] Wilson's disease can be treated with systemic D-penicillamine, which prevents disease progression and reduces the amount of copper already deposited in tissues. Ocular examinations help to document reduction of copper in the tissues of the body.

There is a group of congenital corneal disorders that affect the appearance and structure of the cornea and are apparent at birth. *Sclerocornea* and *cornea plana* are congenital disorders generally associated with scleralization of the cornea and an extremely flat corneal curvature, with keratometry measurements as low as 20 diopters. Although the term cornea plana is generally used in Europe, sclerocornea refers to the same disorder in the United States. These disorders appear to be distinct, with overlapping features, but may represent a spectrum of interrelated clinical findings.[3] *Sclerocornea* is associated with a spectrum of clinical findings, from peripheral cornea opacity to a completely opaque white cornea. Corneal vascularization may be seen in the opaque region, and the curvature of the affected area is typically flatter than normal. *Cornea plana* may resemble sclerocornea, as the majority of cases also exhibit peripheral scleralization of the cornea. As the name denotes, cornea plana is a disorder that exhibits very flat corneal curvatures of 20–30 diopters and hyperopia. Additionally, because the corneal vault is reduced, these individuals also demonstrate shallow anterior chambers. Cornea plana can be associated with diffuse, deep stromal opacities, and so may be difficult to distinguish clinically from sclerocornea.[4] Both disorders can be associated with other ocular anatomic abnormalities.

Table 19.1 Classification of peripheral corneal disorders

1) Congenital/Developmental/Inherited
   - A) Lattice dystrophy type II
   - B) Wilson's disease
   - C) Cornea plana
   - D) Sclerocornea
   - E) Posterior embryotoxin
   - F) Axenfeld–Rieger anomaly
2) Inflammatory/Autoimmune
   - A) Rheumatoid arthritis
   - B) Polyarteritis nodosa
   - C) Wegener's granulomatosis
   - D) Marginal keratitis
   - E) Phlyctenulosis
   - F) Mooren's ulcer
   - G) Vascular pannus
3) Neoplastic
   - A) Pterygium
   - B) Dermoid
   - C) Benign squamous metaplasia
   - D) Carcinoma in situ/intraepithelial neoplasia
   - E) Squamous cell carcinoma
   - F) Melanoma
4) Degenerative

   Degenerative disorders that are not associated with corneal thinning:
   - A) Dry eye/tear film deficiency
   - B) Corneal arcus
   - C) Lipid keratopathy
   - D) Calcific band keratopathy
   - E) White limbal girdle of Vogt
   - F) Furrow degeneration
   - G) Limbal stem cell deficiencies

   Degenerative disorders that are associated with corneal thinning:
   - H) Terrien's marginal degeneration
   - I) Pellucid marginal degeneration
   - J) Dellen
5) Infectious
   - A) Bacterial
   - B) Fungal
   - C) Viral
   - D) Miscellaneous

A group of related congenital corneal localized opacities have been described. The first of these, *posterior embryotoxon*, produces a thickened, prominent Schwalbe's line, which is more anteriorly located than normal. It can be seen with gonioscopy as a fine ground-glass-like membrane and has been estimated to occur in 15% of normal eyes.[5] When posterior embryotoxin exists without additional pathology it does not require treatment. When it is associated with other peripheral corneal abnormalities, including multiple peripheral iris strands, it is termed *Axenfeld–Rieger anomaly*. This and other related congenital diseases are discussed in more detail in their respective chapters.

Inflammatory/Autoimmune Disorders of the Peripheral Cornea

Because of the proximity of the peripheral cornea to the limbal vasculature and conjunctival lymphoid tissue, this region of the cornea is especially susceptible to immunologic disorders. Furthermore, the peripheral cornea may be significantly involved in systemic collagen–vascular disease. Many systemic immune diseases cause a secondary ocular

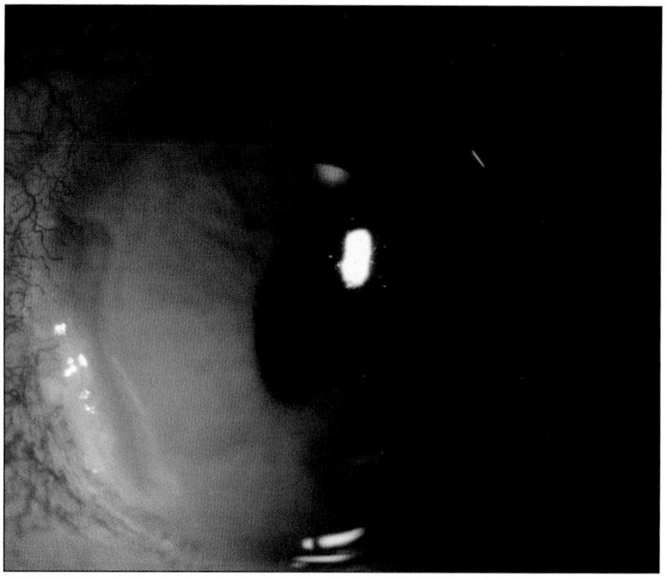

Fig. 19.1 Macroulcerative peripheral keratitis in a patient with rheumatoid arthritis. Observe the deep ulceration concentric with the limbus and the steep, undermined central border of the ulcer.

inflammatory response which results in disorders such as keratoconjunctivitis sicca, scleritis, episcleritis, peripheral corneal disorders and vasculitis. The ophthalmologist should remember that ocular disease can be the presenting sign of these systemic disorders. The most common inflammatory disorders that affect the peripheral cornea are discussed below.

Of the systemic vasculitides, *rheumatoid arthritis* is the most common. Rheumatoid arthritis is a multisystem disease which primarily involves the peripheral joints. Nonarticular vasculitis affects 25% of patients and is associated with cardiac disease, pulmonary disease, splenomegaly, and ocular disease.[6]

The most common ocular disorder associated with rheumatoid arthritis is keratoconjunctivitis sicca. This produces a dry eye, which may result in a mild punctate epithelial keratitis or stromal ulcerations. Dry eyes are discussed more extensively elsewhere in this book. A majority of patients with rheumatoid arthritis have little or no symptomatology; however, more severe immunologic complications include sclerosing keratitis, which manifests as a superficial and mid-stromal peripheral keratitis which is generally associated with a nonnecrotizing scleritis.[7] The associated infiltrates can enlarge or proliferate and produce a breakdown of the corneal epithelium, and a secondary stromal melt may ensue (Fig. 19.1). In addition, a peripheral corneal furrow may develop in an area adjacent to a sclerosing keratitis without the presence of an infiltrate. The area of stromal thinning typically has an intact overlying epithelium and can be differentiated from the more severe form of keratolysis because the furrow may progress but rarely results in perforation of the cornea (Fig. 19.2). Conversely, keratolysis is associated with an acute severe melting of the corneal stroma which can proceed to perforation. Keratolysis is most commonly seen in patients with rheumatoid-associated scleritis. Multiple studies have demonstrated the importance of

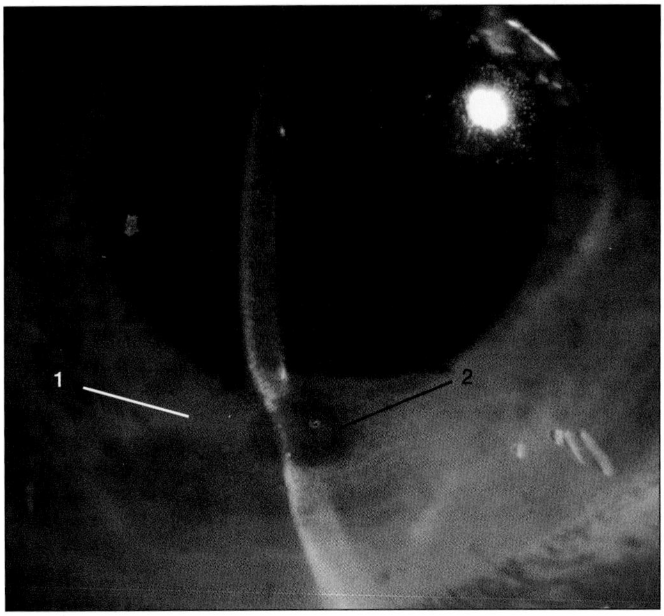

Fig. 19.2 Patient with rheumatoid arthritis and dry eye with typical rheumatoid marginal furrow. Observe the inferior area of corneal melting (1), epithelial defect (2), and lack of associated inflammation. The ulcer healed after treatment with a bandage soft contact lens, punctal occlusion, and frequent artificial tear instillation.

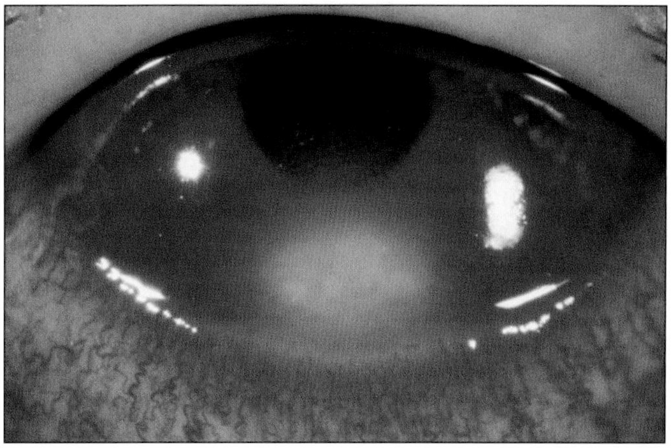

Fig. 19.3 Catarrhal corneal ulcer in a patient with blepharitis. The inferior infiltrate is parallel to the limbus and separated from it by a clear zone.

documenting rheumatoid arthritis-related scleritis, as this heralds the presence of extensive systemic vasculitis. If the systemic vasculitis is untreated, the majority of these patients will die within 5 years.[8]

Like many vasculitis-associated disorders, which are related to the systemic disease, the ultimate treatment involves therapy directed toward control of the systemic vasculitis. This generally entails the use of systemic prednisone or other immunomodulator(s). The addition of topical corticosteroids can be beneficial in the treatment of episcleritis or scleritis; however, they should be used with extreme caution in patients with keratolysis as they can accelerate the 'melting' process. If the keratolysis or scleromalacia progresses, a patch graft may be needed. In severe cases multiple patch grafts will be necessary. Pretibial periosteum has been used for corneal and scleral patch grafts, with success in these severe cases, as it is not susceptible to melting.[9]

Polyarteritis nodosa is a systemic vasculitis which typically affects the eyes in approximately 20% of cases. A bilateral peripheral keratitis typically involves the peripheral cornea and begins with infiltrates located within the mid-stroma.[10] The infiltrates may remain isolated to one region or may coalesce circumferentially and eventually progress to melting of the corneal stroma. The treatment for this disorder requires systemic therapy directed toward control of the vasculitis.

Wegener's granulomatosis may present with corneal signs which are similar to those of the other vascular inflammatory diseases and is usually associated with involvement of the respiratory tract, nasal tissues, glomerulonephritis and other organ systems.[10] Two forms of the ocular disease have been described: a severe progressive disease, which has a 1-year mortality of 82% if untreated; and a limited, less severe form.[11] Additionally, Wegener's granulomatosis may produce a concomitant orbital inflammation with associated proptosis and orbital pain. The diagnosis should include radiographic studies of the chest and sinuses, serum antineutrophil cytoplasmic antigens (ANCA), and possibly tissue biopsy. As in polyarteritis nodosa, ocular involvement may be the initial sign of the vasculitis, and therapy frequently requires systemic immunosuppression.

A group of diseases develop as the result of the subject's own exaggerated hypersensitivity reaction to an antigen. These immune reactions may only cause mild pain, but in severe cases can also result in significant corneal neovascularization and scarring. *Marginal keratitis* is a disorder which is thought to result from ocular hypersensitivity reactions to toxins produced by bacteria that commonly colonize the eyelids. This disorder can produce peripheral corneal infiltrates and ulcerations in severe cases. The peripheral corneal infiltrates generally occur adjacent to the limbus, with a clear intervening zone between the lesion and the limbus (Fig. 19.3). The patient typically complains of redness and pain. The lesions may first appear similar to an infectious infiltrate with an intact corneal epithelium over the infiltrate. These lesions can also be found in patients who wear soft contact lenses. Because the infiltrates associated with the marginal keratitis are not infectious in nature, culture of the lesions results in a diagnosis of a sterile infiltrate. The lesions can be treated effectively with a topical steroid; however, the treatment should also involve reducing the bacterial antigens and toxins that are the underlying cause of the marginal keratitis. Lid hygiene and other treatments for blepharitis can be very effective in reducing the recurrence of this disorder. If there is any question regarding the etiology of a peripheral corneal infiltrate, the initial treatment should include an antibiotic alone or in combination with a steroid, and must include close clinical follow-up.

Phlyctenulosis is an inflammatory disorder which is similar to marginal keratitis but involves a more severe reaction. The immune reaction associated with a phlyctenule can produce significant corneal scarring and significant vascularization of the cornea, but perforation is rare (Fig. 19.4). Current studies have commonly associated staphylococcal disease with phlyctenulosis; however, older studies demonstrated a strong association with tubercular disease.[12] Like marginal keratitis, treatment involves topical steroids or possibly other immunomodulating medications such as topical ciclosporin; however, if tuberculosis is suspected steroids should not be used until a TB test can be performed. Importantly, if the phlyctenular disease is thought to be related to staphyloccocal bacteria, lid hygiene should be a part of any treatment regimen. If long-term treatment is necessary, the author has had success using a commercially available topical ciclosporin emulsion, frequently adding a topical corticosteroid during the initial month of therapy.

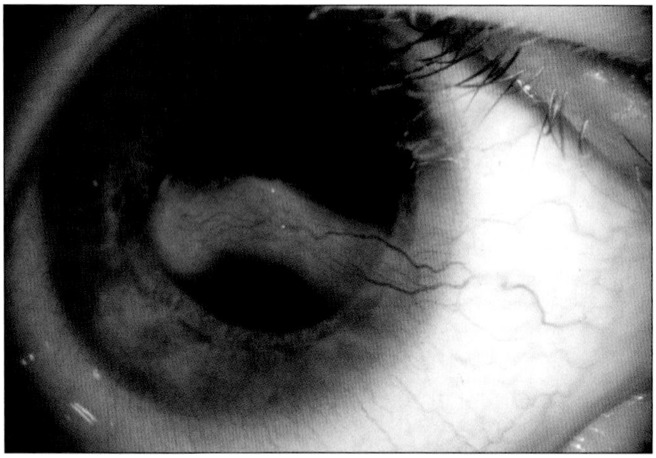

Fig. 19.4 Corneal phlyctenule. These lesions can 'march' across the cornea with progressive vascularization and scarring.

Mooren's ulcer produces a painful progressive peripheral ulceration of the cornea. The cause of Mooren's ulcer is unknown, but there are generally considered to be two clinical types. Patients with the limited type are typically over 40 years old, have unilateral disease, and respond well to medical therapy. A more 'malignant' type of Mooren's ulcer has been described that generally occurs in younger patients and has been seen more commonly in Nigerian men.[13,14] The disorder typically starts with a peripheral corneal infiltrate which slowly progresses. There is generally no clear zone between the infiltrate and the limbus. As the disease progresses, an ulcer develops with a characteristic overhanging edge which has an intact epithelium (Fig. 19.5). If the progression of the disease can be halted, the surface of the ulcer may heal with conjunctivalization over the melted corneal stromal bed. Unfortunately, the severe form of the disease is very difficult to treat and perforation is common. A detailed discussion of the individual medical and surgical treatments for these disorders can be found in the chapters focusing on the specific disease entity.

When blood vessels and fibrous connective tissue from the limbus grow onto the peripheral cornea, secondary to inflammation, the result is a *vascular pannus*. A vascular pannus can occur in any location, depending upon the inciting inflammation. A pannus in an adult may extend from the peripheral cornea towards the central cornea and is generally flat. An exception to this occurs in infants and small children, who may develop a hyperplastic reaction to the inflammation, and the resulting pannus can become extremely exaggerated and elevated.[15]

Superior limbal keratoconjunctivitis (SLK) is an inflammatory disorder of unknown etiology which is associated with

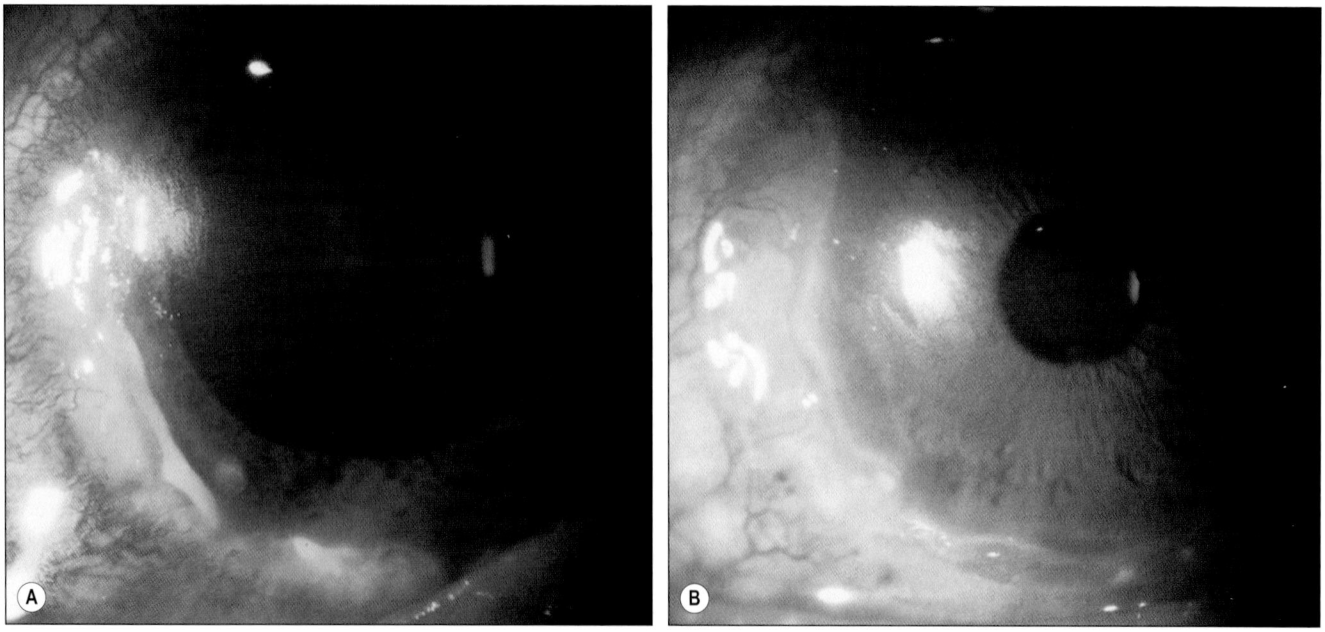

Fig. 19.5 Mooren's ulcer in a young African man. **A**, There are 4 clock hours of dense peripheral infiltration. **B**, Despite treatment, 1 month later the previously infiltrated area is now deeply ulcerated and has extended further circumferentially.

a peripheral corneal pannus, a punctuate keratopathy, a thickened superior conjunctiva which is chemotic and hyperemic, and a filamentary keratitis. As the name states, this is a disorder of the superior limbus and cornea. Patients complain of ocular irritation and a foreign body sensation. It maybe associated with keratitis sicca or thyroid disease. The etiology is unknown. Initial treatment should consist of preservative-free artificial tears. If this eliminates the discomfort, punctate keratopathy and filaments, no further treatment is necessary, although the superior conjunctiva may remain thickened and hyperemic. The clinician can consider a bandage soft contact lens, conjunctival recession, or conjunctival resection with an amniotic membrane graft if further treatment is necessary. Please see the specific chapter concerning SLK if more information is desired.

Neoplastic Disorders of the Peripheral Cornea

Because the surface of the cornea is contiguous with the bulbar conjunctiva, tumors that affect the conjunctiva may also affect the cornea. The differences between the compositions of these tissues alter the range and frequency of neoplasias encountered clinically. Although malignant tumors of the peripheral cornea exist, benign neoplastic growths are far more common in this region.

One of the most common neoplastic growths of the peripheral cornea is a *pterygium*. Some clinicians consider a pterygium a degenerative growth because of the effect of the actinic damage on the substantia propria.[16] Pterygia typically occur in the interpalpebral area owing to its increased actinic exposure. Fibroblasts associated with the pterygium grow onto the surface of the peripheral cornea and eventually penetrate Bowman's layer, resulting over time in a corneal scar.

Because pterygia can recur, we do not remove those that minimally overlap the peripheral cornea. These small pterygia can be treated with artificial tears, and short-term NSAIDs or mild corticosteroids if inflamed. Some clinicians have advocated intralesional corticosteroid injections. When pterygia extend 1.5–2 mm onto the corneal surface or are extremely elevated and inducing astigmatism, we consider surgical excision. Although pterygia are not considered true neoplastic lesions, recent evidence suggests that a significant percentage are associated with squamous cell carcinoma, which is the most common neoplasm of the cornea.[17] Therefore, it is deemed prudent to send pterygia specimens for histopathology examination after their surgical excision. There are a number of methods to remove pterygia, but it is unclear which of the many techniques prevent recurrence with good cosmetic results.

Another fibrovascular growth which may be associated with the peripheral cornea is *pyogenic granuloma*. This reactive tissue response most commonly occurs after surgery, trauma, or infection. Although these lesions are much more common in the conjunctiva, there have been reports of pyogenic granuloma formation in the cornea.[18] Their growth is typically rapid and they are well circumscribed in their appearance. Pyogenic granulomas are composed of fibrovascular tissue and are not true granulomas as the name would imply. Therefore, they are easily excised.

Congenital lesions of the cornea are rare, but there are those that principally affect the peripheral cornea. *Dermoid tumors* are one of the most common congenital growths associated with the peripheral cornea. Dermoids are benign tumors that may grow with the eye but do not substantially enlarge. In addition, they may change in character slightly as the host progresses through puberty. They are most commonly found in the temporal limbal region and are characterized by a thick, firm surface which may contain hair, sebaceous glands, sweat glands, and fat. Dermolipomas are a type of dermoid tumor composed primarily of fat.[19] Dermoid tumors can be associated with other syndromes such as Goldenhar and Proteus syndrome; therefore, the presence of a dermoid should be correlated with other systemic findings.[20] Large dermoids can affect vision either by occluding the pupil or by inducing a significant amount of astigmatism. Dermoids may be excised by performing a superficial lamellar keratectomy; however, they can extend through the full thickness of the cornea and sclera, or peripherally beyond the equator of the globe, which may make their complete removal difficult. If a full thickness or deep dermoid tumor is suspected, careful surgical planning must be undertaken and imaging studies employed to determine its extent. If the surgical plan involves deep excision of the tumor, the surgeon should have sufficient tissue available for a patch graft.

The most common tumors of the limbus and peripheral cornea involve the squamous epithelium. Although the substantia propria of the conjunctiva is not directly continuous within the cornea, it abuts Bowman's layer. Additionally, the epithelium of the cornea and limbal conjunctiva represents a metabolically and mitotically active region. Thus, this location is predisposed to neoplastic transformation. Many types of benign *squamous metaplasia* have been reported, including benign hereditary dyskeratosis, squamous papilloma, pseudoepitheliomatous hyperplasia, and squamous dysplasia. Although these lesions may recur after excision, their potential for developing into a true malignant neoplasm is limited.

There are also *malignant and dysplastic squamous epithelial changes* that arise from this mitotically active limbal region of the eye. Most of these dysplastic lesions arise from the area of the interpalpebral region because of its increased solar exposure.[21] Initially, most dysplastic lesions are gelatinous or clear, thickened, irregular, mildly elevated lesions.[22] Jakobiec[23] found that fewer than 10% of dysplastic lesions initially demonstrated leukoplakia. Interestingly, some studies have demonstrated an association between these lesions and human papilloma virus type 16.[24]

Dysplasia of the corneal epithelium is typically meant to signify a partial epithelial layer involvement by the atypical epithelial cells versus a full-thickness epithelial layer involvement, which is termed *carcinoma in situ or intraepithelial neoplasia (CIN)*. When these limbal lesions spread to the surface of the cornea they typically have a frosted-glass appearance which can be difficult to visualize at the time of surgical excision. Rose Bengal can be used to highlight the extent of the cellular irregularity. Limited areas of squamous dysplasia or carcinoma in situ may be removed mechanically, but larger lesions may require a limbal autograft to supply a new population of limbal corneal stem cells (Fig. 19.6). A relatively new alternative to surgery employs topical

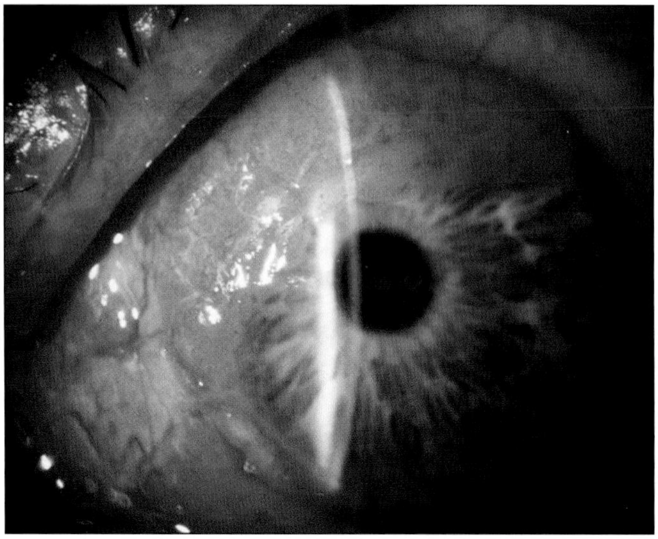

Fig. 19.6 Papillary form of CIN described histopathologically as severe dysplasia with focal areas of carcinoma in situ. The lesion straddles 180° of the corneoscleral limbus. The tumor was treated curatively with a combination of surgical excision and cryotherapy.

interferon-alfa drops, which have been used successfully to treat a number of cases. These lesions have also been treated with topical 5FU and mitomycin C (MMC) with some success. However, treatment with interferon-alfa, 5FU or MMC is not always successful, and surgical excision of the tissue may still ultimately be necessary. Cryoablation of tissue at the time of surgical excision may be required to eliminate abnormal cells from the adherent limbal conjunctiva or to treat an associated fibrovascular pannus.[25] Epithelial squamous carcinomas generally do not penetrate Bowman's layer; however, if this does occur, a wide excision of the affected tissue should be performed. Alcohol or cocaine can be used to facilitate the complete removal of the affected corneal epithelium, with an added excision of the surrounding normal tissue as part of the wide-excision procedure. Cryotherapy has also been employed and has significantly reduced the recurrence rate from 40% to less than 10%.[26]

Other rare peripheral corneal tumors have been identified, such as limbal melanoma and basal cell carcinoma. These entities are discussed in detail in their respective chapters.

Degenerative Disorders of the Peripheral Cornea

This category of ocular disorders comprises a hodgepodge of entities that overlap other categories because they have many causes. Most are not commonly the direct result of other diseases but can be associated with many other disorders.

Several corneal degenerations are not associated with corneal thinning. These disorders are generally benign, but in some instances can become serious.

Corneal arcus is a benign condition that results from lipid deposition within the corneal stroma, Bowman's layer and Descemet's membrane. The corneal epithelium is intact. A white or gray circumferential deposit is seen with an intervening clear space between it and the limbus. Arcus occurs with increasing age and is not considered pathologic; however, it can also be associated with hyperlipoproteinemia, and a lipid profile should be obtained in any patient under 50 who exhibits a corneal arcus.[27]

Lipid keratopathy results in a characteristic dense, yellow-white infiltrate which is usually associated with the presence of an adjacent corneal blood vessel. The lipid deposition can occur suddenly or may progress very slowly over the course of many years. The infiltrate usually has a feathery edge and may or may not have a crystalline appearance. Lipid keratopathy occurs in both primary and secondary forms. The secondary form is associated with peripheral corneal vessels, which may be seen in association with a history of inflammation, infection, trauma, or previous corneal surgery. The primary form is not associated with increased serum lipid levels, inflammation, or adjacent vasculature. It appears as an arcus-like deposition but may be thicker and more prominent. In fact, the lipid is identical to the lipid found in arcus.[28] If this lesion extends more centrally and affects vision, a corneal transplant may be necessary to restore sight. Unfortunately, the lipid deposits may recur in the graft.

White limbal girdle of Vogt was initially described in 1930. Two forms of this degenerative disorder were described. Type I has a characteristic crescent-shaped white or gray opacity near the interpalpebral zones of the limbus. These opacities are located nasally and temporally and are separated from the limbus by a clear zone. Small Swiss cheese-like holes may be evident within the opacity. Vogt also described a second form of the disorder with no clear zone between the opacities and the limbus. The first form of the disease is probably related to early, minor calcific band keratopathy; however, these minor opacities are seen in older individuals and are not related to trauma, intraocular inflammation, or multiple eye surgeries.[29] They are asymptomatic and do not require treatment.[29]

Calcific band keratopathy can be present in the peripheral cornea, the central cornea, or both regions. The corneal calcium may appear as a gray-white haze, with or without a 'Swiss cheese' appearance in mild disease; in advanced disease it can also form dense white-gray plaques (Fig. 19.7). Once the calcium deposits become elevated, it is common for the patient to note a foreign body sensation. If the calcium deposits are centrally located, the patient will typically experience reduced vision. Calcific band keratopathy is frequently associated with intraocular inflammation, trauma, multiple eye surgeries, elevated serum calcium, or other systemic disorders.[30] The calcium can be removed by chelation with EDTA, mechanical debridement, and phototherapeutic keratectomy.[31] For a comprehensive discussion of the topic, please see the specific chapter for the disorder responsible for the calcific band keratopathy.

Unlike other types of epithelium, the corneal epithelium is continuously replenished by new basal epithelial cells from corneal stem cells located at the limbus. The role of limbal stem cells in the turnover of the corneal epithelium

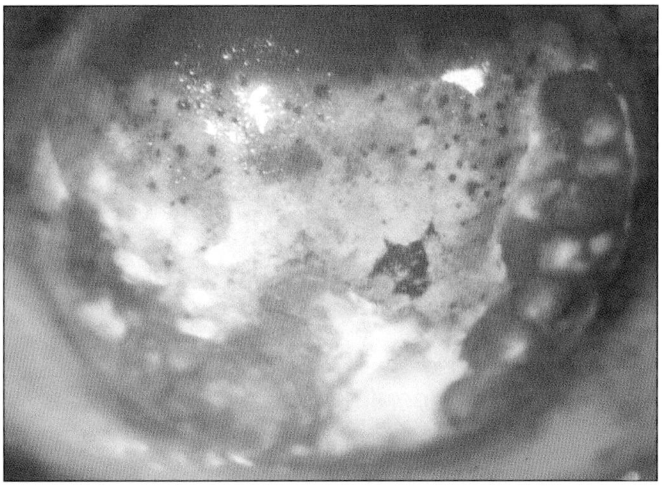

Fig. 19.7 Calcific degeneration. Calcium deposition in the cornea is associated with chronic vascularization or inflammation. Histopathologically, the calcium may be associated with a fibrovascular pannus or may occur deep in the corneal stroma, as opposed to calcific band keratopathy in which the calcium deposition is confined to the region of Bowman's membrane.

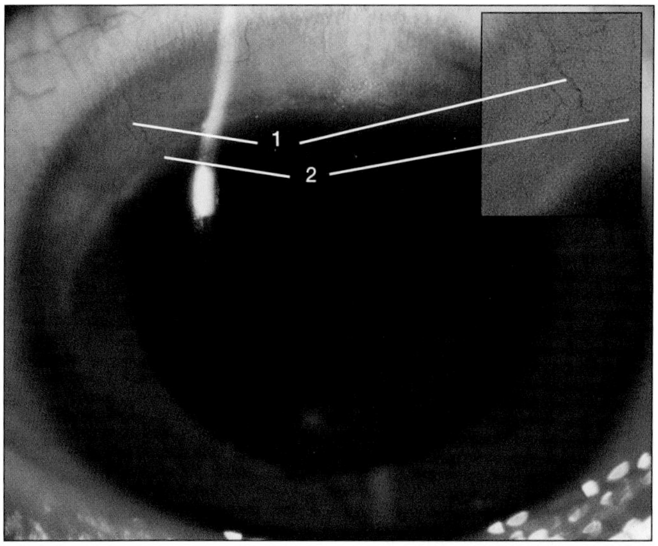

Fig. 19.8 Terrien's marginal degeneration, characterized by superior peripheral thinning, superficial vascularization (1), and lipid infiltration (2).

was recognized as early as 1971.[32] Our understanding of these unique corneal epithelial progenitor cells has evolved, and we have increased our understanding of corneal epithelial stem cells' characteristics. *Corneal epithelial stem cell deficiencies* are seen in genetic as well as acquired disorders. It has been understood for some time that aniridia is frequently associated with limbal stem cell deficiencies. The severity of the deficiency varies from patient to patient, and not all those with aniridia require treatment for limbal stem cell failure. Similarly, the degree of limbal stem cell damage after trauma from a chemical injury or after an acquired disorder such as Stevens–Johnson disease varies from person to person and from eye to eye. Iatrogenic limbal stem cell deficiency may occur in some patients in association with contact lens wear.

In the mildest forms of limbal stem cell deficiency, limbal and peripheral corneal changes with vascularization and slight loss of transparency of the corneal epithelium may be the only signs. In more severe forms of the disorder the entire corneal epithelium may be replaced by a fibrovascular membrane with almost complete loss of transparency of the cornea.[33] Many types of limbal stem cell transplant have been devised, but no single method is universally successful. Generally, autografts have the highest success rate if limbal stem cells can be harvested from the fellow eye, and patients who have small areas of limbal stem cell deficiency appear to have a better long-term prognosis. Patients who suffer from a complete loss of limbal stem cells and have suffered corneal scarring, epithelial defects, and a diffuse fibrovascular membrane covering the cornea are least likely to obtain a good long-term outcome after a limbal stem cell transplant. This may be partly due to acquiring a limbal allograft transplantation with the high potential for graft rejection because of the vascular nature of the limbal region, but also because this severe disorder is frequently associated with loss of accessory lacrimal glands and goblet cells from the conjunctiva.[33] Thus, it is more difficult to maintain a healthy ocular surface, which adversely affects the survival of the newly grafted tissue.

Several disorders result in *corneal thinning* or *apparent corneal thinning*. The following entities are all associated with corneal thinning from differing etiologies.

Terrien's marginal degeneration results in an idiopathic thinning of the peripheral cornea. This usually begins in the superior cornea but may occur in any peripheral region. The disorder typically begins as a fine stromal opacity which has a clear zone between it and the limbus. This area then begins to thin very slowly and becomes vascularized by the limbal vasculature.[34] As the thinning progresses, corneal astigmatism may become evident and cause symptoms of blurry vision.[36] Interestingly, this degeneration is usually not painful even during the active phase of the disorder. The epithelium may remain intact and the cornea may visibly bulge due to the ectasia.[35] The affected area may extend circumferentially without signs of inflammation. This disorder can be associated with episcleritis or scleritis, which generally results in discomfort. The disorder is bilateral in the majority of cases, but can be quite asymmetrical. Peripheral grafts may be necessary if the cornea becomes too thin and perforation or fear of trauma-related perforation exists. Terrien's marginal degeneration can be differentiated from other disorders such as Mooren's ulcer by its characteristic lack of pain, lack of a central undermined edge to the thinning trough, and an intact epithelium (Fig. 19.8). Neither pellucid marginal degeneration nor furrow degeneration have lipid infiltrates associated with the central edge of the thinning region. No current medical treatment is curative.

Pellucid marginal degeneration is a bilateral, inferior corneal thinning. The normal cornea protrudes above an area of abrupt thinning inferiorly (Fig. 19.9). The affected area is clear (pellucid) and eventually results in an against-the-rule astigmatism. Because of the similarities between the entities

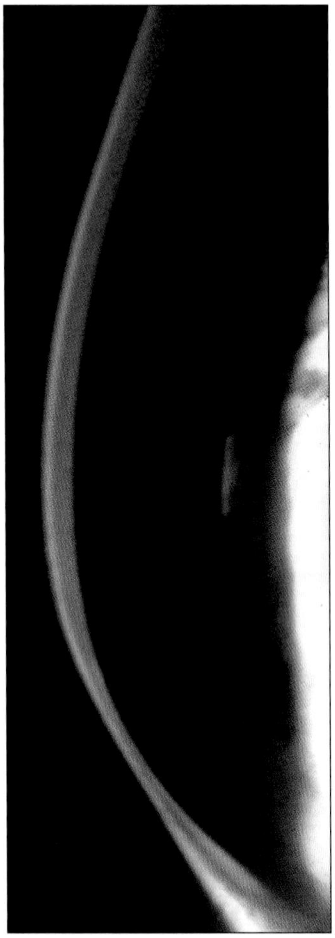

Fig. 19.9 Thin slit-beam view of pellucid marginal degeneration. There is marked thinning of the cornea inferiorly, well below the area of maximal corneal protrusion. In contrast, the thinning in keratoconus is in the area of maximal corneal protrusion.

that comprise the group of corneal ectatic diseases, it is believed that keratoconus, keratoglobus, and pellucid degeneration are related. Rigid gas-permeable (RGP) contact lenses can be used when spectacle correction is not sufficient. Otherwise, the surgeon may perform a tectonic lamellar graft over the thinned periphery, followed many months later by a central penetrating keratoplasty. During the placement of the tectonic graft, removal of a small amount of aqueous humor and reefing sutures may be useful to reduce the degree of steep corneal curvature.

Furrow degeneration is seen in the elderly patient. Although a furrow may be apparent at the slit lamp, careful examination reveals that this is not a true thinning but rather an optical illusion. Occasionally there is some minor thinning present, but this does not substantially progress nor is it associated with perforation of the cornea. No treatment is necessary.

Dellen appear as areas of thinning or excavation. The overlying epithelium is usually intact, but the base can be gray or hazy. Because dellen are the result of tissue thinning due to inadequate tear coverage and tissue drying, they are always associated with an adjacent elevation. Dellen can be seen in association with pingueculae, pterygia, dermoids, filtering blebs, and any other elevated bulbar structure. Treatment is directed toward rehydration, lubrication of the dellen, and elimination of the adjacent elevation. If the epithelium on the surface of the dellen is no longer intact, infection and perforation are critical concerns.

Surgery, surgical complications, and medication-associated (iatrogenic) peripheral corneal damage can mimic the appearance of certain corneal diseases. A careful review of the patient's history will help separate iatrogenic disorders from true corneal diseases.

Infectious Disorders of the Peripheral Cornea

Because the peripheral cornea is adjacent to the rich vascular supply of the limbus, the limbal lymphatic tissue, and inflammatory cells, microbial keratitis maybe thought to be less frequent than in the central cornea. However, other factors increase the likelihood of a peripheral corneal infection.

Contact lens wear can be associated with peripheral corneal disease. Wearing contact lenses reduces the amount of oxygen available to the cellular components of the cornea, the tear flow under the contact lens is less than that which would otherwise pass over the cornea, and contact lenses may increase the temperature of the cornea. Additionally, the insertion and removal of lenses may produce regions of microtrauma to the corneal surface, limbus, and adjacent conjunctiva. Furthermore, if soft contact lenses are worn overnight, the general risk of a corneal infection is increased.[36]

Contact lenses require good maintenance and cleaning. Frequently, patients will not change or clean their contact lens storage cases, which can harbor bacteria and other microorganisms. Also, certain systemic diseases, such as diabetes and other diseases that slow tissue healing, can increase the risk of ocular infections.

In addition, other factors such as dry eye and lagophthalmos serve to compromise the ocular surface. When these conditions are present in an individual who also wears contact lenses, the risk of microbial keratitis increases significantly. Because microbial keratitis is covered extensively elsewhere in this book, only a few specific aspects of infectious peripheral keratitis will be discussed here.

Bacterial and fungal keratitis, which occurs in the inferior third of the cornea, could be secondary to corneal exposure. This should especially be considered in an individual who has suffered multiple ocular infections. Lateral, medial, or both types of tarsorrhaphy may be required to protect the ocular surface and prevent subsequent episodes of infectious keratitis.

Microbial keratitis from specific causes such as syphilis or tuberculosis can produce peripheral corneal changes. Syphilis is associated with a deep corneal inflammation with deep vessels in the peripheral cornea. Conversely, tuberculosis produces an acute inflammation that is more commonly unilateral and involves peripheral sectoral portions of the anterior cornea.

Herpes simplex and zoster can develop peripheral corneal ulcers that do not exhibit typical dendrite formation. Instead, they develop an irregular epithelium or epithelial defect over

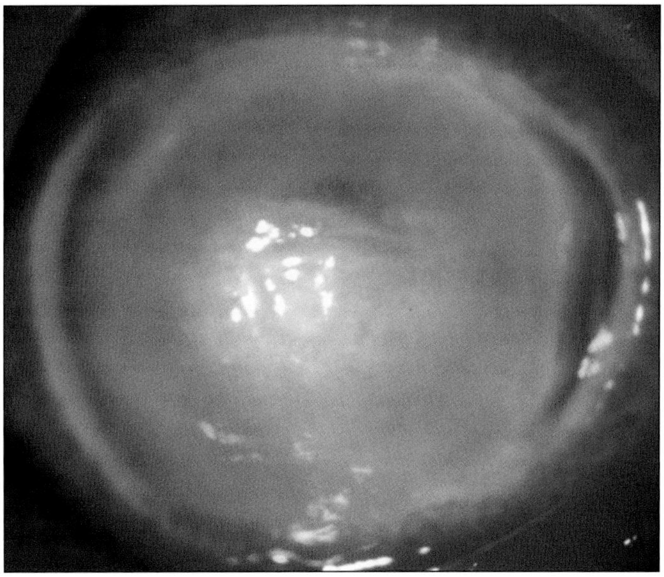

Fig. 19.10 Macroulcerative peripheral keratitis in a patient with herpes zoster keratouveitis.

the affected area, followed by a region of stromal haze that assumes a crescent shape adjacent to the limbus. The associated limbus is typically hyperemic and the eye is painful.[37]

Herpes simplex and zoster may also produce a sterile or an infected neurotropic ulcer (Fig. 19.10). Therefore, corneal sensation should always be tested in patients who experience little pain in association with a corneal ulcer. Treatment is directed at healing the ulcer and protecting the ocular surface with a tarsorrhaphy. A scleral contact lens may protect the corneal surface once the ulcer is healed.

Peripheral corneal diseases are a diverse group of disorders. More information about each individual disorder can be obtained from the chapter on the specific topic.

References

1. Purcell JJ Jr, Rodrigues MM, Chishti MI, et al. Lattice corneal dystrophy associated with familial systemic amyloidosis (Meretoja's syndrome). *Ophthalmology.* 1983;90:1512.
2. Tso MOM, Fine BS, Thorpe HE. Kayser–Fleischer ring and associated cataract in Wilson's disease. *Am J Ophthalmol.* 1975;79:479.
3. Goldstein TE, Cogan DG. Sclerocornea and associated congenital anomalies. *Arch Ophthalmol.* 1962;67:761.
4. Vesaluoma MH, Sankila EM, Gallar J, et al. Autosomal recessive cornea plana: In vivo corneal morphology and corneal sensitivity. *Invest Ophthalmol Vis Sci.* 2000;41:2120.
5. Forsius H, Eriksson A, Fellman J. Embryotoxin corneae posterius in an isolated population. *Acta Ophthalmol (Copenh).* 1964;42:42.
6. Koffler D. The immunology of rheumatoid diseases. *Clin Symp.* 1979;31:1.
7. Brown SI, Grayson M. Marginal furrows: a characteristic corneal lesion of rheumatoid arthritis. *Arch Ophthalmol.* 1968;79:563.
8. Foster CS, Forstot SL, Wilson LA. Mortality rate in rheumatoid arthritis patients developing necrotizing scleritis or peripheral ulcerative keratitis: effects of systemic immunosuppression. *Ophthalmology.* 1980;90:175.
9. Cardona H. Prosthokeratoplasty. *Cornea.* 1983;2:179.
10. Moore JG, Sevel D. Corneoscleral ulceration in polyarteritis nodosa. *Br J Ophthalmol.* 1966;50:651.
11. Straatsma BR. Ocular manifestations of Wegener's granulomatosis. *Am J Ophthalmol.* 1957;44:789.
12. Thygeson PL. The etiology and treatment of phlyctenular keratoconjunctivitis. *Am J Ophthalmol.* 1975;9:446.
13. Wood TO, Kaufman HE. Mooren's ulcer. *Am J Ophthalmol.* 1971;71:417.
14. Kietzman B. Mooren's ulcer in Nigeria. *Am J Ophthalmol.* 1968;65:679.
15. Crowell D, Jakobiec FA. Hemorrhagic corneal pannus simulating a spontaneous expulsive hemorrhage. *Ophthalmology.* 1981;88:693.
16. Austin P, Jakobiec FA, Iwamoto T. Elastodysplasia and elastodystrophy as the pathologic bases of ocular pterygia and pinguecula. *Ophthalmology.* 1983;90:96.
17. Hirst LW, Axelsen RA, Schwab I. Pterygium and associated ocular surface squamous neoplasia. *Arch Ophthalmol.* 2009;127(1):31.
18. Googe JM, Mackman G, Peterson MR, et al. Pyogenic granulomas of the cornea. *Surv Ophthalmol.* 1984;29:188.
19. Grossniklaus HE, Green WR, Luckenbach M, Chan CC. Conjunctival lesions in adults: a clinical and histopathologic review. *Cornea.* 1987;6:78.
20. Bouzas EA, Krasnewich D, Koutroumanidis M, et al. Ophthalmologic examination in the diagnosis of Proteus syndrome. *Ophthalmology.* 1993;100:334.
21. Yanoff M. Hereditary benign intraepithelial dyskeratosis. *Arch Ophthalmol.* 1968;79:291.
22. Reed JW, Cashwell LF, Klintworth GK. Corneal manifestations of hereditary benign intraepithelial dyskeratosis. *Arch Ophthalmol.* 1979;97:297.
23. Odrich MG, Jakobiec FA, Lancaster WD, et al. A spectrum of bilateral squamous conjunctival tumors associated with human papillomavirus type 16. *Ophthalmology.* 1991;98:628.
24. McDonnell J, Mayr A, Martin WJ. DNA of human papillomavirus type 16 in dysplastic and malignant lesions of the conjunctiva and cornea. *N Engl J Med.* 1989;320:1442.
25. Fraunfelder FT, Wingfield D. Management of intraepithelial conjunctival tumors and squamous cell carcinomas. *Am J Ophthalmol.* 1983;95:359.
26. Davanger M, Evensen A. Role of the pericorneal papillary structure in renewal of corneal epithelium. *Nature.* 1971;229:560.
27. Andrews JS. The lipids of arcus senilis. *Arch Ophthalmol.* 1962;68:264.
28. Barchiesi BJ, Eckel RH, Ellis PP. The cornea and disorders of lipid metabolism. *Surv Ophthalmol.* 1991;31:6.
29. Sugar HS, Kobernick S. The white limbus girdle of Vogt. *Am J Ophthalmol.* 1960;50:101.
30. Cursino JW, Fine BS. A histologic study of calcific and noncalcific band keratopathy. *Am J Ophthalmol.* 1976;82:395.
31. Breinin GM, DeVoe AG. Chelation of calcium with EDTA in band keratopathy and corneal calcium affections. *Arch Ophthalmol.* 1954;52:846.
32. Huang AJW, Tseng SCG. Corneal epithelial wound healing in the absence of limbal epithelium. *Invest Ophthalmol Vis Sci.* 1991;32:96.
33. Tsai RJF, Tseng SCG. Human allograft limbal transplantation for corneal surface reconstruction. *Cornea.* 1994;13:389.
34. Wilson SE, Lin DTC, Klyce SD, Insler MS. Terrien's marginal degeneration: corneal topography. *Refract Corneal Surg.* 1990;6:15.
35. Suveges I, Levai G, Alberth B. Pathology of Terrien's disease. *Am J Ophthalmol.* 1972;74:1191.
36. Dart JK, Stapleton F, Minassian D. Contact lenses and other factors in microbial keratitis. *Lancet.* 1991;338:650.
37. Thygeson P. Marginal herpes simplex keratitis simulating catarrhal ulcer. *Invest Ophthalmol.* 1971;10:1006.

Chapter 20

The Corneal Ulcer

Carol L. Karp, Richard K. Forster

An ulcer (Latin *ulcus* or sore) is defined as a lesion 'caused by superficial loss of tissue, usually with inflammation.' Ulcerative keratitis rarely occurs in the normal, healthy eye. A search for the causative agent as well as underlying alterations in corneal structure, immunity, innervation, or defense mechanisms should be considered. Several questions should be asked when managing a patient with a corneal ulcer:

- Is there an infectious agent causing the keratitis?
- What local host factors contribute to increased risk for ulceration?
- What exogenous risk factors exist?
- Are there endogenous factors such as an autoimmune disease, an inflammatory process, or an immunocompromised status?

Diagnosis

One of the first decisions in the diagnostic algorithm is to determine whether the lesion is infectious or sterile. Both historical and clinical features should be considered in this process. Important historical predisposing factors for infectious keratitis include microbial exposure by contact lens use, foreign bodies and trauma, previous ocular surgery including refractive procedures, or exposure to contaminated water. The importance of contact lens use cannot be overemphasized. The use and abuse of contact lenses have played a major role in the epidemiology of keratitis in the United States. In particular, the use of extended (overnight) wear lenses has been clearly associated with an increased risk of keratitis in comparison to daily wear lenses. A history of outdoor trauma, particularly from soil or vegetation, should raise a suspicion for fungi or other fastidious organisms causing the keratitis.

Impaired local host defenses also play a role in the pathogenesis of stromal keratitis. A history of ocular chemical injury, neurotrophic disease, exposure and lid or lash malposition, tear insufficiency, stem cell deficiency, bullous keratopathy, or previous herpetic disease should be elicited. Certain medications such as topical anesthetics and topical corticosteroids also can reduce the local defense mechanisms.

A careful medical history also can be helpful in identifying systemic abnormalities that may predispose to increased risk for keratitis. Such factors could include acquired immunodeficiency syndrome (AIDS), diabetes mellitus, malnutrition, alcoholism, and other chronic debilitating illnesses. Underlying autoimmune diseases such as rheumatoid arthritis, Wegener's granulomatosis, and Sjögren's syndrome, as well as subsequent immunosuppressive treatments are also important.

The clinical evaluation of the patient should be thorough, and an effort should be made not to confine the examination only to the corneal process. Consider why the patient developed a keratitis and whether it is more likely to be sterile or infectious. The cornea and adnexa may provide clues regarding the inciting agent or etiology.

As with all patients, the examination should assess both eyes. Examination of the lids, lashes, and conjunctiva should evaluate for associated skin and adnexal inflammation such as rosacea or seborrhea and mechanical lid dysfunction such as floppy lid syndrome (Fig. 20.1), entropion, or ectropion. Mucous membrane diseases such as ocular cicatricial pemphigoid, Stevens–Johnson syndrome, or chemical injury may lead to symblepharon and trichiasis. Dermatologic cicatricial diseases such as scleroderma or atopic dermatitis or previous surgery may also lead to a compromised ocular surface. The lacrimal system should be examined, in terms of assessing both adequacy of tear function and the possibility that an underlying dacryocystitis or canaliculitis is contributing to the corneal pathology.

When examining the cornea, the epithelium, stroma, and endothelium should be evaluated with the recurring question of why the patient has a corneal ulcer. Most microbial keratitis is precipitated by an epithelial defect, and the epithelium and basement membrane of both eyes should be examined. The presence of reduplicated basement membrane, microcysts, or other findings of anterior basement membrane dystrophy may suggest recurrent erosion as the etiology for the initial epithelial insult. A rolled epithelial edge with an oval central lesion suggests neurotrophic pathology and a persistent epithelial defect (Fig. 20.2). Diffuse epitheliopathy should prompt consideration of a toxic reaction to topical medications such as antibiotics, antivirals, or anesthetics.

The appearance of the corneal stroma is the key to the underlying status of the eye. The classic features of an infectious stromal keratitis include coalescent stromal suppuration and infiltration (Fig. 20.3). The presence of a hypopyon, anterior chamber reaction, or endothelial plaques also

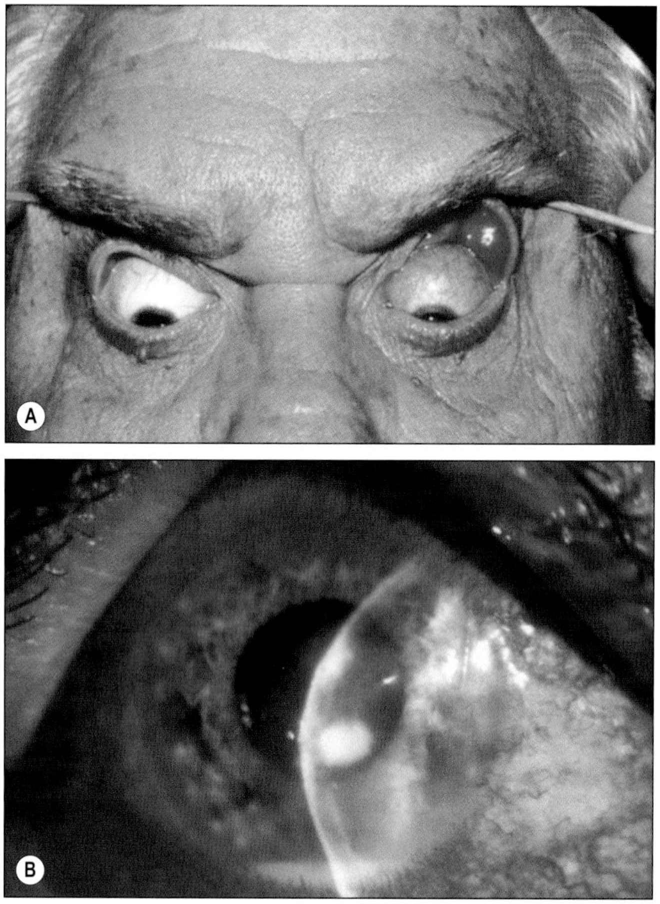

Fig. 20.1 (**A**) Male, obese patient with floppy lids, rosacea, and seborrhea. (**B**) Floppy lid syndrome leading to infectious corneal ulceration secondary to *Candida* sp. (Courtesy of William W. Culbertson MD).

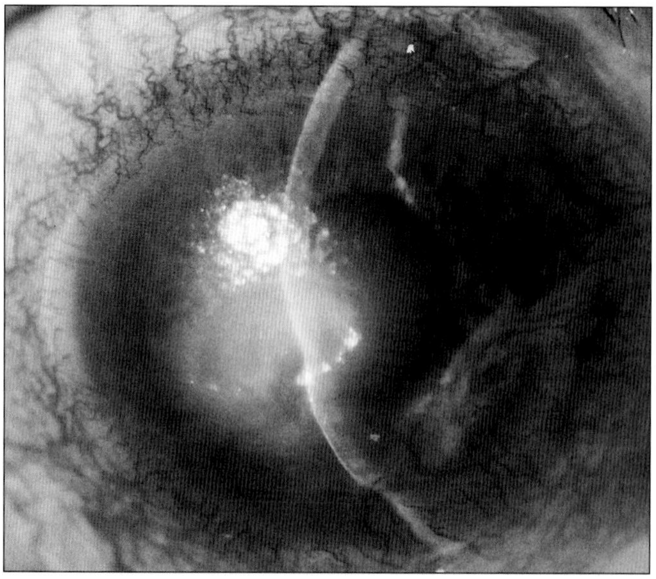

Fig. 20.2 Neurotrophic keratitis, with rolled epithelial edge, epithelial keratopathy, and vascularization.

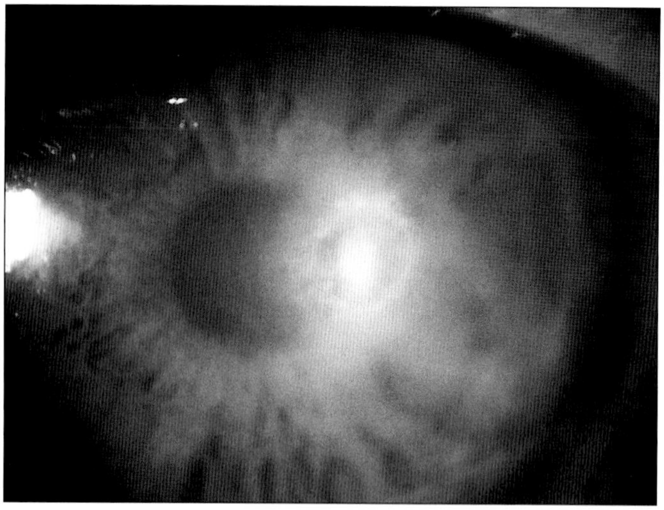

Fig. 20.3 Early *Pseudomonas aeruginosa* keratitis in a soft contact lens user. Note focal infiltrate with overlying epithelial defect and stromal edema.

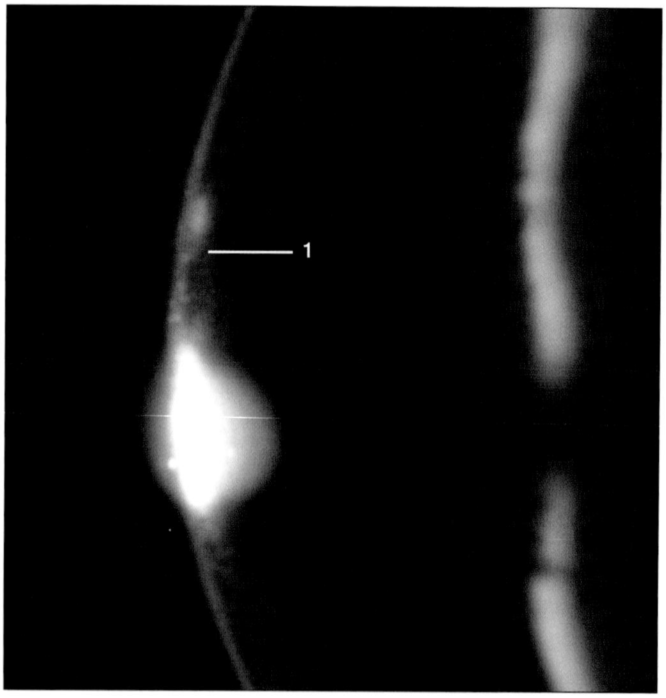

Fig. 20.4 Noninfectious keratitis secondary to a chemical injury. Note discrete midstromal inflammatory cell infiltrate (1), with no overlying epithelial defect.

may suggest infectious etiology. In contrast to the dense suppuration usually seen in infectious keratitis, sterile infiltrates may be characterized by the presence of visibly discrete inflammatory cells adjacent to the infiltrate, with minimal anterior chamber reaction (Fig. 20.4). Furthermore, indications of sterility in a postinfectious or treated keratitis include the presence of a resolved epithelial defect, or one in which the defect is healing over an area of previously dense infiltration (Fig. 20.5). In the setting of AIDS, the inflammatory response may be underwhelming.

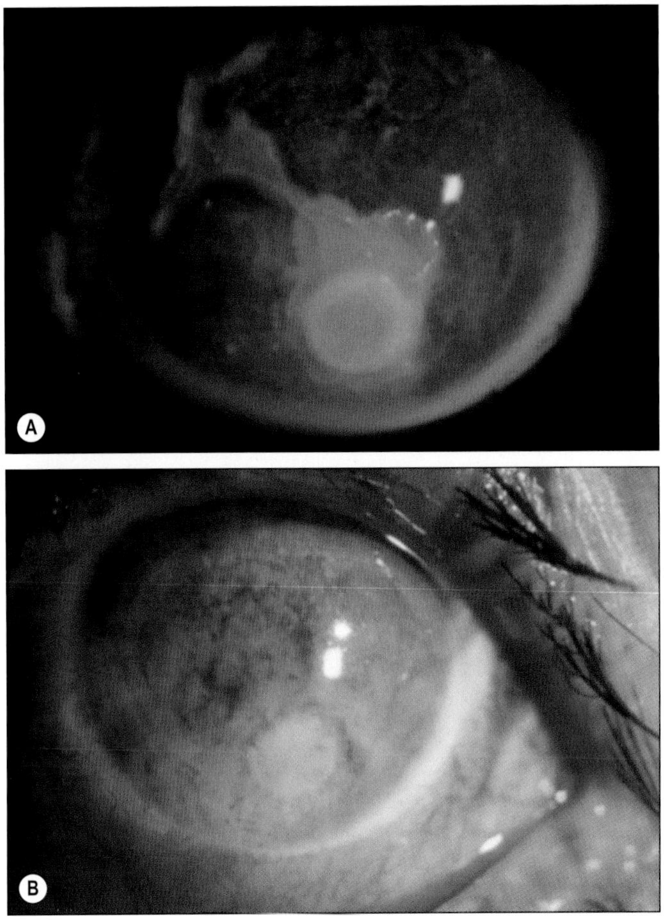

Fig. 20.5 Infectious keratopathy with epithelial defect and infiltrate that was sterilized with 10 days of topical antibiotics. (**A**) Corneal epithelial defect with corneal infiltrate and mucus strands. (**B**) After treatment, residual scarring and a punctate epitheliopathy.

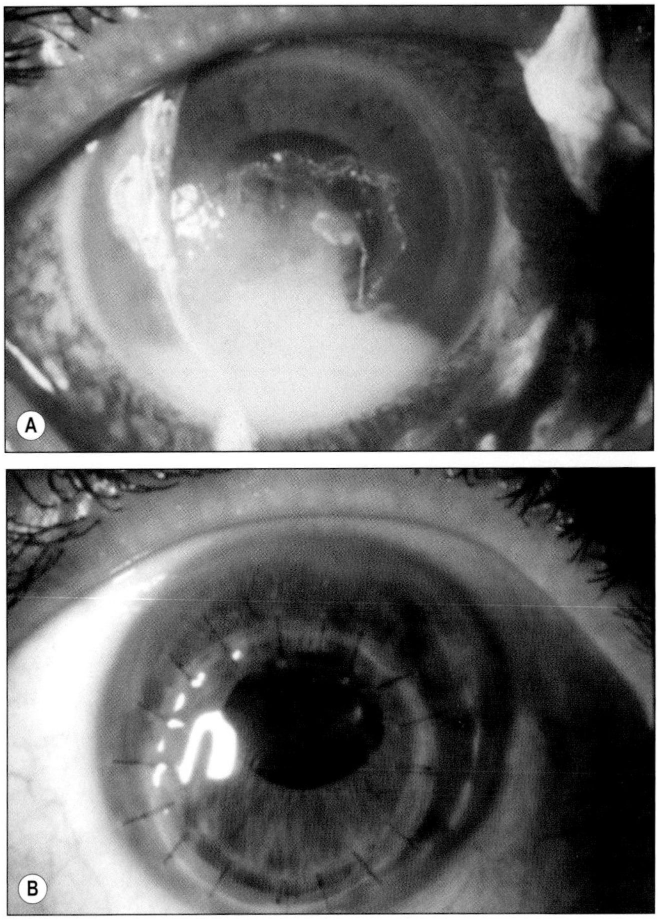

Fig. 20.6 (**A**) *Aspergillus* keratitis. Patient contracted infection while in refugee camp. (**B**) Penetrating keratoplasty for worsening *Aspergillus* keratitis.

Immune-related ulceration of the corneal stroma also may have varying degrees of stromal cellular infiltration. Immune-mediated infiltrates or ulceration may have an associated scleritis, episcleritis, or iritis. Vascularization or scleritis may be localized to the area of corneal pathology. A careful evaluation of the stroma of the other eye should be performed to rule out a possible peripheral immune-mediated marginal keratitis, such as seen in rheumatoid arthritis, Wegener's granulomatosis, and Mooren's ulcer. In general, the peripheral marginal melts, with or without epithelial defects, are rarely infectious. Keratitis associated with Gram-positive organisms is usually characterized by well-circumscribed lesions. *Staphylococcus aureus* usually progresses slowly, and the streptococci elicit an acute and highly suppurative reaction. In addition, the streptococci generally produce a deep central stromal ulceration with an advancing edge of infection, hence the term serpiginous ulceration, and are frequently associated with a sterile hypopyon. A unique presentation of streptococcal infection is the syndrome of infectious crystalline keratopathy (ICK), usually seen at the graft–host junction following keratoplasty and characterized by a paucity of inflammatory cells.

The Gram-negative bacteria usually produce soupy infiltrates, which are less discrete and have abundant conjunctival mucopurulent discharge. Features of less common keratitis include the stromal ring abscess and radial perineuritis of *Acanthamoeba* keratitis, often with complaints of extreme pain. The central 'cracked windshield' and the peripheral 'brush fire' appearance are features of *Nocardia* and *Mycobacterium*. Fungal infections usually have a hyphoid, feathery border and may develop satellite lesions (Fig. 20.6).

In the setting of infectious keratitis following laser-assisted in situ keratomileusis (LASIK), the clinical presentation may be atypical. Infections may initially be thought to be diffuse lamellar keratitis (DLK), delaying diagnosis and treatment. These patients may present without an epithelial defect, since the keratitis may be sequestered in the lamellar interface. In this scenario, the flaps may need to be lifted for culture and irrigation. Management of these cases can also be more difficult, as the antibiotics may not penetrate adequately through the anterior stromal flaps, necessitating flap amputation or penetrating keratoplasty for resolution (Fig. 20.7).

Despite certain classic features, a specific etiologic diagnosis cannot be made by clinical appearance alone. Therefore, when an infectious agent is suspected from the examination,

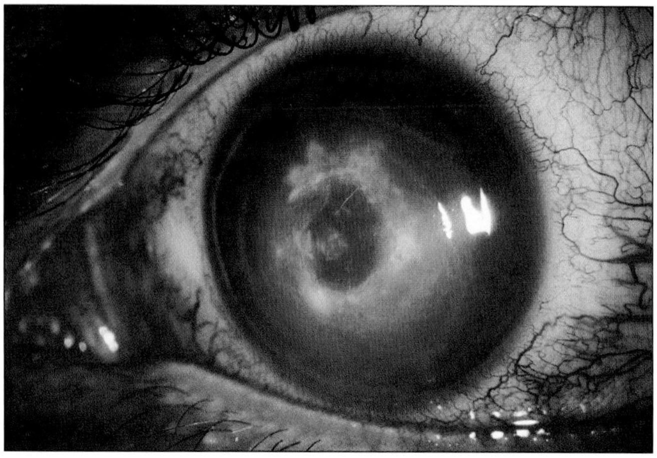

Fig. 20.7 Patient with post-LASIK infection with *Mycobacterium chelonae/abscessus*. Flap was amputated to allow for better antibiotic penetration, but patient ultimately required a penetrating keratoplasty for cure.

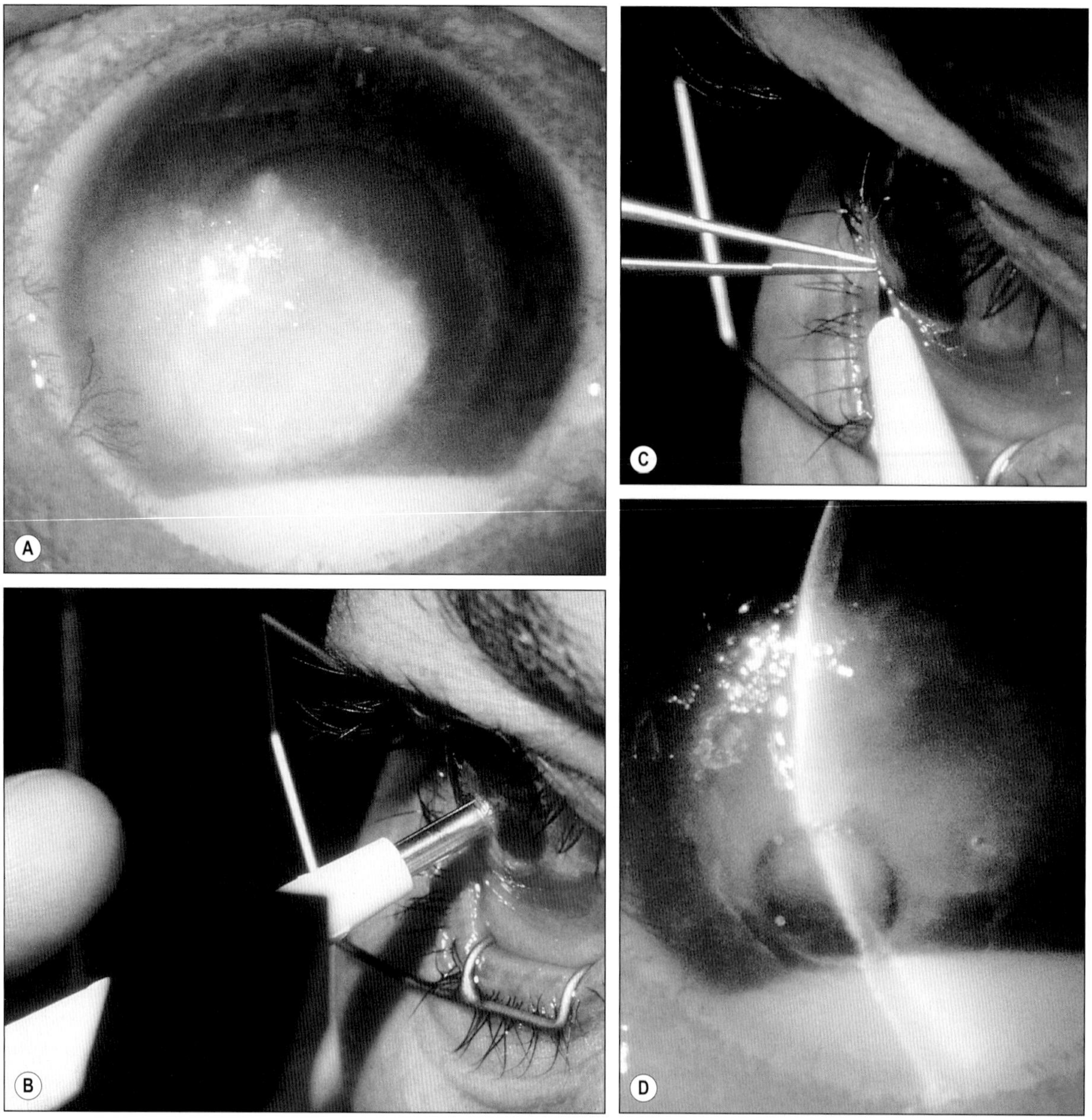

Fig. 20.8 Process of obtaining a corneal biopsy for a worsening keratitis. (**A**) Unresponsive keratitis. (**B**) Using a lid speculum and topical anesthesia, a 2 or 3 mm sterile trephine is used to obtain a superficial biopsy at active edge of the keratitis. If possible, two sites should be selected. (**C**) A sharp No. 75 or 69 Beaver blade may then be used to remove the specimen in a lamellar fashion. (**D**) Post-biopsy appearance of the ulcer.

corneal scrapings for culture and cytology are indicated. When the infection is contact lens related, culture of the contact lenses and case may be helpful. In cases of patients presenting already on topical antibiotics, it may be necessary to discontinue all topical drops for 24 hours prior to culturing. In the setting of a repeatedly negative or equivocal corneal culture in a patient with progressive disease, a corneal biopsy should be performed. A corneal biopsy can also be invaluable in obtaining a microbiologic diagnosis in cases of infectious crystalline keratopathy. Corneal biopsies can be performed easily and rapidly at the slit lamp, are inexpensive, and may provide critical information in the evaluation of the pathologic process. We recommend that the biopsy be performed using a disposable 2-mm dermatologic punch (Fig. 20.8). Two sites should be selected at the active edges of ulceration. Biopsy specimens should be submitted to both microbiology and pathology. Corneal biopsies have also successfully been performed using the femtosecond laser.[1]

In addition to the usual smears and cultures, cases of possible *Acanthamoeba* should have calcofluor white stain and agar plating with an *Escherichia coli* overlay. If *Mycobacterium* is suspected, Lowenstein-Jensen plating should be used and an acid-fast stain performed. Cultures for fungi should be placed on Sabouraud's dextrose agar. Histopathology stains for fungi should include Gram, Giemsa, and Gomori methenamine silver. A new diagnostic tool is the confocal microscope, which may be especially helpful in cases of *Acanthamoeba*[2,3] and possibly fungal keratitis.[4] Future improvements in microscopes and our increasing familiarity with interpreting the confocal images may make this tool increasingly useful.

Treatment

Once the patient is receiving antibiotics, the treating physician must tailor the treatment to the host response. Parameters to judge clinical improvement include resolution of the epithelial defect, decreasing density and size of the infiltrate and inflammation, and decreasing pain. The clinical response should be assessed to modify the treatment. It is important to recognize that many topical antibiotics have toxic effects on the epithelium and may modify the corneal appearance, particularly noted as a punctate epitheliopathy and stromal edema. An important principle in the management of keratitis is that corneal healing takes time. Stabilization or lack of worsening should be interpreted as effective therapy because the reparative process of the cornea may be slow.

Depending on the inciting agent, treatment duration will vary. For example, most fungal infections and *Acanthamoeba* need prolonged treatment. Fungal keratitis seems to benefit from regular debridement. This helps to decrease the infectious load mechanically as well as to maintain an epithelial defect to permit better antifungal medication penetration. We use a sterile No. 69 Beaver blade for this purpose. Additional smears and cultures can be performed easily with the scraped material if necessary.

In infections following LASIK, the treatment of the keratitis can be very prolonged due to poor penetration of the antibiotics through the corneal flap. In several cases of severe keratitis, we have amputated the corneal flap in order to resolve the infection.[5]

In all cases of infectious keratitis, the goal is to sterilize the lesion and enhance corneal healing. In those cases with progressive keratitis or impending perforation, a tectonic or therapeutic penetrating keratoplasty may be needed. Another option for managing a worsening keratitis with failure to heal, especially when there is a component of exposure or lagophthalmos, is a conjunctival flap or amniotic membrane graft. We have seen many cases in which patients have been treated successfully with focal conjunctival flaps for peripheral corneal ulcers, effecting resolution of the corneal ulcer and maintaining a clear central visual axis.

Management of a corneal ulcer is challenging and must include careful history and clinical examination. This information will assist in the tailoring of the microbiologic testing, will direct optimal treatment for the patient, and can be modified as needed, based on the host response.

References

1. Yoo SH, Kyminonis GD, O'Brien TP, et al. Femtosecond-assisted diagnostic corneal biopsy (FAB) in keratitis. *Grafes Arch Clin Exp Ophthalmol.* 2008;246:759–762.
2. Mathers WD, Sutphin JE, Folberg R, et al. Outbreak of keratitis presumed to be caused by *Acanthamoeba*. *Am J Ophthalmol.* 1996;121(2):129–142.
3. Mathers WD, Nelson SE, Lane JL, et al. Confirmation of confocal microscopy diagnosis of *Acanthamoeba* keratitis using polymerase chain reaction analysis. *Arch Ophthalmol.* 2000;118(2):178–183.
4. Winchester K, Mathers WK, Sutphin JE. Diagnosis of *Aspergillus* keratistis in vivo with confocal microscopy. *Cornea.* 1997;16(1):27–31.
5. Solomon A, Karp CL, Miller D, et al. *Mycobacterium* interface keratitis after laser in situ keratomileusis. *Ophthalmology.* 2001;108:2201–2208.

Chapter 21

Corneal Edema

Vahid Feiz

Corneal transparency is an essential aspect of maintaining a clear retinal image. Transparency is dependent on a strict fluid and electrolyte balance within the corneal stroma. When this delicate process is disturbed, accumulation of fluid will lead to an edematous cornea with decreased transparency. The differential diagnosis of corneal edema is fairly extensive, but an understanding of normal physiology, a thorough history and clinical examination, as well as utilization of ancillary tests, will usually lead to the correct diagnosis and a specific plan of treatment.

Physiology

A number of mechanisms regulate corneal hydration. Not all of these are completely understood; however, a simple list, based on corneal anatomy, is discussed below.

Epithelial and endothelial barriers

Using electron microscopy as well as antibody staining against proteins such as ZO-1 and occludin,[1–3] tight junctions have been demonstrated at the epithelial and endothelial layers of the cornea. These tight junctions restrict the flow of electrolytes and fluid through the paracellular route. The integrity of the epithelial barrier can be clinically determined by application of dyes such as fluorescein. Phenomena such as microcystic corneal edema or bullous keratopathy occur when the epithelial barrier is intact, but fluid overload in the cornea leads to entrapment of fluid beneath the epithelium.

Tear evaporation

The role of tear evaporation in maintaining corneal dehydration is controversial. A commonly reported symptom by patients with Fuchs' endothelial dystrophy is worse vision in the morning that may result from decreased tear evaporation and increased corneal edema during sleep.

Studies on the role of tear evaporation on corneal hydration, however, have yielded conflicting results. In one study, the rate of recovery from hypoxic corneal edema was significantly faster with eyes open compared to eyes closed.[4] Another study investigating the effect of humidity on de-swelling of the cornea, however, failed to show any difference in the rate of resolution of edema at different levels of environmental humidity, which suggests a minimal role for tear evaporation on corneal dehydration.[5]

Intraocular pressure

The level of ocular tension can have a profound and variable effect on corneal stromal hydration. Chronic high pressure can lead to endothelial damage and subsequent edema. Acute rises in intraocular pressure (IOP), on the other hand, can lead to either increased or decreased hydration. A common observation in the early postoperative period after corneal transplantation with epithelial defect and high IOP is a clear, non-edematous cornea. High IOP after lamellar refractive surgery such as LASIK, however, can lead to accumulation of fluid in the interface leading to corneal edema, which can be mistaken as interface inflammation.[6]

Metabolically active mechanisms

Both epithelial and endothelial cells have specialized pumps at the cellular level that under normal physiological circumstances regulate the passage of fluid and ions across the cornea. These pumps provide net active transport of fluid out of the corneal stroma either to the ocular surface or into the aqueous. These active processes require oxygen and energy in the form of adenosine triphosphate (ATP). Depletion of either energy or oxygen, as in contact lens-induced hypoxia, can lead to edema at the level of epithelium or stroma. These active transport mechanisms have been studied extensively at both a cellular and biochemical level. For example, treatment of cornea endothelium with ouabain (a pump inhibitor) will result in stromal edema.[7,8]

Diagnosis

The diagnosis of corneal edema depends on obtaining a careful ocular history, clinical examination, and use of ancillary testing. Some of the causes of corneal edema are listed in Table 21.1.

Clinical history

Patients with corneal edema may have a range of presentations, from asymptomatic disease to severe pain and

Table 21.1 Causes of corneal edema

Classification	Etiologies	Characteristics
Primary endothelial failure	Congenital hereditary endothelial dystrophy (CHED), Fuchs' dystrophy, iridocorneal endothelial syndrome (ICE), posterior polymorphous endothelial dystrophy (PPMD)	Primarily stromal, diffuse, progressive
Secondary endothelial failure	Acute or chronic trauma, chemical, inflammatory, hypoxia	Primarily stromal, focal or diffuse, acute or chronic
Normal endothelium	Elevated intraocular pressure	Primarily epithelial, microcystic, central or diffuse, acute
Epithelial failure	Epithelial defect	Stromal, surrounding defect, acute

Box 21.1 Important clinical history elements in diagnosis and management of corneal edema

Age at onset
Duration of symptoms
Unilateral versus bilateral symptoms
Family history of corneal disease
Ocular medications
Previous ocular disease or surgery
Previous refractive surgery
Diurnal variation of symptoms
Environmental effects on symptoms

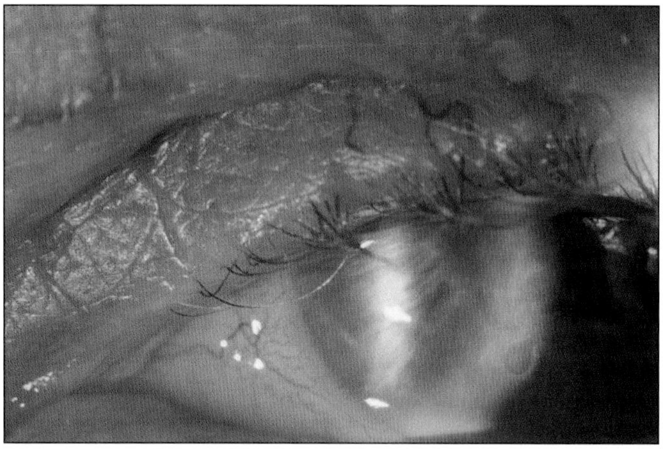

Fig. 21.1 Advanced corneal edema with bullae formation. Note the outline of the bullae highlighted by application of fluorescein.

decreased vision. The location of the edema also influences the symptoms. For example, patients with stromal edema may not have discomfort, while epithelial edema with bulla formation can be very painful. Patients need to be questioned about the duration of symptoms, age of onset, unilaterality versus bilaterality, diurnal variation of the symptoms, use of topical medications, family history of corneal disease, previous ocular disease, and ocular surgeries. Information gathered at this stage can be very useful in determining a cause. For example, patients with corneal edema secondary to endothelial dysfunction often complain of worse vision upon awakening and gradual improvement during the course of the day. Similarly, dystrophies tend to be bilateral, so that unilateral symptoms are less suggestive of dystrophic causes. Box 21.1 has a summary of some of the relevant clinical history and its possible significance.

Examination

A systemic approach to slit lamp examination of the different layers of the cornea will ensure that relevant clinical findings are not missed. Corneal edema can manifest with clinical changes in the epithelium, stroma, and endothelium.

Normal epithelium should have a uniformly smooth surface free of staining with dyes such as fluorescein. This smooth surface turns gray with loss of luster in early, mild edema. As the condition progresses, microcystic changes occur, which can be either diffuse or sectoral. Later in the course, frank bullous keratopathy may develop. The visualization may be enhanced by the application of fluorescein (Fig. 21.1).

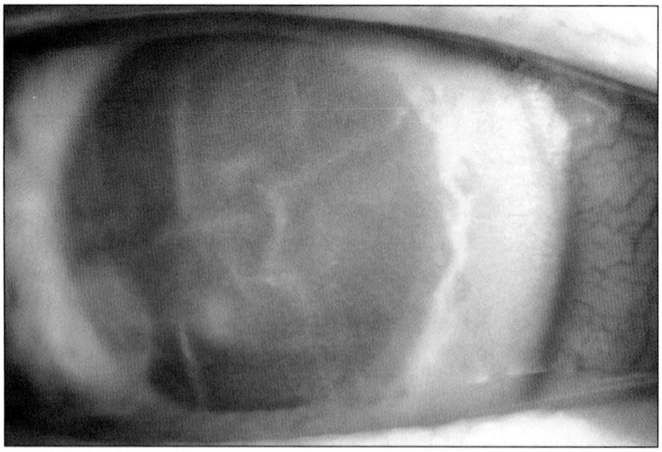

Fig. 21.2 Stromal edema with significant Descemet's fold and loss of corneal transparency due to HSV.

Increased width of the slit beam, as well as presence of folds in the Descemet's membrane, are findings associated with stromal edema (Fig. 21.2). A clear stroma by itself does

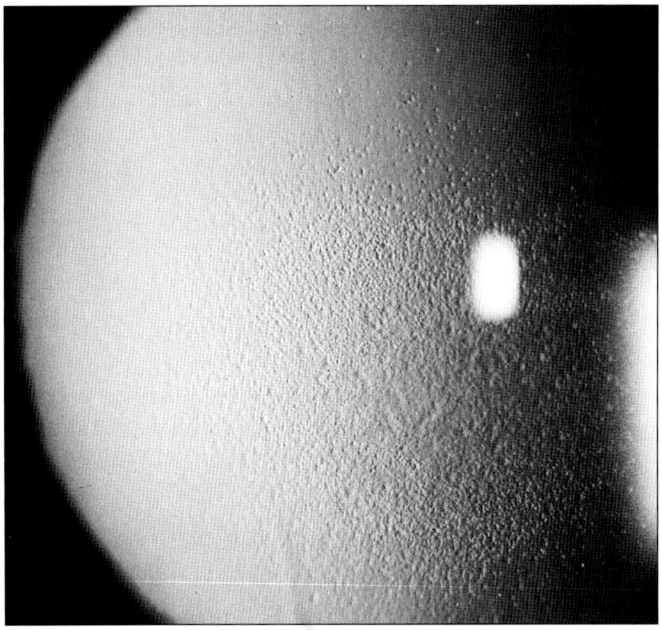

Fig. 21.3 Central corneal endothelial guttae seen against a red reflex in a patient with Fuchs' dystrophy.

not rule out edema, since the cornea may stay optically clear with mild disease.

Using high magnification and a wide angle between the light source and the observer, endothelial abnormalities can be highlighted. Posterior irregularities and pigment may be suggestive of early Fuchs' dystrophy characterized by guttae. These can also be highlighted using retroillumination through a dilated pupil (Fig. 21.3).

Ancillary tests

In addition to the clinical examination, the judicious use of ancillary testing can provide information to determine the stage and severity of the pathological condition and to provide diagnostic clues.

Pachymetry

As corneal hydration increases, the corneal thickness also increases. Pachymetry is the technique of measuring corneal thickness. The two common forms of pachymetry involve the use of ultrasound or optical slit beam measurement. Ultrasound is convenient, since the instruments are easy to use and are commercially available. Optical pachymetry can be performed manually with a slit lamp attachment. Alternatively, a topography unit employs slit beam technology automatically to measure corneal thickness. Although there is usually good agreement between the optical and ultrasound methods, when there is significant loss of cornea clarity, the optical methods become unreliable.

Specular microscopy

Specular microscopy can be used to determine the density and morphology of endothelial cells. The various methods of contact and non-contact specular microscopy as well as analysis of the morphology of endothelial cells provide valuable information that assists the clinician in determining not just the etiology but also the prognosis of corneal edema. In general, most agree that with an endothelial cell count of less than 700 cells/mm^2, corneal edema becomes increasingly likely.

In vivo confocal microscopy

In vivo confocal microscopy can be used to study the microstructural details of different levels of the cornea. The information collected using this modality can be helpful in determining the etiology of corneal edema based on the cellular morphology.[9]

Anterior segment optical coherence tomography

The principle of anterior segment optical coherence tomography (OCT) is analogous to ultrasound but with the emission and reflection of light instead of sound. The anterior segment OCT is an evolution of the retinal OCT. It provides images of anterior segment structures, including the cornea, iris, angle, and anterior lens. Some OCT units have an optical axial resolution of up to 18 μm and optical transverse resolution of up to 60 μm and can scan through an opaque cornea. The software on some units can automatically calculate the central corneal thickness (CCT), the central anterior chamber depth (ACD), the volume of the anterior chamber (AC) and the interspur distance.[10] Although not very useful diagnostically, these instruments can be extremely helpful in following patients after posterior lamellar keratoplasty for treatment of corneal edema (see below).

Treatment

The treatment of corneal edema depends on the specific cause and the symptoms of the individual patient. This can vary from no treatment in an asymptomatic patient with early Fuchs' dystrophy to keratoplasty in a patient with painful bullous keratopathy. A stepwise approach to the treatment of corneal edema is to address any associated ocular abnormality initially and, depending on the result, proceed with additional steps.

Control of associated abnormalities

Inflammation

Treatment of inflammation and the underlying cause of inflammation can be a very powerful tool in resolving corneal edema. Perhaps the most dramatic examples of this are the use of corticosteroids in corneal graft rejection and herpetic stromal keratitis. In the case of a corneal edema due to nonviral infections (bacterial, fungal, etc.), treatment of the underlying infection with appropriate agents will often lead to resolution of edema. In such cases, corticosteroids should be used with extreme caution and only when the infectious component is well under control. The use of corticosteroids in the absence of inflammation will have no effect on corneal edema.[11]

Intraocular pressure

In the setting of either acute or insidious IOP elevation, decreasing the pressure can improve or resolve corneal edema and prevent further damage to endothelial cells. In the past decade there has been a significant increase in the number of new pressure-lowering agents. The specifics of each class are beyond the scope of this text but one class, the carbonic anhydrase inhibitors (CAIs), deserves special attention. Inhibition of corneal carbonic anhydrase pumps may lead to decreased fluid flow from stroma to aqueous and progression to corneal edema. There are several case reports of irreversible corneal edema with the use of topical carbonic anhydrase inhibitors.[12,13] This class of pressure-lowering agents should be used with caution in the setting of corneal edema or compromised endothelial cell function.

Management of epithelial and stromal edema

Hypertonic agents

Use of hypertonic solutions such as 5% sodium chloride drops and ointment facilitates the transition of fluid from epithelium. This in turn will improve microcystic and bullous epithelial keratopathy. Patients should be warned about the stinging associated with the use of these preparations. Glycerin is another hypertonic preparation that can have a dramatic but transient effect on corneal edema. This agent is useful for diagnostic purposes, as it allows better visualization of the corneal layers and the anterior chamber. It should be instilled after application of topical anesthetic, since it is too irritating for use on an unanesthetized eye. Other possibilities include corn syrup and honey, neither of which has practical applications.[14] The use of hypertonic preparations has minimal effect on stromal edema.

Bandage contact lens

Placement of an extended-wear bandage contact lens on the cornea can provide relief from the discomfort of bullous keratopathy and is used in the setting of poor visual potential or when surgical intervention is not recommended or is dealyed. The contact lens chosen should have high oxygen transmissibility. The comfort provided by this modality must be weighed against the risk of contact lens-induced infectious corneal ulcer. Regular follow-up visits and the use of prophylactic topical antibiotics reduce the risk of complications.

Anterior stromal cautery

Application of light burns to Bowman's layer using a thermal cautery (Salleras procedure) leads to formation of scars and firm adhesion between the epithelium and the underlying stroma. This decreases the formation of bullae and microcystic edema. The technique is simple and can provide excellent pain relief. It should be reserved for eyes that have poor visual potential or are poor surgical candidates.

Conjunctival flap

Covering the cornea with vascular conjunctival tissue, after the epithelium has been removed, provides coverage of corneal nerves. Vision is usually worse after the procedure and patients should be warned about this. This modality is usually reserved for eyes with poor visual potential or patients who are not candidates for corneal transplantation.

Amniotic membrane

In the past decade, application of amniotic membrane to rehabilitate the ocular surface has gained popularity. Short-term symptomatic relief of pain after application of amniotic membrane in the setting of corneal edema has been reported.[15,16] Whether or not this method can provide long-term relief is not known.

Excimer laser

Phototherapeutic keratectomy of the anterior corneal stroma using excimer laser has been shown in several studies to provide pain relief for corneal edema with bullous keratopathy. Deeper stromal ablations tend to provide more relief than superficial treatments. Long-term data for this approach are not yet available but it is probably most valuable as a temporizing measure until a definitive treatment can be applied.[17]

Penetrating keratoplasty

Corneal transplantation is the definitive treatment for a range of corneal diseases, especially when the etiology is poor endothelial function. Transplantation provides the eye with a healthy functioning reserve of endothelial cells and new stroma. Adequate use of immunosuppressive agents, as well as modern surgical techniques, has resulted in very high success rates after keratoplasty. The goal of penetrating keratoplasty is both to rehabilitate the eye visually and to relieve symptoms of corneal edema.

Endothelial keratoplasty

Corneal transplant surgery for endothelial dysfunction has evolved over the last decade from penetrating keratoplasty (PKP) to posterior lamellar keratoplasty (PLK).[18] The technological advances have led to the development of a selective endothelial replacement surgery enabling rapid postoperative healing, early visual recovery, and minimal to moderate refractive change. The surgical techniques have further evolved from PLK to deep lamellar endothelial keratoplasty (DLEK), Descemet stripping endothelial keratoplasty (DSEK) and to Descemet stripping automated endothelial keratoplasty (DSAEK).[19,20] At this stage, DSAEK is rapidly becoming the procedure of choice for endothelial dysfunction. The common feature of all these procedures is the transfer of donor tissue, including endothelium, Descemet's membrane, and a thin layer of posterior stroma.

Descemet's membrane endothelial keratoplasty (DMEK) is a new and evolving surgical technique in which only the

Descemet's membrane and the endothelial cell layer are transplanted.[21] This procedure, while technically difficult, may theoretically result in better postoperative visual acuity compared to other endothelial keratoplasty techniques, since it may avoid an irregular interface. Long-term results of DMEK surgery are not yet available.

Collagen Cross-linking

Collagen cross-linking using riboflavin and ultraviolet A (UVA) is an experimental modality that has been utilized for the treatment of corneal ectasia. Some have employed collagen cross-linking for the treatment of cornea and have demonstrated decreased edema in the cross-linked portion of the cornea than in the untreated control area. A recent study evaluated the safety and efficacy of staged UVA cross-linking following intrastromal 0.1% riboflavin administration in eyes with advanced corneal edema.[22] The authors noted significant decrease in corneal edema and increased corneal clarity compared to the control eyes. Long-term follow-up and results from large studies on the use of this modality are not yet available.

References

1. McCartney MD, Wood TO, McLauglin BJ. Freeze-fracture label of functional and dysfunctional human corneal endothelium. *Curr Eye Res.* 1987;6(4):589–597.
2. Sugrue SP, Zieske JD. ZO1 in corneal epithelium: association to the zonula occludens and adherens junctions. *Exp Eye Res.* 1997;64(1):11–20.
3. Petroll WM, Hsu JK, Bean J, et al. The spatial organization of apical junctional complex-associated proteins in the feline and human corneal endothelium. *Curr Eye Res.* 1999;18(1):10–19.
4. O'Neal MR, Polse KA. In vivo assessment of mechanisms controlling corneal hydration. *Invest Ophthalmol Vis Sci.* 1985;26(6):849–586.
5. Bourassa S, Benjamin WJ, Boltz RL. Effect of humidity on the deswelling function of the human cornea. *Curr Eye Res.* 1991;10(6):493–500.
6. Fogla R, Rao SK, Padmanabahn P. Interface fluid after laser in situ keratomileusis. *J Cataract Refract Surg.* 2001;27:1526–1528.
7. Geroski DH, Kies JC, Edelhauser HF. The effect of ouabain on endothelial function in human and rabbit corneas. *Curr Eye Res.* 1984;3(2):331–338.
8. Diecke FP, Zhu Z, Kang F, et al. Sodium, potassium, two chloride cotransport in corneal endothelium: characterization and possible role in volume regulation and fluid transport. *Invest Ophthalmol Vis Sci.* 1998;39(1):104–110.
9. Grupcheva CN, Craig JP, Sherwin T, McGhee CNJ. Differential diagnosis of corneal oedema assisted by in vivo confocal microscopy. *Clin Exp Ophthalmol.* 2001;29:133–137.
10. Konstantopoulos A, Hossain P, Anderson DF. Recent advances in ophthalmic anterior segment imaging: a new era for ophthalmic diagnosis? *Br J Ophthalmol.* 2007;91(4):551–557.
11. Wilson SE, Bourne WM, Brubaker RF. Effect of dexamethasone on corneal endothelial function in Fuchs' dystrophy. *Invest Ophthalmol Vis Sci.* 1988;29:357.
12. Konowol A, Morrison JC, Brown SV, et al. Irreversible corneal decompensation in patients treated with topical dorzolamide. *Am J Ophthalmol.* 1999;127(4):403–406.
13. Domingo Gordo B, Urcelay Segura JL, Conejero Arroyo J, et al. Corneal decompensation in patients with endothelial compromise treated with topical dorzolamide. *Arch Soc Esp Oftalmol.* 2002;77(3):139–144.
14. Mansour AM. Epithelial corneal oedema treated with honey. *Clin Exp Ophthalmol.* 2002;30:149–150.
15. Pires RT, Tseng SC, Prabhavasawat P, et al. Amniotic membrane transplantation for symptomatic bullous keratopathy. *Arch Ophthalmol.* 1999;117(10):1291–1297.
16. Mrukwa-Kominek E, Gierek-Ciaciura S, Rotika-Wala I, Szymkowiak M. Use of amniotic membrane transplantation for treating bullous keratopathy. *Klin Oczna.* 2002;104(1):41–46.
17. Rosa N, Cennamo G. Phototherapeutic keratectomy for relief of pain in patients with pseudophakic corneal edema. *J Refract Surg.* 2002;18(3):276–279.
18. Melles GR, Lander F, Beekhuis WH, et al. Posterior lamellar keratoplasty for a case of pseudophakic bullous keratopathy. *Am J Ophthalmol.* 1999;127(3):340–341.
19. Terry MA, Ousley PJ. Deep lamellar endothelial keratoplasty in the first United States patients: early clinical results. *Cornea.* 2001;20(3):239–243.
20. Price MO, Price FW. Descemet's stripping endothelial keratoplasty. *Curr Opin Ophthalmol.* 2007;18(4):290–294.
21. Melles GR, Ong TS, Ververs B, van der Wees J. Descemet membrane endothelial keratoplasty (DMEK). *Cornea.* 2006;25(8):987–990.
22. Bellini LP. New uses for collagen crosslinking. *J Cataract Refract Surg.* 2008;34(6):879–880.

Chapter 22

Corneal Deposits

David A. Palay

Abnormal deposition of material in the cornea is easily discerned for two reasons. First, the cornea in its normal state is clear, and deposits of any type produce clouding. Second, the details of the cornea can be readily examined with a slit lamp, which magnifies the cornea under conditions of variable illumination.

This chapter presents a systematic approach to the evaluation of the patient with corneal deposits. The focus is on achieving the correct diagnosis by evaluating two major aspects of the deposits: the depth of the deposit in the corneal stroma, and the color of the deposits. Identifying the location and color of the deposits considerably shortens the differential diagnosis.

The cornea can be divided into three depths: superficial, stromal, and deep stromal. The superficial layer corresponds histologically to the epithelium, Bowman's layer, and the very anterior stroma. The stromal layer represents the bulk of the histologic, anatomic stroma. The deep stromal layer is defined as the deep posterior stroma, Descemet's membrane, and the endothelium.

The color of the deposits can be divided into three categories: pigmented, nonpigmented, and refractile/crystalline. Pigmented deposits can be any color, but typically are yellow or brown. Nonpigmented deposits are white or gray. Refractile or crystalline deposits are clear with indirect illumination, but may be white or gray with direct illumination. Occasionally, crystalline deposits may be polychromatic.

The reader is referred to the appropriate nine groupings in Table 22.1. The text highlights further specifics of the deposits.

Superficial Deposits

Pigmented deposits

Cornea verticillata

Cornea verticillata refers to linear opacities located within the corneal epithelium that assume a characteristic whorl-like pattern (Fig. 22.1). The opacities are located primarily in the inferior paracentral cornea and are not elevated. Their color may vary from white to brown. Cornea verticillata is seen in Fabry's disease and as a side effect from multiple systemic medications including amiodarone,[1] chloroquine, quinacrine, chlorpromazinc,[2] indometacin,[3] clofazimine,[4] suramin,[5] naproxen,[6] and tilorone.[7] Fabry's disease is an X-linked lysosomal storage disease, which results in the accumulation of trihexosyl ceramide.[8,9] Corneal changes are found in both the hemizygote male and heterozygote female carriers.[10]

Striate melanokeratosis

Striate melanokeratosis refers to pigment lines located in the epithelium, which extend from the limbus toward the central cornea (Fig. 22.2). These lines normally occur in darkly pigmented individuals but also can occur in lighter pigmented individuals after injury or inflammation. The deposits are probably the result of migration of pigmented limbal stem cells onto the cornea.

Epithelial iron lines

Iron deposits in the epithelium have a yellow-brown coloration (Fig. 22.3). Pooling of tears in the region of topographic irregularities allows iron from the tear film to be deposited within the epithelium. Iron lines can be seen in the palpebral fissure (Hudson-Stahli), at the head of a pterygium (Stocker), surrounding the cone in keratoconus (Fleischer), at the head of a filtering bleb (Ferry), adjacent to areas of corneal elevation such as Salzmann's nodular degeneration, anterior to the sutures in keratoplasty (Mannis), and after keratorefractive surgery.[11,12]

Spheroidal degeneration

Spheroidal degeneration produces golden-yellow globular deposits within the interpalpebral area (Fig. 22.4). The deposits are located within Bowman's layer and the anterior stroma. In primary spheroidal degeneration, the deposits are bilateral and initially located in the nasal and temporal cornea; they can extend onto the conjunctiva. Secondary spheroidal degeneration is associated with ocular injury or inflammation. The deposits in secondary spheroidal degeneration will aggregate near the area of corneal scarring or vascularization.[13]

Adrenochrome deposition

Adrenochrome deposits are usually found within the conjunctiva, but rarely may occur on the corneal surface

Table 22.1 Corneal deposits

	Superficial	Stromal	Deep stromal
Pigmented	Cornea verticillata (Fabry's disease and drug effects) Striate melanokeratosis Epithelial iron lines Spheroidal degeneration Adrenochrome	Phenothiazines Blood staining Bilirubin Siderosis (iron)	Wilson's disease (copper) Chalcosis Chrysiasis (gold) Mottled cyan opacification
Nonpigmented	Subepithelial mucinous dystrophy Coat's white ring Calcific band keratopathy Fluoroquinolones Mucin balls	Granular dystrophy Macular dystrophy Fleck dystrophy Lipid deposition Mucopolysaccharidoses	Cornea farinata Pre-Descemet's dystrophy X-linked ichthyosis Argyrosis (silver)
Refractile/crystalline	Meesmann's dystrophy Gelatinous droplike dystrophy Tyrosinemia II Intraepithelial ointment Gout (urate)	Lattice dystrophy Schnyder's dystrophy Bietti's dystrophy Immunoglobulin Cystinosis	Polymorphic amyloid degeneration

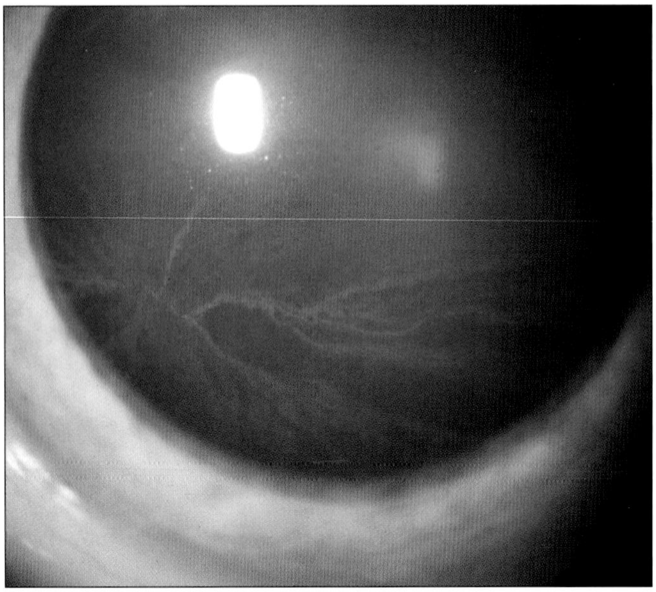

Fig. 22.1 Cornea verticillata (image shown is amiodarone deposits).

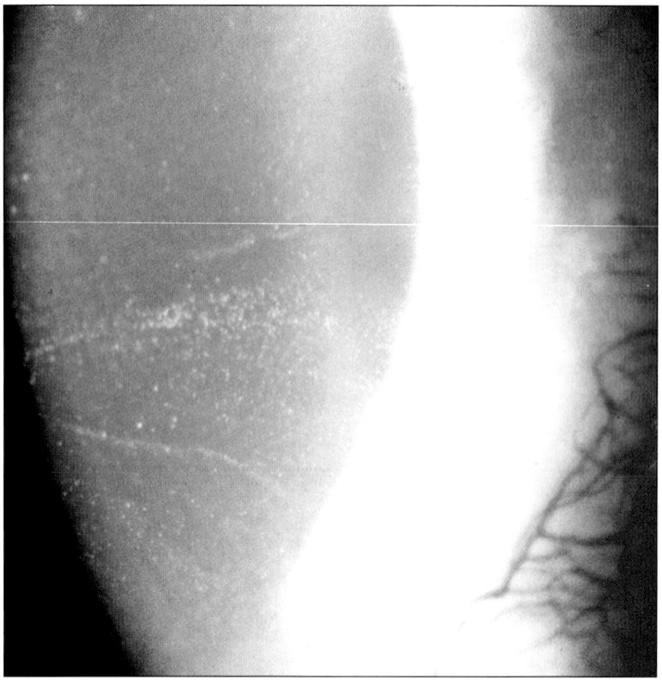

Fig. 22.2 Striate melanokeratosis.

(Fig. 22.5). These brown-black deposits occur in patients treated with epinephrine eye drops for glaucoma.[14]

Nonpigmented deposits

Subepithelial mucinous corneal dystrophy

Subepithelial mucinous corneal dystrophy is an autosomal dominant condition, which results in the deposition of glycosaminoglycans in the subepithelial stroma (Fig. 22.6). Clinically, a diffuse homogeneous subepithelial haze is seen bilaterally. The haze is denser centrally and fades toward the periphery. Irregular gray-white opacities also may be seen centrally; these deposits may be raised.[15]

Coat's white ring

Coat's white ring is a superficial ring of iron deposition that remains after a metallic foreign body is removed (Fig. 22.7).[16] Small white opacities may be seen inside the ring. These rings develop when a rust ring from an iron foreign body is not entirely removed.

Calcific band keratopathy

Hypercalcemia and chronic ocular inflammation are the most common conditions associated with calcific band

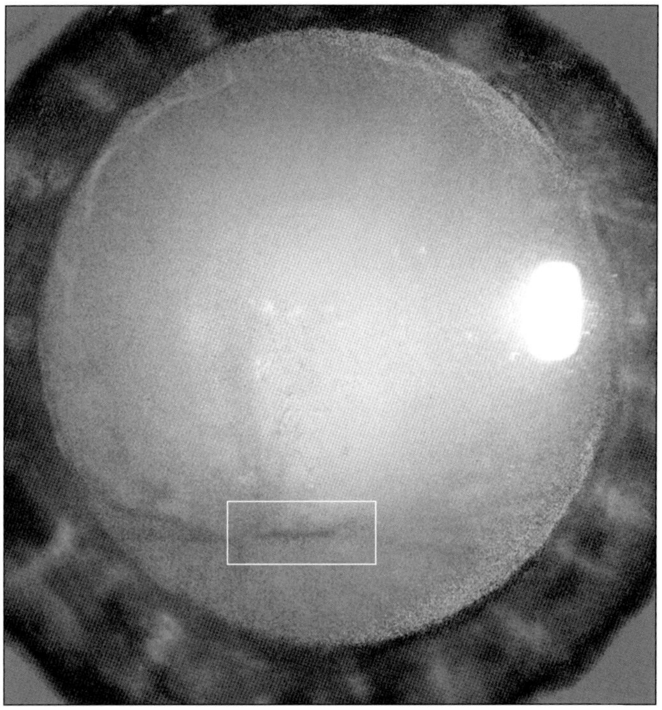

Fig. 22.3 Iron lines (image shown is Hudson-Stahli line).

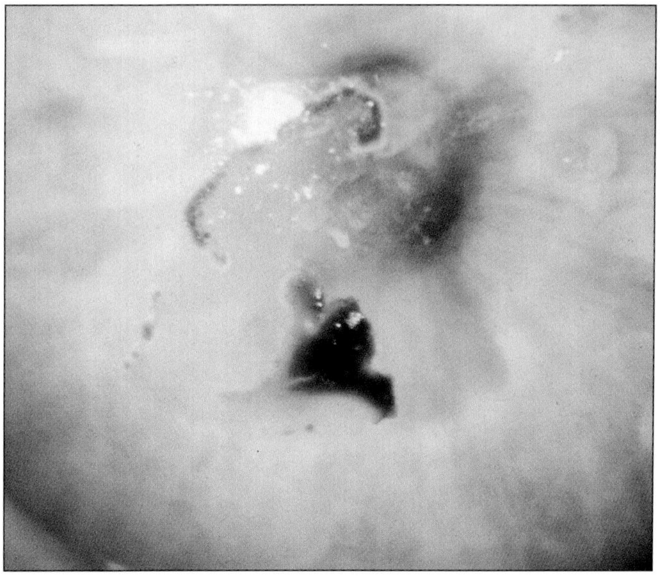

Fig. 22.5 Adrenochrome.

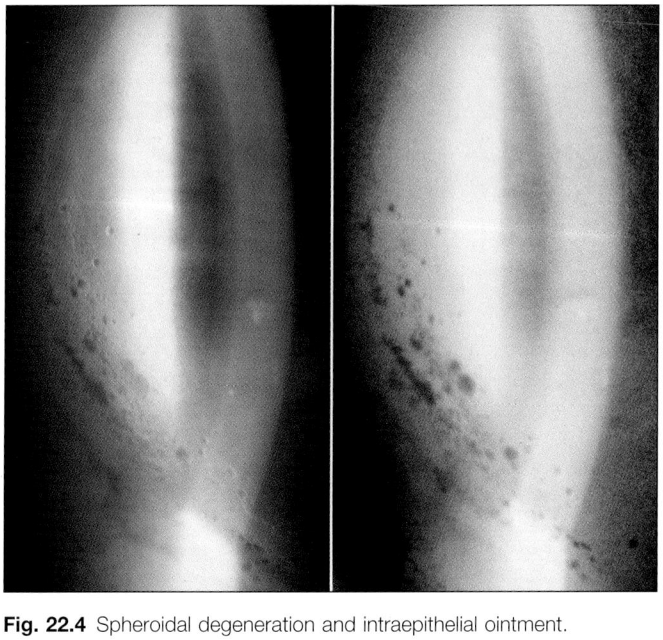

Fig. 22.4 Spheroidal degeneration and intraepithelial ointment.

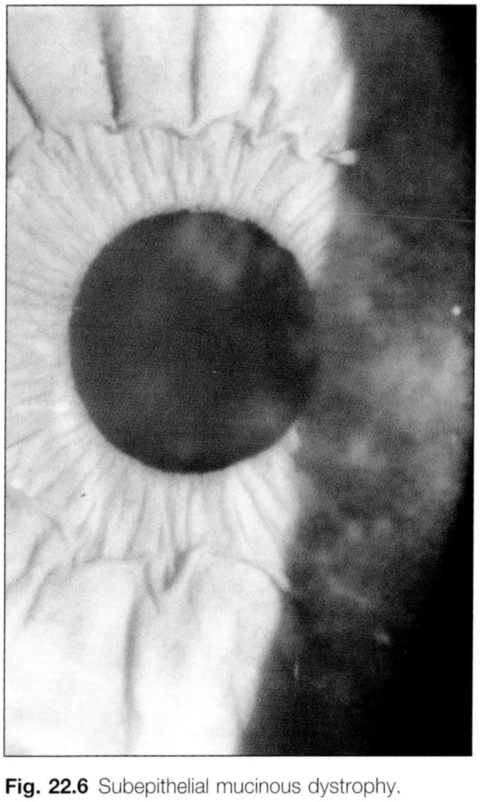

Fig. 22.6 Subepithelial mucinous dystrophy.

keratopathy (Fig. 22.8). The calcium is deposited within the epithelial basement membrane, Bowman's layer, and the anterior stroma. Clinically, subepithelial chalky white deposits are found in the interpalpebral zone. The deposition initially begins in the peripheral cornea, with a clear margin separating the deposit from the limbus. The clear interval is thought to represent the anatomic limit of Bowman's layer. Throughout the band are clear, small holes that give a 'Swiss cheese' appearance. The holes occur at sites where corneal nerves penetrate Bowman's layer.[17]

Fluoroquinolone deposits

Topical ciprofloxacin[18] and norfloxacin[19] therapy can result in the deposition of a chalky white precipitate within an epithelial defect (Fig. 22.9). Although they are predominantly

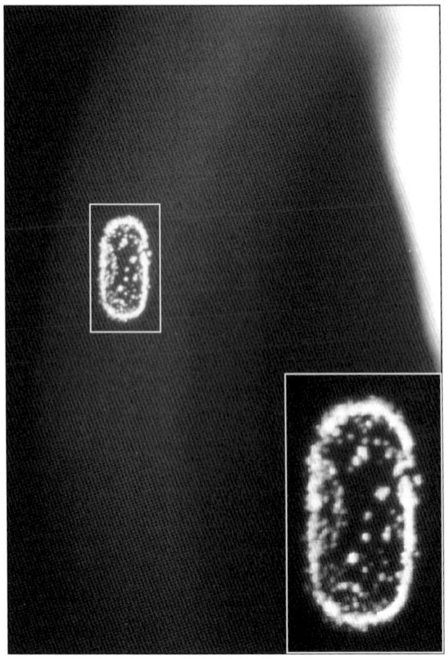

Fig. 22.7 Coat's white ring.

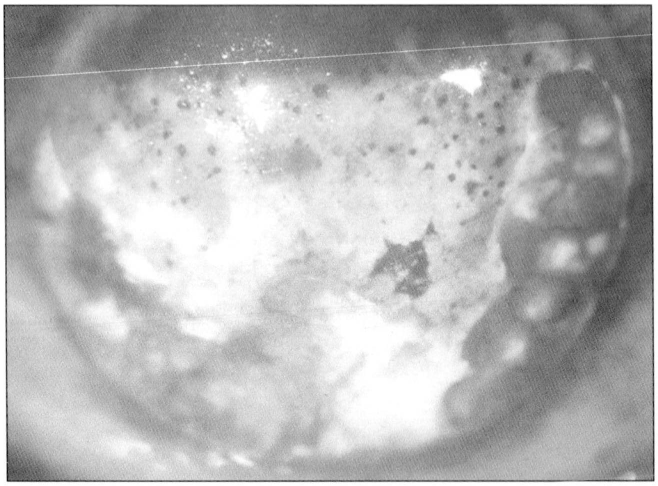

Fig. 22.8 Band keratopathy (image shown is calcific band keratopathy).

white in appearance, a crystalline pattern also may be observed.

Mucin balls

Mucin balls are round white deposits that accumulate between the posterior surface of a contact lens and the corneal epithelium (Fig. 22.10). When the contact lens is removed, the mucin balls may be blinked away, but in some cases they remain adherent to the cornea for several hours. When they are removed they leave a depression in the epithelium. They are more common with rigid soft contact lens material such as high-Dk silicone lenses.[20]

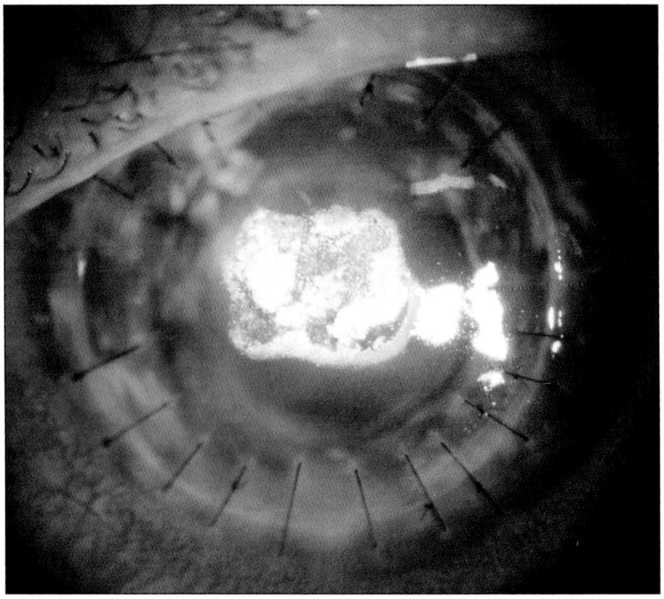

Fig. 22.9 Fluoroquinolone (image shown is ciprofloxacin deposits).

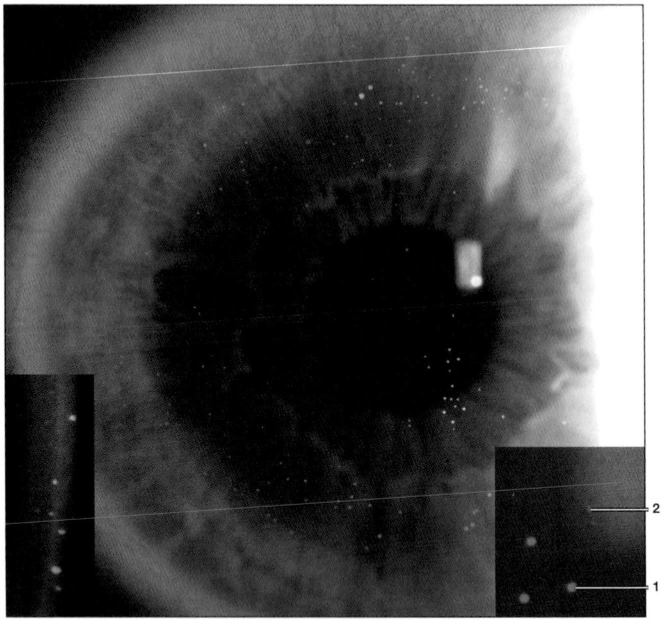

Fig. 22.10 Mucin balls. Mucin ball adherent to cornea (1). Epithelial depression (2) from mucin ball that has been removed. From Krachmer JH, Palay DA (eds). Cornea Atlas, 2nd edn. Mosby, Elsevier Inc, 2005.

Refractile/crystalline deposits

Meesmann's dystrophy

Meesmann's dystrophy is an autosomal dominant disorder that results in the accumulation of bilateral intraepithelial cysts throughout the cornea (Fig. 22.11). These cysts appear gray on direct illumination, but with retroillumination are

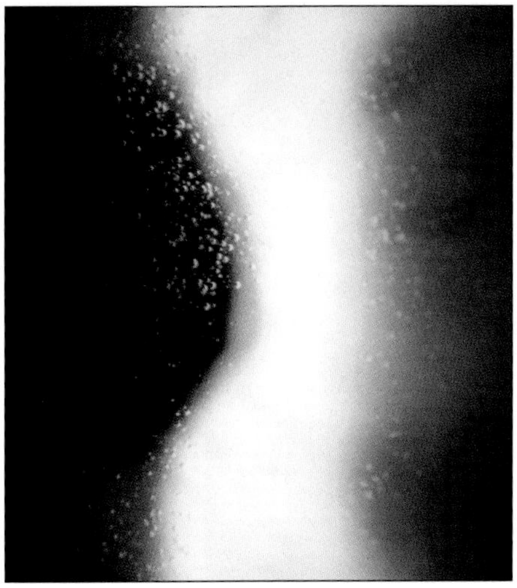

Fig. 22.11 Meesmann's dystrophy.

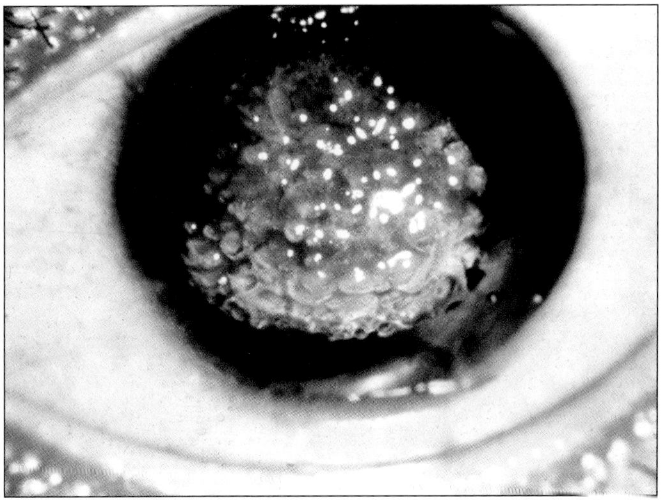

Fig. 22.12 Gelatinous droplike dystrophy.

transparent and are thus better viewed. The cysts are confined to the epithelium and extend to the limbus. The intervening cornea is clear.[21]

Gelatinous droplike dystrophy

Gelatinous droplike dystrophy is an autosomal recessive disorder that results in the bilateral accumulation of amyloid deposits in the anterior corneal stroma (Fig. 22.12). This condition, as well as lattice dystrophy, is a form of primary localized corneal amyloidosis. Clinically, subepithelial raised, gelatinous deposits appear within the first or second decade. These deposits are refractile on indirect illumination, limited to the central cornea, and have been likened to the appearance of a mulberry.[22]

Tyrosinemia II (Richner-Hanhart syndrome)

Tyrosinemia II is an autosomal recessive inborn error of tyrosine metabolism caused by a deficiency of tyrosine aminotransferase. The deposits are located within the

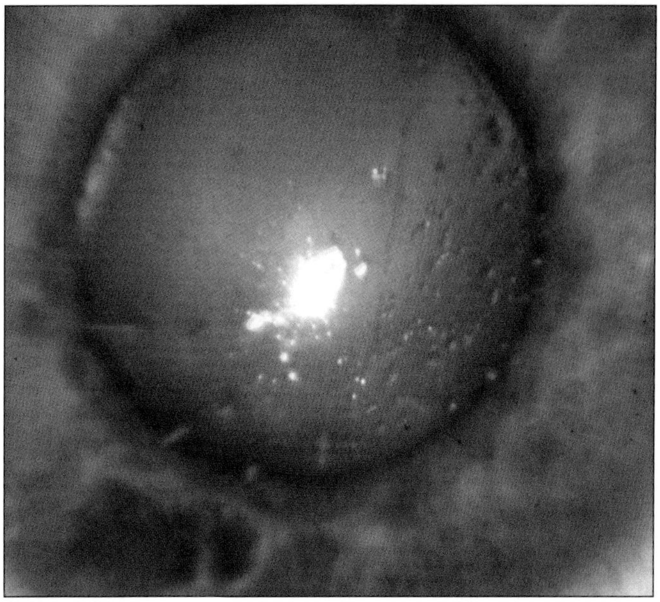

Fig 22.13 Tyrosinemia II. (Courtesy of Gary Foulks MD and Duke University, Durham, NC.)

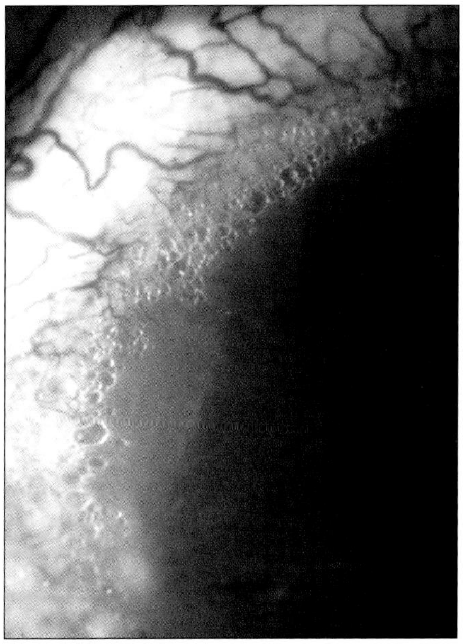

Fig. 22.14 Intraepithelial ointment.

epithelium and subepithelial space of the central cornea (Fig 22.13). They are bilateral and appear as refractile branching linear opacities. The deposits can assume a dendritic pattern and can be confused with herpetic keratitis; however, they do not stain with fluorescein. The opacities may coalesce into a plaque-like configuration. The deposits may clear with appropriate dietary changes.[23]

Intraepithelial ointment

Rarely, ophthalmic ointment preparations can become entrapped in the epithelium after corneal abrasions have healed (Fig. 22.14). The clinical appearance is of clear globules within the epithelium.[24]

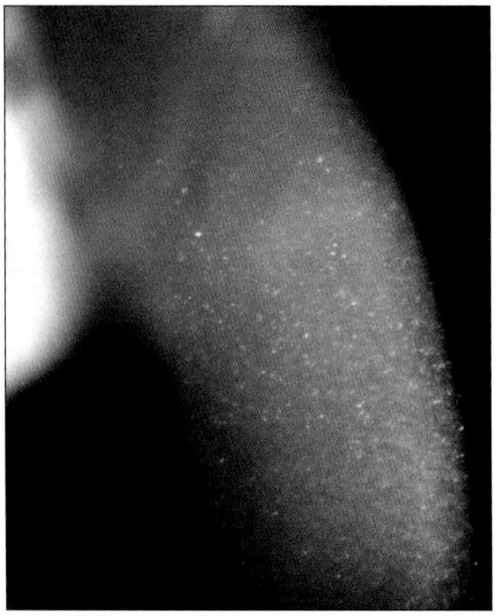

Fig. 22.15 Gout (urate).

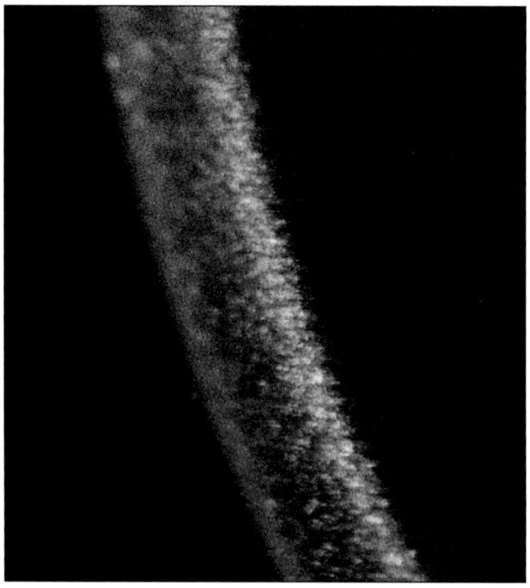

Fig. 22.16 Phenothiazines.

Gout (urate)

Patients with gout may have fine, yellow, scintillating crystals in the superficial cornea (Fig. 22.15).[25] These crystals can become confluent in the interpalpebral region and can form a pigmented band keratopathy.

Stromal Deposits

Pigmented Deposits

Phenothiazines

Phenothiazines are synthetic antipsychotic drugs that can cause numerous toxic side effects when used in high doses. The corneal findings include a diffuse, granular, yellow-brown pigmentation located throughout the stroma, although usually more dense in the deep stroma (Fig. 22.16). Light exposure probably plays a role in the pathogenesis because the deposits are denser in the interpalpebral region. With very high doses, cornea verticillata or conjunctival pigmentation may be seen.[26]

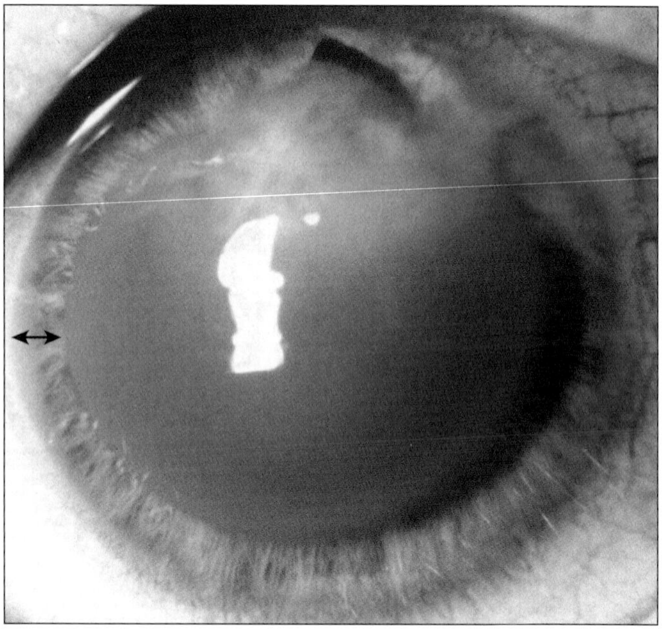

Fig. 22.17 Blood staining. Arrows indicate area where blood has cleared.

Corneal blood staining

Corneal blood staining most commonly occurs in the presence of a hyphema and elevated intraocular pressure. Initially, there are small yellow granules within the posterior stroma. With continued presence of the hyphema, a rust-colored opacity of the stroma develops. With time, the blood in the cornea becomes yellow (Fig. 22.17). This opacity can involve the entire cornea and clears over several years, beginning at the limbus and progressing centrally.[27]

Bilirubin

Elevated levels of bilirubin secondary to advanced liver diseases such as hepatitis, cirrhosis, or biliary obstruction can lead to a yellow staining in the peripheral cornea (Fig. 22.18). The staining is found throughout the corneal stroma but is more extensive in the deep stroma. The bilirubin is thought to diffuse from the limbal circulation. With severe elevations of bilirubin, the entire cornea may be stained.[28] It is almost always associated with conjunctival bilirubin staining.[29]

Siderosis

Ocular siderosis is iron deposition within intraocular structures (Fig. 22.19). It typically occurs in the setting of a metallic intraocular foreign body, although systemic causes of iron overload such as hemochromatosis can also lead to the

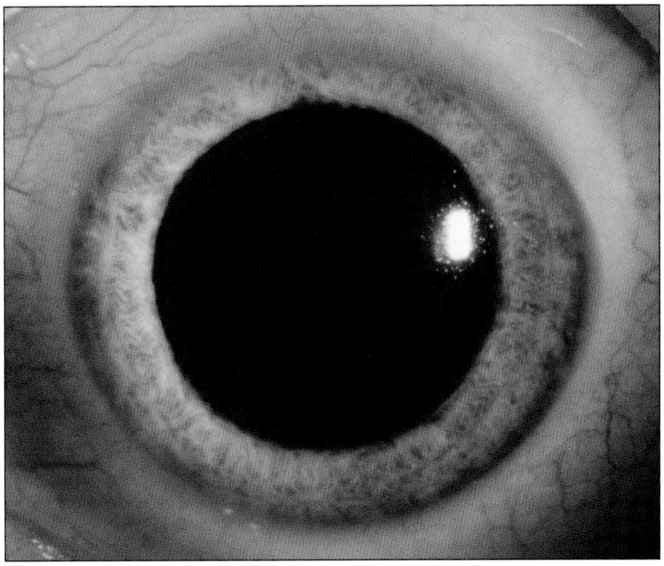

Fig. 22.18 Bilirubin.

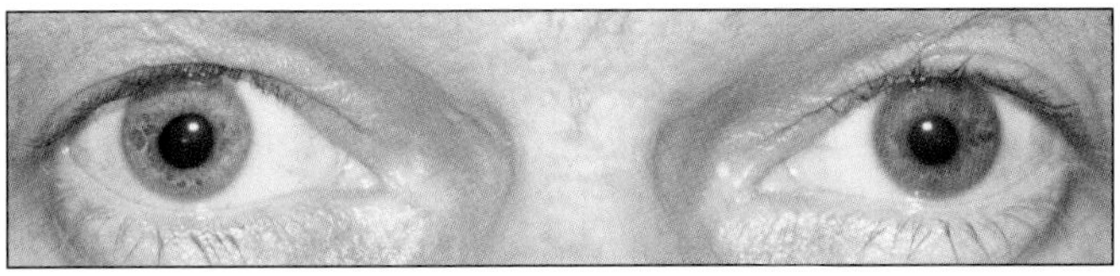

Fig. 22.19 Siderosis.

condition. The cornea can occasionally be affected by siderosis if the foreign body is localized within the anterior chamber. Yellow-brown iron deposits can be seen within the posterior stroma.[30]

Nonpigmented deposits

Granular dystrophy

Granular dystrophy is an autosomal dominant condition that affects the central corneal stroma of both eyes (Fig. 22.20). Focal white 'bread crumb' deposits that assume irregular shapes are located throughout the stroma, but tend to be concentrated anteriorly. A 2–3 mm peripheral clear zone is free of deposits. The deposits initially appear within the first decade of life, and the intervening stroma is clear. Over time, the deposits tend to coalesce, and the intervening stroma assumes a ground-glass appearance. Visual impairment usually begins after the fifth decade.[21]

Macular dystrophy

Macular dystrophy is an autosomal recessive disorder that results in the accumulation of glycosaminoglycans (predominantly keratin sulfate) within stromal keratocytes and the intervening stroma (Fig. 22.21). Clinically, small, gray-white nodular deposits are seen within a diffuse stromal haze. The haze and deposits extend limbus to limbus and throughout

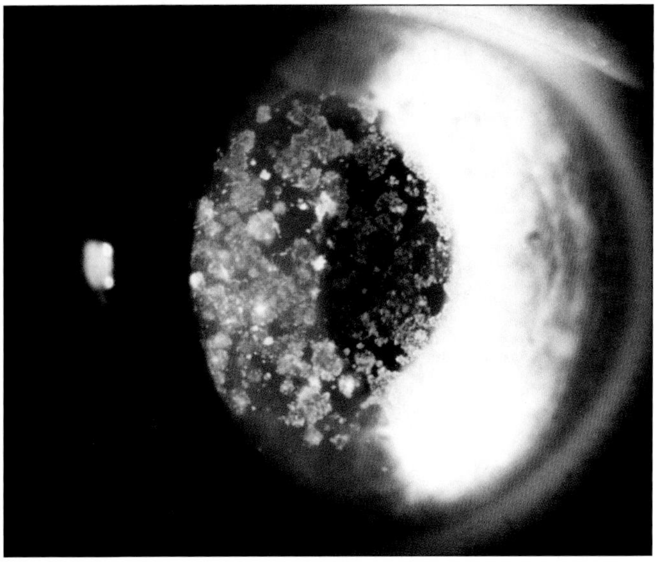

Fig. 22.20 Granular dystrophy.

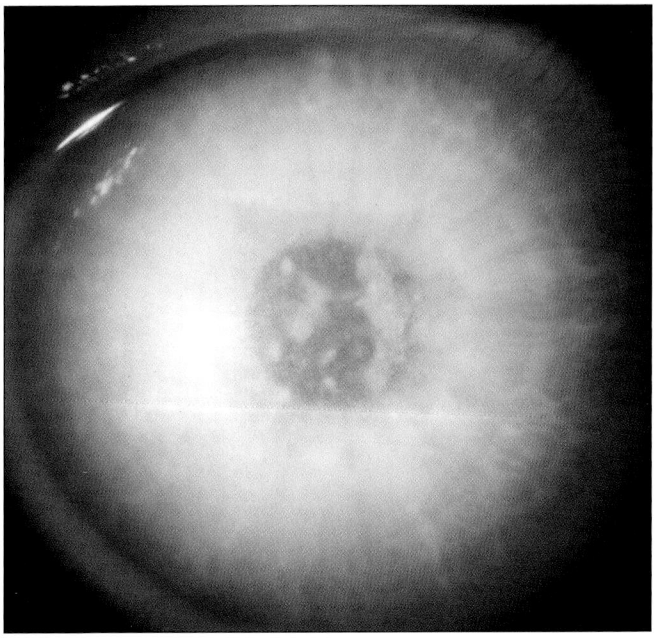

Fig. 22.21 Macular dystrophy.

the corneal stroma. Visual acuity is markedly decreased by the third to fourth decade.[21]

Fleck dystrophy

Fleck dystrophy is an autosomal dominant disorder that results in the bilateral accumulation of glycosaminoglycans and lipid within keratocytes. Clinically, discrete gray-white opacities are seen throughout the stroma (Fig. 22.22). The intervening stroma is clear. Bowman's layer, Descemet's membrane, and the endothelium are uninvolved. The opacities have sharp borders and may be round, oval, or

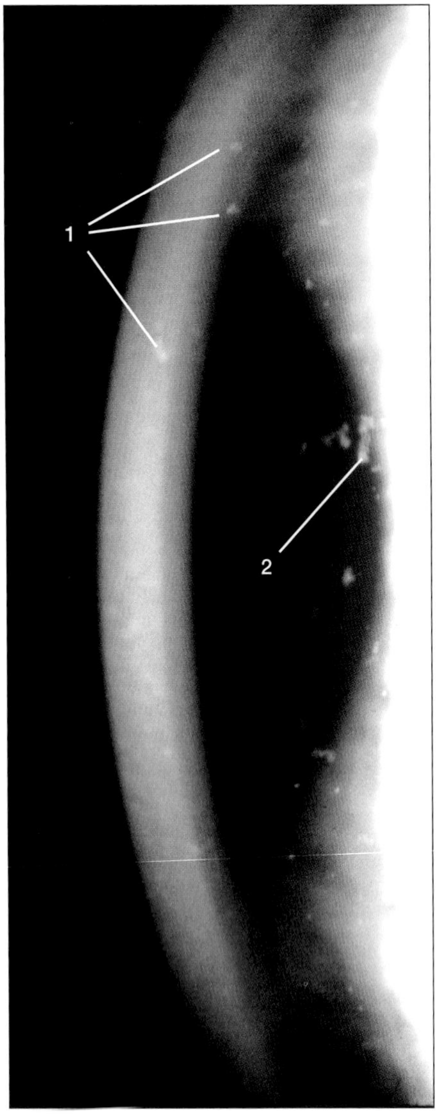

Fig. 22.22 Fleck dystrophy. This autosomal dominant disorder is seen as an incidental finding. There are white, comma-shaped, stellate, circular, and wreathlike opacities at all levels of the corneal stroma. The opacities are white in direct light (1) and gray in indirect light (2). Histologically, the deposits are formed by distended keratocytes filled with complex lipids and glycosaminoglycans. Vision is not affected.

wreathlike. Vision is not affected. Punctate lenticular opacities also may be present.[31]

Lipid deposition

Arcus senilis is lipid deposition within the peripheral cornea, possibly secondary to increased permeability of the limbal vasculature. The lipid is initially deposited in the superior and inferior margins of the cornea. Clinically, the deposits appear as a hazy white circumferential band separated from the limbus by a lucid interval (Fig. 22.23). The outer margin of the deposit is sharply demarcated, and the inner margin is irregular secondary to an arterial diffusion gradient of lipid toward the central cornea and a venous clearing of lipid peripherally.[32]

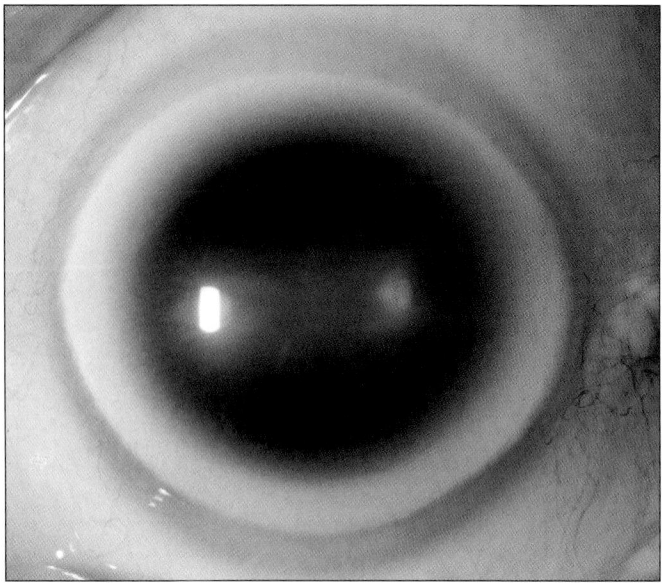

Fig. 22.23 Lipid deposition (image shown is arcus senilis).

Secondary lipid deposition occurs when corneal neovascularization is present. Associated conditions include trauma, interstitial keratitis, and corneal ulceration. Clinically, the lipid may assume either a fan-shaped pattern in front of active neovascularization or a disk-shaped pattern within chronic neovascularization.[33]

Systemic abnormalities in lipid metabolism including lecithin-cholesterol acyl transferase (LCAT) deficiency and fish eye disease, and Tangier disease can result in lipid deposition in the corneal stroma.[34]

Mucopolysaccharidoses

The mucopolysaccharidoses are a group of metabolic disorders that result in the accumulation of mucopolysaccharides secondary to deficiencies of lysosomal acid hydrolases. Corneal clouding is diffuse and composed of fine gray punctate opacities (Fig. 22.24). Hurler's, Scheie's, Morquio's, and Maroteaux-Lamy syndromes all demonstrate progressive corneal clouding. Hunter's and Sanfilippo's syndromes do not demonstrate clouding grossly, but may have slit lamp evidence of clouding at a later age.[35]

Refractile/crystalline deposits

Lattice dystrophy

Lattice dystrophy is an autosomal dominant disorder that results in the accumulation of amyloid within the corneal stroma (Fig. 22.25). There are refractile lines with nodular dilations. The lines are white in direct light and translucent or crystalline in indirect light. The deposits are more common in the anterior stroma. Usually there is a limbal clear zone. The dystrophy is progressive and the stromal haze may obscure the lines and dots. Recurrent epithelial erosions are a common finding in this disease and can lead to subepithelial opacification.[21]

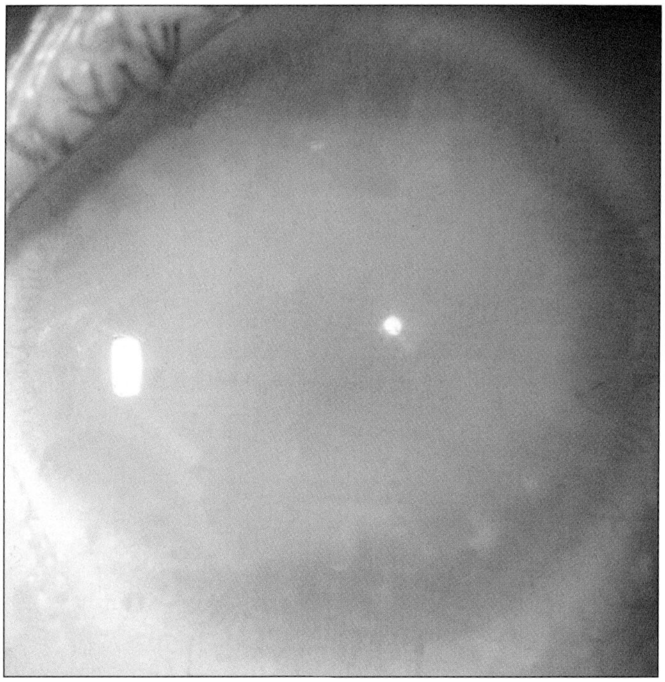

Fig. 22.24 Mucopolysaccharidoses (image shown is Maroteaux-Lamy syndrome).

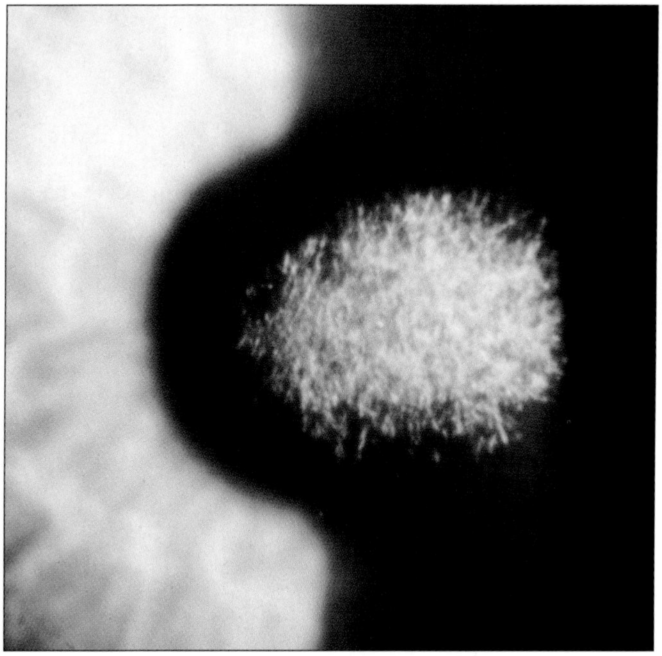

Fig. 22.26 Schnyder's crystalline dystrophy.

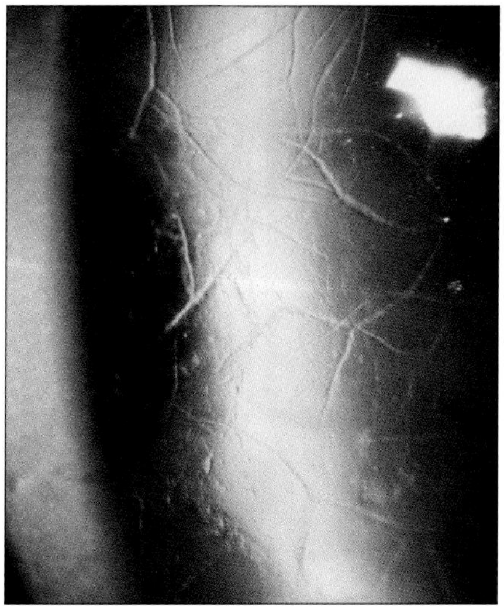

Fig. 22.25 Lattice dystrophy.

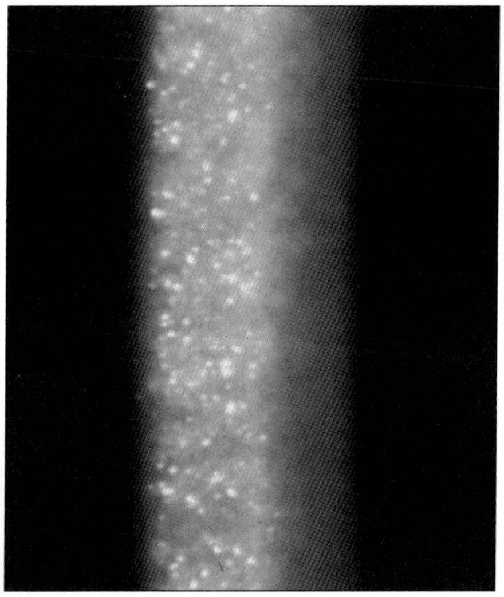

Fig. 22.27 Bietti's crystalline dystrophy.

Schnyder's central crystalline dystrophy

Schnyder's crystalline dystrophy is an autosomal dominant disorder that results in the accumulation of cholesterol and neutral fats within the central stroma (Fig. 22.26). Clinically, a diffuse gray stromal haze is seen with small crystals scattered throughout the haze. A significant number of patients also will have a dense corneal arcus. The haze and crystals usually assume a central disk or ring pattern. The clinical appearance of the dystrophy varies widely, but it typically presents during the first decade, with progressive opacification over time.[21]

Bietti's crystalline dystrophy

Bietti's crystalline dystrophy is a rare autosomal recessive disorder characterized by corneal and retinal crystals associated with retinal pigment epithelial atrophy and choroidal sclerosis (Fig. 22.27). The corneal crystals are small and located in the anterior stroma and subepithelial space in the peripheral cornea. The corneal crystals resemble cholesterol or other lipid deposits histologically, and the disorder may represent a systemic defect in lipid metabolism. This progressive condition usually presents in the third decade with symptoms of nyctalopia, poor dark adaptation, peripheral visual field loss, or central visual acuity loss.[36]

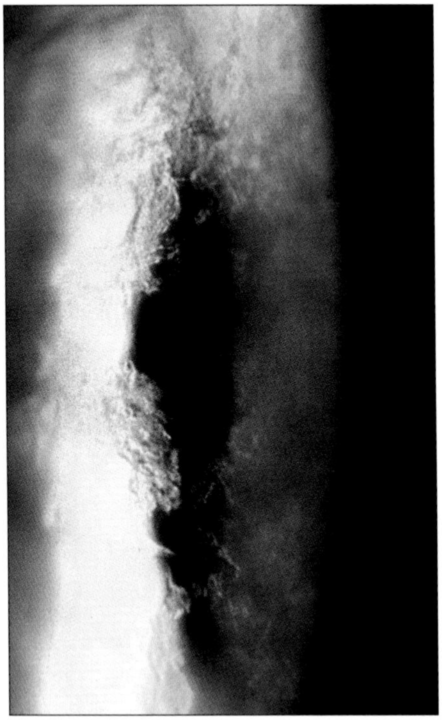

Fig. 22.28 Immunoglobulin deposits (image shown is benign monoclonal gammopathy).

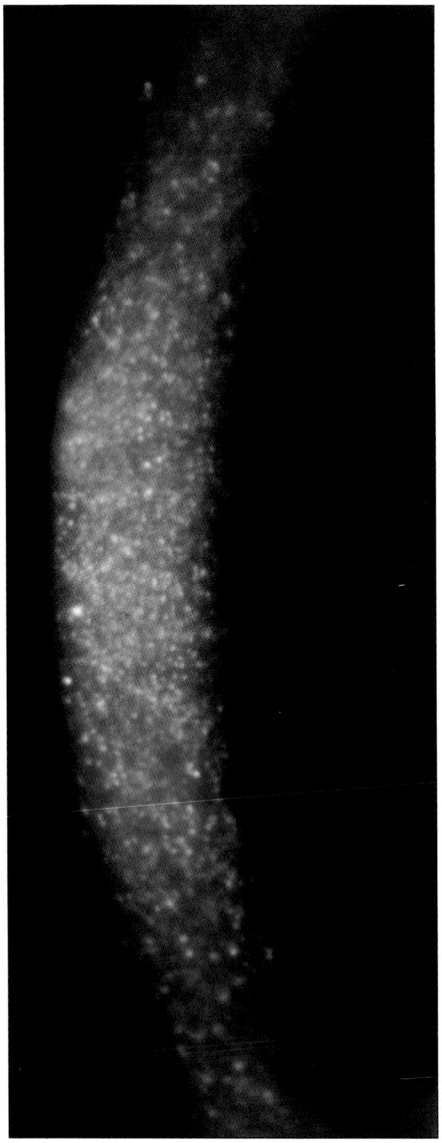

Fig. 22.29 Cystinosis.

Systemic diseases with immunoglobulin deposition

Corneal crystals have been recognized in systemic diseases that result in excessive immunoglobulin production (Fig. 22.28). These diseases include primary amyloidosis, multiple myeloma, Waldenström's macroglobulinemia, lymphoma,[37] benign monoclonal gammopathy,[38] and cryoglobulinemia. The crystals can be seen as the initial clinical sign of these diseases. The crystals are seen throughout the stroma, but may be localized in the posterior stroma in some cases.[38] They are white in direct illumination and crystalline in indirect illumination. The crystals may be refractile or polychromatic. Histologically, the crystals are intracellular immunoglobulin deposition.[37]

Cystinosis

Cystinosis is an autosomal recessive disorder that results in the accumulation of nonprotein cystine in most body tissues. A defect in lysosomal cystine transport allows cystine to accumulate within the lysosomes of the cells. Cystinosis can present as a nephropathic or benign form. The nephropathic form is subdivided into infantile and late-onset groups.

Corneal manifestations are found in all three forms and consist of stromal deposition of iridescent crystals (Fig. 22.29). These crystals are deposited initially in the anterior peripheral stroma and, with time, the deposition proceeds posteriorly and centrally. Deposits of crystals in the cornea can cause severe photophobia and episodes of recurrent erosions. The crystals may also be deposited in the conjunctiva and retina.[39]

Deep Stromal Deposits

Pigmented deposits

Copper deposition associated with Wilson's disease

Wilson's disease is an autosomal recessive disorder that results in the accumulation of copper in most body tissues. The Kayser-Fleischer ring is present in approximately 95% of patients with Wilson's disease. Clinically, it appears as a yellow-brown or green ring located at the level of Descemet's membrane in the peripheral cornea (Fig. 22.30). The copper deposition begins peripherally at Schwalbe's line and progresses centrally. There is no clear interval separating the ring from the limbus. Because of its peripheral location, gonioscopy may be required to locate the ring in its early

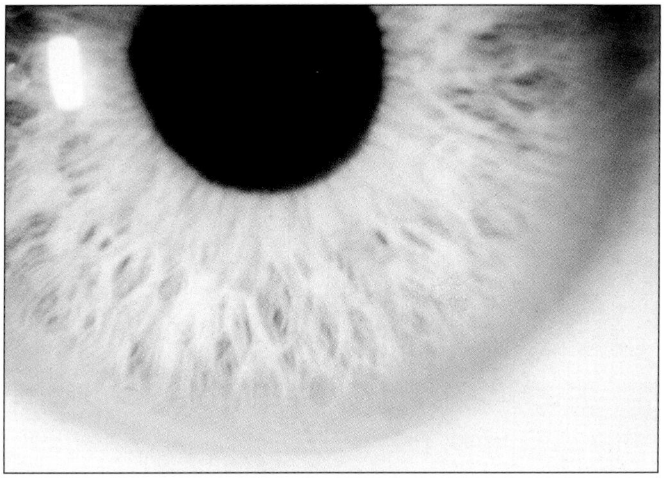

Fig. 22.30 Wilson's disease (copper).

stage.[40] Ocular copper deposition has also been reported with multiple myeloma.[41]

Chalcosis

Ocular chalcosis refers to the deposition of copper within the eye (Fig. 22.31). Deposition typically occurs in the setting of an intraocular foreign body. Copper has an affinity for basement membranes and is preferentially deposited in Descemet's membrane, the lens capsule (characteristically forming a sunflower cataract), and the internal limiting membrane of the retina. The corneal deposition appears as a peripheral greenish discoloration of Descemet's membrane similar to the Kayser-Fleischer ring seen in Wilson's disease.[42]

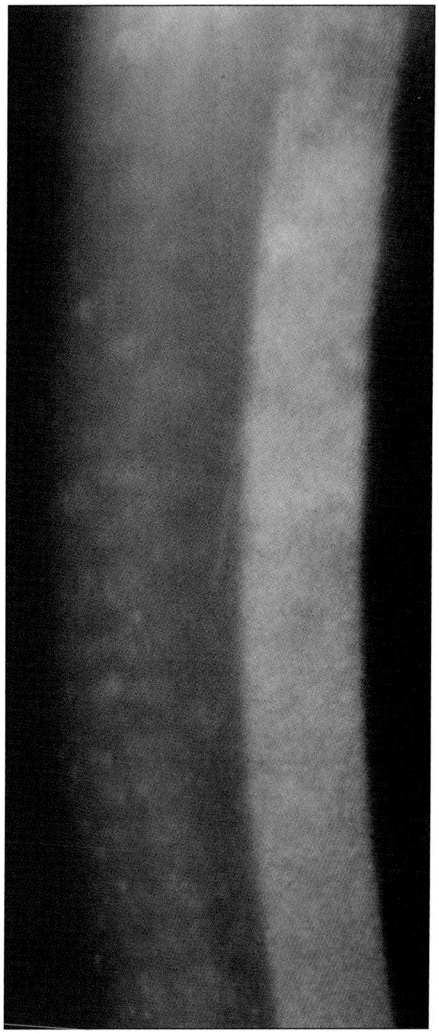

Fig. 22.31 Chalcosis (copper).

Ocular chrysiasis

Ocular chrysiasis occurs in the setting of oral or intramuscular gold therapy for rheumatoid arthritis. Gold deposits may be found in both the cornea and conjunctiva (Fig. 22.32). The deposits are located in the posterior stroma and Descemet's membrane and appear as yellow-brown granules, which may have a metallic sheen.[43] The deposits are visually asymptomatic.

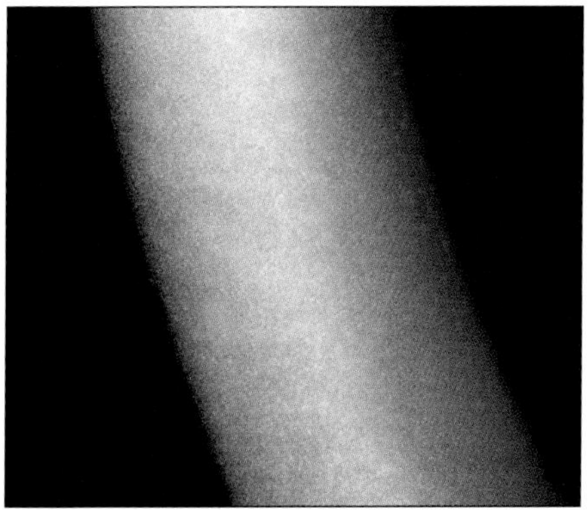

Fig. 22.32 Chrysiasis (gold).

Mottled cyan opacification in contact lens wearers

A mottled cyan-colored opacification at the level of Descemet's membrane has been described in soft contact lens wearers. The opacity is seen in the peripheral and mid-peripheral cornea (Fig. 22.33). The cause is unclear, but it appears to be associated with long-term contact lens wear.[44]

Nonpigmented deposits

Cornea farinata

Cornea farinata is a degenerative disorder characterized by multiple, tan to white, punctate opacities located in the posterior stroma (Fig. 22.34). The opacities are usually bilateral. The deposits are visually asymptomatic.[45]

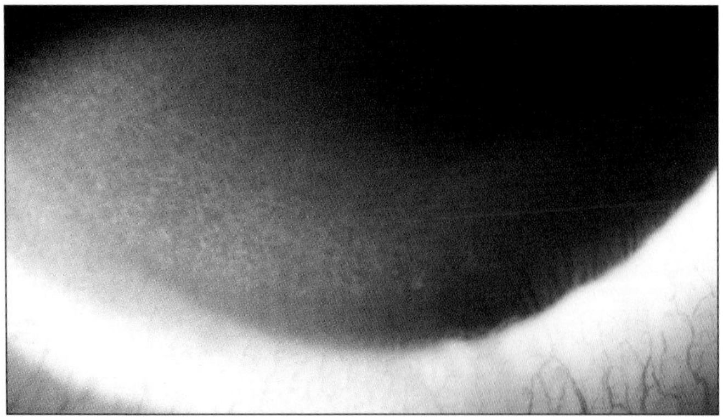

Fig. 22.33 Mottled cyan staining associated with contact lens wear.

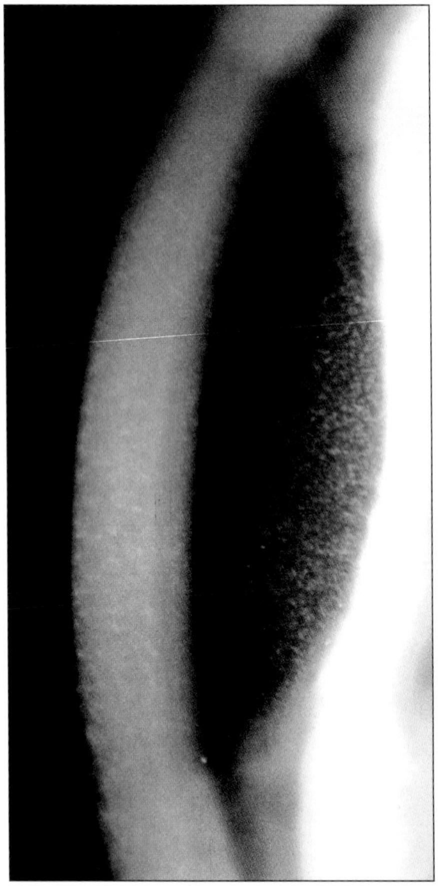

Fig. 22.34 Cornea farinata.

Pre-Descemet's corneal dystrophy

In pre-Descemet's corneal dystrophy, there are fine white punctate opacities within the posterior stroma just anterior to Descemet's membrane (Fig. 22.35). The disorder is familial, although the exact pattern of inheritance has not been established. The deposits are larger than those seen in cornea farinata. They may be located centrally, or in an annular, or diffuse pattern. They are visually asymptomatic.[46]

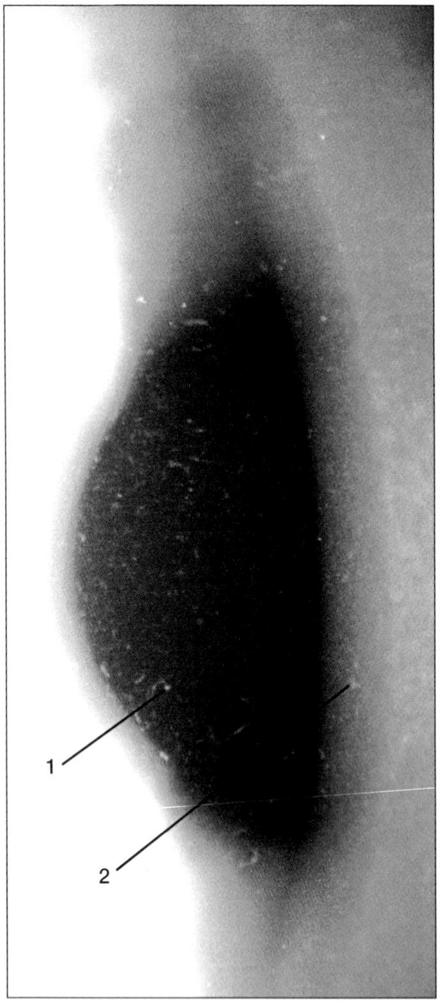

Fig. 22.35 Pre-Descemet's dystrophy. Deep white stromal opacities are seen in indirect light (1) and direct light (2).

X-linked ichthyosis

X-linked ichthyosis is one of a group of hereditary skin disorders that results in hyperkeratosis and scaling of the skin. The disease is inherited in an X-linked recessive pattern, and corneal changes are found in both homozygote males and heterozygote females. These changes consist predominantly of discrete, gray-white, visually asymptomatic opacities located anterior to Descemet's membrane (Fig. 22.36). They are diffusely spread over the cornea and shaped as dots, commas, or filaments.[47]

Ocular argyrosis

Ocular argyrosis is the deposition of silver within the eye (Fig. 22.37). The deposition occurs in the conjunctiva and cornea and is the result of the topical medication Argyrol (a silver nitrate compound rarely used anymore) or industrial exposure to silver. Recent reports of ocular argyrosis have been due to self-application of eyelash tint.[48] The typical corneal change is a diffuse slate-gray discoloration of Descemet's membrane. The deposits may be central or

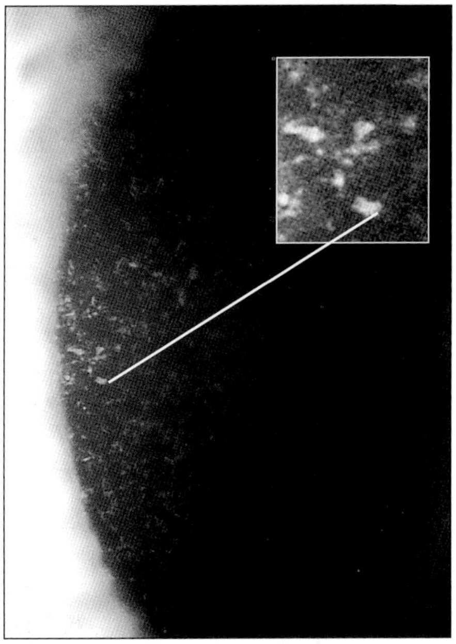

Fig. 22.36 X-linked ichthyosis.

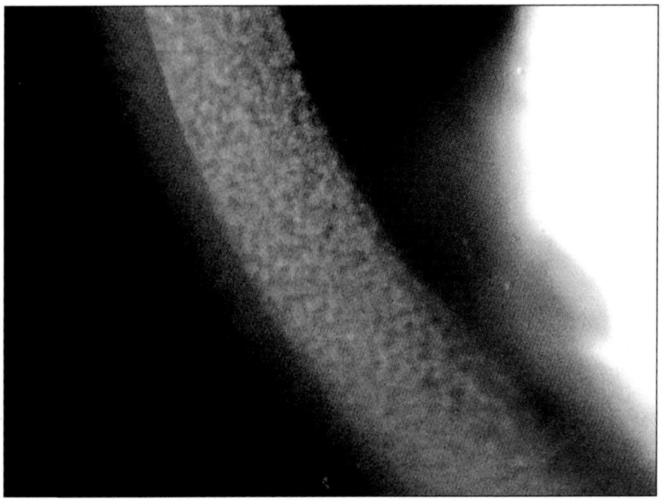

Fig. 22.37 Argyrosis (silver).

peripheral. Almost all cases of corneal deposition are associated with a grayish discoloration of the conjunctiva.[49]

Refractile/crystalline deposits

Polymorphic amyloid degeneration

Polymorphic amyloid degeneration is an age-related change of the cornea that is usually bilateral and does not affect vision. Patients are usually older than 50 years of age at the time of onset. In the deep corneal stroma are polygonal gray-white opacities and lines that are refractile in indirect illumination (Fig. 22.38). The opacities themselves appear similar to those seen in lattice dystrophy; however, they are usually less extensive, located in the deepest level of the

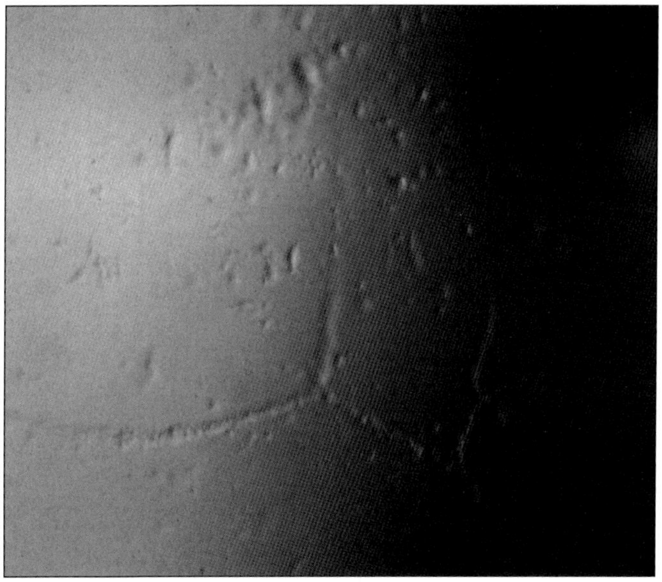

Fig. 22.38 Polymorphic amyloid degeneration.

stroma, and are not associated with the sequelae of lattice dystrophy. These deposits are not associated with any systemic disorder of amyloid deposition.[50]

References

1. Kaplan LJ, Cappaert WE. Amiodarone keratopathy. *Arch Ophthalmol.* 1982;100:601–602.
2. Johnson AW, Buffaloe WJ. Chlorpromazine epithelial keratopathy. *Arch Ophthalmol.* 1966;76:664–667.
3. Burns CA. Indomethacin, reduced retinal sensitivity, and corneal deposits. *Am J Ophthalmol.* 1968;66:825–835.
4. Walinder PE, Gip L, Stempa M. Corneal changes in patients treated with clofazimine. *Br J Ophthalmol.* 1976;60:526–528.
5. Teich SA, et al. Toxic keratopathy associated with suramin therapy. *N Engl J Med.* 1986;314:1455–1456.
6. Szmyd L, Perry HD. Keratopathy associated with the use of naproxen. *Am J Ophthalmol.* 1985;99:598.
7. Weiss JN, Weinberg RS, Regelson W. Keratopathy after oral administration of tilorone hydrochloride. *Am J Ophthalmol.* 1980;89:46–53.
8. Sher NA, Letson RD, Desnick RJ. The ocular manifestations in Fabry's disease. *Arch Ophthalmol.* 1979;97:671–676.
9. Font RL, Fine BS. Ocular pathology in Fabry's disease. *Am J Ophthalmol.* 1972;73:419–430.
10. Weingeist TA, Blodi FC. Fabry's disease: ocular findings in a female carrier. *Arch Ophthalmol.* 1971;85:169–176.
11. Barraquer-Somers E, Chan CC, Green WR. Corneal epithelial iron deposition. *Ophthalmology.* 1983;90:729–734.
12. Gass JD. The iron lines of the superficial cornea. *Arch Ophthalmol.* 1964;71:348–358.
13. Gray RH, Johnson GJ, Freedman A. Climatic droplet keratopathy. *Surv Ophthalmol.* 1992;36:241–253.
14. Green WR, Kaufer GJ, Dubroff S. Black cornea: a complication of topical use of epinephrine. *Ophthalmologica.* 1967;154:88–95.
15. Feder RS, et al. Subepithelial mucinous corneal dystrophy. *Arch Ophthalmol.* 1993;111:1106–1114.
16. Nevins RC, Davis WH, Elliot JH. Coat's white ring of the cornea: unsettled metal fettle. *Arch Ophthalmol.* 1968;80:145–146.
17. O'Connor GR. Calcific band keratopathy. *Trans Am Ophthalmol Soc.* 1972;70:58–81.
18. Kanellopoulos AJ, Miller F, Wittpenn JR. Deposition of topical ciprofloxacin to prevent re-epithelialization of a corneal defect. *Am J Ophthalmol.* 1993;117:258–259.
19. Konishi M, Yamada M, Machima Y. Corneal ulcer associated with deposits of norfloxacin. *Am J Ophthalmol.* 1998;125:258–260.
20. Millar TJ, et al. Clinical appearance and microscopic analysis of mucin balls associated with contact lens wear. *Cornea.* 2003;22(8):740–745.

21. Waring GO, Rodrigues MM, Laibson PR. Corneal dystrophies. I. Dystrophies of the epithelium, Bowman's layer and stroma. *Surv Ophthalmol.* 1978;23:71–122.
22. Weber FL, Babel J. Gelatinous drop-like dystrophy: a form of primary corneal amyloidosis. *Arch Ophthalmol.* 1980;98:144–148.
23. Macsai MS, et al. Tyrosinemia type II: nine cases of ocular signs and symptoms. *Am J Ophthalmol.* 2001;132(4):522–527.
24. Fraunfelder FT, Hanna C, Woods AH. Pseudoentrapment of ointment in the cornea. *Arch Ophthalmol.* 1975;93:331–334.
25. Ferry AP, Safir A, Melikian HE. Ocular abnormalities in patients with gout. *Ann Ophthalmol.* 1985;17:632–635.
26. McClanahan WS, et al. Ocular manifestations of chronic phenothiazine derivative administration. *Arch Ophthalmol.* 1966;75:319–325.
27. McDonnell PJ, et al. Blood staining of the cornea. *Ophthalmology.* 1985;92:1668–1674.
28. Phinney RB, Mondino BJ, Abrahim A. Corneal icterus resulting from stromal bilirubin deposition. *Ophthalmology.* 1989;96:1212–1214.
29. Lipman RM, Deutsch TA. A yellow-green posterior limbal ring in a patient who does not have Wilson's disease. *Arch Ophthalmol.* 1990;108:1385.
30. Talamo JH, et al. Ultrastructural studies of cornea, iris and lens in a case of siderosis bulbi. *Ophthalmology.* 1985;92:1675–1680.
31. Purcell JJ, Krachmer JH, Weingeist TA. Fleck corneal dystrophy. *Arch Ophthalmol.* 1977;95:440–444.
32. Friedlaender MH, Smolin G. Corneal degenerations. *Ann Ophthalmol.* 1979;11:1485–1495.
33. Cogan DC, Kuwabara T. Lipid keratopathy and atheroma. *Circulation.* 1958;18:518.
34. Barchiesi BJ, Eckel RH, Ellis PP. The cornea and disorders of lipid metabolism. *Surv Ophthalmol.* 1991;36:1–22.
35. Sugar J. Corneal manifestations of the systemic mucopolysaccharidoses. *Ann Ophthalmol.* 1979;11:531–535.
36. Kaiser-Kupfer MI, et al. Clinical biochemical and pathological correlations in Bietti's crystalline dystrophy. *Am J Ophthalmol.* 1994;118:569–582.
37. Barr CC, Gelender H, Font RL. Corneal crystalline deposits associated with dysproteinemia. *Arch Ophthalmol.* 1980;98:884–889.
38. Rodrigues MM, et al. Posterior corneal crystalline deposits in benign monoclonal gammopathy. *Arch Ophthalmol.* 1979;97:124–128.
39. Melles RB, et al. Spatial and temporal sequence of corneal crystal deposition in nephropathic cystinosis. *Am J Ophthalmol.* 1987;104:598–604.
40. Tso MO, Fine BS, Thorpe HE. Kayser-Fleischer ring and associated cataract in Wilson's disease. *Am J Ophthalmol.* 1975;79:479–488.
41. Hawkins AS, et al. Ocular deposition of copper associated with multiple myeloma. *Am J Ophthalmol.* 2001;131(2):257–259.
42. Rao NA, Tso MO, Rosenthal AR. Chalcosis in the human eye. *Arch Ophthalmol.* 1976;94:1379–1384.
43. Kincaid MC, et al. Ocular chrysiasis. *Arch Ophthalmol.* 1982;100:1791–1794.
44. Holland EJ, et al. Mottled cyan opacification of the posterior cornea in contact lens wearers. *Am J Ophthalmol.* 1995;119(5):620–626.
45. Grayson M, Wilbrandt H. Pre-Descemet dystrophy. *Am J Ophthalmol.* 1967;64:276–282.
46. Curran RE, Kenyon KR, Green WR. Pre-Descemet's membrane corneal dystrophy. *Am J Ophthalmol.* 1974;77:711–716.
47. Sever RJ, Frost P, Weinstein G. Eye changes in ichthyosis. *JAMA.* 1968;206:2283–2286.
48. Gallardo MJ, et al. Ocular argyrosis after long-term self-application of eyelash tint. *Am J Ophthalmol.* 2006;141(1):198–200.
49. Moss AP, et al. The ocular manifestations and functional effects of occupational argyrosis. *Arch Ophthalmol.* 1979;97:906–908.
50. Mannis MJ, et al. Polymorphic amyloid degeneration of the cornea. *Arch Ophthalmol.* 1981;99:1217–1223.

Chapter 23

Corneal Infiltrates in the Contact Lens Patient

Jennifer H. Kim, Christopher J. Rapuano, Elisabeth J. Cohen

An estimated 36 million Americans are contact lens wearers, comprising nearly 10% of the United States population.[1] While the most feared complication of contact lens wear is infectious corneal ulceration, the ophthalmologist must distinguish several types of sterile contact lens-associated infiltrates from infected ulcers. Current variations in types of contact lenses, disinfection methods, and patterns of use all add to the complexity of managing corneal infiltrates in the contact lens wearer. In addition, contact lens users are subject to problems unrelated to contact lens use, such as staphylococcal hypersensitivity marginal keratitis.

History

A detailed history is the first important step in managing the acutely symptomatic contact lens patient. The onset, duration, and severity of symptoms aid in formulating a diagnosis. The history should include the type of contact lens worn, the pattern of lens usage, the cleaning and disinfection regimen, as well as the type and brand of cleaning solution. Breaks in standard contact lens care, such as exposure of the lenses or case to water, should be specifically sought, as this information is rarely volunteered. Any one of these pieces of information alone will certainly not make the diagnosis, but together, along with careful clinical examination, the information will guide initial diagnosis and management.

Pain

The patient's pain is an important distinguishing feature. As Stein et al.[2] demonstrated, contact lens patients with moderate to severe pain are likely to have a positive corneal culture. Sterile corneal infiltrates tend to be associated with mild discomfort. Increasing pain is consistent with active infection, whereas decreasing pain after contact lens removal favors self-limited inflammation.

Type of contact lens and pattern of wear

It is necessary to determine whether the patient wears disposable (single use), frequent replacement (discards after a few weeks), or conventional lenses, extended- or daily-wear soft contact lenses, or rigid gas-permeable lenses. Daily disposable lenses eliminate standard contact lens hazards such as improper hygiene and storage, when used correctly. Hyper-oxygen transmissible silicone hydrogel lenses were designed to reduce corneal hypoxia, hypothesized to be a major risk factor for corneal infection. However, the relative risk of microbial keratitis with silicone hydrogels was not significantly different compared to planned replacement lenses in a studies by Dart et al.[3] and Stapleton et al.[4] Pure daily-wear use of daily-wear disposable lenses was shown to have the lowest risk of severe microbial keratitis. This was attributed to lack of exposure to pathogens in contact lens cases. Both studies demonstrated that overnight use continues to be the main risk factor for corneal infection. Dart et al. found that overnight wear, of any lens type, increased the risk of corneal infection fivefold. Even occasional overnight wear (less than 1 day per week) was associated with increased risk. Lens usage (daily vs extended wear), not lens type, was the most important risk factor for corneal ulceration.

Designed specifically for overnight wear with lens removal during waking hours, reverse-geometry rigid gas-permeable contact lenses are used to alter corneal shape to temporarily reduce refractive error in orthokeratology. In a series of 123 cases, *Pseudomonas* accounted for 37% of all cases, and *Acanthamoeba* was implicated in 33% of all cases.[5] Most of the cases of microbial keratitis associated with orthokeratology occurred in a relatively short time frame in East Asia, particularly China. In response, the Chinese government intervened to regulate the orthokeratology market. It has also been suggested that the refractive effect was associated with thinning of the central corneal epithelium in addition to the fitting relationship of orthokeratology lenses and that this may compromise the epithelial barrier, thereby increasing the risk of infectious keratitis.

Contact lens solutions and hygeine

Lens care history should include questions about solutions used and any recent changes in solutions. Delayed-type hypersensitivity and toxic reactions to thimerosal were a problem in the past.[6] Newer one-step disinfecting solutions are also associated with reactions including multiple peripheral subepithelial sterile corneal infiltrates, as well as chronic or recurrent follicular conjunctivitis and contact lens keratopathy, manifested by superior corneal epitheliopathy and even superficial scarring due to localized stem cell deficiency.

Multipurpose solutions and no-rub formulas were introduced in recent years to improve patient compliance. There have been two distinct outbreaks of nonbacterial contact lens-related infectious keratitis: first, *Fusarium* keratitis, followed by *Acanthamoeba* keratitis, each associated with the use of a particular contact lens solution – ReNu with MoistureLoc™ and AMO Complete MoisturePlus™, respectively. Although both solutions met all FDA criteria for safety and efficacy, this testing does not include evaluating efficacy against *Acanthamoeba*. Further investigations did not reveal microbial contamination of either solution; however, both solutions were ultimately removed from commercial markets. A study by Chang suggests that exposure to *Fusarium* was likely from the sink area or shower water. Although suboptimal contact lens hygiene practices appear unlikely as the major explanation for the outbreak, one hygiene practice that was statistically significant on univariate analysis was storing lenses by reusing contact lens solution already in the lens case.[7] Only approximately half of *Acanthamoeba* cases were associated with AMO Complete, and the resurgence of *Acanthamoeba* infections continues after its withdrawal. Joslin et al. proposed that additional risk factors may be implicated in this resurgence of contact lens-related *Acanthamoeba* keratitis.[8] Exposure through shower aerosolization may contribute to disease, as recent EPA regulations decreasing the allowable disinfection byproducts in the water supply has resulted in a higher microbial load. Discussions are underway at the FDA to change the standards for contact lens solutions.

Because inadequate lens care hygiene may increase the incidence of microbial keratitis, patients should be questioned about high-risk behaviors, which include topping off of old solutions in the case, infrequent replacement of the contact lens storage case, failure to wash hands before handling lenses, exposure of the lens or lens case to tap water, including swimming or showering while wearing lenses, and elimination of the digital rubbing step. The use of homemade saline and/or tap water to rinse or soak lenses was a problem in the past, associated with *Acanthamoeba* infection.[9] *Acanthamoeba* keratitis continues to be associated with infrequent and/or inadequate disinfection.[10]

Slit Lamp Examination

After taking the history and measuring visual acuity, a careful slit lamp examination is the next step. If the contact lens is in place, the fit should be noted and the lens removed. The presence of acute purulent discharge or evidence of chronic meibomian gland inflammation in the eyelids is noteworthy. The conjunctiva is evaluated for injection and follicles. Eyelid eversion is indicated to determine the presence of giant papillary conjunctivitis. The cornea should be examined carefully for epithelial irregularities, epithelial defects, infiltrates, and corneal edema. The size of the infiltrates and the overlying epithelial defects should be accurately measured and recorded. Abrasions in the acutely symptomatic contact lens wearer, even in the absence of an apparent corneal infiltrate, should be treated cautiously with frequent topical antibiotic ointment such as ciprofloxacin, tobramycin, or bacitracin/polymixin. Patching should be avoided, because severe *Pseudomonas* ulcers have developed overnight in this setting.[11] Topical steroids should not be used upon initial presentation. Anterior chamber reaction should be graded, as the presence of cells in the anterior chamber or a hypopyon are signs of infection.

Diagnosis

Distinguishing noninfectious corneal infiltrates from microbial keratitis is of crucial importance. Stein et al.[2] compared signs and symptoms in contact lens patients with infected and sterile infiltrates. Corneal infiltrates were cultured in all contact lens patients in this prospective study. Patients with positive corneal cultures had pain, anterior chamber reaction, a mucous discharge, and an overlying epithelial defect. It was concluded that patients with some or all of the clinical features associated with infection should be managed as infected cases. Notably, one-third of culture-positive infiltrates were smaller than 1 mm in diameter (Fig. 23.1). When corneal edema surrounds the infiltrate or when there is an anterior chamber reaction, even in the absence of an epithelial defect, infection requiring immediate intensive antibiotic treatment may be present. Small 1-mm peripheral infiltrates may, in fact, be infected (see Fig. 23.1). We agree with Donshik[12] who showed that a large number of patients with peripheral 'sterile' ulcers are in fact culture positive, and should be treated with antibiotics.

In the setting of extended wear of any soft contact lens or a tight lens, signs of acute or chronic hypoxia may be evident. Stromal and epithelial edema without an epithelial defect and a mild to severe anterior chamber reaction, with or without a hypopyon, may be present in acute hypoxia. Chronic hypoxia is often associated with conjunctival injection and superficial and deep corneal neovascularization. Sterile peripheral subepithelial infiltrates may be associated with both acute and chronic hypoxia (Figs 23.2, 23.3). With

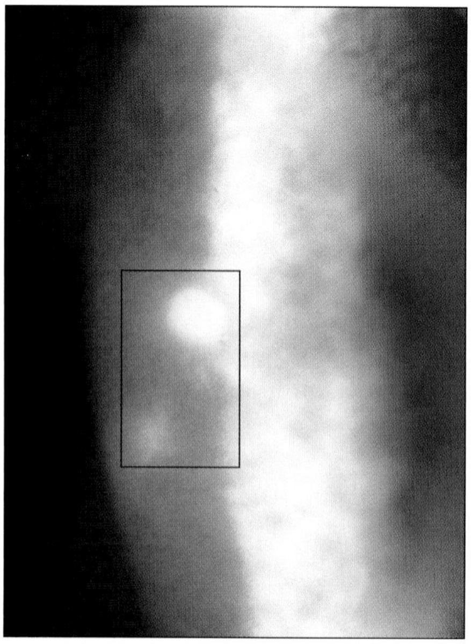

Fig. 23.1 *Pseudomonas* infection was the cause of small infiltrates (*box*) in a patient using disposable lenses for extended wear.

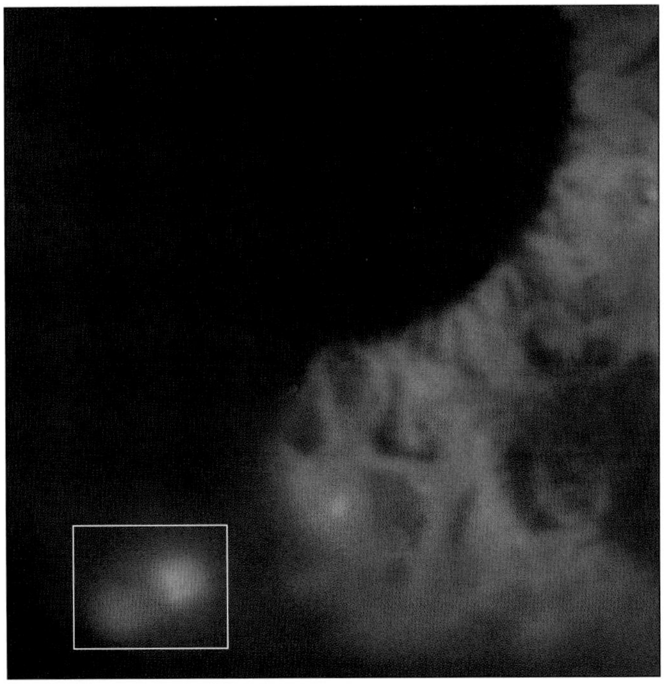

Fig. 23.2 Culture-negative infiltrates (*box*) developed in a patient using disposable contact lenses for extended wear.

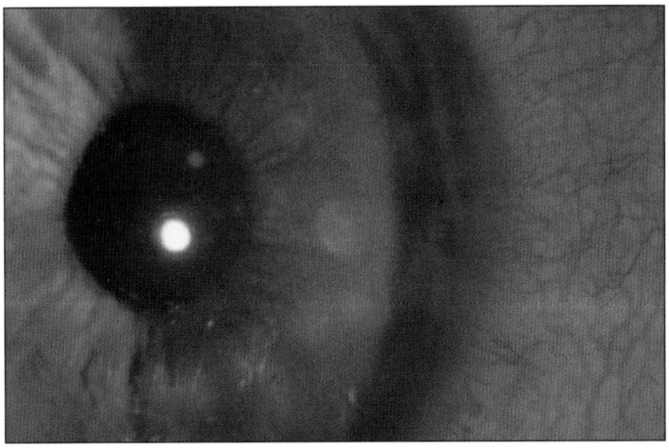

Fig. 23.3 These subepithelial infiltrates were most likely caused by a hypersensitivity to the contact lens solution.

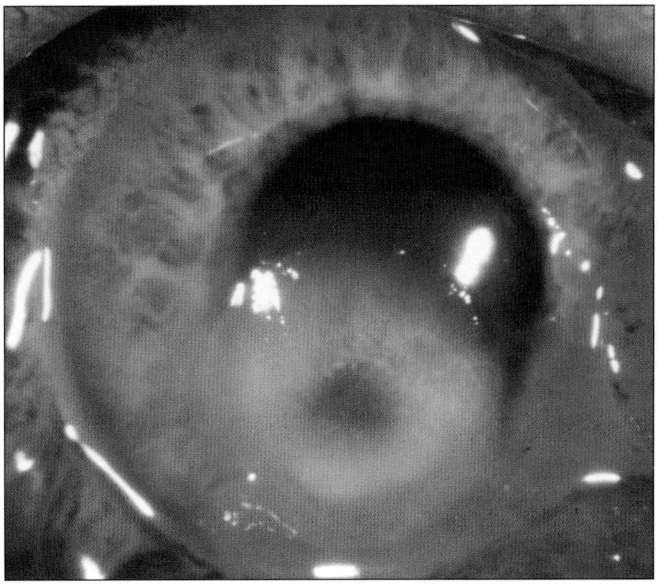

Fig. 23.4 A severe *Pseudomonas* infection occurred in a daily-wear disposable lens user who mistook saline for disinfecting solution.

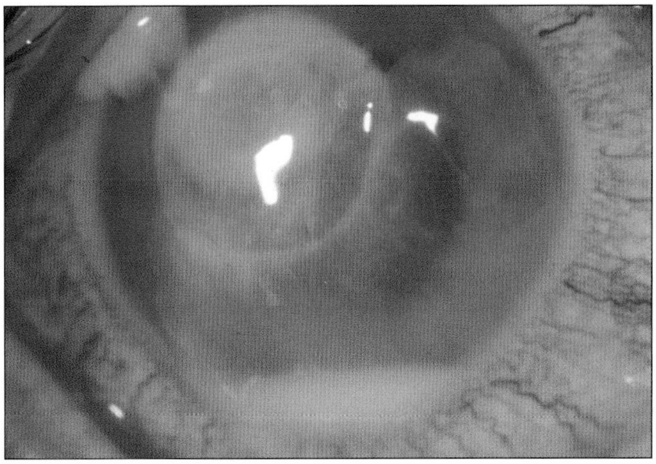

Fig. 23.5 This large, central ulcer initially presented as an abrasion and was treated with tobramycin–dexamethasone combination suspension.

severe chronic hypoxia, deep neovascularization, scarring, and lipid keratopathy can develop.

To diagnose microbial keratitis definitively, cultures are necessary, but are performed less frequently.[13] Small infiltrates are not routinely cultured, but may be infectious (see Fig. 23.1). If the ulcer is getting worse, smears and cultures should be obtained if they were not performed initially, or they should be repeated, if they were negative. Smears and cultures are necessary for the diagnosis of fungal keratitis, which frequently presents as an unresponsive corneal ulcer. Cultures should be obtained if the infiltrate is more than 1 mm, if the keratitis is getting worse on treatment, or if an unusual organism (fungus, *Acanthamoeba*, or atypical mycobacterium) is suspected on the basis of the history or clinical appearance (Figs 23.4–23.6). We treat smaller infiltrates without cultures intensively with fluoroquinolone antibiotics. In contact lens patients, we prefer gatifloxacin or levofloxacin for their possible improved coverage of *Pseudomonas*.

Signs of delayed hypersensitivity or toxic reactions to contact lens solutions include peripheral, subepithelial opacities associated with conjunctival injection with or without follicles. Painful pseudodendrites have been recognized as an early sign of *Acanthamoeba* keratitis.[14] Diagnosis of *Acanthamoeba* keratitis at this early stage is easier to confirm on corneal scrapings and is associated with a better response to medical treatment.

Ring-shaped infiltrates in contact lens wearers can be a diagnostic challenge. Sterile stromal rings are thought to be similar to Wessely rings associated with bacterial endotoxin developing within 7 to 10 days.[15] Rings of acute corneal

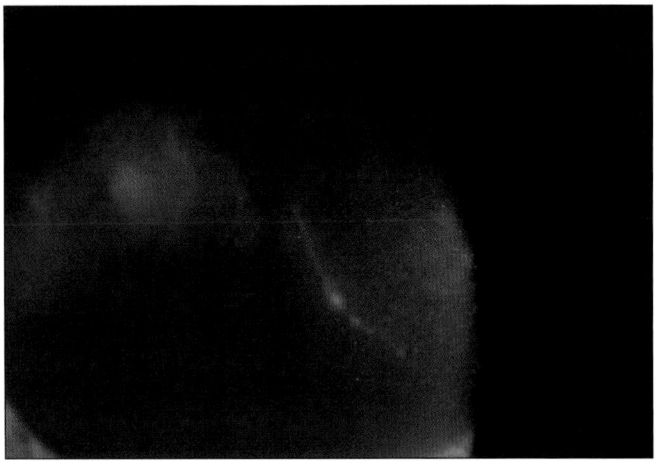

Fig. 23.6 This large paracentral ulcer and radial keratoneuritis presented in a daily-wear lens wearer who correctly cared for her lenses.

suppuration occur in the setting of frank microbial keratitis within 1 to 2 days (see Fig. 23.4). The central area is relatively clear due to corneal melting. Ring infiltrates, which are the hallmark of late *Acanthamoeba* keratitis, typically develop weeks after the onset of symptoms.[16,17] These ring infiltrates are usually associated with the intense pain and severe inflammation characteristic of this devastating infection. Anesthetic abuse is also associated with ring infiltrates similar to those seen in *Acanthamoeba* keratitis. While *Acanthamoeba* keratitis is often misdiagnosed as herpes simplex, HSV stromal keratitis is typically associated with relatively mild discomfort and is responsive to medical therapy.

Ocular conditions unrelated to contact lens use may cause infiltrates in contact lens patients. Patients with blepharitis may present with perilimbal infiltrates related to staphylococcal hypersensitivity. Patients with chronic follicular conjunctivitis may have chlamydial conjunctivitis. Staphylococcal hypersensitivity reactions and chlamydia can be difficult to distinguish from reactions to chemicals in contact lens solutions, but they do not recur with resumption of lens use.

Treatment

Treatment is dictated by the suspected underlying cause determined from the history and clinical examination. Regardless of the presumptive diagnosis, patients must be instructed to return immediately if they have new or increasing pain, a decrease in vision, or if they develop a white spot in their cornea. If a reaction to preservatives in lens solutions is suspected, discontinuing lens wear until symptoms and signs resolve, replacing the contact lenses, and switching to a hydrogen peroxide disinfection system or preferably single-use daily disposable lenses are recommended. Refitting tight lenses and avoiding extended-wear lenses are warranted if hypoxia is thought to be the underlying cause. Topical steroids are best avoided as the initial treatment of infiltrates in contact lens wearers, although there are differences of opinions on their use later. Hypoxic infiltrates and solution reactions often resolve without corticosteroids (see Fig. 23.1). Inappropriate treatment of early infectious infiltrates with topical corticosteroids can have serious adverse effects, especially if the infiltrate proves to be caused by fungal infection. We recommend low-dose antibiotics for suspected sterile infiltrates, although they are not always necessary.

Infectious corneal infiltrates associated with contact lens wear must be treated immediately. The most frequent organisms isolated are *Pseudomonas* and *Staphylococcus aureus*. Standard care for suspected microbial keratitis is intensive broad-spectrum antibiotic therapy. Small infections are treated with fluoroquinolones such as gatifloxacin every 30 minutes after a loading dose every 5 minutes for five doses. For more serious infections, over 1–2 mm in size, broad-spectrum topical fortified tobramycin and cefazolin or vancomycin are given every 30 minutes around the clock. Newer fourth-generation fluoroquinolones, moxifloxacin and gatifloxacin, provide enhanced coverage of both Gram-positive and Gram-negative organisms, respectively. It is unproven that the lower minimal inhibitory concentration (MIC) of gatifloxacin for *Pseudomonas* and *Serratia* is clinically relevant, but we prefer it in contact lens patients. Levofloxacin 1.5% has been shown to reach corneal tissue levels well above the mean for the most common ocular pathogens.[18]

There is controversy regarding the efficacy of fortified drops versus fluoroquinolones. Some data suggest they are equivalent.[19] In our experience, some patients' infections with sensitive organisms progress despite intensive fluoroquinolone therapy but respond to fortified antibiotic drops (see Fig. 23.4). There is increasing resistance to *Staphylococcus* and some recent reports of *Pseudomonas* resistance to fourth-generation fluoroquinolones.[20,21] Patients should be hospitalized if possible if the ulcers are 2 mm or greater in diameter or are worsening on outpatient treatment (see Figs 23.4–23.6). The decision for hospitalization also depends on the patient's or his or her family's ability to comply with frequent medications and follow-up care, and the availability of a hospital that can administer drops at a frequent rate.

Follow-up

After resolution of the corneal ulcer, many patients are anxious to resume contact lens wear. We recommend the use of daily disposable lenses worn for 1 day and then discarded, to avoid the risks of inadequate disinfection and extended wear. If compliance is in doubt, contact lens use should be avoided.

Case Examples

Case 1

A disposable extended-wear lens user presented with three infiltrates measuring 0.2–0.5 mm in diameter (see Fig. 23.1). Because of surrounding corneal edema and moderate anterior chamber reaction, infection was suspected. Cultures were taken, and intensive treatment was begun with fortified tobramycin and cefazolin drops every 30 minutes as an outpatient. Cultures were positive for heavy growth of *Pseudomonas*. The patient responded well to treatment.

Comment: Small infiltrates may be infected. Because small infiltrates may be caused by virulent organisms such as *Pseudomonas*, one should treat them with intensive topical antibiotics and not topical corticosteroids.

Case 2

An extended-wear disposable lens user presented to the emergency room with two peripheral infiltrates (see Fig. 23.2). Cultures were done, and treatment was begun with intensive topical ciprofloxacin. She responded well. Cultures were negative.

Comment: In the absence of anterior chamber reaction, or surrounding corneal edema, these infiltrates were likely to be sterile. Sterile infiltrates improve without topical corticosteroids.

Case 3

A daily-wear frequent replacement lens wearer presented with bilateral redness, pain, foreign body sensation, and tearing (see Fig. 23.3). She used Opti-Free (Alcon Labs, Fort Worth, TX) cleaning solution. Her slit lamp examination revealed central and mid-peripheral subepithelial infiltrates (SEIs) bilaterally, and she had no history of acute conjunctivitis. The SEIs resolved over 1 month with the use of a moderate-strength corticosteroids.

Comment: Patients can manifest a hypersensitivity to their contact lens solutions. If there is no epithelial staining, mild to moderate steroids can carefully be used short term with good effect. Once the reaction has resolved, the patient can resume contact lens use with new lenses and preservative-free contact lens solutions, or switch to daily disposable lenses.

Case 4

A frequent replacement daily-wear lens wearer who used saline instead of disinfecting solution by mistake developed a severe *Pseudomonas* infection (see Fig. 23.4). She was treated initially with intensive topical ciprofloxacin and referred because of worsening. She was hospitalized and treated with fortified tobramycin and mezlocillin. She did well and recovered most of her vision.

Comment: In our experience, intensive fortified antibiotics are more effective than intensive ciprofloxacin, even in *Pseudomonas* infections sensitive to both. Patient education about the types and purposes of various contact lens solutions is critical in preventing infections.

Case 5

A daily-wear frequent replacement lens wearer presented to her local ophthalmologist with a foreign body sensation and pain (see Fig. 23.5). She was diagnosed with a small corneal abrasion and was started on tobramycin–dexamethasone combination suspension twice a day. Two days later she presented to our service with a large, central ulcer and a hypopyon. The ulcer was cultured, and the patient was admitted for frequent fortified topical tobramycin, piperacillin, and vancomycin antibiotics. After 1 month, the ulcer had healed, but her vision only improved to counting fingers at 1 foot due to scarring.

Comment: A small central abrasion in a contact lens wearer should be treated with frequent (every 2 hours) antibiotic ointment with good Gram-negative coverage and watched carefully. Steroids should not be used in the initial management of a contact lens abrasion or ulcer, and patching is contraindicated.

Case 6

A 12-year-old girl presented with a large paracentral ulcer with a radial keratoneuritis (see Fig. 23.6). She was a daily-wear frequent replacement lens wearer who used a multipurpose solution. The patient had been on frequent fluoroquinolone antibiotics for 2 days before being referred. She was cultured and admitted for around-the-clock fortified antibiotics. No organisms grew in the cultures. Two years later, her vision was 20/25 with spectacle correction and she had a mild paracentral stromal scar.

Comment: Presumed infectious keratitis in contact lens wearers can present even in patients who 'do everything right.' Aggressive fortified antibiotics started early in the disease course often result in good outcomes. It should also be noted that radial keratoneuritis is not specific for *Acanthamoeba* keratitis.

References

1. Saviola JF. Contact lens safety and the FDA: 1976 to the present. *Eye Contact Lens.* 2007;33:404–409.
2. Stein RM, et al. Infected sterile corneal infiltrates in contact lens wearers. *Am J Ophthalmol.* 1988;105:632–636.
3. Dart JKG, et al. Risk factors for microbial keratitis with contemporary contact lenses. *Ophthalmology.* 2008;115(10):1647–1654.
4. Stapleton F, et al. Incidence of contact lens-related microbial keratitis. *Ophthalmology.* 2008;115(10):1655–1661.
5. Watt K, et al. Trends in microbial keratitis associated with orthokeratology. *Eye Contact Lens.* 2007;33:373–377.
6. Wilson LA, et al. Delayed hypersensitivity to thimerosal in soft contact lens wears. *Ophthalmology.* 1981;88:804–808.
7. Chang D, et al. Multistate outbreak of *Fusarium* keratitis associated with use of contact lens solution. *JAMA.* 2006;296(8):953–963.
8. Joslin C, et al. The association of contact lens solution use and *Acanthamoeba* keratitis. *Am J Ophthalmol.* 2007;144:169–180.
9. Butcko V, et al. Microbial keratitis and the role of rub and rinsing. *Eye Contact Lens.* 2007;33:421–423.
10. Stehr-Green JK, et al. *Acanthamoeba* keratitis in soft contact lens wearers. *JAMA.* 1987;258:57–60.
11. Radford CF, et al. Risk factors for *Acanthamoeba* keratitis in contact lens users: a case-control study. *Br Med J.* 1995;310:1567–1570.
12. Donshik PC, et al. Peripheral corneal infiltrates associated with contact lens wear. *Trans Am Ophthalmol Soc.* 1995;93:49–64.
13. Clemons CS, et al. *Pseudomonas* ulcers following patching of corneal abrasions associated with contact lens wear. *CLAO J.* 1987;13:161–164.
14. McDonnell PJ, et al. Community care of corneal ulcers. *Am J Ophthalmol.* 1992;114:531–538.
15. Lindquist TD, Sher MA, Doughman DJ. Clinical signs and medical therapy of early *Acanthamoeba* keratitis. *Arch Ophthalmol.* 1988;106:73–77.
16. Kremer I, Cohen EJ. Ring infiltrates associated with contact lens wear. *CLAO J.* 1993;19:192–193.
17. Theodore FH, et al. The diagnostic value of a ring infiltrate in *Acanthamoeba* keratitis. *Ophthalmology.* 1985;92:1471–1479.
18. Hammersmith K, et al. Contact lens-related microbial keratitis: recent outbreaks. *Curr Opin Ophthalmol.* 2008;19:302–306.
19. McDonald MB. Research review and update: IQUIX (Levofloxacin 1.5%). *Int Ophthalmol Clin.* 2006;46(4):47–60.
20. Goldstein MH, et al. Emerging fluoroquinolone resistance in bacterial keratitis. *Ophthalmology.* 1999;106:1313–1318.
21. Kunimoto DY, et al. In vitro susceptibility of bacterial keratitis pathogens to ciprofloxacin. Emerging resistance. *Ophthalmology.* 1999;106:80–85.

Chapter 24

The Red Eye

Christopher R. Croasdale, Michael B. Shapiro

The goal of this chapter is to aid the clinician in using a logical framework for diagnosing a red eye. The target audience is primarily non-cornea-specialized ophthalmologists and optometrists. In-depth discussion of specific conditions can be found elsewhere within *The Cornea*, and other appropriate reference texts.

Defining a Red Eye

Redness is not a symptom, but a nonspecific sign. A red eye from the patient perspective signifies the visible appearance of abnormal redness of the globe, lids, or adnexal structures. The three major processes responsible for the majority of cases are subconjunctival hemorrhages, inflammation, and vascular abnormalities. Of these, conditions with inflammation account for the majority of red eye presentations. Diseases where vascular congestion may give the appearance of the redness of inflammation are the least common. In some instances, two or all mechanisms can occur simultaneously.

Approaching the Patient

Successful diagnosis requires being knowledgeable of the possibilities. One cannot diagnose what one does not know. In training, diseases are studied and organized according to various classification schemes, such as: infectious diseases, inflammatory diseases, diseases of the retina, or diseases of cornea, etc. In practice, the clinician usually determines a number of probable diagnoses based on the initial history. One does not think, 'This is a red eye patient and here is every diagnostic possibility.' Instead, one enters the examination room with specific diagnoses in mind and seeks the additional historical and examination findings which either support the diagnosis or lead to other possibilities. When the diagnosis is not readily forthcoming, one may need to sit back and review the various diagnostic categories (Table 24.1).

Subconjunctival Hemorrhages and Telephone Triage of a Red Eye

This diagnosis is one of the easiest to determine among causes for a red eye, but deserves discussion due to its frequency of occurrence, healthcare utilization costs, and implications when misdiagnosis occurs. This cause usually takes but a moment to diagnose once the clinician sees the patient. Although sometimes dramatic in appearance, the occurrence of a spontaneous subconjunctival hemorrhage alone rarely signifies a risk to the health of the eye or patient. The greater clinical significance of subconjunctival hemorrhages is in the challenge they present to ancillary clinic staff performing telephone triage, and the risk of delaying appropriate treatment for other causes of a red eye if a misdiagnosis is made. Types of patients for whom misdiagnosis over the phone is most critical include patients who have had recent surgery, particularly any type of intraocular surgery where endophthalmitis is a possibility. Additionally, eyes post glaucoma filtering surgeries have a long-term risk of bleb-related infection. Corneal transplant recipients have long-term risk of allograft rejection. A misdiagnosis of 'probable subconjunctival hemorrhage' in such patients can have potentially severe consequences.

The skills and knowledge of the persons likely to be responsible for performing telephone triage will vary widely. In addition to obtaining a history of the present problem, the patient should be asked about prior similar occurrences, other past ocular history, including specifically any recent or past eye surgery, and current medical conditions and medications (specifically anticoagulants and other related agents). Two key symptoms to clarify are whether there is an associated change to or loss of vision, or any significant discomfort or pain of the involved eye. A simple conjunctival hemorrhage alone should not produce an affirmative response to either of these questions. If the response is affirmative, the triage person must strongly consider that another condition may exist.

Even if 'some other condition' is the assessment of the person performing the telephone triage, this does not necessarily indicate the need for emergent or urgent evaluation. The final decision of when or whether the patient needs to be seen will be determined by many factors, chief among which include the knowledge, experience, and self-confidence of the triage person. There is no substitute for experience and knowledge in this process, and this is an area in which most of us can provide helpful training to those in our clinics and healthcare facilities providing such service.

Table 24.1 Causes of a red eye

- **DISORDERS PRIMARILY OF THE GLOBE**
  - **Extraocular**
    - **Conjunctivitis (and keratitis, when mechanism is the same)**
      - Infectious
        - Viral (adenoviral, HSV, VZV, etc.)
        - Bacterial (*Chlamydia*)
        - Fungal, parasitic
      - Inflammatory
        - Idiopathic
          - Superior limbic keratoconjunctivitis
        - Allergic and hypersensitivity reactions
          - Atopic blepharoconjunctivitis
          - Phylectenular (*Staphylococcus*, tuberculosis)
          - Environmental/seasonal allergies
            - Vernal conjunctivitis
          - Medications (brimonidine, apraclonidine, dorzolamide, trifluridine, etc.)
          - Contact lens solutions
          - Contact dermatitis/conjunctivitis
            - (Atropine solution, poison ivy, etc.)
          - Cosmetic products
        - Toxic reactions
          - Chemical exposures (industrial and home cleaning products, etc.)
          - Topical medications (aminoglycosides, neomycin, etc.) and preservatives (e.g., benzalkonium chloride)
          - Molluscum contagiosum (lesion usually on lid)
        - Mechanical/irritant
          - Contact lens related
          - Factitious
          - Foreign body (insect parts, plants debris)
          - Exposed sutures, glaucoma drainage devices, scleral buckle elements
          - Mucus fishing syndrome
          - Any eyelid position/function abnormality
            - Floppy eyelid syndrome
            - Imbrication
            - Trichiasis, lagophthalmos
          - Trauma
        - Systemic immune-mediated
          - Stevens-Johnson syndrome
          - Ocular cicatricial pemphigoid
          - Graft versus host disease
          - Ligneous conjunctivitis
      - Neoplastic lesions causing inflammation and/or increased vascularity of conjunctiva
        - Benign lesions
          - Pinguecula, pterygia, nevi (amelanotic)
        - Malignant lesions
          - Limbal in origin (conjunctival intraepithelial neoplasia, squamous cell carcinoma)
          - Nonlimbal in origin (primary lesion elsewhere, usually the lid: squamous, basal and sebaceous cell carcinoma)
          - Melanoma
    - **Noninflammatory conjunctival redness**
      - Subconjunctival hemorrhage
      - Abnormal vascular engorgement
        - Polycythemia vera
    - **Cornea and/or conjunctiva (dry eye conditions)**
      - Dry eye syndrome (deficient tear syndrome)
        - All combinations of aqueous, mucin or lipid deficiency
      - Evaporative/exposure keratoconjunctivitis
        - Paralytic (Bell's palsy, etc.)
        - Nocturnal
        - Abnormal lid anatomy with inadequate closure
          - Congenital
          - Postsurgical
            - Trauma repair
            - Cosmetic/functional eyelid surgery
            - Reconstruction after tumor excision
        - Proptosis
          - Graves' disease or other orbital process
        - Abnormal blink reflex/frequency (often multifactorial, e.g. Parkinson's disease, systemic medication side effects, especially anti-Parkinson's medications, antipsychotic medications, etc.)
      - Filamentary keratitis
      - Neurotrophic keratoconjunctivitis
        - Postviral (HSV, VZV)
        - Idiopathic
        - Topical medications (anesthetic abuse, excessive nonsteroidal antiinflammatory drugs)
        - Postsurgical (trigeminal nerve ablation)
    - **Cornea**
      - Recurrent corneal erosion/traumatic abrasions
      - Endothelial decompensation of any cause with resultant bullous keratopathy
      - immune-mediated
    - **Episclera/sclera**
      - Infectious episcleritis/scleritis
      - Inflammatory episcleritis/scleritis
  - **Intraocular**
    - Infectious or inflammatory
      - Endogenous/exogenous endophthalmitis
      - Chorioretinitis, retinitis
      - Neovascular glaucoma
      - Acute-angle-closure glaucoma
      - Ocular ischemic syndrome
      - Postsurgical (e.g. retained nucleus, toxic)
      - Postintravitreal injection (toxic)
      - Uveitis (anterior, intermediate, posterior)
    - Neoplastic
      - Any primary or metastatic malignant tumor
      - Masquerade syndromes
- **DISORDERS OF THE EYELIDS AND/OR ADNEXAL STRUCTURES**
  - **Eyelids**
    - Blepharitis
      - Infectious (viral, bacterial, parasitic – lice, *Demodex*)
      - Inflammatory
        - Meibomitis, hordeola, chalazia
        - Rosacea
        - Seborrheic
    - Abnormal anatomy/function
      - Ectropion, entropion, trichiasis/distichiasis
      - Floppy eyelid syndrome
      - Imbrication
    - Neoplasms
      - Benign (keratoacanthoma)
      - Malignant (primarily basal, squamous and sebaceous cell carcinomas)
  - **Nasolacrimal system**
    - Lacrimal gland
      - Infectious/inflammatory (dacryoadenitis)
      - Malignancy
    - Canaliculitis
    - Dacryocystitis
    - Nasolacrimal duct obstruction with secondary conjunctivitis
  - **Orbit/periorbital structures**
    - Infectious
      - Preseptal and orbital cellulitis
    - Inflammatory
      - Idiopathic pseudotumor
      - Sarcoidosis, Wegener's granulomatosis
      - Thryoid-related orbitopathy
      - Myositis
      - Vasculitis
      - Ruptured dermoid cyst
      - Sinus mucocele
    - Neoplastic
      - Malignant
        - Primary
        - Metastatic
    - Abnormal vascular engorgement
      - Arteriovenous malformations
        - Carotid-cavernous fistula
        - Dural shunts
      - Hemangiopericytoma
      - Orbital varix

Redness due to Inflammation

The primary process that produces inflammation and hyperemia can originate with the globe (intra- or extraocular), the orbit, or the lids and adnexal structures. Successful treatment usually requires correctly identifying the etiology, although some conditions are self-limited and will resolve regardless of whether the correct diagnosis is determined or the correct treatment initiated. In other cases, despite the etiology remaining unknown, successful resolution of the inflammation with antiinflammatory medication may occur.

It is important to determine whether inflammation is the primary process, or a secondary reaction, in order to successfully treat the problem. An example of the former is a patient who presents with ocular cicatricial pemphigoid and cicatrizing conjunctivitis. The conjunctivitis may temporarily appear better with topical steroids, but ultimately will worsen unless the correct diagnosis is made and systemic immunosuppression is used to control the systemic disease. An example of inflammation as a secondary reaction can be seen with a missed retained intraocular foreign body. Topical steroids may suppress or temporarily eliminate the inflammatory reaction, but until the primary problem of the foreign body is diagnosed and it is removed, the inflammation will recur with discontinuation of the steroids. The goal is to determine and treat the underlying cause, and not just the symptoms or signs.

Red Eyes due to Vascular Abnormalities

This category includes all noninflammatory conditions that can result in an eye appearing red. In addition to commonly occurring subconjunctival hemorrhages, discussed above, are a heterogeneous number of less common conditions which either increase or reduce the normal vascular pattern of the globe and adnexal structures. An example of the former can occur when a carotid cavernous sinus fistula results in increased venous pressure and dilation of the episcleral and conjunctival vessels. An unusual case of the latter was seen in a patient who received more than a dozen unilateral intravitreal injections of Avastin (bevacizumab) for macular degeneration. The patient wondered why the contralateral eye was red. That eye did not symptomatically feel irritated, or reveal signs of such, but the vessels of the sclera, conjunctiva, and lids were more prominent than the other 'youthful-appearing' eye of this elderly woman. The conclusion was that the Avastin was having an extraocular effect on the vessels of the globe and lids, resulting in a reduction of the caliber of vessels and the asymmetric appearance of the eye redness.

The Medical History and Case Examples

In clinical practice, the greatest barrier to obtaining an adequate history is the decreasing amount of time most spent between most clinicians and their patients. Typically, the history will be obtained by a technician, and often be but a few sentences or less. Depending on the condition, this may suffice. For the auto mechanic with a sore, red eye which started while he was working under a car without protective eyewear, a probable corneal foreign body is a reasonable presumptive diagnosis. One might move quickly to the slit lamp examination. If an offending foreign body is present, the diagnosis is made and treatment rendered. If not, this may be the point when the clinician sits back and begins to ask additional questions.

In general, acute (hours to days) and subacute (days to a few weeks) causes of a red eye are more likely to have a single identifiable cause. Examples include foreign bodies in the cornea or conjunctiva, corneal abrasions and erosions, acute conjunctivitis, and many contact lens-associated problems. Some examples of intraocular conditions include angle-closure glaucoma and uveitis. Most of these acute and subacute conditions do not pose significant diagnostic challenge; with an appropriate history and examination the cause is usually determined.

Chronic (greater than several weeks duration) and recurrent red eye conditions can require greater experience and skill to diagnose. A careful history by the clinician is often necessary, particularly when a patient has seen multiple providers and received multiple treatments over many months or longer. Such an example is the patient with a 6-month history of recurrent, unilateral conjunctivitis who has been treated with multiple courses of topical antibiotics by various providers without improvement. Eventually, a combination of antibiotic and steroid solution is tried for presumed nonspecific viral conjunctivitis, and the redness and irritation improve. But upon discontinuation, the conjunctivitis recurs. Finally, the patient is referred to your office, where a prominent follicular conjunctivitis is found, along with a small umbilicated lesion hidden amongst the upper lid lashes. Molluscum contagiosum is correctly diagnosed, and after curettage of the lesion there is resolution of the follicular conjunctivitis, without recurrence.

Other cases may be far more complex. Take the 76-year-old woman with long-standing glaucoma who has had bilateral filtration surgery, twice in the right eye and once in the left. The initial trabeculectomy in the right eye was 10 years prior, without mitomycin, and failed after 4 years. She was then back on four glaucoma medications for another 4 years until a repeat trabeculectomy with mitomycin-C was done 2 years prior to presentation, with resultant overfiltration and borderline hypotony. The left eye trabeculectomy was done 7 years prior, with partial bleb failure despite needling after 5 years, leading to reinitiation of brimonidine 0.15% three times daily. Both eyes are pseudophakic, and the left also has a history of a retinal detachment with scleral buckle repair before the trabeculectomy. She states that for the last year or longer, both eyes are always red, and painful, with discharge mainly from the right eye. Both eyes itch, and the left eye has had recurrent subconjunctival hemorrhages (per the referring glaucoma specialist). She states that use of artificial tears only brings relief for a few minutes. Her general medical conditions include hypothyroidism, hypertension, depression, osteoarthritis, chronic allergies, and atrial fibrillation. Medications include Synthroid (levothyroxine), hydrochlorothiazide, atenolol, amitryptiline, acetaminophen, Coumadin (warfarin), and Allegra (fexofenadine).

External examination reveals an obese woman with prominent eyes due to a combination of shallow orbits, asymmetric lateral flare, lower lid retraction with several millimeters of scleral show, and mild inferior punctal ectropion. Both upper lids seem moderately floppy, but there is no lash ptosis. The right upper lid is mildly ptotic. On slit lamp examination, all four lids have mild scurf on the lashes, with moderate atrophy and inspissation of the meibomian glands, and prominent telangiectasia of margins. The bulbar conjunctiva of the right eye reveals a large, diffuse bleb at 12 o'clock, with 360 degrees of chemosis from overfiltration. There is mild diffuse injection. An exposed 10-0 nylon suture tail is visible at the medial aspect of the bleb. There is 2+ clear stringy mucus in the inferior cul-de-sac, and a mixed papillary and follicular reaction of the inferior palpebral conjunctiva. Eversion of the right upper lid shows a 4+ papillary reaction of the palpebral conjunctiva. The right cornea has a moderate superficial punctate epitheliopathy of the inferior 30%. Fluoroscein instillation confirms the exposure of the suture tail, and also reveals a moderate amount of fine, diffuse punctate staining of the elevated, chemotic conjunctiva. The tear lake volume seems average.

Additional aspects of the left eye include the following. A mild dull pink appearance of the bulbar conjunctiva, with a small to moderate vascularized and encapsulated bleb at 11 o'clock. Eversion of the upper lid reveals a 1+ papillary reaction. The lower lid palpebral conjunctiva has a 2+ follicular reaction and 1+ papillary reaction. The cornea has diffuse 1+ superficial punctate epitheliopathy. Fluoroscein application does not reveal any additional abnormality of the conjunctiva. The tear lake volume is mildly less than the right eye.

This is not an unusual example in today's practice of a patient referred for chronic red eyes. Obtaining and concisely organizing the pertinent history, which covers many years, would exceed the capabilities of most technicians. The multitude of findings reveals inflammatory changes due to multifactorial processes in each eye. There are the long-term toxic effects of glaucoma medications and their preservatives on the conjunctiva of both eyes, with the additional hypersensitivity reaction to brimonidine in the left eye. Multiple ocular surgeries, including two glaucoma filtering operations on the right eye, and the scleral buckle and filtration surgery on the left eye, cause significant periods of conjunctival inflammation, subsequent fibrosis, and long-term adverse effects on the cells and structures involved in the production and maintenance of a healthy tear film and ocular surface. In the right eye, two additional direct effects of the glaucoma surgery include the abnormal anatomic elevation of the conjunctiva due to overfiltration and chemosis, causing abnormal tear film dynamics with relative exposure and abnormal wetting, as well as the papillary conjunctivitis due to the exposed nylon suture irritating the upper palpebral conjunctiva. Both eyes have mild anterior blepharitis, as well as posterior lid disease, further contributing to the inflammatory milieu of the ocular surface. Amongst the systemic medical conditions was the history of Graves' disease with mild lid signs of flaring of the lateral canthi, and mild lower lid retraction, adding another potential evaporative dry eye component. Obesity is associated with floppy eyelid syndrome. Several of the systemic medications are known contributors to dry eye disease, including the diuretic, the antidepressant, and the antihistamine. The anticoagulant increases the likelihood of subconjunctival hemorrhages.

This example of the complex interaction of numerous conditions with the resultant nonspecific sign of conjunctival injection underscores why one cannot try to follow an algorithmic flowchart to arrive at the correct diagnosis. There are often multiple conditions that must be identified and considered in terms of potential contribution to the overall end result of redness.

Physical Examination

The physical evaluation begins as soon as one encounters the patient. Characteristics such as personal hygiene, body weight, and habitus can provide useful information, especially in patients who are poor historians. Body structures should be observed for structural changes secondary to systemic diseases, such as the hands and skin in rheumatoid arthritis or scleroderma. A light source is used to inspect the external facial features. Many causes of red eye can be overlooked if one immediately 'zooms in' with the high-power view of the slit lamp. The skin of the lids and ocular adnexa is examined for signs of inflammation, past or recent trauma, scarring, unusual pigmentation, scaling, oil content, and texture.

The presence of exophthalmos, either bilateral or unilateral, may be accompanied by injected conjunctival vessels and give definitive clues to the etiology. In addition to the more frequently occurring problem of thyroid-related eye disease, a number of uncommon orbital and intracranial conditions may present as a red eye because of either congestion or exposure of vessels of the globe. A partial list includes hemangiomas, arteriovenous malformations, lacrimal gland tumors, metastatic tumors, and mucoceles.

Palpation for masses as well as for areas of tenderness along the lid margins, lacrimal gland, and lacrimal sac can be performed if entities such as dacryoadenitis, canaliculitis, and dacryocystitis, in addition to tumors of these structures, are suspected. Enlarged preauricular nodes may be present in cases of viral or chlamydial infection or, rarely, in cases of ocular or orbital malignancy.

Examination of the facial features is followed by evaluation of the eyelids for abnormalities in structure or function. Particularly in cases of long-standing unilateral or asymmetric red eye problems it is not rare to detect a problem of the lids or adnexa that has been overlooked by others. Structural abnormalities can be due to past trauma, or prior oculoplastic surgeries (cosmetic or functional), or frequently from age-related involutional changes of the eyelids and adnexal structures.

Lid position is evaluated for ectropion and entropion. The presence of upper eyelid lash ptosis, often accompanied by mild upper lid ptosis, are frequently missed signs of floppy eyelid syndrome. Instructing the patient to squeeze the lids tightly closed can reveal an intermittent, covert spastic entropion or, less commonly, imbrication. Imbrication is the abnormal sliding of the upper lid over the external margin of the lower lid, resulting in mechanical irritation of the palpebral conjunctiva of the upper lid. It is most likely to occur after horizontal lid tightening procedures, particularly if the lower lid tightness is much greater than that of the upper lid. The chronic irritation produces a papillary reaction, increased mucus formation, and ocular surface inflammation.

Another less common, and usually asymmetric condition, is mucus fishing syndrome. The history frequently is of a chronic conjunctivitis with production of stringy white mucus. It can be quite helpful to ask the patient to describe or demonstrate exactly how he removes the mucus. Typically, the patient is mechanically wiping or touching the inferior fornix and palpebral conjunctiva with a cloth, tissue, or cotton-tipped applicator, etc., in order to remove mucus, thereby creating a chronic cycle of irritation and inflammation, which causes continued inceased abnormal mucus production. Findings may include greater distractability of the lower lid of the affected eye, along with a papillary reaction of the inferior palpebral conjunctiva.

Observing for asymmetry of the lower lid tear menisci during the initial general inspection can reveal a clue of underlying nasolacrimal outflow dysfunction. The patient may have a history of recurrent unilateral conjuctivitis, which improves with topical antibiotic treatment. Epiphora may or may not be significant, and sometimes will not be appreciated or mentioned by the patient during episodes because the other signs and symptoms of redness and discharge are of more prominence and concern. If the patient is referred, the episode of conjunctivitis may be resolved by the time of appointment, and the tear meniscus asymmetry may provide one of the few clues that leads to further evaluation of the nasolacrimal drainage system. Although acquired stenosis or obstruction anywhere along the pathway is a more common etiology, a large number of other causes is possible, ranging from infectious canaliculitis, to benign or malignant tumors intrinsic or extrinsic to the nasolacrimal system.

Once the face and ocular adnexa have been examined, one continues without magnification by looking at the globes, fornices, and palpebral conjunctivae. The lower lids are first gently retracted manually, then the upper eyelids are lifted. Abnormal lid laxity should be noted. If floppy eyelid syndrome is suspected, it is easier to demonstrate asymmetric laxity by instructing the patient to gaze inferiorly while the examiner uses the thumb of each hand to lift the upper lids simultaneously. Significantly floppy eyelids will evert rather easily, and usually reveal a marked papillary reaction. Another oft-missed condition that is relatively easily diagnosed with this step is superior limbic keratoconjunctivitis. The classic superior quadrantic bulbar conjunctival injection is much easier to detect without magnification. This is true also for assessing other conjunctival, episcleral, and scleral processes. Areas of scleral thinning may appear bluish-black due to the visibility of the underlying choroid, indicating possible past episodes of scleritis. Signs of ocular cicatricial pemphigoid, such as subconjunctival fibrosis, forniceal shortening, and symblephara are also less easily missed with unaided visual inspection.

Functional eyelid problems refers to conditions where the eyelid anatomy is normal, but function is abnormal. Examples include seventh nerve pareses from any cause (postviral, postsurgical, trauma, stroke, etc.), with a number of possible sequelae: incomplete blink, lagophthalmos, and various degrees of exposure keratoconjunctivitis. Nonparalytic states of dysfunctional blinking and/or closure can also result from use of certain medications or diseases, such as: long-term antipsychotic or other psychiatric medications, advanced Parkinson's disease, or any number of severe chronic medical or end-of-life situations, where the mental state may be declining or subdued, and where frequent narcotic pain relievers may be in usage. Such patients often have multiple possible contributing factors for a red eye or eyes, chief among which include evaporative dry eye and exposure keratoconjunctivitis. One should observe the frequency, symmetry, and completeness of blinking. This is best done unobtrusively while talking with the patient, or in situations where the patient is not communicative, with the attendant family or caregiver. If the patient is conscious that this behavior is being observed, he or she may unintentionally alter the pattern of blinking. Complete closure, without lagophthalmos, should occur with involuntary blinking every 5 to 8 seconds, and there should be good apposition of the lids to the globe, with the punctal openings normally aligned.

Slit lamp biomicroscopy is performed, beginning with low-power magnification and a broad, oblique beam. Blepharitis, with secondary or concomitant ocular surface disease and inflammation, is a common cause of both acute and chronic red eye. Lash cleanliness and quantity are noted. Madarosis can occur with the more common forms of anterior blepharitis, but should also prompt consideration of uncommon eyelid conditions, such as basal cell, sebaceous gland, or squamous cell carcinomas. Infestation of the lashes with parasites such as *Phthirus pubis* may also be the source of red eyes. The umbilicated lid lesions of molluscum contagiosum can be hidden in the lash line.

The tear film is examined, both qualitatively and quantitatively. Dry eye syndrome is commonly either the primary or a contributing cause of red eye. Qualitative abnormalities include the presence of excess mucus or debris. Quantitative assessments can include the height of the tear meniscus along the inferior lid margin and tear breakup time.

Next, a cotton-tipped applicator is used to retract the lower eyelid. This technique is suggested for both patient comfort as well as the examiner's safety. The inferior fornix is examined for discharge. A watery or mucoid discharge suggests a viral process; a more viscid discharge is seen in allergic reactions; and a thick, purulent exudate is commonly seen in bacterial conjunctivitis. Biomicroscopy may also reveal inflammatory membranes. True membranes, when removed, detach the underlying adherent epithelium, leaving a raw and bleeding surface. Pseudomembranes, when removed, cause no epithelial disruption and thus no bleeding. Distinction of the two types can be difficult, and is not highly diagnostic. Membranes in general are uncommon. In the acute setting, viral or bacterial conjunctivitis is the likely cause. Noninfectious conditions include Stevens-Johnson syndrome, alkali injuries and, rarely, ligneous conjunctivitis.

Conjunctival concretions rarely cause inflammation. A careful search for any foreign material, from recent trauma to a more remote injury often forgotten in the history by the patient, should be undertaken. The tear drainage system is also inspected. By rolling the cotton-tipped applicator from the nose outward along the canalicular system, purulent material may be milked from the canaliculi, or a stone may be palpated. Signs of acute dacryocystitis would likely already have been noted on external examination, with redness and swelling over the lacrimal sac, though in a situation where perhaps a prior episode had partially resolved one might illicit pain upon compression of the sac, and sometimes a dramatic reflux of mucopurulent material.

Next is assessment of the inferior palpebral conjunctival surface. The understanding of follicles and papillae in ocular disease can present a challenge but provides major clues in diagnosing the diseases with which they are associated. A follicular reaction consists of aggregates of lymphocytes that appear as whitish bumps surrounded by a red base. Follicles are normally absent in infants, fairly prominent in children, less commonly seen in adults, and bring to mind a specific differential diagnosis. Acute follicular reactions are common with viral infections such as adenovirus and the herpes family. Chronic follicular reactions (present for longer than 3 weeks) can develop with certain infections, such as trachoma, inclusion conjunctivitis, Parinaud's oculoglandular syndrome, and molluscum contagiosum, and as a toxic response to topical medications.

A papillary reaction, characterized by a red velvety appearance in which a central, elevated tuft of vessels is surrounded by a pale base, is seen with nonspecific inflammation and is less specific. Often, however, the palpebral conjunctiva has a 'mixed' papillary and follicular reaction. Prominent papillary hypertrophy may suggest allergic reaction. The superior palpebral conjunctiva is inspected by everting the upper eyelid. Once again, it is important to look for foreign bodies and to assess the palpebral conjunctiva. The appearance of 'cobblestoning' is indicative of giant papillae, which is seen in vernal disease as well as contact lens-induced giant papillary conjunctivitis. A retained suture from previous eye surgery also can cause focal giant papillary conjunctivitis by mechanical irritation of the superior tarsal conjunctiva. Scarring of the superior tarsal conjunctiva also should be documented and may be diagnostic, as in the case of the linear white scarring known as Arlt's lines, which are seen in trachoma.

The bulbar conjunctiva is examined next. Inflamed pingueculae and pterygia are a common cause of red eye visits. Less common are phlyctenules, raised whitish to yellow nodules with surrounding dilated blood vessels that represent a type IV delayed hypersensitivity to a foreign antigen. These lesions occur near the limbus and can invade the cornea. Often, they will partially stain with fluoroscein due to breakdown of the overlying epithelium. Conditions that can cause phlyctenular keratoconjunctivitis include staphylococcal disease, tuberculosis, fungal antigens, lymphogranuloma venereum, and nematodes. Conjunctival tumors, including benign and malignant lesions, can all present with ocular inflammation.

Distinguishing which layer of the ocular surface is inflamed is important but not always easy. Engorgement of the episcleral vessels can be sectorial or diffuse. Episcleral vessels are distinguished from conjunctival and scleral vessels by being thicker, running in a radial direction from the cornea, blanching with the application of topical phenylephrine 2.5%, and being immobile when the overlying conjunctiva is moved. The most common cause of episcleritis is idiopathic inflammation, although it also can be seen with systemic collagen vascular diseases such as rheumatoid arthritis, polyarteritis nodosa, systemic lupus erythematosus, and Wegener's granulomatosis. Scleral vessels are deeper and have a characteristic violaceous hue that does not blanch with phenylephrine.

The cornea often provides critical diagnostic information because clinically significant redness and keratitis often coexist. A broad oblique beam is used to scan the overall appearance. Epithelial punctate keratitis often can be noted even without fluorescein dye. An inferior pattern suggests dryness, exposure, entropion, ectropion, or blepharitis. A more diffuse distribution can be consistent with acute conjunctivitis or keratitis medicamentosa. Filaments are most commonly seen in dry eye states such as keratitis sicca, superior limbic keratoconjunctivitis, or situations where there is limited upper lid excursion due to any cause. Micropannus suggests inclusion conjunctivitis, trachoma, ocular rosacea, contact lens abuse, staphylococcal hypersensitivity, vernal keratoconjunctivitis, superior limbic keratoconjunctivitis, and herpes simplex infection. Subepithelial opacities can be seen in epidemic keratoconjunctivitis, chlamydia, herpes simplex, staphylococcal disease, and nummular keratitis.

Signs of anterior uveitis, such as keratic precipitates, cells in the anterior chamber or anterior vitreous, miosis, posterior synechiae, and injection of the perilimbal blood vessels, usually allow the proper diagnosis to be made with little difficulty. The remainder of the eye examination must not be overlooked. Measurement of the intraocular pressure and a retinal evaluation are crucial to the diagnosis of a variety of other causes of red eye.

Occasionally, ancillary tests are required. Schirmer testing, probing, and irrigation of the lacrimal system, transillumination, exophthalmometry, corneal sensitivity measurements, keratometry, gonioscopy, ultrasonography, fluorescein angiography, and radiology can be considered and may give the extra information needed to make the correct diagnosis. In cases of suspected infection or in cases that have not responded to routine therapy, standard culture techniques and conjunctival scrapings for microscopic examination are indicated. The topical anesthetic test is often useful. If a patient is complaining of ocular irritation or pain accompanying a red eye that is not consistent with the findings, two drops of proparacaine are instilled without the patient being aware of the anesthetic effect. If the patient reports that the pain is not relieved or is actually worse, consideration must be given to factitious disease, hysteria, or a condition that has a more posterior origin. A systemic work-up is sometimes mandatory, especially when malignancies, immunocompromised states, and systemic inflammatory or infectious conditions are contemplated.

Conclusion

It is always gratifying to diagnose and treat a medical condition correctly, especially in a patient referred by another practitioner. Determining the correct diagnosis involves three components. First, one needs an appropriate knowledge base. Second, an accurate and thorough history is usually critical to solve the more complicated or chronic cases of red eye. And finally, avoid rushing to the slit lamp to make the quick diagnosis.

Chapter 25

Minimal Visual Loss: Determining the Role of the Cornea

David Litoff

Evaluating minimal visual loss is a frequent problem for the ophthalmologist. A complete history and ocular examination are essential in determining the cause of any reduction in visual function. Small alterations on the surface of the cornea can have profound effects on visual acuity. In addition, small internal structural changes in the cornea may result in visual loss secondary to light scattering and decreased transparency. In this chapter, we review various techniques for evaluating the role of the cornea in different conditions that may present with minimal visual loss.

There are several categories of corneal abnormalities which can produce minimal visual loss. The first, irregular astigmatism, causes decreased vision because of an irregular optical refracting surface. (Box 25.1 summarizes common causes of irregular astigmatism.) The second, corneal opacities, causes decreased vision from decreased transparency and increased light scattering of the cornea. (Box 25.2 summarizes common causes of corneal opacities.) A third category is irregularity of the posterior corneal surface. Often, these different corneal abnormalities coexist, making evaluation more difficult.

History

A complete history is essential in evaluating patients with minimal visual loss. Family history, recent trauma, or any past ocular surgery can be important in determining the etiology of visual loss. Determining if patterns of visual loss exist can help in the evaulation of these patients. In addition, the ophthalmologist must determine if the visual loss is transient, permanent, or progressive. Table 25.1 outlines ocular symptoms with the corresponding corneal conditions.

Examination Techniques

Visual acuity

When examining patients with minimal visual loss, the ophthalmologist must determine the best corrected visual acuity. One of the most common causes of minimal visual loss is an unrecognized refractive error. The standard method of determining best-corrected visual acuity utilizes a Snellen chart in a dimly lit room and asking the patient to read the letters without pausing.

- Snellen visual acuity measures the patient's ability to resolve fine spatial details on a high-contrast target.[1,2]
- Best-corrected visual acuity only reveals limited information about visual function.

Pinhole aperture

- Increases depth of focus and corrects small amounts of refractive error.
- Reduces irregular astigmatism and light scattering in the cornea.
- Further improvement with pinhole aperture after best refraction suggests irregular astigmatism.

Contrast sensitivity function (CSF)

- Contrast sensitivity is a very important aspect of visual function.
- It is measured with a contrast sensitivity chart such as the CSV-1000E by Vector Vision.
- The method of evaluating visual function is based on sinusoidal patterns of varying spatial frequencies.[3]
- CSF provides a more complete assessment of visual function than Snellen visual acuity.[1]
- CSF can show abnormalities prior to any changes in Snellen visual acuity in patients with corneal edema and early keratoconus.[4,5]

Diagnostic rigid contact lens refraction

- Useful technique in evaluating patients with suspected irregular astigmatism.
- Corrects irregular stigmatism and indicates amount of decrease in vision attributed to this mechanism.

Technique

- Topical anesthesia is placed in eye.
- Contact is fit on the average keratometry reading.
- A large-diameter RGP lens is chosen, within 3 diopters of patient's refraction.
- Over-refraction is performed and compared to the patient's best-corrected spectacle correction.
- If improvement is noted with rigid contact lens, irregular astigmatism is inferred.

Box 25.1 Irregular astigmatism

- Keratoconus
- Postrefractive ectasia
- Post-trauma
- Corneal warpage
- Keratoconjunctivitis sicca
- Recurrent erosion
- Toxic epitheliopathy
- Corneal dystrophies
  - Anterior corneal dystrophies
    - Map-dot-fingerprint dystrophy
    - Meesmann's dystrophy
    - Reis-Bücklers' dystrophy
  - Stromal dystrophies
    - Granular dystrophy
    - Lattice dystrophy
    - Macular dystrophy
- Corneal degenerations
  - Pterygium
  - Pellucid marginal degeneration
  - Band keratopathy
  - Salzmann's degeneration

Table 25.1 Symptoms that often correlate with corneal abnormalities

Symptoms	Corneal abnormalities
Haze and halos	Epithelial edema
Monocular diplopia	Irregular astigmatism
Decreased morning vision	Stromal edema
Glare	Corneal scars
Multiple changes of glasses	Keratoconus
Pain	Epithelial defect
Family history of decreased vision	Corneal dystrophies
Awakening with foreign body sensation	Recurrent erosion

Box 25.2 Corneal opacities

- Traumatic corneal scars
- Postsurgical corneal scars
- Postinfectious corneal scarring
- Corneal dystrophies
  - Anterior corneal dystrophies
    - Reis-Bücklers' dystrophy
  - Stromal dystrophies
    - Granular dystrophy
    - Lattice dystrophy
    - Macular dystrophy
  - Posterior corneal dystrophies
    - Fuchs' endothelial dystrophy
    - Congenital hereditary endothelial dystrophy
    - Posterior polymorphous dystrophy
- Corneal degenerations
  - Pterygium
  - Pellucid marginal degeneration
  - Band keratopathy
  - Salzmann's degeneration
- Keratoconus
- Atopic keratoconjunctivitis
- Ocular ciciatricial pemphigoid
- Corneal infiltrates
- Corneal edema

Potential acuity meter

- The potential acuity meter (PAM) has some use in predicting potential acuity with small corneal scars.
- Small corneal scars can result in scattering of the PAM beam and underestimating the potential visual acuity.
- Although sometimes helpful in evaluating patients with minimal visual loss, the PAM can produce misleading results.[6]

Retinoscopy

- Useful in identifying stromal opacities and irregular astigmatism.[7]
- Careful attention to the quality of the reflex can often demonstrate subtle corneal abnormalities.
- With experience, estimating the degree that the cornea affects vision is possible.

Slit lamp examination

- A complete slit lamp examination is essential in examining patients with minimal visual loss.
- A systematic slit lamp examination of the cornea with low and high magnification, and with various types of illumination, should be performed.

Fluorescein evaluation

- Fluorescein dye forms a thin film over the cornea, visible with a cobalt blue light.
- Fluorescein dye is very useful in evaluating the smoothness of the epithelial surface.
- Unevenness in the distribution of the fluorescein dye is suggestive of irregular astigmatism (Fig. 25.1).

Keratometry

- A keratometer is a useful instrument for measuring the curvature of the central region of the cornea.
- Additional information is obtained from the quality of the reflected mires.
- If the keratometry mires are irregular, irregular astigmatism is present (Fig. 25.2).

Computerized corneal topography

Corneal topography is useful in evaluating patients with minimal visual loss. There are two basic systems currently available: elevation-based topography systems and

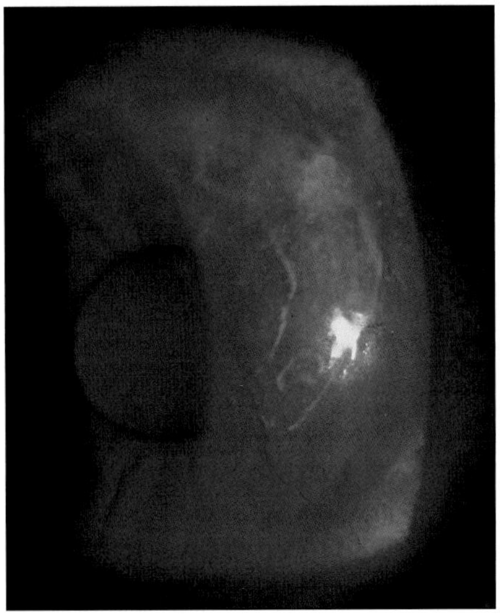

Fig. 25.1 Epithelial surface irregularity demonstrated with topical fluorescein dye in a patient with a recurrent erosion.

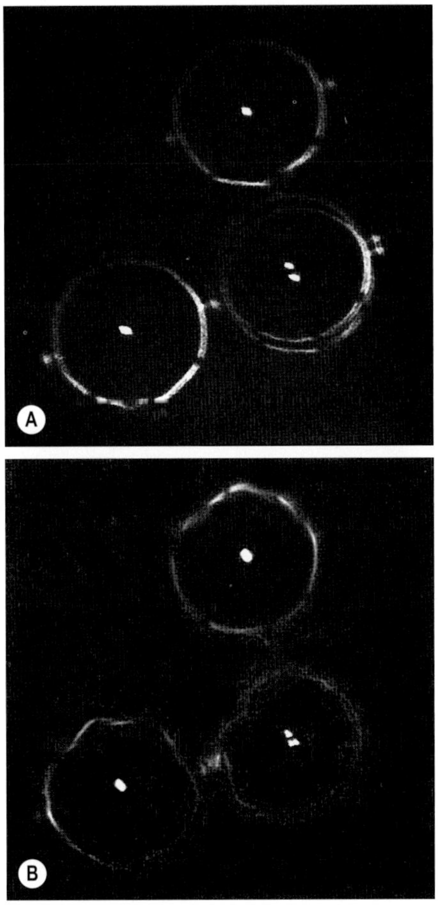

Fig. 25.2 Irregular astigmatism. (**A**) Irregular astigmatism demonstrated with keratometry in a patient with map-dot-fingerprint dystrophy. The central mires cannot be superimposed on each other. (**B**) Irregular astigmatism in a patient with granular dystrophy. Keratometric mires are very irregular, demonstrating surface irregularity.

Placido-based videokeratoscopes. The elevation-based topography systems include the Pentacam, which utilizes Scheimpflug images to determine anterior and posterior corneal topography, corneal pachymetry, and Zernike analysis, which describes wavefronts.[8] The Orbscan employs stereotriangulation to measure the anterior and posterior corneal surface as well as pachymetry. The Placido-based systems work by projecting a Placido disk onto the cornea. The image is photographed and digitized, resulting in curvature maps of the anterior corneal surface. Topography can be used to rule out certain corneal abnormalities which contribute to minimal visual loss. Early keratoconus, pellucid marginal degeneration, or postrefractive ectasia can be extremely difficult to diagnosis without accurate topography. In addition, most of the topography systems can measure corneal irregularity and help confirm etiology of minimal visual loss. The Pentacam has multiple indicies to determine the irregularity of the cornea, including Q-Val (asphericity quotient) and ISV (index of surface variance). The TMS™, made by Tomey, calculates the surface asymmetry index (SAI) and the surface regularity index (SRI) with each topographic evaluation. These measures calculate the degree of asymmetry and the amount of local irregularity in the cornea. The SRI can be useful in predicting optical performance of the anterior corneal surface and has been shown to provide a good correlation with best-spectacle-corrected visual acuity.[9] The Oculus Pentacam topography system utilizes Scheimpflug images to determine information about the cornea (Fig. 25.3). One program, Belin/Ambrosio Enhanced Ectasia, is helpful diagnosing keratoconus and other ectatic corneal abnormalities by looking at front and back elevation and correlating them with corneal thickness maps. Corneal topography can be useful in predicting the best-corrected visual acuity in patients. With the Placido-based videokeratoscopes such as the Humprey Topography System, high values of corneal irregularity measurement (CIM) suggest significant irregular astigmatism and correlate with visual loss. Computerized corneal topography is one of the most sensitive methods of diagnosing early keratoconus, postrefractive ectasia, pellucid marginal degeneration, and contact lens-induced corneal warpage, even in the absence of any slit lamp findings.[10]

Wavefront analysis

Wavefront analyzers are able to measure lower-order errors (sphere, astigmatism, and axis), as well as higher-order aberrations or irregular astigmatism. Wavefront analysis, a relatively new technology, allows for measurement of wavefront errors.[11] There are several methods to measure aberrations of the eye. The most common is the Hartmann-Shack wavefront sensor. In the ideal eye, parallel rays of light are refracted by the eye and form wavefronts that focus exactly on the retina. Aberrations result in wavefronts that do not focus perfectly on the retina. The Hartmann-Shack sensor detects the wavefront leaving the eye though a lenslet array on a charge-coupled device (CCD) camera. By calculating the displacement of the images on the CCD camera, the wavefront error is calculated. Irregular astigmatism or higher-order aberrations can be determined quantitatively as a set of coefficients of the Zernike polynomials.[12] Zernike coefficients of the higher-order aberrations can be derived from

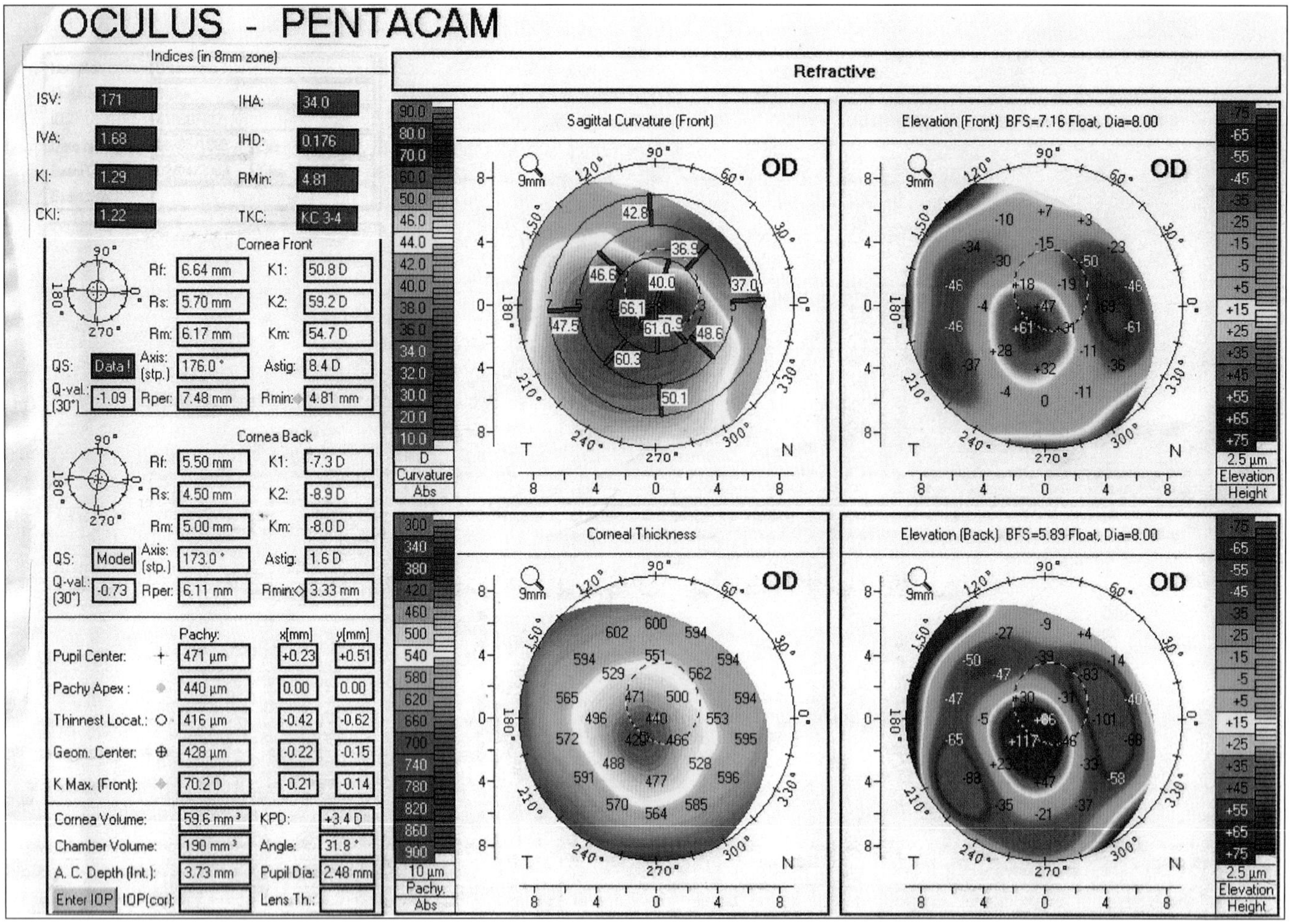

Fig. 25.3 Elevation-based corneal topography from a patient with keratoconus. Note: automatic detection program identified eye as keratoconus and gave a numerical value to the degree of corneal irregularity with an ISV value. The topography map shows a moderate case of keratoconus with a steep cornea thinned to 416 microns (μm) and abnormal indices.

corneal topography. In a normal ametropic eye, defocus (myopia or hyperopia) is the largest aberration followed by astigmatism. The higher-order aberrations are typically small, comprising only about 10–20% of the aberrations of the eye. However, in eyes with significant irregular astigmatism, these higher-order aberrations comprise a much larger percentage of the total aberrations of the eye. Wavefront analysis is an additional tool that can be very powerful in determining the etiology of minimal visual loss.[13] Although wavefront analysis is a relatively new technology, with future developments it may become more common in evaluating patients.

Selected Conditions Causing Minimal Visual Loss

Dry eyes

- Dry eyes are a frequent cause of minimal visual loss.
- The surface dryness results in irregular astigmatism, increased wavefont aberation, and subsequent decreased vision.[14,15]
- Dry eyes often results in a decreased tear film thickness and stability, which can exacerbate any irregularities of the underlying cornea.

Ectatic disorders

Keratoconus

Keratoconus is one of the more common causes of 'unexplained' minimal visual loss that the ophthalmologist encounters. Keratoconus is a noninflammatory corneal thinning disorder characterized by thinning of the central cornea and anterior protrusion of a conical cornea, usually inferiorly.[16,17] This abnormal topography results in irregular corneal astigmatism. In addition, keratoconus results in large amounts of high-order aberrations. Typically, the patient is a young adult with minimal visual loss who has often seen several different medical specialists. The patient has often had frequent spectacle changes, and may be convinced that a serious medical condition is present.

- Symptoms include blurry vision, photophobia, glare, and ocular irritation.

- Findings include prominent corneal nerves, Fleischer ring, stromal thinning, corneal stress lines, and apical scarring.
- Myopic astigmatism is usually present and, with retinoscopy, a scissoring reflex suggestive of irregular astigmatism is commonly seen.[18]

With modern topography, early keratoconus is relatively easy to diagnose.[19–21] Several automated detection programs are currently in use to detect and quantify keratoconus.[21–24] Wavefront analysis in patients with keratoconus has revealed an increase in higher-order aberrations.[12]

Ectasia following refractive surgery

- Corneal ectasia is another cause of minimal visual loss in patients who have had refractive surgery.
- Corneal ectasia is shown by topography: progressive corneal thinning with protrusion and irregular astigmatism.[25]
- Most of these cases probably had unidentified forme fruste keratoconus prior to their refractive surgery.

Pellucid marginal degeneration

- Uncommon cause of minimal visual loss seen in patients 20–40 years of age.
- Keratometry exhibits marked against-the-rule astigmatism.
- Slit lamp examination reveals inferior thinning between 4 and 8 o'clock.[16]
- Corneal topography usually shows a characteristic pattern of marked flattening of the central corneal with inferior peripheral steeping.
- A diagnostic rigid contact lens refraction produces an excellent optical correction and is useful in demonstrating the cause of the decreased vision.

Terrien's marginal degeneration

- A rare cause of minimal visual loss.
- Slit lamp examination reveals peripheral corneal thinning with opacification and superficial vascularization, often superiorly.
- Progression leads to against-the-rule astigmatism and irregular astigmatism.[26]

Punctate epithelial keratitis

Multiple conditions cause punctate epithelial keratitis (PEK) and minimal visual loss. Box 25.3 summarizes common causes of punctate epithelial keratitis.

- PEK results in minimal visual loss secondary to irregular astigmatism.
- Slit lamp examination with fluorescein dye helps confirm the diagnosis.
- Retinoscopy, keratometry, corneal topography, and the use of rigid contact lens refraction are useful in documenting irregular astigmatism as the cause of visual loss.
- Placing a single lubricating drop on the cornea often improves vision in patients with PEK.

Box 25.3 Common causes of punctate epithelial keratitis

Infectious keratitis
- Viral keratitis
  - Herpes simplex keratitis
  - Epidemic keratoconjunctivitis
- Bacterial keratitis
- Chlamydia

Blepharitis

Neurotrophic keratitis

Dry eye condition
- Exposure
- Keratoconjunctivitis sicca

Xerosis

Toxic keratitis

Chemical injury

Allergic reaction

Trauma

Trichiasis

Entropion

Superior limbic keratoconjunctivitis

Thygeson's superficial punctate keratopathy

Corneal scars

- Mild corneal scars can result in minimal visual loss.
- Corneal scars can cause decreased vision due to irregular astigmatism, light scattering, and decreased transparency of the cornea.
- Careful slit lamp examination, retinoscopy, corneal topography, and rigid contact lens refraction are all useful in confirming the cause of the decreased vision.

Corneal dystrophies

Anterior corneal dytrophies

Map-dot-fingerprint dystrophy is a common bilateral epithelial corneal dystrophy. Many patients are asymptomatic. However, minimal visual loss secondary to epithelial irregularity is common. Recurrent erosions can further contribute to irregular astigmatism in these patients.

- Slit lamp examination with a broad oblique beam demonstrates maplike opacities.
- Retroillumination can highlight dots and fingerprints.
- Fluorescein dye can be used to delineate microcysts and areas of elevated epithelium.
- Keratometry is useful in demonstrating irregular mires (see Fig. 25.2).
- Corneal topography can demonstrate areas of irregularity that correspond to the location of the corneal dystrophy.
- Rigid contact lens refraction confirms the visual loss is secondary to irregular astigmatism.

Meesmann's dystrophy

- Meesmann's dystrophy is another anterior corneal dystrophy that can present with minimal visual loss.
- Symptoms include tearing, photophobia, and irritation.
- Slit lamp examination with retroillumination reveals multiple tiny, regular, clear intraepithelial cysts diffusely spread across the entire cornea.[27]

- Tiny vesicles contribute to irregular epithelium, resulting in visual loss.
- Rigid contact lens refraction can be helpful in identifying the amount of irregular astigmatism.

Reis-Bücklers' dystrophy

- Often presents early in life with recurrent erosions.
- Slit lamp examination reveals diffuse reticular opacification in Bowman's membrane.[28]
- With recurrent episodes, subepithelial scarring occurs, which results in irregular astigmatism, decreased corneal transparency, and light scattering.
- Retinoscopy, slit lamp examination, and keratometry are useful in estimating degrees of corneal opacification and irregular astigmatism.

Stromal corneal dystrophies

Stromal corneal dystrophies are relatively uncommon. They can result in visual loss secondary to stromal opacities, causing decreased corneal transparency. If the opacities extend anteriorly, epithelial erosions and irregular astigmatism may occur.

Granular dystrophy

- Generally does not cause a decrease in vision until middle age.
- Slit lamp examination reveals discrete, focal, white granular deposits occurring in the axial portion of the corneal (Fig. 25.4).[29]
- Retinoscopy will overestimate the degree of decreased vision.

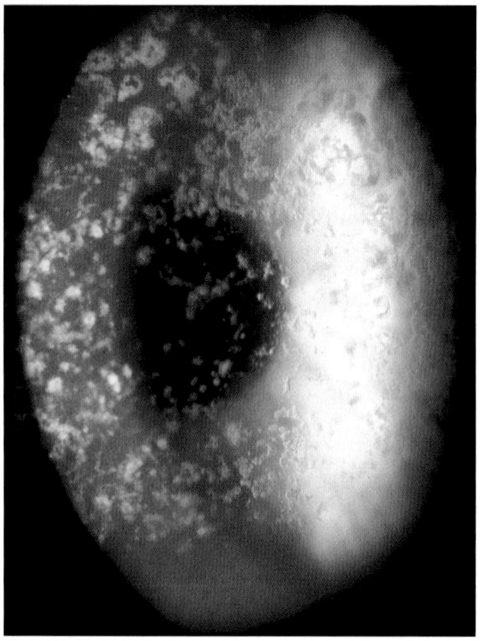

Fig. 25.4 Slit lamp photography using broad oblique illumination and indirect illumination in a patient with granular dystrophy and minimal visual loss.

Lattice dystrophy

- Presents with decreased vision by late adolescence.
- Slit lamp examination reveals refractile lines in a lattice pattern over the central cornea, best seen by retroillumination.[29]
- Recurrent erosions result in subepithelial scarring and irregular astigmatism.

Macular dystrophy

- Macular dystrophy affects visual acuity much earlier than other stromal dystrophies.
- Slit lamp findings include diffuse central stromal clouding with a ground-glass appearance best visualized with diffuse illumination.[29]
- Frequent recurrent erosions result in episodes of pain, photophobia, and visual loss.
- The visual loss is secondary to irregular astigmatism and corneal opacities.

Endothelial disorders

Posterior corneal disorders are common causes of minimal visual loss. The mechanism of decreased visual acuity includes corneal edema, which reduces corneal transparency and increases light scattering. Visual loss depends on the severity of the disease.

Fuchs' endothelial dystrophy

- Bilateral, slowly progressive endothelial dysfunction.
- With slit lamp examination and specular reflection, the endothelial cells are noted to be larger and polymorphic with multiple guttae.[30]
- Early disease is characterized by minimal edema, resulting in minimal visual loss.
- The visual loss is often worse in the morning and improves during the day due to surface evaporation and stromal deturgescence.
- Pachymetry can be useful in detecting early corneal edema.
- Specular microscopy can demonstrate a decreased number of endothelial cells and guttae.
- With progression, epithelial edema results, with marked decrease in vision.

Posterior polymorphous dystrophy (PPMD)

- Bilateral dominant inherited corneal disorder.
- Slit lamp examination reveals scallop-edged endothelial bands or vesicles in Descemet's membrane, best visualized by indirect lateral illumination.[31]
- Progressive stromal and later epithelial edema develop.
- Visual loss worse on awakening and improves during the day.

Iridocorneal endothelial syndrome

- Unilateral condition occurs more commonly in women than men.
- Patients are usually between the ages of 30 and 50.

- Slit lamp findings include corneal endothelial abnormalities, peripheral anterior synechiae, iris atrophy, and iris nodules.[32]
- Visual loss occurs because of progressive corneal edema.

Corneal degenerations

Corneal degenerations can present with minimal visual loss. The mechanisms include decreased corneal transparency due to central corneal opacities and irregular astigmatism. Historical data and careful examination can usually determine when the visual loss is the result of corneal pathology.

Pterygium

- A pterygium can result in minimal visual loss secondary to irregular astigmatism or by growing across the visual axis with decreased corneal transparency.
- The amount of irregular astigmatism can be determined using retinoscopy, keratometry, or corneal topography analysis.
- With-the-rule astigmatism is common, while corneal topography may reveal localized flattening central to the pterygium apex.

Corneal warpage

Contact lens wear can induce changes in the shape of the cornea that result in irregular astigmatism.[33,34] Hard contacts are the most common type; however, both rigid gas permeable contacts lenses and soft contact lenses can induce corneal warpage.

- Typically, visual acuity is normal with contacts but decreased with spectacles.
- Keratometry reveals distortion of mires.
- Corneal topography is a very sensitive aid for the diagnosis of corneal warpage. A typical pattern of central irregular astigmatism, loss of radial symmetry, and loss of the normal pattern of peripheral corneal flattening is often seen.[35]

Keratorefractive surgery

One of the more common causes of minimal visual loss is seen in patients following keratorefractive surgery. Many times, a careful refraction can detect a refractive error that was not previously documented as the cause of the visual loss. A slit lamp evaluation should be performed noting any unusual corneal haze, scarring, or epithelial ingrowth.[36] Irregular astigmatism is one of the most serious and frequent complications of keratorefractive surgery.[37,38] Corneal topography and wavefront analysis can aid in the diagnosis of the irregular astigmatism and variance of the corneal power in the optical zone following keratorefractive surgery.[38] Corneal topography may provide important information on the optical quality of the treated zone, the stability of the procedure over time, and the accuracy of the centration of the optical zone over the pupil.[39,40] Contrast sensitivity function has been shown to be depressed following LASIK.[41] A decrease in contrast sensitivity function after refractive surgery can often explain why the patient's perceived vision is worse than the measured Snellen acuity. A rigid contact lens refraction can aid in the etiology of decreased vision in keratoreactive patients, although some patients have central corneas that are so flat that an inadequate contact lens fitting can result in misleading information.

References

1. Huang F, Tseng S, Shih M, Chen FK. Effects of artificial tears on corneal surface regularity, contrast sensitivity, and glare disability in dry eyes. *Ophthalmology.* 2002;109:1934–1940.
2. Jindra LF, Zemon V. Contrast sensitivity testing: A more complete assessment of vision. *J Cataract Refract Surg.* 1989;15:141–148.
3. Kniestedt C, Stampler RL. Visual acuity and its measurement. *Ophthalmol Clin North Am.* 2003;16:155–170.
4. Mannis MJ, Zadnik K, Johnson CA. The effect of penetrating keratoplasty on contrast sensitivity in keratoconus. *Ophthalmology.* 1984;105: 1513–1516.
5. Miller D, Sanghvi S. Contrast sensitivity and glare testing in corneal disease. In: Nadler MP, Miller D, Nadler DJ, eds. *Glare and contrast sensitivity for clinicians.* New York: Springer-Verlag; 1990:45–52.
6. Minkowski JS, Palese M, Guyton DL. Potential acuity meter using a minute aerial pinhole aperture. *Am J Ophthalmol.* 1983;90:1360–1368.
7. Duke-Elder WS, Abrams D, eds. *System of ophthalmology.* vol. 5. *Ophthalmic optics and refraction.* St Louis: Mosby; 1970.
8. Belin MW, Khachikian SS. Elevation-based topography. *Highlights of Ophthalmology International.* 2008.
9. Wilson SE, Klyce SD. Quantitative descriptors of corneal topography. A clinical study. *Arch Ophthalmol.* 1991;109:349–353.
10. Maguire LJ, Bourne WM. Corneal topography of early keratoconus. *Am J Ophthalmol.* 1989;108:107–112.
11. Brint SF (Moderatator: Presentations from the customized ablation latest advancements). *Supplement to Eyeworld.* October 2002.
12. Maeda N, Fujikado T, Kurada T, et al. Wavefront aberrations measured with Hartmann-Shack sensor in patients with keratoconus. *Ophthalmology.* 2002;109:1996–2003.
13. Kent C. Using wavefront today. *Ophthalmology management.* 2002; 41–48.
14. Montes-Mico R. Role of the tear film in the optical quality of the human eye. *J Cataract Refract Surg.* 2007;33:1631–1635.
15. Ishida R, Kojima T, Dogrun M, et al. The application of a new continuous functional visual acuity measurement system in dry eye syndromes. *Am J Ophthalmol.* 2005;139:253–258.
16. Krachmer JH, Feder RS, Belin MW. Keratoconus and related noninflammatory corneal thinning disorders. *Surv Ophthalmol.* 1984;28:293–322.
17. Rabinowitz YS. Keratoconus. *Surv Ophthalmol.* 1998;42:297–319.
18. Belin MW. *Optical and surgical correction of keratoconus. Focal points: clinical modules for ophthalmologists.* vol. 6. San Francisco: American Academy of Ophthalmology; 1988.
19. Maguire LJ, Bourne WM. Corneal topography of early keratoconus. *Am J Ophthalmol.* 1989;108:107–112.
20. Rabinowitz YS, Mcdonnell PJ. Computer-assisted corneal topography in keratoconus. *Refract Corneal Surg* 1989;5:400–408.
21. Belin MW, Khachikian SS. Corneal diagnosis and evaluation with the Oculus Pentacam. *Highlights of Ophthalmology.* 2007;35:5–8.
22. Maeda N, Klyce SD, Smolek MK, Thompson HW. Automated keratoconus screening with corneal topography analysis. *Invest Ophthalmol Vis Sci* 1994;35:2749–2757.
23. Smolek MK, Klyce SD. Current keratoconus detection methods compared with a neural network approach. *Invest Ophthalmol Vis Sci* 1997;38: 2290–2299.
24. Rabinowitz YS. Videokeratographic indices to aid in screening for keratoconus. *J Refract Surg.* 1995;11:371–379.
25. Randleman JB, Woodward M, Lynn MJ, Stulting RD. Risk assessment for ectasia after corneal refractive surgery. *Ophthalmology.* 2008;115:37–50.
26. Robin JB, Schanzlin DJ, Verity SM, et al. Peripheral corneal disorders. *Surv Ophthalmol.* 1986;31:1–36.
27. Fine BS, Yanoff M, Pitts E, et al. Meesmann's epithelial dystrophy of the cornea. *Am J Ophthalmol.* 1977;83:633–642.
28. Hogan MJ, Wood I. Reis-Bücklers' corneal dystrophy. *Trans Ophthalmol Soc UK.* 1971;91:41–57.
29. Waring GO III, Rodrigues MM, Laibson PR. Corneal dystrophies. I. Dystrophies of the epithelium, Bowman's layer and stroma. *Surv Ophthalmol.* 1978;23:71–122.

30. Miller CA, Krachmer JH. Endothelial dystrophies. In: Kaufman HE et al, eds. *The cornea.* New York: Churchill Livingstone; 1988.
31. Krachmer JH. Posterior polymorphous corneal dystrophy: a disease characterized by epithelial-like endothelial cells which influence management and prognosis. *Trans Am Ophthalmol Soc.* 1985;83:413–475.
32. Shields MB, Campbell DG, Simmons RJ. The essential iris atrophies. *Am J Ophthalmol.* 1978;85:749–759.
33. Hartstein J. Corneal warping due to wearing of corneal contact lenses. A report of 12 cases. *Am J Ophthalmol.* 1965;60:1103–1104.
34. Levenson DS. Changes in corneal curvature with long-term PMMA contact lens wear. *CLAO J.* 1983;9:121–125.
35. Arffa RC. Clinical application of corneal topographic analysis. *Semin Ophthalmol.* 1991;6:122–132.
36. Pasternak J, et al. Corneal haze evaluation after excimer laser photorefractive keratectomy for high myopia. Presented at the Eye Bank Association of America 33rd Scientific Session, Oct 29, 1994.
37. Johnson J, Azar D. Surgically induced topographical abnormalities after LASIK: Management of central islands, cornea ectasia, decentration and irregular astigmatism. *Curr Opin Ophthamol.* 2001;12:309–317.
38. Smokek M, Oshika T, Klyce S, et al. Topographic assessment of irregular astigmatism after photorefractive keratectomy. *J Cataract Refract Surg.* 1998;24:1079–1086.
39. Klyce SD, Smolek MK. Corneal topography of excimer laser photorefractive keratectomy. *J Cataract Refract Surg.* 1993;19(suppl):122–130.
40. Cavanaugh TB, Durrie DS, Riedel SM, et al. Topographical analysis of the centration of excimer laser photorefractive keratectomy. *J Cataract Refract Surg.* 1993;19(suppl):136–143.
41. Chan JWW, Edwards MH, Woo GC, Woo VCP. Contrast sensitivity after laser in situ keratomileusis: One year follow-up. *J Cataract Refract Surg.* 2002;28:1774–1779.

Chapter 26

The Approach to a Patient with Itching and Burning

Joseph D. Iuorno

Patients commonly present with ocular symptoms of itching and burning. Due to their typical self-limiting, non-sight-threatening origin, it is tempting to dismiss these symptoms until the patient has either failed conventional therapy or the condition becomes chronic. Occasionally, more advanced ophthalmic or systemic diseases are hidden in these presenting ocular symptoms. Finding and treating the source of burning and itching is essential to providing excellent care to the patient.

The intent of this chapter is to provide an overview of the clinical approach to a patient referred with burning or itching eyes. Many different causes of burning and itching are listed in Table 26.1. Burning and itching can cohabitate, thereby making it difficult to discern which is the primary symptom associated with the initial cause. Isolating the precipitating factor in a patient with burning and itching eyes starts with listening to the patient's primary symptom.

The Primary Symptom

It is commonly understood that burning is associated with a dry eye condition,[1] whereas itching is linked to allergies.[2] Although these generalizations are not mutually exclusive, they can help direct a concentrated dialogue toward a particular etiology.

Onset

Establishing an onset of symptoms can help identify a potential cause. The introduction of allergens (such as soap, shampoo, perfume, pets, contact lens solution) or a change in environment (employment, housing, or seasons) can precipitate itching and burning. It is important to establish the frequency, duration, and daily occurrence of the primary symptom when investigating a possible cause. Dry eyes upon waking are typically associated with nocturnal exposure or immune-related lacrimal dysfunction, whereas patients with evening symptoms are more likely to have meibomian gland dysfunction.[3] Ocular burning that occurs only while staring at a computer at work[4] on a desk situated below a heating vent is a common clinical scenario with multiple avenues to aggravate a dry eye.[5] Identifying exacerbating or alleviating factors is also helpful in finding a cause for the primary symptom. For example, dry eyes improve with rainy, humid weather and deteriorate in arid, windy conditions.[6] Listening to patients not only is an effective mechanism for identifying aggravating stimuli but also increases patient awareness for future prevention.

Past medical history

Systemic prescription medications (anitidepressants,[7] diuretics,[8] contraceptive pills) and over-the-counter medications (nasal decongestants and antihistamines[9]) can exacerbate aqueous deficiency. Hormone levels in postmenopausal women,[10] men treated for prostate conditions,[11] or women taking estrogen replacement therapy[12] can play a role in chronic dry eye conditions. Previous systemic illness can exacerbate tear production and affect the ocular surface, as is commonly seen in patients following bone marrow transplantation,[13] external beam radiotherapy to the head or neck, or as a sequelae of chronic cicatrizing conjunctivits like Stevens–Johnson syndrome. Active medical diseases such as rheumatoid arthritis can cause lacrimal gland dysfunction producing a dry eye (Sjögren's) syndrome.

A review of positive or negative responses to previous ocular therapies is also valuable information which will assist in diagnosing the cause of the primary symptom. For instance, knowing that a patient's symptom briefly responds to supplemental tear therapy allows the provider to focus additional therapies such as increasing tear volume, retention, adherence, and composition. On the contrary, should symptoms not be relieved at all with pervious therapy, one should reconsider the initial diagnosis.

Contact lens wear

Whereas new technologies in contact lens manufacturing have improved water content and permeability, contact lenses still significantly affect the ocular surface. The amount of contact lens wear, in addition to hygiene and cleaning solutions, are important historical factors which can contribute to possible causes of burning or itching eyes.[14]

Review of systems

Review of systems is an important reminder that many systemic conditions can affect the ocular surface. Rheumatology, dermatology, endocrinology, infectious diseases, and oncology patient can all have conditions which affect the ocular surface and contribute to the primary symptom.

Table 26.1 Differential diagnosis of possible causes of dry eyes

Dry eye syndrome
1. Aqueous tear deficiency
  a. Sjörgren's syndrome
    i. Primary Sjörgren's syndrome
    ii. Secondary Sjörgren's syndrome
      1. Associated with collagen vascular diseases like rheumatoid arthritis, systemic lupus erythematosus, polyarteritis nodosa, scleroderma or Wegener's granulomatosis
  b. Non-Sjögren's aqueous tear deficiency
    i. Congenital
      1. Aplasia or hypoplosia of the lacrimal gland
      2. Anhidrotic ectodermal dysplasia
      3. Aplasia of the lacrimal nerve nucleus
      4. Congenital familial sensory neuropathy with anhidrosis
      5. Cystic fibrosis
      6. Familial autonomic dysfunction (Riley-Day syndrome)
      7. Holmes-Adie syndrome
      8. Multiple endocrine neoplasia
    ii. Acquired
      1. Senile or idiopathic atrophy of lacrimal gland
      2. Associated with systemic illness
        a. Hematopoietic disorders
        b. HIV/AIDS
        c. Graft-versus-host disease
        d. Malignant lymphoma
        e. Lymphosarcoma
        f. Thrombocytopenic purpura
        g. Lymphoid leukemia
        h. Hemolytic anemia
        i. Hypergammaglobulinemia
        j. Waldenström's macroglobulinemia
        k. Chronic hepatitis
        l. Primary biliary cirrhosis
        m. Felty's syndrome
      3. Endocrine dysfunction
        a. Hashimoto's disease
        b. Menopause
      4. Renal disorders
        a. Renal tubular acidosis
        b. Diabetes insipidus
    iii. Obstructive (cicatricial conjunctivitis)
      1. Stevens–Johnson syndrome
      2. Epidermolysis bullosa
      3. Chemical/radiation burns
      4. Ocular cicatricial pemphigoid
      5. Trachoma
      6. Acne rosacea
      7. Chlamydia
      8. Diphtheritic keratoconjunctivitis
      9. Congenital syphilis
      10. Dermatitis herpetiformis
      11. Epidemic keratoconjunctivitis
      12. Syphilis (congenital and acquired)
      13. Exfoliative dermatitis
      14. Impetigo
      15. Scleroderma
      16. Vaccinia
      17. Reiter's syndrome
      18. Linear IgA
      19. Medications
      20. Infiltrative lesions of lacrimal gland
        a. Sarcoidosis
        b. Lymphoma
        c. Hemochromatosis
        d. Amyloidosis
      21. Neuroparalytic
        a. Cranial nerve VII and geniculate ganglion
        b. Greater superficial petrosal nerve
        c. Sphenopalatine ganglion and lacrimal branch
        d. Cranial nerve V and gasserian ganglion
      22. Nutritional/debilitating disorders
        a. Typhus
        b. Cholera
        c. Starvation
        d. Ascorbic acid and vitamin B_{12} deficiency
      23. Postsurgical: partial or total dacryoadenectomies
      24. Medications
        a. Antimuscarinics
        b. Antihistamines
        c. Beta blockers
        d. Phenothiazines
        e. Psychotropics
2. Increased evaporative loss
  a. Exposure
    i. Facial nerve (Bell's) palsy
    ii. Ectropion
    iii. Decreased blink
      1. Altered mental status
      2. Progressive supranuclear palsy
    iv. Proptosis (thyroid eye disease)
    v. Postsurgical (blepharoplasty)
    vi. Arid, warmer climates
    vii. Ptosis
  b. Mucin tear abnormalities
    i. Vitamin A deficiency
      1. Malnutrition
      2. Digestive tract disorders
        a. Colitis
        b. Cystic fibrosis, pancreatitis
        c. Enteritis
      3. Hookworm disease
      4. Chronic cirrhosis
      5. Malaria
      6. Pregnancy
      7. Pulmonary tuberculosis
      8. Thyroid gland disorder
    ii. Cicatricial conjunctivitis (see above listing)
  c. Lipid tear abnormalities
    i. Anterior blepharitis
    ii. Meibomian gland dysfunction
    iii. Acne rosacea
  d. Contact lens related

Advanced age is also a risk factor for dry eyes, as natural hormonal changes and advancing lacrimal dysfunction can affect tear production.[15]

The Examination

External examination

When examining a patient with burning or itching eyes, it is essential to start by stepping away from the slit lamp microscope. Dermatologic nasal telangiectasias, rhinophyma and inflamed posterior lamellae are diagnostic of acne rosacea.[16] The presence of Dennie–Morgan folds or 'allergic shiners' is a classic sign of atopic disease.[17] Proptosis, inferior scleral show, increased palpebral aperture or inflamed muscle insertions are important signs for thyroid eye disease.[18] Masked facies, shuffled gait, and decreased blink rate are seen in patients with Parkinson's syndrome. Many of these conditions can be observed as the patient walks into the examination room.

Lids and lashes

The upper and lower eyelids should be examined for malposition (entropion, ectropion, or ptosis) which could cause exposure keratopathy, tear irregularity or cornea irritation. The unconscious blink effort and rate should be observed at the slit lamp to assess for complete closure and adequate Bell's phenomenon.[19] Chronic exposure and irritation seen in floppy eyelid syndrome can be diagnosed via upper lid double eversion with simple lid elevation.[20] Examining the meibomian glands for inspissation, foamy accumulations, or expression of waxy sebum can help target therapies to improve the lipid tear layer. Inflammation of the posterior lamella can be visualized in dermatologic diseases such as rosacea and localized infections or chalazions. Examination for eyelash misdirection and infestation can be a source of burning or itching. Performing epilation of lashes with cylindrical dandruff has a high incidence of demonstrating *Demodex* mite infestation (Fig. 26.1) when examined under a compound microscope.[21]

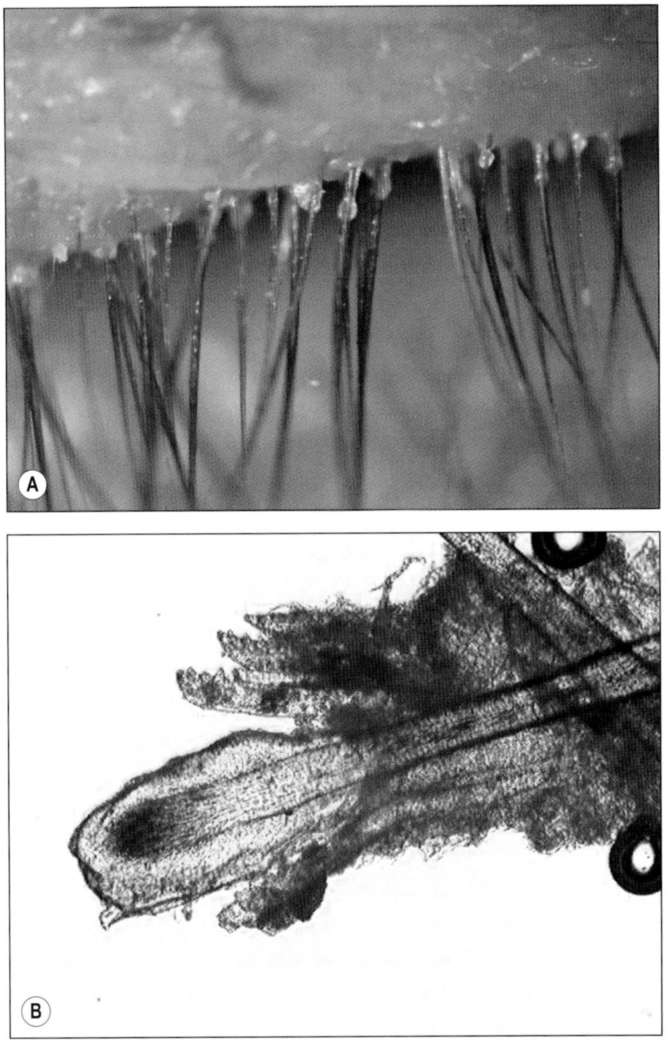

Fig. 26.1 (**A**) Slit lamp photograph of upper eyelid with cylindrical dandruff surrounding lashes. (**B**) Compound microscope demonstrates multiple *Demodex folliculorum* surrounding the lash root and clustered at the hair follicle.

The Ocular Surface

Conjunctiva

Slit lamp examination of the type of conjunctival reaction (papillary or follicular) can assist in developing a differential diagnosis (see Table 26.2). Patients with follicular conjunctivitis, numerous nits (eggs), and active lice infestation of the lashes present with extreme itching (Fig. 26.2). The presence of giant papillary conjunctivitis (GPC) is typically associated with allergic or irritant causes.[22] Seasonally associated Horner-Trantus dots, shield ulcers, and perilimbal pigmentation in the setting of GPC are suggestive of vernal keratoconjunctivitis. Examining the conjunctival fornix for the presence of inflammation, foreshortening, symblepharon, or membranes can reveal systemic immune-mediated cicatrizing illnesses such as ocular cicatricial pemphigoid, linear IgA deficiency, or Stevens–Johnson syndrome. Varying stages of bulbar conjunctival hyperemia can be associated with systemic graft-versus-host disease in bone marrow transplant patients. Common conjunctival staining (rose Bengal, fluorescein, or lissamine green) patterns can be helpful when searching for a cause of burning or itching. Nasal conjunctival vital dye staining can suggest a mucus fishing behavior. Alternatively, an edematous superior bulbar conjunctiva stains positive with lissamine green, indicating a loss of

Table 26.2 Differential diagnosis of follicular and papillary conjunctivitis

A. Acute follicular conjunctivitis
  1. Inclusion conjunctivitis
  2. Adenoviral conjunctivitis
     a. Pharyngoconjunctival fever
     b. Epidemic keratoconjunctivitis
  3. Newcastle disease
  4. Influenza
  5. Herpes zoster
  6. Herpes simplex

B. Chronic follicular conjunctivitis
  1. Medications/toxins
  2. Inclusion conjunctivitis
  3. *Moraxella*
  4. Folliculosis
  5. Molluscum contagiosum
  6. Lyme disease
  7. Pediculosis (lice)
  8. Cat-scratch fever (Parinaud's oculoglandular syndrome)
  9. Trachoma

C. Papillary conjunctivitis
  1. Bacterial conjunctivitis
  2. Allergic conjunctivitis
     a. Atopic keratoconjunctivitis (GPC)
     b. Vernal keratoconjunctivitis (GPC)
  3. Dacryocystitis
  4. Caniculitis
  5. Superior limbic conjunctivitis
  6. Floppy eyelid syndrome (GPC)
  7. Foreign body/toxin (contact lens) (GPC)
  8. Mucous fishing syndrome
  9. Keratoconjunctivitis sicca
  10. Blepharoconjunctivitis

GPC: Giant papillary conjunctivitis.

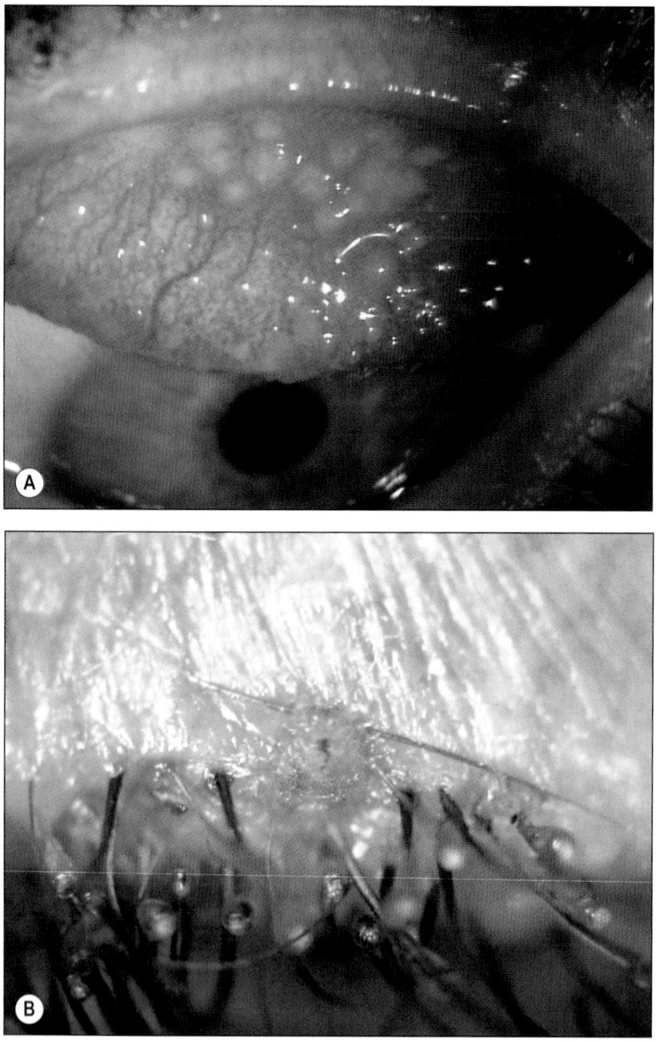

Fig. 26.2 (**A**) Everted upper eyelid demonstrating severe follicular conjunctivitis. (**B**) Note eggs (nits) on lashes and louse with human blood filling its digestive system.

goblet cells typically associated with superior limbic keratoconjunctivitis. Staining the ruggae of redundant conjunctival tissue seen in conjunctivochalasis is an often overlooked diagnosis commonly presenting with symptoms similar to dry eye syndrome. On the contrary, conjunctivochalasis can also obstruct the punctal opening, thereby causing epiphora.[23] Patients with vitamin A deficiency from malabsorption syndromes or specific dietary restriction can present with burning and areas of conjunctival keratinization (Bitot spot), xerosis, and nyctalopia.[24]

Tear film analysis

Investigating the tear film is important when examining a patient with burning or itching eyes. Evaluating the tear meniscus, grading the ocular surface fluorescein stain, establishing a tear film break-up time, and performing a Schirmer's test are all important as clinical investigations in dry eye patients.[25]

Cornea

Slit lamp examination of the ocular surface is pivotal in the work-up of a patient with burning and itching eyes. Extended contact lens wearers may present with limbal neovascularization or central/peripheral cornea edema.[26] Exposure to chronic preservative-based contact lens cleaning solutions and chemical injuries can present with a whirl keratopathy suggestive of limbal stem cell deficiency. Fluorescein staining of discrete white superficial Thygeson granules typically seen in young boys without conjunctival injection is another cause of extreme photophobia and burning. The presence of filaments, dry patches, and punctate erosions indicates keratoconjunctivitis sicca syndrome. Conjunctival or cornea lesions such as pterygia, intraepithelial neoplasia, or squamous cell carcinomas can also cause tear film instability and burning.[27]

While there are many possible causes for burning and itching eyes, the purpose of this chapter is to help clinicians review their approach to these patients. The most important initial step is to listen to each patient's primary symptom and historical events up to presentation. After taking a detailed patient history and reviewing symptoms, narrowing a differential diagnosis can be achieved by performing a focused external and anterior slit lamp examination.

References

1. Bron AJ. Diagnosis of dry eye. *Surv Ophthalmol.* 2001;45(suppl 2):S221–S226.
2. Trocme SD, Sra KK. Spectrum of ocular allergy. *Curr Opin Allergy Clin Immunol.* 2002;2(5):441–445.
3. Rao SK, Basti S, Lin A, et al. The itching, burning eye: diagnostic algorithm and management options. *Comp Ophthalmol Update.* 2006;7(4):1–11.
4. Uchino M, Schaumber DA, Tsubota K, et al. *Ophthalmology.* 2008;115(11):1982–1988.
5. Yee RW, Sperling HG, Hilsenbeck U, et al. Isolation of the ocular surface to treat dysfunctional tear syndrome associated with computer use. *Ocul Surf.* 2007;5(4):308–315.
6. Tsubota K, Yamada M, Urayama K. *Cornea.* 1994;13(3):197–201.
7. Celik L, Kaynak T, Kaynak S, et al. *J Cataract Refract Surg.* 2006;32(10):1775–1776.
8. Bergman MT, Newman BL, Johnson NC. The effect of a diuretic (hydrochlorothiazide) on tear production in humans. *Am J Ophthalmol.* 1985;99:473–475.
9. Bielory L. Ocular toxicity of systemic asthma and allergy treatments. *Curr Allergy Asthma Rep.* 2006;6(4):299–305.
10. Uncu G, Avci R, Develioglu, et al. The effects of different hormone replacement therapy regimens on tear function, intraocular pressure and lens opacity. *Gynecol Endocrinol.* 2006;22(9):501–505.
11. Krenzer KL, Dana MR, Sullivan DA, et al. Effect of androgen deficiency on the human meibomian gland and ocular surface. *J Clin Endocrinol Metab.* 2000;85(12):4874–4882.
12. Erdem U, Ozdegirmenci O, Dagli S. et al. Dry eye in post-menopausal women using hormone replacement therapy. *Maturitas.* 2007;56(3):257–262.
13. Bray LC, Carey PJ, Hamilton PJ, et al. Ocular complications of bone marrow transplantation. *Br J Ophthalmol.* 1991;75(10):611–614.
14. Nichols JJ, Sinnott LT. Tear film, contact lens and patient-related factors associated with contact lens-related dry eye. *Invet Ophthalmol Vis Sci.* 2006;47(4):1319–1328.
15. Damato BE, Allan D, Murray SB, Lee WR. Senile atrophy of the human lacrimal gland: the contribition of chronic inflammatory disease. *Br J Ophthalmol.* 1984;68(9):674–680.
16. Stone DU, Chodosh J. Ocular rosacea: an update on pathogenesis and therapy. *Curr Opin Ophthalmol.* 2004;15(6):499–502.
17. Brenninkmeijer EE, Spuls PI, Bos JD, et al. Clinical differences between atopic and atopiform dermatitis. *J Am Acad Dermatol.* 2008;58(3):407–414.

18. Lim SL, Lim AK, Khir AS, et al. Prevalence, risk factors and clinical features of thyroid-associated ophthalmopathy in multethnic Malaysian patients with Graves' disease. *Thyroid.* 2008;18(12):1297–1301.
19. Doughty MJ, Naase T. Further analysis of the human spontaneous eye blink rate by a cluster analysis-based approach to categorize individuals with 'normal' versus 'frequent' eye blink activity. *Eye Contact Lens.* 2006; 32:294–299.
20. Mastrota KM. Impact of floppy eyelid syndrome in ocular surface and dry eye disease. *Optom Vis Sci.* 2008;85(9):814–816.
21. Kheirkhah A, Casas V, Tseng SC, et al. Corneal manifestations of ocular *Demodex* infestation. *Am J Ophthalmol.* 2007;143(5):743–749.
22. Duke-Elder S, ed. Inflammations of the conjunctiva and associated inflammations of the cornea. In: *Stem of ophthalmology.* vol. VIII. *Diseases of the outer eye.* St. Louis: Mosby; 1961.
23. Wang Y, Dogru M, Tsubota K, et al. The impact of nasal conjunctivochalasis on tear functions and ocular surface findings. *Am J Ophthalmol.* 2007;144(6):930–937.
24. Smtih J, Steinemann TL. Vitamin A deficiency and the eye. *Int Ophthalmol Clin.* 2000;40(4):83–91.
25. Anon. Methodologies to diagnose and monitor dry eye disease: Report of the Diagnostic Methology Subcommittee of the International Dry Eye Workshop. *The Ocular Surface.* 2007;5(2)108–123.
26. Martin R, de Juan V, Martin S, et al. Contact lens-induced corneal peripheral swelling differences with extended wear. *Cornea.* 2008;27(9):976–979.
27. Wilson G, Horner D, Page J, et al. Ocular discomfort from pterygium in men and women. *Eye Contact Lens.* 2008;34(4):201–206.

PART IV

EYE BANKING

Chapter 27

Eye Banking: Structure and Function

Ellen L. Heck, Monty Montoya

Eye Banking: Patient Services and Regulatory Concerns

With over 100 years of successful corneal transplants and over 50 years of history in eye banking with the first formally organized eye bank established in New York in 1944, it may appear there is little new or interesting to discuss about the provision of donor ocular tissues for transplantation. This, however, is not the case. Eye banking is evolving into a physician and patient service delivering more than just corneas for penetrating keratoplasty and sclera for other ocular repair and reinforcement procedures. Endothelial keratoplasty (EK), most commonly referred to as Descemet's stripping endothelial keratoplasty (DSEK) or Descemet's stripping automated endothelial keratoplasty (DSAEK), employ prepared tissues that are now routinely available from multiple eye banks. Femtosecond laser-enabled keratoplasty, in which the femtosecond laser fashions the donor button as well as the recipient site, employs eye banks to provide customized cutting of the donor tissue. Sclera is still utilized for numerous surgeries but glycerol-preserved corneas which meet all transplant requirements except for cell count are also now widely used in repair procedures. New demands and new techniques present new challenges and opportunities, but traditional practices and requirements remain relevant.

Tissue Acquisition

The cornerstone of eye banking and corneal transplantation remains donor tissue availability. This availability is influenced by authorization, screening, recovery, evaluation, and, finally, release. Availability hinges on consent for donation either by first-person consent or, as is more likely, next-of-kin consent at the time of death. Donor registries are also developing throughout the USA, and the impact of these programs is yet to be quantified across the nation. Laws which created these registries generally provide for the first-person intent to donate to be the sole requirement to proceed with donation at the time of death of the registered party. Some states now have several years' history with registry programs, while others are still in early implementation phases. Many programs still make pre-recovery contact with next of kin seeking or confirming permission to proceed. Others contact following recovery for needed medical/social history screening. Development of 'best practices' for dealing with consent concerns and obtaining medical/social history is one major emphasis of the Eye Bank Association of Americas' (EBAA) sponsored 'Cornea Collaborative.' Through this collaborative, eye banks can compare consent conversion, death to retrieval time, and other practices to measure and improve their effectiveness. (With next-of-kin consent, it is important that the individual obtaining the consent verifies the consenter understands the consent process: i.e. what consent covers [e.g. corneas or whole eyes], what is the intended use, what information they will be asked to provide, what testing will be performed, and how the tissue may be directed if not transplantable.) Authorization, as discussed above, can be legally acceptable either by evidence of prior intent or by next-of-kin consent.

Screening

Screening will include two phases. First is the gathering of facts from the hospital related to suitability (i.e. admitting diagnosis or cause of death), medical interventions, possible sepsis, and known or suspected history of communicable disease. Second is the completion of a medical/social history questionnaire with the family. This questionnaire contains inquiries required to comply with FDA Regulation 21 CFR-1271 Donor Eligibility Determination and Good Tissue Banking Practices HCT/Ps. The typical questions in a medical/social screening questionnaire ask about male-to-male sex, sex with prostitutes, drug use, recent piercing or tattoos and the sterility of those processes, and incarceration, to list a few. These questions are precisely designed to elicit history of potential communicable disease, high-risk behaviors for communicable disease, sepsis, and some additional questions that may be specific to tissue suitability (i.e. prior ocular surgery). Once initial screening indicates the potential eligibility of the donation, recovery occurs, followed by a more in-depth screening process. In situations of intent-to-donate legislation, or first-person consent, screening with next of kin or individual or physician knowledgeable of the donor history may not occur until post retrieval. In either circumstance, additional screening parameters will apply.

Retrieval or Recovery

A physical assessment inspection will be performed by the eye bank technician with particular emphasis on any evidence of infection, communicable disease or high-risk behavior.

This includes, but is not limited to:

1. Signs of i.v. drug abuse (nontherapeutic needle marks)
2. Open wounds with drainage or irrathemia
3. Jaundice, hepatomegaly, icterus as possible indications of hepatitis and Kaposi's sarcoma and oral thrush as possible markers for HIV; in both cases serologic testing is also used to identify communicable disease
4. Enlarged lymph nodes
5. Surgical incisions or scars
6. Lesions or growths
7. Tattoos
8. Piercings
9. Abrasions, lacerations or contusions
10. Other observations

Documentation of the physical assessment will often utilize a diagram and reference code as documentation aides as well as defined front-to-back, side-to-side approach to ensure all areas are adequately and consistently reviewed.

Instrumentation for enucleation or excision must be sterile. Instrument kits or retrieval packs should contain sufficient instruments and supplies to perform the surgical removal efficiently with minimal likelihood of contamination or cross-contamination. Many eye banks now utilize sterile, disposable instruments to reduce the possibility of cross-contamination and also to eliminate the requirements for instrument cleaning, packaging, and sterilization. Trephines, scissors, muscle hooks, and speculums are all available as disposable, single-use products.

Tissue Preservation/Storage

Following tissue recovery, corneas are customarily placed in a physiologic media and refrigerated at 2–8°C until needed for transplantation. The acceptable times from death to preservation, as well as death to implantation, may be specified in the eye bank's policy and procedure manuals as approved by the eye bank's medical director. Sclera and corneas may also be preserved for implantation and stored in either glycerol or alcohol. Storage technique will be determined by intended use. Methodology for preservation should be specified in the eye bank's policy and procedures and approved by the bank's medical director.

Donor Eligibility and Tissue Suitability

Donor eligibility is determined by several processes, all designed to ensure the safety of tissue for transplantation. An integral part of this is the medical/social history interview with the donor's next of kin, as previously outlined. In addition, an extensive review of available medical records, medical examiner death investigations and/or autopsies, and any other available medical or social history data pertaining to potential risk factors is performed.

Testing of blood samples from the donor as outlined in FDA Regulation 21 CFR-1271 is also performed. Blood samples must be qualified for testing, utilizing an algorithm for hemodilution by blood products, crystalloid, plasma, and whole blood, when appropriate to insure sample dilution has not occurred which would affect the accuracy of the testing results. Other testing parameters to consider are the type of sample required for specific test (i.e. serum plasma). Whether or not hemolysis is present should be determined and, if so, whether it will affect the test results, usually causing a false-positive reaction. The time of sample collection, sample separation, and sample freezing or refrigeration are also considerations in test sample suitability.

The FDA required testing includes:

- HIV 1–2 antibody
- Hepatitis B & C antibody
- Syphilis testing
- HIV & HCV NAT testing (nucleactic acid DNA/MNA)

Other entities that may require testing include screening for West Nile virus and Chagas' disease. Whenever possible, testing results should be shared among donor retrieval agencies to prevent duplicate testing and discordant results.

Tissue Evaluation

Tissue suitability is an important step in making corneas available for transplant. Following a cursory pen light examination at retrieval to check for trauma, hemorrhage, glass, or other foreign bodies, an evaluation by slit lamp and specular biomicroscopy is performed by a trained technician. Many banks have an EBAA-certified technician responsible for these functions. Medical directors may be consulted to review any unusual or questionable evaluation findings. Final decisions on the acceptance and use of the tissue for transplantation for any intended patient applications rest with the transplanting surgeon. When all screening, testing, and evaluation procedures are complete, acceptable tissue may be distributed for surgery. Records are maintained for all steps in the processes to indicate by whom, where, and when these processes were performed and who was responsible for the tissue release for transplant or its non-use and direction to research or destruction.

Quality Assurance

Federal regulation and peer review accreditation programs have increased the emphasis on eye bank quality assurance programs. While the FDA does not specify the exact components of a bank's quality program, it does state that such a program must be in place.

The added documentation, verification, and record control that has accompanied the expanded emphasis on quality assurance has required most eye banks to direct added resources, both financial and human, to the quality program. One of the most basic yet most important components of a quality program is distribution tracking. There must be traceability from donor to recipient and vice versa. This is essential in the event of any adverse reaction, which may be tissue related or potentially tissue related. Such adverse reactions must be reported to the FDA and the EBAA.

As part of continued quality improvement, the quality program will set and monitor critical eye bank functions for triggers and thresholds that may indicate potential problems. Root cause analysis for problems will be performed and changes implemented as appropriate.

Facilities, Equipment, Instruments, and Supplies

While an eye bank must have a dedicated and secure laboratory environment in which to perform its procedures, these requirements have changed only slightly in the last decade. Likewise, the need for refrigerators, slit lamps, and specular equipment has remained basically unchanged. Instrumentation previously mentioned has moved more toward disposable single-use instruments. Equipment and instrumentation differs to some extent from previous years by now including tissue preparation for endothelial keratoplasty as well as femtosecond laser-assisted keratoplasty.

Distribution

Eye banking continues to develop around the globe with increasing success in developing countries as well as in established programs. With a focus on community-based eye recovery and community-based tissue distribution, there is a rise in sustainable eye banks and eye banking services.

It appears that eye banking, established over a half a century ago, has an ongoing and innovative future in patient care, providing current and new quality services.

Further Reading

Donor eligibility determination. 21 CFR, Food and Drug Administration.
Eye Bank Association of America. *Medical Standard.* Washington, DC, 2002.
Federal Register. Vol. 62, No. 145/Tuesday, July 29, 1997.
Federal Register. March 2002, Guidance for Industry.
Good tissue banking practices HCT/Ps. 21 CFR, Food and Drug Administration.
Rules and regulations human tissue intended for transplant. 21 CFR, Food and Drug Administration.
Validation of procedures for processes of human tissues intended for transplantation. 21 CFR, Food and Drug Administration.

Chapter 28

Medical Standards for Eye Banking

David B. Glasser

The development of modern eye banks, concurrent with intermediate- and long-term preservation techniques, has fundamentally changed the nature of corneal transplant surgery in many areas of the world from that of an urgent procedure, often done after hours and with back-up staff, to that of a regularly scheduled procedure. A body of medical standards and regulations has evolved over the past three decades to keep pace with the increasing sophistication and complexity of eye banking. These regulations are intended to assure the highest possible standards of safety and efficacy for eye tissue intended for human transplantation, while maintaining an adequate donor pool.

The first medical standards in eye or tissue banking were developed by the Eye Bank Association of America (EBAA) in 1979 and were formally adopted in 1980. In the United States, eye banks are also regulated by federal and state laws administered by the Food and Drug Administration (FDA) and state licensing and health departments. The degree of governmental regulation outside of the United States varies from country to country. This chapter will review the standards and regulations applicable to eye banks in the United States, with particular attention to those affecting safety and efficacy of tissue.

Eye Bank Association of America Medical Standards

The EBAA's medical standards are determined by its Medical Advisory Board, a committee composed of transplantation surgeons, eye bankers, and research scientists, with input from an FDA representative.[1] They are based on scientifically obtained information when it is available, and consensus following informed discussion when it is not.[2] The standards are revised twice a year, reviewed and approved by the American Academy of Ophthalmology (AAO), and distributed to EBAA member banks.

The EBAA medical standards are more comprehensive than current federal or state regulations, and cover all aspects of eye banking: consent; recovery of tissue; physical inspection of the donor; preservation of tissue for surgical use, including corneoscleral rim removal and scleral preservation using a laminar flow hood; tissue processing for lamellar or other specific surgical applications; storage of tissue and preservation medium, including quarantine of tissues awaiting determination of surgical suitability; investigation and review of the donor's medical and social history and laboratory evaluation to determine surgical suitability, including autopsy results, next-of-kin and treating physician interviews, and serological testing; evaluation of tissue for surgical use, including slit lamp examination of the whole globe or excised cornea and specular microscopy; distribution, packing, and shipping of tissue for ocular surgery or other uses; and maintenance of donor and recipient case records. Specific standards are discussed in more detail below.

Oversight of eye banking policies and operations by a qualified, corneal fellowship-trained medical director is required. Reporting of adverse reactions, defined as primary graft failure, endophthalmitis, keratitis, corneal dystrophy or degeneration, and transmission of systemic disease has been required since 1990. The EBAA maintains a registry of reported adverse reactions as a means of detecting trends and identifying potential risks. Promulgation of the EBAA medical standards is believed to be a major factor in the remarkably low frequency of adverse reactions associated with ocular tissue transplantation.

Adherence to the medical standards is assured via a time-limited accreditation system. Volunteer inspection teams comprising a corneal surgeon and an eye banker conduct regular, announced site inspections to assess compliance with the medical standards. The findings are presented and eye banks have an opportunity to make corrective actions within specified time limits to address areas of noncompliance. Unannounced inspections may occur when there is evidence of noncompliance with the medical standards that is potentially threatening to eye bank staff or recipient safety. The inspection teams form the EBAA Accreditation Board, which meets semiannually to discuss the results of the site visits and to determine accreditation status. While EBAA membership and accreditation are voluntary, the vast majority of eye banks in North America are EBAA members, and most corneal transplant surgeons use tissue from accredited banks.

Federal and State Regulations

Initially, federal and state regulation of eye, tissue, and organ banks centered on issues of consent and payment. More recent regulations have focused on tissue safety.

The Uniform Anatomical Gift Act (UAGA) of 1968 stated that a signed and witnessed donor card was sufficient legal permission for organ or tissue removal after death. Versions of this law were passed in all 50 states by 1970, substantially simplifying the paperwork necessary to donate body parts for therapeutic, teaching, or research purposes. The UAGA was updated in 1987 and again in 2006 to reflect changes in federal law and regulations as well as changes in donation practices.

In several states, the law allows procurement of organs and tissues with the presumed consent of the next of kin when the family cannot be contacted. The first of these so-called 'medical examiner' or 'legislative consent' laws was passed in Maryland in 1975. They resulted in a significant increase in availability of donor corneas. While presumed consent laws remain controversial in some areas of the United States, in other countries, such as Spain, presumed consent is an accepted policy with a long history of success. The Omnibus Budget Reconciliation Act of 1986 established required request legislation. Hospitals participating in Medicare were required to notify families 'of the option of organ or tissue donation and their option to decline,' again resulting in a substantial increase in donations.[3] Disagreement may arise when next of kin refuse consent despite the presence of a signed donor card. Most recovery agencies defer to the family's wishes in order to avoid controversy and potential legal entanglements. Failure to recover tissue in these cases is not in concert with the wishes of the deceased, though it is unlikely to result in civil or criminal penalties.

The sale or purchase of human tissue was specifically outlawed in 1984 with passage of the National Organ Transplant Act.[4] The Act made it 'unlawful for any person to knowingly acquire, receive, or otherwise transfer any human organ for valuable consideration for use in human transplantation.' Corneas and eyes were included in the definition of human organ. The term 'valuable consideration' was defined to allow reasonable payments for costs associated with recovery, processing, evaluation, and distribution of tissue. A number of bills proposing various means of compensation for both living and cadaveric donors have been introduced in Congress with the intention of increasing solid organ donations, but none has received serious consideration. Pennsylvania currently allows for reimbursement of up to US$300 for food and lodging costs incurred by a donor or a donor's family.

The FDA began a process to formally regulate eye banking practices in the United States in the 1990s. A final rule which spelled out requirements for donor history and physical examination; mandated serological testing for human immunodeficiency virus (HIV) type I and II, hepatitis B, and hepatitis C; and defined regulations pertaining to recalls, inspections, and record retention was adopted as part of the Code of Federal Regulations in 1997. Additional regulations were added in 2004 and 2007, known collectively as the Current Good Tissue Practice (CGTP) rule.[5,6] The stated purpose of the CGTP rule is 'to prevent the introduction, transmission, and spread of communicable disease through the use of human cellular and tissue-based products by helping to insure that: (1) the products do not contain relevant communicable disease agents; (2) they are not contaminated during the manufacturing process; and (3) the function and integrity of the products are not impaired through improper manufacturing.' As noted below, most of these issues are currently addressed by EBAA medical standards.

Table 28.1 Donor eligibility blood tests required by FDA

Human immunodeficiency virus
Antibodies to HIV type 1 (anti-HIV 1)
Nucleic acid test for HIV type 1
Antibodies to HIV type 2 (anti-HIV 2)
Hepatitis B virus
Hepatitis B surface antigen (HBsAg)
Total antibodies to hepatitis B core antigen (anti-HBc, IgG and IgM)
Hepatitis C virus
Antibodies to hepatitis C virus (anti-HCV)
Nucleic acid test for hepatitis C virus
Treponema pallidum
Serologic test for syphilis

Negative screening tests for HIV and hepatitis with test kits approved for cadaveric sera are required prior to release of tissue. Donors with a positive nonspecific serologic test for syphilis may be considered eligible if a specific treponemal test is negative. Nucleic acid testing for West Nile virus has been proposed in an FDA Draft Guidance for Industry[10] and may be required by the time this is in print.

In addition, the FDA has issued 'Guidance for Industry' documents dealing with specific aspects of donor screening and serological testing,[7] the types of test kits that can be used for serological testing of cadaveric blood,[8] and more specific, expanded donor eligibility criteria.[9] Blood tests currently required by the FDA for screening eye donors are listed in Table 28.1. Additional Guidance for Industry recommendations regarding testing for West Nile virus (WNV)[10] and further CGTP requirements[11] were released in draft form in April 2008 and January 2009, respectively. West Nile virus testing may be required by the time this is in print. Although guidance documents are considered nonbinding recommendations, once in final form eye banks must be able to justify any deviations from the recommended practices or face enforcement action from the FDA.

FDA inspectors conduct unannounced site visits. Areas of noncompliance may lead to recalls of tissue and must be addressed within specified time limits. Continued noncompliance can lead to legal action by the FDA. Inspectors' findings are a matter of public record, as are records of tissue recalls. A recall may be ordered by the FDA, or initiated voluntarily by an eye bank, if violations of the Code of Federal Regulations are discovered which indicate a potential risk for transmission of a relevant communicable disease such as HIV or hepatitis. A recall requires notification of the transplanting surgeon of the receipt of positive results for HIV, hepatitis B, or hepatitis C after release of tissue, but it does not require removal of transplanted tissue. Recalls and related market withdrawals are discussed in greater detail below.

Standards Relating to Safety of Tissue

Medical standards relating to the safety and efficacy of tissue are primarily concerned with reducing the risk of disease

Table 28.2 Adverse reactions reported to EBAA, 1991–2007

	Corneas (% of total)*
Primary graft failure	928 (0.12%)
Mated cases	13%
Endophthalmitis	268 (0.035%)
Mated cases	16%
Concordant cultures	40%
Keratitis	88 (0.012%)
Mated cases	9%
Corneal dystrophy or degeneration	25 (0.003%)
Mated cases	32%
Systemic disease	0 (0%)

* *755213 corneas distributed for transplantation by EBAA member banks.*

transmission and insuring that the transplanted tissue is of adequate optical and mechanical integrity for its intended use. The EBAA adverse reaction registry has been tracking reported cases of disease transmission and primary graft failure since 1991 (Table 28.2). Ophthalmic disorders that can be conveyed via corneal transplantation include corneal dystrophies and degenerations, microbial keratitis, and endophthalmitis. Systemic viral infections and prion disease also have the potential for transmission via corneal grafting.

Dystrophies and degenerations

Most corneal dystrophies and degenerations can be easily detected in donor corneas via slit lamp examination of the cornea and specular microscopic examination of the corneal endothelium, both of which are required by EBAA medical standards. Exclusionary criteria include 'congenital or acquired disorders of the eye that would preclude a successful outcome for the intended use, e.g. a central donor corneal scar for an intended penetrating keratoplasty, keratoconus, and keratoglobus,' and 'pterygia or other superficial disorders of the conjunctival or corneal surface involving the central optical area of the corneal button' (EBAA Medical Standard D1.120).[1] It may be difficult to detect subtle signs of keratoconus or anterior basement membrane dystrophy in a donor. However, there have been only 25 cases of transmission of corneal dystrophy or degeneration reported to the EBAA adverse reaction registry since its inception in 1991, a period during which more than 750000 corneas were provided for transplantation (see Table 28.2).

Endophthalmitis and microbial keratitis

The issue of transmission of microbial keratitis or endophthalmitis is more complex. EBAA medical standards exclude tissue from donors with active bacterial, viral, or fungal septicemia; bacterial or fungal endocarditis; or ocular or intraocular inflammation (EBAA Medical Standard D1.120).[1] However, the ocular surface is not sterile. After death, there is a gradual increase in the number and variety of bacteria that can be cultured.[12] Eventually, surface colonization of the donor eye will be followed by bacterial penetration of the epithelium and invasion of the corneal stroma. Short of a visible infiltrate, there are no reliable signs indicating when this has occurred. Lowering the temperature of the ocular surface by refrigerating the body or placing bags of wet ice over the closed lids reduces metabolic demands, prolongs epithelial integrity, and decreases the replication rate of bacteria. There are inadequate scientific data to formulate specific standards relating to death-to-preservation protocols. However, individual eye banks are required to set their own standards for maximum death-to-preservation intervals and to implement procedures for eye maintenance prior to retrieval of tissue (EBAA Medical Standards D1.500 and D1.600). In addition, aseptic technique is stressed throughout the medical standards. To reduce the risk of cross-contamination, corneal excision and other open container tissue processing must be performed under a laminar flow hood meeting ISO Class 5 standards, in an accredited operating room, or in an environment documented to be as free of microbial contaminants as the typical operating room in which corneal transplants are performed (EBAA Medical Standard E1.200). Modern studies report a frequency of bacterial contamination of donor eyes ranging from 5.3% to 19.4%.[12–16] Because corneal tissue is not sterile, when an ocular infection develops in the recipient of a corneal graft, the donor tissue is suspect as a potential source of the pathogen.

The frequency of infectious keratitis following corneal grafting is 4.0% to 4.9% in the United States.[17,18] The vast majority of cases are acquired some time after surgery, and are not related to contamination of donor tissue. Predisposing factors include epithelial defects, exposed sutures, contact lens wear, other ocular surface disorders, trichiasis and other lid disorders, and immune suppression. There have been 88 cases of infectious keratitis reported to the EBAA adverse reaction registry since 1991 (see Table 28.2). Donor tissue was believed to be the source of the pathogen due to the occurrence of infection in an otherwise uninflamed recipient during the immediate postoperative period. In eight of these cases (9% of the total), an infection with the same organism developed in the recipient of the mate cornea. The remainder of the recipients of mate corneas were disease free.

The reported frequency of endophthalmitis after corneal transplantation in several large series ranges from 0.1% to 0.77%.[12–15,19–24] While some of these cases occur long after surgery, and are related to suture manipulations or loss of wound integrity, most occur within a few days or weeks after surgery. The most common organisms isolated in 268 cases of endophthalmitis reported to the EBAA adverse reaction registry were *Streptococcus/Enterococcus* species (40%), followed by fungi (20%), no growth (16%), and *Staphylococcus* species (9%). *Staphylococcus* and *Streptococcus* species are also the most common organisms found in positive donor rim cultures.[13] In 40% of cases reported to the EBAA, the same species was cultured from the donor corneal rim and the recipient's vitreous (see Table 28.2). This rate of species concordance strongly suggests that some of these cases arise from organisms present in or on the donor tissue. However, staphylococcal and streptococcal species are frequently found on the skin, on the ocular surface, and in the upper respiratory tract of recipients. Therefore, identical culture results between donor tissue or storage media and the recipient's vitreous do not necessarily indicate that the donor tissue was the source of the pathogen, particularly when the pathogen is part of the normal flora. A study employing DNA hybridization techniques found that 14 out of 17 (82%) cases of endophthalmitis after intraocular surgery arose from the patient's normal flora.[25] Two of these occurred after penetrating keratoplasty, and in both cases the organisms isolated from the recipient's vitreous were identical to those isolated from the recipient's conjunctiva and nostrils.

Eye banks in the United States are not required to culture donor corneas. In the past, eye banks were required by EBAA standards to recommend that surgeons culture donor material at the time of transplantation. This requirement was rescinded following the publication of two studies indicating a poor correlation between the results of donor cultures and the organisms responsible for endophthalmitis. Everts et al.[14] retrospectively reviewed clinical and culture results in 774 cases of corneal transplantation. Forty-one (5.3%) corneoscleral rim cultures yielded microorganisms, mostly coagulase-negative staphylococci. Two patients developed endophthalmitis within 3 months after transplantation. One was due to *Staphylococcus aureus*; the other was due to *Pseudomonas aeruginosa*. Both donors had negative corneoscleral rim cultures and neither patient's infection was temporally related to the transplant procedure. Everts et al. concluded that donor corneoscleral rim cultures were unreliable predictors of endophthalmitis, and that the discrepancy between the results of corneoscleral rim cultures and subsequent endophthalmitis rendered cultures invalid as a quality assurance procedure. Wiffen et al.[13] retrospectively reviewed clinical and culture results in 1083 consecutive corneal transplants. Corneoscleral rim cultures were positive in 19.4% of the donors, none of which went on to produce endophthalmitis. Donor cultures were negative in the three cases in which endophthalmitis did occur. Wiffen et al. concluded that routine donor corneal rim cultures had no predictive value for infectious complications of penetrating keratoplasty. In contrast, Kloess et al.[15] found three out of four cases of endophthalmitis with concordant donor/recipient cultures in 1010 consecutive keratoplasties, and Cameron et al.[24] found six out of six cases with concordant cultures in 3000 consecutive keratoplasties, but DNA typing was not performed in these studies. Because of the devastating nature of endophthalmitis and the high rate of concordant cultures in their series, these authors advocate culturing the donor corneoscleral rim and/or preservation media at the time of surgery. They point out that positive donor cultures should produce a high level of suspicion for endophthalmitis in cases that demonstrate unexpected or increasing inflammation after surgery, and may give an early indication of the pathogen. While broad-spectrum antibiotic coverage is typically initiated, when a fungus is isolated from the donor material an antifungal regimen is instituted.

Rabies

The first case of rabies transmission via corneal transplant occurred in the United States in 1978.[26,27] Subsequent cases were reported in France, Thailand, India, and Iran.[28–31] All eight recipients died from rabies encephalitis. In one additional case in France, the transplant surgeon was notified one day after surgery that the donor had died from rabies. The recipient was placed on a regimen of interferon, human rabies immunoglobulin, and anti-rabies vaccine, and never developed signs or symptoms of the disease.[32] Most of these cases occurred before it was recognized that rabies could be transmitted via corneal grafting. In each case, the donor had clear signs of encephalitis. Every one of them would have been excluded by current standards precluding the use of tissue from donors with rabies, death from unknown cause, neurological disease of unknown etiology, active viral encephalitis, encephalitis of unknown origin, or progressive encephalopathy (EBAA Medical Standard D1.120). No cases of rabies transmission via corneal grafting have been reported in the United States since 1979.

Hepatitis B

Transmission of hepatitis B virus (HBV) has been documented in two recipients of corneas from two separate donors.[33] Recipients of one cornea from each donor developed clinical and serologic evidence of HBV infection 2 months and 14 weeks after penetrating keratoplasty. The recipient of the fellow cornea from one donor died from a cerebrovascular accident 4 months after surgery without undergoing serologic testing. The recipient of the fellow cornea from the other donor never developed clinical characteristics of hepatitis but tested positive for prior exposure to HBV 2 years after penetrating keratoplasty.

These cases occurred in 1984 and 1985, and were first reported in 1988, before screening for HBV was required or considered the standard of care. The report led the EBAA to require a negative screening test for hepatitis B surface antigen (HBsAg) prior to release of tissue for surgery (EBAA Medical Standards G1.220, G1.240). Since then, there have been no cases of hepatitis B transmission. In addition, the required physical examination and review of the donor's history must specifically seek evidence of hepatitis (EBAA Medical Standards D1.110, D1.120).

HBsAg is usually detectable by enzyme-linked immunosorbent assay (ELISA) or radioimmune assay (RIA) within 2–3 weeks after exposure, approximately 2–4 weeks before elevation of liver enzymes, and 3–5 weeks before onset of symptoms or jaundice. It is the serologic hallmark of HBV infection, and typically disappears within 12 weeks as the patient recovers. Presence of HBsAg beyond 13 weeks is associated with an increased likelihood of chronic carrier status and chronic liver disease. Persistence of HBsAg beyond 6 months defines carrier status. The test kits used for donor screening must be approved by the FDA for use with cadaveric serum.[8] Some noninfectious donors test positive for HBsAg. These false-positive test results are often caused by a

Table 28.3 Interpretation of hepatitis B virus (HBV) serology

HBsAG	Anti-HBc	Anti-HBs	Interpretation
+	+/–	+/–	Infectious
–	+	–	Possibly infectious
–	+	+	Noninfectious (prior infection, immune)
–	–	+	Noninfectious (vaccine-type response)

HBsAg: HBV surface antigen.
Anti-HBc: antibody to HBV core antigen.
Anti-HBs: antibody to HBV surface antigen.

hemolyzed specimen. The EBAA recognizes that these donors with false-positive screening tests can be identified with neutralization assays or confirmatory tests. However, the FDA does not accept the validity of these confirmatory tests for release of tissue, since there is a small risk that a negative confirmatory test could be incorrect.

Donor testing for total antibody to HBV core antigen (anti-HBc, IgG and IgM) is also required. IgM-specific anti-HBc appears with the onset of liver enzyme abnormalities, about 2 months after exposure, and is a marker for ongoing viral replication. It declines whether the disease resolves or becomes chronic, so its absence is no guarantee that the donor is noninfectious. IgG-specific anti-HBc often remains detectable for life, even after resolution of disease. In the clinical setting, a positive anti-HBc is considered a marker for recovery from the disease if the HBsAg is negative and antibodies to hepatitis B surface antigen (anti-HBs) are present. These individuals are not considered infectious (Table 28.3). Even if the anti-HBs is negative, the risk of transmission is probably low, given the presence of a negative HBsAg, the avascular nature of the cornea, the typically hematogenous spread of HBV, and the paucity of reports of transmission prior to the onset of HBV screening. If the donor is a chronic carrier of HBV, a negative hepatitis B e antigen (HBeAg) is associated with a very low risk of transmission, probably less than 1%.[34] A statistical analysis concluded that adding anti-HBc testing to the regimen of HBsAg testing, physical examination of the donor, and medical history screening does not add significantly to the safety of the cornea donor pool.[35] For this reason, the EBAA medical standards do not list anti-HBc as a requirement, and the EBAA has advocated for the ability to qualify an anti-Hbc-positive donor as eligible if HBsAg is negative and anti-HBs is positive. Nevertheless, there is a remote possibility that these donors could harbor infectious virions, and the requirement to disqualify any donor with positive hepatitis B surface or core antigen serology remains.

Hepatitis C

Systemic hepatitis C virus (HCV) infection has never been reported to be transmitted via transplantation of ocular tissues. Polymerase chain reaction (PCR) assays indicate that only 20–26% of seropositive cornea donors have viral RNA in their serum, and initial attempts to detect viral RNA in the cornea were unsuccessful.[36,37] Subsequent efforts have isolated HCV RNA in 24% of corneas obtained from seropositive donors.[38] The risk of contracting hepatitis C after exposure to HCV-positive blood is 1.8% after a percutaneous exposure such as a needle stick, and is considered rare after a mucous membrane exposure.[34] Six recipients of corneas from three HCV-seropositive donors, at least two of whom had viral RNA in their serum, did not seroconvert after surgery.[39] Because of the potential for serious sequelae of hepatitis C infection, negative screening tests for antibodies to HCV and HCV nucleic acid are required prior to release of tissue for surgical use.[9] The antibody tests are limited by a small but significant false-positive rate, and a seronegative window between exposure and seroconversion that may range from 70 to 82 days. Nucleic acid testing (NAT) shortens the seronegative window to 7–11 days, but does not eliminate the loss of donors due to false positives. Given the potential for a prolonged seroconversion window prior to the requirement for NAT in 2007, there have probably been a number of seronegative cornea donors with HCV over the years. Nevertheless, there have been no reported cases of systemic disease transmission.

HIV I and II

HIV has never been reported to be transmitted via transplantation of ocular tissues. Despite the documentation of HIV I in tears[40] and donor corneal tissue,[41–45] the potential for transmission via corneal grafting is probably very low. The incidence of seroconversion after exposure to HIV-positive blood is 0.3% after a percutaneous exposure, and 0.09% after mucous membrane exposure. The risk of seroconversion after exposure to other tissues or fluids, while not quantified, is felt to be considerably lower.[34] There have been nine patients reported in the literature who have received corneas from donors with HIV, and none of them seroconverted or became ill.[46–48]

Screening for HIV I and II antibodies and NAT for HIV 1 is required prior to release of ocular tissue for surgical use.[9] In addition, physical examination of the donor for signs of acquired immunodeficiency syndrome (AIDS) and review of the medical and social history with specific attention to high-risk behavioral criteria are required (EBAA Medical Standards D1.000 and D1.120). Third-generation ELISA tests utilizing sandwich technology to test for both IgG and IgM antibodies to HIV I and II are currently being used. They have a high degree of sensitivity and specificity, and an interval between exposure and seroconversion that typically ranges from 12 to 22 days. NAT shortens the seronegative window to 7–11 days.

Other infectious agents

Human T-lymphotropic virus (HTLV)-I is the cause of an adult-onset T-cell leukemia endemic in Japan, the Caribbean, Melanesia, South America, Iran, and parts of Africa. HTLV-I also causes a slowly progressive myelopathy known in Japan as HTLV-I-associated myelopathy (HAM) and in the Caribbean as tropical spastic paraparesis (TSP), or HAM/TSP. The latent period for leukemia is years to decades, and 2–4 years for HAM/TSP. Routes of transmission include blood transfusion, sexual contact, and breast milk. The prevalence of HTLV-I infection in the United States is estimated at 0.025%.[49] There is no clear association between HTLV-II and human disease. Neither virus has been reported to be transmitted via transplantation of ocular tissues, and testing is not required. However, surgical use of tissue from donors with HTLV-I or HTLV-II infection is precluded (EBAA Medical Standards D1.120, G1.260). OPOs often test for HTLV, so an eye bank could receive notice of donor seropositivity after release of tissue. In such a case, a market withdrawal (see below) would be warranted.

Syphilis has never been transmitted via corneal transplant. Syphilis is thought to be a marker for blood donors at increased risk of HIV infection. Partly for this reason, serologic screening for syphilis used to be required by the EBAA medical standards. Subsequent studies showed a poor correlation between reactive syphilis serology and HIV testing among potential corneal donors.[50] In addition, *Treponema pallidum* could not be transmitted to rabbits via intradermal injection of infected corneal tissue or live organisms after storage in Optisol for 24 hours.[51] This rapid loss of *T. pallidum* infectivity under typical corneal storage conditions makes transmission of syphilis via corneal transplantation extremely unlikely. Based on this information, the EBAA requirement for serologic screening for syphilis was eliminated. Tissue from donors who have had or who have been treated for active syphilis or gonorrhea within the past 12 months are excluded from surgical use (EBAA Medical Standard D.120). However, FDA regulations now require serologic screening for syphilis. Donors with positive nonspecific screening tests may be eligible if they subsequently test negative with a specific treponemal test such as the FTA-Abs or TPI.

No donor screening is currently mandated for cytomegalovirus (CMV), and CMV infection is not a contraindication for surgical use of ocular tissue. CMV infection is common in the United States, with 50–100% of adults demonstrating antibody indicative of prior infection. Most immunocompetent individuals who are infected remain asymptomatic, although they may develop anterior uveitis[52] or a latent infection, which can reactivate or transmit the disease. In contrast, an immunocompromised host is likely to develop clinical disease. Manifestations may include fever, CMV mononucleosis syndrome, retinitis, pneumonitis, hepatitis, encephalitis, disseminated infection, or death. Donor-to-host transmission of CMV is a major risk for immune-suppressed recipients of major organ transplants, so CMV testing of organ donors is routine.[53] There have been no documented reports of symptomatic CMV infection after transplantation of ocular tissues, probably because of the low likelihood of transmission and the immunocompetence of most recipients. In a study of anti-CMV IgG antibodies, 8% of seronegative recipients who received a graft from a seropositive donor seroconverted.[54] In the same study, 9% of seronegative recipients who received a graft from a seronegative donor seroconverted. None of the patients who seroconverted demonstrated signs of clinical disease. Although the sample sizes were small and CMV serology is not always reliable, the authors concluded that transplantation of a corneal graft from a CMV-positive donor does not place the recipient at increased risk of developing CMV infection. CMV has never been documented in the central corneal tissue of immunocompetent patients.[55] However, it has been found in tears and lymphocytes, which may be present in the cornea. CMV also has been identified in the cornea and aqueous humor of patients with AIDS.[56,57] It has been isolated from a failed graft in a case of polymicrobial infection in an immunosuppressed recipient.[58] The role of CMV in the pathogenesis of the graft failure was unclear. Therefore, there is the possibility, however remote, that CMV might be transferred via corneal transplant. CMV transmission could pose a more serious risk to an immunocompromised host, such as the recipient of a limbal stem cell allograft.[59]

Latent herpes simplex virus (HSV) responsible for episodes of dendritic keratitis and uveitis has classically been thought to reside primarily in the trigeminal ganglion. However, HSV may also maintain a latent state within the cornea,[60] giving rise to the possibility that HSV could be transmitted via corneal transplantation. Corneal transplant recipients have an increased likelihood of developing active HSV keratitis, even in the absence of a prior history of herpetic keratitis. But many patients harbor latent HSV with no prior evidence of clinical infection, and corneal surgery itself is a well-known reactivating stimulus.[61] Further, it appears that the latent HSV present in normal-appearing cornea donor buttons is not typically infectious in nature,[62,63] although there has been at least one report ascribing endothelial failure to presumed donor-to-host transmission of HSV.[64] There is no practical screening test for latent HSV, and none is mandated by EBAA medical standards. However, active herpetic dendritic keratitis can be observed in donor corneas.[65] In these cases, as in all cases with active inflammation, the donor is ineligible (EBAA Medical Standard D1.120).

West Nile virus is a blood-borne pathogen with a mosquito vector and human and avian reservoirs. The disease can be transmitted by transplantation of vascular organs and by blood transfusion, but it has not been reported after ocular tissue transplantation. It produces an encephalitis which can be fatal in approximately 3% of cases, although mortality can be as high as 15% in the elderly. Ocular manifestations, when they occur, appear to be limited to the posterior segment of the eye. Corneal involvement has not been reported.[66] The FDA has proposed draft guidelines requiring nucleic acid testing for WNV.[10]

Prion disease

Creutzfeldt–Jakob disease (CJD) is a transmissible spongiform encephalopathy. It is a uniformly fatal, progressive neurological disorder with a clinical latency period measured in years to decades. CJD is caused by an abnormal prion protein which, on contact, induces a conformational change in central nervous system proteins from normal alpha helices to abnormal beta sheets. The beta sheets link to form long dysfunctional chains, with development of amyloid plaques surrounded by vacuoles and spongiform changes within the brain.

The only confirmed case of transmission of CJD via corneal transplantation occurred in the United States in 1974.[67] The recipient became progressively disabled over 18 months, followed by death 26 months after surgery. This case occurred in an era preceding the institution of eye banking medical standards and arose from tissue that was not procured by an eye bank.

Current EBAA medical standards exclude use of tissue for human transplantation from donors with CJD or a history suggestive of an increased risk of CJD or transmissible encephalitis. These exclusionary criteria include death from unknown cause, neurological disease of unestablished diagnosis, dementia, subacute sclerosing panencephalitis, progressive multifocal leukoencephalopathy, congenital rubella, Reye's syndrome, active viral encephalitis, encephalitis of unknown origin, progressive encephalopathy, rabies, recipients of human pituitary-derived growth hormone during the years from 1963 to 1985, and recipients of nonsynthetic dura mater grafts (EBAA Medical Standard D1.120). The latter two exclusions are based on known cases of CJD transmission via these routes. CJD is rare in the United States, with a prevalence of one in one million. The risk of a corneal donor with CJD appearing in the donor pool prior to screening is 0.045 cases per year.[68] Any donor with an established diagnosis of CJD or dementia due to prion disease should be excluded by the current criteria. However, a donor with latent disease would not be detected by these or any additional screening criteria.

A variant form of CJD (vCJD) developed in the United Kingdom and Europe in the 1980s and 1990s, arising from consumption of beef from animals with bovine spongiform encephalopathy (BSE). Fears of a widespread epidemic have waned as time passed and BSE in the food chain was controlled, though the disease's latent period can be measured in decades. Corneal transplantation continues in the UK and Europe, apparently without incident. There was one notorious report of a donor in the UK with biopsy-proven sporadic CJD that went undetected until after the corneas and sclerae had been transplanted into three recipients. Eight years after the event, none of the recipients was showing signs of iatrogenic CJD.[69]

Despite the extremely low prevalence of CJD (one per million) and vCJD (one known case) in the United States, there has been ongoing concern for the potential introduction of the prion agent into the donor pool. There have been nine reported cases worldwide of CJD in patients who were recipients of corneal transplants since the original 1974 report. None was proven to have been transmitted by corneal transplantation. Eight were classified by the original authors as 'probably' due to the corneal tissue, and one was classified as 'possibly' due to the tissue. However, in seven of the 'probable' cases, CJD was biopsy proven in the recipient but not in the donor. In the other 'probable' case, CJD was biopsy proven in the donor but not in the recipient, and in the 'possible' case there was no biopsy material from either the donor or the recipient. Maddox and coworkers at the Centers for Disease Control reviewed these cases and performed an analysis of US eye banking statistics and age-stratified annual mortality rates from CJD versus all causes other than CJD.[70] The authors concluded that sporadic, coincidental CJD unrelated to donor tissue is expected to occur in one cornea recipient in the United States every 1.5 years. They further concluded that it was unlikely that the one 'possible' and eight 'probable' cases were due to corneal tissue, and that there are additional unrelated, coincidental cases of CJD in cornea recipients that remain unreported.

There is no definitive laboratory test currently available for CJD other than open brain biopsy. Because of the short time frame within which corneal tissue remains viable, brain biopsy is not a practical screening test. Due to the rarity of the disease, additional exclusionary criteria would substantially reduce the size of the donor pool without reducing the risk of transmission.[71] While there have been no proven cases of CJD or vCJD transmission via corneal transplant since the initial report in 1974, an accurate, rapid, and cost-effective test for prion disease would be a welcome addition to the screening regimen for cornea donors.

Malignancies

In the history of corneal transplantation, there have only been two reported cases of donor-transmitted malignancies. The first case was a retinoblastoma, reported in Japan in 1939.[72] The second case, reported in New Zealand in 1994, involved a recipient who developed a poorly differentiated adenocarcinoma of the iris 19 months after receiving a corneal graft from a donor who died from disseminated adenocarcinoma.[73] As a result, a donor eye with retinoblastoma cannot be used for transplantation, nor can any eye with a malignant tumor of the anterior segment or known adenocarcinoma in the eye of primary or metastatic origin (EBAA Medical Standard D1.120). In a long-term retrospective study of 86 grafts from donors with systemic malignancies followed for a mean of 10.5 years, there was no evidence of transfer of the same malignancy to any of the recipients.[74] In a retrospective comparison of 47 consecutive corneas transplanted from donor eyes with choroidal melanomas with a matched cohort followed for a median of 2.3 years, no occurrence of melanoma was found in either group.[75] No tumor transmission was found in a 30–86-month follow-up study of 325 recipients of corneas from 204 donors with malignancies, including a small number of donors with metastatic disease to the eye.[76] Despite the lack of reported cases, concern for transmission of nonsolid tumors such as leukemias and lymphomas remains, and these are listed as exclusionary criteria (EBAA Medical Standard D1.120).

Recalls and Market Withdrawals

Eye banks occasionally receive results from other organizations, such as an OPO or tissue bank, of nonrequired screening tests or results that conflict with the eye bank's initial negative results. If this information indicates that there is a possibility that the donor has a transmissible disease, the tissue should be excluded from human transplantation. Because of the need for rapid placement of corneal tissue, however, the additional information may be received after satisfactory completion of the bank's evaluation and release of tissue. In this case, a recall or market withdrawal is required (EBAA Medical Standard G1.290). If the potential pathogen is hepatitis B, hepatitis C, HIV, or syphilis, the eye bank must issue a recall. The recall itself involves notification of the eye bank's medical director, the EBAA, the FDA, and the transplanting surgeon of the test results. There is no requirement for graft removal.

As eye banks have learned to coordinate testing with their sister organizations, the frequency of these discordant test results has decreased. When a positive antibody to hepatitis B core antigen is received, remaining serum should be tested for antibody to hepatitis B surface antigen (see Table 28.3). If the antibody to surface antigen is positive, it is extremely unlikely that the donor was infectious. The recipient should be tested in any case, and infectious disease or gastroenterology consultation obtained. If any other positive donor test for HIV or hepatitis is received and is confirmed as positive on subsequent neutralization testing, repeat antibody, Western blot, and nucleic acid testing can be performed on any remaining serum. While these clinical tests have not been approved for use on cadaveric sera, they may offer insight into the likelihood that the donor was infectious. In the extremely unlikely event that the donor did in fact harbor HIV or hepatitis, the risk of transmission is still likely to be less than 0.3% for HIV, and less than 2% for hepatitis C. The risk for transmission of hepatitis B is probably higher, with seroconversion occurring in up to 62% of those with a percutaneous exposure to infected blood.[34] The avascular cornea should present a much lower risk, and it is notable that only two cases of transmission were reported in all of the years prior to serologic screening. The recipient should be tested and infectious disease consultation obtained.

Receipt of positive tests for pathogens other than hepatitis B, hepatitis C, HIV, or syphilis do not warrant a recall, but a market withdrawal may be necessary in the case of conflicting results for HTLV or other pathogens. FDA notification is not necessary. The eye bank's medical director, the EBAA, and the transplanting surgeon are notified. Confirmatory testing is performed when possible, and the recipient is appropriately evaluated if the results are confirmed.

In the event of a recall or market withdrawal, the surgeon must decide how to proceed, based on the risk of transmission of disease and the potential consequences. In most cases, additional serology testing will confirm that the donor was not infectious. For cases in which the donor may have been infectious, there is no evidence indicating whether graft removal or postexposure prophylaxis has any effect on the risk of transmission of the pathogens discussed in this chapter.

Primary Graft Failure

Primary graft failure occurs when endothelial dysfunction leads to persistent corneal edema after penetrating keratoplasty. The diagnosis is made when the donor cornea is edematous immediately after surgery and remains edematous, with no other identifiable reason for graft failure. Corneas that deturgesce initially but fail thereafter, regardless of etiology, are not examples of primary graft failure.[77] Causes include pre-existing corneal endothelial abnormalities, damage during recovery or storage, and surgical trauma.[78–80] The frequency of primary graft failure has been reported to be between 0% and 10%, and is currently believed to be about 1%.[79–93] The EBAA adverse reaction registry received 928 reports of primary graft failure from 1991 to 2007 (see Table 28.2). This represents 0.12% of the 755 213 corneas distributed for transplantation during this 17-year period. Primary graft failure in mated cases (both corneas from the same donor) accounted for 13% of the reports. A case-control study identified corneal storage for greater than 7 days as a significant risk factor, but no clearly defined donor or eye banking factor accounted for most cases of primary graft failure.[81] Increased intraoperative cell loss and postoperative graft dislocations associated with the learning curve and increasing popularity of Descemet's stripping automated endothelial keratoplasty (DSAEK) may have led to an increase in primary graft failures reported to the EBAA in 2007, but the reporting was not broken down into separate categories for DSAEK versus penetrating keratoplasty. It appears that improvements in surgical techniques have already reduced intraoperative cell loss and the frequency of graft dislocation after DSAEK.

Preservation methods have changed over the years, from whole globe storage in a moist chamber to storage of corneoscleral rims in dextran-based and chondroitin sulfate-based storage media in the United States. Organ culture is the most commonly used storage medium in Europe. There is some evidence that primary graft failure rates were lower with moist chamber whole globe storage, but this effect is probably due to the shorter storage intervals utilized.[81,85,94] EBAA medical standards require the use of an FDA-approved storage medium and stipulate strict maintenance of temperature of 2–8 degrees Celsius for short- or intermediate-term storage (EBAA Medical Standards C3.200, E1.300). FDA-approved corneal storage media currently available in the United States are Optisol GS (Bausch and Lomb), Eusol-C (Alchimia), and Life 4°C (Numedis).

Advanced donor age has been associated with an increased likelihood of primary graft failure in some studies,[89] but not in others.[95–97] Age was not a significant factor for primary or late graft failure in the Cornea Donor Study, a large, prospective, randomized trial designed specifically to answer this question.[98] Endothelial cell density (ECD) may be a more important factor than donor age, though the two are correlated. Yet neither the Cornea Donor Study nor the Australian Graft Registry reported any correlation between cell density or donor age and long-term graft survival.[99,100] Very young donors would be expected to have a high ECD. However, tissue from donors under the age of 2 years tends to be flaccid and prone to excessive and unpredictable steepening after surgery.[101] Since no relationship has been established between the quality of donor tissue and age, the upper and lower age limit is left to the discretion of the eye bank's medical director (EBAA Medical Standard D1.400). Specular microscopy with determination of ECD is required for corneas destined for transplantation. Cell density is measured after tissue processing (e.g. removal of the cornea-scleral rim, performance of a lamellar cut) has been completed (EBAA Medical Standard F1.300).

Mechanical and Optical Integrity

Medical standards require a check for the crystalline lens during excision of the corneoscleral rim and a slit lamp biomicroscope examination of all corneas prior to release (EBAA Medical Standard F1.200). This should be sufficient to detect and exclude all but the most subtle cases of corneal dystrophy, degeneration, or scarring, as well as eyes that have had previous surgery. Corneas from donors with prior anterior segment surgery may be used if the endothelial cell count meets the eye bank's minimum standards for transplantable tissue. Corneas with a prior history of laser photoablation surgery may be used only for tectonic grafting and posterior lamellar procedures; those with a history of radial keratotomy or lamellar inserts may not be transplanted (EBAA Medical Standard D1.120). Evidence of prior photorefractive keratectomy (PRK), phototherapeutic keratectomy (PTK), and laser assisted in situ keratomileusis (LASIK) may be difficult to detect via slit lamp examination. There have been two cases reported of penetrating keratoplasty using tissue from a donor who had undergone LASIK.[102] The surgeons, unaware of the prior history of LASIK, completed the penetrating keratoplasties without complication. A separation of the corneal lamellae was noted during surgery in one of the cases. Both patients were reported to be doing well at 5.5 months after surgery.

References

1. Eye Bank Association of America Medical Advisory Board. *Medical standards*. Washington, DC: Eye Bank Association of America; November 2008.
2. Farge EJ. Eye banking: 1944 to the present. *Surv Ophthalmol.* 1989;33:260–263.
3. United States Code, Title 42, Chapter 7, Subchapter XI, Part A, Section 1320b-8, 2000.
4. United States Code, Title 42, Chapter 6A, Subchapter II, Part H, Section 274e, 2000.
5. United States Code of Federal Regulations, Title 21, Part 1270, Human Tissue Intended for Transplantation, 2008.
6. United States Code of Federal Regulations, Title 21, Part 1271, Human Cells, Tissues, and Cellular and Tissue-Based Products, 2008.
7. U.S. Department of Health and Human Services, Food and Drug Administration, Center for Biologics Evaluation and Research. Guidance for industry. Screening and testing of donors of human tissue intended for transplantation. July 1997. Retrieved February 8, 2009 from http://www.fda.gov/cber/gdlns/tissue2.txt.
8. U.S. Department of Health and Human Services, Food and Drug Administration, Center for Biologics Evaluation and Research. Guidance for industry. Availability of licensed donor screening tests labeled for use with cadaveric blood specimens. June 2000. Retrieved February 8, 2009 from http://www.fda.gov/cber/gdlns/cadbld.pdf.
9. U.S. Department of Health and Human Services, Food and Drug Administration, Center for Biologics Evaluation and Research. Guidance for industry. Eligibility determination for donors of human cells, tissues, and cellular and tissue-based products (HCT/Ps). August 2007. Retrieved February 8, 2009 from http://www.fda.gov/cber/gdlns/tissdonor.pdf.
10. U.S. Department of Health and Human Services, Food and Drug Administration, Center for Biologics Evaluation and Research. Guidance for industry. Use of nucleic acid tests to reduce the risk of transmission of West Nile Virus from donors of whole blood and blood components intended for transfusion and donors of human cells, tissues, and cellular and tissue-based products (HCT/Ps). Draft guidance. April 2008. Retrieved February 8, 2009 from http://www.fda.gov/cber/gdlns/natwnvhctp.pdf.
11. U.S. Department of Health and Human Services, Food and Drug Administration, Center for Biologics Evaluation and Research. Guidance for industry. Current good tissue practice (CGTP) and additional requirements for manufacturers of human cells, tissues, and cellular and tissue-based products (HCT/Ps). Draft guidance. January 2009. Retrieved February 8, 2009 from http://www.fda.gov/cber/gdlns/tissuehctps.pdf.
12. Pardos GJ, Gallagher MA. Microbial contamination of donor eyes. *Arch Ophthalmol.* 1982;100:1611–1613.
13. Wiffen SJ, Weston BC, Maguire LJ, et al. The value of routine donor corneal rim cultures in penetrating keratoplasty. *Arch Ophthalmol.* 1997;115:719–724.
14. Everts RJ, Fowler WC, Chang DH, et al. Corneoscleral rim cultures. Lack of utility and implications for clinical decision-making and infection prevention in the care of patients undergoing corneal transplantation. *Cornea.* 2001;20:586–589.
15. Kloess PM, Stulting RD, Waring GO 3rd, et al. Bacterial and fungal endophthalmitis after penetrating keratoplasty. *Am J Ophthalmol.* 1993;115:309–316.
16. Farrell PL, Fan JT, Smith RE, et al. Donor cornea bacterial contamination. *Cornea.* 1991;10:381–386.
17. Tuberville AW, Wood TO. Corneal ulcers in corneal transplants. *Curr Eye Res.* 1981;1:479–485.
18. Tavakkoli H, Sugar J. Microbial keratitis following penetrating keratoplasty. *Ophthalmic Surg.* 1994;25:356–360.
19. Guss RB, Koenig S, De La Pena W, et al. Endophthalmitis after penetrating keratoplasty. *Am J Ophthalmol.* 1983;95:651–658.
20. Leveille AS, McMullan FD, Cavanagh HD. Endophthalmitis following penetrating keratoplasty. *Ophthalmology.* 1983;90:38–39.
21. Antonios SR, Cameron JA, Badr IA, et al. Contamination of donor cornea: postpenetrating keratoplasty endophthalmitis. *Cornea.* 1991;10:217–220.
22. Kattan HM, Flynn HW Jr, Pflugfelder SC, et al. Nosocomial endophthalmitis survey. Current incidence of infection after intraocular surgery. *Ophthalmology.* 1991;98:227–238.
23. Aiello LP, Javitt JC, Canner JK. National outcomes of penetrating keratoplasty. Risks of endophthalmitis and retinal detachment. *Arch Ophthalmol.* 1993;111:509–513.
24. Cameron JA, Antonios SR, Cotter JB, et al. Endophthalmitis from contaminated donor corneas following penetrating keratoplasty. *Arch Ophthalmol.* 1991;109:54–59.
25. Speaker MG, Milch FA, Shah MK, et al. Role of external bacterial flora in the pathogenesis of acute postoperative endophthalmitis. *Ophthalmology.* 1991;98:639–649.
26. Centers for Disease Control. Human-to-human transmission of rabies by a corneal transplant – Idaho. *MMWR Morb Mortal Wkly Rep.* 1979;28:109–111.
27. Houff SA, Burton RC, Wilson RW, et al. Human-to-human transmission of rabies virus by corneal transplant. *N Engl J Med.* 1979;300:603–604.
28. Centers for Disease Control. Human-to-human transmission of rabies via corneal transplant – France. *MMWR Morb Mortal Wkly Rep.* 1980;29:25–26.
29. Centers for Disease Control. Human-to-human transmission of rabies via corneal transplant – Thailand. *MMWR Morb Mortal Wkly Rep.* 1981;30:473–474.
30. Gode GR, Bhide NK. Two rabies deaths after corneal grafts from one donor. *Lancet.* 1988;2(8614):791.
31. Javadi MA, Fayaz A, Mirdehghan SA, et al. Transmission of rabies by corneal graft, *Cornea.* 1996;15:431–433.
32. Sureau P, Portnoi D, Rollin P, et al. Prevention of inter-human rabies transmission after corneal graft. *C R Seances Acad Sci III.* 1981;293:689–692.
33. Hoft RH, Pflugfelder SC, Forster RK, et al. Clinical evidence for hepatitis B transmission resulting from corneal transplantation. *Cornea.* 1997;16:132–137.
34. Centers for Disease Control and Prevention. Updated U.S. public health service guidelines for the management of occupational exposures to HBV, HCV, and HIV and recommendations for postexposure prophylaxis. *MMWR.* 2001;50(No. RR-11).
35. Mattern RM, Cavanagh HD. Should antibody to hepatitis B core antigen be tested in routine screening of donor corneas for transplant? *Cornea.* 1997;16:138–145.
36. Laycock KA, Wright TL, Pepose JS. Lack of evidence for hepatitis C virus in corneas of seropositive cadavers. *Am J Ophthalmol.* 1994;117:401–402.
37. Laycock KA, Essary LR, Delaney S, et al. A critical evaluation of hepatitis C testing of cadaveric corneal donors. *Cornea.* 1997;16:146–150.
38. Lee HM, Naor J, Alhindi R, et al. Detection of hepatitis C virus in the corneas of seropositive donors. *Cornea.* 2001;20:37–40.
39. Pereira BJ, Milford EL, Kirkman RL, et al. Low risk of liver disease after tissue transplantation from donors with HCV. *Lancet.* 1993;341:903–904.
40. Fujikawa LS, Salahuddin SZ, Palestine AG, et al. Isolation of human T-lymphotropic virus type III from the tears of a patient with the acquired immunodeficiency syndrome. *Lancet.* 1985;2(8454):529–530.
41. Salahuddin SZ, Palestine AG, Heck E, et al. Isolation of the human T-cell leukemia/lymphotropic virus type III from the cornea. *Am J Ophthalmol.* 1986;101:149–152.
42. Doro S, Navia BA, Kahn A, et al. Confirmation of HTLV-III virus in cornea. *Am J Ophthalmol.* 1986;102:390–391.
43. Heck E, Petty C, Palestine A, et al. ELISA HIV testing and viral culture in the screening of corneal tissue for transplant from medical examiner cases. *Cornea.* 1989;8:77–80.

44. Cantrill HL, Henry K, Jackson B, et al. Recovery of human immunodeficiency virus from ocular tissues in patients with acquired immune deficiency syndrome. *Ophthalmology.* 1988;95:1458–1462.
45. Qavi HB, Green MT, Segall GK, et al. The incidence of HIV-1 and HHV-6 in corneal buttons. *Curr Eye Res.* 1991;10(Suppl):97–103.
46. Simonds RJ, Holmberg SD, Hurwitz RL, et al. Transmission of human immunodeficiency virus type 1 from a seronegative organ and tissue donor. *N Engl J Med.* 1992;326:726–732.
47. Pepose JS, MacRae S, Quinn TC, et al. Serologic markers after the transplantation of corneas from donors infected with human immunodeficiency virus. *Am J Ophthalmol.* 1987;103:798–801.
48. Schwarz A, Hoffmann F, L'age-Stehr J, et al. Human immunodeficiency virus transmission by organ donation. Outcome in cornea and kidney recipients. *Transplantation.* 1987;44:21–24.
49. Williams AE, Fang CT, Slamon DJ, et al. Seroprevalence and epidemiological correlates of HTLV-I infection in U.S. blood donors. *Science.* 1988;240:643–646.
50. Goldberg MA, Laycock KA, Kinard S, et al. Poor correlation between reactive syphilis serology and human immunodeficiency virus testing among potential cornea donors. *Am J Ophthalmol.* 1995;119:1–6.
51. Macsai MS, Norris SJ. OptiSol corneal storage medium and transmission of *Treponema pallidum. Cornea.* 1995;14:595–600.
52. Chee SP, Bacsal K, Jap A, et al. Clincal features of cytomegalovirus anterior uveitis in immunocompetent patients. *Am J Ophthalmol.* 2008;145:834–840.
53. Nankervis GA, Kumar ML. Diseases produced by cytomegaloviruses. *Med Clin North Am.* 1978;62:1021–1035.
54. Holland EJ, Bennett SR, Brannian R, et al. The risk of cytomegalovirus transmission by penetrating keratoplasty. *Am J Ophthalmol.* 1988;105:357–360.
55. Pepose JS. The risk of cytomegalovirus transmission by penetrating keratoplasty. *Am J Ophthalmol.* 1988;106:238–240.
56. Wilhelmus KR, Font RL, Lehmann RP, et al. Cytomegalovirus keratitis in acquired immunodeficiency syndrome. *Arch Ophthalmol.* 1996; 114:869–872.
57. Inoue T, Hayashi K, Omoto T, et al. Corneal infiltration and CMV retinitis in a patient with AIDS. *Cornea.* 1998;17:441–442.
58. Wehrly SR, Manning FJ, Proia AD, et al. Cytomegalovirus keratitis after penetrating keratoplasty. *Cornea.* 1995;14:628–633.
59. Holland EJ, Bennett SR, Brannian R, et al. The risk of cytomegalovirus transmission by penetrating keratoplasty (letter). *Am J Ophthalmol.* 1988;106:239–240.
60. Openshaw H, McNeill JI, Lin XH, et al. Herpes simplex virus DNA in normal corneas: persistence without viral shedding from ganglia. *J Med Virol.* 1995;46:75–80.
61. Remeijer L, Doornenbal P, Geerards AJ, et al. Newly acquired herpes simplex virus keratitis after penetrating keratoplasty. *Ophthalmology.* 1997;104:648–652.
62. Morris DJ, Cleator GM, Klapper PE, et al. Detection of herpes simplex virus DNA in donor cornea culture medium by polymerase chain reaction. *Br J Ophthalmol.* 1996;80:654–657.
63. Garweg JG, Boehnke M. Low rate shedding of HSV-1 DNA, but not of infectious virus from human donor corneae into culture media. *J Med Virol.* 1997;52:320–325.
64. Cleator GM, Klapper PE, Dennett C, et al. Corneal donor infection by herpes simplex virus: herpes simplex virus DNA in donor corneas. *Cornea.* 1994;13:294–304.
65. Neufeld MV, Steinemann TL, Merin LM, et al. Identification of a herpes simplex virus-induced dendrite in an eye-bank donor cornea. *Cornea.* 1999;18:489–492.
66. Chan CK, Limstrom SA, Tarasewicz DG, et al. Ocular features of West Nile virus infection in North America: a study of 14 eyes. *Ophthalmology.* 2006;113:1539–1546.
67. Duffy P, Wolf J, Collins G, et al. Possible person-to-person transmission of Creutzfeldt-Jakob disease (letter). *N Engl J Med.* 1974;290:692–693.
68. Hogan RN, Brown P, Heck E, et al. Risk of prion disease transmission from ocular donor tissue transplantation. *Cornea.* 1999;18:2–11.
69. Tullo AB, Buckley RJ, Kelly T, et al. Transplantation of ocular tissue from a donor with sporadic Creutzfeldt-Jakob disease. *Clin Experiment Ophthalmol.* 2006;34:645–649.
70. Maddox RA, Belay ED, Curns AT, et al. Creutzfeldt-Jakob disease in recipients of corneal transplants. *Cornea.* 2008;27:851–854.
71. Kennedy RH, Hogan RN, Brown P, et al. Eye banking and screening for Creutzfeldt-Jakob disease. *Arch Ophthalmol.* 2001;119:721–726.
72. Hata B. The development of glioma in the eye to which the cornea of a patient, who suffered from glioma, was transplanted. *Nippon Ganka Gakkai Zasshi.* 1939;43:1763–1767.
73. McGeorge AJ, Thompson P, Elliot D, et al. Papillary adenocarcinoma of the iris transmitted by corneal transplantation. Eye Bank Association of America Abstracts. *Cornea.* 1994;13:102.
74. Wagoner MD, Dohlman CH, Albert DM, et al. Corneal donor material selection. *Ophthalmology.* 1981;88:139–145.
75. Harrison DA, Hodge DO, Bourne WM. Outcome of corneal grafting with donor tissue taken from eyes with choroidal melanomas. A retrospective cohort comparison. Eye Bank Association of America Abstracts. *Cornea.* 1995;14:115.
76. Lopez-Navidad A, Soler N, Caballero F, et al. Corneal transplantations from donors with cancer. *Transplantation.* 2007;83:1345–1350.
77. Wilson SE, Kaufman HE. Graft failure after penetrating keratoplasty. *Surv Ophthalmol.* 1990;34:325–356.
78. Chipman ML, Willett P, Basu PK, et al. Donor eyes. A comparison of characteristics and outcomes for eye bank and local tissue. *Cornea.* 1989;8:62–66.
79. Buxton JN, Seedor JA, Perry HD, et al. Donor failure after corneal transplantation surgery. *Cornea.* 1988;7:89–95.
80. Mead MD, Hyman L, Grimson R, et al. Primary graft failure: a case control investigation of a purported cluster. *Cornea.* 1994;13:310–316.
81. Wilhelmus KR, Stulting RD, Sugar J, et al. Primary corneal graft failure. A national reporting system. Medical Advisory Board of the Eye Bank Association of America. *Arch Ophthalmol.* 1995;113:1497–1502.
82. Moore TE Jr, Aronson SB. The corneal graft: a multiple variable analysis of the penetrating keratoplasty. *Am J Ophthalmol.* 1971;72:205–298.
83. Payne JW. New directions in eye banking. *Trans Am Ophthalmol Soc.* 1980;78:983–1026.
84. Stainer GA, Brightbill FS, Calkins B. A comparison of corneal storage in moist chamber and McCarey-Kaufman medium in human keratoplasty. *Ophthalmology.* 1981;88:46–49.
85. Halliday BL, Ritten SA. Effect of donor parameters on primary graft failure and the recovery of acuity after keratoplasty. *Br J Ophthalmol.* 1990;74:7–11.
86. Chipman ML, Slomovic AS, Rootman D, et al. Changing risk for early transplant failure: data from the Ontario Corneal Recipient Registry. *Can J Ophthalmol.* 1993;28:254–258.
87. Stark WJ, Maumenee AE, Kenyon KR. Intermediate-term corneal storage for penetrating keratoplasty. *Am J Ophthalmol.* 1975;79:795–802.
88. Mascarella K, Cavanagh HD. Penetrating keratoplasty using McCarey-Kaufman preserved corneal tissue. *South Med J.* 1979;72:1268–1271.
89. Harbour RC, Stern GA. Variables in McCarey-Kaufman corneal storage. Their effect on corneal graft success. *Ophthalmology.* 1983;90:136–142.
90. Bourne WM. Morphologic and functional evaluation of the endothelium of transplanted human corneas. *Trans Am Ophthalmol Soc.* 1983;81:403–450.
91. Bourne WM. Endothelial cell survival on transplanted human corneas preserved at 4°C in 2.5% chondroitin sulfate for one to 13 days. *Am J Ophthalmol.* 1986;102:382–386.
92. Lass JH, Bourne WM, Musch DC, et al. A randomized, prospective, double-masked clinical trial of Optisol vs. DexSol corneal storage media. *Arch Ophthalmol.* 1992;110:1404–1408.
93. Lindstrom RL, Kaufman HE, Skelnik DL, et al. Optisol corneal storage medium. *Am J Ophthalmol.* 1992;114:345–356.
94. Brightbill FS. Primary corneal graft failure. A national reporting system. *Arch Ophthalmol.* 1995;113:1554–1555.
95. Forster RK, Fine M. Relation of donor age to success in penetrating keratoplasty. *Arch Ophthalmol.* 1971;85:42–47.
96. Jenkins MS, Lempert SL, Brown SI. Significance of donor age in penetrating keratoplasty. *Ann Ophthalmol.* 1979;11:974–976.
97. Abbott RL, Forster RK. Determinants of graft clarity in penetrating keratoplasty. *Arch Ophthalmol.* 1979;97:1071–1075.
98. Cornea Donor Study Investigator Group. The effect of donor age on corneal transplantation outcome: results of the cornea donor study. *Ophthalmology.* 2008;115:620–626.
99. Cornea Donor Study Investigator Group. Donor age and corneal endothelial cell loss five years after successful cornea transplantation: specular microscopy ancillary study results. *Ophthalmology.* 2008; 115:627–632.
100. The Australian Corneal Graft Registry: 1990 to 1992 report. *Aust N Z J Ophthalmol.* 1993;21:1–48.
101. Koenig SB. Myopic shift in refraction following penetrating keratoplasty with pediatric donor tissue. *Am J Ophthalmol.* 1986;101:740–741.
102. Michaeli-Cohen A, Lambert AC, Coloma F, et al. Two cases of a penetrating keratoplasty with tissue from a donor who had undergone LASIK surgery. *Cornea.* 2002;21:111–113.

PART V

THE OCULAR ADNEXA

Chapter 29

Eyelid Disorders: Entropion, Ectropion, Trichiasis, and Distichiasis

Cat N. Burkat, Richard K. Dortzbach

The eyelid structures are crucial to corneal surface integrity and maintenance. Precise eyelid margin apposition to the cornea is essential for tear film distribution and maintenance, and removal of debris. Disruption to this interrelationship can result in significant ocular surface irritation and corneal breakdown. Entropion describes an inward rotation of the tarsus such that the eyelid margin, skin, and lashes directly rub against the globe. Without treatment, entropion can lead to keratoconjunctivitis, corneal abrasion, ulceration, and visual loss.[1] In ectropion, the eyelid margin is everted, or rotated away, from its normal apposition to the globe. Ectropion can lead to chronic epiphora, chronic conjunctivitis, exposure keratitis, corneal scarring, and perforation. Trichiasis refers to the posterior misdirection of eyelashes towards the cornea.

Understanding the pathophysiology of these eyelid disorders requires knowledge of eyelid anatomy. The anterior lamella refers to the skin and orbicularis oculi muscle, followed by the middle lamellar orbital septum. The eyelash follicles and associated glandular appendages are located in the anterior lamella. At the eyelid margin, the posterior limit of the anterior lamella is the gray line, which corresponds to the orbicularis muscle of Riolan. The posterior lamella comprises the tarsus and tarsal conjunctiva, with the mucocutaneous junction posterior to the meibomian gland orifices on the margin.

Eyelid malpositions more frequently involve the lower eyelid. The lower eyelid retractor complex originates as aponeurotic expansions of the inferior rectus.[2] These expansions form the capsulopalpebral head, which divides anteriorly around the inferior oblique muscle and then fuses into Lockwood's ligament in front of the inferior oblique to form the capsulopalpebral fascia. This fascia then inserts into the inferior fornix, the inferior tarsal border, and the preseptal orbicularis muscle and skin to create the lower eyelid crease. The capsulopalpebral fascia also contains the inferior tarsal smooth muscle, which is more diffusely distributed than Müller's muscle and does not insert directly onto tarsus. The orbital septum joins with the capsulopalpebral fascia 4–5 mm below the inferior tarsal border, before inserting onto the inferior tarsus (Fig. 29.1).

Entropion

Congenital entropion

Congenital entropion, although rare, can affect both lower and upper eyelids.[3] Pathophysiology often involves dysgenesis of the tarsus (kinked tarsus) or disinsertion of the lower lid retractors, resulting in inversion of the eyelid margin. Ocular anomalies can also be present. In contrast to epiblepharon, in which a fold of skin and orbicularis oculi muscle pushes the lashes inward towards the globe, this condition does not improve spontaneously.

Involutional entropion

The most common type, involutional entropion typically involves the lower eyelids in elderly patients. Several factors in combination can contribute to involutional entropion.[4–6] Horizontal laxity consists of medial canthal tendon laxity, lateral canthal tendon laxity, and tarsal degeneration. Normally, the medial canthal tendon prevents the inferior punctum from being pulled laterally more than 2–3 mm. Lateral displacement of more than 5 mm may warrant surgical correction of the medial canthal tendon (Fig. 29.2). Lateral canthal tendon tone should not allow the lateral canthus to be pulled medially to the limbus. The snapback test is performed by pulling the eyelid down; when released, the eyelid should return sharply to its former apposition against the globe. Failure to do so indicates tarsal attenuation or lateral canthal tendon laxity. The eyelid distraction test is performed by measuring the distance with a ruler from the globe to the eyelid margin when the eyelid is pulled anteriorly from the globe. Distraction more than 6 mm from the cornea would be considered abnormal (Fig. 29.3).

Disinsertion or attenuation of the retractor complex allows the inferior tarsus to move anteriorly and superiorly, causing the eyelid margin to turn inward. A white line corresponding to the leading edge of the disinserted retractor complex may be seen, separated from the inferior tarsus by a pink band that corresponds to the orbicularis visible

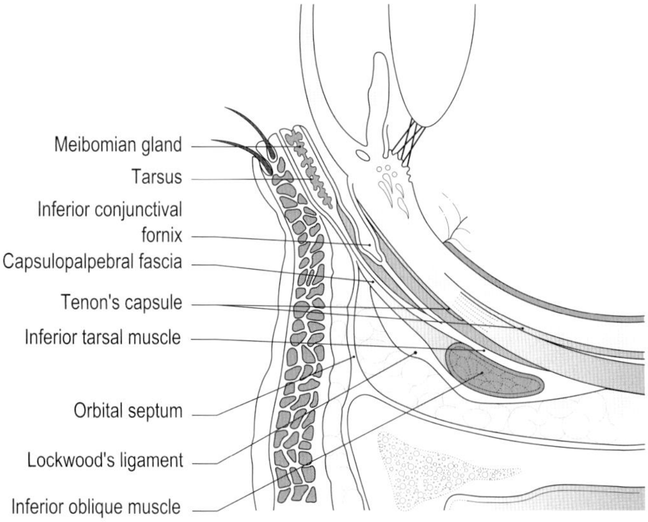

Fig. 29.1 Normal lower lid anatomy in cross-section. (From Lyon DB, Dortzbach RK. Entropion, trichiasis, and distichiasis. In: Dortzbach RK, ed. *Ophthalmic plastic surgery: prevention and management of complications*. New York: Raven Press; 1994.)

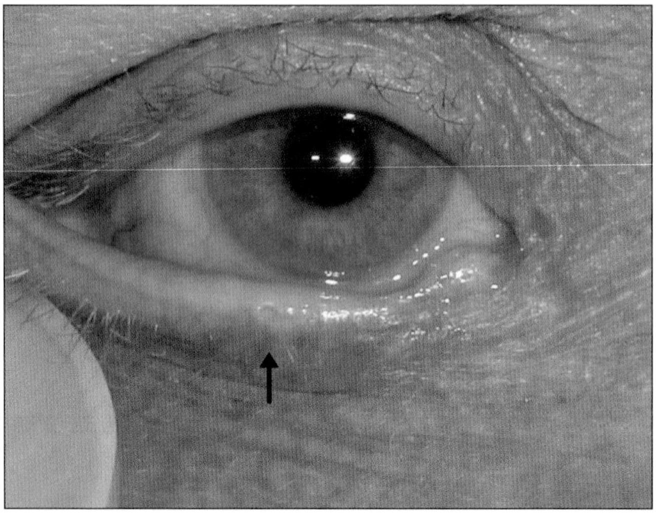

Fig. 29.2 Testing medial canthal tendon tone by distracting the eyelid laterally and measuring the horizontal movement of the punctum.

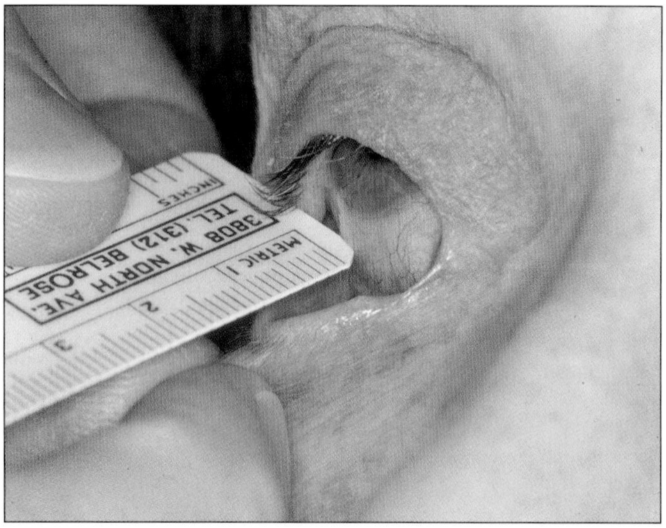

Fig. 29.3 Measuring eyelid distraction away from the globe surface.

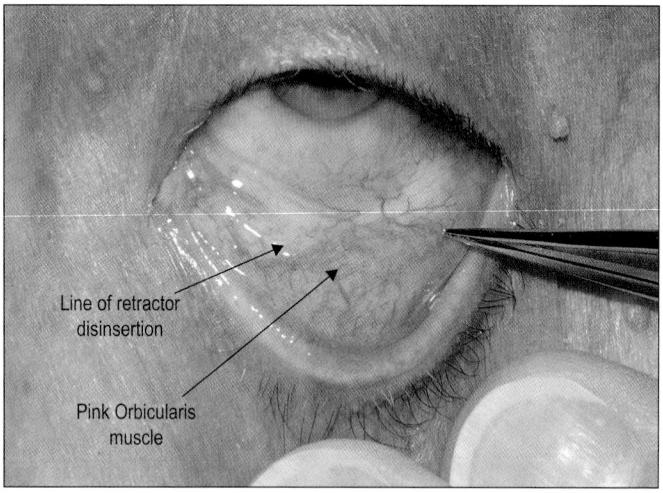

Fig. 29.4 The disinserted inferior retractors are visualized as a white band in the fornix on examination. The pink tissue superior to the leading edge of the retractors is the orbicularis muscle seen through conjunctiva.

through the conjunctiva (Fig. 29.4). Because the capsulopalpebral fascial attachment to the inferior fornix remains intact, the inferior fornix may appear deepened when compared to the normal eye. The affected eyelid may also fail to retract inferiorly during downgaze, in contrast to an intact lid that retracts 3–4 mm in downgaze. It is speculated that resorption of orbital fat may lead to age-related relative enophthalmos and worsened laxity from poor eyelid support.

The previous mechanisms can also cause ectropion. In entropion, a factor that determines whether the unstable lower lid is going to turn inward is the preseptal fibers of the orbicularis muscle overriding the pretarsal fibers. When this occurs, inward pressure is applied to the eyelid margin.

Asians may be more predisposed than Caucasians to involutional entropion due to a more anterior and superior protruding position of orbital fat within the eyelid.[7]

Cicatricial entropion

Contracture of the posterior lamella and subsequent entropion may occur secondary to surgical or trauma-related scarring, chemical burns, and inflammatory conditions such as trachoma, Stevens–Johnson syndrome, ocular cicatricial pemphigoid, acne rosacea, and chronic meibomitis.[8] Any long-standing irritation can induce an added cicatricial component to any type of eyelid malposition. Upper eyelid entropion is typically cicatricial in etiology in contrast to the lower lid, in which involutional entropion is most common.

Acute spastic entropion

Any ocular irritation (e.g. blepharitis, allergies, following cataract or corneal surgery) can induce significant blepharospasm and subsequent entropion. The eyelids are squeezed tightly such that the orbicularis muscle causes inward rotation of the margin.[1] This condition may resolve after several weeks and can affect any age group. In older patients, it may be a manifestation of a latent involutional entropion.

Differential diagnosis

Epiblepharon is a congenital condition that occurs most commonly in Asian patients.[9] The most common presentation is bilateral involvement of the lower eyelids. A thick horizontal fold of eyelid skin and orbicularis is seen overriding the margin, causing the lashes to be pushed backward towards the cornea (Fig. 29.5). In contrast to congenital entropion, the tarsus and posterior margin remain in normal position. The contact of the lashes with the cornea can be present all the time or only in downward gaze. The problem is usually well tolerated, as the lashes in children are fine and soft. However, it should be considered in a child with recurrent ocular irritation or chronic epiphora of unclear etiology.[9]

As the facial bones grow, spontaneous resolution is common, although less often in Asians. Treatment is reserved for cases with significant irritation or a threat to corneal integrity. Similar to the anatomical abnormality in congenital entropion, the anterior insertions of the retractor complex which normally extend through pretarsal orbicularis to insert into the subcutaneous tissues to form the lid crease are absent.[3] This failure to bind skin and orbicularis to the tarsus thus allows them to form the horizontal roll seen clinically. Simple excision of the skin fold and strip of orbicularis muscle is frequently used, but does not directly correct the underlying anatomical defect.[10] Quickert-Rathbun sutures may correct the defect by creating a scar between the skin, muscle, and retractor layers, and creating a lid crease.[3] As many Asians do not normally have a lower lid crease, a rotating suture technique with a skin incision just below the lash line and buried sutures may avoid forming a scar and visible eyelid crease.[11]

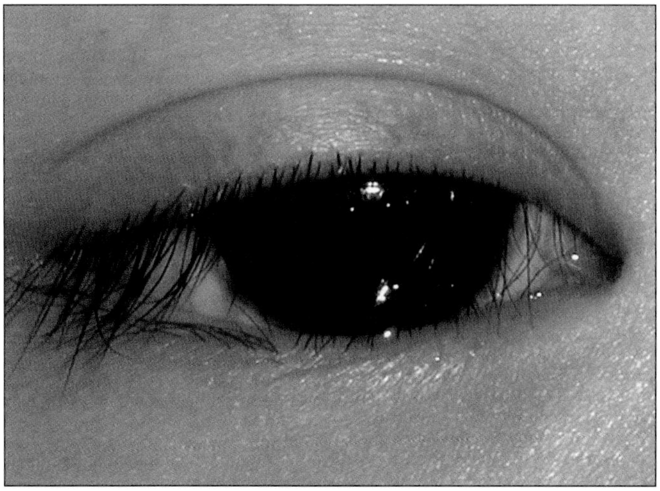

Fig. 29.5 Epiblepharon of medial lower lid with eyelashes oriented vertically and inward towards the cornea.

Medical management

In spastic entropion, conservative management with lubrication, a bandage contact lens, or eyelid taping may break the cycle. Tape is applied near the eyelid margin to pull the margin away from the eye, and horizontally and superiorly to simulate a lateral tarsal strip procedure. Blepharitis and meibomitis require lid hygiene and antibiotic ointment with or without steroid. Acne rosacea responds well to oral doxycycline. Injection of botulinum toxin into the orbicularis muscle can be helpful in treating a spastic entropion. However, injection of botulinum could turn an involutional or spastic entropion into a flaccid ectropion if significant lower lid laxity is also present.

Identifying any irritative triggering factor is important, and care should be taken to trim suture ends on the cornea or conjunctiva after surgery. Eyelid margin sutures can be left long and secured onto the eyelid skin, or cut closely on the knots if absorbable suture is used.

Surgical management

The nonincisional suture technique described by Quickert et al.[3] and modified by Feldstein[12] may be a valuable temporizing measure. One needle of a double-armed 4-0 chromic catgut suture is passed deep into the fornix to secure the dehisced retractors, passes adjacent to the inferior tarsus and exits through the skin at the level of mid-tarsal height. The second needle is passed in the same way 3 mm adjacent to the first. The knot is then tied with enough tension to correct the entropion, without causing ectropion (Fig. 29.6). Three to four sutures can be placed as needed across the eyelid to evert the margin. Resultant subcutaneous inflammatory cicatrix results indirectly in tightening of the retractors to the inferior tarsus, and fibrosis between orbicularis fibers and tarsus that may prevent vertical overriding. This procedure is considered temporary due to high recurrence rates, although one study showed that entropion recurred in 15% with only everting sutures after a mean follow-up of 31 months.[13] Definitive treatment is directed at the specific causes of the entropion.

Congenital entropion

Techniques have included cauterization, everting sutures, skin and muscle excision, blepharotomy, tarsal incision or splitting, and excision of the kinked area or tarsal fracture with reanastomosis of the retractor complex to achieve better margin apposition.[3] Intraoperative findings have suggested dehiscence of normal tarsal–capsulopalpebral fascia attachment, in addition to a lack of cutaneous–capsulopalpebral fascia attachment as in congenital epiblepharon. Thus, definitive repair may include attaching both the retractors to tarsus, and skin to tarsus and retractors, in order to correct the lid malposition and create a normal eyelid crease.[14]

Involutional entropion

The literature is replete with techniques described to correct involutional entropion.[15] Each pathophysiological factor contributing to the entropion can be addressed separately or in combination. Anterior and posterior approaches have

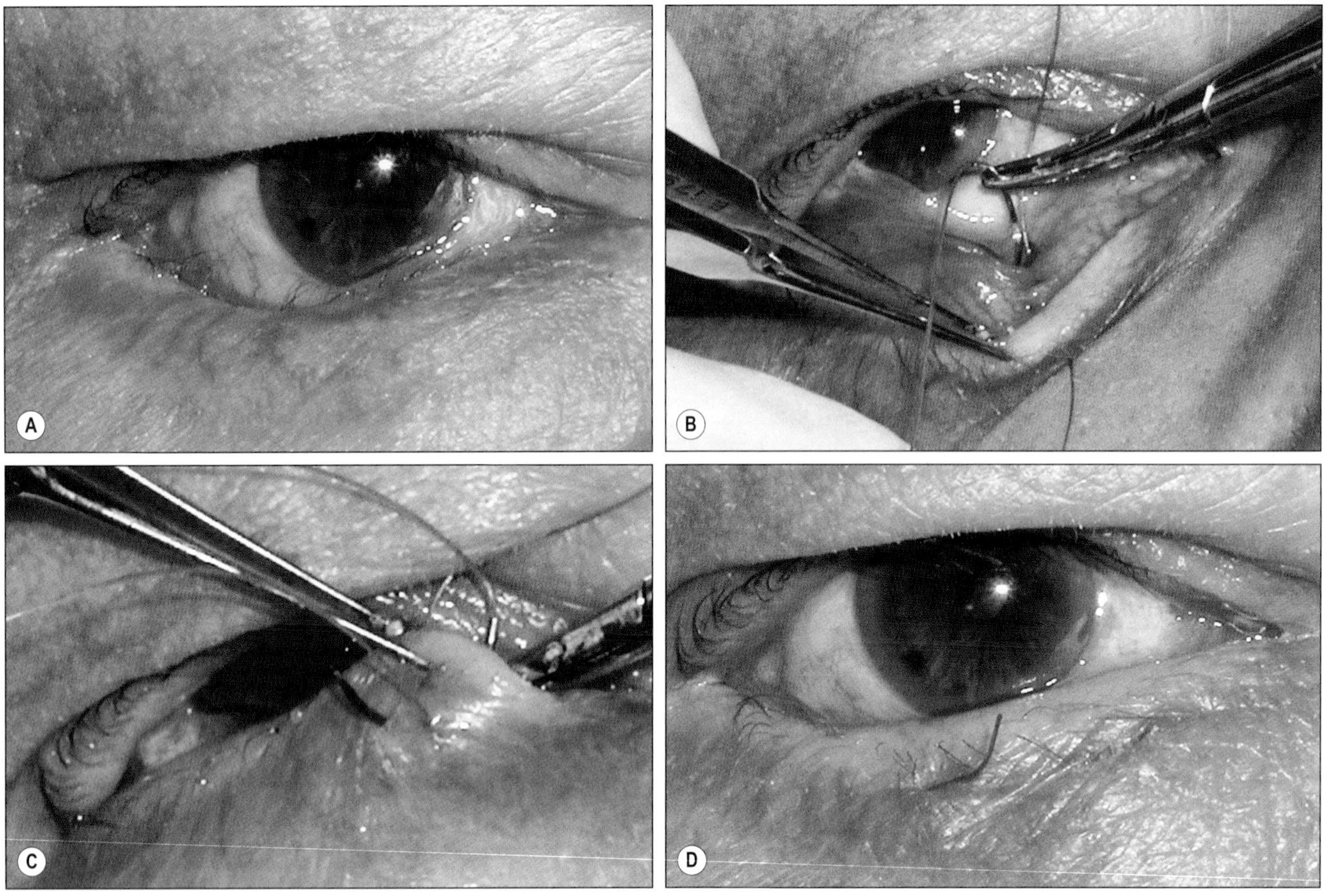

Fig. 29.6 (**A**) Preoperative entropion before placement of Quickert sutures. (**B**) Needle passed deep into fornix to pick up retractors. (**C**) Needle exiting through skin at a level higher than the entry. (**D**) One week after placement of slowly resorbable sutures.

been advocated. The anterior approach has a good success rate, although it involves more tissue dissection.[4,6] The posterior approach avoids a visible scar. Ideally, either approach should address horizontal laxity, disinserted inferior retractors, and orbicularis muscle override.

Medial canthal tendon laxity is repaired first if present.[4] Plication of the anterior crus of the medial canthal tendon can be addressed via a skin incision or a transconjunctival or transcaruncular approach. The medial canthal tendon can also be resuspended with a nonabsorbable horizontal mattress suture (5-0 nylon) to the periosteum of the posterior lacrimal crest to minimize punctal ectropion. Care should be taken to avoid injury to the canaliculi and nasolacrimal sac.

Detached or attenuated lower lid retractors should always be reinserted.[4] In the anterior approach, an infraciliary incision is created and the skin is undermined to the junction of the pretarsal to the preseptal fibers. Dissection then passes through the muscle plane to the orbital septum, which is detached from the tarsus. The detached or attenuated inferior retractors, recognizable by their white color (Fig. 29.7A), are reattached to the inferior tarsal border (Fig. 29.7B) with absorbable or nonabsorbable sutures (e.g. 6-0 Vicryl). It is important to eliminate horizontal laxity in conjunction with retractor repair in order to avoid postoperative ectropion or recurrence.[16,17]

Horizontal laxity is corrected with a lateral tarsal strip procedure.[18,19] A lateral canthotomy is performed and the inferior crus of the lateral canthal tendon lysed. The eyelid is pulled laterally to determine the amount of redundant lid, which is marked on the margin. The eyelid is split into anterior and posterior lamellae up to the mark, and the strip of tarsus denuded of skin, eyelashes, and margin epithelium. The tarsal strip is anchored to the periosteum inside the lateral orbital rim at Whitnall's tubercle using absorbable or nonabsorbable suture (5-0 Vicryl or 5-0 Prolene) (Fig. 29.8). Orbicularis muscle myectomy, performed by excising a narrow horizontal strip of preseptal orbicularis muscle, creates a cicatricial barrier between pretarsal and preseptal orbicularis to prevent orbicularis override postoperatively.

A posterior transconjunctival approach permits all the steps included in the anterior approach and provides a good cosmetic result.[16,20] The radiofrequency unit or cutting monopolar cautery is used to incise the conjunctiva and expose the attenuated retractors at a level 4 mm below the inferior tarsal border. To reduce the overriding orbicularis muscle, a horizontal strip of muscle is excised with the cautery. The retractor complex is reinserted to the inferior tarsal border with absorbable suture, or the sutures may be passed full thickness through the lid to be tied on the skin. Horizontal laxity is repaired similar to the anterior approach.

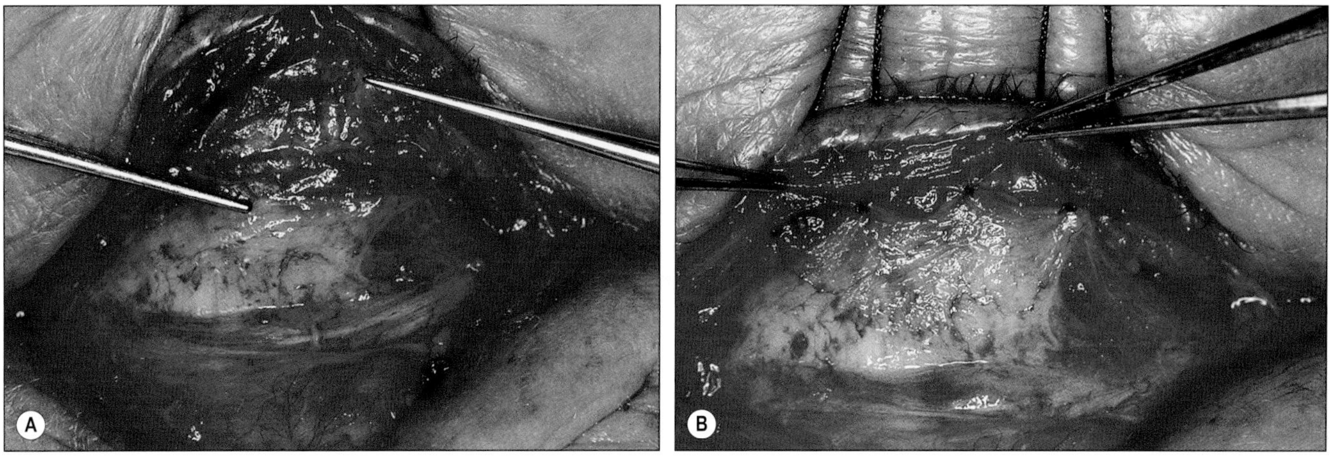

Fig. 29.7 (**A**) Anterior subciliary approach, with the retractors disinserted (left pointer) from the inferior tarsal border (right pointer). (**B**) Edge of the retractors sutured to the inferior tarsal border with permanent sutures. (From Lyon DB, Dortzbach RK. Entropion, trichiasis, and distichiasis. In: Dortzbach RK, ed. *Ophthalmic plastic surgery: prevention and management of complications*. New York: Raven Press; 1994.)

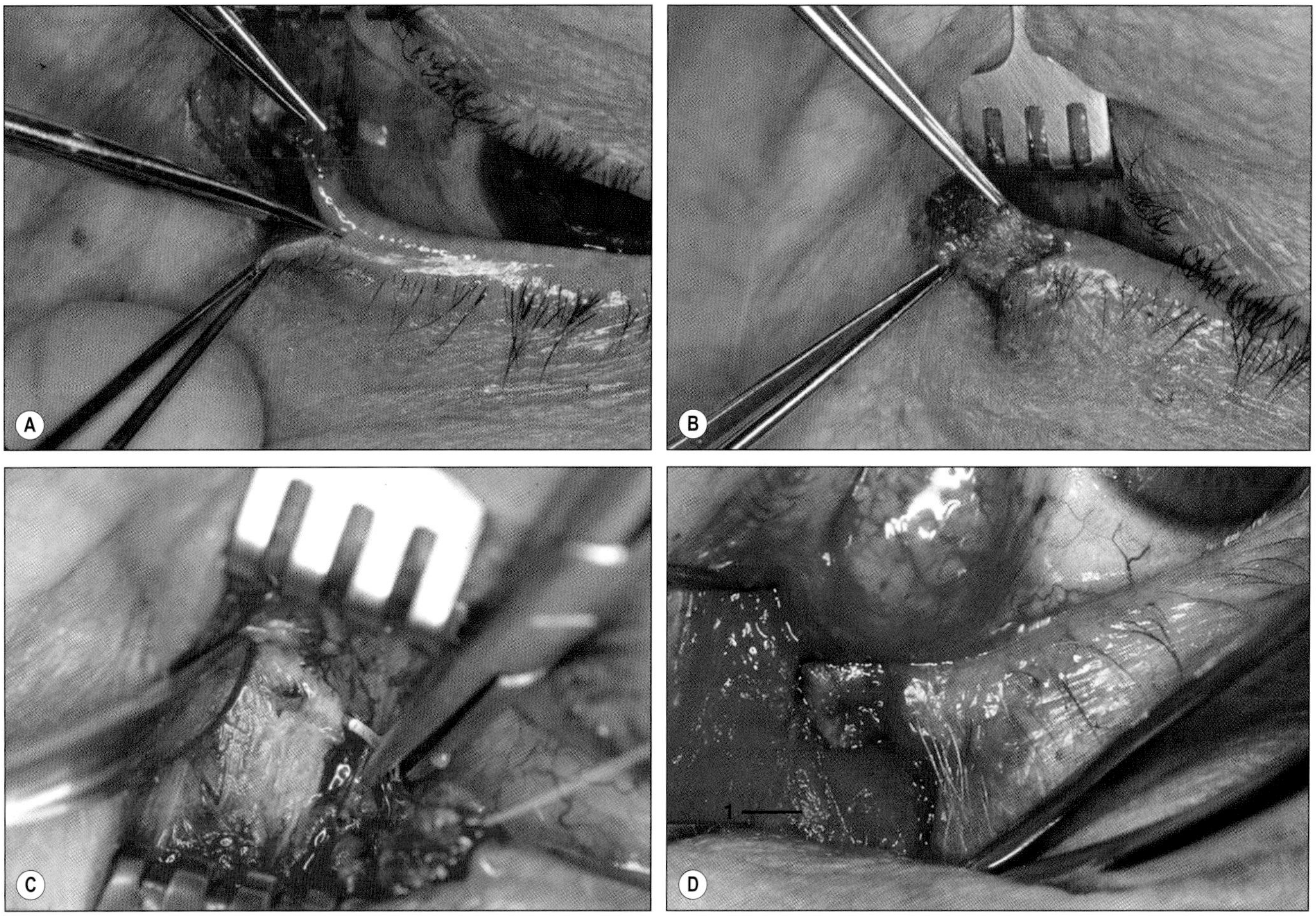

Fig. 29.8 Lateral tarsal strip procedure. (**A**) Splitting the anterior and posterior lamella. (**B**) The tarsal strip denuded of hair follicles, skin, and margin epithelium. (**C**) Passing suture through periosteum at Whitnall's tubercle. (**D**) Completed lateral tarsal strip procedure.

Transconjunctival involutional entropion repair has been reported to have a recurrence rate of 2% to 8.3% in some retrospective studies.[21]

Cicatricial entropion

Before surgery is performed, control of any underlying inflammatory condition is paramount. The severity and extent of posterior lamellar scarring guide the surgical planning.[8] Surgical repair may be considered in three broad categories: margin rotation procedures with a partial- or full-thickness incision through the tarsal plate, eyelid margin splitting procedures with anterior lamellar recession, and those that incorporate a spacer graft to elongate the posterior or middle lamella. Mild cases may require only marginal rotation procedures. A transverse blepharotomy and margin rotation described by Weis can be effective in repairing a cicatricial entropion.[22] A full-thickness horizontal incision inferior to the lower tarsal border along the length of the lid is made; then horizontal mattress sutures are placed through the lower lid retractors, passing anterior to the tarsus, and exiting 1–2 mm inferior to the lash line. In effect, this procedure creates a full-thickness blepharotomy scar between the retractors, the tarsus, and the anterior lamella. Care must be taken to avoid an incision too close to the eyelid margin, as the marginal artery along the inferior tarsal edge could be damaged, resulting in sloughing of the lid margin.

Full-thickness tarsal margin rotation with superadvancement of the posterior lamella 2–3 mm past the new rotated margin may allow for contraction to occur without recurrence of entropion.[23] In the upper lid, a full-thickness posterior tarsal incision is made 3 mm superior to the lash line with back cuts at the incision ends in order to rotate the margin. The remaining posterior lamella is advanced past the rotated margin and secured with horizontal mattress sutures. A horizontal V-wedge resection of anterior tarsus has been described to avoid surgery on the conjunctiva that could reactivate an inflammatory disease.[24] Following an eyelid crease skin incision, the tarsus is exposed down to the lashes. A horizontal V-shaped groove within the tarsus is made at the area of greatest bend using a specialized radiofrequency cutting tip or surgical blades. Closure of the groove using 6-0 polypropylene sutures rotates the lid margin outward.

Additional correction can be achieved with shortening or repositioning of the anterior lamella, such as a lid splitting procedure or tarsoconjunctival advancement.[25] Graft materials are often used for severe scarring or retraction of the posterior lamella. Spacer graft sources include buccal mucosa, tarsoconjunctival flaps, amniotic membrane, nasal chondromucosa, ear cartilage, hard-palate mucosa, and synthetic membranes.

Complications

The most common complication is recurrence.[1] The same involutional mechanisms responsible for the entropion may progress and lead to later recurrence. Proper surgical technique is mandatory to avoid overcorrection, damage to the canaliculus during medial canthopexy, canthal angle dystopia, wound infection, dehiscence, or eyelid necrosis. Complications associated with graft techniques include donor site morbidity, graft failure, symblepharon, and corneal injury induced by a rough posterior eyelid surface.

Ectropion

Congenital ectropion

This rare condition can present alone or combined with other malformations such as blepharophimosis, euryblepharon, ocular anomalies, and trisomy 21. The eyelid ectropion may appear minimal at rest, and become accentuated on upgaze, or when opening the mouth due to a shortage of midfacial skin. Treatment often involves graft techniques to compensate for a deficient anterior lamella. Total bilateral eversion of the upper eyelids in the newborn must be differentiated from congenital ectropion, and conservative treatment with lubrication and patching is usually appropriate.

Involutional ectropion

This condition is most commonly seen in older patients. As in entropion, eyelid instability is a key factor and can be caused by horizontal laxity, vertical laxity with weakness of the retractors, and possibly age-related enophthalmos. Without adequate support, the lower eyelid is pulled further by gravity and the weight of the midface, and constant eye wiping from surface irritation or epiphora stretches the tissues and leads to worsened malposition. In ectropion there is no orbicularis override, which allows the unstable eyelid to turn outward. Focal degeneration of the orbicularis muscle with arteriosclerotic changes of the marginal artery has been found histologically, suggesting chronic muscle ischemia.[26] Patients with ectropion may have larger than age-normal tarsal plates that mechanically overcome the normal or decreased tone of the orbicularis muscle.[27] Preoperative assessment should include documenting eyelid laxity by snapback test, eyelid distraction, medial or lateral canthal tendon laxity, punctal ectropion, inferior scleral show, lagophthalmos, or cicatricial changes.

Cicatricial ectropion

Cicatricial ectropion occurs when there is a shortening of the anterior lamella due to cutaneous or subcutaneous scarring.[28] Trauma, burns, sun damage, inflammatory skin disease, herpes zoster (Fig. 29.9), chemical peels and lasers, and aggressive skin resection from blepharoplasty are frequent causes. Skin contraction can also occur as a result of long-standing ectropion and skin maceration from chronic epiphora. The presence of vertical skin wrinkles, and an ectropion that worsens in upgaze or when the mouth is opened widely, suggest anterior lamellar shortening (Fig. 29.10).

Paralytic ectropion

Paralytic ectropion results from orbicularis oculi paresis or is secondary to facial nerve palsy. More than 80 etiologies of seventh nerve palsy have been described, the most common

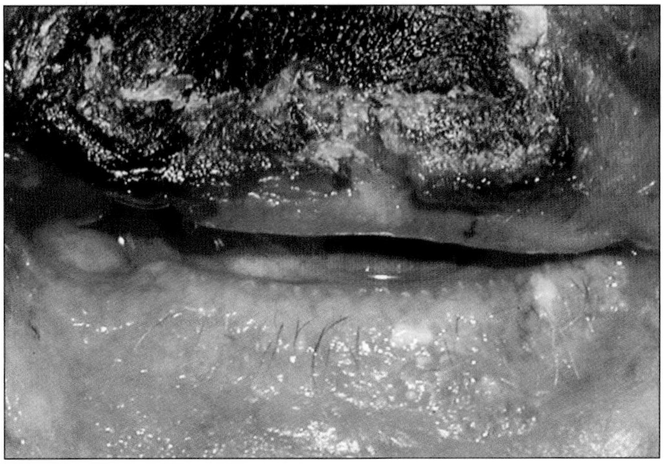

Fig. 29.9 Cicatricial ectropion upper and lower eyelid with large eschar as sequelae of herpes zoster ophthalmicus.

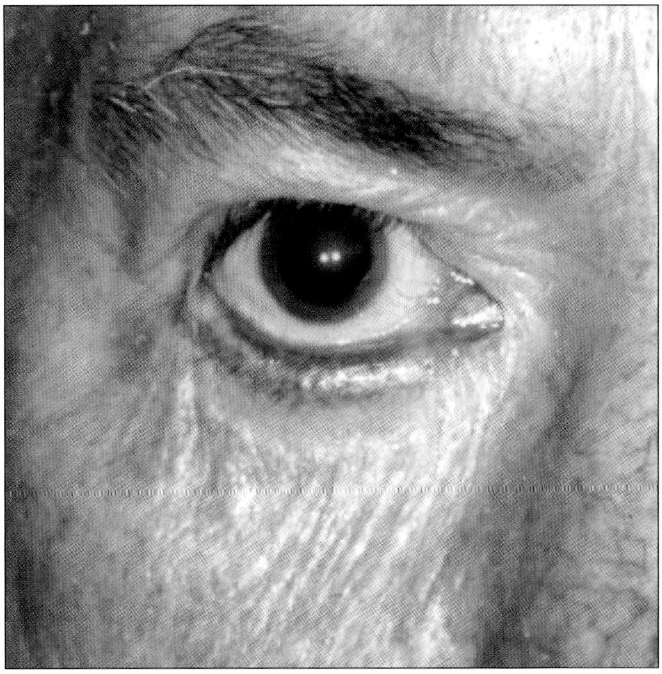

Fig. 29.10 Vertical striae on the lower eyelid skin suggest the presence of cicatricial anterior lamellar tightening.

being traumatic, infection, idiopathic Bell's palsy, and tumor.[29] An atonic lower eyelid is particularly susceptible to gravitational forces and will exacerbate any previous eyelid malposition or result in eventual ectropion and lid retraction with time.

Mechanical ectropion

Mechanical ectropion is caused by the effect of gravity from a large lesion of the eyelid or cheek, pendulous edema, heavy spectacles resting on the cheek, or mechanical weight from significant facial ptosis.[28]

Inflammatory ectropion

Inflammatory ectropion can result from many causes of inflammation or allergy of the eyelids, dermatitis, chronic epiphora, as well as from long-standing ectropion.[28]

Differential diagnosis

In contrast to ectropion, in eyelid retraction the orientation of the tarsal plate is normal rather than turned outward, but the resting position of the margin is retracted beyond the inferior limbus. Eyelid retraction is the most common finding in Graves' ophthalmopathy. Lagophthalmos is present when there is incomplete eyelid closure with normal orbicularis muscle contraction.

Medical management

A thorough history may identify precipitating factors that could be alleviated. In allergic and cicatricial ectropion, cosmetics and ointments or eyedrops may be potential causes of chronic inflammation. Antibiotic-steroid ointment can reduce lid margin and conjunctival inflammation, with surgery delayed until the inflammation has improved adequately. In paralytic ectropion, the incapacitated lacrimal pump disrupts the normal maintenance of a healthy tear film; therefore, lubricating drops and ointments are essential to maintain corneal integrity. Nocturnal eyelid taping or moisture chambers may provide additional protection if there is a poor Bell's phenomenon. In idiopathic facial nerve palsy, orbicularis paresis frequently resolves over a few months, and conservative treatment is indicated as long as corneal exposure is minimal. However, when significant eyelid laxity precedes the paresis, the ectropion is usually permanent and surgical management generally necessary.

Surgical management

Involutional ectropion

Thorough assessment of horizontal laxity, disinsertion or attenuation of the lower lid retractors, or punctal ectropion is essential to selecting the most appropriate surgical management.[30]

When present, medial canthal tendon laxity is corrected first by a plicating or suspension procedure as described for entropion repair. Punctal position is next evaluated. If reposition is indicated, an elliptical or diamond-shaped excision is made in the conjunctiva and retractors inferior to the punctum (Fig. 29.11A).[31] Two or three 6-0 or 7-0 Vicryl buried sutures advance the inferior retractors to the inferior tarsus and close the defect, which rotates the punctum inward (Fig. 29.11B). Lower lid medial ectropion may also be repaired by tightening the posterior limb of the medial canthal tendon.[32] Medial tarsal suspension is a technique in which the medial end of the tarsus is secured to the orbital rim origin of the medial canthal tendon through a transcutaneous or transcaruncular approach.[32,33] This provides vertical support of the eyelid while maintaining posterior apposition of the medial canthus to the globe.

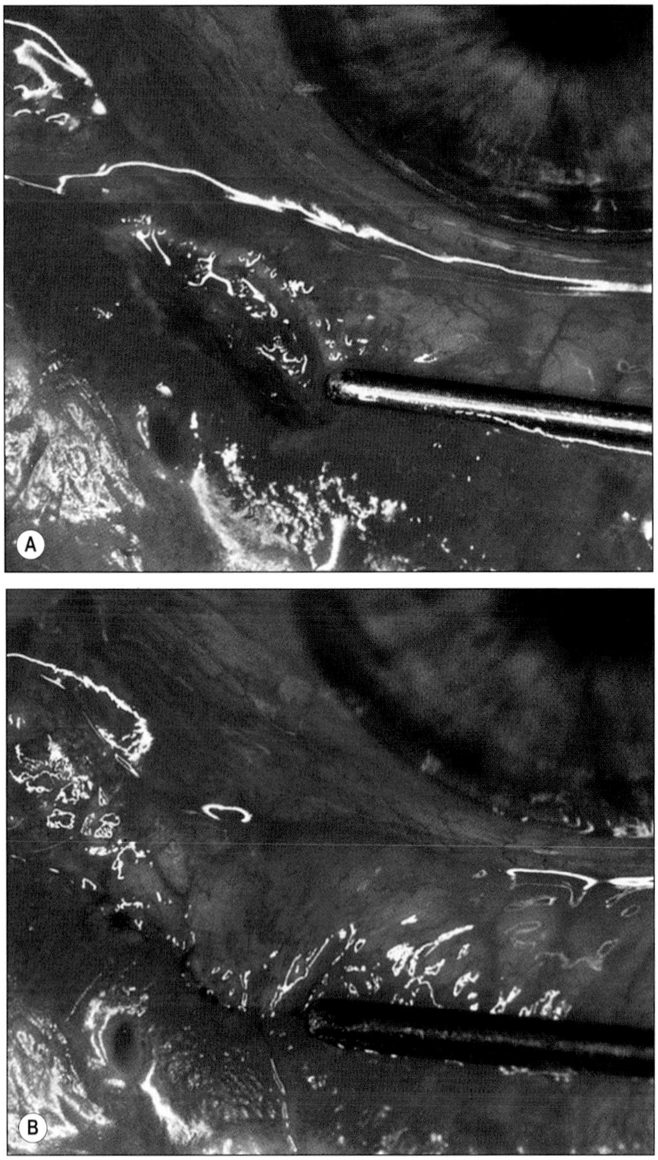

Fig. 29.11 (**A**) Punctal reapposition procedure. Resection of conjunctiva and retractors (pointer) is made below the punctum and canaliculus. (**B**) Vertical closure of the defect achieves reapposition of the punctum to the globe.

Residual horizontal laxity is managed with a tarsal strip procedure or canthus-sparing canthopexy.[19,34] The lateral canthoplasty has been modified in numerous techniques with an interest in avoiding disruption of the lateral commissure. Canthus-sparing techniques performed in combination with upper blepharoplasty and ptosis repair involve dissection of the inferior crus of the lateral canthal tendon performed through the inferolateral portion of the lid crease incision or a horizontally oriented skin incision lateral to the lateral canthus.[34] Attachment of the inferior crus may be secured to a full-thickness periosteal flap.[35] Other approaches include suturing a tarsal strip into an upper lid tarsorrhaphy pocket and tying the sutures over the skin.[36]

A long-standing malposition of the eyelid can induce additional scarring, resulting in shortening of the anterior lamella and secondary cicatricial ectropion. Vertical tightness of the lid skin can be subtle and not immediately detected. Disappearance of horizontal skin wrinkles, or downward traction of the eyelid when the patient opens the mouth widely should alert the physician to cicatricial changes. A shortened anterior lamella requires correction with a skin graft, flap or suborbicularis oculi fat lift.

Congenital ectropion

Shortening of the anterior lamella is corrected with full-thickness skin grafts, and concomitant horizontal laxity is reduced by horizontal lid shortening techniques.

Paralytic ectropion

Conservative treatment with a temporary tarsorrhaphy using nonabsorbable suture (4-0 Prolene, nylon) over bolsters can protect the cornea for weeks. The suture may be tied in a fashion that allows opening for repeated eyedrops or examinations. A lateral tarsorrhaphy may be appropriate and simple to perform. The adjacent lid margins of the lateral upper and lower lids are excised and the eyelids sutured together through the gray line. A more lasting adhesion can be achieved through transposition of a tarsal segment from one lid to the other. The adjacent upper and lower lateral lid margins are split along the gray line for the desired length of closure to a depth of approximately 3 mm. A 3-mm flap of upper lid tarsus and conjunctiva is created laterally and a small matching area is resected from the lower lid tarsus. A double-armed 4-0 chromic suture is passed partial thickness through the upper lid tarsal flap to exit the margin, then through the lower lid tarsal defect margin and tied over the skin. The cut edges of the upper tarsal flap appose the lower tarsal defect for a stronger effect. Horizontal laxity should always be treated if present.[29]

Placement of a gold or platinum weight anterior to the tarsus, or with supratarsal fixation, can facilitate eyelid closure.[37] Different weights are tested preoperatively to ensure adequate closure while minimizing ptosis; a compromise must be agreed upon by both the surgeon and patient. The lower lid may need further support with a fascia lata or temporalis fascia sling. Mid-face ptosis can worsen lower lid ectropion, and correction with a mid-face or suborbicularis oculi fat (SOOF) lift should be considered.[29,38]

Cicatricial ectropion

Depending on the extent of cicatricial involvement, treatment involves scar revision with direct cicatrix excision, Z-plasty, horizontal tightening, and anterior lamella lengthening with pedicle flaps or free skin grafts from the upper lid, preauricular, retroauricular, or supraclavicular areas.[39] Z-plasty transposition flaps camouflage long linear scars and redirect tension along more natural relaxed skin tension lines.

Complications

Complications are similar to those of entropion repair, such as injury to the inferior canaliculus during medial canthal tendon tightening, lateral canthal angle dystopia, asymmetry, dehiscence, infection, hemorrhage, graft failure, and recurrence.

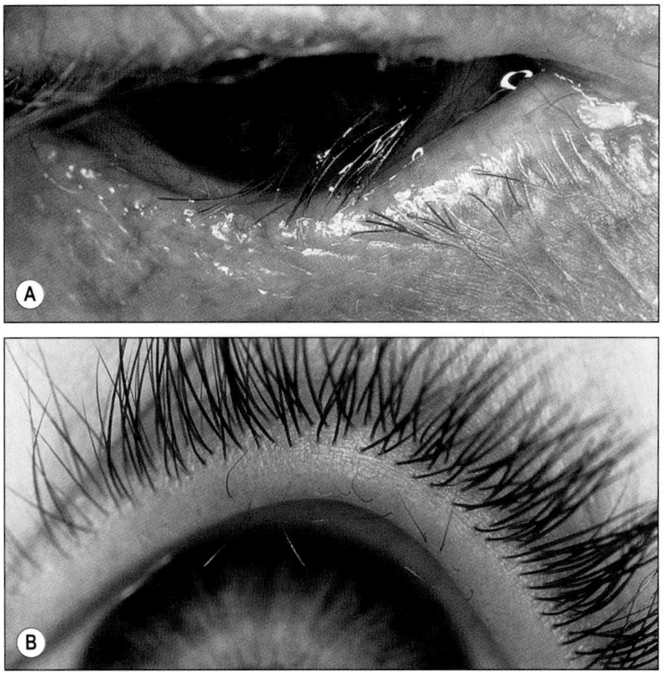

Fig. 29.12 (**A**) Trichiasis of the lower lid with corneal irritation. (**B**) Distichiasis of the upper lid with aberrant lashes originating from the meibomian glands orifices. (From Lyon DB, Dortzbach RK. Entropion, trichiasis, and distichiasis. In: Dortzbach RK, ed. *Ophthalmic plastic surgery: prevention and management of complications*. New York: Raven Press; 1994.)

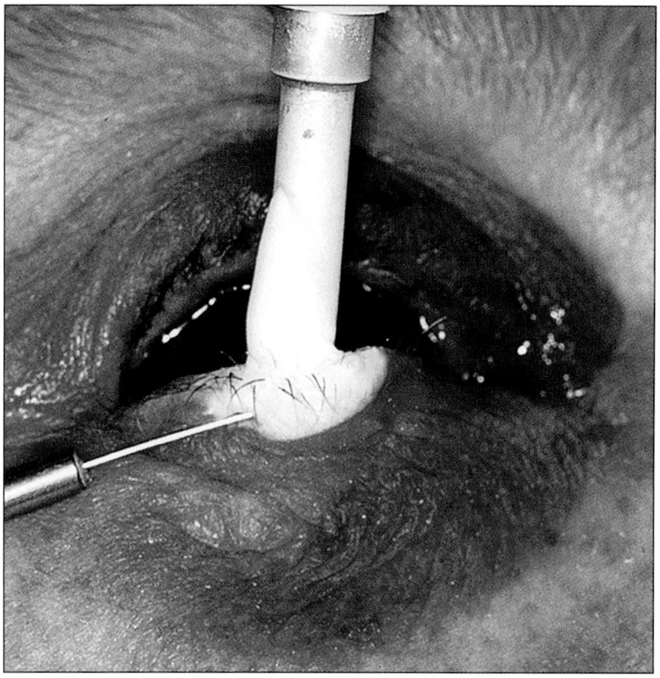

Fig. 29.13 Lash ablation by cryotherapy. A thermocouple needle (left) is placed through the skin adjacent to the lash follicles to monitor the temperature. A cryoprobe is shown freezing the lid margin and offending lashes. (From Lyon DB, Dortzbach RK. Entropion, trichiasis, and distichiasis. In: Dortzbach RK, ed. *Ophthalmic plastic surgery: prevention and management of complications*. New York: Raven Press; 1994.)

Trichiasis and Distichiasis

Trichiasis refers to a condition in which lashes emerging from their normal anterior lamellar origin are misdirected backward toward the cornea, while the tarsal plate maintains a normal apposition to the globe (Fig. 29.12A).[1] It is distinguished from an entropion or an epiblepharon by assessing the lash orientation when the lid is in its normal position. Trichiasis can be idiopathic or secondary to chronic inflammatory conditions such as blepharitis, trachoma, ocular cicatricial pemphigoid, Stevens–Johnson syndrome, or chemical burns.

Distichiasis is a congenital (often autosomal dominant) or acquired condition in which an extra row of eyelashes emerges from the meibomian gland orifices (Fig. 29.12B).[1] In this condition, embryonic common pilosebaceous units differentiate into hair follicles rather than meibomian glands. Trauma and chronic inflammatory conditions of the eyelids and conjunctiva are frequent causes of the acquired type. Distichiatic lashes can be fine and well tolerated, or coarser and a threat to corneal integrity.

Management of trichiasis

Trichiasis may occur diffusely across the entire eyelid margin, or in small segmental distribution. Epilation is appropriate for a few misdirected lashes, although they will usually grow back within 4–6 weeks. Electrolysis can treat individual eyelashes for more permanent results.[1] After local anesthesia, the electrolysis needle is inserted adjacent and parallel to the hairshaft down to the follicle of the eyelash, and the current is applied until a small bubble can be observed at the surface beside the hairshaft. The lash should be able to be wiped away or pulled without resistance. If the lashes recur, retreatment is indicated.

Cryotherapy is effective for groups of eyelashes (Fig. 29.13).[40,41] A nitrous oxide-cooled probe covered with water-soluble petroleum jelly is applied to the margin until a temperature of –20° to –30°C is reached for 30 seconds. After allowing for thawing, a second cycle is applied, and the lashes are epilated. A thermocouple needle placed into the orbicularis close to the targeted follicles can monitor tissue temperature to ensure that adequate treatment temperature is reached. Cryotherapy induces more loss of normal adjacent lashes than electrolysis, and more risks of margin notching, necrosis, skin depigmentation, and recurrence.[1] Treatment can be repeated. Postoperative reaction, consisting mainly of edema and erythema, can be expected up to 1 or 2 weeks.

Blue-green argon laser ablation can be used to treat trichiasis with variable results.[42,43] Thirty shots are typically directed to the lash root, with laser beam variables set at 50–100 μm spot size, 0.3 second duration, and 0.50 watt power. Complications are few but may include mild hypopigmentation and eyelid notching. In a study of trachomatous trichiasis, argon laser ablation was successful in 55.5% of lids after one session, with an increase to 89% after several sessions.[44] Segmental areas of trichiatic lashes can be treated by a full-thickness wedge resection, which offers good cosmesis and few complications.

Management of distichiasis

Focal areas may be treated by epilation or electrolysis. Cryotherapy applied to the posterior lamella can also be used for a few lashes. In the case of more extensive distichiasis, the eyelid can be split along the gray line and the posterior lamella treated with cryotherapy or focal hyfrecation, or the posterior lid margin and tarsal plate containing the distichiatic hair follicles excised directly.[1] Additional steps may involve mucous membrane grafting.

References

1. Lyon DB, Dortzbach RK. Entropion, trichiasis, and distichiasis. In: Dortzbach RK, ed. *Ophthalmic plastic surgery: prevention and management of complications*. New York: Raven Press; 1994.
2. Hawes MJ, Dortzbach RK. The microscopic anatomy of the lower eyelid retractors. *Arch Ophthalmol.* 1982;100:1313–1318.
3. Quickert MH, Wilkes DI, Dryden RM. Nonincisional correction of epiblepharon and congenital entropion. *Arch Ophthalmol.* 1983;101: 778–781.
4. Dortzbach RK, McGetrick JJ. Involutional entropion of the lower eyelid. *Adv Ophthalmic Plast Reconstr Surg.* 1983;2:257–267.
5. Jones LT, Reeh MJ, Wobig JL. Senile entropion: a new concept for correction. *Am J Ophthalmol.* 1972;74:327–329.
6. Dryden RM, Leibsohn JL, Wobig J. Senile entropion. *Arch Ophthalmol.* 1978;96:1883–1885.
7. Carter SR, Chang J, Aguilar GL, Rathbun JE, Seiff SR. Involutional entropion and ectropion of the Asian lower eyelid. *Ophthal Plast Reconstr Surg.* 2000;16:45–49.
8. Dortzbach RK, Callahan A. Repair of cicatricial entropion of upper eyelids. *Arch Ophthalmol.* 1971;85:82–89.
9. Lemke BN, Stasior OG. Epiblepharon. *Clin Pediatr.* 1981;20:661–662.
10. Hayasaka S, Noda S, Setogawa T. Epiblepharon with inverted eyelashes in Japanese children. II: surgical repairs. *Br J Ophthalmol.* 1989;73:128–139.
11. Woo KI, Yi K, Kim YD. Surgical correction for lower lid epiblepharon in Asians. *Br J Ophthalmol.* 2000;84:1407–1410.
12. Feldstein M. Suture correction of senile entropion by inferior lid retractor tuck. *Adv Ophthalmic Plast Reconstr Surg.* 1983;2:269–274.
13. Wright M, Bell D, Scott C. Everting suture correction of lower lid involutional entropion. *Br J Ophthalmol.* 1999;83:1060–1063.
14. Millman AL, Mannor GE, Putterman AM. Lid crease and capsulopalpebral fascia repair in congenital entropion and epiblepharon. *Ophthalmic Surg.* 1994;25:162–165.
15. Benger RS, Frueh BR. Involution entropion: a review of the management. *Ophthalmic Surg.* 1987;18:140–142.
16. Cook T, Lucarelli MJ, Lemke BN, Dortzbach RK. Primary and secondary transconjunctival involutional entropion repair. *Ophthalmology.* 2001;108:989–993.
17. Boboridis K, Bunce C, Rose G. A comparative study of two procedures for repair of involutional lower eyelid entropion. *Ophthalmology.* 2000;107:959–961.
18. Anderson RL, Gordy DD. The tarsal strip procedure. *Arch Ophthalmol.* 1979;97:2192–2196.
19. Jordan DR, Anderson RL. The lateral tarsal strip revisited: the enhanced tarsal strip. *Arch Ophthalmol.* 1989;107:604–606.
20. Dresner SC, Karesh JW. Transconjunctival entropion repair. *Arch Ophthalmol.* 1993;111:1144–1148.
21. Khan SJ, Meyer DR. Transconjunctival lower eyelid involutional entropion repair: long-term follow-up and efficacy. *Ophthalmology.* 2002;109:2112–2117.
22. Weis FA. Spastic entropion. *Trans Am Acad Ophthalmol Otolaryngol.* 1955;59:503–506.
23. Seiff SR, Carter SR, Canales JL, Choo PH. Tarsal margin rotation with posterior lamella superadvancement for the management of cicatricial entropion of the upper eyelid. *Am J Ophthalmol.* 1999;127:67–71.
24. Dutton JJ, Tawfik HA, DeBacker CM, Lipham WJ. Anterior tarsal V-wedge resection for cicatricial entropion. *Ophthal Plast Reconstr Surg.* 2000;16:126–130.
25. Elder MJ, Collin R. Anterior lamella repositioning and grey line split for upper lid entropion in ocular cicatricial pemphigoid. *Eye.* 1996;10: 439–442.
26. Stefanyszyn MA, Hidayat AA, Flanagan JC. The histopathology of involutional ectropion. *Ophthalmology.* 1985;92:120–127.
27. Bashour M, Harvey J. Causes of involutional ectropion and entropion—age-related tarsal changes are the key. *Ophthal Plast Reconstr Surg.* 2000;16:131–141.
28. Bartley GB. Ectropion and lagophthalmos. In: Dortzbach RK, ed. *Ophthalmic plastic surgery: prevention and management of complications.* New York: Raven Press; 1994.
29. Lisman RD, et al. Efficacy of surgical treatment for paralytic ectropion. *Ophthalmology.* 1987;94:671–681.
30. Benger RS, Frueh BR. Involutional ectropion: a review of the management. *Ophthalmic Surg.* 1987;18:136–139.
31. Nowinski TS, Anderson RL. The medial spindle procedure for involutional medial ectropion. *Arch Ophthalmol.* 1985;103:1750–1753.
32. Fante RG, Elner VM. Transcaruncular approach to medial canthal tendon plication for lower eyelid laxity. *Ophthal Plast Reconstr Surg.* 2001;17:16–27.
33. Frueh BR, Su CS. Medial tarsal suspension: a method of elevating the medial lower eyelid. *Ophthal Plast Reconstr Surg.* 2002;18:133–137.
34. Lemke BN, Cook BE, Lucarelli MJ. Canthus-sparing ectropion repair. *Ophthal Plast Reconstr Surg.* 2001;17:161–168.
35. Lemke BN, Sires BS, Dortzbach RK. A tarsal strip-periosteal flap technique for lateral canthal fixation. *Ophthalmic Surg Lasers.* 1999;30:232–236.
36. Hesse RJ. The tarsal sandwich: a new technique in lateral canthoplasty. *Ophthal Plast Reconstr Surg.* 2000;16:39–41.
37. Gilbard SM, Daspit CP. Reanimation of the paretic eyelid using gold weight implantation. *Ophthal Plast Reconstr Surg.* 1991;7:93–103.
38. Seiff SR, Carter SR. Facial nerve paralysis. *Int Ophthalmol Clin.* 2002;42: 103–112.
39. Brown BZ, Beard C. Split-level full-thickness eyelid graft. *Am J Ophthalmol.* 1979;87:388–392.
40. Sullivan JH, Beard C, Bullock JD. Cryosurgery for treatment of trichiasis. *Am J Ophthalmol.* 1976;82:117–121.
41. Sullivan JH. The use of cryotherapy for trichiasis. *Trans Am Acad Ophthalmol Otolaryngol.* 1977;83(4 Pt. 1):708–712.
42. Gossman MD, et al. Experimental comparison of laser and cryosurgical cilia destruction. *Ophthalmic Surg.* 1992;23:179–182.
43. Bartley GB, Lowry JC. Argon laser treatment of trichiasis. *Am J Ophthalmol.* 1992;113:71–74.
44. Unlu K, Aksunger A, Soker S. Prospective evaluation of the argon laser treatment of trachomatous trichiasis. *Jpn J Ophthalmol.* 2000;44: 677–689.

Chapter 30

Lagophthalmos and Other Malpositions of the Lid

Robert C. Kersten

Normal eyelid apposition, blinking, and closure are necessary for maintenance of a healthy ocular surface. In addition to protecting the eye and preventing evaporative loss of surface moisture, the eyelids play a crucial role in resurfacing the tear film through the blink mechanism. With every blink, the eyelid sweeps away lipid-contaminated mucin and allows a new layer of mucin to coat the cornea. The hydrophilic mucin allows for a stable aqueous tear film. Patients with abnormalities of eyelid apposition or closure will develop breakdown of the mucous layer, leading to inadequate surface wetting and subsequent ocular surface pathology.

A separate chapter deals with the problems of entropion and ectropion. This chapter will concentrate on other eyelid abnormalities that affect the ocular surface. These include floppy eyelid syndrome, lid imbrication syndrome, lid retraction, and lagophthalmos.

Floppy Eyelid Syndrome

Floppy eyelid syndrome occurs predominantly in obese males and is characterized by rubbery, floppy, easily everted upper eyelid tarsal plates and a prominent upper palpebral conjunctival papillary reaction. The pathogenesis of the floppy eyelid syndrome is uncertain, but it appears to be primarily a disorder of sleeping position. Patients with floppy eyelid syndrome consistently sleep face down with their eye(s) pressed against the pillow. The disorder may be bilateral or unilateral, but there is close correlation between the side on which the patient preferentially sleeps and the more affected eye.

In the original description of floppy eyelid syndrome by Culbertson and Ostler in 1981,[1] the disorder was thought to be confined to obese males. These patients complained of ocular irritation, mucous discharge, and papillary conjunctivitis. They had significant corneal abnormalities, ranging from punctate keratopathy to gross surface scarring and vascularization. Subsequent studies confirmed that this disorder may also affect women[2] and children,[3] but a face-down sleeping position appears to be consistent.[4]

As this disorder has become more widely recognized, it has been diagnosed more frequently, extending beyond patients with the classic obese male body habitus. Culbertson and Tseng,[4] in a follow-up report on 60 patients diagnosed at the Bascom Palmer Eye Institute over a 10-year period, found that 37% of their patients were women and only 29% of the patients were obese. However, all patients had face-down sleeping position in common.

Patients with floppy eyelid syndrome usually complain of irritation and mattering or discharge from the affected eye(s).[5] The disorder is bilateral in 78% of patients but may be asymmetrical. Typical external findings include a markedly elongated, very lax upper eyelid tarsus, which can be readily everted with upward distraction (Fig. 30.1). Variable degrees of papillary conjunctivitis occur in virtually all patients, and floppy eyelid syndrome should be considered in any case of chronic papillary conjunctivitis of unknown etiology.[6] Eyelash ptosis, although infrequently mentioned, has occurred consistently in patients with this disorder (Fig. 30.2).[7,8] Patients may also have blepharoptosis and dermatochalasis due to repetitive mechanical trauma caused by the lid-to-pillow contact. Lower eyelid involvement has also occurred, with ectropion and frank eversion of the lower lid in conjunction with the typical tarsal conjunctival papillae (Fig. 30.3).[9]

A wide range of corneal abnormalities have been associated with floppy eyelid syndrome. The majority of patients have some degree of corneal abnormality, and the disorder can affect all layers of the cornea.[3–5,9–11] Approximately 50% of patients have punctate epithelial keratopathy, which may be due to trauma associated with globe-to-pillow contact or may be the result of corneal surface irritation from palpebral conjunctival papillae. Parunovic[10] first reported keratoconus occurring in conjunction with the floppy eyelid syndrome in 1983. This association is probably quite common;[11] Culbertson and Tseng also found 18% of their patients to have clinical keratoconus. Surprisingly, five of seven (71%) randomly selected patients with floppy eyelid syndrome who were examined with a videokeratoscope showed subclinical keratoconus.[4] Recurrent corneal erosions, filamentary keratitis, corneal endotheliopathy, and infectious keratitis may also occur in the floppy eyelid syndrome. In addition, one patient had a progressive nonguttate loss of endothelium, and a second had keratoconus and Chandler's variant of an iridocorneal endothelial syndrome in the floppy eyelid eye.[4] Rarely, corneal ulceration and perforation have been reported.[12] Others have found corneal abnormalities to occur less often.[13]

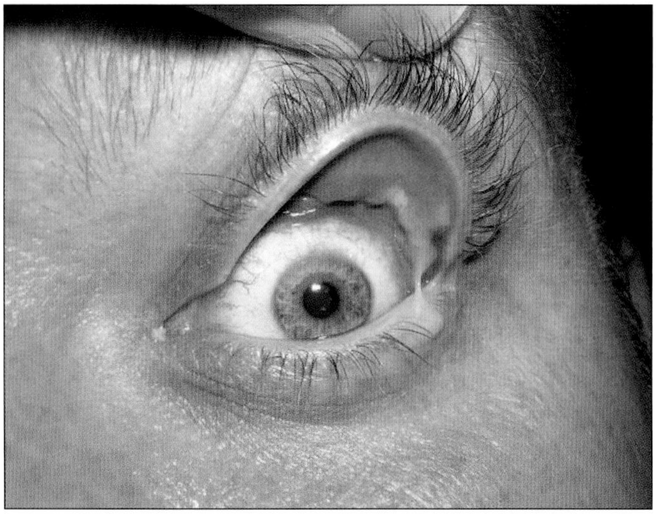

Fig. 30.1 Floppy eyelid syndrome. Note the markedly elongated, easily evertable right upper eyelid with underlying papillary conjunctivitis.

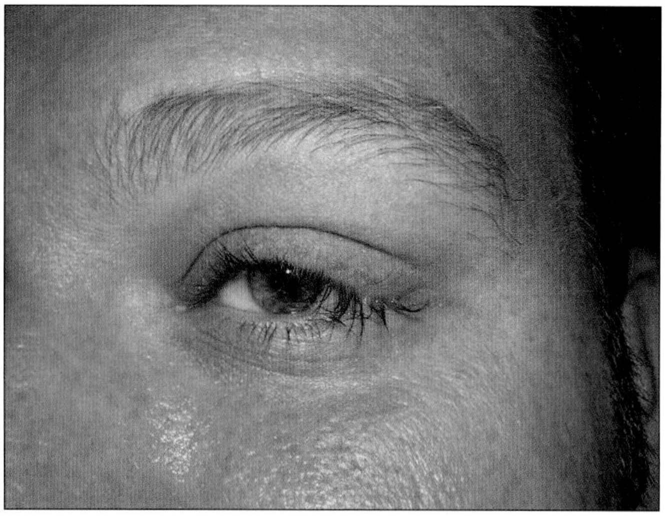

Fig. 30.2 Floppy eyelid syndrome. Eyelash ptosis is a frequent finding and fairly specific for floppy eyelid syndrome.

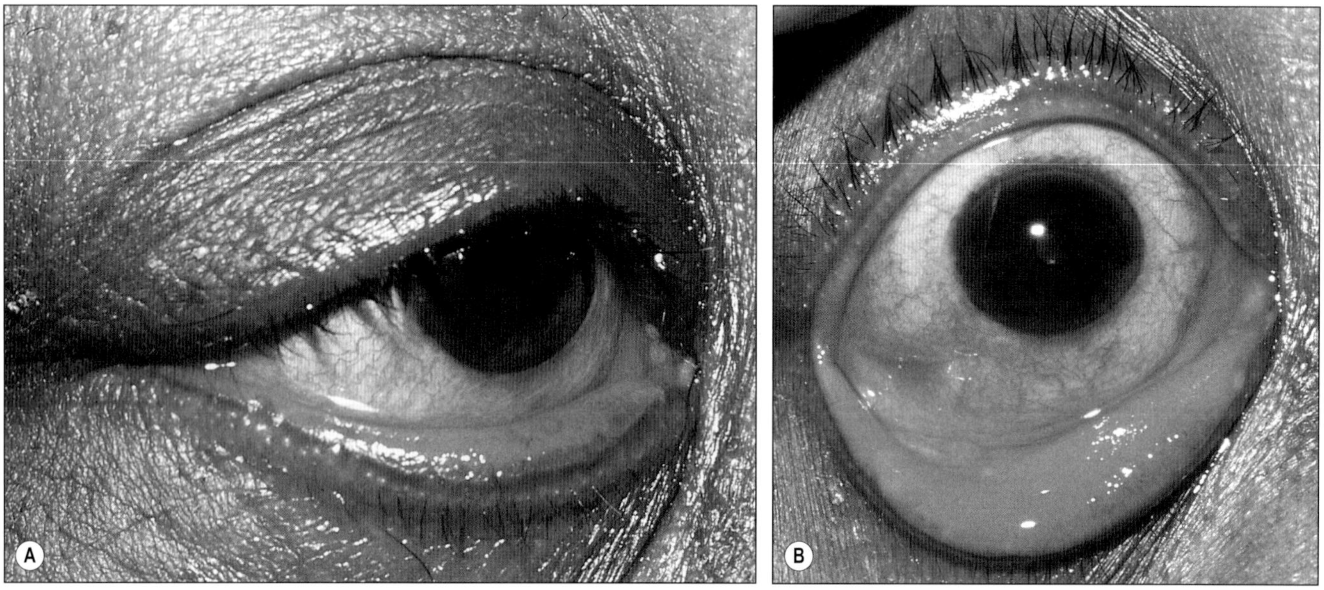

Fig. 30.3 Floppy eyelid syndrome. **A**, Patient with lower lid ectropion that developed when she began to sleep in a prone position with her right side contacting the pillow. **B**, Distraction of the lower lid shows marked elongation, easy eversion, and typical papillary conjunctivitis.

The histopathologic features of the floppy eyelid syndrome point primarily to a marked reduction in eyelid tarsal elastin.[8] Immunohistochemical staining for the distribution of type I and type III collagen has shown no dissimilarity between patients with floppy eyelid syndrome and controls.[14,15] Atrophy of meibomian glands and dysfunction have also been reported.[16]

Because of the high incidence of sleep apnea in the obese males with this syndrome, Culbertson and Tseng have postulated that low oxygen tension during sleep and rapid reoxygenation on awakening may lead to localized free radical-induced damage to the tarsus. However, this mechanism would not explain the similar changes found in the majority of patients who do not have sleep apnea, and it seems more likely that the tarsal changes in floppy eyelid syndrome occur due to the mechanical phenomenon of chronic lid-to-pillow contact.

A number of systemic diseases have been associated with floppy eyelid syndrome. Diabetes mellitus, hyperthyroidism, and hypertension have been noted frequently, but these diseases may correlate better with the preponderance of patients with obesity in this disorder. Obstructive sleep apnea, however, does appear to be a particular risk for the obese males with this syndrome. This disorder is characterized by periods of apnea and hypopnea during sleep that occur as a result of upper airway obstruction. These patients demonstrate partial or complete collapse of the airway during inspiration. Their symptoms include loud snoring, unrefreshing sleep, daytime somnolence, morning headaches, and personality disturbances. Sleep apnea is potentially fatal, and patients have an increased incidence of systemic and pulmonary hypertension, cardiac arrhythmias, and an increased frequency of automobile accidents. It has been recommended that all male patients with floppy eyelid syndrome be evaluated for this sleep disorder.[17] Substance abuse has also been associated with refractory floppy eyelid syndrome.[18]

Recently, van den Bosch and Lemij[19] reported a small group of patients with a clinical picture similar to floppy eyelid syndrome, none of whom reported sleeping face down. They suggested that the more general term lax eyelid syndrome be applied to such patients.

Treatment

Treatment is directed toward interrupting the eversion of the tarsal plate during sleep. Initially treatment consists of mechanically shielding the eyelids. A Fox shield may be used for this purpose, but over time most patients object to repeated taping. An alternative is to use a 'sleep mask,' which can be tied in place. The key to long-term success is interrupting lid–pillow contact during sleep. Surgical procedures to tighten the eyelid will ultimately fail unless the face-down sleeping position is resolved. Identification of sleep apnea and institution of CPAP to allow a supine sleep position is paramount. In fact, the findings of floppy eyelid syndrome have been noted to reverse with appropriate treatment of obstructive sleep apnea.[20] Symptomatic topical lubrication will help alleviate the irritation and discharge. Patients should be cautioned against rubbing the eyelids. Horizontal shortening of the affected eyelid(s) has also been reported to be highly successful,[14] although with prolonged follow-up there may be a disturbing tendency for the lids treated with full-thickness wedge excision to restretch and evert. A lateral canthopexy may be a more effective form of shortening, as it eliminates the lax lateral canthal tendon and allows the broader midportion of the tarsus to be fixed to the periosteum laterally. This seems to make eversion of the lid more difficult around this broader pivot point than around the narrower lateral canthal tendon.

During horizontal tightening, ptosis repair, blepharoplasty, or eyelash repositioning may also be performed. Patients who fail to respond to horizontal tightening may require tarsorrhaphy to prevent lid eversion.[21]

Floppy eyelid syndrome may be difficult to diagnose, especially in patients who do not exhibit the typical body habitus. In a large study[6] atypical body habitus was noted in 2% of patients with chronic conjunctivitis of unknown etiology. In all patients with chronic conjunctivitis, traction of the upper lid should be performed to elicit the rubbery, elongated, everting tarsal plate, which is the hallmark of floppy eyelid syndrome. Examination for lash ptosis may also be highly specific.

Lid Imbrication Syndrome

Lid imbrication syndrome is an abnormality of lid apposition in which the upper lid overrides the lower, thereby allowing the lower lashes and keratinized epithelium to rub chronically against the upper eyelid marginal tarsal conjunctiva. This causes keratinization of the upper lid margin and metaplasia of the distal tarsal conjunctival surface (Fig. 30.4). The resulting abnormal distal superior palpebral surface directly irritates the underlying corneal surface and prohibits normal replenishment of the tear film by blinking. Lid imbrication disrupts tear film mechanics, which results in a poor tear film, symptoms of dryness, and persistent epithelial defects.

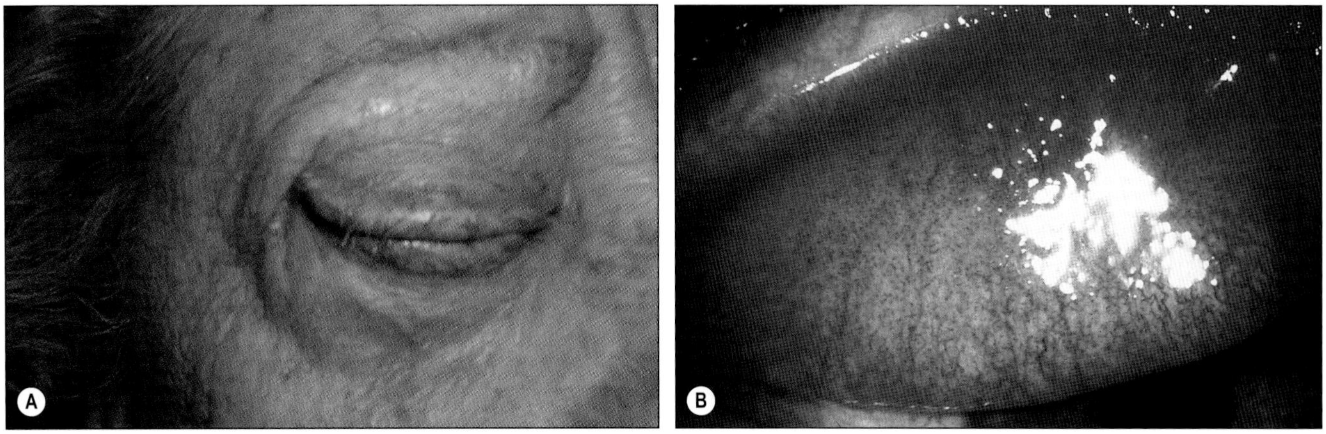

Fig. 30.4 Lid imbrication syndrome. **A**, Patient with lid imbrication syndrome involving the medial half of the upper eyelid. (Courtesy David Tse.) **B**, Eversion of the upper lid revealed keratinization and injection of the lid marginal tarsal conjunctiva. (Courtesy David Tse.)

This rare cause of chronic conjunctivitis was initially described by Karesh and others in 1993.[22] This disorder may have some overlap with floppy eyelid syndrome, and Karesh found that six of his 18 patients also had floppy eyelid syndrome. Patients with this disorder have ocular irritation, foreign body sensation, and burning, which often persists despite the use of copious artificial tears. A significant subset of patients will also have persistent corneal epithelial defects.

Because the upper lid overlies the lower lid, visualization of lid apposition during closure may be difficult and hence this disorder is often missed. Many patients may receive a mistaken diagnosis of dry eye syndrome. On physical examination the condition is best evaluated by having the patient tilt his or her head back and then observing from beneath with a penlight whether the upper lid overrides the lower. Many patients will have a gelatinous thickening of the tarsal marginal conjunctiva.

Donnenfeld and others[23] have reported a high specificity using super vital stains such as 0.5% topical rose Bengal or lissamine green to diagnose lid imbrication. Super vital stains will stain the tarsal conjunctiva along the upper lid margin; in patients with lid imbrication syndrome the severity of staining will correlate to the severity of symptoms. In addition to upper lid laxity, approximately 50% of patients will have concomitant lower lid laxity without frank ectropion. Lid imbrication disorder has also been reported in patients with a history of spontaneously resolved thyroid exophthalmos, where the recession of proptosis results in stretched and lax eyelids.

Lid imbrication disorder should be differentiated from floppy eyelid syndrome, although there is some overlap. Patients with lid imbrication syndrome alone show no predisposition to lid eversion and lack the rubbery, easily distensible upper eyelid tarsal plate. These patients also do not demonstrate upper tarsal giant papillary conjunctivitis, and the eyelid abnormalities are confined to the lid marginal tarsal conjunctiva. Furthermore, approximately two-thirds of patients with lid imbrication syndrome are female.[23]

Treatment

Initial treatment consists of aggressive lubrication with viscous tear substitutes and ointments. Horizontal tightening of the upper lid to prevent the upper tarsal/lower lid apposition has been successful. This can be achieved through full-thickness wedge excision or lateral tarsal periosteal tightening. If the lower lid is lax, it should also be tightened. Patients with persistent epithelial defects due to lid imbrication syndrome may benefit from temporary tarsorrhaphy to prevent the upper lid from overriding the lower lid.

Lagophthalmos

Lagophthalmos is the inability to coapt the eyelids fully during attempted closure. Incomplete closure results in poor tear film replenishment, increased tear evaporation, disruption of the mucin layer, corneal drying, and ocular surface breakdown. The term lagophthalmos comes from the Greek word for hare (*lagos*) because rabbits were thought to sleep with their eyes open. Inability to close the eyelids completely can result from a forward projection of the eye within the orbit, vertical shortening of the upper or lower eyelids, dysfunction of the protractor orbicularis oculi muscle or its seventh cranial nerve motor innervation, or adhesions between the globe and upper lid that limit full eyelid excursion.

Patients complain of irritation, foreign body sensation, and burning. Slit lamp examination characteristically reveals interpalpebral punctate epithelial keratopathy, which is diagnostic of lagophthalmos. In patients with nocturnal lagophthalmos, the distribution of the punctate epithelial keratopathy will depend on the position of the cornea during sleep. Keratopathy may be inferior, central, or even superior, as some patients have been reported to sleep with the globe depressed. Testing for Bell's phenomenon has been a fairly poor predictor of actual globe position during sleep.[24,25] External examination for complete lid closure should be done with the patient gently pressing the lids closed, because subtle degrees of lagophthalmos may not be apparent if the lids are forcefully 'squeezed.'

Acute seventh-nerve dysfunction, due to Bell's palsy or following trauma or iatrogenic injury, is probably the most frequent cause of lagophthalmos presented to the ophthalmologist. In patients with seventh-nerve paralysis, the history and obvious motor dysfunction allow for ready diagnosis. In cases with more subtle orbicularis weakness, manual distraction of the lids during forced closure may expose weakness that may cause nocturnal lagophthalmos or incomplete blink. Patients should be questioned about any history of previous Bell's palsy, as many will show some degree of orbicularis underaction even after apparent clinical recovery. Patients with recovered seventh-nerve palsy should also be evaluated for evidence of aberrant regeneration between the muscles of lower facial expression and the orbicularis oculi muscles. Testing for weakness in other muscle groups innervated by the seventh cranial nerve (forehead, lower face) will help to confirm the diagnosis.

In all patients with lagophthalmos it is crucial to check corneal sensation to ensure that there is also not a component of fifth-nerve dysfunction. Fifth-nerve dysfunction is most likely to occur in patients who have had intracranial trauma, surgery, or a neurovascular accident where multiple cranial nerve palsies may be present.

The protractors may also be weak in various periocular myopathies, including myasthenia gravis, myotonic dystrophy, and chronic progressive external ophthalmoplegia. The associated periocular findings of ptosis and extraocular motility disturbances, and the adynamic facial muscles should indicate the possibility of lagophthalmos in these patients. Leprosy may also cause seventh-nerve dysfunction and lagophthalmos.

The adequacy of the vertical dimension of upper and lower eyelid skin should also be evaluated in patients with suspected lagophthalmos. In the lower eyelids, vertical shortage will usually be apparent and will manifest as scleral show and lid retraction. However, in the upper eyelids the lid margin often rests at a normal height, and only with downward distraction of the lid does the vertical skin shortness become apparent. Vertical shortening usually occurs from accidental or iatrogenic trauma due to scarring or overexcision of the eyelid skin (Fig. 30.5). Some congenital abnormalities, such as type II blepharophimosis syndrome,

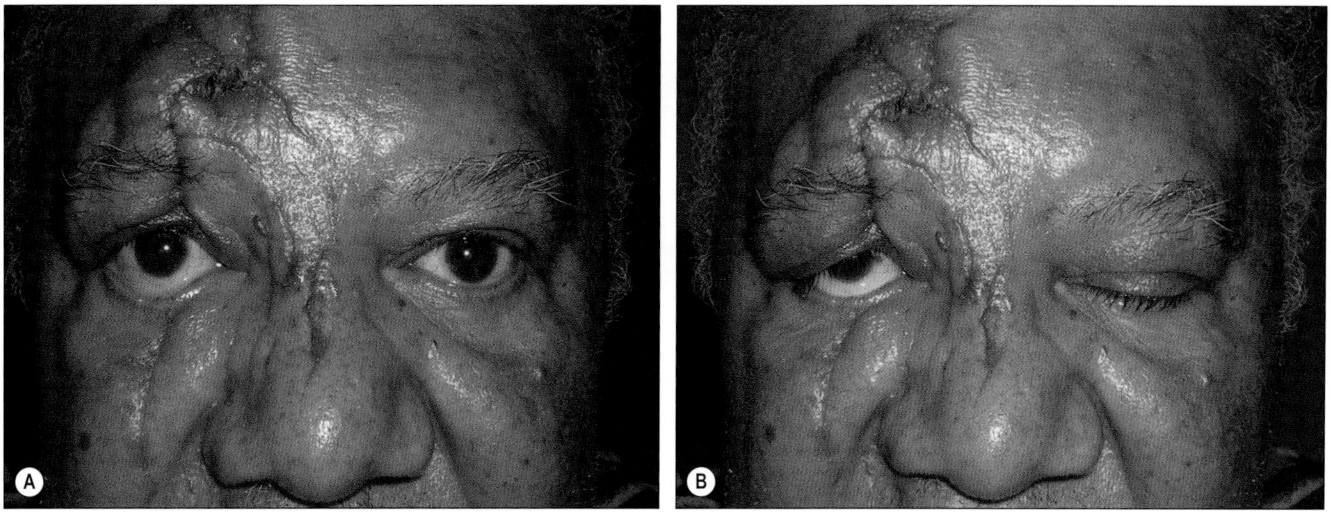

Fig. 30.5 Patient with lagophthalmos due to cicatricial shortening of the upper eyelid. Although the lid remains at reasonably normal height when opened (**A**), the vertical shortage becomes apparent with attempted forced closure (**B**) when the adynamic lid is unable to excurse downward to cover the cornea.

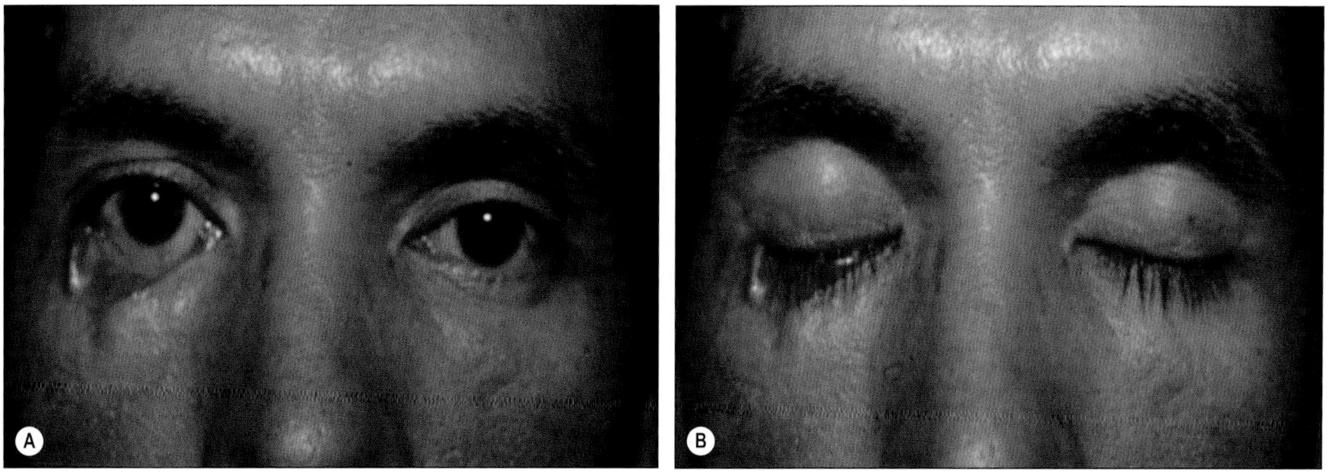

Fig. 30.6 Lagophthalmos. **A**, Patient with long-standing traumatic loss of the entire left lower lid. **B**, Patient demonstrates good corneal cover during closure by downward excursion of the upper lid. Slit lamp examination of this patient revealed no evidence of ocular surface abnormality.

may also have inadequate periocular vertical skin. Measurement of the vertical dimension of skin between the brow and the upper lid margin should demonstrate at least 20 mm to allow complete downward excursion of the upper eyelid during closure.

Closure of the eyelids is primarily a function of the descending upper lid; the lower lid exhibits very little upward movement during closure.[26] For this reason many patients tolerate lower lid retraction or scleral show with minimal or no symptoms as long as the upper lid retains normal excursion (Fig. 30.6). Levator function, or the excursion of the eyelid from up to down, should be measured in all patients in whom lagophthalmos is suspected. Patients with inadequate mobility of the upper eyelid retractors may have lagophthalmos despite a normal vertical amount of skin. This is often observed in patients with congenital ptosis, in whom the stiff, fat-infiltrated levator muscle fails to relax during closure. Vertical shortening of the levator muscle following ptosis surgery further exacerbates this problem. Patients at risk for lagophthalmos from inadequate downward excursion of the lid will have reduced levator function (<15 mm from extreme upgaze to extreme downgaze) and will demonstrate lid lag (a 'hanging up' of the upper eyelid) in downgaze.

Symblepharon between the bulbar and palpebral conjunctiva may also limit downward excursion of the upper eyelid and cause lagophthalmos. The lagophthalmos may actually worsen during closure if there is a prominent Bell's phenomenon, as the lid will be drawn superiorly by the upturning globe. Inspection of the superior fornix reveals the symblepharon, which is invariably quite extensive.

Abnormal globe protrusion is another frequent cause of lagophthalmos. As the globe protrudes forward, it increases the amount of lid excursion necessary to cover the cornea fully during closure. Lagophthalmos associated with proptosis occurs most often in patients with thyroid

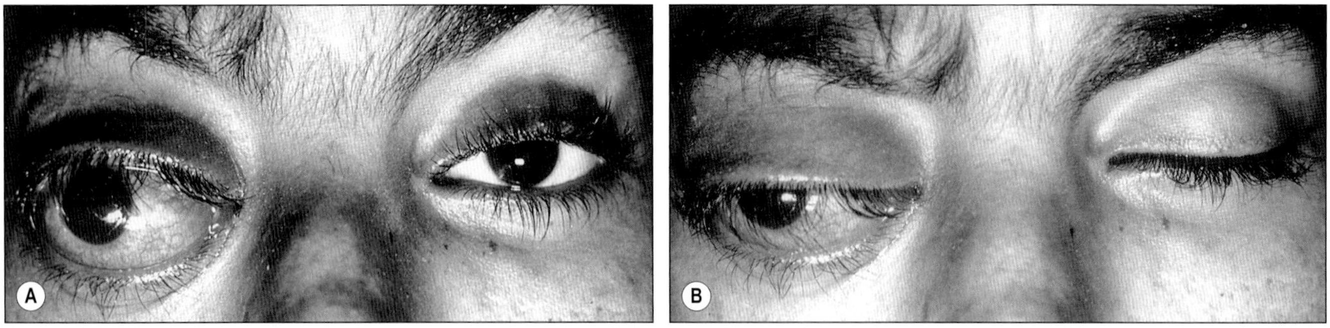

Fig. 30.7 Lagophthalmos. **A**, Patient with posttraumatic subperiosteal orbital hematoma causing proptosis and secondary lid retraction. **B**, Lagophthalmos with attempted closure occurring because the upper lid lacked sufficient vertical height to cover the more protuberant globe.

ophthalmopathy, where fibrosis of the retracting levator muscle may also play a role. Lagophthalmos may also be seen in patients with retrobulbar tumors or hemorrhage displacing the globe forward (Fig. 30.7). Inadequate development of the bony orbit, which occurs in some forms of craniosynostosis, may also result in abnormal globe protrusion. Patients with lid retraction and no proptosis rarely exhibit lagophthalmos.

Several studies of large groups of humans without periocular abnormalities have shown that up to 5% may sleep with their eyes partially open,[27–29] yet very few of these people suffer symptoms of exposure. A majority are probably protected by Bell's phenomenon, by which the cornea moves superiorly beneath the cover of the upper eyelid during sleep. However, a number of patients with nocturnal lagophthalmos will have symptomatic ocular surface breakdown. These patients typically complain of ocular irritation, foreign body sensation, and lacrimation on awakening.[30] Examination reveals typical interpalpebral epithelial keratopathy or breakdown. Lyons and McNab[24] reported on a large series of patients with symptomatic nocturnal lagophthalmos and concluded that this syndrome may be more common than previously thought. Interestingly, in most of their patients the symptoms were unilateral. Testing for Bell's phenomenon did not predict the eye position during sleep as manifested by the distribution of punctate corneal staining. In 42% of these patients no cause could be found, but in 30% alcohol intoxication preceded symptomatic presentation. Use of hypnotics also seemed to predispose to the development of nocturnal exposure symptoms.

Obtunded or comatose patients will often exhibit lagophthalmos because of inadequate central seventh-nerve tone. Staff treating such patients need to be aware of the serious ocular sequela that may result. In addition, unconscious patients with concurrent fifth cranial nerve dysfunction are at particular risk for breakdown of the corneal epithelium.

Treatment

Maintenance of a moist ocular surface is critical. Regardless of etiology, initial symptomatic treatment is directed toward increasing ocular surface lubrication and reducing evaporative drying. Viscous artificial tear substitutes or ointments will often relieve symptoms. Prefabricated moisture chambers are commercially available, or thin polyethylene film can be taped over an exposed eye in acute cases.

Even patients with significant lagophthalmos vary widely in their ability to tolerate it. Differences in tear production and the protective Bell's phenomenon are probably responsible for the variation in corneal breakdown observed in patients with similar degrees of lagophthalmos. Temporary or permanent tarsorrhaphy will sometimes be necessary in some patients to further prevent evaporative drying.

Definitive treatment of lagophthalmos depends on accurate diagnosis of the underlying cause. Whenever possible, address the specific abnormality responsible. It is important to determine whether the lagophthalmos is due to abnormal globe protrusion, inadequate vertical dimensions of the eyelids, inadequate protractor force, or abnormal lid–globe adhesions.

Patients with proptosis are usually best managed by orbital decompression and repositioning of the globe within the orbit. Patients who are not candidates for orbital decompression may undergo lid lengthening procedures in an attempt to reposition the lids anteriorly to the corneal apex during closure. However, if there is significant proptosis it is often difficult to lengthen the lids sufficiently. Proptosis due to craniosynostosis syndromes requires craniofacial surgery and orbital expansion to reposition the globes posteriorly. On occasion, traumatic deformities may cause partial collapse of the orbital skeleton with protrusion of the globe. These patients require reconstruction of the underlying bony abnormality and reexpansion of the orbit. Patients with a retrobulbar mass or hemorrhage displacing the globe anteriorly require removal or drainage of the retrobulbar lesion to allow the globe to be repositioned in the orbit.

Lagophthalmos caused by traumatic or iatrogenic shortening of the eyelids usually requires reconstructive soft tissue surgery. In such cases, symptomatic lagophthalmos almost always results from decreased upper lid excursion. It is important to determine whether the problem is due to inadequate skin, as in patients following eyelid burns or after aggressive skin removal at blepharoplasty, or is due to increased tightness and shortening of the 'middle lamella' (eyelid retractors). The latter is usually seen following ptosis repair or traumatic scar contracture following full-thickness lid lacerations. Measurement of the upper eyelid skin and observing the lid position in both primary and downgaze will help to differentiate between shortage of skin and tight middle lamella. If the lower lid is contributing to incomplete closure, inferior scleral show should be obvious.

Lagophthalmos due to inadequate vertical skin requires anterior lamellar replacement with skin flaps or grafts. Lagophthalmos due to a tight middle lamella that resists complete closure requires recession of the eyelid retractors. Lid lengthening procedures, by releasing either Müller's muscle or the levator aponeurosis, may increase the vertical excursion. Surgeons vary in their use of spacers or simple retractor recession in the upper eyelid. In the lower lid, recessing of the retractors is usually performed in combination with placement of a spacer to counteract the effect of gravity. Lagophthalmos due to lid–globe adhesion by symblepharon must be treated by releasing the symblepharon and reconstructing the appropriate fornix with mucous membrane grafting.

The most commonly encountered cause of lagophthalmos is orbicularis oculi paralysis due to seventh-nerve dysfunction. This may occur due to lesions anywhere along the course of the seventh nerve from the central brain stem nucleus to the distal peripheral nerve. Dysfunction may be caused by local compression, traumatic disruption, or viral or autoimmune inflammation (as in Bell's palsy). In those patients with acute seventh-nerve dysfunction who visit an ophthalmologist, consultation with an otologist may be advisable to determine etiology and to discuss possible treatment strategies that would enhance recovery of the seventh nerve. It is important to determine whether seventh-nerve dysfunction is anticipated to be permanent (e.g., following removal of the nerve as part of radical cancer resection) or temporary (as experienced by over 75% of patients with Bell's palsy). Temporizing measures to reduce evaporation and increase lubrication as described previously may be sufficient in patients with limited exposure of anticipated short duration.

If exposure is severe or anticipated to be long lasting, more permanent surgical corrections should be considered. The importance of testing corneal sensation in patients with seventh-nerve dysfunction of intracranial origin cannot be overemphasized. The combination of a hypesthetic cornea and incomplete closure is particularly threatening to the cornea, and these patients will often require extensive tarsorrhaphy. However, because tarsorrhaphy is cosmetically disfiguring and visually limiting, recent attention has been directed towards finding other means of reintroducing dynamic closure of the paralyzed upper lid.

Various techniques have been used to reanimate the facial musculature in seventh cranial nerve paralysis, including primary facial nerve repair, cross-facial nerve grafting, hypoglossal facial nerve transfer, temporalis muscle transfer, and free innervative muscle transfer.[31] All of these procedures are time-consuming and none will perfectly restore the blink reflex or voluntary closure. Various mechanical aids to eyelid closure have also been used, including eyelid weights, palpebral springs, silastic bands, and permanent eyelid magnets.[32–35] All of these various loading procedures rely on a normally functioning levator muscle to open the eyelid voluntarily. With attempted closure, the levator is inhibited and the gravitational pull exerted on the lid load causes downward excursion and lid closure. Recently, attention has centered chiefly on loading of the upper lid by subcutaneous placement of a gold weight.[31–36] The appropriate size of weight may be determined by taping various weights to the lid preoperatively in order to anticipate the proper weight to minimize ptosis and allow reasonably complete closure. The material consists of 99.9% pure 24 karat gold and is sutured to the tarsus with 7/0 nylon after exposure through an upper eyelid crease incision (Fig. 30.8). It is important to avoid damage to the levator aponeurosis during dissection over the surface of the tarsus to avoid postoperative ptosis. Several series have reported that more than 90% had 'success' with gold weight implantation for paralytic lagophthalmos.[31,37] Although some degree of lagophthalmos may often persist after gold weight implantation, it is usually diminished enough that topical lubrication will control exposure symptoms. Because of this high early success rate many surgeons now consider initial placement of a gold weight even in those patients who are felt likely to recover seventh-nerve function over time. In such patients the weight can be easily removed through a small skin incision when it is no longer required. Alternately, weights may be temporarily fixed to the skin with adhesive while awaiting the return of seventh-nerve function.

Gold weight implantation may be complicated by migration or extrusion of the weight, and lid loading may result in corneal pressure leading to astigmatism. Very rarely, patients may exhibit an allergic reaction to gold, resulting in persistent erythema and swelling. Recently lid loading with platinum chains has been reported. These are reported to be more malleable and to adapt to the tarsal contour better than rigid gold weights. This may reduce migration or exposure. The chains also are more dense, so that for a given weight, the platinum implant is 10% smaller. These are particularly indicated in patients with gold allergy.[38]

Because gold weight implantation of the upper lid often results in diminished but persistent lagophthalmos, elevation of the paralytic lower lid is also important in these patients to further narrow the palpebral aperture and minimize tear film evaporation and exposure. Patients with paralytic ectropion were historically managed by horizontal tightening. Although this procedure will relieve ectropion, it virtually always leaves some degree of residual lower lid retraction and scleral show due to the lack of orbicularis tone. In patients with relative proptosis lower lid retraction may even be exacerbated by horizontal tightening, because this tends to draw the lid beneath the globe. For these reasons, patients with paralytic lower lid laxity and ectropion are best managed by placing a spacer interposed posteriorly between the tarsus and lid retractors to elevate and support the lid.[39] Horizontal tightening is also performed if there is significant laxity of the lid. Many spacer materials have been used, including donor sclera or fascia, polytetrafluoroethylene (Gore-tex), autogenous ear or nasal cartilage, acellular dermis (human or porcine), or hard palate mucosa. The use of hard palate mucosa has become increasingly popular for the relief of lower lid retraction. It results in permanent correction of lower eyelid retraction in 85% of patients.[40] Patients who have unacceptable residual lagophthalmos, despite upper lid loading and placement of a spacer in the lower lid, may benefit from a limited lateral tarsorrhaphy as well.

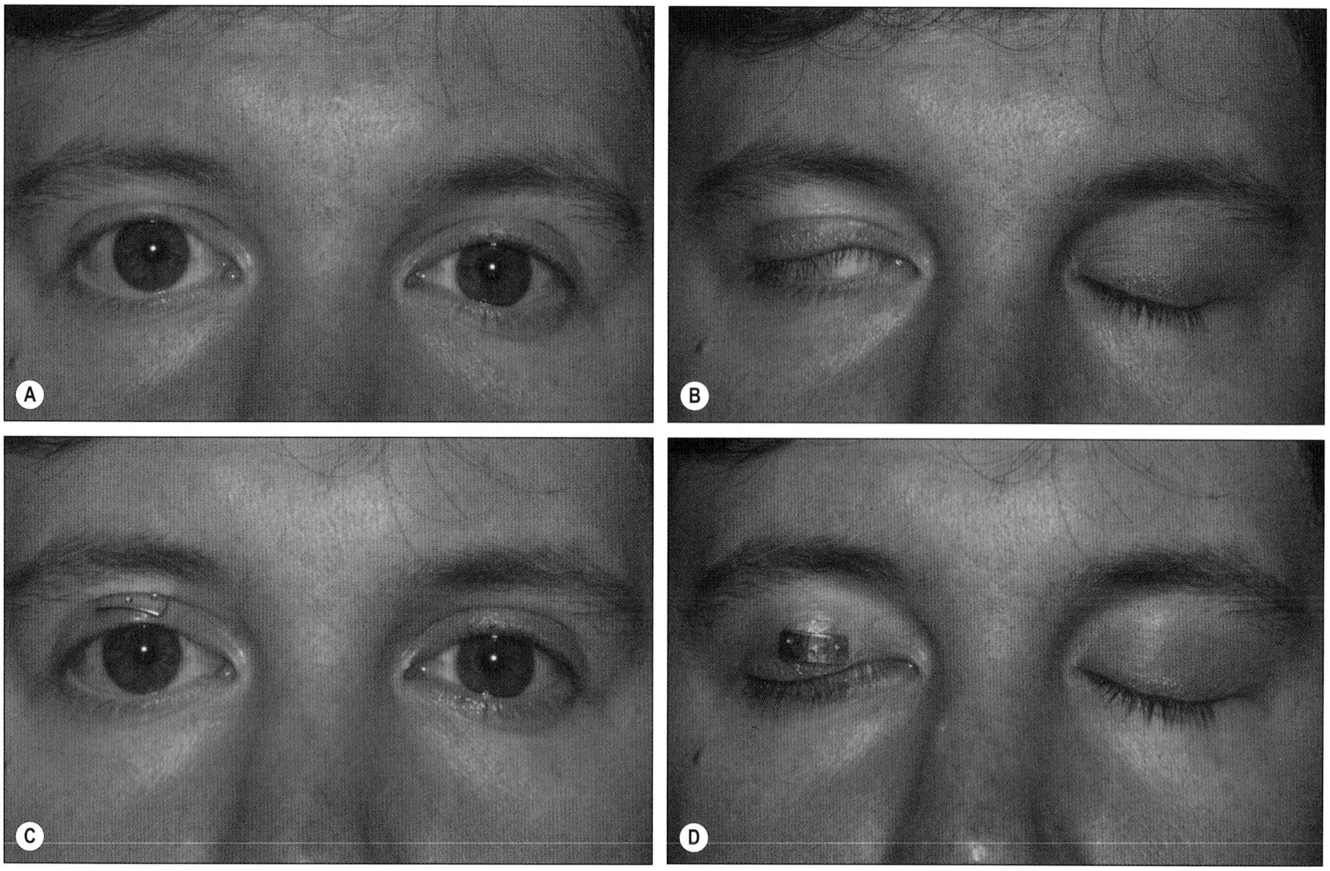

Fig. 30.8 Patient with persistent posttraumatic seventh-nerve palsy demonstrating lagophthalmos (**A** and **B**). Appearance after implantation of a 1 g gold weight through an upper eyelid crease incision (**C**). When closure is attempted, the levator muscle is inhibited and gravity allows the eyelid to close with the aid of the weight (**D**).

Eyelid Retraction

The normal upper eyelid should rest approximately 1–2 mm below the superior limbus and the normal lower eyelid at or just above the inferior limbus. In eyelid retraction the lids are drawn proximally away from the limbus, which results in exposure of the sclera above and below. The upper eyelid disorder occurs most commonly in association with thyroid ophthalmopathy. It may also occur due to tightening of the middle lamella following iatrogenic or traumatic damage; reduced orbicularis tone, which allows unopposed action of the levator muscle; inferior rectus restriction with resultant overstimulation of the superior rectus–levator complex; or lesions of the rostral midbrain. In the lower eyelid, retraction again most often results from thyroid ophthalmopathy. It can also occur following large recessions of the inferior rectus muscle or following lower eyelid surgery, in which scarring of the lower lid retractors (the capsulopalpebral fascia) has occurred. Significant globe protrusion can cause the lids to ride back as the globe comes forward, causing upper and lower eyelid retraction (Fig. 30.7).

Eyelid retraction causes symptoms primarily because of increased evaporation of the tear film. This is due to the broader exposed surface area of the globe and may also be associated with reduced frequency of blinking. Symptoms consist of irritation, foreign body sensation, and increased lacrimation. Slit lamp examination often reveals epithelial keratopathy and reduced tear break-up time. Although lid retraction and lagophthalmos may coexist, these entities need to be distinguished. Most patients with lid retraction do not have lagophthalmos, and most patients with lagophthalmos do not have lid retraction.

Treatment

Treatment depends on the underlying cause. In the absence of proptosis, attention should be directed to surgically lengthening the eyelid retractors to reset the lid margin at the limbus. In the upper eyelid, release of Müller's muscle and the levator aponeurosis is best performed under local anesthesia with intraoperative adjustment of lid contour.[41] Recession of these structures can be achieved with or without an interposed spacer. More recently full-thickness blepharotomy has become popular.[42] This is a reasonably quick and simple procedure which appears to have success comparable to that of more complicated retractor recession. In the lower lid, release of the retractors alone may improve 1–2 mm of lid retraction, but greater degrees usually require placement of a spacer for permanent correction. These techniques are described in the preceding paragraphs.

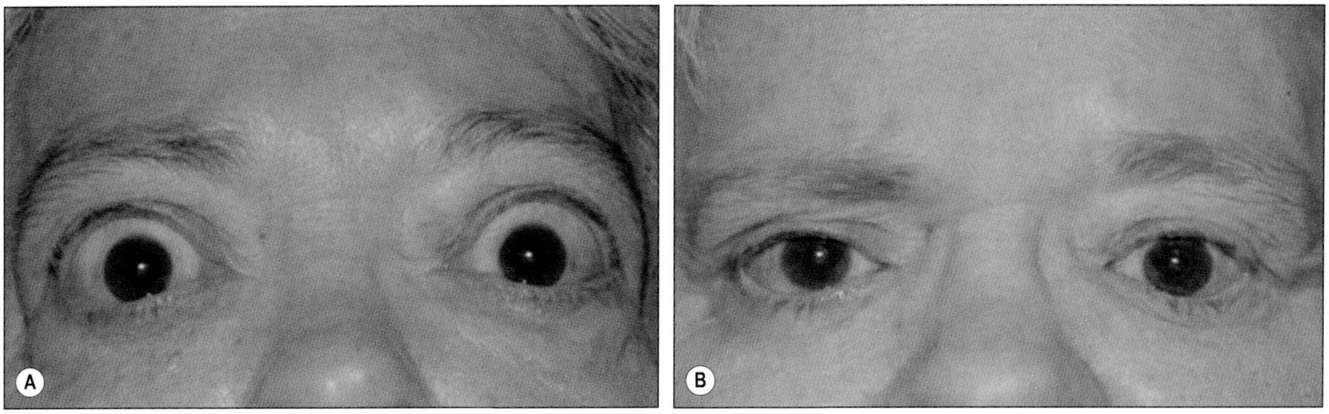

Fig. 30.9 Eyelid retraction. **A**, Patient with upper eyelid retraction following orbital decompression for Graves' ophthalmopathy. **B**, Recession of the inferior rectus muscle bilaterally resulted in correction of the eyelid retraction without the need for eyelid surgery.

In patients with thyroid ophthalmopathy, lid retraction, and proptosis, surgical rehabilitation is complex and must be carried out in an orderly fashion. Patients requiring orbital decompression should have this first, followed by extraocular muscle surgery as necessary, followed by eyelid surgery. Orbital decompression will often paradoxically exacerbate upper lid retraction, especially if the orbital floor is removed. This is due to progressive downward prolapse of the inferior rectus muscle into the maxillary sinus with progressive restriction of globe elevation. Increased neural stimulation to the opposing superior rectus–levator complex results, in order to bring the eye back up to the primary position. When upper eyelid retraction is due to overstimulation of the levator–superior rectus complex in response to a restricted inferior rectus, recession of the tight inferior rectus muscle may relieve the upper lid retraction without the need for eyelid surgery (Fig. 30.9).[41,43]

References

1. Culbertson WW, Ostler HB. The floppy eyelid syndrome. *Am J Ophthalmol.* 1981;92:568–575.
2. Paciuc M, Mier ME. A woman with the floppy eyelid syndrome. *Am J Ophthalmol.* 1982;93:255–256.
3. Eiferman RA, Gossman MD, O'Neill K, et al. Floppy eyelid syndrome in a child. *Am J Ophthalmol.* 1990;109:356–357.
4. Culbertson WW, Tseng SC. Corneal disorders in floppy eyelid syndrome. *Cornea.* 1994;13:33–42.
5. Schwartz LK, Gelender H, Forster RK. Chronic conjunctivitis associated with floppy eyelids. *Arch Ophthalmol.* 1983;101:1884–1888.
6. Rapoza PA, Quinn TC, Terry AC, et al. A systemic approach to the diagnosis and treatment of chronic conjunctivitis. *Am J Ophthalmol.* 1990;109:138–142.
7. Langford JD, Linberg JV. A new physical finding in floppy eyelid syndrome. *Ophthalmology.* 1998;105:1977–1978.
8. Netland PA, Sugrue SP, Albert DM, et al. Histopathologic features of the floppy eyelid syndrome. *Ophthalmology.* 1994;101:174–181.
9. Goldberg R, Seiff S, McFarland J, et al. Floppy eyelid syndrome and blepharochalasis. *Am J Ophthalmol.* 1986;93:184–188.
10. Parunovic A. Floppy eyelid syndrome. *Br J Ophthalmol.* 1983;67:264–266.
11. Donnenfield ED, Perry HD, Gibalter RP, et al. Keratoconus associated with floppy eyelid syndrome. *Ophthalmology.* 1991;98:1674–1678.
12. Rossiter JD, Ellingham R, Hakin KN, et al. Corneal melt and perforation secondary to floppy eyelid syndrome in the presence of rheumatoid arthritis. *Br J Ophthalmol.* 2002;86(4):483.
13. Mojon DS, Goldblum D, Fleischhauer J, et al. Eyelid, conjunctival, and corneal findings in sleep apnea syndrome. *Ophthalmology.* 1999;106:1182–1185.
14. Dutton JJ. Surgical management of floppy eyelid syndrome. *Am J Ophthalmol.* 1985;99:557–560.
15. Arocker-Mettinger E, Haddad R, Konrad K, et al. Floppy eyelid syndrome; licht-und elektronemikroskopische untersuchungen. *Klin Monatsbl Augenheilkd.* 1986;188:596–598.
16. Gonnering RS, Sonneland PR. Meibomian gland dysfunction in floppy eyelid syndrome. *Ophthalmol Plast Reconstruct Surg.* 1987;3(2):99–103.
17. Woog JJ. Obstructive sleep apnea and the floppy eyelid syndrome. *Am J Ophthalmol.* 1990;110:314–315.
18. Riefler DM. Floppy eyelids in crack eye syndrome. *Ophthalmology.* 1993;100:975.
19. van den Bosch WA, Lemij HG. The lax eyelid syndrome. *Br J Ophthalmol.* 1994;78:666–676.
20. McNab AA. Reversal of floppy eyelid syndrome with treatment of obstructive sleep apnoea. *Clin Exp Ophthalmol.* 2000;28:125–126.
21. Bouchard CS. Lateral tarsorrhaphy for a non-compliant patient with floppy eyelid syndrome. *Am J Ophthalmol.* 1992;114:367–368.
22. Karesh JW, Nirankari VS, Hameroff SB. Eyelid imbrication. An unrecognized cause of chronic ocular irritation. *Ophthalmology.* 1993;100:883–889.
23. Donnenfeld ED, Perry HD, Schrier A, et al. Lid imbrication syndrome. Diagnosis with rose Bengal staining. *Ophthalmology.* 1994;101:763–766.
24. Lyons CJ, McNab AA. Symptomatic nocturnal lagophthalmos. *Aust NZ J Ophthalmol.* 1990;18:393–396.
25. Francis IC, Loughhead JA. Bell's phenomenon. A study of 505 patients. *Aust NZ J Ophthalmol.* 1984;12:15–21.
26. Hall AJ. Some observations on the active opening and closing of the eyes. *Br J Ophthalmol.* 1936;20:257–295.
27. Howitt DA, Goldstein JH. Physiological lagophthalmos. *Am J Ophthalmol.* 1969;68:355.
28. Fuchs A, Wu FC. Sleep with half open eyes (physiological lagophthalmos). *Am J Ophthalmol.* 1948;1:717–720.
29. Mueller FO. Lagophthalmos during sleep. *Br J Ophthalmol.* 1957;51:246–248.
30. Sturrock JD. Nocturnal lagophthalmos in recurrent erosion. *Br J Ophthalmol.* 1975;60:97–103.
31. Townsend DJ. Eyelid re-animation for the treatment of paralytic lagophthalmos: historical prospectives in current applications of the gold weight implant. *Ophthalmol Plast Reconstructrg.* 1992;8:196–201.
32. Arion HG. Dynamic closure of the lids in paralysis of the orbicularis muscle. *Int Surg.* 1972;57:48.
33. Morel-Fatio D, Lalardrie JP. Palliative surgical treatment of facial paralysis: the palpebral spring. *Ann Chir Plast Esthet.* 1962;7:275.
34. May M. Gold weight and wire spring implants as alternatives to tarsorrhaphy. *Arch Otolaryngol Head Neck Surg.* 1987;113:656–660.
35. Illig KM. Eine Neue Operationsmethode Gegen Lagophthalmos. *Klin Monatsbl Augenheilkd.* 1988;132:410–411.
36. Pickford MA, Scamp T, Harrison DA. Morbidity after gold weight insertion in the upper eyelid and facial palsy. *Br J Plast Surg.* 1992;45:460–464.
37. Kelley SA, Sharpe DT. Gold eyelid weights in patients with facial palsy. *Plast Reconstruct Surg.* 1992;89:436–440.
38. Berghaus A, Neumann K, Schrom T. The platinum chain: a new upper-lid implant for facial palsy. *Arch Facial Plast Surg.* 2003;5(2):166–170.

39. Kersten RC, Kulwin DR. Management of lower lid retraction with hard palate mucosa grafting. *Arch Ophthalmol.* 1990;108:1339–1343.
40. Wearne MJ, Sandy C, Rose GE, Pitts J, Collin JRO. Autogenous hard palate mucosa: the ideal lower eyelid spacer? *Br J Ophthalmol.* 2001;85: 1183–1187.
41. Wesley RE, Bond JB. Upper eyelid retraction from inferior rectus restriction in disc thyroid orbit disease. *Ann Ophthalmol.* 1987;19:34–36.
42. Elner VM, Hassan AS, Freuh BR. Graded full-thickness anterior blepharotomy for upper eyelid retraction. *Trans Am Ophthalmol Soc.* 2003;101:67–75.
43. Thaller VT, et al. Thyroid lid surgery. *Eye.* 1987;1:609–614.

Chapter 31

Benign Lid Tumors

Richard C. Allen, Michael L. Murphy, Jeffrey A. Nerad

Numerous benign tumors and related noninfectious, noninflammatory lesions arise from the varied structures composing the eyelid. Classification of the lesions discussed in this chapter will be according to the structure of origin: epidermis, dermis, and eyelid adnexa. Melanocytic lesions will be described separately. Many benign eyelid lesions may appear elsewhere on the body as cutaneous lesions. However, when present in the eyelids, their appearance and behavior may differ, due in part to the unique characteristics of the eyelid skin and anatomy. Other eyelid lesions may represent manifestations of systemic disease.

Histology of the Eyelid Skin

The skin of the eyelids is the thinnest on the body, and continues to thin with advancing age. The upper eyelid skin is thinner than the lower eyelid skin. The thin skin characteristic of the eyelids usually extends a short distance beyond the orbital rim. Eyelid skin consists of a keratinized epidermis overlying a poorly defined papillary dermis, which is void of rete ridges. The dermis is separated from the underlying orbicularis oculi muscle by a very thin areolar subcutaneous connective tissue layer void of fat.[1]

The epidermis is composed of two cell types, keratinocytes and dendritic cells. Keratinocytes are arranged in four layers. From deep to superficial, these are the basal, squamous, granular, and horny cell layers.

The basal cell layer consists of a single row of columnar-shaped cells that lie on a basement membrane. This basement membrane is firmly attached to the underlying dermis. The basal layer generates the more superficial layers of the epidermis. The basal keratinocytes contain a variable amount of melanin pigment, which is derived from the adjacent dendritic melanocytes. The degree of skin pigmentation is thus dependent on the amount of pigment present.[1]

The squamous cell layer consists of polygonal cells arranged in a mosaic pattern, usually 5–10 layers thick. The cells become more flattened as they mature and migrate towards the skin surface.

The granular cell layer, also called the prickle-cell layer, consists of a row of elongated, flattened cells. The cytoplasm of the granular cells is filled with basophilic keratohyaline granules.

The horny cell layer consists of flat, anuclear, keratinized cells.

The basal keratinocytes are undifferentiated. As they divide, the cells either remain in the proliferative pool or begin to differentiate. As the cells differentiate, they migrate toward the surface, flatten, and become anucleate. This process terminates as cell death in the superficial horny layer where keratinization occurs.

The second cell type of the epidermis is the dendritic cell. Three types of dendritic cells are present in the epidermis: clear cell melanocytes, Langerhans cells, and undetermined dendritic cells. Histochemistry and electron microscopy are necessary to identify the Langerhans and undetermined cell types.

The epidermal adnexa of the eyelids includes the pilosebaceous unit and the eccrine and apocrine sweat glands. The pilosebaceous unit consists of the eyelid cilia and associated sebaceous glands of Zeis. Sebaceous glands are holocrine glands; thus, their acini possess no lumina, and secretion is via decomposition of their cells. Sebaceous glands may develop from the external root sheath of the hair follicle and empty into the hair follicle. Alternatively, as is the case of the meibomian gland, glandular elements may develop from the epidermis and empty at the skin surface. The meibomian gland is composed of several lobules, which lead to a common secretory duct.[1]

Eccrine and apocrine glands are the two distinct types of sweat glands in humans. Eccrine sweat glands are independent of the hair follicle apparatus. They are found everywhere on the skin surface except the vermilion border of the lip, the glans penis, and the nail bed. Eccrine glands hypersecrete mainly in response to thermal stimuli, thereby aiding in thermoregulation. However, eccrine glands of the axilla, palms, and soles also hypersecrete in response to emotional stimuli. Eccrine glands contain both secretory and ductal components. The secretory cells of the gland are located in the dermis. The ductal cells are located in the dermis and epidermis and function to transport sweat to the skin surface. A wide variety of tumors originate from the pluripotential cells, which normally differentiate into the various components of the eccrine sweat gland unit.

Apocrine sweat glands serve no useful purpose in humans, and function only as scent glands. In the eyelid these glands are referred to as the glands of Moll. They are active only in the years between puberty and senescence. Like sebaceous glands, they are influenced by circulating androgens. Emotional stimuli, mediated through the sympathetic nervous system, stimulate gland secretion. Apocrine glands are larger than sebaceous glands and lie deeper in the skin. They are simple tubular glands that often open above a sebaceous gland orifice in the hair canal. Like the eccrine sweat glands, they have both secretory and ductal components. The sweat from these glands is formed by decapitation and extrusion of the secretory cell cytoplasm into the gland lumen. The sweat is then transported to the skin surface by ductal cells. Tumors of apocrine sweat gland origin are common. Histopathologic examination is frequently required to differentiate between the various benign tumors of the apocrine sweat gland apparatus.

Hair follicles present in the eyelid include the eyelashes and the vellus hairs of the skin. Eyelashes are terminal hair follicles. Vellus hairs cover the remaining skin of the eyelid. These vellus hairs are associated with sebaceous glands.

The dermis of the eyelid is composed of bundles of collagen, variable amounts of elastic and reticulin fibers, and ground substance containing mucopolysaccharide. Nerve fibers, blood vessels, and lymphatics course through the dermis.

Approach to Diagnosis and Management

Many benign tumors of the eyelids may be readily diagnosed on the basis of characteristic clinical appearance, location, and behavior. Some tumors, however, may require biopsy for reliable and definitive differentiation from malignant tumors. Two studies examining the accuracy of clinical diagnosis of eyelid lesions have been reported. One study found that 1.9% of presumed benign lesions proved to be malignant after histopathologic examination; the sensitivity of clinical diagnosis of malignancy was 89.7%, and the specificity was 98.2%.[2] In the other study, 4.6% of presumed benign lesions proved to be malignant; the sensitivity of clinical diagnosis of malignancy was 87.5%, and the specificity was 81.5%.[3] The authors of the first study concluded that all lesions, no matter how apparently benign, should be examined histopathologically.

An incisional biopsy is performed by excising a representative portion of the lesion for histopathologic evaluation. This technique is employed for large-sized lesions. In cases of small tumors, an excisional biopsy may fulfill both diagnostic and treatment goals. Any complete excisional biopsy must include adjacent normal tissue on all margins. The shave biopsy technique is indicated for lesions which involve only the epidermis or upper dermis (e.g. seborrheic keratosis). Shave biopsies are inadequate for pigmented lesions and in cases necessitating differentiation between a keratoacanthoma and squamous cell carcinoma.

Microscopic control with surgical tumor excision can be achieved by either the Mohs' fresh tissue tumor resection technique, or frozen-section controlled excision. In the Mohs' technique, the lesion is shaved into thin sections that are evaluated microscopically. The advantage of this technique is maximum preservation of normal tissue. This technique is especially useful for eyelid lesions. In the frozen-section control method, the lesion and a 3–6-mm margin of normal-appearing tissue are resected, depending on the type of tumor. The margins are then shaved, and the frozen sections are evaluated microscopically by a pathologist to confirm presence or absence of tumor. If margins are involved with a tumor, additional tissue is resected and analyzed until the margins are tumor free.

The majority of the benign lesions discussed here are most appropriately managed by observation or surgical excision. Lesions necessitating alternative treatment modalities will be discussed separately.

Benign Tumors of the Epidermis

As discussed earlier, four types of keratinocytes and three types of dendritic cells exist. Benign epidermal lesions may arise from any of these various cell types in the epidermis. Lesions will be classified and discussed according to epidermal cellular origin. The majority of the lesions described exhibit benign characteristics. Features of malignant transformation include rapid and asymmetric growth pattern, ulceration, color change, and bleeding. Lesions exhibiting any of these characteristics should always be biopsied to rule out malignancy.

Acrochordon

Acrochordon, also called skin tags (Fig. 31.1), are common benign eyelid tumors. Clinically, they appear as small, multiple, flesh-colored lesions attached to the lid margin by a thin pedicle.[4] Occasionally they may be large and pedunculated. These tumors are often ambiguously referred to as papillomata. Papillomata is a descriptive, yet nondiagnostic, term used to describe many cutaneous lesions with various histopathological diagnoses. A common variant is verruca vulgaris, which is an infectious lesion.

Histopathologically, acrochordons are characterized by thickening of the squamous cell layer (acanthosis) and the keratin layer (hyperkeratosis) without loss of polarity or cellular atypia.

Treatment consists of simple surgical excision of the lesion with a sample of the base included. This is easily performed with scissors or scalpel. Sutured closure is usually not necessary.

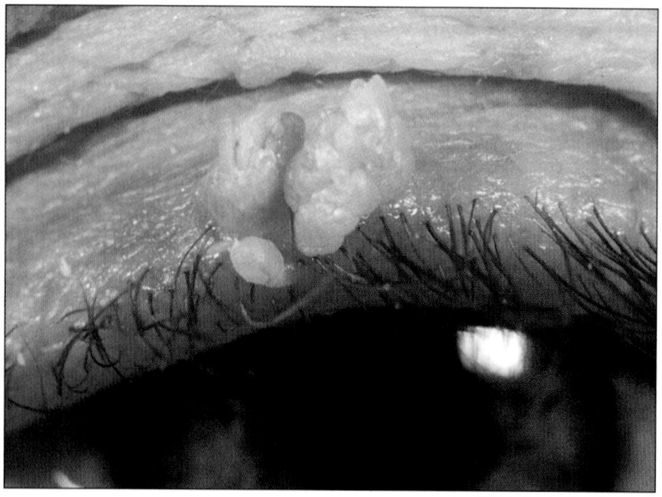

Fig. 31.1 Acrochordon (skin tag) of the upper eyelid.

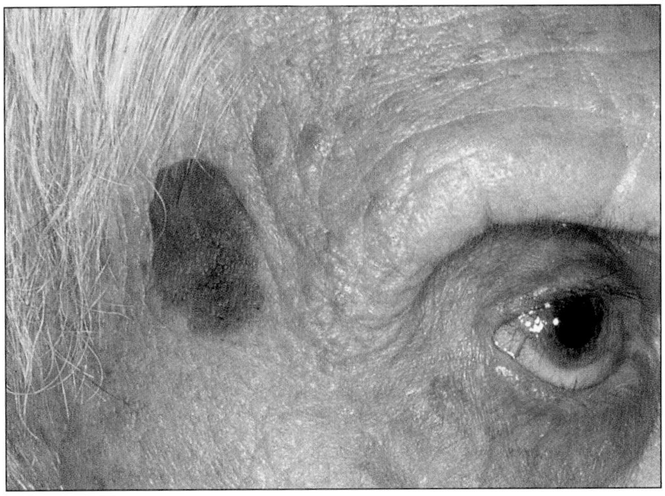

Fig. 31.2 Seborrheic keratosis of the temporal region of an elderly patient.

Milia

Milia are small, raised, round, white, sharply circumscribed cystic lesions of the eyelids.[5] Usually asymptomatic, milia may arise spontaneously, follow trauma, arise in areas of previous radiation, or appear during the healing phase of a bullous disease process. They are particularly common in newborn infants. Histopathologically, these lesions consist of superficial keratin cysts.

Treatment consists of incision of the overlying skin with a sharp blade or needle, and expression of the contents.

Seborrheic keratosis

Seborrheic keratoses are commonly acquired eyelid lesions affecting middle-aged and elderly patients. Clinical appearance varies considerably in terms of size and degree of pigmentation. This variability makes differentiation from nevi, pigmented basal cell carcinomas, and melanoma difficult in some cases (Fig. 31.2).[6] Single or multiple lesions may be present, and hyperpigmentation is common. The lesions have a different appearance when present on the eyelids versus elsewhere on the face. Facial lesions appear smooth and greasy, with elevated and well-demarcated borders producing a 'stuck on' appearance. Eyelid lesions appear lobulated, papillary, or pedunculated, with friable, cerebriform excrescences on the surface (Fig. 31.3A). A sudden eruption of multiple seborrheic keratoses may be a cutaneous manifestation of internal malignant disease (Leser-Trélat sign).[7] A heavily pigmented variant with multiple lesions seen in black individuals has been termed dermatosis papulosa nigra.[8]

Seborrheic keratoses are divided into three major histological types according to the predominant histologic features: hyperkeratotic, acanthotic, and adenoid. Variable degrees of hyperkeratosis and acanthosis are observed in all types. The acanthotic epidermis often contains keratin-filled cystic inclusions. These are referred to as horn cysts when they form within the mass, and pseudohorn cysts when they represent invaginations of surface keratin. Melanin may be abundant in keratinocytes, especially in the adenoid and acanthotic forms. The dermis is uninvolved except in cases of irritated seborrheic keratoses, in which case it is infiltrated by chronic inflammatory cells.

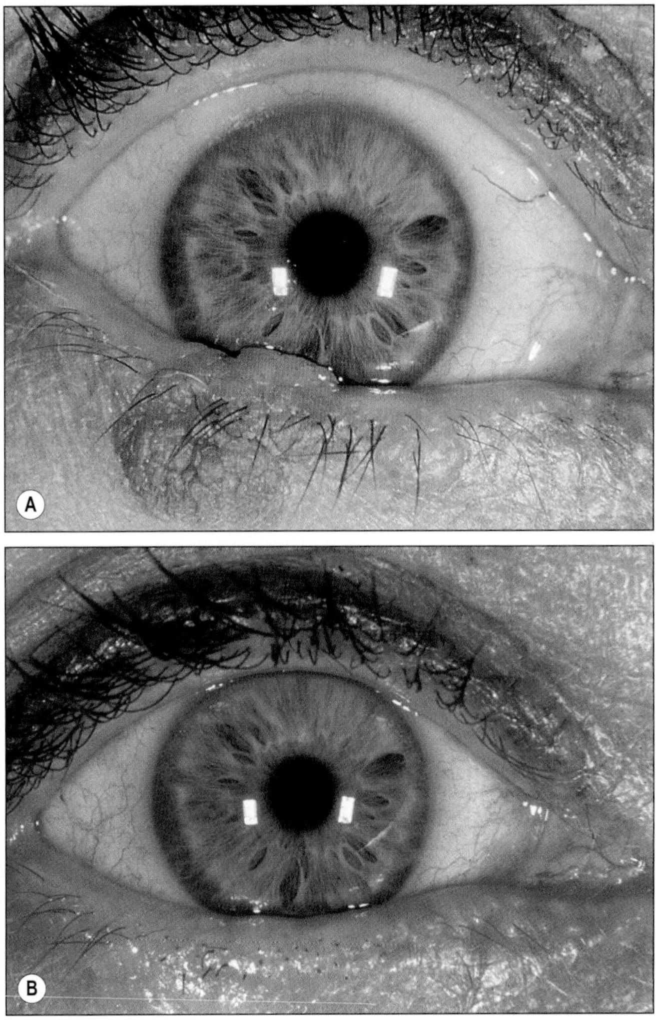

Fig. 31.3 Seborrheic keratosis of the lower eyelid. (**A**) The lesion displays a papillomatous configuration with friable, cerebriform excrescences. (**B**) The same patient following surgical excision of the lesion.

Surgical excision involves shaving the lesions from the skin surface with a scalpel (Fig. 31.3B). Although some lesions are large, the growth pattern is superficial and deep excision is unnecessary. The residual flat surface reepithelializes rapidly.[9]

Keratoacanthoma

Previously, keratoacanthoma was considered a benign, self-limiting lesion. Many authors now regard the tumor as a low-grade squamous cell carcinoma. Although trauma and sunlight exposure have been implicated in pathogenesis, the exact etiology remains unknown. Immunosuppressed patients also exhibit increased risk. Middle-aged or elderly patients are typically affected. Although commonly solitary, multiple lesion cases have been described. The distinctive

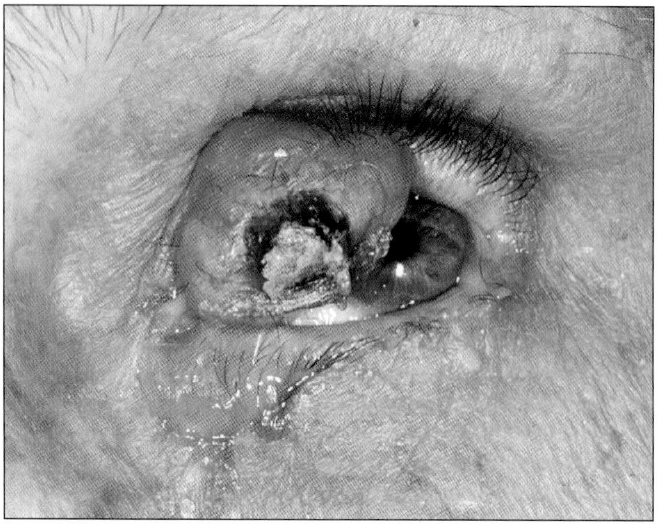

Fig. 31.4 A large keratoacanthoma of the upper eyelid. Note the central ulceration.

clinical appearance and behavior aid in diagnosis. The lesion usually begins as a small flesh-colored papule on the lower lid that develops rapidly over the course of a few weeks into a dome-shaped nodule, with a central, keratin-filled crater and elevated, rolled margins (Fig. 31.4). The lesion often clinically resembles nodular ulcerative basal cell carcinoma. Gradual resolution over the course of approximately 3–6 months ensues, and visible sequelae are rare.

Muir-Torre syndrome is an autosomal dominant disorder in which individuals have a predisposition towards keratoacanthoma, benign and malignant sebaceous tumors, and visceral malignancies. The syndrome is part of the Lynch cancer family syndrome II, which is associated with mutations in the MSH2 and MLH1 genes.[10]

Ferguson-Smith syndrome (multiple self-healing squamous epitheliomas) is an autosomal dominant condition in which multiple keratoacanthomas are observed. Linkage to 9q31 has been demonstrated.[11]

Histologically, a keratoacanthoma typically has a cup-shaped nodular elevation with thickening of the epidermis. The epidermis contains islands of well-differentiated squamous epithelium surrounding a central mass of keratin. Microabscesses may be present within the islands of squamous epithelium. The dermis shows a polymorphous inflammatory infiltrate.

Given the self-limited nature of keratoacanthoma, observation has been advocated. The prolonged healing period and the potential delay in treatment of a misdiagnosed malignancy are reasons to pursue a more definitive treatment strategy.

After incisional biopsy confirms the diagnosis, complete surgical excision is the recommended treatment.[12] Large, aggressive lesions have been treated with radiotherapy.[13] Alternative treatment modalities include cryotherapy, intralesional methotrexate, and topical or intralesional 5-fluorouracil.[14–16]

Pseudoepitheliomatous (pseudocarcinomatous) hyperplasia is a condition often seen in areas of cryosurgery or surgical wounds. It is commonly associated with chronic inflammation and shows an active proliferation of epidermoid or squamous cells that develop into a hyperkeratotic nodule on the skin surface.[17] Keratoacanthoma is considered to be a variant of pseudoepitheliomatous hyperplasia.

Inverted follicular keratosis

The clinical presentation of inverted follicular keratosis may vary. Nodular, papillomatous, verrucous, and cystic forms occur. The lesion is usually solitary, and hyperpigmentation is rare. Although the etiology is unknown, it is generally considered a form of irritated seborrheic keratosis.

The term inverted follicular keratosis describes the histopathological features of this lesion.[18] Epithelial lobular acanthosis with overlying hyperkeratosis and occasional central keratin-filled, cup-shaped invagination is observed. There is a proliferation of uniform basaloid cells with an abrupt transition to concentrically arranged squamoid cells. The dermis is uninvolved.

Treatment is surgical excision.

Cutaneous horn

Cutaneous horn is a clinically descriptive, nondiagnostic term. This lesion may be associated with a variety of benign or malignant lesions, including seborrheic keratosis, verruca vulgaris, and squamous or basal cell carcinoma.

Treatment should be directed at the underlying cutaneous lesion. Biopsy of the base of the cutaneous horn is required to establish the definitive diagnosis. Simple excision of the horn itself provides insufficient tissue for accurate diagnosis.

Epidermal inclusion cyst

This lesion (sebaceous cyst, epidermoid cyst) arises from the infundibulum of the hair follicle. It may occur spontaneously or as a sequela of surgical or traumatic implantation of epidermal tissue into the dermis.[19] Multiple facial inclusion cysts may be seen in patients with Gardner's syndrome, an autosomal dominant disorder characterized by intestinal polyps, multiple facial bone osteomas, fibromas and epithelial inclusion cysts of the skin, fibromatosis (dermoid tumors) of the abdominal wall, mesentery and breasts, and multiple lesions consistent with congenital hypertrophy of the retinal pigment epithelium (CHRPE). Mutations have been demonstrated in the APC gene in patients affected by this disease.[20,21] This slow-growing, elevated, round, smooth, firm, keratin-filled lesion rarely exceeds 1 cm in diameter (Fig. 31.5). It is often attached to the overlying, thinned skin by the remaining pilar duct that may appear as a pore. Rupture of the cyst may cause a foreign body reaction, with the cyst becoming secondarily infected. Malignant degeneration is extremely rare.

Recommended treatment is marsupialization, or if possible, excision of the cyst without violation of the cyst wall.

Linear epidermal nevus

A linear epidermal nevus may be solitary and localized, or multiple and part of the systemic epidermal nevus

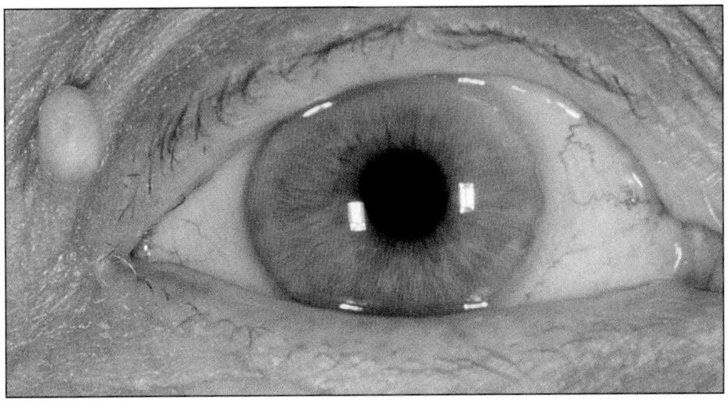

Fig. 31.5 Epidermal inclusion cyst of the right upper eyelid.

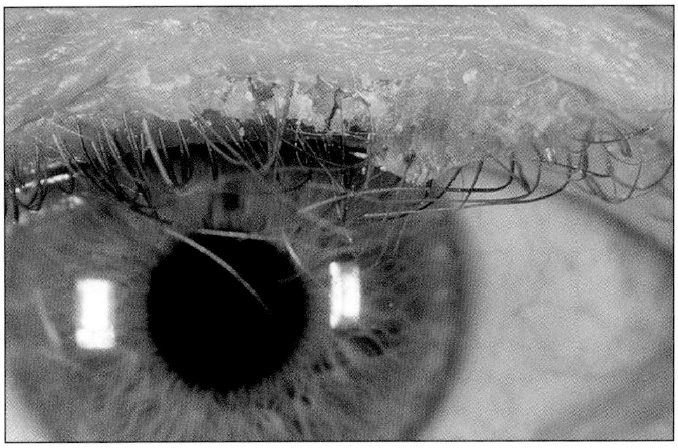

Fig. 31.6 Actinic keratosis of the upper eyelid margin.

syndrome. The lesion consists of multiple closely set, papillomatous, hyperkeratotic papules. Lesion color varies with the degree of pigmentation and hyperkeratosis. Individuals affected with the epidermal nevus syndrome may have associated skeletal deformities and CNS disorders.[22]

Surgical excision is usually curative. Alternate therapeutic modalities include cryotherapy, electrodesiccation, dermabrasion, and topical retinoic acid.

Nodular elastosis with cysts and comedones (Favre-Racouchot syndrome)

This condition occurs in the solar-damaged skin of older, fair-skinned Caucasians. Multiple comedones and yellow nodules with a central comedo occur most commonly near the lateral canthus and extend to the malar eminence and temple. The eyelid and facial skin often reveal other signs of actinic damage. Actinic comedonal plaque is a variant of this condition, in which a solitary plaque with small nodules, dilated follicles, and numerous underlying comedones occurs on the eyelid and facial skin.[23]

Treatment includes topical retinoic acid and mechanical removal of the cysts and comedones.

Actinic keratosis (solar keratosis)

Damage of the epidermal cells of the skin by ultraviolet radiation results in actinic or solar keratoses. Fair-skinned, older patients with a history of sun exposure of significant duration are typically affected. Lesions are multiple and affect the face, scalp, forearms, and dorsum of the hands. The lesions have a yellow-brown or erythematous color, an oval shape, and a white scale.[24] They may occur anywhere on the eyelids (Fig. 31.6). Although a precursor to squamous cell carcinoma, mitotic activity is low, and metastases are rare. Individuals with xeroderma pigmentosum have a predisposition to actinic keratoses and malignancies of the skin. This is an autosomal recessive condition due to a defect in repair of UV light-induced damage to the DNA of epidermal cells.[25] There are at least four different genetic loci.

Histopathology of actinic keratoses shows hyperkeratosis, irregular acanthosis, focal parakeratosis, dyskeratosis, focal atrophy, and atypical keratinocytes.

Treatment modalities include topical liquid nitrogen, electrodesiccation, topical imiquimod, and topical fluorouracil.[26]

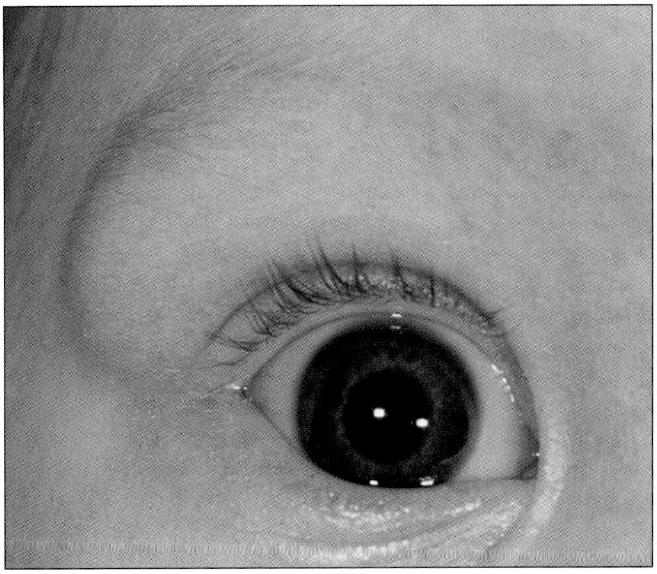

Fig. 31.7 Dermoid cyst of the right brow of an infant. This location at the frontozygomatic suture is the most common site.

Dermoid and epidermoid cysts

Dermoid and epidermoid cysts are choristomas that occur as a result of the sequestration of ectoderm along lines of embryonic closure. They contain dermal and epidermal elements, respectively. Both dermoid and epidermoid cyst walls are lined by keratinizing epidermis. Unlike epidermoid cysts, dermoid cyst walls also contain dermal appendages, including sebaceous glands, sweat glands, and hair follicles. Secretion by contained sebaceous and sweat glands fills the cyst and causes gradual increase in size. In comparison, epidermoid cysts are filled with keratin.

Although present at birth, clinical presentation may not occur until later in life. The lateral brow and upper lid adjacent to the frontozygomatic suture are the most common locations (Fig. 31.7). Dermoid cysts presenting medially at the nasofrontal suture in the orbit must be differentiated from a meningocele or a meningomyelocele. A large dermoid cyst may compress the globe and cause astigmatic amblyopia. Deprivation amblyopia may be caused by a dermoid-induced mechanical ptosis. Extension into the orbit is not uncommon, and large cysts may extend into the cranial vault. Rupture of the cyst releases irritating secretions, which may cause a severe inflammatory reaction. Rupture should be treated intraoperatively with copious irrigation and postoperatively with corticosteroids.

Histologically, the wall of a dermoid cyst is lined with a stratified squamous epithelium. The cyst wall typically possesses dermal appendages including sebaceous and eccrine sweat glands that secrete directly into the lumen of the cyst. Hairs contained in the cyst wall project into the cyst lumen.[27]

Recommended treatment is complete surgical excision without rupture of the cyst wall. Indications for surgical resection include clinical evidence of manifest or threatened amblyopia or cosmetic deformity. Radiologic imaging with CT and MRI is indicated when the entire extent of the cyst cannot be palpated, in the setting of proptosis, or when significant orbital or intracranial extension is suspected. The lesion is nonenhancing and well circumscribed.

Oncocytoma

Oncocytoma is a rare tumor composed of oncocytes or large eosinophilic cells that grow in an adenomatous pattern. Oncocytes are thought to be epithelial cells that undergo transformation with aging. Although the majority of oncocytomas arise from the caruncle, they may also occur at the mucocutaneous border of the eyelid, the lacrimal sac, or the conjunctiva. Rare in patients under the age of 60 years, this benign tumor exhibits slow growth. Rarely exceeding 15 mm in diameter, the color varies from red to yellow and the surface may be smooth or lobulated.[28,29]

Treatment is surgical excision.

Phakomatous choristoma

Phakomatous choristoma is a rare lesion believed to be a congenital neoplasm of lenticular anlage.[30–32] The anteroinferior aspect of the medial lower eyelid is the predominant location (Fig. 31.8). The cells of origin of this lesion are postulated to be surface ectodermal cells induced to form the lens plate and lens vesicle: these cells aberrantly remain external to the optic vesicle as the embryonic fissure closes. The characteristic inferonasal lower eyelid location corresponds to the site of closure of the embryonic fissure. The ectopic cells then proliferate after undergoing rudimentary differentiation. The globe is usually free of developmental defects.

Treatment is surgical excision.

Benign Tumors of the Dermis

The dermis of the eyelid is composed of loose bundles of collagen, variable amounts of elastic and reticulin fibers, and a ground substance containing mucopolysaccharide. The dermis also contains nerves, blood vessels, smooth muscle, monocytes, histiocytes, and macrophages. Benign dermal lesions may arise from any of the tissue types in the dermis. Lesions will be classified and discussed according to dermal cellular origin.

Tumors derived from neural tissue

Neurofibroma

Neurofibromas (plexiform neurofibroma) may occur as solitary cutaneous lesions or as part of the phakomatosis, neurofibromatosis type I (NF-1, von Recklinghausen disease), an autosomal dominant condition in which mutations have been demonstrated in the NF1 gene.[33] Solitary neurofibromas usually occur in adulthood. Multiple cutaneous tumors of neurofibromatosis tend to appear in late childhood or adolescence and gradually increase in size and number. Neurofibromas are soft in consistency, flesh-colored, and often pedunculated. Clinical distinction from dermatofibromas and intradermal nevi may be difficult. A plexiform neurofibroma of the upper lid gives a characteristic S-shaped curve to the lid margin and is pathognomonic for NF-1 (Fig. 31.9).

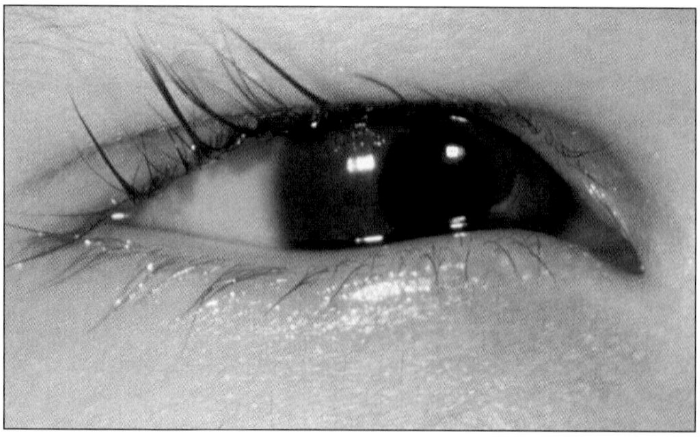

Fig. 31.8 Phakomatous choristoma of the right lower eyelid. This rare tumor most commonly appears at the inferonasal aspect of the lower eyelid.

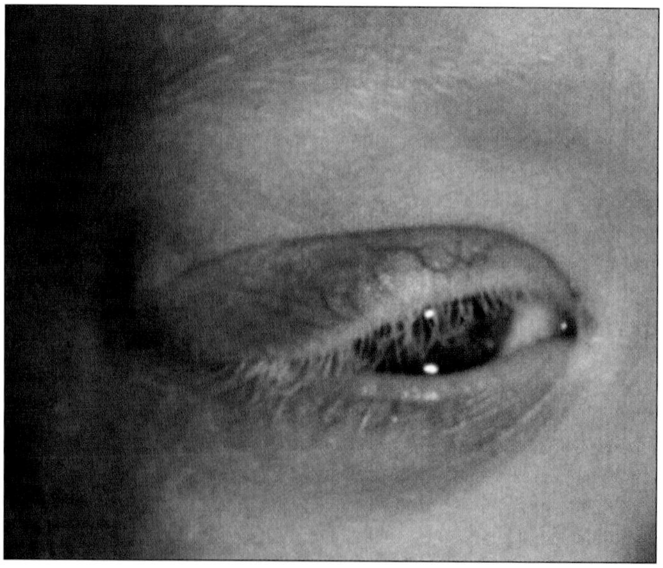

Fig. 31.9 Neurofibroma (plexiform neurofibroma) of the upper eyelid. Note the characteristic S-shaped configuration of the eyelid created by the tumor.

Neurofibromas are tumors resulting from proliferation of all elements of a peripheral nerve. Histologically, the tumors are poorly circumscribed and composed of spindle-shaped cells embedded in a loose myxoid stroma. This pattern represents a proliferation of Schwann cells and endoneural fibroblasts embedded in collagen. Extension of the tumor outside the perineural sheath is not observed. The tumors may be highly vascularized.

Surgical excision is the recommended treatment when solitary lesions cause mechanical lid distortion (upper lid ptosis or lower lid retraction) leading to visual deprivation or exposure keratitis. Cosmetic deformity and establishing a diagnosis are additional indications for excision. The tumors are highly infiltrative; thus, complete excision is often not possible without significant sacrifice of adjacent structures. Recurrence is common.

Neurilemoma

Neurilemomas or schwannomas are derived from Schwann cells of the peripheral nerve sheath. In contrast to neurofibroma, the other components of the peripheral nerve do not proliferate. The lesions are pearly white or yellowish, firm, often painful, intradermal nodules. They occur along the course of peripheral nerves. Occurrence in the eyelid is very rare. Orbital location is more common. Multiple lesions may be seen in neurofibromatosis type II, an autosomal dominant phakomatosis in which mutations have been identified in the NF2 gene.[34]

Histologically, the tumor appears well circumscribed. The Antoni-A pattern is composed of bundles of elongated cells with thin attenuated nuclei that align themselves into compact parallel rows resembling barrel staves. This arrangement of cells, resembling sensory corpuscles, is referred to as Verocay bodies. The Antoni-B pattern, felt to represent tumor degeneration, appears less dense, with myxoid stromal edema.[33]

Excisional biopsy is necessary to establish the histopathologic diagnosis. Incomplete removal may result in recurrence and more aggressive behavior.[36]

Neuroma

Neuromas are proliferation of nerve fascicles. Occurrence in the eyelid is rare. When part of the autosomal dominant multiple endocrine neoplasia syndrome (MEN type IIb), large numbers of small nodular lesions occur on the skin of the face, nose, and eyelid. Mucosal lesions may occur on the lips, tongue, and mouth. MEN type IIb is also associated with prominent corneal nerves, medullary thyroid carcinoma, and pheochromocytoma; mutations have been identified in the RET protooncogene.[37]

Treatment is surgical excision.

Granular cell tumor

Granular cell tumors are rare, benign, Schwann cell tumors. The lesion is a well-circumscribed, yellow, firm, subcutaneous nodule involving the eyelid or eyebrow of adult patients. Clinical differentiation from other nodular subcutaneous nodules is not possible.[38] Histopathologically, the tumor consists of lobules of oval cells with round nuclei. The cytoplasm is granular and eosinophilic.[35]

Surgical excision is the recommended treatment.

Tumors derived from smooth muscle

Leiomyoma

Leiomyomas are benign tumors of smooth muscle origin. Eyelid involvement is rare. The tumor arises from smooth muscle of blood vessels and erector pili muscles. The lesions can be solitary or multiple, pink to brown in color, and may be painful. Differentiation from other nodular subcutaneous lesions, based solely on clinical grounds, is not possible.

Surgical excision is the recommended treatment.

Tumors derived from vascular tissue

Nevus flammeus

Nevus flammeus ('port wine stain') is a lesion composed of dilated capillaries that results from a congenital weakness of capillary walls. It represents a telangiectasia and should not be confused with capillary or cavernous hemangiomas, which are true angiomas. The characteristic lesion appears as one or several dull-red or bluish-red flat patches with an irregular outline, which does not blanch with pressure (Fig. 31.10). Although the lesion may fade in color with age, it does not undergo spontaneous regression or involution. When a facial nevus is associated with leptomeningeal

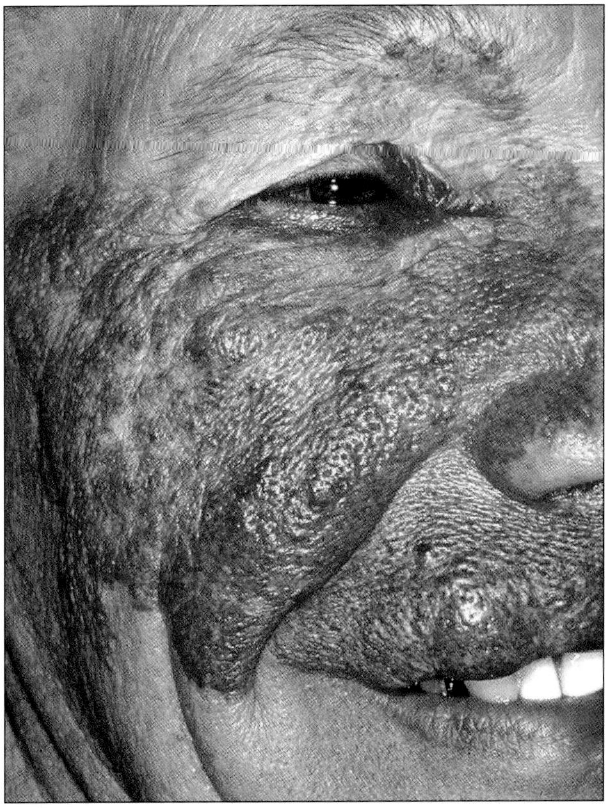

Fig. 31.10 Nevus flammeus ('port wine stain') of the eyelids and face.

angiomatosis or ocular vascular hamartomas, it represents Sturge-Weber syndrome, a sporadic condition. Leptomeningeal angiomatosis may lead to seizures and hemiparesis. When the upper lid is involved, glaucoma may result from ocular vascular hamartomas causing increased episcleral venous pressure.

Other systemic conditions associated with nevus flammeus are Klippel-Trénaunay-Weber syndrome and phakomatosis pigmentovascularis. Klippel-Trénaunay-Weber syndrome consists of hemangiomas, varicosities, and unilateral bony and soft tissue hypertrophy.[39] Phakomatosis pigmentovascularis consists of melanocytic nevi and nevus flammeus.[40]

Histologically, dilated, mature, small capillaries with flattened endothelial lining are present in the papillary dermis.

Treatment goals of nevus flammeus are aesthetic based. Camouflage with cosmetics is the most conservative approach. Carbon dioxide and argon lasers have been employed, but unsatisfactory scarring has resulted.[41] Pulsed dye laser has proven to be more efficacious. Injection with corticosteroids is not effective.

Capillary hemangioma

The capillary hemangioma ('strawberry nevus') is the most common benign periorbital tumor of childhood. This lesion is a vascular hamartoma derived from endothelial cells. Conjunctival and orbital involvement is also characteristic. In most cases, the lesions are not present at birth, but become manifest within the first 2–6 weeks of life. Approximately 95% are evident by age 6 months. Rapid growth occurs over the first 4 months and is followed by slower growth for 8–12 months. The lesion often stabilizes by 18–30 months. Spontaneous involution ensues and, by age 7, 75% of lesions have resolved.[42]

Clinical appearance varies with the depth of the lesion within the skin. The tumor appears bright red when near the surface, and assumes a purple or blue color when deeper in the subcutaneous tissue (Fig. 31.11). The lesion has a spongy consistency, blanches with tactile pressure, and often increases in size with crying or straining. Lid tumors may have extension into the orbit. Fine stellate scarring within the lesion is indicative of resolution.[43]

Although benign, capillary hemangiomas may lead to occlusion or astigmatic amblyopia.[44] In addition, Kasabach-Merritt syndrome, a rare condition of thrombocytopenia with bleeding diathesis due to platelet entrapment with a large capillary hemangioma, may occur.[45]

Histologically, well-circumscribed collections of small, thin-walled capillaries are present in the dermis. The endothelial cell lining is flattened, with occasional presence of endothelial cell buds. The tumor is composed of actively replicating endothelial cells and blood-filled channels. A minimal inflammatory cell infiltrate is often present.

Treatment indications include threatened or manifest amblyopia due to induced astigmatic refractive error or occlusion amblyopia, optic neuropathy due to tumor compression, exposure keratopathy due to massive proptosis, and asymmetry of the facial bony skeleton.[42] Given the natural history of spontaneous resolution, patients and/or parents must be counseled appropriately, because all treatment modalities have significant risks. Small tumors that are not threatening the visual system may be observed. An intralesional steroid injection may be used to induce involution of lid lesions, but should not be injected 'blindly' into orbital lesions.[46,47] Complications of intralesional injection include CRAO, depigmentation, fat atrophy, eyelid necrosis, and adrenal suppression.[48–51] Systemic steroids may be used in selective cases to induce tumor involution, but management of these patients should include pediatric consultation for appropriate monitoring for the development of systemic side effects. Surgical resection is difficult due to the nonencapsulated growth pattern of the tumor. Aggressive resection may sacrifice normal structures. Radiation therapy may also be efficacious, but risk of potential local and systemic side effects must be considered. Success has also been reported with interferon alfa-2b.[52] Recently, promising results have been reported with systemic propranolol.[53]

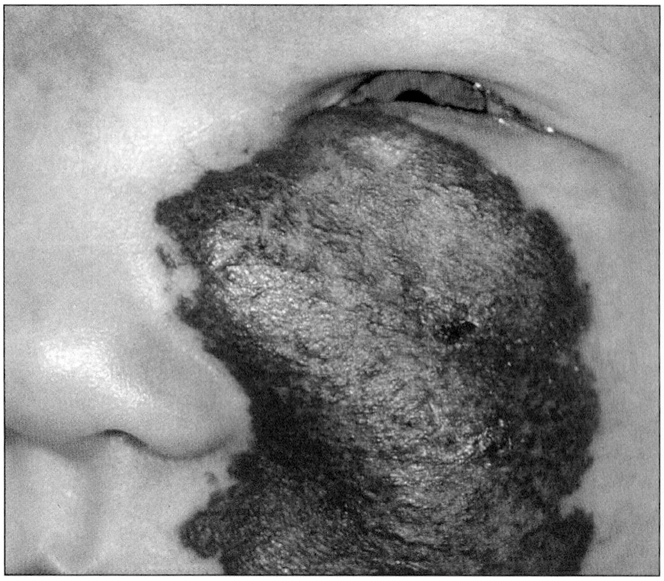

Fig. 31.11 Capillary hemangioma involving the left lower eyelid and face of a 3-month-old infant. Tumor involution was observed after intralesional corticosteroid injection.

Cherry hemangioma

A 'cherry' hemangioma is an acquired capillary hemangioma. These lesions are common in older individuals and appear as bright red nodules, 1–5 mm in diameter. Histopathologically, they are identical to an infantile capillary hemangioma. Treatment is observation or surgical excision for cosmesis.

Cavernous hemangioma

Cavernous hemangioma is the most common benign primary orbital tumor of adults. Eyelid involvement is rare. Eyelid lesions are compressible, solitary, or more commonly, multiple, deep dermal and subcutaneous nodules (Fig. 31.12).[45]

The blue rubber bleb nevus syndrome is characterized by cutaneous cavernous hemangiomas and gastrointestinal hemangiomas.[54]

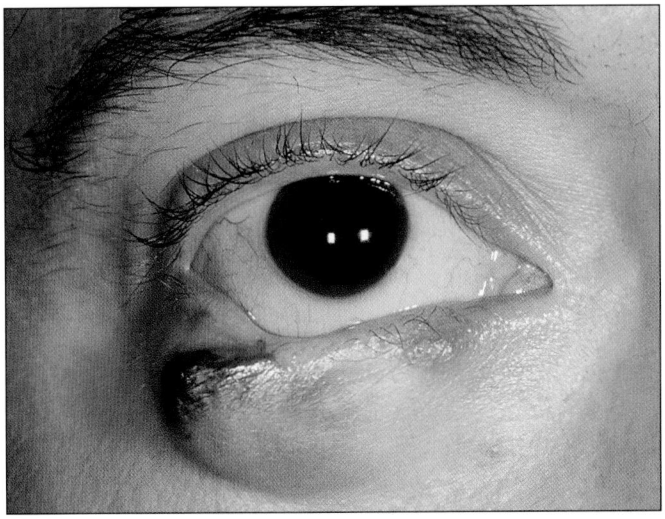

Fig. 31.12 Cavernous hemangioma of the lower eyelid of an adult.

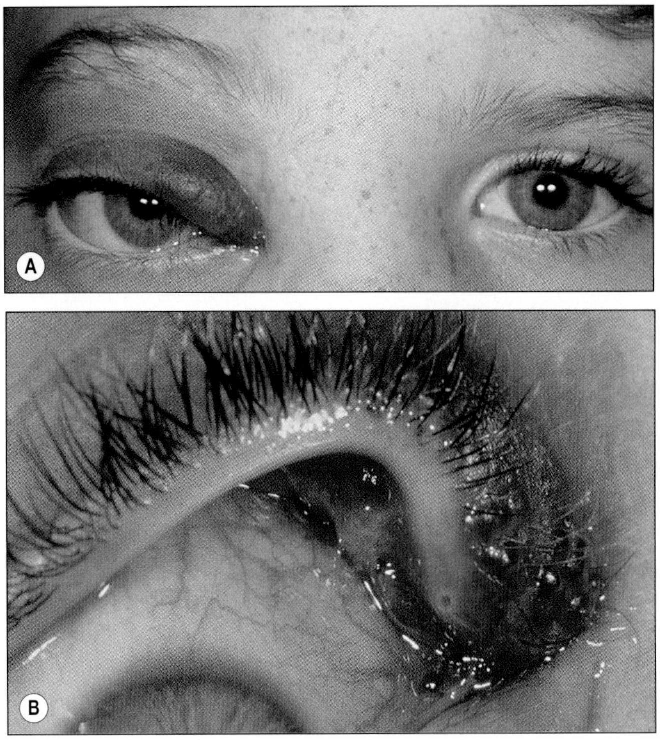

Fig. 31.13 Lymphangioma. (**A**) Lymphangioma of the right upper eyelid of a young woman. (**B**) The color of the vesicles may vary. When filled with clear lymph fluid, they appear clear. The presence of admixed blood may cause a purple coloration.

Histologically, endothelial-lined, dilated, blood-filled vascular spaces are present in the dermis. A thick fibrovascular capsule surrounds the tumor. Unlike a capillary hemangioma, there is no endothelial proliferation. Thrombosis or foci of calcification may be evident.

Surgical excision is the recommended treatment when indicated. Surgical indications are similar to those for capillary hemangioma.

Varix

A varix is a thin-walled, compressible, dilated venule. This lesion, which usually afflicts the elderly patient, appears as an isolated, slightly elevated, dark blue, cystic lesion. Size varies from 2 to 5 mm in diameter, and the lesion increases in size with Valsalva maneuver.

Histologically, the venule wall is thickened with adventitial fibrosis. The lumen contains erythrocytes, scattered monocytes, and fibrin deposits. Partial obliteration by thrombus may be evident; concentric deposition of collagen, hemosiderin deposits, and dystrophic calcification may also be observed.

Recommended treatment is cautious surgical excision, due to the vascularity of the lesion, which may extend into the orbit.

Lymphangioma

Three types of eyelid lymphangioma exist: localized lymphangioma circumscriptum, lymphangioma circumscriptum, and cavernous lymphangioma.[55] Localized lymphangioma circumscriptum presents as a solitary patch of thick-walled vesicles. The vesicles may be filled with clear lymph fluid or with an admixture of blood, giving the lesion a purple color (Fig. 31.13).

In lymphangioma circumscriptum, the characteristic lesion appears as several large patches of vesicles with diffuse edema of the underlying subcutaneous tissue. The lesions may resemble herpetic vesicles when filled with clear transudate. The lesions may break down and exude serous transudate. This may lead to secondary infection.

Cavernous lymphangioma, also referred to as cystic hygroma if present in the neck region, appears as a soft, cystic, circumscribed, or diffuse subcutaneous swelling. The lesion may be either small or large and multifocal.

Associated facial or orbital lymphangioma may be present. Larger lesions may cause lid distortion and malposition. Extensive lid involvement may simulate plexiform neurofibroma.[56]

Histologically, large, thin-walled vascular channels filled with proteinaceous lymph fluid and occasional erythrocytes are present in the dermis. The network of spaces is lined by flattened endothelial cells.

Surgical resection is the recommended treatment, but the infiltrative growth pattern makes complete resection very difficult. The lesions are usually slowly progressive with no tendency for spontaneous regression and are poorly responsive to radiation therapy and steroid therapy. Also, they have a propensity to develop hemorrhages, causing a diffuse hematoma. Treatment indications include functional visual deficit due to lid malposition or optic nerve compromise, and cosmesis. Success has been reported with various sclerosing agents.[57]

Arteriovenous malformation

An arteriovenous malformation (AVM) consists of one or more endothelial-lined channels directly communicating the arterial with venous circulation. They can occur spontaneously as congenital defects, or following accidental or surgical trauma. Occurrence in the eyelids is rare, and usually

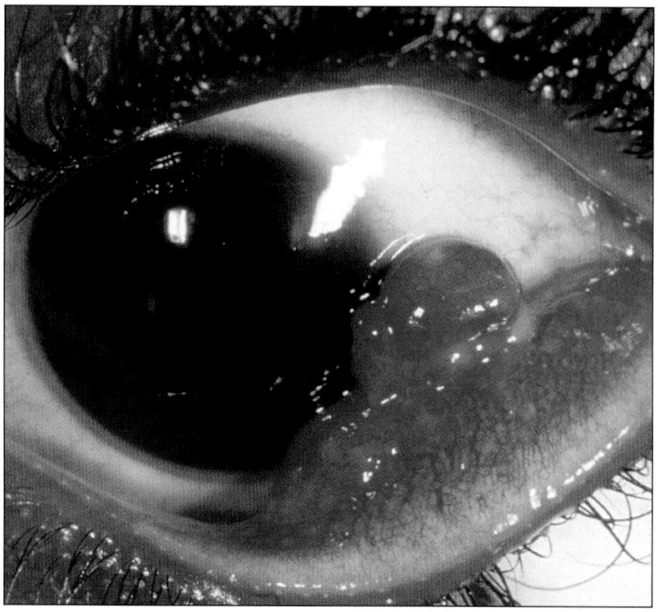

Fig. 31.14 Pyogenic granuloma of the lower eyelid palpebral conjunctiva. This lesion appeared in association with a chronically inflamed chalazion.

appears secondary to orbital involvement.[58] Clinical differentiation from lymphangioma and hemangioma may be difficult and may require ancillary testing to establish the correct diagnosis.

When treatment of isolated eyelid AVMs is required, the feeder vessels are ligated after definitive identification by angiography. Excision to debulk the residual vascular mass may be necessary in selected cases. Embolization, a common treatment for orbital AVMs, is not feasible for lesions confined to the eyelids.

Pyogenic granuloma

Pyogenic granuloma is a misnomer because this lesion is neither pyogenic nor granulomatous. It was assumed incorrectly that this lesion was caused by pyogenic infection of a small wound. Given the histological appearance, eruptive hemangioma or hemangioma of granulation tissue is a more accurate and appropriate term. It is the most commonly acquired vascular lesion of the eyelid, and may be classified as an inflammatory lesion. It appears clinically as a pedunculated, reddish lesion with frequent superficial ulcerations of the overlying epithelium (Fig. 31.14). Rapid growth is characteristic. This lesion most commonly follows minor trauma or surgery, or may be associated with a chalazion.

Histologically, the lesion consists of an exuberant mass of granulation tissue, prominent capillaries, and acute and chronic inflammatory cells.

Recommended treatment is surgical excision; topical or intralesional corticosteroids may also aid in resolution.

Glomus tumor

Glomus bodies are arteriovenous shunts found in distal circulatory regions. They function to regulate blood flow, thereby providing thermoregulation. Glomus cells are similar to pericytes. Two types of glomus tumors are found: the more common solitary glomus tumor and the very rare multiple variety. Both are extremely rare in the eyelid, but they are found more frequently in the extremities, especially in the nail bed where they can be very painful. In the skin they are nonpainful. The solitary type appears as a purplish nodule a few millimeters in diameter. A multiple-type glomus tumor appears as either isolated tumors or as multiple, confluent, bluish, compressible subcutaneous lesions varying from 5 to 20 mm in diameter.[59] The condition is autosomal dominant and mutations have been described in the glomulin gene.[60]

It may be difficult to differentiate this tumor, based on clinical characteristics, from a lymphangioma, blue nevus, melanoma, leiomyoma, and other rare vascular tumors. Diagnostic biopsy is often necessary for definitive diagnosis.

Histologically, a well-circumscribed collection of small vascular channels, surrounded by a dense aggregate of small epithelioid cells are observed in the dermis.

Treatment is surgical excision to establish the diagnosis or for cosmetic concerns. The lesion may be more deeply located and larger than anticipated.

Intravascular papillary endothelial hyperplasia

This benign lesion may be mistaken clinically and histologically for an angiosarcoma.[61] The lesion may or may not have the clinical appearance of a vascular lesion. It can vary in size from a few millimeters to 5 centimeters in diameter. Most of these lesions arise within a vein, but some have been found within a benign vascular lesion such as a venous lake, hemangioma, or lymphangioma. The lesion is usually found in association with a thrombus. As a consequence, most authors regard the lesion as an exaggerated reparative response to thrombosis within a vascular lumen. Spontaneous occurrence has also been reported. Onset and progression may be indolent or rapid. Young female adults are most frequently affected. The lesion has a predilection for the face and extremities. Biopsy is required to establish the diagnosis.[62]

Histologically, the intraluminal mass is intimately attached to the vessel wall. Collagenous cores form papillary tufts, which are lined by a single layer of flat endothelial cells.

Treatment is surgical excision, which, if complete, is curative.

Angiolymphoid hyperplasia with eosinophilia

Angiolymphoid hyperplasia with eosinophilia (ALHE) is an uncommon disorder which presents with one or two nodules involving the dermis or subcutaneous tissue, usually of the head and neck. There has been some confusion in the literature with regards to the correct nomenclature of the disease. The term epithelioid hemangioma has gained favor and is likely preferred. It is unknown whether this is a reactive or neoplastic process.

Kimura's disease and ALHE are believed to be two distinct entities based on clinical and pathologic differences. Kimura's disease occurs almost exclusively in Asian males with lymphadenopathy and increased serum

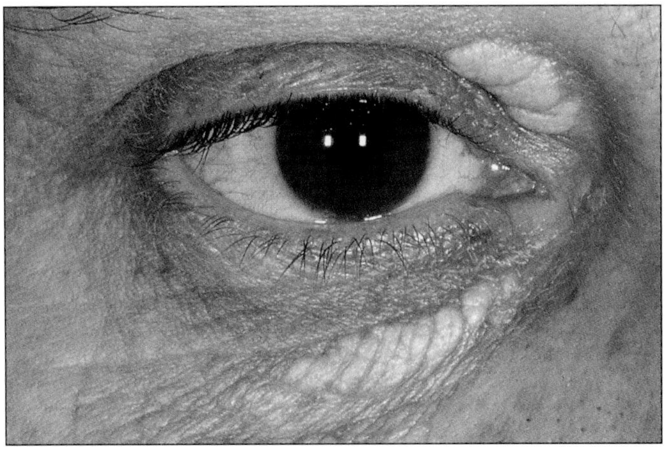

Fig. 31.15 Xanthelasmas of the upper and lower eyelids.

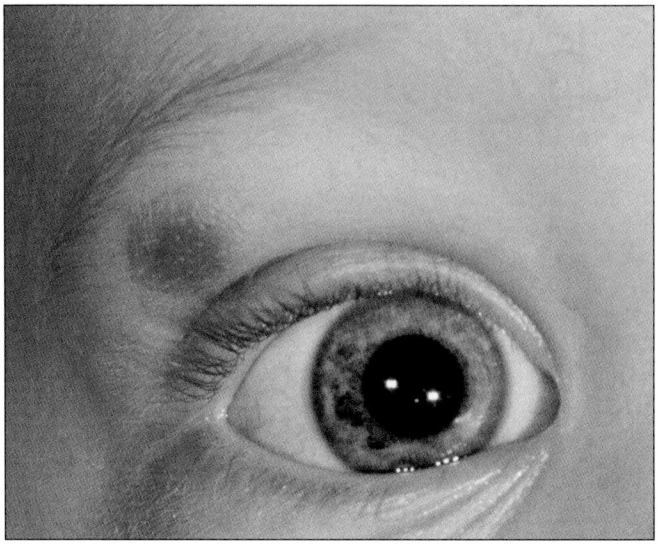

Fig. 31.16 Juvenile xanthogranuloma (nevoxanthoendothelioma) of the right upper eyelid in a 3-year-old child. Note the typical orange color and domed shape.

immunoglobulin E and blood eosinophilia; lesions range in size from 3 to 10 cm and there may be associated nephrotic syndrome and proteinuria. ALHE occurs in males and females of all races, with smaller lesions and no systemic findings.

Histopathologically, the lesions are composed of vascular hyperplasia with plump endothelial cells accompanied by varying degrees of mixed cellular infiltrates dominated by lymphocytes and eosinophils.

Treatment is surgical excision where feasible.

Tumors derived from histiocytes

Xanthelasma

Xanthelasmas are very common dermal lesions of the medial aspects of the upper and lower eyelids occurring in middle-aged to elderly patients. More common in females, they are usually bilateral, plaque-like, yellow, flat or slightly raised deposits composed of foamy histiocytes (Fig. 31.15). Although the lesions are occasionally found in association with diabetes and other hyperlipidemic conditions (especially essential hyperlipidemia types II and III), the majority of patients have no underlying systemic metabolic disorder. Xanthelasmas are also seen in association with Erdheim-Chester disease, a histiocytic inflammation involving the orbit with long bone changes.[63]

Histologically, focal collections of foamy histiocytes are distributed around the vessels and adnexal structures of the dermis. There is no associated inflammation or fibrosis.

The recommended treatment is surgical excision for cosmetic concerns. The full thickness of skin and, in some cases, the underlying orbicularis muscle must be excised. Often, surgical excision can be incorporated into a blepharoplasty incision. Skin grafting may be necessary in cases of large lesions. Recurrences are common. Success has also been reported with numerous lasers, including pulsed dye, argon, CO_2, and erbium:YAG.[64]

Xanthoma

Eyelid xanthomas are more commonly associated with hyperlipidemic states (again, especially essential hyperlipidemia types II and III) than are xanthelasmas.[65]

Histologically, they differ from xanthelasmas. The lesions are situated more deeply in the dermis, and the foamy histiocytes are intermixed with multinucleated Touton-type giant cells, inflammatory cells, and fibrosis.

Treatment recommendations are similar to those for xanthelasmas.

Juvenile xanthogranuloma

Juvenile xanthogranuloma (JXG) or nevoxanthoendothelioma is a histiocytic proliferation of unknown etiology that usually occurs in infants less than 3 years of age. These nonneoplastic lesions most commonly affect the head and neck region. The lesions not only affect the skin but also may affect the eye, including the conjunctiva, iris, or ciliary body. Rare occurrences have been reported in the orbit, testes, and lung.

The skin lesions, which often regress spontaneously, consist of single or multiple elevated, orange or reddish-brown, dome-shaped nodules varying from 5 to 20 mm in diameter (Fig. 31.16). Histologically, the lesions are a mixture of histiocytic foam cells, lymphocytes, histiocytes, Touton-type giant cells, and fibrosis.

Although the skin lesions carry an excellent prognosis, the intraocular lesions may have serious sequelae. Spontaneous hyphema, iritis, and secondary glaucoma may be a consequence of iris involvement. Hyphema is due to rupture of the fragile blood vessels of the iris lesions. It is important to exclude JXG as a cause of hyphema in an infant.[66] Diagnosis of JXG may be aided by a careful skin examination, and typical cutaneous lesions should be biopsied to establish a diagnosis.

Treatment of intraocular lesions consists of systemic corticosteroids, which may expedite regression. The cutaneous lesions resolve spontaneously in 6–12 months.

Tumors derived from fibrous tissue

Dermatofibroma

Also referred to as fibrous histiocytomas, histiocytomas, and sclerosing hemangiomas, dermatofibroma appear in the skin as firm, red to brown, solitary or multiple nodules. Usually only 2–3 mm in diameter, the individual lesions may measure 2–3 cm in diameter following bleeding into the tumor. In the eyelid, the lesion appears as a dome-shaped mass attached to the overlying skin. Histological appearances vary according to the relative contribution of fibrous and cellular elements.[67,68]

Treatment is surgical excision.

Benign Tumors of the Eyelid Adnexa

Tumors of sweat gland origin

The eyelid eccrine and apocrine sweat glands have three major components: the secretory component lying within the dermis, the intradermal duct, and the intraepidermal duct. The eyelid eccrine glands are independent of the hair follicle apparatus. The apocrine glands appear in association with the eyelashes and are referred to as glands of Moll. A wide variety of benign tumors may develop from the pluripotential cells destined to become one of the components of the eccrine sweat gland unit. With the exception of the apocrine hidrocystoma (cyst of Moll), apocrine lesions of the eyelid are relatively uncommon.[1,69]

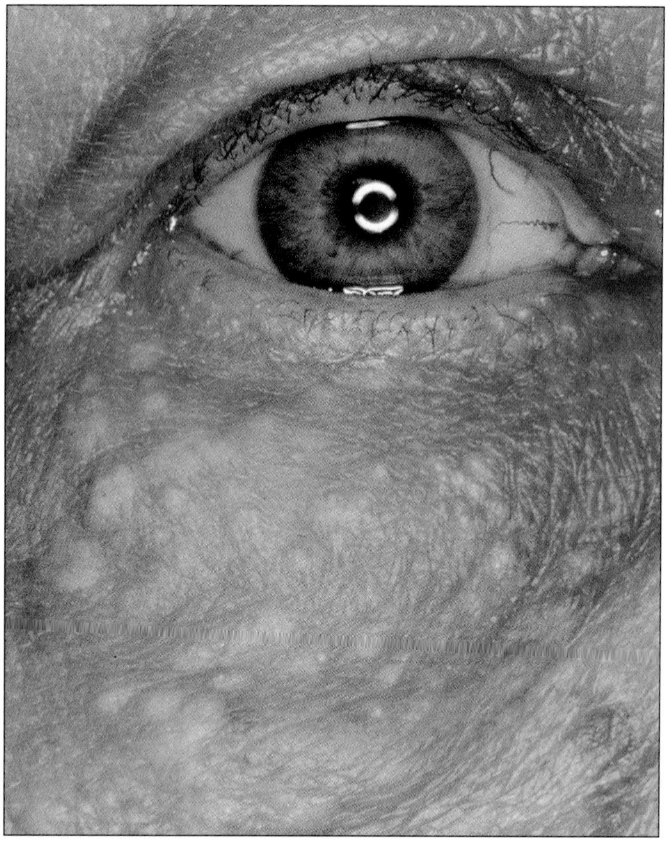

Fig. 31.17 Numerous syringomas of the periocular region of a female. The lesions appear as pale yellow, waxy nodules, 1–2 mm in diameter.

Tumors of eccrine sweat gland origin

Syringoma

Syringomas are benign eccrine sweat gland tumors found most commonly in young females. Clinically, they usually appear as multiple small flesh-colored to yellowish, soft, waxy nodules averaging 12 mm in diameter. The lower eyelids are predominantly affected, but the lesions may also occur on the upper lids, cheeks, and forehead (Fig. 31.17). They are also occasionally found in the axilla, abdomen, and vulva. It may be difficult to differentiate these lesions clinically from other benign lid lesions, and biopsy may be required for an accurate diagnosis. Syringomas have been shown to have an increased incidence in patients with Down's syndrome.[70]

Histologically, the dermis shows poorly circumscribed collections of small basaloid cells lying individually or in nests and strands; many will show duct formation. The ducts contain eosinophilic keratin or amorphous material and may show a tadpole or comma-shaped extension of small basaloid cells.

Since syringomas are located in the dermis, complete removal requires surgical excision. Alternative treatments, such as electrodesiccation, dermabrasion, and carbon dioxide laser treatment may improve the appearance of the lesions.[71–73]

Eccrine spiradenoma

The eccrine spiradenoma shows differentiation toward the secretory portion of the eccrine gland. This benign tumor is an uncommon lesion which appears as a solitary, flesh-colored nodule approximately 1–2 cm in diameter. The nodules may be tender and painful. The tumor tends to occur in early adulthood and has no characteristic location. Familial cases inherited in an autosomal dominant fashion have been reported.[74] Eyelid involvement is rare.[75]

Histologically, the dermis contains well-circumscribed, deeply basophilic lobules composed of cords and islands of two cell types: a peripherally located cell with a small, dense nucleus, and a more centrally located cell with a large, pale nucleus. Eosinophilic hyaline material may be present.

Treatment is surgical excision. Malignant transformation is rare.

Eccrine acrospiroma

The eccrine acrospiroma (clear cell hidradenoma) shows differentiation toward both ductal and secretory portions of the eccrine gland. This tumor appears as a single, nodular, solid or cystic lesion. It is mobile under the skin. Size varies from 0.5 to 2 cm in diameter. The overlying skin is most commonly intact and appears flesh-colored to reddish-blue. Less commonly, the overlying skin may be ulcerated and resembles a keratoacanthoma.[76–78]

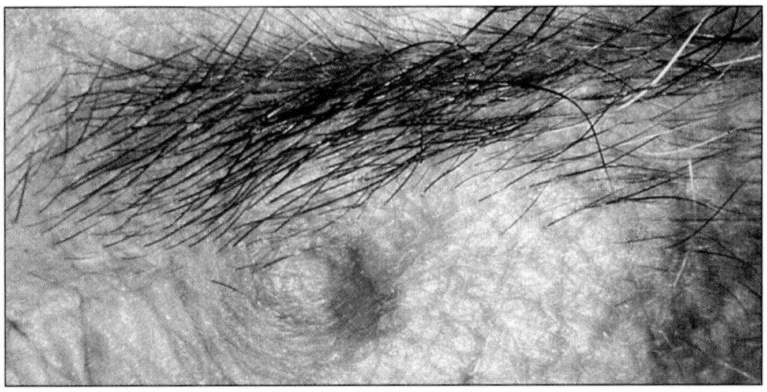

Fig. 31.18 Chondroid syringoma (mixed eccrine tumor) of the upper eyelid. The appearance as a firm, subcutaneous mass is typical.

Histologically, the dermis shows a well-circumscribed, lobular tumor mass composed of sheets and nests of large epithelioid clear cells and smaller cuboidal cells with basophilic cytoplasm. Frequently, tubular lumina containing an amorphous eosinophilic material are found.

Treatment is surgical excision.

Eccrine hidrocystoma

These cystic lesions tend to be small (1–3 mm in diameter) and multiple, and commonly occur clustered around the eyelids and on the face. The lesions are often initiated by heat, humidity, and perspiration, and they may simulate milia. Regarded as ductal retention cysts, there is no connection from the cyst to the overlying surface epidermis.[79]

Histologically, the lesions appear as large dilated cysts. The cysts are lined by a single cuboidal or columnar cell layer surrounded by an outer flattened myoepithelial cell layer. The cysts contain pale eosinophilic granular material.

Treatment is surgical excision.

Pleomorphic adenoma

The pleomorphic adenoma (mixed tumor of skin, chondroid syringoma) occurs most commonly in the head and neck region and may involve the face and eyelids. Clinically, this lesion appears as a firm, intradermal, lobulated mass ranging from 0.5 to 3 cm in diameter (Fig. 31.18).

Histologically, the tumor is identical to the pleomorphic adenoma of the lacrimal gland with epithelial and mesenchymal components. When present in the lateral aspect of the upper lid, differentiation from a lacrimal gland pleomorphic adenoma arising from the palpebral lobe of the lacrimal gland may be difficult.[80]

Treatment is surgical excision due to the potential for malignant transformation.

Tumors of apocrine sweat gland origin

Apocrine hidrocystoma

The apocrine type of hidrocystoma (cyst of Moll) is a true adenoma of the secretory cells of the glands of Moll, rather than a retention cyst. Unlike a retention cyst, the cells lining the cyst are not flattened, and often form papillary projections into the lumen.

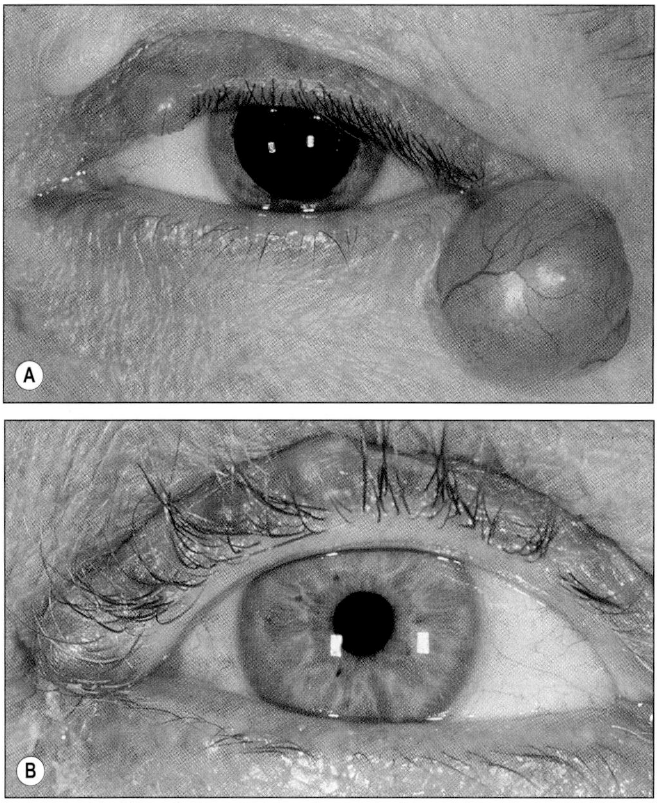

Fig. 31.19 Apocrine hidrocystoma. (**A**) A large, translucent apocrine hidrocystoma (cyst of Moll) of the lateral aspect of the left lower eyelid. (**B**) Multiple apocrine hidrocystoma (cyst of Moll) of the upper eyelid. Note the bluish color due to the cystic nature of the lesion.

The majority of apocrine hidrocystomas occur as solitary lesions near the eyelid margin (Fig. 31.19A). They are usually small, but may reach a size of several centimeters. Because of the cystic nature, they are compressible and may appear translucent or bluish in color (Fig. 31.19B). The major differential diagnostic consideration is cystic basal cell carcinoma.

There are a number of systemic associations, including Schopf-Schulz-Passarge syndrome and focal dermal hypoplasia (Goltz-Gorlin syndrome).[81]

Treatment is surgical excision.

Cylindroma

Although recognized as a tumor of sweat gland origin, the exact origin is uncertain. Solitary or multiple lesions can occur. Cases with multiple lesions are dominantly inherited, and mutations have been demonstrated in the CYLD gene.[82] Solitary lesions affect the adult face or scalp. Multiple lesions appear as dome-shaped, smooth, flesh-colored to reddish nodules of varying size on the scalp. Nodules on the scalp may be present in such large numbers that the scalp is entirely covered. Such lesions are referred to as turban tumors (Fig. 31.20). Malignant degeneration of a cylindroma is rare.

Histologically, the lesions consist of well-circumscribed islands of cells lying in a mosaic pattern. The cells are

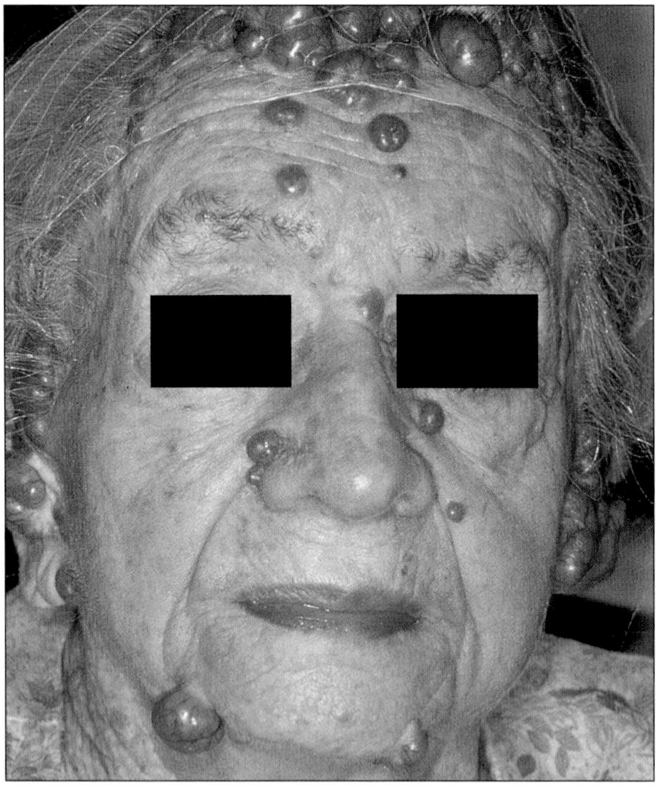

Fig. 31.20 Multiple cylindromas of the scalp, the so-called 'turban tumor.'

surrounded by an eosinophilic hyaline cuticle and sparse amounts of collagen. The islands contain two cell types: a large, pale-staining cell with a vesicular nucleus; and a smaller cuboidal cell with a dark-staining nucleus and with less cytoplasm located at the periphery of the islands.

Treatment is surgical excision. This may prove difficult when multiple lesions are present over a large region.

Syringocystadenoma papilliferum

Appearing at birth or during early childhood, syringocystadenoma papilliferum occurs most commonly on the scalp or face. The lesion appears clinically as a solitary papule or as multiple papules or plaques in a linear arrangement. Size increases at puberty and becomes papillomatous.[83] The eyelid margin is most commonly involved. The lesion appears as a hyperkeratotic papillomatous nodule which may mimic a basal cell carcinoma or keratoacanthoma. It often arises from a nevus sebaceous of Jadassohn, which is a plaque on the face or scalp, that arises secondary to disordered development of epithelial, pilar, sebaceous, and apocrine structures.[84] Patients may also demonstrate epilepsy, mental retardation, and skeletal deformities.

Histologically, the epidermis reveals cystic invagination and a communication with the underlying dermal lesion. The dermal lesion is a poorly circumscribed tumor lobule with large cystic spaces and papillary projections. The cystic spaces are lined by two cell types: a columnar cell with an oval vesicular nucleus and abundant cytoplasm, and a smaller cuboidal cell with a round, dark nucleus and less

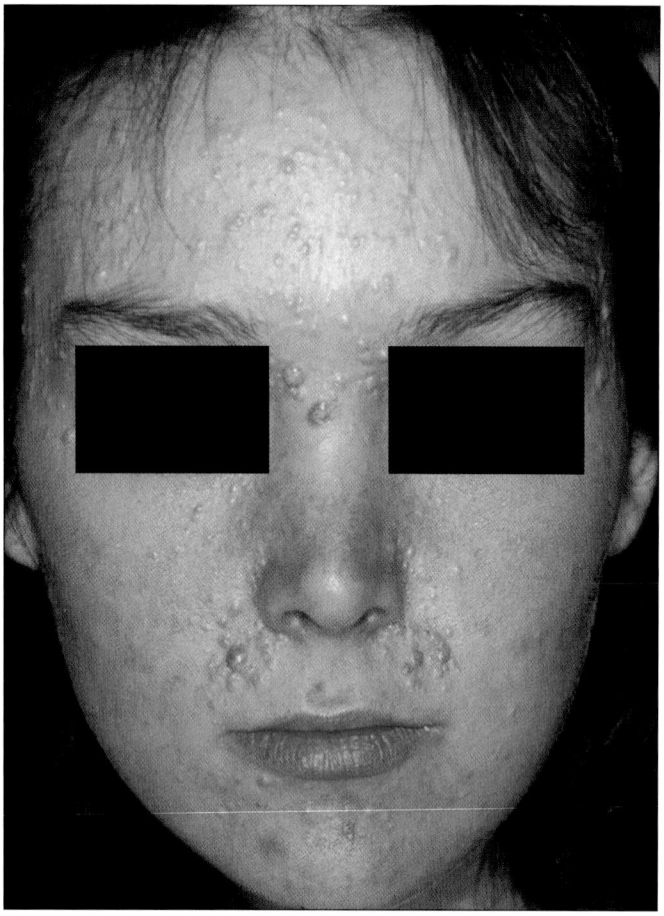

Fig. 31.21 Numerous trichoepitheliomas affecting the face, eyelids, and scalp of a patient with autosomal dominant multiple trichoepitheliomatosis (Brooke's cystic adenoid epithelioma).

cytoplasm. Surrounding the cystic spaces is a fibrous stroma with a dense, predominantly plasmacytic infiltrate.

Treatment is surgical excision.

Tumors of hair follicle origin

Trichoepithelioma

Trichoepithelioma may occur as a solitary lesion, or as multiple lesions inherited in an autosomal dominant manner (Fig. 31.21). The solitary lesion affects older patients, and appears as a firm, elevated, flesh-colored nodule that may ulcerate. Clinically, differentiation from basal cell carcinoma, intradermal nevus, neurofibroma, and other adnexal skin tumors may be difficult.

In contrast, the multiple trichoepitheliomas typically appear in adolescence and commonly increase in size and number. Large numbers of lesions may be present in the nasolabial fold, upper lip, eyelids, and side of the nose. Lesions may also affect the scalp, neck, and upper trunk. Differentiation from adenoma sebaceum (angiofibromas associated with tuberous sclerosis), syringomas, and basal cell nevus syndrome should be made. In contrast to basal cell nevus syndrome, ulceration is rare although transformation to basal cell carcinoma has been described.

Multiple trichoepitheliomas inherited in an autosomal dominant fashion have been linked to 9p21.[85] Mutations have also been found in the CYLD gene in patients with multiple trichoepitheliomas associated with cylindromas (Brooke-Spiegler syndrome), which is in the same gene responsible for multiple cylindromas.[86]

Histologically, the dermis shows well-circumscribed nests of uniform basaloid cells surrounded by a hypercellular stroma.[87] Foci of calcification, foreign body giant cells, and abortive hair follicle forms are observed.

Treatment modalities include simple surgical excision of individual lesions, and dermabrasion or laser therapy for multiple lesions.

Trichoadenoma

Trichoadenomas are rare tumors of the eyelid. Clinically, they are usually solitary, nodular lesions, with superficial telangiectatic vessels and may resemble a basal cell carcinoma or seborrheic keratosis. Histopathologically, the lesion appears less mature than a trichofolliculoma and more mature than a trichoepithelioma, with keratin cysts surrounded by a proliferation of eosinophilic epidermoid cells.

Treatment is surgical excision.[88]

Trichofolliculoma

Trichofolliculoma is often confused with a sebaceous cyst. Clinically, it appears as a solitary, slightly elevated, dome-shaped, flesh-colored nodule (Fig. 31.22). A central umbilicated area representing the opening of a keratin-filled dilated follicle is a diagnostic feature. The observation of white hairs growing from the central pore is strong clinical evidence that the lesion is a trichofolliculoma. The tumor has no reported malignant potential.[89]

Histologically, there is a keratin-filled, cup-shaped invagination of the epidermis with numerous hair shafts. Located around the opening of the hair shafts are poorly to well-differentiated secondary hair bulbs. A hypercellular stroma surrounds the secondary hair follicles.

Treatment is surgical excision.

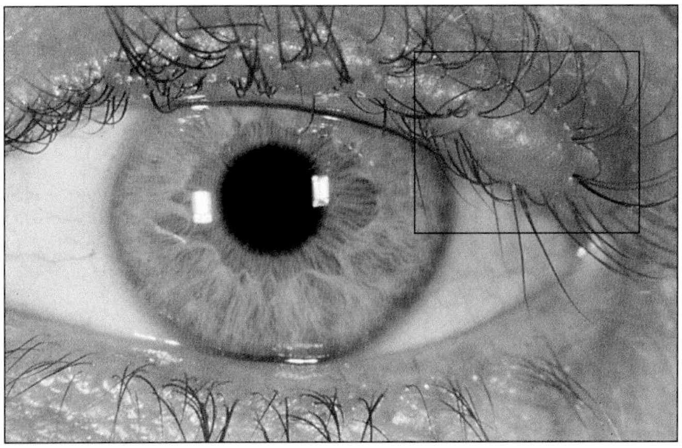

Fig. 31.22 Trichofolliculoma of the left upper eyelid (*box*). The typical features include flesh color, domed shape, and solitary nature.

Trichilemmoma

Trichilemmoma originates from the outer sheath of the hair follicle. Solitary and multiple forms exist. The more common solitary tumor usually occurs in older patients as a flesh-colored, verrucous or papillomatous papule on the face 3–8 mm in diameter. The lesion may mimic a basal cell carcinoma or trichoepithelioma. Most commonly, it appears on the nose and eyelids as a papule, nodule, or cutaneous horn.[90]

Multiple tumors may be a cutaneous marker of Cowden's disease or multiple hamartoma syndrome. In this autosomal dominant condition, trichilemmomas affect the nose, ear, and hands. Affected patients have an increased risk of breast, thyroid, and gastrointestinal carcinoma.[91] In addition, retinal glioma and optic disc drusen have been associated with this syndrome.[92] Lhermitte-Duclos disease consists of Cowden's disease and cerebellar hamartomas. Mutations in the PTEN gene have been described in Cowden's disease and Lhermitte-Duclos disease.[93]

Histologically, the dermis is uninvolved. Sheets of pale-staining to clear epithelioid cells are present in a lobular arrangement. The lobules demonstrate peripheral palisading and thickened basement membranes.

Treatment modalities include surgical excision, curettage, or electrodesiccation.

Pilomatricoma

Pilomatricoma (calcifying epithelioma of Malherbe) develops from hair matrix cells. This solitary tumor tends to affect children, appearing as a pink to purplish, mobile, firm, irregular subcutaneous nodule measuring 0.5–3 cm in diameter (Fig. 31.23). An association has been described with myotonic dystrophy.[94] Pilomatricoma commonly occurs on the eyelid and eyebrow.[95] Malignant transformation has not been reported.

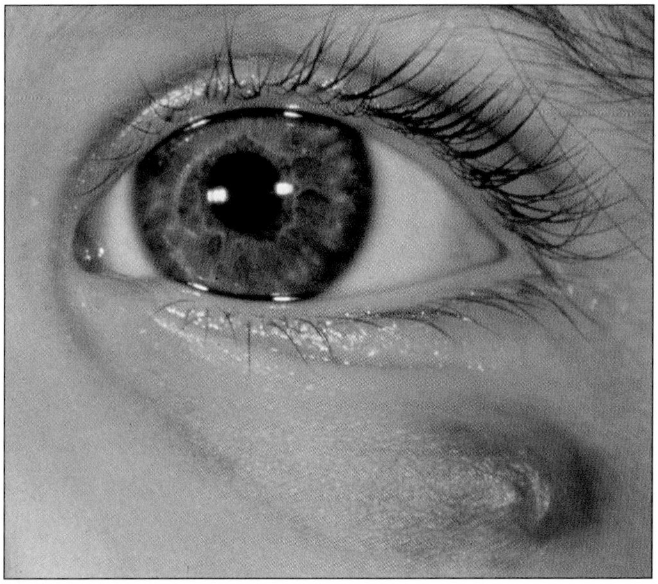

Fig. 31.23 Pilomatricoma (calcifying epithelioma of Malherbe) of the lower eyelid of a child.

Multiple pilomatricomas may be inherited in an autosomal dominant fashion, and mutations have been identified in the CTNNB1 gene in these individuals.[96]

Histologically, the dermis contains well-circumscribed, irregular islands of uniform, small basophilic cells. Foci of calcification, foreign body giant cells, a variable mixed inflammatory infiltrate, and fibrosis are present.

Treatment is surgical excision.

Tumors of sebaceous gland origin

Three subtypes of sebaceous glands are present in the eyelids: meibomian glands, glands of Zeis, and skin sebaceous glands. The meibomian glands are confined to the tarsal plates of the eyelid and contribute an oily surface layer to the tear film that retards its evaporation. The glands of Zeis are sebaceous glands associated with the eyelash follicles.

Sebaceous gland hyperplasia

Hypertrophy or hyperplasia of the meibomian glands may occur in elderly patients. Clinically, this appears as single or multiple small nodules.[97] This is more common on the forehead, cheeks, and nose. The lids may appear thickened and become secondarily ectropic. Chronic blepharitis may coexist. The possibility of sebaceous gland carcinoma must always be included in the differential diagnosis. The lesions may also mimic plexiform neuroma, amyloidosis, and lymphoma. Biopsy may be required to exclude these lesions.

Treatment may be multifaceted, and should address any associated blepharitis. Lid hygiene, topical antibiotics, and, in severe cases, systemic antibiotics and topical steroids may be employed. Surgery may be required if eyelid malposition develops.

Sebaceous adenoma

Sebaceous adenoma is a rare tumor of elderly patients. It appears as a yellowish papule on the face, scalp, or trunk. It may mimic a basal cell carcinoma or a seborrheic keratosis, and may serve as a cutaneous marker for the autosomal dominant Muir-Torre syndrome. As discussed above, patients with Muir-Torre syndrome have multiple sebaceous adenomas and low-grade visceral malignancies.[98,99] Mutations have been identified in two genes: MLH1 and MSH2.

Histology shows a lobular growth pattern composed of an outer one or two layers of germinal basal cells that quickly differentiate centrally into highly vacuolated cells.

Recommended treatment is excisional biopsy to establish the diagnosis. Incomplete excision results in recurrence.

Benign Melanocytic Lesions

Benign cutaneous melanocytic tumors are derived from three sources: nevus cells, epidermal melanocytes, and dermal melanocytes. All three cells are derived embryologically from the neural crest. Nevus cells are considered specialized melanocytes that show a characteristic tendency to organize into focal nests within the skin that do not contain dendritic processes.

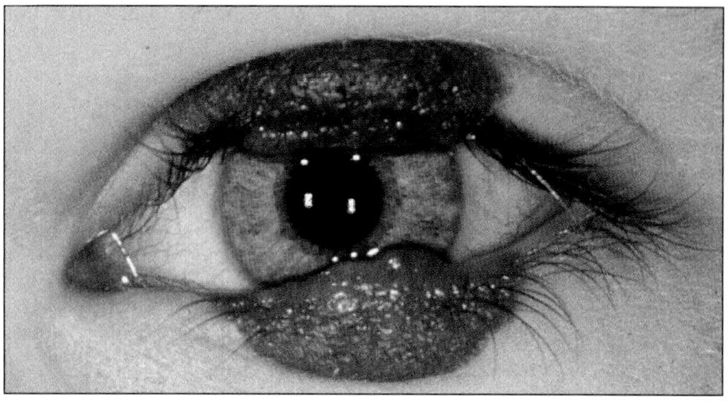

Fig. 31.24 'Kissing nevus' involving the upper and lower eyelids of a child. This is a type of compound nevus that results from deposition of nevus cells in the eyelid fold while the lids are fused during embryogenesis.

Nevocellular nevi

There is considerable variation in the clinical appearance of these lesions. Nevocellular nevi commonly occur on the eyelid skin or margin. Nevi are divided into three histological types: junctional, compound, and intradermal.[1] Although seldom present as congenital lesions, development occurs in childhood. Increased size and pigmentation can be observed at puberty. Histological type may accurately be predicted on the basis of the clinical features.

Junctional nevi

Junctional nevi arise from the deeper layers of the epidermis and do not involve the underlying dermis. The majority of nevi affecting young children are of this type. Clinically, they appear as flat, pigmented macules, round or oval in shape. Growth is slow and may reach 6 mm in diameter.

Compound nevi

Compound nevi possess features of both junctional and intradermal nevi. Nevus cell nests may be seen in the epidermis and dermis. Compound nevi are more common than junctional nevi. Older children and young adults are affected. If an equal portion (mirror image) of the upper and lower eyelid margins are involved, it is termed kissing nevi (Fig. 31.24). The kissing nevi occur when the developing lid folds, which contain embryonic nests of nevus cells, meet and fuse during the eighth week of gestation. They remain fused until the end of the fifth month, then separate.

Melanoma

Although uncommon, junctional and compound nevi have the capacity to evolve into melanoma. Malignant transformation of a purely intradermal nevus, in contrast, is very rare. Signs of malignant degeneration include a large size (greater than 6 mm in diameter), irregular and asymmetric shape, multiple colors, and bleeding.

Intradermal nevi

Intradermal nevi are the most common of the three types of nevi and are most commonly found in adults. Little or no

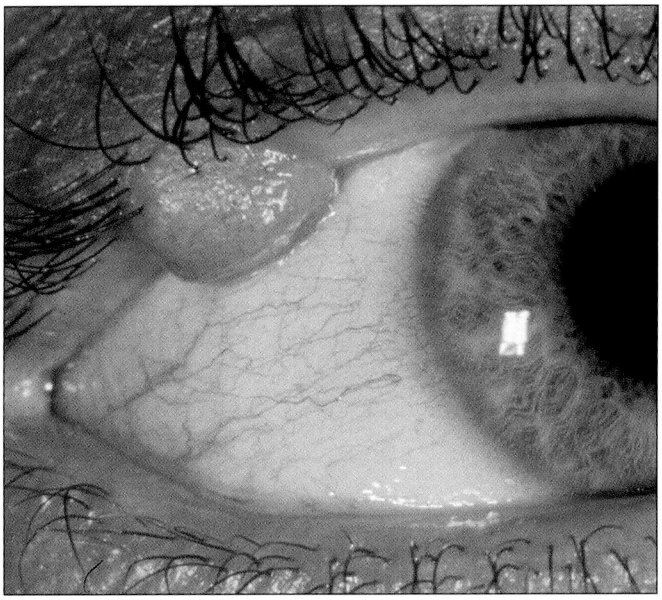

Fig. 31.25 A dome-shaped intradermal nevus of the eyelid margin.

junctional activity is observed. Melanocytes are present in the dermis as discrete nests or sheets of cuboidal cells. Lesions appear as dome-shaped, sessile, verrucous, or even polypoid lesions. Hair may be observed in some lesions. The degree of pigmentation ranges from flesh-colored to light brown. The eyelid margin is commonly involved (Fig. 31.25).

Surgical excision is indicated for cosmesis or concern about malignant change. Complete excision is imperative, as recurrence following incomplete excision may be difficult to differentiate from a melanoma, both clinically and histopathologically.

Variants of nevocellular nevi

There are two special variants of nevocellular nevi which may affect the eyelids: the balloon cell nevus and the spindle or epithelioid nevus ('juvenile melanoma'). The balloon cell nevus is very rare, and possesses no distinguishing clinical features. Histologically, the balloon cells may comprise only a small portion of an intradermal nevus, or they may appear as the major component of the nevus. The balloon cells are larger than conventional nevus cells. Their nuclei are small and pyknotic, located either paracentrally or eccentrically at one pole of the cell. The spindle or epithelioid nevus is a form of compound nevus which mainly affects children and young adults. The lesion appears as a dome-shaped, reddish-pink nodule. Histologically, the lesion has scattered mitotic figures and secondary inflammatory features. Despite this histopathological appearance, the lesion usually pursues an entirely benign clinical course.

Congenital nevus

Congenital nevi may be single or multiple. Generally larger than acquired nevi, these lesions may be 1.5 cm or greater in diameter (Fig. 31.26). Flat papules or nodules may develop over time. The color varies from dark to light brown and lesions often contain dark coarse hairs. These nevi are of

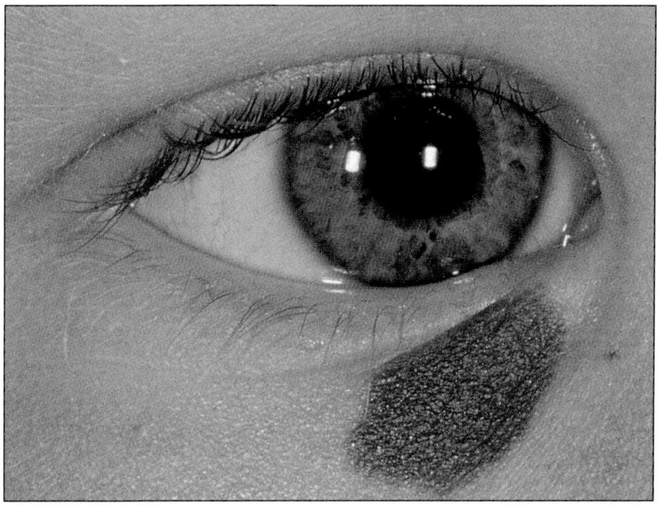

Fig. 31.26 A congenital nevus on the lower eyelid of a child.

concern because of their malignant potential, and malignant potential is greater for larger lesions. Transformation to malignant melanoma is not uncommon, even in childhood.

Surgical excision of large eyelid nevi may necessitate significant tissue loss. For this reason, frequent observation rather than routine excision may be warranted in many cases.

Blue nevus

The blue nevus arises from dermal melanocytes that are deeply located and have been arrested in the dermis before reaching the epidermis. Two types are recognized: the blue nevus and the cellular blue nevus. The blue nevus is a dome-shaped small blue papule or nodule. It has no malignant potential. When a compound nevus is present over a conventional blue nevus, the lesion is termed a combined nevus. Histologically, a proliferation of dermal melanocytes that have been arrested and have not progressed into the dermis is noted. The cellular blue nevus appears as a bluish nodule. Larger than the common blue nevus, it may reach 2–3 cm or larger in diameter. Malignant degeneration with lymph node metastasis is rare.

Surgical excision is recommended for cosmesis or to establish a definitive diagnosis.

Nevus of Ota

The nevus of Ota (oculodermal melanocytosis) occurs as a bluish discoloration of the eyelids and periorbital skin, representing a proliferation of dermal melanocytes. Unilateral involvement is typical, yet bilateral cases may occur. The temple, forehead, malar region, and mucosa of the nose and mouth may also be involved. Patchy bluish discoloration of the sclera and occasionally of the conjunctiva, episclera, uveal tract, and optic disc can be observed. Involvement of the meninges may also be noted. The lesions of the nevus of Ota may appear at birth, or may develop during the first year of life or during adolescence. The lesions tend to gradually extend. Malignant change in the cutaneous lesions of a nevus of Ota is extremely rare. An increased incidence of uveal melanomas is associated with this condition.[100]

Careful observation is the recommended treatment. Frequent follow-up with dilated funduscopy is required to exclude the development of a uveal melanoma.

Freckle

Freckles (ephelis) are small, well-circumscribed, red-brown macules which appear over sun-exposed areas of the skin. Exposure to sunlight causes darkening of the macules. The typical clinical appearance and history of darkening with sun exposure differentiates freckles from junctional nevi and lentigines. Histologic examination shows hyperpigmentation along the basal layer with no change in the number of melanocytes.

Lentigo simplex

The lesions of lentigo simplex are flat, brown to black macules, measuring 1–2 mm in diameter. Clinically indistinguishable from junctional nevi, they are unaffected by sunlight exposure. Multiple lesions of the eyelid may be associated with the autosomal dominant Peutz-Jeghers syndrome of mucocutaneous pigmentation and intestinal polyposis. Mutations have been identified in the STK11 gene.[101] Histology shows hyperpigmentation of the basal layer and an increased number of melanocytes.

Lentigo senilis

The lesions of lentigo senilis are light to dark brown, slowly expanding macules that develop in sun-exposed areas of the skin, including the eyelids. They occur in over 90% of elderly Caucasians. Presenting as small macules 3–5 mm in diameter, the lesions may gradually grow to several centimeters in diameter.[102] Differentiation from lentigo maligna and lentigo malignant melanoma is imperative. Patients with xeroderma pigmentosum develop lentigo senilis during the first decade of life. Histology shows an increase in pigment in the basal cell layer and an increase in melanocytes. Lentigo senilis lesions respond to treatment with liquid nitrogen.

Lentigo maligna

Lentigo maligna (Hutchinson's melanotic freckle, precancerous melanosis) is a slowly enlarging brown patch, frequently found on the malar region in patients over the age of 50. Unlike lentigo senilis, there is a variegated brown pigmentation with an irregular border. Histology shows an uncontrolled, radial, intraepidermal growth of melanocytes. After a variable period of radial extension, nodules of invasive melanoma develop in 30–50% of cases. When this occurs, the lesion is termed lentigo maligna melanoma. Malignant change is suggested by irregular borders, multiple colors, large size, and bleeding. Excision with adequate surgical margins is recommended. Vigilant observation for development of recurrence is warranted in the postoperative period.

Conclusion

The eyelid has numerous structures from which a multitude of benign tumors may occur. The majority of these benign tumors are of cutaneous origin, arising from the structures that make up the eyelid skin. These are the epidermis; dermis; adnexa, including the pilosebaceous unit and the eccrine and apocrine sweat glands; and the associated pigment cells. Many of these cutaneous lesions can appear elsewhere on the skin, but a few more commonly affect the skin of the eyelids.

Benign eyelid tumors may be solid or cystic, solitary or multiple. Occasionally, a diagnosis is readily made on the basis of a characteristic appearance and clinical behavior. In other cases, the diagnosis can only be made with the aid of a biopsy. Appropriate treatment is based upon an accurate diagnosis. Given that some benign eyelid lesions have malignant potential, it is imperative to perform a biopsy if changes in the appearance of an eyelid lesion, such as increase in size, asymmetry or irregular shape, or bleeding, become manifest.

References

1. Nerad JA. *Oculoplastic surgery: the requisites in ophthalmology.* Philadelphia: Mosby; 2001.
2. Kersten RC, Ewing-Chow D, Kulwin DR, et al. Accuracy of clinical diagnosis of cutaneous eyelid lesions. *Ophthalmology.* 1997;104:479–484.
3. Margo CE. Eyelid tumors: accuracy of clinical diagnosis. *Am J Ophthalmol.* 1999;128:635–636.
4. Domonkos AN, Arnold HL, Odom RB, eds. *Andrew's diseases of the skin.* Philadelphia: WB Saunders; 1982.
5. Epstein W, Kligman AM. The pathogenesis of milia and benign tumors of the skin. *J Invest Dermatol.* 1956;26:1–11.
6. Sanderson KV. The structure of seborrheic keratosis. *Br J Dermatol.* 1968;80:588–593.
7. Dantzig PI. Sign of Leser-Trelat. *Arch Dermatol.* 1973;108:700–701.
8. Grimes PE, Arora S, Minus HR, et al. Dermatosis papulosa nigra. *Cutis.* 1983;32:385–386.
9. Scully J. Treatment of seborrheic keratosis. *JAMA.* 1970;213:1498.
10. Bapat BV, Madlensky L, Temple LK, et al. Family history characteristics, tumor microsatellite instability and germline MSH2 and MLH1 mutations in hereditary colorectal cancer. *Hum Genet.* 1999;104:167–176.
11. Goudie DR, Yuille MAR, Leversha MA, et al. Multiple self-healing squamous epitheliomata (ESS1) mapped to chromosome 9q22-q31 in families with common ancestry. *Nat Genet.* 1993;3:165–169.
12. Boynton JR, Searl SS, Caldwell EH. Large periocular keratoacanthoma: the case for definitive treatment. *Ophthalmic Surg.* 1986;17:565–569.
13. Farina AT, Leider M, Newall J, et al. Radiotherapy for aggressive and destructive keratoacanthomas. *J Dermatol Surg Oncol.* 1977;3:177–180.
14. Annest NM, VanBeeek MJ, Arpey CJ, et al. Intralesional methotrexate treatment for keratoacanthoma tumors: a retrospective study and review of the literature. *J Am Acad Dermatol.* 2007;56:989–993.
15. Goette DK, Odom RB, Arrott JW, et al. Treatment of keratoacanthoma with topical application of fluorouracil. *Arch Dermatol.* 1982;118:309–311.
16. Odom RB, Goette DK. Treatment of keratoacanthomas with intralesional fluorouracil. *Arch Dermatol.* 1978;114:1779–1783.
17. Freeman RG. On the pathogenesis of pseudoepitheliomatous hyperplasia. *J Cutan Pathol.* 1974;1:231–237.
18. Boniuk M, Zimmerman LE. Eyelid tumors with reference to lesions confused with squamous cell carcinoma. II. Inverted follicular keratosis. *Arch Ophthalmol.* 1963;69:698–707.
19. McGavran MH, Binnington B. Keratinous cysts of the skin. *Arch Dermatol.* 1966;94:499–508.
20. Groden J, Thliveris A, Samowitz W, et al. Identification and characterization of the familial adenomatous polyposis coli gene. *Cell.* 1991;66:589–600.
21. Kinzler KW, Nilbert MC, Su L-K, et al. Identification of FAP locus genes from chromosome 5q21. *Science.* 1991;253:661–665.

22. Solomon LM, Fretzin DF, Dewald RL. The epidermal nevus syndrome. *Arch Dermatol.* 1968;97:273–285.
23. Wonjo T, Tenzel PR. Actinic comedonal plaque of the eyelid. *Am J Ophthalmol.* 1983;96:687–688.
24. Fu W, Cockerell CJ. The actinic (solar) keratosis: a 21st-century perspective. *Arch Derm.* 2003;139:66–70.
25. Berneburg M, Lehmann AR. Xeroderma pigmentosum and related disorders: defects in DNA repair and transcription. *Adv Genet.* 2001;43:71–102.
26. Weinberg JM. Topical therapy for actinic keratoses: current and evolving therapie. *Rev Recent Clin Trials.* 2006;1:53–60.
27. Jakobiec FA, Bonanno PA, Sigelman J. Conjunctival adnexal cysts and dermoids. *Arch Ophthalmol.* 1978;96:1404–1409.
28. Rodgers IR, Jakobiec FA, Krebs W, et al. Papillary oncocytoma of the eyelid. A previously undescribed tumor of apocrine gland origin. *Ophthalmology.* 1988;95:1071–1076.
29. Thaller VT, Collin JRO, McCartney ACE. Oncocytoma of the eyelid: a case report. *Br J Ophthalmol.* 1987;71:753–756.
30. Filipic M, Silva M. Phakomatous choristoma of the eyelid. *Arch Ophthalmol.* 1972;88:172–175.
31. Tripathi RC, Tripathi BJ, Ringus J. Phakomatous choristoma of the lower eyelid with psammoma body formation. *Ophthalmology.* 1981;88:1198–1206.
32. Zimmerman LE. Phakomatous choristoma of the eyelid, a tumor of lenticular anlage. *Am J Ophthalmol.* 1971;71:169–171.
33. Xu G, O'Connell P, Viskochil D, et al. The neurofibromatosis type 1 gene encodes a protein related to GAP. *Cell.* 1990;62:599–608.
34. Rouleau GA, Merel P, Lutchman M, et al. Alteration in a new gene encoding a putative membrane-organizing protein causes neurofibromatosis type 2. *Nature.* 1993;363:515–521.
35. Brini A, Dhermy P, Sahel J. *Oncology of the eye and adnexa: atlas of clinical pathology.* The Netherlands: Dordrecht, Kluwer; 1990.
36. Shields JA, Guibor PG. Neurilemmoma of the eyelid resembling a recurrent chalazion. *Arch Ophthalmol.* 1984;102:1650.
37. Eng C. The RET proto-oncogene in multiple endocrine neoplasia type 2 and Hirschsprung's disease. *N Engl J Med.* 1996;335:943–951.
38. Friedman Z, Eden E, Neumann E. Granular cell myoblastoma of the eyelid margin. *Br J Ophthalmol.* 1973;57:757–760.
39. Berry SA, Peterson C, Mize W, et al. Klippel-Trenaunay syndrome. *Am J Med Genet.* 1998;79:319–326.
40. DiLandro A, Tadini GL, Marchesi L, et al. Phakomatosis pigmentovascularis: a new case with renal angiomas and some considerations about the classification. *Pediatr Dermatol.* 1999;16:25–30.
41. Noe JM, Barsky SH, Greer DE, et al. Port-wine stains and the response to argon laser therapy: successful treatment and predictive role of color, age, and biopsy. *Plast Reconstr Surg.* 1980;65:130–136.
42. Harris GJ, Massaro BM. Acute proptosis in childhood. In: Tassman W, Jaeger EA, eds. *Clinical ophthalmology.* vol. 2. Philadelphia: JB Lippincott; 1991.
43. Haik BG, Jakobiec FA, Ellsworth RM. Capillary hemangioma of the lids and orbit. *Ophthalmology.* 1979;86:760–789.
44. Stigmar G, Crawford JS, Ward CM, et al. Ophthalmic sequelae of infantile hemangiomas of the eyelids and orbit. *Am J Ophthalmol.* 1978;85:806–813.
45. Jakobiec FA, Jones IS. Vascular tumors, malformations, and degenerations. In: Tassman W, Jaeger EA, eds. *Clinical ophthalmology.* vol. 2. Philadelphia: JB Lippincott; 1991.
46. Glatt HJ, Putterman AM, Van Aalst JJ, et al. Adrenal suppression and growth retardation after injection of periocular capillary hemangioma with corticosteroids. *Ophthalmic Surg.* 1991;22:95–97.
47. Kushner B. Intralesional corticosteroid injection for infantile adnexal hemangioma. *Am J Ophthalmol.* 1982;93:496–506.
48. Ruttum MS, Abrams GW, Harris GJ, et al. Bilateral retinal embolization associated with intralesional corticosteroid injection for capillary hemangioma of infancy. *J Pediatr Ophthalmol Strabismus.* 1993;30:4–7.
49. Droste PJ, Ellis FD, Sondhi N, et al. Linear subcutaneous fat atrophy after corticosteroid injection of periocular hemangiomas. *Am J Ophthalmol.* 1988;105:65–69.
50. Cogan MS, Elsas FJ. Eyelid depigmentation following corticosteroid injection for infantile ocular adnexal hemangioma. *J Pediatr Ophthalmol Strabismus.* 1989;26:35–38.
51. Sutula FC, Glover AT. Eyelid necrosis following intralesional corticosteroid injection for capillary hemangioma. *Ophthalmic Surg.* 1987;18:103–105.
52. Chang F, Boyd A, Nelson CC, et al. Successful treatment of infantile hemangiomas with interferon-alpha-2b. *J Pediatr Hematol Oncol.* 1997;19:237–244.
53. Leaute-Labreze C, Dumas de la Roque E, Hubiche T, et al. Propranolol for severe hemangiomas of infancy. *N Engl J Med.* 2008;358:2649–2651.
54. McCannel CA, Hoenig J, Umlas J, et al. Orbital lesions in the blue rubber bleb nevus syndrome. *Ophthalmology.* 1996;103:933–936.
55. Pang P, Jakobiec FA, Iwamato T, et al. Small lymphangiomas of the eyelids. *Ophthalmology.* 1984;91:1278–1284.
56. Jones IS. Lymphangiomas of the ocular adnexa. An analysis of 62 cases. *Trans Am Ophthalmol Soc.* 1959;57:602–665.
57. Greinwald Jr JH, Burke DK, Sato Y, et al. Treatment of lymphangiomas in children: an update of Picibanil (OK-432) sclerotherapy. *Otolaryngol Head Neck Surg* 1999;121:381–387.
58. Holt JE, Holt GR, Thornton WR. Arteriovenous malformation of the eyelid. *Ophthalmic Surg.* 1980;11:771–777.
59. Charles NC. Multiple glomus tumors of the face and eyelids. *Arch Ophthalmol.* 1976;94:1283–1285.
60. Brouillard P, Boon LM, Mulliken JB, et al. Mutations in a novel factor, glomulin, are responsible for glomuvenous malformations ('glomangiomas'). *Am J Hum Genet.* 2002;70:866–874.
61. Sorenson RL, Spencer WH, Stewart WB, et al. Intravascular papillary endothelial hyperplasia of the eyelid. *Arch Ophthalmol* 1983;101:1728–1730.
62. Clearkin KB, Enzinger FM. Intravascular papillary endothelial hyperplasia. *Arch Pathol Lab Med.* 1976;100:441–444.
63. Amrith S, Hong Low C, Cheah E, et al. Erdheim-Chester disease: a bilateral orbital mass as an indication of systemic disease. *Orbit.* 1999;18:99–104.
64. Rohrich RJ, Janis JE, Pownell PH. Xanthelasma palpebrarum: a review and current management principles. *Plast Reconstr Surg.* 2002;110:1310–1314.
65. Vinger P, Sach B. Ocular manifestations of hyperlipidemia. *Am J Ophthalmol.* 1970;70:563–573.
66. Zimmerman LE. Ocular lesions of juvenile xanthogranuloma (nevoxanthoendothelioma). *Trans Am Acad Ophthalmol Otolaryngol.* 1965;69:412–439.
67. John T, Yanoff M, Scheie HG. Eyelid fibrous histiocytoma. *Ophthalmology.* 1981;88:1193–1195.
68. Jordan DR, Anderson RL. Fibrous histiocytoma. An uncommon eyelid lesion. *Arch Ophthalmol.* 1989;107:1530–1531.
69. Ni C, Dryja TP, Albert DM. Sweat gland tumors in the eyelids: a clinicopathological analysis of 55 cases. *Int Ophthalmol Clin.* 1982;22:1–22.
70. Schepis C, Siragusa M, Palazzo R, et al. Palpebral syringomas and Down's syndrome. *Dermatology.* 1994;189:248–250.
71. Maloney ME. An easy method for removal of syringoma. *J Dermatol Surg Oncol.* 1982;8:973–975.
72. Nerad JA, Anderson RL. CO_2 laser treatment of eyelid syringomas. *Ophthal Plast Reconstr Surg.* 1988;491–494.
73. Roenigk Jr HH. Dermabrasion for miscellaneous cutaneous lesions (exclusive of scarring from acne). *J Dermatol Surg Oncol.* 1977;3:322–328.
74. Ter Poorten MC, Barrett K, Cook J. Familial eccrine spiradenoma: a case report and review of the literature. *Dermatol Surg.* 2003;29:411–414.
75. Kersting DW, Helwig EB. Eccrine spiradenoma. *Arch Dermatol.* 1956;73:199–227.
76. Boniuk M, Halpert B. Clear cell hidradenoma or myoepithelioma of the eyelid. *Arch Ophthalmol.* 1964;72:59–63.
77. Ferry AP, Hadad HM. Eccrine acrospiroma (porosyringoma) of the eyelid. *Arch Ophthalmol.* 1970;83:591–593.
78. Greer CH. Clear-cell hidradenoma of the eyelid. *Arch Ophthalmol.* 1968;80:220–222.
79. Smith JD, Chernosky ME. Hidrocytomas. *Arch Dermatol.* 1973;108:676–679.
80. Hirsch P, Helwig EB. Chondroid syringoma: mixed tumor of the skin, salivary gland type. *Arch Dermatol.* 1961;84:835–847.
81. Alessi E, Gianotti R, Coggi A. Multiple apocrine hidrocystomas of the eyelids. *Br J Dermatol.* 1997;137:642–645.
82. Bignell GR, Warren W, Seal S, et al. Identification of the familial cylindromatosis tumour-suppressor gene. *Nat Genet.* 2000;25:160–165.
83. Jakobiec FA, Streeten BW, Iwamato T, et al. Syringocystadenoma papilliferum of the eyelid. *Ophthalmology.* 1981;88:1175–1181.
84. Prayson RA, Prakash K, Wyllie E, et al. Linear epidermal nevus and nevus sebaceous syndromes: a clinicopathologic study of 3 patients. *Arch Pathol Lab Med.* 1999;123:301–305.
85. Harada H, Hashimoto K, Ko MS. The gene for multiple familial trichoepithelioma maps to chromosome 9p21. *J Invest Dermatol.* 1996;107:41–43.

86. Young AL, Kellermayer R, Szigeti R, et al. CYLD mutations underlie Brooke-Spiegler, familial cylindromatosis, and multiple familial trichoepithelioma syndromes. *Clin Genet.* 2006;70:246–249.
87. Hashimoto K, Lever WF. Histogenesis of skin appendage tumors. *Arch Dermatol.* 1969;100:356–369.
88. Shields JA, Shields CL, Eagle Jr RC. Trichoadenoma of the eyelid. *Am J Ophthalmol.* 1998;126:846–848.
89. Pinkus H, Sutton R. Trichofolliculoma. *Arch Dermatol.* 1965;91:46–49.
90. Hidayat AA, Font RL. Trichilemmoma of eyelid and eyebrow: a clinicopathological study of 31 cases. *Arch Ophthalmol.* 1980;98:844–847.
91. Brownstein MH, Mehregan AH, Bikowski JB, et al. The dermatopathology of Cowden's syndrome. *Br J Dermatol.* 1979;100:667–673.
92. Vantomme N, VanCalenbergh F, Goffin J, et al. Lhermitte-Duclos is a clinical manifestation of Cowden's syndrome. *Surg Neurol.* 2001;56:201–204.
93. DiCristofano A, Pesce B, Cordon-Cardo C, et al. PTEN is essential for embryonic development and tumour suppression. *Nat Genet.* 1998;19:348–355.
94. Geh JL, Moss AL. Multiple pilomatrixomata and myotonic dystrophy: a familial association. *Br J Plast Surg.* 1999;52:143–145.
95. O'Grady RB, Spoerl G. Pilomatrixoma (benign calcifying epithelioma of Malherbe). *Ophthalmology.* 1981;88:1196–1197.
96. Chan EF, Gat U, McNiff JM, et al. A common human skin tumour is caused by activating mutations in beta-catenin. *Nat Genet.* 1999;21:410–413.
97. Yanoff M, Fine BS. *Ocular pathology.* 2nd ed. Philadelphia: Harper and Row; 1982.
98. Jakobiec FA. Sebaceous adenoma of the eyelid and visceral malignancy. *Am J Ophthalmol.* 1974;78:952–960.
99. Torre D. Multiple sebaceous tumors. *Arch Dermatol.* 1968;98:549–551.
100. Dutton JJ, Anderson RL, Schelper RL, et al. Orbital malignant melanoma and oculodermal melanocytosis: report of two cases and review of the literature. *Ophthalmology.* 1984;91:497–506.
101. Jenne DE, Reimann H, Nezu J, et al. Peutz-Jeghers syndrome is caused by mutations in a novel serine threonine kinase. *Nat Genet.* 1998;18:38–43.
102. Hodgson C. Senile lentigo. *Arch Dermatol.* 1963;87:197–207.

Chapter 32

Malignant Eyelid Tumors

David T. Tse, Jennifer I. Hui

Carcinoma of the skin is the most common malignancy in the United States, accounting for half of all cancers.[1] About 500 000 people in the United States are treated annually for basal or squamous cell carcinoma.[2] Forty to 50% of Americans who live to age 65 years will be diagnosed with at least one skin cancer during their lifetime.[3,4] Approximately 5% to 9% of all cutaneous cancers arise in the eyelids. The most common periocular malignancies are basal cell carcinoma, squamous cell carcinoma, sebaceous cell carcinoma, and malignant melanoma. Kaposi's sarcoma is being recognized with increasing frequency among immunosuppressed patients. Systemic diseases such as basal cell nevus syndrome, xeroderma pigmentosum, and Muir-Torre syndrome are associated with periocular cutaneous tumors. The goals in the management of malignant eyelid lesions are to establish early accurate diagnosis, to achieve a permanent cure by total eradication of the tumor, and to preserve or restore eyelid function and cosmesis.

Basal Cell Carcinoma

Basal cell carcinoma (BCC) is the most common skin cancer, with incidence rates between 146 and 317 per 100 000 in the United States[5] and 1 per 100 in tropical regions of Australia.[6] It accounts for 90% of all eyelid malignancies and 20% of all eyelid tumors. The relative frequency of basal cell carcinoma to squamous cell carcinoma (SCC) of the eyelid has been estimated to be as high as 40 : 1. The tumor primarily involves the lower eyelid (50–66%) and the medial canthus (25–30%).

Actinic damage is an important predisposing factor in the genesis of BCC and other epithelial skin tumors. The ultraviolet (UV) rays most responsible for cutaneous carcinogenesis are 290–320 nm (UVB) in wavelength. Individuals with a fair complexion are particularly susceptible to the effects of UV radiation. The majority of patients with BCC are between 50 and 80 years of age; 5–15% are between the ages of 20 and 40 years. Overall, increased UV exposure during childhood and adolescence seems to be a critical risk factor for developing tumors in adulthood.[7] Additionally, positive family history incurs an odds ratio of 2.2 for development of disease.[7,8]

Among young adults with BCC, two distinct groups can be identified. Most young patients tend to be of light complexion and eye coloring without a family history of basal cell carcinoma. A second group possesses characteristics of the basal cell nevus syndrome.[9] The appearance of even a single isolated BCC in a young adolescent should suggest the possibility that the lesion may be a forme fruste of basal cell nevus syndrome.[10] Basal cell carcinomas occurring in younger persons[11] and those with immunodeficiency syndromes[12,13] are usually more aggressive. Patients who have been treated for BCC show a higher risk for developing a subsequent lesion.[14]

Martin et al.[15] noted that approximately 10% of patients with a history of radiation therapy to the head developed cutaneous neoplasm within the treatment field. The median interval between exposure and development of carcinoma was 21 years. Histologically, two-thirds of these radiation-induced skin cancers were BCC and one-third were SCC.

Clinical appearance

Basal cell carcinoma is a tumor with varied clinical and histologic manifestations and develops from the basal layer and epidermal appendages; the malignant character depends on the destructive growth of the primary tumor, rather than on metastasis. The most common clinical presentations include the nodular, noduloulcerative, pigmented, cystic, morpheaform or sclerosing, plaque and superficial varieties.

The typical nodular type appears as a firm, pearly, dome-shaped nodule, often displaying multiple telangiectatic vessels (Fig. 32.1). A hyperkeratotic crust, typical of benign and malignant squamous lesions, is generally not seen with basal cell carcinomas. Some lesions may bleed without pain, whereas others heal spontaneously to form scar tissue as they enlarge. With increasing radial growth, the interior of the tumor may outgrow its blood supply, leading to central ulceration. Eventually, this may appear as a slowly enlarging ulcer, forming the common noduloulcerative variant with characteristic rolled and indurated borders (rodent ulcer) (Fig. 32.2).

Histologically, basal cell carcinoma is composed of solid lobules of small, regularly shaped cells with basophilic and scanty cytoplasm. The most distinctive histopathologic feature of this tumor is the peripheral palisading or 'picket-fence' formation of peripheral nuclei at the edge of the mass.

A variant of the noduloulcerative type, characterized by intermingled crusting, ulceration, erythema, and scarring, is

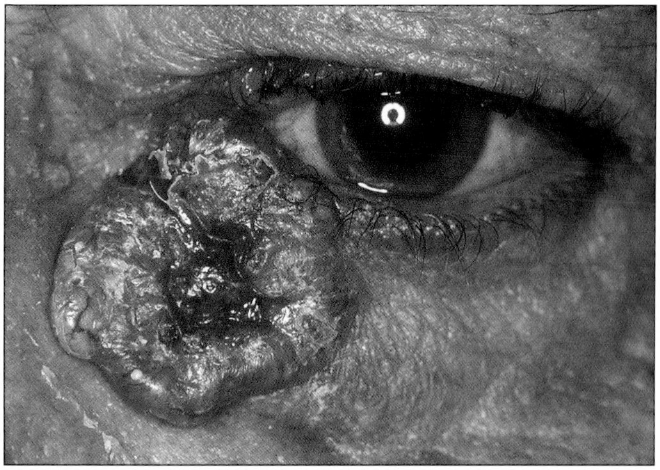

Fig. 32.1 The typical appearance of a nodular basal cell carcinoma. Note exophytic growth and sharp delineation from normal skin.

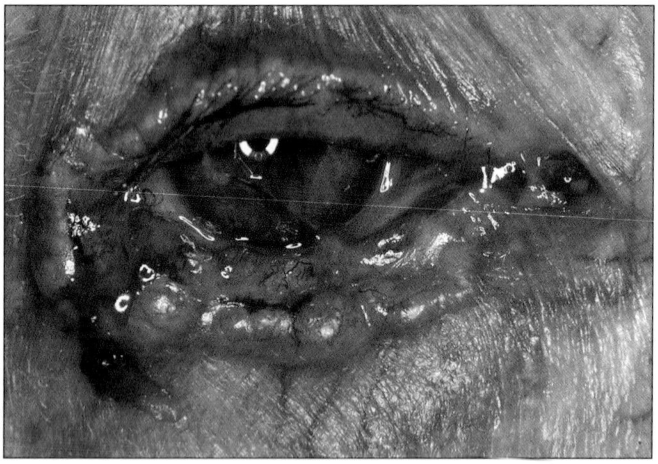

Fig. 32.2 This patient had a nodular lesion of the medial canthus comparable to that shown in Figure 32.1 many years ago. Because of years of neglect, tumor proliferation has caused extensive tissue destruction and ulceration. The term *rodent ulcer* is derived from the resemblance of the lesion to tissue gnawed by a rat.

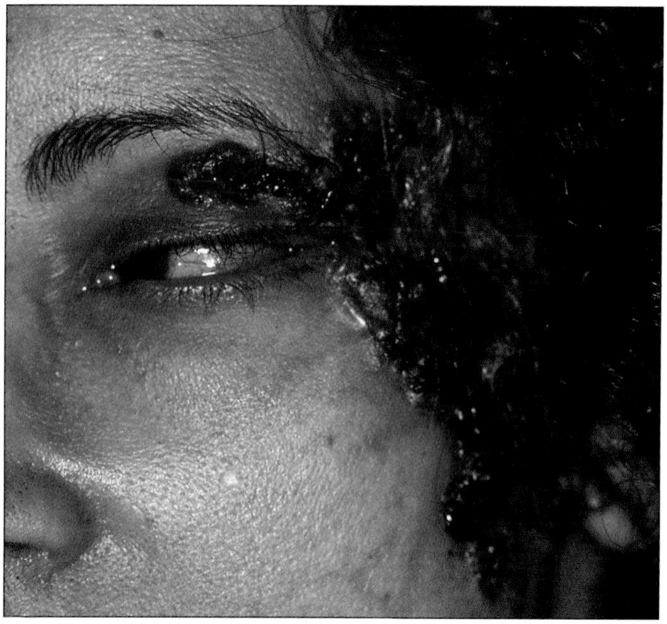

Fig. 32.3 An extensive field-fire lesion involving the eyelids, temple, cheek, and preauricular regions.

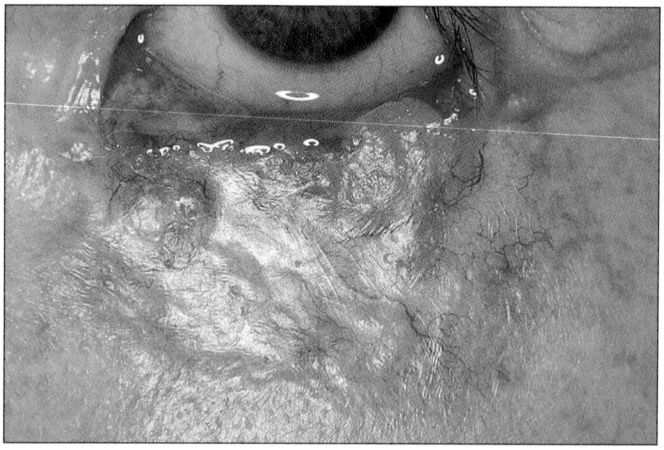

Fig. 32.4 A morpheaform basal cell carcinoma with its centrifugal extensions to the medial and lateral canthal regions. The lesion appears as a flat or slightly depressed indurated plaque of white-pink color. The tumor margins are difficult to decipher by clinical inspection.

referred to as field-fire BCC. It spreads peripherally and may become large (Fig. 32.3). Clinically, it is extremely difficult to determine the margins of this variant. These lesions require extensive surgical extirpation and reconstruction.

Pigmented basal cell carcinomas are rare, accounting for <10% of basal cell carcinomas. They are similar to the nodular type with respect to age, sex, location, duration, and rate of recurrence.[16] Pigmented BCC is seen more often in dark-complexioned individuals,[17] with a spectrum of tumor colors ranging from light brown to black. Melanin pigmentation may occur in all types of basal cell carcinomas with the possible exception of the morpheaform type. These lesions are sometimes misdiagnosed as pigmented nevi or malignant melanomas. The pigmentation is caused by benign melanocytes containing melanin granules that proliferate along with the tumor basal cells.

Cystic basal cell carcinoma may develop with mucin accumulation or degenerative necrosis within solid lobules of proliferating basaloid cells. No particular biologic import is associated with the cystic variety, except that they may be difficult to differentiate from an innocuous, benign epithelial inclusion cyst or apocrine hidrocystoma.

Morpheaform or sclerosing type appears as a flat or slightly depressed, waxy, poorly demarcated, indurated plaque whose pale color has been likened to old ivory (Fig. 32.4). The overlying epidermis remains unaltered for a long time. Ulceration, rolled edges, and crusting are conspicuously absent, but telangiectasias are prominent. If situated along the eyelid margin, the tumor can simulate a localized, chronic blepharitis. Histologically, the morpheaform type is characterized by discrete, elongated islands of basaloid cells encased in a dense, fibrous stroma beneath an intact epidermis. These finger-like cords of tumor can project deep into the dermis and connective tissue, beyond the area of suspected clinical involvement. This subtype often displays a tendency toward invasion of the deeper orbital structures and a propensity for recurrence. The subclinical extension of tumor cells into deep tissue planes and the surgeon's inability to determine the tumor margins render its complete removal difficult. The recurrence rate of an incompletely excised morpheaform tumor is 10 times greater than that of the nodular type.[18] To ensure complete excision, this type is best managed by the Mohs' micrographic technique.

Superficial basal cell carcinoma is a less common variety usually found on the trunk. These flat, superficial lesions appear as erythematous, scaly patches or plaques with well-defined pearly borders. Like the nodular subtype, they are less aggressive and enlarge slowly without tendency to invade or ulcerate. They are often mistaken for psoriatic plaques or Bowen's disease.

Biologic behavior

Regardless of histologic type, basal cell carcinomas are usually only locally invasive. They are typically indolent; however, if neglected, uncontrolled tumor growth can infiltrate nearby structures including the orbit, paranasal sinuses, and cranial cavity. Risk factors for subclinical spread include tumor diameter >2 cm, location on central face or ears, longstanding presence prior to initial treatment, incomplete excision, aggressive subtype, and perineural or perivascular involvement.[1] Tumor deaths resulting from direct intracranial extension of basal cell carcinomas may occur. The reported incidence of basal cell carcinoma metastasis is estimated to be <0.1%.[15] If metastatic disease develops, it is usually found in the regional lymph nodes.[19,20]

Clinical diagnosis

Ophthalmologists are afforded an excellent method of magnified examination of eyelid lesions through the use of slit lamp biomicroscopy. Distortion or destruction of meibomian orifices of the eyelid margin or focal loss of lashes should alert the clinician to the possibility of underlying malignancy. Flaky crust on the surface of a lesion suggests SCC, whereas a more translucent, white, or flesh-colored lesion stretching the skin is likely to represent a BCC.[21] If a lesion attains a diameter of 1 cm in <3 months, a diagnosis of SCC or keratoacanthoma is likely. A careful search for an elevated translucent telangiectatic border is important in differentiating basal cell carcinoma from all other lesions. Despite magnified examination of suspicious lesions, clinical appearance alone may be insufficient to establish a diagnosis and biopsy is required for definitive histologic verification.

Treatment

Biopsy of any suspicious eyelid lesion should be performed to establish a definitive diagnosis. If a lesion is small, excisional biopsy with at least 2–3 mm of margin of normal tissue should be considered. Biopsy can be accomplished by simple elliptical excision and closure of the defect. If the size of the anticipated excisional defect is such that closure will cause eyelid malposition, an incisional biopsy should be performed first. Similarly, if it is anticipated that a graft or flap will be required to repair the defect, the surgical margins must be examined microscopically.

In simple surgical excisions, the specimen should be examined histologically to confirm the margins are clear. Excisional biopsy of even small lesions is controversial because inadequate resection is common. Doxanas et al.[18] reported a 27% incomplete excision rate of basal cell carcinomas managed by excisional biopsy; only 25% of the incompletely excised tumors recurred. This low rate of recurrence is thought to result from local stimulation of the immune system secondary to surgical trauma.[22] Because of the frequency of incomplete excisions, some advocate incisional biopsy to establish the diagnosis first, followed by excision under frozen section control to ensure all surgical margins are free of residual tumor cells.[23]

Several different treatment modalities have been used to manage periocular BCCs. Surgical excision, cryosurgery, radiotherapy, and Mohs' micrographic surgery have been reported to achieve 5-year cure rates of 90%. Currently, the best available options are surgical excision with standard frozen section control or Mohs' micrographic surgery. Reports suggest 5-year cure rates using these two forms of treatment in excess of 95%. Hamada and colleagues found that a 2-mm margin with the nodular subtype and 4 mm for all other subtypes are adequate in preventing recurrences.[24,25] Conventional frozen section control is widely used, but in many instances only a small fraction of the periphery of the excised tumor is actually examined microscopically.

Mohs' micrographic surgery

The fresh tissue technique of micrographic surgery, an adaptation of Mohs' original fixed tissue technique, was developed to maximize examination of margins and conservation of tissue. This resection is best accomplished by dermatologists trained in Mohs' technique. A close working relationship between the Mohs' and reconstructive surgeons results in eradication of periorbital tumor with optimal functional results. The Mohs' fresh tissue technique involves removal of the gross mass of the tumor plus a small peripheral margin of normal tissue. A thin layer of tissue, approximately 2-mm thick, is further excised from the entire base and edges of the wound. The initial specimen is divided into 4–7-μm thick portions on glass slides; the edges are marked with different colored dyes to maintain orientation.[26] Frozen sections are obtained from the undersurface and skin edge of each specimen. Locations of residual tumor are marked on a map and only those areas are re-excised. Surgical resection is continued until there is a microscopically proven tumor-free plane. The defect is then reconstructed by the oculoplastic surgeon. This interdisciplinary collaborative team approach allows two unbiased specialists to offer their shared expertise in achieving the optimum surgical outcome for the patient.

Frozen section control

Excision of BCC using frozen section control can also yield excellent results. Cure rates of 99% have been reported.[27,28] Frozen section control of tumor margins is performed by noting the clinical boundaries of the tumor edges and excising an additional 3-mm cuff of normal-appearing tissue. A pathologist examines each margin; if no tumor cells are noted, immediate repair is undertaken. If tumor remains in the excised portion, further surgery is performed until the margins are tumor free.

Ionizing radiation therapy

A basic principle of cancer surgery is to obtain tumor-free margins. As techniques that ensure the adequacy of tumor-free margins become more popular and available, radiation therapy is used less frequently to treat primary basal cell carcinomas. For individuals with inoperable disease, multiple medical problems, elderly patients unable to tolerate surgical resection, or patients in whom surgery will result in extensive disfigurement with potential loss of useful ocular function, radiation therapy is an acceptable palliative alternative.

Reported cure rates are good but do not approach those of histologically controlled surgical excision. The 5-year tumor control rate of 92–95% for periocular BCCs treated by radiation therapy is slightly less than those associated with histologically monitored surgical excisions.[29,30] When compared to surgical excision with frozen margin control, radiation therapy is associated with higher rates of persistent tumor and recurrences.[31,32]

Despite these encouraging results, this modality has potential disadvantages. It lacks histologic control of the tumor margins beyond the treatment field. Postradiation complications can be potentially vision threatening, and daily treatments for a period of weeks may be necessary. Radiation-induced atrophy and vascular damage to skin may compromise its potential use as flaps for future reconstruction. Side effects and complications after radiotherapy include skin atrophy, ectropion, entropion, nasolacrimal duct stenosis, keratitis, conjunctival keratinization, cataract, loss of eyelashes, and globe perforation.[29] Ocular protection and administration by a well-trained radiation therapist can reduce many of these complications.

Cryosurgery

While surgical excision with frozen section control is preferable, cryosurgery may be an accepted alternative for tumors with well-defined borders.[33-36] Cryotherapy is useful for small lesions, but less effective for larger and deeply invasive tumors. When compared to radiation therapy, cryotherapy is associated with higher rates of recurrence (39% vs 4%).[31,37]

Liquid nitrogen is administered by an open spray or cryoprobes in a closed system. Cryogens such as carbon dioxide and nitrous oxide do not freeze to adequate depths and are not recommended for BCC.[38] Tumor cryonecrosis is achieved through double freeze–thaw cycles while tissue temperature is monitored by a thermocouple. Cryoapplication is applied until a tissue temperature between −25°C and −30°C is reached. The lesion is allowed to thaw to room temperature before repeating the cycle.

Contraindications to cryosurgery of eyelid basal cell carcinomas include: (1) involvement of the conjunctival fornix; (2) fixation of tumor to periosteum; (3) sensory or motor denervation; (4) cold intolerance – cryoglobulinemia or cold urticaria; (5) deeply pigmented skin; (6) indistinct margins; (7) diameter of lesion >10 mm, and (8) sclerosing or multicentric type. Complications include depigmentation, hyperpigmentation, eyelid notching, hypertrophic scar, pseudoepithelial hyperplasia, ectropion, punctal and canalicular stenosis, and lash loss.[35]

Chemotherapy

In patients with extensive, widespread skin cancer that cannot be managed by standard methods of treatment, chemotherapy can be considered as an alternative. Chemotherapy may result in remission of the tumor or induce shrinkage of the lesion, allowing for other forms of treatment or less radical surgery.

Recurrence

Tumor recurrence may be related to the histologic characteristics of the BCC, anatomic site, and failure of cure by the type of previous primary treatment, specifically nonsurgical modalities. Basal cell carcinomas situated in the medial canthal region are more likely to infiltrate deeply than those arising from the central eyelid margin.[39,40] The predilection for deep early penetration of a medial canthal tumor is thought to be related to its proximity to the embryologic fusion planes. These planes offer little resistance to penetration of cutaneous carcinomas and have been implicated in their depth of invasion, horizontal spread, and recurrence. Clinically, the high-risk areas for deep tumor invasion in the midface are depicted as the 'H-zone.' The tissue planes of the inner canthus are formed by embryologic fusion of the frontonasal process with the lateral and maxillary processes.[40] Anatomically, this produces clefts in the subcutaneous fascial planes, allowing tumor cells to follow the 'path of least resistance' to the periosteum of the lacrimal and ethmoid bones, thus gaining access to the posterior orbit.[41] Tumors located in this high-risk zone can invade deeply and ultimately require exenteration.

The increased mortality and morbidity associated with medial canthal lesions may also be attributed to: (1) access to the nose via the nasolacrimal duct, providing a route of tumor extension; (2) an array of arteries, veins, and nerves in this region facilitating tumor extension in multiple directions; (3) an unremarkable external appearance with orbital infiltration along the medial orbital wall, reducing early clinical suspicion; and (4) the surgeon's unwillingness to aggressively resect tumors in this region for fear of damaging a myriad of fine anatomic structures.

Squamous Cell Carcinoma

Squamous cell carcinoma (SCC), a malignant neoplasm of the epidermal keratinizing cells, constitutes approximately 9% of all periocular cutaneous tumors and is the second most common eyelid malignancy. SCC of the eyelids is a potentially lethal tumor that can invade the orbit by direct or perineural extension, spread to regional lymph nodes, and metastasize to distal sites. Regional lymph node metastases have been reported in up to 24% of patients.[42] SCC is also more likely to spread perineurally than BCC, accounting for possible 'skip' lesions.[43] Actinic keratoses and Bowen's disease are considered incipient skin cancers with the potential to progress to invasive SCC.

Ultraviolet UVB rays (290–320 nm) and possibly UVA (320–400 nm) are thought to have carcinogenic effects on skin.[44] Ultraviolet radiation is believed to induce skin cancer by direct DNA damage or alterations in cellular immunity resulting from injury to Langerhans cells within the epidermis.[45,46] Most cutaneous squamous cell carcinomas arise from pre-existing lesions such as actinic keratoses, radiation dermatoses, burn scars, and inflammatory lesions. Photochemotherapy such as psoralen therapy with UVA light has also been implicated in tumor formation.[47] Thermal injuries to the skin have been reported to produce thermal keratoses and squamous cell carcinoma.[48] Other factors implicated in the development of SCC include chemical exposure (arsenic, polycyclic aromatic hydrocarbons, smoking), immunosuppression, prior radiation, and genetic diseases (albinism, xeroderma pigmentosum).[43]

Premalignant Lesions

Actinic keratosis

Actinic keratoses (AKs) are proliferations of transformed, neoplastic keratinocytes confined to the epidermis and are induced by exposure to ultraviolet (UV) radiation. They are extremely prevalent and are seen in most middle-aged to elderly fair-complexioned individuals with a history of significant sun exposure. AKs tend to increase in number with age, and often develop on the face, forearm, scalp, and dorsal hands. They are typically round, flat, scaly, keratotic plaques with an erythematous base, measuring only a few millimeters in diameter (Fig. 32.5). Occasionally, these lesions have a horny or wart-like appearance with the texture of fine sandpaper.

Actinic keratoses are in a state of continual flux.[49] Increased sunlight exposure may activate the lesions, especially in the summer months. Marks et al.[49] reported that 25% of individual actinic keratoses observed over a 12-month period spontaneously resolved, although there was a generalized net increase in total number because of the development of new lesions. The risk of malignant transformation from a single AK lesion has been estimated to be <0.24% per year. Although the risk per lesion per year may be low, a patient with several actinic keratoses followed over a 10-year period may have an expected risk of malignant transformation of 16.9%.[50] SCCs arising from AKs are though to be less aggressive, with lower metastatic potential, than SCC arising de novo.

As mentioned earlier, the literature reflects controversy about the risk of progression. Actinic keratoses are part of a continuum beginning with DNA damage and mutation, neoplastic transformation and proliferation, involvement of

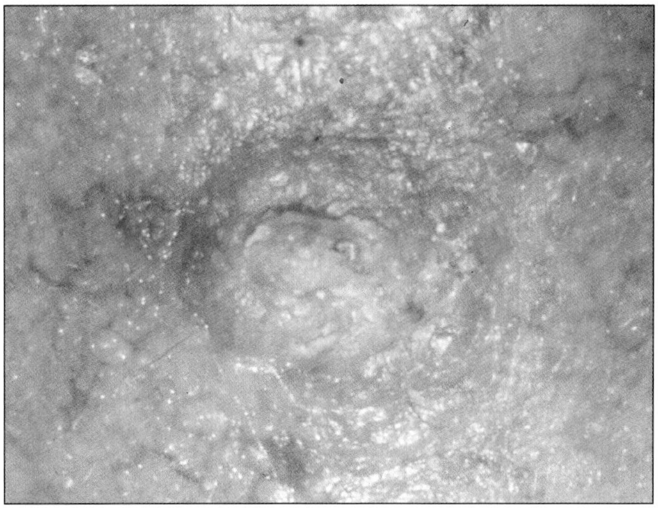

Fig. 32.5 An actinic keratosis on dorsum of nose. A round, flat, scaly keratotic plaque with an erythematous base.

deeper structures, and finally metastasis and death.[51] Most authorities believe that AKs represent squamous cell carcinomas in situ in their earliest stages, as these lesions demonstrate features of malignancy from their inception. These lesions share genetic tumor markers and identical *p53* gene mutations with SCC involving the dermis.[52] Treatment of periocular actinic keratoses depends on size and location of the lesions. Small lesions not involving the eyelid may be observed; however, within the periocular region, biopsy may be performed to establish a definitive diagnosis. With histologic confirmation of actinic keratosis, the remainder of the lesion may be treated with excision or cryotherapy.

Bowen's disease

Bowen's disease is synonymous with carcinoma in situ of the skin and has been implicated as a marker for internal malignancies. In contrast to most other squamous epithelial proliferative lesions that occur predominantly in sun-exposed areas, these lesions can appear in nonexposed regions of the body with a relatively high frequency. Bowen's original description referred only to lesions of the integument. Therefore, application of this designation to mucous membrane growths, such as those of the conjunctiva, should be avoided.

This condition produces a wide variety of clinical appearances. Typically, a patient presents with an isolated, slightly elevated, erythematous lesion with well-demarcated borders that fails to heal. The lesion has the appearance of a red, scaly patch or plaque, does not bleed or itch, and is devoid of hair. The average diameter is 1.3 cm, much larger than a typical AK lesion. Occasionally, Bowen's disease may present as a scaly, crusty, pigmented keratotic plaque.

In Bowen's disease, full-thickness epidermal cellular atypia and loss of polarity of the immature, neoplastic epithelial cell are the constant cytologic findings. The histopathologic hallmark is the lack of penetration of cancerous cells into the dermis. The basement membrane remains intact. Five percent of Bowen's disease lesions may progress to invasive SCC; complete surgical excision is usually curative.

Epidemiology and Differential Diagnosis

Squamous cell carcinoma

Like basal cell carcinomas, the majority of squamous cell carcinomas develop in fair-skinned, elderly individuals with a history of chronic sun exposure.[17,53–55] The average age of presentation is between 68 and 73 years, but primary SCC may be seen in younger patients who are immunosuppressed.[56] The prevalence in males is about twice that in females. The true incidence of squamous cell carcinoma of the eyelids has been debated. There is frequent histopathologic misdiagnosis of squamous cell carcinoma of the eyelid. The most frequent conditions mistaken for SCC are inverted follicular keratosis, benign keratosis, keratoacanthoma, pseudoepitheliomatous hyperplasia, and basal cell carcinoma.

Despite a myriad of predisposing factors, SCC sometimes arises de novo. These de novo lesions are more aggressive than those arising from actinic keratoses. In young patients with disease, underlying genetic predispositions such as xeroderma pigmentosum or albinism should be sought.

Clinical presentation

In the periocular region, SCC affects the lower eyelid more commonly than the upper eyelid, with a propensity for margin involvement.[57] These tumors vary in clinical presentation. They often present as painless plaques or nodules with variable degree of scale, crust, and ulceration (Fig. 32.6). They may also appear as papillomatous growths, cutaneous horns, or cysts along the eyelid margins. The pearly translucent border and the superficial network of telangiectatic vessels, features frequently associated with basal cell carcinomas, are lacking in squamous cell carcinomas. A biopsy is mandatory in all suspicious eyelid lesions to conclusively distinguish SCC from other conditions.

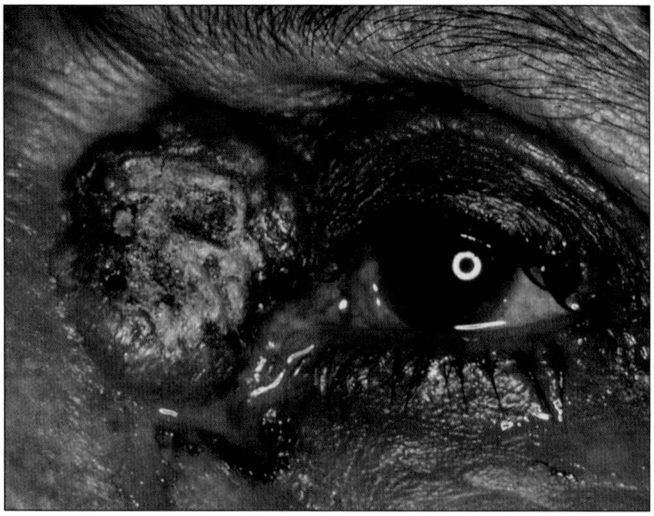

Fig. 32.6 A medial canthal squamous cell carcinoma presenting as a raised nodule with whitish-gray surface crusting.

Biologic behavior

Squamous cell carcinomas proliferate more rapidly than basal cell carcinomas, with a mean duration from onset to time of diagnosis of 9–12 months. Unlike basal cell carcinoma, SCC has greater potential for regional lymph node spread and distant metastases. The probability of metastases is related to: (1) degree of differentiation; (2) etiology – whether chronic osteomyelitis, draining fistulas, or prior radiation; (3) tumor size (>1 cm); and (4) depth of invasion.[58] The more anaplastic the tumor, the more likely it is to metastasize and/or recur. Finally, larger lesions and greater depth of tumor invasion are related to increased risk of tumor spread.[59] A subset of cutaneous tumors arising in areas of previous radiation or osteomyelitic cutaneous fistulas have higher rates of metastases (20% and 44%, respectively) than actinically induced lesions.[60]

Reports of regional lymph node involvement vary from 1.3% to 21.4% in patients with eyelid SCC. Lymphatic spread follows normal anatomic channels, with the outer two-thirds of the upper eyelid and outer one-third of the lower eyelid draining into the ipsilateral preauricular nodes. The medial one-third of the upper eyelid and the medial two-thirds of the lower eyelid drain into the ipsilateral submandibular nodes.

Eyelid squamous cell carcinoma can gain entrance into the orbit by progressive soft tissue destruction with direct contiguous extension. Alternatively, tumor cells can extend locally along fascial planes, perichondrium, lymphatics, blood vessels, or nerve sheaths.[61] Orbital disease may present 2–20 years after initial presentation; thus, lifelong follow-up should be emphasized to the patient.[62] Centripetal perineural spread signals a poor prognosis and should be viewed as similar to lymphatic metastasis. Direct or perineural extension is best treated by orbital exenteration and resection of involved lymph nodes combined with palliative radiation and chemotherapy. Overall, prognosis is generally poor.[63]

Treatment

After an incisional biopsy to confirm the diagnosis, the preferred method of management for primary periocular SCC is surgical excision with microscopic monitoring of tissue margins. Consideration should also be given to concurrent sentinel lymph node biopsy.[42] Excision is followed by immediate reconstruction of the defect.

Radiation therapy may be considered as an alternative primary treatment in patients with contraindications to surgery. Generally, most protocols involve doses greater than that for treatment of basal cell carcinomas.[57] Radiotherapy may also be palliative for patients with orbital extension and metastatic disease. Cryotherapy is another therapy that can be offered to individuals who refuse surgery or are poor surgical candidates. It may be considered for well-demarcated tumors <10 mm in diameter that do not involve the conjunctival fornix, medial canthus, or bone.

Sebaceous cell carcinoma

Sebaceous cell carcinoma has generally been considered the third most common eyelid malignancy. It accounts for approximately 1% of all eyelid tumors and 4.7% of all malignant epithelial eyelid lesions.[64–67] It is a potentially lethal tumor that clinicians must recognize early, as the morbidity and mortality rates approach those of malignant melanoma. Although pagetoid conjunctival spread is associated with higher rates of exenteration, the risk of tumor-related metastases is similar to that of patients without pagetoid disease.[68] The incidence of regional metastases is 17–28%,[69] with a 10-year actuarial tumor death rate of 28%.[70] A key factor for this high mortality rate is delay in establishing diagnosis because this lesion often masquerades as other benign eyelid conditions such as blepharoconjunctivitis, blepharitis, and chalazion.

This tumor tends to affect persons between the fifth and ninth decades of life, with most diagnoses made in the seventh decade.[66,71] Women are affected 1.5–2 times more often than men. Most sebaceous carcinomas arise from the meibomian glands of the eyelid, but may also originate from other sebaceous glands of the ocular adnexa. The upper eyelid is more frequently involved than the lower eyelid,[71] in contradistinction to basal cell carcinoma. This is likely due to the greater number of meibomian glands and Zeis' glands in the upper eyelid.[72] Separate upper and lower eyelid primaries occur in 6–8% of cases, and most likely represent multicentric origin.[66,73]

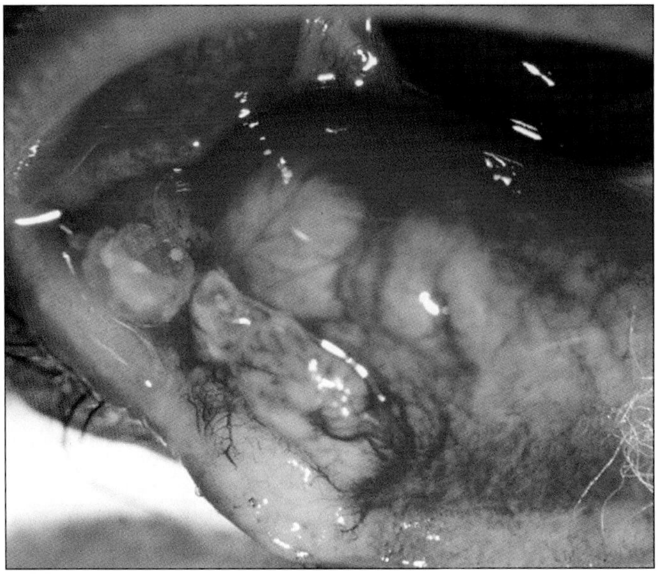

Fig. 32.7 Sebaceous cell carcinoma affecting the tarsal plate and anterior lamella of the lower eyelid. Multiple yellow nodules surrounded by an intense conjunctival reaction in the lower eyelid.

Etiology

The etiology of most cases of sebaceous carcinoma of the eyelid is unknown, but rarely it may be encountered in children who have received prior radiation therapy for tumors such as retinoblastoma or cavernous hemangioma of the face.[74,75]

Clinical presentation

Because of multiple anatomic sites of origin and different growth patterns, sebaceous carcinoma frequently exhibits variable and deceptive clinical presentations. The most common sign of a growth derived from the meibomian glands is a slowly enlarging, firm, and painless mass affecting the tarsal plate or the eyelid margin. These lesions may also exhibit varying degrees of yellow coloration due to the presence of lipid within the mass (Fig. 32.7). This yellow color may exclude other tumors, such as squamous cell or basal cell carcinoma in which lipid is characteristically absent. Lesions originating from the Zeis' glands appear as small, yellowish nodules located at the eyelid margin anterior to the gray line. Tumors arising from sebaceous glands of the caruncle usually appear as a subconjunctival, multi-lobulated, yellow mass.

The sebaceous carcinoma nodule may be mistaken clinically for a chalazion. It is generally rock hard and immobile, whereas a chalazion has a rubbery consistency and is not adherent to skin. As the neoplastic nodule enlarges, it may erupt toward the eyelid skin to initiate the intraepidermal growth phase, wherein the sebaceous cells spread diffusely throughout the epidermis.[19] This 'pagetoid' epidermal invasion is a distinctive feature of sebaceous carcinomas. Clinically, the eyelid is diffusely thickened and the skin appears indurated. With further tumor spread through the eyelid, loss of eyelashes can occur. These surface changes have frequently been misdiagnosed as blepharitis or dermatitis (Fig. 32.8). Similarly, the tumor may erupt onto the conjunctiva and propagate within the conjunctival epithelium. Pagetoid spread has been reported to occur in 40–80% of patients.[68,76] These malignant cells migrate along the conjunctival epithelium, extend onto the epibulbar surface and even the corneal epithelium, resulting in intense conjunctival inflammation and superficial keratitis (Fig. 32.9).[21]

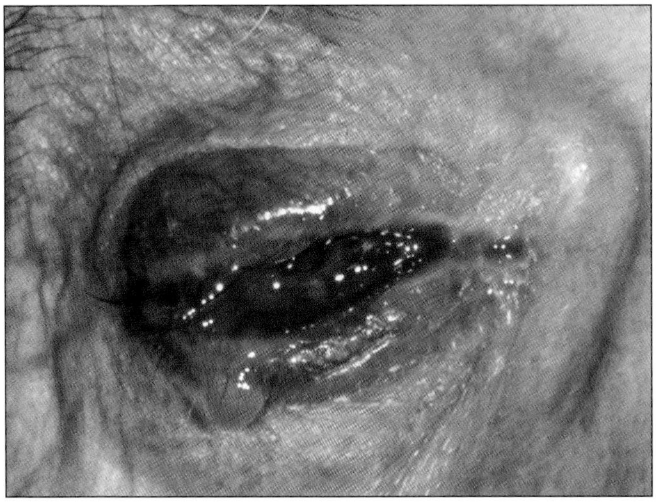

Fig. 32.8 A patient with sebaceous cell carcinoma masquerading as unilateral chronic blepharoconjunctivitis for many years.

Treatment

All cases of unilateral external ocular inflammation or ulcerative eyelid condition that are long-standing and refractory to medical therapy should be suspected occult sebaceous carcinoma. A full-thickness eyelid biopsy followed by direct closure is recommended. If the initial biopsy is negative and the external inflammatory condition persists or worsens, a repeat biopsy is indicated.

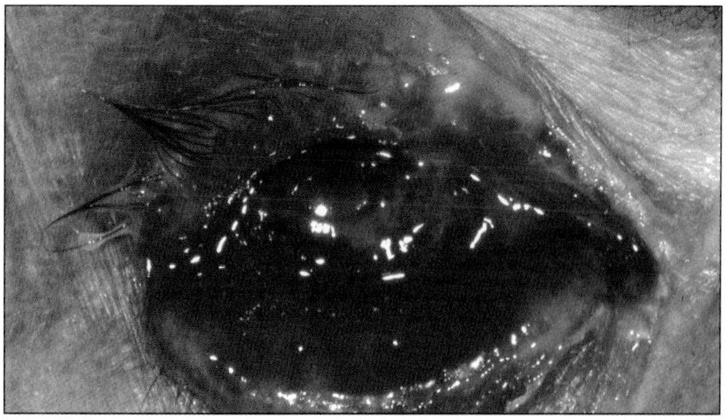

Fig. 32.9 Closer inspection of the involved eyelid (from Fig. 32.8) showed madarosis, hyperemic conjunctiva, symblepharon, and keratitis.

With histologic confirmation of sebaceous carcinoma, the surgeon must consider the extent of possible pagetoid involvement of the bulbar conjunctiva. Nondirected or map conjunctival biopsies[77] are taken in all four quadrants and examined by permanent sections to avoid misinterpretation of subtle intraepithelial spread as can occur with frozen sections. If the bulbar conjunctiva is involved extensively by tumor and reconstruction is not possible, exenteration is recommended. It is important to examine the opposing eyelid for any clinically suspicious areas. If both upper and lower eyelids are involved by tumor without involvement of the conjunctiva, it is possible, although technically difficult, to remove both eyelids and reconstruct the defect. Concomitant involvement of eyelids and conjunctiva may require exenteration. Given the relatively higher rate of regional and systematic metastases for larger/recurrent tumors or those that violate the septum, consideration should be given to sentinel lymph node biopsy at the time of definitive tumor resection. Ten to 15% of sebaceous cell carcinomas eventually present with regional nodal disease.[78] Thus, a negative sentinel lymph node biopsy does not obviate the need for close clinical follow-up and metastatic surveillance.[79]

In a case of nodular sebaceous carcinoma without pagetoid involvement confined to one eyelid, the lesion can be removed by the Mohs' micrographic technique.[80,81] However, the noncontiguous nature of this tumor and the difficulty in evaluating these tumor cells by frozen sections renders its complete removal challenging.[82] Folberg et al.[82] recommend excision of the visible tumor, with a 5-mm margin of clinically normal tissue on either side. The margins are assessed by frozen section and additional tissue is taken until the margins are tumor free.

If the tumor is confined to one eyelid, but there is evidence of pagetoid spread, removal of the entire eyelid and resection of involved conjunctiva are recommended. Lisman et al.[83] have used cryotherapy rather than surgical excision in the management of diffuse intraepithelial pagetoid spread involving the bulbar conjunctiva in patients who refused exenteration. Kass[84] suggested that such cases with residual diffuse intraepithelial neoplasia might be managed with simple periodic observation and repeat biopsy because pagetoid changes have been noted to disappear after resection of the invasive eyelid component. Kass and Hornblass[85] also suggested that wide excision of the primary lid tumor under frozen section control, with or without cryotherapy, might be an alternative to exenteration in one-eyed patients or in those refusing surgery. Radiation therapy and topical mitomycin-C[86] are additional alternative therapies in patients who refuse or are unable to have a surgical resection.

Prognosis

Factors that worsen prognosis include: (1) duration of symptoms >6 months; (2) vascular and lymphatic infiltration; (3) orbital extension; (4) poor tumor differentiation; (5) multicentric origin; (6) intraepithelial carcinomatous changes of the conjunctiva, cornea, or skin; and (7) location in the upper eyelid. Approximately 9–36% of treated sebaceous carcinomas recur, and orbital invasion occurs in 6–17% of all cases. Regional lymph nodes metastases develop in 17–28% of patients. Cervical and supraclavicular nodes may be involved without evidence of preauricular or submandibular enlargement. Remote metastatic sites include the lungs, liver, skull, and brain.

Merkel cell carcinoma (trabecular carcinoma)

Normal Merkel cell

Merkel cells are thought to be derived from the neural crest and are situated in the basal layer of the epidermis adjacent to hair shafts and axon terminals. These specialized epidermal cells are thought to be slowly adapting mechanoreceptors that mediate the sense of touch and direction of hair movement.[87,88]

Merkel cell carcinomas

Merkel cell carcinoma, also known as neuroendocrine carcinoma, is a rare but aggressive primary malignant skin neoplasm. Most lesions occur in elderly patients, with a mean age of 66–73 years.[89] The tumor is found almost exclusively in Caucasians, with an equal distribution between men and women. The cause of Merkel cell carcinoma is unknown, but occurs most frequently in sun-exposed sites of the head and neck region. Occurrence of this tumor is also reported after radiation, immunosuppressive therapy, or in association with other malignancies.[90]

Clinical presentation

Merkel cell carcinoma usually presents as a rapidly growing, firm, nontender, dome-shaped, solitary dermal skin nodule. The tumor is typically red in color, with hues ranging from pink to violaceous and purple (Fig. 32.10). The surface of the tumor is smooth and shiny and may contain multiple telangiectatic vessels. It may clinically resemble an amelanotic melanoma, a primary cutaneous lymphoma, or an angiomatous lesion. The overlying epidermis is usually intact, but ulceration and involvement of the hair follicles may be seen.

Histopathology

Merkel cell carcinoma originates from the papillary dermis and usually extends into the subcutaneous tissue, rarely affecting the overlying epidermis. This finding is curious, as Merkel cells are found mainly in the basal layer of the epi-

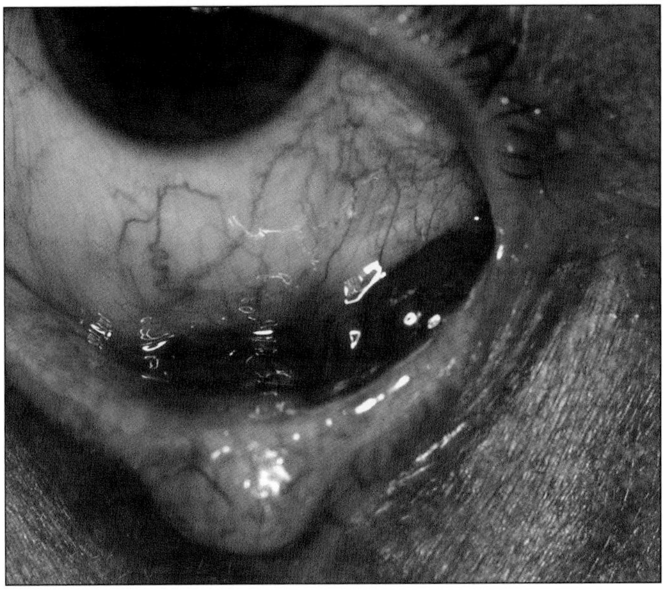

Fig. 32.10 Typical appearance of a Merkel cell carcinoma manifesting as a red, dome-shaped, solitary dermal skin nodule. A portion of the lesion has extended into the fornix.

dermis. The neoplasm lacks a capsule and the cells are compactly arranged in interconnecting trabecular cords separated by connective tissue strands.[91] The individual cells are round, with scant amphophilic cytoplasm with large oval nuclei and prominent nucleoli. Mitotic figures are frequently seen. Many tumors contain a population of small, round to spindle-shaped cells with hyperchromatic nuclei resembling those of bronchial oat cell carcinoma.[87] Included in the histologic differential diagnosis of poorly differentiated round cell tumors are lymphoma, metastatic small cell carcinomas, and carcinoid tumors. Meticulous systemic work-up to exclude other primary tumors is mandatory when confronted with a possible diagnosis of Merkel cell carcinoma.

Although special stains to further characterize the lesion may be helpful, electron microscopy and immunohistochemical studies are needed to conclusively establish the diagnosis. Unlike normal Merkel cells, most Merkel cell tumors express neurofilament proteins.[92] The characteristic electron microscopic finding is the presence of cytoplasmic membrane-bound, dense-core granules ranging between 75 and 240 nm in diameter.

Treatment

Localized disease

Localized disease requires prompt and aggressive initial treatment for potential favorable outcome. Wide surgical excision of the primary tumor is recommended; however, complete removal is difficult due to frequent extension of tumor through lymphatic channels. There are local recurrences in 30–40% of patients within 1 year of initial diagnosis despite apparent complete excision of the primary tumor.[93–95] Radiation therapy may be used as the primary treatment if the patient is unable to tolerate surgery or the tumor encroaches onto vital structures.[96,97] Surgical excision with adjunctive local radiotherapy may be superior to either treatment alone, even when a wide excision has been performed.[94]

Early metastasis is almost always to the regional lymph nodes, with initial hematogenous spread occurring in <2% of patients. If resected lymph nodes contain metastatic tumor, radiotherapy should be administered in a wide field to include the primary site, the soft tissue surrounding the lymphadenectomy, and the intervening regional lymphatic drainage area.[98]

Extraregional disease

Chemotherapy using a combination of drugs that are active against small cell carcinoma of the lung is recommended for patients with unresectable disease.[89,93,99,100] Tumor regression as a result of chemotherapy is often dramatic. However, once the disease progresses, the clinical course often worsens rapidly.

Malignant melanoma

Malignant melanoma represents 5% of all cutaneous cancers. It has been estimated that an American's lifetime risk for developing cutaneous melanoma is 1 in 128.[101] Despite its relatively low incidence, almost two-thirds of all deaths from cutaneous cancer are caused by malignant melanomas.[102] The precise etiology of malignant melanoma is unclear. Multiple factors including genetic predisposition, environmental mutagens, and exposure to sunlight have been implicated. The majority of cutaneous melanomas develop de novo without an antecedent melanocytic nevus.[103]

The subject of malignant melanoma is broad, complex, and controversial. This chapter summarizes some salient features of periocular melanoma. Primary cutaneous malignant melanomas of the eyelid skin are extremely rare, making up only 1% of all eyelid malignancies. The lower eyelid is more frequently involved.[104–106] There are four commonly accepted clinicopathologic forms of cutaneous melanoma: lentigo maligna melanoma, superficial spreading melanoma, nodular melanoma, and acral lentiginous melanoma. Because the last type tends to occur in the volar and subungal regions, and has never been reported to involve the eyelids, it is not discussed here.

Lentigo maligna melanoma

Lentigo maligna (Hutchinson's melanotic freckle) is considered the premalignant lesion of lentigo maligna melanoma. Lentigo maligna melanoma accounts for 10% of all cutaneous melanomas, but 91% of head and neck melanomas.[107] Of these head and neck melanomas, up to 76% occur on the face. Ophthalmologists are in a unique position to diagnose these sometimes long-standing lesions.[104,106,108]

Lentigo maligna usually presents as a flat, nonpalpable, tan to brown macule with irregular borders (Fig. 32.11). Within the lesion, areas of gray and white discoloration may be seen. It occurs predominantly on sun-exposed facial skin of elderly individuals. In the periocular region, the lower eyelid and canthal regions are commonly involved. The lesion may increase slowly in size by centrifugal spread or (radial) growth for many years. Histologically, atypical melanocytes are purely intraepithelial and do not involve

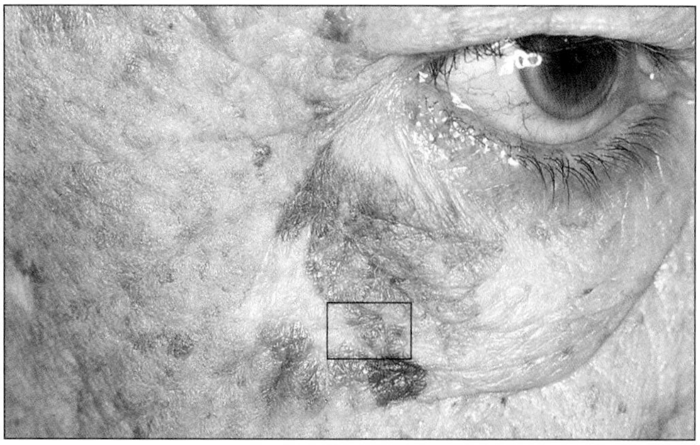

Fig. 32.11 Clinical appearance of lentigo maligna of the face and lower eyelid. Within the lesion, local areas of dark, raised nodules can be seen (*box*). Histologic examination showed the nodules to be lentigo maligna melanoma.

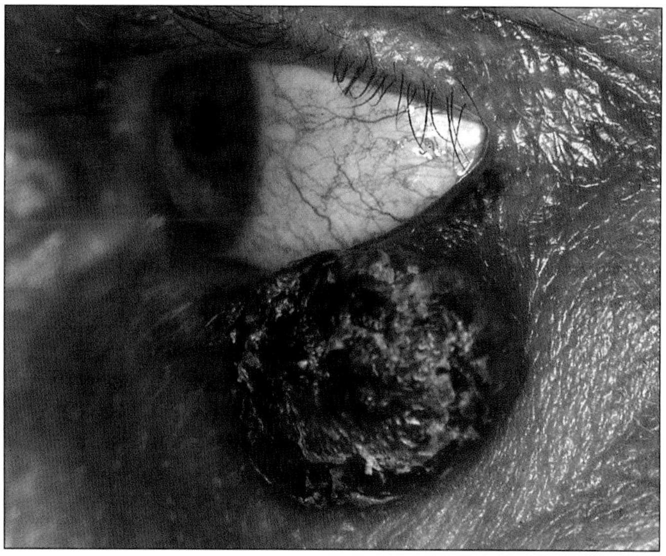

Fig. 32.12 A fully developed malignant melanoma of the lower lid in an elderly man. The nodular component of the lesion measured about 2.5 cm. Note the superficial spreading component of the lesion along the lid margin. The ABCD rule is used in evaluating a pigmented lesion suspicious for melanoma: Asymmetry, Border irregularity, Color variability, and enlarging Diameter. The lesion had clinically enlarged in diameter from only a few millimeters, tan to dark brown, flat pigmentation to the nodule shown in this photograph.

the dermis. After radial spread, invasion (vertical growth) into the dermis occurs, leading to the development of lentigo maligna melanoma.

Clinically, nodule formation and flecks of dark brown or black pigmentation usually mark the invasive areas. The incidence of malignant transformation of lentigo maligna is estimated between 25% and 30%.[109] Once malignant transformation supervenes, local and distant metastasis, though rare, can take place.

For lentigo maligna and lentigo maligna melanoma, surgical excision with careful histologic examination of the margins is the treatment of choice and the only method confirming that the lesion has been removed completely. Transformation of lentigo maligna to melanoma is preventable if the lesion is treated during its prolonged phase of radial growth.

Superficial spreading melanoma

Superficial spreading melanoma is considered the most common variant of melanoma, accounting for 70% of cases. Unlike lentigo maligna and lentigo maligna melanoma, superficial spreading melanoma primarily involves the nonexposed skin surfaces. The upper back and anterior tibia are amongs the most common involved sites. Its location on the nonexposed skin surfaces and its more rapid rate of growth are the distinguishing features of this tumor. The hallmark of this lesion is a round macular lesion with haphazard coloration, including shades of tan, black, or red (Fig. 32.12). The border is often notched by focal regression or asymmetric tumor growth. As the vertical growth phase progresses, focal nodules can be palpated and skin markings disappear. They may be amelanotic and are extremely rare on the eyelids. Histologically, the atypical nests of melanocytes are not restricted to the dermal–epidermal junction but may invade upward to all levels of the epidermis in a pagetoid fashion, mimicking classic Paget's disease of the breast.

Nodular melanoma

Nodular melanoma constitutes about 15% of all cutaneous melanomas. These pigmented papules or nodules with discrete edges typically appear over the course of a few months and occur primarily on sun-exposed areas of the head, neck, and trunk. Nodular melanomas also may be amelanotic and are extremely rare on the eyelids.[110] They arise without a clinically apparent radial growth phase; the vertical growth phase is often the initial and only growth phase of this variant of melanoma.[111]

Treatment

A patient with a suspected eyelid melanoma should have careful slit lamp examination to exclude conjunctival involvement. As eyelid malignant melanomas have a propensity for regional lymph node metastasis (up to 29%),[112] careful palpation of the preauricular and submandibular lymph nodes is important. An incisional biopsy should be performed on all pigmented eyelid lesions suspected as melanoma. Once confirmed histologically, wide surgical excision followed by immediate reconstruction of the defect is recommended. The routine use of 1–3-cm excision margins, a recommendation borne out of treating cutaneous melanomas based on Breslow thickness, on eyelid and periocular skin would yield large surgical defects. In practice, the customary and most tissue-conserving approach is to use either Mohs' micrographic surgery technique or narrow (4–5 mm) margins examined by a well-trained and experienced pathologist.[113–115] Most authorities agree that 5-mm margins are adequate for tumors 1 mm in thickness, and that 10-mm margins may be needed for tumors that are 2 mm in thickness.[116,117]

Lymphatic mapping and sentinel lymph node biopsy is an established technique for the accurate staging of solid tumors with a tendency for regional nodal metastasis. The eyelids drain to the preauricular, submandibular, and deeper cervical nodes. Sentinel lymph node biopsy may be less reliable in patients with previous surgery, radiation, or other causes of lymphatic disruption.[118,119]

The most common approach to detect microscopic metastases in clinically negative regional lymph nodes utilizes two pharmaceuticals – technetium-labeled sulfur colloid and blue dye. The rate of sentinel lymph node identification is enhanced using both an intraoperative gamma-detecting probe and a vital blue dye to visually localize a sentinel node after injection of technetium and blue dye around the tumor site. Mapping begins with a preoperative lymphoscintigraphy to assess the afferent lymphatics. For eyelid and conjunctival malignancies, 0.3 mCi of technetium Tc 99m-labeled sulfur colloid in 0.2 mL of buffered saline is injected around the lesion.[120] Approximately 15–30 minutes after injection of the radiopharmaceutical, lymphoscintigrams of the ipsilateral neck region are taken. Five to ten minutes prior to surgical incision, 0.2 mL of the second mapping agent, a blue dye, is injected into the peritumoral region. Five to ten minutes following blue dye detection, the gamma detector probe is used to survey the skin over the draining lymphatic basin in search of an area of increased radioactivity, representing the sentinel lymph node. A small incision is made over the area of increased activity, and, on entering the subcutaneous tissue, a blue lymphatic can be seen, which represents the affected afferent lymphatic leading to the sentinel node. Using a combination of visualization and the gamma detector probe (sound), the lymphatic basin is explored until the blue sentinel node is identified. It is then removed and sent to the pathologist for evaluation. The use of lymphoscintigraphy with intraoperative gamma probe and vital dye guidance is a valuable tool to better stage malignant tumors of the eyelid because this technique may prevent unnecessary neck dissection.[113] However, close clinical follow-up remains of utmost importance in patients with negative lymph nodes given the relatively high rate of regional and systemic metastatic disease.[79]

Patients with extensive local disease should be referred to medical oncology for consideration of adjuvant interferon-α therapy.[121] Metastatic disease may also be treated systemically with dacarbazine or cisplatin. However, even if both agents are used, meaningful clinical response occurs in <25% of patients.[122]

Kaposi's sarcoma

Kaposi's sarcoma is a malignant vascular tumor that may develop on skin, mucous membranes, lymph nodes, and visceral organs.[123] Before the 1980s, Kaposi's sarcoma was considered a rare, indolent neoplasm affecting primarily the extremities of elderly men of Mediterranean descent. Since acquired immunodeficiency syndrome (AIDS) was first recognized in 1981, the incidence of Kaposi's sarcoma has increased, occurring in approximately 24–35% of AIDS patients.[124,125] Although histologically similar, Kaposi's sarcoma is a much more fulminant disease in AIDS-related patients than the classic form; patients typically have widespread extracutaneous organ involvement.[125,126]

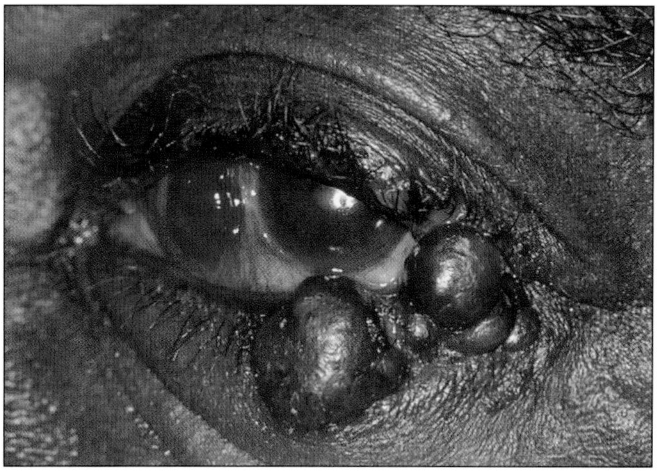

Fig. 32.13 Kaposi's sarcoma presenting as a multilobulated, violet-red subcutaneous nodule along the lid margin. Conjunctival Kaposi's sarcoma manifests as a dark-reddish mass on the medial bulbar conjunctiva.

Clinical presentation

The prevalence of ophthalmic Kaposi's sarcoma in AIDS patients has been estimated at 10–24%.[127–129] Ophthalmic Kaposi's sarcoma is usually localized to the eyelids, conjunctiva, caruncle, and lacrimal sac.[130] The eyelid lesion clinically presents as a flat or raised, nontender, purple-red nodule (Fig. 32.13). It may be mistaken for a pyogenic granuloma, hemangioma, lymphoma, or malignant melanoma. The eyelid tumor mass is capable of causing ocular irritation, recurrent hemorrhage, trichiasis, and visual obstruction from mass effect. Conjunctival Kaposi's sarcoma typically presents as a discrete, dark-reddish mass on the bulbar or palpebral conjunctiva, with the inferior fornix more frequently involved.[129] The lesion often resembles a subconjunctival hemorrhage.

Histopathology

Numerous atypical spindle-shaped cells with prominent ovoid nuclei, interspersed with multiple slitlike vascular channels, characterize the tumor. The stroma contains dense collagenous connective tissue, extravasated erythrocytes, and hemosiderin pigment.

Treatment

Before the AIDS epidemic, local excision of Kaposi's sarcoma was often curative. However, AIDS-related Kaposi's sarcoma is a multifocal disease in which one cannot expect cure with excision of isolated lesions. Because Kaposi's sarcoma of the conjunctiva and eyelid is slow growing and rarely invasive, Shuler et al.[129] suggest that treatment may be unnecessary and observation more appropriate for lesions that are not causing functional or cosmetic problems. Indications for treatment include cosmetically disturbing lesions, ocular discomfort, or visual obstruction by the lesion. For patients with localized, well-delineated conjunctival or eyelid lesions, surgical excision is the best method of treatment. Patients with large lesions, in which excision will require extensive reconstruction, are best treated with radiation therapy. Cryotherapy also has been reported to be effective in treating eyelid or epibulbar lesions that cannot be easily excised.[130] In cases of advanced disease, the use of chemotherapeutic agents has been advocated.[131]

Systemic Associations

Malignant eyelid lesions, particularly basal and squamous cell carcinomas, may be associated with conditions that have multiple systemic manifestations. The discovery of malignant lesions of the eyelid in young patients or those with a positive family history should prompt further inquiry into possible systemic association.[131]

Basal cell nevus syndrome (Gorlin-Goltz syndrome)

The basal cell nevus syndrome is an uncommon, autosomal dominant, multisystem disorder with high penetrance and variable expressivity. In its fullest expression, the disease complex is characterized by multiple nevoid basal cell carcinomas, odontogenic keratocysts of the jaw, congenital skeletal anomalies, ectopic calcification of the falx cerebri, and pitting of the hands and feet. A diagnosis may be established by the presence of any two of these characteristics and is supported by a positive family history.[132] Males and females are affected with equal frequency, and the condition is most commonly found in Caucasians.[133] Genetic counseling is an important aspect of patient management, as are frequent examinations to avoid potentially disfiguring and lethal complications.

Systemic manifestations

Multiple basal cell carcinomas that appear early in life are one of the hallmarks of basal cell nevus syndrome. These cutaneous tumors usually present as pigmented or flesh-colored smooth, round papules between the second and third decades, although they may develop in the first few years of life. These lesions remain quiescent until puberty, when they increase in number and demonstrate more rapid and invasive growth behavior. Their distribution is widespread, unlike the more common acquired BCCs that typically develop in sun-exposed areas. The central facial region and trunk are most often affected; the scalp, neck, and extremities may also be involved. Approximately 50% of affected patients exhibit basal cell carcinomas, which may number from a few to several hundred.

Jaw cysts are found in about 70% of patients and often appear in the first decade of life. Symptoms of pain, swelling, drainage, and displacement of teeth are the presenting complaint in half of cases. Cysts arise in the mandible twice as frequently as in the maxilla. Surgical removal is the treatment of choice.

Various developmental skeletal anomalies are common though nonspecific manifestations of the basal cell nevus syndrome. These include bifurcating ribs, partial agenesis of ribs, and synostosis. Spine deformities such as kyphoscoliosis, spina bifida, and hemivertebrae can also be found.

Ectopic calcification is present in 80% of patients, especially of the falx cerebri, sacrotuberous tissues, subcutaneous tissues, and even the basal cell carcinomas themselves. Pitting of the palms and soles, a unique feature of basal cell nevus syndrome, appears as an erythematous cutaneous depression measuring 2–3 mm in diameter and consists of focal areas of defective keratinization.

Ophthalmic manifestations

The most common and serious ophthalmic manifestation in basal cell nevus syndrome is BCCs of the periocular structures. The cutaneous tumors are multiple and microscopically indistinguishable from actinically induced tumors. Orbital hypertelorism and an associated lateral displacement of the medial canthi are found in a majority of patients. These features, coupled with prominent supraorbital ridges, frontoparietal bossing, broad nasal root, and mild mandibular prognathism, produce a characteristic facies.

Treatment

The potentially invasive and destructive nature of large numbers of basal cell carcinomas may lead to disfigurement and considerable ocular morbidity. Ionizing radiation therapy is contraindicated because of its increased mutagenic potential in these patients. Curettage and electrocoagulation treatment and cryosurgery can be useful in small lesions. For large, invasive, or recurrent lesions, the Mohs' micrographic excision technique is recommended. An experimental method of chemoprevention of basal cell carcinoma and multiple keratoacanthomas with long-term administration of systemic isotretinoin has been reported.[134]

For patients in whom conventional therapy has either failed or cannot be applied, photodynamic therapy (PDT) may be considered. PDT is a technique in which hematoporphyrin derivative (HpD), a photosensitizer, is administered intravenously. This drug is preferentially retained by malignant tissues and initiates a cytotoxic reaction when exposed to red light (630 nm) generated by a dye laser. Normal tissues adjacent to a tumor retain HpD to a much lesser degree and are spared damage from the light-induced reaction.[135] Paclitaxel (Taxol; Bristol-Myers Squibb, Princeton, NJ) has been used successfully to treat an intractable case of hereditary basal cell carcinoma syndrome.[136]

Xeroderma Pigmentosum

Xeroderma pigmentosum (XP) is a rare, autosomal recessive disorder with an estimated incidence of approximately 1 per million persons. This condition is characterized by sun sensitivity and a defective repair mechanism for ultraviolet-induced DNA damage in skin cells.[137,138] Radiation in the ultraviolet spectrum of sunlight induces damage to nuclear DNA by creating dimers between two adjacent pyrimidine molecules. In normal individuals, this defect is repaired by a series of enzymatic steps. In patients with XP, however, the initial step in this reparative process is flawed.[138]

Patients with XP experience cutaneous and ocular abnormalities, including the development of neoplasia at an early age. Skin cancers develop at a frequency more than 1000 times that in the general population.[139] In addition, some patients with XP may have progressive neurologic degeneration.

Cutaneous abnormalities

Patients afflicted with this condition demonstrate an acute sun sensitivity in early childhood. The initial sign is often abnormal skin reaction resembling sunburn in infants with only minimal sun exposure. Freckles, dry and scaly skin, hypopigmentation, cutaneous atrophy, and telangiectasia may develop in the first several years of life. Eventually, premalignant actinic keratoses form in sun-damaged areas. In a review of 830 published XP cases, Kraemer et al.[139] reported that 45% of patients developed basal cell or squamous cell carcinomas by age 8 years, with 97% of the lesions occurring on the face, head, or neck. This young age of onset for first skin neoplasm is nearly 50 years younger than that of the general population of the United States. Malignant melanoma was encountered in 5% of patients. Other types of cutaneous neoplasms were reported, including keratoacanthoma, fibrosarcoma, and angiosarcoma.[139] Two-thirds of patients die before 20 years of age from either metastatic disease or infection.[140]

Ocular abnormalities

Ophthalmic manifestations of XP are confined to the ocular and periocular tissues frequently exposed to ultraviolet radiation. These include the eyelids, interpalpebral zone of the bulbar conjunctiva, cornea, and iris. Common ocular symptoms are photophobia, lacrimation, serous or mucopurulent discharge, and reflexive blepharospasm.[141]

Like skin elsewhere, the eyelids demonstrate similar characteristic dermal changes in XP. In addition to cutaneous neoplasms, madarosis and eyelid malposition are frequently encountered. The most common eyelid manifestation of the disease is progressive atrophy of the lower eyelid. The process begins at the eyelid margin with progressive shrinkage of the anterior lamella, evolving to a total loss of the eyelid. This development can lead to exposure, conjunctival inflammation, symblepharon formation, and corneal ulceration (Fig. 32.14).

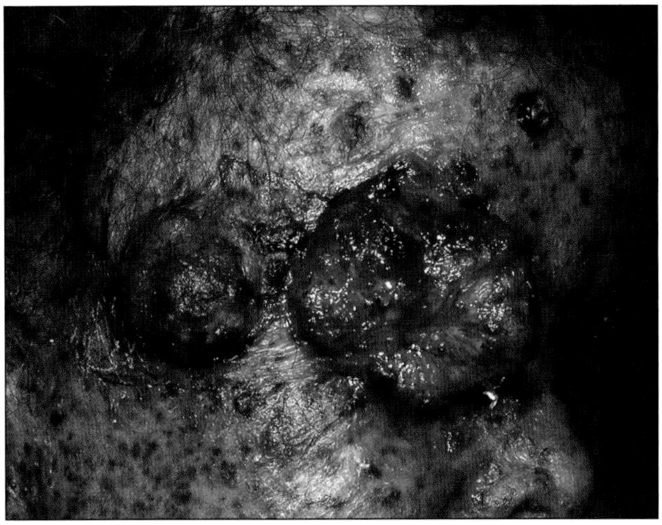

Fig. 32.14 Two large squamous cell carcinomas involving the right temple, upper eyelid, brow, and zygomatic arch region in a child with xeroderma pigmentosum.

The conjunctiva, especially in the interpalpebral fissure, is dry and hyperemic, with areas of pigment deposition and keratin formation. Pingueculae, pseudopterygia, phlyctenules, and epithelial hyperplasia are benign lesions that may also be encountered. SCC of the conjunctiva is seen in approximately 13% of patients.[142]

Neurologic abnormalities

Abnormal neurologic findings consist of progressive mental deterioration, hearing loss, hyporeflexia, ataxia, and quadriparesis. Microcephaly and delayed secondary sexual development have also been described.

Treatment

Treatment of XP is avoidance of sun exposure and protection from UV light with liberal use of sunscreen. Frequent examinations and early detection of cutaneous and ocular malignancies are essential. Isolated BCCs may be managed with conventional excision. Dermabrasion, dermatome shaving, and excision followed by skin grafting of affected facial areas (excluding the periocular region) are surgical options for those with multiple basal cell carcinomas.[143] Recently, high-dose oral isotretinoin was found to be effective in the chemoprophylaxis of skin cancers in patients with XP. However, withdrawal of therapy resulted in a rapid reversal of the chemoprophylactic effect.[144]

Muir-Torre Syndrome

The association of cutaneous keratoacanthomas or sebaceous tumors with visceral malignancy, particularly colonic adenocarcinoma, is known as Muir-Torre syndrome.[143,145] A patient with even one benign sebaceous tumor anywhere on the body may presage the possibility of future internal malignancy.[146,147] Tillawi et al.[148] provided evidence to suggest that solitary meibomian gland lesions of the eyelid, specifically adenoma, epithelioma, and hyperplasia, may represent a marker of underlying visceral malignancy, whereas sebaceous carcinomas of the eyelids are not associated with increased incidence of internal cancers.

Summary

Skin cancers of the periocular region present challenges in diagnosis and management to both ophthalmologists and dermatologists. The potential destructive effects of cutaneous malignant tumors of the periocular region can endanger the protective function of the eyelids. Proper recognition and understanding of the biologic behavior of these tumors are essential in preventing potentially devastating ocular complications. The goals in the management of any malignant eyelid lesion are to establish an early diagnosis, to achieve a permanent cure by total eradication of the tumor, and to preserve or restore both eyelid function and cosmesis.

References

1. Rubin AI, Chen EH, Ratner D. Basal-cell carcinoma. *N Engl J Med.* 2005;353(21):2262–2269.

2. Scotto J, Fears T, Fraumeni JJ. *The incidence of nonmelanoma skin cancer in the United States*. NIH. 1981; Publication No. 82-2433.
3. Batra RS, Kelley LC. Predictors of extensive subclinical spread in nonmelanoma skin cancer treated with Mohs micrographic surgery. *Arch Dermatol*. 2002;138(8):1043–1051.
4. Ries LAB, Kosary LC, Hankey BF, et al. *SEER cancer statistics review, 1973–1996*. National Cancer Institute; 1999.
5. Chuang TY, Popescu A, Su WP, Chute CG. Basal cell carcinoma. A population-based incidence study in Rochester, Minnesota. *J Am Acad Dermatol*. 1990;22(3):413–417.
6. Stenbeck JD, Balanda KP, Williams MJ, et al. Patterns of treated nonmelanoma skin cancer in Queensland: the region with the highest incidence rates in the world. *Med J Aust*. 1990;153:511–515.
7. Wong CS, Strange RC, Lear JT. Basal cell carcinoma. *BMJ*. 2003; 327(7418):794–798.
8. Vitasa BC, Taylor HR, Strickland PT, et al. Association of nonmelanoma skin cancer and actinic keratosis with cumulative solar ultraviolet exposure in Maryland watermen. *Cancer*. 1990;65(12):2811–2817.
9. Nerad JA, Whitaker DC. Periocular basal cell carcinoma in adults 35 years of age and younger. *Am J Ophthalmol*. 1988;106(6):723–729.
10. Milstone EB, Helwig EB. Basal cell carcinoma in children. *Arch Dermatol*. 1973;108(4):523–527.
11. Leffell DJ, Headington JT, Wong DS, Swanson NA. Aggressive-growth basal cell carcinoma in young adults. *Arch Dermatol*. 1991;127(11): 1663–1667.
12. Gupta AK, Cardella CJ, Haberman HF. Cutaneous malignant neoplasms in patients with renal transplants. *Arch Dermatol*. 1986;122(11): 1288–1293.
13. Sitz KV, Keppen M, Johnson DF. Metastatic basal cell carcinoma in acquired immunodeficiency syndrome-related complex. *JAMA*. 1987; 257(3):340–343.
14. Marghoob A, Kopf AW, Bart RS, et al. Risk of another basal cell carcinoma developing after treatment of a basal cell carcinoma. *J Am Acad Dermatol*. 1993;28(1):22–28.
15. Martin H, Strong E, Spiro R. Radiation induced skin cancer of the head and neck. *Cancer*. 1970;25:61–70.
16. Hornblass A, Stefano JA. Pigmented basal cell carcinoma of the eyelids. *Am J Ophthalmol*. 1981;92(2):193–197.
17. Arnold H, Odom R, James D. Epidermal nevi, neoplasms and cysts. In: Arnold HL, Odem RB, James W, eds. *Andrew's diseases of the skin*. 8th ed. Philadelphia: WB Saunders; 1990.
18. Doxanas MT, Green WR, Iliff CE. Factors in the successful surgical management of basal cell carcinoma of the eyelids. *Am J Ophthalmol*. 1981;91(6):726–736.
19. von Domarus H, Stevens PJ. Metastatic basal cell carcinoma. Report of five cases and review of 170 cases in the literature. *J Am Acad Dermatol*. 1984;10(6):1043–1060.
20. Farmer ER, Helwig EB. Metastatic basal cell carcinoma: a clinicopathologic study of seventeen cases. *Cancer*. 1980;46(4):748–757.
21. Jakobiec F. Tumors of the lids. In: Anderson RL, Blodi FC, Boniuk M, eds. *Transactions of the New Orleans Academy of Ophthalmology: symposium on diseases and surgery of the lids, lacrimal apparatus and orbit*. St. Louis: Mosby; 1982.
22. Beard C. Management of malignancy of the eyelids. *Am J Ophthalmol*. 1981;92(1):1–6.
23. Loeffler M, Hornblass A. Characteristics and behavior of eyelid carcinoma (basal cell, squamous cell sebaceous gland, and malignant melanoma). *Ophthalmic Surg*. 1990;21(7):513–518.
24. Nemet AY, Deckel Y, Martin PA, et al. Management of periocular basal and squamous cell carcinoma: a series of 485 cases. *Am J Ophthalmol*. 2006;142(2):293–297.
25. Hamada S, Kersey T, Thaller VT. Eyelid basal cell carcinoma: non-Mohs excision, repair, and outcome. *Br J Ophthalmol*. 2005;89(8):992–994.
26. Lane JE, Kent DE. Surgical margins in the treatment of nonmelanoma skin cancer and Mohs micrographic surgery. *Curr Surg*. 2005;62(5):518–526.
27. Older J, Quickert M, Beard C. Surgical removal of basal cell carcinoma of the eyelids utilizing frozen section control. *Trans Am Acad Ophthalmol Otolaryngol*. 1975:658–663.
28. Perlman GS, Hornblass A. Basal cell carcinoma of the eyelid. *Surg Forum*. 1975;540–542.
29. Fitzpatrick P, Thompson G, Easterbrook W. Basal and squamous cell carcinoma of the eyelids and their treatment by radiotherapy. *J Radiat Oncol Biol Physiol*. 1984;10:449–454.
30. Lederman M. Radiation treatment of cancer of the eyelids. *Br J Ophthalmol*. 1976;60(12):794–805.
31. Bath-Hextall F, Bong J, Perkins W, Williams H. Interventions for basal cell carcinoma of the skin: systematic review. *BMJ*. 2004;329(7468): 705.
32. Petit JY, Avril MF, Margulis A, et al. Evaluation of cosmetic results of a randomized trial comparing surgery and radiotherapy in the treatment of basal cell carcinoma of the face. *Plast Reconstr Surg*. 2000; 105(7):2544–2551.
33. Fraunfelder FT. The indications and contraindications of cryosurgery. *Arch Ophthalmol*. 1978;96(4):729.
34. Fraunfelder F, Wallace T, Farris H. The role of cryosurgery in external ocular and periocular disease. *Trans Am Acad Ophthalmol Otolaryngol*. 1977;713–724.
35. Fraunfelder FT, Zacarian SA, Limmer BL, Wingfield D. Cryosurgery for malignancies of the eyelid. *Ophthalmology*. 1980;87(6):461–465.
36. Fraunfelder FT, Zacarian SA, Wingfield DL, Limmer BL. Results of cryotherapy for eyelid malignancies. *Am J Ophthalmol*. 1984;97(2): 184–188.
37. Hall VL, Leppard BJ, McGill J, et al. Treatment of basal-cell carcinoma: comparison of radiotherapy and cryotherapy. *Clin Radiol*. 1986;37(1): 33–34.
38. Albright SD 3rd. Treatment of skin cancer using multiple modalities. *J Am Acad Dermatol*. 1982;7(2):143–171.
39. Mohs FE, Lathrop TG. Modes of spread of cancer of skin. *AMA Arch Derm Syphil*. 1952;66:427–439.
40. Mora RG, Robins P. Basal-cell carcinomas in the center of the face: special diagnostic, prognostic, and therapeutic considerations. *J Dermatol Surg Oncol*. 1978;4(4):315–321.
41. Monheit GD, Callahan MA, Callahan A. Mohs micrographic surgery for periorbital skin cancer. *Dermatol Clin*. 1989;7(4):677–697.
42. Faustina M, Diba R, Ahmadi MA, Esmaeli B. Patterns of regional and distant metastasis in patients with eyelid and periocular squamous cell carcinoma. *Ophthalmology*. 2004;111(10):1930–1932.
43. Thosani MK, Schneck G, Jones EC. Periocular squamous cell carcinoma. *Dermatol Surg*. 2008;34(5):585–599.
44. Strickland PT. Photocarcinogenesis by near-ultraviolet (UVA) radiation in Sencar mice. *J Invest Dermatol*. 1986;87(2):272–275.
45. Aberer W, Schuler G, Stingl G, Honigsmann H, Wolff K. Ultraviolet light depletes surface markers of Langerhans cells. *J Invest Dermatol*. 1981;76(3):202–210.
46. Robbins JH, Moshell AN. DNA repair processes protect human beings from premature solar skin damage: evidence from studies on xeroderma pigmentosum. *J Invest Dermatol*. 1979;73:102–107.
47. Stern RS, Laird N, Melski J, et al. Cutaneous squamous-cell carcinoma in patients treated with PUVA. *N Engl J Med*. 1984;310(18):1156–1161.
48. Dix C. Occupational trauma and skin cancer. *Plast Reconstr Surg*. 1960;26:546.
49. Marks R, Foley P, Goodman G, Hage BH, Selwood TS. Spontaneous remission of solar keratoses: the case for conservative management. *Br J Dermatol*. 1986;115(6):649–655.
50. Dodson JM, DeSpain J, Hewett JE, Clark DP. Malignant potential of actinic keratoses and the controversy over treatment. A patient-oriented perspective. *Arch Dermatol*. 1991;127(7):1029–1031.
51. Cockerell CJ. Histopathology of incipient intraepidermal squamous cell carcinoma ('actinic keratosis'). *J Am Acad Dermatol*. 2000;42(1 Pt 2):11–17.
52. Schwartz RA. The actinic kertosis: a perspective and update. *J Dermatol Surg*. 1997;23:1009–1019.
53. Aubry F, MacGibbon B. Risk factors of squamous cell carcinoma of the skin. A case-control study in the Montreal region. *Cancer*. 1985; 55(4):907–911.
54. Fry RJ, Ley RD. Ultraviolet radiation-induced skin cancer. *Carcinog Compr Surv*. 1989;11:321–337.
55. Glass AG, Hoover RN. The emerging epidemic of melanoma and squamous cell skin cancer. *JAMA*. 1989;262(15):2097–2100.
56. Hoxtell EO, Mandel JS, Murray SS, Schuman LM, Goltz RW. Incidence of skin carcinoma after renal transplantation. *Arch Dermatol*. 1977;113(4):436–438.
57. Reifler DM, Hornblass A. Squamous cell carcinoma of the eyelid. *Surv Ophthalmol*. 1986;30(6):349–365.
58. Dzubow L, Grossman D. Squamous cell carcinoma and verrucous carcinoma. In: Friedman R, Rigel D, Kopf A, eds. *Cancer of the skin*. Philadelphia: WB Saunders; 1991.
59. Friedman HI, Cooper PH, Wanebo HJ. Prognostic and therapeutic use of microstaging of cutaneous squamous cell carcinoma of the trunk and extremities. *Cancer*. 1985;56(5):1099–1105.
60. Hoxtell EO, Mandel JS, Murray SS, Schuman LM, Goltz RW. Incidence of skin carcinoma after renal transplantation. *Arch Dermatol*. 1977;113(4):436–438.
61. Csaky KG, Custer P. Perineural invasion of the orbit by squamous cell carcinoma. *Ophthalmic Surg*. 1990;21(3):218–220.
62. Soparkar CN, Patrinely JR. Eyelid cancers. *Curr Opin Ophthalmol*. 1998;9:49–53.

63. Shields J. Secondary orbital tumors. In: Shields JA, ed. *Diagnosis and management of orbital tumors*. Philadelphia: WB Saunders; 1989.
64. Aurora AL, Blodi FC. Lesions of the eyelids: a clinicopathological study. *Surv Ophthalmol*. 1970;15:94–104.
65. Bedford MA, Migdal CS. The management of eyelid neoplasms. *Trans Ophthalmol Soc UK*. 1982;102:116–118.
66. Doxanas MT, Green WR. Sebaceous gland carcinoma. Review of 40 cases. *Arch Ophthalmol*. 1984;102(2):245–249.
67. Harvey JT, Anderson RL. The management of meibomian gland carcinoma. *Ophthalmic Surg*. 1982;13(1):56–61.
68. Chao AN, Shields CL, Krema H, Shields JA. Outcome of patients with periocular sebaceous gland carcinoma with and without conjunctival intraepithelial invasion. *Ophthalmology*. 2001;108(10):1877–1883.
69. Maniglia AJ. Meibomian gland adenocarcinoma of the eyelid with neck metastasis. *Laryngoscope*. 1978;88(9 Pt 1):1421–1426.
70. Rao N, McLean J, Zimmerman L. Sebaceous carcinoma of the eyelid and caruncle: correlation of clinicopathologic features with prognosis. In: Jakobiec F, ed. *Ocular and adnexal tumors*. Birmingham: Aesculapius; 1978.
71. Rao NA, Hidayat AA, McLean IW, Zimmerman LE. Sebaceous carcinomas of the ocular adnexa: a clinicopathologic study of 104 cases, with five-year follow-up data. *Hum Pathol*. 1982;13(2):113–122.
72. Wick MR, Goellner JR, Wolfe 3rd JT, Su WP. Adnexal carcinomas of the skin. II. Extraocular sebaceous carcinomas. *Cancer*. 1985;56(5): 1163–1172.
73. McCord CD Jr, Cavanagh HD. Microscopic features and biologic behavior of eyelid tumors. *Ophthalmic Surg*. 1980;11(10):671–681.
74. Lemos L, Santa Cruz D, Baba N. Sebaceous carcinoma of the eyelid following radiation therapy. *Am J Pathol*. 1978;2:305–311.
75. Schlernitzauer DA, Font RL. Sebaceous cell carcinoma of the eyelid following radiation therapy for cavernous hemangioma of the face. *Arch Ophthalmol*. 1977;95:2203–2204.
76. Shields JA, Demirci H, Marr BP, Eagle RC Jr, Shields CL. Sebaceous carcinoma of the eyelids: personal experience with 60 cases. *Ophthalmology*. 2004;111(12):2151–2157.
77. Putterman AM. Conjunctival map biopsy to determine pagetoid spread. *Am J Ophthalmol*. 1986;102(1):87–90.
78. Nijhawan N, Ross MR, Diba R, et al. Experience with sentinel lymph node biopsy for eyelid and conjunctival malignancies at a cancer center. *Ophthal Plast Reconstr Surg*. 2004;20:291–295.
79. Ho VH, Ross MI, Prieto VG, et al. Sentinel lymph node biopsy for sebaceous cell carcinoma and melanoma of the ocular adnexa. *Arch Otolaryngol Head Neck Surg*. 2007;133(8):820–826.
80. Dzubow LM. Sebaceous carcinoma of the eyelid: treatment with Mohs surgery. *J Dermatol Surg Oncol*. 1985;11(1):40–44.
81. Ratz JL, Luu-Duong S, Kulwin DR. Sebaceous carcinoma of the eyelid treated with Mohs' surgery. *J Am Acad Dermatol*. 1986;14(4):668–673.
82. Folberg R, Whitaker DC, Tse DT, Nerad JA. Recurrent and residual sebaceous carcinoma after Mohs' excision of the primary lesion. *Am J Ophthalmol*. 1987;103(6):817–823.
83. Lisman RD, Jakobiec FA, Small P. Sebaceous carcinoma of the eyelids. The role of adjunctive cryotherapy in the management of conjunctival pagetoid spread. *Ophthalmology*. 1989;96(7):1021–1026.
84. Kass LG. Role of cryotherapy in treating sebaceous carcinoma of the eyelid. *Ophthalmology*. 1990;97(1):2–4.
85. Kass LG, Hornblass A. Sebaceous carcinoma of the ocular adnexa. *Surv Ophthalmol*. 1989;33(6):477–490.
86. Shields CL, Naseripour M, Shields JA, Eagle Jr RC. Topical mitomycin-C for pagetoid invasion of the conjunctiva by eyelid sebaceous gland carcinoma. *Ophthalmology*. 2002;109(11):2129–2133.
87. Kivela T, Tarkkanen A. The Merkel cell and associated neoplasms in the eyelids and periocular region. *Surv Ophthalmol*. 1990;35(3):171–187.
88. Merkel F. Tastzellen und tastk-rperchen bei den haustieren und beim menschen. *Arch Mikrosk Anat*. 1875;11:632–652.
89. Hitchcock CL, Bland KI, Laney RG 3rd, et al. Neuroendocrine (Merkel cell) carcinoma of the skin. Its natural history, diagnosis, and treatment. *Ann Surg*. 1988;207(2):201–207.
90. Akhtar S, Oza KK, Wright J. Merkel cell carcinoma: report of 10 cases and review of the literature. *J Am Acad Dermatol*. 2000;43(5 Pt 1): 755–767.
91. Toker C. Trabecular carcinoma of the skin. *Arch Dermatol*. 1972; 105:107–110.
92. Leff E. Expression of neurofilament and neuron specific-enolase in small cell tumors of the skin using immunohistochemistry. *Cancer*. 1985; 56:625–631.
93. Bourne RG, O'Rourke MG. Management of Merkel cell tumour. *Aust N Z J Surg*. 1988;58(12):971–974.
94. Cotlar A, Gates J, Gibbs F. Merkel cell carcinoma: combined surgery and radiation therapy. *Am Surg*. 1986;52:159–164.
95. Tennvall J, et al. Merkel cell carcinoma: management of primary, recurrent and metastatic disease. A clinicopathological study of 17 patients. *Eur J Surg Oncol*. 1989;15:1–9.
96. Know SJ, Kapp DS. Hyperthermia and radiation therapy in the treatment of recurrent Merkel cell tumors. *Cancer*. 1982;62(3):1479–1486.
97. Pople I. Merkel cell tumor of the face successfully treated with radical radiotherapy. *Eur J Surg Oncol*. 1988;14:79–81.
98. Andrew J, Silvers D, Lattes R. Merkel cell carcinoma. In: Friedman R, ed. *Cancer of the skin*. Philadelphia: WB Saunders; 1991.
99. Raaf JH, Urmacher C, Knapper WK, Shiu MH, Cheng EW. Trabecular (Merkel cell) carcinoma of the skin. treatment of primary, recurrent, and metastatic disease. *Cancer*. 1986;57(1):178–182.
100. Wynne CJ, Kearsley JH. Merkel cell tumor. A chemosensitive skin cancer. *Cancer*. 1988;62(1):28–31.
101. Hattis MN, Roses DF. Malignant melanoma: treatment. In: Friedman R, ed. *Cancer of the skin*. Philadelphia: WB Saunders; 1991.
102. Kopf A, et al. *Malignant melanoma*. New York: Masson; 1979.
103. Friedman R, Heilman E, Gottlieb G. Malignant melanoma: clinicopathologic correlations. In: Friedman R, ed. *Cancer of the skin*. Philadelphia: WB Saunders; 1991.
104. Vaziri M, Buffam FV, Martinka M, et al. Clinicopathologic features and behavior of cutaneous eyelid melanoma. *Ophthalmology*. 2002;109(5): 901–908.
105. Grossniklaus HE, McLean IW. Cutaneous melanoma of the eyelid. clinicopathologic features. *Ophthalmology*. 1991;98(12):1867–1873.
106. Chan FM, O'Donnell BA, Whitehead K, Ryman W, Sullivan TJ. Treatment and outcomes of malignant melanoma of the eyelid: a review of 29 cases in Australia. *Ophthalmology*. 2007;114(1):187–192.
107. Clark Jr WH, Elder DE, Guerry 4th D, et al. A study of tumor progression: The precursor lesions of superficial spreading and nodular melanoma. *Hum Pathol*. 1984;15(12):1147–1165.
108. Clark WH Jr, From L, Bernardino EA, et al. The histogenesis and biologic behavior of primary human malignant melanomas of the skin. *Cancer Res*. 1969;29:705–726.
109. Davis J, Pack G, Higgins G. Melanotic freckles of Hutchinson. *Am J Surg*. 1967;113:457–463.
110. Jakobiec F. Tumors of the lids. In: *Transactions of the New Orleans Academy of Ophthalmology: symposium on diseases of the lids, lacrimal apparatus and orbit*. St Louis: Mosby; 1982.
111. Clark WH Jr, Mihm MC. Lentigo maligna and lentigo maligna melanoma. *Am J Pathol*. 1969;55:39–67.
112. Esmaeli B, Wang B, Deavers M, et al. Prognostic factors for survival in malignant melanoma of the eyelid skin. *Ophthal Plast Reconstr Surg*. 2000;16(4):250–257.
113. Cook BE Jr, Bartley GB. Treatment options and future prospects for the management of eyelid malignancies: an evidence-based update. *Ophthalmology*. 2001;108(11):2088–2098; quiz 2099–100, 2121.
114. Coleman WP 3rd, Davis RS, Reed RJ, Krementz ET. Treatment of lentigo maligna and lentigo maligna melanoma. *J Dermatol Surg Oncol*. 1980;6(6):476–479.
115. Zitelli JA, Mohs FE, Larson P, Snow S. Mohs micrographic surgery for melanoma. *Dermatol Clin*. 1989;7(4):833–843.
116. Esmaeli B, Youssef A, Naderi A, et al. Margins of excision for cutaneous melanoma of the eyelid skin: the Collaborative Eyelid Skin Melanoma Group Report. *Ophthal Plast Reconstr Surg*. 2003;19(2):96–101.
117. [Anonymous]. NIH consensus conference. Diagnosis and treatment of early melanoma. *JAMA*. 1992;268(10):1314–1319.
118. Amato M, Esmaeli B, Ahmadi MA, et al. Feasibility of preoperative lymphoscintigraphy for identification of sentinel lymph nodes in patients with conjunctival and periocular skin malignancies. *Ophthal Plast Reconstr Surg*. 2003;19(2):102–106.
119. Bilchik AJ, Giuliano A, Essner R, et al. Universal application of intraoperative lymphatic mapping and sentinel lymphadenectomy in solid neoplasms. *Cancer J Sci Am*. 1998;4(6):351–358.
120. Esmaeli B. Sentinel lymph node mapping for patients with cutaneous and conjunctival malignant melanoma. *Ophthal Plast Reconstr Surg*. 2000;16(3):170–172.
121. Cook BE Jr, Bartley GB. Treatment options and future prospects for the management of eyelid malignancies: an evidence-based update. *Ophthalmology*. 2001;108(11):2088–2098; quiz 2099–100, 2121.
122. Plowman PN. Eyelid tumours. *Orbit*. 2007;26(3):207–213.
123. Safai B, Good RA. Kaposi's sarcoma: a review and recent developments. *CA Cancer J Clin*. 1981;31(1):2–12.
124. Centers for Disease Control. Update: acquired immunodeficiency syndrome. *MMWR*. 1986;35:17–21.
125. Herman D, et al. Ocular manifestations of Kaposi's sarcoma. *Ophthalmol Clin North Am*. 1988;1:73–80.
126. Schuman JS, Orellana J, Friedman AH, Teich SA. Acquired immunodeficiency syndrome (AIDS). *Surv Ophthalmol*. 1987;31(6):384–410.

127. Holland GN, Pepose JS, Pettit TH, et al. Acquired immune deficiency syndrome. Ocular manifestations. *Ophthalmology.* 1983;90(8):859–873.
128. Palestine A, Rodrigues MM, Macher AM, et al. Ophthalmic involvement in acquired immunodeficiency syndrome. *Ophthalmology.* 1984;91:1092–1099.
129. Shuler JD, Holland GN, Miles SA, Miller BJ, Grossman I. Kaposi sarcoma of the conjunctiva and eyelids associated with the acquired immunodeficiency syndrome. *Arch Ophthalmol.* 1989;107(6):858–862.
130. Visser OH, Bos PJ. Kaposi's sarcoma of the conjunctiva and CMV-retinitis in AIDS. *Doc Ophthalmol.* 1986;64(1):77–85.
131. Gelmann EP, Longo D, Lane HC, et al. Combination chemotherapy of disseminated Kaposi's sarcoma in patients with the acquired immune deficiency syndrome. *Am J Med.* 1987;82(3):456–462.
132. Gorlin R, Vickers R, Kelln E. The multiple basal cell nevi syndrome. *Cancer.* 1965;18:89.
133. Olson RA, Stroncek GG, Scully JR, Govin L. Nevoid basal cell carcinoma syndrome: review of the literature and report of a case. *J Oral Surg.* 1981;39(4):308–312.
134. Peck GL, Gross EG, Butkus D, DiGiovanna JJ. Chemoprevention of basal cell carcinoma with isotretinoin. *J Am Acad Dermatol.* 1982;6(4 Pt 2 Suppl):815–823.
135. Tse DT, Kersten RC, Anderson RL. Hematoporphyrin derivative photoradiation therapy in managing nevoid basal-cell carcinoma syndrome. A preliminary report. *Arch Ophthalmol.* 1984;102(7):990–994.
136. El Sobky RA, Kallab AM, Dainer PM, Jillella AP, Lesher JL Jr. Successful treatment of an intractable case of hereditary basal cell carcinoma syndrome with paclitaxel. *Arch Dermatol.* 2001;137(6):827–828.
137. Kraemer KH, Lee MM, Scotto J. DNA repair protects against cutaneous and internal neoplasia: evidence from xeroderma pigmentosum. *Carcinogenesis.* 1984;5(4):511–514.
138. Kraemer KH, Slor H. Xeroderma pigmentosum. *Clin Dermatol.* 1985;3:33–69.
139. Kraemer KH, Lee MM, Scotto J. Xeroderma pigmentosum. Cutaneous, ocular, and neurologic abnormalities in 830 published cases. *Arch Dermatol.* 1987;123(2):241–250.
140. Rook A. Xeroderma pigmentosum. In: Rook A, Wilkinson D, Ebling, ed. *Textbook of dermatology.* Oxford: Blackwell Scientific; 1979.
141. Stenson S. Ocular findings in xeroderma pigmentosum: report of two cases. *Ann Ophthalmol.* 1982;14:580–585.
142. El-Hefnawi H, Mortada A. Ocular manifestations of xeroderma pigmentosum. *Br J Ophthalmol.* 1965;77:261–276.
143. Torre D. Multiple sebaceous tumors. *Arch Dermatol.* 1968;98:549–551.
144. Kraemer KH, DiGiovanna JJ, Moshell AN, Tarone RE, Peck GL. Prevention of skin cancer in xeroderma pigmentosum with the use of oral isotretinoin. *N Engl J Med.* 1988;318(25):1633–1637.
145. Muir E, Bell A, Barlow K. Multiple primary carcinomata of the colon, duodenum and larynx associated with kerato-acanthoma of the face. *Br J Surg.* 1966;54:191–195.
146. Finan MC, Connolly SM. Sebaceous gland tumors and systemic disease: a clinicopathologic analysis. *Medicine (Baltimore).* 1984;63(4):232–242.
147. Rulon DB, Helwig EB. Cutaneous sebaceous neoplasms. *Cancer.* 1974;33:82–102.
148. Tillawi I, Katz R, Pellettiere EV. Solitary tumors of meibomian gland origin and Torre's syndrome. *Am J Ophthalmol.* 1987;104(2):179–182.

Chapter 33

Blepharitis: Overview and Classification

Joseph A. Eliason

Blepharitis is one of the most commonly encountered conditions in the practice of ophthalmology. For both patient and physician, the spectrum of diseases it represents is difficult to understand, frustrating in their chronicity, and tiresome due to the burden of a protracted treatment regimen. Many patients fruitlessly move from doctor to doctor seeking a more satisfying solution to the problem. The mucocutaneous junction along with the numerous follicular and glandular structures that make up the complex lid margin provide a rich environment for the diseases that afflict it. While the lids may be the source of the primary inflammatory process, involvement of the cornea and bulbar conjunctival surfaces produce the most important and significant symptoms and visual consequences for the patient.

Of the many causes of blepharitis, most of the common ones remain ill defined, defying detailed pathophysiologic description and definition. Distinctions among the different clinical manifestations are subtle and can have an important bearing on treatment options, which are limited and, as appropriate to the practice of medicine, depend on diagnostic decisions.[1,2]

Classification

Blepharitis has undergone numerous classifications. Setting aside acute infections, which are usually diagnostically straightforward, the much more common group of chronic, low-grade inflammatory diseases with principally lid margin manifestations has been the object of controversy in classification.

Ostler[3] characterized more than 80 distinct agents responsible for lid infections including both micro- and macro-organisms. Common bacteria[4] such as *Streptococcus*, *Staphylococcus*, *Pseudomonas*, *Moraxella*, and *Actinomyces* and rare agents such as anthrax, *Pasteurella*, *Clostridium*, and *Mycobacterium tuberculosis* can be clinical pathogens. Viral lid infections include some of the most common clinical entities such as verrucae, molluscum contagiosum, herpes simplex, and herpes zoster. A variety of fungal agents have also caused lid infections including *Coccidioides*, *Microsporum*, *Blastomyces*, *Candida*, and *Aspergillus*. Reported parasite infestations include *Ascaris*, *Trichinella*, *Wuchereria*, *Onchocerca*, and *Pediculus*. *Demodex* has a high prevalence, infesting the lash follicles and sebaceous structures of the eyelid. A resurgence of interest in the debate over a pathologic role in blepharitis is refocusing attention on this ectoparasite.[5–10] Protozoan infections, generally rare in developed countries, have been reported, including leishmaniasis and trypanosomiasis.[3]

In addition to lid infections produced by microorganisms and parasites, allergic disorders, including atopy and contact dermatitis, seborrheic dermatitis and other dermatologic diseases such as erythema multiforme (Stevens–Johnson syndrome), toxic epidermal necrolysis (Lyell's disease), and ichthyosis may involve the lids.

Fuchs[11] divided marginal lid disease into two principal groups: *blepharitis squamosa*, which is characterized by small, dry scales covering a hyperemic and intact lid margin; and *blepharitis ulcerosa*, characterized by marginal crusting covering frank ulceration of the surface accompanied by microabscesses of the follicles and sebaceous glands leading to scarring. Fuchs enumerated the principal sequelae of these chronic diseases, particularly the ulcerative form, including madarosis (lash loss), trichiasis (misdirection of the lashes), tylosis (thickening and distortion of the lid margin), punctal misdirection, and poliosis (loss of lash pigmentation). Thygeson[12,13] studied the problem and theorized a central role for the *Staphylococcus* organism, creating and exacerbating chronic inflammation of the lid, and related it and its toxic products to the adjacent inflammation of the conjunctiva and cornea (Fig. 33.1). This work has been validated by subsequent investigators. However, the varying contributions of *S. aureus* and *S. epidermidis* have remained debatable.[14–16]

Duke-Elder and MacFaul[17] added a pathological perspective to Fuchs' classification. They likewise drew a distinction between marginal inflammation and other lid infections. With respect to marginal disease, the first category is simple: *squamous blepharitis*, which they described as a superficial, nondestructive dermatitis with eczema-like inflammation characterized by parakeratosis, acanthosis, vascular congestion, edema, and infiltration. It corresponds to Fuchs' blepharitis squamosa. *Follicular blepharitis* corresponds to Fuchs' blepharitis ulcerosa and was characterized as a deeply seated, purulent process with suppuration of follicles and associated Zeis' glands extending to a perifolliculitis, marginal ulcerations, tylosis, and madarosis.

McCulley et al.[18,19] have expanded the two fundamental categories of marginal lid inflammation into six categories, while at the same time placing a strong emphasis on the role

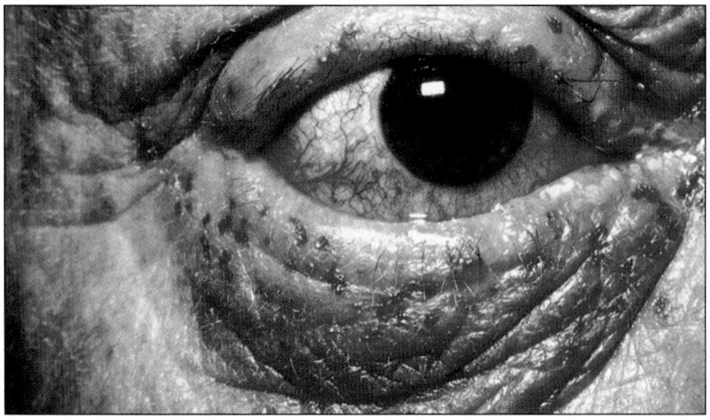

Fig. 33.1 Example of staphylococcus-related chronic disease that has produced extensive marginal lid changes along with generalized lid injection.

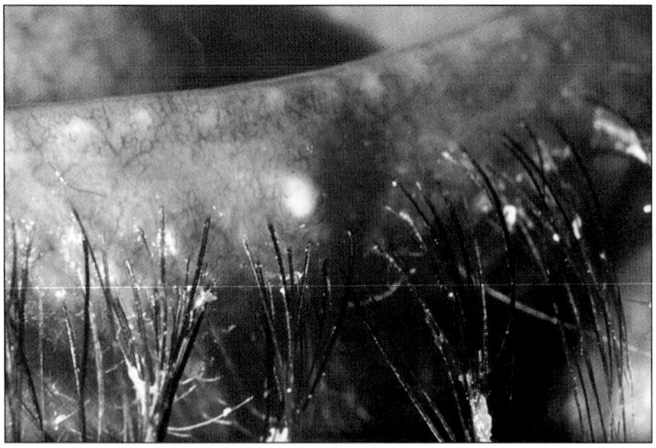

Fig. 33.2 Marginal staphylococcal disease demonstrating the typical crusting, lash misdirection, erythema, and a microabscess in a follicle sebaceous gland.

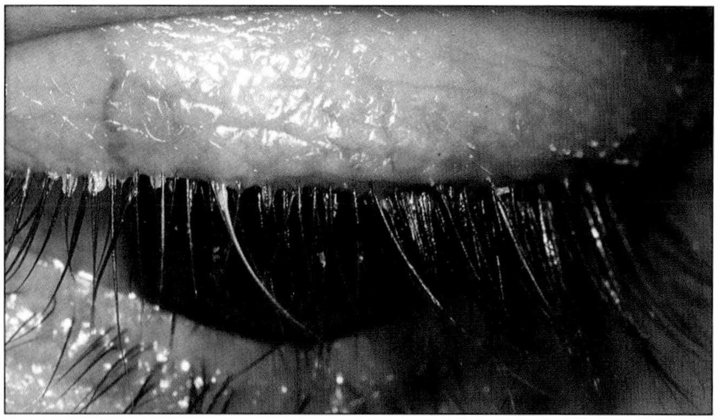

Fig. 33.3 Lid margin with both collarettes and the oily crusting characteristic of a coincidence of staphylococcal and seborrheic marginal disease.

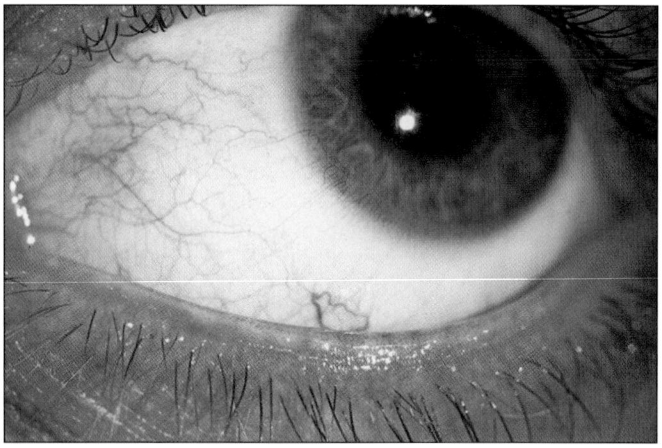

Fig. 33.4 Lid margin demonstrating engorged meibomian glands characteristic of meibomian seborrhea. Note the lack of conjunctival injection.

of the meibomian glands in the inflammatory process. Their first category of staphylococcal disease occurs most commonly in younger patients with a female preponderance and a waxing and waning course. It is manifest by anterior lid inflammation, erythema, telangiectasia, crusts, collarettes, and ulceration associated with a high incidence of positive cultures for *S. aureus* (46%) and nearly all positive for *S. epidermidis* (Fig. 33.2). The second group in McCulley's classification is seborrheic blepharitis. Patients in this group tend to be older than the staphylococcal group, and virtually all have evidence of seborrhea elsewhere on the body. It is a chronic disease and has an equal male and female distribution. It also is an anterior lid process with little erythema and oily, greasy crusting. Cultures of the lid margin match the pattern of normal flora. Therefore, the diagnosis must be made clinically. The coincident occurrence of both staphylococcal and seborrheic diseases represents a third category. The manifestations are a combination of the first two groups and are distinguished from the seborrheic group by a greater level of inflammation (Fig. 33.3). Lid margin cultures demonstrate a high incidence of staphylococcal species (especially *S. aureus,* 80%).

A fourth category, meibomian seborrhea, is a form of seborrhea with the addition of a significant meibomian gland abnormality. It is characterized by dilated meibomian ductules, which are easily expressed, and collections of foam, presumably meibomian secretions, in the tear film. It is associated with prominent symptoms of early morning discomfort. Seborrhea, as well as conjunctival and corneal findings, tends to be a minimal part of the picture (Fig. 33.4). McCulley's fifth and sixth categories are similar. Both are defined by meibomian gland inflammation. They distinguish a meibomitis in localized areas along the lid in conjunction with seborrhea (meibomian seborrhea). In this entity, meibomian secretions are inspissated and difficult to express, resulting in obstruction of the glands. The lid is normal, and efforts to isolate a responsible organism from meibomian secretions have been unsuccessful. The sixth class, meibomitis, is described as generalized inflammation of the posterior lid margin. As with the previous category, the meibomian secretions are inspissated and seem prone to obstruct the glands. Papillary hypertrophy of the tarsal conjunctiva and corneal punctate epitheliopathy are often present, and there are prominent associations with seborrhea and rosacea. A commonly held assumption is that these latter three categories represent one of several functional meibomian gland abnormalities. Although studies have found suggestive alterations in the secretions and described a role for bacterial enzyme activity of flora organisms,[19-22] a definitive picture has yet to be elucidated. Painstaking analysis of meibomian secretions leads to a very complex picture in which Dougherty et al.[23] were able to recognize patterns of fatty acid methyl esters in these six categories by which they could discriminate between them with a 73% probability.

A seventh group is also included in McCulley's classification for forms of blepharitis associated with other conditions such as psoriasis and atopy. From a practical standpoint, many clinicians tend to lump the principal six categories into two groups: anterior blepharitis (comprising the first three) and posterior blepharitis (comprising the remaining meibomian-related groups).

A very different approach to classification was introduced by Mathers et al.[24] who examined the common association of keratitis sicca and blepharitis. They focused upon the tear film as the target of both disease entities, postulating that an elevated tear osmolality is the most important pathophysiologic factor creating injury to epithelial cells. Examining the effect that meibomian gland dysfunction and tear production have on tear osmolarity, they found the highest correlations with the Schirmer test, low lipid volume, high lipid viscosity, meibomian gland drop-out, and tear evaporation. Their classification does not incorporate microbiologic agents; rather, it deals with seborrheic changes and meibomian gland obstruction.

Differential Diagnosis

Several important diagnoses must be considered in the picture of chronic lid margin inflammation. Sebaceous cell carcinoma of the lid lacking significant mass growth can masquerade as a chronic inflammatory process. Although rare, this disease must be kept in mind since its prognosis is so poor, particularly when there is a lack of response to therapy against the common inflammatory lid disorders. Rosacea, a principally dermatologic disease, is often accompanied by lid margin inflammation and peripheral corneal changes. While usually affecting patients in their later decades of life, it has been reported in children as young as 4 years of age.[25-27] Many of the reported pediatric cases failed to show the characteristic dermatologic manifestations. After failing to respond to lid treatment regimens they had good clinical responses to systemic rosacea treatment. In all such cases, recognition of the skin disease is important to direct therapy toward the systemic disease. Poliosis, one of the hallmarks of chronic lid margin inflammation, also can be caused by sympathetic ophthalmia, Vogt-Koyanagi-Harada syndrome, and Waardenburg's syndrome. These diseases usually can be readily differentiated from a local inflammatory process.

Keratitis sicca, while not usually an important differential diagnostic dilemma, is a common accompanying diagnosis to all the forms of blepharitis. McCulley[18] has reported its prominent role in several of his categories of lid marginal disease and, as noted above, Mathers et al.[24] have cast sicca in an etiologic role in forms of blepharitis. The principal importance in recognizing sicca in any of its various presentations is the consequences this will have on therapy plans.

Management

There are four principal arms of therapy for all of the categories of blepharitis: lid hygiene, topical antibiotics, systemic antibiotics (specifically tetracycline), and corticosteroids. In a simple and practical approach to therapeutics, only a few distinctions must be made. All categories of marginal lid inflammation derive benefit from lid hygiene. Warm compresses and detergent-assisted cleansing are the mainstay of treatment. Topical antibiotics are added to this base when a bacterial pathogen is present, usually staphylococcal species, and oral tetracycline (or erythromycin in pediatric cases) when rosacea and meibomitis are a significant component. Although corticosteroids are effective for suppressing acute inflammation, as with allergic disorders, their use in a chronic process can lead to serious side effects. Finer distinctions among categories of lid disease are intellectually satisfying and beneficial in predicting the response to therapy, but do not substantially alter basic treatment choices. Whereas some types of marginal lid disease offer hope for the resolution of an acute process, others require the acceptance and management of a chronic, lifelong disease.

Consistent with the fundamental principles of medicine, a sound diagnosis is the first and most critical step in the management of blepharitis. A clear understanding of the disease greatly enhances the ability of the clinician to educate and provide support to the patient.

References

1. Raskin EM, Speaker MG, Laibson PR. Blepharitis. *Infect Dis Clin North Am.* 1992;6:777–787.
2. Huber-Spitzy V, et al. Blepharitis: a diagnostic and therapeutic challenge. A report on 407 consecutive cases. *Graefes Arch Clin Exp Ophthalmol.* 1991;229:224–227.
3. Ostler HB. *Diseases of the external eye and adnexa.* Baltimore: Williams & Wilkins; 1993.
4. Groden LR, Murphy B, Rodnite J, Genvert GI. Lid flora in blepharitis. *Cornea.* 1991;10:50–53.
5. Clifford CW, Fulk GW. Association of diabetes, lash loss, and *Staphylococcus aureus* with infestation of eyelids by *Demodex folliculorum. J Med Entomol.* 1990;27:467–470.
6. Roth AM. *Demodex folliculorum* in hair follicules of eyelid skin. *Ann Ophthalmol.* 1979;11:37–40.
7. Uyttebroeck W, et al. Incidence of *Demodex folliculorum* on the eyelash follicle in normal people and in blepharitis patients. *Bull Soc Belge Ophthalmol.* 1982;201:83–87.
8. Gao Y-Y, Di Pascuale MA, et al. High prevalence of *Demodex* in eyelashes with cylindrical dandruff. *Invest Ophthalmol Vis Sci.* 2005;46:3089–3094.
9. Gao Y-Y, Di Pascuale MA, et al. In vitro and in vivo killing of ocular *Demodex* by tea tree oil. *Br J Ophthalmol.* 2005;89:1468–1473.
10. Kheirkhah, A, Casas V, et al. Corneal manifestations of ocular *Demodex* infestation. *Am J Ophthalmol.* 2007;143:743–749.
11. Fuchs HE. *Textbook of ophthalmology* [Duane A, Trans.]. Philadelphia: JB Lippincott; 1908.
12. Thygeson P. Bacterial factors in chronic catarrhal conjunctivitis: I. Role of toxin-forming staphylococci. *Arch Ophthalmol.* 1937;18:373–387.
13. Thygeson P. Etiology and treatment of blepharitis: a study in military personnel. *Arch Ophthalmol.* 1946;36:445–477.
14. Hogan MJ, et al. Experimental staphylococcic keratitis. *Invest Ophthalmol.* 1962;1:267.
15. Seal DV, Barrett SP, McGill J. Aetiology and treatment of acute bacterial infection of the external eye. *Br J Ophthalmol.* 1982;66:357–360.

16. Ficker L, et al. Role of cell-mediated immunity to staphylococci in blepharitis. *Am J Ophthalmol.* 1991;111:473–479.
17. Duke-Elder S, MacFaul PA. The ocular adnexa. vol XIII, part I, *System of ophthalmology.* St Louis: Mosby; 1974.
18. McCulley JP. Blepharoconjunctivitis. *Int Ophthalmol Clin.* 1984;24: 65–77.
19. McCulley JP, Dougherty JM, Deneau DG. Classification of chronic blepharitis. *Ophthalmology.* 1982;89:1173–1180.
20. Shine WE, McCulley JP. Role of wax ester fatty alcohols in chronic blepharitis. *Invest Ophthalmol Vis Sci.* 1993;34:3515–3521.
21. Shine WE, Silvany R, McCulley JP. Relation of cholesterol-stimulated *Staphylococcus aureus* growth to chronic blepharitis. *Invest Ophthalmol Vis Sci.* 1993;34:2291–2296.
22. Mathers WD, et al. Meibomian gland dysfunction in chronic blepharitis. *Cornea.* 1991;10:277–285.
23. Dougherty JM, Osgood JK, McCulley JP. The role of wax and sterol ester fatty acids in chronic blepharitis. *Invest Ophthalmol Vis Sci.* 1991;32:1932–1937.
24. Mathers WD, Lane JA, Sutphin JE, Zimmerman MB. Model for ocular tear film function, *Cornea.* 1996;15:110–119.
25. Nazir SA, Murphy S, Siatkowski RM, Cholosh J, Siatkowski RL. Ocular rosacea in childhood. *Am J Ophthalmol.* 2004;137:138–144.
26. Cetinkaya A, Akova YA. Pediatric ocular acne rosacea: long-term treatment with systemic antibiotics. *Am J Ophthalmol.* 2006;142:816–821.
27. McCulley JP, Dougherty JM. Blepharitis associated with acne rosacea and seborrheic dermatitis. *Int Ophthalmol Clin.* 1985;25:159–172.

Chapter 34

Meibomian Gland Dysfunction and Seborrhea

Gary N. Foulks, Michael A. Lemp

Meibomian gland dysfunction (MGD), a major form of blepharitis, is an extremely common, yet often overlooked, chronic condition of the posterior eyelids. It is important to recognize its presence in a patient complaining of dry eye-like symptoms. Lacrimal insufficiency and dermatologic conditions are often concomitant and must be identified and addressed in concert with the treatment of the meibomian gland disease for therapy to be effective.

Seborrhea is defined as hypersecretion of the meibomian glands. An excessive amount of secretion may be expressible from engorged glands secondary to obstruction. However, there is no clear documentation of true meibomian gland hypersecretion in the literature.

This chapter reviews recent developments in the understanding of the histopathology, role of bacteria, and changes in meibomian secretion lipid composition and behavior seen in meibomian gland dysfunction. Effective treatment options for patients with this condition are described.

Normal Anatomy of the Meibomian Glands

The meibomian glands, which number 30 to 40 in the upper lid and 20 to 30 in the lower lid,[1] are arranged in a single row perpendicular to the lid margin. They occupy the full thickness of the tarsal plate. Their orifices emerge posterior to the eyelashes and just anterior to the mucocutaneous junction (Fig. 34.1). The glands are grapelike clusters and yellowish in gross appearance with a main duct with which up to 30 to 40 saccular acini comunicate.

The ducts are lined by four to six layers of at least partially keratinized cells.[2] The acinar cells are nonkeratinized and differentiate in a centripetal direction, with the innermost cells degenerating to form the holocrine lipid secretion.[3] The glands are surrounded by the dense collagen of the tarsus, fibroblasts, lymph spaces, and a network of nerves and blood vessels. Elastic tissue, smooth muscle fibers, and portions of the orbicularis oculi are intimately associated with the glands.

Meibography is a technique that uses transillumination biomicroscopy of the everted eyelid with infrared photography[4] or video imaging.[5] The normal appearance of the meibomian glands using this technique is shown in Figure 34.2A.

Terminology

The term meibomian gland dysfunction was first suggested by Korb and Henriquez.[6a] It is more appropriate than the terms meibomianitis or meibomitis, as inflammation is not necessarily present. The meibomian gland secretion, which is distinct from sebum (skin sebaceous gland secretion) in its composition, has been termed meibum by Nicolaides et al.[7] Meibocyte[5] and meibomiocyte[6] have similarly been proposed for the acinar cells.

Physiology

The lipid layer of the preocular tear film, produced by the meibomian glands, has the following important functions:

1. Retards evaporation from the tear film.
2. Prevents contamination of the tear film by providing a barrier to cutaneous sebum.
3. Lowers the surface tension of tears, allowing water to be drawn into the tear film, thereby thickening it.
4. Provides a seal between the lid margins during sleep.
5. Provides a smooth optical surface.
6. Enhances spreadability and stability of the tear film.

Compromise of the lipid layer leads to increased evaporation with resultant dry eye-like symptoms, despite normal aqueous production.

Studies have shown that the superficial lipid layer retards evaporation of underlying water approximately fourfold in rabbits.[8] In the presence of meibomian gland dropout, there is a threefold increase in evaporative rate in humans.[9] Meibomian gland dysfunction increases tear electrolytes uniformly, consistent with a purely evaporative effect,[10] in contrast to lacrimal gland disease in which sodium ions rise disproportionately in secretion at low flow rates. Increased concentrations of electrolytes are thought to be responsible for changes in conjunctival goblet cell density and corneal epithelial glycogen levels. These changes undoubtedly contribute to the conjunctival and corneal manifestations of meibomian gland disease.

Increasing the concentration of polar lipids in the lipid layer ruptures the tear film. Contamination by a drop of sebum results in immediate tear film dispersal.[11] Thus,

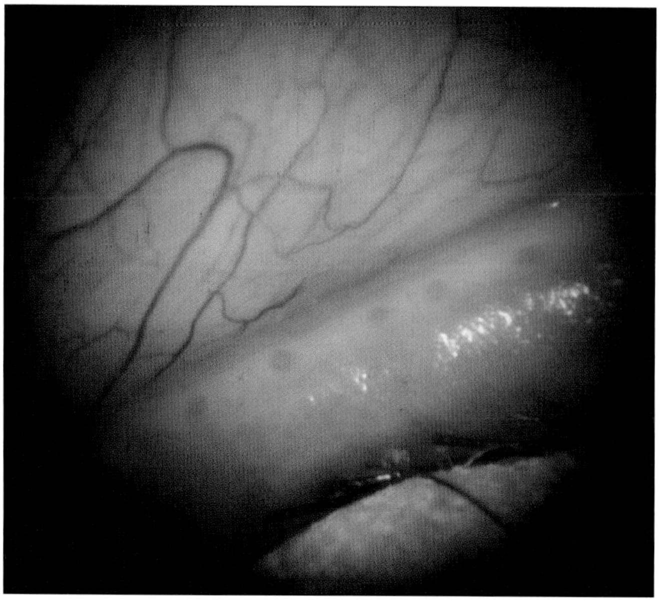

Fig. 34.1 Normal meibomian gland orifices.

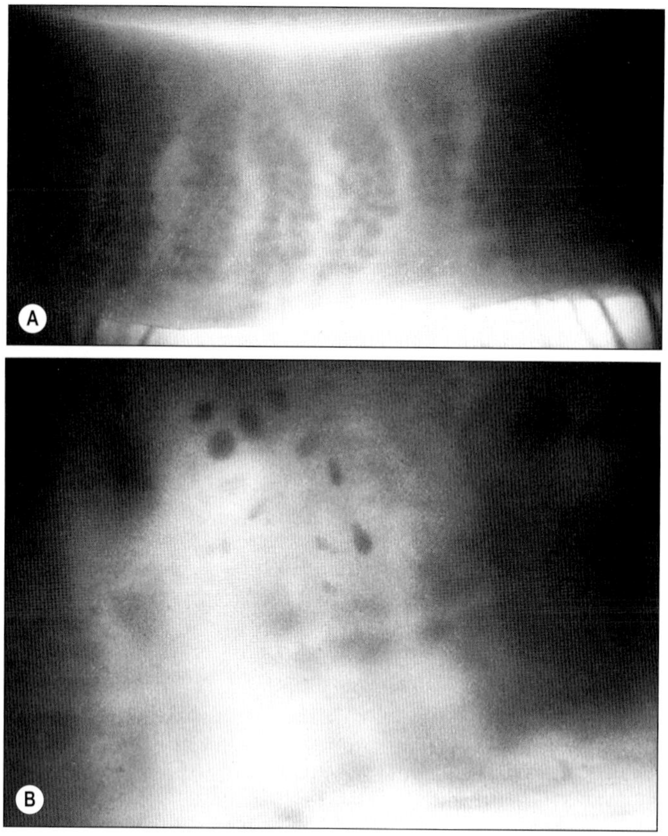

Fig. 34.2 (**A**) Meibography showing normal appearance of meibomian glands. (**B**) Meibography showing meibomian gland dropout.

meibomian gland secretion may provide an important barrier to contamination of the tear film by the highly polar cutaneous sebum. At eye surface temperature, meibomian lipid is more viscous than sebum and able to form a barrier to its entry onto the ocular surface. The melting point of human meibomian secretion is approximately 32°C to 34°C.[12] Normal eye surface temperatures range between 32°C and 36°C.[13] Any decrease in the melting point secondary to abnormal synthesis or the influence of bacterial lipases would result in liquefaction of the meibomian fluid and the loss of the barrier mechanism. Conversely, an increase in melting point would lead to meibomian gland inspissation and a compromised barrier secondary to decreased secretion. A report has linked oleic acid content in meibum with changes in viscosity.[14]

The lipid layer produced by the meibomian glands represents the outermost layer of the tear film and protects the hydrated gel covering the ocular surface. The tear film is thought to be approximately 7 µm thick in the open eye but a recent study indicates that the tear film may be as thick as 40 µm.[15] The lipid layer is about 40–100 nm thick. Thickness is influenced by the width of the interpalpebral opening.

Blinking is important for the excretion of meibomian lipid. Jetting of the oil onto the tear film has been observed with blinking.[16] It has been suggested that the orbicularis muscle milks the glands by contracting during blinking.[17] Meibometry is used to measure the amount of lipid on the lid margin by determining the degree of translucency induced on plastic tape applied to the lid margin. In the absence of blinking, the meibomian glands become engorged and the measurable amount of lipid on the lid margin decreases; it is readily restored by the first few blinks.[18] Levels are greater 1 hour after waking than later in the day and are thought to be due to decreased secretion from the glands during sleep, with glandular engorgement and then discharge of the excess lipid on awakening when blinking resumes. The thickness of the lipid layer increases after forceful blinking.[19] Thus, blinking appears to be important in the release of meibomian gland lipid into the tear film. It is probable that blinking abnormalities contribute to the formation of meibomian gland dysfunction, and studies of those performing prolonged computer work confirm a higher prevalence of MGD.[20]

Tear film break-up time is reduced in meibomian gland dysfunction. Various models have been proposed to explain this phenomenon. One model suggests that with a deficient aqueous subphase, the lipid layer contaminates the hydrophilic mucin layer, making it hydrophobic with resultant disruption of the tear film.[21] Alternatively, it has been postulated that a key step in tear film break-up is the rupture of the mucin layer by van der Waals expulsion forces.[22] Tear film break-up time rapidly returns to normal when the meibomian glands are expressed.[23]

Although the meibomian glands are richly innervated, there is no evidence that meibomian gland secretion in humans is under neural control. Hormones are known to significantly affect the secretion of sebaceous glands of the skin and the meibomian glands. Production is increased by androgens and decreased by antiandrogens and estrogens. Recent studies have demonstrated that the meibomian gland is an androgen target organ and that decreased androgens alter the lipid profile and may lead to meibomian gland dysfunction and evaporative dry eye. There is evidence that meibomian glands are capable of de novo lipid synthesis.[24]

Classification of Meibomian Gland Dysfunction

Blepharitis can be divided into anterior and posterior forms. Meibomian gland dysfunction is a type of posterior blepharitis. Recently, several classification systems for meibomian gland dysfunction have been suggested, but none has been widely adopted (Box 34.1).

McCulley et al.[25] proposed a classification of chronic blepharitis into six entities, based on clinical criteria. The first three groups consist of patients with primarily anterior blepharitis; the last three categories encompass patients with meibomian gland dysfunction. In another classification system, Mathers et al.[26] divided patients with meibomian gland dysfunction into four groups. This classification is based on three objective criteria: tear osmolarity, Schirmer testing, and meibography. Bron et al.[27] classified meibomian gland diseases into seven groups and developed a grading system based on a large number of biomicroscopic features. Foulks and Bron expanded this classification into a clinically oriented schema (Fig 34.3).[28] There is no documentation of primary hyposecretion or of hypersecretion (seborrhea) of the meibomian glands.

Box 34.1 Classifications of meibomian gland disease

McCulley et al. (1982)

Staphylococcal: Anterior lid inflammation with collarettes and madarosis

Seborrheic: Less inflammation with greasy scales on the anterior lid margin

Mixed seborrheic and staphylococcal: A combination of the two above

Seborrheic with meibomian seborrhea: Patients with meibomian gland hypersecretion but without obstruction

Seborrheic with secondary meibomitis: Patients with occluded and inflamed meibomian glands in a spotty distribution

Primary meibomitis (also known as meibomian keratoconjunctivitis): Patients with obstruction and inflammation of all the meibomian glands in association with seborrheic dermatitis or acne rosacea

Mathers et al. (1991)

Seborrheic: Patients with hypersecretion and normal gland morphology and tear osmolarity

Obstructive: Patients with low excretion/high gland dropout on meibography and increased tear osmolarity but normal Schirmer's testing

Obstructive with sicca: Patients with the same findings as for obstructive but with a low Schirmer test result

Sicca: Normal gland morphology; high tear osmolarity and low Schirmer test result

Bron et al. (1991)

Reduced number (congenital deficiency)

Replacement (trichiasis, metaplasia)

Hyposecretion

Obstructive meibomitis subdivided into focal, primary, secondary to local disease or systemic disease, and chalazia

Hypersecretory (seborrhea)

Neoplastic

Suppurative

Foulks and Bron (2003)

Adapted from McCulley JP et al. Ophthalmology. *1982;89:1173; Mathers WD et al.* Cornea. *1991;10:277; Bron AJ et al.* Eye. *1991;5:395; Foulks GN, Bron AJ.* Ocul Surf. *2003;1:107.*

Diagnosis of Meibomian Gland Dysfunction

Symptoms are nonspecific and include burning, irritation, itching, red eyes, and decreased or fluctuating vision; they are often similar to symptoms of dry eye. Findings on examination range from minimal to severe and often do not correlate well with the severity of symptoms. The lid margin is often rounded with thickening, erythema, hyperkeratinization, vascularization, telangiectasia, or notching.[27] Inflammation may or may not be apparent. The meibomian gland orifices are frequently less well defined or may show pouting. An increase or reduction in the number of orifices may be seen. The orifices may be displaced, more often posteriorly. Capping of the orifice with solidified excreta or epithelium is often present. Applying pressure to the lid margin produces little or no expulsion of secretion or secretion that is abnormal in appearance. Instead of being clear, it is turbid, granular, or toothpaste-like (Fig. 34.4). On everting the lid, the yellowish, grape-like appearance of the meibomian glands may appear abnormal with dropout or dilation of the glands.

Using meibography, narrowing or occlusion of the glandular orifices and glandular distortion or dilation are seen in patients with meibomian gland dysfunction (see Fig. 34.2B).[4] In one study using this method of examination, 74% of patients showed meibomian gland loss as compared with only 20% of normal controls.[26] Another technique to diagnose meibomian gland dysfunction measures meibum excretion. Meibum is collected on an adhesive tape placed on the lid margin; this lipid imprint is then analyzed using a density measuring device called a meibometer. The imprint can either be measured directly on the meibometer (direct meibometry) or combined with image-scanning and computer densitometry (integrated meibometry).[29] Patients with meibomian gland dysfunction demonstrate reduced casual lipid levels. Cost and availability limit the use of this technology in the clinical setting.

Corneal and conjunctival staining is often present after application of rose Bengal, lissamine green, or fluorescein solutions. In more severe and chronic cases, there may be corneal pannus, ulceration, or lid abnormalities such as ectropion. Although less common, these more severe manifestations emphasize the importance of diagnosing and treating this condition. The diagnosis of sebaceous cell carcinoma should be considered in unilateral recalcitrant cases of meibomian gland dysfunction, particularly with persistent inflammation in the same area of the lid and when anatomic disturbances are seen (e.g. loss or distortion of lash follicles).

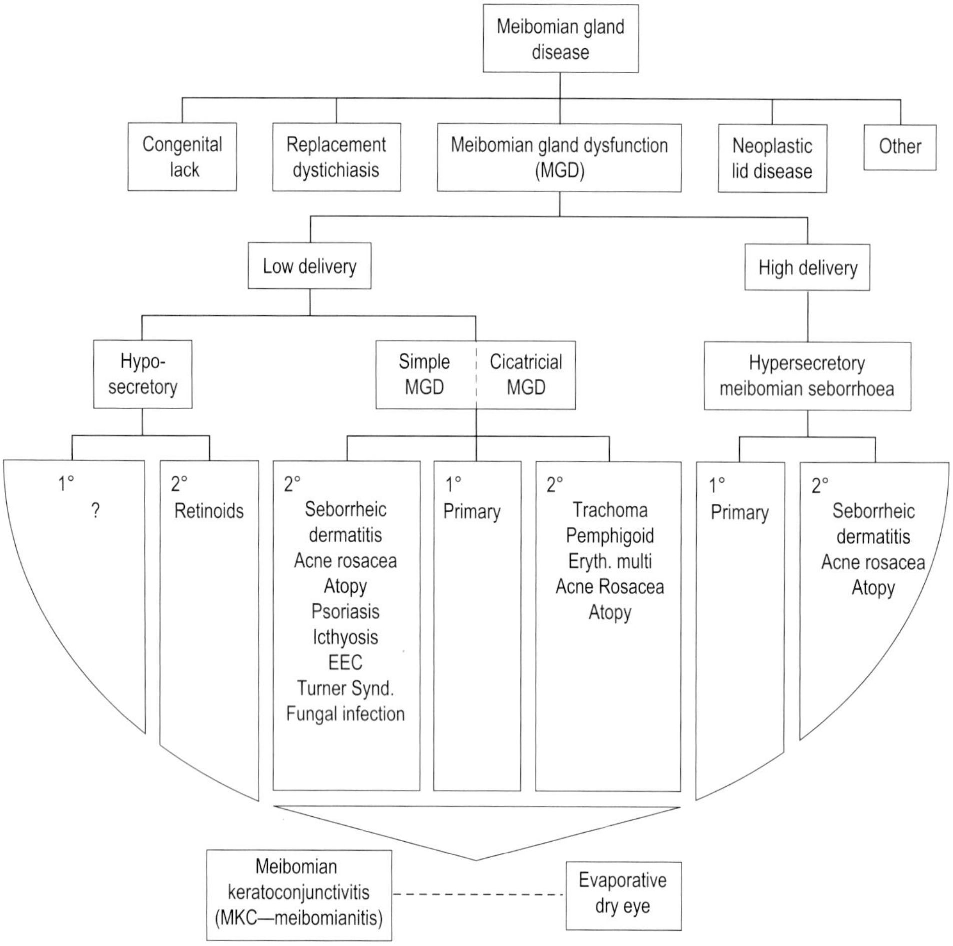

Fig. 34.3 Clinical classification of meibomian gland disease. (Reprinted with permission from Ethis Communication, Inc. from Foulks GN, Bron AJ. *Ocul Suf.* 2003;1:107.)

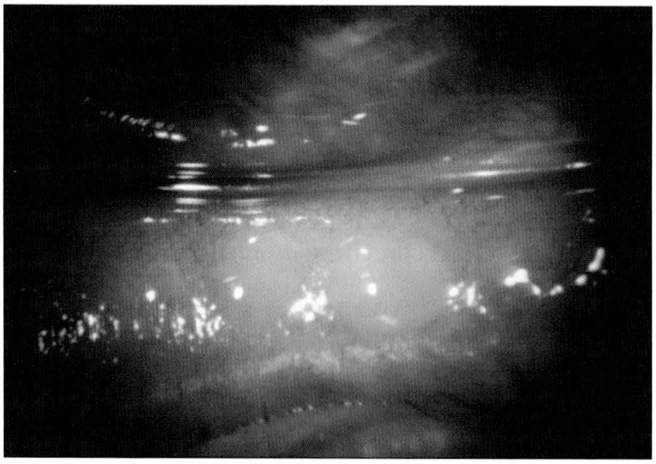

Fig. 34.4 Lid margin in meibomian gland dysfunction. Note turbid secretion and increased vascularity.

Associated Conditions

Meibomian gland dysfunction is frequently associated with lacrimal insufficiency.[30] Patients with both of these entities are likely to have particularly severe dry eye symptoms. Meibomian gland dysfunction causes increased evaporation of the tear film, and this, coupled with decreased aqueous production, results in a severely compromised preocular tear film. Foamy deposits in the tear film are common, especially at the lateral canthus. Approximately 60% of patients with Sjögren's associated aqueous tear deficiency have meibomian gland dysfunction.

Rosacea is common in patients with meibomian gland dysfunction. The pathogenesis of this condition is unknown, but it appears to be primarily a disorder of vasodilation. Histologically, there is often severe elastosis, with disorganization of the dermis and associated edema.[31] Sebum excretion rate is not elevated. Because meibomian glands are modified sebaceous glands, they are affected in a manner similar to the sebaceous glands of the skin in rosacea, with hypertrophy and plugging. Patients with both meibomian gland dysfunction and rosacea appear to have more severe changes when examined with meibography.[4]

It is important to identify these associated conditions when treating meibomian gland dysfunction. Evidence of rosacea and seborrheic dermatitis may be subtle, and a careful history and examination of the skin are necessary.

Meibomian gland dysfunction is found with increasing frequency with age. In some cases, it may represent a senescent degeneration of the meibomian glands or be the result of an abnormal blink mechanism secondary to aging changes affecting the lids. Normal eyelids in the elderly show many of the morphologic changes seen with meibomian gland dysfunction.[32] Secretion decreases with age, but the presence of turbidity or increased viscosity appears to be specific for meibomian gland dysfunction.

Associated sequelae

Contact lens intolerance is common in patients with meibomian gland dysfunction.[33] Contact lenses increase tear evaporation, which exacerbates symptoms in patients who already have a compromised tear film. Giant papillary conjunctivitis (GPC) is also seen with a high frequency in these patients.[34] Any patient with GPC should be examined closely for meibomian gland dysfunction, because treatment of the latter improves GPC and contact lens intolerance.[35]

Chalazia are seen in frequent association with meibomian gland dysfunction. Treatment of the underlying meibomian gland dysfunction will help prevent recurrence of chalazia in these patients.

Histopathology

Obstruction of the meibomian gland orifices is probably the most common cause of meibomian gland dysfunction. Studies indicate that hyperkeratinization is important in the pathogenesis of obstruction.[2,6] Narrowing of the ductule lumen with desquamation of epithelial cells leads to glandular obstruction. Acini dilate or atrophy.

Obstruction of the glandular contents results in increased pressure on the cuboidal cells lining the acini, flattening these cells. Stagnated meibomian secretion leads to lid inflammation and often to the development of chalazia. Cystic degeneration of the glands not associated with inflammation may be seen.[36]

Models of Meibomian Gland Dysfunction

Meibomian gland dysfunction has been replicated in several animal and human models which are useful sources of information about the pathogenesis of these disorders. Systemic polychlorinated biphenyl (PCB) toxicity leads to hyperkeratinization of the meibomian gland ducts and toothpaste-like excreta as seen in meibomian gland dysfunction.[37] Rabbit lids treated topically with epinephrine develop meibomian gland dysfunction.[38] In this model, plugging of the gland orifices occurs with hyperkeratinization of the ductule epithelium, loss of acini, and the development of microcysts. Closure of the meibomian gland orifices by cautery in rabbits increases tear film osmolarity, with an associated reduction in goblet cell number.[10] Isotretinoin (Accutane) taken systemically results in meibomian gland atrophy and hyposecretion, with increased excreta viscosity and tear osmolarity.[39] This effect of isotretinoin on meibomian gland structure and function is reversible when treatment is stopped.

These models of meibomian gland dysfunction support the view that obstructive meibomian gland disease results from hyperkeratinization of the glandular orifice. Hyperkeratinization leads to stasis of the meibomian gland secretion and increased evaporation of the tear film, with the consequent development of ocular surface disease.

Lipid Composition and Behavior of Human Meibomian Secretion

Meibomian gland secretion consists largely of neutral sterol and wax esters with lesser amounts of polar lipids, diesters, triesters, triglycerides, free fatty acids, and free sterols.[7] Studies have found statistically significant differences in each component of meibomian secretion in patients with meibomian gland dysfunction compared to controls.[40–44] Interestingly, cholesterol esters are always present in patients with meibomian gland dysfunction, whereas normal individuals fall into two groups, one with and one without cholesterol esters in their meibomian secretion.[45] Normal subjects who have cholesterol ester in their meibomian secretions have twice as many coagulase-negative staphylococci (CN-S) and *Staphylococcus aureus* strains with cholesterol ester lipase activity as those who do not have cholesterol esters in their meibomian secretions. The presence of cholesterol encourages bacterial growth of *S. aureus*.[46]

Reports have shown considerable variation in lipid composition among normal individuals.[47] There is little doubt, however, that the lipid composition in normal individuals varies greatly from that in patients with meibomian gland dysfunction. Sophisticated spectroscopic studies demonstrate a gradual decline in the phase transition temperature of meibum with age in normal subjects but a marked increase in phase transition temperature in MGD.[48] These changes result in increased viscosity of the lipid secretion.

Unlike meibomian gland secretion, sebum contains more triglycerides and free fatty acids and considerably less sterol esters.[49] Squalene is present in sebum and absent in meibomian gland secretion. The wax ester proportion is similar in both secretions. Overall, sebum is much more polar and will contaminate the tear film when mixed with it. Recently, evidence has been presented suggesting that evaporative tear deficiency is associated with specific lipid changes in meibum secretion, i.e. decreases in phosphatidylethanolamine and sphingomyelin.[50]

Role of Microorganisms

Staphylococcus epidermidis (94%), *Propionibacterium acnes* (87%), and *Corynebacterium* species (64%) are commonly isolated from normal lids.[51] *S. aureus* is found significantly less frequently (13% of normals). The frequency of culture positivity is similar in patients with meibomian gland dysfunction and normal individuals, but growth may be heavier in patients with posterior blepharitis.[52] The meibomian glands yield the same flora as lid cultures, but with decreased frequency. It has been reported that 48% of meibomian gland cultures and only 2% of lid cultures are sterile.

The lid flora is important in the development of meibomian gland dysfunction in many patients. Three of the bacteria commonly isolated from eyelids, *S. aureus*, *Corynebacterium* species (CN-S), and *P. acnes*, produce lipases that can alter the composition of meibomian lipids.[53] Differences in lipase production between normal persons and patients with blepharitis have been associated with *S. epidermidis*, suggesting that certain strains of this bacterium may be responsible for at least some forms of meibomian gland dysfunction. The changes in lipid composition may, in turn, enhance the growth of other local bacteria.

Further evidence for the influence of local bacteria is that meibomian gland dysfunction often responds favorably to topical and systemic antibiotics. Tetracycline reduces lipase production in *S. epidermidis*, *S. aureus*, and *P. acnes*.[54] It also decreases serum cholesterol in mice, has antichemotactic effects on neutrophils, and has activity against collagenase and other metalloproteinases. Any of these properties may produce a marked therapeutic effect in many patients with meibomian gland dysfunction and rosacea.

The role of other microorganisms frequently found on the eyelids, such as *Pityrosporum*[55] and *Demodex*,[56] is unclear. There is no evidence that these ubiquitous organisms cause or worsen the posterior blepharitis seen in meibomian gland dysfunction patients.

Treatment

Treatment of meibomian gland dysfunction consists of lid hygiene, systemic antibiotics, topical antibiotics and antiinflammatories, and treatment of associated conditions.

The mainstay of treatment is lid hygiene, including massage of the eyelid. The patient should be educated that meibomian gland disease is a chronic condition and that lid hygiene should become part of the patient's daily routine. Lid hygiene consists of three steps:

1. Warm compresses: A warm washcloth is placed on the closed lids. As it cools, it is reheated in warm water and reapplied. This regimen is continued for 2 to 10 minutes.
2. Lid massage: This consists of stabilizing the eyelid by pulling the lid horizontally toward the lateral canthus and then massaging the eyelid with the fingertip of the other hand in a horizontal action from the medial canthus towards the lateral canthus.
3. Lid scrubs: If anterior blepharitis is also present, lid scrubs are used along the lid margin to remove deposits and the abnormal oily secretions from the lashes. Commercially available eye scrubs are better tolerated than a dilute solution of baby shampoo applied with a cotton-tipped applicator.[57]

Performing lid hygiene in the morning may be more effective because of the accumulation of secretions overnight.[29] Manual expression of the meibomian glands increases lipid layer thickness with symptomatic relief.[58]

Systemic antibiotic therapy consists of oral tetracycline, 250 mg four times a day; doxycycline, 50–100 mg twice a day, or minocycline, 50 mg twice a day. These lipophilic antibiotics are thought to exert their effect by interfering with bacterial and tissue lipases and their deleterious effects on lipid composition. Doxycycline is preferred over tetracycline because it can be taken twice a day and is not as affected by dairy products and antacids. Minocycline is useful in refractory cases. Tetracycline and doxycycline are also effective in the treatment of rosacea.[59] These antibiotics are generally reserved for patients with prominent symptoms and are used for several months. They take several weeks to show a therapeutic effect. A common side effect is photosensitivity. It is important to warn female patients of reproductive age of the dangers of taking these antibiotics during pregnancy, as they cause tooth enamel abnormalities in children and interfere with oral contraception.

Topical therapy consists of antibiotics and antiinflammatory drugs. Patients with a significant amount of inflammation of the eyelids benefit from a short course of antibiotic–steroid combination ointment while waiting for the systemic antibiotics to take effect. Topical steroids should be used judiciously because of possibile *Candida* superinfection and other ocular side effects. Topical ciclosporin A has been advocated to reduce eyelid inflammation of posterior blepharitis.[60,61] Topical azithromycin has also been reported to reduce inflammation.[62]

Topical 1% metronidazole cream[63] or 1% clindamycin lotion[64] is effective in controlling some of the skin manifestations of rosacea. Antiseborrheic shampoos such as those containing selenium sulfide can be used when seborrheic dermatitis is present. Lubrication should be applied to the eyes in the form of supplemental tears when there is an associated aqueous deficiency.

Other reports detailing the use of lubricants containing low-concentration castor oil or a mix of metastable oil emulsion demonstrate encouraging results in stabilizing the tear film.[65,66]

Conclusion

Meibomian gland dysfunction is an extremely common cause of blepharitis. It is caused most often by an obstruction of the meibomian glands secondary to hyperkeratinization of the duct epithelium or plugging with a solidified secretion. These developments lead to a compromised tear film lipid layer with increased evaporation, decreased tear breakup time, and increased tear osmolarity. The compromised preocular tear film leads to dry eye signs and symptoms.

Recent studies have shown significant abnormalities in the lipid composition and behavior in patients with meibomian gland dysfunction. These differences are thought to be secondary to the influence of lid flora on meibomian gland secretion or abnormal lipid synthesis.

Long-term treatment is aimed at controlling symptoms with lid hygiene and massage. Systemic antibiotics are often used, particularly in patients with rosacea. Topical antibiotic–antiinflammatory combinations can be used when a significant amount of inflammation is present.

References

1. Duke-Elder WS, Wybar KC. *System of ophthalmology.* vol II, *The anatomy of the visual system.* London: H Kimpton; 1961.

2. Jester JV, et al. Meibomian gland studies: histologic and ultrastructural investigations. *Invest Ophthalmol Vis Sci.* 1981;20:537.
3. Weingeist TA. The glands of the ocular adnexa. *Int Ophthalmol Clin.* 1973;13:243.
4. Robin BR, et al. In vivo transillumination biomicroscopy and photography of meibomian gland dysfunction: a clinical study. *Ophthalmology.* 1985;921:423.
5. Mathers WD, et al. Video imaging of the meibomian gland. *Arch Ophthalmol.* 1994;112:448.
6. Gutgesell VJ, et al. Histopathology of meibomian gland dysfunction. *Am J Ophthalmol.* 1982;94:383.
6a. Korb D, Henriquez H. Meibomian gland dysfunction and contact lens intolerance. *J Am Optom Assoc.* 1980;243–251.
7. Nicolaides N, et al. Meibomian gland studies: comparison of steer and human lipids. *Invest Ophthalmol Vis Sci.* 1981;20:522.
8. Iwata S, et al. Evaporation rate of water from the precorneal tear film and cornea in the rabbit. *Invest Ophthalmol Vis Sci.* 1969;8:613.
9. Mathers WD. Ocular evaporation in meibomian gland dysfunction and dry eye. *Ophthalmology.* 1993;100:347.
10. Gilbard JP, et al. Tear film and ocular surface changes after closure of meibomian gland orifices in the rabbit. *Ophthalmology.* 1989;96:1180.
11. McDonald JE. Surface phenomena of the tear film. *Am J Ophthalmol.* 1969;67:56.
12. Tiffany JM. The lipid secretion of the meibomian glands. *Adv Lipid Res.* 1981;22:1.
13. Tiffany JM, Dart JKG. Normal and abnormal functions of meibomian gland secretions. *R Soc Med Int Congr Symp Ser.* 1981;40:1061.
14. Shine WE, McCulley JP. Association of meibum oleic acid with meibomian seborrhea. *Cornea.* 2000;19:72–74.
15. Prydal JI, et al. Study of human precorneal tear film thickness and structure using laser interferometry. *Invest Ophthalmol Vis Sci.* 1992;33: 2006.
16. Norn MS. Lipid tests: tear film interference. In: Lemp MA, Marquardt R, eds. *The dry eye: a comprehensive guide.* Berlin: Springer-Verlag; 1992.
17. Linton RG, et al. The meibomian glands: an investigation into the secretion and some aspects of the physiology. *Br J Ophthalmol.* 1961;45:718.
18. CHew CKS, et al. The casual level of meibomian lipids in humans. *Trans Ophthalmol Soc UK.* 1985;104:374.
19. Korb DR, et al. Tear film lipid thickness as a function of blinking. *Cornea.* 1994;13:354.
20. Yee RW, Sperling HG, Kattek A, et al. Isolation of the ocular surface to treat dysfunctional tear syndrome associated with computer use. *Ocul Surf.* 2007;5(4):308–315.
21. Holly FJ. Physical chemistry of the normal and disordered tear film. *Trans Ophthalmol Soc UK.* 1985;104:374.
22. Sharma A, Ruckenstein H. Mechanism of tear film rupture and formation of dry spots on cornea. *J Colloid Interface Sci.* 1986;111:8.
23. McCulley JP, Sciallis GF. Meibomian keratoconjunctivitis. *Am J Ophthalmol.* 1977;84:788.
24. Kolattukudy PE, et al. Biosynthesis of lipids by bovine meibomian glands. *Lipids.* 1985;20:468.
25. McCulley JP, et al. Classification of chronic blepharitis. *Ophthalmology.* 1982;89:1173.
26. Mathers WD, et al. Meibomian gland dysfunction in chronic blepharitis. *Cornea.* 1991;10:277.
27. Bron AJ, et al. Meibomian gland disease. Classification and grading of lid changes. *Eye.* 1991;5:395.
28. Foulks GN, Bron AJ. Meibomian gland dysfunction: a clinical scheme for description, diagnosis, classification, and grading. *Ocul Surf.* 2003;1: 107–126.
29. Yokoi N, Mossa F, Tiffany JM, et al. Assessment of meibomian gland function in dry eye using meibometry. *Arch Ophthalmol.* 1999;117: 723–729.
30. Bowman RW, et al. Chronic blepharitis and dry eyes. *Int Ophthalmol Clin.* 1987;27:27.
31. Marks R, Harcourt-Webster JN. Histopathology of rosacea. *Arch Dermatol.* 1969;100:682.
32. Hykin PG, et al. Age-related morphologic changes in lid margin and meibomian gland anatomy. *Cornea.* 1992;11:334–342.
33. Henriquez AS, Korb DR. Meibomian glands and contact lens wear. *Br J Ophthalmol.* 1981;65:108.
34. Mathers WD, Billborough M. Meibomian gland function and giant papillary conjunctivitis. *Am J Ophthalmol.* 1992;114:188.
35. Martin NF, et al. Giant papillary conjunctivitis and meibomian gland dysfunction. *CLAO J.* 1992;18:165.
36. Straatsma BR. Cystic degeneration of the meibomian glands. *Arch Ophthalmol.* 1959;61:918.
37. Ohnishi Y, Kohn T. Polychlorinated biphenyls poisoning in monkey eye. *Invest Ophthalmol Vis Sci.* 1979;18:981.
38. Jester JV, et al. Meibomian gland dysfunction. II. The role of keratinization in a rabbit model of MGD. *Invest Ophthalmol Vis Sci.* 1989;30:936.
39. Mathers WD, et al. Meibomian gland morphology and tear osmolarity: changes with Accutane therapy. *Cornea.* 1991;10:286.
40. Osgood JK, et al. The role of wax and sterol esters of meibomian secretions in chronic blepharitis. *Invest Ophthalmol Vis Sci.* 1989;30:1958.
41. Shine WE, McCulley JP. Role of wax ester fatty alcohols in chronic blepharitis. *Invest Ophthalmol Vis Sci.* 1993;34:3515.
42. Dougherty JM, McCulley JP. Analysis of the free fatty acid component of meibomian secretions in chronic blepharitis. *Invest Ophthalmol Vis Sci.* 1986;27:52.
43. Dougherty JM, et al. The role of wax and sterol ester fatty acids in chronic blepharitis. *Invest Ophthalmol Vis Sci.* 1991;32:1932.
44. Shine WE, McCulley JP. The importance of human meibomian secretion triglycerides in the development of chronic blepharitis disease signs. *Invest Ophthalmol Vis Sci.* 1994;35(Suppl):2482.
45. Shine WE, McCulley JP. The role of cholesterol in chronic blepharitis. *Invest Ophthalmol Vis Sci.* 1991;32:2272.
46. Shine WE, et al. Relation of cholesterol-stimulated *Staphylococcus aureus* growth to chronic blepharitis. *Invest Ophthalmol Vis Sci.* 1993;34: 2291.
47. Tiffany JM. Individual variations in human meibomian lipid composition. *Exp Eye Res.* 1978;27:289.
48. Borchman D, Foulks GN, Yappert MC, Ho D. Spectroscopic evaluation of human tear lipids. *Chem Phys Lipids.* 2007;147(2):87–102
49. Greene RS, et al. Anatomical variation in the amount and composition of human skin surface lipids. *J Invest Dermatol.* 1970;54:241.
50. Shine WE, McCulley JP. Keratoconjunctivitis sicca associated with meibomian secretion polar lipid abnormality. *Arch Ophthalmol.* 1998;116:849–852.
51. McCulley JP, Dougherty JM. Bacterial aspects of chronic blepharitis. *Trans Ophthalmol Soc UK.* 1986;105:314.
52. Groden LR, et al. Lid flora in blepharitis. *Cornea.* 1991;10:50.
53. Dougherty JM, McCulley JP. Bacterial lipases and chronic blepharitis. *Invest Ophthalmol Vis Sci.* 1986;27:486.
54. Dougherty JM, et al. The role of tetracycline in chronic blepharitis: inhibition of lipase production in staphylococci. *Invest Ophthalmol Vis Sci.* 1991;32:2970.
55. Parunovic A, Halde C. *Pityrosporum orbiculare:* its possible role in seborrheic blepharitis. *Am J Ophthalmol.* 1962;63:815.
56. Norn MS. *Demodex folliculorum.* Incidence and possible pathogenic role in the human eyelid. *Acta Ophthalmol (Copenh).* 1970;108:1.
57. Polack FM, Goodman DF. Experience with a new detergent lid scrub in the management of chronic blepharitis. *Arch Ophthalmol.* 1988;106:719.
58. Korb DR, Greiner JV. Increase in tear film lipid layer thickness following treatment of meibomian gland dysfunction. In: Sullivan DA, ed. *Tear film and dry eye syndromes.* New York: Plenum Press; 1994.
59. Frucht-Pery J, et al. Efficacy of doxycycline and tetracycline in ocular rosacea. *Am J Ophthalmol.* 1993;116:88.
60. Perry HD, et al. Efficacy of commercially available topical steroid cyclosporine A 0.5% in the treatment of meibomian gland dysfunction. *Cornea.* 2006;25(2):171–175.
61. Rubin M, Rao SN. Efficacy of topical cyclosporine 0.5% in the treatment of posterior blepharitis. *J Ocul Pharmacol Ther.* 2006;22:47–53.
62. John T, Shah AA. Use of azithromycin ophthalmic solution in the treatment of chronic mixed anterior blepharitis. *Ann Ophthalmol.* 2008;40(2): 68–74.
63. Nielson PG. A double blind study of 1% metronidazole cream versus systemic oxytetracycline therapy for rosacea. *Br J Dermatol.* 1983;109:63.
64. Wilkin JK, DeWitt S. Treatment of rosacea: topical clindamycin versus oral tetracycline. *Int J Dermatol.* 1993;32:65.
65. Goto E, Shimazaki J, Monden Y, et al. Low concentration homogenized castor oil drops for non-inflamed meibomian gland dysfunction. *Ophthalmology.* 2002;109: 2030–2035.
66. Korb DR, Scaffidi RC, Greiner JV, et al. The effect of two novel lubricant eye drops on tear film lipid layer thickness in subjects with dry eye symptoms. *Optom Vis Sci.* 2005;82:594–601.

Chapter 35

Eyelid Infections

Andrew L. Moyes, Anthony J. Verachtert

Viral Infections

Most viral infections in humans are self-limiting and relatively asymptomatic. Some viral infections, however, may be associated with high morbidity and mortality. Defects in cell-mediated immunity may render a host even more susceptible to particularly severe manifestations of viral disease. The most common viral infections of the lid include herpes simplex infection, varicella-zoster infection, molluscum contagiosum, and papillomavirus infection. Infections associated with the smallpox virus and the smallpox vaccine are now quite rare, but both were once associated with significant ocular morbidity.

Herpes simplex virus

Herpes simplex virus (HSV) has been subclassified into HSV type I and type II. Although different, these two subtypes share many common antigens. HSV type I is usually associated with infection above the waist, whereas HSV type II is usually associated with infection below the waist. Herpes viruses have a propensity for invasion of neural tissue with the development of latency and associated reactivation.

Clinical manifestations

Herpes simplex virus infection of the eyelids typically presents as multiple vesicles on a raised, edematous, erythematous base. The infection may be limited to the lid margin, or there may be involvement of the periorbital skin. Patients may have concomitant labial or nasal herpetic eruptions. Lid vesicles are more commonly seen in the first week of infection, and lid ulceration is more commonly seen in the second week (Fig. 35.1). Once lid ulceration has occurred, it typically lasts for 2 to 3 weeks but can last for up to 4 to 5 weeks. The involved lid margin is usually swollen and tender to palpation. The conjunctiva adjacent to the lid lesions is usually injected, and a follicular reaction is commonly present on the tarsal conjunctiva. An ipsilateral preauricular adenopathy is present in 60% of ocular HSV disease.[1] An associated follicular conjunctivitis may be seen in as many as 94% of patients with the possible development of pseudomembranes in the fornices.[1]

Herpes simplex blepharitis is usually diagnosed clinically, but the diagnosis can be confirmed in the laboratory. Viral cultures may be obtained from fresh vesicles, with HSV growing in culture in 2–3 days. Viral isolation rate is approximately 70%.

Treatment

Herpes simplex blepharoconjunctivitis is usually a self-limiting disease lasting 3 to 12 days.[2] When limited to the skin, herpes simplex infection does not require any specific therapy. Since it is not possible to predict which patients will develop a herpetic keratitis associated with a blepharoconjunctivitis, prophylactic treatment of eyelid or conjunctival HSV disease with oral antiviral agents may be useful in the treatment of herpes simplex blepharitis. In the United States, where the ophthalmic preparation of acyclovir is not available, care must be taken with the use of the dermatologic preparation because the polyethylene glycol base may be irritating to the conjunctiva and cornea.

In immunocompromised patients and neonates (less than 6 weeks of age), HSV may be associated with severe localized disease, systemic dissemination, and herpetic encephalitis with a high morbidity and mortality.[3,4] In such patients, systemic antiviral therapy is warranted.

Varicella-zoster virus

Primary infection with varicella-zoster virus (VZV)[4] usually presents during childhood as chickenpox. The virus then remains in a latent form, with reactivation presenting as herpes zoster ophthalmicus or shingles. By age 60, nearly 100% of people are seropositive for VZV antibody.

Clinical manifestations of primary VZV infection

Chickenpox is a mild, diffuse exanthematous infection that affects more than 3 million children a year in the United States. Peak incidence is at age 5 to 9 years. The disease is spread by direct contact, droplet, or airborne transmission. It is characterized by a papulovesicular rash, fever, malaise, anorexia, and lethargy. The rash usually begins as a crop of small, red papules that develop into clear vesicles on an erythematous base. The vesicles then break and become scabbed. Crops of vesicles continue to appear for 3 to 4 days, mainly affecting the trunk, face, scalp, and proximal extremities.

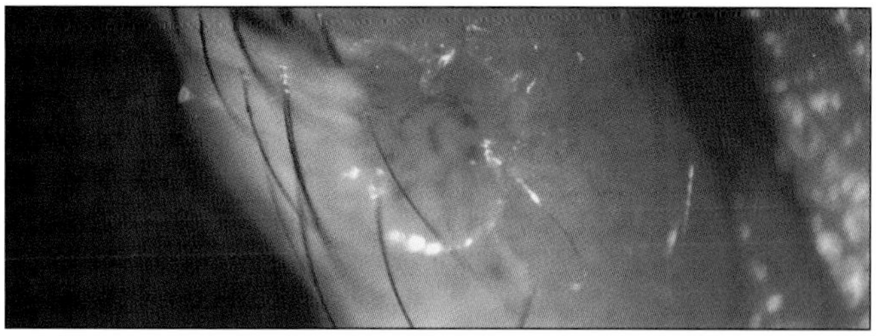

Fig. 35.1 Ulcerative herpes simplex blepharitis.

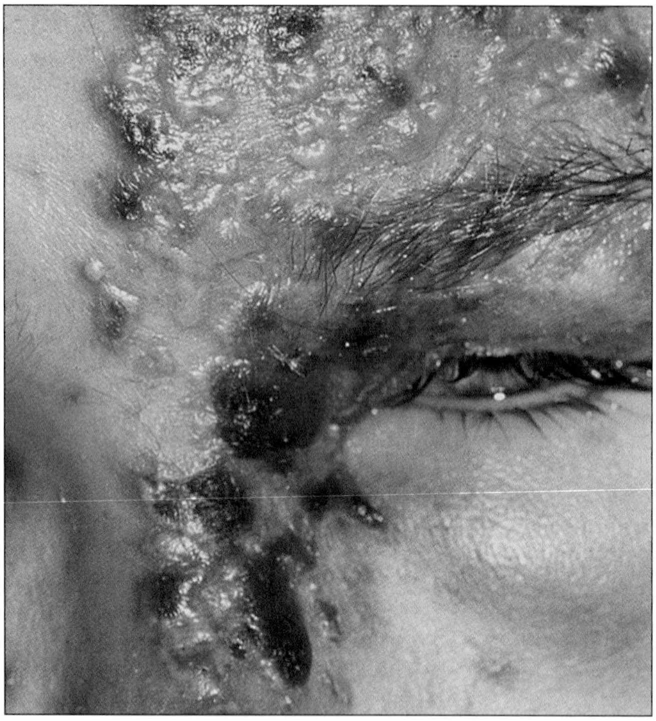

Fig. 35.2 Herpes zoster skin eruption.

Ocular complications from chickenpox are rare. The lids may be affected by vesicular lesions that may become necrotic[5] or secondarily infected. Conjunctival, limbal, and corneal vesicles have been reported, and all are usually associated with a benign course. Rarely, vesicles or phlyctenule-like lesions may be associated with painful ulceration. The cornea may develop dendritic keratitis, immune stromal disease, or a superficial punctate keratitis.[6–8] Uveitis also has been associated with primary VZV infection.[9]

Clinical manifestations of reactivated VZV

The reactivation of latent VZV or contact with exogenous virus from active chickenpox or herpes zoster may result in the development of herpes zoster, a dermatomal, vesicular rash usually associated with severe pain.[10,11] It may occur at all ages, but most commonly after the sixth decade.

The first sign of disease is usually headache, malaise, fever, and chills, followed by pain within the affected dermatome. An erythematous maculopapular rash, which rapidly becomes vesicular, forms within the dermatome 48–72 hours later (Fig. 35.2). Lesions continue to form over 3 to 5 days. Fifty percent to 69% of patients with herpes zoster ophthalmicus (HZO) present with lid margin vesiculation.[12] Active infection usually lasts 7 to 10 days and is followed by crusting of the lesions. Skin ulceration may take several weeks to heal, with resultant cutaneous manifestations ranging from mild scarring to severe sloughing with loss of tissue. Distichiasis, trichiasis, ptosis, and lid deformity interfering with normal lid closure may occur. In addition, dermal and subdermal cicatrization may result in severe ectropion and canalicular obstruction. Unlike herpes simplex, which results in superficial skin changes, herpes zoster forms deep eschars that result in permanent scars.[13]

Diagnosis

The diagnosis of chickenpox and herpes zoster is usually a clinical one. The characteristic rash and a history of recent exposure usually lead to the diagnosis of chickenpox. In the past, however, smallpox and disseminated vaccinia infection could be confused with chickenpox. The observation of unilateral vesicular lesions in a dermatomal pattern usually leads to a diagnosis of herpes zoster. Herpes simplex virus infections and coxsackievirus infections, however, also can cause dermatomal vesicular lesions. Laboratory confirmation of VZV infection may be achieved by viral culture from fresh vesicles. Virus may be cultured from zoster vesicles for up to 1 week in uncomplicated disease and for even longer in immunosuppressed patients.

Treatment of primary VZV infection

Chickenpox usually resolves spontaneously with no major sequelae, and treatment is usually supportive. The daily use of a topical antiseptic solution may help prevent secondary bacterial infection. Itching may be relieved by the use of an antihistamine, and calamine lotion may help to dry the lesions. In a prospective, double-blind, placebo-controlled study, Dunkle et al.[14] showed that a 5-day course of oral acyclovir (20 mg/kg four times a day) begun within 24 hours of rash onset resulted in fewer varicella lesions; reduced incidence and duration of fever, anorexia, and lethargy; less itching; accelerated progression to the crusted and healed stages; and fewer residual hypopigmented lesions.

Patients at an increased risk for severe VZV infection include those on immunosuppressive medications, those immunodeficient from prior therapy, and those with congenital or acquired immunodeficiency. All immunocompromised patients are at increased risk for life-threatening VZV infection and should be treated with a systemic antiviral agent.

The use of topical antivirals for the treatment of a dendritic keratitis or conjunctival, limbal, or corneal vesicles is not effective. Topical antibiotics should be used to prevent bacterial superinfection, and cycloplegic agents should be used to relieve ciliary spasm. Patients with moderate eye involvement who are not at increased risk for life-threatening VZV infection should be treated with oral acyclovir, valacyclovir or famciclovir for 5 to 7 days. In those with severe eye involvement, intravenous acyclovir should be considered. Late-onset immune stromal disease should be treated with a slow taper of topical steroids similar to the treatment of HSV stromal keratitis.

Treatment of reactivated VZV

Three antiviral agents, acyclovir, valacyclovir, and famciclovir, are approved for the treatment of herpes zoster. In a prospective, randomized, double-blind, placebo-controlled study, Cobo et al.[12] showed that a 10-day course of oral acyclovir (600 mg five times a day) resulted in earlier resolution of the signs and symptoms of HZO, particularly in patients treated within 72 hours after onset of the skin lesions. Acyclovir treatment was associated with a shortened duration of viral shedding, decreased development of new skin lesions, and decreased incidence of microdissemination to other dermatomes. The incidence and severity of dendritiform keratopathy, stromal keratitis, and anterior uveitis, three of the more common ocular sequelae of HZO, were reduced with oral acyclovir.

Valacyclovir, a prodrug of acyclovir, produces serum acyclovir levels that are three to five times as high as those achieved with oral acyclovir therapy. Valacyclovir (1000 mg every 8 hours for 7 days) and acyclovir were found to result in equivalent rates of cutaneous healing.[15] Valacyclovir was found to significantly shorten the median time to resolution of zoster-associated pain when compared to acyclovir. Famciclovir (500 mg every 8 hours for 7 days), a prodrug of penciclovir, also reduces the duration of viral shedding, limits the duration of new lesion formation, accelerates cutaneous healing, and shortens the duration of zoster-associated pain.[16]

Immunosuppressed patients and children are at an increased risk for virus dissemination, resulting in increased morbidity and mortality. Treatment with intravenous acyclovir decreases the morbidity associated with viral dissemination.

There is currently no evidence that VZV is clinically responsive to any topical antiviral medication commercially available in the United States. Topical corticosteroids are useful in treating an immune-related keratitis, endothelitiis, or iritis.

The use of systemic corticosteroids in acute HZO is controversial. In two large studies, patients receiving corticosteroids in combination with acyclovir were found to have a more rapid rate of cutaneous healing and alleviation of acute pain, but there was no effect on the incidence or duration of postherpetic neuralgia.[17,18] Because of the risk of disseminated disease and possible side effects, the use of systemic corticosteroids should probably be limited to those nonimmunocompromised patients suffering from vasculitic complications of HZO, including scleritis, episcleritis, corneal immune disease, and uveitis.[19,20] For acute pain in herpes zoster, narcotic and non-narcotic analgesia should be used.

Molluscum contagiosum

Molluscum contagiosum is caused by a virus from the Poxviridae family. Humans are the only known host. Transmission of the virus is by direct contact or through fomites. The incidence is usually greatest in children and young adults. Outbreaks have been reported at swimming pools, saunas, and gymnasiums.[21] Molluscum infection is more common in developing countries and in communities with poor hygiene. In some developing nations, as many as 4.5% of children younger than 10 years of age show evidence of infection with molluscum.[22] In children, lesions are predominantly on the face, head, trunk, and extremities. In young adults, spread occurs primarily through sexual contact with lesions predominantly affecting the genitalia, lower abdomen, and upper thighs.[23]

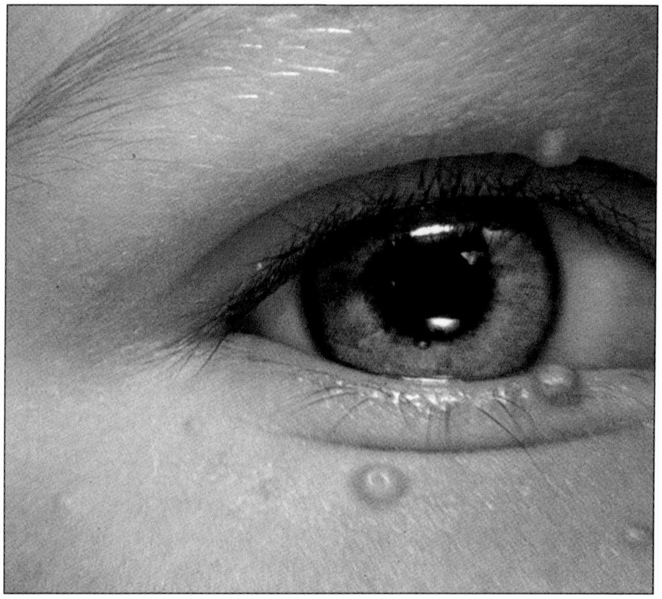

Fig. 35.3 Molluscum contagiosum lesions.

A typical molluscum lesion begins as a small, round, firm, noninflamed papule. The virus replicates in the epithelial cells as the lesion grows to 3–5 mm in diameter. Ultimately, cellular destruction occurs, resulting in central umbilication of the lesion. The lesion then typically appears pearly white, with caseous material in a centrally depressed area (Fig. 35.3).

When molluscum lesions are located in close proximity to the lid margin, virus-laden debris from the center of the lesion may spread into the tear film and conjunctival sac. This spread may result in a secondary follicular conjunctivitis and punctate keratitis with possible subepithelial stromal infiltration and pannus.[24] Secondary corneal ulceration has also been described.[25] Primary molluscum lesions of the conjunctiva and cornea are rare but have also been described.[26–28]

Defects in cell-mediated immunity predispose patients to opportunistic infections including molluscum contagiosum. Disseminated molluscum contagiosum has occurred in patients with defects in cell-mediated immunity. Lesions are usually with more rapid onset, more confluent, increased in number and size, and more likely to be resistant to conventional therapy.[29–34] Recurrences usually appear 6 to 8 weeks after removal of the lesions.

In immunocompetent hosts, molluscum contagiosum is self-limiting with spontaneous resolution in 3 to 12 months.[35,36] There is no effective antiviral treatment for molluscum. Numerous therapies have been described, including excision,[37] incision and curettage,[38] cryotherapy,[38–40] 0.9% cantharidin,[38] electrodessication,[41] and the application of chemical caustics such as liquefied phenol, silver nitrate, and trichloroacetic acid.[37] No method is without complications.

Excision of multiple lid lesions may cause severe scarring. Cryotherapy may result in scarring, depigmentation, and loss of cilia. The use of caustic chemicals to the eyelid can cause accidental corneal scarring. Cases not associated with conjunctivitis or keratitis may be observed for spontaneous regression. Cases associated with chronic conjunctivitis and/or keratitis may result in progressive corneal vascularization and scarring. These cases should be treated. Once the skin lesions are eradicated, the conjunctivitis and/or keratitis usually resolve.

Verruca vulgaris

The human papillomavirus (HPV) causes verruca vulgaris, a hyperkeratotic cutaneous lesion known as the common cutaneous wart. HPV type 16 may be important in the pathogenesis of malignant squamous neoplasms of the conjunctiva, cornea, and eyelid. HPV plays a role in the pathogenesis of proliferative squamous lesions of the male and female genital tracts, particularly the uterine cervix.

Transmission of HPV is usually by direct contact or fomites. Involvement may include the skin of the eyelid, the lid margin, or the conjunctiva. Eyelid skin lesions are usually elevated and irregular with undulating surfaces. They consist of fingerlike projections of papillary dermis covered with epidermis. They may be sessile or pedunculated, and they may be the same color as the adjacent skin, slightly erythematous, or pigmented. Lesions are usually painless, keratinized, and papillomatous. They must be differentiated from actinic keratosis, seborrheic keratosis, basal cell epithelioma, keratoacanthoma, and squamous cell carcinoma.

If lesions are located on the lid margin, virus particles may be shed into the tear film. This shedding may result in the presence of a secondary, subacute papillary conjunctivitis. These patients often experience foreign body sensation and photophobia. A punctate epithelial keratopathy also may occur with or without a conjunctivitis. If untreated, chronic inflammation may lead to the development of peripheral corneal neovascularization.

When viral papillomas occur on the conjunctiva, the most common location is the caruncular region. Conjunctival verrucae also occur at the lid margin, the limbus, and on the bulbar conjunctiva, most commonly in the inferior fornix. Like verrucae involving the skin, they may be sessile or pedunculated. The fibrovascular cores within the fingerlike processes are responsible for the fleshy red strawberry-like appearance. The diagnosis of verruca vulgaris is confirmed by excisional biopsy.

Treatment

Most cases of viral papilloma are self-limiting, and attempted removal may result in recurrence and spread, which is usually more resistant to treatment. If lesions are asymptomatic, observation is recommended. When excision is mandatory, excisional biopsy is the preferred treatment.

Bacterial Infections

Bacterial infections of the eyelid represent a heterogeneous group of disorders ranging from innocuous, self-limiting lesions to life-threatening infections. The infection may be limited to the eyelid or be a local manifestation of a diffuse cutaneous or multisystemic infection.

Hordeolum

A hordeolum is an acute, painful, suppurative, nodular inflammatory lesion of the eyelid. External hordeolum occurs on the anterior eyelid, arising in the glands of Zeis, Moll, or hair follicles, and is usually associated with staphylococcal infection. Internal hordeolum usually occurs on the posterior eyelid, arising from the meibomian glands and can be due to staphylococcal infection or sterile acute inflammation from obstructed meibomian gland orifices. Hordeolum is often associated with blepharitis and can be multiple and recurrent. *Staphylococcus aureus* bacteremia with secondary foci has been associated with hordeolum.[42] Hordeolum usually resolves or ruptures spontaneously with the use of warm compresses. Topical antibiotics are often prescribed. However, they probably offer little benefit. Oral antibiotics are used in cases of eyelid cellulitis. Incision and drainage are reserved for persistent, large, internally bothersome pointing lesions.[43] Treatment of the associated blepharitis may decrease the recurrence rate.

Preseptal cellulitis

Preseptal cellulitis is an infection of the soft tissues of the eyelid located anterior to the orbital septum that extends from the orbital margin to the tarsal plate. Hyperemia and induration are present without the signs of orbital congestion: severe pain, proptosis, and limitation of ocular motility. The major risk factors for preseptal cellulitis are direct inoculation from trauma, extension from infection of the upper respiratory tract and middle ear, and spread from facial skin infections such as impetigo and erysipelas.[44] Preseptal cellulitis is more common in children and young adults during winter.[45]

Post-traumatic suppurative preseptal cellulitis

Post-traumatic preseptal cellulitis occurs after puncture wounds, lacerations, or blunt trauma to the orbital area. The main pathogens are *S. aureus* and *Streptococcus pyogenes*. Human bite injuries are associated with infections by anaerobic pathogens such as *Peptococcus*, *Peptostreptococcus*, and *Bacteroides*, which can produce foul-smelling suppurative discharge, necrotic tissue, and subcutaneous emphysema.[44] Management of traumatic preseptal cellulitis initially involves the exclusion of ocular orbital involvement by careful clinical examination. Computed tomography should be performed if the globe cannot be adequately assessed clinically or penetration of the orbital septum is suspected.[45] However, a subperiosteal abscess can be present with no signs of orbital congestion.[46] Tetanus prophylaxis should be administered according to the Centers for Disease Control (CDC) guidelines.[47] Incision and drainage of an abscess is performed at the site of maximal fluctuance and, if possible, along a skin crease. Smears and cultures are taken of the purulent drainage. Blood cultures should be obtained if the patient is febrile. The wound should then be irrigated and packed with a Penrose drain. The preferred initial therapy for Gram-positive infections is intravenous nafcillin; vancomycin can be used for patients with penicillin allergy. Penicillin G or cefuroxime should be added for anaerobic coverage after bite injuries. Oral cloxacillin or cefaclor may be sufficient in less severe Gram-positive infections. Antimicrobial therapy is later modified, based on the results of the Gram stain and the bacterial cultures.

Nonsuppurative preseptal cellulitis in children

Preseptal cellulitis in children without trauma or facial infections is almost exclusively due to *Haemophilus influenzae* and *Streptococcus pneumoniae*.[45,48]

The preseptal cellulitis begins with a mild upper respiratory tract infection, tends to occur more commonly on the left side, and is often associated with a red or purplish discoloration of the lids. The children are commonly febrile[48] and have leukocytosis. Mild conjunctival hyperemia or chemosis also may be present. Children should be considered for hospitalization because of the rapid progression to orbital cellulitis and the risk of meningitis. Cultures should be performed on the blood and any purulent material from the infected area.

Cefuroxime is the antibiotic of choice because of its high activity against *H. influenzae*, including beta-lactamase-producing strains and other Gram-positive organisms. It also can penetrate the blood–brain barrier to treat meningitis effectively. Intravenous therapy is continued for 5 to 7 days or until definite clinical improvement is noted. Oral agents such as cefuroxime axetil or amoxicillin–clavulanic acid are then continued for 7 to 10 days.

Erysipelas

Erysipelas (St. Anthony's fire) is a febrile skin infection that presents with the sudden onset of a red, indurated, expanding plaque with a distinct border and marked lymphatic involvement.[43] Group A streptococci, particularly *S. pyogenes*, is the pathogen isolated in the majority of cases;[49] however, other groups of streptococci and *S. aureus* also have been cultured from ulcerative lesions.[50] Predisposing factors in erysipelas patients include smoking, alcohol abuse, and venous insufficiency.[50] Complications of the acute infection include septicemia, abscesses, and necrotizing fasciitis. Lid involvement is uncommon.[51]

Localization of erysipelas to the face occurs in approximately 19% of cases.[50] The eyelid lesion presents with an erythematous swelling, crusting, and discharge that develops into a severe necrotizing lesion with secondary cicatrization and contracture.

Initial management of facial erysipelas, particularly in patients with fever or septicemia, is intravenous penicillin or vancomycin for 48 to 72 hours or until clinical improvement is noted. Oral therapy is continued for an additional 7 to 10 days.[52]

Impetigo contagiosa

Impetigo is the most common skin infection of children. Traditionally, it has been divided into the crusted and the bullous forms.[53] *S. aureus* is the pathogen of bullous impetigo. Nonbullous impetigo is caused by both group A streptococci and *S. aureus*.[54] Most cases occur in children younger than 6 years of age.

Impetigo involves exposed areas of the face or the extremities. Small red macules progress to thin-walled serous vesicles that become pustular and rupture to form characteristic soft, golden-yellow, 'honey' crusted lesions. Removal of the crust reveals a weeping red surface.[43]

The diagnosis is made clinically. Smear and culture of the exudate from the lesions can help direct antimicrobial therapy. Precautions should be taken to avoid transmission of this highly contagious disease.[43] Gentle washing of the involved areas followed by application of topical bacitracin or erythromycin ointment is recommended.[55] Oral antibiotic therapy includes cephalexin, erythromycin, or cloxacillin. Penicillin is ineffective treatment for impetigo caused by *S. aureus*.[54] Topical 2% mupirocin is as effective as oral erythromycin.[56] Because neonates and young children have little immunity to this pathogen, prompt and aggressive treatment may be required.[57]

Rare bacterial infections

Anthrax

Most patients in the United States are wool sorters, tanners, cattlemen, and butchers.[55] The lesion begins with a small, pruritic, reddish macule at the site of inoculation, which evolves into an inflammatory papule, vesicle, and pustule. The lesion eventually ruptures to form a necrotic ulcer covered by a black eschar.

Syphilis

Syphilis is a contagious venereal disease caused by *Treponema pallidum*. There has been a recent increase in the reported rate of syphilis in the United States.[58] Syphilis is still considered one of the most common sexually transmitted diseases in developing countries.[59] Involvement of the eyelid with syphilis is rare but can occur in the primary, secondary, tertiary, and congenital forms of this disease.

Mycobacterial Infections

Leprosy is a chronic, disfiguring, crippling, and blinding disease caused by the obligate intracellular parasite *Mycobacterium leprae*. Leprosy is a tropical disease of developing countries.[60] This organism has affinity to the skin, nerves, and the lymphoreticular system. Neural involvement occurs early in the tuberculoid form of leprosy, whereas skin lesions are more numerous in lepromatous leprosy.

Early ocular findings include supraciliary ridge thickening and loss of eyebrows. Infiltration leads to thickening of the eyelids and the skin folds, tylosis, and madarosis. Chronic facial skin thickening results in the characteristic 'leonine facies.' Lacrimal gland involvement results in keratoconjunctivitis sicca. Fifth cranial nerve involvement results in an anesthetic cornea, and the infection may spread to the terminal branches of the seventh cranial nerve, causing paralysis of the orbicularis oculi.[61] Aggressive ocular lubrication and lid procedures may be required to minimize corneal complications.

Mycobacterium tuberculosis may rarely cause a brown-red, soft papule that evolves into an indurated nodule or plaque that may ulcerate. The diagnosis should be suspected in immunocompromised patients.

The atypical mycobacterium *Mycobacterium fortuitum* has been associated with a granulomatous abscess on the eyelid, which was treated successfully by cryotherapy.[62] Bilateral lid abscesses have developed from *Mycobacterium chelonei* infection after blepharoplasty and ptosis surgery, and these abscesses were treated by multiple incision and drainage procedures with intravenous amikacin and doxycycline.[63] *Mycobacterium intracellulare* has caused a lid granuloma with induration and erythema after chalazion incision and curettage.[64]

Actinomycosis

Actinomyces are Gram-positive anaerobic bacteria previously thought to be fungi because of their branching, filamentous morphology. Periocular infection is most commonly a chronic canaliculitis. Often sulfur granules and white, cheeselike material can be expressed out of the lacrimal punctum using firm pressure applied on both sides of the canaliculus with cotton swabs. The lower canaliculus is most commonly involved and only rarely is there an associated eyelid or orbital abscess or dacryocystitis.[65]

Fungal Infections

Blastomycosis

Blastomyces dermatitidis is a dimorphic fungus that is endemic in the southeastern Midwest of the United States. Farmers and other people with outdoor occupations are most commonly affected. The site of primary infection with blastomycosis is almost always the lung.

Extrapulmonary *B. dermatitidis* infection results from hematogenous spread and is characterized by chronic granulomatous and suppurative disease. The most commonly involved ocular structure is the eyelid skin. Skin involvement can begin as small papulopustular lesions and progress to large verrucous lesions with heaped up, erythematous borders and central weeping or crusts.[66,67] The lesions may resemble a papilloma or squamous cell carcinoma as a result of reactive hyperplasia of the epidermis. Early infection is suppurative with microabscesses, but chronic infection is granulomatous, leading to scarring of the eyelid and ectropion. Extrapulmonary involvement requires systemic therapy. Severe infections should be treated with intravenous amphotericin B. Mild to moderate disease can be treated with oral ketoconazole 400–800 mg/day for up to 6 months. Itraconazole may be used in a dose of 200–400 mg/day.[68]

Coccidiomycosis

Coccidiomycosis is caused by the dimorphic fungus *Coccidioides immitis*, which is a normal saprophytic inhabitant of soil in central California, semiarid regions of the southwestern United States, and areas of Central and South America. Infection follows inhalation of airborne arthroconidia. Pulmonary coccidiomycosis is often asymptomatic and may resolve spontaneously, or there may be a mild respiratory flulike illness after a 10- to 14-day incubation period. This condition is referred to as valley fever or desert fever.[69] Erythema nodosum is noted in up to 25% of women. A hypersensitivity reaction of conjunctivitis, episcleritis, or scleritis can accompany the erythema nodosum. Progressive extrapulmonary disease is rare except in patients who are immunosuppressed. Lesions can be noted subcutaneously in the eyelid or eyebrow, as well as subconjunctivally in the eyelid, and can masquerade as a chalazion or basal cell carcinoma.[70]

The diagnosis of coccidiomycosis should be suspected in patients with the appropriate symptoms living in endemic areas. The diagnosis can be confirmed by skin or antibody testing. Disseminated coccidiomycosis should be treated with intravenous amphotericin B, since death may occur in 50% of cases. Less severe cases may benefit from treatment with fluconazole, ketoconazole, or itraconazole.[71]

Cryptococcosis

Cryptococcosis is most commonly caused by the budding yeast *Cryptococcus neoformans*. Many serotypes of this fungus live as a soil saprophyte worldwide. The infection usually results in a mild self-limiting pulmonary disease, but can lead to hematogenous dissemination and extrapulmonary manifestations in immunocompromised patients. The skin of the scalp and face, including that of the eyelids, is the most common site of cutaneous involvement, resulting in erythematous papules, nodules, acneiform pustules, and subcutaneous nodules that can ulcerate.[72]

The diagnosis can be confirmed by culturing a biopsy of the skin lesion. Detection of cryptococcal antigens by latex agglutination also may be helpful. Treatment of skin lesions, which represent hematogenous spread of disease, requires systemic therapy. Five efficacious therapeutic agents are amphotericin B, flucytosine, fluconazole, itraconazole, and ketoconazole.[73]

Dermatophytosis/tinea palpebrum

Dermatophytosis is an infection of keratinized skin by one of three genera of fungi: *Trichophyton*, *Epidermophyton*, or *Microsporum*.[74] They have worldwide distribution and cause ubiquitous disease known as tinea or ringworm. The incidence of infection increases after puberty, except for tinea capitis, a dermatophytosis of the scalp, which is most common in prepubertal children. Infection occurs in immunocompetent people, but can be florid in immunocompromised individuals.[75]

Dermatophytosis is caused by superficial invasion of keratinized tissue, causing an erythematous papule that enlarges to form a red, circular, scaly, pruritic patch that often has a raised border. The center of the lesion clears spontaneously, leaving the classic 'ringworm' pattern. Tinea can involve any keratinized body surface. Eyelid involvement usually results from extension from massive involvement of the scalp. Periocular infection can result in loss of eyebrow hair and eyelashes, marginal blepharitis, and eyelid ulceration. Because the conjunctiva is not keratinized, it is not involved as an infectious conjunctivitis but can develop an allergic reaction to the dermatophytosis.[76] Diagnosis is usually suspected by the clinical presentation and is confirmed by microscopic examination of specimens prepared with 10% potassium hydroxide, but requires culture for confirmation. Treatment of mild infections is with administration of clotrimazole, miconazole, or ketoconazole twice a day for 1 week. Advanced tinea infections require systemic therapy with ketoconazole, fluconazole, itraconazole, or griseofulvin.[77]

Sporotrichosis

Sporotrichosis is caused by the dimorphic fungus *Sporothrix schenckii*, which typically lives on vegetation. The fungus is found worldwide and especially in Central and South America. Primary cutaneous infection is most common and is caused by direct inoculation of the fungus in soil or plant matter through the skin, classically by a rose thorn. Primary cutaneous infection may result in lymphocutaneous spread characterized by subcutaneous nodules along lymphatics to draining lymph nodes.[78]

Eyelid involvement usually occurs from primary inoculation of the eyelid skin, which results in a firm, painless, subcutaneous nodule or pustule that can ulcerate. It may spread in the lymphocutaneous pattern and cause lymph node enlargement and lymphatic spread, with additional nodules forming along the paths of lymphatic drainage. Sporotrichosis also can cause a granulomatous conjunctivitis with preauricular lymph node swelling (Parinaud's oculoglandular syndrome), scleritis, keratitis, and rarely intraocular infection. Sporotrichosis also has been associated with canaliculitis or dacryocystitis with or without a cutaneous fistula. Orbital invasion resembling mucormycosis was reported in a patient with diabetes.[79]

Lymphocutaneous sporotrichosis usually can be diagnosed by its clinical presentation. The diagnosis can be confirmed by immunofluorescence or by culture of the lesions. Treatment is with oral saturated potassium iodide solution for at least 1 month. If infection persists, treatment with oral itraconazole, fluconazole, or intravenous amphotericin B may be necessary.

Mucormycosis

Mucormycosis is a rare, but serious fungal infection of the orbit caused by the fungus *Mucorales*. This infection can be found in patients who are immunocompromised secondary to immunosuppressive medications or hematologic malignancies, but most commonly occurs in diabetic patients with ketoacidosis. The rhino-orbital-cerebral (ROCM) form of infection is the most common.

Parasitic Eyelid Infections

Demodicosis

Demodicosis is caused by infestation of the pilosebaceous units of the eyelid by one of two different species of mites belonging to the class Arachnida or Acarina. *Demodex folliculorum* is a slightly longer mite and is found burrowed in lash and hair follicles. It punctures and consumes epithelial cells and causes a reactive hyperkeratosis that results in the classic clinical finding of semitransparent sleeves around lashes that are composed of keratin and lipid material. *Demodex* is nearly ubiquitous in adults. Roth[80] found 84% of 100 consecutive eyelid biopsies to have lash follicle infestation with *D. folliculorum*. One hundred percent of biopsies from patients 70 years or older were infested.

Despite the near ubiquitous finding of these mites in hair follicles and sebaceous glands, their exact role in the pathogenesis of blepharitis is unclear. The only histopathologic changes noted in association with *Demodex* are hair follicle distention, hyperkeratosis, and occasional mild perifolliculitis.[80] Particularly heavy infiltration has been thought to alter and decrease the lipid component of the tear film sufficiently to cause destabilization of the tear film. Symptoms attributed to heavy mite infestation are burning, itching, crusting, and loss of lashes. Episodic pruritus may be related to the increased activity of the female mite during egg laying.[80–83] The mites can be seen with high-power slit lamp examination of the base of the eyelash follicles. Diagnosis can be confirmed by observing the semitransparent sleeves around lashes or by direct observation of the mites on epilated lashes by light microscopy.[84]

Treatment consists of a rigorous cleaning of the lashes followed by nightly application of sulfacetamide or neomycin/polymyxin B/bacitracin ophthalmic ointment for several weeks. Antibiotic therapy has no effect on mites in the pilosebaceous units, but it does reduce their migration between follicles.

Phthiriasis/pediculosis

Phthiriasis is an infestation by the pubic louse or pubic crab, *Phthirus pubis* (Fig. 35.4). *P. pubis* is a small louse (1–2 mm) with a broad, oval abdomen and stout, clawlike legs, which are adapted for grasping hair and sucking blood.[85] This louse is sedentary and prefers to infest sites where the distance between adjacent hairs is similar to its grasping span. This

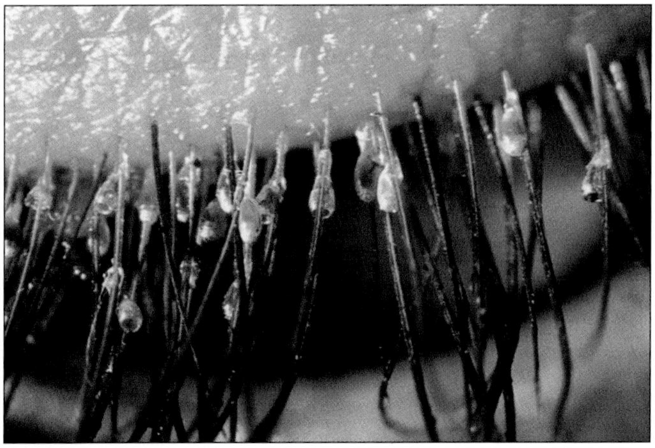

Fig. 35.4 *Phthirus pubis* infestation of eyelashes demonstrating nits on shafts of lashes and pubic lice feces at lash bases.

is most commonly the pubic and inguinal region, but the chest, axilla, beard, eyelashes, and eyebrows also can be infested. Adult, person-to-person contact resulting in infection is usually sexual. Infants can be infested by close contact with chest or axillary hairs of parents.[86] Head-to-head transmission in children has been proposed.[87] Consideration must be given to whether phthiriasis in a child may be due to sexual abuse. Spread of the louse from the genital region to the eyelashes and eyebrows is thought to be caused by manual transmission.

Pediculosis refers to infestation with either *Pediculus humanus corporis* or *capitis*, which are body or head lice, respectively. Body and head lice are similar morphologically and interbreed freely. *Pediculus* organisms are larger (2–4 mm) and have longer legs that afford greater mobility. This allows the louse to move between feedings. Person-to-person transmission is associated with close contact with an infested person or through contact with contaminated bedding or clothing. Both types of lice are often associated with poor personal hygiene and overcrowded conditions.

P. pubis is by far the most common louse to infest the periocular region. The most common symptom of infestation is intense pruritus associated with the injection of louse saliva into the skin during feeding. The associated blepharitis and conjunctivitis can be severe and occasionally associated with preauricular lymphadenopathy. Phthiriasis causes follicular conjunctivitis, and a high index of suspicion is needed to make a prompt diagnosis of this condition. A case of marginal keratitis also has been caused by phthiriasis.[88] The classic sign of phthiriasis is the blue bite marks, maculae caeruleae. Lice may be difficult to see with the unaided eye. However, with careful slit lamp examination the accumulation of nits on the shafts of the lashes and of the reddish-brown feces at the bases of the lashes may be seen (see Fig. 35.4). The transparent lice can be seen near the base of the lashes, and their transparent body can be recognized more easily by following the central reddish dot or line of blood in their body.

Any treatment of phthiriasis or pediculosis is directed at eradicating not only the nymphs and mature lice but also the nits that will hatch over the next 7 to 10 days. Nits are resistant to many therapies that are lethal to the more mature forms. The first line of therapy in mild cases is mechanical removal of adult lice and nits, which may require epilating the involved lashes. Removal of the involved lashes results in immediate removal of both the louse and any ready-to-hatch eggs, as well as destroying hairshaft habitat essential for louse survival and reproduction.[89]

Topical white petrolatum applied twice a day to the lids for 10 days smothers the adult lice and emerging nits. One percent yellow mercuric oxide and 3% ammoniated mercury ophthalmic ointments are effective when used twice per day for 1 week.

A 1% permethrin cream rinse is effective against both pediculosis and phthiriasis. It is not specifically recommended for use around the eyes, but holds some promise as an agent that does not cause ocular irritation.[90] A-200 Pyrinate (pyrethrin ointment) is available without prescription, but should not be used near the eye because it is toxic to the corneal epithelium and has been associated with secondary ulceration and necrosis.[91]

Gamma-benzene hexachloride (Lindane) 1% shampoo is effective in a single application to the head and body and can be repeated, if necessary, after 7 days to treat emerging nits. This agent should not be used near the eyes because of potential ocular irritation and should not be used in infants, children, or pregnant women because of potential central nervous system toxicity from absorption through the skin.

Infected patients must be examined for all sites of infestation. Sexual partners, family members, and close contacts also should be examined. Clothing, linens, and grooming instruments must be sterilized by heating them to 50°C; this is accomplished by washing or drying them at the highest temperature settings of most clothes washers and dryers for 30 minutes. Any cosmetics used around the eyes should be discarded.

Onchocerciasis

Onchocerciasis is an infection with the nematode *Onchocerca volvulus*. Humans are the definitive host, and human-to-human transmission is accomplished by small black flies of the *Simulium* genus. There are endemic foci of disease in Central Africa and Central and South America. These areas are often associated with fast-moving streams and rivers, which are the breeding ground of the black flies; hence the name river blindness. The tiny black flies ingest microfilariae when they bite an infected person. In the fly, the filariae develop into infective larvae and may be introduced into other humans bitten by the fly. Once in the human host, the larvae require 1 year to mature, mate, and produce microfilariae that migrate subcutaneously to other sites. Adult worms found in onchocercomas can live as long as 15 years.

Infection is most often characterized by subcutaneous nodules of adult worms (onchocercomas) that are most commonly found over bony prominences of the extremities and in the scalp. The eyelids and periorbital skin can be involved with the onchocercomas. Microfilariae migrate into the cornea where they induce a massive inflammatory reaction, which leads to progressive corneal scarring and severe anterior uveitis causing photophobia and epiphora. Diagnosis is usually made by identifying microfilaria in skin biopsies, urine, or anterior chamber using biomicroscopy.[92] Ivermectin is the drug of choice for treating onchocerciasis. It kills the microfilariae in the body over a 3-month period, does not result in a massive inflammatory reaction that may further damage the eye, and has been associated with more abrupt microfilaricidal activity.[93–96]

References

1. Darougar S, Wishart MS, Viswalingam ND. Epidemiological and clinical features of primary herpes simplex virus ocular infection. *Br J Ophthalmol.* 1985;69:2–6.
2. Egerer I, Stary A. Erosive-ulcerative herpes simplex blepharitis. *Arch Ophthalmol.* 1980;98:1760.
3. Nahmias AJ, Roizman B. Infection with herpes-simplex virus 1 and 2. *N Engl J Med.* 1973;289:667–674, 719–725, 781–789.
4. Nahmias AJ, Alford CA, Korones SB. Infection of the newborn with herpesvirus hominis. *Adv Pediatr.* 1970;17:185–227.
5. Griffin WP, Searle CWA. Ocular manifestations of varicella. *Lancet.* 1953;2:168.
6. Edwards T. Ophthalmic complications from varicella. *J Pediatr Ophthalmol Strabismus.* 1965;2:37–40.

7. Nesburn AB, et al. Varicella dendritic keratitis. *Invest Ophthalmol Vis Sci.* 1974;13:764–770.
8. DeFreitas D, et al. Delayed onset varicella keratitis. *Cornea.* 1992;11:471–474.
9. Strachman J. Uveitis associated with chicken pox. *J Pediatr.* 1955;46:327.
10. Weller TH. Varicella and herpes zoster. Changing concepts of the natural history, control, and importance of a not-so-benign virus (part 1). *N Engl J Med.* 1983;309:1362.
11. Weller TH. Varicella and herpes zoster (part 2). *N Engl J Med.* 1983;309:1434.
12. Cobo LM, et al. Oral acyclovir in the treatment of acute herpes zoster ophthalmicus. *Ophthalmology.* 1986;93:763–770.
13. Scheie HG. Herpes zoster ophthalmicus. *Trans Ophthalmol Soc UK.* 1970;90:899.
14. Dunkle LM, et al. A controlled trial of acyclovir for chickenpox in normal children. *N Engl J Med.* 1991;325:1539–1544.
15. Beutner KR, Friedman DJ, Forszpaniak C, et al. Valaciclovir compared with acyclovir for improved therapy for herpes zoster in immunocompetent adults. *Antimicrob Agents Chemother.* 1995;39:1546–1553.
16. Tyring S, Barbarash RA, Nahlik JE, et al. Famciclovir for the treatment of acute herpes zoster: effects on acute disease and postherpetic neuralgia: a randomized, double-blind, placebo-controlled trial. *Ann Intern Med.* 1995;123:89–96.
17. Wood MJ, Johnson RW, McKendrick MW, et al. A randomized trial of acyclovir for 7 days and 21 days with and without prednisolone for treatment of acute herpes zoster. *N Engl J Med.* 1994;330:896–900.
18. Whitley RJ, Weiss H, Gnann JW, et al. Acyclovir with and without prednisone for the treatment of herpes zoster: a randomized sample, placebo-controlled trial. *Ann Intern Med.* 1996;125:376–383.
19. Liesegang TJ, et al. Diagnosis and therapy of herpes zoster ophthalmicus. *Ophthalmology.* 1991;98:1216–1229.
20. Merselis JG, Kaye D, Hook EW. Disseminated herpes zoster: a report of 17 cases. *Arch Intern Med.* 1964;113:679–686.
21. Low RC. Molluscum contagiosum. *Edinb Med J.* 1946;53:657–670.
22. Postlethwaite R. Molluscum contagiosum: a review. *Arch Environ Health.* 1970;21:432–452.
23. Becker TM, et al. Trends in molluscum contagiosum in the United States, 1966–1983. *Sex Transm Dis.* 1986;13:88–92.
24. Mathur SP. Ocular complications in molluscum contagiosum. *Br J Ophthalmol.* 1960;44:572–573.
25. Duke-Elder S. *System of ophthalmology. Vol. XIII: The ocular adnexa. Pt. I: diseases of the eyelid.* London: Henry Kimpton; 1974.
26. Sysi R. Molluscum contagiosum corneae. *Acta Ophthalmol (Copenh).* 1941;19:25–27.
27. Quill TH. Molluscum contagiosum of eyelid and cornea: report of a case. *Proc Staff Meet Mayo Clin.* 1940;15:139–142.
28. Redslob E. Molluscum contagiosum a localisation exceptionelle. *Bull Soc Ophthalmol Paris.* 1927;30:315–317.
29. Lombardo PC. Molluscum contagiosum and the acquired immunodeficiency syndrome (letter). *Arch Dermatol.* 1985;121:834–835.
30. Leahey AB, Shane JJ, Listhaus A, et al. Molluscum contagiosum eyelid lesions as the initial manifestation of acquired immunodeficiency syndrome. *Am J Ophthalmol.* 1997;124:240–241.
31. Biswas J, Therese L, Kumarasamy N, et al. Lid abscess with extensive molluscum contagiosum in a patient with acquired immunodeficiency syndrome. *Indian J Ophthalmol.* 1997;45:234–236.
32. Katzman M, Elmets CA, Lederman MM. Molluscum contagiosum and the acquired immunodeficiency syndrome (letter). *Ann Intern Med.* 1985;102:413–414.
33. Sarma DP, Weilbaecher TG. Molluscum contagiosum in the acquired immunodeficiency syndrome (letter). *J Am Acad Dermatol.* 1985;13: 682–683.
34. Kohn SR. Molluscum contagiosum in patients with acquired immunodeficiency syndrome (letter). *Arch Ophthalmol.* 1987;105:458.
35. Duke-Elder S. *System of ophthalmology. Vol. XIII: The ocular adnexa. Pt. I: diseases of the eyelid.* London: Henry Kimpton; 1974.
36. Lever WF, Schaumburg-Lever G. *Histopathology of the skin.* 6th ed. New York: JB Lippincott; 1983.
37. Groden LR, Arentsen JJ. Molluscum contagiosum. In: Fraunfelder FT, Roy FH, Meyer SM, eds. *Current ocular therapy.* 2nd ed. Philadelphia: WB Saunders; 1985.
38. DeLuise VP. Viral conjunctivitis. In: Tabbara KF, Hyndiuk RA, eds. *Infections of the eye.* 2nd ed. Boston/Toronto: Little Brown; 1986.
39. Bardenstein DS, Elmets C. Hyperfocal cryotherapy of multiple molluscum contagiosum lesions in patients with the acquired immune deficiency syndrome. *Ophthalmology.* 1995;102:1031–1034.
40. Luxenberg MN. Molluscum contagiosum. *Arch Ophthalmol.* 1986;104:1390.
41. Ginsburg CM. Management of selected skin and soft tissue infections. *Pediatr Infect Dis J.* 1986;5:735–740.
42. Zimmerman RK. *Staphylococcus aureus* hordeolum as a cause of bacteremia and secondary foci. *J Fam Pract.* 1989;29:433–435.
43. Matoba AY. Acute bacterial infections of the eyelids and tarsal plate. *Ophthalmol Clin North Am.* 1992;5:169–176.
44. Jones DB, Steinkuller PG. Strategies for the initial management of acute preseptal and orbital cellulitis. *Trans Am Ophthalmol Soc.* 1988;86:94–112.
45. Jones DB, Steinkuller PG. Microbial preseptal and orbital cellulitis. In: Tasman W, Jaeger EA, eds. *Duane's clinical ophthalmology.* Vol 4. Philadelphia: JB Lippincott; 1993.
46. Rubin SE, Slavin ML, Rubin LG. Eyelid swelling and erythema as the only signs of subperiosteal abscess. *Br J Ophthalmol.* 1989;73:576–578.
47. ACIP. Tetanus–United States, 1987 and 1988. *MMWR.* 1990;39:37–41.
48. Israele V, Nelson JD. Periorbital and orbital cellulitis. *Pediatr Infect Dis J.* 1987;6:404–410.
49. Bernard P, et al. Streptococcal cause of erysipelas and cellulitis in adults. A microbiologic study using a direct immunofluorescence technique. *Arch Ophthalmol.* 1989;125:779–782.
50. Jorup-Ronstrom C. Epidemiological, bacteriological and complicating features of erysipelas. *Scand J Infect Dis.* 1986;18:519–524.
51. McHugh D, Fison PN. Ocular erysipelas. *Arch Ophthalmol.* 1992;110:1315.
52. Ochs MW, Dolwick MF. Facial erysipelas: report of a case and review of the literature. *J Oral Maxillofac Surg.* 1991;49:1116–1120.
53. Tunnessen WW Jr. Practical aspects of bacterial infections in children. *Pediatr Dermatol.* 1985;2:255–265.
54. Demidovich CW, et al. Impetigo. Current etiology and comparison of penicillin, erythromycin, and cephalexin therapies. *Am J Dis Child.* 1990;144:1313–1315.
55. Glover AT. Eyelid infections. In: Albert DM, Jakobiec FA, eds. *Principles and practice of ophthalmology.* Vol 3. Philadelphia: WB Saunders; 1994.
56. McLinn S. A bacteriologically controlled, randomized study comparing the efficacy of 2% mupirocin ointment (Bactroban) with erythromycin in the treatment of patients with impetigo. *J Am Acad Dermatol.* 1990;22(5 Pt 1):883–885.
57. Wooldridge WE. Managing skin infections in children. *Postgrad Med.* 1991;89:109–112.
58. Margo CE, Hamed LM. Ocular syphilis. *Surv Ophthalmol.* 1992;37: 203–220.
59. Jegakumar W, Chithra A, Shanmugasundararaj A. Primary syphilis of the eyelid, case report. *Genitourin Med.* 1989;3:192–193.
60. Scwab IR. Ocular leprosy. In: Tabbara KF, Hyndiuk RA, eds. *Infections of the eye.* Boston: Little Brown; 1986.
61. Dastur DK. Pathology and pathogenesis of predilective sites of nerve damage in leprous neuritis. Nerves in the arm and face. *Neurosurg Rev.* 1983;6:139–152.
62. Katowitz JA, Kropp TM. *Mycobacterium fortuitum* as a cause for nasolacrimal obstruction and granulomatous eyelid disease. *Ophthalmic Surg.* 1987;18:97–99.
63. Kevitch R, Guyuron B. Mycobacterial infection following blepharoplasty. *Aesthetic Plast Surg.* 1991;15:229–232.
64. Warman ST, Klein RS. Preseptal cellulitis caused by *Mycobacterium intracellulare. Ophthalmology.* 1982;89:499–501.
65. Blanksma LJ, Slijper J. Actinomycotic dacryocystitis. *Ophthalmologica.* 1978;176:145–149.
66. Barr CC, Gamel JW. Blastomycosis of the eyelid. *Arch Ophthalmol.* 1986;104:96–97.
67. Slack JW, Hyndiuk RA, Harris GJ, Simons KB. Blastomycosis of the eyelid and conjunctiva. *Ophthalmol Plast Reconstr Surg.* 1992;8:143–149.
68. Sarosi GA, Davies SF. Blastomycosis. In: Hoeprich PD, Jordan MC, Ronald AR, eds. *Infectious diseases: a treatise of infectious processes.* Philadelphia: JB Lippincott; 1994.
69. Rodenbiker HT, Ganley JP. Ocular coccidioidomycosis. *Surv Ophthalmol.* 1980;24:263–290.
70. Irvine AR Jr. Coccidioidal granuloma of lid. *Trans Am Acad Ophthalmol Otolaryngol.* 1968;72:751–754.
71. Hoeprich PD. Coccidioidomycosis. In: Hoeprich PD, Jordan MC, Ronald AR, eds. *Infectious diseases: a treatise of infectious processes.* Philadelphia: JB Lippincott; 1994.
72. Glover AT. Eyelid infections. In: Albert DM, Jakobiec FA, eds. *Principles and practice of ophthalmology: clinical practice.* Vol 3. Philadelphia: WB Saunders; 1994.
73. Hoeprich PD. Cryptococcosis. In: Hoeprich PD, Jordan MC, Ronald AR, eds. *Infectious diseases: a treatise of infectious processes.* Philadelphia: JB Lippincott; 1994.
74. Rebell G, Taplin D. *Dermatophytes: their recognition and identification.* Coral Gables. Florida: University of Miami Press; 1970.
75. Blumenkranz MS, Penneys NS. Acquired immunodeficiency syndrome and the eye. *Dermatol Clin.* 1992;10:777–783.

76. Ostler HB, Okumoto M, Halde C. Dermatophytosis affecting the periorbital region. *Am J Ophthalmol.* 1971;72:934–938.
77. Elewski BE, Nagashima-Whalen L. Superficial fungal infections of the skin. In: Hoeprich PD, Jordan MC, Ronald AR, eds. *Infectious diseases: a treatise of infectious processes.* Philadelphia: JB Lippincott; 1994.
78. Bullpitt P, Weedon D. Sporotrichosis: a review of 39 cases. *Pathology.* 1978;10:249.
79. Agger WA, Caplan RH, Maki DG. Ocular sporotrichosis mimicking mucormycosis in a diabetic. *Ann Ophthalmol.* 1978;10:767–771.
80. Roth AM. *Demodex folliculorum* in hair follicles of eyelid skin. *Ann Ophthalmol.* 1979;11:37–40.
81. English FP, Nutting WB, Cohn D. Demodedectic infestation of the meibomian glands. *Am J Ophthalmol.* 1983;95:261–262.
82. English FP, Cohn D. *Demodex* infestation of the sebaceous gland. *Am J Ophthalmol.* 1983;95:843–844.
83. English FP, Cohn D, Groeveneveld ER. Demodectic mites and chalazion. *Am J Ophthalmol.* 1985;100:482–483.
84. Coston TO. *Demodex folliculorum* blepharitis. *Trans Am Ophthalmol Soc.* 1967;65:361–392.
85. Couch JM, Green WR, Hirst LW, de la Cruz ZC. Diagnosing and treating phthiris pubis palpebrarum. *Surv Ophthalmol.* 1982;26:219–225.
86. Ronchese F. Treatment of pediculosis ciliorum in an infant. *N Engl J Med.* 1953;249:897–898.
87. Buxton PA. *The louse: an account of the lice which infest man. Their medical importance and control.* London: Arnold; 1947.
88. Ittyerah TP, Fernandez ST, Kutty KN. Marginal keratitis produced by *Phthiris pubis. Ind J Ophthalmol.* 1976;24:21–22.
89. Mansour AM. Phthiriasis palpebrarum. *Arch Ophthalmol.* 2000;118:1458.
90. Kincaid MC. Pediculosis and phthiriasis. In: Fraunfelder FT, Roy FH, eds. *Current ocular therapy.* 4th ed. Philadelphia: WB Saunders; 1995.
91. Péer J, Benezra D. Corneal damage following the use of the pediculocide A-200 Pyrinate. *Arch Ophthalmol.* 1988;106:16–17.
92. Gibson DW, Heggie C, Connor DH. Clinical and pathologic aspects of onchocerciasis. *Pathol Annu.* 1980;15:195–240.
93. Orihel TC. Cutaneous filariasis and dracontiasis. In: Hoeprich PD, Jordan MC, Ronald AR, eds. *Infectious diseases: a treatise of infectious processes.* Philadelphia: JB Lippincott; 1994.
94. Barnett JM, Wolter JR. *Loa loa:* the African eye worm observed in Michigan. *J Pediatr Ophthalmol.* 1971;8:23–25.
95. Farrer WE, Wittner M, Tanowitz HB. African eye worm (*Loa loa*) in a tourist. *Ann Ophthalmol.* 1981;13:1177–1179.
96. Dadzie KY, Bird AC, Awadzi K, et al. Ocular findings in a double-blind study of ivermectin versus diethylcarbamazine versus placebo in the treatment of onchocerciasis. *Br J Ophthalmol.* 1987;71:78–85.

Chapter 36

Dry Eye

Nariman Nassiri, Ali R. Djalilian, Pedram Hamrah, Stephen C. Pflugfelder

Definition

Dry eye disease (DED), or keratoconjunctivitis sicca (KCS), is one of the most common ophthalmologic conditions. According to the International Dry Eye WorkShop (DEWS) in 2007,[1] dry eye is defined as a *multifactorial disease of the tears and ocular surface that results in symptoms of discomfort, visual disturbance, and tear film instability with potential damage to the ocular surface*. It is accompanied by increased osmolarity of the tear film and inflammation of the ocular surface. According to epidemiologic studies in the US, the prevalence of clinically diagnosed DED is 0.4–0.5% overall,[2] and is highest among women and the elderly.[2,3] Tens of millions more have less severe symptoms and probably a more episodic manifestation of the disease that is notable only during adverse contributing conditions, such as low humidity or contact lens wear. Thus, DED is considered a significant public health problem[4] which will have a considerable economic impact in terms of both direct and indirect costs.[2,3]

Lacrimal Functional Unit: Anatomy and Physiology

The lacrimal functional unit (LFU) is an integrated system that comprises the ocular surface (cornea, conjunctiva, accessory lacrimal and meibomian glands), the main lacrimal glands, the blink mechanism that spreads tears, and the sensory and motor nerves that connect them whose parts act together and not in isolation.[5] According to this model, aqueous tear production by the lacrimal gland is largely due to a reflex initiated by subconscious stimulation of the ocular surface[6] and nasal mucosa.[7] This stimulation initiates a sensory afferent signal from conjunctiva and cornea that travels via the trigeminal nerve to the central nervous system in the superior salivary nucleus in the pons area, from whence efferent parasympathetic fibers in the facial nerve pass, in the nervus intermedius, to the pterygopalatine ganglion. Here, postganglionic parasympathetic fibers arise and terminate in the main and accessory lacrimal glands, conjunctival goblet cells, and meibomian glands, where they will secrete tears in response to the efferent signal. Another neural pathway controls the blink reflex, via trigeminal afferents and the somatic efferent fibers of the seventh cranial nerve. Higher centers feed into the brainstem nuclei, and there is a rich sympathetic (paraspinal chain) supply to the epithelia and vasculature of the glands and ocular surface. This entire functional unit controls the major components of the tear film in a regulated fashion and responds to environmental, endocrinologic, and cortical influences. Its overall function is to preserve the integrity of the tear film, the transparency of the cornea, and the quality of the image projected onto the retina.[5,8]

Classically, the tear film was considered to have three major layers, mucous, aqueous, and lipid,[9] but this concept has been substantially revised. The contemporary concept of the tear–ocular surface structure is that of a metastable tear film consisting of an aqueous gel with a gradient of mucin content decreasing from the ocular surface to the undersurface of the outermost lipid layer. The latter structure interacts with the underlying aqueous and mucin components, retarding evaporative loss of aqueous tears and contributing to the stability of the tear film between blinks.[10,11] The normal physiology of the tear film is described in more detail in Chapter 3.

Pathophysiology

Maintaining a healthy and comfortable ocular surface requires stability and renewal of the preocular tear film. DED is a multifactorial disorder involving multiple interacting mechanisms. Dysfunction of any component by causing alterations in the volume, composition, distribution, and/or clearance of the tear film can lead to ocular surface disease that expresses itself as dry eye. Two mutually reinforcing global mechanisms, tear hyperosmolarity and tear film instability, have been identified.[1] Any subclass of dry eye activates these core mechanisms and explains the features of various forms of dry eye.

Tear hyperosmolarity is regarded as the central mechanism causing ocular surface inflammation, damage, and symptoms, and the initiation of compensatory events in dry eye. It can arise from either low aqueous flow or excessive tear film evaporation, or a combination thereof. Hyperosmolar tears can damage the ocular surface epithelium by activating an inflammatory cascade in the epithelial surface cells and releasing inflammatory mediators such as the MAP kinases and NFκB signaling pathways[12] and the generation of inflammatory cytokines (e.g., IL-1α, IL-1β, TNF-α) and MMPs,[13]

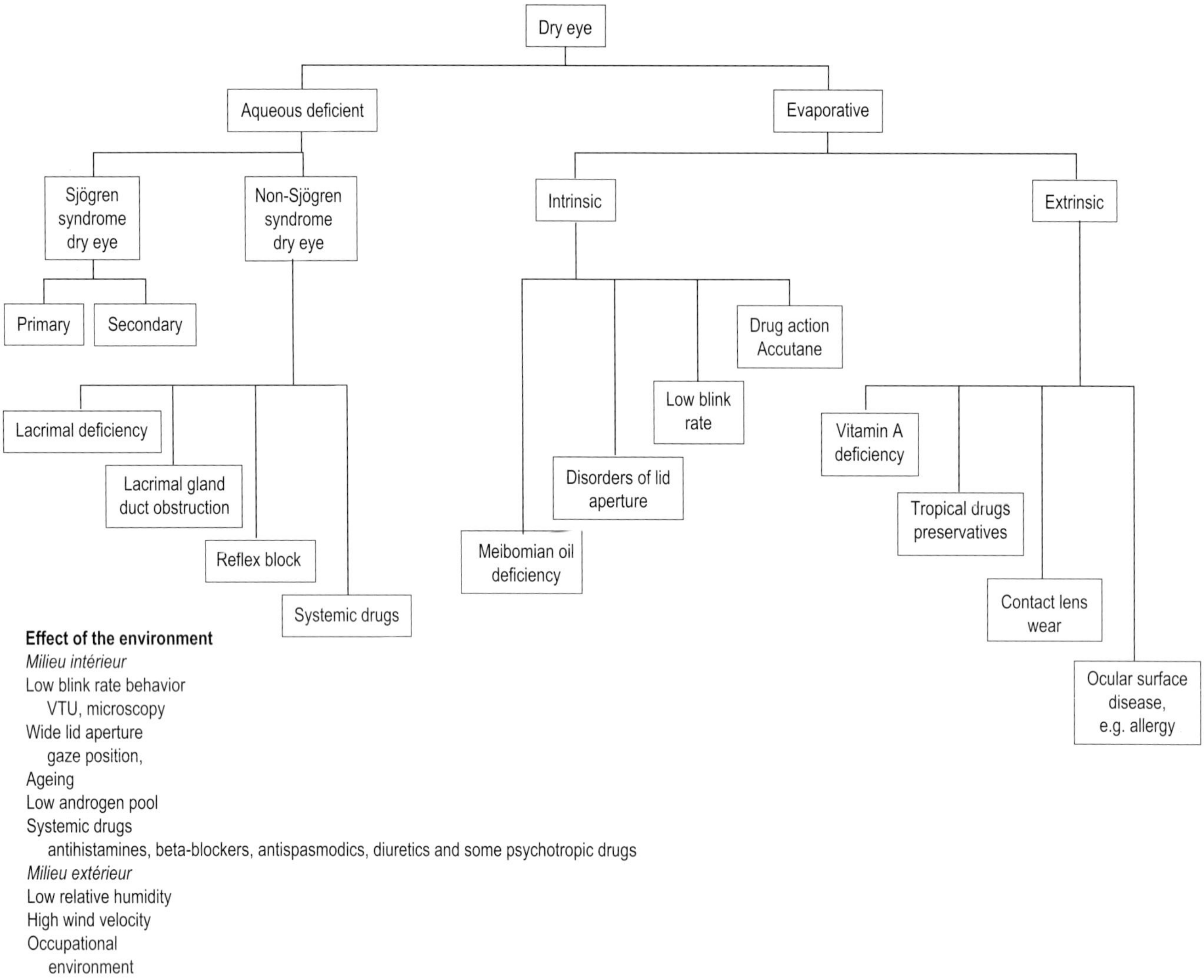

Fig. 36.1 Etiologic classification of dry eye disease. The list (bottom left) illustrates the environmental risk factors for dry eye disease. The scheme indicates the etiologic classification of dry eye disease into aqueous-deficient or evaporative tear deficiency. (From Definition and Classification Subcommittee of the International Dry Eye Workshop. The definition and classification of dry eye disease. *Ocul Surf* 2007;5:75–92.)

which arise from or activate inflammatory cells at the ocular surface.[14] These inflammatory events lead to apoptotic death of surface epithelial cells, including goblet cells,[15] and secondary lacrimal dysfunction. *Tear film instability* can arise secondary to hyperosmolarity, or can be the initiating event (e.g., lipid layer abnormalities in meibomian gland disease). Tear film instability results in increased evaporation, which contributes to tear hyperosmolarity (Fig. 36.1).[1]

Regardless of the initiating event or etiology, inflammation is usually a key factor in perpetuating DED.[16] Chronic inflammation may subsequently result in lacrimal gland insufficiency, reduced corneal sensation (long-term effects of inflammatory mediators on sensory nerve terminals supplying the ocular surface,[17] and morphological changes in the sub-basal nerve plexus,[18] and decreased reflex activity including reflex tearing and blinking, leading to increased evaporation and tear film instability. These postulated interactions, occurring over time, may explain the overlap of findings in dry eyes regardless of the underlying etiology, and reinforce the general concept of a vicious circle in which widely varying influences combine to cause dry eye with a complex profile.[1]

Etiopathogenic Classification

Classically, DED has been divided into major subtypes based on etiology: aqueous tear-deficient dry eye (ADDE) and evaporative dry eye (EDE) (Fig. 36.2). Clinically, however, the distinction between the two is less clear, and both subtypes eventually activate the same final common pathway leading to a dysfunctional tear syndrome. Nonetheless, the classification is useful for categorizing the underlying etiologies of DED.

Aqueous tear-deficient dry eye (ADDE, tear-deficient dry eye; lacrimal tear deficiency)

ADDE has two major subclasses, Sjögren's syndrome dry eye (SSDE) and non-Sjögren's syndrome dry eye (NSSDE).

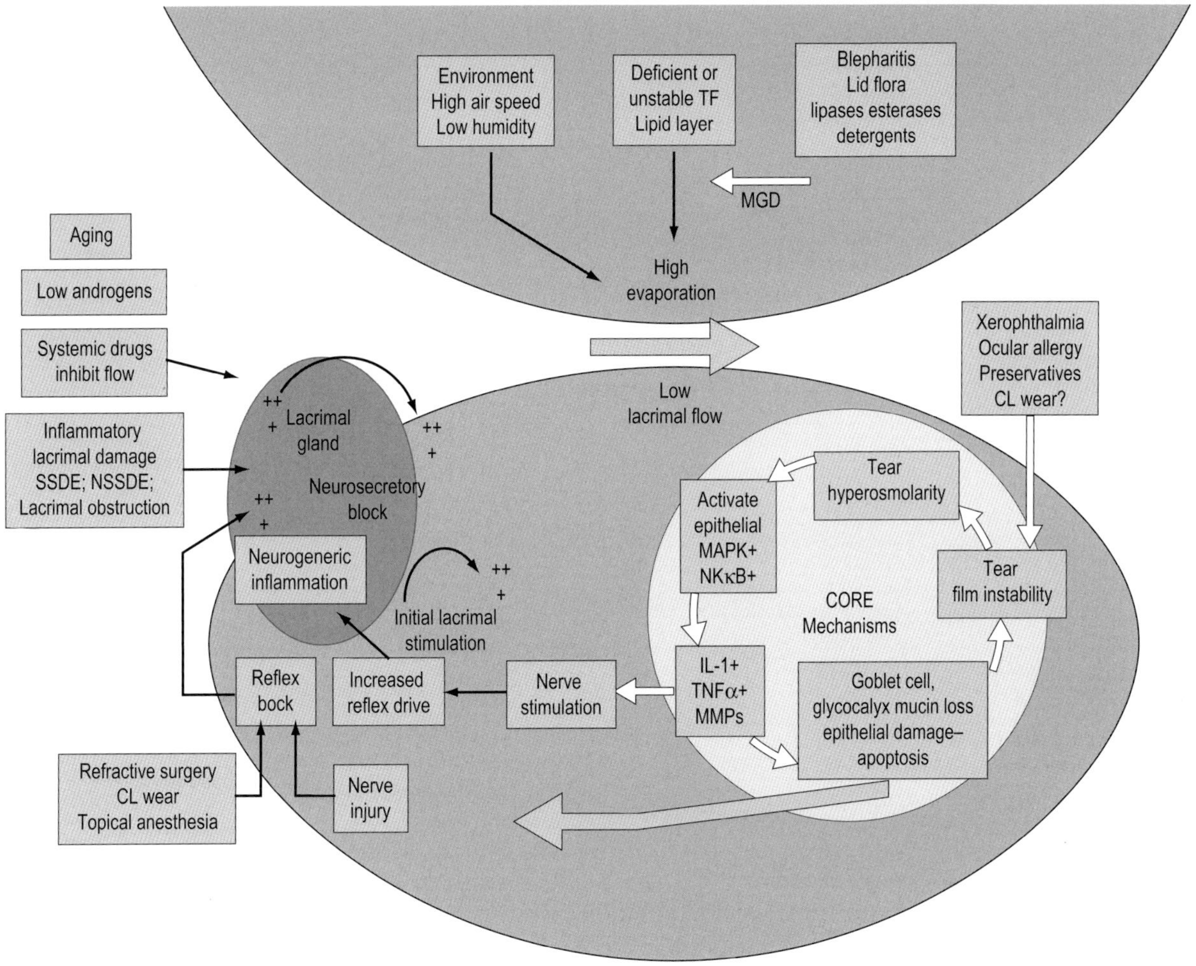

Fig. 36.2 Pathogenesis of dry eye. The core mechanisms responsible for dry eye disease are tear hyperosmolarity and tear film instability. The major causes of tear hyperosmolarity are reduced aqueous tear flow and/or increased tear evaporation. Tear hyperosmolarity induces cascades of inflammatory events that result in damage to the surface epithelium, nerve endings, and ultimately tear film instability. This instability exacerbates ocular surface hyperosmolarity and completes the vicious circle. Tear film instability can also be initiated by other etiologies, including xerophthalmia, ocular allergy, topical preservative use, and contact lens wear. (From Definition and Classification Subcommittee of the International Dry Eye Workshop. The definition and classification of dry eye disease. *Ocul Surf* 2007;5:75–92.) CL, contact lens; SSDE, Sjögren's syndrome dry eye; NSDE, non-Sjögren's syndrome dry eye.

Sjögren's syndrome dry eye

Sjögren's syndrome (SS) is an exocrinopathy in which the lacrimal and salivary glands, as well as other organs, are targeted by an autoimmune process. It is the second most common autoimmune rheumatologic disease, exceeded only by rheumatoid arthritis. There is a strong gender predilection for Sjögren's syndrome, with women representing 95% of patients. It can occur at all ages, with the peak incidence in the fourth and fifth decades. In all cases the lacrimal and salivary glands are progressively infiltrated by activated T cells, which cause acinar and ductular cell death and hyposecretion of the tears or saliva. Inflammatory activation within the glands leads to the expression of autoantigens at the surface of epithelial cells (e.g., fodrin, Ro and La)[19] and the retention of tissue-specific CD4 and CD8 T cells.[20] Hyposecretion is amplified by a potentially reversible neurosecretory block, due to the effects of locally released inflammatory cytokines or to the presence of circulating antibodies (e.g., anti-M3 antibody) directed against muscarinic receptors within the glands.[21] Although there is good agreement about the ocular manifestation of SS (i.e., keratoconjunctivitis sicca), documentation of the oral component (xerostomia) has led to some confusion. Recently a set of criteria for diagnosis of SS (Tables 36.1 and 36.2) has been suggested that requires objective evidence of autoimmune cause for sicca symptoms, including either characteristic damage in a minor salivary gland biopsy or characteristic autoantibodies against antigens such as SS-A or SS-B. There are two forms of SS:[22] *primary SS* refers to cases where there is no other associated systemic connective tissue disease; *secondary SS*, on the other hand, consists of the features of primary SS together with the features of an overt autoimmune connective disease, such as rheumatoid arthritis, which is the most common, or systemic lupus erythematosus, polyarteritis nodosa, Wegener's granulomatosis, systemic sclerosis, primary biliary sclerosis, or mixed connective tissue disease.

The precise triggers leading to autoimmune acinar damage are not known in full, but risk factors include

Table 36.1 Revised international classification criteria for ocular manifestations of Sjögren's syndrome

I. Ocular symptoms: a positive response to at least one of the following questions: 1. Have you had daily, persistent, troublesome dry eyes for more than 3 months? 2. Do you have a recurrent sensation of sand or gravel in the eyes? 3. Do you use tear substitutes more than three times a day?
II. Oral symptoms: a positive response to at least one of the following questions: 1. Have you had a daily feeling of dry mouth for more than 3 months? 2. Have you had recurrently or persistently swollen salivary glands as an adult? 3. Do you frequently drink liquids to aid in swallowing dry food?
III. Ocular signs: that is, objective evidence of ocular involvement defined as a positive result for at least one of the following two tests: 1. Schirmer I test, performed without anesthesia (≤5 mm in 5 minutes) 2. Rose Bengal score or other ocular dye score (≥4 according to van Bijsterveld's scoring system)
IV. Histopathology: in minor salivary glands (obtained through normal-appearing mucosa) focal lymphocytic sialoadenitis, evaluated by an expert histopathologist, with a focus score ≥1, defined as a number of lymphocytic foci (which are adjacent to normal-appearing mucous acini and contain more than 50 lymphocytes) per 4 mm^2 of glandular tissue
V. Salivary gland involvement: objective evidence of salivary gland involvement defined by a positive result for at least one of the following diagnostic tests: 1. Unstimulated whole salivary flow (≤1.5 mL in 15 minutes) 2. Parotid sialography showing the presence of diffuse sialectasias (punctate, cavitary or destructive pattern), without evidence of obstruction in the major ducts 3. Salivary scintigraphy showing delayed uptake, reduced concentration and/or delayed excretion of tracer
VI. Autoantibodies: presence in the serum of the following autoantibodies: 1. Antibodies to Ro(SSA) or La(SSB) antigens, or both

Reprinted with permission from: Vitali C, Bombardieri S, Jonnson R, et al. Classification criteria for Sjögren's syndrome: a revised version of the European criteria proposed by the American-European Consensus Group. Ann Rheum Dis 2002; 1: 554–8.[22]

Table 36.2 Diagnostic and exclusion criteria for primary and secondary Sjögren's syndrome

Primary Sjögren's syndrome In patients without potentially associated disease, primary SS may be defined as follows: • The presence of any four of the six items is indicative of primary SS, as long as either item IV (Histopathology) or VI (Serology) is positive • The presence of any three of the four objective criteria items (that is, items III, IV, V, and VI)
Secondary Sjögren's syndrome In patients with a potentially associated disease (another well-defined connective tissue disease), the presence of item I or item II plus any two from among items III, IV, and V may be considered as indicative of secondary SS
Exclusion criteria 1. Past head and neck radiation treatment 2. Hepatitis C infection 3. Acquired immunodeficiency disease (AIDS) 4. Pre-existing lymphoma 5. Sarcoidosis 6. Graft versus host disease 7. Use of anticholinergic drugs (since a time shorter than four times the half-life of the drug)

genetic profile (whether linked to MHC genes [HLA-DQ genes, specifically DQ1 and DQ2, when associated with the presence of anti-SS-A/Ro and anti-SS-B/La autoantibodies] or non-MHC [e.g. apolipoprotein-E, carbonic anhydrase-2]),[23] androgen status (a low androgen pool favoring an inflammatory environment within the target tissues),[23,24] and exposure to environmental agents ranging from viral infections that affect the lacrimal gland (whether as trigger [herpesvirus, Coxsackiviruses] or mimicking by chronic viral infections [HIV, HBV, HCV, HTLV-1]) to polluted environments.[23–26]

Non-Sjögren's syndrome dry eye

Non-Sjögren's syndrome dry eye is a form of ADDE due to lacrimal dysfunction, where the systemic autoimmune features of SSDE have been excluded. The most common form is age-related dry eye. The different forms of NSSDE are briefly discussed below:

Primary lacrimal gland deficiencies

Age-related dry eye (ARDE): ARDE is a primary disease. With increasing age there is an increase in ductal pathology that could promote lacrimal gland dysfunction by its obstructive effect.[37,38] These alterations include periductal fibrosis, interacinar fibrosis, paraductal blood vessel loss, and acinar cell atrophy.[27] Inflammatory changes have likewise been noted in the lacrimal glands of patients with ARDE. Another contributing factor to these age-related changes may be a decrease in androgen levels. Experimentally, androgens are required for the normal functioning of both the lacrimal[28] and the meibomian glands,[29] and there is clinical evidence that dry eye symptoms are promoted by blockade of androgen receptors.[30]

Schaumberg et al.[31] mentioned that postmenopausal women who use HRT have a higher prevalence of dry eye syndrome than those who have never used HRT, and this is particularly true of women who used estrogen alone. Sex hormone levels may influence both the lacrimal and meibomian glands.[32] Laboratory and preliminary clinical studies suggest that whereas androgens have a beneficial influence on lacrimal and meibomian gland function,[32] estrogen may play a role in exacerbating dry eye syndrome.[32–34] Uncu et al.[35] have similarly shown that HRT reduced tear production and that the decrease was greater in the estrogen-only group. Erdem et al.[36] have shown that the duration of menopause and HRT use in menopausal women may increase the incidence of dry eye. Woman who are taking or considering HRT should be informed of the potential increased risk of dry eye syndrome with this therapy.

Congenital alacrima: This is a rare cause of dry eye in youth resulting from the absence or hypoplasia of the lacrimal gland, or abnormalities of the innervation of the lacrimal gland that normally stimulates lacrimation.[37] True alacrima is usually bilateral, but may also be unilateral.[38] The most common condition associated with alacrima is familial dysautonomia or Riley–Day syndrome, in which decreased tear production may be due to abnormal parasympathetic innervation of the lacrimal gland. Patients with this condition produce a reduced amount of tears when crying. Reflex lacrimation in response to irritants, such as the odor of onions or scratching of the middle nasal turbinate, is absent. Histologically, lacrimal glands from patients with this condition appear to be normal. It is an autosomal recessive disorder in which progressive neuronal abnormality of the cervical sympathetic and parasympathetic innervations of the lacrimal gland and a defective sensory innervation of the ocular surface affects both small myelinated (Aδ) and unmyelinated (C) trigeminal neurons.[39] The chief mutation affects the gene encoding an IκB kinase-associated protein.

Secondary lacrimal gland deficiencies

Lacrimal gland infiltration: Lacrimal secretion may fail because of infiltration of the gland in sarcoidosis (by sarcoid granulomata),[40] lymphoma (by lymphomatous cells),[41] hemochromatosis, and amyloidosis.[42] Dry eye is a common complication in graft versus host disease (GVHD), and may develop in patients with systemic viral infections.[1] DED has been reported after infection by two different retroviruses, HTLV-1 and HIV-1.[43] It is diagnosed in as many as 20% of patients with acquired immunodeficiency syndrome (AIDS),[44] where the lacrimal gland is infiltrated by CD8 suppressor T cells rather than CD4 helper T cells in SSDE.[45] Patients with hepatitis C infection can develop an autoimmune disease with a clinical picture similar to Sjögren's syndrome.[42] Lacrimal gland swelling and dry eye have been associated with primary and persistent Epstein–Barr virus infections.[46] These findings support the notion that certain infections may be a risk factor for the initiation of lacrimal gland inflammation and subsequent development of tear-deficient dry eyes.

Obstruction of the lacrimal gland ducts

Obstruction of the ducts of the main palpebral and accessory lacrimal glands leads to aqueous-deficient dry eye and may be caused by any form of cicatrizing conjunctivitis. In these disorders it is not uncommon for conjunctival scarring to cause a cicatricial obstructive meibomian gland disease (MGD). In addition, lid deformity influences tear film spreading by affecting lid apposition and dynamics. Specific conditions include trachoma, mucous membrane pemphigoid, erythema multiforme major, Stevens–Johnson syndrome, and chemical and thermal burns.

Reflex hyposecretion

Reflex sensory block

When the eyes open, there is an increased reflex sensory drive from the exposed ocular surface. A reduction in sensory drive from the ocular surface is thought to favor the occurrence of dry eye in two ways, first by reducing reflex-induced lacrimal secretion, and second by reducing the blink rate and hence increasing evaporative loss.[47] Bilateral topical proparacaine reduces the blink rate by about 30% and tear secretion by 60–75%.[48] This reflex sensory block is most prominent in the following conditions:

Diabetes mellitus: Diabetes has been identified as a risk factor for dry eye in several studies, including large population studies. An association between poor glycemic control (as indicated by serum HbA1C) and frequency of drop use has been reported. Goebbels[49] found a reduction in reflex tearing (Schirmer test) in insulin-dependent diabetics, but no difference in tear film breakup time or basal tear flow by fluorophotometry. It has been suggested that the association may be due to diabetic sensory or autonomic neuropathy, or to the occurrence of microvascular changes in the lacrimal gland.[50]

Neurotrophic keratitis: Extensive sensory denervation of the anterior segment, involving the cornea and the bulbar and palpebral conjunctiva, as a component of herpes zoster ophthalmicus or induced by trigeminal nerve section, injection, or compression or toxicity, can lead to neurotrophic keratitis. This condition is characterized by features of dry eye, such as tear instability, diffuse punctate keratitis, and goblet cell loss, and also, most importantly, the occurrence of an indolent or ulcerative keratitis, which may lead to perforation.[51] The sensory loss results in a reduction of lacrimal secretion and a reduction in blink rate.[52] In addition, it is envisaged that there is a loss of trophic support to the ocular surface[51] after sensory denervation, owing to a deficient release of substance P or expression of nerve growth factor.[53,54] Two conditions where dry eye disease is predominantly due to neurotrophic disease are *post-refractive surgery* and *congenital corneal anesthesia*, which can be isolated or part of a congenital absence of the trigeminal ganglion.

Reflex motor block

An association between systemic drug use, particularly those with anticholinergic effects, and dry eye has been noted in several studies, with reduced lacrimal secretion being the likely mechanism. Responsible agents include antihistamines, beta-blockers, antispasmodics, and diuretics, and, with less certainty, tricyclic antidepressants, selective serotonin reuptake inhibitors, and other psychotropic drugs.[55]

Evaporative dry eye

Excessive evaporation from the exposed ocular surface has been attributed to intrinsic causes, which are due to intrinsic disease affecting lid structure or dynamics, or extrinsic causes, where ocular surface disease occurs due to some extrinsic exposure. The boundary between these two categories is inevitably blurred.

Intrinsic causes

Meibomian gland dysfunction

Meibomian gland dysfunction, or posterior blepharitis, is a condition of meibomian gland obstruction and is the most common cause of evaporative dry eye.[56,57] It can be both the starting cause and the downstream consequence of dry eye disease. Meibomian gland dysfunction is covered in great detail in Chapter 34.

Disorders of lid aperture and lid/globe congruity or dynamic

An increase in the exposed evaporative surface of the eye occurs in craniostenosis, endocrine (e.g., thyroid) and other forms of proptosis. Lagophthalmos, especially nocturnal, is also a common cause of increase evaporative surface.

Low blink rate

Drying of the ocular surface may be caused by a reduced blink rate, which lengthens the period during which the ocular surface is exposed to water loss before the next blink.[59,60] This may occur as a physiological phenomenon during the performance of certain tasks requiring concentration, e.g., chronic viewing of a video screen[60] or microscope, or it may be a feature of an extrapyramidal disorder, such as Parkinson's disease (PD).[61–63]

Extrinsic causes

Ocular surface disease

Disease of the exposed ocular surface may lead to imperfect surface wetting, early tear film breakup, tear hyperosmolarity, and dry eye. This can occur in any chronic surface disease, such as allergic conjunctivitis, or in nutritional causes such as vitamin A deficiency, where mucin production is disrupted.[64–66] Topical drops can also cause ocular surface toxicity and secondary tear film disruption. The most common etiologic agent is benzalkonium chloride (BAC), which causes surface epithelial cell damage and punctate epithelial keratitis, which interferes with surface wettability.[1] The use of BAC-preserved drops is an important cause of dry eye signs and symptoms in glaucoma patients.[67]

Contact lens wear

The primary reasons for contact lens intolerance are discomfort and dryness.[1] In a large cross-sectional study of contact lens wearers (91% hydrogel and 9% gas permeable lenses), several factors were found to be associated with dry eye diagnosed using the Contact Lens Dry Eye Questionnaire (CLDEQ).[68] Pre-lens tear film thinning time was most strongly associated with dry eye followed by nominal contact lens water content and refractive index.[68] The pre-lens lipid layer was less thick in dry eye subjects and correlated well with the pre-lens tear film thinning time. This, together with poor lens wettability, could be a basis for a higher evaporative loss during lens wear and was attributed to potential changes in tear film lipid composition, rather than to a loss of meibomian gland oil delivery.

Diagnosis of Dry Eye

Making the clinical diagnosis of dry eye disease is not always straightforward, as currently there are no uniform criteria for diagnosis. Traditionally, combinations of questionnaires and diagnostic tests have been used to assess symptoms and clinical signs.[69] The combination of history and examination must be used because some patients have significant symptoms but few findings, whereas others have significant clinical findings with only mild symptoms.[3,16,70] This may be due in part to the subjective nature of symptoms, possible neural hypersensitivity in early cases, and corneal hypersthesia and reduced sensation in more severe and chronic disease.[4,71,72]

History

Subjective symptoms of dry eye are the hallmark of this disease. There may be any number of symptoms, such as foreign body sensation, burning, stinging, itching, dryness, soreness, heaviness of the lids, photophobia, and ocular fatigue. The symptoms reported by patients with dry eyes share some common patterns. An important clue is exacerbation of symptoms by certain activities or environmental conditions.[69] For example, activities that involve prolonged visual effort, such as reading or watching television, can cause worsening of symptoms by reducing the blink rate and promoting ocular surface drying. Fluctuating vision during such activities is an extremely common complaint. Intolerance of the draft from air conditioners, smoky environments, and the low humidity of airplane cabins are other helpful clues when making the diagnosis of dry eye. In general, patients with aqueous tear deficiency tend to get worse as the day progresses, whereas those with predominantly meibomian gland disease are worse in the morning.

Similarly, a symptomatic response to artificial tears supports the diagnosis of dry eye. In addition to the clinical history, use of a validated symptom questionnaire is helpful, particularly for screening as well as follow-up of treatment effect.[11,69] A number of questionnaires are available for evaluating various aspects of dry disease symptomatology, including severity, effect on daily activities, and quality of life.[69]

In addition to the patient's ocular complaints, it is important to obtain a complete past ocular and medical history. Obtaining a complete list of the patient's medications is also important to identify any that may affect tear secretion. The presence of menopause and the use of hormone replacement should also be noted. Finally, a thorough review of systems is necessary to identify patients with a history of dry mouth (xerostomia) or dental and gum disease commonly associated with Sjögren's syndrome, as well as any other signs and symptoms suggestive of systemic diseases that are associated with dry eyes.

Physical examination

After obtaining a thorough history, a careful examination is important for making the diagnosis of dry eye and in order to determine the most likely etiology. Examination should begin by evaluating the face and eyelids for signs of rosacea or floppy lids. The dynamics of blinking and lid position should be observed while taking the history to prevent conscious alterations. Points of interests are: a) frequency of blinking; b) variation of blink intervals; c) size of the palpebral aperature, and d) adequacy of lid closure. Malposition of the lids may influence tear spread and turnover; therefore care should be taken to identify the following malpositions: a) entropion; b) ectropion; c) eversion of the lacrimal puncta; d) cicatrical malposition; e) dermatochalasis; and f) swelling of the temporal aspect of the upper lid, which may imply enlargement of the lacrimal gland.

Slit lamp examination should assess the following anatomical structures and their alterations: a) *Lid margins:* hyperemia, telangiectasia, thickening, scarring, keratinization, ulceration, tear debris, abnormalities of the meibomian orifices, including metaplasia, and the character of expressed meibomian secretions. b) *Eyelashes:* misdirection, malposition, encrustations, collarettes, and staphylococcal blepharitis; c) *Conjunctiva:* erythema, swelling, keratinization, papillary/follicular reaction, pinguecula, lid parallel conjunctival folds (conjunctival chalasis); d) *Cornea:* infiltrates, scars, punctate staining or ulcers, vascularization, pannus, and pterygium. In addition, the tear film should be analyzed for filaments, mucus, and cellular debris and foam. Corneal sensation should likewise be examined in all patients. In many patients with mild to moderate dry eye the slit lamp examination may not be revealing and further diagnostic testing is needed to evaluate and stage patients more objectively.

Diagnostic tests

The diagnostic tests for dry eyes can be divided into four general categories: tear film stability, ocular surface health, tear film composition, and tear flow (Table 36.3).

Table 36.3 Recommended sequence of diagnostic tests for dry eye patients using commonly available tests

1. Fluorescein strip with small non-preserved saline drop:
   a. Measure tear break-up time
   b. Look for staining of the ocular surface
2. Lissamine green strip with small non-preserved saline drop
   a. Look for conjunctival staining
3. Dry excess tears in the eye cul-de-sac
4. Place Schirmer strips in both eyes (no anesthesia): measure wetness after 5 minutes
5. Measure corneal sensation

Tear film stability

Tear film stability, which is reduced in all forms of dry eye, is commonly evaluated by performing a tear breakup time (TBUT) test. A widely used method involves instillation of fluorescein dye in the lower conjunctival sac using a fluorescein-impregnated strip wet with nonpreserved saline solution. The nonpreserved drop is important because preservatives such as benzalkonium chloride (BAC) can artificially speed up tear breakup. After the dye has been distributed throughout the tear film by blinking, the patient is asked to stare straight ahead without blinking. Under slit-lamp examination, the time between the last blink and the appearance of the first break (randomly distributed dry spot or hole) in the precorneal fluorescent tear film is measured.[11,69] Alternatively, tear film stability can be measured in a noninvasive fashion without the use of any dye. This test is known as the noninvasive breakup time, or NIBUT.[69] It involves projecting a target onto the convex mirror surface of the tear film and recording the time following a blink for the image to break up. The test has been performed using custom-built devices such as Tearscope or keratometry devices.

Fluorescein TBUT has been reported to be rapid in different types of dry eye, including keratoconjunctivitis sicca, mucin deficiency, and meibomian gland disease.[69] There is wide variability in the tear breakup time of normal subjects, but an arbitrary cutoff time of 10 s for both fluorescein-added and noninvasive techniques appears quite specific in screening patients for evidence of tear film instability;[69] however, cutoffs as low as <5 s have also been recommended.[69]

Diagnostic dye staining: ocular surface health

Ocular surface damage is commonly assessed by staining with one or more dyes, including fluorescein, rose Bengal, or lissamine green. Fluorescein sodium dye is currently the most commonly used in ophthalmology. When the surface epithelial cells loosen or desquamate, the dye diffuses rapidly in the intercellular spaces and staining indicates increased epithelial permeability.[69] It also penetrates the corneal epithelium when the mucous layer is removed. Fluorescein generally stains the cornea to a greater degree than the conjunctiva. In the clinic setting the best strategy is to place a small drop of nonpreserved saline over the proximal end of

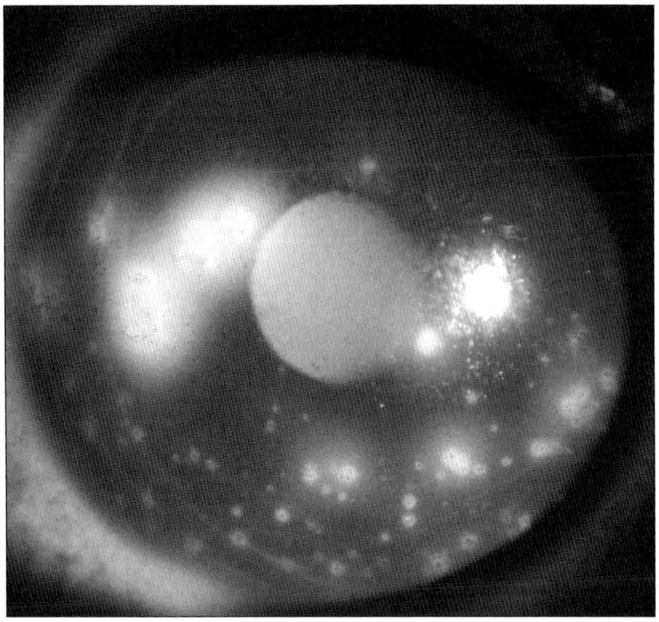

Fig. 36.3 Fluorescein staining of cornea in a patient with Sjögren's syndrome aqueous tear deficiency. Punctate and patchy areas of staining are usually seen and the staining is usually more severe in the inferior cornea.

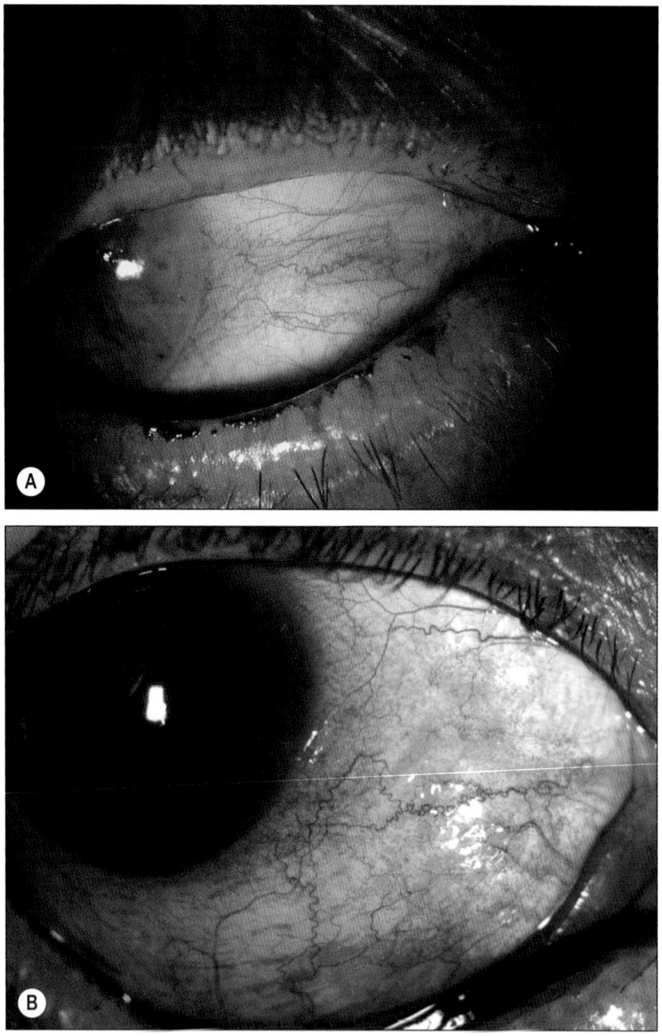

Fig. 36.4 Lissamine green staining in patients with moderate **(A)** and severe **(B)** dry eyes. Typically the conjunctiva stains to a greater extent than the cornea.

the fluorescein strip and let it flow towards the tip, thereby becoming more concentrated. The drop is gently applied to the inferior tarsal conjunctiva below the posterior margin of the lower lid. The patient should be instructed to blink several times to disperse the dye. The amount of staining can be graded using several visual scales as shown in Figure 36.2; viewing the cornea through a yellow intensity filter will enhance the intensity of staining (Fig. 36.3).

Rose Bengal staining of the corneal epithelium is more difficult to visualize than fluorescein, but is definitely more sensitive for staining the conjunctiva; however, it is not tolerated as well and frequently causes irritation and reflex tearing. Rose Bengal stains devitalized epithelial cells as well as epithelial cells that lack a healthy layer of protective mucin coating; rose Bengal is most commonly applied from a dye-impregnated paper strip, but can be formulated as a 1% solution. The interpretation of rose Bengal staining in dry eyes is based on two factors, intensity and location. Van Bijsterveld[73] reported a grading scale that evaluates the intensity of staining based on a scale of 0–3 in three areas: nasal conjunctiva, temporal conjunctiva, and cornea. The maximum possible score with this grading system is 9. The classic location for rose Bengal staining in aqueous tear deficiency is the interpalpebral conjunctiva, which appears in the shape of two triangles whose bases are at the limbus.[69] The conjunctiva usually stains more intensely than the cornea, but in severe cases of dry eye the entire cornea can stain with rose Bengal. It should be noted that the visibility of rose Bengal staining is greatest on the bulbar conjunctiva. Staining may be enhanced when visualized with red-free light.

The intensity of rose Bengal staining correlates well with the degree of aqueous tear deficiency, tear film instability measured by tear breakup time, and with reduced mucus production by conjunctival goblet cells and nongoblet epithelial cells.[69] In a study performed by Pflugfelder et al.,[74] subjects with Sjögren's aqueous tear deficiency had significantly greater van Bijsterveld rose Bengal staining scores than controls and subjects with non-Sjögren's aqueous tear deficiency and meibomian gland disease. Lissamine green B is similar to rose Bengal in its staining characteristics, and produces much less irritation after topical administration than rose Bengal (Fig. 36.4).[69] Several studies have demonstrated the staining pattern with lissamine green to be identical to that of rose Bengal, and therefore it is now commonly used as an alternative.

In summary, vital dye staining is one of the most useful diagnostic tools for assessing the health of the ocular surface. It can be useful as a tool to grade disease severity and the response to therapy. One of the uses of this test is to identify patients with severe staining of the ocular surface (Fig. 36.4) who are at risk for sight-threatening corneal complications, and to also raise suspicion for conditions such as Sjögren's syndrome (Fig. 36.5).

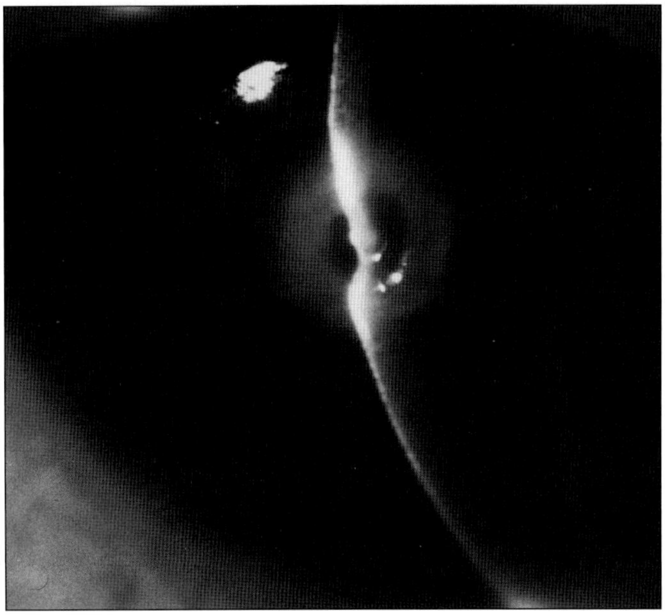

Fig. 36.5 Paracentral corneal ulceration in Sjögren's syndrome patient. Sterile corneal ulcers in Sjögren's syndrome are typically circular or oval, measure less than 3 mm in diameter, are located in the central or paracentral cornea, and resemble paracentral sterile corneal ulcers associated with rheumatoid arthritis. Occasionally, the cornea stroma in the area of ulceration may rapidly thin and perforate.

Corneal sensation

Reduced corneal sensation can be both the cause and the effect of dry eye. Sensory denervation may lead to dry eye by several mechanisms: (1) by reducing the afferent signal that drives aqueous tear secretion, (2) by reducing the blink rate (leading to ocular surface desiccation), and (3) by altering the growth and differentiation of ocular surface epithelia through diminished trophic influences of the trigeminal nerve. Likewise, there is evidence that corneal sensation decreases secondarily in patients with long-standing dry eye. This most likely reflects global dysfunctioning of the ocular surface lacrimal gland functional unit and secondary decreased neural sensitivity. The simplest technique for measuring corneal sensitivity is to take a cotton swab, extend a few fine strands from the tip and gently touch the surface of the cornea and conjunctiva. The patient's objective and subjective response can then be graded. However, the use of an esthesiometer is a more accurate and quantifiable method. Macri and Pflugfelder[54] have used a Cochet–Bonnet esthesiometer which consists of a nylon monofilament that can be extended in length from 0 to 6 cm (Fig. 36.5). Measurements are taken by advancing nylon filament smoothly and perpendicularly toward the center of the cornea. Contact is detected by the slightest bend of the nylon; sensitivity is measured as the length of the filament that gives a 50% positive response from a minimum of four stimuli. The normal cutoff is 4.5 cm, and measurements below this are compatible with decreased sensation. Although the same procedure can be used to measure conjunctival sensation, typically only corneal sensation is measured. Measuring corneal and conjunctival sensation is an important part of the evaluation of the patient with dry eye.

Tear film composition

Osmolarity

Elevated tear film osmolarity is one of the objective features recommended by the National Eye Institute committee to define dry eye.[74–76] Many publications over the last three decades have confirmed the value of tear osmolarity measurements. A recent meta-analysis of 17 published studies performed by Tomlinson et al.[75] has provided a well-validated cutoff value of 316 mmol/L for dry eye disease. Using this value, they reported 89% accuracy for diagnosis of dry eye disease. This degree of accuracy was superior to any other single test for dry eye diagnosis, and comparable with the results of combined tests.

Although tear osmolarity is a sensitive test for identifying dry eye, it lacks specificity. Tear film osmolarity may be elevated secondary to decreased tear secretion (aqueous-deficient dry eye) because of lacrimal gland disease and/or increased tear film evaporation (evaporative dry eye) resulting from exposure, blink abnormalities, or meibomian gland disease.[69] A number of devices for measuring tear osmolarity will soon be available clinically. Tear film osmolarity is discussed in greater detail in the chapter on tear film evaluation (Chapter 8).

Tear protein analysis

Proteins and peptides in tears play an important role in ocular surface disease. Lysozyme accounts for 20–40% of total tear protein and is known to decrease both with age[77] and in patients with dry eyes.[78] van Bijsterveld[72] has reported tear lysozyme concentration to be a more sensitive test for the diagnosis of dry eye than either the Schirmer test or rose Bengal staining, with a sensitivity and specificity >95%. Its main disadvantage is its lack of specificity. Reduced tear lysozyme levels have been measured in patients with herpes simplex virus (HSV) keratitis, bacterial conjunctivitis, smog irritation, and malnutrition.[79]

Lactoferrin is another tear protein with significant antibacterial activity that is normally produced by the lacrimal gland and has been used as a relative indicator of lacrimal gland function. Tear lactoferrin concentrations measured by the Lactocard, a commercially available colorimetric solid phase ELISA technique, have correlated well with clinical diagnosis of severe dry eye based on symptoms, slit lamp examination, Schirmer testing, rose Bengal staining, and TBUT.[80]

Although levels of tear proteins are currently measured primarily for academic purposes, with increasing knowledge and availability, tear protein analysis may become a useful clinical test for both diagnosis and monitoring of response to therapy in dry eye patients.

Aqueous tear flow and turnover

Schirmer test

The most commonly used technique for measuring tear secretion is the Schirmer test. The Schirmer I test is classically done without anesthesia and measures reflex tearing. Van Bijsterveld[72] selected a cutoff value of 5.5 mm strip wetting in 5 minutes for the Schirmer test without anesthesia to diagnose aqueous tear deficiency. Using this cutoff, he reported that the correct diagnosis was made in 83% of dry eye patients tested. Furthermore, those with measures of 6–10 mm and >10 mm were considered as dry eye suspect and normal, respectively. If the Schirmer test is performed after nasal stimulation, it is termed the Schirmer II test. In contrast to non-Sjögren dry eye, in Sjögren's syndrome it has been shown that the ability of nasal stimulation to increase the tear production of the anesthetized eye is greatly reduced, a finding of diagnostic value.[69]

Jones[81] popularized the use of topical anesthesia with a Schirmer test as a measurement of basal tear secretion, independent of reflex tearing. Generally, 3–5 mm of wetting is used as the cutoff when performing 'Schirmer with anesthesia'. In general, for patients with more severe dry eyes such as those with Sjögren's syndrome, it is best to perform the classic Schirmer I test (without anesthesia) to obtain a measure of the patient's reserve of lacrimal function.

The test is performed by placing a Schirmer strip in the lateral one-third of the lower lid. It is important to dry the fornix before placing the strip and to ask the patient to refrain from talking or chewing gum during the procedure. If using an anesthetic, adequate time should be given after the drop to minimize reflex tearing from the burning sensation due to the drop.

The Schirmer test has been criticized for its variability and poor reproducibility. A high degree of variability is seen when the test is repeated, although slightly less when it is performed after topical anesthetic instillation (basic secretion test).[69] The variability is due to different degrees of reflexes elicited by the Schirmer's test which cannot be standardized or controlled even when anesthesia is used. When using a diagnostic cutoff of 1 mm/min (i.e. 5 mm of wetting after 5 minutes), the Schirmer I test is very specific (90%) but only 25% sensitive for diagnosing dry eyes.[82] In a study by Macri and Pflugfelder,[83] significant differences in Schirmer I values were noted between subjects with aqueous tear deficiency and those with meibomian gland disease and normal controls. All eyes of normal controls and subjects with meibomian gland disease had Schirmer I values > 5 mm in both eyes, whereas only 5% of eyes in subjects with Sjögren's syndrome aqueous tear deficiency and 33% of eyes in subjects with non-Sjögren's aqueous tear deficiency had a Schirmer I value >5 mm.

An alternative to the Schirmer I test, the phenol red-impregnated thread test (PRT, Zone-Quick), is another method of functional assessment of tear secretion. Giving a cutoff value of 10 mm at 15 seconds, the sensitivity and specificity of the PRT have been shown to be 56% and 69%, respectively.[84] PRT appears to be mostly a measure of basal tear volume, but it has not been evaluated as extensively as the Schirmer test and therefore clinical data are not as widely available.

Despite its variability and low sensitivity, the Schirmer test continues to be a simple and inexpensive way of measuring aqueous tear production. It is most useful in diagnosing patients with more severe dry eyes who have significant aqueous tear deficiency, but not very useful as a screening test, particularly in patient with mild aqueous deficiency. A more generous cutoff of 10 mm can be used to indicate aqueous tear deficiency. However, the patients with less than 10 mm can be further segregated to document the extent of aqueous tear deficiency. This is especially helpful when trying to differentiate Sjögren's and non-Sjögren's etiologies. Specifically, in patients with Sjögren's syndrome, the Schirmer is usually <5 mm.

Delayed tear clearance

This test measures tear clearance or turnover. Delayed clearance of tears from the eye is a thought to be a contributing factor in the pathogenesis of KCS. Tear turnover is important for removing inflammatory cytokines from the eye and providing a fresh supply of growth factors. Delayed clearance has been associated with increased tear cytokine concentration, which may contribute to chronic inflammation.[85]

One way to objectively measure tear turnover from the ocular surface is with the fluorescein clearance test (FCT). In this test a standardized amount of fluorescein is placed in the conjunctival sac and the tear turnover rate is determined by the persistence of fluorescein in the tears at specific later time points. One method to detect the amount of residual fluorescein is using a Schirmer strip to collect the fluorescein-stained tears. A more precise method is to use a fluorophotometer.

It has been previously reported that the FCT correlates much better than Schirmer I with the severity of corneal epithelial and eyelid disease in both ATD and MGD.[83,85] However, given the time and experience necessary, FCT is not typically used in most office-based practices and its use is limited predominantly to academic centers.

Other noninvasive methods for assessing the tear film

Several diagnostic techniques have been developed to assess the tear film and diagnose dry eye, but many are invasive and modify the parameter they are designed to measure. Noninvasive or minimally invasive tests[86] may overcome this problem and provide more reproducible and objective data.

Tear meniscus height (meniscometry): the tear meniscus can be used to estimate tear volume, either simply by measuring meniscus height using the width of the slit-lamp beam, or in a more sophisticated fashion by reflective meniscometry,[87] or by assessing its profile photographically in slit section.[88] A meniscus radius of curvature <0.25 mm suggests a dry eye condition.

Interferometry of the tear film lipid layer is useful in screening and evaluating dry eye. It is a noninvasive technique for grading the behavior of the tear film lipid layer and estimating its thickness on the basis of the observed interference colors.[89] Instruments which have been used for this purpose include the Tearscope Plus and the Kowa DR-1.

At present there is no single test that is sufficiently sensitive and specific to detect all patients with dry eyes, and instead a combination of tests (alongside history) should be used. This was also recently demonstrated by Khanal et al.,[90] who have shown that a battery of tests employing a weighted comparison of tear turnover, evaporation, and osmolarity measurements derived from discriminant function analysis may be the most effective strategy for diagnosing dry eye disease based on physical examination.

Looking towards the future, newly developed devices that measure tear osmolarity may provide an additional test that could be performed in routine clinical settings and be useful for the diagnosis and management of patients with tear disorders.

Systemic Work-Up

In cases where Sjögren's syndrome is suspected, a thorough review of systems is performed and one or more of the following blood tests may be ordered: anti-SS-A, anti-SS-B, rheumatoid factor, ANA, ESR (sedimentation rate) and C-reactive protein. Additional work-up is best done by a rheumatologist.

Management of Dry Eyes

The main objectives in caring for patients with dry eye disease are to improve their ocular comfort and quality of life, and to return the ocular surface and tear film to the normal homeostatic state. Accurate diagnosis of the underlying cause provides the basis for management.

Tear supplementation: lubricants

Lubricants, including artificial tears, ointments, and gels, are still the mainstay of therapy in all stages of DED, either alone (in mild to moderate disease), or in combination with other treatments (in moderate to severe disease).[91] Most tear supplements act as lubricants; other actions may include replacement of deficient tear constituents, dilution of proinflammatory substances, reduction of tear osmolarity,[91,92] and protection against osmotic stress.[92]

Ocular lubricants are characterized by hypotonic or isotonic buffered solutions containing electrolytes, surfactants, and various types of viscosity agent. In theory, the ideal artificial lubricant should be preservative free, contain electrolytes,[92] particularly potassium[92] and bicarbonate,[92] and have a polymeric system to increase its retention time.[92] Physical properties should include a neutral to slightly alkaline pH. Osmolarities of artificial tears have been measured to range from about 181 to 354 mmol/L.[92] Under osmotic stress the corneal epithelial cells tend to lose water, and may compensate by increasing their internal electrolyte concentration to stabilize their volume. However, elevated electrolyte concentrations can eventually lead to activation of the cellular stress signaling pathway and eventually cellular damage.[92,93] Compatible solutes are small nonionic molecules (e.g., glycerin) that can be taken up by cells, increasing intracellular osmolarity without disrupting cellular metabolism. Artificial tears containing compatible solutes may thus provide protection against osmotic stress.[92] Products containing compatible solutes include Optive and Refresh Endura (with 0.9% and 1% glycerin, respectively).

Colloid osmolality (which relates to macromolecule concentration) also varies among artificial tear products, and may be important because it influences water transport across the ocular surface epithelium. Theoretically, high colloid osmolality may be beneficial in reducing swelling of damaged epithelial cells.[92]

Macromolecular complexes added to artificial lubricants act as viscosity agents. The addition of a viscosity agent increases residence time and slows the rate of clearance from the eye, thus providing a longer interval of patient comfort. Viscous agents may also protect the ocular surface epithelium by either coating and protecting it or by helping restore the protective effect of mucins, thereby reducing frictional stress.[94] Viscosity agents used in artificial tears include carboxymethylcellulose, polyvinyl alcohol, polyethylene glycol, propylene glycol, hydroxypropyl-guar (HP-guar), and lipids such as those that make up castor oil or mineral oil.[92]

Lipid-containing artificial tear products such as Refresh Endura (with castor oil) and Soothe XP (with mineral oil) are intended to reduce tear evaporation by restoring the lipid layer of the tear film;[92] this may be particularly useful in patients with MGD.[92] HP-guar (in products such as Systane) is believed to form a bioadhesive gel when exposed to ocular pH, increasing aqueous retention and protecting the ocular surface by mimicking the mucous layer of the tear film.[92] Hyaluronic acid is a naturally occurring viscoelastic substance.[95] In small randomized trials, artificial tears containing sodium hyaluronate have demonstrated greater improvement of DED signs and/or symptoms compared with normal saline[92] and with other viscosity agents such as CMC19 or hydroxypropyl-methylcellulose/dextran.[95] High-viscosity agents tend to cause visual blurring; therefore, lower-viscosity agents are generally preferred for mild to moderate DED. However, in more severe cases, high-viscosity agents may be needed for symptom control.[91]

Because of the risk of contamination of multidose products, most either contain a preservative or employ some mechanism for minimizing contamination and preventing microbial growth and to prolong shelf-life.[92] There are two main types of preservative: detergent and oxidative.[91] Detergent preservatives act by altering bacterial cell membrane permeability.[91] Detergents have toxic effects on the ocular surface epithelium and, with frequent use, can cause epithelial irritation and damage. Patients with a compromised tear film are at higher risk. Benzalkonium chloride, the most widely used preservative in topical ophthalmic preparations, is an example of a detergent preservative.[91,92] Oxidative preservatives penetrate the bacterial cell membrane and act by interfering with intracellular processes. They are sometimes referred to as 'vanishing' preservatives because they dissipate on contact with the eye and are therefore less likely than detergents to cause ocular damage.[91] However, they may not always dissipate completely in DED patients because of the decreased tear volume.[92] Stabilized oxychloro complex is an example of an oxidative preservative. Preserved tears are usually well tolerated in mild DED, when used no more than four to six times daily[92] (Exposure to preservatives in other topical ophthalmic agents (e.g., glaucoma medications) must also be taken into account.) If more frequent use is necessary, unpreserved tears are recommended.[92]

Ocular ointments and gels are also used in treatment of dry eye disease. Ointments are formulated with a specific mixture of mineral oil and petrolatum. Some contain lanolin, which can be irritating to the eye and delay corneal wound healing.[92] In general, ointments do not support bacterial growth and therefore do not require preservatives. Ophthalmic gels and ointments have higher viscosity and thus a longer contact time than liquids. They also coat the ocular surface during sleep, when aqueous tear production is normally decreased, and are therefore usually reserved for overnight use or to protect the ocular surface in patients with exposure due to reduced lid closure or blink.[92] Gels containing high molecular weight cross-linked polymers of acrylic acid (carbomers) have longer retention times than artificial tear solutions, but have less visual blurring effect than petrolatum ointments – perhaps because carbomer viscosity decreases rapidly on exposure to tear salts.[92]

Tear retention

Punctal occlusion

Punctal occlusion is one of the most useful and practical therapies for conserving tears in patients with aqueous-deficient DED.[92] A number of techniques and approaches have been described. Punctal and intracanalicular plugs generally provide a temporary and reversible means of occlusion, and electrocautery or laser are used for more permanent punctal occlusion. The argon laser has the advantage that the treatment can be titrated to achieve the desired level of punctal stenosis based on the patient's tear function. The wide choice of reversible devices currently available has reduced the need for occlusive surgery.[96] The punctal plugs are divided into two main types: absorbable and nonabsorbable. The former are made of collagen or polymers and last for variable periods (3 days to 6 months). Some newer absorbable materials may last as long as 6 months.[96] The nonabsorbable 'permanent' plugs include the Freeman style, which consists of a surface collar resting on the punctal opening, a neck, and a wider base, and are made of silicone or hydrophilic acrylic.

A variety of clinical studies evaluating the efficacy of punctal plugs have been reported.[92,97,98] Their use has been associated with objective and subjective improvement in patients with both Sjögren's and non-Sjögren's aqueous tear-deficient dry eye. Overall, the clinical utility of punctal plugs in the management of DED has been well documented. It is indicated in patients with symptoms of dry eye having a Schirmer test (with anesthesia) result <5 mm at 5 minutes, and showing evidence of ocular surface dye staining.[92] It has been suggested that plugs may be contraindicated in dry eye patients with clinical ocular surface inflammation, because the occlusion of tear outflow would prolong contact of the abnormal tears containing proinflammatory cytokines with the ocular surface. Treatment of the ocular surface inflammation prior to plug insertion has been recommended.

A common complication of punctal plugs is epiphora (tear overflow). Short-term absorbable plugs may be used initially to predict which patients are likely to tolerate nonabsorbable plugs; however, this test is not completely reliable.[96]

The most common complication of punctal plugs is spontaneous plug extrusion, which is particularly common with the Freeman-style plugs. Over time, an extrusion rate of 50% within 3 months requiring replacement has been reported; but many of these extrusions took place after extensive periods of plug residence. More troublesome complications include internal migration of a plug, biofilm formation and infection,[92] and pyogenic granuloma formation. Intracanalicular plugs are an alternative to punctal plugs with less risk of extrusion or conjunctival irritation. However, canalicular inflammation or infection may occur. Furthermore, removal is more difficult than with punctal plugs, requiring more invasive procedures.[96]

Moisture chamber spectacles

The wearing of moisture-conserving spectacles has for many years been advocated to alleviate ocular discomfort associated with dry eye.[92] They reduce tear evaporation by increasing humidity around the eye. The patient's glasses can be modified using commercially available top and side shields, or for more severe cases swimming goggles can be used.

Contact lenses

Contact lenses may help to protect and hydrate the corneal surface in severe dry eye conditions or when other therapy has failed, to help retain the tear film and/or promote ocular surface healing.[92] However, because contact lenses can also exacerbate DED, patients using them for DED must be monitored closely.[92]

Several different contact lens materials and designs have been evaluated, including silicone rubber lenses and gas-permeable scleral-bearing hard contact lenses with or without fenestration.[92,99] These lenses can protect the ocular surface epithelium by maintaining a tear film near the corneal epithelium and by minimizing frictional forces. Improved visual acuity and comfort, decreased corneal epitheliopathy, and healing of persistent corneal epithelial defects have been reported.[92,99] The Boston scleral lens, designed with a fluid-filled reservoir that eliminates corneal contact, functions as a liquid bandage that is tolerated by even the most severe dry eyes.[92] Although contact lenses can be very effective, because of the risk of bacterial keratitis they are generally reserved only for moderate to severe dry eye in patients who would otherwise become significantly visually debilitated due to severe epitheliopathy or filamentary keratitis. The risk can be lowered by exchanging the lens on a regular basis, avoiding corticosteroids, and using prophylactic antibiotics. Patients with extreme aqueous tear deficiency are not good candidates for contact lenses.

Tarsorrhaphy

A partial tarsorrhaphy is reserved for severe or refractory DED.[92] This surgical approach is used to reduce the area of exposed ocular surface for patients who have developed severe epitheliopathy, persistent epithelial defects, or frank stromal ulceration.

Tear stimulation: secretagogues

Several potential topical pharmacologic agents may stimulate aqueous secretion, mucus secretion, or both. Among several agents which are currently under investigation by pharmaceutical companies, the safety and efficacy of diquafosol (one of the P2Y2 receptor agonists) eye drops has been favorably evaluated in several experimental[102] and clinical trials.[100,101] This agent is capable of stimulating aqueous and mucus secretion in both animals and humans.[102–104]

Orally administered cholinergic agonists, in particular pilocarpine and cevilemine, are sometimes given to treat severe aqueous-deficient DED. They have FDA-approved indications for treatment of dry mouth associated with Sjögren's syndrome, but are off-label for the treatment of dry eye.[92] Several studies have documented the benefits of pilocarpine in patients with Sjögren's syndrome at doses of 5 mg BID[105] and 5–7 mg QID in improvement of DED symptoms.[105,106] The most commonly reported side effect from this medication was excessive sweating,[105,106] which occurred in over 40% of patients. Other adverse effects probably related to pilocarpine included urinary frequency, flushing, and hypersalivation.

Cevilemine is a newer oral cholinergic agonist with high affinity to the muscarinic M1 and M3 that was found to significantly improve symptoms of dryness and aqueous tear production and ocular surface disease compared to placebo when taken in doses of 15 or 30 mg TID.[107] This agent may have fewer adverse systemic side effects than oral pilocarpine. The most common adverse effects were gastrointestinal symptoms (including nausea and diarrhea) and increased sweating, all mild to moderate.[107]

Biological tear substitutes

Serum

Autologous serum tears, produced from the patient's serum, have been used in severe DED. The protocol used for the production of serum eye drops determines their composition and efficacy. Several protocols have been published to date.[92] The tears are typically unpreserved, but can be stored frozen for 3–6 months.[92]

Concentrations between 20% and 100% of serum have been used. Because of significant variations in patient populations, production and storage regimens, and treatment protocols, the efficacy of serum eye drops in dry eyes has varied substantially between studies.[92]

Several small, randomized studies investigating autologous serum tears versus unpreserved saline drops, unpreserved artificial tears, and/or other conventional treatments suggest that autologous serum tears are effective in improving the symptoms and signs of severe or refractory DED.[92] A randomized study in post-LASIK DED demonstrated significant improvement in rose Bengal staining and TBUT, but not in the Schirmer test or symptom scores, with autologous serum tears compared with artificial tears.[92]

Additional reports of successful treatment of persistent epithelial defects – where success is more clearly defined as 'healing of the defect' – with autologous serum substantiate the impression that this is a valuable therapeutic option for ocular surface disease.[108,109] Generally, autologous serum drops showed marked suppression of apoptosis in the conjunctival and corneal epithelium. Albumin, the major protein in serum, improved ocular surface damage in vivo and rescued apoptosis after serum deprivation in vitro.[109]

Few complications have been reported with autologous serum tears; however, circulating antibodies in serum could theoretically cause an inflammatory response.[109]

Salivary gland autotransplantation

Salivary submandibular gland transplantation is capable of replacing deficient mucin and the aqueous tear film phase. This procedure requires collaboration between an ophthalmologist and a maxillofacial surgeon. With appropriate microvascular anastomosis, 80% of grafts survive. In the long term, in patients with absolute aqueous tear deficiency, viable submandibular gland grafts provide significant improvement in the Schirmer test, FBUT, and rose Bengal staining, as well as reduction of discomfort and the need for pharmaceutical tear substitutes. Owing to the hypo-osmolarity of saliva compared to tears, excessive salivary tearing can induce a microcystic corneal edema, which is temporary but can lead to epithelial defects.[92] Hence, this operation is indicated only in end-stage DED with an absolute aqueous tear deficiency (Schirmer-test wetting of 1 mm or less), and persistent severe pain despite punctal occlusion and at least hourly application of unpreserved tear substitutes. For this group of patients, such surgery is capable of substantially reducing discomfort but often has no effect on vision.[92] Transplantation of minor salivary glands is a promising new treatment option for severe dry eyes. The procedure is simple, with minimal surgical risk. These grafts remain viable in over 90% and seem to be capable of sustaining a basal secretion for up to 36 months. As experience with this technique is still very limited, prospective controlled studies have to be performed to establish the long-term survival of the glands and to characterize the salivary tear film and its impact on the ocular surface.[110]

Anti-inflammatory therapy

As inflammation is a key component of the pathogenesis of dry eye, anti-inflammatory agents are considered an important aspect of treatment. Inflammation can be due to hyperosmolarity, chronic irritative stress (e.g., contact lenses), and systemic inflammatory/autoimmune disease (e.g., rheumatoid arthritis).

Ciclosporin

Ciclosporin A (CsA), a fungal-derived peptide, is a calcineurin inhibitor. Topical ciclosporin is currently the only pharmacologic treatment that is FDA approved specifically for DED. In studies of DED patients, ciclosporin reduced proinflammatory cytokines (e.g., conjunctival IL-6 levels), reduced activated lymphocytes in the conjunctiva, reduced conjunctival inflammatory and apoptotic markers, and increased conjunctival goblet cell numbers.[92] The therapeutic efficacy of CsA for treatment of KCS was documented in humans in several clinical trials.[92,111–113] Clinical trials have demonstrated that ciclosporin minimizes the signs and symptoms of dry eye disease and is not associated with any significant systemic or ocular adverse reaction.[112] Perry et al.[114] recently reported that the symptomatic improvement was greatest in the mild group and the best results in improvement of disease signs were in patients with severe DED.

Most adverse effects reported during the phase 3 trials of ciclosporin 0.05% and 0.1% were mild to moderate and transient. The most common treatment-related adverse effects were ocular burning and stinging, occurring in 16.1% and 4.5%, respectively, of the ciclosporin 0.1% group; 14.7% and 3.4% of the ciclosporin 0.05% group; and 6.5% and 1.4% of the vehicle group.[92] The approval of topical CsA for anti-inflammatory therapy of KCS marks the first step in shifting the focus of therapy onto the underlying mechanisms that contribute to the development and progression of this disease. Two additional immunophilins, pimecrolimus and tacrolimus, are being evaluated in clinical trials of KCS.[113]

Corticosteroids

Corticosteroids exert their immunosuppressive effects by nonspecifically inhibiting many aspects of the inflammatory response. Their immunomodulatory actions are due to inhibition of the activity of transcription factors such as activator protein-1 (AP-1) and nuclear factor κB (NFκB), that are involved in the activation of proinflammatory genes. Several randomized trials have demonstrated that short-term topical corticosteroid use (as long as 4 weeks) improves the signs and symptoms of DED.[11,92]

In a 4-week double-masked randomized study of 64 patients with KCS and delayed tear clearance, loteprednol etabonate 0.5% ophthalmic suspension four times a day was found to be more effective than its vehicle in improving some signs and symptoms. Furthermore, the corticosteroid patients had significant improvement in corneal smoothness.[115]

A prospective randomized clinical trial compared the severity of ocular irritation symptoms and corneal fluorescein staining in two groups of patients, one treated with topical nonpreserved methylprednisolone for 2 weeks, followed by punctal occlusion (group 1), and one that received punctal occlusion alone (group 2).[116] After 2 months, 80% of patients in group 1 and 33% of those in group 2 had complete relief of ocular irritation symptoms. Corneal fluorescein staining was negative in 80% of eyes in group 1 and 60% of eyes in group 2 after 2 months. No steroid-related complications were observed.

In an open-label, noncomparative trial, extemporaneously formulated nonpreserved methylprednisolone 1% ophthalmic suspension was found to be clinically effective in 21 patients with Sjögren's syndrome KCS (Fig. 36.6).[117]

Occasionally, in patients with significant inflammatory disease such as Sjögren's syndrome topical steroids may not provide an adequate anti-inflammatory effect and a short pulse of systemic steroids can be very effective. Tabbara and Frayha[119] reported that the majority of patients treated with alternate-day oral prednisone (40 mg) showed improved

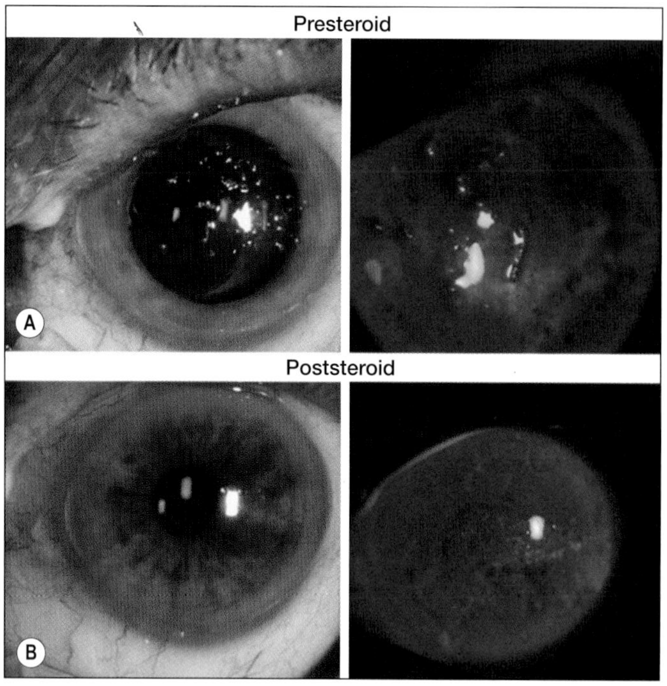

Fig. 36.6 Patient with dry eye disease and filamentary keratitis **(A)** before and **(B)** after a course of preservative-free topical steroids.

aqueous tear production, defined as a 5 mm or greater increase in Schirmer test strip wetting (71% of subjects), decreased rose Bengal staining (86% of subjects), and elevated tear lysozyme levels (64% of subjects).

Overall, topical steroids are very effective for achieving a quick response. Their main limitation is the potential for increasing the risk of infection, elevated intraocular pressure, and posterior subcapsular cataracts. Therefore, this is not a suitable form of therapy for the long-term treatment of KCS. However, corticosteroids may differ in their propensity to cause these complications. For example, some evidence suggests that loteprednol, which is rapidly metabolized to inactive metabolites, may have a better safety profile than other corticosteroids.[115] Thus, it is recommended to use topical steroids mainly as pulse therapy to control exacerbations, followed by change to a low dose (once or twice daily) or to a weaker agent that carries a lower risk of glaucoma and cataract (e.g. loteprednol etabonate and fluorometholone).

Recently, there has been interest in the use of androgenic steroids as therapy for dry eyes. In general, androgens appear to attenuate autoimmune reactions, whereas estrogens have been implicated in the pathogenesis and/or progression of many autoimmune disorders. In murine models of Sjögren's syndrome treatment with systemic androgen also has been reported to reduce the number and size of lacrimal gland lymphocytic foci, reduce the extent of lymphocytic infiltration, and ameliorate the immune-associated effects on lacrimal gland acinar and ductal epithelia.[92]

The immunosuppressive effects of androgens on the lacrimal gland may in part be mediated by stimulating the synthesis of TGF-beta, a potent immunomodulating and anti-inflammatory cytokine, and by reducing the content of IL-1beta and TNF-alfa.

In an epidemiologic study of over 38 000 female health professionals, it was demonstrated that hormone replacement therapy in postmenopausal women is associated with a significant increase in the prevalence of dry eye symptoms and the diagnosed dry eye syndromes. The effects of sex steroids on the tear function are mediated through both meibomian glands and the lacrimal gland. Preparations of topically applied androgen and estrogen steroid hormones are currently being evaluated in randomized clinical trials.

Tetracyclines

The clinical benefits of tetracyclines in DED are most likely due to their *antibacterial, anti-inflammatory and protease inhibitory* properties.[92] Several studies have described the beneficial effects of minocycline and other tetracycline derivatives (e.g., doxycycline) in the treatment of chronic blepharitis.[92] Studies have shown significant changes in the aqueous tear parameters, such as tear volume and tear flow, following treatment with tetracycline derivatives (e.g., minocycline). One study also demonstrated a decrease in aqueous tear production that occurred along with clinical improvement.[119]

Tetracycline derivatives (e.g., minocycline, doxycycline) are generally preferred to tetracycline because of their high concentration in tissues, low renal clearance, long half-life, high level of binding to serum proteins, and decreased risk of photosensitization.[92] The optimal dosing schedule has not been established; however, a variety of dose regimens have been proposed, including 50 or 100 mg doxycycline once a day,[92] or an initial dose of 50 mg a day for the first 2 weeks followed by 100 mg a day for a period of 2.5 months, in an intermittent fashion.[92,119] Others have proposed use of a low dose of doxycycline (20 mg) for treatment of chronic blepharitis on a long-term basis.[92] Tetracyclines are discussed in great detail in Chapter 34.

Essential fatty acids

Essential fatty acids are necessary for complete health, but cannot be synthesized by vertebrates and must be obtained from dietary sources. Among the essential fatty acids are 18 carbon omega-6 and omega-3 fatty acids. In the typical western diet, 20–25 times more omega-6 than omega-3 fatty acids are consumed. Omega-6 fatty acids are precursors for arachidonic acid and certain proinflammatory lipid mediators (PGE2 and LTB4). In contrast, certain omega-3 fatty acids (e.g., EPA found in fish oil) inhibit the synthesis of these lipid mediators and block the production of IL-1 and TNF-alfa.[120] Theoretically, they may benefit DED in two ways: by reducing inflammation and by altering the composition of meibomian lipids.[120,121] There are several EFA nutritional supplements marketed specifically for the treatment of DED that contain omega-3 EFA from flaxseed and fish oil. In some cases, omega-3 EFAs are combined with omega-6 EFAs. A beneficial clinical effect of fish oil omega-3 fatty acids on rheumatoid arthritis has been observed in several double-masked placebo-controlled clinical trials.[120] Epidemiologic data from the Women's Health Study (WHS) showed an association between higher dietary omega-3 fatty acid intake and a lower risk of DED.[120] Omega-6 fatty acid intake was not independently associated with DED; however, a higher omega-6:omega-3 ratio was associated with a significantly greater DED risk.[122] In a mouse model of dry eye,[123] topical application of alfa-linolenic acid omega-3 EFA significantly reduced corneal fluorescent staining and ocular surface inflammation.

Two randomized trials demonstrated significant improvement of DED symptoms and some objective signs with the omega-6 fatty acids linoleic acid (LA) plus GLA, compared to placebo.[120]

Topical vitamin A (retinol)

Vitamin A deficiency is a known cause of xerophthalmia; however, most DED patients are not vitamin A deficient. Because retinol is present in tears, it has been hypothesized that DED may be associated with local retinol deficiency at the ocular surface.[120] Based on this hypothesis, topical retinol has been used to treat various forms of DED, with variable results.[111] Limited data suggest a possible role of vitamin A in reversing conjunctival squamous metaplasia and keratinization in severe DED, for example in cicatrizing conjunctivitis or graft-versus-host disease.[120] However, the efficacy of topical retinol in DED remains to be established.[120]

Mucolytics

Topical acetylcysteine was mentioned in the literature as a DED treatment as early as the 1960s,[120] and is still sometimes used in patients with dense mucus accumulation[119] or filamentary keratitis.[124] Acetylcysteine is not commercially available as a topical ophthalmic agent.[120] Inhalational acetylcysteine (FDA approved for use as a bronchial mucolytic) has been diluted to concentrations of 5–20% (most commonly 10%) for off-label use as a topical ophthalmic agent.

Treatment Guidelines

Previous practice guidelines have used an etiology-oriented approach to DED.[92,120] However, commonly used etiologic classifications (e.g., aqueous-deficient vs evaporative, Sjögren's vs non-Sjögren's) often are not helpful in establishing a treatment plan.[16] International Task Force guidelines, published in 2006, propose a classification of DED severity based on clinical signs and symptoms. In 2007 the Management and Therapy Subcommittee of the International Dry Eye WorkShop (DEWS) adopted a modified form of the ITF severity grading, as shown in Table 36.4.[92] The DEWS treatment recommendations are based on the modified severity grading (Table 36.5).

It is worth mentioning that in the ITF algorithm for treatment of DED without lid margin disease (Table 36.5), topical ciclosporin is recommended as a treatment option for DED at level 2 severity (but only in the presence of clinically evident inflammation), whereas punctal plugs are recommended at level 3 severity (after control of inflammation).[16] In contrast, the DEWS recommendations list both ciclosporin

Table 36.4 Dry eye severity grading scheme

Dry eye severity level	1	2	3	4*
Discomfort, severity & frequency	Mild and/or episodic; occurs under environmental stress	Moderate episodic or chronic, stress or no stress	Severe frequent or constant without stress	Severe and/or disabling and constant
Visual symptoms	None or episodic mild fatigue	Annoying and/or activity-limiting episodic	Annoying, chronic and/or constant, limiting activity	Constant and/or possibly disabling
Conjunctival injection	None to mild	None to mild	+/-	+/++
Conjunctival staining	None to mild	Variable	Moderate to marked	Marked
Corneal staining (severity/location)	None to mild	Variable	Moderate to marked	Severe punctate erosions
Corneal/tear signs	None to mild	Mild debris, ↑↓ meniscus	Filamentary keratitis, mucus clumping, ↑ tear debris	Filamentary keratitis, mucus clumping, ↑ tear debris, ulceration
Lid/meibomian glands	MGD variably present	MGD variably present	Frequent	Trichiasis, keratinization, symblepharon
TBUT (sec)	Variable	≤10	≤5	Immediate
Schirmer score (mm/5 min)	Variable	≤10	≤5	≤2

** Must have signs AND symptoms.*
Reprinted with permission from Behrens A, Doyle JJ, Stern, et al. Dysfunctional tear syndrome. A Delphi approach to treatment recommendations. Cornea 2006;25:900–907.

Table 36.5 Treatment recommendations by severity level

Level 1: Education and counseling Environmental management Elimination of offending systemic medications Preserved tear substitutes, allergy eye drops
Level 2: *If Level 1 treatments are inadequate, add:* Unpreserved tears, gels, ointments Steroids Ciclosporin A Secretagogues Nutritional supplements
Level 3: *If Level 2 treatments are inadequate, add:* Tetracyclines Autologous serum tears Punctal plugs (after control of inflammation)
Level 4: *If Level 3 treatments are inadequate, add:* Topical vitamin A Contact lenses Acetylcysteine Moisture goggles Surgery

Modified from International Task Force dysfunctional tear syndrome treatment algorithm.[19]

and punctal plugs as level 2 options, without specifying the presence or absence of clinical inflammation.[92] Overall, it appears that plugs are more beneficial for immediate relief of dryness, whereas ciclosporin improves ocular surface health over time. The combination of the two treatments produces the greatest overall improvement.[125]

References

1. The definition and classification of dry eye disease: report of the Definition and Classification Subcommittee of the International Dry Eye WorkShop (2007). *Ocul Surf.* 2007;5:75–92.
2. Pflugfelder SC. Prevalence, burden, and pharmacoeconomics of dry eye disease. *Am J Manag Care.* 2008;14(3 Suppl):S102–S106.
3. The epidemiology of dry eye disease: report of the Epidemiology Subcommittee of the International Dry Eye WorkShop (2007). *Ocul Surf.* 2007;5(2):93–107.
4. Miljanovic B, Dana R, Sullivan DA, Schaumberg DA. Impact of dry eye syndrome on vision-related quality of life. *Am J Ophthalmol.* 2007; 143:409–415.
5. Beuerman RW, Mircheff A, Pflugfelder SC, Stern ME. The lacrimal functional unit. In: Pflugfelder SC, Beuerman RW, Stern ME, eds. *Dry eye and ocular surface disorders.* New York: Marcel Dekker; 2004.
6. Jordan A, Baum J. Basic tear flow. Does it exist? *Ophthalmology.* 1980;87:920.
7. Gupta A, Heigle T, Pugfelder SC. Nasolacrimal stimulation of aqueous tear production. *Cornea.* 1997;16:645–648.
8. Stern ME, Gao J, Siemarko KF, et al. The role of the lacrimal functional unit in the pathophysiology of dry eye. *Exp Eye Res.* 2004;78:409–416.
9. Holly FJ, Lemp MA. Tear physiology and dry eyes. *Surv Ophthalmol.* 1977;22(2):69–87.
10. Pflugfelder SC, Liu Z, Monroy D, et al. Detection of sialomucin complex (MUC4) in human ocular surface epithelium and tear fluid. *Invest Ophthalmol Vis Sci.* 2000;41(6):1316–1326.

11. Lemp MA. Report of the National Eye Institute/Industry Workshop on clinical trials in dry eyes. *CLAO J.* 1995;21:221–232.
12. Luo L, Li DQ, Corrales RM, Pflugfelder SC. Hyperosmolar saline is a proinflammatory stress on the mouse ocular surface. *Eye Contact Lens.* 2005;31:186–193.
13. De Paiva CS, Corrales RM, Villarreal AL, et al. Corticosteroid and doxycycline suppress MMP-9 and inflammatory cytokine expression, MAPK activation in the corneal epithelium in experimental dry eye. *Exp Eye Res.* 2006;83:526–535.
14. Baudouin C. The pathology of dry eye. *Surv Ophthalmol.* 2001;45(Suppl 2):S211–S220.
15. Yeh S, Song XJ, Farley W, et al. Apoptosis of ocular surface cells in experimentally induced dry eye. *Invest Ophthalmol Vis Sci.* 2003;44:124–129.
16. Behrens A, Doyle JJ, Stern L, et al. Dysfunctional tear syndrome: a Delphi approach to treatment recommendations. *Cornea.* 2006;25:900–907.
17. Bourcier T, Acosta MC, Borderie V, et al. Decreased corneal sensitivity in patients with dry eye. *Invest Ophthalmol Vis Sci.* 2005;46:2341–2345.
18. Benitez-Del-Castillo JM, Acosta MC, Wassfi MA, et al. Relation between corneal innervation with confocal microscopy and corneal sensitivity with noncontact esthesiometry in patients with dry eye. *Invest Ophthalmol Vis Sci.* 2007;48:173–181.
19. Nakamura H, Kawakamu A, Eguchi K. Mechanisms of autoantibody production and the relationship between autoantibodies and the clinical manifestations in Sjögren's syndrome. *Trans Res.* 2006;148(6):281–288.
20. Hayashi Y, Arakaki R, Ishimaru N. The role of caspase cascade on the development of primary Sjögren's syndrome. *J Med Invest.* 2003;50:32–38.
21. Zoukhri D. Effect of inflammation on lacrimal gland function. *Exp Eye Res.* 2006;82:885–898.
22. Vitali C, Bombardieri S, Jonsson R, et al. Classification criteria for Sjögren's syndrome: a revised version of the European criteria proposed by the American-European Consensus Group. *Ann Rheum Dis.* 2002;61:554–558.
23. Delaleu N, Jonsson MV, Appel S, Jonsson R. New concepts in the pathogenesis of Sjögren's syndrome. *Rheum Dis Clin North Am.* 2008;34(4):833–845.
24. Porola P, Laine M, Virkki L, Poduval P, Konttinen YT. The influence of sex steroids on Sjögren's syndrome. *Ann N Y Acad Sci.* 2007;1108:426–432.
25. Ramos-Casals M, Brito-Zerón P, Font J. Lessons from diseases mimicking Sjögren's syndrome. *Clin Rev Allergy Immunol.* 2007;32(3):275–283.
26. Lee BH, Tudares MA, Nguyen CQ. Sjögren's syndrome: an old tale with a new twist. *Arch Immunol Ther Exp (Warsz).* 2009;57(1):57–66.
27. Obata H, Yamamoto S, Horiuchi H, Machinami R. Histopathologic study of human lacrimal gland. Statistical analysis with special reference to aging. *Ophthalmology.* 1995;102:678–686.
28. Sullivan DA, Krenzer KL, Sullivan BD, et al. Does androgen insufficiency cause lacrimal gland inflammation and aqueous tear deficiency? *Invest Ophthalmol Vis Sci.* 1999;40:1261–1265.
29. Sullivan DA, Sullivan BD, Evans JE, et al. Androgen deficiency, Meibomian gland dysfunction, and evaporative dry eye. *Ann N Y Acad Sci.* 2002;966:211–222.
30. Mantelli F, Moretti C, Micera A, Bonini S. Conjunctival mucin deficiency in complete androgen insensitivity syndrome (CAIS). *Graefes Arch Clin Exp Ophthalmol.* 2006 Nov 2.
31. Schaumberg DA, Buring JE, Sullivan DA, Dana MR. Hormone replacement therapy and dry eye syndrome. *JAMA.* 2001;286(17):2114–2119.
32. Sullivan DA, Wickham LA, Rocha EM, Kelleher RS, da Silveira LA, Toda I. Influence of gender, sex steroid hormones, and the hypothalamic-pituitary axis on the structure and function of the lacrimal gland. *Adv Exp Med Biol.* 1998;438:11–42.
33. Gurwood AS, Gurwood I, Gubman DT, Brzezicki LJ. Idiosyncratic ocular symptoms associated with the estradiol transdermal estrogen replacement patch system. *Optom Vis Sci.* 1995;72:29–33.
34. Nagler RM, Pollack S. Sjögren's syndrome induced by estrogen therapy. *Semin Arthritis Rheum.* 2000;30:209–214.
35. Uncu G, Avci R, Uncu Y, Kaymaz C, Develioğlu O. The effects of different hormone replacement therapy regimens on tear function, intraocular pressure and lens opacity. *Gynecological Endocrinology.* 2006;22:501–505.
36. Erdem U, Ozdegirmenci O, Sobaci E, Sobaci G, Göktolga U, Dagli S. Maturitas. Dry eye in post-menopausal women using hormone replacement therapy. *Maturitas.* 2007;20;56:257–262.
37. Moore BD. Lacrimal system abnormalities. *Optom Vis Sci.* 1994;71(3):182–183.
38. Smith RS, Maddox SF, Collins BE. Congenital alacrima. *Arch Ophthalmol.* 1968;79(1):45–48.
39. Gold-von Simson G, Axelrod FB. Familial dysautonomia: update and recent advances. *Curr Probl Pediatr Adolesc Health Care.* 2006;36:218–237.
40. James DG, Anderson R, Langley D, Ainslie D. Ocular sarcoidosis. *Br J Ophthalmol.* 1964;48:461–470.
41. Heath P. Ocular lymphomas. *Trans Am Ophthalmol Soc.* 1948;46:385–398.
42. Fox RI. Systemic diseases associated with dry eye. *Int Ophthalmol Clin.* 1994;34(1):71–87.
43. Itescu S. Diffuse infiltrative lymphocytosis syndrome in human immunodeficiency virus infection – a Sjögren's-like disease. *Rheum Dis Clin North Am.* 1991;17(1):99–115.
44. Lucca JA, Farris RL, Bielory L, Caputo AR. Keratoconjunctivitis sicca in male patients infected with human immunodeficiency virus type 1. *Ophthalmology.* 1990;97(8):1008–1010.
45. Itescu S, Brancato LJ, Buxbaum J, et al. A diffuse infiltrative CD8 lymphocytosis syndrome in human immunodeficiency virus (HIV) infection: a host immune response associated with HLA-DR5. *Ann Intern Med.* 1990;112:3–10.
46. Pflugfelder SC, Crouse CA, Monroy D, et al. Epstein-Barr virus and the lacrimal gland pathology of Sjögren's syndrome. *Am J Pathol.* 1993;143(1):49–64.
47. Battat L, Macri A, Dursun D, Pflugfelder SC. Effects of laser in situ keratomileusis on tear production, clearance, and the ocular surface. *Ophthalmology.* 2001;108:1230–1235.
48. Jordan A, Baum J. Basic tear flow. Does it exist? *Ophthalmology.* 1980;87:920.
49. Goebbels M. Tear secretion and tear film function in insulin dependent diabetics. *Br J Ophthalmol.* 2000;84:19–21.
50. Kaiserman I, Kaiserman N, Nakar S, Vinker S. Dry eye in diabetic patients. *Am J Ophthalmol.* 2005;139:498–503.
51. Cavanagh HD, Colley AM. The molecular basis of neurotrophic keratitis. *Acta Ophthalmol Suppl.* 1989;192:115–134.
52. Heigle TJ, Pflugfelder SC. Aqueous tear production in patients with neurotrophic keratitis. *Cornea.* 1996;15:135–138.
53. Lambiase A, Rama P, Bonini S, et al. Topical treatment with nerve growth factor for corneal neurotrophic ulcers. *N Engl J Med.* 1998;338:1174–1180.
54. Yamada N, Yanai R, Inui M, Nishida T. Sensitizing effect of substance P on corneal epithelial migration induced by IGF-1, fibronectin, or interleukin-6. *Invest Ophthalmol Vis Sci.* 2005;46:833–839.
55. Moss SE, Klein R, Klein BE. Incidence of dry eye in an older population. *Arch Ophthalmol.* 2004;122: 369–373.
56. Foulks G, Bron AJ. A clinical description of meibomian gland dysfunction. *Ocul Surf.* 2003:107–126.
57. Bron AJ, Tiffany JM. The contribution of Meibomian disease to dry eye. *Cornea.* 2004;2:149–164.
58. Abelson MB, Ousler GW III, Nally LA, et al. Alternative reference values for tear film break up time in normal and dry eye populations. *Adv Exp Med Biol.* 2002;506(Pt B):121–125.
59. Tsubota K, Nakamori K. Effects of ocular surface area and blink rate on tear dynamics. *Arch Ophthalmol.* 1995;113:155–158.
60. Nakamori K, Odawara M, Nakajima T, et al. Blinking is controlled primarily by ocular surface conditions. *Am J Ophthalmol.* 1997;124:24–30.
61. Lawrence MS, Redmond DE Jr, Elsworth JD, et al. The D1 receptor antagonist, SCH23390, induces signs of Parkinsonism in African green monkeys. *Life Sci.* 1991;49:PL229–PL234.
62. Biousse V, Skibell BC, Watts RL, et al. Ophthalmologic features of Parkinson's disease. *Neurology.* 2004;62:177–180.
63. Tamer C, Melek IM, Duman T, Oksuz H. Tear film tests in Parkinson's disease patients. *Ophthalmology.* 2005;112:1795.
64. Tei M, Spurr-Michaud SJ, Tisdale AS, Gipson IK. Vitamin A deficiency alters the expression of mucin genes by the rat ocular surface epithelium. *Invest Ophthalmol Vis Sci.* 2000;41:82–88.
65. Hori Y, Spurr-Michaud S, Russo CL, et al. Differential regulation of membrane-associated mucins in the human ocular surface epithelium. *Invest Ophthalmol Vis Sci.* 2004;45:114–122.
66. Sommer A, Emran N. Tear production in a vitamin A responsive xerophthalmia. *Am J Ophthalmol.* 1982;93:84–87.
67. Pisella PJ, Pouliquen P, Baudouin C. Prevalence of ocular symptoms and signs with preserved and preservative free glaucoma medication. *Br J Ophthalmol.* 2002;86:418–423.
68. Nichols JJ, Sinnott LT. Tear film, contact lens, and patient-related factors associated with contact lens-related dry eye. *Invest Ophthalmol Vis Sci.* 2006;47:1319–1328.

69. Methodologies to diagnose and monitor dry eye disease: report of the Diagnostic Methodology Subcommittee of the International Dry Eye WorkShop (2007). *Ocul Surf.* 2007;5:108–152.
70. Nichols KK, Nichols JJ, Mitchell GL. The lack of association between signs and symptoms in patients with dry eye disease. *Cornea.* 2004;23:762–770.
71. De Paiva CS, Pflugfelder SC. Corneal epitheliopathy of dry eye induces hyperesthesia to mechanical air jet stimulation. *Am J Ophthalmol.* 2004; 137(1):109–115.
72. Rosenthal P, Baran I, Jacobs DS. Corneal pain without stain: is it real? *Ocul Surf.* 2009;7(1):28–40.
73. van Bijsterveld OP. Diagnostic tests in the Sicca syndrome. *Arch Ophthalmol.* 1969;82:10–14.
74. Pflugfelder SC, Tseng SC, Yoshino K, Monroy D, Felix C, Reis BL. Correlation of goblet cell density and mucosal epithelial membrane mucin expression with rose bengal staining in patients with ocular irritation. *Ophthalmology.* 1997;104:223–235.
75. Tomlinson A, Khanal S, Ramaesh K, Diaper C, McFadyen A. Tear film osmolarity: determination of a referent for dry eye diagnosis. *Invest Ophthalmol Vis Sci.* 2006;47:4309–4315.
76. Bron AJ. Diagnosis of dry eye. *Surv Ophthalmol.* 2001;45(suppl 2):S221–S226.
77. Nelson JD. Diagnosis of keratoconjunctivitis sicca. *Int Ophthalmol Clin.* 1994;34:37–56.
78. Prause JU, Frost-Larsen K, Hoj L, et al. Lacrimal and salivary secretion in Sjögren's syndrome: the effect of systemic treatment with bromhexine. *Acta Ophthalmol. (Copenh).* 1984;62:489–497.
79. Watson RR, Reyes MA, McMurray DN. Influence of malnutrition on the concentration of IgA, lysozyme, amylase and aminopeptidase in children's tears. *Proc Soc Exp Biol Med.* 1978;157:215–219.
80. McCollum CJ, Foulks GN, Bodner B, et al. Rapid assay of lactoferrin in keratoconjunctivitis sicca. *Cornea.* 1994;13:505–508.
81. Jones LT. The lacrimal secretory system and its treatment. *Am J Ophthalmol.* 1966;62:47–60.
82. Serin D, Karshoglu S, Kyan A, Alagoz G. A simple approach to the repeatability of the Schirmer test without anesthesia: eyes open or closed? *Cornea.* 2007; 26:903–906.
83. Macri A, Pflugfelder S. Correlation of the Schirmer 1 and fluorescein clearance tests with the severity of corneal epithelial and eyelid disease. *Arch Ophthalmol.* 2000;118:1632–1638.
84. Labetoulle M, Mariette X, Joyeau L, Baudouin C, Kirsch O, Offret H, Frau E. The phenol red thread first results for the assessment of the cut-off value in ocular sicca syndrome. *J Fr Ophtalmol.* 2002; 25:674–680.
85. Afonso AA, Monroy D, Stern ME, Feuer WJ, Tseng SC, Pflugfelder SC. Correlation of tear fluorescein clearance and Schirmer test scores with ocular irritation symptoms. *Ophthalmology.* 1999;106:803–810.
86. Yokoi N, Komuro A. Non-invasive methods of assessing the tear film. *Exp Eye Res.* 2004; 78: 399–407.
87. Yokoi N, Bron AJ, Tiffany JM, Maruyama K, Komuro A, Kinoshita S. Relationship between tear volume and tear meniscus curvature. *Arch Ophthalmol.* 2004;122:1265–1269.
88. Mainstone JC, Bruce AS, Golding TR. Tear meniscus measurement in the diagnosis of dry eye. *Curr Eye Res.* 1996;15:653–661.
89. Yokoi N, Takehisa Y, Kinoshita S. Correlation of tear lipid layer interference patterns with the diagnosis and severity of dry eye. *Am J Ophthalmol.* 1996;122:818–824.
90. Khanal S, Tomlinson A, McFadyen A, Diaper C, Ramaesh K. Dry eye diagnosis. *Invest Ophthalmol Vis Sci.* 2008;49:1407–1414.
91. Asbell PA. Increasing importance of dry eye syndrome and the ideal artificial tear: consensus views from a roundtable discussion. *Curr Med Res Opin.* 2006;22:2149–2157.
92. Management and therapy of dry eye disease: report of the Management and Therapy Subcommittee of the International Dry Eye WorkShop (2007). *Ocul Surf.* 2007;5:163–178.
93. Chen Z, Tong L, Li Z, Yoon KC, Qi H, Farley W, Li DQ, Pflugfelder SC. Hyperosmolarity-induced cornification of human corneal epithelial cells is regulated by JNK MAPK. *Invest Ophthalmol Vis Sci.* 2008;49(2): 539–549.
94. Argueso P, Tisdale A, Spurr-Michaud S, et al. Mucin characteristics of human corneal-limbal epithelial cells that exclude the rose bengal anionic dye. *Invest Ophthalmol V is Sci.* 2006;47:113–119.
95. Prabhasawat P, Tesavibul N, Kasetsuwan N. Performance profile of sodium hyaluronate in patients with lipid tear deficiency: randomised, double-blind, controlled, exploratory study. *Br J Ophthalmol.* 2007;91:47–50.
96. Taban M, Chen B, Perry JD. Update on punctal plugs. *Compr Ophthalmol Update.* 2006;7:205–212; discussion 213–214.
97. Kaido M, Ishida R, Dogru M, Tamaoki T, Tsubota K. Efficacy of punctum plug treatment in short break-up time dry eye. *Optom Vis Sci.* 2008; 85(8):758–763.
98. Boldin I, Klein A, Haller-Schober EM, Horwath-Winter J. Long-term follow-up of punctal and proximal canalicular stenoses after silicone punctal plug treatment in dry eye patients. *Am J Ophthalmol.* 2008; 146(6):968–972.e1.
99. Pullum KW, Whiting MA, Buckley RJ. Scleral contact lenses: the expanding role. *Cornea.* 2005;24:269–277.
100. Tauber J, Davitt WF, Bokosky JE, et al. Double-masked, placebo-controlled safety and efficacy trial of diquafosol tetrasodium (INS365) ophthalmic solution for the treatment of dry eye. *Cornea.* 2004;23:784–792 (CS1)
101. Mundasad MV, Novack GD, Allgood VE, et al. Ocular safety of INS365 ophthalmic solution: a P2Y(2) agonist in healthy subjects. *J Ocul Pharmacol Ther.* 2001;17:173–179.
102. Murakami T, Fujihara T, Horibe Y, Nakamura M. Diquafosol elicits increases in net Cl^- transport through P2Y2 receptor stimulation in rabbit conjunctiva. *Ophthalmic Res.* 2004;36:89–93.
103. Murakami T, Fujita H, Fujihara T, et al. Novel noninvasive sensitive determination of tear volume changes in normal cats. *Ophthalmic Res.* 2002;34:371–374.
104. Yerxa BR, Mundasad M, Sylvester RN, et al. Ocular safety of INS365 ophthalmic solution, a P2Y2 agonist, in patients with mild to moderate dry eye disease. *Adv Exp Med Biol.* 2002;506(Pt B):1251–1257.
105. Tsifetaki N, Kitsos G, Paschides CA, et al. Oral pilocarpine for the treatment of ocular symptoms in patients with Sjögren's syndrome: a randomised 12 week controlled study. *Ann Rheum Dis.* 2003;62: 1204–1207.
106. Vivino FB, Al-Hashimi I, Khan Z, et al, for the P92-01 Study Group. Pilocarpine tablets for the treatment of dry mouth and dry eye symptoms in patients with Sjögren's syndrome: a randomized, placebo-controlled, fixed-dose, multicenter trial. *Arch Intern Med.* 1999;159: 174–181.
107. Ono M, Takamura E, Shinozaki K, et al. Therapeutic effect of cevimeline on dry eye in patients with Sjögren's syndrome: a randomized, double blind clinical study. *Am J Ophthalmol.* 2004;138:6–17.
108. Schulze SD, Sekundo W, Kroll P. Autologous serum for the treatment of corneal epithelial abrasions in diabetic patients undergoing vitrectomy. *Am J Ophthalmol.* 2006;142:207–211.
109. Kojima T, Higuchi A, Goto E, Matsumoto Y, Dogru M, Tsubota K. Autologous serum eye drops for the treatment of dry eye diseases. *Cornea.* 2008;27(Suppl 1):S25–S30.
110. Geerling G, Raus P, Murube J. Minor salivary gland transplantation. *Dev Ophthalmol.* 2008;41:243–254.
111. Kim EC, Choi JS, Joo CK. A comparison of vitamin A and cyclosporine A 0.05% eye drops for treatment of dry eye syndrome. *Am J Ophthalmol.* 2009;147(2):206–213.
112. Ridder WH 3rd. Ciclosporin use in dry eye disease patients. *Expert Opin Pharmacother.* 2008;9:3121–3128.
113. Jap A, Chee SP. Immunosuppressive therapy for ocular diseases. *Curr Opin Ophthalmol.* 2008;19(6):535–540.
114. Perry HD, Solomon R, Donnenfeld ED, Perry AR, Wittpenn JR, Greenman HE, Savage HE. Evaluation of topical cyclosporine for the treatment of dry eye disease. *Arch Ophthalmol.* 2008;126(8):1046–1050.
115. Pflugfelder SC, Maskin SL, Anderson B, et al. A randomized, double-masked, placebo-controlled, multicenter comparison of loteprednol etabonate ophthalmic suspension, 0.5% , and placebo for treatment of keratoconjunctivitis sicca in patients with delayed tear clearance. *Am J Ophthalmol.* 2004;138:444–457.
116. Sainz de la Maza Serra SM, Simon Castellvi C, Kabbani O. Nonpreserved topical steroids and punctal occlusion for severe keratoconjunctivitis sicca. *Arch Soc Esp Oftalmol.* 2000;75:751–756.
117. Marsh P, Pflugfelder SC. Topical nonpreserved methylprednisolone therapy for keratoconjunctivitis sicca in Sjögren's syndrome. *Ophthalmology.* 1999;106:811–816.
118. Tabbara KF, Frayha RA. Alternate-day steroid therapy for patients with primary Sjogren's syndrome. *Ann Ophthalmol.* 1983;15(4): 358–361.
119. Aronowicz JD, Shine WE, Oral D, et al. Short term oral minocycline treatment of meibomianitis. *Br J Ophthalmol.* 2006;90:856–860.
120. Lemp MA. Management of dry eye disease. *Am J Manag Care.* 2008;14:S88–S101.
121. Pinna A, Piccinini P, Carta F. Effect of oral linoleic and gamma-linolenic acid on meibomian gland dysfunction. *Cornea.* 2007;26:260–264.
122. Miljanovic B,Trivedi KA, Dana MR, Gilbard JP, Buring JE, Schaumberg DA. Relation between dietary n-3 and n-6 fatty acids and clinically

diagnosed dry eye syndrome in women. *Am J Clin Nutr.* 2005;82: 887–893.
123. Rashid S, Jin Y, Ecoiffier T, Barabino S, Schaumberg DA, Dana MR. Topical omega-3 and omega-6 fatty acids for treatment of dry eye. *Arch Ophthalmol.* 2008;126(2):219–225.
124. Albietz J, Sanfilippo P,Troutbeck R, Lenton LM. Management of filamentary keratitis associated with aqueous-deficient dry eye. *Optom Vis Sci.* 2003;80:420–430.
125. Roberts CW, Carniglia PE, Brazzo BG. Comparison of topical cyclosporine, punctal occlusion, and a combination for the treatment of dry eye. *Cornea.* 2007;26:805–809.

Chapter 37

Dacryoadenitis, Dacryocystitis, and Canaliculitis

David R. Jordan

Dacryoadenitis

Acute infectious dacryoadenitis is an uncommon, usually unilateral condition that presents with temporal right upper eyelid swelling, pain, and discharge. Patients generally feel unwell and are febrile. On examination, the upper lid typically is ptotic and has an S-shaped curve to it as a result of the inflamed lacrimal gland (Fig. 37.1A). The eyelid skin is red and swollen, while the bulbar conjunctiva is chemotic and erythematous in the superior temporal fornix where the lacrimal ductules exit (Fig. 37.1B). Discharge may also be seen in this area. The globe may be shifted inferiorly and medially, and there is generally discomfort when one tries to palpate the enlarged lacrimal gland through the eyelid. The preauricular lymph node may be enlarged. A hordeolum (stye) should be ruled out by eversion of the lid, which can help to establish the palpebral portion of the lacrimal gland as the seat of the inflammation. In its early stages, acute dacryoadenitis may also be difficult to differentiate from orbital cellulitis. Computed tomography (CT) reveals an enlarged lacrimal gland with irregular margins and no bony defect (Fig. 37.1C). CT scanning also allows one to visualize the sinuses, orbital tissues, and surrounding bone, which should be uninvolved in dacryoadenitis.

The lacrimal gland may be infected exogenously from the skin or as a result of a penetrating trauma, seeded in the course of a bacteremia or as a result of an ascending infection from the conjunctiva. The latter is most common and it is the palpebral lobe of the lacrimal gland that is most often involved.

Infectious dacryoadenitis is usually caused by bacteria. Common organisms are *Staphylococcus aureus* or *Streptococcus pneumoniae*. *Pseudomanas aeruginosa*, *Acanthamoeba*, *Actinomyces* and hematogenous spread from *Neisseria Gonorrhoeae* have been reported.[1–5] Dacryoadenitis may also be seen with some viruses.[1] Many viral infections cause asymptomatic and subclinical lacrimal gland enlargement and inflammation. In children, acute dacryoadenitis may complicate infectious mononucleosis, measles, mumps, and influenza. On rare occasions various fungi, including *Blastomyces*, *Histoplasma*, *Nocardia*, and *Sporotrichum*, may infect the lacrimal gland.[1] Tuberculosis, leprosy, and syphilis can also rarely involve the lacrimal gland.[6–8] Dacryoadenitis secondary to Lyme disease has recently been reported.[9]

Therapy is usually initiated with an oral antibiotic effective against *Staphylococcus* and *Streptococcus* such as cloxicillin (500 mg orally four times a day for 10 days) or an oral cephalosporin such as cephalexin (250 mg to 1 g orally four times a day). For those allergic to penicillin, clindamycin (150–300 mg orally every 6 hours) or erythromycin (500 mg orally four times a day) are also effective. Any conjunctival discharge should be cultured. Hospitalization and intravenous antibiotic therapy is rarely required. Hot compresses and a topical broad-spectrum antibiotic drop such as sulfacetamide, optimyxin, or fucithalmic viscous drops are also helpful. If the infection is thought to be viral in origin, the patient's systemic condition may help with the diagnosis. A complete blood count and appropriate viral antibody titers are useful.

Complications secondary to infectious dacryoadenitis are rare. If a lacrimal gland abscess develops, abscess incision and drainage are indicated.

Nonspecific orbital inflammation (previously known as pseudotumor) may also present acutely as lacrimal gland inflammation and, at times, the clinical picture may be difficult to differentiate from infectious dacryoadenitis.[1,10–12] The patient may have all of the clinical findings one sees with a true infection of the gland: pain; erythema; S-shaped swollen upper lid; tender, palpable lacrimal gland and superotemporal conjunctival chemosis. The CT scan appearance may be identical. With infectious dacryoadenitis, patients commonly have a fever and a feeling of malaise, whereas those with the nonspecific inflammation generally have pain as the major symptom. If there is doubt about whether one is dealing with an infectious or a noninfectious process, it may be preferable to treat the patient with an antibiotic over the first 24–48 hours in conjunction with pain relievers. If there is little or no improvement at this time, a biopsy is required to confirm the diagnosis followed by a course of corticosteroids. Nonspecific idiopathic orbital inflammation involving the lacrimal gland is generally quite sensitive to oral steroids[1,10,12] and should show a response within 24 hours. An initial dose is 60–70 mg prednisone orally, tapered by 5 mg every second day until gone. Antiinflammatory medication such as naproxen or indomethacin may also be of benefit in the treatment. They may be started as the initial medication in a typical case of dacryoadenitis or if there is any flare-up upon tapering of the oral steroids. The usual

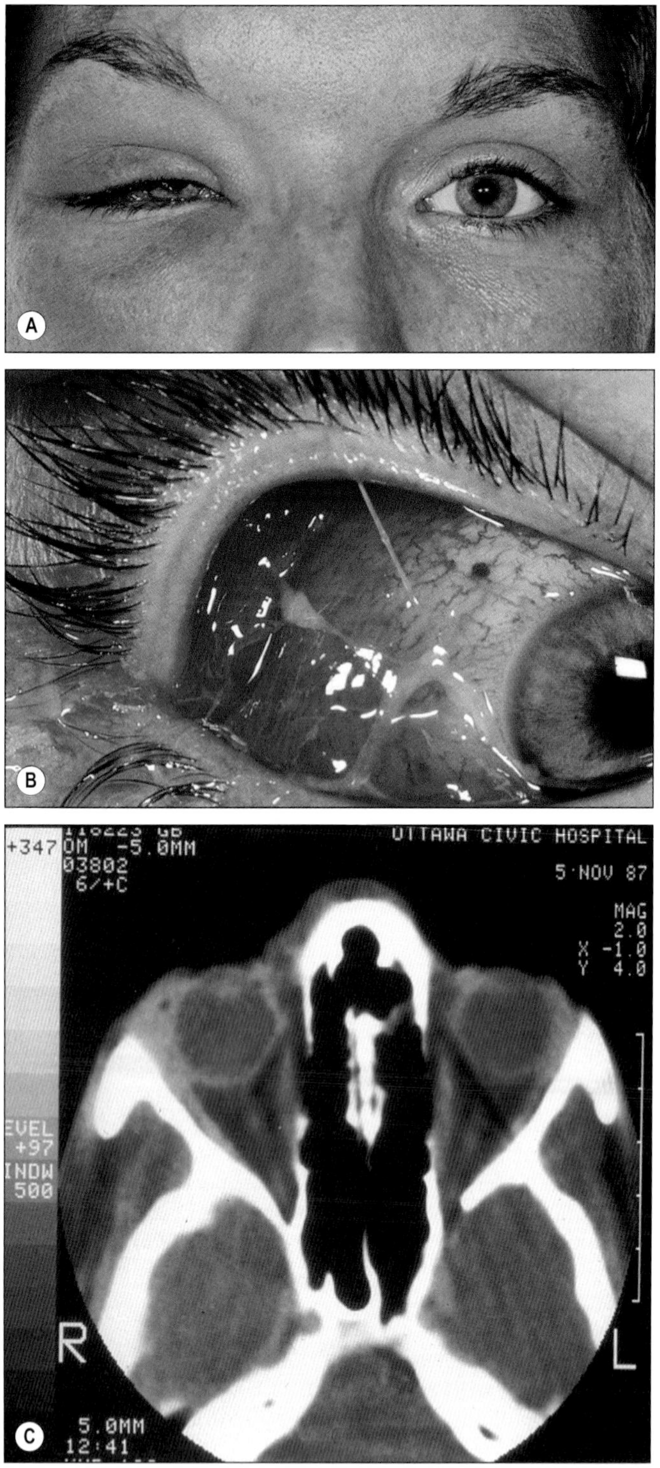

Fig. 37.1 Dacryoadenitis. (**A**) Acute dacryoadenitis with ptosis, upper lid swelling, and conjunctival chemosis. The lateral lid has more droopiness than the medial lid (S-shaped curve) because of the swollen lacrimal gland. (**B**) Temporal bulbar conjunctiva is chemotic and erythematous, with discharge coming from the lacrimal ductule region superiorly and temporally. (**C**) Note enlarged lacrimal gland on right.

dose is naproxen 250 mg twice daily, increasing up to 250 mg four times daily, or indomethacin 25 mg twice daily, increasing up to 25 mg four times daily if needed. If the inflammatory process does not resolve or returns when the steroid course is finished, the addition of methotrexate or azathioprine may be added to help settle the inflammatory process as well as helping to avoid some of the complications associated with long-term steroid use.[13] However, these drugs are nonspecific in their action with respect to inflammatory disease and have potential side effects that may be unacceptable. More recently, biologic agents targeting more specific aspects of the inflammatory process have been introduced.[14] Infliximab is a chimeric (human and mouse) antibody that targets the tumor necrosis factor-α molecule. Its use in orbital inflammatory disorders such as myositis and dacryoadenitis has recently been reported.[15] Low-dose radiotherapy (2000 rads) is also available if the lesion fails to respond to corticosteroids or if the patient has a medical contraindication to the use of corticosteroids.

Dacryocystitis

Acute dacryocystitis (bacterial infection of the nasolacrimal sac) is a result of an obstruction within the nasolacrimal duct. It may begin very quickly during the course of a day and be associated with intense pain as discharge builds up and distends the nasolacrimal sac. Prompt diagnosis and initiation of treatment are important.[16,17]

Acute infection of the nasolacrimal sac may occur at any age but is more commonly encountered in infants, young adults (mid 30s), and the aged (>65 years). A distended noninfected lacrimal sac may be present at birth (congenital dacryocystocele, amniotocele, or amniocele) and is a result of amniotic fluid entering the nasolacrimal sac but not getting out due to a block at the nasolacrimal duct level and a ball-valve effect at the common duct level. The treatment of a dacryocystocele is controversial.[18] Some physicians have advocated conservative treatment with antibiotics and massage, whereas others have recommended early surgical intervention if there is not a rapid response to conservative therapy or recommended prompt surgical therapy.[18] Infants are obligate nasal breathers and airway obstruction from the dacryocystocele may occur in some patients.[19] We generally manage this condition conservatively with digital massage for 2–3 weeks. If resolution does not occur, the child becomes infected (Fig. 37.2A) or if there is any degree of airway obstruction, we move on to surgery, which involves probing the nasolacrimal system with endoscopically guided marsupialization of the dacryocystocele on the nasal side with placement of silicone tubing (stents) within the nasolacrimal system.

Simple congenital nasolacrimal duct obstruction as a result of incomplete nasolacrimal duct canalization at the level of the valve of Hasner is a more common condition than congenital dacryocystocele and few of the affected infants develop acute infections. Infants with simple congenital obstruction have a history of epiphora with mattering of the eyelids (Fig. 37.2B) and minimal if any dilation of the lacrimal sac. It is important to distinguish this common and benign condition from acute dacryocystitis, which presents in a much more dramatic fashion (Fig. 37.2A).

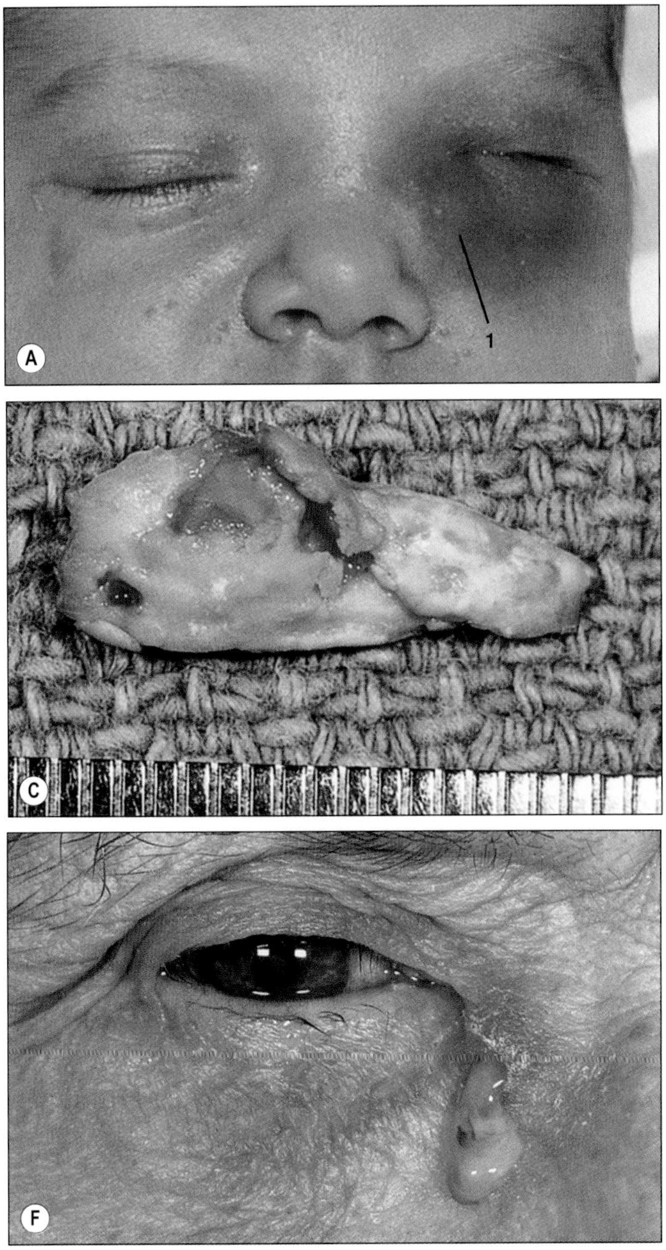

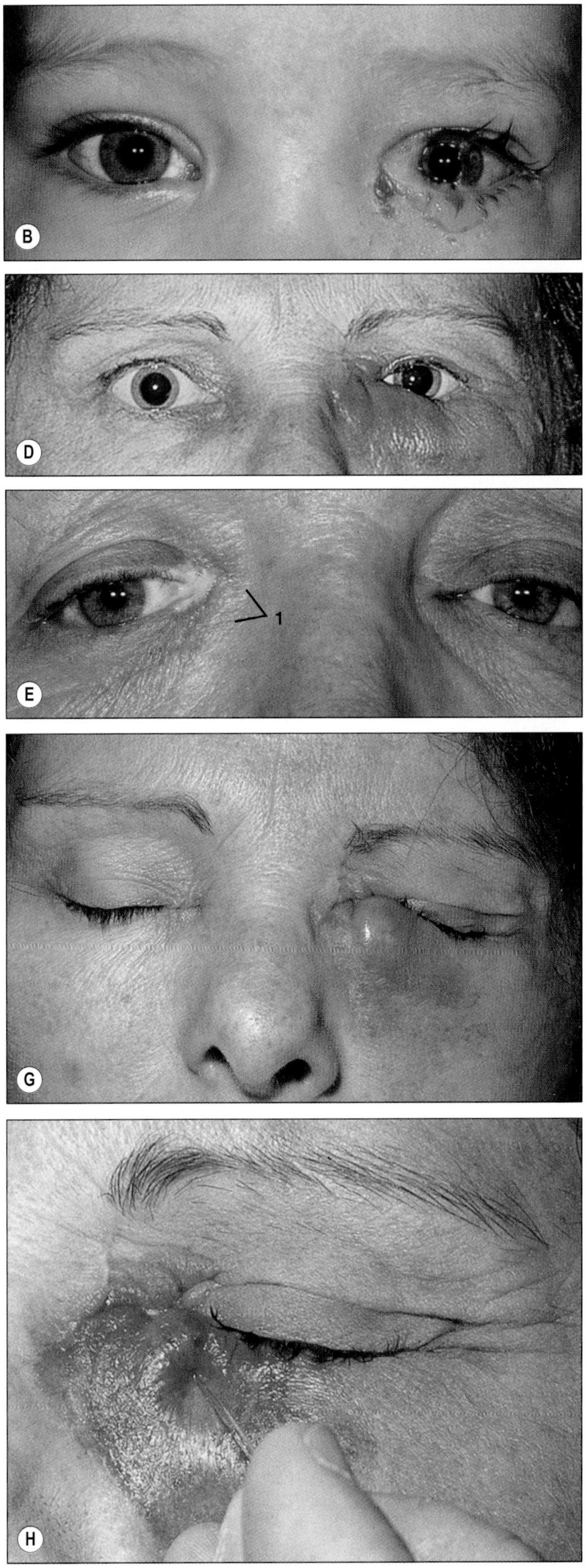

Fig. 37.2 Dacryocystitis. (**A**) Acute dacryocystitis in a 4-week-old child with redness and swelling of left upper and lower lids and a prominent nasolacrimal sac (1). (**B**) Four-year-old child with recurrent purulent discharge resulting from persistent nasolacrimal blockage. (**C**) Example of a dacryolith. (**D**) Acute dacryocystitis in a 45-year-old patient. (**E**) Chronic dacryocystitis with recurrent purulent discharge; a dilated nasolacrimal sac (1) was also present. (**F**) Chronic dacryocystitis with fistulous tract draining onto skin. (**G**) Same patient as in (**D**) developed a fluctuant pointing mass over the nasolacrimal sac. (**H**) A stab incision is being carried out.

In the newborn and young infant, it may be difficult to tell whether one is dealing with dacryocystitis, orbital cellulitis, or both. It may be preferable to hospitalize them for intravenous antibiotic therapy to decrease the chances of orbital abscess or sepsis from occurring. Cefuroxime (in newborns, 30–100 mg/kg per day in two divided doses; and infants, 1 month to 12 years, 30–100 mg/kg per day in three to four divided doses) provides broad-spectrum coverage, including coverage for upper respiratory tract organisms such as *Staphylococcus aureus*, *Streptococcus pneumoniae*, and *Haemophilis influenzae*. Once an organism has been cultured, antibiotic coverage can be adjusted accordingly.

In young adults (30–40 years) and aging individuals (>65 years), any degree of nasolacrimal duct obstruction (from infection, trauma, gradual narrowing with age, etc.) permits stagnation of tears, microorganism accumulation, and desquamated cellular debris to build up within the sac, with potential development of a nasolacrimal infection. In the young adult age group, the most common cause of nasolacrimal duct obstruction is trauma or the presence of a nasolacrimal stone (dacryolith). Individuals with a dacryolith have a characteristic history; females are more commonly affected than males and are usually in their early 30s. Patients complain of a pressure sensation in the medial canthal region followed by tearing discharge and the development of a lump in the nasolacrimal sac area. This is the result of a dacryolith (Fig. 37.2C) that has blocked the tear outflow, causing retention of tears with resultant distension of the nasolacrimal sac and eventually a full-blown dacryocystitis. Symptoms may resolve before developing the dacryocystitis, and patients will be fine until it recurs. Patients generally have a history of similar episodes in the past, lasting 4–7 days and resolving either spontaneously with eye drops or occasionally with antibiotics.

Aging individuals (>65 years) usually demonstrate increasing narrowing of the nasolacrimal duct as they age (primary acquired nasolacrimal duct obstruction [PANDO]).[20] As nasolacrimal duct narrowing develops, the patient develops tearing. With further narrowing, the tearing worsens and dacryocystitis with complete obstruction may occur.

Acute infection of the lacrimal sac presents quickly with redness, swelling, and tenderness of the skin overlying the sac and just inferior to the medial palpebral ligament (Fig. 37.2A and D). Responsible organisms are generally upper respiratory tract organisms such as β-hemolytic *Streptococcus* or *Staphylococcus*. If unchecked, infection may spread into the adjacent soft tissues to become a preseptal cellulitis of the eyelid, orbital cellulitis, or abscess. The infection may also ascend the canaliculus to enter the conjunctival tissue, producing infection or hypersensitivity peripheral corneal ulcers.[21,22]

Chronic infection of the nasolacrimal sac tends to be indolent, producing symptoms of tearing and mild to moderate recurrent unilateral discharge. The patient may apply pressure over the sac, producing reflux of a mucoid or mucopurulent discharge from the punctum recurrently (Fig. 37.2E). The most common organisms responsible for infection are *Streptococcus pneumoniae* or *Haemophilis influenzae*, but various pathogens can be responsible, including other Gram-positive bacteria (*Staphylococcus* species), Gram-negative bacteria (*Klebsiella pneumoniae, Pseudomonas aeruginosa*), anaerobic bacteria (*Arachnia propionica*) and, rarely, *Mycobacterium tuberculosis*, fungi (*Candida, Aspergillus niger, Pityrosporum*), and *Chlamydia trachomatis*.

Complications of chronic dacryocystitis originate either from its reservoir of pathogens, which may cause acute recurrent dacryocystitis, infectious keratitis, or endophthalmitis in the presence of corneal trauma or intraocular surgery. Not uncommonly, the patient develops a fistulous tract draining anteriorly onto the skin (Fig. 37.2F). Medical treatment of chronic dacryocystitis is rarely curative. Dacryocystorhinostomy is the definitive procedure required to reestablish tear flow.

Generally, the diagnosis of acute dacryocystitis in the adult is clinically obvious. Treatment includes pain relief, warm compresses, and topical and systemic antibiotics. Since most of the acute infections in the adult result from Gram-positive upper respiratory organisms (*Streptococcus* or *Staphylococcus*) patients are started on cloxacillin (500–1000 mg orally four times daily), or a cephalosporin such as cephalexin (250–1000 mg four times daily) or cefaclor (250–500 mg four times daily). For those allergic to penicillin, erythromycin (500 mg four times daily) or clindamycin (150–300 mg orally four times daily) is used. If this does not improve the situation within 48–72 hours and the patient remains ill, intravenous therapy with one of the previous oral medications may be required. A broad-spectrum topical antibiotic eyedrop such as sulfacetamide, optimyxin, or fucithalmic viscous drops are also applied four to six times daily to the affected eye. If the acute infection progresses to a superficial fluctuant pointing mass and the patient is uncomfortable, surgical drainage is appropriate (Fig. 37.2 G and H). A stab incision can be made in the office or minor surgical suite with a No. 11 surgical blade. A culture is taken, and one can fill the incision tract with a broad-spectrum antibiotic ointment such as sulfacetamide, optimyxin, or erythromycin. The patient is then instructed to use hot compresses the remainder of the day and is checked the following day to ensure that symptoms are starting to resolve. Once the acute dacryocystitis settles, the majority of patients require dacryocystorhinostomy as a result of scarring within the sac caused by the infection. Rarely, the nasolacrimal system spontaneously opens and no surgery is required.

Canaliculitis

Infections involving the lacrimal canaliculus (canaliculitis), although uncommon, are often overlooked as a cause for a chronic recurrent unilateral conjunctivitis.[23] Although canaliculitis occurs more commonly in the aging population, it should also be included in the differential diagnosis of chronic or recurrent pediatric nasolacrimal duct obstruction as well.[24] Canaliculitis patients usually have a history of unilateral conjunctival inflammation and discharge despite numerous antibiotic drops and several visits to more than one physician. This chronic recurrent history with multiple visits is a clue to the correct diagnosis.

Examination of the patient with canaliculitis usually reveals some typical changes; the patient's redness is

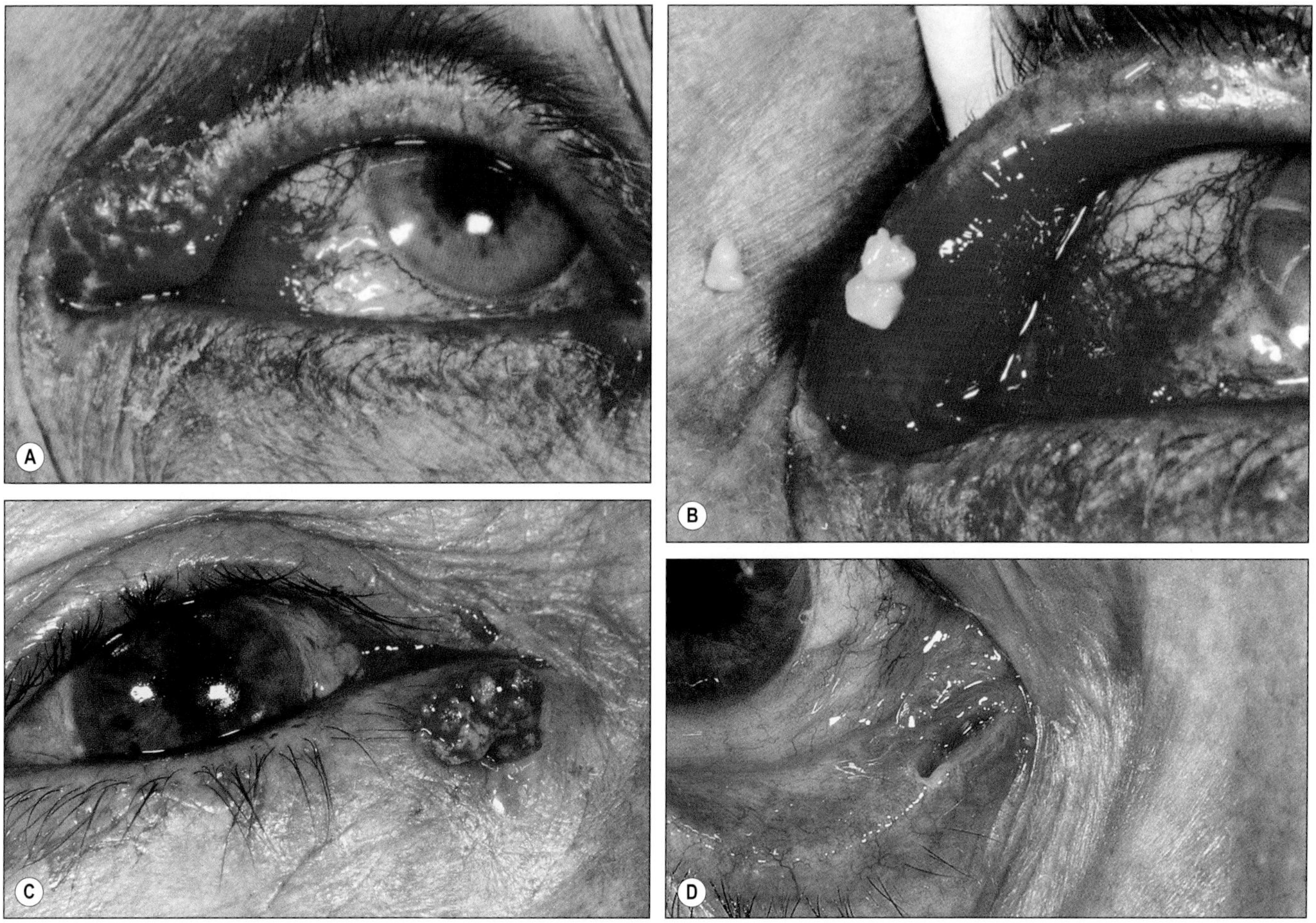

Fig. 37.3 Canaliculitis. (**A**) Canaliculitis involving the superior canaliculus. Notice the swollen canalicular area, medial conjunctival inflammation, and prominent punctum (pouting punctum). (**B**) Concretions having been milked out of the superior punctum. (**C**) A different patient with a right lower lid inferior canaliculitis had an extended three-snip punctoplasty with removal of a large canalicular stone. (**D**) After three-snip punctoplasty the inflammation in the canalicular area has settled, leaving a slitlike canalicular opening.

generally medial, involving the bulbar conjunctiva or caruncular area and possibly the medial eyelid. There is usually swelling in the area of the canaliculus, and the punctum is erythematous and raised (the so-called pouting punctum) (Fig. 37.3A). Posteriorly, directed pressure over the swollen canaliculus produces a milky yellow discharge, often with concretions (sulfur granules) from the punctal orifice (Fig. 37.3B). This confirms the diagnosis of canaliculitis.

Punctal plugs have become an important therapeutic modality in the treatment of tear insufficiency. Tear plugs may have a collar on them and are designed for placement at the punctal level while other plugs have been designed for intracanalicular placement.[25] Either type may lead to chronic canaliculitis with tearing and discharge.[25,26]

The etiology of primary canaliculitis includes viruses (vaccinia, herpes simplex, herpes zoster), a spectrum of bacteria (*Staphylococcus, Pseudomonas, Moraxella, Streptococcus pneumoniae, Actinimyces, Nocardia asteroides*), and fungi, including *Candida albicans* and *Aspergillus niger*.[15,27–35] By far the most commonly described organism has been *Actinomyces*.[32,33] This organism has been mistaken for a fungus because of its branching filaments under the microscope, but it is actually an anaerobic, nonsporulating, higher bacterium. It is part of the normal flora found in mucous membranes and has also been cited as an etiologic agent for dental caries and periodontal disease.[24,33] *Actinomyces* is a strict anaerobic Gram-positive bacillus that is usually arranged in thick filaments. Its colonies appear grossly as glistening white pearls on blood agar plates. *Actinomyces* filaments are easily fragmented into bacillary and coccoid forms with variable Gram-positive and acid-fast staining characteristics. Canaliculitis isolates with these morphologic characteristics have traditionally been assumed to be *Actinomyces* species. It is now clear, however, that other organisms may share some of these characteristics, including *Fusobacterium*,[34] *Arachnia*, and other anaerobic bacteria.[35] Similarly, the yellow sulfur granules or concretions thought to be characteristic of *Actinomyces* have been observed with other organisms, including *Fusobacterium* and *S. aureus*.[34]

Successful treatment of canaliculitis, once it is diagnosed, is surgical and involves opening the canaliculus (Fig. 37.3C and D).[29,32] The responsible organisms reside in diverticula within the dilated canaliculus and may be unexposed to antimicrobial agents administered by drops. It is essential to dilate the punctum and carry out an extended three-snip punctoplasty; that is, the horizontal cut along the canaliculus is longer than one would ordinarily make with a routine three-snip punctoplasty. The canalicular concretions are carefully removed, and the canaliculus is gently irrigated with balanced salt solution. This author strongly recommends against curetting the walls of the canaliculus or syringing with an iodine or antibiotic solution, since it is not necessary. The primary therapy is to open the canaliculus and remove the concretions. Penicillin G has been suggested as the drop of choice against *Actinomyces*, but simply opening the canaliculus and removing the concretions may be the most effective treatment in conjunction with a broad-spectrum steroid–antibiotic combination (tobramycin–dexamethasone, cortisporin, etc.) to settle the inflammation associated with opening the canaliculus. If there is a specific fungus, and the broad-spectrum drop routine is not working, one can use more specific agents such as amphotericin for *Candida* or *Aspergillus*, but this is rarely necessary.

The slit canaliculus is not repaired. In some individuals the redness and discharge settle, but they still tear. This may result from distal canalicular obstruction secondary to the canaliculitis, and, if the patient is symptomatic, a dacryocystorhinostomy may be required.

References

1. Rootman J, Robertson W, Lapoint JS. Orbital inflammatory diseases. In: Rootman J, ed. *Diseases of the orbit: a multidisciplinary approach*. Philadelphia: Lippincott; 2003.
2. Brindley GO. Dacryoadenitis. In: Linberg JV, ed. *Oculoplastic and orbital emergencies*. Norwalk, CT: Appleton & Lange; 1990.
3. Baum J. Antibiotic use in ophthalmology. In: Tasman W, Jaeger EA, eds. *Duane's clinical ophthalmology*. Philadelphia: Lippincott; 1994.
4. Mawn LA, Sanon A, Conlan MR, Nerad JA. Pseudomonas dacryoadenitis secondary to a lacrimal ductile stone. *Ophthal Plas Reconstr Surg*. 1997;13:135–138.
5. Tomita M, Shimmura S, Tsubota K, Shimazaki J. Dacryoadenitis associated with acanthamoeba keratitis. *Arch Ophthalmol*. 2006;124:1239–1242.
6. Duke-Elder S, ed. *System of ophthalmology*. vol XIII: The ocular adnexa. Part 2: Lacrimal, orbital and para-orbital diseases. St Louis: CV Mosby; 1974.
7. Bekir NA, Gungor K. Bilateral dacryoadenitis associated with brucellosis. *Acta Ophthalmol Scand*. 1999;77:357–358.
8. Van Assen S, Lutterman JA. Tuberculosis dacryoadenitis: a rare manifestation of tubeculosis. *Neth J Med*. 2002;60;327–329.
9. Nieto JC, Kim N, Lucarelli MJ. Dacryoadenitis and orbital myositis associated with Lyme disease. *Arch Ophthalmol*. 2008;126(8):1165–1166.
10. Leone CR Jr, Lloyd WC III. Treatment protocol for orbital inflammatory disease. *Ophthalmology*. 1977;92:1325.
11. Jakobiec FA, Yeo JH, Trokel SL. Combined clinical and computed tomographic diagnosis of the lacrimal fossa lesions. *Am J Ophthalmol*. 1982;94:785.
12. Mauriello J Jr, Flanagan JC. Management of orbital inflammatory disease. A protocol. *Surv Ophthalmol*. 1984;29:104–106.
13. Smith JR, Rosenbaum JT. A role for methotrexate in the management of non-infectious orbital inflammatory disease. *Br J Ophthalmol*. 2001;85:1220–1224.
14. Garrity JA, Matteson EL. Biologic response modifiers for ophthalmologists. *Ophthal Plast Reconstr Surg*. 2008;24(5):345–347.
15. Miquel T, Abad S, Badelon I, et al. Succesful treatment of idiopathic orbital inflammation with infliximab: an alternative to conventional steroid-sparing agents. *Ophthal Plast Reconstr Surg*. 2008;24(5):415–416.
16. Tannenbaum M, McCord CD. The lacrimal drainage system. In: Duane TD, ed. *Clinical ophthalmology*. Philadelphia: Harper & Row; 1994.
17. Meyer DM, Linberg JV. Acute dacryocystitis. In: Lindberg JV, ed. *Oculoplastic and orbital emergencies*. Norwalk, CT: Appleton & Lange; 1990.
18. Becker BB. The treatment of congenital dacryocystocele. *Am J Ophthalmol*. 2006;142:835–838.
19. Helper KM, Woodson GE, Kearns DR. Respiratory distress in the neonate. Sequela of a congenital dacrycystocele. *Arch Otolaryngol Head Neck Surg*. 1995;12:1423–1425.
20. Linberg J. Primary acquired nasolacrimal duct obstruction. A clinicopathologic report and biopsy technique. *Ophthalmology*. 1986;93:1055.
21. Scully RE. Case records of the Massachusetts General Hospital. *N Engl J Med*. 1983;309:1171.
22. Cohn H, et al. Marginal corneal ulcers with acute beta streptococcal conjunctivitis and chronic dacryocystitis. *Am J Ophthalmol*. 1979;87:541.
23. Briscoe D, Edelstein E, Zacharopoulos I, et al *Actinomyces* canaliculitis: diagnosis of a masquerading disease. *Graefe's Arch Clin Exp Ophthalmol*. 2004;242:682–686.
24. Park A, Morgensterrn KE, Kahwash SB, Foster JA. Pediatric canaliculitis and stone formation. *Ophthal Plast Reconstr Surg*. 2004;20(3):243–246.
25. Mazow ML, McCall T, Prager TC. Lodged intracanalicular plugs as a cause of lacrimal obstruction. *Ophthal Plast Reconstr Surg*. 2008;23(2):138–142.
26. Fowler AM, Dutton JJ, Fowler CW, Gilligan P. *Mycobacterioum chelonae* canaliculitis associated with smart plug use. *Ophthal Plast Reconstr Surg*. 2008;24(3):241–243.
27. Weil BA. Diseases of the upper excretory system. In: Milder B, Weil BA, eds. *The lacrimal system*. Norwalk, CT: Appleton-Century-Crofts; 1983.
28. Ellis PP, Bausor SC, Fulmer JM. Streptothrix canaliculitis. *Am J Ophthalmol*. 1960;52:36.
29. Jordan DR, Agapitos PJ, McCunn D. *Eikinella corrodens* canaliculitis. *Am J Ophthalmol*. 1993;115(6):823–824.
30. Jones DB, Robinson NM. Anaerobic ocular infections. *Trans Am Acad Ophthalmol Otolaryngol*. 1977;83:309.
31. Moscata EE, Sires BB. Atypical canaliculitis. *Ophthal Plast Reconstr Surg*. 2008;24(1);54–55.
32. Anand S, Hollingworth K, Kumar V, Sandramouli S. Canaliculitis: the incidence of long-term epiphora following canaliculotomy. *Orbit*. 2004;23(1):19–26.
33. McKellar MJ, Aburn NS. Cast-forming *Actinomyces isrealii* canaliculitis. *Aust NZ J Ophthalmol*. 1997;25:301–303.
34. Weinberg RJ, et al. Fusobacterium in presumed *Actinomyces* canaliculitis. *Am J Ophthalmol*. 1977;84:371.
35. Jones DB, Robinson NM. Anaerobic ocular infections. *Trans Am Acad Ophthalmol Otolaryngol*. 1977;83:309.

Chapter 38

Epiphora

Lily Koo Lin, Phillip H. Choo, Sean D. Adrean

Introduction

Tearing is essential for the eye to function normally. Tearing creates not only a protective lubricant layer, but also a refractive surface, and provides immunoglobulins and lysozyme to fight potential infection (see Ch. 3). Excess tearing or lacrimation are often both normal and necessary to flush debris away from the eye or dilute noxious chemicals that may potentially damage the eye. Furthermore, excess tearing may be caused by emotional distress.

Epiphora is an abnormal condition, which describes the chronic overflow of tears onto the cheek. There are many different causes of epiphora. These causes can be divided into three general categories: chronic overproduction of tears, outflow obstruction, and failure of the tear pump.

Etiology

Overproduction

The accessory lacrimal glands (glands of Krause and Wolfring), sometimes called the basal tear secretors, continuously produce tears. However, irritation of the conjunctiva or the corneal surface can activate reflex tearing by the main lacrimal gland. If the response is severe, this may overwhelm the lacrimal outflow system and produce overflow onto the cheek. Therefore, chronic ocular surface irritation can often produce epiphora.

Tear dysfunction can cause chronic ocular irritation, and is a cause of epiphora (see Ch. 36). Ocular surface disorders such as blepharitis, staphylococcal hypersensitivity, allergic, atopic and vernal conjunctivitis, and superior limbic keratoconjunctivitis can also cause epiphora. Conditions that deform the natural contours of the ocular surface can also cause chronic ocular irritation and overflow tearing. Some examples include a large filtering bleb, inflamed pterygium, epibulbar dermoid, conjunctival neoplasm, corneal dellen, and imbedded conjunctival or corneal foreign bodies. Eyelash and eyelid abnormalities can also cause chronic ocular irritation (Fig. 38.1).

In addition, exposure of the ocular surface can lead to epithelial breakdown, chronic eye irritation, pain, and subsequent epiphora. Causes of eye exposure are numerous but can be divided into two broad categories: those that are caused by globe malposition such as proptosis, and those caused by eyelid malposition such as lid retraction. Proptosis can be caused by an intraorbital process such as a tumor, inflammation, or thyroid eye disease. Lid malposition most commonly occurs due to involutional changes with lower lid entropion or ectropion but may occur because of thyroid eye disease, cicatricial changes after facial trauma, or post-surgical changes after facial reconstruction for tumor excision, lower blepharoplasty (especially with skin excision), and laser skin resurfacing.[1] Ptosis repair, especially in patients with congenital ptosis or chronic progressive external ophthalmoplegia, can result in chronic exposure keratopathy.[2] Lastly, facial nerve paralysis and lack of orbicularis muscle tone can cause incomplete eyelid closure and a diminished blink reflex, leading to ocular exposure.[3]

Outflow obstruction

Capillary attraction creates suction at the junction of the tear lake and the eyelid puncta. Tears are then actively pumped into the ampulla and the canaliculus with each blink.[4] From the canaliculus, the tears are pumped into the lacrimal sac through the valve of Rosenmüller and down the nasolacrimal duct to exit out through the valve of Hasner in the inferior meatus underneath the inferior turbinate. An obstruction or a decrease in flow can occur at any point along this route (Fig. 38.2). There may be a congenital absence or dysgenesis of any portion of the lacrimal outflow system.

The punctum is the first possible obstruction site to the outflow of tears. If the punctum is ectropic, stenotic, or completely closed, epiphora can occur (Fig. 38.3). Furthermore, in conjunctivochalasis, a redundant fold of conjunctiva may drape across the punctal opening, blocking the efflux of tears.[5] An enlarged caruncle may also block the punctum, and necessitate a partial carunculectomy.[6] Punctal stenosis can be caused by ocular surface cicatrizing disease, external beam radiation, and chronic exposure.

Obstruction at the canaliculus can also result in epiphora. Causes include prior canalicular injury (e.g. trauma, tumor excision, iatrogenic scarring from intracanalicular plugs), topical ocular medications,[7] and chemotherapeutic agents such as 5-fluorouracil, which can cause sclerosing canaliculitis (Fig. 38.4).[8] Docetaxel, used in the treatment of patients with metastatic breast cancer, can cause canalicular

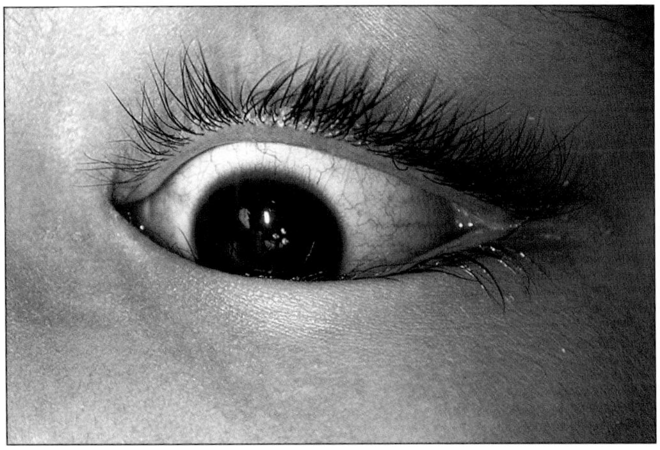

Fig. 38.1 Left lower eyelid epiblepharon causing the eyelashes to rotate in and rub against the cornea. This can cause chronic ocular irritation and overproduction of tears.

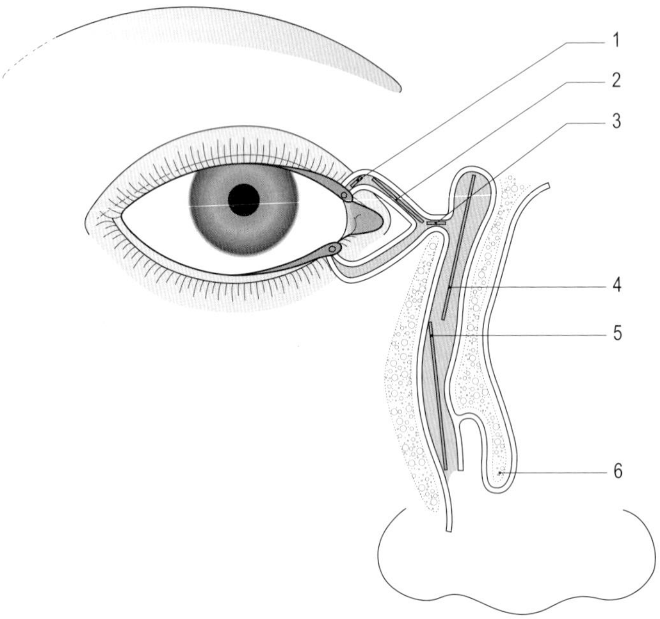

Fig. 38.2 Anatomy of the lacrimal drainage. The common duct occurs in 85% of tracts evaluated. In 15%, the canals enter the sac separately. The schematic shows the following: (*1*) vertical portion of canaliculus (2 mm); (*2*) horizontal portion of canaliculus (8 mm); (*3*) common canaliculus (3 mm); (*4*) lacrimal sac (14 mm); (*5*) nasolacrimal duct (15 mm); (*6*) inferior turbinate.

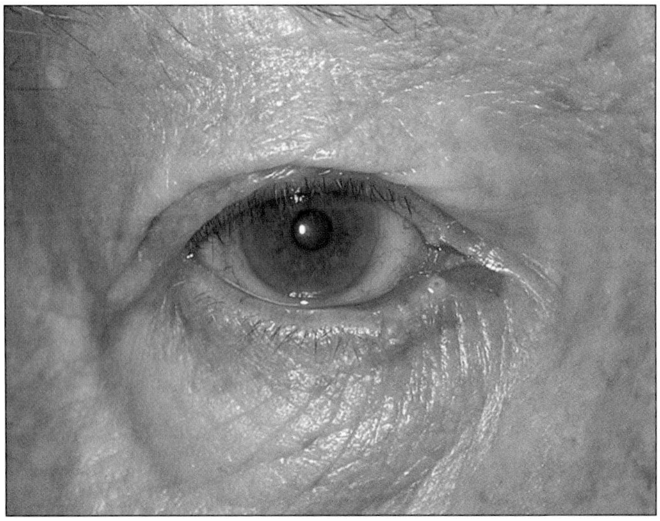

Fig. 38.3 Medial right lower eyelid and punctal ectropion as a cause of epiphora. Patient underwent repair with combined wedge resection of the lower eyelid retractors and conjunctiva underneath the punctum to turn in the punctum, and a lateral tarsal strip procedure to increase lacrimal pump function.

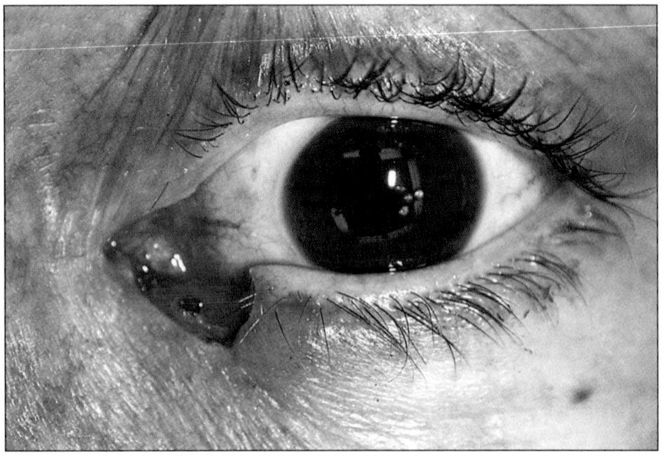

Fig. 38.4 Patient after excision of left lower peripunctal and pericanalicular basal cell carcinoma with Mohs' micrographic surgery. She underwent repair of the defect with placement of silicone tubes within the residual canaliculus.

stenosis.[9,10] Prior infectious canaliculitis can also lead to severe scarring and complete closure of the canaliculus. Lastly, a canalicular diverticulum has also been shown to cause epiphora.[11]

An obstruction can also occur at the lacrimal sac. Tumors within the sac may create resistance to flow or, if large enough, a complete obstruction. Usually, bloody discharge is present and a lacrimal mass is palpable. Malignant tumors are three times more common than benign tumors in the lacrimal sac, and the most common are epithelial tumors including inverted papillomas, squamous cell carcinoma, and adenocarcinomas.[12] Nonepithelial tumors include lymphoma,[13] fibrous histiocytoma, and melanoma (Fig. 38.5). Other conditions such as sarcoidosis and Wegener's granulomatosis may also create an obstruction in the lacrimal sac.

Primary acquired nasolacrimal duct obstruction (PANDO) is a common cause of epiphora in adults. Chronic descending inflammation from the eye or ascending inflammation from the nose and recurrent swelling of the mucous membrane within the duct may eventually lead to fibrous closure of the lumen.[14] When the nasolacrimal duct is completely obstructed, a chronic or an acute dacryocystitis can occur (Fig. 38.6). Secondary causes of nasolacrimal duct obstruction include traumatic nasal injury, iatrogenic causes such as complications from sinus surgery or orbital

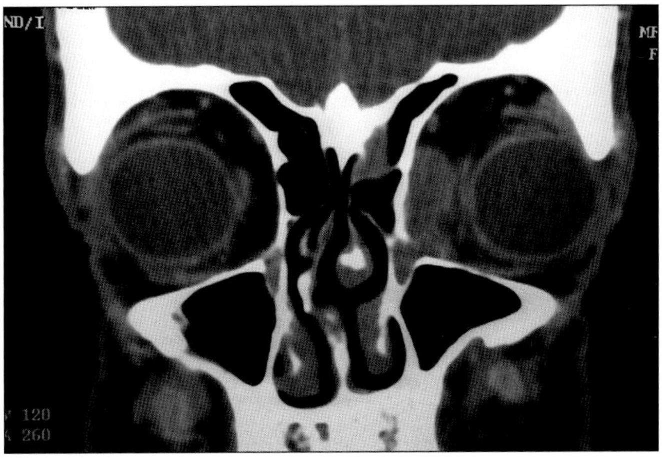

Fig. 38.5 Coronal CT image of the orbits of a patient with left-sided epiphora demonstrates a mass in the left lacrimal sac fossa. Biopsy revealed malignant lymphoma within the lacrimal sac.

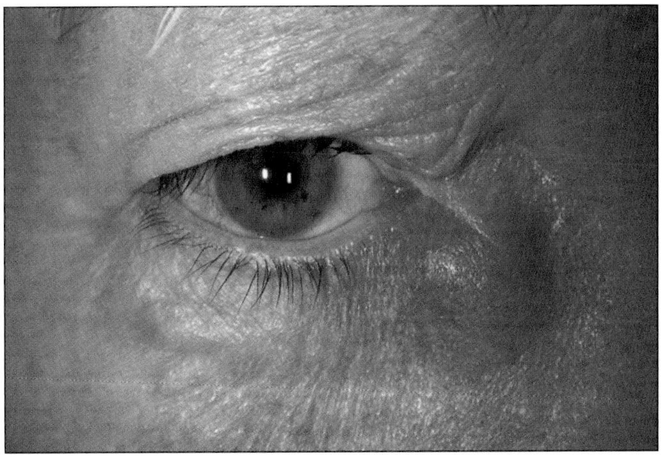

Fig. 38.6 Patient with a right dacryocystitis from PANDO.

decompression, migration of punctal and lacrimal plugs,[15] sarcoidosis, Wegener's granulomatosis, Stevens-Johnson syndrome,[16] and severe nasal polyposis.

A membranous obstruction at the valve of Hasner is the most common cause of congenital tear duct obstruction, although an obstruction can be present anywhere along the outflow system (Fig. 38.7).[17] Lastly, sinus inflammation from upper respiratory disease can obstruct the outflow at the valve of Hasner, and is exacerbated by a lateralized inferior turbinate that crowds the inferior meatus.

Lacrimal pump failure

A patient with an involutional or a paralytic ectropion may tear because of a weak or an absent lacrimal pump. The stretched or paralytic orbicularis fibers (especially the Horner's muscle)[18] of the lower eyelid are unable to create enough negative and positive pressure on the lacrimal sac, and actively pump tears out through the nasolacrimal duct.

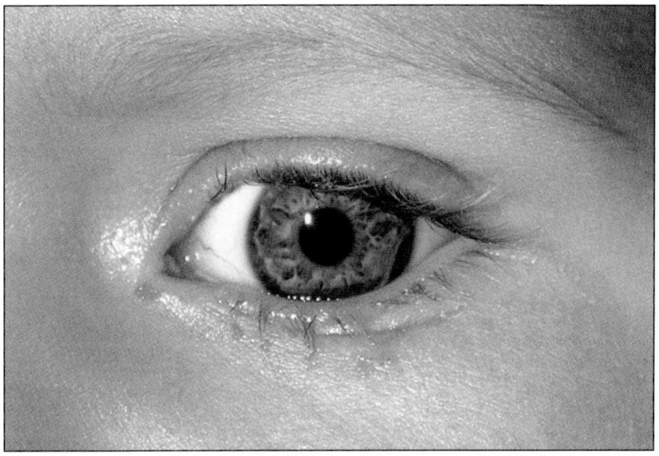

Fig. 38.7 Pediatric patient with an increased tear lake and matted eyelashes on the left side. She underwent probing of the left nasolacrimal duct and an inferior turbinate infracture at 11 months of age with complete resolution of the epiphora.

Differential Diagnosis

The differential diagnosis of epiphora includes a leaking filtering bleb,[19] especially when antimetabolites are used. Patients may also have a ruptured globe with a small penetrating foreign body that may cause leaking of aqueous, although history of trauma and physical examination are confimatory of this diagnosis. Patients may also have leakage of aqueous from a corneal ulcer that has perforated or a corneal melt from autoimmune diseases such as rheumatoid arthritis, Mooren's ulcer, or Wegener's granulomatosis. Congenital glaucoma can often present with tearing, but is also associated with myopia, photophobia, corneal opacity, and blepharospasm. Patients who recover from facial paralysis may have intermittent tearing associated with eating, caused by aberrant regeneration of the facial nerve. Injection of botulinum toxin into the lacrimal gland fossa[20] or into the lacrimal gland[21] can help to alleviate this response.

Evaluation

A thorough medical history, including current and past use of all topical and systemic medications, will often elucidate a cause for the patient's tearing. If overproduction from ocular irritation is suspected, a thorough slit lamp examination is needed as well as an eyelid examination for any eyelash or eyelid abnormalities. One should also look for cicatrizing forces, proptosis, facial nerve function, and lagophthalmos. Laxity of the lower eyelid can be assessed with both the distraction and snap tests.[22] In the distraction test, if the medial eyelid can be pulled 8 mm or more away from the globe, it is positive for eyelid laxity. The snap test is performed by pulling down on the eyelid and instructing the patient not to blink. After letting go, if the eyelid does not return to its original position and a gap is left between the globe and the eyelid margin, the test is positive for eyelid laxity and hypotonicity of the orbicularis oculi muscle.

If decreased outflow is suspected as a cause of epiphora, the lacrimal sac area should first be examined for the presence of dacryocystitis or a mass within the lacrimal sac. Next, the punctum is examined for patency and positioning, and probes can then be passed through both the upper and lower canaliculus to test for canalicular disease. Lastly, the nasolacrimal duct can be irrigated to assess patency. If a patient has some reflux of fluid and limited efflux into the nose, the patient may have a partially open nasolacrimal duct that is functionally closed. Further evaluation with either a functional dacryocystogram or Jones testing may be needed for a definitive diagnosis. Another simpler procedure to screen for PANDO is the microreflux test (MRT).[23] In this test, fluorescein dye is instilled in the inferior fornix, and the patient blinks five times. Excess fluorescein is blotted away and the lacrimal sac is massaged with the index finger in a counterclockwise fashion. Continued reflux of dye from the inferior punctum is positive for lacrimal obstruction.

In children, a dye disappearance test is probably the easiest to perform in the office to assess tear outflow.[24] This test is most helpful when only one side is affected, which may then be compared with the opposite normal side. A 2% fluorescein drop is instilled in the inferior fornix of both eyes. After 5 minutes, a cobalt blue light is used to illuminate the tear lakes. These can be examined for symmetry and only a faint line of fluorescein-tainted fluid should be seen. Otherwise, an outflow obstruction may be present.

The Jones test can be easily performed in the clinic setting, and can offer important information as well as focus the treatment plan.[25] In the Jones 1 primary dye test, 2% fluorescein dye is instilled in the inferior fornix. After 5 minutes, a cotton swab is placed into the nose, near the inferior meatus and swabbed. If dye is found on the swab, the test is positive, and signifies a normal lacrimal outflow system. If, however, no dye is recovered (a negative test result), a Jones 2 secondary dye test is performed. Normal saline without fluorescein dye is irrigated through the canaliculus and into the nasolacrimal duct. If there is complete reflux, the patient has a complete nasolacrimal duct obstruction. If there is efflux into the nose and dye-colored fluid is recovered, the Jones 2 test is positive, and signifies a functional nasolacrimal duct obstruction. If no dye-colored fluid is recovered, this may signify a punctal disorder or a lacrimal pump failure, and not a nasolacrimal duct obstruction.

To further evaluate the lacrimal outflow system, dacryoscintigraphy[26] or dacryocystography[27] can be used. Scintigraphy employs the use of a radionuclide that emits gamma radiation, such as technetium 99, and is placed in inferior fornix. A gammagram then records the gamma-emitting dye 30 minutes later. This examines the physiologic state of the lacrimal outflow system and is useful in diagnosing functional nasolacrimal duct obstruction. In a dacryocystography, radiopaque dye is instilled into the inferior fornix or is irrigated into the lacrimal sac. Dacryocystographs are taken immediately and at 10 minutes. These images can then be used to detect the level and the severity of an outflow obstruction. An orbital computed tomography (CT) is often used to further examine the lacrimal sac and surrounding anatomic structures. This test is crucial in detecting and evaluating neoplastic, inflammatory, and infectious entities in patients with lacrimal drainage obstruction.[28]

Lastly, the use of a rigid endoscope can be extremely helpful. Intranasal abnormalities such as polyps, tumors, and a deviated septum can easily be seen with endoscopy in the office. It can also be used during surgery such as an intranasal dacryocystorhinostomy (DCR) to visualize anatomic structures as well as to assist in the retrieval of silicone tubes.[29] Furthermore, nasal endoscopy can be used postoperatively to assess the effectiveness of surgery in improving lacrimal outflow.[30]

Treatment

Overproduction

Overproduction of tears is best managed by treating the underlying disorder. Treatment of external ocular disease, dry eye, and ocular surface disorders is well described in other chapters. When epiphora is caused by eyelid or eyelash abnormalities, a variety of surgical options exist. Management for a focal area of recurrent trichiasis includes epilation with forceps, electrolysis, and laser surgery.[31] When the eyelash abnormality involves a larger area of the lid margin, cryotherapy can be tried. Distichiasis can be treated with either cryotherapy,[32] lid splitting at the gray line with cryotherapy to the posterior lamella,[33] lid splitting with microhyfrecation of the eyelash follicles,[34] or tarsal resection with mucous membrane grafting.[35] The intermittent inturning of eyelashes against the cornea caused by an epiblepharon usually resolves in children as they age, and can often be followed without surgery. However, when an epiblepharon causes continuous ocular surface irritation and eye pain or impending permanent damage to the cornea, surgical repair should be performed. An infraciliary incision is made and a thin strip of eyelid skin and orbicularis excised. Deep fixation of the wound edges to the anterior surface of the tarsal plate is often effective in permanently turning the eyelashes out and away from the cornea.[36]

Entropion often causes epiphora and should be treated to alleviate eye pain and to prevent a corneal ulcer or scarring. Entropion can be divided into the following categories: congenital, spastic, cicatricial, mechanical, and involutional. Involutional entropion is the most common and is caused by a combination of four factors: override of the preseptal over the pretarsal orbicularis oculi muscle, involutional enophthalmos, eyelid laxity, and dehiscence of the eyelid retractors. The surgical procedures available to treat involutional entropion are too numerous to describe individually and adequately in this chapter. However, many of these procedures include a combination of tightening of the eyelid with a full-thickness resection or with a lateral tarsal strip procedure, reattachment of the lower eyelid retractor layer, rotation of the eyelid margin with Quickert sutures, and excision of the preseptal orbicularis oculi muscle.[37]

Ocular exposure should initially be treated with ocular lubrication. If artificial tears are not adequate, thicker drops such as carboxymethylcellulose and ointments can be tried. If patients have significant lid disease, the inflammatory component may be treated with restasis (ciclosporin 0.05%). Punctal occlusion with collagen or silicone plugs can also be tried. However, permanent occlusion with cautery or laser is discouraged since epiphora may actually worsen after the procedure. For lagophthalmos from facial paralysis, an external gold weight attached to the upper eyelid skin with either tape or tissue glue can be used to improve eyelid closure temporarily.[38] Botulinum toxin injections can also be used to treat upper eyelid retraction in patients with facial paralysis or thyroid eye disease.[39] Lastly, a temporary tarsorrhaphy should always be considered in the early treatment of patients with severe corneal exposure.

When ocular lubrication and temporizing procedures are not effective, or the underlying disease process does not improve, more invasive surgery may be required. For patients with severe proptosis, radiographic studies are needed to direct treatment. Proptosis secondary to an intraorbital tumor or inflammation usually improves with treatment of the underlying disorder. Proptosis secondary to active thyroid eye disease can initially be treated with systemic steroids.[40] However, stable proptosis often requires a surgical procedure to decompress the orbit. Most often, this is done with orbital bone removal. Soft tissue decompression with excision of orbital fat[41] can also be performed or combined with a bony decompression.

Lid malposition or retraction from cicatricial changes after trauma, thyroid eye disease, iatrogenic causes, and facial paralysis can be corrected with various surgical procedures to improve eyelid closure.[42] A müllerectomy can correct upper eyelid retraction, and a lateral tarsal strip procedure combined with a posterior lamellar spacer graft can correct lower eyelid retraction. Procedures to improve eyelid malposition should be performed after orbital decompression surgery or strabismus surgery since these may alter the patient's eyelid position.[43] A patient with lower eyelid retraction after a cosmetic lower blepharoplasty will usually not tolerate the postoperative appearance of a skin graft. Instead, the 'Madame Butterfly' procedure described by Shorr and Fallor uses a midface or suborbicularis oculi fatpad (SOOF) lift to augment the anterior lamellar defect.[44] Along with the SOOF lift, this procedure usually includes lysis of any middle lamellar scarring, placement of a posterior lamellar graft, and lateral canthal suspension. Lastly, a patient with chronic facial nerve paralysis can undergo implantation of a gold weight in the upper eyelid,[45] as well as a lateral tarsal strip procedure to improve eyelid closure. However, some patients with severe lower eyelid paralytic ectropion may require an additional SOOF lift and placement of a posterior lamellar spacer graft.[46]

Outflow obstruction

Treatment of lacrimal outflow dysfunction should be focused on the specific anatomic location.[47] Punctal stenosis can be temporarily treated with dilation. However, a punctoplasty is usually required and is effective in most cases. An ectropic punctum can be inverted back against the tear lake with various procedures. One is to excise an ellipse of both conjunctiva and lower eyelid retractors underneath the punctum.[48] Light electrocautery in the defect will achieve both hemostasis and a mild inversion of the punctum. Approximation of the retractor layer and conjunctiva with suture will further invert the punctum. Lastly, excision of redundant conjunctiva near the punctum in patients with conjunctivochalasis, and partial excision of an abnormally large caruncle, may also improve tear outflow.

Few options remain for patients with canalicular stenosis. For an isolated short segmental obstruction, a canaliculostomy with a 22-gauge intravenous catheter can be tried. The outer sleeve is advanced up to the obstruction site, and the internal needle portion is then advanced. Silicone tube stenting is required to prevent a recurrence of obstruction. Wearne et al. describe a novel approach in patients with proximal and midcanalicular scarring.[49] They describe a retrograde intubation DCR, in which a lacrimal probe is inserted from the common canaliculus towards the punctum during surgery. A slit incision is made over the end of the probe and silicone tubes are inserted through the incision site. For severe canalicular scarring, a conjunctivodacryocystorhinostomy (CDCR) with placement of a Jones tube is often required for resolution of epiphora.[50] Botulinum toxin injections to the lacrimal gland can also provide symptomatic relief and an alternative to a CDCR.[51,52]

Infants with tearing are usually followed without surgery for up to 12 months of age. The parents are instructed to massage the area over the lacrimal sac (in a superior to inferior direction) to create positive pressure at the valve of Hasner, and to open the membranous obstruction. At times, antibiotic drops, ointments, or even systemic antibiotics may be necessary to treat recurrent dacryocystitis. If tearing persists after the first 6 months of life, a probing of the tear duct can be discussed with the parents. Probing of the tear duct can be performed any time between 6 months and 12 months of age. If probing is delayed significantly beyond 12 months of age, there is an increase in the failure to sustain tear duct patency after the procedure. Therefore, older children (more than 18 months of age) may require a more invasive initial procedure such as balloon catheter dilation.[53] At the time of the probing, an inferior turbinate infracture can also be performed if there is crowding in the inferior meatus. If tearing continues to persist after surgery, further surgery is usually indicated: a second probing with inferior turbinate infracture (if not performed initially), probing with silicone tubing, or probing with balloon dacryoplasty. Lastly, if the above procedures fail, Barnes and colleagues have found DCR in children to be both effective (complete cure rate of 96%) and safe.[54]

The procedures above are usually ineffective for adult patients with PANDO, and a DCR is often required for symptomatic relief from epiphora. A DCR is also recommended in these patients to prevent a dacryocystitis (see Ch. 37). An external approach is the gold standard and provides the highest success rate. However, an endonasal DCR using an endoscope can be performed in patients who are concerned about a prominent skin scar.[55] Although the success rate was initially less with the endoscopic approach, the adjuvant use of mitomycin-C[56] during the procedure has improved long-term outcomes.[57] Furthermore, a lacrimal maintainer can also be used to achieve a large patent nasolacrimal communication.[58]

Epiphora from functional nasolacrimal duct obstruction can be difficult to resolve. All attempts to treat the causes of any underlying reflex tearing should be tried first. If no improvement is seen, simple probing, probing with adjunctive mitomycin-C,[59] probing with silicone tubes, or balloon dacryoplasty[60] can be tried. However, some patients may ultimately need a DCR to completely and permanently resolve their epiphora. Botulinum toxin injections to the lacrimal gland can provide palliative relief in patients considered poor surgical candidates.[52]

Lacrimal pump failure

Tightening of the lower eyelid can improve the tear outflow by increasing the force of the pump mechanism. A full-thickness resection can be performed, and subsequent reconstruction to shorten the eyelid. A more common approach is the lateral tarsal strip procedure.[61] Lastly, medial canthal tightening can be performed in patients with medial ectropion to improve tear flow.[62]

Summary

In conclusion, epiphora can have many different causes. These can be classified into overproduction, outflow obstruction, and lacrimal pump failure. Identifying the cause with a thorough history and evaluation including examination of the eye, eyelids, and lacrimal system is important to formulate an effective treatment plan. In some patients, the treatment may be as simple as the removal of an aberrant eyelash. In other patients, there may be multiple factors that require both medical and surgical interventions.

References

1. Sullivan SA, Dailey RA. Complications of laser resurfacing and their management. *Ophthal Plast Reconstr Surg*. 2000;16:417–426.
2. Daut PM, Steinemann TL, Westfall CT. Chronic exposure keratopathy complicating surgical correction of ptosis in patients with chronic progressive external ophthalmoplegia. *Am J Ophthalmol*. 2000;130:519–521.
3. Goldberg R, Seiff S, McFarland J, et al. Floppy eyelid syndrome and blepharochalasis. *Am J Ophthalmol*. 1986;102:376–381.
4. Doane MG. Blinking and the mechanics of the lacrimal drainage system. *Ophthalmology*. 1981;88:844–851.
5. Liu D. Conjunctivochalasis: a cause of tearing and its management. *Ophthal Plast Reconstr Surg*. 1986;2:25–28.
6. Mombaerts I, Colla B. Partial lacrimal caruncolectomy: a simple procedure for epiphora. *Ophthalmology*. 2001;108:793–797.
7. McNab AA. Lacrimal canalicular obstruction associated with topical ocular medication. *Aust NZ J Ophthalmol*. 1998;26:219–223.
8. Lee V, Bentley CR, Olver JM. Sclerosing canaliculitis after 5-fluorouracil breast cancer chemotherapy. *Eye*. 1998;12:343–349.
9. Esmaeli B, Valero V, Ahmadi MA, et al. Canalicular stenosis secondary to docetaxel (Taxotere): a newly recognized side effect. *Ophthalmology*. 2001;108:994–995.
10. Esmaeli B, Hortobagyi GN, Esteva FJ, et al. Canalicular stenosis secondary to weekly versus every-3-weeks docetaxel in patients with metastatic breast cancer. *Ophthalmology*. 2002;109:1188–1191.
11. Adjemian A, Burnstine MA. Lacrimal canalicular diverticulum: a cause of epiphora and discharge. *Ophthal Plast Reconstr Surg*. 2000;16:471–472.
12. Ryan SJ, Font RL. Primary epithelial neoplasms of the lacrimal sac. *Am J Ophthalmol*. 1973;76:73–88.
13. Yip CC, Bartley GB, Habermann TM, et al. Involvement of the lacrimal drainage system by leukemia or lymphoma. *Ophthal Plast Reconstr Surg*. 2002;18:242–246.
14. Paulsen FP, Thale AB, Maune S, et al. New insights into the pathophysiology of primary acquired dacryostenosis. *Ophthalmology*. 2001;108:2329–2336.
15. White WL, Bartley GB, Hawes MJ, et al. Iatrogenic complications related to the use of Herrick lacrimal plugs. *Ophthalmology*. 2001;108:1835–1837.
16. Auran JD, Hornblass A, Gross ND. Stevens-Johnson syndrome with associated nasolacrimal duct obstruction treated with dacryocystorhinostomy and Crawford silicone tube insertion. *Ophthal Plast Reconstr Surg*. 1990;6:60–63.
17. Cassady JV. Developmental anatomy of nasolacrimal duct. *Arch Ophthalmol*. 1952;47:141–158.
18. Reifler DM. Early descriptions of Horner's muscle and the lacrimal pump. *Surv Ophthalmol*. 1996;41:127–134.
19. Kosmin AS, Wishart PK. A full-thickness scleral graft for the surgical management of a late filtration bleb leak. *Ophthalmic Surg Lasers*. 1997;28:461–468.
20. Hofmann R. Treatment of Frey's syndrome (gustatory sweating) and 'crocodile tears' (gustatory epiphora) with purified botulinum toxin. *Ophthal Plast Reconstr Surg*. 2000;16:289–291.
21. Riemann R, Pfennigsdorf S, Riemann E, et al. Successful treatment of crocodile tears by injection of botulinum toxin into the lacrimal gland: a case report. *Ophthalmology*. 1999;106:2322–2324.
22. Stewart JM, Carter SR. Anatomy and examination of the eyelids. *Int Ophthalmol Clin*. 2002;42:1–13.
23. Camara JG, Santiago MD, Rodriguez RE, et al. The micro-reflux test: a new test to evaluate nasolacrimal duct obstruction. *Ophthalmology*. 1999;106:2319–2321.
24. Zappia RJ, Milder B. Lacrimal drainage function: 2. The fluorescein dye disappearance test. *Am J Ophthalmol*. 1972;74:160–162.
25. Jones LT, Linn ML. The diagnosis of the causes of epiphora. *Am J Ophthalmol*. 1969;67:751–754.
26. White WL, Glover AT, Buckner AB, et al. Relative canalicular tear flow as assessed by dacryoscintigraphy. *Ophthalmology*. 1989;96:167–169.
27. Jedrzynski MS, Bullock JD. Radionuclide dacryocystography. *Orbit*. 1998;17:1–25.
28. Francis IC, Kappagoda MB, Cole IE, et al. Computed tomography of the lacrimal drainage system: retrospective study of 107 cases of dacryostenosis. *Ophthal Plast Reconstr Surg*. 1999;15:217–226.
29. Yagci A, Karci B, Ergezen F. Probing and bicanalicular silicone tube intubation under nasal endoscopy in congenital nasolacrimal duct obstruction. *Ophthal Plast Reconstr Surg*. 2000;16:58–61.
30. Linberg JV, Anderson RL, Bumsted RM, et al. Study of intranasal ostium external dacryocystorhinostomy. *Arch Ophthalmol*. 1982;100:1758–1762.
31. Basar E, Ozdemir H, Ozkan S, et al. Treatment of trichiasis with argon laser. *Eur J Ophthalmol*. 2000;10:273–275.
32. Frueh BR. Treatment of distichiasis with cryotherapy. *Ophthalmic Surg*. 1981;12:100–103.
33. Anderson RL, Harvey JT. Lid splitting and posterior lamella cryosurgery for congenital and acquired distichiasis. *Arch Ophthalmol*. 1981;99:631–634.
34. Vaughn GL, Dortzbach RK, Sires BS, et al. Eyelid splitting with excision or microhyfrecation for distichiasis. *Arch Ophthalmol*. 1997;115:282–284.
35. White JH. Correction of distichiasis by tarsal resection and mucous membrane grafting. *Am J Ophthalmol*. 1975;80:507–508.
36. Woo KI, Yi K, Kim YD. Surgical correction for lower lid epiblepharon in Asians. *Br J Ophthalmol*. 2000;84:1407–1410.
37. Choo PH. Distichiasis, trichiasis, and entropion: advances in management. *Int Ophthalmol Clin*. 2002;42:75–87.
38. Shepler TR, Seiff SR. Use of isobutyl cyanoacrylate tissue adhesive to stabilize external eyelid weights in temporary treatment of facial palsies. *Ophthal Plast Reconstr Surg*. 2001;17:169–173.
39. Uddin JM, Davies PD. Treatment of upper eyelid retraction associated with thyroid eye disease with subconjunctival botulinum toxin injection. *Ophthalmology*. 2002;109:1183–1187.
40. Bradley EA. Graves ophthalmopathy. *Curr Opin Ophthalmol*. 2001;12:347–351.
41. Trokel S, Kazim M, Moore S. Orbital fat removal: decompression for Graves orbitopathy. *Ophthalmology*. 1993;100:674–682.
42. Chang EL, Rubin PA. Upper and lower eyelid retraction. *Int Ophthalmol Clin*. 2002;42:45–59.
43. Shorr N, Seiff SR. The four stages of surgical rehabilitation of the patient with dysthyroid ophthalmopathy. *Ophthalmology*. 1986;93:476–483.
44. Shorr N, Fallor MK. 'Madame Butterfly' procedure: combined cheek and lateral canthal suspension procedure for post-blepharoplasty, 'round eye,' and lower eyelid retraction. *Ophthal Plast Reconstr Surg*. 1985;1:229–235.
45. Choo PH, Carter SR, Seiff SR. Upper eyelid gold weight implantation in the Asian patient with facial paralysis. *Plast Reconstr Surg*. 2000;105:855–859.
46. Seiff SR, Carter SR. Facial nerve paralysis. *Int Ophthalmol Clin*. 2002;42:103–112.
47. Weil D, Aldecoa JP, Heidenreich AM. Diseases of the lacrimal drainage system. *Curr Opin Ophthalmol*. 2001;12:352–356.
48. Tse DT. Surgical correction of punctal malposition. *Am J Ophthalmol*. 1985;100:339–341.
49. Wearne MJ, Beigi B, Davis G, et al. Retrograde intubation dacryocystorhinostomy for proximal and midcanalicular obstruction. *Ophthalmology*. 1999;106:2325–2328.

50. Jones LT. Conjunctivodacryocystorhinostomy. *Am J Ophthalmology.* 1965;59:773–783.
51. Tu AH, Chang EL. Botulinum toxin for palliative treatment of epiphora in a patient with canalicular obstruction. *Ophthalmology.* 2005;112: 1469–1471.
52. Whittaker KW, Matthews BN, Fitt AW, Sandramouli S. The use of botulinum toxin A in the treatment of functional epiphora. *Orbit.* 2003;22: 193–198.
53. Tao S, Meyer DR, Simon JW, et al. Success of balloon catheter dilatation as a primary or secondary procedure for congenital nasolacrimal duct obstruction. *Ophthalmology.* 2002;109:2108–2111.
54. Barnes EA, Abou-Rayyah Y, Rose GEi. Pediatric dacryocystorhinostomy for nasolacrimal duct obstruction. *Ophthalmology.* 2001;108:1562–1564.
55. Woog JJ, Kennedy RH, Custer PL, et al. Endonasal dacryocystorhinostomy: a report by the American Academy of Ophthalmology. *Ophthalmology.* 2001;108:2369–2377.
56. You YA, Fang CT. Intraoperative mitomycin C in dacryocystorhinostomy. *Ophthal Plast Reconstr Surg.* 2001;17:115–119.
57. Camara JG, Bengzon AU, Henson RD. The safety and efficacy of mitomycin C in endonasal endoscopic laser-assisted dacryocystorhinostomy. *Ophthal Plast Reconstr Surg.* 2000;16:114–118.
58. Ibrahim HA, Noble JL, Batterbury M, et al. Endoscopic-guided trephination dacryocystorhinostomy (Hesham DCR): technique and pilot trial. *Ophthalmology.* 2001;108:2337–2345.
59. Tsai CC, Kau HC, Kao SC, et al. Efficacy of probing the nasolacrimal duct with adjunctive mitomycin-C for epiphora in adults. *Ophthalmology.* 2002;109:172–174.
60. Perry JD, Maus M, Nowinski TS, et al. Balloon catheter dilation for treatment of adults with partial nasolacrimal duct obstruction: a preliminary report. *Am J Ophthalmol.* 1998;126:811–816.
61. Anderson RL, Gordy DD. The tarsal strip procedure. *Arch Ophthalmol.* 1979;97:2192–2196.
62. Sullivan TJ, Collin JR. Medial canthal resection: an effective long-term cure for medial ectropion. *Br J Ophthalmol.* 1991;75:288–291.

PART VI

THE CONJUNCTIVA

Chapter 39

Squamous Neoplasms of the Conjunctiva

Michael A. Warner, Manisha N. Mehta, Frederick A. Jakobiec

The ectodermally derived nonkeratinized stratified squamous epithelia of the cornea and conjunctiva are contiguous; therefore tumors arising within them are pathologically inseparable. Although contiguous, a significant transition occurs at the corneoscleral limbus. Here, the delicate substantia propria of the conjunctiva becomes condensed into Bowman's layer, a dense acellular connective tissue layer beneath the corneal epithelium.[1] The presence of Bowman's layer provides the cornea with unique protection from deep invasion by epithelial neoplasia. Also at the limbus, the nonsquamous conjunctival cells, including mucin-producing goblet cells and most immunogenic cells, are normally excluded from the corneal epithelium. At the limbus itself, numerous melanocytes are present (see Ch. 60).[2–4] Most important, the limbal epithelium is mitotically active and is the source of all new corneal epithelial cells. If the cornea becomes traumatically de-epithelialized, epithelial cells slide in from the peripheral limbus, filling the defect. As with other body regions with a high mitotic activity (e.g. the uterine cervix), most conjunctival squamous epithelial tumors arise from the limbal zone and spread to include the adjacent conjunctival and corneal surface.[5]

During evaluation of the patient with a suspected squamous neoplasm of the conjunctiva, the clinician should obtain a careful history including time of onset, growth pattern, history of sun exposure, and history of systemic disease or immunosuppression. Clinical evaluation should include careful slit lamp examination, palpation of the orbit, and examination of regional lymph nodes. Clinical photography is also important when following suspicious lesions.

This chapter describes benign and malignant squamous epithelial neoplasms of the conjunctiva and cornea. For completeness, inflammatory and degenerative lesions and nonsquamous neoplasia are also discussed.

Benign Tumefactions

Benign hereditary intraepithelial dyskeratosis

Benign hereditary intraepithelial dyskeratosis (BHID) is an autosomal dominant, bilateral, highly penetrant disorder that usually affects individuals in their first decade of life.[6–8] Molecular analysis in two separate families has demonstrated a duplication of a gene located on chromosome 4 (4 q35).[9] It affects primarily members of the Haliwa Indians, a consanguineous kindred derived from an interracial mixture of black, white, and Native American backgrounds. The Haliwa reside in the Halifax and Washington counties of North Carolina.

The lesions are V-shaped, hyperplastic, translucent, elevations that arise at the limbus (Fig. 39.1). Foci of whiteness and dilated vessels may be present. Although the lesions do not extend centrally, corneal opacity with resultant visual loss can occur. Lesions also may arise in the oropharynx and buccal mucosa.[10]

Biopsy reveals epithelial acanthosis, parakeratosis, and dyskeratosis (premature individual cell keratinization), and the stroma usually contains chronic inflammatory cells. Atypia is not present and there is no dysplastic potential. Complete excision is the treatment of choice, although recurrences are likely because of the inherited nature of these lesions.

Pseudoepitheliomatous hyperplasia and keratoacanthoma

Pseudoepitheliomatous hyperplasia (PEH) is a benign, rapidly growing (usually arising over weeks to months) proliferation of conjunctival or corneal epithelium.[1,11,12] Lesions often occur in response to some preexisting inflammation such as a pterygium. Clinically, the lesion is a white elevated mass with a hyperkeratotic surface. A central umbilication may be present. Pseudoepitheliomatous hyperplasia can mimic ocular surface neoplasia[13] and, when arising at the limbus, differentiation from a squamous cell carcinoma can be difficult. PEH has a more rapid onset and lacks the capillary fronds seen as regular red dots in cases of squamous papillomas and carcinomas.[12]

Histopathologically, massive epithelial acanthosis, without severe cytologic atypia, is present (Fig. 39.2). Mitotic figures are often seen. The acanthotic epithelium may be pushed downward into the substantia propria, forming lobules of squamous cells with keratin whorls (invasive acanthosis). Nongranulomatous inflammatory cells are often present subjacent to the invading epithelium. The lateral margins of the lesion show a smooth transition into the surrounding normal epithelium, in contradistinction to squamous dysplastic processes in which the transition is abrupt.[12]

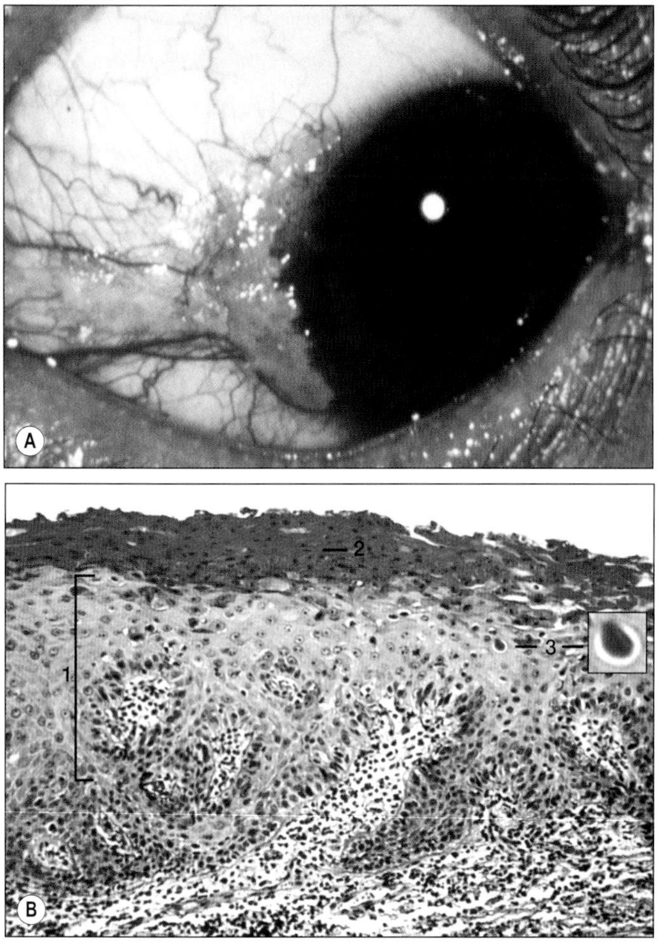

Fig. 39.1 Benign hereditary intraepithelial dyskeratosis. (**A**) A slightly elevated, translucent lesion is located at the nasal limbus. Focal vessel dilation is noted posterior to the lesion. The cornea is clear. (**B**) Histopathology shows epithelial acanthosis (thickening) (*1*), parakeratosis (nuclei within the superficial keratinized epithelial cells) (*2*), and dyskeratosis (the eosinophilic surface cells contain keratin; in addition, eosinophilic keratin is noted within individual cells just subjacent to the corneal surface) (*3*). Cellular dysplasia and atypia are not present. A chronic inflammatory cell infiltrate is present beneath the epithelium.

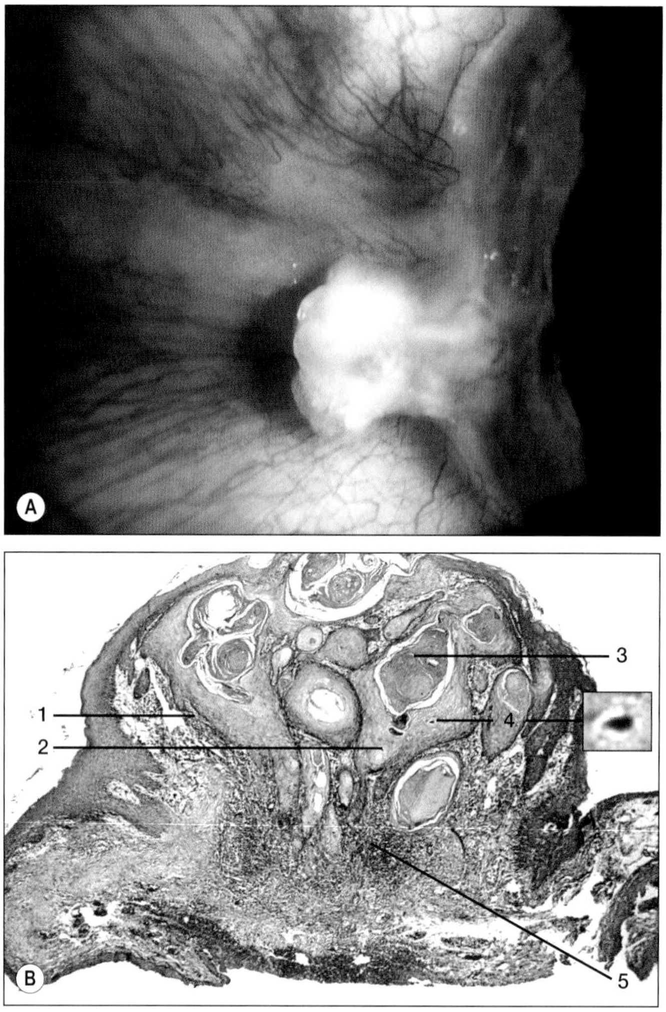

Fig. 39.2 Pterygium with pseudoepitheliomatous hyperplasia. (**A**) These lesions arise from actinically activated fibroblasts which grow onto the peripheral corneal surface. Thus, pterygia are actually subconjunctival degenerative lesions. Frequently, however, conjunctival epithelial atypia also may be present. In this case, differentiation from conjunctival intraepithelial neoplasia was difficult clinically due to the leukoplakic appearance of the lesion. (**B**) Histopathology revealed that the leukoplakic portion contained pseudoepitheliomatous hyperplasia with mild conjunctival epithelial atypia. A lobular pattern of massive epithelial thickening (acanthosis) (*1*) is present. The whorls are composed of squamous cells peripherally (*2*) with keratin debris centrally (*3*). Epithelial keratinization (dyskeratosis) (*4*) and a moderate degree of subepithelial inflammation (*5*) are present.

Although usually of cutaneous origin, keratoacanthomas also may arise in the conjunctiva and caruncle.[14–17] Histopathologically, marked acanthosis is present, but keratoacanthomas grow in a cuplike fashion about a central core of keratin debris.

These lesions are not precarcinomatous and simple excision is usually curative.

Conjunctival squamous papilloma

Conjunctival squamous papillomas are unilateral or bilateral benign lesions that may arise anywhere on the conjunctiva. These lesions are termed papillomas because of the presence of a central vascular core, which is surrounded or covered by squamous epithelium. Clinically, the lesions may be either exophytic or, much more rarely, inverted (see later). Exophytic lesions (termed *pedunculated*) may either arise from a stalk (pedunculated) or be flat, sessile, lesions (Fig. 39.3). Lesions may occur singly or may multiply. The presence of multiple lesions is especially suggestive of an infection with human papillomavirus; subtypes 6, 11, 16, 18, and 33 have been associated with these conjunctival lesions and have been detected using hybrid capture and polymerase chain reaction (PCR) assays.[18–25] Human papillomavirus 45 has also been associated with conjunctival papilloma.[26]

Clinically, the lesions may occur anywhere on the conjunctival surface. Papillomas have a transparent glistening surface through which the clinician can visualize multiple underlying capillaries that supply the connective tissue cores. These capillaries are seen as a characteristically

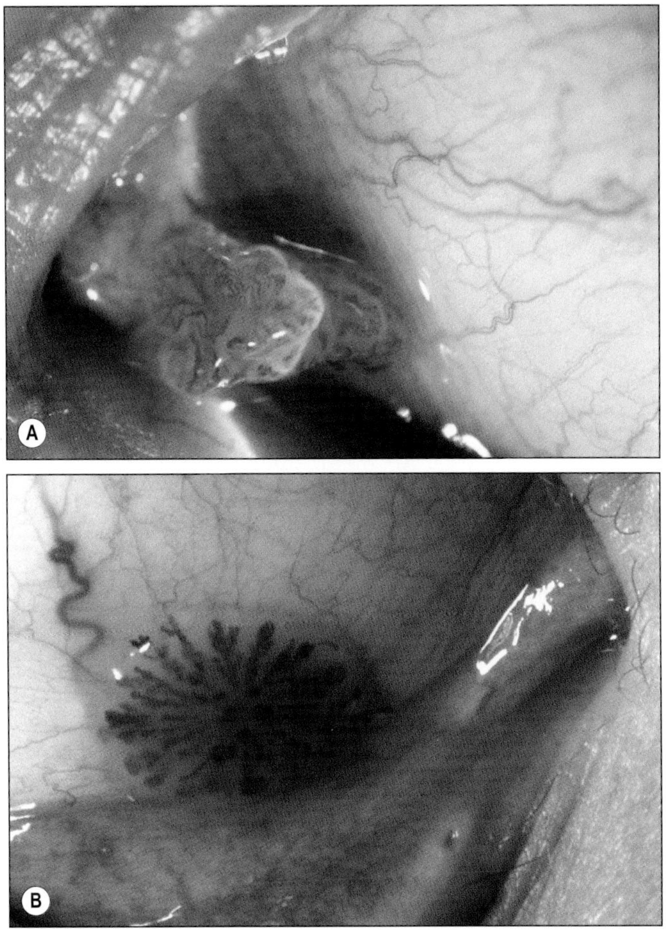

Fig. 39.3 Conjunctival squamous papillomas. Conjunctival papillomas are benign lesions that may arise anywhere on the conjunctival surface. (A) Pedunculated papillomas arise from a central stalk. Fine capillaries can be seen within the central core of the lesion. (B) Sessile papillomas are flat lesions. The papillary vascular pattern is better appreciated in this example. Submucosal connective tissue and conjunctival epithelial tissue surround each of the capillary fronds.

arranged set of red dots. When irritated, focal areas of keratinization may obscure underlying vascular details. Pigmentation may be present in darkly pigmented individuals.[27] When arising next to the cornea, a vascular pannus is present, but the cornea tends not to be invaded.

Most papillomas behave in a benign fashion, with little tendency to undergo malignant transformation. Signs of dysplasia include keratinization, symblepharon formation, inflammation, and palpebral conjunctival involvement.

Histopathologically, the lesions show acanthotic, nonkeratinizing squamous epithelium. Melanocytes and goblet cells are variably present. Viral etiology is suggested by the presence of koilocytotic cells with hyperchromatic nuclei surrounded by clear cytoplasm.

Management of papillomas is difficult and is complicated by multiple recurrences, especially in children.[21] Multiple regimens including α-interferon and mitomycin-C have been tried with variable success; the most effective treatment is simple excision with cryotherapy to the base and surround of the lesion.[28–34] Amniotic membrane transplantation can facilitate complete excisions of large lesions.[35] Oral cimetidine (Tagamet) may act as an immunomodulator and thereby provide a systemic method of treatment.[36,37]

Inverted conjunctival papillomas

Inverted conjunctival papillomas are a rare variant of the aforementioned conjunctival squamous papilloma.[38] Also known as benign mucoepidermoid papilloma of the conjunctiva, the lesion grows in an endophytic manner.[39,40] Clinically, these lesions are benign and not precancerous, in contradistinction to inverted papillomas of the nasal tract, which can be locally destructive with significant malignant potential. Histopathologically, lobules of benign epithelial cells with numerous mucin-secreting cells (hence, the term *mucoepidermoid*) invade into the underlying connective tissue layer. Cellular atypia is not present; inflammatory cells may surround the lesion. Treatment is complete excision; recurrence after excision has not been reported.

Dacryoadenoma

Jakobiec et al.[41] first described dacryoadenoma, a lesion that consists of a benign proliferation of lacrimal secretory-type cells originating from the conjunctival surface epithelium (Fig. 39.4). The lesion presented as a long-standing, asymptomatic, soft, pinkish, mobile mass on the inferior epibulbar surface. Treatment was by wide excision. Histologically, the lesion appeared adenomatous; glands were formed by downward invaginations of the surface epithelium. Thus formed, the tubules then underwent several ramifications. Both the glands and surrounding surface epithelium had similar-appearing cells: cuboidal and columnar cells, some with apical snouts, and nonstaining cytoplasmic vacuoles. There were no mitoses and an abrupt interface with the normal stratified squamous epithelium at the lesion's edges. Electron microscopy revealed large, electron-dense, apical zymogen granules and basilar whorls of rough endoplasmic reticulum similar to lacrimal acinar cells. Goblet cells and scattered myoepithelial cells were present. In contradistinction to ectopic lacrimal gland, a separate duct component and interstitial lymphocytes were absent, and goblet cells and scattered myoepithelial cells were present.

The duration of the lesion was unknown. Thus it is uncertain whether it was congenital or a later metaplasia of squamous epithelium. Because the lacrimal glands arise from conjunctiva embryologically, this lesion is likely a retained segment of conjunctiva, which at one point differentiated into lacrimal-type tissue.

Pterygia and pingueculae

Pterygia and pingueculae are solar-induced lesions that occur within the interpalpebral conjunctiva and result from deposition of abnormal elastic fibers[42] within subepithelial structures. Conjunctival intraepithelial neoplasia has been reported to arise from the site of a pre-existing pterygium[43] and the clinician should consider squamous tumefactions in the differential diagnosis when confronted with an unusual-appearing pterygium or pseudopterygium (see Fig. 39.2).

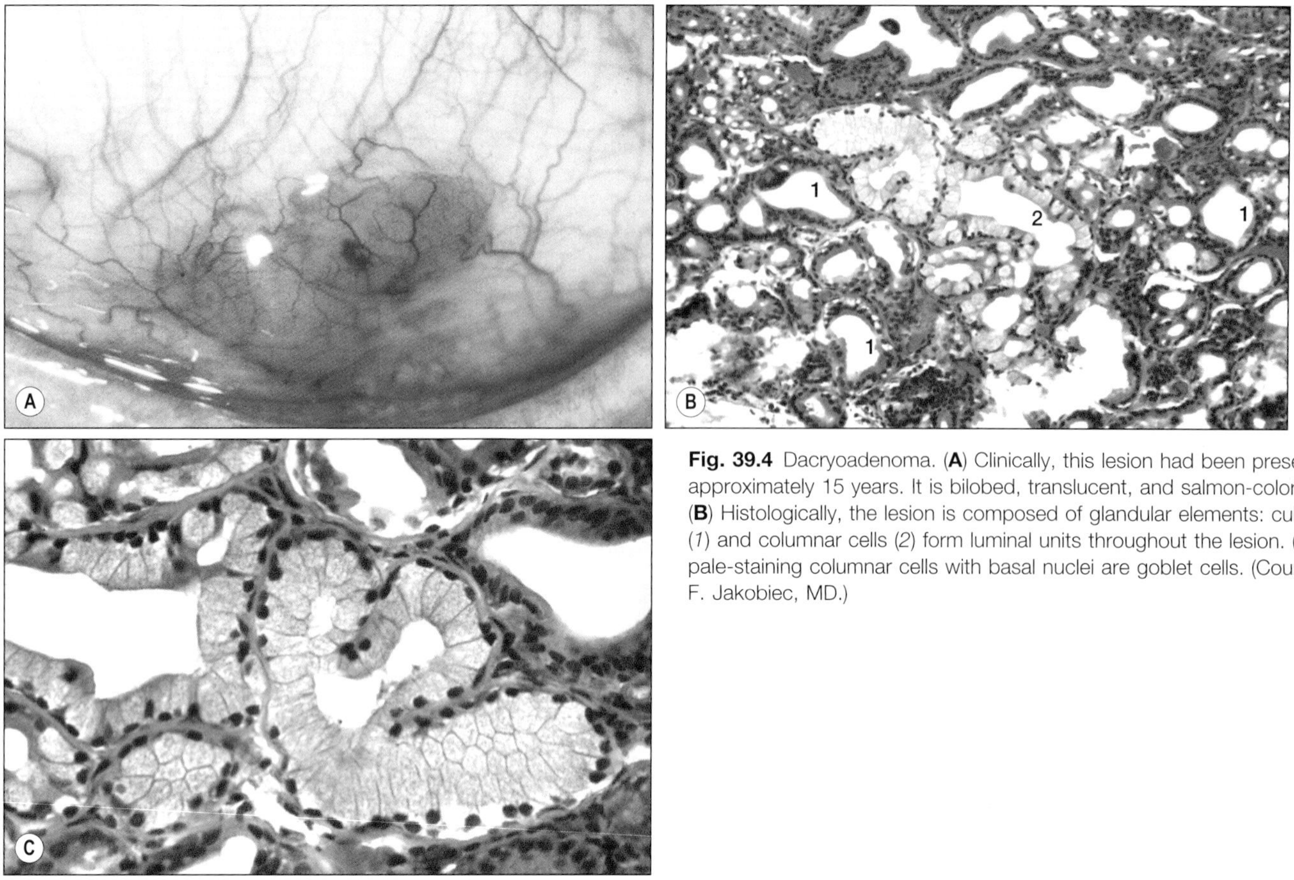

Fig. 39.4 Dacryoadenoma. (**A**) Clinically, this lesion had been present for approximately 15 years. It is bilobed, translucent, and salmon-colored. (**B**) Histologically, the lesion is composed of glandular elements: cuboidal (*1*) and columnar cells (*2*) form luminal units throughout the lesion. (**C**) The pale-staining columnar cells with basal nuclei are goblet cells. (Courtesy F. Jakobiec, MD.)

Malignant Tumefactions

Conjunctival intraepithelial neoplasia

Conjunctival intraepithelial neoplasia (CIN) refers to a neoplastic proliferation of dysplastic squamous epithelium that is noninvasive (i.e. confined to the epithelial layer by an intact basement membrane). CIN has been previously referred to by terms such as *Bowen's disease*, *conjunctival squamous dysplasia*, *intraepithelial epithelioma*, and *dyskeratosis*.[44–52]

The etiology of CIN is uncertain and possibly multifactorial. More than 95% of the lesions occur at the mitotically active limbal region, especially within the sun-exposed interpalpebral fissure.[45,47,53] This, combined with the fact that these lesions are more common in the sun-exposed, white, male population, suggests that actinic exposure is an important pathogenic factor.[46,47,53,54] Ultraviolet radiation produces an upregulation of matrix metalloproteinases in dysplastic conjunctival cells at doses that cause cell death in normal human conjunctival cells, suggesting a potential role of ultraviolet radiation and matrix metalloproteinases in the progression of conjunctival dysplasia.[55] Additional pathogenic factors implicated in CIN include heavy smoking, light skin pigmentation, exposure to petroleum derivatives, immunosuppression/human immunodeficiency virus (HIV) infection, infection with the human papillomavirus (HPV), and xeroderma pigmentosum.[55–69]

Winward and Curtin[62] published a case report in which a young HIV-infected individual was affected by a rapidly growing conjunctival squamous lesion with marked pleomorphism, hyperchromasia, and high mitotic activity. Macarez et al. discussed similar lesions in patients receiving ciclosporin therapy for prevention of organ transplant rejection.[65] As discussed later, this behavior is unusual for CIN and therefore immunosuppression should be considered in unusual cases of CIN.

HPV subtypes 6, 8, and 11 are associated with benign conjunctival epithelial growths while types 16 and 18 are associated with malignant neoplasia.[18–21,56,61,68,70–73] McDonnell et al.[61] used PCR and DNA hybridization techniques to demonstrate the presence of HPV 16 in 37 of 42 (88%) conjunctival biopsies ranging from mild dysplasia to infiltrating conjunctival squamous cell carcinomas. Six control lesions (papillomas and pterygia) were negative for HPV. Four of six (66.7%) patients with unilateral conjunctival dysplasia demonstrated HPV 16 in the contralateral unaffected eye. HPV 16 also was identified in both eyes of a patient who had undergone excision of a unilateral lesion 8 years earlier.[72] HPV 16 has been identified in patients with bilateral squamous conjunctival tumors.[56,71] Despite the strong suggestion of a causative role for HPV in CIN, there is uncertainty as to whether HPV independently produces

CIN or whether it acts as an adjuvant to the environmental factors listed previously. Therefore, further studies are necessary to elucidate the role of HPV in the pathogenesis of CIN.

The aforementioned pathologic factors may cause tumor progression through mutation or deletions of the tumor suppressor gene p53[69,74–76] Mutations and deletions of p53 are said to be the most common genetic abnormality in human cancers.[77] Studies by Dushku et al. suggest that ultraviolet light-induced mutations to the p53 tumor suppressor gene may play a role in the etiology of pterygia and squamous neoplasia.[74] Toth et al. found that p53 gene mutation was a common finding (81%) in corneal squamous neoplasia.[75] In another study, this group found that p53 positivity was associated with adverse clinical behavior, e.g. globe invasion or metastasis.[76]

As previously mentioned, 95% of CIN lesions present at the limbus, usually within the nasal or temporal interpalpebral zone. Lesions also may present at the mucocutaneous junction of the eyelid margin or at the caruncle. Rarely, patients present late, with diffuse involvement over the entire conjunctival surface.

Clinically, the lesions are slow-growing tumefactions (Fig. 39.5). Often, patients are unaware of their presence, and diagnosis is made only after careful routine ophthalmic evaluation. Only 10% of lesions are leukoplakic, a result of surface hyperkeratinization. Leukoplakia refers to the white surface thickening also seen in PEH. Most lesions are translucent or gelatinous thickenings of the conjunctiva. An important sign noted with dysplastic squamous lesions is the fine vascular pattern that has a hairpin configuration. This pattern is in contradistinction to the 'red-dot' pattern seen with squamous papillomas, although infrequently a similar papillomatous pattern may be found within portions of CIN lesions. CIN lesions often spread from the adjacent limbus to involve the adjacent corneal surface, anterior to Bowman's layer. The abnormal epithelium has a frosted appearance with a fimbriated margin.[48] The corneal portion is supported metabolically by a neoplastic pannus consisting of identical hairpin vessels. Varying degrees of corneal involvement are possible, from limited to extensive. The terms *primary corneal dysplasia* and *primary corneal epithelial dysmaturation* have been used to describe cases in which corneal involvement is markedly disproportionate to that of the limbus (see later).[12] Fluorescein or rose Bengal stains may be used both clinically and intraoperatively to demonstrate the extent of disease, as dysplastic epithelium tends to have a diffuse, fine stippling not found with normal conjunctival or corneal epithelium.

Histologically, CIN represents the presence of partial- to full-thickness conjunctival epithelial dysplasia (see Fig. 39.5). Because the basement membrane is not penetrated, CIN does not involve the underlying substantia propria. Individually, cells have a mild to marked increased nuclear–cytoplasmic ratio. Two cell types have been recognized. Spindle cells are small, elongated cells with eosinophilic cytoplasm and a moderately hyperchromatic nucleus; epidermoid cells are larger with large vesicular nuclei and prominent nucleoli. As a group, cells display a lack of normal organization and abnormal polarity (i.e. relationship and orientation to each other). In addition, cells do not mature normally as they approach the epithelial surface. Mitotic figures may be present at all epithelial levels. In general, a sharp demarcation between dysplastic and normal epithelium exists at the lateral edges of the lesion. CIN can manifest as a pigmented tumor, resembling melanoma, due to the presence of intratumoral pigmented dendritic melanocytes.[78] The histologic appearance of CIN is distinguished from squamous papillomata and PEH by the latter's normal or low nuclear–cytoplasmic ratio and the imperceptible blending of hyperplastic epithelium to normal epithelium at the lateral lesional margins.[12]

Because CIN arises from a single cell that has undergone neoplastic transformation, the lesions are only slowly progressive,[47,49,70] despite the degree of dysplasia.[45,47] Because the basement membrane remains intact, there is no metastatic potential. CIN lesions rarely progress to become invasive squamous cell carcinoma.[47,70,79] Despite this apparent unaggressive nature, CIN is difficult to cure.[45,79] Preoperative diagnosis/screening may be possible with the help of exfoliative cytology and impression cytology. However, inability to determine the extent and depth of invasion remain the main caveats.[80–83] Management of lesions depends on whether the lesion is newly diagnosed or a recurrent or inadequately excised lesion. With newly diagnosed lesions, the involved limbal conjunctiva should be excised with 1 to 2 mm of surrounding clinically uninvolved conjunctival margins. The sclera is left bare.[12] The importance for wide margins is demonstrated by the fact that clinically negative conjunctiva can be histopathologically positive.[84] After excision, the corneal epithelial component is removed using a Bard-Parker surgical blade after instilling cocaine solution, which loosens the corneal epithelium. All frosted epithelium and associated fibrovascular pannus should be scraped from the corneal surface. After corneal debridement, cryotherapy should be applied to the involved limbal area, cut conjunctival edges, and bare scleral bed using a nitrous oxide or liquid nitrogen applicator tip with a double or triple freeze–thaw technique. More than 90% long-term tumor control is achieved with this method.[85–87]

Recurrence rates are a function of the adequacy of initial resection. When incompletely excised, recurrence rates may be as high as 50% regardless of the lesion's pre-excisional appearance, cell type, and degree of dysplasia.[45,47,48,51,52] Late recurrences are possible and continuous long-term clinical follow-up is required.[88] When recurrent, CIN tends to be more widespread, and the potential conversion to invasive squamous cell carcinoma is a concern. Recurrent lesions should be treated with identical wide local excision but more aggressive cryotherapy. If the surgeon is concerned about possible deep tissue invasion, a cutaneous cryogun may be used to produce a full-thickness transscleral ice ball. Postoperative inflammation may be treated with oral prednisone, topical steroids, and cycloplegics.[12]

Lesions that involve more than 50% of the corneal limbus tend to have poor visual outcome after excision and cryotherapy because of surface anomalies associated with destruction of the limbal stem cell population. Conjunctival and buccal mucous membrane autografts are usually inadequate. Excision with secondary limbal autografts may provide excellent anatomic and functional results.[89] Topical mitomycin-C is useful for the treatment of incompletely excised or recurrent lesion.[90–98] Mitomycin-C may be associated with iatrogenic punctal stenosis, and some advocate the use of punctal plugs prior to treatment.[97] In addition, topical chemotherapy with 5-flourouracil, interferon alfa-2b, and cidofovir have been reported.[32,99–106] Interferon alfa-2b in particular has been well studied as a treatment for both primary and recurrent lesions.[106] Of note, modified Mohs' techniques, brachyradiation, and phototherapeutic keratectomy have been used with some success.[107–110]

Invasive squamous cell carcinoma

Fortunately, invasive squamous cell carcinoma (SCC) occurs much less frequently than CIN (Fig. 39.6). As with CIN, HPV is thought to play a role in pathogenesis.[56,61,71] CIN is often the precursor of invasive squamous cell carcinoma, occurring when dysplastic epithelial cells penetrate the underlying basement membrane, allowing free access for extension

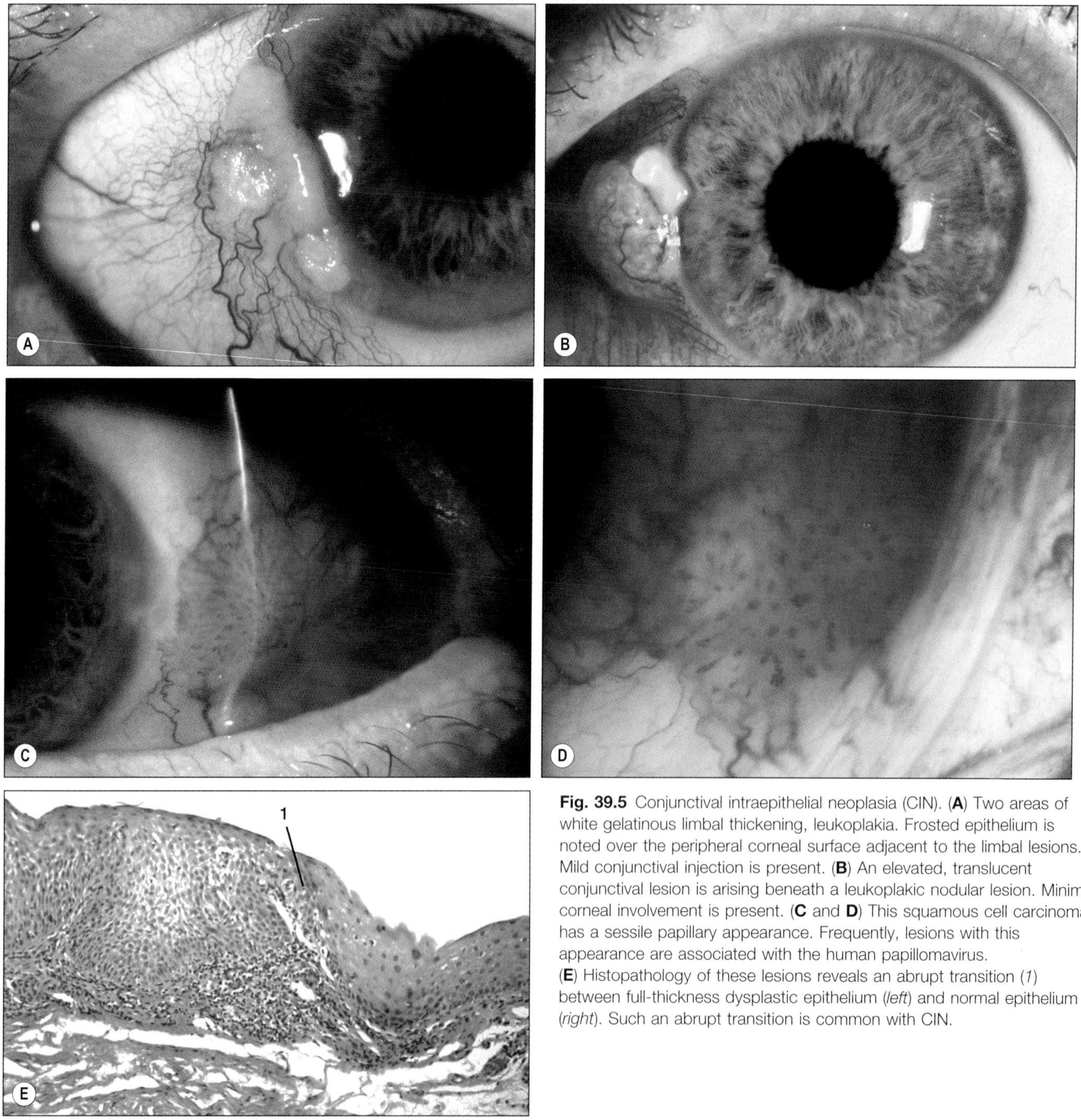

Fig. 39.5 Conjunctival intraepithelial neoplasia (CIN). (**A**) Two areas of white gelatinous limbal thickening, leukoplakia. Frosted epithelium is noted over the peripheral corneal surface adjacent to the limbal lesions. Mild conjunctival injection is present. (**B**) An elevated, translucent conjunctival lesion is arising beneath a leukoplakic nodular lesion. Minimal corneal involvement is present. (**C** and **D**) This squamous cell carcinoma has a sessile papillary appearance. Frequently, lesions with this appearance are associated with the human papillomavirus. (**E**) Histopathology of these lesions reveals an abrupt transition (*1*) between full-thickness dysplastic epithelium (*left*) and normal epithelium (*right*). Such an abrupt transition is common with CIN.

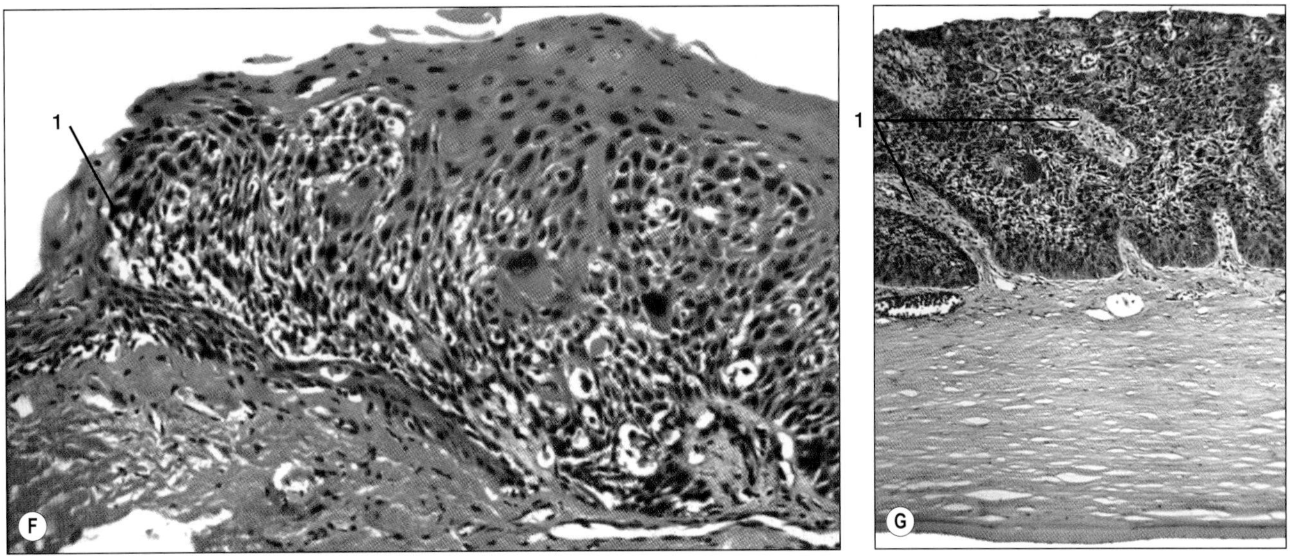

Fig. 39.5, cont'd (**F**) A similar abrupt transition (*1*) between normal epithelium (*left*) and dysplastic epithelium (*right*) is present. (**G**) Full-thickness corneal epithelial dysplasia with associated neoplastic vascular pannus is present. Vascularized papillary stromal projections (*1*) extend within the lesion.

throughout the subconjunctival space. Due to the resistance of Bowman's membrane, invasion occurs virtually exclusively within the conjunctival portion of the lesion.[111] Clinically, the lesions resemble those of CIN but are more elevated; they arise most frequently at the limbus and appear gelatinous, translucent, leukoplakic, or papilliform. Invasive squamous cell carcinoma can present with keratoacanthoma features,[112] while palpebral conjunctival squamous cell carcinoma can appear like a chalazion.[113] Unlike typical unilateral squamous cell carcinoma, bilateral conjunctival lesions possess a verrucous, papillary, keratinized appearance, and may be associated with HPV.[71] Pigmentation may be present in blacks and may be confused clinically with melanoma.[27,114,115] Possibly as a result of neglect, squamous cell carcinomas often involve greater portions of the limbus and are larger than CIN at diagnosis. Some cases may masquerade as chronic blepharitis, delaying diagnosis.[116] Squamous cell carcinomas may demonstrate engorged feeder vessels and may be immobile and firmly fixed to underlying episcleral or scleral tissues, indicating invasion.[47] Diplopia may be present due to involvement of the extraocular muscles.[117] High-frequency ultrasound may help to delineate the extent of scleral and intraocular spread in suspected cases of invasive squamous cell carcinoma.[118] Squamous cell carcinoma has been reported in anophthalmic sockets where they may be concealed by prosthetics.[119] Thus it is important to remove prostheses and examine the conjunctivae of post-enucleation/evisceration patients during routine examinations.

Cutaneous carcinomas (basal cell carcinoma) and visceral malignancies (SCC of the lung, CIS of cervix, carcinoma of the colon and prostate, hepatocellular carcinoma and non-Hodgkin's lymphoma) are known to be associated with conjunctival SCC.[47,120–122]

Histopathologically, lesions closely resemble those of severe CIN. The normal epithelium is replaced by neoplastic cells with high nuclear–cytoplasmic ratios and a combination of spindle- and epithelioid-shaped cells. Cells appear pleomorphic with dyskeratoses, acanthosis, and lack of polarity. The basement membrane, by definition, shows evidence of penetration with subepithelial neoplastic cells.

Conjunctival squamous cell carcinomas may demonstrate especially high concentrations of epidermal growth factor, which may contribute to their aggressive growth pattern.[123]

HLA class I antigens and beta 2-microglubulins may be decreased in conjunctival dysplasias and negative in carcinomas in situ and carcinomas, suggesting a role of cytotoxic T lymphocytes in the pathogenesis, while absence of HLA class II antigen expression in conjunctival squamous cell carcinomas suggests helper T lymphocyte-mediated control of tumor growth.[124,125] Increased glucose uptake by dysplastic cells has been demonstrated by increased immunohistochemical staining for GLUT-1.[126] Genetic ablation (in a mouse model) of alpha v integrin expression, which normally suppresses epithelial cell proliferation in the basal cell epithelium of the conjunctiva, can lead to the formation of malignant epithelial tumor strikingly similar to squamous cell carcinoma.[127]

Invasive conjunctival squamous cell carcinomas usually are not associated with regional or distant metastases; only a few cases have been reported.[11,128] Squamous cell carcinoma appears to be particularly aggressive in HIV-infected individuals, as well as in patients with xeroderma pigmentosum.[46,55,60,61,129] Fortunately, most are minimally invasive and can be treated with wide local excision and aggressive cryotherapy.[86] Often, superficial lamellar sclerectomy or keratectomy is required. The use of cryotherapy extends the effective surgical margin and reduces the recurrence rate from 40% to 10% while maintaining the structural integrity of the eye.[86] Preoperative and postoperative adjunctive topical chemotherapy with mitomycin-C is also useful.[90–95,130] Although successful eye-salvaging treatment has been reported through the use of proton beam

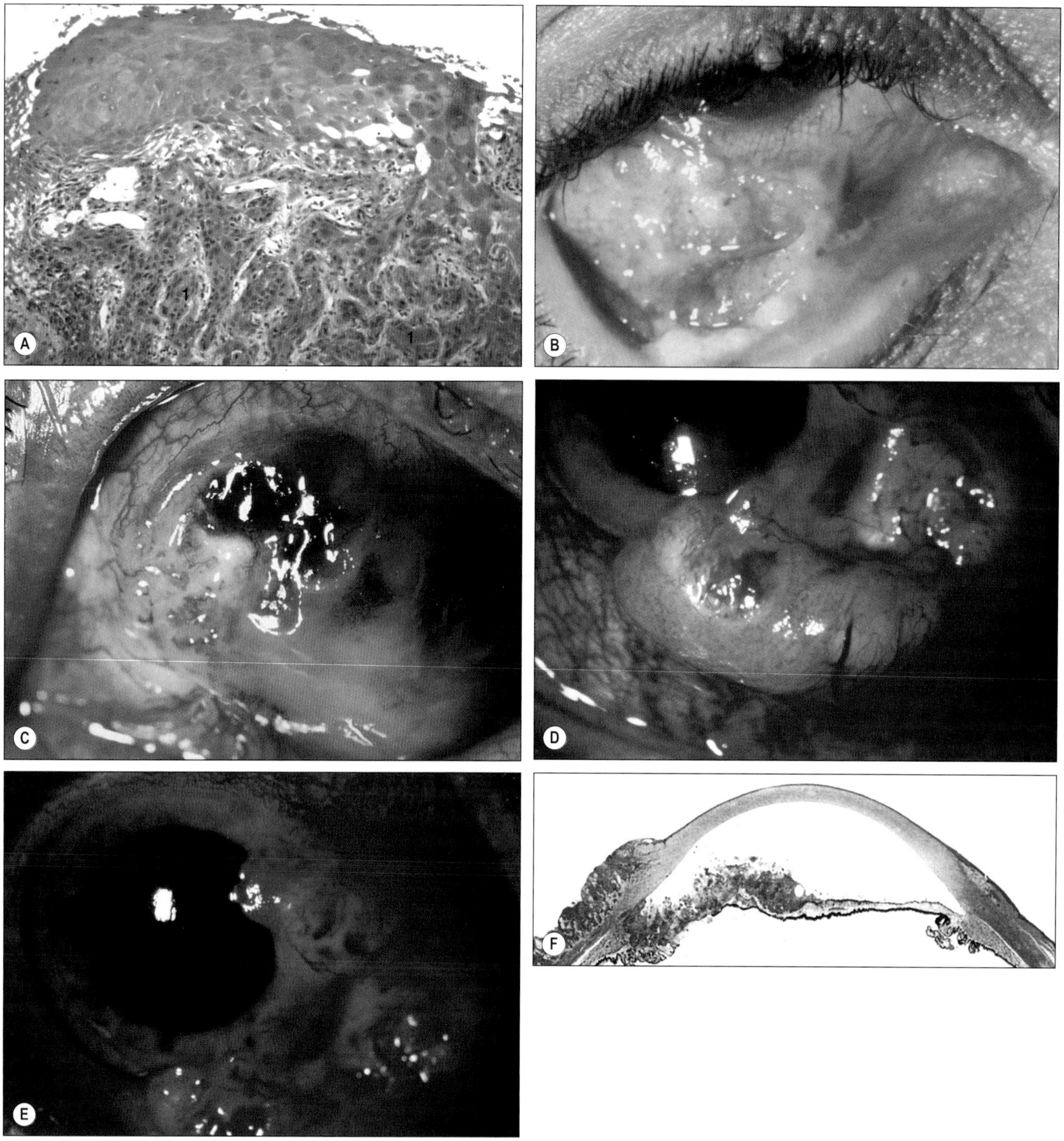

Fig. 39.6 Conjunctival squamous cell carcinoma. Conjunctival squamous cell carcinoma occurs when the dysplastic conjunctival neoplastic process penetrates the underlying basement membrane into the substantia propria. (**A**) Histopathology shows extensive conjunctival squamous cell carcinoma with fimbriae of dysplastic squamous cells (*1*), which are deeply invasive. (**B**) Extensive squamous cell carcinoma fills the inferior fornix. This lesion harbored the human papillomavirus. (**C**) Squamous cell carcinomas may possess extensive pigmentation in pigmented patients. These lesions are frequently diagnosed clinically as malignant melanomas. A frosted corneal epithelium and an extensive leukoplakic limbal component (seen below the pigmented portion) were more consistent with the clinical diagnosis of squamous cell carcinoma. (**D** and **E**) Rarely, intraocular invasion occurs with squamous cell carcinoma. Rapid and diffuse ocular injection is the harbinger of intraocular invasion. When this occurs, enucleation is required. (**F**) Histopathology demonstrates intraocular invasion of a limbal tumor mass and invasion of the chamber angle, iris, and ciliary body.
(**D** and **E**, Courtesy A. Proia, MD; **F**, Courtesy N Rao, MD.)

irradiation, intraocular invasion is usually treated with enucleation, and cases with orbital invasion usually require exenteration.[131–133] Patients refusing invasive treatments, or at risk of developing functional complications after standard treatment for large lesions and recurrent cases, have also been successfully treated with photodynamic therapy,[134] although this therapy may aggravate and promote the growth of lesions in patients with severe DNA disorders such as xeroderma pigmentosum.[135] Successful excision of large lesions is possible with the adjunctive use of amniotic membrane transplants.[35]

Both conjunctival intraepithelial neoplasia and invasive squamous cell carcinoma are associated with HPV. It is possible that the newly developed vaccine for HPV will reduce the incidence of these tumors in a manner similar to that of cervical carcinoma.[136]

Significant predictors for recurrence of conjunctival SSC include the size of the lesion, positive surgical margins,[88] elevated proliferation index measured by Ki-67 index, increased age,[137] and scleral involvement.[122] The incidence of intraocular invasion ranges from 2% to 13% while mortality rates range from 0% to 8%.[120–122,137]

Corneal epithelial dysmaturation and epithelial dysplasia

These lesions tend either to involve exclusively the corneal epithelium or in an amount disproportionate to the components involving conjunctiva or limbus (Fig. 39.7).[48,138] In both conditions, extensive frosted corneal epithelium or individual islands of opalescent epithelium are present. Neoplastic fibrovascular corneal pannus is not present. Epithelial dysmaturation (Fig. 39.7A and B) is a benign and indolent process. Lesions may be unilateral or bilateral, stationary or slowly progressive, and may wax and wane spontaneously. Histologically, lesions consistent with epithelial dysmaturation have benign-appearing epithelial cells with only slight differences in nuclear size. The nuclear–cytoplasmic ratio is normal or only slightly abnormal. Primary corneal epithelial dysplasia (Fig. 39.7C and D) is clinically similar to that of epithelial dysmaturation. Cytologically, however, frank atypia with increased nuclear–cytoplasmic ratio, loss of polarity, and loss of normal epithelial maturation is present. Electron microscopy in cases of primary corneal epithelial dysplasia and epithelial dysmaturation reveals disorganized cytoplasmic tonofilaments that are often clumped about the nucleus. Disorganized desmosomes and electron-dense granules, which may represent keratohyalin or tonofilament degeneration products, are also present. Endocytotic vacuoles containing desmosomes can be found within affected cells.[48,138] These features may indicate changes consistent with cell death (apoptosis). These ultrastructural features are present in both the dysplastic and more benign lesions, and therefore clinical and light microscopic features are more useful in determining the specific diagnosis. It is thought that both lesions occupy a spectrum from benign to malignant. Fortunately, both lesions are indolent and can be treated with simple corneal scraping and, if present, wide excision of limbal components as with CIN. Bowman's membrane should not be surgically excised as in lamellar keratectomy.

Mucoepidermoid carcinoma

Mucoepidermoid carcinoma is a more aggressive variant of squamous cell carcinoma, which is clinically indistinguishable from the more indolent squamous cell carcinoma, and is capable of invading the globe (Fig. 39.8).[139–143] The lesion may occur anywhere on the conjunctival surface in contradistinction to the primarily limbal-based squamous cell carcinoma. It may also arise from the caruncle.[144] Most often, the diagnosis is made retrospectively after recurrence of what was thought to be a simple squamous cell carcinoma. Histologically, lesions consist of squamous cells and mucin-producing goblet cells. In recurrent lesions, mucin-producing goblet cells may be less numerous and therefore initial biopsy specimens should be reviewed. Lesions with predominant mucin-secreting elements tend to behave less aggressively.[141] Mucoepidermoid carcinoma is locally invasive early in its course; most reported cases have either ocular or orbital invasion at the time of diagnosis.[139–142,145] Recurrent lesions are associated with a high risk of regional lymph node metastasis. Treatment is wide local excision with aggressive cryotherapy; if necessary, enucleation or exenteration is used to treat intraocular or intraorbital spread, respectively. Sentinel node biopsy may be helpful for staging the disease to determine appropriate treatment regimens.[146,147]

Spindle cell carcinoma

Like mucoepidermoid carcinoma, spindle cell carcinoma is a highly malignant neoplasm of the epibulbar surface, arising from the conjunctiva, limbus, or cornea (Fig. 39.9).[148–152] The lesion is locally invasive with resultant severe ocular damage. The tumor is composed of pleomorphic elongated or fusiform cells, which may be arranged in spindles or fascicles, features usually suggestive of fibrosarcoma, spindle cell melanoma, leiomyoma, or rhabdomyosarcoma. Monoclonal antibodies to cytokeratins and electron microscopic identification of tonofilaments and desmosomes may be diagnostically helpful. Unlike spindle malignant melanoma, melanosomes are not present on electron microscopy and lesions are S-100 protein negative.[12,148] The treatment options are identical to those for mucoepidermoid carcinoma.

Adenoid squamous carcinoma

Mauriello et al. describe 14 cases of adenoid squamous carcinoma, a variant of squamous cell carcinoma containing adenoid or pseudoglandular spaces arising from acantholysis of cells within islands of neoplastic squamous cells (Fig. 39.10).[153] Unlike mucoepidermoid carcinoma, the mucin within the pseudoglandular spaces is hyaluronidase sensitive. Like mucoepidermoid carcinoma, the tumor is aggressive and tends to recur in spite of wide local excision.[153]

Clear cell carcinoma

Clear cell carcinoma is a rare type of squamous cell carcinoma. Usually found in the head and neck region of white males, it is commonly confused with sebaceous cell carcimoma[154] and rarely can occur in the conjunctiva.[155] It is characterized by extensive cytoplasmic hydropic change

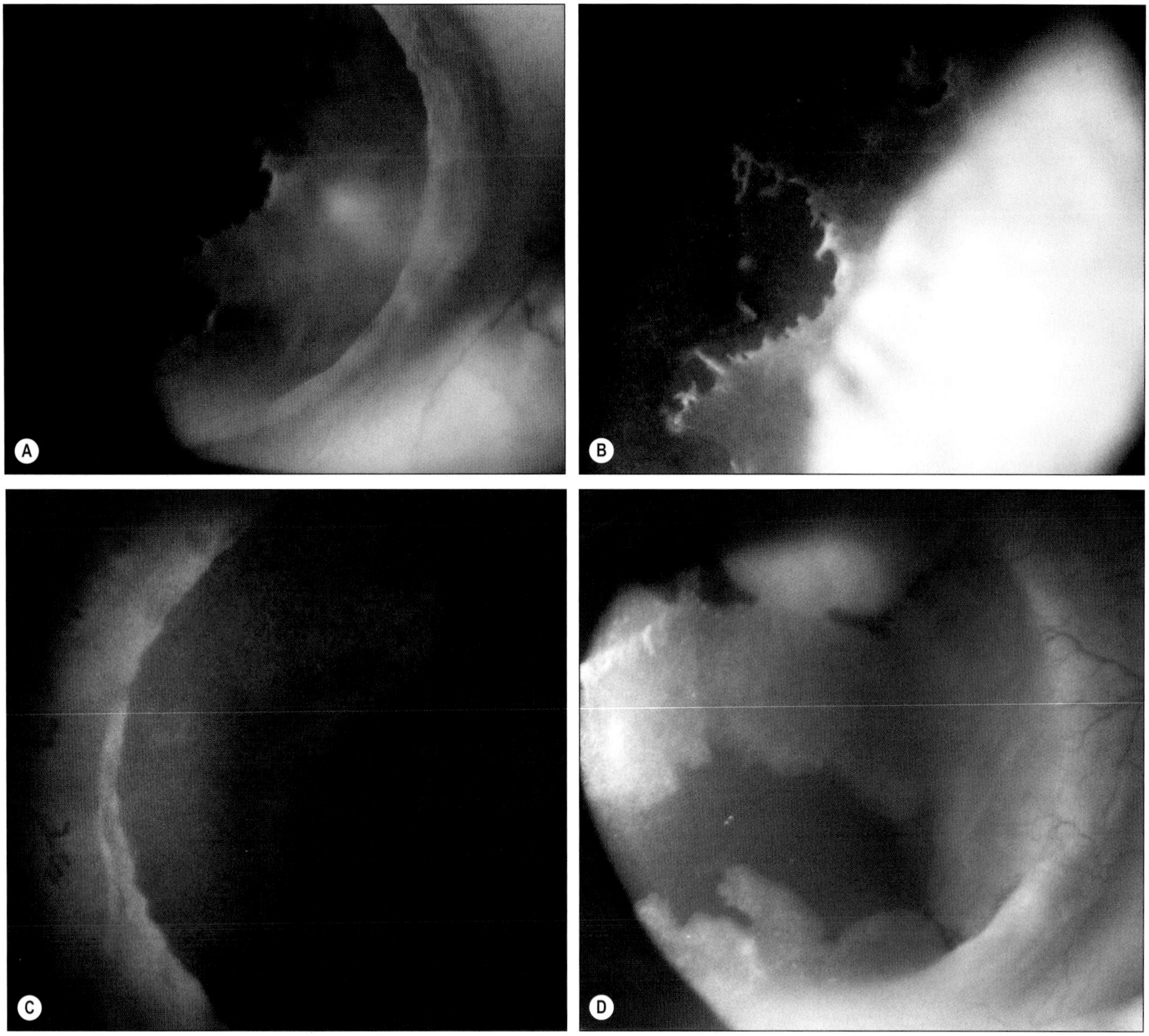

Fig. 39.7 Corneal epithelial dysmaturation and dysplasia. (**A**) The nasal portion of the cornea in dysmaturation shows a scalloped and frosted epithelium without underlying vascularization and without thickening of the limbus. This bilateral and relatively static condition showed minimal progression over several years of follow-up. The absence of connective tissue and elastotic material in the substantia propria of the nasal conjunctiva is a clinical indicator that this is neither a pterygium nor a pingueculum. (**B**) An iron line adjacent to the fimbriated edge of the process underscores its static nature. (**C**) In this corneal dysplasia, frosted epithelium slowly progressed with only the earliest formation of a neoplastic pannus seen at the outer aspect of the lesion. (**D**) A case of corneal epithelial dysplasia. Islands of frosted epithelium now encroach on the visual access without a conspicuous thickening at the limbus. Such lesions are best managed by scraping off the involved epithelium above Bowman's membrane, which is generally a reliable barrier against invasion.

not associated with accumulation of lipid, mucin, or glycogen.

Sebaceous cell carcinoma

Sebaceous cell carcinoma is well known for its ability to spread in a pagetoid (intraepithelial) manner.[156–159] Sebaceous cell carcinoma most often originates in the meibomian glands. Other sebaceous glands, including the Zeis' glands of the eyelash pilosebaceous units, also may give rise to sebaceous cell carcinoma.[160] However, evidence suggests that sebaceous cell carcinoma also may arise de novo in the conjunctiva, especially that of the upper tarsus, thereby presenting as pagetoid spread without a discrete tumor focus.[156–161] These cases probably result from a malignant sebaceous metaplasia of the conjunctiva. Sebaceous cell carcinoma also may arise within the caruncle and lacrimal gland, both embryologic conjunctival outpouchings.[162,163] Cellular DNA content seems to correlate with presence of pagetoid spread. Tumors that are aneuploid demonstrate

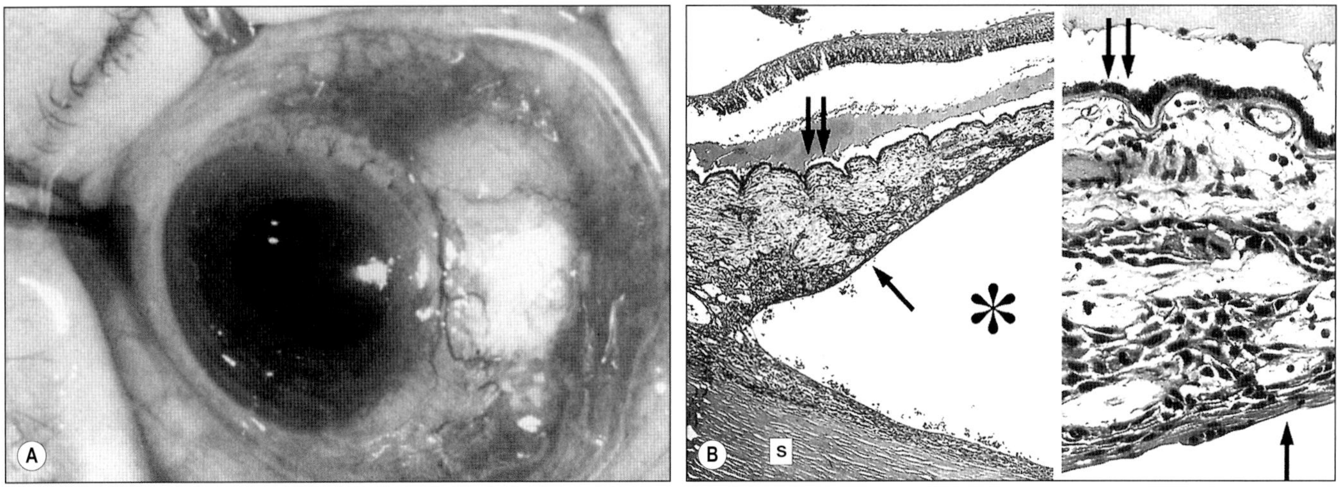

Fig. 39.8 Mucoepidermoid carcinoma of the conjunctiva. (**A**) Clinically, a red elevated epibulbar mass is present with marked ocular inflammation signifying intraocular invasion. (**B**) Histopathology demonstrates extensive intraocular invasion of tumor cells. A cystic space is present (*) lined by squamous epithelium (*single arrows*). *Double arrows* indicate the pigment epithelium of the iris. s, Sclera. (Courtesy K. Gündüz, MD.)

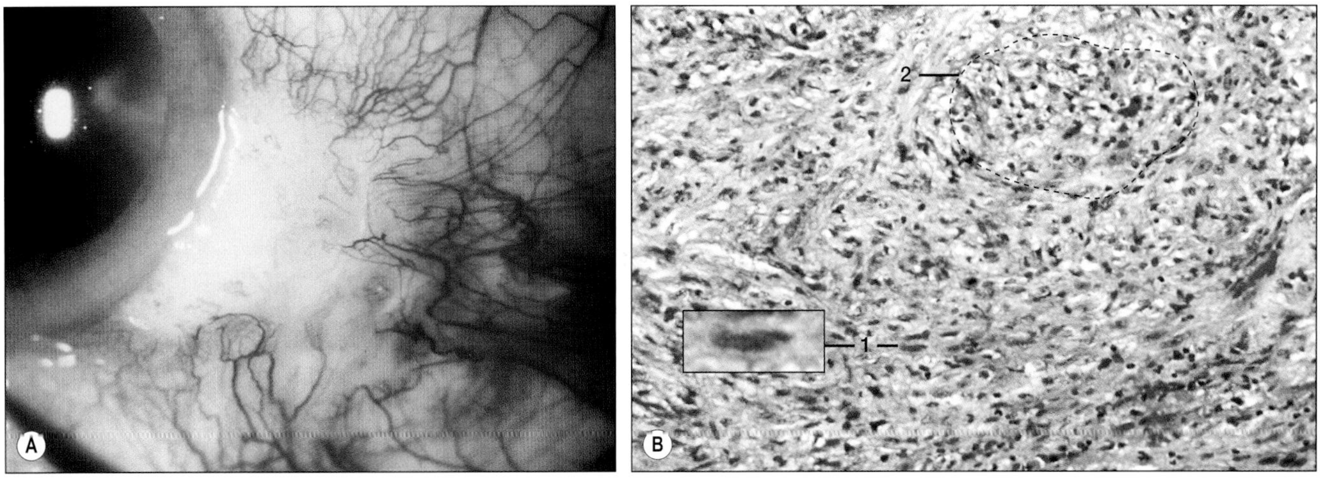

Fig. 39.9 Spindle cell carcinoma. Spindle cell carcinomas are aggressive variants of squamous cell carcinoma. (**A**) Clinically, the lesions are markedly white because of collagen deposition. (**B**) Histopathology of this clinical lesion shows numerous spindle-shaped cells (*1*) arranged in fascicles (*2*). The differential diagnosis of this pathologic appearance includes fibrosarcoma, leiomyoma, rhabdomyosarcoma, sebaceous cell carcinoma, and malignant melanoma. Immunohistochemistry and electron microscopy are often needed to differentiate these lesions. (Courtesy V. Curtin, MD.)

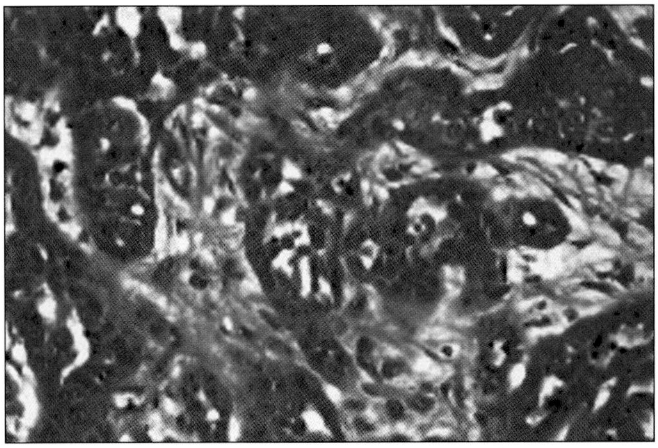

Fig. 39.10 Adenoid squamous carcinoma. Clinically, an irritated red mass is present in the superior bulbar conjunctiva. Histopathology demonstrates proliferating neoplastic squamous cells arranged in lobules, columns, and islands. Lumina are present due to acantholysis of tumor cells leading to a glandular appearance. In contradistinction to mucoepidermoid carcinoma, the mucin present within the acantholytic spaces of adenoid squamous carcinoma is sensitive to hyaluronidase. (Courtesy Joseph Mauriello, MD.)

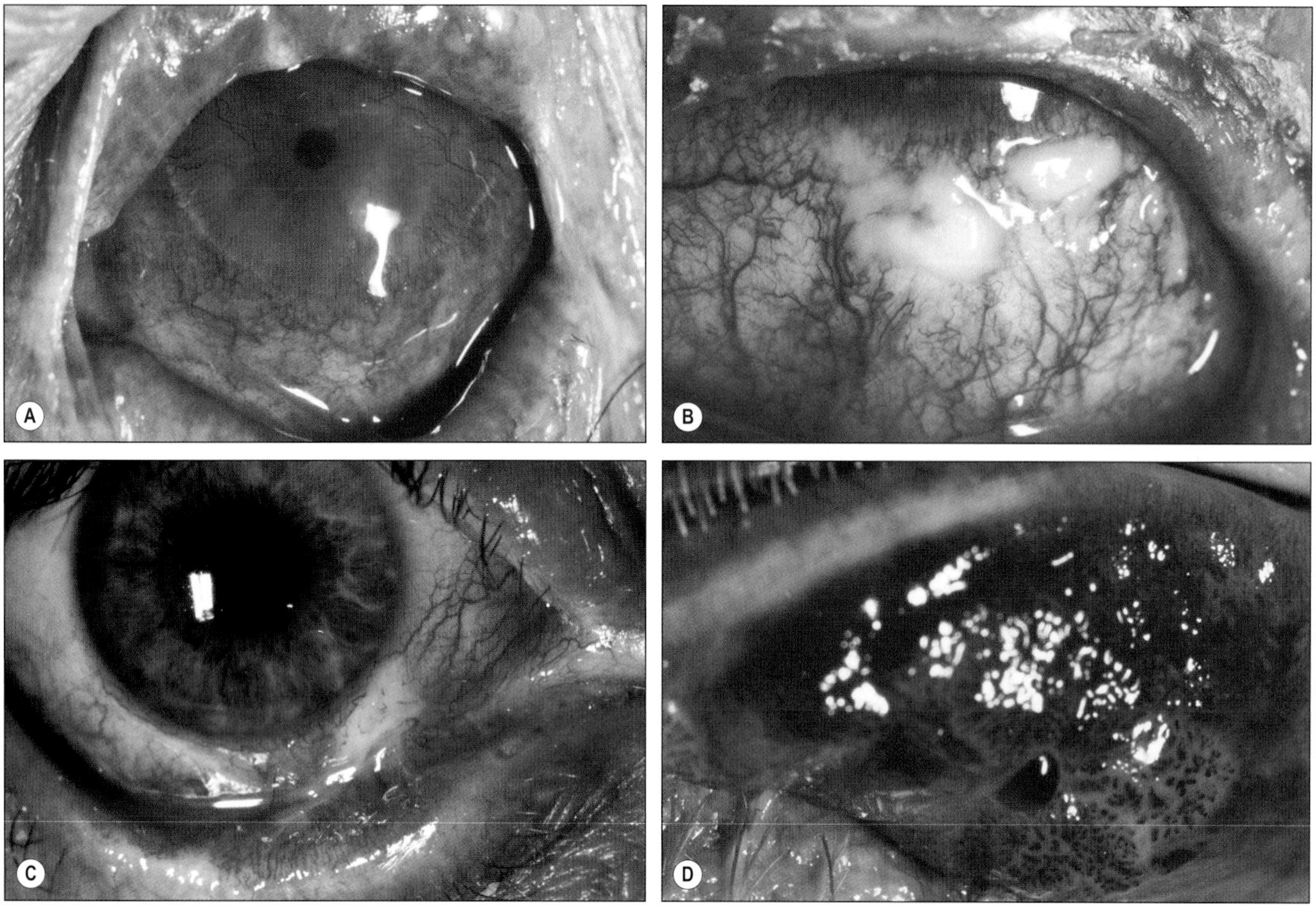

Fig. 39.11 Sebaceous cell carcinoma. Sebaceous cell carcinoma arises from adnexal sebaceous glands including the meibomian glands, Zeis' glands, and, rarely, the lacrimal gland. Sebaceous cell carcinoma often presents as unilateral blepharoconjunctivitis. (**A**) Significant findings in this case include conjunctival injection, neovascular pannus, thickened lid margin, and eyelash loss. (**B**) In addition to lash loss and conjunctival injection, white nodules composed of neoplastic sebaceous cells are present near the limbus. (**C**) Neoplastic symblepharon is present nasally. (**D**) Marked thickening of the upper palpebral conjunctiva. Papillary fronding is present in the lower portion of the lesion.

pagetoid spread and more severe anaplasia than do diploid cells that are less anaplastic and nonpagetoid.[156,160–164]

The rare condition of autosomal dominant Muir-Torre syndrome should always be considered and a systemic evaluation for visceral malignancies, mainly colon cancer, should be performed in patients with sebaceous carcinomas without history of radiotherapy or immunosuppression.[165,166] Rishi and Font found that the sebaceous tumors of the ocular adnexa in patients with Muir-Torre syndrome were immunohistochemically positive for mismatch repair gene (MSH2).[165] Merkel cell carcinoma has been reported to be associated with sebaceous cell carcinoma of the conjunctiva.[167]

Patients with conjunctival pagetoid sebaceous cell carcinoma present with unilateral inflamed red eyes (Fig. 39.11). The etiology of the inflammation is believed secondary to sebaceous breakdown products released by the sebaceous cells.[156,157,159–164,168] Indeed, clinically, sebaceous cell carcinoma may masquerade as conjunctivitis, superior limbic keratitis, blepharitis, and chalazia,[116,161,169–171] in part explaining why the average duration between initial presentation and diagnosis ranges from 1 to 3 years.[172–174] In a 2004 study by Shields et al., sebaceous cell carcinoma was correctly suspected in only 32% of patients upon initial examination and was correctly diagnosed histopathologically in only 50% of cases.[115] Therefore, it is important to consider the diagnosis of sebaceous cell carcinoma in any patient with unilateral conjunctival or eyelid inflammation, with or without lid thickening or lash loss, that does not respond completely to conventional therapy. Impression cytologic analysis may facilitate the early diagnosis in suspicious cases.[175]

When confronted with suspected sebaceous cell carcinoma, biopsy should be performed. During biopsy, care should be taken because the sebaceous cells are easily rubbed off the specimen's surface. Indeed, whenever a biopsy shows extensive denuded epithelium, sebaceous cell carcinoma should be suspected.[12,159] Histopathologically, the diagnosis can be confused with squamous cell carcinoma.[176,177] In contrast to squamous cell carcinoma, which evolves from the basal layer outward, sebaceous cell carcinoma often involves the superficial layers of the conjunctiva and spares the normal epithelium in the basal regions. Indeed, sebaceous cell carcinoma should be suspected whenever superficial anaplastic cells overlie a normal-appearing basal cell layer. When well differentiated, individual cells contain vacuolated, frothy cytoplasm. Less well-differentiated specimens contain more anaplastic basophilic-staining cells with multiple mitoses. In addition, sebaceous elements may be appreciated with lipid stains and electron microscopy if routine stains are inadequate for diagnosis.

Management is directed at first identifying the extent of disease with map biopsy. If disease is extensive (i.e. greater than 50% of the epibulbar surface) treatment is exenteration.[178] If disease is less extensive, wide local excision of the primary lesion with adjunctive cryotherapy is effective.[179] A pilot study of four patients with pagetoid sebaceous cell carcinoma, including some with extensive disease, suggested that topical mitomycin-C is effective treatment.[157] If orbital invasion is present, exenteration is indicated. Radiation treatment is associated with an unacceptably high recurrence rate and should be reserved for patients unable to undergo surgery.[180] If present, lymph node metastases should be treated aggressively, as long-term survival is possible.[158,181] Sentinel lymph node biopsy may be helpful for staging purposes.[146,147] Close postexcisional follow-up and, if necessary, rebiopsy should be carried out.

Prognostically, the importance of early diagnosis cannot be overemphasized. Rao et al.[181] noted that potential survival is reduced from 87% to 57% if diagnosis is delayed by 6 months or more. Other features related to poor prognosis include diameter greater than 10 mm, involvement of both lids, orbital invasion, vascular invasion, and multicentric origin.[181] Recent studies report significantly lower mortality rates, possibly as low as 18%.[177] In one study, no deaths were reported in patients diagnosed after 1970,[177] after which more thorough surgical treatments were used. The improved prognosis is likely a result of increased vigilance for the disease and aggressiveness in treatment.

Basal cell carcinoma

Basal cell carcinoma (BCC), arising from the basal germinal layer of the squamous epithelium, is the commonest carcinoma occurring in the eyelid and is very rarely seen in the conjunctiva.[182] BCC can arise primarily from the caruncle[183,184] or secondary to local invasion from an adjacent skin lesion,[185] and can appear papillomatous, nodular or pedunculated.[185,186]

References

1. Spencer WZL, ed. *Conjunctiva*. Vol. 1. Philadelphia: WB Saunders; 1985.
2. Jakobiec FA. The ultrastructure of conjunctival melanocytic tumors. *Trans Am Ophthalmol Soc.* 1984;82:599–752.
3. Sacks E, Rutgers J, Jakobiec FA, et al. A comparison of conjunctival and nonocular dendritic cells utilizing new monoclonal antibodies. *Ophthalmology.* 1986;93(8):1089–1097.
4. Sacks EH, Wieczorek R, Jakobiec FA, Knowles DM 2nd. Lymphocytic subpopulations in the normal human conjunctiva. A monoclonal antibody study. *Ophthalmology.* 1986;93(10):1276–1283.
5. Richard R. Cervical intraepithelial neoplasia. *Pathol Annu.* 1973;8.
6. Reed JW, Cashwell F, Klintworth GK. Corneal manifestations of hereditary benign intraepithelial dyskeratosis. *Arch Ophthalmol.* 1979; 97(2):297–300.
7. Yanoff M. Hereditary benign intraepithelial dyskeratosis. *Arch Ophthalmol.* 1968;79(3):291–293.
8. McLean IW, Riddle PJ, Schruggs JH, Jones DB. Hereditary benign intraepithelial dyskeratosis. A report of two cases from Texas. *Ophthalmology.* 1981;88(2):164–168.
9. Allingham RR, Seo B, Rampersaud E, et al. A duplication in chromosome 4q35 is associated with hereditary benign intraepithelial dyskeratosis. *Am J Hum Genet.* 2001;68(2):491–494.
10. Witkop CJ Jr, Shankle CH, Graham JB, et al. Hereditary benign intraepithelial dyskeratosis. II. Oral manifestations and hereditary transmission. *Arch Pathol.* 1960;70:696–711.
11. Zimmerman L. The cancerous, precancerous, and pseudocancerous lesions of the cornea and conjunctiva: corneoplastic surgery. *Proceedings of the Second Annual International Corneoplastic Conference.* London: Pergamon Press; 1969.
12. McLean I. *Tumors of the eye and ocular adnexis.* Washington, DC: Armed Forces Institute of Pathology; 1995.
13. Fatima A, Matalia HP, Vemuganti GK, et al. Pseudoepitheliomatous hyperplasia mimicking ocular surface squamous neoplasia following cultivated limbal epithelium transplantation. *Clin Experiment Ophthalmol.* 2006;34(9):889–891.
14. Freeman R. Keratoacanthoma of the conjunctiva: a case report. *Arch Ophthalmol.* 1961;65.
15. Roth AM. Solitary keratoacanthoma of the conjunctiva. *Am J Ophthalmol.* 1978;85(5 Pt 1):647–650.
16. Bellamy ED, Allen JH, Hart NL. Keratoacanthoma of the bulbar conjunctiva. *Arch Ophthalmol.* 1963;70:512–514.
17. Kaeser PF, Uffer S, Zografos L, Hamedani M. Tumors of the caruncle: a clinicopathologic correlation. *Am J Ophthalmol.* 2006;142(3):448–455.
18. McDonnell PJ, McDonnell JM, Kessis T, et al. Detection of human papillomavirus type 6/11 DNA in conjunctival papillomas by in situ hybridization with radioactive probes. *Hum Pathol.* 1987;18(11): 1115–1119.
19. Pfister H, Fuchs PG, Volcker HE. Human papillomavirus DNA in conjunctival papilloma. *Graefes Arch Clin Exp Ophthalmol.* 1985;223(3): 164–167.
20. Naghashfar Z, McDonnell PJ, McDonnell JM, et al. Genital tract papillomavirus type 6 in recurrent conjunctival papilloma. *Arch Ophthalmol.* 1986;104(12):1814–1815.
21. Lass JH, Grove AS, Papale JJ, et al. Detection of human papillomavirus DNA sequences in conjunctival papilloma. *Am J Ophthalmol.* 1983; 96(5):670–674.
22. Miller DM, Brodell RT, Levine MR. The conjunctival wart: report of a case and review of treatment options. *Ophthalmic Surg.* 1994;25(8): 545–548.
23. Sjo NC, Heegaard S, Prause JU, et al. Human papillomavirus in conjunctival papilloma. *Br J Ophthalmol.* 2001;85(7):785–787.
24. Buggage RR, Smith JA, Shen D, Chan CC. Conjunctival papillomas caused by human papillomavirus type 33. *Arch Ophthalmol.* 2002; 120(2):202–204.
25. Takamura Y, Kubo E, Tsuzuki S, Akagi Y. Detection of human papillomavirus in pterygium and conjunctival papilloma by hybrid capture II and PCR assays. *Eye.* 2008;22(11):1442–1445.
26. Sjo NC, von Buchwald C, Cassonnet P, et al. Human papillomavirus in normal conjunctival tissue and in conjunctival papilloma: types and frequencies in a large series. *Br J Ophthalmol.* 2007;91(8):1014–1015.
27. Kremer I, Sandbank J, Weinberger D, et al. Pigmented epithelial tumours of the conjunctiva. *Br J Ophthalmol.* 1992;76(5):294–296.
28. Wilson FM. In: Fraunfelder FT, Roy FH, eds. *Current ocular therapy.* Philadelphia: WB Saunders; 1990.
29. Burns RP, Wankum G, Giangiacomo J, Anderson PC. Dinitrochlorobenzene and debulking therapy of conjunctival papilloma. *J Pediatr Ophthalmol Strabismus.* 1983;20(6):221–226.
30. Petrelli R, Cotlier E, Robins S, Stoessel K. Dinitrochlorobenzene immunotherapy of recurrent squamous papilloma of the conjunctiva. *Ophthalmology.* 1981;88(12):1221–1225.
31. Hawkins AS, Yu J, Hamming NA, Rubenstein JB. Treatment of recurrent conjunctival papillomatosis with mitomycin C. *Am J Ophthalmol.* 1999;128(5):638–640.
32. Schechter BA, Rand WJ, Velazquez GE, et al. Treatment of conjunctival papillomata with topical interferon Alfa-2b. *Am J Ophthalmol.* 2002; 134(2):268–270.
33. Morgenstern KE, Givan J, Wiley LA. Long-term administration of topical interferon alfa-2beta in the treatment of conjunctival squamous papilloma. *Arch Ophthalmol.* 2003;121(7):1052–1053.
34. Muralidhar R, Sudan R, Bajaj MS, Sharma V. Topical interferon alpha-2b as an adjunctive therapy in recurrent conjunctival papilloma. *Int Ophthalmol.* 2009;29(1):61–62.
35. Chen Z, Yan J, Yang H, et al. Amniotic membrane transplantation for conjunctival tumor. *Yan Ke Xue Bao.* 2003;19(3):165–167, 45.

36. Shields CL, Lally MR, Singh AD, et al. Oral cimetidine (Tagamet) for recalcitrant, diffuse conjunctival papillomatosis. *Am J Ophthalmol.* 1999;128(3):362–364.
37. Chang SW, Huang ZL. Oral cimetidine adjuvant therapy for recalcitrant, diffuse conjunctival papillomatosis. *Cornea.* 2006;25(6):687–690.
38. Chang T, Chapman B, Heathcote JG. Inverted mucoepidermoid papilloma of the conjunctiva. *Can J Ophthalmol.* 1993;28(4):184–186.
39. Streeten BW, Carrillo R, Jamison R, et al. Inverted papilloma of the conjunctiva. *Am J Ophthalmol.* 1979;88(6):1062–1066.
40. Jakobiec FA, Harrison W, Aronian D. Inverted mucoepidermoid papillomas of the epibulbar conjunctiva. *Ophthalmology.* 1987;94(3): 283–287.
41. Jakobiec FA, Perry HD, Harrison W, Krebs W. Dacryoadenoma. A unique tumor of the conjunctival epithelium. *Ophthalmology.* 1989;96(7): 1014–1020.
42. Austin P, Jakobiec FA, Iwamoto T. Elastodysplasia and elastodystrophy as the pathologic bases of ocular pterygia and pinguecula. *Ophthalmology.* 1983;90(1):96–109.
43. Pournaras JA, Chamot L, Uffer S, Zografos L. Conjunctival intraepithelial neoplasia in a patient treated with tacrolimus after liver transplantation. *Cornea.* 2007;26(10):1261–1262.
44. McGavie J. Intraepithelial epithelioma of the cornea and conjunctiva (Bowen's disease). *Am J Ophthalmol.* 1942;25:167.
45. Pizzarello LD, Jakobiec FA. Bowen's disease of the conjunctiva: a misnomer. In: Jakobiec FA, ed. *Ocular and adnexal tumors.* New York: Aesculapius; 1978.
46. Zimmerman LE. Squamous cell carcinoma and related lesions of the bulbar conjunctiva. In: Bonuik M, ed. *Ocular and adnexal tumors.* St Louis: Mosby; 1964.
47. Erie JC, Campbell RJ, Liesegang TJ. Conjunctival and corneal intraepithelial and invasive neoplasia. *Ophthalmology.* 1986;93(2):176–183.
48. Waring GO 3rd, Roth AM, Ekins MB. Clinical and pathologic description of 17 cases of corneal intraepithelial neoplasia. *Am J Ophthalmol.* 1984;97(5):547–559.
49. Ni C, Searl SS, Kriegstein HJ, Wu BF. Epibulbar carcinoma. *Int Ophthalmol Clin.* 1982;22(3):1–33.
50. Dark AJ, Streeten BW. Preinvasive carcinoma of the cornea and conjunctiva. *Br J Ophthalmol.* 1980;64(7):506–514.
51. Carroll JM, Kuwabara T. A classification of limbal epitheliomas. *Arch Ophthalmol.* 1965;73:545–551.
52. Irvine AR. Dyskeratotic epibulbar tumors. *Trans Am Ophthalmol Soc.* 1963;61:243–273.
53. Ash JE, Wilder HC. Epithelial tumors of the limbus. *Am J Ophthalmol.* 1942;25.
54. Clear AS, Chirambo MC, Hutt MS. Solar keratosis, pterygium, and squamous cell carcinoma of the conjunctiva in Malawi. *Br J Ophthalmol.* 1979;63(2):102–109.
55. Ng J, Coroneo MT, Wakefield D, Di Girolamo N. Ultraviolet radiation and the role of matrix metalloproteinases in the pathogenesis of ocular surface squamous neoplasia. *Invest Ophthalmol Vis Sci.* 2008;49(12): 5295–5306.
56. Odrich MG, Jakobiec FA, Lancaster WD, et al. A spectrum of bilateral squamous conjunctival tumors associated with human papillomavirus type 16. *Ophthalmology.* 1991;98(5):628–635.
57. Hertle RW, Durso F, Metzler JP, Varsa EW. Epibulbar squamous cell carcinomas in brothers with xeroderma pigmentosa. *J Pediatr Ophthalmol Strabismus.* 1991;28(6):350–353.
58. Lauer SA, Malter JS, Meier JR. Human papillomavirus type 18 in conjunctival intraepithelial neoplasia. *Am J Ophthalmol.* 1990;110(1): 23–27.
59. Kim RY, Seiff SR, Howes EL Jr, O'Donnell JJ. Necrotizing scleritis secondary to conjunctival squamous cell carcinoma in acquired immunodeficiency syndrome. *Am J Ophthalmol.* 1990;109(2):231–233.
60. Napora C, Cohen EJ, Genvert GI, et al. Factors associated with conjunctival intraepithelial neoplasia: a case control study. *Ophthalmic Surg.* 1990;21(1):27–30.
61. McDonnell JM, Mayr AJ, Martin WJ. DNA of human papillomavirus type 16 in dysplastic and malignant lesions of the conjunctiva and cornea. *N Engl J Med.* 1989;320(22):1442–1446.
62. Winward KE, Curtin VT. Conjunctival squamous cell carcinoma in a patient with human immunodeficiency virus infection. *Am J Ophthalmol.* 1989;107(5):554–555.
63. Goyal JL, Rao VA, Srinivasan R, Agrawal K. Oculocutaneous manifestations in xeroderma pigmentosa. *Br J Ophthalmol.* 1994;78(4):295–297.
64. Muccioli C, Belfort R Jr, Burnier M, Rao N. Squamous cell carcinoma of the conjunctiva in a patient with the acquired immunodeficiency syndrome. *Am J Ophthalmol.* 1996;121(1):94–96.
65. Macarez R, Bossis S, Robinet A, et al. Conjunctival epithelial neoplasias in organ transplant patients receiving cyclosporine therapy. *Cornea.* 1999;18(4):495–497.
66. Fogla R, Biswas J, Kumar SK, et al. Squamous cell carcinoma of the conjunctiva as initial presenting sign in a patient with acquired immunodeficiency syndrome (AIDS) due to human immunodeficiency virus type-2. *Eye.* 2000;14 (Pt 2):246–247.
67. Rouberol F, Burillon C, Kodjikian L, et al. [Conjunctival epithelial carcinoma in a 9-year-old child with xeroderma pigmentosum. Case report]. *J Fr Ophtalmol.* 2001;24(6):639–642.
68. Scott IU, Karp CL, Nuovo GJ. Human papillomavirus 16 and 18 expression in conjunctival intraepithelial neoplasia. *Ophthalmology.* 2002;109(3):542–547.
69. Mahomed A, Chetty R. Human immunodeficiency virus infection, Bcl-2, p53 protein, and Ki-67 analysis in ocular surface squamous neoplasia. *Arch Ophthalmol.* 2002;120(5):554–558.
70. Char D. Conjunctival malignancies: diagnosis and management. In: Char D, ed. *Clinical ocular oncology.* New York: Churchill Livingstone; 1989.
71. Odrich MG, Kornmehl E, Kenyon K. Two cases of bilateral conjunctival squamous cell carcinoma with associated human papillomavirus. *Ophthalmology.* 1989;(suppl).
72. McDonnell JM, McDonnell PJ, Sun YY. Human papillomavirus DNA in tissues and ocular surface swabs of patients with conjunctival epithelial neoplasia. *Invest Ophthalmol Vis Sci.* 1992;33(1):184–189.
73. Moubayed P, Mwakyoma H, Schneider DT. High frequency of human papillomavirus 6/11, 16, and 18 infections in precancerous lesions and squamous cell carcinoma of the conjunctiva in subtropical Tanzania. *Am J Clin Pathol.* 2004;122(6):938–943.
74. Dushku N, Hatcher SL, Albert DM, Reid TW. p53 expression and relation to human papillomavirus infection in pingueculae, pterygia, and limbal tumors. *Arch Ophthalmol.* 1999;117(12):1593–1599.
75. Toth J, Karcioglu ZA, Moshfeghi AA, et al. The relationship between human papillomavirus and p53 gene in conjunctival squamous cell carcinoma. *Cornea.* 2000;19(2):159–162.
76. Karcioglu ZA, Toth J. Relation between p53 overexpression and clinical behavior of ocular/orbital invasion of conjunctival squamous cell carcinoma. *Ophthal Plast Reconstr Surg.* 2000;16(6):443–449.
77. Bartek J, Bartkova J, Vojtesek B, et al. Aberrant expression of the p53 oncoprotein is a common feature of a wide spectrum of human malignancies. *Oncogene.* 1991;6(9):1699–1703.
78. Shields CL, Manchandia A, Subbiah R, et al. Pigmented squamous cell carcinoma in situ of the conjunctiva in 5 cases. *Ophthalmology.* 2008;115(10):1673–1678.
79. Nicholson DH, Herschler J. Intraocular extension of squamous cell carcinoma of the conjunctiva. *Arch Ophthalmol.* 1977;95(5):843–846.
80. Tsubota K, Kajiwara K, Ugajin S, Hasegawa T. Conjunctival brush cytology. *Acta Cytol.* 1990;34(2):233–235.
81. Tseng SC. Staging of conjunctival squamous metaplasia by impression cytology. *Ophthalmology.* 1985;92(6):728–733.
82. Tole DM, McKelvie PA, Daniell M. Reliability of impression cytology for the diagnosis of ocular surface squamous neoplasia employing the Biopore membrane. *Br J Ophthalmol.* 2001;85(2):154–158.
83. Tananuvat N, Lertprasertsuk N, Mahanupap P, Noppanakeepong P. Role of impression cytology in diagnosis of ocular surface neoplasia. *Cornea.* 2008;27(3):269–274.
84. Prezyna AP, Monte JF, Satchidanand SK. Unilateral corneal intraepithelial neoplasia: management of the recurrent lesion. *Ann Ophthalmol.* 1990;22(3):103–105.
85. Peksayar G, Soyturk MK, Demiryont M. Long-term results of cryotherapy on malignant epithelial tumors of the conjunctiva. *Am J Ophthalmol.* 1989;107(4):337–340.
86. Fraunfelder FT, Wingfield D. Management of intraepithelial conjunctival tumors and squamous cell carcinomas. *Am J Ophthalmol.* 1983;95(3):359–363.
87. Divine RD, Anderson RL. Nitrous oxide cryotherapy for intraepithelial epithelioma of the conjunctiva. *Arch Ophthalmol.* 1983;101(5): 782–786.
88. Tabin G, Levin S, Snibson G, et al. Late recurrences and the necessity for long-term follow-up in corneal and conjunctival intraepithelial neoplasia. *Ophthalmology.* 1997;104(3):485–492.
89. Copeland RA Jr, Char DH. Limbal autograft reconstruction after conjunctival squamous cell carcinoma. *Am J Ophthalmol.* 1990;110(4): 412–415.
90. Frucht-Pery J, Rozenman Y. Mitomycin C therapy for corneal intraepithelial neoplasia. *Am J Ophthalmol.* 1994;117(2):164–168.
91. Frucht-Pery J, Sugar J, Baum J, et al. Mitomycin C treatment for conjunctival-corneal intraepithelial neoplasia: a multicenter experience. *Ophthalmology.* 1997;104(12):2085–2093.

92. Heigle TJ, Stulting RD, Palay DA. Treatment of recurrent conjunctival epithelial neoplasia with topical mitomycin C. *Am J Ophthalmol.* 1997;124(3):397–399.
93. Khokhar S, Soni A, Singh Sethi H, et al. Combined surgery, cryotherapy, and mitomycin-C for recurrent ocular surface squamous neoplasia. *Cornea.* 2002;21(2):189–191.
94. Frucht-Pery J, Rozenman Y, Pe'er J. Topical mitomycin-C for partially excised conjunctival squamous cell carcinoma. *Ophthalmology.* 2002; 109(3):548–552.
95. Shields CL, Naseripour M, Shields JA. Topical mitomycin C for extensive, recurrent conjunctival-corneal squamous cell carcinoma. *Am J Ophthalmol.* 2002;133(5):601–606.
96. Di Pascuale MA, Espana EM, Tseng SC. A case of conjunctiva-cornea intraepithelial neoplasia successfully treated with topical mitomycin C and interferon alfa-2b in cycles. *Cornea.* 2004;23(1):89–92.
97. Khong JJ, Muecke J. Complications of mitomycin C therapy in 100 eyes with ocular surface neoplasia. *Br J Ophthalmol.* 2006;90(7):819–822.
98. Hirst LW. Randomized controlled trial of topical mitomycin C for ocular surface squamous neoplasia: early resolution. *Ophthalmology.* 2007;114(5):976–982.
99. Schechter BA, Schrier A, Nagler RS, et al. Regression of presumed primary conjunctival and corneal intraepithelial neoplasia with topical interferon alpha-2b. *Cornea.* 2002;21(1):6–11.
100. Midena E, Boccato P, Angeli CD. Conjunctival squamous cell carcinoma treated with topical 5-fluorouracil. *Arch Ophthalmol.* 1997;115(12): 1600–1601.
101. Vann RR, Karp CL. Perilesional and topical interferon alfa-2b for conjunctival and corneal neoplasia. *Ophthalmology.* 1999;106(1):91–97.
102. Midena E, Angeli CD, Valenti M, et al. Treatment of conjunctival squamous cell carcinoma with topical 5-fluorouracil. *Br J Ophthalmol.* 2000;84(3):268–272.
103. Yeatts RP, Engelbrecht NE, Curry CD, et al. 5-Fluorouracil for the treatment of intraepithelial neoplasia of the conjunctiva and cornea. *Ophthalmology.* 2000;107(12):2190–2195.
104. Karp CL, Moore JK, Rosa RH Jr. Treatment of conjunctival and corneal intraepithelial neoplasia with topical interferon alpha-2b. *Ophthalmology.* 2001;108(6):1093–1098.
105. Sherman MD, Feldman KA, Farahmand SM, Margolis TP. Treatment of conjunctival squamous cell carcinoma with topical cidofovir. *Am J Ophthalmol.* 2002;134(3):432–433.
106. Schechter BA, Koreishi AF, Karp CL, Feuer W. Long-term follow-up of conjunctival and corneal intraepithelial neoplasia treated with topical interferon alfa-2b. *Ophthalmology.* 2008;115(8):1291–1296, 6 e1.
107. Cerezo L, Otero J, Aragon G, et al. Conjunctival intraepithelial and invasive squamous cell carcinomas treated with strontium-90. *Radiother Oncol.* 1990;17(3):191–197.
108. Dausch D, Landesz M, Schroder E. Phototherapeutic keratectomy in recurrent corneal intraepithelial dysplasia. *Arch Ophthalmol.* 1994; 112(1):22–23.
109. Jones DB, Wilhelmus KR, Font RL. Beta radiation of recurrent corneal intraepithelial neoplasia. *Trans Am Ophthalmol Soc.* 1991;89:285–298; discussion 98–301.
110. Buus DR, Tse DT, Folberg R, Buuns DR. Microscopically controlled excision of conjunctival squamous cell carcinoma. *Am J Ophthalmol.* 1994;117(1):97–102.
111. Cha SB, Shields CL, Shields JA, et al. Massive precorneal extension of squamous cell carcinoma of the conjunctiva. *Cornea.* 1993;12(6):537–540.
112. Grossniklaus HE, Martin DF, Solomon AR. Invasive conjunctival tumor with keratoacanthoma features. *Am J Ophthalmol.* 1990;109(6):736–738.
113. Motegi S, Tamura A, Matsushima Y, et al. Squamous cell carcinoma of the eyelid arising from palpebral conjunctiva. *Eur J Dermatol.* 2006;16(2):187–189.
114. Jauregui HO, Klintworth GK. Pigmented squamous cell carcinoma of cornea and conjunctiva: a light microscopic, histochemical, and ultrastructural study. *Cancer.* 1976;38(2):778–788.
115. Shields JA, Shields CL, Eagle RC Jr, et al. Pigmented conjunctival squamous cell carcinoma simulating a conjunctival melanoma. *Am J Ophthalmol.* 2001;132(1):104–106.
116. Akpek EK, Polcharoen W, Chan R, Foster CS. Ocular surface neoplasia masquerading as chronic blepharoconjunctivitis. *Cornea.* 1999;18(3): 282–288.
117. Cervantes G, Rodriguez AA Jr, Leal AG. Squamous cell carcinoma of the conjunctiva: clinicopathological features in 287 cases. *Can J Ophthalmol.* 2002;37(1):14–19; discussion 9–20.
118. Char DH, Kundert G, Bove R, Crawford JB. 20 MHz high frequency ultrasound assessment of scleral and intraocular conjunctival squamous cell carcinoma. *Br J Ophthalmol.* 2002;86(6):632–635.
119. Nguyen J, Ivan D, Esmaeli B. Conjunctival squamous cell carcinoma in the anophthalmic socket. *Ophthal Plast Reconstr Surg.* 2008;24(2): 98–101.
120. Iliff WJ, Marback R, Green WR. Invasive squamous cell carcinoma of the conjunctiva. *Arch Ophthalmol.* 1975;93(2):119–122.
121. Lee GA, Hirst LW. Ocular surface squamous neoplasia. *Surv Ophthalmol.* 1995;39(6):429–450.
122. Tunc M, Char DH, Crawford B, Miller T. Intraepithelial and invasive squamous cell carcinoma of the conjunctiva: analysis of 60 cases. *Br J Ophthalmol.* 1999;83(1):98–103.
123. Shepler TR, Prieto VG, Diba R, et al. Expression of the epidermal growth factor receptor in conjunctival squamous cell carcinoma. *Ophthal Plast Reconstr Surg.* 2006;22(2):113–115.
124. Krishnakumar S, Lakshmi SA, Pusphparaj V, et al. Human leukocyte class I antigen and beta2-microglobulin expression in conjunctival dysplasia, carcinoma in situ, and squamous cell carcinoma. *Cornea.* 2005;24(3):337–341.
125. Abhyankar D, Lakshmi SA, Pushparaj V, et al. HLA class II antigen expression in conjunctival precancerous lesions and squamous cell carcinomas. *Curr Eye Res.* 2003;27(3):151–155.
126. Gurses I, Doganay S, Mizrak B. Expression of glucose transporter protein-1 (Glut-1) in ocular surface squamous neoplasia. *Cornea.* 2007;26(7):826–830.
127. McCarty JH, Barry M, Crowley D, et al. Genetic ablation of alpha v integrins in epithelial cells of the eyelid skin and conjunctiva leads to squamous cell carcinoma. *Am J Pathol.* 2008;172(6):1740–1747.
128. Tabbara KF, Kersten R, Daouk N, Blodi FC. Metastatic squamous cell carcinoma of the conjunctiva. *Ophthalmology.* 1988;95(3):318–321.
129. Guech-Ongey M, Engels EA, Goedert JJ, et al. Elevated risk for squamous cell carcinoma of the conjunctiva among adults with AIDS in the United States. *Int J Cancer.* 2008;122(11):2590–2593.
130. Shields CL, Demirci H, Marr BP, et al. Chemoreduction with topical mitomycin C prior to resection of extensive squamous cell carcinoma of the conjunctiva. *Arch Ophthalmol.* 2005;123(1):109–113.
131. Char DH, Crawford JB, Howes EL Jr, Weinstein AJ. Resection of intraocular squamous cell carcinoma. *Br J Ophthalmol.* 1992;76(2):123–125.
132. Ramonas KM, Conway RM, Daftari IK, et al. Successful treatment of intraocularly invasive conjunctival squamous cell carcinoma with proton beam therapy. *Arch Ophthalmol.* 2006;124(1):126–128.
133. Kaines A, Davis G, Selva D, et al. Conjunctival squamous cell carcinoma with perineural invasion resulting in death. *Ophthalmic Surg Lasers Imaging.* 2005;36(3):249–251.
134. Sears KS, Rundle PR, Mudhar HS, Rennie IG. The effects of photodynamic therapy on conjunctival in situ squamous cell carcinoma – a review of the histopathology. *Br J Ophthalmol.* 2008;92(5):716–717.
135. Procianoy F, Cruz AA, Baccegã A, et al. Aggravation of eyelid and conjunctival malignancies following photodynamic therapy in DeSanctis-Cacchione syndrome. *Ophthal Plast Reconstr Surg.* 2006;22(6):498–499.
136. Hughes DS, Powell N, Fiander AN. Will vaccination against human papillomavirus prevent eye disease? A review of the evidence. *Br J Ophthalmol.* 2008;92(4):460–465.
137. McKelvie PA, Daniell M, McNab A, et al. Squamous cell carcinoma of the conjunctiva: a series of 26 cases. *Br J Ophthalmol.* 2002;86(2): 168–173.
138. Campbell RJ, Bourne WM. Unilateral central corneal epithelial dysplasia. *Ophthalmology.* 1981;88(12):1231–1238.
139. Rao NA, Font RL. Mucoepidermoid carcinoma of the conjunctiva: a clinicopathologic study of five cases. *Cancer.* 1976;38(4):1699–1709.
140. Brownstein S. Mucoepidermoid carcinoma of the conjunctiva with intraocular invasion. *Ophthalmology.* 1981;88(12):1226–1230.
141. Herschorn BJ, Jakobiec FA, Hornblass A, et al. Mucoepidermoid carcinoma of the palpebral mucocutaneous junction. A clinical, light microscopic and electron microscopic study of an unusual tubular variant. *Ophthalmology.* 1983;90(12):1437–1446.
142. Lacour S, Legeais JM, D'Hermies F, et al. [Mucoepidermoid carcinoma of the conjunctiva with intraocular invasion. Apropos of a case]. *J Fr Ophtalmol.* 1991;14(5):349–352.
143. Gunduz K, Shields CL, Shields JA, et al. Intraocular neoplastic cyst from mucoepidermoid carcinoma of the conjunctiva. *Arch Ophthalmol.* 1998;116(11):1521–1523.
144. Rodman RC, Frueh BR, Elner VM. Mucoepidermoid carcinoma of the caruncle. *Am J Ophthalmol.* 1997;123(4):564–565.
145. Hwang IP, Jordan DR, Brownstein S, et al. Mucoepidermoid carcinoma of the conjunctiva: a series of three cases. *Ophthalmology.* 2000; 107(4):801–805.

146. Wilson MW, Fleming JC, Fleming RM, Haik BG. Sentinel node biopsy for orbital and ocular adnexal tumors. *Ophthal Plast Reconstr Surg.* 2001;17(5):338–344; discussion 44–5.
147. Esmaeli B. Sentinel node biopsy as a tool for accurate staging of eyelid and conjunctival malignancies. *Curr Opin Ophthalmol.* 2002;13(5): 317–323.
148. Huntington AC, Langloss JM, Hidayat AA. Spindle cell carcinoma of the conjunctiva. An immunohistochemical and ultrastructural study of six cases. *Ophthalmology.* 1990;97(6):711–717.
149. Wise AC. A limbal spindle-cell carcinoma. *Surv Ophthalmol.* 1967; 12(3):244–246.
150. Cohen BH, Green WR, Iliff NT, et al. Spindle cell carcinoma of the conjunctiva. *Arch Ophthalmol.* 1980;98(10):1809–1813.
151. Seregard S, Kock E. Squamous spindle cell carcinoma of the conjunctiva. Fatal outcome of a plerygium-like lesion. *Acta Ophthalmol Scand.* 1995;73(5):464–466.
152. Shields JA, Eagle RC, Marr BP, et al. Invasive spindle cell carcinoma of the conjunctiva managed by full-thickness eye wall resection. *Cornea.* 2007;26(8):1014–1016.
153. Mauriello JA Jr, Abdelsalam A, McLean IW. Adenoid squamous carcinoma of the conjunctiva – a clinicopathological study of 14 cases. *Br J Ophthalmol.* 1997;81(11):1001–1005.
154. Kuo T. Clear cell carcinoma of the skin. A variant of the squamous cell carcinoma that simulates sebaceous carcinoma. *Am J Surg Pathol.* 1980;4(6):573–583.
155. Margo CE, Groden LR. Primary clear cell carcinoma of the conjunctiva. *Arch Ophthalmol.* 2008;126(3):436–438.
156. Chao AN, Shields CL, Krema H, Shields JA. Outcome of patients with periocular sebaceous gland carcinoma with and without conjunctival intraepithelial invasion. *Ophthalmology.* 2001;108(10):1877–1883.
157. Shields CL, Naseripour M, Shields JA, Eagle RC Jr. Topical mitomycin-C for pagetoid invasion of the conjunctiva by eyelid sebaceous gland carcinoma. *Ophthalmology.* 2002;109(11):2129–2133.
158. Rao NA, McLean IW. Zimmerman LE. Sebaceous carcinoma of eyelids and caruncle. Correlation of clinicopathologic features with prognosis. In: Jakobiec FA, ed. *Ocular and adnexal tumors.* New York: Aesculapius; 1978.
159. Jakobiec FA. Sebaceous tumors of the ocular adnexa. In: Albert DM, Jakobiec FA, ed. *Principles and practice of ophthalmology.* Philadelphia: WB Saunders; 1994.
160. Ni C. Sebaceous cell carcinoma of the ocular adnexa. *Int Ophthalmol Clin.* 1981;22:23.
161. Margo CE, Lessner A, Stern GA. Intraepithelial sebaceous carcinoma of the conjunctiva and skin of the eyelid. *Ophthalmology.* 1992;99(2):227–231.
162. Levinson AW, Jakobiec FA, Reifler DM, Hornblass A. Ectopic epibulbar Fordyce nodules in a buccal mucous membrane graft. *Am J Ophthalmol.* 1985;100(5):724–727.
163. Boniuk M, Zimmerman LE. Sebaceous carcinoma of the eyelid, eyebrow, caruncle and orbit. *Int Ophthalmol Clin.* 1972;12(1):225–257.
164. Sakol PJ, Simons KB, McFadden PW, et al. DNA flow cytometry of sebaceous cell carcinomas of the ocular adnexa: introduction to the technique in the evaluation of periocular tumors. *Ophthal Plast Reconstr Surg.* 1992;8(2):77–87.
165. Rishi K, Font RL. Sebaceous gland tumors of the eyelids and conjunctiva in the Muir-Torre syndrome: a clinicopathologic study of five cases and literature review. *Ophthal Plast Reconstr Surg.* 2004;20(1):31–36.
166. Demirci H, Nelson CC, Shields CL, et al. Eyelid sebaceous carcinoma associated with Muir-Torre syndrome in two cases. *Ophthal Plast Reconstr Surg.* 2007;23(1):77–79.
167. Tanahashi J, Kashima K, Daa T, et al. Merkel cell carcinoma co-existent with sebaceous carcinoma of the eyelid. *J Cutan Pathol.* 2008.
168. Jakobiec FA, Brownstein S, Albert W, et al. The role of cryotherapy in the management of conjunctival melanoma. *Ophthalmology.* 1982; 89(5):502–515.
169. Condon GP, Brownstein S, Codere F. Sebaceous carcinoma of the eyelid masquerading as superior limbic keratoconjunctivitis. *Arch Ophthalmol.* 1985;103(10):1525–1529.
170. Wagoner MD, Beyer CK, Gonder JR, Albert DM. Common presentations of sebaceous gland carcinoma of the eyelid. *Ann Ophthalmol.* 1982;14(2):159–163.
171. Miyagawa M, Hayasaka S, Nagaoka S, Mihara M. Sebaceous gland carcinoma of the eyelid presenting as a conjunctival papilloma. *Ophthalmologica.* 1994;208(1):46–48.
172. Ginsberg J. Present status of meibomian gland carcinoma. *Arch Ophthalmol.* 1965;73:271–277.
173. Straatsma BR. Meibomian gland tumors. *AMA Arch Ophthalmol.* 1956;56(1):71–93.
174. Sweebe E, Cogan D. Meibomian gland tumors. *Arch Ophthalmol.* 1956;61.
175. Sawada Y, Fischer JL, Verm AM, et al. Detection by impression cytologic analysis of conjunctival intraepithelial invasion from eyelid sebaceous cell carcinoma. *Ophthalmology.* 2003;110(10):2045–2050.
176. Yeatts RP, Waller RR. Sebaceous carcinoma of the eyelid: pitfalls in diagnosis. *Ophthal Plast Reconstr Surg.* 1985;1(1):35–42.
177. Doxanas MT, Green WR. Sebaceous gland carcinoma. Review of 40 cases. *Arch Ophthalmol.* 1984;102(2):245–249.
178. Callahan MA, Callahan A. Sebaceous carcinoma of the eyelids. In: Jakobiec FA, ed. *Ocular and adnexal tumors.* New York: Aesculapius; 1978.
179. Lisman RD, Jakobiec FA, Small P. Sebaceous carcinoma of the eyelids. The role of adjunctive cryotherapy in the management of conjunctival pagetoid spread. *Ophthalmology.* 1989;96(7):1021–1026.
180. Nunery WR, Welsh MG, McCord CD Jr. Recurrence of sebaceous carcinoma of the eyelid after radiation therapy. *Am J Ophthalmol.* 1983;96(1):10–15.
181. Rao NA, Hidayat AA, McLean IW, Zimmerman LE. Sebaceous carcinomas of the ocular adnexa: a clinicopathologic study of 104 cases, with five-year follow-up data. *Hum Pathol.* 1982;13(2):113–122.
182. Cable MM, Lyon DB, Rupani M, et al. Case reports and small case series: primary basal cell carcinoma of the conjunctiva with intraocular invasion. *Arch Ophthalmol.* 2000;118(9):1296–1298.
183. Ostergaard J, Boberg-Ans J, Prause JU, Heegaard S. Primary basal cell carcinoma of the caruncle with seeding to the conjunctiva. *Graefes Arch Clin Exp Ophthalmol.* 2005;243(6):615–618.
184. Meier P, Sterker I, Meier T. Primary basal cell carcinoma of the caruncle. *Arch Ophthalmol.* 1998;116(10):1373–1374.
185. Grossniklaus HE, Green WR, Luckenbach M, Chan CC. Conjunctival lesions in adults. A clinical and histopathologic review. *Cornea.* 1987;6(2):78–116.
186. Husain SE, Patrinely JR, Zimmerman LE, Font RL. Primary basal cell carcinoma of the limbal conjunctiva. *Ophthalmology.* 1993;100(11): 1720–1722.

Chapter 40

Melanocytic Neoplasms of the Conjunctiva

Ian W. McLean, J. Douglas Cameron

This chapter is the work of the late Ian W. McLean, MD, which required little updating because of the quality of the original chapter. Dr. McLean was an outstanding ophthalmic pathologist who contributed to many areas of ophthalmic pathology including conjunctival melanoma. His absence is definitely felt, particularly by colleagues who knew him personally.

J. Douglas Cameron

Introduction

The conjunctiva is a mucous membrane that may be affected by several types of melanocytic neoplasia, including potentially fatal conjunctival melanoma.

Melanocytes are specialized cells capable of producing the complex protein melanin. Melanocytes are a normal constituent of the conjunctival epithelium. Melanin is distributed through delicate dendritic (branching) cellular processes to neighboring epithelial cells. Melanin production is stimulated by several means, including exposure to ultraviolet light. The additional melanin produced plays a role in protecting epithelial cells from the harmful effects of ultraviolet light. Melanin production may also be stimulated by inflammation, trauma, and various hormones. In their normal location at the base of the conjunctival epithelium melanocytes do not contain pigment and are difficult to identify by light microscopy without the use of special immunohistochemical stains such as S-100, HMB-45, and melanin A.[1]

Melanocytic nevus cells are developmentally abnormal cells that do not have dendritic processes and retain rather than distribute melanin. Certain subgroups of nevus cells are found at the junction of the conjunctival epithelium and the conjunctival stroma. Over time, the nevus cells tend to lose pigment and move deeper into the conjunctival stroma. Other types of nevus cells that are stationary in location are found and remain at deeper sites in the conjunctival stroma, even to the level of episcleral tissue. Clinical clues to the tissue location of the nevus cells are often indicated by the apparent color of the melanin: superficial golden brown to deep blue-gray.

Not all cells containing melanin are melanocytes. Damaged or senescent melanocytes may discharge melanin into the surrounding matrix to be phagocytized by macrophages (melanophages). Increasing pigmentation of a melanocytic lesion may be due to melanin in macrophages rather than melanin in the neoplastic cells.

Both melanocytes and nevus cells have the potential to undergo malignant transformation to malignant melanoma. Melanophages have no potential for malignant transformation.

Conjunctival Nevus

The melanocytic nevi of the conjunctiva are classified by tissue location relative to the surface epithelium, as are types of nevi of the skin, with only minor modifications in terminology: junctional (at the dermal–epidermal junction), subepithelial (limited to the stroma), combined (junctional and subepithelial), blue (oval to round melanocytes in episcleral tissue), and cellular blue (spindle-shaped melanocytes in the episcleral tissue).

Most conjunctival nevi are compound or subepithelial. Pure intraepithelial nevi (junctional nevi) are present most commonly in younger individuals.[2] Blue and cellular blue nevi are seldom encountered in the conjunctiva. In patients with the nevus of Ota, the discrete bluish episcleral spots may be considered special examples of blue nevi. When there is a combination of an intraepithelial, subepithelial, or compound nevus with a blue or cellular blue nevus, the lesion may be designated a combined nevus.

Subepithelial and compound nevi of the conjunctiva are similar in their clinical and histologic characteristics. The amount of junctional activity (histologic signs of cellular proliferation) varies considerably in compound nevi and most subepithelial nevi can be shown to have a small junctional component if adequately sampled. Inclusions of conjunctival epithelium in the form of solid islands or cysts are usually observed with conjunctival nevi (Figs 40.1–40.3). These epithelial inclusions may represent an anomalous development of the conjunctival epithelium. The junctional component of the nevus may be observed only within the subsurface inclusions of conjunctival epithelium. In young individuals, great cytologic pleomorphism (a histologic sign of cell growth instability) may be present in conjunctival nevi, and large spindle- or epithelioid-shaped melanocytes characteristic of 'Spitz nevi' may be encountered.[3,4] The Spitz nevus is a variant of a compound nevus that can mimic a malignant melanoma but generally has a benign course. Subepithelial and compound nevi typically elevate the

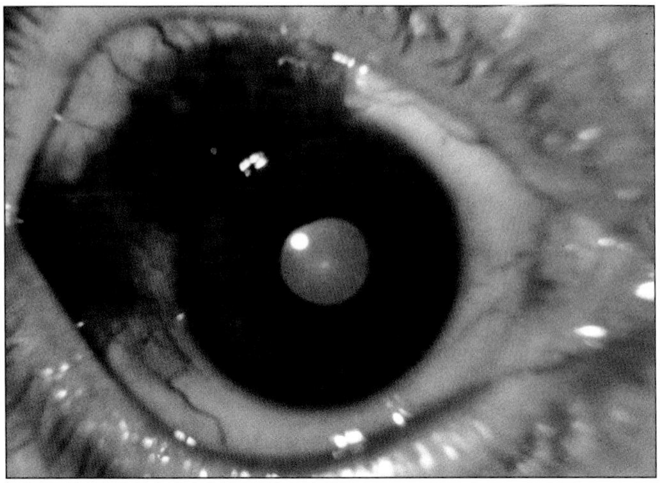

Fig. 40.1 Cystic compound nevus. Clinically, the lesion is sharply demarcated, sightly elevated, vascularized, and moderately pigmented. Intralesional cysts are present that are clearly seen by slit lamp examination.

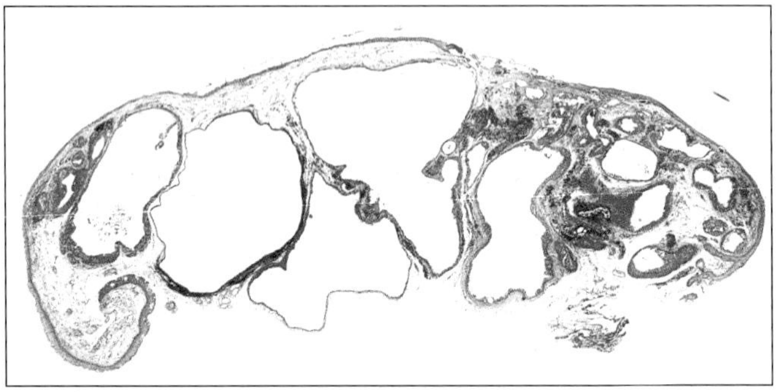

Fig. 40.2 Cystic compound nevus. Multiple cystic spaces lined by squamous epithelium are clearly evident in this section of a compound nevus. The cysts are developmental abnormalities of the surface epithelium and not the melanocytes. Elevation of the surface contour of the conjunctiva will be affected by the number and volume of epithelial inclusion cysts (hematoxylin & eosin stained section) (AFIP Neg. 73-4253, ×11).

conjunctival surface (see Fig. 40.1), whereas junctional nevi, like melanosis (see following), characteristically do not thicken the conjunctiva.[5]

Conjunctival nevi may become more noticeable at the time of puberty. With growth spurts and tissue maturation, melanocytes may proliferate or increase pigment production. Conjunctival epithelial cells within inclusions may proliferate and secrete extracellular material, enlarging the size of the cysts. As the nevus increases in volume, changes in hydration of the ocular surface causes irritation with secondary inflammation. Inflammatory cell infiltration further increases the size, elevation, and vascularity of the nevus. These alterations tend to provoke clinical concern that a malignant melanoma has arisen from the nevus, which has led to surgical excision of a large number of benign conjunctival nevi.[6] The degree of pigmentation is variable in conjunctival nevi. Some nevi are totally amelanotic and, when the lesion is small, the epithelial inclusions may

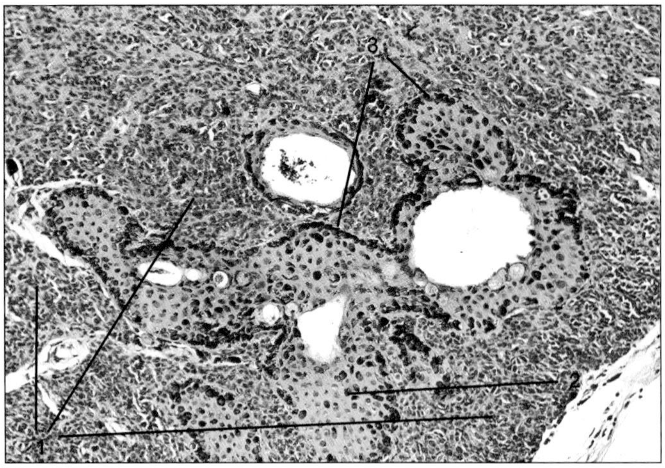

Fig. 40.3 Cystic compound nevus. The lesion is composed of small nevus cells (prominent homogeneous nucleus with a small amount of clear cytoplasm), in this case arranged in a sheetlike distribution (*1*) around a central inclusion cyst. The cyst (*2*) is lined by squamous epithelial cells that are identical to the surface epithelial cells. In this case, the squamous cells have proliferated to partially fill the cyst. The nevus cells have transferred melanin pigment (*3*) to the cytoplasm of the epithelial cells (hematoxylin & eosin stain) (AFIP Neg. 64-4595).

predominate. As they enlarge or become inflamed, they may be confused with epithelial neoplasia such as squamous cell carcinoma.[7,8] Inflamed juvenile conjunctival nevi contain epithelial cysts and solid epithelial islands associated with discrete lymphocytic aggregates, plasma cells, and eosinophils. There is often a history of allergy.[9] Occasionally, an amelanotic nevus may develop reactive vascularization that may be mistaken for an angiomatous neoplasm of the conjunctiva.[5]

Conjunctival Melanosis

Melanosis refers to excessive melanin production and retention of pigment by epithelial melanocytes. This process, however, does not elevate the surface of the conjunctiva. Nevi usually will cause elevation of the surface. Classification of conjunctival melanosis is based on three main characteristics: whether the abnormality is congenital or acquired; whether the melanosis is epithelial or subepithelial; and whether the melanosis is primary or secondary. Congenital melanoses are primary and divided into epithelial and subepithelial types. The acquired melanoses are epithelial and are divided into primary and secondary types. Thus, a good history and a careful clinical biomicroscopic examination are essential for accurate classification of conjunctival melanosis.

Epithelial congenital melanosis

An ephelis (freckle) is a discrete, stationary lesion (present since birth or early childhood) characterized by excessive melanin production in the basal epithelium by a normal number of melanocytes. The melanocytes in an ephelis are cytologically normal. This lesion is not a precursor of malignant melanoma.

Subepithelial congential melanosis

Subepithelial congenital melanosis is not a lesion of the conjunctiva but the episclera. Ocular melanocytosis or melanosis oculi is pigment change limited to tissues of the eye. In addition to increased numbers of pigmented melanocytes in the sclera and episclera, this condition is characterized by a congenital increase in the number, size, and degree of pigmentation of melanocytes of the uvea. Ocular melanocytosis is almost invariably unilateral. Heterochromia iridis with episcleral pigmentation in the more heavily pigmented uveal tract are visible clinical signs of melanosis oculi (Fig. 40.4).

The nevus of Ota (oculodermal melanocytosis) is the combination of melanosis oculi along with ipsilateral melanosis of the deep dermal tissues of the lids or periocular facial skin or both. In both forms of congenital subepithelial melanosis, the deeply located affected tissues have a slate blue-gray discoloration. Individual and small clusters of melanocytes are interspersed with the connective tissue of the sclera, episclera, and dermis of the eyelid. Bilateral oculodermal melanocytosis is rare, but is more common than bilateral melanosis oculi. In bilateral nevus of Ota, the degree of pigmentation is usually not symmetric. Oculodermal melanocytosis is observed with relatively greater frequency in Asians and blacks than in whites. Both conditions may also be associated with melanosis of the orbital tissues and the meninges of the optic nerve or brain.

Subepithelial congenital melanosis predisposes to the development of malignant melanoma not only in the conjunctiva but also in intraocular uveal tract and extraocularly in the soft tissues of the orbit. There have been only a few reports of the occurrence of malignant change in the nevus of Ota.[10] Any of the tissues affected by congenital melanosis may develop a malignant melanoma, but most melanomas have arisen in the uveal tract followed in frequency by melanoma of the orbit.

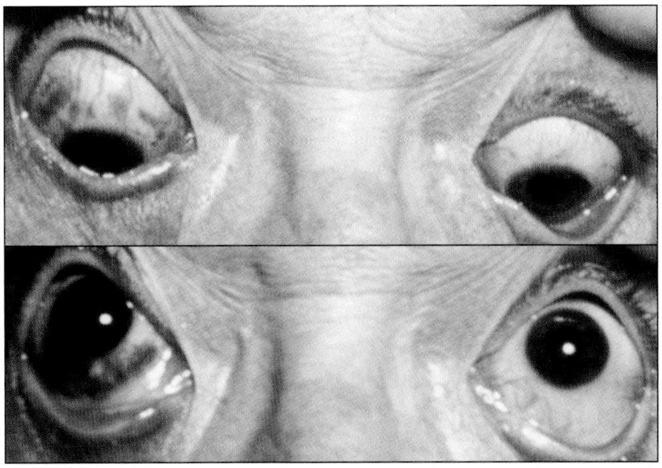

Fig. 40.4 Congenital melanosis. The bulbar conjunctiva and the episcleral areas contain irregular areas of gray to brown patches of melanin pigment. The brown areas represent melanin located superficially in the bulbar conjunctiva above and below the cornea. The gray areas represent melanin pigment in the superficial layers of episcleral tissue. Generalized hyperpigmentation of the iris is also present.

Secondary acquired melanosis

Bilateral acquired melanoses are usually secondary, i.e. caused by extraocular factors. Increased pigmentation is attributed to racially associated genetic, metabolic, or toxic factors and do not predispose to the development of malignant melanoma. The most frequent form is the acquired melanosis of the limbal and perilimbal conjunctival epithelium. In darkly pigmented individuals, progressive bilateral pigmentation of the conjunctiva is generally considered a normal aspect of aging.

Unilateral secondary acquired melanosis, like bilateral melanosis, is observed most frequently in nonwhites. Secondary melanosis occurs in varying degrees in association with any subepithelial or epithelial mass (e.g. a cyst, foreign body, or mound of scar tissue) that elevates the conjunctival surface, causing irritation. Because of secondary melanosis, epithelial tumors (e.g. papilloma, actinic keratosis, squamous cell carcinoma, and mucoepidermoid carcinoma) of the conjunctiva in blacks may be mistaken for malignant melanomas.[11]

Primary acquired melanosis

Primary acquired melanosis (PAM) is a neoplastic proliferation with potential for malignant transformation of melanocytes within the conjunctival epithelium. This condition is most often observed as a unilateral lesion in middle-aged whites.

The classification of cutaneous acquired melanoses,[12] has generally not been applied to conjunctival acquired melanosis.[13,14] One reason for using a unique classification for conjunctival lesions is because primary acquired melanosis of the conjunctiva without further stratification into high-risk groups has historically been overtreated. Clinical/pathologic studies of biopsied cases of PAM indicate that only one-third of conjunctival primary acquired melanosis diagnosed by clinical criteria alone progress to melanoma.[15] Histological characterization from a conjunctival biopsy is required to further stratify those clinically pigmented lesions that are likely to progress to malignant melanoma of the conjunctiva.

Primary acquired melanosis of the conjunctiva typically begins insidiously in middle age (median age 56 years, range 15–91 years)[16] as a subtle, yellow-brown stippling of the epithelium (Fig. 40.5). Although bulbar conjunctival involvement is most common (most often in the temporal and inferior quadrants),[16] any part of the conjunctiva, including that of the non-sun-exposed forniceal, palpebral, and canthal regions, may be affected. Conjunctival melanosis may extend onto cutaneous surfaces, particularly at the lid margin or in the region of the canthus. Primary acquired melanosis of the conjunctiva is initially a flat lesion, as opposed to nevi and melanomas, which are elevated (see Figs 40.1 and 40.5). Acquired thickening of tissue affected by primary acquired melanosis is a risk factor for the presence of transformation to melanoma. Shields et al. have observed that 35% of lesions will progress over a 10-year interval and 12% will

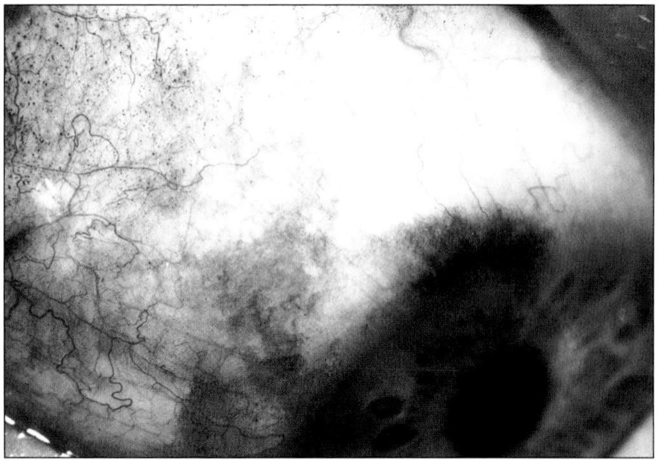

Fig. 40.5 Primary acquired melanosis. Ill-defined granular, golden brown pigmentation of the bulbar conjunctiva is more intense at the limbus. The pigmented region is not elevated above the surrounding nonpigmented tissue (AFIP Acc. 1441952).

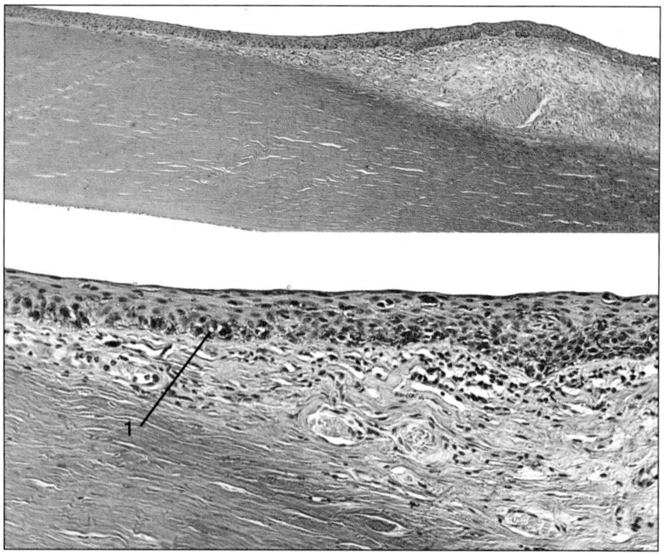

Fig. 40.6 Primary acquired melanosis. Basilar hyperplasia of melanocytes is present at the dermal–epidermal junction seen at low magnification of limbal tissue (*top*). In the higher magnification (*bottom*) the melanocytes can be seen to be mildly to moderately atypical, characterized by increased nuclear to cytoplasmic ratio and nuclear pleomorphism) (*1*). (*Top*: hematoxylin & eosin stain, original magnification ×35. *Bottom*: hematoxylin & eosin stain, original magnification ×130.)

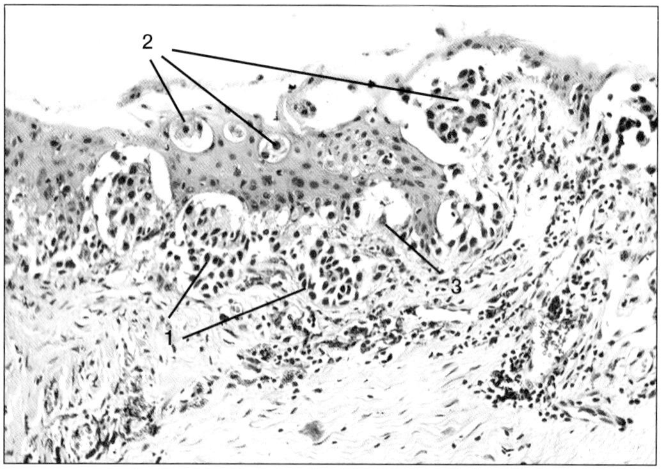

Fig. 40.7 Primary acquired melanosis. A carcinoma-in-situ pattern is present with the surface epithelium almost totally replaced with spindle-shaped cells (*1*). The proliferating melanocytes are moderately to markedly atypical. Because of the intense inflammatory infiltrate of the superficial stroma (*2*), it is difficult to determine if the proliferating melanocytes have invaded across the basement membrane of the surface epithelium (AFIP Neg. 596300) (hematoxylin-eosin stain, original magnification ×220).

undergo malignant transformation.[16] The greater the extent of primary acquired melanosis in clock hours, the greater the risk for transformation to melanoma.[16] However, in some unusual cases discrete nodular masses composed entirely of inflammatory cells may simulate a malignant melanoma.[17]

The natural history of primary acquired melanosis is unpredictable. The condition often progresses slowly, but may wax and wane, i.e. disappearance of pigmentation in one area with simultaneous increase of pigmentation in another area. Clinical evaluation by simple inspection and slit lamp examination may not reveal the full extent of the melanosis. An ultraviolet light (Wood's light) or confocal microscopy[18] may identify areas of subclinical melanosis extending beyond the edges of the lesion as observed by ambient light. The rate of progression from acquired melanosis to melanoma is extremely variable, but typically is measured in years. In a series of 41 cases of biopsied primary acquired melanosis, 13 (32%) progressed to malignant melanoma, but none of the patients who were followed for 10 years without progression to malignant melanoma subsequently developed a malignant melanoma.[13]

Maly et al., utilizing cytological criteria such as nest cohesion, melanocytic hyperplasia, nuclear features, and pagetoid spread, have suggested a standardized protocol for grading atypia in melanocytic conjunctival lesions.[19]

The histologic features of primary acquired melanosis are also extremely variable, both in comparing different cases and in comparing different areas within a lesion. The melanocytes vary in size, shape, and degree of atypia. There may be small polyhedral cells, with little or no atypia, polyhedral or spindle-shaped cells, with moderate atypia (Figs 40.6, 40.7), or large epithelioid cells with extensive atypia (Fig. 40.8). The pattern of involvement also varies. Individual melanocytes may line up along the basal lamina of the epithelium (Fig. 40.6), form nests of melanocytes that extend into the epithelium (Fig. 40.7) or invade the epithelium in a pagetoid fashion (malignant cells replacing normal epithelial cells without elevating the surface of the tissue in a manner similar to that found in the cutaneous spread of carcinoma of the breast) (Fig. 40.7), or completely replace the epithelium with atypical melanocytes mimicking an in situ carcinoma (Fig. 40.8). Two helpful features are extent of involvement of the epithelium: basal layer only, 20% progression to melanoma (Fig. 40.6), pagetoid invasion, 90% progression to melanoma (Figs 40.7 and 40.8), and the presence of epithelioid cells (Fig. 40.7).[13]

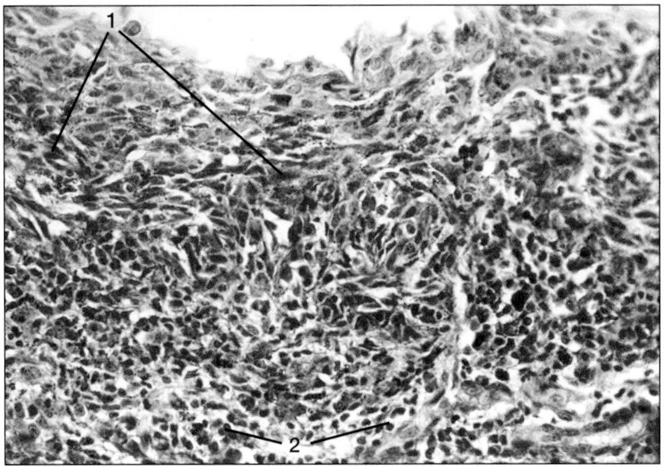

Fig. 40.8 Primary acquired melanosis. A nestlike pattern of melanocytic proliferation is present at the basal epithelium (*1*) and in the epithelium closer to the surface (*2*). Moderate to servere atypia is present (*3*) (AFIP Neg. 669136) (hematoxylin & eosin stain, original magnification ×115).

All lesions, especially those with the histological features that are indicative of high risk, should be completely resected, if feasible, without damaging the eye. Cryotherapy[20] and mitomycin-C[21–23] have also been used.

Primary acquired melanosis of the conjunctiva is associated with a nevus in about 20% of cases. The presence of a nevus, however, does not appear to increase significantly the chances of melanoma developing in acquired melanosis or affect the prognosis once a melanoma has developed.[24]

Malignant Melanoma

Conjunctival melanoma may arise from primary acquired melanosis (Fig. 40.9), from pre-existing nevi (Figs 40.10, 40.11), or may arise de novo from apparently normal conjunctiva (Fig. 40.12). The presence or absence of a nevus associated with a conjunctival melanoma does not appear to significantly affect survival. Primary acquired melanosis is the primary risk factor.[24]

Most conjunctival malignant melanomas occur in white adults and at least two-thirds arise in acquired melanosis. Only 28 cases of malignant melanoma have been reported in individuals under age 15 years.[25] The incidence in blacks is exceedingly small.[26] The incidence of melanoma arising in ocular sites has remained stable in the Danish Cancer Registry between 1943 and 1997.[27] In the United States between 1974 and 1998 the incidence of conjunctival melanoma in males has increased. The incidence of intraocular melanoma has remained relatively stationary.[28] For these reasons, any change in a pigmented lesion of the conjunctiva in a white adult, but particularly growth with increasing elevation, should be suspected of being a malignant melanoma and treated accordingly.[17] Other pigmented lesions that may occur at the limbus include pigmented squamous carcinoma[8] and iris herniated through a dehisced cataract wound.[29] Melanoma may arise in unusual circumstances such as in the anophthalmic socket of an 8-month-old child following chemotherapy and radiation for retinoblastoma.[30]

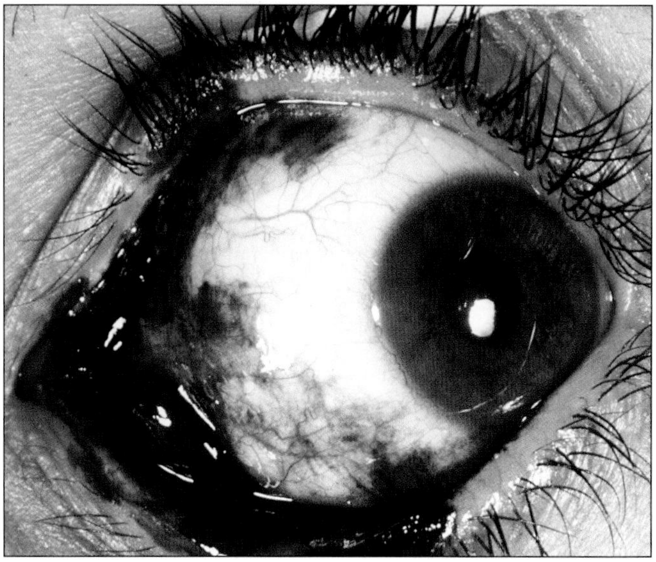

Fig. 40.9 Malignant melanoma. Malignant melanoma has arisen from an extensive area of primary acquired melanosis in the conjunctival fornix. The thickness of the lesion and its location in the forniceal tissue rich with lymph channels are both poor prognostic signs.

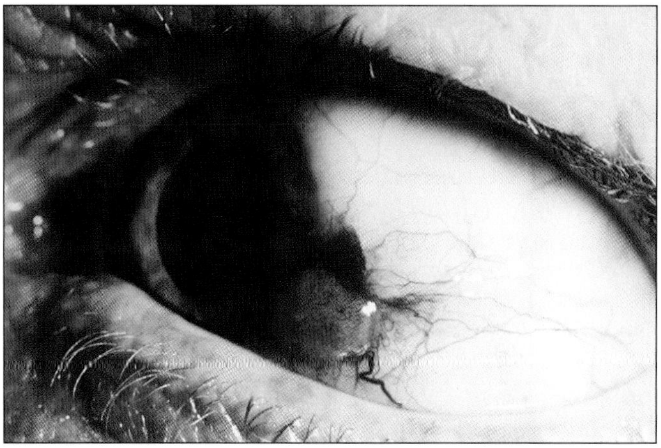

Fig. 40.10 Malignant melanoma. Malignant melanoma has arisen in a compound nevus near the limbus. The region of malignant transformation is less intensely pigmented than the original compound nevus.

In a malignant melanoma, atypical melanocytes invade from the epithelium into the substantia propria of the conjunctiva. Conjunctival melanomas, like uveal melanomas, vary cytologically, with spindle-type cells or epithelioid-type cells (Fig. 40.13). The cytological composition of conjunctival melanomas does not have prognostic significance, unlike that of uveal melanomas.[24] The presence of mitotic activity, large clusters of atypical cells, and lack of maturation and infiltrative growth at the deep margin are helpful in differentiating melanomas from nevi. Spindle-shaped melanoma cells (Figs 40.13, 40.14) are often amelanotic, and they may induce a desmoplastic stroma. They can be highly invasive, with involvement of nerves and extension posteriorly into the orbit. Such tumors in the orbit can mimic a malignant schwannoma.

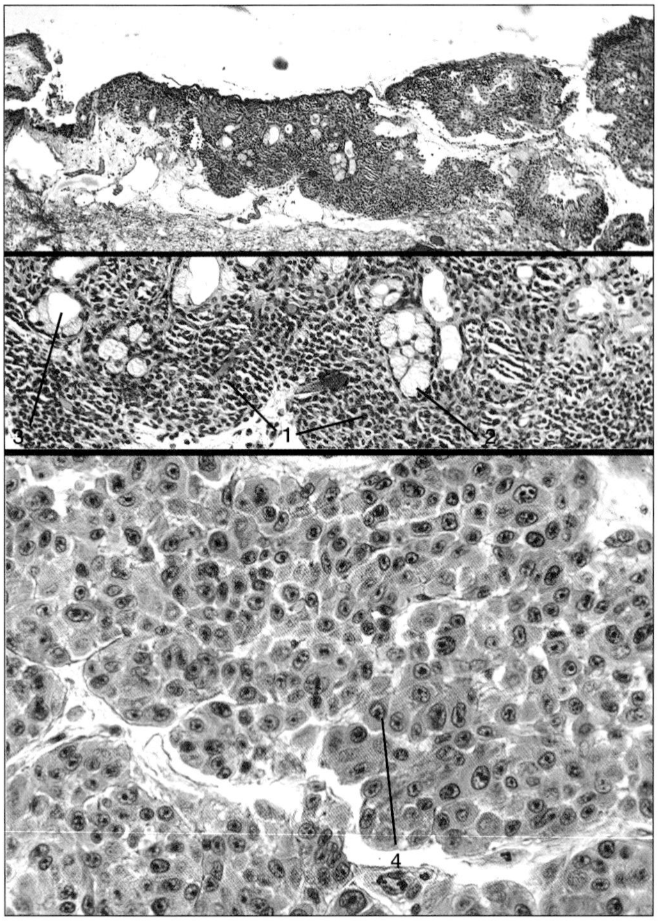

Fig. 40.11 Malignant melanoma. This melanoma originated in a compound nevus. **Top**: The original nevus is characterized by inclusion of squamous epithelial cells (hematoxylin & eosin stain, original magnification ×35). **Middle**: The remaining nevus is characterized by nests of small polyhedral cells with homogeneously staining small nuclei (*1*). Goblet cells (*2*) are present within the conjunctival inclusion cysts (*3*) (hematoxylin & eosin stain, original magnification ×115). **Bottom**: The cells of the melanoma are larger, with prominent large nucleoli with marked margination chromatin and prominent central nucleoli (*4*) (hematoxylin & eosin stain, original magnification ×265).

At times, because of the complete absence of pigmentation, the melanocytic nature of a lesion may be totally unsuspected clinically and difficult to establish beyond reasonable doubt by light microscopy of routinely stained sections. In such cases, positive immunohistochemical reactivity for HMB-45, MELAN-A, and S-100 and negative staining for cytokeratin provide a reliable method for distinguishing amelanotic melonoma from epithelial tumors.[31]

Thickness of the melanomas of the conjunctiva, like melanomas of the skin, is the most important prognostic feature.[32] Silvers found that a thickness of about 1.8 mm (from the surface of the epithelium to the deepest level of invasion) separated most lethal from nonlethal conjunctival melanomas.[33] Several studies have confirmed a positive relationship between increasing tumor thickness and a fatal outcome,[24,34–37] but Folberg et al.[24] and Crawford[38] found that even flat melanomas less than 0.8 mm thick are able to

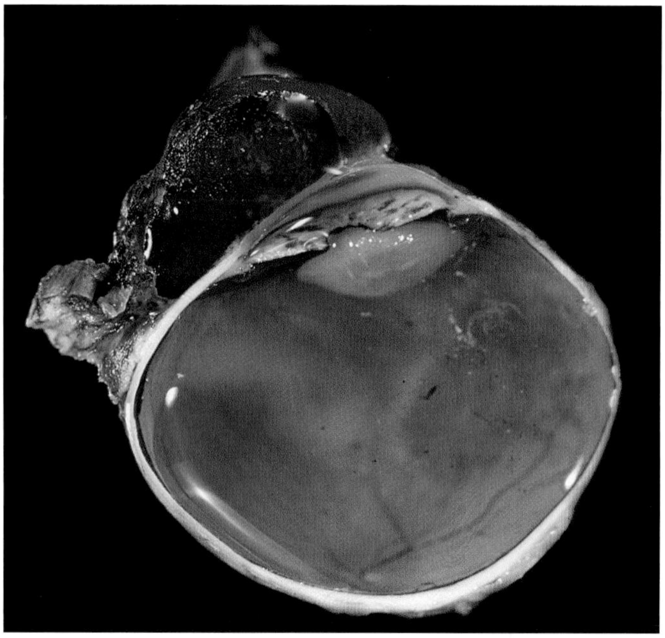

Fig. 40.12 Malignant melanoma. A large exophytic conjunctival melanoma began in the region of the limbus. Lesions of this size have an unpredictable natural history but are more likely to be associated with metastasis of tumor cells than are smaller tumors. However, the correlation between size and metastasis is highly variable (AFIP Neg. 624854).

metastasize, possibly because of the proximity of conjunctival lymph channels to the epithelium (Fig. 40.14).

Additional risk factors for metastasis of conjunctival melanoma include lesions located in nonbulbar conjunctiva, involvement of the eyelid margin, invasion of sclera or orbit, pagetoid or in situ invasion of the epithelium, high mitotic rate, and recurrence.[24,36,37,39,40]

Favorable features include inflammatory cells invading among invasive tumor cells and limbal tumors (see Fig. 40.12).[24]

The behavior of conjunctival melanomas is more like cutaneous than uveal melanomas. Both conjunctival and cutaneous melanomas arise in the surface epithelium. In sharp contrast with uveal melanomas, which almost never metastasize to the regional lymph nodes, conjunctival melanomas share with cutaneous melanomas the ability to invade lymphatics (see Fig. 40.14) and spread initially to the regional lymph nodes (Fig. 40.15).[41] The preauricular and intraparotid nodes are more often affected than the submandibular and cervical lymph nodes.[42] Lymphatic spread to regional nodes indicates a poor prognosis, but it does not always denote widespread dissemination or a lethal outcome. In several cases, simple excision of metastatic malignant melanoma to preauricular lymph nodes has resulted in an apparent cure even without radical surgery or supplemental therapy.[43]

Intraocular extension may occur, particularly in those cases where multiple excisions are necessary and Bowman's membrane has been breached.[44] Conjunctival melanoma may extend into the soft tissues of the orbit.[45] Robertson et al. reported spread of conjunctival melanoma to nasal

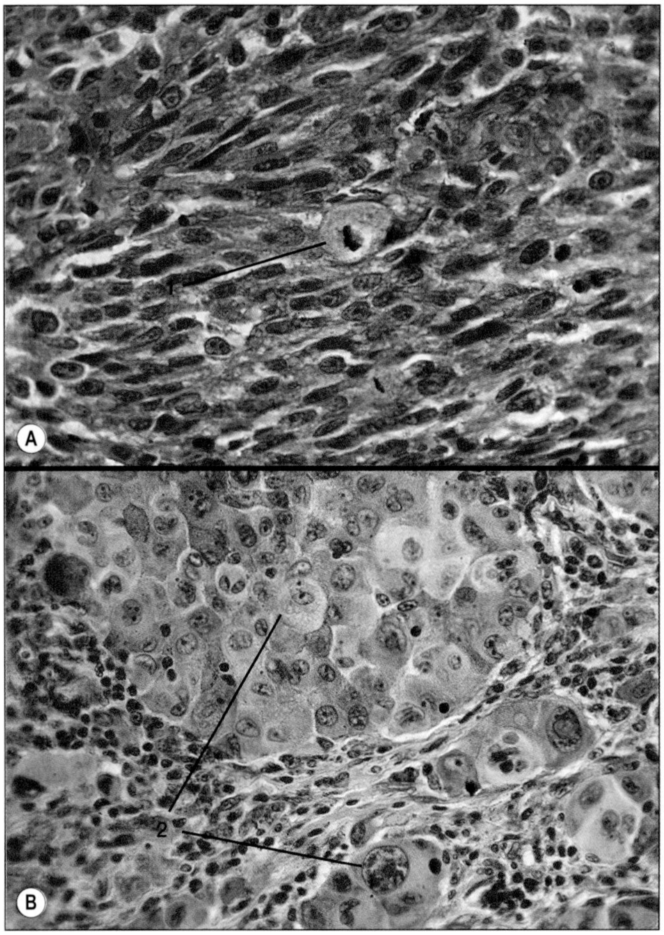

Fig. 40.13 Malignant melanoma. (**A**) This portion of the tumor is composed of spindle-shaped cells, generally of uniform shape and size. Mitotic figures are present (*1*) (AFIP Accession number 790958) (hematoxylin-eosin stain, original magnification ×305). (**B**) This portion of the tumor is composed of epithelioid cells (*2*) that are variable in size and nuclear to cytoplasmic ratio (AFIP Neg. 57 6310) (hematoxylin & eosin stain, original magnification ×305).

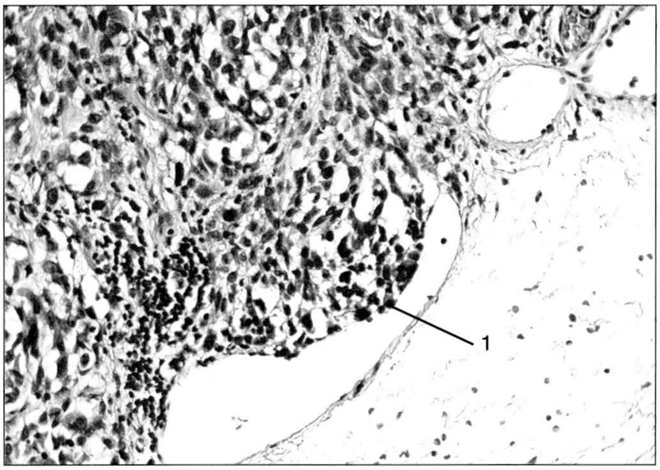

Fig. 40.14 Malignant melanoma. Melanoma cells are invading a lymphatic vessel (*1*) in the process of metastasizing to regional lymph nodes and other distant sites (AFIP Neg. 63-1809) (hematoxylin & eosin stain, original magnification ×145).

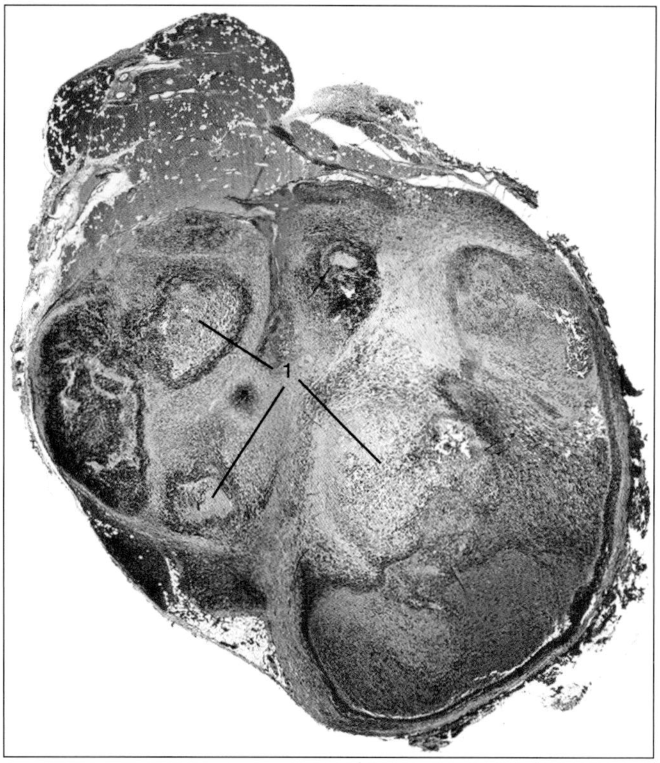

Fig. 40.15 Malignant melanoma. Melanoma cells have spread to a preauricular lymph node. The metastatic tumor site has undergone extensive necrosis (*1*) (AFIP Acc. 609918) (hematoxylin & eosin stain, original magnification ×6).

cavity and paranasal sinuses, probably via the nasolacrimal epithelium.[39]

Generally, conjunctival melanoma metastasizes to the liver; however, metastasis to other organ systems have occurred.[46] The tumor node and metastasis (TNM) T stage has been determined by Coupland in a series of 40 patients with conjunctival melanoma treated between 1993 and 2006.[47] The majority of patients were found in T stages I and II.

The mortality rate has been reported to be between 8%[36] and 26%.[24,37] Treatment options for primary lesions include surgical excision and cryotherapy. Metastatic lesions have been treated with lymph node dissection, chemotherapy, radiotherapy, and immunotherapy.[36] Proton radiation may serve as an alternative to exenteration in advanced cases of conjunctival melanoma.[48]

References

1. Iwamoto S, et al. Immunophemotype of conjunctival melanoma. *Archives of Ophthalmology.* 2000;120:1625–1629.
2. Shields C, et al. Conjunctival nevi: clinical features and natural course in 410 consecutive patients. *Archives of Ophthalmology.* 2004;122:167–175.
3. Kantelip B, et al. A case of conjunctival Spitz nevus: review of the literature and comparison with cutaneous locations. *Annals of Ophthalmology.* 1989;21:176–179.
4. Vervaet N, et al. A rare conjunctival Spitz nevus: a case report and literature review. *Bulletin de la Societe Belge d Ophtalmologie.* 2007;303:63–67.
5. Folberg R, Jakobiec F. Benign conjunctival melanocytic lesions: clinicopathologic feature. *Ophthalmology.* 1989;96:436–461.

6. Lommatzsch P, et al. Inflammatory juvenile conjunctival nevus (IJCN). *Klinische Monatsblatter fur Augenhielkunde*. 2007;224:422–446.
7. Shields JA, et al. Differentiation of pigmented conjunctival squamous cell carcinoma from melanoma. *Ophthalmic Surgery, Lasers & Imaging*. 2003;34:406–408.
8. Shields CL, et al. Pigmened squamous cell carcinoma in situ of the conjunctiva in 5 cases. *Ophthalmology*. 2008;115:1673–1678.
9. Zamir E, et al. Inflamed juvenile conjunctival naevus: clinicopathological characterisation. *British Journal of Ophthalmology*. 2002;86:28–30.
10. Nik N, Glew W, Zimmerman L. Malignant melanoma of the choroid in the nevus of Ota. *Archives of Ophthalmology*. 1982;100:1641–1643.
11. Jauregui H, Klintworth G. Pigmented squamous cell carcinoma of the cornea and conjunctiva. *Cancer*. 1976;38:778–788.
12. Clark W. A classification of malignant melanomas in man correlated with histogenesis and biologic behavior. In: Montagnev W, Hu F, eds. *Advances in biology of the skin. The pigmentary system*. London: Pergamon Press; 1967.
13. Folberg R, McLean IW, Zimmerman L. Primary acquired melanosis of the conjunctiva. *Human Pathology*. 1985;16:129–135.
14. Folberg R, McLean IW. Primary acquired melanosis and melanoma of the conjunctiva: terminology, classification, and biologic behavior. *Human Pathology*. 1986;17:652–654.
15. Folberg R, et al. Is primary acquired melanosis of the conjunctiva equivalent to melanoma in situ? *Modern Pathology*. 1992;5:2–5.
16. Shields J, et al. Primary acquired melanosis of the conjunctiva: risks for progression to melanoma in 311 eyes. The 2006 Lorenz E Zimmerman Lecture. *Ophthalmology*. 2008.
17. Jakobiec F, Folberg R, Iwamoto T. Clinicopathologic characteristics of premalignant and malignant melanocytic lesions of the conjunctiva. *Ophthalmology*. 1989;96:147–166.
18. Messmer EM, et al. In vivo confocal microscopy of pigmented conjunctival tumors. *Graefe's Arch Clin Exp Ophthalmol*. 2006;244:1437–1445.
19. Maly A, et al. Histological criteria for grading of atypia in melanocytic conjunctival lesions. *Pathology*. 2008;40:676–681.
20. Brownstein S, et al. Cryotherapy for precancerous melanosis (atypical melanocytic hyperplasia) of the conjunctiva. *Archives of Ophthalmology*. 1981;99:1224–1231.
21. Groh M, et al. Management of conjunctival malignant melanoma associated with primary acquired melanosis (PAM) using 0.02% mitomycin C eyedrops. *Ophthalmologe*. 2003;100:708–712.
22. Pe'er J, Frucht-Pery J. The treatment of primary acquired melanosis (PAM) with atypia by topical mitomycin C. *American Journal of Ophthalmology*. 2005;139:229–234.
23. Chalasani R, Giblin M, Conway RM. Role of topical chemotherapy for primary acquired melanosis and malignant melanoma of the conjunctiva and cornea. *Clinical & Experimental Ophthalmology*. 2006;343:708–714.
24. Folberg R, McLean I, Zimmerman L. Malignant melanoma of the conjunctiva. *Human Pathology*. 1985;16:136–143.
25. Taban M, Traboulsi EI. Malignant melanoma of the conjunctiva in children: a review of the international literature. *Journal of Pedicatric Ophthalmology & Strabismus*. 2007;44:277–282.
26. Colby KA, Nagel D. Conjunctival melanoma arising from diffuse priamry acquired melanosis in a young black woman. *Cornea*. 2005;24:352–355.
27. Isager P, et al. Unveal and conjunctival malignant melanoma in Denmark, 1943–1997. *Ophthalmic Epidemiology*. 2005;12:223–232.
28. Inskip PD, Devesa SS, Fraumeni JFJ. Trends in the incidence of ocular melanoma in the United States, 1974–1998. *Cancer Causes & Control*. 2003;15:251–257.
29. Marr B, et al. Uveal prolapse following cataract extraction simulating melanoma. *Ophthalmic Surgery, Lasers & Imaging*. 2008;39:250–251.
30. Mahajan A, et al. Conjunctival melanoma 3 years after radiation and chemotherapy for retinoblastoma. *Journal of Pedicatric Ophthalmology & Strabismus*. 2007;44:300–302.
31. McDonnell J, Sun Y, Wagner D. HMB-45 immunohistochemical staining of conjunctival melanocytic lesions. *Ophthalmologe*. 1991;98:453–458.
32. Breslow A. Tumor thickness, level of invasion and node dissection in stage I cutaneous melanoma. *Annals of Surgery*. 1975;182:572–575.
33. Silvers D. Melanoma of the conjunctiva: a cilnicopathologic study. In: Jakobiec F, ed. *Ocular and adnexal tumors*. Birmingham, Alabama: Aesculapius; 1978.
34. Fuchs U, et al. Prognosis of conjunctival melanomas in relation to histological features. *British Journal of Cancer*. 1989;59:261–267.
35. Uffer S. Melanomes malins de la conjunctive: etude histopathologique. *Klinische Monatsblatter fur Augenhielkunde*. 1990;196:290–294.
36. Shields CL. Conjunctival melanoma: risk factors for recurrence, exenteration, metastasis and death in 150 consecutive patients. *Archives of Ophthalmology*. 2000;118:1497–1507.
37. Anastassiou G, et al. Prognostic value of clinical and histologic parameters in conjunctival melanomas: a retrospective study. *British Journal of Ophthalmology*. 2002;86:163–167.
38. Crawford J. Conjunctival melanomas: prognostic factors, a review and analysis of a series. *Transactions of the American Ophthalmological Society*. 1980;78:467–502.
39. Robertson D, Hungerford J, McCartney A. Pigmentation of the eyelid margin accompanying conjunctival melanoma. *American Journal of Ophthalmology*. 1989;108:435–439.
40. Seregard S, Kock E. Conjunctival malignant melanoma in Sweden 1969–1991. *Acta Ophthalmologica (Copenh)*. 1992;70:289–296.
41. Cuthbertson F, Luck J, Rose S. Malignant melanoma of the conjunctiva metastasising to the partoid gland. *British Journal of Ophthalmology*. 2003;87:1428–1429.
42. Lim M, et al. Patterns of regional head and neck lymph node metastasis in primary conjunctival malignant melanoma. *British Journal of Ophthalmology*. 2006;90:1468–1471.
43. Folberg R, McLean I, Zimmerman L. Conjunctival melanosis and melanoma. *Ophthalmology*. 1984;91:673–678.
44. Sandinha T, et al. Malignant melanoma of the conjunctiva with intraocular extension: a clinicopathlogoical study of three cases. *Graefe's Arch Clin Exp Ophthalmol*. 2007;245:431–436.
45. Gokmen SH, F A. Malignant conjunctival tumors invading the orbit. *Ophthalmologica*. 2008;222:338–343.
46. Koklu S, et al. Diffuse gastroduodenal metastasis of conjunctival melanoma. *American Journal of Gastroenterology*. 2008;103:1321–1323.
47. Coupland DB. Clinical mapping of conjunctival melanomas. *British Journal of Ophthalmology*. 2008;92:1545–1549.
48. Wuestemeyer H, et al. Proton radiotherapy as an alternative to exenteration in the management of extended conjunctival melanoma. *Graefe's Arch Clin Exp Ophthalmol*. 2006;244:438–446.

Chapter 41

Subepithelial Neoplasms of the Conjunctiva

Michael A. Warner, Pooja V. Bhat, Frederick A. Jakobiec

The substantia propria of the conjunctiva is a loose network of connective tissue composed of fibroblasts, blood vessels, nerves, and lymphatics.[1] Rather than arising from mesodermal somites, which are absent in the head and neck region, the cells of this layer are derived from migration from the neural crest (mesectoderm or ectomesenchyme). A wide range of tumors may arise from this rich tissue layer.[1–3] This chapter discusses subepithelial neoplasms of the conjunctiva; for completeness, certain congenital, inflammatory, and degenerative lesions are also mentioned.

During evaluation of a patient with a subepithelial lesion, the clinician should obtain a careful history, especially concerning the time of onset, rapidity of growth, history of trauma, and history of systemic disease. Complete ocular examination, including palpation of regional lymph nodes, should be performed. Photographic documentation should be obtained.

Congenital Lesions

Congenital lesions are primarily choristomas, tumor-like growths composed of elements not normally indigenous to the affected area. There are three types of choristomas: dermoids and dermolipomas, ectopic lacrimal gland, and epibulbar osseous and neuroglial choristomas.

Choristomas

Dermoid and dermolipoma

Dermoids most commonly involve the inferotemporal limbal corneal and epibulbar region (Fig. 41.1).[1] Bilateral, congenital ring dermoids rarely affect 360 degrees of both limbal areas.[4] Small dermoids appear clinically as tan, rather inconspicuous lesions, whereas larger lesions are whiter and may protrude from the ocular surface. Clinically, most dermoids are asymptomatic; however, they may produce significant astigmatism with secondary amblyopia and ocular irritation due to poor lid closure, tear film anomalies, or trauma from fine hairs that may grow from their surface. Histologically, dermoids are solid, placoid tumors that arise from the outer third of the sclera and consist of thick dermis-like collagen within which may be hair follicles, sebaceous glands, sweat glands, and fat lobules. In rare cases, the entire cornea is involved with white, corneal opacifications and disorganized stroma with adnexal glands.[5]

Clinically, dermolipomas are similar to dermoids, but are somewhat yellow in color and arise near the insertion of the lateral rectus muscle. The lesion may extend upward to the superior fornix. Because of the location and color of dermolipomas, the differential diagnosis of this lesion includes prolapsed orbital fat (Fig. 41.2), prolapse of the palpebral lobe of the lacrimal gland, and lymphoma. These last three lesions, however, are freely mobile over the underlying sclera, unlike dermolipomas which are firmly fixed. With computed tomography (CT) or magnetic resonance imaging (MRI), dermolipomas have features that may be indistinguishable from prolapsed orbital fat.[6] Dermolipomas are similar to dermoids histopathologically except that the former usually lack pilosebaceous units and have more fat.

Both dermoids and dermolipomas may occasionally coexist with other systemic malformations including Goldenhar's syndrome (with preauricular appendages, hemifacial microsomia, and vertebral body anomalies), mandibulofacial dysostosis (Treacher Collins syndrome, Franceschetti syndrome), and bandlike cutaneous nevus and central nervous system dysfunction (Solomon's syndrome, linear sebaceous nevus of Jadassohn).[7–14] Both lesions are occasionally associated with lid colobomas, suggesting that limbal dermoids and dermolipomas may arise from entrapment of dermal elements within the sclera at the time of eyelid development. Indeed, choristomas have also been associated with microphthalmos; in some of these cases dermal appendages are found within the vitreous cavity.[15,16]

Dermoids and dermolipomas tend to grow with the patient and tend not to undergo neoplastic transformation. Indications for removal include astigmatism with or without amblyopia, irritation, and cosmetic deformity. Because the outer third of the sclera is often involved, a lamellar excision is usually required. When the cornea is involved exclusively, the surgeon should anticipate lamellar or penetrating keratoplasty. Amniotic membrane transplantation may assist with the closure of large conjunctival defects.[17] Complications of excision include globe penetration, reduced motility from scarring or surgical injury of a rectus muscle, and increased astigmatism. Some dermoids and most dermolipomas extend to the fornices and may become entangled in extraocular muscles and orbital fat. Care should be taken to excise all

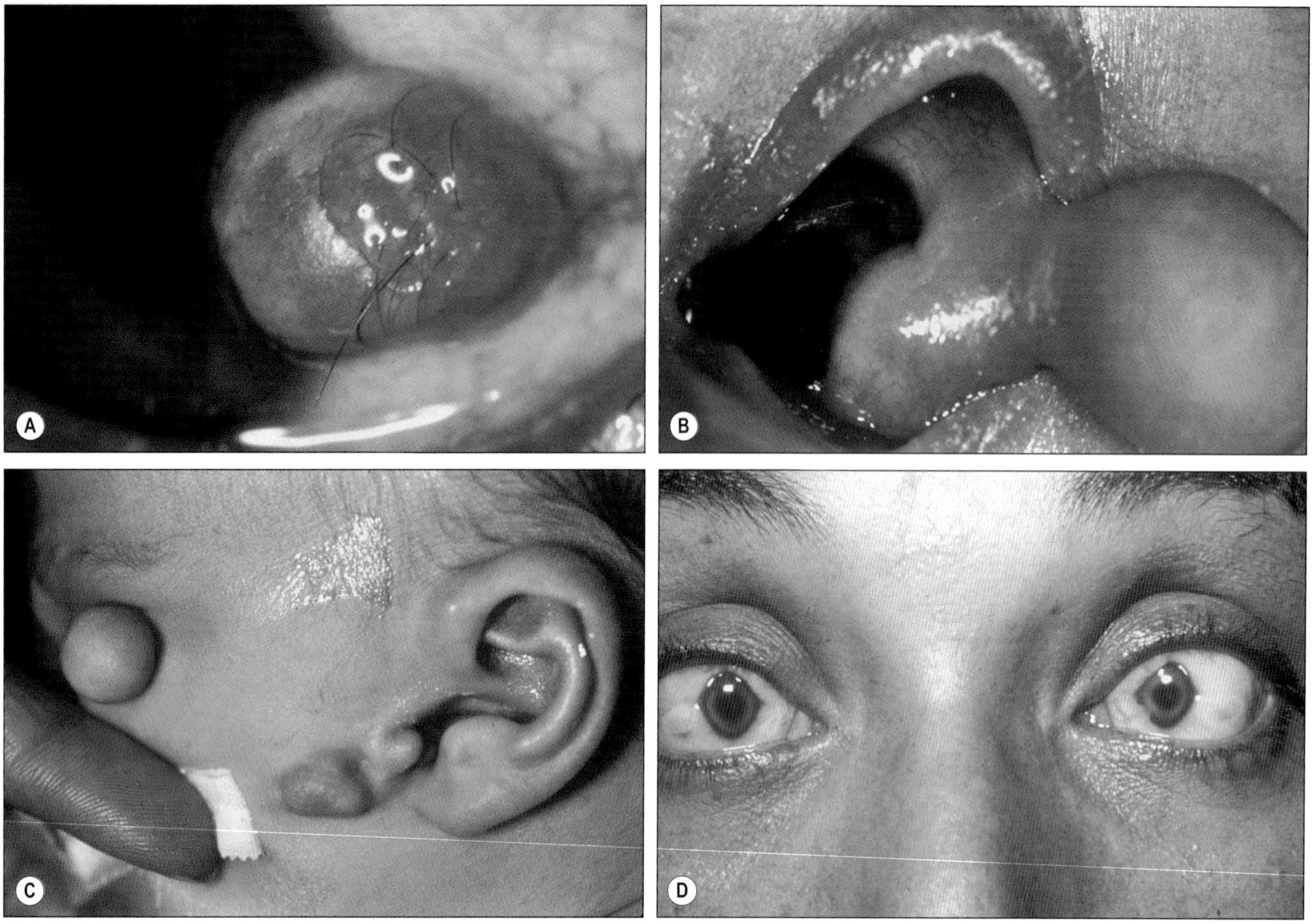

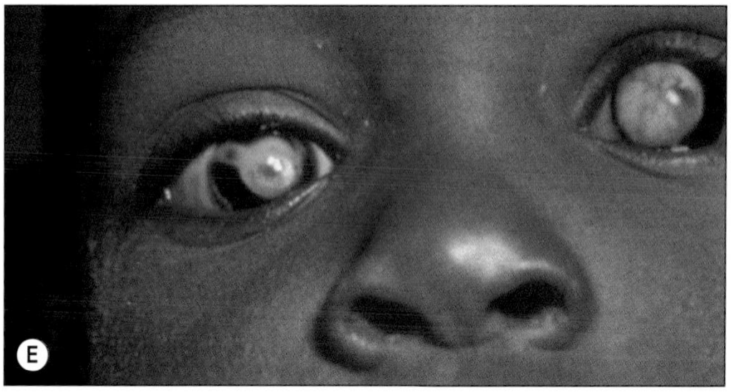

Fig. 41.1 Conjunctival dermoid. Dermoids are choristomatous congenital lesions which most commonly occur in the inferotemporal limbal corneal and epibulbar region. (**A**) Typical appearance of a limbal dermoid. The lesion is tan and has fine hairs protruding from its surface. Moderate conjunctival injection is noted to surround the lesion. (**B** and **C**) Large, tan pedunculated limbal dermoid in a neonate with ipsilateral preauricular appendages. (**D**) Bilateral ring dermoids involve 360 degrees of both limbal areas. (Courtesy W.R. Green, MD.) (**E**) Central corneal dermoids are present bilaterally. (Courtesy L.E. Zimmerman, MD.)

remnants, since exposed elements may incite a significant inflammatory response.[1,18,19]

Ectopic lacrimal gland; simple and complex choristomas

Ectopic lacrimal gland is the second most common choristoma that affects the epibulbar surface (Fig. 41.3).[20–24] Simple choristomas are composed only of acinar lacrimal gland tissue, whereas complex choristomas also possess other elements, such as smooth muscle, nerve elements, cartilage, sweat glands, or pilosebaceous units. The frequent presence of smooth muscle suggests that the lesions may represent the ectopic palpebral lobe of the lacrimal gland, which is intermixed with the smooth Müller's muscle. Clinically, the lesions tend to have a fleshy pink appearance with raised translucent nodules; they are well vascularized. If the lesion extends onto the corneal surface, associated corneal scarring may be present. Occasionally, the palpebral portion of the lacrimal gland may prolapse into the subconjunctival space at the upper temporal bulbar conjunctiva and may consequently be misdiagnosed as ectopic lacrimal gland tissue. Incorrect diagnosis with consequent surgical intervention can jeopardize the excretory ducts of the prolapsed lacrimal gland tissue, leading to dry eye.[21,24] Choristomas

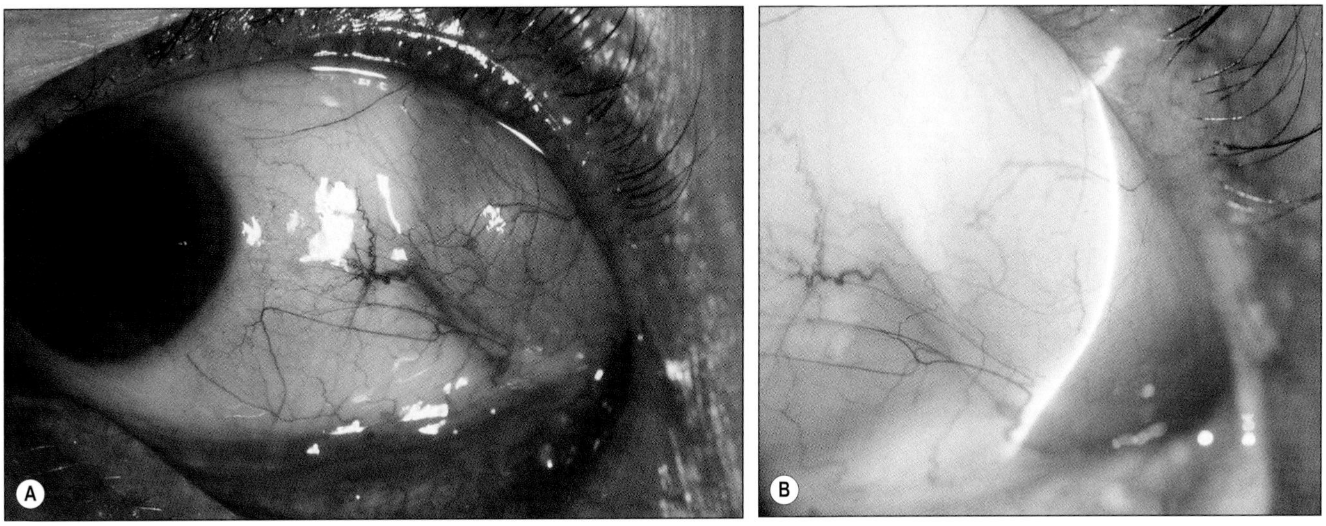

Fig. 41.2 Herniated orbital fat. (**A** and **B**) Clinically, prolapsed orbital fat appears similar to dermolipoma, lymphoma, fibrous histiocytoma, histiocytic tumors, and amyloid. Unlike dermolipomas, prolapsed orbital fat is freely mobile over the underlying sclera.

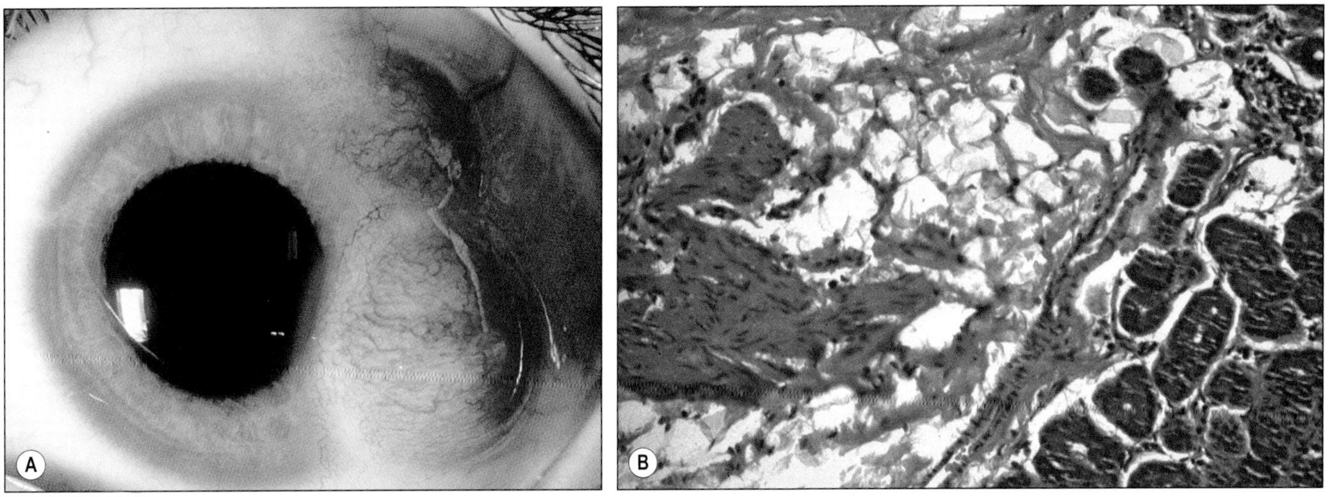

Fig. 41.3 Ectopic lacrimal gland. Ectopic lacrimal gland may represent ectopic rests of the palpebral lobe of the lacrimal gland. (**A**) Clinically, these lesions are fleshy-pink, well-vascularized nodules. In this case, two lesions are present. (**B**) Eosinophilic glandular elements (*lower right*). Smooth muscle cells are intermixed with fat and connective tissue (*left*).

have been reported in cases of encephalocraniocutaneous lipomatosis, which is associated with hemifacial microsomia, subcutaneous lipomas, and central nervous system lipomas.[25,26] Complex and simple choristomas may slowly grow under the hormonal influence of puberty; however, unlike orbital ectopic lacrimal gland, there is exceedingly rare malignant potential, with only one reported case in the literature.[27] Because the lesion may extend quite deeply into the sclera and cornea, only partial excision may be possible.

Epibulbar osseous and neuroglial choristomas

Osseous choristomas, the rarest of the epibulbar choristomas,[28] are solitary nodules that resemble conjunctival dermoids[29,30] but are much more discrete and spare the underlying cornea, as they are characteristically located 5–10 mm posterior to the limbus (Fig. 41.4). Since the first description by von Graefe in 1863, 55 cases of epibulbar osseous choristoma have been reported.[31–33] Most frequently, they present as isolated epibulbar lesions in the superotemporal quadrant, but may occur in other locations on the surface of the globe or in association with other choristomatous tissue in 10% of cases.[32] Extensive tumors have simulated extraocular extension of retinoblastoma.[34] Histologically, they are composed of mature, compact bone surrounded by additional choristomatous elements as outlined previously. The osteocytes appear normal and Haversian canals are present.[35] Epibulbar neuroglial choristomas may represent ectopic neural tissue from the anterior lip of the optic cup or

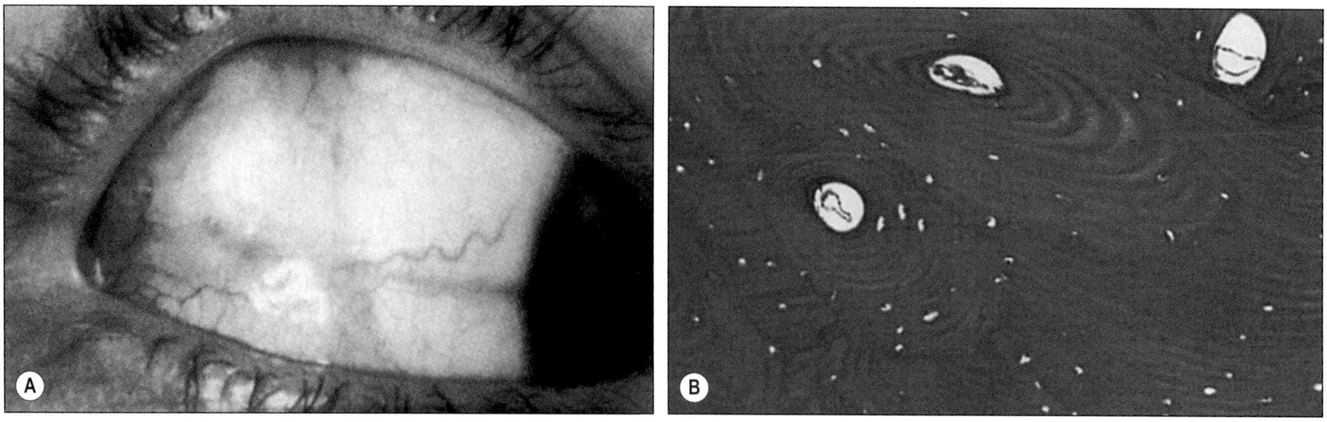

Fig. 41.4 Epibulbar osseous choristoma. Epibulbar osseous choristoma represents choristomatous epibulbar nodules of bone surrounded by connective tissue. (**A**) Clinically, these lesions are fleshy, yellow subconjunctival nodules that are soft and not associated with hair growth. (**B**) Bone formation with Haversian canals. (Courtesy Jonathan Dutton, MD, PhD.)

vesicle.[36,37] Both lesions are stationary, and removal is indicated only for diagnostic and cosmetic purposes.

Hamartomas

Unlike choristomas, hamartomas are composed of elements normally found in the affected area. Examples of subepithelial hamartomas that occur rarely include neurofibromas and fibrous hamartomas. Neurofibromas are solid, nodular, tan or gray-white lesions occurring on the bulbar or palpebral conjunctiva. The lesions may be of plexiform, solitary, or diffuse types and are almost always associated with neurofibromatosis type 1 or 2.[38–41] At times, diagnosis of the conjunctival lesion may antedate the diagnosis of neurofibromatosis by at least 10 years.[40,41] Neurofibromas must be distinguished from neuromas of the conjunctiva which can occur in association with multiple endocrine neoplasias (MEN).[40] Fibrous hamartomas have been reported in patients with the Proteus syndrome, a rare hamartomatous syndrome associated with epibulbar tumors, skeletal anomalies, plantar or palmar gyriform hyperplasia, subcutaneous tumors, epidermal nevi, and visceral abnormalities. These lesions are isolated, temporal epibulbar lesions that contain abundant mature elastic fibers intermixed with fibrous tissue.[42,43] Smooth muscle hamartomas can arise from vascular smooth muscle and from smooth muscle in the eyelid retractor complexes (Müller's muscle superiorly and capsulopapebral muscle inferiorly). Periocular congenital smooth muscle hamartomas have rarely been reported but should be considered in the differential diagnosis of a cystic-appearing conjunctival fornix lesion.[44]

First described by Leber in 1880, hemorrhagic lymphangiectasia may be a developmental anomaly or may occur in association with trauma or inflammation. In contradistinction to lymphangiomas, which are cellular proliferations of lymphatic channel elements, hemorrhagic lymphangiectasias are irregularly dilated, periodically hemorrhage-filled, lymphatic channels of the bulbar conjunctiva. Surrounding conjunctival edema or subconjunctival hemorrhage may be present (Fig. 41.5). Treatment is local excision or diathermy.[1] The preceding condition must be distinguished from ataxia telangiectasia (Louis-Bar syndrome), Bloom syndrome, and hereditary hemorrhagic telangiectasia (Rendu-Osler-Weber disease) in which there are epibulbar and interpalpebral telangiectasias of the arteries without an associated lymphatic component. The conjunctival lesions of the Louis-Bar syndrome are a marker for associated cerebellar abnormalities and immunologic derangements (e.g. hypogammaglobulinemia), which are conducive to sinopulmonary infection and lymphoreticular proliferations, particularly T-cell leukemias. Bloom syndrome is an autosomal recessive condition caused by a mutation of the *BLM* gene on chromosome 15 (15q26.1). Most common in Ashkenazi Jews, it is associated with increased susceptibility to cancer and infections, photosensitivity, and growth retardation. Patients with hereditary hemorrhagic telangiectasia, or Rendu-Osler-Weber disease, have dilated vessels due to abnormalities in vascular wall repair which increases susceptibility to bleeding from the skin and mucous membranes, CNS, lungs, and other vital organs. It is an autosomal dominant disorder produced by an abnormality in one of two genes (chromosomes 9q33–34 and 12q13) involved in vessel wall repair. In these conditions, the epibulbar vascular lesions do not acquire a tumefactive character (hamartia) because they are simple telangiectasias that grow with the patient and the eyeball. Episodic events such as hemorrhage or swelling also are not encountered.[45–47]

Conjunctival cysts

Conjunctival cysts may be congenital or acquired; the latter occur in the setting of inflammation or following inflammatory processes such as vernal conjunctivitis or Stevens-Johnson syndrome or after traumatic or surgical subconjunctival implantation of epithelium and are much more common than congenital cysts.[48–50] Usually stable, conjunctival cysts may rarely enlarge or, if intracorneal, cause intracorneal pseudohypopyon.[51,52] Histologically, cysts are lined by nonkeratinizing conjunctival epithelium with goblet cells. The center contains cellular debris and inflammatory cells. If double-layer cuboidal epithelium is present, the cyst is of ductal origin. Rarely, corneal intrastromal cysts may result

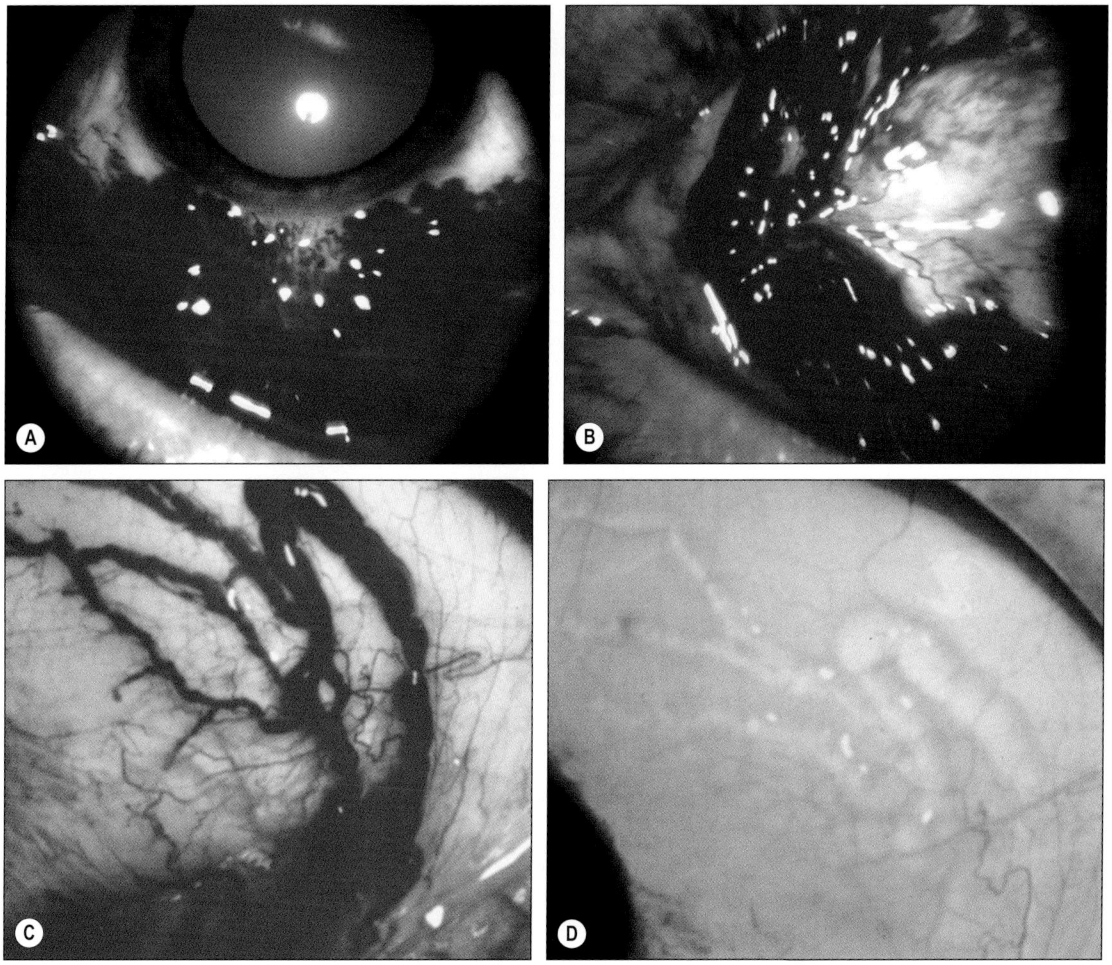

Fig. 41.5 Leber's hemorrhagic lymphangiectasia. These lesions occur in children and spontaneously in adults or may be associated with trauma, inflammation, or lymphatic and vascular malformations in the parotid gland and eyelid. The anomalous lymphatic vessels may arise on either the bulbar or palpebral conjunctival surfaces. The hemorrhagic episodes wax and wane with resolution between episodes. Local excision and/or cautery is the treatment of choice for symptomatic lesions. Histopathology shows dilated, thin-walled, endothelial-lined vascular channels with a mild chronic inflammatory cell infiltrate. Hemorrhage occurs because of anomalous communications between the lymphatic and venous channels. (**A**) Spontaneous hemorrhage produced a large hemorrhagic subconjunctival mass. Engorged blood-filled lymphatic vessels are visible overlying the surface of this edematous and hemorrhagic lesion. (**B** and **C**) With time, the hemorrhagic episode cleared. (**D**) After the hemorrhagic episode cleared, lymph-filled, dilated, tortuous channels remained. (Courtesy W. Beebe, MD.)

from penetrating or perforating wounds to the cornea (Fig. 41.6).[52] Such wounds implant epithelium within the stroma where it proliferates between the lamellae. Spontaneous, acquired epibulbar mucogenic subconjunctival cysts have been described. These lesions are freely movable and may arise because of a mucosecretory abnormality of both goblet cells and conjunctival epithelial cells.[53] Rarely, conjunctival cysts may enlarge sufficiently to involve substantial portions of the orbital cavity.[54] Primary conjunctival cysts of the orbit are most frequently located in the superonasal quadrant of the orbit, while dermoid and epidermoid cysts of the orbit are most commonly located superotemporally.[54] Conjunctival cysts can develop after the sequestration of conjunctival epithelium into the orbital soft tissues during embryonic development.[55] The cysts may be treated with simple excision; visualization of the cyst may be enhanced by preoperative injection of a dye such as trypan blue or indocyanine green.[56–58] In postenucleation patients, conjunctival cysts of the orbit have been successfully treated with intralesional injections of 20% trichloroacetic acid solution.[59]

Reactive, Degenerative, and Inflammatory Lesions

Pyogenic granuloma/capillary hemangioma

The term *pyogenic granuloma* is a misnomer because the lesion does not represent granulomatous inflammation but is rather a reactive proliferation of vascular endothelial cells and granulation tissue. These lesions (Fig. 41.7A) usually develop rapidly over days to weeks, often in response to some inciting event including strabismus surgery, inflammation (from chalazia or infection), chemical burn, phthisis

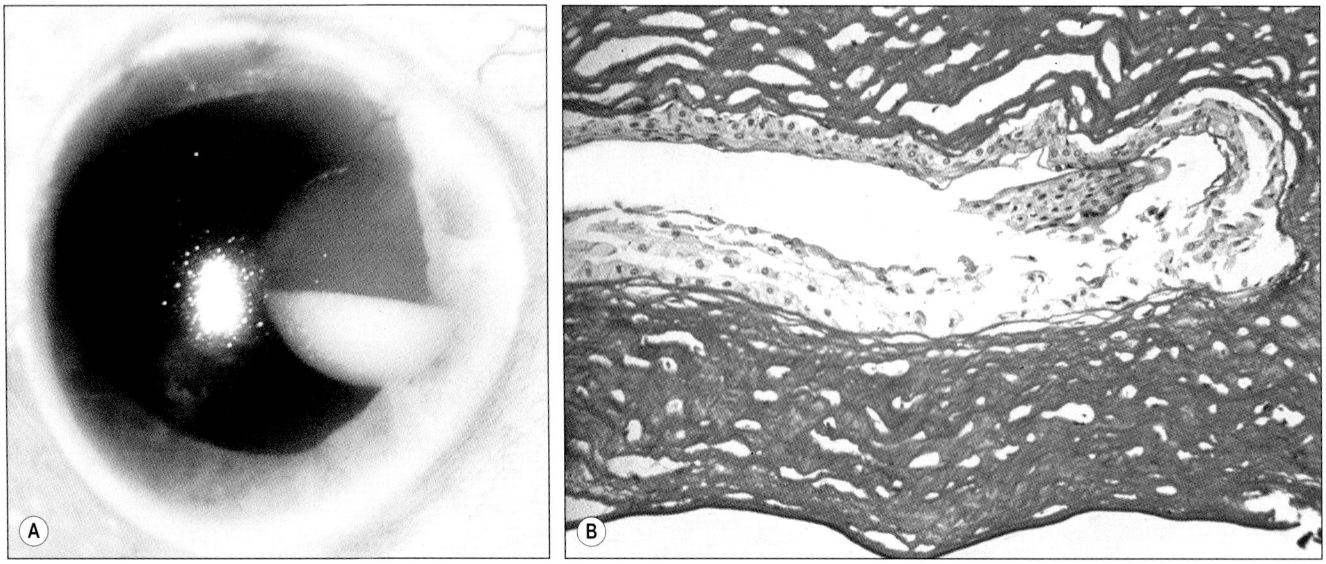

Fig. 41.6 Intrastromal corneal cyst. (**A**) A midstromal cystic lesion containing cellular debris after penetrating trauma. After the cyst slowly grew to occlude the visual axis, penetrating keratoplasty was performed. (**B**) Histopathology shows a midstromal cystic lesion lined with nonkeratinizing squamous epithelium. Descemet's membrane is noted on the lower part of the specimen. (Courtesy A. Boruchoff, MD.)

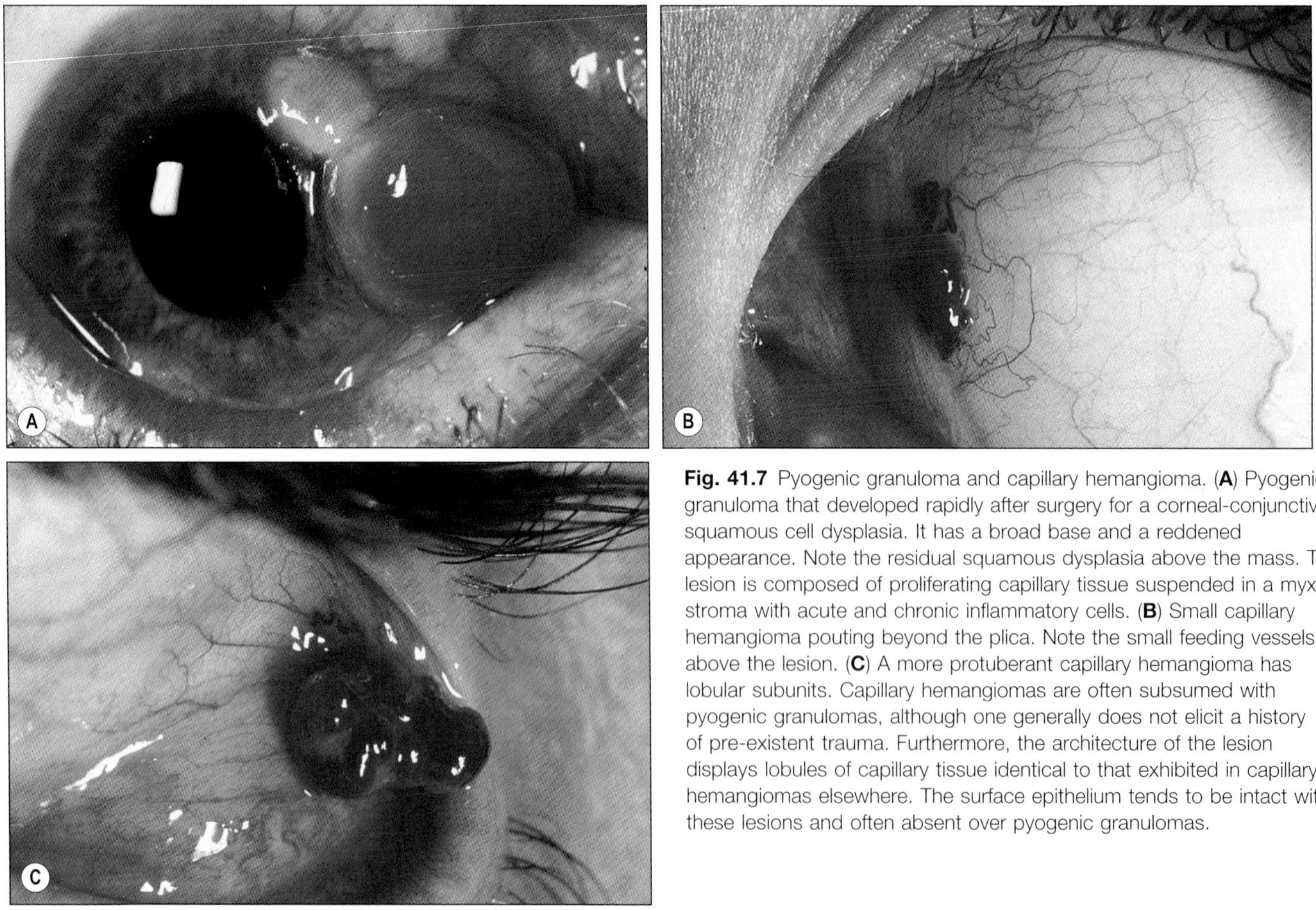

Fig. 41.7 Pyogenic granuloma and capillary hemangioma. (**A**) Pyogenic granuloma that developed rapidly after surgery for a corneal-conjunctival squamous cell dysplasia. It has a broad base and a reddened appearance. Note the residual squamous dysplasia above the mass. This lesion is composed of proliferating capillary tissue suspended in a myxoid stroma with acute and chronic inflammatory cells. (**B**) Small capillary hemangioma pouting beyond the plica. Note the small feeding vessels above the lesion. (**C**) A more protuberant capillary hemangioma has lobular subunits. Capillary hemangiomas are often subsumed with pyogenic granulomas, although one generally does not elicit a history of pre-existent trauma. Furthermore, the architecture of the lesion displays lobules of capillary tissue identical to that exhibited in capillary hemangiomas elsewhere. The surface epithelium tends to be intact with these lesions and often absent over pyogenic granulomas.

bulbi, penetrating keratoplasty, foreign bodies, previous limbal surgery (e.g. for pterygium or squamous cell carcinoma excision), or even after transconjunctival blepharoplasty.[60–64] These lesions are variably reddened and may be placoid or molded to surrounding tissues and surfaces (Fig. 41.7C). When arising after excision of a squamous cell carcinoma, a pyogenic granuloma can be confused with recurrent disease.[65] In addition, pyogenic granulomas may be confused with Kaposi's sarcoma.[66,67] The rate of onset and inciting circumstances help differentiate the two lesions. Although spontaneous involution after a protracted period can occur from progressive fibrosis, simple excisional biopsy with cautery of the base can be both diagnostic and curative.[63] The prevention of recurrence depends on the rapidity with which the raw surface can be re-epithelialized to prevent the extrusion of any persistent granulation tissue. Therefore, primary closure of the surrounding conjunctiva is recommended. Histopathologically, pyogenic granuloma is a double misnomer. It is not pyogenic, because it is not caused by an underlying bacterial infection, nor is it granulomatous, unless it is somewhat penetrated by an underlying chalazion. The lesion is composed of a profusion of immature capillary channels, which are normally oriented perpendicular to the surface of the lesion. The interstitium is variably myxoid, displaying polymorphonuclear leukocytes, lymphocytes, plasma cells, and a loose population of fibroblasts. The surface is frequently denuded of epithelium; the latter may cause a constriction of the base of the lesion, where it can form a collaret.

Capillary hemangiomas are also rapidly developing lesions of the conjunctiva; however, these lesions develop in the absence of any clear-cut pre-existent trauma.[63,64] These lesions can appear in the young and old and tend to be intensely reddened and protuberant (Fig. 41.7B and C). Histopathologically, the lesion is composed of lobules of capillary tissue without significant interstitial inflammation or a myxoid stroma; the surface epithelium is usually intact. Many individuals regard this lesion as a variant of pyogenic granuloma, except that it has the more regular lobular architecture of a true capillary hemangioma. It is not associated with deeper orbital lesions. In fact, the more extensive infantile capillary hemangiomas of the orbit and lid tend to spare the conjunctiva, in contradistinction to orbital lymphangioma, which frequently has expressions in the conjunctival sac. These lesions may be treated with simple excision or with cryotherapy.

Pinguecula/pterygium

Pingueculae are yellowish, raised growths on the epibulbar conjunctiva within the palpebral fissure.[1] Pingueculae are thought to be the precursors of pterygia. Both lesions arise from actinically activated fibroblasts that grow onto the peripheral corneal surface with secondary blood vessel ingrowth and destruction of Bowman's layer.[68–70] They are more common on the nasal epibulbar surface, but may occur both temporally and nasally at the same time. An isolated temporal lesion should be suspected of being either a hamartoma or choristoma. Histologically, there are increased fibroblasts, hyalinization of the subepithelial connective tissue, increased thick and tortuous fibers that stain positive for elastin, diffuse and lobulated eosinophilic granular areas, and basophilic concretions within the granular and hyalinized areas. The term *pseudoelastosis* has been applied to these changes. Evidence suggests that the abnormal elastin material is produced by actinically transformed fibroblasts.[70,71] The treatment of pterygium is discussed in Chapter 144; one should consider the diagnosis of pterygium within the context of other lesions discussed in this chapter as well as Chapter 53.

Elastofibroma oculi

Elastofibroma oculi is a rare pseudotumorous lesion composed of thick collagen bundles, linear elastinophilic material, and adipose tissue.[72–74] These lesions occur on the temporal epibulbar surface where they may imitate a pterygium, hamartoma, or choristoma. The etiology is uncertain, but the lesion may be either a response to some inciting trauma or, because adipose tissue is present, a hamartomatous lesion. The collagen and elastic fibers are probably produced by activated fibroblasts. Treatment is complete excision.

Nodular fasciitis

Nodular fasciitis is a rapidly developing lesion composed of reactive immature connective tissue (Fig. 41.8).[74,75] Histologically, the lesions are highly cellular, displaying zonal architecture, with immature fibroblasts in some areas and extracellular mucinous material in others. Plump vascular endothelial cells, plasma cells, and lymphocytes are also present. Rarely, lesions may behave aggressively and extend into the eye. Simple excision is usually curative.

Granulomatous and histiocytic lesions

Conditions associated with subconjunctival granuloma formation include parasitic and mycotic infection, acne rosacea, systemic vasculitis, foreign bodies, lupus erythematosus, allergy, and inflammatory bowel disease.[76–86] Granulomatous conjunctivitis is also a rare manifestation of Vogt-Koyanagi-Harada syndrome and Wegener's granulomatosis; in the latter it may be associated with life-threatening subglottic stenosis.[87,88] Additional conditions that deserve some attention are sarcoidosis, rheumatoid nodulosis, leprosy, and juvenile xanthogranuloma. Sarcoid nodules with noncaseating granulomata may involve the bulbar or palpebral conjunctiva. Clinically, the lesions appear as small, tan-yellow nodules that can resemble follicles.[89] These lesions are more common in patients under the age of 35 years. Conjunctival sarcoid also may result in symblepharon and cicatricial entropion.[90] Biopsy of these nodules can be helpful in suspected cases of sarcoid. Even blind biopsy of clinically normal conjunctiva reveals granulomatous inflammation in up to 50% of patients with sarcoid.[91,92] Subconjunctival granulomatous nodules may rarely be associated with rheumatoid arthritis. In a case report by Lebowitz et al.,[93] a 61-year-old woman with quiescent rheumatoid arthritis developed multiple, bilateral, translucent, raised, yellow lesions approximately 2 mm in diameter. The term *epibulbar rheumatoid nodulosis* was coined to describe the condition.

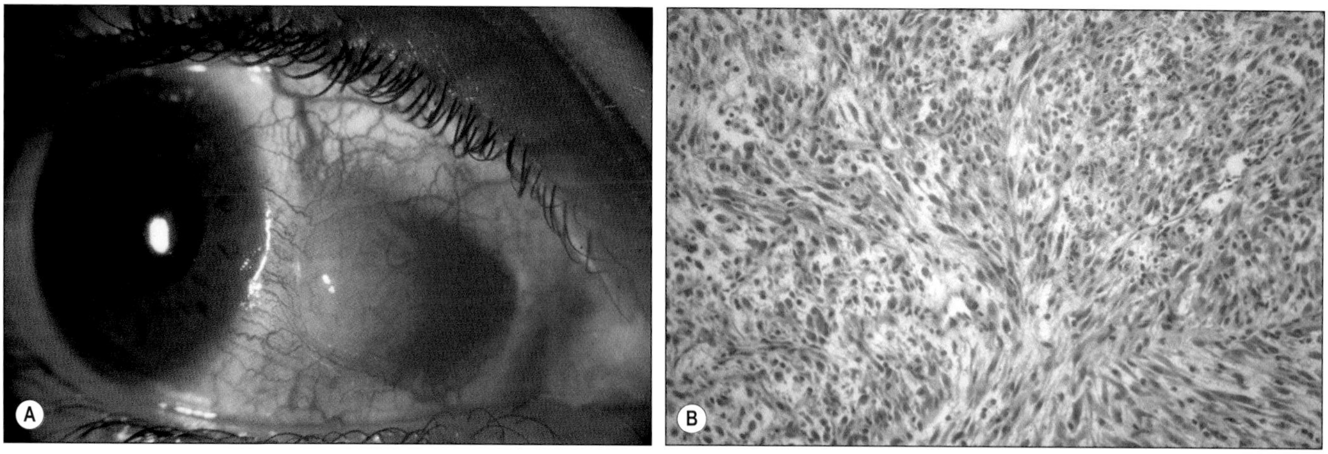

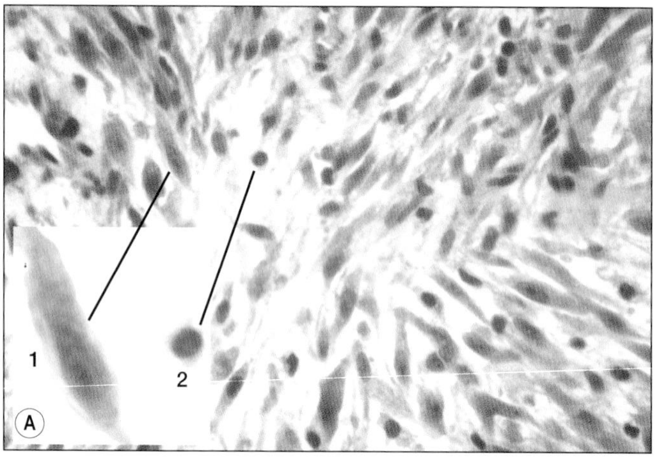

Fig. 41.8 Nodular fasciitis. (**A**) This epibulbar lesion arose rapidly over a few weeks. The patient noted an antecedent history of a foreign body sensation. The lesion itself is firm and is surrounded by dilated conjunctival and episcleral vessels. (**B**) Histopathology demonstrates sheets of immature spindle-shaped fibroblasts with copious cytoplasm. (**C**) In portions of the specimen, plump fibroblasts (*1*) and inflammatory cells (*2*) are present.

Pathologic examination of the specimens revealed zonal granulomatous inflammation surrounding necrobiotic foci similar to subcutaneous rheumatoid nodules. Granulomas associated with lepromatous leprosy are potentially confused with fibrous histiocytoma, except that in leprosy the abundant and highly vacuolated histiocytes contain copious numbers of acid-fast bacilli (Virchow cells).[94]

In addition to involving the uveal tract, juvenile xanthogranuloma also may produce Touton giant cells containing granulomas within the conjunctiva and cornea.[95–97] Touton giant cells exhibit a central eosinophilic cytoplasm surrounded by an annulus of nuclei, which is in turn surrounded by peripheral vacuolated cytoplasm. Other histiocytic-granulomatous conditions that may also have corneal or conjunctival involvement include subcutaneous xanthogranulomatosis, sinus histiocytosis with massive lymphadenopathy, reticulohistiocytoma (Fig. 41.9), Churg-Strauss syndrome, histiocytosis X, and xanthoma disseminatum.[98–107] Secondary subconjunctival involvement may occur in Erdheim-Chester disease, adult periocular xanthogranulomas associated with asthma (Fig. 41.10), and tuberous xanthoma.[108] Additional nodular subconjunctival inflammatory lesions include limbal inflammatory pseudotumor and nodular hypersensitivity conjunctivitis (Splendore-Hoeppli reaction).[109] The latter lesion is of uncertain etiology and is composed of periodically occurring small, nodular, yellowish to white subconjunctival lesions with surrounding hyperemia. Similar but more extensive nodular allergic granulomatous nodules have been described in the setting of human immunodeficiency virus infection.[84]

Epibulbar molluscum contagiosum

Molluscum contagiosum, a large ovoid, double-stranded DNA poxvirus, typically produces nodular eyelid lesions with secondary keratoconjunctivitis (Fig. 41.11). Direct conjunctival involvement in molluscum contagiosum is rare and usually occurs in patients with immunosuppression.[110–112] Only 10 cases have been reported in the world literature in immunocompetent individuals.[110] The lesions are white nodules that are freely mobile. The lesions may be treated with excision.

Keloid

Unlike skin keloids, which are pink, corneal keloids are chalky white, glistening, solid tumors that may occur as a result of injury or primarily as a congenital corneal mass.[113,114] Penetrating trauma often precedes the development of some keloids. In these cases, microscopic evaluation shows lens fragments or portions of iris within the lesion. In these cases, the iris tissue itself rather than corneal stroma may be the source of the keloid tissue. Histologically, keloids are composed of exuberant fibrous tissue. Treatment is by excision

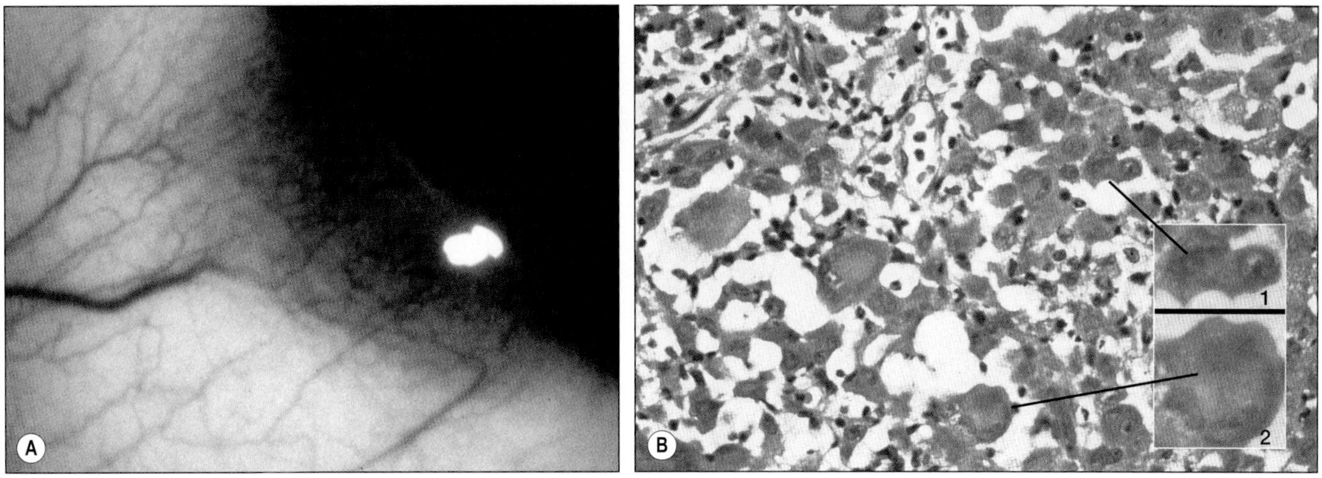

Fig. 41.9 Reticulohistiocytoma. Reticulohistiocytomas are rare, benign histiocytic lesions that usually occur as isolated skin nodules or as a finding of multicentric reticulohistiocytosis. Two cases of limbal reticulohistiocytomas have been reported by Allaire et al.[103] (**A**) A translucent, salmon-pink mass arises from the limbus. This lesion, which resembled lymphoma, had been present for 2 months before excision in this 21-year-old patient. (**B**) Histopathology revealed mononuclear cells (*1*) and multiple multinucleated histiocytes (*2*). No Touton giant cells were seen. Electron microscopy and immunohistochemical stains confirmed the histiocytic nature of the lesion. (Courtesy A.A. Hidayat, MD.)

with an understanding that further keloids may form. Rarely, congenital glaucoma can lead to buphthalmos and corneal keloid formation.

Amyloid

Amyloid has two biochemical forms.[115–119] Amyloid-B is derived from immunoglobulins and is found in primary amyloidosis and plasma cell dyscrasias. Amyloid-A is composed of an unknown substance and occurs in the remaining types of amyloidosis. Clinically, both forms appear as firm, yellowish subconjunctival deposits (Fig. 41.12). Conjunctival primary localized amyloidosis is virtually never associated with systemic disease. Conjunctival amyloidosis may be associated with spontaneous hemorrhage resulting from vascular fragility from perivascular deposition.[120] Secondary localized amyloidosis occurs in response to previous conjunctival disease including tumors, infections (including trachoma), and trauma. Histologically, amyloid is an extracellular accumulation of pale, amorphous, glassy, eosinophilic, hyaline material, which is birefringent with polarized light. Amyloid stains positively with Congo red. If ocular irritation is present, the treatment of choice is surgical extirpation.

Hematic cyst

Hematic cysts are pseudocystic or loculated collections of blood breakdown products that may accumulate either post-surgically or post-traumatically.[121] Clinically, hematic cysts rarely occur subconjunctivally and appear as dark-brown masses that may mimic melanocytic tumors. Histologically, they are composed of blood breakdown products including hemosiderin-laden macrophages, lipid-laden histiocytes, and cholesterol clefts, with granulomatous inflammation most often present. The lesion is pseudocystic, encased within a fibrous pseudocapsule that lacks an endothelial or epithelial lining. Treatment is surgical excision, especially to rule out melanoma.

Neoplastic Lesions

Fibrous histiocytoma

Although the most common mesenchymal orbital tumor in adults, fibrous histiocytoma may rarely arise from the conjunctiva, episclera, and sclera.[122–128] Interestingly, fibrous histiocytoma may have a higher incidence in patients with xeroderma pigmentosum.[129,130] Fibrous histiocytoma is a yellow to white lesion that may grow to produce a subconjunctival nodular lesion (Fig. 41.13). If nodular, they may grow at the limbus and extend over the peripheral cornea; if infiltrative, they may infiltrate the corneal stroma. The lesion is cytologically bland, consisting of a predominance of fibrous tissue within which are two morphologically distinct populations of cells: spindle-shaped fibroblasts and round lipidized histiocytes. Rarely, some lesions may have characteristics of juvenile xanthogranuloma with Touton giant cells. Fibrous histiocytoma lesions do not have the inflammatory response and systemic findings associated with juvenile xanthogranuloma. The cellular elements are arranged in bundles that weave throughout the fibrous tissue in a storiform or cartwheel pattern. Electron microscopy of the two cell types reveals abundant rough endoplasmic reticulum within fibroblasts and smooth endoplasmic reticulum, curvilinear inclusions, and lysosomes within the histiocytes. Both cell types have numerous lipid vacuoles.[125,126] Treatment involves complete surgical excision. Malignant varieties also occur.[131] Malignant tumors may be treated with excision and either adjunctive radiation therapy or cryotherapy.[132,133] If these malignancies are extensive, exenteration is required, as lesions can be aggressive locally and may in rare instances metastasize.[134,135]

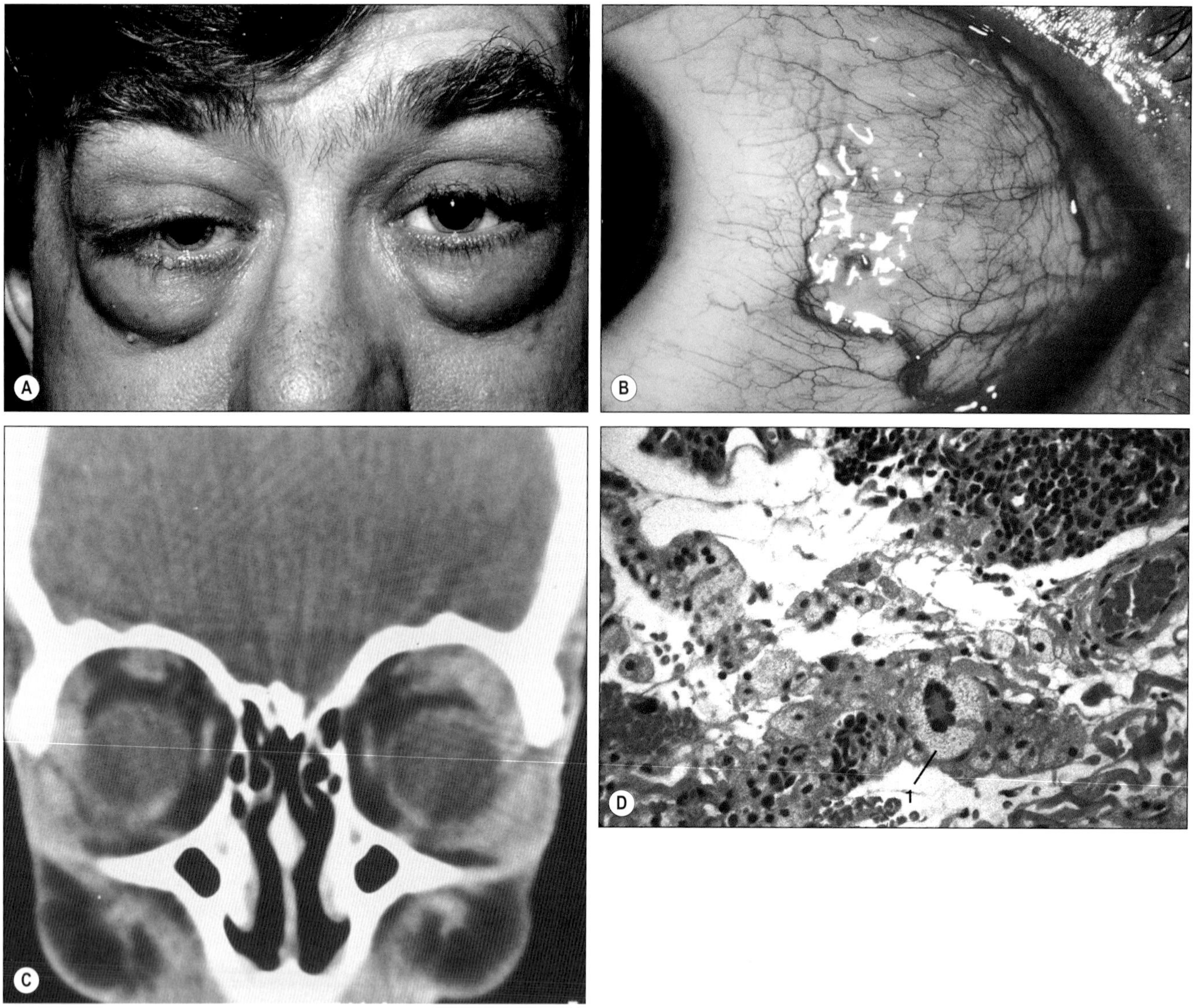

Fig. 41.10 Adult periocular xanthogranulomas associated with asthma. Xanthogranulomatous disorders are included within the differential of acquired yellow subconjunctival lesions. This disorder is included in the differential diagnosis of xanthogranulomatous disorders, which frequently have severe systemic manifestations. Included within the differential are Erdheim-Chester, necrobiotic xanthogranuloma, xanthoma disseminatum, and sinus histiocytosis with massive lymphadenopathy. (**A**) Yellow diffuse masses have developed in all four lids over many years. The patient developed asthma nearly concomitantly with the onset of eyelid swelling. (**B**) Evaluation of the ocular surface revealed a slightly elevated, yellow subconjunctival mass. The conjunctiva was not markedly injected. (**C**) CT evaluation revealed tracking of the lesional subconjunctival and subcutaneous tissue along the lateral orbital wall and recti muscle involvement (bilateral lateral and inferior recti; left superior rectus muscle). (**D**) Histopathology demonstrates a Touton giant cell (*1*) with a central annulus of nuclei that encloses a central eosinophilic cytoplasm; the outer cytoplasm is pale and vacuolated.

Kaposi's sarcoma

This once rare neoplasm is now a major cause of morbidity and mortality for patients with acquired immunosuppression, especially for those infected with HIV. Although it may rarely occur in the setting of a normal immune status, Kaposi's sarcoma is the most common tumor in the setting of HIV infection.[136–138] First described by Kaposi in 1872 as 'idiopathic multiple pigmented sarcoma of the skin,' Kaposi's sarcoma now affects the ocular adnexa, including the conjunctiva, in approximately 20% of patients with AIDS; approximately 7% affect the conjunctiva.[139–141] Clinically, conjunctival lesions are nodular or diffuse, blue-red or deep-brown, and often elevated (Fig. 41.14).[142,143] They are commonly found in the inferior fornix. The lesions are slow growing and may cause secondary entropion, vision obstruction, and discomfort. Kaposi's sarcoma arises from vascular elements, including endothelial cells and pericytes.[143] Dugel et al.[144] have described three histologic types: type 1 has dilated endothelial cell-lined vascular spaces without spindle cells; type 2 has plump fusiform endothelial cells containing hyperchromatic nuclei with spindle cell patches; type 3 is composed of densely packed spindle cells with abundant slitlike spaces. Types 1 and 2 are less than 3 mm high and

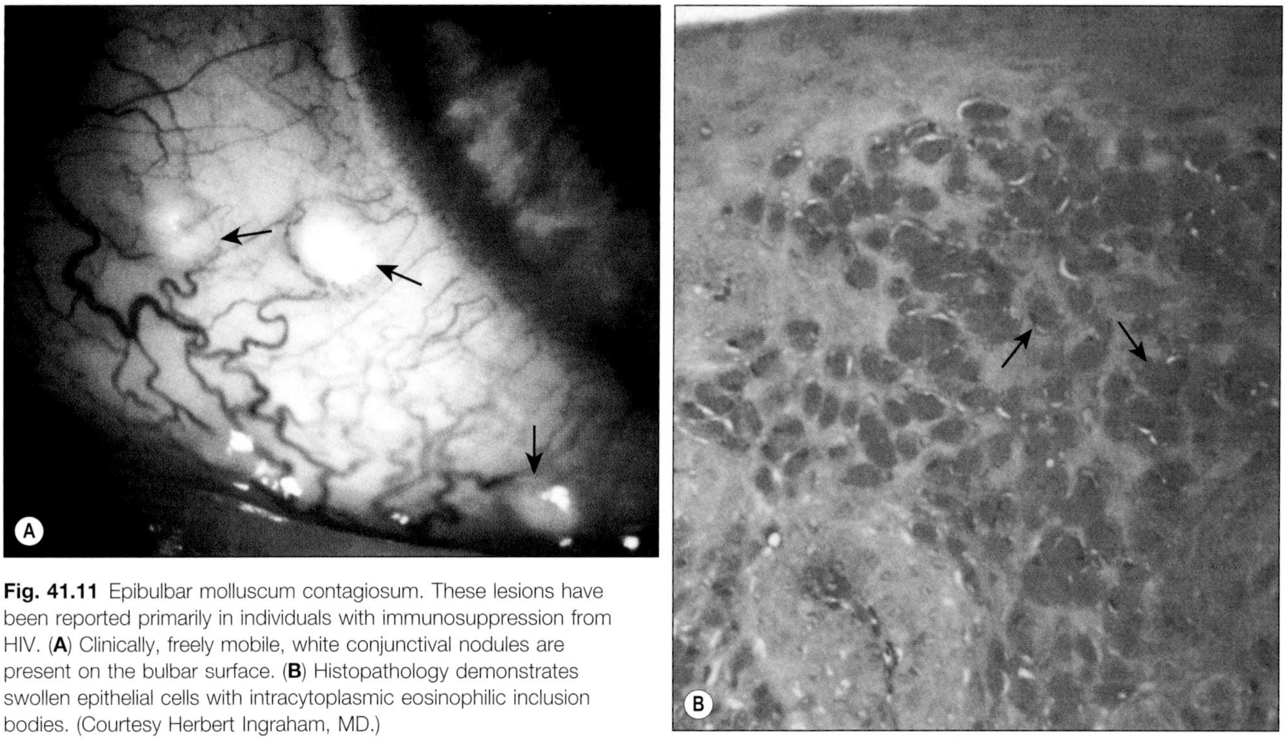

Fig. 41.11 Epibulbar molluscum contagiosum. These lesions have been reported primarily in individuals with immunosuppression from HIV. (**A**) Clinically, freely mobile, white conjunctival nodules are present on the bulbar surface. (**B**) Histopathology demonstrates swollen epithelial cells with intracytoplasmic eosinophilic inclusion bodies. (Courtesy Herbert Ingraham, MD.)

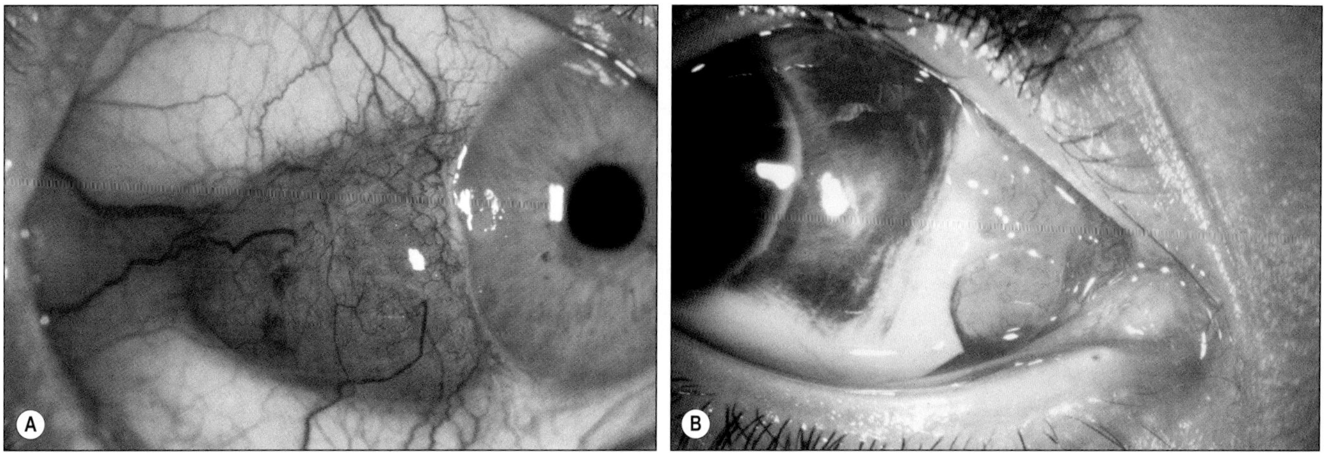

Fig. 41.12 Amyloidosis. Like xanthogranulomatous disorders and herniated orbital fat, amyloidosis should be included within the differential diagnosis of acquired yellow orbital lesions. (**A** and **B**) Clinical examples of primary localized subconjunctival amyloidosis. Acquired amyloidosis is composed of amyloid-A. (**A**) Lesion is elevated, well-vascularized, and a translucent-pink color. (**B**) Lesion is a more typical yellow color. Associated subconjunctival hemorrhage, seen in this case, is common in amyloidosis because of vascular fragility. (**C**) Gelatinous droplike dystrophy is an autosomally dominant inherited form of corneal primary localized amyloidosis. Like other inherited corneal dystrophies, bilateral involvement is the rule. When vision loss occurs, lamellar keratectomy may be performed. (**D**) Hematoxylin and eosin stain of the lamellar keratectomy specimen demonstrates copious glassy, amorphous, eosinophilic deposits between the corneal lamellae. (**E**) The deposits stain red with the Congo red stain. (**F**) With polarized light, the green birefringence is noted. (**G** and **H**) Peripheral subepithelial deposits of amyloid-B are present in this patient with systemic B-cell lymphoma. The deposits in amyloid-A appear similar histologically to that of primary localized amyloid (amyloid-A). However, this secondary systemic form of amyloid substance is derived from immunoglobulins.

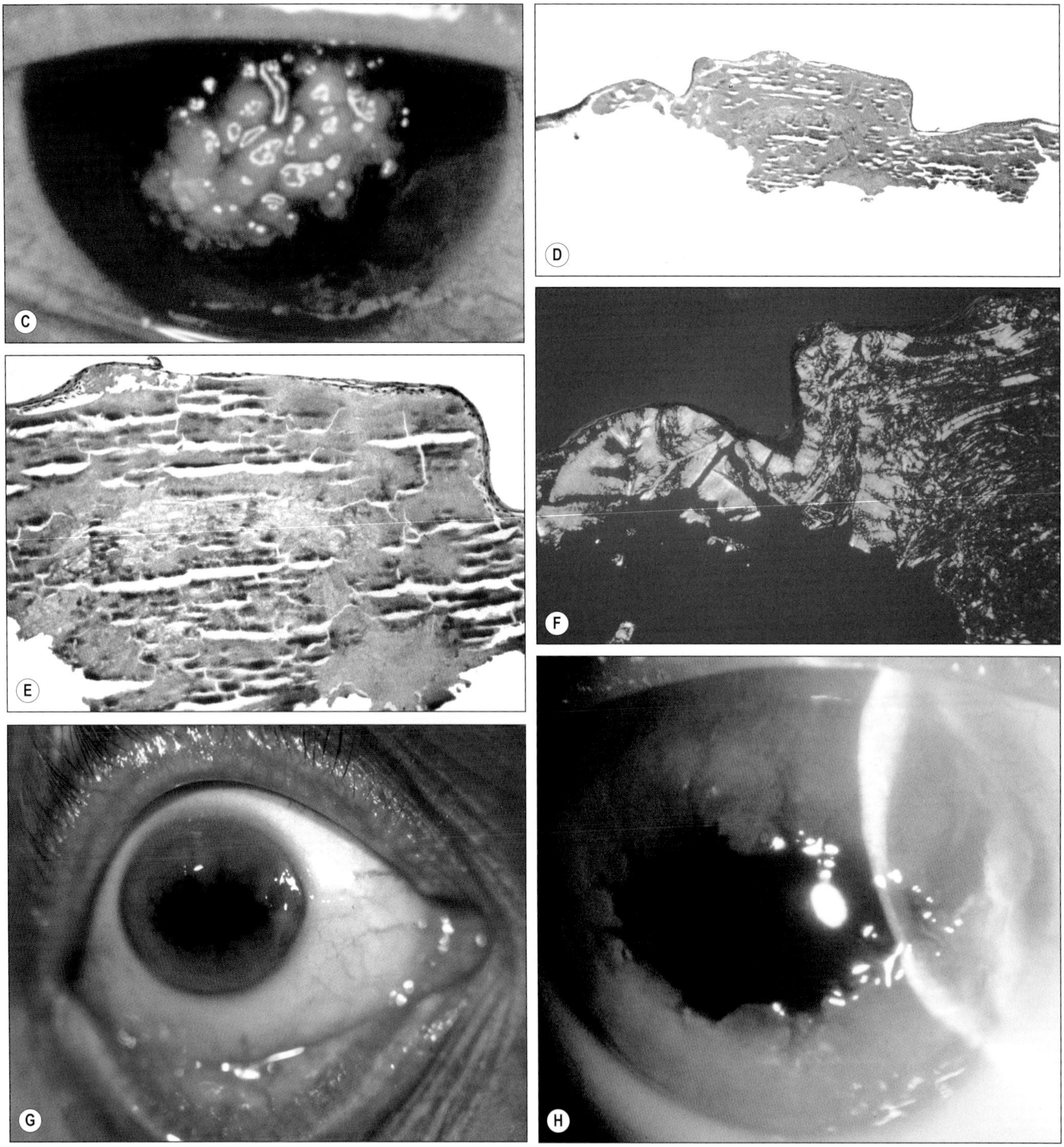

Fig. 41.12, cont'd

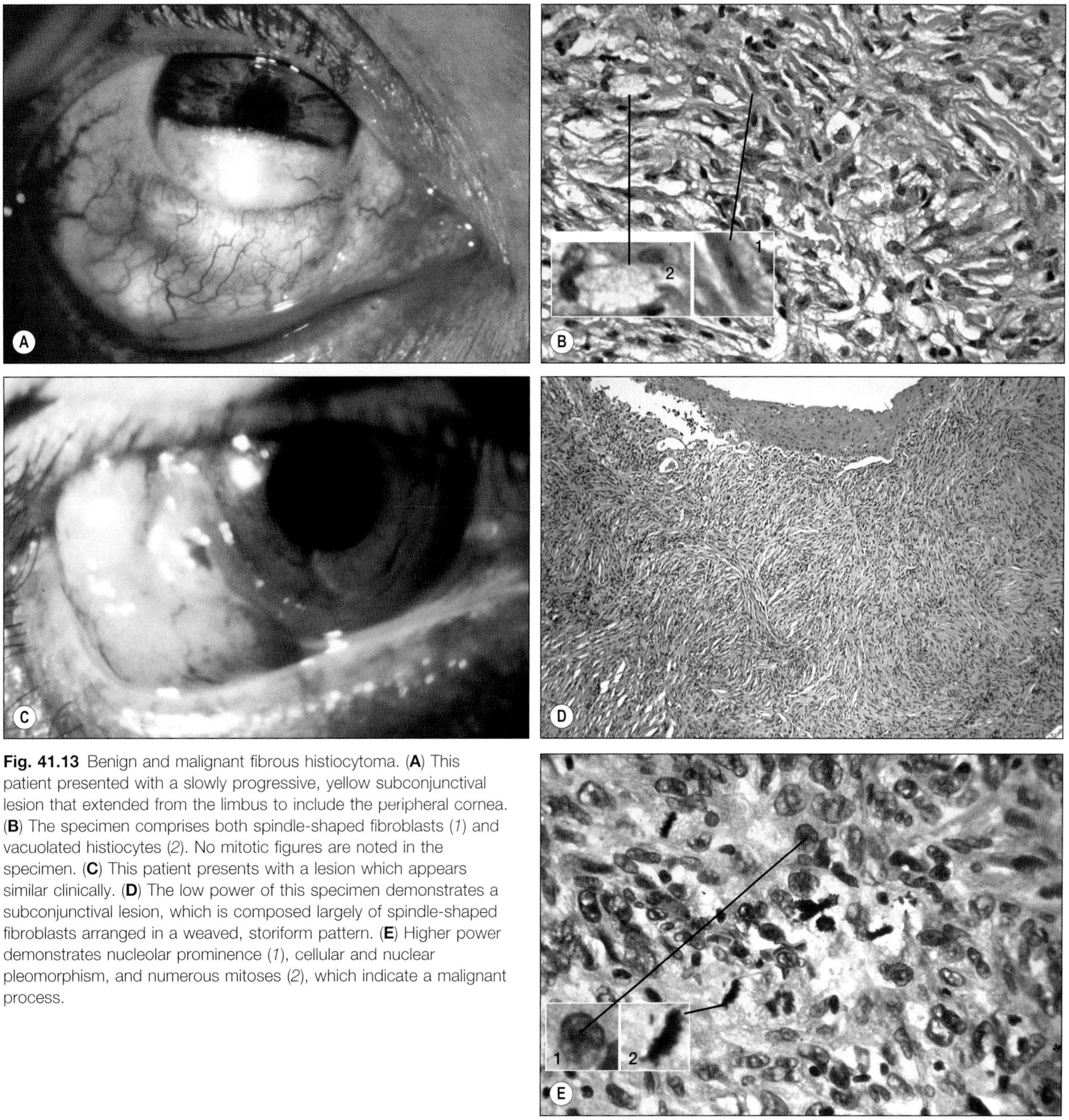

Fig. 41.13 Benign and malignant fibrous histiocytoma. (**A**) This patient presented with a slowly progressive, yellow subconjunctival lesion that extended from the limbus to include the peripheral cornea. (**B**) The specimen comprises both spindle-shaped fibroblasts (*1*) and vacuolated histiocytes (*2*). No mitotic figures are noted in the specimen. (**C**) This patient presents with a lesion which appears similar clinically. (**D**) The low power of this specimen demonstrates a subconjunctival lesion, which is composed largely of spindle-shaped fibroblasts arranged in a weaved, storiform pattern. (**E**) Higher power demonstrates nucleolar prominence (*1*), cellular and nuclear pleomorphism, and numerous mitoses (*2*), which indicate a malignant process.

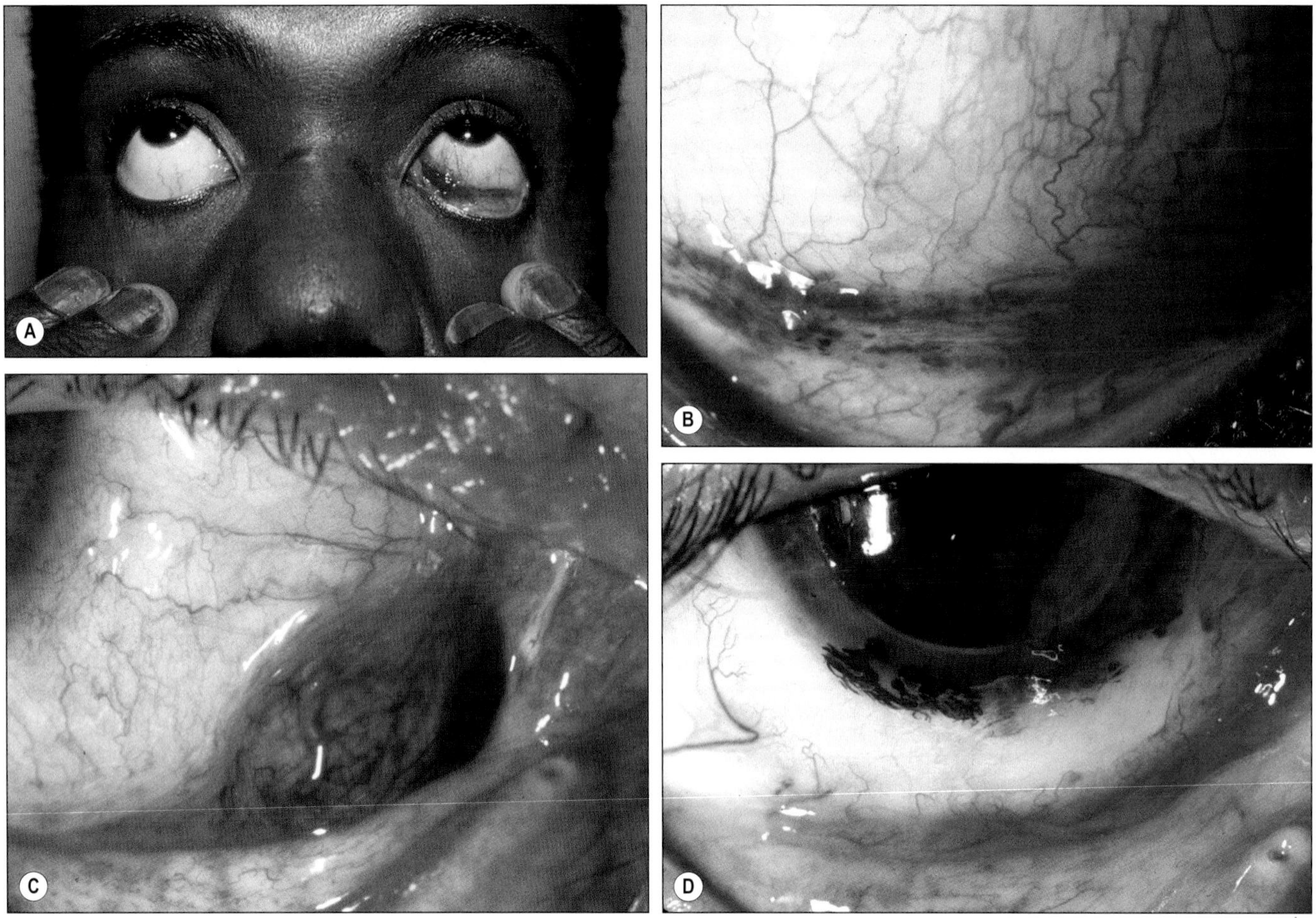

Fig. 41.14 Kaposi's sarcoma. Once rare, Kaposi's sarcoma is now a major cause of morbidity and mortality in patients infected with HIV. (**A** and **B**) This patient presents with a red, slightly elevated mass located in the inferonasal fornix of the left eye. The lesion is noted to diffusely involve the subconjunctival tissue of the inferior fornix. Numerous fine vessels and petechial hemorrhages are present. (**C**) This patient developed a more nodular lesion. Larger dilated vessels are noted to overlie a dark, maroon-colored subconjunctival mass. (**D**) A perilimbal, brownish-red, slightly elevated mass is noted in this patient who experienced a recurrence. The white sclera with overlying scarred conjunctiva marks the location of the previously excised mass.

patchy; type 3 is nodular and more than 3 mm high. Type 1 may appear similar to subconjunctival hemorrhage, foreign body granulomas, cavernous hemangiomas, and pyogenic granuloma.[144] One current model for the pathogenesis of Kaposi's sarcoma implicates the human herpesvirus 8, also referred to as the Kaposi's sarcoma herpesvirus (KSHV).[145,146] Following an initial event, possibly infection with KSHV, normal mesenchymal cells are transformed such that they become abnormally sensitive to the elevated levels of cytokines present during HIV infection. Subsequent mutational events and proliferation result in clinically apparent disease. For most cases of Kaposi's sarcoma, the appropriate treatment is observation. Excision may be necessary for diagnostic purposes or debulking. Chemotherapy or immunotherapy is appropriate for systemic disease.[147–150] Local control may be obtained with improvement of the immune status, as can be achieved with highly active antiretroviral therapy.[151] In cases in which systemic therapy is not curative, local control may be obtained with local irradiation, cryotherapy, or local injection with vinblastine, interferon alfa-2a, or human chorionic gonadotropin.[152–159]

Oncocytoma (oxyphilic adenoma)

Oncocytomas are rare tumors derived from lacrimal ductal epithelium in the caruncle, lacrimal gland, and accessory conjunctival lacrimal glands; lid apocrine glands and the lacrimal sac also may be sources.[160–162] They account for 3–8% of all caruncular lesions.[163] Systemically, oncocytomas usually arise from the salivary glands and rarely from other glands including the thyroid, parathyroid, adrenal, breast, and pituitary.[161] They do not arise on the epibulbar surface because of the absence of accessory lacrimal tissue in this site. Clinically, the caruncle tumors are small (2–5 mm), red to yellow, tan, or rusty and cystic. There is an increased prevalence in women and older patients. Generally, caruncular lesions are benign. There are rare reports of malignancy in extracaruncular oncocytomas, including cases of orbital extension from lacrimal gland and sac lesions. Histologically, cells, which contain eosinophilic, granular cytoplasm, are arranged together forming sheets and cystic, ductlike spaces.[164] Electron microscopy reveals copious mitochondria with fragmented cristae. The mito-

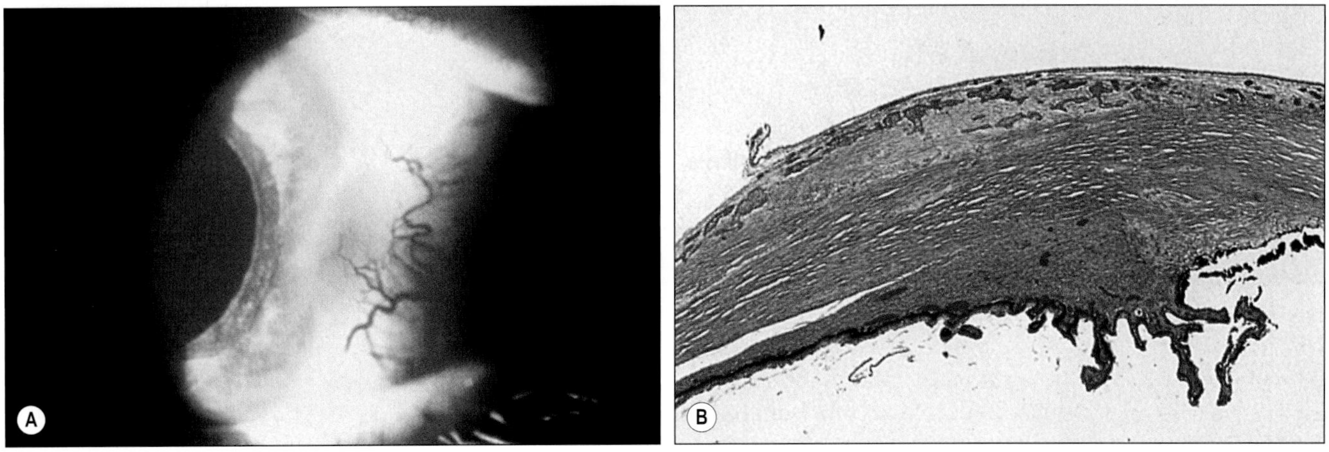

Fig. 41.15 Conjunctival basal cell carcinoma. (**A**) Clinically, a slightly elevated, hyperemic, nodular limbal lesion is present at the temporal limbus. (**B**) Histopathologically, basaloid tumor cells are located in the anterior stroma of the cornea. (Courtesy Melissa Cable, MD.)

chondria may push the nucleus eccentrically, whereupon it becomes pyknotic, possibly a prelude to cell death.[161,165,166] Removal is usually indicated for cosmesis; wide local excision is usually curative.

Basal cell carcinoma

Most cases of subconjunctival basal cell carcinoma result from local spread of a primary skin lesion. Husain et al.[167] described a case of primary basal cell carcinoma of the nasal epibulbar conjunctiva. A multiloculated, yellowish-pink, nonulcerated mass measuring 4 × 3 × 2 mm was excised. Histopathologic examination showed classic basal cell carcinoma. Because the lesions typically arise nasally, they may arise in caruncular adnexal structures, which is consistent with the belief that basal cell carcinoma can originate from pilosebaceous units.[168–171] Cable et al. have described a morpheaform basal cell carcinoma that likely arose from the temporal limbal conjunctiva (Fig. 41.15).[172] A slightly elevated limbal nodule with hyperemia was noted. Intraocular extension of the tumor was present at the time of diagnosis. Because primary subconjunctival basal cell carcinoma is rare, prognosis after complete excision is unknown.

Malignant melanoma

Conjunctival neoplasia of melanocytic origin is discussed in Chapter 40. Amelanotic malignant melanoma of the conjunctiva, however, should be considered in the differential diagnosis of any unusual nonpigmented, well-vascularized, subconjunctival mass. Conversely, when confronted with a pigmented conjunctival mass, one also should consider nonmelanocytic processes such as papillomas, hematic cysts, foreign bodies, and adrenochrome deposition.

Lymphoid lesions

Similar to all mucous membranes, the conjunctiva contains moderate amounts of lymphoid tissue from which both benign and malignant neoplasia may arise.[168] In the recent largest series of 353 cases of ocular adnexal lymphoma (OAL) published in the pathology literature by Ferry and associates,[173,174] 78% of all OALs had no prior history of lymphoma, and overall, 12% had bilateral lesions. Of the lymphoid proliferations that occur in the ocular adnexa, approximately 20–30% arise within the conjunctiva.[175–178] At presentation, bilateral disease is present in up to 38% of patients, but systemic lymphoma usually is not present.[175–179] In addition, among all ocular adnexal lymphomas, conjunctival tumors have the lowest incidence of extraocular lymphoma – 20–37.5% compared to 35–54% for orbital lesions and 67–100% for lid skin tumors.[175,176,179,180] The relatively low incidence of nonocular spread from conjunctival lymphoma may be related to the fact that the conjunctiva normally has its own lymphocytic population, which may support, and thus contain, polyclonal hyperplasia or even primary localized lymphoma better than other tissues normally devoid of an indigenous lymphocytic population.

In another large series, 84% of patients presented at 50 years or older; however, conjunctival lymphoma has been reported in patients as young as 12 years old.[175,176,179–181] Clinically, conjunctival lymphoid tumors are asymptomatic, sharply demarcated, salmon-pink colored masses of insidious onset (Fig. 41.16). They are nontender and nonulcerated and lack apparent feeder vessels. They tend to be freely movable on the globe; any lesion fixed to the sclera should be suspected of being uveal lymphoid hyperplasia with extraocular extension.[182] Sigelman and Jakobiec[177] described the clinical features, which suggest a benign conjunctival lymphoid process, including 'surface nodularity or follicularity, multifocality, and minimal elevation.' Malignancy is suggested by more diffuse involvement of the conjunctiva. A biopsy should be performed in all suspected cases.

Histologically, well-differentiated lymphoid tumors consist of masses of small, mature, monotonous lymphocytes, with multiple nuclear chromatin clumps located within a delicate vascular stroma and composed of reticulum cells and devoid of fibrous tissue. Intermediate or mantle-zone lymphomas consist of somewhat larger cells with nuclear membrane irregularities. Large-cell lymphomas have larger, more anaplastic, often cleaved nuclei. Cytomorphologic features

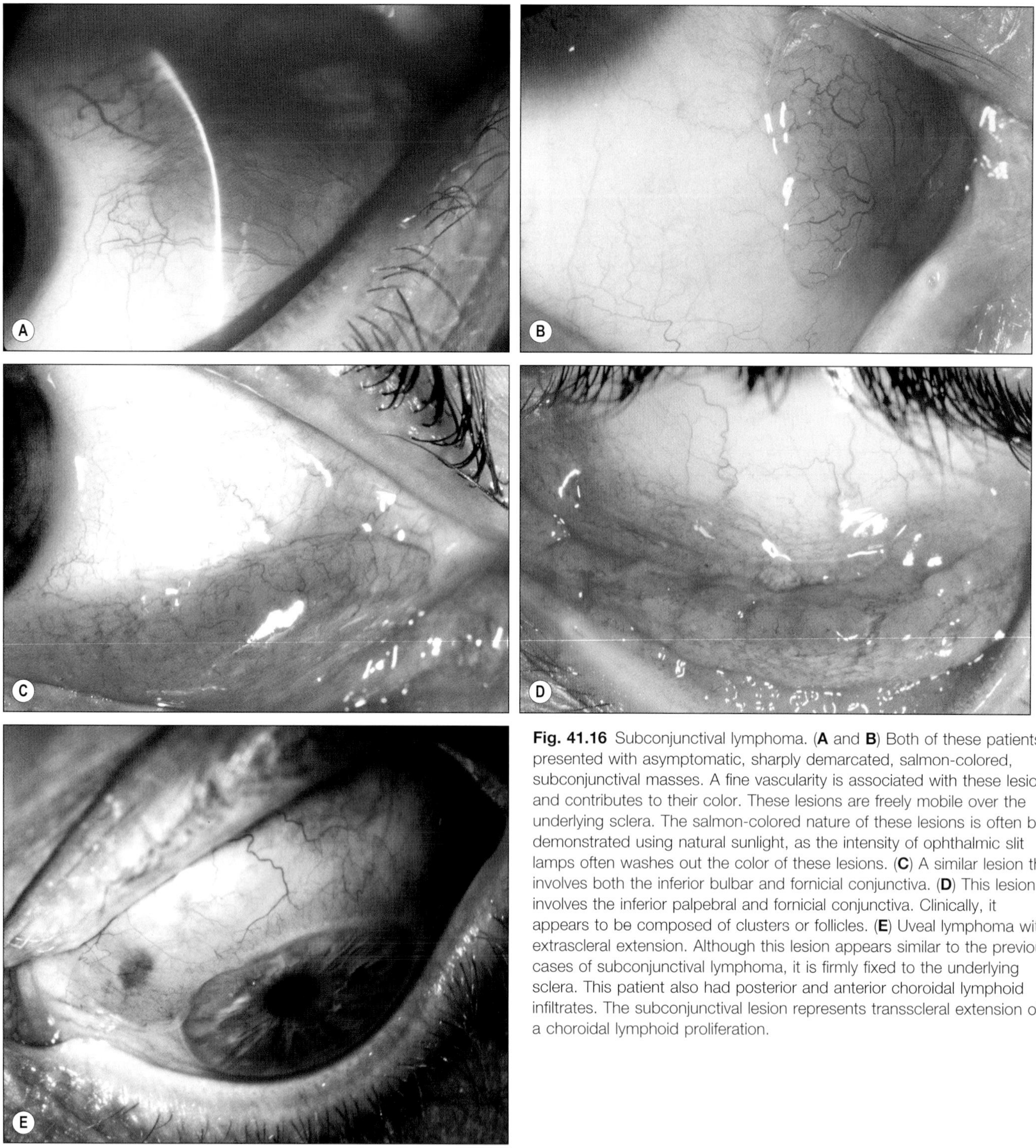

Fig. 41.16 Subconjunctival lymphoma. (**A** and **B**) Both of these patients presented with asymptomatic, sharply demarcated, salmon-colored, subconjunctival masses. A fine vascularity is associated with these lesions and contributes to their color. These lesions are freely mobile over the underlying sclera. The salmon-colored nature of these lesions is often best demonstrated using natural sunlight, as the intensity of ophthalmic slit lamps often washes out the color of these lesions. (**C**) A similar lesion that involves both the inferior bulbar and fornicial conjunctiva. (**D**) This lesion involves the inferior palpebral and fornicial conjunctiva. Clinically, it appears to be composed of clusters or follicles. (**E**) Uveal lymphoma with extrascleral extension. Although this lesion appears similar to the previous cases of subconjunctival lymphoma, it is firmly fixed to the underlying sclera. This patient also had posterior and anterior choroidal lymphoid infiltrates. The subconjunctival lesion represents transscleral extension of a choroidal lymphoid proliferation.

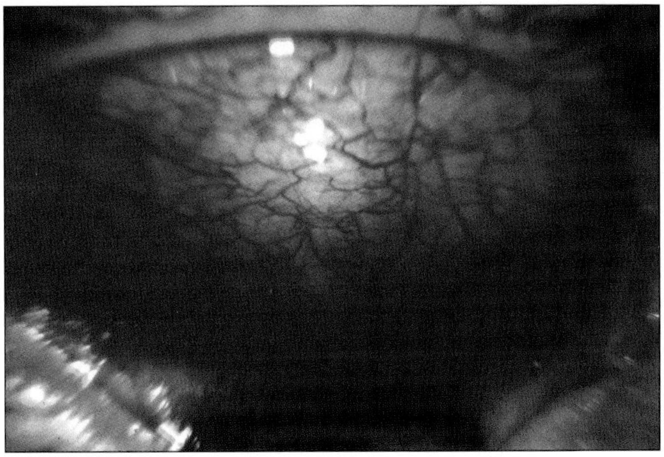

Fig. 41.17 Subconjunctival plasmacytoma. This beefy-red subconjunctival lesion arose in a patient with a history of plasmacytoma. Subconjunctival plasmacytomas are highly vascular collections of plasma cells. After diagnosis, this patient underwent radiation treatment. Over the course of 2 years, the lesion slowly resolved. (Courtesy R.L. Dallow, MD.)

are useful in determining the diagnosis and are correlated to outcome.[176–178] Small lymphocytic and intermediate lymphocytic lymphomas are less often associated with extraocular disease than are other morphologic types. Immunohistochemical separation into polyclonal lymphoid hyperplasia or B-cell lymphoma has not proven useful in predicting individual patient outcomes.[175,177,183,184] Immunohistochemistry has been used in one large series to demonstrate the makeup of conjunctival lesions at presentation; approximately 26% are polyclonal lymphoid hyperplasia, 71% are monoclonal B-cell lymphomas, and 3% are indeterminate.[175] Hodgkin's and T-cell lymphomas are both exceedingly rare.[185,186] Cases of extramedullary plasmacytoma presenting as subconjunctival masses also have been reported, and these lesions are often beefy red clinically (Fig. 41.17).[187–189] In the OAL series,[174] the most common form was the marginal zone lymphoma, accounting for 52%, followed by follicular lymphoma (23%). The marginal zone OALs predominantly anatomically involved the orbital soft tissues and lacrimal gland (112/182 cases) and then the conjunctiva (60/182 cases); the follicular lymphomas were situated in 50 of 80 cases in the orbit and 24 of 80 in the conjunctiva.[190]

The overall prognosis for conjunctival lymphoid lesions is excellent. Important prognostic factors include extent and location of disease at time of presentation. Extensive disease and fornicial or midbulbar conjunctival location is associated with a higher incidence of systemic lymphoma.[179] As previously mentioned, up to 37% of patients with conjunctival lymphoma develop systemic disease at some point over the course of their disease.[180] If no sign of systemic disease is present after initial evaluation, approximately 10–15% of patients will later develop systemic disease at 5 years while 28% will have systemic disease at 10 years.[175,179] A somewhat less significant prognostic factor relates to the degree of differentiation of the lesion determined by histopathology, with small and intermediate cell types faring better than other cell types.[175,176] Bilaterality of disease at presentation and local recurrence after treatment do not adversely affect the prognosis or indicate malignancy. Significantly, up to 20% of patients with initially diagnosed 'benign' polyclonal lymphoid lesions develop systemic lymphoma; therefore, the recommended work-up and treatment for both benign and malignant lymphoid lesions are often identical.[175] This clinical finding is consistent with immunohistochemical findings that an immunoregulatory defect is present in polyclonal proliferations, in which T-helper cells outnumber T-suppressor cells by a greater than normal ratio. Furthermore, many polyclonal lesions have been found to harbor a few populations of B-lymphocytic clones and, therefore, are oligoclonal from early stages.[175,176] Thus, polyclonal lesions might best be thought of as representing a prelymphomatous state, just as primary acquired melanosis with atypia may precede malignant melanoma.

As is the case with systemic lymphoma, some have suggested a role of infectious agents, such as *Chlamydia psittaci* and *Helicobacter pylori*, in the etiology of conjunctival and ocular adnexal lymphoma. To date, these studies have been inconclusive.[191–193]

The treatment after confirmed biopsy diagnosis is outlined as follows. Patients should first be fully evaluated for the presence of systemic disease. Evaluation should include lymph node palpation, chest radiograph, whole-body computed tomography, complete blood count, sedimentation rate, antirheumatoid factor, serum protein immunoelectrophoresis, bilateral bone marrow biopsy, antinuclear antibodies, bone scan, and liver-spleen scan. Positron emission tomography may also be useful in the staging process.[194] Systemic lymphoma usually involves lymph nodes and bone marrow; however, blood and other sites may be involved. If this evaluation reveals systemic disease, systemic chemotherapy is indicated.[195,196] If the disease is localized to the conjunctiva, the gold standard treatment of radiotherapy in a dose of 1500–2000 rads for polyclonal, small lymphocytic lesions or 2000–3000 rads for higher-grade lesions is recommended to prevent systemic dissemination of disease.[197] Cryotherapy is an effective and less costly alternative to radiation therapy and is useful in less extensive lesions and in those for whom radiation therapy is not appropriate.[198] In addition, some have proposed local chemotherapy with interferon alfa-2b or topical mitomycin-C.[199–202] After treatment, patients should be monitored by the ophthalmologist and oncologist for development of local and systemic disease. After treatment, patients should be followed every 6 months for 5 years and then yearly thereafter. Since disease may not develop for months to years, long-term follow-up is necessary.

Other Subconjunctival Neoplastic Lesions

The palpebral conjunctiva may be secondarily involved in capillary hemangiomas of the lids and orbit.[203] Lymphangiomas may be exclusively conjunctival lesions or also involve the orbits and lids (Fig. 41.18). Spontaneous hemorrhage may occur within these lesions, making differentiation from capillary hemangioma difficult. Subconjunctival peripheral nerve sheath tumors include schwannomas, neurofibromas,

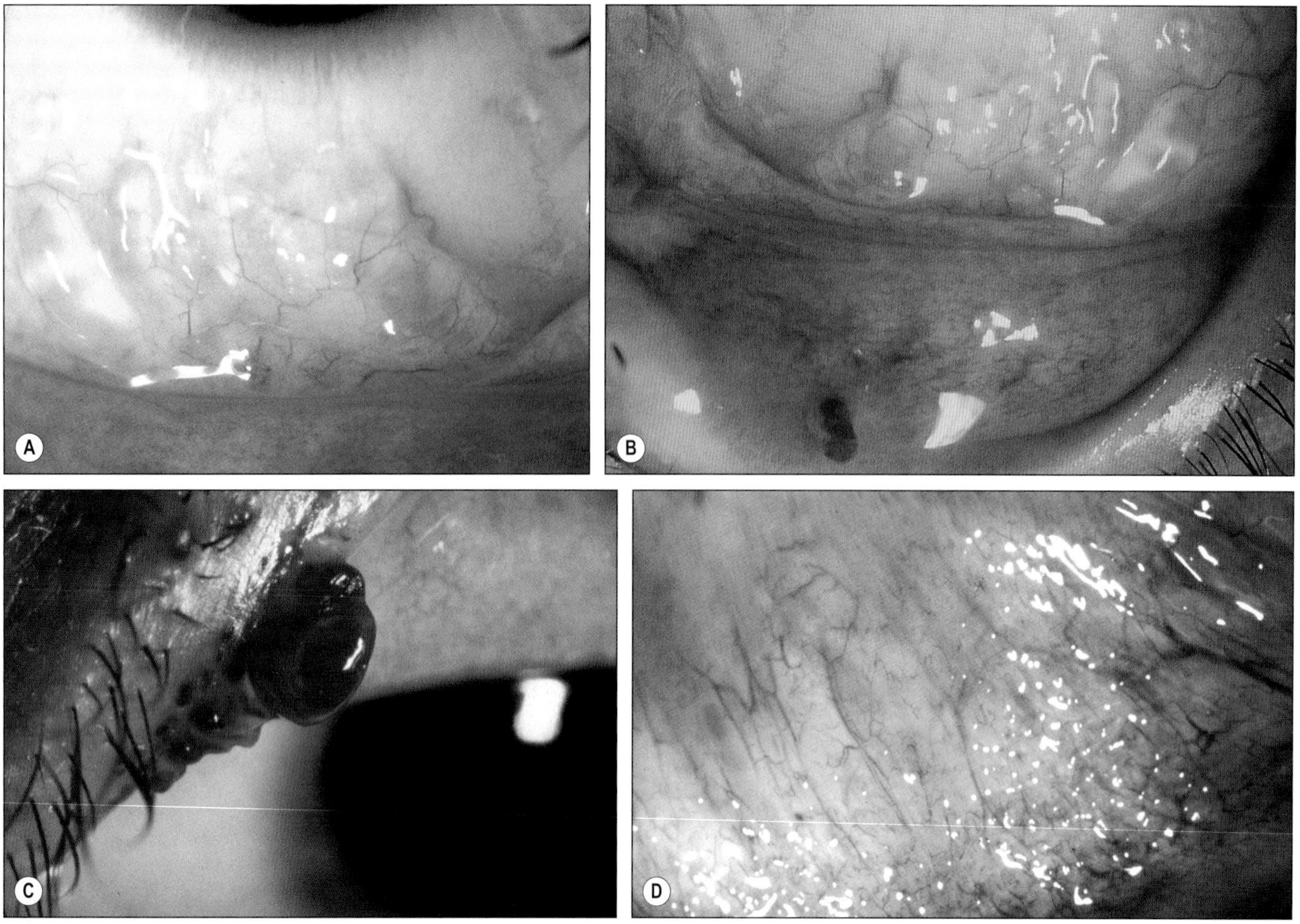

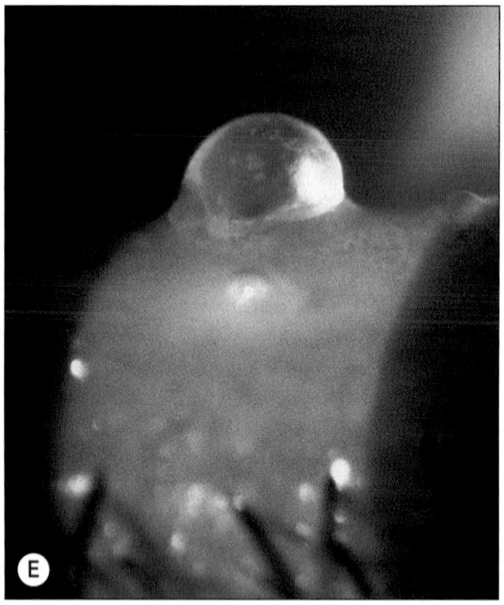

Fig. 41.18 Lymphangioma. (**A**, **B**, and **C**) Numerous dilated, lymph-filled lymphatic vessels are noted over the inferior bulbar surface. They represent the anterior-most extension of an orbital lymphangioma. Because of the fragility of the lymphatic vessels, spontaneous hemorrhage is common, especially in the setting of respiratory infections or Valsalva maneuvers. (**B**, **C**, and **D**) Spontaneous hemorrhage within the lesion. Numerous microlobulated lymph-filled vessels are noted along the inferior bulbar surface in this patient. (**E**) This patient also had lid and orbital involvement.

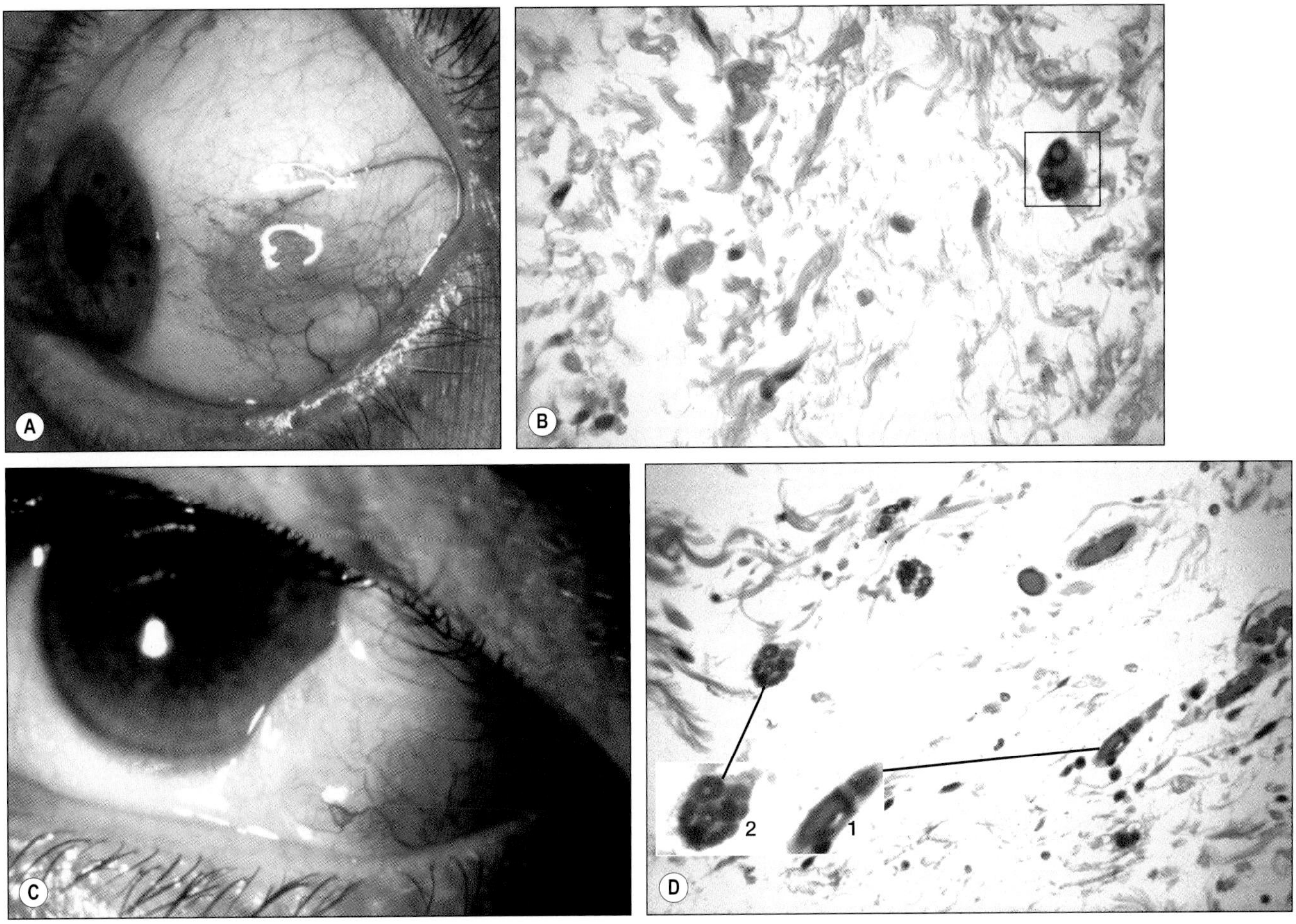

Fig. 41.19 Pleomorphic lipoma and myxoma. Pleomorphic lipomas most commonly occur in the subcutaneous tissue of the neck, back, or shoulder. Only one case has been reported within the conjunctiva.[217] (**A**) This patient noted a 1-month history of a gelatinous, soft, elevated tumor on the temporal bulbar conjunctiva. The lesion, pink in color, was movable over the underlying sclera but somewhat attached. (**B**) Underlying an unremarkable conjunctiva was a collection of cells scattered in a myxoid stroma with loosely arranged collagen fibers. A few multinucleated cells (florets[217]) are noted throughout the lesion. One such cell (*box*) is present in the right side of the specimen. (Courtesy T.P. Dryja.) (**C**) This patient has a larger but similar-appearing lesion arising from the temporal limbus. (**D**) Histopathology shows capillaries (*1*) and multinucleated cells (*2*) (i.e. florets), within a loose myxoid connective tissue background. (Courtesy B. Streeten, MD.)

and neuromas (especially in multiple endocrine neoplasia types III and IIb).[38–41,204,205] Non-neoplastic corneal nerve thickening may be present in Refsum's disease and multiple endocrine neoplasia type IIb (with medullary thyroid carcinoma and pheochromocytoma).[205–208] Krause's end-bulb microtumor is a rare subconjunctival tumor composed of axons and proliferating perineural cells.[209] Adenoid cystic carcinoma may arise from subconjunctival accessory lacrimal glands or ectopic lacrimal gland.[27] Steatocystoma simplex may arise from the pilosebaceous units of the caruncle producing a benign, yellow, soft mass in the medial portion of the globe.[210] Additional mesenchymal tumors that may arise include liposarcoma, pleomorphic lipoma (Fig. 41.19), angiosarcoma, leiomyosarcoma, rhabdomyosarcoma, myxoma, and subconjunctival hemangiopericytoma.[2,211–217] The Carney complex is an autosomal dominantly inherited syndrome in which affected individuals may have two or more of the following: myxomas (cardiac, cutaneous, or mammary), spotty skin pigmentation (often periocular, conjunctival, or caruncular lentigines or blue nevi), Cushing's syndrome, acromegaly or gigantism, sexual precocity (from Leydig cell tumor of the testes, Sertoli cell tumor, or adrenocortical rest tumor), or psammomatous melanotic schwannomas (Fig. 41.20).[218] All patients with eyelid myxomas should be referred for medical evaluation to rule out potentially life-threatening cardiac myxomas. Orbital processes may extend to produce subconjunctival masses; usually complete evaluation reveals the presence of a more extensive process. The conjunctiva is rarely the site of metastatic neoplasia and leukemic infiltration.[219–225]

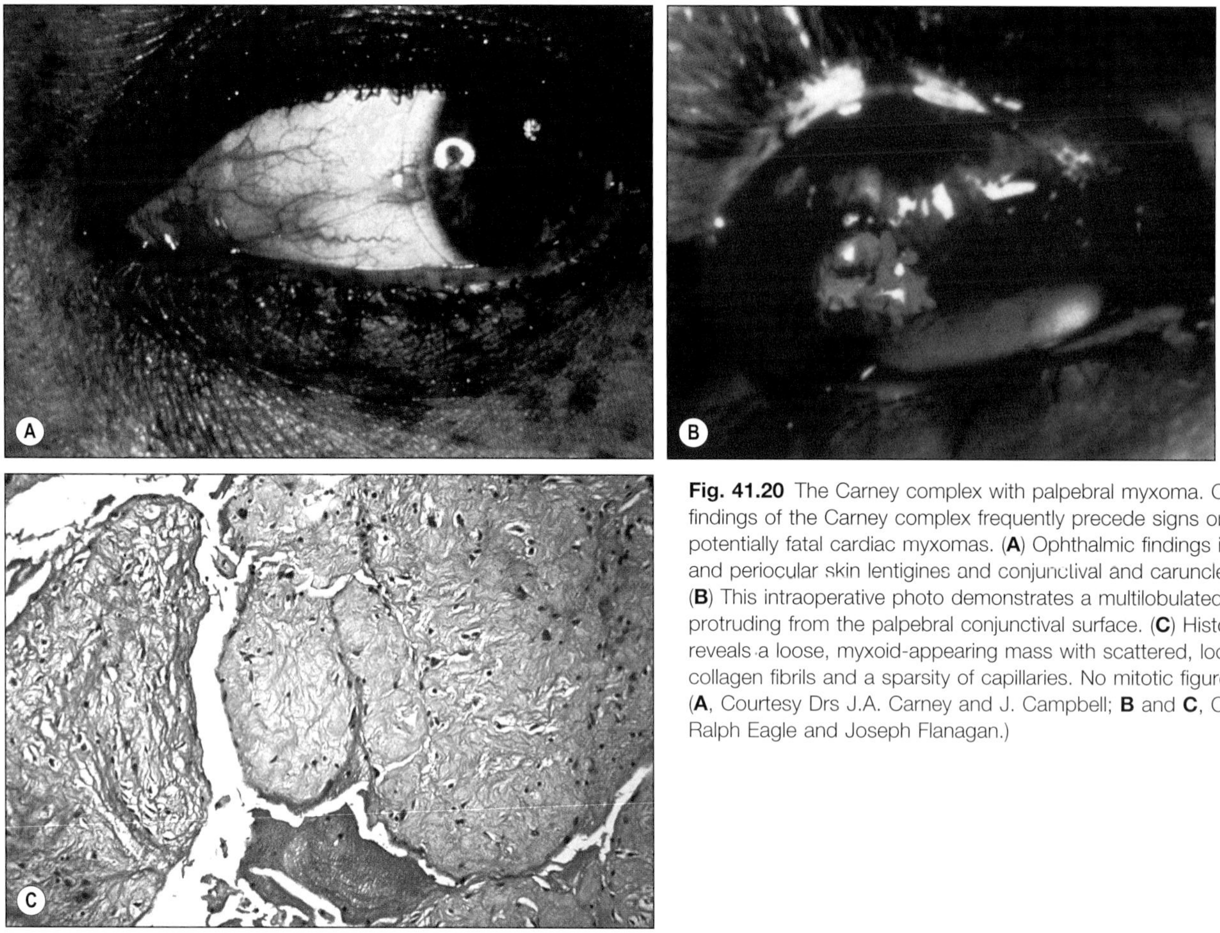

Fig. 41.20 The Carney complex with palpebral myxoma. Ophthalmic findings of the Carney complex frequently precede signs or symptoms of potentially fatal cardiac myxomas. (**A**) Ophthalmic findings include facial and periocular skin lentigines and conjunctival and caruncle pigmentation. (**B**) This intraoperative photo demonstrates a multilobulated, yellow mass protruding from the palpebral conjunctival surface. (**C**) Histopathology reveals a loose, myxoid-appearing mass with scattered, loosely arranged collagen fibrils and a sparsity of capillaries. No mitotic figures are present. (**A**, Courtesy Drs J.A. Carney and J. Campbell; **B** and **C**, Courtesy Drs Ralph Eagle and Joseph Flanagan.)

References

1. Spencer WH, Zimmerman LE. Conjunctiva. In: Spencer WH, ed. *Ophthalmic pathology: an atlas and textbook*. Philadelphia: WB Saunders; 1985.
2. Elsas FJ, Green WR. Epibulbar tumors in childhood. *Am J Ophthalmol*. 1975;79:1001.
3. Grossniklaus HE, et al. Conjunctival lesions in adults: a clinical and histopathologic review. *Cornea*. 1987;6:78.
4. Mattos J, Contreras F, O'Donnell FE. Ring dermoid syndrome: a new syndrome of autosomal dominantly inherited, bilateral, annular limbal dermoids with corneal and conjunctival extension. *Arch Ophthalmol*. 1980;98:1059.
5. Henkind P, et al. Bilateral corneal dermoids. *Am J Ophthalmol*. 1973;76:972.
6. Shields CL, Shields JA. Tumors of the conjunctiva and cornea. *Surv Ophthalmol*. 2004;49(1):3–24.
7. Goldenhar M. Associations malformations de l'oeil et de l'orielle, fistula auris congenita et ses relations avec le dyostose mandibulofacial. *J Genet Hum*. 1952;1:243.
8. Gorlin R, et al. Oculoauriculovertebral dysplasia. *J Paediatr*. 1963;63:991.
9. Collins ET. Cases 8 and 9 with symmetrical congenital notches in the outer part of each lower lid and defective development of the malar bones. *Trans Ophthalmol Soc UK*. 1900;20:190.
10. Quayle SA, Copeland KC. 46, XX gonadal dysgenesis with epibulbar dermoid. *Am J Med Genet*. 1991;40:75.
11. Franceschetti A. Malformations oculaires et suriculaires familiales. *Rev Otoneurophtalmol*. 1946;18:500.
12. Franceschetti A, Zwahlen P. Un nouveau syndrome; la dysostose mandibulofacile. *Bull Schweiz Akad Med Wiss*. 1944;1:60.
13. Solomon L, Fretzin D. An unusual neurocutaneous syndrome. *Arch Dermatol*. 1967;96:732.
14. Kucukoduk S, et al. A new neurocutaneous syndrome: nevus sebaceous syndrome. *Cutis*. 1993;51:437.
15. Murata T, et al. Corneal choristoma with microphthalmos. *Arch Ophthalmol*. 1991;109:1130.
16. Casey RJ, Garner A. Epibulbar choristoma and microphthalmia: a report of two cases. *Br J Ophthalmol*. 1991;75:247.
17. Sangwan VS, Sridhar MS, Vemuganti GK. Treatment of complex choristoma by excision and amniotic membrane transplantation. *Arch Ophthalmol*. 2003;121:278.
18. Grove AS. Dermoid. In: Fraunfelder FT, Roy FH, eds. *Current ocular therapy*. 3rd ed. Philadelphia: WB Saunders; 1990.
19. Panton RW, Sugar J. Excision of limbal dermoids. *Ophthalmic Surg*. 1991;22:85.
20. Pokorny KS, et al. Epibulbar choristomas containing lacrimal tissue: clinical distinction from dermoids and histologic evidence of an origin from the palpebral lobe. *Ophthalmology*. 1987;94:1249.
21. Green WR, Zimmerman LE. Ectopic lacrimal gland tissue: report of eight cases with orbital involvement. *Arch Ophthalmol*. 1967;78:318.
22. Pfaffenbach DD, Green WR. Ectopic lacrimal gland. *Int Ophthalmol Clin*. 1971;11:149.
23. Roth DB, et al. Lacrimal gland choristoma of the conjunctiva simulating a squamous cell carcinoma. *J Pediatr Ophthalmol Strabismus*. 1994;31:62.
24. Alyahya GA, et al. Occurrence of lacrimal gland tissue outside the lacrimal fossa: comparison of clinical and histopathologic findings. *Acta Ophthalmol Scand*. 2003;83:100.
25. Grimalt R, et al. Encephalocraniocutaneous lipomatosis: case report and review of the literature. *Pediatr Dermatol*. 1993;10:164.
26. Kodsi SR, et al. Ocular and systemic manifestations of encephalocraniocutaneous lipomatosis. *Am J Ophthalmol*. 1994;118:77.

27. Font RL, et al. Primary adenoid cystic carcinoma of the conjunctiva arising from the accessory lacrimal glands: a clinicopathologic study of three cases. *Cornea*. 2008;27:494.
28. Cunha RP, Cunha MC, Shields JA. Epibulbar tumors in children: a survey of 282 biopsies. *J Pediatr Ophthalmol Strabismus*. 1987;24:249.
29. Dreizen NG, et al. Epibulbar osseous choristoma. *J Pediatr Ophthalmol Strabismus*. 1983;20:247.
30. Melki TS, et al. A unique epibulbar osseous choristoma. *J Pediatr Ophthalmol Strabismus*. 1990;27:252.
31. von Graefe A. Tumor in submucosen gewebe lid-bindehaut von eigenthumlicher, beschaffenheit. *Klin Monatsbl Augenheilkd {German}*. 1863;1:23.
32. Gayre GS, Proia AD, Dutton JJ. Epibulbar osseous choristoma: case report and review of the literature. *Ophthalmic Surg Lasers*. 2002;33:410–415.
33. Kim BJ, Kazim M. Bilateral symmetrical epibulbar osseous choristoma. *Ophthalmology*. 2006;113(3):456–458.
34. Marback EF, Stout TJ, Rao NA. Osseous choristoma of the conjunctiva simulating extraocular extension of retinoblastoma. *Am J Ophthalmol*. 2002;133:825.
35. Gayre GS, Proia AD, Dutton JJ. Epibulbar osseous choristoma: case report and review of the literature. *Ophthalmic Surg Lasers*. 2002;33:416.
36. Hutchinson DS, Green WR, Iliff CE. Ectopic brain tissue in a limbal dermoid associated with a scleral staphyloma. *Am J Ophthalmol*. 1973;76:984.
37. Emamy J, Ahmadian H. Limbal dermoid with ectopic brain tissue. *Arch Ophthalmol*. 1977;95:2201.
38. Perry HD. Isolated episcleral neurofibroma. *Ophthalmology*. 1982;89:1095.
39. Dabezies OH Jr, Penner R. Neurofibroma or neurilemmoma of the bulbar conjunctiva. *Arch Ophthalmol*. 1961;66:73.
40. Kalina PH, et al. Isolated neurofibromas of the conjunctiva. *Am J Ophthalmol*. 1991;111:694.
41. Perry HD. Isolated neurofibromas of the conjunctiva [comment]. *Am J Ophthalmol*. 1992;113:112.
42. Burke JP, Bowell R, O'Doherty N. Proteus syndrome: ocular complications. *J Pediatr Ophthalmol Strabismus*. 1988;25:99.
43. Bouzas EA, et al. Ophthalmic examination in the diagnosis of Proteus syndrome. *Ophthalmology*. 1993;100:334.
44. Roper GL, Smith MS, Lueder GT. Congenital smooth muscle hamartoma of the conjunctival fornix. *Am J Ophthalmol*. 1999;128:643.
45. Harley RD, Baird HW, Craven EM. Ataxia telangiectasia: report of seven cases. *Arch Ophthalmol*. 1967;77:582.
46. Sahn EE, Hussey RH 3rd, Christmann LM. A case of Bloom syndrome with conjunctival telangiectasia. *Pediatr Dermatol*. 1997;14:120.
47. Soong HK, Pollock DA. Hereditary hemorrhagic telangiectasia diagnosed by the ophthalmologist. *Cornea*. 2000;19:849.
48. Lee SW, Lee SE, Jin KH. Conjunctival inclusion cysts in long-standing chronic vernal keratoconjunctivitis. *Korean J Ophthalmol*. 2007;21:251.
49. Sing G, et al. Bilateral conjunctival retention cysts in the aftermath of Stevens-Johnson syndrome. *Indian J Ophthalmol*. 2008;56:70.
50. Vishwanath MR, Jain A. Conjunctival inclusion cyst following sub-Tenon's local anaesthetic injection. *Br J Anaesth*. 2005;95:825.
51. Boynton JR, et al. Primary nonkeratinized epithelial ('conjunctival') orbital cysts. *Arch Ophthalmol*. 1992;110:1238.
52. Bloomfield SE, Jakobiec FA, Iwamoto T. Traumatic intrastromal corneal cyst. *Ophthalmology*. 1980;87:951.
53. Srinivasan BD, Jakobiec FA, Iwamoto T, DeVoe AG. Epibulbar mucogenic subconjunctival cysts. *Arch Ophthalmol*. 1978;96:857.
54. Imaizumi M, et al. Primary conjunctival epithelial cyst of the orbit. *Int Ophthalmol*. 2007;27:269.
55. Shields JA, Shields CL. Orbital cysts of childhood – classification, clinical features, and management. *Surv Ophthalmol*. 2004;49:281–299
56. Kobayashi A, et al. Visualization of conjunctival cyst by indocyanine green. *Am J Ophthalmol*. 2002;133:827.
57. Kobayashi A, Sugiyama K. Successful removal of a large conjunctival cyst using colored 2.3% sodium hyaluronate. *Ophthalmic Surg Lasers Imaging*. 2007;38:81.
58. Kobayashi A, Sugiyama K. Visualization of conjunctival cyst using Healon V and trypan blue. *Cornea*. 2005;24:759.
59. Owji N, Aslani A. Conjunctival cysts of the orbit after enucleation: the use of trichloroacetic acid. *Ophthal Plast Reconstr Surg*. 2005;21:264.
60. Ferry AP. Pyogenic granulomas of the eye and ocular adnexa: a study of 100 cases. *Trans Am Ophthalmol Soc*. 1989;87:327.
61. Soll SM, et al. Pyogenic granuloma after transconjunctival blepharoplasty: a case report. *Ophthal Plast Reconstr Surg*. 1993;9:298–301.
62. DePotter P, et al. Pyogenic granuloma of the cornea after penetrating keratoplasty. *Cornea*. 1992;11:589–591.
63. Jakobiec FA. Corneal tumors. In: Kaufman H, et al, eds. *The cornea*. New York: Churchill Livingstone; 1988.
64. Patten JT, Hydiuk RA. Granuloma pyogenicum of the conjunctiva. *Ann Ophthalmol*. 1975;7:1588.
65. Ferry AP, Zimmerman LE. Granuloma pyogenicum of limbus: simulating recurrent squamous cell carcinoma. *Arch Ophthalmol*. 1965;74:229.
66. Howard G, Jakobiec FA, DeVoe AG. Kaposi's sarcoma of the conjunctiva. *Am J Ophthalmol*. 1975;79:420.
67. Weiter JJ, Jakobiec FA, Iwamoto T. The clinical and morphologic characteristics of Kaposi's sarcoma of the conjunctiva. *Am J Ophthalmol*. 1980;89:546.
68. Fraunfelder FW, Fraunfelder FT. Liquid nitrogen cryotherapy of a conjunctival vascular tumor. *Cornea*. 2005;24:116.
69. Clear AS, Chirambo MC, Hutt MSR. Solar keratosis, pterygium, and squamous cell carcinoma of the conjunctiva in Malawi. *Br J Ophthalmol*. 1979;63:102.
70. Austin P, Jakobiec FA, Iwamoto T. Elastodysplasia and elastodystrophy as the pathologic basis of pterygia and pinguecula. *Ophthalmology*. 1983;90:96.
71. Bouissou H, et al. The elastic tissue of the skin: a comparison of spontaneous and actinic (solar) aging. *Int J Dermatol*. 1988;27:327.
72. Austin P, et al. Elastofibroma oculi. *Arch Ophthalmol*. 1983;101:1575.
73. Hsu JK, Cavanagh HD, Green WR. An unusual case of elastofibroma oculi. *Cornea*. 1997;16:112.
74. Font RJ, Zimmerman LE. Nodular fasciitis of the eye and adnexa: a report of 10 cases. *Arch Ophthalmol*. 1966;75:475.
75. Holds JB, Mamalis N, Anderson RL. Nodular fasciitis presenting as a rapidly enlarging episcleral mass in a 3-year-old. *J Pediatr Ophthalmol Strabismus*. 1990;27:157.
76. Austin P, et al. Peripheral corneal degeneration and occlusive vasculitis in Wegener's granulomatosis. *Am J Ophthalmol*. 1978;85:311.
77. Ashton N, Cook C. Allergic granulomatous nodules of the eyelid and conjunctiva. *Am J Ophthalmol*. 1979;87:1.
78. Cameron ME, Greer H. Allergic conjunctival granulomas. *Br J Ophthalmol*. 1980;64:494.
79. Purcell JJ, Birkenkamp K, Tsai CC. Conjunctival lesions in periarteritis nodosa: a clinical and immunopathologic study. *Arch Ophthalmol*. 1984;102:736.
80. Blase WP, Knox DL, Green WR. Granulomatous conjunctivitis in a patient with Crohn's disease. *Br J Ophthalmol*. 1984;68:901.
81. Albert DL, Brownstein S, Jackson WB. Conjunctival granulomas in rosacea [letter]. *Am J Ophthalmol*. 1992;113:108.
82. Slack JW, Hyndiuk RA, Harris GJ. Blastomycosis of the eyelid and conjunctiva. *Ophthal Plast Reconstr Surg*. 1992;8:143.
83. Rathinam S, et al. An outbreak of trematode-induced granulomas of the conjunctiva. *Ophthalmology*. 2001;108:1223.
84. Godfrey DG, Carr JD, Grossniklaus HE. Epibulbar allergic granulomatous nodules in a human immunodeficiency virus positive patient. *Am J Ophthalmol*. 1998;126:844.
85. Ashton N, Cook C. Allergic granulomatous nodules of the eyelid and conjunctiva. *Am J Ophthalmol*. 1979;87:1.
86. Knox DL, O'Brien TP, Green WR. Histoplasma granuloma of the conjunctiva. *Ophthalmology*. 2003;110:2051.
87. Nakao K, et al. Conjunctival nodules associated with Vogt-Koyanagi-Harada disease. *Graefes Arch Clin Exp Ophthalmol*. 2007;245:1383.
88. Robinson MR, et al. Tarsal-conjunctival disease associated with Wegener's granulomatosis. *Ophthalmology*. 2003;110:1770.
89. Hegab SM, al-Mutawa SA, Sheriff SM. Sarcoidosis presenting as multilobular limbal corneal nodules. *J Pediatr Ophthalmol Strabismus*. 1998;35:323.
90. Geggel HS, Mensher JH. Cicatricial conjunctivitis in sarcoidosis: recognition and treatment. *Ann Ophthalmol*. 1989;21:92.
91. Nichols CW, et al. Conjunctival biopsy as an aid in the evaluation of the patient with suspected sarcoidosis. *Ophthalmology*. 1980;87:287.
92. Leavitt JA, Campbell RJ. Cost-effectiveness in the diagnosis of sarcoidosis: the conjunctival biopsy. *Eye*. 1998;12:959.
93. Lebowitz MA, Jakobiec FA, Donnenfeld ED, Starr M. Bilateral epibulbar rheumatoid nodulosis. *Ophthalmology*. 1988;95:1256.
94. Wedemeyer LL, et al. Fibrous histiocytoid leprosy of the cornea. *Cornea*. 1993;12:532.
95. Cogan DG, Kuwabara T, Parke D. Epibulbar nevo-xantho-endothelioma. *Arch Ophthalmol*. 1958;59:717.
96. Zimmerman LE. Ocular lesions of juvenile xanthogranuloma. *Trans Am Acad Ophthalmol Otolaryngol*. 1965;69:412.
97. Kobayashi A, et al. Adult-onset limbal juvenile xanthogranuloma. *Arch Ophthalmol*. 2002;120:96.
98. Fleischmajer R, et al. Normolipemic subcutaneous xanthomatosis. *Am J Med*. 1983;75:1076.

99. Winkelmann RK, Oliver GF. Subcutaneous xanthogranulomatosis: an inflammatory non-X histiocytic syndrome (subcutaneous xanthomatosis). *J Am Acad Dermatol.* 1989;21:924.
100. Foucar E, Rosai J, Dorfman RF. The ophthalmologic manifestations of sinus histiocytosis with massive lymphadenopathy. *Am J Ophthalmol.* 1979;87:354.
101. Zimmerman LE, et al. Atypical cases of sinus histiocytosis (Rosai-Dorfman disease) with ophthalmological manifestations. *Trans Am Ophthalmol Soc.* 1988;86:113.
102. Friendly DS, Font RL, Rao NA. Orbital involvement in 'sinus' histiocytosis: a report of four cases. *Arch Ophthalmol.* 1977;95:2006.
103. Allaire GS, et al. Reticulohistiocytoma of the limbus and cornea. *Ophthalmology.* 1990;97:1018.
104. Giller RH, et al. Xanthoma disseminatum. *Am J Pediatr Hematol Oncol.* 1988;10:252.
105. Margolis R, et al. Conjunctival involvement in Churg-Strauss syndrome. *Ocul Immunol Inflamm.* 2007;15:113.
106. Ooi KG, et al. Churg-Strauss syndrome presenting with conjunctival nodules in association with *Candida albicans* and ankylosing spondylitis. *Clin Experiment Ophthalmol.* 2004;32:441.
107. Shields CL, Shields JA, Rozanski TI. Conjunctival involvement in Churg-Strauss syndrome. *Am J Ophthalmol.* 1986;102:601.
108. Jakobiec FA, et al. Periocular xanthogranulomas associated with severe adult-onset asthma. *Trans Am Ophthalmol Soc.* 1993;91:99.
109. Mullaney J. Peculiar ophthalmic proliferations. *Eye.* 1990;4:79.
110. Charles NC, Friedberg DN. Epibulbar molluscum contagiosum in acquired immune deficiency syndrome. *Ophthalmology.* 1992;99:1123.
111. Merisier H, et al. Multiple molluscum contagiosum lesions of the limbus in a patient with HIV infection. *Br J Ophthalmol.* 1995;79:393.
112. Ingraham HJ, Schoenleber DB. Epibulbar molluscum contagiosum. *Am J Ophthalmol.* 1998;125:394.
113. O'Grady RB, Kirk HQ. Corneal keloids. *Am J Ophthalmol.* 1972;73:206.
114. Parikh JG, et al. Keloid of the conjunctiva simulating a conjunctival malignancy. *Br J Ophthalmol.* 2007;91:1251.
115. Lampkin JC, Jakobiec FA. Amyloidosis and the eye. In: Albert DM, Jakobiec FA, eds. *Principles and practice of ophthalmology.* Philadelphia: WB Saunders; 1994.
116. Howes EL. Basic mechanisms in pathology. In: Spencer WH, ed. *Ophthalmic pathology.* 3rd ed. Philadelphia: WB Saunders; 1985.
117. Brownstein MH, Elliott R, Helwig EB. Ophthalmic aspects of amyloidosis. *Am J Ophthalmol.* 1970;69:423.
118. Smith ME, Zimmerman LE. Amyloidosis of the eyelid and conjunctiva. *Arch Ophthalmol.* 1966;75:42.
119. Pepys MB. Amyloidosis. In: Samter M, ed. *Immunological disease.* 4th ed. Boston: Little Brown; 1988.
120. Lee HM, et al. Primary localized conjunctival amyloidosis presenting with recurrence of subconjunctival hemorrhage. *Am J Ophthalmol.* 2000;129:245.
121. Lieb WE, et al. Postsurgical hematic cyst simulating a conjunctival melanoma. *Retina.* 1990;10:63.
122. Lahoud S, Brownstein S, Laflamme MY. Fibrous histiocytoma of the corneoscleral limbus and conjunctiva. *Am J Ophthalmol.* 1988;106:579.
123. Albert DM, Smith RS. Fibrous xanthomas of the conjunctiva. *Arch Ophthalmol.* 1968;80:474.
124. Jakobiec FA. Fibrous histiocytoma of the corneoscleral limbus. *Am J Ophthalmol* 78:700, 1974.
125. Faludi JE, Kenyon KR, Green WR. Fibrous histiocytoma of the corneoscleral limbus. *Am J Ophthalmol.* 1975;80:619.
126. Iwamoto T, Jakobiec FA, Darrell RW. Fibrous histiocytoma of the corneoscleral limbus: the ultrastructure of a distinctive inclusion. *Ophthalmology.* 1981;88:1260.
127. Grayson M, Pieroni D. Solitary xanthoma of the corneo-scleral limbus. *Br J Ophthalmol.* 1970;54:562.
128. Jakobiec FA, et al. Infantile subconjunctival and anterior orbital fibrous histiocytoma. *Ophthalmology.* 1988;95:516.
129. Pe'er J, et al. Malignant fibrous histiocytoma of the skin and conjunctiva in xeroderma pigmentosa. *Arch Pathol Lab Med.* 1991;115:910.
130. Pe'er J, et al. Malignant fibrous histiocytoma of the conjunctiva. *Br J Ophthalmol.* 1990;74:624.
131. Allaire CS, Corriveau C, Teboul N. Malignant fibrous histiocytoma of the conjunctiva. *Arch Ophthalmol.* 1999;117:685.
132. Kim HJ, et al. Fibrous histiocytoma of the conjunctiva. *Am J Ophthalmol.* 2006;142:1036.
133. Arora R, et al. Malignant fibrous histiocytoma of the conjunctiva. *Clin Experiment Ophthalmol.* 2006;34:275.
134. Balestrazzi E et al. Malignant conjunctival epibulbar fibrous histiocytoma with orbital invasion. *Eur J Ophthalmol.* 1991;1:23.
135. Margo CE, Horton MB. Malignant fibrous histiocytoma of the conjunctiva with metastasis. *Am J Ophthalmol.* 1989;107:433.
136. Reiser BJ, et al. Non-AIDS-related Kaposi sarcoma involving the tarsal conjunctiva and eyelid margin. *Arch Ophthalmol.* 2007;125:838.
137. Fogt F, et al. Conjunctival Kaposi's sarcoma in a nonimmunocompromised patient. *Can J Ophthalmol.* 2007;42:310.
138. Curtis TH, Durairaj VD. Conjunctival Kaposi sarcoma as the initial presentation of human immunodeficiency virus infection. *Ophthal Plast Reconstr Surg.* 2005;21:314.
139. Kaposi M. Idiopathisches multiple pigmentsarkom der haut. *Arch Dermatol Syphilol.* 1872;4:265.
140. Shuler JD, et al. Kaposi sarcoma of the conjunctiva and eyelids associated with the acquired immunodeficiency syndrome. *Arch Ophthalmol.* 1989;107:858.
141. Kurumety UR, Lustbader JM. Kaposi's sarcoma of the bulbar conjunctiva as an initial clinical manifestation of acquired immunodeficiency syndrome. *Arch Ophthalmol.* 1995;113:978.
142. Macher AM, et al. Multicentric Kaposi's sarcoma of conjunctiva in a male homosexual with acquired immunodeficiency syndrome. *Ophthalmology.* 1983;90:879.
143. Weiter JJ, Jakobiec FA, Iwamoto T. The clinical and morphologic characteristics of Kaposi's sarcoma of the conjunctiva. *Am J Ophthalmol.* 1980;89:546.
144. Dugel PU, et al. Ocular adnexal Kaposi's sarcoma in acquired immunodeficiency syndrome. *Am J Ophthalmol.* 1990;110:500.
145. Miles S. Pathogenesis of AIDS-related Kaposi's sarcoma: evidence of a viral etiology. *Hematol Oncol Clin North Am.* 1996;10:1011.
146. Chang Y, et al. Identification of herpesvirus-like DNA sequences in AIDS-associated Kaposi's sarcoma. *Science.* 1994;266:1865.
147. Lee F, Mitsuyau R. Chemotherapy of AIDS-related Kaposi's sarcoma. *Hematol Oncol Clin North Am.* 1996;10:1051.
148. Gill P, et al. Systemic treatment of AIDS-related Kaposi's sarcoma: results of a randomized trial. *Am J Med.* 1991;90:427.
149. Heimann H, et al. Regression of conjunctival Kaposi's sarcoma under chemotherapy with bleomycin. *Br J Ophthalmol.* 1997;81:1019.
150. Scadden D, et al. Granulocyte-macrophage colony-stimulating factor mitigates the neutropenia of combined interferon alpha and zidovudine treatment of acquired immune deficiency syndrome – associated Kaposi's sarcoma. *J Clin Oncol.* 1991;9:802.
151. Leder HA, et al. Resolution of conjunctival Kaposi sarcoma after institution of highly active antiretroviral therapy alone. *Br J Ophthalmol.* 2008;92:151.
152. Berson AM, et al. Radiation therapy for AIDS-related Kaposi's sarcoma. *Int J Radiat Oncol Biol Phys.* 1990;19:569.
153. Glynne-Jones R, et al. Epidemic Kaposi's sarcoma of the conjunctiva: considerations for radiotherapy. *Clin Oncol.* 1990;2:358.
154. Brunt AM, Phillips RH. Strontium-90 for conjunctival AIDS-related Kaposi's sarcoma: the first case report. *Clin Oncol.* 1990;2:118.
155. Ghabrial R, et al. Radiation therapy of acquired immunodeficiency syndrome-related Kaposi's sarcoma of the eyelids and conjunctiva. *Arch Ophthalmol.* 1992;110:1423.
156. Kirova YM, et al. Radiotherapy in the management of epidemic Kaposi's sarcoma. A retrospective study of 643 cases. *Radiother Oncology.* 1998;46:19.
157. Palestine A, Palestine R. External ocular manifestations of the acquired immunodeficiency syndrome. *Ophthalmol Clin North Am.* 1992;5:319.
158. Hummer J, Gass JD, Huang AJ. Conjunctival Kaposi's sarcoma treated with interferon alpha-2A. *Am J Ophthalmol.* 1993;116:502.
159. Gill P, et al. The effects of preparations of human chorionic gonadotropin on AIDS-related Kaposi's sarcoma. *N Engl J Med.* 1996;335:1261.
160. Hamperl H. Benign and malignant oncocytomas. *Cancer.* 1962;15:303.
161. Rodgers IR, et al. Papillary oncocytoma of the eyelid: a previously undescribed tumor of apocrine gland origin. *Ophthalmology.* 1988;95:1071.
162. Biggs SL, Font RL. Oncocytic lesions of the caruncle and other ocular adnexa. *Arch Ophthalmol.* 1977;95:474.
163. Shields CL, et al. Types and frequency of lesions of the caruncle. *Am J Ophthalmol.* 1986;102:771.
164. Kurli M, et al. Peribulbar oncocytoma: high-frequency ultrasound with histopathologic correlation. *Ophthalmic Surg Lasers Imaging.* 2006;37:154.
165. Freddo TF, Leibowitz HM. Oncocytoma of the caruncle: a case report and ultrastructural study. *Cornea.* 1991;10:175.
166. Orcutt JC, Matsko TH, Milam AH. Oncocytoma of the caruncle. *Ophthal Plast Reconstr Surg.* 1992;8:300.
167. Husain SE, et al. Primary basal cell carcinoma of the limbal conjunctiva. *Ophthalmology.* 1993;100:1720.
168. Meier P, Sterker I, Meier T. Primary basal cell carcinoma of the caruncle. *Arch Ophthalmol.* 1998;116:1373.
169. Rossman D, et al. Basal cell carcinoma of the caruncle. *Ophthal Plast Reconstr Surg.* 2006;22:313.

170. Mencia-Gutierrez E, Gutierrez-Diaz E, Perez-Martin ME. Lacrimal caruncle primary basal cell carcinoma: case report and review. *J Cutan Pathol.* 2005;32:502.
171. Ostergaard J, et al. Primary basal cell carcinoma of the caruncle with seeding to the conjunctiva. *Graefes Arch Clin Exp Ophthalmol.* 2005; 243:615.
172. Cable MM, et al. Primary basal cell carcinoma of the conjunctiva with intraocular invasion. *Arch Ophthalmol.* 2000;118:1296.
173. Sacks E, et al. Lymphocyte subpopulations in the normal human conjunctiva: a monoclonal antibody study. *Ophthalmology.* 1986;93:1276.
174. Ferry JA, Fung CY, Zukerberg L, et al. Lymphoma of the ocular adnexa: a study of 353 cases. *Am J Surg Pathol.* 2007;31:170 -184
175. Knowles DM, et al. Lymphoid hyperplasia and malignant lymphoma occurring in the ocular adnexa (orbit, conjunctiva, and eyelids): a prospective multiparametric analysis of 108 cases during 1977 to 1987. *Hum Pathol.* 1989;21:959.
176. Jakobiec FA, Knowles DM. An overview of ocular adnexal lymphoid tumors. *Trans Am Ophthalmol Soc.* 1990;87:420.
177. Sigelman J, Jakobiec FA. Lymphoid proliferations of the conjunctiva: relation of histopathology to clinical outcome. *Ophthalmology.* 1978; 85:818.
178. McNally L, Jakobiec FA, Knowles DM II. Clinical, morphological, immunophenotypic, and molecular genetic analysis of bilateral ocular adnexal lymphoid neoplasms in 17 patients. *Am J Ophthalmol.* 1987; 103:555.
179. Shields CL, et al. Conjunctival lymphoid tumors: clinical analysis of 117 cases and relationship to systemic lymphoma. *Ophthalmology.* 2001;108:979.
180. Johnson TE, et al. Ocular-adnexal lymphoid tumors: a clinicopathologic and molecular genetic study of 77 patients. *Ophthal Plast Reconstr Surg.* 1999;15:171.
181. Karadeniz C, et al. Primary subconjunctival lymphoma: an unusual presentation of childhood non-Hodgkin's lymphoma. *Med Pediatr Oncol.* 1991;19:204.
182. Jakobiec FA, et al. Multifocal static creamy choroidal infiltrates: an early sign of lymphoid neoplasia. *Ophthalmology.* 1987;94:397.
183. Ellis JM, et al. Clinical correlation with the working formulation classification and immunoperoxidase staining of paraffin sections. *Ophthalmology.* 1985;92:1311.
184. Medeiros LJ, Harris NL. Immunohistologic analysis of small lymphocytic infiltrates of the orbit and conjunctiva. *Hum Pathol.* 1990;21:1126.
185. Shields CL, Shields JA, Eagle RC. Rapidly progressive T-cell lymphoma of the conjunctiva. *Arch Ophthalmol.* 2002;120:508.
186. Hu FR, et al. T-cell malignant lymphoma with conjunctival involvement. *Am J Ophthalmol.* 1998;125:717.
187. Kremer I, Flex D, Manor R. Solitary conjunctival extramedullary plasmacytoma. *Ann Ophthalmol.* 1990;22:126.
188. Tetsumoto K, Iwaki H, Inoue M. IgG-kappa extramedullary plasmacytoma of the conjunctiva and orbit. *Br J Ophthalmol.* 1993;77:255.
189. Lugassy G, et al. Primary lymphoplasmacytoma of the conjunctiva. *Eye.* 1992;6:326.
190. Jakobiec FA. Ocular adnexal lymphoid tumors: progress in need of clarification. *Am J Ophthalmol.* 2008;145(6):941–950.
191. Ferreri AJ, et al. *Chlamydophila psittaci* is viable and infectious in the conjunctiva and peripheral blood of patients with ocular adnexal lymphoma: results of a single-center prospective case-control study. *Int J Cancer.* 2008;123:1089.
192. Lee SB, Yang JW, Kim CS. The association between conjunctival MALT lymphoma and *Helicobacter pylori*. *Br J Ophthalmol.* 2008;92:534.
193. Sjo NC, et al. Role of *Helicobacter pylori* in conjunctival mucosa-associated lymphoid tissue lymphoma. *Ophthalmology.* 2007;114:182.
194. Valenzuela AA, et al. Positron emission tomography in the detection and staging of ocular adnexal lymphoproliferative disease. *Ophthalmology.* 2006;113:2331.
195. Zinzani PL, et al. Rituximab in primary conjunctiva lymphoma. *Leuk Res.* 2005;29:107.
196. Salepci T, et al. Conjunctival malt lymphoma successfully treated with single agent rituximab therapy. *Leuk Res.* 2009;33:e10.
197. Jereb B, et al. Radiation therapy of conjunctival and orbital lymphoid tumors. *Int J Radiat Oncol Biol Phys.* 1984;10:1013.
198. Eichler MD, Fraunfelder FT. Cryotherapy for conjunctival lymphoid tumors. *Am J Ophthalmol.* 1994;118:463.
199. Lachapelle KR. Treatment of conjunctival mucosa-associated lymphoid tissue lymphoma with intralesional interferon alpha-2b. *Arch Ophthalmol.* 2000;118:284.
200. Blasi MA, et al. Local chemotherapy with interferon-a for conjunctival mucosa-associated lymphoid tissue lymphoma. *Ophthalmology.* 2001; 108:559.
201. Ross JJ, Tu KL, Damato BE. Systemic remission of non-Hodgkin's lymphoma after intralesional interferon alpha-2b to bilateral conjunctival lymphomas. *Am J Ophthalmol.* 2004;138:672.
202. Yu CS, et al. Localized conjunctival mucosa-associated lymphoid tissue (MALT) lymphoma is amenable to local chemotherapy. *Int Ophthalmol.* 2008;28:51.
203. Goble RR, Frangoulis MA. Lymphangioma circumscriptum of the eyelids and conjunctiva. *Br J Ophthalmol.* 1990;74:574.
204. Vincent NJ, Cleasby GW. Schwannoma of the bulbar conjunctiva. *Arch Ophthalmol.* 1968;80:641.
205. Nassir MA, et al. Multiple endocrine neoplasia Type III. *Cornea.* 1991;10:454.
206. Robertson DM, Sizemore GW, Gordon H. Thickened corneal nerves as a manifestation of multiple endocrine neoplasia. *Trans Am Acad Ophthalmol Otolaryngol.* 1975;79:772.
207. Spector B, Klintworth GK, Wells SA. Histologic study of the ocular lesions in multiple endocrine neoplasia syndrome type IIb. *Am J Ophthalmol.* 1981;91:204.
208. Baum JL, Tannenbaum M, Kolodny EH. Refsum's syndrome with corneal involvement. *Am J Ophthalmol.* 1965;60:699.
209. Figols J, Hanuschik W, Cervos-Navarro J. Krause's end-bulb microtumor of the conjunctiva: optic and ultrastructural description of a case. *Graefes Arch Clin Exp Ophthalmol.* 1992;230:206.
210. Kim NJ, Moon KC, Khwarg SI. Steatocystoma simplex of the caruncle. *Can J Ophthalmol.* 2006;41:83.
211. Miyashita K, Abe Y, Osamura Y. Case of conjunctival liposarcoma. *Jpn J Ophthalmol.* 1991;35:207.
212. Hufnagel T, Ma L, Kuo TT. Orbital angiosarcoma with subconjunctival presentation: report of a case and literature review. *Ophthalmology.* 1987;94:72.
213. White VA, et al. Leiomyosarcoma of the conjunctiva. *Ophthalmology.* 1991;98:1560.
214. Pe'er J, Hidayat AA. Myxomas of the conjunctiva. *Am J Ophthalmol.* 1986;102:80.
215. Lo GG, et al. Corneal myxoma: case report and review of the literature. *Cornea.* 1990;9:174.
216. Grossniklaus HE, et al. Hemangiopericytoma of the conjunctiva: two cases. *Ophthalmology.* 1986;93:265.
217. Bryant J. Pleomorphic lipoma of the bulbar conjunctiva. *Ann Ophthalmol.* 1987;19:148.
218. Kennedy RH, et al. The Carney complex with ocular signs suggestive of cardiac myxoma. *Am J Ophthalmol.* 1991;111:699.
219. Ferry AP, Font RL. Carcinoma metastatic to the eye and orbit: a clinicopathological study of 227 cases. *Arch Ophthalmol.* 1974;92: 276.
220. Gritz DC, Rao NA. Metastatic carcinoid tumor diagnosis from a caruncular mass. *Am J Ophthalmol.* 1991;112:470.
221. Tsumura T, et al. A case of acute myelomonocytic leukemia with subconjunctival tumor. *Jpn J Ophthalmol.* 1991;35:226.
222. Kincaid MC, Green WR. Ocular and orbital involvement in leukemia. *Surv Ophthalmol.* 1983;27:211.
223. Shields JA, et al. Conjunctival metastasis as the initial manifestation of lung cancer. *Am J Ophthalmol.* 1997;124:399.
224. Ortiz JM, Esterman B, Paulson J. Uterine cervical carcinoma metastasis to subconjunctival tissue. *Arch Ophthalmol.* 1995;113:1362.
225. Tokuyama J, et al. Rare case of early mucosal gastric cancer presenting with metastasis to the bulbar conjunctiva. *Gastric Cancer.* 2002;5: 102.

Chapter 42

Conjunctivitis: An Overview and Classification

Thomas D. Lindquist

The conjunctiva is a thin, translucent mucous membrane whose palpebral portion lines the posterior surface of the eyelids, and whose bulbar portion lines the anterior surface of the globe. The conjunctiva is firmly adherent to the lids over the tarsal plates and loosely attached in the fornices and over the globe, with the exception of the limbus.

As with other mucous membranes, the conjunctiva has an epithelial layer and a submucosal substantia propria. The conjunctival epithelium is contiguous with the corneal epithelium and also lines the lacrimal passages and glands, a fact that has significant clinical implications. The substantia propria is composed of a superficial adenoid layer and a deeper fibrous layer. The adenoid layer contains lymphoid tissue from which follicles are formed. Within the lymphoid tissue are germinal centers with lymphoblasts in the center. The fibrous layer is composed of connective tissue, which attaches to the tarsal plate and contributes to the characteristic appearance of papillae.[1]

The formation of papillae is a nonspecific sign of conjunctival inflammation resulting from edema and polymorphonuclear (PMN) cell infiltration of the conjunctiva. Papillae can form only where the conjunctiva is attached to the underlying tissue by anchoring septae, such as over the tarsus or the bulbar limbus. Fibroblasts, macrophages, mast cells, and PMNs are found extravascularly within the substantia propria. Mast cells (5000 mm^3) and plasma cells are normally present in the substantia propria, but not in the conjunctival epithelium. Neutrophils and lymphocytes (100 000 mm^3) are routinely found in both conjunctival epithelium and substantia propria, whereas basophils and eosinophils are not normally present in either conjunctival epithelium or substantia propria.[2,3]

Conjunctival Injection

The conjunctival vessels are derived from the anterior ciliary and palpebral arteries. Conjunctival injection is characterized by superficial bright red blood vessels, which are most conspicuous in the fornices and fade toward the corneoscleral limbus. These vessels move as the conjunctiva is mechanically manipulated and are blanched by topical instillation of phenylephrine.

Conjunctival hyperemia is secondary to dilation of the conjunctival blood vessels without accompanying exudation or cellular infiltration. Hyperemia may be caused by a multiplicity of environmental factors including smoke, smog or chemical fumes, wind, ultraviolet radiation, and prolonged topical instillation of vasoconstrictors.

Conjunctivitis

Conjunctivitis implies inflammation of the conjunctiva and is characterized by cellular infiltration and exudation in addition to vascular dilation. Chemosis, an accumulation of fluid within or beneath the conjunctiva, is frequently present. The patient may complain of eyelid fullness and a diffuse, gritty foreign body sensation. Frequently, patients may notice a discharge that causes the eyelids to stick together. The condition may be unilateral or bilateral.

The diagnosis of conjunctivitis may be based on one or more of the following: (1) the history and clinical examination; (2) Gram and Giemsa stains of conjunctival scrapings; and (3) culture and identification of conjunctival scrapings. Patient history can be helpful. Infectious disease is often bilateral and may involve other members of the family or community. Most cases of acute viral conjunctivitis initially involve one eye, followed a few days later by involvement of the other eye. The presence of an enlarged preauricular lymph node suggests a viral etiology. Unilateral involvement may suggest a toxic, pharmacological, mechanical, or lacrimal origin.

Several diagnostic criteria are helpful in determining the underlying etiology of conjunctivitis. Chronicity plays an important role and is the most widely used criterion for classification of conjunctivitis. An acute conjunctivitis is arbitrarily defined as having a duration of less than 3 weeks, whereas chronic conjunctivitis has a longer duration of symptoms.[4,5] The morphologic appearance, type of exudate, and principally affected areas of the conjunctiva are the other most important physical findings that help define the etiology of conjunctivitis.

In addition to the chronicity of conjunctivitis, five morphologic responses can be identified that help define algorithms for acute or chronic conjunctivitities (Figs 42.1, 42.2): papillary, follicular, membranous/pseudomembranous, cicatrizing, granulomatous. Proper identification of the morphologic response is crucial to the correct diagnosis.

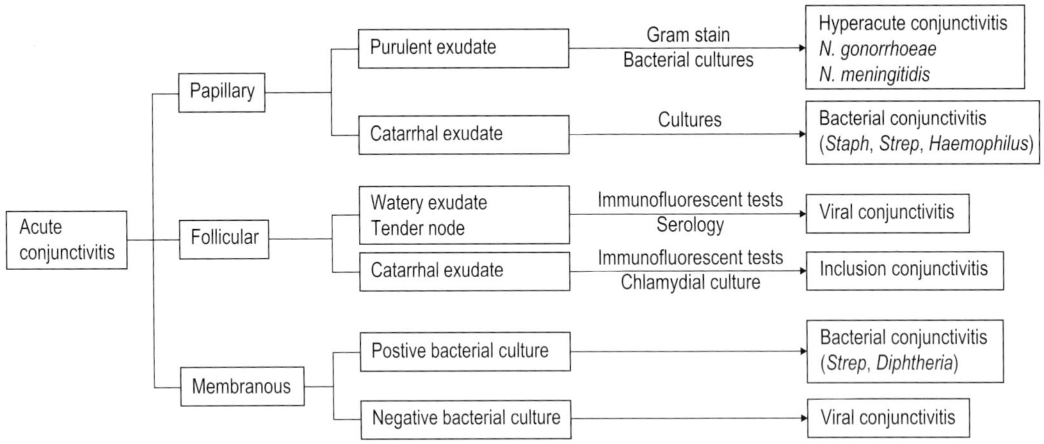

Fig. 42.1 An algorithm for diagnosing acute conjunctivitis. (Adapted from Buttross M, Stern GA: Acute conjunctivitis. In: Margo C, Hamed LM, Mames RN, editors: *Diagnostic problems in clinical ophthalmology.* Philadelphia: WB Saunders; 1994. Copyright Elsevier 1994.)

Morphologic responses

Papillae

Papillae are found only where the conjunctiva is attached to the underlying tissue by anchoring septae. The anchoring septae normally divide the conjunctiva into a mosaic pattern of polygonal papillae, each less than 1 mm in diameter.[6] Papillae are characterized by folds or projections of hypertrophic epithelium that contain a central fibrovascular core whose blood vessels arborize on reaching the surface (Fig. 42.3). A papillary response is a nonspecific sign of conjunctival inflammation resulting from edema and PMN cell infiltration of the conjunctiva. Papillae in the tarsal conjunctiva tend to be flat-topped, whereas those at the limbus tend to be dome-shaped. When the upper tarsal conjunctiva is everted, the superior edge may contain large papillae, which may be a normal finding resulting from the paucity of anchoring septae in this area.

Giant papillae may develop from breakdown of the fine, fibrous strands that make up the anchoring septae. Giant papillae are greater than 1 mm in diameter and are most commonly found in the upper tarsal conjunctiva. They can be seen in vernal conjunctivitis, atopic keratoconjunctivitis, and as a foreign body reaction to suture material, contact lenses, or prostheses.

Follicles

Follicles are yellowish-white, discrete, round elevations of conjunctiva produced by a lymphocytic response. Unlike a papilla, the central portion of the follicle is avascular, with blood vessels sweeping up over the convexity from the base (Fig. 42.4). Follicles are most readily appreciated in the upper tarsal conjunctiva and the lower cul-de-sac; however, they also can be seen at the limbus. Follicles are typically 0.5–2.0 mm in diameter, although follicles larger than 2 mm in diameter are seen, particularly in chlamydial disease.[1] Follicles are lymphoid germinal centers with fibroblasts in the center, and may be seen in the normal conjunctiva, especially temporally in young patients. Folliculosis of childhood is not a disease entity but a physiologic change of childhood and adolescence in which follicles tend to be prominent in the fornix and fade out toward the lid margin. A follicular response is extremely important to identify because it is a relatively specific inflammatory response with a well-defined differential diagnosis (Box 42.1).

Box 42.1 Follicular conjunctivitis

I. Acute follicular conjunctivitis
   - A. Adenovirus
     1. Epidemic keratoconjunctivitis
     2. Pharyngeal conjunctival fever
     3. Acute, nonspecific follicular conjunctivitis
   - B. Inclusion conjunctivitis
   - C. Herpesviruses
     1. Herpes simplex (primary)
     2. Epstein-Barr virus
   - D. Paramyxoviruses (measles, mumps, Newcastle disease)
   - E. Poxviruses (smallpox, vaccinia and monkeypox)
   - F. Picornaviruses (acute hemorrhagic conjunctivitis)
   - G. Orthomyxoviruses (influenza)
   - H. Togaviruses (rubella, yellow fever, dengue, and sandfly fever)

II. Chronic follicular conjunctivitis
   - A. Chlamydial infections
     1. Trachoma
     2. Inclusion conjunctivitis
   - B. Molluscum contagiosum
   - C. *Moraxella*
   - D. Parinaud's oculoglandular syndrome
   - E. Lyme disease
   - F. Toxic conjunctivitities
   - G. Folliculosis

Membranes

Membranes are composed primarily of fibrin that has attached to the epithelial conjunctival surface. True membranes leave a raw surface and cause bleeding when peeled

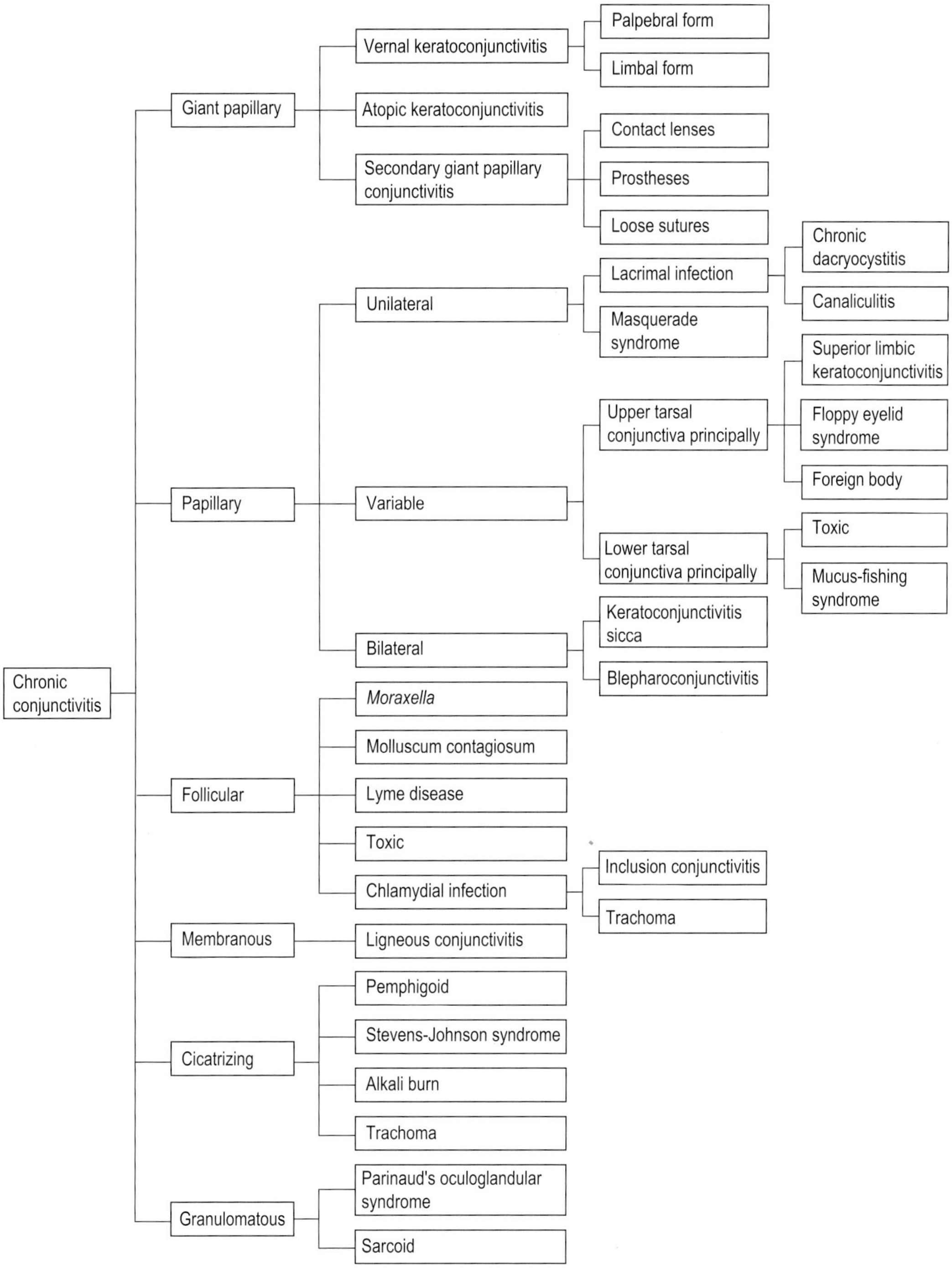

Fig. 42.2 An algorithm for diagnosing chronic conjunctivitis. (Adapted from Buttross M, Stern GA: Acute conjunctivitis. In: Margo C, Hamed LM, Mames RN, editors: *Diagnostic problems in clinical ophthalmology.* Philadelphia: WB Saunders; 1994. Copyright Elsevier, 1994.)

off, which differentiates them from pseudomembranes. The distinction between the two, however, really reflects the degree of the inflammatory response, as true membranes signify more intense conjunctival inflammation. Historically, *Corynebacterium diphtheriae* and β-hemolytic streptococci were the principal causes of membranous/pseudomembranous conjunctivitis;[6] however, adenoviral conjunctivitis is now the most common cause in Western countries (Fig. 42.5), followed by primary herpes simplex virus conjunctivitis.[1,4] Other causes include vernal conjunctivitis, inclusion conjunctivitis, and *Candida*. Stevens-Johnson syndrome (SJS) and toxic epidermal necrolysis (TEN) affect mucous membranes and skin. Bilateral pseudomembranous conjunctivitis is common in these conditions and may lead to severe conjunctival scarring, loss of goblet cells, entropion, trichiasis, and limbal stem cell failure.[7]

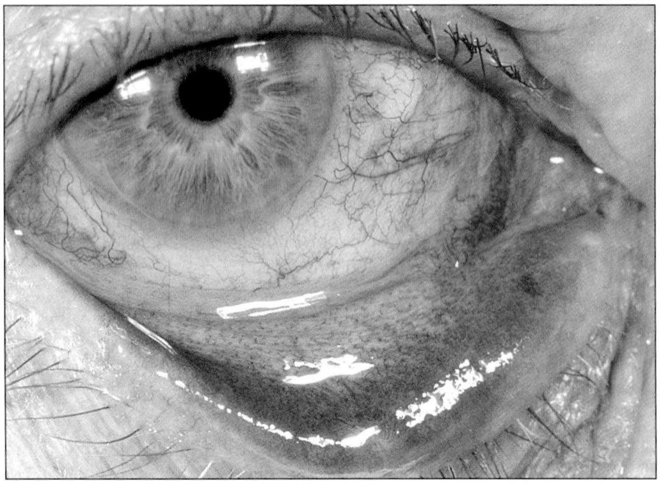

Fig. 42.3 Fine papillary conjunctivitis. Note the fibrovascular core in which the blood vessels arborize on reaching the surface.

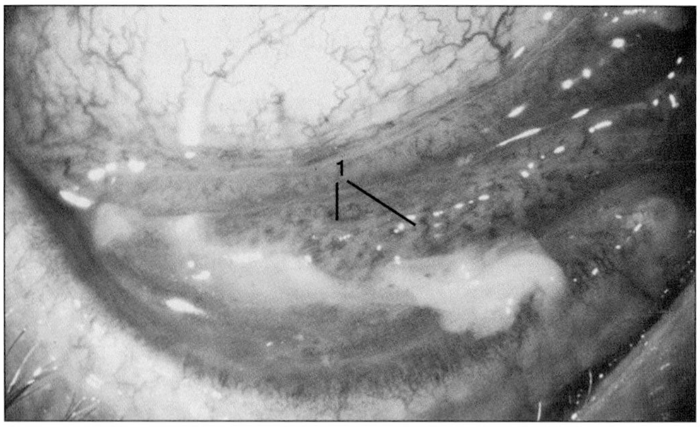

Fig. 42.5 Membranous conjunctivitis secondary to epidemic keratoconjunctivitis. The pseudomembrane is composed of fibrin and polymorphonuclear leukocytes obscuring much detail of the palpebral conjunctiva. Petechial hemorrhages (*1*) can be seen.

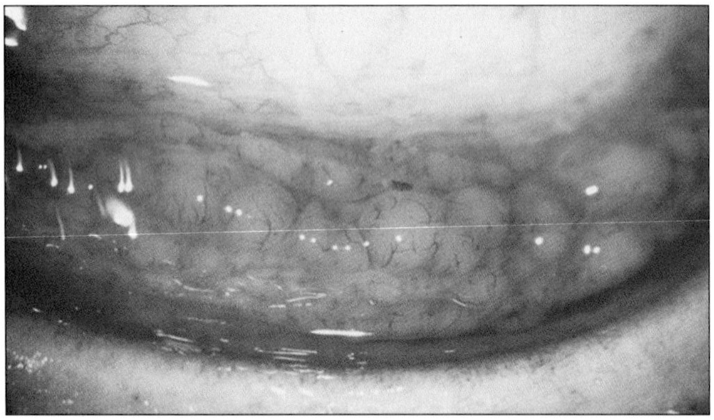

Fig. 42.4 Follicular conjunctivitis involving the lower palpebral conjunctiva secondary to culture-proven chlamydial disease. Note the large follicles with blood vessels sweeping up from the base over the convexity.

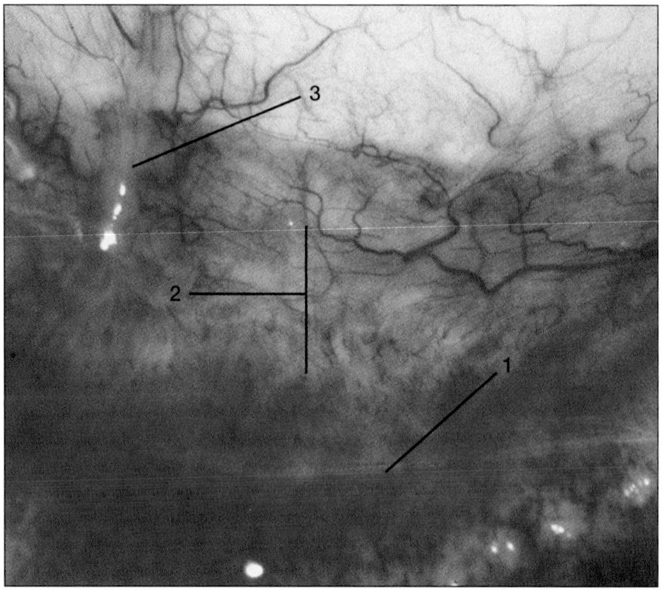

Fig. 42.6 Cicatrizing conjunctivitis secondary to cicatrical ocular pemphigoid. Note the fine, lacy subepithelial fibrosis (*1*), foreshortening of the inferior fornix (*2*), and symblepharon formation (*3*).

Cicatrizing changes

Injury to the conjunctival epithelium does not provoke scar formation. Scar formation ensues only when there is destruction of stromal tissue. The early stages of cicatrization consist of foreshortening of the conjunctival fornix and stellate or linear, lacey, subepithelial fibrosis. Subconjunctival cicatrization and scarring may have long-standing complications, including cicatricial entropion and trichiasis. If the process continues, foreshortening of the conjunctival fornix worsens and symblepharon develops (Fig. 42.6). End stages of chronic cicatrizing disease as seen in cicatricial ocular pemphigoid include obliteration of the conjunctival fornix, keratinization of the epithelium, and fusion of the eyelids known as ankyloblepharon.[8]

Membranous conjunctivitis is generally an acute condition, but may result in subepithelial fibrosis and limited symblepharon formation. Scarring after membranous conjunctivitis shows no predilection for any portion of the conjunctiva.

Scarring from atopic keratoconjunctivitis tends to be focal and located in the centers of giant papillae. Diffuse shrinkage of the lower fornix may be seen, but entropion and trichiasis tend not to occur.

Scarring from trachoma is quite specific. The pathognomonic sign is the cicatricial remains of a limbal follicle known as Herbert's peripheral pit. A line of cicatricial subepithelial fibrosis may be seen near the superior border of the upper tarsus known as Arlt's line.[9,10] Arlt's line may be seen in other diseases, but is an important finding in trachoma. The disease process in trachoma always involves the upper lid more severely than the lower lid. Dermatitis herpetiformis, epidermolysis bullosa, SJS and TEN, and exfoliative dermatitis also may result in conjunctival scarring.

Granulomas

Conjunctival granulomas always affect the stroma. A conjunctival granuloma may be seen in sarcoidosis or from a

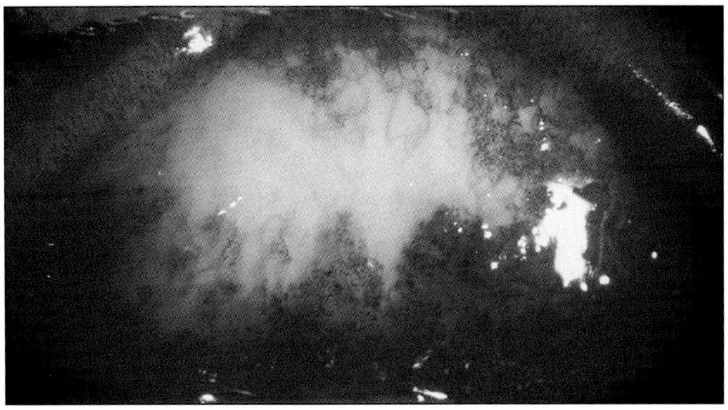

Fig. 42.7 Granulomatous conjunctivitis secondary to Parinaud's oculoglandular syndrome. Conjunctival granulomas always affect the conjunctival stroma.

retained foreign body. Parinaud's oculoglandular syndrome is a unilateral granulomatous conjunctivitis (Fig. 42.7) with a localized follicular response, often associated with a visibly swollen preauricular or submandibular lymph node. Fever and other systemic signs may be present. A variety of infectious agents may cause this syndrome, including cat-scratch disease, tularemia, sporotrichosis, tuberculosis, syphilis, lymphogranuloma venereum, and rickettsiosis.[11] A biopsy may be required to establish the diagnosis.

Type of exudate

Conjunctival exudates may be classified as: (1) purulent or hyperacute; (2) mucopurulent or catarrhal; and (3) watery.[1,4,6] Hyperacute conjunctivitis has a rapidly progressive course, with grossly purulent discharge. When the discharge is irrigated from the eye, it tends to re-form in minutes. A mucopurulent or catarrhal discharge consists of a mixture of mucus and pus and is most commonly seen in bacterial or chlamydial conjunctivitis. A mucopurulent discharge adheres firmly to the lashes, causing the eyelids to stick together. A copious, watery discharge is more typical of viral conjunctivitis.

Anatomic localization

The most severely affected area of the conjunctiva can be helpful in determining a differential diagnosis. Trachoma affects the upper tarsus more severely than the lower tarsus. Follicles also may be seen at the upper limbus in trachoma. Other disorders involving the upper palpebral conjunctiva predominantly include superior limbic keratoconjunctivitis and the floppy eyelid syndrome.

Vernal keratoconjunctivitis (VKC) is a chronic, allergic conjunctival inflammation with seasonal exacerbations, particularly in the spring and early summer. Giant papillae may be seen on the upper pretarsal conjunctiva. In black patients, the papillae have predilection for the limbus. In atopic keratoconjunctivitis (AKC), giant papillary hypertrophy predominates in the upper lid, but also can be seen in the lower lid. In contrast to symptoms of VKC, symptoms of AKC may be present throughout the year. The chronicity of AKC may lead to corneal vascularization and scarring and, in some cases, conjunctival cicatrization.

Giant papillae also may be seen secondarily on the upper tarsus in contact lens wearers, patients wearing prostheses, or from exposed suture material. Secondary giant papillae may be difficult to differentiate from follicles, as they tend to have rounder apices, are more spherical, and have pale centers. In follicular conjunctivitis, however, both the upper and lower palpebral conjunctivae are affected, whereas in secondary giant papillary conjunctivitis, only the upper palpebral conjunctiva is typically affected.

Conditions principally affecting the lower tarsal conjunctiva include toxic papillary conjunctivitis and the 'mucus-fishing syndrome.' The follicular response in inclusion conjunctivitis is more pronounced inferiorly than superiorly.

Acute Conjunctivitis

Acute papillary conjunctivitis

The morphologic response and type of exudate are the most important considerations in acute conjunctivitis. Acute papillary conjunctivitis is nearly always bacterial. Hyperacute conjunctivitis is most likely caused by *Neisseria gonorrhoeae* or *N. meningitidis* and is characterized by a rapidly progressive course with grossly purulent discharge. Corneal ulceration with resultant scarring is the major cause of visual loss and can lead to corneal perforation. With the exception of neonatal conjunctivitis, gonococcal conjunctivitis is nearly always associated with genital infection where transmission occurs by autoinoculation from the patient's dominant hand.[6] Gonococcal conjunctivitis is more common than meningococcal conjunctivitis, but the two are clinically indistinguishable. Systemic dissemination, including septicemia, can occur with either organism. Gram stain of conjunctival scrapings should be carefully examined for the presence of intracellular Gram negative diplococci. Specific identification of the organism can be established by culture and sugar fermentation tests. Antimicrobial susceptibility studies are essential because of the emergence of resistant strains of *Neisseria* to penicillin.

Treatment of hyperacute conjunctivitis includes frequent saline lavage of the corneas, topical antibiotic, and parenteral antibiotics. Public health screening of sexual contacts is mandatory when *N. gonorrhoeae* is identified. If *N. meningitidis* is isolated, close contacts must be treated with prophylactic antibiotics.

Acute papillary conjunctivitis with a catarrhal or mucopurulent exudate characterizes the majority of cases of bacterial conjunctivitis. One or both eyes may be involved, and the onset is acute. Signs include papillary hypertrophy, conjunctival injection, a mucopurulent discharge, and crusting of the eyelashes. The cornea may be involved by a secondary punctate epitheliopathy that may affect vision. *Staphylococcus aureus*, *Haemophilus influenzae*, and streptococci are the most frequently isolated organisms.[2,12,13] Cytologic examination using Giemsa or Wright's stain reveals a preponderance of PMNs in bacterial conjunctival infections. A specific diagnosis can be established only by performing conjunctival cultures. Broad-spectrum topical antibiotic therapy, in general, results in rapid resolution.

Acute follicular conjunctivitis

Acute follicular conjunctivitis has a well-defined differential diagnosis that includes viral infections and the early phase of chlamydial inclusion conjunctivitis. Papillae may be seen in addition to follicles, since papillae simply represent a nonspecific response of conjunctival tissue to any acute or chronic inflammatory condition.

Adenovirus

Adenovirus is responsible for the majority of cases of acute viral conjunctivitis. Adenoviral infection may present as epidemic keratoconjunctivitis (EKC), pharyngeal conjunctival fever (PCF), or nonspecific follicular conjunctivitis. Epidemic keratoconjunctivitis is a highly contagious infection principally caused by adenovirus serotypes 8 and 19.[14] Transmission commonly occurs by direct contact. Clinical symptoms are seen approximately 8 days after exposure. Symptoms of EKC include a sudden onset of an acute, watery discharge associated with foreign body sensation, and mild photophobia. The infection generally involves first one eye and the second eye a few days later, which typically has a milder course. Preauricular node enlargement and tenderness is common and is more prominent on the side initially involved. The distinguishing feature of EKC is the pattern of corneal involvement.

A few days after the onset of conjunctivitis, diffuse punctate epithelial erosions develop on the cornea. These coalesce into larger, coarse, epithelial infiltrates 7 to 10 days after onset. Approximately 2 weeks after onset, the coarse, epithelial infiltrates are replaced by focal subepithelial infiltrates, which are randomly distributed throughout the central cornea. The subepithelial infiltrates grow in intensity during the third to fourth week of infection and may number from 1 to 50 or more. The subepithelial infiltrates indicate a delayed hypersensitivity response and may significantly decrease vision for months. Because subepithelial infiltrates and EKC are immunologic phenomena, treatment with topical corticosteroids is indicated.

Transmission of EKC may occur in eye clinics where the virus may be spread by unwashed hands or improperly cleaned instruments. Adenovirus serotype 8 is resistant to 70% isopropyl alcohol.[15] Adequate sterilization can be achieved with 500 to 5000 parts per million (PPM) sodium hypochlorite. Alternatively, disposable tonometer tips may be used with any patient who has follicular conjunctivitis. The Centers for Disease Control recommends that infected healthcare personnel avoid direct patient contact up to 14 days after onset of epidemic keratoconjunctivitis.[16]

Pharyngoconjunctival fever is an acute illness characterized by follicular conjunctivitis, pharyngitis, and fever. This syndrome is most commonly caused by adenovirus types 3 and 7. Submandibular lymph node enlargement is frequently present. Membrane formation is unusual, and corneal involvement is distinctly absent. Nonspecific follicular conjunctivitis may be seen in children or adults and is typically a mild disease without an associated keratitis. It may be caused by many serotypes of adenovirus.

Inclusion conjunctivitis

Inclusion conjunctivitis caused by *Chlamydia trachomatis* is an oculogenital disease that most commonly occurs in sexually active young adults.[10,17,18] Unlike trachoma, inclusion conjunctivitis is rarely transmitted through eye-to-eye contact. The incubation period ranges from 2 to 19 days, but an acute follicular conjunctivitis begins approximately 5 days after exposure.[7,17] Onset tends to be more insidious than with viral infections. Inclusion conjunctivitis is generally a unilateral condition. Fully developed follicles do not present until the second or third week of disease and become considerably larger and more opalescent than follicles seen in viral disease. Without treatment, the conjunctivitis may persist for months. Yellowish-white subepithelial infiltrates may be seen in the corneal periphery and can be confused with the subepithelial infiltrates of adenovirus. Micropannus may develop at the superior limbus of the cornea, and a superficial punctate epithelial keratitis may be noted.

Conjunctival scrapings reveal a preponderance of PMNs with lymphocytes and plasma cells. Basophilic intracytoplasmic inclusions may be seen in epithelial cells, although this finding is more common in neonatal chlamydial conjunctivitis than in adult inclusion conjunctivitis. Because inclusion conjunctivitis is a manifestation of a systemic disease, therapy should be systemic. Doxycycline, 100 mg twice a day for 7 to 14 days, is recommended; however, a single oral dose of 1 g azithromycin has provided adequate treatment for genital chlamydial disease.[19] In chronic cases, therapy for several weeks to months may be required.

Ocular herpes infections

Primary herpes simplex keratoconjunctivitis and Epstein-Barr virus (EBV) may cause an acute follicular conjunctivitis. Primary herpes simplex infection is frequently associated with a vesicular lesion on the lid margin, which helps establish the diagnosis. The disease typically occurs in children and may include fever, upper respiratory symptoms, and a vesicular stomatitis or dermatitis. The conjunctivitis characteristically has a watery discharge with preauricular lymphadenopathy. Small ecchymoses may be seen on the conjunctiva. Within 2 weeks of onset, 50% of patients with primary herpes simplex virus (HSV) involving the lid margin will develop corneal epithelial manifestations,[18,20] which may range from fine, punctate epithelial staining to dendritic ulceration. Unlike the prominent dendritic figures seen in recurrent disease, fine microdendrites are more common and may involve both the cornea and conjunctiva.

In patients with vesicles on the eyelid or dendritic corneal lesions, the clinical diagnosis is rarely in question. In the absence of these findings, however, conjunctival scrapings can be obtained for fluorescent antibody testing or enzyme-linked immunosorbent assay (ELISA), as well as for cultures. A rising antibody titer also may provide confirmatory evidence of primary herpes simplex infection.

Children with primary herpes ocular infections may have such profuse tearing that topical trifluorothymidine may be washed out rapidly. In such cases, the use of vidarabine ointment five times a day to the conjunctival sac and eyelids may provide better delivery of antiviral therapy. Neonates who develop herpes simplex primary conjunctivitis also should receive intravenous treatment with vidarabine or acyclovir.

EBV may cause a follicular or membranous conjunctivitis with or without subconjunctival hemorrhage. The clinical manifestations of primary EBV may range from silent seroconversion to the classic syndrome of infectious mononucleosis characterized by fever, sore throat, and lymphadenopathy. Serologic testing in patients with symptoms of acute EBV infection manifest elevated IgM and IgG antibody levels against viral capsid antigen, and IgG response to Epstein-Barr early antigen. Antibodies against Epstein-Barr nuclear antigen do not develop until several weeks or months after the onset of clinical disease. Discrete, granular subepithelial infiltrates may be seen with overlying punctate epithelial keratitis. The corneal disease from EBV may closely mimic that seen in adenoviral keratitis.[21]

RNA-containing viruses

The Paramyxoviridae include measles, mumps, and Newcastle disease, all of which are capable of eliciting a follicular conjunctivitis.[22] Measles infection of the eye may result in a mucopurulent conjunctivitis, mild epithelial keratitis, and occasionally the development of whitish Koplik's spots on the conjunctiva or semilunar fold. Newcastle disease is unique because it is a unilateral follicular conjunctivitis with preauricular adenopathy. It is limited almost exclusively to contact with poultry but is self-limited and does not require therapy.

The Picornaviridae cause an acute hemorrhagic conjunctivitis associated with a follicular conjunctivitis, which initially affects one eye and rapidly spreads to the other. All patients develop a hemorrhagic bulbar conjunctival reaction that is more pronounced temporally and takes 1 to 2 weeks to resolve. The causative agents include enterovirus type 70 or coxsackievirus type A24. Preauricular adenopathy may be seen in 60% of affected individuals.[22]

The Orthomyxoviridae include the influenza virus, which may cause severe bronchopneumonia, particularly in elderly people. A follicular conjunctivitis with a mucopurulent discharge may be noted.[22]

The Togaviridae include the causative agent of rubella and the group B arboviruses responsible for yellow fever, dengue, and sandfly fever. These viruses cause hyperemia of the conjunctiva, lid swelling, photophobia, and lacrimation in association with the development of conjunctival follicles.[22]

Poxviruses

The Poxviridae include variola (smallpox), vaccinia (cowpox), monkeypox, and molluscum contagiosum. The poxviruses are dermatotrophic DNA viruses that cause lesions of the eyelids, conjunctiva, and rarely the cornea.[22] Ocular complications have been reported in 5–9% of patients with smallpox.[23] Variola has been eradicated because of the efforts of the World Health Organization; however, concerns have been raised about the use of smallpox as a biological weapon.

Vaccinia virus, used for mass smallpox inoculation, may be associated with eyelid and conjunctival infection, corneal ulceration, disciform keratitis, iritis, optic neuritis, and blindness.[23–25] About 10 to 20 patients per million smallpox immunizations develop ocular complications, usually through accidental autoinoculation with fingers or fomites from the vaccination site to the eye.[24,25]

Monkeypox, like variola and vaccinia, is an orthopox virus and was first isolated from a colony of sick monkeys. It was identified to cause disease in humans in 1970 in central Africa, but an outbreak occurred in the United States in the summer of 2003, during which one patient developed severe ocular involvement.[26,27] The virus is acquired through contact with an animal's blood or through a bite. Secondary attack rates from person-to-person are less than 10%, whereas for smallpox they are 70% with a mortality as high as 50%.[24,25] Monkeypox appears as a pustular rash affecting the head, trunk, and extremities. The rash of monkeypox is exactly like that of smallpox, although monkeypox is associated with more lymphadenopathy than is smallpox.[26] Unlike varicella, where vesicular lesions are characteristically in different stages of development and healing, monkeypox lesions are all essentially at the same stage.

Molluscum contagiosum may cause a chronic follicular conjunctival reaction (see Chronic Conjunctivitis).

Acute membranous conjunctivitis

Acute membranous or pseudomembranous conjunctivitis develops as fibrin coagulates on the epithelial surface, which may obscure the underlying morphologic response of the conjunctiva, making further classification difficult. Acute membranous conjunctivitis may be caused by both viral and bacterial organisms. Adenoviral conjunctivitis caused by EKC is now the most common cause, followed by HSV conjunctivitis.[22] β-hemolytic streptococci and *S. aureus* are the most common bacterial causes for membranous conjunctivitis. *C. diphtheriae* was previously the most common bacterial cause,[6] but is now rarely seen. Nevertheless, because of the potential for bacteria to cause membranous conjunctivitis, cultures need to be obtained when there is any question about the etiology of the infection. Noninfectious causes of membranous conjunctivitis, such as chemical injury, Stevens-Johnson syndrome, or vernal conjunctivitis, are readily distinguished, based on the history or associated systemic findings.

Chronic Conjunctivitis

In chronic conjunctivitis, the conjunctival morphology and anatomic localization are the most important variables.[5] Unlike most causes of acute conjunctivitis, the diseases causing chronic conjunctivitis are not usually self-limited. In contrast to the majority of cases of acute conjunctivitis, which are infectious in nature, the causes of chronic conjunctivitis include immunologic, traumatic, toxic, neoplastic, as well as infectious factors.

Clinical evaluation of a patient with chronic conjunctivitis begins with a detailed history. The onset of chronic conjunctivitis is usually insidious, and the progression of the disease may be slow. Symptoms generally include ocular discomfort, conjunctival injection, and perhaps a discharge. Symptoms of severe pain or photophobia generally suggest some corneal involvement. Many patients have used a variety of medications to treat the disorder; therefore, a careful medication history is essential. A history of animal exposure, trauma, surgery, and foreign travel are all important considerations.

The clinician should ask the patient to describe ocular discomfort in some detail. Itching is the most prominent feature of allergic disease. Irritation that is worse in the morning may suggest blepharoconjunctivitis, whereas a gritty sensation that worsens later in the day may suggest keratoconjunctivitis sicca.

A thorough eye examination is important, but particular attention should be paid to the skin and eyelids. The skin should be examined for signs of atopic dermatitis, seborrheic dermatitis, or rosacea. Preauricular and submandibular nodes should be palpated for the presence of lymphadenopathy. The eyelids should be inspected for the loss of eyelashes; the presence of tumors, papillomas, and molluscum contagiosum lesions; and for signs of blepharitis. The lacrimal drainage system should be evaluated for obstructive disease or for signs of infection. The conjunctiva is examined carefully for the presence of follicles or foreign bodies, and the upper lid should be everted to examine the pretarsal conjunctiva. The corneal examination should include the use of both fluorescein and rose bengal dyes, as well as careful evaluation of any keratitis, vascularization, peripheral scarring, or stromal inflammation. Morphologic responses critical to establishing a correct diagnosis include papillary, giant papillary, follicular, membranous, cicatrizing, and granulomatous responses.

Laboratory investigation may be invaluable in some cases of chronic conjunctivitis. Conjunctival scrapings can help identify inflammatory and infectious microorganisms. The presence of eosinophils is a reliable indicator of an allergic disorder such as atopic or vernal keratoconjunctivitis. In chronic chlamydial infection, conjunctival scrapings stained with Giemsa may reveal basophilic intracytoplasmic inclusion bodies within epithelial cells. Immunofluorescent studies may be confirmatory for chlamydial or herpes simplex disease. Gram stain or culture of a scraping may identify *Moraxella*, which is an unusual bacterial cause of chronic follicular conjunctivitis. Cultures also can be crucial in establishing a diagnosis of dacryocystitis or canaliculitis.

A conjunctival biopsy may reveal a neoplastic etiology, identify a noncaseating or foreign body granuloma, or uncover microorganisms. Immunofluorescence microscopy of a conjunctival biopsy may confirm suspicion of mucous membrane pemphigoid (ocular cicatricial pemphigoid) in which immunoglobulin or complement may be seen bound to the conjunctival basement membrane.

Giant papillary conjunctivitis

Giant papillae are >1 mm in diameter by definition. Vernal and atopic keratoconjunctivitis compose the two primary forms of giant papillary conjunctivitis (GPC). Secondary forms of GPC are related to contact lenses, ocular prostheses, or exposed sutures. In allergic disorders, such as vernal keratoconjunctivitis, giant papillae may measure several millimeters in diameter and assume a flat top and polygonal shape, giving rise to the description of 'cobblestone' papillae. Secondary forms of giant papillae assume a rounder shape with pale centers. Although these secondary giant papillae may be confused with follicles, the lower fornix is never involved in secondary GPC.

Vernal keratoconjunctivitis

Vernal keratoconjunctivitis (VKC) is a seasonally recurrent, bilateral conjunctival inflammation of youth; boys are affected twice as often as girls. The most prominent symptom is itching, which can become worse toward evening and is exacerbated by rubbing. Tearing is characteristic and macerates the skin about the corner of the eye. A characteristic thick, mucoid, ropy discharge is noted.[28]

Clinically, VKC may be divided into a palpebral and limbal form. These two forms may occur together, although the limbal form is more common in blacks. Palpebral VKC is characterized by the formation of giant papillae on the upper pretarsal conjunctiva. The conjunctiva of the lower eyelid shows a diffuse, fine papillary reaction. In limbal VKC, both the upper and lower papillary conjunctiva reveal a fine, diffuse papillary reaction. The limbal form is marked by thickened, broad, gelatinous opacification of the upper limbus. Within the thickened areas are whitish chalklike excrescences called Trantas' dots, which are concretions of eosinophils that may be evanescent. Corneal involvement may range from a punctate epithelial keratitis to a 'vernal ulcer,' which is a sterile shield-shaped epithelial defect at the junction of the upper and middle third of the cornea.

The diagnosis of VKC may be made by examination of conjunctival scrapings of the upper tarsus. Greater than two eosinophils per high-power field is diagnostic of VKC.

Atopic keratoconjunctivitis

Unlike VKC, atopic keratoconjunctivitis (AKC) shows no seasonal variation. Onset is generally during the late teens; in most cases AKC improves or 'burns out' by the fourth or fifth decade.

The lid margins may be indurated and lichenified. Giant papillary hypertrophy is noted in the upper and lower lids. Corneal scarring and foreshortening of the conjunctival fornix may occur secondary to the chronicity of the disorder. Conjunctival scrapings reveal mast cells, basophils, eosinophils, and possible lymphocytes.[28]

Secondary giant papillary conjunctivitis

Secondary giant papillary conjunctivitis occurs most commonly in soft contact lens wearers.[28] Patients complain of a foreign body sensation and ocular discomfort. Mucinous and proteinaceous deposits are frequently present on the contact lenses. Similar complaints and findings may be noted in patients with ocular prostheses or loose or broken sutures.

Chronic papillary conjunctivitis

Chronic papillary conjunctivitis has several different etiologies. Anatomic localization and the differentiation of unilateral or bilateral involvement can be helpful in establishing a correct diagnosis.[5]

Masquerade syndrome

A chronic, unilateral papillary conjunctivitis should arouse the suspicion of a masquerade syndrome caused by an underlying ocular surface malignancy. Chronic conjunctival inflammation may be associated with intraepithelial neoplasia, pigmented or amelanotic melanoma, and sebaceous cell carcinoma.

Intraepithelial neoplasia

Squamous dysplasia or intraepithelial neoplasia of the conjunctiva nearly always arises at the limbus and, more commonly, in the intrapalpebral area. The lesions appear as raised, somewhat gelatinous masses, which may be gray or slightly red.[29] The extent of the lesion is best visualized by application of rose bengal dye. Treatment involves conjunctival excision and scraping of the epithelial extension onto the cornea. The limbus, base, and conjunctival margin are frozen with a retinal cryoprobe in a rapid, double freeze–thaw manner.[30]

Malignant melanoma

Malignant melanoma can arise in clear conjunctiva in 10% of cases, from a pre-existing nevus in 20–30% of cases, or from primary acquired melanosis in 60–70% of cases.[31] It is particularly rare before the third decade of life. Clinically, lesions can be pigmented or nonpigmented, are elevated, and can affect any portion of the conjunctiva.[32] Treatment is by wide local excision followed by freeze–thaw–freeze cryotherapy.[33] Topical interferon-alfa has been shown to cause regression of conjunctival and corneal melanoma.[34] Topical mitomycin-C may be used as an adjuvant therapy for conjunctival melanoma.[35]

Sebaceous cell carcinoma

Sebaceous cell carcinoma arises from meibomian glands most commonly, although it can also develop in Zeis' glands or from sebaceous glands in the caruncle. Patients with an unexplained unilateral conjunctivitis should undergo biopsy that includes the tarsus and conjunctiva or skin. Sebaceous cell carcinoma often spreads in a pagetoid fashion within the epithelium, requiring multiple conjunctival biopsies. Clues to the correct diagnosis include eyelid thickening and deformity, focal loss of eyelashes, unilateral involvement, and an abnormal papillary conjunctival inflammation. A full-thickness wedge biopsy should be performed to definitively diagnose this disorder. Sebaceous cell carcinoma is a life-threatening disorder, and early diagnosis may be lifesaving.[33]

Lacrimal drainage system infection

Chronic dacryocystitis

Chronic dacryocystitis or chronic canaliculitis may lead to a chronic papillary conjunctivitis secondary to infectious organisms. Chronic dacryocystitis occurs in the presence of lacrimal outflow obstruction distal to the lacrimal sac.[34] This obstruction causes stasis of tears within the lacrimal sac, which leads to secondary bacterial colonization and infection. An acute lacrimal sac abscess may develop; however, if the common canaliculus remains patent, a chronic conjunctivitis may develop as purulent material drains in a retrograde fashion. Patients may initially complain of epiphora before the onset of chronic conjunctival irritation and a mucopurulent discharge. Examination typically reveals a unilateral, diffuse papillary conjunctivitis with a mucopurulent discharge. When pressure is applied over the lacrimal sac, reflux of purulent material can be observed through the punctum and is diagnostic of dacryocystitis. The skin overlying the lacrimal sac may be quite tender and swollen. Conjunctival cultures are necessary to identify the infectious etiology. Staphylococci and streptococci are the most common organisms isolated; however, a wide variety of bacterial and fungal organisms have been noted. Treatment involves oral and topical antibiotics. Once the infection is resolved, obstruction distal to the lacrimal sac needs to be further investigated and patency established to avoid recurrence.

Chronic canaliculitis

Chronic canaliculitis is frequently due to a diverticulum of the canaliculus in which organisms proliferate. Symptoms are similar to that of chronic dacryocystitis, except that epiphora is absent.[34] Examination reveals a papillary conjunctivitis with mucopurulent discharge. Frequently, there is a discharge from the punctal orifice. The punctum is often enlarged and pouts externally. Mechanical expression of infected material from the canaliculus is accomplished by applying pressure using cotton-tipped applicators to both the inner and outer surfaces of the medial aspect of the eyelid while rolling the applicators toward the punctum. Cheesy concretions may be expressed from the punctum. The expressed material should be cultured for aerobic and anaerobic bacteria and fungi. Gram stain of the exudate often reveals a filamentous, branching, Gram-positive bacterium, which may be identified as *Actinomyces israelii*, the most common cause of canaliculitis.[35]

The differential diagnosis of chronic papillary conjunctivitis involving both eyes includes keratoconjunctivitis sicca, blepharoconjunctivitis, and disorders that specifically have a predilection for the upper palpebral conjunctiva, including superior limbic keratoconjunctivitis, the floppy eyelid syndrome, and a retained foreign body.

Superior limbic keratoconjunctivitis

Superior limbic keratoconjunctivitis is a noninfectious inflammatory disease characterized by: (1) velvety papillary hypertrophy of the upper palpebral conjunctiva; (2) hyperemia and rose bengal staining of the upper bulbar conjunctiva; (3) micropannus and punctate rose bengal staining of the superior limbus; (4) thickening and keratinization of the superior limbal, bulbar, and palpebral conjunctiva; and (5) superior filamentary keratitis in about 50% of patients.[36,37] Scrapings of the superior bulbar conjunctiva reveal keratinized epithelial cells.

Floppy eyelid syndrome

The floppy eyelid syndrome is a distinct entity seen more commonly in obese people and in those who sleep on their stomachs. It is characterized by a rubbery, redundant upper tarsus, which everts with minimal pressure. A chronic papillary conjunctivitis is seen over the upper palpebral conjunctiva and may be associated with corneal changes ranging from mild punctate keratitis to superficial pannus.[38] During sleep, the upper eyelid is thought to evert, resulting in mechanical contact with the pillow or other bed clothes accounting for the chronic irritation. Treatment consists of a protective metal shield or taping the eyelids while asleep. Surgical treatment is directed toward eyelid-tightening procedures.

Blepharoconjunctivitis

Bilateral chronic papillary conjunctivitis is most frequently caused by blepharoconjunctivitis or keratoconjunctivitis sicca, which often coexist. Patients with blepharitis complain of chronic burning, irritation, and foreign body sensation associated with photophobia if the cornea is involved. Symptoms are frequently worse early in the morning. Blepharitis may be classified as (1) staphylococcal, (2) seborrheic, and (3) meibomian, although patients with blepharitis frequently exhibit signs from more than one category.[39]

Staphylococcal and seborrheic

Staphylococcal and seborrheic forms are frequently categorized as 'anterior blepharitis,' whereas meibomian gland dysfunction is characterized as 'posterior blepharitis.' Staphylococcal blepharitis is characterized by ulcerations surrounding the lash follicle, which become crusted. As the crusts are exfoliated, they surround the eyelash like a collar from which the term collarette is derived. Seborrheic blepharitis is probably the most common cause of chronic lid inflammation and is part of a generalized sebaceous gland abnormality in which hard, oily scales may be seen clinging to the eyelashes.

Meibomian gland dysfunction

Meibomian gland dysfunction is characterized by thickening of the eyelid margin, inspissated and thickened secretions of the glands, dilation of the ducts of the glands, a foamy secretion on the lid margins, and recurrent chalazia. Not uncommonly, meibomian gland dysfunction is associated with ocular rosacea.[40] Secondary colonization of meibomian glands by staphylococcal organisms may further destabilize the tear film. Treatment of blepharoconjunctivitis includes mechanical cleansing of the eyelids, application of warm compresses, systemic tetracyclines, oral supplementation of essential fatty acids, and use of erythromycin or bacitracin antibiotic.[41]

Keratoconjunctivitis sicca

The other principal cause of chronic, bilateral papillary conjunctivitis is keratoconjunctivitis sicca. This disorder occurs when the quantity or quality of the precorneal tear film is insufficient to ensure the well-being of the ocular epithelial surface.[41] Symptoms include ocular discomfort, foreign body sensation, and burning, all of which are worsened by wind, smoke, low humidity, and environmental pollutants. Symptoms tend to become worse as the day progresses. Clinical signs of keratoconjunctivitis sicca include a decreased tear lake, mucous debris in the tear film, and corneal and conjunctival staining with rose Bengal, most prominent in the interpalpebral fissure. Schirmer testing may be performed with or without topical anesthesia. Wetting <5 mm when performed without anesthesia is highly specific for the diagnosis of keratoconjunctivitis sicca.[42] Treatment is directed toward artificial tear substitutes, antiinflammatory agents including short-term topical steroids and topical ciclosporin, damming of the lacrimal outflow system, and in severe cases, reducing the rate of evaporation through tarsorrhaphy.

Mucus-fishing syndrome

A mechanically induced, chronic papillary conjunctivitis has been described in patients with various underlying, external ocular diseases, including keratoconjunctivitis sicca, blepharitis, and allergic conjunctivitis. These patients exacerbate their conjunctival irritation by the frequent mechanical removal of excess mucus from the surface of the globe or from the inferior fornix. The entity has been called the 'mucus-fishing' syndrome and exacerbates the findings in external ocular diseases in which the treatment might otherwise be appropriate.[43]

Toxic papillary keratoconjunctivitis

Toxic papillary keratoconjunctivitis is the most common of all adverse reactions to topical medications.[44] The toxic effects usually take at least 2 weeks to develop. Punctate staining, best identified with rose Bengal dye, is more pronounced on the inferonasal conjunctiva and cornea where medications gravitate on their way to the lacrimal outflow system. Hyperemia, nonspecific papillary conjunctivitis, and scant mucoid discharge are noted clinically. Itching is absent, and eosinophils are not seen in conjunctival scrapings. The principal causes of toxic papillary reactions are aminoglycoside antibiotics, antiviral agents, and the preservative benzalkonium chloride (Box 42.2). Benzalkonium is a particularly frequent offender, not only because of its

Box 42.2 Principal causes of toxic papillary reactions

- Aminoglycoside antibiotics
  - Neomycin
  - Gentamicin
  - Tobramycin
- Nearly all 'concentrated' or 'fortified' antibiotics and antifungal agents
- Antiviral agents
  - Idoxuridine
  - Vidarabine
  - Trifluorothymidine
- Topical anesthetic agents
  - Proparacaine
  - Tetracaine
- Preservatives
  - Benzalkonium chloride

frequent use as a preservative but also because it is a surfactant with detergent-like properties.[44]

Factors predisposing to toxic papillary reactions include keratoconjunctivitis sicca and other ocular surface disorders, the prolonged use of medications, and the use of multiple preparations. The mainstay of treatment is withdrawal of offending medications and preservatives, the use of preservative-free artificial tears, and substitution with nonpreserved medications that can be formulated by pharmacists.

Chronic follicular conjunctivitis

Chlamydial

Chlamydia trachomatis is the etiologic agent most frequently responsible for chronic follicular conjunctivitis.[5,10] Chlamydial disease may manifest as trachoma or inclusion conjunctivitis.

Trachoma

Trachoma is endemic in most developing countries of the world, and is the most common cause of blindness.[17,18] In endemic areas, children are affected within the first 2 years of life and frequent reinfection associated with bacterial superinfection prolongs the course of the disease.[9,10,17,18] Active inflammation decreases with age, but the cicatricial changes result in progressive lid deformity and corneal changes for many years. Trachoma is a bilateral, chronic, follicular conjunctivitis that causes conjunctival and corneal scarring.[9] During the infectious stage of the disease, large follicles are seen most prominently in the upper fornix and pretarsal conjunctiva. Limbal follicles also may be seen, and as they eventually necrose and heal, shallow depressions described as Herbert's peripheral pits are left. Limbal involvement also results in a superficial vascular pannus, which is most prominent superiorly.

Inclusion conjunctivitis

Inclusion conjunctivitis, which is often unilateral, is characterized by follicles that are more pronounced in the inferior conjunctival fornix. Fully developed follicles do not present until the second or third week of the disease and may persist for many months when untreated. The disease is generally regarded as benign and self-limited in adults but can persist for 6 months or longer.[5,7,10]

Moraxella

Moraxella organisms are large, Gram-negative diplobacilli that can cause either a chronic follicular conjunctivitis or an angular blepharoconjunctivitis. The latter is characterized by ulceration of the lateral lid margin associated with conjunctival injection. Proteases, produced by the *Moraxella* bacterium, are thought to be responsible for the conjunctival follicular responses.[1]

Molluscum contagiosum

Molluscum contagiosum is one of the DNA poxviruses that may cause a chronic, follicular conjunctivitis. It is more common in children and young adults, but can affect all age groups. The typical lesions of molluscum contagiosum are pink, umbilicated, seen on the eyelid margin of periocular skin, and measure 2–3 mm in diameter. These lesions secrete large quantities of virus, which spill onto the cornea or the lower conjunctival fornix. Clinically, a chronic follicular conjunctivitis is seen, which may involve both the upper and lower fornix and is associated with superficial punctate keratitis and corneal pannus.[45] These responses are most likely a toxic reaction to the viral particles. The disease is spread by close personal contact and may be transmitted sexually. Treatment involves simple excision, curetting, or cryotherapy of the lesions.

Box 42.3 Principal causes of drug-induced toxic follicular conjunctivitis

Antiviral agents	Dipivefrin epinephrine
Idoxuridine	Carbachol
Vidarabine	Apraclonidine
Trifluorothymidine	Brimonidine tartrate
Antiglaucoma agents	Cycloplegic agents
Pilocarpine	Atropine
Echothiophate	Homatropine
Epinephrine	

Toxic follicular conjunctivitis

Toxic follicular conjunctivitis may result from chronic exposure to topical medications, eye make-up, and various environmental pollutants. Follicles develop slowly, usually requiring at least several weeks to develop.[44] The mechanism by which toxic follicular conjunctivitis develops is not thought to be allergic, but most likely results from the ability of certain drugs to act as nonantigenic mitogens that induce mitotic and lymphoblastic transformations of lymphocytes by nonimmunologic means.[44] Nevertheless, true lymphoid follicles with germinal centers containing lymphoblasts are present. The follicles are most prominent in the lower fornix and inferior palpebral conjunctiva. Hyperemia and punctate staining are usually mild, if present. Principal causes of toxic follicular conjunctivitis are shown in Box 42.3.[45–47]

Lyme disease

Lyme disease is the most common tick-transmitted illness in the United States. Ocular manifestations include blepharitis, conjunctivitis, keratitis, iritis, choroiditis, macular and disc edema, and pseudotumor cerebri syndrome. The conjunctivitis has now been described as follicular in nature and is bilateral.[48,49] Lyme disease is caused by the spirochete *Borrelia burgdorferi*. The transient conjunctivitis is seen in early stages of this disease. However, bilateral follicular conjunctivitis, eyelid swelling, and regional lymphadenopathy may be the only manifestation of Lyme disease if the tick bite is located in the periorbital region.[49] Therefore, inclusion of Lyme disease as a cause of a chronic follicular conjunctivitis may help establish an early diagnosis.

Chronic membranous conjunctivitis

The only chronic membranous conjunctivitis is ligneous conjunctivitis.[5] This rare, chronic conjunctivitis of unknown origin occurs predominantly in young girls. Persistent whitish membranes 1–2 mm thick form on the upper and less frequently on the lower tarsal conjunctiva. Systemic illnesses including fever, urinary tract, or upper respiratory tract infections may precede the onset of ocular involvement. The disease begins as a subacute inflammation of the tarsal conjunctiva. An initial, subacute, membranous conjunctivitis is followed by the development of sessile or pedunculated masses of the tarsal conjunctiva.[50,51] Infrequently, the bulbar conjunctiva and cornea may be involved. These membranes or masses may recur rapidly when excised.

Cicatrizing and granulomatous conjunctivitis

Cicatrizing and granulomatous conjunctivities are additional types of chronic inflammation and have been discussed in detail earlier in this chapter under morphologic responses. Establishing the correct diagnosis of conjunctivitis requires a deliberate history and a careful ocular and adnexal examination. Particular attention to chronicity, conjunctival morphology, anatomic distribution, and unilateral versus bilateral involvement can help establish a working differential diagnosis. Specific laboratory findings may further identify the etiologic diagnosis.

References

1. Arffa RC, ed. Conjunctivitis. I. Follicular, neonatal, and bacterial. In: *Grayson's diseases of the cornea.* 3rd ed. St Louis: Mosby; 1991.
2. Allansmith MR, Ross RN. Ocular allergy and mast cell stabilizers. *Surv Ophthalmol.* 1986;30:229.
3. Abelson MB, Madiwale N, Weston JH. Conjunctival eosinophils in allergic ocular disease. *Arch Ophthalmol.* 1983;101:631.
4. Buttross M, Stern GA. Acute conjunctivitis. In: Margo C, Hamed LM, Mames RN, eds. *Diagnostic problems in clinical ophthalmology.* Philadelphia: WB Saunders; 1994.
5. Bozkir N, Stern GA. Chronic conjunctivitis. In: Margo C, Hamed LM, Mames RN, eds. *Diagnostic problems in clinical ophthalmology.* Philadelphia: WB Saunders; 1994.
6. Duke-Elder S, ed. Inflammations of the conjunctiva and associated inflammations of the cornea. In: *System of ophthalmology, vol. VIII, Diseases of the outer eye.* St Louis: Mosby; 1961.
7. Gregory DG. The ophthalmologic management of acute Stevens-Johnson syndrome. *Ocul Surf.* 2008;6:87–95.
8. Chan LS, et al. The first international consensus on mucous membrane pemphigoid: definition, diagnostic criteria, pathogenic factors, medical treatment and prognostic indicators. *Arch Dermatol.* 2002;138:370–379.
9. MacCallan A. The epidemiology of trachoma. *Br J Ophthalmol.* 1931;15:369.
10. Arffa RC, ed. Chlamydial infections. In: *Grayson's diseases of the cornea.* 3rd ed. St Louis: Mosby; 1991.
11. Chin GA. Parinaud's oculoglandular conjunctivitis. In: Tasman W, Jaegar EA, eds. *Duane's clinical ophthalmology.* Philadelphia: JB Lippincott; 1994.
12. Locatcher-Khorazo D, Seegal BC. *Microbiology of the eye.* St Louis: Mosby; 1972.
13. Perkins RE, et al. Bacteriology of normal and infected conjunctiva. *J Clin Microbiol.* 1975;1:147.
14. O'Day DM, et al. Clinical and laboratory evaluation of epidemic keratoconjunctivitis due to adenovirus types 8 and 19. *Am J Ophthalmol.* 1976;81:207.
15. Corboy JM, Goucher CR, Parnes CA. Mechanical sterilization of the applanation tonometer. Part 2: Viral study. *Am J Ophthalmol.* 1971;71:891.
16. Centers for Disease Control. Epidemic keratoconjunctivitis in an ophthalmology clinic – California. *MMWR.* 1990;39:598.
17. Schachter J. Chlamydia infections. *West J Med.* 1990;153:523.
18. Hammerschlag MR. Chlamydia infections. *J Pediatr.* 1989;114:727.
19. Schachter J, et al: Azithromycin in control of trachoma. *Lancet.* 1999;354:630–635.
20. Glasser DB, Hyndiuk RA. Herpes simplex keratitis. In: Tabbara KF, Hundiuk RA, eds. *Infections of the eye.* Boston: Little Brown; 1986.
21. Matoba AY, Jones DB. Corneal subepithelial infiltrates associated with systemic Epstein-Barr viral infection. *Ophthalmology.* 1987;94:1669.
22. Vastine DW. Viral diseases: adenovirus and miscellaneous viral infections. In: Smolin G, Thoft RA, eds. *The cornea.* Boston: Little Brown; 1987.
23. Semba RD. The ocular complications of smallpox and smallpox immunization. *Arch Ophthalmol.* 2003;121:719.
24. Lane JM, et al. Complications of smallpox vaccination, 1968: national surveillance in the United States. *N Engl J Med.* 1969;281:1201.
25. Pepose JS, et al. Ocular complications of smallpox vaccination. *Am J Ophthalmol.* 2003;136:343.
26. Centers for Disease Control. Multistate outbreak of monkeypox – Illinois, Indiana, and Wisconsin, 2003. *MMWR Morb Mortal Wkly Rep.* 2003;52:537.
27. Croasdale CR et al. Human monkeypox ocular infection; first western hemisphere case report, The Cornea Federated Societies Scientific Session, Anaheim, CA, Nov. 15, 2003.
28. Abelson MB, Allansmith MR. Ocular allergies. In: Smolin G, Thoft RA, eds. *The cornea.* Boston: Little Brown; 1987.
29. Waring GO, Roth AM, Skins MB. Clinical and pathologic description of 17 cases of corneal intraepithelial neoplasia. *Am J Ophthalmol.* 1984;97:547.
30. Fraunfelder FT, Wingfield D. Management of intraepithelial conjunctival tumors and squamous cell carcinomas. *Am J Ophthalmol.* 1983;95: 359.
31. McLean FR, McLean IW, Zimmerman LE. Malignant melanoma of the conjunctiva. *Hum Pathol.* 1985;16:136.
32. Shields JA, Shields CL, Mashayekhi A, et al. Primary acquired melanosis of the conjunctiva: risks for progression to melanoma in 311 eyes. The 2006 Lorenz E. Zimmerman lecture. *Ophthalmology.* 2008;115:511–519.
33. Shields CL. Conjunctival melanoma. *Br J Ophthalmol.* 2002;86:127.
34. Finger PT, Sedeek RW. Topical interferon alfa in the treatment of conjunctival melanoma and primary acquired melanosis complex. *Am J Ophthalmol.* 2008;145:124–129.
35. Schallenberg M, Niederdraing N, Steuhl KP, et al. Topical mitomycin C as a therapy of conjunctival tumours. *Ophthalmologe.* 2008;1056: 777–784.
36. Kivela T, Tarkkanen A. The Merkel cell and associated neoplasms in the eyelids and periocular region. *Surv Ophthalmol.* 1990;35:171–187.
37. Jones LT. The lacrimal secretory system and its treatment. *Am J Ophthalmol.* 1966;62:47.
38. Duke-Elder WS, MacFaul PA. Canaliculitis. Actinomycosis. In: Duke-Elder WS, ed. *System of ophthalmology.* vol. 13. St Louis: Mosby; 1974.
39. Bainbridge JW, Mackie IA, Mackie I. Diagnosis of Theodore's superior limbic keratoconjunctivitis. *Eye.* 1998;12:748–749.
40. Cher I. Superior limbic keratoconjunctivitis: multifactorial mechanical pathogenesis. *Clin Experiment Ophthalmol.* 2000;28:181–184.
41. Behrens A, Doyle JJ, Stern L, et al. Dysfunctional tear syndrome: a Delphi approach to treatment and recommendations. *Cornea.* 2006;25: 900–907.
42. Goren MB, Goren SB. Diagnostic tests in patients with symptoms of keratoconjunctivitis sicca. *Am J Ophthalmol.* 1988;106:570.
43. McCulley JP, Moore MB, Matoba AY. Mucus fishing syndrome. *Ophthalmology.* 1985;92:1262.
44. Wilson FM II. Toxic and allergic reactions to topical ophthalmic medications. In: Arffa RC, ed. *Grayson's diseases of the cornea.* 3rd ed. St Louis: Mosby; 1991.
45. Curtin BJ, Theodore FH. Ocular molluscum contagiosum. *Am J Ophthalmol.* 1955;39:302.
46. Theodore J, Leibowitz HM. External ocular toxicity of dipivalyl epinephrine. *Am J Ophthalmol.* 1979;88:1013.
47. Wilkerson M, Lewis RA, Shields MB. Follicular conjunctivitis associated with apraclonidine. *Am J Ophthalmol.* 1991;111:105.
48. Flach AJ, LaVoie PE. Episcleritis, conjunctivitis and keratitis as ocular manifestations of Lyme disease. *Ophthalmology.* 1990;97:973.
49. Mombaerts IM, Maudgal PC, Knockaert DC. Bilateral follicular conjunctivitis as a manifestation of Lyme disease. *Am J Ophthalmol.* 1991;112:96.
50. Ramsby ML, Donshik PC, Makowski GS. Ligneous conjunctivitis: biochemical evidence for hypofibrinolysis. *Inflammation.* 2000;24:45–71.
51. Chen S, Wishart M, Hiscott P. Ligneous conjunctivitis: a local manifestation of a systemic disorder? *J AAPOS.* 2000;4:313–315.

Chapter 43

Bacterial Conjunctivitis

Sarkis H. Soukiasian, Jules Baum

The incidence of bacterial conjunctivitis is difficult to determine because most patients with conjunctivitis are treated empirically without cultures by physicians other than ophthalmologists. The large majority of cases of acute bacterial conjunctivitis are of a limited duration, even without specific therapy. With effective topical treatment, both the morbidity and duration of disease are reduced. In the preantibiotic era, bacterial conjunctivitis generally ran its course in several weeks, even with a pathogen as virulent as *Neisseria gonorrhoeae*. Two exceptions to this rule are *Staphylococcus* and *Moraxella*. In each instance, the bacterium has a proclivity for colonizing the skin of the eyelid, which may be a risk factor for chronicity. Because it is the exceptional case of acute bacterial conjunctivitis that does not respond to antibiotic therapy, the choice of drug should be determined in large part by cost and propensity for adverse reactions and to a lesser degree by host immunosuppression, in which case, bactericidal rather than bacteriostatic agents are preferred.

Nonspecific and Specific Natural Defenses

Although the normal conjunctiva is exposed to various types of microorganisms from the lids, air, and hand contact, the tissue is remarkably resistant to infection. Nonspecific (innate) and specific (adaptive) natural defenses of the ocular surface operate in synergy, preventing and limiting infections.[1,2] In addition to the anatomic mechanical barriers of the ocular surface, toll-like receptors (TLRs), which are transmembrane proteins on local inflammatory and immunoregulatory cells, form the first line of defense against pathogens and function to both trigger and modulate the activation of the adaptive immune system (reviewed in Ref. 2). The tears both mechanically flush the ocular surface and also contain immunoglobulins,[3–5] including secretory IgA,[6–8] components of the classic and alternative complement pathways,[9] lysozyme,[5,10–12] β-lysin,[13] lactoferrin.[12,14,15] and other antimicrobial peptides including cathelicidin.[2,16,17] These agents help kill microorganisms and prevent bacterial adhesion to mucosal surfaces, thus limiting colonization and subsequent infection.[18,19]

Both aerobic and anaerobic bacteria, qualitatively similar to those of the eyelid margins, compose the normal (commensal) bacterial flora of the conjunctiva.[20–23] An organism may be isolated in as many as 90% of normal subjects, with more than one organism found in up to 35%.[21,24] In most subjects, the flora is composed of aerobic staphylococci (>60%) (mostly *Staphylococcus epidermidis*), diphtheroids (>35%), and the anaerobe *Propionibacterium acnes*,[21,24] but the spectrum of bacteria and sensitivity to antibiotics varies among major age groups.[25,26] The presence of indigenous bacteria on the conjunctival surface may reduce the colonization of more pathogenic microorganisms by releasing antibiotic-like substances (bacteriocins)[27] or metabolic waste products.[1,28,29] The cellular immune defenses are provided largely by the abundant lymphoid tissue in the conjunctival substantia propria including the conjunctival-associated lymphoid tissue (CALT).[30,31] Polymorphonuclear leukocytes (PMNs) and macrophages in tears are acute inflammatory response effector cells.[32] Finally, the low temperature[33] of the exposed ocular surface is generally not conducive to bacterial growth, and mucus from goblet cells traps bacteria.[1,2] Thus, in most instances of bacterial conjunctival infection, local host defenses combine to contain the pathogen, resulting in a self-limited, acute inflammatory process.

Disruption of the host's defense mechanisms are predisposing factors for the development of bacterial conjunctivitis (Box 43.1). Conjunctival inflammation associated with systemic conditions such as ocular cicatricial pemphigoid, Stevens-Johnson syndrome, and atopic and vernal conjunctivitis may affect the conjunctival bacterial flora and the epithelial integrity and result in secondary infections. Localized infections by virus or *Chlamydia* may compromise the conjunctival epithelial barrier and allow bacterial invasion. In addition, the composition of the normal conjunctival bacterial flora will typically change to a more pathogenic bacterial population that includes *Staphylococcus aureus* or Gram-negative bacilli in hospitalized patients,[34] those with immunodeficiency syndromes,[35,36] severe burns,[37] and certain ocular diseases.[38]

Bacterial conjunctival infections are sometimes caused by virulent bacteria capable of disrupting the intact conjunctival epithelial surface integrity (*N. gonorrhoeae*, *Listeria monocytogenes*, *Corynebacterium diphtheriae*, and *Haemophilus* species). Some bacteria may overcome the host defense mechanisms by enhanced surface attachment by bacterial pili (*N. gonorrhoeae*)[19,39] or by glycocalyx adherence (*Pseudomonas*),[40] evasion of the host immune defenses by intracellular invasion to hinder phagocytosis (*Listeria*),[41] or by the

Box 43.1 Risk factors for the development of bacterial conjunctivitis

Disruption of host defense mechanisms caused by

Dry eye

Exposure due to:
- Lid retraction
- Exophthalmos
- Lagophthalmos
- Inadequate blinking

Nutritional deficiency/malabsorption
- Avitaminosis A

Local or systemic immune deficiency often after topical and systemic immunosuppressive therapy
- Nasolacrimal duct obstruction and infection
- Radiation damage
- Trauma
- Surgery
- Prior conjunctival inflammation or infection
- Systemic infection
- Exogenous inoculation

production of IgA protease (*Haemophilus influenzae, Streptococcus pneumoniae, N. gonorrhoeae,* and *N. meningitidis*).[42,43]

Bacterial conjunctivitis is frequently caused by inoculation from an exogenous source,[44] but can also result from the invasion and the proliferation of indigenous organisms or be secondary to a systemic infection.[45]

Bacterial conjunctivitis is frequently bilateral, but localized disruption of ocular surface integrity or immunity may produce unilateral disease. There may be concomitant involvement of the lid margin (blepharoconjunctivitis).

Manifestations of Conjunctivitis

Discharge

After bacterial invasion of the conjunctiva, there is a nonspecific PMN response. Initially, a scanty serous discharge is observed. With increased secretion of mucus by goblet cells and the accumulation of inflammatory and epithelial cells, the exudate becomes more mucoid and then purulent.

The most common organisms causing purulent discharge are gonococci and meningococci. Most other infections cause a mucopurulent discharge (Fig. 43.1).

Membranes and pseudomembranes

Infections by certain organisms may produce either membranes or pseudomembranes. A true membrane is formed after more severe inflammation in which coagulation occurs in the tissue and on the conjunctival surface. The exudate has a high fibrin content, and coagulation occurs in the epithelium so that if a membrane is stripped, the epithelium remains attached to the membrane, leaving a raw, bleeding surface. The lids may become more rigid because of the fibrin coagulation in the subepithelial conjunctival tissues.

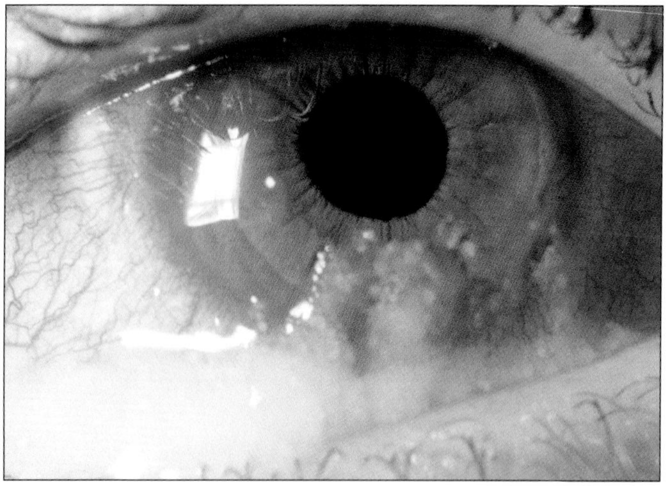

Fig. 43.1 Conjunctivitis with purulent discharge. (Courtesy John Dart, MA, DM, FRCS.)

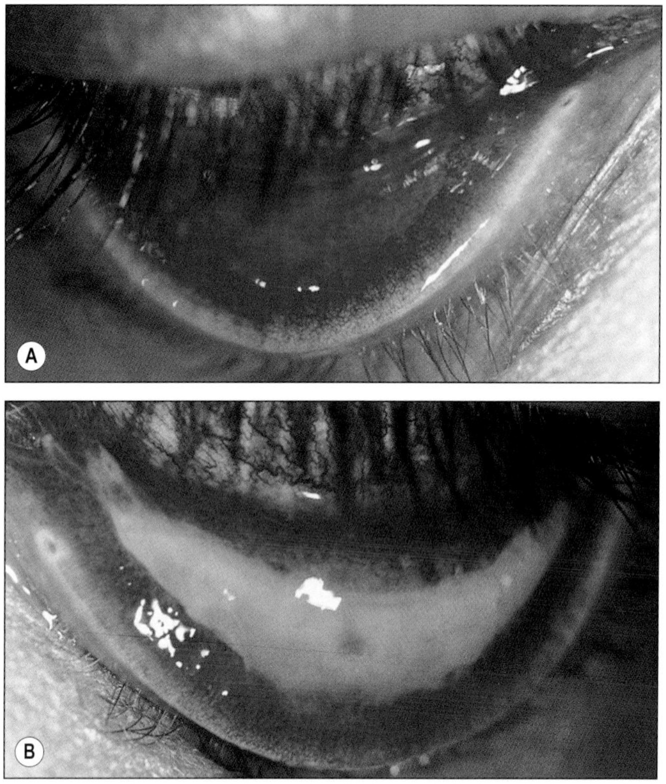

Fig. 43.2 Pseudomembranous conjunctivitis in the (**A**) right and (**B**) left eyes.

A pseudomembrane consists of coagulation of an exudate on the surface of the epithelium (Fig. 43.2). A pseudomembrane can be stripped off without underlying bleeding. The most common bacterial causes of membranes and pseudomembranes are *C. diphtheriae* and *Streptococcus pyogenes*,[46,47] but they may be caused by other organisms, especially in compromised hosts.

Papillae and follicles

Papillary hypertrophy and rare follicular hyperplasia may be seen in response to a bacterial conjunctival infection. Bacte-

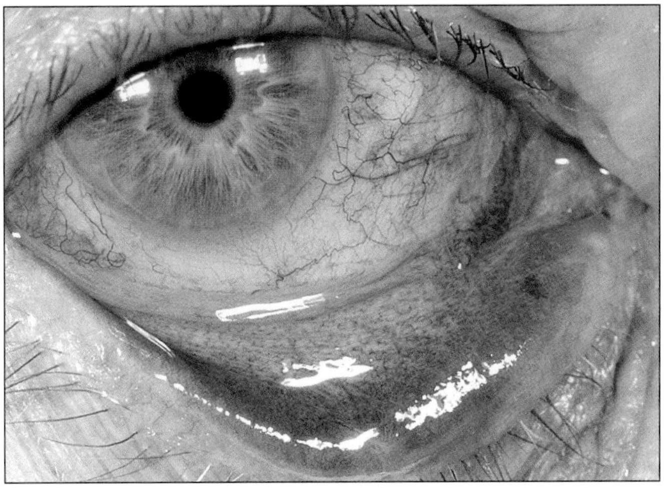

Fig. 43.3 Papillary conjunctivitis. Note the diffuse vascular dotlike appearance.

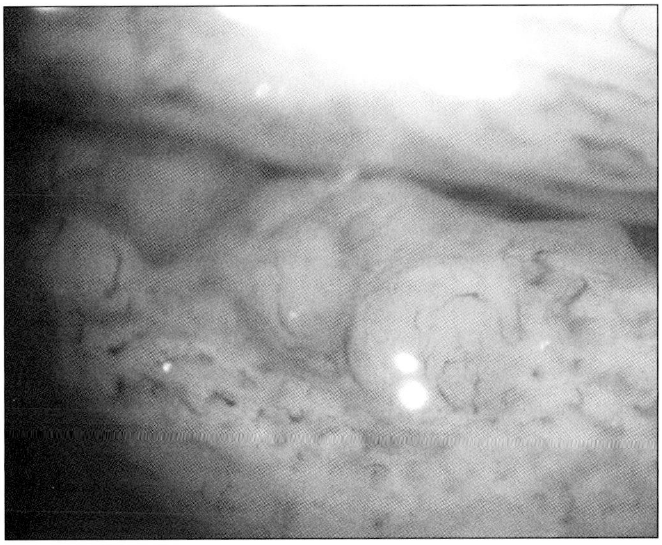

Fig. 43.4 Follicular conjunctivitis. Follicles are subepithelial mounds of rounded tissue surrounded by vessels.

rial virulence, including invasiveness, determines the extent of these changes.

Papillae, which are found more frequently on the palpebral than on the bulbar conjunctiva, have a velvety appearance (Fig. 43.3). Although a nonspecific finding, they are commonly seen in bacterial conjunctivitis.

Follicles (Fig. 43.4) are slightly larger (1–2 mm in diameter) than papillae and may be seen along the superior tarsal border conjunctiva in many normal subjects and throughout the tarsal conjunctiva in children. Follicles are of significance when found on the lower two-thirds of the superior tarsal conjunctiva or the inferior tarsal conjunctiva. Although follicles are associated with viral, chlamydial, and certain types of toxic conjunctivitis, they also are seen with *Moraxella* conjunctivitis and have been reported in *Neisseria meningitidis* conjunctivitis.[48]

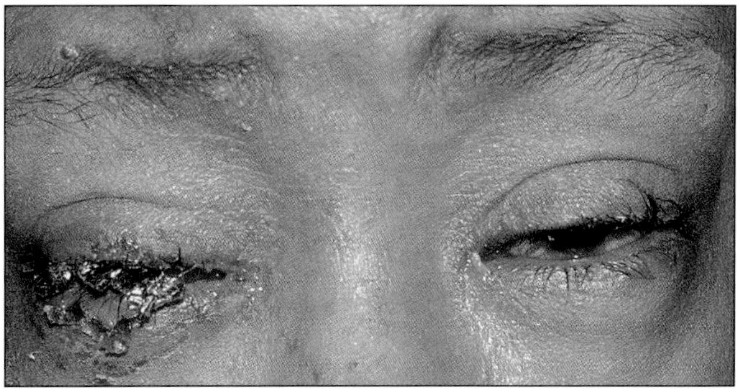

Fig. 43.5 Hyperacute conjunctivitis caused by *N. gonorrhoeae*. Note the lid edema, hyperemia, and copious discharge. (Courtesy Keith Walter, MD.)

Classification

Bacterial conjunctivitis can be classified on the basis of duration of illness (hyperacute, acute, chronic) and severity or appearance of the clinical findings (i.e. degree and type of exudation [purulent or mucopurulent] and presence of membranes or granulomas). The clinical presentation may at times be characteristic of the causative organism (e.g. *N. gonorrhoeae* is a frequent cause of hyperacute purulent conjunctivitis); however, Gram stains and cultures are the definitive traditional methods of identifying the pathogen.

Hyperacute bacterial conjunctivitis

Hyperacute purulent conjunctivitis is a rapidly progressive condition characterized by lid edema, marked conjunctival hyperemia, chemosis, and copious amounts of purulent discharge (Fig. 43.5). The infection usually starts unilaterally but often becomes bilateral. A membrane or pseudomembrane may be present and associated with preauricular adenopathy, as in the case of *N. gonorrhoeae* and *N. meningitidis*.[49,50] Ocular discomfort is characteristic. Ocular pain is seen in association with membrane formation and the onset of keratitis.

The most common causative pathogens are *N. gonorrhoeae* and *N. meningitidis*. Although ocular infection with these agents is relatively uncommon in developed countries, complications can be devastating if the disease is not diagnosed and treated rapidly. In rare instances (e.g. the immunosuppressed host or if the eye is patched), organisms that usually produce a mucopurulent conjunctivitis may produce a purulent conjunctivitis, albeit less purulent than the typical *Neisseria* organism.[50]

N. gonorrhoeae is the most common bacterial pathogen associated with hyperacute bacterial conjunctivitis. In 1841, Piringer[51] showed that gonorrheal conjunctivitis was caused by contamination from urethritis. In 1879, Neisser[52] discovered the gonococcus in both urethral and conjunctival pus. However, the conjunctivitis in adults may be associated with concomitant asymptomatic genital infection.[53] The incubation periods in ocular disease range from a few hours to 3 days, with rapidly reaccumulating copious purulent discharge seen around day 5; however, probable incubation periods of up to 19 days have been reported.[54,55] Local inoculation by the instillation of urine as a folk remedy[55–57] and accidental inoculations[54,58] have been reported as causes of the disease.

N. gonorrhoeae, an important cause of ophthalmia neonatorum, is acquired during transit through the infected birth canal. The incidence is approximately 0.04% of all births.[59] It presents as a hyperacute purulent conjunctivitis, with chemosis beginning 2 to 4 days after birth. Corneal ulceration and perforation may develop in untreated or poorly treated cases. A more detailed account of ocular infections in neonates is presented in Chapter 46.

N. meningitidis conjunctivitis has a similar clinical presentation to that seen after infection by *N. gonorrhoeae*. As with *N. gonorrhoeae*, *N. meningitidis* is seen more often in children than adults. Although relatively rare, the infection has important implications because the conjunctiva, pharynx, and upper respiratory tract are potential portals of entry leading to meningococcemia and meningitis.[60,61] The disease is transmitted by respiratory secretions but orogenital transmission has been reported.[62] Hematogenous dissemination is the most frequently reported cause of ocular infection by *N. meningitidis*,[63,64] although exogenous dissemination is well described.[61,65] The process is frequently bilateral, but a significant proportion of exogenous (primary) cases may be unilateral.[61] Multiple family members may be affected.[63]

Associated ocular and systemic complications

Serious corneal involvement may accompany untreated or undertreated *Neisseria* infections of the conjunctiva or develop when treatment is delayed.[66,67] Rapid development of corneal haze and peripheral infiltrates followed by peripheral or central ulcerations is not uncommon after infection by *N. gonorrhoeae*.[66,68–70] A hypersensitivity reaction has been suggested for the peripheral infiltrates.[67] Corneal perforation resulting from an infectious ulcer, in contrast to that caused by peripheral infiltrates, may occur within a few days of the onset of the conjunctivitis in untreated cases (Fig. 43.6).[46] Hypopyon iritis, dacryoadenitis, and lid abscess may rarely develop.[46,48,49] A risk factor for the development of microbial keratitis caused by *N. gonorrhoeae* is pressure necrosis of the corneal epithelium resulting from the increasing volume of pus trapped under the eyelids that are kept closed by severe eyelid edema. Keratitis and iritis also have been reported to occur with infection from *N. meningitidis*.[61]

Nearly one-fifth of patients with exogenous (primary) *N. meningitidis* conjunctivitis may develop systemic meningococcal disease, including meningitis, with the portal of entry being the conjunctiva.[60] The risk of developing systemic meningococcal disease is nearly 20 times higher in patients treated with topical therapy alone than in those who receive systemic therapy.[61] Thus, systemic therapy is mandatory.

Diagnosis

When hyperacute conjunctivitis is diagnosed in an adult, a Gram stain and confirmatory culture are mandatory because of the systemic and therapeutic implications. In *Neisseria* conjunctivitis, the Gram stain demonstrates Gram-negative intracellular diplococci, often within PMNs. Gonococci may be more readily identified from scrapings of the inferior tarsal conjunctiva than from smears. Material for culture should be placed on chocolate agar media in a 4–8% CO_2 environment. Although historically *N. gonorrhoeae* has been sensitive to penicillin, the incidence of strains resistant to both penicillins and tetracyclines has increased, thus influencing therapeutic preferences.[71–76] Penicillinase-producing *N. gonorrhoeae* strains account for about 10% of all cases of gonorrhea seen in the United States today, with substantially higher rates in coastal areas.[75,76] It is endemic in some parts of the developing world, with some areas of the Philippines and Russia reporting rates of over 70%.[77–79] There is also a significant increase in chromosomal resistance to the penicillins and tetracyclines, especially in homosexual men.[68]

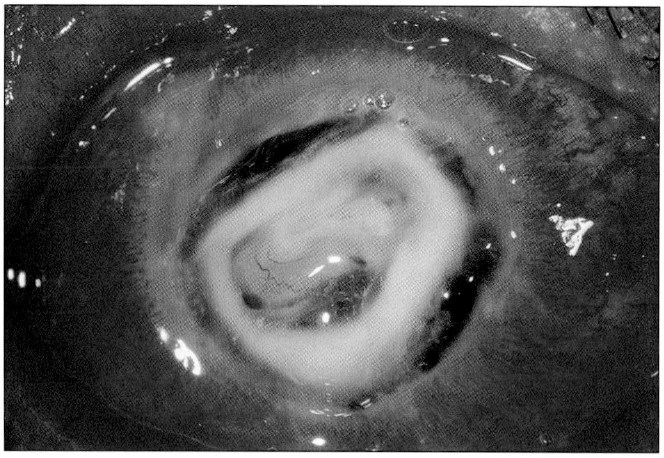

Fig. 43.6 Extensive corneal ulceration with perforation in the right eye of patient in Figure 43.5. The patient experienced an expulsive hemorrhage, and the retina plugs the perforation site. (Courtesy Keith Walter, MD.)

Sexual partners of patients with gonorrhea and mothers of neonates with gonococcal conjunctivitis should be referred for evaluation and treatment because of the public health implications (epidemiologic treatment). Patients being treated for gonorrhea should be screened for syphilis by serology.[80] Contacts of patients with *N. meningitidis* conjunctivitis should be evaluated to identify carriers for consideration of prophylactic therapy.

Treatment

Systemic treatment is mandatory for patients with *Neisseria* conjunctivitis; concomitant topical antibiotic therapy is optional. Treatment should be instituted immediately after collection of material for diagnostic testing in order to reduce the potential for corneal involvement and systemic infection.

Recent studies evaluating the specific treatments for adult gonococcal conjunctivitis are limited.[56,81] In one study, a single-dose intramuscular (IM) regimen of 1 g of ceftriaxone was effective in 13 of 13 patients with gonococcal conjunctivitis.[56] This drug regimen was also effective in another case report.[82] Other single-dose regimens with cefotaxime,[54,71] spectinomycin,[66,67] and norfloxacin[83] for gonococcal conjunctivitis also have demonstrated effectiveness. The use of spectinomycin to treat gonococcal infections, however, has become increasingly limited because of the occurrence of spectinomycin-resistant gonococci and the drug's ineffectiveness in eradicating pharyngeal infection. The sole remaining indication for the use of spectinomycin is in the treatment of pregnant women with disease who have histories of rapid-onset allergic reactions to penicillin or documented cephalosporin allergy.[77] The current regimen recommended by the US Public Health Service for gonococcal conjunctivitis is an initial single IM dose of 1 g ceftriaxone with a one-time saline lavage of the conjunctiva.[81] Because of the frequent incidence of coinfection with *Chlamydia trachomatis*,[84] this regimen should be followed by either a single dose of 1 g of oral azithromycin or 100 mg of oral doxycycline twice a day for 7 days.[56,81] This combined therapy not only treats concomitant chlamydial infection but also reduces the risk of postgonococcal urethritis and salpingitis. This regimen also may reduce the potential for selection of gonococci with increased antimicrobial resistance.[77]

Other regimens have been found effective for uncomplicated gonococcal genital and anal infections in adults. The Centers for Disease Control and Prevention recommends either an initial single dose of 125 mg of IM ceftriaxone or 400 mg of oral cefixime, 500 mg of oral ciprofloxacin, or 400 mg of oral ofloxacin. This treatment should be followed by the same regimens effective against *C. trachomatis* described previously. Studies using the aforementioned antibiotics have not been published for the treatment of gonococcal conjunctivitis, although they may be effective. For complicated gonorrhea in adults, such as pelvic inflammatory disease, acute epididymitis, and disseminated gonococcal infection, a more intensive course of antibiotics in either an inpatient or outpatient setting is required.[81]

To treat *N. gonorrhoeae* conjunctivitis in the newborn, 25–50 mg/kg intravenous (IV) or IM ceftriaxone administered in a single dose not exceeding 125 mg is currently recommended.[81,85] Concurrent saline irrigation of the conjunctiva should be used.[81,86] The use of tetracycline and its congeners is contraindicated in infants and young children.

Treatment of *N. meningitidis* conjunctivitis consists of penicillin administered IV or IM. The recommended dosage for meningitis is 300 000 IU/kg per day, with an upper limit of 24 million units/day as 2 million units every 2 hours.[87] Chloramphenicol is an effective substitute for the penicillin-allergic patient. Dramatic improvement may be seen within 2 days. When *N. meningitidis* conjunctivitis was the initial or only clinical manifestation, concomitant topical administration of 100 000 IU/mL per hour of penicillin G has been prescribed.[63] Prophylactic antimicrobial therapy is mandatory for contacts because these people are at risk of contracting or carrying the disease. Orally administered rifampin should be prescribed twice a day for 2 days.[88,89] The recommended dose is 600 mg in adults, and 10 mg/kg in children.

Acute conjunctivitis

Acute conjunctivitis has a rapid onset but is less severe than hyperacute bacterial conjunctivitis. Symptoms usually have been present less than a week when the fellow eye commonly becomes involved. The discharge is characteristically mucopurulent, but may at times be mucoid (catarrhal) or purulent. The bulbar conjunctiva is characteristically more inflamed than the palpebral conjunctiva. Most frequently, a velvety papillary reaction is seen on the palpebral conjunctiva. Symptoms generally subside in 10 to 14 days, in many instances even without treatment. When the pathogen is *Staphylococcus* or *Moraxella*, however, the conjunctivitis may become chronic because of the potential for these organisms to induce a blepharitis. Most cases of bacterial conjunctivitis are caused by Gram-positive cocci (aerobic and anaerobic),[21,90] but with prior abnormalities of the conjunctiva caused by exposure (e.g. thyroid exophthalmos, coma), keratinization (e.g. after irradiation) and hospitalization of greater then 2 days in neonates[26] the incidence of infection from Gram-negative bacilli increases. In children, *H. influenzae*, *S. pneumoniae*, and *S. aureus* are common causes of bacterial conjunctivitis (Box 43.2) with recent publications also reporting a high incidence of *Moraxella* species.[91–95] Anaerobes have been isolated in a significant number of pediatric cases but less frequently than in adults with acute conjunctivitis.[21,93] A seasonal variation may be seen, with one study demonstrating culture-proven bacterial conjunctivitis

Box 43.2 Common bacterial pathogens causing conjunctivitis[21,90–97]

Hyperacute purulent
- *Neisseria gonorrhoeae*
- *N. meningitidis*

Acute conjunctivitis (adults)
- *Staphylococcus aureus*
- *S. pneumoniae*
- Gram-positive anaerobes (*Peptostreptococcus* spp.)
- *Haemophilus* spp.
- *H. influenzae*
- *H. influenzae* biogroup *aegyptius*
- *S. pyogenes*
- Gram-negative (rare)

Acute conjunctivitis (children)
- *H. influenzae*
- *S. pneumoniae*
- Anaerobic bacteria (*Peptostreptococcus* spp. and *Peptococcus* spp.)
- *S. aureus*
- *Moraxella* spp.

Chronic conjunctivitis
- *S. aureus*
- *Moraxella lacunata*
- *S. pyogenes*
- *Klebsiella pneumoniae*
- *Serratia marcescens*
- *Escherichia coli*

predominating in the winter and spring and viral conjunctivitis predominating in the summer.[96] The incidence of infection with *S. pneumoniae* is greater in colder weather. *H. influenzae* conjunctivitis is seen more frequently during the warmer months.

S. aureus, the most frequent cause of bacterial conjunctivitis worldwide, is common in any age group.[97] Although it is a more frequent cause of chronic conjunctivitis and is associated with a characteristic blepharitis, it can cause an acute purulent conjunctivitis from the elaboration of exotoxins and biologically active substances such as hemolysin, fibrinolysin, and coagulase. The mucopurulent discharge may produce stickiness of the lids upon awakening. *S. epidermidis* is an infrequent cause of conjunctivitis.

Streptococcus species are a common cause of acute conjunctivitis. *S. pneumoniae* conjunctivitis is usually self-limited and may occur in epidemics. It occurs more frequently in temperate climates and in winter months. It is also more commonly seen in children than in adults.[91] The incubation period is approximately 2 days, followed by the acute onset of conjunctival hyperemia and a mucopurulent discharge that causes sticky eyelids on awakening. Maximum severity is reached by 2 to 3 days after onset. Subconjunctival hemorrhages are frequently seen and usually involve the upper tarsal conjunctiva[98] or fornix.[99] Chemosis also may be seen (see Fig. 43.2). Severe purulent conjunctivitis rarely develops. Pneumonia is rare, even if upper respiratory symptoms are present.[49] A case of pneumococcal sepsis has been reported that developed 72 hours after the onset of pneumococcal conjunctivitis and resulted in the death of a previously healthy 70-year-old woman.[49]

Other streptococcal species are infrequent causes of conjunctivitis. *S. pyogenes* (β-hemolytic streptococcus) may present with an acute purulent conjunctivitis with chemosis and occasionally membranes or pseudomembranes. The appearance may be similar to diphtheria, although the membranes in streptococcal disease are more likely to involve the bulbar conjunctiva. The source may be exogenous or endogenous. Scarlet fever may provoke an associated toxic conjunctivitis, and streptococcal impetigo can spread from the skin of the lids, particularly in children, and produce severe conjunctivitis and corneal ulceration.[46]

H. influenzae (nonencapsulated) is the most common cause of bacterial conjunctivitis in young children,[91,93,100] but may also be seen in adults (see Box 43.2). Humans are the only natural host with the nonencapsulated strains of *H. influenzae*, being a normal commensal of the upper respiratory tract in up to 80% of adults. The encapsulated *H. influenzae* type b rarely causes conjunctivitis, although this species is associated with serious invasive infections such as meningitis, septic arthritis, epiglottitis, and cellulitis with associated bacteremia. *Haemophilus* spp. are likely associated with two different clinical types of conjunctivitis, each caused by a different bacterium.[101] For some decades, investigators often failed to differentiate between *H. influenzae* and *H. influenzae*, biogroup *aegyptius*, thus making a critical evaluation of the ophthalmic literature difficult. Further, as diagnostic techniques for species discrimination improved, the need for culture identification of the pathogen became less important because of the rapid resolution of the infection after effective antibiotic therapy.

Haemophilus infections of the conjunctiva have been recognized since 1883 when Koch[102] observed the organism as a cause of a purulent infection in Egypt while he was investigating cholera. In 1886, Weeks[103] identified the organism from patients with conjunctivitis in New York City. Although the organism causing this conjunctivitis has been considered a distinct species because it has unique phenotypic characteristics, biotype III, *H. aegyptius*, and the 'Koch-Weeks bacillus' are the same species and are now referred to as *H. influenzae*, biogroup *aegyptius*. The conjunctivitis is often epidemic but may be endemic in regions with a warmer climate, such as the southern United States. It can be seasonal (i.e. from May to September in Egypt, and from May to October in Georgia, Texas, and southern California).[101] The high degree of contagion is manifested by its rapid spread within families. In a study of inoculated volunteers,[104] symptoms developed after an incubation period of about 24 hours, with maximal clinical findings occurring in 3 to 4 days. Clinical disease resolved within 7 to 10 days after initiation of antibiotic therapy.[102] Hyperemia, chemosis, and subconjunctival hemorrhages are present, and the discharge is purulent or mucopurulent. Without therapy, relapses and recurrences are possible.[46]

Nonencapsulated *H. influenzae* (not biogroup *aegyptius*) is more prevalent in temperate climates and during spring and may be seen in association with upper respiratory infections. The ocular infection is usually subacute and the discharge less purulent and at times thinner and more watery than that caused by *H. influenzae*, biogroup *aegyptius*. Conjunctival hemorrhages occur less frequently. The palpebral conjunctiva and fornices are most frequently involved. Many cases are self-limited and resolve within 7 to 10 days.[46,101] Recurrent episodes of *H. influenzae* conjunctivitis may be associated with *H. influenzae* otitis media.[91,105,106]

In Brazil, a fulminant and often fatal childhood illness, known as Brazilllian purpuric fever, may develop following a purulent conjunctivitis caused by a particular clone of *H. influenzae*, biogroup *aegyptius*.[107–110]

C. diphtheriae produces an acute membranous or pseudomembranous conjunctivitis. Although common in the nineteenth century, *C. diphtheriae* infections began to decline in the early twentieth century after the introduction of diphtheria toxoid. *C. diphtheriae* conjunctivitis, which is now extremely rare,[111] usually occurs in children following diphtheritic membranous pharyngitis. Although the nasopharynx and larynx may become involved before or after the appearance of the conjunctivitis, cutaneous diphtheria seems to be more frequently associated with ocular surface involvement.[112] During the initial stage, the lids are red, brawny, hot, tender, and swollen. Preauricular lymphadenopathy may be present. In severe cases, the grayish-yellow membrane or pseudomembrane can spread over the bulbar conjunctiva. Necrosis and sloughing of the conjunctiva may be seen with cicatrizing changes as a late sequela. Fever and toxic symptoms may not be severe in the absence of nasal and pharyngeal diphtheria.[50] The disease is highly contagious, and systemic antibiotic therapy with erythromycin and antitoxin therapy is required.

Moraxella species, which more commonly cause chronic conjunctivitis (see Chronic Conjunctivitis) and are often associated with angular blepharitis, rarely cause an acute mucopurulent conjunctivitis without blepharitis.[113,114] Although *M. lacunata* historically was a frequent cause of conjunctivitis, especially in urban sites associated with a high prevalence of alcoholism, the incidence of this infection had decreased by 1972.[115] In 1989, however, an outbreak was reported in New Mexico.[114] Sharing of eye make-up was the significant risk factor. Recent publications have also reported a high incidence of *Moraxella* species in acute childhood conjunctivitis.[94,95]

Branhamella catarrhalis may present as an acute conjunctivitis.[116] Its morphologic characteristics are similar at times to *Neisseria* and *Moraxella* species on Gram stain. It is prudent to treat this infection as one caused by gonococci if the clinical picture suggests this etiology and to modify the therapy when the pathogenic organism is identified on culture.[49] *N. cinerea* may be a rare cause of acute purulent conjunctivitis.[117]

Other pathogens that can cause acute purulent conjunctivitis include *Pseudomonas* species, *Escherichia coli*, *Shigella* species, *Borrelia vincentii*, and *Fusobacterium bacilli*. *Shigella* species may induce a concomitant diarrhea. *B. vincentii* and *Fusobacterium* bacilli, which are infrequently seen, are associated with unilateral infection, lid swelling, chemosis, an occasional pseudomembrane, and may rarely involve the cornea.[98] Rare cases presumably caused by *Capnocytophaga* or *Vibrio alginolyticus*, a marine organism, have been reported.[118,119]

Associated ocular and systemic complications

Corneal opacities, marginal corneal ulceration, and phlyctenular keratoconjunctivitis may develop with *H. influenzae*, biogroup *aegyptius* conjunctivitis. In young children, associated periorbital cellulitis caused by *H. influenzae* may have a characteristic blue to purple skin discoloration.[120,121] Malaise, fever, upper respiratory infection, otitis media, and meningitis may be associated with *H. influenzae*, especially in the winter months.[122]

Corneal involvement is rare following *Streptococcus* species conjunctivitis, but was more common in the preantibiotic era. However, corneal haze, infiltration, and necrosis progressing occasionally to perforation has been reported to follow keratitis from β-hemolytic streptococcus (*S. pyogenes*),[46] especially when there is a severe purulent discharge, membrane or pseudomembrane formation involving the inferior tarsal conjunctiva and eyelid induration. Iritis and hypopyon also have been reported as complications of erysipelas and in a rare case of *S. pneumoniae*.[46]

Moraxella species can cause bacterial corneal ulcers, especially in an alcoholic, derelict, and nutritionally deficient population in which there is poor hygiene (see Chronic Conjunctivitis).[123,124]

Xerosis, symblepharon formation, trichiasis, and entropion are common complications of severe *C. diphtheriae* conjunctivitis. Corneal ulcerations are rare but may rapidly progress to perforation.[46] *C. diphtheriae* toxin may cause paralysis of the extraocular muscles and accommodation, airway obstruction, and cardiac toxicity. Concomitant systemic antitoxin therapy is required to prevent these complications. For other ocular complications associated with staphylococcal infection, see Chronic Conjunctivitis.

Diagnosis

The diagnosis of acute bacterial conjunctivitis is usually made by observing clinical symptoms and signs and without the aid of laboratory studies. However, the clinical differentiation between bacterial and other infectious causes of conjunctivitis may be difficult.[91,125] Because laboratory cultures for bacteria and viruses are expensive, time-consuming, and may not be definitive, they should be reserved for cases of acute conjunctivitis refractory to treatment, severe conjunctivitis in infants and children, and hyperpurulent conjunctivitis in an adult. Blood cultures should be obtained in patients with Brazilian purpuric fever and infants with systemic symptoms associated with *H. influenzae* conjunctivitis.

Treatment

Many milder cases of acute conjunctivitis are self-limited. A recent systematic review reported clinical cure or significant improvement occurring in 2 to 5 days in 64% of patients treated with placebo.[126,127] However, topical antibiotic therapy hastens resolution, improves microbiologic cure, and may reduce morbidity, especially in culture-proven cases.[126–131] The exceptions are *Staphylococcus* and *Moraxella* infections, which may become chronic if not adequately treated. Eyedrops are generally preferred over ointments for adults because ointments blur vision. By contrast, ointments are preferred for infants and children because eyedrops are squeezed out and diluted by tearing. Ointments are acceptable for adults at bedtime and are useful because of their increased contact time when compared to solutions. A variety of broad-spectrum antibiotic eyedrops and ointments are commercially available and are adequate for most cases of bacterial conjunctivitis (Table 43.1).[130] There does not appear to be a significant difference in clinical response or microbiologic cure between various antibiotics.[126,128,132–136] Drops can be instilled initially every 2 to 4 hours and ointments about four times a day. Less frequent administration may potentially be as effective with some antibiotics, with a recent report finding no clinical difference between twice a day and four times a day administration of gatifloxacin.[137] Additionally, azithromycin 1% solution, a new topical macrolide antibiotic in a gel-forming drop, was approved for twice a day administration for the first 2 days, followed by daily administration for only 3 additional days.[136,137] Topical antibiotics do vary considerably in cost, which should be considered when prescribing them. The aminoglycosides continue to have good broad-spectrum coverage and are relatively inexpensive,[139] but they may be less effective in the treatment of streptococcal ocular infections.[140] Polymyxin B–trimethoprim eyedrops and bacitracin–polymyxin B ointment are effective broad-spectrum antibiotic combinations, which may be alternative choices. There has not been a trend toward increased bacterial resistance toward these antibiotics over the last decade.[141] The fluoroquinolone eyedrops, ciprofloxacin and ofloxacin, have been shown to be comparable in clinical outcome to the aminoglycosides (a recent study also found levofloxacin (the L-isomer of ofloxacin) comparable to ofloxacin).[132,134,135,139,142,143] Their initial broad-spectrum coverage and low toxicity was appealing. However, over the first decade of use, there was

Table 43.1 Commercial topical antibiotics for bacterial conjunctivitis

Antibiotic/concentration[131]	Brand Name	Formulation	Size	AWP[182]
Recommended				
Single antibiotic preparations				
Azithromycin 1%	AzaSite®	Solution	2.5 mL	$75.13
Bacitracin 500 IU/g		Ointment †	3.5 g	$2.55
(G)Erythromycin 0.5%*		Ointment†	3.5 g	$3.13
(G)Gentamicin 0.3%		Ointment†	3.5 g	$19.67
(G)		Solution†	5 mL	$8.17
(G)Tobramycin 0.3%	Tobrex™	Ointment	3.5 g	$75.38
(Br)	Tobrex™	Solution	5 mL	$64.44
		Solution†	5 mL	$14.25
Ciprofloxacin 0.3%	Ciloxan™	Ointment	3.5 g	$82.69
	Ciloxan™	Solution	5 mL	$66.13
		Solution†	5 mL	$47.3
Ofloxacin 0.3%		Solution†	5 mL	$42.17
Levofloxacin 0.5%	Quixin®	Solution	5 mL	$73.50
Moxifloxacin 0.5%	Vigamox®	Solution	3 mL	$73.63
Gatifloxacin 0.3%	Zymar®	Solution	5 mL	$77.65
Combination antibiotic preparations				
Polymyxin B (10000 IU) + trimethoprim (1 mg/mL)	Polytirm®	Solution	10 mL	$34.55
		Solution†	10 mL	$17.42
Polymyxin B (10000 IU) + bacitracin (500 IU)/ointment		Ointment†	3.5 g	$18.00
Other‡				
Sulfacetamide* 10%	Bleph®-10	Solution	15 mL	$18.71
		Solution†	15 mL	$5.08
Polymyxin B (10000 IU) + neomycin (1.75 mg) + gramicidin (0.025 mg/mL)		Solution†	10 mL	$25.30
Polymyxin B (10000 IU) + neomycin (3.5 mg) + bacitracin (400 IU/g)	Neosporin®	Ointment	3.5g	$52.10
		Ointment†	3.5 g	$4.20

** Bacteriostatic.*
† Available as a generic product.
‡ These antibiotics may be used in the treatment of bacterial conjunctivitis, but have more adverse effects or clinical limitations:
Sulfacetamide: bacteriostatic with increasing resistance by S. aureus *noted*
Compounds with neomycin have a significant risk of punctate keratitis
AWP, average wholesale price.

increasing resistance to these antibiotics, especially by Gram-positive bacteria (which has been documented in both conjunctivitis and keratitis isolates).[144–146] A recent study reviewing bacterial conjunctivitis isolates reported a threefold increase in resistance of Gram-positive bacteria to ciprofloxacin and ofloxacin between the years 1994 and 2004.[147] The introduction of fourth-generation fluoroquinolones (moxifloxacin and gatifloxacin) which have an expanded spectrum of activity to cover the bacterial resistance seen with second- and third-generation fluoroquinolones, with more potent activity against Gram-positive organisms and equivalent potency against Gram-negative organisms, has expanded the treatment options for bacterial conjunctivitis.[148] However, there has also been a significant increase in methicillin-resistant *Staphylococcus aureus* (MRSA) from conjunctivitis isolates, with recent studies reporting between four- and tenfold increase over a 10-year period,[147,149] and with about 85% having in vitro resistance to the fluoroquinolones,[149,150] MRSA conjunctivitis does not appear to be clinically different than conjunctivitis caused by methicillin-sensitive strains.[149] In special situations, specially formulated antibiotic eyedrops should be considered. For cases of refractory or severe methicillin-resistant staphylococcal conjunctivitis, vancomycin eyedrops, 5 mg/mL, may be used. A new fluoroquinolone developed specifically for ophthalmic use, and still in phase III clinical trials, may for the time being overcome some of the current microbial resistance issues.[151] Recently, a double-masked, controlled, prospective clinical trial reported that povidone-iodine 1.25% ophthalmic solution (an antiseptic agent) was as effective as neomycin–polymyxin B–gramicidin for the treatment of bacterial conjunctivitis in children.[95] Low cost, effectiveness, availability, and lack of microbial resistance make this agent a desirable drug to treat ocular infections, especially in developing countries.

Systemic antibiotics are rarely used for the treatment of uncomplicated acute conjunctivitis; however, they are required for infants and children with acute conjunctivitis caused by *H. influenzae* when there are associated systemic signs and symptoms, and for acute conjunctivitis resulting from the Brazilian clone of *H. influenzae*, biogroup *aegyptius*. A patient with relapsing *H. influenzae* conjunctivitis with nasopharyngeal carriage was successfully treated with oral cefixime and rifampin.[152]

Chronic conjunctivitis

By definition, chronic conjunctivitis has a more indolent and prolonged course than more acute forms of conjunctivitis. Symptoms are variable and frequently include foreign body sensation, mild stickiness and matting of the lashes, and minimal discharge. Symptoms characteristically outweigh clinical objective findings, which consist of diffuse conjunctival hyperemia, papillae formation (although follicles are characteristic of *Moraxella* infections), and a mild mucopurulent discharge. Until recently, *S. aureus* and *M. lacunata* have been the two most common causes of chronic bacterial conjunctivitis.[153] The incidence of *Moraxella* infection seems to be decreasing in the United States, probably because of decreased clustering and improved nutrition of alcoholics in some of the largest cities.

S. aureus is the most commonly isolated organism in chronic bacterial conjunctivitis.[97] Blepharoconjunctivitis, with concurrent lid margin involvement with loss of lashes, trichiasis, erythema, telangiectasis, and hordeola are suggestive of staphylococcal infection. Conjunctival inflammation may be the result of direct infection or release of toxins.[154] Usually, only low numbers of the organism are demonstrated. The agent may survive in the tear film. A dermonecrotic toxin is thought to produce the ulcerations of the medial and lateral canthus skin and lid margin. Hypersensitivity to the *S. aureus* cell wall, in particular the ribitol teichoic acid, may play a role in the etiology of staphylococcal blepharitis.[155]

Exotoxins may produce a nonspecific conjunctivitis or superficial punctate keratitis, usually inferiorly. The patient often complains of an intense, gritty sensation on eyelid opening in the morning, and the mucopurulent discharge may produce lid stickiness on awakening and crusting on their margins. Lid closure not only provides a better climate for bacterial growth but also permits concentrated toxin to act on the corneal and conjunctival surfaces with decreased dilution and irrigation by the tears.[156] Symptoms decrease during the day as the toxins are diluted and washed away and as the ocular surface heals.

S. epidermidis is a common component of the normal ocular surface flora. Pathogenic strains may cause a chronic blepharoconjunctivitis through the elaboration of toxins similar to *S. aureus*.[157]

M. lacunata, characterized by Morax in 1896,[158] may cause an isolated chronic conjunctivitis, although frequently the infection is associated with an ulcerative inner and outer canthal blepharitis. Although common in the United States during the early years of the last century and frequently associated with alcoholics and the poorly nourished, the incidence of this condition has decreased significantly in recent years. A study published in 1986 identified *Moraxella* in only 2.4% of bacterial cultures isolated from patients with external ocular infections.[159] The pathogen causes a follicular conjunctivitis and may be incorrectly diagnosed as epidemic keratoconjunctivitis, herpes simplex, or chlamydial infection.[159] Preauricular lymphadenopathy may be present. Patients may have symptoms for months before seeking medical evaluation. A Gram stain of specimens obtained by conjunctival swab may often be teeming with bacteria when clinical signs are minimal. It has been postulated that, after conjunctival infection, the disease progresses to involve the lid margin and canthal skin, because of a proteolytic enzyme that ultimately dominates the clinical picture.[113]

Enteric Gram-negative rods more frequently cause chronic than acute conjunctivitis, partly because of their association with ocular surfaces previously compromised by chronic exposure, prior disease, or past treatment with irradiation. *Proteus* species is most frequently encountered, but infection with *Klebsiella pneumoniae*, *Serratia marcescens*, and *E. coli* is also seen. These infections may at times be caused by self-inoculation in the elderly as the result of poor hygiene.[97]

Neisseria catarrhalis, streptococci, and pneumococci may rarely produce a chronic mucopurulent conjunctivitis. Even *N. gonorrhoeae* may produce a similar clinical picture on rare occasions, probably related to the specific strain.[48,160]

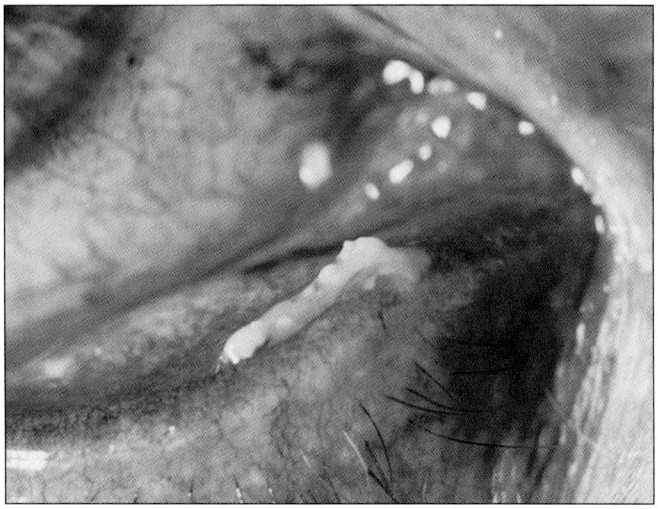

Fig. 43.7 Chronic unilateral conjunctivitis caused by *Actinomyces israelii*. The thick granular material ('sulfur granules') can be expressed from the canaliculus.

Chronic unilateral conjunctivitis also should suggest the possibility of a silent chronic canaliculitis or dacryocystitis (Fig. 43.7). Careful evaluation of the canaliculi and lacrimal sac is important because each may be a chronic reservoir of organisms such as *S. pneumoniae*. The most common canalicular pathogen is *A. israelii*, although viral, chlamydial, and other *Actinomyces* bacterial infections have been described.[161] The lower canaliculus is affected more frequently. Symptoms include unilateral itching, tearing, and irritation. The nasal conjunctiva may be more inflamed, with possible swelling and pouting of the punctum. Mucopurulent material may be present near the puncta. Milking of the canaliculi often expresses yellow granular material ('sulfur granules') from the punctum (see Fig. 43.7) that demonstrates the Gram-positive filaments on smears. Oral anaerobic bacteria may cause chronic unilateral conjunctivitis associated with periodontal disease.[162]

Associated ocular complications

Corneal complications associated with *S. aureus* conjunctivitis are not uncommon. Inferior corneal epithelial punctate erosions occur because of liberated exotoxins, as demonstrated experimentally.[163] In more severe cases, the punctate keratitis may involve the entire corneal surface. Marginal corneal infiltrates and ulcerations also can be seen in chronic *S. aureus* blepharoconjunctivitis. They are frequently found near the limbus at the 4 and 8 o'clock positions with associated paralimbal conjunctival injection and are most likely the results of a hypersensitivity reaction to *S. aureus* toxin or cell wall products (ribitol).[164,165] Infrequently, a phlyctenular keratitis may be seen. The phlyctenules, gelatinous nodular lesions, may be limbal, on the conjunctiva, or on the cornea where a trailing branch of vessels may be seen (migrating phlyctenule). They are most frequently caused by a hypersensitivity reaction to staphylococcal cell wall antigens.[164,165] Punctate keratitis, subepithelial infiltrates, and scleral nodules near the lateral canthus have been reported with *Moraxella*.[159]

Diagnosis

Diagnosis is based most often on the history and clinical findings. Culturing of the lid margin and conjunctiva in refractory situations may be necessary, giving attention to evidence of heavy growth of a suspected pathogen but recognizing that *S. aureus* is a common inhabitant of the lid margin in normal eyes. Gram and Giemsa staining of conjunctival scrapings and bacterial cultures may be clinically important in chronic follicular conjunctivitis cases when *Chlamydia* and *Moraxella* infections are suspected.

Treatment

Treatment of chronic conjunctivitis should be based on similar principles as in acute conjunctivitis. However, because chronic staphylococcal conjunctivitis may be frequently associated with lid involvement, short-term topical therapy is often ineffective. Long-term therapy is required and, if there is concomitant blepharitis, the therapeutic regimen should include lid hygiene, lid margin cleansing with a mild baby shampoo diluted 50% with water, and the nightly application of an antibiotic ointment with good Gram-positive coverage, such as bacitracin, to the lid margins. Adjunctive oral therapy with 100 mg doxycycline one to two times a day, often administered for many months, may be required in refractory cases or when acne rosacea is present. Lack of compliance is a frequent cause of treatment failures. Topical antistaphylococcal antibiotics such as trimethoprim–polymyxin B, gentamicin, tobramycin, erythromycin, gatifloxacin, moxifloxacin, and azithromycin also can be administered. In refractory cases, therapy can be modified based on culture results if resistant organisms are identified. Although *Moraxella* is usually sensitive to most ophthalmic antibiotics, a significant increase in in vitro antibiotic resistance has been reported to the staphylococcus.[166,167]

Unusual Causes of Bacterial Conjunctivitis

Treponema pallidum may rarely cause conjunctival disease. The most frequent manifestation is a severe diffuse papillary conjunctivitis with marked injection, chemosis, and regional lymphadenopathy seen in early secondary syphilis and usually accompanied by skin or mucous membrane manifestations.[168] Treponemal organisms may be identified by conjunctival biopsy even when the biopsied skin lesions are negative.[45] A conjunctival chancre may be found on the bulbar conjunctiva associated with conjunctival and lid edema. Conjunctival gummata may be seen in tertiary syphilis.[169]

Conjunctival tuberculosis is extremely rare. Most earlier cases have been in young patients with primary exogenous *Mycobacterium tuberculosis* following a recent exposure.[170–173] Conjunctival tuberculosis can also occur as the result of an exogenous or endogenous *M. bovis* infection (the bovine equivalent of *M. tuberculosis*).[174,175] *M. bovis* has virtually been eradicated in North America.[176] Conjunctival tuberculosis usually presents as unilateral palpebral conjunctival lesions, including nodules that can ulcerate, with associated lymphadenopathy.

Immunodeficiency and AIDS

Bacterial conjunctivitis does not appear to be more prevalent in patients infected with the human immunodeficiency virus (HIV). *Gonococcus* should be considered as a potential pathogen even in an uncharacteristic conjunctivitis when seen in patients with acquired immunodeficiency syndrome (AIDS), and even in the absence of anogenital symptoms.[53,177] *Pseudomonas* species may be especially virulent.[178]

The incidence of bacterial conjunctivitis may be greater in patients with primary immunodeficiency syndromes (particularly those with deficiencies of B-cell immunity), than in patients with AIDS.[35,179] *H. influenzae* type b has been a frequent pathogen.[180]

Malacoplakia, a chronic persistent bacterial infection, may present as a granulomatous conjunctival lesion.[181] The most common organism seen in this condition is *E. coli*, although other pathogens have been identified. The disease is believed to be the result of a defect in intracellular bacteriolysis. Although medical management succeeds infrequently, a case with conjunctival involvement was successfully treated with systemic ciprofloxacin.[181] Sepsis following *S. aureus* conjunctivitis has been reported in a patient with AIDS and chemotherapy-induced neutropenia.[179]

References

1. Chandler JW, Gillette TE. Immunologic defense mechanisms of the ocular surface. *Ophthalmology.* 1983;90:585.
2. Gilger BC. Immunology of the ocular surface. *Vet Clin North Am Small Anim Pract.* 2008;38:223.
3. Dawson CR. How does the external eye resist infection? *Invest Ophthalmol.* 1976;15:971.
4. McClellan BH, Whitney CR, Newman LP, Allansmith MR. Immunoglobulins in tears. *Am J Ophthalmol.* 1973;76:89.
5. Selinger DS, Selinger RC, Reed WP. Resistance to infection of the external eye: the role of tears. *Surv Ophthalmol.* 1979;24:33.
6. Williams RC, Gibbons RJ. Inhibition of bacterial adherence by secretory immunoglobulin A: a mechanism of antigen disposal. *Science.* 1972;177:697.
7. Mongomery P, Rockey J, Majumdar A, et al. Parameters influencing the expression of IgA antibodies in tears. *Invest Ophthalmol Vis Sci.* 1984;25:369.
8. Knop E, Knop N, Claus P. Local production of secretory IgA in the eye-associateed lymphoid tissue (EALT) of the normal human ocular surface. *Invest Ophthalmolo Vis Sci.* 2008;49:2322–2329.
9. Yamamoto GK, Allansmith MR. Complement in tears from normal humans. *Am J Ophthalmol.* 1979;88:758.
10. Ridley R. Lysozyme: an antimicrobial present in great concentrations in tears, and its relation to infection of the human eye. *Proc R Soc Med.* 1978;21:1495.
11. Rotkis WM. Lysozyme: its significance to external ocular disease. In: O'Connor GR, ed. *Immunologic diseases of the mucous membranes: pathology, diagnosis, and treatment.* New York: Masson; 1980.
12. Stuchell RN, Farris RL, Mandel ID. Basal and reflex human tear analysis. II. Chemical analysis: lactoferrin and lysozyme. *Ophthalmology.* 1981;88:858.
13. Ford LC, DeLange RJ, Petty RW. Identification of a nonlysozymal bactericidal factor (beta lysine) in human tears and aqueous humor. *Am J Ophthalmol.* 1976;81:30.
14. Broekhuyse RM. Tear lactoferrin: a bacteriostatic and complexing protein. *Invest Ophthalmol.* 1974;13:550.
15. Kijlstra A, Jeuissen SHM, Koning KM. Lactoferrin levels in normal human tears. *Br J Ophthalmol.* 1983;67:199.
16. McIntosh RS, Cade JE, Al-Abed M, et al. The spectrum of antimicrobial peptide expression at the ocular surface. *Invest Ophthalmol Vis Sci.* 2005;46:1379–1385.
17. Paulsen FP, Varaga D, Steven P. Antimicrobial peptides at the ocular surface. In: Zierhut M, Stern M, Sullivan D, eds. *Immunology of the lacrimal gland, tear film, and ocular surface.* New York: Taylor & Francis; 2005:97–104.
18. Lemp MA, Blackman HJ. Ocular surface defense mechanisms. *Ann Ophthalmol.* 1981;13:61.
19. Ward ME, Watta PJ. The role of specific and nonspecific factors in the interaction of gonococci with host cells. *FEMS symposium.* Vol 2. New York: Academic Press; Gonorrhea – Epidemiology and Pathogenesis, 1977.
20. Gutierrez-Khorazo D, Gutierrez EH. The bacterial flora of the healthy eye. In: Locatcher-Khorazo D, Seegal BC, eds. *Microbiology of the eye.* St Louis: Mosby; 1972.
21. Perkins RE, Kundsin RB, Abrahamsen I, Leibowitz HM. Bacteriology of normal and infected conjunctiva. *J Clin Microbiol.* 1975;1:147.
22. McNatt J, Allen SD, Wilson CA, Dowell VR Jr. Anaerobic flora of the normal conjunctival sac. *Arch Ophthalmol.* 1978;96:1448.
23. Locatcher-Khorazo D, Guitierrez EH. Ocular flora of 1,024 children (1–10 years old), 1,786 young adults (20–35 years old), and 7,461 patients awaiting ocular surgery with no known infection. In: Locathcer-Khorazo D, Seegal BC, eds. *Microbiology of the eye.* St Louis: Mosby; 1972.
24. Khorazo F, Thompson R. The bacterial flora of the normal conjunctiva. *Am J Ophthalmol.* 1935;18:1114.
25. Hautala N, Koskela M, Hautala T. Major age group-specific differences in conjunctival bacteria and evolution of antimicrobial resistance revealed by laboratory data surveillance. *Curr Eye Res.* 2008;33:907.
26. Tarabishy AB, Hall GS, Procop GW, et al. Bacterial culture isolates from hospitalized pediatric patients with conjunctivitis. *Am J Ophthalmol.* 2006;142:678.
27. Barefoot SF, Harmon KM, Grinstead DA, Nettles CG. Bacteriocins, molecular biology. In: Lederberg H, ed. *Encyclopedia of microbiology.* Vol 1. New York, 1992, Academic Press.
28. Hsu C, Wiseman GM. Antibacterial substances from staphylococci. *Can J Microbiol.* 1967;13:947.
29. Fredrickson AG. Behavior of mixed cultures of microorganisms. *Annu Rev Microbiol.* 1977;31:63.
30. Chandler JW, Axelrod AJ. Conjunctival-associated lymphoid tissue. In: O'Connor GR, ed. *Immunologic diseases of the mucous membranes.* New York: Masson; 1980.
31. Knop N, Knop E. Conjunctiva-associated lymphoid tissue in the human eye. *Invest Ophthalmolo Vis Sci.* 2000;41:1270.
32. Friedlander MH, West C, Cyr R. The role of the eosinophil, basophil and mast cell in conjunctival immunopathology. In: O'Connor GR, ed. *Immunologic diseases of the mucous membranes: pathology, diagnosis and treatment.* New York: Masson; 1980.
33. Smolin G, Tabbara K, Whitcher J. The conjunctiva. In: *Infectious diseases of the eye.* Baltimore: Williams & Wilkins; 1984.
34. Valenton MJ, Tan RV. The changing ocular 'microflora' in compromised patients. *Philippine J Ophthalmol.* 1972;4:149.
35. Friedlander MH, et al. Ocular microbial flora in immunodeficient patients. *Arch Ophthalmol,* 1980;98:1211.
36. Franklin R, Winkelstein J, Seto D. Conjunctivitis and keratoconjunctivitis associated with primary immunodeficiency diseases. *Am J Ophthalmol.* 1977;84:563.
37. Pramhus C, Runyan TE, Lindberg RB. Ocular flora in the severely burned patients. *Arch Ophthalmol.* 1978;96:1421.
38. Suie T, Havener WH. Bacteriologic studies of socket infections. *Am J Ophthalmol.* 1964;57:749.
39. Pearce WA, Buchanan TM. Attachment role of gonococcal pili. *J Clin Invest.* 1978;61:931.
40. Hyndiuk RA. Experimental *Pseudomonas* keratitis. *Trans Am Ophthalmol Soc.* 1981;79:541.
41. Zimianski CM, Dawson CR, Togni B. Epithelial cell phagocytosis of *L. monocytogenes* in the conjunctiva. *Invest Ophthalmol Vis Sci.* 1974;13:623.
42. Mulks MH, Kornfeld SJ, Plaut AG. Specific proteolysis of human IgA by *Streptococcus pneumoniae* and *Haemophilus influenzae. J Infect Dis.* 1980;141:450.
43. Plaut A. Microbial IgA proteases. *N Engl J Med.* 1978;298:1459.
44. Fahmy JA, Moller S, Bentzon MW. Bacterial flora of the normal conjunctiva. 1. Topographical distribution. *Acta Ophthalmol (Copenh).* 1974;52:786.
45. Spector FE, Eagle RC Jr, Nichols CW. Granulomatous conjunctivitis secondary to *Treponema pallidum. Ophthalmology.* 1981;88:863–865.
46. Duke-Elder S, ed. *System of ophthalmology, vol. 8. Part 1. Diseases of the outer eye, Bacterial conjunctivitis.* St Louis: Mosby; 1965.
47. Kluever HC. Streptococci in inflammations of the eye: report of 18 cases. *Arch Ophthalmol.* 1935;14:805.
48. Givner I. Purulent, membranous, and pseudomembranous conjunctivitis. In: *Infectious diseases of the conjunctiva and cornea: Symposium of the New Orleans Academy of Ophthalmology.* St Louis: Mosby; 1963.
49. Syed NA, Hyndiuk RA. Infectious conjunctivitis. In: Barza M, Baum J, eds. *Infectious disease clinics of North America, ocular infections.* Philadelphia: WB Saunders; 1992.

50. Ostler HB, Thygeson P, Okumoto M. Infectious diseases of the eye. Part II. Infections of the conjunctiva. *J Contin Educ Ophthalmol.* 1978;40:11.
51. Piringer JF. *Die Blenorrhoe am Menschenauge.* Eline von dem deutschen ärztlichen Vereime in St. Petersburg gekrönte, Preisschrift. 80. Grätz, 1841.
52. Neisser A. *Ueber eine der Gonorrhoe eigentumliche Micrococcusfrom, viorlaufige Mitteilung. Centralblatt fur die medicinischen.* Berlin: Wissenschaften, Jahrg; 1879.
53. Handsfield HH, et al. Asymptomatic gonorrhea in men. *N Engl J Med.* 1974;290:117.
54. Bruins SC, Tight RR. Laboratory-acquired gonococcal conjunctivitis. *JAMA.* 1979;241:274.
55. Valenton MJ, Abendanio R. Gonorrheal conjunctivitis. *Can J Ophthalmol.* 1973;8:421.
56. Haimovici T, Roussel TJ. Treatment of gonococcal conjunctivitis with single-dose intramuscular ceftriaxone. *Am J Ophthalmol.* 1989;107:511–514.
57. Alfonso E, et al. *Neisseria gonorrhoeae* conjunctivitis: an outbreak during an epidemic of acute hemorrhagic conjunctivitis. *JAMA.* 1983;250:794.
58. Diena BB, et al. Gonococcal conjunctivitis: accidental infection. *Can Med Assoc J.* 1976;115:609.
59. Rothenberg R. Ophthalmia neonatorum due to *Neisseria gonorrhoeae*: prevention and treatment. *Sex Transm Dis.* 1979;6(suppl):187.
60. Fuerst R, ed. *Frobisher and Fuerst's microbiology in health and disease.* Philadelphia: WB Saunders; 1983.
61. Barquet N, et al. Primary meningococcal conjunctivitis: report of 21 patients and review. *Rev Infect Dis.* 1990;12:838.
62. De Souza AL, Seguro A. Conjunctivitis secondary to *Neisseria meningitidis*: a potential vertical transmission pathway. *Clin Pediatr.* 2009;48:119.
63. Al-Mutlaq F, Byrne-Rhodes KA, Tabbara KF. Neisseria meningitis conjunctivitis in children. *Am J Ophthalmol.* 1987;104:280.
64. Hedges TR Jr, McAllister RM, Coriell LL, Moore W. Metastatic endophthalmitis as a complication of meningococcal meningitis. *Arch Ophthalmol.* 1956;55:503.
65. Brisner JH, Hess JB. Meningococcal endophthalmitis without meningitis. *Can J Ophthalmol.* 1981;16:100.
66. Kestelyn P, Bogaerts J, Meheus A. Gonorrheal keratoconjunctivitis in African adults. *Sex Transm Dis.* 1987;14:191.
67. Ullman S, et al. *Neisseria gonorrhoeae* keratoconjunctivitis. *Ophthalmology.* 1987;94:525.
68. Hyndiuk RA, Skorich DN, Burd EM. Bacterial keratitis. In: Tabbara KF, Hyndiuk RA, eds. *Infections of the eye.* Boston: Little Brown; 1986.
69. Allen JH, Erdman GH. Meningococcic keratoconjunctivitis. *Am J Ophthalmol.* 1946;29:21.
70. Thatcher RW, Pettit TH. Gonorrheal conjunctivitis. *JAMA.* 1971;215:1494.
71. Faruki H, Kohmescher RN, McKinney WP, Sparking PF. A community-based outbreak of infection with penicillin-resistant *Neisseria gonorrhoeae* not producing penicillinase (chromosomally mediated resistance). *N Engl J Med.* 1985;313:607.
72. Plasmid-mediated tetracycline-resistant *Neisseria gonorrhoeae*: Georgia, Massachusetts, Oregon. *MMWR.* 1986;35:304.
73. Knapp JS, et al. Frequency and distribution in the United States of strains of *Neisseria gonorrhoeae* with plasmid-mediated, high-level resistance to tetracycline. *J Infect Dis.* 1987;155:819.
74. Boslego JW, et al. Effect of spectinomycin use on the prevalence of spectinomycin-resistant and of penicillinase-producing *Neisseria gonorrhoeae. N Engl J Med.* 1978;317:272.
75. Division of STD/HIV prevention. *Sexually transmitted disease surveillance, 1992.* US Department of Health and Human Services, Public Health Service. Atlanta: Centers for Disease Control and Prevention; 1993.
76. Schwarcz SK, et al. National surveillance of antimicrobial resistance in *Neisseria gonorrhoeae. JAMA.* 1990;264:1413.
77. Handfield HH, Sparling PF. *Neisseria gonorrhoeae.* In: Mandell GL, Bennet JE, Dolin RP, eds. *Principles and practice of infectious diseases.* 4th ed. New York: Churchill Livingstone; 1995.
78. Perrine PL, Morton RS, Piot P, et al. Epidemiology and treatment of penicillinase-producing *Neisseria gonorrhoeae. Sex Transm Dis.* 1979;6(Z suppl):152.
79. Kubanova A, Frigo N, Kubanova A, et al. National surveillance of antimicrobial susceptibility in *Neisseria gonorrhoeae* in 2005–2006 and recommendation of first-line antimicrobial drugs for gonorrhoea treatment in Russia. *Sex Transm Infect.* 2008;84:285.
80. Handsfield HH, et al. Correlation of autotype and penicillin susceptibility of *Neisseria gonorrhoeae* with sexual preference and clinical manifestations of gonorrhea. *Sex Transm Dis.* 1980;7:1.
81. Centers for Disease Control and Prevention. 1993 Sexually transmitted disease treatment guidelines. *MMWR.* 1993;42(Suppl RR-14):47.
82. Zajdowicz TR, Kerbs SB, Berg SW, Harrison WO. Laboratory acquired gonococcal conjunctivitis: successful treatment with single-dose ceftriaxone. *Sex Transm Dis.* 1984;11:28.
83. Kestelyn P, et al. Treatment of adult gonococcal keratoconjunctivitis with oral norfloxacin. *Am J Ophthalmol.* 1989;108:516.
84. Judson FN. The importance of coexisting syphilitic, chlamydial, mycoplasmal, and trichomonal infections in the treatment of gonorrhea. *Sex Transm Dis.* 1979;6:112.
85. Laga M, et al. Single-dose therapy of gonococcal ophthalmia neonatorum with ceftriaxone. *N Engl J Med.* 1986;315:1382.
86. Alexander ER. Gonorrhea in the newborn. *Ann NY Acad Sci.* 1988;549:180.
87. Berkow R, ed. *The Merck manual of diagnosis and therapy.* Rahway, NJ: Merck Sharp & Dohme; 1977.
88. Klein JO, ed. *Report of the Committee on Infectious Disease.* Evanston, IL: American Academy of Pediatrics; 1982.
89. Centers for Disease Control and Prevention. *MMWR.* 1976;25:56.
90. Brook I, Pettit TH, Martin WJ, Finegold SM. Anaerobic and aerobic bacteriology of acute conjunctivitis. *Ann Ophthalmol.* 1979;11:389.
91. Gigliotti F, et al. Etiology of acute conjunctivitis in children. *J Pediatr.* 1981;98:531.
92. Locatcher-Khorazo D, Seegal BC, eds. *Microbiology of the eye.* St Louis: Mosby; 1972.
93. Brook I. Anaerobic and aerobic bacterial flora of acute conjunctivitis in children. *Arch Ophthalmol.* 1980;98:833.
94. Weiss A, Brinser JH, Nazar-Stewart V. Acute conjunctivitis in childhood. *J Pediatr.* 1993;122:10.
95. Isenberg SJ, et al. Controlled trial of povidone-iodine to treat infectious conjunctivitis in children. *Am J Ophthalmol.* 2002;134:681.
96. Fitch CP, et al. Epidemiology and diagnosis of acute conjunctivitis at an inner-city hospital. *Ophthalmology.* 1989;96:1215.
97. Mannis MJ. Bacteria conjunctivitis. In: Tasman W, Jaeger EA, eds. *Duane's clinical ophthalmology.* Vol 4. Philadelphia: JB Lippincott; 1990.
98. Givner I. Catarrhal conjunctivitis. In: *Infectious diseases of the conjunctiva and cornea: symposium of the New Orleans Academy of Ophthalmology.* St Louis: Mosby; 1963.
99. Fedukowicz HB, Stenson S, eds. *External infections of the eye, bacteria.* Norwalk, CT: Appleton, Century, Crofts; 1985.
100. Davis DJ, Pittman M. Acute conjunctivitis caused by *Haemophilus. Am J Dis Child.* 1950;79:211.
101. Gingrich WD. *Haemophilus*-type infections. In: *Infectious diseases of the conjunctiva and cornea: symposium of the New Orleans Academy of Ophthalmology.* St Louis: Mosby; 1963.
102. Koch R. Berichte über die Tätigkeit der Deutchen Cholerakomission in aegypten und Ostindien. *Wien Med Wochenschr.* 1883;33:1548.
103. Weeks JE. The bacillus of acute conjunctival catarrhal or pink eye. *Arch Ophthalmol.* 1886;15:1441.
104. Davis P, Pittman M. Effectiveness of streptomycin in treatment of experimental conjunctivitis caused by *Haemophilus* sp. *Am J Ophthalmol.* 1949;32:111.
105. Bodor FF. Conjunctivitis-otitis syndrome. *Pediatrics.* 1982;69:695.
106. Bodor FF, et al. Bacterial etiology of conjunctivitis-otitis media syndrome. *Pediatrics.* 1985;76:26.
107. Harrison LA, et al. Epidemiology and clinical spectrum of Brazilian purpuric fever. Brazilian Purpuric Fever Study Group. *J Clin Microbiol.* 1989;27:599.
108. Centers for Disease Control: Epidemic fatal purpuric fever among children-Brazil. *MMWR.* 1985;34:217.
109. Brazilian Purpuric Fever Study Group. Epidemic purpura fulminans associated with antecedent purulent conjunctivitis. *Lancet.* 1987;2:758.
110. Brazilian Purpuric Fever Study Group. *Haemophilus aegyptius* bacteremia in Brazilian purpuric fever. *Lancet.* 1987;2:761.
111. Boralkar AN. Diphtheritic conjunctivitis: a rare case report in Indian literature. *Ind J Ophthalmol.* 1989;101:437.
112. Chandler JW, Milam DF. Diphtheria corneal ulcers. *Arch Ophthalmol.* 1978;96:53.
113. van Bijsterveld OP. Acute conjunctivitis and *Moraxella. Am J Ophthalmol.* 1968;63:1702.
114. Schwartz B, et al. Investigation of an outbreak of *Moraxella* conjunctivitis at a Navajo boarding school. *Am J Ophthalmol.* 1989;107:341.
115. van Bijsterveld OP. The incidence of *Moraxella* on mucous membranes and the skin. *Am J Ophthalmol.* 1972;74:72.
116. Romberger JA, Wald ER, Wright PF. *Branhamella catarrhalis* conjunctivitis. *South Med J.* 1987;80:926.
117. Au Y-K, Reynolds MD, Rambin ED, Mahjoub SB. *Neisseria cinerea* acute purulent conjunctivitis. *Am J Ophthalmol.* 1990;109:96.
118. Parenti DM, Snydman DR. *Capnocytophaga* species: infections in nonimmunocompromised and immunocompromised hosts. *J Infect Dis.* 1985;151:140.
119. Lessner AM, Webb RM, Rabin B. *Vibrio alginolyticus* conjunctivitis. *Arch Ophthalmol.* 1985;103:229.

120. Feingold M, Gellis SS. Cellulitis due to *Haemophilus influenzae* type B. *N Engl J Med.* 1965;272:788.
121. Londer L, Nelson DL. Orbital cellulitis due to *Haemophilus influenzae*. *Arch Ophthalmol.* 1974;91:89.
122. Bodor FF. Conjunctivitis-otitis media syndrome: more than meets the eye. *Contemp Pediatr.* 1989;6:55.
123. von Bijsterveld OP. Host-parasite relationship and taxonomic position of *Moraxella* and morphologically related organisms. *Am J Ophthalmol.* 1973;76:545.
124. Baum J, Fedukowicz HB, Jordan A. A survey of *Moraxella* corneal ulcers in a derelict population. *Am J Ophthalmol.* 1980;90:476.
125. Leibowitz HM, et al. Human conjunctivitis. I. Diagnostic evaluation. *Arch Ophthalmol.* 1976;94:1747.
126. Sheikh A, Hurwitz B, Cave J. Antibiotics for acute bacterial conjunctivits. *Cochrane Database Syst Rev.* 2006;2:CD001211.
127. Sheikh A, Hurwitz B. Topical antibiotics for acute bacterial conjunctivitis, a systematic review. *Br J Gen Pract.* 2001;467:473.
128. Liebowitz HM. Antibacterial effectiveness of ciprofloxacin 0.3% ophthalmic solution in the treatment of bacterial conjunctivitis. *Am J Ophthalmol.* 1991;112:29S.
129. Gigliotti F, et al. Efficacy of topical antibiotic therapy in acute conjunctivitis in children. *J Pediatr.* 1984;104:623.
130. Glasser DB, Hyndiuk RA. Ophthalmic antibiotics. In: Lamberts DW, Potter D, eds. *Clinical ophthalmic pharmacology.* Boston: Little Brown; 1987.
131. Ofloxacin Study Gorup III. A placebo-controlled clinical study of the fluoroquinolone ofloxacin in patients with external infection. *Invest Ophthalmol Vis Sci.* 1990;31:572.
132. Gross RD, Hoffman RO, Lindsay RA. A comparison of ciprofloxacin and tobramycin in bacterial conjunctivitis in children. *Clin Pediatr.* 1997;36:435.
133. Lohr JA, Austin RD, Grossman M, et al. Comparison of three topical antimicrobials for acute bacterial conjunctivitis. *Pediatr Infect Dis J.* 1988;7:626.
134. Miller IM, Vogel R, Cook TJ, Wittreich J. Topically administered norfloxacin compared with topically administered gentamicin for the treatment of external ocular bacterial infections. The Worldwide Norfloxacin Ophthalmic Study Group. *Am J Ophthalmol.* 1992;113:638.
135. Schwab IR, Friedlaender M, McCulley J, et al. Levofloxacin Bacterial Conjunctivitis Active Control Study Group: A phase III clinical trial of 0.5% levofloxacin ophthalmic solution versus 0.3% ofloxacin ophthalmic solution for the treatment of bacterial conjunctivitis. *Ophthalmology.* 2003;110:457.
136. Protzko E, Bowman L, Abelson M, et al. Phase 3 safety comparisons of 1.0% azithromycin in polymeric mucoadhesive eye drops versus 0.3% tobramycin eye drops for bacterial conjunctivitis. *Invest Ophthalmol Vis Sci.* 2007;48:3425.
137. Yee RW, Tepedino M, Bernstein P, et al. A randomized, investigator-masked clinical trial comparing the efficacy and safety of gatifloxacin 0.3 % administered BID versus QID for the treatment of acute bacterial conjunctivitis. *Curr Med Tes Opin.* 2005;21:425.
138. Abelson MB, Heller W, Shapiro AM, et al. Clinical cure of bacterial conjunctivitis with azythromycin 1%: vehicle-controlled, double-masked clinical trial. *Am J Ophthalmol.* 2008;145:959.
139. Leibowitz HM, et al. Tobramycin in external eye disease: a double-masked study vs. gentamycin. *Curr Eye Res.* 1981;1:259.
140. Mehta NJ, Webb RM, Krohel GB, Smith RS. Clinical inefficacy of tobramycin and gentamicin sulfate in the treatment of ocular infections. *Cornea.* 1984;3:228.
141. Kowalski RP, Karenchak LM, Romanowski MS. Infectious disease: changing antibiotic susceptibility. *Ophthalmol Clin N Am.* 2003;16:1–9.
142. Gwon A, the Ofloxacin Study Group. Topical ofloxacin compared with gentamicin in the treatment of external ocular infection. *Br J Ophthalmol.* 1992;76:714.
143. Gwon A, the Ofloxacin Study Group II. Ofloxacin vs tobramycin for the treatment of external ocular infection. *Arch Ophthalmol.* 1992;110:1234.
144. Block SL, Hedrick J, Tyler R, et al. Increasing bacterial resistance in pediatric acute conjunctivitis. *Antimicrob Agents Chemother.* 2000; 44:1650.
145. Goldstein ML, Kowalski RP, Gordon YJ. Emerging fluoroquinolone resistance in bacterial keratitis: a 5-year review. *Ophthalmology.* 1999; 106:1313.
146. Kowalski RP, Pandya AN, Karenchak LM, et al. An in vitro resistance study of levofloxacin, ciprofloxacin, and ofloxacin using keratitis isolates of *Staphylococcus aureus* and *Pseudomonas aeruginosa*. *Ophthalmology.* 2001;108:1826.
147. Cavuoto K, Zutshi D, Karp CL, et al. Update on bacterial conjunctivitis in South Florida. *Ophthalmology.* 2008;115;51.
148. Mather R, Karenchak LM, Romanowski EG, et al. Fourth generation fluoroquinalones. New weapons in the arsenal of ophthalmic antibiotics. *Am J Opahthalmol.* 2002;133:463.
149. Freidlin J, Acharua M, Lietman TA, et al. Spectrum of eye disease caused by methicillin-resistant *Staphylococcus aureus*. *Am J Ophthalmol.* 2007;144:313.
150. Asbell PA, Colby KA, Deng S, et al. Ocular TRUST: nationwide antimicrobial susceptibility patterns in ocular isolates. *Am J Ophthamol.* 2008;145:951.
151. Cambau E, Matrat S, Pan XS, et al. Target specificity of the new fluoroquinolone besifloxacin in *Streptococcus pneumoniae, Staphylococcus aureus* and *Escherichia coli*. *J Antimicrob Chemother.* 2009;63:443.
152. Hwang D. Systemic antibiotic therapy for relapsing *Haemophilus influenzae* conjunctivitis. *Am J Ophthalmol.* 1993;115:814.
153. Thygeson P, Kimura S. Chronic conjunctivitis. *Trans Am Acad Ophthalmol Otolaryngol.* 1963;67:494.
154. Thygeson P. Bacterial factors in chronic catarrhal conjunctivitis. *Arch Ophthalmol.* 1973;18:373.
155. Mondino BJ, Caster AI, Dethlefs B. A rabbit model of staphylococcal blepharitis. *Arch Ophthalmol.* 1987;105:409.
156. Gunderson T. In discussion of Thygeson P: Clinical signs of diagnostic importance in conjunctivitis. *Trans Sect Ophth AMA.* 1946;95:76.
157. Valenton MJ, Okumoto M. Toxin-producing strains of *Staphylococcus epidemidis* (albus): isolates from patients with staphylococcal blepharoconjunctivitis. *Arch Ophthalmol.* 1973;89:186.
158. Morax V. Note sur un diplobacille pathogene pour la conjunctivite humaine. *Ann Inst Pasteur (Paris).* 1896;10:337.
159. Kowalski RP, Harwick JC. Incidence of *Moraxella* conjunctivitis infection. *Am J Ophthalmol.* 1986;101:437.
160. Podgore JK, Holmes KK. Ocular gonococcal infection with little or no inflammatory response. *JAMA.* 1981;246:242.
161. Boruchoff SA, Boruchoff SA. Infections of the lacrimal system. In: Barza M, Baum J, eds. *Infectious diseases of North America, ocular infections.* Philadelphia: WB Saunders; 1992.
162. Van Winkelhoff AJ, Abbas F, Pavicic MJ, de Graaff J. Chronic conjunctivitis caused by oral anaerobes and effectively treated with systemic metronidazole plus amoxicillin. *J Clin Microbiol.* 1991;29:723.
163. Allen JH. Staphylococcic conjunctivitis: experimental reproduction with staphyloccic toxin. *Am J Ophthalmol.* 1937;20:1025.
164. Mondino BJ, Kowalski RP. Phlyctenulae and catarrhal infiltrates: occurrence in rabbits immunized with staphylococcal cell walls. *Arch Ophthalmol.* 1982;100:1968.
165. Mondino BJ, Dethlefs B. Occurrence of phlyctenules after immunization with ribitol teichoic acid of *Staphylococcus aureus*. *Arch Ophthalmol.* 1984;102:461.
166. McCullun JP. Blepharoconjunctivitis. *Int Ophthalmol Clin.* 1984;24:65.
167. Bowman RW, Dougherty JM, McCully JP. Chronic blepharitis and dry eye. *Int Ophthalmol Clin.* 1987;27:27.
168. Woods AC. *Endogenous uveitis.* Baltimore: Williams & Wilkins; 1956.
169. Duke-Elder S. *Systems of ophthalmology, vol. IX: Diseases of the uveal tract.* St Louis: Mosby; 1966.
170. Bruce GM, Locatcher-Khorazo D. Primary tuberculosis of the conjunctiva. *Arch Ophthalmol.* 1947;37:375.
171. Goldfarb AA, Seltzer I. Primary tuberculosis of the conjunctiva. *Am J Child.* 1946;72:211.
172. Anhalt EF, et al. Conjunctival tuberculosis. *Am J Ophthalmol.* 1960;50:265.
173. Chandler AC Jr, Locatcher-Khorazo D. Primary tuberculosis of the conjunctiva. *Arch Ophthalmol.* 1964;71:202.
174. Blegvard O. Fortgesetzte Untersuchungen über die conjunctivaltuberkulose. *Acta Ophthalmol (Copenh).* 1936;14:200.
175. Liesegang TJ, Cameron D. *Mycobacterium bovis* infection of the conjunctiva. *Arch Ophthalmol.* 1980;98:1764.
176. Meyers JA. *Tuberculosis: a half century of study and conquest.* St Louis: Warren H Green; 1970.
177. Lau RKW, et al. Adult gonococcal keratoconjunctivitis with AIDS. *Br J Ophthalmol.* 1990;42:52.
178. Nanda M, Pflugfelder SC, Holland S. Fulminant pseudomonal keratitis and scleritis in human immunodeficiency virus-infected patients. *Arch Ophthalmol.* 1991;109:503.
179. Wolf MD, Pfaller MA, Hollis RJ, Weingeist TA. *Staphylococcus aureus* conjunctivitis and sepsis in a neutropenic patient. *Am J Ophthalmol.* 1989;107:87.
180. Franklin RM, Winkelstein JA, Seto DSY. Conjunctivitis and keratoconjunctivitis with primary immunodeficiency diseases. *Am J Ophthalmol.* 1977;84:563.
181. Simpson C, Dickinson J, Sandford-Smith JH. Medical management of ocular malacoplakia. *Ophthlomology.* 1992;99:192.
182. Amerisource wholesaler (address pending)

Chapter 44

Viral Conjunctivitis

Lênio Alvarenga, Marinho Scarpi, Mark J. Mannis

Viral conjunctivitis is a common form of ocular morbidity. The severity of the disease may range considerably, and a number of viruses have been identified as causes. The differentiation of these causes is important, since therapy may not only be based on symptomatic relief but also may include antiviral and/or antiinflammatory drugs, the use of which requires a specific diagnosis.

The clinical hallmark of most viral conjunctivitis is the follicular reaction of the conjunctiva, although this feature may also be present in chlamydial infection and toxic conjunctivitis as well. Follicles are the macroappearance of aggregates of lymphocytes surrounded by plasma and mast cells in the superficial conjunctival stroma of the conjunctiva (Fig. 44.1). During its enlargement, the cluster of immune cells displaces the blood vessels peripherally. As such, the biomicroscopic finding is a yellowish-white oval mound with dilated blood vessels in the periphery.

Both RNA- and DNA-containing viruses can infect the conjunctiva. The former usually cause more benign forms of conjunctivitis, while the latter are more frequently associated with vision-threatening forms of inflammation.

DNA Viruses

Adenoviruses

Adenoviruses (Ad) are the most common cause of viral conjunctivitis. Fifty-one distinct human adenoviral serotypes have been described[1,2] and are classified into six subgenera (A–F). More than half of all adenoviral serotypes (32) belong to subgenus D. With few exceptions, most adenoviral conjunctivitis is caused by this subgenus. The application of restriction endonucleases and the analysis of cleavage patterns have led to the identification of different genotypes of a single serotype (e.g. eight different genotypes of adenovirus 8 have been described (Ad8A–Ad8H).[3]

Classically, ocular Ad infection is grouped into four different clinical presentations: (1) pharyngoconjunctival fever (PCF); (2) epidemic keratoconjunctivitis (EKC); (3) acute nonspecific follicular conjunctivitis; and (4) chronic keratoconjunctivitis.

Pharyngoconjunctival fever (PCF) is characterized by pharyngitis, follicular conjunctivitis, fever, and adenopathy (preauricular and cervical). Diarrhea and rhinitis are often associated symptoms. Ad 3, 4, and 7 are the causative agents in most of the reported cases, although Ad 1, 2, 5, and 14 have also been implicated. This highly infectious disease occurs in small outbreaks. It is transmissible by three routes: personal contact, fomites, or through swimming pools or ponds. PCF is one of the most common illnesses seen by physicians at children's summer camps.[4] The communicability is extremely high during the first several days and might last for 2 weeks after the onset of the symptoms.

The onset is acute, after 5 to 14 days of incubation. Most of the patients present with symptoms 6 to 9 days after exposure, especially when contaminated water is the source of infection.[5] Pharyngitis varies from a mild sore throat to severe and painful inflammation causing difficult and painful swallowing. Examination of the posterior oropharynx reveals reddened mucosa without exudates. The pharyngitis as well as the fever may last up to 10 days. Lower respiratory tract infection, hepato- or splenomegaly, and rash are uncommon and may suggest a nonadenoviral etiology.

The ocular findings are often present at the onset of the disease. Initial symptoms vary in severity even within the same outbreak. PCF is most commonly bilateral, and the eyes may be affected simultaneously or in sequence up to 3 days apart. Normally, the second eye is clinically less severe. Initially, the patient complains of the abrupt onset of itching and irritation. The serous discharge may be abundant and often leads to crusting of the superior and inferior lashes, causing difficulty with opening the eyes on awakening. The hyperemia involves the entire conjunctiva but is more prominent in the inferior fornix. Mild punctate keratitis may be detectable by 2 days to 1 week after onset of symptoms. Minute punctate dots that stain poorly with rose Bengal and fluorescein are the initial finding. These dots may become diffuse and persist for up to a week. The subepithelial infiltrates (SEIs) of the type seen in EKC are not frequent in patients with PCF.

Epidemic keratoconjunctivitis (EKC) is the severest ocular disease caused by adenoviruses.[6] Ad 8, 19, and 37 are the serotypes most commonly associated with EKC, but many other types have been documented.[7] Mixed infection can occur. Ad 8 is the classic cause of EKC, and its clinical picture is the prototype of ocular changes induced by adenoviral disease.[8] Transmissibility is high during the first days of symptoms, and hospital outbreaks are not uncommon. In

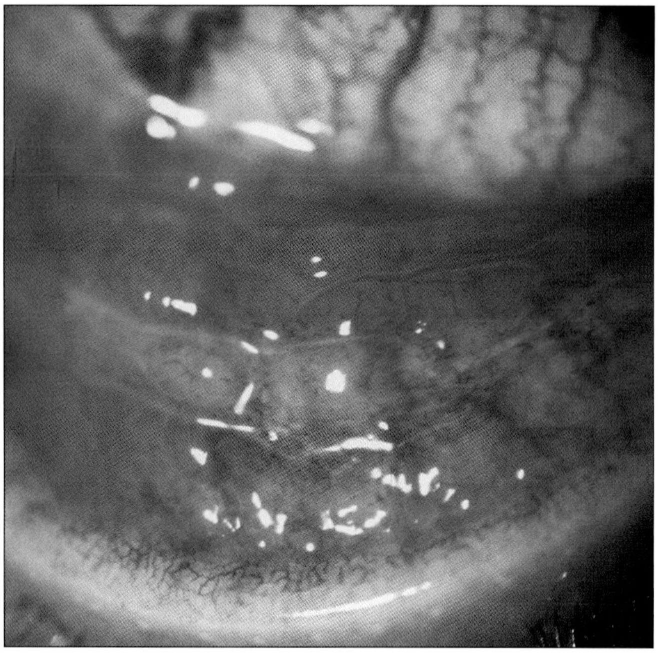

Fig. 44.1 Follicles in a patient with adenoviral infection. Fluorescein demarcates the elevated follicles.

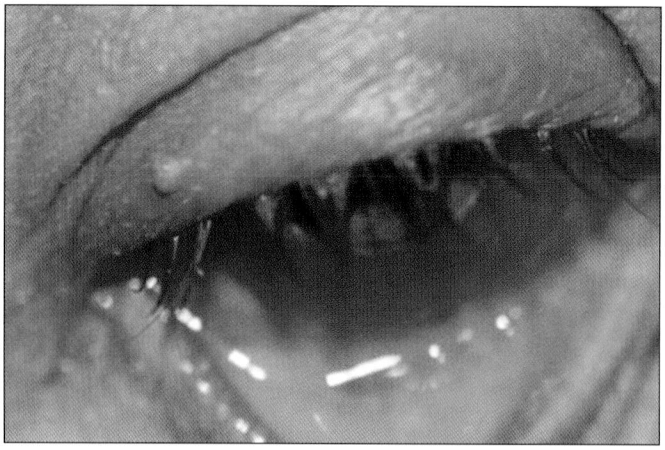

Fig. 44.2 Epidemic keratoconjunctivitis. Lid edema, crusting of the eyelashes, and membrane.

communities with epidemics, the transmission occurs by contaminated fingers or objects, sexual contact, and swimming pool water. Instruments (such as tonometer tips) can also spread the disease along with hand contact in the doctor's office.

Ocular signs and symptoms are often more severe than those found in patients with PCF, but the two conditions may be indistinguishable on biomicroscopy. The absence of extraocular manifestations and severe stromal infiltrates in EKC are the differentiating features. EKC has a higher prevalence (up to half of patients) of unilateral disease when compared to PCF. Conjunctival involvement ranges from mild inflammation with diffuse hyperemia and a mixed follicular and papillary reaction (both more intense in the lower fornix) to a severe response with subconjunctival hemorrhages and intense inflammation. Pseudomembranes (inflammatory debris and fibrin) or true membranes (Fig. 44.2) are a marker of severe conjunctival involvement. True membranes bleed when removed, and their presence makes the patient uncomfortable. Membranes can also rub against the cornea, causing mechanical, geographic ulcers that can mimic herpetic keratitis.

The initial corneal alteration in EKC can be detected as early as two days after the onset of the disease, as epithelial vesicle-like elevations of about 25–30 μm in diameter, hardly perceptible at the slit lamp, develop. By day 5, these elevations are easily visible both with and without fluorescein (the epithelial protrusions causing dark 'holes' in the stained tear film).[8] These findings are classified as stage 0 and stage I adenoviral keratitis, respectively. Histological preparations of these focal lesions obtained at this stage have demonstrated scattered swollen cells and round or globular cells with various shapes and sizes, some fused to syncytia. These fused cells may exhibit necrosis and alterations in the cell surface.[9] The next stage (II) persists for 2 to 5 days and is characterized by a coalescence of the lesions and involvement of the deep epithelium.

The incidence of stage 0–II keratitis ranges from as low as 13% to as high as 70% of patients with EKC.[3,10] This broad range is apparently related to the serotype as well as the genotype of the virus (e.g. Ad8H has a higher incidence of keratitis when compared to Ad8C and Ad8E).[3] Marked worsening of photophobia, tearing, and discomfort heralds the presence of keratitis. The duration of the superficial keratitis is usually less than 2 weeks but, in Ad8 infections is typically longer (over 3 weeks) and with a higher incidence of both coarse lesions and progression to subepithelial infiltrates (SEIs). The superficial keratitis may resolve or progress to SEIs in 43% of patients with EKC.[10] In stage III, besides the deep epithelial punctate keratitis, faint SEIs just beneath the compromised areas of the epithelium are present (Fig. 44.3). Stage III is typically detected during the second week. These infiltrates must be differentiated from immune-mediated SEIs as a manifestation of graft rejection. In the latter case, there is no conjunctivitis, and SEIs are limited to the donor.

Stages IV and V are detected in or after the third week. No staining is seen. Stage IV is characterized by the classic SEIs that may be present for weeks or months after the infection (Fig. 44.4). Stage V is characterized by punctate epithelial granularity, often overlying subepithelial opacities. The highest incidence of SEIs is associated with Ad 5 and 8. SEIs most commonly diminish with time; however, even with treatment, SEIs may cause photophobia and blurred vision for many months and, in some cases, may lead to visually significant scarring. SEIs are lymphocytic infiltrates in the superficial corneal stroma and the overlying (deep) epithelium and represent an immune reaction against Ad antigens.

The keratitis is usually central, but the periphery can also be affected. Visual acuity is often diminished, especially when there is coalescence of the SEIs in the visual axis. These opacities may cause a decrease in contrast sensitivity and the presence of haloes and/or glare. Paracentral opacities may cause visual disturbances (haloes and/or glare) only in low-lit rooms and during the night, especially when

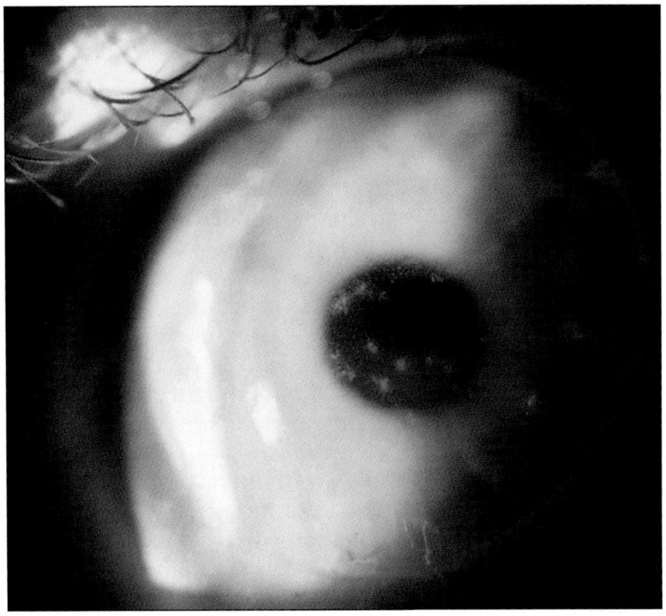

Fig. 44.3 Stage III adenoviral keratitis (second week) in a patient with previous penetrating keratoplasty.

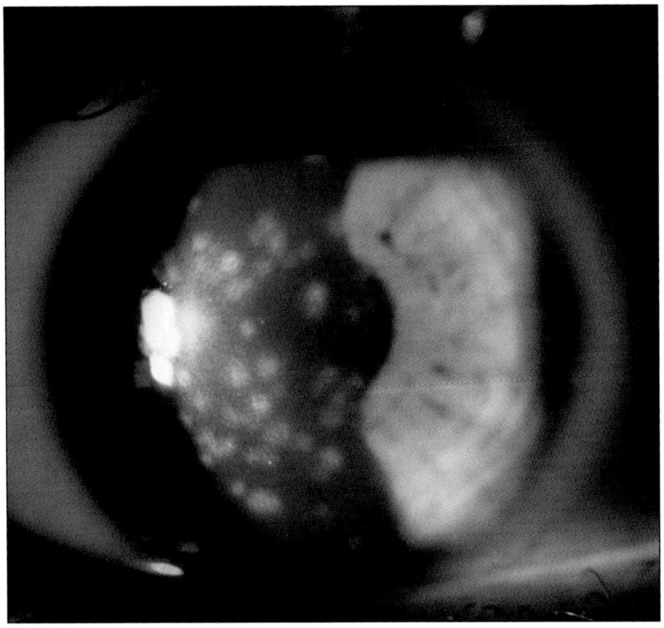

Fig. 44.4 Stage IV adenoviral keratitis (third week). (Courtesy of Dr Denise de Freitas.)

driving. Quantifying the visual discomfort (interview, contrast sensitivity charts, visual acuity) is important when deciding whether or not treat the patient. Nevertheless, there is no standardization of any of these indices regarding eligibility for treatment.

Subconjunctival hemorrhage can be seen in the bulbar and palpebral conjunctiva. It has been described in 33.3% of patients with Ad8 infection,[3] but the incidence is probably lower in infection from other serotypes.

Uveitis is a rare finding in adenovirus conjunctivitis and has been described only in patients with EKC and severe keratitis due to Ad8 infection.[10] It was characterized by a mild flare and small numbers of cells in the aqueous of the anterior chamber. Resolution without complication within few days is the rule.

Acute nonspecific follicular conjunctivitis may be caused by many serotypes of adenovirus, including those classically associated with PCF and EKC. The conjunctival involvement is milder, and keratitis is limited to the epithelium or most commonly is not present. Ocular signs are limited to a mild follicular reaction, mild conjunctival hyperemia, and discrete lid edema. Preauricular adenopathy may be present. The resolution of the signs and symptoms is usually more rapid than in PCF and EKC, and patients are often cured by the beginning of the third week. Some patients infected during an outbreak of EKC will present a mild disease compatible with nonspecific follicular conjunctivitis. The identification of these patients is important, because they might not seek medical assistance, and despite the benign presentation they can serve as a virus reservoir, spreading a not always benign disease in the community.

Chronic conjunctivitis is the least common form of adenovirus conjunctivitis. It was described in 1965[11] and has been reported infrequently.[12,13] Ad 2, 3, 4, and 5 have been isolated. The symptoms persist longer than expected for typical cases of adenoviral disease, and the virus can be recovered many months or years after the onset of symptoms. The conjunctivitis presents with intermittent bouts of ocular irritation with a waxing and waning superficial punctate epithelial keratitis and with SEIs. Both eyes can be affected, and the conjunctiva may present a follicular or a papillary reaction. Spontaneous resolution is the rule.

Adenovirus infection cases considered to be typical, on clinical grounds, are commonly treated without laboratory confirmation.[7] The clinical diagnosis of viral conjunctivitis can be based on the presence of acute conjunctivitis and one of the following features: follicles on the inferior tarsal conjunctiva, preauricular lymphadenopathy, an associated upper respiratory infection, and a recent contact with a person with a red eye.[14]

After performing a systematic literature search and concluding that there was no evidence that signs and symptoms could differentiate viral from bacterial conjunctivitis,[15] Rietveld et al. performed a prospective study involving 184 patients presenting with red eye and either (muco-) purulent discharge or glued eyelid(s), not wearing contact lenses. They identified that patients with early morning glued eye(s) were more likely to present with bacterial conjunctivitis, whereas those with itchy eyes and reporting previous conjunctivitis were more likely diagnosed with non-bacterial etiology.[16] However these findings have been contested by other authors.[17,18]

Identification of the virus is not always necessary, and treatment in most cases will not depend on it. Nevertheless, objective data are important in public health and surveillance programs and in atypical cases. Analysis of conjunctival scrapings and serology are the methods used in adenoviral identification.

The historical gold standard for adenovirus conjunctivitis is cell culture with confirmatory immunofluorescence staining (CC-IFA). Despite being costly and time consuming, the isolation is definitive and allows further characterization.[19]

However, other issues affect the test results (e.g. virus survival after collection/transportation and growth in the medium). Therefore, a trend toward the newer and more rapid PCR techniques, which are more sensitive without losing specificity,[20–22] has been reported.[23,24] PCR undoubtedly achieves the accuracy needed for diagnosis of adenoviral conjunctivitis. Nevertheless, the method lacks the speed and simplicity required for an office-based test. The ideal test, besides providing high accuracy, should also provide the result in a short time (10–30 minutes[19]), so that the practitioner can confirm the diagnosis at the first visit.

Traditional cytology is considered insensitive and subjective by some authors;[25] however, meticulous analysis (quantitative/qualitative) of Giemsa staining can be of help. Paired blood specimens (acute and convalescent titers: first week/one week after cure) revealing a fourfold increase in specific humoral antibody is considered an indication of infection, but absence does not exclude it. Serologic diagnosis based on IgM detection is not always possible, and false-positive results may arise because of cross-reactivity with related pathogens.

Antigen detection techniques are less time consuming and do not require the presence of viable organisms. The sensitivity and specificity are highly variable among the available methods (enzyme immunoassay, immunofluorescence, immunochromatography, specific latex agglutination, immunofiltration, and immune dot-blot). The variation among the methods' results (sensitivity and specificity) is due to different cut-off values for positive results, the experience of the observer in discriminating specific and nonspecific staining (immunofluorescence), cross-reactivity leading to false-positive results (enzyme immunoassays), and different gold standards (culture or clinical diagnosis).

Rapid diagnostic tests are available for Ad detection. The Adenoclone™ test (Cambridge BioScience, Worcester, MA) is an enzyme immunoassay applied directly to conjunctival swabs of infected eyes. In a retrospective analysis,[26] this test showed low sensitivity (38%) with a better result (65%) for samples positive in culture during the first week. The RPS Adeno Detector (Rapid Pathogen Screening Inc., South Williamsport, PA) is based on the principle of lateral flow immunochromatography in which two antigen-specific antibodies capture viral antigens or particles (common epitopes among the serotypes).[23] In this test, tear fluid is collected directly onto a detachable part of the detector, which is then assembled to the other part containing the test strip. In the SAS Adenotest™ Immunochromatography (SA Scientific Ltd., San Antonio, TX) there are additional steps: following a brief extraction step using a buffer containing 0.1% sodium azide, the sample is added to a sample well in a plastic device.[27] When compared to PCR, rapid immunochromatography tests showed the following sensitivity/specificity: RPS = 89% / 94%;[23] SAS 54% / 97%[28] and 72% / 100% in a cohort of patients with epidemic keratoconjunctivitis.[29]

A recent analysis of cost-effectiveness using US data indicated that the incorporation of RPS could avoid much of the cost to society caused by acute conjunctivitis.[30] Nevertheless, besides possible different regional costs associated with each intervention, many assumptions used in the study need to be verified in each setting (e.g. all patients receive antibiotic treatment when no test is used; relationship between number of days absent from work/school and diagnosis).

Treatment

The treatment of adenoviral conjunctivitis includes preventing the transmission and complications as well as providing symptomatic relief. Suspected cases should be examined in a separate area. After the clinical diagnosis, patients must be advised to avoid personal contacts, to wash the hands after touching the eyes, and to avoid sharing towels, pillows, and any personal item that could be contaminated by ocular secretions. Children must be warned to avoid social activities for the duration of the illness. Adults should also avoid any close contact, at least during the period of intense discharge. Restriction of activity of healthcare professionals (direct hand-to-patient contact) for a minimum of 14 days (after onset) is recommended. The examiner should wash hands before and after each examination with use of paper towels. Moreover, cleaning and disinfection are mandatory for all the equipment handled during the examination. In a recent reported nosocomial outbreak[31] the detection rate of adenoviral DNA in environmental swabs was 81%. Chlorine-releasing solutions (e.g. 2% solution of sodium hypochlorite) and povidone-iodine are effective against viruses.[32] Recently prepared chlorine solutions should be used because activity is rapidly lost after dilution.

Cold compresses may provide a temporary relief of symptoms, but some patients will not benefit from them. Considering that the manipulation of the eye and adnexa is not advisable in patients with viral conjunctivitis (to avoid hand contamination and secondary infection) patients can use compresses but should discontinue them if no improvement is noticed. Multidose eyedrop bottles given to patients with adenoviral conjunctivitis are a possible vector for adenoviral transmission, especially to the family members of infected patients.[33] Single-dose medications are preferred. Sunglasses can be of help in patients with photophobia.

Pseudomembranes and membranes should be removed when detected. Cotton-swabs may be used in the procedure but forceps (Fig. 44.5) are usually necessary.

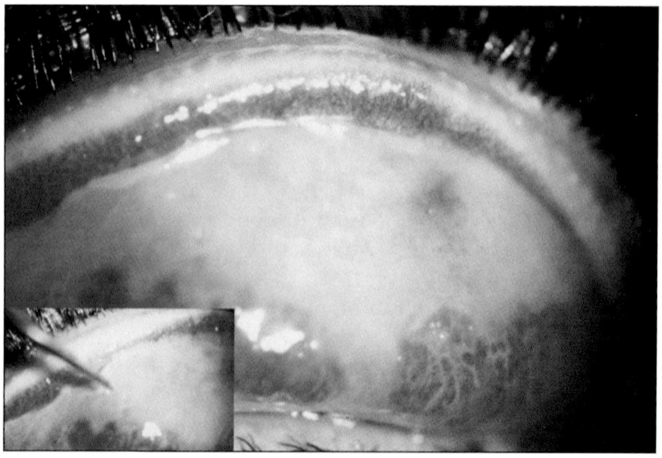

Fig. 44.5 Membrane in a patient with epidemic keratoconjunctivitis (first week). Detail, removal with forceps.

Topical treatment of adenoviral conjunctivitis is controversial. Antiinflammatory agents are of interest, because inflammation of the conjunctiva is an essential feature of viral conjunctivitis, and it is believed to cause many of the symptoms of the infection.[14]

The influence of antiinflammatory drugs on viral replication should be considered. Corticosteroids enhance viral replication and increase the duration of viral shedding. These effects have been demonstrated for both potent (1% prednisolone acetate)[34] and limited potency (0.12% prednisolone acetate, 0.1% fluorometholone, and 1% rimexolone)[35] topical corticosteroids, even when used for a short period. Corticosteroids can also reverse the effect of topical antivirals.[36] Topical nonsteroidal antiinflammatory drugs (NSAIDs) (0.5% ketorolac tromethamine and 0.1% diclofenac sodium), in contrast, do not promote significant differences with respect to viral replication and viral shedding.

The administration of corticosteroids promotes a decrease in inflammation and significant symptomatic relief, but these agents should be judiciously prescribed. Topical corticosteroid use is justified in cases with membranous or pseudomembranous conjunctivitis, iridocyclitis, severe keratitis (exclude grade 0 and I), and persistent SEIs with visual loss. Limited-potency eyedrops (0.12% prednisolone acetate, 0.1% fluorometholone, 1% rimexolone, and dexamethasone 0.001%, loteprednol etabonate) should be instilled three to four times daily for 1 to 3 weeks. Apparently, 0.12% prednisolone is the least potent of these preparations, with the possible advantage of limited interference with viral clearance.[36] In cases of moderate to severe keratitis, a more potent topical steroid (1% prednisolone or 0.5% loteprednol) may be required. Slow tapering of the medication (half dose every 3–7 days) is mandatory, especially when dealing with infiltrates. Patients with SEIs must be warned of the potential risks of chronic corticosteroid therapy (cataract, glaucoma). With cessation of the treatment, the infiltrates often recur. It has been postulated, but not proved, that patients treated with corticosteroids in the acute phase of adenoviral conjunctivitis are more likely to develop SEIs. The increased incidence of SEIs may be due to the enhancement in virus replication that provides a bigger load of viral antigens or a prolonged wash-out time of such antigens.

The routine use of steroidal antiinflammatory agents is discouraged in general for adenoviral conjunctivitis. In patients with mild adenoviral conjunctivitis the side effects of such drugs clearly outweigh the benefits. Misdiagnosis (herpes simplex) and the probability of superinfection are also of concern. Chronic adenoviral conjunctivitis has been associated with the use of corticosteroids.[13]

Besides the implications for the individual patient, the use of corticosteroids delays the viral clearance and can lead to a much higher number of patients in community epidemics.

NSAIDs have limited action in the inflammation cascade. One mechanism of action of these agents is to inhibit the cyclooxygenase arm of the arachidonic acid metabolic pathway. This inhibition prevents the formation of prostacyclins, thromboxanes, and prostaglandins that contribute to inflammation. The efficacy of one of these topical agents (0.5% ketorolac tromethamine) in patients with viral conjunctivitis was tested in a randomized, controlled trial, and no difference in relieving the symptoms was detected when compared to artificial tears. The efficacy of oral NSAIDs is not well established but certainly carries the risk of the systemic adverse effects of NSAIDs (gastritis, coagulation disorder, etc.).

Patients with SEIs are usually initially treated with corticosteroids. NSAIDs can be administered if the patient is still symptomatic after tapering. Severe cases will demand a new course of corticosteroids, however. The use of excimer laser ablation in such cases is controversial. There are two case reports with conflicting results regarding recurrence of opacities.[37,38]

Topical ciclosporin was reported to be valuable in the treatment of SEIs.[39] Further studies are warranted to better demonstrate efficacy (compared to corticosteroids and NSAIDs), the ideal concentration, and the frequency of administration. The use of this drug in the acute phase of viral conjunctivitis (1% ciclosporin q.i.d.) has not been correlated with a significant improvement of the symptoms, and some patients complained of mild local burning associated with the instillation. In this group, the drug was also associated with a weak tendency toward drier eyes.[40] In a rabbit model, the use of 2% or 0.5% ciclosporin was associated with significantly reduced formation of SEIs; however, viral shedding was prolonged.[41]

An efficient topical antiviral would be helpful in shortening the course of the disease, decreasing viral replication, and lowering the amount of viral antigens. Trifluridine has been tested, but no difference between the treatment group and control (artificial tears) was detected.[42]

The use of povidone-iodine as a topical antiviral in acute conjunctivitis is appealing. This low-cost antiseptic has an extremely broad spectrum of antimicrobial activity, including bacteria, fungi, and viruses.[32,43] A controlled trial using 1.25% povidone-iodine in acute conjunctivitis in children demonstrated that the drug is useful in bacterial conjunctivitis but is ineffective against viral conjunctivitis.[44] Data from in vitro experiments show that povidone-iodine is active against free virus but less effective against intracellular adenovirus,[45] and this limits its effectiveness in already established infections. However, povidone-iodine may play a role in preventing transmission within households and for controlling community epidemics. Confirmation of this assumption will require additional studies.

The anti-adenoviral activity of cidofovir, a nucleotide analog, was tested in vivo, initially in the New Zealand rabbit ocular model, and demonstrated significant antiviral activity against Ad1, Ad5, and Ad16.

The cidofovir controlled trials demonstrated that the therapeutic effect of the drug is not achieved in 0.2% concentration,[40] but is detected when a 1% concentration is used four times daily.[46] The toxicity of the latter preparation limits its clinical use. Whether or not cidofovir will have a place in the management of adenoviral conjunctivitis depends on the identification of a lower concentration and/or lower frequency of administration and/or shorter treatment in which the efficacy is still present and toxicity is not a problem.

In vitro studies have shown that some anti-HIV drugs are active against Ad. Zalcitabine, stavudine, and stampidine[47,48] are nucleoside reverse transcriptase inhibitors with different degrees of anti-Ad activity including differential effects on serotypes.[48] Future studies are warranted to evaluate their potential as topical treatment for Ad conjunctivitis.

Antibiotics are not necessary, and most cases of conjunctivitis can be managed without them.[49] Secondary infection is rare in adenoviral conjunctivitis, and antibiotics cannot be recommended based on that occurrence. The best approach for avoiding superinfection is the cautious use of corticosteroids, since corneal superinfection following viral conjunctivitis is almost always related to corticosteroid use.[50] Antibiotics should be prescribed only for patients with large epithelial defects and after the removal of pseudomembranes or membranes.

Herpes simplex virus (HSV)

Conjunctivitis may be a component of both primary and recurrent herpetic disease (Fig. 44.6). It is usually a benign condition except in neonates when the herpetic infection can be associated with fatal disease and should be promptly treated.

HSV infection is commonly diagnosed in dendritic/geographic ulcers, disciform keratitis, and keratouveitis. Herpetic conjunctivitis may be associated with typical lid and/or corneal lesions, but the virus is rarely implicated as a cause of conjunctivitis alone without other lesions. In such cases, patients may be misdiagnosed as having adenoviral conjunctivitis.

Cell culture of conjunctival samples from a large consecutive series of patients with follicular conjunctivitis and no lid lesions or dendritic ulceration were positive for HSV in 4.8% of patients.[51] None of the patients with herpetic conjunctivitis in that series had a history of previous herpetic ocular infection. The possibility of a herpetic etiology should always be remembered when treating follicular conjunctivitis.

The clinical course of the conjunctivitis is usually limited to 2 weeks. Initial signs are similar to adenovirus conjunctivitis, but the majority of the patients will present unilateral disease. Mucous discharge, conjunctival hyperemia, follicular reaction, and enlarged preauricular nodes are usually present at the first visit. Membranes and dendritic or dendrogeographic conjunctival ulcers are uncommon findings. The most frequent complaints are itching, foreign body sensation, and lacrimation. The clinical features of HSV conjunctivitis are usually different from those in severe cases of conjunctivitis caused by subgenera D (Ad8, Ad19, and Ad37), which are associated with pseudomembrane/membrane and SEIs. However, HSV conjunctivitis presents features similar to those caused by subgenera B serotypes (Ad3, Ad7, and Ad11) but with a shorter duration and a lower rate of bilateral illness.[51]

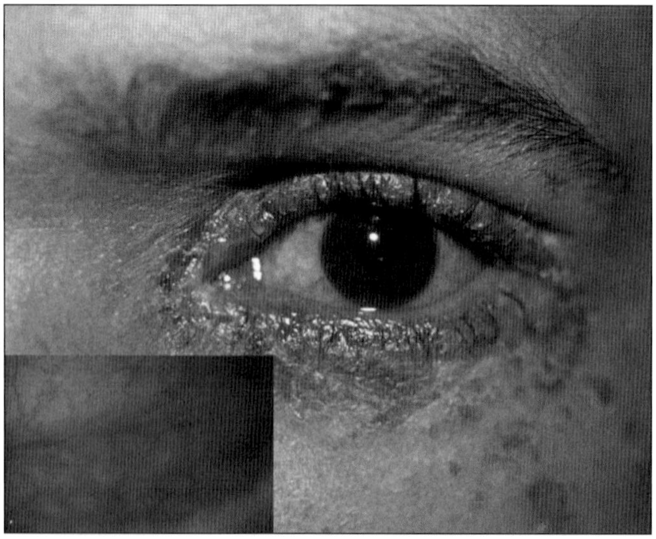

Fig. 44.6 Recurrent herpetic ocular disease (blepharoconjunctivitis). Detail, follicular conjunctival reaction.

Corneal involvement, such as typical dendritic keratitis, may be present at the first visit or develop later, especially in the immunocompromised patient or in those treated with corticosteroids. Superficial punctate keratitis may be detected in patients without dendritic lesions.

Typical cases of HSV conjunctivitis may be treated without laboratory confirmation. However, testing for HSV virus is important in atypical cases.[52]

Cell cultures are the gold standard method for detecting HSV. Cells used for culture isolation of HSV (Vero, HEK, and PRK) are different from those used for adenovirus isolation (culture Hep-2, HeLa, and A549). Therefore, the culture method selected for processing a conjunctival sample from a patient with follicular conjunctivitis should include HSV-sensitive cells; otherwise it will not be isolated.

A diagnosis based on a positive cell culture can delay therapy since the detection of cytopathic effects generally requires more than 48 hours. The use of an enzyme-linked inducible system allows the detection of HSV in a 24-hour procedure and is apparently a reliable alternative to traditional cultures.[53] Commercially available antigen detecting methods can be processed in less than 24 hours. Rapid results can also be obtained by PCR, where available.

Treatment of HSV conjunctivitis in the neonate is mandatory and should include both topical antiviral and intravenous acyclovir. A pediatric consultation should be obtained.

Non-neonatal HSV conjunctivitis usually resolves even when not treated. When a dendritic corneal lesion is present, topical therapy should be administered. In patients without corneal involvement, the treatment is controversial. There is no evidence that treatment with topical antivirals will shorten the duration of the disease or prevent and/or attenuate the keratitis. Nevertheless, treatment with a topical antiviral (3% vidarabine or 3% acyclovir ointment, for 10–14 days) is usually prescribed, based on relative safety and potential benefit. One should also consider a course of oral antiviral agents. Corticosteroids should not be administered for HSV conjunctivitis.

Varicella-zoster virus (VZV)

Varicella (chickenpox) is the infection caused by VZV. This highly contagious disease is characterized by a mucocutaneous exanthem. Typically, lesions in various stages are present simultaneously. The infectious period ends only when all lesions are crusted.

The conjunctiva is rarely involved. Small, ulcerative, phlyctenule-like lesions at the limbus are the most common finding. When the cornea is not affected, the patient can be either carefully observed without treatment or treated with topical antiviral ointments (3% vidarabine or 3% acyclovir, 10–14 days). If keratitis is detected, treatment is recommended.

VZV gains access to the sensory ganglia during the primary disease (varicella). Infection might present subtle symptoms (fever and malaise) without rash, and patients may, therefore, be unaware of it. After reaching the ganglia, VZV enters a latent stage. The reactivation of latent virus in the trigeminal ganglion leads to the involvement of V1 (ophthalmic nerve) dermatome and is referred to as herpes zoster ophthalmicus. The conjunctiva may be involved, but this will not modify the treatment (discussed elsewhere).

Epstein-Barr virus (EBV)

Epstein-Barr virus is a ubiquitous virus with a high prevalence in the adult population. The virus is transmitted by airborne droplets of upper respiratory secretions. It is the most common agent of infectious mononucleosis syndrome. This syndrome is characterized by fever, sore throat, lymphadenopathy, lymphocytosis, polyarthritis, myositis, and occasionally follicular conjunctivitis.[54] Membranes should be treated as described for adenoviral membranous conjunctivitis.

The anterior ocular manifestations of EBV infection also include episcleritis, subconjunctival hemorrhages, uveitis, and keratitis. Treatment is generally unnecessary and the conjunctivitis resolves without specific treatment.

Cytomegalovirus (CMV)

Follicular conjunctivitis can be a feature of CMV infection (mononucleosis) in otherwise healthy individuals.[55] CMV is a common cause of chorioretinitis in immunosuppressed individuals. Conjunctivitis has been reported,[56] but is not frequent in these patients.[57] The treatment of CMV conjunctivitis is symptomatic. The corneal epithelium and stroma are usually spared. Endothelial deposits are usually associated with CMV retinitis.[57]

Variola and vaccinia virus

Ocular involvement in smallpox was uncommon. Conjunctivitis was usually the initial sign of ocular disease, with pustules on the bulbar conjunctiva and purulent discharge. Extension to the cornea and a severe inflammatory reaction were the most devastating complications. Vaccinia virus (cowpox disease), used in immunization and in laboratory research, can cause similar findings as well as corneal involvement.

Human vaccinia is usually related to laboratory infection or immunization. Contamination from infected animals had been postulated.[58] The treatment of ocular vaccinia should include hyperimmune vaccinia immune globulin and topical antivirals.

Molluscum contagiosum virus (MC)

Molluscum contagiosum is a human host-specific poxvirus. Transmission may be direct or through fomites. In

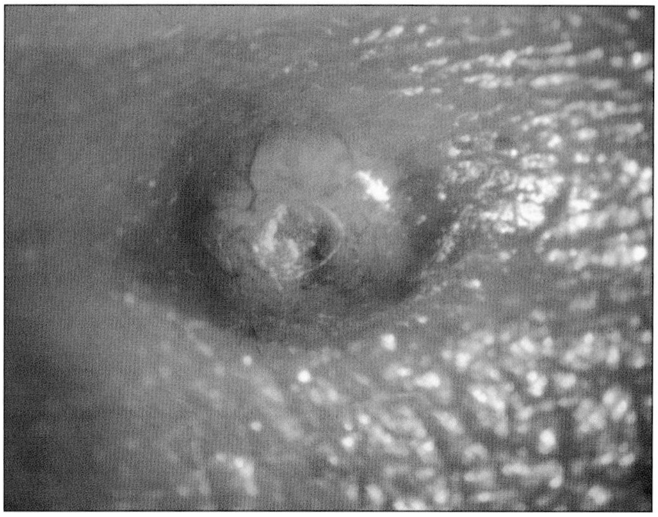

Fig. 44.7 Molluscum contagiosum lesion on the upper lid of a patient with chronic follicular conjunctivitis. The lesion was hidden in the lid fold and could be seen only when the patient closed her eye.

immunocompetent patients, the disease has a predilection for the head and neck. The typical presentation of ocular involvement is a follicular conjunctivitis and lid margin lesions. MC lesions are often raised, umbilicated, waxy, and flesh colored (Fig. 44.7). The disease may resolve spontaneously (months or years) without complication. Treatment is often indicated to shorten the duration of the disease, hinder additional autoinoculation, and ameliorate the conjunctivitis. Cryotherapy is effective, but depigmentation of the treated area is a risk. Surgical removal (simple excision, curettage) of the lesions is curative in most cases. AIDS patients may present with exuberant and/or recalcitrant MC. Meticulous surgical removal,[59] electron beam radiation,[60] carbon dioxide laser,[61] and topical cidofovir[62] can be effective in these patients. Remission can also be observed with administration of highly active antiretroviral therapy.[63]

RNA Viruses

Picornaviruses

Enterovirus type 70 (EV70) and coxsackievirus A type 24 variant (CA24v) (picornavirus family) are the most common causes of acute hemorrhagic conjunctivitis (AHC).[64,65] Similar clinical findings have been reported in infections caused by Ad19 and Ad37.[66]

The syndrome begins with the sudden onset of pain, tearing, foreign body sensation, conjunctival injection, subconjunctival hemorrhages (Fig. 44.8), and periorbital swelling. The second eye becomes involved within 1 to 2 days in the majority of the cases. The superficial punctate keratitis is usually mild. Although EKC with prominent subconjunctival hemorrhages may resemble AHC, the latter has a shorter incubation time, a more rapid disease course, and less corneal involvement.

The diagnosis is often based on clinical findings. Cultures and PCR are the tools most commonly used in diagnosing the pathogen of a viral ACH. To detect the common agents

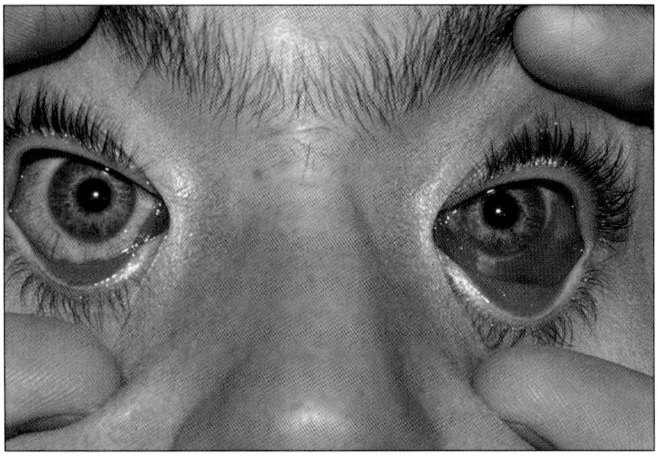

Fig. 44.8 Bilateral acute hemorrhagic conjunctivitis with more advanced stage in the left eye.

(EV70 and CA24v) and rule out Ad infection, three different sets of primers and conditions should be used.[66] A one-step, single-tube, real-time RT-PCR has been developed and may be helpful in identifying CA24v-related epidemics.[67]

The disease is often self-limiting and only symptomatic treatment (e.g. cold compress, artificial tears) and contagion precautions should be prescribed. The use of corticosteroids is a predisposing factor for the development of corneal ulceration.[50] A potential therapeutic use of small interference RNA has been shown in vitro.[68]

Paramyxoviruses

This family includes the viruses of measles, Newcastle disease, and mumps.

Measles is a highly contagious viral infection. Transmission is via large respiratory droplets. The clinical features are high fever, cough, runny nose, and a generalized maculopapular rash. Its incidence in the United States has been reduced by widespread vaccination.

Catarrhal conjunctivitis, superficial keratitis, and photophobia are the most common clinical features in healthy individuals. Subconjunctival hemorrhages may be present.[69] Keratitis is usually severe in patients with vitamin A deficiency. This sight-threatening keratitis is an important cause of blindness in developing nations.[70] Potentially fatal systemic complications (pneumonia, encephalitis, and myocarditis) may be encountered in immunocompromised patients. No specific treatment is available. Prophylactic topical antibiotics should be prescribed if large epithelial defects are noticed. Superficial keratitis in healthy patients is unresponsive to topical diclofenac drops,[69] but spontaneous resolution is observed within 3 to 5 days.

Newcastle disease is limited to poultry workers and laboratory personnel. Infection is usually acquired when dealing with infected poultry or directly with infected material. Ocular disease is characterized by mild follicular conjunctivitis and tearing. Subepithelial infiltrates might be present.[71] No specific treatment is required and resolution without sequelae is observed in 7 to 10 days.

Mumps is an acute viral infection characterized by swelling (more commonly bilateral) of the parotid salivary glands. Orbital pain and a mass are present when the lacrimal gland is affected. Superficial punctate keratitis or stromal keratitis may be present.[72] No specific treatment is required.

Togaviruses

Rubella (German measles) occurs worldwide and is normally a mild childhood disease. Self-limiting follicular conjunctivitis and punctate keratitis (located primarily in the central cornea[73]) can be detected. Topical lubricants can be prescribed in more symptomatic patients, but the findings usually resolve without specific treatment. Infection during early pregnancy may cause fetal death or congenital rubella syndrome.

Flaviviruses

Yellow fever is the prototype virus of this family that also includes dengue. These viruses are arthropod-borne and are more common in tropical areas. They may cause conjunctival injection, lid edema, and photophobia. Discharge is unusual. Conjunctival hemorrhages are likely to occur in patients who develop a coagulopathy disorder, especially during the toxic phase of yellow fever when vomiting (black vomit) is frequent.

References

1. Shenk T. Adenoviridae. In: Fields B, Knipe D, Howley P, eds. *Fields virology*. Philadelphia: Lippincott-Raven; 1996:2111–2148.
2. De Jong JC, Wermenbol AG, Verweij-Uijterwaal MW, et al. Adenoviruses from human immunodeficiency virus-infected individuals, including two strains that represent new candidate serotypes Ad50 and Ad51 of species B1 and D, respectively. *J Clin Microbiol*. 1999;37:3940–3945.
3. Chang C, Sheu M, Chern C, et al. Epidemic keratoconjunctivitis caused by a new genotype of adenovirus type 8 (Ad8)—a chronological review of Ad8 in Southern Taiwan. *Jpn J Ophthalmol*. 2001;45:160–166.
4. McMillan N, Martin S, Sobsey M, et al. Outbreak of pharyngoconjunctival fever at a summer camp – North Carolina, 1991. *MMWR Morb Mortal Wkly Rep*. 1992;41:342–344.
5. Harley D, Harrower B, Lyon M, et al. A primary school outbreak of pharyngoconjunctival fever caused by adenovirus type 3. *Commun Dis Intell*. 2001;25:9–12.
6. Pavan-Langston D, Dunkel E. Major ocular infections: herpes simplex, adenovirus, Epstein-Barr virus, pox. In: Galasso G, Merigan T, Whitley R, eds. *Antiviral agents and viral diseases of man*. Philadelphia: Lippincott-Raven; 1997:187–228.
7. Cooper RJ, Hallett R, Tullo AB, et al. The epidemiology of adenovirus infections in Greater Manchester, UK 1982–96. *Epidemiol Infect*. 2000;125:333–345.
8. Tabery H. Corneal epithelial changes due to adenovirus type 8 infection, *Acta Ophthalmol Scand*. 2000;78:45–48.
9. Maudgal PC. Cytopathology of adenovirus keratitis by replica technique, *Br J Ophthalmol*. 1990;74:670–675.
10. Darougar S, Grey RH, Thaker U, et al. Clinical and epidemiological features of adenovirus keratoconjunctivitis in London. *Br J Ophthalmol*. 1983;67:1–7.
11. Boniuk M, Phiilips A, Friedman JB. Chronic adenovirus type 2 keratitis in man. *N Engl J Med* 1965;273:924–925.
12. Darougar S, Quinlan PM, Gibson JA, et al. Epidemic keratoconjunctivitis and chronic papillary conjunctivitis in London due to adenovirus type 19. *Br J Ophthalmol*. 1977;61:76–85.
13. Pettit T, Holland G. Chronic keratoconjunctivitis associated with ocular adenovirus infection. *Am J Ophthalmol*. 1979;99.

14. Shiuey Y, Ambati BK, Adamis AP. A randomized, double-masked trial of topical ketorolac versus artificial tears for treatment of viral conjunctivitis. *Ophthalmology.* 2000;107:1512–1517.
15. Rietveld RP, van Weert HC, ter Riet G, et al. Diagnostic impact of signs and symptoms in acute infectious conjunctivitis: systematic literature search. *BMJ.* 2003;327:789.
16. Rietveld RP, ter Riet G, Bindels PJ, et al. Predicting bacterial cause in infectious conjunctivitis: cohort study on informativeness of combinations of signs and symptoms. *BMJ.* 2004;329:206–210.
17. Robbie SJ, Qureshi K, Kashani S, et al. Managing conjunctivitis in general practice: research into management strategies for acute infective conjunctivitis. *BMJ.* 2006;333:446–447.
18. Davies RL. Predicting bacterial cause in infectious conjunctivitis: why say itching counts against bacterial infection in conjunctivitis? *BMJ.* 2004;329:625; author reply 625.
19. Elnifro E, Cooper RJ, Klapper PE, et al. Diagnosis of viral and chlamydial keratoconjunctivitis: which laboratory test? *Br J Ophthalmol.* 1999;83: 622–627.
20. Saitoh-Inagawa W, Oshima A, Aoki K, et al. Rapid diagnosis of adenoviral conjunctivitis by PCR and restriction fragment length polymorphism analysis. *J Clin Microbiol.* 1996;34:2113–2116.
21. Elnifro EM, Cooper RJ, Klapper PE, et al. Multiplex polymerase chain reaction for diagnosis of viral and chlamydial keratoconjunctivitis. *Invest Ophthalmol Vis Sci.* 2000;41:1818–1822.
22. Cooper RJ, Yeo AC, Bailey AS, et al. Adenovirus polymerase chain reaction assay for rapid diagnosis of conjunctivitis. *Invest Ophthalmol Vis Sci.* 1999;40:90–95.
23. Sambursky R, Tauber S, Schirra F, et al. The RPS adeno detector for diagnosing adenoviral conjunctivitis. *Ophthalmology.* 2006;113:1758–1764.
24. Sambursky RP, Fram N, Cohen EJ. The prevalence of adenoviral conjunctivitis at the Wills Eye Hospital Emergency Room. *Optometry.* 2007;78: 236–239.
25. Kobayashi TK, Sato S, Tsubota K, et al. Cytological evaluation of adenoviral follicular conjunctivitis by cytobrush. *Ophthalmologica.* 1991;202:156–160.
26. Wiley LA, Roba LA, Kowalski RP, et al. A 5-year evaluation of the Adenoclone test for the rapid diagnosis of adenovirus from conjunctival swabs. *Cornea.* 1996;15:363–367.
27. Levent F, Greer JM, Snider M, et al. Performance of a new immunochromatographic assay for detection of adenoviruses in children. *J Clin Virol.* 2009;44:173–175.
28. Uchio E, Aoki K, Saitoh W, et al. Rapid diagnosis of adenoviral conjunctivitis on conjunctival swabs by 10-minute immunochromatography. *Ophthalmology.* 1997;104:1294–1299.
29. Mielke J, Grub M, Freudenthaler N, et al. Keratoconjunctivitis epidemica. Nachweis von Adenoviren. *Ophthalmologe.* 2005;102:968–970.
30. Udeh BL, Schneider JE, Ohsfeldt RL. Cost effectiveness of a point-of-care test for adenoviral conjunctivitis. *Am J Med Sci.* 2008;336:254–264.
31. Hamada N, Gotoh K, Hara K, et al. Nosocomial outbreak of epidemic keratoconjunctivitis accompanying environmental contamination with adenoviruses. *J Hosp Infect.* 2008;68:262–268.
32. Kawana R, Kitamura T, Nakagomi O, et al. Inactivation of human viruses by povidone-iodine in comparison with other antiseptics. *Dermatology.* 1997;195:29–35.
33. Uchio E, Ishiko H, Aoki K, et al. Adenovirus detected by polymerase chain reaction in multidose eyedrop bottles used by patients with adenoviral keratoconjunctivitis. *Am J Ophthalmol.* 2002;134:618–619.
34. Romanowski EG, Yates KA, Gordon YJ. Short-term treatment with a potent topical corticosteroid of an acute ocular adenoviral infection in the New Zealand white rabbit. *Cornea.* 2001;20:657–660.
35. Romanowski E, Yates KA, Gordon YJ. Topical corticosteroids of limited potency promote adenovirus replication in the Ad5/NZW rabbit ocular model. *Cornea.* 2002;21:289–291.
36. Romanowski EG, Araullo-Cruz T, Gordon YJ. Topical corticosteroids reverse the antiviral effect of topical cidofovir in the Ad5-inoculated New Zealand rabbit ocular model. *Invest Ophthalmol Vis Sci.* 1997;38: 253–257.
37. Starr MB. Recurrent subepithelial corneal opacities after excimer laser phototherapeutic keratectomy. *Cornea.* 1999;18:117–120.
38. Fite SW, Chodosh J. Photorefractive keratectomy for myopia in the setting of adenoviral subepithelial infiltrates. *Am J Ophthalmol.* 1998; 126:829–831.
39. Reinhard T, Godehardt E, Pfahl HG, et al. Lokales cyclosporin A bei nummuli nach keratokonjunktivitis epidemica. *Ophthalmologe.* 2000;97: 764–768.
40. Hillenkamp J, Reinhard T, Ross R, et al. Topical treatment of acute adenoviral keratoconjunctivitis with 0.2% cidofovir and 1% cyclosporine. *Arch Ophthalmol.* 2001;119:1487–1491.
41. Romanowski EG, Pless P, Yates KA, et al. Topical cyclosporine A inhibits subepithelial immune infiltrates but also promotes viral shedding in experimental adenovirus models. *Cornea.* 2005;24:86–91.
42. Ward JB, Siojo LG, Waller SG. A prospective, masked clinical trial of trifluridine, dexamethasone, and artificial tears in the treatment of epidemic keratoconjunctivitis. *Cornea.* 1993;12:216–221.
43. Benevento WJ, Murray P, Reed CA, et al. The sensitivity of *Neisseria gonorrhoeae, Chlamydia trachomatis*, and herpes simplex type II to disinfection with povidone-iodine. *Am J Ophthalmol.* 1990;109:329–333.
44. Isenberg SJ, Apt L, Valenton M, et al. A controlled trial of povidone-iodine to treat infectious conjunctivitis in children. *Am J Ophthalmol.* 2002;134:681–688.
45. Monnerat N, Bossart W, Thiel MA. Povidoniod zur Behandlung von Adenoviruskonjunktivitis: eine In-vitro-Studie. *Klin Monatsbl Augenheilkd.* 2006;223:349–352.
46. Hillenkamp J, Reinhard T, Ross R, et al. The effects of cidofovir 1% with and without cyclosporin A 1% as a topical treatment of acute adenoviral keratoconjunctivitis. *Ophthalmology.* 2002;109:845–850.
47. Uchio E, Fuchigami A, Kadonosono K, et al. Anti-adenoviral effect of anti-HIV agents in vitro in serotypes inducing keratoconjunctivitis. *Graefes Arch Clin Exp Ophthalmol.* 2007;245:1319–1325.
48. D'Cruz OJ, Uckun FM. Stampidine: a selective oculo-genital microbicide. *J Antimicrob Chemother.* 2005;56:10–19.
49. Rautakorpi U-M, Klaukka T, Honkanen P, et al. Antibiotic use by indication: a basis for active antibiotic policy in the community. *Scand J Infect Dis.* 2001;33:920–926.
50. Vajpayee RB, Sharma N, Chand M, et al. Corneal superinfection in acute hemorrhagic conjunctivitis. *Cornea.* 1998;17:614–617.
51. Uchio E, Takeuchi S, Itoh N, et al. Clinical and epidemiological features of acute follicular conjunctivitis with special reference to that caused by herpes simplex virus type 1. *Br J Ophthalmol.* 2000;84:968–972.
52. Kowalski RP, Gordon YJ, Romanowski EG, et al. A comparison of enzyme immunoassay and polymerase chain reaction with the clinical examination for diagnosing ocular herpetic disease. *Ophthalmology.* 1993;100: 530–533.
53. Crist GA, Langer JM, Woods GL, et al. Evaluation of the ELVIS plate method for the detection and typing of herpes simplex virus in clinical specimens. *Diagn Microbiol Infect Dis.* 2004;49:173–177.
54. Slobod KS, Sandlund JT, Spiegel PH, et al. Molecular evidence of ocular Epstein-Barr virus infection. *Clin Infect Dis.* 2000;31:184–188.
55. Garau J, Kabins S, DeNosaquo S, et al. Spontaneous cytomegalovirus mononucleosis with conjunctivitis. *Arch Intern Med.* 1977;137: 1631–1632.
56. Brown HH, Glasgow BJ, Holland GN, et al. Cytomegalovirus infection of the conjunctiva in AIDS. *Am J Ophthalmol.* 1988;106:102–104.
57. Brody JM, Butrus SI, Laby DM, et al. Anterior segment findings in AIDS patients with cytomegalovirus retinitis. *Graefes Arch Clin Exp Ophthalmol.* 1995;233:374–376.
58. Marennikova SS, Wojnarowska I, Bochanek W, et al. [Cowpox in man]. *Zh Mikrobiol Epidemiol Immunobiol.* 1984;64–69.
59. Wheaton AF, Timothy NH, Dossett JH, et al. The surgical treatment of molluscum contagiosum in a pediatric AIDS patient. *Ann Plast Surg.* 2000;44:651–655.
60. Scolaro MJ, Gordon P. Electron-beam therapy for AIDS-related molluscum contagiosum lesions: preliminary experience. *Radiology.* 1999;210: 479–482.
61. Nehal KS, Sarnoff DS, Gotkin RH, et al. Pulsed dye laser treatment of molluscum contagiosum in a patient with acquired immunodeficiency syndrome. *Dermatol Surg.* 1998;24:533–535.
62. Zabawski EJ Jr, Cockerell CJ. Topical and intralesional cidofovir: a review of pharmacology and therapeutic effects. *J Am Acad Dermatol.* 1998;39:741–745.
63. Cattelan AM, Sasset L, Corti L, et al. A complete remission of recalcitrant molluscum contagiosum in an AIDS patient following highly active antiretroviral therapy (HAART). *J Infect.* 1999;38:58–60.
64. Kuo PC, Lin JY, Chen LC, et al. Molecular and immunocytochemical identification of coxsackievirus A-24 variant from the acute haemorrhagic conjunctivitis outbreak in Taiwan in 2007. *Eye.* 2009.
65. Wu D, Ke CW, Mo YL, et al. Multiple outbreaks of acute hemorrhagic conjunctivitis due to a variant of coxsackievirus A24: Guangdong, China, 2007. *J Med Virol.* 2008;80:1762–1768.
66. Chang CH, Sheu MM, Lin KH, et al. Hemorrhagic viral keratoconjunctivitis in Taiwan caused by adenovirus types 19 and 37: applicability of polymerase chain reaction-restriction fragment length polymorphism in detecting adenovirus genotypes. *Cornea.* 2001;20:295–300.
67. Leveque N, Lahlou Amine I, Tcheng R, et al.: Rapid diagnosis of acute hemorrhagic conjunctivitis due to coxsackievirus A24 variant by real-time one-step RT-PCR. *J Virol Methods.* 2007;142:89–94.

68. Tan EL, Marcus KF, Poh CL. Development of RNA interference (RNAi) as potential antiviral strategy against enterovirus 70. *J Med Virol.* 2008;80:1025–1032.
69. Kayikcioglu O, Kir E, Soyler M, et al. Ocular findings in a measles epidemic among young adults. *Ocul Immunol Inflamm.* 2000;8:59–62.
70. Bowman R, Faal H, Dolin P, et al. Non-trachomatous corneal opacities in the Gambia – aetiology and visual burden. *Eye.* 2002;16:27–32.
71. Hales RH, Ostler HB. Newcastle disease conjunctivitis with subepithelial infiltrates. *Br J Ophthalmol.* 1973;57:694–697.
72. Mickatavage R, Amadur J. A case report of mumps keratitis. *Arch Ophthalmol.* 1963;69:758–759.
73. Hara J, Fujimoto F, Ishibashi T, et al. Ocular manifestations of the 1976 rubella epidemic in Japan. *Am J Ophthalmol.* 1979;87:642–645.

Chapter 45

Chlamydial Infections

Neera Singal, David S. Rootman

Introduction

Chlamydial infections remain an important diagnostic and therapeutic challenge for the physician. Worldwide, they represent the most common cause of infectious blindness.[1] The genus *Chlamydia* is composed of three species, *C. trachomatis, C. pneumoniae,* and *C. psittaci*. Humans are the natural host for *C. trachomatis* and *C. pneumoniae*, whereas birds and some mammals are the natural hosts of *C. psittaci*, although all three may have clinical manifestations in humans. Each species causes a distinct constellation of clinical findings, and an understanding of these is crucial to identify the underlying etiologic species.

In humans the largest burden of ocular disease is caused by *C. trachomatis*. Traditionally, this species has been subclassified into immunotypes or 'serovars.' Serovars A, B, and C are associated with trachoma. Serovars D–K are causative of adult or neonatal inclusion conjunctivitis as well as urogenital diseases. Finally, serovars L1–3 are associated with lymphogranuloma venereum.

C. psittaci may also have ocular manifestations, albeit with far less frequency than *C. trachomatis*. This species is divided into avian and mammalian strains, the avian being a potential cause of conjunctivitis in humans. Although *C. pneumoniae* may be a cause of significant systemic disease, no ocular complications in humans have so far been identified.

This chapter will focus exclusively on the major ocular syndromes caused by each distinct species of *Chlamydia*. This chapter will address trachoma, neonatal inclusion conjunctivitis, adult inclusion conjunctivitis, lymphogranuloma venereum, and psittacosis.

Basic Science

Chlamydia is an obligate intracellular bacterium with a unique life cycle.[2] Being unable to synthesize its own ATP, it is forced to exist within cells, utilizing the cellular machinery of the host to provide it with energy for metabolic activity. *Chlamydia* may exist in two forms: a reticulate or initial body (RB) and an elementary body (EB). The RB is the classic metabolically active intracellular form. In contrast, the EB exists only in an extracellular form.[3] This form is metabolically inactive, possessing a rigid cell wall which is relatively impermeable to stimuli in its extracellular environment. This wall contains disulfide bond cross-linking, which contributes to the rigidity and low permeability, enhancing the ability of the elementary body to survive outside the cell. The EB is the infectious particle of chlamydia, and is the only way that it may spread from cell to cell.

The life cycle begins when the infectious EB attaches to the surface of a susceptible host cell, then enters by way of parasite-induced endocytosis (Fig. 45.1). Once inside the cell, the vesicle resists fusion with the host cell's lysosomes and is therefore protected from digestion. The mechanism by which this takes place is not yet completely understood. The vesicle that has formed within the host cell is referred to as an inclusion body. This inclusion body then travels to the Golgi region, where it intercepts metabolites being transported from the Golgi apparatus to the cell membrane. It is thought that these nutrients are used by the EB for maturation. The EB ultimately metamorphoses into an RB, and several important changes take place: it grows from 300 nm in diameter to approximately 800 nm in diameter; it loses its infectious nature; and there is an increase in the ratio of DNA to RNA from 1:1 to 3:1. In addition, there is a reduction of disulfide bond cross-linking, thereby increasing the permeability and reducing the rigidity of the cell wall. This is important, as the increased permeability allows nutrients and ATP from the host cell to be taken up by the rapidly dividing RB. From infection of the EB to metamorphosis into an RB is thought to take approximately 8 hours. The RB is metabolically active, dividing through the process of binary fission. In response to subtle changes in the intracellular milieu, replication ceases approximately 24–72 hours after infection. The RBs condense with one another to form the metabolically inactive EBs. Approximately 72 hours after infection, the host cell rife with organisms is lyzed, releasing thousands of elementary bodies into the extracellular environment to begin anew the cycle of infection, replication, and lysis.[4]

Trachoma

Epidemiology

Trachoma is the leading cause of preventable blindness worldwide and remains the third most common cause of

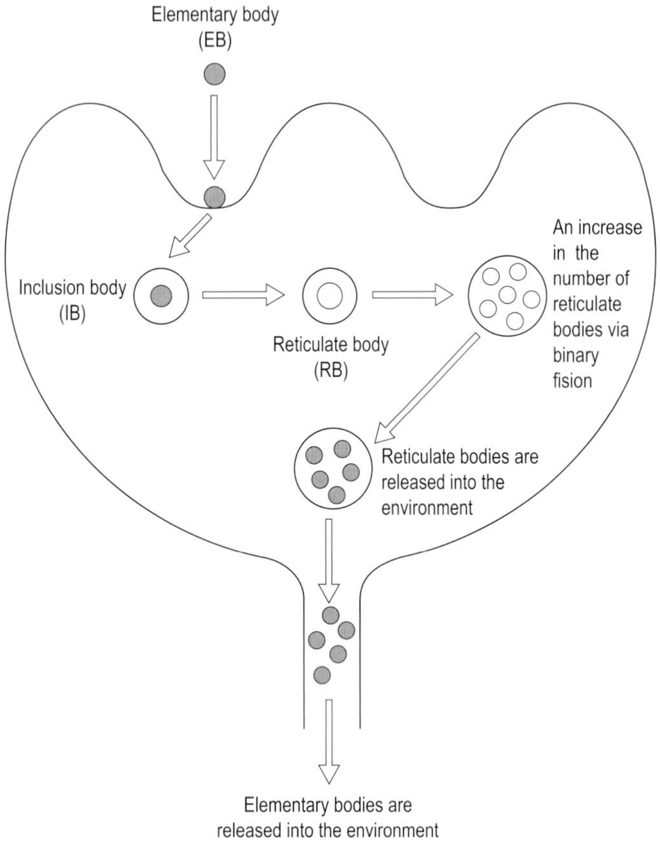

Fig. 45.1 The life cycle of *Chlamydia*.

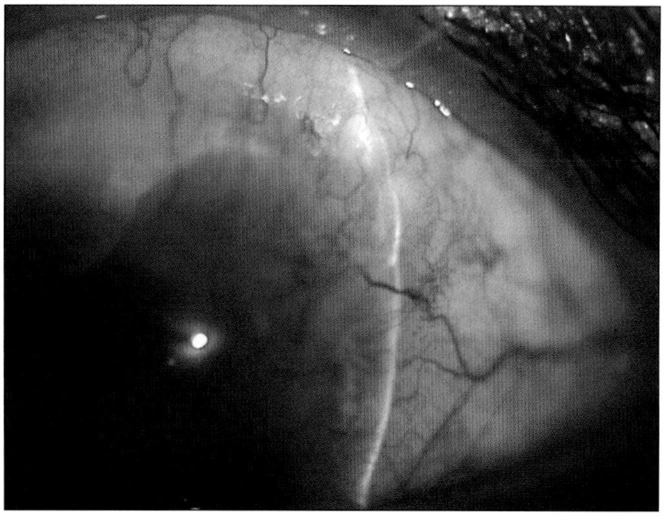

Fig. 45.2 Herbert's pits.

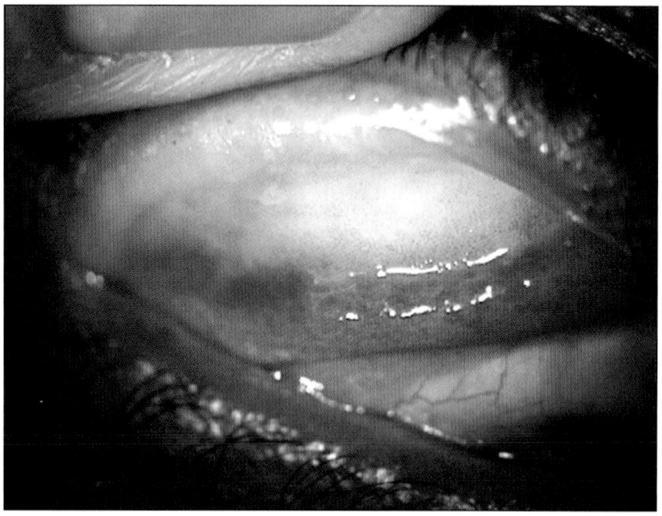

Fig. 45.3 Arlt's line.

blindness worldwide after cataract and glaucoma. Overall, active trachoma affects an estimated 84 million people; another 7.6 million have end-stage disease, of whom 1.3 million are blind.[5] Although trachoma has virtually disappeared from Western Europe and North America, efforts are being made to eliminate it from Africa, Southeast Asia, Central and South America, Australia and the Middle East, where it remains a significant problem. Trachoma is most prevalent between the ages of 1 and 5 years.[6] Although most infections are thought to be transmitted directly from eye to eye, other routes of transmission may also play a role. These less common routes include fomites, flies, and eye make-up. Moreover, low socioeconomic status, lack of water, and poor hygiene are also thought to be important risk factors for acquiring trachoma.[5,7,8]

Clinical manifestations

Trachoma initially presents as a follicular conjunctivitis with hyperemia, irritation, and discharge. Associated rhinitis, preauricular lymphadenopathy, and upper respiratory tract infection have been reported during the acute phase of the infection. During the initial disease process, follicles and papillae on the upper palpebral conjunctiva may be present. The follicles around the limbus may eventually break down, and necrosis of the tissue can occur with subsequent scarring. These scars are referred to as Herbert's pits (Fig. 45.2). Linear or stellate scarring on the upper tarsus can coalesce and form an 'Arlt's line', which is suggestive of prior trachoma infection (Fig. 45.3).[6] As the scarring progresses, chronic changes develop. Cicatricial lid changes with tarsal plate contraction may occur along with accompanying trichiasis, leading to superior corneal pannus, scarring, or opacification of the cornea (Fig. 45.4).[7]

Of the many classifications of trachomatous disease, the World Health Organization (WHO) classification is the most commonly accepted. This has the advantage over previous classification systems because it is simpler and encompasses both the inflammatory as well as the cicatricial stages. Allied health personnel such as nurses and assistants can easily use this system. More importantly, it provides a universal way of measuring, scoring, and guiding treatment for trachoma.

This classification involves five stages as follows:[5,9]

1. Trachomatous inflammation – follicular (TF): the presence of five or more follicles in the upper tarsal conjunctiva. Follicles must be at least 0.5 mm in diameter to be considered.

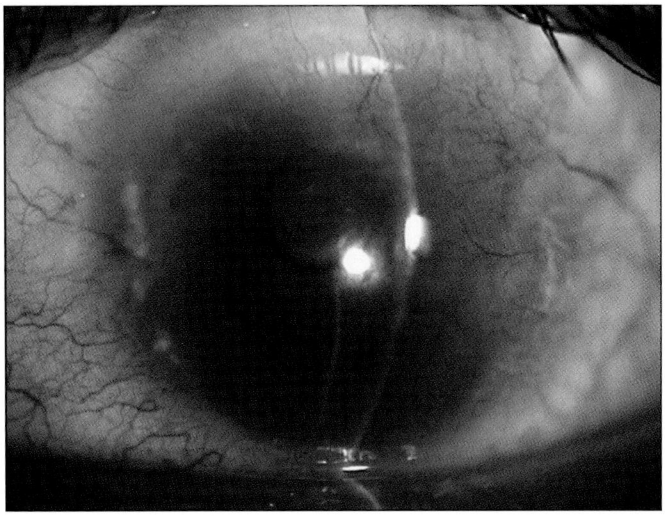

Fig. 45.4 Superior corneal pannus and corneal opacification.

2. Trachomatous inflammation – intense (TI): pronounced inflammatory thickening of the tarsal conjunctiva that obscures more than half of the normal deep tarsal vessels.
3. Trachomatous scarring (TS): the presence of scarring in the tarsal conjunctiva.
4. Trachomatous trichiasis (TT): at least one eyelash rubs on the eyeball. Evidence of recent removal of inturned eyelashes should also be graded as trichiasis.
5. Corneal opacity (CO): easily visible corneal opacity over the pupil.

Pathophysiology

Although the pathogenesis of trachoma has not been well elucidated, the establishment of a persistent and recurrent infection is an important step in the pathogenesis of conjunctival and corneal scarring that is seen with trachomatous infection. This scarring is what eventually leads to the sight-threatening complications. Recent evidence suggests that following the initial infection with ocular *C. trachomatis*, a hypersensitive state occurs such that subsequent infections results in more intense inflammation.[10] Candidate antigens for inducing this hypersensitive state include the 60 kDa chlamydial heat shock protein, the major outer membrane protein surface antigen, and lipopolysaccharide from the bacterial cell membrane, although none of these in isolation is sufficient to induce progressive disease.[11] Most data suggest that reduced cell-mediated immunity and high levels of T-helper (Th)2 cell-like responses are correlated with conjunctival scarring and evidence of persistent chlamydial infection in individuals with trachoma. Specifically, reduced interferon (IFN), interleukin (IL)-2, and increased IL-4 secretion have been found to exist in subjects who progress to develop significant scarring from trachoma. Also, serum antichlamydial antibody titers have been found to be significantly higher in subjects with scarring trachoma than in matched controls. Interestingly, similar evidence showing an inverse relationship between low cell-mediated responses and high humoral responses has been reported in patients with reproductive tract sequelae of *C. trachomatis* infection.[12]

The cellular involvement can be broken down by the different clinical stages. Early on, in the TF and TI stages, the main cell type is the polymorphonuclear leukocyte (PMN). As the infection progresses during this stage, the number of PMNs decrease and lymphocytes start to become more numerous. These lymphocytes develop clusters that later develop into the distinct lymphoid follicles that are seen superiorly as well as around the limbus. Other cell types that are present during the TF and TI stages are plasma cells, eosinophils, and macrophages.[11] As the trachomatous infection progresses to the TS stage, cicatricial changes start to occur. Histologically, subepithelial fibrous membrane formation, squamous metaplasia, and loss of goblet cells occur. These changes produce the pathognomonic Arlt's line on the tarsus as well as decreased mucin production that can predispose to chronic corneal ulceration. The contraction of the subepithelial fibrous tissue formed by collagen fibers and anterior surface drying are the main factors contributing to the chronic cicatrization and entropion formation.[12] The presence of cicatricial entropion leads to trichiasis and the TT stage of trachoma. With the presence of trichiasis, there is an eightfold increase in risk of developing corneal opacity (CO).[9] It is this final stage of trachoma that results in the major loss of vision.

Treatment

The ultimate goal of treatment is to prevent the ocular sequelae of chlamydia infection. Primary prevention strategies are of paramount importance. Many are widely in place, and will be discussed later in this section. Because the clinical stage determines the treatment, they will be discussed in order.

In the TF stage acute infection is present, and therefore treatment is directed at eliminating the chlamydia organism. There are numerous antibiotic regimens available, and generally the tetracyclines and macrolide antibiotics such as erythromycin are effective. Antibiotic resistance has not yet been a well-documented problem, although there is some theoretical concern with respect to mass treatment protocols, as discussed below.[13] Topical therapy with erythromycin ointment twice daily for 6 weeks is effective in eliminating the acute infection. It has been shown that a single dose of oral azithromycin is as effective as 6 weeks of topical therapy.[14,15] As a result, in areas where the drug is available and affordable, single-dose therapy is preferred, as compliance with a prolonged course of topical therapy is known to be quite poor. The standard systemic therapy has traditionally consisted of a 2-week course of oral tetracycline 250 mg four times daily or doxycycline 100 mg twice daily. Recently, single-dose azithromycin has been shown to be as effective as a 2-week course of either tetracycline or doxycycline, and is becoming the standard therapy.[16] In children under the age of 8 or pregnant women, oral erythromycin should be used.

The TI stage is managed in a similar manner to TF; however, the threshold for using systemic therapy is lower. In the TS stage the infection is no longer present, and consequently antimicrobial therapy is not useful. Treatment is conservative, with ocular lubricants as well as close observation for the development of trachomatous trichiasis (TT) and chronic ulcerations.

During the TT stage, treatment is aimed at managing trichiasis in order to avoid subsequent bacterial ulcers and corneal scarring. In patients who have gone on to develop trichiasis, surgical intervention to avoid repeated corneal injury becomes necessary. Bilamellar tarsal rotation is the surgical procedure of choice when there are multiple lashes involved, and in experienced hands it has an overall success rate of 80%.[17] If only a few lashes are aberrant, other forms of permanent lash removal, such as hyfercation, radiofrequency epilation, or cryotherapy may be effective. Finally, if corneal opacification (CO) has already occurred, the goal is to manage the disability and to restore vision. Treatment options for improving vision are limited and essentially consist of penetrating keratoplasty (PKP) once the lids and lashes have been managed. In patients who have significant corneal scarring, the outcome of penetrating keratoplasty remains less than optimal because these patients usually have extensive corneal vascularization, as well as ocular surface problems. Nevertheless, PKP may be helpful for visual rehabilitation.[18] Because of the coexistent ocular surface problems, punctal occlusion and lateral tarsorrhaphy may be useful adjuncts to consider for increasing the success of the surgery.

Blindness due to trachomatous infection is preventable. Primary prevention strategies are crucial in alleviating the huge socioeconomic burden of blindness. In response to this, in 1997 the World Health Organization (WHO), along with several nongovernmental organizations and national health services, began implementing a program designed to eliminate blinding trachoma.[15] The WHO's GET 2020 program (Global Elimination of Trachoma by the year 2020) has adopted the so called 'SAFE' strategy (Surgery for entropion/trichiasis, Antibiotics for infectious trachoma, Facial cleanliness to reduce transmission, and Environmental improvements such as access to clean water and control of disease-spreading flies) to help eliminate blindness due to trachoma.[19] Because the reinfection rate from personal contact is high in certain regions, a key component to this program is the elimination of chlamydia by mass treatment of endemic and hyperendemic communities. Single-dose azithromycin is the current treatment of choice. The currently accepted WHO guidelines include community-wide antibiotic treatment if there is >10% active trachoma in children aged 1–9 years. This treatment should be reinstituted annually for 3 years, with reassessment at that time.[20] To date, the results have been encouraging, with data consistently showing that high treatment coverage among communities may result in sustained reduction of infection and disease.[11]

The administration of a single dose of azithromycin along with the other treatment modalities of the SAFE strategy is a major advance in eliminating trachoma from those areas where it remains a significant problem.

Neonatal Inclusion Conjunctivitis

Neonatial inclusion conjunctivitis (NIC), also known as ophthalmia neonatorum, is an uncommon but easily treatable cause of blindness. Early diagnosis is the key to preventing progression. Its incidence is estimated to be between 0.4% and 5% in industrialized countries.[21] *C. trachomatis* is the single most common etiologic agent, accounting for up to 40% of cases.[22] Other causes include *Neisseria gonorrhoeae*, other bacterial infections, herpes simplex virus (HSV), and chemical toxins. By far, the most important microorganism to rule out is *N. gonorrhoeae* because of its sight-threatening sequelae. Consequently, all ophthalmia neonatorum must be considered gonococcal until proven otherwise. Silver nitrate, once widely used as prophylaxis against chlamydial ocular infection, is well known to cause a toxic conjunctivitis. Because of this, many developed countries have switched to erythromycin ointment. Nevertheless, worldwide, silver nitrate toxicity still remains a common cause of ophthalmia neonatorum.

In contrast to trachoma, which is associated with serovars A–C, NIC is associated with serovars D–K. Most evidence suggests that infants acquire chlamydial infections from the birth canal during delivery.[23] The incidence of genital chlamydial infections in pregnant women in the United States is approximately 8%.[24] In addition to NIC, intrapartum chlamydia infection is known to cause a number of neonatal sequelae, including pneumonia, otitis media, and infections of the nasopharynx, rectum, or vagina.[25] A mother who harbors this organism has a 50–75% chance of passing one of these infections to her baby. The risk of acquiring NIC is 30–50%.[26] Whereas infection after cesarean section is rare, situations in which there has been a premature rupture of membranes do increase the likelihood of chlamydial infection.

Clinically, the first manifestation is often bilateral conjunctival hyperemia, occurring 5–14 days after birth. Other typical yet nonspecific signs include mucoid or mucopurulent discharge, lid edema, pseudomembranes, papillary reaction and not a follicular reaction, all occurring within the same timeframe. In severe cases, conjunctival and corneal scarring can occur. Although most cases are self-limiting, correct diagnosis and treatment are critical to rule out other pathologies, as well as to treat any possible concurrent systemic infection.

Clinically, the precise timing of symptoms may be helpful in distinguishing the different causes of conjunctivitis in the neonate (Table 45.1). Microbiologic data, however, are

Table 45.1 Causes of ophthalmia neonatorum

Ophthalmia neonatorum: etiology and time of onset (postpartum)	
Etiology	***Time of onset***
Chemical	1–36 hours
Neisseria gonorrhoeae	1–2 days
Bacterial (*Staphylococcus, Streptococcus, Haemophilus*)	2–5 days
Viral	3–15 days
Chlamydia	5–14 days

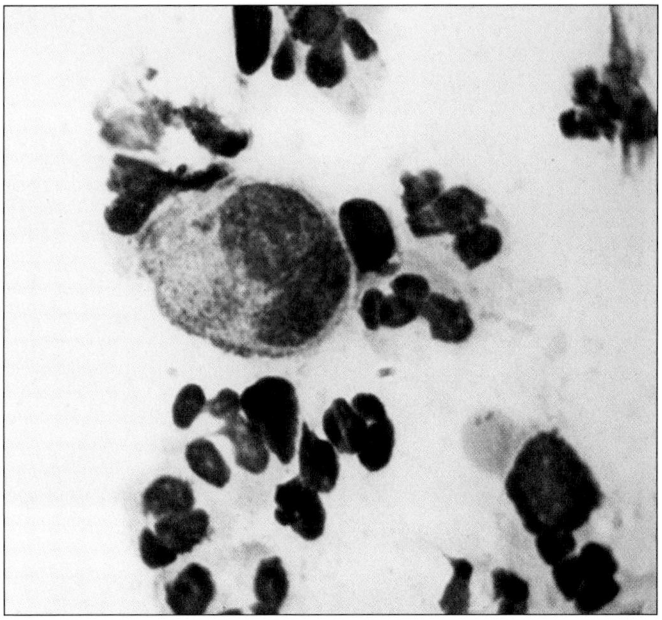

Fig. 45.5 Giemsa stain showing intracytoplasmic inclusion bodies.

essential in ruling out other causes. Gram staining, swabs, and cultures are the cornerstone of bacteriologic diagnosis. The appropriate media to rule out GC should be used, preferably Thayer–Martin media. To assess for chlamydia, routine conjunctival swabs are inadequate. Because *C. trachomatis* is an obligate intracellular organism, conjunctival scraping of the tarsal conjunctiva using a Kimura spatula must be performed to acquire cells. This material should be stained with Giemsa to look for intracytoplasmic inclusion bodies, which are pathognomonic for chlamydial infection (Fig. 45.5). Although the Giemsa stain has been reported to have >90% specificity, its sensitivity is only 36% and therefore it should not be relied upon as the sole investigation.[27] Culture using McCoy cells can also be performed. This method has a >95% specificity and 50–70% sensitivity.[28] Although this has been considered the gold standard, it is not widely available for general use. Polymerase chain reaction (PCR) testing is now replacing the McCoy culture test as the gold standard of diagnosis. It is known to have both a high sensitivity and specificity for the detection of chlamydia. Compared to traditional culture methods, which have only a 50–70% sensitivity, PCR has been shown to have 92% sensitivity.[28] Fluorescein-labeled monoclonal tests have also become popular, and in a recent study were shown to be as sensitive and specific as PCR (Figs 45.6, 45.7).[29] The main drawback is that this is a meticulous examination and requires a fluorescent microscope and an experienced reader. Until PCR becomes more widely available, one must continue to be familiar with the traditional methods of diagnosis. It should be emphasized, however, that because of the higher specificity of traditional McCoy cell culture techniques, for medicolegal reasons this is still considered the gold standard in cases that involve children.

For decades, topical silver nitrate, erythromycin, or tetracycline drops have been used prophylactically to reduce the chance of developing neonatal chlamydial conjunctivitis.

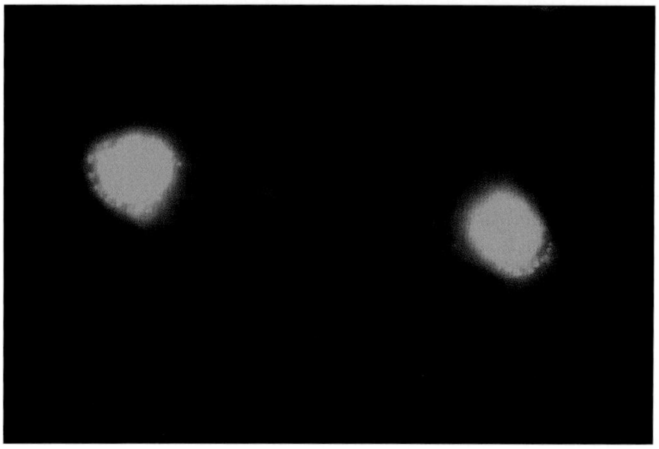

Fig. 45.6 Fluorescein-labeled monoclonal test showing intracytoplasmic inclusion bodies.

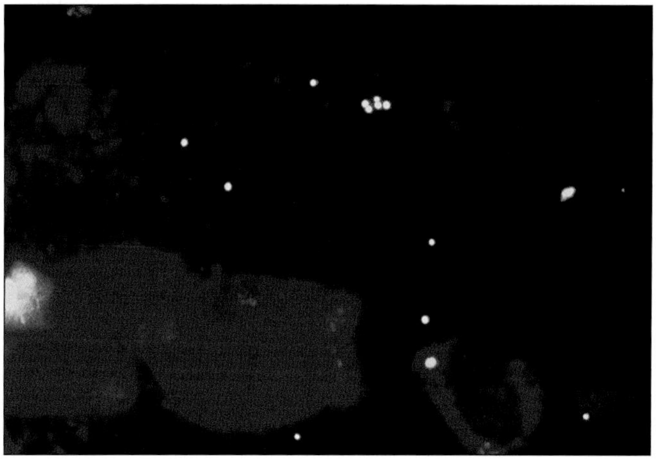

Fig. 45.7 Fluorescein-labeled monoclonal test showing elementary bodies.

Topical therapy for confirmed cases should not be used in isolation, as there is a high incidence of concomitant systemic involvement. For example, a neonate diagnosed with NIC has a 1 in 3 chance of having concurrent chlamydial pneumonia.[30] Because of the systemic risk, the treatment for NIC should include systemic antibiotics. The current recommended therapy is oral erythromycin 50 mg/kg/day in four divided doses for 10–14 days.[25] Topical treatment is not necessary. The mother and her sexual partners must also be treated with the appropriate recommended therapy (see Adult Inclusion Conjunctivitis below). Currently trials are evaluating single-dose azithromycin for the treatment of NIC. To date, the best treatment remains prevention, which begins with good prenatal care. It has been well established that the diagnosis and treatment of chlamydial disease during pregnancy can significantly reduce the transmission rate.

Adult Inclusion Conjunctivitis

Chlamydia trachomatis serotypes D–K are primarily responsible for urogenital disease. Chlamydia remains the most

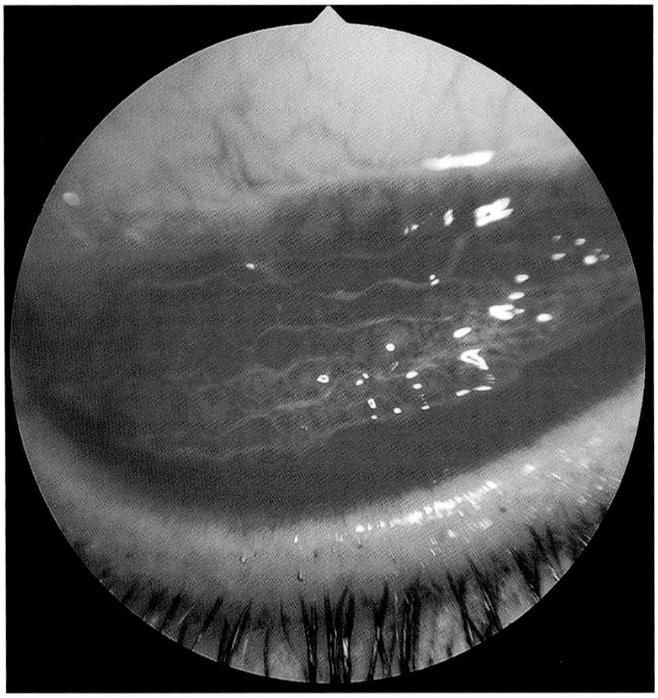

Fig. 45.8 Follicular response.

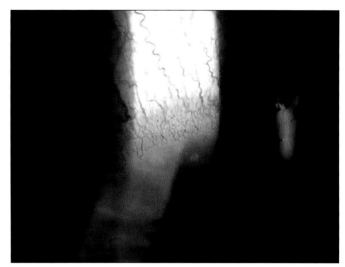

Fig. 45.9 Subepithelial infiltrates.

common sexually transmitted disease and a significant cause of urogenital disability in adults.[31] Its clinical manifestations include pelvic inflammatory disease, ectopic pregnancy, and infertility in women, and it may result in urethral stricture disease in men.[32] This is a disease that occurs predominantly in sexually active young adults and, in contrast to trachoma, is more common in economically developed countries. Although the exact prevalence is unknown, the Centers for Disease Control and Prevention estimates that more than 4 million cases of urogenital chlamydia infection occur annually.[31] Adult inclusion conjunctivitis (AIC) is the ocular manifestation of this disease and is seen in about 0.3–2% of patients with urogenital disease.[33] Its route of spread is via direct inoculation, either genital–hand–eye or genital–eye. Although it is uncommon to develop AIC with the urogenital disease, in patients with documented AIC urogenital disease is common, seen in 54% of men and 74% of women.[34] It is therefore important to think of AIC as a systemic disease with ocular involvement; thus, systemic therapy is required.

Typically, ocular manifestations begin approximately 5–14 days following inoculation with an acute follicular conjunctivitis. This ultimately becomes chronic, and often patients delay seeking medical attention until this point. The follicular response is most prominent in the lower palpebral conjunctiva and fornix (Fig. 45.8). Complaints of redness, scant mucopurulent discharge, and matting of the lids are typical. On clinical examintaion there is usually a nontender preauricular lymph node on the ipsilateral side. Whereas most infections begin unilaterally, bilateral involvement often develops. With time, the cornea may be affected, and yellowish subepithelial infiltrates as well as micropannus may be seen, most often in the superior cornea (Fig. 45.9). Although these findings appear dramatic, with appropriate treatment they resolve completely and without sequelae.

The differential diagnosis of follicular conjunctivitis may be classified as either acute or chronic. Sometimes differentiation from other disease entities is difficult, and a careful history, clinical examination, and laboratory evaluation are crucial in determining the etiology. The microbiologic evaluation of AIC is similar to that of NIC. If AIC is suspected, the appropriate conjunctival scrapings should be obtained, stained using Giemsa, and cultured using McCoy cells. As with NIC, the gold standard for diagnosis is becoming PCR, if available. In children, the gold standard still remains McCoy cell culture owing to its superior specificity compared to nonculture tests.[35]

All patients with AIC need to be treated systemically. The current recommended regimen is a 3-week course of oral doxycycline 100 mg twice a day or oral tetracycline 250–500 mg four times a day. The use of single-dose azithromycin may be equally efficacious but has not so far been clinically proven in the treatment of AIC. Additional topical therapy is not necessary, and all sexual partners should receive treatment as well.[30]

Lymphogranuloma Venereum

Lymphogranuloma venereum (LGV) is a sexually transmitted disease caused by *C. trachomatis*, serovars L1–3. The rate of reported disease in the United States has been steadily decreasing, with only 113 documented cases in 1997.[36] Nevertheless, it may still account for 2–10% of genital ulcer diseases in focal geographic regions, particularly in areas of India and Africa.[37]

An important distinction between the serovars responsible for LGV and those causing other chlamydial diseases is the type of cell infected. LGV serovars infect macrophages, whereas other serovars infect squamocolumnar cells. This is important because the former tends to produce more systemic disease whereas the latter results in a more limited superficial infection of the mucous membranes.[38,39]

Ocular involvement with LGV is extremely uncommon. When present, it can manifest as Parinaud's oculoglandular syndrome, a condition in which patients present with a severe papillary conjunctivitis as well as massive tender posterior cervical and preauricular lymphadenopathy.[40] In 1947, a series of five patients with inguinal scars and a peripheral infiltrate in the superior cornea was published, with the cause attributed to LGV. In this series, however, the causative organism was never isolated.[41] In addition to Parinaud's, LGV-associated iridocyclitis, episcleritis, and optic neuritis have also been reported.[4]

The diagnosis of LGV is based on clinical grounds as well as laboratory results. The definitive diagnosis can be achieved with the isolation of the organism on culture and cell typing of the isolate.[42] An aspirate of the involved lymph node is the best source for diagnosis.[43] A swab of the infected tissue can also be obtained. Culture of *C. trachomatis* has limitations and at best will be positive only 30% of the time.[44] Consequently, other laboratory methods that can be used for diagnosis have been sought. Currently, the diagnosis is best obtained with serology. Along with the characteristic clinical presentation, a complement fixation antibody titer >1:64 is considered diagnostic.[43,45] Immunofluorescent testing with monoclonal antibodies and PCR have also been described for diagnosis, but they are not readily available for routine use.[45–48]

The current recommended treatment is doxycycline 100 mg twice a day for 3 weeks, erythromycin 500 mg four times a day for 3 weeks, or azithromycin 1 g every week for 3 weeks. In addition, aspiration of the affected lymph nodes may be required to relieve pain and to prevent ulcer formation.[40,42]

Chlamydia psittaci

Chlamydia psittaci is an organism that can be spread from its natural host, birds and mammals, to humans. In humans the resulting infection is referred to as psittacosis, whereas in birds and mammals it is known as avian chlamydiosis. The main groups at risk are those with exposure to birds.[49]

Infection usually occurs when a person inhales the organism, which has been aerosolized from dried feces or respiratory secretions of infected birds. Although pneumonia is the most frequent presentation (the so-called bird fancier's lung), ocular involvement in humans has been reported, albeit rarely. The usual presentation is a chronic follicular conjunctivitis that is equally prominent on both the superior and inferior palpebral conjunctiva. Bulbar follicles may also be present. In addition, a punctate epithelial keratitis and macropannus may be found.[49]

Unlike patients who present with AIC, sexual activity is not a risk factor and may be an important clue in helping to differentiate this from the more common AIC. In cases of psittacosis, a history of bird or mammalian contact is crucial to help make the diagnosis. In 1997, the Centers for Disease Control and the Council of State and Territorial Epidemiologists established case definitions for confirmed and probable psittacosis. A patient is considered to have a confirmed case of psittacosis if clinical illness is compatible with psittacosis and the case is laboratory confirmed by one of three methods: (1) *C. psittaci* is cultured from respiratory secretions; (2) antibody against *C. psittaci* is increased fourfold or more, as demonstrated by complement fixation or microimmunofluorescence (MIF); or (3) immunoglobulin M antibody against *C. psittaci* is detected by MIF. A probable case of psittacosis is defined as either: (1) clinically compatible illness that is epidemiologically linked to a confirmed case, or (2) an antibody titer of at least 32 by CF or MIF in at least one serum specimen after the onset of symptoms.[49] The serologic diagnosis of ocular infections remains difficult owing to the difficulty of obtaining acute and convalescent titers in chronic diseases, the variability in the systemic response to local infections, and the cross-reactivity found between other *Chlamydia* species. PCR remains the most effective diagnostic tool to help differentiate *C. psittaci* from other infections.[49,50] Ocular psittacosis is generally treated with oral tetracycline. The optimum duration of therapy is unknown, although most experts agree that a prolonged course is necessary.

Conclusion

Chlamydia is responsible for a large spectrum of human ocular infections. Early diagnosis is important so that treatment can be initiated to prevent the development of long-term sequelae.

References

1. Resnikoff S, Pascolini D, Etya'ale D, et al. Global data on visual impairment in the year 2002. *Bull WHO.* 2004;82:844–851.
2. Tabbara KF. Trachoma: a review. *J Chemother.* 2001;13(Suppl 1):18–22.
3. Peeling RW, Brunham RC. Chlamydiae as pathogens: New species and new issues. *Emerging Infect Dis.* 1996;2:307–319.
4. Albert DM, Jakobiec FA. *Principles and practice of ophthalmology.* ed. 2. Philadelphia: WB Saunders; 2000: 115–116, 1960.
5. Wright HR. Trachoma. *Lancet.* 2008;371(9628):1945–1954.
6. Lansign VC, Weih LM, Keeffe JE, et al. Assessment of trachoma prevalence in a mobile population in Central Australia. *Ophthalmic Epidemiol.* 2001;8:97–108.
7. Lietman T, Porco T, Dawson C. Global elimination of trachoma: How frequently should we administer mass chemotherapy? *Nature Med.* 1999;5:572–576.
8. Schemann JF. Risk factors for trachoma in Mali. *Int J Epidemiol.* 2002;31(1):194–201.
9. Bowman RJC, Jatta B, Cham B. Natural history of trachomatous scarring in Gambia. *Ophthalmology.* 2001;12:2219–2224.
10. Bailey R, Cuong T, Carpenter R, et al. The duration of human ocular *Chlamydia trachomatis* infection is age dependent. *Epidemiol Infect.* 1999;123:479–486.
11. Gambhir M, Basanez M-G, Turner F. Trachoma: transmission, infection, and control. *Lancet.* 2007;7:401–427.
12. Yang X, Brunham RC. T lymphocyte immunity in host defence against *Chlamydia trachomatis* and its implication for vaccine development. *Can J Infect Dis.* 1998;9(2):99–109.
13. Fry AM, Jha HC, Lietman TM. Adverse and beneficial secondary effects of mass treatment with azithromycin to eliminate blindness due to trachoma in Nepal. *Clin Infect Dis.* 2002;35:395–402.
14. Bailey RL, Arullendran P, Whittle HC, et al. Randomized controlled trial of single-dose azithromycin in the treatment of trachoma. *Lancet.* 1993;342:453–456.
15. World Health Organization. *Report of the first meeting of the WHO Alliance for the Global Elimination of Trachoma.* Geneva: World Health Organization; 1997.
16. Dawson C. Flies and the elimination of blinding trachoma. *Lancet.* 1999;353:1376–1377.
17. Reacher MH, Munoz B, Alghassany A, et al. A controlled trial of surgery for trachomatous trichiasis of the upper lid. *Arch Ophthalmol.* 1992; 110:667–674.

18. Kocak-Midillioglu I. Penetrating keratoplasty in patients with corneal scarring due to trachoma. *Ophthalmic Surg Lasers.* 1999;30(9):734–741.
19. World Health Organization. *Report of the second meeting of the WHO Alliance for the Global Elimination of Trachoma.* Geneva: World Health Organization; 1998.
20. International Council of Ophthalmology International Clinical Guidelines, Trachoma, April 2007.
21. Yip T, Chan WH, Yip KT, et al. Incidence of neonatal chlamydial conjunctivitis and its association with nasopharyngeal colonization in a Hong Kong hospital assessed by polymerase chain reaction. *Hong Kong Med J.* 2007;13(1):22–26.
22. Hammerschlag M, Roblin P, Gelling M, et al. Use of polymerase chain reaction for the detection of *Chlamydia trachomatis* in ocular and nasopharyngeal specimens from infants with conjunctivitis. *Pediatr Infect Dis J.* 1997;16:293–297.
23. Alexander E, Harrison H. Role of *Chlamydia trachomatis* in perinatal infection. *Rev Infect Dis.* 1983;5:713–719.
24. Newton ER, Piper JM, Shain RN, et al. Predictors of the vaginal microflora. *Am J Obstet Gynecol.* 2001;184(5):845–853.
25. Workowski KA, Levine WC. Sexually transmitted diseases treatment guidelines 2002. *Morbidity Mortality Weekly Report.* 2002;51:RR6.
26. Hammerschlag M. *Chlamydia trachomatis* in children. *Pediatr Ann.* 1994;23:349–353.
27. Madhavan HN. Evaluation of laboratory tests for diagnosis of chlamydial infections in conjunctival specimens. *Indian J Med Res.* 1994;100:5–9.
28. Quinn TC. DNA amplification assays: a new standard for diagnosis of *Chlamydia trachomatis* infections. *Ann Acad Med Singapore.* 1995;24(4):627–633.
29. Yip PP. The use of polymerase chain reaction assay versus conventional methods in detecting neonatal chlamydial conjunctivitis. *J. Pediatr Ophthalmol Strabismus.* 2008;45(4):234–239.
30. Hammerschlag M. Chlamydial infections. *J Pediatr.* 1989;114:724–734.
31. Centers for Disease Control and Prevention. Recommendations for the prevention and management of *Chlamydia trachomatis* infections. *MMWR.* 1993;42:RR-12.
32. Centers for Disease Control and Prevention. *Chlamydia trachomatis* genital infections – United States. *MMWR.* 1997;46:193–198.
33. Stenberg K, Maardh PA. Genital infection with *Chlamydia trachomatis* in patients with chlamydial conjunctivitis: Unexpected results. *Sex Transm Dis.* 1991;18:1–4.
34. Postema E, Remeijer L, van der Meijden W. Epidemiology of genital chlamydial infections in patients with chlamydial conjunctivitis: A retrospective study. *Genitourin Med.* 1996;72:203–205.
35. Hammerschlag MR, Stephen AJL, Laraque D. Inappropriate use of nonculture tests for the detection of *Chlamydia trachomatis* in suspected victims of child sexual abuse: a continuing problem. *Pediatrics.* 1999;104(5):1137–1139.
36. Division of STD Prevention. *Sexually Transmitted Disease Surveillance, 1997. US Department of Health and Human Services, Public Health Service.* Atlanta: Centers for Disease Control; September 1998.
37. Rosen T, Dhir A. Chancroid, granuloma inguinale, and lymphogranuloma venereum. In: Arndt KA, ed. *Cutaneous medicine and surgery, an integrated program in dermatology.* Philadelphia: WB Saunders; 1996: 973–982.
38. Schachter J, Osoba AO. Lymphogranuloma venereum. *Br Med Bull.* 1983;39:151–154.
39. Schachter J. Chlamydial infections. *N Engl J Med.* 1978;298:428–435.
40. Czelusta A, Yen-Moore A, Van der Straten M. An overview of sexually transmitted diseases. Part III. Sexually transmitted diseases in HIV-infected patients. *J Am Acad Dermatol.* 2000;43(3):409–432.
41. Scheie HG, Crandall AS, Henle W. Keratitis associated with lymphogranuloma venereum. *JAMA.* 1947;135:333–339.
42. Brown TJ, Yen-Moore A, Tyring SK. An overview of sexually transmitted diseases. Part I. *J Am Acad Dermatol.* 1999;41(4):511–532.
43. Buntin DM, Rosen T, Lesher JL, et al. Sexually transmitted diseases: bacterial infections. *J Am Acad Dermatol.* 1999;25:287–299.
44. Van Dyck E, Piot P. Laboratory techniques in the investigation of chancroid, lymphogranuloma venereum and donovanosis. *Genitourin Med.* 1992;68:130–133.
45. Joseph AK, Rosen T. Laboratory techniques used in the diagnosis of chancroid, granuloma inguinale, and lymphogranuloma venereum. *Dermatol Clin.* 1994;12:1–8.
46. Mittal A, Sachdeva KG. Monoclonal antibody for the diagnosis of lymphogranuloma venereum: a preliminary report. *Br J Biomed Sci.* 1993;50:3–7.
47. Stephens RS, Kuo CC, Tam MR. Sensitivity of immunofluorescence with monoclonal antibodies for detection of *Chlamydia trachomatis* inclusions in cell culture. *J Clin Microbiol.* 1982;16:4–7.
48. Aldridge KE, Cammarata C, Martin DH. Comparison of the in vitro activities of various parenteral and oral antimicrobial agents against endemic *Haemophilus ducreyi*.3. *Antimicrob Agents Chemother.* 1993;37: 1986–1988.
49. Centers for Disease Control and Prevention. Compendium of measures to control *Chlamydia psittaci* infection among humans (psittacosis) and pet birds (avian chlamydiosis), 2000 and Compendium of animal rabies prevention and control, 2000: National Association of State Public Health Veterinarians, Inc. *MMWR.* 2000;49(No. RR-8):3–17.
50. Dean D. Molecular identification of an avian strain of *Chlamydia psittaci* causing severe keratoconjunctivitis in a bird fancier. *Clin Infect Dis.* 1995;20(5):1179–1185.

Chapter 46

Ophthalmia Neonatorum

Thomas D. Lindquist

Ophthalmia neonatorum, or neonatal conjunctivitis, is defined as inflammation of the conjunctiva during the first month of life. It is characterized by injection and swelling of the eyelids and conjunctiva, coupled with purulent discharge in which one or more polymorphonuclear cells are seen per high-power field on a Gram-stained conjunctival smear.[1]

Neonatal conjunctivitis manifests as a diffuse, often hyperacute conjunctivitis with a papillary reaction. A follicular response is not seen prior to 6 to 8 weeks of life and, therefore, is not a helpful finding in establishing a differential diagnosis. Neonatal conjunctivitis may result from exposure to silver nitrate prophylaxis or from infection by a variety of bacterial, chlamydial, viral, or fungal pathogens. The severity of the inflammatory response depends largely on the inciting agent. The reported incidence ranges from 1.6% to 12% of newborns.[2]

Pathogenesis

Understanding the incubation times of the different etiologic agents can be useful clinically; however, the onset of neonatal conjunctivitis postpartum can be affected by many other factors.[3] All infants delivered vaginally are exposed to many different bacteria. Isenberg and colleagues[4] cultured the conjunctiva of 100 eyes of newborns within 15 minutes of delivery. (Bacteria were isolated from 75% of the 100 eyes that were cultured.) Microaerophilic bacteria including *Lactobacillus* species and diphtheroids accounted for 62% of all bacteria isolated, whereas true anaerobes including *Bifidobacterium* species, *Propionibacterium acnes*, and *Bacteroides* species accounted for 28%. However, these organisms rarely cause neonatal conjunctivitis. Aerobic bacteria accounted for only 10% of all bacteria isolated. *Staphylococcus epidermidis* was the most common aerobic organism followed by *Corynebacterium*, *Streptococcus* species, and *Escherichia coli*. The conjunctival bacteria of infants born by vaginal delivery reflect the bacterial flora of the vagina.

Isenberg and colleagues[5] found sterile conjunctival cultures in more than 75% of infants delivered by Caesarean section within 3 hours of membrane rupture. In neonates delivered by Caesarean section more than 3 hours after membrane rupture, the number of positive conjunctival cultures began to increase.

In cases of premature rupture of membranes or during a difficult delivery, the infant may have prolonged exposure to infectious agents.[6] Premature rupture of membranes allows retrograde spread of organisms to the conjunctiva and cornea. Prolonged intrauterine exposure to infectious organisms may be largely responsible for the errors in relating the time of onset of neonatal conjunctivitis to the etiologic agent.

Any trauma to the ocular tissues during delivery may further facilitate invasion by infectious organisms.[3] Epithelial trauma may result from abrasions, exposure, or secondary to chemical prophylaxis, particularly with silver nitrate. *Neisseria gonorrhoeae* is an important exception to the rule that epithelial trauma predisposes to infection, because this organism is capable of penetrating intact epithelium.[7]

The neonate's immune system is immature, which increases the susceptibility to infection. Inadequate antibody synthesis is largely compensated by the passive transfer of maternal IgG. However, local secretory IgA is lacking unless the infant ingests breast milk.[8] In most premature infants and in 20% of full-term infants, the tear secretory rate is abnormally low.[9] Lysozyme, which catalyzes the breakdown of bacterial cell membranes, has a higher concentration in tears than in serum.[10] However, the concentration of lysozyme in tears is decreased in premature infants compared to full-term infants and adults.[9]

After birth, a caregiver who has a 'cold sore' or who harbors bacteria in the nasopharynx may inadvertently infect a neonate. Prolonged neonatal intensive care increases the potential of nosocomial infection.

The Role of Sexually Transmitted Diseases

The increasing prevalence of sexually transmitted disease accounts for the finding that *Chlamydia trachomatis* is now the most common cause of infectious neonatal conjunctivitis in industrialized countries.[11] In the United States, more than 4 million new infections are estimated annually.[12] Whereas chlamydial infections are common in higher socioeconomic groups, gonorrhea is seldom encountered. When students were screened at private colleges, chlamydial infection exceeded gonococcal infection by a factor of five- to tenfold in symptomatic men or in asymptomatic women having routine pelvic examinations. In contrast, in urban venereal disease clinics, chlamydial and gonococcal infections occur at the same rate.[13] The most important factor for *C. trachomatis* infection is age. Younger women have the highest infection rates.[14] In the United States it is estimated that 5% of pregnant women have cervical chlamydial infection, placing their infants at risk.[11] Approximately 60% of infants exposed to *C. trachomatis* during birth contract the infection.[15] The incidence of neonatal conjunctivitis caused by *C. trachomatis* is between 5 and 60 per 1000 live births in the United States and as high as 80 per 1000 live births in Kenya.[16]

In the United States, 335 104 gonococcal infections were reported in 2003.[17] The incidence of gonococcal neonatal conjunctivitis is 0.3 per 1000 live births in the United States, whereas in Kenya the incidence is 40 per 1000 live births.[16] More than 50% of the infants with neonatal conjunctivitis in Kenya were found to be co-infected with both *Neisseria gonorrhoeae* and *C. trachomatis*.[18] A study conducted in Kenya suggested that 42% of neonates exposed to N. *gonorrhoeae* during delivery developed gonococcal conjunctivitis.[16]

In the United States, 500 000 new genital infections with herpes simplex virus are estimated annually.[19] Between 1500 and 2000 cases of neonatal herpes infection occur annually in the United States, giving an incidence of one in approximately 3500 deliveries.[19,20] Four percent of these cases are acquired transplacentally prior to birth, 86% during birth, and 10% postnatally.[19] Seventy to eighty percent of neonatal herpetic infections are caused by the genital strain, herpes simplex virus (HSV) II, as the infant's abraded skin or mucosal surfaces contact the infected maternal genital secretions.[19] However, 60–80% of these mothers have asymptomatic or unrecognized infection at the time of delivery and have a negative history of genital herpes.[21] Neonatal infection from herpes simplex virus occurs in 40–60% of neonates exposed to active genital herpes virus.[22] The greatest risk of neonatal herpes simplex infection occurs when the mother has primary genital herpes involving the cervix at delivery, and the infant is premature and delivered with instrumentation such as scalp electrodes.[19]

Approximately 10% of infants acquire HSV-I postnatally through close contact with relatives or hospital personnel with active mucocutaneous herpes infections.[19]

Causes of Neonatal Conjunctivitis

Chemical

In 1881, Credé[23] recommended cleansing of the eyelids immediately after birth and instillation of 2% silver nitrate into the conjunctival fornix. Silver nitrate is a surface-active chemical that agglutinates gonococci and inactivates them. This prophylaxis has played a major role in reducing severe vision loss due to gonococcal neonatal conjunctivitis. However, a chemical conjunctivitis characterized by mild and transient conjunctival injection and tearing is common and usually resolves in 24 to 48 hours.[24] It develops rapidly and is seen in as many as 90% of treated eyes.[25]

Silver nitrate is available as a buffered 1% solution in a single-use wax ampule, which ensures its safety. Previously, more highly concentrated solutions of silver nitrate (most likely secondary to evaporation) were instilled, which caused a potentially severe chemical irritation with lid edema, chemosis, exudate, membranes or pseudomembranes, and even conjunctival or corneal scarring.

Bacterial

Neisseria gonorrhoeae was a major cause of blindness among children 100 years ago as evidenced by the finding that 24% of children enrolled in schools for the blind between 1906 and 1911 were blinded by complications of gonococcal ophthalmia.[26]

Conjunctivitis due to *N. gonorrhoeae* typically appears 2 to 5 days after birth.[27] Later onset of gonococcal conjunctivitis suggests postnatal exposure to the organism. An initial serosanguineous discharge progresses to a thick and purulent discharge within 24 hours, associated with markedly edematous eyelids and prominent chemosis (Fig. 46.1). Conjunctival membranes may be seen. Gonococci have the ability to penetrate intact epithelial cells and replicate rapidly.[28] Any delay in diagnosis can lead to corneal ulceration, which may progress rapidly to corneal perforation.

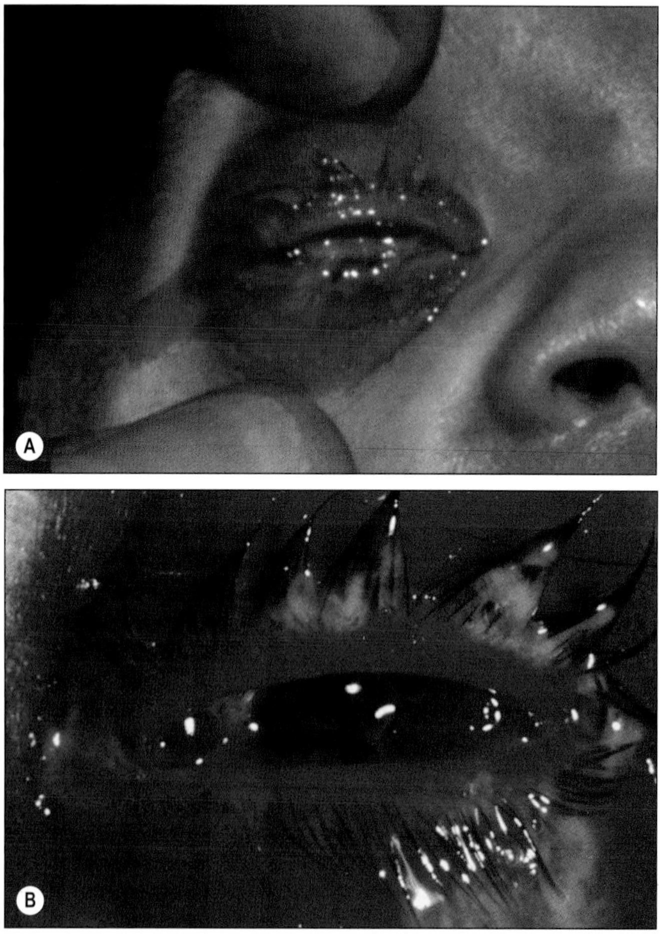

Fig. 46.1 Hyperacute neonatal conjunctivitis caused by *Neisseria gonorrhoeae*. (**A**) Markedly edematous eyelids and grossly purulent discharge. (**B**) Note thick, purulent discharge, conjunctival chemosis, and papillary hypertrophy.

Other bacteria implicated in neonatal conjunctivitis principally include *Haemophilus* species, *Streptococcus pneumoniae*, and *Staphylococcus aureus*.[16,29] Methicillin-resistant *Staphylococcus aureus* (MRSA) can be passed from mother to preterm infant through contaminated breast milk, even in the absence of maternal infection.[30] Neonates may be colonized with MRSA in a newborn intensive care unit, and a significant number may develop purulent conjunctivitis.[31]

Although *Pseudomonas aeruginosa* is a rare cause of neonatal conjunctivitis, this organism can rapidly progress from conjunctivitis to corneal ulceration and perforation. Microaerophilic and anaerobic bacteria are most frequently isolated from conjunctival cultures taken at birth; however, these organisms are rarely responsible for neonatal conjunctivitis.[4]

Historically, the latent period for development of bacterial conjunctivitis other than *N. gonorrhoeae* has been 5 to 8 days after birth.[3,29] However, the onset of bacterial conjunctivitis may occur any time in the immediate postpartum period. Lid edema, chemosis, conjunctival injection, and purulent discharge are variable and are frequently indistinguishable from other causes of neonatal conjunctivitis.

Chlamydial

The Chlamydiae are nonmotile, Gram-negative, obligate intracellular bacteria whose unique developmental cycle differentiates them from all other microorganisms.[11] Replication occurs within the cytoplasm of host cells, where characteristic basophilic intracellular inclusions can be identified for diagnostic purposes.

Neonatal inclusion conjunctivitis, or inclusion blennorrhea caused by *C. trachomatis*, is the most common cause of infectious neonatal conjunctivitis in industrialized nations.[11] Because of the long growth cycle, the incubation period of chlamydia ranges from 5 to 14 days, although premature rupture of membranes with exposure to the pathogen may herald the onset of disease earlier than 5 days postpartum. Clinically, inclusion conjunctivitis is accompanied by a mild mucopurulent palpebral conjunctivitis, moderate lid edema, and mild chemosis (Fig. 46.2). It may be unilateral or bilateral. In some cases, the inflammation may be severe, causing a hyperacute conjunctivitis with swollen lids, marked injection, and purulent discharge.[3,24,29]

The development of large conjunctival follicles so characteristic of chlamydial ocular disease[6] is not seen in the neonate because of the immaturity of the lymphoid system. Follicular hypertrophy is not seen in the infant prior to 6 to 8 weeks of age and, therefore, is not a helpful diagnostic sign unless the disease becomes chronic.[3,6,24]

Pseudomembranes or true membranes may develop and can lead to conjunctival scarring.[32] In the peripheral cornea, punctate epithelial erosions may develop and subepithelial infiltrates and areas of stromal haze may be seen infrequently.[6] Corneal micropannus and scarring are uncommon but may be seen, particularly in untreated cases.

If left untreated, the disease may persist for up to a year or more. However, neonatal inclusion conjunctivitis is generally considered benign and self-limiting. The average duration is 4.5 months.[33] However, this fact does not eliminate the need for treatment.

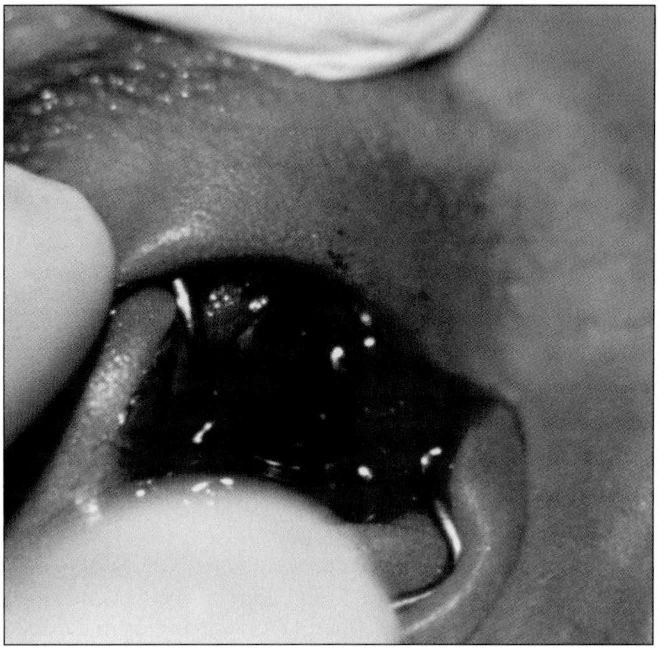

Fig. 46.2 Neonatal chlamydial conjunctivitis in a 13-day-old infant with conjunctival hyperemia, papillary hypertrophy, and mucopurulent discharge.

Systemic disease may develop and involve the pharynx, rectum, or vagina, but the major nonocular complication is chlamydial pneumonia. The reported incidence of pneumonia ranges from 11% to 20% of infected infants who present between 1 and 3 months of age with nasal congestion, prolonged cough, normal temperature, tachypnea, and rales on auscultation. It is the systemic nature of this disease that dictates the systemic treatment.[15,34]

Viral

Neonatal conjunctivitis due to HSV typically occurs within 6 to 14 days after birth and may be unilateral or bilateral.[19] The conjunctivitis is associated with eyelid edema and a serous discharge. Unless there are vesicular lesions on the skin or lid margins, the conjunctivitis is indistinguishable from other causes of ophthalmia neonatorum.[3] However, 80% of neonates with herpes will have typical herpetic lesions of the skin, eye, or mouth.[19] Microdendrites or geographic ulcers are the more prominent signs of corneal involvement, rather than the typical herpetic dendrites seen in recurrent disease.[24] Although primary ocular HSV infection in children typically causes a follicular conjunctival response, follicles are not seen prior to 6 to 8 weeks of life because of the immaturity of the infant's immune system.

It is important for the ophthalmologist to bear in mind that, although neonatal keratoconjunctivitis may be the sole manifestation of herpes infection, it is frequently associated with systemic infection. The mortality rate for disseminated disease is 50%.[20] El Azazi and colleagues[35] examined 32 children after virologically verified neonatal HSV infection and found ocular morbidity in 40%. The incidence of the ophthalmic findings was as follows: chorioretinal scarring, 69%; optic atrophy, 54%; corneal scars, 15%; and cataract, 8%.

Twelve of thirteen (93%) severely handicapped children in the study had impaired vision, mainly from cortical blindness.

Fungal

An infrequent cause of neonatal conjunctivitis is *Candida*, which may present in the eye as a pseudomembranous conjunctivitis or as a white conjunctival plaque. The time of onset after exposure is 5 days or more.[36]

Laboratory Diagnosis

Because of the potentially disastrous complications of untreated neonatal conjunctivitis, determination of the specific etiologic agent is mandatory. Multiple factors influence the onset and etiology of neonatal conjunctivitis and, because more than one agent can be present, conjunctival smears and cultures are imperative.[3,24,37]

Preliminary diagnosis of the etiologic agent of neonatal conjunctivitis can be made from Gram- and Giemsa-stained conjunctival smears (Table 46.1). A Papanicolaou-stained smear is necessary for suspected HSV infection.[37]

Scraping of the conjunctiva is optimally done with a Kimura spatula, since epithelial cells must be obtained to assess the cytologic aspects of the inflammatory response. Cultures may be obtained with a calcium alginate swab, prewetting with sterile liquid media.[38] Recommended media for aerobic bacteria include reduced blood agar, thioglycolate, or brain-heart infusion broth, as well as chocolate agar in CO_2 or Thayer-Martin media to rule out *Neisseria gonorrhoeae*.[37] Fungal cultures can be obtained using a Sabouraud's slant without antibiotic supplementation.

A smear from an infant with chemical conjunctivitis should demonstrate neutrophils and occasional lymphocytes, whereas a smear from neonatal bacterial conjunctivitis would reveal neutrophils and bacteria. Intracellular Gram-negative diplococci are demonstrated in up to 95% of culture-positive cases of *N. gonorrhoeae* conjunctivitis.[29] A conjunctival smear from an infant with *Chlamydia* would show neutrophils, lymphocytes, plasma cells, and basophilic intracytoplasmic inclusions in epithelial cells. Although intracytoplasmic inclusion bodies are infrequently seen in adult inclusion conjunctivitis, they are frequently found in neonatal inclusion conjunctivitis. A smear from an infant with herpes simplex conjunctivitis would be expected to demonstrate lymphocytes, plasma cells, multinucleate giant cells, and eosinophilic intranuclear inclusions.[24] Lastly, a smear from a neonate with *Candida* conjunctivitis would show neutrophils and pseudohyphal budding yeast forms.[36]

Nonculture tests of gonococcal infections are widely available and may use urine samples rather than more invasive swabs and permit evaluation of *C. trachomatis* with the same specimen. Non-amplified DNA–DNA hybridization probe tests are based on a single-stranded DNA probe complimentary to gonococcal rRNA. Nucleic acid amplification tests are as sensitive as culture, have specificities of at least 99%, and can be used to evaluate first-void urine specimens.[17] Confirmation of *C. trachomatis* conjunctivitis has traditionally been performed by McCoy cell culture, but this technique is expensive and requires at least 2 to 3 days for results. Enzyme immunoassays (EIA) use enzyme-labeled chlamydial-specific antibodies to detect chlamydial lipopolysaccharides. Direct fluorescent antibody (DFA) assays use fluorescein-conjugated monoclonal antibodies to stain chlamydial antigens in smear, and results can be obtained within hours.[39,40] DFA yields 100% sensitivity and 94% specificity.[39] Highly sensitive nucleic acid amplification tests (NAATS) are commercially available for the diagnosis of genital chlamydial infection in adolescents and adults.[41] As with other nonculture tests, NAATS do not require viable organisms. Preliminary data suggest these test are equivalent to culture for the detection of *C. trachomatis* in the conjunctiva and nasopharynx of infants, but these are not yet FDA-approved due to limited evaluation.[41]

In addition to collecting ocular specimens, dermal or mucosal vesicular lesions should be scraped for cytologic evaluation with Papanicolaou stain, viral culture, or immunologic testing.[11,37] Viral isolation of HSV in human cell culture can provide a definitive diagnosis. However, growth takes at least 2 to 4 days and the culture technique is expensive. Viral antigens can be detected rapidly using immunologic tests. Direct immunofluorescent, enzyme-linked immunosorbent assay (ELISA), and immunofiltration methods are available. Direct immunofluorescent testing can also differentiate HSV-I from HSV-II.[42]

Table 46.1 Cytologic characteristics of Giemsa-stained conjunctival smears

Etiologic agent	Cytology
Chemical	Neutrophils, occasional lymphocytes
Bacterial	Neutrophils, bacteria
Chlamydial	Neutrophils, lymphocytes, plasma cells, basophilic intracytoplasmic inclusions in epithelial cells
Viral	Lymphocytes, plasma cells, multinucleated giant cells, eosinophilic intranuclear inclusions
Fungal (yeast)	Neutrophils, pseudohyphal budding yeast forms

Treatment

No treatment is necessary for chemical conjunctivitis, which typically resolves within 24 to 48 hours.

Bacterial conjunctivitis from Gram-positive cocci is appropriately treated with tetracycline 1% or erythromycin 0.5% ointment every 4 hours for 7 days.[37,39] MRSA neonatal conjunctivitis may be treated with bacitracin 500 IU/g ointment, chloramphenicol 1% ointment (no longer available in the USA) or vancomycin 5–31 mg/ml depending upon bacterial sensitivity.[40,43] Gram-negative bacilli causing conjunctivitis may be treated with tobramycin 0.3% or ciprofloxacin 0.3% ointment every 4 hours for 7 days.[44] Only rarely are these regimens ineffective.

Until recently, treatment of *N. gonorrhoeae* neonatal conjunctivitis consisted of intravenous aqueous penicillin G, 100 000 units/kg/day in divided doses for 7 days.[24,37] However,

Table 46.2 Treatment of neonatal conjunctivitis

Etiologic agent	Treatment
Chemical	None required
Bacterial: Gram-positive cocci	Tetracycline 1%, bacitracin 500 IU/g or erythromycin 0.5% ointment, every 4 hours for 7 days
Gram-negative bacilli	Tobramycin 0.3% OR ciprofloxacin 0.3% ointment every 4 hours for 7 days
Neisseria gonorrhoeae	Ceftriaxone 125 mg IM once, plus saline irrigation, OR cefotaxime 25 mg/kg IV or IM every 8–12 hours for 7 days plus saline irrigation, OR penicillin G 100 000 U/kg/day IV in 4 divided doses ×7 days for susceptible strains plus saline irrigation
Chlamydial	Erythromycin ethylsuccinate 12.5 mg/kg/day orally or IV in 3–4 divided doses, for 14 days, OR sulfisoxazole 100 mg/kg/day orally or IV in divided doses for 14 days in infants greater than 4 weeks old OR azithromycin suspension 20 mg/kg once daily for 3 days plus erythromycin 0.5% ointment 4 times daily until the conjunctivitis resolves
Viral (herpes simplex)	Acyclovir 30 mg/kg/day for 10 days OR vidarabine 30 mg/kg/day for 10 days plus trifluorothymidine 1% topically every 2 hours for 7 days or until the cornea reepithelializes, OR adenosine arabinoside 3% ointment or acyclovir 5% ointment 5 times daily for 7 days or until the cornea reepithelializes
Fungal (yeast)	Natamycin 5% drops hourly for 10–14 days, OR flucytosine 1% drops hourly for 10–14 days.

three major types of antimicrobial resistance in *N. gonorrhoeae* are now recognized: penicillinase production, chromosomally mediated resistance to the penicillins or tetracyclines, and plasmid-mediated tetracycline resistance.[45,46] Because of the emergence of resistant strains to as high as 53% in some areas of the world,[16] ceftriaxone has become the recommended treatment. A single intramuscular dose of ceftriaxone 125 mg is highly effective against neonatal gonococcal conjunctivitis and also simultaneously treats extraocular infection.[47] Cefotaxime in an intramuscular dose of 100 mg is also effective against resistant *N. gonorrhoeae* organisms,[48] but the recommended dose for neonatal ophthalmia is 25 mg/kg IV or IM every 8 to 12 hours for 7 days. Cefixime is an orally absorbed cephalosporin with excellent activity against resistant gonococci, and single doses of 400–800 mg orally are highly effective for adults.[49] Single oral doses of the fluoroquinolones are also effective, but have the potential disadvantage of inducing antibiotic resistance.[50] Caregivers and relatives with *N. gonorrhoeae* should also be treated with doxycycline 100 mg orally twice daily for 7 days or a single oral dose of 1.0 g azithromycin because of the high risk of concomitant chlamydial infection.[24,34,51]

In addition to intravenous antibiotics, infant eyes with gonococcal conjunctivitis should be irrigated hourly with saline.[37] The in vitro minimal inhibitory concentration of the fluoroquinolones to *N. gonorrhoeae* is extremely low, and, therefore, consideration may be given to topical fluoroquinolone use in the early treatment of gonococcal neonatal conjunctivitis[50] in addition to systemic therapy.

The treatment of choice for neonatal chlamydial conjunctivitis is oral erythromycin ethylsuccinate suspension, 50 mg/kg/day in three or four divided doses for 14 days.[34] Topical erythromycin ointment may be clinically effective against chlamydial conjunctivitis, but this treatment does not eradicate nasopharyngeal colonization, which can exceed 50% in infants with neonatal chlamydial conjunctivitis.[34] If not treated systemically, a number of infants may develop chlamydial pneumonia. Systemic treatment with erythromycin has been associated with a 20–30% failure rate. Infants may be treated alternatively with azithromycin suspension 20 mg/kg either as a single dose or once daily for 3 days.[34] As discussed above, caregivers and relatives with *C. trachomatis* infection should be treated with oral doxycycline for 7 days or with a single dose of azithromycin.

All infections caused by herpes simplex in the neonatal period should be treated with systemic acyclovir or vidarabine.[19,52–54] No differences in outcome were observed between intravenous acyclovir or vidarabine in the treatment of neonatal HSV infections in a multicenter, randomized, and masked study.[55] Infants with HSV keratoconjunctivitis should also be treated with topical antivirals. Trifluorothymidine 1% solution may be given topically every 2 hours for 7 days or until the cornea has reepithelialized, but no longer than 21 days.[36,37] Infants who are tearing profusely may be more efficiently treated with the use of adenine arabinoside 3% ointment or acyclovir 5% ointment given five times daily because drug availability may be increased by the use of ointment (Table 46.2). Neonates with HSV keratitis may also be treated with topical cycloplegic agents for the relief of ciliary spasm. Topical corticosteroids should be avoided in neonatal or primary HSV keratoconjunctivitis.

Ocular Prophylaxis

Ocular prophylaxis is directed principally toward preventing infected genital secretions of the mother from contaminating the neonate's eyes at birth.[56] To that end, Caesarean section is advised for women who have active herpes lesions at delivery.[3,18,57] Surveillance of women during the third trimester of pregnancy for evidence of herpetic, chlamydial, or gonococcal infection is critical in the prevention of neonatal conjunctivitis.[56]

Neonatal ocular prophylaxis should be directed primarily against gonococcal ophthalmia since this agent poses the greatest risk of eye injury.[56] Immediately after birth, the infant's eyes should be carefully cleansed. Topical 1% silver nitrate solution, 1% tetracycline ointment, or 0.5% erythromycin ointment were formerly recommended for prophylaxis, but have largely been replaced by povidone-iodine. Povidone-iodine (2.5% ophthalmic solution) has been shown to be as effective as the three commonly used prophylactic preparations in reducing conjunctival bacterial colonies in neonates and causes less toxicity than silver nitrate.[58,59] Because of the broad spectrum of povidone-iodine which includes fungi, chlamydia, viruses, and all bacteria, this agent is becoming the most widely used for ocular prophylaxis.[60]

References

1. Fransen L, Klauss V. Neonatal ophthalmia in the developing world: epidemiology, etiology, management and control. *Int Ophthalmol.* 1988;11:189.
2. Armstrong JH, Zacarias F, Rein MF. Ophthalmia neonatorum: a chart review. *Pediatrics.* 1976;57:884.
3. Isenberg SJ, Apt L, Wood M. The influence of perinatal factors on ophthalmia neonatorum. *J Pediatr Ophthalmol Strabismus.* 1996;33:185.
4. Isenberg SJ, et al. Bacterial flora of the conjunctiva at birth. *J Pediatr Ophthalmol Strabismus.* 1986;23:284.
5. Isenberg SJ, et al. Source of the conjunctival bacterial flora at birth and implications for ophthalmia neonatorum prophylaxis. *Am J Ophthalmol.* 1988;106:458.
6. Yetman RJ, Coody DK. Conjunctivitis: a practice guideline. *J Pediatr Health Care.* 1997;11:238.
7. Buchanan TM. Surface antigens pili. In: Roberts RB, ed. *The gonococcus.* New York: John Wiley & Sons; 1974.
8. Miller ME, Stiehm ER. Immunology and resistance to infection. In: Remington JS, Klein JO, eds. *Infectious diseases of the fetus and newborn infant.* Philadelphia: WB Saunders; 1983.
9. Etches PC, Leahy F, Harris D. Lysozyme in the tears of newborn babies. *Arch Dis Child.* 1979;54:218.
10. Gillette TE, Greiner JV, Allansmith MR. Immunohistochemical localization of human tear lysozyme. *Arch Ophthalmol.* 1981;99:298.
11. Rours GIJG, Hammerschlag MR, Ott A, et al. *Chlamydial trachomatis* as a cause of neonatal conjunctivitis in Dutch infants. *Pediatrics.* 2008; 121:321–326.
12. *Chlamydia trachomatis* genital infections – United States, 1995. *MMWR Morb Mortal Wkly Rep.* 1997;193–198.
13. McCormack WM, et al. Sexually transmitted conditions among women college students. *Am J Obstet Gynecol.* 1981;139:130.
14. Schachter J, Stone E, Moncada J. Screening for chlamydial infections in women attending family planning clinics: evaluations of presumptive indicators for therapy. *West J Med.* 1983;138:375.
15. Alexander ER, Harrison HR. Role of *Chlamydia trachomatis* in perinatal infection. *Rev Infect Dis.* 1983;5:713.
16. Laga M, et al. Epidemiology of ophthalmia neonatorum in Kenya. *Lancet.* 1986;2:1145.
17. Woods CR. Gonococcal infections in neonates and young children. *Semin Pediatr Infect Dis.* 2005;16:258–270.
18. Fransen L, et al. Ophthalmia neonatorum in Nairobi, Kenya: the roles of *Neisseria gonorrhoeae* and *Chlamydia trachomatis.* *J Infect Dis.* 1986;153:862.
19. Overall JC Jr. Herpes simplex virus infection of the fetus and newborn. *Pediatr Ann.* 1994;23:131.
20. Gutierrez KM, et al. The epidemiology of neonatal herpes simplex virus infections in California from 1985 to 1995. *J Infect Dis.* 1999;180:199.
21. Whitley RJ. Herpes simplex virus infections. In: Remington JS, Klein JO, eds. *Infectious diseases of the fetus and newborn infant.* 3rd ed. Philadelphia: WB Saunders; 1990.
22. Nahmias AJ, et al. Perinatal risk associated with maternal genital herpes simplex virus infection of fetus and newborn. *Obstet Gynecol.* 1974;44:63.
23. Credé CSR. Die Verhutuna der augenentzundung der Neugeborenen. *Arch Gynakol.* 1881;18:367.
24. Grosskreutz C, Smith LBH. Neonatal conjunctivitis. *Int Ophthalmol Clin.* 1992;32(1):71.
25. Nishida H, Rosenberg HM. Silver nitrate ophthalmic solution and chemical conjunctivitis. *Pediatrics.* 1975;56:368.
26. Barsam PC. Specific prophylaxis of gonorrheal ophthalmia neonatorum: a review. *N Engl J Med.* 1966;274:731.
27. Glasgow LA, Overall JC Jr. Infections of the newborn. In: Behrman RE, et al, eds. *Textbook of pediatrics.* Philadelphia: WB Saunders; 1983.
28. Duke-Elder S, ed. Inflammations of the conjunctiva and associated inflammations of the cornea. In: *System of ophthalmology, diseases of the outer eye.* Vol VIII. St Louis: Mosby; 1965.
29. Chandler JW, Rapoza PA. Ophthalmia neonatorum. *Int Ophthalmol Clin.* 1990;30:36.
30. Behari P, Englund J, Alcasid G, et al. Transmission of methicillin-resistant *Staphyloccoccus aureus* to preterm infants through breast milk. *Infect Control Hosp Epidemiol.* 2004;25:778–780.
31. Cimolai N. Ocular methicillin-resistant *Staphyloccoccus aureus* infections in a newborn intensive care cohort. *Am J Ophthalmol.* 2006;142: 183–184.
32. Ostler HB. Oculogenital disease. *Surv Ophthalmol.* 1976;20:233.
33. Thygeson P, Stone W Jr. Epidemiology of inclusion conjunctivitis. *Arch Ophthalmol.* 1942;27:91.
34. Hammerschlag MR, Gelling M, Roblin PM, et al. Treatment of neonatal chlamydial conjunctivitis with azithromycin. *Pediatr Infect Dis J.* 1998; 17:1049–1050.
35. el Azazi M, Malm G, Forsgren M. Late ophthalmologic manifestations of neonatal herpes simplex virus infection. *Am J Ophthalmol.* 1990; 109:1.
36. Arffa RC, ed. Conjunctivitis. I. Follicular, neonatal, and bacterial. In: *Grayson's diseases of the cornea.* 3rd ed. St Louis: Mosby; 1991.
37. DeToledo AR, Chandler JW. Conjunctivitis of the newborn. *Infect Dis Clin North Am.* 1992;4:807–813.
38. Benson WH, Lanier JD. Comparison of techniques for culturing corneal ulcers. *Ophthalmology.* 1992;99:800.
39. Hammerschlag MR. Diagnosis of chlamydial infection in the pediatric population. *Immunol Invest.* 1997;26:151–156.
40. Teoh DL, Reynolds S. Diagnosis and management of pediatric conjunctivitis. *Pediatr Emerg Care.* 2003;19:48–55.
41. Darville T. *Chlamydial trachomatis* infections in neonates and young children. *Semin Pediatric Infect Dis.* 2005;16:235–244.
42. Kowalski RP, Gordon YJ. Evaluation of immunologic tests for the detection of ocular herpes simplex virus. *Ophthalmology.* 1989;96:1583.
43. Freidlin J, et al. Spectrum of eye disease caused by methicillin-resistant *Staphylococcus aureus. Am J Ophthalmol.* 2007;144:313.
44. Leibowitz HM. Antibacterial effectiveness of ciprofloxacin 0.3% ophthalmic solution in the treatment of bacterial conjunctivitis. *Am J Ophthalmol.* 1991;112:29S.
45. Schwarcz SK, et al. National surveillance of antimicrobial resistance in *Neisseria gonorrhoeae. JAMA.* 1990;264:1413.
46. Centers for Disease Control. Plasmid-mediated antimicrobial resistance in *Neisseria gonorrhoeae* – United States, 1988 and 1989. *MMWR.* 1990;39:284, 294.
47. Laga M, et al. Single-dose therapy of gonococcal ophthalmia neonatorum with ceftriaxone. *N Engl J Med.* 1986;315:1382.
48. Lepage P, et al. Single-dose cefotaxime intramuscularly cures gonococcal ophthalmia neonatorum. *Br J Ophthalmol.* 1988;72:518.
49. Handsfield HH, et al. A comparison of single-dose cefixime with ceftriaxone as treatment for uncomplicated gonorrhea. *N Engl J Med.* 1991;325:1337.
50. Hooper DC, Wolfson JS. Fluoroquinolone antimicrobial agents. *N Engl J Med.* 1991;324:384.
51. Lau CY, Qureshi AK. Azithromycin versus doxycycline for genital chlamydial infections: a meta-analysis of randomized clinical trials. *Sex Transm Dis.* 2002;29:497.
52. Whitley RJ. Herpes simplex virus infections of women and their offspring: implications for a developed society. *Proc Natl Acad Sci USA.* 1994;91:2441.
53. Garland SM, Doyle L, Kitchen W. Herpes simplex virus type 1 infections presenting at birth. *J Paediatr Child Health.* 1991;27:360.
54. Whitley RJ. Herpes simplex virus infections of the central nervous system. Encephalitis and neonatal herpes. *Drugs.* 1991;42:406.
55. Whitley R, et al. A controlled trial comparing vidarabine with acyclovir in neonatal herpes simplex virus infection. Infectious Diseases Collaborative Antiviral Study Group. *N Engl J Med.* 1991;324:444.
56. Reimer K, et al. Antimicrobial effectiveness of povidone-iodine and consequences for new application areas. *Dermatology.* 2002;204:114.
57. Jeffries DJ. Intrauterine and neonatal herpes simplex virus infection. *Scand J Infect Dis Suppl.* 1991;80:21.
58. Isenberg SJ, Apt L, Campeas D. Ocular applications of povidone-iodine. *Dermatology.* 2002;204:92.
59. Isenberg SJ, Apt L, Wood M. A controlled trial of povidone-iodine as prophylaxis against ophthalmia neonatorum. *N Engl J Med.* 1995;332: 562.
60. Rotta AT. Povidone-iodine to prevent ophthalmia neonatorum. *N Engl J Med.* 1995;333:126.

Chapter 47

Parinaud's Oculoglandular Syndrome

William D. Gruzensky

History

In 1889 Henri Parinaud described two patients with unilateral nodular or ulcerative conjunctivitis associated with regional lymphadenopathy.[1] These patients had close contact with animals and Parinaud suspected a relationship. As clinicians recognized similar cases and added to the literature, this constellation of findings became known as Parinaud's oculoglandular syndrome.

Although the underlying cause of the disease originally described by Parinaud is unknown, we now know that the combination of granulomatous conjunctivitis and preauricular or cervical adenopathy can be caused by more than one infectious agent. Laboratory studies, which can now culture or identify the causative agents through PCR, serology and other technologies, played a key role in clarifying our current understanding of the causes of this syndrome. The syndrome is now known to be a common pathway for several infectious agents. Table 47.1 shows an extended list of the known infectious causes of Parinaud's oculoglandular syndrome.[2]

The most common bacterial cause, *Bartonella henselae,* is particularly difficult to culture. Thus the association of cat-scratch disease (CSD) with Parinaud's oculoglandular syndrome was suspected long before the infectious agent was identified and characterized. In 1950, Pesme and Marchand[3] reported a 6-year-old patient with a positive cat-scratch skin test and Parinaud's oculoglandular syndrome. This association was further supported when Cassady and Culbertson[4] published a report of four patients with Parinaud's oculoglandular syndrome and positive cat-scratch skin tests. However, it was not until 1985 that Wear and associates demonstrated the cat-scratch bacillus in conjunctival specimens.[5] And although the bacterial agents were cultured from lymph nodes of patients with cat-scratch disease by Gerber and associates[6] in 1985, it was not until 1999 that Grando and associates[7] reported culturing *Bartonella henselae* from a conjunctival specimen in Parinaud's oculoglandular syndrome. The identity of this organism was confirmed with PCR studies.

Directed Work-up

The history and physical findings should assist in directing laboratory testing and treatment for patients with Parinaud's oculoglandular syndrome. Table 47.2 shows a recommended approach to work-up and treatment based on symptoms and findings. Most notably, a more aggressive approach is indicated in patients who are immunocompromised or have more severe symptoms.

Patient history should include questions about pets and wild animals. Any history of exposure to cats, dogs, rabbits, prairie dogs, squirrels, and ticks is important. A history of rabbit or tick exposure or high fever, for example, warrants special emphasis on work-up for tularemia. Cats are known vectors for *Bartonella henselae,* coccidioidomycosis[8], and sporotrichosis.[9] Ticks can be involved in transmission of both tularemia and cat-scratch disease. A family or exposure history for tuberculosis should be sought, and any history of sexually transmitted disease should prompt a more extensive work-up for syphilis and lymphogranuloma venereum. A history of soil or vegetable matter contamination would suggest the need to test for sporotrichosis. Unusual animal exposures, including contact with caterpillar hairs, should also be sought.

Because a fourfold rise in antibody titers is strongly suggestive of causation, serum drawn early in the course of Parinaud's oculoglandular syndrome may be helpful in establishing a diagnosis. In some cases convalescent serum titers may also be useful to demonstrate this rise in serum titer. Immunofluorescent antibody (IFA) and/or enzyme immunoassay (EIA) serum titers are useful in identifying *Bartonella henselae, Francisella tularensis, Coccidioides immitis,* Epstein–Barr virus, and may also be useful in the lymphogranuloma strain of *Chlamydia trachomatis.* A serum test for syphilis should be included in the work-up.

Several authors have described polymerase chain reaction (PCR) techniques for identifying *Bartonella henselae*[10], *Coccidioides immitis*[11], and *Francisella tularensis.*[12] Because the availability of these tests may vary in different laboratories, PCR may be most helpful in cases where serum titers are equivocal and cultures are negative.

Skin testing in patients with Parinaud's oculoglandular syndrome is no longer as important in diagnosis as it once was. Certainly, patients should have appropriate skin tests for tuberculosis if TB is suspected, but cat-scratch skin tests have been supplanted by serum titers. Skin testing has also been used historically in sporotrichosis and coccidioidomycosis.

Conjunctival scrapings should include acid-fast, Gram, and fungal stains. When culture is performed, suitable media

Table 47.1 Causes of Parinaud's oculoglandular syndrome (Adapted from Chin GN, Hyndiuk RA: Parinaud's oculoglandular conjunctivitis. In Tasman W, Jaeger EA, editors, *Duane's Clinical Ophthalmology*, Philadelphia, 1993, JB Lippincott)

More frequent causes	Organism
Cat-scratch disease	*Bartonella henselae*
Tularemia	*Francisella tularensis*
Sporotrichosis	*Sporotrichum schenckii*
Occasional causes	
Tuberculosis	*Mycobacterium tuberculosis*
Syphilis	*Treponema pallidum*
Coccidioidomycosis	*Coccidioides immitis*
Rare causes	
Sarcoidosis	Unknown
Chancroid	*Haemophilus ducreyi*
Pasteurellosis	*Pasteurella multocida*
Yersinia sp.	*Yersinia enterocolitica* *Yersinia pseudotuberculosis*
Hansen's disease	*Mycobacterium leprae*
Glanders	*Pseudomonas mallei*
Lymphogranuloma venereum (LGV)	*Chlamydia trachomatis* – LGV subtype
Listeria	*Listeria monocytogenes*
Actinomycosis	*Actinomyces israelii*
Blastomycosis	*Blastomyces dermatitidis*
Mumps	Mumps virus
Infectious mononucleosis	Epstein–Barr virus
Mediterranean fever	*Rickettsia conorii*
Vaccinia	Smallpox vaccine
Herpes simplex	Herpes virus
Paracoccidioidomycosis	*Paracoccidioides brasiliensis*
Possible causes	
Ophthalmia nodosa (caterpillar hair)	Urticarial hairs of *Macrothylacia rubi, Arctia caja, Thaumetopoea* sp.

for the growth of fungus and *Mycobacterium* should be included. *Francisella tularensis* can be grown on cysteine-enriched medium, but the yield is low and titers are a helpful supplementary test. In cat-scratch disease, *Bartonella henselae* can be cultured from conjunctival scrapings plated on chocolate blood agar in 5% CO_2.[7] Again, the yield is low. Thus, in uncomplicated cat-scratch disease, with high clinical suspicion, routine culture may be unnecessary.

In some cases biopsy produces rapid resolution of the conjunctival granuloma. Histopathologic examination from atypical or complicated patients will usually confirm the diagnosis of granulomatous conjunctivitis but may at times suggest an incorrect diagnosis of lymphoma.[13] Biopsy material should be cultured. A Warthin–Starry, Steiner silver stain or Brown–Hopp's stain will sometimes demonstrate Gram-negative pleomorphic bacilli in biopsies from patients with cat-scratch disease.[5]

Individual Etiologies

Cat-scratch disease

The most common cause of Parinaud's oculoglandular syndrome is cat-scratch disease (CSD). Earlier literature on CSD predates the identification of *Bartonella henselae* as the etiologic agent. In one of the most extensive publications of over 1200 cases, Carithers[14] outlined criteria for the diagnosis of CSD. Although Carithers' original criteria included the less reliable cat-scratch skin test, these criteria still serve as a basis for suspicion. In this modification of Carithers' original criteria, the diagnosis of CSD is based on the following:

1. Lymphadenopathy
2. A history of cat contact or recent cat scratch or bite
3. The presence of a primary inoculation site
4. Positive IFA titer or PCR test for *B. henselae*
5. Absence of other causes of lymphadenopathy.

Bartonella henselae has been established as the causative agent of CSD through Warthin–Starry-stained conjunctival specimens,[5] culture from conjunctival scrapings,[7] and PCR techniques.[15] Wear and colleagues[5] first identified the organisms on Warthin–Starry silver-stained conjunctival specimens in 1985 (Fig. 47.1 A and B).

In oculoglandular CSD the organism may gain entry to the eye through the conjunctiva or from facial scratches. Usually a history of cat contact can be obtained. However, a cat bite or scratch is not always present.[16] This suggests that the mechanism of entry in some cases may be direct transmission by the cat flea, which usually only acts as an intermediate vector.[17] In addition to cat scratches and bites, dogs and ticks have been implicated in the transmission of *Bartonella henselae*.[18,19] Following inoculation, DNA of *Bartonella henselae* can be detected in serum samples for as long as 3–4 months.[20]

Within 1–3 weeks after exposure, conjunctival lesions measuring 3–4 mm in diameter appear. These occur anywhere in the palpebral or bulbar conjunctiva. Conjunctival nodules vary in appearance from red to whitish, yellow, or gray, and may be surrounded locally by inflamed conjunctiva. Purulent discharge is absent or minimal.[4,14,21] Eyelid swelling is mild, and conjunctival ulceration may occur over

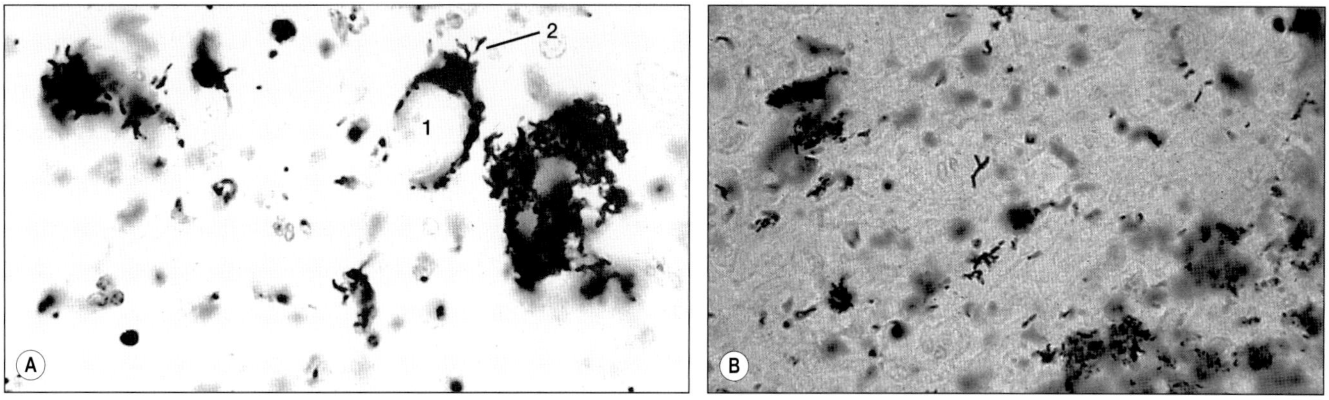

Fig. 47.1 Cat-scratch disease bacillus from conjunctival biopsies. **A,** Clumps of bacilli (2) surround blood vessels (1). **B,** Intracellular and extracellular organisms from necrotic conjunctiva. (From Wear DJ et al.: Cat scratch disease bacilli in the conjunctiva of patients with Parinaud's oculoglandular syndrome, *Ophthalmology* 1985;92:1282–1287. Copyright Elsevier, All rights reserved.)

Table 47.2 Directed work-up based on clinical findings and history

Clinical findings and symptoms	Diagnostic tests	Treatment
Uncomplicated		
History of cat contact, no fever, no immunocompromise, no other historical triggers	Save serum for IFA. TB skin test, VDRL, ± cultures	Hot packs, consider fluoroquinolone or sulfamethoxazole if tender lymphadenopathy present
Complicated		
Fever, lethargy, conjunctival or corneal vascularization or ulceration, historical triggers (hunter, rabbit, tick, STDs, TB, etc.)	Conjunctival culture on blood, chocolate, Lowenstein–Jensen and Sabouraud's agar, thioglycolate and BHI, glucose–cysteine–tellurite. Blood cultures if febrile, IFA for CSD, tularemia, Epstein–Barr virus, PPD or ELISpot, FTA-ABS, VDRL. Consider fungal IFA, biopsy, Warthin–Starry	Initial treatment: 1) Historical flags for tularemia – fluoroquinolone. 2) History for CSD or TB – rifampin. 3) STD symptoms or history – penicillin, tetracycline. 4) Lymphangitis – posaconazole, ketoconazole. Subsequent treatment: based on lab and response to therapy
Immunocompromised		
Kaposi-like skin and conjunctival lesions, HIV positive. Hepatic involvement	Cultures and titers as in complicated Parinaud's oculoglandular syndrome	Azithromycin, fluoroquinolone or tetracycline

the underlying granuloma.[21] Over the long term, chronic recurrent peripheral corneal ulceration can be seen following repeated treatment for Parinaud's oculoglandular syndrome caused by *Bartonella henselae*.[22]

In Parinaud's oculoglandular disease due to CSD enlarged preauricular, cervical, or submaxillary lymph nodes accompany the conjunctival granulomas. About 10% of these become fluctuant and suppurate.[23]

The incidence of CSD follows a seasonal pattern that mirrors the breeding and maturation cycle of cats and fleas. The cat flea, *Ctenocephalides felis*, is largely responsible for transmitting *B. henselae* from cat to cat.[21,24]

In the broader context of all cases of cat-scratch disease, Parinaud's oculoglandular syndrome is an uncommon presentation. Estimates of its frequency are around 4–8% of CSD cases.[14,17,23] Although death from encephalitis and meningitis due to CSD has been reported,[25] most patients follow a benign and self-limited clinical course.[26] Headache, anorexia, fever, and malaise occur in up to 30% of patients, but severe symptoms occur infrequently.[27]

A generalized rash is present in some patients. This is most commonly maculopapular, but may be petechial, papulovesicular, purpuric, or urticarial. Purpura may be accompanied by immune thrombocytopenia.[28] Erythema annulare and erythema nodosum occur rarely.

Systemic spread of the cat-scratch bacillus can occur during bacteremia, and cases of mesenteric lymph node involvement and pulmonary hilar adenopathy can occur. Albeit unusual, Parinaud's oculoglandular syndrome accompanied by osteomyelitis has been reported.[29]

Unlike the often self-limited course in immunocompetent patients, cat-scratch disease can follow a more aggressive

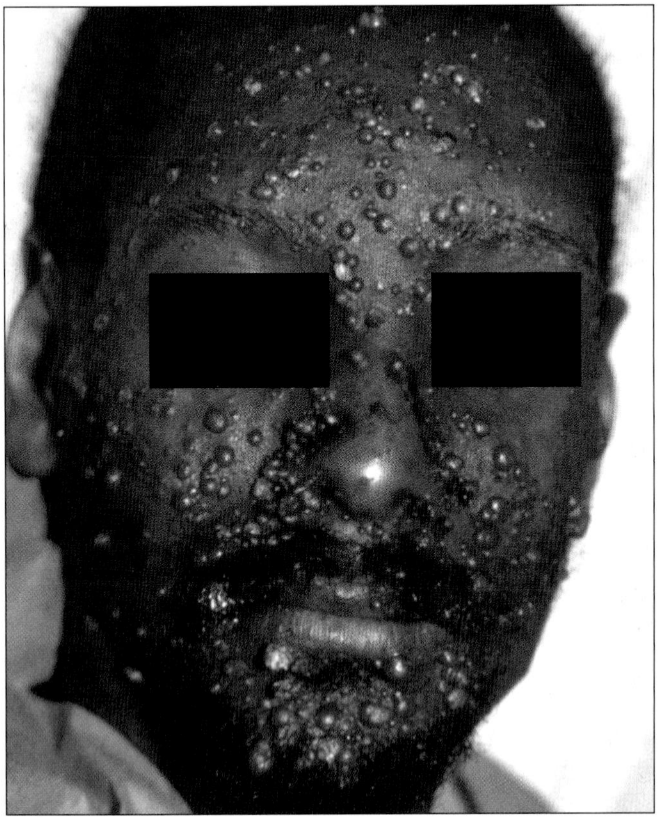

Fig. 47.2 AIDS patient with lesions of epithelioid angiomatosis associated with disseminated cat-scratch disease. (Reproduced from Szaniawski WK et al.: Epithelioid angiomatosis in patients with AIDS, *J Am Acad Dermatol* 1990;23:41–45 with permission from the American Academy of Dermatology.)

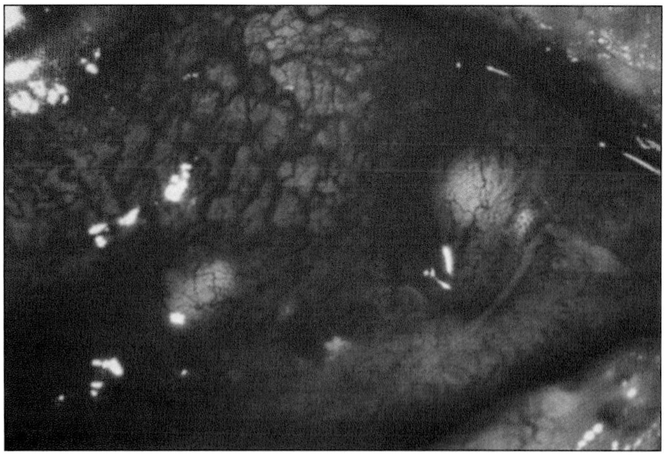

Fig. 47.3 Conjunctival nodules in Parinaud's oculoglandular syndrome secondary to tularemia. (Reproduced from Steinemann TL et al.: Oculoglandular tularemia, *Arch Ophthalmol* 1999;117:132–133. Copyright 1999 American Medical Association. All rights reserved.)

progression in AIDS patients and the immunocompromised. Disseminated *B. henselae* produces hepatic infection (bacillary peliosis) or cutaneous spread. In the skin, vascularized papillary skin lesions which resemble Kaposi's sarcoma are called epithelioid angiomatosis or bacillary angiomatosis[30] (Fig. 47.2). This dissemination, probably transmitted through unchecked bacteremia, is responsible for acute illness in the immunocompromised patient. These conditions can respond dramatically to systemic antibiotics.[31]

Treatment, when required for severe symptoms or immunocompromise, consists of fluoroquinolones, azithromycin, trimethoprim and sulfamethoxazole or rifampin.[31]

Tularemia

Unlike cat-scratch disease, severe systemic symptoms are more frequent in tularemia. The presenting symptoms and complications include high fever, constitutional symptoms, prostration, and death. In the preantibiotic era the mortality rate was as high as 9%.[32] With antibiotic treatment, however, this has fallen to about 2.5%.[33] Because of the risk of systemic involvement and the higher mortality rate, an infectious disease consultant may be a valuable asset in suspected tularemia.

Most patients with tularemia contract the infection through contact with ticks, rabbits, and squirrels. The patient need not be bitten by the tick for infection to occur: tularemia can be acquired by crushing ticks found on domestic dogs.[34] Cat bites, mosquitoes, deerflies, muskrats, beavers, woodchucks, hamsters, prairie dogs, sheep, and game birds are other possible vectors.[35–37] Contaminated water has also been implicated in outbreaks of tularemia.[38] Hunters in endemic areas have a higher level of seropositivity than nonhunters, suggesting that subclinical infection may lead to immunity.[39] Infection with tularemia is reportable to the Center for Disease Control and is considered one of the potential agents of bioterrorism.

The most important feature of oculoglandular syndrome in tularemia is ulceration of the conjunctiva. Conjunctival nodules appear on tarsal or bulbar conjunctiva (Fig. 47.3) and frequently progress to necrosis and ulceration. Less common findings include dacryocystitis, purulent discharge, corneal ulceration, and corneal perforation with endophthalmitis.[32,40] Angle closure due to ciliary body involvement has been reported and may lead to high intraocular pressure and corneal edema.[41] Preauricular, submaxillary, or cervical lymphadenopathy is present (Fig. 47.4). Lymph node tenderness, pharyngeal lesions, and tonsillitis may also be found.

As with cat-scratch disease, Parinaud's oculoglandular syndrome is a rare presentation of tularemia. Oculoglandular syndrome represents only 1% of all tularemia patients, whereas ulceroglandular, typhoidal, glandular, and oropharyngeal presentations are more common.

Laboratory confirmation of tularemia is best accomplished by serum titers. Although in some cases tularemia can occur without a serological response,[42] a fourfold rise in serum titer is diagnostic. When titers are borderline or equivocal, PCR-based techniques may be needed to supplement immunofluorescent antibody titers. Culture of the organism is difficult and requires cysteine-enriched media. *Francisella tularensis*, the responsible organism, is a nonmotile, Gram-negative pleomorphic coccobacillus. Safe handling of tularemia cultures requires special laboratory techniques, as injection or inhalation of as few as 10–50 bacilli may produce disease in the laboratory worker. Histopathology on conjunctival specimens shows granulomatous conjunctivitis (Fig. 47.5A) and multinucleated giant cells (Fig. 47.5B).

Topical broad-spectrum antibiotics should be combined with systemic antibiotic therapy. Moxifloxacin, ciprofloxacin, levofloxacin, doxycycline, and systemic gentamicin are attractive alternatives to traditional 7-day IM streptomycin injections.[43,44]

Tuberculosis

Although tuberculosis is quite uncommon in developed countries, primary conjunctival tuberculosis should be considered in the differential diagnosis of Parinaud's oculoglandular syndrome. The agent of pulmonary tuberculosis, *Mycobacterium tuberculosis*, can infect the conjunctiva either primarily or as a secondary reactivation. In addition, atypical *Mycobacterium* species can involve the conjunctiva and regional lymph nodes.

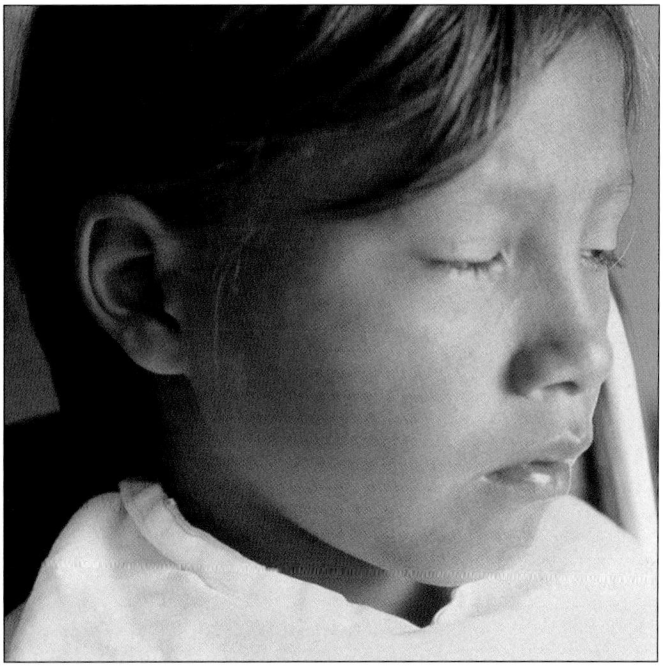

Fig. 47.4 Regional lymphadenopathy in Parinaud's oculoglandular syndrome secondary to tularemia. (Photo courtesy of E. Holland, MD.)

Conjunctival tuberculosis with regional lymphadenopathy can have varied appearances. The conjunctiva can manifest hyperemic ulceration, multiple nodules, hypertrophic granulations, or a pedunculated conjunctival mass.[45] Nodules and granulations may progress to ulceration. Regional lymph nodes in tuberculous Parinaud's oculoglandular syndrome often suppurate.

Testing for TB should include appropriate TB tests. The purified protein derivative (PPD) skin test is the most widely used screening skin test. It is, however, limited by variable and false-positive results in patients who have had bacille Calmette–Guérin (BCG) vaccination. Alternatives to PPD testing include enzyme-linked immunosorbent assay (ELISA) and enzyme-linked immunospot (ELISpot) blood tests.[46] These are based on measurement of T-cell interferon (IFN)-gamma release in response to unique antigens that are not present in BCG. Thus they are most useful in patients where prior BCG immunization is a confounding factor.

Further diagnostic testing can involve scraping of conjunctival lesions for culture and acid-fast staining. In addition, the lymph node may be aspirated or conjunctival lesions biopsied. Biopsy material should be cultured, and acid-fast and other tissue stains should be performed. Histology of conjunctival tissue shows granulomatous changes with Langhans' giant cells and caseating granulomas.

Treatment consists of isoniazid, rifampin, streptomycin, para-aminosalicylic acid, or ethambutol. Ocular examinations should be monitored both for resolution of the infection and for ocular toxicity from medications. Infectious disease consultation may be helpful.

Sporotrichosis

Skin changes in ocular sporotrichosis, along with historical information, help to distinguish it from other forms of Parinaud's oculoglandular syndrome. This fungal infection,

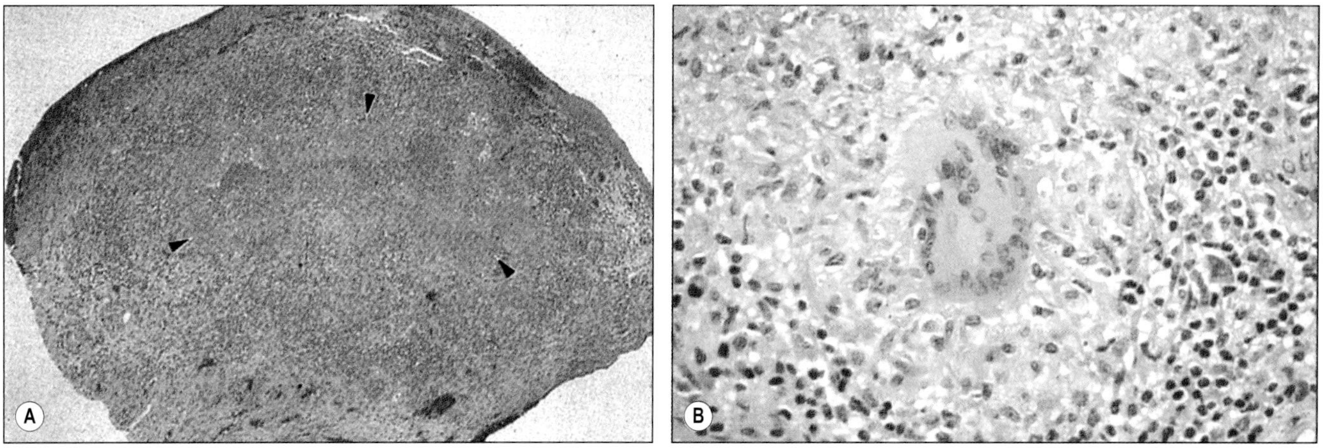

Fig. 47.5 Histopathology of oculoglandular tularemia. **A,** Granulomatous conjunctival nodule. **B,** Multinucleated giant cell from granuloma. (Reproduced from Steinemann TL et al.: Oculoglandular tularemia, *Arch Ophthalmol* 1999;117:132–133. Copyright 1999 American Medical Association. All rights reserved.)

caused by *Sporothrix schenckii*, is initiated by trauma from contaminated vegetable matter or dirt. The conjunctiva can be affected either primarily or in association with lesions of the face and eyelids. The most common presentation is lymphangitis. Along the course of the lymphatic channels subcutaneous nodules develop and may ulcerate.[47] Typically the condition remains localized to the skin and lymphatics. Systemic or pulmonary involvement is rare.

A history of trauma and agricultural contamination should raise suspicion for sporotrichosis or other fungal infections. Preceding trauma is not always present, however. Human transmission of sporotrichosis from infected cats has also been reported.[48] A characteristic lesion called a sporotrichotic chancre is helpful in suggesting the diagnosis. Biopsy is required to obtain material for culture on Sabouraud's agar and for fungal stains.

Itraconazole is effective in treatment.[48] In vitro testing indicates that ketoconazole is also effective; amphoteracin B is more variable but is effective in some strains of *S. schenckii*.[49] Potassium iodide (SSKI) has been used extensively in the past and is also effective, but well-designed in vivo comparison studies of antifungal medications are not currently available.[50]

Syphilis

Treponema pallidum is a motile spirochete responsible for syphilis. In primary syphilis, conjunctival chancres can be seen.[51] Nodular conjunctivitis, injection, and chemosis are frequently associated with skin and mucous membrane involvement in secondary syphilis. Gummatous tarsitis is an uncommon manifestation of tertiary syphilis.[52] The lymphadenopathy of Parinaud's oculoglandular syndrome may occur in all three stages of syphilis.

Systemic signs are protean and include maculopapular or ichthyosis-like rashes and alopecia. Generalized lymphadenopathy may be present. Mucocutaneous ulceration is common in secondary syphilis. Ocular complications include scleritis, uveitis, retinitis, and trachoma-like corneal vascularization. Papilledema, neurologic abnormalities, and Argyll Robertson pupils are found in tertiary neurosyphilis. The differential diagnosis includes sarcoidosis, and the laboratory work-up should include angiotensin-converting enzyme and serum lysozyme. Serum tests for syphilis (VDRL, FTA-ABS) should be performed on all patients. Dark-field examination of scrapings and fluid specimens may be useful.

Penicillin is the treatment of choice. Penicillin-allergic patients may be treated with azithromycin, but resistance, conferred by a genetic mutation that affects macrolide binding to the 50s ribosome, has been reported.[53] Syphilis is a reportable disease, and contacts should be traced and treated.

Other causes

Lymphogranuloma venereum produces prolonged conjunctivitis and may lead to corneal perforation or opacity.[54] Chlamydial culture and serology aid in the diagnosis. Treatment is tetracycline 500 mg four times a day for 10–14 days.

Coccidioides immitis, *Blastomyces dermatitidis*, and *Paracoccidioides brasiliensis* are fungal agents that have been reported in Parinaud's oculoglandular syndrome.[55,56] Biopsy, skin tests, and serology are helpful in diagnosing these rare conditions. Posaconazole[57] and voriconazole[58] are reported to be effective in systemic fungal infections, but therapy should be guided by laboratory studies and clinical response along with infectious disease consultation.

Actinomycosis is caused by a filamentous bacterium that is acquired from trauma.[2] Lesions contain characteristic yellow clumps called sulfur granules. Treatment consists of penicillin or tetracycline.

Among the more unusual causes of Parinaud's oculoglandular syndrome are the zoonoses caused by *Yersinia pseudotuberculosis*,[59] *Y. enterocolitica*, *Actinobacillus mallei* (glanders), *Listeria monocytogenes*, *Rickettsia conorii*,[60] and *Pasteurella multocida*.[2] These infections are acquired through contact with an animal source.

Epstein–Barr virus, the agent of mononucleosis, produces lymphadenopathy, fever, and pharyngitis.[61] Conjunctival inflammation as well as membranous conjunctivitis and follicular conjunctivitis are possible. EB virus-specific serology, heterophil antibody testing, and exclusion of other causes of lymphadenopathy help make the diagnosis. Treatment is nonspecific.

Herpes simplex may be diagnosed by history, viral culture, and immunofluorescence studies of infected tissue.[62] Treatment consists of oral and topical antiviral medications.

Mumps, caused by a paramyxovirus, produces parotitis. Rarely, it can be accompanied by granulomatous conjunctivitis. Ocular complications are rare, and the disease can be prevented by immunization.[63]

Listed as a possible cause is the unusual case of a biopsied conjunctival specimen in which caterpillar hairs were found. This patient also had a positive CSD skin test and exposure to a cat bite.[64]

References

1. Parinaud H. Conjonctivite infectieuse paraissant transmise a l'homme par les animaux. *Recueil Ophtal.* 1889;11:176.
2. Chin GN, Hyndiuk RA. Parinaud's oculoglandular syndrome. In: Tasman W, Jaeger FA, eds. *Duane's clinical ophthalmology*. Vol 4. Philadelphia: JB Lippincott; 1993:4:1–6.
3. Pesme P, Marchand E. Sur un nouveau type de conjonctivite infectieuse probablement transmise par un chat. *J Med Bordeaux*. 1950;127:127–131.
4. Cassady JV, Culbertson CS. Cat-scratch disease and Parinaud's oculoglandular syndrome. *Arch Ophthalmol*. 1953;50:68–74.
5. Wear DJ, Malaty RH, Zimmerman LE, et al. Cat scratch disease bacilli in the conjunctiva of patients with Parinaud's oculoglandular syndrome. *Ophthalmology*. 1985;92:1282–1287.
6. Gerber MA, Sedgwick AK, MacAlister TJ, et al. The aetiological agent of cat scratch disease. *Lancet*. 1985;1:1236–1239.
7. Grando D, Sullivan LJ, Flexman JP, et al. *Bartonella henselae* associated with Parinaud's oculoglandular syndrome. *Clin Infect Dis*. 1999;28:1156–1158.
8. Gaidici A, Saubolle MA. Transmission of coccidioidomycosis to a human via a cat bite. *J Clin Microbiol*. 2009;47:505–506.
9. Xavier MH, Teixeira Ade L, Pinto JM, et al. Cat-transmitted cutaneous lymphatic sporotrichosis. *Dermatol Online J*. 2008;14:4.
10. Anderson B, Sims K, Regnery R, et al. Detection of *Rochalimaea henselae* DNA in specimens from cat scratch disease patients by PCR. *J Clin Microbiol*. 1994;32:942–948.
11. Brilhante RS, Cordeiro RA, Rocha MF, et al. Coccidioidal pericarditis: a rapid presumptive diagnosis by an in-house antigen confirmed by mycological and molecular methods. *J Med Microbiol*. 2008;57:1288–1292.
12. Johansson A, Ibrahim A, Goransson I, et al. Evaluation of PCR-based methods for discrimination of *Francisella* species and subspecies

and development of a specific PCR that distinguishes the two major subspecies of *Francisella tularensis*. *J Clin Microbiol.* 2000;38:4180–4185.

13. Fanous MM, Margo CE. Parinaud's oculoglandular syndrome simulating lymphoma. *Am J Ophthalmol.* 1991;112:344–345.
14. Carithers HA. Cat-scratch disease: an overview based on a study of 1200 patients. *Am J Dis Child.* 1985;139:1124–1133.
15. Vermeulen MJ, Herremans M, Verbakel H, et al. Serological testing for *Bartonella henselae* infections in The Netherlands: clinical evaluation of immunofluorescence assay and ELISA. *Clin Microbiol Infect.* 2007;13: 627–634.
16. Tobin EH, McDaniel H. Oculoglandular syndrome. Cat-scratch disease without the cat scratch. *Postgrad Med J.* 1992;91:207–208, 210.
17. Ridder GJ, Boedeker CC, Technau-Ihling K, Sander A. Cat-scratch disease: Otolaryngologic manifestations and management. *Otolaryngol Head Neck Surg.* 2005;132:353–358.
18. Cotté V, Bonnet S, Le Rhun D, et al. Transmission of *Bartonella henselae* by *Ixodes ricinus*. *Emerg Infect Dis.* 2008;14:1074–1080.
19. Chen TC, Lin WR, Lu PL, et al. Cat scratch disease from a domestic dog. *J Formos Med Assoc.* 2007;106(2 Suppl):S65–S68.
20. Arvand M, Schäd SG. Isolation of *Bartonella henselae* DNA from the peripheral blood of a patient with cat scratch disease up to 4 months after the cat scratch injury. *J Clin Microbiol.* 2006;44:2288–2290.
21. Cunningham ET, Koehler JE. Ocular bartonellosis. *Am J Ophthalmol.* 2000;130:340–349.
22. Prasher P, Di Pascuale M, Cavanagh HD. Bilateral chronic peripheral ulcerative keratitis secondary to cat-scratch disease. *Eye Contact Lens.* 2008;34:191–193.
23. Huang MC, Dreyer E. Parinaud's oculoglandular conjunctivitis and cat-scratch disease. *Int Ophthalmol Clin.* 1996;36:29–36.
24. Chomel BB, Kasten RW, Floyd-Hawkins K, et al. Experimental transmission of *Bartonella henselae* by the cat flea. *J Clin Microbiol.* 1996;34:1952–1956.
25. Gerber JE, Johnson JE, Scott MA, et al. Fatal meningitis and encephalitis due to *Bartonella henselae* bacteria. *J Forensic Sci.* 2002;47: 640–644.
26. Margileth AM. Antibiotic therapy for cat-scratch disease: clinical study of therapeutic outcome in 268 patients and a review of the literature. *Pediatr Infect Dis J.* 1992;11:474–478.
27. Margileth AM. Cat scratch disease: No longer a diagnostic dilemma. *Semin Vet Med Surg.* 1991;6:199–202.
28. Palumbo E, Sodini F, Boscarelli G, et al. Immune thrombocytopenic purpura as a complication of *Bartonella henselae* infection. *Infez Med.* 2008;16:99–102.
29. Karpathios T, Fretzayas A, Kakavakis C, et al. Maladie des griffes du chat accompagnée d'ostéomyélite. *Arch Fr Pediatr.* 1990;47:369–371.
30. Szaniawski WK, Don PC, Bitterman SR, et al. Epithelioid angiomatosis in patients with AIDS: report of seven cases and review of the literature. *J Am Acad Dermatol.* 1990;23:41–48.
31. Conrad DA. Treatment of cat-scratch disease. *Curr Opin Pediatr.* 2001; 13:56–59.
32. Francis E. Oculoglandular tularemia. *Arch Ophthalmol.* 1942;28: 711–741.
33. Rohrbach BW, Westerman E, Istre GR. Epidemiology and clinical characteristics of tularemia in Oklahoma, 1979 to 1985. *South Med J.* 1991;84:1091–1096.
34. Ohara Y, Sato T, Homma M. Arthropod-borne tularemia in Japan: clinical analysis of 1374 cases observed between 1924 and 1996. *J Med Entomol.* 1998;35:471–473.
35. Nigrovic LE, Wingerter SL. Tularemia. *Infect Dis Clin North Am.* 2008;22:489–504.
36. Centers for Disease Control and Prevention (CDC). Tularemia associated with a hamster bite – Colorado, 2004. *MMWR Morb Mortal Wkly Rep.* 2005;53:1202–1203.
37. Avashia SB, Petersen JM, Lindley CM, et al. First reported prairie dog-to-human tularemia transmission, Texas, 2002. *Emerg Infect Dis.* 2004;10: 483–486.
38. Willke A, Meric M, Grunow R, et al. An outbreak of oropharyngeal tularaemia linked to natural spring water. *J Med Microbiol.* 2009;58: 112–116.
39. Jenzora A, Jansen A, Ranisch H, et al. Seroprevalence study of *Francisella tularensis* among hunters in Germany. *FEMS Immunol Med Microbiol.* 2008;53:183–189.
40. Steinemann TL, Sheikholeslami MR, Brown HH, et al. Oculoglandular tularemia. *Arch Ophthalmol.* 1999;117:132–133.
41. Parssinen O, Rummukainen M. Acute glaucoma and acute corneal oedema in association with tularemia. *Acta Ophthalmol Scand.* 1997;75:732–734.
42. Johansson A, Berglund L, Eriksson U, et al. Comparative analysis of PCR versus culture for diagnosis of ulceroglandular tularemia. *J Clin Microbiol.* 2000;38:22–26.
43. Meric M, Willke A, Finke EJ, et al. Evaluation of clinical, laboratory, and therapeutic features of 145 tularemia cases: the role of quinolones in oropharyngeal tularemia. *APMIS.* 2008;116:66–73.
44. Kantardjiev T, Padeshki P, Ivanov IN. Diagnostic approaches for oculoglandular tularemia: advantages of PCR. *Br J Ophthalmol.* 2007;91: 1206–1208.
45. Archer D, Bird A. Primary tuberculosis of the conjunctiva. *Br J Ophthalmol.* 1967;51:679–684.
46. Lalvani A. Diagnosing tuberculosis infection in the 21st century: new tools to tackle an old enemy. *Chest.* 2007;131:1898–1906.
47. McGrath H, Singer JI. Ocular sporotrichosis. *Am J Ophthalmol.* 1952;35:102–105.
48. Barros MB, Costa DL, Schubach TM, et al. Endemic zoonotic sporotrichosis: profile of cases in children. *Pediatr Infect Dis J.* 2008;27:246–250.
49. Alvarado-Ramirez E, Torres-Rodriguez JM. In vitro susceptibility of *Sporothrix schenckii* to six antifungal agents determined using three different methods. *Antimicrob Agents Chemother.* 2007;51:2420–2423.
50. Xue SL, Li L. Oral potassium iodide for the treatment of sporotrichosis. *Mycopathologia* Epub Jan 8, 2009.
51. Maxey EE. Primary syphilis of palpebral conjunctiva. *Am J Ophthalmol.* 1965;65(Suppl):13–17.
52. Spektor FE, Eagle RC, Nichols CW. Granulomatous conjunctivitis secondary to *Treponema pallidum*. *Ophthalmology.* 1981;88:863–865.
53. Katz KA, Klausner JD. Azithromycin resistance in *Treponema pallidum*. *Curr Opin Infect Dis.* 2008;21:83–91.
54. Buus DR, Pflugfelder SC, Schachter J, et al. Lymphogranuloma venereum conjunctivitis with a marginal corneal perforation. *Ophthalmology.* 1988;95:799–802.
55. Wood TR. Ocular coccidioidomycosis: report of a case presenting as Parinaud's oculoglandular syndrome. *Am J Ophthalmol.* 1967;64(Suppl): 587–590.
56. Costa PS, Hollanda BV, Assis RV, et al. Parinaud's oculoglandular syndrome associated with paracoccidioidomycosis. *Rev Inst Med Trop Sao Paulo.* 2002;44:49–52.
57. Langner S, Staber PB, Neumeister P. Posaconazole in the management of refractory invasive fungal infections. *Ther Clin Risk Manag.* 2008;4: 747–758.
58. Freifeld A, Proia L, Andes D, et al. Voriconazole use for endemic fungal infections. *Antibicrob Agents Chemother.* 2009;53:1648–1651.
59. Chin GN, Noble RC. Ocular involvement in *Yersinia enterocolitica* infection presenting as Parinaud's oculoglandular syndrome. *Am J Ophthalmol.* 1977;83:19–23.
60. Pinna A, Sotgiu M, Carta F, et al. Oculoglandular syndrome in Mediterranean spotted fever acquired through the eye. *Br J Ophthalmol.* 1997;81:172.
61. Matoba AY. Ocular disease associated with Epstein–Barr virus infection. *Surv Ophthalmol.* 1990;35:145–150.
62. Caputo GM, Byck H. Concomitant oculoglandular and ulceroglandular fever due to herpes simplex virus type I. *Am J Med.* 1992;93:577–580.
63. Wilhelmus KR. Mumps. In: Gold DH, Weingeist TA, eds. *The eye in systemic disease.* Philadelphia: JB Lippincott; 1990:262–265.
64. Martin X, Uffer S, Gailloud C. Ophthalmia nodosa and the oculoglandular syndrome of Parinaud. *Br J Ophthalmol.* 1986;70:536–542.

Chapter 48

Seasonal and Perennial Allergic Conjunctivitis

Jason S. Rothman, Michael B. Raizman, Mitchell H. Friedlaender

Ocular allergy is a common disorder which can be debilitating for patients and, at times, challenging for physicians to diagnose and treat. Ocular allergy and non-allergic ocular surface disease can occur simultaneously; each can exacerbate surface inflammation. For unclear reasons, the prevalence of allergy in developed countries has increased during the past few decades.[1] The popular hygiene hypothesis suggests that a reduction of allergen exposure during childhood may offset the balance of T cells. Other theories include genetic influence, increased industrialization, and pollution. The financial impact of ocular allergy on the healthcare system is substantial and increasing; the expenditure for prescription medications used to treat allergic rhinoconjunctivitis in the United States was recently estimated at $1.5 billion.[2] Ocular allergy may be classified into five categories – seasonal and perennial allergic conjunctivitis, vernal keratoconjunctivitis, atopic keratoconjunctivitis, giant papillary conjunctivitis, and contact allergic conjunctivitis.

Allergic disease affects 30–50% of the population, while ocular symptoms are present in 40–60% of allergic individuals.[3,4] Seasonal allergic conjunctivitis, typically accompanied by seasonal allergic rhinitis, is the most prevalent form of ocular allergic disease. The seasonal incidence of seasonal allergic conjunctivitis is closely related to the cycles of released plant-derived airborne allergens, or aeroallergens. The signs and symptoms of perennial allergic conjunctivitis are more likely to occur year-round, although about 79% of patients may still have seasonal exacerbations.[5] The gradual development of ocular and nasal allergic signs and symptoms after exposure to plant products was initially described by Blackley in 1873.[6] Since that time, both seasonal and perennial allergic conjunctivitis have been recognized as conditions which can cause significant morbidity, but rarely permanent visual impairment. Vernal keratoconjunctivitis is a rare condition primarily seen in children in the arid regions of the world. It is a recurrent self-limiting inflammatory disease. Atopic keratoconjunctivitis is a chronic condition associated with atopic dermatitis or eczema, including inflammation of the eyelids, which occurs in about 3% of the population.[7] Nearly all the patients will have other manifestations of systemic atopy. Both vernal and atopic keratoconjunctivitis can threaten sight secondary to corneal scarring. Giant papillary conjunctivitis (GPC) is a reversible condition, most commonly associated with contact lens wear, exposed sutures, or prostheses. GPC appears to be in response to chronic microtrauma and not from an allergic mechanism, but is often included as a type of ocular allergy. Contact allergic conjunctivitis occurs after sensitization to ocular medications and their preservatives. This chapter focuses on seasonal and perennial allergic conjunctivitis.

Immunopathophysiology

The conjunctiva is a very vascular and immunologically active component of the external eye. Mast cells (predominantly MC_{TC} phenotype), the primary inflammatory cells involved in ocular allergy, normally reside within the vascular stroma (substantia propria), but can be present within the conjunctival epithelium in pathologic situations. The number of mast cells present within the stroma may be increased up to 61% in patients with seasonal allergic conjunctivitis compared with normal patients.[8] Both seasonal and perennial allergic conjunctivitis are examples of a type I IgE-mediated allergic response. Clinically, the immediate response lasts for 20–30 minutes. However, evidence from allergen challenge studies has demonstrated two separate allergic responses, an early-phase response (EPR) and a dose related late-phase response (LPR).[9] Although the late-phase response is frequently seen in allergic respiratory, nasal, and skin disease, its clinical relevance in ocular allergy is unclear.[10]

In sensitized individuals, environmental allergens dissolve in the tear film and traverse the conjunctival epithelium.[11] Ultimately they bind to cytrotropic antibodies (antibodies which are responsible for the immediate hypersensitivity reaction) on the surface of conjunctival mast cells within the stroma. Although IgE is considered to be the principal cytotropic antibody in humans, an IgG-type antibody (typically IgG_4 in humans) with cytotropic properties has also been reported.[12] When mast cell Fc receptors are cross-linked by allergens, signals are sent through the cell membrane and into the cytoplasm, resulting in the release of allergic mediators. Bridging of less than 1% of the total IgE molecules on the surface of the mast cell is required for signal production. This signal begins with an influx of calcium and microtubule assembly, resulting in the fusion of granules to the cell membrane and, ultimately, granule release. It is important to recognize two components of mast cell activation. The first is the release of preformed mediators, including histamine. The second is the synthesis of

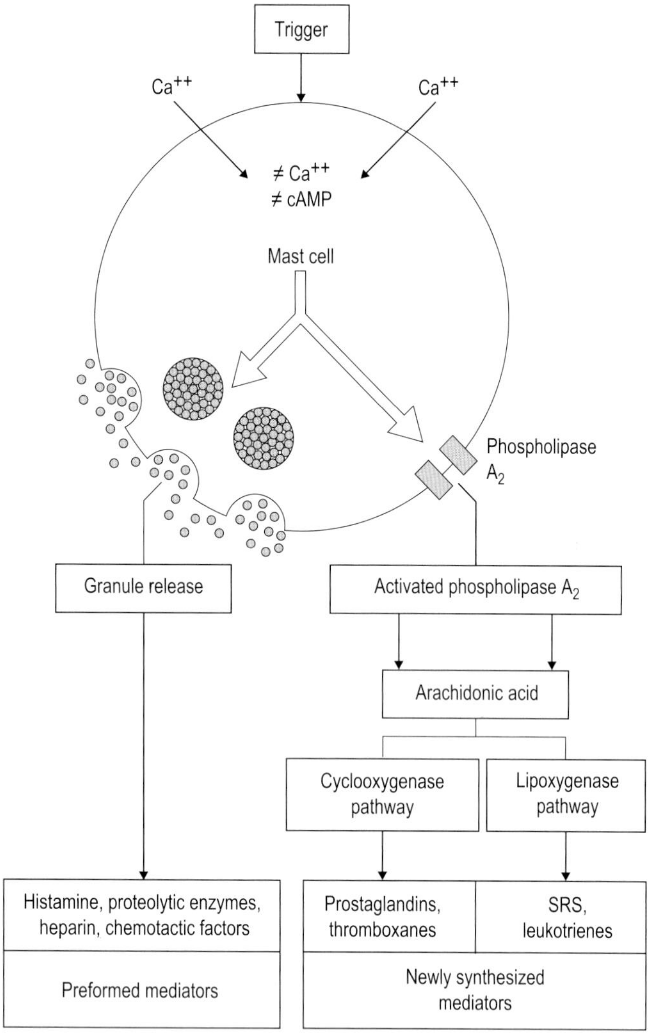

Fig. 48.1 When activated, mast cells in the conjunctiva and eyelid release preformed mediators of inflammation from their granules and newly synthesized mediators from their cell membranes via the arachidonic acid cascade. (Raizman MB: Update on ocular allergy. *Focal Points: Clinical Modules for Ophthalmologists* 12(5):1, 1994.)

arachidonic acid and the subsequent metabolic cascade, resulting in the production of prostaglandins and leukotrienes (Fig 48.1). The released histamine binds H_1 and H_2 receptors on the target tissue cell surfaces. Binding to the H_1 receptor results in vasodilation, increased vascular permeability, pruritus, burning, and stinging, while binding to the H_2 receptor also results in mucus production.[7] The exocytosis of preformed mediators leads to the early-phase response. This acute phase (EPR) results in the primary allergic symptom, ocular itching, along with burning and tearing. The leukotrienes and prostaglandins stimulate mucus production and increase vascular permeability. After the mast cells are activated, cytokines are released. These include IL-4, IL-6, IL-8, IL-13, and eosinophil chemotactic factor. These cytokines attract eosinophils, lymphocytes, and neutrophils. Eosinophil infiltration of the conjunctiva is present in about 43% of patients with seasonal allergic conjunctivitis, and about 25–84% of patients with perennial allergic conjunctivitis.[5] The role of eosinophils is paramount in the allergic response. Degranulating eosinophils release toxic proteins, including eosinophil major basic protein (MBP) and eosinophil cationic protein (ECP). These proteins, which have been detected in tear samples in patients with allergic conjunctivitis,[5] can have profound cytotoxic effects and further enhance mast cell degranulation. These products of eosinophils are toxic to the corneal epithelium and, if present chronically, may result in ulceration. Interferon (IFN)-gamma, a Th1 cytokine, may act as a regulator of conjunctival inflammation. Substance P has been identified in the tears of patients with ocular allergy, which may contribute to the ocular inflammation through the release of cytokines.[13] Altering the balance of Th1 and Th2 cells and their cytokines may contribute to allergic sensitization and response. Recent research suggests that CD8+ T cells may aid IgE production and cytokine generation, while CD4+ CD25+ T cells may suppress the development of experimental allergic conjunctivitis.[14,15]

Studies have shown a late-phase reaction can occur from 6 to 24 hours after an allergen challenge.[16] About 6 hours after conjunctival challenge, elevated levels of histamine, ECP, E-selectin and intercellular adhesion molecule 1 (ICAM-1),[17–19] which promotes eosinophil migration into the conjunctival tissue, have been detected. This correlates with increased lymphocyte and granulocyte activity. Given the absence of tryptase in tear samples about 6 hours after the acute allergic response, it is hypothesized that granulocytes may be responsible for the elevated levels of histamine.[9] The late-phase response is characterized by an influx of multiple inflammatory cells, including eosinophils, basophils, neutrophils, and macrophages, along with CD4+ and CD8+ cells.[19] Conjunctival epithelial cells may also prolong the allergic inflammatory response by releasing chemotactic mediators. Stimulated conjunctival epithelium may induce a chemotactic response, producing IL-8 and the regulated upon activation, normal T cell expressed and secreted (RANTES) chemokine.[20] The role of epithelial cells during allergic inflammation is an active area of research. Lymphocytes are instrumental in causing the chronic signs and symptoms of allergy seen in both atopic and perennial allergic conjunctivitis. Chronic inflammation may lead to a loss of goblet cells, resulting in dry eye and surface dysregulation. In atopic individuals, this unremitting inflammation can result in fibrosis with symblepharon formation, as well as vision-threatening conditions resulting from corneal neovascularization, corneal scarring, and shield ulcers. Continued immunohistopathological studies may help further elucidate the pathophysiology responsible for the ocular allergic reaction.

Clinical Features of Seasonal Allergic Conjunctivitis

Seasonal allergic conjunctivitis (SAC) is the most common form of ocular allergy, affecting up to 22% of the population.[3,4] A wide variety of aeroallergens have been associated with seasonal allergic conjunctivitis. Tree and flower pollen

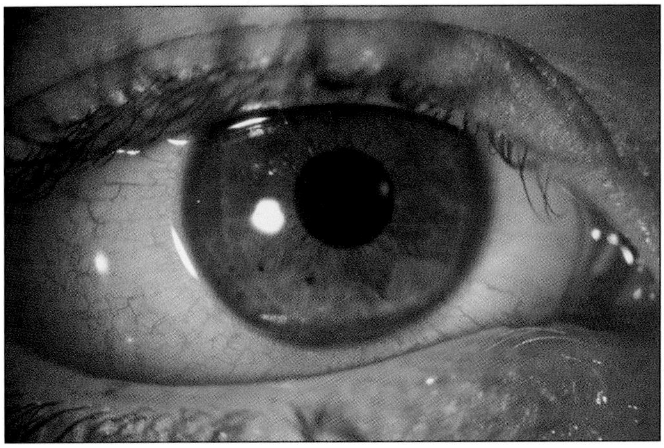

Fig. 48.2 Chemosis and injection of allergic conjunctivitis.

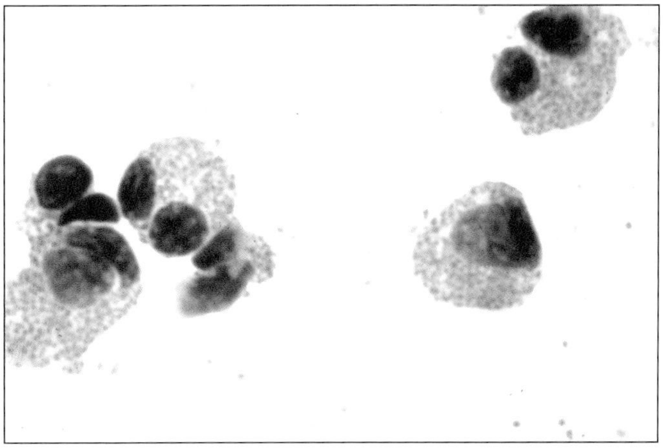

Fig. 48.3 Eosinophils in a conjunctival scraping taken from an allergic patient.

in the spring, grass pollen in the late spring and early summer, and ragweed during the late summer and early fall are the common allergens implicated in SAC. Historically, the most significant allergic reactions in the United States are from ragweed. Allergens and seasonal timing may differ in various parts of the world, but the clinical features are consistent. The onset of symptoms is seasonally related, although cooler or rainy days may provide some relief. SAC is characterized by the hallmark symptom, ocular itching. The itching is usually mild, but can be severe. Patients may also present with ocular burning, stinging, redness, photophobia, or increased lacrimation. Itchy, red eyes are the usual presentation. Symptoms are typically bilateral, although they may be asymmetric. Patients may present with a mild papillary reaction. Chemosis may be apparent in the bulbar and lower tarsal conjunctiva. Subtle chemosis can often be detected along the plica semilunaris, but frequently signs may be absent or consist of faint hyperemia. When patients rub their eyes, the chemosis may be more dramatic with occasional conjunctival ballooning (Fig. 48.2).[21] Discharge, if present, can vary between serous and mucopurulent, but a clear, ropy discharge is characteristic. Fortunately, SAC is seldom followed by permanent visual impairment. The ocular symptoms are usually accompanied by seasonal rhinitis and pharyngeal symptoms. The inflammation within the nasal mucosa may be exacerbated by inflammatory mediators released into the tears, which drain through the nasolacrimal ducts. In certain individuals, asthma may also be a serious component.

A careful history (including a family history of atopy) and examination are usually sufficient for diagnosing allergic conjunctivitis. Many patients are aware of their 'allergen triggers,' although allergen testing may be prudent in some individuals for a definitive diagnosis. It is helpful to ask about nasal and pulmonary symptoms, as the same allergens could trigger rhinitis and asthma. Provocative conjunctival challenge testing is helpful but rarely necessary for obtaining diagnostic information. Abelson et al. have described a novel and successful method of conjunctival challenge; it has proven to be a safe and reliable method to evaluate ocular therapeutics.[22] Skin testing, both prick and intradermal methods, is the most widely accepted method for allergy testing. Prick skin testing is the favored method because it is more sensitive, less variable, and more comfortable than intradermal testing.[23] The presence of eosinophils in conjunctival scrapings may be helpful (Fig. 48.3), although their absence should not rule out the diagnosis.[24] Even one eosinophil or eosinophil granule is consistent with a diagnosis of allergy. About 25% of patients with diagnosed SAC have eosinophils on cytologic examination.

Clinical Features of Perennial Allergic Conjunctivitis

Perennial allergic conjunctivitis (PAC) is a year-round variant of seasonal allergic conjunctivitis. Historically, the prevalence of PAC is lower than SAC, but has increased over the past few decades.[1] In contrast to patients with SAC, where there is a clear time of onset and termination, patients with PAC will have symptoms throughout the year. About 79% of these patients have seasonal exacerbations.[5] The most common aeroallergens implicated in PAC are found indoors, and include animal dander, dust mites, and feathers. Other associated allergens include mold spores and fungi. Both home and occupational exposures need to be determined. The majority of patients will have serum- and tear-specific IgE for house dust. Not surprisingly, perennial rhinitis is more prevalent in PAC than in SAC. The ocular features of PAC are similar to those of SAC. Patients typically present with itching, although burning, tearing, and photophobia are common associated symptoms. On examination, patients typically have mild conjunctival hyperemia, along with a variable amount of chemosis. If severe enough, the chemosis may result in lower lid swelling and possible dellen formation. The diagnosis is typically made by history and examination alone, although measuring serum-specific IgE, conjunctival scraping (looking for eosinophils), allergen challenge testing, and skin testing may be useful in ambiguous situations.

Treatment of Seasonal and Perennial Allergic Conjunctivitis

Advisory interventions

Treatment for seasonal or perennial allergic conjunctivitis depends on the degree and expected duration of the allergic response. Avoiding known allergen triggers is critical. Possible strategies for avoiding allergens include staying indoors during times of high pollen counts, using both room and car air conditioners, keeping windows closed when possible, and washing hair and clothes after being outdoors. Patients with perennial allergic conjunctivitis may benefit from covering bedding with plastic covers, removing carpets, and avoiding pets. At a minimum, pets should be barred from the bedroom. When eyes itch, the natural response is to rub. The temporary relief of itching achieved from rubbing is followed by a more exuberant inflammatory response.[25] Eye rubbing may bring large quantities of allergens in direct contact with the conjunctiva from the hands and mechanically disrupt cell membranes, resulting in further release of inflammatory mediators.[21,25] This, in turn, may result in an itch–rub cycle that is difficult to break. Encouraging patients to stop rubbing their eyes should be a fundamental goal. Cool artificial tears may provide some relief by diluting both inflammatory mediators and allergens. Cold compresses may reduce swelling and provide some additional relief. For many patients, nonmedical treatments alone are not sufficient.

Medical therapy

When choosing a medical therapy, it is important to remember that the efficacy of an individual medication will vary among patients. Selection of an antiallergy medication should be based on the severity, symptoms, and projected duration of a patient's allergic disease. For example, a patient with a severe allergic response may initially benefit from a topical corticosteroid, while a patient with moderate symptoms from complex allergies or who requires extended treatment may do well with mast cell stabilizers or dual-action agents (mast cell stabilizer and antihistamine).

Over-the-counter topical decongestants containing vasoconstrictors with or without antihistamines are generally well tolerated and effective for patients with mild allergic symptoms.[26,27] Although the antihistamine component is weak, the vasoconstrictor component is very effective in reducing conjunctival hyperemia via alpha-adrenoceptor stimulation. In the United States, either pheneramine or antazoline, the common antihistamines, is combined with naphazolin, a vasoconstrictor. Using these drops over time may result in tachyphylaxis, requiring patients to use the drops more frequently to obtain the same vasoconstrictor effect. Furthermore, discontinuation of vasoconstricting eyedrops may result in rebound hyperemia. Depending on the underlying condition, artificial tears, corticosteroid drops, or long-term therapy with mast cell stabilizers and/or immunotherapy may help alleviate dependence on the vasoconstricting eyedrops.[28] Due to their mydriatic effect, topical decongestants are contraindicated in patients with narrow angles.

The more potent topical antihistamines, levocabastine hydrochloride 0.05% and emedastine difumarate 0.05%, selectively block H_1 receptors.[29,30] Controlled studies have shown these antihistamines to be effective in reducing redness and itching associated with allergic conjunctivitis.[31] They have a rapid onset of action, but have a short duration of action, requiring up to four times daily dosing. Patients with pure seasonal allergic conjunctivitis who develop symptoms during peak pollen counts may benefit from using a potent topical antihistamine alone. This is in contrast to patients with perennial allergic conjunctivitis or complex seasonal allergic conjunctivitis, who may benefit more from mast cell stabilizers or the dual-acting (antihistamine and mast cell stabilizer) agents.

The dual-acting medications, including olopatadine hydrochloride 0.1% and 0.2%, azelastine hydrochloride 0.05%, ketotifen fumarate 0.025% (available over the counter), and epinastine hydrochloride 0.05%, have antihistamine and mast cell stabilizing properties. Ketotifen, epinastine, and azelastine have additional modes of action, including eosinophil and basophil inhibition.[32,33] These medications are usually effective for the treatment and prevention of signs and symptoms of allergic conjunctivitis.[34–36] Olopatadine 0.1% is indicated to treat the signs and symptoms of allergic conjunctivitis, while azelastine and olopatadine 0.2%, are indicated to treat itching associated with allergic conjunctivitis. Epinastine and ketotifen are indicated for the prevention of itching secondary to allergic conjunctivitis. Olopatadine 0.2% is the only antiallergy eyedrop approved for once-daily dosing. These dual-action medications are appropriate choices for patients with acute seasonal exacerbations as well as those with chronic perennial symptoms.

Traditional mast cell stabilizers include sodium cromoglycate 4% and lodoxamide tromethamine 0.1%. Lodoxamide is about 2500 times more potent than sodium cromoglycate in an animal model,[37] although their efficacy in controlling the symptoms of allergic conjunctivitis is similar. Their effects are not seen until 2 to 5 days after initiation of therapy, while their maximum benefit is achieved 15 days after initiating therapy. Thus, if patients have allergic symptoms during a defined season, they should begin these medications about two weeks prior to their allergy season. Given that these medications inhibit the release of histamine rather than block histamine receptors, they are better at preventing than treating allergic signs and symptoms. Newer mast cell stabilizers include pemirolast potassium 0.1% and nedocromil sodium 2% solutions. Both have proven to be safe and effective for treating signs and symptoms of allergic conjunctivitis.[38,39] Nedocromil, originally thought to be just a mast cell stabilizing agent, is recognized to have multiple actions resulting in rapid relief of symptoms. This includes antihistaminic (H_1 antagonist) effects, reduction of ICAM-1 expression, and inhibitory effects on eosinophils and neutrophils.[40]

Ketorolac tromethamine 0.5% and diclofenac are nonsteroidal antiinflammatory agents which decrease the activity of cyclooxygenase, an enzyme responsible for arachidonic acid metabolism. This, in turn, reduces prostaglandin production, most notably the highly pruritic PGE_2 and PGI_2.[41] Topical ketorolac tromethamine, the only approved nonsteroidal antiinflammatory drug for managing ocular allergies, has been shown to provide relief of the signs and symptoms of allergic conjunctivitis.[42,43] Some patients have transient stinging upon instillation. The newer agents discussed above have largely replaced the nonsteroidal antiinflammatory agents.

Topical corticosteroids are highly effective therapy for ocular allergy, blocking most allergic inflammatory cascades (including the late-phase mediators). They are seldom used for the treatment of seasonal or perennial allergic conjunctivitis, but may be necessary for a short period if the allergic response is severe and conservative therapy has failed. Given their propensity to induce cataracts, elevate intraocular pressure in susceptible individuals, and potentiate ocular infections, their judicious use is indicated.[44] Loteprednol, an ester corticosteroid which is metabolized in the aqueous humor, is effective in treating seasonal allergic conjunctivitis. In a recent retrospective study, Loteprednol 0.2% was well tolerated with no reports of adverse reactions in patients treated for SAC or PAC for at least 12 months.[45] Intranasal corticosteroids, when used to treat allergic rhinitis, may also improve concurrent ocular symptoms.[46] If corticosteroids are necessary, patients should be given the lowest concentration for the shortest duration with appropriate follow-up.

Oral antihistamines are seldom used to treat isolated seasonal or perennial allergic conjunctivitis, but are frequently used to treat systemic allergy. They should be used with caution in patients with cardiac arrhythmias, or in combination with erythromycin, ketoconazole, itraconazole, and troleandomycin. These medications may improve systemic symptoms, but ocular symptoms may worsen. Symptoms of dry eye may be induced or compounded by the propensity of antihistamines to reduce tear production. Topical antihistamines have muscarinic binding properties which, in theory, may also cause or worsen dry eye syndrome. The data on their effect on tear production are conflicting.[47,48]

Contact Lens Wearers

Contact lens wearers often do not want to discontinue wearing their lenses, despite having symptomatic allergic conjunctivitis. After insertion, contact lenses become coated with a biofilm which can act as a base for antigen deposition. Patients should maintain meticulous contact lens hygiene or switch to a daily disposable type. Theoretically, when contact lenses are worn while eye drops are used, the pharmacokinetics of the drug's active ingredient and preservative can be altered, allowing for prolonged ocular exposure to these chemicals.[49] Thus, putting in contacts at least 20 minutes after drop instillation is recommended. Allergic conjunctivitis can adversely affect tear film stability, which may be why patients with a history of ocular allergy often have contact lens-related discomfort.[50]

Research in Diagnosis and Treatment

Noninvasive methods to quantify the ocular allergic response when diagnosis is unclear or to assess treatment response are being researched. These include measuring cytokine levels and IgE concentration in the tear film.[51,52] Researchers are also exploring the role of confocal microscopy to quantify the severity of conjunctival inflammation.[53]

New therapies are being investigated which may be more effective and have safer side-effect profiles than current treatment modalities. Sublingual allergen immunotherapy holds promise as a new form of hyposensitization therapy.[54] Various cytokine antagonists are being evaluated and may offer novel methods for modulating the inflammatory response. Antibodies to lymphocyte function associated antigen-1 (LFA-1) and ICAM-1,[55] and treatment with an IL-1 receptor antagonist[56] have immunomodulating effects in animal models. A recombinant humanized monoclonal anti-IgE antibody, omalizumab, has promising results for the treatment of allergic rhinitis and rhinoconjunctivitis.[57] This antibody binds to the Fc epsilonRI site on the IgE molecule, thereby blocking the binding of the IgE molecule to mast cells and basophils. Further research is necessary to better understand the ocular allergic response as well as provide better diagnostic and treatment modalities.

References

1. Bremond-Gignac D. The clinical spectrum of ocular allergy. *Curr Allergy Asthma Rep*. 2002;2:321–324.
2. Bielory L. Update on ocular allergy treatment. *Expert Opin Pharmacother.* 2002;3(5):541–543.
3. Friedlaender MH. Current concepts in ocular allergy. *Ann Allergy.* 1991;67:5–10.
4. Ono SJ, Abelson MB. Allergic conjunctivitis: update on pathophysiology and prospects for future treatment. *J Allergy Clin Immunol.* 2005; 115:118–122.
5. Bielory L. Allergic and immunologic disorders of the eye. Part II: Ocular allergy. *J Allergy Clin Immunol.* 2000;106:1019–1032.
6. Blackley CH. *Experimental researches on causes and cure of Catarrhus Aestiuus.* London: Trindall and Cox Ltd; 1873:77.
7. Allansmith MR, Ross RN. Ocular allergy and mast cell stabilizers. *Surv Ophthalmol.* 1986;30:229–244.
8. Anderson DF, Macleod JDA, Baddeley SM, et al. Seasonal allergic conjunctivitis is accompanied by increased mast cell numbers in the absence of leucocyte infiltration. *Clin Exp Allergy.* 1997;27:1060–1066.
9. Bacon AS, Ahluwalia P, Irani A. Tear and conjunctival changes during the allergen-induced early- and late-phase responses. *J Allergy Clin Immunol.* 2000;106:948–954.
10. Hansen I, Klimek L, Mosges R, Hormann K. *Curr Opin Allergy Clin Immunol.* 2004;4(3):159–163.
11. Trocme SD, Raizman MB, Bartley GB. Medical therapy for ocular allergy. *Mayo Clin Proc.* 1992;67:557–565.
12. Bryant DH, Burns MW, Lazarus L. Identification of IgG antibody as a carrier of reaginic activity in asthmatic patients. *J Allergy Clin Immunol.* 1975;56:417–428.
13. Stern ME, Siemasko K, Gao J, et al. Role of interferon-gamma in a mouse model of allergic conjunctivitis. *Invest Ophthalmol Vis Sci.* 2005;46(9): 3239–3246.
14. Sumi T, Fukushima A, Fukuda K, et al. Thymus-derived CD4+ CD25+ T cells suppress the development of murine allergic conjunctivitis. *Int Arch Allergy Immunol.* 2007;143(4):276–281.
15. Fukushima A, Yamaguchi T, Fukuda K, et al. CD8+ T cells play disparate roles in the induction and the effector phases of murine experimental allergic conjunctivitis. *Microbiol Immunol.* 2006;50(9):719–728.
16. Zuber P, Pecoud A. Effect of levocabastine, a new H1 antagonist, in a conjunctival provocation test with allergens. *J Allergy Clin Immunol.* 1988;82:590–594.
17. Bacon AS, McGill JI, Anderson DF, et al. Adhesion molecules and relationship to leukocyte levels in allergic eye disease. *Invest Ophthalmol Vis Sci.* 1998;39:322–330.
18. Ciprandi G, Buscaglia S, Pesce G, et al. Allergic subjects express intercellular adhesion molecule-1 (ICAM-1 or CD54) on epithelial cells of conjunctiva after allergen challenge. *J Allergy Clin Immunol.* 1993;91: 783–792.

19. Nomura K, Takamura E, Murata M, et al. Quantitative evaluation of inflammatory cells in seasonal allergic conjunctivitis. *Ophthalmologica.* 1997;211: 1–3.
20. Smit EE, Sra SK, Grabowski CR, et al. Modulation of IL-8 and RANTES release in human conjunctival epithelial cells. *Cornea.* 2003;224:322–337.
21. Raizman MB, Rothman JS, Maroun F, et al. Effect of eye rubbing on signs and symptoms of allergic conjunctivitis in cat-sensitive individuals. *Ophthalmology.* 2000;107:2158–2161.
22. Abelson MB, Chambers WA, Smith LM. Conjunctival allergen challenge. A clinical approach to studying allergic conjunctivitis. *Arch Ophthalmol.* 1990;108:84–88.
23. Imber WE. Allergic skin testing: a clinical investigation. *J Allergy Clin Immunol.* 1977;60:47–55.
24. Friedlaender MH, Okumoto M, Kelley J. Diagnosis of allergic conjunctivitis. *Arch Ophthalmol.* 1984;102:1198–1199.
25. Greiner JV, Peace DG, Baird RS, et al. Effects of eye rubbing on the conjunctiva as a model of ocular inflammation. *Am J Ophthalmol.* 1985;100:45–50.
26. Abelson MB, Allansmith MR, Friedlaender MH. Effects of topically applied ocular decongestant and antihistamine. *Am J Ophthalmol.* 1980;90:254–257.
27. Greiner JV, Udell IJ. A comparison of the clinical efficacy of pheneramine solution and olopatadine hydrochloride ophthalmic solution in the conjunctival allergen challenge model. *Clin Ther.* 2005;27(5):468–577.
28. Spector SL, Raizman MB. Conjunctivitis medicamentosa. *J Allergy Clin Immunol.* 1994;94:134–136.
29. Noble S, McTravish D. Levocabastine. An update of its pharmacology, clinical efficacy and tolerability in the topical treatment of allergic rhinitis and conjunctivitis. *Drugs.* 1995;50:1032–1049.
30. Sharif NA, Su SX, Yanni JM. Emedastine: a potent, high affinity histamine H1-receptor-selective antagonist for ocular use: receptor binding and second messenger studies. *J Ocul Pharmacol.* 1994;10:653–664.
31. Secchi A, Leonardi A, Discepola M, et al. An efficacy and tolerance comparison of emedastine difumarate 0.05% and levocabastine 0.05%: reducing chemosis and eyelid swelling in subjects with seasonal allergic conjunctivitis. Emadine Study Group. *Acta Ophthalmol Scand Suppl.* 2000;230:48–51.
32. Hasala H, Malm-Erjefalt M, Erjefalt J, et al. Ketotifen induces primary necrosis of human eosinophils. *J Ocul Pharmacol Ther.* 2005;21(4): 318–327.
33. Randley BW, Sedgwick J. The effect of azelastine on neutrophils and eosinophil generation of superoxide. *J Allergy Clin Immunol.* 1989;83: 400–405.
34. Whitcup SM, Bradford R, Lue J, et al. Efficacy and tolerability of ophthalmic epinastine: a randomized, double-masked, parallel-group, active-and vehicle-controlled environmental trial in patients with seasonal allergic conjunctivitis. *Clin Ther.* 2004;26(1):29–34.
35. Greiner JV, Michaelson C, McWhirter CL, et al. Single dose of ketotifen fumarate .025% vs 2 weeks of cromolyn sodium 4% for allergic conjunctivitis. *Adv Ther.* 2002;19:185–193.
36. Spangler DL, Bensch G, Berdy GJ. Evlauation of the efficacy of olopatadine hydrochloride 0.1% ophthalmic solution and azelastine hydrochloride 0.05% ophthalmic solution in the conjunctival allergen challenge model. *Clin Ther.* 2001;23(8):1272–1280.
37. Johnson HG, White GJ. Development of new antiallergic drugs (cromolyn sodium, lodoxamide tromethamine). What is the role of cholinergic stimulation in the biphasic dose response? *Monogr Allergy.* 1979;14: 299–306.
38. Abelson MB, Berdy GJ, Mundorf T, et al. Pemirolast potassium 0.1% ophthalmic solution is an effective treatment for allergic conjunctivitis: a pooled analysis of two prospective, randomized, double-masked, placebo-controlled, phase III studies. *J Ocul Pharmacol Ther.* 2002;18: 475–488.
39. Stockwell A, Easty DL. Group comparative trial of 2% nedocromil sodium with placebo in the treatment of seasonal allergic conjunctivitis. *Eur J Ophthalmol.* 1994;4(1):12–23.
40. Corin RE. Nedocromil sodium: a review of the evidence for dual mechanism of action. *Clin Exp Allergy.* 2000;30(4):461–468.
41. Woodward DF, Nieves AL, Hawley SB, et al. The pruritogenic and inflammatory effects of prostanoids in the conjunctiva. *J Ocul Pharmacol Ther.* 1995;11:339–347.
42. Raizman MB. Results of a survey of patients with ocular allergy treated with topical ketorolac tromethamine. *Clin Ther.* 1995;17:882–890.
43. Donshik PC, Pearlman D, Pinnas J, et al. Efficacy and safety of ketorolac tromethamine 0.5% and levocabastine 0.05%: a multicenter comparison in patients with seasonal allergic conjunctivitis. *Adv Ther.* 2000;17: 94–102.
44. Friedlaender MH. Corticosteroid therapy of ocular inflammation. *Int Ophthalmol Clin.* 1983;23(1):175–182.
45. Ilyas H, Slonim CB, Braswell GR, et al. Long-term safety of loteprednol etabonate 0.2% in the treatment of seasonal and perennial allergic conjunctivitis. *Eye Contact Lens.* 2004;(30):10–13.
46. Bernstein DI, Levy AL, Hampel FC, et al. Treatment with intranasal fluticasone propionate significantly improves ocular symptoms in patients with seasonal allergic rhinitis. *Clin Exp Allergy.* 2004;34(6): 592–597.
47. Lekhanont K, Park CY, Combs JC, et al. Effect of topical olopatadine and epinastine in the botulinum toxin B-induced mouse model of dry eye. *J Ocul Pharm Ther.* 2007;23(1):83–88.
48. Villareal AL, Farley W, Pflugfelder SC, et al. Effect of topical epinastine and olopatadine on tear volume in mice. *Eye Contact Lens.* 2006;32(6):272–276.
49. Jain MR. Drug delivery through soft contact lenses. *Br J Ophthalmol.* 1988;72:150–154.
50. Suzuki S, Goto E, Dogru M, et al. Tear film layer alterations in allergic conjunctivitis. *Cornea.* 2006;25(3):277–280.
51. Leonardi A. In-vivo diagnostic measurements of ocular inflammation. *Curr Opin Allergy Clin Immunol.* 2005;5:464–472.
52. Ono T, Kawamura M, Arao S, et al. Quantitative analysis of antigen specific IgE in tears in comparison to serum samples. *Asian Pac J Allergy Immunol.* 2005;23(2–3):93–100.
53. Lim LL, Hoang L, Wong T, et al. Intravital microscopy of leukocyte-endothelial dynamics using the Heidelberg confocal laser microscope in scleritis and allergic conjunctivitis. *Mol Vis.* 2006;12:1302–1305.
54. Dahl R, Kapp A, Columbo G, et al. Efficacy and safety of sublingual immunotherapy with grass allergen tablets for seasonal allergic rhinoconjunctivitis. *J Allergy Clin Immunol.* 2006;118:434–440.
55. Whitcup SM, Chan CC, Kozhich AT, et al. Blocking ICAM-1 (CD54) and LFA-1 (CD11a) inhibits experimental allergic conjunctivitis. *Clin Immunol.* 1999;93:107–113.
56. Keane-Myers AM, Miyazaki D, Liu G, et al. Prevention of allergic eye disease by treatment with IL-1 receptor antagonist. *Invest Ophthalmol Vis Sci.* 1999;40:3041–3046.
57. Okubo K, Ogino S, Nagakura T, et al. Omalizumab is effective and safe in the treatment of Japanese cedar pollen-induced seasonal allergic rhinitis. *Allergol Int.* 2006;55:379–386.

Chapter 49

Vernal and Atopic Keratoconjunctivitis

Neal P. Barney

Atopy refers to hypersensitivities in persons with a hereditary background of allergic diseases as first described by Cocoa and Cooke.[1] The major, most commonly recognized atopic conditions include eczema (atopic dermatitis), asthma, hay fever, and allergic rhinitis. Atopic conditions affect 28–32% of the population.[2] Atopic ocular disease includes seasonal allergic conjunctivitis (SAC), perennial allergic conjunctivitis (PAC), vernal keratoconjunctivitis (VKC), atopic keratoconjunctivitis (AKC), and giant papillary conjunctivitis (GPC). VKC and AKC may cause significant complications and lead to loss of vision. Type I hypersensitivity reactions of the ocular surface are important in AKC and VKC but are not considered the only pathophysiologic mechanism in these similar, yet distinct entities. VKC and AKC are discussed separately and compared and contrasted.

Vernal Keratoconjunctivitis

Definition

Vernal keratoconjunctivitis (VKC) is a chronic, bilateral, conjunctival inflammatory condition found in individuals predisposed by their atopic background. An excellent review of the history and description of this disease was published by Kumar in 2008.[3] Beigelman's 1950 monograph *Vernal Conjunctivitis* continues to be the most exhaustive compilation of this disease and is unmatched in current times.[4] The list of easily recognized names in ophthalmology to have published regarding this entity is formidable: Arlt,[5] Desmarres,[6] von Graefe,[7] Axenfeld,[8] Trantas,[9] and Herbert.[10] In 2000, Bonini et al. reviewed a series of 195 patients with VKC as the only allergic manifestation in 58.5% of patients.[11]

Demographics

The onset of disease is generally before age 10, it lasts 2 to 10 years, and it usually resolves during late puberty. Only 11% of patients were greater than 20 years of age in the Bonini series.[11] Males predominate in the younger ages but the male to female ratio is nearly equal in older patients. Young males in dry, hot climates are those primarily affected. The Mediterranean area and West Africa are areas with the greatest numbers of patients. VKC is relatively unusual in most of North America and Western Europe. There is a significant history of other atopic manifestations, such as eczema or asthma in 40–75% of patients with VKC.[12] A family history of atopy is found in 40–60% of patients.[11] Seasonal exacerbation, as the name implies, is common, but patients may have symptoms year-round.

Symptoms

Severe itching and photophobia are the main symptoms. Associated foreign body sensation, ptosis, thick mucus discharge, and blepharospasm occur.

Signs

The signs are confined mostly to the conjunctiva and cornea; the skin of the lids and lid margin are relatively uninvolved compared to AKC. The conjunctiva develops a papillary response, principally of the limbus or upper tarsus. The tarsal papillae are discrete, greater than 1 mm in diameter, have flattened tops that may stain with fluorescein, and occur more frequently in European and North American patients.[13] Thick, ropy mucus tends to be associated with the tarsal papilla (Fig. 49.1). These are the classic 'cobblestone' papillae.

Limbal papillae tend to be gelatinous and confluent, and they occur more commonly in African and West Indian patients.[14] Horner-Trantas dots, which are collections of epithelial cells and eosinophils, may be found at any meridian around the limbus.[9] These changes may lead to superficial corneal neovascularization. The forniceal conjunctiva usually does not show foreshortening or symblepharon formation.

The corneal findings may be sight threatening. Buckley describes in detail the sequence of occurrence of corneal findings.[13] Mediators from the inflamed tarsal conjunctiva cause a punctate epithelial keratitis. Coalescence of these areas leads to frank epithelial erosion, leaving Bowman's membrane intact. If, at this point, inadequate or no treatment is rendered, a plaque containing fibrin and mucus deposits over the epithelial defect.[15] Epithelial healing is then impaired, and new vessel growth is encouraged. This so-called shield ulcer (Fig. 49.2) usually has its lower border in the upper half of the visual axis. With resolution, the ulcerated area leaves a subepithelial ringlike scar. The

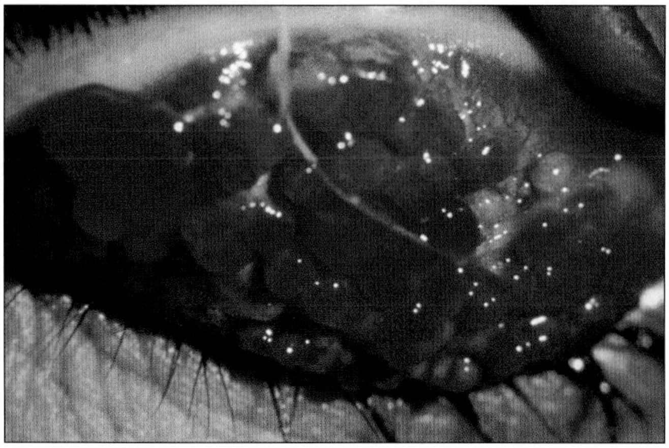

Fig. 49.1 Upper tarsal conjunctiva of patient with VKC. Note the flat-topped 'cobblestone' papillae and thick ropy mucus.

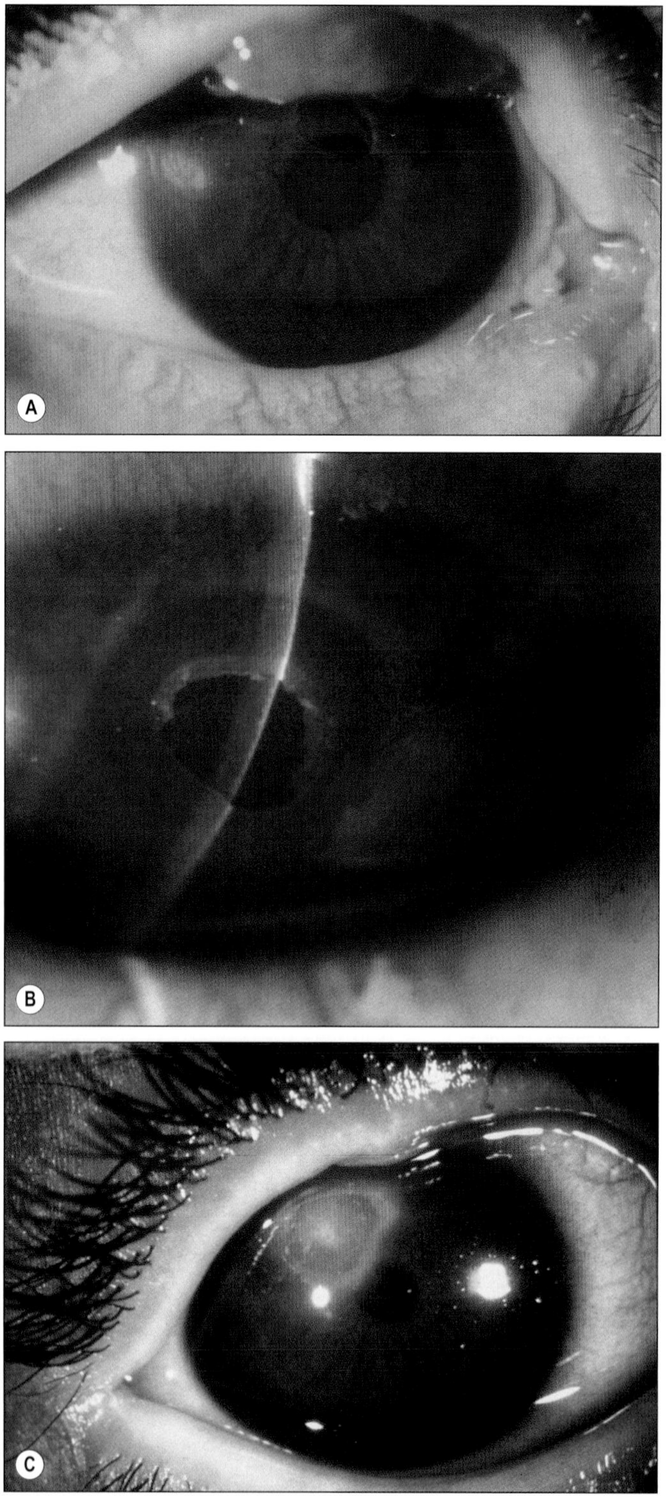

Fig. 49.2 Shield ulcer in VKC. (**A**) Large papilla visible just below the upper lid margin. The border of an epithelial defect of the cornea is seen just inferior to the papilla. (**B**) Slit lamp view of the epithelial defect. (**C**) The same defect with progressive ulceration of the stroma. (All photos courtesy of Devon Harrison, MD.)

peripheral cornea may show a waxing and waning, superficial stromal, gray-white deposition termed pseudogerontoxon. Iritis is not reported to occur in VKC.

Pathophysiology

Biopsy of a tarsal conjunctival papilla in VKC reveals distinct findings. The epithelium contains large numbers of mast cells and eosinophils, neither of which are found in normal individuals.[16,17] Human mast cells may be categorized based on the presence of neutral proteases.[18] The epithelium of VKC patients contains mast cells predominantly of the type containing the neutral proteases tryptase and chymase.[19] Basophils are found in the epithelium, and may indicate that one form of a delayed-type hypersensitivity reaction is occurring. Leonardi et al. demonstrated eosinophils, neutrophils, and mononuclear cells in the hyperplastic epithelium.[17] Brush cytology of the conjunctival epithelium from patients with VKC showed more eosinophils and neutrophils in patients with corneal erosion or ulcer than in those without.[20] Goblet cell density is not found to be elevated in the conjunctival epithelium of VKC.[21] Some neurotransmitters, their receptors, integrins, growth factors, Toll-like receptor 2, and the inflammation modulating peptide thymosin-beta 4 are found in greater amount in VKC epithelium compared to normals.[22–25] Eosinophil major basic protein is deposited diffusely throughout the conjunctiva of VKC patients, including the epithelium.[26]

The substantia propria contains elevated numbers of mast cells compared to normal individuals.[16,17] The predominant mast cell subtype found contains tryptase and chymase. Forty-six percent of the mast cells in the substantia propria contain basic fibroblast growth factor (bFGF).[27] This may serve as a stimulus for fibroblast growth and production of collagens. Eosinophil major basic protein granules are found close to mast cells in VKC.[26] As in the epithelium, the substantia propria contains increased numbers of eosinophils and basophils compared to normal tissue.[16] A unique profile of lymphocytes is found. T-cell clones can be isolated from biopsy specimens of VKC tarsal conjunctiva. These CD4+ T-cell clones show helper function for IgE synthesis in vitro and produce interleukin-4 (IL-4).[28] Calder et al., in separate work, found IL-5 expressed in T-cell lines from vernal biopsy specimen.[29] Cognate interaction with T cells and the presence of IL-4 are needed for B-cell production of IgE.[28] This would support the suggestion that IgE is produced locally. The substantia propria stains positive for metalloprotease 9, EGFR, VEGF, TGF-beta, bFGF, PDGF, and thymosin-beta 4 associated with inflammatory cells.[23,24,30] The substantia propria also has an increased amount of collagen. Fibroblasts from the tarsal conjunctival biopsy of VKC patients can be induced to proliferate by histamine and epithelium-derived growth factor.[17] Alpha-SMA-positive cells are found in papillae of VKC.[31] Ciclosporin A, often used in VKC, has been shown in vitro to reduce collagen production and induce apoptosis of conjunctival fibroblasts from VKC patients.[32]

The corneal epithelium of VKC patients has been shown to express intercellular adhesion molecule-1, an important cell adhesion molecule.[33] Eosinophil peroxidase, in contact with human corneal epithelial cells, causes disruption of cell adhesion.[34] Eosinophil major basic protein (EMBP) and cationic protein (ECP) are proinflammatory, and EMBP has been shown to be cytotoxic to corneal epithelium.[35] In vitro, both of these damage monolayers of human corneal epithelial cells but not the stratified corneal epithelial cells in culture.

Specific IgE and IgG have been isolated from the tears of VKC patients.[36,37] Histamine and tryptase are elevated in the tears of VKC patients.[38,39] The serum of VKC patients has been found to contain decreased levels of histaminase and increased levels of nerve growth factor.[40,41] Finally, VKC is reported to occur in patients with the hyperimmunoglobulin E syndrome.[42]

Diagnosis

The diagnosis is relatively easily arrived at, based on the history and presentation of findings. As indicated previously, VKC occurs predominantly in young boys living in warm climates. These patients have intense photophobia, ptosis, and the characteristic finding of giant papillae. The principal differential diagnostic entity is AKC. The two are compared and contrasted in Table 49.1. Tear fluid analysis and cytology, conjunctival scraping for cytology, and biopsy are rarely needed to assist in establishing the diagnosis.

Treatment

As with any atopic condition, avoidance of allergens is important although many afflicted are skin test negative. Often, this is difficult for VKC patients because of the possible large number of antigens to which they react. Seasonal removal of affected children from their home to a reduced allergen climate is usually not practical for most families. What is practical and should not be overlooked is alternate occlusive therapy, as allergen avoidance strategy. Hyposensitization in VKC has limitations. It is not feasible to desensitize these children to all of the allergens to which they are responsive. Moreover, some suggest that while skin and lung are responsive to hyposensitization, the conjunctiva is not.[13]

For the patient with a significant seasonal exacerbation, a short-term, high-dose pulse regimen of topical steroids is necessary. Usually, dexamethasone 0.1% or prednisolone phosphate 1% eight times daily for 1 week brings excellent relief of symptoms. This should be tapered rapidly to as little as is needed to maintain patient comfort. As in any chronic ocular inflammatory disease, the risks of prolonged use of corticosteroids are cataract and glaucoma. Thus, any limited use of steroids should include additional measures to sustain a decreased state of inflammation. Cromolyn sodium, a mast cell stabilizer, has repeatedly been shown to be effective in VKC.[43–45] At the time of an exacerbation, the patient should be given a steroid pulse dose and begin using a mast cell stabilizing drug topically or a dual-acting drug such as olopatadine, ketotifen, epinastine, or azelastine concurrently to begin mast cell stabilization and antihistamine treatment. Oral medications that have a variable role include steroids, antihistamines, and nonsteroidal antiinflammatory agents.[38,46] For the care of severe bilateral vision-threatening disease, oral steroids may be used, but using this treatment for VKC alone is unusual. Maximizing the use of nonsedating antihistamines is often helpful.

Topical calcineurin inhibitors of ciclosporin A (CsA) and tacrolimus have been demonstrated effective in the treatment of VKC.[47–56] The corneal shield ulcer is a vision-threatening complication of VKC. Treatment may include antibiotic–steroid ointment and occlusive therapy. If a plaque forms in the ulcer bed, a superficial keratectomy is sometimes beneficial in promoting epithelial healing.[57] Recently, phototherapeutic keratectomy and keratectomy with amniotic membrane graft placement have been shown to be effective.[58,59]

Climatotherapy may be beneficial. This may involve simple measures, such as cool compresses over the closed lids. Maintenance of an air-conditioned environment or relocation to a cool, dry climate is most helpful during seasonal exacerbations. The economic and geographic restrictions of these measures are obvious.

Table 49.1 Comparison of VKC and AKC

	VKC	AKC
Age	Younger	Older
Sex	Males > females	No predilection
Duration of disease	Limited; resolves at puberty	Chronic
Time of year	Spring	Perennial
Conjunctival involvement	Upper tarsus	Lower tarsus
Conjunctival cicatrization	Rare	Common
Cornea	Shield ulcer	Persistent epithelial defects
Corneal scar	Common; not vision threatening	Common; vision threatening
Corneal vascularization	Rare	Common

Cryoablation of upper tarsal cobblestones is reported to render short-term improvement. However, scar formation from this may lead to lid and tear film abnormalities. The risk of these adverse permanent changes is probably not warranted in this usually self-limiting disease.[13] Surgical removal of the upper tarsal papilla in combination with forniceal conjunctival advancement or buccal mucosal grafting may result in obliteration of the fornix.[4,60] Injection of short- or long-acting steroids into the tarsal papilla has been shown effective at reducing their size.[61–63] Excision of upper tarsal papillae with or without adjunctive use of mitomycin-C is reported to be helpful.[64,65]

The therapy of the future will be directed toward diminishing mast cell numbers or function and immunomodulation of the cell-mediated response.

Atopic Keratoconjunctivitis

Definition

Atopic keratoconjunctivitis (AKC) is a bilateral, chronic inflammation of the conjunctiva and lids associated with atopic dermatitis. Hogan, in 1953, was the first to describe the findings of chronic conjunctivitis and keratitis in patients with atopic dermatitis.[66] Three percent of the population has atopic dermatitis.[67,68] From 15% to 67.5% of patients with atopic dermatitis have ocular involvement, usually AKC.[67–69]

Demographics

The onset of disease is usually in the second through fifth decade although the majority of patients with atopic dermatitis are diagnosed by age 5 years. Recent series of patients report the onset of symptoms between the ages of 7 and 76.[70–72] The male:female ratio is reported as 2.4:1 and less than 1.[70,72] No racial or geographic predilection is reported.

Symptoms

Itching is the major symptom of AKC. This may be more pronounced in certain seasons or it may be perennial. Other symptoms, in decreasing order of frequency, include watering, mucus discharge, redness, blurring of vision, photophobia, and pain.[72] Exacerbation of symptoms most frequently occurs in the presence of animals.[72]

Signs

Signs of AKC include skin, lid margin, conjunctival, corneal, and lens changes (Table 49.2). The periocular skin often shows a scaling, flaking dermatitis with a reddened base (Fig. 49.3). The lids may become lichenified and woody, developing cicatricial ectropion and lagophthalmos. Lateral canthal ulceration, cracking, and madarosis may also be present. This may be the principal manifestation in a minority of cases. The lid margins may show loss of cilia, meibomianitis, keratinization, and punctal ectropion. The conjunctiva of the tarsal surfaces has a papillary reaction, follicles, and possibly a pale white edema (Fig. 49.4). In contrast to VKC, the papillary hypertrophy of AKC is more prominent in the inferior conjunctival fornix. Subepithelial fibrosis is present in many, fornix foreshortening in some, and symblepharon in a few. The bulbar conjunctiva may have few findings besides erythema and chemosis. A perilimbal, gelatinous hyperplasia may occur (Fig. 49.5). Horner-Trantas dots have been reported to occur in AKC.[73]

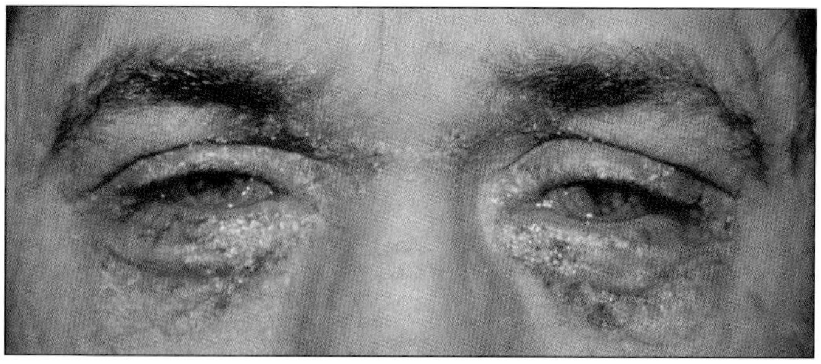

Fig. 49.3 Severe periocular and lid involvement of AKC.

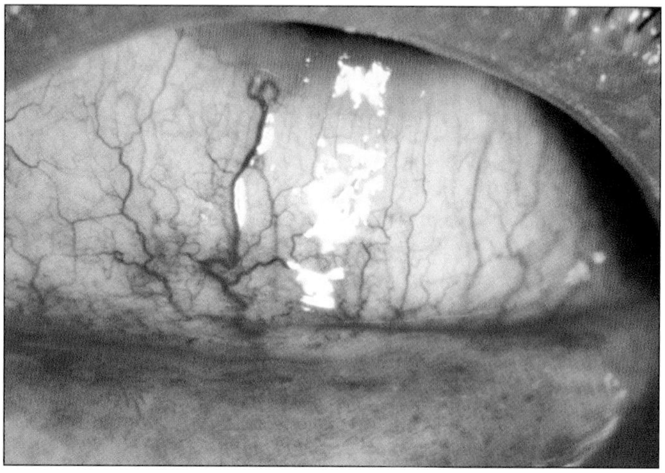

Fig. 49.4 Lower tarsal conjunctiva in AKC. Note the fornix foreshortening and pale edema.

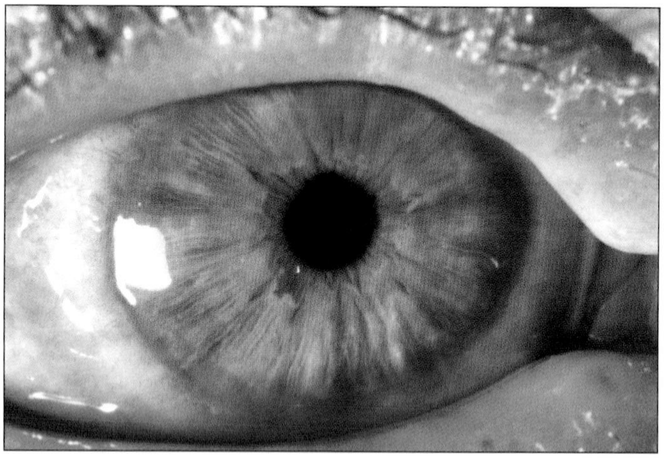

Fig. 49.5 Limbal gelatinous hyperplasia in AKC.

Significant vision loss in this disease usually results from pathologic conditions of the cornea. Punctate epithelial keratopathy is the most common corneal finding. Persistent

Table 49.2 Clinical signs in patients with AKC

	Foster and Calonge[70] (N = 45)		Tuft et al[72] (N = 37)	
Condition	**No. of patients**	**%**	**No. of patients**	**%**
Lids				
Eczema	28	62.2	30	81.1
Blepharitis	25	55.6	33	89.2
Meibomianitis	25	55.6	–	–
Tarsal margin keratinization	13	28.9	–	–
Trichiasis	8	17.8	6	16.2
Madarosis	6	13.3	–	–
Punctal ectropion	–	–	18	48.6
Ectropion	5	11.1	–	–
Entropion	2	4.4	–	–
Conjunctiva				
Subepithelial fibrosis	26	57.8	26	70.3
Fornix foreshortening	13	28.9	–	–
Symblepharon	12	26.7	10	27.0
Giant papillae	11	24.4	11	29.7
Follicles	6	13.3	5	13.5
Cornea				
Superficial punctate keratitis	24	53.3	37	100
Neovascularization	17	37.8	24	64.9
Persistent epithelial defects	17	37.8	4	10.8
Filamentary keratitis	2	4.4	1	2.7

epithelial defects, scarring, microbial ulceration, and neovascularization are the main corneal causes for decreased vision (see Table 49.2). Penetrating keratoplasty typically results in similar surface problems but has been shown to improve vision in some.[74] Herpetic keratitis is reported to occur in 14–17.8% of patients.[70,72] Keratoconus occurs in 6.7–16.2% of patients.[70,72]

Anterior uveitis and iris abnormalities are not reported. The prevalence of cataract associated with AKC is difficult to determine, since steroids are so frequently used in the treatment of the disease. The lens opacity typically associated with AKC, however, is an anterior or subcapsular cataract. This cataract often has the configuration of a Maltese cross. Retinal detachment with or without previous cataract surgery is the principal posterior manifestation of AKC reported.[75–77]

Pathophysiology

Atopic keratoconjunctivitis is thought to consist of both type I and type IV hypersensitivity mechanisms. Evidence of the pathologic process comes from histologic and immunohistochemical analysis of conjunctival biopsy specimens and from tear fluid analysis for mediators and cells.

Mast cells and eosinophils are found in the conjunctival epithelium of AKC patients but not in normal individuals.[78] Mast cells in the epithelium of AKC patients contain predominantly tryptase as the neutral protease. Goblet cell density and squamous metaplasia are then examined by impression cytology.[79] The epithelium may become involuted, allowing pseudotubule structures to form.[80] Antibodies to HLA-DR stain diffusely throughout the epithelium.[80] This suggests an up-regulation of antigen presentation. There is an increase in the CD4:CD8 ratio in AKC over normal conjunctival epithelium.[80] This increase of CD4 or helper T cells (Th) probably serves to amplify the immune response that is occurring. In vivo confocal microscopy reveals fewer basal epithelial cells in the cornea.[81] Mucin proteins and mRNA are increased in the epithelium.[82,83]

The substantia propria in AKC has an increased number of mast cells compared to normal. Conjunctival inflammatory cell density showed a negative correlation with tear stability and corneal sensitivity and a positive correlation with the vital staining scores.[84] Eosinophils, never found in normal structures, are present in the substantia propria in AKC. These eosinophils are found to have increased numbers of activation markers on their surface.[85] A large number of mononuclear cells is present in the substantia propria. Fibroblast number is increased, and there is an increased amount of collagen compared to normal individuals. In addition, the substantia propria demonstrates increased CD4/CD8, B cells, HLA-DR staining, and Langerhans cells.[80] The T-cell receptor on lymphocytes in the substantia propria is predominantly of the α or β subtype.[80] The T-cell population of the substantia propria includes CD4 and memory cells.[86,87] Th2 cytokines predominate in allergic disease yet lymphocytes with Th1 cytokines have been found in the substantia propria of AKC patients.[87]

Tears of AKC patients contain increased levels of IgE, eosinophil cationic protein (reduced following papillae resection), activated B cells, eotaxin, eosinophil neurotoxin, soluble IL-2 receptor, IL-4, IL-5, specific sIgA, and osteopontin.[27,65,69,70,88–94] AKC has reduced tear break-up time and decreased Schirmer's values (56% less than 5 mm) compared to controls.[83,95] Serum of AKC patients has been found to contain increased levels of IgE, eosinophil cationic protein, eosinophil neurotoxin, and IL-2 receptor.[69,96–98] Tabbara et al. report adoptive transfer of AKC in bone marrow recipients.[99] Messmer and colleagues show eosinophils and their products deposited in the ulcers and stroma of corneas from AKC patients.[100]

In summary, AKC patients demonstrate an increased number of conjunctival mast cells and evidence of mast cell activation. Furthermore, a complex immune cell profile implicates more than the mast cell alone, but the details of these cellular interactions remain speculative.

Diagnosis

Paramount to both diagnosis and treatment in AKC is a careful history. The patient typically describes severe, persistent, periocular itching associated with dermatitis. There is usually a family history of atopic disease in one or both parents and commonly other atopic manifestations in the patient, such as asthma (65%) or allergic rhinitis (65%).[71] A history of seasonal or exposure-related exacerbations is usually present. History and examination reveal features to help differentiate AKC from other atopic ocular conditions. The lack of contact lens wear aids in differentiating AKC from GPC. AKC patients are usually older and have major lid involvement compared to patients with VKC. SAC patients have no or markedly diminished symptoms out of their season and show no evidence of chronic inflammation in the conjunctiva. The significant past history or concurrent presence of eczema cannot be emphasized enough as a finding in patients with AKC. The serum level of IgE is often elevated in patients with AKC. A Giemsa stain of a scraping of the upper tarsal conjunctiva may reveal eosinophils.

Treatment

The approach to treatment is multifaceted and includes environmental controls as well as topical and systemic medications. It is unlikely that the AKC patient will see the ophthalmologist without also being under the care of a medical physician. However, the patient must remove environmental irritants in both the home and the employment or school setting. The nature of the irritants may be better defined through skin testing.

The topical application of a vasoconstrictor–antihistamine combination may bring transient relief of symptoms but is unlikely to intervene in the immunopathologic process or its sequelae. There is potential for overuse due to the chronic nature of the disease. The potent topical antihistamines offer much greater H_1 receptor antagonism than over-the-counter antihistamines. The topical administration of steroids such as prednisolone acetate eight times per day for 7 to 10 days is clearly beneficial in controlling symptoms and signs. These agents, of course, must be used judiciously, since the chronic nature of the disease may encourage overuse. The patient must be instructed that steroid use must be transient only and must be carefully monitored for efficacy; he or she must also be warned of the potential for causing cataract and glaucoma. Nonsteroid medications have been shown to be effective in reducing itching, tearing, and photophobia.[101–103] Mast cell stabilizers two to four times daily is recommended year-round in patients with perennial symptoms. If an exacerbation occurs and the patient is not taking a mast cell stabilizing agent topically, its use should be initiated two to four times daily concurrent with a short burst of topical steroids (for 7–10 days). Mast cell stabilizers alone such as cromolyn, nedocromil, lodoxamide, or mast cell stabilizer combination antihistamines such as olopatadine, azelastine, epinastine, and ketotifen may be helpful. Ciclosporin A and tacrolimus, both orally and topically, have been shown effective in treating AKC as well as reducing the amount of topical steroid use.[55,104–108] Foster and Calonge recommend maximizing the use of systemic antihistamines.[70] H_1 receptors seem most responsible for the symptoms of AKC, and newer antagonists are fairly specific for the H_1 receptor. Only in rare cases of uncontrolled dermatitis with vision-threatening complications are oral steroids indicated. The role of systemic desensitization is similar to that in VKC. Plasmapheresis has been shown effective in the treatment of AKC.[109]

Lid and ocular surface abnormalities may require treatment other than that directed toward the underlying pathologic condition of AKC. Trichiasis or lid position abnormalities, if contributing in any way to corneal compromise, must be corrected. Any staphylococcal blepharitis should receive adequate antibiotic treatment. If, despite adequate control of signs and symptoms of AKC, corneal punctate staining persists, artificial tears should be used to aid in avoiding the development of corneal epithelial defects. It may be extremely difficult to achieve reepithelialization in these defects and surgical approaches have been attempted.[110] Lid or ocular surface herpes simplex virus (HSV) infection should be treated with topical antiviral agents. Care should be taken in using these to achieve viral eradication without sustained use and subsequent epithelial toxicity. If there are frequent recurrent episodes of epithelial HSV keratitis, one may consider oral acyclovir (400 mg orally twice daily) as prophylaxis against recurrences.

In summary, topical steroids will control most patients with AKC. The chronic use of steroids must be avoided and, early in treatment, steroid-sparing strategies must be considered.

References

1. Cocoa AF, Cooke RA. On the classification of the phenomena of hypersensitiveness. *J Immunol.* 1923;8:163–182.
2. Dorner T, Lawrence K, Rieder A, Kunze M. Epidemiology of allergies in Austria. Results of the first Austrian allergy report. *Wien Med Wochenschr.* 2007;157(11–12):235–242.
3. Kumar S. Vernal keratoconjunctivitis: a major review. *Acta Ophthalmol.* 2008.
4. Beigelman MN. *Vernal conjunctivitis.* Los Angeles: University of Southern California Press; 1950.
5. Arlt F. Physiologisch and pathologisch anatomische Bemerkungen uber die bindehaut des Auges. *Prager Vierteljahrschrift.* 1846;4:73.
6. Desmarres LA. *Hypertrophie perikeratique de la conjonctive. Traite theorie et pratique des maladies des yeus.* 2nd ed. Paris: Germer Baillere; 1855.
7. von Graefe A. Klinische Vortrage uber Augenheilkunde. *Journal Hirshberg.* 1871;21.
8. Axenfeld T. Rapport sur le catarrhe printanier. *Bull Mem Soc Fr Ophthalmol.* 1907;24:1.
9. Trantas A. Sur le catarrhe prntanier. *Arch D'opht.* 1910;30:593–621.
10. Herbert H. Preliminary note on the pathology and diagnosis of spring catarrh. *Br Med J* 1903:735.
11. Bonini S, Lambiase A, Marchi S, et al. Vernal keratoconjunctivitis revisited: a case series of 195 patients with long-term followup. *Ophthalmology.* 2000;107(6):1157–1163.
12. Bonini S, Coassin M, Aronni S, Lambiase A. Vernal keratoconjunctivitis. *Eye.* 2004;18(4):345–351.
13. Buckley RJ. Vernal keratoconjunctivitis. *Int Ophthalmol Clin.* 1988;28(4):303–308.
14. Verin PH, Dicker ID, Mortemousque B. Nedocromil sodium eye drops are more effective than sodium cromoglycate eye drops for the long-term management of vernal keratoconjunctivitis. *Clin Exp Allergy.* 1999;29(4):529–536.
15. Rahi AHS. Pathology of Corneal plaque in vernal keratoconjunctivitis. In: O'Connor GR, Chandler JW, eds. *Advances in immunology and immunopathology of the eye.* New York: Masson; 1985.
16. Allansmith MR, Baird RS, Greiner JV. Vernal conjunctivitis and contact lens-associated giant papillary conjunctivitis compared and contrasted. *Am J Ophthalmol.* 1979;87(4):544–555.
17. Leonardi A, Abatangelo G, Cortivo R, Secchi AG. Collagen types I and III in giant papillae of vernal keratoconjunctivitis. *Br J Ophthalmol.* 1995;79(5):482–485.
18. Irani AA, Schechter NM, Craig SS, et al. Two types of human mast cells that have distinct neutral protease compositions. *Proc Natl Acad Sci U S A.* 1986;83(12):4464–4468.
19. Irani AM, Butrus SI, Tabbara KF, Schwartz LB. Human conjunctival mast cells: distribution of MCT and MCTC in vernal conjunctivitis and giant papillary conjunctivitis. *J Allergy Clin Immunol.* 1990;86(1):34–40.
20. Miyoshi T, Fukagawa K, Shimmura S, et al. Interleukin-8 concentrations in conjunctival epithelium brush cytology samples correlate with neutrophil, eosinophil infiltration, and corneal damage. *Cornea.* 2001;20(7):743–747.
21. Allansmith MR, Baird RS, Greiner JV. Density of goblet cells in vernal conjunctivitis and contact lens-associated giant papillary conjunctivitis. *Arch Ophthalmol.* 1981;99(5):884–885.
22. Motterle L, Diebold Y, Enriquez de Salamanca A, et al. Altered expression of neurotransmitter receptors and neuromediators in vernal keratoconjunctivitis. *Arch Ophthalmol.* 2006;124(4):462–468.
23. Micera A, Bonini S, Lambiase A, et al. Conjunctival expression of thymosin-beta4 in vernal keratoconjunctivitis. *Mol Vis.* 2006;12:1594–1600.
24. Abu El-Asrar AM, Al-Mansouri S, Tabbara KF, et al. Immunopathogenesis of conjunctival remodelling in vernal keratoconjunctivitis. *Eye.* 2006;20(1):71–79.
25. Bonini S, Micera A, Iovieno A, Lambiase A. Expression of Toll-like receptors in healthy and allergic conjunctiva. *Ophthalmology.* 2005;112(9):1528; discussion 48–49.
26. Trocme SD, Kephart GM, Allansmith MR, et al. Conjunctival deposition of eosinophil granule major basic protein in vernal keratoconjunctivitis and contact lens-associated giant papillary conjunctivitis. *Am J Ophthalmol.* 1989;108(1):57–63.
27. Leonardi A, Borghesan F, Faggian D, et al. Tear and serum soluble leukocyte activation markers in conjunctival allergic diseases. *Am J Ophthalmol.* 2000;129(2):151–158.
28. Romagnani S. Regulation and deregulation of human IgE synthesis. *Immunol Today.* 1990;11(9):316–321.
29. Calder VL, Jolly G, Hingorani M, et al. Cytokine production and mRNA expression by conjunctival T-cell lines in chronic allergic eye disease. *Clin Exp Allergy.* 1999;29(9):1214–1222.
30. Leonardi A, Brun P, Di Stefano A, et al. Matrix metalloproteases in vernal keratoconjunctivitis, nasal polyps and allergic asthma. *Clin Exp Allergy.* 2007;37(6):872–879.
31. Kato N, Fukagawa K, Dogru M, et al. Mechanisms of giant papillary formation in vernal keratoconjunctivitis. *Cornea.* 2006;25(10 Suppl 1):S47–S52.
32. Leonardi A, DeFranchis G, Fregona IA, et al. Effects of cyclosporin A on human conjunctival fibroblasts. *Arch Ophthalmol.* 2001;119(10):1512–1517.
33. Temprano J. Corneal epithelial expression of ICAM-1 in vernal keratoconjunctivitis. *Invest Ophthalmol Vis Sci.* 1995;36(4):s1024.
34. Hallberg CK. Eosinophil peroxidase and eosinophil-derived neurotoxin toxicity on cultured human corneal epithelium. *Invest Ophthalmol Vis Sci.* 1995;36(4):s698.
35. Ward SL. The barrier properties of an in vitro human corneal epithelial model are not altered by eosinophil major basic protein or eosinophil cationic protein. *Invest Ophthalmol Vis Sci.* 1995;36(4):s699.
36. Sompolinsky D. A contribution to the immunopathology of vernal keratoconjunctivitis. *Documenta Ophthalmologica.* 1982;53:61–92.
37. Ballow M, Mendelson L. Specific immunoglobulin E antibodies in tear secretions of patients with vernal conjunctivitis. *J Allergy Clin Immunol.* 1980;66(2):112–118.
38. Abelson MB, Baird RS, Allansmith MR. Tear histamine levels in vernal conjunctivitis and other ocular inflammations. *Ophthalmology.* 1980;87(8):812–814.
39. Butrus SI, Ochsner KI, Abelson MB, Schwartz LB. The level of tryptase in human tears. An indicator of activation of conjunctival mast cells. *Ophthalmology.* 1990;97(12):1678–1683.
40. Bonini S, Lambiase A, Levi-Schaffer F, Aloe L. Nerve growth factor: an important molecule in allergic inflammation and tissue remodelling. *Int Arch Allergy Immunol.* 1999;118(2–4):159–162.
41. Mukhopadhyay K, Pradhan SC, Mathur JS, Gambhir SS. Studies on histamine and histaminase in spring catarrh (vernal conjunctivitis). *Int Arch Allergy Appl Immunol.* 1981;64(4):464–468.
42. Butrus SI, Leung DY, Gellis S, et al. Vernal conjunctivitis in the hyperimmunoglobulinemia E syndrome. *Ophthalmology.* 1984;91(10):1213–1216.
43. El Hennawi M. Clinical trial with 2% sodium cromoglycate (Opticrom) in vernal keratoconjunctivitis. *Br J Ophthalmol.* 1980;64(7):483–486.
44. Foster CS, Duncan J. Randomized clinical trial of topically administered cromolyn sodium for vernal keratoconjunctivitis. *Am J Ophthalmol.* 1980;90(2):175–181.
45. Tabbara KF, Arafat NT. Cromolyn effects on vernal keratoconjunctivitis in children. *Arch Ophthalmol.* 1977;95(12):2184–2186.
46. Chaudhary KP. Evaluation of combined systemic aspirin and cromolyn sodium in intractable vernal catarrh. *Ann Ophthalmol.* 1990;22(8):314–318.
47. Avunduk AM, Avunduk MC, Erdol H, et al. Cyclosporine effects on clinical findings and impression cytology specimens in severe vernal keratoconjunctivitis. *Ophthalmologica.* 2001;215(4):290–293.

48. BenEzra D, Pe'er J, Brodsky M, Cohen E. Cyclosporine eyedrops for the treatment of severe vernal keratoconjunctivitis. *Am J Ophthalmol.* 1986;101(3):278–282.
49. Gupta V, Sahu PK. Topical cyclosporin A in the management of vernal keratoconjunctivitis. *Eye.* 2001;15(Pt 1):39–41.
50. Holland EJ, Olsen TW, Ketcham JM, et al. Topical cyclosporin A in the treatment of anterior segment inflammatory disease. *Cornea.* 1993;12(5):413–419.
51. Mendicute J, Aranzasti C, Eder F, et al. Topical cyclosporin A 2% in the treatment of vernal keratoconjunctivitis. *Eye.* 1997;11(Pt 1):75–78.
52. Pucci N, Novembre E, Cianferoni A, et al. Efficacy and safety of cyclosporine eyedrops in vernal keratoconjunctivitis. *Ann Allergy Asthma Immunol.* 2002;89(3):298–303.
53. Secchi AG, Tognon MS, Leonardi A. Topical use of cyclosporine in the treatment of vernal keratoconjunctivitis. *Am J Ophthalmol.* 1990;110(6):641–645.
54. Tomida I, Schlote T, Brauning J, et al. [Cyclosporin a]. *Ophthalmologe.* 2002;99(10):761–767.
55. Miyazaki D, Tominaga T, Kakimaru-Hasegawa A, et al. Therapeutic effects of tacrolimus ointment for refractory ocular surface inflammatory diseases. *Ophthalmology.* 2008;115(6):988–992 e5.
56. Vichyanond P, Tantimongkolsuk C, Dumrongkigchaiporn P, et al. Vernal keratoconjunctivitis: result of a novel therapy with 0.1% topical ophthalmic FK-506 ointment. *J Allergy Clin Immunol.* 2004;113(2):355–358.
57. Jones BR. Vernal keratitis. *Trans Ophthalmol Soc UK.* 1961;81:215–228.
58. Autrata R, Rehurek J, Holousova M. [Phototherapeutic keratectomy in the treatment of corneal surface disorders in children]. *Cesk Slov Oftalmol.* 2002;58(2):105–111.
59. Sridhar MS, Sangwan VS, Bansal AK, Rao GN. Amniotic membrane transplantation in the management of shield ulcers of vernal keratoconjunctivitis. *Ophthalmology.* 2001;108(7):1218–1222.
60. Nishiwaki-Dantas MC, Dantas PE, Pezzutti S, Finzi S. Surgical resection of giant papillae and autologous conjunctival graft in patients with severe vernal keratoconjunctivitis and giant papillae. *Ophthal Plast Reconstr Surg.* 2000;16(6):438–442.
61. Holsclaw DS, Whitcher JP, Wong IG, Margolis TP. Supratarsal injection of corticosteroid in the treatment of refractory vernal keratoconjunctivitis. *Am J Ophthalmol.* 1996;121(3):243–249.
62. Saini JS, Gupta A, Pandey SK, et al. Efficacy of supratarsal dexamethasone versus triamcinolone injection in recalcitrant vernal keratoconjunctivitis. *Acta Ophthalmol Scand.* 1999;77(5):515–518.
63. Sethi HS, Wangh VB, Rai HK. Supratarsal injection of corticosteroids in the treatment of refractory vernal keratoconjunctivitis. *Indian J Ophthalmol.* 2002;50(2):160–161; discussion 1.
64. Tanaka M, Takano Y, Dogru M, et al. A comparative evaluation of the efficacy of intraoperative mitomycin C use after the excision of cobblestone-like papillae in severe atopic and vernal keratoconjunctivitis. *Cornea.* 2004;23(4):326–329.
65. Tanaka M, Dogru M, Takano Y, et al. Quantitative evaluation of the early changes in ocular surface inflammation following MMC-aided papillary resection in severe allergic patients with corneal complications. *Cornea.* 2006;25(3):281–285.
66. Hogan MJ. Atopic keratoconjunctivitis. *Am J Ophthalmol.* 1953;36:937–947.
67. Garrity JA, Liesegang TJ. Ocular complications of atopic dermatitis. *Can J Ophthalmol.* 1984;19(1):21–24.
68. Rich LF, Hanifin JM. Ocular complications of atopic dermatitis and other eczemas. *Int Ophthalmol Clin.* 1985;25(1):61–76.
69. Dogru M, Nakagawa N, Tetsumoto K, et al. Ocular surface disease in atopic dermatitis. *Jpn J Ophthalmol.* 1999;43(1):53–57.
70. Foster CS, Calonge M. Atopic keratoconjunctivitis. *Ophthalmology.* 1990;97(8):992–1000.
71. Power WJ, Tugal-Tutkun I, Foster CS. Long-term follow-up of patients with atopic keratoconjunctivitis. *Ophthalmology.* 1998;105(4):637–642.
72. Tuft SJ, Kemeny DM, Dart JK, Buckley RJ. Clinical features of atopic keratoconjunctivitis. *Ophthalmology.* 1991;98(2):150–158.
73. Friedlaender MH. Diseases affecting the eye and skin. In: Friedlaender MH, ed. *Allergy and immunology of the eye.* Hagerstown: Harper and Row; 1979.
74. Ghoraishi M, Akova YA, Tugal-Tutkun I, Foster CS. Penetrating keratoplasty in atopic keratoconjunctivitis. *Cornea.* 1995;14(6):610–613.
75. Hurlbut WB, Damonkos AN. Cataract and retinal detachment associated with atopic dermatitis. *Arch Ophthalmol.* 1961;52:852–857.
76. Klemens F. Dermatose, Kataradt und ablatio retinae. *Klin Monatsbl Augenheilkd.* 1966;152:921–927.
77. Yoneda K, Okamoto H, Wada Y, et al. Atopic retinal detachment. Report of four cases and a review of the literature. *Br J Dermatol.* 1995;133(4):586–591.
78. Baddeley SM, Bacon AS, McGill JI, et al. Mast cell distribution and neutral protease expression in acute and chronic allergic conjunctivitis. *Clin Exp Allergy.* 1995;25(1):41–50.
79. Dogru M, Katakami C, Nakagawa N, et al. Impression cytology in atopic dermatitis. *Ophthalmology.* 1998;105(8):1478–1484.
80. Foster CS, Rice BA, Dutt JE. Immunopathology of atopic keratoconjunctivitis. *Ophthalmology.* 1991;98(8):1190–1196.
81. Hu Y, Matsumoto Y, Adan ES, et al. Corneal in vivo confocal scanning laser microscopy in patients with atopic keratoconjunctivitis. *Ophthalmology.* 2008;115(11):2004–2012.
82. Dogru M, Okada N, Asano-Kato N, et al. Alterations of the ocular surface epithelial mucins 1, 2, 4 and the tear functions in patients with atopic keratoconjunctivitis. *Clin Exp Allergy.* 2006;36(12):1556–1565.
83. Hu Y, Matsumoto Y, Dogru M, et al. The differences of tear function and ocular surface findings in patients with atopic keratoconjunctivitis and vernal keratoconjunctivitis. *Allergy.* 2007;62(8):917–925.
84. Hu Y, Adan ES, Matsumoto Y, et al. Conjunctival in vivo confocal scanning laser microscopy in patients with atopic keratoconjunctivitis. *Mol Vis.* 2007;13:1379–1389.
85. Hingorani M, Calder V, Jolly G, et al. Eosinophil surface antigen expression and cytokine production vary in different ocular allergic diseases. *J Allergy Clin Immunol.* 1998;102(5):821–830.
86. Metz DP, Bacon AS, Holgate S, Lightman SL. Phenotypic characterization of T cells infiltrating the conjunctiva in chronic allergic eye disease. *J Allergy Clin Immunol.* 1996;98(3):686–696.
87. Metz DP, Hingorani M, Calder VL, et al. T-cell cytokines in chronic allergic eye disease. *J Allergy Clin Immunol.* 1997;100(6 Pt 1):817–824.
88. Avunduk AM, Avunduk MC, Dayanir V, et al. Pharmacological mechanism of topical lodoxamide treatment in vernal keratoconjunctivitis: a flow-cytometric study. *Ophthalmic Res.* 1998;30(1):37–43.
89. Avunduk AM, Avunduk MC, Dayioglu YS, Centinkaya K. Flow cytometry tear analysis in patients with chronic allergic conjunctivitis. *Jpn J Ophthalmol.* 1997;41(2):67–70.
90. Fukagawa K, Nakajima T, Tsubota K, et al. Presence of eotaxin in tears of patients with atopic keratoconjunctivitis with severe corneal damage. *J Allergy Clin Immunol.* 1999;103(6):1220–1221.
91. Montan PG, van Hage-Hamsten M. Eosinophil cationic protein in tears in allergic conjunctivitis. *Br J Ophthalmol.* 1996;80(6):556–560.
92. Uchio E, Matsuura N, Kadonosono K, et al. Tear osteopontin levels in patients with allergic conjunctival diseases. *Graefes Arch Clin Exp Ophthalmol.* 2002;240(11):924–928.
93. Uchio E, Ono SY, Ikezawa Z, Ohno S. Tear levels of interferon-gamma, interleukin (IL) -2, IL-4 and IL-5 in patients with vernal keratoconjunctivitis, atopic keratoconjunctivitis and allergic conjunctivitis. *Clin Exp Allergy.* 2000;30(1):103–109.
94. Inada N, Shoji J, Hoshino M, Sawa M. Evaluation of total and allergen-specific secretory IgA in tears of allergic conjunctival disease patients. *Jpn J Ophthalmol.* 2007;51(5):338–342.
95. Leonardi A, Fregona IA, Plebani M, et al. Th1- and Th2-type cytokines in chronic ocular allergy. *Graefes Arch Clin Exp Ophthalmol.* 2006;244(10):1240–1245.
96. Akova YA, Jabbur NS, Neumann R, Foster CS. Atypical ocular atopy. *Ophthalmology.* 1993;100(9):1367–1371.
97. Geggel HS. Successful penetrating keratoplasty in a patient with severe atopic keratoconjunctivitis and elevated serum IgE level treated with long-term topical cyclosporin A. *Cornea.* 1994;13(6):543–545.
98. Leonardi A, Brun P, Tavolato M, et al. Growth factors and collagen distribution in vernal keratoconjunctivitis. *Invest Ophthalmol Vis Sci.* 2000;41(13):4175–4181.
99. Tabbara KF, Nassar A, Ahmed SO, et al. Acquisition of vernal and atopic keratoconjunctivitis after bone marrow transplantation. *Am J Ophthalmol.* 2008;146(3):462–465.
100. Messmer EM, May CA, Stefani FH, et al. Toxic eosinophil granule protein deposition in corneal ulcerations and scars associated with atopic keratoconjunctivitis. *Am J Ophthalmol.* 2002;134(6):816–821.
101. Avunduk AM, Avunduk MC, Kapicioglu Z, et al. Mechanisms and comparison of anti-allergic efficacy of topical lodoxamide and cromolyn sodium treatment in vernal keratoconjunctivitis. *Ophthalmology.* 2000;107(7):1333–1337.
102. Jay JL. Clinical features and diagnosis of adult atopic keratoconjunctivitis and the effect of treatment with sodium cromoglycate. *Br J Ophthalmol.* 1981;65(5):335–340.
103. Ostler HB, Martin RG, Dawson CR. The use of disodium cromoglycate in the treatment of atopic ocular disease. In: Leopold JG, Burns RD, eds. *Symposium on ocular therapy.* New York: John Wiley; 1977.
104. Rikkers SM, Holland GN, Drayton GE, et al. Topical tacrolimus treatment of atopic eyelid disease. *Am J Ophthalmol.* 2003;135(3):297–302.

105. Hoang-Xuan T, Prisant O, Hannouche D, Robin H. Systemic cyclosporine A in severe atopic keratoconjunctivitis. *Ophthalmology.* 1997;104(8):1300–1305.
106. Hingorani M, Moodaley L, Calder VL, et al. A randomized, placebo-controlled trial of topical cyclosporin A in steroid-dependent atopic keratoconjunctivitis. *Ophthalmology.* 1998;105(9):1715–1720.
107. Stumpf T, Luqmani N, Sumich P, et al. Systemic tacrolimus in the treatment of severe atopic keratoconjunctivitis. *Cornea.* 2006;25(10):1147–1149.
108. Anzaar F, Gallagher MJ, Bhat P, et al. Use of systemic T-lymphocyte signal transduction inhibitors in the treatment of atopic keratoconjunctivitis. *Cornea.* 2008;27(8):884–888.
109. Aswad MI, Tauber J, Baum J. Plasmapheresis treatment in patients with severe atopic keratoconjunctivitis. *Ophthalmology.* 1988;95(4):444–447.
110. Thoft RA. Keratoepithelioplasty. *Am J Ophthalmol.* 1984;97(1):1–6.

Chapter 50

Giant Papillary Conjunctivitis

Steven P. Dunn, David G. Heidemann

Giant papillary conjunctivitis (GPC) is a noninfectious inflammatory disorder involving the superior tarsal conjunctiva. The disorder was originally named for the presence of 'giant' papillae (1.0 mm or greater in diameter) along the upper tarsal surface, though papillae measuring 0.3 mm or greater are now considered abnormal and a feature of this condition.[1] While most frequently occurring in association with hydrophilic contact lens wear, rigid gas-permeable contact lenses, glaucoma filtering blebs,[2] exposed sutures,[3,4] ocular prosthetics,[5] and extruded scleral buckles[6] have been implicated. MacIvor was the first to report a GPC-like condition associated with ocular prosthetics in 1950.[7] Other reports followed. It acquired its present name in 1977 with the work of Allansmith et al.[1]

In patients with contact lens-associated giant papillary conjunctivitis, a variety of factors such as contact lens type, wearing schedule, cleaning routine, and length of time contacts have been worn seem to influence the incidence of giant papillary conjunctivitis. It has been estimated that 1–5% of soft contact lens wearers and 1% of hard contact lens wearers have clinically significant signs or symptoms of GPC.[1,8] The incidence among extended wear contact lens wearers is unknown but generally thought to be higher than that of daily wear soft contact lens wearers. Symptomatic GPC due to filtering blebs, exposed sutures, and extruding scleral buckling elements is comparatively rare.

The onset of signs and symptoms of GPC (currently defined as papillae greater than 0.3 mm in diameter) depends on the type of contact lens being worn. The average length of time that patients had worn soft contact lenses before developing GPC was 8 months as compared with 8 years for hard contact lenses.[1,9] The syndrome may occur as early as 3 weeks after the start of soft contact lens wear and 14 months after the start of hard contact lenses. It may occur at any age and is seen with equal frequency among males and females.

Symptoms and Signs

Symptoms of giant papillary conjunctivitis are low grade at their onset, consisting of mild irritation, scant mucous discharge, and occasionally mild itching. Many patients take only passing notice of the disease at this early stage and rarely present for evaluation because of these symptoms alone. Undetected and untreated, giant papillary conjunctivitis progresses with gradual development of more significant symptoms. Blurring of vision due to lens surface debris, the accumulation of mucus in the medial canthal region, and a persistent foreign body sensation while wearing lenses inevitably lead to decreased contact lens wearing time. Itching of the eyes even when the lenses are removed is a frequent complaint. As these problems intensify, patients cease wearing their contact lenses altogether or seek ophthalmologic evaluation.

The slow, progressive character of giant papillary conjunctivitis has been described in detail by Allansmith et al.[1] Mild hyperemia of the upper tarsal conjunctiva is the earliest finding and is frequently accompanied by subtle conjunctival thickening. Conjunctival translucency is unaltered during this early phase, but gradually, as the disease progresses and increased inflammatory cell infiltrates develop, conjunctival thickening and increased opacification become evident (Fig. 50.1). Small strands of mucus are frequently evident early in the course of giant papillary conjunctivitis. A ropy, whitish, mucoid discharge develops (Fig. 50.2) as the condition worsens and is usually concentrated medially and in the inferior fornix.

Persistent contact lens wear or continued exposure to the inciting material leads to increased conjunctival hyperemia and inflammation. Opacification of the conjunctiva and the development and enlargement of tarsal conjunctival papillae ensue. Papillae normally measure less than 0.3 mm in diameter. In giant papillary conjunctivitis, papillae greater than 0.3 mm (often ranging from 0.6 to 1.75 mm) in diameter can be seen (Fig. 50.3). The presence of giant papillae, defined as papillae greater than 1.0 mm in diameter, give giant papillary conjunctivitis its name (Fig. 50.4).

The appearance and location of papillae may vary considerably. The upper tarsal conjunctiva may be covered by a uniform pattern of small to medium papillae proximally and distally, a nonhomogeneous-zonal pattern may develop, or large, cobblestone-like giant papillae may be seen (Fig. 50.5). One must be careful when evaluating the superior tarsal surface to 'ignore' the far lateral, medial, and superior borders of the tarsal plate since these areas respond unpredictably to adverse stimuli. Allansmith[1] has divided the superior tarsal surface into three zones (Fig. 50.6). Zone 1 is located proximally along the uppermost edge of the tarsal plate; zone 3 is located distally adjacent to the lid margin. Papillae

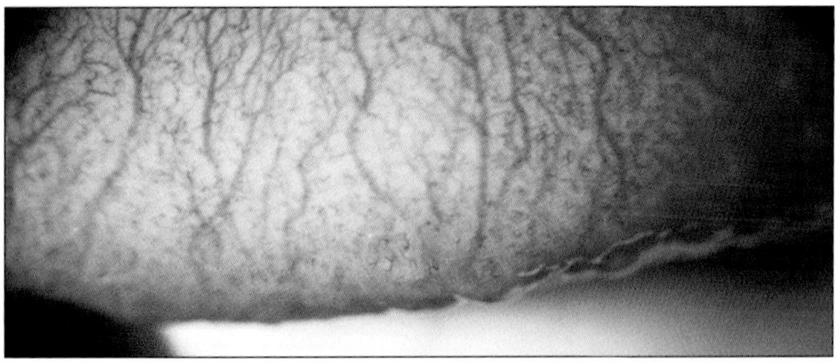

Fig. 50.1 Early giant papillary conjunctivitis with mild conjunctival hyperemia and thickening.

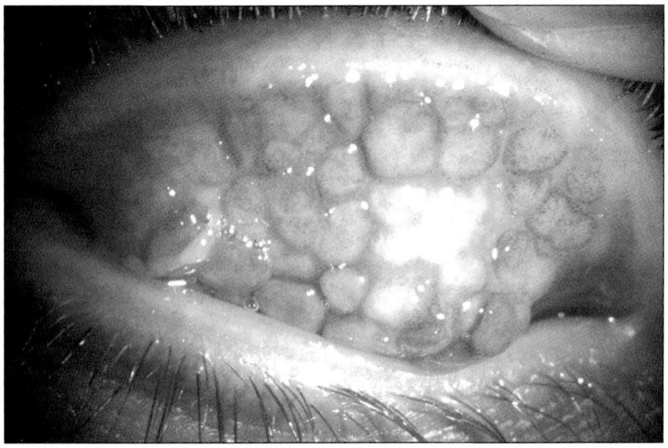

Fig. 50.2 Giant papillary conjunctivitis with ropy, whitish, mucoid discharge.

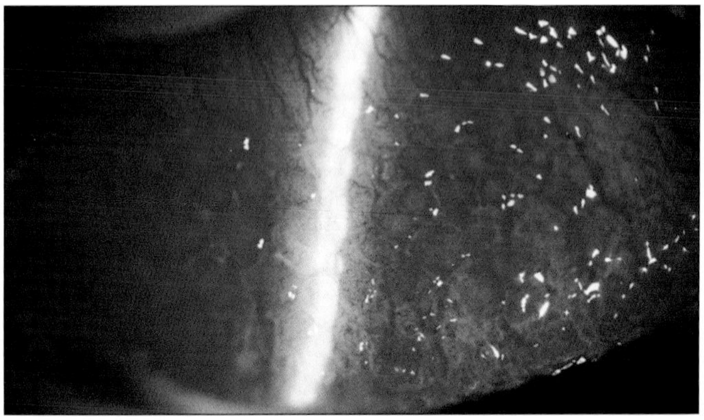

Fig. 50.3 Advancing conjunctival thickening and papillary formation.

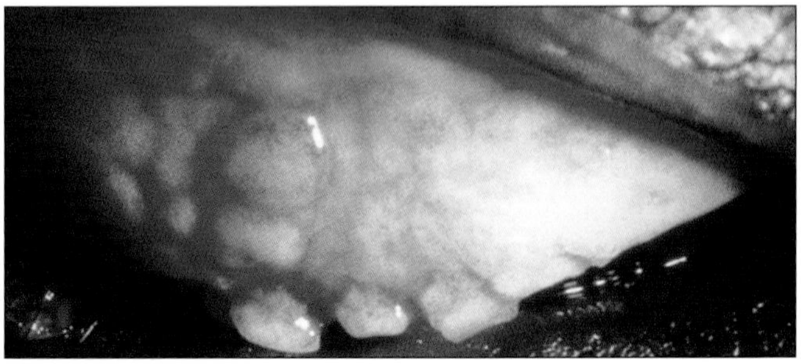

Fig. 50.4 Giant papillae.

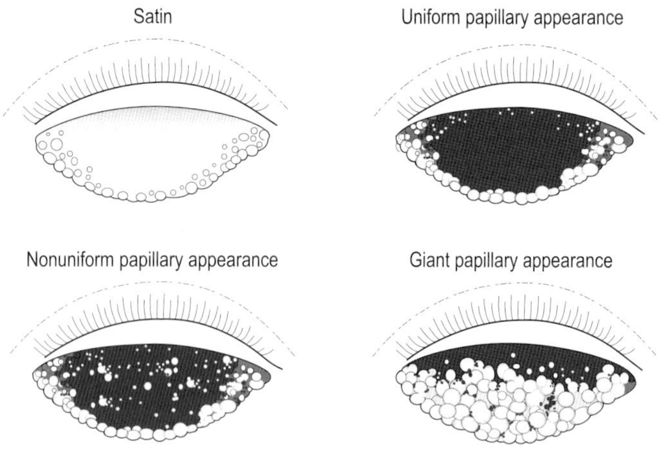

Fig. 50.5 Diagrammatic representation of the upper tarsal surface in GPC. (After Allansmith MR et al. Giant papillary conjunctivitis in contact lens wearers, *Am J Ophthalmol* 83:697–698, 1977. Copyright Elsevier 1977.)

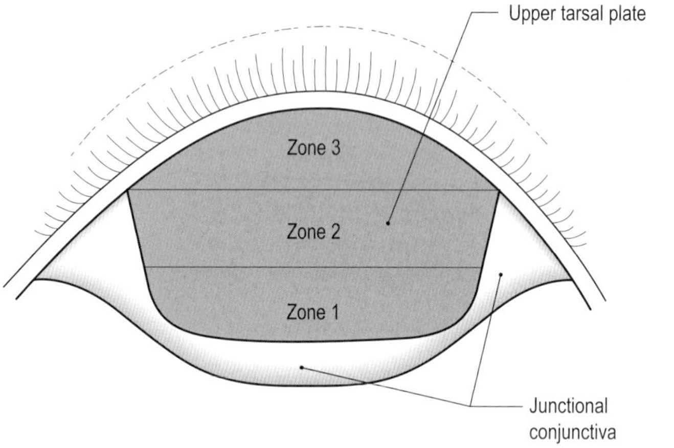

Fig. 50.6 Topographic division of upper tarsal conjunctiva into zones. (After Allansmith MR et al. Giant papillary conjunctivitis in contact lens wearers, *Am J Ophthalmol* 83:697–698, 1977. Copyright Elsevier 1977.)

associated with soft contact lens-related giant papillary conjunctivitis first appear in zone 1 and progress toward zones 2 and 3. The pattern is reversed in giant papillary conjunctivitis related to rigid gas-permeable contact lenses. Papillae associated with rigid gas-permeable contact lens wear are typically seen in zone 3, adjacent to the lid margin or the distal half of the lid. These papillae are usually fewer in number and craterlike or flattened in appearance. The topographic variation between GPC associated with large-diameter soft contact lenses and smaller-diameter rigid gas-permeable lenses is consistent with current theories related to a mechanical and/or immunologic stimulus for giant papillary conjunctivitis.

Giant papillary conjunctivitis associated with exposed suture material, elevated band keratopathy, and filtering blebs is usually characterized by large clusters of giant papillae overlying the inciting area (Fig. 50.7).[2] The topographic character of these changes suggests that chronic mechanical trauma may be a strong factor in the development of giant papillary conjunctivitis in these cases. Large clusters of

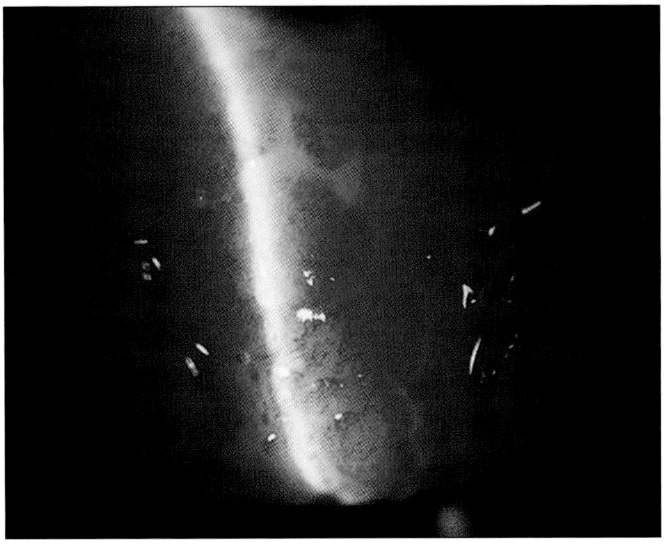

Fig. 50.7 Giant papillary conjunctivitis secondary to an exposed limbal suture.

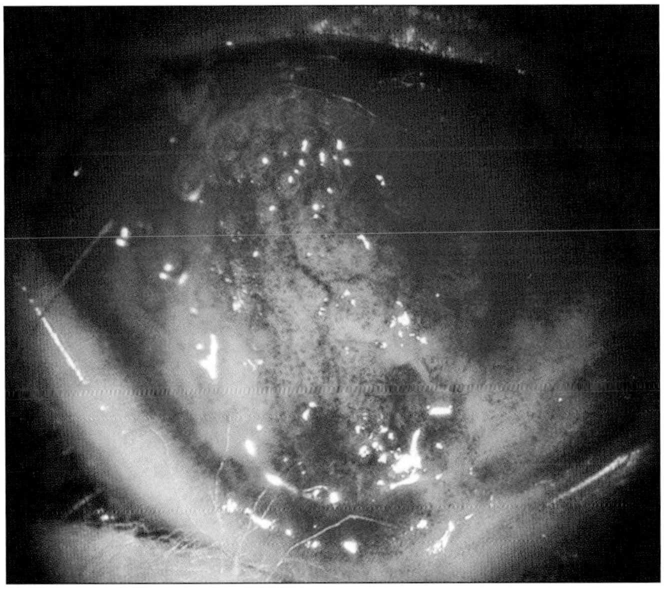

Fig. 50.8 Giant papillary conjunctivitis secondary to an ocular prosthesis.

papillae are seen on the tarsal surface and in the superior fornix when scleral lenses or prosthetic shells are the stimulus (Fig. 50.8). A granulomatous-like thickening may occasionally be seen in the superior fornix. Fluorescein staining of the apex of the papillae is not uncommon. It is not uncommon to see a white, scarlike cap covering larger papillae (Fig. 50.9). These changes regress as the conjunctival inflammation resolves, suggesting that inflammatory infiltrates may be partially responsible for these findings. Horner-Trantas dots have been reported in some patients with giant papillary conjunctivitis.[10] Rarely, the disease may be confined to the limbus with no inflammation of the tarsal surface. An association between giant papillary conjunctivitis and meibomian gland dysfunction has been described,[11]

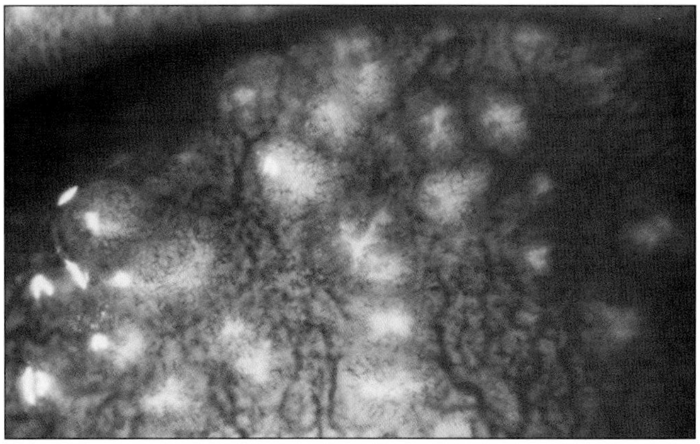

Fig. 50.9 Irregular, white, papillary capping in giant papillary conjunctivitis.

with increased meibomian gland dropout and an increased viscosity of the meibomian gland excreta being noted.[12]

Histopathology and Immunopathology

Histologic changes are seen at many levels of the conjunctiva in giant papillary conjunctivitis. Giant papillae are covered by a thickened and irregular conjunctival epithelium that contains numerous invaginations. Superficial epithelial erosion and corresponding fluorescein staining is seen in many cases. Ultrastructurally, scanning electron microscopy shows variability of epithelial cell size as well as a loss of the normal polygonal cell shape. Flattening, tufting, and branching of surface microvilli can also be seen.[13,14]

The increased mucus secretion associated with giant papillary conjunctivitis is not related to an increased density of goblet cells. The actual number of goblet cells appears to be increased due to an increased overall conjunctival surface area. The interpapillary crypts also frequently contain increased numbers of nongoblet mucus-secreting cells with increased numbers of secretory vesicles per cell.[15,16] Changes in both the quantity and distribution of inflammatory cells are seen throughout the conjunctiva in GPC. Infiltration of the conjunctival substantia propria by eosinophils and basophils, and increased numbers of lymphocytes, mast cells, and plasma cells are findings typical of giant papillary conjunctivitis. Increased numbers of eosinophils, mast cells, and basophils in the conjunctival epithelium, however, are a feature that readily differentiates giant papillary conjunctivitis from normal. The presence of these cell types within the conjunctiva is a strong indication of the immunologic character of this disease.

The role of mast cells in giant papillary conjunctivitis remains unclear. The absence of epithelial mast cells in the normal conjunctiva and their presence in the conjunctiva of patients with giant papillary conjunctivitis has been noted by a number of investigators.[17,18] There is not a significant increase in mast cells in the substantia propria as compared with normal conjunctiva. Recent work has shown that mast cells in giant papillary conjunctivitis are from the subset of mast cells (MCtc) that contain tryptase, chymase, and a cathepsin G-like protein. This type of mast cell is independent of T lymphocytes and is the predominant type observed in skin and in the mucosa of the small intestine. A large percentage (30%) of these cells have already undergone degranulation in patients with giant papillary conjunctivitis.[15] Correspondingly, elevated tear tryptase levels, an indicator of mast cell activation, has been demonstrated in patients with giant papillary conjunctivitis.[19] Interestingly, histamine, which is found in mast cells and basophils, is not found in higher concentrations in the tear film.[20] Whether mast cell degranulation is a primary event or a result of eye rubbing is still not known.

Eosinophils and basophils are increased in both the conjunctival epithelium and substantia propria in giant papillary conjunctivitis. Eosinophil granule major basic protein, a potent cytotoxin released by eosinophils, has been demonstrated within the conjunctiva of patients with giant papillary conjunctivitis and in contact lens coatings of patients with concurrent atopy and giant papillary conjunctivitis.[21] Soft contact lenses from patients with giant papillary conjunctivitis alone, however, did not demonstrate measurable amounts of major basic protein. Tear levels of eosinophil granule major basic protein have not been elevated in patients with giant papillary conjunctivitis.[22] Despite its presence within the conjunctiva, most evidence suggests that eosinophil granule major basic protein is probably not a major pathogenic factor in the development of giant papillary conjunctivitis.

Studies analyzing tear samples from patients with giant papillary conjunctivitis have shown increased levels of IgE and in some cases IgG and IgM.[23,24] Higher IgE levels were found in the more symptomatic eye of a group of patients with bilateral giant papillary conjunctivitis and asymmetric symptomatology.[20] Donshik et al.[46] reported a drop in elevated tear immunoglobulin levels to normal upon discontinuation of contact lenses in patients with GPC. Meisler[4] demonstrated IgA, IgD, IgE, IgG, and IgM specific plasma cells in conjunctival tissue obtained from a patient with an ocular prosthesis-induced giant papillary conjunctivitis. A high percentage (27%) of these were IgE-containing cells. It is unclear as to whether the increased immunoglobulin levels reflect local production alone (conjunctival biopsy has demonstrated increased numbers of plasma cells in the substantia propria in patients with giant papillary conjunctivitis[1]), or are also secondary to transudation brought on by the vasodilatory effect of mast cell degranulation. These findings lend support to an IgE-mediated, type I, immediate hypersensitivity reaction playing a role in giant papillary conjunctivitis.

Cytologic and immunohistopathologic evaluation of the conjunctiva and tear film has demonstrated an increased number of CD4+, CD45RO+, and HLA-DR+ T cells in patients with GPC.[43] The expression of surface antigens such as adhesion molecules (ICAM-1, HLA-DR) on conjunctival epithelial cells and the synthesis of cytokines suggest that the conjunctival epithelium actively participates in the immune process. Cytokines IL-2, IL-4, IL-6, IL-8, IL-11, RANTES, GM-CSF, and interferon transcripts are upregulated in GPC.[44,47] Elevated tear fluid leukotriene C4 levels (responsible for conjunctival redness, edema, increased mucus production, and papillary development) have also been found in soft contact lens wearers with GPC.[40–42]

Pathophysiology

The pathogenesis of giant papillary conjunctivitis is unknown but is most frequently attributed to the combined effect of mechanical trauma and the subsequent immune response to antigens in the form of contact lens surface deposits or environmental factors. The trauma has typically been associated with the use of soft, rigid, and hard contact lenses but has also been reported to be triggered by glaucoma-filtering blebs,[2] elevated subepithelial calcium plaques, limbal dermoids, exposed corneal and conjunctival sutures,[3,4] ocular prosthetics,[5] and scleral buckling elements.[6]

The accumulation of lens surface deposits on soft and hard contact lenses predisposes to the development or exacerbation of giant papillary conjunctivitis. Ballow and Donshik[25] demonstrated the importance of surface deposits in the pathogenesis of giant papillary conjunctivitis in monkeys when they showed an enhanced ocular allergic response to contact lenses from patients with giant papillary conjunctivitis compared with the response to lenses from normal and asymptomatic contact lens wearers. Common tear constituents such as IgA, IgG, IgE, lactoferrin, and lysozyme have been demonstrated in similar amounts on the lens surface of patients with and without giant papillary conjunctivitis. These findings would suggest that the stimulus is not from the deposits of normal tear proteins, but rather some other substance(s) produced by the conjunctiva or present in the environment and adherent to the lens surface.[26–28] Elevated levels of neutrophil chemotactic factor, a factor associated with conjunctival tissue injury, in giant papillary conjunctivitis further emphasize the role that trauma (presumably mechanical) plays in this condition.[48]

The presence of elevated levels of cytokines, chemokines, and locally produced immunoglobulins underscores the immunologic side to this condition. What actually triggers the production of these agents and why is still unclear. It has been shown by Xingwu et al.[49] that cells similar to the membranous antigen processing cells (M cells) that are typically found atop mucosa-associated lymphoid tissue (MALT), play a role in the binding, uptake, and translocation of soluble and particulate antigens in giant papillary conjunctivitis. They postulated that overproliferation of M cells and the accumulation of lymphocytes lead to the structural changes that are characteristic of GPC. Antigens from the surface coatings of contact lenses are first processed by these cells (M cells) in areas of conjunctival-associated lymphoid tissue (CALT) before being presented to B lymphocytes, which then mediate the subsequent immune response.

Differential Diagnosis

Giant papillary conjunctivitis and vernal keratoconjunctivitis have frequently been compared with each other because there are a number of similarities clinically and histopathologically. These similarities, however, rarely lead to confusion in the differential diagnosis. Vernal keratoconjunctivitis is typically seen in children, most often before puberty, and resolves by the late teens or early twenties. It is most active in the spring and summer, with symptoms resolving in the fall and winter. Allergic rhinitis, atopic dermatitis, and asthma are frequently seen in conjunction with vernal keratoconjunctivitis. Cobblestone-like giant papillae and limbal Horner-Trantas dots are seen clinically and are associated with increased levels of tear histamine, IgE, and eosinophilic major basic protein. Histologically, increased numbers of eosinophils and mast cells are found in the conjunctiva. Giant papillary conjunctivitis shares some but not all of these features and can be easily differentiated in most cases. Since vernal keratoconjunctivitis usually presents prior to the age that most adolescents begin wearing contact lenses, this group of patients is usually bothered sufficiently by their ocular symptoms that cosmetic contact lenses have limited appeal.

Treatment

The goal of treatment in giant papillary conjunctivitis is to reduce and eventually eliminate the burning, itching, and excess mucus production that are characteristic symptoms of this condition. When an ocular prosthetic or contact lenses are the underlying stimulus, restoring the patient to a normal or near normal wearing schedule is the ultimate measure of success.

Attention to the dual pathogenic mechanisms of mechanical trauma and antigenic stimulation in giant papillary conjunctivitis provides a guide to managing this disease. There is little question that removal of the inciting agent leads to resolution of the signs and symptoms of giant papillary conjunctivitis. This is easily achieved when there is a suture barb or exposed scleral buckle. Discontinuing contact lens wear also is quite effective, although many patients have difficulty accepting this, especially for prolonged periods. Others, such as patients with anisometropia or keratoconus, may be significantly handicapped if they have to limit or discontinue contact lens wear.

Modifying the patient's contact lens care routine and wearing schedule will often relieve many of the signs and symptoms of giant papillary conjunctivitis. This is often the easiest and most acceptable 'first step' in treating this problem when lenses cannot be discontinued completely.

The relationship between lens deposits and giant papillary conjunctivitis is well established. The use of daily disposable soft contact lenses is the best solution to this problem. When this is not possible due to cost or the need to use specialty lenses or rigid gas-permeable lenses, the daily use of an appropriate surfactant cleaner and a 'rub' routine becomes mandatory. Careful examination of the contact lens surface rarely gives a true indication as to the extent of surface deposits. Routines using enzymatic cleaners should be encouraged in all patients. Those who build up deposits easily may need to consider enzymatic cleaning as often as three to five times a week.[26] Cleaning, rinsing, and storage solutions should be carefully reassessed to minimize preservative-related toxicity. Disinfection by hydrogen peroxide appears to be the method least likely to further traumatize the conjunctiva.

Reducing contact lens wearing time is an important component of treatment in giant papillary conjunctivitis. Extended wear patients should be converted to a daily wear schedule. Daily wear should be limited, when lens wear is still necessary, to those situations where the patient cannot function without the lens (i.e. at work and while driving). Wearing time can be gradually increased according to the patient's treatment response.

The decision as to whether a different lens material or design should be utilized is probably of lesser importance as long as a good fit is maintained. The importance of edge design is unclear, though most practitioners feel that a thick or poorly manufactured edge may cause localized trauma and should be avoided. Scheduled contact lens replacement offers theoretical advantages for both the prevention and treatment of giant papillary conjunctivitis. Donshik and Porazinski[45] showed that the frequency of contact lens replacement is an important variable in the development of GPC. Patients on a 1-day to 3-week replacement cycle had a significantly lower risk of developing GPC than patients who replaced their lenses on a longer interval. Minimizing the build-up of lens deposits appears to reduce the chance of mechanical and immunologic stimuli developing. A change from soft contact lens wear to a rigid gas-permeable contact lens is a treatment strategy often tried when other approaches have not succeeded. The smaller diameter of these lenses and their reduced tendency to develop adherent deposits may be helpful in these situations.

The relationship between meibomian gland disease and giant papillary conjunctivitis is unclear.[11,12,31] The suggestion that one should look for evidence of meibomian gland disease in patients with giant papillary conjunctivitis and treat it when found is sound advice and may help to control the GPC as well as reduce the risk of secondary problems.

The pharmacologic management of giant papillary conjunctivitis focuses on the reduction of histamine release from mast cells and inhibition of local inflammation. Topical corticosteroids, nonsteroidal antiinflammatory drugs (NSAIDs), mast cell stabilizers, histamine receptor blockers, and vasoconstrictors have all been used alone or in combination.

Histamine antagonists and receptor blocking agents have, to date, been of limited benefit. While histamines are contained within mast cells and basophils, tear levels do not appear to be significantly elevated.[18]

Topical corticosteroids, while frequently utilized to reduce tarsal hyperemia and inflammation, have not proved particularly effective in the management of other aspects of giant papillary conjunctivitis. Their use should be restricted to the acute phase of giant papillary conjunctivitis. The need for corticosteroids usually signifies a level of disease severity requiring discontinuation of contact lens wear until the corticosteroids are no longer required. The risks of secondary infection outweigh the benefits of using corticosteroids with contact lenses in giant papillary conjunctivitis. Long-term use of topical corticosteroids has no role in the treatment of GPC.

Suprofen, an NSAID, has been studied topically in contact lens-associated GPC. A twofold reduction (as compared with placebo) in ocular signs (papillae) and symptoms was noted in a study of patients after a treatment course of 2 to 4 weeks.[33] Its mode of action appears to be inhibition of mast cell-stimulated prostaglandin biosynthesis.[34] Chronic use of topical NSAIDs in giant papillary conjunctivitis has not been reported.

Cromolyn sodium has been studied extensively and has been shown to promote resolution of early giant papillary conjunctivitis when combined with meticulous lens hygiene.[35,36] Relief of dryness, grittiness, and lens movement problems as well as a reduction in conjunctival hyperemia, mucus production, and papillary size have been reported.[37,38] No adverse effects have been noted when cromolyn sodium is applied with the contact lens on the eye. Advanced giant papillary conjunctivitis does not respond to cromolyn sodium and usually will require discontinuation of the contact lens for a period of time, refitting, and then gradual reintroduction of the contact lens with adjunctive cromolyn sodium treatment. This medication and its relatives, lodoxamide tromethamine and nedocromil, stabilize the mast cell membrane and inhibit type I immediate hypersensitivity reactions. While similar pharmacologically, the role of lodoxamide tromethamine, which has been released for use in vernal keratoconjunctivitis, in the management of giant papillary conjunctivitis has yet to be determined.[39]

Prognosis

The prognosis for giant papillary conjunctivitis is good. Permanent visual loss has not been reported with this condition. All patients will show symptomatic improvement if they stop wearing their contact lenses. Early recognition and aggressive treatment of the signs and symptoms of giant papillary conjunctivitis are key to ensuring a patient's contact lens comfort and continued ability to wear lenses. Mild cases of giant papillary conjunctivitis may respond to modification of lens care and wearing routines alone. The successful treatment of advanced giant papillary conjunctivitis is more problematic and usually requires discontinuation of contact lenses combined with a short course of topical steroids. Recurrences are possible.

References

1. Allansmith MR, Korb DR, Greiner JV, et al. Giant papillary conjunctivitis in contact lens wearers. *Am J Ophthalmol.* 1977;83:697–708.
2. Heidemann DG, Dunn SP. Unusual causes of giant papillary conjunctivitis. *Cornea.* 1993;12:78–80.
3. Sugar A, Meyer RF. Giant papillary conjunctivitis after keratoplasty. *Am J Ophthalmol.* 1981;92:368–371.
4. Jolson AS, Jolson SC. Suture barb giant papillary conjunctivitis. *Ophthalmic Surg.* 1984;15:139.
5. Meisler DM, Krachmer JH, Goeken MD. An immunopathologic study of giant papillary conjunctivitis associated with an ocular prosthesis. *Am J Ophthalmol.* 1981;92:368–371.
6. Robin JB, Regis-Pacheco LF, May WN, et al. Giant papillary conjunctivitis associated with extruded scleral buckle. *Arch Ophthalmol.* 1987;105:619.
7. MacIvor J. Contact allergy to plastic artificial eyes: preliminary report. *Can Med Assoc J.* 1950;62:164.
8. Korb DR, Allansmith MR, Greiner JV, et al. Prevalence of conjunctival changes in wearers of hard contact lenses. *Am J Ophthalmol.* 1980;90:336.
9. Allansmith MR, Ross RN, Greiner JV. Giant papillary conjunctivitis: diagnosis and treatment. In: *Contact lenses, update 5.* Boston, MA: Little, Brown; 1989:1 [Chapter 43].
10. Meisler DM, Zaret CR, Stock EL. Trantas dots and limbal inflammation associated with soft contact lens wear. *Am J Ophthalmol.* 1980;89:66.
11. Martin NF, Rubinfeld RS, Malley JD, et al. Giant papillary conjunctivitis and meibomian gland dysfunction blepharitis. *CLAO J.* 1992;18: 165–169.
12. Mathers WD, Billborough M. Meibomian gland function and giant papillary conjunctivitis. *Am J Ophthalmol.* 1992;114:188–192.
13. Greiner JV, Gladstone L, Covington HI, et al. Branching of microvilli in the human conjunctival epithelium. *Arch Ophthalmol.* 1980;98:1253.
14. Greiner JV, Covington HI, Allansmith MR. Surface morphology of giant papillary conjunctivitis in contact lens wearers. *Am J Ophthalmol.* 1978;85:242.
15. Greiner JV, Weidman TA, Korb DR, et al. Histochemical analysis of secretory vesicles in non-goblet conjunctival epithelial cells. *Acta Ophthalmol (Copenh).* 1985;63:89.
16. Greiner JV, Henriquez AS, Weidman TA, et al. 'Second' mucus secretory system of the human conjunctiva. *Invest Ophthalmol Vis Sci.* 1979;18 (Suppl):123.
17. Allansmith M, Greiner JV, Baird RS. Number of inflammatory cells in the normal conjunctiva. *Am J Ophthalmol.* 1978;86:250.
18. Irani A, Butrus SL, Tabbara K, et al. Mast cell subtypes in vernal and giant papillary conjunctivitis. *J Allergy Clin Immunol.* 1990;86:34–39.
19. Butrus SL, Ochsner K, Abelson M, et al. The level of tryptase in human tears. *Ophthalmology.* 1990;97:1678.
20. Fukagawa K, Saito H, Asuma N, et al. Histamine and tryptase levels in allergic conjunctivitis and vernal keratoconjunctivitis. *Cornea.* 1994; 13:345–348.
21. Trocme SD, Kephart GM, Bourne WM, et al. Eosinophil granule major basic protein in contact lenses of patients with giant papillary conjunctivitis. *CLAO J.* 1990;16:219–222.
22. Udell IJ, Gleich GJ, Allansmith MR, et al. Eosinophil granule major basic protein and Charcot-Leyden crystal protein in human tears. *Am J Ophthalmol.* 1981;92:824.
23. Donshik PC, Ballow M. Tear immunoglobulins in giant papillary conjunctivitis induced by contact lenses. *Am J Ophthalmol.* 1983; 96:460–466.
24. Barishak Y, Zavoro A, Samra Z, et al. An immunological study of papillary conjunctivitis due to contact lenses. *Curr Eye Res.* 1989;3:1161–1167.
25. Ballow M, Donshik PC. Immune responses in monkeys to lenses from patients with contact lens induced giant papillary conjunctivitis. *CLAO J.* 1989;15:64–70.
26. Normand RR, Anderson JA, Tasevska ZG, et al. Evaluation of tear protein deposits on contact lenses from patients with and without giant papillary conjunctivitis. *CLAO J.* 1992;18:143–147.
27. Fowler SA, Greiner JV, Allansmith MR. Attachment of bacteria to soft contact lenses. *Arch Ophthalmol.* 1979;97:659.
28. Allansmith MR, Baird RS, Askenase PW. Conjunctival basophil hypersensitivity: a model of vernal conjunctivitis. *J Allergy Clin Immunol.* 1984;73:148.
29. Kosmos MA, Gabiarrelli EB. Heat implicated in giant papillary conjunctivitis. *Invest Ophthalmol Vis Sci (Suppl).* 1990;31:549.
30. Kosmos MA, Gabiarrelli EB. Daily enzyme cleaning for giant papillary conjunctivitis. *Eur J Ophthalmol.* 1992;2:98.
31. Robin J, Nobe JR, Suarez E, et al. Meibomian gland evaluation in patients with extended wear soft contact lens deposits. *CLAO J.* 1986;12:95.
32. Bucci FA, Lopatiynsky MO, Jenkins PL, et al. Comparison of the clinical performance of the Acuvue disposable contact lens and CSI lens in patients with giant papillary conjunctivitis. *Am J Ophthalmol.* 1993; 115:454–459.
33. Wood TS, Stewart RH, Bowman RW, et al. Suprofen treatment of contact lens-associated giant papillary conjunctivitis. *Ophthalmology.* 1988; 95:822–826.
34. Capteola RJ, Argentieri D, Weintraub HS, et al. Suprofen. In: Goldberg ME, ed. *Pharmacological and biochemical properties of drug substances.* Washington, DC: American Pharmaceutical Association of the Academy of Pharmaceutical Science; 1981.
35. Meisler DM, Bersins UJ, Krachmer JH, et al. Cromolyn treatment of giant papillary conjunctivitis. *Am J Ophthalmol.* 1982;100:1608.
36. Iwasaki W, Kosaka Y, Momose T, et al. Absorption of topical disodium cromoglycate and its preservative by soft contact lenses. *CLAO J.* 1988;14:155–158.
37. Matter M, et al. Sodium cromoglycate in the treatment of contact lens-associated giant papillary conjunctivitis. Proceedings of the seventh Congress of the European Society of Ophthalmology. Finland: Helsinki; 1984.
38. Donshik PC, Ballow M, Lustro A, et al. Treatment of contact lens-induced giant papillary conjunctivitis. *CLAO J.* 1984;10:346.
39. Alcon Laboratories, Fort Worth, Texas: Alomide Ophthalmic Solution 0.1% (lodoxamide tromethamine ophthalmic solution), FDA Drug Application – NDA 20–191.
40. Hingorani M, Calder VL, Buckley RJ, Lightman SL. The role of conjunctival epithelial cells in chronic ocular allergic disease. *Exp Eye Res.* 1998;67:491–500.
41. Irkee MT, ORhan M, Erderner U. Role of tear inflammatory mediators in contact lens-associated giant papillary conjunctivitis in soft contact lens wearers. *Ocul Imm Infl.* 1999;7:35–38.
42. Sengor T, Irkec M, Gulen Y, Taseli M, Erker H. Tear LTC4 levels in patients with subclinical contact lens related giant papillary conjunctivitis. *CLAO J.* 1995;21:159–162.

43. Metz DP, Bacon AS, Holgate S, Lightman SL. Phenotypic characterization of T cells infiltrating the conjunctiva in chronic allergic eye disease. *J Allergy Clin Immunol.* 1996;98:686–696.
44. Calder VL, Jolly G, Hingorani M, et al. Cytokine production and mRNA expression by conjunctival T-cell lines in chronic allergic eye disease. *Clin Exp Allergy.* 1999;29:1155–1157.
45. Donshik PC, Porazinski AD, Giant papillary conjunctivitis in frequent-replacement contact lens wearers: a retrospective study. *Trans Am Ophthalmol Soc.* 1999;97:205–216.
46. Donshik PC, Ehlers WH, Ballow M. Giant papillary conjunctivitis. *Immunol Allergy Clin North Am.* 2008;28:83–103.
47. Shoji J, Inada N, Sawa M. Antibody array generated cytokine profiles of tears of patients with vernal keratoconjunctivitis and giant papillary conjunctivitis. *Jpn J Ophthalmol.* 2006;50:195–204.
48. Ehlers WH, Fishman JB, Donshik PC, et al. Neutrophil chemotactic factor in the tears of giant papillary conjunctivitis patients. *CLAO J.* 1991; 17:65–68.
49. Xingwu Z, Hongshan L, et al. M cells are involved in pathogenesis of human contact lens-associated giant papillary conjunctivitis. *Arch Immunol Ther Exp.* 2007;55:173–177.

Chapter 51

Cicatricial Pemphigoid

C. Stephen Foster

Definition

Mucous membrane pemphigoid (MMP) is a chronic cicatrizing autoimmune disease of the mucous membranes and skin.[1] MMP is a heterogeneous group of disorders with varying clinical manifestations and target autoantigens. Bullous pemphigoid, for example, affects primarily skin and, to a lesser extent oral mucosa, with an antibody-mediated autoimmune attack on glycoproteins in the epithelial basement membrane zone, BP1 (BP230) and BP2 (BP180, also shown to be type XVII collagen). Ocular cicatricial pemphigoid (OCP) affects primarily the conjunctiva (and the mucosae, including oral, nasal, and esophageal, in lesser frequency), with the β4 subunit of α6β4 integrin the target of attack. The average age at onset of OCP is 65 years. However, this figure does not report the true epidemiologic features of this disease, because the reported cases are usually not in their earliest stages.[2] Females are affected two to three times as frequently as males. Conjunctival involvement may occur as early as 10 years before other mucosal or skin lesions develop, or it may occur as much as 20 years following the onset of other lesions; the disease may be limited to the conjunctiva. Scarring (Brusting-Perry) dermatitis occurs in approximately 25% of cases (Fig. 51.1), and cicatrizing conjunctivitis develops in 70–75%.[3,4] Involvement of other mucosa may lead to scarring of the soft palate and oral and nasal mucosa; and esophageal, urethral, vaginal, and anal strictures may develop. Laryngeal involvement may cause pain and hoarseness.[5] The esophageal scarring can be lethal; asphyxiation can occur if a food bolus lodges during attempted swallowing by a patient with dysphagia from esophageal strictures that have been neglected by both the patient and physician.

Lever[6] credits Wichmann[7] with the first description of pemphigoid affecting the conjunctiva. Wichmann[7] and Cooper[8] considered the disease affecting the eyes to be pemphigus, and Thost[9] continued to use the word pemphigus in describing the ocular manifestations of what is now known to be ocular cicatricial pemphigoid (OCP). Walter Lever, a Boston dermatologist, made the clinical and histopathologic distinction between pemphigoid and pemphigus in 1953.[6]

Franke[10] published a report in 1900 summarizing the clinical course of 107 patients with cicatricial pemphigoid affecting the conjunctiva. Since that description, many other authors have published their observations, and all agree that the disease is invariably progressive and that the ultimate prognosis is quite poor. Unfortunately, it seems to take each new generation of ophthalmologists some personal experience to appreciate this fact. Because few ophthalmologists have the opportunity to observe significant numbers of patients with this disease over a sustained period, and because the disease does not progress inexorably and continuously but rather in fits and starts, there are still many ophthalmologists who have the mistaken belief that cicatricial pemphigoid affecting the conjunctiva can be treated with drops (steroid, vitamin A, ciclosporin) or with subconjunctival injections (steroid, mitomycin-C). It may take the disease 10 to 30 years or more to reach end stage, with bilateral blindness as the result. However, if one follows patients with cicatricial pemphigoid on conventional therapy long enough, one will invariably observe the long-term devastating consequences.[11] The progression of the disease, although usually slow, may be punctuated by periods of remission or by periods of explosive exacerbation with rampant progression of conjunctival scarring and associated keratopathy.[12] It is also clear that the more advanced the disease is, the more likely it is to progress significantly within 2 years.[13]

Histologically, the conjunctival lesions show submucosal scarring, chronic inflammation, perivasculitis, and squamous metaplasia of the epithelium, with loss of goblet cells; mast cell participation in the inflammation is surprisingly great.

Tissue-fixed immunoglobulins and complement components are present in the epithelial basement membrane zone (BMZ) in patients with CP. Indeed, this immunoreactant deposition is the sine qua non for definitive establishment of the diagnosis.[14] Circulating antibodies to the basement membrane of conjunctiva are found in all of these patients if ultrasensitive radio immunoassay techniques are employed,[15] and circulating antibodies to conjunctival epithelium have been found.[16] Circulating antinuclear antibodies (ANA) have also been demonstrated in patients with CP.[17]

Epidemiology

Ocular cicatricial pemphigoid is probably not as rare as published incidence figures indicate. Bettelheim et al.[18] estimated 1 in 15 000 ophthalmic patients. Hardy and Lamb[19]

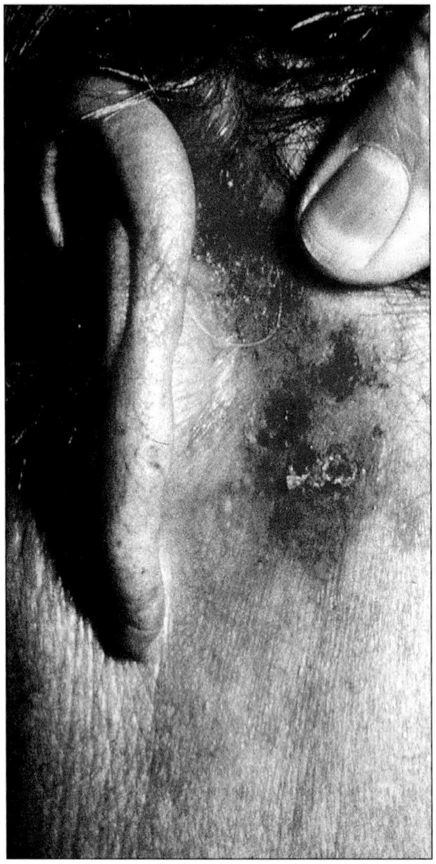

Fig. 51.1 Brusting-Perry dermatitis, typical of the dermatologic manifestations of patients with cicatricial pemphigoid.

and others[20] estimated an incidence of 1 in 20000 patients. Smith and colleagues[21] estimated 1 in 46000. Bedell[22] estimated 1 in 8000, and Lever and Talbott[23] stated frankly that it is impossible to make an accurate estimate from available data; they guessed that the incidence of OCP is somewhere between 1 in 12000 and 1 in 60000 ophthalmic patients. However, these figures estimate the incidence of relatively advanced OCP. Diagnosis of this disorder in its early stages is difficult,[2] and most cases are not recognized as OCP until they reach what could be categorized as stage III disease. There are, therefore, patients with stage I and stage II OCP uncounted in the epidemiologic estimates.

Data on the average age of OCP patients are also somewhat distorted by subtleties of the diagnostic signs. OCP is said in many publications to be a disease of older people, with average age given as 60[24] or 70[25] years. Although reports of OCP in children may, in fact, represent cases of localized erythema multiforme, it certainly is now recognized that OCP can begin at least as early as the third decade of life.

Most reports describe a slight but clear female predilection. Klauder and Cowan[26] reported eight females and three males, Lever[6] reported three females for every male, and Hardy and Lamb[19] reported 52 females and 29 males with OCP; 62 of these patients had ocular involvement, but Hardy and Lamb[19] did not report the sex distribution for this subset of patients. No racial or geographic predilection is reported.[2]

Pathogenesis

Ocular cicatricial pemphigoid is clearly an autoimmune disease, with a genetic predisposition and probably a 'second-hit' environmental requirement to trigger the onset of the disease. An increase in frequency in the HLA-DR4 and HLA-DQw3 alleles was the first reported association in patients with OCP.[27] Subsequently, in patient and family studies employing restriction fragment length polymorphism analysis of the DQ3 haplotypes, we determined that the HLA-DQ7 (HLA-DQβ1*0301) gene is linked to enhanced susceptibility of OCP development.[28] However, DQβ chain sequencing studies from patients with the HLA-DQβ1*0301 gene affected by cicatricial pemphigoid and from their unaffected relatives with the HLA-DQ identical gene HLA-DQβ1*0301 disclosed that the amino acid sequences of the HLA-DQβ chains from patient and unaffected relatives were identical. These identical genes suggest, therefore, that it is not the HLA-DQβ1*0301 gene itself, but rather a different gene, in close linkage disequilibrium with HLA-DQβ1*0301, that is truly the susceptibility gene.[29]

The second-hit environmental trigger that stimulates the genetically susceptible individual to develop OCP may be microbial, as is suspected for idiopathic OCP, or may be chemical, as in the case of so-called drug-induced OCP or pseudo-OCP, which develops in some individuals exposed to practolol[30] or to a limited variety of ocular medications.[31–33] Patients with pseudo-OCP carry the same susceptibility gene (HLA-DQβ1*0301) in addition to another.[34] But the autoantigens in these two forms of OCP are different. We have identified a 205 kilodalton (kDa) protein molecule in the BMZ of conjunctiva and epidermis as the relevant target antigen in idiopathic OCP.[35] This target autoantigen is the β4 peptide of α6β4 integrin.[36] Further, the autoantibodies in the sera of patients with OCP directed against this autoantigen are directed (predominantly) against epitopes within the large cytoplasmic domain of the β4 peptide.[37] Additionally, these autoantibodies produce lesions in conjunctiva in an in vitro organ culture system, indicating their very likely pathogenic role in OCP.[38] Sera from patients with pseudo-OCP bind to 97 and 290 kDa proteins in conjunctiva and epidermis lysates, and to 45, 150, 290, and 400 kDa proteins in dermal lysates.[39] None of these autoantigen protein targets is absorbed from the tissue lysates by sera from patients with bullous pemphigoid, pemphigus vulgaris, or OCP, indicating that the autoantigens in OCP, pseudo-OCP, and bullous pemphigoid are distinct from each other.

The autoantibodies that develop in patients with OCP[15] can be detected in all of these patients when the disease is active. The autoantibodies are probably pathogenic, just as they are in patients with pemphigus.[40,41] The binding of the autoantibody to the autoantigen at the epithelial basement membrane then sets in motion a complex series of events.[2] CD4 (helper) T lymphocytes far outnumber CD8 (suppressor) T cells in the inflammatory cell population, which develops in the substantia propria of the conjunctiva. Plasma cells, histiocytes, and mast cells are present in very large numbers, and a panoply of cytokines are elaborated from these cells, including macrophage migration inhibitory factor, interferon-γ and TGF-β, the effects of which are only now being dissected by molecular biologic techniques.[42,43]

The result of this complex activity is corneal epithelial damage from inflammatory cytokines and from the xerosis, meibomian gland dysfunction, and trichiatic trauma developing as a consequence of cytokine-induced conjunctival fibroblast proliferation and activation, with resultant subepithelial fibrosis.

Diagnosis

The diagnosis of OCP is extremely important, given the natural history of the disease, the effective but potentially toxic therapy, and the potential confusion in differentiation from other causes of chronic cicatrizing conjunctivitis (Box 51.1). The clinical diagnosis requires immunohistochemical confirmation before the institution of therapy.[2] The diagnosis is confirmed by the demonstration of one or more immunoreactants at the epithelial BMZ (Fig. 51.2). Additional confirmation can be sought from immunoblot analysis of patient serum, an identifying autoantibody that binds to the 205-kDa protein band from conjunctival or epidermal lysates: anti-β4 antibody.

Box 51.1 Causes of chronic cicatrizing conjunctivitis

Cicatricial pemphigoid	Progressive systemic sclerosis
Stevens–Johnson syndrome	Sarcoidosis
Lyell's syndrome	Trachoma
Rosacea	Epidemic keratoconjunctivitis
Atopic keratoconjunctivitis	Diphtheria conjunctivitis
Sjögren's syndrome	'Pseudopemphigoid'

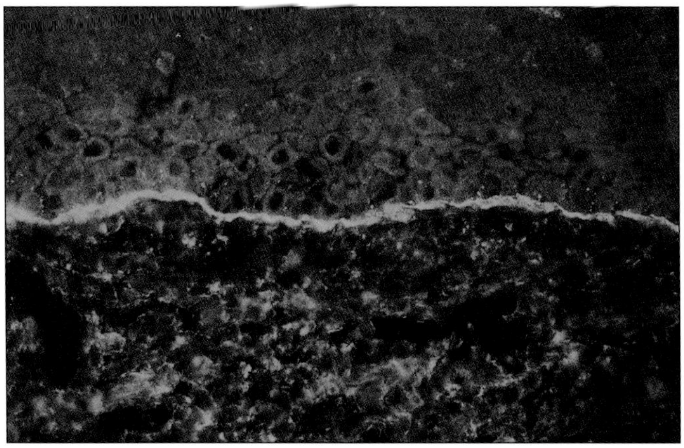

Fig. 51.2 Immunofluorescence microscopy, 40×, conjunctival biopsy from the inflamed bulbar conjunctiva of a patient suspected of having cicatricial pemphigoid. The cryopreserved tissue has been sectioned at 4 μm and incubated with a rabbit antibody directed against human IgG, fluorescein-labeled. Note the bright apple-green linear pattern of fluorescence at the conjunctival epithelial basement membrane zone, indicating the deposition of IgG at the basement membrane, providing immunohistopathologic confirmation of the suspected clinical diagnosis.

And as important as the definitive establishment of the diagnosis is, given the type of therapy required to prevent OCP from progressing to blindness, the sad fact is that few laboratories (even dermatopathology labs) are sufficiently equipped and experienced to process small pieces of conjunctiva, snap freezing and cryostat sectioning and performing not only immunofluorescent probing studies but also the much more tedious yet more sensitive immunoperoxidase avidin–biotin complex studies which are often positive even when the immunofluorescent studies are negative.[44] Yet the definitive diagnosis is quite critical, since many other diseases can cause chronic cicatrizing conjunctivitis.[45]

Ocular Manifestations

The ocular disease in OCP typically presents as a chronic, recurrent unilateral conjunctivitis. Subepithelial fibrosis is characteristic of stage I of OCP (Fig. 51.3), with stage II showing fornix foreshortening (Fig. 51.4). Symblepharon formation is the hallmark of stage III (Fig. 51.5). Stage IV,

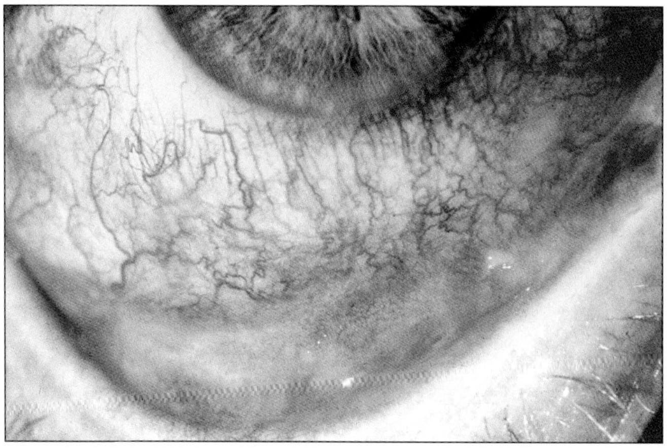

Fig. 51.3 Stage I pemphigoid with subepithelial fibrosis. Note the subepithelial fibrotic stria, some of which have coalesced into a net or 'feltwork.'

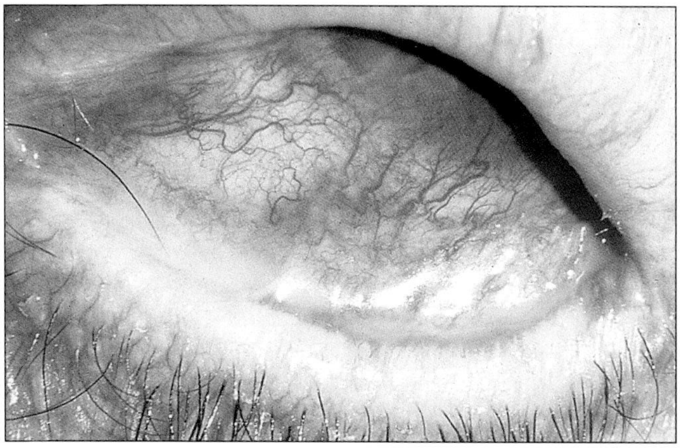

Fig. 51.4 Stage II pemphigoid. Note that the subepithelial fibrosis process has progressed and contracted, producing foreshortening of the inferior fornix.

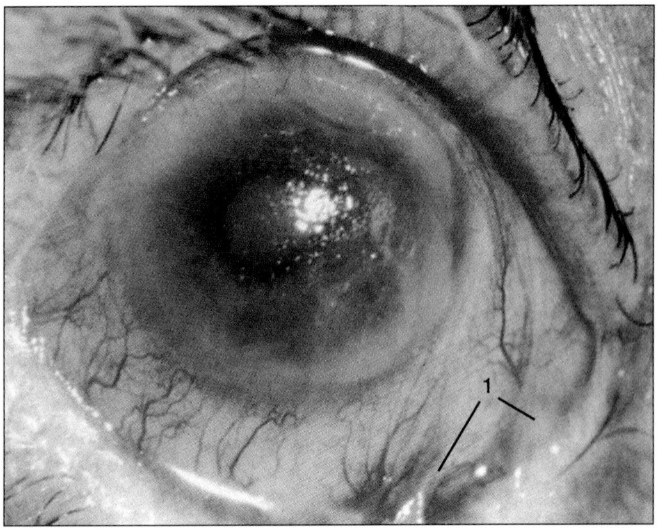

Fig. 51.5 Stage III pemphigoid. Note that the fornix has foreshortened further in this patient, and that, additionally, two symblephara (*1*) have appeared.

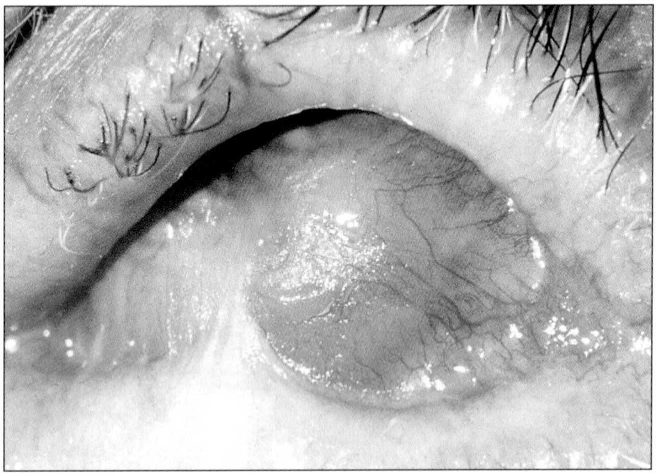

Fig. 51.6 Stage IV pemphigoid. Note the total obliteration of the inferior fornix, the ankyloblepharon formation, and the total 'leatherization,' or keratinization, of the ocular surface.

end-stage disease, is characterized by ankyloblepharon and surface keratinization (Fig. 51.6). Obstruction of the lacrimal ductules and meibomian gland ducts eventually produces an unstable tear film and progressive sicca syndrome, but it is to be emphasized that OCP is not a dry eye syndrome until relatively late in the course of the disease.[2] Trichiasis and entropion occur because of the subepithelial fibrosis, with eventual keratopathy, corneal neovascularization, and corneal ulceration and scarring.[2] Twenty-one of 81 patients with cicatricial pemphigoid were blind at the time of the report of a series from the Mayo Clinic; 17 were blind in both eyes.[20] Sixty-two of the 81 patients had ocular involvement. Approximately 88% of the 62 patients had the ocular disease bilaterally.[20] It must be emphasized again that 'ocular' cicatricial pemphigoid is truly a systemic autoimmune disease, is eventually invariably progressive, and is blinding when only local ocular treatment is employed. High-dose systemic prednisone therapy can be effective, but every series reported to date discloses the unacceptably high, life-threatening complication rate from this therapeutic strategy.[20]

Therapy

Medical treatment of the ocular complications of cicatricial pemphigoid was once difficult, protracted, and not very effective. Herron reported on the management of a case with ocular, skin, and mucosal involvement of the pharynx and larynx. Oral triamcinolone was used, along with injections of the drug into the areas of symblepharon. The skin and mucosal lesions responded in 10 weeks, but the ocular disease did not.[46]

Dave and Vickers[47] successfully treated four patients with progressive cicatricial pemphigoid with azathioprine after systemic prednisone therapy resulted in the development of diabetes mellitus in two patients and failed to control the disease in the other two. Brody and Perozzi[48] reported on an additional patient who failed to achieve control of inflammation while on azathioprine therapy, but whose disease came under perfect control with cyclophosphamide therapy; eye, mouth, and esophageal lesions all vanished. Person and Rogers[49] extended dapsone therapy to 24 patients with cicatricial pemphigoid, 17 of whom had ocular involvement. Twelve of these 17 patients responded well, in that active conjunctival inflammation was substantially reduced.

In 1982, Foster and associates reported the results of an uncontrolled study on the efficacy of cyclophosphamide therapy for cicatricial pemphigoid affecting the conjunctiva.[50] I reported the results of two randomized, masked, controlled trials for this disease, one comparing the efficacy of cyclophosphamide with prednisone versus prednisone alone in the treatment of progressive cicatricial pemphigoid affecting the conjunctiva, and the other comparing the efficacies of cyclophosphamide with dapsone in 1986.[2] Additional immunomodulatory modalities employed by us over the succeeding 15 years in our care of patients with OPC include azathioprine, methotrexate, mycophenolate mofetil, cytosine arabinoside, intravenous immunoglobulin, rituximab monoclonal antibody B cell depletion, and humanized antibody directed against CD25 glycoprotein on the surface of activated CD4 helper T cells.[51] Based on the results of these studies, and additional experience, I now make the therapeutic recommendations expressed below.

Current Status of Medical Therapy Program for Ocular Cicatricial Pemphigoid

Our current approach to medical treatment of patients with active OCP may be summarized as follows:

1. Sicca syndrome is treated aggressively. We favor ointment lubricants without preservatives, applied at a frequency sufficient to maintain adequate surface lubrication and protection (e.g. every 2 to 4 hours and at bedtime). Artificial tears without preservatives are employed as needed between ointment applications. Punctal occlusion is performed if Schirmer values are below 5 mm/5 min. Topical retinoid (0.01% tretinoin) ointment is used once or twice

daily in one eye; we compare objective and subjective responses to retinol ointment, and continue treatment beyond 4 weeks of therapy only if we and/or the patient conclude that there is a distinct therapeutic benefit from this agent. Fewer than 30% of our OCP patients have shown an apparent benefit from topical retinoids. The author strongly cautions against inappropriate enthusiasm for the efficacy of this component of the therapeutic plan. The author has observed the unfortunate results of such inappropriate preoccupation with topical therapy for this systemic disease in three patients who are now functionally blind because the disease progressed while they were on topical retinoids without concomitant appropriate systemic therapy.

2. Chronic blepharitis and meibomitis are treated with vigorous warm compresses and lid hygiene (with massage to keep oil flowing through the ductules) and oral doxycycline, 100 mg once or twice daily. Microbial colonization of the lids and meibomian glands by any organism, including *Staphylococcus*, is treated with appropriate topical and/or systemic antimicrobial agents.
3. Immunomodulatory therapy for cases that are extremely active and rapidly progressive is begun with prednisone 1 mg/kg/day, and cyclophosphamide 2 mg/kg/day. The cyclophosphamide dose is adjusted according to therapeutic response, bone marrow response, and drug tolerance. My current preference is intravenous cyclophosphamide therapy for 6 months, with subsequent conversion to orally administered immunomodulatory therapy with less potential toxicity than that of cyclophosphamide. Prednisone is gradually tapered, with a switch to alternate-day dosing by 8 to 12 weeks, and subsequent taper and discontinuation by 4 to 6 months. The goal is the elimination of all conjunctival inflammation (Fig. 51.7). Patients are presently maintained on immunomodulatory therapy for a minimum of 2 years. It is to be emphasized that the direct management of patients treated with immunosuppressive agents must be by an individual who is, by virtue of training and experience, expert in chemotherapy, recognition of early, subtle drug-induced side effects, and treatment of same. The authors find that a 'hand-in-glove' relationship between the ophthalmologist and an oncologist works best, with the ophthalmologist appraising the oncologist of the ocular status and the oncologist determining drug dose changes. It is also important for the ophthalmologist to remember that external confounding variables can aggravate conjunctiva, producing vascular dilation and a 'red eye' in the absence of immunologically active pemphigoid. Increasing chemotherapy in such a setting is clearly inappropriate. One can judge the presence or absence of true inflammation only after the elimination of such confounding variables as trichiasis, distichiasis, meibomian gland dysfunction, ocular surface drying, entropion, exposure, and tarsal conjunctival keratinization.

Methotrexate (15–25 mg once weekly) and mycophenolate mofetil (1–3 g/day) are used for cases that are less active and are not rapidly progressing. Dapsone and prednisone can also be used for such cases; the initial daily dose of dapsone employed is 1 mg/kg/day; the maximum dose ever employed is 200 mg/day. The author emphasizes that dapsone is not a benign drug. The patients on dapsone are followed as often and as carefully as those who are on cyclophosphamide. Patients who are not glucose-6-phosphate dehydrogenase deficient, as determined by the screening test, may still hemolyze when treated with dapsone. Therefore, the hemoglobin, hematocrit, reticulocyte count, and net hemoglobin, in addition to the white blood count and liver enzymes, are important monitoring parameters for these patients. A low degree of hemolysis is acceptable if dapsone is achieving the desired therapeutic response, but reticulocytosis must adequately compensate for such hemolysis; a steadily falling hematocrit level is unacceptable.

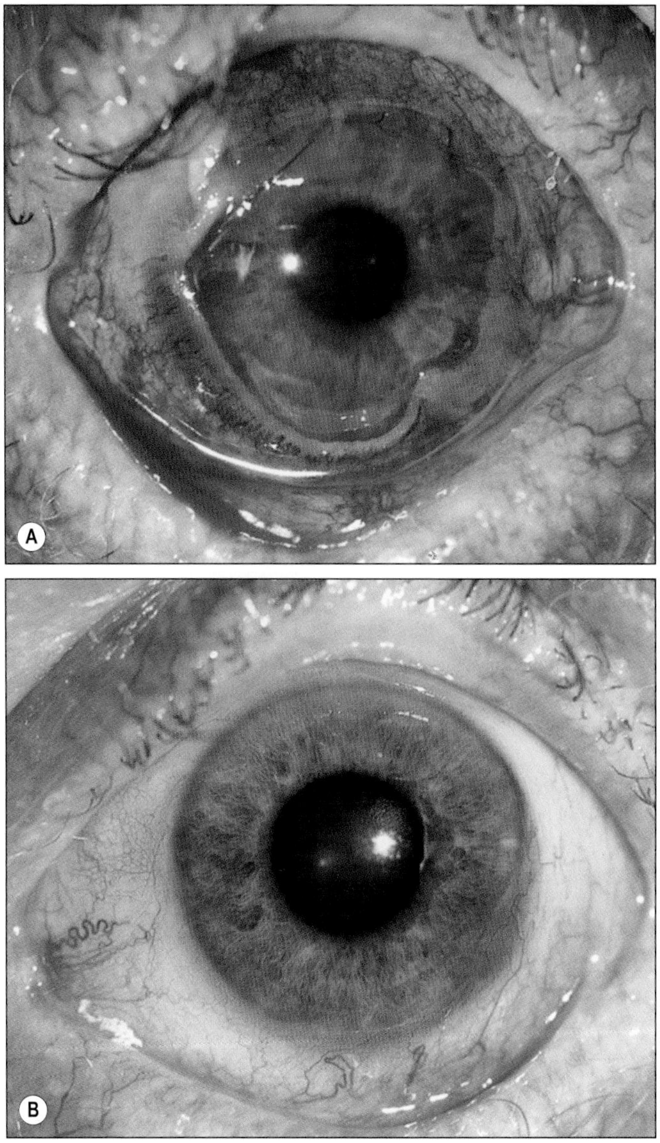

Fig. 51.7 Cicatricial pemphigoid. (**A**) Active cicatricial pemphigoid before institution of therapy. (**B**) Same eye, same patient, 10 weeks after the institution of systemic therapy with cyclophosphamide. Note the complete abolition of all active conjunctival inflammation.

Approximately 70% of patients will respond well to dapsone. A large proportion of these (41% in our

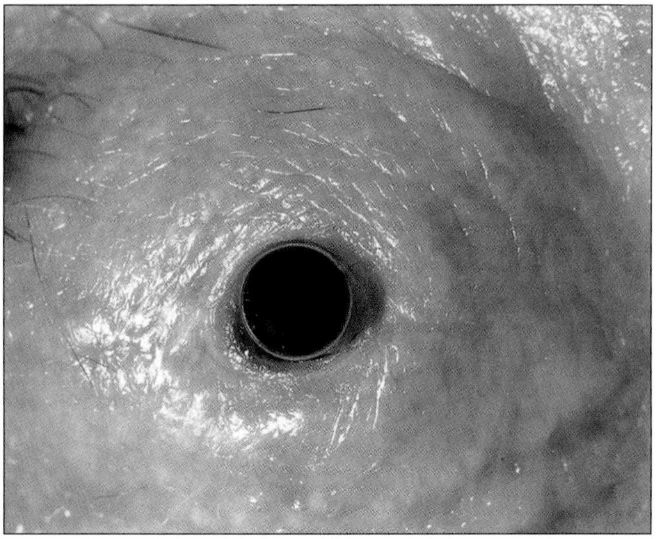

Fig. 51.8 Keratoprosthesis in a patient whose pemphigoid had progressed to stage IV before referral for chemotherapy. Chemotherapy is inappropriate for patients with stage IV disease, as is any form of corneal surgery. The only technique available for successful visual rehabilitation in selected individuals with this end-stage disease is keratoprosthesis as shown here.

experience), will relapse within 6 months of cessation of dapsone therapy.[51] It is for these reasons that, for me, methotrexate or mycophenolate mofetil have supplanted dapsone in my care of patients with ocular cicatricial pemphigoid.[52] These patients are treated with dapsone, methotrexate, azathioprine, or mycophenolate mofetil. Azathioprine, 2 mg/kg/day initial dose, methotrexate (7.5 mg once/week) or mycophenolate mofetil (1 g bid) are also second-choice agents for the 30% of patients who do not respond adequately to dapsone. Adjustment of dose is accomplished, as in the case of other agents, through the judgment of the skilled chemotherapist, who, by virtue of training and experience, is the expert in the use of these agents.

Note should also be made of the exceptional safety and efficacy of intravenous immunoglobulin (IVIG) alone and especially in combination with rituximab therapy in the care of patients with OCP and other ocular inflammatory disorders.[53–55] This approach would probably become the preferred therapy for all cases were it not for the expense and administration inconvenience of it.

Some authors have advocated surgical treatment in the early or 'moist' phase of the disease: tarsectomy for correction of entropion, strip peritomy to provide an avascular barrier against corneal neovascularization, superficial keratectomy for removal of corneal vascular and scar tissue, and fornix incision for release of symblepharon. These approaches will not only fail but, in fact, will make the disease worse if the patient is not adequately immunosuppressed before surgery. Mucous membrane grafting may be of benefit in cases of cicatricial entropion and lid marginal keratinization associated with this disease.[56] Contact lenses and shells with concurrent use of lubricants may aid in the management of the chronic, dry phase of the disease with corneal involvement. Keratoprosthesis (Fig. 51.8) is the measure of last resort in patients with bilateral end-stage disease.

References

1. Chan L, Ahmed AR, Anhalt G, et al. The first international consensus on mucous membrane pemphigoid: definition, diagnostic criteria, pathogenic factors, medical treatment, and diagnostic indicators. *Arch Dermatol.* 2002;138:370–379.
2. Foster CS. Cicatricial pemphigoid. *Trans Am Ophthalmol Soc.* 1986;84:527.
3. Person JR, Rogers RS. Bullous and cicatricial pemphigoid: clinical histopathological and immunopathological correlations. *Mayo Clin Proc.* 1977;52:54.
4. Hardy KM, et al. Benign mucous membrane pemphigoid. *Arch Dermatol.* 1971;1–4:467.
5. Hanson RD, Olsen KD, Rogers RS. Upper aerodigestive tract manifestations of cicatricial pemphigoid. *Ann Otol Rhinol Laryngol.* 1988;97:493.
6. Lever WF. Pemphigus. *Medicine.* 1953;32:1.
7. Wichmann JE. *Ideen zur diagnostic.* Vol 1. Hannover: Helwing; 1793:89.
8. Cooper W. Pemphigus of the conjunctivae. *Ophthalmol Hosp Rep Lond Hosp Res.* 1857;1:155.
9. Thost A. Falle von Schleimhautpemphigus. *Deutsche Med Wochenschr.* 1919;45:477.
10. Franke E. *Pemphigus und de essential le Schrumpfung der Bindehart per des Auges.* Wiesdbaden JF: Bergmann; 1900.
11. Duke-Elder S, Leigh AG. Diseases of the outer eye. *Syst Ophthalmol.* 1965:8L502.
12. Mondino BJ, et al. The acute manifestations of ocular cicatricial pemphigoid: diagnosis and treatment. *Ophthalmology.* 1979;86:543.
13. Mondino BJ, Brown SI. Ocular cicatricial pemphigoid. *Ophthalmology.* 1981;95:88.
14. Find JD. Epidermolysis bullosa: variability of expression of cicatricial pemphigoid, bullous pemphigoid and epidermolysis acquisita antigens in clinically uninvolved skin. *J Invest Dermatol.* 1985;85:47.
15. Ahmed AR, et al. Preliminary serological studies comparing immunofluorescence assay with radioimmunoassay. *Curr Eye Res.* 1989;8:1011.
16. Mondino BJ, Brown SI, Rabin BS. Autoimmune phenomena of the external eye. *Ophthalmology.* 1978;85:801.
17. Waltman SR, Yarian D. Circulating antibodies in ocular pemphigoid. *Am J Ophthalmol.* 1974;77:891.
18. Bettelheim H, Kraft D, Zehetbauer G. [On the so-called ocular pemphigus (pemphigus ocularis, pemphigus conjunctivae)]. *Klin Monbl Augenheilkd.* 1972;160:65–75.
19. Hardy WF, Lamb HD. Essential shrinking of the conjunctiva with reports of two cases. *Am J Ophthalmol.* 1917;34:289.
20. Hardy KM, et al. Benign mucous membrane pemphigoid. *Arch Dermatol.* 1971;104:467.
21. Smith RC, Myers EA, Lamb HD. Ocular and oral pemphigus: report of case with anatomic findings in eyeball. *Arch Ophthalmol.* 1934;11:635.
22. Bedell AJ. Ocular pemphigus: a clinical presentation. *Trans Am Ophthalmol Soc.* 1964;62:109.
23. Lever WF, Talbott JH. Pemphigus: a historical study. *Arch Dermatol Syph.* 1942;46:800.
24. Chalkely TH. Chronic cicatricial conjunctivitis. *Am J Ophthalmol.* 1964;67:526.
25. Claussen WT. Zur klinik des pemphigus conjunctivae. *Ber Zusammenkunft Dtsch Ophthalmol Des.* 1922;43:251.
26. Klauder JV, Cowan A. Ocular pemphigus and its relation to pemphigus of the skin and mucous membranes. *Am J Ophthalmol.* 1942;25:643.
27. Zaltas MM, Ahmed AR, Foster CS. Association of HLA-DR4 with ocular cicatricial pemphigoid. *Curr Eye Res.* 1989;8:184.
28. Ahmed AR, et al. Association of DQW7 (DQβ1*0301) with ocular cicatricial pemphigoid. *Proc Nat Acad Sci USA.* 1992;88:11579.
29. Haider N, et al. Report on the sequence of DQβ1*0301 gene in ocular cicatricial pemphigoid patients. *Curr Eye Res.* 1992;11:1233.
30. Rahi AH, et al. Pathology of practolol-induced ocular toxicity. *Br J Ophthalmol.* 1976;60:312.
31. Patten JT, Cavanagh HD, Allansmith MR. Induced ocular pseudopemphigoid. *Am J Ophthalmol.* 1976;82:272.
32. Hirst LW, Werblin T, Novak M. Drug induced cicatrizing conjunctivitis simulating ocular pemphigoid. *Cornea.* 1982;1:121.
33. Norn MS. Pemphigoid related to epinephrine treatment. *Am J Ophthalmol.* 1977;83:138.
34. Yunis JJ, et al. Common major histocompatibility complex class II markers in clinical variants of cicatricial pemphigoid. *Proc Natl Acad Sci USA.* 1994;91:7747.
35. Mohimen A, et al. Detection and partial characterization of ocular cicatricial pemphigoid antigens on COLO and SCaBER tumor cell lines. *Curr Eye Res.* 1993;12:741.

36. Tyagi S, Bhol K, Natarajan K, et al. Ocular cicatricial pemphigoid antigen: partial sequence and characterization. *Proc Nat Acad Sci USA.* 1996;93:14714–14719.
37. Bhol KC, Dans MJ, Simmons RK, et al. The autoantibodies to α6β4 integrin of patients affected by ocular cicatricial pemphigoid recognize predominantly epitopes within the large cytoplasmic domain of human β4. *J Immunol.* 2000;165:2824–2829.
38. Chan R, Bhol K, Tesavibul N, et al. The role of antibody to human β4 integrin in conjunctival basement membrane separation: possible in vitro model for ocular cicatricial pemphigoid. *Invest Ophthalmol Vis Sci.* 1999;40:2283–2290.
39. Bhol K, Mohimen A, Neumann R, et al. Differences in the anti-basement membrane zone antibodies in ocular and pseudo-ocular cicatricial pemphigoid. *Curr Eye Res.* 1996;15:521.
40. Anhalt GJ, et al. Induction of pemphigus in neonatal mice by passive transfer of IgG from patients with the disease. *N Engl J Med.* 1982;306: 1189.
41. Rashid KA, Gurcan HM, Ahmed AR. Antigen specificity in subsets of mucous membrane pemphigoid. *J Invest Dermatol.* 2006;126:2631–2636.
42. Razzaque MS, Chu DS, Kumari S, et al. Role of macrophage colony stimulating factor in local proliferation of macrophages in ocular cicatricial pemphigoid. *Invest Ophthalmol Vis Sci.* 2004;45:1174–1181.
43. Razzaque MS, Foster CS, Ahmed AR. Role of macrophage migration inhibitory factor in conjunctival pathology in ocular cicatricial pemphigoid. *Invest Ophthalmol Vis Sci.* 2004;45:1174–1181.
44. Eschle-Menicone ME, Ahmed SR, Foster CS. Mucous membrane pemphigoid: an update. *Curr Opin Ophthalmol.* 2005;16:303–307.
45. Letko E, Bhol K, Anzaar F, et al. Chronic cicatrizing conjunctivitis in a patient with epidermolysis bullosa acquisita. *Arch Ophthalmol.* 2006; 124:1615–1618.
46. Herron BE. Immunologic aspects of cicatricial pemphigoid. *Am J Ophthalmol.* 1975;79:271.
47. Dave VK, Vickers CFH. Azathioprine in the treatment of mucocutaneous pemphigoid. *Br J Dermatol.* 1974;90:183.
48. Brody HJ, Pirozzi DJ. Benign mucous membrane pemphigoid: response to therapy with cyclophosphamide. *Arch Dermatol.* 1977;113: 1598.
49. Person JR, Rogers RS III. Bullous pemphigoid responding to sulfapyridine and the sulfones. *Arch Dermatol.* 1977;13:610.
50. Foster CS, Wilson LA, Ekins MB. Immunosuppressive therapy for progressive ocular cicatricial pemphigoid. *Ophthalmology.* 1982;89:340.
51. Foster CS, Ahmed AR. Intravenous immunoglobulin therapy for ocular cicatricial pemphigoid: a preliminary study. *Ophthalmology.* 1999;106: 2136–2143.
52. Thorne JE, Jabs DA, Qazi FA, et al. Mycophenolate mofetil therapy for inflammatory eye disease. *Ophthalmology.* 2005;112:1472–1477.
53. Letko E, Miserocchi E, Daoud YJ, et al. A nonrandomized comparison of the clinical outcome of ocular involvement in patients with mucous membrane (cicatricial) pemphigoid between conventional immunosuppressive and intravenous immunoglobulin therapies. *Clin Immunol.* 2004;111:303–310.
54. Sami N, Letko E, Androudi S, et al. Intravenous immunoglobulin therapy in patients with ocular cicatricial pemphigoid: a long-term follow-up. *Ophthalmology.* 2004;111:1380–1382.
55. Iaccheri B, Roque M, Fiori T, et al. Ocular cicatricial pemphigoid, keratomycosis, and intravenous immunoglobulin therapy. *Cornea.* 2004;23: 819–822.
56. Shore JW, Faster CS, Westfall CT, Rubin PA. Results of buccal mucosal grafting for patients with medically controlled ocular cicatricial pemphigoid. *Ophthalmology.* 1992;99:383.

Chapter 52

Erythema Multiforme, Stevens-Johnson Syndrome, and Toxic Epidermal Necrolysis

Florentino E. Palmon, Harilaos S. Brilakis, Guy F. Webster, Edward J. Holland

Erythema multiforme (EM), Stevens-Johnson syndrome (SJS), and toxic epidermal necrolysis (TEN) have traditionally been regarded as across-the-spectrum manifestations of the same clinical entity, affecting the skin and mucous membranes. Confusion, however, has ruled in the nomenclature, especially until the international classification was adopted in 1993. All three conditions are thought to be precipitated by certain drugs or, particularly for EM, by infection, often viral, though no precipitating factor can be identified in several cases. Erythema multiforme has in the past been classified as having a minor and major form. Erythema multiforme minor primarily involves the skin and often no or, at most, one mucosal surface. It usually does not involve the eye. Erythema multiforme major has been used interchangeably with Stevens-Johnson syndrome. It is characterized by both skin lesions and involvement of two or more mucosal surfaces; systemic symptoms are much more common. A distinction has been made between EM major (or bullous EM) and SJS, both in their clinical picture and in their etiology.[1] Toxic epidermal necrolysis is the most severe, potentially life-threatening disease of the three and the most difficult to manage. Patients with toxic epidermal necrolysis have involvement of over 30% of their epidermis, and skin can be sloughed from the body in sheets.[2,3] The ocular sequelae of SJS, and particularly TEN, can be severe, involving pathologic changes of the bulbar and palpebral conjunctiva, eyelids, and cornea. This chapter will describe the clinical findings and management options available to the clinician.

History

Ferdinand von Hebra, in 1866, first described erythema multiforme. He coined the term erythema exudativum multiforme to describe a cutaneous disease with erythematous lesions of the skin.[4] His findings included a severe stomatitis and a purulent conjunctivitis associated with erythema multiforme. Von Hebra was very accurate in specifying the disease's clinical course, distribution, and evolution of skin findings as well as systemic symptoms. Fuchs later (in 1876) described a generalized cutaneous eruption of the herpes virus type in association with pseudomembranous conjunctivitis.[5] Fiessinger and Rendu, in 1917, noted that the classic dermatologic presentation could accompany severe mucosal involvement.[6] Two American physicians, Stevens and Johnson, reported two classic cases in children and named the disease eruptive fever with stomatitis and ophthalmia in 1922.[7] That nomenclature was not adopted, but since that time erythema multiforme major has most commonly been referred to as Stevens-Johnson syndrome. Thomas, in 1950, coined the terms erythema multiforme minor and major: EM minor referred to the disease described by von Hebra as erythema multiforme, while EM major was applied to patients with oral mucosal involvement, similar to what Stevens and Johnson described. Lyell, in 1956, introduced the term toxic epidermal necrolysis to describe four patients with large amounts of skin loss in conjunction with mucous membrane involvement.[8] A shift has been made recently by international collaborators to differentiate between EM and SJS; they are felt to share mucosal but have different patterns of cutaneous lesions.[9]

- Herpes simplex virus (HSV)-induced EM major is characterized by mucosal erosions, typical target lesions or atypical raised targets, and detachment of the epidermis involving less than 10% of the body surface area, usually on the face and the extremities.
- Drug-induced SJS is characterized also by mucosal erosions and atypical flat target lesions or macular purpuric lesions and epidermal detachment, again involving less than 10% of the body surface; the face, extremities, and the trunk may be involved.

Incidence and Prevalence

Erythema multiforme minor, Stevens-Johnson syndrome, and toxic epidermal necrolysis are not common disease entities. Chan et al., in an American study, reported an incidence of erythema multiforme, Stevens-Johnson syndrome, or toxic epidermal necrolysis resulting from all causes at 4.2 per million person-years.[10] They also described the incidence of toxic epidermal necrolysis as 0.5 per million person-years. Schöph et al. found an overall risk of 0.93 per million person-years for toxic epidermal necrolysis and 1.1 per million person-years for Stevens-Johnson syndrome.[11] Roujeau et al.

described an incidence of 1.2 to 1.3 cases per million per year.[12] An incidence of 0.6 cases per million per year was described in an Italian population.[13] Bottinger et al. reported an incidence of 5 to 10 cases per million persons per year in a Swedish population for erythema multiforme and toxic epidermal necrolysis.[14] Combined SJS, TEN, and SHS/TEN overlap have an incidence estimated at 1.89 per million per year.[15,16] Erythema multiforme may be more common in patients with acquired immunodeficiency syndrome (AIDS).[17,18] Rzany et al. calculated in a German population an incidence of 0.95 to 1.0 per 1000 AIDS cases.[19] Males have a higher incidence of erythema multiforme by a ratio of 3:1. Peak incidence is in the second and third decades of life.[20] Conversely, toxic epidermal necrolysis is slightly more common in women, with a ratio ranging from 1.5:1 to 2.0:1.[11–13] The elderly have an increased incidence of toxic epidermal necrolysis and also have a higher rate of morbidity and mortality.[11,21]

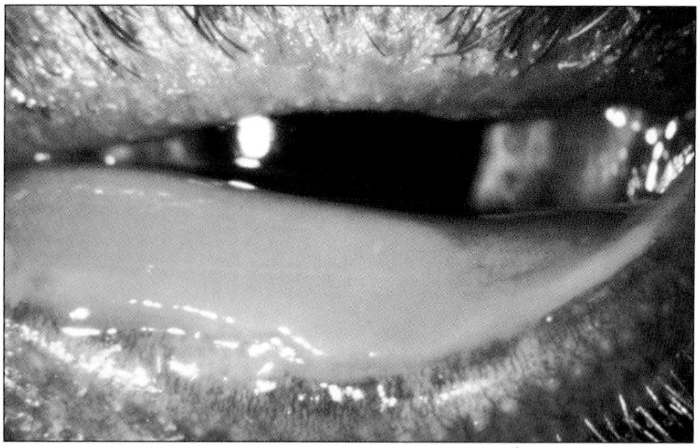

Fig. 52.1 Erythema multiforme with acute pseudomembranous conjunctivitis.

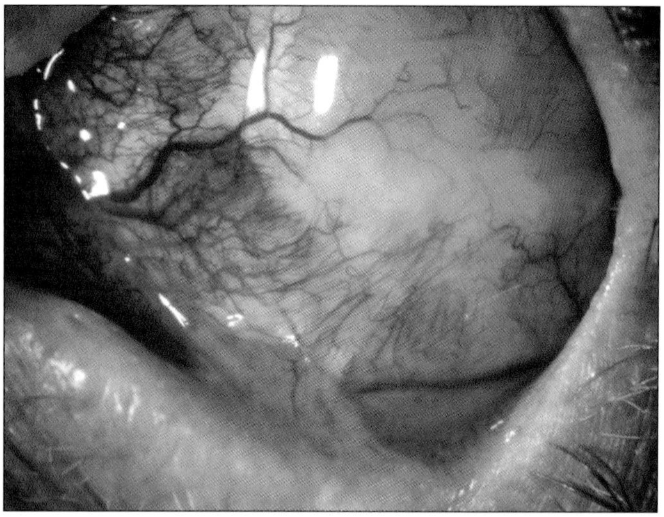

Fig. 52.2 Chronic corneal scarring, neovascularization, and symblepharon formation after toxic epidermal necrolysis.

Clinical Findings

Initial presentation

Drugs and infections are the most frequent identifiable precipitating factors in the erythema multiforme disease spectrum. A systemic prodrome of malaise, fever, and headache or symptoms of an upper respiratory tract infection may precede the ocular and dermatologic manifestations and can begin 1 to 3 weeks after initial exposure and within hours after reexposure to an inciting agent. The prodrome may be more severe in Stevens-Johnson syndrome and in toxic epidermal necrolysis and can include high fever, muscular pain, nausea, vomiting, diarrhea, migratory arthralgias, and pharyngitis.[20,22] Within days, the typical dermatologic and mucosal lesions begin to break out. In Stevens-Johnson syndrome, mucosal involvement begins at the same time as, or succeeding, the skin manifestations. The disorder is usually self-limited, with a typical total duration of 4 to 6 weeks.

Eye findings

The ocular findings in erythema multiforme are best divided into two categories: acute and chronic.

Acute eye findings

Initially, in Stevens-Johnson syndrome and toxic epidermal necrolysis, a nonspecific conjunctivitis usually occurs at the same time as lesions on the skin and other mucous membranes. The conjunctivitis may, however, precede the skin eruption.[23–25] The bilateral conjunctivitis may be catarrhal or pseudomembranous and occurs in 15–75% of patients with Stevens-Johnson syndrome (Fig. 52.1).[26–29] Secondary purulent bacterial conjunctivitis can complicate the initial ocular involvement. In some patients, a severe anterior uveitis may occur. Uncommonly, corneal ulceration occurs during the acute stage of the disease. The initial eye findings usually resolve in 2 to 4 weeks.[29] Monocular involvement is unusual and should raise questions about the diagnosis.[26]

Chronic eye findings

Scarring, symblepharon formation, and cicatrization of the conjunctiva may result from the initial inflammatory process. This leads to entropion formation, trichiasis, and instability of the tear film.[23,25,30] Breakdown of the ocular surface leads to corneal scarring, neovascularization, and, in severe cases, keratinization (Fig. 52.2). Keratin often accumulates not only on the corneal surface but also along the posterior lid margin, characteristically extending onto normally nonkeratinized palpebral conjunctiva and further abrading the ocular surface. Subepithelial fibrosis of the conjunctiva can be seen, as in ocular cicatricial pemphigoid. An orbital cyst may occur when epithelial cells become trapped between adhesions of the tarsal and bulbar conjunctiva.[23] Cicatrization of the lacrimal ducts in association with destruction of the conjunctival goblet cells may lead to a severe dry eye state.[30–33] If there is no scarring of the lacrimal ducts, patients may have considerable photophobia and lacrimation. With loss of goblet cells and their mucus secretion, the tear film becomes unstable, with poor wetting of the cornea.[23] The entropion, trichiasis, and lid margin keratinization mentioned earlier can result in chronic irritation of the cornea and resultant persistent epithelial defects.[34] Patients may develop a degenerative pannus that can be stripped from Bowman's membrane, with little effect to the underlying stroma.[23] These corneal manifestations are not the result of the initial acute inflammation but rather of goblet cell dysfunction, trichiasis, and dry eye. The degree of corneal scarring correlates with the severity of eyelid margin and tarsal pathology.[35] A new grading system has been proposed to provide an objective method for evaluating eye involvement in patients with Stevens-Johnson syndrome. Loss of the palisades of Vogt and meibomian gland involvement were the most ominous signs.[36]

Not all patients with ocular findings of erythema multiforme end up with severe loss of vision. The clinical spectrum ranges from a mild surface dysfunction and blurred vision to hand-motions-only vision caused by severe corneal scarring and neovascularization.

Nonocular findings

The clinical spectrum of erythema multiforme accounts for the majority of severe cutaneous reactions after drug therapy. There has been much debate over the proper diagnostic criteria for these three diseases.[37,38] Box 52.1 delineates a useful diagnostic schema to subdivide erythema multiforme, Stevens-Johnson syndrome, and toxic epidermal necrolysis.[39] A multinational consensus classification system (Table 52.1) has been proposed to further subdivide the overlap area between Stevens-Johnson syndrome and toxic epidermal necrolysis.[40]

The rash of erythema multiforme appears suddenly and is typically found on the dorsal aspect of the hands and feet and on the extensor surfaces of forearms, legs, palms, and soles, but not the trunk (Fig. 52.3).[41] Single lesions are usually less than 3 cm in diameter, and less than 20% of the body surface area is involved. The skin changes evolve over the course of the disease process. Initially, they are erythematous annular macules and papules, which may undergo concentric alterations, producing lesions described as resembling a target, iris, or bull's eye.[42,43] Some of the lesions may coalesce or may become vesicular or bullous, particularly in the center. In addition, urticarial plaques may also appear. This eruption usually lasts less than 4 weeks. Erythema multiforme minor is the name given to the disease process when lesions are limited to the skin.

Cutaneous lesions in Stevens-Johnson syndrome usually start off as erythematous macules, and then develop central necrosis to form vesicles, bullae, and areas of denudation on the face, trunk, and extremities. Two or more mucosal surfaces are involved, including the conjunctiva, oral cavity, upper airway or esophagus, gastrointestinal tract, or

Box 52.1 Diagnostic criteria for bullous skin diseases

Erythema multiforme minor
- Target (iris) lesions (typical or atypical)
- Individual lesions less than 3 cm in diameter
- No or minimal mucous membrane involvement
- Less than 20% of body area involved in reaction
- Biopsy specimen compatible with erythema multiforme minor

Stevens-Johnson syndrome (erythema multiforme major)
- Less than 20% of body area involved in first 48 hours
- Greater than 10% body area involvement
- Target (iris) lesions (typical or atypical)
- Individual lesions <3 cm in diameter (lesions may coalesce)
- Mucous membrane involvement (at least two areas)
- Fever
- Biopsy specimen compatible with erythema multiforme major

Toxic epidermal necrolysis
- Bullae and/or erosions over 20% of body area
- Bullae develop on erythematous base
- Occurs on non-sun-exposed skin
- Skin peels off in >3 cm sheets
- Mucous membrane involvement frequent
- Tender skin within 48 hours of onset of rash
- Fever
- Biopsy specimen compatible with toxic epidermal necrolysis

Adapted from Chan HL et al: Arch Dermatol *126:43–47, 1990.*

Table 52.1 Overlap classification of erythema multiforme/toxic epidermal necrolysis

Classification	Detachment	Typical targets	Atypical targets	Spots
Bullous EM	<10% BSA	Yes	Raised	
SJS	<10% BSA		Flat	Yes
Overlap				
SJS-TEN	10–30% BSA		Flat	Yes
TEN with spots	>30% BSA		Flat	Yes
TEN without spots	10% BSA			

Adapted from Bastuji-Garin S et al: Arch Dermatol *129:92–96, 1993.*
EM, Erythema multiforme; SJS, Stevens-Johnson syndrome; TEN, toxic epidermal necrolysis; BSA, basal surface area.

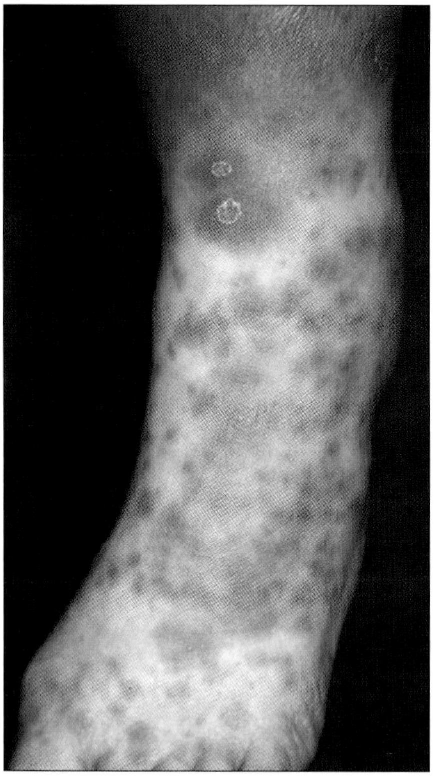

Fig. 52.3 Typical rash of erythema multiforme.

anogenital mucosa. The lesions are generally more widespread than in EM. A frequent presentation begins with a burning sensation, edema, and erythema of the lips and buccal mucosa. Bullae, ulceration, and hemorrhagic crusting then form. Lesions may be preceded by a flulike upper respiratory illness. Severe pain may accompany mucosal ulceration; skin tenderness, however, is minimal, in contrast to toxic epidermal necrolysis.[43–45] The incidence of oral lesions varies from 40% to 60%.[46] Skin involvement is typically less than 20% of the total body surface area in Stevens-Johnson syndrome. Associated risks depending on the extent of the bullae could be significant blood and insensible fluid loss, as well as a high risk of bacterial superinfection and sepsis. Laboratory abnormalities in Stevens-Johnson syndrome are nonspecific: leukocytosis, elevated erythrocyte sedimentation rate and liver transaminase levels, and decreased serum albumin values.

Involvement of more than 30% of body surface area is characteristic of toxic epidermal necrolysis, and it is frequently preceded by constitutional symptoms.[41] The extent of skin involvement has been estimated in one series at 45% of body surface area with TEN compared to less than 10% with SJS.[47] The rash is initially morbilliform, typically involving the trunk, along with the face and extremities. Smaller bullous lesions quickly coalesce, leading to huge bulla formation and epidermal sloughing (Fig. 52.4). A positive Nikolsky's sign is seen frequently in toxic epidermal necrolysis and is elicited when friction is applied to healthy areas of the skin, causing the epidermis to wrinkle and separate. The mucosae are usually involved, with severe erosions of the lips, oral surface, conjunctiva, and genital areas. Systemic features are more prominent and can be life threatening, with fever, leukocytosis, renal dysfunction, sepsis, pulmonary embolism, or gastrointestinal bleeding.[48]

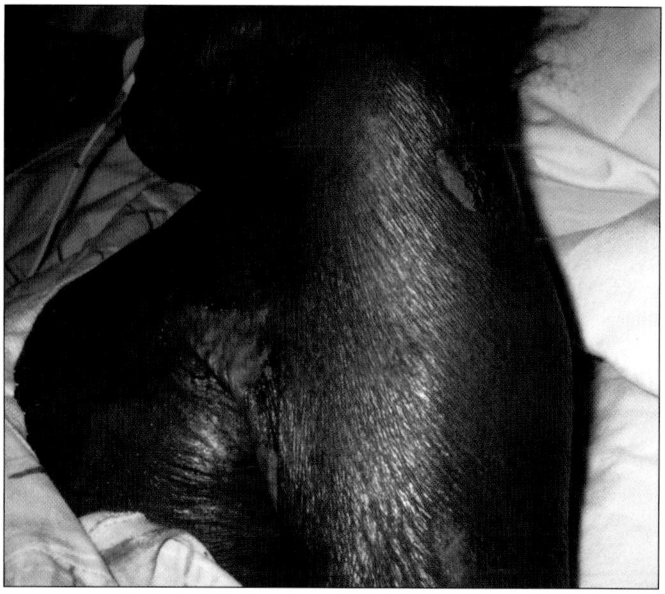

Fig. 52.4 Epidermal sloughing seen in toxic epidermal necrolysis.

Recurrent Disease

Recurrent erythema multiforme is not uncommon. Most people avoid reexposure to the precipitating agent. However, Schofield et al., in a British population, described the largest series of patients with this condition.[49] Most cases in their study (71%) were secondary to reactivation of herpes simplex. The mean number of attacks was six per year, and the mean duration of disease was 9.5 years. Herpetic erythema multiforme does not usually involve the mucosa, although the herpes infection is typically mucosal.

A small number of Stevens-Johnson syndrome patients develop recurrent conjunctival inflammation not associated with trichiasis, entropion, keratoconjunctivitis sicca, or lid margin keratinization.[50] In these patients, recurrent conjunctival inflammation lasting from 8 days to 5 weeks occurs without the typical skin lesions of erythema multiforme. One patient had recurrent oral mucosal ulcers, but these were not concurrent with the development of episodes of conjunctivitis.

Incidence of ocular complications

Ocular complications from erythema multiforme major and toxic epidermal necrolysis vary with the degree of severity of the systemic disease. In a series of 366 patients with EM, SJS, or TEN, an average of 24% had ocular manifestations during their hospitalization: 9% of EM, 69% of SJS, and 5% of TEN patients,[51] and those rates were not affected by administration of steroids. Prendiville et al. found ocular involvement in 17 of 21 patients hospitalized with Stevens-Johnson syndrome or toxic epidermal necrolysis.[52] In more severe cases, acute ocular involvement may cause keratitis, corneal perforation, and endophthalmitis.[25,53] Chronic complications, including conjunctival scarring, symblepharon, entropion, and dry eye syndrome, may cause late corneal damage, which represents the most significant long-term complication for survivors of toxic epidermal necrolysis and Stevens-Johnson syndrome.[25,30,53] In other reports of Stevens-Johnson syndrome and toxic epidermal necrolysis, 43–81% of patients may undergo acute ocular involvement, with up to 35% experiencing permanent visual changes.[28,30,54] Because patients with AIDS may already have decreased lacrimation, they may be at increased risk for ocular complications of Stevens-Johnson syndrome and toxic epidermal necrolysis.[55,56]

Differential Diagnosis

Ocular disorders

The differential diagnosis of erythema multiforme encompasses both the ocular and the cutaneous manifestations of the disease. The chronic ocular findings can most closely resemble cicatricial pemphigoid. The symblepharon is rarely as extensive in erythema multiforme as in ocular cicatricial pemphigoid.[23] Other diseases in the differential diagnosis include severe chronic keratoconjunctivitis caused by bacteria or viruses, medications, allergies, chemical burns, avitaminosis A, and trachoma.[23] A history of a drug reaction with the typical skin lesions of erythema multiforme, accompanied by mucosal symptoms, often points toward the diagnosis. Progressive scarring of the ocular mucosae that appears clinically similar to ocular cicatricial pemphigoid can occur.[10] Biopsy of the involved mucosa in ocular cicatricial pemphigoid patients demonstrates linear immune deposits along the basement membrane and differentiates it from erythema multiforme.

Dermatologic manifestations

The differential diagnosis of the dermatologic manifestations of erythema multiforme is broad. Erythema multiforme may range from urticarial to bullous lesions or even epidermal sloughing, as is seen in toxic epidermal necrolysis. One such entity is staphylococcal scalded-skin syndrome, which can be confused with toxic epidermal necrolysis or Stevens-Johnson syndrome.[2] This diagnosis is important to make quickly because the management and prognosis are different. Staphylococcal scalded-skin syndrome is rare in adults and most commonly occurs in neonates.[57–60] These patients show intense cutaneous erythema and a more superficial desquamation with less severe systemic toxicity. The epidermis quickly regenerates and effectively restores its barrier functions in the staphylococcal scalded-skin syndrome. In erythema multiforme the damage is deeper and regeneration may not be quick.

Other dermatologic diseases in the differential diagnosis include urticarial viral exanthema, drug reaction, toxic shock syndrome, Kawasaki disease, Leiner disease, erythroderma secondary to other causes, contact dermatitis, thermal burns, or poisonings.[61,62] The history will sometimes provide clues necessary to make the correct diagnosis, but biopsy is often required.

Etiology

Drug-related cases of erythema multiforme have a clinical spectrum that typically arises within 3 weeks after initiation of drug therapy.[39] If the patient is reexposed to the inciting drug, a reaction may begin within hours of restarting drug therapy. From 50% to 60% of erythema multiforme cases are secondary to drugs.[27,63] The sulfonamides are the best documented agents causing erythema multiforme in healthy patients as well as in patients with human immunodeficiency virus (HIV) infection or AIDS.[64–67] Chan estimated the frequency of reaction to sulfonamides to be 26 per 1 million person-years.[39] Although any medication may cause erythema multiforme, a number of other medications are linked to erythema multiforme, including phenytoin, barbiturates, phenylbutazone, penicillin, and salicylates.[41,68] Box 52.2 lists the drugs that have been implicated in erythema multiforme or toxic epidermal necrolysis. HIV-positive patients taking the newer antiretroviral medications have demonstrated an increased risk of developing erythema multiforme.[69,70]

Erythema multiforme can be caused by oral, intravenous, or topical application of various medications. Commonly used ophthalmic drops such as scopolamine, sulfonamide, dorzolamide, or tropicamide have all been associated with erythema multiforme.[71–76] Erythema multiforme can follow certain infections, such as herpes simplex, *Mycoplasma pneumoniae*, measles infection, *Mycobacterium*, group A streptococci, Epstein-Barr virus, *Yersinia*, enterovirus, smallpox vaccination, and malignancy.[22,24,63,77] Viral antigens have been seen in skin lesions of patients with erythema multiforme.[78–81] An attempt to differentiate erythema multiforme major from SJS and TEN has been made based on the distribution of etiologic factors: herpetic infection was found to be more prevalent in cases of EM major, while drugs tended to be linked more to SJS and TEN.[1,9] Unlike SJS and TEN, EM was not linked to HIV, collagen vascular diseases, or cancer in that study.

Pathogenesis

Erythema multiforme and toxic epidermal necrolysis appear to be immune-mediated responses to certain drugs and infectious organisms. A definitive mechanism of action has yet to be determined. Histologically, keratinocyte death occurs from extensive apoptosis.[82] Some studies have shown that the apoptosis is induced by a suicidal interaction between Fas and Fas ligand (FasL) which is either membrane bound on keratinocytes or soluble.[83] Abe et al. have postulated that soluble FasL is secreted by peripheral blood mononuclear cells and is elevated in erythema multiforme and toxic epidermal necrolysis patients.[84] Cytokines released by T lymphocytes, macrophages, or keratinocytes may enhance the expression of Fas and FasL on keratinocytes or enhance skin recruitment of lymphocytes by up-regulating adhesion molecules.[85] Apoptosis may also occur from drug-specific CD8+ and cytotoxic T cells using a perforin/granzyme B trigger.[85] Chung et al. have found blister fluid from skin lesions contained cytotoxic T lymphocytes and natural killer cells. These cells release the cytotoxic molecule granulysin in high concentrations and may be a primary cause for cell

Box 52.2 Drugs associated with erythema multiforme

- Antimicrobials
  - Sulfonamides
  - Sulfones
  - Penicillins
  - Cephalosporins
  - Griseofulvin
  - Rifampicin
  - Tetracyclines
  - Ethambutol
  - Isoniazid
  - Streptomycin
  - Thiacetazone
  - Vancomycin
  - Choramphenicol
  - Chloroquine
  - Ciprofloxacin
  - Clindamycin
  - Quinine
  - Fluconazole
  - Lincomycin
  - Nystatin
- Nonsteroidal antiinflammatory drugs
  - Salicylates
  - Fenbufen
  - Ibuprofen
  - Sulindac
  - Pyrazolone derivatives
  - Isoxicam
- Metals
  - Arsenic
  - Bromides
  - Mercury
  - Gold
  - Iodides
  - Lithium
- Anticonvulsants
  - Barbiturates
  - Carbamazepine
  - Hydantoin derivatives
  - Trimethadione
- Central nervous system drugs
  - Mianserin
  - Phenothiazines
  - Trazodone
- Cardiovascular drugs
  - Captopril
  - Acetazolamide
  - Enalapril
  - Iopamidol
  - Propranolol
  - Quinidine
  - Furosemide
  - Hydralazine
  - Minoxidil
  - Thiazide diuretics
  - Diltiazem
  - Verapamil
- Miscellaneous agents
  - Adrenocorticotropin
  - Alkylating agents
  - Allopurinol
  - Atropine
  - Bismuths
  - Cimetidine
  - Chlorpropamide
  - Codeine
  - Cyclophosphamide
  - Clofibrate
  - Danazol
  - Dipyridamole
  - Estrogens
  - Ethanol
  - Methaqualone
  - Nitrogen mustard
  - Pentazocine
  - Phenolphthalein
  - Progesterone
  - Vaccinating agents
  - Ethosuximide
  - Glucagon
  - Glucocorticoids
  - Hydroxyurea
  - Methotrexate
  - Methylthiouracil
  - Indapamide
  - Methenamine
  - Nalidixic acid
  - Novobiocin
  - Theophylline
  - Vitamin A
  - Tolbutamide
  - Dorzolamide
  - Nevirapine
  - lamotrigine
  - Tipranavir
  - Darunavir
  - Etravirine
  - Enfuvirtide
  - Raltegravir
  - Maroviroc

death.[86] Further work in pathogenesis is ongoing and will hopefully afford a better understanding of the erythema multiforme group of diseases.

Herpes-associated EM may represent a cell-mediated immune reaction to HSV antigen, affecting HSV-expressing keratinocytes. Apoptosis of keratinocytes is induced by cytotoxic T cells. Neighboring epidermal cells are HLA-DR positive.

Certain HLA markers have been associated with different forms of erythema multiforme. Patients with the ocular lesions of Stevens-Johnson syndrome have a significantly increased incidence of HLA-B12, HLA-Aw33, and DRw53.[87,88] Herpes simplex-induced erythema multiforme is related to HLA-DQw3.[88] HLA association for recurrent EM has been established with HLA types A33, B35, B62 (B15), DR4, DQB10301, DQ3, and DR53. HLA DQ3 has been proven to be especially related to recurrent EM and may be a helpful marker for distinguishing herpes-related EM from other diseases with EM-like lesions. An increased incidence of HLA-B12 was also seen in white patients with toxic epidermal necrolysis.[89] Patients with sulfonamide-induced toxic epidermal necrolysis showed a significant increase in the frequency of HLA-A29, B12, and DR7.[87] An association between HLA-B44 and the ocular lesions of Stevens-Johnson syndrome has been reported.[88] Japanese who develop Stevens-Johnson syndrome have a strong association with HLA-A*0206.[90] Thai patients with HLA-D*1502 have an association with carbamazepine and phenytoin-induced Stevens-Johnson syndrome.[91]

Histopathology

Skin

Briefly, biopsy shows a lymphocytic infiltrate at the dermal–epidermal junction with a characteristic vacuolization of epidermal cells and necrotic keratinocytes within the epidermis. The dermal infiltrate has been found to be more pronounced in EM major than in SJS or TEN.[92]

In erythema multiforme major, separation of the epidermis and basement membrane from the dermis occurs.[41,43] Initial lesions show vasodilation in the superficial dermis with endothelial swelling, lymphohistiocytic perivascular infiltration, and papillary dermal edema. Orfanos et al. have described two different histologic patterns.[93] In the first type, pure dermal damage occurs with dermal edema, intradermal bulla formation, and erythematous papular lesions. Epidermal damage characterizes the second type, resulting in bulla formation at the dermal–epidermal junction with the basal laminae at the floor of the bullae in 'target lesions.' Hydropic degeneration of keratinocytes with focal necrosis of epitheliocytes can be seen. Eosinophils can be seen in skin lesions of drug-induced Stevens-Johnson syndrome but are not considered to be diagnostic.[94]

Toxic epidermal necrolysis has a histopathologic picture similar to that of the epidermal type of erythema multiforme major.[93] Eosinophilic necrosis of the epidermis occurs with a cleavage plane above the basement membrane at the basal cell layer. Endothelial swelling may be seen in the dermal vessels, although they do not undergo major histopathologic change. The earliest changes seen are vacuolar changes at the dermal–epidermal junction; these progress to dermoepidermal separation and subepidermal blister formation.[95] The epidermis becomes dyskeratotic and then necrotic. The majority of the inflammatory cells of the dermal infiltrate are of the helper/inducer T-lymphocyte subsets.[96] Deposition of immunoglobulins and/or complement can be seen using immunofluorescent techniques but is nonspecific.[20,97]

Eye

A nonspecific inflammatory response is seen in the acute phases in enucleated eyes of patients with erythema multiforme.[98,99] Widespread necrosis of arterioles and venules occurs with fibrinoid degeneration of the associated collagen.[100] During the chronic phase, the effects of cicatrization on the cornea, conjunctiva, and eyelids are most prominent. Conjunctival biopsies in Stevens-Johnson syndrome show an absence of the mucus-producing goblet cells as a sequelae of cicatrization.[23,32] Conjunctival goblet cells are decreased to 1–2% of normal when measured by impression cytologic techniques.[101] Nonspecific mononuclear inflammation can characterize the acute phase of Stevens-Johnson syndrome, affecting the subepithelial layers of the conjunctiva.[102] Circulating immune complexes and immune complexes in the microvasculature of the mucosal subepithelial tissue have been found.[103–106] Increased proliferation of basal epithelial cells has been demonstrated in Stevens-Johnson syndrome, and an increased percentage of proliferating conjunctival cells appears to be correlated with the severity of disease.[107]

Management

Systemic disease

Taking proper care of patients with severe erythema multiforme is challenging and difficult. These patients are critically ill and require specialized nursing and medical care. Careful monitoring of fluid balance, respiratory function, nutritional requirements, and wound care is crucial.[2] A number of studies support the idea that these patients are best managed in an intensive burn care unit.[62,108–112] Adequate control of environmental temperature is needed to decrease caloric loss through the skin and should be increased from 30°C to 32°C.[113] Proper fluid balance management is crucial because of the loss of the stratum corneum.[109] Dehydration can occur easily without close fluid management through insensible losses. More than half of all deaths occurring in toxic epidermal necrolysis are secondary to sepsis, so control of infection is critical.[111] It is generally felt that antibiotics should be reserved for culture-proven sepsis, and prophylactic antibiotic coverage is not needed.[24,110,111] Silver nitrate solution can be used as an antibacterial on the denuded skin.[62] Biologic dressings such as cadaver or porcine skin, amniotic membrane, and iodoplex can be used to reduce pain and evaporative loss as well as protect against infection.[108,110,111,114,115] Nanocrystaline silver dressings were shown to be beneficial.[116] Any potentially offending drug should be discontinued immediately.[40] Early cessation decreases the mortality rate.[117] Agents that are common causes of erythema multiforme, such as silver sulfalazine, a sulfa agent, which is often used in burn centers, should be avoided.[113,112]

The use of systemic corticosteroids in patients with Stevens-Johnson syndrome and toxic epidermal necrolysis is controversial.[38,48,118–126] There are a number of potential beneficial reasons to use steroids. High-dose corticosteroids may arrest the necrolysis and benefit the patient's systemic recovery.[118,125,127] Recent studies indicating an immune disease mechanism logically point toward steroid use.[66,83–86] The course of toxic epidermal necrolysis and Stevens-Johnson syndrome is quite variable and unpredictable, which casts doubt on uncontrolled observations of steroid use. The disadvantages of employing systemic steroids include increased susceptibility to infection, masking of the early signs of sepsis, gastrointestinal hemorrhage, impaired wound healing, and prolonged recovery. Because evidence for the beneficial effects of steroids is lacking, most authors now agree that the use of corticosteroids in severe cutaneous drug reactions does not outweigh the potential risks involved and does not positively affect the final outcome.[38,111,120–122,124,126,128,129] A well-designed, prospective, randomized, controlled study is needed to answer the question definitively.

There has been a case report of ciclosporin therapy that showed the progression of toxic epidermal necrolysis after failure of high-dose steroid therapy.[130] This patient developed no permanent sequelae on follow-up examination. The use of ciclosporin in this disease requires further delineation. Cases of plasma exchange and plasmapheresis therapy in patients with toxic epidermal necrolysis have also been reported, although there are no controlled clinical trials.[131–134] Most small series have shown benefit for high-dose IVIG at reducing overall mortality.[135–140] IVIG does contain natural anti-Fas antibodies. A large prospective randomized, controlled trial is the logical next step.

Acyclovir and cimetidine each have been shown effective in cases of erythema multiforme secondary to herpes simplex virus.[49,141]

Ophthalmic disease

Management of the ocular effects of erythema multiforme can be divided into acute and chronic stages.

Acute stage

During the acute stage, ocular surface hygiene should be maintained. This includes frequent conjunctival irrigation and installation of prophylactic antibiotics to combat secondary infection.[23,28–30] Frequent preservative-free artificial tear supplements should be used to lubricate the corneal and conjunctival epithelium. Cycloplegics are employed for the anterior uveitis that is often associated with the external inflammation in Stevens-Johnson syndrome and toxic epidermal necrosis.

The use of topical steroids, like systemic steroids, is controversial and can be associated with secondary infection. Topical steroids tend to decrease ocular inflammation, although symblepharon can form despite their use.[23] If steroids are used, the patient should be followed closely to monitor for secondary bacterial infection. Bacterial keratitis in this setting can lead to rapid corneal perforation. If a keratitis does occur, careful cultures should be obtained, and vigorous antimicrobial therapy should be started with fortified antibiotics.

Lamellar or penetrating keratoplasty can be used if perforation is impending or occurs. A conjunctival flap is also a valuable option for treatment of an impending perforation in the acute stage. Daily lysis of the symblepharon can be attempted, but it is usually ineffective in preventing recurrence of the symblepharon. Robin and Dugel have suggested using clear plastic wrap or a symblepharon ring in association with a bandage soft contact lens to line the palpebral surface and prevent symblepharon formation.[142] Stabilizing the ocular surface and stopping the inflammatory process are of paramount importance. Cryopreserved amniotic membrane can be applied to the bulbar and tarsal conjunctiva and the cornea. Three reports have shown promising data for suturing amniotic membrane over the inflamed surface during the acute phase.[143–145]

The role of topical ciclosporin has not been studied, although one case in which systemic treatment was employed suggested that it may be useful in this disease.[130]

Chronic stage

Management of the chronic stages of erythema multiforme usually proves to be very challenging and involved. Goals of treatment are to:

1. restore eyelid and forniceal anatomy and function
2. supply tear function
3. restore ocular surface.

Trichiasis is a constant and recurring problem in patients with this disorder. Epilation, cryotherapy, argon laser treatment, electrolysis, or blepharotomy can be used to destroy lashes.[146,147] Rotation of the entire lid margin can be performed in some patients. A rapid freeze of the eyelid margin of −20 to 30°C, followed by a slow thaw, will irreversibly damage approximately 80% of the eyelash follicles.[147] A period of 40 to 60 seconds of freezing is required to reach the appropriate tissue temperature. A double freeze–thaw technique is recommended for best results. Cicatricial entropion and epidermalization of the conjunctiva can lead to mechanical trauma to the cornea. This in turn leads to corneal scarring and neovascularization. Entropion repair, possibly combined with mucous membrane grafting, should be performed to correct lid problems.[53,148–150] Foreshortening of the fornices and restoration of the conjunctiva can be addressed either through mucous membrane grafts such as hard palate,[151,152] nasal,[153,154] or buccal[155–157] mucosa or with the use of amniotic membrane grafts,[158,159] or at the time of a keratolimbal allograft.

Nasolacrimal duct and/or canalicular obstruction or stenosis can occur, which is not always a bad result. Sometimes this offsets the relatively dry eye state and may not need correction. But if dacryocystitis or chronic epiphora occurs, dacryocystorhinostomy and silicone tube insertion may become necessary.[160]

Frequent artificial tear supplementation should be used to treat the keratoconjunctivitis sicca that develops after scarring of the conjunctiva and lacrimal ducts in erythema multiforme. Loss of goblet cells contributes greatly to the dry eye state. The extent of the compromise of the tear function preoperatively, before ocular surface restoration procedures, has been inversely correlated with the success rates of those procedures.[161] Nonpreserved methylcellulose lubricants should be used because of the toxicity that can be seen with preservatives in patients with such severe dry eye states. Conjunctival impression cytology can be used to assess the ocular surface and to monitor response to treatment.

Mucolytic agents such as 10% *N*-acetylcysteine can be used to control filament formation or abnormal mucous discharge. A lateral and/or medial tarsorrhaphy can be used to improve the status of the ocular surface by decreasing the surface area available for evaporation. Bandage soft or gas-permeable contact lenses can be used to manage persistent epithelial defects; high oxygen permeability and provision of an optically regular ocular surface are the major advantages of rigid contact lenses emphasized by their proponents.[162–164] Care should be taken to watch these patients for tight lens syndrome because of their compromised ocular surface and low mucin production.[165] Microbial keratitis is also a risk with bandage lenses.

Different types of keratoprostheses have been described for use in patients with Stevens-Johnson syndrome who have poor epithelial healing.[166–169] Anatomical success ranges around 85%,[167,168] vision obtained in successful cases from 20/20 to 20/200. Potential complications associated with keratoprosthesis use include eyelid cellulitis, extrusions of the keratoprosthesis, aqueous leaks, retroprosthetic membranes, endophthalmitis, retinal detachment, and progressive glaucoma.[167,168,170,171] The prognosis with SJS is worse than with other preoperative indications for keratoprosthesis.[168,170] Improved results have recently been seen with the Boston K Pro. The largest study showed 75% at 20/200 or better and 50% at 20/40 or better with no extrusions or endophthalmitis. This is due to the prophylactic use of vancomycin and more aggressive treatment of glaucoma.[172] For more advanced cases with extremely dry eye osteo-odonto keratoprosthesis (OOKP) may be the only option.[173] This two-stage procedure involves the use of an autologous canine tooth modified to accept an optical cylinder and implanted in the cheek. At the same time, the ocular surface is replaced with oral buccal mucosa. In stage 2, a few months later, the cornea is trephined, the iris and lens are removed, and the tooth cylinder is implanted in the cornea. The largest series reported a 73.3% at 20/40 or better with 100% anatomic success.[174] Mean follow-up was short at 19.1 months. Liu et al. reported a longer follow-up and 72% anatomic success.[175] Failure was mostly due to resorption of the OOKP lamina.

Keratolimbal allograft (keratoepithelioplasty) is a procedure first described by Thoft, then improved by others, that can be useful in the treatment of persistent epithelial dysfunction resulting from various causes, including erythema multiforme.[176] Lenticules of cadaveric keratolimbal,[177–180] living-related conjunctivolimbal,[181–184] combination of the above, or cultivated allo-epithelial[185–187] donor limbal tissue, with or without amniotic membrane, are transplanted to the limbus of an affected eye after superficial keratectomy to remove the abnormal damaged surface cells. HLA matching increases the rates of success of living-related tissue.[188] Conjunctivolimbal autografts from the fellow eye do not apply in cases of bilateral disease, such as SJS. A combined keratolimbal allograft and living-related conjunctivolimbal allograft combines the benefits of both procedures and improves chances of success in cases of total or near-total limbal stem cell deficiency, such as SJS. Amniotic membrane transplantation has been reported to produce acceptable results with

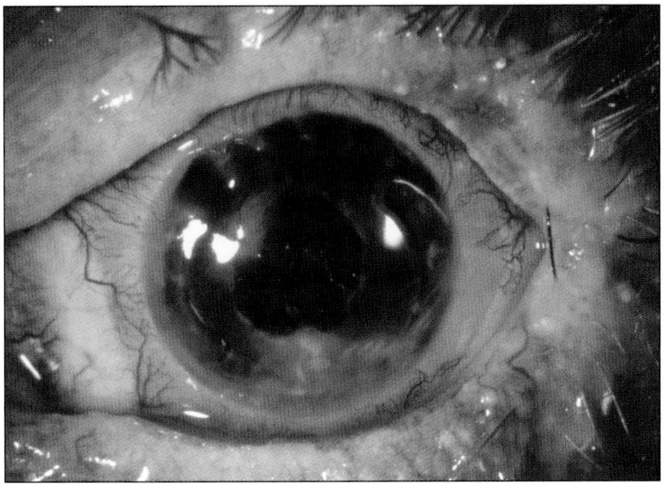

Fig. 52.5 Clear corneal graft after keratoepithelioplasty and penetrating keratoplasty.

limited partial stem cell deficiency.[189] Immunosuppression is necessary to ensure the survival of the transplanted surface cells.[190,191] Cultivated human limbal epithelium heals faster and may represent a longer-lasting source for surface cells.[192–194] Another promising technique uses serum-derived autologous cultivated oral epithelium for transplantation,[195–197] Healthy transplanted limbal stem cells can then multiply and spread to cover the cornea.[176,198,199] Once the epithelium has been stabilized by performing the keratolimbal graft, penetrating keratoplasty can be performed to improve vision (Fig. 52.5). Penetrating keratoplasty produces better results if performed months after the keratolimbal allograft.[177] Satisfactory results have also been achieved in children with SJS-related ocular surface disease.[200] A diagnosis of SJS or TEN carries a greater challenge and a worse prognosis than other indications for those procedures, such as chemical or thermal burns and aniridia.[177,193,201] The most common postoperative complications in these patients are related to epithelial toxicity from medications, trichiasis, and mucin deficiency. Short-term results of patients with erythema multiforme treated with this technique are promising. Long-term stability of the epithelial surface remains a question.

Topical transretinoic acid can be used to reverse conjunctival transdifferentiation seen after ocular surface injury.[202,203] Topical and systemic vitamin A was used to treat a 9-year-old child with Stevens-Johnson syndrome and achieved improvement in his ocular surface appearance.[204] Improvement in clinical symptoms, visual acuity, rose Bengal staining, and Schirmer's test results, and the degree of squamous metaplasia, have been seen after treatment with topical retinoids.[205] Topical vitamin A in a 0.01% or 0.025% ointment is commercially available and can be used twice daily. Autologous serum has also been reported to provide factors that improve transdifferentiation and maintenance of a healthy epithelium.[182] Topical bevacizumab can reduce corneal neovascularization and opacification.[206] Blepharitis or ocular inflammation may increase after the initiation of topical vitamin A, and this agent's dosage can be tapered to minimize these side effects.[207]

Prognosis

The two most serious forms of erythema multiforme, Stevens-Johnson syndrome and toxic epidermal necrolysis, are potentially fatal disease processes with a 25–40% mortality in toxic epidermal necrolysis patients.[15,112,113,208] AIDS patients who develop erythema multiforme do not have a worse prognosis.[113] Elderly patients have a worse prognosis, and children have the best.[21,209]

The chronic ocular disease may often be the most devastating result for survivors of the acute reaction. The outcome depends on the severity of the initial event much more than it does on the initial treatment. To minimize visual impairment, prevention of complications is the key to success. Careful attention to ophthalmic examinations during the early period of the skin reaction and recognizing the complications of trichiasis, epithelial surface disease, and secondary infection can improve the outcome. Systemic steroids are falling out of favor because of their significant systemic side effects and the potential for secondary infection. If topical steroids are used, careful monitoring of the ocular surface should be performed for early detection of secondary infections. Preserving the ocular surface is the main goal during the acute phase. Early cryopreserved amniotic membrane transplantation may be the key.[143–145] If the ocular surface is destroyed, procedures to transplant limbal stem cells in conjunction with the generous use of tarsorrhaphy, nonpreserved artificial lubricants, and treatment of trichiasis may improve the prognosis of this disease. As high as the cost may be of those procedures, the benefit of restoring functional vision and rehabilitating those incapacitated individuals outweighs the cost.[210] Improvements in keratoprosthesis for end-stage disease provides hope for those most severely affected.

References

1. Auquier-Dunant A, et al. Correlations between clinical patterns and causes of erythema multiforme majus, Stevens-Johnson syndrome, and toxic epidermal necrolysis: results of an international prospective study. *Arch Dermatol.* 2002;138(8):1019–1024.
2. Rohrer TE, Ahmed AR. Toxic epidermal necrolysis. *Int J Dermatol.* 1991;30:457–466.
3. Ghislain PD, Roujeau JC. Treatment of severe drug reactions: Stevens-Johnson syndrome, toxic epidermal necrolysis and hypersensitivity syndrome. *Dermatol Online J.* 2002;8(1):5.
4. Hebra F. *On diseases of the skin, including the exanthemata.* Translated and edited by CH Fagge. London: New Sydenham Society; 1866.
5. Fuchs E. Herpes iris conjunctivae. *Klin Monatsbl Augenheilkd.* 1876; 14:333–351.
6. Fiessinger N, Rendu R. Sur un syndrome caracterise par l'inflammation simultanee de toutes les muqueuses coexistant avec une eruption vesiculeuse des quatres membres. *Paris Med.* 1917;25:54.
7. Stevens AM, Johnson FC. A new eruptive fever associated with stomatitis and ophthalmia. *Am J Dis Child.* 1922;24:526–533.
8. Lyell A. Toxic epidermal necrolysis: an eruption resembling scalding of the skin. *Br J Dermatol.* 1956;68:355–361.
9. Assier H, et al. Erythema multiforme with mucous membrane involvement and Stevens-Johnson syndrome are clinically different disorders with distinct causes. *Arch Dermatol.* 1995;131(5):539–543.
10. Chan LS, et al. Ocular cicatricial pemphigoid occurring as a sequela of Stevens-Johnson syndrome. *JAMA.* 1991;266:1543–1546.
11. Schöph E, et al. Toxic epidermal necrolysis and Stevens-Johnson syndrome. An epidemiologic study from West Germany. *Arch Dermatol.* 1991;127:839–842.
12. Roujeau JC, et al. Toxic epidermal necrolysis (Lyell syndrome). Incidence and drug etiology in France, 1981–1985. *Arch Dermatol.* 1990; 126:37–42.

13. Nadli L, et al. Incidence of toxic epidermal necrolysis in Italy. *Arch Dermatol.* 1990;126:1103–1104.
14. Bottinger LE, Strandberg I, Westerholm B. Drug induced febrile mucocutaneous syndrome. *Acta Med Scand.* 1975;198:229–233.
15. Mockenhaupt M, Schöpf E. Epidemiology of drug-induced severe skin reactions. *Semin Cutan Med Surg.* 1996;15(4):236–243.
16. Rzany B, et al. Epidemiology of erythema exudativum multiforme majus, Stevens-Johnson syndrome, and toxic epidermal necrolysis in Germany (1990–1992): structure and results of a population-based registry. *J Clin Epidemiol.* 1996;49(7):769–773.
17. Miller L, Cohn D. High rates of recurrent pneumocystis pneumonia and toxicity in AIDS patients taking pyrimethamine-sulfadoxine (abstract number T.B.P. 317). *Int Conference AIDS.* 1989;5:294.
18. Breathnach SM, Phillips WG. Epidemiology of bullous drug eruptions. *Clin Dermatol.* 1993;11:441–447.
19. Rzany B, et al. Incidence of Stevens-Johnson syndrome and toxic epidermal necrolysis in patients with acquired immunodeficiency syndrome in Germany. *Arch Dermatol.* 1993;129:1059.
20. Fabbri P, Panconesi E. Erythema multiforme ('minus' and 'maius') and drug intake. *Clin Dermatol.* 1993;11:479–489.
21. Bastuji-Garin S, et al. Toxic epidermal necrolysis (Lyell syndrome) in 77 elderly patients. *Age Ageing.* 1993;22:450–456.
22. Behrman RE, Kliegman RM, Jenson HB. In: *Nelson textbook of pediatrics.* Philadelphia: Saunders; 2000.
23. Dohlman CH, Doughman DJ. The Stevens-Johnson syndrome. *Trans New Orleans Acad Ophthalmol.* 1972;24:236–252.
24. Ostler HB, Conant MA, Groundwater J. Lyell's disease, the Stevens-Johnson syndromes, and exfoliative dermatitis. *Trans Am Acad Ophthalmol Otolaryngol.* 1970;74:1254–1265.
25. Wright P, Collin JR. The ocular complications of erythema multiforme (Stevens-Johnson syndrome) and their management. *Trans Ophthalmol Soc UK.* 1983;103:338–341.
26. Ashby DW, Lazar T. Erythema multiforme exudativum major (Stevens-Johnson syndrome), *Lancet.* 1951;260:1091–1095.
27. Bianchine JR, et al. Drugs as etiologic factors in the Stevens-Johnson syndrome. *Am J Med.* 1968;44:390–405.
28. Howard GM. The Stevens-Johnson syndrome. Ocular prognosis and treatment. *Am J Ophthalmol.* 1963;55:893–900.
29. Patz A. Ocular involvement in erythema multiforme. *Arch Ophthalmol.* 1950;43:244–256.
30. Arstikaitis MJ. Ocular aftermath of Stevens-Johnson syndrome. Review of 33 cases. *Arch Ophthalmol.* 1973;90:376–379.
31. Desai VN, Shields CL, Shields JA. Orbital cyst in a patient with Stevens-Johnson syndrome. *Cornea.* 1992;11:592–594.
32. Mondino BJ, Brown SI. Ocular cicatricial pemphigoid. *Ophthalmology.* 1981;88:95–100.
33. Ralph RA. Conjunctival goblet cell density in normal subjects and in dry eye syndromes. *Invest Ophthalmol Vis Sci.* 1975;14:299–302.
34. Stark HH. Membranous conjunctivitis of over four years' duration. *Am J Ophthalmol.* 1918;1:91.
35. Di Pascuale MA, et al. Correlation of corneal complications with eyelid cicatricial pathologies in patients with Stevens-Johnson syndrome and toxic epidermal necrolysis syndrome. *Ophthalmology.* 2005;112: 904–912.
36. Sotozono C, et al. New grading system for the evaluation of chronic ocular manifestations in patients with Stevens-Johnson syndrome. *Ophthalmology.* 2007;114:1294–1302.
37. Crosby SS, et al. Management of Stevens-Johnson syndrome. *Clin Pharm.* 1986;5:682–689.
38. Ruiz-Maldonado R. Acute disseminated epidermal necrosis types 1, 2, and 3. Study of sixty cases. *J Am Acad Dermatol.* 1985;13:623–635.
39. Chan HL, et al. The incidence of erythema multiforme, Stevens-Johnson syndrome, and toxic epidermal necrolysis. A population-based study with particular reference to reactions caused by drugs among outpatients. *Arch Dermatol.* 1990;126:43–47.
40. Bastuji-Garin S, et al. Clinical classification of cases of toxic epidermal necrolysis, Stevens-Johnson syndrome, and erythema multiforme. *Arch Dermatol.* 1993;129:92–96.
41. Raviglione MC, Pablos-Mendez A, Battan R. Clinical features and management of severe dermatological reactions to drugs. *Drug Saf.* 1990;5:39–64.
42. Ackerman AB, Penneys NS, Clark WH. Erythema multiforme exudativum: distinctive pathological process. *Br J Dermatol.* 1971;84:554–566.
43. Elias PM, Fritsch PO. Erythema multiforme. In: Fitzpatrick TB, et al, eds. *Dermatology in general medicine.* New York: McGraw-Hill; 1987.
44. Araujo OE, Flowers FP. Stevens-Johnson syndrome. *J Emerg Med.* 1984;2:129–135.
45. Benichou C, et al. Lesions oculopalpebrales dans les erythè mes polymorphes graves: prevention du symblepharon. *Bull Soc Ophthalmol Fr.* 1988;88:391–396.
46. Laskaus G, Satriano RA. Drug-induced blistering oral lesions. *Clin Dermatol.* 1993;11:545–550.
47. Wong KC, Kennedy PJ, Lee S. Clinical manifestations and outcomes in 17 cases of Stevens-Johnson syndrome and toxic epidermal necrolysis. *Australas J Dermatol.* 1999;40(3):131–134.
48. Revuz J, et al. Toxic epidermal necrolysis: clinical findings and prognosis factors in 87 patients. *Arch Dermatol.* 1987;123:1160–1165.
49. Schofield JK, Tatnall FM, Leigh IM. Recurrent erythema multiforme: clinical features and treatment in a large series of patients. *Br J Dermatol.* 1993;128:542–545.
50. Foster CS, et al. Episodic conjunctival inflammation after Stevens-Johnson syndrome. *Ophthalmology.* 1988;95:453–462.
51. Power WJ, et al. Analysis of the acute ophthalmic manifestations of the erythema multiforme/Stevens-Johnson syndrome/toxic epidermal necrolysis disease spectrum. *Ophthalmology.* 1995;102(11):1669–1676.
52. Prendiville JS, et al. Management of Stevens-Johnson syndrome and toxic epidermal necrolysis in children. *J Pediatr.* 1989;115:881–887.
53. Beyer CK. The management of special problems associated with Stevens-Johnson syndrome and ocular pemphigoid. *Trans Am Acad Ophthalmol Otolaryngol.* 1977;83:701–707.
54. Yetiv JZ, Bianchine JR, Owen JA. Etiologic factors of the Stevens-Johnson syndrome. *South Med J.* 1980;73:599–602.
55. Belfort R Jr, et al. Ocular complications of Stevens-Johnson syndrome and toxic epidermal necrolysis in patients with AIDS, *Cornea.* 1991; 10:536–538.
56. Schiodt M, et al. Parotid gland enlargement and xerostomia associated with labial sialoadenitis in HIV-infected patients. *J Autoimmunol.* 1989;2:415–425.
57. Hawley HB, Aronson MD. Scalded-skin syndrome in adults. *N Engl J Med.* 1973;288:1130.
58. Levine G, Norden CW. Staphylococcal scalded-skin syndrome in an adult. *N Engl J Med.* 1972;287:1339–1340.
59. Reid L, Weston WL, Humbert JR. Staphylococcal scalded-skin syndrome. Adult onset in a patient with deficient cell-mediated immunity. *Arch Dermatol.* 1974;109:239–241.
60. Rothenberg R, et al. Staphylococcal scalded skin syndrome in an adult. *Arch Dermatol.* 1973;108:408–410.
61. Lyell A. Toxic epidermal necrolysis (the scalded-skin syndrome): a reappraisal. *Br J Dermatol.* 1979;100:69–86.
62. Parsons JM. Management of toxic epidermal necrolysis. *Cutis.* 1985;36:305–311.
63. Tonnesen MG, Soter NA. Erythema multiforme. *J Am Acad Dermatol.* 1979;1:357–364.
64. Fischel MA, Dickinson GM. Fansidar prophylaxis of *Pneumocystis* pneumonia in the acquired immunodeficiency syndrome. *Ann Intern Med.* 1986;105:629.
65. Kovacs JA, Masur H. *Pneumocystis carinii* pneumonia: therapy and prophylaxis. *J Infect Dis.* 1988;158:254–259.
66. Miller KD, et al. Severe cutaneous reactions among American travelers using pyrimethamine-sulfadoxine (Fansidar) for malaria prophylaxis. *Am J Trop Med Hyg.* 1986;35:451–458.
67. Navin TR, et al. Adverse reactions associated with pyrimethamine-sulfadoxine prophylaxis for *Pneumocystis carinii* infections in AIDS. *Lancet.* 1985;1:1332.
68. Dunagin WG, Millikan LE. Drug eruptions. *Med Clin North Am.* 1980;64:983–1003.
69. Jain V, et al. Nevirapine-induced Stevens-Johnson syndrome in an HIV patient. *Cornea.* 2008;27:366–367.
70. Borras-Blasco J, et al. Adverse cutaneous reactions associated with the newest antiretroviral drugs in patients with human immunodeficiency virus infection. *J Antimicrob Chemother.* 2008;62:879–888.
71. Genvert GI, et al. Erythema multiforme after use of topical sulfacetamide. *Am J Ophthalmol.* 1985;99:465–468.
72. Gottschalk HR, Stone OJ. Stevens-Johnson syndrome from ophthalmic sulfonamide. *Arch Dermatol.* 1976;112:513–514.
73. Guill MA, et al. Erythema multiforme and urticaria. *Arch Dermatol.* 1979;115:742–743.
74. Margolis DJ, Bondi EE. Toxic epidermal necrolysis associated with sulfonamides. *Int J Dermatol.* 1990;29:153.
75. Rubin Z. Ophthalmic sulfonamide-induced Stevens-Johnson syndrome. *Arch Dermatol.* 1977;113:235–236.
76. Munshi V, et al. Erythema multiforme after use of topical dorzolamide. *J Ocul Pharmacol Ther.* 2008;24:91–93.
77. Shelley WB. Herpes simplex virus as a cause of erythema multiforme. *JAMA.* 1967;201(3):71–74.

78. Major PP, Morriset R, Kustak C. Isolation of herpes simplex virus type 1 from lesions of erythema multiforme. *Can Med J.* 1978;118:821–822.
79. MacDonald A, Peiwel M. Isolation of herpes virus for erythema multiforme. *Br J Med.* 1972;2:570–571.
80. Brice SL, Krzemien D, Weston WL. Detection of herpes simplex virus DNA in cutaneous lesions of erythema multiforme. *J Invest Dermatol.* 1989;93:183–187.
81. Darragh T, Egbert B, Berger T. Identification of herpes simplex virus DNA in lesions of erythema multiforme by polymerase chain reaction. *J Am Acad Dermatol.* 1991;24:23–26.
82. Paul C, et al. Apoptosis as a mechanism of keratinocyte death in toxic epidermal necrolysis. *Br J Dermatol.* 1996;134:710–714.
83. French LE. Toxic epidermal necrolysis and Stevens-Johnson syndrome: our current understanding. *Allergol Int.* 2006;55:9–16.
84. Abe R, et al. Toxic epidermal necrolysis and Stevens-Johnson syndrome are induced by soluble Fas ligand. *Am J Pathol.* 2003;162:1515–1520.
85. Borchers AT, et al. Stevens-Johnson syndrome and toxic epidermal necrolysis. *Autoimmun Rev.* 2008;7:598–605.
86. Chung WH, et al. Granulysin is a key mediator for disseminated keratinocyte death in Stevens-Johnson syndrome and toxic epidermal necrolysis. *Nat Med.* 2008;14:1343–1350.
87. Mondino BJ, Brown SI, Biglan AW. HLA antigens in Stevens-Johnson syndrome with ocular involvement. *Arch Ophthalmol.* 1982; 100:1453–1454.
88. Mobini N, Ahmed AR. Immunogenetics of drug-induced bullous diseases. *Clin Dermatol.* 1993;11:449–460.
89. Roujeau JC, et al. Genetic susceptibility to toxic epidermal necrolysis. *Arch Dermatol.* 1987;123:1171–1173.
90. Ueta M, et al. Strong association between HLA-A*0206 and Stevens-Johnson syndrome in the Japanese. *Am J Ophthalmol.* 2007; 143:367–368.
91. Locharernkul C, et al. Carbamazepine and phenytoin induced Stevens-Johnson syndrome is associated with HLA-B*1502 allele in Thai population. *Epilepsia.* 2008;49:2087–2091.
92. Rzany B, et al. Histopathological and epidemiological characteristics of patients with erythema exudativum multiforme major, Stevens-Johnson syndrome and toxic epidermal necrolysis. *Br J Dermatol.* 1996;135(1):6–11.
93. Orfanos CE, Schaumburg-Lever G, Lever WF. Dermal and epidermal types of erythema multiforme: a histopathologic study of 24 cases. *Arch Dermatol.* 1974;109:682–688.
94. Patterson JW, et al. Eosinophils in skin lesions of erythema multiforme. *Arch Pathol Lab Med.* 1989;113:36–39.
95. Merot Y, Saurat JH. Clues to pathogenesis of toxic epidermal necrolysis. *Int J Dermatol.* 1985;24:165–168.
96. Merot Y, et al. Lymphocyte subsets and Langerhan's cells in toxic epidermal necrolysis: report of a case. *Arch Dermatol.* 1986;122:455–458.
97. Wilkins J, Morrison L, White CL. Oculocutaneous manifestations of the erythema multiforme/Stevens-Johnson syndrome/toxic epidermal necrolysis spectrum. *Derm Clin.* 1992;10:571–582.
98. Ginandes GJ. Eruptive fever with stomatitis and ophthalmia; atypical erythema exudativum multiforme (Stevens-Johnson). *Am J Dis Child* 1935;49:1148–1160.
99. Richards JM, Romaine HH. Keratoconjunctivitis sicca: a sequela to purulent erythema exudativum multiforme (Stevens-Johnson's disease). *Am J Ophthalmol.* 1946;29:1121–1125.
100. Alexander MK, Cope S. Erythema multiforme exudativum major (Stevens-Johnson syndrome). *J Path Bact.* 1954;68:373–380.
101. Nelson JD, Wright JC. Conjunctival goblet cell densities in ocular surface disease. *Arch Ophthalmol.* 1984;102:1049–1051.
102. Bedi TR, Pinkus H. Histopathological spectrum of erythema multiforme. *Br J Dermatol.* 1976;95:243–250.
103. Kazmierowski JA, Wuepper KD. Erythema multiforme: immune complex vasculitis of the superficial cutaneous microvasculature. *J Invest Dermatol.* 1978;71:366.
104. Safai B, Good RA, Day NK. Erythema multiforme: report of two cases and speculation on immune mechanisms involved in the pathogenesis. *Clin Immunol Immunopathol.* 1977;7:379–385.
105. Swinehart JM, et al. Identification of circulating immune complexes in erythema multiforme. *Clin Res.* 1978;26:577A.
106. Wuepper KD, Watson PA, Kazmierowski JA. Immune complexes in erythema multiforme and the Stevens-Johnson syndrome. *J Invest Dermatol.* 1980;74:368–371.
107. Weissman SS, et al. Alteration of human conjunctival proliferation. *Arch Ophthalmol.* 1992;110:357–359.
108. Demling RH, Ellerbe S, Lowe NJ. Burn unit management of toxic epidermal necrolysis. *Arch Surg.* 1978;113:758–759.
109. Finlay AY, Richards J, Holt PJ. Intensive therapy unit management of toxic epidermal necrolysis: practical aspects. *Clin Exp Dermatol.* 1982;7:55–60.
110. Heimbach DM, et al. Toxic epidermal necrolysis: a step forward in treatment. *JAMA.* 1987;257:2171–2175.
111. Revuz J, et al. Treatment of toxic epidermal necrolysis. Créteil's experience. *Arch Dermatol.* 1987;123:1156–1158.
112. Green D, Law E, Still JM. An approach to the management of toxic epidermal necrolysis in a burn centre. *Burns.* 1993;19:411–414.
113. Roujeau J. Drug induced toxic epidermal necrolysis. I Current aspects. *Clin Dermatol.* 1993;11:493–500.
114. Artz CP, Rittenbury MS, Yarbrough DR. An appraisal of allografts and xenografts as biological dressings for wounds and burns. *Ann Surg.* 1972;175:934–938.
115. Kaufman T, et al. Topical treatment of toxic epidermal necrolysis with iodoplex. *J Burn Care Rehab.* 1991;12:346–348.
116. Dalli RL, et al. Toxic epidermal necrolysis/Stevens-Johnson syndrome: current trends in management. *ANZ J Surg.* 2007;77:671–676.
117. Garcia-Doval I, et al. Toxic epidermal necrolysis and Stevens-Johnson syndrome: does early withdrawal of causative drugs decrease the risk of death? *Arch Dermatol.* 2000;136:323–327.
118. Garabiol B, Touraine R. Syndrome de Lyell de l'adulte: éléments de prognostic et déductions thérapeutiques: étude de 27 cas. *Ann Med Interne.* 1976;127:670–672.
119. Ginsburg CM. Stevens-Johnson syndrome in children. *Pediatr Infect Dis J.* 1982;1:155–158.
120. Halebian PH. Improved burn center survival of patients with toxic epidermal necrolysis managed without corticosteroids. *Ann Surg.* 1986;204:503–512.
121. Kim PS, et al. Stevens-Johnson syndrome and toxic epidermal necrolysis: a pathophysiologic review with recommendations for a treatment protocol. *J Burn Care Rehab.* 1983;4:91–100.
122. Kint A, Geerts ML, de Weert J. Le syndrome de Lyell. *Dermatologica.* 1981;163:433–454.
123. Lyell A. A review of toxic epidermal necrolysis in Britain. *Br J Dermatol.* 1967;79:662–671.
124. Nethercott JR, Choi BCK. Erythema multiforme (Stevens-Johnson syndrome) – chart review of 123 hospitalized patients. *Dermatologica.* 1985;171:383–396.
125. Simons HW. Acute life-threatening dermatologic disorders. *Med Clin North Am.* 1981;65:227–243.
126. Ting HC, Adam BA. Erythema multiforme – response to corticosteroid. *Dermatologica.* 1984;169:175–178.
127. Björnberg A. Fifteen cases of toxic epidermal necrolysis (Lyell). *Acta Derm Venereol.* 1973;53:149–152.
128. Marvin JA, et al. Improved treatment of the Stevens-Johnson syndrome. *Arch Surg.* 1984;119:601–605.
129. Rasmussen JE. Erythema multiforme in children: response to treatment with systemic corticosteroids. *Br J Dermatol.* 1976;95:181–186.
130. Renfro L, Grant-Kels JM, Daman LA. Drug-induced toxic epidermal necrolysis treated with cyclosporine. *Int J Dermatol.* 1989;28:441–444.
131. Kamanabroo D, Schmitz-Landgraf W, Czarnetzki BM. Plasmapheresis in severe drug-induced toxic epidermal necrolysis. *Arch Dermatol.* 1985;121:1548–1549.
132. Sakellariou G, et al. Plasma exchange (PE) treatment in drug-induced toxic epidermal necrolysis. *Int J Artif Organs.* 1991;14:634–638.
133. Yamada H, Takamori K. Status of plasmapheresis for the treatment of toxic epidermal necrolysis in Japan. *Ther Apher Dial.* 2008;12:355–359.
134. Yamane Y, et al. Analysis of Stevens-Johnson syndrome and toxic epidermal necrolysis in Japan from 2000 to 2006, *Allergol Int.* 2007; 56:419–425.
135. Cazzola G, et al. High-dose i.v. 7S immunoglobulin treatment in Stevens-Johnson syndrome. *Helv Paediatr Acta.* 1986;41:87–88.
136. Amato GM, et al. The use of intravenous high-dose immunoglobulins (IGIV) in a case of Stevens-Johnson syndrome. *Pediatr Med Chir.* 1992;14:555–556.
137. Moudgil A, et al. Treatment of Stevens-Johnson syndrome with pooled human intravenous immune globulin. *Clin Pediatr.* 1995;34:48–51.
138. Tan AW, et al. High-dose intravenous immunoglobulins in the treatment of toxic epidermal necrolysis: an Asian series. *J Dermatol.* 2005;32:1–6.
139. Mittmann N, et al. Intravenous immunoglobulin use in patients with toxic epidermal necrolysis and Stevens-Johnson syndrome. *Am J Clin Dermatol.* 2006;7:359–368.
140. Stella M, et al. Toxic epidermal necrolysis (TEN) and Stevens Johnson syndrome (SJS): experience with high-dose intravenous immunoglobulins and topical conservative approach. A retrospective analysis. *Burns.* 2007;33:452–459.

141. Kurkcuoglu N, Alli N. Cimetidine prevents recurrent erythema multiforme major resulting from herpes simplex virus infection. *J Am Acad Dermatol.* 1989;1:814–815.
142. Robin JB, Dugel R. Immunologic disorders of the cornea and conjunctiva. In Kaufman HE, et al, eds. *The cornea.* Edinburgh: Churchill Livingstone; 1988.
143. Gregory DG. The ophthalmologic management of acute Stevens-Johnson syndrome. *Ocul Surf.* 2008;6:87–95.
144. Tandon A, et al. Amniotic membrane grafting for conjunctival and lid surface disease in the acute phase of toxic epidermal necrolysis. *J AAPOS.* 2007;11:612–613.
145. Mugit MM, et al. Technique of amniotic membrane transplant dressing in the management of acute Stevens-Johnson syndrome. *Br J Ophthalmol.* 2007;91:1536.
146. Bartley GB, Lowry JC. Argon laser treatment of trichiasis. *Am J Ophthalmol.* 1992;113:71–74.
147. Hecht SD. Cryotherapy of trichiasis with use of the retinal cryoprobe. *Ann Ophthalmol.* 1977;9:1501–1503.
148. Callahan A. Correction of entropion from Stevens-Johnson syndrome, use of nasal septum and mucosa for severely cicatrized eyelid entropion. *Arch Ophthalmol.* 1976;94:1154–1155.
149. Leone CR Jr. Mucous membrane grafting for cicatricial entropion. *Ophthalmic Surg.* 1974;5(2):24–28.
150. McCord CD Jr, Chen WP. Tarsal polishing and mucous membrane grafting for cicatricial entropion, trichiasis and epidermalization. *Ophthalmic Surg.* 1983;14:1021–1025.
151. Naumann GO, Rummelt V. Hard-palate mucosa graft in Stevens-Johnson syndrome. *Am J Ophthalmol.* 1995;119(6):817–819.
152. Mannor GE, et al. Hard-palate mucosa graft in Stevens-Johnson syndrome. *Am J Ophthalmol.* 1994;118(6):786–791.
153. Callahan A. Correction of entropion from Stevens-Johnson syndrome: use of nasal septum and mucosa for severely cicatrized eyelid entropion *Arch Ophthalmol.* 1976;94(7):1154–1155.
154. Naumann GO, et al. Autologous nasal mucosa transplantation in severe bilateral conjunctival mucus deficiency syndrome. *Ophthalmology.* 1990;97(8):1011–1017.
155. Heiligenhaus A, et al. Long-term results of mucous membrane grafting in ocular cicatricial pemphigoid. Implications for patient selection and surgical considerations. *Ophthalmology.* 1993;100(9):1283–1288.
156. Shore JW, et al. Results of buccal mucosal grafting for patients with medically controlled ocular cicatricial pemphigoid. *Ophthalmology.* 1992;99(3):383–395.
157. McCord CD Jr, Chen WP. Tarsal polishing and mucous membrane grafting for cicatricial entropion, trichiasis and epidermalization. *Ophthalmic Surg.* 1983;14(12):1021–1025.
158. Solomon A, Espana EM, Tseng SC. Amniotic membrane transplantation for reconstruction of the conjunctival fornices. *Ophthalmology.* 2003;110(1):93–100.
159. Honavar SG, et al. Amniotic membrane transplantation for ocular surface reconstruction in Stevens-Johnson syndrome. *Ophthalmology.* 2000;107(5):975–979.
160. Auran JD, Hornblass A, Gross WD. Stevens-Johnson syndrome with associated nasolacrimal duct obstruction treated with dacryocystorhinostomy and Crawford silicone tube insertion. *Ophthal Plast Reconstr Surg.* 1993;6:60–63.
161. Shimazaki J, et al. Association of preoperative tear function with surgical outcome in severe Stevens-Johnson syndrome. *Ophthalmology.* 2000;107(8):1518–1523.
162. Brown SI, Weller CA, Akiya S. Pathogenesis of ulcers of the alkali-burned cornea. *Arch Ophthalmol.* 1970;83:205–208.
163. Rosenthal P, Cotter JM, Baum J. Treatment of persistent corneal epithelial defect with extended wear of a fluid-ventilated gas-permeable scleral contact lens. *Am J Ophthalmol.* 2000;130(1):33–41.
164. Tappin MJ, Pullum KW, Buckley RJ. Scleral contact lenses for overnight wear in the management of ocular surface disorders. *Eye.* 2001;15(Pt 2):168–172.
165. Bouchard CS, Lemp MA. Tight lens syndrome associated with a 24-hour disposable collagen lens: a case report. *CLAO J.* 1991;17:141–142.
166. Kozarsky AM, Knight SH, Waring GO III. Clinical results with a ceramic keratoprosthesis placed through the eyelid. *Ophthalmology.* 1987;94:904–911.
167. Kim MK, et al. Seoul-type keratoprosthesis: preliminary results of the first 7 human cases. *Arch Ophthalmol.* 2002;120(6):761–766.
168. Yaghouti F, et al. Keratoprosthesis: preoperative prognostic categories. *Cornea.* 2001;20(1):19–23.
169. Khan B, Dudenhoefer EJ, Dohlman CH. Keratoprosthesis: an update. *Curr Opin Ophthalmol.* 2001;12(4):282–287.
170. Dohlman CH, Terada H. Keratoprosthesis in pemphigoid and Stevens-Johnson syndrome. *Adv Exp Med Biol.* 1998;438:1021–1025.
171. Nouri M, et al. Endophthalmitis after keratoprosthesis: incidence, bacterial causes, and risk factors. *Arch Ophthalmol.* 2001;119(4):484–489.
172. Sayegh RR, et al. The Boston keratoprosthesis in Stevens-Johnson syndrome. *Am J Ophthalmol.* 2008;145:438–444.
173. Falcinelli G, et al. Modified osteo-odonto-keratoprosthesis for treatment of corneal blindness: long-term anatomical and functional outcomes in 181 cases. *Arch Ophthalmol.* 2005;123:1319–1329.
174. Tan DT, et al. Keratoprosthesis surgery for end-stage corneal blindness in Asian eyes. *Ophthalmology.* 2008;115:503–510.
175. Liu C, et al. Visual rehabilitation in end-stage inflammatory ocular surface disease with the osteo-odonto-keratoprosthesis: results from the UK. *Br J Ophthalmol.* 2008;92:1211–1217.
176. Thoft RA. Keratoepithelioplasty. *Am J Ophthalmol.* 1984;97:1–6.
177. Solomon A, et al. Long-term outcome of keratolimbal allograft with or without penetrating keratoplasty for total limbal stem cell deficiency. *Ophthalmology.* 2002;109(6):1159–1166.
178. Tsubota K, et al. Treatment of severe ocular-surface disorders with corneal epithelial stem-cell transplantation. *N Engl J Med.* 1999;340(22):1697–1703.
179. Holland EJ. Epithelial transplantation for the management of severe ocular surface disease. *Trans Am Ophthalmol Soc.* 1996;94:677–743.
180. Tsai RJ, Tseng SC. Human allograft limbal transplantation for corneal surface reconstruction. *Cornea.* 1994;13(5):389–400.
181. Dua HS, Azuara-Blanco A. Allo-limbal transplantation in patients with limbal stem cell deficiency. *Br J Ophthalmol.* 1999;83(4):414–419.
182. Tsubota K, et al. Clinical application of living-related conjunctival-limbal allograft. *Am J Ophthalmol.* 2002;133(1):134–135.
183. Daya SM, Ilari FA. Living related conjunctival limbal allograft for the treatment of stem cell deficiency. *Ophthalmology.* 2001;108(1):126–133; discussion 133–134.
184. Rao SK, et al. Limbal allografting from related live donors for corneal surface reconstruction. *Ophthalmology.* 1999;106(4):822–828.
185. Shimazaki J, et al. Transplantation of human limbal epithelium cultivated on amniotic membrane for the treatment of severe ocular surface disorders. *Ophthalmology.* 2002;109(7):1285–1290.
186. Koizumi N, et al. Cultivated corneal epithelial transplantation for ocular surface reconstruction in acute phase of Stevens-Johnson syndrome. *Arch Ophthalmol.* 2001;119(2):298–300.
187. Koizumi N, et al. Cultivated corneal epithelial stem cell transplantation in ocular surface disorders. *Ophthalmology.* 2001;108(9):1569–1574.
188. Kwitko S, et al. Allograft conjunctival transplantation for bilateral ocular surface disorders. *Ophthalmology.* 1995;102(7):1020–1025.
189. Tseng SC, et al. Amniotic membrane transplantation with or without limbal allografts for corneal surface reconstruction in patients with limbal stem cell deficiency. *Arch Ophthalmol.* 1998;116(4):431–441.
190. Solomon A, et al. Long-term outcome of keratolimbal allograft with or without penetrating keratoplasty for total limbal stem cell deficiency. *Ophthalmology.* 2002;109:1159–1166.
191. Liang L, et al. Limbal stem cell transplantation: new progresses and challenges. *Eye.* 2009;23(10):1946–1953.
192. Nakamura T, et al. Transplantation of autologous serum-derived cultivated corneal epithelial equivalents for the treatment of severe ocular surface disease. *Ophthalmology.* 2006;113:1765–1772.
193. Shimazaki J, et al. Factors influencing outcomes in cultivated limbal epithelial transplantation for chronic cicatricial ocular surface disorders. *Am J Ophthalmol.* 2007;143:945–953.
194. Higa K, Shimazaki J. Recent advances in cultivated epithelial transplantation. *Cornea Suppl.* 2008;1:S41–S47.
195. Nakamura T, et al. Transplantation of cultivated autologous oral mucosal epithelial cells in patients with severe ocular surface disorders. *Br J Ophthalmol.* 2004;88:1280–1284.
196. Ang LP, et al. Autologous serum-derived cultivated oral epithelial transplants for severe ocular surface disease. *Arch Ophthalmol.* 2006;124:1543–1551.
197. Nakamura T, et al. Phenotypic investigation of human eyes with transplanted autologous cultivated oral mucosal epithelial sheets for severe ocular surface diseases. *Ophthalmology.* 2007;114:1080–1088.
198. Kinoshita S, et al. Long-term results of keratoepithelioplasty in Mooren's ulcer. *Ophthalmology.* 1991;98:438–445.
199. Turgeon PW, et al. Indications for keratoepithelioplasty. *Arch Ophthalmol.* 1990;108:233–236.
200. Tsubota K, Shimazaki J. Surgical treatment of children blinded by Stevens-Johnson syndrome. *Am J Ophthalmol.* 1999;128(5):573–581.
201. Samson CM, et al. Limbal stem cell transplantation in chronic inflammatory eye disease. *Ophthalmology.* 2002;109(5):862–868.
202. Tseng SC, et al. Inhibition of conjunctival transdifferentiation by topical retinoids. *Invest Ophthalmol Vis Sci.* 1987;28:538–542.
203. Tseng SCG, Farazdaghi M. Reversal of conjunctival transdifferentiation by topical retinoic acid. *Cornea.* 1988;7:273–279.

204. Singer L, et al. Vitamin A in Stevens-Johnson syndrome. *Ann Ophthalmol.* 1989;21:209–210.
205. Tseng SCG, et al. Topical retinoid treatment for various dry eye disorders. *Ophthalmology.* 1985;92:717–727.
206. Uy HS, et al. Topical bevacizumab and ocular surface neovascularization in patients with Stevens-Johnson syndrome. *Cornea.* 2008;27:70–73.
207. Soong HK, et al. Topical retinoid therapy for squamous metaplasia of various ocular surface disorders. A multicenter, placebo-controlled double-masked study. *Ophthalmology.* 1988;95:1442–1446.
208. Westly ED, Wechsler HL. Toxic epidermal necrolysis. Granulocytic leukopenia as a prognostic indicator. *Arch Dermatol.* 1984;120(6):721–726.
209. Giannetti A, Malmus M, Girolomomi G. Vesiculobullous drug eruptions in children. *Clin Dermatol.* 1993;11:551–555.
210. Geerling G, et al. Costs and gains of complex procedures to rehabilitate end stage ocular surface disease. *Br J Ophthalmol.* 2002;86(11):1220–1221.

Chapter 53

Toxic Conjunctivitis

Charles D. Reilly, Mark J. Mannis

Introduction

Toxic conjunctivitis has been known since antiquity, but descriptions of this entity were not typical until a case of keratoconjunctivitis caused by topical atropine was described by Von Graefe in 1864.[1] This chapter reviews the subject of toxic keratoconjunctivitis primarily due to the use of topical ophthalmic preparations. Other chapters in this text will address other causes of toxic reactions of the ocular surface, although other causes of toxic keratoconjunctivitis are mentioned here, including cosmetics, hair care products, tear gas weapons, and industrial chemical exposures.

Toxicity versus Allergy

Topical medications can confuse the clinical picture, since patients are often helped by the medications initially, but as the medications are continued the condition being treated appears to worsen as a result of medication toxicity. This poses the question for the clinician as to whether signs and symptoms are due to the worsening underlying disease process or to medication toxicity. Very often, both toxic and allergic mechanisms are active to varying degrees, depending on the frequency, duration, and strength of the medication. However, certain characteristics of the allergic and toxic reactions help to distinguish the two in most situations in which one or the other is dominant.

Cellular mechanisms

Toxicity implies damage to the structure of the ocular tissues, or disturbance of function, with or without an accompanying inflammatory response. This damage may occur as a direct result of the drug itself, the accompanying preservatives, or from breakdown products of the drug.

Allergic reactions may be of the anaphylactoid (type 1) or of the delayed (type IV) hypersensitivity type. The type 1 reaction is characterized by the union of allergen, IgE antibody, and mast cells, leading to the degranulation of the mast cell and the release of multiple mediators, including histamine, various chemotactic factors, and others. These mediators are responsible for the signs and symptoms of the acute allergic reaction. In the delayed hypersensitivity reaction, drugs act as haptens that conjugate with proteins. This conjugate combines with T lymphocytes, leading to the elaboration of various lymphokines, which mediate the inflammatory response.

Signs and symptoms

In general, allergic reactions are characterized by chronicity. Repeated exposure to the agent and adequate sensitization time are needed for the reaction to develop. The development of this reaction may require an amount of time ranging from days to years. On the other hand, a toxic reaction, although also often requiring repeated exposure, may occur with the first exposure to the agent.

Conjunctival redness, chemosis, lid or periorbital swelling, mucous discharge, papillary palpebral conjunctival reaction, and itching are common manifestations of allergy. Itching may be the strongest indication of allergic conjunctivitis. Many of the available topical medications may cause this type of reaction, perhaps the most common being idoxuridine (IDU), gentamicin, atropine, and neomycin.[1,2]

In allergic conjunctivitis, a papillary reaction of the tarsal conjunctiva may occur, as well as a milky chemosis with hyperemia. Papillary reactions are common in toxic conjunctivitis also, but in addition, a follicular component may be present. Follicles are generally not seen in allergy alone, and may be a key sign suggesting toxicity. Table 53.1 lists medications associated with follicular conjunctivitis.[3,4]

In addition, the hyperemia and chemosis that may occur with toxicity may not be as diffusely distributed on the bulbar conjunctiva as in the allergic reaction, but may spare the superior aspect relatively. It is often more prominent in the inferonasal cornea and conjunctiva from the natural Bell's phenomena and the locus of the direct placement of topical drops (Figs 53.1, 53.2, 53.3).

Allergic conjunctivitis is often associated with a mucous discharge that is typically thin and clear. A more purulent or mucopurulent discharge may be associated with toxicity.

The cornea in allergic conjunctivitis is often unaffected or may show punctate staining with fluorescein, more prominent inferiorly. The cornea in toxic reactions, on the other hand, may demonstrate a broad range of involvement, from mild punctate keratitis to severe ulcerative keratopathy. As described by Wilson, the most common manifestations are coarse and punctate epithelial lesions. Heaps and swirls of

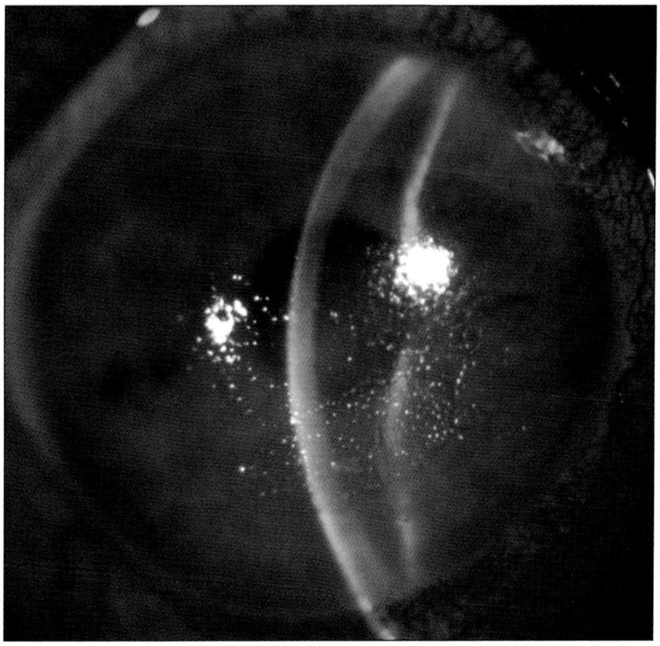

Fig. 53.1 Toxic ulcerative keratopathy secondary to preservatives in artificial tear solutions. Note the oval epithelial defect with coarse surrounding keratitis, resembling a 'comet's impact' crater. The epithelial defect has a well-defined, rolled margin. Marked inferior and inferonasal conjunctival injection is present, as well as intense ciliary flush. (Courtesy of Ivan R. Schwab.)

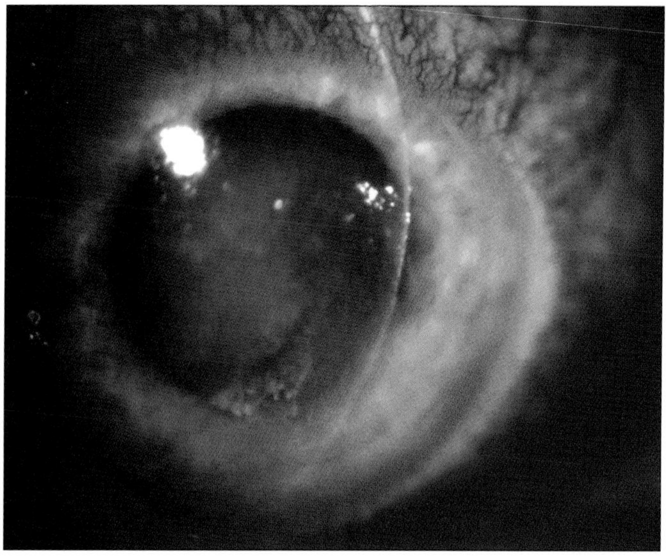

Fig. 53.2 Toxic keratoconjunctivitis secondary to topical gentamicin. The epithelium is diffusely irregular, but more so inferiorly. The increased conjunctival injection inferiorly and inferonasally is characteristic. (Courtesy of Ivan R. Schwab.)

Table 53.1 Topical ophthalmic medications associated with follicular conjunctivitis

Physostigmine	Demecarium
Echothiophate	Isoflurophate
Diisopropylfluorophosphate	Gentamicin
Neostigmine	Framycetin
Furtrethonium iodide	Neomycin
Pilocarpine	Sulfacetamide
Atropine	Sulfamethizole
Idoxuridine	Sulfisoxazole
Aproclonidine	Amphotericin B
Bromonidine	Scopolamine
Carbachol	Diatrizoate
Epinephrine	Hyaluronidase
Dipivefren	Meglumine

Adapted from Wilkerson M, Lewis RA, Shields MB: Follicular conjunctivitis associated with apraclonidine, Am J Ophthalmol 111(1):105–106, 1991; Watts P, Hawksworth N. Delayed hypersensitivity to brimonidine tartate 0.2% associated with high intraocular pressure, Eye 16(2):132–135, 2002; and Cai F, Backman Ha, Baines MG: Thimerosal. an ophthalmic preservative which acts as a hapten to elicit specific antibodies and cell mediated immunity, Curr Eye Res 7;341–351, 1988.

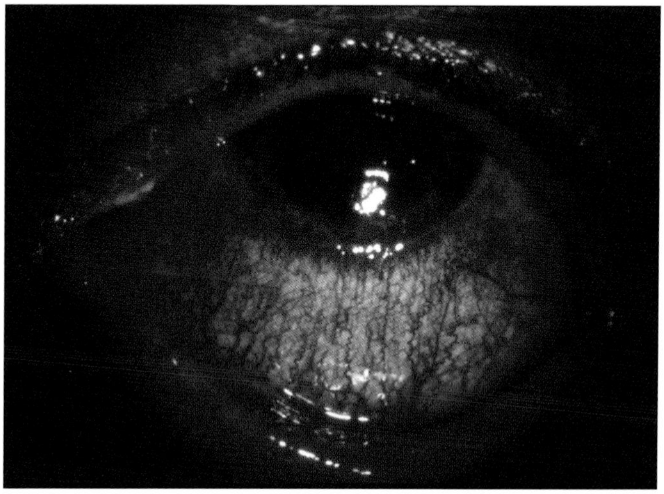

Fig. 53.3 Toxic keratoconjunctivitis secondary to topical trifluorothymidine (Viroptic). Once again, seen here is the characteristic corneal epithelial irregularity and conjunctival injection more prominent in the inferior aspect of the eye. (Courtesy of Ivan R. Schwab.)

opaque epithelium may occur as well, which may lead to large erosions. Pseudodendrites may develop, resembling herpetic dendrites.[2] Schwab and Abbott emphasized the importance of the largely unrecognized problem of toxic ulcerative keratopathy.[5] They described a series of patients with similar findings secondary to inappropriate use of topical medications, including anesthetic abuse. All of these patients had oval epithelial defects located primarily in the inferonasal quadrants, with coarse surrounding keratitis, resembling a 'comet's impact' crater (see Fig. 53.1). Mucous threads, intense ciliary flush, papillary tarsal response, chemosis, and marked inferior or inferonasal injection were also common (see Figs 53.1, 53.2, 53.3). The epithelial defects typically had rolled, but not heaped, margins. These findings were observed in patients with iatrogenic toxic keratopathy as well as in factitious, self-induced keratoconjunctivitis.

Diagnostic testing

Various clinical tests are available, although not often performed, which may help to distinguish allergy from toxicity. The standard clinical test for the diagnosis of type 1 hypersensitivity is the intradermal skin test, in which injection of the agent intradermally elicits a wheal and flare reaction within seconds or minutes. The ocular equivalent of this – application of the substance into the conjunctival fornix – may yield a positive result with immediate chemosis, hyperemia, itching, and eyelid swelling.[2] The standard test for type IV hypersensitivity, or contact dermatitis, is the patch test. Here, the substance is applied to the skin and covered. Examination of the skin 24 to 48 hours later may reveal a contact dermatitis if positive. However, false negatives and false positives may both occur, and a careful history is often more helpful in making this diagnosis. Conjunctival scrapings may show eosinophils in allergic conjunctivitis and not in toxic reactions. In addition, large toxic granules may be present in the cytoplasm of epithelial, mononuclear, and polymorphonuclear cells. These are large basophilic granules that differ from the usual smaller neutrophilic granules. However, they are not specific for toxicity, and may be found in allergic responses as well.[2]

Toxic Keratoconjunctivitis Related to Topical Medications

Topical medications of all therapeutic categories may cause external ocular irritation, either from a direct effect of the active chemical or from degradation products and preservatives. Topical drugs produce higher concentrations in the cornea and conjunctiva than in the other ocular tissues and may, therefore, more easily affect the function and structure of the epithelial cells adversely.[6]

Methods of assessing toxicity

Many techniques have been devised to measure the adverse effects of topical agents to the external eye quantitatively or qualitatively. Animal testing has long been a standard method of evaluating the acceptability of drugs for safe human use. A modified Draize test uses rabbits, whose eyes are more sensitive to many chemicals than are monkey or human eyes. In this ocular irritation test, the rabbit eye is treated with topical agents for 3 weeks, evaluated for 1 week, and then sacrificed for histological study. As pointed out by Burstein, however, this method cannot reliably detect surface defects, because epithelial defects are able to heal in less than 3 days.[6] Other tests include wound healing models to evaluate the adverse or beneficial effects of drugs on reepithelialization and corneal permeability measurements with fluorometry, electrophysiologic monitoring, and isotope localization. Morphologic evaluation is possible with specular and confocal microscopy, transmission electron microscopy, and scanning electron microscopy. Pfister and Burstein have looked at the effects of many drugs, vehicles, and preservatives on the corneal epithelium with the scanning electron microscope, demonstrating effects ranging from changes in the cellular microvilli position to frank loss of superficial layers of epithelial cells.[7] In vivo tandem scanning confocal microscopy has been used to detect desquamation of superficial epithelial cells secondary to benzalkonium chloride in rabbits.[8] Cell culture techniques allow in vitro assessment of cytologic effects of drugs but are not an accurate depiction of the in vivo environment. Efforts are being made to avoid testing of damaging chemicals and drugs on animals, a potentially advantageous but difficult proposition; many recent publications are concerned with developing alternatives to testing on animal eyes. Investigators are now using cultured rabbit and human conjunctival cell lines in vitro to collect data concerning toxicity of topical ophthalmic preparations.

Toxicity of specific agents

The specific effects of all topical medications have been catalogued in other comprehensive sources.[9] The following is a review of some of the more common medications associated with toxic keratoconjunctivitis.

Antivirals

The three common topical antiviral preparations are IDU (Stoxil, Herplex, Dendrid), vidarabine (Vira-A), and trifluorothymidine (Viroptic). Although all three are associated with toxic keratoconjunctivitis, IDU may cause more severe irritation than the others. In the treatment of herpes simplex keratitis, IDU not uncommonly produces a punctate keratitis, epithelial edema, and corneal erosions with heaped opaque epithelium and pseudodendrites. Overtreatment with IDU may produce the clinical appearance of continued or worsened herpetic disease because of its ability to perpetuate postherpetic defects or indolent ulcers. IDU is also one of several medications known to elicit a follicular response on the palpebral conjunctiva with occasional conjunctival scarring and punctal occlusion (pseudotrachoma *or pseudopemphigoid* syndrome).[2] Although IDU probably does not retard epithelial healing, wounds involving the corneal stroma exhibit abnormally slow healing.[9]

Trifluorothymidine and vidarabine also may produce punctate keratitis and corneal erosions, but to a lesser degree. These medications are generally not associated with a *pseudopemphigoid* syndrome. Corneal epithelial dysplasia may develop with trifluorothymidine use.[10] Although not available in the United States, topical acyclovir is also an effective antiviral agent with low toxicity that has been very well tolerated.[11,12]

Glaucoma medications

The miotic alkaloids, such as pilocarpine and carbachol, are fairly common causes of nonspecific irritative conjunctivitis, most likely related to the fact that these drugs form toxic degradation products.[2] Pilocarpine is also one of the topical medications known to cause conjunctival follicles.[13] It may also be involved in a drug-induced cicatricial pemphigoid.[14]

Epinephrine, not commonly in current use, is associated with contact sensitivity as well as an actual toxic effect on the epithelium. Follicular conjunctivitis and occasionally cicatricial pemphigoid are also associated with long-term use. Adrenomelanin (adrenochrome) deposits, tiny black or brown specks in the conjunctiva, are commonly produced by chronic use of epinephrine eye drops, and are not associated with discomfort or inflammation.[15] These deposits represent material produced by oxidation and polymerization of epinephrine. A black cornea, in which the cornea appears coated with a black plaque of amorphous material, may occur as a result of the same adrenomelanin accumulating in the anterior cornea; this usually occurs in cases in which the corneal epithelium is already abnormal from edema or trauma.

Dipivefrin (Propine), an ophthalmic adrenergic designed to minimize some of the adverse effects of epinephrine, is also associated with a follicular conjunctivitis that resolves with discontinuation of the drug.[16]

Topical beta-adrenergic blockers such as timolol are generally associated with little external ocular irritation, although systemic and cardiovascular effects are well documented. Timolol has been associated with corneal hypoesthesia, punctate epithelial keratopathy, and pseudodentrites.[17] Corneal epithelial erosions have been reported with timolol use and concomitant contact lens wear.[18]

Dorzolamide has been associated with the development of a mucopurulent sterile conjunctivitis as a toxic side effect of this newer class of antiglaucoma medication.[19]

Apraclonidine hydrochloride (Iopidine) and brimonidine (Alphagan), alfa-2-adrenergic agonists, have as their most common adverse effect allergic blepharoconjunctivitis that occurs in up to 20–30% of patients.[20] The discontinuation rate of Iopidine 0.5% has been reported at 15%. It has also been reported to cause a follicular conjunctivitis.[3] Brimonidine has undergone a change in its preservative from benzalkonium chloride (BAK) to Purite™ in an attempt to limit toxic side effects of the medication. A study by Katz demonstrated a 41% lower incidence of allergic conjunctivitis in the brimonidine with Purite™ group versus the brimonidine with BAK group.[21]

The prostaglandin group of antiglaucoma medications has become a major new class of medications with known toxicity to conjunctiva. Latanoprost, travoprost, bimatoprost, and unoprostone isopropyl are included in this class of medication. A common side effect is conjunctival hyperemia but true toxicity has been reported with latanoprost (Xalatan).[22] As clinical experience with this class of medications becomes greater, the incidence of allergic and toxic reactions to these medications will become better defined.

Antibiotics and antifungals

Of the aminoglycoside antibiotics, tobramycin may be the least irritative, with generally less ocular toxicity than gentamicin.[23] Localized ocular toxicity and hypersensitivity, eyelid itching, eyelid swelling, and conjunctival hyperemia have occurred occasionally with tobramycin, as well as gentamicin.

Fortified cefazolin (5%) is commonly used in the empiric treatment of infectious keratitis, often in conjunction with fortified gentamicin or tobramycin. It is relatively nontoxic and affects corneal epithelial wound healing less than tobramycin, gentamicin, chloramphenicol, sulfacetamide, and neomycin.[21]

Topical bacitracin, in a dose of 500 units/g, is not irritating to the conjunctiva or cornea and does not interfere with epithelial healing. Contact sensitivity, however, is frequently associated with bacitracin.[24]

Neomycin commonly causes an allergic reaction of the eye with prolonged use, as well as a toxic conjunctivitis, with cutaneous and conjunctival sensitization reported to occur in 5–15% of patients.[23]

Topical penicillin is rarely used because of its well-known allergenic tendency and it may cause anaphylaxis in a sensitized person. Allergic blepharitis is noted in as many as 16% of patients.[23]

Chloramphenicol is another rarely used topical antibiotic. Although it is generally very well tolerated, with very little effect on epithelial integrity and wound healing, it has been associated with bone marrow suppression and aplastic anemia, and for this reason is used uncommonly.[25–28]

Polymyxin B is generally nonirritating to the eye, but repeated applications can lead to irritation and low-grade conjunctivitis; allergic reactions are rare.[29]

Topical sulfonamides may produce an allergic reaction, and the more serious may rarely induce Stevens-Johnson syndrome or toxic epidermal necrolysis.[30–32] Circumscribed sunburn of the lid margin has occurred from local photosensitization after topical sulfisoxazole ointment application.[33]

The fluoroquinolones, the most commonly employed topical antimicrobial agents, are generally less toxic than aminoglycosides. Agents associated with corneal epithelial toxicity, ranked from least to most, are as follows: ciprofloxacin and temafloxacin, norfloxacin, ofloxacin, pefloxacin.[34] A relatively common finding in patients treated with ciprofloxacin for corneal ulcers is a white crystalline precipitate located in the superficial aspect of the ocular surface defect (17%).[35] The latest generation of the fluoroquinolones, moxifloxacin and gatifloxacin, are gaining more widespread use in the ophthalmic and primary care communities. Clinical experience with toxicity from these newer-generation quinolones is limited but, as with other antibiotics of this class, epithelial toxicity will continue to be a concern. Gatifloxacin is being produced with the preservative benzalkonium chloride, which is a well-known preservative that can cause toxic reactions. Benzalkonium chloride toxicity is discussed below. Moxifloxacin has no added chemical preservatives and instead relies on its own pH and inherent stability to maintain potency.

A topical macrolide antibiotic, azithromycin 1%, has been recently approved for ophthalmic use in the United States. It appears to be well tolerated, but it does contain benzalkonium chloride at a concentration of 0.003%, so toxicity from the preservative may be observed.

There are three major classes of antifungal medications: polyenes, pyrimidines, and imidazoles. Amphotericin B and Natamycin (pimaricin) are polyenes. Although not available in ophthalmic preparations, a topical solution of amphotericin B may be prepared by diluting the intravenous form to strengths from 0.05% to 0.2%. One percent amphotericin causes corneal epithelial defects and may impair epithelial healing.[36] Subconjunctival injection of amphotericin B has been associated with permanent conjunctival yellowing and the formation of a raised nodule.[37] Natamycin, which is commercially available in topical ophthalmic preparations, is generally nonirritating.[38] In the pyrimidine group, flucytosine as a 1.0% solution has relatively low toxicity.[39] None of the imidazoles – clotrimazole, miconazole, econazole, and ketoconazole – are commercially available for ophthalmic use, but topical preparations may be adapted. These seem to be well tolerated in general, although miconazole may be severely irritating to the epithelium and has produced punctate keratitis with pinpoint vesicular epithelial elevations in one patient with *Acanthamoeba* keratitis.[39] Ketoconazole may cause transient epithelial disturbances.[36]

Anesthetics

Repeated use or abuse of topical anesthetic agents is a well-known cause of severe corneal damage. Numerous reports exist in the literature implicating different local anesthetics in toxic keratopathy of varying degrees.[18] Single application of a topical anesthetic, for diagnostic purposes, may produce stinging, as well as spotty drying of the corneal epithelium from decreased blinking.[2] The syndrome of anesthetic abuse is rather characteristic. A traumatic corneal epithelial injury or other disorder leads to the indiscriminate use of topical anesthetics for the instant relief provided. The patient may take the anesthetic from the doctor's office after instillation by the physician produces welcomed relief. However, pain control becomes increasingly more difficult, as the period of relief decreases with continued anesthetic use. Conjunctival hyperemia, photophobia, lid swelling, and erythema develop. Corneal epithelial defects appear with rolled, heaped-up edges. The stroma may become edematous and infiltrated, often with a ring-shaped infiltrate. This ring infiltrate may mislead the clinician to the diagnosis of *Acanthamoeba* keratitis, which may present with the same clinical signs and symptoms. Iridocyclitis, hypopyon, and hyphema may occur. In one case, abuse of topical proparacaine following a corneal transplant for HSV keratitis led ultimately to necrosis of the graft, wound dehiscence, and uveal prolapse requiring a repeat corneal transplant and full conjunctival flap.[40] Many local anesthetics have been responsible for toxic keratopathy, including proparacaine, tetracaine, lidocaine, buracaine, cornecaine, and benoxinate.[18] Topical anesthetics destabilize the tear film, interfere with cell metabolism and cell membrane permeability, directly damage cytoskeletal proteins, and decrease epithelial wound healing.[2,18,41–44] The potentially devastating effects of prolonged anesthetic use have been amply demonstrated in the literature, and it is clear that they do not have a place in the long-term treatment of eye disease.

Preservatives

The US Food and Drug Administration requires the use of preservatives for multiple-dose containers. In addition, some drugs require an antioxidant as a preservative to prevent oxidation. Although preservatives play an important role in reducing the incidence of ocular infections related to topical medications, they might be quite toxic to the corneal and conjunctival epithelium. Therefore, in situations in which the drug itself is relatively well tolerated, the preservative accompanying the drug may produce an unwanted keratopathy that improves only with cessation of the agent. A number of chemicals have been used as preservatives in eye drops, including benzalkonium chloride, benzethonium chloride, cetylpyridinium chloride, chlorhexidine, chlorobutanol, edetate, paraben esters, phenyl mercuric salts, and thimerosal. Of these, the agents that are in principal use are benzalkonium, benzalkonium with edetate, chlorobutanol, and thimerosal.[18]

Benzalkonium chloride (BAK) is a quaternary ammonium cationic agent that is widely used as a preservative in eye drops. It is also highly toxic to the eye. In higher concentrations, such as 2% or 10%, a single drop of BAK may cause very significant damage to the cornea, including the endothelium, with resulting edema and clouding.[45] In topical preparations, BAK is commonly used in dilutions from 0.005% to 0.033%. At these concentrations, the drug is generally not irritating. However, with frequent or extended use, lacrimation, edema, hyperemia, and punctate keratitis may result. Wilson suggests that this may be related to the instability of the tear film induced by BAK.[46] Epithelial wound healing is also retarded. When used with soft contact lenses, epithelial toxicity is augmented as a result of the binding of BAK to the lenses.[45]

Chlorobutanol is another commonly used preservative in topical medications, usually in concentrations of 0.5%. This preservative is generally very well tolerated and in rat studies has been found to be less toxic than BAK, chlorhexidine, and thimerosal at their usual concentrations.[47] However, experiments in which the corneal epithelium was exposed continuously to solutions containing chlorobutanol for prolonged periods of time have produced a transient keratitis with punctate changes and light haze.[18] Animal experiments have demonstrated that chlorobutanol reduces epithelial cohesion, inhibits oxygen uptake, and reduces adhesion of epithelium to the corneal stroma.[18] Chlorobutanol tends to be unstable with long-term storage.[48]

Thimerosal is a mercury-containing preservative in eye drops. In artificial tear solutions, it has been a frequent cause of irritation and inflammation in eyes of contact lens wearers, with hyperemia and punctate epithelial keratopathy resulting in some cases.[49] In addition to irritative reactions, thimerosal commonly produces hypersensitivity reactions, especially in contact lens wearers, with anterior stromal infiltrates and conjunctival follicles resulting.[50] In fact, the incidence of thimerosal hypersensitivity in the United States has been reported to be from 6.6% to 8%.[46] Historically, mercury-containing compounds, specifically those containing phenylmercuric nitrate or phenylmercuric acetate, have been known to cause a calcific band-shaped keratopathy similar to that seen in workers exposed to mercury vapors. These agents also caused deposition of mercury in the cornea at the level of Descemet's membrane, and in the central aspect of the anterior lens capsule, an entity known as mercurialentis.[1] However, clinically, thimerosal has not been found to produce these problems.

Follicular conjunctivitis

As mentioned before, a number of ophthalmic preparations are capable of causing a follicular conjunctivitis (see Table 53.1), which is presumably irritative in nature rather than allergic. The lack of itching, conjunctival eosinophilia, or dermatitis supports a toxic mechanism over an allergic one.[2] Follicles appear on the tarsal conjunctiva, with a greater distribution in the lower tarsal conjunctiva than the upper. In addition, follicles may occasionally be found on the bulbar conjunctiva, particularly with dipivefrin (Propine) use.[16] When on the bulbar conjunctiva, the reaction is often more severe in the area of the semilunar plica or around the limbus.[16] Perhaps the drugs most often associated with a follicular response are the antivirals (idoxuridine, vidarabine, trifluorothymidine) and dipivefrin.[16,51] Regardless of the inciting agent, the follicles are similar both clinically and histopathologically, although they have not been shown to have fully developed germinal centers.[2,52] The same medications that cause a follicular conjunctivitis may also produce a '*pseudopemphigoid* syndrome,' with conjunctival scarring, keratitis, and pannus; Herbert's pits are absent, however.[52] Punctal and even canalicular occlusion can develop.[2] In general, the follicles gradually resolve with cessation of the medication. Corticosteroids tend to have little or no effect on the conjunctivitis.[2]

Hurricane keratitis

A characteristic pattern of epithelial keratopathy occurs frequently in postoperative corneal transplant patients as a result of the toxicity of topical medications. A whorl-shaped punctate keratopathy develops as early as 1 week postoperatively, extending from the peripheral graft inward (Fig. 53.4).[54] The presumed mechanism is related to the intrinsic pattern of corneal epithelial repair, which appears to be a spiral or whorl-shaped epithelial slide.[55,56] The epithelium of the corneal graft is highly sensitive to the toxic effects of topical medications. Hurricane keratitis usually resolves completely following cessation of offending toxic agents, which may include antibiotics, cycloplegics, antiglaucoma medications, or preservatives (especially benzalkonium chloride).[54]

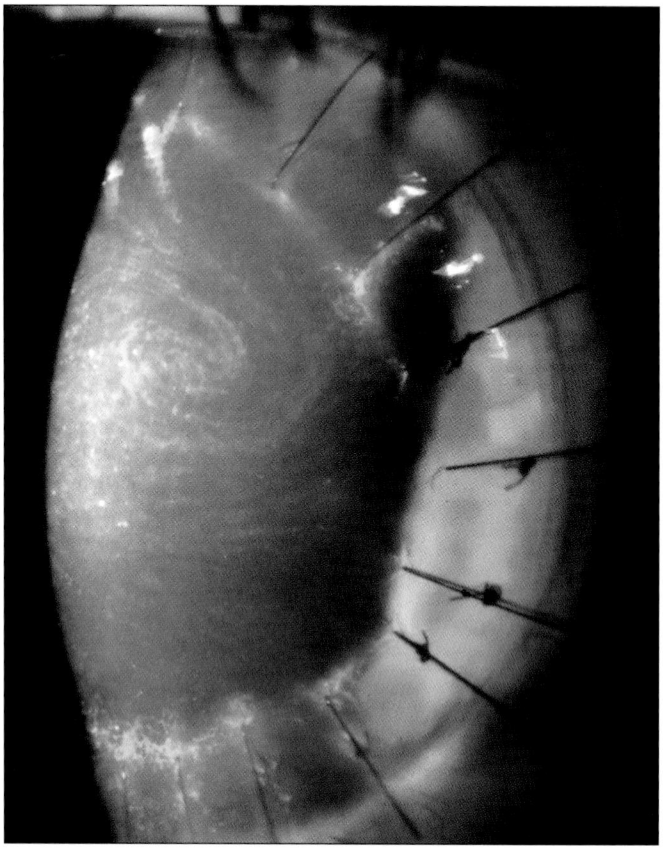

Fig. 53.4 Hurricane keratitis in a corneal graft. The whorl-shaped punctate epithelial keratopathy seen here may in part be due to medications in corneal transplant patients. (Courtesy of Mark J. Mannis.)

Drug-induced cicatricial pemphigoid

A number of topical ophthalmic medications have been implicated in causing a clinical syndrome very similar to idiopathic ocular cicatricial pemphigoid. The idiopathic form, presumably of autoimmune etiology, is characterized by chronic conjunctivitis, conjunctival shrinkage, symblepharon formation, trichiasis, keratopathy, keratitis sicca, and ocular surface keratinization. Drugs identified as causing physical findings indistinguishable from this syndrome include antivirals (IDU[57] and trifluorothymidine), miotics (echothiophate iodide[58] and pilocarpine[59]), sympathetic agents (epinephrine and dipivefrin hydrochloride[60]), and beta blockers (timolol[14]). As in the idiopathic, autoimmune form of the disease, patients may even demonstrate immunoglobulins bound to the basement membrane of the conjunctiva,[57,58,61] with light and electron microscopy revealing findings identical to those in idiopathic pemphigoid.[14] As outlined by Mondino, there are five possible explanations offered for the role of topical medications in the development of cicatricial pemphigoid: (1) the drug may cause nonprogressive scarring that mimics cicatricial pemphigoid, which is progressive; (2) the relationship may be purely coincidental; (3) the drug may somehow catalyze the development of pemphigoid that may have developed anyway; (4) the drug may be a cause of cicatricial pemphigoid; or (5) cicatricial pemphigoid may cause glaucoma by scarring the outflow pathway, requiring topical glaucoma medication.[62,63] A reasonable therapeutic approach set forth by Mondino is to stop any drug that has been implicated in its development and to watch for further signs of progression. If progression occurs, immunosuppressive agents (corticosteroids, dapsone, cyclophosphamide) may be used; if no progression occurs, the patient is simply followed.

Others Causes of Toxic Keratoconjunctivitis

Cosmetics and skin care products

Mascara or eyeliner can produce an asymptomatic follicular response on the tarsal conjunctiva. Often, darkly pigmented granules of cosmetic material accumulate in the tarsal conjunctiva and in the follicles. Typically, the pigment deposits are found at the upper margin of the tarsus of the everted upper lid.[18] The bulbar conjunctiva and cornea are generally not affected. Cessation of the cosmetic is not required unless the condition is symptomatic.[2,18,53] Eye cosmetics have been reported to cause other types of irritation in addition to pigment deposits and follicular conjunctivitis. Certain skin moisturizers, eye creams, and wrinkle creams can cause ocular discomfort, burning, and stinging when applied to the face some distance from the eyes. This results presumably from the chemical spreading over the skin to the eye, known as the eye area sensitivity syndrome.[64] Mannis and Sandler reported a case of keratitis from the use of a skin polishing agent, an abrasive cleansing material used on the facial skin. In this case, tiny beads of the abrasive agent were visible in the corneal epithelium on slit lamp examination.[65]

Hair care products

Hair sprays are occasionally directed into the eyes inadvertently, causing temporary discomfort and stinging. The sprays are usually composed of a resin that has been dissolved in alcohol and packaged under pressure for spraying. MacLean reported a large series of 'spray keratitis,' described as a punctate epithelial keratitis that involves 'a foreign-body reaction to the implantation into the corneal epithelium of small particles of relatively noncorrosive organic compounds by force of a pressurized spray.'[66] The keratitis is typically delayed in onset, mild in severity, and temporary, resolving in 1 to 3 days. Interestingly, in this series of patients, relief of irritation was aided by the use of IDU drops.

Hair groom gel has been implicated in at least one case as a cause of bilateral corneal edema. Satterfield and Mannis reported a case of a 57-year-old man observed over a period of 4 years to have intermittent bilateral corneal edema, occurring in warm weather with exertion, and spontaneously resolving within 24 to 36 hours (Fig. 53.5).[67] The corneal edema was eventually linked to the use of a hair grooming gel containing anionic detergent compounds that are known to cause corneal edema, discomfort, hyperemia, and punctate keratitis. In this case, the patient's perspiration carried the offending hair groom gel into his eyes. Cessation of the hair gel provided the cure.

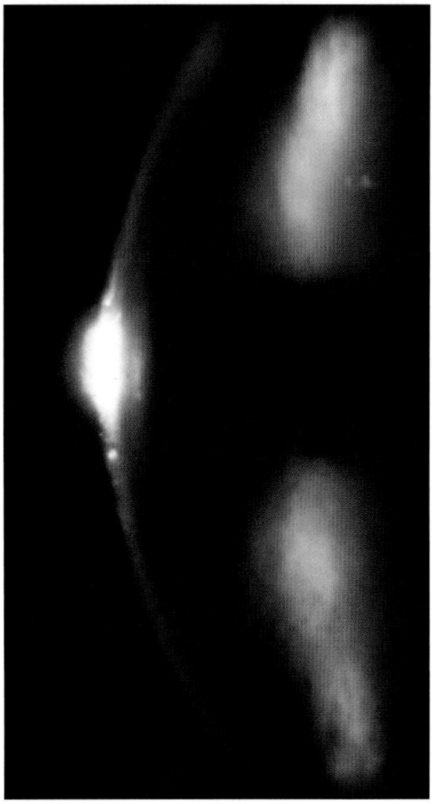

Fig. 53.5 Episodic bilateral corneal edema caused by hair groom gel. Appearance of both corneas during an acute episode of diffuse stromal and epithelial edema, punctate epithelial keratopathy, and hyperemic conjunctiva. The epithelial edema blurs iris details. (Courtesy of Mark J. Mannis and Denise Satterfield.)

Tear gas weapons and lacrimating agents

Chemical Mace is a potent solvent spray-type tear gas weapon that is commonly carried as a self-defense instrument. The active ingredient is chloroacetophenone, a powerful lacrimator, which is mixed in a solvent and kept under high pressure in a metal container. When sprayed, droplets of the solution are effectively delivered to the skin and eyes, causing an intense burning and stinging sensation, copious tearing and watering of the nose, spontaneous closing of the eyes, and a burning sensation on the skin. The spray-type tear gas is the newer and safer type; the earlier weapons were explosive and would send particles of solid concentrated chemical (lacrimator) flying at high speeds. Severe corneal damage with edema, scarring, and opacification often resulted.[68] The newer type of solvent spray weapons, of which Mace is the prototype, deliver the lacrimator in much more dilute concentrations at lower pressures and speeds. Chemical Mace generally produces temporary injury to the corneal and conjunctival epithelium which resolves within hours to days. However, certain conditions, if present, may lead to more serious and slowly healing corneal injuries. Specifically, if the victim has reduced corneal sensation and diminished protective reflexes of eye closing and lacrimation, permanent corneal opacities may result secondary to inadequate washing away of the chemical.[18] In addition, when the chemical is delivered at very close range (less than 6 feet), more serious damage may be done.[18] Inadvertent exposure to chemical Mace is best treated with copious irrigation.

Recently, the use of pepper spray has become more popular among law enforcement officers and private individuals as a nonlethal means of subduing hostile attackers. Pepper spray is an aerosolized form of oleoresin capsicum, a chemical irritant. Zollman et al. followed 11 patients who were exposed to pepper spray in a training environment and found the most significant features of ocular exposure to be pain, punctate epithelial erosions, and reduced corneal sensitivity at 10 minutes postexposure. All patient eyes returned to baseline, including normal corneal sensitivity at 1 week, with no sequelae.[69]

Therapeutic Considerations

As mentioned before, in any case in which topical medication is the cause of a persistent keratoconjunctivitis, recognition of the diagnosis of toxicity is the key to treatment. If the relationship between the offending agent and the clinical condition is overlooked, the physician is apt to continue the medication and, even worse, add others. This, of course, leads only to worsening of the toxic keratoconjunctivitis. Therefore, it is always extremely important to consider the possibility of toxicity in any chronic ocular irritation or inflammation that does not improve with seemingly appropriate treatment, or whose clinical diagnosis is not readily apparent. Likewise, one must be aware of the possibility of factitious keratoconjunctivitis and should investigate the possibility of anesthetic abuse, if suspected. This is invariably difficult and should be approached with tact and sympathy.[5] In cases of suspected chronic anesthetic abuse, measures such as extended patching, partial or complete tarsorrhaphy, or observation as an inpatient may be helpful.

Management of toxicity secondary to topical medications is cessation of the offending agent. A good first step in addressing possible toxicity is to stop as many topical medications as is feasibly permissible. Often, if the irritation is related to an expired solution that has undergone degradation, simply replacing the solution with a fresh preparation is curative. Replacement is also a diagnostic aid in distinguishing allergy from toxicity; if a fresh preparation relieves the conjunctivitis, the process is more likely to be irritative or toxic.[2] If the specific topical medication is required for treating an underlying disorder, and it cannot be feasibly discontinued, one might substitute a preservative-free preparation to eliminate the possibility of preservative toxicity. In addition, substituting an alternative medication that addresses the same problem may be helpful. Similarly, oral preparations may be practical in situations in which the topical agent is not tolerated. Once the responsible agent is stopped, nonpreserved lubricating solutions or ointments may be helpful in providing symptomatic relief.

When an epithelial defect is present, cessation of the toxic medication and patching for 1 or more days is often very effective. If necessary, partial or complete tarsorrhaphy should be considered in cases of persistent epithelial defects. Therapeutic soft contact lenses may be effective in some cases, although caution must be used in situations of coexisting dry eye or ocular adnexal disease. It is also important to remember that contact lenses may act as a repository for toxic drugs if drops are continued. In very severe cases, with large defects and/or significant thinning, conjunctival flap procedures may be warranted, particularly in cases of factitious keratoconjunctivitis or anesthetic abuse. Penetrating keratoplasty or tectonic keratoplasty is occasionally necessary when stromal perforation or impending perforation is present.

References

1. Wilson FM II. Adverse external ocular effects of topical ophthalmic therapy: an epidemiologic, laboratory, and clinical study. *Trans Am Ophthalmol Soc.* 1983;81:854–965.
2. Wilson FM II. Adverse external ocular effects of topical ophthalmic medications. *Surv Ophthalmol.* 1979;24(2):57–88.
3. Wilkerson M, Lewis RA, Shields MB. Follicular conjunctivitis associated with apraclonidine. *Am J Ophthalmol.* 1991;111(1):105–106.
4. Watts P, Hawksworth N. Delayed hypersensitivity to brimonidine tartate 0.2% associated with high intraocular pressure. *Eye.* 2002;16(2): 132–135.
5. Schwab IR, Abbott RL. Toxic ulcerative keratopathy. An unrecognized problem. *Ophthalmology.* 1989;96:1187.
6. Burstein NL. Corneal cytotoxicity of topically applied drugs, vehicles and preservatives. *Surv Ophthalmol.* 1980;25(1):15–30.
7. Pfister RR, Burstein N. The effects of ophthalmic drugs, vehicles, and preservatives on corneal epithelium: a scanning electron microscope study. *Invest Ophthalmol.* 1976;15:246–259.
8. Ichijima H, et al. Confocal microscopic studies of living rabbit cornea treated with benzalkonium chloride. *Cornea.* 1992;11(3):221–225.
9. Langston RHS, Pavan-Langston D, Dohlman CH. Antiviral medication and corneal wound healing. *Arch Ophthalmol.* 1974;92:509–513.
10. Maudgal PC, Van Damme B, Misotten L. Corneal epithelial dysplasia after trifluridine use. *Graefe's Arch Ophthalmol.* 1983;220:6–12.
11. Collum LMT, Benedict-Smith A, Hillary IB. Randomized double-blind trial of acyclovir and idoxuridine in dendritic corneal ulceration. *Br J Ophthalmol.* 1980;64:766–769.
12. Lass JH, Pavan-Langston D, Park NH. Acyclovir and corneal wound healing. *Am J Ophthalmol.* 1979;88:102–108.
13. Cvetkovic D, Parunovic A, Kontic D. Conjunctival changes in local long-term glaucomatous therapy. *Fortschr Ophtalmol.* 1986;83:407–409 (German).
14. Pouliquen Y, Patey A, Foster CS, et al. Drug-induced cicatricial pemphigoid affecting the conjunctiva. *Ophthalmology.* 1986;93:775–783.
15. Ferry AP, Zimmerman LE. Black cornea: a complication of topical use of epinephrine. *Am J Ophthalmol.* 1964;58:205–210.
16. Liesegang TJ. Bulbar conjunctival follicles associated with dipivefrin therapy. *Ophthalmology.* 1985;92:228–233.
17. Van Buskirk EM. Adverse reactions from timolol administration. *Ophthalmology.* 1980;87:447.
18. Grant WM, Schuman JS. *Toxicology of the eye.* 4th ed. Springfield, IL: Charles C. Thomas; 1993.
19. Schnyder CC, et al. Sterile mucopurulent conjunctivitis associated with the use of dorzolamide eyedrops. *Arch Ophthalmol.* 1999;117:1429–1431.
20. Nagasubramanian S, Hitchings RA, Demailly P, et al. Comparison of apraclonidine and timolol in chronic open-angle glaucoma. A three-month study. *Ophthalmology.* 1993;100(9):1318–1323.
21. Katz LJ. Twelve-month evaluation of brimonidine-purite versus brimonidine in patients with glaucoma or ocular hypertension. *J Glaucoma.* 2002;11(2):119–126.
22. Jerstad KM, Warshaw E. Allergic contact dermatitis to latanoprost. *Contact Dermat.* 2002;13(1):39–41.
23. Lass JH, Mack RJ, et al: An in vitro analysis of aminoglycoside corneal epithelial toxicity. *Curr Eye Res.* 1989;8:299–304.
24. Stern GA, Shemmer GB, Farber RD. Effect of topical antibiotic solutions on corneal epithelial wound healing. *Arch Ophthalmol.* 1983; 101:644–647.
25. Apt L, Gaffney WL. Toxic effects of topical eye medication in infants and children. In: Tasman W, Jaeger EA, eds. *Duane's foundations of clinical ophthalmology*, vol. 3. Philadelphia: JB Lippincott; 1994,.
26. Burstein NL, Klyce SD. Electrophysiologic and morphologic effects of ophthalmic preparations on rabbit corneal epithelium. *Invest Ophthalmol Vis Sci.* 1977;16:899–911.
27. Petroutsos G, Guimaraes R, et al. Antibiotics and corneal epithelial wound healing. *Arch Ophthalmol.* 1983;101:1775–1778.
28. Rosenthal RL, Blackman A. Bone-marrow hypoplasia following use of chloramphenicol eyedrops. *JAMA.* 1965;191:136–137.
29. Hatinen A, Terasvirta M, Fraki JE. Contact allergy to components in topical ophthalmologic preparations. *Acta Ophthalmol. (Copenh).* 1985;63: 424–426.
30. Rubin Z. Ophthalmic sulfonamide-induced Stevens-Johnson syndrome. *Arch Dermatol.* 1977;113:235–236.
31. Gottschalk HR, Stone OJ. Stevens-Johnson syndrome from ophthalmic sulfonamide. *Arch Dermatol.* 1976;112:513.
32. Fine HF, et al. Toxic epidermal necrolysis induced by sulfonamide eyedrops. *Cornea.* 2008;27:1068–1069.
33. Flach AJ, Peterson JS, Mathias CGT. Photosensitivity to topically applied sulfisoxazole ointment. *Arch Ophthalmol.* 1982;100:1286–1287.
34. Cutarelli PE, Lass JH, Lazarus HM, et al: Topical fluoroquinolones: antimicrobial activity and in vitro corneal epithelial toxicity. *Curr Eye Res.* 1991;10:557–563.
35. Weisbecker CA, Fraunfelder FT, Arthur A, et al, eds. *Physicians' desk reference for ophthalmology.* 23rd ed. Montvale, NJ: Medical Economics; 1995.

36. Foster CS, Lass JH, Moran-Wallace K, et al. Ocular toxicity of topical antifungal agents. *Arch Ophthalmol* 1981;99:1081–1084.
37. Bell RW, Ritchey JP. Subconjunctival nodules after amphotericin B injection. *Arch Ophthalmol.* 1973;90:402–404.
38. Levinskas GJ, Ribelin WA, Shaffer CB. Acute and chronic toxicity of pimaricin. *Toxicol Appl Pharmacol.* 1966;8:97–109.
39. Zaidman GW. Miconazole corneal toxicity. *Cornea.* 1991;10:90–91.
40. Mannis MJ. Personal communication, 1994.
41. Higbee RG, Hazlett LD. Topical ocular anesthetics affect epithelial cytoskeletal proteins of wounded cornea. *J Ocular Pharmacol.* 1989;5:241.
42. Hermann H, Moses SG, Friedenwald JS. Influence of pontocaine hydrochloride and chlorobutanol on respiration and glycolysis of cornea. *Arch Ophthalmol.* 1942;28:652–660.
43. Rossenwasser GOD, Holland S, Pflugfelder SC, et al. Topical anesthetic abuse. *Ophthalmology.* 1990;97:967–972.
44. Dass BA, Soong HK, Lee B. Effects of proparacaine on actin cytoskeleton of corneal epithelium. *J Ocular Pharmacol.* 1988;4:187.
45. Gasset AR. Benzalkonium chloride toxicity to the human cornea. *Am J Ophthalmol.* 1977;84:169–171.
46. Wilson WS, Duncan AJ, Jay JL. Effect of benzalkonium on the stability of the precorneal tear film in rabbit and man. *Br J Ophthalmol.* 1975;59:667–669.
47. Neville R, Dennis P, Sens D, et al. Preservative cytotoxicity to cultured corneal epithelial cells. *Curr Eye Res.* 1986;5:367–372.
48. Mondino BJ, Salamon SM, Zaidman GW. Allergic and toxic reactions in soft contact lens wearers. *Surv Ophthalmol.* 1982;26(6):337–344.
49. Wilson LA, McNatt J, Reitschel R. Delayed hypersensitivity to thimerosal in soft contact lens wearers. *Ophthalmology.* 1981;88:804–809.
50. Cai F, Backman HA, Baines MG. Thimerosal: an ophthalmic preservative which acts as a hapten to elicit specific antibodies and cell mediated immunity. *Curr Eye Res.* 1988;7:341–351.
51. Fraunfelder FT, Meyer SM. *Drug-induced ocular side effects and drug interactions,* ed. 2. Philadelphia: Lea & Febiger; 1982.
52. Thygeson P, Dawson CR. Pseudotrachoma caused by molluscum contagiosum virus and various chemical irritants. *Excerpta Medica International Congress Series.* 1970;222:1894–1897.
53. Dawson CR, Sheppard JD. Follicular conjunctivitis. In: Tasman W, Jaeger EA, eds. *Duane's clinical ophthalmology.* vol. 4. Philadelphia: JB Lippincott; 1994.
54. Mackman GS, Polack FM, Sydrys L. Hurricane keratitis in penetrating keratoplasty. *Cornea.* 1983;2:31–34.
55. Kuwabara T, Perkins DG, Cogan DG. Sliding of the epithelium in experimental corneal wounds. *Invest Ophthalmol.* 1976;14:4–14.
56. Bron AJ. Vortex patterns of the corneal epithelium. *Trans Ophthalmol Soc UK.* 1973;93:455–472.
57. Lass JH, Thoft RA, Dohlman CH. Idoxuridine-induced conjunctival cicatrization. *Arch Ophthalmol.* 1983;101:747.
58. Patten JT, Cavanaugh HD, Allansmith MR. Induced ocular pseudopemphigoid. *Am J Ophthalmol.* 1976;82:262–276.
59. Hirst LW, Werblin T, Novak M, et al. Drug-induced cicatrizing conjunctivitis simulating ocular pemphigoid. *Cornea.* 1982;1:121.
60. Kristensen EB, Norn MS. Benign mucous membrane pemphigoid. I. Secretion of mucus and tears. *Acta Ophthalmol.* 1974;52:266.
61. Leonard JN, Hobday CM, Haffenden GP. Immunofluorescent studies in ocular cicatricial pemphigoid. *Br J Dermatol.* 1988;118:209.
62. Mondino BJ. Discussion of drug-induced cicatricial pemphigoid affecting the conjunctiva. *Ophthalmology.* 1986;93:782.
63. Mondino BJ. Bullous diseases of the skin and mucous membranes. In: Tasman W, Jaeger EA, eds. *Duane's clinical ophthalmology.* vol. 4. Philadelphia: JB Lippincott; 1994.
64. Stephens TJ, McCulley JP, Tharpe M, et al: Localized eye area sensitivity syndrome. *J Toxicol Cutaneous Ocul Toxicol.* 1989/1990;92:569–570.
65. Mannis MJ, Sandler BJ. Keratitis induced by skin polish. *Am J Ophthalmol.* 1988;106:104–105.
66. MacLean AL. Spray keratitis: a common epithelial keratitis from noncorrosive household sprays. *Trans Am Acad Ophthalmol Otol.* 1967;71: 330–339.
67. Satterfield D, Mannis MJ. Episodic bilateral corneal edema caused by hair groom gel. *Am J Ophthalmol.* 1992;113:107–108.
68. Laibson PR, Oconor J. Explosive tear gas injuries of the eye. *Trans Am Acad Ophthalmol Otol.* 1970;74:811–819.
69. Zollman TM, Bragg RM, Harrison DA. Clinical effects of oleoresin capsicum (pepper spray) on the human cornea and conjunctiva. *Ophthalmology.* 2000;107(12):2186–2189.

Chapter 54

Superior Limbic Keratoconjunctivitis

William T. Driebe Jr, Monali V. Sakhalkar

Historical Perspective and Epidemiology

In January 1963, Frederick Theodore published the first clinical description of a specific keratoconjunctivitis that he termed superior limbic keratoconjunctivitis (SLK).[1] His initial paper contained 11 patients who were characterized by the following: (1) marked inflammation of the tarsal conjunctiva of the upper lid, (2) inflammation of the upper bulbar conjunctiva, (3) fine punctate staining of the cornea at the upper limbus and the adjacent conjunctiva above the limbus, (4) superior limbic proliferation, and (5) filaments on the superior limbus or upper fourth of the cornea in about half of the patients. Impaired tearing was observed in 50% of Theodore's patients, and corneal hypoesthesia was another frequent finding. Theodore was unable to recover any significant bacterial pathogens by means of culture.

Thygeson and Kimura had both presented elements of this entity before Theodore's complete description in January 1963.[2,3] Theodore himself later updated his observations in a larger number of patients he had followed.[4] Cases that have been reported are almost always nonfamilial, but the disorder has been documented in identical twins.[5] Collective observations and reports suggest a mean age of 50 years and a female:male ratio of approximately 3 : 1.[6]

Clinical Presentation

Superior limbic keratoconjunctivitis eventually runs its course, but only after years of flares and remissions.[1,4] Visual prognosis in most patients remains excellent, since the process is usually limited to the superior fourth of the cornea. Typical complaints include foreign body sensation, photophobia, and pain. Some present with blepharospasm, particularly if filaments are present. Patients with filaments often complain of a mucoid discharge.

The clinical signs of SLK bear further discussion.[4,6,7] Eversion of the upper lid characteristically demonstrates hyperemia of the palpebral conjunctiva and a fine papillary reaction (Fig. 54.1). The superior bulbar and limbal conjunctiva shows sectoral injection and appears thickened and redundant (Fig. 54.2). The affected conjunctiva may appear keratinized. There is generally a superior punctate epithelial keratitis, and application of rose Bengal often shows coarse punctate staining of the superior bulbar and limbal conjunctiva as well (Fig. 54.3). Superior corneal and limbic filaments are another frequently associated finding (Fig. 54.4). Advanced cases may also present with inflammatory ptosis and increased mucus production. A useful diagnostic maneuver is to have the patient look down while lifting the upper lid in order to demonstrate the superior sectoral leash of bulbar conjunctival hyperemia so characteristic of this syndrome. Another diagnostic technique is to document the redundancy of the superior bulbar conjunctiva. After instillation of topical anesthetic, a cotton-tipped applicator can be used to slide the superior bulbar conjunctiva over the superior cornea. This should not be possible in the normal eye.

Histopathology

Histopathologic evaluation of the disorder has been reported by a number of investigators. Theodore and Ferry showed that scraping the superior bulbar conjunctiva often reveals keratinized epithelium as well as the presence of polymorphonuclear leukocytes.[8] Scraping the palpebral conjunctiva shows normal epithelium, but, like the bulbar conjunctiva, a polymorphonuclear exudate is present. Theodore also reported the results of biopsy specimens of the superior bulbar and palpebral conjunctiva. The superior bulbar conjunctiva shows obvious keratinization as well as acanthosis, dyskeratosis, and balloon degeneration of nuclei. The palpebral conjunctiva reveals normal epithelium but infiltration with polymorphonuclear leukocytes, lymphocytes, and plasma cells. The superior palpebral conjunctiva shows goblet cell hypertrophy, while the bulbar conjunctiva, which is thickened and keratinized, shows very few goblet cells.[7]

Collin et al. reported the results of electron microscopy of superior bulbar conjunctival tissue in patients with SLK.[9,10] Aside from demonstrating prominent keratinization of the superior bulbar conjunctiva, they found abnormal distribution and aggregation of nuclear chromatin. Filaments were found within nuclei, as well as in the cytoplasm surrounding nuclei, resulting in a description of 'nuclear strangulation.' These findings were considered unique to SLK.

Donshik et al. studied conjunctival resection specimens by light and transmission electron microscopy.[11] They demonstrated intracellular accumulation of glycogen in the bulbar conjunctiva. Wander and Masukawa later reported an

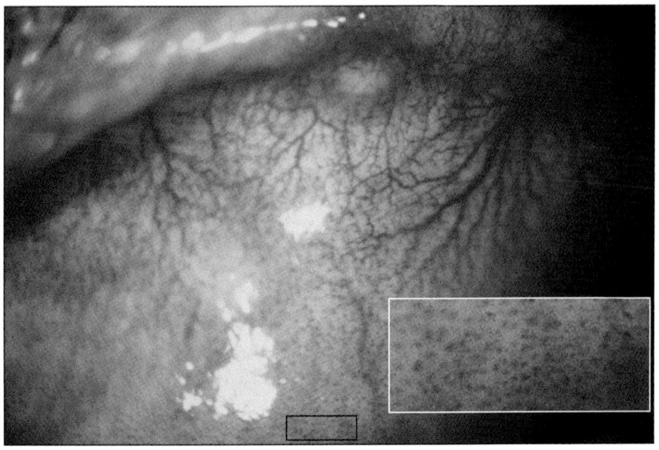

Fig. 54.1 Diffuse papillary reaction of the superior tarsal conjunctiva in a patient with SLK. A magnified example is seen in the inset.

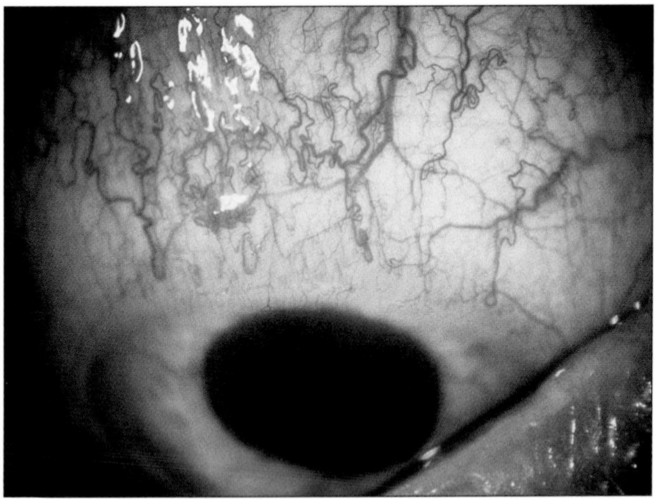

Fig. 54.2 Superior sectoral bulbar conjunctival injection in a patient with SLK.

unusual pattern of condensed chromatin in the nuclei of epithelial scrapings taken from the superior bulbar conjunctiva of patients affected with SLK. This finding was present in all 13 cases studied.[12] Watanabe et al. observed markedly diminished levels of a 'mucin-like glycoprotein' believed to participate in mucin–apical epithelial interaction of conjunctiva. These glycoprotein levels normalized after successful treatment of SLK.[13] Matsuda et al. also observed abnormal differentiation and hyperproliferation of conjunctival epithelium in patients with SLK by examining expression of cytokeratins and proliferating cell nuclear antigen.[14] Furthermore, they also reinforced the theory of mechanical trauma as an inciting factor in SLK by the observation that there is an up-regulation of TGF-beta2 and tenascin, both of which are induced by mechanical trauma.[15]

Origin and Pathogenesis

The origin of SLK has not been determined. A viral etiology has been suspected but has never been proven. An

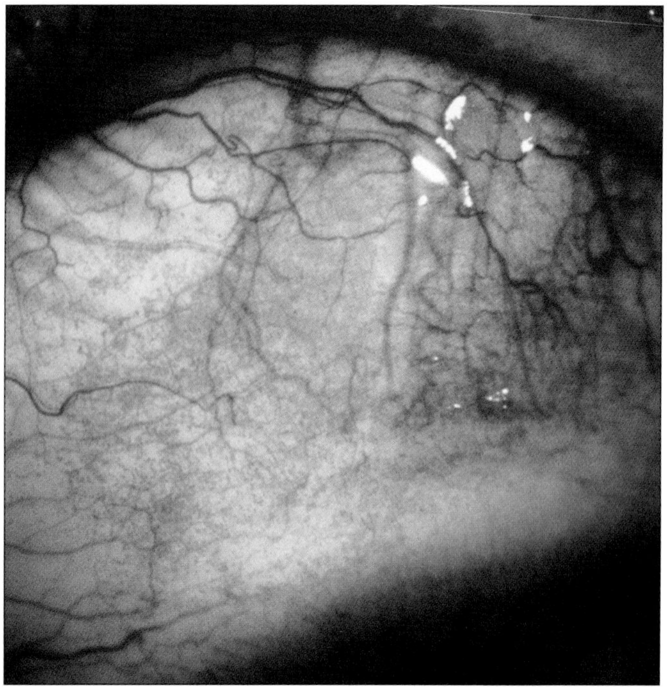

Fig. 54.3 Rose Bengal staining of the superior bulbar conjunctiva in a patient with SLK.

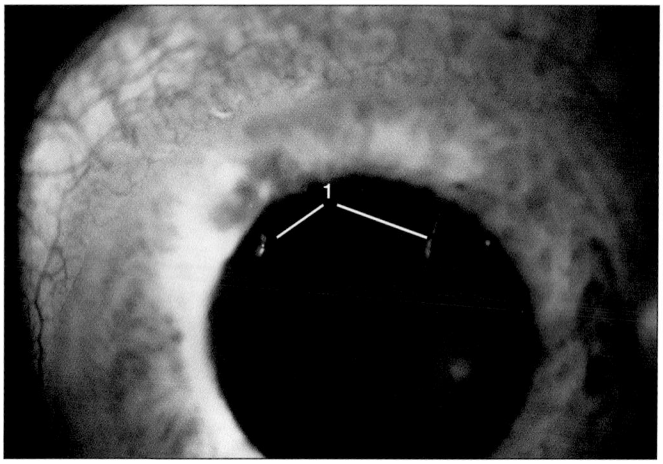

Fig. 54.4 Superior corneal filaments (1) in a patient with SLK.

immunologic basis has also been suspected but has not been confirmed. Eiferman and Wilkins reported the results of three patients with SLK who underwent conjunctival resection and immunologic evaluation.[16] They were unable to find any specific immune defects and therefore concluded that there was no immunologic basis for this disorder.

Although the etiology is not clear, there are a number of interesting associations. The one most frequently mentioned is thyroid disease. Tenzel was the first to mention this association when he reported a number of his patients with SLK who had elevated serum protein-bound iodine.[17] This association was later confirmed by Cher, who reported patients with SLK who had thyrotoxicosis.[18] Theodore endorsed

Tenzel's observation when he reported a number of his patients with laboratory evidence of thyroid disease.[19] The association of SLK with thyroid dysfunction, particularly hyperthyroidism, is present in patients with SLK in at least 30% of cases.[6,20]

Another abnormality found among patients with SLK is keratoconjunctivitis sicca. Theodore noticed this finding in half of the patients he originally reported.[1] A summary of the clinical findings of patients with SLK from seven different reports found this association in 25% of cases.[20] Hyperparathyroidism has also been reported in association with SLK.[20]

The exact pathogenesis of this disorder continues to be debated. Theodore suspected the primary abnormality lay in the region of the superior limbal area, hence the term SLK.[1] Wright felt the superior palpebral conjunctiva was the initiating tissue in the sequence of events.[7] Donshik et al., reporting results of the pathologic evaluation of conjunctival specimens, felt the site of abnormality was the superior bulbar conjunctiva.[11] Regardless of the exact initiating site, the mechanical theory advocated by Wright is attractive.[7] He postulated that the problem in SLK is a continual rubbing of the superior palpebral conjunctiva against the superior bulbar conjunctiva secondary to tight apposition. This theory fits nicely in patients who present with tight upper lids or in those with exophthalmos, as in thyroid eye disease. The redundant appearance of the superior bulbar conjunctiva also suggests a mechanical factor.[6]

Patients with chronic ocular inflammatory disease can develop a picture of SLK because of increased friction between the superior palpebral and bulbar conjunctiva. Those with keratoconjunctivitis sicca may also have a drying effect between the upper lid and the bulbar conjunctiva, which enhances friction. Wright hypothesized that a chronically inflamed palpebral conjunctival surface could lead to changes in viscosity that prevent the normal maturation and replacement of bulbar conjunctiva epithelium, thereby causing the clinical picture of SLK.[7]

Treatment Options

A number of different treatment modalities have been suggested for SLK. Which modality will be most beneficial may be based on the underlying inciting factors. An attempt should be made to assess for common comorbid conditions such as tear function, lid tension, and thyroid status. This can help guide the direction of initial therapy.

Theodore originally recommended local application of 0.5–1% silver nitrate solution to the anesthetized superior palpebral conjunctiva.[1] Others have advocated applying silver nitrate solution to both the palpebral conjunctiva and the affected superior bulbar conjunctiva.[20] After treatment, care should be taken to irrigate the ocular surface thoroughly to avoid excessive contact of silver nitrate with the corneal surface, since it is slightly irritating even at this concentration. Unfortunately, the patient may only improve for a matter of months.[20] While at lower concentrations of 0.5–1%, silver nitrate probably works by chemical debridement, serious chemical burns of the cornea may result from the use of solid silver nitrate applicators.[21]

Conjunctival resection is another recommended therapeutic approach. Passons and Wood reported that superior bulbar conjunctival resection was effective for treating SLK patients with normal Schirmer tear results before surgery. They postulated that conjunctival resection improves the mechanical interface between the superior palpebral and bulbar conjunctiva.[22] Tenzel had previously reported improvement of symptoms in patients with SLK by recessing the superior bulbar conjunctiva.[23] Conjunctival resection is generally done by performing a superior peritomy at the limbus, along the involved superior bulbar conjunctiva. A 3–4-mm wide strip of conjunctiva is then excised. In our experience, conjunctival resection has been one of the best therapeutic modalities in patients who have failed to respond to silver nitrate therapy. In 2003, Yokoi and associates adequately treated SLK by removing the redundant conjunctiva adjacent and distant from the diseased area.[24] Yi Chen Sun and associates reported success with superior bulbar conjunctival resection combined with Tenon layer excision.[25]

Mondino et al. reported their experience with pressure patching and/or soft contact lenses in eight patients with SLK.[26] Two patients were treated with pressure patching alone, while the other six patients were fitted with therapeutic soft contact lenses after the initial use of pressure patching. Mondino et al. found this treatment particularly useful in patients with filaments and postulated that interruption of mechanical factors existing between the superior tarsus and bulbar conjunctiva accounted for the improvement. They suggest this treatment be considered in patients in whom silver nitrate or conjunctival resection or recession has failed. Wright had also advocated the use of therapeutic soft contact lenses in patients with filaments, but noted difficulty in maintaining their long-term use because of associated mucus production.[7]

In a further attempt at reducing the mechanical malinteraction of the superior tarsus and bulbar conjunctiva, botulinum toxin injection of the orbicularis was reported to have beneficial effects in 16 of 21 patients.[27] Mackie injected a botulinum toxin solution consisting of 200 units/mL and injected 0.1–0.2 mL into the superior orbital rim and inferior orbicularis at a total of four sites. Two of his patients did not require repeat injections whereas the others did. Furthermore, patients experienced symptomatic relief only, without clinical improvement of findings.

In 1986, Udell et al. reported the results of treating SLK with thermal cauterization.[28] They treated 13 eyes of 11 patients with thermal cautery applied to the inflamed superior bulbar conjunctival tissue after subconjunctival lidocaine (Xylocaine). Seventy-three percent of their patients showed an improvement in symptoms and findings. Five of the eight patients who improved had been considered silver nitrate treatment failures. Over half of the patients studied were also diagnosed with coexistent keratitis sicca. The authors also demonstrated return of bulbar conjunctival goblet cells after successful treatment. It has been postulated that alteration of the bulbar conjunctival surface with thermal cautery somehow improves the interaction between the superior palpebral and the bulbar conjunctival tissue. The authors suggest that this modality be employed before conjunctival resection. They also advocate punctal occlusion in patients with SLK who have coexisting keratitis sicca.

Yang and colleagues found resolution of SLK symptoms in 22 eyes after permanent punctal occlusion. In addition, they found reversal of squamous metaplasia and an increase in goblet cell number (by impression cytology) after punctal occlusion.[29]

Confino and Brown reported improvement after topical use of cromolyn sodium in six of eight patients with SLK in whom standard therapy failed.[30] Grutzmacher et al. also found lodoxamide four times a day to be effective in three patients with SLK refractory to topical silver nitrate, topical steroids, antibiotics, and conjunctival cautery.[31]

Ohashi et al. advocated the use of topical vitamin A for SLK.[32] They treated 12 patients with SLK with vitamin A (retinol palmitate) eye drops. Their patients were followed for at least 3 months. Treatment was effective in 83% of patients. The authors also noted their patients did not have recurrent disease while they continued topical vitamin A therapy.

Udell et al. reported subjective improvement in five patients having bilateral SLK with the use of topical ketotifen fumarate twice daily.[33] Topical autologous serum drops have been advocated by Goto et al. They determined that 20% diluted autologous serum drops ten times a day in addition to the routine dry eye regimen provided symptomatic and objective improvement based on rose Bengal and fluorescein staining in 9 of 11 patients.[34]

Perry et al. advocated the use of 0.5% topical ciclosporin A as a primary or adjunctive therapy for SLK. The authors treated five patients previously managed with prednisolone acetate 1% drops and topical silver nitrate 0.5% application with 0.5% topical ciclosporin four times a day in both eyes. All five patients had long-term (6 months to 3 years) improvement of irritation and foreign body sensation, as well as improvement of injection and filamentary keratitis. Aside from burning on instillation, there were no side effects related to this therapy.[35] Similar success was reported by Sahin et al. who used topical ciclosporin A 0.05% (Restasis; Allergan, Irvine, CA) as an adjunctive therapy mainly after treatment failure with topical corticosteroid drops.[36]

Supratarsal triamcinolone injection has been efficacious in resolving the signs and symptoms of SLK. Shen et al. treated 20 patients unresponsive to artificial tears and topical steroids with triamcinolone acetonide 3 mg/0.3 mL injected in the temporal supratarsal conjunctiva with a 27-gauge needle. They proposed that SLK is suppressed by the antiinflammatory effects of triamcinolone.[41]

Liquid nitrogen cryotherapy of SLK performed using a Brymill E tip spray (0.013-inch aperture) with a double freeze–thaw technique is another approach described by Frederick Fraunfelder. Liquid nitrogen cryotherapy acts by causing a scar similar to that produced by chemocautery to form between the superior bulbar conjunctiva and the underlying Tenon's capsule and sclera.[38]

Other therapies have also been recommended. N-acetylcysteine, a mucolytic agent, is felt to be useful for patients with filamentary keratitis and excessive mucus production. Vasoconstrictors have been tried with limited success, and topical steroids may be of value in some patients.[7]

Differential Diagnosis

If there is close adherence to the clinical criteria originally described by Theodore when diagnosing this entity, the differential diagnosis is rather limited. However, there is a syndrome associated with the use of cosmetic soft contact lenses that closely resembles SLK. Stenson reported four soft contact lens wearers who developed lens intolerance and irritation and were subsequently found to have clinical findings suggestive of SLK.[39] Her patients had mild papillary hypertrophy of the tarsal conjunctiva, as well as injection and inflammation of the superior bulbar conjunctiva. They demonstrated fluorescein staining of the superior bulbar conjunctiva and upper corneal punctate staining. Hypertrophy of the superior limbus was also noted. Symptoms and findings cleared after discontinuance of contact lens wear, although one patient had mild continuing signs for 2 years. Subsequently, three of the four patients reported were able to resume lens wear on a more limited basis.

Sendele et al. reported 40 patients who, while wearing cosmetic soft contact lenses, developed a clinical picture resembling SLK.[40] Each patient studied was using a thimerosal-preserved solution. They felt that exposure to thimerosal was the causative factor in what they described as contact lens-superior limbic keratoconjunctivitis (CL-SLK). Bulbar conjunctival specimens submitted for transmission electron microscopy demonstrated decreased goblet cells and signs of acute and chronic inflammation. Keratinization of the conjunctiva was not a prominent feature, and filaments were present in only 13% of cases. Interestingly, a number of these patients presented with substantially decreased vision and had more diffuse inflammation of the bulbar conjunctiva than is usually seen in Theodore's SLK. The corneal epithelial irregularity and punctate keratitis were more substantial than in typical SLK and were considered the source of the decreased vision.

A close comparison of Theodore's SLK and CL-SLK indicates that the two are clearly separate entities. Theodore himself objected to the use of the aforementioned terminology.[37] He pointed out that SLK offers a more clear-cut picture, while the presentation of CL-SLK varies. Also, CL-SLK is not always bilateral and has no relationship with thyroid disease. SLK is more commonly seen in females, while CL-SLK is not. CL-SLK also occurs in younger patients than does SLK. While vision with SLK is usually not decreased, it can be severely decreased in patients with CL-SLK, since corneal involvement is greater. Corneal filaments are usually not seen with CL-SLK, but they are frequently seen with SLK. While there is some similarity in terms of the cytologic conjunctival characteristics between the two, Theodore advocated the use of the term contact lens keratoconjunctivitis for these patients, rather than CL-SLK. A final distinction between the two is that contact lens keratoconjunctivitis often improves quickly after cessation of lens wear, whereas SLK goes on with remissions and recurrences for many years. One possible etiology suggested for the syndrome of contact lens keratoconjunctivitis is that of a superior-riding soft contact lens that may have a mechanical effect on the bulbar conjunctival tissue and superior cornea.[42]

Considering the aforementioned discussion, the term contact lens-induced keratoconjunctivitis is a more accurate description of the changes that can occur in contact lens wearers, which are similar to Theodore's superior limbic keratoconjunctivitis. The term Theodore's superior limbic keratoconjunctivitis should be reserved for those patients who develop SLK without the use of contact lenses.

Summary

Superior limbic keratoconjunctivitis is a distinct clinical entity that was originally described in 1963 by Frederick Theodore. Once patients are correctly diagnosed, they may benefit from a number of therapeutic modalities, including silver nitrate therapy, pressure patching, therapeutic soft contact lenses, N-acetylcysteine, superior bulbar conjunctival thermal cautery, topical mast cell stabilizers or NSAIDs, autologous serum drops, botulinum injection of eyelids, punctal occlusion, and superior bulbar conjunctival resection or recession surgery. New treatment modalities such as topical ciclosporin A 0.5%, supratarsal triamcinolone injection, and liquid nitrogen cryotherapy may benefit patients.[35,38,41] The disease itself eventually burns out, but its course can be protracted, with multiple recurrences and remissions. There is a definite association with thyroid disorders, and this diagnosis should be considered in any patient with Theodore's SLK. Patients with SLK may also have associated keratitis sicca, which can be addressed via improved lubrication or punctal occlusion. This disease is an interesting entity probably produced by mechanical factors existing between the tarsal conjunctiva and the superior bulbar conjunctival and corneal tissues. Its exact etiology remains unknown. Various inciting factors may be present which lead to a common end point, i.e. inflammation of the tarsal and bulbar conjunctiva with squamous metaplasia and goblet cell loss of the bulbar conjunctiva resulting in a cycle of inflammation and pain.

References

1. Theodore FH. Superior limbic keratoconjunctivitis. *Eye Ear Nose Throat Mon.* 1963;42:25–28.
2. Thygeson P. Further observations on superficial punctate keratitis. *Arch Ophthalmol.* 1961;66:158–162.
3. Thygeson P, Kimura SJ. Chronic conjunctivitis. *Trans Am Acad Ophthalmol Otolaryngol.* 1963;67:494–517.
4. Theodore FH. Further observations on superior limbic keratoconjunctivitis. *Trans Am Acad Ophthal Otolaryngol.* 1967;71:341–351.
5. Darrell RW. Superior limbic keratoconjunctivitis in identical twins. *Cornea.* 1992;11(3):262–263.
6. Wilson FM, Ostler HB. Superior limbic keratoconjunctivitis. *Int Ophthalmol Clin.* 1986;26:99–112.
7. Wright P. Superior limbic keratoconjunctivitis. *Trans Ophthalmol Soc UK.* 1972;92:555–560.
8. Theodore FH, Ferry AP. Superior limbic keratoconjunctivitis. Clinical and pathological correlations. *Arch Ophthalmol.* 1970;84:481–484.
9. Collin HB, et al. Keratinization of the bulbar conjunctival epithelium in superior limbic keratoconjunctivitis in humans: an electron microscopic study. *Acta Ophthalmologica Copenh.* 1978;56:531–543.
10. Collin HB, et al. The fine structure of nuclear changes in superior limbic keratoconjunctivitis. *Invest Ophthalmol Vis Sci.* 1978;17:79–84.
11. Donshik PC, et al. Conjunctival resection treatment and ultrastructural histopathology of superior limbic keratoconjunctivitis. *Am J Ophthalmol.* 1978;85:101–110.
12. Wander AH, Masukawa T. Unusual appearance of condensed chromatin in conjunctival cells in superior limbic keratoconjunctivitis. *Lancet.* 1981;2(8236):42–43.
13. Watanabe H, Maeda N, Kiritoshi A, et al. Expression of a mucin-like glycoprotein produced by ocular surface epithelium in normal and keratinized cells. *Am J Ophthalmol.* 1997;124(6):751–757.
14. Matsuda A, Tagawa Y, Matsuda H. Cytokeratin and proliferative cell nuclear antigen expression in superior limbic keratoconjunctivitis. *Curr Eye Res.* 1996;15(10):1033–1038.
15. Matsuda A, Tagawa Y, Matsuda H. TGF-beta2, tenascin, and integrin beta1 expression in superior limbic keratoconjunctivitis. *Jpn J Ophthalmol.* 1999;43(4):251–256.
16. Eiferman RA, Wilkins EL. Immunological aspects of superior limbic keratoconjunctivitis. *Can J Ophthalmol.* 1979;14:85–87.
17. Tenzel RR. Comments on superior limbic filamentous keratitis: part II. *Arch Ophthalmol.* 1968;79:508.
18. Cher I. Clinical features of superior limbic keratoconjunctivitis in Australia. A probable association with thyrotoxicosis. *Arch Ophthalmol.* 1969;82:580–586.
19. Theodore FH. Comments on findings of elevated protein-bound iodine in superior limbic keratoconjunctivitis: part I. *Arch Ophthalmol.* 1968;79:508.
20. Nelson JD. Superior limbic keratoconjunctivitis (SLK). *Eye.* 1989;3(Pt 2):180–189.
21. Laughrea PA, Arentsen JJ, Laibson PR. Iatrogenic ocular silver nitrate burn. *Cornea.* 1985–1986;4:47–50.
22. Passons GA, Wood TO. Conjunctival resection for superior limbic keratoconjunctivitis. *Ophthalmology.* 1984;91:966–968.
23. Tenzel RR. Resistant superior limbic keratoconjunctivitis. *Arch Ophthalmol.* 1973;89:439.
24. Yokoi N, Komuro A, et al. New surgical treatment for superior limbic keratoconjunctivitis and its association with conjunctivochalasis. *Am J Ophthalmol.* 2003;135:303–308.
25. Sun YC, Hsiao CH, Chen WL, et al. Conjunctival resection combined with tenon layer excision and the involvement of mast cells in superior limbic keratoconjunctivitis. *Am J Ophthalmol.* 2008;145:445–452.
26. Mondino BJ, Zaidman GW, Salamon SW. Use of pressure patching and soft contact lenses in superior limbic keratoconjunctivitis. *Arch Ophthalmol.* 1982;100:1932–1934.
27. Mackie IA. Management of superior limbic keratoconjunctivitis with botulinum toxin. *Eye.* 1995;9(Pt 1):143–144.
28. Udell IJ, et al. Treatment of superior limbic keratoconjunctivitis by thermocauterization of the superior bulbar conjunctiva. *Ophthalmology.* 1986;93:162–166.
29. Yang HY, Fujishima H, Toda I, et al. Lacrimal punctal occlusion for the treatment of superior limbic keratoconjunctivitis. *Am J Ophthalmol.* 1997;124(1):80–87.
30. Confino J, Brown SI. Treatment of superior limbic keratoconjunctivitis with topical cromolyn sodium. *Ann Ophthalmol.* 1987;19:129–131.
31. Grutzmacher RD, Foster RS, Feiler LS. Lodoxamide tromethamine treatment for superior limbic keratoconjunctivitis. *Am J Ophthalmol.* 1995;120(3):400–402.
32. Ohashi Y, et al. Vitamin A eye drops for superior limbic keratoconjunctivitis. *Am J Ophthalmol.* 1988;105:523–527.
33. Udell IJ, Guidera AC, Madani-Becker J. Ketotifen fumarate treatment of superior limbic keratoconjuctivitis. *Cornea.* 2002;21(8):778–780.
34. Goto E, Shimmura S, Shimazaki J, Tsubota K. Treatment of superior limbic keratoconjunctivitis by application of autologous serum. *Cornea.* 2001;20(8):807–810.
35. Perry HD, Doshi-Carnevale S, Donnenfeld ED, Kornstein HS. Topical cyclosporine A 0.5% as a possible new treatment for superior limbic keratoconjunctivitis. *Ophthalmology.* 2003;110:1578–1581.
36. Sahin A, Bozhurt B, Irkec M. Topical cyclosporine A in the treatment of superior limbic keratoconjunctivitis: a long-term follow-up. *Cornea.* 2008;27:193–195.
37. Theodore FH. Superior limbic keratoconjunctivitis. *Arch Ophthalmol.* 1983;101:1627–1629.
38. Fraunfelder F. Liquid nitrogen cryotherapy of superior limbic keratoconjunctivitis. *Am J Ophthalmol.* 2009;147:234–238.
39. Stenson S. Superior limbic keratoconjunctivitis associated with soft contact lens wear. *Arch Ophthalmol.* 1983;101:402–404.
40. Sendele DD, et al. Superior limbic keratoconjunctivitis in contact lens wearers. *Ophthalmology.* 1983;90:616–622.
41. Shen YC, et al. Supratarsal triamcinolone injection in the treatment of superior limbic keratoconjunctivitis. *Cornea.* 2007;26:423–426.
42. Carpel EF. Superior limbic keratoconjunctivitis. *Arch Ophthalmol.* 1983;102:662, 664.

Chapter 55

Ligneous Conjunctivitis

Kristiana D. Neff, Edward J. Holland, Gary S. Schwartz

Ligneous conjunctivitis (LC) is a rare disorder characterized by a protracted course of recurrent, membranous, conjunctival lesions, which has been associated with a systemic plasminogen deficiency. This ocular manifestation of a systemic disorder typically presents in childhood, although can occur at any age. It may be associated with lesions of other mucous membranes including the mouth, ear, nasopharynx, trachea and respiratory tract, gastrointestinal tract, or female genital tract. Rarely, it is seen in conjunction with congenital occlusive hydrocephalus or juvenile colloid milium.

In 1847, Bouisson[1] described a 46-year-old man with bilateral pseudomembranous conjunctivitis in what is thought to be the first published case of ligneous conjunctivitis. Borel,[2] in 1933, assigned the name ligneous, meaning 'woody,' to this disorder because of the charateristic wood-like consistency of the membranes in severe cases. Most patients under active treatment have thinner, softer, membranous lesions (Fig. 55.1).

Epidemiology

Ligneous conjunctivitis is rare. Since the introduction of the term, more than 150 cases have been described in the literature.[3–35] In a recent study of 50 patients with severe type I plasminogen deficiency, the median age of first clinical manifestation was 9.75 months (range, 3 days to 61 years) with a female to male ratio of 1.27 to 1. Due to unknown factors, LC has been reported in the literature to be more common in females than males.[36,37] The most common manifestation in this group was ligneous conjuctivitis (80%), followed by ligneous gingivitis (34%), with 14% of patients suffering from both. More rare extraocular manifestations included involvement of the ears, upper and lower respiratory tract (sinus, larynx, bronchi, lungs; 30%), the female genital tract (8%), the gastrointestinal tract (duodenal ulcer; 2%), congenital occlusive hydrocephalus (8%), and juvenile colloid milium of the skin (2%). Two of the patients with congenital occlusive hydrocephalus had Dandy-Walker malformation.[38] Several studies have shown extraocular manifestations of severe plasminogen deficiency without ocular involvment.[26,36,38]

Numerous case reports have described this condition after infection or trauma. Abnormal inflammatory response to conjunctival injury is likely a factor in the development of this disease. Of interest are cases that occurred after surgery to the conjunctiva, including surgery for pterygium,[20,33] pingueculum,[9] strabismus,[3,22] cataract,[22] keratoplasty,[39] ptosis,[22] and even conjunctival autograft from a healthy donor eye for the fellow eye which had LC.[40]

Clinical Findings

Patients typically present with a chronic conjunctivitis. Discharge or membranes are not seen in the early stages. The earliest true ligneous lesion appears as a highly vascularized, raised, friable lesion. This lesion can be removed easily with forceps, although it tends to bleed on removal. Although this lesion is referred to as pseudomembranous in the literature, in actuality, it is a true membraneous lesion.

With continued inflammation, a white, thickened, avascular mass appears above the neovascular membrane. Attempts at removal of this lesion without appropriate anti-inflammatory therapy often results in recurrence of the lesion to its original size within days. These lesions are most often seen on the palpebral conjunctiva of the upper and lower lids but may also be found on the bulbar conjunctiva, including the limbus. Bulbar conjunctival involvement may occur either from extension of a palpebral lesion or de novo. Limbal lesions may extend over the surface of the cornea and, in the most severe cases, lead to corneal neovascularization and scarring.

From time to time, despite appropriate therapy, inflammation continues, and the chronic lesions become thickened, vascularized, and firm, giving rise to the name 'ligneous,' meaning woody.

Early in the course of the disease, patients may complain of chronic tearing, mild discomfort, and redness. As the lesions grow, almost all patients complain of pain and photophobia. Severe cases result in almost constant discomfort, making it difficult for patients to carry out activities of daily living. The more severe lesions extend beyond the lid margin, giving rise to one of the worst complications of the disorder, the cosmetic deformity (Fig. 55.2).

Pathophysiology/Histopathology

Before the identification of a type I plasminogen deficiency as the disorder underlying LC, numerous causes had been

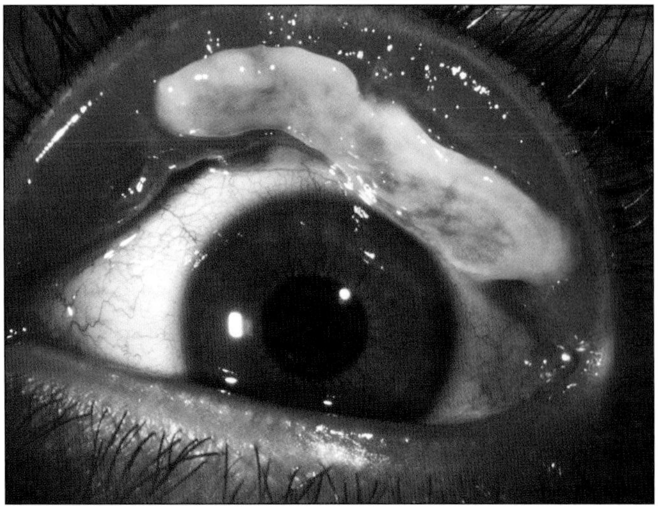

Fig. 55.1 Ligneous conjunctivitis of the superior palpebral conjunctiva. Note the white, avascular lesion at the perimeter and the vascularized base.

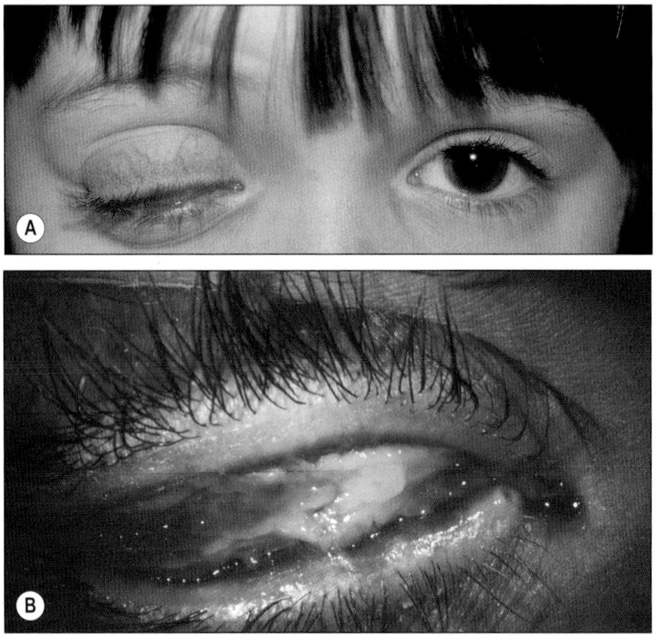

Fig. 55.2 Ligneous conjunctivitis in an 8-year-old girl. (**A**) The ligneous lesions involve the entire palpebral and bulbar conjunctiva of the right eye. (**B**) Note that the limbal lesions have grown to completely obscure the cornea.

proposed including autoimmune reaction, trauma, hypersensitivity reaction, genetic disorder, and secondary response to a viral or bacterial infection. Histologic examination of pseudomembranes shows superficial or subepithelial deposits of eosinophilic amorphous hyaline, amyloid-like material with a variable proportion of granulation tissue, and inflammatory cells (lymphocyes, plasma cells, and granulocytes).[36,41–43] Previous reports describe mucopolysaccharide as a major component of these lesions.[7,12] This response is postulated to be the result of a disturbance in conjunctival metabolism or may result from an exaggerated tissue response to trauma. Schuster and Seregard postulated that conjunctivitis is the most common manifestation of planminogen deficiency due to frequent exposure to ocular irritants.[36] These irritants may start or perpetuate local inflammation and create ligneous pseudomembranes. Other studies[13,21] indicate that the hyaline material is largely made up of fibrin, and the acid mucopolysaccharide present is located only in adjacent granulation tissue. Abnormal vascular permeability also has been suggested as the source of the various components of the ligneous lesion. Melikian[14] postulated that a serofibrinous transudate from the conjunctival neovascularization undergoes subsequent coagulation, with the resulting formation of granulation tissue and accumulation of the hyaline material, which becomes hardened in forming the ligneous membranes.

Immunohistochemical evaluation of ligneous conjunctivitis lesions was first performed in 1988.[11] In this study, a cellular infiltrate was seen that was composed mainly of T lymphocytes, seen again in later studies.[33] The ratio of T-helper/inducer to T-suppressor/cytotoxic cells was approximately 3:1. Immunofluorescent techniques demonstrated that the major components of the hyaline material in the substantia propria were immunoglobulins. IgG was the most prominent, with staining for both light and heavy chains, but primarily for κ-light chains. A subsequent immunohistochemical study revealed similar findings in the T-cell populations.[3]

Etiology

There has been definitive evidence to support that LC is the result of plasminogen deficiency.[23,27,29,34,35,38] The case of ligneous conjunctivitis reported by Mingers et al. was also the first report of plasminogen deficiency in humans.[35] There are two types of inherited plasminogen deficiency: type I hypoplasminogenemia shows reduction in plasminogen level and activity, and type II dysplasminogenemia shows only a reduction in plasminogen activity with normal levels. Only type I plasminogen deficiency has been reported to cause any form of pseudomembranous disease. Development of ligneous lesions is most commonly caused by sporadic mutations in the plasminogen gene; however, compound-heterozygous or homozygous mutations have been reported.[29,34–36,38] Tefts et al. found the K19E mutation to be the most common genetic cause of type I plasminogen deficiency (34%) in a series of 50 patients.[38] Knowledge of the genetics of the disease allows for prenatal diagnosis in known carrier families, which could be crucial in cases of obstructive congenital hydrocephalus.[30]

Although plasminogen is primarily synthesized by liver tissue, plasminogen activators on the ocular surface would normally be produced in the cornea,[44] to convert plasminogen to plasmin, which in turn will clear fibrin deposits off the cornea through fibrinolysis. With plasminogen deficiency, fibrin-rich membranes or mucus strands accumulate, stimulating inflammatory cells and fibroblasts, while desiccation of the fibrin leads to the ligneous consistency of the conjunctival lesions. Supplementing plasminogen has reversed those findings.[23,31,34,35]

While in extravascular spaces fibrinolysis with low to nonexistent levels of plasminogen activity is impaired, intravascularly this is not the case, as can be inferred from the fact that thrombotic phenomena are absent in patients with LC and plasminogen deficiency. It has been suggested that nonplasmin-induced fibrinolysis is intensified in patients with plasminogen deficiency and LC, through, among other factors, elevated polymorphonuclear elastase levels.[31,34]

With regards to extraocular manifestations of LC and plasminogen deficiency, pathogenetic mechanisms similar to LC have been proposed in other tissues: the middle ear,[45] the cilia in the respiratory tract,[37,46–49] and the ventricles and the aqueduct of Sylvius in cases of congenital obstructive hydrocephalus.[35,37,47,50]

From the appearance, histopathology, clinical course, and response to treatment, the authors also believe that ligneous conjunctivitis results from an exaggerated inflammatory response to tissue injury. This injury may arise from infection or physical trauma, including surgery. These factors may be inciting a genetic predisposition such as plasminogen deficiency to develop this response. Many cases of antecedent viral or bacterial infections have been described in the literature, including staphylococcal, streptococcal, and *Haemophilus* conjuctivitis.[4,15,18]

In these cases, it appears that ligneous conjunctivitis in genetically susceptible individuals develops as an abnormal response to the conjunctival trauma elicited by the infecting organisms.

Trauma, especially from surgery, is also thought to be a cause of ligneous conjunctivitis. The authors have reported a case of a 24-year-old woman with ligneous conjunctivitis of the left upper eyelid who underwent a conjunctival autograft from her left lower to left upper eyelid. Ligneous conjunctivitis subsequently developed at the previously unaffected donor site and became resistant to treatment in the original site of disease in the palpebral conjunctiva of the upper lid.[19] Later studies reported the same negative experience in previously unaffected fellow eyes.[33] In these cases, ligneous conjunctivitis appears to develop as an abnormal response of the immune system to the conjunctival trauma.

Topical ciclosporin A has been reported to be more effective than other topical agents short of plasminogen preparations in the treatment of this disorder in several studies.[11,18,19] Ciclosporin A interferes with IL-2 production, thus preventing the activation and recruitment of the T-cell response. Immunohistochemical analysis of a lesion resected after 6 months of topical ciclosporin A therapy supports the immune role of this entity.[11] A significant decrease in the total number of T lymphocytes was found, with the greatest decrease occurring in the T-suppressor/cytotoxic cell subpopulation. Also of interest was the absence of IL-2 receptors on the T cells. Finally, a decrease in the number of B lymphocytes and plasma cells occurred. These results indicate the local effect ciclosporin A has on the immune response. The marked reduction of T-suppressor/cytotoxic cells was a secondary effect, as these cells are recruited by activated T cells. The clinical response and histopathologic confirmation of the effect of ciclosporin A further support the inflammatory nature of this disease.

Treatment

Plasminogen substitution is presently being investigated as the primary treatment for LC.[23,31,34,35] Mingers et al. first proposed the theory of plasminogen deficiency and attempted supplementing plasminogen.[35] Higher doses of intravenous lysine-conjugated plasminogen, 1000 units/day continuous infusion for 2 weeks, have been used successfully in an infant with LC, followed by 1000-unit daily bolus injections thereafter.[8] Topical plasminogen preparations extracted from fresh frozen plasma have successfully been employed in the treatment of LC; three patients remained free of recurrences for over 12 months with topical administration as frequently as every 2 hours.[23] Another patient with hourly plasminogen drop administration had resolution of pseudomembranes in 3 weeks; after tapering, the disease reoccurred and was again quieted with readministration of plaminogen drops. Chronic low-dose maintenance treatment with topical plasminogen was thought necessary for this patient.[51] A combination of systemic or subconjuctival fresh frozen plasma (FFP) and topical FFP have shown success in two patients.[52,53] These modes of treatment bypass the need for plasminogen concentrate alone which has a very short half-life and is difficult to have readily available. No reoccurrence of disease was noted 12 months after pseudomembrane excision in either of these patients.

Early histologic studies had shown that the three major components of ligneous lesions are (1) an acellular, eosinophilic, periodic acid–Schiff-positive, hyaline material; (2) areas of granulation tissue; and (3) areas of cellular infiltration.[7,10,12,14,21] Based on those early observations, topical medical regimens geared toward these nonspecific findings were developed, although treatment of this disorder, for the most part, was unsuccessful. Topical hyaluronidase in conjunction with α-chymotrypsin, was reported to be effective,[7] but in other studies it was not beneficial.[12,14,21] Other forms of topical therapy, including antibiotics, corticosteroids, sodium cromoglycate, fibrinolysin, heparin, and silver nitrate, have met with limited success. Ciclosporin had been the most promising element in the therapeutic armamentarium before plasminogen.[51,55] Recently, oral contraceptives have been noted to show a marked increase in plasminogen levels due to hormonal up-regulation of plasminogen synthesis. In two patients, Sartori et al. showed treatment to be associated with a rise in plasminogen levels and improvement in clinical findings with resolution of disease in one patient.[56] This therapy may be useful in selected female patients with hypoplasminogenemia.

Because trauma to the conjunctiva is likely to be an etiologic factor in ligneous conjunctivitis, conjunctival surgery must be performed only with the utmost forethought and care. The authors recommend against performing conjunctival autograft for ligneous conjunctivitis. Recently, Barabino and Rolando performed amniotic membrane transplantation for conjuctival reconstruction of LC.[57] Following surgery, the patient was given a 6-month course of heparin eyedrops (5000 U/mL) with dexamethasone and tobramycin for 2 weeks postoperatively. The patient had small recurrences at 8 months, necessitating regrafting of the amniotic membrane. At 36 months post-procedure, the patient was disease free. The authors would advise pretreating any

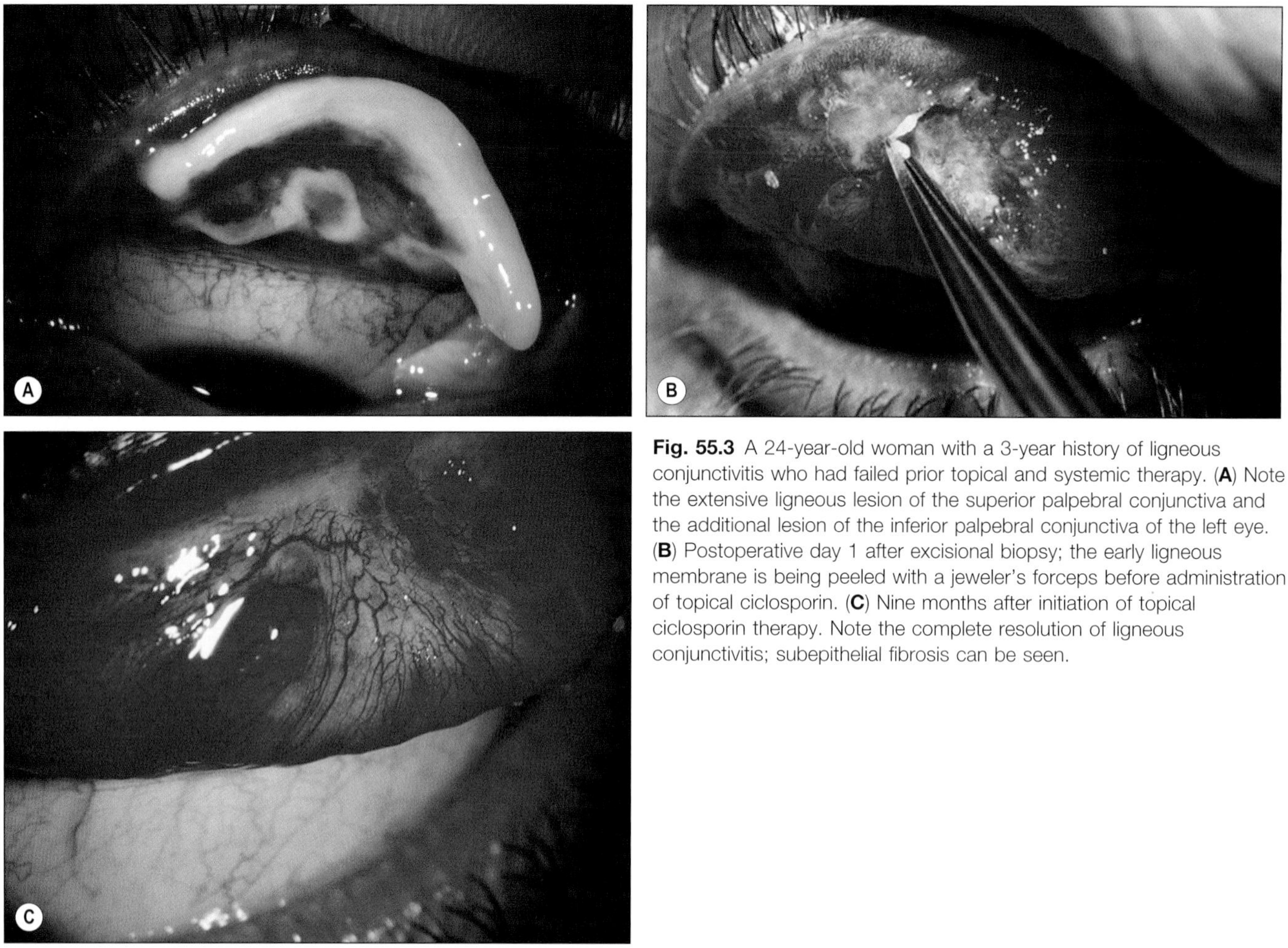

Fig. 55.3 A 24-year-old woman with a 3-year history of ligneous conjunctivitis who had failed prior topical and systemic therapy. (**A**) Note the extensive ligneous lesion of the superior palpebral conjunctiva and the additional lesion of the inferior palpebral conjunctiva of the left eye. (**B**) Postoperative day 1 after excisional biopsy; the early ligneous membrane is being peeled with a jeweler's forceps before administration of topical ciclosporin. (**C**) Nine months after initiation of topical ciclosporin therapy. Note the complete resolution of ligneous conjunctivitis; subepithelial fibrosis can be seen.

patient with plasminogen therapy prior to surgery with slow postoperative tapering. Otherwise, cryosurgery, electrocoagulation, and surgical resection of ligneous lesions typically result in rapid recurrence of the lesions within days to weeks.

Based on the literature and the authors' clinical experience, the authors recommend the following approach with these patients. All patients should receive a thorough, dilated ocular examination. Otolaryngology and anesthesia are consulted to evaluate the patient's respiratory tract, not only to search for concomitant disease but also because many patients need to be debrided under anesthesia, and any tracheal or laryngeal abnormalities must be discovered before induction. Systemic and topical plasminogen or FFP treatment is started, as described above, possibly in combination with a plasminogen activator (uPA or tPA) to help soften the pseudomembrane and facilitate removal. If patients do not respond to this approach, consideration may be given to therapeutic options other than plasminogen treatment.

The next step would be a complete excisional biopsy of all ocular ligneous lesions. General anesthesia may be used in adults with significant disease and in all children. In advanced disease, excision will require extensive surgery to dissect the substantia propria of the conjunctiva. Eversion of the eyelid is mandatory. Significant bleeding should be expected, and topical epinephrine and cautery may prove helpful. Failure to completely remove the lesion results in rapid recurrence because the retained lesion acts as a physical barrier to topical medical treatment.

Immediately after surgery, the patient is continued on systemic and topical FFP and started on a corticosteroid and broad-spectrum antibiotic four times daily with topical ciclosporin A 2% twice daily. These medications must be given after surgery, as early recurrence is the hallmark of this disorder.

Early in the postoperative period, patients must be seen at least once a day. A small but significant amount of recurrence will be seen daily in every patient, and every recurrent lesion must be debrided daily with a jeweler's forceps (Fig. 55.3). If abnormal tissue is allowed to collect for even 1 to 2 days, it will act as a barrier and prevent the topical medications from reaching the basal tissue, which is the origin of the ligneous membranes. Pediatric patients are placed in a restraining papoose for their daily examinations, and their parents are taught to debride the lesions with cotton-tipped applicators while they are applying the ciclosporin A.

Within the first few weeks of therapy, the rate and severity of recurrences lessen, and the topical medications can be tapered slowly. Some lesions progress despite this aggressive

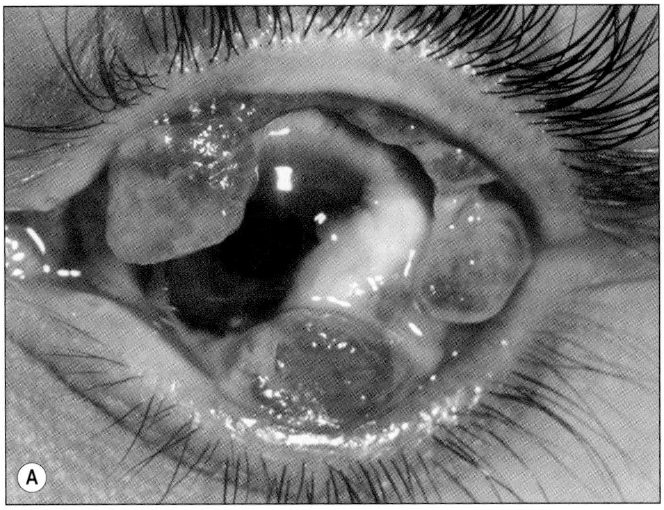

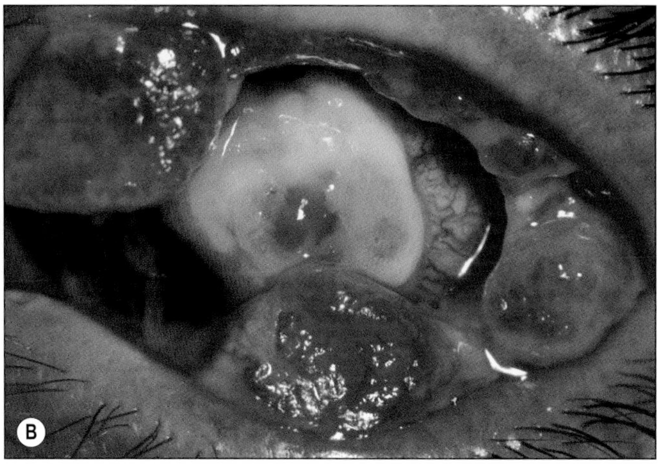

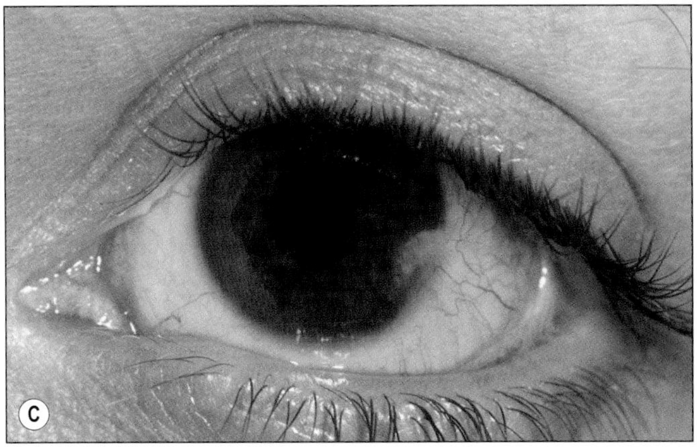

Fig. 55.4 A 20-year-old woman with a 10-year history of ligneous conjunctivitis of the left eye. (**A**) Extensive vascularized ligneous lesions of the superior and inferior palpebral conjunctiva. (**B**) Note the fleshy ligneous lesion at the 3 o'clock meridian extending over the cornea. (**C**) The same patient showing complete resolution after 9 months of topical ciclosporin and serial excisional biopsies.

topical therapy. Patients with these lesions must be brought back to the operating room for repeat excisional biopsy. After this surgical procedure, the patient must be placed back on the initial, topical regimen described previously. Results with repeated excisions and aggressive topical management have been satisfactory (Fig. 55.4).

As we continue to refine plasminogen therapy, more light is being shed on the pathophysiology of this disease. Overall, the development of systemic and topical plasminogen preparations as a treatment of ligneous conjunctivitis carries a new promise for patients with ligneous conjuctivitis.

References

1. Bouisson M. Ophthalmie sur-aigue avec formation de pseudomembranes a la surface de la conjonctive. *Ann Ocul (Paris)*. 1847;17:100–104.
2. Borel MG. Un nouveau syndrome palpebral. *Bull Soc Ophthalmol Fr.* 1933;46:168–180.
3. Bierly JR, et al. Ligneous conjunctivitis as a complication following strabismus surgery. *J Pediatr Ophthalmol Strabismus*. 1994;31:99–103.
4. Chambers JD, et al. Ligneous conjunctivitis. *Trans Am Acad Ophthalmol Otolaryngol*. 1969;73:996–1004.
5. Cohen SR. Ligneous conjunctivitis: an ophthalmic disease with potentially fatal tracheobronchial obstruction. *Ann Otol Rhinol Laryngol.* 1990;99:509–512.
6. Diamond JP, et al. Tranexamic acid-associated ligneous conjunctivitis with gingival and peritoneal lesions. *Br J Ophthalmol.* 1991;75:753–754.
7. Francois J, Victoria-Troncoso V. Treatment of ligneous conjunctivitis. *Am J Ophthalmol.* 1968;65:674–678.
8. Frimodt-Moller J. Conjunctivitis lignosa combined with a dental affection. *Acta Ophthalmol (Copenh)*. 1973;51:34–38.
9. Girard LJ, Veselinovic A, Font RL. Ligneous conjunctivitis after pinguecula removal in an adult. *Cornea*. 1989;8:7–14.
10. Hidayat AA, Riddle PJ. Ligneous conjunctivitis: a clinicopathologic study of 17 cases. *Ophthalmology*. 1987;94:949–959.
11. Holland FJ, et al. Immunohistologic findings and results of treatment with cyclosporine A in ligneous conjunctivitis. *Am J Ophthalmol.* 1989;107:160–166.
12. Kanai A, Polack FM. Histologic and electron microscopic studies of ligneous conjunctivitis. *Am J Ophthalmol.* 1971;72:909–916.
13. McGrand JC, Rees DM, Harry J. Ligneous conjunctivitis. *Br J Ophthalmol.* 1969;53:373–381.
14. Melikian HE. Treatment of ligneous conjunctivitis. *Ann Ophthalmol.* 1985;17:763–765.
15. Newcomer V, Klein A. Ligneous conjunctivitis. *Arch Dermatol.* 1977;113:511–512.
16. Nussgens Z, Roggenkamper P. Ligneous conjunctivitis: ten-year follow-up. *Ophthalmic Paediatr Genet.* 1993;14:137–140.
17. Rubin A, Buck D, MacDonald MR. Ligneous conjunctivitis involving the cervix. *Br J Obstet Gynaecol.* 1989;96:1228–1230.
18. Rubin BI, et al. Response of reactivated ligneous conjunctivitis to topical cyclosporine. *Am J Ophthalmol.* 1991;112:95–96.
19. Schwartz GS, Holland EJ. Induction of ligneous conjunctivitis by conjunctival surgery. *Am J Ophthalmol.* 1995;120:253–254.
20. Weinstock SM, Kielar RA. Bulbar ligneous conjunctivitis after pterygium removal in an elderly man. *Am J Ophthalmol.* 1975;79:913–915.
21. Eagle RC, et al. Fibrin as a major constituent of ligneous conjunctivitis. *Am J Ophthalmol.* 1986;101:493–494.
22. De Cock R, et al. Topical heparin in the treatment of ligneous conjunctivitis. *Ophthalmology.* 1995;102:1654–1659.
23. Watts P, et al. Effective treatment of ligneous conjunctivitis with topical plasminogen. *Am J Ophthalmol.* 2002;133(4):451–455.

24. Ozcelik U, et al. Pulmonary involvement in a child with ligneous conjunctivitis and homozygous type I plasminogen deficiency. *Pediatr Pulmonol.* 2001;32(2):179–183.
25. Chang BY, et al. An interesting case of ligneous conjunctivitis. *Eye.* 2001;15(Pt 6):806–807.
26. Scully C, et al. Oral lesions indicative of plasminogen deficiency (hypoplasminogenemia). *Oral Surg Oral Med Oral Pathol Oral Radiol Endod.* 2001;91(3):334–337.
27. Ramsby ML, Donshik PC, Makowski GS. Ligneous conjunctivitis: biochemical evidence for hypofibrinolysis. *Inflammation.* 2000;24(1):45–71.
28. Chowdhury MM, Blackford S, Williams S. Juvenile colloid milium associated with ligneous conjunctivitis: report of a case and review of the literature. *Clin Exp Dermatol.* 2000;25(2):138–140.
29. Schuster V, et al. Compound-heterozygous mutations in the plasminogen gene predispose to the development of ligneous conjunctivitis. *Blood.* 1999;93(10):3457–3466.
30. Schuster V, et al. Prenatal diagnosis in a family with severe type I plasminogen deficiency, ligneous conjunctivitis and congenital hydrocephalus. *Prenat Diagn.* 1999;19(5):483–487.
31. Mingers AM, et al. Human homozygous type I plasminogen deficiency and ligneous conjunctivitis. *Apmis.* 1999;107(1):62–72.
32. Klebe S, et al. Immunohistological findings in a patient with unusual late onset manifestations of ligneous conjunctivitis. *Br J Ophthalmol.* 1999;83(7):878–879.
33. Rao SK, et al. Ligneous conjunctivitis: a clinicopathologic study of 3 cases. *Int Ophthalmol.* 1998;22(4):201–206.
34. Mingers AM, et al. Polymorphonuclear elastase in patients with homozygous type I plasminogen deficiency and ligneous conjunctivitis. *Semin Thromb Hemost.* 1998;24(6):605–612.
35. Mingers AM, et al. Homozygous type I plasminogen deficiency. *Semin Thromb Hemost.* 1997;23(3):259–269.
36. Schuster V, Seregard S. Ligneous conjunctivitis. *Surv Ophthalmol.* 2003;48(4):369–388.
37. Cooper TJ, Kazdan JJ, Cutz E. Lingeous conjunctivitis with tracheal obstruction. A case report, with light and electron microscopy findings. *Can J Ophthalmol.* 1979;14(1):57–62.
38. Tefts K, et al. Molecular and clinical spectrum of type I plasminogen deficiency: a series of 50 patients. *Blood.* 2006;108(9):3021–3026.
39. Trojan H. Histology of conjuctivitis lignosa. *Klin Monatsbl Augenheilkd.* 1971;158(4):551–554.
40. Schwartz GS, Holland EJ. Induction of ligneous conjunctivitis by conjunctival surgery. *Am J Ophthalmol.* 1995;120(2):253–254.
41. Rodriguez-Ares MT, et al. Ligneous conjuctivitis: a clinicopathological, immunohistochemical, and genetic study including the treatment of two sisters with multiorgan involvement. *Virchows Arch.* 2007;451(4): 815–821.
42. McCullough K, et al. Ligneous conjuctivitis: a case report with multiorgan involvement. *Histopathology.* 2007;50(4):511–513.
43. Gokbuget AY, et al. Amyloidaceous ulcerated gingival hyperplasia: a newly described entity related to ligneous conjunctivitis. *J Oral Pathol Med.* 1997;26(2):100–104.
44. Mirshahi M, et al. Production of proteases type plasminogen activator and their inhibitor in cornea. *Biochem Biophys Res Commun.* 1989; 160(3):1021–1025.
45. Marcus DM, et al. Ligneous conjunctivitis with ear involvement. *Arch Ophthalmol.* 1990;108(4):514–519.
46. Ridley CM, Morgan H. Ligneous conjunctivitis involving the fallopian tube. *Br J Obstet Gynaecol.* 1993;100(8):791.
47. Babcock MF, Bedford RF, Berry FA. Ligneous tracheobronchitis: an unusual cause of airway obstruction. *Anesthesiology.* 1987;67(5):819–821.
48. Hidayat AA, Riddle PJ. Ligneous conjunctivitis. A clinicopathologic study of 17 cases. *Ophthalmology.* 1987;94(8):949–959.
49. Cohen SR. Ligneous conjunctivitis: an ophthalmic disease with potentially fatal tracheobronchial obstruction. Laryngeal and tracheobronchial features. *Ann Otol Rhinol Laryngol.* 1990;99(7 Pt 1):509–512.
50. Nussgens Z, Roggenkamper P. Ligneous conjunctivitis. Ten years' follow-up. *Ophthalmic Paediatr Genet.* 1993;14(3):137–140.
51. Heidemann DG, et al. Treatment of ligneous conjuctivitis with topical plasmin and topical plasminogen. *Cornea.* 2003;22(8):760–762.
52. Gurlu VP, et al. Systemic and topical fresh-frozen plasma treatment in a newborn with ligneous conjuctivitis. *Cornea.* 2008;27(4):501–503.
53. Tabbara KF. Prevention of ligneous conjuctivitis by topical and subconjuctival fresh frozen plasma. *Am J Ophthalmol.* 2004;138(2):299–300.
54. Rubin BI, et al. Response of reactivated ligneous conjunctivitis to topical cyclosporine. *Am J Ophthalmol.* 1991;112(1):95–96.
55. Holland EJ, et al. Topical cyclosporin A in the treatment of anterior segment inflammatory disease. *Cornea.* 1993;12(5):413–419.
56. Sartori MT, et al. Contrceptive pills induce an improvement in congential hypoplasminogenemia in two unrelated patients with lignous conjuctivitis. *Thromb Haemost.* 2003;90(1)86–91.
57. Barabino S, Rolando M. Amniotic membrane transplantation in a case of ligneous conjuctivitis. *Am J Ophthalmol.* 2004;137(4):752–753.

Chapter 56

Conjunctivochalasis

Julie H. Tsai

Introduction

Conjunctivochalasis (CCh), defined as redundant conjunctiva, is most often located between the eyeball and the lower eyelid. In general, CCh is a bilateral condition, and is often asymptomatic and thus generally overlooked as a normal variant of age. The term was first coined by Hughes in 1942, though the findings of loose, nonedematous conjunctiva had been reported as early as 1908 by Elschnig, and later in 1921 and 1922 by Braunschweig and Wollenberg, respectively.[1,2] These early cases often presented with symptoms of pain, corneal ulceration, and subconjunctival hemorrhage. Treatment described during this period was predominantly medical, including frequent lubrication, and nighttime patching to prevent nocturnal exposure.

In some cases, the loose conjunctiva can be interposed between the globe and lower eyelid, and the protrusion of this tissue can lead to occlusion of the lower punctum. This mechanical obstruction could lead to intermittent tearing, notably worse in nasal gaze. The loose conjunctiva could also cause tearing secondary to mechanical disruption of the tear meniscus. This description was reported later, in 1986 by Liu, who proposed that the disruption of the tear meniscus would be more common than mechanical displacement of the inferior punctum.[3]

Since then, the relationship between conjunctivochalasis and the tear film was further elucidated by Rieger in 1990, Grene in 1991, and Höh et al. in 1995.[4] These authors found a high correlation with the degree of conjunctivochalasis and the symptoms of dry eye, or keratoconjunctivitis sicca (KCS), and the grading of the degree of CCh was found to have a high predictive value for diagnosis of KCS. In these cases, the degree of conjunctivochalasis was often mild, though it is unclear whether the presence of this redundant tissue definitively causes dry eye as defined by the current criteria.

Epidemiology

Conjunctivochalasis may be one of the most common changes related to the aging eye. There have been reports of conjunctivochalasis in patients in the first decade of life, though the majority of cases are seen in the elderly (Fig. 56.1). Mimura et al. conducted a prospective, nonrandomized consecutive case study to evaluate the prevalence of conjunctivochalasis and found that, beyond 30 years of age, the presence and severity of conjunctivochalasis became more extensive with each successive decade.[5] There were no significant differences between females and males from each age group. Interestingly, the regions of conjunctivochalasis – such as nasal, medial, and temporal regions – differed by gender, though this has not been noted in other studies.

Histopathology

Initially, a senile process related to conjunctival laxity was suggested in the nineteenth century, and to date it has continued to receive some support. Eye movements were also suggested as a possible cause of conjunctivochalasis in 1921, when Braunschweig noted that ductions often produced conjunctival displacement and laxity. Eye rubbing from irritation or allergy may also contribute to this laxity. Abnormalities in lid position were also suggested as an underlying etiology during the early twentieth century. Entities such as ectropion often present with similar clinical findings of epiphora and irritation, and thus were considered possible etiologies for conjunctivochalasis.[2]

However, the underlying etiology of conjunctivochalasis remains unknown, though several recent studies suggest that abnormalities in the extracellular components may contribute to the pathogenesis. Some clinicopathologic studies have found signs of elastosis and chronic nongranulomatous inflammation, in addition to collagenolysis.[6] These can also be seen in other ocular surface degenerations (i.e. pinguecula, pterygium), and have been associated with conjunctivochalasis.[7,8] Matrix metalloproteinases (MMPs), enzymes that modify or degrade the extracellular matrix, have been found to be up-regulated in tissue culture; specifically, MMP-1 and MMP-3 were found to be overexpressed in the conjunctivochalasis fibroblasts when compared to normal conjunctival fibroblasts in cell culture.[9] However, tissue inhibitors of metalloproteinases (TIMPs) expression remains unchanged, particularly TIMP-1 and TIMP-2, when compared to normal conjunctival fibroblasts. This change in the ratio of MMPs to TIMPs may facilitate the breakdown of the extracellular matrix and result in the clinical changes observed in conjunctivochalasis. Furthermore, inflammatory cytokines such as interleukin-1 (IL-1) and tumor necrosis factor alpha (TNF-

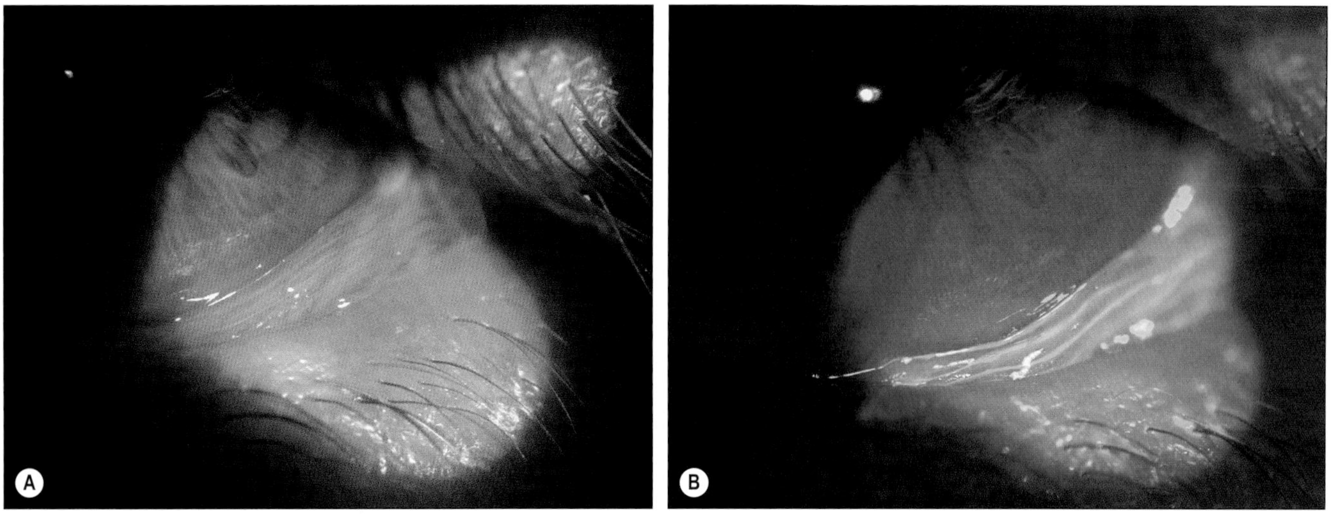

Fig. 56.1 Temporal conjunctivochalasis in a patient with symptoms of irritation, tearing, and occasional pain. (**A**) Clinical photograph depicting temporal conjunctivochalasis and (**B**) note that instillation of fluorescein highlights the redundant folds seen on examination.

α) may initiate increased expression of MMPs and increasing degradation of the extracellular milieu.[9] Inflammatory cytokines in the tear film, specifically interleukin-6 (IL-6) and interleukin-8 (IL-8) have been found to be elevated in the tear film of patients with CCh. The severity of disease has been positively correlated with elevated levels of these inflammatory markers.[10]

Another etiology has been revisited and studied recently by Watanabe et al., who suggest that the pressure from the lids affects the conjunctival lymphatics, and that this may contribute to the development of conjunctivochalasis (Fig. 56.2).[11] Histopathologic sections comparing the conjunctiva of an affected area to that of normal conjunctiva revealed large areas of lymphangiectasia in the conjunctivochalasis sample. In addition, the authors found fragmented elastic fibers with loss of collagen in the affected samples as compared to controls. They postulate that this, along with a lack of inflammation in their study population, supports the hypothesis that underlying histopathologic changes in conjunctivochalasis may be related to the aging process rather than a proinflammatory milieu, as suggested by other groups.

Symptoms and Clinical Presentation

Conjunctivochalasis is generally asymptomatic, though the clinical presentation can range from irritation in mild stages, marked tearing due to obstruction of the lower punctum in the moderate stage, and ocular surface exposure in more severe stages. The location of the redundant tissue lies along the inferior lid margin, and in mild cases, disruption or aggravation of the tear film may be the only contribution to the patient's symptoms. Patients often note irritation, watery eyes, and redness. Other complaints may include blurring of the vision while reading, and minimal improvement upon instillation of ocular lubricants. Untreated patients may complain of worsening epiphora and persistent foreign body sensation. In more moderate cases, nasal CCh can impede tear outflow through the inferior punctum, resulting in epiphora.[3,11–13]

Once the patient has reached the advanced stages of the disease, the complaints may include severe pain and blurry vision upon awakening in addition to an increase in the severity of the aforementioned symptoms. In these instances, the protrusion of the affected tissue can cause corneal exposure, irritation, and pain when the conjunctiva is caught between the eyelids upon closure or blink. These dramatic presentations often go hand in hand with the associated symptoms of blurred vision, irritation, and excessive tearing. In most cases, visual prognosis remains excellent, though in some individuals acuity may be limited by concomitant ocular surface or lid diseases. It is important to note that these symptoms can be found in the setting of aqueous tear deficiency, and they can also be found with conjunctivochalasis alone, without concomitant tear deficiency.[14] The difficulty lies in the determination of the full extent of involvement of the redundant conjunctiva as it relates to tear film dysfunction, or dry eye.

Diagnosis

In evaluating these complaints of tearing and irritation, lid pathology such as horizontal laxity, entropion, ectropion trichiasis, punctual stenosis, and nasolacrimal obstruction should be ruled out. Other systemic causes of tearing, including allergy, thyroid orbitopathy, and dry eye should also be excluded. In severe cases, the areas of redundant conjunctiva are easily visualized upon biomicroscopy. There may be prolapse of the conjunctiva over the lower lid margin in the temporal, medial, or nasal regions, or all three regions may be affected. The diagnostic dilemma lies in elucidating the more subtle presentations of CCh, which are associated with vague complaints. The patient often notes irritation, watery eyes, and redness. These findings are often attributed to dry eye syndrome or tear film instability. Conjunctivochalasis is often mild and may not appear to be disrupting the tear meniscus. In these cases, the difficulty lies in determining the extent to which the redundant conjunctival tissue contributes to the patient's symptoms. The grading systems

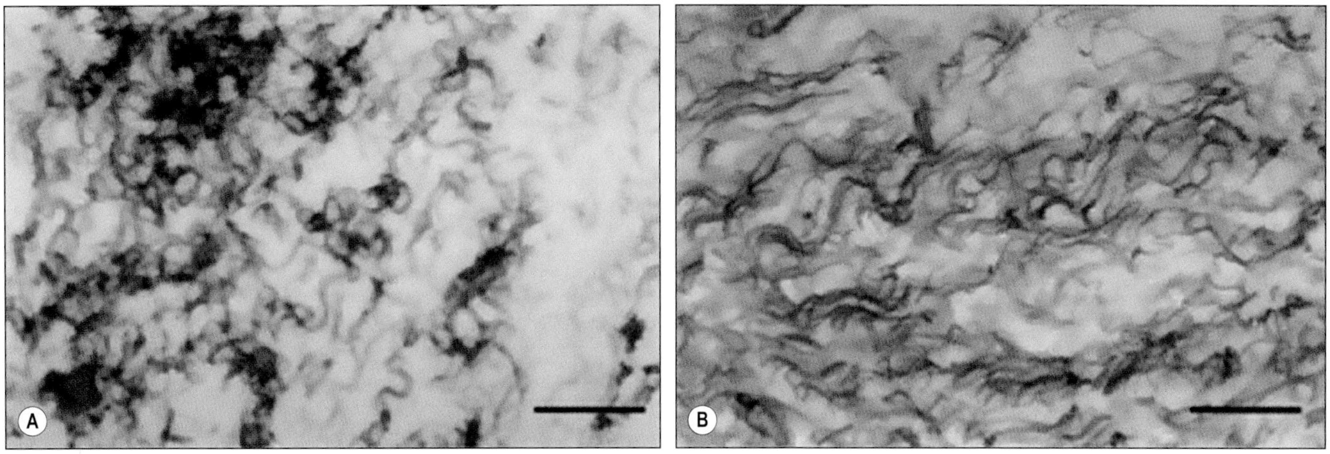

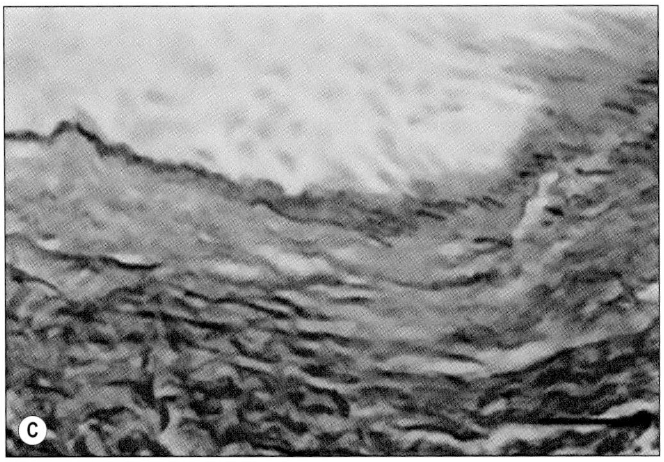

Fig. 56.2 Elastica van Gieson (EVG) staining of a representative example of excited redundant conjunctiva (**A**) and supposed normal conjunctiva from a 32-year-old woman (**B**) and a 13-year-old boy (**C**). (Scale bars = 100 μm). (**A**) Fragmentation of elastic fibers and sparsely assembled collagen fibers. (**B**) There is slight fragmentation of elastic fibers. Collagen fibers are plentiful. (**C**) There is no fragmentation of elastic fibers. Collagen fibers are plentiful and arranged regularly. (Reprinted with permission from: Watanabe A, Yokoi N, Kinoshita S, Hino Y, Tsuchihashi Y. Clinicopathologic study of conjunctivochalasis. *Cornea*. 2004;23:294–298.)

Table 56.1 Classification of conjunctivochalasis using the lid-parallel folds method grading of conjunctivochalasis by LIPCOF*

Grade	Number of folds and relationship to the tear meniscus height
0	No persistent fold
1	Single, small fold
2	More than two folds and not higher than the tear meniscus
3	Multiple folds and higher than the tear meniscus

* *Modified from Höh et al.[4] with permission of the authors and* Ophthalmologe. *Reprinted with permission from: Meller D, Tseng SC. Conjunctivochalasis: literature review and possible pathophysiology.* Surv Ophthalmol. *1998;43: 225–232. Copyright Elsevier, 1998.*

proposed by Höh et al. and Meller and Tseng offer objective and reliable criteria for diagnosis (Tables 56.1, 56.2).[4,15]

The standard work-up for dry eye syndrome can be employed, though such testing may be low yield if the patient does not have concomitant aqueous-deficient dry eye. In cases where there is tear film instability, the presence of the parallel lid folds may mechanically disrupt the tear film and thus confound results of diagnostic testing. These cases can often go undiagnosed for months, and trials of topical medications such as corticosteroids and antihistamines are often needed to determine if the patient's symptoms are related to ocular surface inflammation or are secondary to the mechanical effects of the boggy conjunctiva. The hallmark finding in these cases is the refractory nature of the patient's symptoms to medical therapy.

Treatment

No treatment is recommended if the patient is asymptomatic. For those patients with severe disease, medical therapy can be suggested. This often includes the use of surface lubricants, antihistamines, and topical corticosteroids. In mild cases, these medications can often relieve the symptoms on a temporary basis. Patching of the eye may be suggested for cases of nocturnal exposure or ulceration. In cases where medical management remains largely unsuccessful, or if there is worsening of symptoms despite patient compliance with the topical regimen, surgical treatment becomes necessary.

Surgical management often involves the resection of the redundant tissue. Several methods have been described, including crescent resection with or without suture, suture

Table 56.2 Proposed new grading system for conjunctivochalasis*

Different aspects, including location, height of tear meniscus, presence of punctual occlusion, position of gaze, and pressure from the lids can affect the degree of conjunctivochalasis.

Location	Folds versus tear meniscus height	Punctal occlusion	Changes in downgaze	Changes by digital pressure
0	A	O +	G ↑	P ↑
1	B	O −	G ⇌	P ⇌
2	C		G ↓	P ↓
3				
0: none	A: < tear meniscus	O ≥ nasal location with punctal occlusion	G ↑ = height/extent of chalasis increases in downgaze	P ↑ = height/extent of chalasis increases on digital pressure
1: one location	B: = tear meniscus			
2: two locations	C: > tear meniscus			
3: whole lid		O ≤ nasal location without punctal occlusion	G ⇌ = no difference G ↓ = height/extent of chalasis decreases in downgaze	P ⇌ = no difference P ↓ = height/extent of chalasis decreases on digital pressure

* *The new grading system defines the extension of redundant conjunctiva as grade 1 = one location, 2 = 2 locations, 3 = whole lid. For 1 and 2, it is further specified as T, M, and N if conjunctivochalasis is found in the temporal, the middle (or inferior to the limbus), and the nasal aspect of the lower lid, respectively. For each location (T, M, and N), further notation is given to indicate if the height of folds is less than (A), equal to (B), or greater than (C) the tear meniscus height. If it is found in the nasal (N) location, the extent of chalasis is further determined as to whether it occludes the inferior puncta. For each location, it is further graded as G ↑ if its height is greater than, as G ⇌ if equal to, and as G ↓ if less than the tear meniscus height. Likewise it is further graded as P ↑, P ⇌, and P ↓ if it is worse, no difference, or better with digital pressure (P), respectively.*

Reprinted with permission from: Meller D, Tseng SC. Conjunctivochalasis: literature review and possible pathophysiology. Surv Ophthalmol. *1998;43:225–232. Copyright Elsevier, 1998.*

fixation of the redundant conjunctiva to the globe, and amniotic membrane with or without the use of fibrin tissue glue.[1,15–20] The most common involves a crescent excision of the affected area 5 mm posterior to the limbus (Fig. 56.3A,B). Closure is completed with absorbable sutures. Serrano and Mora describe a modification which includes a peritomy made close to the limbus along with two radial relaxing incisions (Fig. 56.3C,D).[16] This was proposed to avoid visible scarring or retraction of the inferior conjunctival fornix. Another modification developed to avoid these same complications involves the use of amniotic membrane transplantation to resurface the defect after excision of the involved conjunctiva (Fig. 56.3E,F). In all instances, aggressive resection of conjunctiva should be avoided in order to reduce complications such as cicatricial entropion, retraction of the lower fornix, and restriction of motility. Other findings can include suture-induced granulomas, scar formation, and focal inflammation of the conjunctiva surrounding an amniotic graft, though the graft itself remains uninflamed. The latter can be managed successfully with subconjunctival injections of triamcinolone (20–40 mg).[20]

Success rates with each method are similar. Initial reports of these surgical techniques suggest satisfactory results, and in more recent years more data have been published which support these approaches to treatment. In a study of the impact of conjunctivochalasis on the ocular surface, Yokoi and colleagues found an improvement in symptoms in 88.2% (104 eyes) with resection of the affected tissue and subsequent suturing of the resultant defect in the bulbar conjunctiva.[19] Meller et al. report that 46 eyes (97.8%) that underwent sutured amniotic membrane transplantation for symptomatic CCh refractory to medical therapy recovered smooth conjunctival surfaces, which remained stable and quiet over a follow-up period of 6.9 ± 4.3 months.[20] Specific symptoms including episodic epiphora, pain, redness, itching, blurry vision, and burning were also reduced. Lastly, in cases where amniotic membrane and fibrin glue have been utilized, 100% of treated cases (25 eyes) recovered smooth conjunctival surfaces and 44–56% of those patients noted a reduction in their symptoms of pain, blurred vision, and epiphora.[18]

Conclusion

Conjunctivochalasis is a common age-related finding that may contribute to symptoms such as irritation and excessive tearing. It is important to consider this entity during the diagnostic work-up of chronic irritation and epiphora. In cases where medical therapy is suboptimal, surgical reconstruction of the affected areas should be considered.

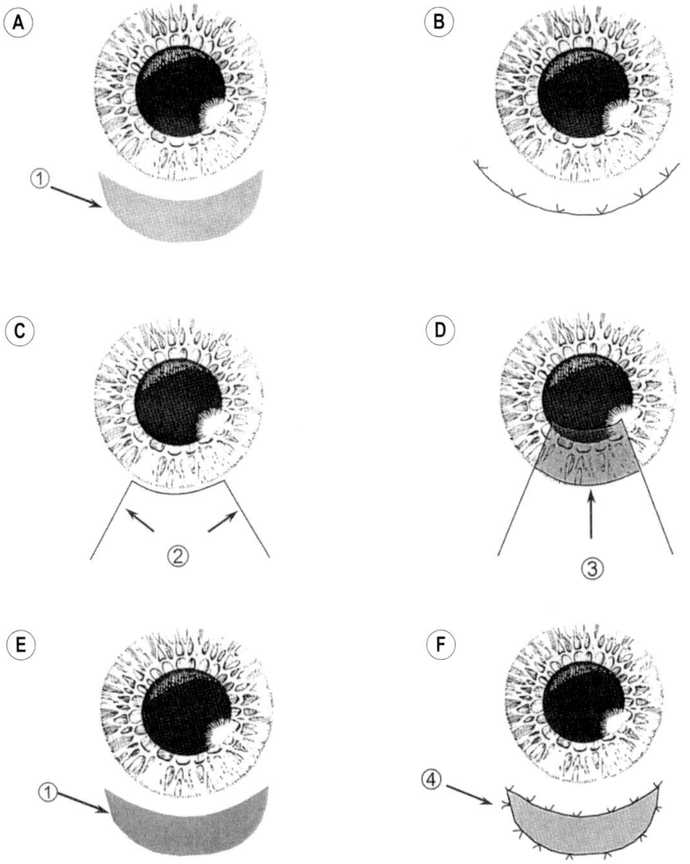

Fig. 56.3 Methods for excising redundant conjunctiva. (**A**) Crescentic resection with (**B**) use of absorbable suture for closure. (**C**) Peritomy with relaxing incisions. (**D**) The redundant conjunctiva is pulled toward the limbus, excised, and the remaining conjunctiva sutured in position. (**E**) Crescentic resection with (**F**) use of amniotic membrane for resurfacing the inferior bulbar conjunctival defect. This can be accomplished with suture fixation or with the use of fibrin tissue glue. (Reprinted with permission from: Meller D, Tseng SC. Conjunctivochalasis: literature review and possible pathophysiology. *Surv Ophthalmol.* 1998;43:225–232. Copyright Elsevier, 1998.)

References

1. Hughes WL. Conjunctivochalasis. *Am J Ophthalmol.* 1942;25:48–51.
2. Murube J. Characteristics and etiology of conjunctivochalasis: historical perspective. *Ocul Surf.* 2005;3:7–14.
3. Liu D. Conjunctivochalasis: a cause of tearing and its management. *Ophthal Plast Reconstr Surg.* 1986;2:25–28.
4. Höh H, Schirra F, Kienecker C, Ruprecht KW. Lidparrallele konjunktivale Falten (LIPCOF) sind ein sicheres diagnostisches Zeichen des trockenen Auges. *Ophthalmologe.* 1995;92:802–808.
5. Mimura T, Yamagami S, Usui T, et al. Changes of conjunctivochalasis with age in a hospital-based study. *Am J Ophthalmol.* 2009;147:171–177.
6. Chan DG, Francis IC, Filipic M, Coroneo MT, Yong J. Clinicopathologic study of conjunctivochalasis. *Cornea.* 2005;24:634.
7. Jaros PA, DeLuise VP. Pingueculae and pterygia. *Surv Ophthalmol.* 1988;33:41–49.
8. Wollenberg A. Pseudopterygium mit Faltenbildung der Conjunctiva bulbi. *Klin Monatsbl Augenheilkd.* 1922;68:221–224.
9. Li DQ, Meller D, Liu Y, Tseng SC. Overexpression of MMP-1 and MMP-3 by cultured conjunctivochalasis fibroblasts. *Invest Ophthalmol Vis Sci.* 2000;41:404–410.
10. Erdogan-Poyraz C, Mocan MC, Bozkurt B, et al. Elevated tear interleukin-6 and interleukin-8 levels in patients with conjunctivochalasis. *Cornea.* 2009;28:189–193.
11. Watanabe A, Yokoi N, Kinoshita S, Hino Y, Tsuchihashi Y. Clinicopathologic study of conjunctivochalasis. *Cornea.* 2004;23:294–298.
12. Erdogan-Poyraz C, Mocan MC, Irkec M, Orhan M. Delayed tear clearance in patients with conjunctivochalasis is associated with punctal occlusion. *Cornea.* 2007;26:290–293.
13. Wang Y, Dogru M, Matsumoto Y, et al. The impact of nasal conjunctivochalasis on tear functions and ocular surface findings. *Am J Ophthalmol.* 2007;144:930–937.
14. Meller D, Tseng SC. Conjunctivochalasis: literature review and possible pathophysiology. *Surv Ophthalmol.* 1998;43:225–232.
15. Di Pascuale MA, Espana EM, Kawakita T, Tseng SC. Clinical characteristics of conjunctivochalasis with or without aqueous tear deficiency. *Br J Ophthalmol.* 2004;88:388–392.
16. Serrano F, Mora LM. Conjunctivochalasis: a surgical technique. *Ophthalmic Surg.* 1989;20:883–884.
17. Otaka I, Kyu N. A new surgical technique for management of conjunctivochalasis. *Am J Ophthalmol.* 2000;129:385–387.
18. Kheirkhah A, Casas V, Blanco G, et al. Amniotic membrane transplantation with fibrin glue for conjunctivochalasis. *Am J Ophthalmol.* 2007;144:311–313.
19. Yokoi N, Komuro A, Nishii M, et al. Clinical impact of conjunctivochalasis on the ocular surface. *Cornea.* 2005;24:S24-S31.
20. Meller D, Maskin SL, Pires RT, Tseng SC. Amniotic membrane transplantation for symptomatic conjunctivochalasis refractory to medical treatments. *Cornea.* 2000;19:796–803.

PART VII

DISEASES OF THE CORNEA

Chapter **57**

Developmental Corneal Anomalies of Size and Shape

Preeya K. Gupta, Terry Kim

This chapter is devoted to specific diseases appearing predominantly in early infancy or childhood as the result of disruption in the normal development of the cornea and its associated structures. These developmental abnormalities may arise because of one or a combination of various genetic, infectious, inflammatory, toxic, metabolic, traumatic, or mechanical processes and may occur at any time during tissue induction, differentiation, and maturation. Most of the etiologic factors are believed to exert their influence either during the period of organogenesis (between the fourth and sixth gestational weeks) or during the period of anterior segment differentiation (between the sixth and sixteenth gestational weeks). Developmental insults with an earlier onset result in more severe and extensive injury than those that take place at a later intrauterine date. Therefore, not only the nature but also the timing of these insults contributes to determining the degree of damage and may aid the clinician in deducing the chronology of embryologic events. The exact time points of developmental insult as well as the pathophysiologic mechanisms and specific causative elements involved are often speculative and unknown.

An additional point of clarification should be made regarding the definition and implication of the term developmental. Developmental disorders may be manifest at birth and refer to those conditions occurring secondary to some alteration(s) of normal growth and differentiation (Box 57.1). The descriptive term congenital refers to any condition that is evident at the time of birth and carries no implications as to etiologic process, mechanism of injury, or hereditary status. Therefore, developmental abnormalities of the cornea should be considered as a separate and distinct subcategory of congenital disorders, since not all congenital corneal anomalies result from errors in development.

Although rarely encountered in routine ophthalmic practice, developmental corneal abnormalities are important to recognize in the newborn or child for several reasons. Providing the correct diagnosis can inform the clinician concerning the natural history of the condition, indicate the necessary medical or surgical treatment, and determine appropriate scheduling of follow-up care. Prompt examination can also alert the physician to the various ocular and systemic complications that may accompany the disorder and warrant additional investigation by other subspecialists. Finally, accurate identification and analysis of the disease help parents deal with the realities of the prognosis and guide them in seeking the proper genetic counseling when indicated.

The multitude of other congenital anomalies causing corneal opacities that are not considered to be truly developmental in origin are addressed in Chapter 19. The distinctive assortment of developmental conditions known to produce corneal opacities have been labeled as the anterior chamber cleavage syndromes and are discussed in Chapter 58. The present chapter will focus on the developmental corneal anomalies of size and shape.

Developmental corneal anomalies of size and shape represent an interesting collection of conditions caused by a defect in development resulting in a departure from normal corneal structure. These alterations in normal development often involve the neighboring structures of the anterior chamber angle, iris, and lens. Some of the ocular and systemic associations with the various corneal anomalies involve the anterior segment and occur because of the close embryologic relationship between these structures and the cornea. However, some of these associations do not have any connection with the developmental process and merely reflect reported cases of various accompanying characteristics.

Absence of the Cornea

Although absence of the cornea does not reflect an actual anomaly of size or shape, it is discussed in this chapter because it represents an extreme deviation of normal corneal structure. True absence of the cornea is a very rare condition that is always accompanied by agenesis of various other anterior segment structures. Manschot described a case of primary congenital aphakia that was associated with a missing cornea.[1] True absence of the cornea can never be an isolated finding simply because of its close relation to the embryologic differentiation of other anterior segment structures.[2] The absence of the cornea, iris, lens, and other anterior structures lies on a spectrum of agenesis, with anophthalmos (absence of the entire eye) representing the most extreme example.

True cryptophthalmos, otherwise known as complete cryptophthalmos or ablepharon, occurs when skin replaces the normal eyelid architecture and connects to the underlying globe, leaving the cornea and part of the conjunctiva unprotected and exposed (Fig. 57.1).[3] The cornea and

Box 57.1 Developmental corneal anomalies of size and shape

Absence of the cornea
- True absence of the cornea
- True cryptophthalmos (ablepharon)
- Pseudocryptophthalmos (total ankyloblepharon)

Anomalies of corneal size
- Megalocornea
- Microcornea

Anomalies of corneal shape
- Oval cornea
  - Horizontal
  - Vertical
- Astigmatism
- Sclerocornea (cornea plana)
- Posterior keratoconus
  - Generalized
  - Circumscribed
- Keratoglobus
- Congenital anterior staphyloma and keratectasia

conjunctiva are present in this condition but undergo metaplastic change (termed dermoid transformation) to form skin.[3] This condition is also very rare, with only approximately 50 reported cases in the literature.[4] It is usually bilateral although it can be asymmetric and is commonly transmitted as an autosomal recessive trait.[3] It is also accompanied by the absence of any lashes or brows, with the lacrimal glands and canaliculi frequently absent as well.[3,5] The eye itself usually contains a small or absent anterior chamber; the iris, lens, trabecular meshwork, and Schlemm's canal are frequently nonexistent or otherwise replaced by connective tissue.[6] Of the reported associated systemic abnormalities, craniofacial anomalies are the most common; others include syndactyly, spina bifida, deformed ears and teeth, cleft lip or palate, laryngeal or anal atresia, ventral hernias, nipple or umbilicus displacement, basal encephalocele, genitourinary anomalies, cardiac anomalies, and mental retardation.[4,6,7] The term cryptophthalmos syndrome, also termed Fraser syndrome, has been used to describe patients who meet specific criteria as outlined by Thomas (Table 57.1).[5,8]

Pseudocryptophthalmos (total ankyloblepharon) is a related condition in which the eyelids form but fail to separate, leaving a normal cornea and conjunctiva totally covered by skin. Unlike its true counterpart, both lashes and brows are present with an otherwise normal eye, and vision is restored by surgically creating a palpebral fissure.[9]

With the exception of pseudocryptophthalmos, the two former conditions are associated with a very dismal visual prognosis with no indicated treatment. Besides proper education and counseling, the only warranted intervention may be for cosmetic purposes.[10] While pseudocryptophthalmos is associated with an excellent visual potential after surgery, the newly opened eyelids pose a continued challenge in terms of preventing lid reclosure and maintaining a functionally normal eyelid.

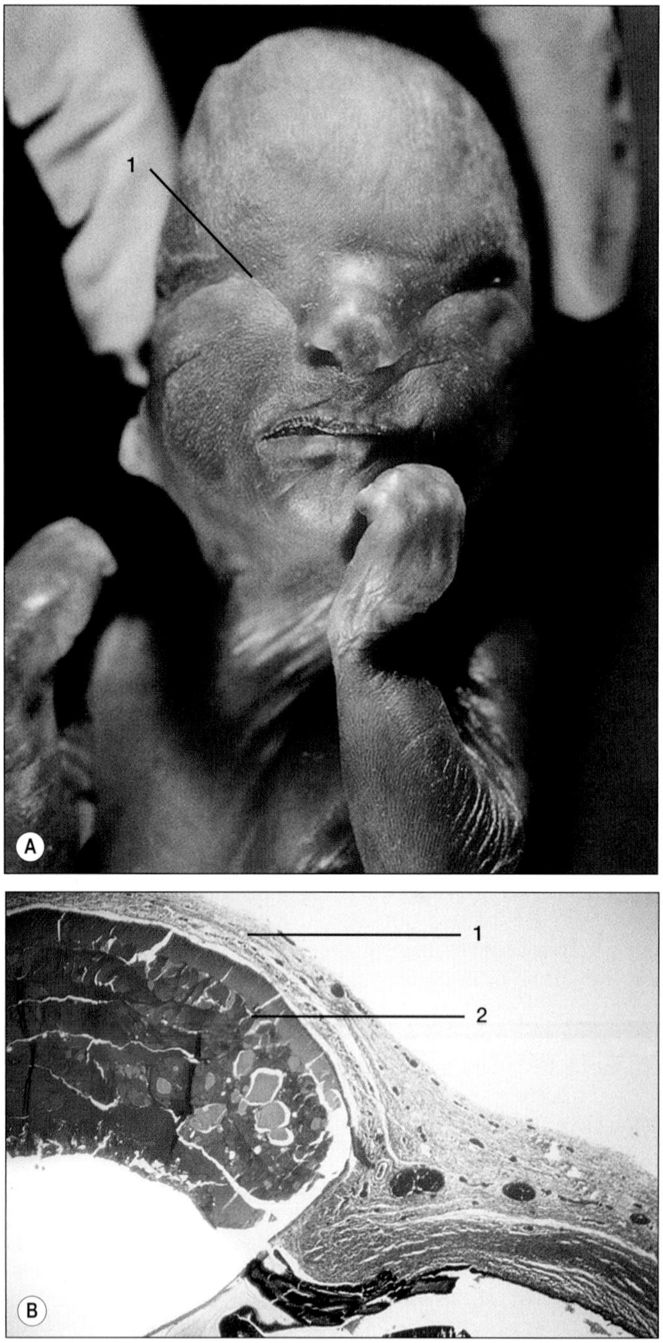

Fig. 57.1 Cryptophthalmos. (**A**) Twenty-one-week-old fetus with multiple congenital anomalies including cryptophthalmos. The lids are completely fused, and the eyes are not visible. Note the fold of skin running from the brow to the cheek (*1*). (**B**) Same case. The histopathology shows superficial fibrovascular tissue (*1*) with an absence of the normal corneal tissue. Posterior to the fibrovascular tissue, lens material (*2*) is seen.

Anomalies of Size

The size of a normal newborn cornea measures approximately 10 mm in horizontal diameter, whereas the size of a normal adult cornea measures approximately 12 mm in horizontal diameter. The measured horizontal diameter of

Table 57.1 Diagnostic criteria for cryptophthalmos syndrome

Major criteria	Minor criteria
1. Cryptophthalmos	1. Congenital malformation of the nose
2. Syndactyly	2. Congenital malformation of the ears
3. Abnormal genitalia	3. Congenital malformation of the larynx
4. Sibling with cryptophthalmos syndrome	4. Cleft lip and/or palate
	5. Skeletal defects
	6. Umbilical hernia
	7. Renal agenesis
	8. Mental retardation

For diagnosis of cryptophthalmos syndrome, patients must have at least two major criteria and one minor criterion, or they may have one major criterion and four minor criteria.

Box 57.2 Ocular and systemic associations of megalocornea

Ocular
- Arcus juvenilis[74]
- Astigmatism (with-the-rule)[74]
- Cataract (usually posterior subcapsular)[74]
- Congenital glaucoma[74]
- Congenital miosis[75]
- Ectopia lentis[75]
- Ectopia lentis et pupillae[15]
- Excess mesenchymal tissue in angle[74]
- Iridodonesis[74]
- Iris stromal hypoplasia[74]
- Iris transillumination defects[74]
- Krukenberg's spindle[75]
- Mosaic corneal dystrophy[76]
- Myopia (mild to severe)[74]
- Open angle glaucoma[74]
- Phacodonesis[74]
- Pigmentation of trabecular meshwork[74]
- Posterior embryotoxon[74]
- Prominent iris processes[74]
- Rieger's anomaly[38]

Systemic
- Albinism[77]
- Apert's syndrome[78]
- Arachnodactyly[79]
- Craniosynostosis[74]
- Down's syndrome[74]
- Dwarfism[15]
- Facial hemiatrophy[74]
- Lamellar ichthyosis[74]
- Marfan's syndrome[80,81]
- Mucolipidosis type II[82]
- Neuhauser syndrome[83,84]
- Osteogenesis imperfecta[85]

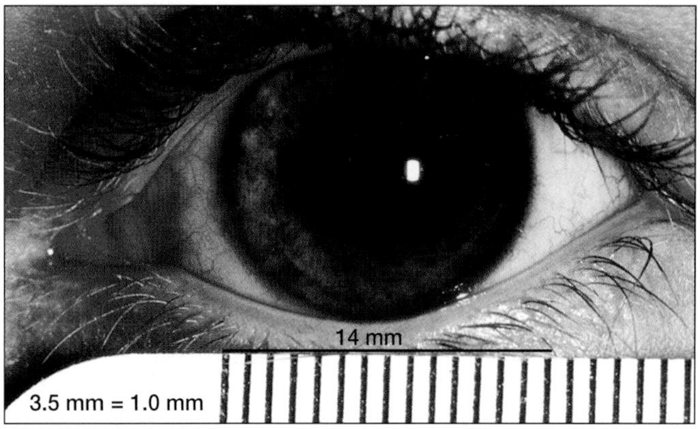

Fig. 57.2 Megalocornea. The corneal diameter measures approximately 14 mm.

the normal cornea virtually always exceeds the vertical diameter by approximately 1 mm because of the prominent scleral encroachment present in the superior and inferior limbus. The cornea usually reaches adult size by 2 years of age.[11]

Megalocornea

Megalocornea, as the name implies, refers to an enlarged cornea defined as having a horizontal diameter greater than or equal to 13 mm. It is a nonprogressive condition that is usually bilateral and symmetrical. Because of its predominant transmission as an X-linked recessive trait, 90% of cases are found in the male population.[12,13] Megalocornea has been mapped to the long arm of the X-chromosome (Xq21.3-q22 and Xq12-q26).[14] Autosomal dominant, autosomal recessive, and sporadic cases have also been reported.[15]

The clinical characteristics that have been described for megalocornea include an enlarged but clear cornea of slightly below normal or normal thickness (Fig. 57.2). The cornea usually possesses a greater than normal steepness but can be normal by keratometry.[16] It has been shown to be histologically normal in all respects with a normal endothelial cell density.[17] Although megalocornea is most frequently seen as an isolated condition, many ocular and systemic associations have been documented (Box 57.2). The steeper cornea usually results in with-the-rule astigmatism and myopia.[16] Many of the ocular associated findings involving the lens, iris, and iridocorneal angle are thought to exist secondary to the coexisting anatomic changes of an enlarged anterior segment and ciliary ring, sometimes referred to as a separate condition known as anterior megalophthalmos.[18] The widened ciliary ring presumably causes zonular stretching, resulting in phacodonesis, iridodonesis, and ectopia lentis. The iris also undergoes anatomic stress manifesting in stromal hypoplasia and transillumination defects along with subsequently increased trabecular meshwork pigmentation and Krukenberg's spindle formation.[19] These changes, coupled with an abnormal angle containing excess mesenchymal tissue and prominent iris processes, may predispose the eye to glaucoma.[20]

The etiology of megalocornea is not exactly known, but many theories have been proposed. The most popular belief holds that the condition occurs because of a defect in the growth of the optic cup where the anterior tips of the cup fail to close, thereby leaving a larger space to be taken up by the cornea.[21] Other explanations that have been postulated include a spontaneous arrest in the development of congenital glaucoma and exaggerated growth of the cornea relative to the rest of the eye. Abnormal collagen production may play a role in the pathogenesis, since this entity can be associated with systemic disorders of collagen synthesis (see Box 57.2).[22]

The differential diagnosis is limited mainly to buphthalmos from congenital glaucoma. The diagnosis of congenital glaucoma can easily be made in the presence of the obvious and classic signs of elevated intraocular pressure, Haab's striae, and optic disk changes.[23] However, in milder cases of congenital glaucoma where these findings may not be evident, the differentiation may be difficult but possible by finding a sharply demarcated limbal region, a distinguishing feature of megalocornea not seen in eyes with congenital glaucoma.[21] Furthermore, Topouzis et al. reported the first known case of megalocornea and ocular hypertension in a 10-year-old male who remained stable after 10 years of follow-up and demonstrated an autosomal dominant mode of inheritance.[24] The measurement of ocular axial length with A scan ultrasonography may also be helpful to rule out buphthalmos, in which the entire globe as well as the cornea is enlarged. Recent studies have also suggested using biometric examination to highlight the pathognomonic biometric findings of X-linked megalocornea not present in congenital glaucoma or other forms of megalocornea: markedly increased anterior chamber depth, posterior lens and iris positioning, and a short vitreous length.[16] Careful examination skills and use of ancillary studies can make the crucial distinction between megalocornea and congenital glaucoma, a condition in which early diagnosis and surgical intervention can help prevent severe visual loss and other complications.

No definite treatment besides correction of the refractive error is indicated when megalocornea presents as an isolated anomaly. However, ophthalmic examinations should be performed regularly after diagnosis to detect and monitor the various associated findings. Cataract formation, especially of the posterior subcapsular type, has been reported to occur in adults age 30–50 with megalocornea.[14,25,26] Surgical intervention is often challenging; complicating factors reported include possible poor iris dilation, lens subluxation, vitreous loss, posterior capsule rupture, and intraocular lens dislocation (Fig. 57.3).[25–28] The large anterior chamber and capsular bag size often makes intraocular lens selection difficult; the use of iris-claw intraocular lens and Artisan lens implantation (not currently approved by the FDA for this use) has shown promising results.[26,29]

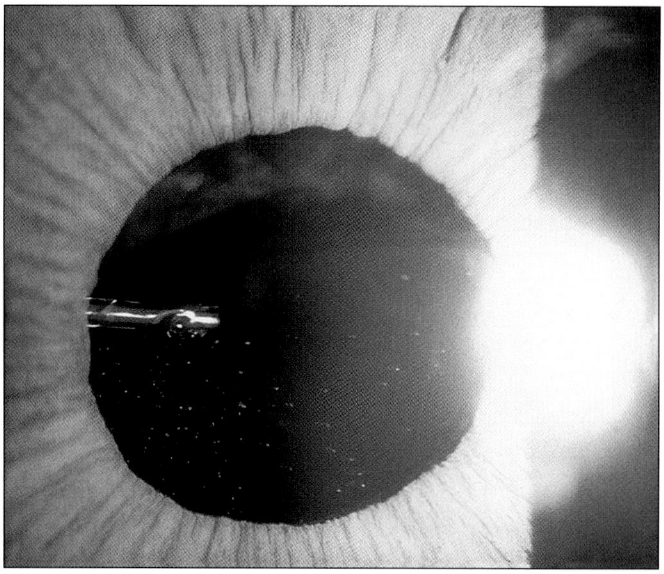

Fig. 57.3 Posterior chamber intraocular lens dislocation in a patient with megalocornea.

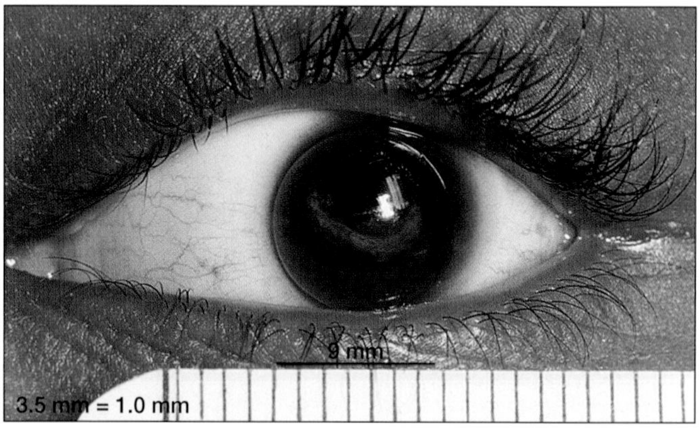

Fig. 57.4 Microcornea. The corneal diameter measures approximately 9 mm. The patient is aphakic and is wearing an aphakic contact lens.

Microcornea

Microcornea is defined as a cornea having a horizontal diameter less than or equal to 10 mm in an otherwise normal-sized globe (Fig. 57.4). Other terms that are not to be confused with microcornea are anterior microphthalmos (entire anterior segment is small), microphthalmos (entire eye is small and disorganized), and nanophthalmos (if the entire eye is small but otherwise normal). The condition is nonprogressive and may be unilateral or bilateral. There is no sex predilection, and most cases are inherited in an autosomal dominant or recessive fashion with very rare sporadic cases.[30,31]

The small cornea is clear with normal thickness but usually flatter than the normal cornea. Histologic specimens have shown the microcornea to be normal in all other respects. Unlike megalocornea, microcornea is rarely an isolated condition and can have many ocular and systemic anomalies associated with it (Box 57.3). The flatter cornea usually gives rise to hyperopia, but any refractive error can exist, depending on the axial length of the eye. It is thought that the anatomic changes produced by the smaller cornea contribute to the development of glaucoma, whether it be the narrow or closed angle type, resulting from a shallow and crowded anterior chamber, or the open angle type, caused by angle remnants left during goniodysgenesis.[32] Twenty percent of patients with microcornea develop glaucoma, with angle closure being most common.[33]

Box 57.3 Ocular and systemic associations of microcornea

Ocular
- Aniridia[86]
- Autosomal dominant vitreoretinochoroidopathy[87]
- Axenfeld's syndrome[74]
- Choroidal coloboma[32]
- Closed angle glaucoma[34]
- Congenital cataract[30,88,89]
- Corectopia[90]
- Corneal leukoma[91]
- Cornea plana[91]
- Hyperopia[74]
- Infantile glaucoma[91]
- Iris coloboma[92]
- Mesodermal angle remnants[74]
- Microblepharon[91]
- Microphakia[91]
- Narrow angle glaucoma[91]
- Nystagmus[93]
- Open angle glaucoma[91]
- Persistent pupillary membrane[94]
- Retinal pigmentary changes[87]
- Retinopathy of prematurity[95]
- Rieger's anomaly[96]
- Small orbit[91]
- Uveal coloboma[97]

Systemic
- Alagille syndrome[98]
- Alport syndrome[99]
- Cornelia de Lange syndrome[36]
- De Grouchy's syndrome[100]
- Ehlers-Danlos syndrome[101]
- Goltz syndrome[36]
- Grieg's hypertelorism[102]
- Hallerman-Streiff syndrome[103]
- Kohn-Romano syndrome[104]
- Meckel syndrome[105]
- Meyer-Schwickerath syndrome[106]
- Nance-Horan syndrome[107]
- Norrie's disease[36]
- Onycho-osteodysplasia[108]
- Progeria[109]
- Rubella[110]
- Sjögren-Larsson syndrome[36]
- Smith-Lemli-Opitz syndrome[111]
- Trisomy 3p,[112] 13,[113,114] 18[114]
- Turner's syndrome[39]
- Waardenburg's syndrome[115]
- Weill-Marchesani syndrome[116]
- Weyers syndrome[74]

Microcornea is possibly caused by an arrest in the growth of the cornea, which begins after the fifth gestational month when differentiation is complete. Another hypothesis attributes the condition to an overgrowth of the anterior tips of the optic cup, thereby leaving less space for the cornea.[34]

The differential diagnosis includes the other conditions listed that may involve a disorganized eye. In addition to slit lamp examination, use of both A and B scan ultrasonography may help differentiate microcornea from these other conditions.[35] When present as an isolated finding, visual prognosis is excellent, especially with the help of spectacles. However, because of the frequent associated findings, additional treatment may be indicated, with a variable prognosis for vision.

Anomalies of Shape

Oval cornea

Oval cornea is a general term used to describe the apparent shape of a normal-sized cornea when viewed from the front and presents in both a horizontal and a vertical form. While the normal cornea is horizontally oval, the use of the term horizontal oval cornea is reserved for cases where there is an exaggeration of scleral encroachment in the superior and inferior horizontal meridians. Horizontal oval cornea indicates the presence of some degree of sclerocornea and has no other associated findings.

Vertical oval cornea exists when the vertical diameter of the cornea exceeds the horizontal diameter. It merely refers to the shape of an otherwise normal cornea and has been reported to occur with iris coloboma, microcornea,[36] intrauterine keratitis (usually secondary to syphilis),[37] Rieger's anomaly,[38] and Turner's syndrome.[39]

Astigmatism

Corneal astigmatism is considered to be a fairly common refractive error caused by an anomaly in corneal curvature where the radius of curvature in one meridian differs from that in another meridian. Diagnostic tools and techniques such as manifest refraction, keratometry, and corneal topography have aided in identifying and quantifying different patterns of astigmatism.[40] Conventional treatment with corrective spectacles and contact lenses along with the contemporary techniques of astigmatic keratotomy and laser refractive surgery have given patients various options for improved vision.

The normal pattern of corneal development shows a trend from with-the-rule astigmatism in the first decade of life progressing to against-the-rule astigmatism in later years.[41] However, against-the-rule astigmatism appears to be more common in low birth weight and premature infants regardless of the presence or severity of retinopathy of prematurity according to a recent study.[42] Periorbital lesions, such as hemangiomas, may also induce astigmatism via direct compression of the globe.[43] Genetic studies suggest an autosomal dominant mode of inheritance.[44,45]

Sclerocornea (cornea plana)

In sclerocornea, the cornea is flat with a curvature of less than 43 diopters (D). While the curvature in this condition commonly ranges from 30 to 35 D, some cases have been reported with keratometry readings as low as 20 D.[46] Corneal curvatures that are the same or even lower than that of the sclera are a pathognomonic finding.[47] The observation that all cases of cornea plana were noted to have some degree of

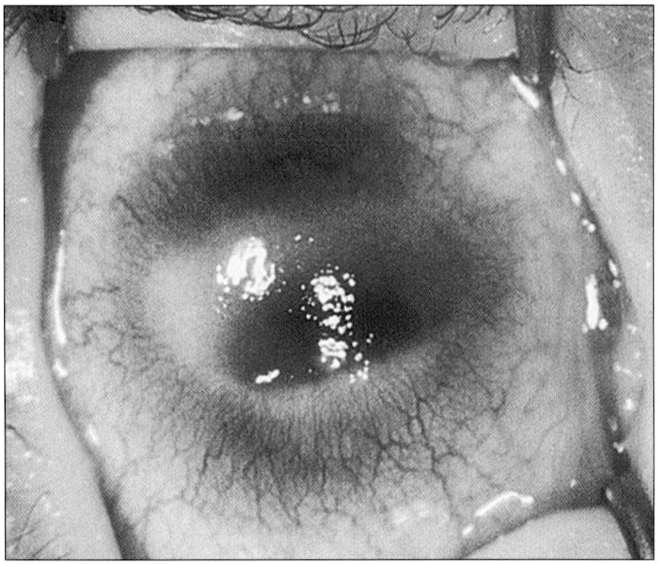

Fig. 57.5 Peripheral sclerocornea. There is peripheral scleralization of the cornea with vascularization. The central cornea is clear relative to the peripheral cornea.

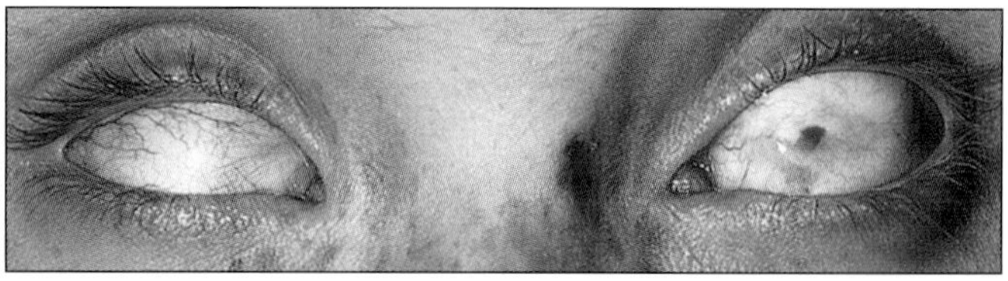

Fig. 57.6 Diffuse sclerocornea. There is complete scleralization and vascularization of the cornea.

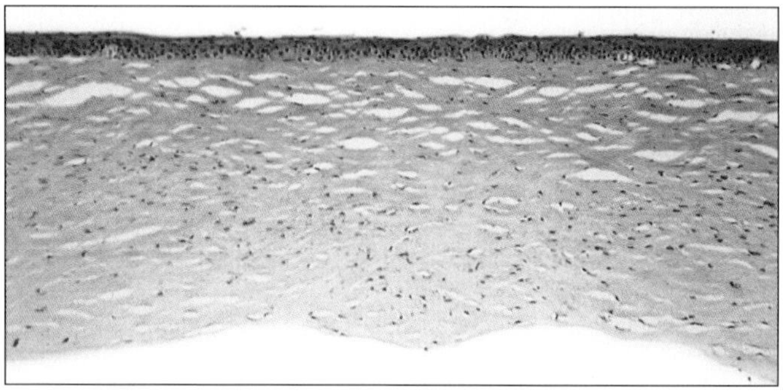

Fig. 57.7 Histopathology of sclerocornea. There is an absence of Bowman's layer, increased cellularity of the corneal stroma, and loss of the normal collagen lamellar architecture.

either peripheral or central scleralization[46] led to the argument that cornea plana and sclerocornea are, in fact, the same entity. The similarities in clinical and histopathologic characteristics, inheritance pattern, and ocular and systemic associations between these two entities have certainly strengthened this argument. However, some authorities still separate the two conditions to emphasize the anomalous flat shape of cornea plana versus the anomalous transparency of sclerocornea.

The embryologic explanation for sclerocornea lies in the absence of the limbal anlage, the structure responsible for both limbal differentiation and corneal curvature. The formation of the limbal anlage during the seventh to tenth gestational weeks allows mesenchymal cells of neural crest origin to differentiate into either sclera or cornea and also allows corneal curvature to exceed scleral curvature. With its absence, the normal interface between sclera and cornea is disrupted and the normal surface curvature is flattened. This very plausible developmental concept not only illustrates the close relationship between limbal differentiation and corneal curvature but also provides further evidence of why sclerocornea and cornea plana could be considered as a single entity.[48] This chapter will consider cornea plana and sclerocornea as interchangeable descriptive terms for the same condition.

Sclerocornea is more commonly bilateral (and asymmetric) than unilateral. Most cases are sporadic, with the remaining cases showing a familial transmission. There is an equal incidence in males and females.[49] Pedigrees have demonstrated both autosomal dominant and recessive patterns of inheritance, with the autosomal recessive cases exhibiting a more severe manifestation of total sclerocornea, and autosomal dominant cases presenting with a more benign form of peripheral sclerocornea (see later discussion).[50,51] The autosomal recessive form of sclerocornea has been mapped to the proximal part of the long arm of chromosome twelve.[50]

Scleralization occurs in varying degrees and progresses from the periphery toward the center. Therefore, the peripheral cornea alone (Fig. 57.5) or the entire cornea (Fig. 57.6) can be involved. When scleralization is complete (total sclerocornea), the central cornea tends to be less opaque than the peripheral cornea. The affected areas appear as if sclera has extended onto the cornea, contributing to the opacification as well as the deep and superficial vascularization arising from the normal conjunctival and episcleral vessels.[52] Histopathologic studies of sclerocornea have revealed morphologic features resembling scleral tissue (Fig. 57.7). Specimens have revealed an irregular epithelium, a variably thickened basement membrane, and a fragmented or absent Bowman's layer.[53] In addition, the vascularized stroma consists of irregularly arranged collagen fibrils of variable and increased diameter present anteriorly and of smaller-diameter fibrils present posteriorly (the reverse order is more typical for the normal cornea). Because these fibrils lack precise lamellar organization and also have accompanying blood vessels, optical transparency is lost. Descemet's membrane and endothelium have been found to be normal, abnormal, or absent.[53] The anterior chamber angle is occasionally difficult to visualize through the opaque cornea and is frequently abnormal, with multiple anterior chamber abnormalities often contributing to the development of glaucoma.[54] Ultrasound biomicroscopy has been used to assist in diagnosis, highlight potential associated structural anomalies, and to help guide surgical management.[55] Box 57.4 outlines the many ocular and systemic conditions associated with sclerocornea.

Besides neutralizing any refractive error, treatment is limited to penetrating keratoplasty for cases involving central corneal opacification.[54,56] However, the prognosis is guarded because of complications related to glaucoma, the

Box 57.4 Ocular and systemic associations of sclerocornea (cornea plana)

Ocular
- Aniridia[91]
- Arcus juvenilis[91]
- Blue sclera[91]
- Cataract[91]
- Closed angle glaucoma[117]
- Congenital anterior synechiae[52]
- Ectopia lentis[91]
- Hyperopia[91]
- Microcornea[91]
- Microphthalmos[52]
- Narrow angle glaucoma[117]
- Nonspecific corneal opacities[91]
- Open angle glaucoma[117]
- Pseudoptosis (Streiff's sign)[74]
- Retinal aplasia[91]
- Retinal coloboma[52]
- Uveal coloboma[52]

Systemic
- Cerebellar anomalies[52]
- Cranial dystrophies[52]
- Cryptorchidism[52]
- Dandy-Walker cyst[118]
- Ear deformities[52]
- Epidermolysis bullosa dystrophica[119]
- Hallerman-Streiff syndrome[120]
- Hereditary onycho-osteodysplasia[108]
- Hurler's syndrome[121]
- Lobstein's syndrome[47]
- Lohmann syndrome[122]
- Maroteaux-Lamy syndrome[74]
- Melnick-Needles syndrome[123]
- Mieten's syndrome[124]
- Monosomy 21[53]
- Osteogenesis imperfecta[85]
- Polydactyly[52]
- Smith-Lemli-Opitz syndrome[125]
- Trisomy 13, 18[56]
- Unbalanced translocation (17p, 10q)[126]

frequent association with other severe ocular abnormalities, and the increased risk of allograft rejection.[54]

Posterior keratoconus

Because anterior keratoconus is not considered to be a true developmental anomaly, it is not addressed in this chapter but instead discussed in detail in Chapter 74. Posterior keratoconus is considered to be a rare developmental condition that bears no relationship to anterior keratoconus and is sometimes classified as one of the anterior chamber cleavage syndromes. The condition is usually unilateral, nonprogressive, and noninflammatory, and is associated with a normal visual acuity. The condition may occur in a generalized or circumscribed form.[57]

Generalized posterior keratoconus exists when the entire posterior corneal surface has an increased curvature with a shorter radius of curvature and a normal anterior corneal surface.[57] Although the central cornea may be thinned, the cornea is almost always clear, with only rare instances of corneal clouding. This pattern of posterior keratoconus is less common and thought to occur sporadically as a result of a developmental arrest. Although there has been no documentation of hereditary transmission, all reported cases have occurred in females.

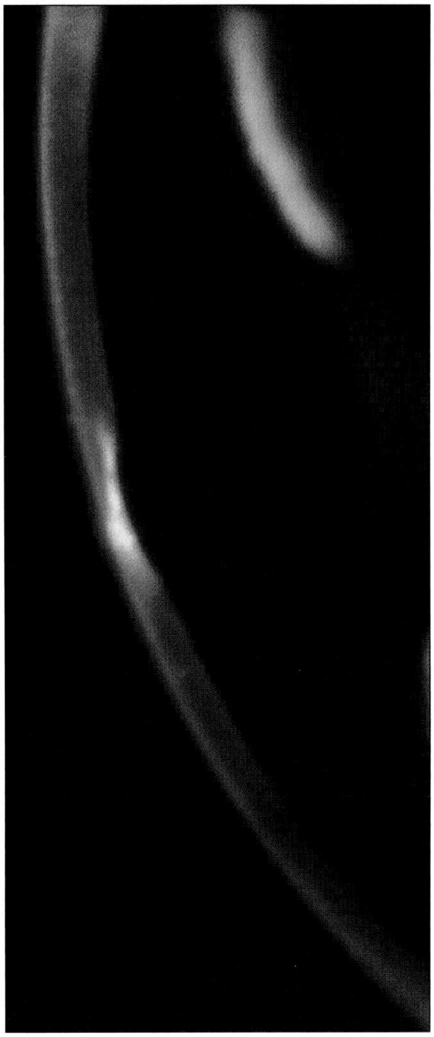

Fig. 57.8 Circumscribed posterior keratoconus. A focal indentation of the posterior cornea with overlying stromal scarring is seen.

The more common circumscribed form of posterior keratoconus is characterized by one or more localized, crater-like lesions in the central or eccentric posterior cornea (but usually presents as a single, central lesion) (Fig. 57.8).[57] Corneal clouding with variable corneal thinning is frequently encountered overlying the posterior corneal defect, which is commonly surrounded by endopigment.[58] This condition may accompany a host of ocular and systemic anomalies, which are listed in Box 57.5. While the majority of cases are sporadic, a few familial cases have been cited.[59–61] It is also thought to represent a mild variant of Peters' anomaly, thereby implying intrauterine inflammation or some other anterior segment dysgenesis as an etiologic factor. Some attribute the cause to an abnormal migration

Box 57.5 Ocular and systemic associations of circumscribed posterior keratoconus

Ocular
- Aniridia[74]
- Anterior lenticonus[127]
- Anterior polar cataract[127]
- Anterior segment dysgenesis[127]
- Choroidal/retinal sclerosis[60]
- Ectopia lentis[128]
- Ectropion uveae[128]
- Glaucoma[128]
- Iris atrophy[128]
- Iron lines in epithelium[129]
- Optic nerve hypoplasia[129]
- PPMD with iris adhesions[130]
- Ptosis[131]
- Retinal coloboma[131]
- Superior lateral canthus displacement[63]

Systemic
- Brachydactyly[61]
- Broad, flat nasal bridge[63]
- Bull or webbed neck[63]
- Cleft lip/palate[131]
- Genitourinary anomalies[131]
- Growth retardation[131]
- Hypertelorism[63]
- Mental retardation[131]

or differentiation of the secondary mesenchyme that normally forms the corneal stroma.[58]

The histopathologic and ultrastructural characteristics of posterior keratoconus include a present but altered Descemet's membrane and endothelium in the area of the defect.[62,63] Some of the alterations in Descemet's membrane may involve thinning, abnormal anterior banding, multilamination, and posterior excrescences.[57] Other changes may consist of an irregularly thickened basement membrane, focal disruption of Bowman's layer, and stromal irregularity.[63,64]

Posterior keratoconus rarely affects visual acuity but may cause myopic astigmatism that should be corrected with spectacles to prevent amblyopia. When marked corneal clouding limits functional vision, penetrating keratoplasty is the treatment of choice.

Keratoglobus

Unlike anterior keratoconus, which typically develops during the first 20 years of life and rarely manifests as a congenital condition, keratoglobus is more frequently present at birth and is considered a developmental anomaly.

Keratoglobus is a bilateral, noninflammatory, ectatic disorder in which the entire cornea becomes thinned and takes on a globular shape, with keratometry readings as high as 60–70 D. The cornea has been shown to be clear, normal in size, and diffusely thinned to approximately one-third to one-fifth of the normal corneal thickness. The thinning may be more pronounced in the mid-peripheral cornea. Histopathologic studies have revealed an absent or fragmented Bowman's layer, a thinned stroma with normal lamellar orientation, a thinned Descemet's membrane with focal breaks in the anterior layers, a normal endothelium, and a thinned sclera. Its globular shape creates a very deep anterior chamber with otherwise normal anterior segment structures and a normal-sized globe. The cornea does not exhibit stress lines, iron rings, or subepithelial scarring characteristic of keratoconus but may become opaque and edematous from spontaneous breaks in Descemet's membrane. These breaks usually heal over several weeks to months. When associated with connective tissue disorders, corneal rupture has been reported to occur spontaneously. Ruptured globe is also associated with minor blunt trauma to the eye or head in these patients.[65] Keratoglobus has a strong association with Ehlers-Danlos syndrome type VI, a systemic collagen disorder characterized by hyperextensible joints, skeletal abnormalities, blue sclerae, mottled teeth, and neurosensory deafness (Fig. 57.9).[66] Associations with Rubenstein-Taybi syndrome[67] and Leber's congenital amaurosis[68] have also been described.

The differential diagnosis includes keratoconus, pellucid marginal degeneration, megalocornea, and buphthalmos. Treatment is centered on correcting the accompanying high myopia with spectacles to prevent amblyopia. Lamellar/penetrating keratoplasty and epikeratoplasty are technically challenging procedures in this setting[65,66] and should only be attempted when absolutely necessary. Some success has been achieved with a two-stage approach, performing an epikeratoplasty or tectonic lamellar corneoscleral graft first, followed by a penetrating keratoplasty weeks to months later.[69,70] The prognosis accompanying a ruptured globe is very guarded because of the complications involved in surgically repairing a thin cornea and sclera. The use of protective eye wear in a safe environment should be strongly encouraged and reinforced.

Congenital Anterior Staphyloma and Keratectasia

Congenital anterior staphyloma is defined as an ectatic condition in which a bulging, opaque cornea lined posteriorly with uveal tissue protrudes through the palpebral fissure beyond the plane of the normal eyelids.[71] This disorder can be unilateral or bilateral and shows variable corneal thinning and scarring along with a deep and disorganized anterior segment.[72] The lens may even become adherent to the protuberant cornea, mimicking one of the features found in Peters' anomaly.[73] Characteristic histopathologic findings include an irregular epithelium, attenuated Bowman's layer, increased stromal thickness with vascular ingrowth, absent Descemet's membrane and endothelium along with a posterior uveal lining, representing the remaining pigmented epithelium of an atrophic iris.[72] The cornea is vulnerable to perforation in utero and subsequently undergoes dermoid transformation to resemble the stratified squamous epithelium of skin; however, unlike cryptophthalmos, the metaplastic change is limited to the cornea and does not involve the conjunctiva or eyelids.[71] Congenital anterior staphyloma is believed to result from the abnormal migration of

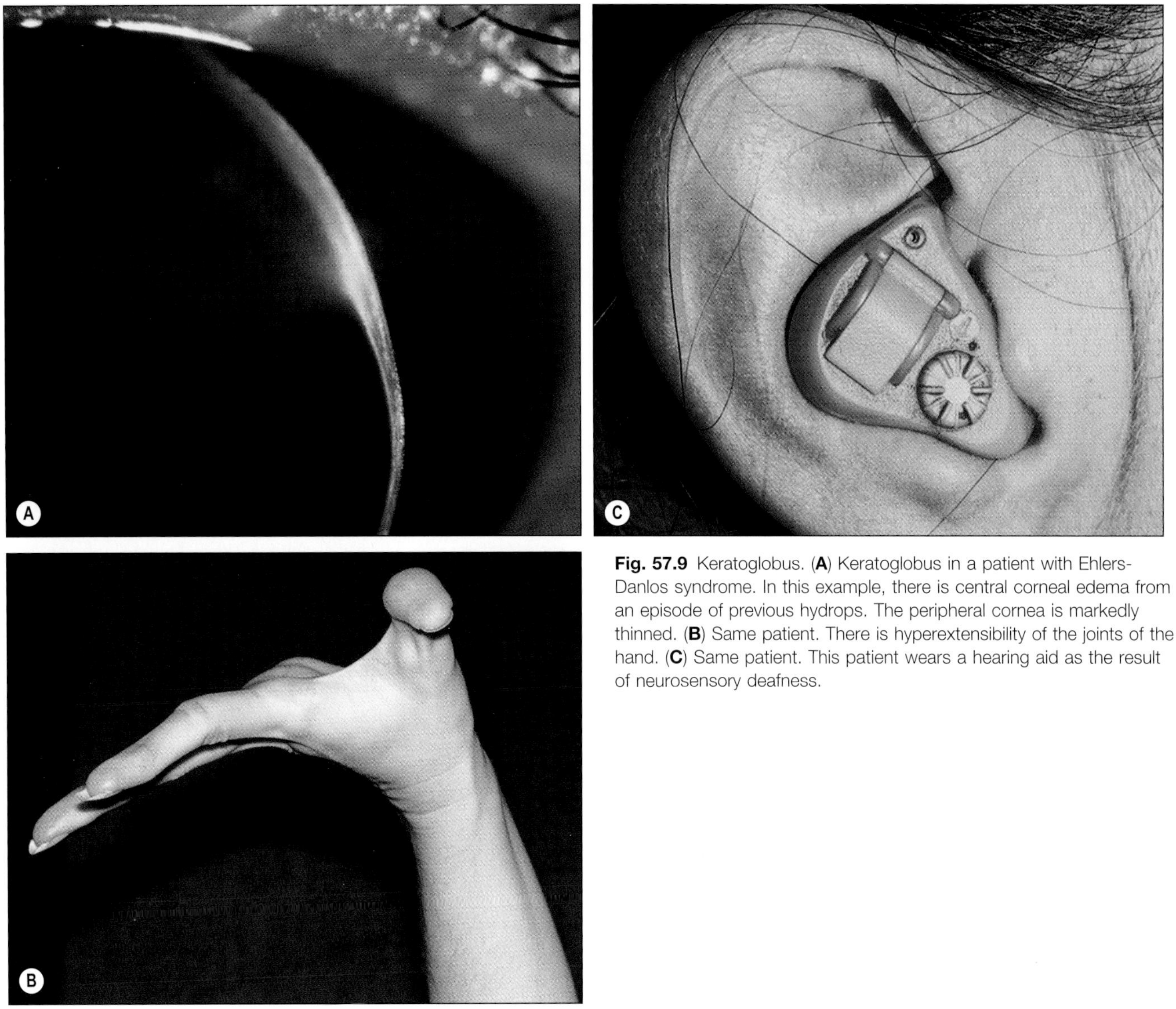

Fig. 57.9 Keratoglobus. (**A**) Keratoglobus in a patient with Ehlers-Danlos syndrome. In this example, there is central corneal edema from an episode of previous hydrops. The peripheral cornea is markedly thinned. (**B**) Same patient. There is hyperextensibility of the joints of the hand. (**C**) Same patient. This patient wears a hearing aid as the result of neurosensory deafness.

neural crest cells into the developing cornea. This factor puts the disorder in the same group of diseases as Peters' anomaly, i.e. an extreme form of anterior segment dysgenesis. The visual prognosis is poor because of the severe damage incurred by the anterior segment structures. Although a few patients with milder cases are reported to have undergone penetrating keratoplasty with variable degrees of success, enucleation remains the recommended surgical procedure in the setting of a blind, glaucomatous, and painful eye.[72]

Keratectasia is essentially congenital anterior staphyloma minus the posterior uveal lining. The condition is otherwise clinically identical to congenital anterior staphyloma, and has similar proposed embryologic origins.

References

1. Manschot WA. Primary congenital aphakia. *Arch Ophthalmol.* 1963;69:571.
2. Duke-Elder S. *System of ophthalmology.* Vol. 3. *Normal and abnormal development: congenital deformities.* St. Louis: Mosby; 1955.
3. Waring GO, Shields JA. Partial unilateral cryptophthalmos with syndactyly, brachycephaly, and renal anomalies. *Am J Ophthalmol.* 1975;79:437–440.
4. Ide CH, Wollschlaeger PB. Multiple congenital abnormalities associated with cryptophthalmos. *Arch Ophthalmol.* 1969;81:638.
5. Kündüz K, Günalp I. Congenital symblepharon (abortive cryptophthalmos) associated with meningoencephalocele. *Ophthalmic Plast Reconstr Surg.* 1997;13:139–141.
6. Codere F, Brownstein S, Chen MF. Cryptophthalmos syndrome with bilateral renal agenesis. *Am J Ophthalmol.* 1981;91:737–742.
7. Goldhammer Y, Smith JL. Cryptophthalmos syndrome with basal encephaloceles. *Am J Ophthalmol.* 1975;80:146–149.
8. Thomas TT, Frias JL, Felix V, et al. Isolated and syndromic cryptophthalmos. *Am J Med Genet.* 1986;25:85–98.
9. Reinecke RD. Cryptophthalmos. *Arch Ophthalmol.* 1971;85:376.
10. Ferri M, Harvey JT. Surgical correction for complete cryptophthalmos: case report and review of the literature. *Can J Ophthalmol.* 1999;34:233–236.
11. Friede R. Surface area of cornea and sclera in embryos and in newborn infants and its relation to megalocornea in adults. *Z Augenheilkd.* 1933;81:213.
12. Kayser B. Megalokornea oder Hydrophthalmus? *Klin Monatsbl Augenheilkd.* 1914;52:226.
13. Meire FM, Bleeker-Wagemakers EM, Oehler M, et al. X-linked megalocornea: ocular findings and linkage analysis. *Ophthalmic Paediatr Genet.* 1991;12:153–157.

14. Mackey CA, Buttery RG, Wise GM, et al. Description of X-linked megalocornea with identification of the gene locus. *Arch Ophthalmol.* 1999;829–833.
15. Meire FM. Megalocornea. Clinical and genetic aspects. *Doc Ophthalmol.* 1994;87:1–121.
16. Meire FM, Delleman JW. Biometry in X linked megalocornea: pathognomonic findings. *Br J Ophthalmol.* 1994;78:781.
17. Wood WJ, Green WR, Marr WG. Megalocornea: a clinicopathologic clinical case report. *Md State Med J.* 1974;23:57.
18. Vail DT. Adult hereditary anterior megalophthalmos sine glaucoma: a definite disease entity. *Arch Ophthalmol.* 1931;6:39.
19. Friede R. Megalocornea congenita, a phylogenetic anomaly. *Arch Ophthalmol.* 1948;148:716.
20. Malbran E, Dodds R. Megalocornea and its relation to congenital glaucoma. *Am J Ophthalmol.* 1960;49:908.
21. Mann I. *Developmental abnormalities of the eye.* 2nd ed. Philadelphia: JB Lippincott; 1957.
22. Maumenee IM. The cornea in connective tissue diseases. *Trans Am Acad Ophthalmol Otolaryngol.* 1978;85:1014.
23. Pollack A, Oliver M. Congenital glaucoma and incomplete congenital glaucoma in two siblings. *Acta Ophthalmol.* 1984;62:359.
24. Topouzis F, Karadimas P, Gatzonis S, et al. Autosomal-dominant megalocornea associated with ocular hypertension. *J Pediatr Ophthalmol Strabismus.* 2000;37:173–175.
25. Berry-Brincat A, Chan TKJ. Megalocornea and bilateral developmental cataracts. *J Cataract Refract Surg.* 2008;34:168–170.
26. Lee GA, Hann JV, Braga-Mele R. Phacoemulsification in anterior megalophthalmos. *J Cataract Refract Surg.* 2006;32:1081–1084.
27. Sharan S, Billson FA. Anterior megalophthalmos in a family with 3 female siblings. *J Cataract Refract Surg.* 2005;31:1433–1436.
28. Ugo de Sanctis MD, Grignolo FM. Cataract extraction in X-linked megalocornea: a case report. *Cornea.* 2004;23:533.
29. Oetting TA, Newsom TH. Bilateral Artisan lens for aphakia and megalocornea: long-term follow-up. *J Cataract Refract Surg.* 2006;32:526–528.
30. Salmon J, Wallis C, Murray A. Variable expressivity of autosomal dominant microcornea with cataract. *Arch Ophthalmol.* 1988;106:505.
31. Vingolo E, et al. Autosomal dominant simple microphthalmos. *J Med Genet.* 1994;31:721.
32. Eida H, Ohira A, Amemiya T. Choroidal coloboma in two members of a family. *Ophthalmologica.* 1998;212:208–211.
33. Chandler PA, Grant WM. *Lectures on glaucoma.* Philadelphia: Lea & Febiger; 1965.
34. Sugar S. Oculodentodigital dysplasia syndrome with angle closure glaucoma. *Am J Ophthalmol.* 1978;86:36.
35. Tane S, Sakuma Y, Ito S. The studies on the ultrasonic diagnosis in ophthalmology. Ultrasonic biometry in microphthalmos and buphthalmos. *Acta Soc Ophthalmol Jpn.* 1977;81:1112.
36. Warburg M. The heterogeneity of microphthalmos in the mentally retarded. In: Bergsma D, ed. *The eye.* Baltimore: Williams & Wilkins; 1971.
37. Thomas C, Cordier J, Reny A. Les manifestations ophthalmologiques du syndrome de Turner. *Arch Ophthalmol.* 1969;29:565.
38. Alkemade PPH. *Dysgenesis mesodermalis of the iris and the cornea.* Springfield, IL: Charles C Thomas; 1961.
39. Lessel S, Forbes AP. Eye signs in Turner's syndrome. *Arch Ophthalmol.* 1966;76:211.
40. Maloney RK, Bogan SJ, Waring GO. Determination of corneal image-forming properties from corneal topography. *Am J Ophthalmol.* 1993;115:31.
41. Fledelius HC, Stubgaard M. Changes in refraction and corneal curvature during growth and adult life. A cross-sectional study. *Acta Ophthalmol.* 1986;64:487.
42. Holmström G, el Azazi M, Kugelberg U. Ophthalmological long-term follow up of preterm infants: a population based, prospective study of the refraction and its development. *Br J Ophthalmol.* 1998;82:1265–1271.
43. Metry DW, Hebert AA. Benign cutaneous vascular tumors of infancy: when to worry, what to do. *Arch Dermatol.* 2000;136:905–914.
44. Hammond CJ, Snieder H, Gilbert CE, Spector TD. Genes and environment in refractive error: the Twin Eye Study. *Invest Ophthalmol Vis Sci.* 2001;42:1232–1236.
45. Clementi M, Angi M, Forabosco P, et al. Inheritance of astigmatism: evidence for a major autosomal dominant locus. *Am J Human Gen.* 1998;63:825–830.
46. Erikkson AW, Lehmann W, Forsius H. Congenital cornea plana in Finland. *Clin Genet.* 1973;4:301.
47. Desvignes P, et al. Aspect iconographique d'une cornea plana dans une maladie de Lobstein. *Arch Ophthalmol (Paris).* 1967;72:585.
48. Friedman AH, et al. Sclerocornea and defective mesodermal migration. *Br J Ophthalmol.* 1975;59:683.
49. Howard RO, Abrahams IW. Sclerocornea. *Am J Ophthalmol.* 1971;71:1254.
50. Tahvanainen E, Forsius H, Kolehmainen J, et al. The genetics of cornea plana congenita. *J Med Genet.* 1996;33:116–119.
51. McKusick VA. *Mendelian inheritance in man.* 12th ed. Baltimore: Johns Hopkins University Press; 1998.
52. Goldstein JE, Cogan DG. Sclerocornea and associated congenital anomalies. *Arch Ophthalmol.* 1962;67:761.
53. Doane JF, Sajjadi H, Richardson WP. Bilateral penetrating keratoplasty for sclerocornea in an infant with monosomy 21. *Cornea.* 1994;13:454–458.
54. Freuh BE, Stuart I. Transplantation of congenitally opaque corneas. *Br J Ophthalmol.* 1997;81:1064–1069.
55. Kim T, Cohen EJ, Schnall BM, et al. Ultrasound biomicroscopy and histopathology of sclerocornea. *Cornea.* 1998;17:443–445.
56. Kolbert GS, Seelenfreund M. Sclerocornea, anterior cleavage syndrome, and trisomy 18. *Ann Ophthalmol.* 1970;2:26.
57. Krachmer JH, Feder RS, Belin MW. Keratoconus and related noninflammatory corneal thinning disorders. *Surv Ophthalmol.* 1984;28:293.
58. Rao SK, Padmanabhan P. Posterior keratoconus. An expanded classification scheme based on corneal topography. *Ophthalmology.* 1998;105:1206–1212.
59. Butler TM. Keratoconus posticus. *Trans Ophthalmol Soc UK.* 1930;50:551.
60. Collier M. Le kératocône postérieur. *Arch Ophthalmol.* 1962;22:376.
61. Haney WP, Falls HF. The occurrence of congenital keratoconus posticus circumscriptus. *Am J Ophthalmol.* 1961;52:53.
62. Townsend WM. Congenital corneal leukomas. I. Central defect in Descemet's membrane. *Am J Ophthalmol.* 1974;77:80.
63. Streeten BW, Karpik AG, Spitzer KH. Posterior keratoconus associated with systemic abnormalities. *Arch Ophthalmol.* 1983;101:616.
64. Wolter JR, Haney WP. Histopathology of keratoconus posticus circumscriptus. *Arch Ophthalmol.* 1963;69:357.
65. Cameron JA. Keratoglobus. *Cornea.* 1993;12:124.
66. Cameron JA. Corneal abnormalities in Ehlers-Danlos syndrome type VI. *Cornea.* 1993;12:54.
67. Nelson ME, Talbot JF. Keratoglobus in the Rubinstein-Taybi syndrome. *Br J Ophthalmol.* 1989;73:385.
68. Elder MJ. Leber congenital amaurosis and its association with keratoconus and keratoglobus. *J Pediatr Ophthalmol Strabismus.* 1994;31:38.
69. Jones DH, Kirkness CM. A new surgical technique for keratoglobus-tectonic lamellar keratoplasty followed by secondary penetrating keratoplasty. *Cornea.* 2001;20:885–887.
70. Macsai MS, Lemley HL, Schwarz T. Management of oculus fragilis in Ehlers-Danlos type VI. *Cornea.* 2000;19:104–107.
71. Schanzlin DJ, et al. Histopathologic and ultrastructural analysis of congenital anterior staphyloma. *Am J Ophthalmol.* 1983;95:506.
72. Leff SR, et al. Congenital anterior staphyloma: clinical, radiological, and pathological correlation. *Br J Ophthalmol.* 1986;70:427.
73. Olson JA. Congenital anterior staphyloma. Report of two cases. *J Pediatr Ophthalmol.* 1971;8:177.
74. Wilson FM. Congenital anomalies of the cornea and conjunctiva. In: Smolin G, Thoft RA, eds. *The cornea. Scientific foundations and clinical practice.* 3rd ed. Boston: Little Brown and Company; 1994.
75. Meire FM, Delleman JW. Autosomal dominant congenital miosis with megalocornea. *Ophthalmic Ped Genet.* 1992;13:123–129.
76. Malbran E. Megalocornea with mosaic-like dystrophy in identical twins. *Am J Ophthalmol.* 1968;66:734.
77. Awaya S, Tsunekawa F, Koizumi E. Studies of X-linked recessive ocular albinism of the Nettleship-Falls type. *Acta Soc Ophthalmol Jpn.* 1988;92:146.
78. Calamandrei D. Megalocornea in due pazienti con syndrome craniosinotoscia. *Q Ital Ophthalmol.* 1950;3:278.
79. Bloch N. Megalocornea associated with multiple skeletal anomalies: a new genetic syndrome? *J Genet Hum.* 1973;21:67.
80. Allen RA, et al. Manifestations of the Marfan syndrome. *Trans Am Acad Ophthalmol Otolaryngol.* 1967;71:18.
81. Calder CA. Marfan's syndrome with bilateral megalocornea and subluxated cataractous lenses. *J All India Ophthalmol Soc.* 1966;14:262.
82. Libert J, Van Hoof F, Farriaux JP, Toussaint D. Ocular findings in I-cell disease (mucolipidosis type II). *Am J Ophthalmol.* 1977;83:617.
83. Verloes A, et al. Heterogeneity versus variability in megalocornea-mental retardation (MMR) syndromes: report of new cases and delineation of 4 probable types. *Am J Med Genet.* 1993;46:132.
84. Neuhauser GE, et al. Syndrome of mental retardation, seizures, hypotonic cerebral palsy and megalocornea, recessively inherited. *Z Kinderheilk.* 1975;120:1.
85. Chan CC, et al. Ocular findings in osteogenesis imperfecta congenita. *Arch Ophthalmol.* 1982;100:1459.

86. David R, MacBeath L, Jenkins T. Aniridia associated with microcornea and subluxated lenses. *Br J Ophthalmol.* 1978;62:118.
87. Lafaut BA, Loeys B, Leroy B, et al. Clinical and electrophysiological findings in autosomal dominant vitreoretinochoroidopathy: report of a new pedigree. *Graefe's Arch Clin Exp Ophthalmol.* 2001;239:575–582.
88. Devi RR, Vijayalakshmi P. Novel mutations in GJA8 associated with autosomal dominant congenital cataract and microcornea. *Mol Vis.* 2006;12:190–195.
89. Willoughby CE, Shafiq A, Ferrini W, et al. CRYBB1 mutation associated with congenital cataract and microcornea. *Mol Vis.* 2005;11:587–593.
90. Ghose S, Mehta U. Microcornea with corectopia and macular hypoplasia in a family. *Jpn J Ophthalmol.* 1984;28:126.
91. Arffa R. *Grayson's diseases of the cornea.* 4th ed. St Louis: Mosby; 1997.
92. Hornby SJ, Gilbert AS, Foster DL. Visual acuity in children with coloboma: clinical features and a new phenotypic classification system. *Ophthalmology.* 2000;107:511–520.
93. Cebon L, West RH. A syndrome involving congenital cataracts of unusual morphology, microcornea, abnormal irides, nystagmus, and congenital glaucoma, inherited as an autosomal dominant trait. *Aust J Ophthalmol.* 1982;10:237.
94. Waardenburg PJ. Gross remnants of the pupillary membrane, anterior polar cataract and microcornea in a mother and her children. *Ophthalmologica.* 1949;118:828.
95. Kelly SP, Fielder AR. Microcornea associated with retinopathy of prematurity. *Br J Ophthalmol.* 1987;71:201.
96. Henkind P, Siegel IM, Carr RE. Mesodermal dysgenesis of the anterior segment: Rieger's anomaly. *Arch Ophthalmol.* 1965;73:810.
97. Bateman JB, Maumenee IH. Colobomatous macrophthalmia with microcornea. *Ophthalmic Pediatr Genet.* 1984;4:59.
98. Brodsky MC, Cunniff C. Ocular anomalies in the alagille syndrome (arteriohepatic dysplasia). *Ophthalmology.* 1993;100:1767.
99. Colville DJ, Savige J. Alport syndrome. A review of the ocular manifestations. *Ophthalmic Genet.* 1997;18:161–173.
100. Levenson J, Crandall B, Sparkes R. Partial deletion syndromes of chromosome 18. *Ann Ophthalmol.* 1971;3:756.
101. Durham DG. Cutis hyperelastica (Ehlers-Danlos syndrome) with blue scleras, microcornea, and glaucoma. *Arch Ophthalmol.* 1953;49:229.
102. Friede R. Uber physiologische Euryopie und pathologischen hypertelorismus ocularis. *Graefes Arch Klin Exp Ophthalmol.* 1954;155:359.
103. Sugar A, Bigger JF, Podos SM. Hallerman-Streiff-Francois syndrome. *J Pediatr Ophthalmol.* 1971;8:234.
104. Kohn R, Romano R. Ptosis, blepharophimosis, epicanthus inversus and telecanthus – the syndrome with no name. *Am J Ophthalmol.* 1971;72: 625.
105. McRae D, et al. Ocular manifestations of Meckel syndrome. *Arch Ophthalmol.* 1972;88:106.
106. Meyer-Schwickerath G, Gruterich E, Weyers H. Mikrophthalmussyndrome. *Klin Monatsbl Augenheilkd.* 1957;131:18.
107. Lewis RA, Nussbaum RL, Stambolian D. Mapping X-linked ophthalmic diseases. IV. Provisional assignment of the locus for X-linked congenital cataracts and microcornea (the Nance-Horan syndrome to Xp22.2-p22.3). *Ophthalmology.* 1990;97:110.
108. Fenske HD, Spitalny LA. Hereditary onycho-osteodysplasia. *Am J Ophthalmol.* 1970;70:604.
109. Francois J. *Hereditary in ophthalmology.* St Louis: Mosby; 1961.
110. Boniuk V, Boniuk M. Congenital rubella syndrome. *Int Ophthalmol Clin.* 1968;8:487.
111. Gold JD, Pfaffenbach DD. Ocular abnormalities in the Smith-Lemli-Opitz syndrome. *J Pediatr Ophthalmol.* 1975;12:228.
112. Ginocchio VM, De Brasi D, Genesio R, et al. Sonic Hedgehog deletion and distal trisomy 3p in a patient with microphthalmia and microcephaly, lacking cerebral anomalies typical of holoprosencephaly. *Eur J Med Genet.* 2008;51:658–665.
113. Ginsberg J, Boue KE. Ocular pathology of trisomy 13. *Ann Ophthalmol.* 1974;6:113.
114. Butera C, Plotnik J, Bateman JB, et al. Ocular genetics. *Pediatric Ophthalmology: A Clinical Guide.* 2000;85.
115. Goldberg G: Waardenburg's syndrome with fundus and other anomalies. *Arch Ophthalmol.* 1966;76:797.
116. Feiler-Ofry V, Stein R, Godel V. Marchesani's syndrome and chamber angle anomalies. *Am J Ophthalmol.* 1968;65:862.
117. Barkan H, Borley WE. Familial cornea plana congenita complicated by cataracta nigra and glaucoma. *Am J Ophthalmol.* 1936;19:307.
118. March WF, Chalkley TH. Sclerocornea associated with Dandy-Walker cyst. *Am J Ophthalmol.* 1974;78:54.
119. Sharkey JA, et al. Cornea plana and sclerocornea in association with recessive epidermolysis bullosa dystrophica. *Cornea.* 1992;11:83.
120. Schanzlin DJ, Goldberg DB, Brown SI. Hallerman-Streiff syndrome associated with sclerocornea, aniridia, and a chromosomal abnormality. *Am J Ophthalmol.* 1980;90:411.
121. Kanai A, et al. The fine structure of sclerocornea. *Invest Ophthalmol Vis Sci.* 1971;9:687.
122. Lepri G. Un caso di malformazioni oculari ed extraoculari congenite (sindrome di Lohmann). *Arch Ottal.* 1949;53:203.
123. Perry LD, Edwards WS, Bramson RT. Melnick-Needles syndrome. *J Pediatr Ophthalmol Strabismus.* 1978;15:226.
124. Waring GO, Rodrigues MM. Ultrastructure and successful keratoplasty of sclerocornea in Mieten's syndrome. *Am J Ophthalmol.* 1980;90:469.
125. Harbin RL, et al. Sclerocornea associated with the Smith-Lemli-Opitz syndrome. *Am J Ophthalmol.* 1977;84:72.
126. Rodrigues MM, Calhoun J, Weinreb S. Sclerocornea with an unbalanced translocation (17p 10q). *Am J Ophthalmol.* 1974;78:49.
127. Greene CB. Keratoconus posticus circumscriptus. *Arch Ophthalmol.* 1945;34:432.
128. Hagedoorn A, Velzeboer CM. Postnatal partial spontaneous correction of a severe congenital anomaly of the anterior segment of the eye. *Arch Ophthalmol.* 1959;62:685.
129. Krachmer JH, Rodrigues MM. Posterior keratoconus. *Arch Ophthalmol.* 1978;96:1867.
130. Grayson M. The nature of hereditary deep polymorphous dystrophy of the cornea: its association with iris and anterior chamber dysgenesis. *Trans Am Ophthalmol Soc.* 1974;72:516.
131. Young ID, et al. Keratoconus posticus circumscriptus, cleft palate, genitourinary abnormalities, short stature, and mental retardation in sibs. *J Med Genet.* 1982;19:332.

Chapter 58

Axenfeld-Rieger Syndrome and Peters' Anomaly

Mansi Parikh, Wallace L.M. Alward

Disorders related to anterior segment development include a wide range of diseases such as primary congenital glaucoma, aniridia, and posterior polymorphous dystrophy. This chapter will focus only on Axenfeld-Rieger syndrome and Peters' anomaly. As will be discussed later, some feel they are part of a single disease spectrum.[1] Rarely, they are both found in the same patient or within the same family.[2] There have also been reports of patients with Peters' anomaly having *PITX2* and *FOXC1* gene mutations, both of which are known to cause Axenfeld-Rieger syndrome.[2,3] Despite this overlap, this chapter will treat Axenfeld-Rieger syndrome and Peters' anomaly as separate diseases because, although they may occur together, it is not common.

Terminology

The terminology of Axenfeld-Rieger syndrome, Peters' anomaly, and related diseases is an area of much confusion. These diseases have variably been lumped into large groups or split into small entities, both of which have the potential for causing confusion.

Several terms have been used to lump these conditions and other anterior segment developmental disorders. 'Anterior chamber cleavage syndrome' was popularized by Reese and Ellsworth in 1966.[4] This name is no longer considered accurate because there is no evidence that the anterior segment develops by cleavage of the cornea from the iris and lens. It also does not account for the nonocular features of Axenfeld-Rieger syndrome. 'Anterior segment dysgenesis'[5] fails to separate these diseases from other diseases such as primary congenital glaucoma and aniridia and, again, does not account for the nonocular features. 'Mesodermal dysgenesis' is inaccurate because the embryonic origin of the angle structures is from neural crest cells, not mesoderm. The neural crest origin has led some to suggest the term neurocristopathy.[6]

Splitting the diseases can also be confusing. Often, cases with features of Axenfeld-Rieger syndrome, but minor variations from the typical picture, have been given entirely new disease names. This has led to terms such as iridogoniodysgenesis anomaly,[7] iridogoniodysgenesis syndrome,[8] and familial glaucoma iridogoniodysplasia.[9] Some consider Axenfeld-Rieger syndrome by its component pieces (Table 58.1): Axenfeld anomaly (if changes are confined to the angle without iris abnormalities), Rieger anomaly (if there are iris as well as angle abnormalities), and Rieger syndrome (if there are associated nonocular features such as dental, maxillary, or umbilical abnormalities). Adding to the confusion is the term Axenfeld syndrome, which is Axenfeld anomaly with glaucoma. While the word 'syndrome' means systemic abnormalities in 'Rieger syndrome,' it means glaucoma when used in 'Axenfeld syndrome.'

Special mention should be made of the word goniodysgenesis, devised by Kluyskens in 1950[10] and expanded upon by Jerndal et al.[11] Goniodysgenesis is based upon the theory that mutations in a single gene cause different ranges of glaucoma: a severe mutation would cause congenital glaucoma, a less severe mutation would cause juvenile-onset glaucoma, and mild mutations would cause adult-onset primary open-angle glaucoma.[11] Even milder mutations might require a second insult, such as pigment dispersion, to cause glaucoma. A single genetic etiology, however, is not supported by the multiple genes that have been linked to the various types of glaucoma to date.[12]

In 1985, Shields et al. made a strong argument for lumping together Axenfeld anomaly, Rieger anomaly, Rieger syndrome, and related diseases (not including Peters' anomaly) under the heading of Axenfeld-Rieger syndrome, based on their overlapping clinical features.[13] We repeated this recommendation based on the molecular genetics of these conditions.[14]

Axenfeld-Rieger Syndrome

History

Vossius published the first known report of a patient with probable Axenfeld-Rieger syndrome in 1883.[15] He described a 9-year-old girl with ectopic pupils and full-thickness iris stromal defects. This patient was also missing several teeth. In 1920, Axenfeld reported a patient with a white line in the peripheral cornea approximately 1 mm from the limbus, which he called 'ringlinie.'[16] He also noted iris strands adherent to this peripheral corneal line. Axenfeld termed this condition 'embryotoxon cornea posteriorius.' This patient also had iris stromal hypoplasia with an iris defect.

In 1934, Rieger described two patients with iris hypoplasia and other ocular and systemic abnormalities.[17] One of the patients had abnormal tissue in the iridocorneal angle. This patient also had elevated intraocular pressure, which was

Table 58.1 Divisions of Axenfeld-Rieger syndrome

Disease	Posterior embryotoxon	Angle abnormalities	Iris stroma abnormalities	Systemic abnormalities	Glaucoma risk
Posterior embryotoxon	+	–	–	–	–
Axenfeld anomaly	+	+	–	–	+
Rieger anomaly	+	+	+	–	+
Rieger syndrome	+	+	+	+	+

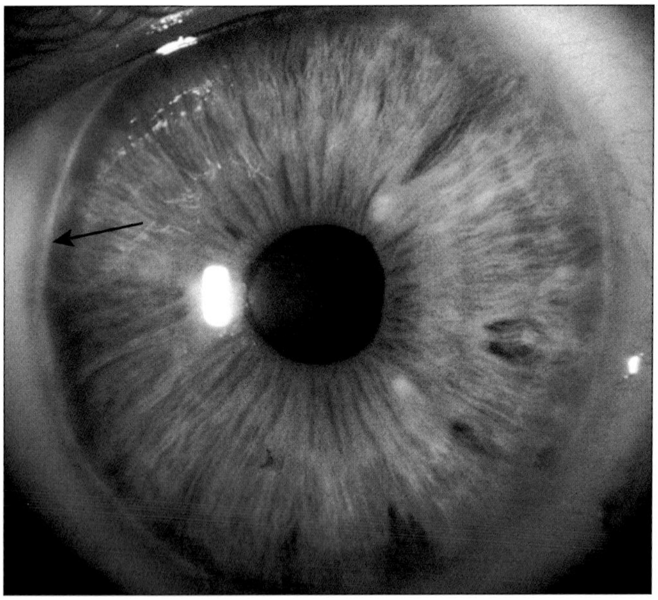

Fig. 58.1 Posterior embryotoxon is seen as a distinct white line in the far periphery of the cornea (*arrow*). This is an anterior and prominent Schwalbe's line.

treated with a cyclodialysis procedure. In 1935, Rieger provided a detailed report of the ocular features of the disease that bears his name and also provided excellent illustrations.[18] He described a mother and two children who had hypoplasia of the anterior iris stroma and ectopic pupils, which he called 'dysgenesis mesodermalis corneae et iridis.'

Clinical features

Cornea

A clear to white line in the peripheral cornea is a hallmark of Axenfeld-Rieger syndrome. This line, considered to be a prominent and anterior Schwalbe's line, is termed posterior embryotoxon (Fig. 58.1). It can appear over the entire circumference of the cornea or can be confined to a few clock hours. At the slit lamp, posterior embryotoxon is most readily seen in the temporal cornea. Sometimes, adherent strands of iris can be observed on slit lamp examination. Rarely, the embryotoxon can detach from the cornea and hang into the anterior chamber. On histopathological examination, the embryotoxon consists of collagen with ground substance that is covered by spindle-shaped cells (Fig. 58.2).[13] While most patients with Axenfeld-Rieger syndrome have a visible posterior embryotoxon on slit lamp examination, this is not universal. In a large series reported by Shields, 5 of 24 patients with Axenfeld-Rieger syndrome had no embryotoxon visible on slit lamp examination, but all had embryotoxon visible on gonioscopy.[19] The corneal endothelium is normal.

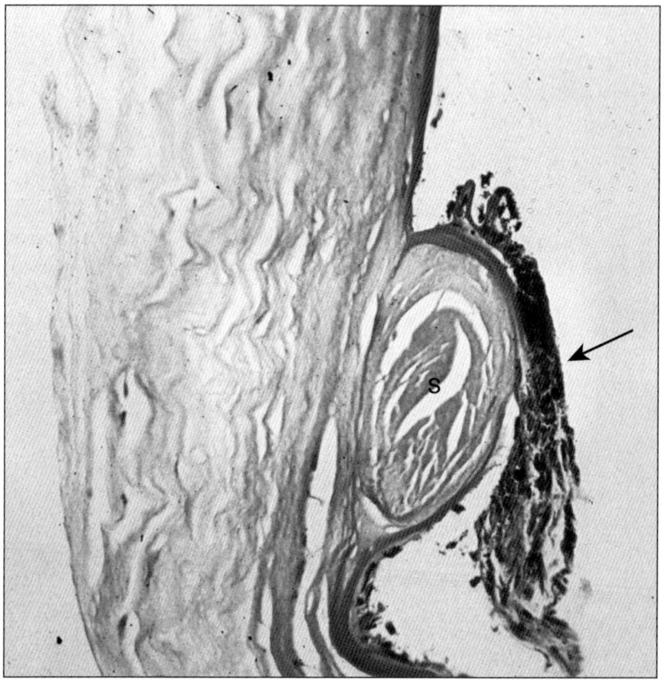

Fig. 58.2 Histopathology of posterior embryotoxon. Markedly thickened Schwalbe's line is noted with the letter 'S', and adherent iris tissue is seen at the arrow. (From Alward, WLM: *Color atlas of gonioscopy*, San Francisco, 2001, American Academy of Ophthalmology. Courtesy Robert Folberg, MD. © University of Iowa.)

Posterior embryotoxon can also be seen in otherwise normal eyes. Up to 15% of normal eyes will have this finding on slit lamp examination.[20] These rings, however, are usually much less prominent than those seen in Axenfeld-Rieger syndrome. Patients with isolated posterior embryotoxon are at no increased risk of developing glaucoma.[19]

Iridocorneal angle

The iridocorneal angle in patients with Axenfeld-Rieger syndrome can be striking on gonioscopic examination. There may be bands of iris extending across the iridocorneal angle to the trabecular meshwork and to the posterior embryotoxon. These strands are called iris processes but are usually not the fine processes seen in normal iridocorneal angles. They can range from discreet strands (Fig. 58.3) to broad sheets covering several clock hours (Fig. 58.4). The level of iris insertion tends to be high enough to obscure the scleral spur (Fig. 58.5).

Iris

Many patients with Axenfeld-Rieger syndrome have iris hypoplasia. The iris stroma may be very thin, allowing easy visualization of the iris sphincter (Fig. 58.6). These patients often have a characteristic slate-gray to chocolate-brown color to their irides. This peculiar appearance is so characteristic that some family members are able to determine who is at risk for glaucoma by the color of the iris.[21] Patients may also develop displacement of the pupil from the central position (corectopia) (Fig. 58.7). In eyes with corectopia, the pupil is often drawn towards an accumulation of iris process adhesions (Fig. 58.8). Some eyes may develop extra holes in the iris (polycoria) (Fig. 58.9). The iris changes are usually stationary, but have been reported to progress in some patients.[22]

Iris hypoplasia can also be an isolated finding. The iris appearance may be identical to Axenfeld-Rieger syndrome; however, there are no other ocular or systemic findings. Despite the lack of associated features, the two are related because both have been found in a single family.[23]

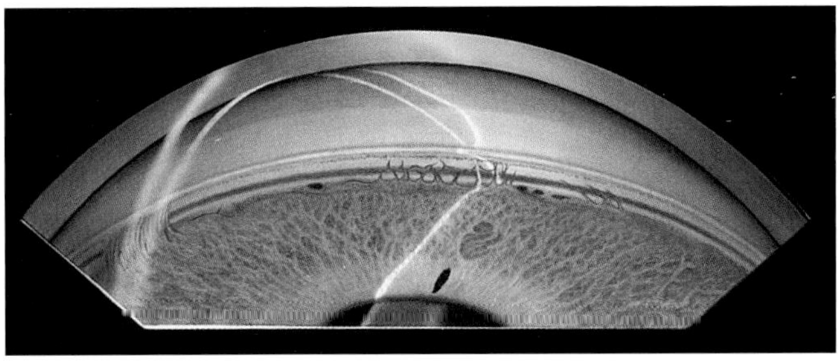

Fig. 58.3 Iris processes in the iridocorneal angle of a patient with Axenfeld-Rieger syndrome. Multiple connections are noted between the iris and the prominent Schwalbe's line. There is a broader adhesion to Schwalbe's line on the left portion of the illustration. (Burian HM et al: *Transactions of the American Ophthalmological Society* 1954:52:389-428. Copyright American Medical Association. All rights reserved.)

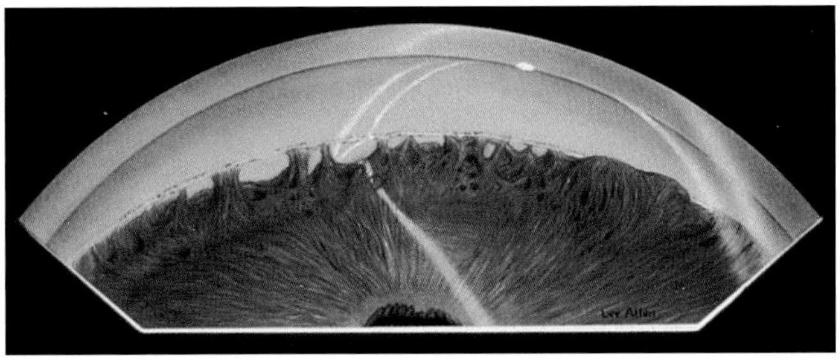

Fig. 58.4 The iris processes in this patient with Axenfeld-Rieger syndrome are much denser and more confluent than those seen in Figure 58.3. They cover much of the trabecular meshwork. (Burian HM et al: *Transactions of the American Ophthalmological Society* 1954:52:389–428. Copyright American Medical Association. All rights reserved.)

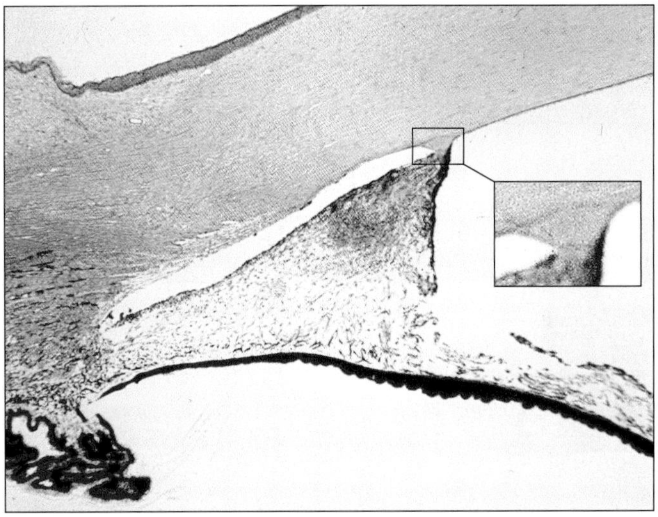

Fig. 58.5 Histopathology of the iridocorneal angle in Axenfeld-Rieger syndrome. There is an area of adhesion between the iris and Schwalbe's line (*inset*). The iris inserts high into the trabecular meshwork. (Krachmer JH, Palay DA: *Cornea color atlas,* St. Louis, 1995, CV Mosby.)

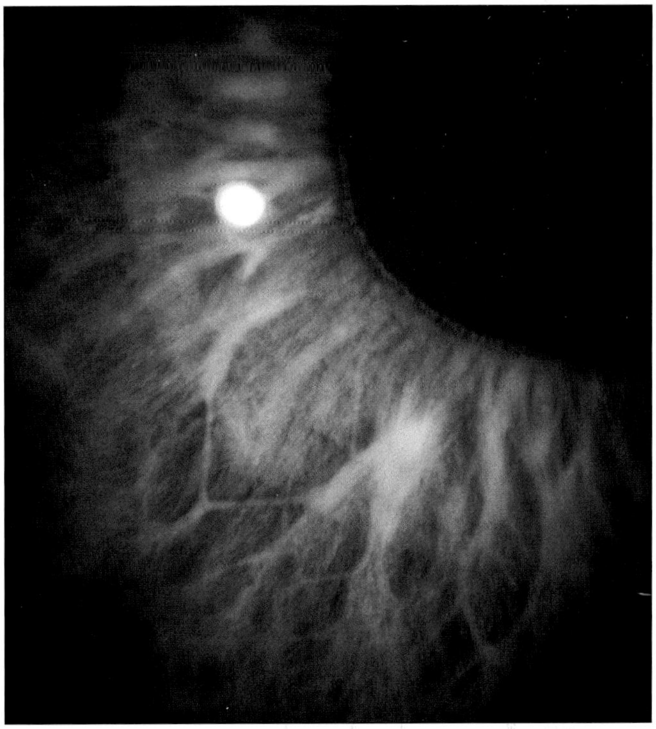

Fig. 58.6 Iris hypoplasia. The iris sphincter is seen clearly in this eye due to the hypoplastic iris stroma.

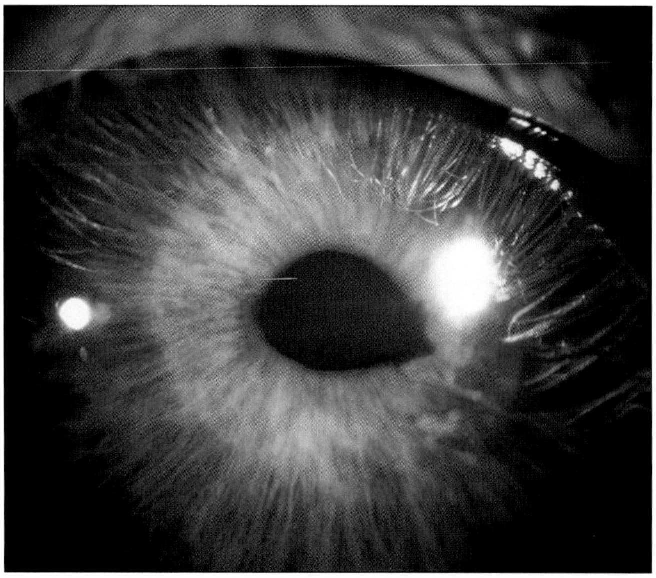

Fig. 58.7 Mild corectopia in a patient with Axenfeld-Rieger syndrome.

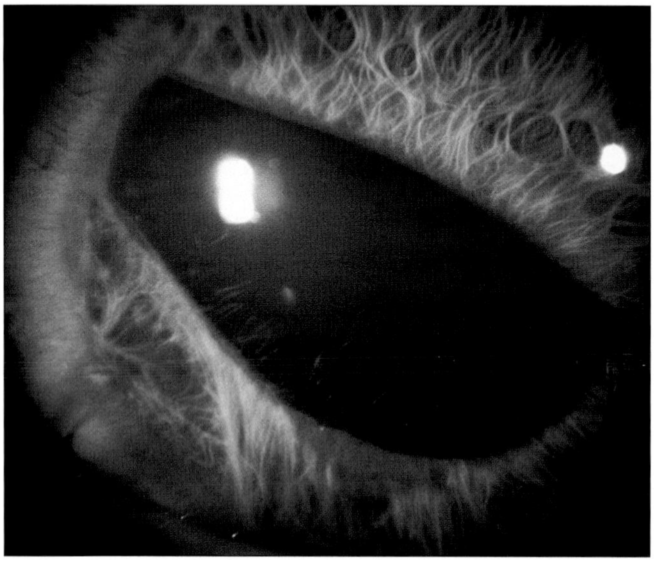

Fig. 58.8 Axenfeld-Rieger syndrome. There is iris hypoplasia. Note the corectopia, with the iris being pulled towards material in the iridocorneal angle at ten o'clock and four o'clock.

Additionally, some patients with isolated iris hypoplasia have mutations in the RIEG1 (*PITX2*) gene, which is one of the Axenfeld-Rieger syndrome genes.[24]

Glaucoma

Glaucoma develops in about 50% of patients with Axenfeld-Rieger syndrome.[19] The risk of developing glaucoma does not appear to correlate with the extent of iris processes but is related to the height of their insertion into the iridocorneal angle. Patients with more anterior iris insertions have a higher risk of developing glaucoma.[13] Affected patients usually develop glaucoma in their teens to twenties.

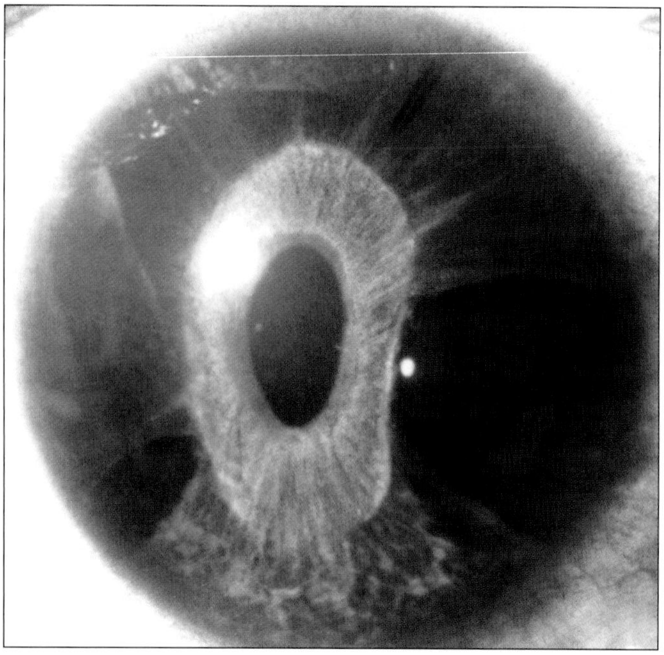

Fig. 58.9 The eye of a patient with Axenfeld-Rieger syndrome demonstrating iris hypoplasia with polycoria. (Alward WLM: *Requisites in ophthalmology: glaucoma,* St. Louis, 2000, CV Mosby.)

Other ocular findings

Other reported ocular findings include strabismus, limbal dermoids, cataract, retinal degeneration, chorioretinal colobomas, and optic nerve hypoplasia.[13] None of these has been seen with enough frequency to be considered part of the disease.

Slit lamp video of typical anterior segment and gonioscopic findings in Axenfeld-Rieger syndrome are available online at www.gonioscopy.org/axenfeldRieger.html.

Nonocular findings

Face

Patients may have maxillary hypoplasia with mid-face flattening, hypertelorism, telecanthus, a broad flat nasal bridge, and a prominent lower lip (Figs 58.10, 58.11). These features give patients with Axenfeld-Rieger syndrome a distinctive and characteristic appearance.

Teeth

Typical dental anomalies include too few teeth (hypodontia) and small teeth (microdontia) (Fig. 58.12). Besides examining the patient, it is important to ask whether he or she has had previous dental reconstructive work.

Umbilical

Patients often have redundant periumbilical skin (Fig. 58.13). This is frequently mistaken for an umbilical hernia that may have been repaired early in the patient's life.

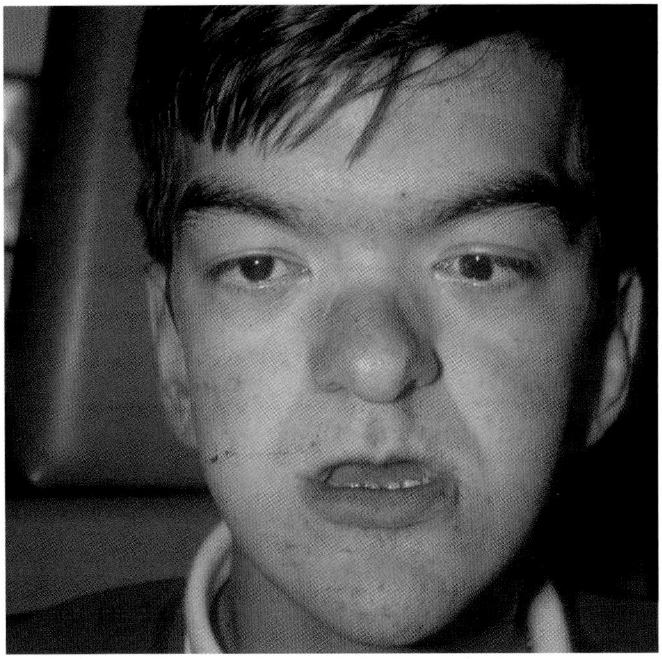

Fig. 58.10 A patient with Axenfeld-Rieger syndrome demonstrating telecanthus and a right esotropia.

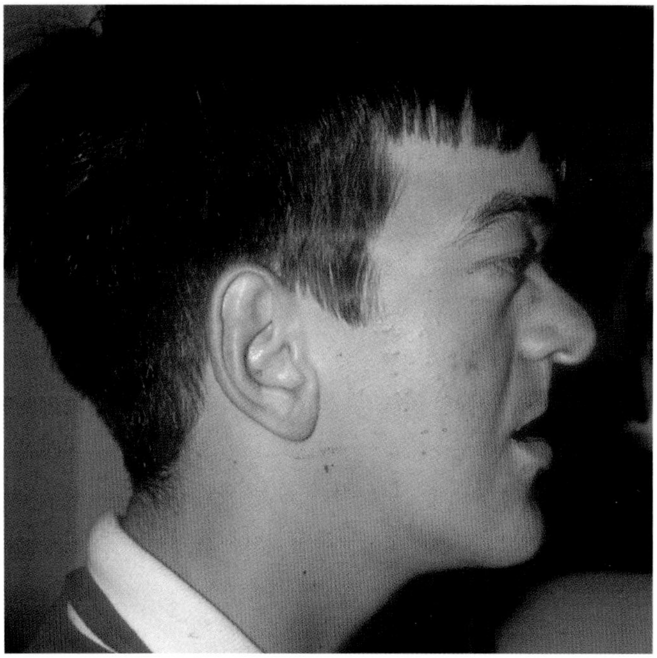

Fig. 58.11 Side view of a patient with Axenfeld-Rieger syndrome. Note the poorly developed maxilla, the flattened appearance of the face, and the protruding lower lip.

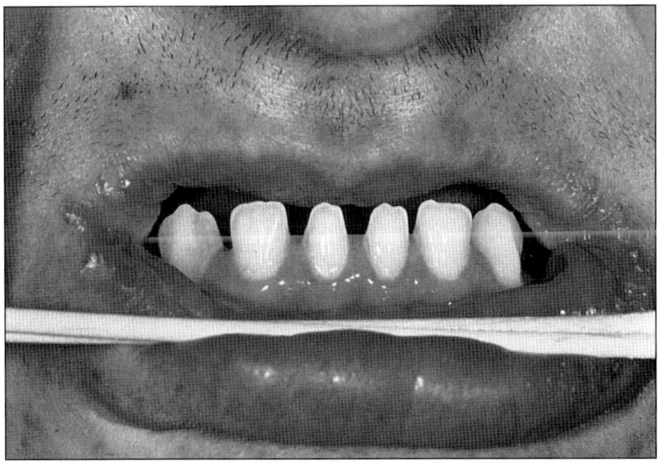

Fig. 58.12 View of the teeth of a patient with Axenfeld-Rieger syndrome demonstrating abnormally small teeth (microdontia) and an abnormally small number of teeth (hypodontia).

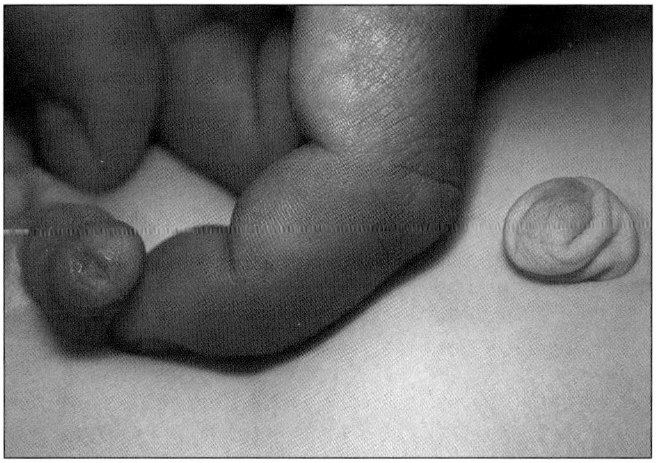

Fig. 58.13 A photograph of a young male child with Axenfeld-Rieger syndrome demonstrating the urethra opening on the underside of the penis (hypospadias) and redundant periumbilical skin.

Genital

Among males, the urethra may exit from the underside of the penis (hypospadias) (see Fig. 58.13).

Others

Patients with Axenfeld-Rieger syndrome can have other associated nonocular features. The most commonly reported ones are listed in Box 58.1. Of note, some patients may have empty sella syndrome with growth hormone deficiency. The growth of Axenfeld-Rieger syndrome patients should be monitored with referral to an endocrinologist if there is concern about growth hormone deficiency.

Differential diagnosis

The disease that may be confused with Axenfeld-Rieger syndrome is the iridocorneal endothelial (ICE) syndrome. Both syndromes can have corectopia and polycoria as prominent features and both commonly cause glaucoma. The iris

Box 58.1 Nonocular abnormalities that occur frequently enough in Axenfeld-Rieger syndrome to be considered a part of the disease

Head and neck
- Maxillary hypoplasia
- Telecanthus
- Hypodontia
- Microdontia
- Prominent lower lip
- Hearing loss (especially RIEG2)

Central nervous system
- Empty sella syndrome
- Mental retardation

Endocrine
- Growth hormone deficiency

Cardiovascular
- Valvular abnormalities (especially *FOXC1*)

Genital
- Hypospadias

Other
- Redundant periumbilical skin

atrophy in the ICE syndrome can look very much like the iris hypoplasia in Axenfeld-Rieger syndrome. In both diseases, broad sheets of iris may cover the iridocorneal angles. In Axenfeld-Rieger syndrome these are iris processes, and in the ICE syndrome they are broad synechiae.

Despite these similarities, separating the diseases is not difficult. Axenfeld-Rieger syndrome is almost always bilateral and typically has a family history, while ICE syndrome is almost always unilateral and acquired. Axenfeld-Rieger syndrome is present at birth, while ICE syndrome typically develops during adulthood. Posterior embryotoxon is almost always seen in Axenfeld-Rieger syndrome and is not a feature of ICE syndrome. The ICE syndrome has corneal findings of a hammered silver endothelium with abnormalities seen on specular microscopy. The cornea in Axenfeld-Rieger syndrome is normal unless there are Haab's striae from early-onset glaucoma.

Pathogenesis

Some of the early theories regarding pathogenesis were reviewed in the terminology section. More recently, Shields has postulated that residual primordial neuroectodermal cells remain on the iris and in the iridocorneal angle.[19] Contraction of these cells and their secreted basement membrane can lead to the adhesion of the iris to the trabecular meshwork and also to the distortion of the iris and pupil. Studies in transgenic mice have pointed to the critical role that corneal endothelial cells play in anterior segment development.[25] The pathogenesis of Axenfeld-Rieger syndrome is not fully elucidated.

Table 58.2 Genes and genetic loci for Axenfeld-Rieger syndrome

Chromosomal locus	Gene	MIM number
4q25 (*RIEG1*)	*PITX2*	601542
6p25	*FOXC1*	601090
13q14 (*RIEG2*)	Not identified	601499

MIM, Mendelian Inheritance in Man (http://www3.ncbi.nlm.nih.gov/Omim/)

Genetics

Axenfeld-Rieger syndrome is typically inherited in an autosomal dominant fashion. There are now three genetic loci and two genes at these loci that have been described for Axenfeld-Rieger syndrome (Table 58.2).

Chromosome 4q, RIEG1, *PITX2*

In the literature, there have been several cases of individuals with chromosome 4q deletions and translocations who also had Axenfeld-Rieger syndrome.[26] Using this information, Murray and colleagues performed linkage analysis on three small families with autosomal dominant Axenfeld-Rieger syndrome and found linkage to chromosome 4q.[26] This site was designated RIEG1. Later studies by the same group found the gene at this locus, *PITX2*.[27] Mutations in *PITX2* have been shown to cause Axenfeld-Rieger syndrome,[27] iris hypoplasia,[24] iridogoniodysgenesis syndrome,[28] and Peters' anomaly.[3]

Chromosome 13q, RIEG2

The second linkage site was discovered by Phillips and coworkers on chromosome 13q14.[29] They studied a four-generation family with eleven affected family members. These patients all had anterior segment abnormalities and nine of eleven had glaucoma. Ten of eleven had nonocular abnormalities that included hearing loss and dental abnormalities, but did not include redundant periumbilical skin. To date, no gene has been isolated from this region.

Chromosome 6p, *FOXC1*

Nishimura and associates identified two unrelated children with chromosomal translocations that involved chromosome 6p.[30] A number of anterior segment disorders have been linked to this area.[30] These children had many nonocular abnormalities but also had congenital glaucoma. Studying the break point in chromosome 6 led to the discovery of a gene that was originally called *FKHL7* and is now called *FOXC1*.[30] This gene may be responsible for a wide range of disease severity. A report of one family with a *FOXC1* mutation included patients with Rieger anomaly, Rieger syndrome, and Peters' anomaly.[2] This family also had one member with cardiac valvular abnormalities. *FOXC1* is expressed in the heart, and there is evidence that

Axenfeld-Rieger syndrome patients can have cardiac valvular abnormalities.[31]

The *PITX2* and *FOXC1* genes both function by regulating the expression of other genes in time and space. They do not code for structural proteins but rather regulate phases in embryonic development. This explains the wide variety of systems affected by mutations in these genes.

Natural history

The iris abnormalities are usually stationary but have been documented to worsen over time in some patients.[22] Glaucoma develops in about 50% of patients.[13]

Treatment

The cornea rarely presents a problem in Axenfeld-Rieger syndrome. If patients have early-onset glaucoma they can develop buphthalmos with Haab's striae and secondary corneal changes, but this is uncommon. In these cases, it is important to address possible amblyopia as well as the glaucoma.

More commonly, glaucoma develops later in childhood or in early adulthood and is managed much like primary open-angle glaucoma. First-line treatment is with aqueous suppressants. Laser trabeculoplasty is usually not an option because of obscuration of the trabecular meshwork by iris processes. Angle surgeries are often not applicable in Axenfeld-Rieger syndrome. Even in early-onset cases, goniotomy and trabecultomy can be very difficult because of extensive angle adhesions. Ultimately, patients may require trabeculectomy or tube-shunt surgery.

Peters' Anomaly

Peters' anomaly is a rare disease in which patients are born with opaque central corneas. Sometimes included with Axenfeld-Rieger syndrome under the umbrella of the anterior chamber cleavage syndromes, it is probably best considered separately. Others have called the disease posterior keratoconus and primary mesodermal dysgenesis of the cornea. Some authors divide the disease into type I (without lens involvement) and type II (with lens involvement).

History

In 1897, von Hippel was the first to report a patient with Peters' anomaly.[32] He described an 'ulcer internum corneae,' which he felt was due to intrauterine keratitis. In 1906, Peters postulated that the disease resulted from the incomplete separation of the lens from the surface ectoderm.[33]

Clinical features

Cornea

Peters' anomaly is characterized by a central white opacity (leukoma) with a lucent periphery (Fig. 58.14). This finding is bilateral in 80% of cases.[34] There may be overlying corneal edema, especially early in the course of the disease or if there is elevated intraocular pressure. The size and density of the central defect is variable. It can range from a small, faint opacity to a dense leukoma precluding visualization of the anterior chamber (Fig. 58.15). In rare cases, the leukoma may be vascularized and bulge forward similar to an anterior staphyloma.[35] More commonly, the affected cornea does not become vascularized.

There are frequently adhesions of iris tissue to the edge of the corneal opacity. These adhesions appear to extend from the iris collarettes to the periphery of the posterior corneal defect and may be present for 360 degrees or segmentally. In addition, there may be keratolenticular adhesions.

Histopathologically, there are abnormalities in all layers of the cornea (Fig. 58.16). Anterior changes include disorganized epithelium and may include loss of Bowman's layer. The affected stroma may demonstrate edema. Posteriorly, there is an abrupt absence or marked attenuation of the endothelium and Descemet's membrane underlying the corneal opacity. Peripheral to the opacity, the endothelium is normal.

Anterior chamber

The anterior chamber may be quite shallow, with the iris and lens shifted anteriorly towards the corneal defect. The cause of the shallowing is not known.

Lens

Cataract is a frequent finding in Peters' anomaly. In some, this may be from a primary lens anomaly, and in others it may be a secondary change as the lens is pushed forward against the cornea. The lens may touch or be adherent to the cornea, but can also be in its normal position and yet be cataractous.

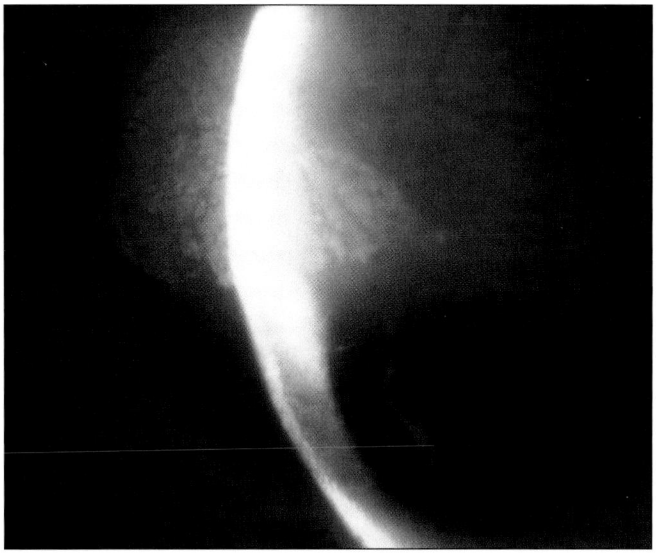

Fig. 58.14 A photograph of patient with Peters' anomaly demonstrating a central white opacity (leukoma) in the cornea. (Alward WLM: *Requisites in ophthalmology: glaucoma,* St. Louis, 2000, CV Mosby.)

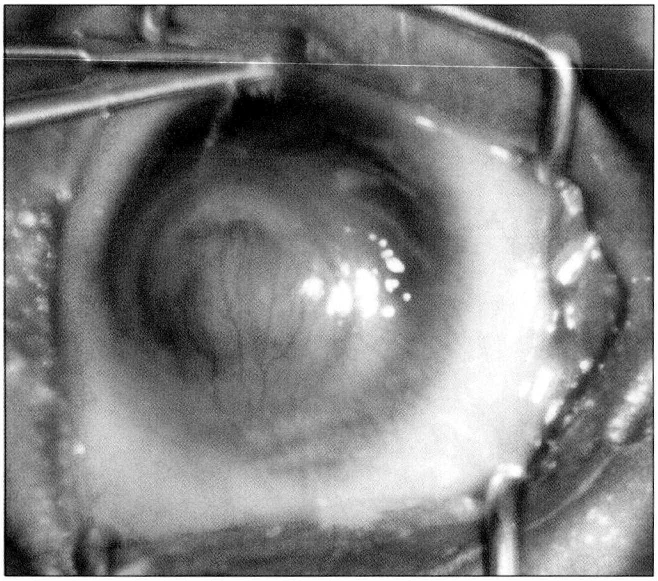

Fig. 58.15 Severe Peters' anomaly demonstrating marked opacification of the cornea. There is also a superficial vascular pannus. (Krachmer JH, Palay DA: *Cornea color atlas*, St. Louis, 1995, CV Mosby.)

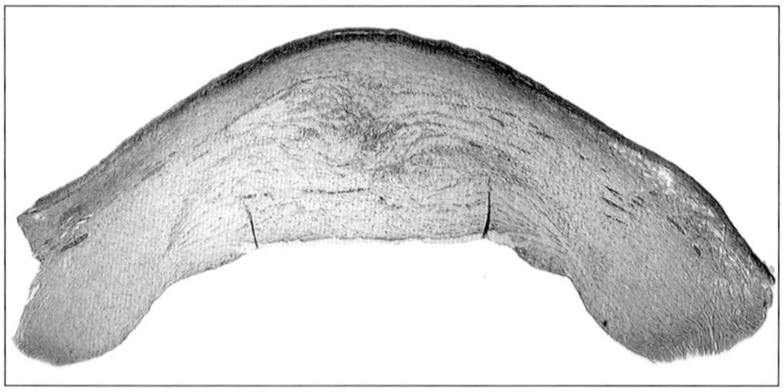

Fig. 58.16 Histopathology of Peters' anomaly demonstrating a defect in the posterior cornea with absent endothelium and Descemet's membrane. The central corneal stroma is thickened and scarred.

Glaucoma

Glaucoma develops in approximately 50–70% of patients.[34] While glaucoma can develop at any time, it most commonly develops soon after birth. Most patients with Peters' anomaly appear to have a normal trabecular meshwork. Kuper and colleagues postulated a failure of proper neural crest differentiation into corneal and trabecular endothelial cells as a possible disease mechanism.[36] Patients should have regular monitoring of intraocular pressure and other signs of infantile glaucoma such as buphthalmos. The glaucoma associated with Peters' anomaly is typically very difficult to control.

Other ocular findings

In 1992, Traboulsi and Maumenee reviewed the malformations associated with Peters' anomaly in 29 patients.[37] They found colobomatous microphthalmia in 7 (24%), persistent hyperplastic primary vitreous in 3 (10%), and retinal detachment (not related to ocular surgery) in 3 (10%).

Nonocular findings

Of the 29 Peters' anomaly patients studied by Traboulsi and Maumenee, developmental delay was found in 15 (52%), congenital heart disease in 8 (28%), external ear abnormalities in 5 (17%), central nervous system structural abnormalities in 4 (14%), genitourinary abnormalities in 4 (14%), hearing loss in 3 (10%), cleft lip and palate in 3 (10%), and spinal defects in 2 (7%).[37] A host of other anomalies have been reported in isolated cases. A condition called Peters'-plus syndrome refers to patients with Peters' anomaly associated with cleft lip and palate, short stature, abnormal ears, and mental retardation.[37,38] This syndrome is usually inherited in an autosomal recessive pattern. Traboulsi and Maumenee noted that associated defects tend to affect midline structures and suggested evaluating patients with Peters' anomaly for abnormalities of the heart and pituitary gland.[37]

Differential diagnosis

Peters' anomaly needs to be differentiated from other diseases that can cause corneal opacities such as primary congenital glaucoma, the mucopolysaccharidoses, congenital hereditary endothelial dystrophy (CHED), and birth trauma. Birth trauma is usually unilateral and should demonstrate breaks in Descemet's membrane. Primary congenital glaucoma may also demonstrate breaks in Descemet's membrane (Haab's striae) as well as buphthalmos. In both primary congenital glaucoma and CHED, the cornea is usually diffusely hazy as opposed to centrally hazy.

Pathogenesis

In Peters' anomaly, the corneal endothelium does not develop properly. Corneal endothelium and Descemet's membrane are absent beneath the corneal opacity. Peters felt that the underlying process was a failure of the lens and cornea to separate during embryogenesis. Against this theory are cases where there are no keratolenticular adhesions and the lens is well developed. Additionally, there is evidence that the lens epithelium is intact even in cases where the lens and cornea are closely apposed. Von Hippel suggested that intrauterine infection was the underlying etiologic factor, giving rise to the term von Hippel's internal corneal ulcer. Reese and Ellsworth found evidence of prenatal rubella infection in five of 21 patients with Peters' anomaly and associated iris adhesions.[4] While there are several theories, the true underlying pathogenesis is not known.

Genetics

Most cases are sporadic; however, there are autosomal recessive pedigrees and rare autosomal dominant pedigrees reported in the literature. Genetic mutations have been described in four genes to date among patients with Peters' anomaly. These genes include the *PAX6* gene associated with aniridia,[39] the *PITX2*[3] and *FOXC1*[2] genes associated with Axenfeld-Rieger syndrome, and the *CYP1B1* gene associated with primary congenital glaucoma.[40] The wide range of genes capable of causing Peters' anomaly, and the widely variable clinical picture suggest that there are a number of pathways that can lead to this central corneal defect.

Natural history

Corneal edema may be present early in the course of the disease and may persist or recur in the face of elevated intraocular pressure. The edema may progressively resolve as peripheral endothelial cells migrate over the posterior defect, leaving an overlying corneal scar. Corneal edema may recur later in life secondary the natural attrition of already compromised endothelial cells.

Treatment

The main issue in Peters' anomaly is poor visual development secondary to an opaque visual axis. In cases with a small central opacity and a clear lens, a large peripheral iridectomy may permit a formed retinal image.[41] In more severe cases, penetrating keratoplasty may be required to clear the visual axis. There have been varying success rates reported after keratoplasty for Peters' anomaly. In general, the prognosis is poorer if there is coexistent glaucoma. In a series of 144 penetrating keratoplasties in 72 eyes with a median follow-up of 11.1 years, Yang and colleagues showed that the prognosis for graft survival was highest for the first surgery and fell markedly for subsequent surgeries.[42] In their series, 35% of first grafts maintained clarity for 10 years compared to <10% of second or subsequent grafts. When primary grafts failed, they were most likely to do so in the first 2 years. They found that several features placed patients at increased risk for graft failure: severe disease, anterior synechiae, large corneal grafts, and central nervous system abnormalities. The most common postoperative complications were cataract, glaucoma, retinal detachment, and phthisis.[34] Phthisis developed in up to one-third of eyes.[34] Overall, the final visual outcome for these eyes was poor, with only 20% of patients achieving a visual acuity of 20/200 or better.[34] The patients who had a more favorable course had milder disease. A more recent series by Zaldman and colleagues reported on 30 eyes of 24 patients with type 1 Peters' anomaly (no lens abnormalities) undergoing penetrating keratoplasy with a mean follow-up of 6.5 years.[43] In their series, 90% of all eyes had clear grafts. Of the 24 eyes of 18 verbal children, 50% achieved a visual acuity of 20/200 of better. This supports the previous observation of higher success rates in patients with milder disease. Even if the visual axis can be successfully cleared, visual rehabilitation can be difficult secondary to associated developmental delay and other central nervous system abnormalities.

Glaucoma can be managed with topical medications, oral carbonic anhydrase inhibitors, or glaucoma surgery. The glaucoma associated with Peters' anomaly frequently requires surgical intervention such as trabeculectomy, tube-shunt procedures, or cyclodestructive procedures.[34] Even with these procedures, attaining pressure control is very difficult.[34]

References

1. Waring III GO, Rodrigues MM, Laibson PR. Anterior chamber cleavage syndrome. A stepladder classification. *Surv Ophthalmology.* 1975;20:3–27.
2. Honkanen RA, Nishimura D, Swiderski R, et al. A family with Axenfeld-Rieger syndrome and Peters' anomaly caused by a point mutation (Phe112Ser) in the FOXC1 gene. *Am J Ophthalmol.* 2003;135:368–375.
3. Doward W, Perveen R, Lloyd IC, et al. A mutation in the RIEG1 gene associated with Peters' anomaly. *J Med Genet.* 1999;36:152–155.
4. Reese AB, Ellsworth RM. The anterior chamber cleavage syndrome. *Arch Ophthalmol.* 1966;75:307–318.
5. Henkind P, Siegel IM, Carr RE: Mesodermal dysgenesis of the anterior segment: Rieger's anomaly. *Arch Ophthalmol.* 1965;73:810–817.
6. Tripathi BJ, Tripathi RC. Neural crest origin of the human trabecular meshwork and its implication for the pathogenesis of glaucoma. *Am J Ophthalmol.* 1989;107:583–590.
7. Mears AJ, Mirzayans F, Gould DB, et al. Autosomal dominant iridogoniodysgenesis anomaly maps to 6p25. *Am J Hum Genet.* 1996;59:1321–1327.
8. Pearce WG, Mielke BC, Kulak SC, Walter MA. Histopathology and molecular basis of iridogoniodysgenesis syndrome. *Ophthalmic Genet.* 1999;20:83–88.
9. Jordan T, Ebenezer N, Manners R, et al. Familial glaucoma iridogoniodysplasia maps to a 6p25 region implicated in primary congenital glaucoma and iridogoniodysgenesis anomaly. *Am J Hum Genet.* 1997;61:882–888.
10. Kluyskens J. Le glaucome congenital. *Bulletin de la Societe Belge d'Ophtalmologie.* 1950;94:3–248.
11. Jerndal T, Hansson HA, Bill A. *Goniodysgenesis – a new perspective on glaucoma.* Copenhagen: Scriptor Publisher ApS; 1990.
12. Sheffield VC, Alward WLM, Stone EM. The glaucomas. In: Scriver CR, Beaudetal AL, Sly SS, Valle D, eds. *The metabolic and molecular bases of inherited disease (in 4 volumes).* edn. 8. New York: McGraw-Hill; 2001.
13. Shields MB, Buckley E, Klintworth GK, Thresher R. Axenfeld-Rieger syndrome. A spectrum of developmental disorders. *Surv Ophthalmol.* 1985;29:387–409.
14. Alward WLM. Axenfeld-Rieger syndrome in the age of molecular genetics. *Am J Ophthalmol.* 2000;130:107–115.
15. Vossius A. Congenitale abnormalien der iris. *Klin Monatsbl Augenheilkd.* 1883;21:233–237.
16. Axenfeld TH. Embryotoxon cornea posterius. *Klin Monatsbl Augenheilkd.* 1920;65:381–382.
17. Rieger H. Verlagerung und Schlitzform der Pupille mit Hypoplasie des Irisvorderblattes. *Z Augenheilkd.* 1934;84:98–103.
18. Rieger H. Beiträge zur Kenntnis seltener Mißbildungen der Iris. II. Über Hypoplasie des Irisvorderblattes mit Verlagerung und Entrundung der Pupille. *Albrecht von Graefe's Arch Klin Exp Ophthalmol.* 1935;133:602–635.
19. Shields MB. Axenfeld-Rieger syndrome: a theory of mechanism and distinctions from the iridocorneal endothelial syndrome. *Trans Am Ophthalmol Soc.* 1983;81:736–784.
20. Burian HM, Rice MH, Allen L. External visibility of the region of Schlemm's canal. *Arch Ophthalmol.* 1957;57:651–658.
21. Martin JP, Zorah FC. Familial glaucoma in nine generations of a South Hampshire family. *Br J Ophthalmol.* 1974;58:536–542.
22. Judisch GF, Phelps CD, Hanson J. Rieger's syndrome – a case report with a 15-year follow-up. *Arch Ophthalmol.* 1979;97:2120–2122.
23. Héon E, Sheth B, Kalenak J, et al. Linkage of autosomal dominant iris hypoplasia to the region of the Rieger syndrome locus (4q25). *Hum Mol Genet.* 1995;4:1435–1439.
24. Alward WLM, Semina EV, Kalenak JW, et al. Autosomal dominant iris hypoplasia is caused by a mutation in the Rieger syndrome (RIEG/PITX2) gene. *Am J Ophthalmol.* 1998;125:98–100.
25. Reneker LW, Silversides DW, Xu L, Overbeek PA. Formation of corneal endothelium is essential for anterior segment development – a transgenic mouse model of anterior segment dysgenesis. *Development.* 2000;127:533–542.
26. Murray JC, Bennett SR, Kwitek AE, et al. Linkage of Rieger syndrome to the region of the epidermal growth factor gene on chromosome 4. *Nat Genet.* 1992;2:46–49.
27. Semina EV, Reiter R, Leysens NJ, et al. Cloning and characterization of a novel bicoid-related homeobox transcription factor gene, RGS, involved in Rieger syndrome. *Nat Genet.* 1996;14:392–399.
28. Kulak SC, Kozlowski K, Semina EV, et al. Mutation in the RIEG1 gene in patients with iridogoniodysgenesis syndrome. *Hum Mol Genet.* 1998;7:1113–1117.
29. Phillips JC, del Bono EA, Haines JL, et al. A second locus for Rieger syndrome maps to chromosome 13q14. *Am J Hum Genet.* 1996;59:613–619.
30. Nishimura DY, Swiderski RE, Alward WLM, et al. The forkhead transcription factor gene FKHL7 is responsible for glaucoma phenotypes which map to 6p25. *Nat Genet.* 1998;19:140–147.
31. Swiderski RE, Reiter RS, Nishimura DY, et al. Expression of the Mf1 gene in developing mouse hearts: implication in the development of human congenital heart defects. *Dev Dyn.* 1999;216:16–27.
32. von Hippel E. Über Hydrophthalmos Congenitus nebst Bemerkungen über die Verfarbund der Cornea durch Blufarbstoff; Pathologisch-

anatomische Untersuchungen. *Graefe's Arch Clin Exp Ophthalmol.* 1897;4: 539–564.
33. Peters A. Über angeborene Defekbildung der Descemetschen Membran. *Klin Monatsbl Augenheilkd.* 1906;44:27–41.
34. Yang LL, Lambert SR. Peters' anomaly: a synopsis of surgical management and visual outcome. *Ped Ophthalmol.* 2001;14:467–477.
35. Zaidman GW, Juechter K. Peters' anomaly associated with protruding corneal pseudo-staphyloma. *Cornea.* 1998;17:163–168.
36. Kuper C, Kuwabara T, Stark WJ. The histopathology of Peters' anomaly. *Am J Ophthalmol.* 1975;80:653–660.
37. Traboulsi EI, Maumenee IH. Peters' anomaly and associated congenital malformations. *Arch Ophthalmol.* 1992;110:1739–1742.
38. van Schooneveld MJ, Delleman JW, Beemer FA, Bleeker-Wagemakers EM. Peters'-plus: a new syndrome. *Ophthalmic Paediatr Genet.* 1984;4:141–145.
39. Hanson IM, Fletcher JM, Jordan T, et al. Mutations at the PAX6 locus are found in heterogeneous anterior segment malformations including Peters' anomaly. *Nat Genet.* 1994;6:168–173.
40. Vincent A, Billingsley G, Priston M, et al. Phenotypic heterogeneity of CYP1B1: mutations in a patient with Peters' anomaly. *J Med Genet.* 2001;2001:324–326.
41. Jünemann A, Gusek GC, Naumann GO. Optical sector iridectomy: an alternative to perforating keratoplasty in Peters' anomaly. *Klin Monatsbl Augenheilkd.* 1996;209:117–124.
42. Yang LL, Lambert SR, Lynn MJ, Stulting RD. Long-term results of corneal graft survival in infants and children with Peters' anomaly. *Ophthalmology.* 1999;106:833–848.
43. Zaidman GW, Flanagan FK, Furey CC. Long-tern visual prognosis in chicldren after corneal transplant surgery for Peters' anomaly type 1. *Am J Ophthalmol.* 2007;144:104–108.

Chapter 59

Corneal Manifestations of Metabolic Diseases

Sathish Srinivasan, Raneen Shehadeh-Mashor, Allan R. Slomovic

Introduction

The cornea serves as the external gateway into the eye. It, together with the sclera, forms the outer shell of the eyeball. The cornea not only serves as the major refracting structure for light entering the eye but also, with its epithelial barrier, plays a major role in the ocular biodefense system. Maintenance of the corneal shape and transparency is of paramount importance. The optical properties of the cornea are determined by its transparency, surface smoothness, contour, and its refractive index. The absence of corneal blood vessels and the regular arrangement of the stromal collagen fibers play an important role in the transparency of the cornea. The uniform arrangement and the continuous slow production and degradation of the stromal collagen fibers are essential for corneal transparency.

The corneal stroma is made up of extracellular matrix, keratocytes, and nerve fiber bundles. The extracellular matrix composed of collagen (type 1) and glycosaminoglycans (GAGs) make up the entire corneal stroma, with the cellular components contributing to only 2–3% of the total stromal volume.[1] Not only are the collagen fibers in the corneal stroma highly uniform[2] but also the distance between them is highly uniform.[3] Several glycosaminoglycans are present among the stromal collagen fibers. The most abundant GAG is keratan sulphate, which constitutes about 65% of the total GAG content. The remaining GAGs include chondroitin sulfate and dermatan sulfate. Although the corneal hydration is predominantly controlled by the endothelial pump, it is also influenced by the intraocular pressure, stromal swelling pressure, and the epithelial barrier function. The GAG content of the stroma plays a substantial role in this homeostatic process. Metabolic changes intrinsic to the cornea or from secondary involvement due to a systemic disorder can lead to abnormal accumulation of storage products within the cornea, which can interfere with both the clarity and the function of the cornea. Abnormalities in the carbohydrate, lipid, and lipoprotein metabolism can significantly affect the structure and function of the cornea. Ever since the discovery of lysosomes by de Duve[4] there has been an interest in their role in systemic diseases. Lysosomal storage disorders, of which over 40 are now known, are caused by the defective activity of lysosomal proteins, which result in the intralysosomal accumulation of undegraded metabolites. Of these, the mucopolysaccharidoses (MPS) are a group of disorders caused by inherited defects in lysosomal enzymes resulting in widespread intra- and extracellular accumulation of glycosaminoglycans. In this chapter, we summarize the major systemic metabolic diseases that affect the cornea.

Disorders of Carbohydrate Metabolism

Diabetes mellitus – diabetic keratopathy

Diabetes mellitus (DM) is a syndrome of chronic hyperglycemia due to relative insulin deficiency, resistance, or both. The number of cases of diabetes worldwide in 2000 among adults over 20 years of age is estimated to have been over 171 million.[5] This figure is 11% higher than the previous estimate of 154 million.[6]

With the evidence that the 'diabetic epidemic' will continue, one would expect the prevalence and the incidence of diabetic eye disease to increase as well. Although diabetes does not have a classic corneal manifestation, several ultrastructural and functional changes occur in a diabetic cornea, resulting in diabetic keratopathy (DK). DK encompasses a clinical spectrum which includes superficial punctuate epitheliopathy, persistent epithelial erosions, corneal hypoesthesia, nonhealing persistent epithelial defects (PEDs), and corneal edema (Fig. 59.1).[7,8] The reported prevalence of DK is around 50–70% among diabetic patients.[9,10] Before DK clinically sets in, several subclinical abnormalities develop in diabetic corneas. These abnormalities affect both the structure (anatomical changes) and the function of the cornea.

Ultrastructural changes in DK include a decrease in the epithelial barrier function,[11,12] abnormalities in shape of the epithelial cells,[13,14] basement membrane thickening,[15,16] decreased corneal sensations,[17,18] and abnormalities of the endothelial cells.[19,20] These subclinical abnormalities often have a close temporal relationship to the development of symptomatic DK. In addition to the ultrastructural changes, several enzymatic and neural changes contribute to the development of DK (Table 59.1). Studies have proposed that three enzymatic dysregulations contribute to DK: an activated polyol pathway,[21,22] accumulation of advanced glycation end products (AGEs),[23] and increased nonenzymatic

Table 59.1 Factors contributing to diabetic keratopathy

Structural and functional abnormalities	Enzymatic dysregulation
1. Decreased corneal epithelial basal cell density	1. Increase in polyol metabolism
2. Thickening of the epithelial basement membrane	2. Increased accumulation of polyol in corneal epithelial and endothelial cells
3. Decreased penetration of anchoring fibrils	3. Increased nonenzymatic glycation of protein components
4. Reduction in hemidesmosome density	4. Advanced glycation end products
5. Decrease in epithelial barrier function	

Diabetic keratopathy

Neural dysregulation
1. Decreased corneal sensation
2. Decrease in the number and density of corneal nerve bundles
3. Loss of nerve-derived growth factors (IGF-1, substance P)

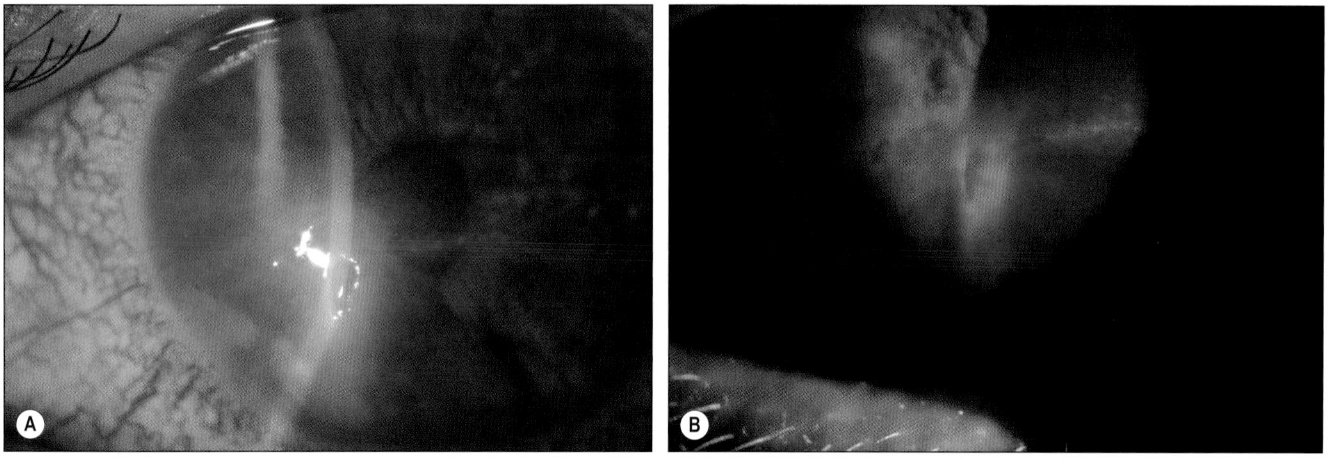

Fig. 59.1 (**A**) Slit lamp photograph of a 31-old-year old type I diabetic with diabetic keratopathy. Note the persistent epithelial defect, stromal haze, and corneal thinning. (Courtesy Pankaj Gupta, MD.) (**B**) Higher magnification view of the persistent epithelial defect with surrounding stromal haze. (Courtesy Pankaj Gupta, MD.)

glycation of protein components[24] in the basement membrane of the corneal epithelium. Efficacies of pharmacologically inhibiting the aldose reductase, the first enzyme in the polyol pathway, have been evaluated. Both oral (ONO-2235) and topical (CT-112) aldose reductase inhibitors (ARIs) have been shown to decrease the corneal epithelial changes in diabetic patients through recovery of corneal sensation and tear production.[18,25] In addition, ARIs have been shown to improve corneal epithelial wound healing,[26] prevent breakdown of the corneal epithelial barrier function,[27] and inhibit the accumulation of polyol.[28] Nakahara et al., in a randomized, placebo-controlled trial, showed that topical ARI treatment was effective in restoring the corneal epithelial barrier function but not in the prevention of superficial punctuate keratopathy.[29]

Decrease in corneal sensation and loss of nerve-derived trophic factors have been postulated as causative factors in the development of DK. Confocal microscopy has become

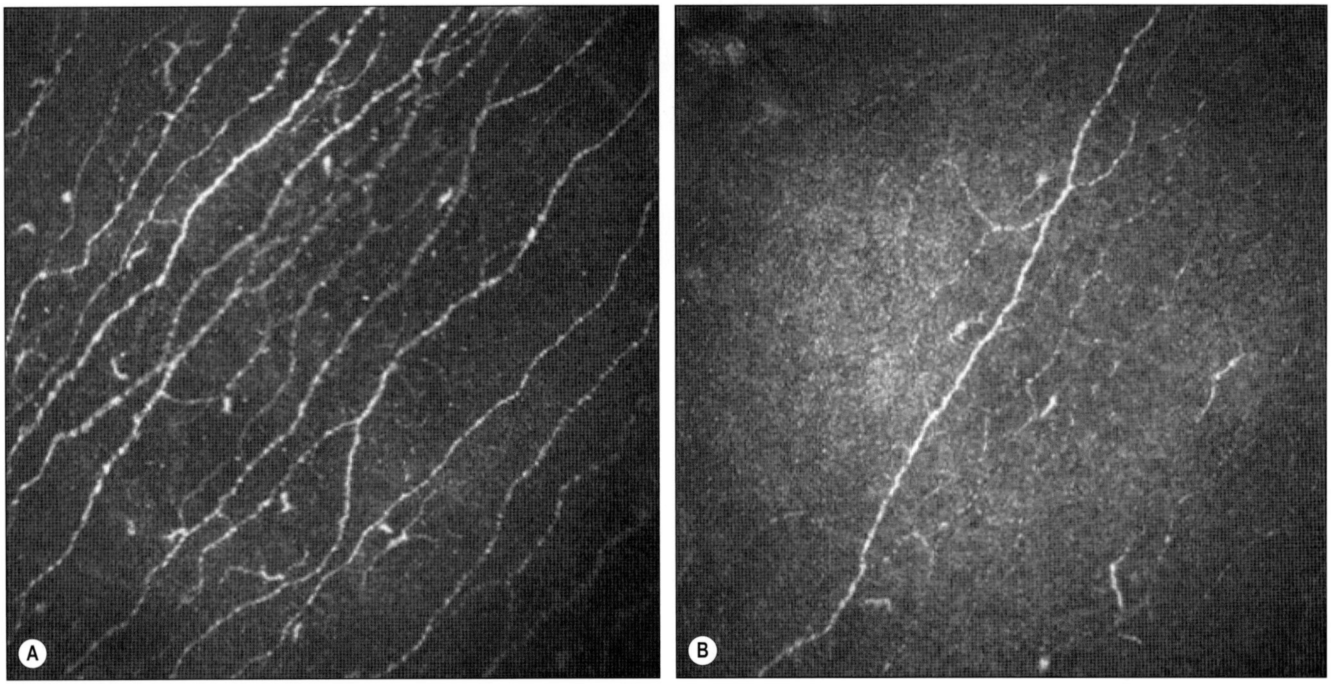

Fig. 59.2 (**A**) Confocal microscopy images of corneal nerves in Bowman's layer from a healthy subject. (**B**) Confocal microscopy images of the corneal nerves in Bowman's layer from a diabetic patients with severe neuropathy. Note the marked reduction in the density of the corneal nerves. (Courtesy Mitra Tavakoli, PhD.)

the tool of choice to quantify the corneal nerve density and morphology in diabetic corneas. These measurements can be correlated with the severity of neuropathy in diabetic patients.[30,31] Confocal studies on corneas in patients with diabetes have shown a reduction in the number of corneal nerve bundles, reduction in the density of nerve fiber suggestive of enhanced degeneration, and reduction in the branching of nerve bundles suggestive of limited regeneration (Fig. 59.2). These changes seem to precede the impairment of corneal sensitivity when measured clinically, and they also relates to the measures of somatic neuropathy in diabetic patients.[30,31] Insulin-like growth factor 1 (IGF-1) and substance P, a neuropeptide present in sensory nerves, have been shown to accelerate corneal epithelial wound healing.[32] Thus, topical applications of IGF-1 and substance P have been shown to promote regeneration of corneal nerve fibers in patients with diabetic neurotrophic keratopathy.[33]

Lysosomal storage disorders

Introduction

Lysosomes are membrane-bound organelles that function as the 'stomachs' of eukaryotic cells. First discovered by de Duve in 1949,[34] this intracellular membrane consists of a limiting external membrane and intralysosomal vesicles. The lysosomes contain about 50 different digestive enzymes that break down all types of biological molecules including proteins, nucleic acids, lipids, and carbohydrates. Both extracellular materials brought into the cell by endocytosis and obsolete intracellular materials are degraded in the lysosome. It is estimated that there are at least 50–60 soluble hydrolases[35] and at least seven integral membrane proteins in lysosomes.[36] In theory, mutations in the genes that encode any of these proteins can lead to lysosomal storage diseases (LSDs) (Fig. 59.3).

LSDs can be grouped according to various classifications, but perhaps the most useful is based on the characterization of the defective enzymes or protein, rather than of the nature of the accumulated substrate(s) (Table 59.2). Classification based on the accumulated substrate(s) can lead to erroneous characterization of a number of diseases as the accumulating substrate was identified many years before the enzymatic defects were known.[37] However, the classification of many LSDs can still be made based on the nature of the substrate that accumulates. For example, in mucopolysaccharidoses (MPS), GAGs accumulate due to the impaired function of the lysosomal enzymes, which are required for the sequential degradation of GAGs. In sphingolipidoses, unmetabolized sphingolipids accumulate due to defective enzyme activity, and oligosaccharides accumulate in oligosaccharidoses. In some cases, because of a common determinant, a deficiency of a single enzyme can result in the accumulation of different substrates.

Mucopolysaccharidoses

The mucopolysaccharidoses (MPS) are a group of LSDs, each of which is produced by an inherited deficiency of an enzyme

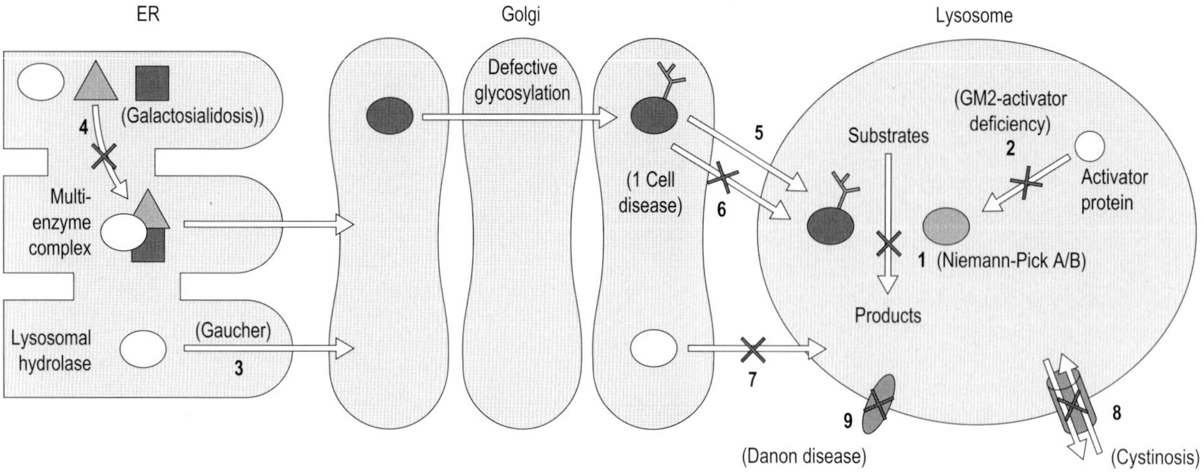

Fig. 59.3 The biochemical and cellular basis of lysosomal storage disorders (LSDs). Most mutations in LSD result in the delivery of a defective enzyme that has a reduced catalytic activity to lysosomes (*1*). In some case, a protein that is required for optimal hydrolase activity is defective or absent (*2*). LSD can be caused by defective transport of a lysosomal hydrolase out of the endoplasmic reticulum (ER) due to a mutation that causes misfolding (*3*). A defective transport of a lysosomal hydrolase out of the ER due to the lack of a required multienzyme complex can also lead to LSD (*4*). In the Golgi, defective glycosylation could result in an enzyme with reduced catalytic activity (*5*). Alternatively, defective glycosylation in the Golgi could produce an enzyme that cannot reach lysosomes, as it cannot bind to mannose-6-phosphatase receptors (*6*). Defects in other transport steps from the Golgi could also lead to LSD (*7*). Several LSDs are caused by defects in the integral lysosomal membrane proteins. These include defects in transporters (*8*), or in proteins involved in vital regulatory events of lysosomal function (*9*). In this figure lysosomal hydrolases are shown in various shades of blue, and a relevant LSD example is shown for each defect when one is known. (Published with permission from *Nat Rev Mol Cell Biol* 5:554–65, 2004.)

involved in the degradation of glycosaminoglycans. This condition is clinically progressive and has many common features that result from the accumulation of partially degraded GAGs in various tissues. They have a combined incidence of about 1 per 10000 births and their current nomenclature, biochemistry, screening, and diagnostic tests are summarized in Table 59.2. Each lysosomal enzyme is specific for a specific linkage. An inherited deficiency of any enzyme involved disrupts the sequential degradative process and leads to the accumulation of partially degraded GAGs within the lysosomes. The accumulation is progressive and eventually disrupts the cellular architecture and function. The tissue and organs affected and the severity will depend on the degree of enzyme deficiency (i.e. partial or total).

Deposition of these substances in the connective tissue leads to connective tissue laxity manifest by inguinal and umbilical hernias. Connective tissue thickening secondary to GAG accumulation and collagen deposition leads to coarse facial features, peripheral nerve entrapments, thickened meninges, spinal cord compression, and hydrocephalus. Deposition of GAGs in the heart valve leaflets, endocardium, and myocardium leads to symptomatic heart disease which is the common cause of death in these patients. Most of these disorders produce short stature, secondary to impaired long bone growth and vertebral abnormalities. These and other changes in the bony skelton are referred to as *dysostosis multiplex*. Central nervous system storage may produce progressive mental retardation, especially in disorders involving the impaired degradation of heparan sulfate (MPS I, II, and III). Corneal clouding and visual handicap result from the storage of the partially degraded GAGs within the corneal stroma, especially in disorders involving impaired degradation of dermatan sulfate and keratan sulfate (MPS I, IV, and VI). The corneal stroma, which constitutes more than 90% on the corneal thickness, is composed of extracellular matrix, keratocytes, and stromal nerve fibers. Over 97% of the stroma is made up of collagen (type I) and GAGs. Various GAGs are present between the collagen fibers in the corneal stroma. With the exception of hyaluronan, all these GAGs bind to core proteins to form proteoglycans. The most abundant GAG in the cornea is keratan sulfate, constituting about 65% of the total GAG content. The remainder is made up by dermatan sulfate and chondroitin sulfate. Abnormal, excessive accumulation of GAGs within the corneal stroma in MPS interferes with the regular arrangement of the collagen–GAG matrix, thus causing corneal clouding. Except for Hunter's syndrome (MPS II) in which the missing enzyme is specified by a gene on the X chromosome and the inheritance is X linked, all of the other MPS are inherited as autosomal recessive. In most cases, the affected offspring have heterozygous carrier parents, both of whom have about half the normal level of the enzyme for which the affected individual is deficient.

MPS I

MPS type I is further subdivided into three subtypes based on the phenotypic expression (MPS I-H [Hurler's] syndrome, MPS I-S [Scheie's] syndrome, and MPS I-HS [Hurler-Scheie] syndrome). It was first described by Gertrud Hurler in 1919.

In this subtype, approximately 90 mutations in the gene coding for the lysosomal enzyme α-1-iduronidase are known to cause deficiency or absence of the enzyme.[38] The deficiency of α-1-iduronidase leads to intracellular and extracellular accumulation of the GAGs dermatan and heparan

Table 59.2 Lysosomal storage disorders

Disease	Defective protein	Storage material	Screening test	Diagnostic test
Mucopolysaccharidoses (MPS)				
MPS I (Hurler, Scheie, Hurler/Scheie)	α-iduronidase	Dermatan and heparan sulfate	Urine GAGs	WBC enzyme assay
MPS II (Hunter)	Iduronate-2-sulfatase	Dermatan and heparan sulfate	Urine GAGs	Plasma enzyme assay
MPS IIIA (Sanfilippo)	Heparan *N*-sulfatase (sulphamidase)	Heparan sulfate	Urine GAGs	WBC enzyme assay
MPS IIIB (Sanfilippo)	*N*-Acetyl-α-glucosaminidase	Heparan sulfate	Urine GAGs	Plasma enzyme assay
MPS IIIC (Sanfilippo)	Acetyl-CoA, α-glucosamide *N*-acetyltransferase	Heparan sulfate	Urine GAGs	WBC enzyme assay
MPS IIID (Sanfilippo)	*N*-acetylglucosamine-6-sulfatase	Heparan sulfate	Urine GAGs	WBC enzyme assay
MPS IV (Morquio) IVA	*N*-acetyl galactosamine-6-sulfatase	Keratan sulfate	Urine GAGs	WBC enzyme assay
MPS IV (Morquio) IVB	β-galactosidase	Keratan sulfate	Urine GAGs	WBC enzyme assay
MPS VI (Maroteaux-Lamy)	*N*-acetylgalactosamine-4-sulfatase	Dermatan sulfate	Urine GAGs	WBC enzyme assay
MPS VII (Sly)	β-glucuronidase	Heparan, dermatan and chondroitin sulfate	Urine GAGs	WBC enzyme assay
MPS IX (Natowicz)	Hyaluronidase	Hyaluronic acid	None	Cultured cells
Sphingolipidoses				
Fabry's disease	α-galactosidase A	Globotriaosylceramide and blood group B substances	None	WBC enzyme assay
Farber lipogranulomatosis	Ceramidase	Ceramide	None	WBC enzyme assay
Gaucher disease	β-glucosidase, saposin C activator	Glucosylceramide	None	WBC enzyme assay
Niemann-Pick A and B	Sphingomyelinase	Sphingomyelin	None	WBC enzyme assay
GM1 gangliosidosis	β-glucosidase	GM1 ganglioside	Urine oligosaccharides	WBC enzyme assay
GM2 gangliosidosis (Tay-Sachs)	β-hexosaminidase A	GM2 ganglioside and related glycolipids	None	WBC enzyme assay
GM2 gangliosidosis (Sandhoff)	β-hexosaminidase A and B	GM2 ganglioside and related glycolipids	None	WBC enzyme assay
GM2 gangliosidosis (Gm2 activator deficiency)	GM2-activator protein	GM2 ganglioside and related glycolipids	None	Cultured cells and natural substrate
Globoid cell leucodystrophy Krabbe	Galactocerebrosidase	Galactosylceramides	None	WBC enzyme assay
Mucolipidoses				
ML I (sialidosis I)	Neuraminidase	Sialic acid	Urine sialic acid	Cultured cells
MLII (I cell)	Transferase	Many	Urine oligosaccharides	Plasma enzyme assay

Table 59.2 Lysosomal storage disorders—cont'd

Disease	Defective protein	Storage material	Screening test	Diagnostic test
Mucolipidoses—cont'd				
ML III (pseudo-Hurler)	Transferase	Many	Urine oligosaccharides	Plasma enzyme assay
ML IV	Mucolipin-1	Lipids and mucopolysaccharides	Urine oligosaccharides	Histology
Glycoproteinoses				
α-mannosidosis	α-mannosidase	α-mannosides	Urine oligosaccharides	WBC enzyme assay
β-mannosidosis	β-mannosidase	β-mannosides	Urine oligosaccharides	WBC enzyme assay
Fucosidosis	Fucosidase	Fucosides glycolipids	Urine oligosaccharides	WBC enzyme assay
Aspartylglucosaminuria	Aspartylglucosaminidase	Aspartylglucosamine	Urine oligosaccharides	WBC enzyme assay
Schindler disease	α-galactosidase B	*N*-acetyl-galactosamide glycoprotein	Urine oligosaccharides	WBC enzyme assay
Glycogen				
Pompe disease	α-glucosidase	Glycogen	ECG characteristic	Lymphocyte enzyme assay
Lipid				
Wolman disease and cholesterol ester storage disease (CESD)	Acid lipase	Cholesterol ester	None	WBC enzyme assay
Niemann-Pick C (NPC)	NPC 1 and 2	Cholesterol and sphingolipids	Filipin staining of cultured cells	Cholesterol esterification studies
Diseases caused by defects in integral membrane proteins				
Cystinosis	Cystinosin	Cystine	Renal function	WBC cystine
Danon disease	Lysosome associated membrane protein 2 (LAMP 2)	Cytoplasmic debris and glycogen	Unknown	Unknown
Infantile sialic acid storage disease and Salla disease	Sialin	Sialic acid	Urine oligosaccharides	Cultured cells
Others				
Galactosialidosis	Cathepsin	Sialyloligosaccharides	Urine oligosaccharides	Cultured cells
Multiple sulfatase deficiency	Cα –formylglycine-generating enzyme	Sulfatides	Urine GAGs	WBC and plasma enzyme assay
Neuron ceroid-lipofuscinosis (Batten disease)				
NCL 1	CLN-1 (protein palmitoylthioesterase-1)	Lipidated thioesters	Histology	Cultured cells and DNA
NCL 2	CLN 2 (tripeptidyl amino peptidase-1)	Subunit C of mitochondrial ATP synthase	Histology	Cultured cells and DNA
NCL 3	Arginine transporter	Subunit C of mitochondrial ATP synthase	Histology	DNA

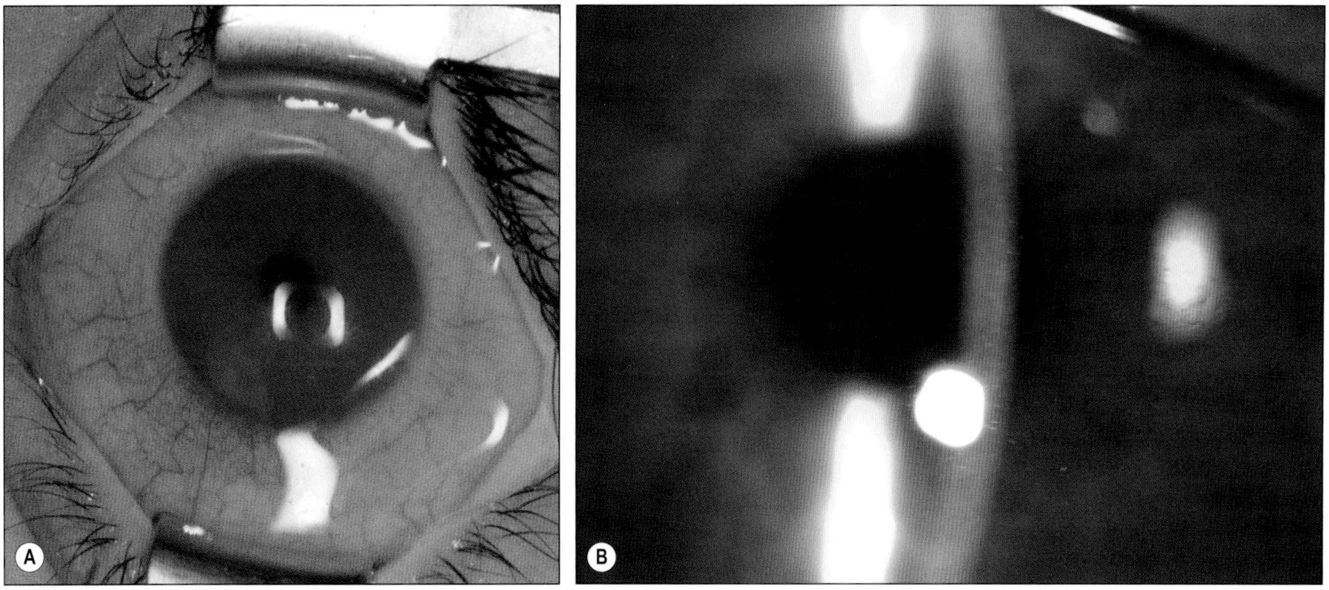

Fig. 59.4 (**A**) Intraoperative picture showing a cloudy cornea in a 7-year-old boy with Hurler's syndrome. (Courtesy Peter Meyer, MD.) (**B**) Slit lamp photograph of a 14-year-old girl with Hurler's syndrome. Note the marked stromal clouding within the slit beam.

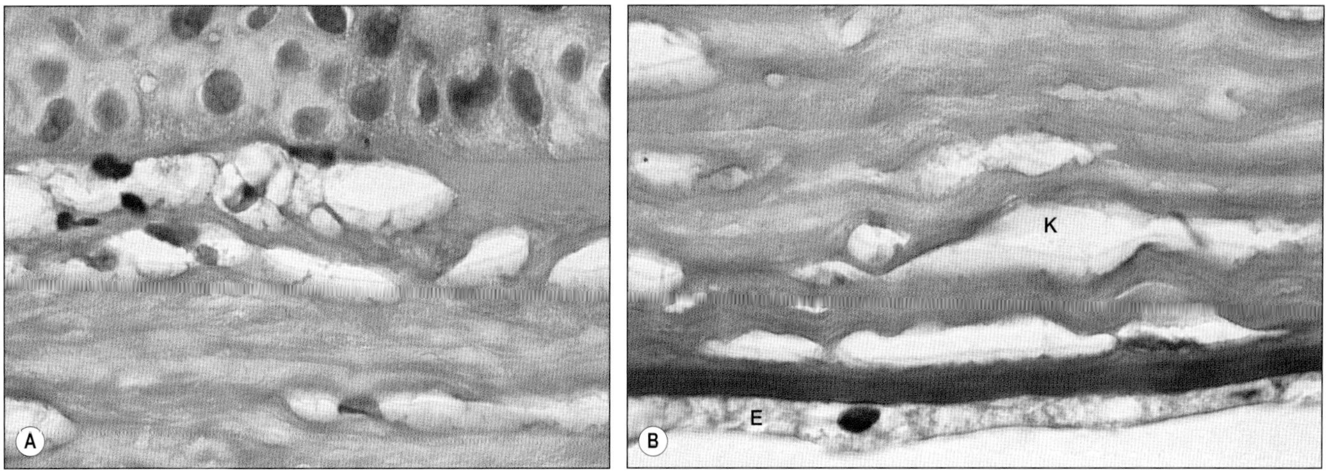

Fig. 59.5 (**A**) Anterior cornea from a case of Hurler's syndrome (PAS, magnification ×400). (Courtesy Peter Meyer, MD.) (**B**) Posterior corneal stroma in Hurler's syndrome showing granular deposits within keratocytes (*K*) and the endothelium (*E*) (PAS, magnification ×400). (Courtesy Peter Meyer, MD.)

sulfate, causing cell death, tissue damage, and excessive excretion of GAGs in the urine. There is a wide phenotypic variation of MPS I with the severe form being described as Hurler's syndrome, the milder form Scheie's syndrome, and the intermediate form Hurler-Scheie syndrome. Ocular features are common in all MPS I subtypes.

Hurler's syndrome (MPS I-H)

Infants with MPS I grow normally until 6–12 months of age, when they begin to manifest coarsening of facial features, skeletal deformities, and other systemic manifestations. Skeletal problems include dysostosis multiplex, odontoid dysplasia, spondyololisthesis, thoracolumbar gibbus, and joint contractures. Other systemic manifestations include large head circumference, communicating hydrocephalus, mental retardation, hepatosplenomegaly, and cardiac complications (cardiomyopathy, coronary artery disease, and heart valvular disease).[39] Intellectual impairment is a prominent feature of MPS I-H. Untreated children usually die during the first decade of life.[40] Bone marrow transplantation in MPS I-H has a significant impact on the life span and the systemic health of the patient.[41]

The main ocular manifestations of MPS I include severe corneal clouding (Figs 59.4–59.6),[42] retinal pigmentary degeneration,[43] glaucoma and optic nerve head swelling, and optic atrophy.[44] Prominent, wide-set eyes (shallow orbits, hypertelorism) may be seen in severely affected

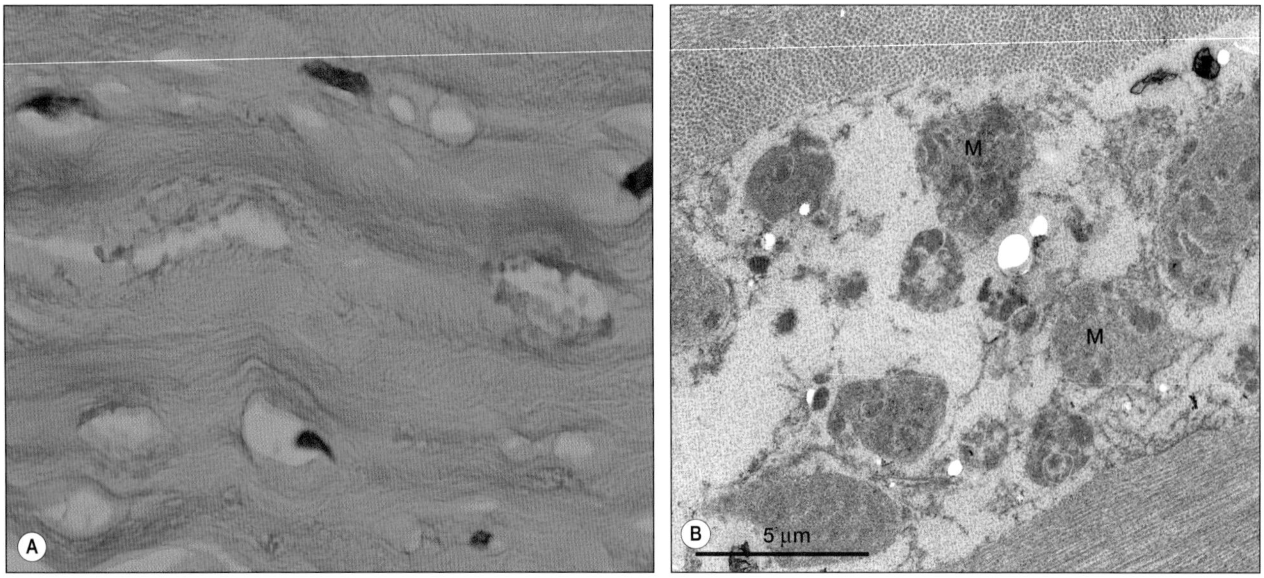

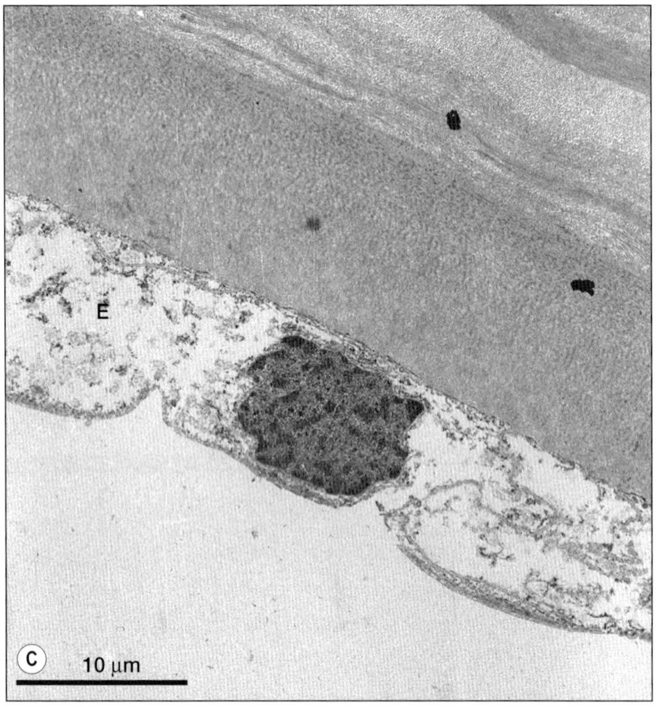

Fig. 59.6 (**A**) Mid corneal stroma in case of Hurler's syndrome showing granular deposits in within keratocytes (*arrows*) (Masson, magnification ×400). (Courtesy Peter Meyer, MD.) (**B**) Transmission electron microscopy showing keratocyte in Hurler's syndrome containing cytoplasmic deposits of mucopolysaccharide (*M*). (Courtesy Peter Meyer, MD.) (**C**) Transmission electron microscopy of endothelial cells (*E*) with granular cytoplasm in Hurler's syndrome. (Courtesy Peter Meyer, MD.)

patients. The retinal and optic nerve involvement may limit the success of corneal transplantation in these patients. In addition to posterior segment pathology, open-angle glaucoma has also been reported.[45]

Scheie's syndrome (MPS I-S)

This rare disorder is also due to the deficiency of α-1-iduronidase and is characterized by severe corneal clouding, deformity of the hands, and aortic valvular disease. Symptoms usually appear between the ages of 5 and 15. The striking joint stiffness of the hands is similar to that seen in Hurler's syndrome but is complicated by carpal tunnel syndrome due to median nerve entrapment. These subgroups of patients have normal height and intelligence. Life expectancy may be nearly normal. Although the corneal clouding is severe and affects the entire cornea, there are reports of dense peripheral corneal clouding with almost clear central corneas in subgroups of MPS.[46,47] Although the deposition of proteoglycan material among the stromal lamella is characteristic of all MPS, histological appearance of epithelial breaks with peglike undulations, marked attenuation of the Bowman's layer, and the appearance of fibrous long-spacing (FLS) collagen may present histopathological changes unique to Scheie's syndrome.[48]

Hurler-Scheie (MPS I-HS)

Some patients with a phenotype that is intermediate between that of Hurler's and Scheie's syndromes are thought to represent compound heterozygotes, having inherited one Hurler and one Scheie gene from each parent. They usually have normal intelligence and only mild facial changes and die in their twenties or later of associated cardiorespiratory disease. Diffuse corneal opacification and retinopathy occur.[49]

Hunter's syndrome (MPS II)

This results from defective function of iduronate-2-sulfatase, resulting in deposition of the GAGs dermatan and heparan sulfate. Hunter's syndrome is distinguished from Hurler's syndrome by three features: (1) slow progression with longer survival,[50] (2) lack of corneal clouding, and (3) X-linked rather than autosomal recessive inheritance. Unlike MPS I, seizures are more common in MPS II and patients develop learning difficulties with progressive neurodegeneration.

Ocular abnormalities in MPS II Hunter's syndrome include exophthalmos, hypertelorism, disk swelling and optic atrophy,[51] and retinopathy.[43] In contrast to MPS I, the corneal changes in MPS II do not usually significantly impair vision.[52,53]

Sanfilippo's syndrome (MPS III)

MPS III (Sanfilippo) results from deficiency of at least four different enzymes that result in the deposition and accumulation of heparan sulfate (see Table 59.2). Clinically, the four types (MPS III A–D) are indistinguishable. Patients with MPS III (Sanfilippo) present with learning difficulties and severe behavioral disturbance, but have mild systemic manifestations. Early development is normal but slows or halts between the ages of 2 and 6 years, after which mental deterioration is often rapid. They often have a large head, coarse hair, and hirsutism. The clinical diagnosis may be suspected from severe mental retardation, which appears disproportionate with relatively mild somatic and radiological abnormalities. Moderate to severe retinopathy with pigmentary retinal degeneration and associated electroretinogram changes are prominent features of MPS III.[54,55]

Morquio's syndrome (MPS IV)

MPS IV (Morquio) is caused by mutations in *N*-acetylgalactosamine-6-sulfatase, resulting in deposition and accumulation of keratan sulfate (Figs 59.7, 59.8). The main feature of MPS IV is the severe skeletal changes and features of spinal cord compression resulting from neck instability.[56] At a very early age (around 2 years), patients start developing pigeon chest deformity, genu valgum, and gait disturbances. Diagnosis depends on the clinical and radiological features, which are characteristic; the finding of keratan sulfaturia and the deficiency of *N*-acetylgalactosamine-6-sulfatase, which is active on both Gal*N*Ac6-S in chondroitin sulfate and Gal 6-S in keratan sulfate. The corneal opacification in MPS IV (Morquio) is usually mild.[56,57] Retinopathy also occurs.[58,59]

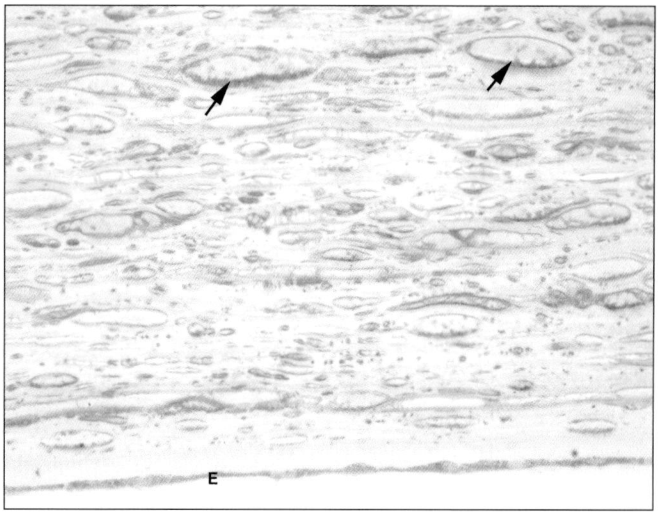

Fig. 59.7 Posterior cornea from a case of Morquio's syndrome showing accumulation of mucopolysaccharide within keratocytes (*arrows*) as well as within the endothelium (*E*) (Hale's colloidal iron, magnification ×200). (Courtesy Fiona Roberts, MD.)

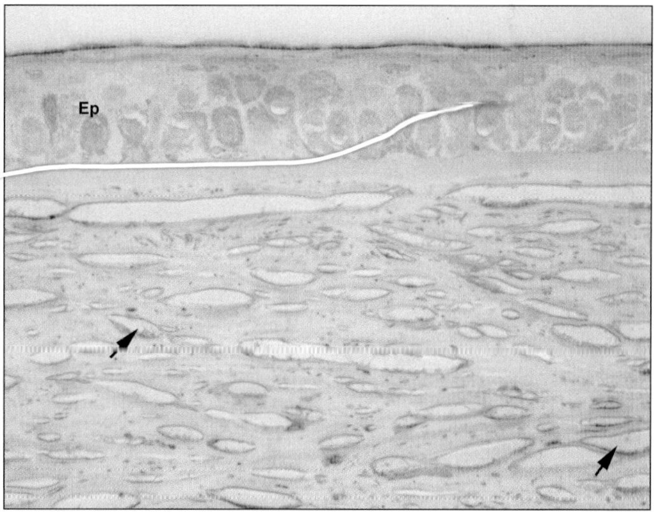

Fig. 59.8 Anterior cornea from a case of Morquio's syndrome showing accumulation of mucopolysaccharide within keratocytes (*arrows*) as well as within the epithelium (*Ep*) (Hale's colloidal iron, magnification ×200). (Courtesy Fiona Roberts, MD.)

Pseudoexophthalmos may be seen secondary to shallow orbits.[59] Penetrating keratoplasty has limited success to reopacification of the graft and also the poor visual outcome due to retinal changes (Figs 59.9, 59.10).

Maroteaux-Lamy syndrome (MPS VI)

In 1963, Maroteaux and colleagues recognized a new form of MPS that resembled Hurler's but was different in that the patients were intellectually normal, the urinary GAG was exclusively dermatan sulfate, and the leukocytes exhibited striking metachromatic inclusions. MPS VI (Maroteaux-Lamy) results from deficiencies of *N*-acetylgalactosamine-

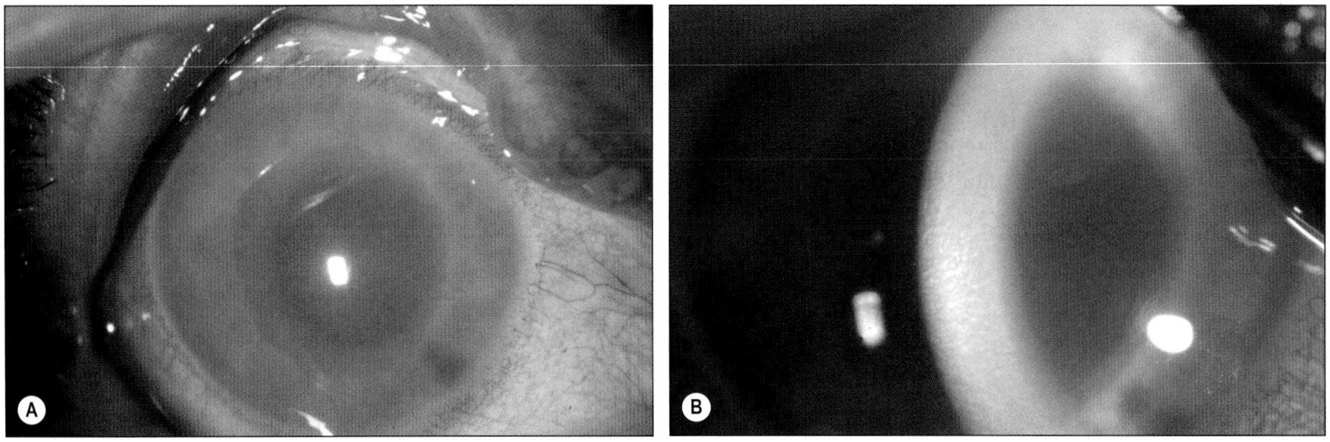

Fig. 59.9 (**A**) Anterior segment photograph of the right eye showing an opaque, cloudy cornea in a patient with Morquio's syndrome. (Courtesy Fiona Roberts, MD.) (**B**) Slit lamp photograph of the same patient showing marked corneal clouding involving all the layers of the cornea. (Courtesy Fiona Roberts, MD.)

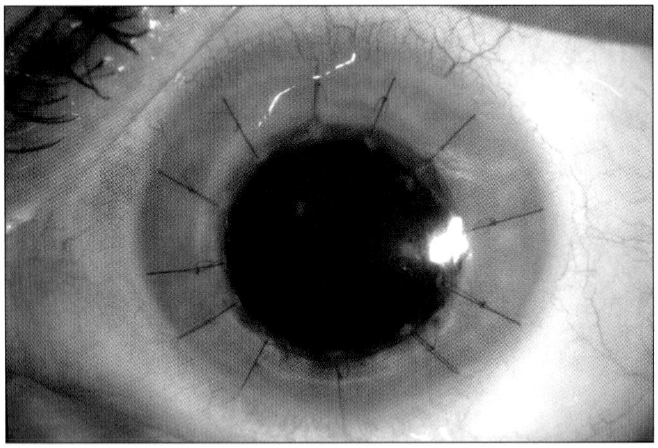

Fig. 59.10 Slit lamp photograph showing a clear full-thickness corneal transplant in a case of Morquio's syndrome. Note the cloudy stroma in the peripheral host cornea. (Courtesy Fiona Roberts, MD.)

4-sulfatase, causing deposition of the GAG dermatan sulfate. Patients develop coarse facial features, a large head, short neck, restriction of joint movement, claw hand, hepatosplenomegaly, hernias, and carpal tunnel syndrome. Significant progressive corneal opacification occurs in MPS VI,[53,60] associated with increased corneal thickness (Figs 59.11, 59.12).[56] However, early cases may have clear corneas.[61] Patients affected with marked corneal clouding may benefit from corneal transplantation.

Sly's syndrome (MPS VII)

MPS VII is a very rare disease, with approximately only 33 cases reported since its initial description by Sly in 1973.[62] This syndrome is caused by the deficiency of β-glucuronidase, which has been mapped to 7q21.I-7q22. Although hydrops fetalis from severe β-glucuronidase deficiency has been reported, patients with milder deficiency may survive into adulthood.[62] Corneal opacification is associated with MPS VII and may necessitate penetrating keratoplasty.[63]

Natowicz's syndrome (MPS IX)

MPS IX (Natowicz) is due to the deficiency of hyaluronidase, resulting in accumulation of chondroitin sulfate. There has only been a single patient reported so far who demonstrated a mild clinical phenotype with periauricular soft tissue masses and mild short stature, but no neurological or ocular manifestations.[64]

Corneal histopathology in MPS

Progressive corneal opacification (ground-glass cornea) affects all the MPS I subgroup (MPS I-H, I-S, I-HS)[49,65] and MPS VI (Maroteaux-Lamy),[66] due to the accumulation of dermatan sulfate within the cornea, which is not present in the normal cornea. Corneal opacification is also seen in MPS IV (Morquio) due to keratan sulfate deposition.[57] Progressive corneal opacification is also seen in MPS VII (Sly).[63] Corneal opacification is mild in MPS I-S and MPS II (Hunter), and rarely requires corneal transplantation,[52,67] and is not a prominent feature of MPS III (Sanfillipo).[66] This GAG deposition in the corneal stroma can lead to increased corneal thickness.[56] Ultrastructural and histochemical studies have demonstrated GAG accumulation in the conjunctiva,[68] cornea,[69] lens epithelial cells, and sclera.[70]

All layers of the cornea are infiltrated with intracellular and extracellular GAG (see Figs 59.5, 59.7). The accumulation of the GAG leads to vacuolation changes in the epithelium, breaks, and peglike undulations affecting the epithelial basement membrane,[47,48] and attenuation of Bowman's layer.[48] Glycosaminoglycans accumulate within corneal stroma and stromal keratocyte lysosomes and vacuoles, causing distension of keratocytes (see Figs 59.5, 59.6). Anterior stromal scarring occurs with abnormal keratocytes in the middle and posterior stroma.[71,72] The posterior layers of the cornea, namely Descemet's membrane and endothelium, remain unaffected, although thinning of Descemet's membrane with excrescences has been described in MPS VI.[73] The corneal endothelial cells usually have normal morphology in MPS but may contain vacuolated lysosomal inclusion materials.[67]

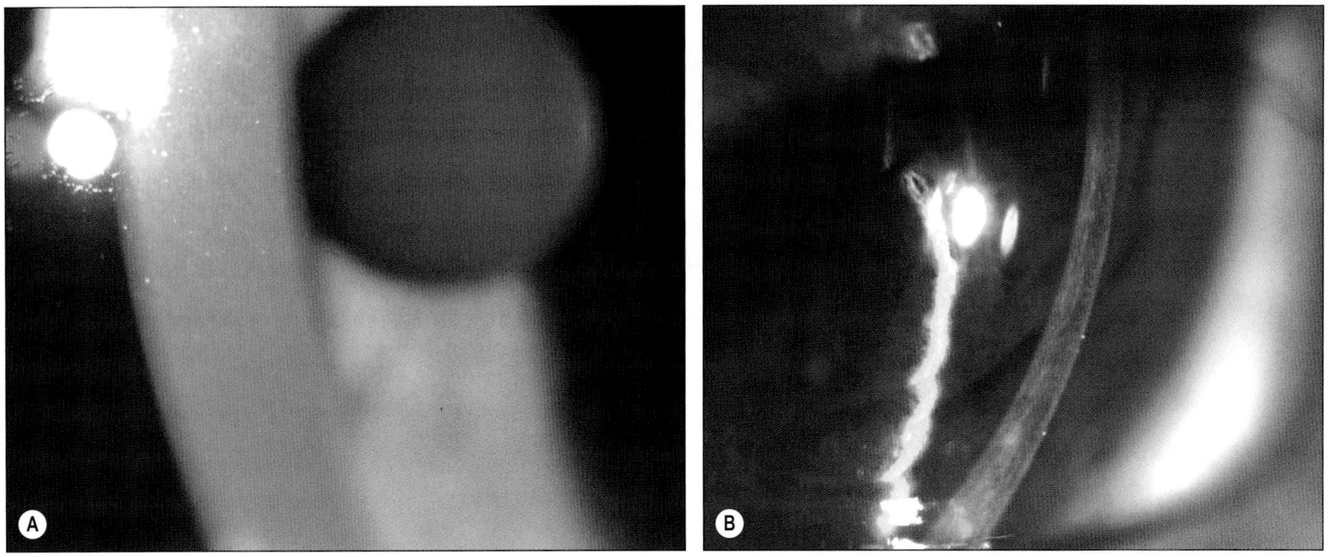

Fig. 59.11 (**A**) Slit lamp biomicroscopy of a 7-year-old male with mucopolysaccharidosis type IVA, demonstrating a diffuse granular appearance of the corneal stroma. (Courtesy of Dipika Patel, MD and Charles McGhee, MD.) (**B**) Slit lamp biomicroscopy of a 17-year-old female with mucopolysaccharidosis type VI, highlighting mild stromal haze predominantly involving the posterior corneal stroma. (Courtesy of Dipika Patel, MD and Charles McGhee, MD.)

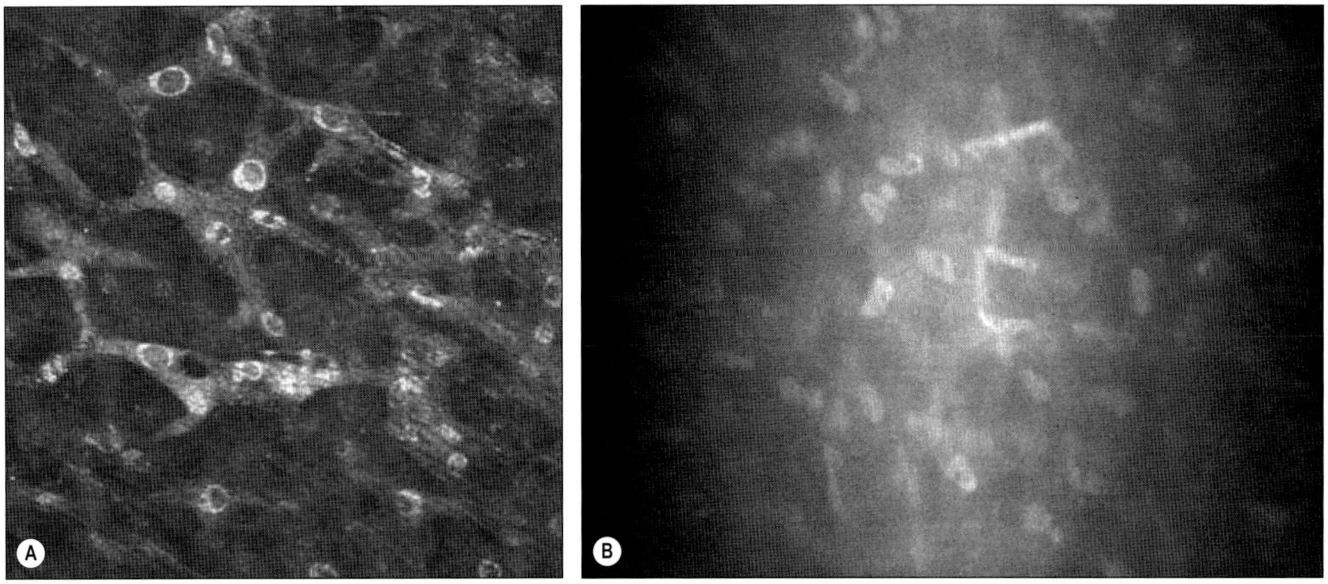

Fig. 59.12 (**A**) Laser scanning in vivo confocal microscopy of the cornea with MPS IVA at the level of the mid stroma demonstrates vacuolated keratocyte nuclei and reflective keratocyte cytoplasm with visible cell processes (frame size 400 μm × 400 μm). (Courtesy of Dipika Patel, MD and Charles McGhee, MD.) (**B**) Slit scanning in vivo confocal microscopy of the cornea with MPS VI demonstrating the posterior stroma with vacuolated keratocytes (frame size 340 μm × 255 μm). (Courtesy of Dipika Patel, MD and Charles McGhee, MD.)

Disorders of Lipid and Lipoprotein Metabolism

Dyslipoproteinemias

The important clinical relevance of dyslipoproteinemias is their potential association with premature-onset coronary artery and peripheral vascular disease.[74–76] From the ophthalmic perspective, their ocular manifestation might not affect vision significantly but rather provide the first clue for a genetic systemic disease and alert to potential risk for coronary disease that warrant medical and laboratory investigation.[77–80] Dyslipoproteinemias affect the cornea via lipid deposition and can be divided into hyperlipoproteinemias and hypolipoproteinemias. Hyperlipoproteinemias in general are associated with accelerated bilateral corneal arcus and xanthelasma, whereas diffuse bilateral opacification with or without corneal arcus is a feature of hypolipoproteinemias.[81]

Hyperlipoproteinemias and Schnyder crystalline dystrophy

Five patterns of abnormal elevations of plasma lipoproteins are associated with systemic and ocular abnormalities.[74–78]

- *Type I hyperlipoproteinemia (hyperchylomicronemia)* is characterized by marked elevation of triglycerides and chylomicrons, resulting in recurrent attacks of acute pancreatitis, eruptive xanthoma, hepatosplenomegaly, and lipemia retinalis in which the retinal arterioles and venules become distended and white because of scattering of light by the large chylomicrons. Accelerated atherosclerosis and corneal arcus are not features.[82]
- *Type II hyperproteinemia (hyperbetalipoproteinemia)* is associated with high betalipoprotein and LDL levels, and manifests a xanthelasmas, arcus cornesa, and premature mortality from cardiovascular complications.[81]
- *Type III hyperlipoproteinemia (familial dysbetalipoproteinemia)* is associated with elevated beta-VLDL. Clinical manifestations include coronary and peripheral vascular disease, xanthomas, lipemia retinalis, xanthelasma, and occasionally corneal arcus.[81]
- *Type IV hyperlipoproteinemia (hyperprebetalipoproteinemia)* involves elevated levels of VLDL. Clinical manifestation comprises vascular disease, pancreatitis, lipemia retinalis, xanthelasma, and corneal arcus, thought less common than in type 1.[81]
- *Type V hyperlipoproteinemia (hyperprebetalipoproteinemia and hyperchylomicronemia)* results in elevations of triglycerides, cholesterol, chylomicron, and VLDL. Clinical manifestations include vascular disease, pancreatitis, xanthomas, lipemia retinalis, xanthelasma, and occasionally corneal arcus[81]

Schnyder's crystalline corneal dystrophy (Fig. 59.13) is a dominantly inherited corneal dystrophy discussed in Chapter 72. It is characterized by bilateral deposition of lipid and/or cholesterol crystals mostly in the superficial to mid-stroma, but full-thickness corneal involvement is not uncommon[83,84] The clinical appearance is of central corneal disciform opacity apparent during the first two decades of life; prominent corneal arcus develops later and diffuse corneal haze is usually seen in all the patients by age 40. Only 50% of affected individuals have corneal crystalline deposits.[85] Although this dystrophy is considered a localized defect of lipid metabolism, some patients demonstrate hypercholesterolemia, xanthelasma, and genu valgum;[86,87] thus, the importance of performing serum lipid studies. Schnyder's dystrophy can be managed by laser phototherapeutic keratectomy (PTK)[88] and lamellar or penetrating keratoplasty, with recurrence infrequent in grafts.[89]

Hypolipoproteinemias

The hypolipoproteinemias result from abnormal reductions of serum lipoprotein levels and include Lecithin-cholesterol acyltransferase (LCAT) deficiency, Tangier disease, fish eye disease, familial hypobetalipoproteinemia, and Bassen-Kornzweig disease. Since the latter two exhibit retinal changes but lack corneal manifestations, only the former three diseases are reviewed here.[78]

Familial LCAT deficiency is an autosomal recessive condition characterized by a major reduction of plasma cholesterol esters and lysolecithin with an increase of unesterified cholesterol, triglycerides, and phospholipids. This causes the

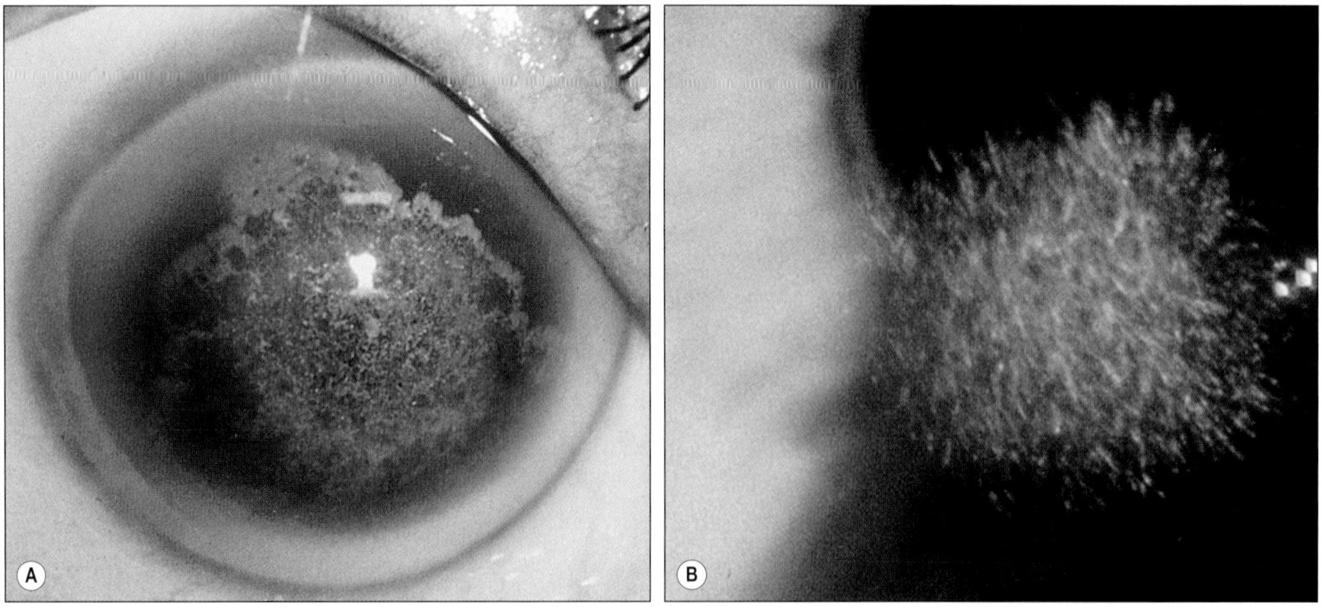

Fig. 59.13 Schnyder's crystalline dystrophy. (**A**) The clinical appearance of the advanced stage demonstrates visually significant crystalline opacity involving the central cornea plus dense peripheral arcus. (**B**) Slit lamp photography at earlier stage of the dystrophy demonstrates fine refractile crystals in the anterior stroma.

accumulation of unesterified cholesterol within tissues and is associated with atherosclerosis, renal insufficiency, and corneal opacity. Corneal findings comprise a peripheral arcus along with a nebular stromal haze composed of myriad minute focal deposits of lipid.[78,90–92] Histopathological evaluations disclosed extracellular vacuoles with acid mucopolysaccharide contents and secondary amyloidal deposits in the stroma and pre-Descemet's membrane.[93] Other ocular changes include retinal venous dilation, angioid streaks, and peripapillary hemorrhages.

Tangier disease (familial high-density lipoprotein deficiency) is a rare autosomal recessive disease resulting in complete absence of HDLs, with other concomitant lipid abnormalities resulting in accumulation of cholesterol in various tissues and prevalent atherosclerosis. Presenting features include large yellow-orange tonsils, neuropathies, hepatosplenomegaly, corneal opacifications and cardiovascular disease.[94] Corneal manifestations include diffuse clouding with dense posterior stromal opacities, but no arcus, with no or little visual impairment.[95,96] The corneal manifestation might be complicated with reduced corneal sensation and exposure, resulting from neuropathy and leading to visual impairment.[96]

Fish eye disease is an autosomal recessive disease in which LCAT function is only partially impaired, such that the enzyme is unable to esterify cholesterol in HDL particles, but retains its activity in the presence of cholesterol on VLDL and LDL, resulting in a reduction of HDL but the generation of near-normal levels of plasma cholesteryl esters. This may account for the clinical differences between fish eye and familial LCAT deficiency, including a lesser expression of premature coronary disease in fish eye disease. The corneal manifestation results from lipid depositions and is characterized by visually significant diffuse opacification accentuated peripherally.[97–99]

Lipidoses

Lipidoses are inherited disorders of complex lipids, predominantly gangliosides and sphingomyelin, and include generalized gangliosidosis (GM1 gangliosidosis type I), juvenile gangliosidosis (GM1 gangliosidosis type II), Tay-Sachs disease (GM2 gangliosidosis type I), Sandhoff disease (GM2 gangliosidosis type II), several Niemann-Pick disease variants, Gaucher disease, Fabry's disease, metachromatic leukodystrophy, multiple sulfatase deficiency, and Farber lipogranulomatosis. Corneal manifestations are usually limited to Fabry's disease, multiple sulfatase deficiency, and generalized gangliosidosis. The discussion here is, therefore, limited to these disorders.

Fabry's disease

Fabry's disease is an X-linked recessive disorder derived from the deficiency of the enzyme α-galactosidase A, with progressive deposition of sphingolipids within the lysosomes of most visceral tissues, blood vessels, and ocular tissues including the epithelium of conjunctiva, cornea, lens capsule, ciliary and iris sphincter muscle, and connective tissue fibroblasts. As resolved by electron microscopy, the lipids appear within lysosomes as concentrically arranged membranous lamellae.[100,101]

The disease is expressed in hemizygous males by cutaneous angiokeratomas, febrile crises with peripheral extremity pain, renal failure, cardiovascular disease, and neurologic changes. Heterozygous females may also develop complications related to the disease such as cardiac, renal, or neurological symptoms, although with later onset and less severity.[102,103]

Corneal changes are the earliest and most consistent ocular abnormality, occurring in most affected males and carrier females (Fig. 59.14). It presents as a whorl-shaped biomicroscopically visible opacity, consisting of fine lines emanating from a central nodal point. Cornea verticillata is visually insignificant but may represent a sign with high sensitivity and specificity for the early diagnosis of Fabry's disease, as it is rare in individuals not suffering from it. In the differential diagnosis is the verticillate keratopathy occurring in the drug-induced lipidoses related to amiodarone and chloroquine.[104] In vivo confocal laser scanning microscopy revealed the same pattern of hyper-reflective deposits in the basal cell layer of corneal epithelium in

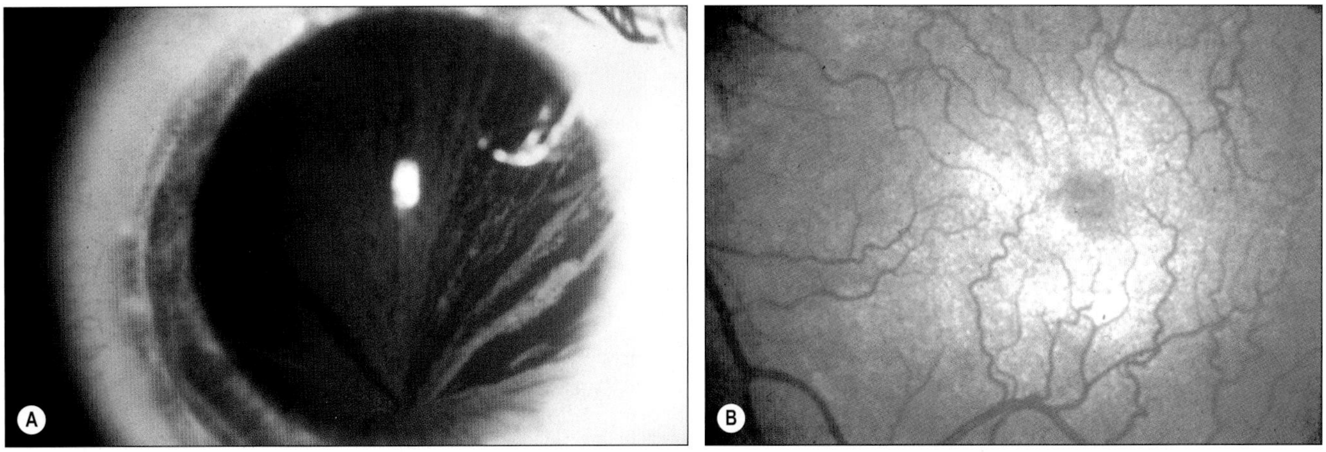

Fig. 59.14 Fabry's disease. (**A**) Slit lamp appearance of cornea verticillate. (**B**) Retinal vascular tortuosity in Fabry's disease.

patients with Fabry's disease and drug-induced verticillate keratopathy.[105] Both affected males and carrier females exhibit other ocular changes, including aneurysmal dilations and tortuosity of the conjunctival and retinal vessels and a characteristic spokelike posterior capsular cataract.[104]

Once the disease is suspected, diagnosis can be made in men by screening for greatly deficient or absent α-galactosidase A activity in plasma or peripheral leukocytes, or by gene sequencing.[106] A broad range of α-galactosidase A values up to normal exist in heterozygotes; thus, only gene sequencing and identification of disease-causing mutations has proven reliable for confirming the diagnosis in women.[107]

Kidney transplantation has proven to be of systemic and renal benefit in patients experiencing end-stage renal failure, but the storage process may recur.[108] Enzyme replacement therapy has been available for several years and received approval in Europe in 2001 and the USA in 2003. Despite the fact that enzyme replacement therapy has shown improvement in different symptoms, especially when started early, this treatment does not resolve all symptoms, and the evidence is not strong enough to show long-term benefit.[107] Other treatment approaches are being developed in trials, including pharmacological chaperones (stabilizes any native enzyme that makes the potential for residual activity maximum), and substrate inhibition (decreases the production of globotriaosylceramide to prevent storage), but are still not available for clinical use.[109–111]

Multiple sulfatase deficiency

This autosomal recessive disorder is the result of multiple sulfatase deficiencies (specifically arylsulfatases A, B, and C), resulting in abnormal accumulations of sulfatide within various tissues. Clinical features become manifest in infancy as neuromuscular retardation, coarse facies, organomegaly, and ichthyosis. Ocular involvement includes subtle diffuse corneal opacities, macular changes, optic atrophy, and opacity of the peripheral anterior lens capsule.[112] Death usually occurs within the first decade.

Generalized gangliosidoses

Variable deficiencies of β-galactosidases A, B, and C in this autosomal recessive disorder result in the accumulation of gangliosides in the central nervous system (CNS) and the deposition of keratan sulfate in somatic tissues.[113,114] Clinical aspects are apparent early in life as psychomotor retardation, facial and skeletal dysmorphism, and organomegaly. Ocular findings include mild, diffuse corneal clouding, nystagmus, macular cherry-red spots, retinal hemorrhages, and optic atrophy. Corneal opacity in the Shiba dog with generalized gangliosidosis was shown to be caused by neutral carbohydrate accumulation in lysosomes resulting in swelling and dysfunction of keratocytes, and subsequent irregular arrangement of collagen fibrils in the corneal proper substance.[115] Death usually occurs by the age of 2 years.

Drug-induced lipidoses

In contrast to inherited disorders, a second broad category of lysosomal dysfunction may be characterized by abnormal inclusions from exogenous causes. Because drugs are the most common precipitating cause, these conditions have been referred to as drug-induced lipidoses.[116,117] In the inborn disorders such as Fabry's disease, one may anticipate an abnormality in a specific intralysosomal hydrolase in contrast with the possibly more generalized interference with lysosomal enzymes induced by drug toxicity and accumulation. Nevertheless, striking parallels have been discovered clinically and ultrastructurally between Fabry's disease and the drug-induced lipidoses.[105,118]

Many drugs that cause lipid inclusions share the physicochemical property of cationic amphiphilia[116] As hypothesized by Lüllmann et al.,[116,117] cationic amphiphilic drugs are able to penetrate freely into lysosomes, where they are protonated and complexed with polar lipids. These complexes are then unable to pass from the lysosomes or be degraded, resulting in progressive accumulation.

Corneal deposits are typical manifestations of drug-induced lipidoses (Fig. 59.15).[119] Frequently, a verticillate pattern is apparent and might be a result of the centripetal migration of deposit-laden limbal epithelial cells,[120] although many cases may present as linear opacities. Conjunctival biopsy is an invaluable and simple technique that permits ultrastructural examination even though this tissue appears clinically normal in most conditions.[119] The diagnosis is important, as the corneal manifestation is often dose related and may reflect the potential risk for retinal changes.

The drug-induced cornea verticillata was first observed with amiodarone and chloroquine. At present, a wide array of systemic medications are known to induce intralysosomal accumulation of lipids and a vortex keratopathy.

Chloroquine

Members of the chloroquine family (chloroquine, hydroxychloroquine, amodiaquine), used in the management of malaria and rheumatoid arthritis, may lead to ocular manifestations involving the cornea (vortex keratopathy, decreased corneal sensation), ciliary body (accommodative weakness), lens (posterior subcapsular cataracts), and retina (bull's eye maculopathy).[121–123]

The bilateral keratopathy occurs in a higher percentage of patients taking chloroquine (28–95%) than hydroxychloroquine (1–28%), often developing within 2 to 3 weeks,[121,122,124–126] and strongly resembles the keratopathy of Fabry's disease.[118,127] It has been reported that by using confocal microscopy, corneal alterations could be detected prior to becoming apparent with slit lamp biomicroscopy.[128] These subepithelial deposits can gradually be eliminated after discontinuation of the drug. Thus, in contrast with retinopathy, the keratopathy is reversible and its presence is not an indication for cessation of therapy,[129] though it is associated with a greater risk of retinopathy.[130] Although the corneal change does not usually produce symptoms, patients occasionally complain of halos or blurry vision in the absence of detectable retinopathy or visual acuity change. Corneal sensation has also been reported to be diminished by this drug.

Ultrastructural examination of conjunctival and corneal epithelium discloses numerous concentrically lamellated cytoplasmic inclusions in basal epithelial cells of both tissues.[123,131]

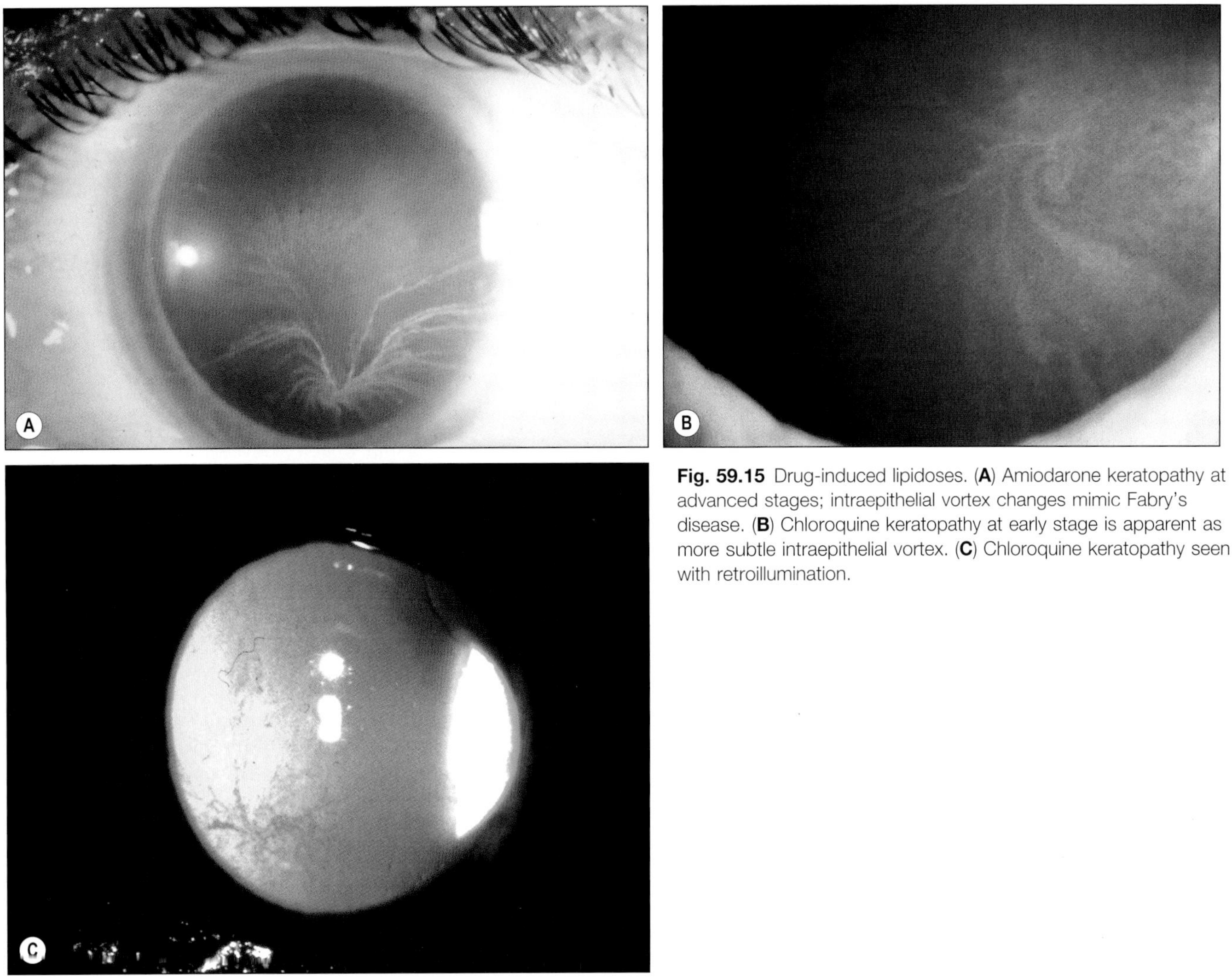

Fig. 59.15 Drug-induced lipidoses. (**A**) Amiodarone keratopathy at advanced stages; intraepithelial vortex changes mimic Fabry's disease. (**B**) Chloroquine keratopathy at early stage is apparent as more subtle intraepithelial vortex. (**C**) Chloroquine keratopathy seen with retroillumination.

Amiodarone

Amiodarone, an antiarrhythmic agent, is frequently associated with a vortex keratopathy. Cornea verticillata is present in 69–100% of patients on 200–1400 mg daily,[132] typically developing within a few weeks to months, although it has been reported as early as 6 days (1000 mg/d) following initiation of therapy.[133]

Corneal deposition is typically bilateral and symmetric, and develops in a characteristic fashion, related to both dosage and duration.[134,135] In the early stages (grade 1), brown punctate opacities are deposited in the basal epithelium at the inferior pupillary margin. Gradually, these coalesce into horizontal lines that extend toward the limbus (grade II). Arborization and extension of these lines results in a whorl-like pattern involving the pupillary axis (grade III). An additional stage (grade IV) was proposed in which 'clumps' of golden-brown deposits are present.[133] Low dosages (200 mg/d or less) may show limited progression, while grade III keratopathy has been correlated with both treatment duration (>1 year) and daily dosage (400 mg or greater).[133,134] The corneal deposits rarely lead to visual symptoms or visual loss, though patients may report halos and colored rings around lights. The development of vortex keratopathy is not an indication for discontinuation of therapy, though it typically resolves within 3 to 20 months following discontinuation of the medication.[132]

Electron microscopy has demonstrated lipid-bearing intralysosomal inclusions in the basal layer of corneal epithelium, as well as in normal-appearing conjunctiva.[136,137] Confocal microscopy has demonstrated anterior stromal changes, including microdeposits (resembling the epithelial deposition), reduction in keratocyte density, and irregular nerve fibers.[138]

Amiodarone has also been associated with the development of anterior subcapsular lens opacities,[139] retinopathy (choroidal neovascularization),[140] and irreversible vision loss from optic neuropathy.[141] Discontinuation or reduction of the medication should be considered if optic neuropathy is observed, although a causal relationship is not well established.[142]

Other agents

Tamoxifen, an estrogen antagonist commonly used in the treatment of breast carcinoma, has been associated with keratopathy and retinopathy with high-dose therapy of 180–200 mg/d.[143] However, low-dose therapy may also lead to ocular toxicity (keratopathy, retinopathy, optic neuritis).[144,145] In a prospective study of 65 women receiving 20 mg/d, reversible corneal verticillata was present in seven patients (10.8%), with pigmentary retinopathy in three.[145]

Suramin was originally developed as an antitrypanosomal agent and more recently has been employed in trials for AIDS and unresectable adrenal and prostate cancer. The use of higher doses (total dose 3.2–15.8 g) in recent trials has been associated with a vortex keratopathy, as well as rare reports of subepithelial opacities, superficial punctate keratopathy, and peripheral epithelial erosions.[146,147] Electron microscopic examination has demonstrated inclusion bodies in the basal epithelial cells.[147]

Additional agents capable of producing cornea verticillata include phenothiazines[148] and clofazimine,[149] which produce also corneal stromal deposition, atovaquone, used in the treatment of *Pneumocystis carinii* pneumonia,[150] perhexilene maleate, an antianginal drug,[151] tilorone hydrochloride, an antineoplastic agent,[152] oral nonsteroidal antiinflammatory medications, including naproxen, indometacin, and ibuprofen,[153–155] as well as topical skin application of monobenzone for vitiligo.[156]

Two patients with AIDS were reported with electron microscopic evidence of drug-induced lipidoses.[157] They presented with translucent vacuoles within the corneal epithelium and mild conjunctival hyperemia. Corneal epithelial debridement and conjunctival biopsy revealed intracellular, electron-dense lipoidal bodies and multilaminated lysosomal inclusions. The ocular surface changes resolved within 1–3 months after dosage reduction of systemic ganciclovir and acyclovir, but the responsible agent remains to be identified.[158]

Gentamicin, an aminoglycoside antibiotic, has been shown to induce lamellated cytoplasmic inclusions in the conjunctiva of human subjects as early as 3 days after its subconjunctival injection.[159]

Disorders of Glycosaminoglycan and Lipid Metabolism

Mucolipidoses

The mucolipidoses comprise a group of usually autosomal recessive metabolic storage diseases with features common to both mucopolysaccharidoses and lipidoses.

Mucolipidosis I (dysmorphic sialidosis) is the result of glycoprotein sialidase deficiency.[160,161] Two variants have been described – a mild form (type I) and a severe form (type II) – exhibiting a spectrum of psychomotor retardation, mucopolysaccharidosis-like facial and skeletal dysmorphism and organomegaly. Corneal abnormalities include clinically insignificant fine epithelial and stromal opacities that result from intralysosomal inclusions of fibrillogranular and membranous lamellar materials. Conjunctival and retinal vascular tortuosity, spokelike lenticular changes, and macular cherry-red spots also occur.

Mucolipidosis II (inclusion cell [I-cell] disease) is caused by an abnormality of *N*-acetylglucosamine phosphotransferase, resulting in marked intracellular deficiency of multiple acid hydrolases as a result of the secretion of abnormal lysosomal enzymes that are not recognized and taken up by either normal or I-cell fibroblasts.[162,163] The name of the disease derives from the inclusion cell (or I-cell) phenomenon of cultured skin fibroblasts, which display many birefringent lysosomal inclusions. Conjunctival ultrastructure resolves similar pathologic alterations.[164] The severity of the conjunctival abnormality is in contrast to the relatively mild corneal changes where similar inclusions develop within keratocytes.[165] The cornea appears clear initially, but in older patients a mild granular stromal opacity develops.[162] Megalocornea, glaucoma, and orbital hypoplasia have also been described. Clinical features appear soon after birth as dysostosis multiplex, coarse facies, and mental retardation, but without mucopolysacchariduria. Death usually occurs between ages 2 and 8 years as a result of congestive heart failure.

Mucolipidosis III (pseudo-Hurler polydystrophy) is biochemically indistinguishable from mucolipidosis II, and the I-cell phenomenon in tissue culture is also evident.[164,166,167] Clinically, it appears as a mild phenotype of mucolipidosis II and it is compatible with normal life expectancy. Corneal clouding is biomicroscopically visible but visually insignificant. Disc edema and retinal inner limiting membrane changes have also been noted.[168]

Mucolipidosis IV was initially described in Ashkenazi Jewish Israeli children, although it is not exclusive to that group.[169,170] It occurs as a result of a ganglioside sialidase deficiency that results in the accumulation of mucopolysaccharides and sialogangliosides.[171,172] Clinically evident early in life, it presents as profound psychomotor retardation in the absence of skeletal or facial deformity,[173] organomegaly, or excessive mucopolysacchariduria. The striking ocular aspect is diffuse corneal clouding, sometimes associated with episodic pain that results from marked corneal surface irregularities,[174] corresponding to massive accumulations of intracytoplasmic storage material in the epithelium of the cornea and conjunctiva.[175,176] Hence, corneal epithelial debridement temporarily diminishes the corneal haze until the defect is healed by epithelium of similar translucency. In this situation, limbal allograft transplantation might afford long-lasting improvement in corneal clarity,[177] whereas lamellar or penetrating keratoplasty is certain to be of no benefit. Mucolipidosis IV is seemingly unique in demonstrating the intraepithelial storage phenomenon as the cause of clinically significant corneal clouding. Other ocular findings have included cataract, retinal degeneration, attenuated retinal vessels, and optic atrophy.[178] The mucolipidosis IV gene was localized to chromosome 19p13.2–13.3.[179,180] The gene encodes a protein, called mucolipin, important for the maintenance of cellular integrity, and the absence of this protein results in an accumulation of solutes in intracellular vesicles.[181] Cases with clinical abnormalities restricted to the eye with lack of generalized symptoms have been described.[182,183]

Galactosialidosis

Galactosialidosis is an autosomal recessive disorder that demonstrates a combined deficiency of sialidase and β-galactosidase. Systemic findings evident by age 5 years comprise skeletal and facial dysmorphism, psychomotor retardation, seizures, hearing loss, ataxia, and myoclonus. Ocular involvement includes mild corneal clouding and macular cherry-red spot.[184]

Disorders of Amino Acid, Nucleic Acid, and Protein Metabolism

Cystinosis

Cystinosis is an autosomal recessive lysosomal storage disease caused by a defect in the cystine transporter cystinosin,[185] encoded by the gene CTNS.[186] This defect results in intralysosomal cystine accumulation and crystal formation in many tissues of the body, mainly the kidney and the eye, including the conjunctiva, cornea, iris, choroid, retinal pigment epithelium, and optic nerve.[187] Based on age of onset and severity of symptoms, cystinosis is divided into nephropathic and non-nephropathic. Nephropathic cystinosis further divides to infantile (classic) and intermediate (juvenile-onset or adolescent).[188] Non-nephropathic cystinosis was formerly called benign or adult-type cystinosis.[189] Although the corneal findings are identical for all three variants, the range of systemic manifestations extends from absent in the adult form to lethal in infantile cystinosis.

The most severe and common form, infantile cystinosis, generally appears between 6 and 12 months with the renal Fanconi syndrome and can proceed to end-stage renal disease (ESRD) by 10 years. Corneal cystine crystals appear from the first year of life and result in photophobia and blepharospasm, leading to varying degrees of visual discomfort and impairment in the first or second decade. Retinal depigmentation appears by 3–7 years and can evolve into blindness between 13 and 40 years in 15% of cases.[188,190] Patients with infantile cystinosis might be predisposed to glaucoma because of a distinct angle and ciliary body configuration as well as crystals in the trabecular meshwork.[162] Renal transplantation can prolong life expectancy significantly but does not prevent the progressive accumulation of cystine in other tissues, including the retina and cornea.[191] Thus, cystinosis patients are living longer and manifesting long-term complications of the disease.

In the adult form, corneal crystals identical to those of the nephropathic form are present, but renal disease is subclinical. Retinoschisis and retinal detachment have been reported in association with adult cystinosis,[192] but in most cases the patient is asymptomatic except for photophobia. The adolescent form is intermediate between the infantile and adult forms. Nephropathy may be present with much slower progression to ESRD, and corneal crystals are present but retinopathy is absent.[193,194]

Crystal accumulation in the conjunctiva and cornea is the pathognomonic ophthalmic manifestation of cystinosis (Fig. 59.16). Corneal crystals present as myriad needle-shaped, highly reflectile opacities easily seen by slit lamp examination. They appear to be present in the corneal epithelium, stroma, and endothelium. Accumulation of crystals in the cornea starts in infancy and is definitely evident by 16 months of age. Deposition begins in the anterior periphery and proceeds posteriorly and centripetally. By approximately 7 years of age, the entire peripheral stroma and endothelium accumulates crystals. By approximately 20

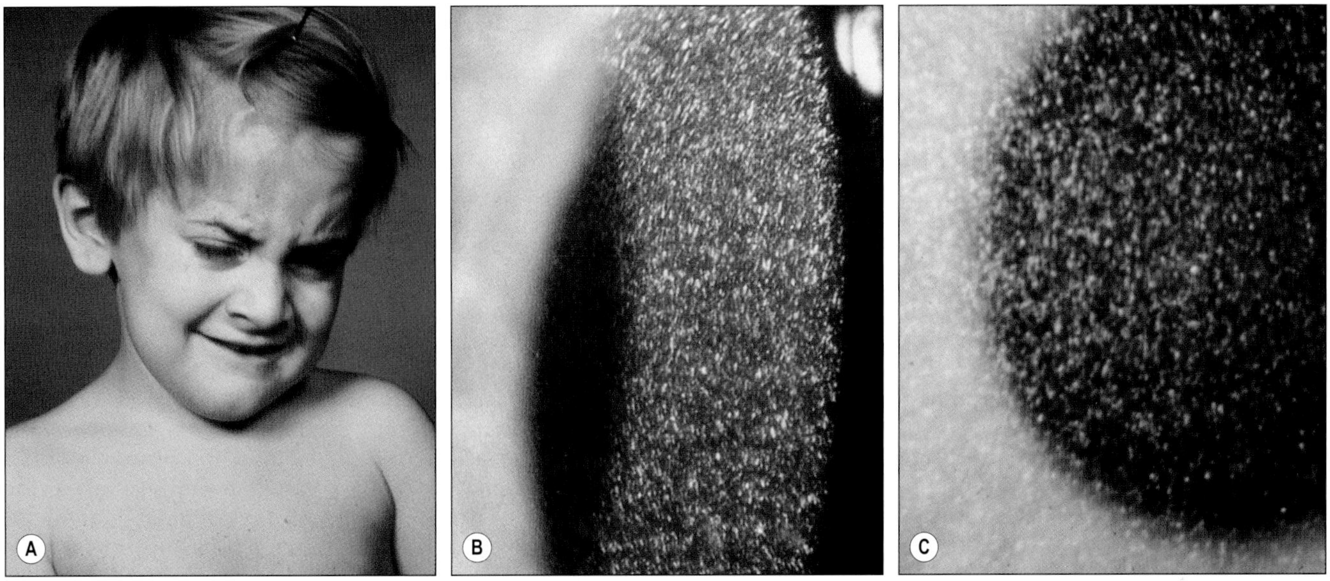

Fig. 59.16 Cystinosis. (**A**) A childhood nephropathic cystinosis patient displays typical fair features and photophobia. (**B**) Slit lamp appearance of adolescent cystinosis exhibits myriad fine refractile crystals, predominantly in the anterior stroma. (**C**) Adult cystinosis demonstrates more diffuse crystalline stromal involvement.

years of age, crystals can be seen in the entire corneal stroma. Increased density of cystine crystals results in a hazy cornea. Breaks in the Bowman's membrane were also reported. A different form of cystine accumulation in the cornea has been described lately in a 35-year-old patient who suffered from infantile cystinosis. These consisted of large polygonal angular-shaped electron-transparent areas different from the needle-shaped crystals reported in mostly younger patients. Corneal crystals are thought to acquire their needle shape as they are forced from the tightly packed corneal stromal lamellae. The reason for the unusual shape of the corneal crystals might be related to prolonged survival with therapy and thus increased accumulation of cystine over the years, which disrupted the normal corneal stromal architecture, allowing the cystine to assume this shape.[187]

Corneal crystals are initially asymptomatic, but photophobia can develop within the first few years of life. The severity of photophobia varies but nearly all patients have some degree of discomfort with bright illumination after the first decade of life and some have significant blepharospasm. Corneal complications reported in older nephropathic cystinosis patients include superficial punctate keratopathy with associated foreign body sensation assumed to be caused by the breaks in a thinned Bowman's membrane with the deposition of cystine crystals and filamentary keratopathy. Band keratopathy and peripheral corneal neovascularization are most commonly reported in post-transplant patients.[187] The anterior location of the crystals also predisposes to recurrent erosion.[195] Katz et al. documented loss of contrast sensitivity, increased glare disability, decreased corneal sensitivity, and increased corneal thickness in patients with nephropathic cystinosis, speculated to result from crystal deposition.[196–198]

The presence of typical corneal crystals on slit lamp examination is characteristic of cystinosis, although crystals may be absent before 1 year of age. The diagnosis can be confirmed by measuring the leukocyte cystine content. The diagnosis can also be made by conjunctival biopsy to measure the extracted free cystine or to detect the characteristic crystals by electron microscopy, but these invasive tests are usually unnecessarily.[199]

Treatment for infantile nephropathic cystinosis was initially addressing only the disease complications including renal transplantation for renal failure. Few corneal transplants were performed, with recurrence of crystals in the transplanted cornea.[200] The introduction of therapy with cysteamine in the 1970s has revolutionized the treatment and prognosis of cystinosis. Cysteamine (β-mercaptoethylamine) is a simple aminothiol that depletes cystinotic cells of cystine. After traversing the plasma and lysosomal membranes, cysteamine reacts with cystine to produce cysteine and the mixed disulfide cysteine-cysteamine, both of which freely exit the lysosome.[201] Cysteamine treatment, if started early, can stabilize glomerular function, and decrease the frequency of cystinotic retinopathy.[202] Although oral cysteamine alleviates most of the symptoms associated with cystinosis, it has no effect on the corneal crystal accumulation, most likely due to inadequate local cysteamine concentrations. Topical cysteamine treatment has proven safe and efficient in dissolving corneal crystals in both young and old cystinosis patients; it also significantly alleviates the symptoms of photophobia, blepharospasm, and eye pain. The recommended regimen is a 0.55% cysteamine hydrochloride solution with benzalkonium chloride 0.01% as a preservative, used 10–12 times per day. At room temperature, the active free thiol, cysteamine, oxidizes to the disulfide form, cystamine, requiring shipping and storage of the topical solution in the frozen state. The formulation may be used at room temperature for up to 1 week.[187]

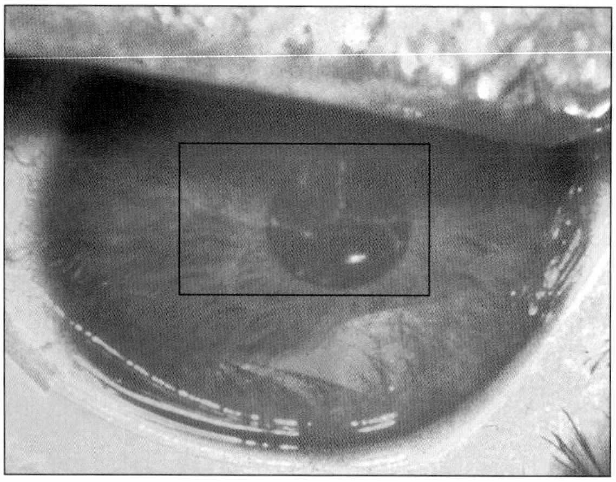

Fig. 59.17 Tyrosinemia: a pseudodendrite corneal lesion in tyrosinemia.

Tyrosinemia II

Tyrosinemia is an autosomal recessive disease caused by either fumarylacetoacetate hydrolase deficiency (type I) or a deficiency of hepatic tyrosine aminotransferase (type II). Both are associated with elevated levels of tyrosine in the blood and urine. Only the latter, however, is associated with corneal changes.

Tyrosinemia II (Richner-Hanhart syndrome) is an oculocutaneous syndrome that manifests skin findings, which usually begin the same time or after the eye lesions develop, and present as painful blisters on the palms and soles that crust and become hyperkeratotic.[203] There are families with skin lesions but no eye lesions. Central nervous system involvement is variable and may include mental retardation, nystagmus, and convulsions.[204]

Ocular symptoms include epiphora, photophobia, and blepharospasm. Ocular signs include pseudodendritic corneal lesions (usually bilateral) (Fig. 59.17), dendritic ulcers and, rarely, corneal or conjunctival plaques. Because ocular symptoms can occur in isolation and may be the initial manifestation of tyrosinemia II, ophthalmologists must be able to differentiate it from other, more common causes of keratitis, most notably herpes simplex virus keratitis. The lack of terminal bulbs and absent or poor staining should arouse suspicion. Other findings suggesting tyrosinemia II include bilateral involvement (rare with herpes simplex virus keratitis), lack of history of herpetic infection, consistent inferocentral location of the pseudodendrites, normal corneal sensitivity, negative viral cultures, exacerbation of symptoms with increased dietary protein, and lesions persisting for longer than 6 weeks despite antiviral therapy.[205] Chronic keratitis may develop and cause

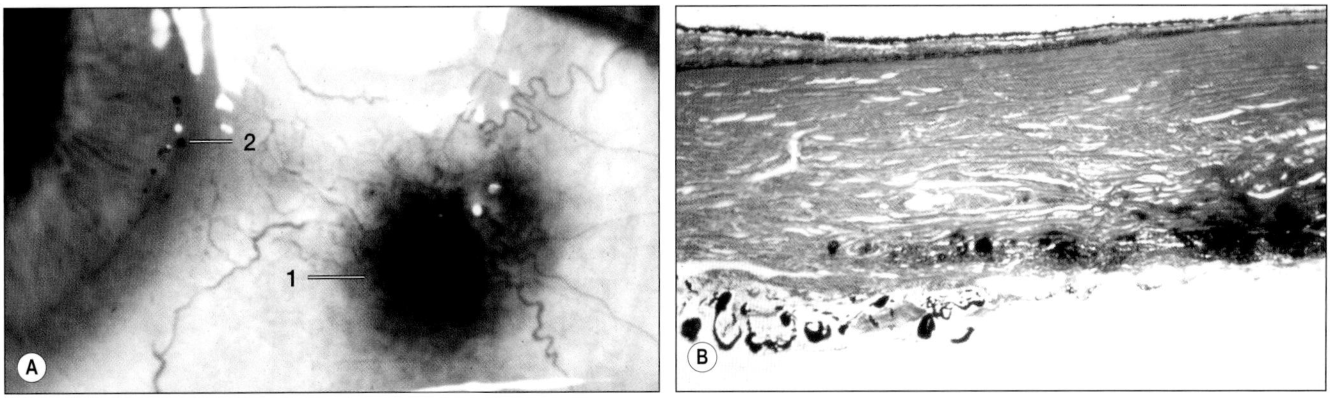

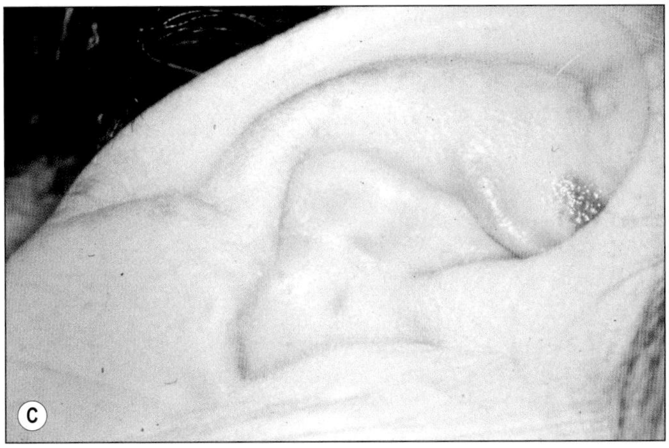

Fig. 59.18 Alkaptonuria: (**A**) Black-blue discoloration of the interpalpebral sclera. (**B**) Extracellular pigment deposition in the sclera. (**C**) Pigmentation of the ear lobe in alkaptonuria.

marked neovascularization and scarring.[206,207] Lesions can recur in a corneal transplant, particularly if systemic steroids are used.[208]

The diagnosis is based on the finding of hypertyrosinemia and hypertyrosinuria. Initiation of a tyrosine- and phenylalanine-restricted diet in infancy is currently the most effective therapy available to resolve symptoms, including clearing of corneal lesions and prevention of visual and developmental impairment. Long-term follow-up demonstrates recurrence of ocular lesions with the cessation of dietary therapy, indicating the need for continued dietary restrictions.[205]

Alkaptonuria

Alkaptonuria is an extremely rare, autosomal recessive disorder caused by deficient homogentisic acid oxidase.[209] The enzymatic deficiency results in accumulation of homogentisic acid, an intermediate breakdown product in the catabolism of phenylalanine and tyrosine. The excess metabolite is excreted in the urine, but its oxidized, pigmented derivatives (alkapton) deposit in collagen-rich tissues. Clinical manifestations include ochronotic arthropathy, ocular and cutaneous pigmentation, genitourinary tract obstruction by ochronotic calculi, and cardiovascular ochronosis, especially stenosis of the aortic valve.[210]

Ocular changes occur in about 70% of alkaptonurics.[211] These consists of blue-black discoloration of the conjunctiva and intrapalpebral sclera, just anterior to the insertions of the horizontal rectus muscles. The cornea may also develop brownish-black 'oil droplet' pigmentation just inside the limbus (Fig. 59.18).[212] Vision is usually not impaired although a case in which marked, late-onset bilateral astigmatism, related to sclerolimbic ochronotic pigment was reported.[213] Ultrastructural examination reveals the pigment to be extracellular, associated with collagen and fibrocytes[211] Unfortunately, no treatment exists, and the pigmentation gradually increases throughout adulthood.

Amyloidosis

Amyloid denotes a family of proteins identified by their unique histologic properties: (1) homogeneous granular to filamentous eosinophilia with hematoxylin and eosin stain; (2) metachromasia with crystal violet; (3) ultraviolet fluorescence (yellow-green) with thioflavin T; and (4) orange-red staining with Congo red, which exhibits two additional properties – birefringence (ability to rotate plane-polarized light 90°) and dichroism (red to green shift under polarized light).

Amyloidosis denotes a spectrum of heterogeneous disorders that have in common an extracellular amyloid deposition, both localized and systemic. The cornea is involved in systemic a well as in localized amyloidosis, either secondarily or as a site of primary amyloid deposition.

Localized primary corneal amyloidosis consists of two localized inherited corneal involvements, gelatinous droplike dystrophy and lattice corneal dystrophy types I and III.[214] In

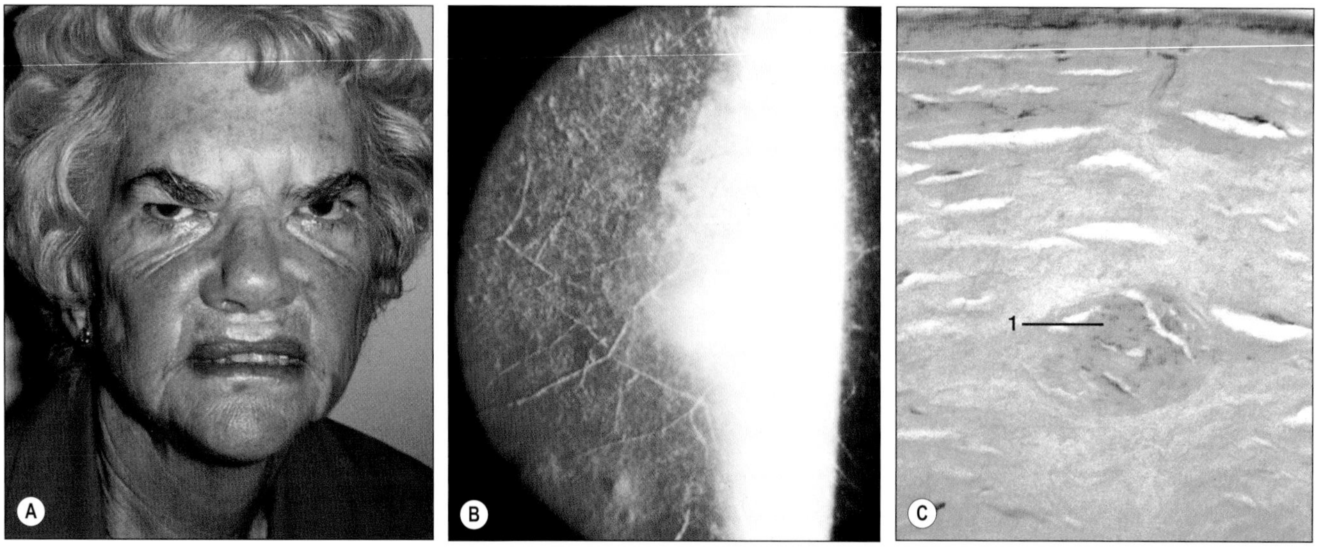

Fig. 59.19 Systemic amyloidosis associated with lattice corneal dystrophy (Meretoja syndrome). (**A**) Facial features typically comprise facial nerve palsy and brow ptosis plus incomplete blink. (**B**) Retroillumination slit lamp biomicroscopy highlights typical lattice line features of stromal deposits. (**C**) Immunoperoxidase staining of keratoplasty specimen identifies deposits (*1*) containing amyloid protein (**C**, ×200).

these dystrophies the amyloidosis is localized to the cornea without systemic manifestations and thus they are discussed with the stromal corneal dystrophies.

Systemic primary amyloidosis is known as lattice dystrophy type II (LCD II), familial amyloidotic polyneuropathy type V, or Meretoja syndrome. A rare dominantly inherited disorder, it appears in early adulthood and is only rarely described in patients of other than those of Finnish origin.[215] A similar syndrome has been reported with an idiopathic, nonfamilial occurrence.[216]

This dystrophy is caused by a mutation of the GLN ('gelsolin') gene located on chromosome 9.[217,218] Gelsolin is an actin severing protein and the abnormality in the gelsolin molecule eventually leads to release, polymerization, and deposition throughout the body of the highly amyloidogenic protein.[219]

The cardinal features of amyloidosis type V are a triad of ophthalmic (LCD II, glaucoma), neurological (cranial, peripheral, and autonomic neuropathies), and dermatological manifestations.[220] Renal and cardiac involvement have been described.[221–223]

The corneal changes resemble those seen in lattice type I, except that the lattice lines are branching with a radial distribution and are maximal peripherally, in contradiction to the findings in type I and IIIA LCD (Fig. 59.19). Progressive loss of corneal sensory nerves, resulting in reduced corneal sensitivity has been shown[224] and might contribute to the dry eye syndrome in these patients.[225] Epithelial erosions occur less and later in life compared to type I LCD.[226,227] Visual acuity is usually retained until the sixth decade but visual loss after 60 years of age is not uncommon.[228]

Associated findings include cranial blepharochalasis[229] and glaucoma resulting in part from low-outflow facility related to amyloid deposition.[230]

Penetrating keratoplasty was reported to be complicated by neurotrophic persistent epithelial defect. The integrity of a corneal graft is dependent on an intact nerve supply to the cornea which is absent in amyloidosis type V.[231,232] Excimer laser phototherapeutic keratectomy has been successfully used to treat patients who have had recurrences after lamellar keratoplasty.[233]

Localized secondary corneal amyloidosis usually follows chronic diseases such as neoplasms, infections, connective tissue disorders, and trauma and is discussed under corneal degenerations.

Secondary systemic amyloidosis does not affect the cornea.

Gout

Hyperuricemia may arise from a heterogeneous group of metabolic disorders and may accumulate in the joints and kidneys, causing gout. The disease occurs predominantly in men in the fourth and fifth decades. Gout may less commonly occur with hyperuricemia secondary to myeloproliferative disorders, alcohol consumption, cytotoxic chemotherapy, and obesity.

The eye may be acutely inflamed in gout, in relationship with acute arthritis, giving rise to the 'hot eye of gout'.[234] Scleritis and episcleritis may also be associated with deposits of urate crystals in these tissues.[235] Even in the absence of inflammation, fine refractile crystals may be present in the corneal stroma and epithelium of both the conjunctiva and the cornea.[236] Multiple chalky deposits on the corneal stroma representing urate crystals have been reported in a patient with long-standing untreated gout.[237]An orange-brown band keratopathy may also be seen;[238] however, other cases may closely resemble the whitish form seen with calcium deposition. Interestingly, urate keratopathy may occur in the absence of systemic hyperuricemia. It is postulated to be caused by a localized abnormality of urate metabolism.[239]

Antiinflammatory agents such as colchicine, indometacin, and phenylbutazone are used to treat acute attacks of gouty arthritis. Long-term therapy includes drugs that lower the serum urate level. These include probenecid, salicylates, sulfinpyrazone, and allopurinol. The latter agent may have a cataractogenic action.[240] The ocular manifestations can be improved with the medical treatment.[237] Superficial scraping or keratectomy effectively removes the corneal deposits.

Porphyria

The porphyrias are a group of disorders that have in common the excessive excretion of porphyrins – pigments involved in heme biosynthesis.

Porphyria cutanea tarda (PCT) is the most common form. It occurs sporadically or in autosomal dominant inheritance, and is caused by a partial deficiency of uroporphyrinogen decarboxylase. The disease is characterized by sun-induced skin lesions, liver disease, hypertrichosis, and urinary excretion of porphyrins. Presentation is usually in middle life, and is aggravated by concurrent compromise of liver metabolism by alcohol or drugs. Skin abnormalities include increased facial pigmentation, increased fragility to trauma, erythema, scleroderma-like changes, and vesicular and ulcerative lesions.

Congenital erythropoietic porphyria (CEP), a very rare type of porphyria, is inherited as an autosomal recessive trait and becomes manifest shortly after birth. It is characterized by intense itching and erythema of sun-exposed skin, leading to bullous lesions. Hemolytic anemia and splenomegaly are prominent features.

Conjunctival and corneal manifestations parallel those of exposed skin. The interpalpebral conjunctiva can be hyperemic and chemotic, and vesicles can form, leading to necrosis, scarring, and symblepharon formation.[241] Similarly, the cornea may be involved primarily by blistering lesions or secondarily to exposure resulting from cicatricial ectropion. Thinning and perforation may occur.[242,243] In one case, white-tan nonrefractile crystals were present in Bowman's layer in addition to deep stromal opacification.[244] In addition, incidence of pinguecula and pterygium were eight and two times higher, respectively, in PCT patients than in the control group.[245] Scleral involvement has been described as painless, slowly progressing, noninflammatory lesions at the interpalpebral areas akin to scleromalacia perforans.[246,247] Acute scleritis has also been reported.[247,248]

Systemic manifestations, along with the detection of excreted porphyrins, make the diagnosis.

Sunlight should be avoided, and phlebotomy and subcutaneous desferrioxamine may be successful in reducing the systemic iron load[249] Frequent application of artificial tears for a mechanical washing effect on the accumulating porphyrins, as well as systemic and topical antiinflammatory medications including steroids and ciclosporin A have been used to improve healing of scleral tissue.[246,247] In addition, amniotic membrane grafting over areas of scleromalacia has been reported.[247]

References

1. Otori T. Electrolyte content of rabbit corneal stroma. *Exp Eye Res.* 1967;6:356–367.
2. Giraud JP, Pouliquen Y, Giranud JP, et al. Statistical morphometric studies in normal human and rabbit corneal stroma. *Exp Eye Res.* 1975;21:221–229.
3. Hamada R, Pouliquen Y, Giranud JP, et al. Quantitative analysis on the ultrastructure of human fetal cornea. In: Yamada E, Mishima S, eds. *The structure of the eye III.* Tokyo, 1976; *Jpn J Ophthalmol*, pp 49–62.
4. de Duve, C. Exploring cells with a centrifuge. *Science.* 1975;189: 186–194.
5. Wild S, Roglic G, Green A, Sicree R, King H. Global prevalence of diabetes: estimates for the year 2000 and projections for 2030. *Diabetes Care.* 2004;27:1047–1053.
6. King H, Aubert RE, Herman WH. Global burden of diabetes, 1995–2025: prevalence, numerical estimates, and projections. *Diabetes Care.* 1988;21:1414–1431.
7. Kaji Y. Prevention of diabetic keratopathy. *Br J Ophthalmol.* 2005;89:254–255.
8. Chikamma T, Wakuta M, Liu Y, Nishida T. Deviated mechanism of wound healing in diabetic corneas. *Cornea.* 2007;26(Suppl 1):S75–S81.
9. Schultz RO, Van Horn DL, Peters MA, Klewin KM, Schutten WH. Diabetic keratopathy. *Trans Am Ophthalmol Soc.* 1981;79:180–199.
10. Didenko TN, Smoliakova GP, Sorokin EL, et al. Clinical and pathogenetic features of neurotrophic corneal disorders in diabetes. *Vestn Oftalmol.* 1999;115:7–11.
11. Gekka M, Miyata K, Nagai Y, et al. Corneal epithelial barrier function in diabetic patients. *Cornea.* 2004;23:35–37.
12. Gobbels M, Spitzans M, Oldendoerp J. Impairment of corneal epithelial barrier function in diabetics. *Graefe's Arch Clin Exp Ophthalmol.* 1989;227:142–144.
13. Tsubota K, Yamada M. The effect of aldose reductase inhibitor on the corneal epithelium. *Cornea.* 1993;12:161–162.
14. Hosotani H, Ohashi Y, Yamada M, et al. Reversal of abnormal corneal epithelial cell morphologic characteristics and reduced corneal sensitivity in diabetic patients by aldose reductase inhibitor, CT-112. *Am J Ophthalmol.* 1995;119:288–294.
15. Azar DT, Spurr-Michaud SJ, Tisdale AS, et al. Decreased penetration of anchoring fibrils into the diabetic stroma. A morphometric analysis. *Arch Ophthalmol.* 1989;107:1520–1523.
16. Azar DT, Spurr-Michaud SJ, Tisdale AS, et al. Altered epithelial–basement interactions in diabetic corneas. *Arch Ophthalmol.* 1992;110; 537–540.
17. Schultz RO, Peters MA, Sobocinski K, et al. Diabetic keratopathy as a manifestation of peripheral neuropathy. *Am J Ophthalmol.* 1983;96; 368–371.
18. Fujishima H, Shimazaki J, Yagi Y, et al. Improvement of corneal sensation and tear dynamics in diabetic patients by oral aldose reductase inhibitor, ONO-2235: a preliminary study. *Cornea.* 1996;15:368–375.
19. Meyers LA, Ubels JL, Eldelhauser HF. Corneal endothelial morphology in the rat. Effect of aging, diabetes, and topical aldose reductase inhibitor treatment. *Invest Ophthalmol Vis Sci.* 1988;29:940–948.
20. Ohguro N, Matsuda M, Ohashi Y, et al. Topical aldose reductase inhibitor for correcting corneal endothelial changes in diabetic patients. *Br J Ophthalmol.* 1995;79:1074–1077.
21. Cogan DG, Kinoshita JH, Kador PR, et al. Aldose reductase and complications of diabetes. *Ann Intern Med.* 1984;101:82–91.
22. Akagi Y, Yajima Y, Kador PR, et al. Localization of aldose reductase in the human eye. *Diabetes.* 1984;33:562–566.
23. Kaji Y, Usui T, Oshika T, et al. Advanced glycation end products in diabetic corneas. *Invest Ophthalmol Vis Sci.* 2000;41:362–368.
24. McDermott Am, Xiao TL, Kern TS, et al. Non-enzymatic glycation in corneas from normal and diabetic donors and its effects on epithelial cell attachment in vitro. *Optometry.* 2003;74:443–452.
25. Fujishima H, Tsubota K. Improvement of corneal fluorescein staining in post cataract surgery of diabetic patients by an oral aldose reductase inhibitor, ONO-2235. *Br J Ophthalmol.* 2002;86:860–863.
26. Awata T, Sogo S, Yamagami Y, et al. Effect of an aldose reductase inhibor, CT-112, on healing of the corneal epithelium in galactose-fed rats. *J Ocul Pharmacol.* 1988;4:195–201.
27. Yokoi N, Niiya A, Komuro A, et al. Effects of aldose reductase inhibitor CT-112 on the corneal epithelial barrier of galactose-fed rats. *Curr Eye Res.* 1997;16;595–599.
28. Awata T, Sogo S, Yamamoto Y. Effects of aldose reductase inhibitor, CT-112, on sugar alcohol accumulation in corneal epithelium of galactose-fed rats. *Jpn J Ophthalmol.* 1986;30:245–250.
29. Nakahara N, Miyata K, Otani S, et al. A randomised, placebo controlled clinical trial of the aldose reductase inhibitor CT-112 as management of corneal epithelial disorders in diabetic patients. *Br J Ophthalmol.* 2005;89:266–268.

30. Malik RA, Kallinikos P, Abbott CA, et al. Corneal confocal microscopy: a non-invasive surrogate of nerve fiber damage and repair in diabetic patients. *Diabetologia*. 2003;46;683–688.
31. Kallinikos P, Berhanu M, O'Donnell C, et al. Corneal nerve tortuosity in diabetic patients with neuropathy. *Invest Ophthalmol Vis Sci*. 2004;45:418–422.
32. Nakamura M, Kawahara M, Morishige N, et al. Promotion of corneal epithelial wound healing in diabetic rats by the combination of a substance P-derived peptide (FGLM-NH2) and insulin-like growth factor-1. *Diabetologia*. 2003;46:839–842.
33. Morishige N, Komatsubara T, Chikama T, Nishida T. Direct observation of corneal nerve fibers in neurotrophic keratopathy by confocal biomicroscopy. *Lancet*. 1999;354:1613–1614.
34. de Duve, C. Exploring cells with a centrifuge. *Science*. 1975; 189:186–194.
35. Journet A, Chapel A, Kieffer S, Roux F, Garin J. Proteomic analysis of human lysosomes: application to monocytic and breast cancer cells. *Proteomics*. 2002;2:1026–1040.
36. Eskelinen EL, Tanaka Y, Saftig P. At the acidic edge: emerging functions for lysosomal membrane proteins. *Trends Cell Biol*. 2003;13:137–145.
37. van Meer G, Futerman AH. The cell biology of lysosomal storage disorders. *Nat Rev Mol Cell Biol*. 2004;5:554–565.
38. Neufeld E, Muenzer J. The mucopolysaccharidoses. In: Scriver CR, Beaudet AR, Sly WS, Valle D, eds. *The metabolic and molecular bases of inherited disease*. New York: McGraw-Hill; 2001:3421–3452.
39. Wraith JE. The mucopolysaccharidoses: a clinical review and guide to management. *Arch Dis Child*. 1995;72:263–267.
40. Wraith JE. The first 5 years of clinical experience with laronidase enzyme replacement therapy for mucopolysaccharidosis I. *Expert Opin Pharmacother*. 2005;6:489–506.
41. Muenzer J, Fisher A. Advances in the treatment of mucopolysaccharidosis. Type I. *N Eng J Med*. 2004;350:1932–1934.
42. Kenyon KR, Quigley HA, Hussels IE, et al. The systemic mucopolysaccharidoses. Ultrastructural and histochemical studies of conjunctiva and skin. *Am J Ophthalmol*. 1972;73:811–833.
43. Caruso RC, Kaiser-Kupfer MI, Muenzer J, et al. Electroretinographic findings in the mucopolysaccharidoses. *Ophthalmology*. 1986; 93:1612–1616.
44. Collins ML, Traboulsi EI, Maumenee IH. Optic nerve head swelling and optic atrophy in the systemic mucopolysaccharidoses. *Ophthalmology*. 1990;97:1445–1449.
45. Nowaczyk MJ, Clarke JT, Morin JD. Glaucoma as an early complication of Hurler's disease. *Arch Dis Child*. 1988;63:1091–1093.
46. Summers CG, Whitley CB, Holland EJ, Purple RL, Krivit W. Dense peripheral corneal clouding in Scheie syndrome. *Cornea*. 1994;13: 277–279.
47. Quigley HA, Kenyon KR. Ultrastructural and histochemical studies of a newly recognized form of systemic mucopolysachharidosis (Maroteaux-Lamy syndrome, mild phenotype). *Am J Ophthalmol*. 1974;77: 809–818.
48. Zabel RW, MacDonald IM, Mintsioulis G, Addison DJ. Scheie's syndrome. An ultrastructural analysis of the cornea. *Ophthalmology*. 1989;96:1631–1638.
49. Girard B, Hoang-Xuan T, D'Hermies F, et al. Mucopolysaccharidosis type I, Hurler-Scheie phenotype with ocular involvement. Clinical and ultrastructural study. *J Fr Ophtalmol*. 1994;17:286–295.
50. Lorincz AE. The mucopolysaccharidoses: advances in understanding and treatment. *Pediatr Ann*. 1978;7:104–122.
51. Collins ML, Traboulsi EI, Maumenee IH. Optic nerve head swelling and optic atrophy in the systemic mucopolysaccharidoses. *Ophthalmology*. 1990;97:1445–1459.
52. François J. Metabolic disorders and corneal changes. *Dev Ophthalmol*. 1981;4:1–69.
53. François J. Ocular manifestations of the mucopolysaccharidoses. *Ophthalmologica*. 1974;169:345–361.
54. Caruso RC, Kaiser-Kupfer MI, Muenzer J, et al. Electroretinographic findings in the mucopolysaccharidoses. *Ophthalmology*. 1986;93: 1612–1616.
55. Del Monte MA, Maumenee IH, Green WR, et al. Histopathology of Sanfilippo's syndrome. *Arch Ophthalmol*. 1983;101:1255–1262.
56. Northover H, Cowie RA, Wraith JE. Mucopolysaccharidosis type IVA (Morquio syndrome): a clinical review. *J Inherit Metab Dis*. 1996; 19:357–365.
57. Ghosh M, McCulloch C. The Morquio syndrome – light and electron microscopic findings from two corneas. *Can J Ophthalmol*. 1974;9:445–452.
58. Dangel ME, Tsou BH. Retinal involvement in Morquio's syndrome (MPS IV). *Ann Ophthalmol*. 1985;17:349–354.
59. Käsmann-Kellner B,Weindler J, Pfau B, et al. Ocular changes in mucopolysaccharidosis IV A (Morquio A syndrome) and long-term results of perforating keratoplasty. *Ophthalmologica*. 1999;213:200–205.
60. Naumann GO, Rummelt V. [Clearing of the para-transplant host cornea after perforating keratoplasty in Maroteaux-Lamy syndrome (type VI-A mucopolysaccharidosis)]. *Klin Monatsbl Augenheilkd*. 1993;203: 351–360.
61. Shigematsu Y, Hori C, Nakai A, et al. Mucopolysaccharidosis VI (Maroteaux-Lamy syndrome) with hearing impairment and pupillary membrane remnants. *Acta Paediatr Jpn*. 1991;33:476–481.
62. Spranger J. The mucopolysaccharidoses. In: Emery AEH, Rimoin D, eds. *Principle and practise of medical genetics*. Edinburgh: Churchill Livingstone; 1990:2077–2079.
63. Bergwerk KE, Falk RE, Glasgow BJ, Rabinowitz YS. Corneal transplantation in a patient with mucopolysaccharidosis type VII (Sly disease). *Ophthalmic Genet*. 2000;21:17–20.
64. Natowicz MR, Short MP, Wang Y, et al. Clinical and biochemical manifestations of hyaluronidase deficiency. *N Engl J Med*. 1996;335: 1029–1033.
65. Jensen OA, Pedersen C, Schwartz M, et al. Hurler/Scheie phenotype. Report of an inbred sibship with tapeto-retinal degeneration and electron-microscopic examination of the conjuctiva. *Ophthalmologica*. 1978;176:194–204.
66. Alroy J, Haskins M, Birk DE. Altered corneal stromal matrix organization is associated with mucopolysaccharidosis I, III and VI. *Exp Eye Res*. 1999;68:523–530.
67. Goldberg MF, Duke JR. Ocular histopathology in Hunter's syndrome. Systemic mucopolysaccharidosis type II. *Arch Ophthalmol*. 1967;77: 503–512.
68. Kenyon KR. Conjunctival biopsy for diagnosis of lysosomal disorders. *Prog Clin Biol Res*. 1982;82:103–122.
69. Süveges I. Ocular symptoms and histopathology in mucopolysaccharidoses. *Bull Soc Belge Ophtalmol*. 1987;224:23–25.
70. Topping TM, Kenyon KR, Goldberg MF, Maumenee AE. Ultrastructural ocular pathology of Hunter's syndrome. Systemic mucopolysaccharidosis type II. *Arch Ophthalmol*. 1971;86:164–177.
71. Grupcheva CN, Craig JP, McGhee CN. In vivo microstructural analysis of the cornea in Scheie's syndrome. *Cornea*. 2003;22:76–79.
72. Tabone E, Grimaud JA, Peyrol S, et al. Ultrastructural aspects of corneal fibrous tissue in the Scheie syndrome. *Virchows Arch B Cell Pathol*. 1978;27:63–67.
73. Laver NM, Friedlander MH, McLean IW. Mild form of Maroteaux-Lamy syndrome: corneal histopathology and ultrastructure. *Cornea*. 1998;17:664–668.
74. Frederickson D, Levy R, Lees F. Fat transport in lipoproteinemias – an integrated approach to mechanisms and disorders, *N Engl J Med*. 1967;276:34, 94, 148, 215, 273.
75. Breckenridge W, et al. Lipoprotein abnormalities associated with a familial deficiency of hepatic lipase. *Atherosclerosis*. 1982;45:161.
76. Motulsky A. The genetic hyperlipidemias. *N Engl J Med*. 1976;294:823.
77. Vinger P, Sachs B. Ocular manifestations of hyperlipoproteinemia. *Am J Ophthalmol*. 1970;70:563.
78. Barchiese B, Eckel R, Ellis P. The cornea and disorders of lipid metabolism. *Surv Ophthalmol*. 1991;36:1.
79. Pe'er J, et al. Association between corneal arcus and some of the risk factors for coronary artery disease. *Br J Ophthalmol*. 1983;67:795.
80. Segal P, et al. The association of dyslipoproteinemia with corneal arcus and xanthelasma. The Lipid Research Clinics Program Prevalence Study. *Circulation*. 1986;73:1108–1118.
81. Crispin SM. Lipid deposition at the limbus. *Eye*. 1989;3:240–250.
82. Sugandhan S, Khandpur S, Sharma VK. Familial chylomicronemia syndrome. *Pediatr Dermatol*. 2007;24:323–325.
83. Weiss JS, Rodrigues MM, Kruth HS, et al. Panstromal Schnyder's corneal dystrophy: ultrastructural and histochemical studies. *Ophthalmology*. 1992;99:1072–1081.
84. McCarthy M, Innis S, Dubord P, White V. Panstromal Schnyder corneal dystrophy: a clinical pathologic report with quantitative analysis of corneal lipid composition. *Ophthalmology*. 1994;101:895–901.
85. Weiss JS. Schnyder's dystrophy of the cornea: a Swede–Finn connection. *Cornea*. 1992;11:93–101.
86. Hoang-Xuan T, Pouliquen Y, Gasteau J. Schnyder's crystalline dystrophy. II. Association with genu valgum. *J Fr Ophtalmol*. 1985;8: 743–747.
87. Gjone E, Bergaust B. Corneal opacity in familial plasma cholesterol ester deficiency. *Acta Ophthalmol (Copenh)*. 1969;47:222.
88. Paparo LG, Rapuano CJ, Raber IM, Grewal S, Cohen EJ, Laibson PR. Phototherapeutic keratectomy for Schnyder's crystalline corneal dystrophy. *Cornea*. 2000;19:343–347.

89. Marcon AS, Cohen EJ, Rapuano CJ, Laibson PR. Recurrence of corneal stromal dystrophies after penetrating keratoplasty. *Cornea.* 2003;22:19–21.
90. Vrabec M, et al. Ophthalmic observations in lecithin cholesterol acyltransferase deficiency. *Arch Ophthalmol.* 1988;106:225.
91. Bethell W, McCulloch C, Ghosh M. Lecithin cholesterol acyltransferase deficiency: light and electron microscopic findings from two corneas. *Can J Ophthalmol.* 1975;10:494.
92. Cogan DG, et al. Corneal opacity in LCAT disease. *Cornea.* 1992;11:595–599.
93. Viestenz A, et al. Histopathology of corneal changes in lecithin-cholesterol acyltransferase deficiency. *Cornea.* 2002;21:834–837.
94. Kolovou GD, Mikhailidis DP, Anagnostopoulou KK, Daskalopoulou SS, Cokkinos DV. Tangier disease four decades of research: a reflection of the importance of HDL. *Curr Med Chem.* 2006;13(7):771–782.
95. Winder AF, Alexander R, Garner A, et al. The pathology of cornea in Tangier disease (familial high density lipoprotein deficiency). *J Clin Pathol.* 1996;49:407–410.
96. Pressly TA, Scott WJ, Ide CH, Winkler A, Reams GP. Complications of Tangier disease. *Am J Med.* 1987;83(5):991–994.
97. Winder AF, Owen JS, Pritchard PH, et al. A first British case of fish-eye disease presenting at age 75 years: a double heterozygote for defined and new mutations affecting LCAT structure and expression. *J Clin Pathol.* 1999;52:228–230.
98. Kuivenhoven JA, van Voorst tot Voorst EJ, Wiebusch H, et al. A unique genetic and biochemical presentation of fish-eye disease. *J Clin Invest.* 1995;96:2783–2791.
99. Koster H, Savoldelli M, Dumon MF, Dubourg L, Clerc M, Pouliquen Y. A fish-eye disease-like familial condition with massive corneal clouding and dyslipoproteinemia. Report of clinical, histologic, electron microscopic, and biochemical features. *Cornea.* 1992;11(5):452–464.
100. Frost P, Tanaka Y, Spaeth G. Fabry's disease – glycolipid lipidosis. Histochemical and electron microscopic studies of two cases. *Am J Med.* 1966;40:618–627.
101. Font R, Fine B. Ocular pathology in Fabry's disease. Histochemical and electron microscopic observations. *Am J Ophthalmol.* 1972;73:419–430.
102. Wang RY, Lelis A, Mirocha J, Wilcox WR. Heterozygous Fabry women are not just carriers, but have a significant burden of disease and impaired quality of life. *Genet Med.* 2007;9:34–45.
103. Wilcox WR, Oliveira JP, Hopkin RJ, et al. Females with Fabry disease frequently have major organ involvement: lessons from the Fabry Registry. *Mol Genet Metab.* 2008;93:112–128.
104. Sodi A, Ioannidis AS, Mehta A, Davey C, Beck M, Pitz S. Ocular manifestations of Fabry's disease: data from the Fabry Outcome Survey. *Br J Ophthalmol.* 2007;91(2):210–214.
105. Falke K, Büttner A, Schittkowski M, et al. The microstructure of cornea verticillata in Fabry disease and amiodarone-induced keratopathy: a confocal laser-scanning microscopy study. *Graefe's Arch Clin Exp Ophthalmol.* 2009;247:523–534.
106. Desnick RJ, Brady R, Barranger J, et al. Fabry disease, an underrecognized multisystemic disorder: expert recommendations for diagnosis, management, and enzyme replacement therapy. *Ann Intern Med.* 2003;138:338–346.
107. Zarate YA, Hopkin RJ. Fabry's disease. *Lancet.* 2008;372(9647):1427–1435.
108. Maizel S, et al. Ten-year experience in renal transplantation for Fabry's disease. *Transplant Proc.* 1981;13:57.
109. Yam GH, Bosshard N, Zuber C, Steinmann B, Roth J. Pharmacological chaperone corrects lysosomal storage in Fabry disease caused by trafficking – incompetent variants. *Am J Physiol Cell Physiol.* 2006;290:C1076–C1082.
110. Frustaci A, Chimenti C, Ricci R, et al. Improvement in cardiac function in the cardiac variant of Fabry's disease with galactose-infusion therapy. *N Engl J Med.* 2001;345:25–32.
111. Shin SH, Murray GJ, Kluepfel-Stahl S, et al. Screening for pharmacological chaperones in Fabry disease. *Biochem Biophys Res Commun.* 2007;359:168–173.
112. O'Brien JS. The gangliosidoses. In: Stanbury JB, Wyngaarden JB, Fredrickson DS, eds. *The metabolic basis of inherited disease.* New York: McGraw-Hill; 1983.
113. Godtfredsen E. New aspects of the classification and pathogenesis of lipidoses with neuro-ophthalmological manifestations. *Acta Ophthalmol.* 1971;49:489.
114. Emery JM, et al. GM1-gangliosidosis: ocular and pathological manifestations. *Arch Ophthalmol.* 1971;85:177.
115. Nagayasu A, Nakamura T, Yamato O, et al. Morphological analysis of corneal opacity in Shiba dog with GM1 gangliosidosis. *J Vet Med Sci.* 2008;70(9):881–886.
116. Lüllmann H, Lüllmann-Rauch R, Wassermann O. Drug-induced phospholipidoses. II. Tissue distribution of the amphiphilic drug chlorphentermine. *CRC Crit Rev Toxicol.* 1975;4:185–218.
117. François J. Cornea verticillata. *Bull Soc Belge Ophthalmol.* 1968;150:656.
118. Calkins LL. Corneal epithelial changes occurring during chloroquine therapy. *Arch Ophthalmol.* 1958;60:981.
119. D'Amico DJ, Kenyon KR. Drug-induced lipidoses of the cornea and conjunctiva. *Int Ophthalmol.* 1981;4:67.
120. Dua HS, Singh A, Gomes JA, et al. Vortex or whorl formation of cultured human corneal epithelial cells induced by magnetic fields. *Eye.* 1996;10:447–450.
121. Bernstein HN. Chloroquine ocular toxicity. *Surv Ophthalmol.* 1967;12:415–447.
122. Shearer RV, Dubois EL. Ocular changes induced by long-term hydroxychloroquine (plaquenil) therapy. *Am J Ophthalmol.* 1967;64:245–252.
123. Hirst LW, Sanborn G, Green WR, et al. Amodiaquine ocular changes. *Arch Ophthalmol.* 1982;100:1300–1304.
124. Easterbrook M. Is corneal deposition of antimalarial any indication of retinal toxicity? *Can J Ophthalmol.* 1990;25:249–251.
125. Grierson DJ. Hydroxychloroquine and visual screening in a rheumatology outpatient clinic. *Ann Rheum Dis.* 1997;56:188–190.
126. Jeddi A, Ben Osman N, Daghfous F, et al. The cornea and synthetic antimalarials. *J Fr Ophtalmol.* 1994;17:36–38.
127. Nylander V. Ocular damage in chloroquine therapy. *Acta Ophthalmol.* 1967;92:1.
128. Slowik C, et al. Detection of morphological corneal changes caused by chloroquine therapy using confocal in vivo microscopy. *Ophthalmologe.* 1997;94:147–151.
129. Jeddi A, et al. The cornea and synthetic antimalarials. *J Fr Ophthalmol.* 1994;17:36–38.
130. Neubauer AS, Samari-Kermani K, Schaller U, et al. Detecting chloroquine retinopathy: electro-oculogram versus colour vision. *Br J Ophthalmol.* 2003;87:902–908.
131. Pulhorn G, Thiel HJ. Ultrastructural aspects of chloroquine-keratopathy. *Albrecht Von Graefe's Arch Klin Exp Ophthalmol.* 1976;201:89–99.
132. Hollander DA, Aldave AJ. Drug-induced corneal complications. *Curr Opin Ophthalmol.* 2004;15(6):541–548.
133. Orlando RG, Dangel ME, Schaal SF. Clinical experience and grading of amiodarone keratopathy. *Ophthalmology.* 1984;91:1184–1187.
134. Kaplan LJ, Cappaert WE. Amiodarone keratopathy. Correlation to dosage and duration. *Arch Ophthalmol.* 1982;100:601–602.
135. Mantyjarvi M, Tuppurainen K, Ikaheimo K. Ocular side effects of amiodarone. *Surv Ophthalmol.* 1998;42:360–366.
136. D'Amico DJ, Kenyon KR, Ruskin JN. Amiodarone keratopathy: drug-induced lipid storage disease. *Arch Ophthalmol.* 1981;99:257–261.
137. Haug SJ, Friedman AH. Identification of amiodarone in corneal deposits. *Am J Ophthalmol.* 1991;111:518–520.
138. Ciancaglini M, Carpineto P, Zuppardi E, et al. In vivo confocal microscopy of patients with amiodarone-induced keratopathy. *Cornea.* 2001;20:368–373.
139. Dolan BJ, Flach AJ, Peterson JS. Amiodarone keratopathy and lens opacities. *J Am Optom Assoc.* 1985;56:468–470.
140. Thystrup JD, Fledelius HC. Retinal maculopathy possibly associated with amiodarone medication. *Acta Ophthalmol (Copenh).* 1994;72:639–641.
141. Feiner LA, Younge BR, Kazmier FJ, et al. Optic neuropathy and amiodarone therapy. *Mayo Clin Proc.* 1987;62:702–717.
142. Mantyjarvi M, Tuppurainen K, Ikaheimo K. Ocular side effects of amiodarone. *Surv Ophthalmol.* 1998;42:360–366.
143. Kaiser-Kupfer MI, Lippman ME. Tamoxifen retinopathy. *Cancer Treat Rep.* 1978;62:315–320.
144. Pavlidis NA, Petris C, Briassoulis E, et al. Clear evidence that long-term, low-dose tamoxifen treatment can induce ocular toxicity. A prospective study of 63 patients. *Cancer.* 1992;69:2961–2964.
145. Noureddin BN, Seoud M, Bashshur Z, et al. Ocular toxicity in low-dose tamoxifen: a prospective study. *Eye.* 1999;13:729–733.
146. Teich SA, Handwerger S, Mathur-Wagh U, et al. Toxic keratopathy associated with suramin therapy. *N Engl J Med.* 1986;314:1455–1456.
147. Holland EJ, Stein CA, Palestine AG, et al. Suramin keratopathy. *Am J Ophthalmol.* 1988;106:216–220.
148. Johnson AW, Buffaloe WJ. Chlorpromazine epithelial keratopathy. *Arch Ophthalmol.* 1996;76:664–667.
149. Walinder PE, Gip L, Stempa M. Corneal changes in patients treated with clofazimine. *Br J Ophthalmol.* 1976;60:526–528.
150. Shah GK, Cantrill HL, Holland EJ. Vortex keratopathy associated with atovaquone. *Am J Ophthalmol.* 1995;120:669–671.
151. Gibson JM, Fielder AR, Garner A, Millac P. Severe ocular side effects of perhexilene maleate: case report. *Br J Ophthalmol.* 1984;68:553–560.

152. Weiss JN, Weinberg RS, Regelson W. Keratopathy after oral administration of tilorone hydrochloride. *Am J Ophthalmol.* 1980;89:46–53.
153. Burns CA. Indomethacin, reduced retinal sensitivity, and corneal deposits. *Am J Ophthalmol.* 1968;66:825–835.
154. Szmyd Jr L, Perry HD. Keratopathy associated with the use of naproxen. *Am J Ophthalmol.* 1985;99:598.
155. Fitt A, Dayan M, Gillie RF. Vortex keratopathy associated with ibuprofen therapy. *Eye.* 1996;10:145–146.
156. Hedges TR 3rd, Kenyon KR, Hanninen LA, Mosher DB. Corneal and conjunctival effects of monobenzone in patients with vitiligo. *Arch Ophthalmol.* 1983;101:64–68.
157. Wilhelmus KR, et al. Corneal lipidosis in patients with the acquired immunodeficiency syndrome. *Am J Ophthalmol.* 1995;119:14–19.
158. Wilhelmus KR, Keener MJ, Jones DB, Font RL. Corneal lipidosis in patients with the acquired immunodeficiency syndrome. *Am J Ophthalmol.* 1995;119(1):14–19.
159. Libert J, et al. Cellular toxicity of gentamicin. *Am J Ophthalmol.* 1979;87:405.
160. Rapin I, et al. The cherry red spot-myoclonus syndrome. *Am J Neurol.* 1978;3:234.
161. O'Brien J. Neuraminidase deficiency in the cherry red spot-myoclonus syndrome. *Biochem Biophys Res Commun.* 1977;79:1136.
162. Hickman S, Neufeld EF. A hypothesis for I-cell disease. Defective hydrolases that do not enter lysosomes. *Biochem Biophys Res Commun.* 1977;49:992–999.
163. Neufeld E, McKusick V. Disorders of lysosomal enzyme synthesis and localization: I-cell disease and pseudo-Hurler polydystrophy. In Stanbury JB, Wyngaarden J, Fredrickson OO, eds. *The metabolic basis of inherited disease.* New York: McGraw-Hill; 1983.
164. Kenyon KR, Sensenbrenner JA. Mucolipidosis II (I-cell disease): ultrastructural observations of conjunctiva and skin. *Invest Ophthalmol.* 1971;10:555–567.
165. Libert J, et al. Ocular findings in I-cell disease (mucolipidosis type II). *Am J Ophthalmol.* 1977;83:617–628.
166. Stein H, et al. Pseudo-Hurler polydystrophy (mucolipidosis III). A clinical, biochemical and ultrastructural study. *Isr J Med Sci.* 1974;10:463–475.
167. Berman ER, et al. Acid hydrolase deficiencies and abnormal glycoproteins in mucolipidosis III (pseudo-Hurler polydystrophy). *Clin Chim Acta.* 1974;52:115–124.
168. Traboulsi E, Maumenee IH. Ophthalmologic finding in mucolipidosis III (pseudo-Hurler polydystrophy). *Am J Ophthalmol.* 1986;102:592.
169. Berman ER, et al. Congenital corneal clouding with abnormal systemic storage bodies. A new variant of mucolipidosis. *J Pediatr.* 1979;84:519–526.
170. Noffke AS, et al. Mucolipidosis IV in an African-American patient with new findings in electron microscopy. *Cornea.* 2001;20:536–539.
171. Merin S, et al. Mucolipidosis IV. Ocular, systemic and ultrastructural findings. *Invest Ophthalmol.* 1975;14:437–448.
172. Bach G, Cohen M, Kohn G. Abnormal ganglioside accumulation in cultured fibroblasts from patients with mucolipidosis IV. *Biochem Biophys Res Commun.* 1975;66:1483–1490.
173. Merin S, et al. The cornea in mucolipidosis IV. *J Pediatr Ophthalmol.* 1976;13:289–295.
174. Newman NJ, et al. Corneal surface irregularities and episodic pain in a patient with mucolipidosis IV. *Arch Ophthalmol.* 1990;108:251–254.
175. Kenyon KR, et al. Mucolipidosis IV. Histopathology of conjunctiva, cornea and skin. *Arch Ophthalmol.* 1979;97:1106–1111.
176. Riedel K, Zwann J, Kenyon KR. Ocular abnormalities in mucolipidosis IV. *Am J Ophthalmol.* 1985;99:125.
177. Dangel M, Bremer D, Rogers G. Treatment of corneal opacification in mucolipidosis IV with conjunctival transplantation. *Am J Ophthalmol.* 1985;99:137.
178. Goldberg MF, et al. Macular cherry-red spot, corneal clouding, and beta-galactosidase deficiency. Clinical, biochemical and electron microscopic study of a new autosomal recessive storage disease. *Arch Intern Med.* 1971;128:387.
179. Slaugenhaupt SA, et al. Mapping of the mucolipidosis type IV gene to chromosome 19p and definition of founder haplotypes. *Am J Hum Genet.* 1999;65:773–778.
180. Bargal R, et al. Identification of the gene causing mucolipidosis type IV. *Nat Genet.* 2000;26:118–123.
181. Sun M, et al. Mucolipidosis type IV is caused by mutations in a gene encoding a novel transient receptor potential channel. *Hum Mol Genet.* 2000;9:2471–2478.
182. Goldin E, Caruso RC, Benko W, Kaneski CR, Stahl S, Schiffmann R. Isolated ocular disease is associated with decreased mucolipin-1 channel conductance. *Invest Ophthalmol Vis Sci.* 2008;49(7):3134–3142.
183. Dobrovolny R, Liskova P, Ledvinova J, et al. Mucolipidosis IV: report of a case with ocular restricted phenotype caused by leaky splice mutation. *Am J Ophthalmol.* 2007;143(4):663–671.
184. Wenger DA, Tarly TJ, Wharton C. Macular cherry red spots and myoclonus with dementia: coexistent neuraminidase and beta-galactosidase deficiencies. *Biochem Biophys Res Commun.* 1978;82:589.
185. Kalatzis V, Cherqui S, Antignac C, Gasnier B. Cystinosin, the protein defective in cystinosis, is a H(+)-driven lysosomal cystine transporter. *EMBO J.* 2001;20:5940–5949.
186. Town M, Jean G, Cherqui S, et al. A novel gene encoding an integral membrane protein is mutated in nephropathic cystinosis. *Nat Genet.* 1998;18:319–324.
187. Tsilou E, Zhou M, Gahl W, Sieving PC, Chan CC. Ophthalmic manifestations and histopathology of infantile nephropathic cystinosis: report of a case and review of the literature. *Surv Ophthalmol.* 2007;52(1):97–105, Review.
188. Gahl WA, Thoene JG, Schneider J. Cystinosis. *N Engl J Med.* 2002;347:111–121.
189. Cogan DG, Kuwabara T, Kinoshita J, et al. Cystinosis in an adult. *JAMA.* 1957;164:394–396.
190. Dufier JL, Dhermy P, Gubler MC, Gagnadoux MF, Broyer M. Ocular changes in long-term evolution of infantile cystinosis. *Ophthalm Paediatr Genet.* 1987;8:131–137.
191. Gahl WA, Kaiser-Kupfer MI. Complications of nephropathic cystinosis after renal failure. *Pediatr Nephrol.* 1987;1:260–268.
192. Goldman H, et al. Adolescent cystinosis: comparison with infantile and adult forms. *Pediatrics.* 1971;47:979.
193. Zimmerman TJ, Hood I, Gasset AF. 'Adolescent' cystinosis: a case report and review of the literature. *Arch Ophthalmol.* 1974;92:265.
194. Yamamoto GK, et al. Long-term ocular changes in cystinosis: observations in renal transplant recipients. *J Pediatr Ophthalmol.* 1979;16:16–21.
195. Alsuhaibani H, Wagoner MD, Khan AO. Confocal microscopy of the cornea in nephropathic cystinosis. *Br J Ophthalmol.* 2005;89:1530–1531.
196. Katz B, Melles RB, Schneider JA, et al. Corneal thickness in nephropathic cystinosis. *Br J Ophthalmol.* 1989;73:665–668.
197. Katz B, Melles RB, Schneider JA. Contrast sensitivity function in nephropathic cystinosis. *Arch Ophthalmol.* 1987;105:1667–1669.
198. Katz B, Melles RB, Schneider JA. Corneal sensitivity in nephropathic cystinosis. *Am J Ophthalmol.* 1987;104:413–416.
199. Cruz-Sanchez FF, et al. The value of conjunctival biopsy in childhood cystinosis. *Histol Histopathol.* 1989;4:305–308.
200. Gahl WA, Thoene JG, Schneider JA. Cystinosis. *N Engl J Med.* 2002;347(2):111–121.
201. Katz B, Melles RB, Schneider JA. Recurrent crystal deposition after keratoplasty in nephropathic cystinosis. *Am J Ophthalmol.* 1987;104:190–191.
202. Tsilou ET, Rubin BI, Reed G, et al. Nephropathic cystinosis: posterior segment manifestations and effects of cysteamine therapy. *Ophthalmology.* 2006;113:1002–1009.
203. Goldsmith LA, Kang E, Bienfang DC, et al. Tyrosinemia with planter and palmer keratosis and keratitis. *J Pediatr.* 1973;83:798–805.
204. Kato M, Suzuki N, Koezda T. A case of tyrosinemia type II with convulsion and EEG abnormality. *No To Hattatsu.* 1993;25:558–562.
205. Macsai MS, Schwartz TL, Hinkle D, Hummel MB, Mulhern MG, Rootman D. Tyrosinemia type II: nine cases of ocular signs and symptoms. *Am J Ophthalmol.* 2001;132(4):522–527.
206. Herre F, et al. Incurable keratitis and chronic palmoplantar hyperkeratosis with hypertyrosinemia. Cure using a tyrosine-restricted diet. *Arch Fr Pediatr.* 1986;43:19.
207. Burns RP. The tyrosine aminotransferase deficiency: an unusual cause of corneal ulcers. *Am J Ophthalmol.* 1972;73:400.
208. Sayar RB, et al. Clinical picture and problems of keratoplasty in Richner-Hanhart syndrome (tyrosinemia type II). *Ophthalmologica.* 1988;197:1–6.
209. Rosenberg LE. Storage diseases of amino acid metabolism. In: Petersdorf RG et al, eds. *Harrison's principles of internal medicine.* New York: McGraw Hill; 1987.
210. Van Offel JF, et al. The clinical manifestations of ochronosis: a review. *Acta Clin Belg.* 1995;50(6):358–362.
211. Kampik A, Sani JN, Green WR. Ocular ochronosis clinicopathological, histochemical and ultrastructural studies. *Arch Ophthalmol.* 1980;98:1441–1447.
212. Carlson DM, Helgeson MK, Hiett JA. Ocular ochonosis from alkaptonuria. *J Am Optom Assoc.* 1991;62:854–856.
213. Ehongo A, Schrooyen M, Pereleux A. Important bilateral corneal astigmatism in a case of ocular ochronosis. *Bull Soc Belge Ophtalmol.* 2005;295:17–21.

214. Seitz B, Weidle E, Naumann GO. Unilateral type III (Hida) lattice stromal corneal dystrophy. *Klin Monatsbl Augenheilkd.* 1993;203: 279–285.
215. Starck T, et al. Clinical and histopathologic studies of two families with lattice corneal dystrophy and familial systemic amyloidosis (Meretoja syndrome). *Ophthalmology.* 1991;98:1197–1206.
216. Tsunoda I, et al. Idiopathic AA amyloidosis manifested by autonomic neuropathy, vestibulocochelopathy, and lattice corneal dystrophy. *J Neurol Neurosurg Psychiatry.* 1994;57:635–637.
217. de la Chapelle A, et al. Familial amyloidosis, Finnish type: G654-a mutation of the gelsolin gene in Finnish families and an unrelated American family. *Genomics.* 1992;13:898–901.
218. Steiner RD, et al. Asp187Asn mutation of gelsolin in an American kindred with familial amyloidosis, Finnish type (FAP IV). *Hum Genet.* 1995;95:327–330.
219. Maury CPJ, Nurmiaho-Lassila E-L. Creation of amyloid fibrils from mutant Asnl87 gelsolin peptides. *Biochem Biophys Res Commun.* 1992;183:227–231.
220. Kiuru S. Gelsolin-related familial amyloidosis, Finnish type (FAF) and its variants found worldwide. *Amyloid Int J Exp Clin Invest.* 1998;5: 55–66.
221. Kiuru S, Matikainen E, Kupari M, et al. Autonomic nervous system and cardiac involvement in familial amyloidosis, Finnish type (FAF). *J Neurol Sci.* 1994;126:40–48.
222. Maury CP. Homozygous familial amyloidosis, Finnish type: demonstration of glomerular gelsolin-derived amyloid and non-amyloid tubular gelsolin. *Clin Nephrol.* 1993;40:53–56.
223. Fernandez AL, Herreros JM, Monzonis AM, et al. Heart transplantation for Finnish type familial systemic amyloidosis. *Scand Cardiovasc J.* 1997;31:357–359.
224. Rosenberg ME, Tervo TM, Gallar J, et al. Corneal morphology and sensitivity in lattice dystrophy type II (familial amyloidosis, Finnish type). *Invest Ophthalmol Vis Sci.* 2001;42:634–641.
225. Meneray MA, Bennett DJ, Nguyen DH, Beuerman RW. Effect of sensory denervation on the structure and physiologic responsiveness of rabbit lacrimal gland. *Cornea.* 1998;17:99–107.
226. Meretoja J. Familial systemic paramyloidosis with lattice dystrophy of the cornea, progressive cranial neuropathy, skin changes and various internal symptoms: a previously unrecognized heritable syndrome. *Ann Clin Res.* 1969;1:314–324.
227. Meretoja J. Comparative histopathological and clinical findings in eyes with lattice corneal dystrophy of two different types. *Ophthalmologica.* 1972;165:15–37.
228. Kiuru, S. Gelsolin-related familial amyloidosis, Finnish type (FAF), and its variants found worldwide. *Int J Exp Clin Invest.* 1998;5:55–66.
229. Kiuru S. Familial amyloidosis of the Finnish type (FAF). A clinical study of 30 patients. *Acta Neurol Scand.* 1992;86:346–353.
230. Kivela T, Tarkkanen A, Frangione B, et al. Ocular amyloid deposition in familial amyloidosis, Finnish: an analysis of native and variant gelsolin in Meratoja's syndrome. *Invest Ophthalmol Vis Sci.* 1994;35:3759–3769.
231. Stark T, Kenyon KR, Hanninen LA, et al. Clinical and histopathologic studies of two families with lattice corneal dystrophy and familial systemic amyloidosis (Meretoja syndrome). *Ophthalmology.* 1991;98(8): 1197–1206.
232. Stewart HS, Parveen R, Ridgway AE, Bonshek R, Black GC. Late onset lattice corneal dystrophy with systemic familial amyloidosis, amyloidosis V, in an English family. *Br J Ophthalmol.* 2000;84:390–394.
233. John ME, et al. Excimer laser photoablation of primary familial amyloidosis of the cornea. *Refract Corneal Surg.* 1993;9:138–141.
234. Hutchinson J. The relation of certain diseases of the eye to gout. *Br Med J.* 1884;2:995.
235. McWilliams JR. Ocular findings in gout. *Am J Ophthalmol.* 1952;35:1778.
236. Slansky HH, Kuwabara T. Intranuclear urate crystals in corneal epithelium. *Arch Ophthalmol.* 1969;80:338.
237. Bernad B, Narvaez J, Diaz-Torné C, Diez-Garcia M, Valverde J. Clinical image: corneal tophus deposition in gout. *Arthritis Rheum.* 2006; 54(3):1025.
238. Fishman RS, Sunderman FW. Band keratopathy in gout. *Arch Ophthalmol.* 1966;75:367.
239. Weve HJM. *Uric acid keratitis and other ocular findings in gout.* Rotterdam: Van Hengel; 1924.
240. Lerman S, Megaw J, Fraunfelder FT. Further studies on allopurinal therapy and human cataractogenesis. *Am J Ophthalmol.* 1984;97: 205.
241. Mohan M, et al. Corneoscleral ulceration in congenital erythropoietic porphyria (a case report). *Jpn J Ophthalmol.* 1988;32:21–25.
242. Ueda S, et al. Corneal and conjunctival changes in congenital erythropoietic porphyria. *Cornea.* 1989;8:286–294.
243. Sevel D, Burger D. Ocular involvement in cutaneous porphyrias. *Arch Ophthalmol.* 1971;85:580.
244. Sevel D, Burger D. Ocular involvement in cutaneous porphyria: a clinical and histological report. *Arch Ophthalmol.* 1971;85:580.
245. Hammer H, Korom I, Morvay M, Simon M. [Ocular manifestations in porphyria cutanea tarda]. *Orv Hetil.* 1992;133(46):2971–2973.
246. Altiparmak UE, Oflu Y, Kocaoglu FA, Katircioglu YA, Duman S. Ocular complications in 2 cases with porphyria. *Cornea.* 2008;27(9):1093–1096.
247. Veenashree MP, Sangwan VS, Vemuganti GK, Parthasaradhi A. Acute scleritis as a manifestation of congenital erythropoietic porphyria. *Cornea.* 2002;21(5):530–531.
248. Salmon JF, Strauss PC, Todd G, et al. Acute scleritis in porphyria cutanea tarda. *Am J Ophthalmol.* 1990;109:400–406.
249. Gibertini P, et al. Advances in the treatment of porphyria cutanea tarda. *Liver.* 1984;4:280.

Chapter 60

Skeletal and Connective Tissue Disorders with Anterior Segment Manifestations

Elias I. Traboulsi

The corneal extracellular matrix is composed predominantly of collagen and proteoglycans. The types and organization of these constituents influence the cornea's clarity and tensile strength. Similarly, the functional anatomy of the sclera and anterior chamber angle depend on the same connective tissue elements. Olsen and McCarthy have provided a superb overview of the molecular structure of collagens and other components of the extracellular matrix of the cornea, sclera, and vitreous.[1] Table 60.1 lists the different types of collagen and proteoglycans within the corneal layers.

Fibrillin[2] and the microfibrillar glycoproteins[3] make up the microfibrillar system of the extracellular matrix. Fibrillin molecules are associated with elastin. In the cornea, fibrillin is localized predominantly at the level of the epithelial basement membrane (Fig. 60.1). Other ocular structures that are rich in fibrillin include the suspensory zonules of the lens, the lens capsule, and the sclera.[4] It follows that diseases that involve collagen or other connective tissue components can have adverse structural and functional implications for corneal and lenticular structures. Conditions such as microcornea, megalocornea, and corneal opacification may be present at birth. Alternatively, connective tissue abnormalities of the cornea may become manifest later in life as progressive disorders, such as keratoconus and keratoglobus, or as manifestations of such diseases as Ehlers-Danlos syndrome or Marfan syndrome. Robertson found that 50% of 44 consecutive patients with keratoconus who were examined for hypermobile joints, blue sclerae, hyperextensible skin, fragile tissues, bleeding diathesis, and a family history of keratoconus had hypermobile joints suggestive of Ehlers-Danlos syndrome type II, as compared to none of 44 age-matched controls without keratoconus.[5] Beardsley and Foulks found that 28% of 32 patients with keratoconus had mitral valve prolapse, compared to 13% of control individuals.[6,7] These examples highlight the generalized nature of connective tissue abnormalities and the involvement of the cornea in many.

The sclera is not excluded from global effects of connective tissue disorders. Scleral weakness can allow enlargement of an eye, or its thinning with exposure of the underlying uvea, leading to so-called 'blue sclera.' Similarly,

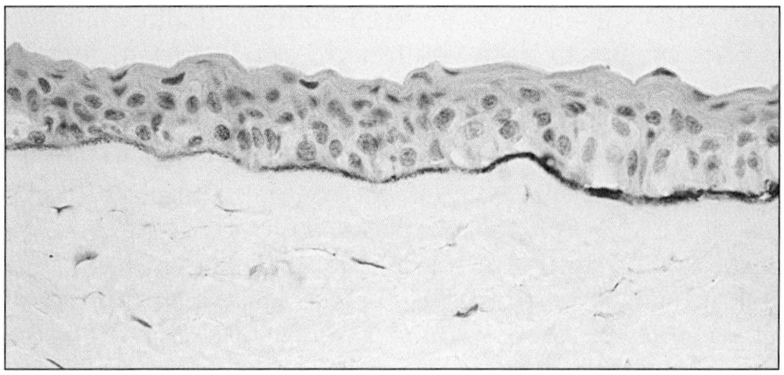

Fig. 60.1 Immunohistochemical study of cornea for distribution of fibrillin shows staining in the epithelial basement membrane zone. (Original magnification ×50. Counterstain: Harrys hematoxylin.) (Wheatley HM et al: Immunohistochemical localization of fibrillin in human ocular tissues. Relevance to the Marfan syndrome. *Arch Ophthalmol* 113:103, 1995. Copyright © (1995) American Medical Association. All rights reserved.)

Table 60.1 Extracellular matrix composition of corneal layers

Corneal layer	Extracellular matrix components
Basement membrane of epithelium	Type VII collagen (anchoring fibrils)
Bowman's layer	Type VII collagen Type I collagen
Stroma	Type I collagen (predominant) Type V collagen (abundant) Type XII collagen Type III collagen (minor) Keratan sulfate proteoglycan Dermatan sulfate proteoglycan Decorin Biglycan
Descemet's membrane	Type VIII collagen in anterior (banded) Type IV collagen in posterior (nonbanded)

abnormalities of the corneoscleral limbal structures, including the anterior chamber angle structures, may lead to collapse of filtering channels and glaucoma. When present in a fetus or very young infant, glaucoma leads to stretching of the globe, causing megalophthalmos and a large cornea. If Descemet's membrane ruptures, Haab striae are observed and corneal clouding ensues. In contrast, the conjunctiva is usually normal in appearance in patients with connective tissue disease, and in those with skeletal dysplasias. An exception occurs in hypophosphatasia, or other disorders involving calcium deposition.

Classification of Skeletal Disorders

There is no single easy method of classifying skeletal disorders, especially for the purpose of remembering their ocular manifestations. The International Working Group on Constitutional Diseases of Bone recently revised its classification of osteochondrodysplasias in 2006.[8] This clinical classification will undoubtedly undergo further modifications as molecular genetic data continue to be elucidated. Rimoin et al. provide an excellent overview of the current clinical and molecular aspect of the skeletal dysplasias.[9]

Abnormalities of procollagen and collagen genes result in such skeletal dysplasias as Stickler syndrome, Kniest dysplasia, spondyloepiphyseal dysplasia, and osteogenesis imperfecta. Abnormalities in fibrillin result in Marfan syndrome and in congenital contractual arachnodactyly. A number of enzyme defects cause lysosomal storage diseases such as the mucopolysaccharidoses and their skeletal abnormalities, collectively known as dysostosis multiplex in regard to their radiologic characteristics. Finally, abnormalities of the fibroblast growth factor receptors (FGFRs) lead to the phenotypes of Crouzon, Apert, Jackson-Weiss, and Saethre-Chotzen syndromes and to achondroplasia. Numerous skeletal and craniofacial malformation syndromes, however, remain characterized only at the clinical level, and further insight into their pathogenesis remains to be elucidated. Table 60.2 lists some of the skeletal disorders of special interest to the ophthalmologist because of their ocular manifestations.

Craniofacial dysostosis syndromes

Although clinically distinguishable on the basis of cranial morphology and the presence or absence of hand malformations such as polydactyly (supernumerary digits) and syndactyly (fused digits), molecular genetic studies have shown that mutations of individual fibroblast growth factor receptor genes may lead to a number of clinically distinct phenotypes.[10–14] Allelic mutations in the fibroblast growth factor receptor-2 (*FGFR2*) gene on chromosome 10 lead to Apert, Crouzon, or Jackson-Weiss syndrome. *FGFR2* has two alternative gene products: keratinocyte growth factor receptor (*KGFR*) and bacterially expressed kinase (*BEK*). Mutations in *FGFR1*, located on 8p11.2-p12, lead to the Pfeiffer syndrome, characterized by premature fusion of several sutures of the skull, broad thumbs and great toes, short fingers and toes, and variable degrees of syndactyly. It is now known that Pfeiffer syndrome can be caused by mutations in *FGFR2* or *FGFR1*.[15] Mutations in *FGFR3* lead to achondroplasia and to

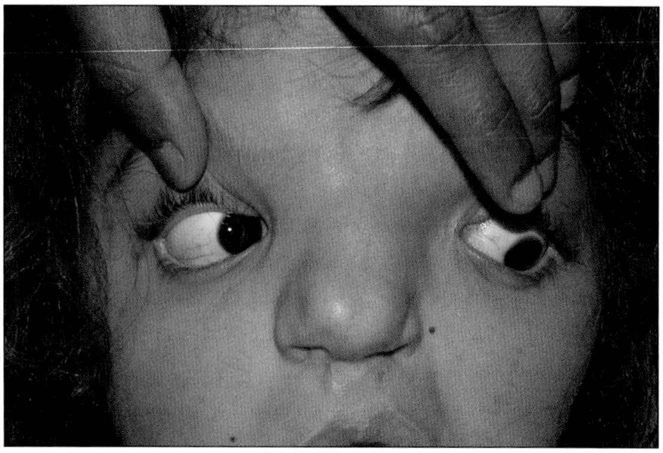

Fig. 60.2 Limited movement in the field of action of the right superior oblique from its absence in this patient with craniofacial malformation syndrome.

Crouzon syndrome with acanthosis nigricans.[16] Thus, there is tremendous genetic and allelic heterogeneity among the various craniofacial malformation syndromes. The blur between the craniofacial dysostoses has become even greater, but intermediate phenotypes are easier to explain. Clinical differentiation remains possible in most cases, and is based primarily on distal limb findings. In the absence of syndactyly, a diagnosis of Crouzon syndrome is most likely. If an extra digit is present in association with syndactyly and the cranial findings, Carpenter syndrome is suggested. Patients with the Pfeiffer syndrome have broad thumbs and great toes. The absence of obesity and hypogenitalism in patients with Pfeiffer syndrome allow its differentiation from the Summitt type of acrocephalopolysyndactyly, a syndrome characterized by obesity and hypogenitalism with normal intelligence and the premature closure of the cranial sutures which is likely identical with Carpenter and Goodman syndromes, displaying a continuum in phenotypic expression.[17]

In Crouzon syndrome there is craniosynostosis, maxillary hypoplasia, and shallowing of the orbits with proptosis. The cranial deformity is variable and depends on the order and rate of sutural stenosis. Premature closure of the cranial sutures leads to increased intracranial pressure with secondary mental retardation and optic atrophy. Some patients have true hypertelorism. The eyelids usually have an antimongoloid slant. The proptosis, which may be severe, is caused by the shallow orbits and may lead to exposure keratitis. Rarely, the eyes may spontaneously subluxate. V-pattern exotropia secondary to overacting inferior oblique muscles is frequently present.[18] Diamond and colleagues reported the absence of various extraocular muscles in some patients with strabismus.[19] More recent case reports have recognized a pattern of multiple missing, vestigial, or anomalous extraocular muscles in craniosynostosis patients (Fig. 60.2).[20] Patients with Crouzon syndrome can have optic nerve involvement; optic atrophy may result from long-standing papilledema secondary to elevated intracranial pressure. Intraocular abnormalities such as iris coloboma,

Table 60.2 Skeletal disorders of interest to the ophthalmologist

Name (OMIM #)	Corneal findings	Other ocular findings	Genetics/map/other information
Albright hereditary osteodystrophy (103580)	None	Zonular cartaracts with multicolored flecks in 25% of patients	AD Loss of function of the paternal allele of the *GNAS* gene on 20q13.2
Apert syndrome (101200)	Exposure keratitis with severe proptosis Keratoconus (very rare) Megalocornea (very rare)	Strabismus (exotropia with V pattern) Absence of extraocular muscles, proptosis, ocular hypopigmentation, optic atrophy Rare: nystagmus, ptosis, cataract, ectopia lentis, coloboma of iris	AD Gene maps to 10q26 Mutations in *FGFR2*
Carpenter syndrome; acrocephalo-polysyndactyly type II (201000)	Exposure keratitis secondary to severe proptosis Microcornea (rare) Corneal leukoma (rare)	Epicanthal folds, antimongoloid slant, hyper- or hypotelorism, optic atrophy, strabismus Rare: coloboma of the iris and choroid, congenital cataract, lens subluxation, nystagmus, retinal detachment	AR Mutations in *RAB23* gene
Cockayne syndrome (Type A: 216400 Type B: 133540)	Raised inferior corneal lesion, band keratopathy, recurrent erosions	Cataracts, retinal dystrophy, nystagmus, iris atrophy, hyperopia, enophthalmos, strabismus	AR Type A: chromosome 5; mutations in *ERCC8* gene Type B: 10q11; mutations in *ERCC6* gene
Crouzon syndrome (123500)	Exposure keratitis with severe proptosis Keratoconus (very rare) Microcornea (very rare)	Strabismus (exotropia with V pattern) Exophthalmos, hypertelorism, optic atrophy in 30% Rare: nystagmus, glaucoma, cataract, ectopia lentis, aniridia, anisocoria, myelinated nerve fibers	AD Gene maps to 10q26 Mutations in *FGFR2*
Ehlers-Danlos syndrome (EDS I: 130000 EDS II: 130010 EDS III: 130020 EDS IV: 130050 EDS V: 305200 EDS VI: 225400 EDS VII: AD – 130060 EDS VII: AR – 225410 EDS VIII: 130080)	Brittle cornea in type VI Keratoconus in types I and VI Keratoglobus in type VI	Epicanthal folds, blue sclerae, retinal detachment, glaucoma, ectopia lentis, angioid streaks (rare)	See text
Goldenhar-Gorlin syndrome; oculo-auriculo-vertebral sequence; hemifacial microsomia (164210)	Limbal dermoid	Upper > lower lid coloboma, strabismus (25%), Duane's retraction syndrome, microphthalmia, anophthalmia, lacrimal system dysfunction, optic nerve hypoplasia, tortuous retinal vessels, macular hypoplasia and heterotropia, choroidal hyperpigmentation, iris and retinal colobomas	Sporadic Rarely AD and AR
Hallermann-Streiff-Francois syndrome; oculo-mandibulo-dyscephaly (234100)	One case of sclerocornea	Congenital cataracts, spontaneous resorption of lens cortex with secondary membranous cataract formation, glaucoma, uveitis, retinal folds, optic nerve dysplasia, microphthalmia	Sporadic Rarely AD Increased anesthetic risk secondary to tracheomalacia

Table 60.2 Skeletal disorders of interest to the ophthalmologist—cont'd

Name (OMIM #)	Corneal findings	Other ocular findings	Genetics/map/other information
Hypophosphatasia (Infantile: 241500 Childhood: 241510 Adult: 146300)	Band keratopathy with conjunctival calcifications in infantile form	Blue slcerae, cataracts, optic atrophy secondary to craniostenosis, atypical retinitis pigmentosa. Ocular complications present only in infantile and childhood forms, not in adult form	Infantile: AR Childhood: AR, AD Adult: AD *ALPL* gene maps to 1p36-p34
Marfan syndrome (154700)	Megalocornea Flat cornea Keratoconus (uncommon)	Ectopia lentis, strabismus, cataracts, myopia, retinal detachment, glaucoma, flat cornea	AD Gene maps to 15q21.1 Mutations in *FBN1*
Nail-patella syndrome; onycho-osteodysplasia (161200)	Microcornea	Cataracts, microphthalmia	AD Gene maps to 9q34.1 Mutations in *LMX1B* gene
Oculo-dento-osseous dysplasia (AD – 164200 AR – 257850)	Microcornea	Hypotelorism, convergent strabismus, anterior segment dysgenesis, glaucoma, cataracts, remnants of the hyaloid system	AD Mutations in Connexin-43 (*GJA1*) gene on 6q21-23.2
Osteogenesis imperfecta (Type I: 259400 Type II: 166200 Type III: 259420 Type IV: 166220)	Decreased central corneal thickness Keratoconus Megalocornea (rare) Posterior embryotoxon (rare)	Blue sclerae Rare: congenital glaucoma, cataract, choroidal sclerosis, subhyaloid hemorrhage, hyperopia, ectopia lentis	See text
Parry-Romberg syndrome; progressive facial hemiatrophy (141300)	Neuroparalytic keratitis	Enophthalmos, oculomotor palsies, pupillary abnormalities, Horner syndrome, heterochromia, intraocular inflammation, optic nerve hypoplasia, choroidal atrophy	Sporadic 5% bilateral, left > right
Pierre Robin malformation (261800)	Megalocornea (rare)	Congenital glaucoma, high myopia, vitreoretinal degeneration, retinal detachment, esotropia, congenital cataracts, microphthalmia	Sporadic Stickler syndrome in one-third of cases Other syndromes N.B.: increased anesthetic risk secondary to glossoptosis
Rothmund-Thomson syndrome (268400)	Degenerative lesions of cornea	Cataracts	AR 70% female Mutations in DNA helicase (*RECQL4*) gene on 8q24.3
Treacher Collins syndrome; mandibulo-facial dysostosis (154500)	Microcornea	Coloboma of lower lids, dysplasia of bony orbit, absent lower lid cilia, absent lower lid lacrimal punctae, iris coloboma, microphthalmia, strabismus, antimongoloid slant	AD Mutations in treacle (*TCOF1*) gene on 5q32-q33.1
Werner syndrome (277700)	Corneal edema secondary to endothelial decompensation following cataract surgery Poor wound healing	Presenile posterior subcapsular cataracts (20s–30s), proptosis, blue sclerae Rare: nystagmus, astigmatism, telangiectasia of iris, macular degeneration, pigmentary retinopathy	AR Mutations in DNA helicase (*RECQL2*) gene on 8p12-p11

For more information and bibliography on disorders listed in this table consult On-line Mendelian Inheritance in Man (OMIM) at http://www.ncbi.nlm.nih.gov/omim/. The numbers given in column 1 after the disease name(s) are the OMIM entry numbers.
AD, autosomal dominant; AR, autosomal recessive.

cataract, and ectopia lentis are noted infrequently. Wolter reported a patient with Crouzon syndrome and bilateral keratoconus associated with unilateral acute hydrops.[21] Crouzon syndrome is transmitted as an autosomal dominant trait with complete penetrance and a characteristic variability of expression. Approximately one-third of all cases result from new mutations that are highly correlated with advanced paternal age.[22] The gene for this disorder was mapped to 10q26 in the region of the gene coding for the fibroblast growth factor receptor-2 (*FGFR2*).[23] Mutations were soon identified in *FGFR2*.[10,14]

The treatment of Crouzon syndrome consists of craniosynostectomy to relieve increased intracranial pressure. Major cosmetic surgery is often performed in infancy. Strabismus surgery is frequently necessary. Diamond et al. have shown that it is not necessary to delay the strabismus surgery until the extensive facial reconstruction has been completed.[24]

Patients with Apert syndrome have craniosynostosis (abnormal development and premature fusion of the cranial sutures) and symmetric syndactyly of the hands and feet involving at least digits two, three, and four. There may be fusion of the nails as well as the bones of the digits. Premature closure of the coronal suture is typically present. The anterior fontanelle may remain open longer than normal. Sutural involvement is variable and so is skull shape. The occiput is usually flat and the forehead steep. The midface is flat, and the ears may be low-set. The palate is high and arched. Most patients are of normal intelligence but may have learning disabilities. A minority are mentally retarded. Although controversial, craniectomy early in life may have a positive effect on intelligence. Hydrocephalus may be present. In the Apert syndrome, hypertelorism is common. The orbits are flat and shallow with significant proptosis which predisposes to exposure keratopathy. Exotropia with a V-pattern is a common finding. Antimongoloid lid slant and optic atrophy have also been reported. Jadico et al. carried a retrospective review of 18 children carrying either the S252W or the P253R mutations in the *FGFR2* gene and found some differentiating features suggesting phenotype/genotype correlation.[25] Cohen and Kreiborg commented on the cutaneous manifestations on a large series of Apert patients. Hyperhidrosis was characteristic of all patients in their series.[26] Most cases arise from new autosomal dominant mutations, and the disorder has a birth prevalence of 1 in 65 000.[27] Paternal age effect is well documented. In stark contrast with the wide range of mutations in Crouzon syndrome, the spectrum of mutations in Apert syndrome is quite narrow.[28] Two principal mutations in *FGFR2* appear to have differential phenotypic effects, with syndactyly more severe with the P253R mutation and cleft palate more common in S252W patients.[29,30] Although most cases of the Apert syndrome are sporadic (fresh mutations), 11 instances of direct transmission of the disease have been reported,[31] and affected females have given birth to affected children. Increased paternal age and an equal number of affected males and females is compatible with autosomal dominant inheritance.

The Saethre-Chotzen syndrome is characterized by craniosynostosis leading to an asymmetrical skull shape with frontal and parietal bossing. Limb abnormalities include brachydactyly, broad great toes, and cutaneous syndactyly of the second and third digits of the hands and feet. The head circumference is reduced, and the anterior hairline is low. In Saethre-Chotzen syndrome, ptosis and hypertelorism are common and optic atrophy may be seen. Both esotropia and exotropia have been described.[32] Because of phenotypic variability and occasional mild expression, those patients without limb abnormalities may be confused with Crouzon syndrome.[33] Saethre-Chotzen syndrome is an autosomal dominant disorder, maps to chromosome 7p21,[34] and results from mutations in the *TWIST* gene. Mutations in *FGFR2* and *FGFR3* are causative in a minority of patients. *TWIST*, a transcription factor, may affect expression of *FGFRs*, and these genes may be part of a common developmental pathway.[35,36] Surgical correction of skull and digital anomalies may be indicated. Patients are carefully monitored for hydrocephalus. Strabismus surgery should be done as indicated, even before facial reconstructive surgery.

Goldenhar syndrome

The characteristic features of the Goldenhar syndrome, a variant of the oculo-auriculo-vertebral sequence, include malformations of the external ear with preauricular skin tags and pits, vertebral hypoplasia, micrognathia, and epibulbar dermoids (Fig 60.3). The malformations result from errors in morphogenesis of the first and second branchial arches. The presence of epibulbar dermoids is necessary for the diagnosis. Over 70% of patients are males, and when the defect is unilateral, it tends to involve the right side more often than the left. Most patients are of normal intelligence. Hearing loss is frequent, and auditory testing should be performed at an early age. Seventy percent of cases are unilateral and the rest asymmetric. There is hypoplasia of the maxilla and, in some cases, of the mandible. There may be a lateral cleftlike extension of the mouth with a bandlike structure bridging the corner of the mouth to the ear. The parotid and soft palate may be involved with deficient function. Cleft lip and/or palate is occasionally present, as are various abnormalities of the heart, kidneys, limbs, and ribs. Epibulbar dermoids are almost invariably located at the limbus

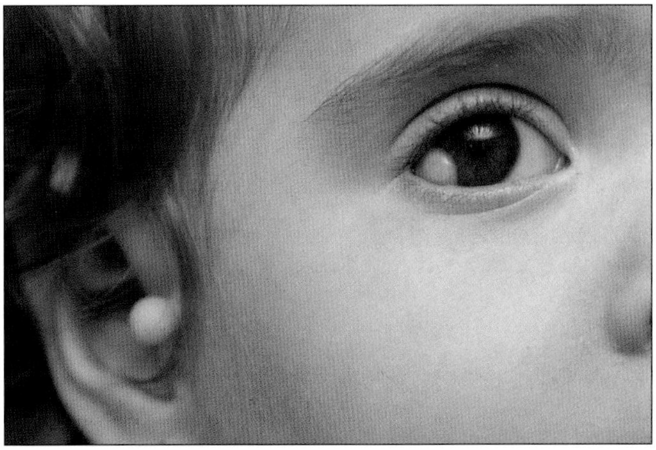

Fig. 60.3 Right preauricular tag and limbal epibulbar dermoid in a patient with Goldenhar syndrome.

inferotemporally in one or both eyes. Baum and Feingold found bilateral limbal dermoids in 23% of cases and unilateral in 53%.[37] Dermoids may cause irregular astigmatism. Anisometropic amblyopia must be constantly suspected and errors of refraction corrected early in life. Subconjunctival dermolipomas are frequently present and occur bilaterally in the superotemporal quadrants of the globe and orbit.

Colobomas of the upper lid are present in about one-fourth of patients with Goldenhar syndrome.[37] The association of Goldenhar syndrome and Duane retraction syndrome has been reported on numerous occasions.[38] Except for one familial report, Goldenhar syndrome is not heritable. In one family, linkage analysis placed the gene at 14q32; however, genetic allelism was suspected.[39]

Indications for the removal of epibulbar dermoids using a superficial keratectomy include continued growth, persistent irritation, and restoration of a more normal ocular appearance. Excision of a lipodermoid may be complicated by its adherence to the conjunctiva, its extension posteriorly around the globe, and its occasional intermixture with lacrimal gland tissue. A lamellar graft may be necessary if the tumor is exceedingly large. Incomplete excision of an extensive lesion is recommended over exploratory surgery in the orbit.[40,41]

Hallermann-Streiff syndrome (oculomandibulodyscephaly, Francois dyscephalic syndrome)

Patients with the Hallermann-Streiff syndrome have a receding chin resulting from hypoplasia of the mandible. They have a pinched, thin nose and a bulging head.[42,43] Scalp and facial hair is scanty. The skin over the scalp, face, nose, and, at times, extremities is strikingly atrophic, revealing the underlying dermal vasculature.[44] Malocclusion, absent or malformed teeth, persistence of deciduous teeth, and the presence of teeth at birth have all been observed. Proportional dwarfism is the rule, with an average adult height of around 5 feet. Mental retardation is present in about 15% of affected individuals. Respiratory infections and pulmonary insufficiency may cause death in infancy. However, a normal life span is possible. Cases are most often sporadic, and chromosome analysis is unrevealing.

Bilateral microphthalmos and congenital cataracts are present in almost every patient and usually account for the first visit to a physician. Microcornea or a small anterior segment may be present with a normal-sized posterior segment.[44] Spontaneous rupture and resorption of the crystalline lens occur frequently,[44,45] and a phacoanaphylactic reaction has been demonstrated histopathologically.[46] Late iridocyclitis, angle closure, rubeosis iridis, retinal neovascularization, and retinal detachment may occur after lens resorption. Hopkins and Horan reviewed five patients with glaucoma from the literature and presented two new cases.[47] They found that glaucoma usually occurred after cataract surgery or after resorption of the lens with persistent granulomatous uveitis. Posterior and peripheral anterior synechiae are common. Intraocular pressure is particularly high when the uveitis is active. Chorioretinal atrophy, retinal dystrophy with an abnormal ERG,[44] retinal folds, blue sclerae, and antimongoloid lid fissures have been reported occasionally.[47] Newell et al. reported the unique occurrence of bilateral Coats disease in a patient with Hallermann-Streiff syndrome.[48]

Cataracts should be extracted as soon as they are diagnosed to circumvent spontaneous lens rupture and phacolytic complications. Intraocular inflammation should be treated promptly with topical steroids and cycloplegic agents. Glaucoma in these patients has responded in some to miotics and carbonic anhydrase inhibitors. A review of potential anesthetic problems in these patients is strongly recommended before ocular surgery.[49]

Treacher Collins syndrome (mandibulofacial dysostosis; Franceschetti syndrome)

Patients with this condition have antimongoloid slanting of the palpebral fissures, mandibular and malar hypoplasia, malformed external ears, and colobomas of the lower lids. Deafness occurs in 50% of patients. The face has been described as being 'bird-like' in appearance. There may be grooves, clefts, or pits on the cheek between the mouth and the ear.[50] Most patients are of normal intelligence. Other common clinical findings include macrostomia, dental malocclusion, high-arched palate, and a high nasal root. The clinical features of this syndrome result from an abnormality in development of structures derived from the first branchial arch. The mode of inheritance is autosomal dominant with full penetrance and wide variability in expression in families.[51] Sixty percent of cases result from new mutations in the *TCOF-1* gene at 5q32-q33.1.[52–54]

Ophthalmic abnormalities include antimongoloid slanting of the lids and lower lid colobomas, with partial to total absence of the eyelashes. Occasionally, colobomas may involve the upper lid, but this is more characteristic of Goldenhar syndrome. Orbital lipodermoids and corneoscleral dermoids may be present, making the differentiation from Goldenhar syndrome sometimes difficult. Microphthalmia and defects of the orbital rim are occasionally present.[55] Intraocular structures are rarely affected.[56]

Ehlers-Danlos syndrome

Ehlers-Danlos syndrome (EDS) comprises a heterogeneous group of connective tissue disorders characterized by hyperextensibility of the joints (Fig. 60.4) and skin and easy bruisability with formation of peculiar 'cigarette paper' scars (Fig. 60.5). A number of distinct clinical types are recognized on the basis of biochemical, genetic, and clinical findings (Table 60.3). The identification of underlying genetic defects will continue to elucidate the relationships among the various EDS forms.

EDS type I (gravis type) is the most common severe form. The skin is remarkably hyperextensible and bruises easily. Cigarette paper-like scarring is present over the forehead, chin, elbows, knees, and shins. Generalized tissue friability makes healing difficult. The eyelids are easily stretched and everted. Mutations in collagen genes *COL5A1* (9q34.2-q34.3), *COL5A2* (2q31), and *COL1A1* (17q21.31-q22) account for this most severe form of EDS.[57] EDS type II resembles type I but has milder clinical findings and was hence called

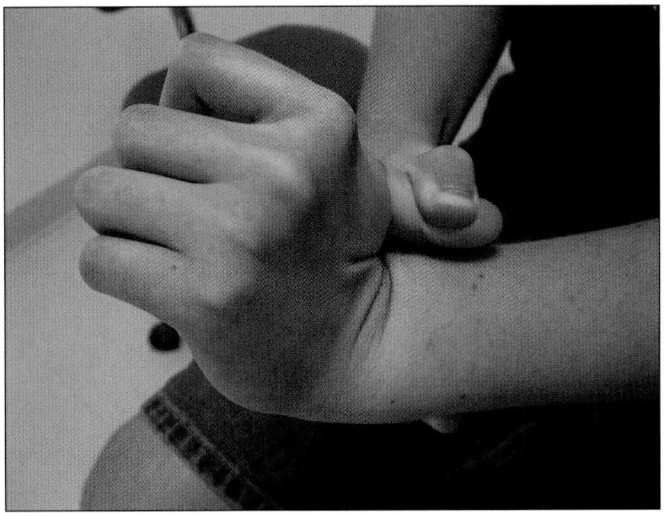

Fig. 60.4 Hyperextension of thumb in a patient with Ehlers-Danlos syndrome.

'mitis' type. It is now recognized that types I and II are part of a clinical and molecular spectrum and demonstrate genetic heterogeneity.[58] In fact, a new descriptive classification scheme proposed by Beighton et al. consider type I and II together as the 'classic' form of EDS.[59] Both adhere to autosomal dominant inheritance patterns. In EDS type III (hypermobility type) there is severe hypermobility of all joints without other musculoskeletal abnormalities. Skin changes are minimal. Inheritance is autosomal dominant. Mutations in the *COL3A1* gene (2q31) cause at least some cases of the hypermobility type of EDS.[60] Mutations in *COL3A1* also cause EDS type IV, or 'vascular' type.[61] EDS type IV is transmitted in an autosomal dominant manner. Various abnormalities of the large to medium-sized arterial vessels predominate. Spontaneous arterial rupture may occur at a young age. Spontaneous carotid-cavernous fistula at presentation has been reported several times.[62] Ocular complications of EDS type IV relate exclusively to carotid-cavernous fistulas, which give rise to subjective ocular bruits, proptosis, conjunctival hyperemia/chemosis, blurred vision, diplopia, and orbital pain. Compromised perfusion can lead to ocular ischemia.[63] Perforation of the bowel is an associated finding. The skin is very thin and transparent and may show elastosis perforans serpiginosa. Hyperextensibility of the joints and skin laxity are minimal. Patients with EDS type V have minimal joint hypermobility and a markedly hyperextensible skin. Floppy mitral valve may be an associated feature. EDS type V is inherited in an X-linked recessive fashion. EDS type VII is characterized by short stature and extreme generalized joint hypermobility. Subluxation of the hips, knees, and feet is common. The skin is moderately stretchable and easily bruisable. Hypertelorism and epicanthal folds are common in EDS type VII. EDS type VII is further divided into autosomal dominant and autosomal recessive forms. Autosomal dominant forms are caused by mutations in at least two loci, *COL1A1* (17q21.31-q22) and *COL1A2* (7q22.1), each with differential phenotypic effects.[64] Autosomal recessive EDS type VII result from mutations in the *ADAMTS2* gene (5q23), or procollagen I N-proteinase (*NPI*), the enzyme that excises the N-propeptide of type I and type II procollagens.[65]

Of most interest to the ophthalmologist is EDS type VI, characterized by severe scoliosis with moderate joint and skin involvement. The hyperextensibility and joint laxity are not as severe as in EDS type I (gravis type). Rupture of the globe or retinal detachment in type VI may occur from minor trauma. EDS type VI-A results from deficiency of the enzyme lysyl hydroxylase (1p36.3-p36.2) and subsequent abnormality in the cross-linking of collagen.[66] Spontaneous rupture of the globe, however, has been observed in the absence of lysyl hydroxylase deficiency.[67] This type is now designated EDS type VI-B, which includes the once separate brittle cornea syndrome. Both forms are inherited in an autosomal recessive manner. Patients with EDS type VI-B may have macrocephaly. The patients reported by Judisch et al. apparently have EDS type VI with macrocephaly.[67] Even within the EDS type VI classification, there is marked genetic heterogeneity. One example has been described in Tunisian Jews[68] and in a Syrian girl.[69] This form is characterized by blue sclerae, large cloudy, thin, fragile, bulging corneas with normal intraocular pressure, dental anomalies similar to those of osteogenesis imperfecta, predisposition to bone fractures, long slender hyperextensible fingers, hernias, and red hair. Farag and Schimke reported a Bedouin brother and sister with EDS type VI and polyneuropathy and proposed that this was another variant of the oculoscoliotic type of the disease, and further evidence of heterogeneity.[70] These last patients had blue sclerae, myopia, ocular fragility, and retinal detachment. May and Beauchamp reported a 15-year-old patient with type I or type VI EDS who had microcornea, cornea plana, posterior embryotoxon, and keratoconus posticus.[71] Cameron found a halo sign at the limbus in 11 patients with EDS type VI; corneal rupture occurred in seven patients, bilateral microcornea in one patient, megalocornea as a result of glaucoma in two patients, peripheral sclerocornea in five patients, and abnormalities of corneal curvature such as cornea plana, keratoconus, or keratoglobus in all patients.[72,73] Heim et al. described an Iranian patient with kyphoscoliosis, glaucoma, microcornea, myopia, brownish sclerae, and tortuous retinal arteries.[74] Keratoglobus with brittle cornea and blue sclera may result in acute hydrops and in corneal rupture, either spontaneously or from minor trauma.[75,76] Biglan et al. reported corneal perforations in 15 of 20 patients before the age of 18 years.[77] Repair proved difficult, and many eyes needed to be eviscerated or enucleated. Cameron and co-workers performed prophylactic epikeratophakia in six patients with good tectonic results in five.[73] All their patients had keratoglobus (Fig. 60.6) and joint hyperextensibility. Four had previous corneal rupture in one eye; one had scarring from hydrops; and one had a sister with the disease. These authors advocated the use of a 12.5-mm lenticule sutured onto the intact recipient cornea. The edge of the lenticule is covered by the recipient limbal conjunctiva. Macsai et al. applied a novel surgical technique to treat a ruptured globe in a patient with keratoglobus, successfully combining onlay epikeratoplasty with a delayed full-thickness corneal graft.[78] Nakazawa and colleagues used preserved sclera to patch a post-traumatic scleral staphyloma in a 38-year-old woman with type VI EDS.[79]

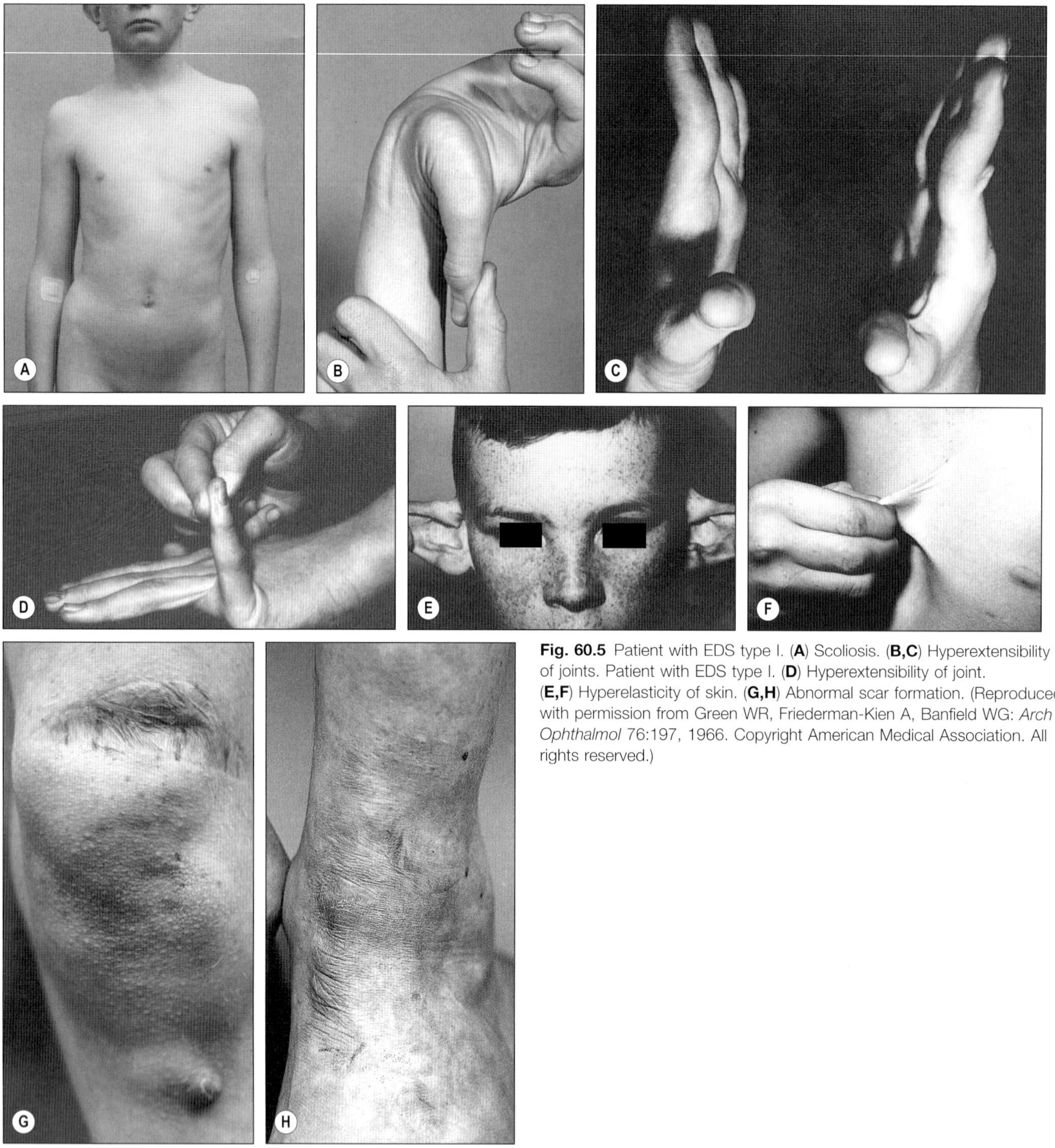

Fig. 60.5 Patient with EDS type I. (**A**) Scoliosis. (**B,C**) Hyperextensibility of joints. Patient with EDS type I. (**D**) Hyperextensibility of joint. (**E,F**) Hyperelasticity of skin. (**G,H**) Abnormal scar formation. (Reproduced with permission from Green WR, Friederman-Kien A, Banfield WG: *Arch Ophthalmol* 76:197, 1966. Copyright American Medical Association. All rights reserved.)

Table 60.3 Clinical and genetic classification of EDS

Type and MIM No.	Clinical features	Inheritance/genetic defect/gene map
Type I: gravis, classic, severe (130000)	Most common; hyperextensible skin; easy bruisability; cigarette-paper scarring; mitral valve prolapse; joint dislocation; spontaneous bowel rupture; premature rupture of fetal membranes	Autosomal dominant/*COL5A1*, *COL5A2* or *COL1A1*/17q21.31-q22, 9q34.2-q34.3, or 2q31
Type II: mitis, mild, classic (130010)	Like type I but milder	Autosomal dominant/*COL5A1* or *COL5A2*/9q34.2-q34.3
Type III: benign hypermobility syndrome (130020)	Severe hypermobility of all joints without musculoskeletal abnormalities; minimal skin changes	Autosomal dominant/*COL3A1*, Tenascin-XB/2q31
Type IV: arterial, ecchymotic, of Sack (130050, 225350, 225360)	Abnormalities of medium and large arteries with spontaneous arterial rupture at a young age; bowel perforation; thin and transparent skin; minimal hyperextensibility of joints and skin laxity; recessive more severe than dominant type	Autosomal dominant, autosomal recessive, genetic heterogeneity/*COL3A1*/2q31
Type V: X-linked (305200)	Minimal joint hypermobility; marked skin hyperextensibility; mitral valve prolapse	X-linked recessive/?lysyl oxidase deficiency
Type VI-A: oculo-scoliotic (225400, 153454)	Mitral valve prolapse; multiple arterial aneurysms; kyphoscoliosis; distal interphalangeal joint hypermobility; blue sclerae; retinal detachment; myopia	Autosomal recessive/lysyl hydroxylase deficiency/1p36.3-p36.2
Brittle cornea syndrome (229200)	Joint hypermobility; blue sclerae; spontaneous perforation of the globe; keratoconus; keratoglobus	May be same as type VI-A
Type VI-B: brittle cornea with macrocephaly (229200)	Blue sclerae; spontaneous perforation of the globe; keratoconus	Autosomal recessive/normal lysyl hydroxylase
Type VII-A and B: (130060)	Arthrochalasis multiplex congenita; short stature; skin hyperextensibility and bruisability	Autosomal dominant/*COL1A1*, *COL1A2*/17q21.31-q22, 7q22.1
Type VII-C (225410)	Short stature; extreme generalized joint hypermobility; hypertelorism; very fragile tearable skin (dermatosparaxis type)	Autosomal recessive/*ADAMTS2* gene/5q23
Type VIII (130080)	Cigarette-paper scars; periodontal disease; mitral valve prolapse; joint hypermobility of distal interphalangeal joints	Autosomal dominant
Type IX (304150)	Cutis laxa, not EDS; previously EDS with occipital horns	X-linked recessive
Type X (225310)	Defective platelet aggregation with collagen; striae distensae; loose joints; hyperelastic skin	Possible fibronectin defect
Type XI (147900)	Familial joint laxity; recurrent joint dislocation	Autosomal dominant
Unclassified (130090)	Hernias; foot deformities; thoracic deformities; stretchable and thin skin; facial asymmetry; kyphoscoliosis; cystic medial necrosis of aorta	Autosomal dominant
Progeroid (130070)	Short stature; osteopenia; bone dysplasia; periodontosis; nevi; loose and elastic skin; scanty hair; hypermobile joints; lack of progeric features such as diminished subcutaneous fat, prominent scalp veins, and joint contractures	Autosomal dominant/xylosylprotein 4-β-galactosyltransferase/5q35.2-q35.3

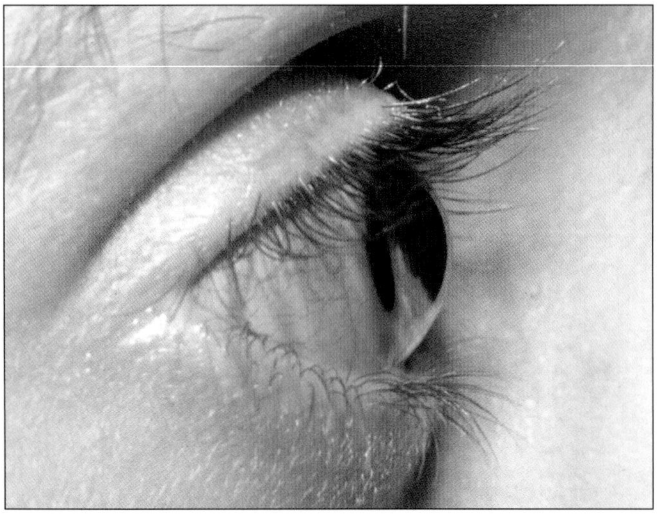

Fig. 60.6 Keratoglobus in a patient with EDS type VI. (Courtesy Jay Krachmer, MD.)

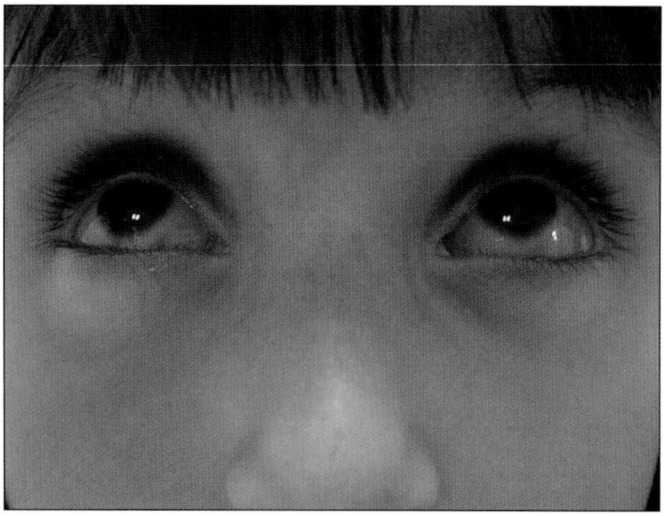

Fig. 60.8 Blue sclerae in a patient with osteogenesis imperfecta.

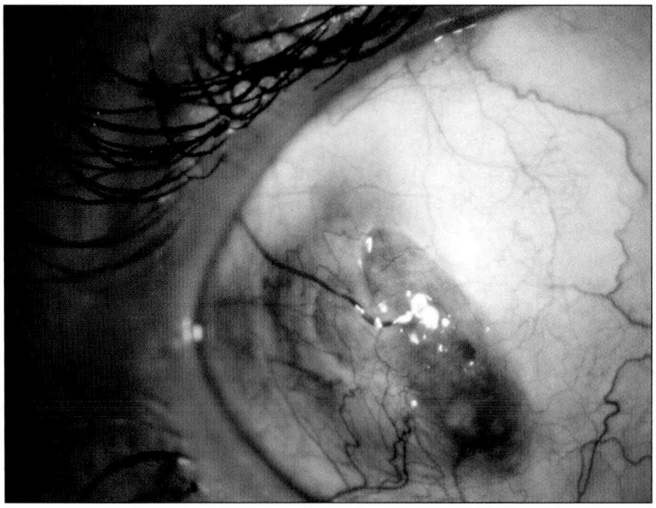

Fig. 60.7 Severe scleral thinning in area of previous strabismus surgery in patient with EDS.

Epicanthal folds are the most common ocular finding in EDS but are of little functional significance. Strabismus may also be found. Repair of strabismus may be complicated by severe thinning of the sclera at the site of the original muscle insertion (personal observation) (Fig. 60.7). Subluxation of the crystalline lens has been described in patients with EDS but is extremely uncommon; its occurrence in a patient suspected of having EDS probaly indicates a diagnosis of Marfan syndrome. Myopia is very prevalent. Spontaneous and traumatic retinal detachment most frequently occur in EDS type VI.[80] Green et al. described the occurrence of angioid streaks in a mother and daughter with a dominant form of EDS.[81] Other affected and nonaffected family members were examined and did not have angioid streaks. Pouliquen et al. reported a 6-year-old boy with a benign form of EDS (type unspecified), megalocornea, and fine, lamellar, nonhomogeneous opacities in the deep corneal stroma with 'microcraters' in Descemet's membrane and a few subepithelial opacities.[82] The significance of these findings is unclear. They may result from the collagen abnormalities or may be coincidental. In this era of keratorefractive surgery, a high suspicion of connective tissue defects such as EDS should be maintained by the refractive surgeon, as its presence could potentially have a negative impact on the outcome of surgery.[83]

Osteogenesis imperfecta

Four clinical types of osteogenesis imperfecta (OI) are recognized and are caused by abnormalities of the a_1 or a_2 chains of type I collagen.[84,85] There is failure of type I collagen fibers to mature to their normal diameter. Mutations in the *COL1A1* (17q21.31-q22) and *COL1A2* genes (7q22.1) account for most cases in all four types. The location of the mutation in the gene seems to determine the clinical phenotype.[86,87] OI occurs in about 1 in 20 000 live births. The skeleton, ears, eyes, teeth, skin, and joints are involved. Conductive or mixed-type hearing loss occurs in about 50% of families and begins in the late teens. This gradually leads to profound deafness, tinnitus, and vertigo by the fourth or fifth decades.[88,89] The diagnosis of OI is based on clinical, dental, and radiologic criteria.

Individuals with type I OI have bright-blue sclerae that remain intensely blue throughout life (Fig. 60.8). In types III and IV, the sclerae may be blue at birth, but the intensity of the discoloration decreases with time and the sclera is of normal color by adulthood. The blue coloration results from visualization of the underlying choroid through a thin sclera. Kaiser-Kupfer et al. found ocular rigidity to be reduced in a group of 16 patients with different types of OI.[90] The perilimbal region is often whiter than the remaining sclera, resulting in the so-called 'Saturn's ring.'

Electron microscopy reveals reduction in the diameter of collagen fibers and change in their cross-striation pattern.[91] Blue sclerae are also present in EDS type VI and in small children with hypophosphatasia. Optic nerve damage may result from deformities or fractures of calvarial bones. Posterior embryotoxon, keratoconus, and megalocornea may be present. Rare ocular findings include congenital glaucoma, cataracts, choroidal sclerosis, and subhyaloid hemorrhage. In a series of 53 patients, central corneal thickness was reduced to a mean 0.443 mm as compared to 0.522 mm in normal control groups ($p < 0.001$).[89] Hyperopia is common. Spontaneous rupture of the globe is very rare.

Patients with OI need aggressive orthopedic management of fractures to prevent extensive deformities of the extremities and spine. Patients with the severe congenital form rarely survive beyond the first few years of life. Many become wheelchair bound because of extensive limb and spine deformities. Promising new therapy with intravenous bisphosphonates has resulted in striking reduction in the frequency of new fractures in OI patients.[92] Bisphosphonates inhibit osteoclastic bone resorption, and have been used successfully to treat osteoporosis, Paget disease of bone, and fibrous dysplasia. Moreover, the safety and efficacy for the use of bisphosphonates in children has been established.[93–95]

Stickler syndrome (hereditary progressive arthro-ophthalmopathy), Wagner syndrome, and Marshall syndrome

There is extensive clinical heterogeneity in Stickler syndrome, the most common dominantly inherited disorder of collagen.[96–100] Until recently, the disorder was divided into a number of clinical subtypes including a marfanoid variant, a variant with the Pierre Robin anomaly, and patients with a classic phenotype consisting of a flattened face and a depressed bridge of the nose. A new classification is now based on genotypic diversity. Furthermore, the relationship of Stickler syndrome to Wagner and Marshall syndromes has been clarified. The incidence of Stickler syndrome is estimated at 1:20000 live births. Opitz et al. believe that Stickler syndrome is more common than Marfan syndrome.[99] Sensorineural hearing loss occurs in about 25% of patients and cleft palate in 25% of patients. A progressive arthropathy that is commonly subtle early in life becomes most pronounced in the fourth or fifth decade in many patients, with stiffness, soreness, and sometimes arthritic changes. Some patients have hyperextensible joints. Radiologic evidence of flattened epiphyseal centers is noted early in life and, together with congenital myopia, constitutes the minimal diagnostic criteria for the Stickler syndrome. Mitral valve prolapse occurs in up to 45% of patients.[101] Patients with Wagner disease have ocular abnormalities that resemble those of Stickler syndrome, but lack skeletal abnormalities. Marshall syndrome is typically associated with high myopia, vitreoretinal degeneration, cataract, characteristic mid-facial hypoplasia, but a lack of arthropathy. Stickler et al. analyzed questionnaire replies and concluded that there is significant clinical heterogeneity in Stickler syndrome, even within a single family.[102]

Stickler syndrome type I (STL1) is due to mutations in the *COL2A1* gene. Descriptively referred to as the 'membranous vitreous type,' this form represents two-thirds of Stickler syndrome cases. *COL2A1* localizes to 12q13.11-q13.2,[103] and mutations have been identified in the *COL2A1* gene in several families with the Stickler syndrome.[104] The gene responsible for the disease in Wagner's original pedigree[105] was excluded from the *COL2A1* location, and later mapped to 5q13-14 by Brown et al.[106] The disease was discovered to be caused by mutations in the *GSPG2* gene that encodes versican, a large proteoglycan, which is an extracellular matrix component of the human vitreous and participates in the formation of the vitreous gel.[107] The same year, Kloeckener-Gruissem discovered a splice site mutation in *GSPG2* in the original family reported by Wagner.[108] The significance of the genetic allelism with STL1 described by Korkko et al. in a family with Wagner vitreoretinal degeneration is unclear.[109] Subsequent to the discovery of *COL2A1* linkage with Sticker syndrome type I,[110] mutations in *COL11A1* (1p21) were shown to cause a second form of Stickler syndrome, referred to as type II or the 'beaded vitreous type.'[111] Stickler syndrome type II is allelic with Marshall syndrome, and there is significant clinical overlap as well. While some believe the syndromes are clinically distinct,[112] Marshall emphasized ectodermal abnormalities, specifically in sweat glands and dentition, in the original description of the syndrome.[113] Shanske et al. described a similar family with ectodermal dysplasia and ocular hypertelorism.[114] These features are not consistent with Stickler syndrome. There is no uncertainty that Stickler syndrome type I differs from Marshall syndrome; however, phenotypic overlap in *COL11A1* mutations raise questions about the separateness of the type II Stickler and Marshall syndromes.[115,116] Hence, Marshall-Stickler syndrome is sometimes advocated in the literature.

A third form of Stickler syndrome, type III, is also descriptively named the 'nonocular type.' Brunner et al. recognized this phenotype in a Dutch kindred.[117] In this family, affected individuals manifested the facial features of Stickler syndrome, hearing deficits, and skeletal abnormalities. However, high myopia and vitreoretinal abnormalities were nonexistent. Brunner found close linkage in the 6p21.3 region, and Vikkula et al. later identified a nonsense mutation in the *COL11A2* gene in the same family.[118] Others have discovered similar *COL11A2* mutations causing the Stickler phenotype.[119]

The ocular findings in Stickler syndrome include congenital and generally stable high myopia,[120] presenile cataracts, and vitreoretinal degeneration; retinal detachment is common.[121,122] Vitreous phenotypes differ between types I and II Stickler syndrome. In patients with *COL2A1* mutations (type I) the vitreous is described as 'membranous,' whereas patients with *COL11A1* mutations manifest a different 'beaded' vitreous type.[123] Richards et al. noted that vitreous slit lamp biomicroscopy alone is able to distinguish the two types.[124] Radial perivascular patches of lattice degeneration are present in the posterior pole and midperiphery. Glaucoma develops in a significant number of patients. Rarely, patients develop subluxation of the lens. In Marshall syndrome, spontaneous rupture of the anterior and posterior lens capsule has been observed associated with acute glaucoma.[125] Lastly, in both Stickler and Marshall-Stickler syndromes, there may be an association with retinal capillary hemangiomas that is unrelated to von Hippel-Lindau syndrome.[126,127]

Retinal detachment in Stickler syndrome is prevented by repeated careful ophthalmoscopic examinations and prophylactic treatment of retinal holes.[128] Screening for hearing loss is mandatory in infants with Stickler syndrome. The diagnosis of Stickler syndrome should be suspected in patients with the Pierre Robin malformation complex, in those with dominantly inherited myopia[129] with or without retinal detachment and deafness, in patients with dominantly inherited cleft palate, in those with mild spondyloepiphyseal dysplasia, and in patients with dominantly inherited mitral valve prolapse syndrome. It should be emphasized that the main ocular manifestations of Stickler syndrome can be identified at an early age, which should allow for proper counseling and help to prevent grave visual outcomes.[120]

Kniest dysplasia

Kniest dysplasia is a bone dysplasia characterized by short stature, prominent wide joints, a short trunk with a broad thorax and protrusion of the sternum, and a flat midface with depressed nasal bridge (Fig. 60.9).[130] Cleft palate is present in about 40% of patients, and 75% of patients have hearing loss.

There is severe vitreoretinal degeneration with a high rate of retinal detachment (five eyes of seven patients in one series).[131] The retinal detachments frequently result from giant tears or retinal dialysis. All patients have congenital stable severe myopia and oblique astigmatism. Cataracts may develop in the first or second decade of life. Subluxation of the lens and glaucoma are rare findings.

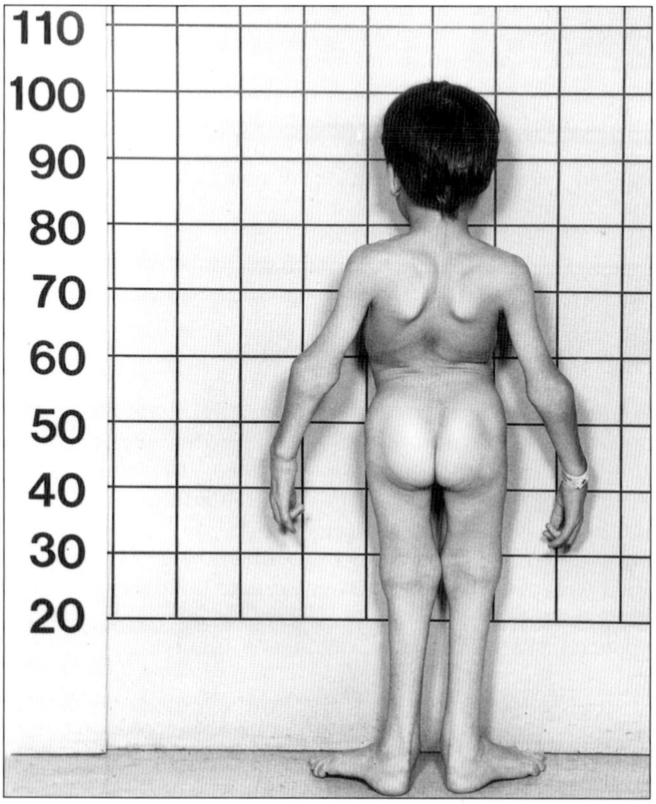

Fig. 60.9 Patient with Kniest dysplasia. The trunk is short, and the epiphyses are broad. There is contracture of the fingers.

Inheritance is autosomal dominant. Mutations in the *COL2A1* gene (12q13.11-q13.2) are causative for Kniest dysplasia.[132–134]

Marfan syndrome

Marfan syndrome is a systemic connective tissue disorder caused by mutations in the fibrillin-1 gene. It was originally believed that Marfan syndrome results exclusively from the production of abnormal fibrillin-1 that leads to structurally weaker connective tissue when incorporated into the extracellular matrix. This effect seemed to explain many of the clinical features of Marfan syndrome, including aortic root dilatation and acute aortic dissection, which represent the main causes of morbidity and mortality in Marfan syndrome. Recent molecular studies, most based on genetically defined mouse models of Marfan syndrome, have challenged this paradigm. These studies established the critical contribution of fibrillin-1 haploinsufficiency and dysregulated transforming growth factor-β (TGF-β) signaling to disease progression. It seems that many manifestations of Marfan syndrome are less related to a primary structural deficiency of the tissues than to altered morphogenetic and homeostatic programs that are induced by altered transforming growth factor-beta signaling. Most important, TGF-β antagonism, through TGF-β neutralizing antibodies or losartan (an angiotensin II type 1 receptor antagonist), has been shown to prevent and possibly reverse aortic root dilatation, mitral valve prolapse, lung disease, and skeletal muscle dysfunction in a mouse model of Marfan syndrome. There are indicators that losartan, a drug widely used to treat arterial hypertension in humans, offers the first potential for primary prevention of clinical manifestations in Marfan syndrome.[135]

Marfan syndrome[136] is characterized by abnormalities in three systems: ocular (ectopia lentis), cardiovascular (dilation of the aortic root and aneurysm of the ascending aorta, and aortic aneurysm), and skeletal (dolichostenomelia, upper segment/lower segment ratio two standard deviations below mean for age, pectus excavatum, and kyphoscoliosis).[137] In addition to these three major criteria, auxiliary signs include myopia, mitral valve prolapse, arachnodactyly, joint laxity, tall stature, pes planus, striae distensae, pneumothorax, and dural ectasia in a large number of patients.[138] Dural ectasia can be reliably identified by CT or MRI. The disease has a frequency of 1 per 20 000 persons. Using linkage analysis, the gene for Marfan syndrome was mapped to chromosome 15 in the region of the fibrillin-1 gene.[139] Soon after, mutations were detected in the fibrillin-1 gene in a number of patients with Marfan syndrome.[140]

The most characteristic and diagnostic ocular abnormality in the Marfan syndrome is subluxation of the crystalline lens (Fig. 60.10).[141,142] Lens zonules are abnormally weak because of their defective fibrillin component.[143,144] Immunohistochemical techniques have recently elucidated a potential role of matrix metalloproteinases and the dysregulation of protease inhibitors in fibrillin degradation in Marfan patients.[145] It is intriguing to hypothesize future therapies based on these findings. In Marfan syndrome, the degree of subluxation varies from mild superior and

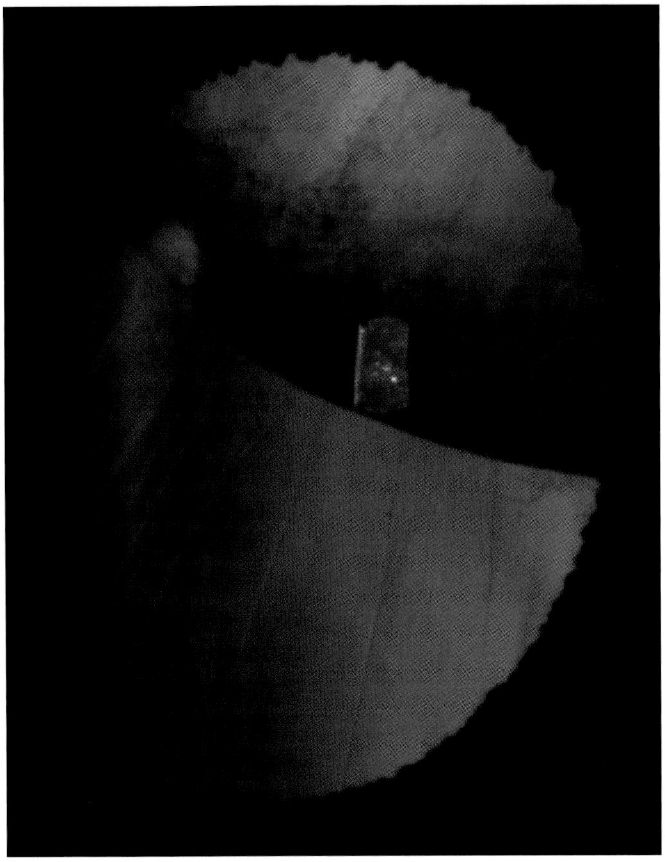

Fig. 60.10 Superotemporal dislocation of lens in a 40-year-old patient with Marfan syndrome. Note stretched zonules.

posterior displacement, evident only on maximal pupillary dilation, to significant subluxation, placing the equator of the lens in the pupillary axis. Although superior and temporal displacement of the lens is most common, inferior, nasal, or lateral movement also occurs. Subluxation of the lens is slowly progressive in some patients and most noticeable in the first few years of life or in the late teens and early twenties; in most patients, however, no progression of the displacement is noted over the years. Total dislocation into the vitreous cavity is unusual in young patients but occurs in older patients, where it may rarely be complicated by phacolytic glaucoma. Lens dislocation into the pupil or the anterior chamber is much more characteristic of untreated homocystinuria.

In Marfan syndrome, stretched zonular fibers can be seen through the dilated pupil. In places where zonules have ruptured, a straightening of the lens contour is noted and has been referred to as a coloboma of the lens. Microspherophakia is present in about 15% of patients and results in high myopia. The cornea is flat with keratometric readings in the high 30s in about 20% of patients.[141] Sultan et al. noted that Marfan syndrome is associated with corneal thinning, and that reduced pachymetric readings were highly correlated with ectopia lentis.[146] More recently, I explored the utility of keratometry and central corneal thickness (CCT) measurements in diagnosis of Marfan syndrome.[147] I reviewed the charts of 211 patients referred for ocular examination to rule out Marfan syndrome. Sixty-two patients met the diagnostic criteria for Marfan syndrome and 98 patients were assigned to the control group. Marfan patients had significantly lower keratometry and CCT values than controls (40.8 D Marfan vs 43.3 D controls) (Fig. 60.11); and

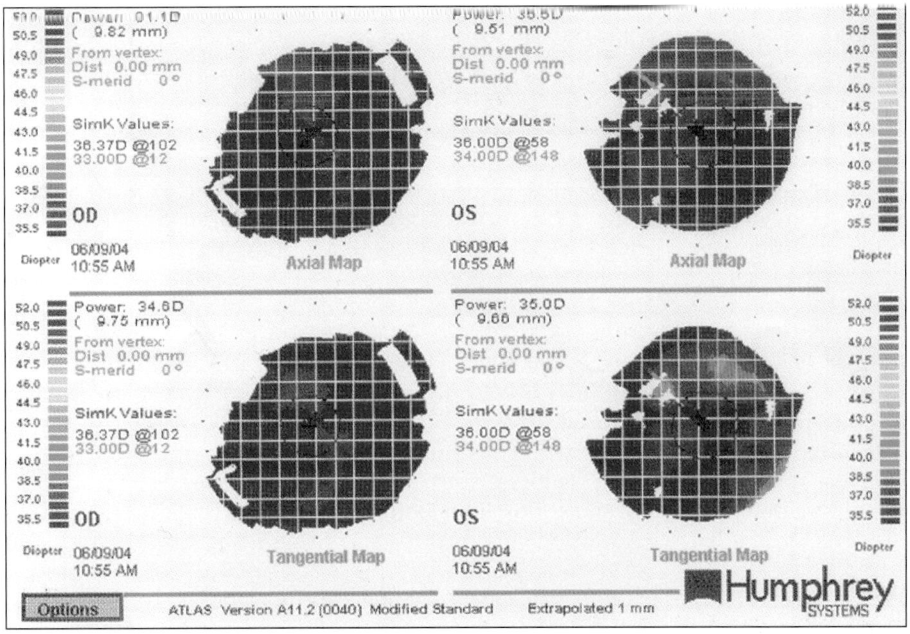

Fig. 60.11 Flat corneas in a patient with Marfan syndrome.

543.5 microns (μm) Marfan vs 564.2 microns (μm) controls). In Marfan syndrome patients without ectopia lentis, these values were 41.5 D (p = 0.00026 vs control) and 542.0 microns (μm). I concluded that there was a highly significant difference in keratometry values between Marfan and control patients, and values less than 42 D could be used as a clinical diagnostic criterion for Marfan syndrome. Significant overlap in CCT values between Marfan and control patients suggested that further investigations were necessary to determine their clinical utility.[147] Megalocornea (corneal diameter measuring more than 13.5 mm) may be present in some patients. The iris has a thin velvety texture, and the pupil is difficult to dilate in some patients. This results from atrophy of the dilator muscle fibers. Exotropia occurs in about 10% and esotropia in 2% of patients.[148] Strabismic and/or anisometropic or ametropic amblyopia may be present and responds surprisingly well to optical correction and penalization despite years of uncorrected high errors of refraction. Open-angle glaucoma is significantly more common in patients with Marfan syndrome in all age groups as compared to the general population, and it becomes more prevalent in this disease with increasing patient age.[149] Pupillary block is unusual but has been documented. Phacolytic glaucoma has been noted in older patients with mature dislocated lenses and carries a guarded prognosis because of the complex vitreoretinal surgery needed to extract the hard cataractous lenses. Retinal detachment may occur spontaneously in eyes with axial myopia or after cataract extraction, especially in longer eyes. Cataracts develop earlier than in the general population and, in most cases, are the indication for lens extraction. Occasionally, poor vision from high astigmatic errors of refraction from lenses whose equator is in the middle of a small pupillary area leads to a surgical decision. Sometimes, lens removal is necessary at an early age to avoid development of amblyopia. Finally, the very rare recurrent dislocation into the anterior chamber may prompt lens extraction.

The surgical management of ectopia lentis is varied and controversial, and beyond the scope of this chapter to discuss all available techniques. Some prefer complete pars plana lensectomy with vitrectomy, which avoids traction on the vitreous base.[150] Others favor the preservation of the posterior capsule with anterior lensectomy techniques. Limbal approaches are often deemed necessary when a lens dislocates into the anterior chamber.[151] Transscleral fixation of the intraocular lens has been used in adults when capsular support is inadequate.[152] Anterior chamber lenses are considered safe and effective by some.[150] In the pediatric population, many feel that intraocular lenses of either type have unpredictable and potentially hazardous outcomes, and consider aphakic correction to be a more sound alternative.[151] I favor a clear corneal incision with total lensectomy and leaving the children aphakic. To date, there are no large-scale studies that compare the various available treatments for lens subluxation.

Some infants with Marfan syndrome can be severely affected and present major orthopedic and cardiovascular therapeutic challenges.[153,154] The use of beta-blockers and complex surgical procedures has allowed patients with Marfan syndrome to survive longer than into the third or fourth decade.[155] In fact, there has been more than a 25% increase in the life expectancy in Marfan since 1972.[156] In 1998, Gray et al. reported the median survival as 53 years for men and 72 for women.[157]

Progressive enlargement of the aortic root, leading to dissection, is the main cause of premature death in patients with Marfan syndrome. Following the discovery by Habashi et al.[158] that aortic root enlargement in mouse models of Marfan syndrome is caused by excessive signaling by TGF-β that can be mitigated by treatment with TGF-β antagonists, including angiotensin II-receptor blockers (ARBs). Brooke et al. evaluated the clinical response to ARBs in 18 pediatric patients with Marfan syndrome who had severe aortic root enlargement. They found that the mean rate of change in aortic root diameter decreased significantly from 3.54 ± 2.87 mm per year during previous medical therapy to 0.46 ± 0.62 mm per year during ARB therapy ($p < 0.001$). They also found that the sinotubular junction, which is prone to dilation in Marfan syndrome as well, also showed a reduced rate of change in diameter during ARB therapy ($p < 0.05$), whereas the distal ascending aorta, which does not normally become dilated in Marfan syndrome, was not affected by ARB therapy.[159] Multicenter treatment trials are under way to confirm these findings.

Oculo-dento-osseous dysplasia

Oculo-dento-osseous dysplasia (ODOD) is a malformation syndrome involving the hair, face, eyes, teeth, and bones (Fig. 60.12).[160,161] It is inherited in an autosomal dominant fashion, but a recessive variety probably exists.[162,163] Linkage studies have mapped the locus for ODOD to chromosome 6.[164] The connexin-43 gene, which is on 6q21-q23.2, was analyzed as a candidate for ODOD and identified mutations in all 17 families studied.[165] Patients have a characteristic physiognomy: facies with scarce eyebrows, narrow and short palpebral fissures, microcornea or microphthalmia, and a small nose with hypoplastic alae nasae and a prominent columella. The dental enamel is dysplastic, and microdontia or hypodontia may be present. The most conspicuous skeletal abnormalities are camptodactyly or syndactyly of the ulnar two or three digits. The toes are short and frequently lack second metatarsals. Other skeletal abnormalities include calvarial hyperostosis, a heavy mandible with an obtuse angle between the body and rami, plump clavicles, thickened ribs, and poorly tubulated long bones. Patients have hypotrichosis, trichorrhexis, and dry, lusterless hair, brows, and lashes. Patients are of normal intelligence but have neurological abnormalities. Norton et al. documented progressive paraplegia with associated leukodystrophic brain findings on MRI in a family with ODOD.[166] Neurologic symptoms may be more frequent in ODOD than previously recognized. Noted manifestations include dysarthria, neurogenic bladder disturbances, spastic paraparesis, ataxia, anterior tibial muscle weakness, and seizures.[167] These neurologic associations may not be surprising in light of the new discovery of abnormal gap junctions in ODOD.[168]

Most patients have telecanthus and epicanthal folds. Hypotelorism is present in 40% of cases.[169] Esotropia is common. The eye may be microphthalmic with anterior segment dysgenesis, or the abnormalities may be restricted to the anterior segment with normal ocular size. Anterior

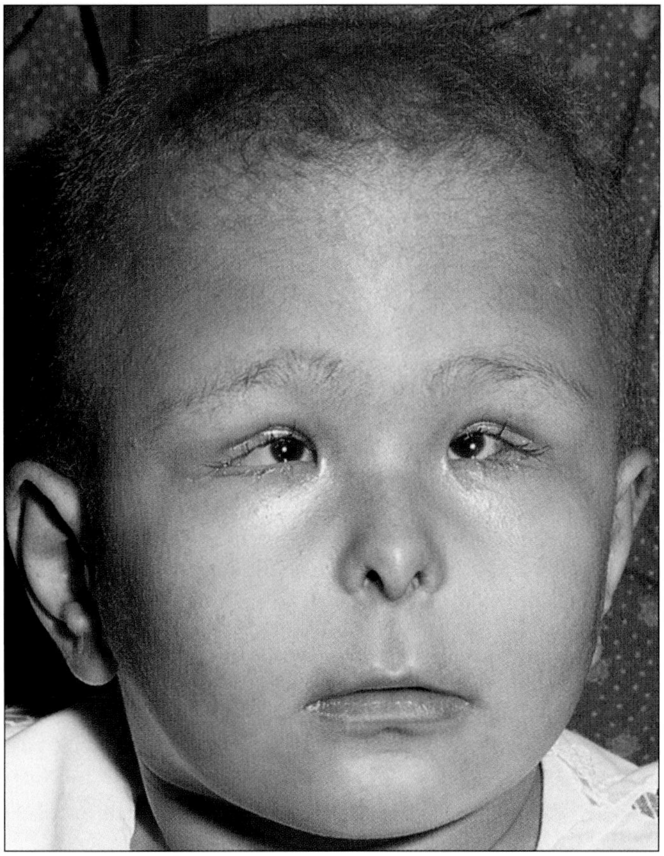

Fig. 60.12 Eighteen-month-old girl with oculo-dento-osseous dysplasia with typical pinched nose and small alae nasae as well as sparse hair and eyebrows. (Traboulsi EI, Faris BM, Der Kaloustian VM: Persistent hyperplastic primary vitreous and recessive oculo-dento-osseous dysplasia. *Am J Med Genet* 24:95, 1986. Copyright © (1986). Reprinted with permission of Wiley-Liss, Inc., a subsidiary of John Wiley & Sons, Inc.)

segment dysgenesis may be more severe in the rarer, presumably recessive form of ODOD.[163] Remnants of the pupillary membrane are frequently present. Cataracts have been reported in two cases.[170,171] Posterior segment abnormalities have included remnants of the hyaloid system[171,172] and increased numbers of retinal vessels at the optic disk.[173]

Glaucoma can develop in ODOD at different ages and may be caused by various mechanisms. In infancy the pathogenesis appears similar to that of infantile glaucoma: namely, trabeculodysgenesis. Anterior segment dysgenesis also predisposes to the development of glaucoma in childhood or early adulthood as in patients with the Axenfeld-Rieger spectrum of anomalies. The patients reported by Meyer-Schwikerath et al.,[161] Weintraub et al.,[174] and Dudgeon and Chisholm[175] fall into this second category of glaucoma in ODOD. An adult-onset open-angle type of glaucoma may occur and was present in one affected member of the family reported by Dudgeon and Chisholm.[175] Finally, an angle-closure mechanism has been reported by Sugar in one eye of one patient who had infantile glaucoma in the other eye.[176] In that same report, Sugar updated the information on a patient he had previously reported who also developed angle-closure glaucoma in mid-adulthood. Glaucoma is the most common cause of visual loss in patients with ODOD.[177] Regular intraocular pressure measurements should be initiated as early as possible after diagnosis, especially in the presence of symptoms or signs suggesting the presence of glaucoma, such as tearing, photophobia, and hazy or enlarged corneas.

Sotos syndrome

Sotos syndrome, or cerebral gigantism, is characterized by a typical craniofacial appearance, increased birth weight and length, excessive growth in the first few years of life, advanced bone age, and a nonprogressive developmental delay in some patients.[178,179] A predisposition to tumors has been identified in patients with Sotos syndrome.[180] Ocular abnormalities include esotropia, nystagmus,[181] hypertelorism,[181] and a juvenile type of macular degeneration.[182] Koenekoop et al. reported a mother and two daughters with this condition.[183] The mother had presenile nuclear sclerotic cataracts, megalophthalmos, hypo-orbitism, and exotropia. One of her daughters had megalocornea, exophoria, and iris hypoplasia. Her other daughter had megalocornea. Yen et al. reported a case of unilateral glaucoma associated with Sotos syndrome. It is not clear whether or not this represents an incidental finding or a possible genetic link.[184]

Most cases of Sotos appear to have been sporadic. After the identification of chromosome 5 as the probable genetic locus for this disorder, 77% of individuals with Sotos syndrome were found to have mutations in the *NSD1* gene at 5q35 as the cause of Sotos syndrome.[185] Since then, numerous other cases have been reported with mutations in *NSD1* and Sotos syndrome.

Dermo-chondro-corneal dystrophy of Francois

An autosomal recessive condition, dermo-chondro-corneal dystrophy of Francois is characterized by abnormal ossification of the cartilage of the hands and feet, leading to marked deformities.[186,187] Patients have dermal nodules that resemble xanthomas. These nodules appear on the dorsal surface of the fingers, posterior surface of the elbows, and pinnae of the ears. The corneal lesions consist of a central collection of epithelial white, irregular opacities. The opacities lead to moderate reduction of visual acuity. The stroma, endothelium, and periphery of the cornea remain clear. Some patients have hypercholesterolemia. The entire skeleton may become involved, except for the vertebrae and skull. Remky and Engelbrecht reported on two patients who also had seizures and an abnormal electroencephalogram.[188] Ruiz-Maldonado et al. reported two Mexican brothers who had clinical findings indistinguishable from those of the patients reported by Francois.[189,190]

Werner syndrome

Werner syndrome is a rare autosomal recessive disease characterized by a phenotype of progeria without true accelerated aging.[172] There is arrest of growth at puberty along with premature graying of the hair and balding, scleroderma-like involvement of the limbs, marked reduction of muscle mass and subcutaneous fat, chronic ulcerations over pressure points, premature arteriosclerosis, diabetes mellitus, hypogonadism, and localized soft tissue calcifications. Patients die in their fourth to fifth decade from coronary artery disease or cancer. Patients with Werner syndrome develop cataracts in the second to fourth decades of life.[191] In a series of nine patients with this disease who had undergone intracapsular cataract surgery, Jonas et al. reported a high incidence of postoperative complications, including corneal wound dehiscence in ten eyes, peripheral anterior synechiae in four, epiretinal gliosis in four, unplanned filtering bleb in two, postoperative anterior optic neuropathy in one, and cystoid macular edema in three.[192] Corneal endothelial decompensation occurred in eight eyes. These authors recommend small-incision cataract surgery because of the apparent reduced ability of endothelial and other cells to handle the trauma of surgery and because of the high incidence of wound dehiscence.

The gene locus for Werner syndrome was mapped to chromosome 8p12-p11.2.[193] The molecular pathology of Werner syndrome has been linked to mutations in the *WRN* gene (a.k.a. *RECQL2*), which encodes a homolog of a DNA helicase in *Escherichia coli*. The helicase that is defective in Werner syndrome is missing the nuclear localization signal (NLS) which impairs nuclear import.[194] It has been demonstrated that Werner syndrome fibroblast cell lines are particularly sensitive to certain DNA-damaging agents. In one study, forced expression of telomerase Werner syndrome fibroblasts confered extended cellular life span, which suggested a potential future therapy for this human progeroid syndrome.[195]

Syndrome of acromegaly, cutis verticis gyrata, and corneal leukoma of Rosenthal and Kloepfer

Rosenthal and Kloepfer described an autosomal dominant syndrome of cutis verticis gyrata, acromegaloid features, and progressive corneal opacification in 13 members of a large African-American family.[169] Patients have large hands and feet, tall stature, and prominent frontal bones. The scalp is enlarged, causing a gyri-like formation. Corneal opacification starts in the inferior epithelium, and the flat gray lesions enlarge and thicken to become chalky white and involve the whole cornea except for the most peripheral millimeter. Histopathologic examination of one button showed changes compatible with keratitis and lipoidal degeneration.

Hypophosphatasia

Hypophosphatasia is a rare inborn error of metabolism that results in a disease with onset in the first year of life in the infantile form.[170,171] The infantile and childhood forms are autosomal recessive and allelic. A mild adult-onset form of the disease exists and is dominantly inherited.[173] Both are caused by mutations in the *ALPL* gene (1p36.1-p34), which encodes alkaline phosphatase.[196] Patients may have various symptoms, including irritability, vomiting, anorexia, and fever. They develop progressive orthopedic deformities characteristic of rickets with costochondral bending and prominence of the ends of long bones. Growth is retarded, and height and weight are below normal values. Craniosynostosis is common, and in adults there is a beaten copper appearance of the skull on X-rays. There is diminished activity or absence of alkaline phosphatase and hypercalcemia. Death results from nephrocalcinosis.

Ocular findings include prominent eyes, blue sclerae,[197] band keratopathy and conjunctival calcification,[198] and optic nerve complications of craniostenosis.

Treatment of Ocular and Corneal Abnormalities in Skeletal Disorders

Errors of refraction are common in skeletal dysplasia and result from abnormalities in corneal curvature, axial length, lens contour, or subluxation of the lens. Careful refraction and correction with spectacles or contact lenses is essential to ensure good vision and to prevent ametropic and anisometropic amblyopia. Because of the progressive nature of some of the diseases, refraction is repeated biannually or yearly. Aphakic correction is often necessary in patients with Marfan syndrome and significantly dislocated lenses; this usually provides clearer images than those obtained through spherophakic tilted and dislocated lenses. Hard contact lenses are useful in patients with keratoconus. Soft lenses may be used in those with a very high error of refraction. There is no experience to date with keratorefractive or excimer laser surgery in patients with connective tissue disease, but this type of therapy seems intuitively contraindicated because of the abnormalities in corneal thickness and tensile strength in such patients. Protective eye wear and avoidance of contact sports and other activities that predispose to ocular trauma are indicated in patients with EDS type VI because of the very high rate of corneal rupture in these patients. There is no evidence that sports activities increase the likelihood of ocular complications in Marfan syndrome, but recommended guidelines for such activities are not available. Complications of keratoconus and keratoglobus are managed per guidelines in other sections of this book. The connective tissue abnormalities, however, lead to poor wound healing and wound dehiscence. Surgeons should be alert to immediate postoperative complications, and frequent examinations are necessary to detect wound leaks and cheesewiring of sutures.

Glaucoma is common in Marfan syndrome, Stickler syndrome, and some of the skeletal dysplasias such as oculo-dento-osseous dysplasia. Although data are not available, the optic nerve fibers may be more susceptible to mechanical damage from relatively low intraocular pressure in these eyes with a more deformable lamina cribrosa, if the mechanical theory of optic nerve damage in glaucoma is accepted. Visual field testing is indicated if optic nerve head configuration is suggestive of glaucomatous damage, even in the presence of normal intraocular pressure.

Surgical correction of lid colobomas and ptosis is performed as needed and is tailored to the specific patient.

The management of strabismus in patients with connective tissue disorders is similar to that in patients with normal connective tissue. Amblyopia is corrected as needed, and extraocular muscle surgery is planned, depending on the type of ocular deviation. There is one notable exception to this rule. Absence and misinsertion of extraocular muscles are common in patients with craniofacial dysostosis such as Apert and Crouzon syndromes. Imaging studies may be helpful in the preoperative identification of such anatomic variations.

Finally, and most importantly, ophthalmic surgeons should be aware of the possible complications of local and general anesthesia in patients with connective tissue disease. Cardiac abnormalities are common. Hematoma formation may be problematic in some patients with EDS. Fragile cartilaginous structures may pose a problem in the endotracheal intubation of these patients, and laryngeal masks may be a good alternative. Furthermore, due to the high rate of cervical fusions in craniosynostosis syndromes, radiographic analysis of the cervical spine is recommended before general anesthesia in these patients.[199] Dolan et al. give general recommendations for anesthesia in patients with EDS.[200] Appropriate consideration should be given to the possible anesthetic complications in individual diseases.

References

1. Olsen BR, McCarthy MT. Molecular structure of the sclera, cornea and vitreous body. In: Albert DM, Jakobiec FA, eds. *Principles and practice of ophthalmology.* Philadelphia: Saunders; 1994.
2. Sakai LY, Keene DR, Engvall E. Fibrillin, a new 350-kD glycoprotein, is a component of extracellular microfibrils. *J Cell Biol.* 1986;103(6 Pt 1):2499–2509.
3. Gibson MA, Sandberg LB, Grosso LE, Cleary EG. Complementary DNA cloning establishes microfibril-associated glycoprotein (MAGP) to be a discrete component of the elastin-associated microfibrils. *J Biol Chem.* 1991;266(12):7596–7601.
4. Wheatley HM, Traboulsi EI, Flowers BE, et al. Immunohistochemical localization of fibrillin in human ocular tissues. Relevance to the Marfan syndrome. *Arch Ophthalmol.* 1995;113(1):103–109.
5. Robertson I. Keratoconus and the Ehlers-Danlos syndrome: a new aspect of keratoconus. *Med J Aust.* 1975;1(18):571–573.
6. Traboulsi EI, Aswad MI, Jalkh AE, Malouf JF. Ocular findings in mitral valve prolapse syndrome. *Ann Ophthalmol.* 1987;19(9):354–357, 359.
7. Beardsley TL, Foulks GN. An association of keratoconus and mitral valve prolapse. *Ophthalmology.* 1982;89(1):35–37.
8. Superti-Furga A, Unger S. Nosology and classification of genetic skeletal disorders: 2006 revision. *Am J Med Genet A.* 2007;143(1):1–18.
9. Rimoin DL, Cohn D, Krakow D, et al. The skeletal dysplasias: clinical-molecular correlations. *Ann NY Acad Sci.* 2007;1117:302–309.
10. Jabs EW, Li X, Scott AF, et al. Jackson-Weiss and Crouzon syndromes are allelic with mutations in fibroblast growth factor receptor 2. *Nat Genet.* 1994;8(3):275–279.
11. Reardon W, Winter RM, Rutland P, et al. Mutations in the fibroblast growth factor receptor 2 gene cause Crouzon syndrome. *Nat Genet.* 1994;8(1):98–103.
12. Rousseau F, Bonaventure J, Legeai-Mallet L, et al. Mutations in the gene encoding fibroblast growth factor receptor-3 in achondroplasia. *Nature.* 1994;371(6494):252–254.
13. Rutland P, Pulleyn LJ, Reardon W, et al. Identical mutations in the FGFR2 gene cause both Pfeiffer and Crouzon syndrome phenotypes. *Nat Genet.* 1995;9(2):173–176.
14. Wilkie AO, Slaney SF, Oldridge M, et al. Apert syndrome results from localized mutations of FGFR2 and is allelic with Crouzon syndrome. *Nat Genet.* 1995;9(2):165–172.
15. Schell U, Hehr A, Feldman GJ, et al. Mutations in FGFR1 and FGFR2 cause familial and sporadic Pfeiffer syndrome. *Hum Mol Genet.* 1995;4(3):323–328.
16. Meyers GA, Orlow SJ, Munro IR, et al. Fibroblast growth factor receptor 3 (FGFR3) transmembrane mutation in Crouzon syndrome with acanthosis nigricans. *Nat Genet.* 1995;11(4):462–464.
17. Cohen DM, Green JG, Miller J, et al. Acrocephalopolysyndactyly type II – Carpenter syndrome: clinical spectrum and an attempt at unification with Goodman and Summit syndromes. *Am J Med Genet.* 1987;28(2):311–324.
18. Gray TL, Casey T, Selva D, et al. Ophthalmic sequelae of Crouzon syndrome. *Ophthalmology.* 2005;112(6):1129–1134.
19. Diamond GR, Katowitz JA, Whitaker LA, et al. Variations in extraocular muscle number and structure in craniofacial dysostosis. *Am J Ophthalmol.* 1980;90(3):416–418.
20. Greenberg MF, Pollard ZF. Absence of multiple extraocular muscles in craniosynostosis. *J AAPOS.* 1998;2(5):307–309.
21. Wolter JR. Bilateral keratoconus in Crouzon's syndrome with unilateral acute hydrops. *J Pediatr Ophthalmol.* 1977;14(3):141–143.
22. Glaser RL, Jiang W, Boyadjiev SA, et al. Paternal origin of FGFR2 mutations in sporadic cases of Crouzon syndrome and Pfeiffer syndrome. *Am J Hum Genet.* 2000;66(3):768–777.
23. Preston RA, Post JC, Keats BJ, et al. A gene for Crouzon craniofacial dysostosis maps to the long arm of chromosome 10. *Nat Genet.* 1994;7(2):149–153.
24. Diamond GR, Katowitz JA, Whitaker LH, et al. Ocular alignment after craniofacial reconstruction. *Am J Ophthalmol.* 1980;90(2):248–250.
25. Jadico SK, Young DA, Huebner A, et al. Ocular abnormalities in Apert syndrome: genotype/phenotype correlations with fibroblast growth factor receptor type 2 mutations. *J AAPOS.* 2006;10(6):521–527.
26. Cohen MM Jr, Kreiborg S. Cutaneous manifestations of Apert syndrome. *Am J Med Genet.* 1995;58(1):94–96.
27. Cohen MM Jr, Kreiborg S, Lammer EJ, et al. Birth prevalence study of the Apert syndrome. *Am J Med Genet.* 1992;42(5):655–659.
28. Moloney DM, Slaney SF, Oldridge M, et al. Exclusive paternal origin of new mutations in Apert syndrome. *Nat Genet.* 1996;13(1):48–53.
29. Slaney SF, Oldridge M, Hurst JA, et al. Differential effects of FGFR2 mutations on syndactyly and cleft palate in Apert syndrome. *Am J Hum Genet.* 1996;58(5):923–932.
30. von Gernet S, Golla A, Ehrenfels Y, et al. Genotype-phenotype analysis in Apert syndrome suggests opposite effects of the two recurrent mutations on syndactyly and outcome of craniofacial surgery. *Clin Genet.* 2000;57(2):137–139.
31. Lewanda AF, Cohen MM Jr, Hood J, et al. Cytogenetic survey of Apert syndrome. Reevaluation of a translocation (2;9)(p11.2;q34.2) in a patient suggests the breakpoints are not related to the disorder. *Am J Dis Child.* 1993;147(12):1306–1308.
32. Reardon W, Winter RM. Saethre-Chotzen syndrome. *J Med Genet.* 1994;31(5):393–396.
33. Dollfus H, Biswas P, Kumaramanickavel G, et al. Saethre-Chotzen syndrome: notable intrafamilial phenotypic variability in a large family with Q28X TWIST mutation. *Am J Med Genet.* 2002;109(3):218–225.
34. Brueton LA, van Herwerden L, Chotai KA, Winter RM. The mapping of a gene for craniosynostosis: evidence for linkage of the Saethre-Chotzen syndrome to distal chromosome 7p. *J Med Genet.* 1992;29(10):681–685.
35. Paznekas WA, Cunningham ML, Howard TD, et al. Genetic heterogeneity of Saethre-Chotzen syndrome, due to TWIST and FGFR mutations. *Am J Hum Genet.* 1998;62(6):1370–1380.
36. Johnson D, Horsley SW, Moloney DM, et al. A comprehensive screen for TWIST mutations in patients with craniosynostosis identifies a new microdeletion syndrome of chromosome band 7p21.1. *Am J Hum Genet.* 1998;63(5):1282–1293.
37. Baum JL, Feingold M. Ocular aspects of Goldenhar's syndrome. *Am J Ophthalmol.* 1973;75(2):250–257.
38. Marshman WE, Schalit G, Jones RB, et al. Congenital anomalies in patients with Duane retraction syndrome and their relatives. *J AAPOS.* 2000;4(2):106–109.
39. Kelberman D, Tyson J, Chandler DC, et al. Hemifacial microsomia: progress in understanding the genetic basis of a complex malformation syndrome. *Hum Genet.* 2001;109(6):638–645.
40. Coster DJ, Aggarwal RK, Williams KA. Surgical management of ocular surface disorders using conjunctival and stem cell allografts. *Br J Ophthalmol.* 1995;79(11):977–982.
41. Kaufman A, Medow N, Phillips R, Zaidman G. Treatment of epibulbar limbal dermoids. *J Pediatr Ophthalmol Strabismus.* 1999;36(3):136–140.
42. Streiff EB. Dysmorphie mandibulofaciale (tete d'oiseau) et alterations oculaires. *Ophthalmologica.* 1950;120:79.
43. Hallerman W. Vogelgesicht und cataracta congenita. *Klin Mbl Augenheilk.* 1948;113:315.
44. Francois J, Pierard J. The Francois dyscephalic syndrome and skin manifestations. *Am J Ophthalmol.* 1971;71(6):1241–1250.
45. Wolter JR, Jones DH. Spontaneous cataract absorption in Hallermann-Streiff syndrome. *Ophthalmologica.* 1965;150(6):401–408.
46. Sugar A, Bigger JF, Podos SM. Hallermann-Streiff-Francois syndrome. *J Pediatr Ophthalmol.* 1971;8:234.
47. Hopkins DJ, Horan EC. Glaucoma in the Hallermann-Streiff syndrome. *Br J Ophthalmol.* 1970;54(6):416–422.

48. Newell SW, Hall BD, Anderson CW, Lim ES. Hallermann-Streiff syndrome with Coats disease. *J Pediatr Ophthalmol Strabismus*. 1994; 31(2):123–125.
49. Ravindran R, Stoops CM. Anesthetic management of a patient with Hallermann Streiff syndrome. *Anesth Analg*. 1979;58(3):254–255.
50. Treacher Collins E. Case with symmetrical congenital notches in the outer part of each lower lid and defective development of the malar bones. *Trans Ophthalmol Soc UK*. 1900;20:191.
51. Rovin S, Dachi SF, Borenstein DB, Cotter WB. Mandibulofacial dysostosis, a familial study of five generations. *J Pediatr*. 1964;65: 215–221.
52. Splendore A, Silva EO, Alonso LG, et al. High mutation detection rate in TCOF1 among Treacher Collins syndrome patients reveals clustering of mutations and 16 novel pathogenic changes. *Hum Mutat*. 2000; 16(4):315–322.
53. Dixon MJ. Treacher Collins syndrome. *Hum Mol Genet*. 1996;5 Spec No:1391–1396.
54. Positional cloning of a gene involved in the pathogenesis of Treacher Collins syndrome. The Treacher Collins Syndrome Collaborative Group. *Nat Genet*. 1996;12(2):130–136.
55. Hertle RW, Ziylan S, Katowitz JA. Ophthalmic features and visual prognosis in the Treacher-Collins syndrome. *Br J Ophthalmol*. 1993;77(10): 642–645.
56. Prenner JL, Binenbaum G, Carpentieri DF, et al. Treacher Collins syndrome with novel ophthalmic findings and visceral anomalies. *Br J Ophthalmol*. 2002;86(4):472–473.
57. Michalickova K, Susic M, Willing MC, et al. Mutations of the alpha2(V) chain of type V collagen impair matrix assembly and produce Ehlers-Danlos syndrome type I. *Hum Mol Genet*. 1998;7(2):249–255.
58. Wenstrup RJ, Langland GT, Willing MC, et al. A splice-junction mutation in the region of COL5A1 that codes for the carboxyl propeptide of pro alpha 1(V) chains results in the gravis form of the Ehlers-Danlos syndrome (type I). *Hum Mol Genet*. 1996;5(11):1733–1736.
59. Beighton P, De Paepe A, Steinmann B, et al. Ehlers-Danlos syndromes: revised nosology, Villefranche, 1997. Ehlers-Danlos National Foundation (USA) and Ehlers-Danlos Support Group (UK). *Am J Med Genet*. 1998;77(1):31–37.
60. Narcisi P, Richards AJ, Ferguson SD, Pope FM. A family with Ehlers-Danlos syndrome type III/articular hypermobility syndrome has a glycine 637 to serine substitution in type III collagen. *Hum Mol Genet*. 1994;3(9):1617–1620.
61. Superti-Furga A, Gugler E, Gitzelmann R, Steinmann B. Ehlers-Danlos syndrome type IV: a multi-exon deletion in one of the two COL3A1 alleles affecting structure, stability, and processing of type III procollagen. *J Biol Chem*. 1988;263(13):6226–6232.
62. Fox R, Pope FM, Narcisi P, et al. Spontaneous carotid cavernous fistula in Ehlers Danlos syndrome. *J Neurol Neurosurg Psychiatry*. 1988;51(7): 984–986.
63. Pollack JS, Custer PL, Hart WM, et al. Ocular complications in Ehlers-Danlos syndrome type IV. *Arch Ophthalmol*. 1997;115(3):416–419.
64. Byers PH, Duvic M, Atkinson M, et al. Ehlers-Danlos syndrome type VIIA and VIIB result from splice-junction mutations or genomic deletions that involve exon 6 in the COL1A1 and COL1A2 genes of type I collagen. *Am J Med Genet*. 1997;72(1):94–105.
65. Colige A, Sieron AL, Li SW, et al. Human Ehlers-Danlos syndrome type VII C and bovine dermatosparaxis are caused by mutations in the procollagen I N-proteinase gene. *Am J Hum Genet*. 1999;65(2):308–317.
66. Pinnell SR, Krane SM, Kenzora JE, Glimcher MJ. A heritable disorder of connective tissue. Hydroxylysine-deficient collagen disease. *N Engl J Med*. 1972;286(19):1013–1020.
67. Judisch GF, Waziri M, Krachmer JH. Ocular Ehlers-Danlos syndrome with normal lysyl hydroxylase activity. *Arch Ophthalmol*. 1976;94(9): 1489–1491.
68. Zlotogora J, BenEzra D, Cohen T, Cohen E. Syndrome of brittle cornea, blue sclera, and joint hyperextensibility. *Am J Med Genet*. 1990;36(3): 269–272.
69. Royce PM, Steinmann B, Vogel A, et al. Brittle cornea syndrome: an heritable connective tissue disorder distinct from Ehlers-Danlos syndrome type VI and fragilitas oculi, with spontaneous perforations of the eye, blue sclerae, red hair, and normal collagen lysyl hydroxylation. *Eur J Pediatr*. 1990;149(7):465–469.
70. Farag TI, Schimke RN. Ehlers-Danlos syndrome: a new oculo-scoliotic type with associated polyneuropathy? *Clin Genet*. 1989;35(2):121–124.
71. May MA, Beauchamp GR. Collagen maturation defects in Ehlers-Danlos keratopathy. *J Pediatr Ophthalmol Strabismus*. 1987;24(2):78–82.
72. Cameron JA. Corneal abnormalities in Ehlers-Danlos syndrome type VI. *Cornea*. 1993;12(1):54–59.
73. Cameron JA, Cotter JB, Risco JM, Alvarez H. Epikeratoplasty for keratoglobus associated with blue sclera. *Ophthalmology*. 1991;98(4): 446–452.
74. Heim P, Raghunath M, Meiss L, et al. Ehlers-Danlos Syndrome Type VI (EDS VI): problems of diagnosis and management. *Acta Paediatr*. 1998; 87(6):708–710.
75. Izquierdo L Jr, Mannis MJ, Marsh PB, et al. Bilateral spontaneous corneal rupture in brittle cornea syndrome: a case report. *Cornea*. 1999;18(5): 621–624.
76. Arkin W. Blue scleras with keratoglobus. *Am J Ophthalmol*. 1964;58: 678–682.
77. Biglan AW, Brown SI, Johnson BL. Keratoglobus and blue sclera. *Am J Ophthalmol*. 1977;83(2):225–233.
78. Macsai MS, Lemley HL, Schwartz T. Management of oculus fragilis in Ehlers-Danlos type VI. *Cornea*. 2000;19(1):104–107.
79. Nakazawa M, Tamai M, Kiyosawa M, Watanabe Y. Homograft of preserved sclera for post-traumatic scleral staphyloma in Ehlers-Danlos syndrome. *Graefe's Arch Clin Exp Ophthalmol*. 1986;224(3): 247–250.
80. Pemberton JW, Freeman HM, Schepens CL. Familial retinal detachment and the Ehlers-Danlos syndrome. *Arch Ophthalmol*. 1966;76(6):817–824.
81. Green WR, Friedman-Kien A, Banfield WG. Angioid streaks in Ehlers-Danlos syndrome. *Arch Ophthalmol*. 1966;76(2):197–204.
82. Pouliquen Y, Petroutsos G, Papaioannou D. [Corneal dystrophy and Ehlers-Danlos syndrome]. *J Fr Ophtalmol*. 1983;6(4):387–389.
83. Pesudovs K. Orbscan mapping in Ehlers-Danlos syndrome. *J Cataract Refract Surg*. 2004;30(8):1795–1798.
84. Sillence DO, Barlow KK, Garber AP, et al. Osteogenesis imperfecta type II delineation of the phenotype with reference to genetic heterogeneity. *Am J Med Genet*. 1984;17(2):407–423.
85. Byers PH. Osteogenesis imperfecta. In: Ryce BM, Steinmann B, eds. *Connective tissue and its heritable disorders: molecular, genetic and medical aspects*. New York: Wiley-Liss; 1993.
86. Byers PH, Wallis GA, Willing MC. Osteogenesis imperfecta: translation of mutation to phenotype. *J Med Genet*. 1991;28(7):433–442.
87. Wenstrup RJ, Willing MC, Starman BJ, Byers PH. Distinct biochemical phenotypes predict clinical severity in nonlethal variants of osteogenesis imperfecta. *Am J Hum Genet*. 1990;46(5):975–982.
88. Riedner ED, Levin LS, Holliday MJ. Hearing patterns in dominant osteogenesis imperfecta. *Arch Otolaryngol*. 1980;106(12):737–740.
89. Pedersen U, Bramsen T. Central corneal thickness in osteogenesis imperfecta and otosclerosis. *ORL J Otorhinolaryngol Relat Spec*. 1984;46(1): 38–41.
90. Kaiser-Kupfer MI, McCain L, Shapiro JR, et al. Low ocular rigidity in patients with osteogenesis imperfecta. *Invest Ophthalmol Vis Sci*. 1981;20(6):807–809.
91. Chan CC, Green WR, de la Cruz ZC, Hillis A. Ocular findings in osteogenesis imperfecta congenita. *Arch Ophthalmol*. 1982;100(9): 1458–1463.
92. Bembi B, Parma A, Bottega M, et al. Intravenous pamidronate treatment in osteogenesis imperfecta. *J Pediatr*. 1997;131(4):622–625.
93. Plotkin H, Rauch F, Bishop NJ, et al. Pamidronate treatment of severe osteogenesis imperfecta in children under 3 years of age. *J Clin Endocrinol Metab*. 2000;85(5):1846–1850.
94. Lee YS, Low SL, Lim LA, Loke KY. Cyclic pamidronate infusion improves bone mineralisation and reduces fracture incidence in osteogenesis imperfecta. *Eur J Pediatr*. 2001;160(11):641–644.
95. Glorieux FH, Bishop NJ, Plotkin H, et al. Cyclic administration of pamidronate in children with severe osteogenesis imperfecta. *N Engl J Med*. 1998;339(14):947–952.
96. Vintiner GM, Temple IK, Middleton-Price HR, et al. Genetic and clinical heterogeneity of Stickler syndrome. *Am J Med Genet*. 1991;41(1): 44–48.
97. Maumenee IH. Vitreoretinal degeneration as a sign of generalized connective tissue diseases. *Am J Ophthalmol*. 1979;88(3 Pt 1):432–449.
98. Herrmann J, France TD, Spranger JW, et al. The Stickler syndrome (hereditary arthroophthalmopathy). *Birth Defects Orig Artic Ser*. 1975;11(2):76–103.
99. Opitz JM, France T, Herrmann J, Spranger JW. The Stickler syndrome. *N Engl J Med*. 1972;286(10):546–547.
100. Stickler GB, Belau PG, Farrell FJ, et al. Hereditary progressive arthro-ophthalmopathy. *Mayo Clin Proc*. 1965;40:433–455.
101. Liberfarb RM, Goldblatt A. Prevalence of mitral-valve prolapse in the Stickler syndrome. *Am J Med Genet*. 1986;24(3):387–392.
102. Stickler GB, Hughes W, Houchin P. Clinical features of hereditary progressive arthro-ophthalmopathy (Stickler syndrome): a survey. *Genet Med*. 2001;3(3):192–196.

103. Takahashi E, Hori T, O'Connell P, et al. R-banding and nonisotopic in situ hybridization: precise localization of the human type II collagen gene (COL2A1). *Hum Genet.* 1990;86(1):14–16.
104. Ritvaniemi P, Hyland J, Ignatius J, et al. A fourth example suggests that premature termination codons in the COL2A1 gene are a common cause of the Stickler syndrome: analysis of the COL2A1 gene by denaturing gradient gel electrophoresis. *Genomics.* 1993;17(1):218–221.
105. Wagner H. Ein bisher unbekanntes Erbleiden des Aunges (Degeneratio hyaloideretinalis hereditaria), beobachtet im Kanton Zurich. *Kiln Montasbl Augenheilkd.* 1938;100:840–857.
106. Brown DM, Graemiger RA, Hergersberg M, et al. Genetic linkage of Wagner disease and erosive vitreoretinopathy to chromosome 5q13–14. *Arch Ophthalmol.* 1995;113(5):671–675.
107. Mukhopadhyay A, Nikopoulos K, Maugeri A, et al. Erosive vitreoretinopathy and Wagner disease are caused by intronic mutations in CSPG2/Versican that result in an imbalance of splice variants. *Invest Ophthalmol Vis Sci.* 2006;47(8):3565–3572.
108. Kloeckener-Gruissem B, Bartholdi D, Abdou MT, et al. Identification of the genetic defect in the original Wagner syndrome family. *Mol Vis.* 2006;12:350–355.
109. Korkko J, Ritvaniemi P, Haataja L, et al. Mutation in type II procollagen (COL2A1) that substitutes aspartate for glycine alpha 1–67 and that causes cataracts and retinal detachment: evidence for molecular heterogeneity in the Wagner syndrome and the Stickler syndrome (arthro-ophthalmopathy). *Am J Hum Genet.* 1993;53(1):55–61.
110. Francomano CA, Liberfarb RM, Hirose T, et al. The Stickler syndrome: evidence for close linkage to the structural gene for type II collagen. *Genomics.* 1987;1(4):293–296.
111. Richards AJ, Yates JR, Williams R, et al. A family with Stickler syndrome type 2 has a mutation in the COL11A1 gene resulting in the substitution of glycine 97 by valine in alpha 1 (XI) collagen. *Hum Mol Genet.* 1996;5(9):1339–1343.
112. Ayme S, Preus M. The Marshall and Stickler syndromes: objective rejection of lumping. *J Med Genet.* 1984;21(1):34–38.
113. Marshall D. Ectodermal dysplasia; report of kindred with ocular abnormalities and hearing defect. *Am J Ophthalmol.* 1958;45(4, Part 2):143–156.
114. Shanske AL, Bogdanow A, Shprintzen RJ, Marion RW. The Marshall syndrome: report of a new family and review of the literature. *Am J Med Genet.* 1997;70(1):52–57.
115. Majava M, Hoornaert KP, Bartholdi D, et al. A report on 10 new patients with heterozygous mutations in the COL11A1 gene and a review of genotype-phenotype correlations in type XI collagenopathies. *Am J Med Genet A.* 2007;143(3):258–264.
116. Annunen S, Korkko J, Czarny M, et al. Splicing mutations of 54-bp exons in the COL11A1 gene cause Marshall syndrome, but other mutations cause overlapping Marshall/Stickler phenotypes. *Am J Hum Genet.* 1999;65(4):971–983.
117. Brunner HG, van Beersum SE, Warman ML, et al. A Stickler syndrome gene is linked to chromosome 6 near the COL11A2 gene. *Hum Mol Genet.* 1994;3(9):1561–1564.
118. Vikkula M, Mariman EC, Lui VC, et al. Autosomal dominant and recessive osteochondrodysplasias associated with the COL11A2 locus. *Cell.* 1995;80(3):431–437.
119. Sirko-Osadsa DA, Murray MA, Scott JA, et al. Stickler syndrome without eye involvement is caused by mutations in COL11A2, the gene encoding the alpha2(XI) chain of type XI collagen. *J Pediatr.* 1998;132(2):368–371.
120. Wilson MC, McDonald-McGinn DM, Quinn GE, et al. Long-term follow-up of ocular findings in children with Stickler's syndrome. *Am J Ophthalmol.* 1996;122(5):727–728.
121. Spallone A. Stickler's syndrome: a study of 12 families. *Br J Ophthalmol.* 1987;71(7):504–509.
122. Knobloch WH, Layer JM. Clefting syndromes associated with retinal detachment. *Am J Ophthalmol.* 1972;73(4):517–530.
123. Ang A, Ung T, Puvanachandra N, et al. Vitreous phenotype: a key diagnostic sign in Stickler syndrome types 1 and 2 complicated by double heterozygosity. *Am J Med Genet A.* 2007;143(6):604–607.
124. Richards AJ, Baguley DM, Yates JR, et al. Variation in the vitreous phenotype of Stickler syndrome can be caused by different amino acid substitutions in the X position of the type II collagen Gly-X-Y triple helix. *Am J Hum Genet.* 2000;67(5):1083–1094.
125. Sabti K, Chow D, Fournier A, Aroichane M. Spontaneous rupture of the lens capsule in a case of Marshall syndrome. *J Pediatr Ophthalmol Strabismus.* 2002;39(5):298–299.
126. Gray RH, Gregor ZJ. Acquired peripheral retinal telangiectasia after retinal surgery. *Retina.* 1994;14(1):10–13.
127. Shields JA, Shields CL, Deglin E. Retinal capillary hemangioma in Marshall-Stickler syndrome. *Am J Ophthalmol.* 1997;124(1):120–122.
128. Leiba H, Oliver M, Pollack A. Prophylactic laser photocoagulation in Stickler syndrome. *Eye.* 1996;10(Pt 6):701–708.
129. Marr JE, Halliwell-Ewen J, Fisher B, et al. Associations of high myopia in childhood. *Eye.* 2001;15(Pt 1):70–74.
130. Siggers DC. Kniest disease. *Birth Defects Orig Artic Ser.* 1974;10(12):432–442.
131. Maumenee IH, Traboulsi EI. The ocular findings in Kniest dysplasia. *Am J Ophthalmol.* 1985;100(1):155–160.
132. Wilkin DJ, Bogaert R, Lachman RS, et al. A single amino acid substitution (G103D) in the type II collagen triple helix produces Kniest dysplasia. *Hum Mol Genet.* 1994;3(11):1999–2003.
133. Spranger J, Menger H, Mundlos S, et al. Kniest dysplasia is caused by dominant collagen II (COL2A1) mutations: parental somatic mosaicism manifesting as Stickler phenotype and mild spondyloepiphyseal dysplasia. *Pediatr Radiol.* 1994;24(6):431–435.
134. Winterpacht A, Hilbert M, Schwarze U, et al. Kniest and Stickler dysplasia phenotypes caused by collagen type II gene (COL2A1) defect. *Nat Genet.* 1993;3(4):323–326.
135. Matt P, Habashi J, Carrel T, et al. Recent advances in understanding Marfan syndrome: should we now treat surgical patients with losartan? *J Thorac Cardiovasc Surg.* 2008;135(2):389–394.
136. Marfan A. Un cas de deformation congenitale des quatre membres, plus prononcee aux extremites, characterisee par l'allongement des os, avec un certain degre d'amaincissement. *Bull Mem Soc Med Hop (Paris).* 1896;13:220–226.
137. Pyeritz RE, McKusick VA. The Marfan syndrome: diagnosis and management. *N Engl J Med.* 1979;300(14):772–777.
138. Pyeritz RE, Fishman EK, Bernhardt BA, Siegelman SS. Dural ectasia is a common feature of the Marfan syndrome. *Am J Hum Genet.* 1988;43(5):726–732.
139. Kainulainen K, Pulkkinen L, Savolainen A, et al. Location on chromosome 15 of the gene defect causing Marfan syndrome [see comments]. *N Engl J Med.* 1990;323(14):935–939.
140. Dietz HC, Pyeritz RE. Mutations in the human gene for fibrillin-1 (FBN1) in the Marfan syndrome and related disorders. *Hum Mol Genet.* 1995;4 Spec No:1799–1809.
141. Maumenee IH. The eye in the Marfan syndrome. *Trans Am Ophthalmol Soc.* 1981;79:684–733.
142. Hamod A, Moodie D, Clark B, Traboulsi EI. Presenting signs and clinical diagnosis in individuals referred to rule out Marfan syndrome. *Ophthalmic Genet.* 2003;24(1):35–39.
143. Mir S, Wheatley HM, Hussels IE, et al. A comparative histologic study of the fibrillin microfibrillar system in the lens capsule of normal subjects and subjects with Marfan syndrome. *Invest Ophthalmol Vis Sci.* 1998;39(1):84–93.
144. Traboulsi EI, Whittum-Hudson JA, Mir SH, Maumenee IH. Microfibril abnormalities of the lens capsule in patients with Marfan syndrome and ectopia lentis. *Ophthalmic Genet.* 2000;21(1):9–15.
145. Sachdev NH, Di Girolamo N, McCluskey PJ, et al. Lens dislocation in Marfan syndrome: potential role of matrix metalloproteinases in fibrillin degradation. *Arch Ophthalmol.* 2002;120(6):833–835.
146. Sultan G, Baudouin C, Auzerie O, et al. Cornea in Marfan disease: Orbscan and in vivo confocal microscopy analysis. *Invest Ophthalmol Vis Sci.* 2002;43(6):1757–1764.
147. Heur M, Costin B, Crowe S, et al. The value of keratometry and central corneal thickness measurements in the clinical diagnosis of Marfan syndrome. *Am J Ophthalmol.* 2008;145(6):997–1001.
148. Izquierdo NJ, Traboulsi EI, Enger C, Maumenee IH. Strabismus in the Marfan syndrome. *Am J Ophthalmol.* 1994;117(5):632–635.
149. Izquierdo NJ, Traboulsi EI, Enger C, Maumenee IH. Glaucoma in the Marfan syndrome. *Trans Am Ophthalmol Soc.* 1992;90:111–117; discussion 8–22.
150. Koenig SB, Mieler WF. Management of ectopia lentis in a family with Marfan syndrome. *Arch Ophthalmol.* 1996;114(9):1058–1061.
151. Halpert M, BenEzra D. Surgery of the hereditary subluxated lens in children. *Ophthalmology.* 1996;103(4):681–686.
152. Omulecki W, Nawrocki J, Palenga-Pydyn D, Sempinska-Szewczyk J. Pars plana vitrectomy, lensectomy, or extraction in transscleral intraocular lens fixation for the management of dislocated lenses in a family with Marfan's syndrome. *Ophthalmic Surg Lasers.* 1998;29(5):375–379.
153. Gruber MA, Graham TP Jr, Engel E, Smith C. Marfan syndrome with contractural arachnodactyly and severe mitral regurgitation in a premature infant. *J Pediatr.* 1978;93(1):80–82.
154. Morse RP, Rockenmacher S, Pyeritz RE, et al. Diagnosis and management of infantile marfan syndrome. *Pediatrics.* 1990;86(6):888–895.
155. Gott VL, Pyeritz RE, Magovern GJ Jr, et al. Surgical treatment of aneurysms of the ascending aorta in the Marfan syndrome. Results of composite-graft repair in 50 patients. *N Engl J Med.* 1986;314(17):1070–1074.

156. Silverman DI, Burton KJ, Gray J, et al. Life expectancy in the Marfan syndrome. *Am J Cardiol.* 1995;75(2):157–160.
157. Gray JR, Bridges AB, West RR, et al. Life expectancy in British Marfan syndrome populations. *Clin Genet.* 1998;54(2):124–128.
158. Habashi JP, Judge DP, Holm TM, et al. Losartan, an AT1 antagonist, prevents aortic aneurysm in a mouse model of Marfan syndrome. *Science.* 2006;312(5770):117–121.
159. Brooke BS, Habashi JP, Judge DP, et al. Angiotensin II blockade and aortic-root dilation in Marfan's syndrome. *N Engl J Med.* 2008;358(26):2787–2795.
160. Gorlin RJ, Miskin LH, St Geme JW. Oculodentodigital dysplasia. *J Pediatr* 1963;63:69–75.
161. Meyer-Schwikerath G, Gruterch E, Weyers H. Mikrophthalmus-syndrome. *Klin Mbl Augenheilk.* 1957;131:18.
162. Frasson M, Calixto N, Cronemberger S, et al. Oculodentodigital dysplasia: study of ophthalmological and clinical manifestations in three boys with probably autosomal recessive inheritance. *Ophthalmic Genet.* 2004;25(3):227–236.
163. Traboulsi EI, Faris BM, Der Kaloustian VM. Persistent hyperplastic primary vitreous and recessive oculo-dento-osseous dysplasia. *Am J Med Genet.* 1986;24(1):95–100.
164. Gladwin A, Donnai D, Metcalfe K, et al. Localization of a gene for oculodentodigital syndrome to human chromosome 6q22–q24. *Hum Mol Genet.* 1997;6(1):123–127.
165. Paznekas WA, Boyadjiev SA, Shapiro RE, et al. Connexin 43 (GJA1) mutations cause the pleiotropic phenotype of oculodentodigital dysplasia. *Am J Hum Genet.* 2003;72(2):408–418.
166. Norton KK, Carey JC, Gutmann DH. Oculodentodigital dysplasia with cerebral white matter abnormalities in a two-generation family. *Am J Med Genet.* 1995;57(3):458–461.
167. Loddenkemper T, Grote K, Evers S, et al. Neurological manifestations of the oculodentodigital dysplasia syndrome. *J Neurol.* 2002;249(5): 584–595.
168. Amador C, Mathews AM, Del Carmen Montoya M, et al. Expanding the neurologic phenotype of oculodentodigital dysplasia in a 4-generation Hispanic family. *J Child Neurol.* 2008;23(8):901–905.
169. Rosenthal JW, Kloepfer HW. An acromegaloid, cutis verticis gyrata, corneal leukoma syndrome. A new medical entity. *Arch Ophthalmol.* 1962;68:722–726.
170. Whyte MP. Heritable metabolic and dysplastic bone diseases. *Endocrinol Metab Clin North Am.* 1990;19(1):133–173.
171. Whyte MP. Hypophosphatasia and the role of alkaline phosphatase in skeletal mineralization. *Endocr Rev.* 1994;15(4):439–461.
172. Adoue DP. Images in clinical medicine. Werner's syndrome. *N Engl J Med.* 1997;337(14):977.
173. Fraser D. Hypophosphatasia. *Am J Med.* 1957;22(5):730–746.
174. Weintraub DM, Baum JL, Pashayan HM. A family with oculodentodigital dysplasia. *Cleft Palate J.* 1975;12:323–329.
175. Dudgeon J, Chisholm IA. Oculo-dento-digital dysplasia. *Trans Ophthalmol Soc UK.* 1974;94:203.
176. Sugar HS. Oculodentodigital dysplasia syndrome with angle-closure glaucoma. *Am J Ophthalmol.* 1978;86(1):36–38.
177. Traboulsi EI, Parks MM. Glaucoma in oculo-dento-osseous dysplasia. *Am J Ophthalmol.* 1990;109(3):310–313.
178. Bale AE, Drum MA, Parry DM, Mulvihill JJ. Familial Sotos syndrome (cerebral gigantism): craniofacial and psychological characteristics. *Am J Med Genet.* 1985;20(4):613–624.
179. Cole TR, Hughes HE. Sotos syndrome: a study of the diagnostic criteria and natural history. *J Med Genet.* 1994;31(1):20–32.
180. Lapunzina P. Risk of tumorigenesis in overgrowth syndromes: a comprehensive review. *Am J Med Genet C Semin Med Genet.* 2005;137C(1): 53–71.
181. Goldstein DJ, Ward RE, Moore E, et al. Overgrowth, congenital hypotonia, nystagmus, strabismus, and mental retardation: variant of dominantly inherited Sotos sequence? *Am J Med Genet.* 1988;29(4): 783–792.
182. Ferrier PE, de Meuron G, Korol S, Hauser H. Cerebral gigantism (Sotos syndrome) with juvenile macular degeneration. *Helv Paediatr Acta.* 1980;35(1):97–102.
183. Koenekoop RK, Rosenbaum KN, Traboulsi EI. Ocular findings in a family with Sotos syndrome (cerebral gigantism). *Am J Ophthalmol.* 1995; 119(5):657–658.
184. Yen MT, Gedde SJ, Flynn JT. Unilateral glaucoma in Sotos syndrome (cerebral gigantism). *Am J Ophthalmol.* 2000;130(6):851–853.
185. Kurotaki N, Imaizumi K, Harada N, et al. Haploinsufficiency of NSD1 causes Sotos syndrome. *Nat Genet.* 2002;30(4):365–366.
186. Caputo R, Sambvani N, Monti M, et al. Dermochondrocorneal dystrophy (Francois' syndrome). Report of a case. *Arch Dermatol.* 1988;124(3): 424–428.
187. Jensen VJ. Dermo-chondro-corneal dystrophy; report of a case. *Acta Ophthalmol (Copenh).* 1958;36(1):71–78.
188. Remky H, Engelbrecht G. [Dystrophia dermo-chondro-cornealis (Francois)]. *Klin Monatsbl Augenheilkd.* 1967;151(3):319–331.
189. Francois J. Dystrophie dermo-chondro-corneene familiale. *Ann Oculist (Paris).* 1949;182:409.
190. Ruiz-Maldonado R, Tamayo L, Velazquez E. [Familial dermo-chondrocorneal dystrophy (Francois' syndrome)]. *Ann Dermatol Venereol.* 1977;104(6–7):475–478.
191. Rosenthal G, Assa V, Monos T, et al. Werner's syndrome. *Br J Ophthalmol.* 1996;80(6):576–577.
192. Jonas JB, Ruprecht KW, Schmitz-Valckenberg P, et al. Ophthalmic surgical complications in Werner's syndrome: report on 18 eyes of nine patients. *Ophthalmic Surg.* 1987;18(10):760–764.
193. Goto M, Rubenstein M, Weber J, et al. Genetic linkage of Werner's syndrome to five markers on chromosome 8. *Nature.* 1992;355(6362): 735–738.
194. Yu CE, Oshima J, Fu YH, et al. Positional cloning of the Werner's syndrome gene. *Science.* 1996;272(5259):258–262.
195. Wyllie FS, Jones CJ, Skinner JW, et al. Telomerase prevents the accelerated cell ageing of Werner syndrome fibroblasts. *Nat Genet.* 2000;24(1): 16–17.
196. Greenberg CR, Taylor CL, Haworth JC, et al. A homoallelic Gly317→Asp mutation in ALPL causes the perinatal (lethal) form of hypophosphatasia in Canadian Mennonites. *Genomics.* 1993;17(1):215–217.
197. Lessell S, Norton EW. Band keratopathy and conjunctival calcification in hypophosphatasia. *Arch Ophthalmol.* 1964;71:497–499.
198. Brenner RL, Smith JL, Cleveland WW, et al. Eye signs of hypophosphatasia. *Arch Ophthalmol.* 1969;81(5):614–617.
199. Kreiborg S, Barr M Jr, Cohen MM Jr. Cervical spine in the Apert syndrome. *Am J Med Genet.* 1992;43(4):704–708.
200. Dolan P, Sisko F, Riley E. Anesthetic considerations for Ehlers-Danlos syndrome. *Anesthesiology.* 1980;52(3):266–269.

Chapter 61

Inflammatory Bowel Disease and Other Systemic Inflammatory Diseases

Terry L. Kaiura, Glenn L. Stoller, George J. Florakis

Inflammatory Bowel Disease

Inflammatory bowel disease (IBD) refers to both ulcerative colitis and Crohn's disease (regional enteritis), which are chronic, recurrent, inflammatory disorders of the gastrointestinal tract of unknown etiology. IBD is also characterized by a number of extraintestinal manifestations that occur in 25–36% of patients.[1] The most commonly involved organs are the skin, joints, eye, and biliary tract.[2]

Etiology and pathogenesis

The cause of IBD remains uncertain. Observed differences in the incidence of the disease among ethnic groups and the occasional familial occurrence, including monozygotic twins, have led investigators to suggest that genetic factors play a role.[3–5] Recently, the *Nod2* gene on chromosome 16 has been associated with an increased susceptibility to Crohn's disease.[6,7] These *Nod2* genetic variants appear to have an altered innate immune response to bacteria.[8] Researchers have also proposed infectious origins for IBD, given the similar gastrointestinal manifestations caused by certain microbial pathogens; however, consistent specific agents have yet to be isolated.[9] In addition, immunologic dysregulation with abnormal expression of cytokines such as tumor necrosis factor-alpha (TNF-α) and interferon gamma (INF-γ) results in tissue damage in patients with IBD.[10] A positive response to immunosuppressive agents also supports an immunologic association. It is likely that the genetics of IBD are complex with more than one susceptibility locus and that many gene–gene and gene–environment interactions are pivotal in the pathogenesis of IBD.[11]

Pathology and clinical manifestations

Ulcerative colitis is a recurrent inflammatory disease of the colon and rectum and is characterized by rectal bleeding, diarrhea, cramping abdominal pain, anorexia, and weight loss. The acute lesion is diffuse (without skip areas) and involves the superficial layers of the bowel wall (mucosa and submucosa). Ulcerations, crypt abscesses, diminished goblet cell numbers, and cellular infiltration with lymphocytes, plasma cells, eosinophils, and polymorphonuclear cells may be seen.

Crohn's disease is a subacute and chronic inflammation that may affect any part of the gastrointestinal tract. It is prevalent in the distal ileum, colon, and anorectal area. The inflammation may be discontinuous (with skip areas) and is transmural (involving all layers of the bowel wall and serosal surface). Symptoms include fever, diarrhea, cramping, abdominal pain, and weight loss. The bowel wall inflammation is focal, with microerosions, fissuring, ulcerations, lymphoid aggregates, and dilation of submucosal lymphatic vessels.[12] Multiple granulomas are seen in 60% of patients, and their presence is diagnostic of Crohn's disease.[12]

Differentiation between ulcerative colitis and Crohn's disease may be difficult in 20–25% of cases[13] because of a number of factors, including a limited morphologic response of the colon to disease, an incomplete expression of IBD,[12] and the occurrence of an 'indeterminate' colitis with features of both ulcerative colitis and Crohn's disease.[14] Although neither disease has pathognomonic findings that are consistently present, the rectum is typically involved in ulcerative colitis and spared in Crohn's disease. Rectal bleeding is more common in ulcerative colitis, whereas fever and abdominal pain are more prominent in Crohn's disease. Patients with IBD have increased risk of cancer, Crohn's disease carcinoma being more proximally distributed than ulcerative colitis carcinoma. In IBD, carcinoma develops at earlier ages than de novo colorectal carcinoma[15]

In general, treatment of all forms of uncomplicated IBD is primarily medical, consisting of various regimens of diet, vitamin replacement, azulfidine, corticosteroids, and other immunosuppressive agents. Surgery is reserved for disease complications or for intractability.

Ocular manifestations

Ocular manifestations of IBD are relatively uncommon, involving fewer than 10% of patients with Crohn's disease and an even smaller percentage of patients with ulcerative colitis.[16] Ocular involvement may occur before or after bowel symptoms.[17] However, there appears to be a strong correla-

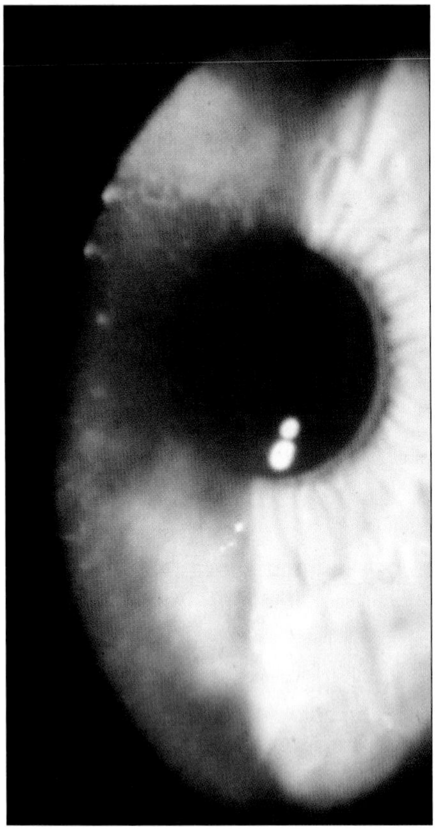

Fig. 61.1 Subepithelial keratopathy, in this case scarring, in Crohn's disease patient. (Courtesy David L. Knox, MD.)

tion between clinical attacks of the colitis and the development of eye lesions.[18]

The presence of ocular involvement in IBD is almost always associated with at least one other extraintestinal manifestation. In patients with both Crohn's disease and arthritis, the incidence of eye involvement increases to approximately 33%.[18] There is an increased prevalence of HLA-B27-type leukocytes in this subset of patients.[19] Another risk factor for ocular inflammation in patients with Crohn's disease includes colitis or ileocolitis versus those with only ileitis.[20]

Ocular complications in IBD can be divided into primary, secondary, and coincidental.[16] Primary complications are those that occur with increased activity of the bowel disease and respond to treatments directed at the gut disease itself. These can affect the anterior and posterior segments of the eye as well as the orbital contents. Anterior segment manifestations include episcleritis, scleritis, uveitis (acute iritis, chronic iridocyclitis, or panuveitis), conjunctivitis (granulomatous), and keratopathy.[1,2,16,17,21–23] It has also been observed that active episcleritis is closely correlated with active Crohn's disease in contrast to scleritis and uveitis.[16,18]

The keratopathy of Crohn's disease is felt to be so distinctive that Knox et al.[24] reported a patient who had no gastrointestinal symptoms but whose corneal findings were so suggestive of Crohn's disease that the correct diagnosis was ultimately made. These investigators describe two forms of keratopathy that likely represent a spectrum of corneal involvement: (1) an epithelial or subepithelial infiltration with an elevation characterized as small gray, pale dots, and (2) later finding of lamellar nebulous subepithelial infiltrates or scarring (Fig. 61.1). These seem to be more marked inferiorly but may appear superiorly as well. The keratopathy tends to be bilateral, symmetrical, nonstaining, and located 2–3 mm inside the entire corneoscleral limbus. The keratopathy typically does not affect vision because the lesions spare the central cornea; however, it has been reported that progressive peripheral thinning of the cornea secondary to a possible vasculitic mechanism may induce astigmatism and progressive visual deterioration.[25]

Primary complications associated with the posterior segment and the orbit include macular edema, central serous retinopathy (CSR), retinal vasculitis, retrobulbar neuritis, papillitis, and proptosis from orbital myositis.[26–28]

Secondary ocular complications of IBD result from a primary gastrointestinal complication such as poor diet or surgical resection of the affected gut, leading to malabsorption and malnutrition. Hypovitaminosis A may result from diminished absorption of vitamin A and can lead to decreased tear film production and night blindness. Additional secondary complications include cataracts, which are presumed to be the result of uveitis and steroid use, scleromalacia occurring as a result of repeated bouts of scleritis, and optic disc edema caused by peripapillary scleritis.

Some ocular manifestations may be categorized as coincidental.[16] These changes occur so frequently in the general population that a causal relationship with IBD is difficult to establish. Coincidental ocular findings include dry eye syndrome, recurrent corneal erosion, corneal ulcer, and subconjunctival hemorrhage.[22]

Treatment

Therapeutic plans for the ocular manifestations of IBD include topical steroids and/or sub-Tenon's corticosteroid injections for anterior uveitis and scleritis. Systemic nonsteroidal antiinflammatory agents may be considered if approved by a gastroenterologist. Systemic corticosteroids are indicated in the presence of severe inflammation not responsive to local therapy, optic neuropathy, or orbital disease. If inflammation does not decrease, azathioprine or other cytotoxic immunosuppressive agents should be considered, especially in patients who are HLA-B27 positive. Additionally, anti-TNF monoclonal antibody therapy is considered safer than cytotoxic immunosuppression and has been used with some success in patients who are refractive to conventional treatment.[29] Infliximab, an anti-TNF-α antibody, has been used to treat difficult acute, chronic, and refractory ocular inflammatory cases associated with inflammatory bowel disease.[30,31]

Whipple's Disease

Whipple's disease (WD) (intestinal lipodystrophy)[32] is an adult-onset, multisystem chronic inflammatory disease caused by a bacterial infection. The gastrointestinal tract, joints, heart, lung, muscles, brain, and eyes may be affected. Diarrhea associated with fat malabsorption (steatorrhea) develops as the disease progresses.

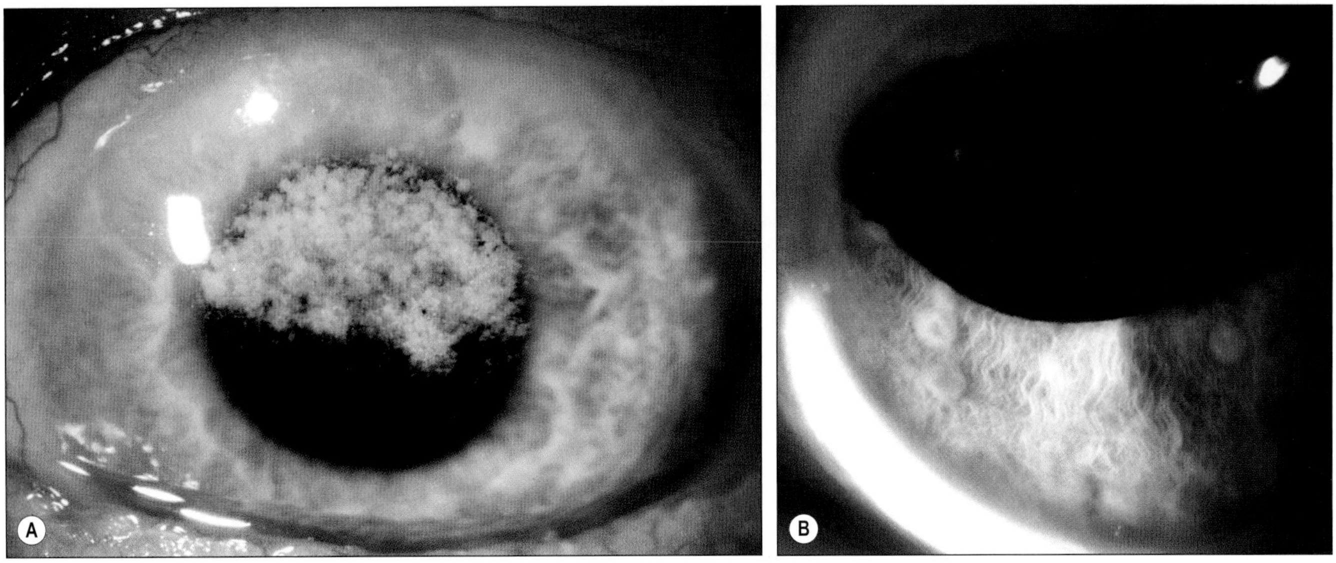

Fig. 61.2 Whipple's disease. (**A**) White, 'greasy,' flocculent precipitates on the back of the cornea. (**B**) Multiple tan iris nodules. (Courtesy Sandy Feldman, MD.)

Systemic manifestations

Whipple's disease is rare, having a predilection for HLA-B27-positive, middle-aged white men. Intestinal features include abdominal pain, diarrhea, steatorrhea, anorexia, and weight loss. Extraintestinal symptoms include fever, arthritis, generalized lymphadenopathy, skin hyperpigmentation, chronic pericarditis, and central nervous system disorders.[33,34] After review of the literature of 77 cases of ocular Whipple's disease, Chan et al. found migratory polyarthralgias to be the most common and specific extraintestinal presenting manifestation.[35]

Etiology and pathogenesis

Jejunal mucosal biopsy reveals the presence of periodic acid–Schiff (PAS)-positive macrophages.[36,37] A Gram-positive bacilli, *Tropheryma whippelii*,[37] has been identified using polymerase chain reaction (PCR) on bacterial ribosomal RNA from duodenal tissue. Abnormalities in host immunologic competence may be a contributing factor. Patients with WD have suppressed delayed-type hypersensitivity responses in vivo and decreased in vitro T-cell responses.[38] In addition, the organism has a cytotoxic effect on immunoglobulin A plasma cells which may allow it to resist local gut immune defenses.[39]

Ocular manifestations

Ophthalmic involvement in WD approaches 2.7% and may occur with or without the presence of intestinal symptoms.[33,40,41] Ophthalmic manifestations may be divided into three groups:[42] (1) ocular involvement secondary to central nervous system (CNS) damage – ophthalmoplegia,[43] nystagmus, gaze palsy, ptosis, and papilledema;[42] (2) CNS involvement together with intraocular signs; and (3) intraocular signs without CNS involvement. Such ocular signs may include stromal keratitis,[44] superficial punctate keratitis,[44] uveitis,[41] glaucoma,[44] inflammatory vitreous opacities,[40] vitreous or retinal hemorrhage, diffuse retinal and choroidal vasculitis,[42] and orbital inflammation.[46] A report described white endothelial precipitates, tan iris nodules, pars plana exudation, retinal nodular precipitates, and disk neovascularization (Fig. 61.2).[41] These findings were felt to be similar to those seen in sarcoidosis. An immune mechanism has been proposed for the ocular findings.[47] Others have reported bacterial invasion of the eye by the Whipple's bacillus, as supported by identification of the bacterium in vitrectomy samples using PCR.[40,46]

The keratitis in WD is associated with conjunctival hyperemia and slight chemosis of the perilimbal area. An inflammatory pannus may occur as a deep fibrovascular corneal infiltrate supplied by vessels from the anterior chamber angle and a distinctly separate superficial fibrovascular pannus supplied by limbal vessels.[44] Leland and Chambers described the corneal involvement as a 'grey white opacity of the stroma sandwiched between vascular membranes.'[44]

CNS involvement (which is reported in 10% of cases of WD) may produce a vertical saccadic palsy or a global saccadic palsy.[48,49] WD should be considered in the presence of any supranuclear gaze paralysis and uveitis even in the absence of gastrointestinal symptoms.[49] In addition, a distinctive oculomasticatory myorhythmia has been described as a unique pendular vergence oscillation of the eye with concurrent contractions of the masticatory muscles.[48] This movement disorder is only seen in WD. It should be used to make the presumptive diagnosis even if jejunal biopsy is normal. It is recommended that treatment for Whipple's disease be instituted in the presence of ocular masticatory myorhythmia.[48]

Treatment

The organism implicated in WD is responsive to broad-spectrum antibiotics such as tetracycline, erythromycin, ampicillin, penicillin, or chloramphenicol. Tetracycline is most commonly used, but has a 43% failure rate.[50] As a result, 2 weeks of IV therapy with ceftriaxone, streptomycin, or penicillin followed by 1 year of trimethoprim-sulfamethoxazole double strength twice a day is currently recommended as first-line treatment for improved central nervous system penetration.[51]

Antibiotic therapy usually induces a remission in WD, although if left untreated, it can be fatal. Jejunal biopsies and/or PCR analysis may be used to follow disease activity and will demonstrate decreasing number of macrophages and bacilli with response to antibiotic treatment.[50]

Recurrences up to 11 years after initial therapy have been reported.[51] Ocular inflammation, however, may persist or recur even after antibiotic therapy has 'cleared' the intestinal bacilli. Intraocular inflammation should be considered to herald possible recurrence of the systemic disease and, in its presence, antibiotic therapy should be reinstituted or the antibiotic dose increased.[41]

Chronic Granulomatous Disease

Chronic granulomatous disease (CGD) is a rare disorder associated with neutrophil dysfunction. Intrinsic neutrophil defects may be the result of impaired chemotaxis, neutrophil granule function, phagocytosis, or intracellular killing.[52] It is characterized by recurrent life-threatening infections of the lung, liver, lymph nodes, and skin with catalase-positive bacteria and fungi.[53] Excessive inflammatory reactions lead to granuloma formation.[54] The disease probably represents a group of congenital disorders that have a variety of biochemical defects but share the inability to mount a respiratory burst (the generation of microbicidal oxygen metabolites: hydrogen peroxide, hydroxyl radical, and superoxide anion).[55] In addition to altered oxidative metabolism, abnormalities in neutrophil complement (C3b)-receptor expression, antibody-dependent cellular cytotoxicity, and microtubule metabolism have all been demonstrated. The disease is inherited, and most cases are transmitted in an X-linked recessive fashion, although autosomal dominant and recessive patterns have been reported.[55]

Systemic manifestations

Infection in CGD often presents in an indolent manner with only a low-grade fever. A leukocytosis may be seen; however, the most reliable blood test to detect the presence of infection is an elevated erythrocyte sedimentation rate.[56] Patients with 'classic' CGD develop infections early in life, sometimes even within the first week, but usually during the first year. Common clinical findings include hepatosplenomegaly, dermatitis, generalized lymphadenopathy, suppurative lymphadenitis, pneumonitis, anemia, and hypergammaglobulinemia.[52] Despite aggressive medical and surgical care, a fatal outcome before adolescence frequently occurs. In addition to the classic form of the disease, adult-onset variants have been described that may be milder and not invariably fatal.[57]

Patients with CGD are most susceptible to infections by both bacteria and fungi. The frequently observed bacterial pathogens are of the staphylococcal species and the Gram-negative enteric bacilli.[52] Catalase-positive organisms are the usual offending agents because catalase-negative organisms supply their own hydrogen peroxide, thus compensating for the inability of the CGD neutrophil to produce active oxygen metabolites. Since the cell is otherwise functionally replete, intracellular killing occurs normally.[56]

Despite prompt sterilization of wounds, patients often develop continually draining sites.[56] Chronic inflammation may lead to granuloma formation throughout the body, which lead to further morbidity by occluding vital structures.[54] Histologically, the granulomas consist of plasma cells, lymphocytes, macrophages, and occasionally multinucleated giant cells.[58]

Patients who demonstrate a susceptibility to recurrent staphylococcal, fungal, or Gram-negative bacterial infections should be suspected of having CGD. Evaluation of neutrophil function in these patients will reveal normal chemotaxis and phagocytosis, but abnormal respiratory burst function.[55]

The mainstay of therapy remains aggressive treatment of the associated infections. Prophylactic antibiotics such as trimethoprim-sulfamethoxazole may be used, as well as itraconazole and INF-γ for antimycotic protection.[56,59] Recently, some investigators have reported success with bone marrow transplant and gene transfer into bone marrow stem cells.[60,61]

Ocular manifestations

Ocular findings involving both the anterior and posterior segments affect approximately 25% of CGD patients.[62] Anterior segment findings may be secondary to the inability to control normal eyelid flora. Chronic blepharoconjunctivitis and marginal or punctate keratitis have been reported, frequently accompanied by pannus formation and perilimbal immune infiltrates.[63] Patients with CGD who have chronic staphylococcal blepharitis require rigorous lid hygiene and selective use of topical antibiotics and corticosteroids to prevent corneal neovascularization and scarring. In these patients, an anterior fungal infection may also initially masquerade as staphylococcal marginal keratitis (Fig. 61.3).[64]

Typically, posterior segment findings have been described as inactive peripheral and peripapillary chorioretinal scars or optic nerve atrophy.[65] Some investigators have speculated that these scars result from bacterial microemboli or the residua of granulomas without an infectious etiology.[63] Recent reports of active inflammatory mass lesions of the retina with associated vitritis and retinal edema have been described in toddlers. CGD should be included in this differential diagnosis.[62,66]

Wegener's Granulomatosis

Wegener's granulomatosis (WG) classically includes the presence of necrotizing granulomatous inflammation of the upper or lower respiratory tract, a focal necrotizing glomerulonephritis, and a focal necrotizing vasculitis involving both arteries and veins.[67] More recently, a limited form of WG that spares the kidneys and has a better prognosis than the classic form has been recognized.[68] The granulomatous

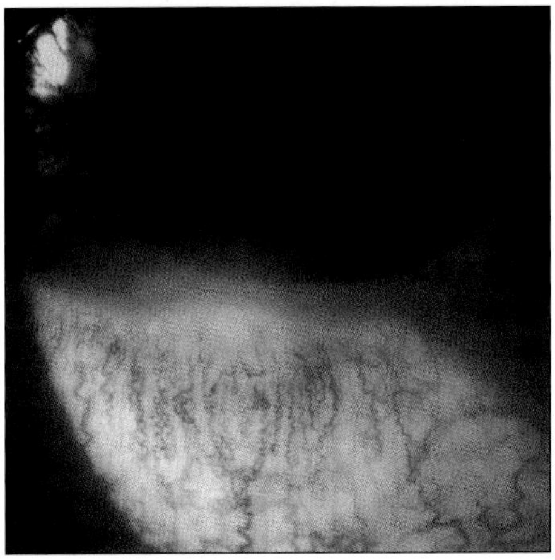

Fig. 61.3 Focal conjunctival injection with an adjacent peripheral corneal infiltrate OD in a patient with chronic granulomatous disease. (From Djalilian AR, Smith JA, Walsh TJ et al: Keratitis caused by *Candida glabrata* in a patient with chronic granulomatous disease. *Am J Ophthalmol* 132:782, 2001. Copyright Elsevier 2001.)

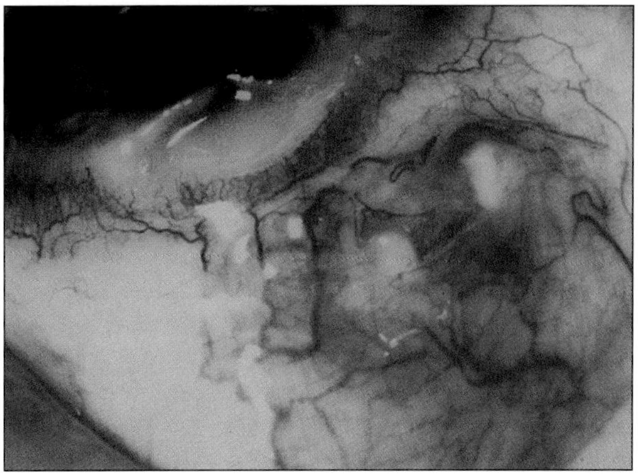

Fig. 61.4 Severe necrotizing disease affecting the cornea and sclera in a patient with Wegener's granulomatosis. (From Harper SL, Letko E, Samson CM et al: Wegener's granulomatosis: the relationship between ocular and systemic disease. *J Rheumatol* 28:1029, 2001.)

lesions consist of fibrinoid or granular necrosis surrounded by palisading histiocytes and multinucleated giant cells.[69]

Systemic manifestations

Classic Wegener's granulomatosis

Patients with classic WG may present at any age; however, the disease most commonly occurs during the fourth to fifth decades of life. There is no racial or sex predilection. The upper and lower respiratory tracts, followed by the kidney, are most commonly affected.[70]

Patients may initially have mild upper respiratory tract symptoms, night sweats, and arthralgias or show fulminant symptoms such as respiratory insufficiency and rapidly progressing renal failure. Necrotizing inflammation of the upper respiratory mucosa can lead to destruction of the nasal septum, nasal arch, and bones of the paranasal sinuses, with resultant extension into the orbits.[70–73] Involvement of the lower respiratory tract leads to a productive cough and hemoptysis. Chest roentgenograms characteristically show multiple bilateral infiltrates and nodules that may cavitate. Renal involvement usually occurs late in the course of the disease; however, in approximately 10% of patients this may be the presenting sign. Apart from the typical pulmonary and renal disease, a focal vasculitis affecting the smaller arteries and occasionally the veins of other organ systems is frequently observed.[73]

The diagnosis of WG is facilitated by the detection of antineutrophil cytoplasmic autoantibodies (ANCA) in patients with systemic vasculitis.[74–77] Two types of autoantibodies have been identified and are characterized by their pattern of staining neutrophils: c-ANCA (cytoplasmic staining) and p-ANCA (perinuclear staining).[75,76] The former appears to be specific for WG, but not all patients positive for c-ANCA can be clinically identified to have the disease and 5% of patients with WG have a positive p-ANCA.[77–80] Additionally, because a small group of patients with active, generalized disease and those with limited forms of WG may be ANCA negative, a negative blood test is not exclusive.[81]

The clinical course of classic WG is one of rapid progression. The average survival time after diagnosis in untreated patients is 5 months, with a 1-year mortality of 82% and a 2-year mortality of 90%.[82]

Limited Wegener's granulomatosis

In limited WG, the characteristic necrotizing upper and lower respiratory tract lesions are present without renal disease.[68] In addition, other forms of extrapulmonary involvement are less common and less severe than those seen in the classic form of the disease.[68,83]

The prognosis in limited WG is more favorable, with a 5-year mortality of only 20% and a greater response to immunosuppressive therapy.[83] However, ocular involvement may be as severe as in the classic form.[84]

Pathogenesis

Wegener's granulomatosis is considered a hypersensitivity disorder on the basis of its histologic manifestations. The etiology remains obscure, although inhaled and autoimmune antigens have been postulated.[85,86]

Ocular manifestations

The ocular manifestations of classic WG were first described by Cutler and Blatt in 1956.[87] The incidence of ocular involvement is generally reported to be about 40%.[88] Ranges of 28% to 58% have been cited.[89,90] This high prevalence results partly from the proximity of the orbit to the upper airways, but isolated ocular involvement may occur as part of a focal necrotizing vasculitis.

The anterior segment is the most common site of focal ocular involvement.[88] Affected patients may have conjunctivitis, marginal conjunctivitis, corneoscleral ulceration, episcleritis, and/or scleritis (Fig. 61.4).[90,91] Corneoscleral involvement is most often bilateral and usually begins with perilimbal infiltrates similar to those seen in staphylococcal hypersensitivity.[88] These infiltrates may ulcerate, with the process extending concentrically to form a ring ulcer or centrally ultimately causing perforation.[92–94]

The pathogenesis of the marginal corneal ulcers is uncertain but is believed to involve hypersensitivity, collagenase production, or local ischemia. The perilimbal keratitis is often associated with an adjacent scleritis[93] resulting from an occlusive vasculitis of intrascleral portions of the anterior ciliary arteries, perilimbal arteries, or both.[93]

The histopathology of marginal keratitis in WG involves necrosis of the epithelium and superficial stroma, along with formation of chronic granulation tissue lining the ulcer base.[93] The corneal stroma is filled with acute and chronic inflammatory cells. Occasional epithelioid and giant cells surround the ulcer.[95]

Scleritis is a frequent ocular manifestation of WG and is another example of a focal vasculitis.[91] The scleritis is usually nodular and necrotizing. The anterior sclera is primarily involved, and the inflammation is often adjacent to an area of marginal keratitis.[93] Necrotizing granulomas of the ciliary body are also seen and may be a distinctive feature of the disease.[95]

In general, local treatment of the anterior segment in WG is unsuccessful. Management should be directed at systemic therapy; however, corneal perforation may be managed acutely with cyanoacrylate glue, conjunctival flap, lamellar patch graft, or penetrating keratoplasty.[94]

WG may also cause posterior segment, orbital, and neuro-ophthalmic disease.[91,92,96] Posterior segment involvement is uncommon, but, when it is present, usually takes the form of a retinal vasculitis.[89] Other posterior segment complications include disseminated retinitis, posterior uveitis, and serous choroidal and retinal detachments.[97,98] Orbital disease is common, accounting for up to 50% of the ocular manifestations, and is characteristically bilateral. It is usually a result of contiguous spread from diseased paranasal sinuses.[89] Patients most often present with proptosis, often accompanied by chemosis and other signs or symptoms of orbital congestion.[90] Adnexal involvement may take the form of dacryoadenitis,[99] eyelid necrosis, nasolacrimal duct obstruction, or discrete granulomas of the eyelid. Neuro-ophthalmic disease presents in the form of an optic neuropathy secondary to orbital disease, a posterior ciliary vasculitis, or increased intracranial pressure secondary to cerebral involvement.[91]

Harper et al. recently explored the relationship between ocular and systemic disease and found that at the time of presentation of ocular symptoms, most patients had systemic manifestations of WG, but only 50% of these patients carried a prior diagnosis of this disease. In addition, ocular inflammation led to the diagnosis of WG in 68% of patients. This emphasizes the importance of recognizing this potentially fatal disease in patients with scleritis or ocular inflammatory lesions with or without obvious systemic manifestations of WG.[91]

Management

Currently, the first-line treatment of combined corticosteroid and cyclophosphamide successfully induces remission in 75–93% of the patients.[90,100] Rituximab, a humanized monoclonal antibody against CD20, a marker expressed by all B cells prior to maturing into plasma cells, is a novel treatment that has been used to treat patients whose symptoms are refractory to steroid and cyclophosphamide. It has been successful in treatment of progressive peripheral ulcerative keratitis and scleritis.[101,102] Rituximab is fast acting with resolution of epithelial defects and scleritis in 1 to 2 weeks. Additionally, it has a reasonable side-effect profile, making it a palatable alternative.

Kawasaki disease

Kawasaki disease (KD), or the mucocutaneous lymph node syndrome (MCLS), is an acute febrile multisystem vasculitis of unknown etiology that occurs mainly in infants and young children. The diagnosis of KD is a clinical one because, at present, no diagnostic tests or pathognomonic histologic or laboratory findings exist. The differential diagnosis includes juvenile rheumatoid arthritis, erythema multiforme minor, Stevens-Johnson syndrome, scarlet fever, toxic shock syndrome, measles, leptospirosis, tick typhus, sarcoidosis, and Reiter's syndrome.[103]

Epidemiology

Kawasaki disease occurs both endemically and epidemically and has a monomodal age distribution. Peak incidence is between the ages of 6 months and 2 years, with a range of 2 weeks to 11 years. KD is more commonly observed in males than in females, with a ratio of approximately 1.5 to 1.[104,105] The incidence of KD varies by country; however, the highest attack rates are reported in Asian countries, where an incidence of 40 to 150 cases per 100 000 children has been reported. The incidence of KD among US children less than 5 years of age is 6 to 10 cases per 100 000 children.[105]

Etiology and pathogenesis

The etiology of KD is unknown. The clinical presentation (acute onset of fever and aseptic meningitis) and the epidemiology (occurrence of epidemics) strongly suggest an infectious etiology. Viruses, bacteria, and fungi have all been implicated.[105] However, no infectious entity has been consistently isolated.

The pathogenesis of the vasculitis is believed to have an immunologic origin. Evidence for this is based on elevated acute-phase reactants, elevated immunoglobulin concentrations,[104,106] elevated levels of B- and T-helper cells, a depression of suppressor T cells, the presence of circulating immune complexes,[104] increased cytokine elaboration,[107] and the clinical response to intravenous immune globulin (IVIG).

Systemic manifestations

A patient who fulfills five of the following six criteria should be considered to have KD:[104,107]

1. Fever persisting for more than 5 days
2. Bilateral conjunctival injection
3. Changes in the mouth consisting of
   a. Erythema and fissuring of the lips
   b. Diffuse oropharyngeal erythema
   c. Strawberry tongue

4. Changes in the peripheral extremities consisting of
   a. Induration of the hands and feet
   b. Erythema of the palms and soles
   c. Desquamation of finger and toe tips approximately 2 weeks after onset
   d. Transverse grooves across fingernails, 2 to 3 months after onset
5. Erythematous rash of torso
6. Enlarged lymph node mass greater than 1.5 cm in diameter

The clinical course of KD is triphasic,[104,106] consisting of an acute febrile phase, a subacute phase, and a convalescent phase. During the acute febrile phase, leukocytosis with a predominance of polymorphonuclear leukocytes is observed. There is also an elevation in the C-reactive protein and erythrocyte sedimentation rate, which gradually normalizes. Thrombocytosis occurs, with platelet counts peaking at levels of 600 000 to 1.8 million between the fifteenth and twenty-fifth days after onset of the illness.[106] As the fever, rash, and lymphadenopathy subside, the second phase commences with features of persistent anorexia, irritability, thrombocytosis, and desquamation. In addition, arthritis, arthralgia, aseptic meningitis, and various forms of cardiac disease may be seen during this phase.[106] The period of thrombocytosis is associated with the highest risk of coronary artery thrombosis. The convalescent phase lasts from the period when all signs of illness have disappeared until the sedimentation rate has returned to normal, usually 6 to 8 weeks from onset.

The illness is usually self-limited and without sequelae; however, the prognosis depends on the presence and extent of cardiac involvement.[104] A fatal outcome is reported in 1–2.8% of cases.[108,109] Recurrence is uncommon, with less than 3% of children experiencing more than one episode.[104,105]

Ocular manifestations

Bilateral conjunctival injection, present in greater than 95% of cases,[108] appears within 2 days of the onset of fever, persists throughout the febrile course, and may last for as long as 3 to 5 weeks. It consists of a mild to moderate symmetrical vascular injection of the bulbar conjunctiva that is more severe than that seen in the tarsal or palpebral conjunctiva.[104,110] It is not a true conjunctivitis, since the conjunctival tissue itself demonstrates little or no inflammation.[110] There is an absence of chemosis, follicles, papillae, membrane, or pseudomembrane formation. Exudate and discharge, if present, are minimal. The conjunctival changes generally resolve without sequelae. However, a case of an infant who developed bilateral scarring of the superior and inferior conjunctival fornices has been reported.[111]

The presence of an anterior uveitis was reported in 66–100% of cases in three small series.[110,112] The inflammation of anterior chamber vessels is believed to be another example of systemic vasculitis[112] and reaches a maximal intensity at 5 to 8 days after the onset of fever.[110] The iritis is mild, bilateral, nongranulomatous, and symmetrical. It is self-limited, resolving without the use of pharmacologic agents and without any of the usual sequelae of uveitis.[110]

Additional, less frequently observed ocular findings in KD include superficial punctate keratitis, vitreous opacities, papilledema, and subconjunctival hemorrhage.[110] Rare ocular manifestations include chorioretinal inflammation and retinal ischemia associated with thrombosis of the ophthalmic artery.[113,114] Retinal vascular involvement is surprisingly rare, given the systemic vasculitis associated with KD.

Management

Early diagnosis and treatment of KD have been shown to decrease cardiac complications.[115] When IVIG and aspirin therapy are initiated within the first 10 days after the onset of fever, the formation of coronary artery dilation and aneurysm is decreased. It is recommended that IVIG and aspirin be initiated as early as possible.[106]

References

1. Danzi T. Extraintestinal manifestations of idiopathic inflammatory bowel disease. *Arch Intern Med.* 1988;148:297–302.
2. Das KM. Relationship of extraintestinal involvements in inflammatory bowel disease. *Dig Dis Sci.* 1999;44:1–13.
3. Satsangi J, et al. Genetics of inflammatory bowel disease. *Clin Sci.* 1998;94(5):473–478.
4. Pena AS, Crusius JB. Genetics of inflammatory bowel disease: implications for the future. *World J Surg.* 1998;22(4):390–393.
5. Binder V, Orholm M. Familial occurrence and inheritance studies in inflammatory bowel disease. *Neth J Med.* 1996;48(8):53–56.
6. Hugot JP, Laurent-Puig P, Gower-Rousseau C, et al: Mapping susceptibility locus for Crohn's disease on chromosome 16. *Nature.* 1996;29: 821–823.
7. Karban A, Ellakim R, Brant SR. Genetics of inflammatory bowel disease. *Isr Med Assoc J.* 2002;4(10):798–802.
8. Cho JH. The Nod2 gene in Crohn's disease: implications for future research into the genetics and immunology of Crohn's disease. *Inflamm Bowel Dis.* 2001;7(3):271–275.
9. Kleessen B, et al. Mucosal and invading bacteria in patients with inflammatory bowel disease compared with controls. *Scand J Gastroenterol.* 2002;37(9):1034–1041.
10. Abreu MT. The pathogenesis of inflammatory bowel disease. *Curr Gastroenterol Rep.* 2002;4(6):506–512.
11. Duerr RH. The genetics of inflammatory bowel disease. *Gastroenterol Clin North Am.* 2002;31(1):63–73.
12. Kirsner JB, Shorter RG. Recent developments in 'nonspecific' inflammatory bowel disease. *N Engl J Med.* 1982;306:779–785, 837–848.
13. Kirsner JB. Problems in the differentiation of ulcerative colitis and Crohn's disease of the colon: the need for repeated diagnostic evaluation. *Gastroenterology.* 1975;68:187–191.
14. Rudolph WG, et al. Intermediate colitis: the real story. *Dig Colon Rectum.* 2002;45(11):1528–1534.
15. Bernstein CN, et al. Cancer risk in patients with inflammatory bowel disease: a population based study. *Cancer.* 2001;91:854–862.
16. Knox DL, Schachat AP, Mustonen E. Primary, secondary, and coincidental ocular complications of Crohn's disease. *Ophthalmology.* 1984;91:163–173.
17. Petrelli EA, McKinley M, Troncale FJ. Ocular manifestations of inflammatory bowel disease. *Ann Ophthalmol.* 1982;14:356.
18. Hopkins DDJ, Horan E, Burton EL, et al. Ocular disorders in a series of 332 patients with Crohn's disease. *Br J Ophthalmol.* 1974;58:732–737.
19. Mallas EG, et al. Histocompatibility antigens in inflammatory bowel disease; their clinical significance and their association with arthropathy with special reference to HLA-B27. *Gut.* 1976;17:906–910.
20. Salmon JF, Wright JP, Murray AD. Ocular inflammation in Crohn's disease. *Ophthalmology.* 1991;98:480–484.
21. Mintz R, et al. Ocular manifestations of inflammatory bowel disease. *Inflamm Bowel Dis.* 2004;10(2):135–139.
22. Felekis T, et al. Spectrum and frequency of ophthalmologic manifestations in patients with inflammatory bowel disease: a prospective single-center study. *Inflamm Bowel Dis.* 2009;15(1):29–34.
23. Blase WP, Knox DL, Green WR. Granulomatous conjunctivitis in a patient with Crohn's disease. *Br J Ophthalmol.* 1984;68:901–903.
24. Knox DL, Snip RC, Stark WJ. The keratopathy of Crohn's disease. *Am J Ophthalmol.* 1980;90:862–865.

25. Geerards AJM, Beekhuis WH, Remeyer L, et al. Crohn's colitis and the cornea. *Cornea.* 1997;16:227–231.
26. Durno CA, et al. Keeping an eye on Crohn's disease: orbital myositis as the presenting symptom. *Can J Gastroenterol.* 1991;11:497–500.
27. Ernst BB, Lowder CY, Meisler DM, et al: Posterior segment manifestations of inflammatory bowel disease. *Ophthalmology.* 1991;98:1272–1280.
28. Ruby AJ, Jampol LM. Crohn's disease and retinal vascular disease. *Am J Ophthalmol.* 1990;110:349–353.
29. D'Haens G, Daperno M. Advance in medical therapy for Crohn's disease. *Curr Gastroenterol Rep.* 2002;4(6):506–512.
30. Ally MR, Veerapa GR, Koff JM. Treatment of recurrent Crohn's uveitis with infliximab. *Am J Gastro.* 2008;103:2150–2151.
31. Hale S, Lightman S. Anti-TNF therapies in the management of acute and chronic uveitis. *Cytokine.* 2006;33:231–237.
32. Whipple GH. A hitherto undescribed disease characterized anatomically by deposits of fat and fatty acids in the intestinal and mesenteric lymphatic tissues. *Bull Johns Hopkins Hosp.* 1907;18:382–391.
33. Frohman L, Lama P. Annual update of systemic disease – 1999: emerging and re-emerging infections. *J Neuro-Ophthalmol.* 1999;19(4):263–273.
34. Fleming JL, Wiesner RH, Shorter RG. Whipple's disease: clinical biochemical and histopathologic features and assessment of treatment in 29 patients. *Mayo Clin Proceed.* 1988;63:539–551.
35. Chan RY, Yannuzzi LA, Foster CS. Ocular Whipple's disease. *Ophthalmology.* 2001;108:2225–2231.
36. Maiwald M, Ditton HJ, von Herbay A, et al. Reassessment of the phylogenetic position of the bacterium associated with Whipple's disease and determination of the 16S-23S ribosomal intergenic spacer sequence. *Int J Syst Bacteriol.* 1996;46:1078–1082.
37. Relman DA, Schmidt TM, MacDermott RP, et al. Identification of the uncultured bacillus of Whipple's disease. *J Med.* 1992;327(5):293–301.
38. Marth T, Neurath M, Cuccherini BA, et al. Defects of monocyte interleukin 12 production and humoral immunity in Whipple's disease. *Gastroenterology.* 1997;113:442–448.
39. Eck M, Kreipe H, Harmsen D, et al. Invasion and destruction of mucosal plasma cells by *Tropheryma whippelii. Hum Pathol.* 1996;28:1424–1428.
40. Selsky EJ, Knox DL, Maumenee E, et al. Ocular involvement in Whipple's disease. *Retina.* 1984;4:103–106.
41. Rickman LS, Freeman WR, Green WR, et al. Uveitis caused by *Tropheryma whippelii* (Whipple's bacillus). *N Engl J Med.* 1995;332:363–366.
42. Avila MP, Jalkh AE, Feldman E, et al. Manifestations of Whipple's disease in the posterior segment of the eye. *Arch Ophthalmol.* 1984;102:384–390.
43. Knox DL, Green WR, Troncoso JC, et al. Cerebral ocular Whipple's disease: a 62-year odyssey from death to diagnosis. *Neurology.* 1995;45:617–625.
44. Leland TM, Chambers JK. Ocular findings in Whipple's disease. *South Med J.* 1978;71:335–338.
45. Lieger O, et al. Orbital manifestations of Whipple's disease: an atypical case. *J Craniomaxillofac Surg.* 2007;35(8):393–396.
46. Nishimura JK, Cook BE, Pach JM. Whipple disease presenting as posterior uveitis without prominent gastrointestinal symptoms. *Am J Ophthalmol.* 1998;126:130–132.
47. Adams M, et al. Whipple's disease confined to the central nervous system. *Ann Neurol.* 1987;21:104–108.
48. Schwartz MA, Selhorst JB, Ochs AL, et al. Ocular masticatory myorhythmia: a unique movement disorder occurring in Whipple's disease. *Ann Neurol.* 1986;20:677–683.
49. Simpson DA, Wishnow R, Gargulinski RB, et al. Oculofacial-skeletal myorhythmia in central nervous system Whipple's disease: additional case and review of the literature. *Movement Disorders.* 1995;10(2):195–200.
50. Keinath RD, et al. Antibiotic treatment and relapse in Whipple's disease. Long-term follow-up of 88 patients. *Gastroenterology.* 1985;88:1867–1873.
51. Schnider PJ, et al: Treatment guidelines in central nervous system Whipple's disease (letter). *Ann Neurol.* 1997;41:561–562.
52. Johnston RB Jr. Clinical aspects of chronic granulomatous disease. *Curr Opin Hematol.* 2001;8(1):17–22.
53. Buggage RR, et al. Uveitis and a subretinal mass in a patient with chronic granulomatous disease. *Br J Ophthalmol.* 2006;90:514–515.
54. Foster CB, et al. Host defense molecule polymorphisms influence the risk for immune-mediated complications in chronic granulomatous disease. *J Clin Invest.* 1998;102:2146–2155.
55. Winkelstein JA, et al. Chronic granulomatous disease. Report on a national registry of 368 patients. *Medicine.* 2000;79:155–169.
56. Gallin JI, et al. Recent advances in chronic granulomatous disease. *Ann Intern Med.* 1983;99:657–674.
57. Perry HB, et al. Chronic granulomatous disease in an adult with recurrent abscesses. *Arch Surg.* 1980;115:200–202.
58. Nakhleh RE, Glock M, Snover DC: Hepatic pathology of chronic granulomatous disease of childhood. *Arch Pathol Lab Med.* 1992;116:71–75.
59. Goldblatt D. Current treatment options for chronic granulomatous disease. *Expert Opin Pharmacother.* 2002;3(7):857–863.
60. Horwitz ME, et al. Treatment of chronic granulomatous disease with nonmyeloablative conditioning and a T-cell depleted hematopoietic allograft. *N Engl J Med.* 2001;344:881–888.
61. Baehner RL. Chronic granulomatous disease of childhood: clinical, pathological, biochemical, molecular, and genetic aspects of the disease. *Pediatr Pathol.* 1990;10:143–153.
62. Buggage RR, et al. Uveitis and a subretinal mass in a patient with chronic granulomatous disease. *Br J Ophthalmol.* 2006;90:514–515.
63. Palestine AG, et al. Ocular findings in patients with neutrophil dysfunction. *Am J Ophthalmol.* 1983;95:598–604.
64. Djalilian AR, et al: Keratitis caused by *Candida glabrata* in a patient with chronic granulomatous disease. *Am J Ophthalmol.* 2001;132:782–783.
65. Valluri S, Chu FC, Smith ME. Ocular pathologic findings of chronic granulomatous disease of childhood. *Am J Ophthalmol.* 1995;120:120–123.
66. Mansour AM, et al. Chronic granulomatous disease presenting as retinal mass. *Cases J.* 2008;1(1):257.
67. Godman GC, Chung J. Wegener's granulomatosis. Pathology and review of the literature. *Arch Pathol.* 1954;58:533–553.
68. Carrington CB, Liebow AA. Limited forms of angiitis and granulomatosis of the Wegener's type. *Am J Med.* 1966;41:497–527.
69. Grove AS. Wegener's disease. In: Gold DH, Weingeist TA, eds. *The eye and systemic disease.* Philadelphia: Lippincott; 1990.
70. Leavitt RY, et al. The American College of Rheumatology 1990 criteria for the classification of Wegener's granulomatosis. *Arthritis Rheum.* 1990;33:1101–1107.
71. Rasmussen N. Management of the ear, nose, and throat manifestations of Wegener granulomatosis: an otorhinolaryngologist's perspective. *Curr Opin Rhuematol.* 2001;13:3–11.
72. Robin JB, et al. Ocular involvement in the respiratory vasculitides. *Surv Ophthalmol.* 1985;30:127–140.
73. Stone JH, Nousari HC. 'Essential' cutaneous vasculitis: what every rheumatologist should know about vasculitis of the skin. *Curr Opin Rheumatol.* 2001;13:23–34.
74. van der Woude FJ, et al. Autoantibodies against neutrophils and monocytes: tool for diagnosis and marker for disease activity in Wegener's granulomatosis. *Lancet.* 1985;i:425–429.
75. Savage COS, et al. Prospective study of radioimmunoassay for antibodies against neutrophil cytoplasm in the diagnosis of systemic vasculitis. *Lancet.* 1987;i:1389–1393.
76. Goldschmeding R, et al. Identification of the ANCA antigen as a novel myeloid lysosomal serine protease. *APMIS.* 1989;97(suppl 6):46.
77. Falk RJ, Jennett JC. Anti-neutrophil cytoplasmic autoantibodies with specificity for myeloperoxidase in patients with systemic vasculitis and idiopathic necrotizing and crescenteric glomerulonephritis. *N Engl J Med.* 1989;318:1651–1657.
78. Jenett JC, et al. Antineutrophil cytoplasmic autoantibody associated glomerulonephritis. *Am J Pathol.* 1989;135:921.
79. Jacobs DS, Foster CS. Wegener's granulomatosis. In: Albert DM, Jakobiec FA, eds. *Principles and practice of ophthalmology.* Philadelphia: Saunders; 1994.
80. Hauschild S, et al. ANCA in systemic vasculitides, collagen vascular diseases, rheumatic disorders and inflammatory bowel disease. *Adv Exp Med Biol.* 1993;336:245–251.
81. Musashir E, et al. Wegener granulomatosis: a case report and update. *S Med Ass.* 2006;99(9).
82. Walton EW. Giant cell granuloma of the respiratory tract. *Br Med J.* 1958;2:265.
83. Cassan SM, Coles DT, Harrison EG Jr. The concept of limited forms of Wegener's granulomatosis. *Am J Med.* 1966;41:497–526.
84. Coutu RE, et al. Limited form of Wegener's granulomatosis: eye involvement as a major sign. *JAMA.* 1975;233:868–871.
85. Blatt IM, et al. Fatal granulomatosis of the respiratory tract. *Arch Otolaryngol.* 1959;70:707–749.
86. Haynes BF. Wegener's granulomatosis and midline granuloma. In: Hyngaarden JB, Smith LH, Bennett JC, eds. *Cecil's textbook of medicine.* Philadelphia: Saunders; 1988.
87. Cutler WM, Blatt IM. The ocular manifestations of lethal midline granuloma (Wegener's granulomatosis). *Am J Ophthalmol.* 1956;42:21–35.
88. Spalton DJ, et al. Ocular changes in limited forms of Wegener's granulomatosis. *Br J Ophthalmol.* 1981;65:553–563.

89. Fauci AS, et al. Wegener's granulomatosis: prospective clinical and therapeutic experience with 85 patients in 21 years. *Ann Intern Med.* 1983;98:76.
90. Harper SL, et al. Wegener's granulomatosis: the relationship between ocular and systemic disease. *J Rheumatol.* 2001;28:1025–1032.
91. Bullen CL, et al. Ocular complications of Wegener's granulomatosis. *Ophthalmology.* 1983;90:279–290.
92. Hanada K, et al. Therapeutic keratoplasty for corneal perforation: clinical results and complications. *Cornea.* 2008;27(2): 156–160.
93. Austin P, et al. Peripheral corneal degeneration and occlusive vasculitis in Wegener's granulomatosis. *Am. J Ophthalmol.* 1978;85:311–317.
94. Messmer EM, Foster CS. Vasculitic peripheral ulcerative keratitis. *Surv Ophthalmol.* 1999;43:379–396.
95. Frayer WC. The histopathology of perilimbal ulceration in Wegener's granulomatosis. *Arch Ophthalmol.* 1960;64:58–64.
96. Haynes BF, et al. The ocular manifestations of Wegener's granulomatosis: fifteen years experience and review of the literature. *Am J Med.* 1977;63:131–141.
97. Jaben SL, Morton EW. Exudative retinal detachment in Wegener's granulomatosis: case report. *Ann Ophthalmol.* 1982;14:717–720.
98. Leveille AS, Morse PH. Combined detachments in Wegener's granulomatosis. *Br J Ophthalmol.* 1981;65:564–567.
99. Leavitt JA, Butrus SI. Wegener's granulomatosis presenting as dacryoadenitis. *Cornea.* 1991;10(6):542–545.
100. Langford CA. Wegner granulomatous. *Am J Sci.* 2001;321:76–82.
101. Freidlin J, Wong IG, Acharya N. Rituximab treatment for peripheral ulcerative keratitis associated with Wegener's granulomatosis. *Br J Ophthalmol.* 2007;91:1414.
102. Cheung CMG, Murray PI, Savage COS. Successful treatment of Wegener's granulomatosis associated scleritis with rituximab. *Br J Ophthalmol.* 2005;89:1542.
103. Smith LBH, Newburger JW, Burns JC. Kawasaki syndrome and the eye. *Pediatr Infect Dis J.* 1989;8:116–118.
104. Melish ME, Hicks RV. Kawasaki syndrome: clinical features. Pathophysiology, etiology and therapy. *J Rheumatol.* 1990;17(suppl 24):2–10.
105. Dajani AS, et al. Diagnosis and therapy of Kawasaki disease in children. *Circulation.* 1993;87:1776–1780.
106. Melish ME. Kawasaki syndrome (the mucocutaneous lymph node syndrome). *Ann Rev Med.* 1982;33:569–585.
107. Leung DYM, et al. Ism antibodies present in the acute phase of Kawasaki syndrome lyse cultured vascular endothelial cells stimulated by gamma interferon. *J Clin Invest.* 1986;77:1428–1435.
108. Morens DM, Anderson LJ, Hurwitz ES. National surveillance of Kawasaki disease. *Pediatrics.* 1980;65:21–25.
109. Puglise JV, et al. Ocular features of Kawasaki's disease. *Arch Ophthalmol.* 1982;100:1101–1103.
110. Ohno S, et al. Ocular manifestations of Kawasaki's disease, (mucocutaneous lymph node syndrome). *Am J Ophthalmol.* 1982;93:713–717.
111. Ryan EH, Walton DS. Conjunctival scarring in Kawasaki disease: a new finding? *J Pediatr Ophthalmol Strabismus.* 1983;20:106–108.
112. Burns JC, et al. Anterior uveitis associated with Kawasaki syndrome. *Pediatr Infect Dis.* 1985;4:258–261.
113. Font RL, et al. Bilateral retinal ischemia in Kawasaki disease. *Ophthalmology.* 1983;90:569–577.
114. Favardin M, et al: Sudden unilateral blindness in a girl with Kawasaki disease. *J Pediatr Ophthalmol Strabismus.* 2007;44(5):303–304.
115. Newburger JW, et al. The treatment of Kawasaki syndrome with intravenous gamma globulin. *N Engl J Med.* 1986;315:341–347.

Chapter 62

Nutritional Disorders

Deval R. Paranjpe, Christopher J. Newton, Andrew A. E. Pyott, Colin M. Kirkness

All tissues throughout the body depend on adequate levels of nutrition, and the cornea is no exception. Deficiency or excess of various substances can lead to altered corneal metabolism but, with few exceptions, only one is of clinical importance. This striking example is given by inadequate levels of vitamin A.

It is estimated that as many as 140 million children worldwide are vitamin A deficient,[1] making it the second most prevalent nutritional disorder after protein calorie malnutrition. Of these, 4.4 million are xerophthalmic.[2] Between 250 000 and 500 000 xerophthalmic children become blind annually, and up to half will die within 1 year of losing their vision.[1] Improving the vitamin A status of all deficient children could prevent between 1 and 3 million deaths,[3] with the cost of 2 days of supplementation being about 10 US cents per child.[4] If the scale of the problem is impressive, so too is the behavior of an individual cornea, which, when faced with a sudden decompensation of vitamin A levels, can undergo complete colliquative necrosis within a matter of hours.

While this tragedy is largely borne by the impoverished of developing countries, it is occasionally encountered in so-called developed nations. Thus, clinical xerophthalmia has been observed in food fadists,[5] psychiatric patients,[6–8] and alcoholics.[9,10] Particularly important is the recognition that conditions that can lead to fat malabsorption, such as cystic fibrosis[11,12] or surgical procedures involving jejunoileal bypass,[13] can lead to xerophthalmia and that ocular problems can be overlooked for many years because the diagnosis is not entertained.[14]

Metabolism of Vitamin A

The storage capacity of the human body is greater for fat-soluble than for water-soluble vitamins and, accordingly, under normal conditions the liver can maintain a 1 to 2 years' supply of vitamin A. Thus, when intake exceeds 300 to 1200 µg/day of retinol or its equivalent, stores are laid down. When intake falls below this level, liver stores are drained to maintain serum retinol levels above 0.7 µmol/L.[15] Vitamin A is found in animal foods and dairy products, usually esterified as retinyl palmitate. After ingestion, hydrolysis occurs in the small intestine, producing retinol, which is then incorporated into mixed micelles and absorbed into mucosal cells.[16] Carotene is a naturally occurring progenitor of vitamin A produced by plants. However, the efficiency of carotenoid conversion varies among individuals,[17] and only 50 or 60 of the 400 known carotenoids have provitamin activity.[18] The most important of these is beta-carotene, which is present in dark green leafy vegetables and certain colored fruits. Carotene, when absorbed into mucosal cells, is split into two molecules of retinaldehyde, which are then reduced to retinol. Retinol travels to the liver largely in the re-esterified form. Retinol is a highly active, membrane-toxic molecule. It is released from the liver in combination with a specific transport protein called apo-RBP (retinol-binding protein). The complex of apo-RBP and retinol is known as holo-RBP16 (Fig. 62.1). Associated deficiencies of fat or protein can interfere with the metabolism of both carotene and vitamin A. However, these deficiencies seem to play a relatively minor role compared with actual vitamin A deficiency, In areas prone to kwashiorkor, even the small amounts of carotene in bananas and other produce can prevent the development of xerophthalmia.[19] Xerophthalmia is particularly prevalent in areas such as Southeast Asia where rice is the staple food.[20] In all areas of endemic xerophthalmia, the diet is deficient in sources of the preformed vitamin, such as milk, eggs, and meat, and reliance is on limited amounts of the provitamin.[19]

Historical Considerations

Xerophthalmia is one of the oldest recorded medical afflictions, and both nyctalopia (night blindness) and keratomalacia were recognized by the ancient Egyptians and Greeks. Interestingly, their treatments for these conditions frequently involved the use of animal livers.[21] The celebrated Scottish ophthalmologist William Mackenzie was familiar with the disease, and in 1830 he published *A Practical Treatise on the Diseases of the Eye*, where he refers to 'conjunctiva arida.' He also elaborated on the beautifully descriptive term myiocephalon (head of a fly) to describe the prolapse of the iris through a softened cornea.[22]

Probably the first person to produce xerophthalmia experimentally was the French physiologist Magendie. In 1816, he fed dogs a restrictive diet of wheat gluten, starch, and olive oil, and he mentions the development of corneal ulcers.[23] Such animal experiments have since often been

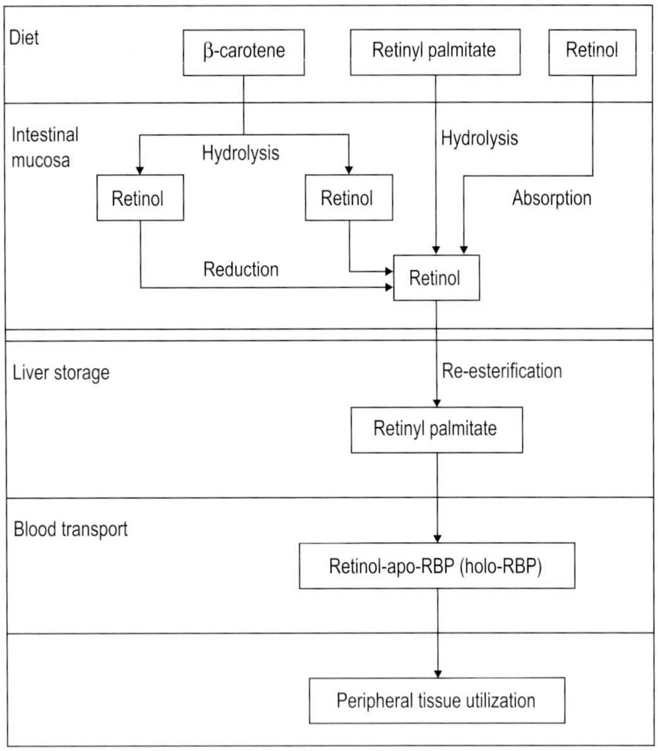

Fig. 62.1 Metabolism of vitamin A.

repeated. Only in 1925 in the work of Wolbach and Howe, using selectively vitamin A-deficient diets in rats, was the primacy of the vitamin's role in the development of keratomalacia established.[24] It was, however, a European epidemic of keratomalacia and painstaking observations by the Danish physician Bloch that confirmed the parallels in humans.[25,26]

Classification and Clinical Manifestations of Xerophthalmia

Vitamin A deficiency results in changes in mucosal surfaces throughout the body, and the resulting keratinizing metaplasia in the lining epithelia of the lungs and intestines is responsible for the respiratory and gastrointestinal symptoms of severely depleted children. It is in the eye that the classic signs of vitamin A deficiency can be readily observed. Because of the importance of being able to screen and evaluate treatment regimens in communities at risk, considerable care has been taken to draw up a classification of the different stages of the disease (Box 62.1).[27] This classification scheme remains the standard for assessment of xerophthalmia to date.

Night blindness (XN)

Retinol is essential for the production by the rod photoreceptors of the visual pigment rhodopsin. In mild cases, nyctalopia or 'night blindness' is apparent only after photic stress, but all patients respond rapidly to therapy with vitamin A, usually within 48 hours.[15]

Box 62.1 Classification of xerophthalmia (1982 revision)

XN Night blindness
X1A Conjunctival xerosis
X1B Bitot's spots
X2 Corneal xerosis
X3A Corneal ulceration/keratomalacia < ⅓ of corneal surface
X3B Corneal ulceration/keratomalacia > ⅓ of corneal surface
XS Corneal scar
XF Xerophthalmic fundus

Adapted from Control of vitamin A deficiency and xerophthalmia. *Report of a joint WHO/USAID/UNICEF/HKI/IVACG meeting (WHO Technical Report Series, No. 672), Geneva, 1982, World Health Organization.*

Conjunctival xerosis (X1A) and Bitot's spots (X1B)

Conjunctival xerosis and Bitot's spots should be considered together. The diagnosis of 'Bitot's spots' is dogged with controversy. The first description was by Hubbenet (1860)[28] but Bitot (1863)[29] made the observation of dry scaly patches on the bulb of the eye and their association with nyctalopia and lack of 'corneal luster.' The observation that some Bitot's spots appear in isolation (without coexisting clinical or biochemical evidence) and fail to respond to vitamin A therapy has led some to claim that they bear no relationship to vitamin A deficiency at all.[30,31]

Histologically, xerosis represents metaplasia of the conjunctival epithelium from its normal columnar to a stratified squamous type. A prominent granular layer is apparent, but most significant is the loss of goblet cells and the formation of a metaplastic, keratinized surface.[16] In inverse relationship with the depletion of goblet cells is an increase in the mitotic rate of the epithelial cells, although, unlike ocular cicatricial pemphigoid where this also occurs, there is no subepithelial scarring.[32] As an example of the extreme lengths to which the keratinizing effect can occur, there is a documented case of a calf born to a vitamin A-deficient cow that had a thick patch of hair in the center of its cornea.[33]

Histologically, Bitot's spots are tangles of keratin admixed with saprophytic bacteria and sometimes fungi.[16] Often *Corynebacterium* xerosis is present, and it is suggested that since this is a gas-forming organism, it is responsible for the typical 'foamy' appearance of other spots.[31] The material can be easily scraped off. The base, however, remains xerotic and the 'spot' will recur within a few days. The deposit can be very extensive, involving the cornea as well as the conjunctiva.[19]

The real confusion regarding the significance of Bitot's spots has arisen because sometimes they are observed in individuals who have no supportive evidence of vitamin A deficiency, nor do they always disappear with supplemental vitamin therapy. Sommer[16] has carried out a careful investigation comparing lesions responsive and those unresponsive to retinol. While numerically far less prevalent, nasally situated lesions are a more reliable sign of active deficiency. They are always less prominent than temporal lesions.

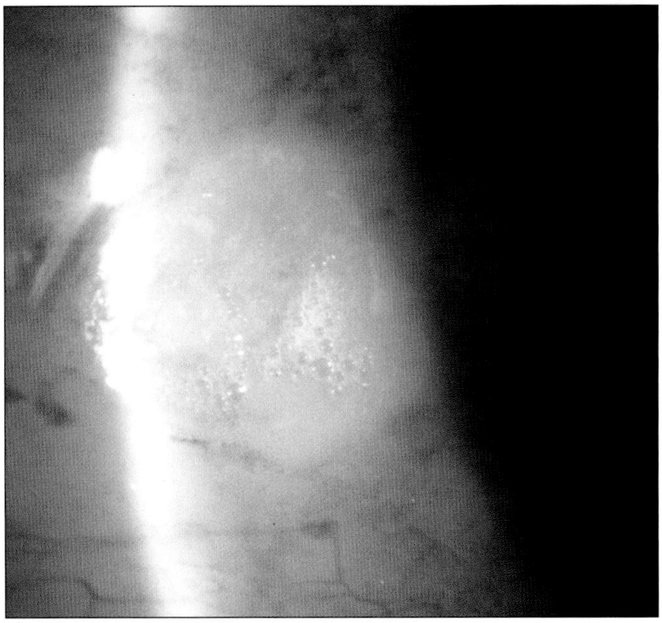

Fig. 62.2 Typical 'foamy' Bitot's spot.

A far more significant indicator is the age of the patient. Sommer found that in those under 6 years of age, 97% of lesions disappeared rapidly; xerosis resolves within 2 to 5 days, and most spots resolve in 2 weeks. In children over 10 years of age, 60% were unresponsive. The general principle applies that in a child under 6, especially when a history of night blindness can be established, a Bitot's spot should be regarded as evidence of vitamin A deficiency. In older children it is evidence of past or chronic suboptimal levels of retinol. From a practical point of view, given the tendency for clustering of vitamin A deficiency,[34] when an older child is found with Bitot's spots, it is probably the younger siblings who are in greater need of examination and treatment.

The development and persistence of Bitot's spots are almost certainly related to exposure.[35] Although histologic evidence is widespread early in the disease, clinically obvious xerosis is seen just on the temporal conjunctiva (Fig. 62.2), then nasally, then inferiorly, and finally superiorly. If excised, lesions do not recur, providing an adequate diet is maintained.[36]

In adults, the presence of thickening, wrinkling, and pigmentation of the conjunctiva can be caused by chronic ultraviolet (UV) exposure, smoke, dust, and eye infections and should not be seen as pathognomonic of vitamin A deficiency.[19] In children, however, dryness of the conjunctiva is always significant. While it is usual for conjunctival xerosis to precede or coexist with more severe ocular involvement, it should not be regarded as a sine qua non. Inflammation may mask (or possibly even reverse) conjunctival xerosis. In general, however, when 180 degrees of the conjunctiva is involved, then there is either established or incipient corneal disease.[37]

Corneal xerosis (X2)

Careful slit lamp examination may reveal superficial punctate, fluorescein-staining lesions in eyes that otherwise have no obvious clinical evidence of conjunctival xerosis. Initially, these lesions are seen inferonasally, but later they progress to involve the entire corneal surface. Sometimes nonstaining, water-repellant microcysts are seen. They respond readily to vitamin A therapy, often being replaced by fluorescein-positive punctate defects.[15] In more established disease, it is possible to use a penlight to detect localized or generalized edema with a typical dry, 'lackluster' appearance (Fig. 62.3). Later, the cornea may develop a 'peau d'orange' appearance from keratinization (Fig. 62.4). Sometimes, fluorescein staining reveals pooling between plaques of keratinized epithelium, giving rise to a tree-bark appearance.[16] Accumulated keratin debris and bacteria resembling Bitot's spots may form; these peel off with treatment, often leaving a small superficial erosion that heals rapidly.[15] Many of the early changes of corneal xerosis resemble localized exposure and dellen formation.[38] Vitamin A deficiency has been shown to reduce aqueous tear production.[39] Loss of mucus-producing goblet cells leads to localized drying and epithelial loss.[40] Furthermore, vitamin A deficiency has been

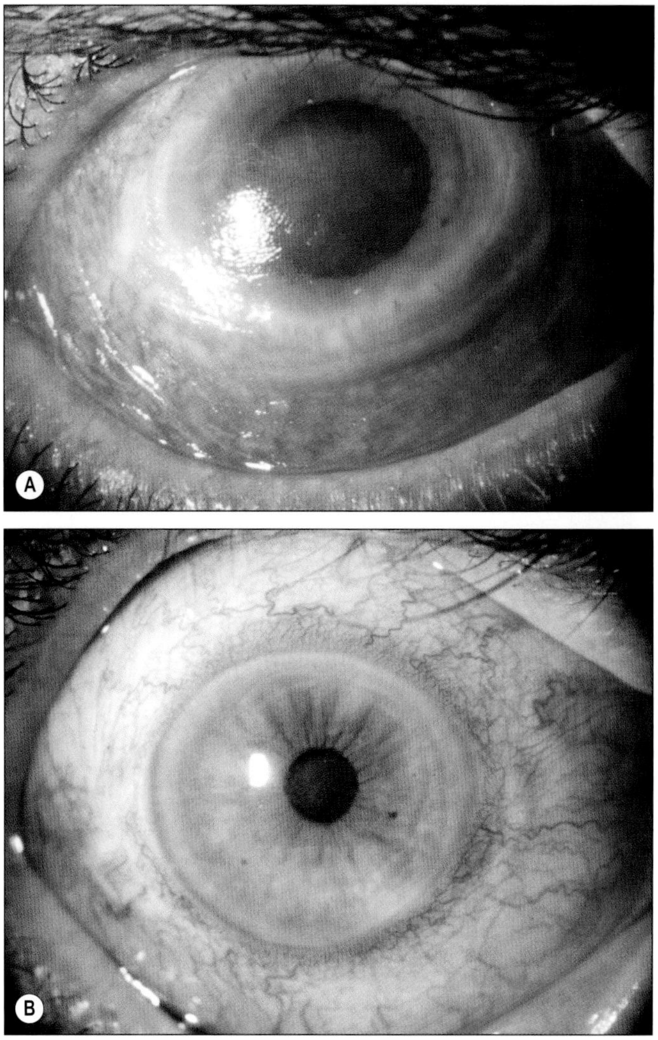

Fig. 62.3 Corneal xerosis. (**A**) Dry lusterless appearance of corneal xerosis (X2). (**B**) Appearance of cornea from Figure 62.3A after vitamin A supplementation.

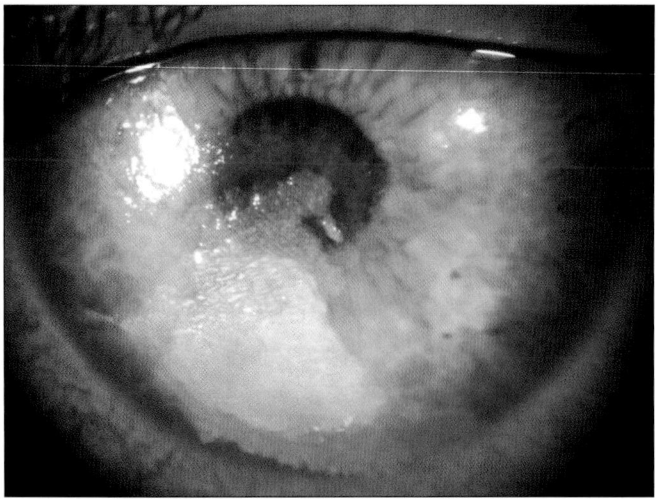

Fig. 62.4 Marked keratinization of the inferior cornea.

shown to alter both the expression of mucin genes in rat ocular surface epithelium[41] and the balance of rat corneal matrix metalloproteinases.[42]

Corneal ulceration/keratomalacia (X3A/X3B)

Uncomplicated corneal ulcers typically have very sharp margins, as if they have been cut with a trephine. Superficial ulcers may result from the rupture of subepithelial bullae, but their depth can vary. They tend to form in the lower half of the cornea and may be multiple. Smaller ones tend to be peripheral and, if both eyes are involved, are frequently symmetrical.[43] Uninvolved cornea, although xerotic, is clear and lacks the gray infiltration typical of bacterial keratitis. Superficial ulcers frequently heal with remarkably little scarring. Deeper ulcers may perforate, often with the anterior chamber being maintained by a plug of iris. This will obviously result in a dense peripheral leukoma. Eyes with ulcers frequently have a hypopyon.[16] In more severe lesions there is frank necrosis or sloughing of the corneal stroma, and these deserve the term keratomalacia. The lesions may be gray or yellow and vary in size from 2 mm to involvement of almost the entire cornea. The lesions may appear elevated but with treatment may collapse to reveal an area of stromal loss with sharp boundaries. Occasionally, the borders so produced are much smaller than otherwise anticipated, which may indicate that a central area of necrosis is bounded by a region of potential reversibility.[16] Deep stromal loss results in the production of descemetoceles. With minimal pressure, these can rupture, resulting in loss of the ocular contents, although frequently they scar and form anterior staphylomata. Prompt treatment when ulceration or keratomalacia involves less than one-third of the corneal surface (X3A) often restores useful vision, since the visual axis may be uninvolved (Fig. 62.5). When corneal involvement is more extensive (X3B) (Figs 62.6–62.9), treatment may not only prevent loss of the globe but, more importantly, may preserve useful vision in the fellow eye as well as the life of the child.

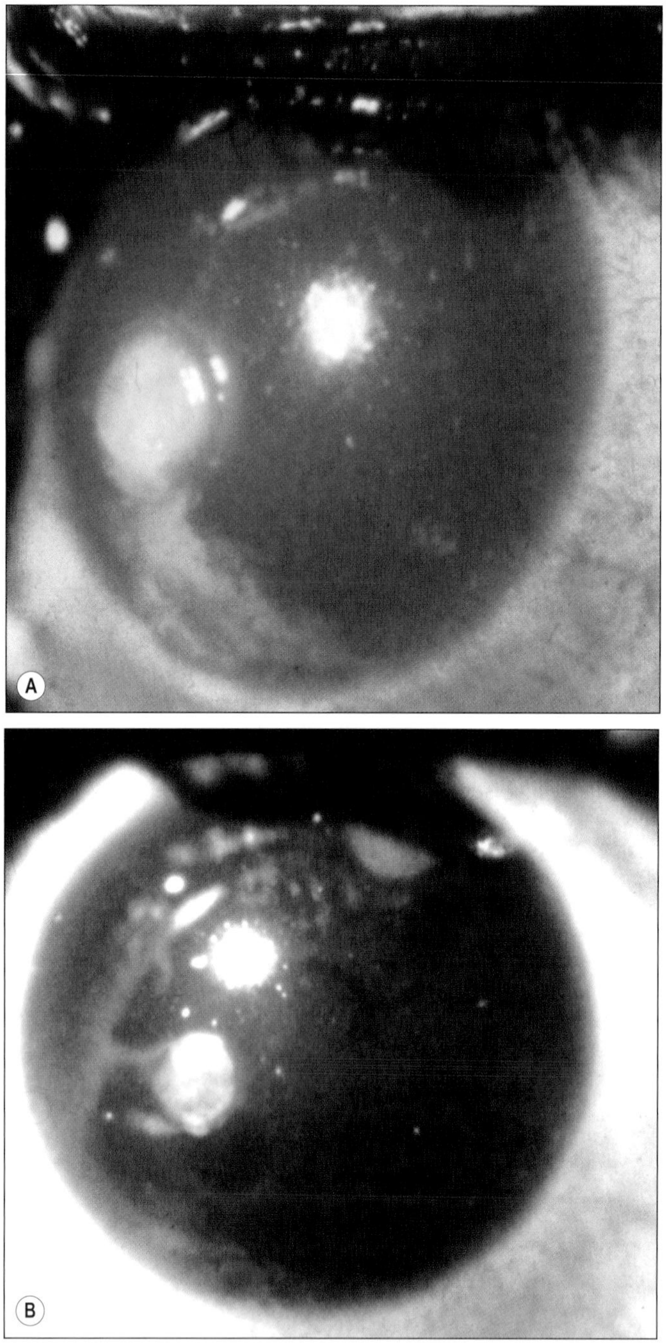

Fig. 62.5 Corneal ulceration/keratomalacia. (**A**) Corneal xerosis progressing to a small ulcer involving less than one-third of the cornea (X3A). (**B**) Same patient after three doses of 200000 IU vitamin A, 5 days later. (Courtesy Dr. Allen Foster.)

Pathogenesis of corneal ulceration

Although the role of vitamin A deficiency in xerophthalmia is undoubted, the mechanisms by which this occurs are not clear. Vitamin A is involved in corneal metabolism,[44] and specific retinol-binding proteins are present in the epithelium, keratocytes, and endothelium.[45] Vitamin A is merely a necessary but not sufficient factor. Additional components in the pathogenesis of vitamin A deficiency keratopathy are

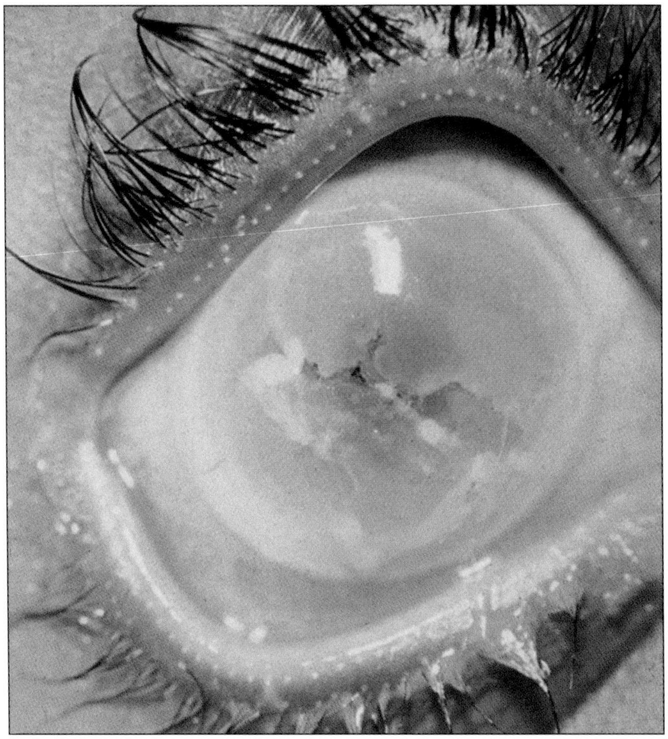

Fig. 62.6 Keratomalacia involving the whole corneal surface (X3B). (Courtesy Dr. Allen Foster.)

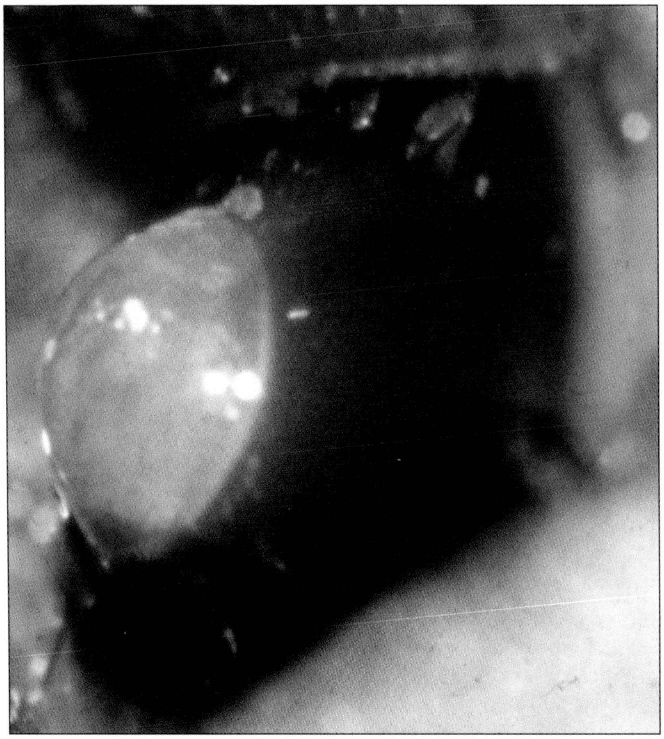

Fig. 62.7 Keratomalacia progressing to descemetocele formation (X3B). (Courtesy Dr. Allen Foster.)

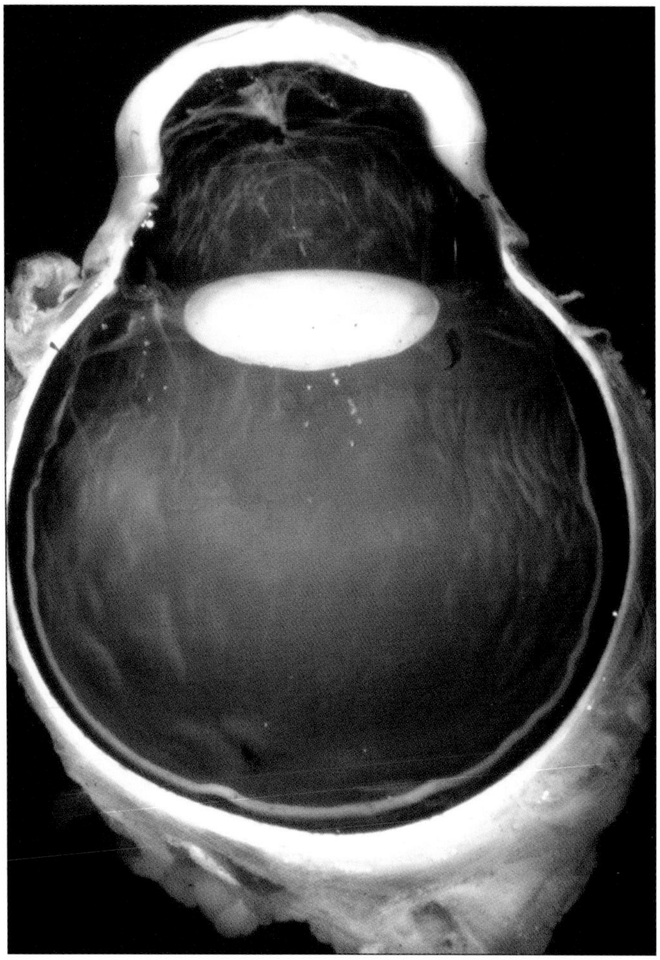

Fig. 62.8 Gross pathologic specimen illustrating descemetocele complicating keratomalacia. (Courtesy Professor W.R. Lee.)

trauma and infection. Sloughing of cornified epithelium by lid action could remove a deep epithelial plug,[43] and animal studies suggest that this might be caused by a reduction in hemidesmosomes.[46] Inflammatory cells, particularly polymorphonuclear leukocytes (PMNs), are visibly involved in keratomalacic corneas and release destructive proteases such as collagenase.[47–49] Collagenase may also be released by regenerating epithelium.[50] Elevated levels of chemoattractant factors for PMNs, such as interleukin-1, have been identified in rat models of corneal injury in vitamin A deficiency.[50] Sommer notes the relative lack of inflammatory change in humans when compared with animal models.[43] Furthermore, rat studies showed that despite heavy PMN infiltration provoked by corneal abrasion, it took stromal injury to produce frank keratomalacia.[51] However, a more recent study demonstrated keratomalacia after epithelial scraping alone and correlated its development with the degree of xerosis at the time of injury.[52] In addition, clinical reports suggest that xerophthalmic dissolution can proceed beneath an intact epithelium.[53]

Infection complicates many cases. One study suggested that nearly 90% of xerophthalmic eyes harbored either pathogenic (*Pseudomonas*, *Pneumococcus*, *Moraxella*) or potentially pathogenic (*Streptococcus viridans*, *Staphylococcus aureus*)

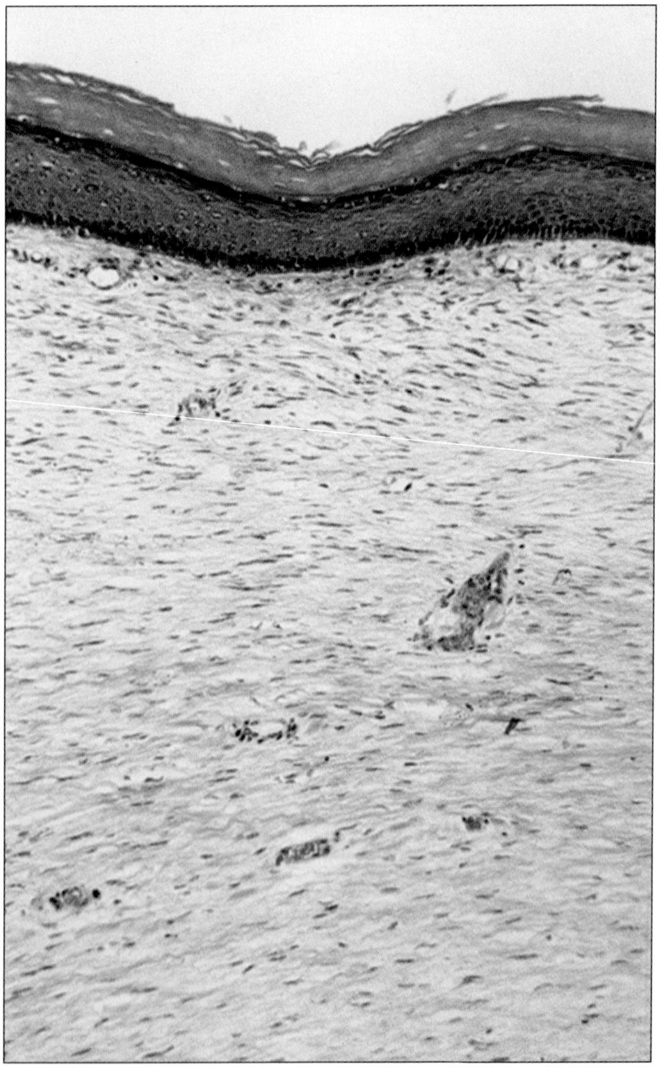

Fig. 62.9 Histologic section illustrating a heavily keratinized epithelial surface in a xerophthalmic patient. (Courtesy Professor W.R. Lee.)

organisms.[54] Other studies have shown that the cultures of organisms from ulcerated and nonulcerated xerophthalmic eyes are very similar.[55] Although eyes may harbor organisms such as *Pseudomonas* without corneal ulceration,[56] a breach in epithelial integrity can produce a devastating result. Experiments with the germ-free rat in which corneal liquefaction fails to occur argue for a central role of infection.[57] Others, particularly Sommer,[51] maintain that metabolic derangement of the cornea caused by vitamin A deficiency can by itself lead to the rapid colliquative process. This is supported by demonstration that prompt dosing with vitamin A can bring about dramatic reversal in a way that is not achievable with antibiotics alone.

Interactions with Other Factors

Vitamin A deficiency rarely occurs in isolation; it usually occurs with generalized protein energy malnutrition (PEM). Approximately 43%, or 230 million children under 5 years of age in the developing world, have stunted growth due to PEM.[58] Due to the frequent coexistence of these two conditions, there has been confusion as to which is the more important factor in corneal disease.[55,59,60] Vitamin A deficiency and PEM are clearly interrelated. The malabsorption that accompanies PEM may reduce retinol levels both directly and by impaired conversion of beta-carotene, while reduced protein synthesis (and, in particular, reduced synthesis of RBP) prevents release of vitamin A from the liver.[61–63] Protein status may also in some way influence the metabolism of vitamin A at the level of the target cell.[64] Attempts have been made to control for the influence of PEM by using serum albumin and transferrin as indices of protein status, along with basic weight-for-height measurements.[64] Furthermore, the observation that massive dosing with vitamin A can sometimes promote some healing of xerophthalmic corneas even in the presence of severe PEM would argue for the primacy of vitamin A.[65,66]

Vitamin E and zinc have also been investigated in regards to potential interactions with vitamin A. The administration of intraperitoneal vitamin E yielded a significant protective effect against corneal changes observed in rats fed a vitamin A deficient diet. These changes specifically included decreased microvilli and clear cells in the superficial corneal epithelium and conjunctiva, fewer secretory granules in goblet cells, and keratinization of the corneal surface.[67] Similarly, zinc may be a factor in corneal epithelial health. A recent in vivo rat study demonstrated a synergistic interaction between zinc and vitamin A by showing amelioration of effects caused by deficiency of one nutrient via supplementation with the other. Effects caused by deficiency of either nutrient included changes in corneal epithelial microvilli, conjunctival goblet cells, and keratinization.[68]

Infectious processes may interact with vitamin A in a number of ways. Vitamin A deficiency is a well-recognized risk factor for severe measles infection associated with increased morbidity and mortality,[69,70] as well as an increased rate of maternal–fetal HIV transmission.[71] Vitamin A deficiency may reduce normal cellular immunity by causing an alteration in T-cell subsets and, in particular, by reducing CD4 cell numbers. This is reversible when retinol levels are restored.[72] Fever from any cause can depress vitamin A levels by reducing the hepatic synthesis of RBP, and prolonged anorexia may diminish absorption.[19]

The disease most closely associated with vitamin A deficiency is rubeola (measles).[73,74] Corneal involvement after measles keratoconjunctivitis was a significant problem in Europe until the mid-twentieth century.[75] However, general improvement in nutrition, immunization, and a possible decrease in the virulence of the organism has led to only rare reports of late.[76] The same is not true in developing countries, where several studies highlight the devastating effect of postmeasles xerophthalmia.[77–79] A mild keratoconjunctivitis is an almost universal finding in patients with rubeola. Punctate superficial keratopathy occurs, resulting from direct viral involvement in the cornea and causing lacrimation and photophobia.[80,81] This usually resolves as the skin rash fades, leaving no scarring sequelae. On occasion, areas of punctate involvement may become confluent, leading to a central epithelial defect.[82] Generally, these heal readily, but can become secondarily infected.

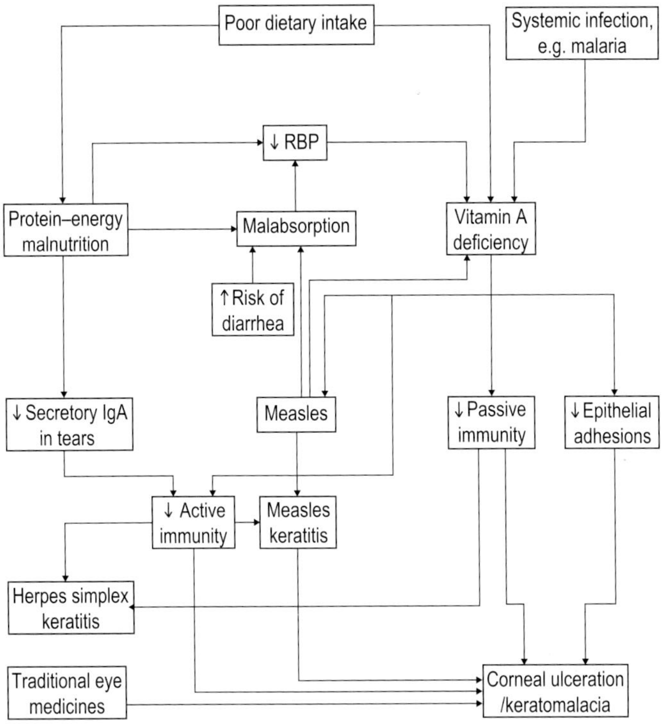

Fig. 62.10 Vitamin A deficiency and its interaction with other factors.

Response to early *Pseudomonas* infection can be compromised by vitamin A deficiency. Vitamin A deficient corneas developed pseudomonal ulcers in the presence of normally subthreshold bacterial loads, and demonstrated inflammatory cells with unusual characteristics and increased concentrations of cysteine protease inhibitors. Other major alterations to the corneal response to *Pseudomonas aeruginosa* infection included decreased tear film, epithelial keratinization, impaired corneal wound healing, and changes in polymorphonuclear leukocyte function.[83]

A further infection that can affect children with measles and/or malnutrition involves herpes simplex virus (HSV). Probably, these children are rendered more susceptible by suppression of their cell-mediated immunity.[82,84] Foster and Sommer found vitamin A deficiency to be responsible for half of the measles-associated corneal ulcers, HSV for a fifth, and PEM for about 17%.[82] The longer the duration between onset of measles and the development of the ulcer, the more likely the ulcer was hypovitaminosis-related. HSV infection was associated with features of immunosuppression, with 50% of the ulcers being geographic and nearly a quarter bilateral. In general, bilaterality was more suggestive of vitamin A deficiency. Figure 62.10 illustrates how the various factors mentioned can conspire to result in keratomalacia.

Epidemiology

The vitamin A reserves of the neonate are limited,[85] and initially the child depends on vitamin A supplied by mother's milk. Except for colostrum (which has a higher concentration), vitamin A in breast milk is equivalent to plasma levels (40 μg/100mL), although this tends to drop with the progression of breastfeeding.[86] If the mother herself is deficient, the situation becomes precarious; examples exist of xerophthalmic children whose mother's milk contained no vitamin A at all.[87] Currently, it is estimated that 7.2 million pregnant women are vitamin A deficient, and an additional 13.5 million have reduced vitamin A levels.[2] Annually, over six million pregnant women develop night blindness, usually during the third trimester when maternal and fetal demands are greatest. Southeast and South Asia account for over 60% of all maternal night blindness, with three-fourths of this number located in India.

Table 62.1 Criteria for assessing the public health significance of xerophthalmia and vitamin A deficiency, based on the prevalence among children less than 6 years old (1982 revision)

Criterion	Minimum prevalence
Clinical	
Night blindness (XN)	1%
Bitot's spots	0.5%
Corneal xerosis and/or ulceration/ keratomalacia (X2 + X3A + X3B)	0.01%
Xerophthalmic-related corneal scars (XS)	0.05%
Biochemical	
Serum retinol level less than 100 μg/L (0.35 μg/L)	5.0%

From Control of vitamin A deficiency and xerophthalmia. *Report of a joint WHO/USAID/UNICEF/HKI/IVACG meeting, (WHO Technical Report Series, No. 672), Geneva, 1982, World Health Organization.*

Despite these figures and the previously mentioned decrease in breast milk vitamin A levels over time, studies have demonstrated reduced risk of xerophthalmia resulting from delayed weaning and prolonged breastfeeding.[88,89] The age group most at risk of blinding corneal disease (X2, X3) is between 6 months and 3 years of age. These children are often severely malnourished and, as mentioned, there is frequently a precipitating illness. Both sexes are at equal risk. Conversely, conjunctival disease (X1A, X1B) is more common in older children (between 3 and 6 years) and reflects a chronic nutritional problem. Signs of PEM are milder, and a precipitating illness is less likely. In males, the metabolism of vitamin A is less efficient; night blindness and Bitot's spots are, therefore, encountered more frequently in boys.[15] Xerophthalmia is most frequently a problem among the poorest, most disadvantaged groups within a society with limited access to medical services. To assist health administrators in assessing which communities are most at risk, the World Health Organization (WHO) has established prevalence criteria of the various stages of xerophthalmia (Table 62.1).

Xerophthalmia can also be found among more affluent patient subsets, especially in the developed world. Malabsorption related to gastric bypass procedures for bariatric surgery is a notable cause of iatrogenic hypovitaminosis A. Xerophthalmia, nyctalopia, and corneal scarring have been described in the setting of inadequate vitamin A supplementation in a post-gastric bypass patient. Psychiatrically induced severe self-imposed dietary restrictions have been associated with keratomalacia, and bilateral corneal ulcers and melting. Chronic alcoholics are also vulnerable to hypovitaminosis A and its ocular complications via nutritional deficiency.

Attempts have been made to improve the detection of conjunctival xerosis using vital dyes such as lissamine green; however, they have not been found to be particularly specific.[90] Much more encouraging is the use of impression cytology (IC).[91–96] The technique involves application of a strip of cellulose acetate filter paper to the ocular surface to remove the superficial layers of the conjunctival epithelium. Active deficiency is evident by loss of goblet cells and both enlargement and partial keratinization of epithelial cells. Abnormal cytology is a sensitive marker of early disease, and the reliability of the test has been improved by the use of a specific 'disk applicator.'[94] IC is a noninvasive test, which is well tolerated, and most significantly does not require the large population samples of clinical or biochemical surveys, since 50% abnormal cytology is proposed as a marker of significant risk.[92] A recent IC study revealed abnormal cytology results in children aged 6 months to 10 years with subclinical vitamin A deficiency based on serum retinol levels. These children were retested after supplementary vitamin A and reversal of the abnormalities was seen.[97] Results should be interpreted carefully, since the specificity will be compromised by coexisting conjunctival disease such as trachoma.[91] The presence of PMNs in a sample is more likely to lead to its being read as abnormal. Presumably, the PMNs and accompanying mucin tend to lie as a surface layer, which is lifted by the cellulose paper, leaving the epithelium behind.[94]

Treatment

The diagnosis of xerophthalmia constitutes a medical emergency, and prompt treatment with massive supplementation of vitamin A is required. World Health Organization standard doses vary with the age of the patient. In children over 12 months of age and in all women of childbearing age with severe xerophthalmia, this should be given orally, either as 110 mg of retinol palmitate or as 66 mg retinol acetate (200 000 IU vitamin A) immediately and again the following day. An additional dose should be given 2 weeks later to boost liver reserves. Oil-miscible injections should not be given because they are poorly absorbed, but if parenteral replacement is essential, 55 mg of water-miscible retinol palmitate (100 000 IU) can replace the first oral dose.[15] Parenteral administration is indicated in children with severe anorexia, edematous malnutrition, septic shock, or inability to take oral supplementation. For children aged 6 to 12 months, half dosage is appropriate, while for children less than 6 months of age quarter dosage is recommended. While this regimen can result in swift corneal healing, protein-deficient children do not handle massive vitamin A dosages adequately, and holo-RBP levels may decline rapidly with return of corneal lesions within 1 to 3 weeks.[98] This is especially likely to occur if only a single dose is given, rather than two doses. It is apparent, therefore, that adequate treatment includes correction of PEM. Until this has been achieved, vitamin A supplementation should continue every 1 or 2 weeks.[98] Women of reproductive age with night blindness or Bitot's spots should receive 5000–10 000 IU daily for 4 weeks, not exceeding 10 000 IU daily. A weekly dose of 25 000 IU is acceptable. Figure 62.3A,B illustrates the dramatic response of xerophthalmia to vitamin A therapy.

Some studies suggest a link between vitamin A supplementation and an increased prevalence of acute lower respiratory tract infections.[99,100] Several animal studies have suggested that vitamin A excess can have an immunosuppressive effect.[101,102] Vitamin A overdosage can be toxic,[18] and 4% of patients developed transient diarrhea and vomiting on a 300 000 IU dosing regimen.[103] This discouraged community support, so the lower dose of 200 000 IU is recommended. These factors are important because our concern is not only to treat individuals but also whole communities that are at risk. Children at highest risk should receive repeated dosing at 4–6-month intervals. Studies suggest that priming doses 1 week before the full dose can extend the protection conferred by such supplementation.[104] Vitamin E deficiency can impair the absorption and storage of vitamin A,[19] and combined supplementation with vitamin E may have the additional benefit of reducing the toxicity of hypervitaminosis A.[105] To avoid the risk of teratogenesis,[18] supplementation should be avoided in pregnancy but should be given to the mother at childbirth (400 000 IU) to augment milk vitamin A levels.

Vitamin A supplementation programs have been undertaken in numerous developing nations and have been shown to be effective in reducing the incidence of xerophthalmia. Vehicles for supplementation include capsules given out during national immunization days, fortified beverages, as well as other food products.[106,107]

Such supplementation regimens usually form part of a general mother and child health program and are short-term solutions to the problems of vitamin A deficiency and xerophthalmia. Certain risk factors can be removed by measures such as measles immunization and the prevention of diarrhea. Undoubtedly, the most effective measure is education about adequate nutrition and the benefits of foods rich in vitamin A and carotenoids. While vitamin A capsules are inexpensive, distribution systems may be suboptimal; dietary vitamin A has been shown superior to supplementation programs in reducing rates of xerophthalmia.[108]

Topical retinoic acid is of benefit in the treatment of xerophthalmic animals,[109,110] and limited trials in humans have suggested that it might induce more rapid healing. In vivo rabbit studies have suggested that topical application of a 0.05% all-*trans* retinoic acid emulsion shortens healing time after corneal abrasion.[111] The role of retinoic acid in corneal wound healing is likely complex. Retinoic acid has been shown to inhibit collagenase.[112] In vitro studies have demonstrated that retinoic acid is instrumental in stimulating the normal differentiation of limbal stem cells and also inhibits abnormal terminal differentiation.[113]

Fibronectin has been found to aid in corneal epithelial wound healing in vitamin A deficient rats when applied topically.[114] No human studies using only fibronectin in this situation have been reported to date.

Surgery has only a limited role in the management of xerophthalmia and none at all when complete corneal necrosis is present. Ben-Sira et al. reported the successful use of 'covering grafts' in restoring anterior chambers.[115] However, Sommer[16] questions whether this represents a great advance, as medical therapy often results in a similar reformed anterior chamber, albeit with a corneal defect plugged by iris. Singh and Malik[116] claim restoration of useful vision by penetrating keratoplasty, but no mention is made of the follow-up period. Of necessity, the trephines were large, which even in less compromised situations carries with it the risk of postoperative problems. In a 2003 study involving 29 young children, Vajpayee et al. agree with the conclusion that keratoplasty for keratomalacia is associated with poor visual outcome even in the unlikely instance when the graft survives.[117] Amniotic membrane transplantation for corneal perforation in xerophthalmia has been described as a reasonable option in conjunction with oral vitamin A supplementation as an alternative to primary corneal grafting.[118]

Other Nutritional Deficiencies

Vitamin B (riboflavin)

Various animal studies have reported corneal vascularization as a result of riboflavin deficiency.[119–121] Riboflavin-deficient rats show markedly decreased goblet cells and conjunctival epithelial layers, findings reversible with riboflavin repletion. No convincing evidence exists for similar pathology in humans, although reports exist from the southern USA that initially suggested that circumcorneal injection and corneal vascularization were pathognomonic of riboflavin deficiency.[122] Experiments with human volunteers on restricted diets have failed to reproduce these findings,[123,124] and it is possible that Sydenstricker et al.[122] were describing dilated vessels in the limbal capillary plexus.[19] While nutritional amblyopia was frequently reported among inmates of Japanese prisoner-of-war (POW) camps,[125,126] there is a paucity of recorded corneal problems. Métivier, in the West Indies, described a 'corneal epithelial dystrophy,' comprising grayish-white spots on the cornea, which he attributed to vitamin B deficiency.[127] Similar lesions occurred in POWs treated in a single military hospital.[128]

Vitamin C

There is no convincing evidence that deficiency of other vitamins can lead to corneal problems, although in a vitamin C deprivation trial extending over approximately 3 months, some subjects developed xerosis.[129] In animal studies, scorbutic guinea pig corneas healed less well when subjected to injury.[130] Ascorbic acid promotes healing by stimulating collagen production from fibroblasts, and topical ascorbate has been shown to reduce the incidence of perforating corneal ulcers in rabbit eyes subjected to alkali burns.[131–134] Although endogenous delivery to the cornea will be less than that which can be supplied topically, it is not unreasonable to suppose that effective corneal healing is enhanced by adequate circulating levels of vitamin C. The ascorbate concentration in the normal cornea is 14 times that of the aqueous humor, and there is some evidence to suggest that vitamin C protects the basal epithelium by absorbing UV radiation.[135]

Other nutrients

Animal studies of deprivation of individual amino acids have produced nonspecific corneal vascularization.[19] Prolonged zinc deprivation, as mentioned earlier, has produced a similar picture in a rat model.[136] Zinc-deficient rats show decreased goblet cells and decreased conjunctival vitamin C levels. Although no human studies have been reported, magnesium-deficient rats show corneal alterations as well. These include decreased epithelial microvilli and microplicae as well as deposits in the subepithelial stroma and pentagonal or square endothelial cells.[137] Such highly artificial diets are unlikely to have counterparts in human clinical practice, although a recent study claimed reduced serum magnesium levels in a group of keratoconic patients.[138] The significance of this is unclear.

Discrete colliquative keratopathy

One final condition that may have a nutritional basis is the so-called discrete colliquative keratopathy (DCK). First described by Blumenthal in 1950 as 'malnutritional keratoconjunctivitis,'[139] it is a somewhat mysterious disease, having only been described in the South African Bantu. Frequently confused with keratomalacia, it would appear to be distinct in that the softening of the cornea occurs from within out, culminating in nonulcerating perforation in an otherwise 'quiet eye.' Affected children tend to be slightly older than those whose corneas perforate with keratomalacia, being generally of preschool age. Typically, they suffer from early PEM rather than being marasmic. There is, however, no clear evidence that it is primarily a nutritional problem, and seasonal and annual fluctuations suggest that other unknown factors play a more important role.[19]

Summary

The most important nutritional disorder by far giving rise to corneal blindness is deficiency of vitamin A. While it is critical that ophthalmologists be able to recognize and effectively treat keratomalacia, perhaps more important is their role in directing action for those communities most at risk. The remedy may be inexpensive, but the communication infrastructure for capsules, vaccines, and, above all, mass education is all too often sadly lacking. Vitamin A deficiency is primarily associated with poverty. The unfortunate truth is that vitamin A capsule distribution programs will largely fail, since they are essentially not self-sustaining. It is not until there is a major shift in political will to unlock the cycle of 'the poverty trap' that we will see the scourge of keratomalacia relegated to the history books.

References

1. WHO website. www.who.int/vaccines-diseases/en/vitamina
2. West KP Jr. Extent of vitamin A deficiency among preschool children and women of reproductive age. *J Nutr.* 2002;132:2857S–2866S.

3. Sommer A. Vitamin A, infectious disease, and childhood mortality: a 2 solution? *J Infect Dis.* 1993;167(5):1003–1007.
4. Sommer A. Xerophthalmia, keratomalacia and nutritional blindness. *Int Ophthalmol.* 1990;14(3):195–199.
5. Buchanan NM, et al. A case of eye disease due to dietary vitamin A deficiency in Glasgow. *Scott Med J.* 1987;32(2):52–53.
6. Bors F, Fells P. Reversal of the complications of self-induced vitamin A deficiency. *Br J Ophthalmol.* 1971;55:210–214.
7. Olver J. Keratomalacia on a 'healthy diet.' *Br J Ophthalmol.* 1986; 70(5):357–360.
8. Clark JH, Rhoden DK, Turner DS. Symptomatic vitamin A and D deficiencies in an eight-year-old with autism. *J Parenter Enteral Nutr.* 1993;17(3):284–286.
9. Nicolai U, Rochels R. Bilateral severe keratomalacia after acute pancreatitis. *Cornea.* 1993;12(2):171–173.
10. Suan EP, et al. Corneal perforation in patients with vitamin A deficiency in the United States. *Arch Ophthalmol.* 1990;108(3):350–353.
11. Brooks HL Jr, Driebe WT Jr, Schemmer GG. Xerophthalmia and cystic fibrosis. *Arch Ophthalmol.* 1990;108(3):354–357.
12. Raynor RJ, et al. Night blindness and conjunctival xerosis caused by vitamin A deficiency in patients with cystic fibrosis. *Arch Dis Child.* 1989;64(8):1151–1156.
13. Tripathi RC, et al. Iatrogenic ocular complications in patients after jejunoileal bypass surgery. *Int Surg.* 1993;78(1):68–72.
14. Ettl A, Daxecker F. Xerophthalmia in liver cirrhosis. Correct diagnosis after 15 years. *Ophthalmologica.* 1992;204(2):63–66.
15. Sommer A. *Field guide to detection and control of xerophthalmia.* Geneva: WHO; 1982.
16. Sommer A. *Nutritional blindness: xerophthalmia and keratomalacia.* New York: Oxford University Press; 1982.
17. Olsen JA. Vitamin A. In: *Nutrition reviews. Present knowledge in nutrition.* 5th ed. Washington, DC: The Nutrition Foundation; 1984.
18. Bendich A, Langseth L. Safety of vitamin A. *Am J Clin Nutr.* 1989;49:358–371.
19. McLaren DS. *Nutritional ophthalmology.* 2nd ed. London: Academic Press; 1980.
20. Oomen HPAC. Hypovitaminosis A. III. Clinical experience of hypovitaminosis A. *Fed Proc Fed Am Socs Exp Biol.* 1958;17(Suppl 2):111–128.
21. Wolf G. An historical note on the mode of administration of vitamin A for the cure of night blindness. *Am J Clin Nutr.* 1978;31:290–292.
22. Mackenzie W. *A practical treatise on the diseases of the eye.* London: Longman, Ree, Orme, & Green; 1830.
23. Magendie F. *Ann Chim Phys 3:66 1816.* Cited in McLaren DS: *Nutritional ophthalmology,* ed 2. London: Academic Press; 1980.
24. Wolbach SB, Howe PR. Tissue changes following deprivation of fat soluble A vitamin. *J Exp Med.* 1925;42:753–778.
25. Bloch CE. Blindness and other diseases in children arising from deficient nutrition (lack of fat-soluble A factor). *Am J Dis Child* 1924;27: 139–148.
26. Bloch CE. Further clinical investigations into the diseases arising in consequence of a deficiency in the fat-soluble A factor. *Am J Dis Child* 1924;28:659–667.
27. Hubbenet M. *Ann Oculist, Paris, 44:293.* Cited in McLaren DS: *Nutritional ophthalmology.* 2nd ed. London: Academic Press; 1980.
28. Bitot C. Sur une lesion conjonctivale non encore décrite, coincidant avec l'héméralopie, *Gas Hebd Med Chir 10:284, 1863.* Cited in McLaren DS: *Nutritional ophthalmology.* 2nd ed. London: Academic Press; 1980.
29. Control of vitamin A deficiency and xerophthalmia. Report of a joint WHO/USAID/UNICEF/HKI/IVACG meeting, Geneva, 1982 (WHO Technical Report Series, No. 672), World Health Organization.
30. Paton D, McLaren DS. Bitot's spots. *Am J Ophthalmol.* 1960;50: 568–574.
31. Roger FC, et al. A reappraisal of the ocular lesion known as Bitot's spots. *Br J Nutr.* 1963;17:475–485.
32. Rao V, et al. Conjunctival goblet cells and mitotic rate in children with retinol deficiency and measles. *Arch Ophthalmol.* 1987;105: 378–380.
33. Schmidt H. Vitamin A deficiencies in ruminants. *Am J Vet Res.* 1941;2:373–389.
34. Katz J, et al. Clustering of xerophthalmia within households and villages. *Int J Epidemiol.* 1993;22(4):709–715.
35. Appelmans M, Lebas P, Missotten L. Vitamin A deficiency and its ocular manifestations. *Scalpel (Brux).* 1957;110:217–234.
36. Semba RD, et al. Response of Bitot's spots in preschool children to vitamin A treatment. *Am J Ophthalmol.* 1990;110(4):416–420.
37. Sommer A. Conjunctival appearance in corneal xerophthalmia. *Arch Ophthalmol.* 1982;100:951–952.
38. Baum JL, Mishima S, Boruchoff A. On the nature of dellen. *Arch Ophthalmol.* 1968;79:657–662.
39. Sommer A, Emran N. Tear production in vitamin A responsive xerophthalmia. *Am J Ophthalmol.* 1982;93:84–87.
40. Sommer A, Green WR. Goblet cell response to vitamin A treatment for corneal xerophthalmia. *Am J Ophthalmol.* 1982;94:213–215.
41. Tei M, Spurr-Michaud SJ, Tisdale AS, Gipson IK. Vitamin A deficiency alters the expression of mucin genes by the rat ocular surface epithelium. *Invest Ophthalmol Vis Sci.* 2000;41:82–88.
42. Twining SS, Schulti DP, Zhou X, et al. Changes in rat corneal matrix metalloproteinases and serine proteinases under vitamin A deficiency. *Curr Eye Res.* 1997;16:158–165.
43. Sommer A, Sugana T. Corneal xerophthalmia and keratomalacia. *Arch Ophthalmol.* 1982;100:404–411.
44. Hayashi K, et al. Metabolic changes in the cornea of vitamin A deficient rats. *Invest Ophthalmol Vis Sci.* 1989;30(4):769–772.
45. Wiggert B, et al. Retinol receptors in corneal epithelium, stroma, and endothelium. *Biochem Biophys Acta.* 1977;491:104–113.
46. Shams NBK, et al. Effect of vitamin A deficiency on the adhesion of rat corneal epithelium and the basement membrane complex. *Invest Ophthalmol Vis Sci.* 1993;34(9):2646–2654.
47. Pirie A, Werb Z, Burleigh M. Collagenase and other proteases in the cornea of the retinol deficient rat. *Br J Nutr.* 1975;34:297–309.
48. Pirie A. Effect of vitamin A deficiency on cornea. *Trans Ophthalmol Soc UK.* 1978;98:357–360.
49. Leonard MC, Maddison LK, Pirie A. A comparison between the enzymes in the cornea of the vitamin A deficient rat and those of rat leukocytes. *Exp Eye Res.* 1981;33:479–495.
50. Shams NBK, et al. Increased interleukin-1 activity in the injured vitamin A deficient cornea. *Cornea.* 1994;13(2):156–166.
51. Hayashi K, et al. Stromal degradation in vitamin A deficient rat cornea, comparison of epithelial abrasion and stromal incision. *Cornea.* 1990;9(3):254–265.
52. Haddox JL, Pfister RR, Daniel RL, et al. A new classification system predicting keratomalacia after trauma in vitamin A deficiency: sodium citrate does not prevent disease progression. *Cornea.* 1997;16:472–479.
53. Sommer A, Green R, Kenyon KR. Clinicopathologic correlations in xerophthalmic ulceration and necrosis. *Arch Ophthalmol.* 1982;100: 953–963.
54. Valenton MT, Tan RV. Secondary ocular bacterial infection in hypovitaminosis A xerophthalmia. *Am J Ophthalmol.* 1975;80(4):673–677.
55. Kuming BS, Politzer WM. Xerophthalmia and protein malnutrition in Bantu children. *Br J Opthalmol.* 1967;51:649–665.
56. Pramhus C, Runyan TE, Lindberg RB. Ocular flora in the severely burned patient. *Arch Ophthalmol.* 1978;96:1421–1424.
57. Rogers NE, Bieri JG, McDaniel EG. Vitamin A deficiency in the germ-free rat. *Fed Proc Fed Am Socs Exp Biol.* 1971;30:1773–1778.
58. De Onis M, Monteiro C, Akre J, Clugston G. The worldwide magnitude of protein-energy malnutrition: an overview from the WHO world database on child growth. www.who.int/nut/documents/pem_bulletin_1995.htm
59. Yap KT. Protein deficiency in keratomalacia. *Br J Ophthalmol.* 1956;40:502–503.
60. Emiru VP. The cornea in kwashiorkor. *J Trop Pediatr.* 1971;17: 117–134.
61. Arroyave G, et al. Serum and liver vitamin A and lipids in children with severe protein malnutrition. *Am J Clin Nutr.* 1961;9:180–185.
62. Smith FR, et al. Serum vitamin A, retinol-binding protein and prealbumin concentration in protein and calorie malnutrition. *Am J Clin Nutr.* 1973;26:973–981.
63. Zaklama MS, et al. Liver vitamin A in protein-calorie malnutrition. *Am J Clin Nutr.* 1972;25:412–418.
64. Sommer A, Muhilal H. Nutritional factors in corneal xerophthalmia and keratomalacia. *Arch Ophthalmol.* 1982;100:399–403.
65. Sommer A, et al. Oral vs intramuscular vitamin A in the treatment of xerophthalmia. *Lancet.* 1980;1:557–559.
66. Sommer A. Vitamin A, xerophthalmia and diarrhoea. *Lancet.* 1980;1:1411–1412.
67. Fujikawa A, Gong H, Amemiya T. Vitamin E prevents changes in cornea and conjunctiva due to vitamin A deficiency. *Graefe's Arch Clin Exp Ophthalmol.* 2003;241:287–297.
68. Kanazawa S, Kitaoka T, Ueda Y, Gong H. Amemiya: interaction of zinc and vitamin A on the ocular surface. *Graefe's Arch Clin Exp Ophthalmol.* 2002;240:1011–1021.
69. D'Souza RM, D'Souza R. Vitamin A for the treatment of children with measles – a systematic review. *J Trop Ped.* 2002;48:323–327.
70. Rosales FJ. Vitamin A supplementation of vitamin A deficient measles patients lowers the risk of measles-related pneumonia in Zambian children. *J Nutr.* 2002;132:3700–3703.
71. Semba RD. Overview of the potential role of vitamin A in the mother-to-child transmission of HIV-1. *Acta Paediatr Suppl.* 1997;421:107–112.

72. Semba RD, et al. Abnormal T-cell subset proportions in vitamin-A-deficient children. *Lancet*. 1993;341:5–8.
73. Latham MC. Vitamin A and childhood mortality. *Lancet*. 1993;342:5–8.
74. Bhandari N, Bhan MK, Sazawal S. Impact of massive dose of vitamin A given to preschool children with acute diarrhoea on subsequent respiratory and diarrhoeal morbidity. *Br Med J*. 1994;309:1404–1407.
75. Duke-Elder WS. *System of ophthalmology*, vol. 8, Part 1. London: Kimpton; 1965:338.
76. Blatz G. Hornhauteinschmelzung nach Masern. *Klin Monatsbl Augenheilkd*. 1956;129:763–772.
77. Sandford-Smith JH, Whittle HC. Corneal ulceration following measles in Nigerian children. *Br J Ophthalmol*. 1979;63:720–724.
78. Frederique G, Howard R, Boniuk V. Corneal ulcers in rubeola. *Am J Ophthalmol*. 1969;68:996–1003.
79. BenEzra D, Chirambo MC. Incidence and causes of blindness among the under 5 age group in Malawi. *Br J Ophthalmol*. 1977;61: 154–157.
80. Trantas M. Complications oculaires rares de la rougéole. *Ann Oculist (Paris)*. 1900;123:300.
81. Dekkers NWHM. *The cornea in measles*. The Hague: Junk; 1981.
82. Foster A, Sommer A. Corneal ulceration, measles, and childhood blindness in Tanzania. *Br J Ophthalmol*. 1987;71:331–343.
83. Twining SS, Zhou X, Schulte DP, et al. Effect of vitamin A deficiency on the early response to experimental *Pseudomonas* keratitis. *Invest Ophthalmol Vis Sci*. 1996;37:511–512.
84. Templeton AC. Generalised herpes simplex in malnourished children. *J Clin Pathol*. 1970;23:24–30.
85. Moore T. *Vitamin A*. Amsterdam: Elsevier; 1957.
86. Thanangkul O, et al. Comparison of the effects of a single high dose of vitamin A given to mother and infant upon the plasma levels in the infant. Joint/WHO/USAID meeting on the control of vitamin A deficiency: priorities for research and action programmes, Jakarta, Indonesia (Nov 25–29, 1974).
87. Meulemans O, De Haas JH. Over het gehalte aan carotine en vitamine A van moedermeld in Batavia. *Geneesk Tijdschr Ned-IndiÅe*. 1936;76:1538–1571.
88. Mahalanabis D. Breast feeding and vitamin A deficiency among children attending a diarrhoea treatment centre in Bangladesh: a case-control study. *Br Med J*. 1991;303(6801):493–496.
89. West KP, et al: Breast feeding, weaning patterns, and the risk of xerophthalmia in Southern Malawi. *Am J Clin Nutr*. 1986;44(5): 690–697.
90. Emran N, Sommer A. Lissamine green staining in the clinical diagnosis of xerophthalmia. *Arch Ophthalmol*. 1979;97:2332–2335.
91. Resnikoff S, et al. Impression cytology with transfer in xerophthalmia and conjunctival diseases. *Int Ophthalmol*. 1992;16(6):445–451.
92. Carlier C, et al. Conjunctival impression cytology with transfer as a field applicable indicator of vitamin A status for mass screening. *Int J Epidemiol*. 1992;21(2):373–380.
93. Usha N, et al. Assessment of preclinical vitamin A deficiency in children with persistent diarrhoea. *J Paediatr Gastroenterol Nutr*. 1991;13(2): 168–175.
94. Keenum DG, et al. Assessment of vitamin A status by a disk applicator for conjunctival impression cytology. *Arch Ophthalmol*. 1990; 108(10):1436–1441.
95. Nelson JD. Impression cytology. *Cornea*. 1988;7(1):71–81.
96. Wittpenn JR, Tseng SC, Sommer A. Detection of early xerophthalmia by impression cytology. *Arch Ophthalmol*. 1986;104(2):237–239.
97. Chowdhury S, Kumar R, Ganguly NK, et al. Dynamics of conjunctival impression cytologic changes after vitamin A supplementation. *Br J Nutr*. 1997;77:863–869.
98. Sommer A, Muhilal H, Tarwatjo I. Treatment of xerophthalmia. *Arch Ophthalmol*. 1982;100:785–787.
99. Dibley MJ, Sadjimin T, Kjolhede CL. Impact of high dose vitamin A supplementation on incidence and duration of episodes of diarrhoea and acute respiratory infections in preschool Indonesian children. *FASEB J*. 1992;6(Abstract 4923):A1787.
100. Standsfield SK, et al. Vitamin A supplementation and increased prevalence of childhood diarrhoea and acute respiratory infections. *Lancet*. 1993;342:578–582.
101. Friedman A, Sklan D. Antigen-specific immune response impairment in the chick as influenced by dietary vitamin A. *J Nutr*. 1989;119: 790–795.
102. Friedman A, et al. Decreased resistance and immune response to *Escherichia coli* in chicks with low and high intakes of vitamin A. *J Nutr*. 1991;121:395–400.
103. Swaminathan MC, Susheela TP, Thimmayamma BVS. Field prophylactic trial with a single annual oral dose of vitamin A. *Am J Clin Nutr*. 1970;23:119–122.
104. Humphrey JH, et al. A priming dose of oral vitamin A given to preschool children may extend protection conferred by a subsequent large dose of vitamin A. *J Nutr*. 1993;123(8):1363–1369.
105. Bauernfeind JC. *The safe use of vitamin A: a report of the International Vitamin A Consultative Group*. Washington DC: The Nutrition Foundation; 1980.
106. Djunaedi E, Sommer A, Pandji A, et al. Impact of vitamin A supplementation on xerophthalmia. *Arch Ophthalmol*. 1998;106:218–222.
107. Ash DM, Tatala SR, Frongillo EA, et al. Randomized efficacy trial of a micronutrient-fortified beverage in primary school children in Tanzania. *Am J Clin Nutr*. 2003;77:891–898.
108. Fawzi WW, et al. Vitamin A supplementation and dietary vitamin A in relation to the risk of xerophthalmia. *Am J Clin Nutr*. 1993;58(3): 385–391.
109. Ubel JL, Rismondo V, Edelhauser HF. Treatment of corneal xerophthalmia in rabbits with micromolar doses of topical retinoic acid. *Curr Eye Res*. 1987;6(5):735–737.
110. Van Horn DL, et al. Topical retinoic acid in the treatment of experimental xerophthalmia in the rabbit. *Arch Ophthalmol*. 1981;99: 317–321.
111. Johansen S, Heegaard S, Prause JU, Rask-Pedersen E. The healing effect of all-trans retinoic acid on epithelial corneal abrasions in rabbits. *Acta Ophthalmol Scand*. 1998;76:401–404.
112. Wolf G. The molecular basis of the inhibition of collagenase by vitamin A. *Nutr Rev*. 1992;50:292–297.
113. Kruse FE, Tseng SCG. Retinoic acid regulates clonal growth and differentiation of cultured limbal and peripheral corneal epithelium. *Invest Ophthalmol Vis Sci*. 1994;35:2405–2420.
114. Watanabe K, Frangieh G, Reddy CV, Kenyon KR. Effect of fibronectin on corneal epithelial wound healing in the vitamin A deficient rat. *Invest Ophthalmol Vis Sci*. 1991;32:2159–2162.
115. Ben-Sira I, Ticho U, Yassur Y. Surgical treatment of active keratomalacia by 'covering graft.' *Isr J Med Sci*. 1972;8:1209–1211.
116. Singh G, Malik SRK. Therapeutic penetrating keratoplasty in keratomalacia. *Br J Ophthalmol*. 1973;57:638–640.
117. Vajpayee RB, Vanathi M, Tandon R, et al. Keratoplasty for keratomalacia in preschool children. *Br J Ophthamol*. 2003;87:538–542.
118. Su WY, Chang SW, Huang SF. Amniotic membrane transplantation for corneal perforation related to vitamin A deficiency. *Ophthalm Surg Las Imag*. 2003;34:140–144.
119. Day PL, Langston WC, O'Brien CS. Cataract and other ocular changes in vitamin G deficiency: experimental study on albino rats. *Am J Ophthalmol*. 1931;14:1005–1009.
120. Bessey OA, Wolbach SB. Vascularisation of the cornea of the rat in riboflavin deficiency, with a note on corneal vascularisation in vitamin A deficiency. *J Exp Med*. 1939;69:1–12.
121. Bowles LL, et al. The development and demonstration of corneal vascularisation in rats deficient in vitamin A and riboflavin. *J Nutr*. 1946;32:19–35.
122. Sydenstricker VP, et al. The ocular manifestations of ariboflavinosis. *J Am Med Assoc*. 1940;114:2437–2445.
123. Gordon OE, Vail D. XVI Conc Ophthal Br Acta 2:438.
124. Boehrer JJ, Stanford CE, Ryan E. Experimental riboflavin deficiency in man. *Am J Med Sci*. 205:544–549, 1943.
125. Ridley H. Ocular manifestations of malnutrition in released prisoners-of-war from Thailand. *Br J Ophthalmol*. 1945;29:613–618.
126. Dansey-Browning GC, Rich WM. Ocular signs in the prisoner-of-war returned from the Far East. *Br Med J*. 1946;1:20–21.
127. Métivier VM. Eye disease due to vitamin deficiency in Trinidad; tropical nutritional amblyopia; essential corneal epithelial dystrophy; conjunctival bleeding in newborn. *Am J Ophthalmol*. 1941;24:1265–1280.
128. Smith DA, Woodruff MFA. Deficiency diseases in Japanese prison camps. *Spec Rep Ser Med Res*. Coun No. 274, 1951.
129. Campbell FW, Ferguson ID. The role of ascorbic acid in corneal vascularisation. *Br J Ophthalmol*. 1950;34:329–334.
130. Hood J, Hodges RE. Ocular lesions in scurvy. *Am J Clin Nutr*. 1969;22:559–567.
131. Levinson RA, Paterson CA, Pfister RR. Ascorbic acid prevents corneal ulceration and perforation following experimental alkali burns. *Invest Ophthalmol Vis Sci*. 1976;15:986.
132. Pfister RR, Paterson CA. Additional clinical and morphological observations on the favourable effect of ascorbate in experimental ocular alkali burns. *Invest Ophthalmol Vis Sci*. 1977;16:478.
133. Pfister RR, et al. The efficacy of ascorbate treatment after severe experimental alkali burns depends on the route of administration. *Invest Ophthalmol Vis Sci*. 1980;19:1526.
134. Pfister RR, Haddox JL, Yuille-Barr D. The combined effect of citrate/ascorbate treatment in alkali-injured rabbit eyes. *Cornea*. 1991; 10(2):100–104.

135. Brubaker RF, Bourne WM, Bachman LA, McLaren JW. Ascorbic acid content of human corneal epithelium. *Invest Ophthalmol Vis Sci.* 2000;41:1681–1683.
136. Leure-Dupree AE. Vascularisation of the rat cornea after prolonged zinc deficiency. *Anat Rec.* 1986;216(1):27–32.
137. Gong H, Takami Y, Kitaoka T, Amemiya T. Corneal changes in magnesium-deficient rats. *Cornea.* 2003;22:448–456.
138. Thalasselis A, et al. Keratoconus, magnesium deficiency, type A behavior, and allergy. *Am J Optom Physiol Opt.* 1988;65(6):499–505.
139. Blumenthal CJ: Malnutritional keratoconjunctivitis disease of South African Bantu. *S Afr Med J.* 1950;24:191–198.

Chapter 63

Hematologic Disorders

Michael R. Grimmett

The ophthalmologist who is aware of the various ocular manifestations of systemic disease is in a position to identify serious systemic disorders based on a 'routine' ophthalmic examination. Knowledge of the various ocular manifestations of hematologic disease may lead to the early diagnosis and treatment of a potentially life-threatening disorder in those patients who have not yet developed overt systemic clinical symptoms. Furthermore, the familiarity of the ophthalmologist with such secondary ocular findings additionally benefits those patients with established hematologic disorders who are referred for ophthalmic consultation and care.

Hematopoiesis

After 7 months' gestation the primary site for hematopoiesis is the bone marrow. Giving rise to all cell lines in the marrow is the pluripotential stem cell, which can undergo self-renewal and differentiation into myeloid or lymphoid stem cells. Myeloid cell lines include: (1) erythroid progenitor cells that ultimately form erythrocytes; (2) granulocyte-macrophage progenitor cells that ultimately form basophils, neutrophils, peripheral blood monocytes/tissue macrophages, and eosinophils; and (3) megakaryocyte progenitor cells that ultimately form platelets.

Evidence suggests that the marrow pluripotential stem cell can also differentiate into the lymphoid line of cells, including B-lymphocyte precursors and T-lymphocyte precursors. However, in contradistinction to the marrow's primary role in the production of the other hematopoietic cell lines, the usual sites of production for lymphocytes are the lymph nodes, thymus, and spleen. Plasma cells are differentiated forms of B lymphocytes that produce antibodies.

Miscellaneous Disorders of the Erythroid Line

Iron deficiency anemia

An estimated 15% of the world's population has iron deficiency anemia.[1] The prevalence in the United States is estimated to be less than 1% in men, and 2–5% in women.[2] The usual causes of iron deficiency in adults include chronic blood loss (e.g. gastrointestinal tract loss and menstruation), malabsorption, and poor dietary intake. The effects of iron deficiency can be profound: decreased exercise tolerance, increased perinatal morbidity, decreased mental and motor function in childhood, and increased susceptibility to various infections.

Systemic manifestations

In severe cases of iron deficiency anemia, a peripheral blood smear reveals erythrocyte morphologic changes that include microcytosis and hypochromia. Additional systemic manifestations may include cold intolerance, thrombocytosis, nail changes, atrophy of the gastrointestinal mucosa with dysphagia, gastric achlorhydria, and pica. Furthermore, severe iron deficiency may be associated with the following abnormal laboratory values: reduced serum iron level, elevated iron-binding capacity, reduced hemoglobin level, reduced serum ferritin level, and elevated free erythrocyte protoporphyrin level. These laboratory values may vary with mild iron-deficient states. Prussian blue staining of a bone marrow aspirate is rarely necessary to establish iron stores.

Ophthalmic manifestations

There are few specific anterior segment manifestations of iron deficiency anemia, although severe iron deficiency may be associated with blue sclera.[3] While pallor of the inferior palpebral conjunctiva is a known sign to screen for anemia, the sensitivity of the technique is poor. In contrast, discontinuous blood columns within the bulbar conjunctival vasculature are easily viewed with a slit lamp and are a highly sensitive screening tool.[2] With worsening anemia, there is an increasing chance that the blood column will develop a gap between the erythrocytes.

Iron overload

While hemochromatosis is not specifically a disorder of erythrocytes, iron metabolism is directly linked to the production of red blood cells. Idiopathic hemochromatosis describes a systemic disorder of iron overload secondary to the breakdown of the normal control of iron absorption from the gastrointestinal tract. The disease is inherited as a recessive trait, and the prevalence may approach 2 to 5 persons per 1000 population.

Systemic manifestations

Clinical symptoms generally appear between 40 and 60 years of age and primarily in homozygous males. As the total body iron stores increase, iron is deposited in the liver, joints, gonads, pancreas, heart, and skin. This abnormal deposition of iron may cause hepatic fibrosis and macronodular cirrhosis, hypogonadism leading to impotence or decreased libido, hypothyroidism, diabetes, cardiomyopathies, arthropathy, skin discoloration, and abdominal pain.

Ophthalmic manifestations

Little literature exists regarding the anterior segment manifestations of systemic iron overload. Hudson[4] in 1953 examined five patients with hemochromatosis, finding no corneal abnormalities, but described the occurrence of conjunctival microaneurysms in four of the patients with coexisting diabetes mellitus. Maddox[5] in 1933 described four patients with hemochromatosis who were found to have grayish-blue retinal discoloration. Brodrick[6] commented that transfusional iron overload never results in the deposition of iron in the eye either as iron dextran, hemosiderin, or ferritin. Overall, systemic hemochromatosis rarely has significant corneal manifestations.

Lazzaro and colleagues described a diffuse pattern of fine brown corneal pigmentation in the intraepithelial and anterior third of the stroma in a patient with acquired hemochromatosis.[7]

Leukemia

The term leukemia defines a group of disorders characterized by the proliferation of a clone of abnormal hematopoietic cells. These abnormal clones are typically characterized by the following: (1) decreased responsiveness to normal regulatory mechanisms, (2) abnormal cellular differentiation, and (3) proliferation at the expense of other normal hematopoietic cells. The leukemias are classified by the cell type involved and whether the disease is acute or chronic. Without appropriate diagnosis and treatment, the leukemias are generally fatal.

Overall, the percentage of patients with any type of ocular involvement from leukemia at the time of autopsy ranges from 28% to 80%.[8] In general, the major manifestations of leukemic ophthalmopathy are hemorrhage (primarily retinal) and leukemic tissue infiltration. Intraretinal hemorrhages are considered a poor prognostic sign and may portend a shorter overall survival time.[9] The avascular cornea is generally spared from these leukemic complications. Should the anterior segment and iris become infiltrated with leukemic cells, associated symptoms and physical findings may include decreased vision, ocular discomfort, headache, photophobia, epiphora, conjunctival injection, abnormal cells in the aqueous, fine keratic precipitates on the endothelium, hypopyon, gray-yellow discoloration of the iris, loss of the normal iris architecture with a gelatinous material filling the iris crypts, spontaneous hyphema, and glaucoma. The eye is considered a 'pharmacologic sanctuary' and may be the primary site of recurrence in previously treated leukemia. Anterior chamber paracentesis may be considered for any patient presenting with uveitis and a recent history of leukemia.[10]

Acute myeloid leukemias

Disorders of the erythroid line

Erythroleukemia

Systemic manifestations

Acute erythroleukemia, a variant of acute myeloblastic leukemia, usually occurs in elderly patients either as a spontaneous disorder or as a consequence of prior alkylator therapy. Primary manifestations are pancytopenia and ineffective erythropoiesis. In one study, complete remission after chemotherapy occurred in 6 of 14 patients (43%) with erythroleukemia.[11]

Ophthalmic manifestations

Allen and Straatsma[12] reported that only one of three patients with erythroleukemia had histopathologic evidence of ocular involvement. The specific ocular structures with leukemic infiltration included the conjunctiva, the sclera and episclera, the choroid, the retina, and the retrobulbar optic nerve. In this isolated case, the iris and cornea showed no pathologic evidence of neoplastic infiltration.

Disorders of the granulocyte-macrophage progenitor line

Acute myeloblastic, acute promyelocytic, acute myelomonocytic, and acute monocytic leukemia

Systemic manifestations

Patients with acute myeloblastic leukemia generally have a prodrome of weakness, bleeding, and fever associated with infections. In these patients, a general physical examination may reveal petechiae and sternal tenderness. Occasionally, lymphadenopathy, hepatosplenomegaly, and testicular, cutaneous, and meningeal involvement may occur. Because of bone marrow infiltration, patients may develop anemia, thrombocytopenic hemorrhage, and neutropenic infections. Leukemic infiltration into the gums, skin, perineum, and central nervous system may occur in patients with monoblastic cellular morphology. A diagnosis of acute myeloblastic leukemia is confirmed by bone marrow examination.

Ophthalmic manifestations

Allan and Straatsma[12] described ocular involvement in seven of ten patients with acute myelogenous leukemia. Regarding the specific anterior segment findings in these seven patients, three had conjunctival leukemic infiltration, five had scleral and episcleral leukemic infiltration, and no patient had iris involvement. The cornea was not involved in any patient. Clinically, the conjunctival involvement manifested itself as a slight thickening of the perilimbal epibulbar tissue. Occasionally, this conjunctival involvement progressed to yellow or flesh-colored small gelatinous nodules at the limbus.

Corneal abnormalities are rare in patients with acute myelogenous leukemia. Bhadresa[13] reported a patient with acute myeloblastic leukemia who had a sterile corneal ring ulcer, pannus, iritis, and limbal stromal infiltrates. Wood and Nicholson[14] described the occurrence of a bilateral corneal ring ulcer as the presenting sign of acute monocytic leukemia in a patient with red eyes and decreased vision for 1 week. Rootman and Gudauskas[15] reported a patient with acute myelomonocytic leukemia presenting with corneal edema, perilimbal injection, a sterile hypopyon of myeloblasts, and a mild elevation of intraocular pressure.

Chronic myeloid leukemia

Chronic myeloid leukemia, also known as chronic granulocytic leukemia or chronic myelocytic leukemia, arises from an abnormal stem cell that gives rise to erythrocytes, neutrophils, eosinophils, basophils, monocyte-macrophages, platelets, T cells, and possibly B cells. Almost all cases of chronic myeloid leukemia are characterized by the presence of the Philadelphia chromosome, which is produced by a reciprocal translocation between chromosomes 9 and 22.

Systemic manifestations

Three phases of chronic myeloid leukemia are described: a chronic phase, an accelerated phase, and a blast crisis phase. The chronic phase is characterized by symptoms of weight loss and fatigue. The patient displays hepatosplenomegaly along with laboratory findings of moderate anemia and an elevated white blood cell count (ranging from 50000 to 300000/mm^3). Variably, abnormalities of the platelets may occur. Bone marrow examination displays hypercellularity with a granulopoietic left shift. The accelerated phase follows this period of stability and is characterized by symptoms of bone pain, fever, night sweats, and weight loss. The spleen and liver show progressive enlargement, and laboratory examination reveals progressive anemia and thrombocytopenia. There is no clear demarcation between this accelerated phase and the ensuing blast crisis phase in which all the previously mentioned symptoms and findings worsen. In the blast phase the peripheral blast count increases, with one-fourth to one-third of patients exhibiting lymphoid morphologic characteristics.

Ophthalmic manifestations

In general, the eye is involved much more often in the acute leukemias than in the chronic leukemias.[12] Regarding the specific type of ocular involvement with chronic myeloid leukemia, Allen and Straatsma[12] reported histologic evidence of conjunctival, scleral, episcleral, and choroidal leukemic infiltration in two of six cases. No corneal abnormalities were described. Chronic myelogenous leukemia has been reported as a cause of glaucoma as a result of presumed leukemic infiltration of the trabecular meshwork.[16] Rarely, hyperviscosity due to extreme leukocytosis may lead to anterior segment ischemia.[17]

Disorders of the lymphoid line

Acute lymphocytic leukemia

Systemic manifestations

The clinical manifestations of acute lymphocytic leukemia are similar to those of acute myelogenous leukemia (see earlier discussion) with one exception: the incidence of central nervous system involvement is higher in acute lymphocytic leukemia. An oculomotor nerve palsy has been described as a rare manifestation of leukemic invasion.[18]

Ophthalmic manifestations

Ridgway et al.[19] reported 41 cases of ocular involvement in patients with acute lymphoblastic leukemia (retinal hemorrhages and leukemic infiltration of the optic nerve, retina, iris, or orbit). No corneal abnormalities were identified in any patient. Similarly, Allen and Straatsma[12] found no evidence of corneal leukemic infiltration in 17 cases of acute lymphocytic leukemia, although one unexplained case of corneal edema was identified histologically. However, leukemic tissue infiltration may occur in the choroid, optic nerve, sclera, episclera, retina, conjunctiva, ciliary body, iris, and orbit.

A review by Bunin et al.[20] of 723 children with recurrent leukemia found 11 cases of acute lymphoblastic leukemia with anterior chamber involvement (nine with hypopyon, two with iris involvement). No corneal involvement was described. Several other isolated case reports describe the occurrence of iritis and hypopyon in acute lymphocytic leukemia.[8,15,20–22] Acute lymphoblastic leukemia may involve the conjunctiva.[8] In these cases, biopsy of a diffuse or focal conjunctival mass revealed blast cell infiltration, ultimately leading to a diagnosis of lymphocytic leukemia.

Chronic lymphocytic leukemia

Chronic lymphocytic leukemia is characterized by the abnormal proliferation of relatively mature lymphocytes. The majority of the time the abnormal clone arises from B cells. T-cell chronic lymphocytic leukemia accounts for 5% of cases and is clinically similar to the B-cell variants except for an increased frequency of skin involvement. Because normal B cells are replaced by the abnormal clone, immunoglobulin levels may be depressed, leading to impaired humoral immunity. Second malignancies occur frequently in patients with chronic lymphocytic leukemia.

Systemic manifestations

Signs and symptoms vary widely in chronic lymphocytic leukemia. Certain cases may be uncovered on a routine physical examination with generalized nontender lymphadenopathy or hepatosplenomegaly. Other cases may be found with recurrent infections secondary to extensive leukemic marrow infiltration and its resultant neutropenia and impaired humoral immunity. Peripheral pancytopenia may be exacerbated by autoimmune hemolytic anemia or splenic trapping of cells. In most cases, systemic symptoms with chronic lymphocytic leukemia are absent. As time progresses, some patients with chronic lymphocytic leukemia develop weight loss, fever, night sweats, and rapidly enlarging nodal and extranodal masses (Richter's syndrome).

The diagnosis of chronic lymphocytic leukemia is established by a peripheral blood smear, a bone marrow evaluation, and a lymph node biopsy.

Ophthalmic manifestations

Specific corneal manifestations of chronic lymphocytic leukemia are rare because the cornea is avascular. However, isolated cases have been reported with corneal involvement. Eiferman et al.[23] described an 83-year-old woman with a long-standing history of chronic lymphocytic leukemia who had numerous superficial light-gray circular infiltrates just below an intact epithelium in a corneal graft. A subsequent corneal biopsy disclosed sheets of well-differentiated lymphocytes invading the superficial corneal stroma. A systemic evaluation revealed hepatosplenomegaly and bone marrow infiltration. The authors stressed that these infiltrates may be the initial sign of an acute leukemic exacerbation. Moller et al.[24] described a bilateral paraproteinemic crystalline keratopathy as a result of an abnormal serum cryoglobulin (IgG κ) in a patient with chronic lymphocytic leukemia. The corneal opacities were white and were located just beneath the epithelium in the superficial stroma, with a distribution in both the center and the periphery of the cornea. The authors likened the appearance of these opacities to granular corneal dystrophy. Other ocular involvement may include local tissue infiltration (e.g. scleral, episcleral, orbit, optic nerve, iris, extraocular muscles).

Infectious complications of leukemia

Patients with leukemia are at risk for a wide variety of bacterial, viral, fungal, and protozoal opportunistic infections as a result of altered immunity. Overall, posterior pole infectious complications predominate in patients with leukemia, including cytomegalovirus retinitis, herpes simplex retinitis, herpes zoster retinitis, measles retinitis, *Candida* retinitis/uveitis, and *Aspergillus* choroiditis/vitritis. Other opportunistic infections reported to involve the eye include *Mucor*, *Cryptococcus*, *Toxoplasma*, and bacterial retinitis.[8]

General diagnostic techniques in leukemia

No matter what the actual variant of leukemia encountered, an ophthalmic diagnosis of leukemic anterior segment infiltration rests largely on a high degree of clinical suspicion and knowledge of the wide variety of clinical presentations possible. In general, tissue biopsy of clinically involved areas usually yields the diagnosis (e.g. lid conjunctiva, and cornea). Cytologic analysis of a corneal scraping has yielded the diagnosis of leukemia in a case of acute myelogenous leukemia.[14] When a uveitis-like picture predominates, a paracentesis aspirate of the aqueous may be sent for cytology to obtain the diagnosis. A complete ophthalmic examination may disclose other supporting features for a diagnosis of leukemia: leukemic retinopathy (venous dilation, hemorrhages, and cotton-wool spots), choroidal leukemic infiltration (with secondary retinal pigment epithelial alterations and/or serous retinal detachment), papilledema and/or direct optic nerve head infiltration, extraocular muscle palsies from cranial nerve involvement, and orbital infiltration (exophthalmos, lid edema, chemosis, and pain).

Ocular treatment in leukemia

The eye is considered a 'sanctuary' for leukemic relapses after adequate systemic therapy because cranial irradiation used for central nervous system prophylaxis does not include the anterior pole of the eye and chemotherapeutic agents may not achieve adequate therapeutic levels in the anterior segment.[20] Since anterior segment ocular involvement is uncommon, large-scale studies of different treatment modalities are not currently available.

Local radiation therapy is generally advocated to control anterior segment leukemic infiltration (iris infiltration, uveitis, elevated intraocular pressure).[8] Optic nerve infiltration with decreased vision is a recognized ophthalmic emergency and requires urgent local radiation of 700 to 2000 rads.[8] There is a limited role for topical corticosteroids and subconjunctival medications (e.g. methotrexate, cytarabine, corticosteroids) in select cases. With any ocular relapse, systemic evaluation and treatment is required because concomitant meningeal leukemia can coexist with ocular relapses.[19]

Many chemotherapeutic agents have ocular toxicity. Busulfan has been linked with posterior subcapsular cataracts.[11] Vincristine and vinblastine can induce cranial nerve oculomotor palsies, including corneal hypoesthesia.[25] Cytarabine can induce corneal epithelial opacities and microcysts when administered systemically or topically.[8]

After bone marrow transplantation, acute and chronic graft-versus-host disease may occur. Ocular manifestations include dry eyes, pseudomembranous conjunctivitis, ectropion, and uveitis.[8]

Bruton's Hypogammaglobulinemia

Bruton's disease, described in 1952, is a rare X-linked condition of abnormal B-cell maturation with resultant hypogammaglobulinemia.[26] Young males typically present between the ages of 4 months and 2 years with severe respiratory tract infections, generally caused by encapsulated bacteria (e.g. *Streptococcus pyogenes*, *Haemophilus influenzae*, or *Neisseria meningitidis*). Maternal transplacental passive transfer of antibody is protective for the affected individual in the first few months of life. Treatment consists of lifelong immunoglobulin therapy and intermittent courses of antibiotics as necessary.

Ocular manifestations of Bruton's disease concern complications from infectious conjunctivitis, blepharitis, and keratitis.

Plasma Cell Dyscrasias

Multiple myeloma

Plasma cell myeloma, or multiple myeloma, is characterized by the uncontrolled proliferation of a single clone of plasma cells with altered immunoglobulin production. Normally, the synthesis of immunoglobulins by plasma cells has a synchronized production of both light (κ or λ) and heavy chains (γ, α, μ, δ, or ε). Some of the clinical features of multiple myeloma depend on the specific type of immunoglobulin overproduction or underproduction by the malignant plasma cell clone. Possibilities for the malignant clone include: (1) matched production of heavy chains and light chains with overproduction of monoclonal immunoglobulins known as M proteins; (2) excess production of light chains with respect to heavy chains, with these excess light chains appearing in the urine (Bence Jones proteins) or in low concentrations in the serum; (3) lack of production of heavy chains altogether with only light-chain production, causing Bence Jones proteinuria and proteinemia; (4) excess production of heavy chains with respect to light chains, producing a so-called heavy-chain disease (γ, α, or μ); and (5) lack of the ability to synthesize either light or heavy chains with the possibility of producing panhypogammaglobulinemia. In multiple myeloma, the production of normal immunoglobulins by normal B cells is typically suppressed.

Systemic manifestations

The malignant transformation of plasma cells probably occurs 4 to 6 years before clinically apparent disease. Anorexia, weight loss, and weakness may precede the actual diagnosis of multiple myeloma in many cases. The vast majority of the many other clinical manifestations of multiple myeloma are ultimately related to direct tissue tumor infiltration or the presence of an abnormal protein in the serum.

Bone involvement is a hallmark of multiple myeloma. Direct marrow infiltration by malignant plasma cells may cause a peripheral pancytopenia. Additionally, generalized osteoporosis or focal bone destruction in the form of plasmacytomas occurs commonly in the axial skeleton and may cause painful fractures and vertebral collapse. Hypercalcemia occurs because of this bone destruction, with possible symptoms of nausea, vomiting, somnolence, polydipsia, polyuria, and coma. Other complications of multiple myeloma may include extramedullary sites of infiltration, renal disease, and hyperviscosity syndrome.

Ophthalmic manifestations

In general terms, ocular involvement is secondary to myelomatous infiltration in and around the eye or is secondary to serum and hematologic disturbances. Myeloma has been reported to involve almost every ocular structure, including the cornea (crystalline and copper deposition, prominent corneal nerves), conjunctiva (crystalline deposition and sludging of blood flow), uvea (proteinaceous pars plana cysts, choroidal tumors, infiltrates, and chorioretinal destruction), retina (subretinal deposits, dysproteinemic fundus consisting of venous dilation and retinal hemorrhages), sclera (infiltration), optic nerve (infiltration, papilledema), lacrimal gland (infiltration), lacrimal sac (infiltration), and orbit (invasion of orbital bones with proptosis and compression of cranial nerves).[27,28]

The presence of numerous, delicate, scintillating, polychromatic crystals within the corneal stroma has been recognized as a manifestation of hypergammaglobulinemia since Burki's original description in 1958.[29] These deposits

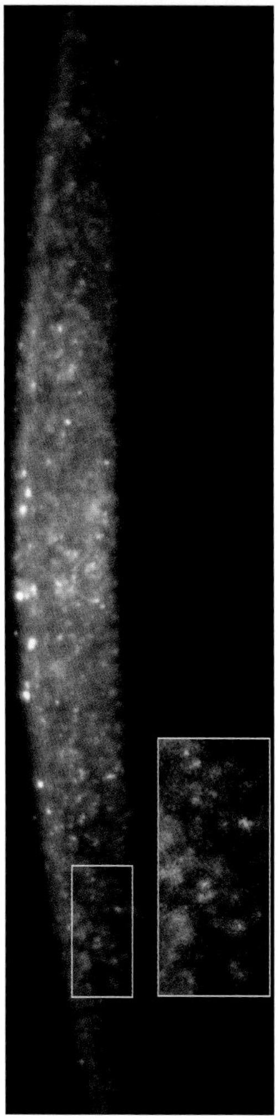

Fig. 63.1 Corneal deposits in multiple myeloma. In this case, crystals are found throughout the stroma. Inset shows varying sizes of crystals.

may occur at all levels in the cornea (Fig. 63.1) and are composed of immunoglobulin resembling that found in the serum.[30] While most reports indicate that vision is minimally affected by these deposits, others have reported visual decline to the 20/400 level.[28] Although penetrating keratoplasty, lamellar keratoplasty, and excimer phototherapeutic keratectomy are options for marked visual decline, recurrence of crystal deposition can happen, especially if the systemic condition worsens. The precise incidence of the crystalline deposition in patients with multiple myeloma is largely unknown. Other reported corneal findings in patients with myeloma include central corneal copper deposition at the level of Descemet's membrane and band keratopathy associated with hypercalcemia.[31–33]

Other authors have described noncrystalline corneal opacities in association with multiple myeloma. Beebe et al.[28] reported the bilateral corneal deposition of a monoclonal IgG κ-type immunoglobulin that appeared as epithelial and subepithelial amorphous gray-white 'candle wax drippings' causing focal epithelial elevation. In this patient, the anterior third of the corneal stroma also displayed a diffuse noniridescent granular haze. After penetrating keratoplasty the proteinaceous deposits eventually recurred in the graft and caused visual impairment. Hill and Mulligan[30] described the bilateral corneal deposition of an IgG λ-type immunoglobulin in a patient with multiple myeloma. The deposits were described as translucent subepithelial peripheral corneal deposits with a lucid zone of normal cornea separating them from the limbus. Perry et al.[34] described a 52-year-old man with bilateral asymptomatic intraepithelial opacities (nonstaining) that were secondary to the deposition of IgG κ. These linear thin opacities were more numerous in the central cornea than in the periphery. Auran et al.[35] noted that the epithelial manifestations of multiple myeloma may present in a vortex pattern.

Conjunctival findings have included crystalline deposition similar to that of the cornea. Pinkerton et al. described them as fine iridescent crystalline bodies appearing as glistening specks on the bulbar conjunctiva.[36] Aronson and Shaw described crystals throughout the superficial layers of the bulbar conjunctiva with minimal involvement of the tarsal conjunctiva.[37] Erythrocyte sludging within the conjunctival vessels can be observed as well.[36] Franklin et al. described the unusual occurrence of a unilateral plasmacytoma of the bulbar conjunctiva in a man with long-standing multiple myeloma.[38] The authors speculated that IgA-producing tumors may have a 'homing' mechanism to mucosal surfaces.

Overall, corneal and conjunctival crystalline deposition in multiple myeloma is a relatively rare event. Since structurally normal intact immunoglobulins do not easily crystallize under physiologic conditions, it has been proposed that most corneal deposits consist of incomplete monoclonal proteins (e.g. light chains).[39] Overall, the precise pathophysiologic mechanisms leading to paraprotein tissue deposition are poorly understood but may include local tissue factors such as the temperature of the cornea, pH, water transport mechanisms, and various components of the corneal extracellular matrix. Two clinical factors increase the likelihood that corneal paraprotein deposition will occur: (1) a gammopathy of IgG κ light-chain type is present (approximately 70% of all monoclonal gammopathies are IgG in type), and (2) chronicity.[40,41] Of note, IgG shows greater diffusibility within the cornea than other immunoglobulin classes.[41] While paraprotein levels have been documented in tears and aqueous humor, corneal deposition most likely derives from transport of immunoglobulins across the limbal microvasculature.[41]

Waldenström's macroglobulinemia

Waldenström's macroglobulinemia is characterized by the uncontrolled growth and proliferation of a malignant plasma cell clone that primarily secretes IgM, causing increased serum viscosity. Older men are affected most commonly.[42]

Systemic manifestations

Typical presenting features include weakness, fatigue, bleeding gums, and epistaxis. Recurrent infections, congestive heart failure, dyspnea, weight loss, and neurologic symptoms may also occur.[42] The marrow is infiltrated with malignant cells, and, typically, the liver, spleen, and lungs are involved. On examination, pallor, peripheral adenopathy, hepatosplenomegaly, and purpura are commonly identified.

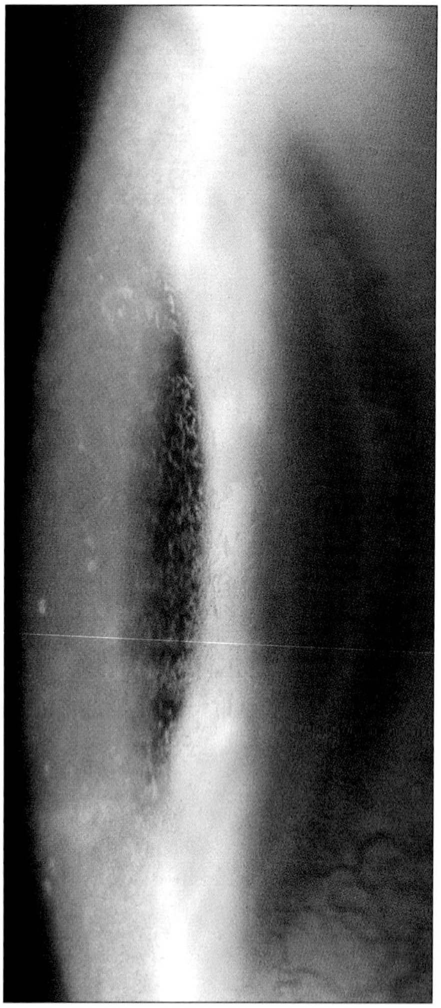

Fig. 63.2 Corneal deposits in Waldenström's macroglobulinemia. In this case, crystals are needle-like and are located at all stromal levels.

Ophthalmic manifestations

The majority of the ocular findings in patients with Waldenström's macroglobulinemia are secondary to hyperviscosity and primarily involve the retina (venous congestion, hemorrhages, retinal edema, exudates, branch or central vein occlusion, and disk edema). Specific anterior segment findings include erythrocyte sludging in the conjunctival vessels, conjunctival crystal deposition, and keratoconjunctivitis.[42] Deposition of periodic acid–Schiff-positive material between the corneal epithelium and Bowman's layer and within the epithelium has been demonstrated histopathologically in patients with Waldenström's macroglobulinemia.[42] Deposits may occur at any level in the cornea (Fig. 63.2).

Cryoglobulinemia

Cryoglobulins are proteins that precipitate on exposure to cold. The cryoglobulinemias are typically associated with autoimmune disorders, immunoproliferative disorders, or hepatitis B infection. It is common for the abnormal immunoglobulins to form immune complexes, leading to complement activation and inflammation.

Systemic manifestations

Clinically, the patient may initially present with Raynaud's phenomenon, vascular purpura, urticaria, ulceration of the skin, and peripheral gangrene. Hyperviscosity is common. Coagulation disorders are secondary to platelet aggregation and consumption of clotting factors by the cryoglobulins. Renal and neurologic problems also occur with cryoglobulinemia. Plasmapheresis is beneficial for complications of hyperviscosity.

Ophthalmic manifestations

As with other hyperviscosity states, retinal vascular disease is common with cryoglobulinemia. Palm described superficial crystalline corneal deposits in a patient with cryoglobulinemia (as cited by Kremer et al.[43]). Other authors have reported noncrystalline corneal findings as well. Kremer et al.[43] described bilateral, raised, gelatinous, gray-white, subepithelial, noncrystalline, avascular nodules in the corneal periphery that were subsequently proven to be a monoclonal IgG κ paraprotein by histopathology in a patient with essential IgG κ cryoglobulinemia. Oglesby[44] described the occurrence of bilateral, gray, irregular, geographic deposits in the posterior corneal stroma in a patient with cryoglobulinemia and reticulohistiocytosis.

Benign monoclonal gammopathy (monoclonal gammopathy of undetermined significance)

The incidence of benign monoclonal gammopathy is as high as 6% in persons from 60 to 80 years of age when immunofixation techniques are used to make the diagnosis.[45] The diagnosis of benign monoclonal gammopathy assumes that a complete systemic work-up has excluded the possibility of multiple myeloma or other disorders.

Systemic manifestations

Patients with a diagnosis of benign monoclonal gammopathy have no osteolytic lesions, minimal marrow plasmacytosis, less than 3 g/dL of a paraprotein, little to no Bence Jones proteinuria, minimal anemia, no azotemia, no hypoalbuminemia, and stable levels of M protein. One study showed that 19% of 241 patients with a diagnosis of benign monoclonal gammopathy developed myeloma, macroglobulinemia, amyloidosis, or a related disorder when followed for 10 years or more.[46] No specific factor is known to predict later malignant conversion. It must be recognized that gammopathies can also be found in patients with lymphoma, leukemia, chronic inflammations of the gallbladder or bile ducts, hepatic cirrhosis, and neoplasms of the intestine, kidney, nasopharynx, biliary tract, lungs, and thymus.[42] A thorough systemic work-up is therefore mandatory for patients with abnormal immunoglobulin levels.

Ophthalmic manifestations

The anterior segment findings in patients with benign monoclonal gammopathy mimic those of multiple myeloma because the underlying abnormality is similar: the serum contains an abnormally elevated immunoglobulin fraction.

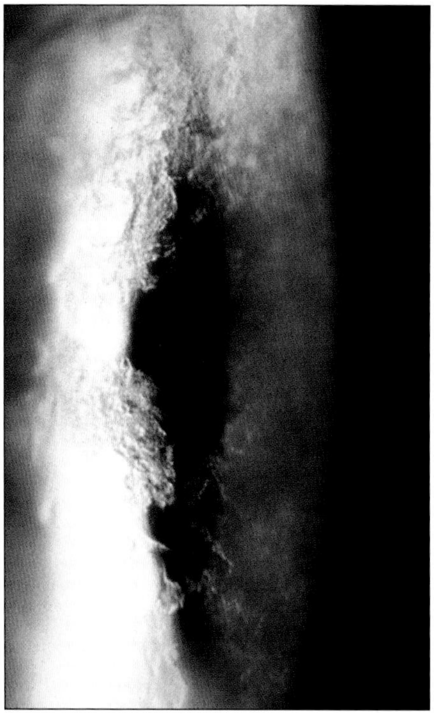

Fig. 63.3 Corneal deposits in benign monoclonal gammopathy. In this case, proteinaceous deposits are pre-Descemet's membrane.

As such, iridescent crystalline deposition has been reported to occur within the cornea in a diffuse pattern, in the posterior stroma (Fig. 63.3), or in the anterior stroma in patients with benign monoclonal gammopathy.[47,48] The deposits may be central, midperipheral, or paralimbal and may appear as gray-white, yellow, gray-brown, or polychromatic iridescent dotlike opacities with a diffuse, fine stippled appearance.[48] Irregular geographic configurations and patches are reported as well. Corneal sensation is usually normal, and corneal neovascularization associated with the deposits is absent.[48]

In addition to crystalline deposition, paraproteinemic corneal deposition may appear as discrete nonrefractile opacities in various patterns or as a diffuse haze. Eiferman and Rodrigues[49] reported the occurrence of a circumferential dense gray-white band at the level of Bowman's membrane associated with severe photophobia and tearing as the initial signs of an IgG κ monoclonal gammopathy. Spiegel et al.[50] described counting-fingers vision and diffusely hazy corneas bilaterally along with small grayish opacities forming a reticular pattern that resembled end-stage lattice dystrophy in a patient with an IgG κ monoclonal peak. Cherry et al.[51] described a patient that later progressed to multiple myeloma with diffuse small grayish spots throughout the corneal stroma bilaterally.

Slit lamp screening for corneal crystals in patients with a monoclonal gammopathy is not a useful procedure, as demonstrated by Bourne et al.,[52] who found corneal crystals in only 1 of 100 patients with a confirmed diagnosis of monoclonal gammopathy. There was, however, a positive correlation between erythrocyte sludging in the conjunctival vessels and the concentration of the monoclonal protein in the serum.

Differential Diagnosis of the Crystalline Keratopathies

In general, corneal crystalline deposition can be divided into several categories: (1) lipid keratopathies such as Schnyder's crystalline dystrophy, Tangier disease, lecithin-cholesterol acyltransferase deficiency, and familial lipoprotein disorders; (2) errors of protein metabolism such as tyrosinemia, cystinosis, hyperuricemia, and gout; (3) acquired immunoprotein keratopathies, including multiple myeloma, benign monoclonal gammopathy, cryoglobulinemia, Waldenström's macroglobulinemia, and rheumatoid arthritis; (4) infectious crystalline keratopathies including those resulting from viral, bacterial, and fungal causes; (5) miscellaneous dystrophies and metabolic abnormalities such as posterior crystalline corneal dystrophy, Bietti's corneal dystrophy, calcium deposition, porphyria, and oxalosis; and (6) drug deposition, including chrysiasis, and deposits of chlorpromazine and chloroquine.[41] Histopathologic analysis of the crystalline deposition, the clinical appearance of the deposits, and a directed systemic evaluation will aid in determining the correct underlying diagnosis.

References

1. Cook JD, Lynch SR. The liabilities of iron deficiency. *Blood*. 1986;68:803.
2. Kent AR, Elsing SH, Hebert RL. Conjunctival vasculature in the assessment of anemia. *Ophthalmology*. 2000;107(2):274–277.
3. Kalra L, Hamlyn AN, Jones BJM. Blue sclerae: a common sign of iron deficiency? *Lancet*. 1986;2:1267.
4. Hudson JR. Ocular findings in haemochromatosis. *Br J Ophthalmol*. 1953;37:242.
5. Maddox K. The retina in haemochromatosis. *Br J Ophthalmol*. 1933;17:393.
6. Brodrick JD. Pigmentation of the cornea: review and case history. *Ann Ophthalmol*. 1979;11:855.
7. Lazzaro DR, Lin K, Stevens JA. Corneal findings in hemochromatosis. *Arch Ophthalmol*. 1998;116:1531–1532.
8. Kincaid MC, Green WR. Ocular and orbital involvement in leukemia. *Surv Ophthalmol*. 1983;27:211.
9. Reddy SC, Quah SH, Low HC, Jackson N. Prognostic significance of retinopathy at presentation in adult acute leukemia. *Ann Hematol*. 1998;76(1):15–18.
10. MacLean H, Clarke MP, Strong NP, et al. Primary ocular relapse in acute lymphoblastic leukemia. *Eye*. 1996;10:719–722.
11. Tamura K, Preisler HD. Treatment of erythroleukemia with anthracycline antibiotics and cytosine arabinoside. *Cancer*. 1983;51:1795.
12. Allen RA, Straatsma BR. Ocular involvement in leukemia and allied disorders. *Arch Ophthalmol*. 1961;66:68.
13. Bhadresa GN. Changes in the anterior segment as a presenting feature in leukemia. *Br J Ophthalmol*. 1971;55:133.
14. Wood WJ, Nicholson DH. Corneal ring ulcer as the presenting manifestation of acute monocytic leukemia. *Am J Ophthalmol*. 1973;76:69.
15. Rootman J, Gudauskas G. Treatment of ocular leukemia with local chemotherapy. *Cancer Treat Rep*. 1985;69:119.
16. Mehta P. Ophthalmologic manifestations of leukemia. *J Pediatr*. 1979; 95:156.
17. Cullis CM, Hines DR, Bullock JD. Anterior segment ischemia: classification and description in chronic myelogenous leukemia. *Ann Ophthalmol*. 1979;11:1739.
18. Jinnai K, Hayashi Y. Hemorrhage in the oculomotor nerve as a complication of leukemia. *Neuropathology*. 2001;21(3):241–244.
19. Ridgway EW, Jaffe N, Walton D. Leukemic ophthalmopathy in children. *Cancer*. 1976;38:1744.
20. Bunin N, et al. Ocular relapse in the anterior chamber in childhood acute lymphoblastic leukemia. *J Clin Oncol*. 1987;5:299.
21. Jankovic M, et al. Recurrences of isolated leukemic hypopyon in a child with acute lymphoblastic leukemia. *Cancer*. 1986;57:380.
22. Gruenewald RL, Perry MC, Henry PH. Leukemic iritis with hypopyon. *Cancer*. 1979;44:1511.
23. Eiferman RA, Levartovsky S, Schulz JC. Leukemic corneal infiltrates. *Am J Ophthalmol*. 1988;105:319.
24. Moller HU, et al. Differential diagnosis between granular corneal dystrophy Groenouw type I and paraproteinemic crystalline keratopathy. *Acta Ophthalmol*. 1993;71:552.
25. Albert DW, Wong VG, Henderson ES. Ocular complications of vincristine therapy. *Arch Ophthalmol*. 1967;78:709.
26. Hansel TT, et al. Infective conjunctivitis and corneal scarring in three brothers with sex linked hypogammaglobulinaemia (Bruton's disease). *Br J Ophthalmol*. 1990;74:118.
27. Maisel JM, et al. Multiple myeloma presenting with ocular inflammation. *Ann Ophthalmol*. 1987;19:170.
28. Beebe WE, Webster RG, Spencer WB. Atypical corneal manifestations of multiple myeloma. A clinical, histopathologic, and immunohistochemical report. *Cornea*. 1989;8:274.
29. Klintworth GK, Bredehoeft SJ, Reed JW. Analysis of corneal crystalline deposits in multiple myeloma. *Am J Ophthalmol*. 1978;86:303.
30. Hill JC, Mulligan GP. Subepithelial corneal deposits in IgGγ myeloma. *Br J Ophthalmol*. 1989;73:552.
31. Lewis RA, Falls HF, Troyer DO. Ocular manifestations of hypercupremia associated with multiple myeloma. *Arch Ophthalmol*. 1975;93:1050.
32. Wilson KS, Alexander S, Chisholm IA. Band keratopathy in hypercalcemia of myeloma. *Can Med Assoc J*. 1982;126:1314.
33. Hawkins AS, Stein RM, Gaines BI, Deutsch TA. Ocular deposition of copper associated with multiple myeloma. *Am J Ophthalmol*. 2001; 131(2):257–925.
34. Perry HD, Donnenfeld ED, Font RL. Intraepithelial corneal immunoglobulin crystals in IgG-kappa multiple myeloma. *Cornea*. 1993;12:448.
35. Auran JD, Donn A, Hyman GA. Multiple myeloma presenting as vortex crystalline keratopathy and complicated by endocapsular hematoma. *Cornea*. 1992;11:584.
36. Pinkerton RMH, Robertson DM. Corneal and conjunctival changes in dysproteinemia. *Invest Ophthalmol*. 1969;8:357.
37. Aronson SB, Shaw R. Corneal crystals in multiple myeloma. *Arch Ophthalmol*. 1959;61:541.
38. Franklin RM, et al. Epibulbar IgA plasmacytoma occurring in multiple myeloma. *Arch Ophthalmol*. 1982;100:451.
39. Green ED, et al. A structurally aberrant immunoglobulin paraprotein in a patient with multiple myeloma and corneal crystal deposits. *Am J Med*. 1990;88:304.
40. Steuhl KP, et al. Paraproteinemic corneal deposits in plasma cell myeloma. *Am J Ophthalmol*. 1991;111:312.
41. Henderson DW, et al. Paraproteinemic crystalloidal keratopathy: an ultrastructural study of two cases, including immunoelectron microscopy. *Ultrastruct Pathol*. 1993;17:643.
42. Orellana J, Friedman AH. Ocular manifestations of multiple myeloma, Waldenström's macroglobulinemia and benign monoclonal gammopathy. *Surv Ophthalmol*. 1981;26:157.
43. Kremer I, et al. Corneal subepithelial monoclonal kappa IgG deposits in essential cryoglobulinaemia. *Br J Ophthalmol*. 1989;73:669.
44. Oglesby RB. Corneal opacities in a patient with cryoglobulinemia and reticulohistiocytosis. *Arch Ophthalmol*. 1961;4:63.
45. Crawford J, Eye MK, Cohen HJ. Evaluation of monoclonal gammopathies in the 'well' elderly. *Am J Med*. 1987;82:39.
46. Kyle RA: 'Benign' monoclonal gammopathy: a misnomer? *JAMA*. 1984;251:1849.
47. Grossniklaus HE, Stulting RD, L'Hernault N. Corneal and conjunctival crystals in paraproteinemia. *Hum Pathol*. 1990;21:1181.
48. Rodrigues MM, et al. Posterior corneal crystalline deposits in benign monoclonal gammopathy. A clinicopathologic case report. *Arch Ophthalmol*. 1979;97:124.
49. Eiferman RA, Rodrigues MM. Unusual superficial stromal corneal deposits in IgG κ monoclonal gammopathy. *Arch Ophthalmol*. 1980;98:78.
50. Spiegel P, et al. Unusual presentation of paraproteinemic corneal infiltrates. *Cornea*. 1990;9:81.
51. Cherry PMH, et al. Corneal and conjunctival deposits in monoclonal gammopathy. *Can J Ophthalmol*. 1983;18:142.
52. Bourne WM, et al. Incidence of corneal crystals in the monoclonal gammopathies. *Am J Ophthalmol*. 1989;107:192.

Chapter 64

Endocrine Disease and the Cornea

Rebecca M. Bartow

Diabetes Mellitus

Diabetes mellitus is the most common endocrine disorder an ophthalmologist will encounter. The anterior segment findings of this disorder are less extensively described than the retinopathy. Before the 1970s, descriptions of diabetic changes in the anterior segment included conjunctival microaneurysms, ectropion uveae, an increased incidence of Descemet's folds, and pigment deposition on the corneal endothelium, anterior iris surface, and trabecular meshwork. Extensive corneal pathology was not noticed.[1] However, in the 1970s Schwartz[2] and Hyndiuk[3] noted a decreased corneal sensitivity and sterile neurotrophic corneal ulcers in diabetics. The advent of vitrectomy heightened interest in the diabetic cornea, since diabetics were found to have increased problems with epithelial healing and stromal edema after vitrectomy.[4–6] Since this time, research has focused on the biochemical and anatomic changes in the cornea.

Biochemistry

Past studies of the biochemistry of the diabetic cornea have examined the role of the sorbitol pathway. In this pathway, glucose is metabolized to sorbitol by aldose reductase and further to fructose by sorbitol dehydrogenase. More recent studies have focused on factors that can alter cell adhesion and tissue repair. Findings include changes in the adhesive molecules of the extracellular matrix and basement membrane.[7–10]

Animal studies

Many investigators have identified the presence of aldose reductase and by-products of the sorbitol pathway in various animal models, including in the corneal epithelium and endothelium of dogs,[11] the corneal epithelium of normal[12] and diabetic[13] rabbits, and the corneal endothelium of rats.[14]

The next level of investigation focused on whether aldose reductase inhibitors could improve epithelial healing problems in diabetic animals. Reepithelialization of corneal defects occurred faster in one study when animals were treated with an aldose reductase inhibitor.[15] Another study compared morphologic changes in rats treated with and without aldose reductase inhibitors.[16] The epithelium of treated rats not only healed more quickly but also showed a thicker multilayered epithelium. Untreated rats had an irregularly shaped epithelium that was not as transparent. Finally, endothelial changes were less significant in diabetic rats treated with aldose reductase inhibitor compared to controls.[17,18]

Despite these studies, questions remain about precisely how the sorbitol pathway contributes to abnormalities. Unlike diabetes-induced cataract formation, osmotic forces do not seem to be important.[12,13] In addition, not all studies demonstrate abnormal epithelial healing in diabetic animals[13] or find high enough levels of by-products of the sorbitol pathway to account for problems.[19]

Degradative enzymes known as matrix metalloproteinases are elevated in healing corneal epithelium of diabetic rats as compared to control.[20] This finding suggests that these enzymes are responsible for the slowed epithelial healing in a high glucose state. Finally, cytokines and Ki-67-positive cells are increased as corneal epithelial wounds heal in GK rats.[9,10] Changes in the structural and proliferative capacity of the epithelial cells result.

Human studies

Biochemical studies in humans are scarce. Aldose reductase has been found in the diabetic conjunctiva and corneal epithelium and endothelium.[4,15,21] Epithelial healing in humans has been enhanced by aldose reductase inhibitors.[22] These effects have included resolution of poorly healing epithelial abrasions and reduction in the number of recurrent erosions. The oxygen consumption of the epithelium is reduced compared to normal individuals,[24] and insulin does not seem to be present in the human cornea.[25]

Studies of epithelial cells in diabetic humans focus on the components of the extracellular matrix and basement membrane. Findings include an increase in both matrix metalloproteinases and advanced glycolation end products,[26] a decrease in major epithelial basement membrane components including nidogen-1/entactin, lamin-1, laminin-10, and lamin binding integrin,[27,28] and an abnormal expression of several proteinases and growth factors.[29]

Morphology

Animal models of diabetes mellitus include the rat, the rabbit, and the dog. The rat has been extensively studied, and corneal epithelial changes include calcium deposition, degeneration of basal epithelial cells, and an increase in glycogen granules.[16,19] Cell membranes appear to be broken down adjacent to the basal lamina,[16] and the interactions of hemidesmosomes with the basement membrane are not normal.[29] The subepithelial basement membrane is thickened, with infoldings of the basement membrane into the epithelial cell layer. Cytoplasmic lipid vacuoles with deposition of amorphous material are found in the stroma.[30]

Abnormalities in the corneal nerves are evident as irregularities in the basal lamina of Schwann cells.[31] These changes increase with the duration of diabetes. Finally, there is a decreased percentage of hexagonal cells and an increased coefficient of variation for cell size in the corneal endothelium.[17,18]

The rabbit has been another useful model for diabetic corneal change. In addition to findings similar to those seen in the rat,[32] it is evident that the epithelial basement membrane in diabetic rabbits is more easily damaged than in control animals.[33] The only endothelial changes described are functional; stromal hydration and corneal thickness in diabetic rabbits increase after stress.[34] Finally, endothelial changes have been noted in diabetic dogs. Descemet's membrane is unaltered in dogs regardless of diabetic control. However, there is marked pleomorphism and polymegathism in diabetic compared to normal dogs.[35]

Many descriptions of the morphologic changes in human diabetics exist, although explanation of their etiology remains unclear. Microscopic examination of the epithelium and stroma reveal many changes that could account for clinical findings of poor epithelial adhesion. As in animals, there is a thickened, multilayered basement membrane that is discontinuous.[31,32,36–40] The basal epithelium and Bowman's membrane easily detach from the stroma in a sheet.[34,40,44] Filamentary structures similar to anchoring fibrils are present, but not in their normal positions, and do not penetrate as deeply into the anterior stroma.[32,36,40] Hemidesmosomes are fewer in number than in control groups.[31,32,36] Stromal changes are similar to those in animals and consist of cytoplasmic lipid vacuoles with deposition of an amorphous material adjacent to cells. In addition, there are long spaced collagen fibers of variable thickness noted in the stroma and next to Descemet's membrane.[30]

Specular microscopy of the corneal epithelium shows many irregularities in diabetics compared to control groups. There is more irregularity of cell arrangements[31,32] and greater variation in cell size, with a shift in the ratio of large to small cells.[31]

The conjunctiva demonstrates increased thickness of the basement membrane of capillaries and many collagen-like fibrils.[41] The nerves in human diabetics show irregularity in the basal lamina of Schwann cells, but no decrease in nerve density.[31]

The corneal endothelium of diabetics has more polymegathism and pleomorphism than in nondiabetics.[42,43,46] The baseline corneal thickness is found to be increased in most studies[44,48,49] but not in all.[42] These morphologic studies are paralleled by changes in the permeability characteristics of the cornea. There is more autofluorescence of the diabetic cornea,[51] and the corneas of diabetics thin more slowly after stress than those of normal individuals.[32]

Clinical correlations

In 1974, Schwartz noted a decrease in corneal sensation when comparing age- and sex-matched control groups with diabetics.[2] In 1977, Hyndiuk reported that a possible consequence of reduced corneal sensation was sterile neurotrophic corneal ulcers.[3]

Since these initial reports, many cases of reduction of corneal sensation have been noted. Although the amount of reduction seems to correlate with the extent of diabetic retinopathy,[12,53] it can occur in the absence of retinopathy. This decrease seems to be a part of the polyneuropathy of diabetes. The keratopathy resulting from reduced corneal sensation correlates directly with a decrease in the vibratory sense in the great toe. Other related factors may be age, type of diabetes, and duration of diabetes.[54] Of clinical significance, these changes are associated with problems of epithelial healing after vitrectomy[4,36] and with more problems involving contact lens wear.[55]

The tear film in diabetics is also abnormal. There is decreased tearing, and 23% of those with decreased tearing have decreased corneal sensation. In addition, glucose levels in the tears are elevated. A worsening of dry eye symptoms correlates with severity of diabetic retinopathy.[56] Abnormalities exist in the tear lipid layer, tear break-up time, tear quantity, and impression cytology.[57,58]

Diabetics are much more susceptible to damage to the epithelium and to epithelial healing problems. These problems were first noted with the advent of vitrectomy. Clouding of the corneal epithelium in diabetics during vitrectomy frequently requires scraping of the epithelium during surgery.[5] Postoperatively, there were significantly more healing problems in these diabetic patients, including slow healing of abrasions, superficial punctate keratitis, and recurrent epithelial erosions.[4–6]

Recent improvements in vitrectomy technique have eliminated many postoperative epithelial problems. In addition, some investigators question whether the problem is one of slow healing or rather of abnormal epithelial adhesion.[59,60] Morphologic findings that the epithelium comes off as a sheet and that there are abnormalities in adhesion complexes support the latter view. The role of the sorbitol pathway continues to be an issue, since by-products of this pathway are found in the epithelium scraped at the time of surgery, and healing has been promoted by treatment with aldose reductase inhibitors.[22]

The final abnormality in the epithelium is an increase in permeability. This is found more often after anesthetic use[61] and correlates with the severity of retinopathy.[62] The basis for this is unknown but is presumed to be secondary to either abnormal tight junctions or biochemical changes.

The fragility of the corneal epithelium is important when considering refractive surgery in diabetics. Complications involving the epithelium after LASIK occur in 47% of diabetics compared to 6.9% in controls. The overall refractive result tends not to be as good in diabetics.[63]

Although mean cell density is not different in diabetics compared to control groups,[64] there are indications of endothelial dysfunction. These findings are not unexpected, given the abnormal morphology of corneal endothelial cells in diabetes. The cornea is thicker than in disease-free, age-matched control groups.[50] This seems to correlate with retinopathy[45,65,66] but not with fasting blood sugar levels, laser therapy, duration of diabetes, or insulin dose.[47,49]

Changes in the endothelial cells vary after surgical stress. Although the numbers of cells are not reduced after vitrectomy in diabetics compared to others, the stroma remains swollen longer in diabetics.[66,67] Measurements of endothelial change show no difference in barrier function or cell density after cataract extraction,[68,69] in some studies but not in others.[70] Recovery of corneal edema after wearing a contact lens with a closed eye shows similar amounts of swelling in diabetics versus control groups, but recovery from the edema takes a longer period of time in diabetics.[14]

Parathyroid Disease

The parathyroid gland regulates calcium metabolism by causing release of calcium and phosphorus from bone, increasing resorption of calcium from the renal tubule, and increasing renal excretion of phosphorus. Disorders causing both hypoparathyroidism and hyperparathyroidism have been associated with anterior segment findings.

Hypoparathyroidism

Corneal findings are present in autoimmune polyendocrinopathy syndrome, type 1 (APS1). Two of these three features of Addison's disease, hypoparathyroidism or chronis mucocutaneous candidiasis, must be present to diagnose this recessive disorder. Mucocutaneous candidiasis has an average onset at age 5 years, hypoparathyroidism by age 9, and Addison's disease by age 14.[71] Other organs may fail, and patients may have chronic active hepatitis, pernicious anemia, autoimmune thyroid disease, insulin-dependent diabetes mellitus, vitiligo, gonadal failure, and alopecia. The male:female ratio is approximately 1:1.35. The disease is autosomal recessive and the responsible gene locus is 21q22.3.[72] A mutation at this locus results in malfunction of the autoimmune regulator gene (AIRE).[73]

Gass first described ocular findings in this syndrome in 1962. Many more cases have since been reported.[71,74] The incidence of eye findings is 25–50%, with the average age of onset being 5.75 years of age (range: 2–9 years). Patients present with blepharospasm and photophobia. Visual acuity is usually reduced. External eye findings consist of pseudoptosis, conjunctival injection, and superficial corneal vascularization, which is usually most prominent superiorly. Some patients have elevated nodular opacities similar to phlyctenules or anterior stromal scarring. Although the corneal disease may be self-limiting, some cases progress to significant corneal scarring. Shah et al. believe limbal stem cell deficiency is casuative and report successful vision rehabilitation with keratolimbal stem cell transplant.[75]

Hyperparathyroidism

Regulation of calcium levels depends on parathyroid hormone secretion, which is determined by serum calcium levels. A low serum calcium level promotes parathyroid hormone formation, whereas a high level suppresses it. Changes in the anterior segment can result from either primary or secondary hyperparathyroidism or other problems with increased calcium absorption. The site of calcium deposition seems to depend on the etiology of hypercalcemia.

Primary hyperparathyroidism usually results from benign tumors of the parathyroid gland. These patients may be symptomatic, with muscle weakness, gastrointestinal complaints, neuropathy, pseudogout, renal stones, bone pain, and fractures. The vast majority of patients have an elevated serum calcium level. Radiologic examination often shows signs of bone resorption.

Parathyroid hyperplasia and secondary hyperparathyroidism may occur in the presence of hypercalcemia and hypophosphatemia. The most common causes include milk alkali syndrome, sarcoidosis, and excessive intake of vitamin D. An additional mechanism is the hypocalcemia and hyperphosphatemia of chronic kidney disease. History, physical examination, and laboratory studies can usually identify these disorders.

Ocular findings in hypercalcemia vary and may be the earliest sign of the disorder.[76] Findings range from the microscopic evidence of calcium deposition only[77,78] to clinical symptoms of foreign body sensation.[77,79,80] Conjunctival changes are less uniform than corneal changes and include superficial crystalline deposits or whitish plaques (Fig. 64.1). The deposits are usually superficial to conjunctival blood vessels, and the conjunctiva may be tented over them.[81] Corneal changes are more specific than conjunctival findings. Descriptions of band keratopathy in the ophthalmic literature are similar despite the varying etiologies. The calcium deposits are within the interpalpebral area and are in the superficial cornea. They are grayish and start concentric with the 3 and 9 o'clock limbus. Calcification is generally denser in the peripheral cornea and often fades more centrally. The deeper corneal stroma is unaffected.

Calcific changes may also occur in the absence of hyperparathyroidism or increased serum calcium levels. These findings occur in patients with renal insufficiency and a calcium-phosphorus product of 70 or greater.[81,82] The conjunctival and corneal findings are as noted previously. In addition, some individuals with renal failure can develop conjunctival irritation, with red eyes and foreign body sensation. These symptoms are secondary to calcium crystals within the conjunctiva. Renal transplantation, but not

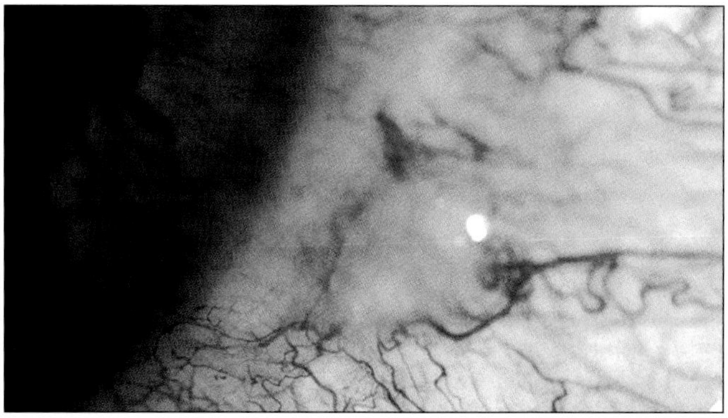

Fig. 64.1 Calcific plaque in the conjunctiva of a patient with renal insufficiency.

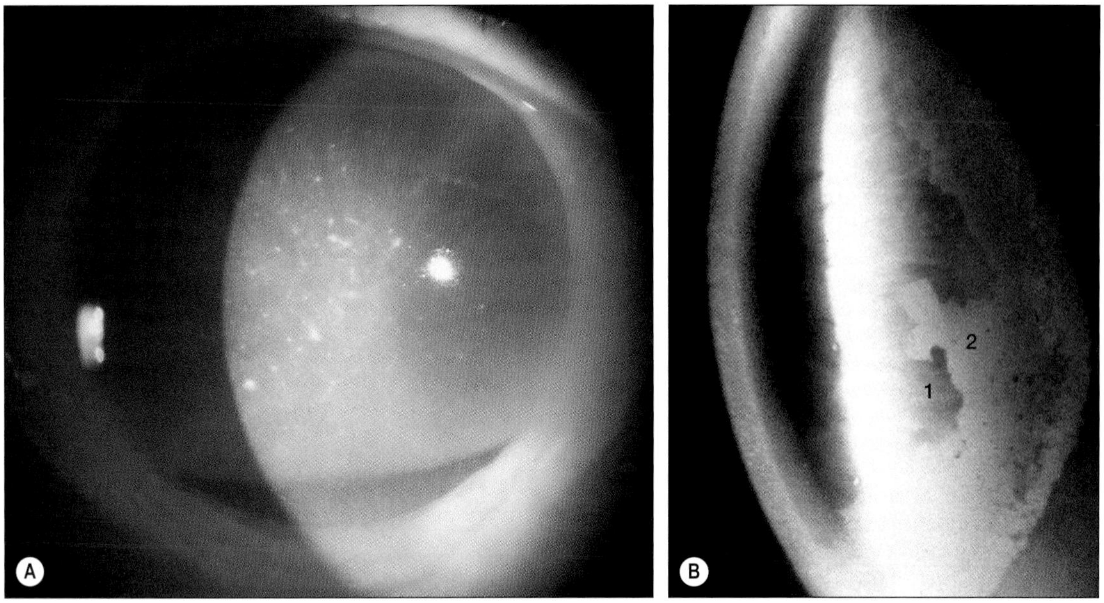

Fig. 64.2 (**A**) Band keratopathy before treatment with EDTA. (**B**) Band keratopathy after treatment with EDTA. The area where calcium has been chelated (*1*) is in sharp contrast to the periphery (*2*) where calcium was purposely allowed to remain.

necessarily dialysis, may reduce the conjunctival and corneal deposition.[71,80–83]

Microscopic evidence of calcium deposition differs, depending on the etiology of the calcium abnormality. Microscopic studies in primary or secondary hyperparathyroidism show positive stains for calcium in the conjunctival epithelium and substantia propria, cornea, anterior sclera, pigment epithelium and iris processes, ciliary muscle, and ciliary processes.[77] Calcium is particularly prominent in the basal cells of the corneal and conjunctival epithelium and is especially found within cell nuclei. It is also found within stromal keratocytes and the corneal endothelium. Bowman's and Descemet's membranes are usually calcium free.

Electron microscopy in these patients demonstrates intracellular deposits of needle-like crystals. The crystals are prominent in the basal cells of the corneal epithelium, and most are seen within cell nuclei. X-ray diffraction studies reveal the crystalline structure to be identical to hydroxyapatite.[77]

The histologic changes in calcium deposition secondary to renal failure differ from those of hyperparathyroidism. The calcium in these disorders is noted within the epithelial and subepithelial layers of the conjunctiva and cornea.[81,84] Unlike cases of hyperparathyroidism, the calcium can be deposited within Bowman's membrane. The calcium is found both intracellularly and extracellularly. Electron microscopy shows these deposits to be spherical or ovoid bodies with an electron-dense core and periphery.[77,78] They tend to form large aggregates and not smaller crystals.

It is not known why the calcium deposition in hyperparathyroidism differs from that in other disturbances of calcium metabolism. Berkow et al.[77] and Jensen[78] propose that the parathyroid hormone itself must have an effect on cell membranes. This is plausible, since parathyroid hormone does exert its regulatory effects by activation of membrane-bound adenylate cyclases, which in turn produce cyclic adenosine monophosphate.

The deposition of large aggregates of calcium hydroxyapatite in the interpalpebral areas seems to be secondary to local changes in pH. As carbon dioxide evaporates from the surface of the eye, the pH in the superficial tissues drops. This provides an ideal environment for the deposition of calcium phosphorus salts.

If calcium deposits interfere with vision or produce irritative symptoms, they can be removed with sodium ethylenediamine tetraacetic acid (EDTA) as described by Golan et al.[85] Local anesthetic is applied to the eye, and a solution of EDTA is dropped on the eye. Calcium can generally be removed either by rubbing it away using a cotton-tipped applicator soaked in EDTA or by gently scraping it away with a Beaver blade (Fig. 64.2).

Thyroid Disease

After diabetes mellitus, the most common endocrine disease encountered by the ophthalmologist is hyperthyroidism, especially Graves' disease. Eye findings in hyperthyroidism alone are usually minimal, while in Graves' disease, they may vary from minimal to vision threatening. As one might expect, the presentation of Graves' disease varies, and the diagnosis can be quite difficult.

Graves' disease is a specific form of hyperthyroidism that includes diffuse toxic goiter, ophthalmopathy, and infiltrative dermopathy. It is a disorder of immune regulation or of autoimmunity; this hypothesis is supported by the presence of circulating thyroid-stimulating antibodies and by the finding that ophthalmopathy often develops after patients have been rendered euthyroid. In addition, an occasional patient may be euthyroid when he or she first comes for treatment. Patients generally have symptoms of hyperthyroidism, including weight loss despite a good appetite, insomnia, nervousness, palpitations, and diarrhea. Women are affected more frequently than men, and the disease onset is usually in the fourth to fifth decades.

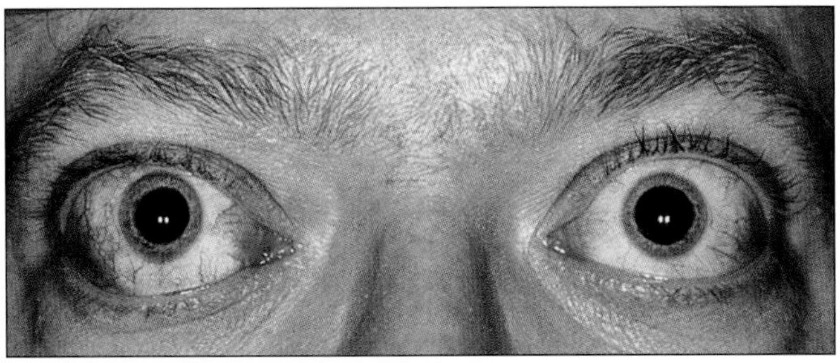

Fig. 64.3 Patient with lid retraction and proptosis secondary to Graves' disease.

Diagnosis can generally be confirmed by the finding of elevated total and free thyroxine (T4) levels.

Eye findings in Graves' disease are quite variable. In 1969, Werner suggested classifying thyroid eye disease, and the acronym 'NO SPECS' was introduced.[86] The 'NO' portion of the acronym refers to no problems or signs in the absence of symptoms, whereas the remaining portion of the acronym notes increasing tissue involvement. The NO SPECS designation does not imply that patients with Graves' disease progress from one symptom or sign to another. Many patients have only some findings and never develop others.

Anterior segment findings in Graves' disease result from many factors. Lid retraction is common and has been described in up to 92% of patients. Exophthalmos is also common and again has been reported in 34–94% of patients.[87] The combination of lid retraction and proptosis can lead to corneal exposure, which is the most commonly described anterior segment abnormality (Fig. 64.3). Patients with corneal exposure typically complain of grittiness, photophobia, and watering.[88] Patients have conjunctival injection and punctate keratopathy that usually appears inferiorly. Rose Bengal staining is often the first clinical sign associated with exposure.[89] Nocturnal lagophthalmos may be a particular problem, and patients should be observed during sleep. Inadequate treatment of corneal exposure can lead to corneal ulcers and compromise of vision.

Damage to the ocular surface does correlate with the extent of orbitopathy. Khalil et al.[90] found increased permeability of the corneal epithelium, even in the absence of corneal changes on slit lamp examination. There was a positive correlation between these increased permeability values and exophthalmos. In addition, tear osmolarity increases with increasing palpebral width.[88] Recent studies also suggest possible abnormalities in the composition of tears, especially elevations of tear protein levels, which may be related to infiltrative changes within the lacrimal gland.[91] All of these findings can be present in patients without clinical evidence of corneal exposure.

Treatment of corneal findings depends on the severity of the changes. Mild exposure can often be treated with lubricants, paying special attention to possible nocturnal lagophthalmos. More persistent changes may lead to the need for eyelid surgery, and this may include tarsorrhaphy and correction of eyelid retraction. Corneal exposure secondary to more malignant exophthalmos is usually also accompanied by optic nerve compromise, and various measures, including medication, radiation, or orbital decompression, are used to control the problem.

Multiple Endocrine Neoplasia

Multiple endocrine neoplasia refers to a group of familial disorders that consist of hyperplasia or malignant tumors of organs of neural crest origin. These syndromes are autosomal dominant and have a high penetrance with variable expressivity. Although classically described as multiple endocrine neoplasia 1 (MEN 1) and multiple endocrine neoplasia 2a and 2b (MEN 2a and MEN 2b), the latter two are now recognized as separate clinical entities with different, though linked, genetic lesions on chromosome 10.[92]

MEN 1, or Werner's syndrome, involves changes in the pituitary gland, the parathyroid glands, and the islet cells of the pancreas. The genetic abnormality has been localized to a small area of chromosome 11.[93] The major ophthalmologic manifestations are visual field defects caused by pituitary gland tumors.

MEN 2a, or Sipples' syndrome, is a familial disorder consisting of medullary carcinoma of the thyroid, pheochromocytoma, and parathyroid adenomas. The disease entity is autosomal dominant and has been localized to chromosome 10.[94]

MEN 2b (or MEN 3) is often referred to as multiple mucosal neuroma syndrome.[95] The notable characteristics of this syndrome are medullary carcinoma of the thyroid, pheochromocytoma, mucosal neuromas, and intestinal neurogangliomas. MEN 2b is also autosomal dominant, localized to chromosome 10, and is caused by a defect in the RET (rearranged during transfection) proto-oncogene.[96] The genetic lesions causing MEN 2a and MEN 2b are distinct, and there is no allelism of the genes.[92]

The diagnosis of MEN 2a or 2b depends on family history. Although sporadic forms of these problems may exist, they are usually autosomal dominant[96] and also involve the RET proto-oncogene. Ninety-five percent of MEN 2b cases are caused by a single point mutation with a substitution of threonine for methionine at codon 918.[96,97] Laboratory investigations are usually directed at the detection of elevated calcitonin levels, a sign of medullary carcinoma of the thyroid, and vanillylmandelic acid levels, which indicate the presence of pheochromocytoma. If elevated calcitonin level is not noted in individuals suspected to have this disorder, provocative testing with an infusion of calcium, glucagon, or pentagastrin can sometimes increase the diagnostic yield.

Ocular manifestations of MEN are classically described only in MEN 2b. The major finding is prominence of the corneal nerves in a clear corneal stroma.[98,99] Prominent nerves are thought to be present in all cases, and it is therefore an important early diagnostic sign (Fig. 64.4). When corneal nerves are present in other conditions, they are usually less prominent (Box 64.1). These other disease entities can usually be ruled out on the basis of clinical signs.[100]

Additional ocular findings in MEN 2b include conjunctival neuroma (87%), eyelid neuroma (80%), dry eye (67%), and prominent perilimbal blood vessels (40%).[98,99] Less frequent findings are prominent eyebrows, impaired pupillary dilation, ectopic lacrimal punctum, and thick iris nerves.

The ocular pathology of MEN 2b has been well described.[99] The thickened conjunctival nerves contain numerous Schwann cells and partially myelinated axons. Conjunctival neuromas consist of discrete masses composed of Schwann

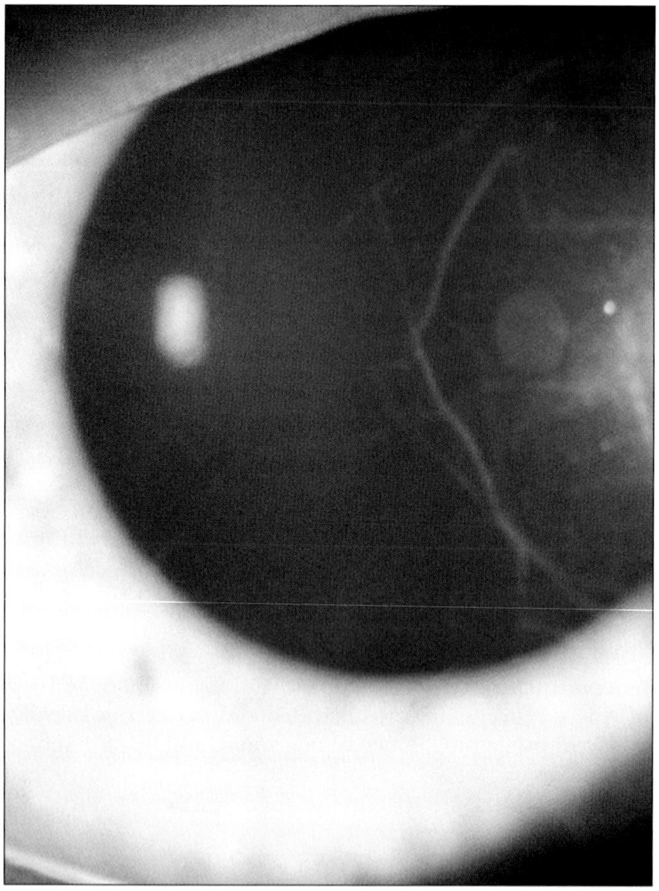

Fig. 64.4 Prominent corneal nerves in a patient with MEN 2b.

Box 64.1 Conditions with increased visibility of corneal nerves

Fuchs' dystrophy
Keratoconus
Ichthyosis
Posterior polymorphous dystrophy
Leprosy
Refsum's syndrome
Neurofibromatosis
MEN 2a
MEN 2b

From Mensher JH. Surv Ophthalmol *19:1; 1974. Copyright Elsevier 1974.*

cells and poorly myelinated axons. Corneal nerves consist of Schwann cells and unmyelinated nerve fibers. Finally, prominent nerves with a mixture of myelinated and unmyelinated fibers were found in the ciliary body, iris, anterior ciliary muscle, and uveal meshwork.

The pathophysiology of the prominent nerves in these syndromes is not well understood. Only affected family members have prominent corneal nerves. Kinoshita et al. speculate that the abnormal nerves appear during corneal development.[94] This idea is supported by the fact that MEN 2a and 2b is thought to originate as a genetic defect leading to abnormalities in organs of neural crest origin.

References

1. Armaly MF, Baloglou PJ. Diabetes mellitus and the eye I. Changes in the anterior segment. *Arch Ophthalmol.* 1967;77:485.
2. Schwartz DE. Corneal sensitivity in diabetes. *Arch Ophthalmol.* 1974;91:174.
3. Hyndiuk RA, et al. Neurotrophic corneal ulcers in diabetes mellitus. *Arch Ophthalmol.* 1977;95:2193.
4. Foulks JN, et al. Factors related to corneal epithelial complications after closed vitrectomy in diabetics. *Arch Ophthalmol.* 1979;97:1076.
5. Brightbill FS, Myers FL, Bresnick JH. Post vitrectomy keratopathy. *Am J Ophthalmol.* 1978;85:651.
6. Perry HD, et al. Corneal complications after closed vitrectomy through the pars plana. *Arch Ophthalmol.* 1978;96:1401.
7. Saghizadeh M, et al. Overexpression of matrix metalloproteinase-10 and matrix metallproteinase-3 in human diabetic corneas. *Am J Pathol.* 2001;158(2):723.
8. Ljubimov A, et al. Human corneal epithelial basement membrane and integrin alterations in diabetics and diabetic retinopathy. *J Histochem Cytochem.* 1998;46:1033.
9. Wakuta M, et al. Delayed wound closure and phenotypic changes in corneal epithelium of the spontaneously diabetic Goto-Kakizaki rat. *Inv Ophthalmol Vis Sci.* 2007;48:590.
10. Chikami T,Wakuta M, Liu Y, Nishada T. Deviated mechanisms of wound healing in diabetic corneas. *Cornea.* 2007;26(9 Suppl 1):575–581.
11. Kern TS, Engerman RL. Distribution of aldose reductase in ocular tissues. *Exp Eye Res.* 1981;33:175.
12. Friend J, et al. Insulin insensitivity and sorbitol production of the normal rabbit corneal epithelium in vitro. *Invest Ophthalmol Vis Sci.* 1980;19:913.
13. Friend J, Kiorpes TC, Thoft RA. Diabetes mellitus and the rabbit corneal epithelium. *Invest Ophthalmol Vis Sci.* 1981;21:317.
14. Ludvigson MJ, Sorenson RL. Immunohistochemical localization on aldolase reductase II. Rat eye and kidney. *Diabetes.* 1980;29:450.
15. Kinoshita JH, et al. Aldose reductase and diabetic complications of the eye. *Metabolism.* 1979;28:462.
16. Fukushi S, et al. Reepithelization of denuded corneas in diabetic rats. *Exp Eye Res.* 1980;31:611.
17. Matsuda M, et al. The effects of aldose reductase inhibitor on the corneal endothelial morphology in diabetic rats. *Curr Eye Res.* 1987;6:391.
18. Meyer LA, Ubels JL, Edelhauser HF. Corneal endothelial morphology in the rat. *Invest Ophthalmol Vis Sci.* 1988;29:940.
19. Friend J, Ishii Y, Thoft RA. Corneal epithelial changes in diabetic rats. *Ophthalmol Res.* 1982;14:269.
20. Takahashi H, et al. Matrix metalloproteinase activity is enhanced during corneal wound repair in high glucose conditions. *Curr Eye Res.* 2000; 21(2):608.
21. Akagi Y, et al. Localization of aldose reductase in the human eye. *Diabetes.* 1984;33:562.
22. Ohasi Y, et al. Aldose reductase inhibitor (CT112) eye drops for diabetic corneal epitheliopathy. *Am J Ophthalmol.* 1988;105:233.
23. Nakahara M, et al. A randomised, placebo controlled clinical trial of the aldose reductase inhibitor CT-112 as management of corneal epithelial disorders in diabetic patients. *Br J Ophthalmol.* 2005;89:254.
24. Rubinstein MP, Parrish ST, Vernona SA. Corneal epithelial oxygen uptake rate in diabetes mellitus. *Eye.* 1990;4:757.
25. Larsen HW, Rerner AU. Immunohistochemical studies on human diabetic and nondiabetic eyes II. Autoradiography I^{125}-labeled insulin, and application of histochemical procedures. *Acta Ophthalmol.* 1969;47:956.
26. Kaji Y, et al. Advanced glycation end products in diabetic corneas. *Inves Ophthalmol Vis Sci.* 2000;41:362.
27. Ljubimov A, et al. Human corneal epithelial basement membrane and integrin alterations in diabetics and diabetic retinopathy. *J Histochem Cytochem.* 1998;46:1033.
28. Lyubimov A, et al. Basement membrane abnormalities in human eyes with diabetic retinopathy. *J Histochem Cytochem.* 1996;44(12):1468.
29. Azar DT. Altered epithelial basement membrane interactions in diabetic corneas. *Arch Ophthalmol.* 1992;110:537.
30. Ishii Y, Lahav M, Mukai Y. Corneal changes in diabetic patients and streptozotocin diabetic rats: an ultrastructural correlation. *Invest Ophthalmol Vis Sci.* 1981;20(Suppl):154.
31. Yao GN. Diabetic keratopathy. *Indian J Ophthalmol.* 1987;35:16.
32. Azar TA, Gipson IK. Repair of corneal epithelial adhesion structures following keratectomy wounds in diabetic rabbits. *Acta Ophthalmol.* 1989;67(Suppl):72.

33. Hatchell DL, et al. Damage to the epithelial basement membrane in the corneas of diabetic rabbits. *Arch Ophthalmol*. 1983;101:469.
34. Herse PR. Corneal hydration control in normal and alloxan-induced diabetic rabbits. *Invest Ophthalmol Vis Sci*. 1990;31:2205.
35. Yee RW, et al. Corneal endothelial changes in diabetic dogs. *Curr Eye Res*. 1985;4:759.
36. Tababy CA, et al. Reduced number of hemidesmosomes in the corneal epithelium of diabetics with proliferative vitreoretinopathy. *Graefes Arch Clin Exp Ophthalmol*. 1988;226:389.
37. Azar DT, et al. Decreased penetration of anchoring fibrils into the diabetic stroma. *Arch Ophthalmol*. 1989;107:1520.
38. Taylor HR, Kimsey RA. Corneal epithelial basement membrane changes in diabetes. *Invest Ophthalmol Vis Sci*. 1981;20:548.
39. Kenyon K, et al. Corneal basement membrane abnormality in diabetes mellitus. *Invest Ophthalmol Vis Sci*. 1978;17(Suppl):245.
40. Tsubota K, Chiba K, Shimaszaki J. Corneal epithelium in diabetic patients. *Cornea*. 1991;10:156.
41. Kern P, Regnault F, Robert L. Biochemical and ultrastructural study of human diabetic conjunctiva. *Biomedicine*. 1976;24:32.
42. Keoleian JM, et al. Structural and functional studies of the corneal endothelium and diabetes mellitus. *Am J Ophthalmol*. 1992;113:64.
43. Schultz RO, et al. Corneal endothelial changes in type I, type II diabetes mellitus. *Am J Ophthalmol*. 1984;98:401.
44. Busted N, Olsen T, Schmitz O. Clinical observations on the corneal thickness and the corneal endothelium in diabetes mellitus. *Br J Ophthalmol*. 1981;65:687.
45. Matsuda M, et al. Relationship of corneal endothelial morphology to diabetic retinopathy, duration of diabetes and glycemic control. *Jpn J Ophthalmol*. 1990;34:53.
46. Itoi M, et al. Specular microscopic studies of the corneal endothelia of Japanese diabetics. *Cornea*. 1989;8:2.
47. Olsen T, Busted N. Corneal thickness in eyes with diabetic and nondiabetic neovascularization. *Br J Ophthalmol*. 1981;65:691.
48. Lee JS, Oum BS, Choie HY, et al. Differences in corneal thickness and corneal endothelium related to duration in diabetes. *Eye*. 2006;20:315–318.
49. Pierro L, Brancato R, Zaganelli E. Correlation of corneal thickness with blood glucose control in diabetes mellitus. *Acta Ophthalmol*. 1993;71:169.
50. Olsen T, Busted N, Schmitz O. Corneal thickeness in diabetes mellitus. *Lancet*. 1980;1:883.
51. Stolwijk T, et al. Corneal autofluorescence in diabetic and penetrating keratoplasty patients as measured by fluorophotometry. *Exp Eye Res*. 1990;51:403.
52. McNamara N, et al. Corneal function during normal and high serum glucose levels in diabetics. *Invest Ophthalmol Vis Sci*. 1998;39:3.
53. Rogell JD. Corneal hypesthesia and retinopathy in diabetes mellitus. *Ophthalmology*. 1980;87:229.
54. Schultz RO, et al. Diabetic keratopathy as a manifestation of peripheral neuropathy. *Am J Ophthalmol*. 1983;96:368.
55. Schultz RO, et al. Diabetic keratopathy. *Trans Am Ophthalmol Soc*. 1981;74:108.
56. Nepp J, et al. Is there a correlation between the severity of diabetic retinopathy and keratoconjunctivitis sicca? *Cornea*. 2000;19(14):487.
57. Inoue K, et al. Ocular and systemic factors relevant to diabetic keratopathy. *Cornea*. 2001;20:798.
58. Dogru M, et al. Tear function and ocular surface changes in noninsulin dependent diabetes mellitus. *Ophthalmology*. 2001;108:586.
59. Snip RC, Thoft RA, Tolentino FI. Similar epithelial healing rates of the corneas of diabetic and nondiabetic patients. *Am J Ophthalmol*. 1980;90:463.
60. Snip RC, Thoft RA, Tolentino FI. Epithelial healing rates of the normal and diabetic human cornea. *Invest Ophthalmol Vis Sci*. 1979;18(Suppl):73.
61. Stolwijk TR, et al. Corneal epithelial barrier function after oxybuprocaine provocation in diabetes. *Invest Ophthalmol Vis Sci*. 1990;31:436.
62. Gobbels M, Spitznas M, Oldendoerp J. Impairment of corneal epithelial barrier function in diabetes. *Graefes Arch Clin Exp Ophthalmol*. 1989;227:142.
63. Fraunfelder F, Rich LF. Laser assisted in situ keratomileusis complications in diabetes mellitus. *Cornea*. 2002;21(3):246.
64. Shetlar GJ, Bourne WM, Campbell RJ. Morphological evaluation of Descemet's membrane and corneal endothelium in diabetes mellitus. *Ophthalmology*. 1989;96:247.
65. Aaberg TM. Correlation between corneal endothelial morphology and function. *Am J Ophthalmol*. 1984;98:510.
66. Friberg TR, Doran DL, Lazenby FL. The effect of vitreous and retinal surgery on corneal endothelial density. *Ophthalmology*. 1984;91:1166.
67. Diddie KR, Schanzlin DJ. Specular microscopy in pars plana vitrectomy. *Arch Ophthalmol*. 1983;101:408.
68. Furuse N, et al. Corneal endothelial changes after posterior chamber intraocular lens implantation in patients with or without diabetes mellitus. *Br J Ophthalmol*. 1990;74:258.
69. Gobbels M, Spitznas M. Endothelial barrier function after phacoemulsification: a comparison between diabetic and nondiabetic patients. *Graefes Arch Clin Exp Ophthalmol*. 1991;229:254.
70. Moridubo S, et al. Corneal changes after small incision cataract srugery in patients with diabetes mellitus. *Arch Ophthalmol*. 2004;122:966.
71. Wagman RD. Keratitis associated with multiple endocrine deficiency, autoimmune disease and candidiasis syndrome. *Am J Ophthalmol*. 1987;103:569.
72. Aaltonen J, et al. An autosomal locus causing autoimmune disease: autoimmune polyglandular disease type 1 assigned to chromosome 21. *Nat Genet*. 1994;8:83.
73. Pearce SHS, et al. A common and recurrent 13-bp deletion in the autoimmucne regulator gene in British kindreds with autoimmune polyendocrinopathy type 1. *Am J Hum Genet*. 1998;63:1675.
74. Traboulsi EI, et al. Ocular findings in the candidiasis-endocrinopathy syndrome. *Am J Ophthalmol*. 1985;99:486.
75. Shah M, Holland E, Chan C. Resolution of autoimmune polyglandular syndrome-keratopathy with keratolimabl stem cell transplantation. *Cornea*. 2007;26(5):632.
76. Porter R, Crombi AL. Corneal calcification as a presenting and diagnostic sign in hyperparathyroidism. *Br J Ophthalmol*. 1973;57:665.
77. Berkow JW, Fine BS, Zimmerman LE. Unusual ocular calcification in hyperparathyroidism. *Am J Ophthalmol*. 1968;66:812.
78. Jensen OA. Ocular calcification in primary hyperparathyroidism. *Acta Ophthalmol*. 1975;53:173.
79. Cogan DG, Albright F, Bartter FC. Hypercalcemia and band keratopathy. *Arch Ophthalmol*. 1948;40:624.
80. Porter R, Crombi AL. Corneal and conjunctival calcification in chronic renal failure. *Br J Ophthalmol*. 1973;57:339.
81. Berlyne GM. Microcrystalline conjunctival calcification in renal failure. *Lancet*. 1968;2:366.
82. Hareis LS, et al. Conjunctival and corneal calcific deposits in uremic patients. *Am J Ophthalmol*. 1971;72:130.
83. Caldeira JAF, Sabbaga E, Ianhez LE. Conjunctival and corneal changes in renal failure. *Br J Ophthalmol*. 1970;54:399.
84. Demco TA, McCormick AQ, Richards JSF. Conjunctival and corneal changes in chronic failure. *Can J Ophthalmol*. 1974;9:208.
85. Golan A, et al. Band keratopathy due to hyperparathyroidism. *Ophthalmologica*. 1975;171:119.
86. Werner SC. Classification of the eye changes of Graves' disease. *J Clin Endocrinol Metab*. 1969;29:982.
87. Duke-Elder S. *System of ophthalmology*. Vol 13. St. Louis: Mosby; 1974.
88. Gilbard JP, Farris RL. Ocular surface drying and tear film osmolarity in thyroid eye disease. *Acta Ophthalmol*. 1983;61:108.
89. Foster CS, Yee M. Corneal scleral manifestations of Graves' disease, the acquired connective tissue disorders and systemic vasculitis. *Int Ophthalmol Clin*. 1983;23:131.
90. Khalil HA, van Best JA, de Keizer RJ. The permeability of the corneal epithelium of Graves' ophthalmopathy as determined by fluorophotometry. *Doc Ophthalmol*. 1990;73:249.
91. Khalil HA, de Keizer RJW, Kiglstra A. Analysis of tear proteins in Graves' ophthalmopathy by high performance liquid chromatography. *Am J Ophthalmol*. 1988;106:186.
92. Jackson CE, et al. Update on linkage of the multiple endocrine neoplasia Type IIB gene (MEN 2b) to chromosome 10 markers linked to MEN 2a. *Am J Hum Genet*. 1990;47(Suppl):A10.
93. Nakamura Y, et al. Localization of the genetic defect in multiple endocrine neoplasia type I within a small region of chromosome 11. *Am J Hum Genet*. 1989;44:751.
94. Kinoshita S, et al. Incidence of prominent corneal nerves in multiple endocrine neoplasia type IIA. *Am J Ophthalmol*. 1991;111:307.
95. Schimke RN, et al. Syndrome of bilateral pheochromocytoma, medullary thyroid carcinoma and multiple neuromas. *N Engl J Med*. 1968;279:1.
96. Lee NC, Norton JC. Multiple endocrine neoplasia type 2B – genetic basis and clinical expression. *Surg Oncol*. 2000;9:111.
97. Jacobs JM, Hawes MJ. From eyelid bumps to thyroid lumps: report of a MEN type IIb family and review of literature. *Ophthal Plast Reconstr Surg*. 2001;17(3):195.
98. Robertson DM, Sizemore JW, Gordon H. Thickened corneal nerves as a manifestation of multiple endocrine neoplasia. *Trans Am Acad Ophthalmol Otolaryngol*. 1975;79:OP772.
99. Spector B, Clintworth JK, Wells SA Jr. Histologic study of the ocular lesions in multiple endocrine neoplasia syndrome type IIb. *Am J Ophthalmol*. 1981;91:204.
100. Mensher JH. Corneal nerves. *Surv Ophthalmol*. 1974;19:1.

Chapter 65

Dermatologic Disorders and the Cornea

Alan E. Sadowsky

Dermatologic disorders often have manifestations involving the eyelids, conjunctiva, and cornea. Inflammatory and papulosquamous, immunobullous, genetic, and miscellaneous disorders are presented with attention to skin and ocular findings, histopathology, inheritance, etiology, and treatment.

Inflammatory and Papulosquamous Disorders

Psoriasis

Psoriasis is a common, chronic, recurrent, inflammatory disease characterized by well-demarcated, erythematous plaques covered by dry, silvery white scales.

Psoriasis occurs with equal frequency in both sexes[1] and affects 1–2% of the population.[2] Age of onset can range from infancy to the seventies, with a mean age of 27 years.[1] Histopathologically, epidermal hyperplasia with atrophy over the dermal papillae, parakeratosis, and inflammatory cell infiltrates are seen.[3] Accelerated epidermopoiesis is the hallmark event in psoriasis. Although various immunologic abnormalities have been described, the specific biochemical cause responsible for the high turnover rate remains unknown.[4] One-third of patients report a relative with the disease.[1] The genetic inheritance is presumed to be multifactorial. Psoriasis is associated with a number of different HLA haplotypes, especially -Cw6, -B57, -DR7, and -Cw2.[2]

Typical lesions of psoriasis vulgaris occur on the scalp, nails, knees, shins, elbows, and gluteal cleft and usually are symmetric. The course of the disease fluctuates, with a tendency to recur and persist. Removal of the psoriatic scale results in pinpoint bleeding sites (Auspitz sign). Lesions can occur at the site of mechanical trauma (Koebner phenomenon). Involvement may vary from mild to severe generalized disease. Spontaneous remission can occur. Stress,[5] acute streptococcal infections,[6] drugs,[7] and human immunodeficiency virus (HIV) infection[8] have been implicated in inducing or exacerbating the disease.

Ocular signs occur in up to 10% of patients with psoriasis.[9] The periorbital skin, eyebrow, and eyelid can show typical scaly lesions (Fig. 65.1). Blepharitis characterized by scaling, edema, erythema, trichiasis, or madarosis may be present. Ectropion, usually cicatricial, can occur. Conjunctivitis may result from the lid scales or from primary involvement of the conjunctiva with whitish-yellow plaque lesions. Corneal changes are less common and include peripheral infiltrates and vascularization, punctate epithelial keratopathy, erosions, superficial or deep opacities (Fig. 65.2), and chronic ulceration and melting.[10] Iritis occurs most often in the 6% of patients with psoriatic arthritis and may be clinically distinct from other types of anterior uveitis.[11] Contrary to previous thinking, cataract risk is not increased in patients undergoing PUVA (psoralen photochemotherapy) who use eye protection.[12]

Treatment of skin lesions includes both topical and systemic modalities. Topical therapy includes skin hydration, glucocorticoids, tar preparations, anthralin, tazarotene, and exposure to midrange ultraviolet radiation. Systemic therapies include oral retinoids, PUVA treatments, and, in severe psoriasis, methotrexate, ciclosporin,[13] or bioimmunomodulators.[14]

Ocular therapy is directed to the involved site. Artificial tears and lubricating ointments for keratitis sicca, hygiene for blepharitis, topical corticosteroid drops for conjunctivitis and iritis, cycloplegics and oral prednisone for severe iritis, and surgical repair of symptomatic ectropion. Biologic agents may prove beneficial.[15]

Seborrheic dermatitis

Seborrheic dermatitis is a common, chronic, superficial inflammatory disorder characterized by oily scales and plaques on an erythematous base. The disease affects 2–5% of the population.[16] It is localized to sites containing large numbers of sebaceous glands, including the scalp, eyebrows, eyelids, glabella, nasolabial folds, retroauricular skin, external ear canal, chest, and back. An infantile form occurs that is generally self-limiting. The etiology is unknown, but hypersecretion of sebum may not actually be involved.[17] A pathogenic role for *Pityrosporum* species has been postulated.[16] Seborrheic blepharitis is very common in this disease and may be associated with a keratoconjunctivitis.

Treatment of the dermatitis includes shampoos containing tar, zinc pyrithione or ketoconazole, topical corticosteroids, topical antifungal agents, and topical calcineurin inhibitors. Blepharitis is controlled with eyelid hygiene, intermittent topical antibiotic–steroid preparations, and ocular lubricants.

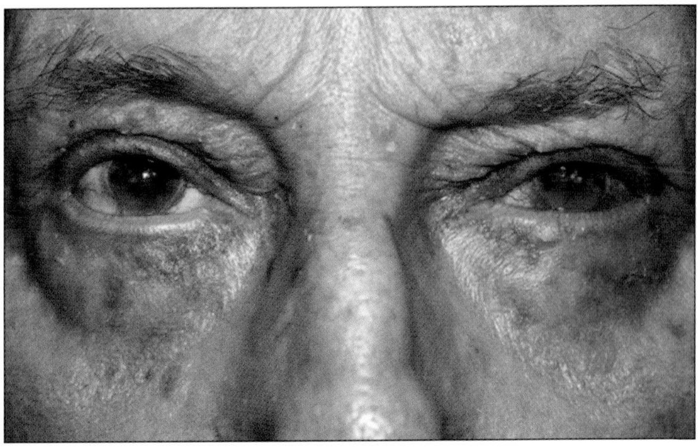

Fig. 65.1 Psoriasis: skin and eyelid involvement.

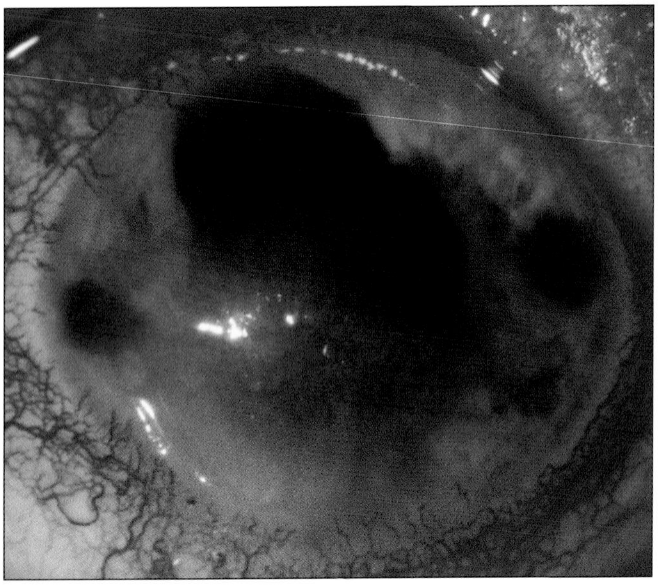

Fig. 65.2 Psoriasis: corneal scar.

Exfoliative dermatitis (erythroderma)

Exfoliative dermatitis refers to a universal or very extensive scaling and itching erythroderma, often associated with loss of hair.[3] Etiologies include various chronic dermatoses (e.g. psoriasis), drug reactions, and underlying malignancies. Fifty percent of cases may be idiopathic. Conjunctival irritation can occur from desquamated scales, and cicatricial ectropion caused by chronic lower eyelid inflammation can occur.[18]

Rosacea

Rosacea is a common, chronic inflammatory eruption of the flush areas (forehead, nose, cheeks) of the face. It occurs mostly in middle-aged and older individuals and is more common in women than men.[3] Ten percent of the population may demonstrate the disease.[19] Rosacea is often overlooked as an important cause of ocular disease.

The facial skin lesions are characterized by erythema, papules, pustules, and telangiectasia. In contrast to acne vulgaris, comedones are rare in rosacea. The onset is often subtle and generally becomes more severe with time. Although disease activity can wax and wane, spontaneous remission is rare. Patients with advanced rosacea, especially males, may develop rhinophyma. This process involves hypertrophy and hyperemia of the distal nose (Fig. 65.3).

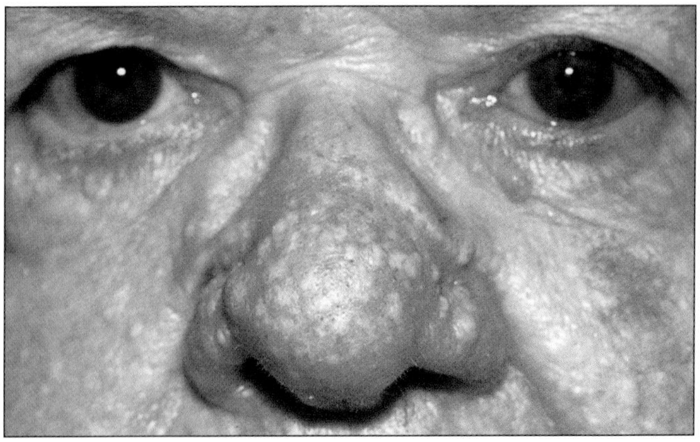

Fig. 65.3 Rosacea: rhinophyma.

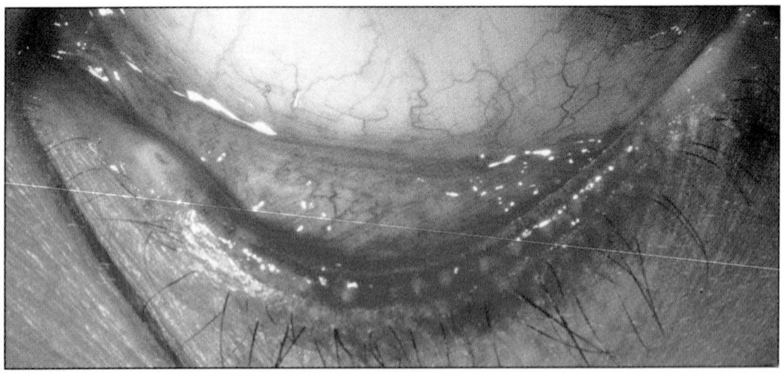

Fig. 65.4 Rosacea: posterior lid inflammation.

Ocular manifestations occur in about 50% of patients with rosacea at some point in the course of their disease.[20] Symptoms of ocular rosacea include burning, photophobia, and foreign body sensation. The lids, conjunctiva, cornea, and episclera may be involved. Blepharitis and meibomian dysfunction are the most common associated findings (Fig. 65.4). The lid margins are hyperemic, thickened, and telangiectatic. The meibomian glands secrete excess sebum, and the orifices may be inspissated and inflamed. Chalazia and hordeola are common,[21] and in some patients staphylococcal lid infections can be demonstrated. Eyelid lymphedema has also been reported.[22]

Chronic, diffuse conjunctival injection may occur, with vascular dilation and edema most prominently seen in the interpalpebral area. Less often, small, gray, vascularized nodules that resemble phlyctenules arise on the interpalpebral limbal conjunctiva.

Corneal involvement is seen in approximately 5–30% of cutaneous rosacea patients.[23,24] A superficial punctate keratopathy is common with meibomianitis or blepharitis. A marginal vascular infiltration (Fig. 65.5) can occur with vessels extending into grayish-white peripheral corneal tissue. As the keratitis progresses, subepithelial infiltrates

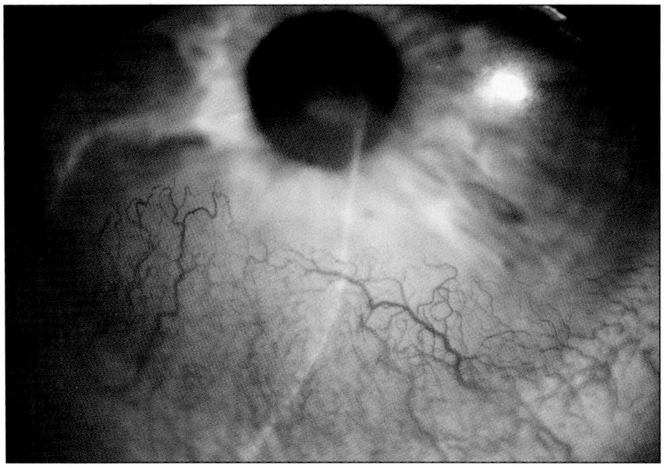

Fig. 65.5 Rosacea: keratitis.

may form at the leading edge of a leash of vessels. These lesions are more common inferiorly but can advance toward the central cornea. Ulceration and, rarely, perforation can occur. Chronic rosacea keratitis results in broad areas of pannus, usually inferior, 'spade-shaped' peripheral scars, and stromal thinning.

Nodular episcleritis,[25] keratitis sicca,[26] pseudokeratoconus,[24] dendritic keratopathy,[27] cicatrizing conjunctivitis,[28] and bilateral herpetic keratitis[29] have also been described with ocular rosacea.

Skin findings usually precede the eye findings, but on occasion the eye may be involved first. Although ocular involvement is usually bilateral, patients may have a unilateral red eye. The skin changes may be subtle and can be masked by facial make-up.

Histopathologic changes in the skin involve disorganization of the upper dermis with vasodilation, edema, solar elastosis, and a nonspecific nongranulomatous inflammatory infiltrate. With rhinophyma, there is epidermal epithelial hyperplasia and sebaceous gland hyperplasia with fibrosis, inflammation, and telangiectasia.[3] Ocular pathologic findings include conjunctival and corneal infiltration with chronic inflammatory cells, including lymphocytes, epithelioid cells, plasma cells, and giant cells.[30]

The etiology of rosacea is unknown. Vasomotor lability is easily induced and appears to be aggravated by coffee, tea, other hot beverages and foods, alcohol, spicy foods, endocrine abnormalities, menopause, and anxiety. The demonstration of the mite *Demodex folliculorum* in the facial lesions of rosacea has implied a pathogenic role, although the significance of this is not known. An immunopathologic study of conjunctival inflammation suggested a type IV hypersensitivity reaction.[31] Recent studies show conjunctival epithelium-derived protease activity, especially matrix metalloproteinases, is elevated in ocular rosacea patients. Doxycycline has been demonstrated to reduce the levels and activity of this inflammatory marker in tears.[32]

Treatment of rosacea begins with avoidance of food, beverages, and environments that exacerbate flushing. Both cutaneous and ocular rosacea respond well to oral tetracycline, doxycycline,[33,34] or azithromycin. Because antibiotic therapy is suppressive rather than curative, many patients require daily maintenance indefinitely. The mechanism of action of tetracycline is unknown, but it may affect the secretion of sebum or influence the interaction of the sebaceous glands with bacteria. Patients resistant to tetracycline may respond to low-dose isotretinoin but caution must be used as this can worsen the ocular disease.

Topical metronidazole cream and gel are beneficial remission-maintaining agents for cutaneous rosacea.[19] Low-potency topical corticosteroids also may be of benefit.

Although ocular manifestations usually respond well to antibiotic therapy, additional measures may be beneficial. Frequent preservative-free artificial tears help in patients with dryness. Eyelid hygiene and antibiotic ointment may help control blepharitis. Topical corticosteroids may be useful for conjunctivitis and keratitis. If corneal ulceration is present, scrapings for smears and cultures to rule out microbial involvement must be performed. Corticosteroids must be used judiciously, as some patients may be susceptible to corneal melt and perforation. Small perforations may be treated with cyanoacrylate adhesive and contact lens or by lamellar keratoplasty. Large corneal perforations or extensive scarring and vascularization may require amniotic membrane transplantation,[35] conjunctival advancement pedicles,[36] or penetrating keratoplasty.

Contact dermatitis

Contact dermatitis is an inflammatory disorder that frequently involves the thin skin of the eyelids. The inflammation may result from an allergic hypersensitivity response or from direct irritation of the skin by an offending topical agent. Acutely, the eyelids are erythematous, edematous, and may show scaling and crusting. When the disorder is chronic, lichenification and hyperpigmentation are seen. Chemosis, papillary conjunctivitis, and punctate keratopathy can occur. A careful history is essential in attempting to identify a cause. Cosmetics, ocular medications, and agents transferred from the hands to the eyelids are frequently implicated. Removal of the offending agent and judicious use of topical corticosteroids are beneficial.

Atopic dermatitis

Atopic dermatitis (see Ch. 49) is a common, chronic, pruritic, erythematous, inflammatory disorder associated with various ocular manifestations.

Pityriasis rubra pilaris

Pityriasis rubra pilaris is a rare, chronic dermatosis characterized by small follicular papules, disseminated yellowish-pink scaling patches, and palmoplantar hyperkeratosis.[3] There are distinctive islands of normal skin within affected areas. Various childhood and adult forms have been described. There is no gender predilection. The disease may be autosomal dominant in transmission or sporadic. The etiology is unknown.

Skin lesions involving the eyelid can produce ectropion.[37] Thickening of the bulbar conjunctiva, keratinization of the conjunctiva and cornea, corneal epithelial erosions, pannus, and interstitial keratitis can occur.[38]

Isotretinoin alone or in combination with methotrexate is the treatment of choice.

Impetigo

Impetigo is a superficial skin infection caused by streptococcus species or *Staphylococcus aureus* characterized by vesicles that become pustular, rupture, and form a golden crust. The disease occurs most frequently in early childhood and usually involves the face, hands, and neck. Ocular involvement is usually secondary to periocular skin involvement. Blepharitis, conjunctivitis, and keratitis have been described.[39] Systemic antibiotics are generally the most effective treatment.

Immunobullous Disorders

Pemphigus

Pemphigus vulgaris

Pemphigus is a group of clinical syndromes characterized by intraepithelial bullae of the skin or mucous membranes. Pemphigus vulgaris (PV) is the most common form of pemphigus in North America and usually occurs in the fifth and sixth decades.[40] It occurs in all ethnic groups, with equal frequency in men and women. The primary lesions are thin-walled, flaccid, easily ruptured bullae on normal skin or mucosa or on an erythematous base. The bullae may rupture spontaneously, forming erosions, or extend with pressure on rubbing (Nicolsky's sign). The denuded areas become crusted and heal slowly; scarring does not occur. The groin, scalp, neck, face, and axillae may be involved. Oral lesions are the presenting sign in the majority of cases, and mucous membrane involvement often predominates.

Active eyelid cutaneous involvement can occur in PV, and medial lid margin erosions have been described.[41] A mucus-producing conjunctivitis is not uncommon, but conjunctival bullae and erosions are rare.[42] Conjunctival scarring does not occur, and corneal involvement is uncommon but keratolysis has been reported.[43] Ocular manifestations may be underdiagnosed, may not correlate with disease severity, and may persist chronically.[44]

Characteristic skin histopathologic changes consist of acantholysis, intraepidermal cleft and blister formation just above the basal cell layer, and the presence of acantholytic cells lining the bullae. A subepithelial inflammatory infiltrate of plasma cells and lymphocytes is seen.

PV is an autoimmune disease that results from the binding of circulating IgG autoantibodies to a glycocalyx antigen in the intercellular spaces of stratified squamous epithelium. This binding inhibits the adhesive function of desmogleins, thereby diminishing adhesion of [illegible] in blister formation. Immunofluorescent testing is of great value in diagnosing PV. PV responds well to systemic prednisone. Immunosuppressive agents and plasmapheresis are also useful. Therapy can be adjusted based on serum pemphigus antibody titers. Conjunctivitis usually responds to topical corticosteroids, topical immunomodulators, or to the systemic treatment of the disease. The ocular side effects of chronic steroid usage may pose a greater ocular disease threat than that caused by PV.

Pemphigus foliaceus

Pemphigus foliaceus is a relatively mild, chronic variety of pemphigus also characterized by flaccid bullae but with more prominent exfoliation. Histologically, the bullae are more superficial in the subcorneal epidermis. Conjunctivitis may be seen, and corneal pannus and infiltration secondary to entropion and trichiasis have been described.[45]

Paraneoplastic pemphigus

Paraneoplastic pemphigus is an autoimmune inflammatory mucocutaneous disease described in association with a number of different underlying neoplasms.[46–48] Histopathologic and direct immunofluorescence findings are consistent with PV. However, indirect immunofluorescence and immunoprecipitation studies are unique.[46] The conjunctivitis, in distinction to PV, is severe and may be cicatrizing.[47,48]

Pemphigoid

Bullous pemphigoid

Bullous pemphigoid (BP), ocular cicatricial pemphigoid, and pemphigoid gestationis are diseases characterized by a subepidermal vesiculobullous eruption and deposition of immunoglobulin within the lamina lucida of the epithelial basement membrane.

BP is characterized by large, tense, subepidermal blisters with a predilection for the flexor surfaces of the forearms, axillae, and groin. The disease usually occurs in the seventh and eighth decades and occurs with equal frequency in both sexes. There is no racial or HLA haplotype association.[49] The bullae may rupture and heal spontaneously without scarring. Oral lesions are seen in 10–40% of patients, but other mucous membranes, including the conjunctiva, are only rarely involved.

Histopathology shows subepidermal bullae, the absence of acantholysis, and a superficial dermal infiltrate containing eosinophils. IgG autoantibodies bind to the BP antigen in the lamina lucida of the basement membrane zone. Immunoelectron microscopy can differentiate these antibodies from those of epidermolysis bullosa acquisita, which are found in a similar location.[50]

BP tends to be a self-limiting disorder that responds well to prednisone and immunosuppressive agents.

Cicatricial pemphigoid

Cicatricial pemphigoid (see Ch. 51) is a chronic subepithelial bullous disease of mucous membranes and skin. The eye is involved in approximately 90% of patients.

Drug-induced ocular pemphigoid (pseudopemphigoid)

Various topical ophthalmic drugs have been reported to cause conjunctival scarring clinically indistinguishable from idiopathic cicatricial pemphigoid. Pilocarpine, echothiophate,

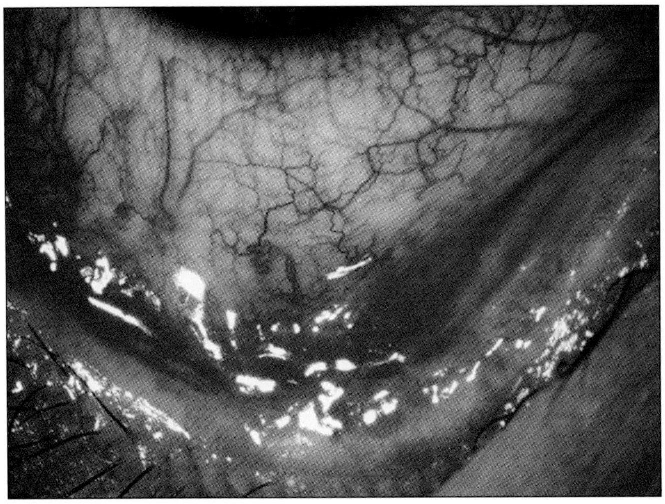

Fig. 65.6 Linear IgA bullous dermatosis: symblephora.

demecarium bromide, epinephrine, timolol, and idoxuridine have been implicated in this disease.[51] Histopathologic changes are similar to those seen in cicatricial pemphigoid. Immunofluorescence testing is negative or nonspecific. Although progression usually ceases once the offending drug is discontinued, some believe that drug-induced pemphigoid may represent a spectrum from a clearly self-limiting disorder to a progressive, unrelenting disease.[51]

Linear IgA bullous dermatosis

Linear IgA bullous dermatosis (LABD) is characterized by medium-sized blisters in an annular or rosette distribution. Skin lesions heal without scarring. The disease bears resemblance to BP and dermatitis herpetiformis but shows a unique linear distribution of IgA in either the lamina lucida or the sublamina densa of the epidermal basement membrane.[52] Chronic bullous disease of childhood is probably the same entity as LABD found in the pediatric age group.[53] Childhood LABD usually remits within 2–4 years.

Oral lesions are a common finding in LABD, and conjunctival inflammation can occur in 50% of patients.[54–56] A cicatrizing conjunctivitis with symblepharon formation (Fig. 65.6), entropion, and secondary corneal scarring can occur.

Epidermolysis bullosa acquisita

Epidermolysis bullosa acquisita (EBA) is a nonhereditary, acquired disorder that may occur either as a noninflammatory blistering disease similar to inherited dystrophic epidermolysis bullosa, with increased skin fragility, trauma-induced blistering with erosions, atrophic scarring, and milia over extensor surfaces, or as an inflammatory, generalized bullous disease similar to BP. Sodium chloride split skin techniques can help differentiate these disorders by demonstrating antibodies on the floor of the blister (lamina densa) in EBA rather than on the roof (lamina lucida) in BP.[57] The EBA antigen is a portion of type VII collagen.

Mucous membrane involvement is common in EBA, and ocular changes similar to those of cicatricial pemphigoid can be seen with symblepharon formation, corneal subepithelial vesiculation, primary peripheral corneal ulceration, and corneal opacification and perforation.[58–61]

Intravenous immunoglobulin therapy may be effective against the chronic cicatrizing conjunctivitis associated with EBA.[62]

Genetic Disorders

Acrodermatitis enteropathica

Acrodermatitis enteropathica is an autosomal recessive disorder that appears in early infancy and is characterized by acral and periorofacial dermatitis, alopecia, diarrhea, failure to thrive, and impaired immune function.[63] The skin lesions are vesiculobullous and symmetric and are also found around the eyes, occiput, elbows, hands, knees, and feet. Paronychial lesions and secondary infections are common. The syndrome is a result of intestinal malabsorbtion of zinc and is successfully treated with oral zinc supplementation.[64]

Ocular symptoms include photophobia, blurred vision, and abnormal dark adaptation. Findings include pericanthal dermatitis, loss of eyebrows and eyelashes, conjunctivitis, punctal stenosis, cataract, and retinal pigment epithelial abnormalities. Linear subepithelial corneal opacities, corneal epithelial thinning, anterior corneal scarring and vascularization, and prominent corneal nerves have been reported.[65–67]

Nevoid basal cell carcinoma syndrome (Gorlin syndrome)

Nevoid basal cell carcinoma syndrome is an autosomal dominant disorder characterized by multiple basal cell epitheliomata, odontogenic keratocysts of the jaw, congenital skeletal anomalies, calcification of the falx cerebri, and distinctive pits of the palms and soles.[68] The epitheliomata can occur in childhood but usually proliferate after puberty. The distribution is widespread and not limited to sun-exposed areas.

The most common ocular manifestation is involvement of the eyelids and periorbital areas with basal cell carcinomas. Controlled surgical excision and eyelid reconstruction is the recommended treatment. Other abnormalities include hypertelorism, strabismus, cataract, colobomata, glaucoma, and optic nerve anomalies.[69]

Darier's disease (keratosis follicularis)

Darier's disease is an autosomal dominant disorder characterized by firm, brown, papular excrescences that tend to coalesce into patches on symmetrical areas of the scalp, face, trunk, and flexures of the extremities.[3] The nails and mucous membranes may be involved. The usual onset is in childhood. All races and both genders are affected equally.

Histopathologic skin findings are hyperkeratosis, parakeratosis, acanthosis, formation of suprabasal lacunae, and upward proliferation of villi into the lacunae. In the lacunae, distinctive dyskeratotic cells are present.

The Darier gene has been localized to 12q23-24.1 and codes for a calcium ATPase (*SERCA2*).[70] A mutation results in inadequate filling of the endoplasmic reticulum calcium stores, stimulating a cascade of events that lead to acantholysis and apoptosis.

Ocular manifestations are common and include keratotic eyelid plaques, blepharoconjunctivitis, corneal opacities, and pannus. The corneal lesions seen in 75% of patients in one study[71] were distinctive, peripheral, flat, avascular, waxy, intraepithelial, variously shaped opacities[72] combined with a central corneal whorling epithelial irregularity. While the corneal changes are usually asymptomatic and helpful in diagnosing the disease, corneal ulceration and perforation have been reported, presumed related to chronic dryness and corneal erosion.[73] Histopathology of the peripheral corneal opacities showed basal epithelial cell edema and decreased desmosomes.

Treatment can include systemic vitamin A; isotretinoin, etretinate, and topical tretinoin; and corticosteroids. Treatment does not affect the corneal lesions.

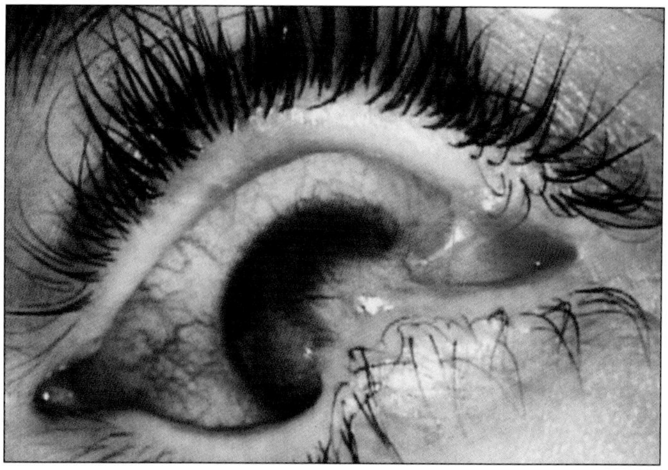

Fig. 65.7 Ectodermal dysplasia: lid–cornea adhesion.

Dyskeratosis congenita

Dyskeratosis congenita is a syndrome characterized by atrophy and reticulated pigmentation of the skin, nail dystrophy, and leukoplakia, together with multisystem ectodermal and some mesodermal changes.[3] The most common inheritance pattern is X-linked recessive, with males almost exclusively affected.

Ocular manifestations include epiphora, ectropion, madarosis, blepharitis, conjunctivitis, and leukokeratotic conjunctival plaques. The epiphora occurs in about 75% of patients and results from closure of the lacrimal puncta by epithelial hyperplasia.[74] Retinal hemorrhages can develop as a result of pancytopenia.[75]

Ectodermal dysplasias

The ectodermal dysplasias are a heterogeneous group of conditions with various inheritance patterns. They are characterized by the presence of abnormalities at birth, by being nonprogressive, by diffuse disease, and by involvement of the epidermis plus at least one of its appendages (hair, nails, teeth, sweat glands).[3]

Hypohidrotic (anhidrotic) ectodermal dysplasia is usually an X-linked recessive disorder consisting of hypotrichosis, anodontia, and hypohidrosis. Sweating is almost completely lacking, and hyperpyrexia is a common problem in childhood. Atopic disease is often an associated finding.[76]

Hidrotic ectodermal dysplasia is an autosomal dominant disorder characterized by a distinctive alopecia, dystrophic nails, and hyperkeratosis of the palms and soles.

The ectrodactyly–ectodermal dysplasia–cleft lip/palate (EEC) syndrome is an association of ectodermal dysplasia, cleft lip and/or palate, and a clefting deformity of the hands and/or feet ('lobster claw deformity').

Many ocular abnormalities have been described in the ectodermal dysplasias. These include sparse lashes and brows, blepharitis, ankyloblepharon (Fig. 65.7), hypoplastic lacrimal ducts, diminished tear production, abnormal meibomian glands, dry conjunctivae, pterygia, corneal scarring, neovascularization and perforation, cataract, panuveitis, and glaucoma.[77,78] Cicatrizing conjunctivitis with anti-basement membrane autoantibodies has been described.[79] Keratolimbal autograft transplantation performed with penetrating keratoplasty has been beneficial.[80]

Ehlers-Danlos syndrome

Ehlers-Danlos syndrome comprises a group of distinct connective tissue disorders that may affect the skin, eyes, vasculature, and joints. The skin is excessively elastic and the joints hyperextensible. The many subtypes are classified by inheritance pattern, clinical findings, and specific ultrastructural and biochemical abnormalities of collagen and connective tissue synthesis.[81]

Ocular manifestations include epicanthal folds, lax eyelid skin, strabismus, myopia, blue sclera, and angioid streaks. Ocular fragility may be present with corneal thinning (keratoconus, keratoglobus), lens dislocation, or retinal detachment. Corneal or scleral rupture may occur with minor trauma.[82] Carotid-cavernous fistula and spontaneous retrobulbar hemorrhage have been described.[83,84]

Epidermolysis bullosa

Epidermolysis bullosa (EB) refers to a heterogeneous group of heritable disorders characterized by the formation of blisters after minor physical injury. Onset is at birth or in early childhood. These diseases are distinct from EBA, which is an acquired autoimmune condition. The three major categories of EB are defined by electron microscopic[85] and immunofluorescence[86] findings and by their mode of inheritance. EB simplex is an autosomal dominant disorder characterized by intraepidermal breakdown of the basal cells. The clinical course is generally benign except in the Dowling-Meara type, which is caused by a mutation in the epidermal keratin genes. Junctional EB is an autosomal recessive disorder in which blisters form in the lamina lucida of the basement membrane complex. Many specific genetic defects have now been identified in various forms of junctional EB. Severe generalized blistering of the skin (Fig. 65.8) and mucous membranes that eventually heals without scarring can occur. There are both recessive and dominant forms of dystrophic EB, in which blisters occur below the lamina densa in the superficial dermis. Anchoring fibrils are reduced in number,

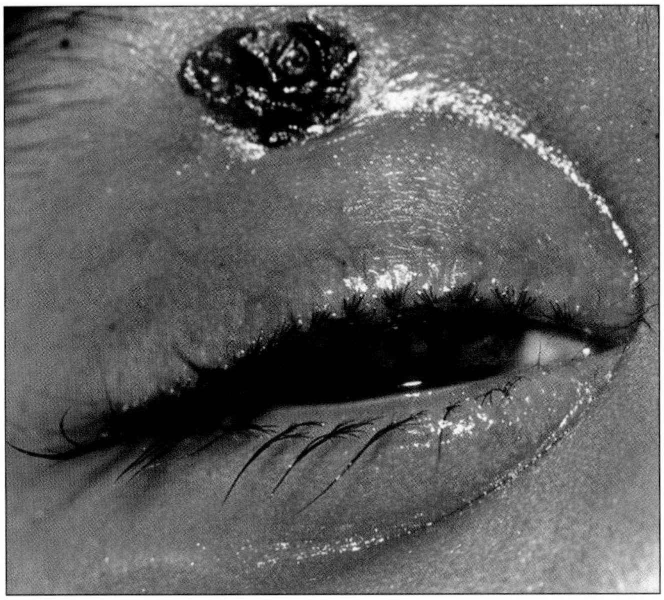

Fig. 65.8 Junctional epidermolysis bullosa: lid lesion.

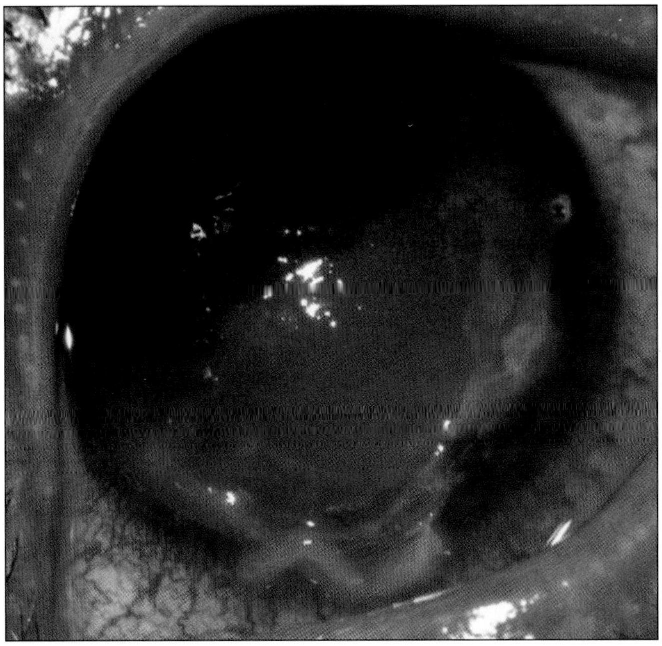

Fig. 65.9 Junctional epidermolysis bullosa: corneal erosion.

absent, or abnormal.[85] Skin and mucous membrane involvement is usually severe, with scarring and limb deformities.

Ocular involvement is uncommon in EB simplex. Small basal epithelial corneal bullae[87] and redundant, multilaminar basement membrane have been described.[88] In junctional EB, 40% of patients have ocular findings, including recurrent corneal erosions (Fig. 65.9), corneal scarring, and ectropion.[89] Dominant dystrophic EB patients may have corneal abrasions and eyelid blisters, but these occur in only 15% of cases. In contrast, the ocular findings in the recessive dystrophic variant are common (50%) and severe.[90] Corneal abrasions lead to pannus and scarring. Conjunctival injury may result in symblepharon formation, and eyelid scarring can cause ectropion and exposure keratitis. Lamellar keratoplasty and symblepharolysis, along with amniotic membrane transplantation,[91,92] may be necessary.

Focal dermal hypoplasia

Focal dermal hypoplasia is most often an X-linked dominant disorder characterized by multiple abnormalities of mesodermal and ectodermal tissues. Skin lesions, often present at birth, are linear, serpiginous, reddish-tan atrophic patches on the buttocks, axillae, and thighs.[93] Subcutaneous fat may herniate through atrophic areas, resulting in soft, yellow nodules. Angiofibromas may develop at mucous membrane borders. Skeletal and dental abnormalities are common.

Ocular manifestations occur in 40% of cases. Photophobia is a common symptom. Abnormalities include colobomas of the iris, retina, choroid, or optic nerve; microphthalmos; anophthalmos; aniridia; lipodermoid of the conjunctiva; corneal opacities; blue sclera; lens subluxation; abnormal retinal pigmentation; strabismus; nystagmus; ptosis; and dacryostenosis.[94]

Ichthyosis

Ichthyosis is a general term used to describe a diverse group of skin disorders characterized by excessively dry skin and the accumulation of scale. The major ichthyoses are ichthyosis vulgaris (IV), epidermolytic hyperkeratosis (EHK), X-linked ichthyosis (XLI), lamellar ichthyosis (LI), and congenital ichthyosiform erythroderma (CIE). There are also forms of ichthyosis that are acquired and several miscellaneous syndromes that have scaling skin as part of the disorder. Almost 17 000 people are born with some type of ichthyosis each year in the United States. Except for the X-linked recessive type, there is a 1:1 ratio of affected males to females in the population.[95]

IV is the most common hereditary scaling disorder, affecting 1 in 250 to 300 persons.[95] It is an autosomal dominant trait and usually first occurs or appears between 3 and 12 months of age. Scales are fine and white and frequently involve the trunk and the extensor surfaces of the extremities. Hyperkeratosis of the palms and soles is a consistent feature. Patients commonly show follicular accentuation (keratosis pilaris), and some may show atopic tendencies. The expression of the disease varies widely, and features often abate by the time adulthood is reached.

EHK is also an autosomal dominant disorder but is much less common than IV, affecting 1 in 250 000 people. At birth the skin is blistered, red, and peeling. Shortly thereafter, thick, ridged scales appear on the face, trunk, flexural surfaces of the extremities, and intertriginous areas. Pyogenic infection and sepsis are not uncommon problems. The disease tends to become less severe with age.

XLI is transmitted only to males as an X-linked recessive trait. It affects 1 in 6000 men.[95] The clinical features are apparent within a month of birth, with the development of large, brown scales especially prominent on the anterior neck, extensor surfaces of the extremities, and trunk. The palms and soles are spared. There is a 12–25% incidence of

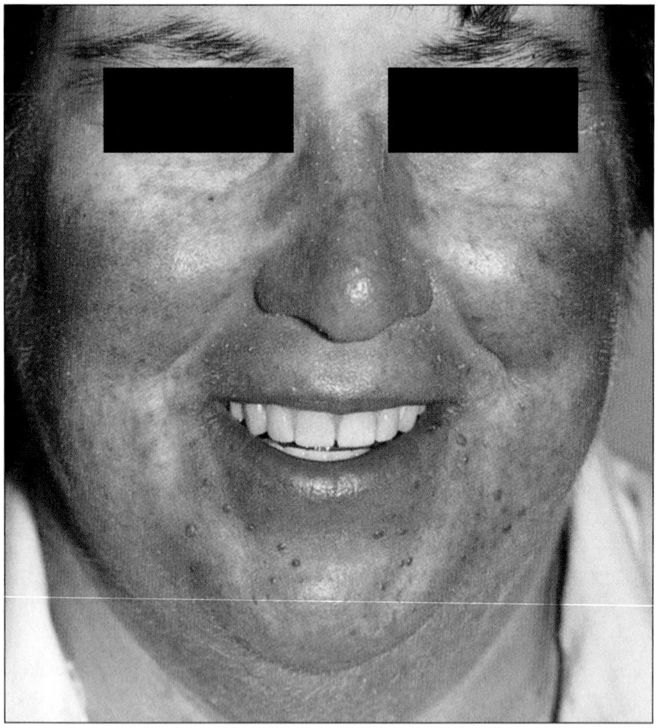

Fig. 65.10 Congenital ichthyosiform erythroderma: lid and facial scales.

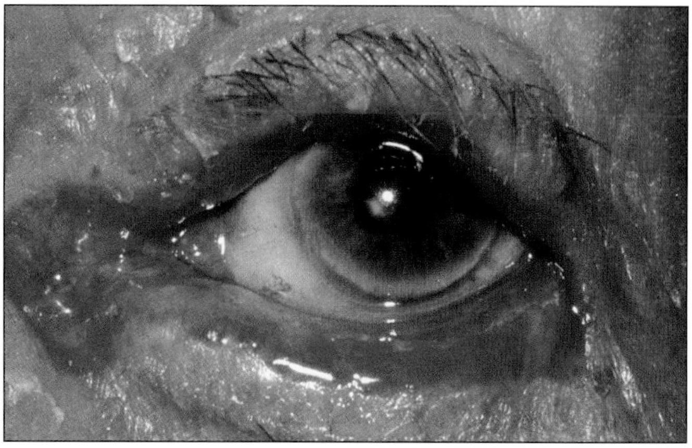

Fig. 65.11 Lamellar ichthyosis: lid thickening and ectropion.

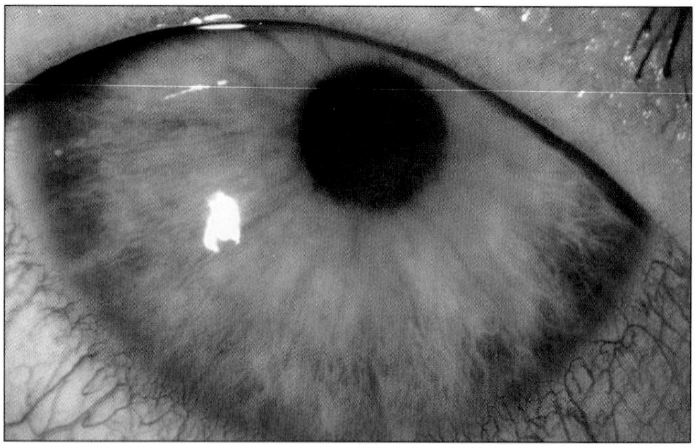

Fig. 65.12 Congenital ichthyosiform erythroderma: corneal scarring.

cryptorchidism and an independently increased risk of testicular cancer.[96] This disease gradually worsens in both extent and severity with age.

LI is a rare autosomal recessive disorder affecting 1 in 300000 persons.[95] It is apparent at birth and almost always involves the entire skin surface. A collodion-like membrane encases these babies at birth but sloughs over the first 2 to 3 weeks of life. Subsequent scales are large, platelike, and grayish brown.

CIE is also inherited as an autosomal recessive disease with about the same incidence as LI.[95] The collodion baby phenotype is seen at birth. As the membrane is shed, pronounced erythroderma may be apparent. Scales are generalized and tend to be finer and whiter than those of LI.

Acquired ichthyosis clinically similar to IV has been reported in Hodgkin's disease and various other malignancies, hypothyroidism, sarcoidosis, acquired immuno deficiency syndrome (AIDS), lupus erythematosus, dermatomyositis, and secondary to various drugs.[3]

Ichthyosis is a prominent feature in several genetic syndromes, including Sjögren-Larsson, Rud's, keratitis-ichthyosis-deafness (KID), Refsum's, Conradi-Hünermann-Happle, and congenital hemidysplasia with ichthyosiform erythroderma and limb defects (CHILD).

Ocular involvement with ichthyosis varies with the form of the disease. Eyelid scales are seen in IV, XLI, and CIE (Fig. 65.10). Ectropion is seen commonly in LI (Fig. 65.11) and CIE.[97] The ectropion is cicatricial and may require surgical correction.[98] Occasionally, the congenital ectropia seen in collodion babies can resolve spontaneously.[99] Conjunctival involvement with thickening and hyperemia can be seen in LI, CIE, and IV.[100]

Secondary corneal changes (Fig. 65.12) from severe ectropion can develop as a result of exposure, leading to vascularization and scarring.[101] Primary corneal opacities are seen in 50% of patients with XLI and rarely in IV.[96] In XLI, dot- or filament-shaped opacities are seen diffusely located in pre-Descemet's membrane or in deep stroma. The opacities become more apparent with age, although they cause no decrease in visual acuity.[101] Less pronounced, similar opacities are seen in carrier females. An epithelial and subepithelial stromal keratopathy has also been described in XLI.[102] In IV, white or gray stromal opacities, epithelial refractive bodies, nodular corneal degeneration, and band keratopathy have all been described.[101,103] Vascularizing keratitis is a prominent feature of the KID syndrome and may manifest as a punctate epithelial keratopathy, intraepithelial cysts, pannus, thinning, and stromal opacification. Limbal stem cell deficiency is presumed to be an etiological factor.[104] The corneal vascularization may worsen with isotretinoin therapy.[105]

Sjögren-Larsson syndrome is caused by an inherited enzymatic defect in the fatty alcohol cycle. Ocular findings include blepharoconjunctivitis, keratitis, and abnormalities in the retinal pigment epithelium. Refsum's disease, caused by phytanic acid accumulation, is characteristically associated with a form of retinitis pigmentosa. Rud's syndrome patients may develop a pigmentary retinopathy, and cataracts may be seen in Conradi-Hünermann-Happle disease.

The histopathology in these diseases varies. In IV, there is only moderate hyperkeratosis and a reduced or absent granular layer. By contrast, in EHK, dense, compact, hyperkeratosis is marked, as is the thickening of the granular layer. In XLI the epidermis is hyperplastic and hyperkeratotic with a normal granular layer. In LI and CIE there is marked hyperkeratosis and a prominent granular layer. LI is a retention disorder, with normal epidermal turnover, whereas CIE is hyperproliferative, with an increased epidermal turnover rate.

Among these diseases, molecular studies have provided a way to categorize them on the basis of their underlying genetic defects. For example, in EHK, mutations in the genes that code for either keratin 1 (chromosome 12) or keratin 10 (chromosome 17) have been found.[106] Mutation screening of these genes is commercially available. In XLI, the underlying biochemical defect is a deficiency of steroid sulfatase, an enzyme whose gene is located on the X-chromosome.[96]

Treatment for the ichthyoses is aimed at hydrating the skin, removing scale, and slowing epidermal turnover rates when appropriate. While these disorders are not steroid responsive, some respond well to oral retinoids.

Incontinentia pigmenti

Incontinentia pigmenti is an X-linked dominant disorder of females that presents in the first weeks of life. The initial lesions are vesicular, followed by verrucous changes. Eventually, a characteristic pigmentary phase occurs with whorling, dendritic, irregularly shaped eruptions scattered over the trunk, upper arms, and upper legs. The pigmentary changes often last for a few years and then fade away, leaving atrophic, hypopigmented patches and streaks. Extracutaneous manifestations occur in about 80% of patients.[107] Most common are skeletal, dental, ocular, and central nervous system abnormalities. Mutations of the *NEMO* gene have been described.[108]

Ocular manifestations occur in about 35% of patients.[107] Focal conjunctival hyperpigmentation with histopathologic changes similar to those seen in the skin can occur.[109] A vortex epithelial keratitis characterized by epithelial microcysts has been reported.[110] Microphthalmos, optic atrophy, cataracts, and strabismus have been described. The retinal abnormalities include peripheral retinal vascular nonperfusion, preretinal and optic nerve neovascularization, infantile retinal detachment, foveal hypoplasia, and persistent fetal vasculature.[111–113]

Histologic findings in the skin in the later stages of the disease are a decreased amount of melanin in the epithelium and an increased amount of pigment in the upper dermis.

There is no treatment for the skin manifestations. Photocoagulation, cryotherapy, and vitrectomy may be beneficial in some patients with advanced retinal disease.[111]

Keratosis follicularis spinulosa descalvans

Keratosis follicularis spinulosa descalvans is a disorder characterized by follicular hyperkeratosis of the face, scalp, neck, arms, and soles, and eventually scarring alopecia of the scalp.[3]

Ocular manifestations include the prominent feature of loss or absence of eyebrows and eyelashes, hyperkeratosis of the eyelids, and corneal changes accompanied by photophobia.[114] The corneas can show circumferential pannus with diffuse, superficial, farinaceous opacities.[115] Female carriers may manifest mild similar corneal findings.

Melkersson-Rosenthal syndrome

The Melkersson-Rosenthal syndrome is characterized by the triad of recurring facial paralysis, swelling of the lips, and furrowed tongue. The etiology is unknown. Ocular manifestations include eyelid edema, lagophthalmos, exposure keratitis, keratitis sicca, and 'crocodile tear' formation.[116] Peripheral corneal opacities,[116] thickening of Bowman's membrane with a whorling keratopathy, and uveitis[117] have been described.[118]

Pachyonychia congenita

Pachyonychia congenita is an autosomal dominant disorder characterized by excessively thickened, discolored nails of all fingers and toes, follicular keratosis of the knees and elbows, friction blisters of the palms and soles, and leukokeratosis of the mucous membranes.[3]

Ocular manifestations can include cataracts and corneal changes, described in one case as bilateral, faint, rust-colored, superficial opacities in a pinwheel configuration.[119]

Richner-Hanhart syndrome

The Richner-Hanhart syndrome is an autosomal recessive disorder characterized clinically by bilateral subepithelial dendritic corneal lesions, hyperkeratotic and erosive lesions of the palms and soles, and, in most cases, mental retardation. The disease is caused by a deficiency of cytoplasmic tyrosine aminotransferase with consequent hypertyrosinemia.

Corneal lesions generally appear in the first few months of life, resulting in photophobia, tearing, and redness. The keratitis varies from mild epithelial branching to deep ulcerations that may involve the anterior stroma. Nystagmus, cataract, strabismus, and thickened conjunctiva have also been described.[120]

Serum tyrosine levels confirm the diagnosis. Dietary restriction of tyrosine and phenylalanine can cause regression of skin and eye lesions. Rarely, penetrating keratoplasty is required for corneal scarring and vascularization.

Rothmund-Thomson syndrome

Rothmund-Thomson syndrome is an autosomal recessive disease characterized by reticular erythematous skin changes of the hands and face that develop in the months shortly after birth.[121] In time, atrophy and hyperpigmentation occur. Other manifestations include short stature, hypogonadism, bony defects, and sun sensitivity.[121] Some patients demonstrate abnormal DNA helicase activity.[122]

Ocular manifestations include sparse eyebrows and eyelashes, bilateral juvenile cataracts, band keratopathy, keratoconus, prominence of Schwalbe's line, strabismus,[123] and infantile glaucoma.[124]

Werner's syndrome

Werner's syndrome is an autosomal recessive disorder of premature aging (progeria) in which cessation of growth at puberty, premature balding and graying, scleropoikiloderma, trophic ulcerations of the legs, and atrophy of subcutaneous tissues are hallmark characteristics. Hypogonadism, diabetes, sarcomatous tumors, and diffuse metastatic calcification are also frequently seen. Abnormalities on chromosome 8 have been described.[3]

The primary ocular finding is early-onset cataract, which is seen almost universally. Cataracts appear between the ages of 10 and 35 years and are described as posterior cortical or posterior subcapsular opacities.[125] Other reported findings include keratoconjunctivitis, blue sclera, corneal clouding, iris telangiectasis, and retinitis pigmentosa.[126] Bullous keratopathy[125] and wound dehiscence[127] have been reported as complications of cataract extraction. Corneal metastatic calcification has been seen after both cataract extraction and penetrating keratoplasty.[128]

Xeroderma pigmentosum

Xeroderma pigmentosum is a rare autosomal recessive disorder characterized by solar injury to exposed skin and ocular tissues. Patients with this disease have an enzymatic defect in the ability to repair DNA damage induced by shortwave ultraviolet light. Skin sensitivity appears in early infancy, and freckling appears within the first several years of life. Eventually, telangiectasia, hypopigmentation, atrophy, and premalignant and malignant lesions form on the face, neck, hands, and arms.[129] Basal cell carcinomas, squamous cell carcinomas, and melanomas are the most common tumors. Although mild forms of the disease are occasionally seen, death often occurs in early adulthood as a result of metastatic disease or infection.

Ocular symptoms and findings occur in most patients with xeroderma pigmentosum. Photophobia, epiphora, and blepharospasm are early complaints. Eyelids show atrophy, madarosis, ectropion, malignant degeneration, and eventually loss of tissue. Conjunctivae become hyperemic, xerotic, and keratinized. Symblepharon formation and ankyloblepharon may ensue. Corneal scarring is common and usually secondary to exposure and dryness. Tumors of the conjunctiva and limbus, especially squamous cell carcinoma, are seen.[130–132]

Treatment consists of wearing sunscreen lotions, clothing, and eyewear to shield the skin and eyes from ultraviolet light. Malignancies should be excised in a manner that maximizes normal eyelid function. Corneal involvement may require complex medical and surgical strategies.[133]

Miscellaneous Disorders

Acanthosis nigricans

Acanthosis nigricans is characterized by hyperpigmentation and papillary hypertrophy, which may symmetrically affect the face, neck, axillae, groin, antecubital and popliteal fossae, umbilicus, and anus. Histopathology primarily shows papillomatosis and hyperkeratosis with only mild acanthosis.[134] Three clinical forms of the disease are described. A rare autosomal dominant type presents during childhood. A second common type occurs in association with obesity, insulin-resistant states, endocrine disorders, and certain drugs. The third form is the 'malignant' form of acanthosis nigricans and may precede, accompany, or follow the onset of internal adenocarcinomas of various organs. Acanthosis nigricans is probably caused by elevated levels of a factor stimulating keratinocytes and dermal fibroblasts at the cell receptor level.[134]

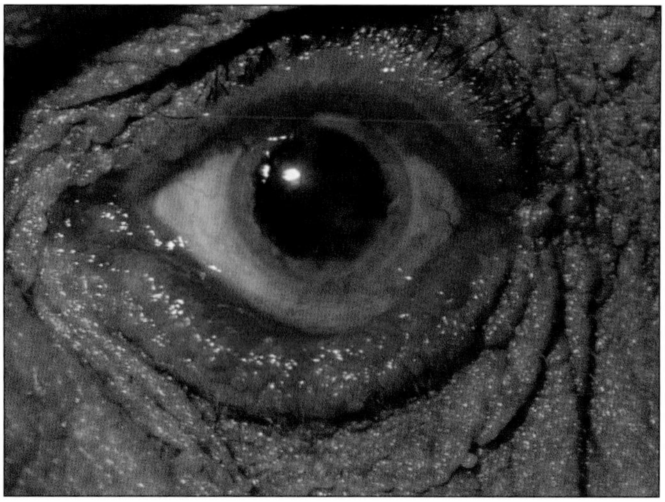

Fig. 65.13 Acanthosis nigricans: skin and lid changes.

Ocular manifestations include eyelid thickening and pigmentation (Fig. 65.13), canalicular obstruction with epiphora, conjunctival hypertrophy, and corneal opacification and vascularization.[135–137]

Epidermal nevus syndrome

The epidermal nevus syndrome is usually a noninherited disorder characterized by linear plaques of pigmented verrucous hyperplasia on the head, neck, or trunk with anomalies of the central nervous system, skeleton, skin, and cardiovascular system. Ocular abnormalities occur in 33% and include ocular melanocytic nevus, cloudy cornea, colobomata, strabismus, and conjunctival lipodermoid.[138]

Hydroa vacciniforme

Hydroa vacciniforme is a self-limited, recurrent vesiculobullous disease of childhood affecting the sun-exposed skin of the face, ears, neck, arms, and hands. Stinging and burning occur hours after sun exposure, followed by the development of tense erythematous papules, which, over a period of days, develop into discrete vesicles and eventually umbilicate and necrose, leaving hypopigmented depressed scars.[139] The cause of this disorder is unknown.

Tearing and photophobia are often present. Ocular findings are less common and include cicatricial ectropion, conjunctival chemosis, hyperemia, vesiculation and scarring, and corneal opacification and vascularization.[140,141] Rarely, the ocular findings may be the presenting sign of the disease.[142]

Juvenile xanthogranuloma

Juvenile xanthogranuloma is an idiopathic, noninherited histiocytic inflammatory disorder affecting infants and children. The skin and eye are the two most commonly involved sites. Cutaneous lesions are reddish-yellow, firm papules or nodules that appear on the face, scalp, trunk, and extensor surfaces. Histopathology shows lipid-laden histiocytes, foreign body giant cells, Touton giant cells, lymphocytes, and eosinophils.[3] Skin lesions usually involute spontaneously within 3 to 6 years.

Ocular involvement occurs in 10% of patients.[143] Xanthogranulomas most frequently occur in the iris and ciliary body. Fluoroscein angiography can be useful in diagnosing iris lesions.[144] Spontaneous hemorrhage from these lesions into the anterior chamber may occur and cause secondary glaucoma or corneal blood staining.[145] Less commonly involved sites are the eyelids, orbit, corneoscleral limbus, vitreous, choroid, and optic nerve.[146] Treatment of uveal lesions includes topical, subconjunctival,[147] or systemic steroids; irradiation; and surgery.

Kaposi's sarcoma

Kaposi's sarcoma is a multicentric vascular neoplasm or hyperplasia that usually begins with red-blue macules on the lower extremity and progresses to involve the upper extremities, face, ears, trunk, and soft palate. There are several classifications of the disease, including those seen in immunosuppressed and HIV-infected patients (see Ch. 67). Human herpesvirus-8 is the implicated agent in all clinical variants.[148,149] Lesions affecting the eyelid margin, conjunctiva, or, rarely, the orbit are seen in 18% of patients with AIDS-associated systemic Kaposi's sarcoma.[150] Treatment options include surgical excision, cryotherapy, irradiation, chemotherapy, and immunotherapy.[151,152]

Malignant atrophic papulosis (Degos' syndrome)

Malignant atrophic papulosis is a rare systemic disease usually presenting with distinctive skin lesions and often later advancing to fatal involvement of the gastrointestinal and central nervous systems. Most patients are young or middle-aged. Initially, the dermatosis is characterized by pale rose, round, edematous papules, 2–10 mm in diameter, occurring mostly on the trunk and upper body. Later, the lesions form a distinctive porcelain-white central depression with a peripheral telangiectatic border.[3] Gastrointestinal symptoms usually appear months or years after the skin eruption and include cramps, pain, distension, and hematemesis. Fulminant peritonitis may ensue, caused by multiple perforations of the intestine. Central nervous system manifestations are wide ranging, and death from cerebral infarction and hemorrhage is not uncommon. Other organ systems may also be involved.

Ocular involvement includes characteristic skin lesions on the eyelid; conjunctival microaneurysms, telangiectasia, and atrophic plaques; and cataract.[153] Episcleritis, choroiditis, and neuro-ophthalmologic signs of cerebral lesions may be seen.[154]

The etiology of this disease is unknown. Histopathology shows a lymphocyte-mediated obliterative arteriolitis or endovasculitis with resultant thrombosis and necrosis common to all involved tissues.[155] Impaired fibrinolytic activity and platelet aggregation and antiphospholipid antibodies have been reported.

Treatment with aspirin and dipyridamole and fibrinolytic agents have some reported success.[156] Topical and systemic steroids are not of benefit.

References

1. Farber EM, Nall ML. The natural history of psoriasis in 5,600 patients. *Dermatologica.* 1974;148:1.
2. Elder JT, et al. The genetics of psoriasis. *Arch Dermatol.* 1994;130:216.
3. Odom RB, James WD, Berger TG. *Andrews' diseases of the skin: clinical dermatology.* 9th ed. Philadelphia: Saunders; 2000.
4. Gottlieb AB. Immunologic mechanisms in psoriasis. *J Am Acad Dermatol.* 1988;18:1376.
5. Seville RH. Psoriasis and stress I & II. *Br J Dermatol.* 1977;97:297;98:151.
6. Whyte HJ, et al. Acute guttate psoriasis and streptococcal infection. *Arch Dermatol.* 1964;89:350.
7. Abel EA, et al. Drugs in exacerbation of psoriasis. *J Am Acad Dermatol.* 1986;15:1007.
8. Sadick NS, NcNutt MS, Kaplan MH. Papulosquamous dermatoses of AIDS. *J Am Acad Dermatol.* 1990;22:1270.
9. Kaldeck R. Ocular psoriasis. *Arch Dermatol.* 1953;68:44.
10. Eustace P, Pierce D. Ocular psoriasis. *Br J Ophthalmol.* 1970;54:810.
11. Durrani K, Foster CS. Psoriatic uveitis: a distinct clinical entity? *Am J Ophthalmol.* 2005;139(1):106.
12. Malanos D, Stern RS. Psoralen plus ultraviolet A does not increase the risk of cataracts: a 25-year prospective study. *J Am Acad Dermatol.* 2007;57:231.
13. Wentzell JM, et al. Cyclosporin in psoriasis. *Arch Dermatol.* 1987;123:163.
14. Gottlieb AB, et al. Infliximab induction therapy for patients with severe plaque-type psoriasis: a randomized, double-blind placebo-controlled trial. *J Am Acad Dermatol.* 2004;51:534.
15. Huynh N, et al. Biologic response modifier therapy for psoriatic ocular inflammatory disease. *Ocul Immunol Inflamm.* 2008;16:89.
16. Faergemann J. Pityrosporum infections. *J Am Acad Dermatol.* 1994;31(3):18
17. Borton JL, Pye RJ. Seborrhea is not a feature of seborrheic dermatitis. *Br Med J.* 1983;286:1169.
18. Ostler HB, Conant MA, Groundwater J. Lyell's disease, the Stevens-Johnson syndrome, and exfoliative dermatitis. *Trans Am Acad Ophthalmol Otolaryngol.* 1970;74:1254.
19. Wilkin JK. Rosacea. *Arch Dermatol.* 1994;130:359.
20. Starr PAJ, McDonald A. Oculocutaneous aspects of rosacea. *Proc R Soc Med.* 1969;62:9.
21. Lempert SL, Jenkins MS, Brown SI. Chalazia and rosacea. *Arch Ophthalmol.* 1979;97:1652.
22. Bernardini FP, et al. Chronic eyelid lymphedema and acne rosacea. Report of two cases. *Ophthalmology.* 2000;107:2220.
23. Thygeson P. Dermatoses with ocular manifestations. In: Sorsby A, ed. *Systemic ophthalmology.* 2nd ed. London: Butterworths; 1958.
24. Durson D, Piniella AM, Pflugfelder SC. Pseudokeratoconus caused by rosacea. *Cornea.* 2001;20:668.
25. Watson PG, Hayreh SS. Scleritis and episcleritis. *Br J Ophthalmol.* 1976;60:163.
26. Lemp MA, Mahmood MA, Weiler HH. Association of rosacea and keratoconjunctivitis sicca. *Arch Ophthalmol.* 1984;102:556.
27. Lee WB, et al. Dendritic keratopathy in ocular rosacea. *Cornea.* 2005;24:632.
28. Ravage ZB, et al. Ocular rosacea can mimic trachoma: a case of cicatrizing conjunctivitis. *Cornea.* 2004;23:630.
29. Souza PM, Holland EJ, Huang AJ. Bilateral herpetic keratoconjunctivitis. *Ophthalmology.* 2003;110:493.

30. Foster CS. Ocular surface manifestations of neurological and systemic disease. *Int Ophthalmol Clin.* 1979;19(2):207.
31. Hoang-Xuan T, et al. Ocular rosacea. *Ophthalmology.* 1990;97:1468.
32. Maatta M, et al. Tear fluid levels of MMP-8 are elevated in ocular rosacea – treatment effect of oral doxycycline. *Graefe's Arch Clin Exp Ophthalmol.* 2006;244:957.
33. Sneddon IB. A clinical trial of tetracycline in rosacea. *Br J Dermatol.* 1966;78:649.
34. Jenkins MS, et al. Ocular rosacea. *Am J Ophthalmol.* 1979;88:1618.
35. Jain AK, Sukhija J. Amniotic membrane transplantation in ocular rosacea. *Ann Ophthalmol.* 2007;39:71.
36. Sandinha T, et al. Superior forniceal conjunctival advancement pedicles (SFCAP) in the management of acute and impending corneal perforations. *Eye.* 2006;20:84.
37. Gelmetti C, et al. Pityriasis rubra pilaris in childhood: a long-term study of 29 cases. *Pediatr Dermatol.* 1986;3:446.
38. Duke-Elder S. Diseases of the outer eye: conjunctiva. In: *System of ophthalmology.* vol. 8. St. Louis: Mosby; 1965.
39. Sugar A. Impetigo. In: Fraunfelder FT, Roy FH, eds. *Current ocular therapy.* 4th ed. Philadelphia: Saunders; 1995.
40. Ahmed AR. Pemphigus vulgaris: clinical features. *Dermatol Clin.* 1983;1:171.
41. Nelson ME, Rennie IG. Symmetrical lid margin erosions: a condition specific to pemphigus vulgaris. Case report. *Arch Ophthalmol.* 1988;106:1652.
42. Hodak E, et al. Conjunctival involvement in pemphigus vulgaris: a clinical, histopathological and immunofluorescence study. *Br J Dermatol.* 1990;123:615.
43. Suami M, et al. Keratolysis in a patient with pemphigus vulgaris. *Br J Ophthalmol.* 2001;85:1263.
44. Palleschi GM, Giomi B, Fabbri P. Ocular involvement in pemphigus. *Am J Ophthalmol.* 2007;144:149.
45. Amendola F. Ocular manifestations of pemphigus foliaceus. *Am J Ophthalmol.* 1949;32:35.
46. Anhalt GJ, et al. Paraneoplastic pemphigus: an autoimmune mucocutaneous disease associated with neoplasia. *N Engl J Med.* 1990;323: 1729.
47. Meyers SJ, et al. Conjunctival involvement in paraneoplastic pemphigus. *Am J Ophthalmol.* 1992;114:621.
48. Lam S, et al. Paraneoplastic pemphigus, cicatricial conjunctivitis, and acanthosis nigricans with pachydermatoglyphy in a patient with bronchogenic squamous cell carcinoma. *Ophthalmology.* 1992;99:108.
49. Stanley JR. Bullous pemphigoid. *Dermatol Clin.* 1983;1:205.
50. Gammon WR, et al. Direct immunofluorescence studies of sodium chloride-separated skin in the differential diagnosis of bullous pemphigoid and epidermolysis bullosa acquisita. *J Am Acad Dermatol.* 1990;22:664.
51. Fiore PM, Jacobs IH, Goldberg DB. Drug induced pemphigoid: a spectrum of diseases. *Arch Ophthalmol.* 1987;105:1660.
52. Zone JJ, et al. Identification of the cutaneous basement membrane antigen and isolation of the antibody in linear immunoglobulin A bullous disease. *J Clin Invest.* 1990;85:812.
53. Wojnarowska F, et al. Chronic bullous disease of childhood, childhood cictricial pemphigoid, and linear IgA disease of adults: a comparative study demonstrating clinical and immunopathologic overlap. *J Am Acad Dermatol.* 1988;19:792.
54. Aultbrinker EA, Starr MB, Donnenfeld ED. Linear IgA disease. The ocular manifestations. *Ophthalmology.* 1988;95:340.
55. Kelly SE, et al. A clinicopathological study of mucosal involvement in linear IgA disease. *Br J Dermatol.* 1988;119:161.
56. Webster GF, et al. Cicatrizing conjunctivitis as a predominant manifestation of linear IgA bullous dermatosis. *J Am Acad Dermatol.* 1994;30: 355.
57. Gammon WR, et al. Differentiating anti-lamina lucida and anti-sublamina densa anti-BMZ antibodies by indirect immunofluorescence on 1.0 M sodium chloride-separated skin. *J Invest Dermatol.* 1984;82:139.
58. Lang PG Jr, Tapert MJ. Severe ocular involvement in a patient with epidermolysis bullosa acquisita. *J Am Acad Dermatol.* 1987;16:439.
59. Zierhut M, et al. Ocular involvement in epidermolysis bullosa acquisita. *Arch Ophthalmol.* 1989;107:398.
60. Aclimandos WA. Corneal perforation as a complication of epidermolysis bullosa acquisita. *Eye.* 1995;9:633.
61. Dantas PEC, et al. Bilateral corneal involvement in epidermolysis bullosa acquisita. *Cornea.* 2001;20:664.
62. Letko E, et al. Chronic cicatrizing conjunctivitis in a patient with epidermolysis bullosa acquisita. *Arch Ophthalmol.* 2006;124:1615.
63. Cameron JD, McClain CJ, Doughman DJ. Acrodermatitis enteropathica. In: Gold DH, Weingeist TA, eds. *The eye in systemic disease.* Philadelphia: Lippincott; 1990.
64. Moynahan EJ, Barnes PM. Zinc deficiency and a synthetic diet for lactose intolerance. *Lancet.* 1973;1:676.
65. Matta CS, Felker GV, Ide CH. Eye manifestations in acrodermatitis enteropathica. *Arch Ophthalmol.* 1973;93:140.
66. Warshawsky RS, et al. Acrodermatitis enteropathica. Corneal involvement with histochemical and electron micrographic studies. *Arch Ophthalmol.* 1975;93:194.
67. Cameron JD, McClain CJ. Ocular histopathology of acrodermatitis enteropathica. *Br J Ophthalmol.* 1986;70:662.
68. Gorlin, RJ. Nevoid basal-cell carcinoma syndrome. *Medicine.* 1987;66:98.
69. Tse DT. Basal cell nevus syndrome. In: Gold DH, Weingeist TA, eds. *Color atlas of the eye in systemic disease.* Philadelphia: Lippincott Williams & Wilkins; 2001.
70. Sakuntabhai A, et al. Mutations in ATP2A2, encoding a Ca^{2+} pump, cause Darier's disease. *Nat Genet.* 1999;21:271.
71. Blackman HJ, Rodrigues MM, Peck GL. Corneal epithelial lesions in keratosis follicularis (Darier's disease). *Ophthalmology.* 1980;87:931.
72. Krachmer JH. The discussion of corneal epithelial lesions in keratosis follicularis (Darier's disease). *Ophthalmology.* 1980;87:942.
73. Mielke J, et al. Recurrent corneal ulcerations with perforation in keratosis follicularis (Darier-White disease). *Br J Ophthalmol.* 2002;86:1192.
74. Sirinavin C, Trowbridge AA. Dyskeratosis congenita: clinical features and genetic aspects. *J Med Genet.* 1975;12:339.
75. Nazir S, Sayani N, Phillips PH. Retinal hemorrhages in a patient with dyskeratosis congenita. *J AAPOS.* 2008;12:415.
76. Clarke A, et al. Clinical aspects of x-linked hypohidrotic ectodermal dysplasia. *Arch Dis Child.* 1987;62:989.
77. Moyes AL, Hordinsky M, Holland EJ. Ectodermal dysplasia. In: Mannis MJ, Macsai MS, Huntley AC, eds. *Eye and skin disease.* Philadelphia: Lippincott; 1996.
78. Rodriguez N, et al. Bilateral panuveitis in a child with hypohidrotic ectodermal dysplasia. *Am J Ophthalmol.* 2002;134:443.
79. Saw VP, et al. Cicatrising conjunctivitis with anti-basement membrane autoantibodies in ectodermal dysplasia. *Br J Ophthalmol.* 2008;92:1403.
80. Anderson NJ, Hardten DR, McCarty TM. Penetrating keratoplasty and keratolimbal allograft transplantation for corneal perforations associated with the ectodermal dysplasia syndrome. *Cornea.* 2003;22:385.
81. Johnson DS, Kolansky G, Whitaker DC. Ehlers-Danlos syndrome. In: Gold DH, Weingeist TA, eds. *Color atlas of the eye in systemic disease.* Philadelphia: Lippincott Williams & Wilkins; 2001.
82. Beighton P. Serious ophthalmological complications in the Ehlers-Danlos syndrome. *Br J Ophthalmol.* 1970;54:263.
83. Pollack JS, et al. Ocular complications in Ehlers-Danlos syndrome type IV. *Arch Ophthalmol.* 1997;115:416.
84. Shaikh S, Braun M, Eliason J. Spontaneous retrobulbar hemorrhage in type IV Ehlers-Danlos syndrome. *Am J Ophthalmol.* 2002;133:422.
85. Smith LT. Ultrastructural findings in epidermoloysis bullosa. *Arch Dermatol.* 1993;129:1578.
86. Hintner H, et al. Immunofluorescence mapping of antigenic determinants within the dermal–epidermal junction in mechanobullous diseases. *J Invest Dermatol.* 1981;76:288.
87. Granek H, Howard B. Corneal involvement in epidermolysis bullosa simplex. *Arch Ophthalmol.* 1980;98:469.
88. Adamis AP, Schein OD, Kenyon KR. Anterior corneal disease of epidermolysis bullosa simplex. *Arch Ophthalmol.* 1993;111:499.
89. Lin AN, et al. Review of ophthalmic findings in 204 patients with epidermolysis bullosa. *Am J Ophthalmol.* 1994;118:384.
90. Tong L, et al. The eye in epidermolysis bullosa. *Br J Ophthalmol.* 1999;83:323.
91. Altan-Yaycioglu R, Akova YA, Oto S. Amniotic membrane transplantation for treatment of symblepharon in a patient with recessive dystrophic epidermolysis bullosa. *Cornea.* 2006;25:971.
92. Goyal R, et al. Amniotic membrane transplantation in children with symblepharon and massive pannus. *Arch Ophthalmol.* 2006;124: 1435.
93. Goltz RW, et al. Focal dermal hypoplasia syndrome: a review of the literature and report of two cases. *Arch Dermatol.* 1970;101:1.
94. Thomas JV, et al. Ocular manifestations of focal dermal hypoplasia syndrome. *Arch Ophthalmol.* 1977;95:1997.
95. Bale SJ, Doyle SZ. The genetics of ichthyosis: a primer for epidemiologists. *J Invest Dermatol.* 1994;102:495.
96. Lykkesfeldt G, et al. Steroid sulfatase deficiency disease. *Clin Genet.* 1985;28:231.
97. Sever R, Frost P, Weinstein G. Eye changes in ichthyosis. *JAMA.* 1968;206:2283.
98. Shindle RD, Leone CR. Cicatricial ectropion associated with lamellar ichthyosis. *Arch Ophthalmol.* 1975;89:62.
99. Oestreicher JH, Nelson CC. Lamellar ichthyosis and congenital ectropion. *Arch Ophthalmol.* 1990;108:1772.

100. Cordes FC, Hogan MJ. Ocular ichthyosis. *Arch Ophthalmol.* 1939;22:590.
101. Jay B, Blach R, Wells R. Ocular manifestations of ichthyosis. *Br J Ophthalmol.* 1968;52:217.
102. Haritoglou C, et al. Corneal manifestations of X-linked ichthyosis in two brothers. *Cornea.* 2000;19:861.
103. Friedman B. Corneal findings in ichthyosis. *Am J Ophthalmol.* 1955;39:575.
104. Messmer EM, et al. Ocular manifestations of keratitis-ichthyosis-deafness (KID) syndrome. *Ophthalmology.* 2005;112:1.
105. Hagen PG, et al. Corneal effect of isotretinoin. *J Am Acad Dermatol.* 1986;14:141.
106. Cheng J, et al. The genetic basis of epidermolytic hyperkeratosis: a disorder of differentiation-specific epidermal keratin genes. *Cell.* 1992;70:811.
107. Carney RG. Incontinentia pigmenti. *Arch Dermatol.* 1976;112:535.
108. Fusco F, et al. Molecular analysis of the genetic defect in a large cohort of IP patients and identification of novel NEMO mutations interfering with NF-kappaB activation. *Hum Mol Genet.* 2004;13:1763.
109. McCrary J, Smith JL. Conjunctival and retinal incontinentia pigmenti. *Arch Ophthalmol.* 1968;79:417.
110. Ferreira RC, et al. Corneal abnormalities associated with incontinentia pigmenti. *Am J Ophthalmol.* 1997;123:549.
111. Goldberg MF, Curtis PH. Retinal and other manifestations of incontinentia pigmenti: Bloch-Sulzberger syndrome. *Ophthalmology.* 1993;100:1645.
112. Shah GK, et al. Optic nerve neovascularization in incontinentia pigmenti. *Am J Ophthalmol.* 1997;124:410.
113. Fard AK, Goldberg MF. Persistence of fetal vasculature in the eyes of patients with incontinentia pigmenti. *Arch Ophthalmol.* 1998;116:682.
114. Rand R, Baden HP. Keratosis follicularis spinulosa decalvans. *Arch Dermatol.* 1983;119:22.
115. Forgacs J, Franceschetti A. Histologic aspect of corneal changes due to hereditary metabolic and cutaneous affections. *Am J Ophthalmol.* 1959;47:191.
116. Paton D. The Melkersson-Rosenthal syndrome. *Am J Ophthalmol.* 1965;59:705.
117. Ates O, Yoruk O. Unilateral anterior uveitis in Melkersson-Rosenthal syndrome: a case report. *J Int Med Res.* 2006;34:428.
118. Mulvihill JJ, et al. Melkersson-Rosenthal syndrome, Hodgkin disease, and corneal keratopathy. *Arch Intern Med.* 1973;132:116.
119. Buckley WR, Cassuto J. Pachyonychia congenita. *Arch Dermatol.* 1962;85:397.
120. Goldsmith LH, Reed J. Tyrosine induced skin and eye lesions: a treatable genetic disease. *JAMA.* 1976;236:382.
121. Bey E, et al. Rothmund-Thomson syndrome. *J Am Acad Dermatol.* 1987;17:332.
122. Kitao S, et al. Mutations in RECQL4 cause a subset of cases of Rothmund-Thomson syndrome. *Nat Genet.* 1999;22:82.
123. Kirkham TH, Werner EB. The ophthalmologic manifestations of Rothmund's syndrome. *Can J Ophthalmol.* 1975;10:1.
124. Turacli ME, Tekeli O. Infantile glaucoma in a patient with Rothmund-Thomson syndrome. *Can J Ophthalmol.* 2004;39:671.
125. Petrohelos M. Werner's syndrome. *Am J Ophthalmol.* 1963;56:941.
126. Bullock J, Howard R. Werner's syndrome. *Arch Ophthalmol.* 1973;90:53.
127. Ruprecht KW. Ophthalmological aspects in patients with Werner's syndrome. *Arch Gerontol Geriatr.* 1989;9:263.
128. Kremer I, Ingber A, Ben-Sira I. Corneal metastatic calcification in Werner's syndrome. *Am J Ophthalmol.* 1988;106:221.
129. Kraemer KH, Lee MM, Scotto J. Xeroderma pigmentosum. *Arch Dermatol.* 1987;123:241.
130. El-Hefnawi H, Mortada A. Ocular manifestations of xeroderma pigmentosum. *Br J Dermatol.* 1965;77:261.
131. Goyal JL, et al. Oculocutaneous manifestations in xeroderma pigmentosum. *Br J Ophthalmol.* 1994;78:295.
132. Riley FC, Teichmann KD. Conjunctival necrobiotic granuloma in xeroderma pigmentosum. *Cornea.* 2001;20:543.
133. Calonge M, et al. Management of corneal complications in xeroderma pigmentosum. *Cornea.* 1992;11:173.
134. Schwartz RA. Acanthosis nigricans. *J Am Acad Dermatol.* 1994;31:1.
135. Groos EB, et al. Eyelid involvement in acanthosis nigricans. *Am J Ophthalmol.* 1993;115:42.
136. Lamba P, Lal S. Ocular changes in benign acanthosis nigricans. *Dermatologica.* 1970;140:356.
137. Tabandeh H, et al. Conjunctival involvement in malignancy-associated acanthosis nigricans. *Eye.* 1993;7:648.
138. Solomon LM, et al. The epidermal nevus syndrome. *Arch Dermatol.* 1968;97:272.
139. Kirkland C Jr, Lanier JD. Hydroa vacciniforme. In: Gold DH, Weingeist TA, eds. *The eye in systemic disease.* Philadelphia: Lippincott; 1990.
140. Stokes WH. Ocular manifestations in hydroa vacciniforme. *Arch Ophthalmol.* 1940;23:1131.
141. Crews SJ. Hydroa vacciniforme affecting the eye. *Br J Ophthalmol.* 1959;43:629.
142. Jeng BH, et al. Ocular findings as a presenting sign of hydroa vacciniforme. *Br J Ophthalmol.* 2004;88:1478.
143. Roper SS, Spraker MK. Cutaneous histiocytosis syndromes. *Pediatr Dermatol.* 1985;3:19.
144. Danzig CJ, et al. Fluorescein angiography of iris juvenile xanthogranuloma. *J Pediatr Ophthalmol Strabism.* 2008;45:110.
145. Zimmerman LE. Ocular lesions of juvenile xanthogranuloma. *Am J Ophthalmol.* 1965;60:1011.
146. Berrocal AM, Davis JL. Chorioretinal involvement and vitreous hemorrhage in a patient with juvenile xanthogranuloma. *J Pediatr Ophthalmol Strabism.* 2005;42:241.
147. Treacy KW, Letson RD, Summers CG. Subconjunctival steroid in the management of uveal juvenile xanthogranuloma: a case report. *J Pediatr Ophthalmol Strabismus.* 1990;27:126.
148. Weiss RA, et al. Human herpesvirus type 8 and Kaposi's sarcoma. *J Natl Cancer Inst Monogr.* 1998;23:51.
149. Minoda H, et al. Human herpesvirus-8 in Kaposi's sarcoma of the conjunctiva in a patient with AIDS. *Jap J Ophthalmol.* 2006;50:7.
150. Holland GN, et al. Acquired immune deficiency syndrome: ocular manifestations. *Ophthalmology.* 1983;90:859.
151. Hummer J, Gass JDM, Huang AJW. Conjunctival Kaposi's sarcoma treated with interferon alpha-2a. *Am J Ophthalmol.* 1993;116:502.
152. Brasnu E, et al. Efficacy of interferon-alpha for the treatment of Kaposi's sarcoma herpesvirus-associated uveitis. *Am J Ophthalmol.* 2005;140:746.
153. Egan R, Lessell S. Posterior subcapsular cataract in Degos' disease. *Am J Ophthalmol.* 2000;129:806.
154. Lee DA, Su WPD, Liesegang TJ. Ophthalmic changes of Degos' disease (malignant atrophic papulosis). *Ophthalmology.* 1984;91:295.
155. Soter NA, Murphy GF, Mihm MC Jr. Lymphocytes and necrosis of the cutaneous microvasculature in malignant atrophic papulosis: a refined light microscope study. *J Am Acad Dermatol.* 1982;7:620.
156. Delaney TJ, Black MM. Effect of fibrinolytic treatment in malignant atrophic papulosis. *Br Med J.* 1975;3:415.

Chapter 66

Infectious Disease: Corneal Manifestations

Zachary J. Berbos, Jay H Krachmer

Infectious disease affects the entirety of the human body, often presenting with a myriad of nonspecific, subjective complaints and symptoms ascribable to the innate immune response. The eye serves as a diagnostic window into the diseased body, providing clinical insight by demonstrating signs suggestive of certain disease processes. For this reason, the ophthalmologist may be consulted for input regarding systemic disease processes. The ocular examination can be used to develop (or limit) a differential diagnosis, direct diagnostic evaluation, provide tissue and/or fluid for definitive diagnostic studies, make a definitive diagnosis, and direct therapeutic intervention.

Alternatively, systemic infection may first present to the ophthalmologist due to the immense impact of visual dysfunction on an individual's daily activities. Impaired vision limits an individual's independence by decreasing mobility, impairing/preventing occupational capabilities, and preventing participation in recreational activities. Further, visual impairment renders the patient less capable of compliance with treatment regimens for systemic illness. Clearly, this represents a significant socioeconomic burden for both the individual and the healthcare system at large.

This chapter will discuss several systemic diseases that may be encountered by the ophthalmologist as a primary care provider or as a member of a multidisciplinary treatment team.

Lyme Disease

History

The first recorded case of Lyme borreliosis dates back to 1883 when Alfred Buchwald described its association with degenerative dermatologic findings (now termed acrodermatis chronica atrophincans).[1] The disease gained public interest in 1975, when Allen Steere reported a peculiar rash and swollen joints among 50 children in Lyme, Connecticut, which he erroneously termed 'Lyme arthritis,' believing it to be a form of juvenile rheumatoid arthritis.[2] On the insistence of two skeptical mothers, further research by Steere's group revealed a similarity between the children's rash and a lesion described in 1909 Europe, termed erythema migrans (EM).[3] The etiologic spirochete was eventually isolated from the *Ixodes dammini* tick in 1982 by Dr. Burgdofer. A causal relationship between *Borrelia burgdorferi* and Lyme disease was established when the organism was isolated from the blood and cerebrospinal fluid of patients with Lyme disease.[4]

Epidemiology

With 248074 cases reported in the United States between 1992 and 2006, and 27444 in 2007 alone, Lyme disease ranks as the most common vector-borne disease in the United States and Europe.[5] Incidence is highest among 5–14 year olds, with a slight male preponderance. Despite population admixture and the commonplace nature of travel, Lyme disease demonstrates a highly focused geographical distribution. The disease clusters in three distinct US regions: Northeast (Massachusetts, Maryland), Midwest (Minnesota, Wisconsin), and West (California, Oregon). While Lyme disease has been reported in all 50 states, 10 states account for 93% of all reported cases. Distinct seasonal patterns occur as well, with 87% of cases having their onset in the summer months.[6]

Transmission

Lyme disease is transmitted via the bite of the *Ixodes* tick infected with one of three spirochetes of the *Borrelia burgdorferi sensu lato* group. Variation within this group is thought to account for differing clinical manifestations reported in Europe, Asia, and the United States.[7] The *Ixodes* tick has a three-stage life cycle consisting of larval, nymph, and adult stages, the latter two being responsible for human infection.[8] Ninety percent of Lyme disease is transmitted by the nymph. The bite typically goes unnoticed due to the innocuous nature of the tiny nymph bite.[9] The remaining 10% of Lyme disease is transmitted by the conspicuous adult tick. Recognition and subsequent removal of the tick is critical to avoidance of Lyme disease, as the spirochete is not typically transmitted during the first 72 hours of tick attachment.[10]

Clinical manifestations

While Lyme disease is traditionally divided into three distinct stages, considerable overlap exists among stages, and they need not proceed chronologically.[11] Patients may present with stage 2 or 3 Lyme disease without a history of 'earlier' stage signs/symptoms.

Early localized (stage 1)

Early localized Lyme disease presents with the characteristic erythema migrans (EM) skin lesion along with a variety of nonspecific constitutional symptoms (fatigue, myalgias, arthralgias, headache, etc.).[12] EM develops in 60–80% of infected individuals within 1 month of the tick bite.[13] The rash begins as a warm pruritic red macule or papule that expands circumferentially over days to weeks, reaching a diameter of up to 20 cm.[11] Central clearing may produce a classic 'targetoid' appearance.[14] Spirochetemia may lead to multiple EM lesions, giving the false impression of multiple bites.[15] At this stage, *B. burgdorferi* can be cultured from peripheral blood; however, commercial culture is currently unavailable.[16] Identification and proper treatment of Lyme disease at this stage prevents progression to systemic manifestations described below.

Early disseminated (stage 2)

Weeks to months after transmission, dissemination of *B. burgdorferi* produces widespread signs and symptoms involving multiple organ systems. Neurologic involvement develops in 15% of affected individuals. The classic triad of neuroborreliosis includes meningitis, cranial neuropathy, and motor/sensory radiculoneuropathy.[17] Bell's palsy (CN VII) (unilateral or bilateral) is the most common cranial neuropathy, and most relevant to ophthalmologic evaluation.[18] Cardiac involvement occurs in 4–10% of untreated individuals, most often causing variable degrees of A-V block.[19] Myocarditis and pericarditis occur in a minority of patients.

Late (stage 3)

Months to years following infection, untreated individuals develop a chronic migratory oligoarthritis, most commonly involving the knees.[20] Joint swelling, pain, and inflammation may lead to permanent structural joint damage. Late neurologic sequelae include encephalopathy,[21] chronic polyneuropathy, and relapsing radiculopathy.[22]

Ocular manifestations

Conjunctivitis, which occurs in about 10% of infected individuals, is the most common ocular finding in Lyme disease.[23] Less common associations include keratitis, iridocyclitis, retinal vasculitis, choroiditis, uveitis, temporal arteritis, Horner's syndrome, pseudotumor cerebri, and optic nerve involvement.[24–31]

Early localized

Early Lyme disease may produce mild nonspecific follicular conjunctival inflammation.[24] Estimates suggest that conjunctivitis occurs in about 10% of affected individuals.[32] Given the mild nature of the inflammatory symptoms, this likely underestimates true incidence, as many patients do not seek ophthalmologic care at this stage.

Early disseminated

Stage 2 Lyme disease can present with a variety of ocular findings, ranging in severity, and is the most likely stage at which patients seek ophthalmologic care. Acute-onset CN VII neuropathy (Bell's palsy) is the most common neurologic manifestation of early disseminated Lyme disease, accounting for up to 25% of new-onset Bell's palsy in endemic regions.[17,18] One prospective study found CN VII palsy (one-quarter bilateral) in 10.6% of 951 patients diagnosed with Lyme disease.[33] Ninety-nine percent of these resolved spontaneously within 1 month. Diplopia, headache, and blurred vision may result secondary to involvement of cranial nerves III, IV, or VI. Among these, CN VI is most common, and dysfunction can be secondary to direct infection, inflammation, or increased intracranial pressure (ICP).[34] The possibility of increased ICP mandates optic nerve evaluation, and steroid treatment of 'idiopathic Bell's palsy' should proceed only after consideration of possible infection.[35] Optic nerve involvement (nerve swelling, optic neuritis, optic atrophy, papilledema, pseudotumor cerebri) presents with blurry vision and/or headache, and may be accompanied by symptoms of concurrent meningitis.[26,34]

Late stage 2/stage 3

A wide range of ocular inflammatory conditions can occur in late Lyme disease, the most common being keratitis, vitritis, and intermediate uveitis.[24,36–38] Keratitis typically presents years after initial infection with bilateral patchy immune-mediated stromal inflammation (Fig. 66.1).[37]

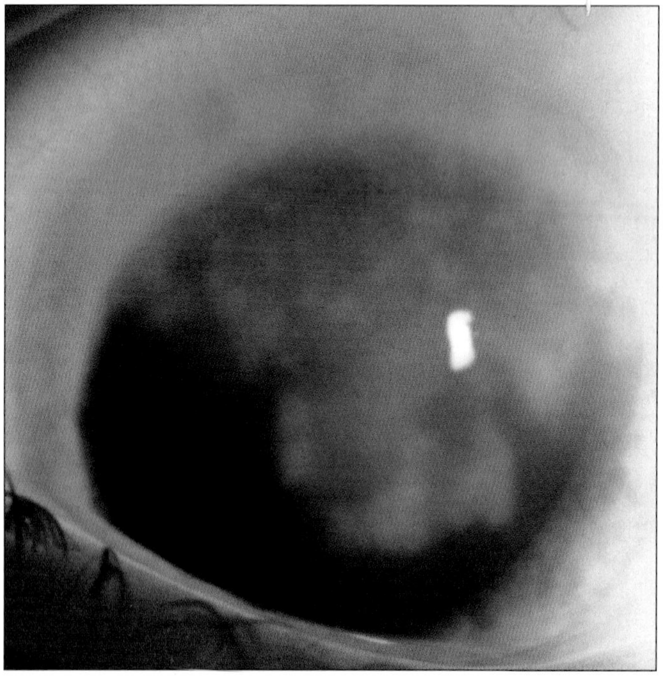

Fig. 66.1 Lyme disease. Caused by a spirochete (*Borrelia burgdorferi*), Lyme disease is transmitted by ticks. In the acute infection, patients develop fever, chills, malaise, and an enlarging red rash on the thighs, buttocks, or trunk (chronicum migrans). Months later, patients may experience a relapsing migratory polyarthritis. Patients may develop an interstitial keratitis characterized by multiple corneal infiltrates with indistinct borders in all levels of the stroma. Corneal vascularization is limited, and the conjunctiva is usually uninflamed. (From Krachmer JH, Palay DA (eds). Cornea Atlas, 2nd edn. Mosby, Elsevier Inc, 2005. Copyright Elsevier 2005).

Scattered nummular infiltrates are seen throughout the stroma, with intact overlying epithelium. Less common corneal findings in Lyme disease include peripheral keratitis, peripheral stromal edema, and an ulcerative interstitial keratitis.[37,39,40]

Intermediate uveitis (typically bilateral) is the most common posterior segment finding in Lyme disease.[41] Of diagnostic significance, mutton-fat keratic precipitates and posterior synechiae may be seen in Lyme-related intermediate uveitis, while these are atypical of alternate etiologies.[38] Progression of inflammation posteriorly may produce retinal vasculitis, choroiditis, exudative retinal detachment, vitreous hemorrhage, and branch retinal artery occlusion (BRAO).[9,42,43]

Diagnosis

Early localized

Because antibodies to *B. burgdorferi* appear at 1–2 weeks (IgM) and 2–6 weeks (IgG)[44] only 20–40% of patients presenting with early localized Lyme disease can be diagnosed serologically.[45] Therefore, early Lyme disease is a clinical diagnosis made by history of tick bite with exposure to an endemic region in the presence of erythema migrans. A detailed history is imperative as only 25% of patients recall a tick bite, and EM is frequently misdiagnosed as cellulitis, and inadequately treated.[11]

Early disseminated/late

Diagnosis of early disseminated and late-stage Lyme disease is made by compatible history together with confirmatory serologic testing. A two-tiered serologic approach is recommended;[46] however, given the high rate of false positives, a history consistent with Lyme disease is critical for diagnosis. The first step is a highly sensitive enzyme-linked immunosorbent assay (ELISA) (immunofluorescent assay [IFA] may be substituted), which, if positive or equivocal, is followed by a highly specific Western Blot. To be considered seropositive, both ELISA and Western Blot must be positive.[47]

Treatment of Lyme disease

Treatment of Lyme disease is directed by clinical presentation and organ system involvement, and should be co-managed with a neurologist, rheumatologist, cardiologist, or infectious disease specialist, as necessary.

Early localized

Patients presenting with erythema migrans (single or multiple lesions) and constitutional symptoms soon after contracting Lyme disease can be treated with a single course of oral antibiotics. Multiple randomized, controlled trials demonstrate equal efficacy of oral doxycycline, cefuroxime, or amoxicillin/probenecid. A single 3-week course achieves clinical resolution of symptoms in 90–95% of cases regardless of regimen chosen.[48,49] Doxycyline is considered first line, as it is also effective against the human pathogens *Anaplasma phagocytophilum*, and *Babesia microti*, commonly carried by *Ixoides* ticks infected with *B. burgdorferi*.[50,51] Signs and symptoms of infection typically resolve within 20 days among successfully treated individuals.[52] Of equal importance, successful treatment prevents progression to late Lyme disease, and its myriad sequelae.

Early disseminated

When neurologic or cardiac manifestations of Lyme disease are present, patients typically benefit from parenteral antibiotic therapy. Isolated facial nerve (CN VII) palsy is the exception. Patients with isolated CN VII palsy can be treated successfully with oral doxycycline.[33,53] Beyond this situation, intravenous antibiotics are indicated for central nervous system (CNS) or cardiac involvement. A 14-day course of IV ceftriaxone, cefotaxime, or penicillin G is recommended.[54]

Late

Ninety percent of late Lyme-associated arthritis with objective joint swelling resolves with a 28-day course of oral doxycycline or amoxicillin.[55] Cases of incomplete resolution are given a second course of oral antibiotics. Parenteral ceftriaxone is recommended for patients unresponsive to oral antibiotics.

Late neurological manifestations (encephalopathy, peripheral neuropathy, encephalomyelitis) are treated as per early disseminated neurological complications. In late disease, intravenous ceftriaxone is superior to penicillin G.[56]

Jarisch-Herxheimer reaction

Treating physicians should be aware that approximately 15% of patients develop transient worsening of symptoms following initiation of therapy as a result of massive spirochete death.[11,57] Steroids have been used to combat this reaction, but studies suggest steroid therapy may prolong disease course or result in treatment failure.[33,58]

Lyme disease prevention

Individuals at greatest risk for Lyme disease include those with occupational or recreational exposure to wooded areas in endemic regions (campers, hunters, hikers, forestry workers). In 1998, a vaccine was approved for Lyme disease prevention.[59] However, post-vaccination arthritis and neurologic concerns, compounded by poor sales, led to discontinuation of the vaccine in 2002.[60] At the present time, the best preventive methods include protective clothing, chemical repellants, and post-exposure screening of persons and pets.[61] Light-colored (improves tick visibility) long-sleeved shirts and pants reduce tick attachment by 40%. *N,N*-Diethyl-*meta*-toluamide (DEET)-containing repellants reduced tick exposure by 20% in a case-control study.[62] Post-exposure inspection and tick removal is important, as *B. burgdorferi* is rarely transmitted prior to 72 hours of tick attachment.[63] The Infectious Disease Society of America recommends antibiotic prophylaxis with single-dose doxycycline for patients meeting the following criteria: tick acquired in Lyme-endemic region, tick identified as *Ixodes*, attachment of tick >36 hours, treatment can be instituted with 72 hours of tick bite.[55]

Tuberculosis

Epidemiology

Tuberculosis (TB) is the number-one cause of infectious disease-related morbidity and mortality on the planet. Worldwide, it is estimated that 2 billion individuals are infected, with 2–3 million tuberculosis-related deaths occurring annually.[64] The disease reemerged as a worldwide threat in the wake of rising HIV infection rates during the 1980s.[65] While primarily a disease of indigent and malnourished regions, 13 293 cases of TB and 644 TB-related deaths were reported in the United States in 2007.[64] Fifty-eight percent of these cases were among foreign-born citizens. Risk factors include immune compromise, residence or travel to endemic regions, intravenous drug use, and low socioeconomic status.[65,66] While these numbers represent a trend toward decreased worldwide disease burden, continued efforts are needed to address this global disease.

Systemic tuberculosis overview

The causative organism of TB is the acid-fast *Mycobacterium tuberculosis*. Transmission occurs by airborne droplets acquired from an infected individual. In most cases, the infection is destroyed by an intact immune system, or rendered dormant and sequestered within bodily tissues. Reactivation of latent infection may occur years later following systemic insult resulting in relative immune compromise. The systemic manifestations of tuberculosis are myriad, and beyond the scope of this chapter. In general, TB should be suspected in at-risk individuals who present with fever, chills, weight loss, cough, and/or chest pain, which are common symptoms among patients with pulmonary TB.[67] Extrapulmonary TB presents with similar constitutional symptoms along with signs and symptoms reflecting the site of infection.

Ocular manifestations

The true incidence of ocular TB is unknown due to difficulty obtaining specimens, laborious microdiagnostic procedures, and inexact diagnostic criteria.[68] Estimates range from 1% to 18%, with higher incidence among HIV-infected individuals.[69]

External ocular involvement

Orbit

Orbital tuberculosis is more common among children than adults. It develops via direct extension from sinus disease or hematogenous dissemination. Often presenting as nonspecific inflammation or as a mass lesion akin to orbital pseudotumor, it may initially respond to steroid treatment.[70] Diagnosis requires biopsy-proven histopathology with AFB infiltration.

Eyelids

Eyelid involvement presents as a superficial infection, discrete abscess, or lupus vulgaris.[71] Superficial lesions may consist of a scaly plaque, subepithelial nodule, or ulcer.[72] Deeper involvement of the tarsus presents similar to chalazion, and suspicion of TB should prompt histopathologic examination of the specimen obtained on incision and curettage.

Lacrimal gland

Lacrimal gland tuberculosis most commonly presents as a nonspecific dacryoadenitis with or without abscess.[73] If risk factors exist, failure of empiric antibiotic treatment should prompt diagnostic biopsy.

Conjunctiva

Tuberculous conjunctivitis may appear as a subconjunctival nodule, ulcer, polyp, or firm, nonulcerative mass (tuberculoma).[71,74] Phlyctenulosis (discussed below) may involve the conjunctiva.

Cornea

Classically, phlyctenular keratoconjunctivitis has been associated with ocular tuberculosis. While TB remains the most common etiology of phlyctenule in endemic regions, many other causes exist. The lesion begins at the limbus as a small pink nodule with local hyperemia and a range of tearing, foreign body sensation, and photophobia (Fig. 66.2).[75,76] The phlyctenule progresses centrally with time, accompanied by superficial vascularization and eventual epithelial erosion with fluorescein staining.[77] The pathogenesis of phlyctenulosis is thought to be related to hypersensitivity to tuberculoproteins, rather than a direct effect of active disease.[68]

Corneal involvement may also present as interstitial keratitis (IK). As in phlyctenulosis, IK is postulated to be a

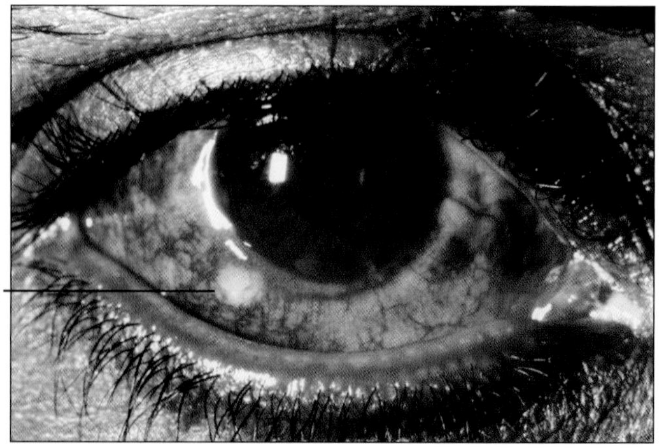

Fig. 66.2 Tuberculosis. Tuberculosis is caused by *Mycobacterium tuberculosis*. Many ocular manifestations of tuberculosis have been described, but the characteristic lesion is the conjunctival (*1*) or, in some cases, corneal phlyctenule. This is presumed to be an allergic hypersensitivity of the conjunctival or corneal epithelium to an endogenous toxin. (From Helm CJ, Holland GN. Ocular Tuberculosis. *Surv Ophthalmol* 38:229;1993. Copyright Elsevier 1993).

hypersensitivity reaction to *M. tuberculosis* antigen within the cornea. TB-associated interstitial keratitis is characterized by a unilateral, sectoral, peripheral stromal infiltrate with vascularization. Relative to interstitial keratitis seen in syphilis, TB-related IK tends to be more anterior and recur more often. Both IK and phlyctenular keratoconjunctivitis may be associated with anterior uveitis and regional lymphadenopathy.[77]

Sclera

Tuberculosis can present with nonspecific scleral inflammation, and should be included in the differential diagnosis of scleritis in a patient with risk factors.[78]

Intraocular involvement

Posterior segment

The earliest described case of intraocular tuberculosis was one of choroidal tubercle/tuberculoma, and the choroid remains the most common site of intraocular involvement.[79] Infection occurs by hematogenous dissemination, giving the organism a predilection for the high-flow choroid.[80] However, any aspect of the uveal tract may be involved. Tubercles appear as poorly defined, elevated, gray-white nodules with or without hemorrhage,[81] and may be associated with serous retinal detachment. Alternatively, a miliary pattern of choroidal involvement may be seen with multiple (up to 60) lesions scattered throughout the fundus.[80]

Retinal involvement is typically by extension from adjacent choroidal infection; however, cases of primary retinitis have been reported.[82] Isolated retinal vasculitis may be seen in patients with systemic tuberculosis.[83] Reports of optic nerve involvement include optic nerve tubercle, papillitis, papilledema, optic neuritis, retrobulbar neuritis, and neuroretinitis.[77]

Anterior segment

Tuberculosis has long been identified as an etiology of acute and/or chronic, typically unilateral, iridocyclitis. Patients present with visual deterioration and various levels of pain/irritation. Characteristic findings include granulomatous inflammation with mutton-fat keratic precipitates, iris nodules, posterior synechiae, and ciliary body inflammation/nodules.[77] Untreated, anterior chamber inflammation can progress to panophthalmitis, with eventual necrosis and scleral perforation.[84]

Diagnosis

Definitive diagnosis of orbital, adnexal, and external ocular tuberculosis is made via tissue biopsy and/or corneal scraping for culture and histopathological evaluation. Characteristic findings include caseating granulomatous inflammation with acid-fast bacillus organism infiltration.[72] Intraocular tuberculosis is most often diagnosed presumptively, based on characteristic ocular findings in a patient with systemic tuberculosis. Definitive diagnosis by chorioretinal biopsy has been reported,[85] but it is rarely performed, as treatment would likely proceed in the event of a negative result. Less invasive methods of establishing diagnosis include aqueous/vitreous fluid aspiration for culture, stain, and/or polymerase chain reaction for *Mycobacterium tuberculosis*.[86]

Treatment

Treatment of ocular tuberculosis is identical to systemic chemotherapy recommended for extraocular tuberculosis by current infectious disease literature. In addition, judicious topical corticosteroids are employed against inflammatory ocular manifestations.[87] Dosing is titrated to control ocular signs and symptoms. Co-administration of systemic corticosteroids together with standard chemotherapy is recommended for cases of tuberculous retinitis.[82]

Leprosy

Introduction

Long feared for its propensity to cause gross bodily dysmorphism, leprosy is an ancient disease, with its first recorded mention dating back to 600 BC.[88] Despite millennia of accrued knowledge, the disease remains marginally understood, and carries significant stigma among the lay public. However, recent advancements in therapeutic infrastructure have greatly improved prognosis among the afflicted, quelling fears and blunting associated social stigmata.

Epidemiology

While leprosy is found worldwide, in 2005, 75% of reported cases clustered in nine countries throughout Asia, Africa, and Latin America. Global efforts toward eradication of leprosy have achieved steady declines in overall disease burden and newly detected cases. The World Health Organization (WHO) reported global incidence of leprosy at 254 525 in 2007, a decrease from 763 262 in 2001. In the United States, 137 new cases of leprosy were detected in 2006, 85% of which occurred among immigrants.[89] The male to female ratio was 1.5 : 1. Risk factors for acquiring leprosy in the United States include exposure to infected individuals and travel to endemic areas. Cases of transmission from infected armadillos have been reported.[90]

Pathogenesis

Leprosy is caused by the obligate intracellular acid-fast bacillus (AFB) *Mycobacterium leprae*. The organism is slow-growing (12.5-day doubling time) and thrives in cool temperatures (<37°C), giving it a predilection for skin, cutaneous nerves, and respiratory mucous membranes.[91,92] *M. leprae* has never been cultured on artificial media, but an armadillo animal model exists. Other nonhuman primates have recently been reported as potential reservoirs of disease.[93]

Transmission

The definitive route of leprosy transmission has never been proven; however, respiratory droplets are most likely, given their high AFB content. Less commonly, the organism may be directly acquired through broken skin in the setting of trauma or infection.[94]

Classification

In 1998, the World Health Organization divided leprosy into two categories based on number of cutaneous lesions and AFB load. This system replaced the traditional tuberculoid and lepromatous classification scheme. Individuals with five or fewer skin lesions and low AFB load are said to have paucibacillary (PB) leprosy, while those with six or more lesions are termed multibacillary (MB). PB leprosy encompasses cases previously termed indeterminate, tuberculoid, and borderline tuberculoid leprosy, while MB leprosy includes midborderline, borderline lepromatous, and lepromatous leprosy.[88]

Clinical manifestations

Most immunocompetent individuals who contract *M. leprae* will never manifest clinical disease. Risk factors for development of clinical leprosy include intimate contact with an infected individual, impaired cellular immunity, old age, and possibly use of tumor necrosis factor (TNF) antagonists.[95,96]

Dermatologic

Cutaneous involvement varies from hypopigmented, erythematous macules with or without raised borders and desquamation, to frank granulomatous lesions. Peripheral nerve enlargement is common, and sensation varies from mild hypoesthesia to frank anesthesia.[97]

Ocular

Ocular leprosy is protean in its manifestation, and can involve any part of the eye or adnexa. Estimates of the incidence of ocular involvement among affected individuals range from 5% to 95%, with 5–15% of these resulting in blindness.[98] Ocular involvement is twice as common among those with MB leprosy.[99] Ocular manifestations of leprosy range from incidental to vision-threatening. Loss of vision results primarily from lagophthalmos, corneal hypoesthesia, iridocyclitis, and cataract. These processes cause potentially blinding sequelae in 20% of affected individuals despite successful treatment of systemic disease.[100]

Adnexa

Loss of eyelash and brow hair (madarosis) is a relatively benign ocular manifestation of early leprosy (Fig. 66.3).[101]

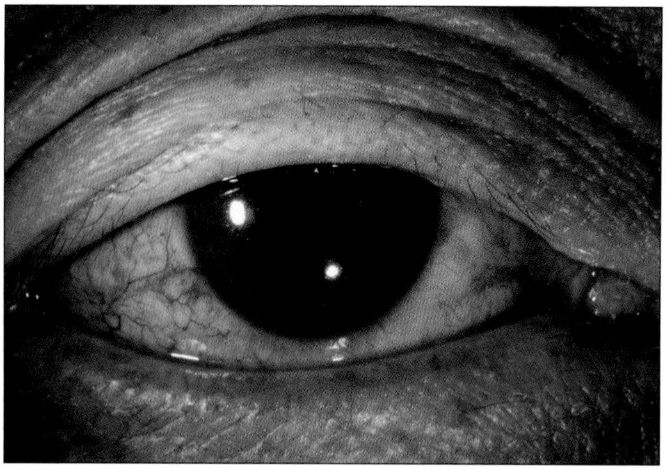

Fig. 66.3 Leprosy. Worldwide, it is estimated that there are six to eight million people with leprosy, with most cases occurring in Asia, Africa, and Latin America. The causative agent, *Mycobacterium leprae*, is an acid-fast bacillus that has a predilection for skin and peripheral nerves. Madarosis, loss of the eyelashes or eyebrows, is one of the earliest and most universal signs of leprosy. (From Krachmer JH, Palay DA (eds). Cornea Atlas, 2nd edn. Mosby, Elsevier Inc. 2005. Copyright Elsevier 2005).

Cornea

Lagophthalmos/corneal exposure

Facial nerve (CN VII) damage represents the most common leprosy-related threat to the cornea. Zygomatic and temporal branches are most commonly affected by leprous neuritis, resulting in lagophthalmos and lower lid ectropion.[102] This sets the stage for exposure keratopathy, secondary infectious keratitis, and possible endophthalmitis, producing devastating vision loss. Interestingly, onset of CN VII damage appears to depend on which class of leprosy predominates. One study reported 59% of PB patients developed lagophthalmos within 4 years of diagnosis, while 70% of MB patients remained unaffected until 10 years following diagnosis.[102,103] These data further emphasize the need for long-term follow-up of infected individuals.

Leprosy-related corneal hypoesthesia as a result of CN V damage is reported to occur in 8–60% of diseased individuals.[98,104,105] This complicates lagophthalmos via loss of the physiologic blink reflex. Studies demonstrate that patients with decreased corneal sensation have increased incidence of avascular keratitis, uveitis, iris atrophy, and blindness.[105]

Leprosy-related ocular surface disease is further amplified by tear film dysfunction. AFB and inflammatory cell infiltration of lacrimal and meibomian glands, and destruction of conjunctival goblet cells, leads to keratoconjunctivitis sicca. Clinical evidence of this process includes tear film instability (decreased tear break-up time) and decreased tear production as measured by Schirmer's testing.[106,107]

Management of leprosy-related ocular surface disease and lagophthalmos requires education of at-risk populations to ensure early detection and minimize complications. Individuals should be encouraged to blink regularly, inspect the cornea and lids for foreign bodies, and tape eyelids closed during sleep. Aggressive ocular lubrication is essential. Regarding lagophthalmos, one study demonstrated potential for medical intervention, with resolution of acute inflammatory CN VII-related lagophthalmos in 58% of patients treated with 6 months of oral steroids.[108] Surgical management studies are lacking, but in general, tarsorrhaphy and lateral eyelid shortening procedures are reasonable strategies, given the resources available in endemic regions.

Corneal infiltration

Corneal nerve opacification is an early asymptomatic, transitory manifestation of ocular leprosy. Acid-fast bacillus and

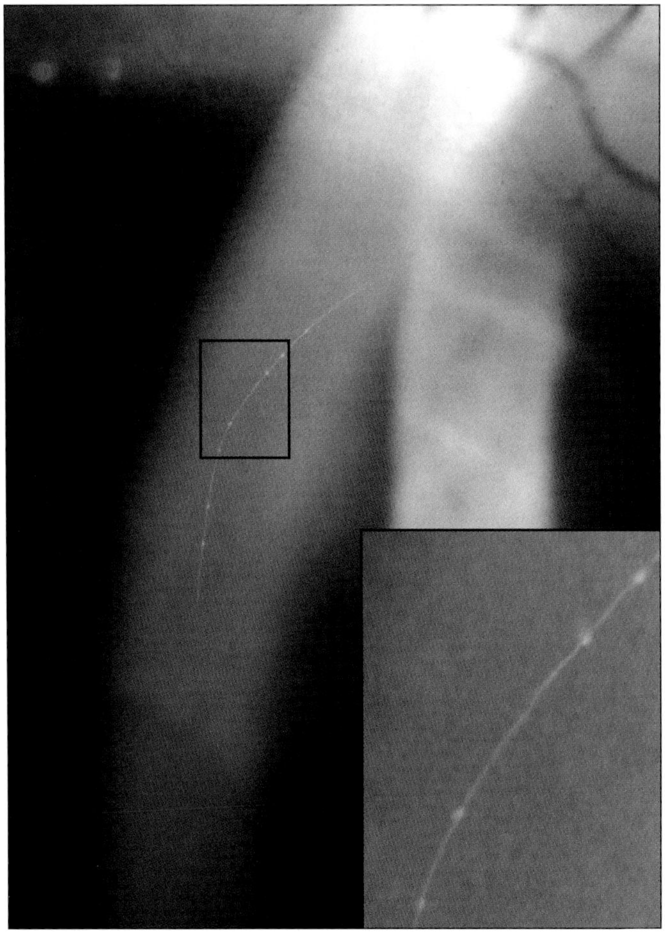

Fig. 66.4 Leprosy. Inflammation of the corneal nerves in leprosy causes the nerves to enlarge. There are focal areas of nerve beading (*inset*) from inflammatory cell aggregation near active bacillus. (From Krachmer JH, Palay DA (eds). Cornea Atlas, 2nd edn. Mosby, Elsevier Inc. 2005. Copyright Elsevier 2005).

inflammatory cell infiltration results in perineural edema, producing stromal opacification with a beaded nerve appearance (Fig. 66.4).[109] Nerve swelling begins in the superolateral quadrant due to its relatively low-temperature environment. With time, a diffuse gray-white inflammatory haze-termed avascular keratitis-develops in the anterior stroma, radiating centrally from the corneal periphery.[110] The diffuse stromal haze resolves with time, leaving punctate, white opacities ('chalk-dust' or 'flour-dust') composed of *M. leprae* deposits and focal cellular infiltration beneath Bowman's membrane (Fig. 66.5).[91,109] These lesions involve the entire stroma at the limbus, becoming progressively more superficial centrally.[111] Destruction of Bowman's membrane leads to limbal vessel ingrowth centrally between the epithelium and Bowman's membrane, producing a vascular pannus (Fig. 66.6).[112] Stromal vascularization can occur, producing a clinical picture similar to that seen in syphilis, although the process is more often sectoral in leprosy.[113]

Intraocular disease

Acute and/or chronic uveitis represent the most common intraocular manifestations of leprosy. The acute form typically presents shortly after institution of treatment with acute-onset anterior and/or posterior uveitis with hypopion and possible hyphema. A concomitant systemic hypersensitivity reaction termed erythema nodosum leprosum may occur, producing fever, joint pain, orchitis, and an erythematous macular rash.[114] More commonly, evidence of a chronic uveitic process including anterior and/or posterior synechiae, old keratic precipitates, posterior subcapsular cataract, and iris atrophy are found.[115] Iris pearls (lepromas) consisting of milky-white aggregates of *M. leprae*, epithelioid cells, and monocytes are classically associated with lepromatous chronic uveitis. These lesions have been reported throughout the iris, but most often near the papillary

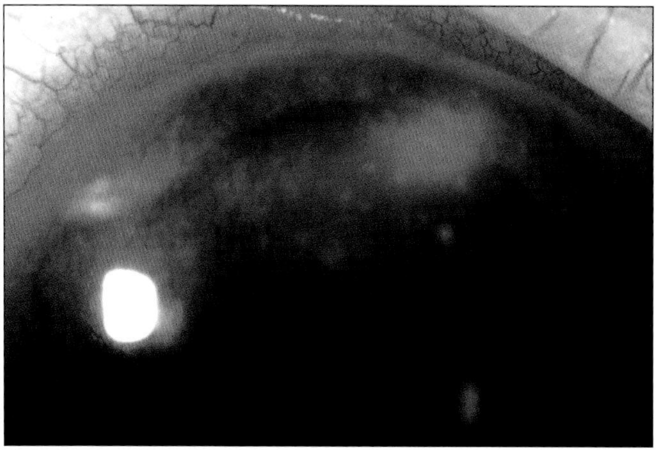

Fig. 66.5 Leprosy. The keratitis in leprosy usually begins in the superior temporal cornea. This is the coolest area of the cornea and the bacillus replicates better in a cooler environment. The inflammation is mostly subepithelial and the lesions have a chalky-white coloration. The initial inflammation is avascular. (From Krachmer JH, Palay DA (eds). Cornea Atlas, 2nd edn. Mosby, Elsevier Inc. 2005. Copyright Elsevier 2005).

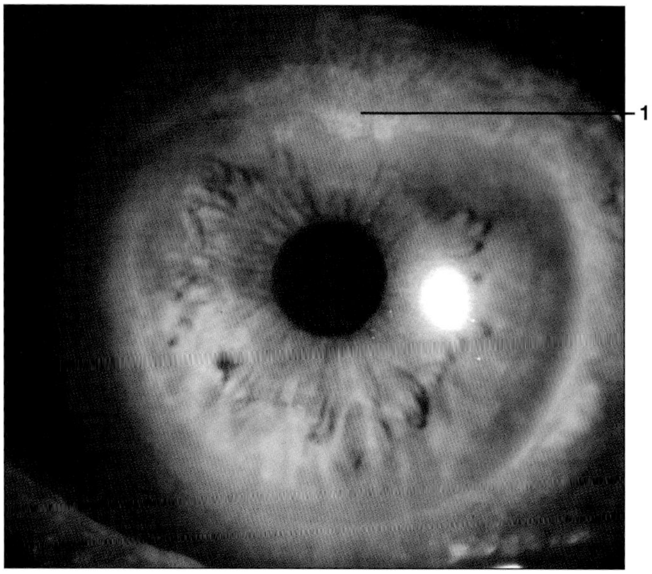

Fig. 66.6 Leprosy. With repeated bouts of inflammation there is destruction of Bowman's layer, and a superficial pannus develops. The pannus (*1*) begins in the superficial temporal cornea. Calcium deposition may also occur. (From Krachmer JH, Palay DA (eds). Cornea Atlas, 2nd edn. Mosby, Elsevier Inc. 2005. Copyright Elsevier 2005).

margin.[116] In addition, glaucoma may result as a late sequela of long-standing inflammation.

Diagnosis

Diagnosis of leprosy is made by physical examination of skin lesions with palpation for enlarged nerves, and sensory examination. Identified lesions can be biopsied for histopathologic diagnosis. Polymerase chain reaction (PCR) and antibody detection modalities are also available.[117,118]

Treatment

Treatment recommendations for leprosy are dependent on the form of disease present. Most patients are successfully managed with dapsone, rifampin, and clofazimine per infectious disease treatment recommendations.[88]

Brucellosis

Introduction

Brucellosis (also known as 'undulant fever,' 'Malta fever,' and 'Mediterranean fever') was first described by Martson in 1860. The causative organism was isolated in 1886 by Sir David Bruce, and in his honor the bacterium bears his name.[119,120]

The genus *Brucella* contains six species, of which four cause human disease. *B. melitensis* is the predominant human pathogen.[121] The small Gram-negative aerobic coccobacilli require special laboratory conditions for isolation.[122,123]

Epidemiology

Brucellosis causes human disease worldwide. Endemic areas include the Mediterranean basin, Arabian Gulf, India, Central and South America, and parts of Mexico.[124,125] One to two hundred cases are reported annually in the United States.[126] Infection occurs most commonly in California and Texas, which accounted for greater than 50% of reported cases between 1993 and 2002.[127] Humans acquire disease through several mechanisms. Transmission may occur while handling infected animal carcasses or placentas, via infected fluids contacting the conjunctiva, inhalation of infected aerosols, or ingestion of raw/unpasteurized milk or cheese.[124] Venereal transmission has been reported, but the data are inconclusive.[128] Finally, brucellosis is among the most commonly reported laboratory-acquired infections.[123]

Clinical manifestations

Clinical illness has variable presentation and course depending on the immune status and comorbidities of the infected individual, as well as the particular strain of *Brucella* causing infection.[129]

Systemic

Constitutional symptoms predominate early in brucellosis. More than 90% of symptomatic infections result in diurnal fever peaking in the afternoon, hence the term 'undulant fever.'[130] In addition, patients may present with fatigue, malaise, night sweats, anorexia, arthralgias, and weight loss.[125] Organ system involvement includes: articular (sacroiliitis) 20–30%,[131] genitourinary 2–40%,[131,132] neurologic (meningitis, papilledema, optic neuropathy, etc.) 1–2%,[133–135] endocarditis 1%, and hepatic abscess 1%.[131]

Ocular

Corneal involvement manifests as a uni- or bilateral nummular (coin-shaped) keratitis. Patients present with decreased vision, foreign body sensation, and photophobia. On examination, multiple 1–3-mm circular subepithelial and/or anterior stromal infiltrates are seen.[136] The lesions may ulcerate, but generally heal spontaneously, leaving a slight depression. These infiltrates are believed to be due to immune-mediated inflammation. *Brucella* has never been demonstrated histopathologically. Occasionally, sectoral corneal vascularization may occur.[136,137]

Uveitis (anterior, posterior, or intermediate) is the most common ocular manifestation of brucellosis. The inflammation can be granulomatous or nongranulomatous. With respect to the anterior segment, ocular involvement can present as an acute anterior uveitis with hypopion. The inflammation is responsive to topical steroids, and may clear spontaneously.[130]

Diagnosis

Given that brucellosis most often presents with nonspecific symptoms, a focused history is imperative to establish a diagnosis. Specific questioning regarding occupational exposure, travel, and raw meat or milk product consumption is important. One should suspect the disease in an at-risk individual with unexplained chronic fever and nonspecific constitutional symptoms. Serology and blood/tissue culture are helpful in the acute stages, with 80% positivity early in disease.[138] As disease becomes chronic, laboratory testing and organism isolation become difficult.[139] Because of the special laboratory conditions necessary for isolation, lab personnel should be alerted to the suspicion of brucellosis. Combination PCR–ELISA testing for *Brucella* appears to be a highly sensitive and specific method for diagnosis.[140]

Treatment

Many treatment regimens have been described, none of which is 100% effective, and 10% of patients suffer relapses. First-line treatment includes co-administration of oral doxycycline and rifampin for 6 weeks. For severe cases involving the CNS, 3 weeks of intramuscular streptomycin or gentamicin combined with 6 weeks of oral doxycycline is recommended.[141]

Onchocerciasis

Introduction

Identified in 1891 by Rudolph Leuckart, onchocerciasis is a chronic parasitic infection caused by the filarial nematode *Onchocerca volvulus*.[142] Worldwide, it represents a major cause of skin disease and visual impairment. The moniker 'river blindness' is associated with the disease because the

Simulium black fly vector lives and breeds near rivers and fast-moving streams.[143]

Epidemiology

It is estimated that roughly 18 million people are infected with *O. volvulus* worldwide, 99% of whom reside in sub-Saharan Africa. Of these individuals, 3–4 million manifest skin disease, while 1–2 million suffer visual impairment and/or blindness.[143,144] Two distinct *O. volvulus* strains exist in Africa. Those breeding in the savanna are more commonly associated with ocular morbidity.[145] Infection rates peak around 20 years of age; however, clinical symptoms lag infection, with visual impairment occurring 20–30 years later.[142,143] Individuals blinded by onchocerciasis have a fourfold increased risk of mortality and life expectancy is reduced by 7–12 years.[142]

Life cycle

O. volvulus larvae are transmitted into human skin via the bite of *Simulium* black fly. They require 6–12 months to mature into adult form. Female worms (20–80 cm) live in subcutaneous tissues, isolated from the immune system within fibrous capsules. Males (3–5 cm) migrate among these nodules to fertilize females.[146] Ten to twelve months following fertilization, females produce microfilariae (1000–3000/day), which migrate subcutaneously, where they may be picked up by a *Simulium* fly feeding on an infected human, completing the life cycle.[147]

Pathogenesis

Adult worms are isolated from the immune system, encapsulated within fibrous subcutaneous/intramuscular nodules, while microfilariae migrate though subcutaneous and ocular tissues. Clinical signs/symptoms manifest following microfilarial death, which incites variable degrees of inflammatory response. Intensity of the inflammation depends on microfilarial burden, host immune factors, and duration of disease.[146,148–150] In addition, release of antigens from the common bacterial endosymbiont *Wolbachia* may exacerbate the inflammatory response.[151]

Clinical manifestations

Infection with *O. volvulus* manifests as dermatologic and ocular disease. Given the scope of this chapter, we will focus on the ocular findings, providing only a brief outline of the dermatologic manifestations.

Dermatologic

Subcutaneous nodule

Harboring adult worms, these 0.5–3.0-cm firm nodules ('onchocercoma') are typically asymptomatic, as they are not associated with inflammation.[152]

Dermatitis

Inflammation resulting from microfilarial death causes an intensely pruritic papulonodular rash in 50% of infected individuals living in endemic areas.[149] Cutaneous excoriation frequently leads to secondary bacterial infection and lymphadenopathy. Chronic lymphatic obstruction results from fibrosis of enlarged nodes, producing elephantiasis.[153] The dermatitis is further subdivided into acute, chronic, lichenified, and atrophic forms.[154]

Ocular

Ocular disease most often results upon migration of microfilariae from periocular skin into the conjunctiva. Thereafter, the organism may penetrate posteriorly, affecting any ocular structure, save the lens.[155] Alternatively, the organism may gain access to the posterior segment via ciliary vessels and/or nerves.[156] Live microfilariae can cause intense pruritus, while their death results in inflammation and fibrotic scarring. Reported ocular sequelae include conjunctivitis, keratitis, uveitis, chorioretinitis, and optic neuritis.[142,157]

Anterior segment

Migration of microfilariae into the conjunctiva is heralded by conjunctival inflammation with injection, chemosis, and limbal-based phlyctenular lesions. Irritation, lacrimation, and foreign body sensation may be present, but without corneal involvement these symptoms are minimal.

Corneal manifestations

Entrance of *O. volvulus* microfilariae into the cornea initially results in a reversible punctate keratitis termed 'snowflake opacity.' These opacities are 0.5–1.5 mm in diameter, located in temporal and nasal corneal stroma with intact overlying epithelium (Fig. 66.7).[158] Clinically, there is little associated inflammation. Histologically, these opacities represent focal infiltration of neutrophils and eosinophils in response to microfilarial invasion.[159,160] Untreated, the condition progresses to an irreversible sclerosing keratitis[161] with infiltration of sensitized neutrophils (T cells) and eosinophils beneath Bowman's membrane.[162–164] The inflammatory infiltrate begins in the corneal periphery and proceeds centrally. Chronic infection results in stromal opacification and neovascularization with ingress of a fibrovascular pannus.[165] Ultimately, fibrotic and degenerative stromal changes result in stromal opacification and vision loss (Fig. 66.8).[160–163] Inflammation may proceed posteriorly to involve the anterior and posterior chambers, resulting in chorioretinitis, subretinal fibrosis, optic neuritis, optic atrophy, glaucoma, and blindness.[142,157,166–168]

Diagnosis

Diagnosis of systemic onchocerciasis is made by history of exposure to endemic areas, characteristic dermatologic and/or ocular manifestations, and supportive laboratory markers.

Serology

Complete blood count (CBC) classically demonstrates peripheral eosinophilia and/or hypergammaglobulinemia. However, studies have shown CBC to be normal in up to 30% of infected individuals in endemic regions.[169]

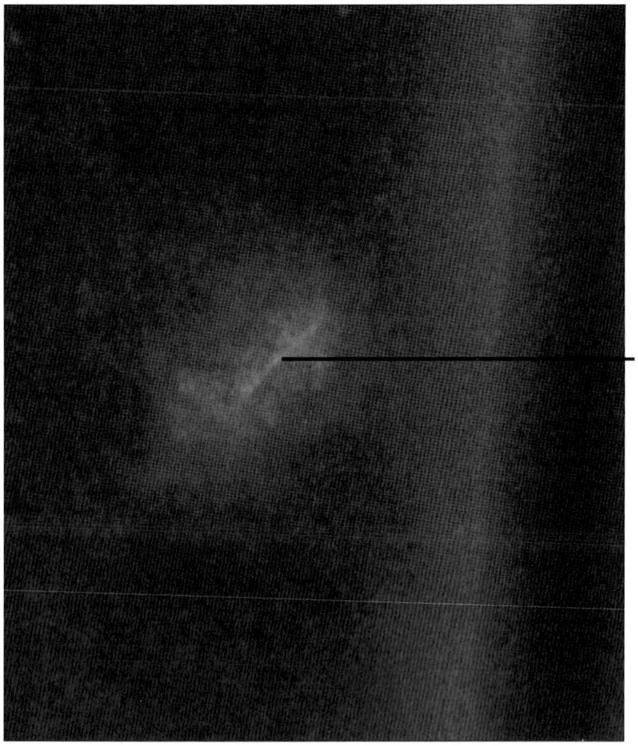

Fig. 66.7 Onchocerciasis. Onchocerciasis or 'river blindness' is a parasitic infection caused by the nematode *Onchocerca volvulus*, which is spread between human hosts by the *Simulium* black fly. Once established in the host, the worm produces 10 000 microfilariae a day. These microfilariae spread throughout the body, causing an intense host inflammatory reaction. Seen here is an inflammatory reaction surrounding dead microfilariae (*1*) in the cornea. (From Krachmer JH, Palay DA (eds). Cornea Atlas, 2nd edn. Mosby, Elsevier Inc, 2005. Copyright Elsevier 2005).

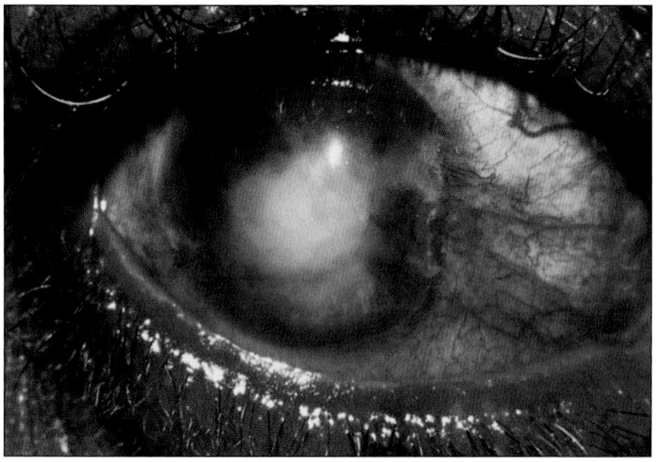

Fig. 66.8 Onchocerciasis. In patients with high skin counts of disease, blindness results from corneal scarring. Shown here is sclerosing keratitis of the cornea. This inflammation begins peripherally and spreads centrally as a reaction to dead microfilariae. (From Krachmer JH, Palay DA (eds). Cornea Atlas, 2nd edn. Mosby, Elsevier Inc, 2005. Copyright Elsevier 2005).

Skin snip

Biopsy of dermatologic lesions can be performed with a needle or corneoscleral punch for staining and evaluation for motile microfilariae.[170] While highly specific, this method has a high false-negative rate during early infection with low worm burden.[171]

Slit lamp examination

Direct visualization of *O. volvulus* microfilariae circulating in the anterior chamber and/or vitreous is possible when present.[172] To maximize the chance of visualization, the patient should be face down with the head in a dependent position (e.g. head between knees) for approximately 5 minutes prior to examination to bring microfilariae behind the central cornea.

Mazzotti test

Diethylcarbamazine, given as a topical patch or orally, results in an inflammatory reaction following microfilarial death among infected individuals. Pruritus developing 3–24 hours after administration is considered diagnostic of onchocerciasis. Sensitivity is greater than 90%.[173] However, as severe systemic reactions can occur, this test has fallen out of favor, and should be performed only after negative skin snip and eye examination with continued clinical suspicion.

Antigen testing

Detection of *O. volvulus* antigen has shown diagnostic promise with reported sensitivities of 92% for serum,[174] 86% for urine, 96% for tears, and 100% for skin, along with excellent specificity.[175] A dipstick antigen detection assay demonstrated 92% sensitivity for tears and 100% for skin, with 100% specificity.[176] These tests have the advantage of being positive only during active disease, while serologic antibody studies may remain positive as a result of past infection.[177] Unfortunately, at the current time, these antigen kits are unavailable for clinical use.

Ultrasonography

Ultrasound of subcutaneous nodules can aid in diagnosis by detection of adult worms within the nodules.[178] The organism can thereafter be removed and studied for diagnostic speciation. Ultrasound has also been used for following treatment to confirm death of adult worms within subcutaneous nodules.[179]

Treatment

Ivermectin is the drug of choice for treatment of onchocerciasis.[178] It inhibits release of microfilariae from female worms and has some antihelmenthic activity, but will not eradicate infection.[180] Microfilarial load is reduced by 85–95% 1 week after a single dose.[181] Ivermectin is given as a single oral dose every 6 months until the patient is asymptomatic, which may require treatment for more than 10 years.[182]

Loa loa coinfection

Administration of ivermectin to patients coinfected with *Loa loa* may result in serious neurologic issues by facilitating entrance of the worm into the CNS.[183] Therefore, in areas endemic for *Loa loa*, evaluation for coinfection is imperative prior to treatment.

Wolbachia coinfection

Doxycycline is effective against the common endosymbiont *Wolbachia*, and can eradicate the bacteria with 6 weeks of oral therapy.[184] To minimize inflammation secondary to release of the *Wolbachia* following microfilarial death, doxycycline pretreatment is advisable prior to institution of ivermectin therapy.[185]

References

1. Herxheimer K, Hartmann K. Uber Acrodermatitis chronica atrophicans. *Arch Derm Syph*. 1902;(61):57–76, 255–300.
2. Steere AC. *Borrelia burgdorferi* (Lyme disease, Lyme borreliosis). In: Bennett JC, Dolin R, Mandell GL, eds. *Principles and practice of infections diseases*. 4th ed. New York: Churchill Livingstone; 1994.
3. Burgdorfer W, Barbour AG, Hayes SF, et al. Lyme disease – a tick born spirochetosis? *Science*. 1982;(216):1317–1319.
4. Preac-Murisic V, et al. Repeated isolation of spirochetes from the cerebrospinal fluid of a patient with meningoradiculitis. *Eur J Clin Microbiol*. 1984;(3):564–565.
5. Bacon R, Kugeler K, Mead P. Surveillance for Lyme disease – United States 1992–2006. *MMWR*. 2008;57(SS10):1–9.
6. Centers for Disease Control. Lyme desease – United States, 2003–2005. *MMWR*. CDC; 2007.
7. Pachner AR, et al. Genotype determines phenotype in experimental Lyme borreliosis. *Ann Neurol*. 2004 Sep;56(3):361–370.
8. Spielman A. The emergence of Lyme disease and human babesiosis in a changing environment. *Ann NY Acad Sci*. 1994;(740):146–156.
9. Zaidman GW. The ocular manifestations of Lyme disease. *Int Ophthalmol Clin*. 1993;(33):9–22.
10. Nadelman RB, et al. Prophylaxis with single-dose doxycycline for the prevention of Lyme disease after an *Ixodes scapularis* tick bite. *N Engl J Med*. 2001;2(345):79–84.
11. Steere AC. Lyme Disease. *N Engl J Med*. 1989;9(321):586–596.
12. Nadelman RB, Nowakowski J, Forseter G, et al. The clinical spectrum of early Lyme borreliosis in patients with culture-confirmed erythema migrans. *Am J Med*. 1996;100(5):502–508.
13. Steere AC, et al. Lyme arthritis: an epidemic of oligoarticular arthritis in children and adults in three Connecticut communities. *Arthritis Rheum*. 1977;20(1):7–17.
14. Smith RP, et al. Clinical characteristics and treatment outcome of early Lyme disease in patients with microbiologically confirmed erythema migrans. *Intern Med*. 2002;136(6):421–428.
15. Wormser GP, et al. J Brief communication: hematogenous dissemination in early Lyme disease. *Ann Intern Med*. 2005;142(9):751–755.
16. Berger BW, et al. Isolation and characterization of the Lyme disease spirochete from the skin of patients with erythema chronicum migrans. *J Am Acad Dermatol*. 1985;13:444–449.
17. Pachner AR, Steere AC. The triad of neurologic manifestations of Lyme disease: meningitis, cranial neuritis, and radiculoneuritis. *Neurology*. 1985;35:47–53.
18. Halperin JJ. Nervous system lyme disease. *Infect Dis Clin North Am*. 2008;22(2):261–274.
19. McAlister HF, et al. Lyme carditis: an important cause of reversible heart block. *Ann Intern Med*. 1989;110(5):339–345.
20. Steere AC, Schoen RT, Taylor E. The clinical evolution of Lyme arthritis. *Ann Intern Med*. 1987;107(5):725–731.
21. Logigian EL, Kaplan RF, Steere AC. Chronic neurologic manifestations of Lyme disease. *N Engl J Med*. 1990;323(21):1438–1444.
22. Logigian EL, Steere AC. Clinical and electrophysiologic findings in chronic neuropathy of Lyme disease. *Neurology*. 1992;42(2):303–311.
23. Steere AC, et al. The early clinical manifestation of Lyme disease. *Ann Intern Med*. 1988;99:76.
24. Flach AJ, Lavoie PE. Episcleritis, conjunctivitis, and keratitis as ocular manifestations of Lyme disease. *Ophthalmology*. 1990;97:973–975.
25. Pachner AR. Spirochetal disease of the CNS. *Neurol Clin*. 1986;4:207–222.
26. Farris BK, Webb RM. Lyme disease and optic neuritis. *J Clin Neuro-Ophthalmol*. 1988;8:73–78.
27. Jacobson DM, Frens DB. Pseudotumor cerebri syndrome associated with Lyme disease. *Am J Ophthalmol*. 1989;107:81–82.
28. Pizzarello LD, et al. Temporal arteritis associated with *Borrelia* infection: a case report. *J Clin Neuro-Ophthalmol*. 1989;9:3–6.
29. Schechter SL. Lyme disease associated with optic neuropathy. *Am J Med*. 1986;81:143–145.
30. Glauser TA, Brennan PJ, Galetta SI. Reversible Horner's syndrome and Lyme disease. *J Clin Neuro-Ophthalmol*. 1989;9:225–228.
31. Stanek G, Strle F. Lyme borreliosis. *Lancet*. 2003;362(9396):1639–1647.
32. Lesser RL. Ocular manifestations of Lyme disease. *Am J Med*. 1995; 98:605–625.
33. Clark JR, et al. Facial paralysis in Lyme disease. *Laryngoscope*. 1985; 95:1341–1345.
34. Lesser RL, Kornmehl EW, Pachmer AR, et al. Neuroophthalmologic manifestations of Lyme disease. *Ophthalmology*. 1990;97:609–706.
35. Lesser R. Ocular manifestations of Lyme disease. *Am J Med*. 1995;98: 60–62.
36. Orlin SE, Lauffer JL. Lyme disease keratits. *Am J Ophthalmol*. 1988; 107:678–680.
37. Baum J, et al. Bilateral keratitis as a manifestations of Lyme disease. *Am J Ophthalmol*. 1988;105:75–77.
38. Winward KE, et al. Ocular Lyme borreliosis. *Am J Ophthalmol*. 108: 651–657.
39. Deluise VP, O'Leary MJ. Peripheral ulcerative keratitis related to Lyme. *Am J Ophthalmol*. 1991;111:244–245.
40. Miyashiro MJ, Yee RW, Patel G, Ruiz RS. Lyme disease associated with. *Cornea*. 1999;18:115–116.
41. Bergloff J, Gasser R, Feigl B. Ophthalmic manifestations in Lyme borreliosis. A review. *J Neuroophthalmol*. 1994;14(1):15–20.
42. Bialasiewicz AA, et al. Bilateral diffuse chorioditis and exudative retinal. *Am J Ophthalmol*. 1988;105:419–420.
43. Mikkila HO, et al. The expanding clinical spectrum of ocular lyme borreliosis. *Ophthalmology*. 2000;107(3):581–587.
44. Steere AC, et al. Prospective study of serologic tests for lyme disease. *Clin Infect Dis*. 2008;47(2):188–195.
45. Nowakowski J, et al. Laboratory diagnostic techniques for patients with early Lyme disease associated with erythema migrans: a comparison of different techniques. *Clin Infect Dis*. 2001;33(12):2023–2027.
46. CDC. Recommendations for test performance and interpretation from the Second National Conference on Serologic Diagnosis of Lyme Disease. MMWR. Centers for Disease Control; 1995.
47. Brown SL, Hansen SL, Langone JJ. Role of serology in the diagnosis of Lyme disease. *JAMA*. 1999;282(1):62–66.
48. Dattwyler RJ, et al. Amoxycillin plus probenecid versus doxycycline for treatment of erythema migrans borreliosis. *Lancet*. 1990;336(8728): 1404–1406.
49. Luger SW, et al. Comparison of cefuroxime axetil and doxycycline in treatment of patients with early Lyme disease associated with erythema migrans. *Antimicrob Agents Chemother*. 1995;39(3):661–667.
50. Swanson SJ, Neitzel D, Reed KD. Coinfections acquired from *Ixodes* ticks. *Clin Microbiol Rev*. 2006;19(4):708–727.
51. Steere AC, et al. Prospective study of coinfection in patients with erythema migrans. *Clin Infect Dis*. 2003;36(8):1078–1081.
52. Luft BJ, et al. Azithromycin compared with amoxicillin in the treatment of erythema migrans. A double-blind, randomized, controlled trial. *Ann Intern Med*. 1996;124(9):785–791.
53. Dotevall L, Hagberg L. Successful oral doxycycline treatment of Lyme disease-associated facial palsy and meningitis. *Clin Infect Dis*. 1999; 28(3):569–574.
54. Halperin JJ, et al. Practice parameter: treatment of nervous system Lyme disease (an evidence-based review): report of the Quality Standards Subcommittee of the American Academy of Neurology. *Neurology*. 2007;69(1):91–102.
55. Wormser GP, et al. The clinical assessment, treatment, and prevention of lyme disease, human granulocytic anaplasmosis, and babesiosis: Clinical Practice Guidelines by the Infectious Diseases Society of America. *Clin Infect Dis*. 2006;43(9):1089–1134.
56. Halperin JJ, et al. Practice parameter: treatment of nervous system Lyme disease (an evidence-based review): report of the Quality Standards Subcommittee of the American Academy of Neurology. *Neurology*. 2007;69(1):91–102.
57. Luger SW, et al. Comparison of cefuroxime axetil and doxycycline in treatment of patients with early Lyme disease associated with erythema migrans. *Antimicrob Agents Chemother*. 1995;39(3):661–667.

58. Kalish RA, et al. Evaluation of study patients with Lyme disease, 10–20-year follow-up. *J Infect Dis.* 2001;183(3):453–460.
59. Steere AC, Sikand VK, Meurice F, et al. Vaccination against Lyme disease with recombinant *Borrelia burgdorferi* outer-surface lipoprotein A with adjuvant. *N Engl J Med.* 1998;339:209–215.
60. The Pink Sheet, FDC Reports, Inc. *FDA Lymerix study to test potential genetic marker for adverse events.* Chevy Chase, Maryland; 2001.
61. Hayes EB, Piesman J. How can we prevent Lyme disease? *N Engl J Med.* 2003;348(24):24–30.
62. Vazquez M, et al. Effectiveness of personal protective measures to prevent Lyme disease. *Emerg Infect Dis.* 2008;14(2):210–216.
63. CDC. Lyme disease knowledge, attitudes, and behaviors. *MMWR Morb Mortal Wkly Rep.* 1992;41(28):505–507.
64. Pratt R, Robison V, Navin T. Trends in tuberculosis – United States, 2007. *MMWR Morb Mortal Wkly Rep.* 2008;57(11):281–285.
65. Schneider E, Moore M, Castro KG. Epidemiology of tuberculosis in the United States. *Clin Chest Med.* 2005;26(2):183–195.
66. Maher D, Raviglione M. Global epidemiology of tuberculosis. *Clin Chest Med.* 2005;26(2):167–182.
67. Tead WW, Kerby GR, Schlueter DP, Jordahl CW. The clinical spectrum of primary tuberculosis in adults. Confusion with reinfection in the pathogenesis of chronic tuberculosis. *Ann Intern Med.* 1968;68:731.
68. Helm CJ, Holland GN. Ocular tuberculosis. *Surv Ophthalmol.* 1993; 38(3):229–256.
69. Beare NA, et al. Ocular disease in patients with tuberculosis and HIV presenting with fever in Africa. *Br J Ophthalmol.* 2002;86(10):1076–1079.
70. Madge D, Prabhakaran SN, Shome VC, et al. Orbital tuberculosis: a review of the literature. *Orbit.* 2008;27(4):267–277.
71. Cook CD, Hainsworth M. Tuberculosis of the conjunctiva occurring in association with a neighbouring lupus vulgaris lesion. *Br J Ophthalmol.* 1990;74(5):315–316.
72. Dinning WJ, Marston S. Cutaneous and ocular tuberculosis: a review. *J R Soc Med.* 1985;78:576.
73. Madhukar K, et al. Tuberculosis of the lacrimal gland. *J Trop Med Hyg.* 1991;94(3):150–151.
74. Singh I, Chaudhary U, Arora B. Tuberculoma of the conjunctiva. *J Indian Med Assoc.* 1989;87:265.
75. Philip RN, Comstock GW, Shelton JH. Phlyctenular keratoconjunctivitis among Eskimos in southwestern Alaska. *Am Rev Respir Dis.* 1965; 91:171–187.
76. Sheu SJ, Shyu JS, Chen LM, et al. Ocular manifestations of tuberculosis. *Am J Ophthalmol.* 2001;108:1580–1585.
77. Thompson MJ, Albert DM. Ocular tuberculosis. *Arch Ophthalmol.* 2005;123:844–849.
78. Nanda M, Pflugfelder SC, Holland S. *Mycobacterium tuberculosis* scleritis. *Am J Ophthalmol.* 1989;108(6):736–737.
79. Tejada P, Mendez MJ, Negreira S. Choroidal tubercles with tuberculous meningitis. *Int Ophthalmol.* 1994;18(2):115–118.
80. Fernández CC, Garcia JJ, Moro BD, et al. Choroidal tubercles in miliary tuberculosis. *Arch Soc Esp Oftalmol.* 2000;75:355–358.
81. Shiono T, Abe S, Horiuchi T. A case of miliary tuberculosis with disseminated choroidal haemorrhages. *Br J Ophthalmol.* 1990;74(5):317–319.
82. Saini JS, Mukherjee AK, Nadkarni N. Primary tuberculosis of the retina. *Br J Ophthalmol.* 1986;70:533–535.
83. Reny JL, et al. Tuberculosis-related retinal vasculitis in an immunocompetent patient. *Clin Infect Dis.* 1996;22(5):873–874.
84. McMoli TE, et al. Tuberculous panophthalmitis. *J Pediatr Ophthalmol Strabismus.* 1978;15(6):383–385.
85. Barondes MJ, Sponsel WE, Stevens TS, Plotnik RD. Tuberculous choroiditis diagnosed by chorioretinal endobiopsy. *Am J Ophthalmol.* 1991; 112:460.
86. Ortega-Larrocea G, et al. Nested polymerase chain reaction for *Mycobacterium tuberculosis* DNA detection in aqueous and vitreous of patients with uveitis. *Arch Med Res.* 2003;34(2):116–119.
87. Rohatgi J, Dhaliwal U. Phlyctenular eye disease: a reappraisal. *Jpn J Ophthalmol.* 2000;44:146–150.
88. WHO Expert Committee on Leprosy. *Seventh Report. WHO Tech Rep Ser No 874.* Geneva: World Health Organization; 1998.
89. *Weekly epidemiological record – Global leprosy situation, beginning of 2008.* World Health Organization; 2008. Report No.: 33.
90. *Progress towards leprosy elimination.* World Health Organization; 1998.
91. Gelber RH. Leprosy (Hansen's disease). In: Bennett JC, Dolin R, Mandell GL, eds. *Principles and practice of infectious disease.* 4th ed. New York: Churchill Livingstone; 1994.
92. Schwab IR, et al. Leprosy in a trachomatous population. *Arch Ophthalmol.* 1984;69:24–244.
93. Valverde CR, et al. Spontaneous leprosy in a wild-caught cynomolgus macaque. *Int J Lepr Other Mycobact Dis.* 1998;66(2):140–148.
94. Abraham S, et al. Epidemiological significance of first skin lesion in leprosy. *Int J Lepr Other Mycobact Dis.* 1998;66(2):131–139.
95. Keane J, Gershon S, Wise RP, et al. Tuberculosis associated with infliximab, a tumor necrosis factor-neutralizing agent. *N Engl J Med.* 2001;345: 1098–1104.
96. van Beers SM, Hatta M, Klatser PR. Patient contact is the major determinant in incident leprosy: implications for future control. *Int J Lepr Other Mycobact Dis.* 1997;67(2):119–128.
97. Lawn SD, Lockwood DN. Leprosy after starting antiretroviral treatment. *BMJ.* 2007;334:217.
98. Dana MR, et al. Ocular manifestations of leprosy in a noninstitutionalized community in the United States. *Arch Ophthalmol.* 1994;112: 626–629.
99. Courtright P, Lewallen S. Ocular manifestations of leprosy. In: Minassian DC, Weale RA, Johnson GJ, et al, eds. *The epidemiology of eye disease.* London: Arnold; 2003:306–317.
100. Lewallen S, Tungpakom NC, Kim SH, Courtright P. Progression of eye disease in 'cured' leprosy patients: implications for understanding the pathophysiology of ocular disease and for addressing eyecare needs. *Br J Ophthalmol.* 2000;84(4):817–821.
101. Choyce DP. Diagnosis and management of ocular leprosy. *Br J Ophthalmol.* 1969;53:217–223.
102. Courtright P, Lewallen S, Li HY, et al. Lagophthalmos in a multibacillary population under multidrug therapy in the Peoples Republic of China. *Lepr Rev.* 1995;66:214–219.
103. Yan LB, Chang GD, Li WZ. Analysis of 2114 cases of lagophthalmos in leprosy. *China Lepr J.* 1993;9:6–8.
104. Tcho U, Sira IB. Ocular leprosy in Malawi: clinical and therapeutic survery of 8325 leprosy patients. *Br J Ophthalmol.* 1970;54:107–112.
105. Karacorlu MA, Cakiner T, Saylan T. Corneal sensitivity and correlations between decreased sensitivity and anterior segment pathology in ocular leprosy. *Br J Ophthalmol.* 1991;75:117–119.
106. Saint Andre A, Blackwell NM, Hall LR, et al. Pathogenesis of dry eye in leprosy and tear functions. *Int J Lepr Other Mycobact Dis.* 2001;69(3): 215–218.
107. Lamba PA, Rohatgi J, Bose S. Factors influencing corneal involvement in leprosy. *Int J Leprosy.* 1987;55:667–671.
108. Kiran KU, Hogeweg M, Suneetha S. Treatment of recent facial nerve damage with lagophthalmos, using a semistandardized steroid regimen. *Lepr Rev.* 1991;62:150–154.
109. Allen JH, Byers JL. The pathology of ocular leprosy: cornea. *Arch Ophthalmol.* 1960;64:80–84.
110. Lewallen S, Courtright P. *A Overview of ocular leprosy after 2 decades of multidrug therapy.* Philadelphia: Lippincott Williams & Wilkins; 2007.
111. Duke-Elder S, MacFaul PA. *System of ophthalmology.* St. Louis: Mosby; 1965.
112. Prendergast JJ. Ocular leprosy in the United States. *Am J Ophthalmol.* 1942;23:112–137.
113. Daniel E, David A, Rao PS. Quantitative assessment of the visibility of unmyelinated corneal nerves in leprosy. *Int J Leprosy.* 1994;62: 374–379.
114. Gibson JB. Eye complications of leprosy. *Med J Aust.* 1950;1:8–11.
115. Shields JA, Waring GO, Monte LG. Ocular findings in leprosy. *Am J Ophthalmol.* 1974;77:880–890.
116. Prendergast JJ. Ocular leprosy in the United States. *Am J Ophthalmol.* 1942;23:112–137.
117. Buhrer SS, et al. A simple dipstick assay for the detection of antibodies to phenolic glycolipid-I of *Mycobacterium leprae. Am J Trop Med Hyg.* 1998;58(2):133–136.
118. Job CK, et al. Role of polymerase chain reaction in the diagnosis of early leprosy. *Int J Lepr Other Mycobact Dis.* 1997;65(4):461–464.
119. Acha PN, Szyfres B. Brucellosis. In: *Zoonoses and communicable diseases common to man and animals.* 3rd ed. Washington, DC: Pan American Health Organization; 2001:40.
120. Brucem D. Note on the discovery of a microorganism in Malta fever. *Arch Ophthalmol.* 1939;2:51–67.
121. Da Costa M, et al. Specificity of six gene sequences for the detection of the genus *Brucella* by DNA amplification. *J Appl Bacteriol.* 1996;81(3): 267–275.
122. Koneman EN, Allen SD, Janda WM, et al. Other miscellaneous fastidious Gram-negative bacteria. In: *Color atlas and textbook of diagnostic microbiology.* 5th ed. Philadelphia: Lippincott-Raven Publishers; 1997:431.
123. Robichaud S, et al. Prevention of laboratory-acquired brucellosis. *Clin Infect Dis.* 2004;38(12):119–122.
124. Young EJ. An overview of human brucellosis. *Clin Infect Dis.* 1995;21(2): 283–289.
125. Pappas G, et al. Brucellosis. *N Engl J Med.* 2005;352(22):2325–2336.

126. Donch DA, Gertonson AA, Rhyan JH, Gilsdorf MJ. *U.S. Cooperative State–Federal Brucellosis Eradication Program status report – fiscal year 2005.* Washington DC: USDA; 2006.
127. Pappas G, et al. The new global map of human brucellosis. *Lancet Infect Dis.* 2006;6(2):91–99.
128. Mantur BG, Mangalgi SS, Mulimani M. Brucella melitensis – a sexually transmissible agent? *Lancet.* 1996;347:1763.
129. Braude AI. Studies in the pathology and pathogenesis of experimental brucellosis. A comparson of the pathogenicity of *Brucella abortus, Brucella melitensis* and *Brucella suis* for guinea pigs. *J Infect Dis.* 1951; 89:76–82.
130. al-Kaff AS. Ocular brucellosis. *Int Ophthalmol Clin.* 1995;35(3):139–145.
131. Colmenero JD, et al. Complications associated with *Brucella melitensis* infection: a study of 530 cases. *Medicine.* 1996;75(4):195–211.
132. Afsar H, Baydar I, Sirmatel F. Epididymo-orchitis due to brucellosis. *Br J Urol.* 1993;72(1):74–75.
133. McLean DR, Russell N, Khan MY. Neurobrucellosis: clinical and therapeutic features. *Clin Infect Dis.* 1992;15(4):582–590.
134. Bouza E, et al. Brucellar meningitis. *Rev Infect Dis.* 1987;9(4):810–822.
135. Rolando I, et al. Ocular manifestations associated with brucellosis: a 26-year experience in Peru. *Clin Infect Dis.* 2008;46(9):1338–1345.
136. Woods AC. Nummular keratitis and ocular brucellosis. *Arch Ophthalmol.* 1946;35:490.
137. Valenton MJ. Deep stromal involvement in Dimmer's nummular keratitis. *Am J Ophthalmol.* 1974;78:897.
138. Ariza J, et al. Characteristics of and risk factors for relapse of brucellosis in humans. *Clin Infect Dis.* 1995;20(5):1241–1249.
139. Young EJ. Serologic diagnosis of human brucellosis. Analysis of 214 cases by agglutination tests and review of the literature. *Rev Infect Dis.* 1991;13:359.
140. Morata P, et al. Development and evaluation of a PCR-enzyme-linked immunosorbent assay for diagnosis of human brucellosis. *J Clin Microbiol.* 2003;41(1):144–148.
141. Ariza J, et al. Treatment of human brucellosis with doxycycline plus rifampin or doxycycline plus streptomycin. A randomized, double-blind study. *Ann Intern Med.* 1992;117(1):25–30.
142. Malatt AE, Taylor HR. Onchocerciasis. *Infec Dis Clin North Am.* 1992;6(4):963–977.
143. Taylor HR. Onchocerciasis. *Int Ophthalmol.* 1990;14(3):189–194.
144. Control, Report of a WHO Expert Committee on Onchocerciasis. Onchocerciasis and its control. *World Health Organ Tech Rep Ser.* 1995;852:1.
145. Ogunrinade A, et al. Distribution of the blinding and nonblinding strains of *Onchocerca volvulus* in Nigeria. *J Infect Dis.* 1999;179(6): 1577–1579.
146. Brattig NW. Pathogenesis and host responses in human onchocerciasis: impact of *Onchocerca* filariae and *Wolbachia* endobacteria. *Microbes Infect.* 2004;6(1):113–128.
147. Nelson GS. Human onchocerciasis: notes on the history, the parasite and the life cycle. *Ann Trop Med Parasitol.* 1991;85(1):83–95.
148. Ottesen EA. Immune responsiveness and the pathogenesis of human onchocerciasis. *J Infect Dis.* 1995;171(3):659–671.
149. Burnham G. Onchocerciasis. *Lancet.* 1998;351(9112):1341–1346.
150. King CL, Nutman TB. Regulation of the immune response in lymphatic filariasis and onchocerciasis. *Immunol Today.* 1991;12(3):54–58.
151. Saint Andre A, et al. The role of endosymbiotic *Wolbachia* bacteria in the pathogenesis of river blindness. *Science.* 2002;295(5561):1892–1895.
152. Stingl P. Onchocerciasis: clinical presentation and host parasite interactions in patients of southern Sudan. *Intern J Derm.* 1997;36(1):23–28.
153. Connor DH, George GH, Gibson DW. Pathologic changes of human onchocerciasis: implications for future research. *Rev Infect Dis.* 1985; 7(6):809–819.
154. Murdoch ME, et al. A clinical classification and grading system of the cutaneous changes in onchocerciasis. *Br J Dermatol.* 1993;129(3):260–269.
155. Budden F. Route of entry of *Onchocerca volvulus* microfilariae into the eye. *Trans R Soc Trop Med Hyg.* 1976;70:265–266.
156. Neumann G. Pathogenesis of post segment lesion of ocular onchocerciasis. *Am J Ophthalmol.* 1973;(75):82–89.
157. Grove D. Tissue nematodes (trichinosis, dracunculiasis, filariass). In: Bennett JC, Dolin R, Mandell GL, eds. *Principles and practice of infectious disease.* 4th ed. New York: Churchill Livingstone; 1994.
158. Tonjum AM, Thylefora B. Aspects of corneal changes in onchocerciasis. *Br J Ophthalmol.* 1978;62:458–461.
159. Sakla AA, et al. Punctate keratitis induced by subconjunctivally injected microfilariae of *Onchocerca lienalis. Arch Ophthalmol.* 1986;104:894–898.
160. Duke-Elder S, MacFaul PA. *System of ophthalmology.* St Louis: Mosby; 1965.
161. Budden F. Natural history of onchocerciasis. *Br J Ophthalmol.* 1957;41: 214–227.
162. Von Noorden GK, Buck AA. Ocular onchocerciasis. *Arch Ophthalmol.* 1968;80:26–34.
163. Pearlman E, Hall LR. Immune mechanisms in *Onchocerca volvulus*-mediated corneal disease (river blindness). *Parasite Immunol.* 2000; 22(12):625–631.
164. Pearlman E. Immunopathology of onchocerciasis: a role for eosinophils in onchocercal dermatitis and keratitis. *Chem Immunol.* 1997;66: 26–40.
165. Ottensen E. Immune responsiveness and the pathogenesis of human onchocerciasis. *J Infect Dis.* 1995;171:659–671.
166. Semba RD, et al. Longitudinal study of lesions of the posterior segment in onchocerciasis. *Ophthalmology.* 1990;97:1334–1341.
167. Newland HS, et al. Ocular manifestations of onchocerciasis in a rain forest of West Africa. *Br J Ophthalmol.* 1991;75:163–169.
168. Thylefors B, Tonjum AM. Visual field defects in onchocerciasis. *Br J Ophthalmol.* 62:462–467.
169. Boatin BA, Toe L, Alley ES, et al. Diagnostics in onchocerciasis: future challenges. *Ann Trop Med Parasitol.* 1998;92(Suppl 1):S41-S45.
170. [Online]. Available from: www.emro.who.int/publications/RegionalPublications/Specimen_Collection/Spcec_Coll_Body_Surface_Skin_Snips.htm.
171. Lipner EM, et al. Field applicability of a rapid-format anti-Ov-16 antibody test for the assessment of onchocerciasis control measures in regions of endemicity. *J Infect Dis.* 2006;194(2):216–221.
172. Lelij AV. Analysis of aqueous humor in ocular onchocerciasis. *Curr Eye Res.* 1991;10:169–176.
173. Stingl P, et al. A diagnostic 'patch test' for onchocerciasis using topical diethylcarbamazine. *Trans R Soc Trop Med Hyg.* 1984;78(2):254–258.
174. Schlie-Guzman MA, Rivas-Alcala AR. Antigen detection in onchocerciasis: correlation with worm burden. *Trop Med Parasitol.* 1989;40(1): 47–50.
175. Ngu JL, et al. Novel, sensitive and low-cost diagnostic tests for 'river blindness' – detection of specific antigens in tears, urine and dermal fluid. *Trop Med Int Health.* 1998;3(5):339–348.
176. Ayong LS, et al. Development and evaluation of an antigen detection dipstick assay for the diagnosis of human onchocerciasis. *Trop Med Int Health.* 2005;10(3):228–233.
177. Weil GJ, et al. IgG4 subclass antibody serology for onchocerciasis. *J Infect Dis.* 1990;161(3):549–554.
178. Udall DN. Recent updates on onchocerciasis: diagnosis and treatment. *Clin Infect Dis.* 2007;44(1):53–60.
179. Mand S, et al. Frequent detection of worm movements in onchocercal nodules by ultrasonography. *Filaria J.* 2005;4(1):1.
180. Van Laethem Y, Lopes C. Treatment of onchocerciasis. *Drugs.* 1996; 52(6):861–869.
181. Goa KL, McTavish D, Clissold SP. Ivermectin. A review of its antifilarial activity, pharmacokinetic properties and clinical efficacy in onchocerciasis. *Drugs.* 1991;42(4):640–658.
182. Freedman D. Onchocerciasis. In: Walker R, Weller DH, Guerrant PF, eds. *Tropical infectious diseases: principles, pathogens and practice.* Philadelphia: Churchill Livingstone; 2005:1176.
183. Twum-Danso NA, Meredith SE. Variation in incidence of serious adverse events after onchocerciasis treatment with ivermectin in areas of Cameroon co-endemic for loiasis. *Trop Med Int Health.* 1993;8(9):820–831.
184. Johnston KL, Taylor MJ. *Wolbachia* in filarial parasites: targets for filarial infection and disease control. *Curr Infect Dis Rep.* 2007;9(1):55–59.
185. Hoerauf A, et al. Doxycycline in the treatment of human onchocerciasis: kinetics of *Wolbachia* endobacteria reduction and of inhibition of embryogenesis in female *Onchocerca* worms. *Microbes Infect.* 2003;5(4): 261–273.

Chapter 67

Corneal and External Ocular Infections in Acquired Immunodeficiency Syndrome (AIDS)

Christopher T. Hood, Bennie H. Jeng, Careen Y. Lowder, Gary N. Holland, David M. Meisler

The eye is a target organ for many of the secondary disorders that occur in individuals infected with human immunodeficiency virus (HIV). Attention has been focused primarily on retinal pathology (cotton-wool spots, microvasculopathy, and cytomegalovirus retinitis), but with the introduction of highly active antiretroviral therapy (HAART) patients are less likely to fall victim to blinding posterior segment infections, and in these individuals care can be focused on numerous HIV-related disorders involving the cornea, ocular surface, and adnexa of the eye. Both infectious and noninfectious disorders can occur in a spectrum of severity that ranges from asymptomatic problems to painful and vision-threatening disease. This chapter will address infectious disorders of the cornea and adjacent surfaces.

Viral Infections

Human immunodeficiency virus

Human immunodeficiency virus has been identified in tears, cornea, and conjunctiva.[1–4] It has not been associated with local ocular inflammatory disease, but its presence in the external ocular environment has caused concern regarding the transmissibility of virus from these sites. As a result, corneal donor tissue is routinely screened before distribution. Donor history is reviewed for evidence of acquired immunodeficiency syndrome (AIDS) or high-risk factors for HIV infection, and cadaveric blood is tested for HIV antibodies before corneal tissue is offered for transplantation.[5–8] To date, no documented cases of HIV transmission or seroconversion after keratoplasty have been reported, despite the fact that corneal grafts inadvertently taken from HIV-seropositive individuals have been transplanted into recipients without known risk factors for HIV infection before the status of the donor was discovered. Lack of seroconversion may reflect the avascular nature of the cornea and/or an extremely low inoculum.

Proper precautions regarding possible contamination of contact lenses, tonometers, and other instruments by tears or surface-infected cells have become the concern of all ophthalmologists and ophthalmic personnel.[9–13] Contact lenses appear to be disinfected adequately by heat and hydrogen peroxide disinfection systems, but the efficacy of other chemical disinfection systems to inactivate HIV has not been established. Tonometer tips are effectively disinfected by swabbing with a 70% isopropyl alcohol-soaked pledget followed by air drying.[11] Contaminated instruments should be cleaned mechanically to remove blood, mucus, and other particulate organic matter. Disinfection may be achieved by heat or by 10-minute soaks in 3% hydrogen peroxide, 70% ethanol, 70% isopropyl alcohol, or a 1:10 solution of household bleach.[9,14] To date, there have been no reports of HIV transmission in the practice of ophthalmology.

Cytomegalovirus

Cytomegalovirus (CMV) is the most common opportunistic pathogen of the eye in individuals with AIDS; in 30–40% of severely immunocompromised individuals it causes a necrotizing retinopathy and is usually associated with a CD4+ T-lymphocyte count <50 cells/μL. Although the virus is not associated with clinical findings consistent with conjunctivitis, histopathologic examination of conjunctival tissue obtained from an individual with AIDS showed edema, inflammation, and cytomegalic cells containing prominent intranuclear inclusions.[15] Immunohistochemical studies demonstrated positive staining for CMV antigen, and electron microscopy showed intranuclear and intracytoplasmic viral particles consistent with a herpes group virus and intracytoplasmic membrane-bound homogeneous dense bodies characteristic of CMV. CMV DNA has also been dectected by polymerase chain reaction (PCR) in the conjunctiva of AIDS patients diagnosed clinically with CMV retinitis,[16,17] as well as HIV-positive patients without evidence of CMV retinitis.[18] Additionally, CMV was demonstrated by histopathologic and immunohistochemical studies to be present in a biopsy specimen obtained from a hyperemic caruncle in an individual with AIDS.[19] A suspected association between CMV infection and decreased aqueous tear production, which is common in HIV-infected individuals, has not been proven.

In the cornea, CMV has been reported as a cause of corneal epithelial keratitis.[20] These lesions were characterized by a slightly elevated, opaque, branching, nonulcerative epitheliopathy that recurred after corneal scrapings and persisted despite oral and topical antiviral therapy. A stromal keratouveitis also subsequently developed. Other investigators have described an isolated stromal keratitis that was presumed to be secondary to CMV infection. The lesion resolved with systemic ganciclovir administration in this patient, who had typical CMV retinitis and a positive PCR test for detection of CMV DNA in the aqueous humor. There was, however, no direct evidence linking CMV to the corneal infiltrate.[21]

Corneal endothelial deposits are routinely seen with CMV retinitis,[22–25] although they have also been reported in HIV-positive and CMV-positive patients without concomitant ocular disease.[26] These fairly distinct deposits have been described as being diffuse, fine, refractile, and stellate, and are best seen with retroillumination.[25] They have also been described as microscopic, opaque, linear flecks arranged in a reticular-like fashion.[23] They usually have no direct effect on vision. Histologically, these corneal deposits have been found to be composed of macrophages and fibrin material without lymphocytes and without evidence of endothelial cell CMV infection.[25] It has been suggested that they are the result of mild ocular inflammation associated with CMV infection of the retina. Recent evidence has also suggested that CMV may be an etiologic factor in corneal endotheliitis in patients who have received local or systemic immunosuppression without evidence of HIV,[27] as well as in patients without evidence of systemic immunodeficiency.[28] Additionally, CMV is suspected to be the cause of some cases of chronic anterior uveitis in HIV-negative patients.[29] Based on this finding, it could be speculated that some cases of chronic anterior uveitis of undetermined cause in patients with AIDS[30] might be related to CMV, in view of its ubiquitous nature in this population. This issue would be an appropriate subject for future study.

Varicella-zoster virus

Herpes zoster ophthalmicus

Herpes zoster ophthalmicus is probably the most common external ocular infection affecting patients with HIV disease.[31–35] Herpes zoster infection usually affects individuals older than 50 years and has been attributed to waning immunocompetency. Like non-HIV-infected individuals, HIV-infected individuals can develop a classic vesiculobullous rash in the distribution of the ophthalmic branch of the trigeminal nerve; however, ocular involvement with maxillary herpes zoster has been reported in an HIV-infected pregnant woman.[36] Herpes zoster virus causes a necrotizing vasculitis and can be associated with conjunctival injection, pseudodendrites, keratitis, episcleritis, scleritis, iridocyclitis with an associated elevation of intraocular pressure, retinal vasculitis, retinitis, optic neuritis, and ocular motor palsies.[37] Dendriform lesions of the cornea occur in up to 51% of cases of ocular involvement.[38]

Herpes zoster ophthalmicus (HZO) occurs with a greater prevalence in individuals with HIV infection than in those without. It has been found to be a true opportunistic infection in such individuals, with a relative prevalence risk ratio of 6.6:1.[39] In a prospective study of 100 consecutive patients with HZO in Ethiopia, 95% of all those who underwent testing and 100% of those aged under 45 were found to be HIV positive.[40] Other studies in Africa have demonstrated that 40–50% of patients presenting with HZO were infected with HIV.[41,42]

In another study,[35] of 112 patients with herpes zoster ophthalmicus in the United States, 29 (26%) had HIV infection or AIDS. All were younger than 50 years of age. The authors therefore recommended that all individuals younger than 50 years who have HZO be tested for HIV at initial examination.[35] Therefore, HIV infection should be strongly suspected in young individuals with no other known risk factors for immune suppression (e.g., malignancy or chronic corticosteroid therapy) who present with HZO.[31] HZO has even been reported as an initial manifestation of HIV infection.[31,32,34]

The occurrence of cutaneous herpes zoster lesions in an asymptomatic HIV-infected individual appears to predict an increased risk for the subsequent development of AIDS. One study found that 61% of unselected individuals with HZO who were younger than 44 years in New York City were members of groups at high risk for AIDS, and over a 2.5-year follow-up period 21% of these individuals developed AIDS.[34]

HZO associated with HIV infection can be especially severe.[31] In the series of young individuals with HZO followed in New York City, those with risk factors for AIDS had a higher rate of ocular complications than those who did not have such risk factors (57% vs 38%).[34] In addition, when HIV infection is present there is also a higher incidence of corneal involvement (89% vs 65%).[43]

In a retrospective cohort study of 48 eyes in 48 HIV-infected individuals who were treated for HZO, 35% of individuals developed stromal keratitis and 50% developed anterior uveitis. The authors attributed the low rates of complications to the aggressive antiviral therapy that was used, and to the compromised cellular immunity of the individuals (mean CD4+ T-lymphocyte count 48 cells/μL).[44] A prospective study in South Africa demonstrated a 63.6% incidence of complications in HIV-infected patients, including uveitis, punctate corneal staining, corneal ulcer, nummular keratitis, and elevated intraocular pressure.[45] Interestingly, among HIV-positive patients the rate of complications was statistically lower in those with CD4+ T-lymphocyte counts <200 than in those with counts >200. Again, this suggests that most clinically evident complications are secondary to the host immune response rather than viral cellular destruction.

HZO in HIV-infected individuals should be treated aggressively with systemic aciclovir, valaciclovir, or famciclovir to promote healing and to prevent or reduce the severity of ocular lesions.[44] These antiviral agents may be administered intravenously with prolonged subsequent oral maintenance to avoid or minimize recurrence as well as the sequelae of subsequent disseminated varicella-zoster virus infection, such as contralateral hemiplegia caused by cerebral arteritis,[14,46,47] and necrotizing retinitis.[35]

In individuals with AIDS, systemic corticosteroid therapy should be avoided as it could potentiate a more disseminated varicella-zoster virus infection or facilitate the emergence of another opportunistic infection elsewhere. In one case of HZO occurring in an individual with AIDS-related complex, systemic corticosteroid treatment was associated with the reemergence of toxoplasmic retinochoroiditis.[46]

The efficacy of VZV vaccination in preventing HZO in HIV-infected individuals has not been proven, but limited data from a clinical trial in HIV-infected children indicated that the vaccine was well tolerated and that >80% of subjects had detectable VZV-specific immune response 1 year after immunization.[48] Hardy and associates[49] have shown that VZV vaccination in leukemic children reduced incidence of herpes zoster from 15% to 3%. Currently, the vaccine should be considered for HIV-infected children with age-specific CD4+ T-lymphocyte percentages >15%, and may be considered for adolescents and adults with CD4+ T-lymphocyte counts >200/μL.[50]

Ophthalmologists must be suspicious for atypical presentations of HZO in HIV-infected individuals, and must be aware of the treatment that is required and be prepared for a longer course of the disease. Although the presentation of HZO in a young individual should raise suspicion for an underlying immune disorder such as HIV infection, and although the proportion of individuals with HIV disease is higher in younger than in older individuals, it should be remembered that HZO may occur in young individuals who are not HIV infected.[51]

Varicella-zoster virus keratitis

HIV-infected individuals are at risk for chronic, productive varicella-zoster virus keratitis, which is characterized by a gray, elevated, dendriform epithelial lesion with variable fluorescein and rose bengal staining (Fig. 67.1).[51,52] Most commonly, these lesions are found in the midperipheral and peripheral cornea, and often they cross the limbus.[51] They may occur in individuals who have only mild transient skin lesions or in those with no obvious history of skin disease. VZV has been recovered in culture from corneal scrapings taken 11 weeks after the onset of the keratitis, suggesting that the immunodeficiency of HIV infection may allow persistence of active viral infection in the corneal epithelium.[52] Treatment of chronic VZV keratitis has met with variable success, but the disease may respond to debridement and topically applied aciclovir.[52] Often, the disease course is prolonged and extremely painful.[51] Before the AIDS epidemic this disorder had not been reported.

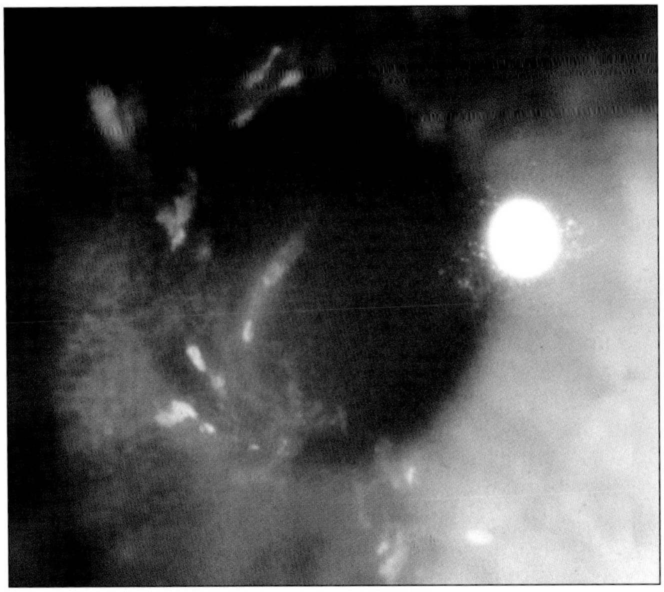

Fig. 67.1 Chronic dendriform lesions of the cornea caused by active varicella-zoster virus infection in an individual with AIDS. (Published with permission from *Am J Ophthalmol* 1988;105:556–558. Copyright Elsevier, All rights reserved.)

Although previously described in individuals with debilitating systemic disorders such as drug-induced immunosuppression, advanced diabetes, and neoplasias,[53] peripheral ulcerative keratitis associated with HZO has also been described in association with HIV disease. In the reported series, all three individuals had skin involvement and bilateral keratouveitis. All three responded to oral aciclovir, but one developed progressive outer retinal necrosis syndrome upon discontinuation of therapy.[54]

Immune recovery stromal keratitis presumed to be secondary to VZV antigen has been reported in a patient with AIDS.[55] The keratitis was not associated with skin or corneal epithelial disease, and occurred despite aciclovir prophylaxis. VZV has also been implicated by PCR as the cause of disciform corneal edema in an AIDS patient without a history of varicella-zoster dermatitis.[56]

Herpes simplex virus

Herpes simplex virus (HSV) keratitis has been reported in HIV-infected individuals, but has not been shown to occur at a greater frequency than in healthy individuals.[57,58] Whereas herpetic infections of the cornea are usually caused by HSV-1, HSV-2 has also been recovered from the same infected cornea of an individual with AIDS.[59] Infection is usually characterized by epithelial dendriform lesions but, as one study showed, the dendrites may have somewhat atypical characteristics compared to those in immunocompetent individuals.[59] HIV-seropositive individuals appeared to have a predilection for marginal, as opposed to central, HSV infection; peripheral corneal involvement is relatively uncommon in immunocompetent individuals. Individuals with HIV infection can subsequently develop large dendrites covering extensive areas of the cornea (Fig. 67.2), and can have frequent recurrences. Of five individuals followed for longer than 3 months, two to three recurrences occurred per individual over an average of 17 months, with the median dendrite-free interval being 7 months. This course is unlike that for keratitis occurring in immunocompetent individuals, in which a median dendrite-free interval of 18 months has been reported.[58] A more recent report found no difference between HIV-infected and HIV-negative individuals with regard to the incidence of HSV keratitis, lesion type (epithelial versus stromal), lesion location (central versus peripheral), and treatment time.[57] The recurrence rate, however, was found to be 2.48 times higher in HIV-infected individuals.[57] A retrospective study in India also demonstrated that patients with recurrent herpes simplex keratitis were significantly more likely to be HIV-infected than matched patients with first-episode herpes simplex keratitis (16.7% vs 3.3%).[60]

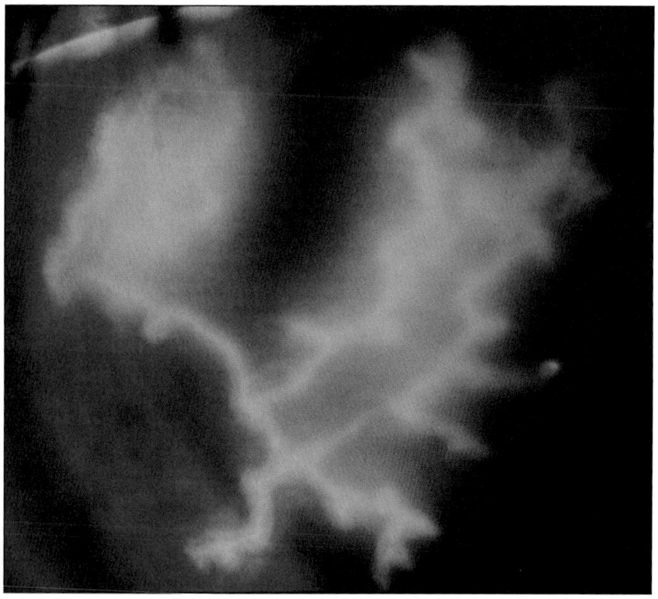

Fig. 67.2 Fluorescein-stained cornea of an individual with AIDS with severe HSV keratitis. The keratitis at the limbus extends over the central cornea. (Published with permission from *Int Ophthalmol Clin* 1989;29:98–104.)

In a small case series of HIV-infected individuals with HSV keratitis, corneal stromal disease was less common than expected, based on the incidence of stromal keratitis observed in the general population.[58] Although the CD4+ T-lymphocyte counts were not reported in this series, all patients had AIDS at the time of HSV keratitis diagnosis. In contrast, a more recent retrospective cohort study reported no difference in lesion type (epithelial versus stromal) among patients with and without HIV infection who had HSV keratitis.[57] It is possible that patients in the latter study study were, on average, less immunocompromised than those in the earlier series, which might explain the apparent discrepancy in the prevalence of HSV stromal disease. The incidence of HSV stromal disease in HIV-infected patients overall may be similar to that in the general population, but when immunodeficiency becomes severe, T-lymphocyte depletion and dysfunction associated with AIDS may actually protect these individuals against the development of immune-mediated stromal disease.

HSV epithelial keratitis in individuals with HIV infection appears to be more resistant to treatment with commercially available topical antiviral agents and systemic aciclovir than in otherwise healthy individuals; as a result, HIV-infected individuals with HSV keratitis can have prolonged infectious episodes.[61] In one report, the median healing time after initiation of topical antiviral therapy was 3 weeks, compared to less than 2 weeks in immunocompetent individuals.[58] In another report, HSV keratitis in an individual with AIDS responded only to treatment with topical interferon-α.[62] Because individuals with cell-mediated immune dysfunction (as in HIV disease) have a subsequent lack of endogenous interferon, the addition of exogenous interferon, as in these cases, may be efficacious for treating antiviral-resistant HSV keratitis.

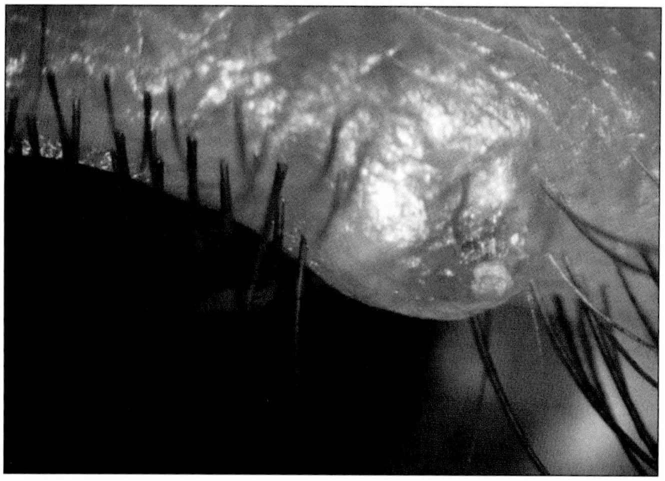

Fig. 67.3 Molluscum contagiosum lesion on the eyelid margin of an individual with AIDS.

In one HIV-infected patient, an unusual exophytic tumor of the bulbar conjunctiva and eyelid that resembled squamous cell carcinoma was shown by immunohistochemistry to be positive for HSV I/II antigens.[63] The exophytic lesion responded to oral valaciclovir and corticosteroids, initially recurred upon discontinuation, but subsequently rapidly resolved with reinitiation of oral valaciclovir. In HIV-infected patients, severe mucocutaneous HSV reactivation can be seen with CD4+ T-lymphocyte counts <100 μL,[64] and this case illustrates that HSV infection of the eyelid and conjunctiva can be especially severe in an HIV-positive patient and should be considered in the differential of a tumor-like growth.

Although studies may differ in their conclusions, the course and presentation of HSV keratitis among HIV-infected and noninfected individuals appears to be no different except for an increased risk of recurrence in HIV-infected individuals. Therefore, clinicians may wish to consider long-term suppressive therapy with a systemic antiviral agent for HIV-infected individuals presenting with HSV keratitis. In immunocompromised individuals with HSV keratitis refractory to antiviral therapy, the addition of interferon may prove to be useful.

Molluscum contagiosum virus

Molluscum contagiosum, caused by a DNA virus of the poxviridae group, causes nodular skin lesions approximately 2–3 mm in diameter with a central umbilication filled with a cheesy-appearing material (Fig. 67.3).[65] It is generally believed that molluscum contagiosum is more common in individuals with HIV infection than in noninfected individuals, as the profound dysfunction of the T-lymphocyte-mediated immune response caused by HIV infection causes individuals to be susceptible to many viral infections. Because of this, some authors have recommended that the appearance of molluscum contagiosum lesions in adult men should prompt an evaluation for an immunocompromised state.[66]

In the immunocompetent individual there may be an associated follicular conjunctivitis or keratitis with involvement of the eyelids; it usually is a self-limited infection that involves the face and eyelids with fewer than 10 lesions, and resolution occurs spontaneously within 3–12 months, although simple excision, curettage, or cryotherapy of lesions generally is curative.

Molluscum contagiosum infection in individuals with depressed cell-mediated immunity follows a more aggressive course, with extensive dissemination of lesions over skin surfaces, including the eyelids.[65,67–69] The lesions tend to be more numerous and larger than in immunocompetent hosts. Follicular conjunctivitis may be absent, and individuals remain asymptomatic until mechanical problems arise. In patients with AIDS, molluscum contagiosum has also been reported to affect the limbal conjunctiva,[70,71] a rare finding in healthy individuals. These lesions are notable for their lack of surrounding conjunctival inflammation, which probably reflects the inability of the patient to mount an immune response. Molluscum contagiosum lesions of the eyelid have even been reported as the initial clinical manifestation of HIV disease.[72]

In HIV-infected patients, eradication of lesions is difficult; in a report on two individuals, removal of the lesions by surgical excision or cryotherapy was followed by recurrences within 6–7 weeks, which corresponds to the incubation period of the virus.[69] In contrast, a later study reported successful eradication of molluscum contagiosum lesions in individuals with AIDS using focal cryotherapy.[73] Reconstitution of immune function with HAART can result in the resolution of existing lesions even without therapy specifically directed toward the virus. A report of three individuals with AIDS who were being followed for molluscum contagiosum infection that was recalcitrant to therapy demonstrated that their cutaneous lesions cleared 5–6 months after beginning HAART.[74] A single limbal conjunctival molluscum lesion has also been seen to regress 6 months after starting HAART.[75] In this case, pronounced conjunctival inflammation ensued until the lesion regressed. Immune reconstitution does not necessarily prevent recurrence of molluscum, but if new lesions develop they will most likely be less severe, as seen in immunocompetent patients.[76]

Other viruses

Other viruses have been found to play a role in the development of certain malignancies associated with HIV infection that can affect the ocular surface. Squamous cell carcinoma of the conjunctiva occurs more frequently in patients with HIV/AIDS;[77–80] it tends to affect younger patients and have a more aggressive course than in noninfected individuals.[81–84] In sub-Saharan Africa, conjunctival squamous neoplasia has been reported as the primary and only apparent manifestation of HIV.[85] Squamous cell carcinoma can also present on the eyelids.[86] Although the pathogenesis of HIV-associated squamous cell carcinoma has not been definitely established,[79] it has been linked to infection with the human papillomavirus.[80,81,86] Interestingly, a review of autopsy cases in Uganda revealed that individuals who died of AIDS-related complications were no more likely to have conjunctival HPV infection than were controls.[87] It remains unclear whether immunosuppression or HIV itself plays a role in the pathogenesis,[79] although complete regression of invasive squamous cell carcinoma with orbital invasion has been reported with immune reconstitution using HAART.[88]

Human herpes virus-8 (HHV-8) has been found to represent an important, if not essential, factor in the pathogenesis of Kaposi's sarcoma (KS).[79,89] Up to 30% of all patients with AIDS in the United States will develop KS, with eyelid, conjunctival, or orbital involvement in approximately 10–20%.[90] Adnexal and conjunctival KS has been described as the presenting feature for HIV infection[91] and can be the AIDS-defining illness. One study found that approximately one-third of individuals infected with both HIV and HHV-8 developed KS within 10 years of HIV seroconversion. In this study, higher antibody titers to HHV-8 appeared to be associated with faster progression to KS, but not to other AIDS-defining illnesses.[92] In another study, evidence of HHV-8 was found in 95% of all tissue samples from individuals with AIDS-associated KS, from HIV-negative homosexual males with KS, and from individuals with classic KS.[93]

In the eyelid and conjunctiva, HHV-8 has been identified in Kaposi's sarcoma in HIV-positive patients.[91,94] A recent report from Japan on a man infected with HIV provides histological, DNA, and serological evidence of HHV-8 in a case of bilateral conjunctival Kaposi's sarcoma.[95] Although the exact mechanism by which HHV-8 mediates oncogenesis has not been fully elucidated, molecular biology studies have identified a number of HHV-8 viral oncogenes that may contribute to neoplasia.[96] Recently, complete resolution of conjunctival KS was reported with immune reconstitution under HAART, without the use of systemic or local chemotherapy.[97] Nevertheless, Kaposi's sarcoma can still occur in HIV-infected patients with high CD4+ T-lymphocyte counts and low HIV blood levels.[98]

Bacterial Infections

Although it is generally believed that infection with HIV alone does not predispose to bacterial keratitis,[99] many cases of spontaneous corneal infections in individuals with HIV infection have been published.[99–103] Conventional risk factors for infectious keratitis, such as contact lens wear, trichiasis, topical corticosteroid use, and trauma, may undoubtedly also be present in HIV-infected individuals. However, other risk factors, such as underlying immunodeficiency, as well as HIV-associated keratoconjunctivitis sicca,[104] herpetic eye disease, and anatomical eyelid abnormalities secondary to molluscum contagiosum lesions and KS, could also theoretically predispose to colonization or penetration of the ocular surface by bacteria in HIV-infected individuals.[37] The use of crack cocaine by HIV-infected individuals could also predispose to corneal ulcers and epithelial defects: its anesthetic qualities may numb the cornea, giving rise to neurotrophic corneal surface abnormalities. The smoke itself may be toxic and cause a breakdown of the epithelial barrier. Furthermore, its alkaline nature may cause a chemical insult to the epithelium.[105]

There have been several studies comparing the ocular flora in HIV-infected and immunocompetent patients. Increased numbers of colonies of bacterial flora have been cultured from the eyelids of asymptomatic HIV-positive patients compared to controls.[106] Other authors demonstrated that anerobic organisms are common in the conjunctival sacs of patients with HIV as well as normal controls, but the spectrum of organisms was different in the two groups.[107] High levels of pathogenic flora cultured from the conjunctiva of inpatients with AIDS in another study may have been related to their hospitalization, and the results may not be generalizable to all HIV-infected patients.[108] Other studies have shown no difference in ocular flora between patients infected with HIV and immunocompetent patients.[109,110] Based on a study involving 40 individuals with AIDS and 42 HIV-negative individuals, no qualitative or quantitative differences were found in the ocular flora obtained by cultures of the conjunctiva and eyelids. The study also found that the presence of keratoconjunctivitis sicca and the level of immunosuppression do not appear to affect the ocular flora in individuals with AIDS.[109]

The effect of prophylactic systemic antibiotics on the ocular flora in patients with HIV is not entirely clear. Gritz and associates[109] found that the use of systemic antibiotics in patients with AIDS did not appear to affect the conjunctival flora. In contrast, other studies suggest that systemic antibiotic use may exert a selection pressure on the ocular flora. Fontes and associates[111] reported more negative cultures and increased bacterial resistance associated with chronic systemic use of trimethoprim-sulfamethoxasole in patients infected with HIV. Another group of authors reported that systemic treatment with clarithromycin reduced the prevalence of bacteria from the conjunctivae of HIV-infected individuals, even in the setting of a low CD4+ T-lymphocyte count.[110] Another recent study, however, suggests that nearly all bacterial culture isolates from HIV-infected patients are sensitive to topical gentamicin, even though the majority of patients were receiving systemic antibiotic prophylaxis.[112]

The clinical presentation of bacterial keratitis in individuals with HIV infection may differ from that in individuals without HIV; the ulcerative processes may be more aggressive, recalcitrant to treatment, and characterized by a fulminant course that may lead, particularly in cases of *Pseudomonas aeruginosa* infections (Fig. 67.4), to corneal perforation[99] and require enucleation.[102] In one case of pseudomonal scleritis[102] the diagnosis was unrecognized for several weeks secondary to the lack of contiguous spread and to the lack of inflammatory signs that are normally present in immunocompetent individuals with such infections.[113]

A case of Parinaud's oculoglandular syndrome caused by *Chlamydia trachomatis* serotype L2 (the causative agent of lymphogranuloma venereum) was reported in an HIV-seropositive individual.[114] The ocular manifestations included a mixed papillary–follicular conjunctivitis and fleshy superior limbal lesions in both eyes. A superior marginal corneal perforation occurred, requiring a therapeutic corneal graft. The ocular disease resolved after 6 weeks of oral tetracycline therapy. There have been no other similar reports.

Because of the potential lack of typical inflammatory signs and symptoms in immunosuppressed individuals, bacterial infections of the anterior segment in those infected with HIV may be diagnosed later in the course of the disease. Therefore, it is important for the ophthalmologist to recognize these atypical presentations in order to institute prompt and intensive therapy.

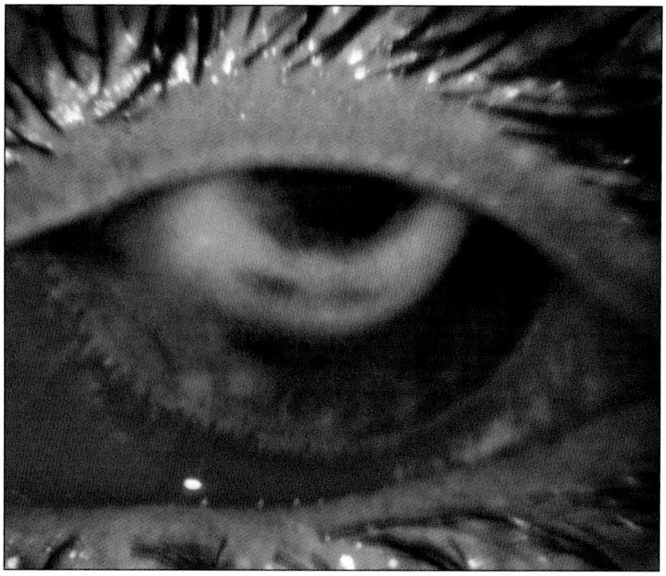

Fig. 67.4 Ring-shaped stromal infiltrate caused by *Pseudomonas aeruginosa* in an individual with AIDS.

Fungal Infections

Fungal corneal ulcers are rare in the absence of preceding trauma, ocular surface disease, or corticosteroid use,[115,116] and most reported cases of fungal infection have involved *Candida* species.[99,117–119] It has been suggested that fungal corneal ulcers may be among the opportunistic infections associated with HIV disease,[118,119] as fungal ulcers of the cornea have been reported in HIV-infected individuals who do not otherwise have risk factors for this condition.[99,117–119] In one study in Africa, 20 of 32 (81.2%) of individuals who presented with fungal keratitis were HIV infected.[120] A more recent study in the United States examining 61 cases of fungal keratitis reported that serologic positivity for HIV was the most common associated risk factor.[121] In another report, nonsimultaneous bilateral corneal ulcers secondary to *Candida albicans* were reported in an individual who later tested positive for antibodies to HIV.[119]

Infection with *Cryptococcus neoformans* has also been reported on the ocular surface[122,123] and adnexae[124] and should be considered as a possible anterior segment lesion in an AIDS patient. Clinical manifestations have included a focal subconjunctival granuloma that was fixed to the sclera[122] and a large conjunctival lesion resembling squamous cell carcinoma; [125] in both cases the lesions preceded the diagnosis of HIV infection. In two other cases in patients with a known diagnosis of AIDS, cryptococcus infection manifested as granulomatous lesions of the corneoscleral limbus[123] and as painless scleral ulceration.[126] An eyelid lesion that clinically resembled molluscum contagiosum in a known HIV-infected patient also proved to be a sentinel lesion of disseminated cryptococcosis.[124]

Because immunocompetent individuals without risk factors such as previous ocular trauma, ocular surface disease, or corticosteroid therapy rarely develop fungal infections of the ocular surface, such presentations should prompt ophthalmologists to consider evaluation for latent HIV infection or other underlying immunologic disorders. Culture or biopsy of suspicious lesions is necessary to establish the diagnosis of fungal infections.

Parasitic Infections

Microsporidia are obligate intracellular parasites that have emerged as important opportunistic pathogens in individuals with AIDS. There are two clinical presentations of ocular microsporidial infections: a corneal stromal keratitis occurs in immunocompetent individuals,[127,128] and an epithelial keratopathy and conjunctivitis occurs in individuals with AIDS (Fig. 67.5). The infectious agents are of different genera: genus *Nosema* is the causative agent of stromal keratitis, and *Encephalitozoon* and *Septata* have been associated with keratoconjunctivitis.[129–135] In individuals with AIDS, the conjunctivitis may consist of a mild to marked papillary reaction. The corneal infection appears as a unilateral or bilateral coarse epithelial keratopathy that stains irregularly with fluorescein; it may become chronic and severely compromise vision. Upper respiratory colonization may be concurrent with the eye infection.

In patients infected with HIV, severe immunosuppression appears to be required for microsporidial infection to occur. In one study, all seven individuals with ocular microsporidiosis had depressed CD4+ T-lymphocyte counts (mean, 26 cells/μL).[136] However, another report on a single

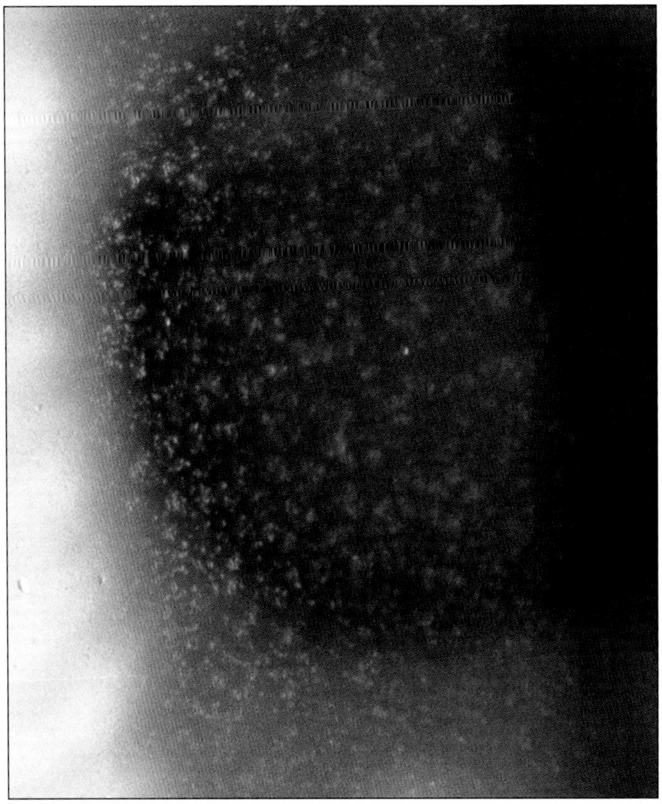

Fig. 67.5 Coarse punctate epithelial keratopathy in an individual with microsporidial corneal infection.

patient suggests that ocular surface disease may be less severe when CD4+ T-lymphocyte counts are low; with immune reconstitution, signs and symptoms became more pronounced.[137]

Although microsporidial epithelial keratitis has been the pattern of disease seen in association with HIV infection, reports have described this presentation in HIV-negative individuals.[138–141] In many of these cases, topical or systemic corcitosteroid use was a predisposing factor to the development or persistence of infection, presumably by effectively creating an immunocompromised state.

Microsporidia are fastidious and difficult to recover in culture. Diagnosis is made by histopathologic studies of infected tissue obtained by corneal or conjunctival scraping. By light microscopy, the organisms stain a deep blue color with Giemsa stain, and they are Gram positive. A polar body is seen on periodic acid–Schiff-stained sections. Little or no inflammatory response is associated with the organisms. Definitive identification is made by electron microscopic studies,[129,132,134,136] which reveal the intracytoplasmic coiled polar tubule characteristic of this organism. Confocal microscopy in vivo may also aid in the diagnosis,[142] and an immunofluorescent antibody technique has been used for species identification in tissue.[136] PCR may eventually prove useful in the diagnosis, but still requires validation.[143]

Management of microsporidial keratitis has been difficult. Case reports have suggested variable benefit with oral itraconazole and topical propamidine drops.[134,135] Fumadil B (Fumagillin) is a commercial preparation used to control nosematosis, a microsporidial infection in honeybees. A topical solution of fumadil B has been reported effective in the treatment of epithelial keratopathy.[144–146] When therapy is discontinued, however, reinfection and recrudescence occur. Albendazole, a benzimidazole, given orally, has also been reported to be effective in two cases of ocular microsporidiosis.[147,148] Oral itraconazole treatment has also been successful in one patient after albendazole treatment was unsuccessful.[149] Lastly, immune reconstitution by the initiation of HAART resulted in the resolution of microsporidia keratoconjunctivitis over 1 month in an individual with AIDS, without specific treatment for microsporidia.[150]

Summary

There is a broad spectrum of corneal and external ocular disorders that occur in HIV-infected individuals. Most are uncommon, but when they do occur they can be severe, leading to pain and visual loss. Infections in these individuals tend to be more severe than those in immunocompetent hosts, and more difficult to treat. An appreciation of these disorders facilitates diagnosis and management and, in some cases, prevents their occurrence.

HIV-infected individuals share the same risk factors for infections as the general population, such as contact lens wear or other forms of trauma. In addition, they may develop specific risk factors such as severe dry eyes, neurotrophic corneas after HSV or varicella-zoster virus keratitis, eyelid deformities, or trichiasis from lesions such as KS. Although most eye care practitioners do not absolutely advise against contact lens wear by HIV-infected individuals, such people should be encouraged to use daily-wear rigid gas-permeable lenses and to practice meticulous hygiene. If infections do occur, they may present with atypical features and have a prolonged or more severe course. Immediate and aggressive treatment should be undertaken. In contrast to many retinal infections, there is little need for chronic, suppressive ('maintenance') therapy once a corneal or external infection is under control. In fact, chronic use of topical antibiotics may select for resistant bacteria or fungi.

It should be remembered that patients can have multiple infections, and even asymptomatic patients can shed infectious agents in their tears. Special attention must be paid to the prevention of nosocomial spread of disease. As HIV-infected individuals may show no overt manifestations of their disease, universal precautions must be employed in all patient encounters.

HAART has substantially reduced the rates of opportunistic infections in individuals with HIV disease, but has not eliminated them altogether, and these drugs are not available to many individuals worldwide. Furthermore, serious problems may reappear as resistance to antiretroviral agents develops. Thus, knowledge about AIDS-related corneal and external ocular infections by clinicians remains important.

References

1. Doro S, Navia BA, Kahn A, et al. Confirmation of HTLV-III virus in cornea. *Am J Ophthalmol.* 1986;102(3):390–391.
2. Fujikawa LS, Salahuddin SZ, Ablashi D, et al. Human T-cell leukemia/lymphotropic virus type III in the conjunctival epithelium of a patient with AIDS. *Am J Ophthalmol.* 1985;100(4):507–509.
3. Fujikawa LS, Salahuddin SZ, Ablashi D, et al. HTLV-III in the tears of AIDS patients. *Ophthalmology.* 1986;93(12):1479–1481.
4. Salahuddin SZ, Palestine AG, Heck E, et al. Isolation of the human T-cell leukemia/lymphotropic virus type III from the cornea. *Am J Ophthalmol.* 1986;101(2):149–152.
5. O'Day DM. The risk posed by HTLV-III-infected corneal donor tissue. *Am J Ophthalmol.* 1986;101(2):246–247.
6. Pepose JS, Buerger DG, Paul DA, et al. New developments in serologic screening of corneal donors for HIV-1 and hepatitis B virus infections. *Ophthalmology.* 1992;99(6):879–888.
7. Pepose JS, Mac Rae S, Quinn TC, Holland GN. The impact of the AIDS epidemic on corneal transplantation. *Am J Ophthalmol.* 1985;100(4):610–613.
8. Pepose JS, MacRae S, Quinn TC, Ward JW. Serologic markers after the transplantation of corneas from donors infected with human immunodeficiency virus. *Am J Ophthalmol.* 1987;103(6):798–801.
9. Centers for Disease Control. Recommendations for preventing possible transmission of human T-lymphotropic virus type III/lymphadenopathy-associated virus from tears. *MMWR – Morbidity & Mortality Weekly Report.* 1985;34(34):533–534.
10. Pepose JS. Contact lens disinfection to prevent transmission of viral disease. *CLAO J.* 1988;14(3):165–168.
11. Pepose JS, Linette G, Lee SF, MacRae S. Disinfection of Goldmann tonometers against human immunodeficiency virus type 1. *Arch Ophthalmol.* 1989;107(7):983–985.
12. Vogt MW, Ho DD, Bakar SR, et al. Safe disinfection of contact lenses after contamination with HTLV-III. *Ophthalmology.* 1986;93(6):771–774.
13. Tervo T, Lahdevirta J, Vaheri A, et al. Recovery of HTLV-III from contact lenses. *Lancet.* 1986;1(8477):379–380.
14. Holland GN. Acquired immunodeficiency syndrome and ophthalmology: the first decade. *Am J Ophthalmol.* 1992;114(1):86–95.
15. Brown HH, Glasgow BJ, Holland GN, Foos RY. Cytomegalovirus infection of the conjunctiva in AIDS. *Am J Ophthalmol.* 1988;106(1):102–104.
16. Liu JH, Hsu WM, Wong WW, et al. Using conjunctival swab with polymerase chain reaction to aid diagnosis of cytomegalovirus retinitis in AIDS patients. *Ophthalmologica.* 2000;214(2):126–130.
17. Pathanapitoon K, Ausayakhun S, Kunavisarut P, et al. Detection of cytomegalovirus in vitreous, aqueous and conjunctiva by polymerase chain reaction (PCR). *J Med Assoc Thai.* 2005;88(2):228–232.
18. Lee-Wing MW, Hodge WG, Diaz-Mitoma F. The prevalence of herpes family virus DNA in the conjunctiva of patients positive and negative for human immunodeficiency virus using the polymerase chain reaction. *Ophthalmology.* 1999;106(2):350–354.
19. Espana-Gregori E, Vera-Sempere FJ, Cano-Parra J, et al. Cytomegalovirus infection of the caruncle in the acquired immunodeficiency syndrome. *Am J Ophthalmol.* 1994;117(3):406–407.
20. Wilhelmus KR, Font RL, Lehmann RP, Cernoch PL. Cytomegalovirus keratitis in acquired immunodeficiency syndrome. *Arch Ophthalmol.* 1996;114(7):869–872.
21. Inoue T, Hayashi K, Omoto T, et al. Corneal infiltration and CMV retinitis in a patient with AIDS. *Cornea.* 1998;17(4):441–442.
22. Althaus C, Best J, Hintzmann A, et al. Endothelial precipitates and laser flare photometry in patients with acquired immunodeficiency syndrome: a screening test for cytomegalovirus retinitis? *German J Ophthalmol.* 1996;5(6):443–448.
23. Brody JM, Butrus SI, Laby DM, et al. Anterior segment findings in AIDS patients with cytomegalovirus retinitis. *Graefes Arch Clin Exp Ophthalmol.* 1995;233(6):374–376.
24. Mitchell SM, Barton K, Lightman S. Corneal endothelial changes in cytomegalovirus retinitis. *Eye.* 1994;8(Pt 1):41–43.
25. Walter KA, Coulter VL, Palay DA, et al. Corneal endothelial deposits in patients with cytomegalovirus retinitis. *Am J Ophthalmol.* 1996;121(4):391–396.
26. Miedziak AI, Rapuano CJ, Goldman S. Corneal endothelial precipitates in HIV- and CMV-positive patients without concomitant ocular disease. *Eye.* 1998;12(Pt 4):743–745.
27. Chee SP, Bacsal K, Jap A, et al. Corneal endotheliitis associated with evidence of cytomegalovirus infection. *Ophthalmology.* 2007;114(4):798–803.
28. Koizumi N, Suzuki T, Uno T, et al. Cytomegalovirus as an etiologic factor in corneal endotheliitis. *Ophthalmology.* 2008;115(2):292–297 e3.
29. Chee SP, Bacsal K, Jap A, et al. Clinical features of cytomegalovirus anterior uveitis in immunocompetent patients. [see comment]. *Am J Ophthalmol.* 2008;145(5):834–840.
30. Rosberger DF, Heinemann MH, Friedberg DN, Holland GN. Uveitis associated with human immunodeficiency virus infection. [see comment]. *Am J Ophthalmol.* 1998;125(3):301–305.
31. Cole EL, Meisler DM, Calabrese LH, et al. Herpes zoster ophthalmicus and acquired immune deficiency syndrome. *Arch Ophthalmol.* 1984;102(7):1027–1029.
32. Kestelyn P, Stevens AM, Bakkers E, et al. Severe herpes zoster ophthalmicus in young African adults: a marker for HTLV-III seropositivity. *Br J Ophthalmol.* 1987;71(11):806–809.
33. Sandor E, Croxson TS, Millman A, Mildvan D. Herpes zoster ophthalmicus in patients at risk for AIDS. *N Engl J Med.* 1984;310(17):1118–1119.
34. Sandor EV, Millman A, Croxson TS, Mildvan D. Herpes zoster ophthalmicus in patients at risk for the acquired immune deficiency syndrome (AIDS). *Am J Ophthalmol.* 1986;101(2):153–155.
35. Sellitti TP, Huang AJ, Schiffman J, Davis JL. Association of herpes zoster ophthalmicus with acquired immunodeficiency syndrome and acute retinal necrosis. *Am J Ophthalmol.* 1993;116(3):297–301.
36. Omoti AE, Omoti CE. Maxillary herpes zoster with corneal involvement in a HIV positive pregnant woman. *Afr J Reprod Health.* 2007;11(1):133–136.
37. Ryan-Graham MA, Durand M, Pavan-Langston D. AIDS and the anterior segment. *Int Ophthalmol Clin.* 1998;38(1):241–263.
38. Pavan-Langston D. Viral disease of the cornea and external eye. In: Albert DM, Jakobiec FA, eds. *Principles and practice of ophthalmology.* Vol. 1. Philadelphia: WB Saunders; 1994.
39. Hodge WG, Seiff SR, Margolis TP. Ocular opportunistic infection incidences among patients who are HIV positive compared to patients who are HIV negative. *Ophthalmology.* 1998;105(5):895–900.
40. Bayu S, Alemayehu W. Clinical profile of herpes zoster ophthalmicus in Ethiopians. *Clin Infect Dis.* 1997;24(6):1256–1260.
41. Owoeye JF, Ademola-Popoola DS. Herpes zoster infection and HIV seropositivity among eye patients – University of Ilorin Teaching Hospital experience. *West Afr J Med.* 2003;22(2):136–138.
42. Palexas GN, Welsh NH. Herpes zoster ophthalmicus: an early pointer to HIV-1 positivity in young African patients. *Scand J Immunol Suppl.* 1992;11:67–68.
43. Stenson SM. Anterior segment manifestations of AIDS. In: Stenson SM, Friedberg DN, eds. *AIDS and the eye.* Vol. 1. New Orleans: Contact Lens Association of Ophthalmologists; 1995.

44. Margolis TP, Milner MS, Shama A, et al. Herpes zoster ophthalmicus in patients with human immunodeficiency virus infection. *Am J Ophthalmol.* 1998;125(3):285–291.
45. Richards JC, Maartens, G, Davidse, AJ. Course and complications of varicella zoster ophthalmicus in a high HIV seroprevalence population (Cape Town, South Africa). *Eye.* 2009;23(2):376–381.
46. Pillai S, Mahmood MA, Limaye SR. Herpes zoster ophthalmicus, contralateral hemiplegia, and recurrent ocular toxoplasmosis in a patient with acquired immune deficiency syndrome-related complex. *J Clin Neuro-Ophthalmol.* 1989;9(4):229–233; discussion 34–5.
47. Seiff SR, Margolis T, Graham SH, O'Donnell JJ. Use of intravenous acyclovir for treatment of herpes zoster ophthalmicus in patients at risk for AIDS. *Ann Ophthalmol.* 1988;20(12):480–482.
48. Levin MJ, Gershon AA, Weinberg A, et al. Administration of live varicella vaccine to HIV-infected children with current or past significant depression of CD4(+) T cells. *J Infect Dis.* 2006;194(2):247–255.
49. Hardy I, Gershon AA, Steinberg SP, LaRussa P. The incidence of zoster after immunization with live attenuated varicella vaccine. A study in children with leukemia. Varicella Vaccine Collaborative Study Group. [see comment]. *N Engl J Med.* 1991;325(22):1545–1550.
50. Marin M, Guris D, Chaves SS, et al. Prevention of varicella: recommendations of the Advisory Committee on Immunization Practices (ACIP). *Morbid Mortal Wkly Rep Recommendations & Reports.* 2007;56(RR-4):1–40.
51. Chern KC, Conrad D, Holland GN, et al. Chronic varicella-zoster virus epithelial keratitis in patients with acquired immunodeficiency syndrome. *Arch Ophthalmol.* 1998;116(8):1011–1017.
52. Engstrom RE, Holland GN. Chronic herpes zoster virus keratitis associated with the acquired immunodeficiency syndrome. *Am J Ophthalmol.* 1988;105(5):556–558.
53. Mondino BJ, Brown SI, Mondzelewski JP. Peripheral corneal ulcers with herpes zoster ophthalmicus. *Am J Ophthalmol.* 1978;86(5):611–614.
54. Neves RA, Rodriguez A, Power WJ, et al. Herpes zoster peripheral ulcerative keratitis in patients with the acquired immunodeficiency syndrome. *Cornea.* 1996;15(5):446–450.
55. Naseri A, Margolis TP. Varicella zoster virus immune recovery stromal keratitis in a patient with AIDS. *Br J Ophthalmol.* 2001;85(11):1390–1391.
56. Silverstein BE, Chandler D, Neger R, Margolis TP. Disciform keratitis: a case of herpes zoster sine herpete. *Am J Ophthalmol.* 1997;123(2):254–255.
57. Hodge WG, Margolis TP. Herpes simplex virus keratitis among patients who are positive or negative for human immunodeficiency virus: an epidemiologic study. *Ophthalmology.* 1997;104(1):120–124.
58. Young TL, Robin JB, Holland GN, et al. Herpes simplex keratitis in patients with acquired immune deficiency syndrome. *Ophthalmology.* 1989;96(10):1476–1[illegible].
59. Rosenwasser GO, Greene WH. Simultaneous herpes simplex types 1 and 2 keratitis in acquired immunodeficiency syndrome. *Am J Ophthalmol.* 1992;113(1):102–103.
60. Pramod NP, Hari R, Sudhamathi K, et al. Influence of human immunodeficiency virus status on the clinical history of herpes simplex keratitis. *Ophthalmologica.* 2000;214(5):337–340.
61. Bodaghi B, Mougin C, Michelson S, et al. Acyclovir-resistant bilateral keratitis associated with mutations in the HSV-1 thymidine kinase gene. *Exp Eye Res.* 2000;71(4):353–359.
62. McLeish W, Pflugfelder SC, Crouse C, et al. Interferon treatment of herpetic keratitis in a patient with acquired immunodeficiency syndrome. *Am J Ophthalmol.* 1990;109(1):93–95.
63. Milazzo L, Trovati S, Pedenovi S, et al. Recurrent herpes simplex virus (HSV) eyelid infection in an HIV-1 infected patient. *Infection.* 2007;35(5):393–394.
64. Stewart JA, Reef SE, Pellett PE, et al. Herpesvirus infections in persons infected with human immunodeficiency virus. *Clin Infect Dis.* 1995;21(Suppl 1):S114–S120.
65. Kohn SR. Molluscum contagiosum in patients with acquired immunodeficiency syndrome. *Arch Ophthalmol.* 1987;105(4):458.
66. Gur I. The epidemiology of molluscum contagiosum in HIV-seropositive patients: a unique entity or insignificant finding? *Int J STD AIDS.* 2008;19(8):503–506.
67. Hughes WT, Parham DM. Molluscum contagiosum in children with cancer or acquired immunodeficiency syndrome. *Pediatr Infect Dis J.* 1991;10(2):152–156.
68. Pelaez CA, Gurbindo MD, Cortes C, Munoz-Fernandez MA. Molluscum contagiosum, involving the upper eyelids, in a child infected with HIV-1. *Pediatr AIDS HIV Infect.* 1996;7(1):43–46.
69. Robinson MR, Udell IJ, Garber PF, et al. Molluscum contagiosum of the eyelids in patients with acquired immune deficiency syndrome. *Ophthalmology.* 1992;99(11):1745–1747.
70. Charles NC, Friedberg DN. Epibulbar molluscum contagiosum in acquired immune deficiency syndrome. Case report and review of the literature. *Ophthalmology.* 1992;99(7):1123–1126.
71. Merisier H, Cochereau I, Hoang-Xuan T, et al. Multiple molluscum contagiosum lesions of the limbus in a patient with HIV infection. *Br J Ophthalmol.* 1995;79(4):393–394.
72. Leahey AB, Shane JJ, Listhaus A, Trachtman M. Molluscum contagiosum eyelid lesions as the initial manifestation of acquired immunodeficiency syndrome. *Am J Ophthalmol.* 1997;124(2):240–241.
73. Bardenstein DS, Elmets C. Hyperfocal cryotherapy of multiple molluscum contagiosum lesions in patients with the acquired immune deficiency syndrome. *Ophthalmology.* 1995;102(7):1031–1034.
74. Calista D, Boschini A, Landi G. Resolution of disseminated molluscum contagiosum with highly active anti-retroviral therapy (HAART) in patients with AIDS. *Eur J Dermatol.* 1999;9(3):211–213.
75. Schulz D, Sarra GM, Koerner UB, Garweg JG. Evolution of HIV-1-related conjunctival molluscum contagiosum under HAART: report of a bilaterally manifesting case and literature review. *Graefes Arch Clin Exp Ophthalmol.* 2004;242(11):951–955.
76. Albini T, Rao N. Molluscum contagiosum in an immune reconstituted AIDS patient. *Br J Ophthalmol.* 2003;87(11):1427–1428.
77. Guech-Ongey M, Engels EA, Goedert JJ, et al. Elevated risk for squamous cell carcinoma of the conjunctiva among adults with AIDS in the United States. *Int J Cancer.* 2008;122(11):2590–2593.
78. Kestelyn P, Stevens AM, Ndayambaje A, et al. HIV and conjunctival malignancies. *Lancet.* 1990;336(8706):51–52.
79. Verma V, Shen D, Sieving PC, Chan CC. The role of infectious agents in the etiology of ocular adnexal neoplasia. *Surv Ophthalmol.* 2008;53(4):312–331.
80. Waddell KM, Lewallen S, Lucas SB, et al. Carcinoma of the conjunctiva and HIV infection in Uganda and Malawi. [see comment]. *Br J Ophthalmol.* 1996;80(6):503–508.
81. Lewallen S, Shroyer KR, Keyser RB, Liomba G. Aggressive conjunctival squamous cell carcinoma in three young Africans. *Arch Ophthalmol.* 1996;114(2):215–218. [erratum appears in *Arch Ophthalmol.* 1996; 114(7):855].
82. Muccioli C, Belfort R Jr, Burnier M, Rao N. Squamous cell carcinoma of the conjunctiva in a patient with the acquired immunodeficiency syndrome. *Am J Ophthalmol.* 1996;121(1):94–96.
83. Soong HK, Feil SH, Elner VM, et al. Conjunctival mucoepidermoid carcinoma in a young HIV-infected man. *Am J Ophthalmol.* 1999;128(5):640–643.
84. Tulvatana W, Tirakunwichcha S. Multifocal squamous cell carcinoma of the conjunctiva with intraocular penetration in a patient with AIDS. *Cornea.* 2006;25(6):745–747.
85. Spitzer MS, Batumba NH, Chirambo T, et al. Ocular surface squamous neoplasia as the first apparent manifestation of HIV infection in Malawi. *Clin Exp Ophthalmol.* 2008;36(5):422–425.
86. Maclean H, Dhillon B, Ironside J. Squamous cell carcinoma of the eyelid and the acquired immunodeficiency syndrome. *Am J Ophthalmol.* 1996;121(2):219–221.
87. Ateenyi Agaba C, Weiderpass E, Tommasino M, et al. Papillomavirus infection in the conjunctiva of individuals with and without AIDS: an autopsy series from Uganda. *Cancer Lett.* 2006;239(1):98–102.
88. Holkar S, Mudhar HS, Jain A, et al. Regression of invasive conjunctival squamous carcinoma in an HIV-positive patient on antiretroviral therapy. *Int J STD AIDS.* 2005;16(12):782–783.
89. Boivin G, Gaudreau A, Routy JP. Evaluation of the human herpesvirus 8 DNA load in blood and Kaposi's sarcoma skin lesions from AIDS patients on highly active antiretroviral therapy. *AIDS.* 2000;14(13):1907–1910.
90. Biswas J, Sudharshan S. Anterior segment manifestations of human immunodeficiency virus/acquired immune deficiency syndrome. *Indian J Ophthalmol.* 2008;56(5):363–375.
91. Schmid K, Wild T, Bolz M, et al. Kaposi's sarcoma of the conjunctiva leads to a diagnosis of acquired immunodeficiency syndrome. *Acta Ophthalmol Scand.* 2003;81(4):411–413.
92. Rezza G, Andreoni M, Dorrucci M, et al. Human herpesvirus 8 seropositivity and risk of Kaposi's sarcoma and other acquired immunodeficiency syndrome-related diseases. [see comment]. *J Natl Cancer Inst.* 1999;91(17):1468–1474.
93. Moore PS, Chang Y. Detection of herpesvirus-like DNA sequences in Kaposi's sarcoma in patients with and without HIV infection. [see comment]. *N Engl J Med.* 1995;332(18):1181–1185.
94. Tunc M, Simmons ML, Char DH, Herndier B. Non-Hodgkin lymphoma and Kaposi sarcoma in an eyelid of a patient with acquired immunodeficiency syndrome. Multiple viruses in pathogenesis. *Arch Ophthalmol.* 1997;115(11):1464–1466.

95. Minoda H, Usui N, Sata T, et al. Human herpesvirus-8 in Kaposi's sarcoma of the conjunctiva in a patient with AIDS. *Jpn J Ophthalmol.* 2006;50(1):7–11.
96. Moore PS, Chang Y. Kaposi's sarcoma-associated herpesvirus-encoded oncogenes and oncogenesis. *J Natl Cancer Inst Monographs.* 1998(23): 65–71.
97. Leder HA, Galor A, Peters GB, et al. Resolution of conjunctival Kaposi sarcoma after institution of highly active antiretroviral therapy alone. *Br J Ophthalmol.* 2008;92(1):151.
98. Maurer T, Ponte M, Leslie K. HIV-associated Kaposi's sarcoma with a high CD4 count and a low viral load. [see comment]. *N Engl J Med.* 2007;357(13):1352–1353.
99. Aristimuno B, Nirankari VS, Hemady RK, Rodrigues MM. Spontaneous ulcerative keratitis in immunocompromised patients. *Am J Ophthalmol.* 1993;115(2):202–208.
100. Hemady RK. Microbial keratitis in patients infected with the human immunodeficiency virus. *Ophthalmology.* 1995;102(7):1026–1030.
101. Maguen E, Salz JJ, Nesburn AB. Pseudomonas corneal ulcer associated with rigid, gas-permeable, daily-wear lenses in a patient infected with human immunodeficiency virus. *Am J Ophthalmol.* 1992;113(3): 336–337.
102. Nanda M, Pflugfelder SC, Holland S. Fulminant pseudomonal keratitis and scleritis in human immunodeficiency virus-infected patients. *Arch Ophthalmol.* 1991;109(4):503–505.
103. Ticho BH, Urban RC Jr, Safran MJ, Saggau DD. Capnocytophaga keratitis associated with poor dentition and human immunodeficiency virus infection. *Am J Ophthalmol.* 1990;109(3):352–353.
104. Lucca JA, Farris RL, Bielory L, Caputo AR. Keratoconjunctivitis sicca in male patients infected with human immunodeficiency virus type 1. *Ophthalmology.* 1990;97(8):1008–1010.
105. Sachs R, Zagelbaum BM, Hersh PS. Corneal complications associated with the use of crack cocaine. [see comment]. *Ophthalmology.* 1993;100(2):187–191.
106. Comerie-Smith SE, Nunez J, Hosmer M, Farris RL. Tear lactoferrin levels and ocular bacterial flora in HIV positive patients. *Adv Exp Med Biol.* 1994;350:339–344.
107. Campos MS, Campos e Silva Lde Q, Rehder JR, et al. Anaerobic flora of the conjunctival sac in patients with AIDS and with anophthalmia compared with normal eyes. *Acta Ophthalmol.* 1994;72(2):241–245.
108. Gumbel H, Ohrloff C, Shah PM. Die Konjunktivalflora HIV-positiver Patienten in fortgeschrittenen Stadien. *Fortschr Ophthalmol.* 1990;87(4):382–383.
109. Gritz DC, Scott TJ, Sedo SF, et al. Ocular flora of patients with AIDS compared with those of HIV-negative patients. *Cornea.* 1997;16(4): 400–405.
110. Yamauchi Y, Minoda H, Yokoi K, et al. Conjunctival flora in patients with human immunodeficiency virus infection. *Ocul Immunol Inflamm.* 2005;13(4):301–304.
111. Fontes BM, Muccioli C, Principe AH, et al. Effect of chronic systemic use of trimethoprim-sulfamethoxazole in the conjunctival bacterial flora of patients with HIV infection. *Am J Ophthalmol.* 2004;138(4): 678–679.
112. Chaidaroon W, Ausayakhun S, Pruksakorn S, et al. Ocular bacterial flora in HIV-positive patients and their sensitivity to gentamicin. *Jpn J Ophthalmol.* 2006;50(1):72–73.
113. Alfonso E, Kenyon KR, Ormerod LD, et al. *Pseudomonas* corneoscleritis. *Am J Ophthalmol.* 1987;103(1):90–98.
114. Buus DR, Pflugfelder SC, Schachter J, et al. Lymphogranuloma venereum conjunctivitis with a marginal corneal perforation. *Ophthalmology.* 1988;95(6):799–802.
115. Forster RK, Rebell G. The diagnosis and management of keratomycoses. I. Cause and diagnosis. *Arch Ophthalmol.* 1975;93(10):975–978.
116. Thygeson P, Okumoto M. Keratomycosis: a preventable disease. *Trans Am Acad Ophthalmol Otolaryngol.* 1974;78(3):OP433–OP439.
117. Hemady RK, Griffin N, Aristimuno B. Recurrent corneal infections in a patient with the acquired immunodeficiency syndrome. *Cornea.* 1993;12(3):266–269.
118. Parrish CM, O'Day DM, Hoyle TC. Spontaneous fungal corneal ulcer as an ocular manifestation of AIDS. *Am J Ophthalmol.* 1987;104(3): 302–303.
119. Santos C, Parker J, Dawson C, Ostler B. Bilateral fungal corneal ulcers in a patient with AIDS-related complex. *Am J Ophthalmol.* 1986;102(1): 118–119.
120. Mselle J. Fungal keratitis as an indicator of HIV infection in Africa. *Tropical Doctor.* 1999;29(3):133–135.
121. Ritterband DC, Seedor JA, Shah MK, et al. Fungal keratitis at the New York Eye and Ear Infirmary. *Cornea.* 2006;25(3):264–267.
122. Balmes R, Bialasiewicz AA, Busse H. Conjunctival cryptococcosis preceding human immunodeficiency virus seroconversion. *Am J Ophthalmol.* 1992;113(6):719–721.
123. Muccioli C, Belfort Junior R, Neves R, Rao N. Limbal and choroidal *Cryptococcus* infection in the acquired immunodeficiency syndrome. *Am J Ophthalmol.* 1995;120(4):539–540.
124. Coccia L, Calista D, Boschini A. Eyelid nodule: a sentinel lesion of disseminated cryptococcosis in a patient with acquired immunodeficiency syndrome. *Arch Ophthalmol.* 1999;117(2):271–272.
125. Waddell KM, Lucas SB, Downing RG. Case reports and small case series: conjunctival cryptococcosis in the acquired immunodeficiency syndrome. *Arch Ophthalmol.* 2000;118(10):1452–1453.
126. Garelick JM, Khodabakhsh AJ, Lopez Y, et al. Scleral ulceration caused by *Cryptococcus albidus* in a patient with acquired immune deficiency syndrome. *Cornea.* 2004;23(7):730–731.
127. Ashton N, Wirasinha PA. Encephalitozoonosis (nosematosis) of the cornea. *Br J Ophthalmol.* 1973;57(9):669–674.
128. Pinnolis M, Egbert PR, Font RL, Winter FC. Nosematosis of the cornea. Case report, including electron microscopic studies. *Arch Ophthalmol.* 1981;99(6):1044–1047.
129. Cali A, Meisler DM, Rutherford I, et al. Corneal microsporidiosis in a patient with AIDS. *Am J Trop Med Hyg.* 1991;44(5):463–468.
130. Didier ES, Didier PJ, Friedberg DN, et al. Isolation and characterization of a new human microsporidian, *Encephalitozoon hellem* (n. sp.), from three AIDS patients with keratoconjunctivitis. *J Infect Dis.* 1991;163(3):617–621.
131. Friedberg DN, Stenson SM, Orenstein JM, et al. Microsporidial keratoconjunctivitis in acquired immunodeficiency syndrome. *Arch Ophthalmol.* 1990;108(4):504–508.
132. Lowder CY, McMahon JT, Meisler DM, et al. Microsporidial keratoconjunctivitis caused by *Septata intestinalis* in a patient with acquired immunodeficiency syndrome. *Am J Ophthalmol.* 1996;121(6):715–717.
133. Lowder CY, Meisler DM, McMahon JT, et al. Microsporidia infection of the cornea in a man seropositive for human immunodeficiency virus. *Am J Ophthalmol.* 1990;109(2):242–244.
134. Metcalfe TW, Doran RM, Rowlands PL, et al. Microsporidial keratoconjunctivitis in a patient with AIDS. *Br J Ophthalmol.* 1992;76(3): 177–178.
135. Yee RW, Tio FO, Martinez JA, et al. Resolution of microsporidial epithelial keratopathy in a patient with AIDS. *Ophthalmology.* 1991;98(2): 196–201.
136. Schwartz DA, Visvesvara GS, Diesenhouse MC, et al. Pathologic features and immunofluorescent antibody demonstration of ocular microsporidiosis (*Encephalitozoon hellem*) in seven patients with acquired immunodeficiency syndrome. [see comment]. *Am J Ophthalmol.* 1993;115(3): 285–292.
137. Gajdatsy AD, Tay-Kearney ML. Microsporidial keratoconjunctivitis after HAART. *Clin Exp Ophthalmol.* 2001;29(5):327–329.
138. Chan CM, Theng JT, Li L, Tan DT. Microsporidial keratoconjunctivitis in healthy individuals: a case series. *Ophthalmology.* 2003;110(7): 1420–1425.
139. Silverstein BE, Cunningham ET Jr, Margolis TP, et al. Microsporidial keratoconjunctivitis in a patient without human immunodeficiency virus infection. *Am J Ophthalmol.* 1997;124(3):395–396.
140. Sridhar MS, Sharma S. Microsporidial keratoconjunctivitis in a HIV-seronegative patient treated with debridement and oral itraconazole. *Am J Ophthalmol.* 2003;136(4):745–746.
141. Theng J, Chan C, Ling ML, Tan D. Microsporidial keratoconjunctivitis in a healthy contact lens wearer without human immunodeficiency virus infection. *Ophthalmology.* 2001;108(5):976–978.
142. Shah GK, Pfister D, Probst LE, et al. Diagnosis of microsporidial keratitis by confocal microscopy and the chromatrope stain. *Am J Ophthalmol.* 1996;121(1):89–91.
143. Conners MS, Gibler TS, Van Gelder RN. Diagnosis of microsporidia keratitis by polymerase chain reaction. *Arch Ophthalmol.* 2004;122(2): 283–284.
144. Diesenhouse MC, Wilson LA, Corrent GF, et al. Treatment of microsporidial keratoconjunctivitis with topical fumagillin. [see comment]. *Am J Ophthalmol.* 1993;115(3):293–298.
145. Rosberger DF, Serdarevic ON, Erlandson RA, et al. Successful treatment of microsporidial keratoconjunctivitis with topical fumagillin in a patient with AIDS. *Cornea.* 1993;12(3):261–265.
146. Wilkins JH, Joshi N, Margolis TP, et al. Microsporidial keratoconjunctivitis treated successfully with a short course of fumagillin. *Eye.* 1994;8(Pt 6):703–704.
147. Gritz DC, Holsclaw DS, Neger RE, et al. Ocular and sinus microsporidial infection cured with systemic albendazole. *Am J Ophthalmol.* 1997;124(2):241–243.

148. Lecuit M, Oksenhendler E, Sarfati C. Use of albendazole for disseminated microsporidian infection in a patient with AIDS. *Clin Infect Dis.* 1994;19(2):332–333.
149. Rossi P, Urbani C, Donelli G, Pozio E. Resolution of microsporidial sinusitis and keratoconjunctivitis by itraconazole treatment. *Am J Ophthalmol.* 1999;127(2):210–212.
150. Martins SA, Muccioli C, Belfort R Jr, Castelo A. Resolution of microsporidial keratoconjunctivitis in an AIDS patient treated with highly active antiretroviral therapy. *Am J Ophthalmol.* 2001;131(3):378–379.

Chapter 68

Ocular Graft-versus-Host Disease

Stella K. Kim

Introduction

Blood and marrow transplantation is one of the most important advancements in the treatment of hematologic/immune disorders, metabolic disorders, and malignancies. Types of transplantation depend on the source of the donor cells: autologous (self), syngeneic (twin), and allogeneic (another individual). Classically referred as bone marrow transplantation (BMT), donor cells can now be harvested not only from the bone marrow but also from peripheral blood as well as cord blood from the placenta. Graft-versus-host disease (GVHD) is observed in the allogeneic transplant setting, and unlike graft rejection in a solid organ transplantation, where the host immune system responds to the transplanted organ, in GVHD the donor cells (graft) mount an immune response against the recipient (host patient), precipitating immunologic attack typically to the skin, gastrointestinal system, liver, mouth, lungs, and eyes.[1–3]

The incidence of GVHD varies greatly, ranging from 10% to 90%, and multiple factors influence its prevalence, such as histocompatibility, age, prophylaxis, and host environment among others.[2,4] There may also be a difference in the incidence of GVDH between bone marrow transplantation and peripheral blood stem cell transplantation (PBSC).[5–10] GVHD is described as 'acute' versus 'chronic,' purely by an arbitrary division of events occurring either before or 100 days post transplantation, respectively. Grading of GVHD serves as an important tool for assessing patients' morbidity and mortality; the current grading system for acute GVHD has been updated,[11] and more recently efforts are being made to reorganize the classification system so that it may be applicable for prospective clinical trials.

A similar effort for chronic GVHD led by the National Institute of Health/National Cancer Center has been completed and the consensus reports published in six separate papers.[12–17] Of these, four are relevant to chronic ocular GVHD[12–15] and describe the diagnostic criteria, histology, and management, all of which were written for a target audience of BMT transplantation specialists.[12–15] GVHD remains a significant limiting factor for successful blood and marrow transplantation.[1,2,18]

Ocular Graft-versus-Host Disease

Ocular complications in transplant patients can range from 60% to 90% of patients with GVHD and may affect all layers of the eyes, from lid to nerve, in both acute and chronic settings.[19–22] As is the case for systemic GVHD, acute ocular GVHD is a clinical event that occurs between days 1 and 100 post BMT, whereas the same ocular manifestation are considered chronic GVHD after day 100 post transplantation. Ocular complications such as infections, cataracts, and dry eye syndrome in BMT patients are not called ocular GVHD but are commonly observed, given the overall immunocompromised status of these patients and their cancer treatments, such as chemotherapy, radiation, and steroid administration.

Ocular GVHD is an umbrella term to describe a post-allogeneic transplantation condition that can cause a spectrum of ocular disorders, typically of the ocular surface and the lacrimal glands, such as conjunctival inflammation, lacrimal gland dysfunction resulting in keratoconjunctivitis sicca, meibomian gland dysfunction, and cicatricial conjunctival scarring, all of which may result in ocular surface diseases.[20,23–25] Without proper intervention, patients may experience debilitating conditions such as chronic filamentary keratitis, shield ulcers, or even corneal perforations.[26–28] Unusual presentations such as bloody epiphora have also been observed in patients with chronic ocular GVHD, with a possible association with granulomatous growth in the punctum and on the palpebral conjunctiva.[29] Uveitis has been rarely observed, though this is a diagnosis of exclusion in patients who often have the diagnosis of lymphoma or leukemia and are severely immunocompromised.[30,31] Posterior chamber ocular GVHD is rare,[20,32,33] and there are even more unexpected presentations, such as posterior scleritis.[34] Ocular GVHD may have similarities in clinical manifestation to any autoimmune/collagen vascular disease that affects the eye. This chapter will focus on ocular surface disease.

Conjunctival Disease: Spectrum and Diagnosis

In order to make a clinical diagnosis of ocular GVHD, a thorough ocular history and examination are required so as to understand the patient's history of their transplantation course, systemic GVHD, and systemic medication changes. For example, systemic GVHD symptoms such as abdominal pain, diarrhea, rash, shortness of breath, recent infection, or fever may all represent active or recent flare of the patient's disease.

Ocular GVHD typically involves the conjunctiva. Jabs et al.[35] described a clinical staging for conjunctival ocular GVHD: hyperemia alone for stage I; hyperemia with chemosis and/or serosanguineous exudates for stage II; pseudomembranous conjunctivitis for stage III; and corneal epithelial sloughing for stage IV. The level of hyperemia may be subtle for stage I (Fig. 68.1). Even if the clinical findings are subtle, the diagnosis of ocular GVHD should be considered when accompanied by symptoms such as photophobia, foreign body sensation, and clinical signs of a decrease in aqueous tear function concurrently with systemic GVHD. Conjunctival swabs for viral culture must be considered to rule out other causes of mild hyperemia. For stage II, conjunctival hyperemia is associated with a spectrum of moderate chemosis to exuberant serosanguineous exudates (Fig. 68.2A). Systemic fluid retention can occur in BMT patients who are usually immunosuppressed with steroids, and it can be challenging to decide whether a chemotic conjunctiva is the result of fluid status or ocular GVHD. Assessing the patient's overall fluid status along with other causes of increased fluid retention should be considered, such as systemic electrolytes (particularly sodium) and albumin levels. The presence of systemic GVHD, recent change in immunosuppressive medications, reduction in aqueous tear function, and conjunctival biopsies may also aid in the diagnosis.

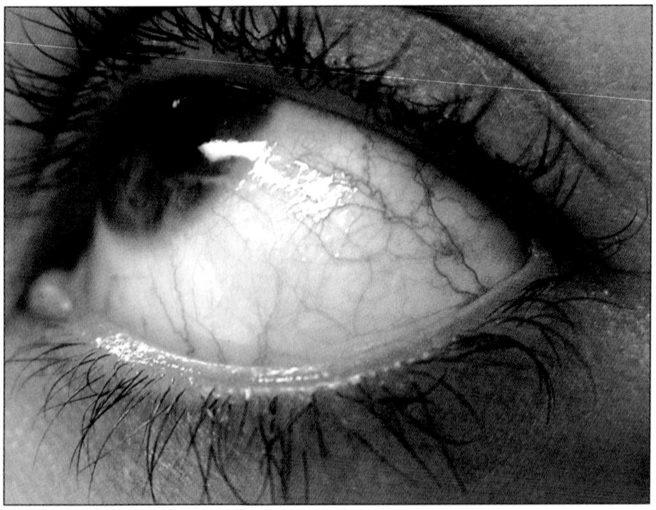

Fig. 68.1 Mild conjunctival hyperemia. Patient also had complete lack of aqueous tear function. Stage I.

Severe hyperemia can also be seen in stage II ocular GVHD (Fig. 68.2B). Despite its aggressively inflamed appearance, symptoms may vary from severe pain to only mild photophobia. When conjunctival hyperemia is accompanied by conjunctival epithelial sloughing leading to pseudomembranous changes, the staging becomes III (Fig. 68.3). The term 'pseudomembranous' conjunctivitis is not entirely accurate, given that the pseudomembrane of GVHD can quickly become 'membranous' as it scars. Attempts to remove them from the palpebral conjunctiva, even in the 'pseudomembranous' stage, can cause bleeding, even in the setting of a normal platelet count. Stage III, therefore, is best characterized by pseudomembranous/membranous conjunctivitis and occurs in 12–17% of acute GVHD patients and 11% of chronic GVHD patients.[21,22,35] In the most severe cases the corneal epithelium is also involved, resulting in nearly complete corneal epithelial sloughing (Fig. 68.4). Stage IV ocular GVHD resembles severe skin GVHD (with generalized erythema progressing to bullous formation and desquamation)[36] and GI GVHD (with crypt dropouts, epithelial necrosis, and sloughing).[1,36] Approximately one-third of patients who have pseudomembranes will have corneal sloughing,[35] although with current aggressive local treatment of stage III ocular GVHD this number may vary between institutions.

Conjunctival biopsy may aid in the diagnosis and management of ocular GVHD[12,37] for patients who have clinical findings of conjunctival disease. Routine biopsies, however,

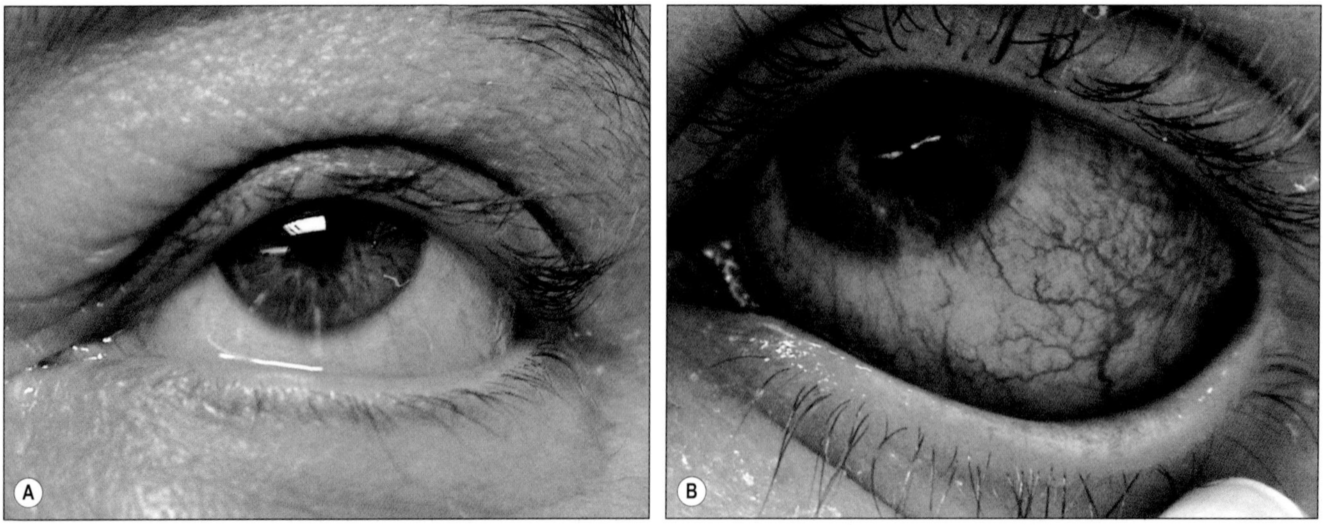

Fig. 68.2 Conjunctival disease. **A,** Ocular GVHD with mild hyperemia and chemosis with +3 serosanguineous exudates. Stage II. **B,** Ocular GVHD with severe hyperemia with mild chemosis. Stage II.

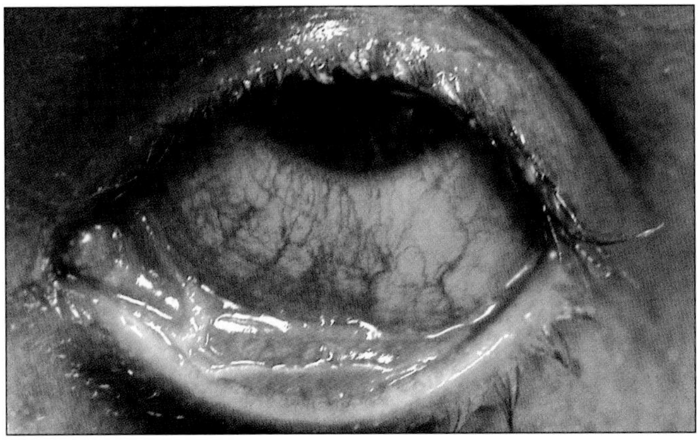

Fig. 68.3 Pseudomembranous/membranous conjunctivitis. Stage III conjunctival ocular GVHD.

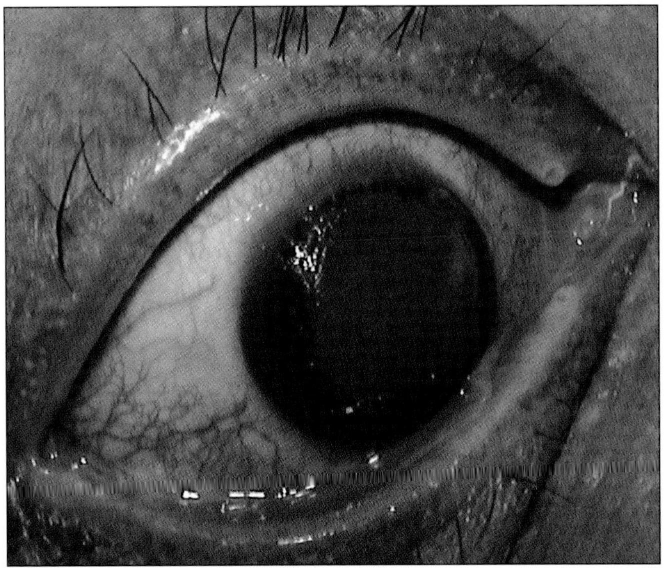

Fig. 68.4 Nearly complete corneal epithelial sloughing with fluorescein uptake. Notice the pseudomembranous changes of the lower tarsal conjunctiva, which also stains with fluorescein. Stage IV conjunctival ocular GVHD scale.

are thought to be less useful for early GVHD.[22,38] Histologically, the features of conjunctival GVHD include lymphocyte exocytosis, satellitosis, and epithelial cell necrosis, which may have been describing, in part, apoptotic cells which are currently thought to be the hallmark of GVHD in the skin, bile ducts, and GI tract.[12,24,37,39–51] Nonspecific features can also be observed, including epithelial attenuation and goblet cell depletion; these findings alone are not sufficient for the diagnosis of ocular GVHD.[37] Depolarization of the epithelial layer and loss of goblet cells may also be observed (Fig. 68.5). T-cell analysis performed on one acute conjunctival GVHD biopsy specimen showed an abundance of CD4+ helper T-lymphocytes,[35] whereas a conjunctival specimen from a patient with chronic GVHD showed predominantly suppressor/cytotoxic cells,[43] the significance of which remains unclear. The histology of pseudomembrane/membrane (Fig.

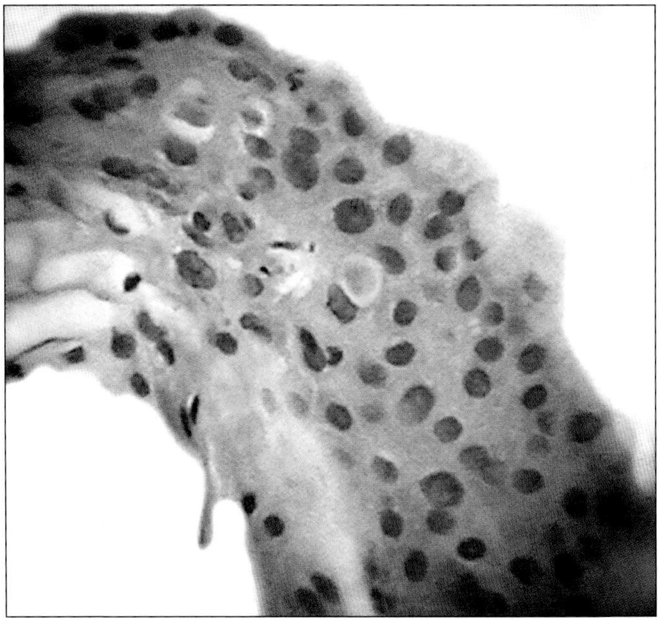

Fig. 68.5 Conjunctival specimen for ocular GVHD. Note the apoptotic cells that are reminiscent of apoptotic keratinocytes of skin GVHD. Vacuolization of the basal epithelial cells is also present. Loss of goblet cells and depolarization of the epithelium are present in this specimen.

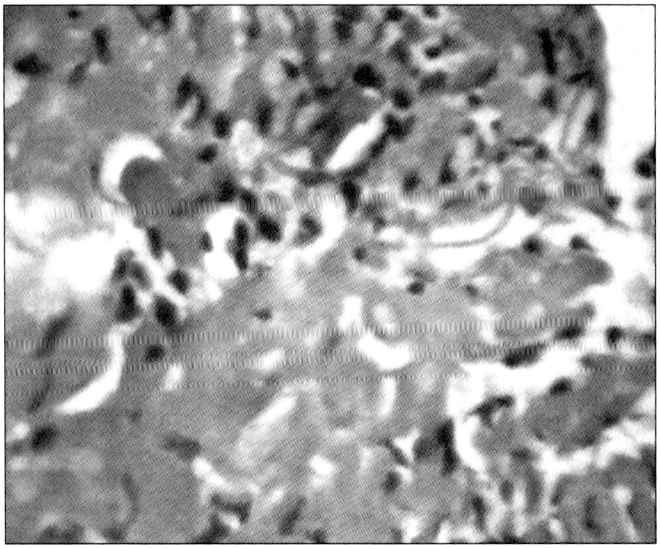

Fig. 68.6 Histopathology of conjunctival pseudomembrane. Note the inflammatory cells, fibrinous material, and cellular debris.

68.6) consists of inflammatory cells, fibrinous material, and cellular debris,[35] and one case report has shown that T cells in the pseudomembrane are donor derived.[44]

It has been suggested that conjunctival ocular GVHD may serve as a marker for the severity of acute GVHD and may reflect the course of systemic GVHD.[35,45] In those affected by acute systemic GVHD and conjunctival involvement, the ocular GVHD occurred approximately 2 weeks after the onset of the acute systemic ocular GVHD. These patients had worse survival than those with same grade of acute GVHD without conjunctival involvement, suggesting that the presence of conjunctival disease indicates worse disease. Observations have also been made that conjunctival ocular GVHD occurs only in the setting of systemic GVHD.[35,46] Experience at MD Anderson Cancer Center, however, suggests that conjunctival acute ocular GVHD may be present without systemic GVHD and may be the initial presenting GVHD in BMT patients. Further studies are needed to elucidate the role of conjunctival ocular GVHD in predicting the presence and/or progression of systemic GVHD.

Other conjunctival clinical manifestations have been observed in ocular GVHD. Cicatricial scarring is commonly seen in chronic ocular GVHD patients,[20,52–54] and superior limbic keratoconjunctivitis has also been observed in patients with chronic ocular GVHD who have reduced tear function and cicatricial lid scarring.[55]

Keratoconjunctivitis Sicca/Dry Eye Syndrome

Keratoconjunctivitis sicca (KCS) or dry eye syndrome (DES) (Fig. 68.7) is one of the most common forms of ocular complication in BMT patients.[21,22,24,46–50] It has been observed in the earliest BMT patients,[42,51] and studies have shown that in most patients with sicca syndrome the aqueous tear dysfunction does not recover.[22,39] The incidence of KCS post BMT, however, varies greatly, ranging from 22% to 80%,[21,22,46,48,49,56] and it is equally challenging to decipher the clinical variables used to diagnose KCS. Most studies have shown that ocular GVHD with KCS is more common in patients who have chronic systemic GVHD (69–77%). In one retrospective study[49] KCS was observed in over 80% of patients with chronic systemic GVHD, whereas a large multicenter retrospective evaluation for KCS[50] noted 19% overall. Of interest, this study also showed that female gender and older age are independent risk factors for developing KCS post BMT, as observed in de novo Sjögren's syndrome. On the other hand, in prospective studies,[22,47,48] KCS ranges from 40% to 44%. Using a set of most comprehensive clinical

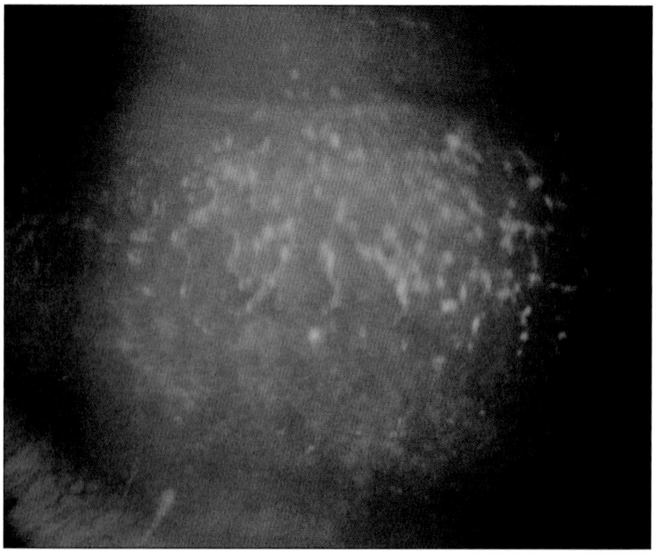

Fig. 68.7 Severe keratoconjunctivitis sicca with diffuse fluorescein uptake on the cornea. Chronic ocular GVHD.

variables for DES in a prospective study,[24] 50% of allogeneic stem cell transplantation patients developed dry eye syndrome with aqueous tear deficiency and severe meibomian gland dysfunction.

Histopathological studies of the lacrimal glands strongly suggest a relationship between KCS ocular GVHD and lacrimal gland dysfunction. A postmortem study of lacrimal glands in patients with acute GVHD[38] described the presence of 'lacrimal gland stasis,' with accumulation of PAS-positive material in the acini and distended ductules, and obliteration of the lumina. The 'stasis' was significantly associated with acute GVHD and dry eye syndrome, and it was proposed that it may represent a similar process seen in liver GVHD with involvement of the bile ducts.[1,37] In studies of lacrimal glands in chronic ocular GVHD, the glands of symptomatic dry eye patients show marked fibrosis of the glandular interstitium, similar to the chronic skin GVHD changes with generalized sclerodermal lichenoid changes.[57,58] There were increased stromal fibroblasts associated with T cells found in periductal areas, which is thought to be the primary site of T-cell activation.[58,59]

Lacrimal gland dysfunction can be assessed with Schirmer's test, which is the gold standard for the diagnosis of chronic ocular GVHD. New onset of KCS with a Schirmer score of 6–10 mm or a symptomatic patient with a Schirmer score of ±5 mm in the presence of at least one other organ affected by GVHD is sufficient to make the diagnosis of chronic ocular GVHD. Lacrimal gland dysfunction/KCS is also commonly observed in the acute setting.[22,36,39,52] Lacrimal gland dysfunction can be the result of many factors, such as a preparatory regimen, dehydration, systemic medication, or pre-existing dry eye syndrome. Therefore, the diagnosis, as for acute ocular GVHD, must be made in the context of the patient's overall GVHD status, transplantation course, and medication history. Recent study has shown that the ocular surface disease index (OSDI)[60] is statistically higher in patients with chronic ocular GVHD than in patients who are pre-transplant or in those who are post-transplant with no ocular GVHD.[61] Also, chronic ocular GVHD patients showed higher aberrations on the videokeratoscopic indices than those without chronic ocular GVHD and pretransplantation patients.[62] These facts may help in evaluating patients for ocular GVHD.

Ocular surface disease in GVHD patients is partly due to meibomian gland dysfunction (MGD).[23,24,46,63] In one study, 63% of chronic GVHD patients had MGD, and this showed a significant correlation with the severity of KCS symptoms.[24] A recent study[63] also suggested that MGD may have a role in early diagnosis of DES associated with chronic GVHD. Meibomian and lacrimal gland dysfunction is commonly observed in pretransplantation patients, although they may not be symptomatic. Ideally, a pretransplant examination can be helpful to document these existing ocular surface conditions and to assess the patient's Schirmer scores, tear breakup time, fluorescein staining for the cornea and conjunctiva, and overall status of the eyelids (palpebral conjunctival keratinization, trichiasis, cicatricial ectropion, and lagophthalmos).[39,64] These findings can also be the sequela of ocular GVHD, as shown in Figure 68.8, and establishing the patient's existing ocular surface disease can help in assessing ocular GVHD.

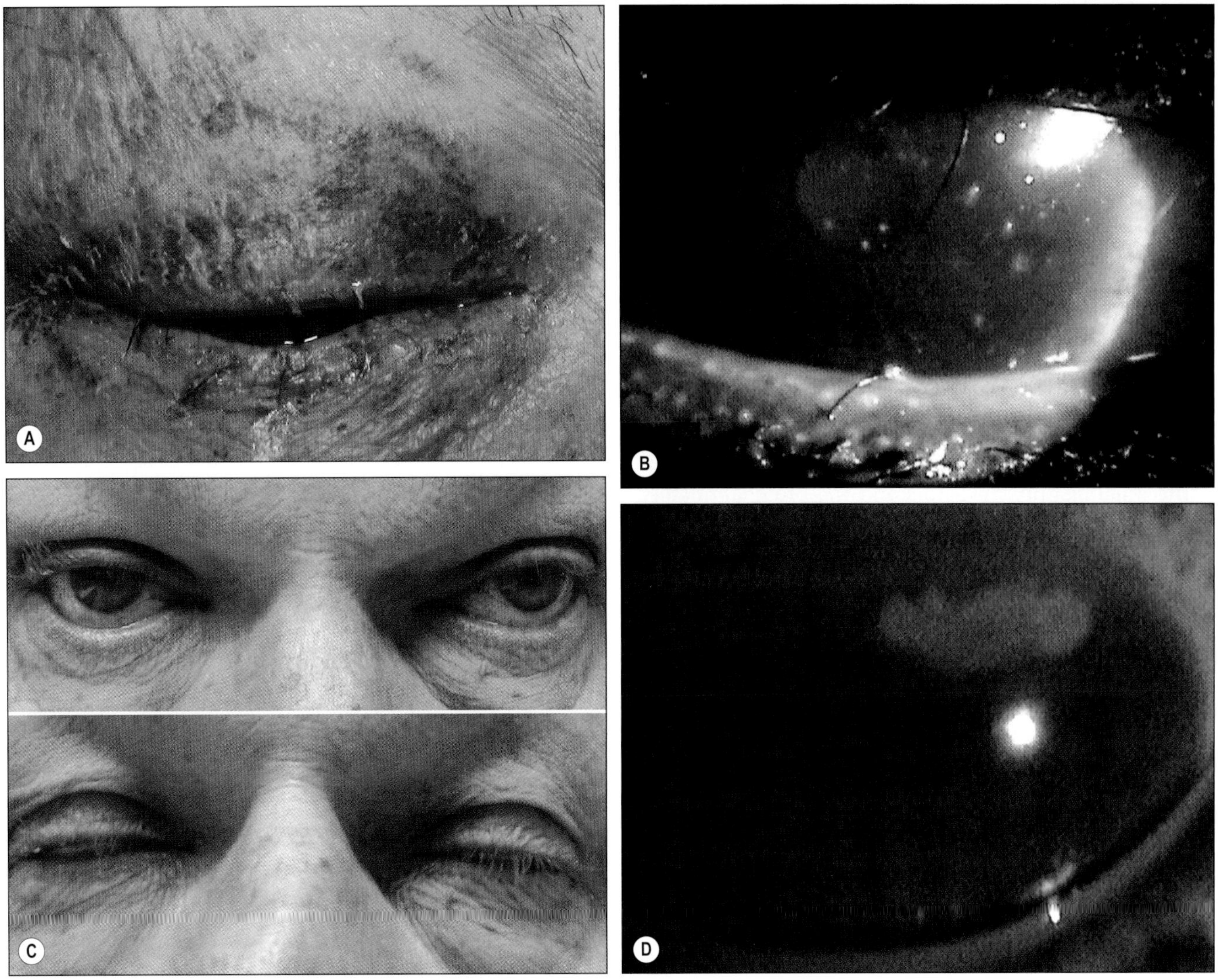

Fig. 68.8 Common ocular manifestations of chronic ocular GVHD. **A,** Lid changes of skin GVHD. **B,** Filamentary keratitis with trichiasis. **C,** Cicatricial, ectropion with lagophthalmos. **D,** Shield ulcer from upper lid conjunctival scarring with sicca.

Management of Ocular GVHD

A consideration for ocular GVHD is to coordinate treatment with the BMT team. Increasing systemic immunosuppression may not necessarily be the optimal approach for treating organ-specific GVHD in the era in which the graft versus tumor (GVT) effect is important in keeping patients in cancer-free remission. There is a greater emphasis on treating organ-specific GVHD with organ-specific treatment (such as topical steroid cream for mild skin GVHD, and steroid inhalers for chronic lung GVHD).[15,65] Depending on the level of systemic GVHD, immunosuppressive medications such as tacrolimus or ciclosporin may be increased in dosage, with or without systemic steroids. If GVHD is of higher grade or shows multiple organ involvement, the first line of treatment is typically high-dose systemic steroids along with tacrolimus or ciclosporin and/or methotrexate. Ocular GVHD often improves with the increase in systemic steroid, but the clinical benefit is less impressive with secondary systemic immunosuppressive therapy.[15,66–68] If GVHD is refractory to steroid treatment, patients are often treated with a variety of adjuvant therapies (e.g., photopheresis, rituximab, mycophenolate mofetil, infliximab, and others) with a variable response, often on GVHD protocols.[1,15,67,69–74] Tapering systemic immunosuppressive medications may trigger systemic GVHD. A slower taper and/or maintenance of systemic immunosuppression to control signs and symptoms of chronic GVHD, including chronic ocular GVHD, is a clinical judgment that must be made with the multidisciplinary team. The clinical approach is to address organ-specific GVHD with organ-specific treatment so that systemic immunosuppression can be relatively unaltered from its stable or tapering schedule. Organ-specific treatment (intended for the BMT audience) has been summarized as part of the chronic GVHD Consensus Workshop.[15]

The management of chronic ocular GVHD has three main strands: lubrication, controlling evaporation, and most importantly, reducing ocular surface inflammation. Medication (topical and oral), surgery, and environmental strategies should all be tried in order to achieve and maintain optimal health in the ocular surface of GVHD patients.

For both acute and chronic ocular GVHD with severe aqueous tear deficiency, frequent topical lubrication with preservative-free artificial tears is the obvious treatment, but equally important is punctal occlusion by silicon plugs or thermal cauterization. Typically, if there is no detectable tear production on Schirmer tests performed without anesthetic, and the patient has severe DES symptoms, it is reasonable to occlude all four lids in one session, in both acute and chronic settings. The threshold for punctal occlusion by silicone plugs should be low, especially in chronic ocular GVHD, where the lacrimal gland dysfunction is thought to be virtually irreversible. Copious lubrication is crucial, especially in acute ocular GVHD, not only for the purpose of lubrication but also to achieve a theoretical benefit by diluting the inflammatory mediators and the proinflammatory milieu of the tears, and on the ocular surface affected by GVHD.[4,52]

Topical ciclosporin A has been used successfully for a series of systemically immunosuppressed patients with chronic ocular GVHD with KCS who were refractory to conventional treatment of lubrication and topical steroids.[75,76] Topical retinoic acid has also been tried in one patient with chronic ocular GVHD, with beneficial effects.[77] Topical autologous serum to treat chronic ocular GVHD with KCS has been described in two patients,[78] and more recently a larger study has been published to reveal the benefit of 20% autologous serum in chronic ocular GVHD patients[59] as a safe and effective modality for the treatment of severe dry eye syndrome. Recently, allogeneic serum has also been used in two chronic ocular GVHD patients with good outcome.[79] The role of autologous serum in the treatment of acute ocular GVHD has not been determined.

The role of topical steroid in acute ocular GVHD has been controversial. It has been suggested that topical steroid or removing pseudomembranes may not have a role in the treatment of acute conjunctival ocular GVHD.[22,35,46] Clinical experience at MD Anderson Cancer Center suggests that topical steroid may be beneficial in these settings.[52,80] Depending on the level of clinical findings at stage II conjunctival GVHD, pulse topical steroid with a rapid taper and prophylactic topical antibiotics, with or without topical ciclosporin, is initiated. Stage III and IV ocular GVHD with severe pseudomembranous/membranous conjunctivitis and corneal sloughing are treated aggressively with frequent lubrication using preservative-free artificial tears and ointment, topical steroid, topical ciclosporin (if tolerated), punctal occlusion, and prophylactic topical antibiotic. In our experience, this approach has improved the rate of corneal epithelial defect healing and reduced palpebral conjunctival scarring, with less symblepharon and cicatricial change of the tarsal conjunctiva.[52,80] Topical steroid has been used in the chronic setting for cicatricial chronic ocular GVHD with positive effect.[53]

The use of a bandage contact lens to treat refractory chronic ocular GVHD has its place,[81] but must be done with judicious follow-up. In the acute setting, however, there are compelling reasons against the use of bandage contact lenses for large corneal epithelial defects in stage IV ocular GVHD: risk of infection, ischemia and other CTL-related problems, extreme inflamed ocular surface, and severe immunosuppression.[20] For patients who are unable to tolerate the soft lenses, scleral lenses can be beneficial.[82,83]

A variety of oral medications can be tried to optimize the ocular surface, though their benefit is unclear. Doxycyline or tetracycline can be used to address MGD, along with lid hygiene. Secretagogues such as oral pilocarpine can be tried to increase tear function. Flaxseed oil tablets may also aid in reducing the ocular surface inflammation.[15]

In summary, maximizing organ-specific ocular treatment for acute and chronic ocular GVHD and balancing systemic immunosuppression must be done in a multidisciplinary fashion with the BMT team in order to optimize the quality of life of the transplant patient.

References

1. Sullivan KM. Graft-versus-host-disease. In: Forman SJ, ed. *Hematopoietic cell transplantation*. Oxford: Blackwell; 1999:515–536.
2. Ferrara JL, et al. Graft-versus-host disease. *Lancet*. 2009;373(9674):1550–1561.
3. Vogelsang GB. Acute and chronic graft-versus-host disease. *Curr Opin Oncol*. 1993;5(2):276–281.
4. Ferrara J, Antin J. The pathophysiology of graft-versus-host disease. In: Forman SJ, ed. *Hematopoietic cell transplantation*. Oxford: Blackwell; 1999:305–315.
5. Schmitz N, et al. Allogeneic bone marrow transplantation vs filgrastim-mobilised peripheral blood progenitor cell transplantation in patients with early leukaemia: first results of a randomised multicentre trial of the European Group for Blood and Marrow Transplantation. *Bone Marrow Transplant*. 1998;21(10):995–1003.
6. Vigorito AC, et al. A randomised, prospective comparison of allogeneic bone marrow and peripheral blood progenitor cell transplantation in the treatment of haematological malignancies. *Bone Marrow Transplant*. 1998;22(12):1145–1151.
7. Powles R, et al. Allogeneic blood and bone-marrow stem-cell transplantation in haematological malignant diseases: a randomised trial. *Lancet*. 2000;355(9211):1231–1237.
8. Blaise D, et al. Randomized trial of bone marrow versus lenograstim-primed blood cell allogeneic transplantation in patients with early-stage leukemia: a report from the Société Française de Greffe de Moelle. *J Clin Oncol*. 2000;18(3):537–546.
9. Bensinger WI, et al. Transplantation of bone marrow as compared with peripheral-blood cells from HLA-identical relatives in patients with hematologic cancers. *N Engl J Med*. 2001;344(3):175–181.
10. Heldal D, et al. A randomised study of allogeneic transplantation with stem cells from blood or bone marrow. *Bone Marrow Transplant*. 2000;25(11):1129–1136.
11. Przepiorka D, et al. 1994 Consensus Conference on Acute GVHD Grading. *Bone Marrow Transplant*. 1995;15(6):825–828.
12. Shulman HM, et al. Histopathologic diagnosis of chronic graft-versus-host disease: National Institutes of Health Consensus Development Project on Criteria for Clinical Trials in Chronic Graft-versus-Host Disease: II. Pathology Working Group Report. *Biol Blood Marrow Transplant*. 2006;12(1):31–47.
13. Filipovich AH, et al. National Institutes of Health Consensus Development Project on Criteria for Clinical Trials in Chronic Graft-versus-Host Disease: I. Diagnosis and Staging Working Group Report. *Biol Blood Marrow Transplant*. 2005;11(12):945–956.
14. Pavletic SZ, et al. Measuring therapeutic response in chronic graft-versus-host disease: National Institutes of Health Consensus Development Project on Criteria for Clinical Trials in Chronic Graft-versus-Host Disease: IV. Response Criteria Working Group Report. *Biol Blood Marrow Transplant*. 2006;12(3):252–266.
15. Couriel D, et al. Ancillary therapy and supportive care of chronic graft-versus-host disease: National Institutes of Health Consensus Development Project on Criteria for Clinical Trials in Chronic Graft-versus-Host Disease: V. Ancillary Therapy and Supportive Care Working Group Report. *Biol Blood Marrow Transplant*. 2006;12(4):375–396.
16. Schultz KR, et al. Toward biomarkers for chronic graft-versus-host disease: National Institutes of Health Consensus Development Project on Criteria

for Clinical Trials in Chronic graft-versus-Host Disease: III. Biomarker Working Group Report. *Biol Blood Marrow Transplant.* 2006;12(2):126–137.

17. Martin PJ, et al. National Institutes of Health Consensus Development Project on Criteria for Clinical Trials in Chronic Graft-versus-Host Disease: VI. Design of Clinical Trials Working Group report. *Biol Blood Marrow Transplant.* 2006;12(5):491–505.
18. Murphy WJ, Blazar BR. New strategies for preventing graft-versus-host disease. *Curr Opin Immunol.* 1999;11(5):509–515.
19. Thomas E, et al. Bone-marrow transplantation (first of two parts). *N Engl J Med.* 1975;292(16):832–843.
20. Franklin RM, et al. Ocular manifestations of graft-vs-host disease. *Ophthalmology.* 1983;90(1):4–13.
21. Bray LC, et al. Ocular complications of bone marrow transplantation. *Br J Ophthalmol.* 1991;75(10):611–614.
22. Hirst LW, et al. The eye in bone marrow transplantation. I. Clinical study. *Arch Ophthalmol.* 1983;101(4):580–584.
23. Kim SK. Update on ocular graft versus host disease. *Curr Opin Ophthalmol.* 2006;17(4):344–348.
24. Ogawa Y, et al. Dry eye after haematopoietic stem cell transplantation. *Br J Ophthalmol.* 1999;83(10):1125–1130.
25. Claes K, Kestelyn P. Ocular manifestations of graft versus host disease following bone marrow transplantation. *Bull Soc Belge Ophtalmol.* 2000(277):21–26.
26. Millar MJ, et al. *Mycobacterium hemophilum* infection presenting as filamentary keratopathy in an immunocompromised adult. *Cornea.* 2007;26(6):764–766.
27. Yoshida A, et al. Apoptosis in perforated cornea of a patient with graft-versus-host disease. *Can J Ophthalmol.* 2006;41(4):472–475.
28. Yeh PT, et al. Recurrent corneal perforation and acute calcareous corneal degeneration in chronic graft-versus-host disease. *J Formos Med Assoc.* 2006;105(4):334–339.
29. Cornelison AM, et al. Bloody epiphora in patients with chronic ocular graft vs. host disease; a case series. *Invest Ophthalmol Vis Sci.* 2009;50S:2615.
30. Hettinga YM, et al. Anterior uveitis: a manifestation of graft-versus-host disease. *Ophthalmology.* 2007;114(4):794–797.
31. Wertheim M, Rosenbaum JT. Bilateral uveitis manifesting as a complication of chronic graft-versus-host disease after allogeneic bone marrow transplantation. *Ocul Immunol Inflamm.* 2005;13(5):403–404.
32. Cheng LL, et al. Graft-vs-host-disease-associated conjunctival chemosis and central serous chorioretinopathy after bone marrow transplant. *Am J Ophthalmol.* 2002;134(2):293–295.
33. Alvarez MT, et al. Multifocal choroiditis after allogenic bone marrow transplantation. *Eur J Ophthalmol.* 2002;12(2):135–137.
34. Kim RY, et al. Scleritis as the initial clinical manifestation of graft-versus-host disease after allogenic bone marrow transplantation. *Am J Ophthalmol.* 2002;133(6):843–845.
35. Jabs DA, et al. The eye in bone marrow transplantation. III. Conjunctival graft-vs-host disease. *Arch Ophthalmol.* 1989;107(9):1343–1348.
36. Jabs DA, Ocular complications of bone marrow transplantation. In: Pepose J. Wilhelmus K, eds. *Ocular infection and immunity.* St. Louis: Mosby; 1996:426–434.
37. West RH, Szer J, Pedersen JS. Ocular surface and lacrimal disturbances in chronic graft-versus-host disease: the role of conjunctival biopsy. *Aust NZ J Ophthalmol.* 1991;19(3):187–191.
38. Jabs DA, et al. The eye in bone marrow transplantation. II. Histopathology. *Arch Ophthalmol.* 1983;101(4):585–590.
39. Jack MK, et al. Ocular manifestations of graft-v-host disease. *Arch Ophthalmol.* 1983;101(7):1080–1084.
40. Sale GE, et al. Oral and ophthalmic pathology of graft versus host disease in man: predictive value of the lip biopsy. *Hum Pathol.* 1981;12(11):1022–1030.
41. Fisk JD, et al. Gastrointestinal radiographic features of human graft-vs.-host disease. *AJR Am J Roentgenol.* 1981;136(2):329–336.
42. Shulman HM, et al. Chronic graft-versus-host syndrome in man. A long-term clinicopathologic study of 20 Seattle patients. *Am J Med.* 1980;69(2):204–217.
43. Bhan AK, Fujikawa LS, Foster CS. T-cell subsets and Langerhans cells in normal and diseased conjunctiva. *Am J Ophthalmol.* 1982;94(2):205–212.
44. Saito T, et al. Ocular manifestation of acute graft-versus-host disease after allogeneic peripheral blood stem cell transplantation. *Int J Hematol.* 2002;75(3):332–334.
45. Vogelsang GB, et al. Thalidomide for the treatment of chronic graft-versus-host disease. *N Engl J Med.* 1992;326(16):1055–1058.
46. Johnson DA, Jabs DA. The ocular manifestations of graft-versus-host disease. *Int Ophthalmol Clin.* 1997;37(2):119–133.
47. Calissendorff B, el Azazi M, Lonnqvist B. Dry eye syndrome in long-term follow-up of bone marrow transplanted patients. *Bone Marrow Transplant.* 1989;4(6):675–678.
48. Mencucci R, et al. Ophthalmological aspects in allogenic bone marrow transplantation: Sjogren-like syndrome in graft-versus-host disease. *Eur J Ophthalmol.* 1997;7(1):13–18.
49. Livesey SJ, Holmes JA, Whittaker JA. Ocular complications of bone marrow transplantation. *Eye.* 1989;3(Pt 3):271–276.
50. Tichelli A, et al. Late-onset keratoconjunctivitis sicca syndrome after bone marrow transplantation: incidence and risk factors. European Group or Blood and Marrow Transplantation (EBMT) Working Party on Late Effects. *Bone Marrow Transplant.* 1996;17(6):1105–1111.
51. Lawley TJ, et al. Scleroderma, Sjogren-like syndrome, and chronic graft-versus-host disease. *Ann Intern Med.* 1977;87(6):707–709.
52. Kim SK, et al. Ocular graft vs. host disease experience from MD Anderson Cancer Center: Newly described clinical spectrum and new approach to the management of stage III and IV ocular GVHD. *Biol Blood Marrow Transplant.* 2006;12(2S1):49.
53. Robinson MR, et al. Topical corticosteroid therapy for cicatricial conjunctivitis associated with chronic graft-versus-host disease. *Bone Marrow Transplant.* 2004;33(10):1031–1035.
54. Karwacka E, et al. Pemphigoid-like ocular lesions in patients with graft-versus-host disease following allogeneic bone marrow transplantation. *Transplant Proc.* 2006;38(1):292–294.
55. Kim SK, et al. Superior limbic keratoconjunctivitis in chronic ocular graft vs. host disease. *Invest Ophthalmol Vis Sci.* 2005;46S:2661.
56. Kerty E, et al. Ocular findings in allogeneic stem cell transplantation without total body irradiation. *Ophthalmology.* 1999;106(7):1334–1338.
57. Shulman HM, et al. Chronic cutaneous graft-versus-host disease in man. *Am J Pathol.* 1978;91(3):545–570.
58. Ogawa Y, et al. A significant role of stromal fibroblasts in rapidly progressive dry eye in patients with chronic GVHD. *Invest Ophthalmol Vis Sci.* 2001;42(1):111–119.
59. Ogawa Y, et al. Autologous serum eye drops for the treatment of severe dry eye in patients with chronic graft-versus-host disease. *Bone Marrow Transplant.* 2003;31(7):579–583.
60. Schiffman RM, et al. Reliability and validity of the Ocular Surface Disease Index. *Arch Ophthalmol.* 2000;118(5):615–621.
61. Agomo E, et al. Role of ocular surface disease index (OSDI) in chronic ocular graft vs. host disease (OGVHD). *Invest Ophthalmol Vis Sci.* 2008; 49S:2369.
62. Chang-Strepka J, et al. Videokeratoscopic indices in chronic ocular graft versus host disease (OGVHD). *Invest Ophthalmol Vis Sci.* 2009;50S:2610.
63. Ban Y, et al. Tear function and lipid layer alterations in dry eye patients with chronic graft-vs-host disease. *Eye.* 2009;23(1):202–208.
64. Arocker-Mettinger E, et al. Manifestations of graft-versus-host disease following allogenic bone marrow transplantation. *Eur J Ophthalmol.* 1991;1(1):28–32.
65. Kim SK, Ocular graft vs. host disease. *Ocul Surf.* 2005;3(4):177–179.
66. Wang Y, et al. First-line therapy for chronic graft-versus-host disease that includes low-dose methotrexate is associated with a high response rate. *Biol Blood Marrow Transplant.* 2009;15(4):505–511.
67. Teshima T, et al. Rituximab for the treatment of corticosteroid refractory chronic graft versus host disease. *Int J Hematol,* 2009.
68. Couriel D, et al. Extracorporeal photopheresis for acute and chronic graft-versus-host disease: does it work? *Biol Blood Marrow Transplant.* 2006;12(1 Suppl 2):37–40.
69. Couriel DR, et al. Extracorporeal photochemotherapy for the treatment of steroid-resistant chronic GVHD. *Blood.* 2006;107(8):3074–3080.
70. Cutler C, et al. Rituximab for steroid-refractory chronic graft-versus-host disease. *Blood.* 2006;108(2):756–762.
71. Basara N, et al. Mycophenolate mofetil for the treatment of acute and chronic GVHD in bone marrow transplant patients. *Bone Marrow Transplant.* 1998;22(1):61–65.
72. Baudard M, et al. Mycophenolate mofetil for the treatment of acute and chronic GVHD is effective and well tolerated but induces a high risk of infectious complications: a series of 21 BM or PBSC transplant patients. *Bone Marrow Transplant.* 2002;30(5):287–295.
73. Krejci M, et al. Mycophenolate mofetil for the treatment of acute and chronic steroid-refractory graft-versus-host disease. *Ann Hematol.* 2005;84(10):681–685.
74. Jacobsohn DA, et al. Infliximab for steroid-refractory acute GVHD: a case series. *Am J Hematol.* 2003;74(2):119–124.
75. Kiang E, et al. The use of topical cyclosporin A in ocular graft-versus-host-disease. *Bone Marrow Transplant.* 1998;22(2):147–151.
76. Lelli GJ Jr, et al. Ophthalmic cyclosporine use in ocular GVHD. *Cornea.* 2006;25(6):635–638.
77. Murphy PT, et al. Successful use of topical retinoic acid in severe dry eye due to chronic graft-versus-host disease. *Bone Marrow Transplant.* 1996;18(3):641–642.
78. Rocha EM, et al. GVHD dry eyes treated with autologous serum tears. *Bone Marrow Transplant.* 2000;25(10):1101–1103.

79. Chiang CC, et al. Allogeneic serum eye drops for the treatment of severe dry eye in patients with chronic graft-versus-host disease. *Cornea.* 2007;26(7):861–863.
80. Kim SK, et al. Early topical steroid treatment for Grade IV acute ocular graft vs. host disease (GVHD) with corneal epithelial sloughing. *Invest Ophthalmol Vis Sci.* 2003;44S:1387.
81. Russo PA, Bouchard CS, Galasso JM. Extended-wear silicone hydrogel soft contact lenses in the management of moderate to severe dry eye signs and symptoms secondary to graft-versus-host disease. *Eye Contact Lens.* 2007;33(3):144–147.
82. Takahide K, et al. Use of fluid-ventilated, gas-permeable scleral lens for management of severe keratoconjunctivitis sicca secondary to chronic graft-versus-host disease. *Biol Blood Marrow Transplant.* 2007;13(9): 1016–1021.
83. Schornack MM, et al. Jupiter scleral lenses in the management of chronic graft versus host disease. *Eye Contact Lens.* 2008;34(6):302–305.

Chapter 69

Corneal Manifestations of Local and Systemic Therapies

Carol J. Hoffman, Peter R. Laibson

Physicians are fortunate to have available a multitude of drugs and chemical solutions to fight infection and treat disease. Many of these agents are of interest to the ophthalmologist because of their effects on the cornea, lids, and conjunctiva. Although some of these drugs are used routinely by ophthalmologists, many are not. The purpose of this chapter is to familiarize the ophthalmologist with the adverse effects of local and systemically administered therapies on ocular tissue. This discussion will include agents that are prescribed by the ophthalmologist as well as those the patient is taking under the guidance of other physicians.

It is useful to divide medications that affect the cornea, conjunctiva, and lids into three categories: topical medications, systemic medications, and drugs used during ophthalmic surgery.

Topical Ophthalmic Medications

Topical ophthalmic medications are used routinely as diagnostic aids and in the prevention and treatment of infection, inflammation, and glaucoma. The effect of topical medications on the cornea and adnexa may result from the drug itself or its preservative.

Topical anesthetics

Commonly used topical anesthetics are benoxinate (Fluress™), proparacaine (Alcaine™, Ophthaine, Ophthetic™), tetracaine, and cocaine. All of these agents act by blocking afferent nerve conduction. Epithelial toxicity occurs with repeated instillation of these agents and may manifest as a nonhealing epithelial defect. This occurs as a result of decreased epithelial cell motility, which retards healing and may be aggravated by an anesthetic-induced decrease in reflex tearing and blinking.[1] Left undetected, anesthetic abuse may lead to persistent epithelial defects, corneal ulceration with stromal ring infiltrates, and secondary microbial infection (Figs 69.1, 69.2).[2,3] It is frequently difficult to detect topical anesthetic abuse because of the patient's denial, often induced by psychological problems. Psychiatric referral may be necessary.

Topical antimicrobials

The most common local effect of these agents, which include antibiotics, antivirals, and antifungals, is delayed hypersensitivity leading to dermatitis, conjunctivitis, and keratitis. The reaction may be induced by the active drug itself or by chemical preservatives. Benzalkonium chloride, a common preservative, is a well-documented offender.[4] Manifestations include an eye that is injected more inferiorly where the medication gravitates, follicular and papillary conjunctivitis, mucoid discharge, and inferior punctate epithelial keratitis. These findings occur within 24 to 72 hours of repeated doses. A punctate marginal keratitis, including small perilimbal subepithelial and anterior stromal sterile infiltrates, may also occur. The lids manifest the same injection, crusting, and scaling as with acute eczema.[5] A chronic follicular and papillary conjunctivitis may occur with prolonged use of these drugs. Deposition of topical antimicrobial drugs in the cornea is unusual; one exception is the superficial white grainy precipitate seen in approximately 16% of patients using topical ciprofloxacin (Fig. 69.3).[6]

The antiviral agents idoxuridine (IDU), no longer manufactured in the United States, adenine arabinoside (vidarabine, Ara-A), and trifluridine (Viroptic™) are known to be toxic to the corneal and conjunctival epithelium. Toxicity is most commonly seen with idoxuridine applications but does occur with the other antivirals as well. Conjunctival and limbal hyperemia and punctate epithelial keratitis are most commonly encountered. Nonhealing epithelial defects and stromal inflammation are less common (Figs 69.4, 69.5).[7] With chronic use, conjunctival hyperplasia around the punctum can occlude the punctal opening, causing epiphora. It is important to consider antiviral toxicity in a patient who initially improves on antiviral therapy only to worsen after 14 or more days of continued therapy.

Delayed epithelial wound healing has been studied with antibiotics and antifungals. Stern et al.[8] found that gentamicin and tobramycin retarded epithelial healing, whereas cefazolin had the least undesirable effect when rabbit corneas were studied. The authors note that the preservative used in the preparations may have been the primary offender as opposed to the drug itself. Foster et al.[9] found that

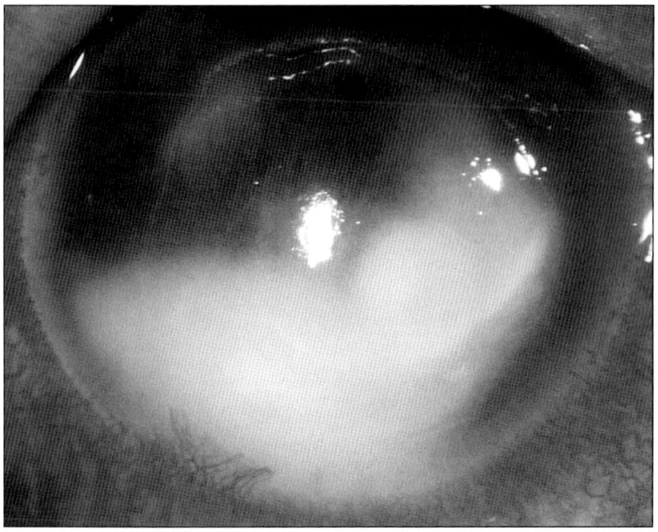

Fig. 69.1 Corneal ulcer has developed in a patient with a ring abscess after Ophthaine abuse. Patient used proparacaine for 4 weeks starting two or three times/day and progressing to use every 30 minutes.

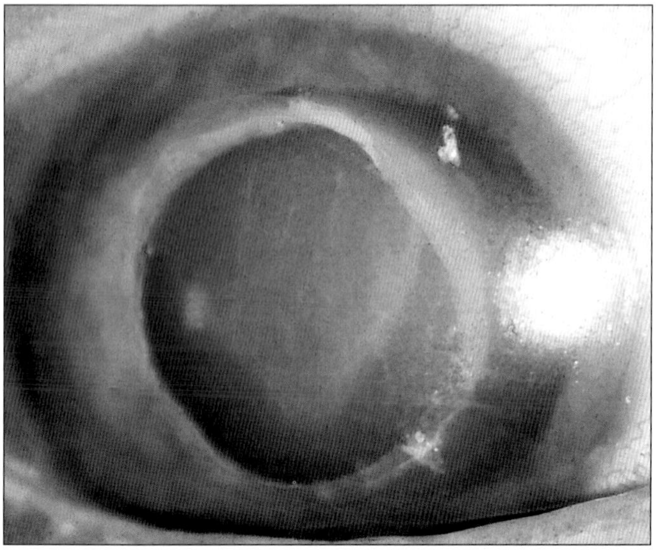

Fig. 69.2 Proparacaine (Ophthaine) abuse in a patient who had used this anesthetic every hour for 3 days. Central epithelial defect with ring infiltrate typical of Ophthaine abuse.

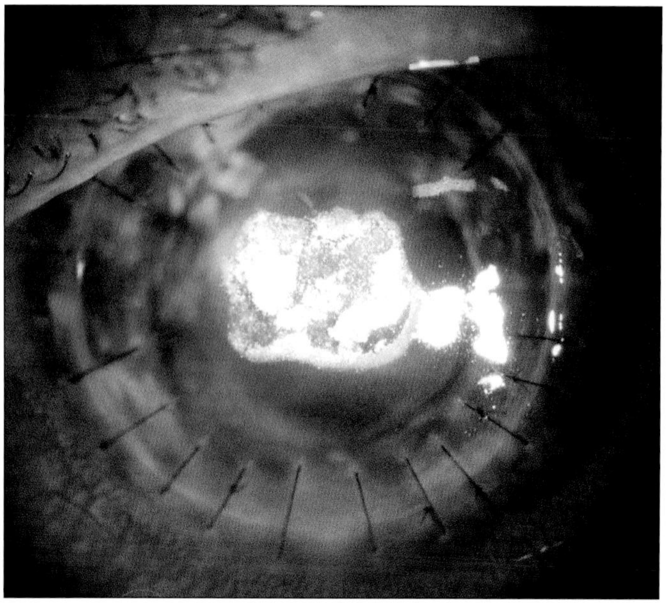

Fig. 69.3 Ciprofloxacin deposits. Topical ciprofloxacin will precipitate at physiologic pH. Chalky white deposits accumulate in areas of absent epithelium.

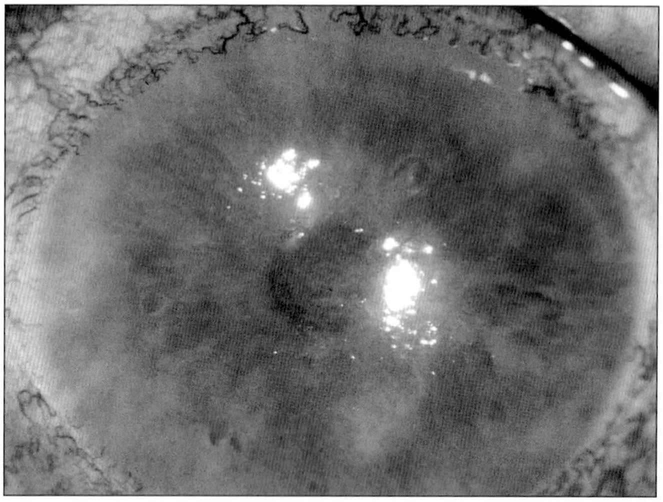

Fig. 69.4 Topical antiviral toxicity. Patient had used trifluridine drops on several occasions for recurrent herpes. Eventually, marked punctate epithelial keratitis, corneal haze, conjunctival injection, and perilimbal vascularization occurred. Patient also had swollen conjunctiva and epiphora.

amphotericin B in 1% concentration markedly reduced epithelial wound healing, whereas flucytosine, miconazole nitrate, and ketoconazole did not. Natamycin appeared to have little epithelial toxicity.[5] Sulfacetamide, topically, has been known to trigger Stevens-Johnson disease.

Topical corticosteroid preparations may delay epithelial wound healing and may cause degeneration of epithelial and stromal cells. Topical steroids are known to facilitate recrudescence of *Pseudomonas* corneal infections and to make fungal corneal infections worse; they are contraindicated with active epithelial herpes simplex virus infections. Caution should be exercised when using these agents in the setting of any pre-existing epithelial defect.

While discussing hypersensitivity and toxic reactions to these commonly used drugs, it is important to note that these agents may cause keratitis medicamentosa. This condition has a variety of clinical presentations, including punctate epithelial keratitis, filamentary keratitis, pseudodendrites, and complete loss of the epithelium with stromal edema, scarring, and neovascularization.[5] The history is very important in making this diagnosis. Typically, a patient is treated for a minor irritation with a topical antimicrobial or combination preparation. When the patient's condition fails to

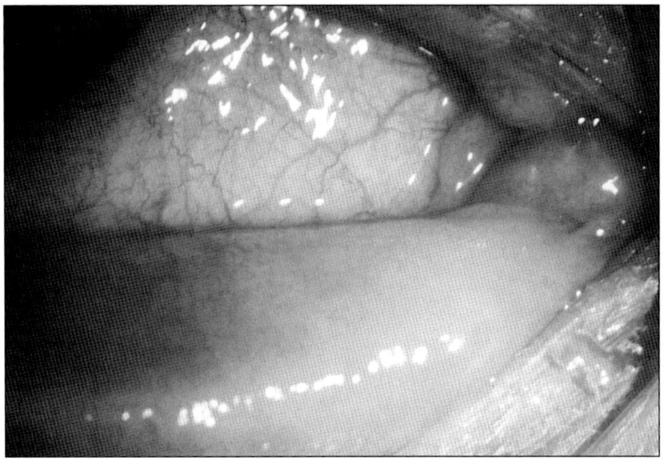

Fig. 69.5 Idoxuridine toxicity with markedly swollen conjunctiva, closure of the puncta, and severe epiphora. This patient also had bulbar conjunctival chemosis and injection, and marked punctate epithelial keratitis. The epiphora was this patient's chief complaint. Patient had used idoxuridine on several occasions for recurrent ocular inflammation resulting from recurrent herpes simplex dendritic lesions.

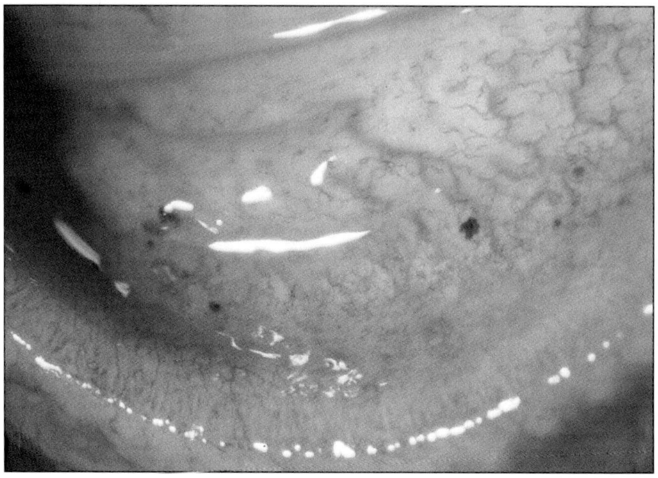

Fig. 69.6 Adenochrome deposits. These dark black deposits are commonly found in the conjunctiva of patients treated with epinephrine eyedrops for glaucoma.

improve or worsens, other medications are substituted or added. The diagnosis of hypersensitivity/toxic reaction may not be considered, and additional topical agents are added. An escalation in the variety and number of drops occurs until there is significant cumulative toxicity. The distinction between the true diagnosis of keratoconjunctivitis medicamentosa and another diagnosis such as herpes simplex, *Mycobacterium* infection, *Acanthamoeba* keratitis, and endothelial dysfunction becomes difficult. The ophthalmologist must consider medication toxicity in patients who are not responding to treatment or who are worsening while continuing therapy.

Antiglaucoma medications

Although no longer commonly employed, epinephrine compounds frequently cause innocuous brownish-black pigmentation of the inferior palpebral conjunctiva after prolonged use (adrenochrome deposits) (Fig. 69.6). This is thought to result from the accumulation of oxidative products of the epinephrine in conjunctival cysts.[10] Rarely, brown or black deposits may occur in the corneal stroma and in Bowman's membrane, leading to the designation 'black cornea.' This has been misdiagnosed in some patients as uveal prolapse.[11]

Pilocarpine, physostigmine, and atropine after prolonged use may lead to follicular conjunctivitis. This is thought to be a toxic or irritative effect and not a true allergic reaction.[7]

Topical beta-blockers have caused a dendriform keratopathy in some patients. Resolution usually occurs within 2 weeks of discontinuing the medication. The mechanism is thought to be epithelial toxicity with subsequent epithelial regeneration.[12] Latanoprost, a topical prostaglandin analog, has induced dendriform epitheliopathy in some patients. This tends to resolve with discontinuation of the medication (Fig. 69.7).[13]

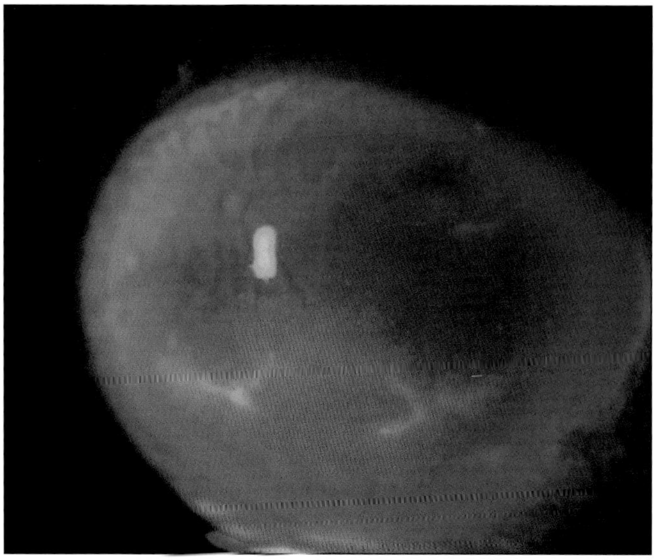

Fig. 69.7 Pseudodendrites with latanoprost therapy.

Several antiglaucoma medications are commonly implicated in drug-induced ocular cicatrization. As in ocular cicatricial pemphigoid (OCP), signs range from chronic conjunctivitis to end-stage conjunctival scarring with symblepharon formation, corneal vascularization, and scarring with keratinization (Fig. 69.8). Epinephrine, pilocarpine, timolol, and echothiophate iodide have all been implicated in ocular cicatrization, in addition to the antiviral medication idoxuridine.[14] A careful history of long-term use of these medications and the exclusion of other causes of cicatrization, including trauma, OCP, past infections (trachoma, membranous conjunctivitis, primary herpes simplex, diphtheria, and β-hemolytic streptococcal infection), and Stevens-Johnson syndrome, is important in this diagnosis.[14]

Although the cause of cicatrization is not entirely clear, some investigators have shown that these drugs induce

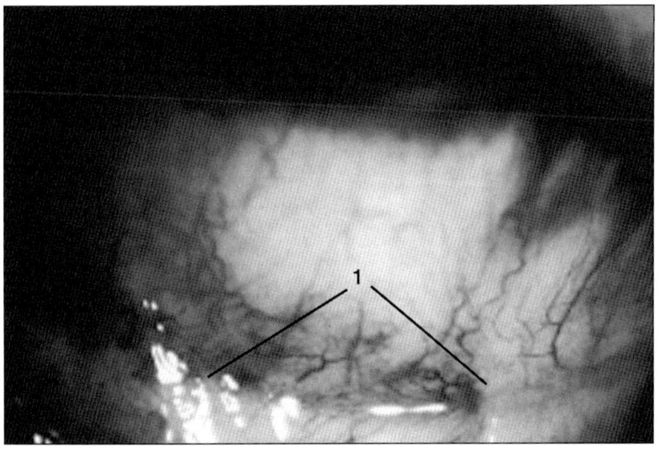

Fig. 69.8 Unilateral shortening of the cul-de-sac (*1*) in a patient who had used physostigmine for glaucoma. This patient had no other signs of ocular cicatricial pemphigoid and had the symblepharon only in the eye where the drug was used.

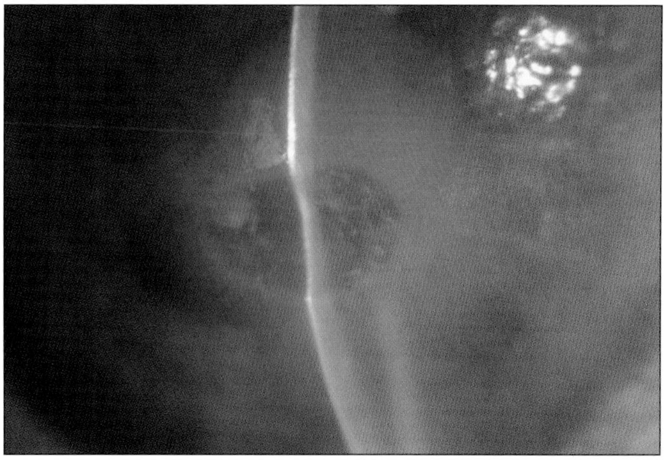

Fig. 69.9 Corneal melt after NSAID use.

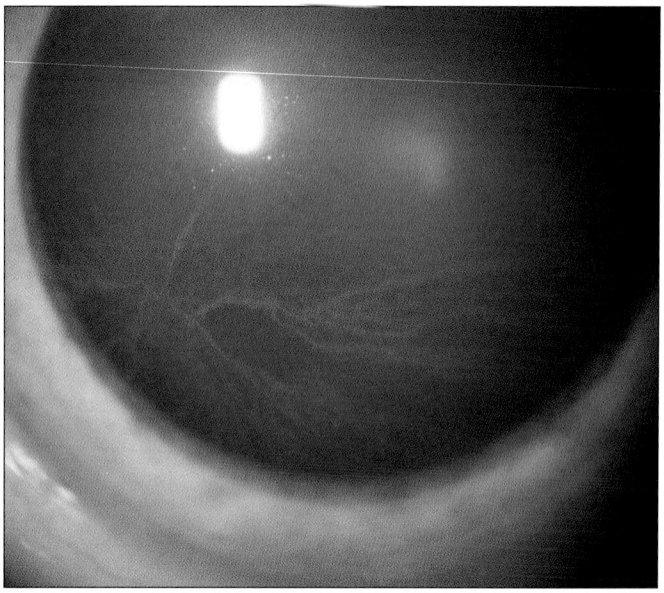

Fig. 69.10 Amiodarone deposits. This example of cornea verticillata occurred after a cumulative dose of 219 g of amiodarone.

conjunctival metaplasia.[15] Drug-induced pemphigoid may be self-limiting, resolving, or stabilizing when the offending agent is discontinued, or it may be chronic and progressive.[16] It is unclear whether drug-induced pemphigoid is truly a separate entity from OCP or whether it represents the unmasking of a predisposition to OCP in a particular patient.

Nonsteroidal antiinflammatory drugs (NSAIDs)

Cyclooxygenase inhibitors are commonly used in the postoperative cataract and refractive surgery patient to provide analgesia, mediate inflammation, and prevent and treat cystoid macular edema. Since their introduction in the early 1990s, there have been several reports of severe corneal toxicity, ulceration, and perforation following their use.[17–19] Cyclooxygenase inhibitors, such as diclofenac and ketorolac, block conversion of arachidonic acid to prostaglandin. This reduces the presence of important mediators of inflammation. However, excess arachidonic acid may then be metabolized by an alternate pathway, resulting in the increased production of substances that attract and promote the degranulation of neutrophils.[18] These conditions, in concert with concomitant steroid use, coexisting ocular surface disease, and underlying systemic pathology, such as diabetes mellitus and collagen vascular disease, may favor the development of stromal infiltrates as well as corneal melting and perforation.[18] However, there are also instances of severe complications where no underlying medical conditions or use of steroids exist (Fig. 69.9).[17]

Systemic Therapies

The cornea, conjunctiva, and lids may be affected by systemic agents, either in the form of drug deposition or from toxic effects. A complete history, including systemic medications in current or past use, is essential when evaluating patients with drug-induced deposits and toxicities.

Drug deposition

Drugs can reach the cornea by three routes: via the tear film, perilimbal vasculature, or aqueous fluid. Access from the tear film leads to deposition in the epithelium, whereas entrance from the aqueous accounts for posterior layer accumulation. When the perilimbal vasculature is the source, deposits generally occur in the corneal stroma.[20] Drugs deposited in the corneal epithelium may produce a verticillate or whorl-like pattern and seldom affect vision. This pattern may be produced by the aminoquinolones, clofazimine, indometacin, naproxen, perhexiline, suramin, tamoxifen, thioxanthines, tilorone,[20] and amiodarone (Fig. 69.10). Electron microscopic sections of corneas with drug-related vortex keratopathy have demonstrated lipid deposition particles arranged concentrically in the corneal epithelium.[21] Some of these are discussed in more detail later.

Antimalarial agents

The antimalarial agents include chloroquine, hydroxychloroquine, quinacrine, and amodiaquine. Chloroquine and hydroxychloroquine cause harmless corneal deposits that can occur at doses ranging from 100 mg/day over several years to 1000 mg over as little as 3 weeks. The deposits usually abate and disappear after cessation of treatment. Corneal deposits are concentrated in the epithelium of the central cornea with a less dense concentration toward the periphery. The opacities are described as fine punctate gray deposits that in the early stages are diffuse but later develop curvilinear or swirl-like lines of deposition that may later coalesce and leave green-yellow pigment lines in the center of the cornea.[10] Quinacrine deposition is reversible and causes pigmentation of the conjunctiva, plica semilunaris, and caruncle, described as blue-gray in color, in addition to yellow pigmentation of the cornea and sclera.[10]

Phenothiazines

Phenothiazine ocular toxicity affecting the cornea, conjunctiva, and lens was first described by Greiner and Berry in 1964.[22] Since then, numerous authors have described similar changes in patients on long-term chlorpromazine therapy.

Asymptomatic corneal deposits are found in the posterior stroma, Descemet's membrane, and endothelium, and are described as yellow-brown dustlike granules occurring only in the exposed cornea of the interpalpebral fissures.[23] The interpalpebral conjunctiva and the lids may also develop brown discoloration. Biopsies of the conjunctiva have revealed pigment thought to be melanin.[24] In a series by DeLong et al.[25] lenticular changes were noted in about half of the patients with cumulative doses of 1000 g. At higher doses, about 18% showed corneal and conjunctival changes.[25] It is hypothesized that chlorpromazine denatures protein when exposed to light, then the protein, in turn, becomes opacified and is deposited in the lens, corneal stroma, conjunctiva, and skin.[26] These ocular changes are found to persist after discontinuation of the drug.[27]

Gold

Systemic gold therapy is used in the treatment of collagen vascular disease, particularly rheumatoid arthritis. Gold deposition in the cornea, called corneal chrysiasis, occurs at cumulative doses exceeding 1500 mg. These gold-to-violet fine deposits, which are symptomless and reversible, are scattered from the epithelium to the deep stroma but may occur in the bulbar conjunctiva as well.[10] Deposits tend to clear after cessation of therapy but may also be found to persist years later.[10]

Silver

Argyrosis is less common now that topical silver preparations, Argyrol in particular, are rarely used. Today, it is more commonly associated with industrial exposure to organic silver salts. The lids and conjunctiva have a light to dark slate-gray appearance, whereas the cornea develops peripheral deep stromal and Descemet's deposits of blue-gray, green, or gold-like material (Figs 69.11, 69.12).[10] Visual acuity remains normal.

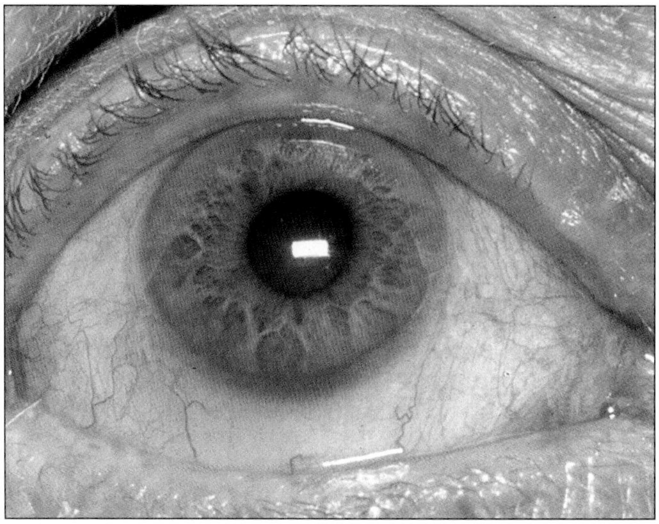

Fig. 69.11 Argyrosis. Silver deposits may also occur in the conjunctiva. The conjunctiva is gray when compared with the white card on the left. Here and in Figure 69.12, the silver deposits are secondary to the topical medication Argyrol, a silver nitrate compound.

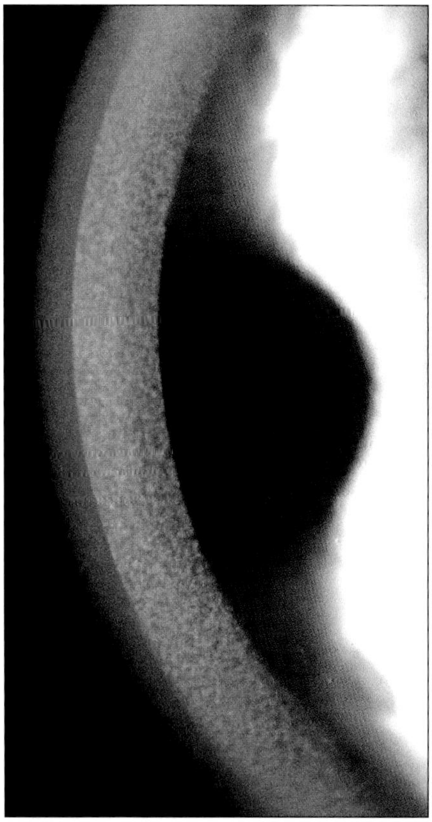

Fig. 69.12 Argyrosis. This is the accumulation of silver in tissues in the body. Silver deposits in the cornea occur in the deepest portion, near Descemet's membrane; they have a slate-gray appearance.

Other drugs associated with stromal corneal deposits include antacids, indomethacin, phenylbutazone, practolol, and retinoids.[20]

Oral contraceptives

Garmizo and Frauens[28] report hypercupremia and pigment deposition with oral contraceptive use. Blue-green pigment deposition at the level of the endothelium or Descemet's membrane, in a 2–3-mm band in the peripheral cornea, is described. A 2-mm clear space from the limbus, with deposition greater inferiorly, was found.

Toxic effects

Several systemic medications have toxic or irritative effects on the cornea, conjunctiva, and lids. Although the mechanism is poorly understood, it is believed that these agents become concentrated in the tears and then exert a local toxic effect.

Chemotherapeutic agents

A regimen of cyclophosphamide, methotrexate, and 5-fluorouracil (5-FU) is commonly used to treat breast carcinoma and some types of lymphoma. In one series, conjunctivitis was reported in 25% of patients.[29] Loprinzi et al.[30] reported symptoms of foreign body sensation and tearing in 42.3% of patients, usually 2 weeks into the chemotherapy cycle. Although complaints were significant, ophthalmic examination failed to reveal significant anterior segment pathology. Cytosine arabinoside (cytatabine) used systemically to treat acute myelogenous leukemia has been reported to cause conjunctival injection, dense central punctate epithelial keratitis, refractile epithelial microcysts, subepithelial opacities, and corneal edema.[31,32] Because these medications concentrate in the tears,[31,32] the toxicity of cytosine arabinoside as well as 5-FU is not surprising. The topical forms of these medications have well-described local toxic effects.

Tetracycline and minocycline

Tetracycline and minocycline are common antibiotics used to treat infection and acne vulgaris. Intracystic concretions ranging in color from unpigmented to dark brown in the lower tarsal conjunctiva have been reported and are thought to represent oxidation products of tetracycline. Patients with these findings had been on drug therapy for 10 years or more.[33] Infants and children should not be treated with tetracycline or minocycline to avoid dental pigmentation. Teenagers using tetracycline for acne can develop black molars.

Isotretinoin

Isotretinoin is an oral agent used to treat severe cystic acne. Fraunfelder et al.[34] reviewed reports of 236 patients who developed adverse ocular affects occurring 1 to 34 weeks after beginning therapy. Twelve patients developed subepithelial opacities in the central or peripheral cornea, 47 patients developed dry eyes, 19 became contact lens intolerant, 88 developed blepharoconjunctivitis or meibomianitis, and 6 had photodermatitis involving the lids. The authors hypothesized that decreased lipid content of the tear film led to increased evaporation of tears. This may account for the dry eye and contact lens intolerance symptoms. With discontinuation of the medication, signs and symptoms usually resolve.

Amantadine

Amantadine hydrochloride (Symmetrel™) is an oral agent used in the treatment of Parkinson's disease, tardive dyskinesia, and prophylaxis of influenza A_2. Diffuse white subepithelial punctate opacities, occasionally with overlying punctate keratitis associated with corneal epithelial edema and significantly reduced vision, have been reported 1 to 2 weeks after the beginning of therapy at doses of 200–400 mg/day.[35] Signs and symptoms resolve with discontinuation of therapy.

Stevens-Johnson syndrome

Stevens-Johnson syndrome, also known as erythema multiforme major (described in detail elsewhere in this text), may be associated with an inciting topical or systemic drug. Systemic drugs that have been associated include sulfonamides, salicylates, penicillin, phenytoin sodium, barbiturates, isoniazid, and phenylbutazone. Topical scopolamine, tropicamide, proparacaine, and sulfonamides have also been inciting agents (Figs 69.13, 69.14).[36,37]

Medications may indirectly cause irritative effects on the cornea and conjunctiva by decreasing tear production, thus exacerbating or causing dry eye syndrome. This has been demonstrated with hydrochlorothiazide and the antihistamine chlorpheniramine maleate.[38,39]

Conjunctival irritation, conjunctivitis, and occasionally punctate keratitis have also been described with the systemic use of chloral hydrate, barbiturates, morphine, antipyrine, salicylate, reserpine, and digitalis.[10]

Ophthalmic Surgical Solutions

With the advent of advanced microsurgical techniques have come various intraocular agents to make these procedures

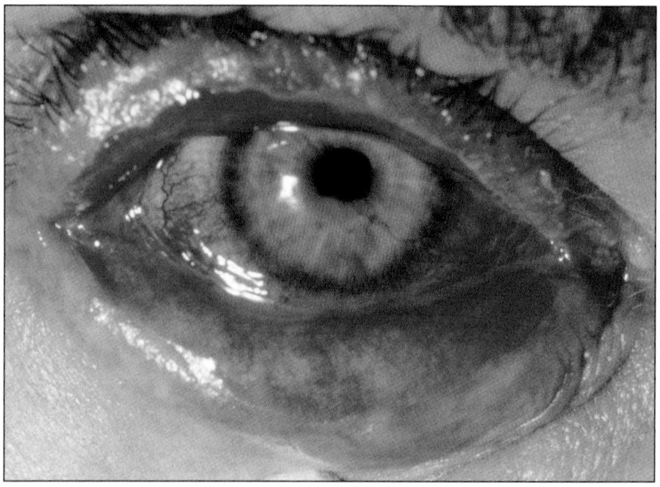

Fig. 69.13 Active Stevens-Johnson syndrome. The conjunctiva is diffusely injected and thickened. Corneal vascularization occurs in severe cases.

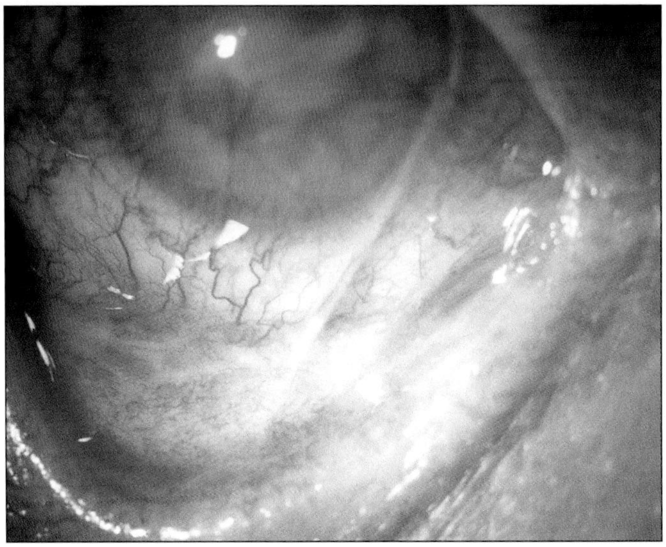

Fig. 69.14 Stevens-Johnson syndrome. Corneal scarring, conjunctival scarring, and symblepharon formation may occur after the acute stage.

possible. Many of these agents have effects other than those intended on the anterior ocular tissues.

Irrigating solutions

Irrigating solutions used intraocularly at the time of surgery require a formulation similar to that of aqueous and vitreous to help reduce the risk of postoperative corneal edema. Solutions containing sodium, potassium, calcium, bicarbonate, glucose, and glutathione in concentrations similar to aqueous and vitreous are essential in maintaining normal cell function, especially during long surgical procedures. Irrigating solutions such as sodium chloride and lactated Ringer's solution cause endothelial cell loss and subsequent corneal edema.[40]

Solutions used in treating traumatic injuries may also have undesirable effects. Kompa et al.[41] found, in a retrospective review of eye burns, that eye drops and ointments containing phosphate buffer increase the risk of corneal calcification twofold.

Viscoelastics

Viscoelastics have greatly reduced trauma to the corneal endothelium and increased the safety of many intraocular procedures. Despite this, prolonged exposure of these substances to the endothelium may be damaging. Human donor corneas exposed to Healon have shown significant endothelial cell death after 30 minutes of exposure and complete cell death after 2 hours.[40] Viscoelastics may also elevate intraocular pressure if left in place after use. This is a temporary problem only. For these reasons, as complete a washout of the viscoelastic as possible is recommended to avoid postoperative corneal edema.

Epinephrine

The intraocular use of epinephrine is common in situations of poor pupillary dilation. Irreversible corneal edema caused by endothelial toxicity may occur when epinephrine solutions containing sodium bisulfite are used.[42] Commercial preparations of epinephrine without sodium bisulfite are currently available and may be used safely.

Miotics

Intraocular miotics are often used at the conclusion of cataract and other intraocular surgeries. Both 1% acetylcholine and 0.01% carbachol chloride are commercially available for this use. Comparison studies of these two agents have demonstrated mild to marked adverse effects on the corneal endothelium when using 1% acetylcholine preparations, and caution is advised when using this agent in corneas already at risk for corneal decompensation.[40]

5-Fluorouracil

5-Fluorouracil, an antimetabolite that impedes normal cell mitosis, is used to increase the success of glaucoma filtering surgery. Since corneal epithelial cells are constantly being replaced, 5-FU is toxic to the corneal epithelium. Mild corneal complications, including punctate epithelial keratitis, filaments, and small epithelial defects, can occur during active drug administration or after its completion. Moderate changes, including larger epithelial defects, may fail to heal even after discontinuation of the drug. Severe complications, including microbial and sterile ulceration sometimes leading to perforation, may occur months after completion of 5-FU administration.[43] Reduction in doses of 5-FU have reduced the rate of complications, but serious side effects still occur at the reduced doses.[44]

Mitomycin-C

Mitomycin-C is an alkylating agent used to increase the success of glaucoma filtering surgery, decrease recurrence after pterygium excision, and reduce the incidence of corneal haze formation after photorefractive keratectomy (PRK). Serious corneal complications can occur at the recommended dosage levels in certain patients. Rubinfeld et al.[45] have reported a series of patients in whom complications occurred after pterygium excision, with adjunctive mitomycin-C given topically either intraoperatively, postoperatively, or both. These complications included corneal perforation, corectopia, iritis, scleral calcification, and incapacitating photophobia and pain (Fig. 69.15). The authors recommend a 0.02% or less concentrated topical solution given either as a single application at the time of surgery or twice daily for 5 days. Avoiding the use of mitomycin-C in patients with pre-existing Sjögren's syndrome, severe keratitis sicca, acne rosacea, atopic keratoconjunctivitis, or herpetic keratitis is also recommended, since these conditions predispose the patient to poor wound healing and ulceration. Despite the dominance of LASIK as a refractive surgical procedure, PRK has recently regained popularity. Mitomycin-C is a common adjunctive therapy used at the time of PRK surgery. Nassiri et al.[46] found a significant decrease in central endothelial cell density 6 months postoperatively in eyes treated with 0.02% mitomycin-C for PRK haze prevention.

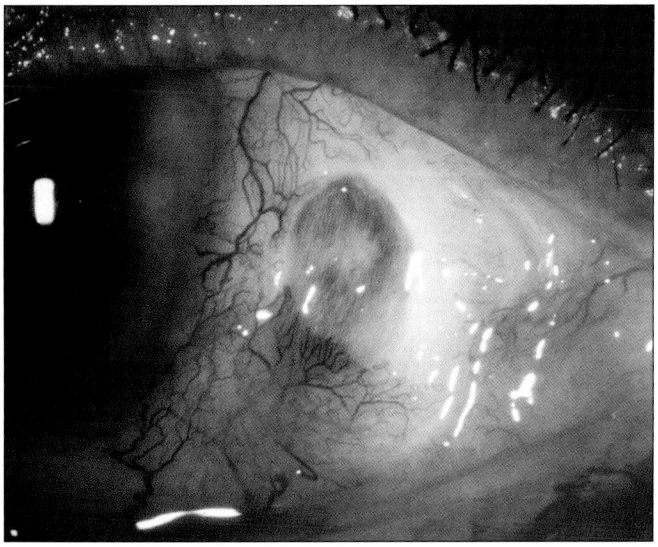

Fig. 69.15 Pterygium excision with mitomycin-C application to the scleral bed. Approximately 1 year after the excision, there was continued scleral melting and a lack of vascularity in the necrotic scleral bed. Uveal tissue is seen at the base of the ulcer.

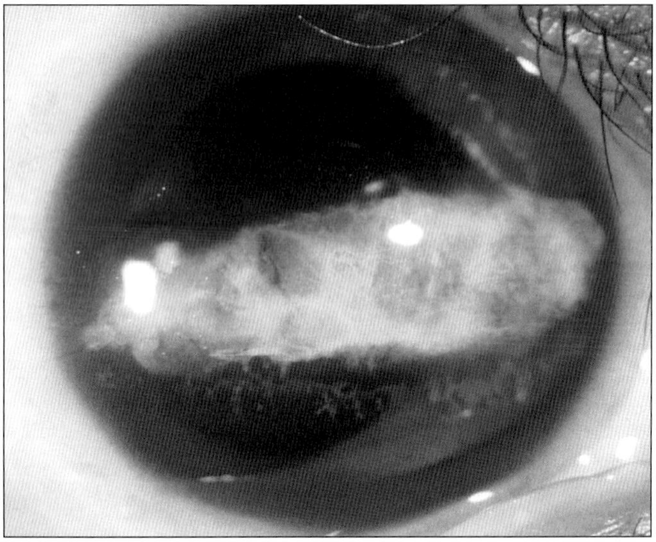

Fig. 69.16 Band keratopathy developed in a patient who had major vitreal retinal surgery with silicone oil. Band keratopathy occurs frequently in patients who have this surgery with the use of silicone oil. Despite EDTA removal of band keratopathy, it can recur with this surgery. (Courtesy of Irving Raber, MD.)

Silicone oil

Silicone oil is an important adjunctive tool in the treatment of complicated retinal detachment. Corneal band keratopathy may occur when the silicone oil comes in contact with the corneal endothelium either as an intact large silicone oil bubble or as emulsified droplets.[47] The keratopathy is thought to result from pH changes caused by reduced flow across the cornea (Figs 69.16, 69.17).[48]

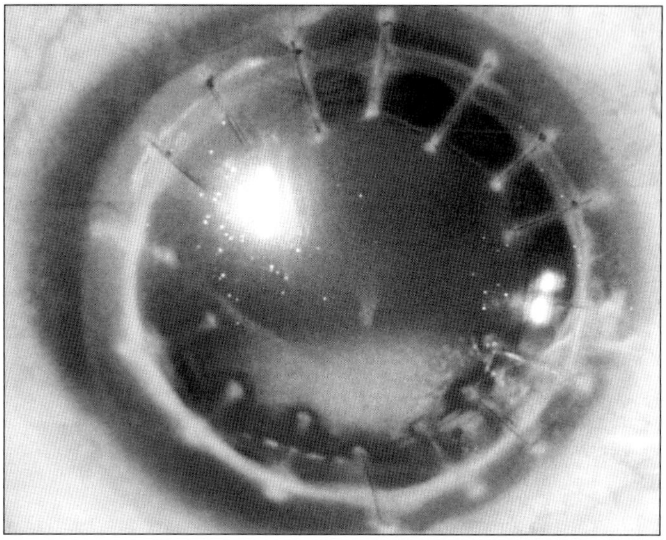

Fig. 69.17 Band keratopathy recurrent in corneal transplant done for the patient in Figure 69.16. (Courtesy of Irving Raber, MD.)

Conclusion

Drugs and chemical solutions currently used locally and systemically provide physicians with a multitude of therapeutic choices for the treatment of disease not thought possible in the recent past. For the ophthalmologist, recognizing the side effects and toxicities of these agents is of great importance to the proper care of patients. Of equal importance is recognizing new side effects and toxicities and reporting them to agencies such as the National Registry of Drug-Induced Ocular Side Effects, which can evaluate and disseminate this information.

References

1. Burstein NL. Corneal cytotoxicity of topically applied drugs, vehicles, and preservatives. *Surv Ophthalmol*. 1980;25(1):15–30.
2. Rosenwasser GOD, et al. Topical anesthetic abuse. *Ophthalmology*. 1990;97(8):967–972.
3. Berns RP, et al. Chronic toxicity of local anesthesia on the cornea. *Drug Symp*. 1976.
4. Pfister RR, Burstein N. The effects of ophthalmic drugs, vehicles, and preservatives on the corneal epithelium: a scanning electron microscope study. *Invest Ophthalmol*. 1976;15:246–259.
5. Stern GA, Killingsworth DW. Complications of topical antimicrobial agents. *Int Ophthalmol Clin*. 1989;29(3):137–142.
6. Leibowitz HM. Clinical evaluation of ciprofloxacin 0.3% in the treatment of bacterial conjunctivitis. *Am J Ophthalmol*. 1991;112:34s.
7. Wilson FM II. Adverse external ocular effects of topical ophthalmic medications. *Surv Ophthalmol*. 1979;24(2):57–88.
8. Stern GA, et al. The effect of topical antibiotic solutions on corneal epithelial wound healing. *Arch Ophthalmol*. 1983;101:644–647.
9. Foster CS, et al. Ocular toxicity of topical antifungal agents. *Arch Ophthalmol*. 1981;99:1081–1084.
10. Goldstein JH. Effects of drugs on cornea, conjunctiva, and lids. *Int Ophthalmol Clin*. 1971;11(2):13–34.
11. Kaiser PK, et al. 'Black cornea' after long-term epinephrine use. *Arch Ophthalmol*. 1992;110:1273–1275.
12. Wilhelmus KR, et al. Dendritic keratopathy associated with β-blocker eye drops. *Cornea*. 1990;9(4):335–337.
13. Sudesh S, et al. Corneal toxicity associated with latanoprost. *Arch Ophthalmol*. 1999;117:539–540.
14. Fiore PM. Drug induced ocular cicatrization. *Int Ophthalmol Clin*. 1989;29(3):147–150.

15. Brandt JD, et al. Conjunctival impression cytology in patients with glaucoma using long-term topical medications. *Am J Ophthalmol.* 1991;112: 297–301.
16. Hirst LW, et al. Drug induced cicatrizing conjunctivitis simulating ocular pemphigoid. *Cornea.* 1982;1:121–128.
17. Lin JC, et al. Corneal melting associated with use of topical nonsteroidal anti-inflammatory drugs after ocular surgery. *Arch Ophthalmol.* 2000; 118(8):1129–1132.
18. Guidera AC, et al. Keratitis, ulceration, and perforation associated with topical nonsteroidal anti-inflammatory drugs. *Ophthalmology.* 2001; 108(5):936–944.
19. Congdon NG, et al. Corneal complications associated with topical ophthalmic use of nonsteroidal anti-inflammatory drugs. *J Cataract Refract Surg.* 2001;27(4):622–631.
20. Arffa RC, Eve FR. Systemic associations of corneal deposits. *Int Ophthalmol Clin.* 1991;31(3):89–110.
21. Holland EJ, et al. Suramin keratopathy. *Am J Ophthalmol.* 1988;106: 216–220.
22. Greiner AC, Berry K. Skin pigmentation and corneal and lens opacities with prolonged chlorpromazine therapy. *Can Med Assoc J.* 1964;90: 663–665.
23. Siddal JR. Ocular toxic findings with prolonged and high dosage of chlorpromazine intake. *Arch Ophthalmol.* 1965;74:460–464.
24. Hays GB, Lyle CB Jr, Wheeler CE Jr. Slate gray color in patients receiving chlorpromazine. *Arch Dermatol.* 1964;90:471–476.
25. DeLong SL, Poley BJ, McFarlane JR. Ocular changes associated with long-term chlorpromazine therapy. *Arch Ophthalmol.* 1965;73:611–617.
26. Howard RO, et al. Experimental chlorpromazine cataracts. *Invest Ophthalmol.* 1969;8:413–421.
27. Petrohelos MA, Tricoulis D. Ocular complications of chlorpromazine therapy. *Ophthalmologica.* 1969;159:31–38.
28. Garmizo G, Frauens BJ. Corneal copper deposition secondary to oral contraceptives. *Optom Vis Sci.* 2008;85(9):E802–E807.
29. Bonadonna G, et al. Combination chemotherapy as an adjuvant treatment in operable breast cancer. *N Engl J Med.* 1976;294:405–410.
30. Loprinzi CL, et al. Cyclophosphamide, methotrexate, and 5-fluorouracil (CMF) induced ocular toxicity. *Cancer Invest.* 1990;8(5):459–465.
31. Friedland S, Loya N, Shapiro A. Handling punctate keratitis resulting from systemic cytarabine. *Ann Ophthalmol.* 1993;25:290–291.
32. Barletta JP, Fanous MM, Margo CE. Corneal and conjunctival toxicity with low-dose cytosine arabinoside. *Am J Ophthalmol.* 1992;113(3): 587–588.
33. Messmer E, et al. Pigmented conjunctival cysts following tetracycline/minocycline therapy. *Ophthalmology.* 1983;90(12):1462–1468.
34. Fraunfelder FT, LaBraico JM, Meyer SM. Adverse ocular reactions possibly associated with isotretinoin. *Am J Ophthalmol.* 1985;100:534–537.
35. Fraunfelder FT, Meyer SM. Amantadine and corneal deposits. *Am J Ophthalmol.* 1990;110(1):96–97.
36. Guill MA, et al. Erythema multiforme and urticaria. *Arch Dermatol.* 1979;115:742.
37. Ward B, McCulley JP, Segal RJ. Dermatologic reaction in Stevens-Johnson syndrome after ophthalmic anesthesia with proparacaine hydrochloride. *Am J Ophthalmol.* 1978;86:133.
38. Bergmann MT, Newmann BL, Johnson NC Jr. The effect of a diuretic (hydrochlorothiazide) on tear production in humans. *Am J Ophthalmol.* 1985;99:473–475.
39. Koffler BH, Lemp MA. The effect of an antihistamine (chlorpheniramine maleate) on tear production in humans. *Ann Ophthalmol.* 1980;12:217.
40. Hyndiuk RA, Schultz RO. Overview of the corneal toxicity of surgical solutions and drugs and clinical concepts in corneal edema. *Lens, Eye Toxic Res.* 1992;9(3&4):331–332.
41. Kompa S, et al. Corneal calcification after chemical eye burns caused by eye drops containing phosphate buffer. *Burns.* 2006;32(6):744–747.
42. Edelhauser HF, et al. Corneal edema and the intraocular use of epinephrine. *Am J Ophthalmol.* 1982;93:327.
43. Loane ME, Weinreb RN. Reducing corneal toxicity of 5-fluorouracil in the early postoperative period following glaucoma filtering surgery. *Aust NZ J Ophthalmol.* 1991;19(3):197–202.
44. Hickey-Dwyer M, Wishart PK. Serious corneal complications of 5-fluorouracil. *Br J Ophthalmol.* 1993;77:250–251.
45. Rubinfeld RS, et al. Serious complications of topical mitomycin-C after pterygium excision. *Ophthalmology.* 1992;99(11):1647–1654.
46. Nassiri N, et al. Corneal endothelial cell injury induced by mitomycin-C in photorefractive keratectomy: nonrandomized controlled trial. *J Cataract Refract Surg.* 2008;34(6):902–908.
47. Bennett SR, Abrams GW. Band keratopathy from emulsified silicone oil. *Arch Ophthalmol.* 1990;108:1387.
48. Breekhuis WH, van Rij G, Zivojnovic R. Silicone oil keratopathy: indications for keratoplasty. *Br J Ophthalmol.* 1985;69:247–253.

Chapter 70

Corneal Dystrophy Classification

Jayne S. Weiss

History

The word *dystrophy* derived from the Greek (*dys* = wrong, difficult; *trophe* = nourishment)[1] was introduced into the ophthalmology literature in 1890 by Arthur Groenouw when he published his classic paper describing two patients with 'Noduli Corneae.'[2] In the pre-slit lamp era, Groenouw did not initially appreciate the differences between the two conditions described, one patient having granular dystrophy and the other macular dystrophy. Nevertheless, the two diseases later became known as corneal dystrophies.[3] The word dystrophy continued to be used by Ernst Fuchs,[4] Wilhelm Uhthoff[5] and later Yoshiharu Yoshida.[6]

Corneal Dystrophy Definition

The words 'corneal dystrophy' typically refer to a group of inherited corneal diseases that are usually bilateral, symmetric, slowly progressive and not related to environmental or systemic factors.[7] However, exceptions to each part of this definition exist. Hereditary pattern is not present in most patients with epithelial basement membrane dystrophy (EBMD). Unilateral corneal changes may be found in some patients with posterior polymorphous corneal dystrophy (PPCD). Systemic changes are found in macular dystrophy, in which the level of antigenic serum keratan sulfate correlates with the immunophenotypes of the disease.

Corneal Dystrophy Classification in the Literature

The first classification by Bücklers of corneal dystrophies described the differences between granular, macular, and lattice dystrophy.[8] The most commonly used classification system is anatomically based.[7] The dystrophies are typically classified by level of the cornea that is involved, which separates these entities into epithelial and subepithelial, Bowman layer, stromal, and endothelial dystrophies.[9,10]

Shortcomings of Corneal Dystrophy Nomenclature and Classification

There have been many misconceptions and errors in the corneal dystrophy nomenclature and classification. For example, the dystrophy previously called, Schnyder crystalline corneal dystrophy (SCD) is a rare dystrophy often misdiagnosed precisely because of the deceptive name. While many publications emphasize the necessity of demonstrating corneal crystals to make the diagnosis of SCD,[11–13] examination of large pedigrees of affected individuals demonstrates that only 50% of affected patients actually have corneal crystals.[11]

Errors in the dystrophy literature include the fact that some of the early papers describing the ultrastructure of Reis-Bücklers corneal dystrophy had actually analyzed tissue from patients with Thiel-Behnke corneal dystrophy.[14] Some entities described as corneal dystrophies may actually be corneal degenerations and have no hereditary tendency. The original publication on central cloudy dystrophy of François[15] indicated this corneal opacification was inherited, but there have been only a few other publications that have described an entire family with this disease.[16,17] Furthermore, central cloudy dystrophy of François appears clinically indistinguishable from the degenerative condition, posterior crocodile shagreen.[18] Without additional affected pedigrees or genetic studies, it is possible that central cloudy dystrophy of François and posterior crocodile shagreen are the same entity.

Another flaw in the corneal dystrophy classification is the relative lack of scrutiny that has been required to call something a new corneal dystrophy. Prior to the 1970s, new corneal dystrophies were identified and characterized almost exclusively by their clinical appearance, and sometimes the report of a single family signaled the creation of a new dystrophy.[19] In some such cases, a variant of a previously described dystrophy was instead given a different name and misclassified as a new dystrophy. For example, the dystrophy named Waardenburg and Jonkers[20] was not a unique entity and was actually identical to the previously described Thiel-Behnke dystrophy.[21]

The Impact of Genotyping on Corneal Dystrophy Nomenclature

Genotypic analysis has revealed other inaccuracies of dystrophy nomenclature. Different genes (KRT3 and KRT12) can result in a single dystrophy phenotype such as Meesmann dystrophy, and one single gene (TGFBI) can cause multiple allelic dystrophy phenotypes (Reis-Bücklers, Thiel-Behnke, granular type 1, granular type 2, lattice type 1). Newer genetic information has clearly demonstrated the flaws in the older system of phenotypic classification of corneal dystrophies.

Since the first descriptions of granular, macular, and lattice dystrophies over a century ago, the word dystrophy has lost significance as the distinctive name of many of the individual dystrophies has become less meaningful. While a more meaningful classification would be called 'inherited corneal diseases,' it is likely that 'the popular designation of corneal dystrophy will probably keep its place.'[22]

The International Committee for Classification of Corneal Dystrophies

The International Committee for Classification of Corneal Dystrophies (IC3D) was created in 2005 in order to revise the corneal dystrophy nomenclature and create a current and accurate corneal dystrophy classification system. An international panel of interested world experts possessing firsthand experience with the clinical, genetic, and histopathologic findings of all the corneal dystrophies was recruited to evaluate critically the past literature and to distill the facts and remove outdated inaccurate information. The goal was to establish a new nomenclature which would reflect current clinical, pathologic, and genetic knowledge, be easily adaptable to advances in understanding from the continued discovery of new genes and mutations, and be linked to the old nomenclature for ease of use. The revised dystrophy classification was published in 2008.[23]

The IC3D Classification – an Anatomically Based Classification System

The IC3D corneal dystrophy classification system is anatomically based, with dystrophies divided according to the layer chiefly affected, similar to the former classification system. They are: epithelial and subepithelial, Bowman layer, stromal, and those affecting Descemet's membrane and the endothelium. For ease of use, the majority of the dystrophy names are identical or similar to those in the current nomenclature. However, dystrophies with a known common genetic basis, i.e. TGFBI dystrophies, have been grouped together.

The IC3D Category System to Denote the Evolution of a Corneal Dystrophy

One challenge in revising the dystrophy nomenclature was how to devise a classification that would be flexible enough to facilitate the expansion of knowledge from other sources, including genotyping.

When a corneal dystrophy is first described, there is usually a predictable chain of events. First, an entity is identified and characterized clinically. Subsequently, if tissue evaluations of the diseased cornea are available, these may lead to the establishment of distinct clinicopathologic entities. Finally, genetic linkage studies lead to the mapping of the chromosomal locus of the disorder, especially if the condition has a simple Mendelian inheritance pattern. This task becomes more complex when more than one gene is involved or if there is an interaction between genetic and environmental factors. Ultimately, there is identification of the relevant gene and isolation of specific mutations that are responsible for different phenotypical forms of the disorder. Finally, the mechanism of the disorder will eventually be understood, with identification of the gene product.

In order to reflect the natural evolution of a corneal dystrophy and indicate the level of evidence supporting the existence of a given dystrophy, four descriptive, evidential categories were created in the IC3D classification (Box 70.1).[23] While the category assigned to a specific corneal dystrophy will change as knowledge advances, all valid corneal dystrophies should eventually have a category 1 classification. Conversely, as further information is gathered over time, some category 4 dystrophies may be shown not to be distinct entities and may be removed (Box 70.2).

The IC3D Templates

Each corneal dystrophy is assigned a template in the IC3D system, which includes a brief summary of the current genetic, clinical, and pathologic information about the disease and includes representative clinical images (Box 70.3). To facilitate investigation online, Mendelian Inheritance Online (MIM) numbers are included for each dystrophy in addition to MIM abbreviations and newer revised abbreviations (Table 70.1).

Box 70.1 Evidential categories for IC3D classification

Category 1. A well-defined corneal dystrophy in which the gene has been mapped and identified and specific mutations are known.

Category 2. A well-defined corneal dystrophy that has been mapped to one or more specific chromosomal loci, but the gene(s) remains to be identified.

Category 3: A clinically well-defined corneal dystrophy in which the disorder has not yet been mapped to a chromosomal locus.

Category 4. This category is reserved for a suspected new, or previously documented, corneal dystrophy, where the evidence for it being a distinct entity is not yet convincing.

From: Weiss JS, Møller H, Lisch W, et al. The IC3D classification of the corneal dystrophies. Cornea *2008;27:S1–S42, S4.*

Box 70.2 The IC3D classification

Epithelial and subepithelial dystrophies

1. Epithelial basement membrane dystrophy (EBMD) – majority degenerative, some C1
2. Epithelial recurrent erosion dystrophy (ERED) C4 (Smolandiensis variant)
3. Subepithelial mucinous corneal dystrophy (SMCD) C4
4. Mutation in keratin genes
   Meesmann corneal dystrophy (MECD) C1
5. Lisch epithelial corneal dystrophy (LECD) C2
6. Gelatinous drop-like corneal dystrophy (GDLD) C1

Bowman layer dystrophies

1. Reis-Bücklers corneal dystrophy (RBCD) – granular corneal dystrophy type 3 C1
2. Thiel-Behnke corneal dystrophy (TBCD) C1, potential variant C2
3. Grayson-Wilbrandt corneal dystrophy (GWCD) C4

Stromal dystrophies

1. TGFBI corneal dystrophies
   A. Lattice corneal dystrophy
      i. Lattice corneal dystrophy, TGFBI type (LCD)
         Classic lattice corneal dystrophy (LCD1) C1, variants (III, IIIA, I/IIIA, IV) are C1
      ii. Lattice corneal dystrophy, gelsolin type (LCD2) C1
         This is not a true corneal dystrophy but is included here for ease of differential diagnosis
   B. Granular corneal dystrophy C1
      i. Granular corneal dystrophy, type 1 (classic) (GCD1) C1
      ii. Granular corneal dystrophy, type 2 (granular-lattice) (GCD2) C1
      iii. Granular corneal dystrophy, type 3 (RBCD) = Reis-Bücklers) C1
2. Macular corneal dystrophy (MCD) C1
3. Schnyder corneal dystrophy (SCD) C1
4. Congenital stromal corneal dystrophy (CSCD) C1
5. Fleck corneal dystrophy (FCD) C1
6. Posterior amorphous corneal dystrophy (PACD) C3
7. Central cloudy dystrophy of Francois (CCDF) C4
8. Pre-Descemet's corneal dystrophy (PDCD) C4

Descemet membrane and endothelial dystrophies

1. Fuchs' endothelial corneal dystrophy (FECD) C1, C2 or C3
2. Posterior polymorphous corneal dystrophy (PPCD) C1 or C2
3. Congenital hereditary endothelial dystrophy 1 (CHED 1) C2
4. Congenital hereditary endothelial dystrophy 2 (CHED 2) C1
5. X-linked endothelial corneal dystrophy (XECD) C2

C, Category.
From: Weiss JS, Møller H, Lisch W, et al. The IC3D classification of the corneal dystrophies. Cornea *2008;27:S1–S42, S5.*

Box 70.3 Schnyder corneal dystrophy (SCD)

MIM # 21800

Alternative Names, Eponyms

Schnyder crystalline corneal dystrophy (SCCD)

Schnyder crystalline dystrophy sine crystals

Hereditary crystalline stromal dystrophy of Schnyder

Crystalline stromal dystrophy

Central stromal crystalline corneal dystrophy

Corneal crystalline dystrophy of Schnyder

Schnyder corneal crystalline dystrophy

Genetic Locus
1p36

Gene
UBIAD1-UbiA prenyltransferase domain containing 1

Inheritance
Autosomal dominant

Onset
May be as early as childhood, but diagnosis usually made by the 2nd or 3rd decade. Diagnosis may be further delayed in patients who have the a crystalline form of the disease.

Signs
Corneal changes are predictable on the basis of age. Patients 23 years of age or less have central corneal haze and/or subepithelial crystals. Between 23 and 38 years of age, arcus lipoides is noted. After age 38, mid-peripheral panstromal haze develops causing the entire cornea to appear hazy. Despite the name, only 50% of patients demonstrate corneal crystals. Crystals may be unilateral, may rarely regress, and can occur late in the disease.

Symptoms
Visual acuity decreases with age. Complaints of glare increase with age. While scotopic vision may be remarkably good (considering the slit lamp appearance), photopic vision may be disproportionately decreased. Corneal sensation decreases with age. Both affected and unaffected members of the pedigrees may have hyperlipoproteinemia (type IIa, III or IV).

Course
Slowly progressive, although majority of patients above age 50 may require keratoplasty for decreased photopic vision.

Light Microscopy
Abnormal deposition of intra- and extracellular esterified and unesterified phospholipids and cholesterol in basal epithelial cells, Bowman layer, and stroma. Organic solvents and resins can dissolve lipids. Consequently, in order to process the corneal specimen to allow special lipid stains such as oil red O or sudan black to be performed, the ophthalmologist should inform the pathologist, prior to placing the corneal specimen in solution, that lipid stains are requested.

Transmission Electron Microscopy
Abnormal accumulation of intracellular and extracellular esterified and unesterified phospholipids and cholesterol are deposited in the epithelium, Bowman layer, and throughout the stroma. Endothelial lipid has rarely been reported.

Confocal Microscopy
Intracellular and extracellular highly reflective deposits may lead to eventual disruption of the basal epithelial/subepithelial nerve plexus.

Category
1

From: Weiss JS, Møller H, Lisch W, et al. The IC3D classification of the corneal dystrophies. Cornea *2008;27:S1–S42.*

Table 70.1 The IC3D classification – abbreviations and MIM number

	MIM abbreviation	IC3D abbreviation	MIM#
Epithelial basement membrane dystrophy	EBMD	EBMD	121820
Epithelial recurrent erosion dystrophy	none	ERED	122400
Subepithelial mucinous CD	none	SMCD	none
Meesmann CD	none	MECD	122100
Lisch epithelial CD	none	LECD	none
Gelatinous drop-like CD	GDLD, CDGDL	GDLD	204870
Reis-Bücklers CD	CDB1, CDRB, RBCD	RBCD	608470
Thiel-Behnke CD	CDB2, CDTB,	TBCD	602082
Grayson-Wilbrandt CD	none	GWCD	none
Classic lattice CD	CDL1	LCD1	122200
Lattice CD, Meretoja type	none	LCD2	105120
Granular CD, type 1	CGDD1	GCD1	121900
Granular CD, type 2 (granular-lattice)	CDA, ACD	GCD2	607541
Macular CD	MCDC1	MCD	217800
Schnyder CD	none	SCD	121800
Congenital stromal CD	CSCD	CSCD	610048
Fleck CD	none	FCD	121850
Posterior amorphous CD	none	PACD	none
Central cloudy dystrophy of François	none	CCDF	217600
Pre-Descemet CD	none	PDCD	none
Fuchs' endothelial CD	FECD1	FECD	136800
Posterior polymorphous CD	PPCD1	PPCD	122000
Congenital hereditary endothelial CD 1	CHED1	CHED1	121700
Congenital hereditary endothelial CD 2	CHED2	CHED2	217700
X-linked endothelial CD	none	XECD	none

CD, corneal dystrophy; MIM; Mendelian Inheritance In Man.
Online Mendelian Inheritance in Man: McKusick VA et al. http://www.ncbi.nlm.nih.gov/sites/entrez
From: Weiss JS, Møller H, Lisch W, et al. The IC3D classification of the corneal dystrophies. Cornea 2008;27:S1–S42, S6 (Table 1).

Summary

The IC3D corneal dystrophy classification system is a revision of the corneal dystrophy nomenclature which is accurate, easy to use, and can be updated with new discoveries. The original IC3D article with photographs is easily accessible on the web at www.corneasociety.org. This system should facilitate more scientific and objective criteria for determining whether a new corneal dystrophy has indeed been discovered.

References

1. Warburg M, Møller HU. Dystrophy: a revised definition. *J Med Genet.* 1989;26:769–771.
2. Groenouw A. Knötchenförmige Hornhauttrübungen 'Noduli Corneae.' *Arch Augenheilkd.* 1890;21:281–289.
3. Møller HU. Granular corneal dystrophy Groenouw type I. Clinical and genetic aspects. *Acta Ophthalmol (Copenh).* 1991;69(Suppl 198):1–40.
4. Fuchs E. Dystrophia epithelialis corneae. *Albrecht von Graefe's Arch Clin Exp Ophthalmol.* 1910;76:478–508.
5. Uhthoff W. Ein Fall von doppelseitiger zentraler, punktförmiger, supepithelialer knötchenförmiger Keratitis. Groenouw mit anatomischem Befunde. *Klin Monatsbl Augenheilkd.* 1915;54:377–383.
6. Yoshida Y. Über eine neue Art der Dystrophia corneae mit histologischem Befunde. *Albrecht von Graefe's Arch Clin Exp Ophthalmol.* 1924; 114:91–100.
7. American Academy of Ophthalmology. External diseases and cornea. In: *Basic and Clinical Sciences Course 2007–2008.* San Francisco: American Academy of Ophthalmology; 2007.
8. Bücklers M. Die erblichen Hornhaut-dystrophie. *Klin Monatsbl Augenheilkd.* 1938;3:1–135.
9. Waring GO 3rd, Rodrigues MM, Laibson PR. Corneal dystrophies. I. Dystrophies of the epithelium. Bowman's layer and stroma. *Surv Ophthalmol.* 1978;23:71–122.
10. Waring GO 3rd, Rodrigues MM, Laibson PR. Corneal dystrophies. II. Endothelial dystrophies. *Surv Ophthalmol.* 1978;23:147–168.
11. Weiss JS. Schnyder's dystrophy of the cornea. A Swede–Finn connection. *Cornea.* 1992;11:93–100.
12. Weiss JS. Schnyder crystalline dystrophy sine crystals. Recommendation for a revision of nomenclature. *Ophthalmology.* 1996;103:465–473.
13. Weiss JS. Visual morbidity in thirty-four families with Schnyder's crystalline corneal dystrophy. *Trans Am Ophthamol Soc.* 2007;105:616–648.
14. Kanai A, Kaufman HE, Polack FM. Electron microscopic study of Reis-Bücklers dystrophy. *Ann Ophthalmol.* 1973;5:953–962.
15. François J. Une nouvelle dystrophie heredo-familiale de la cornee. *J Genet Hum.* 1956;5:189–196.
16. Strachan IM. Cloudy central corneal dystrophy of François. Five cases in the same family. *Br J Ophthalmol.* 1969;53:192–194.
17. Bramsen T, Ehlers N, Baggesen LH. Central cloudy corneal dystrophy of François. *Acta Ophthalmol (Copenh).* 1976;54:221–226.
18. Meyer JC, Quantock AJ, Thonar EJ, et al. Characterization of a central corneal cloudiness sharing features of posterior crocodile shagreen and central cloudy dystrophy of François. *Cornea.* 1996;15:347–354.
19. Reis W. Familiäre, fleckige Hornhautentartung. *Dtsch Med Wochenschr.* 1917;43:575.
20. Waardenburg PJ, Jonkers GH. A specific type of dominant progressive dystrophy of the cornea, developing after birth. *Acta Ophthalmol (Copenh).* 1961;39:919–923.
21. Thiel H-J, Behnke H. Fine bisher unbekannte subepitheliale hereditäre Hornhaut-dystrophie. *Klin Monatsbl Augenheilkd.* 1967;150:862–874.
22. Kintworth GK. Genetic disorders of the cornea: from research to practical diagnostic testing. *Graefe's Arch Clin Exp Ophthalmol.* 2005;33:231–232.
23. Weiss JS, Møller H, Lisch W, et al. The IC3D classification of the corneal dystrophies. *Cornea.* 2008;27:S1-S42.

Chapter 71

Anterior Corneal Dystrophies

Peter R. Laibson

A corneal dystrophy is defined as a corneal opacity or alteration which is most often bilateral and progressive, occurs after birth, and is not inflammatory. Located in the central cornea, it is generally less evident at the limbus. Most corneal dystrophies are dominantly inherited.

The anterior corneal dystrophies or anterior membrane dystrophies include dystrophies that involve only the corneal epithelium, the epithelium and epithelial basement membrane, and Bowman's membrane. The dystrophies involving Bowman's membrane usually exhibit pathologic changes of the superficial stroma as well as the epithelial basement membrane and epithelium.

Meesmann's dystrophy and Lisch epithelial corneal dystrophy are exclusively within the corneal epithelium. Dystrophies involving the epithelial layer and the epithelial basement membrane generally have been called epithelial or anterior basement membrane dystrophy. (Synonyms are map-dot-fingerprint dystrophy, Cogan's microcystic dystrophy, and fingerprint corneal dystrophy.) All of these dystrophies have in common involvement of the epithelial basement membrane, a product of the basal layer of epithelium, and, in many cases, epithelial changes.

Dystrophies in the region of Bowman's membrane and superficial stroma include Reis–Bücklers' dystrophy (now considered by some to be a superficial variant of granular dystrophy), and Thiel-Behnke honeycomb dystrophy. There has been considerable misunderstanding in the ophthalmic literature concerning Reis–Bücklers' dystrophy, first described by Reis[1] in 1917 and later by Bücklers[2] in 1949. Unfortunately, their descriptions did not include light or electron microscopy, which has contributed to the problem.

The somewhat similar appearance and location of the dystrophies of Bowman's layer, which in general have a common clinical course, have further confused our understanding of them. Fortunately, in the last 10 years, authors in Europe and most recently the United States have redefined and reclassified these dystrophies. Two different dystrophic entities that are called CDB-I and CDB-II (corneal dystrophy of Bowman's layer and the superficial stroma, I and II) can be differentiated both clinically and by light and electron microscopy. New methods in molecular genetics have resulted in improved diagnosis and understanding of the pathogenesis of corneal dystrophies and will require new classification.

A new classification system for corneal dystrophies has been proposed in a recent supplement to the journal *Cornea*. An International Committee for Classification of Corneal Dystrophies was created (IC3D), and based on current phenotypic description, genetic analysis, and pathologic examination this new classification system was described.[3]

Meesmann's Juvenile Epithelial Dystrophy (IC3D, MECD, Category 1)

Meesmann's juvenile epithelial dystrophy is a rare, bilaterally symmetric, hereditary epithelial dystrophy that is inherited in an autosomal dominant pattern.[4] A mutation in corneal keratin (K3 or K12) has been shown to underlie Meesmann's corneal dystrophy.[5] This dystrophy is seen in the first few years of life as intraepithelial microcysts or vesicles visible only at the slit lamp. The epithelial microcysts are present primarily in the visual axis and in the mid-periphery. They may be seen best with indirect illumination from the iris (Fig. 71.1), or in retroillumination against the red reflex of the dilated pupil (Fig. 71.2). Vision is usually good in the first few years of life but may diminish gradually if the cysts increase in number and cause slight irregularity of the corneal surface. Recurrent erosion is not common with this dystrophy, and neither superficial keratectomy nor lamellar corneal transplantation is appropriate.

The epithelial microcysts consist of degenerated epithelial cell products with cytoplasmic and nuclear debris found in epithelial cells. There is a thickened basement membrane and the basal epithelial cells have increased glycogen.[6] Transmission electron microscopic findings have been described as collections of granular and filamentary material ('peculiar substance') within the cytoplasm of epithelial cells.

The cause of the cysts is unknown, but the hereditary nature of this dystrophy has been recognized. Burns[7] mentioned the possibility of an anterior stromal cause for this dystrophy based on corneal superficial biopsy (including some anterior stroma) and epithelium removal. Even years later, no microcystic changes occurred above the area of biopsy. This opinion was reinforced by Wittebol-Post et al.,[8] who found a slightly thinned stroma in three families with Meesmann's dystrophy. As with other hereditary

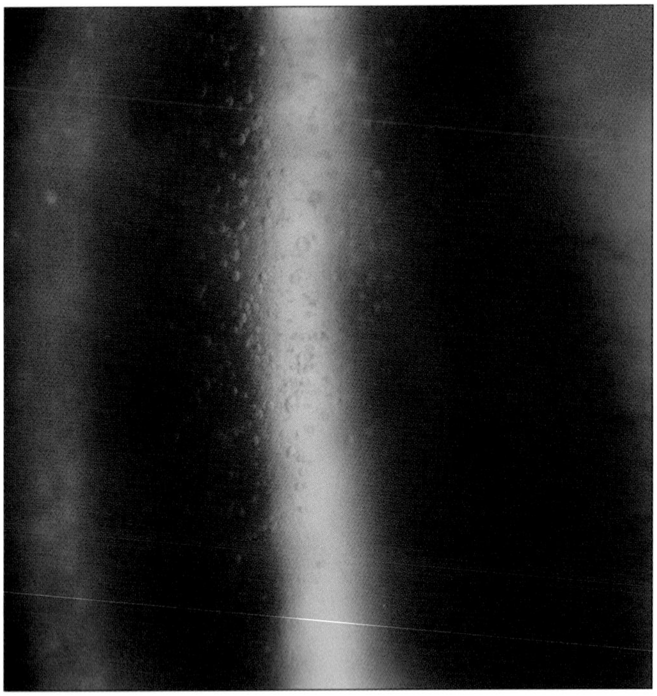

Fig. 71.1 Meesmann's corneal dystrophy. Notice the microvacuoles in retroillumination. These are fine vacuolar changes in the epithelium.

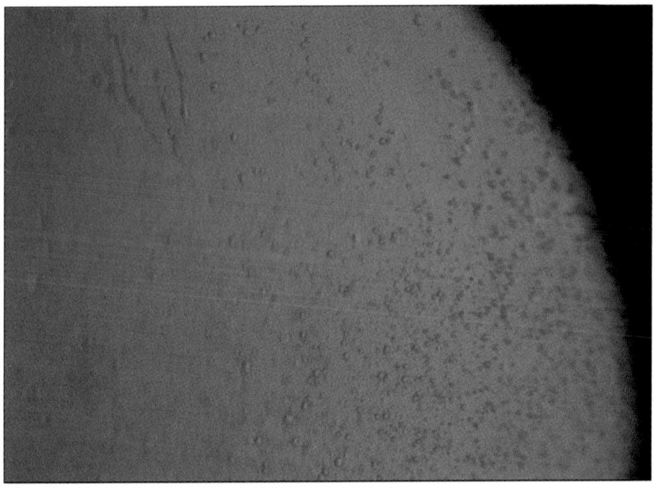

Fig. 71.2 Meesmann's corneal dystrophy with retroillumination against the dilated red reflex of the fundus. These vacuoles stand out a little better than the vacuoles in Figure 71.1.

dystrophies, there was a difference between families in the progression of the disease: one family had progression and one family did not.

Symptoms related to Meesmann's dystrophy are usually mild or nonexistent. Because pathologic findings are limited to the corneal epithelium and the individual microcysts are small, the corneal surface is usually smooth. Even though the pathologic findings are seen well with retroillumination, there may be little disturbance of visual acuity. Patients may require lubricating ointments for minute erosions, which occur when the cysts surface, but surgical intervention is rarely necessary. Bourne[9] used soft contact lenses for patients

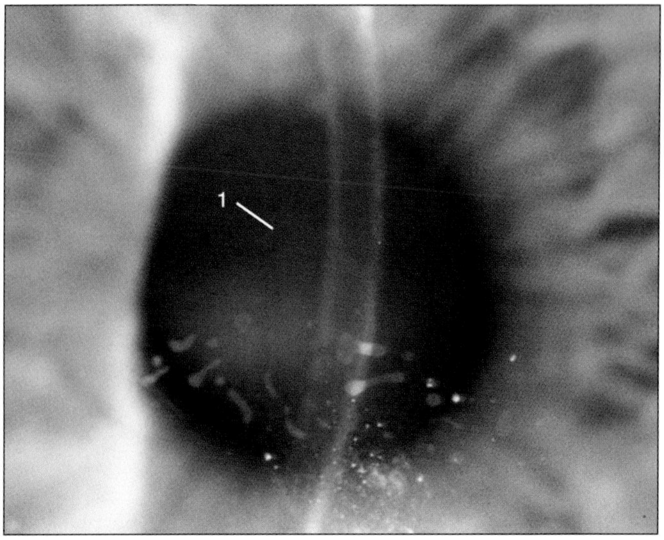

Fig. 71.3 Epithelial basement membrane dystrophy (map-dot-fingerprint, Cogan's microcystic dystrophy). Notice the intraepithelial microcysts in the slit just at the inferior margin of the visual axis. There is also an iron line superiorly (1).

with Meesmann's dystrophy for 1, 3, and 8 years of daily use. No adverse long-term consequences were seen, and the microcysts decreased beneath the soft lens.

Although dystrophies of the cornea are usually unique, a rare case combining Meesmann's, anterior epithelial basement membrane, and posterior polymorphous corneal dystrophies has recently been described.[10]

In 1983 Lisch and Lisch[11] described an epithelial corneal dystrophy genetically distinct from Meesmann's and epithelial basement membrane corneal dystrophies. This consisted of a band-shaped and whorl microcystic dystrophy specific to the corneal epithelium.[12] There were few recurrent erosive symptoms, but blurred vision occurred if the cornea over the pupil was involved (IC3D, LECD, Category 2).

Epithelial Basement Membrane Dystrophy (IC3D, EBMD, Some Category 1)

Epithelial basement membrane dystrophy is the most common anterior corneal dystrophy and is classified as a corneal dystrophy because these changes occur more in some families than in the general population.[13] Others have found it more generally prevalent in the community and do not consider it a corneal dystrophy.[14] In a study of 250 normal individuals, however, these changes were seen in only 5% of normal corneas when observed by corneal fellowship-trained ophthalmologists.[15]

Cogan et al.[16] first described the characteristic microcystic changes in the corneal epithelium in this disorder. They found minute pinpoint and larger, oval, and irregularly shaped grayish-white opacities in the superficial corneal epithelium (Fig. 71.3) of women who were mildly symptomatic with transient blurred vision and, in one case, a recurrent erosion. The maplike changes around these microcysts, which are the characteristic and pathophysiologic feature of this dystrophy, were not described by Cogan et al.[16] It was

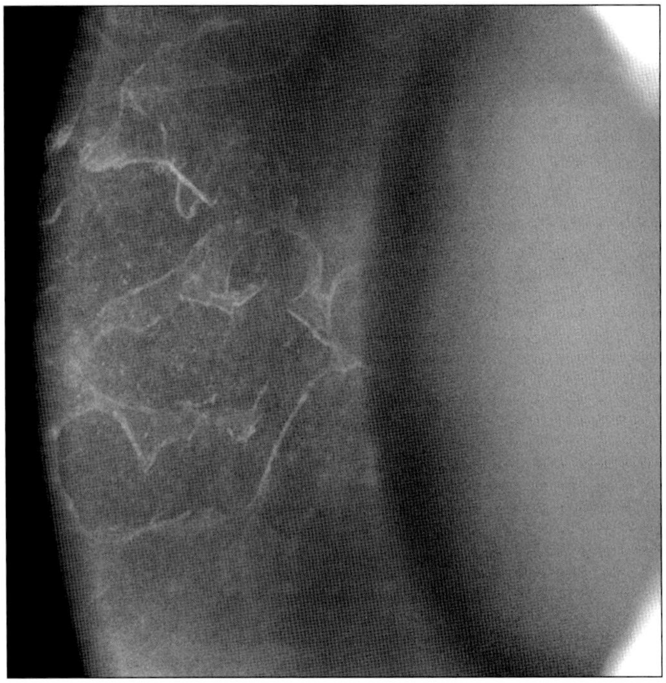

Fig. 71.4 Maplike changes in epithelial basement membrane dystrophy are not apparent in Figure 71.3. There are no microcysts. Most patients with epithelial basement membrane dystrophy have only the map changes as seen in Figure 71.4, which represent basement membrane within the epithelium.

Guerry[17] who pointed out the maplike changes (Fig. 71.4) in nine cases of Cogan's microcystic dystrophy the next year.

Guerry[17] found irregular, faintly grayish areas, sharply demarcated from one to several millimeters in size, with clear zones interspersed between the grayish patches. He called these findings maplike areas and also reported seeing putty-gray dots (microcysts) previously described by Cogan et al.[16] (Fig. 71.5).

Vogt,[18] in his slit lamp atlas of 1930, described fingerprint lines in the corneal epithelium, which are parallel lines like the furrows in a plowed field (Fig. 71.6). He also mentioned corneal changes, which were later described as microcysts by Cogan et al.[16] Microcysts were also reported in two additional cases by Guerry in 1950[19] and by DeVoe in 1962.[20] Devoe thought they were easily overlooked unless the observer was particularly interested in corneal disease.

In 1972, Trobe and Laibson[21] found map changes, microcysts (dots), and fingerprints in various combinations in the patient; in a few instances all were present in the same cornea. They coined the phrase map-dot-fingerprint corneal dystrophy for this condition.

A more unusual corneal change, which is also seen in the corneal epithelium, particularly the basal layer of epithelium, was described by Bron and Brown.[22] These bleblike changes (Fig. 71.7) were linked to the maps and fingerprints in some patients, and are the most unusual finding in this condition. They are seen best on retroillumination and may be found with other pathology such as maps, fingerprints, and dots, or may occur alone.

The term epithelial basement membrane dystrophy, which is now generally used to include map, dot, and

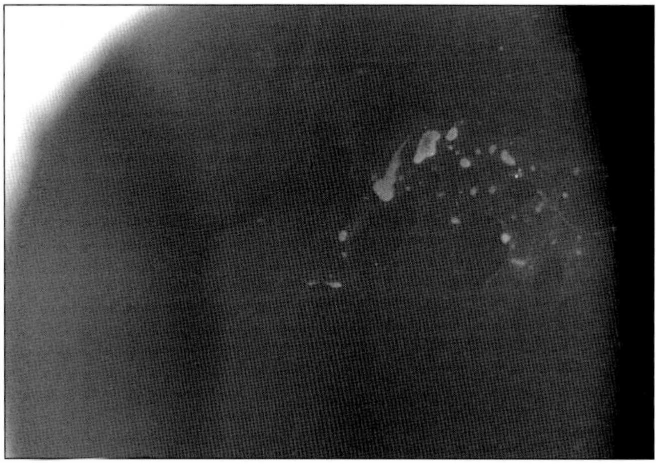

Fig. 71.5 Both microcystic changes of Cogan and maplike changes together. Usually, the microcysts are in the area of basement membrane and not in the clear lacuna as noted here.

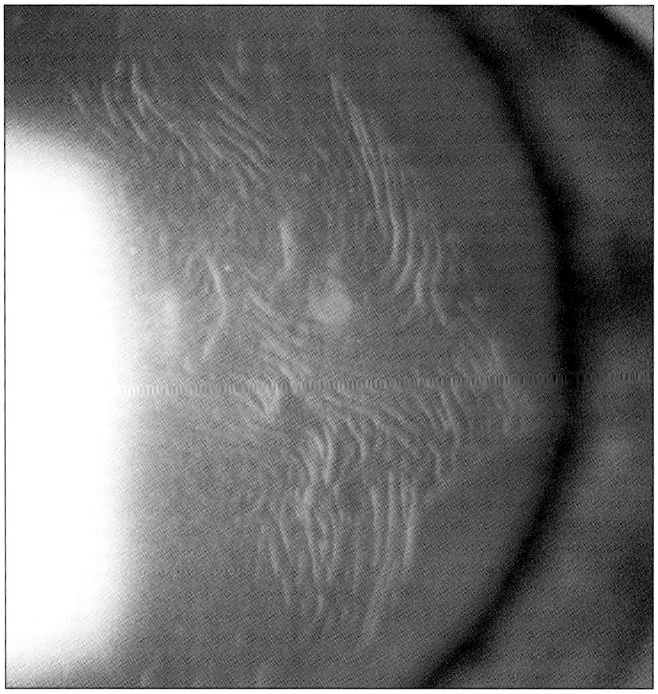

Fig. 71.6 Retroillumination of highlighted basement membrane dystrophy seen as fingerprint lines and map patterns. It is easier to see fingerprint lines and map changes against the dilated pupil and red reflex of the fundus.

fingerprint pathology, derives its name from the maplike changes that represent corneal epithelial basement membrane present within the epithelium itself. Rodrigues et al.[23] and Cogan et al.[24] described the pathology of these changes in 1974. These authors found sheetlike areas of basement membrane originating from the basement membrane of the basal epithelial cells of the corneal epithelium and extending superficially into the substance of the epithelium (Fig. 71.8).

Maturing epithelial cells migrating from the deeper to the superficial layers of epithelium, which would eventually be

Fig. 71.7 Bleb pattern is seen in retroillumination against the fundus red reflex. The bleblike deposits beneath the basal epithelium are seen to the right of the slit lamp light reflex.

discharged from the corneal surface, become trapped beneath the sheets of basement membrane and are prevented from surfacing (Fig. 71.9).[25] These cysts contain cellular and nuclear debris and may be two to three epithelial cells in size, or may be quite large and irregular, measuring up to 1 mm (Fig. 71.9). They are usually found beneath the basement membrane, but may be seen within the epithelial layer alone if epithelial debridement is performed to rid the patient of the cysts, and if the basement membrane is not removed with debridement (Fig. 71.10). In other cases, where maplike changes or fingerprint lines are noted, large

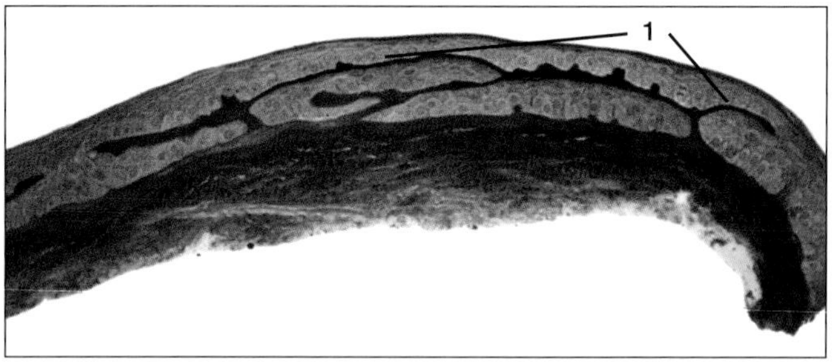

Fig. 71.8 Biopsy specimen of a patient with recurrent corneal erosion with map changes and fingerprint lines. Extra sheets of basement membrane material (1) grow into the epithelium. The biopsy specimen in the peripheral cornea includes Bowman's membrane and superficial stroma.

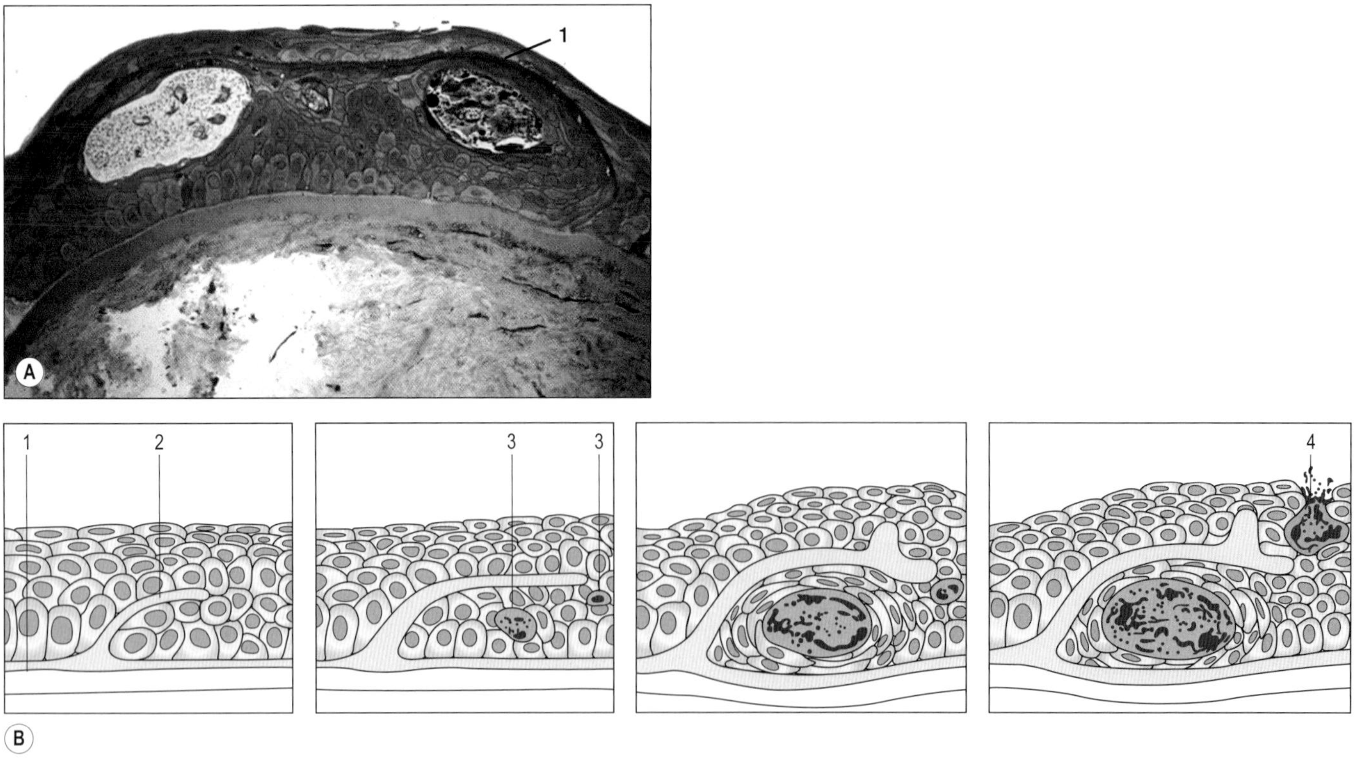

Fig. 71.9 Epithelial basement membrane dystrophy. **A,** Two large epithelial microcysts trapped beneath extensions of epithelial basement membrane (1) coming forward from the basal epithelium. This superficial corneal biopsy of a patient with recurrent erosion and epithelial basement membrane dystrophy also shows some anterior stromal elements beneath Bowman's membrane. **B,** Theoretical pathogenesis of epithelial basement membrane dystrophy. Epithelial cells produce abnormal multilaminar basement membrane, both in normal location (1) and intraepithelially (2). As the intraepithelial basement membrane thickens, it blocks normal migration of epithelial cells toward the surface. Trapped epithelial cells degenerate to form intraepithelial microcysts (3) that slowly migrate to the surface (4). Abnormal basement membrane produces map and fingerprint changes, and microcysts produce the dot pattern seen clinically. (From Waring GO et al. *Surv Ophthalmol* 1978;23:71–122. Copyright Elsevier, All rights reserved.)

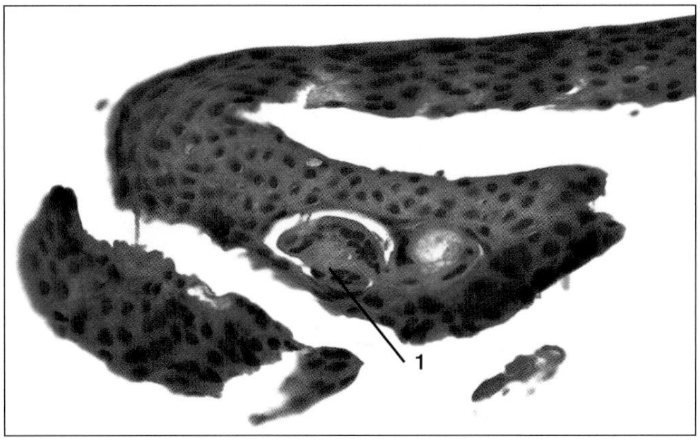

Fig. 71.10 Debridement specimen of epithelium showing intraepithelial microcyst (1) (Cogan) but no aberrant basement membrane, which remained attached to Bowman's membrane when the debridement was performed. The patient had multiple recurrent erosions in the symptomatic eye and epithelial basement membrane dystrophy but no erosions in the asymptomatic fellow eye.

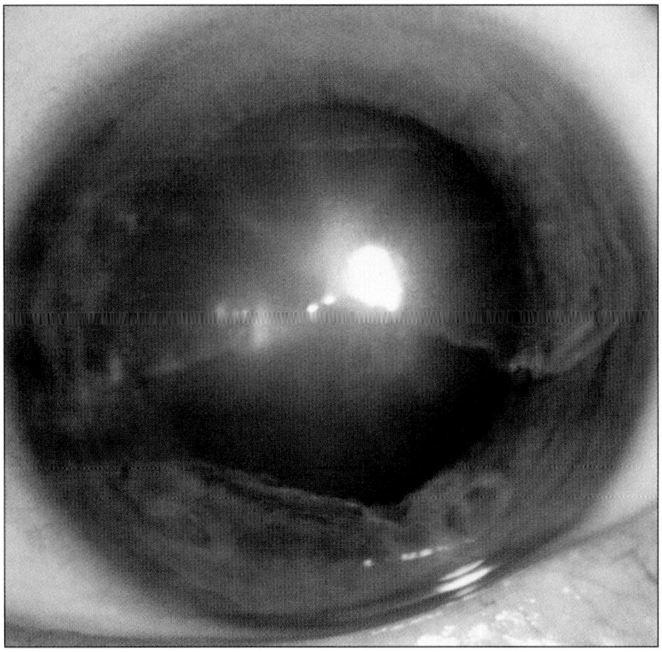

Fig. 71.11 Marked epithelial basement membrane changes photographed by diffuse illumination. No microcysts were seen in either eye. This pathology in the visual axis caused irregular astigmatism. Notice the irregular light reflex in the center of the cornea, which caused blurred vision. Removing the epithelium and basement membrane restored reasonable vision in this patient.

areas of abnormally thickened basement membrane may be present within the epithelium and microcysts may be absent (Fig. 71.11). The fingerprint lines are parallel rows of thickened basement membrane within the epithelium. These areas may be seen in conjunction with microcysts and map changes, or may be present without these changes. The parallel rows of thickened basement membrane are best seen on retroillumination (Fig. 71.12).

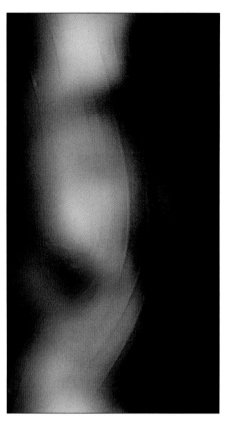

Fig. 71.12 Parallel lines and fingerprint lines in broad slit retroillumination are evidence of epithelial basement membrane changes or shift lines in this patient. This patient had recurrent corneal erosion and required continued use of lubricating ointment at bedtime for several years before symptoms were alleviated.

The pathology of the bleblike changes may consist of individual small mounds of thickened basement membrane beneath the basal layer of epithelium and are not continuous. They are generally viewed best by retroillumination (see Fig. 71.7).

The primary symptoms of epithelial basement membrane dystrophy are spontaneous recurrent corneal erosions and blurred vision. The erosions may be mild and transient, lasting minutes, or occasionally characterized by more severe pain. This pain can persist for hours or even days, but more characteristically it is transient and lasts for only a few minutes. Pain may be present on awakening, or it can awaken the patient when the eyelids are opened during sleep.

Patients with epithelial basement dystrophy who have traumatic abrasions are more likely to have recurrent epithelial erosions. Patients who have recurrent epithelial erosions and no history of trauma should be examined carefully for signs of the presence of epithelial basement membrane dystrophy in both the eye with the recurrent erosion and in the asymptomatic opposite eye.

Hykin et al.[26] prospectively examined 117 patients with a history of recurrent corneal erosions and found that 23 had only epithelial basement membrane dystrophy with no history of trauma; eight patients had both epithelial basement membrane dystrophy and trauma. Seventy-five patients had a history of trauma, but no slit lamp evidence of

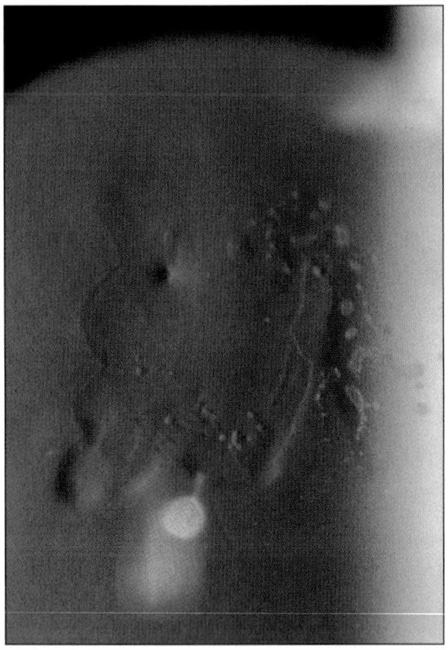

Fig. 71.13 Retroillumination of epithelial basement membrane dystrophy seen as map patterns and microcysts. The light highlight to one side, which is the slit lamp beam, throws light across the corneal surface, highlighting one side of the map changes and shadowing the other side. This picture indicates a slight epithelial elevation.

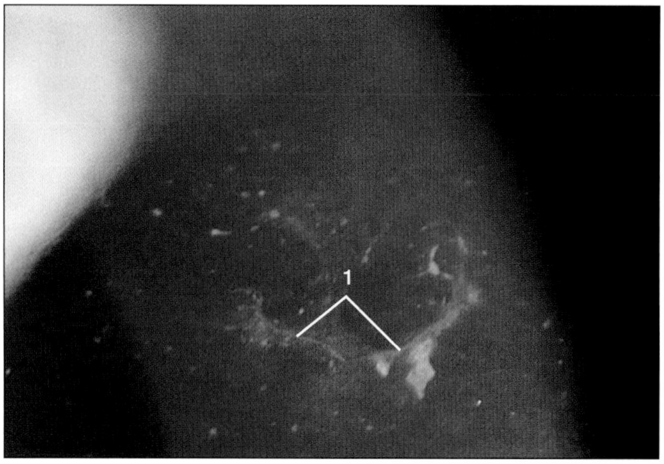

Fig. 71.14 Epithelial basement membrane dystrophy and recurrent corneal erosion in the lower third of the cornea. Fluorescein stains the lack of epithelial integrity (1), which leads to continued symptoms from recurrent corneal erosion.

dystrophy; 11 had neither trauma nor epithelial basement membrane dystrophy. Williams and Buckley[27] stated that map-dot-fingerprint dystrophy is the most common cause of recurrent erosion in general ophthalmic practice.

When the basement membrane and microcystic changes are concentrated in the visual axis, blurred vision occurs because of the minimal, but irregular, astigmatism produced by the slightly elevated corneal epithelium (Fig. 71.13). Thus, some patients may be relatively asymptomatic except for mildly blurred vision.

When examining patients who have recurrent erosions or slightly decreased vision because of irregular astigmatism, a meticulous search of the corneal epithelium may reveal either epithelial microcysts, maplike basement membrane changes, or parallel lines of aberrant basement membrane, which are the fingerprint lines. A careful examination of the uninvolved fellow eye may show similar changes in an eye that is otherwise asymptomatic. The cause of recurrent corneal erosion may be loosening of the epithelium secondary to faulty epithelial adhesion. Any signs of minute pinpoint epithelial staining or microcysts indicate that recurrent erosion may still occur (Fig. 71.14). Symptoms alone cannot distinguish the cause of a recurrent corneal erosion, whether traumatic, dystrophic, or idiopathic.

Treatment for epithelial basement membrane corneal dystrophy is directed at either alleviating blurred vision or managing recurrent corneal erosion. The treatment has been similar for recurrent corneal erosion, whether traumatic or dystrophic.[28,29] It consists of lubricating ointments at bedtime and patching as necessary. One study showed no difference between bland ointment and hypertonic saline ointment prophylactically for recurrent erosion.[26] Some physicians prefer patching, and others have used collagen shields or bandage contact lenses. The long-term use of collagen shields and bandage lenses is not indicated in this disease because there is concern about corneal infection with overnight use of soft contact lenses, and bland ointments work in the great majority of erosions.[26,27] Treatment of recalcitrant recurrent corneal erosions with topical corticosteroids and doxycycline, inhibitors of matrix metalloproteinase-9, has been effective in a small nonprospective study.[30]

With the more severe corneal erosions, whether they are based on an epithelial basement membrane dystrophy or traumatic recurrent erosion, mechanical debridement of the loosened epithelium, with or without diamond burr polishing, has been recommended.[31] This treatment can cause significant unpleasant symptoms until epithelial regrowth occurs, which can take 2–3 days. The use of nonsteroidal drops in conjunction with bandage soft lenses and antibiotics has helped.

McLean et al.[32] recommended the use of an 18-gauge needle to perform anterior stromal reinforcement or puncture for recurrent corneal erosion, but not for anterior basement membrane dystrophy without erosions. This technique, although seemingly traumatic to the cornea, works well for recalcitrant recurrent erosions. The loose epithelium should not be debrided before anterior stromal reinforcement. Rubinfeld et al.[33] suggested the use of a bent 24- or 25-gauge needle to prevent corneal perforation, and this technique worked as well as the 18-gauge needle originally used. Other forms of treatment for recurrent erosions include Nd:YAG laser micropuncture,[34] cautery to the region of erosion, and, most recently, excimer laser phototherapeutic keratectomy (PTK).[35] PTK works well because ablations are superficial, just into Bowman's layer, ensuring that all abnormal epithelial basement membrane is removed.

Considering comfort, cost, and length of time to recovery, anterior stromal reinforcement (puncture) seems to be the best way to treat recalcitrant recurrent erosions below the visual axis. It is effective in 80% of cases the first time it is done; however, re-treatment of adjacent areas where erosion may occur beyond the puncture spots is sometimes necessary. If recurrent erosion or blurred vision from map-dot-fingerprint changes are in the visual axis, excimer laser PTK has been effective.[36–38]

Epithelial debridement with diamond burr polishing works best for anterior basement membrane dystrophy in the visual axis causing either blurred vision or recurrent erosion. Several recent studies have shown that debridement of the intraepithelial pathology in map-dot-fingerprint dystrophy, whether for blurred vision and/or recurrent erosion, followed by diamond burr polishing of Bowman's membrane to remove any remaining abnormal basement membrane complexes, seems to be the best way to treat these changes from the standpoint of efficacy and economy.[39,40] Even a recent prospective randomized control trial testing diamond burr debridement versus simple debridement found the diamond burr addition a better choice.[41] In another recent publication, debridement alone was helpful, but there was no comparison with diamond burr use.[42]

Corneal Dystrophies of Bowman's Layer

In 1917, Reis[1] described a condition in a family with painful recurrent corneal erosions leading to moderate or severe reduction of vision in the first and second decades of life characterized by dominant autosomal inheritance. In 1949, Bücklers[2] described members of the same family that had been described 30 years previously. Since then, the term Reis–Bücklers' anterior membrane dystrophy has been common in the literature. Unfortunately, histopathology was not reported in these papers, and confusion has arisen because of varying descriptions of a least two disparate dystrophies involving the superficial region of the cornea. The first dystrophy was termed Reis–Bücklers' dystrophy (IC3D, RBCD, type 3 C1) and the second was referred to as honeycomb-shaped dystrophy described by Thiel and Behnke in 1967 (IC3D, TBCD, C1).[43] Generally, patients with honeycomb-shaped dystrophy are born with normal corneas. In the first and second decades of life they develop corneal opacification, severe recurrent erosion, reticular corneal scarring, and honeycomb changes in the region of Bowman's layer. All of these entities were labeled Reis–Bücklers' dystrophy, but it is now apparent that there are at least two distinctly different disorders that have a similar clinical picture and response to treatment. What was originally Reis–Bücklers' dystrophy is now considered to be a superficial variant of granular dystrophy because of 'rod-shaped bodies' seen by electron microscopy and band-shaped granular, Masson-positive, subepithelial deposits.

Recently, Küchle et al.[44] described eight eyes of six patients with honeycomb-shaped, Thiel-Behnke corneal dystrophy. They reviewed the literature and offered a classification that seems valid, based on clinical appearance and light and electron microscopy. Winkelman et al.,[45] Weidle,[46] and Wittebol-Post et al.[47] all tried to elucidate the differences between these superficial corneal dystrophies. Bron[48] also made careful note of the two different causes of this pathology but stated that, as Reis–Bücklers' dystrophy was so entrenched in the literature, this nomenclature probably could not be changed.

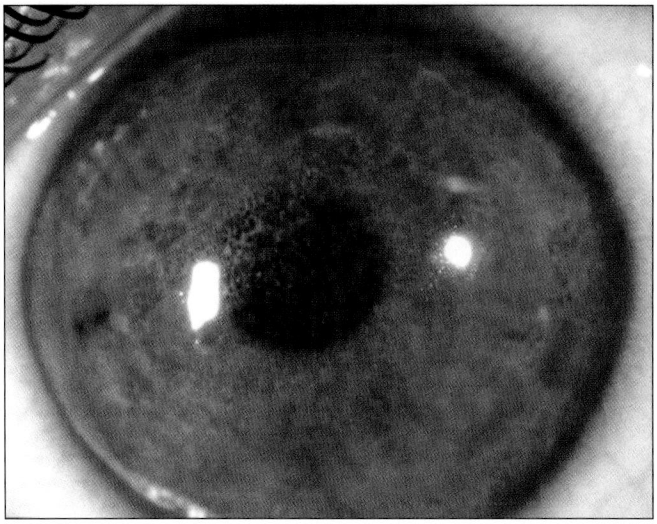

Fig. 71.15 CDB-I or 'true' Reis–Bücklers' corneal dystrophy. Rodlike granules, seen by transmission electron microscopy in the superficial stroma and in the region of Bowman's layer, indicate that this may be a superficial variant of granular dystrophy.

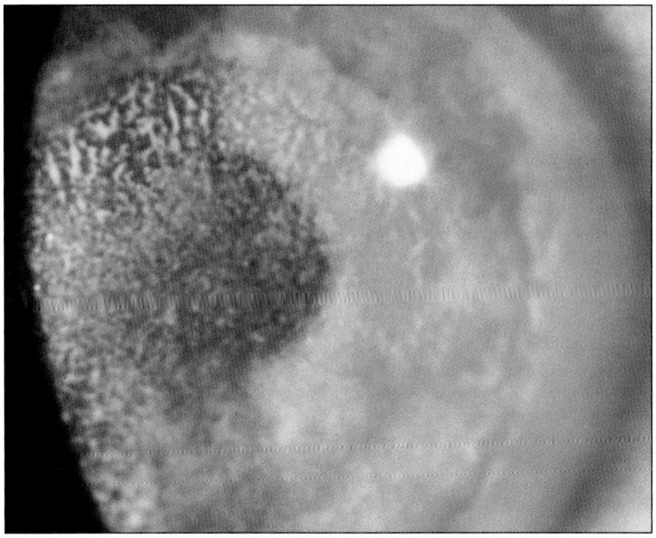

Fig. 71.16 Two years after phototherapeutic keratectomy on the patient in Figure 71.15, there is recurrence of pathology in the ablated area. This patient had improved vision compared to the pre-excimer state.

Küchle et al.[44] divided the anterior membrane dystrophies into two classifications: corneal dystrophy of Bowman's layer types I (CDB-I) and II. Type I is synonymous with Reis–Bücklers' original dystrophy and equivalent to what has been called the superficial variant of granular dystrophy. It has an autosomal dominant inheritance, recurrent corneal erosions beginning in childhood, and is marked by early and fairly marked visual loss (Figs 71.15–71.17).

Corneal dystrophy of Bowman's layer type II (CDB-II), which many people have confused with the Reis–Bücklers' dystrophy, is honeycomb-shaped and should be known as Thiel–Behnke corneal dystrophy. Similar to CDB-I, CDB-II's inheritance is dominant, with recurrent erosions starting early in childhood, but visual acuity is reduced later in life

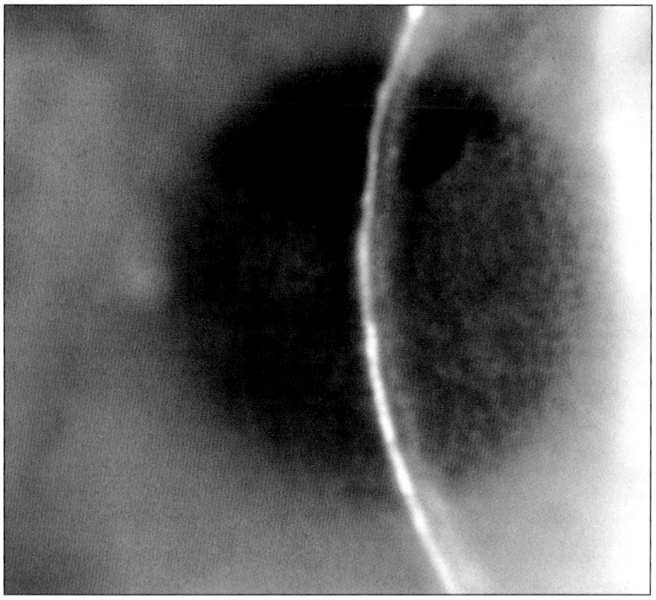

Fig. 71.17 Slit view to show the corneal irregularity in the uncle of the patient in Figure 71.15. Note the partially clear cornea but surface irregularity 1.5 years after excimer laser phototherapeutic keratectomy.

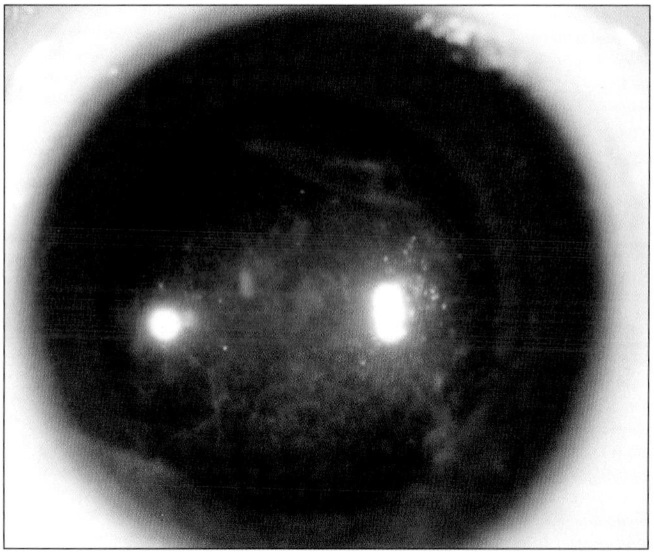

Fig. 71.18 CDB-II (Thiel–Behnke honeycomb dystrophy). Slightly irregular corneal surface with grayish opacities, which are superficial in the region of Bowman's membrane and superficial stroma. This dystrophy is characterized by curly filaments seen by transmission electron microscopy in the region of Bowman's layer.

than with CDB-I (Figs 71.18, 71.19). The clinical appearance of these dystrophies is similar, and differentiation can be made only with light and, particularly, electron microscopy. Interestingly, CDB-I stains positively with Masson's stain, whereas CDB-II is only equivocally positive to Masson's stain (honeycomb-shaped, Thiel–Behnke dystrophy).

Transmission electron microscopy differentiates these two dystrophies. The region of Bowman's membrane and basement membrane have been replaced with a fibrocellular

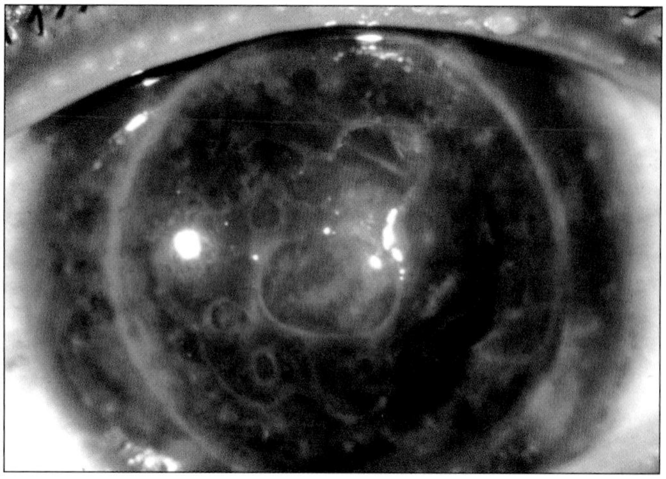

Fig. 71.19 After corneal transplantation in the father of the patient in Figure 71.13, there is recurrence of the pathology in the region of Bowman's membrane and superficial cornea. Notice the ringlike or honeycomb appearance.

scar tissue that has an undulating 'sawtooth' configuration. This configuration, however, is not specific for CDB-I or II and may be seen with both dystrophies. In CDB-I, ultrastructural deposits of rodlike bodies are present, similar to those seen in granular dystrophy (Fig. 71.20). These changes are not seen in CDB-II. Instead, 'curly' fibers appear in the region of Bowman's membrane. These fibers are arcuate or rounded and measure 9–15 mm in diameter (Fig. 71.21). They were first described by Perry et al.,[49] who incorrectly thought these changes were characteristic of Reis–Bücklers' dystrophy. In three of the eight specimens described by Küchle et al., there were variably sized empty vacuoles consistent with some type of lipid keratopathy in the deeper stroma.[44]

Treatment of these two dystrophies has varied. Early in the course of the disease, when only recurrent erosions occur, they can be managed similarly to the therapy of recurrent erosion due to epithelial basement membrane dystrophy. With significant superficial corneal scarring and opacification, superficial keratectomy with blade and peeling can be performed (Fig. 71.22). Phototherapeutic keratectomy (PTK) with the excimer laser is now the treatment of choice when vision is disturbed sufficiently or painful erosions occur, despite recurrences after PTK.[49–52] Later, with deeper scarring and opacities, lamellar and penetrating keratoplasty can be performed. Recurrence of the dystrophy in the graft is frequent (see Fig. 71.19).

Although recurrences are common, treatment can be repeated several times.[53] The addition of topical mitomycin-C with PTK has helped (see Figs 71.16, 71.17).

The literature has confused the two dystrophies in the region of Bowman's membrane, Thiel–Behnke and Reis–Bücklers' dystrophies. This confusion stems from a similar clinical course and failure to demonstrate histopathology in early papers, as well as the loss of family records from two world wars and the passage of time. Even in a recent article by Chan et al.,[53] CDB-I and CDB-II were misdiagnosed in the same family. Küchle et al.[44] corrected this error when they

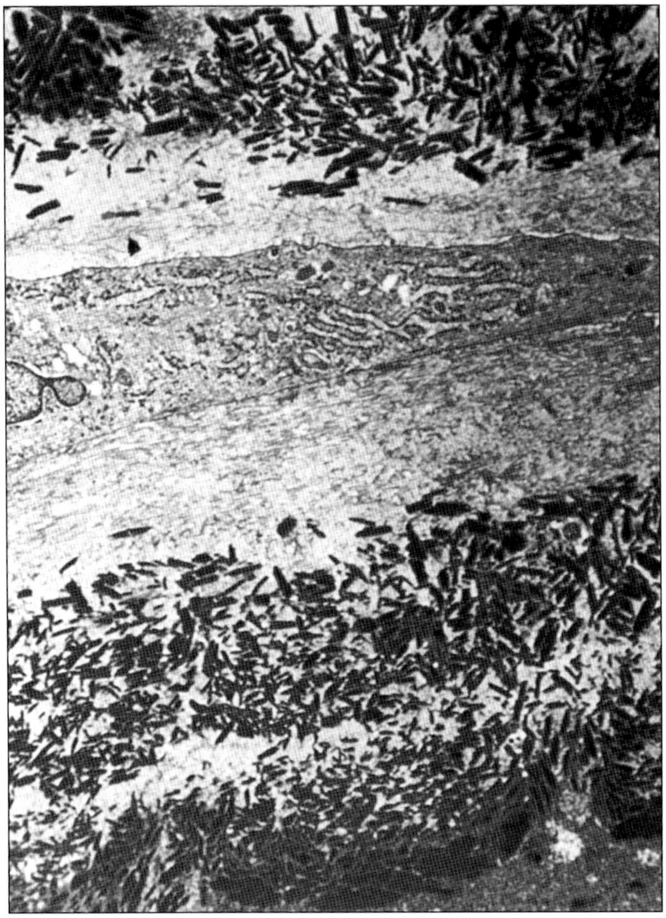

Fig. 71.20 Rodlike bodies seen by transmission electron microscopy in a patient with opacities in the region of Bowman's layer. This patient at first was thought to have Reis–Bücklers' dystrophy, but pathology indicated a superficial variant of granular dystrophy. It now appears that this was the dystrophy first described by Reis and later Bückler, and is now referred to as CDB-I or 'true' Reis–Bücklers' dystrophy, and by some still as a superficial variant of granular dystrophy. (Courtesy Merlyn Rodrigues, MD.)

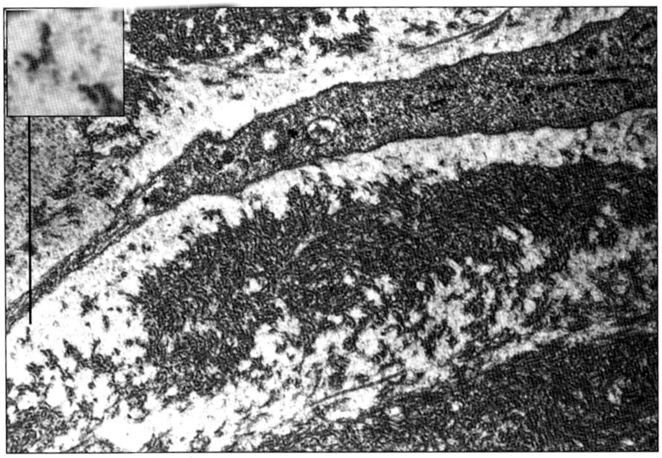

Fig. 71.21 Curly filaments seen on transmission electron microscopy in a patient with Thiel–Behnke honeycomb dystrophy. This has been confused with Reis–Bücklers' dystrophy, but transmission electron microscopy defines it probably as a separate dystrophy, CDB-II. (Courtesy Merlyn Rodrigues, MD.)

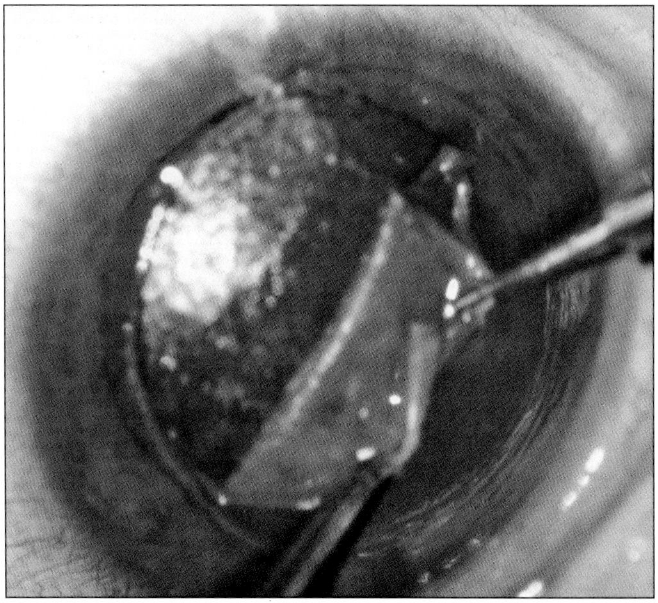

Fig. 71.22 Superficial keratectomy was once used to help restore vision in patients with CDB-I and CDB-II. Now excimer laser phototherapeutic keratectomy is the treatment of choice.

reviewed the corneal tissue specimens of two sisters and found that both had CDB-II.

The electron microscopic changes hold up for two specific entities involving the same region of the superficial cornea. Although some authors like to group these together and state that the curly fibers may be degenerative products of the rodlike granules, until further evidence is accumulated these two similar dystrophies should be reviewed as separate dystrophies. The nomenclature defining two dystrophies, CDB-I and CDB-II, involving Bowman's layer seems reasonable. Molecular genetics in the future will answer many of these questions.

References

1. Reis W. Familiare, fleckige Hornhautentartung. *Dtsch Med Wochenschr.* 1917;43:575.
2. Bücklers M. Uber eine weitere familiare Hornhautdystrophie (Reis)? *Klin Monatsbl Augenheilkd.* 1949;114:386–397.
3. Weiss JS, Møller HU, Lisch W, et al. The IC3D classification of the corneal dystrophies. *Cornea.* 2008;27(10) (Suppl 2).
4. Meesmann A, Wilke F. Klinische und anatomische untersuchungen uber eine bisher unbekannte, dominant verebte epitheldystrophie der hornhaut. *Klin Monatsbl Augenheilkd.* 1939;103:361–391.
5. Coleman CM, Hannush S, Covello SP, et al. A novel mutation in the helix termination motif of keratin K12 in a US family with Meesmann corneal dystrophy. *Am J Ophthalmol.* 1999;128(6):687–691.
6. Kuwabara T, Ciccarelli EC. Meesmann's corneal dystrophy. A pathological study. *Arch Ophthalmol.* 1964;71: 676–682.
7. Burns RP. Meesmann's corneal dystrophy. *Trans Am Ophthalmol Soc.* 1968;66:530–636.
8. Wittebol-Post D, van Bijsterveld OP, Delleman JW. Meesmann's epithelial dystrophy of the cornea. *Ophthalmologica.* 1987;194:44–49.
9. Bourne W. Soft contact lens wear decreases epithelial microcysts in Meesmann's corneal dystrophy. *Trans Am Ophthalmol Soc.* 1986;84:170–181.
10. Cremona FA, Ghosheh FR, Laibson PR, et al. Meesman corneal dystrophy associated with epithelial basement membrane and posterior polymorphous corneal dystrophies. *Cornea.* 2008;27(3):374–377.
11. Lisch W, Lisch C. Die epitheliale Hornhaut basal membrane dystrophie. *Klin Monatsbl Augenheilkd.* 1983;183:251–255.

12. Lisch WB, Buttner A, Offner F, et al. Lisch corneal dystrophy is genetically distinct from Meesman corneal dystrophy and maps to xp22.3. *Am J Ophthalmol.* 2000;130:461–468.
13. Laibson PR, Krachmer JH. Familial occurrence of dot (micro-cystic) map fingerprint dystrophy of the cornea. *Invest Ophthalmol.* 1975; 14:397–400.
14. Werblin TP, Hirst LW, Stark WJ, Maumenee IH. Prevalence of map-dot-fingerprint dystrophy of the cornea. *Br J Ophthalmol.* 1981;65:401–409.
15. Laibson PR. Microcystic corneal dystrophy. *Trans Am Ophthalmol Soc.* 1976;74:488–531.
16. Cogan DG, Donaldson DD, Kuwabara T, Marshall D. Microcystic dystrophy of the corneal epithelium. *Trans Am Ophthalmol Soc.* 1964;63:213.
17. Guerry D. Observations on Cogan's microcystic dystrophy of the corneal epithelium. *Trans Am Ophthalmol Soc.* 1965;63:320–334.
18. Vogt A. Lehrbuch und Atlas Spaltlampenmikroskopie des Lebenden Auges. *Julius Spring.* 1930;1:264–265.
19. Guerry D. Fingerprint lines in the cornea. *Am J Ophthalmol.* 1950;33:724–726.
20. DeVoe A. Certain abnormalities in Bowman's membrane with particular reference to fingerprint lines in the cornea. *Trans Am Ophthalmol Soc.* 1962;60:195–201.
21. Trobe JD, Laibson PR. Dystrophic changes in the anterior cornea. *Arch Ophthalmol.* 1972;87:378–382.
22. Bron AJ, Brown NA. Some superficial corneal disorders. *Trans Ophthalmol Soc UK.* 1971;91:13–29.
23. Rodrigues MM, Fine B, Laibson PR, Zimmerman L. Disorders of the corneal epithelium: a clinical pathological study of dot, geographic and fingerprint patterns. *Arch Ophthalmol.* 1974;92:475–482.
24. Cogan DG, Kuwabara T, Donaldson DD, Collins E. Microscopic dystrophy of the cornea. A partial explanation for its pathogenesis. *Arch Ophthalmol.* 1974;92:470–474.
25. Waring GO, Rodrigues MM, Laibson PR. Corneal dystrophies. I. Dystrophies of the epithelium, Bowman's layer, and stroma. *Surv Ophthalmol.* 1978;23:71–122.
26. Hykin PG, Foss AE, Pavesio C, Dart JKG. The natural history and management of recurrent corneal erosion: a prospective randomized trial. *Eye.* 1994;8:35–40.
27. Williams R, Buckley RJ. Pathogenesis and treatment of recurrent erosion. *Br J Ophthalmol.* 1985;69:435–437.
28. Brown J, Bron A. Recurrent erosion of the cornea. *Br J Ophthalmol.* 1976;60:84–96.
29. Laibson PR. Recurrent corneal erosions. In: Reinecke RD, ed. *Diagnosis and management, ophthalmology annual.* New York: Raven Press; 1989.
30. Dursun D, Kim MC, Solomon A, Pflugfelder SC. Treatment of recalcitrant recurrent corneal erosions with inhibitors of matrix metalloproteinase-9, doxycycline and corticosteroids. *Am J Ophthalmol.* 2001;132:8–13.
31. Wood TO, Griffith ME. Surgery for corneal epithelial basement membrane dystrophy. *Ophthalmic Surg.* 1988;19:20–24.
32. McLean EN, MacRae SM, Rich LF. Recurrent erosion: treatment by anterior stromal puncture. *Ophthalmology.* 1986;93:784–788.
33. Rubinfeld RS, Laibson PR, Cohen EJ, Arentsen JJ, Eagle RC Jr. Anterior stromal puncture for recurrent erosion: further experience and new instrumentation. *Ophthalmic Surg.* 1990;21:318–326.
34. Geggel HS. Successful treatment of recurrent corneal erosion with Nd:YAG anterior stromal puncture. *Am J Ophthalmol.* 1990;110: 404–407.
35. Stark WJ, Chamon W, Kamp MT, et al. Clinical follow-up of 193-nm ArF excimer laser photokeratectomy. *Ophthalmology.* 1992;99:805–812.
36. Rapuano CJ, Laibson PR. Lasers in corneal surgery. In: Benson WE, Coscas G, Katz LJ, eds. *Current techniques of ophthalmic laser surgery* Philadelphia: Current Medicine; 1994.
37. Orndahl MJ, Fagerholm PP. Phototherapeutic keratectomy for map-dot-fingerprint corneal dystrophy. *Cornea.* 1998;17(6):595–599.
38. Bourges JL, Dighiero P, Assaraf E, et al. Phototherapeutic keratectomy for the treatment of Cogan's microcystic dystrophy. *J Fr Ophthalmol.* 2002;25(6):594–598.
39. Sridhar MS, Rapuano CJ, Cosar CB, Cohen EJ, Laibson PR. Phototherapeutic keratectomy versus diamond burr polishing of Bowman's membrane in treatment of recurrent corneal erosions associated with anterior basement membrane dystrophy. *Ophthalmology.* 2002;109:674–679.
40. Tzelikis PF, Rapuano CJ, Hammersmith KM, Laibson PR, Cohen EJ. Diamond burr treatment of poor vision from anterior basement membrane dystrophy. *Am J Ophthalmol.* 2005;140:308–310.
41. Wong VWY, Chi Stanley CC, Lam DS. Diamond burr polishing for recurrent corneal erosions: Results from a prospective randomized controlled trial. *Cornea.* 2009;28:152–156.
42. Itty S, Hamilton SS, Baratz KH, Diehl NN, Maguire LJ. Outcomes of epithelial debridement for anterior basement membrane dystrophy. *Am J Ophthalmol.* 2007;144:217–221.
43. Thiel HJ, Behnke H. Eine bisher unbekannte, subepitheliale hereditare Hornhaut dystrophie, *Klin Monatsbl Augenheilkd.* 1967;150:862–874.
44. Küchle M, Green WR, Volcker HE, Barraquer J. Reevaluation of corneal dystrophies of Bowman's layer and the anterior stroma (Reis–Bücklers' and Thiel–Behnke types): a light and electron microscopic study of eight corneas and a review of the literature. *Cornea.* 1995;14:333–354.
45. Winkelman JE, Wittelbol-Post D, Delleman JW. Ein beitrag zur Hornhaut dystrophie Reis–Bücklers'. *Klin Monatsbl Augenheilkd.* 1986;188: 143–147.
46. Weidle EG. Differential diagnose der Hornhaut dystrophien vom Type Groenouw I, Reis–Bücklers' and Thiel–Behnke. *Fortschr Ophthalmol.* 1989;86:265–271.
47. Wittebol-Post D, van Bijsterveld OP, Delleman JW. The honeycomb type of Reis–Bücklers' dystrophy of the cornea: biometrics and an interpretation. *Ophthalmologica.* 1987;194:65–70.
48. Bron AJ. The corneal dystrophies. *Curr Opin Ophthalmol.* 1990;1: 333–346.
49. Perry HD, Fine BS, Caldwell DR. Reis–Bücklers' dystrophy. A study of eight cases. *Arch Ophthalmol.* 1979;97:664–670.
50. Orndahl M, Fagerholm P, Fitzsimmons T, Tengroth B. Treatment of corneal dystrophies with excimer laser. *Acta Ophthalmol (Copenh).* 1994;72:235–240.
51. Rapuano CJ, Laibson PR. Excimer laser phototherapeutic keratectomy. *CLAO J.* 1993;19:235–240.
52. Dinh R, Rapuano CJ, Cohen EJ, Laibson PR. Recurrence of corneal dystrophy after excimer phototherapeutic keratectomy. *Ophthalmology.* 1999;106(8):1490–1497.
53. Chan CC, Cogan DG, Bucci FS, et al. Anterior corneal dystrophy with dyscollagenosis (Reis–Bücklers' type?). *Cornea.* 1993;12:451–460.

Chapter 72

The Stromal Dystrophies

Luciene B. De Sousa, Mark J. Mannis

The clinical manifestations of the corneal dystrophies depend largely on the layer of the cornea that is affected. Accordingly, the anterior membrane dystrophies are characteristically symptomatic with recurrent corneal erosions and/or the presence of irregular corneal astigmatism resulting from abnormalities in the epithelium, the corneal basement membrane, or Bowman's layer. The posterior membrane dystrophies are characterized ultimately by the development of corneal edema from dystrophic interference with normal endothelial pump function. In general, the mechanism by which the stromal dystrophies cause dysfunction is opacification, in some degree, from the deposition of metabolically generated abnormal material. With the advances in the molecular genetics, our understanding of the role of specific genes on corneal transparency and of the pathogenesis of the disorders has advanced, leading to a new classification of the dystrophies. The International Committee for Classification of the Corneal Dystrophies (IC3D) has revised the corneal dystrophy nomenclature considering clinical findings, pathologic characteristics, and genetic patterns (Table 72.1). Mutations in seven genes of ten human chromosomes are responsible for some of the findings. This chapter describes the dystrophic disorders of the corneal stroma, its mendelian inheritance in man, and the status of our knowledge about molecular genetics of the dystrophies.

Granular Dystrophy

Using the IC3D classification, granular dystrophy is TGFBI corneal dystrophy, with three different subtypes, all of them representing *Category 1* (C1), which means a well-defined corneal dystrophy in which the gene has been mapped and identified and for which specific mutations are known.[1]

- Granular corneal dystrophy, type 1 (classic) (GCD1) C1
- Granular corneal dystrophy, type 2 (granular-lattice) (GCD2) C1
- Granular corneal dystrophy, type 3 (RBCD Reis-Bücklers) C1

Granular corneal dystrophy, type 1 (classic) (GCD1) (dystrophy Groenouw type 1)

Clinical features

First described in 1890 by Groenouw[2] and later differentiated from macular dystrophy with which it was initially linked,[3] granular dystrophy (Groenouw type I) is a bilateral corneal disorder characterized by the deposition of small, discrete, sharply demarcated, grayish-white opacities in the anterior central stroma (Fig. 72.1). The opacities of granular dystrophy may vary in shape, but are usually grouped into three basic morphologic types: drop-shaped, crumb-shaped, and ring-shaped. The overall pattern of deposition is ray- or disk-shaped.[4] Individual deposits can be round or may resemble snowflakes; they can take the form of a 'Christmas tree;' and they have often been described as resembling popcorn (Fig. 72.2). Initially, the stroma between the opacities remains clear. Vision is usually not affected in the early stages of the disease, and there is no associated discomfort. Some patients may have mild photophobia from light scattering by the corneal lesions. In a certain subset of patients, erosive episodes are more common and tend to occur among affected family members.

As the condition advances, individual lesions increase in size and number and may coalesce. They frequently extend into the deeper and more peripheral stroma. However, 2–3 mm of the peripheral cornea usually remain free of deposits. With more advanced disease, the intervening cornea develops a diffuse, ground-glass appearance. Although the lesions can involve Bowman's layer and result in superficial irregularity, recurrent erosions are unusual. Visual impairment is rare before the fifth decade and usually occurs secondary to the opacification of the intervening stroma. Corneal sensation is variably affected. Homozygotes have more severe manifestations.[1]

Atypical, more severe forms have been reported with an earlier onset around 6 years of age, with diffuse subepithelial opacification, a higher frequency of erosive episodes, and more severe eventual visual impairment. Some investigators

Table 72.1 The IC3D classification – abbreviations, MIM number, gene, and genetic locus for stromal dystrophy

	MIM abbreviation	IC3D abbreviation	MIM #	Gene	Genetic locus
Lattice – classic	CDL1	LCD1	122200	*TGFBI*	5q31
Lattice – Meretoja type	None	LCD2	105120	*GSN*	9q34
Granular CD, type 1	CGDD1	GCD1	121900	*TGFBI*	5q31
Granular CD, type 2	CDA,ACD	GCD2	607541	*TGFBI*	5q31
Macular CD	MCDC1	MCD	217800	*CHST6*	16q22
Schnyder CD	None	SCD	121800	*UBIAD1*	1p36
Congenital stromal CD	CSCD	CSCD	610048	*DCN*	12q21.33.
Fleck CD	None	FCD	121850	*PIP5K3*	2q35
Posterior amorphous CD	None	PACD	None	Unknown	Unknown
Central cloudy dystrophy of François	None	CCDF	217600	Unknown	Unknown
Pre-Descemet CD	None	PDCD	None	Unknown	Unknown

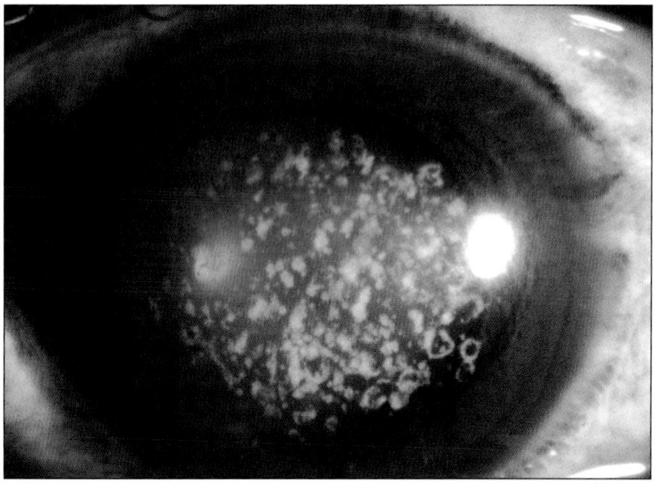

Fig. 72.1 Granular dystrophy with discrete stromal opacities with intervening clear stroma and sparing of the periphery.

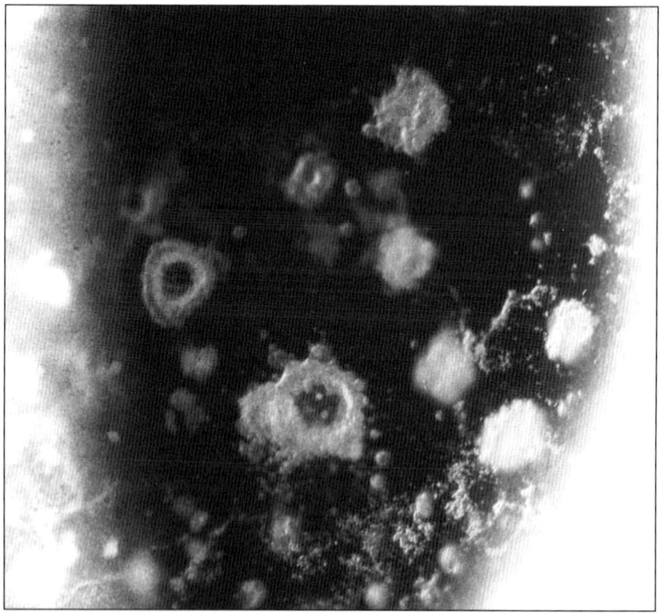

Fig. 72.2 Macrophotographic image of the opacities in granular dystrophy demonstrating the variation in the shape of the lesions and the difference in appearance with direct focal illumination versus retroillumination. With focal illumination, the lesions appear opaque, but are translucent in retroillumination. Note the annular figure.

have classified this form as a separate dystrophy: the progressive corneal dystrophy of Waardenburg and Jonkers.[5] Variants of granular dystrophy with atypical appearance[6–8] and the association of the dystrophy and lesions of the fundus, consistent with cone dystrophy,[9] have also been described.

Slit lamp examination in early stages of the disease reveals fine dots and radial lines in the superficial stroma. The dots are opaque on focal illumination and may appear translucent on retroillumination. The lesions usually occur in a random distribution and may be individual or may aggregate into different patterns (Fig. 72.3). The intervening stromal opacification that develops can best be seen as a slight haze with oblique illumination or as a discrete granularity on retroillumination. The surface may stain negatively with fluorescein over the superficial lesions, or there may be areas of rapid tear film break-up.

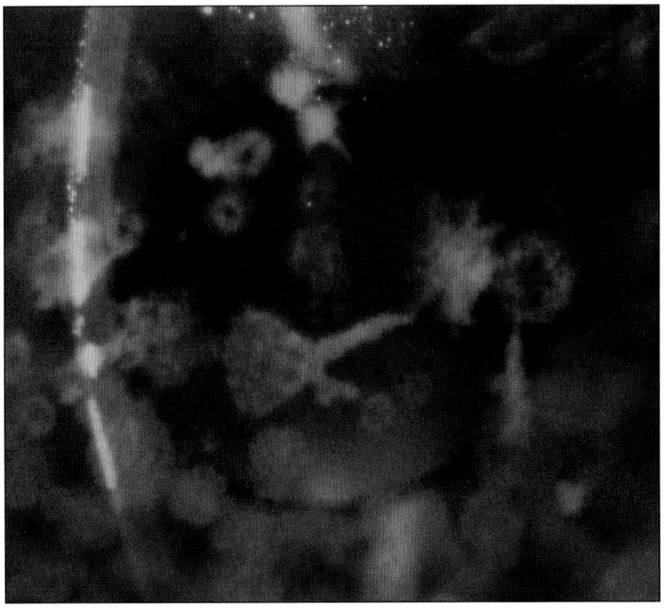

Fig. 72.3 Slit lamp photograph demonstrating the shapes of the lesions and their primarily anterior stromal location.

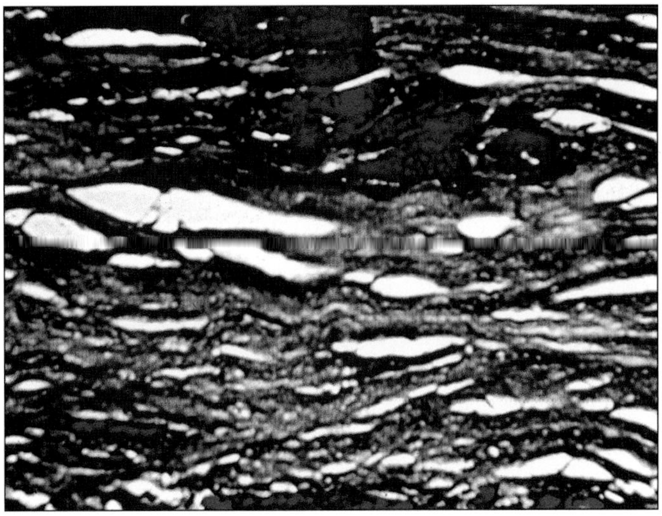

Fig. 72.4 Light microscopy of granular dystrophy stained with Masson's trichrome.

Epidemiology and heritability

Granular dystrophy is transmitted as an autosomal dominant trait and appears in the first or second decade of life; isolated cases have been reported.[5,10] It is a *TGFBI* gene-related dystrophy, with a mutation of Arg555Trp at 5q31 gene locus and it is MIM 121900 (mendelian inheritance in man number).[11,12]

Histopathology

The histopathology of granular dystrophy is characteristic. Light microscopy demonstrates eosinophilic, rod, or trapezoidal-shaped hyaline deposits in the stroma and beneath

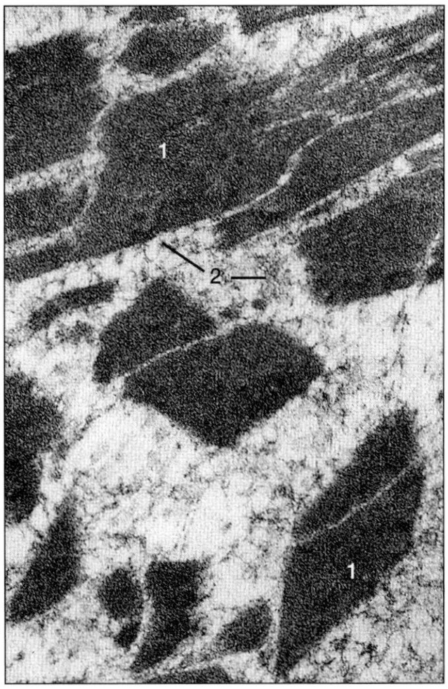

Fig. 72.5 Transmission electron micrograph of granular dystrophy demonstrating dense amorphous deposits (*1*) and microfibrillar protein (*2*).

the epithelium. These deposits stain bright red with Masson's trichrome and stain weakly with periodic acid-Schiff (PAS) (Fig. 72.4).[13] The peripheral portions of the deposits also may stain with Congo red.[14,15] Immunohistochemical stains reveal reactivity with antibodies to transforming growth factor beta (TGF-β)-induced protein (keratoepithelin).[16,17] Histochemical studies indicate that the deposits are probably noncollagenous protein containing tryptophan, tyrosine, arginine, and sulfur-containing amino acids.[14] Phospholipids also have been demonstrated in addition to microfibrillar protein.[16] Electron microscopy demonstrates rod-shaped or trapezoidal extracellular structures 100–500 μm wide, and they can display a homogeneous, filamentous, or moth-eaten pattern in their inner structure (Fig. 72.5).[15,18–21] Surrounding these lesions may be 8–10-nm tubular microfibrils that usually lack the typical orientation of amyloid, despite the Congo red staining.[16] Stromal keratocytes may be normal in appearance or may be in various stages of degeneration, with dilation of the endoplasmic reticulum and Golgi apparatus as well as vacuolation of the cytoplasm.[18]

The exact nature and source of the deposits in granular dystrophy remain unclear. It is probably the result of abnormal synthesis or handling of protein or phospholipids that are the principal components of cell membranes.[22] It is unknown whether these deposits are produced by epithelium, stromal keratocytes, or both. These characteristic rod-shaped structures have been seen within both type of cells.[21] Some suggest that because epithelial findings are prominent in recurrent granular dystrophy, the disorder has an epithelial genesis.[14,19,23–26]

The confocal microscopy shows hyper-reflective opacities.[1]

Management

Most patients with granular dystrophy do not require treatment. Recurrent epithelial erosions should be managed routinely with therapeutic contact lenses and artificial tears. If vision is markedly reduced, surgery can be considered. Surgical management varies based on the depth and extent of the stromal lesions. The traditional surgical approach has been penetrating keratoplasty, which is uncommonly performed before the fifth decade. If the opacities are extremely superficial, epithelial scraping, superficial keratectomy, or lamellar keratoplasty can be performed.[26–29] Phototherapeutic keratectomy (PTK) with the argon-fluoride excimer laser has been used to treat superficial granular dystrophy with good results.[30–32] The laser is used to ablate superficial deposits in the optical zone or to smooth irregular surfaces. This new treatment modality can be used in patients in whom the postoperative corneal thickness is predicted to be at least 250 μm based on preoperative ultrasonic pachymetry.[30,31] With deeper stromal lesions and significant visual loss, penetrating keratoplasty is the indicated procedure.

Granular dystrophy can recur in the grafts as early as 1 year after surgery, and the recurrence-free interval seems to be independent of size and type of graft performed.[26,33–37] Recurrent lesions often appear different from those seen in primary disease and clinically are seen as diffuse, subepithelial lesions coming from the periphery (Fig. 72.6). Recurrence also may appear like more typical granular lesions in the middle and posterior portions of the donor stroma.[25] The recurrence of the dystrophy first appears centrally and superficially, occasionally producing a vortex pattern suggesting epithelial involvement.[26] More superficial lesions can be removed by phototherapeutic keratectomy with restoration of good vision.[28]

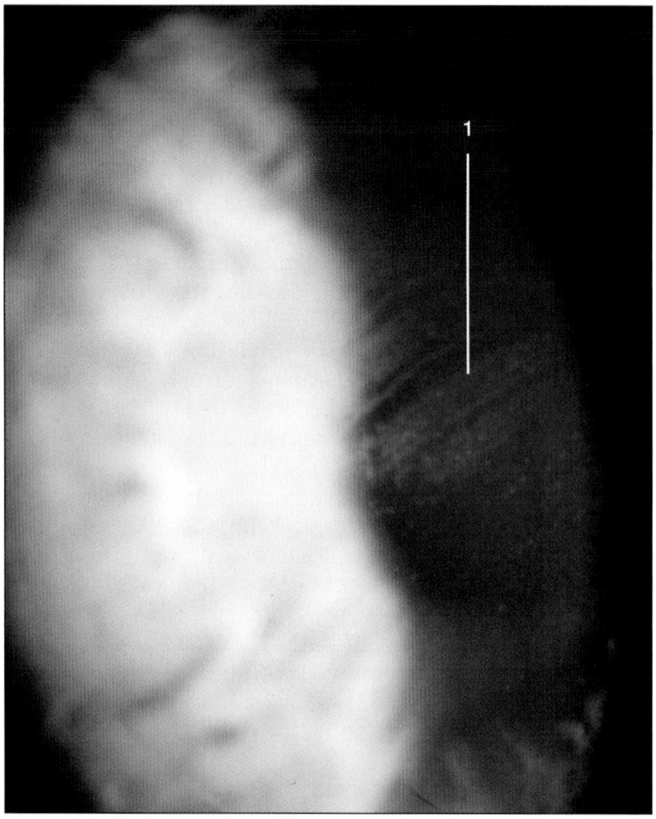

Fig. 72.6 Early recurrence of granular dystrophy in a corneal graft (*1*).

Granular corneal dystrophy, type 2 (granular-lattice) (GCD2)

(Combined granular-lattice corneal dystrophy, Avellino corneal dystrophy)

Clinical features

Avellino corneal dystrophy (Fig. 72.7) is a variant of granular dystrophy in which there are lattice deposits in addition to the characteristic granular lesions. Folberg et al.[38] reported on four patients from three families who had histologic features of both granular and lattice dystrophies. Clinically, these patients had evidence of well-circumscribed central stromal opacities similar to those seen in granular dystrophy. On histologic examination, however, they had lattice-like deposits in addition to the granular lesions.

Holland et al.[39] described the clinical manifestations and natural history of this disorder. They reported the three clinical signs that characterized Avellino corneal dystrophy: (1) anterior, stromal, discrete gray-white granular deposits; (2) mid to posterior stromal lattice lesions; and (3) anterior stromal haze. The earliest clinical evidence of this condition is discrete granular deposits. Lattice lesions develop after the granular deposits appear. No patient was seen with lattice lesions without granular opacities. The last clinical sign to emerge is stromal haze. All patients with stromal haze had both granular and lattice lesions. With increasing age, the granular lesions become larger and more prominent and often coalesce to form linear opacities, espe-

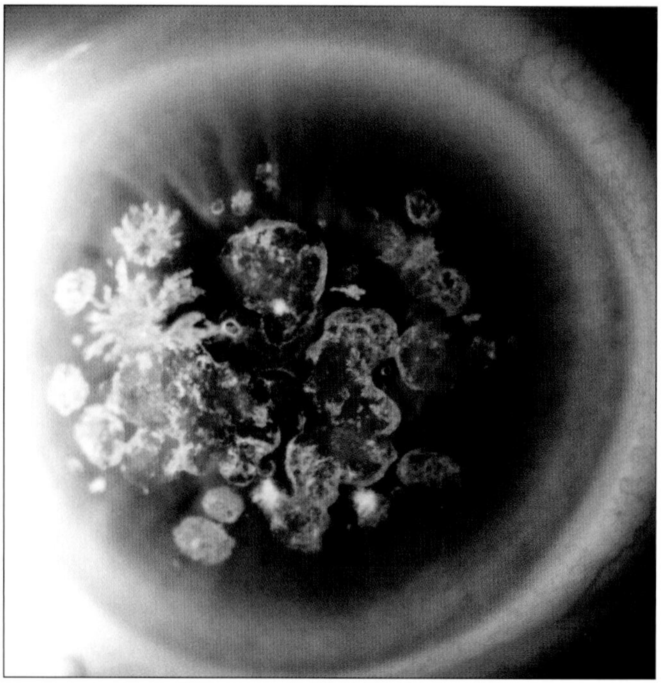

Fig. 72.7 Avellino corneal dystrophy. (Photograph courtesy Edward J. Holland, MD.)

cially in the inferior cornea. The lattice lesions also become more prominent with age. Initially, they are found in the mid and deep stroma and later involve the entire stroma. The stromal haze is seen only in patients with advanced granular and lattice opacities and becomes more prominent with age.

Patients with Avellino corneal dystrophy experience foreign body sensation, pain, and photophobia, most likely secondary to recurring erosion. More patients with Avellino corneal dystrophy appear to experience recurring erosions than patients with typical granular corneal dystrophy. Homozygous patients have earlier onset, as early as 3 years of age, and demonstrate more rapid progression.[1] Recurrent granular deposits have been noted in donor corneal tissue after penetrating keratoplasty for this condition.[39]

Epidemiology and heritability

This is an autosomal dominant dystrophy expressing the clinical and histologic features of both granular and lattice dystrophies. In a recent study, Stone et al.[40] mapped the disease-causing gene of lattice corneal dystrophy type I, granular dystrophy, and Avellino dystrophy all to chromosome 5q. It is possible that more than one gene in this interval is responsible for these diseases, but it is more likely that they are allelic. If allelic, the different phenotypes could result from different mutations in the single gene, the effect of other genes on the expression of a single mutation, or both. It is a *TGFBI* gene-related dystrophy, with genetic locus at 5q31 and MIM number 607541.[1] It is caused by an Arg124His mutation in the βig-h3.[41–43]

Histopathology

The opacities stain with either Masson trichrome or Congo red, indicating deposition of both typical GCD1 deposits and amyloid. Transmission electron microscopy shows deposits similars to GCD1 and LCD. The opacities extend from the basal epithelium to the deep stroma and the confocal microscopy can show findings as a combination of GCD1 and LCD, with reflective linear and branching deposits and breadcrumb-like round deposits in the stroma.[1]

Granular corneal dystrophy, type 3 (RBCD – Reis-Bücklers) C1

Type III ('true' Reis-Bücklers corneal, superficial granular dystrophy, corneal dystrophy of Bowman's layer type I, geographic corneal dystrophy; MIM 121900): The rod-shaped deposits accumulate mainly in Bowman's layer and beneath the corneal epithelium. Rings and disk-shaped opacities form within the superficial cornea and gradually progress, creating a central ring or geographic pattern. This variant of granular dystrophy is caused by a mutation in βig-h3 (Arg-124Leu; Arg555Gln).[43,44]

This dystrophy will be describe with the Bowmans's layer dystrophies.

Macular Dystrophy (MCD)

(Groenouw corneal dystrophy type II; Fehr spotted dystrophy)

Using the IC3D classification, macular dystrophy is a TGFBI corneal dystrophy, representing *Category 1* (C1), i.e. a well-defined corneal dystrophy in with the gene has been mapped and identified and specific mutations are known.[1]

Clinical features

Macular corneal dystrophy (Groenouw type II) is characterized by corneal opacities resulting from intracellular and extracellular deposits within the corneal stroma.[45] Of the three classic stromal dystrophies, macular dystrophy is the least common and the most severe. Patients experience progressive loss of vision as well as attacks of irritation and photophobia. Vision is usually severely affected by the time the patient reaches the twenties or thirties. There are reports of unusually severe photophobia and recurrent erosions.[46] Macular dystrophy also has been associated with cornea guttata.[47] The symmetric changes of macular dystrophy are usually first noted between 3 and 9 years of age, characterized by a diffuse, fine, superficial clouding in the central stroma. This opacification extends to the periphery and usually involves the entire thickness of the cornea by the second decade of life. Multiple, irregular, dense, gray-white nodules with indistinct borders can protrude anteriorly, resulting in irregularity of the corneal surface. In the corneal periphery, deep posterior focal plaques, grayness, and a guttate appearance of Descemet's membrane may be seen.[48] Macular dystrophy is often associated with reduced central corneal thickness.[49–51]

In the early stages of the disease, slit lamp examination demonstrates a ground-glasslike haze in the central and superficial stroma, which is best observed with oblique illumination. With progression of the dystrophy, small, multiple, gray-white, pleomorphic opacities with irregular borders are seen (Fig. 72.8). These opacities are more superficial and prominent in the central cornea and are deeper and more discrete in the periphery (Fig. 72.9). They are opaque to focal illumination and are easily visualized with indirect illumination. In later stages, the stroma is diffusely involved, Descemet's membrane takes on a gray appearance, and surface irregularity may become prominent.

In very early stages of disease, the clinical distinction between macular and granular dystrophies may be difficult. The recessive family history, decreased corneal thickness, involvement of the peripheral and deep stroma, and the early intervening stromal haze will help to identify macular dystrophy.

Epidemiology and heritability

Macular corneal dystrophy (MIM 217800) is inherited as an autosomal recessive trait. The least common of the classic stromal dystrophies, it is clinically more severe and often occurs in pedigrees with consanguinity.[52]

A gene for macular corneal dystrophy is located on chromosome 16 (16q22.1),[53] and three immunotypes of the dystrophy are recognized, based on the reactivity of the serum and corneal tissue to an antibody that recognizes sulfated keratan sulfate. Type I has no detectable antigenic keratan sulfate; type II has normal amounts of antigenic keratan sulfate; in type IA the serum lacks detectable antigenic keratan sulfate, but the keratocytes react with

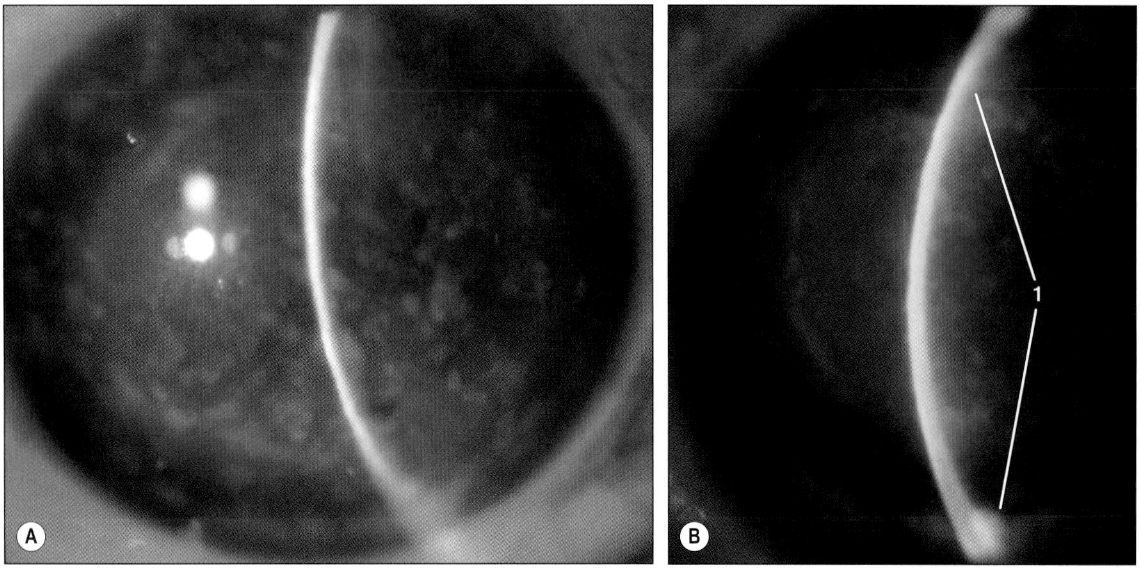

Fig. 72.8 Macular dystrophy. (**A**) Macular dystrophy with diffuse opacification of the stroma and multiple, irregular, gray-white opacities extending to the limbus. (**B**) Slit lamp photograph demonstrating deep peripheral lesions (*1*).

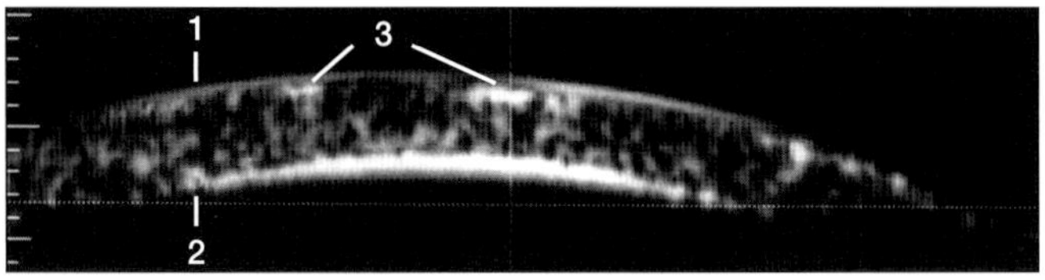

Fig. 72.9 Ultrasound biomicroscopy in macular dystrophy. Central cornea demonstrating anterior echo (*1*) epithelium and Bowman's membrane, posterior echo (*2*) Descemet's membrane and endothelium, and stroma containing highly reflective opacities (*3*) at a depth of 93 μm from the surface. (Courtesy of Norma Allemann, MD, São Paulo, Brazil.)

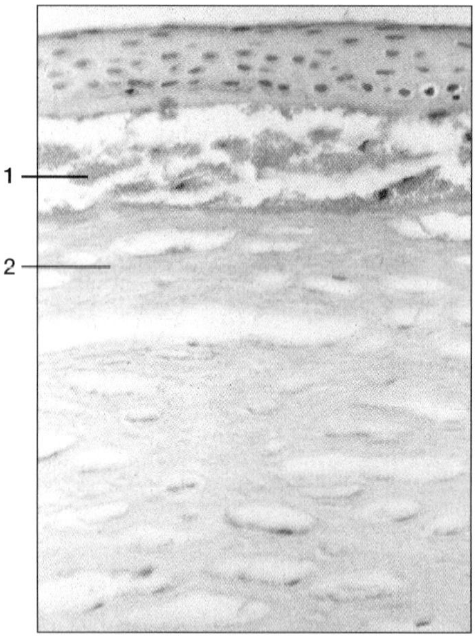

Fig. 72.10 Light microscopy of macular dystrophy stained with Alcian blue. Note both thick (*1*) and diffuse (*2*) staining for acid mucopolysaccharides (×500).

antibodies to keratan sulfate.[54,55] Recently, a mutation in a new carbohydrate sulfotransferase gene (*CHST6*) has been identified as the cause of macular dystrophy.[56,57]

Histopathology

Histologically, macular dystrophy is characterized by the accumulation of glycosaminoglycans between the stromal lamellae, underneath the epithelium, and within keratocytes and endothelial cells.[13,58–61] The glycosaminoglycans stain with Alcian blue, colloidal iron, metachromatic dyes, and PAS (Fig. 72.10). Guttae are commonly present on Descemet's membrane.[1]

Light microscopy demonstrates degeneration of the basal epithelial cells, and focal epithelial thinning is seen over the accumulated material. Bowman's membrane may be irregular, thinned, or absent in some areas. Electron microscopy shows accumulation of mucopolysaccharide within stromal keratocytes, which are distended by numerous intracytoplasmic vacuoles with pyknotic nuclei.[60–63] The stromal keratocytes are normal in number, and the more involved cells usually concentrate in the superficial or the deeper layers of the stroma. In the mid and peripheral stroma they are generally less involved.[63] The vacuoles may appear clear or may contain a granular or fibrillar material of moderate electron density as well as lamellar bodies.[62–64] The anterior banded portion of Descemet's membrane is normal, but the posterior, nonbanded portion is infiltrated by vesicular and granular material deposited by the abnormal endothelium.[58–62,64]

A possible pathologic mechanism of the dystrophy is that the keratocytes and endothelial cells synthesize abnormal fibrillogranular material consisting of glycosaminoglycan, glycoprotein, and lipid instead of mature keratan sulfate proteoglycans. The precise enzyme defect in this process has not been determined but may involve specific sulfotransferases active in sulfation of the lactosaminoglycan backbone of the chains.[65–67] Alterations in corneal stromal glycoconjugates also have been detected using biotinylated lectins showing the presence of oligosaccharides with terminal α-fucose, β-galactose, *N*-acetylglucosamine, and *N*-acetylgalactosamine residues, and oligosaccharide chains with a β-galactose-*N*-acetylgalactosamine sequence.[59,68,69] Some studies suggest that the defect in keratan sulfate synthesis in macular dystrophy is only one manifestation of a systemic disorder of keratan sulfate.[70–72] The activity of α-galactosidase, which cleaves sugar molecules from complex glycopolymers, is significantly lower in corneal tissue and keratocytes from patients with macular corneal dystrophy than in normal corneas.[73]

Macular dystrophy appears to manifest heterogeneity with at least two distinct varieties based on differences in the storage material: keratan sulfate negative (type 1) and keratan sulfate positive (type 2).[74] There are also differences in the serum keratan sulfate levels, the packing of the collagen fibrils, and the distribution of chondroitin/dermatan sulfate proteoglycans, confirming a heterogeneity within the macular dystrophies.[75]

Macular dystrophy differs from other disorders involving glycosaminoglycans such as the systemic mucopolysaccharidoses. In macular dystrophy, there appears to be a localized abnormality in the synthesis of mucopolysaccharide, whereas in the systemic disorders, there is a generalized abnormality in the breakdown of mucopolysaccharides, resulting in their accumulation and deposition in a variety of tissues.[76] In the systemic mucopolysaccharidoses, the abnormal material accumulates in lysosomal vacuoles, whereas in macular dystrophy it accumulates in endoplasmic reticulum. Clinically, in the systemic disorder, epithelial involvement is prominent, and Descemet's membrane is usually not affected. The systemic mucopolysaccharidoses are most easily differentiated from macular corneal dystrophy by associated clinical features, involvement of extracorneal tissue, and abnormalities of urinary excretion.[76] Few cases of macular dystrophy with an accompanying systemic mucopolysaccharidosis have been reported.[77]

Management

The treatment of macular dystrophy depends on the patient's symptoms. Tinted cosmetic lenses can be used to reduce photophobia. Recurrent erosions are treated with therapeutic contact lenses or lubricant drops. Phototherapeutic keratectomy has been used in early stages of the disease.[30,31,78] In selected cases, lamellar keratoplasty may be performed for restoration of vision. Most commonly, however, penetrating keratoplasty is the surgical modality of choice. Although the surgical success rate is fairly good, recurrences are seen in both lamellar and penetrating grafts.[79–81]

The clinical manifestation of recurrent disease has the same pattern as the primary disorder, usually involving the peripheral donor stroma in the superficial and deep layers. Host keratocytes invade the graft and produce abnormal glycosaminoglycan. The endothelium and Descemet's membrane are also affected,[80,81] and the size of the graft seems to be inversely related to the recurrence.[79,81]

Lattice Dystrophy

Using the IC3D classification, lattice dystrophy is a TGFBI corneal dystrophy, with two different types, both representing *Category 1* (C1), indicating a well-defined corneal dystrophy in with the gene has been mapped and identified, and specific mutations are known.[1]

- Lattice corneal dystrophy, TGFBI type (LCD): classic lattice corneal dystrophy (LCD1) C1, variants (III, IIIA, I/IIIA, and IV) are C1
- Lattice corneal dystrophy, gelsolin type (LCD2) C1

Lattice corneal dystrophy, TGFBI type (LCD): classic (LCD1) and variants

Clinical features

Lattice dystrophy is a bilateral, inherited, primary, localized corneal amyloidosis. Published descriptions of families with lattice dystrophy of the cornea reveal variation in both the corneal manifestations and the clinical course.[82] Early features of lattice dystrophy include discrete ovoid or round subepithelial opacities, anterior stromal white dots, and small refractile filamentary lines that may appear in the first decade of life (Fig. 72.11).[17,83] With time, patients also may develop a diffuse central anterior stromal haze.

With further progression, the lesions can appear as small nodules, dots, threadlike spicules, or thicker, radially oriented branching lines. The lines can extend into deep stroma and epithelium and may opacify. The stroma between the lines and dots is clear initially. With time, the opacities coalesce, and a diffuse ground glass haze may develop in the anterior and mid stroma (Fig. 72.12). The predominant anterior involvement of this dystrophy commonly leads to recurrent erosions and irregularity of the epithelial surface, with accompanying decreased visual acuity (Fig. 72.13). In extreme cases, vascularization may be present. Central corneal sensitivity also can be decreased.

At the slit lamp, the lattice lines are typically refractile with a double contour and a clear core on retroillumination. The filaments are opaque with irregular margins. They are radially oriented with dichotomous branching near their central terminations (Fig. 72.14). The lines overlap one another, creating a latticework pattern. In more advanced stages, the lattice depositions may also autofluoresce with slit lamp illumination using the cobalt-blue filter.

Clinically and histologically, there are different types of lattice dystrophy (Table 72.2). Lattice corneal dystrophy type I is characterized by branching stromal lattice figures with subepithelial opacities and anterior stromal haze.[84] Lattice dystrophy with late onset of decreasing vision, no recurrent epithelial erosions, and lattice lines much thicker than those usually observed in lattice corneal dystrophy types I and II has been described as lattice corneal dystrophy type III.[85]

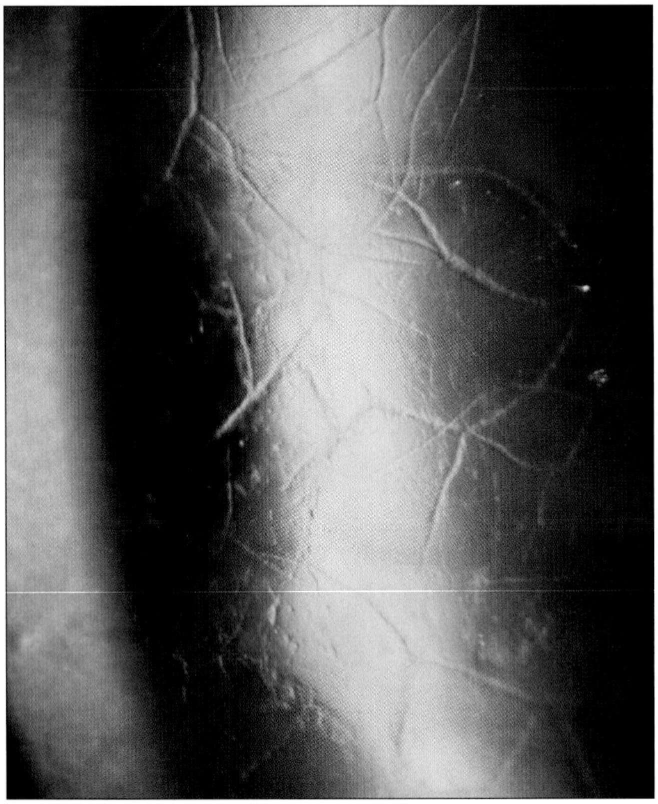

Fig. 72.11 Indirect illumination of punctiform and linear lesions seen in lattice dystrophy.

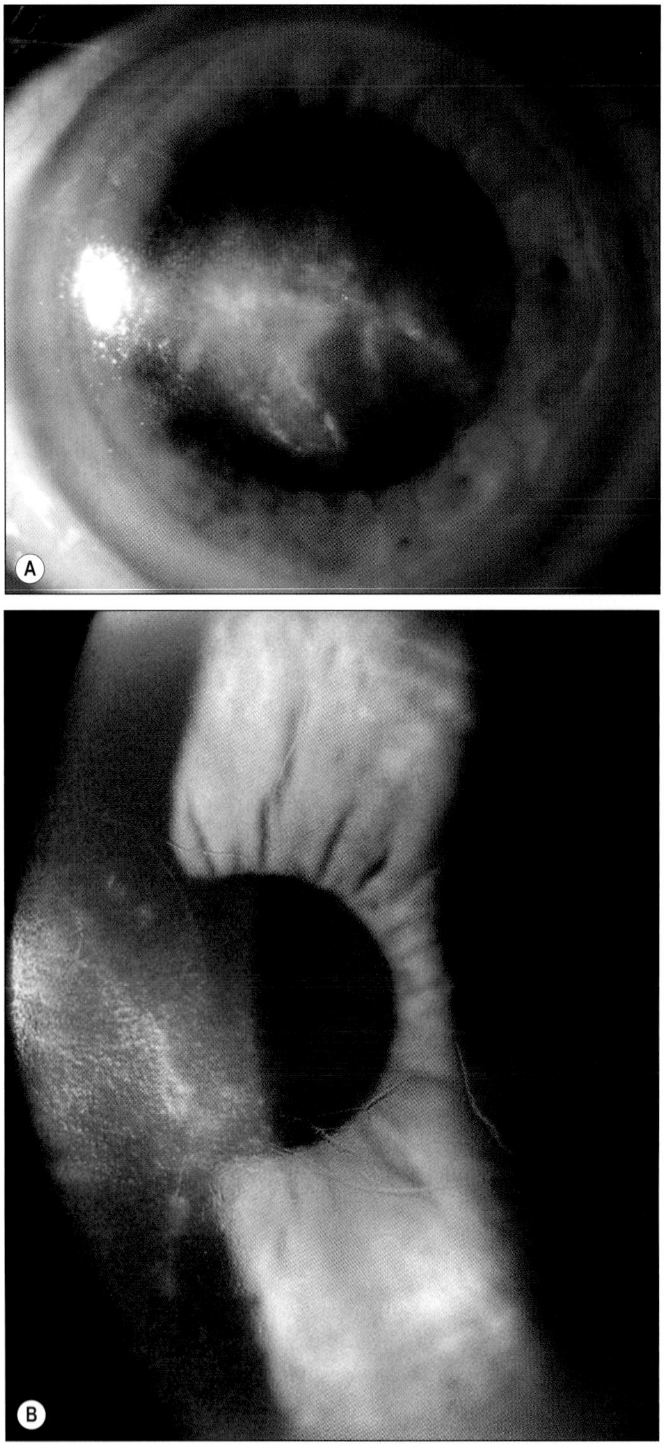

Fig. 72.12 Examples of the central corneal haze seen in diffuse (**A**) and slit (**B**) illumination that is often seen in long-standing lattice dystrophy.

Histopathology

Lattice dystrophy is a primary, localized corneal amyloidosis.[20] Possible sources of the amyloid include leakage from serum, extracellular breakdown of corneal collagen, and, most probably, localized intracellular production.[86]

Histologically, corneas with lattice dystrophy have an atrophic and disarrayed epithelium with degeneration of the basal epithelial cells, degenerative pannus, and focal disruption in the thickness or absence of Bowman's layer that is progressive with age.[13,87,88] An eosinophilic layer separating the epithelial basement membrane from Bowman's layer is present and is composed of amyloid and collagen (Fig. 72.15).[89] Irregular, eosinophilic deposits that distort the configuration of the corneal lamellae are seen in the stroma (Fig. 72.16). The central, superficial corneal stroma may have a crater-like appearance with fine, short, branching or criss-crossing lines.[90]

Because of the structure of amyloid in which the fibrils are highly aligned with a diameter of 8–10 nm (Fig. 72.17A), the histochemical staining and polarization microscopy of these deposits are characteristic.[89] The deposits stain orange-red with Congo red, and also stain with PAS, Masson's trichrome, and fluorochrome thioflavin T. When viewed with a polarizing filter, amyloid deposits demonstrate green birefringence (Fig. 72.17B). Red-green dichroism is also a characteristic feature when the tissue is examined with a green filter and a polarization filter. With crystal violet staining, metachromasia is apparent. Positive staining with antisera to human amyloid has been shown using immunofluorescence techniques.[91]

Amyloid is a noncollagenous, fibrous protein with 2–5% carbohydrate. The structure of the amyloid deposits varies in the different forms of amyloidosis, which is commonly

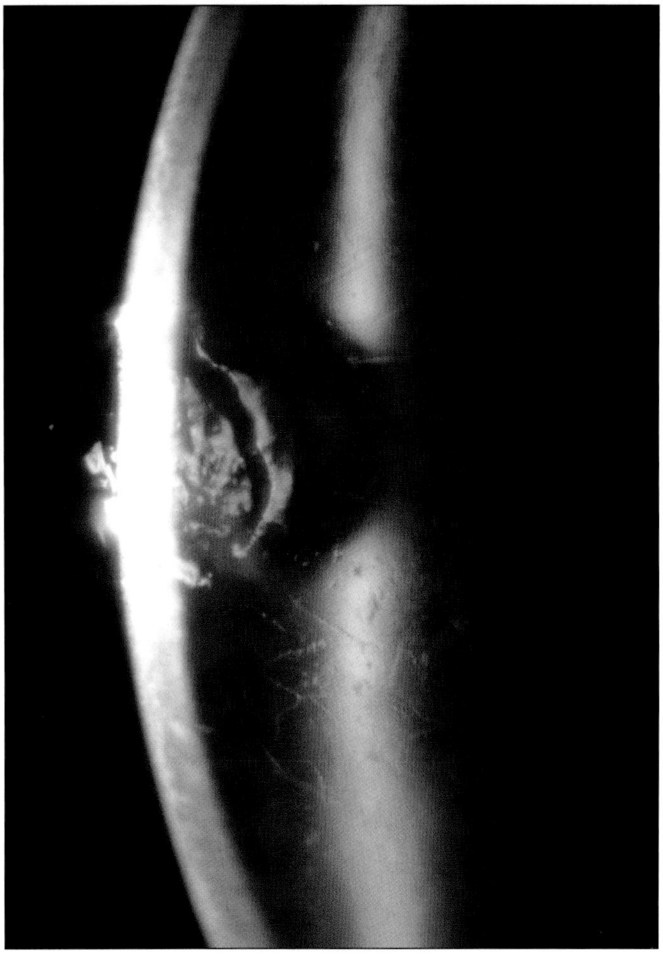

Fig. 72.13 Recurrent central corneal erosion in a patient with lattice dystrophy.

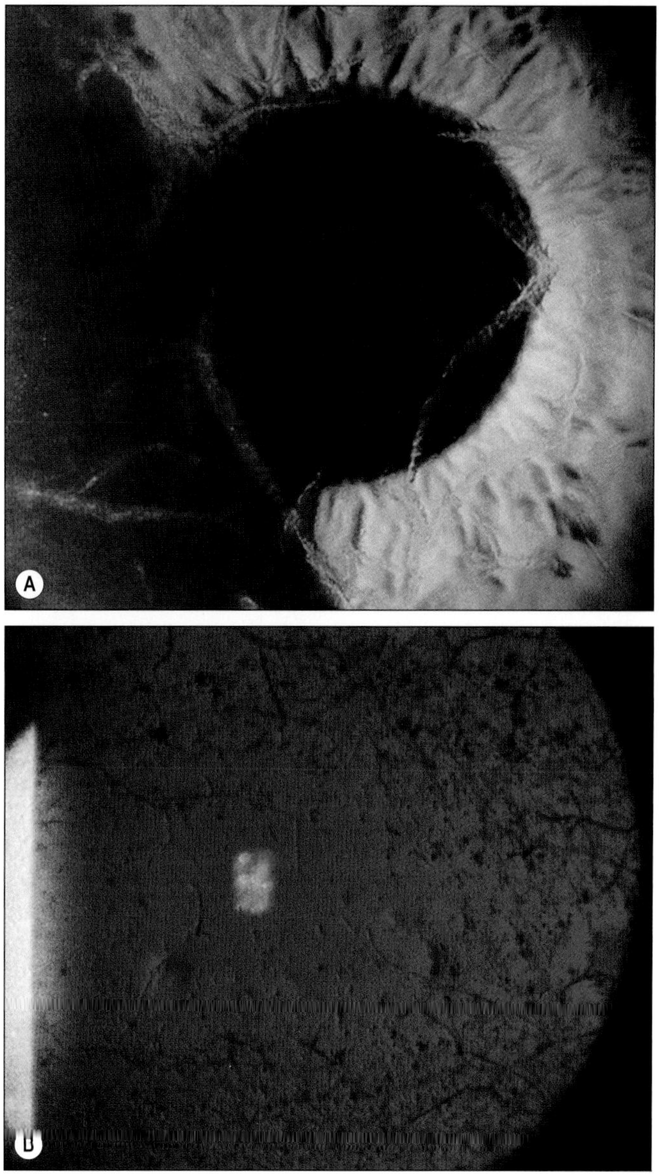

Fig. 72.14 Lattice dystrophy. (**A**) Branching, doubly relucent lines of lattice dystrophy in the central cornea. (**B**) Diffusely involved cornea with lattice dystrophy seen in red-reflex illumination.

Table 72.2 Comparison of different types of lattice corneal dystrophy

Characteristic	Type I	Type II (Meretoja)
Inheritance	Autosomal dominant	Autosomal dominant
Onset	<10 years	20–35 years
Visual acuity	Poor after age 40	Good until age 65
Erosions	Frequent	Infrequent
Cornea	Numerous, delicate lines; many amorphous deposits; few amorphous deposits; periphery clear	Few thick lines; extend to periphery; few amorphous deposits
Systemic involvement	None	Amyloidosis involving skin, arteries, and other organs
Face	Normal	Facial paresis and blepharochalasis after age 40

classified into systemic and localized forms and further subdivided into primary and secondary forms. In the primary systemic form of amyloidosis, the amyloid contains fragments of immunoglobulin light chains. In secondary systemic amyloidosis, the major component of amyloid deposits is a nonimmunoglobulin protein (protein AA) that appears to be a degradation product of a serum acute-phase reactant (serum AA).[92] In both primary and secondary amyloid, deposits are associated with a protein (protein AP), which is present in normal serum. In lattice dystrophy, only protein AP is present.[93–95] Electron microscopy shows elastotic degeneration (elastin) within the amyloid deposits that stains positive with Verhoeff-van Gieson and Movat pentachrome stains and shows autofluorescence.[87,91,96,97]

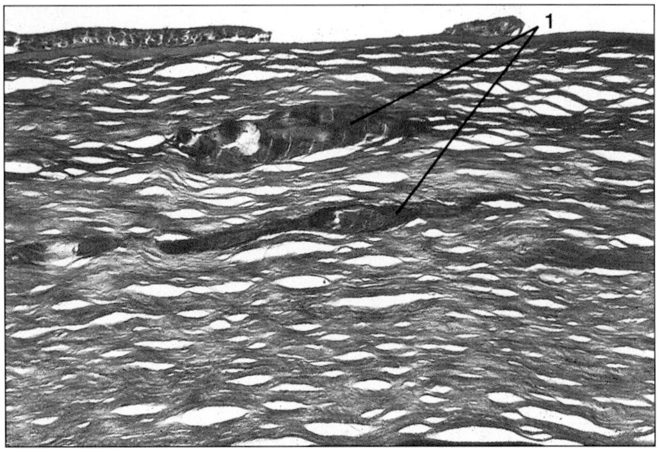

Fig. 72.15 Light microscopy of lattice dystrophy with PAS stain (×80) demonstrating fusiform deposits (*1*) in the anterior stroma and subepithelium.

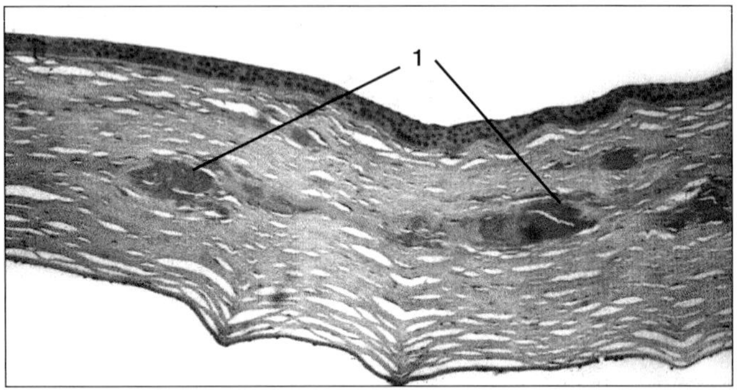

Fig. 72.16 Fusiform lesions (*1*) of the anterior stroma stained with Congo red (×125).

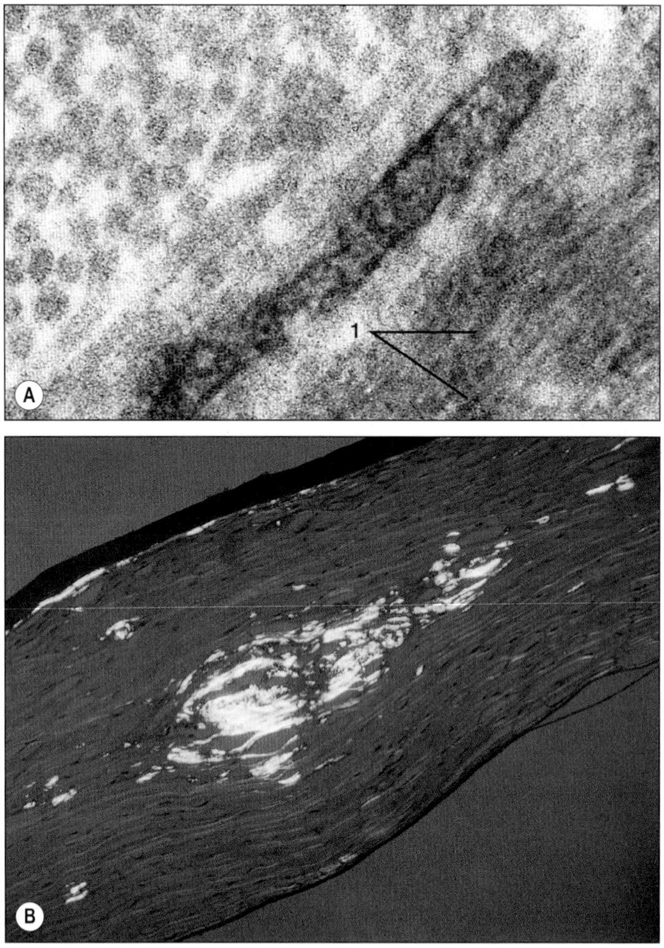

Fig. 72.17 Lattice dystrophy. (**A**) Transmission electron micrograph of lattice dystrophy demonstrating amyloid filaments (*1*) (10-nm diameter). (**B**) Characteristic birefringence seen with polarized light in amyloid deposits.

Abnormal glycoconjugates are also present in corneas with lattice dystrophy.[68,98]

Ultrastructural examination in lattice corneal dystrophy type 1 shows extracellular masses of fine, electron-dense fibrils with a diameter of 80–100 Å.[62,99] Keratocytes in the involved areas are decreased in number and may show cytoplasmic vacuolation and degeneration, whereas others appear metabolically active.[100–102] Descemet's membrane and endothelium are usually normal.[89,101]

In type III lattice dystrophy, numerous amyloid deposits are scattered throughout the corneal stroma. These deposits are predominantly located midway between the epithelium and the endothelium. Bowman's membrane usually has only one or two small disruptions and beneath the membrane, in the superficial stroma, a discontinuous band of amyloid (15–25 μm wide) can be seen.[85,103] Descemet's membrane and the endothelium are normal. The deposits stain positively with Congo red, and immunohistochemical studies indicate that only some deposits react weakly with antibodies to amyloid protein AA, positively with antibodies to protein AP, and negatively with antibodies to kappa and lambda immunoglobulin light chains.[103]

Amyloid deposits in the cornea also may occur in association with local ocular disease and trauma,[104] gelatinous droplike dystrophy,[105,106] and polymorphic amyloid degeneration.[107]

The confocal microscopy shows linear and branching structures in the stroma, with poorly demarcated margins and changing reflectivity.[1]

Epidemiology and heritability

Lattice dystrophy (Biber-Haab-Dimmer dystrophy) was first described by Biber,[108] Haab,[109] and Dimmer[110] in the 1890s. Mutations in the βig-h3 gene cause amyloid deposition in different patterns. Opaque areas with different shapes from the filamentous opacities may appear within the corneal stroma of both eyes in conditions in which amyloid has not been detected in other tissues. Lattice corneal dystrophy type I (MIM 122200) has an autosomal dominant mode of inheritance, and the disease results from mutations at 5q31 gene locus (Arg124Cys; Ala546Asp; Pro551Gln and Leu518Pro).[43,44,111,112] Lattice corneal dystrophy type III is an autosomal recessive disorder, associated with thick, midstromal, lattice-like lines that extend from limbus to limbus,[113,114] and the condition presents between the ages of 60 and 80 years. Recurrent erosions are infrequent. The gene has not yet been mapped. Lattice corneal dystrophy type IIIA has an autosomal dominant pattern, and the clinical findings are due to a mutation at 5q31(Pro501Thr; Ala622His; His-626Ala).[112,115,116] The lattice corneal dystrophy type IV is associated with a Leu527Arg mutation in the βig-h3 and is a dominant form of late-onset, deep lattice dystrophy.[117]

Lattice dystrophy is inherited as an autosomal dominant trait and varies in both penetrance and expression; some members of the same family may show only dystrophic recurrent erosions with little or no clinically visible opacification. Cases of unilateral lattice dystrophy, generally asymptomatic, with a firm clinical diagnosis, have been reported in the same family.[118–121]

Interestingly, an association between lattice dystrophy and keratoconus has been described.[122,123] An atypical corneal dystrophy with stromal amyloid deposits, with an autosomal dominant pattern resembling Reis-Bücklers dystrophy, also has been documented.[96] There is an association between patients wearing hydroxyethyl methacrylate (HEMA) contact lenses and an asymptomatic lattice-like corneal pattern, normal visual acuity, and normal or slightly reduced corneal sensitivity.[124] Finally, lattice dystrophy must be distinguished from polymorphic amyloid degeneration (PAD). In PAD, polymorphic punctate and filamentous opacities appear in the deep stroma of the axial cornea in patients in the fourth decade of life or older. The intervening stroma is normal.[107] There is no pattern of heritability in these patients, and they have no visual dysfunction.

Management

Treatment of lattice dystrophy depends on the patient's symptoms. Recurrent erosions are treated in a routine fashion: patching, hypertonic agents, artificial tears, or a therapeutic contact lens. Excimer laser phototherapeutic keratectomy has been described as an optional treatment for recurrent erosions and superficial opacities. Selection of patients should follow the same guidelines as described for those with granular dystrophy.[30,31]

If visual acuity is impaired, lamellar or penetrating keratoplasty can be performed.[125,126] Penetrating keratoplasty has a high rate of success in these patients. However, lattice dystrophy recurs more frequently than does granular or macular dystrophy, and the recurrence can appear in the graft in as few as 3 years after keratoplasty.[31,127,128] Recurrence of lattice lines, however, is unusual.[125,126] More commonly, diffuse, dotlike, or filamentous subepithelial opacities, elevated subepithelial opacities, or diffuse anterior stromal haze are seen (Fig. 72.18).[92,125,126] Table 72.3 summarizes the characteristics of the three major stromal dystrophies.

Lattice corneal dystrophy, gelsolin type (LCD2)

(Familial amyloidosis, Finnish (FAF); Meretoja's syndrome, amyloidosis V, familial amyloidotic polyneuropathy IV (FAP-IV))

Clinical features

Lattice-like dystrophy or lattice dystrophy type II (Meretoja's syndrome or familial amyloid polyneuropathy type IV) is a systemic amyloidosis associated with corneal dystrophic changes.[129] Clinical corneal changes are later in onset, recurrent erosions are unusual, and the visual outcome is more favorable than in type I. Systemic manifestations, including cranial and peripheral neuropathies such as facial paresis, bulbar palsy, and dermatologic involvement with laxity of the facial skin, appear with age. Peripheral polyneuropathy affecting mainly senses of vibration and touch, carpal tunnel syndrome, autonomic disturbance as orthostatic hypotension, cardiac conduction abnormalities, and dysfunction of perspiration also can be seen. Glaucoma and pseudoexfoliation with or without glaucoma are common.[130] In lattice dystrophy type II, lattice lines are fewer and more radially oriented and involve

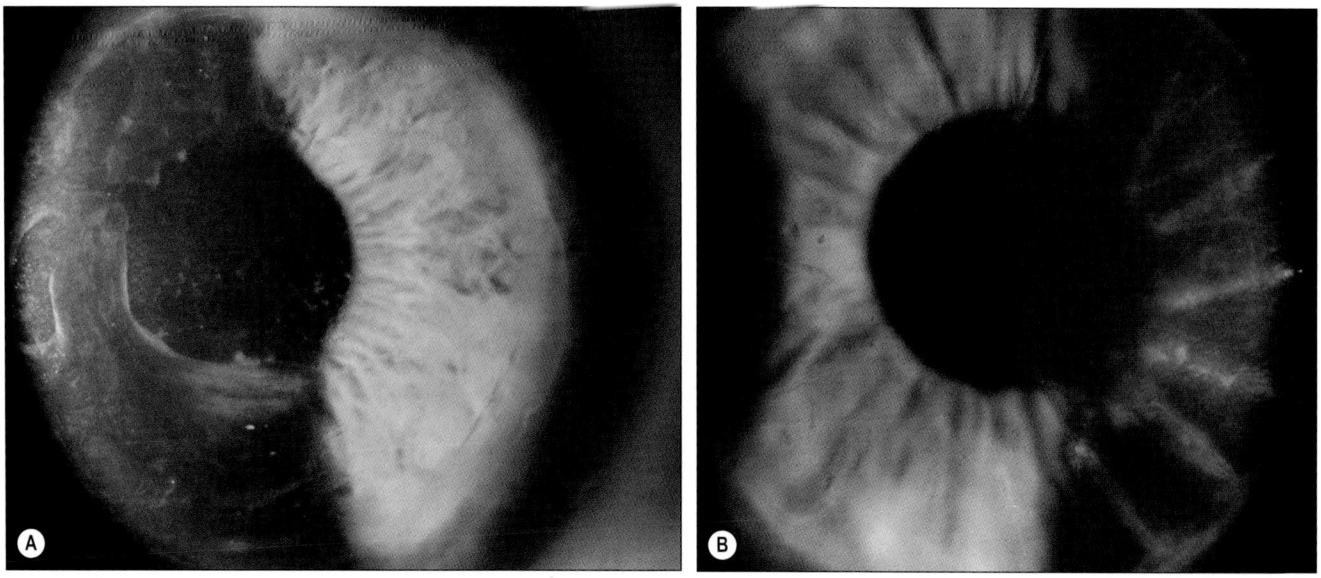

Fig. 72.18 Lattice dystrophy. (**A**) Recurrent lattice in a corneal graft. (**B**) Recurrent lattice seen along suture tracks in a corneal graft.

Table 72.3 Characteristics of the three major stromal dystrophies

Feature	Granular dystrophy	Macular dystrophy	Lattice dystrophy
Age of onset Deposits Symptoms	 1st decade 3rd decade or asymptomatic	 1st decade 1st decade	 1st decade 2nd decade
Heredity	Autosomal dominant	Autosomal recessive	Autosomal dominant
Reduced vision	By 4th or 5th decade	1st or 2nd decade	By 2nd or 3rd decade
Erosions	Uncommon	Common	Frequent
Opacities	Discrete, sharp borders Intervening stroma clear early but becomes hazy Subepithelial spots Not to limbus	Indistinct margins Hazy intervening stroma Extends to limbus Endothelium affected Central lesions more anterior, peripheral lesions more posterior	Early Refractile tiny lines and dots Diffuse central haze Limbal zone clear except in extreme cases
Corneal thickness	Normal	Thinned	Normal
Histochemical stains	Masson's trichrome Luxol fast blue Antibodies to microfibrillar protein Thioflavine-T (fluorescence)	PAS Colloidal iron Alcian blue Metachromatic dyes	PAS Congo red Crystal violet (metachromasia)
Material accumulated	Hyaline	Glycosaminoglycans	Amyloid
Distinguishing clinical characteristics	Clear limbal zone	Opacities reach limbus Cornea thinned unless decompensated	Lattice lines

primarily the peripheral cornea, with relative central sparing. The amorphous dots are fewer and more confined in distribution.

In lattice dystrophy type II (Meretoja's syndrome or familial amyloid polyneuropathy type IV), histopathology demonstrates mutated gelsolin deposited in arteries, skin, peripheral nerves, sclera, and other tissues.[131] A regular amyloid layer lies beneath a normal-appearing Bowman's membrane, in contrast to type I in which Bowman's membrane is disrupted.[92]

It is important to stress that is not a true corneal dystrophy but it is listed to avoid uncorrected diagnosis with true lattice dystrophy.

Epidemiology and heritability

This variety of lattice dystrophy is caused by mutations in the gelsolin gene (*GSN*) on the long arm of chromosome 9 (9q34).[132–135] It is MIM 105120, and the mutation involves a G to A substitution at nucleotide 654, resulting in a Asn-187 variant of gelsolin[133–135] or a G to T transversion in position 654 at codon 187, resulting the substitution of tyrosine for aspartic acid.[54,132]

Schnyder's Crystalline Dystrophy (SCD)

In the IC3D classification, Schnyder's dystrophy represents a *Category 1* (C1) dystrophy: that is, a well-defined corneal dystrophy in which the gene has been mapped and identified and for which specific mutations have been identified. It is also commonly referred to as Schnyder crystalline corneal dystrophy (SCCD), Schnyder crystalline dystrophy sine crystals, hereditary crystalline stromal dystrophy of Schnyder, crystalline stromal dystrophy, central stromal crystalline corneal dystrophy, and corneal crystallline dystrophy of Schnyder.

Clinical features

This rare stromal dystrophy was first described in three generations of a single family by Van Went and Wibaut,[136] and the characteristics were further clarified by Schnyder.[137,138] Schnyder's crystalline dystrophy has previously been reported to be nonprogressive after childhood, but recent reports have documented significant progression.[139] No regression of lesions has been reported.[140] A variety of symmetric, bilateral corneal lesions are seen in this dystrophy. Bilateral gray, disclike opacities are seen, primarily in the anterior stroma. These opacities are often central and also may include fine polychromatic cholesterol crystals in the anterior stroma, which are more prominent in the earlier phases of the disease. These crystals may be deposited in a geographic, annular, or disciform pattern and may extend to the deeper stromal layers (Fig. 72.19A).[141] The intervening stroma is usually clear but sometimes demonstrates diffuse, small punctate opacities.[142,143] Arcus lipoides or senilis is

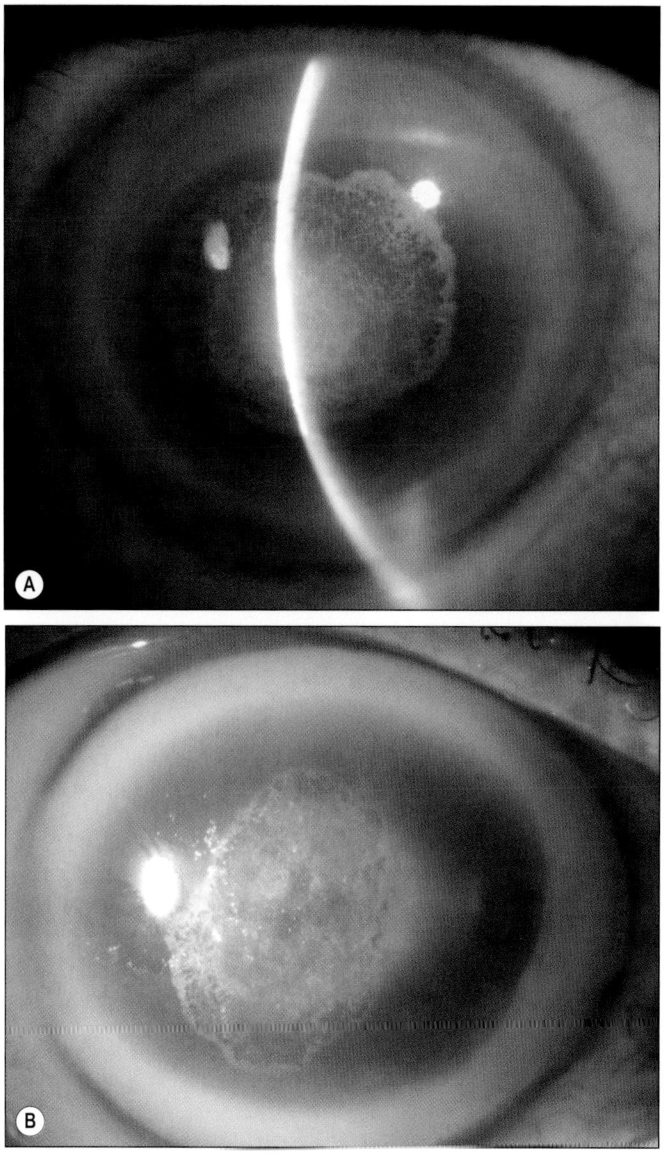

Fig. 72.19 Schnyder's crystalline dystrophy. (**A**) Anterior disciform lipid deposition in Schnyder's central crystalline dystrophy. (**B**) Central crystalline deposit associated with characteristic dense arcus. The visual acuity in this eye was 20/70.

often a prominent finding in the peripheral cornea in patients over the age of 23 with this dystrophy (Fig. 72.19B). The differential diagnosis of corneal stromal crystals includes Bietti's peripheral crystalline dystrophy, cystinosis, and dysproteinemias such as multiple myeloma, Waldenstrom's macroglobulinemia, Hodgkin's disease, benign monoclonal gammopathy, and cryoglobulinemia. A detailed clinical history will readily distinguish these entities. Bietti's dystrophy is the most similar histopathologically, with deposits of cholesterol and complex lipids in corneal and conjunctival fibroblasts and circulating lymphocytes in association with retinal degeneration.

A diffuse, progressive stromal haze also can be seen in Schnyder's dystrophy, which may affect all levels of the stroma. Some studies have reported this haze in nearly all patients older than 40.[144] Corneal sensation may decrease progressively over the lesions. The epithelium, endothelium, and Descemet's membrane remain largely uninvolved, and patients rarely demonstrate epithelial erosions.

The clinical variations of the corneal opacities have been divided into five types, any of which may be present in the same family:[145] (1) a central discoid lesion without crystals; (2) a crystalline discoid central lesion with a garland-like margin; (3) a crystalline discoid central lesion with a poorly defined edge; (4) a crystalline annular opacity with a clear center; and (5) an annular opacity with crystal collections and a clear center.

Epidemiology and heritability

This rare autosomal dominant condition is strongly associated with hypercholesterolemia with or without hypertriglyceridemia and less commonly with genu valgum, which may be inherited as a separate trait.[145] There is no direct association with primary hyperlipidemias, and the serum lipid levels do not correlate with the density of the corneal opacities.[140] It likely represents a localized defect in cholesterol metabolism, which may be exacerbated by systemic hyperlipidemia. Burns et al.[146] investigated this theory using intravenous labeled cholesterol, which was concentrated in the corneas of patients with Schnyder's dystrophy before keratoplasty. This finding suggested either active deposition of cholesterol or decreased serum cholesterol turnover rates. Fewer than 100 cases have been reported in the literature, but a large cohort of patients was identified in central Massachusetts.[8] Many of these patients have ancestors from Scandinavian countries such as Sweden and Finland. Animal models have been reported with similar corneal lesions in mice fed high-cholesterol diets[147] and spontaneously in Siberian husky dogs.[20]

Schnyder's crystalline dystrophy, MIM 121800, is an autosomal dominant diseases, related with gene *UbiA* prenyltransferase domain containing 1_UBIAD1, at the genetic locus 1p36.[54,148,149]

Histopathology

Lipid, neutral globular fat and cholesterol deposition have been identified at all levels of the corneal stroma.[150–153] Free fatty acid and triglyceride stains are often negative.[154] Cholesterol has been identified as birefringent crystals, noncrystalline cholesterol, and cholesterol esters.[141,154–157] Consequently, to process the specimen special lipid stains such as oil red O or Sudan black are necessary. Epithelial changes include increased glycogen stores, with subepithelial glycogen deposits and focal or complete destruction of Bowman's layer (Fig. 72.20).[155,157] The overlying epithelial basement membrane also may be missing on pathologic examination. The stroma demonstrates focal round empty spaces, which are likely to be the site of neutral fat deposits that have dissolved because of tissue processing. These deposits likely correlate with the punctate dots seen on slit lamp examination. Fibrillar or granular electron-dense material can be seen in patches near these spaces and may correspond to the stromal haze noted on clinical examination.[143] Macrophages, which have ingested lipid, have been found

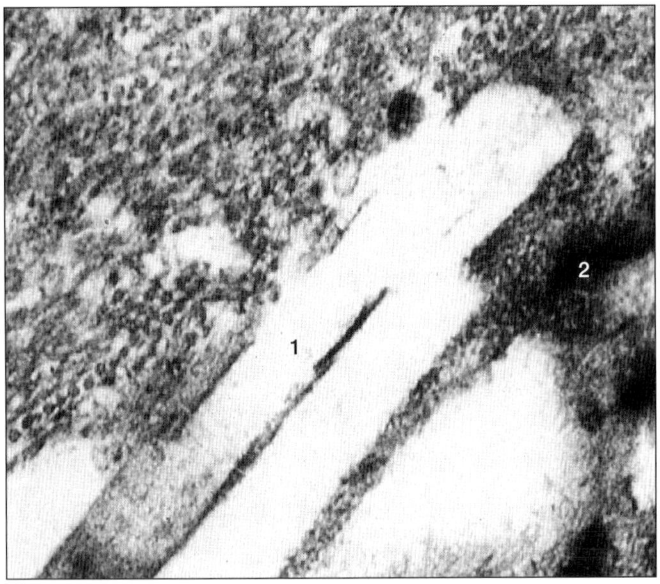

Fig. 72.20 Electron microscopy of central crystalline dystrophy. Note the crystals (*1*) and the fibrogranular deposits surrounding them (*2*).

in the stroma and uncommonly in the basal epithelium.[158] Rarely, focal degeneration of the endothelial cell layer has been noted with discontinuities.[151]

Management

Identification of cholesterol crystals and differentiation from other conditions can be facilitated by the use of specular microscopy.[159] Investigation of systemic hyperlipidemia should include a fasting blood level of cholesterol and triglyceride and a lipoprotein electrophoresis.

Few patients in the early phases of the disease have visual impairment significant enough to warrant a penetrating keratoplasty. Both visual acuity and corneal sensation, however, may deteriorate as the disease progresses, necessitating surgical intervention. Recurrence of cholesterol crystals may occur in both lamellar or penetrating grafts.[140,145,155]

Fleck Corneal Dystrophy (FCD)

Using the IC3D classifications, fleck corneal dystrophy represents a *Category 1* (C1) dystrophy: that is, a well-defined corneal dystrophy in which the gene has been mapped and identified and specific mutations are known.[1]

Clinical features

This usually bilateral but often asymmetric condition also has been called speckled or mouchetée dystrophy and was originally described by Francois and Neetans.[160] Visual acuity is often unaffected because of the small stromal opacities and lack of involvement of the epithelial surface, which remains optically smooth. Occasionally, patients complain of photophobia, but most have no symptoms. No epithelial erosions are found. Flat, gray-white, discrete

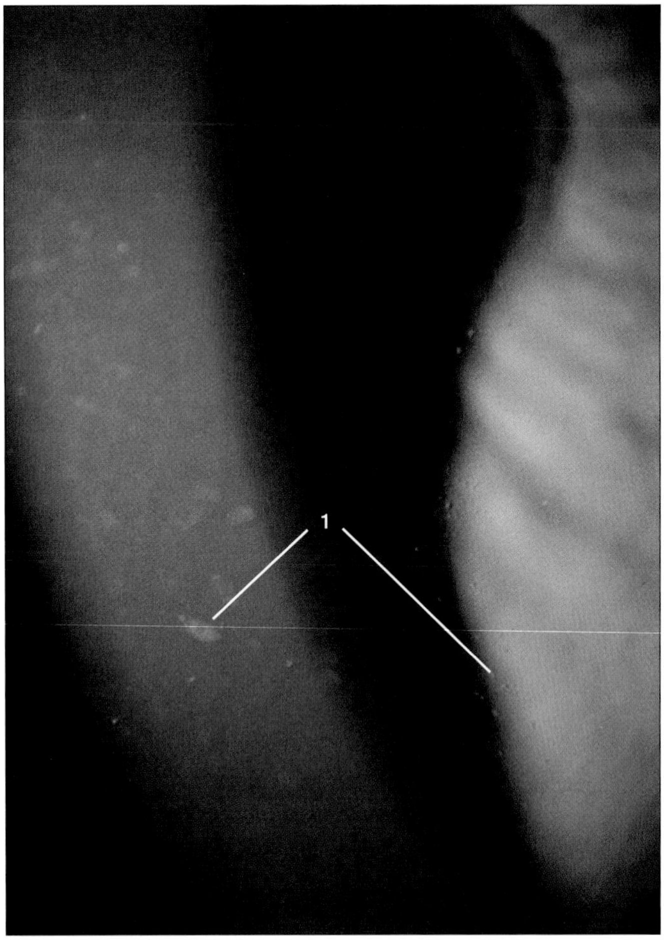

Fig. 72.21 Fleck dystrophy demonstrating multiple small grayish pleomorphic deposits (*1*) at all stromal layers with clear intervening stroma. The lesions are present from limbus to limbus.

flecks are seen throughout the stroma and are present from limbus to limbus, sparing Bowman's layer (Fig. 72.21).[161] The flecks may surround the clear central cornea in a ring and may have comma, oval, circular, or stellate shapes. Some opacities may have a ring shape with clear centers.[162] The flecks have a fine granular texture with discrete or scalloped borders.[20] On retroillumination, they may appear refractile. There is little progression, and the condition is often only discovered on careful biomicroscopic examination. Punctate cortical lens opacities also may be present.[163] Corneal sensation may be reduced.[164] This dystrophy has been rarely associated with keratoconus, atopic disease,[165] central cloudy dystrophy, pseudoxanthoma elasticum, and limbal dermoid.[163] However, these associations may also be due to chance. There may be asymmetric or unilateral corneal involvement.

Epidemiology and heritability

Fleck dystrophy is autosomal dominant and may be present at birth. It is related to the gene phosphatidylinositol-3-phosphate/phosphatidylinositol 5-kinase type III – *PIP5K3*, at gene locus 2q35. Its MIM number is 121850.[1]

Histopathology

Only certain keratocytes are involved in this dystrophy; the remainder of the stromal, epithelial, and endothelial architecture remains intact. The abnormal keratocytes contain both excess glycosaminoglycan in membrane-bound vacuoles with fibrogranular substance and lipids in smaller membrane vacuoles with electron-dense lamellar bodies.[163,166] The glycosaminoglycans are demonstrated with Alcian blue or colloidal iron stains, and the lipids with Sudan black B and oil red O stains. Cytoplasmic vacuoles, pleomorphic electron-dense material, and membranous inclusions in involved keratocytes are seen on electron microscopy and are similar to those seen in macular dystrophy and mucopolysaccharidoses.[20,166,167] Macular dystrophy differs in the presence of abnormal extracellular glycosaminoglycans. No underlying mechanism or mucopolysaccharide abnormality has been discovered in fleck dystrophy.

Management

Patients with this dystrophy are asymptomatic, and treatment is not necessary.

Central Cloudy Dystrophy of François (CCDF)

Using the IC3D classifications, central cloudy dystrophy of François represents a *Category 4* (C4) dystrophy, indicating a suspected new or previously documented corneal dystrophy, although the evidence for it being a distinct entity is not yet convincing.[1]

Clinical features

François originally described this bilaterally symmetric dystrophy.[166] Unilateral cases have rarely been reported.[168] It is generally a nonprogressive dystrophy with faint, cloudy, gray snowflake-like lesions with ill-defined edges deep in the stroma. The lesions do not involve the superficial stroma and do not extend to the periphery. They may appear polygonal (cracked ice) in shape and can be confused with anterior mosaic dystrophy (Fig. 72.22). The stroma is of normal thickness, and no loss of sensation has been noted. These cloudy lesions are most often in the central one-third of the cornea and are separated by cracklike areas of clear stroma. The epithelium is uninvolved, and erosions do not occur. Clinically, the lesions are identical to those in posterior crocodile shagreen, and this diagnosis should be considered, especially if there is no strong autosomal dominant inheritance pattern.[162,169,170] Posterior crocodile shagreen, however, is more commonly peripheral and anterior stromal. Collagen lamellae at right angles with interspersed abnormal collagen with 100-nm banding has been found in posterior crocodile shagreen,[170] and it is possible that these same lesions are present in central cloudy dystrophy, although histopathologic specimens are lacking. Other ocular disorders have been reported in these patients including spherophakia, fleck and pre-Descemet's dystrophies, and glaucoma.[27,162] It appears in the first decade, and is mostly asymptomatic and nonprogressive.

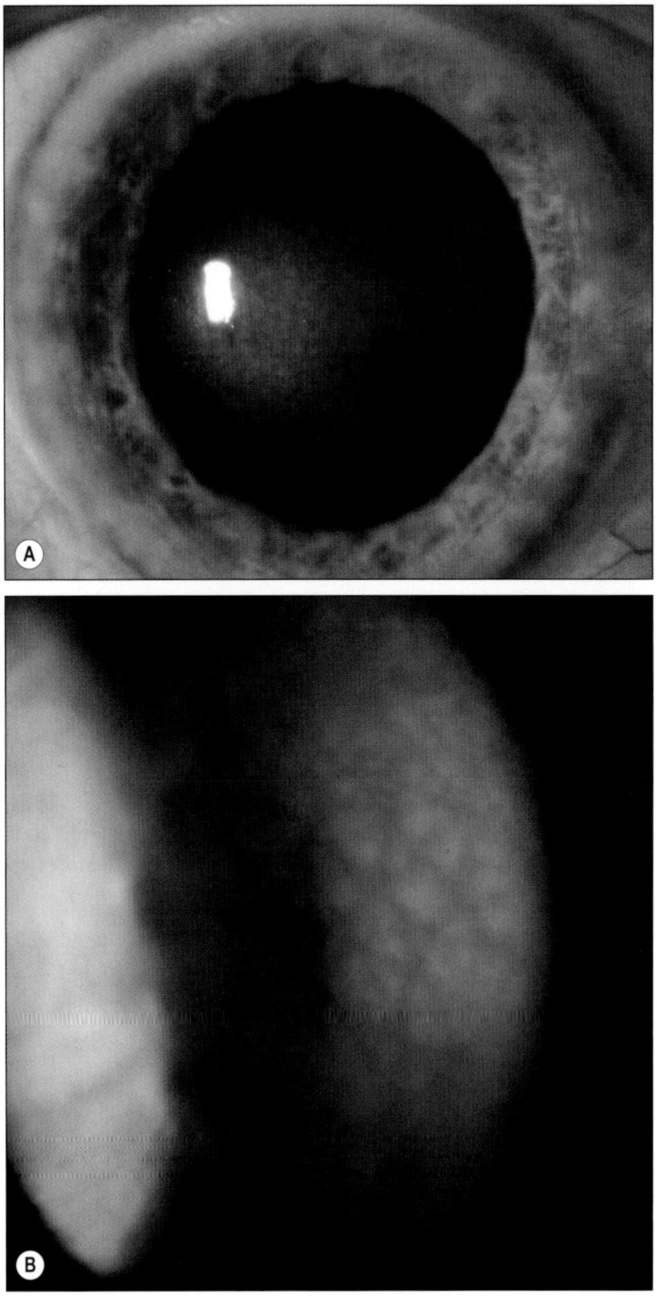

Fig. 72.22 Central cloudy dystrophy of François. (**A**) Diffuse illumination. (**B**) Broad oblique illumination highlighting the 'cracked ice' appearance of the corneal lesion.

The differential diagnosis includes corneal edema, which would demonstrate thickening by pachymetry, and posterior amorphous corneal dystrophy, which results in peripheral involvement and corneal thinning. Pre-Descemet's dystrophy and cornea farinata have discrete lesions unlike those in central cloudy dystrophy.

Epidemiology and heritability

This dystrophy has an unknown inheritance, but an autosomal dominant pattern is reported.[170] It has an MIM number of 217600 and the envolved gene and genetic locus are not described.

Histopathology

The pathologic abnormality has yet to be elucidated. The abnormal collagen found in posterior crocodile shagreen may represent the same defect.[171]

Management

No treatment is required.

Posterior Amorphous Corneal Dystrophy (PACD)

Using the IC3D classifications, posterior amorphous corneal dystrophy represents a *Category 3* (C3) dystrophy: i.e. a well-defined clinical corneal dystrophy in which the disorder has not yet been mapped to a chromosomal locus (Fig. 72.23).[1]

Clinical features

This dystrophy is characterized by bilateral, symmetric opacification with central stromal thinning. It often appears in the first decade of life and shows slow progression. Visual acuity is often only mildly affected (usually better than 20/40) as the stroma thins from the normal thickness of 0.5 mm centrally to as thin as 0.3 mm. The thinning does not appear to induce irregular astigmatism,[172] and keratometry and topography reflect this central flattening.[173] Patches of gray sheets with indistinct borders are seen in the deep stroma from limbus to limbus (Fig. 72.24).[173] Alternatively, they may be found peripherally or centrally. Clear stromal breaks between these sheets are best seen with focal illumination or retroillumination. These lesions may extend to Descemet's membrane with posterior bowing, and endothelial disruption has been described. Gonioscopy may demonstrate a prominent Schwalbe's line and fine iris processes.[162] Glaucoma has not been a reported association.

The differential diagnosis includes posterior polymorphous dystrophy, which has refractile Descemet's membrane changes; pre-Descemet's dystrophy, which has punctate filiform opacities; congenital hereditary stromal or endothelial dystrophies, which have normal or thickened stroma, respectively; and interstitial keratitis, which has inflammation and deep active or ghost vessels. Posterior crocodile shagreen may have a similar appearance to the peripheral form but retains normal corneal thickness. Macular dystrophy may also demonstrate stromal thinning but is easily distinguishable on clinical grounds.

Reported associations with posterior polymorphous dystrophy include corectopia, pseudopolycoria, iridocorneal adhesions,[172] other iris abnormalities such as anterior stromal tags and sponginess of the stroma, and hypermetropia.[173] No iris atrophy, however, has been reported in posterior amorphous dystrophy. The combination of iris abnormalities, possible congenital onset, and nonprogressive stromal lesions has generated the theory that this condition may be a dysgenesis or abnormality of growth of embryonic mesoderm.[173] Because of the location of the lesions, this involvement would most likely be in the second wave of corneal mesoderm.

Epidemiology and heritability

This dystrophy is autosomal dominant and was originally described in three generations of a single pedigree.[172] This pattern was confirmed in a study spanning five generations of a single pedigree.[173] The condition may be congenital in some cases. At this time, no gene has been identified and no MIM classification has been assigned.[1]

Histopathology

The few reported pathologic cases of this dystrophy have demonstrated findings similar to posterior crocodile shagreen, sclerocornea, Peters' anomaly, and congenital hereditary endothelial dystrophy.[174,175] Another report of a single case by Roth et al.[176] showed more extensive disease with subepithelial deposits of electron-dense fibrils and a thick collagenous layer posterior to Descemet's membrane. Stromal thinning to 0.3 mm centrally was noted with focal disorganization and a relative absence of keratocytes, as had been noted in the only previous histopathologic report.[175] Some of the keratocytes had focal vacuolization. The fibers were uniform and 23 nm in diameter with focal bands of long-spaced collagen. Descemet's membrane was greatly thickened (14 μm [normally 4–5 μm]), and the endothelium was normal in appearance.

Management

No treatment is generally required. The thinning is not severe enough to compromise the integrity of the globe.

Congenital Hereditary Stromal Dystrophy (CSCD)

Using the IC3D classifications, congenital hereditary stromal dystrophy represents a *Category 1* (C1) dystrophy: i.e. a well-defined corneal dystrophy in which the gene has been mapped and identified and specific mutations are known.[1] It is also known as congenital hereditary stromal dystrophy and congenital stromal dystrophy of the cornea.

Clinical features

This bilateral, congenital, inherited opacification of the cornea is not related to abnormal endothelial cell function. The disorder is nonprogressive or slowly progressive and must be distinguished from other causes of congenital corneal opacification such as congenital hereditary endothelial dystrophy, congenital glaucoma, and posterior polymorphous dystrophy. This unique stromal dystrophy is probably due to disordered stromal fibrogenesis.[177,178] A diffuse haze made up of flaky lesions is seen primarily in the central anterior stroma, but also may involve the deeper layers. The lesions are often less dense peripherally. Follow-up of more than 10 years has shown no changes in the density or char-

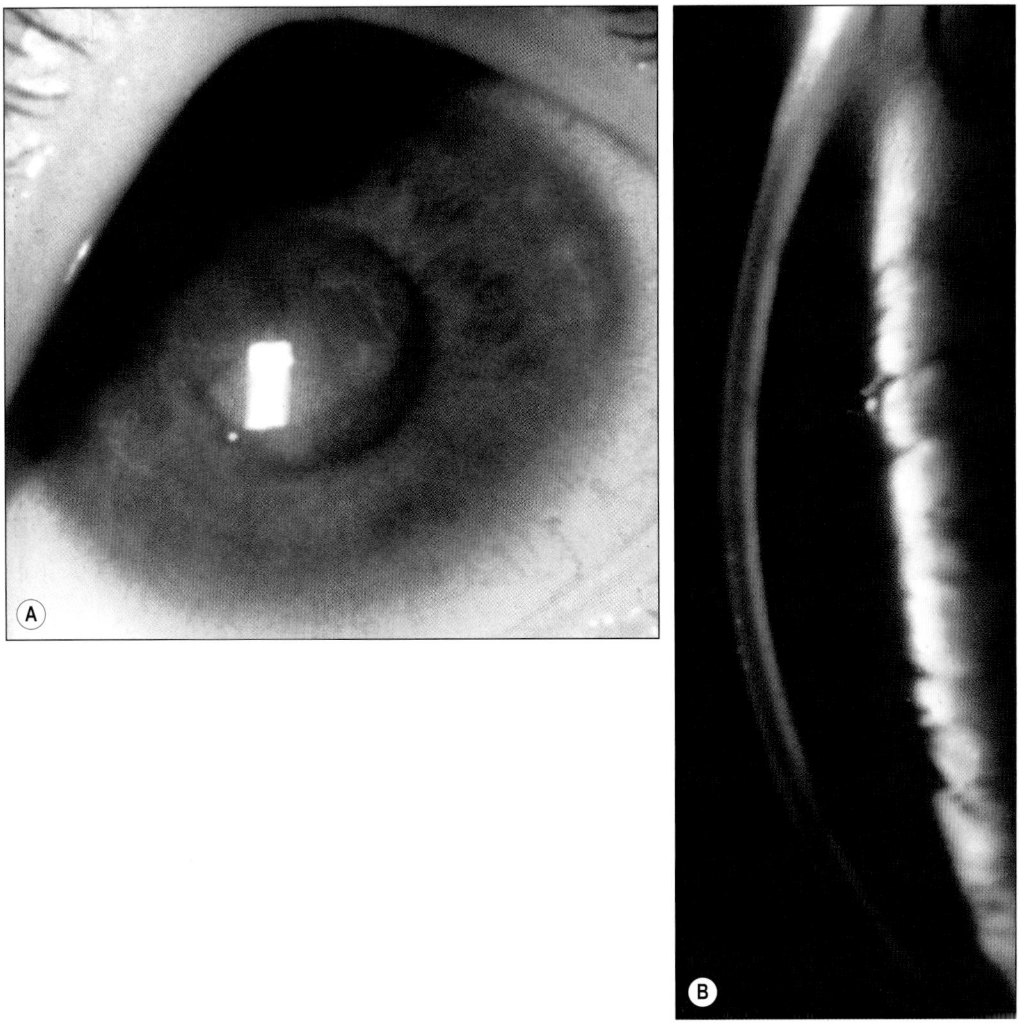

Fig. 72.23 (A) Posterior amorphous stromal dystrophy in a 6-month-old infant. There is central corneal opacification (*1*). (B) Posterior amorphous stromal dystrophy. This thin slit-beam view demonstrates deep stromal opacification. The corneas in this disorder are thin, and the corneal topography is flat, leading to hyperopia. Iris anomalies may be present. The inheritance pattern is autosomal dominant. The presence of anomalies in infants and occasional iris abnormalities suggest that this may be a congenital disorder of anterior segment differentiation. Vision is not usually greatly affected but rarely can be reduced enough to require corneal transplantation.

acter of these lesions. The stromal thickness is not increased, or can show increased thickness. The epithelium is intact without erosions, edema, or decreased sensation. Visual acuity is depressed, and dense amblyopia and searching nystagmus may develop.[178] Esotropia also has been reported.[20]

Epidemiology and heritability

Autosomal dominant inheritance was found in two families with congenital hereditary stromal dystrophy documented by electron microscopy, with the Decorin_*DCN* gene involved, and a 12q21.33. genetic locus. The MIM number is 610048.[1,177,178]

Histopathology

The epithelium and Bowman's layer are uninvolved. Abnormalities of the stromal lamellae are noted, with clefting and layering. All collagen fibrils in the stroma have a diameter of about 15 nm, which is one-half the normal diameter of 30 nm. Densely packed and aligned collagen lamellae, with a pattern similar to normal lamellae, alternate with layers of collagen fibrils that are arranged randomly, have lucent centers, and are packed less densely. Smaller than normal diameter collagen fibrils are also found in lattice and granular dystrophies, but the alternating pattern is unique to congenital hereditary stromal dystrophy. No stromal edema has been identified on histopathologic sections. The endothelium is of normal architecture and function.[178] Descemet's membrane is of normal thickness with a poorly developed anterior band. The significance of the abnormal anterior Descemet's band is unknown. It is possible that early abnormal endothelial cell function may play a role in the disease pathogenesis.[162] The appearance of congenital hereditary endothelial dystrophy is much different, with a very thin Descemet's membrane and multiple layers of collagenous tissue between Descemet's membrane and the abnormal endothelium.

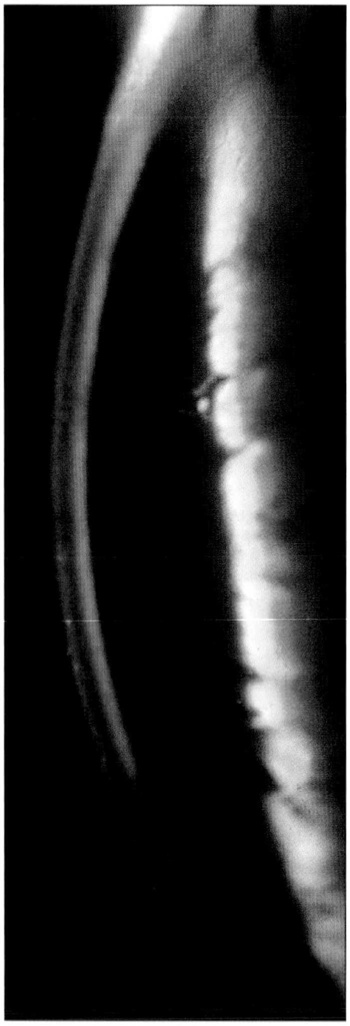

Fig. 72.24 Posterior amorphous corneal dystrophy demonstrating deep corneal opacification.

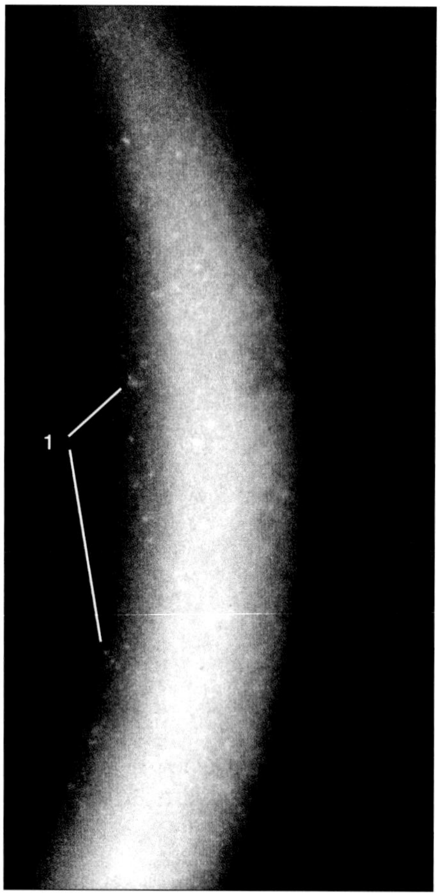

Fig. 72.25 Pre-Descemet's dystrophy demonstrating deep, fine pre-Descemet's punctiform deposits (*1*).

Management

To save useful vision, penetrating keratoplasty is often indicated at an early age. Earlier intervention may prevent dense amblyopia. No recurrences of the dystrophy in the donor graft have been reported. Final visual acuity is rarely better than 20/200,[20] but acuities as good as 20/30 have been reported.[178]

Pre-Descemet Corneal Dystrophy (PDCD)

In the IC3D classifications, pre-Descemet corneal dystrophy represents a *Category 4* (C4) dystrophy—that is, a suspected new, or previously documented corneal dystrophy—although the evidence for it as a distinct entity is not yet convincing.[1]

Clinical features

In pre-Descemet's dystrophy, focal fine gray dots are seen in the posterior stroma in a variety of punctate and linear shapes (Fig. 72.25). Less commonly, larger lesions occur with circular, comma, boomerang, wormlike, and dendritic shapes.[179] These lesions are most often bilateral and symmetric and occur after age 30. They may be diffuse, central, or form a ring, sparing the peripheral and central cornea. Visual acuity is usually not affected. Other entities included in the group of disorders with deep punctiform lesions include polymorphic amyloid degeneration; cornea farinata, which is a fine flourlike speckling of the deep stroma associated with aging; and deep filiform dystrophy. Another variant is punctiform and polychromatic pre-Descemet's dominant dystrophy, which has more uniform deep stromal lesions or filaments that extend to the limbus and do not demonstrate annular or other patterns. The lesions in this variant are polychromatic. Pre-Descemet's opacities also may be associated with systemic diseases such as pseudoxanthoma elasticum[180] and X-linked recessive ichthyosis.[181] Other associations include keratoconus,[179,182,183] posterior polymorphous dystrophy,[179] epithelial membrane dystrophy,[183] and central cloudy dystrophy.[184] The punctiform and polychromatic lesions of pre-Descemet's dystrophy are generally nonprogressive, although some forms demonstrate progression.

Epidemiology and heritability

No definite pattern of inheritance has been determined because of the paucity of cases reported in the same family. Grayson and Wilbrandt[179] reported this dystrophy in siblings, and it has been described in three pedigrees over two generations. This group of dystrophies may be a collection of both sporadic and age-related degenerative lesions.[20]

Punctiform and polychromatic pre-Descemet's dominant dystrophy was recently described in four generations of a single pedigree in 46 family members.[185] Autosomal dominant inheritance is probable, but further studies are needed for confirmation. The gene is unknown and there is no MIM number for the dystrophy.

Histopathology

Curran et al.[186] described a single case with a normal cornea except for enlarged keratocytes near Descemet's membrane, which contained PAS-positive material and vacuolation. This abnormal material also stained for lipid with oil red O, Sudan black B, and Baker's phospholipid.[186] Electron microscopy revealed membrane-bound vacuoles in the cytoplasm containing electron-dense lamellar bodies and fibrillogranular material. This finding was consistent with phospholipid and neutral fat deposition, suggesting a degenerative process that may be age related.

Management

No therapy is required.

References

1. Weiss JS, et al. The IC3D classification of the corneal dystrophies. *Cornea*. 2008;27:S2.
2. Groenouw A. Knötchenförmige Hornhauttrübungen (noduli corneae). *Arch Augenheilkd*. 1890;21:281.
3. Bücklers M. *Die erblichen Hornhautdystrophie: dystrophiae corneae hereditariae*. Stuttgart: Ferdinand Enke Verlag; 1938.
4. Weidle EG, Lisch W. Various forms of opacities of granular corneal dystrophy. *Klin Monatsb Augenheilkd*. 1984;185:167.
5. Waardenburg PJ, Jonkers GH. A specific type of dominant progressive dystrophy of the cornea, developing after birth. *Acta Ophthalmol (Copenh)*. 1961;39:919.
6. Haddad R, Font RL, Fine BS. Unusual superficial variant of granular dystrophy of the cornea. *Am J Ophthalmol*. 1977;83:213.
7. Rodrigues MM, Gaster RN, Pratt MV. Unusual superficial confluent form of granular corneal dystrophy. *Ophthalmology*. 1984;91:1507.
8. Forsius H, et al. Granular corneal dystrophy with late manifestations. *Acta Ophthalmol (Copenh)*. 1983;61:514.
9. Sekimoto M, Hayasaka S, Furuse N, Stogawa T. Concomitant granular dystrophy of the cornea and cone dystrophy. *Ophthalmologica*. 1988;197:57.
10. Duke-Elder SS. *System of ophthalmology. Diseases of the outer eye*. St Louis: Mosby; 1965.
11. Munier FL, Korvatska E, Djemai A, et al. Kerato-epithelin mutations in four 5q31-linked corneal dystrophies. *Nat Genet*. 1997;15:247–251.
12. Korvatska E, Munier FL, Djemai A, et al. Mutation hot spots in 5q31-linked corneal dystrohies. *Am J Hum Genet*. 1998;62:320–324.
13. Jones ST, Zimmerman LE. Histopathologic differentiation of granular, macular, and lattice dystrophies of the cornea. *Am J Ophthalmol*. 1961;51:394.
14. Garner A. Histochemistry of corneal granular dystrophy. *Br J Ophthalmol*. 1969;8:475.
15. Iwamoto T, et al. Ultrastructural variations in granular dystrophy of the cornea. *Graefe's Arch Clin Exp Ophthalmol*. 1975;194:1.
16. Rodrigues MM, Streeten BW, Krachmer JH. Microfibrillar protein and phospholipid in granular corneal dystrophy. *Arch Ophthalmol*. 1983;101:802.
17. Rodrigues MM, Krachmer JH. Recent advances in corneal stromal dystrophies. *Cornea*. 1988;7:19.
18. Sornson ET. Granular dystrophy of the cornea. An electron microscopic study. *Am J Ophthalmol*. 1965;59:1001.
19. Akiya S, Brown SI. Granular dystrophy of the cornea. *Arch Ophthalmol*. 1970;84:179.
20. Waring GO, Rodrigues MM, Laibson PR. Corneal dystrophies. 1. Dystrophies of the epithelium, Bowman's layer and stroma. *Surv Ophthalmol*. 1978;23:71–122.
21. Wittebol-Post D, van der Want JJ, van Bijsterveld OP. Granular dystrophy of the cornea (Groenouw type I): is the keratocyte the primary source after all? *Ophthalmologica*. 1987;195:169.
22. Li YP, Yi YZ, Zheng HL. Macular, lattice and granular dystrophy of the cornea: ultra-histochemistry and ultrastructure study. *Yen Ko Hsueh Pao Eye Science*. 1989;5:122.
23. Johnson BL, Brown SI, Zaidman GW. A light and electron microscopic study of recurrent granular dystrophy of the cornea. *Am J Ophthalmol*. 1981;92:49.
24. Klintworth GK. Proteins in ocular disease. In: Garner A, Klintworth GK. *Pathology of ocular disease: a dynamic approach, Part B*. New York: Marcel Dekker; 1982.
25. Witschel H, Sundmacher R. Bilateral recurrence of granular corneal dystrophy in the grafts. *Graefe's Arch Clin Exp Ophthalmol*. 1979;209:179.
26. Lyons CJ, et al. Granular corneal dystrophy. Visual results and pattern of recurrence after lamellar or penetrating keratoplasty. *Ophthalmology*. 1994;101:1812.
27. Bramsen T, Ehlers N, Baggeson LH. Central cloudy dystrophy of Francois. *Acta Ophthalmol (Copenh)*. 1976;36:395–417.
28. Lempert SL, et al. A simple technique for removal of recurring granular dystrophy in the grafts. *Am J Ophthalmol*. 1978;86:89.
29. Moller HU, Ehlers N. Early treatment of granular dystrophy (Groenouw type I). *Acta Ophthalmol (Copenh)*. 1985;63:597.
30. Stark W, et al. Clinical follow-up of 193-nm ArF excimer laser photokeratectomy. *Ophthalmology*. 1992;99:805.
31. Stein HA, Cheskes A, Stein RM, eds. *Phototherapeutic keratectomy*. In: *The excimer: fundamentals and clinical use*. Thorofare, NJ: Slack; 1994.
32. Hahn TW, Sah WJ, Kim JH. Phototherapeutic keratectomy in nine eyes with superficial corneal diseases. *Refract Corneal Surg*. 1993;9:115.
33. Brownstein S, et al. Granular dystrophy of the cornea: electron microscopic confirmation of recurrence in a graft. *Am J Ophthalmol*. 1974;77:701.
34. Herman SJ, Hughes WF. Recurrence of hereditary corneal dystrophy following keratoplasty. *Am J Ophthalmol*. 1973;75:689.
35. Pouliquen Y, et al. Ophthalmology clinic, Hotel-Dieu. *Exp Eye Res*. 1974;18:163.
36. Rodrigues MM, McGavic JS. Recurrent corneal granular dystrophy: a clinicopathologic study. *Trans Am Ophthalmol Soc*. 1975;73.
37. Stuart JC, Mund ML. Recurrent granular dystrophy. *Am J Ophthalmol*. 1975;79:18.
38. Folberg R, et al. Clinically atypical granular corneal dystrophy with pathologic features of lattice-like amyloid deposits: a study of these families. *Ophthalmology*. 1988;95:46.
39. Holland EJ, et al. Avellino corneal dystrophy: clinical manifestations and natural history. *Ophthalmology*. 1992;99:1564–1568.
40. Stone EM, et al. Three autosomal dominant corneal dystrophies map to chromosome 5q. *Nat Genet*. 1994;6:47–51.
41. Weidel EG. Granular corneal dystrophy: two variants. In: Ferraz de Oliveira FN, ed. *Ophthalmology today. Proceedings of the Eighth Congress of the European Society of Ophthalmology*. Amsterdam (International Congress Series No. 803): Excepta Medica; 1989:617–619.
42. Konishi M, Yamada M, Nakamura Y, et al. Varied appearance of cornea of patients with corneal dystrophy associated with R124H mutation in the BIGH3 gene. *Cornea*. 1999;18:424–429.
43. Munier F, Korvatska E, Djemai A, et al. 5Q31-linked corneal dystrophies: genotype-phenotype correlation at the kerato-epithelin gene locus (ARVO abstract 4454). *Invest Ophthalmol Vis Sci*. 1997;38(suppl):S961.
44. Sommer JR, Wong F, Klintworth GK. Phenotypic variations of corneal dystrophies caused by different mutations in the BIGH3 gene (ARVO abstract 2347). *Invest Ophthalmol Vis Sci*. 1998;39(suppl):S513.
45. SundarRaj N, et al. Macular corneal dystrophy: immunochemical characterization using monoclonal antibodies. *Invest Ophthalmol Vis Sci*. 1987;28:1678.
46. Jonasson F, Johannsson JH, Garner A, Rice NS. Macular corneal dystrophy in Iceland. *Eye*. 1989;3(Pt4):446.
47. Pouliquen Y, et al. Combined macular dystrophy and cornea guttata: an electron microscopic study. *Graefe's Arch Clin Exp Ophthalmol*. 1980;212:149.

48. Francois J. Heredo-familial corneal dystrophies. *Trans Ophthalmol Soc UK*. 1966;86:367.
49. Ehlers N, Bramsen T. Central thickness in corneal disorders. *Acta Ophthalmol (Copenh)*. 1978;56:412.
50. Donnenfeld ED, et al. Corneal thinning in macular corneal dystrophy. *Am J Ophthalmol*. 1986;101:112.
51. Quantock AJ, et al. Macular corneal dystrophy: reduction in both corneal thickness and collagen interfibrillar spacing. *Curr Eye Res*. 1990;9:393.
52. Klintworth GK. Corneal dystrophies. In: Nicholson DK, ed. *Ocular pathology update*. New York: Masson; 1980.
53. Vance JM, Jonasson F, Lennon F, et al. Linkage of a gene for macular corneal dystrophy to chromosome 16, *Am J Hum Genet*. 1996;58: 757–762.
54. Bron AJ. Genetics of the corneal dystrophies. What we have learned in the past twenty-five years. *Cornea*. 2000;19(5):699–711.
55. Klintworth GK, Oshima E, Al-Rajhi A, et al. Macular corneal dystrophy in Saudi Arabia: a study of 56 cases and recognition of new immunophenotype. *Am J Ophthalmol*. 1997;124:9–19.
56. Akama TO, Nishida K, Nakayama J, et al. Macular corneal dystrophy type I and type II are caused by distinct mutations in a new sulfotransferase gene. *Nat Genet*. 2000;26:237–241.
57. El-Ashry AF, et al. Identification of novel mutations in the carbohydrate sulfotransferase gene (CHST6) causing macular corneal dystrophy. *Invest Ophthalmol Vis Sci*. 2002;43(2):377–382.
58. Garner A. Histochemistry of corneal macular dystrophy. *Invest Ophthalmol*. 1969;8:473.
59. Livni N, Abraham FA, Zauberman H. Groenouw's macular dystrophy: histochemistry and ultrastructure of the cornea. *Doc Ophthalmol*. 1973;37:327.
60. Snip RC, Kenyon KR, Green WR. Macular corneal dystrophy. Ultrastructural pathology of corneal endothelium and Descemet's membrane. *Invest Ophthalmol*. 1973;12:88.
61. Teng CC. Macular dystrophy of the cornea. A histochemical and electron microscopic study. *Am J Ophthalmol*. 1966;62:436.
62. Francois J, Hanssens M, Teuchy H, Sbruyns M. Ultrastructural findings in corneal macular dystrophy (Groenouw II type). *Ophthalmic Res*. 1975;7:80.
63. Klintworth GK, Vogel FS. Macular corneal dystrophy. An inherited acid mucopolysaccharide storage disease of the corneal fibroblast. *Am J Pathol*. 1964;45:565.
64. Tremblay M, Dubé I. Macular dystrophy of the cornea: ultrastructure of two cases. *Can J Ophthalmol*. 1973;8:47.
65. Ghosh M, McCulloch C. Macular corneal dystrophy. *Can J Ophthalmol*. 1973;8:515.
66. Nakazawa K, et al. Defective processing of keratan sulfate in macular corneal dystrophy. *J Biol Chem*. 1984;259:13751.
67. Klintworth GK, Reed J, Stainer GA, Binder PS. Recurrence of macular corneal dystrophy within grafts. *Am J Ophthalmol*. 1983;95:60.
68. Panjwani N, Baum J. Lectin receptors of normal and dystrophic corneas. *Acta Ophthalmol (Copenh)*. 1989;192(suppl):171.
69. Panjwani N, et al. Alterations in stromal glycoconjugates in macular corneal dystrophy. *Invest Ophthalmol Vis Sci*. 1986;27:1211.
70. Klintworth GK, et al. Macular corneal dystrophy. Lack of keratan sulfate in serum and cornea. *Ophthalmic Paediatr Genet*. 1986;7:139.
71. Thonar EJ, et al. Quantification of keratan sulfate in blood as a marker of cartilage catabolism. *Arthritis Rheum*. 1985;28:1367.
72. Hassell JR, Newsome DA, Krachmer JH, Rodrigues MM. Macular corneal dystrophy: failure to synthesize a mature keratan sulfate proteoglycan. *Proc Natl Acad Sci USA*. 1980;77:3705.
73. Brune WE, et al. Corneal alphagalactosidase deficiency in macular corneal dystrophy. *Ophthalmic Paediatr Genet*. 1985;5:179.
74. Yang CJ, SundarRaj N, Thonar EJ, Klintworth GK. Immunohistochemical evidence of heterogeneity in macular corneal dystrophy. *Am J Ophthalmol*. 1988;106:65.
75. Meek KM, et al. Macular corneal dystrophy: the macromolecular structure of the stroma observed using electron microscopy and synchrotron X-ray diffraction. *Exp Eye Res*. 1989;49:941.
76. Quigley HA, Goldberg MF. Scheie syndrome and macular corneal dystrophy. *Arch Ophthalmol*. 1971;85:553.
77. Akova YA, et al. Recurrent macular corneal dystrophy following penetrating keratoplasty. *Eye*. 1990;4(Pt5):698.
78. Niesen U, Thomann U, Schipper I. Phototherapeutic keratectomy. *Klin Monatsbl Augenheilkd*. 1994;205:187.
79. Klintworth GK, Smith CF. Abnormalities of proteoglycans and glycoproteins synthesized by corneal organ cultures derived from patients with macular corneal dystrophy. *Lab Invest*. 1983;48:603.
80. Robin AL, et al. Recurrence of macular corneal dystrophy after lamellar keratoplasty. *Am J Ophthalmol*. 1977;84:457.
81. Newsome DA, et al. Biochemical and histological analysis of 'recurrent' macular corneal dystrophy. *Arch Ophthalmol*. 1982;100:1125.
82. Sturrock GD. Lattice corneal dystrophy: a source of confusion. *Br J Ophthalmol*. 1983;67:629.
83. Dubord PJ, Krachmer JH. Diagnosis of early lattice corneal dystrophy. *Arch Ophthalmol*. 1982;100:788.
84. Durand L, Resal R, Burillon C. Focus on an anatomoclinical entity: Biber-Haab-Dimmer lattice dystrophy. *J Fr Ophtalmol*. 1985;8:729.
85. Hida T, et al. Clinical features of a newly recognized type of lattice corneal dystrophy. *Am J Ophthalmol*. 1987;104:241.
86. Skrypuch OW, Willis NR. Lattice dystrophy of the cornea: a clinicopathological case report. *Can J Ophthalmol*. 1987;22:181.
87. Zechner EM, Croxatto JO, Malbran ES. Superficial involvement in lattice corneal dystrophy. *Ophthalmologica*. 1986;193:193.
88. Yanoff M, Fine BS, Colosi NJ, Katowitz JA. Lattice corneal dystrophy. Report of an unusual case. *Arch Ophthalmol*. 1977;95:651.
89. François J, Feher J. Light microscopy and polarization optical study of the lattice dystrophy of the cornea. *Ophthalmologica*. 1972;164:1.
90. Takahashi N, Sasaki K, Nakaizumi H, Konishi F. Specular microscopic findings of lattice corneal dystrophy. *Int Ophthalmol*. 1987;10:47.
91. Bowen RA, et al. Lattice dystrophy of the cornea as a variety of amyloidosis. *Am J Ophthalmol*. 1970;7:822.
92. Miller CA, Krachmer JH. Epithelial and stromal dystrophies. In: Kaufman HE, McDonald MB, Waltman SR, eds. *The cornea*. New York: Churchill Livingstone; 1988.
93. Rodrigues MM, et al. Lack of evidence for AA reactivity in amyloid deposits of lattice corneal dystrophy and corneal amyloid degeneration. *Invest Ophthalmol Vis Sci*. 1984;25.
94. Arffa RC. Dystrophies of the epithelium, Bowman's layer, and stroma. In: Arffa RC, ed. *Grayson's diseases of the cornea*. St Louis: Mosby; 1991.
95. Meretoja J. Comparative histopathological and clinical findings in eyes with lattice corneal dystrophy of two different types. *Ophthalmologica*. 1972;165:15.
96. Malbran ES, Meijide RF, Croxatto JO. Atypical corneal dystrophy with stromal amyloid deposits. *Cornea*. 1988;7:210.
97. Pe'er J, Fine BS, Dixon A, Rothberg DS. Corneal elastosis within lattice dystrophy lesions. *Br J Ophthalmol*. 1988;72:183.
98. Panjwani N, et al. Lectin receptors of amyloid in corneas with lattice dystrophy. *Arch Ophthalmol*. 1987;105:688.
99. McTigue JW, Fine BS. The stromal lesion in lattice dystrophy of the cornea. A light and electron microscopic study. *Invest Ophthalmol*. 1964;3:355.
100. François J, Hanssens M, Teuchy H. Ultrastructural changes in lattice dystrophy of the cornea. *Ophthalmic Res*. 1975;7:321.
101. Klintworth GK. Lattice corneal dystrophy. An inherited variety of amyloidosis restricted to the cornea. *Am J Pathol*. 1967;50:371.
102. Hogan MJ, Alvarado J. Ultrastructure of lattice dystrophy of the cornea. A case report. *Am J Ophthalmol*. 1967;64:656.
103. Hida T, et al. Histopathologic and immunochemical features of lattice corneal dystrophy type III. *Am J Ophthalmol*. 1987;104:249.
104. Garner A. Amyloidosis of the cornea. *Arch Ophthalmol*. 1969;53:73.
105. Akiya S, Ito I, Matsui M. Gelatinous drop-like dystrophy of the cornea: light and electron microscopic study of superficial stromal lesion. *Jpn J Clin Ophthalmol*. 1972;26:815.
106. Weber FL, Babel J. Gelatinous drop-like dystrophy. *Arch Ophthalmol*. 1980;98:144.
107. Mannis MJ, Krachmer JH, Rodrigues MM, Pardos GJ. Polymorphic amyloid degeneration of the cornea. A clinical and histopathologic study. *Arch Ophthalmol*. 1981;99:1217.
108. Biber H. Ueber einige seltene Horhautkrankungan (Diss.). Zurich, 1890.
109. Haab O. Die gittrige Keratitis. *Z Augenheilkd*. 1899;2:235.
110. Dimmer F. Ueber oberflächliche gittrige Hornhauttrübung. *Z Augenheilkd*. 1899;2:354.
111. Mashima Y, Imamura Y, Konishi M, et al. Homogeneity of keratoepithelin codon 124 mutations in Japanese patients with either of two types of corneal stromal dystrophy. *Am J Hum Genet*. 1997;61: 1448–1450.
112. Yamamoto S, Maeda N, Watanabe H, et al. The spectrum of BIGH, R gene mutations among patients with corneal dystrophy in Japan (ARVO abstract 2971). *Invest Ophthalmol Vis Sci*. 1999;40(suppl):S563.
113. Hida T, Tsubota K, Kgasawa K, et al. Clinical features of a newly recognized type of lattice corneal dystrophy. *Am J Ophthalmol*. 1987;104: 241–248.
114. Hida T, Proia AD, Kigasawa K, et al. Histopathologic and immunochemical features of lattice corneal dystrophy type III. *Am J Ophthalmol*. 1987;104:249–254.
115. Stewart H, Black GC, Donnai D, et al. A mutation within exon 14 of the TGFBI(BIGH3) gene on chromosome 5q31 causes an asymmetric,

late-onset form of lattice corneal dystrophy. *Ophthalmology.* 1999;106: 964–970.
116. Stock EL, Feder RS, O'Grady RB, et al. Lattice corneal dystrophy type IIIA: clinical and histopathologic correlations. *Arch Ophthalmol.* 1991;109:354–358.
117. Fujiki K, Hotta Y, Nakayasu K, et al. A new L527 mutation of the BIGH3 gene in patients with lattice corneal dystrophy with deep stromal opacities. *Hum Genet.* 1998;103:286–289.
118. Mehta RF. Unilateral lattice dystrophy of the cornea. *Br J Ophthalmol.* 1980;64:53.
119. Ramsey RM. Familial corneal dystrophy, lattice type. *Trans Am Ophthalmol Soc.* 1957;60:701.
120. Ramsey MS, Fine BS. Localized corneal amyloidoses. *Am J Ophthalmol.* 1972;75:560.
121. Reshmi CS. Unilateral lattice dystrophy of the cornea: report of a case. *Med J Aust.* 1971;1:966.
122. Hoang-Xuan T, et al. Association of a lattice dystrophy and keratoconus: anatomo-clinical study of a case. *Bull Soc Ophtalmol Fr.* 1989;89:35.
123. Sassani JW, Smith G, Rabinowitz YS. Keratoconus and bilateral lattice-granular corneal dystrophies. *Cornea.* 1992;11:343.
124. Pinckers A, Eggink F, Aandekerk AL, van't Pad Bosch A. Contact lens-induced pseudo-dystrophy of the cornea? *Doc Ophthalmol.* 1987;65: 433.
125. Meisler DM, Fine M. Recurrence of clinical signs of lattice corneal dystrophy (type I) in corneal transplants. *Am J Ophthalmol.* 1984;97: 210.
126. Klintworth GK, Ferry AP, Sugar A, Reed J. Recurrence of lattice corneal dystrophy type 1 in the corneal grafts of two siblings. *Am J Ophthalmol.* 1982;94:540.
127. Lanier JD, Fine M, Togni B. Lattice corneal dystrophy. *Arch Ophthalmol.* 1976;94:921.
128. Lorenzetti DWC, Kaufman HE. Macular lattice dystrophies and their recurrences after keratoplasty. *Trans Am Acad Ophthalmol Otolaryngol.* 1967;71:112.
129. Donders PC, Blanksma LJ. Meretoja syndrome. Lattice dystrophy of the cornea with hereditary generalized amyloidosis. *Ophthalmologica.* 1979; 178:173.
130. Meretoja J, Tarkkanen A. Pseudoexfoliation syndrome in familial systemic amyloidosis with lattice corneal dystrophy. *Ophthalmic Res.* 1975;7:194.
131. McMullan FD, et al. Corneal amyloidosis: an immunohistochemical analysis. *Invest Ophthalmol Vis Sci.* 1984;25(suppl):6.
132. De la Chapelle A, Kere J, Sack GH Jr, et al. Familial amyloidosis caused by asparagine or tyrosine substitution for aspartic acid at residue 187. *Nat Genet.* 1992;2:157–160.
133. De al Chapelle A, Kere J, Sack GH Jr, et al. Familial amyloidosis, Finnish type:G654-a mutation of the gelsolin gene in Finnish families and an unrelated American family. *Genomics.* 1992;13:898–901.
134. Steiner RD, Paunio T, Uemichi T, et al. Asp187Asn mutation of gelsolin in an American kindred with familial amyloidosis, Finnish type (FAP IV). *Hum Genet.* 1995;95:327–330.
135. Hiltunen T, Kiuru S, Hogell V, et al. Finnish type of familial amyloidosis: cosegregation of Asp187-Asn mutation of gelsolin with the disease in three large families. *Am J Hum Genet.* 1991;49:522–528.
136. Wibaut F, Van Went JM. Een Zeldzame Erfelijke Hoornvliesaandoening. *Ned Tijdschr Geneeskd.* 1924;1:2996–2997.
137. Schnyder WF. Mitteiltung uber einen neuen Typus von familiarer Hornhauterkrankung. *Schweiz Med Wochenschr.* 1929;59:559–571.
138. Schnyder WF. Scheibenformige Krystallienlagerungen in der Hornhautmitte als Erbleiden. *Klin Monatsbl Augenheilkd.* 1939;103:494–502.
139. Ingraham HJ, Perry HD, Donnenfeld ED, Donaldson DD. Progressive Schnyder's corneal dystrophy. *Ophthalmology.* 1993;100:1824–1827.
140. Lisch W, et al. Schnyder's dystrophy. *Ophthalmic Paediatr Genet.* 1986;7:45–56.
141. Bron AJ, Williams HP, Carruthers ME. Hereditary crystalline stromal dystrophy of Schnyder. I. Clinical features of a family with hyperlipoproteinemia. *Br J Ophthalmol.* 1972;56:383–399.
142. Luxenberg M. Hereditary crystalline dystrophy of the cornea. *Am J Ophthalmol.* 1967;63:507–511.
143. Ehlers N, Mathiessen M. Hereditary crystalline corneal dystrophy of Schnyder. *Acta Ophthalmol (Copenh).* 1973:316–324.
144. Weiss JS. Schnyder's dystrophy of the cornea. *Cornea.* 1992;1:93–101.
145. Delleman JW, Winkleman JF. Degeneratio corneae cristallinea hereditaria: a clinical, genetical, and histologic study. *Ophthalmologica.* 1968; 155:409–426.
146. Burns RP, Connor W, Gipson I. Cholesterol turnover in hereditary crystalline corneal dystrophy of Schnyder. *Trans Am Ophthalmol Soc.* 1978;76:184–196.
147. Kim KS, et al. Effects of cholesterol feeding on corneal dystrophy in mice. *Biochem Biophys Acta.* 1991;1085:343–349.
148. Shearman AM, Hudson TJ, Andresen JM, et al. The gene for Schnyder's crystalline corneal dystrophy maps to human chromosome 1p34.1-p36, *Hum Mol Genet.* 1996;5:1667–1672.
149. Takeuchi T, Furihata M, Heng HH, et al. Chromosomal mapping and expression of the human B120 gene. *Gene.* 1998;213:189–193.
150. Rodrigues MM, Kruth HS, Krachmer JH, Willis R. Unesterified cholesterol in Schnyder's crystalline dystrophy of the cornea. *Am J Ophthalmol.* 1987;104:157–163.
151. Freddo TF, Polack FM, Leibowitz HM. Ultrastructural changes in the posterior layers of the cornea in Schnyder's crystalline dystrophy. *Cornea.* 1989;8:170–177.
152. Weiss JS, Rodrigues M, Rajagopalan S, Kruth H. Atypical Schnyder's crystalline dystrophy of the cornea: a light and electron microscopic study. *Proc Int Soc Eye Res.* 1990;6:198.
153. Weiss JS, Rodrigues M, Rajagopalan S, Kruth H. Schnyder's corneal dystrophy: clinical, ultrastructural, and histochemical studies. *Ophthalmology.* 1990;97(suppl):141.
154. Weller RO, Rodger FC. Crystalline stromal dystrophy: histochemistry and ultrastructure of the cornea. *Br J Ophthalmol.* 1980;64:46–52.
155. Garner A, Tripathi RC. Hereditary crystalline stromal dystrophy of Schnyder. II. Histopathology and ultrastructure. *Br J Ophthalmol.* 1972;56:400–408.
156. Rodrigues MM, et al. Cholesterol localization in ultrathin frozen sections in Schnyder's corneal crystalline dystrophy. *Am J Ophthalmol.* 1990;110:513–517.
157. Hoang-Xuan T, Pouliquen Y, Salvoldelli M, Gasteau J. Schnyder's crystalline dystrophy. I. Study of a case by light and electron microscopy. *J Fr Ophthalmol.* 1985;8:735–742.
158. Ghosh M, McCulloch C. Crystalline dystrophy of the cornea: a light and electron microscopic study. *Can J Ophthalmol.* 1977;12:321–329.
159. Brooks AMV, Grant G, Gillies WE. Differentiation of posterior polymorphous dystrophy from other posterior corneal opacities by specular microscopy. *Ophthalmology.* 1989;96:1639–1646.
160. Francois J, Neetans A. Nouvelle dystrophy heredo-familiale du parenchyme corneen (heredo-dystrophie Mouchettee), *Bull Soc Belge Ophtalmol.* 1957;114:641–646.
161. Stankovic I, Stojanovic D. L'heredodystrophie mouchettee du parenchyme corneen. *Ann Ocul (Paris).* 1964;197:52–57.
162. Miller CA, Krachmer JH. Epithelial and stromal dystrophies. In: Kaufman HE, Barron BA, McDonald MB, eds. *The cornea.* New York: Churchill Livingstone; 1993.
163. Purcell JJJ, Krachmer JH, Weingeist TA. Fleck corneal dystrophy. *Arch Ophthalmol.* 1977;95:440–444.
164. Birndorf LA, Ginsberg SP. Hereditary fleck dystrophy associated with decreased corneal sensitivity. *Am J Ophthalmol.* 1972;73:670–672.
165. Patten JT, Hundiak RA, Donaldson DD. Fleck (mouchetee) dystrophy of the cornea. *Ann Ophthalmol.* 1976;8(1):25–32.
166. Nicholson DH, Green WR, Cross HE. A clinical and histopathological study of Francois-Neetans speckled corneal dystrophy. *Am J Ophthalmol.* 1977;83:554–560.
167. Kiskaddon BM, Campbell RJ, Waller RR, Bourne W. Fleck dystrophy of the cornea: case report. *Ann Ophthalmol.* 1980;12:700–704.
168. Francois J. Une novelle dystrophie heredofamiliale de la cornee. *J Genet Hum.* 1956;5:189–196.
169. Goodside V. Posterior crocodile shagreen. *Am J Ophthalmol.* 1958; 46:748–750.
170. Strachan IM. Cloudy central corneal dystrophy of François. Five cases in the same family. *Br J Ophthalmolol.* 1969;53:192–194.
171. Krachmer JH, Dubord PJ, Rodrigues MM, Mannis MJ. Corneal posterior crocodile shagreen and polymorphic amyloid degeneration. *Arch Ophthalmol.* 1983;101:54–59.
172. Carpel EF, Sigelman RJ, Doughman DJ. Posterior amorphous corneal dystrophy. *Am J Ophthalmol.* 1977;83:629–632.
173. Dunn SP, Krachmer JH, Ching SST. New findings in posterior amorphous corneal dystrophy. *Arch Ophthalmol.* 1984;102:236–239.
174. Kenyon KR. Mesenchymal dysgenesis in Peters' anomaly, sclerocornea, and congenital endothelial dystrophy. *Exp Eye Res.* 1975;21:125–142.
175. Johnson AT, et al. The pathology of posterior amorphous corneal dystrophy [see comments]. *Ophthalmology.* 1990;97:104–109.
176. Roth SI, Mittelman D, Stock EL. Posterior amorphous corneal dystrophy. An ultrastructural study of a variant with histopathological features of an endothelial dystrophy. *Cornea.* 1992;11:165–172.
177. Desvignes P, Vigo A. A propos d'un cas de dystrophie corneenne parenchymateuse familiale a heredite dominate. *Bull Soc Ophtalmol Fr.* 1955;55:220–225.

178. Witschel H, Fine BS, Grutzner P, McTigue JW. Congenital hereditary stromal dystrophy of the cornea. *Arch Ophthalmol.* 1978;96:1043–1051
179. Grayson M, Wilbrandt H. Pre-Descemet dystrophy. *Am J Ophthalmol.* 1967;64:276–282.
180. Collier M. Elastorrhexie systematisee et dystrohes corneenes chez deux soeurs. *Bull Soc Ophthalmol.* 1965;65:301–310.
181. Sever RJ, Frost P, Weinstein G. Eye changes in ichthyosis. *JAMA.* 1968;206:2283–2286.
182. Collier M. Dystrophie filiforme profonde de la cornee. *Bull Soc Ophtalmol Fr.* 1964;64:1034–1036.
183. Maeder G, Danis P. Sur une nouvelle forme de dystrophie corneenne (dystrophia filiformis profunda corneaea) associee a us keratocone. *Ophthalmologica.* 1947;114:246–248.
184. Collier M. Dystrophie nuageuse centrale et dystrophie pontiforme predescemetique dans une meme famille. *Bull Soc Ophtalmol Fr.* 1966;66:575–579.
185. Fernandez-Sasso D, Acosta JEP, Malbran E. Punctiform and polychromatic pre-Descemet's dominant corneal dystrophy. *Br J Ophthalmol.* 1979;63:336–338.
186. Curran RE, Kenyon KR, Green WR. Pre-Descemet's membrane corneal dystrophy. *Am J Ophthalmol.* 1974;77:711–716.

Chapter 73

Descemet's Membrane and Endothelial Dystrophies

Robert W. Weisenthal, Barbara W. Streeten

Posterior Polymorphous Corneal Dystrophy

MIM PPCD1 #122000 – PPCD2 #609140 – PPCD3 #609141

Posterior polymorphous corneal dystrophy (PPCD), initially described by Koeppé[1] in 1916, encompasses a broad spectrum of corneal and anterior segment abnormalities (Table 73.1). The clinical expression of this autosomal dominant disorder varies considerably, even within the same family.[2] For example, one family member may be asymptomatic with only a single endothelial lesion whereas a sibling might have corneal decompensation, broad peripheral synechiae, and advanced glaucoma.

PPCD is a bilateral disease, although it may be asymmetrical. In the vast majority of cases it is asymptomatic and stable, diagnosed incidentally on routine examination, but in certain patients it is a progressive, debilitating condition. PPCD typically occurs in the second or third decade of life, although in rare instances it may manifest as a cloudy cornea in the first decade of life.

Clinical presentation and course

The corneal abnormalities in PPCD occur at the level of Descemet's membrane and endothelium and can be divided into three patterns: vesicle-like lesions, band lesions, and diffuse opacities.[2–6] The hallmark of PPCD is the vesicular lesion, which occurs in almost all patients with the disorder. This lesion may not truly be a vesicle, as discussed later, but its original designation continues to be used. In one study of 48 patients, the vesicular lesion was the sole finding in 42% of cases.[4] Forty-eight percent of patients had a combination of band and vesicular lesions, and 10% had a diffuse opacity in addition to vesicular lesions. On slit lamp examination the vesicular lesion appears as a transparent cyst surrounded by a gray halo at the level of Descemet's membrane and endothelium (Fig. 73.1). The vesicles can be found anywhere on the posterior cornea and may appear as isolated lesions or in lines, clusters, or confluent groups.[2–6]

By specular microscopy, the vesicular lesions range in diameter from 0.10 to 1.00 mm.[4–8] They appear as sharply demarcated large round areas that contain lighter thick ridges or cell aggregates (Fig. 73.2) or as black spots that interrupt the endothelial mosaic (Fig. 73.3). Using specular microscopy with a relief mode, Laganowski et al.[4] observed that the vesicles appear as pits or excavations in the posterior aspect of Descemet's membrane, filled with fibrillar or collagenous material and not as fluid-filled spaces as the term 'vesicle' would imply. Enlarged and pleomorphic endothelial cells may overlie or line the vesicular lesion, but can be masked or distorted.[4,8] The endothelial cells between the involved areas may have three appearances: normal-sized cells with a typical mosaic pattern, cells smaller than normal and crowded together, or most often, enlarged pleomorphic cells.[4,5,7,8]

Band lesions are typically horizontal, have parallel scalloped edges, and do not taper toward the ends (Fig. 73.4).[2–6] Like the vesicular lesions, band lesions may be seen on any area of the posterior cornea, although the most frequent location is just inferior to the central cornea.[4] The band lesions are easily differentiated from the tapered smooth-edged tears seen in congenital glaucoma, trauma, and hydrops.[9] Specular microscopy of the band lesions demonstrates shallow trenches and ridges arising from a large number of confluent vesicles (Fig. 73.5).[4,8] The endothelial cells that line the bands appear enlarged and pleomorphic.

Diffuse opacities are either small, macular, gray-white lesions or larger sinuous geographic lesions at the level of Descemet's membrane (Fig. 73.6). With direct illumination there is a haze in the posterior stroma adjacent to the lesions. In retroillumination, the opacities have a peau d'orange texture.[2,4–8] They range in size from 0.5 to 2.0 mm in diameter and by specular microscopy appear as well-demarcated areas of enlarged and pleomorphic cells with indistinct borders and multiple reflective highlights surrounded by normal or small endothelial cells (Fig. 73.7). Endothelial guttae can also be seen in PPCD.[5,6] The guttae are similar to those in macular corneal dystrophy, interstitial keratitis, and Fuchs' dystrophy but can be distinguished by other features of each condition.

Corneal edema occurs infrequently and ranges from minimal stromal thickening to bullous keratopathy.[2–8] The edema can appear at any age and be rapidly progressive or remain stable. In advanced cases there may be associated stromal lipid deposition or superficial calcific (band) keratopathy.

Peripheral anterior synechiae (PAS) are also a characteristic feature of PPCD and an important prognostic indicator

Table 73.1 Chief clinical characteristics and genetics of Descemet's membrane and endothelial dystrophies

	PPCD1 MIM #122000 PPCD2 MIM #609140 PPCD3 MIM #609141	**FECD MIM #136800**	**CHED 1 MIM #121700 CHED 2 MIM 217700**
Onset	Teens to 20s Rarely at birth	40s to 50s: classic 1st to 3rd decade: early onset	Birth to 10 years
Heredity Genetic locus Gene	AD PPCD1 – 20p11.2-q11.2 Unknown gene PPCD2—1p34.3-p32.3 Gene – collagen type VIII alpha 2, COL8A2 PPCD3—10p11.2 Gene – two-handed zinc-finger homeodomain transcription factor 8-ZEB1	AD, many with no inheritance pattern Classic FECD 13pTel-13q12.13 18q21.2-q21.32 possible SLC4A11 Early-onset FECD 1p34.3-p32 Gene—type VIII, Alpha 2 – COL8A2 L450W, Q455K	CHED 1 – AD 20p11.2-q11.2 Unknown gene CHED 2 – AR 20p13 Gene—solute carrier family 4, sodium borate transporter member 11 – SLC4A11
Corneal findings	Vesicles bands Diffuse opacities Corneal edema Corneal guttae Corneal steepening (rare)	Guttae Stromal thickening Epithelial edema Map-dot and other anterior basement membrane changes Subepithelial fibrosis Corneal steepening (rare)	Marked corneal thickening and opacification Endothelium rarely visible
Other ocular abnormalities	Broad peripheral synechiae Increased intraocular pressure Iris atrophy/corectopia	Increased intraocular pressure Narrow angles	None
Specular microscopy	Vesicles – well-demarcated dark areas with central light ridge or cell clusters Bands – fusion of linearly arranged vesicles Diffusely abnormal mosaic Endothelial cells usually enlarged	Polymorphism Polymegathism Decreased endothelial cell count Small dark areas with central bright spot in mild disease May coalesce and increase in size with multiple highlights Late severely disorganized endothelial mosaic	Not applicable
Differential diagnosis	ICE syndrome Posterior corneal vesicle syndrome Early-onset CHED	Pseudoguttae Chandler's syndrome Herpes simplex keratitis Other guttae (e.g. interstitial keratitis, macular dystrophy)	Congenital glaucoma CHSD Metabolic Peters' anomaly Infectious (e.g. rubella, syphilis) Forceps injury Early-onset PPCD X-Linked endothelial dystrophy
Prognosis for surgery	Good, if no synechiae or increased intraocular pressure	Very good; long-term, more guarded	Fair to good Guarded in early-onset age group

AD, Autosomal dominant; AR, autosomal recessive; CHSD, congenital hereditary stromal dystrophy.
Note: X-linked endothelial corneal dystrophy (XECD) MIM: none is not included in chart—see text at end of chapter.

for the outcome of transplant surgery, as will be discussed later. In one study, PAS were present in 27% of patients with PPCD.[5] These can range from fine adhesions visible only by gonioscopy to large, broad-based membranes with a glassy surface (Fig. 73.8) obvious without gonioscopy. The iris may be normal or may show broad areas of atrophy. Corectopia may also be present. Elevated intraocular pressure was found in 14% of patients in one series, associated with either anatomically open angles or angle closure.[2,5] Angle closure is thought to result from endothelial cell migration across the trabecular meshwork onto the iris, forming synechiae.[10] The mechanism of open angle glaucoma has been suggested to be compression of the trabecular meshwork secondary to a high iris insertion.[11]

Corneal steepening and apical corneal thinning reminiscent of keratoconus have been described in patients with PPCD.[12,13] It is unclear whether this is coincidental or relates to a common pathogenesis.

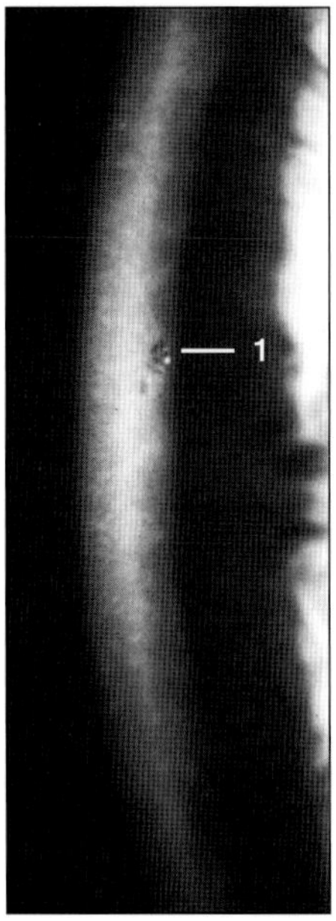

Fig. 73.1 Slit lamp photomicrograph of vesicular lesion (*1*) in PPCD.

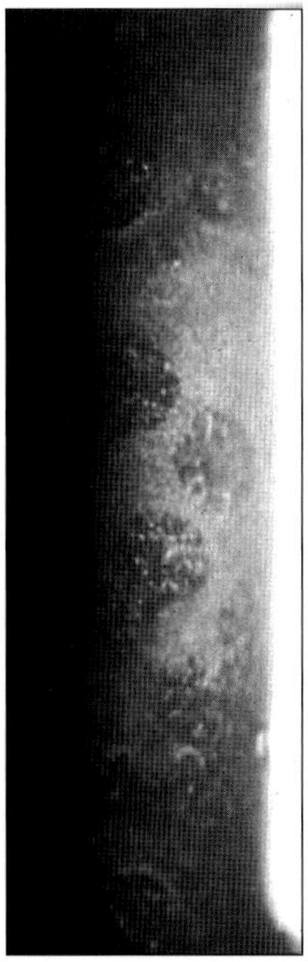

Fig. 73.2 Specular photomicrograph of vesicular lesions in PPCD showing well-demarcated areas containing curvilinear lines and highlighted dots. (Courtesy Jay Krachmer, MD.)

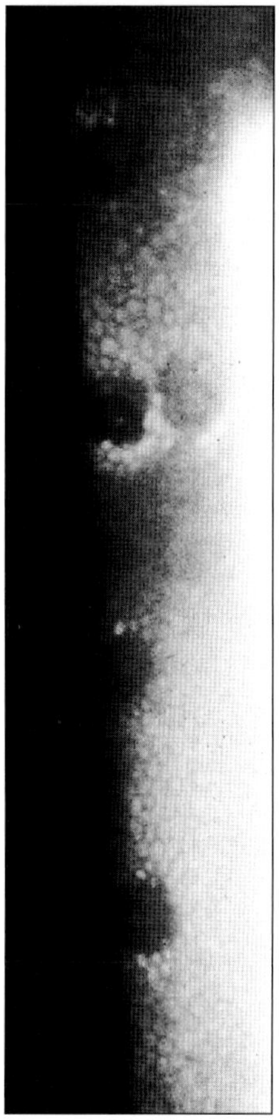

Fig. 73.3 Specular photomicrograph of vesicular lesions in PPCD appearing as rounded black areas that interrupt the dotted white endothelial mosaic. (Courtesy Mark Mannis, MD.)

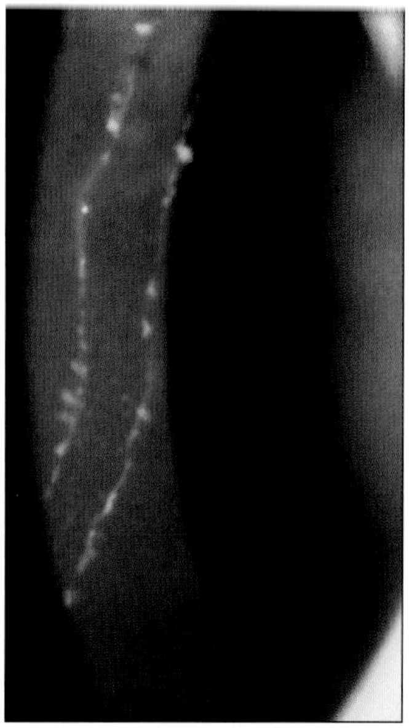

Fig. 73.4 Slit lamp appearance of a linear band lesion in PPCD. (Courtesy Richard Yee, MD.)

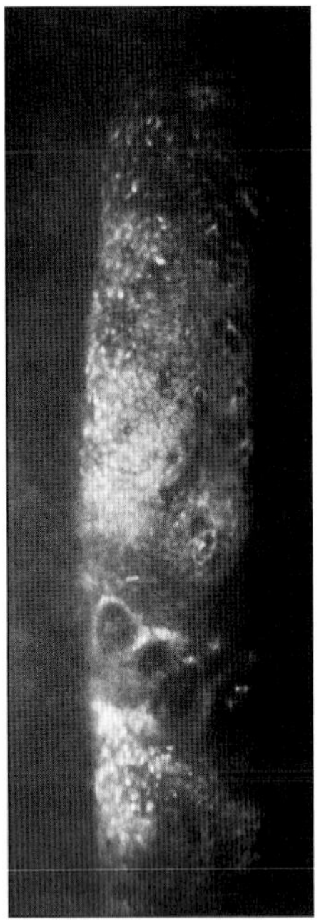

Fig. 73.5 Specular microscopy of confluent vesicles in a shallow trench representing a band lesion in PPCD. Above, there is an area with a mildly abnormal endothelial mosaic. (Courtesy Mark Mannis, MD.)

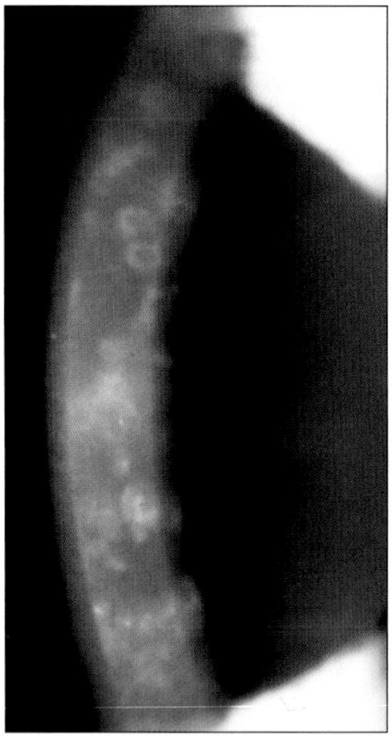

Fig. 73.6 Slit lamp photomicrograph of diffuse opacities in PPCD. (From Krachmer JH: *Trans Am Ophthalmol Soc* 83:413–475, 1985.)

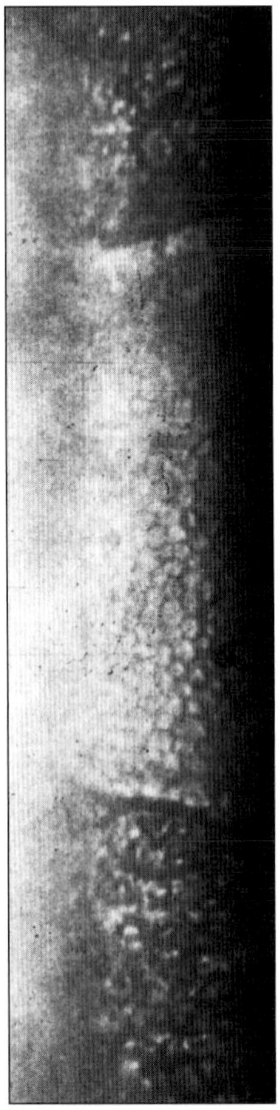

Fig. 73.7 Specular microscopy of a diffuse opacity, showing two well-demarcated dark areas with grossly abnormal-appearing cells and a large central area of normal endothelial mosaic intervening. (From Krachmer JH: *Trans Am Ophthalmol Soc* 83:413–475, 1985.)

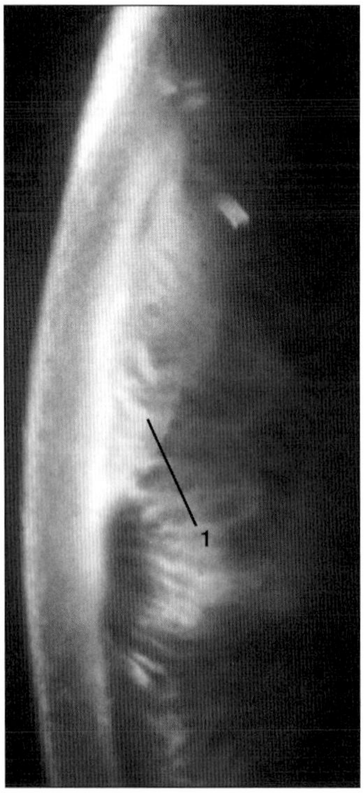

Fig. 73.8 A glasslike membrane (*1*) is seen between the iris and cornea. This peripheral anterior synechia is seen without gonioscopy.

Differential diagnosis

Posterior polymorphous corneal dystrophy and the iridocorneal endothelial (ICE) syndrome share many clinical features, including iridocorneal adhesions, glassy membranes over the angle and anterior surface of the iris, iris atrophy, corectopia, increased intraocular pressure, and corneal edema.[14–16] Traditionally, a dystrophy such as PPCD is by definition bilateral with familial inheritance, in contrast to the sporadic occurrence and unilateral presentation seen in the ICE syndrome. However, this distinction is less clear as a result of several case reports of patients with the presumptive diagnosis of the ICE syndrome but with bilateral involvement,[15–17] most of whom had the clinical diagnosis of essential iris atrophy. In one report a patient had clinical features of both the ICE syndrome and PPCD.[16]

Specular microscopy may be helpful in differential diagnosis.[8,18] The involved cells in the ICE syndrome classically appear as dark areas with a central highlight and light peripheral borders, although there may be variations in this appearance. Sherrard et al.[18] classified the pattern of the endothelial mosaic in the ICE syndrome into diffuse and partial forms. In the diffuse form the entire cornea is involved, while in the partial form there is only focal involvement. Sherrard et al.[18] believe it is possible to differentiate the endothelial cellular characteristics in the ICE syndrome from those in PPCD, but there is no unanimity about making this distinction on the basis of specular microscopy alone.[17,19] Histopathologic studies of ICE syndrome tissues also reveal differences from PPCD, as discussed later in this chapter.

The term *posterior corneal vesicle syndrome* has been coined to describe patients who have unilateral vesicular or band lesions similar to PPCD, but which is not found in other family members.[20] These patients typically have the onset at a younger age than is usual in PPCD (age range 7–24 years), with good vision, and without other ocular abnormalities. The lesions are stable. Specular microscopy of these lesions reveals changes similar to those seen in PPCD.[20,21]

PPCD can also present with a cloudy cornea at birth,[22,23] and should be included in the differential diagnosis of corneal opacification along with metabolic disorders, congenital hereditary endothelial dystrophy, congenital hereditary stromal dystrophy, congenital glaucoma, sclerocornea, congenital infections, and X-linked endothelial corneal dystrophy.[24]

Prognosis and management

In the great majority of patients, PPCD is stable and asymptomatic. However, in a small number of cases the dystrophy may be very extensive and progressive, necessitating surgical intervention. In the largest series of PPCD cases reported, including eight families with 120 individuals, only 13 patients required corneal transplantation surgery.[5] Risk factors for severe disease included the presence of iridocorneal adhesions and increased intraocular pressure. Only 27% of patients had iridocorneal adhesions, yet 57% of patients with iridocorneal adhesions required corneal transplantation. Similarly, only 14% of patients in this series had increased intraocular pressure, yet 62% of patients with increased intraocular pressure required corneal transplantation.

The prognosis for surgery also correlated with the presence of PAS and elevated intraocular pressure.[5] Fifty percent of patients undergoing transplantation attained 20/40 vision postoperatively and 55% of patients maintained clear grafts in this study. However, in the patients with PAS visible without gonioscopy on slit lamp examination, 80% had postoperative vision worse than 20/400. In contrast, 91% of patients with PAS visible only by gonioscopy, or with no synechiae, maintained a clear graft, and 82% attained 20/40 vision postoperatively.

In this same study, all patients with increased intraocular pressure preoperatively had problems with pressure control postoperatively.[5] Medical management with carbonic anhydrase inhibitors and topical medications, or surgical intervention with filtering procedures or cryotherapy, had limited success. In nine of 13 patients with elevated intraocular pressure preoperatively, the postoperative vision was worse than 20/400. Conversely, patients with normal intraocular pressure preoperatively did not encounter pressure problems postoperatively and had a good prognosis for visual recovery with transplantation. In summary, the presence of PAS visible without gonioscopy and increased intraocular pressure must be considered relative contraindications to corneal transplantation in PPCD.

PPCD can recur after transplantation. In the 22 corneal transplants in Krachmer's series, four corneas developed retrocorneal membranes, three of which led to opacified grafts.[5] Histologic examination was performed on only one cornea, which showed an epithelial-like endothelial membrane across the posterior aspect of the graft. Similar membranes were also reported on failed grafts in two patients with PPCD by Boruchoff et al.[25] and on two regrafted corneas from a single PPCD eye by Sekundo et al.[26]

Histopathology

The corneal epithelium and stroma show no remarkable features in PPCD, except for evidence of chronic edema, subepithelial fibrosis, and band keratopathy, depending on its duration and severity (Table 73.2). Descemet's membrane and the endothelium hold the most interest in PPCD pathologically as well as clinically. By light microscopy the abnormalities may vary from some thickening of Descemet membrane with rare foci of bilayered large endothelial cells (Fig. 73.9A), to 3–4 layered broad patches of flattened endothelial cells and irregular thickness of Descemet's membrane with focal absences (Fig. 73.9B).

Electron microscopy

Ultrastructurally, Boruchoff and Kuwabara[27] made the surprising finding that in focal areas the endothelium contained large squamous epithelial cells like those seen in epithelial downgrowth after penetrating injury. They contained large numbers of 8–10 nm intermediate filaments (tonofilaments), some in bundles and attached to prominent desmosomal intercellular junctions as in epithelial cells, but no cells had the tight junctions characteristic of endothelium (Fig. 73.10). Mitochondria, endoplasmic reticulum, and Golgi apparatus were sparse in the cytoplasm. Apical cell surfaces were densely covered by microvilli (Fig. 73.11).

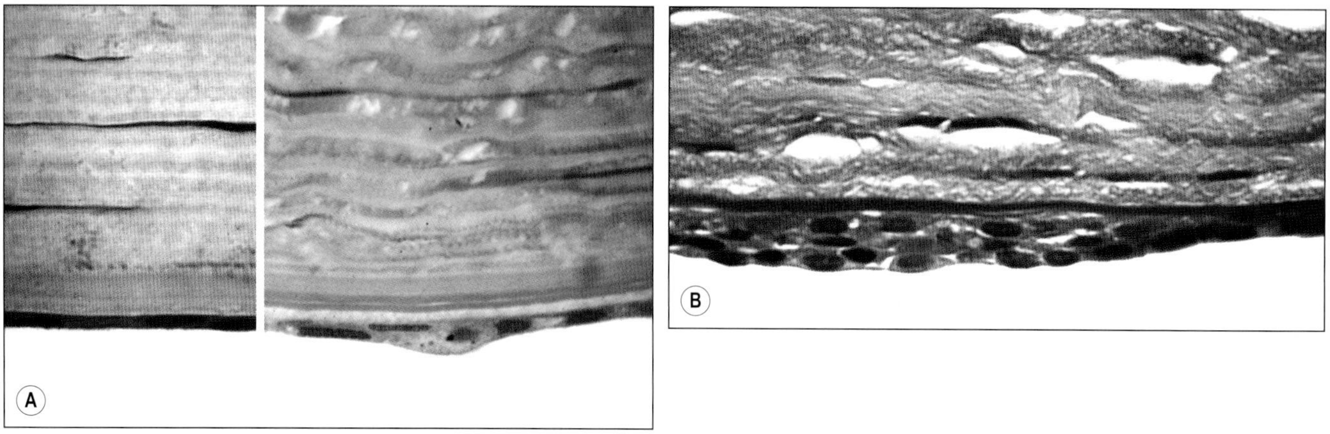

Fig. 73.9 Light microscopy of the endothelium in PPCD. (**A**) *Left*: Deep cornea showing dark enlarged endothelial cells with a thick Descemet's membrane. *Right*: Small area of multilayered cells with a multilaminar Descemet's membrane. (Courtesy T Kuwabara, MD.) (**B**) Large area of multilayered endothelial cells, with irregular thickness of Descemet's membrane. (PAS stain.) (Courtesy of M Rodrigues, MD.)

Table 73.2 Chief histopathologic characteristics of posterior membrane dystrophies

	PPCD	FECD	CHED1/CHED2
Epithelium	No edema, or late	Late edema Map-dot and fingerprint Scarring	Edema from early stage
Subepithelium	Late subepithelial fibrosis Late band keratopathy	Subepithelial fibrosis, thick in advanced disease	Subepithelial fibrosis Defects in Bowman's membrane
Superficial stroma			Spheroidal degeneration
Deeper stroma	Mild thickening, edema	Moderate thickening, edema	Marked thickening, edema, disrupted lamellar pattern
Descemet's membrane ABZ PNBZ	 Normal, thinner in early onset Absent or minimal Changes to a thick PCL-like layer with scant BM*	 Normal Thin and irregular Followed by a thick banded layer similar to the ABZ, also composing the guttae	 Normal Absent to poorly demarcated Replaced by thick mixed collagen components, some banded, and strands of BM
PCL (where present)	Fibrillar and banded Laminated	Fibrillar and banded, with wide and narrow spacing collagen, and oxytalan	Fibrillar Laminated
Endothelium	Epithelial-like metaplasia Multilayering, microvilli, cytokeratin-positive intermediate filaments, desmosomes Fibroblast-like metaplasia Degenerating endothelium	Thinned over guttae Low cell density Enlarged cells Fibroblast-like metaplaria, in end stage	Absent, markedly reduced, or dystrophic cells Rare multilayering, or microvilli
Trabeculum and iris	Can become covered by epithelial-like cells and BM	Normal	Normal

BM, Basement membrane; ABZ, anterior banded zone; PNBZ, posterior nonbanded zone; PCL, posterior collagenous layer.

The presence of this unusual epithelial-like cell type was confirmed in many reports over the next decade, using both transmission and scanning electron microscopy.[3,27–31] Normal endothelial cells with minimal or no microvilli over their free surfaces were also present, as well as fibroblast-like cells containing prominent endoplasmic reticulum[25,28,31,32] resembling the metaplastic endothelial cells common in reactive conditions.[33] Attenuated and degenerated endothelial cells were always present, showing a contracted appearance with blebs or holelike pits on their surface by scanning electron microscopy.

The epithelial-like nature of the new endothelial cell type in PPCD was strongly supported by the report of Rodrigues et al.[34] that its intermediate filaments stained positively with antibodies to human epidermal cytokeratins. These alternated with nonstaining patches appearing to represent

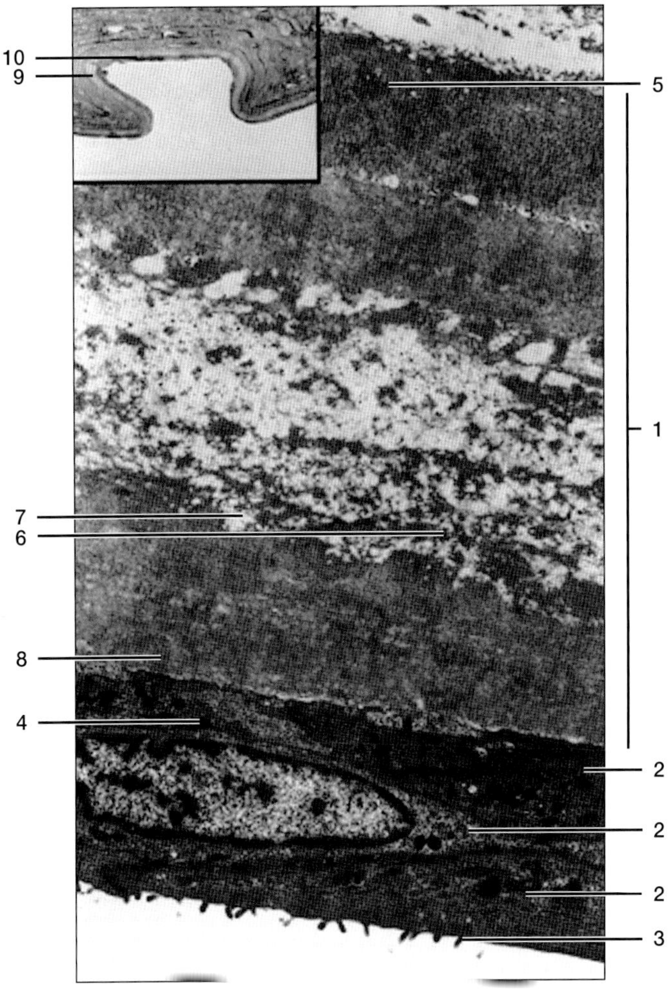

Fig. 73.10 Multilayered Descemet's membrane (*1*) and three layers of epithelial-like endothelium (*2*) with a microvillous surface (*3*) in PPMD. Endothelium has many desmosomal junctions (*4*). The outer layer of Descemet's membrane at the top of the figure has normal fetal banding (*5*), but the posterior nonbanded layer has mixed banded material (*6*), vacuolated areas (*7*) containing collagen fibers, and a compact basement membrane-like zone (*8*) next to the endothelium. *Inset*: Marked thickness of Descemet's membrane (*9*) and abnormal endothelial cells (*10*) on light microscopy. (Original magnification ×3000.) (Courtesy M. Rodrigues, MD).

normal endothelium. In tissue culture, the epithelial-like cells were also like epithelium in their more rapid growth rate, showing outgrowth from 2 to 3 days faster than endothelium from normal donor eyes.[35] In primary cultures, the epithelial-like and normal endothelium grew out as two cell lines, with cytokeratin positivity limited to the epithelial-like cells. A few fibroblast-like spindle cells were seen, but the majority were the large epithelial-like cells.[5]

Cockerham et al.[36] reported evidence that the epithelial-like PPCD endothelial cells do not represent a simple change from endothelium to normal surface epithelium. In seven PPCD corneas and five controls, the surface epithelium was positive with antibodies for cytokeratins (CKs) typically found in the cytoplasmic filaments of squamous epithelium, including panCK (pancytokeratin) AE1 and AE3. The endothelium in controls did not react with any of these

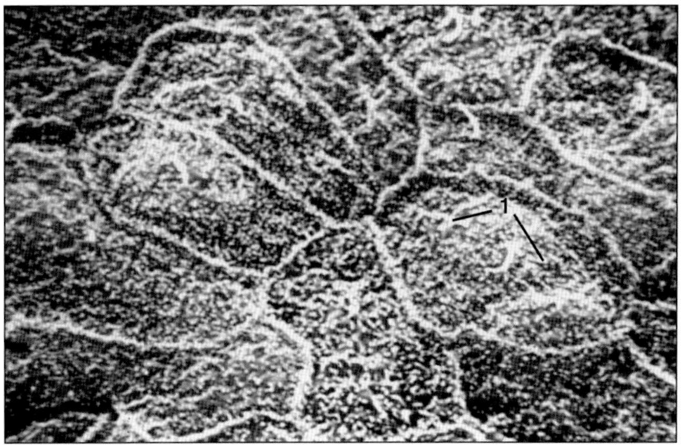

Fig. 73.11 Patch of metaplastic epithelial-like endothelial cells showing pleomorphism and polymegathism, intensely covered by microvilli (*1*) (Scanning electron micrograph). (Courtesy M. Rodrigues, MD.)

antibodies, but the endothelium in PPCD reacted strongly with panCK, less consistently with AE1 and AE3. Of interest was that the endothelium in all PPCD cases was diffusely positive for another cytokeratin, CK7, which did not react with the surface epithelium of either PPCD or controls. CK7 is a cytokeratin related to glandular epithelium, and known to be negative on stratified squamous epithelium and normal endothelium. The strong reactivity for CK7 in PPCD endothelium (also in CHED, see later discussion) may be of help in differentiating these entities from other abnormal endothelial processes and also in investigating further the nature of the aberrant cells.

Descemet's membrane in most PPCD cases has a normal 100–110 nm anterior banded zone (ABZ) approximately 3 μm in thickness,[3,5] as is normal for this zone throughout life. The wide banding in this zone is formed primarily by collagen type VIII,[37] a collagen common in fetal life, especially around blood vessels. Since the ABZ is secreted between 3 and 4 months of fetal life and term, with full banding of the basement membrane lamellae evident by the seventh month of gestation, a normal ABZ is strong evidence that the endothelial cells prenatally were functioning normally in this regard. It is noteworthy, however, that in many PPCD patients who had cloudy and edematous corneas at birth, the ABZ of Descemet's membrane was partially or in focal areas completely absent, thinned, or had nonhomogeneous banding,[22,23] suggesting endothelial dysfunction can occur even before 12 weeks' gestation.[22]

The next layer of normal Descemet's membrane, the posterior nonbanded zone (PNBZ), is slowly synthesized throughout postnatal life as a homogeneous basement membrane.[38] In PPCD there is little or no normal PNBZ, but only an abnormal mixture of collagenous components, often appearing multilaminated (see Fig. 73.10). These laminae contain aggregates of small collagen fibrils, 100 nm banded material resembling the ABZ, and large bundles of 50 and 100 nm banded collagen. Relatively normal, homogeneous type IV collagenous basement membrane may be admixed in deeper portions of this posterior collagenous layer (PCL), sometimes giving the appearance of a second thin Descemet's membrane (see Fig. 73.10).

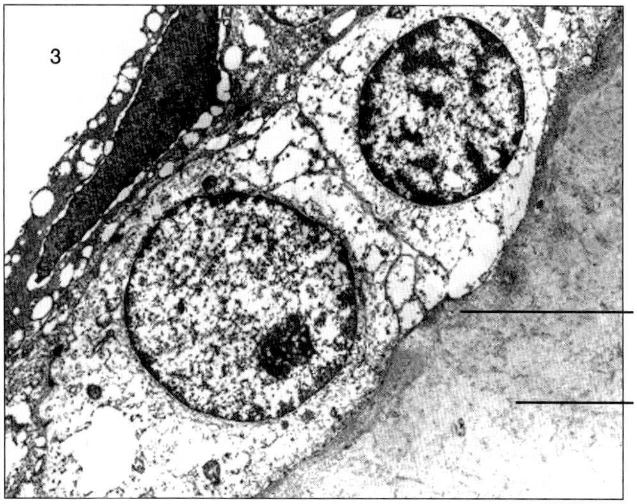

Fig. 73.12 An epithelial-like cell layer three cells deep, growing over the iris in PPCD, producing basement membrane (*1*) and a thick layer of new matrix (*2*) containing collagen fibers and bundles of microfibrils. Many dark desmosomal junctions between cells are visible. Anterior chamber (*3*) at upper left. (Original magnification ×14 560.)

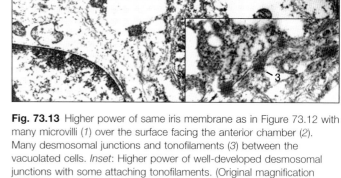

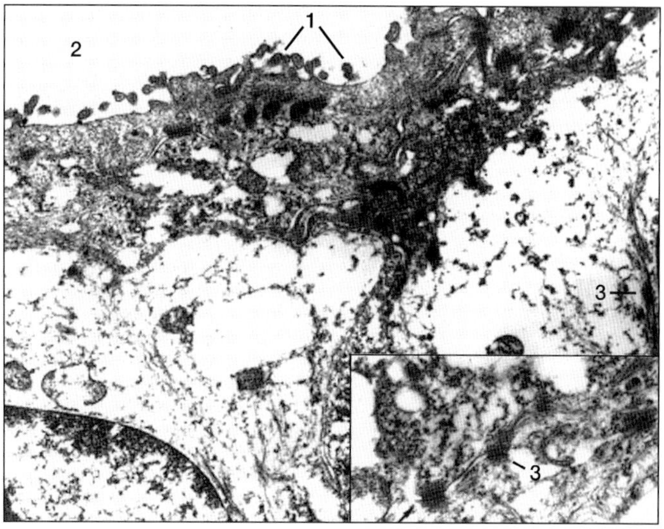

Fig. 73.13 Higher power of same iris membrane as in Figure 73.12 with many microvilli (*1*) over the surface facing the anterior chamber (*2*). Many desmosomal junctions and tonofilaments (*3*) between the vacuolated cells. *Inset*: Higher power of well-developed desmosomal junctions with some attaching tonofilaments. (Original magnification ×33 800. *Inset*: Original magnification ×54 600.)

The vesicles so characteristic of PPCD clinically have not had a completely satisfactory explanation pathologically. Some studies suggest they represent vacuolar degeneration within or between dying endothelial cells, often covered by a layer of epithelial-like cells.[39] Others infer that the multilayered epithelial-like cell clumps are themselves responsible.[27] Fusiform protuberances from Descemet's membrane that might appear vesicular were found to be dense plaques between two laminae of Descemet's membrane,[31] or gutta-like aggregates in the PCL.[5,39]

In some cases, the multilayered epithelial-like cells migrate back over the trabecula and iris, causing extensive peripheral synechiae and glaucoma (Fig. 73.12).[10,28] The thick membrane they elaborate over the trabecula resembles the abnormal Descemet's membrane – PCL. On the iris there is less basement membrane and a matrix of looser collagen fibrils, granular material, and tubular bundles suggestive of elastic system microfibrils (Fig. 73.13). The epithelium is multilayered with prominent desmosomal intercellular connections, unlike the monolayer of endothelial cells in the migrating cells of the ICE syndrome, connected by normal junctional complexes with a thinner basement membrane.[10] Recurrence of PPCD as a multilayered epithelial-like membrane on four corneas after grafting was a striking confirmation of the ability of these cells to migrate while maintaining their aberrant phenotype.[5,25,26]

Molecular genetics

Posterior polymorphous corneal dystrophy is a genetically heterogeneous disease. In the IC3D classification of corneal dystrophies three distinct genetic loci have been identified: two of which are category 1 (gene mapped and identified with a specific mutation known) and one listed as category 2 (mapped to a specific chromosome without a gene identified).[40] However, only one of the three loci has been validated in case-control studies.

In 1995, Heon et al.[41] performed a genome-wide linkage analysis in a large family with PPCD and found linkage to the long arm of chromosome 20 (20p11.2-q11.2) that is now designated as PPCD 1. Subsequently the VSX1 gene was mapped to this region by the same group and was considered a candidate gene for PPCD. They found two sequence changes in a severely affected proband (G160 and P247R).[42] However, the role of VSX1 is not clear as case-control studies on families with PPCD by Aldave,[43] Krafchak,[44] and Gwilliam[45] have not demonstrated the previously identified mutations.

Biswas et al.[46] performed a genome-wide search on several families with early-onset Fuchs' corneal dystrophy, and one two-generational family with PPCD, discovering a missense mutation common to both disease processes on the short arm of chromosome 1p34.3-p32 now classified as PPCD 2. The mutated gene codes for the alpha 2 chain of collagen VIII (COL8A2). However, additional screening of affected individuals with PPCD has failed to confirm similar mutations.[43,44,47]

Shimizu et al. recently identified a third genetic locus (10p11.2) now designated as PPCD 3 in a family initially described by Moroi.[48,49] Subsequent testing revealed four different nonsense and frameshift mutations in a gene that encodes the two-handed zinc-finger homeodomain transcription factor TCF8.[44] TCF8 is involved in the repression of the epithelial cell phenotype.[50] Two unusual features in this family are the aggressive growth of a retrocorneal membrane after surgical intervention and the presence of guttae in many members of the family with and without PPCD.[49] In addition, a recent study of four unrelated families by Liskova revealed four novel pathogenic mutations within the ZEBI gene located at the same loci (10p11.2).[51]

Aldave and colleagues performed additional screening for the TCF8 gene and identified eight different pathogenic mutations in eight probands without any mutations noted in 200 control chromosomes.[52] Thus, TCF8 mutations were found in 25% of affected families and were also associated with abdominal and inguinal hernias. TCF8 is involved in the repression of the epithelial cell phenotype and so its role in the pathogenesis of a disease that is associated with epithelial-like endothelial cells is interesting.[50,53]

Both vesicles and patches of dysmorphic endothelium similar to those in PPCD have been described in Alport's syndrome.[54] Examination of families with PPCD has revealed some individuals with Alport-like renal abnormalities, hematuria, and sensorineural hearing loss.[54] Also, one patient with PPCD and Alport's syndrome has been reported.[39] Classic Alport's syndrome is an X-linked dominant disease, resulting in some families from mutations in the $\alpha5$ chain of collagen IV, the prime basement membrane collagen, and one of three collagen IV α-chains with restricted distribution to the eye, ear, and kidney.[55] Krafchak et al. demonstrated a shared molecular component between the two diseases. They identified a binding site for TCF8 in the promotor of Alport syndrome gene COL4A3 as well as immunohistochemical evidence of COL4A3 in the corneal endothelium of a member of the original PPCD3 family.[44]

Fuchs' Endothelial Corneal Dystrophy

MIM #136800

In 1910, Fuchs[56] initially described bilateral corneal stromal and epithelial edema in elderly patients, without the benefit of slit lamp microscopy (see Table 73.1). Fuchs' endothelial corneal dystrophy (FECD) is a slowly progressive disease with initial onset in the fifth through seventh decades in life. Fifty percent of the time there is family clustering with an autosomal dominant inheritance pattern.[57–61] Females are predisposed to Fuchs' dystrophy and develop corneal guttae 2.5 times more frequently than males, progressing to corneal edema 5.7 times more often than males.[57] Magovern et al. described a family with early-onset FECD that recently has been found to have a distinct genetic loci and mutations from adult-onset FECD (see below).[59,62]

Clinical presentation and course

The initial manifestation in FECD is central corneal guttae. The guttae appear as dark spots on the posterior corneal surface by direct illumination (Fig. 73.14), which are highlighted in retroillumination and resemble dewdrops (Fig. 73.15). Pigment dusting is often present on the endothelium and, to the inexperienced observer, may be difficult to differentiate from guttae (Fig. 73.16). Patients at this early stage of disease are not symptomatic. Over time, the guttae spread peripherally and may also coalesce centrally, producing a beaten metal appearance associated with increased pigmentation (Fig. 73.17). Descemet's membrane becomes visibly thickened, gray, and irregular. A more advanced FECD may have 'buried guttae' centrally, where fibrous thickening of Descemet's membrane masks the presence of guttae.[61,63]

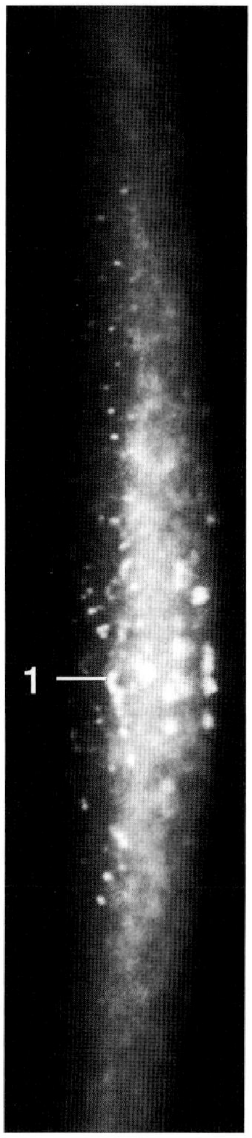

Fig. 73.14 Slit lamp photomicrograph of cornea guttata (*1*) in Fuchs' corneal dystrophy. (Courtesy Jay Krachmer, MD.)

Corneal edema is initially manifest in the posterior stroma adjacent to Descemet's membrane and just behind Bowman's membrane, causing a fine gray haze best seen with sclerotic scatter. In addition, swelling of the corneal stroma can produce fine vertical wrinkles or striae in Descemet's membrane. Microcystic epithelial edema may follow and is seen as a stippled pattern that stands out in sclerotic scatter. Using fluorescein stain, the microcystic pattern is highlighted as a disruption in the tear film. At this point, the patient's vision will be reduced, most prominently in the morning. Progressive stromal edema results in a ground-glass opacification with marked thickening of the central cornea. The epithelial microcystic changes may coalesce to form bullae, which can lead to epithelial erosions and fingerprint lines (Fig. 73.18). Irregularity of the corneal surface and stromal haze further reduce vision. Confocal microscopy has aided in the diagnosis of advanced FECD where corneal edema may obscure visualization of the endothelium.[64]

In end-stage disease, infrequently seen today because of improved success with corneal transplantation, avascular subepithelial fibrous scarring occurs between the epithelium and Bowman's membrane, best seen with tangential

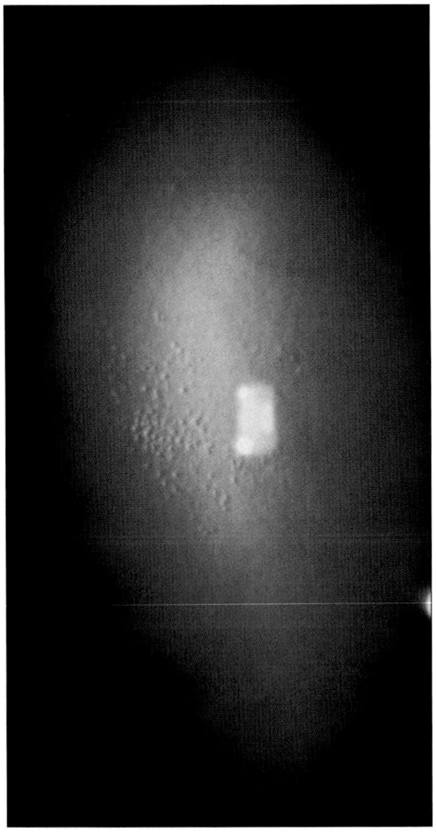

Fig. 73.15 Slit lamp photograph of highlighted corneal guttae in retroillumination resembling dewdrops, in Fuchs' dystrophy. (Courtesy Jay Krachmer, MD.)

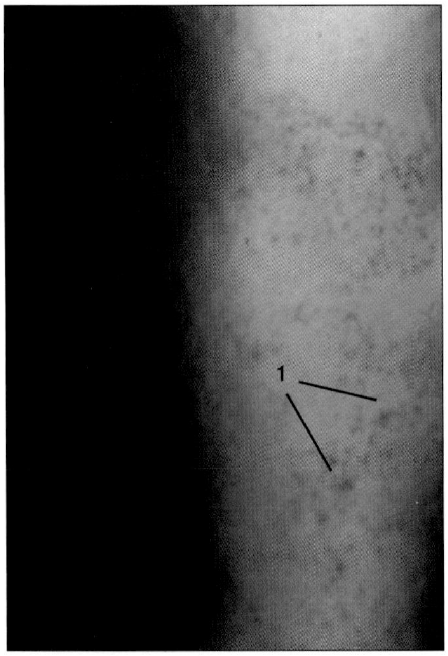

Fig. 73.16 Slit lamp photomicrograph of corneal guttae with melanin granule pigmentation (*1*) in Fuchs' dystrophy.

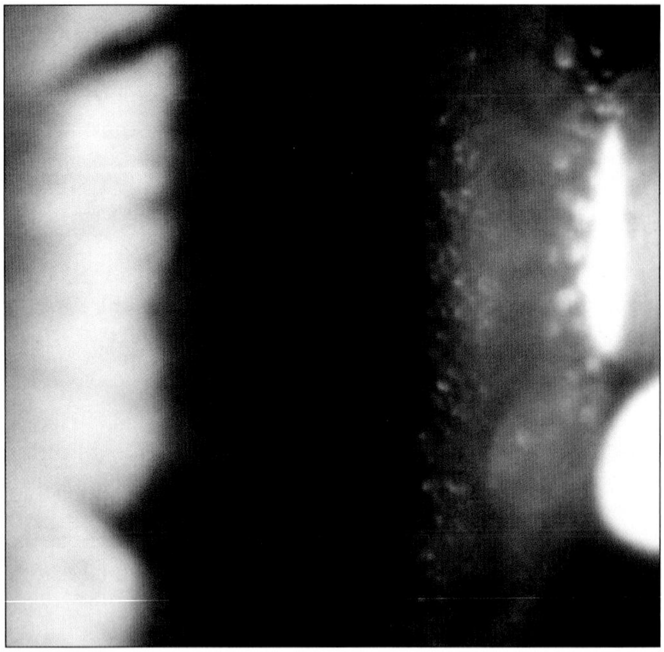

Fig. 73.17 Slit lamp photomicrograph of beaten metal appearance of confluent guttae in Fuchs' dystrophy.

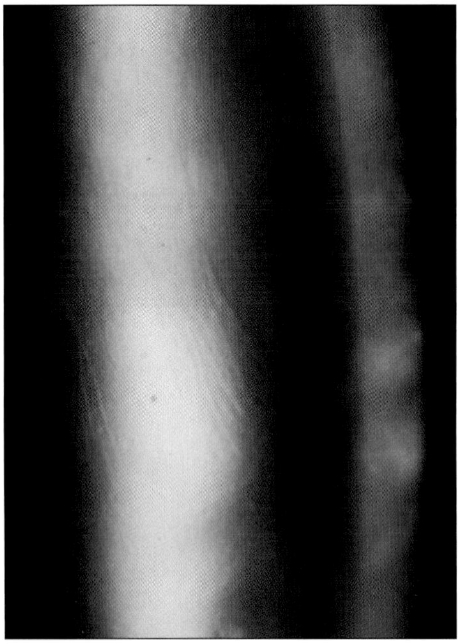

Fig. 73.18 Slit lamp photomicrograph of fingerprint changes secondary to corneal edema in Fuchs' dystrophy. (Courtesy Jay Krachmer, MD.)

illumination (Fig. 73.19). Peripheral superficial corneal neovascularization can also occur. Subepithelial scarring may eliminate the recurrent erosions, but the irregularity of the surface and loss of transparency further reduce vision.

Magovern first identified a family with early-onset FECD.[59] In this subtype of FECD the guttae present within the first decade of life and as early as age 3 years. On slit lamp examination with retroillumination there is a fine, patchy distribution of guttae in contrast to the coarse and distinct guttae

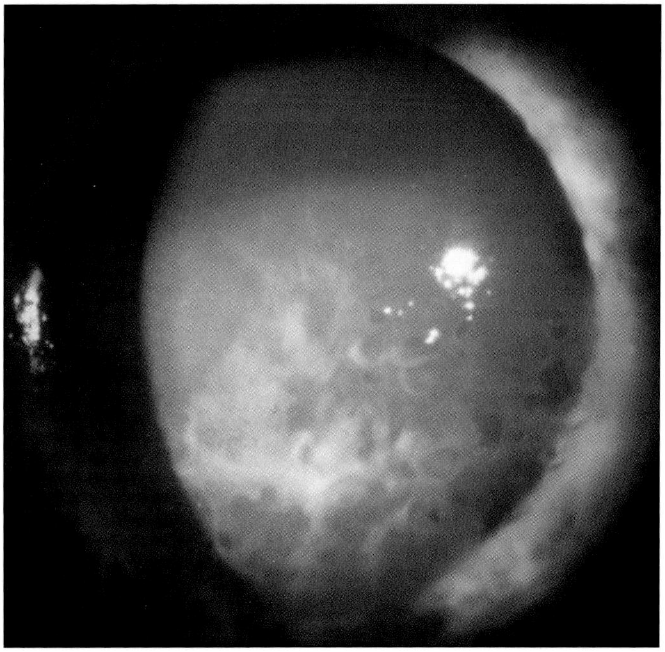

Fig. 73.19 Slit lamp micrograph of subepithelial fibrosis and bullae in Fuchs' dystrophy.

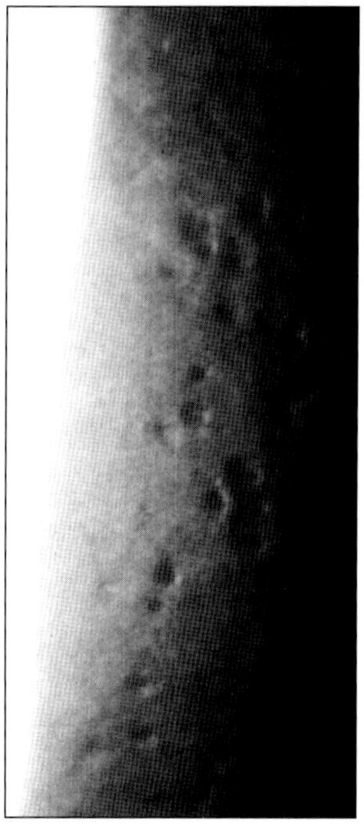

Fig. 73.20 Slit lamp photomicrograph of corneal pseudoguttae secondary to intraocular inflammation, which resolved after cessation of the uveitis.

seen in late-onset FECD. Specular microscopy shows small, shallow guttae in the center of the endothelial cell in contrast to the larger guttae seen in late-onset FECD. There is a similar temporal progression as late-onset FECD but with an earlier onset. There is high penetrance without a sexual predilection.

Abbott et al.[65] described a nonguttate corneal endothelial degeneration in six phakic patients who had unilateral edema, with only polymorphic corneal endothelial cells in the opposite eye. The endothelial cell counts were decreased (840 to 1992/mm^2), with no evidence of corneal guttae in either eye clinically or histologically. While these cases may be a variant of FECD as suggested by Abbott et al.,[65] the ultrastructural differences seem significant enough to make it a distinct entity. The accumulation of more clinical data about age of onset, family history, specular microscopy, and course, with immunologic and genetic correlation, will help to define whether this is a clinical entity distinguishable from classic FECD.

In one recent report, FECD was the most common corneal dystrophy associated with typical signs and topographic evidence of keratoconus. Patients with decreased vision and FECD should be evaluated carefully for corneal steepening or irregularity secondary to keratoconus as the cause of the reduced acuity.[13] It is not known if there is a common pathogenesis between the two dystrophies.

Differential diagnosis

Focal gutta formation without corneal edema has been observed in interstitial keratitis, particularly in linear arrangement under the deep vessels.[66] Guttae have also been observed in macular dystrophy and posterior polymorphous dystrophy.[2] In each instance, associated corneal and anterior segment findings make differential diagnosis straightforward.

Corneal pseudoguttae can be seen after trauma, intraocular inflammation, infection, toxins, and thermokeratoplasty (Fig. 73.20). These apparent guttae are transient, representing edema of the endothelial cells, and disappear with resolution of the underlying condition.[67]

Central herpetic disciform keratitis can mimic FECD; however, the presence of underlying keratic precipitates (KP) helps to differentiate the conditions. With acute corneal inflammation, the KP may be difficult to see, but with resolution of the edema they become more prominent.

Chandler's syndrome, one of the triad in the ICE syndrome, can be confused with corneal guttae since its endothelial pattern has a prominent beaten-bronze appearance with overlying corneal edema. However, it is typically unilateral, which helps to differentiate the two conditions.

Prognosis and management

The medical management of patients with FECD with visually significant edema includes topical hypertonic saline solutions, dehydration of the cornea by a blow dryer in the morning or throughout the day, and reduction of intraocular pressure. Bandage lenses may be helpful in the treatment of recurrent erosion caused by epithelial bullae.

FECD is a common indication for corneal transplantation. According to the Eye Bank statistical report, 9.2% of patients who underwent corneal transplantation in 2007 had FECD.[68] However, this may be an underestimate, as postcataract corneal edema was the preoperative diagnosis in an additional 15.7% of patients who had transplants. These patients may have had undiagnosed FECD preoperatively or were diagnosed with FECD but not felt to be at risk for corneal decompensation following surgery.

It is difficult to predict the risk of corneal decompensation with cataract surgery in patients with corneal guttae. Measuring the endothelial cell count with specular microscopy may be helpful; however, there is only an indirect statistical correlation between endothelial cell count and corneal hydration. When the cell count is between 2000 and 750 cells/mm^2 the compensatory mechanisms of increased metabolic activity and increasing number and density of pump sites may prevent significant corneal swelling.[69,70] However, at 500 cell/mm^2 the endothelial cells become so spread out that the normal compensatory mechanisms fail and corneal edema results.[71] The American Academy of Ophthalmology guidelines, as outlined in the *External Disease and Corneal* textbook (Section 8 in the Basic and Clinical Science Course) suggests that an endothelial cell count of less than 1000 should raise concern about the possibility of corneal decompensation with intraocular surgery.[72]

Another option is to perform corneal pachymetry. The American Academy of Ophthalmology guideline found in Section 8 of the Basic and Clinical Science Course[72] and a recent study from Wilmer Eye Institute[73] both suggest that a corneal thickness of over 640 microns (μm) increases the risk of corneal decompensation with cataract surgery. The difficulty with the corneal pachymetry measurements is that there is a significant amount of individual variation in corneal thickness. One helpful technique is to compare the mid-peripheral corneal thickness with the central corneal thickness. If the central corneal thickness exceeds the mid-peripheral thickness, this may be a indication of clinically significant corneal thickening.

It is also important to use clinical signs in the decision-making process, such as symptomatic blurring in the morning or evidence of epithelial edema on slit lamp examination. In general, the decision to perform a cataract surgery alone versus a triple procedure is based upon many factors, including the patient's expectations and visual requirements, and is best made in consultation with the patient after a thorough discussion of the alternatives.

The prognosis for corneal transplant surgery in FECD is good. To date, the best long-term data are from patients undergoing full-thickness penetrating keratoplasty. In one study from Price et al. the postoperative period required for good visual function was found to be slightly slower than, but comparable to, keratoconus, with 98% of patients maintaining clear grafts with follow-up from 3 to 84 months.[74] Today, endothelial transplantation is the treatment of choice for patients with FECD. To this point, there have been no long-term studies on graft survival with endothelial transplantation.

Histopathology

The primary site of pathology in Fuchs' dystrophy is the endothelial cell that lays down abnormal Descemet's membrane and, as its barrier and pumping action wane, leads to stromal and epithelial edema (see Table 73.2). Far more corneas with Fuchs' dystrophy have been examined than with any other dystrophy because of its frequency and early recognition, with extensive light and ultrastructural pathology providing confirmation that this is an endothelial disease (see reference 60). Changes in the deep cornea will be described first, then the progression of secondary effects in the anterior cornea and stroma.

By light microscopy, flat preparations of the endothelium show increase in cellular size and irregularity of shape as they are stretched and their nuclei are pushed into the valleys between the developing guttate bodies, compared with the regular hexagonal mosaic of normal endothelial cells (Fig. 73.21). On cross-section, there is generalized cellular thinning over the apices of the guttate excrescences as they protrude into the anterior chamber at an early stage, with an overall reduction in number of cells. Descemet's membrane becomes two to three times thicker than the

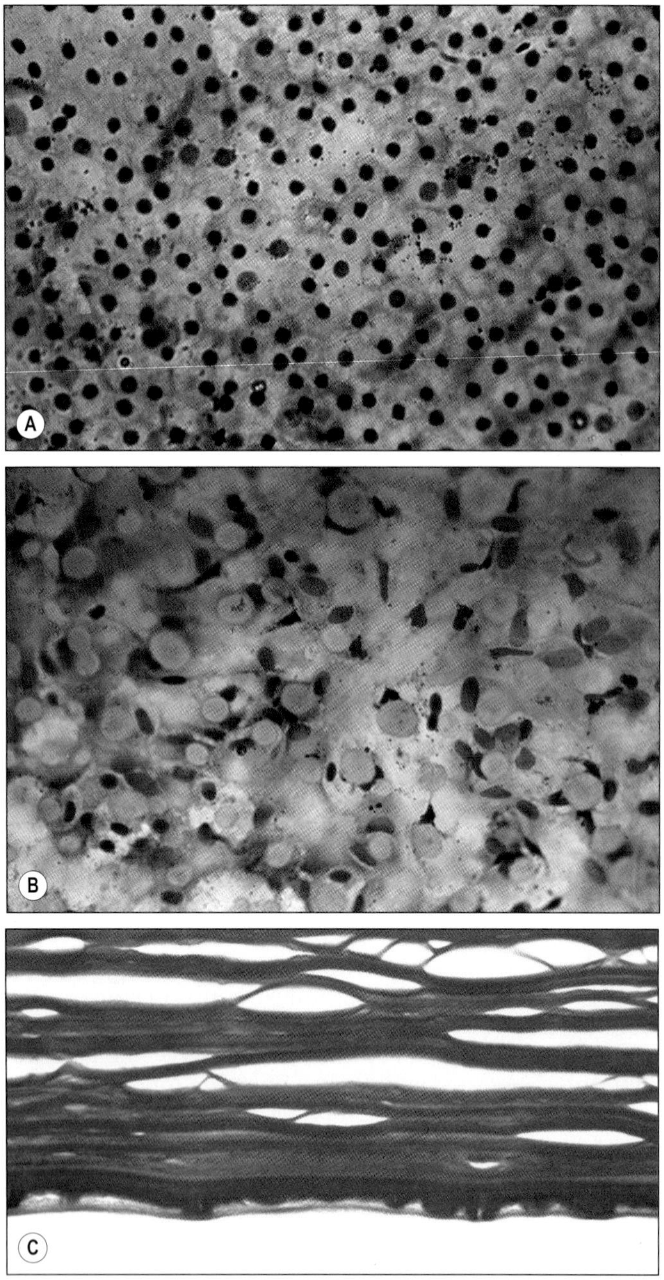

Fig. 73.21 Flat preparations and cross-sections of endothelium and Descemet's membrane in Fuchs' dystrophy. (**A**) Regular pattern of hexagonal endothelial cells with small round nuclei in normal adult eye bank eye. (**B**) Completely disrupted endothelial pattern in moderately advanced Fuchs' dystrophy. Marked decrease in cells, with large and small polymorphic nuclei, displaced to the side by the larger, round guttate bodies under them. (**C**) Many large guttae 'buried' in a less PAS-positive fibrous membrane (PCL). (PAS stain.)

normal 10–12 μm for the age group affected and, even by light microscopy, may show a lamellar pattern in this thickening as it progresses. Often the guttae become buried and almost invisible as a result of the synthesis of new fibrous components around them. Since Descemet's membrane is a basement membrane, it is intensely PAS positive, as are the guttate bodies, but the new fibrous tissue is usually less positive and makes the lamellar pattern more evident. Both hematoxylin and eosin and PAS stains demonstrate well the mushroom-shaped hemispherical or flat-topped anvil-like profiles of the guttate bodies.[61,63]

Electron microscopy

Electron microscopy has made FECD an important model for the study of aberrant Descemet's membrane synthesis by the endothelium. In FECD the 100–110 nm anterior banded zone (ABZ) of Descemet's membrane, secreted during the fourth fetal month until close to term, is entirely normal in banding and thickness (3 μm) (Fig. 73.22).[75,76] The banded fibers are largely composed of type VIII collagen,[77] a collagen commonly found in fetal tissues, especially around blood vessels. About the time of birth the endothelial cells should switch to synthesis of a homogeneous, amorphous type IV basement membrane collagen, which will compose the posterior nonbanded zone (PNBZ) of Descemet's membrane. Unlike the ABZ, the PNBZ increases slowly throughout life at a fairly constant rate to become the major portion of Descemet's membrane. The width of these two layers can thus be used to date approximately when synthesis of an abnormal Descemet's membrane began.

Many investigators have noted or illustrated a thinner than normal PNBZ of Descemet's membrane in FECD. In 11 FECD corneas, Bourne et al.[76] found the PNBZ absent in four eyes, with thinning in the rest to a mean of 1.8 μm compared with a normal 7.8 μm for this age group, concluding that the onset of FECD begins before the age of 20 years in most cases.

Besides a thin or absent PNBZ, the most typical finding in FECD is an abnormal posterior collagenous layer (PCL) (Fig. 73.23).[63,76,78] This layer is present in all cases and is responsible for most of the thickness in Descemet's

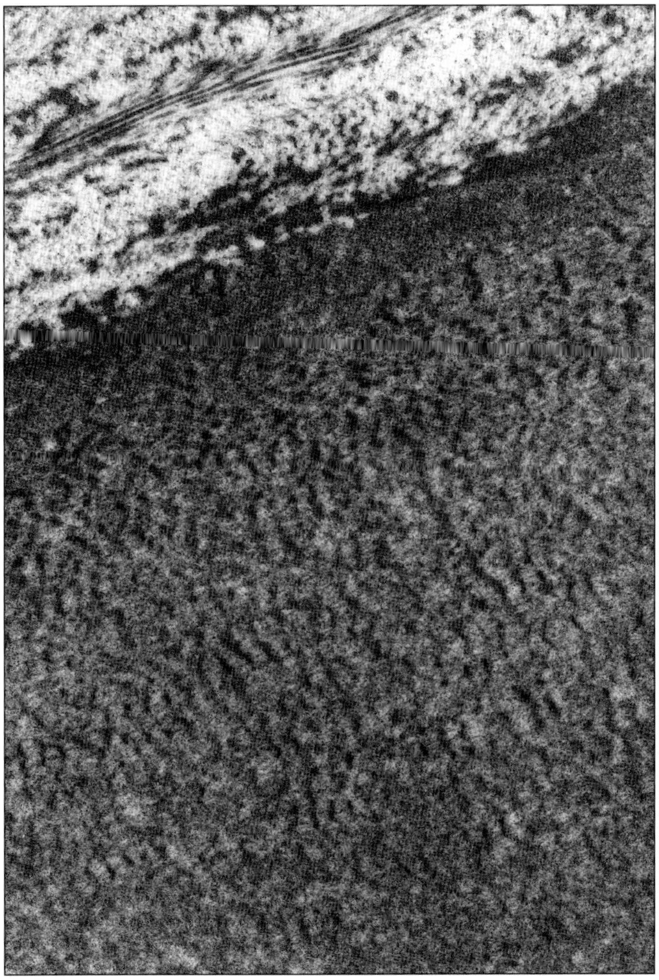

Fig. 73.22 Relatively normal columns of wide-banding collagen in ABZ of Fuchs' dystrophy. (Original magnification ×40 770.)

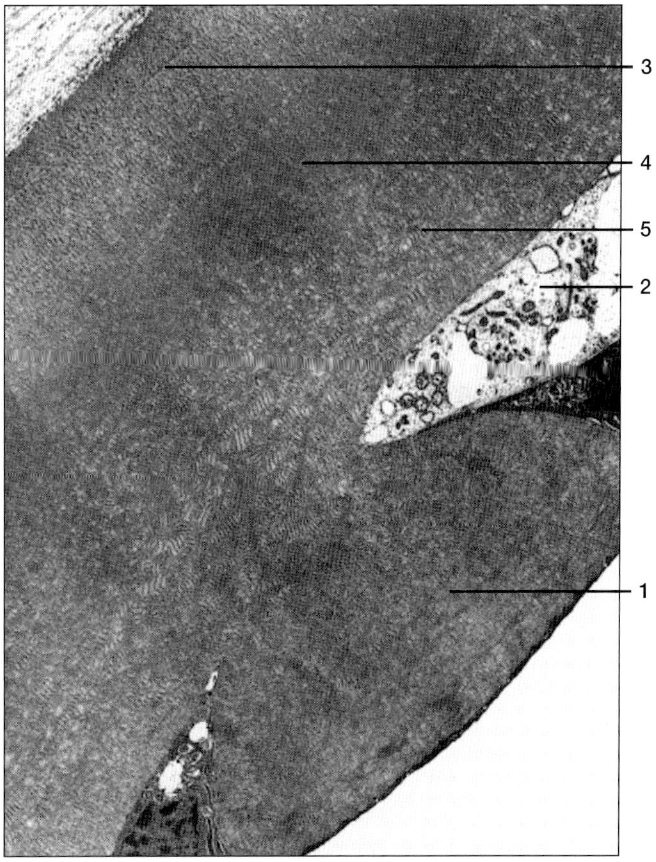

Fig. 73.23 Electron micrograph of Descemet's membrane and endothelium in Fuchs' dystrophy in a 38-year-old woman. Flat anvil-like guttate body (*1*) covered by thin endothelium with a pale dystrophic cell (*2*) at one edge. Normal ABZ (*3*). Irregular thin PNBZ (*4*), mostly replaced by a thick ABZ-like PCL layer showing homogeneous basement membrane with a variety of wide-spacing collagen forms (*5*) composing most of Descemet's membrane, including the guttate body. (Original magnification ×8200.)

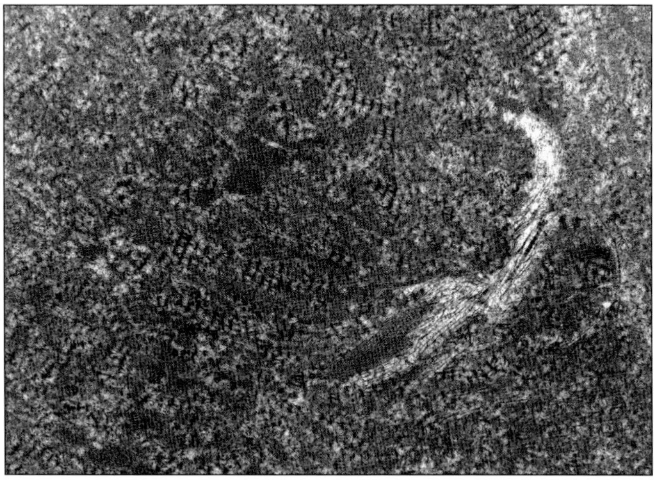

Fig. 73.24 Detail of guttate body. Wide-spacing and narrow-banded fibrillar bundles with scanty homogeneous basement membrane are seen. (Original magnification ×24 840.)

membrane as well as composing the guttate bodies, giving a mean Descemet's total thickness of 16.6 µm in one study.[76] The PCL is filled with 100 nm banded fibers similar to those in the normal ABZ and continuous with the thin PNBL, but more irregular because amorphous basement membrane is also scattered through it. The guttae are continuous with this layer (Fig. 73.24) and may be reduplicated, one lying on top of the other, surrounded by spindled bundles of 100 nm wide-spacing collagen and bundles with a narrower 50 nm periodicity. These lie in a 'border layer'[78] which may have some amorphous basement membrane also, and 10 nm thin filaments that probably represent oxytalan (elastic system microfibrils) around the guttate bodies.[79] These fibrillin-containing microfibrils are not a normal component of Descemet's membrane but do serve as attachment fibers to other basement membranes.

The posterior border layer may be added to by a simpler loose fibrous layer whose thickness increases with greater corneal edema (Fig. 73.25).[76] This fibrous layer contains primarily 20–30 nm collagen fibrils and bundles (Fig. 73.26) and is most like the undifferentiated PCLs in aphakic bullous keratopathy. None of these components is specific for FECD, since they can be seen in other diseases and conditions involving the corneal endothelium, but their varying proportions and locations can help to identify the different entities (see Table 73.2).

With advancing disease, the endothelial cells in FECD become increasingly dedifferentiated from their normal morphology as well as function. This alteration or metaplasia makes them appear more fibroblast-like cytologically, with increased rough endoplasmic reticulum, cytoplasmic filaments, lysosomes, membrane-bound vacuoles, phagocytosed pigment granules, and some desmosomal intercellular junctions. Increasingly degenerate changes occur (see Fig. 73.23) with swollen mitochondria, widened intercellular spaces, larger vacuoles, and finally pyknotic nuclei and death of many cells. The continuous loss of endothelial

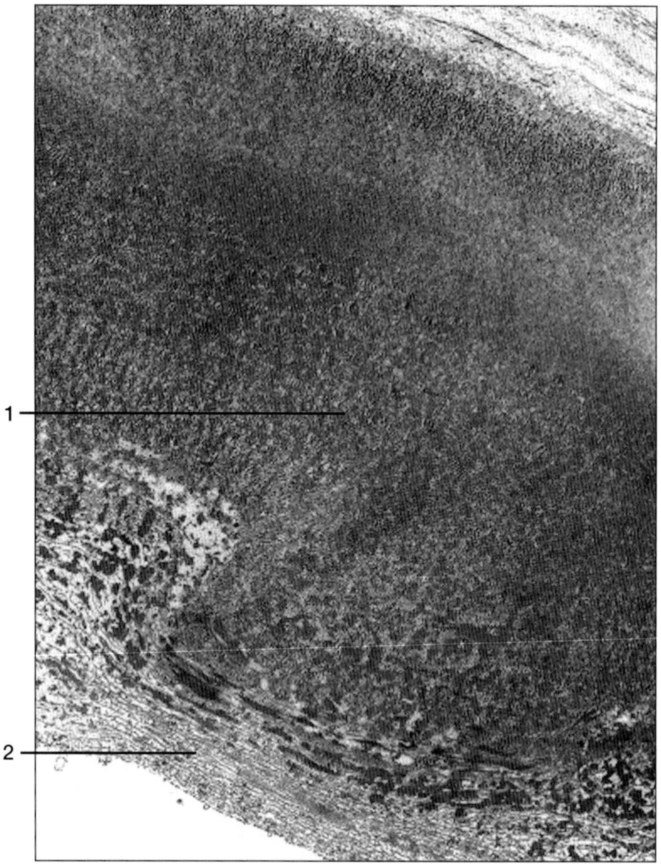

Fig. 73.25 Advanced Fuchs' dystrophy with almost identical morphology to Figure 73.23, but the guttate body (*1*) is 'buried' by development of a simple fibrillar posterior collagenous layer (*2*) in a 65-year-old woman. (Original magnification ×5800.)

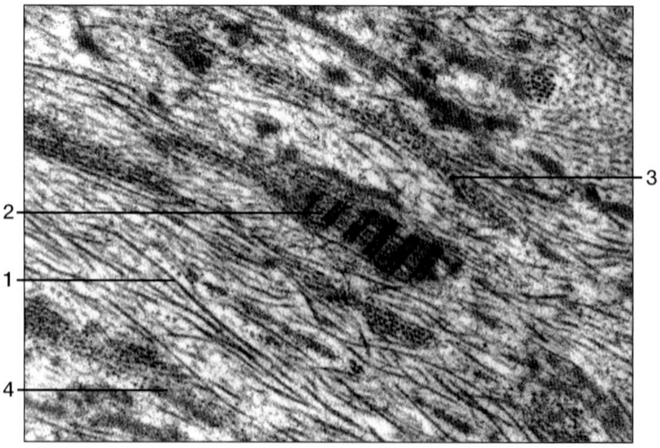

Fig. 73.26 Details of PCL from cornea with advanced Fuchs' dystrophy in Figure 73.23, showing large numbers of small collagen fibers (*1*), wide-spacing collagen ellipsoids (*2*), narrow-banded material (*3*), and a minimum of basement membrane-like clumps (*4*). (Original magnification ×67 500.)

cells is very evident in FECD, with cell counts of 5–10 per high-power microscopic field in advanced disease, compared with counts of 15–20 in a similar age group of normal corneas.

Thinning of the endothelium over the enlarging guttate bodies may result in complete baring of these bodies as the disease progresses, seen most dramatically by scanning electron microscopy. While some of this baring may be artifact, the cells are undoubtedly more fragile than usual, separate more easily from Descemet's membrane, and are markedly decreased in number. Occasionally, long endothelial cell processes extend into the guttate bodies in cleftlike spaces, like those in peripheral Hassal-Henle warts. Warts have a composition similar to that of guttae except for scanty banded components. In advanced cases of FECD the endothelial cells produce almost entirely fibrous components, and the few remaining endothelial cells have an elongated or stellate fibroblast-like shape.

Gottsch and colleagues[80] used immunohistochemistry and transmission electron microscopy to study early-onset FECD patients and found many similarities to late-onset FECD including a markedly thicker Descemet's membrane, refractile strands and blebs staining intensely for COL8A2, alpha 1 and alpha 2 subtypes of collagen VIII along the anterior edge of Descemet's membrane (DM), and deposition of collagen IV, fibronectin, and laminin. In later work by the same group there were also significant differences observed.[81] The DM in early-onset FECD was considerably thicker than commonly observed in late-onset FECD even though the patients tended to be younger at the time of surgical intervention. In addition, the guttae were much flatter, appearing as structural discontinuities buried deep within DM, correlating with the clinical findings of fine, shallow guttae. As the disease progressed, increased secretion of collagen VIII by the stressed endothelium produced buried guttae. The most anterior layer of DM showed unusually high levels of collagen VIII, indicating that the mutation may have been present prior to birth.

Molecular genetics

In adult-onset FECD many patients have no known inheritance pattern, placing it in category 3 of the IC3D classification (see Table 73.1). However, Sundin et al.[82] studied a single family with adult-onset FECD who had an autosomal dominant mendelian inheritance with high penetrance. A whole-genome linkage scan mapped to a single locus at 13pTel-13q12.13 with significant two-point LOD scores of 3.91 at D13S1236 and 3.80 at D13S1304. They were unable to find a gene mutation. Sundin et al.[83] later studied three additional families, also with autosomal dominant inheritance, but with an incomplete penetrance and high phenocopy. They identified a second genetic locus FCD2, at 18q21.2-q21.3, again without a gene mutation identified. The presence of a known chromosome loci without a gene mutation identified place it in category 2 in the IC3D classification.

However, Vithana and colleagues[84] recently identified four heterozygous and one deletion mutations in the SLC4A11 gene in 89 patients with classic late-onset FECD. The missense mutations involved amino acid residues showing high interspecies conservation, suggesting that the aberrant misfolded protein may play an important role in the pathology of FECD. This mutation was also found in AR CHED (CHED2) which will be discussed later.

Early-onset FECD is considered category 1 in the IC3D classification as it has been associated with both a genetic locus and specific gene mutation. Biswas and colleagues[46] first identified a mutation in the gene for the alpha 2 chain of collagen VIII (COL8A2 -Q455K) on chromosome 1 p34.3-p32. This three-generational family had 13 affected members, all of whom shared the same missense mutation of a glutamine substitution by lysine in codon 455 (Gln455Lys). Gottsch et al.[62] performed genetic linkage analysis on the original family with early-onset FECD identified by Magovern and found a second COL8A2 mutation L450W. The clinical presentation of the L450 W and Q455K COL8A2 patients is similar with small, shallow guttae.

Case-control studies by Kobayashi et al.[85] and Aldave et al.[86] demonstrated that the gene mutations found in early-onset FECD (COLA81 and COL8A2) were not present in adult-onset FECD. Further, Mehta and colleagues[87] investigated whether the TCF8 gene implicated in the pathogenesis of PPCD could be associated with FECD. A genome-wide analysis on 74 unrelated Chinese patients found that only one patient had a novel missense mutation in TCF8, demonstrating that TCF8 probably does not play a role in the pathogenesis of FECD.

Congenital Hereditary Endothelial Dystrophy

Congenital hereditary endothelial dystrophy (CHED) is a rare corneal dystrophy except in Saudi Arabia[88] and south India.[89] It is bilateral, symmetric, noninflammatory corneal clouding without other anterior segment abnormalities that is usually evident at birth or within the early postnatal period (see Table 73.1). The corneal opacification extends to the limbus without clear zones (Fig. 73.27). It is associated with marked corneal clouding, often two to three times normal. It is primarily a diagnosis of exclusion, so other causes of corneal clouding must be ruled out first.

Cases consistent with CHED were described sporadically in the European literature under many different names, from the first report by Laurence[90] in 1893 of 'corneitis interstitialis in utero.' In 1960, Maumenee[91] suggested that the disease arises from an abnormality in the endothelial cells, strengthened by evidence of an abnormal Descemet's membrane on electron microscopy.[92,93] Kenyon and Maumenee gave the disease its current name.[94]

Recent genetic analysis confirms that the autosomal recessive and autosomal dominant disease are two distinct entities.[95–101] In early reports, some series attempted to separate the autosomal dominant from autosomal recessive disease on the basis of clinical presentation, consanguinity, apparent familial inheritance, or geographic location,[91–93,102,103] while in other series the authors did not distinguish between inheritance as they felt the clinical presentation was too similar.[103–105] As a result, a review of CHED is partially confounded by the lack of reports based upon genetic analysis clearly delineating the two groups.

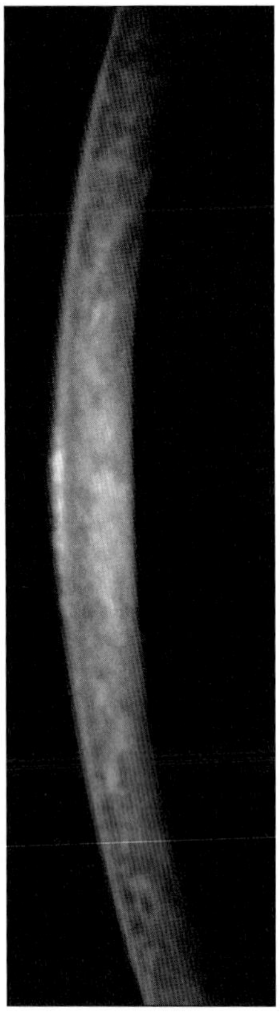

Fig. 73.27 Slit lamp photomicrograph of congenital hereditary endothelial dystrophy. (Courtesy A Sugar, MD.)

Differential diagnosis

The most common systemic metabolic abnormality associated with corneal opacification in childhood is one of the mucopolysaccharidoses. However, in these diseases, corneal clouding is not present at birth, typically developing within the first few years of life. Since the opacification results from infiltration of the tissues by mucopolysaccharides rather than edema, the cornea is not thickened. Except in the Scheie syndrome, other systemic stigmata are typically present. A urinalysis or corneal biopsy will usually identify the abnormal metabolic product to confirm the diagnosis.

Differentiation from congenital glaucoma should not be difficult because of the increased intraocular pressure in glaucoma, often an increase in corneal diameter, Haab's striae, and, in severe disease, buphthalmos. Anterior segment dysgenesis such as Axenfeld's syndrome or Peters' anomaly can also present with elevated intraocular pressure and corneal opacification. However, these have other associated anterior segment abnormalities.

Transient corneal edema can occur in congenital rubella, but, in contrast to CHED, there is episcleral injection, typically a nuclear cataract, increased intraocular pressure, posterior synechiae, miosis, and chorioretinopathy. Syphilitic interstitial keratitis also produces an inflamed eye with corneal clouding, deep stromal vascularization, and iris atrophy, but it rarely occurs within the first year of life. After resolution, there is corneal scarring rather than edema. Systemic abnormalities such as Hutchinson's teeth or saddle nose may also aid in the diagnosis.

Forceps injury results in localized corneal edema overlying the break or breaks in Descemet's membrane, typically unilateral. The edema is transitory, leaving a double linear scar in Descemet's membrane at the rupture edges.

Most corneal dystrophies are not evident at birth, developing only after the first decade. Besides CHED, the only exceptions are PPCD and congenital hereditary stromal dystrophy (CHSD). PPCD may be differentiated from CHED by the presence of other anterior segment abnormalities such as endothelial vesicles and bands, a characteristic endothelial pattern on specular microscopy (if possible), and bridging synechiae in the patient or family. In CHSD the corneal opacification appears as full-thickness, feathery clouding of the stroma with a normal corneal thickness.[106] In addition, the histopathology in CHSD shows a normal epithelium, Bowman's layer, endothelium, and Descemet's membrane. The stroma consists of tightly packed lamellae with rigidly ordered small-diameter collagen fibrils alternating with loosely aligned and haphazardly arranged larger-diameter collagen fibrils, distinctive for CHSD.

Autosomal Dominant Congenital Hereditary Endothelial Dystrophy 1 (CHED 1)

MIM #121700

Patients with autosomal dominant inheritance are very rare and most of the information on clinical presentation derives from two large pedigrees reported by Maumenee[91] and Pearce,[93] later reviewed by Judisch.[102] Photophobia and tearing may be the presenting symptoms prior to the onset of corneal clouding. The corneal clouding is not present at birth, developing late in the first year or in the second year of life and may be stable or slowly progressive. It is often asymmetric. Corneal clouding manifests as a ground-glass, milky appearance with profound thickening of the cornea. As the opacification worsens, the symptoms of photophobia and tearing recede. The vision tends to be better (20/60 to 20/400) than in the recessive cases, without nystagmus, allowing patients to learn to read and write during the school years. No definite sexual predilection has been recognized.

Toma et al.[95] initially showed linkage of AD CHED to chromosome 20p11.2-q11.2, within the larger 30cM pericentric interval where PPCD had been localized. The pericentrometric region of chromosome 20 colocalizes with VSX1, although as discussed under PPCD it is unclear whether this plays a pathogenic role in the development of disease. As such, it is considered category 2 in the IC3D classification. Although AD CHED is a more severe a disease than the usual PPCD, with more stromal and Bowman's level involvement, there are similarities in abnormalities of their Descemet's PNB and PCL zones. The endothelial cell loss is much more severe as well, and there is no migratory activity in AD CHED. The endothelial cells, however, can show focal ultrastructural epithelial phenotypia, and have a similar epithelial cytokeratin profile to PPCD, including positivity for CK7.[36]

Autosomal Recessive Congenital Hereditary Endothelial Dystrophy 2 (CHED 2)

MIM #217700

The most common history is of a gray-blue, ground-glass haziness of the corneal stroma noted within the first week to 6 months of age that shows no change or very slow progression over the next few decades. In some, however, there can be more rapid progression to a milky cornea by 1 year of age, or the onset may be delayed to the end of the first decade. The corneal epithelium has an irregular or roughened appearance suggestive of edema. The stromal haziness involves all layers of the thickened cornea, although it may be greater in the deeper layers and centrally. Stromal dots and flakes of greater opacification in the deeper cornea are sometimes mentioned. When visible, Descemet's membrane may appear thickened, but the endothelium is usually not seen. A fine nystagmus is often described in patients with significantly reduced vision, but functional reading vision may be present at close range even with a visual acuity of less than 20/100. There is no vascularization in these corneas except following ulceration in some older patients, after years of chronic corneal edema. No other anterior or posterior segment abnormalities are associated. No definite sexual predilection has been recognized.

CHED 2 is considered category 1 in the IC3D classification as both the gene has been mapped and a mutation identified. Toma and colleagues initially mapped AR CHED to chromosome 20p13-12.[95] Subsequently Vithana et al. discovered seven different missense and nonsense mutations in the SLC4A11 gene, which encodes a membrane-bound sodium borate cotransporter.[96] This genetic mutation was validated by numerous investigators who identified additional homozygous and heterozygous mutations in Burmese, Indian, Pakistani, and Chinese families with AR CHED.[97–100] The transporter that supposedly regulates intracellular boron concentration is felt to play a key role in the growth and terminal differentiation of neural crest cells. Loss of function of this transporter may impact the normal restrictive pattern of corneal endothelial synthesis and secretion, leading to failure of growth regulation during the terminal differentiation and reorganization of the endothelium. Subsequent endothelial cell death may lead to loss of barrier function and progressive corneal edema.

Harboyan syndrome (CHED 2 and perceptive deafness (CDPD)) is an autosomal recessive disease mapped at overlapping loci 20p13. Novel SLC4A11 mutations have been found in seven families.[101]

Prognosis and management

The prognosis for graft clarity and visual rehabilitation is dependent upon the age of onset. In general, patients with autosomal recessive disease tend to have an earlier onset, have transplants at younger age, and as a result have reduced graft survival and worse postoperative visual acuity. A multicenter retrospective study of penetrating keratoplasty for CHED by Schaumberg et al.[107] on patients with presumed autosomal recessive disease had a first graft survival rate of 71%. The median age of first keratoplasty was 40 months, ranging from 3 months to 10 years. Visual acuity was 20/200 in only 4 of 10 eyes where assessment was possible. In a more recent series by Pandrowala from south India on presumed autosomal recessive patients, there was only a 75% graft survival at 4 years.[89] In another series performed by Al-Rajhi and Wagoner,[105] a similar low rate of graft survival was found, with 62.5% of graft survival beyond 3 years. These authors found a clear difference between operating on patients with congenital-onset CHED and 'delayed-onset' CHED, the later defined by corneal clouding which did not start until at least 4 months of age. In the congenital-onset group there was only a 56% success rate as compared to the 'delayed-onset' group with a success rate of 92%. They speculated that the prognosis in these corneal transplantations was related to either the earlier age of onset of the disease or to the increased severity of disease necessitating earlier surgical intervention, due to dense corneal opacification, nystagmus, or amblyopia.

In contrast, in the series reported by Kirkness,[103] Kirkness et al.,[104] and Sajjadi[108] the patients had corneal grafts at a later age. This may have been a result of milder disease allowing the patient to function with less compromise of visual function until older. In the series by Sajjadi the mean age of surgery was 9.5 years of age, with the youngest at 2 years. In this series the graft survival was approximately 90% after 3 years with 19 of 37 eyes obtaining 20/60 vision or better. In the series reported by Kirkness et al., 90% of grafts were clear and 66% of eyes obtained best corrected acuity of 6/18 or better.

Histopathology

By light microscopy[39,91–93,109,110] the corneal epithelium in all reports showed alterations secondary to chronic corneal edema, appearing thin or atrophic with hydropic changes of the basal epithelium, vacuolization of intercellular spaces, and occasional microbullae (see Table 73.2). Kirkness et al.[104] noted subepithelial fibrosis with some calcification in 60% of autosomal dominant cases and 3% of autosomal recessive cases, perhaps related to the older age of the dominant patients. Some loss of Bowman's membrane occurred in most patients, varying from minute disruptions, areas of partial loss with other areas of thickening in an irregular manner, to absence.[39,103] As the most characteristic feature of CHED, the stroma was generally thickened to two to three times normal and severely disorganized with disruption of the lamellar pattern, most marked posteriorly. The collagen fibers appeared more dispersed, sometimes with visible pockets of interstitial fluid. Antine[109] observed a fibrillar type of stromal collagen degeneration in a newborn. Kirkness et al.[104] found spheroidal degeneration of the superficial stroma in six of 10 corneas from patients with autosomal dominant disease, but in only one of 16 corneas from patients with recessive disease.

Descemet's membrane was usually observed to be thickened. Where a genetic pattern was specified, the thickness was said to be more variable in autosomal dominant disease, from 6 to 10 μm up to 21 μm in some cases.[104] In autosomal recessive cases a more homogeneous 20–24 μm thickening was described. Using the PAS stain, a less

PAS-positive posterior collagenous layer was often detectable, more characteristic of the autosomal recessive cases.[104] No other special stains have proven useful to date.

The endothelial cells were absent, markedly reduced in number, or showed evidence of significant degeneration. Contributions of surgical artifact to this loss of endothelium were mentioned in many cases, and in some, Descemet's membrane had a tendency to strip away artifactually as well.[93] Melanin granules were present within some endothelial cells,[39,93,104] particularly in a large dominant kindred.

Electron microscopy

Descemet's membrane in CHED has as its most characteristic feature a normal 110 nm ABZ of approximately 3 μm thickness, but an abnormal, poorly demarcated PNBZ merging into, or mixed with, a PCL. This abnormal PNBZ was not composed of homogeneous basement membrane, as it should be in a young cornea, but rather was a variable mixture of basement membrane-like material, fine fibrils 12 nm in diameter, medium-sized collagen fibrils 25–48 nm in diameter, and 55–100 nm banded bundles.[110] Others have referred to this complex in recessive CHED as an abnormal mixture of basement membrane-like material, focal long-spacing collagen, and fine fibrillar collagen.[104] In dominant CHED, as studied by two groups,[104,109] the PNBZ had even less resemblance to normality, because it contained little basement membrane material, but primarily aggregates of matted collagen fibrils with some foci of long-spacing collagen. This zone was more than twice as thick in a 63-year-old dominant CHED patient as in a 37-year-old patient, suggesting continuous excess secretion.[109]

The endothelium in all reported cases of CHED has been either absent (Fig. 73.28) or has a greatly reduced number of cells, many vacuolated and dystrophic. Although artifact may contribute, the extent of Descemet's abnormality has usually correlated well with the degree of cell loss, even when extreme.[110] Sometimes, more normal-appearing cells with a greater number of organelles lay over the vacuolated cells as though replacing them.[104] Multilayering of this double cell type was found, apparently focally, in 25–33% of these CHED cases.[39,103,104] Frank multilayering, like that in PPCD, was seen in only one of the younger patients with recessive disease.[104] Microvilli in limited numbers were present on some endothelial cells in 20% of the autosomal recessive cases but in none of the dominant ones. No cytofilaments suggestive of epithelial-like metaplasia were seen in any of the endothelial cells.

CHED appears to result from a primary dysfunction of the endothelial cells. The healthy anterior banded portion of Descemet's membrane seen in most cases indicates that the endothelial cells were capable of secreting some normal products in utero, from the fourth through the eighth month of gestation. The abnormal posterior non-banded portion of Descemet's membrane points to dysfunction beginning in the late prenatal period. As previously discussed, it is unknown what triggers the normal change in secretory product of the endothelial cells from fetal banded type VIII collagen to the normal amorphous basement membrane type IV collagen during this period, or what other changes in secretion may also be associated. Kirkness et al.[104]

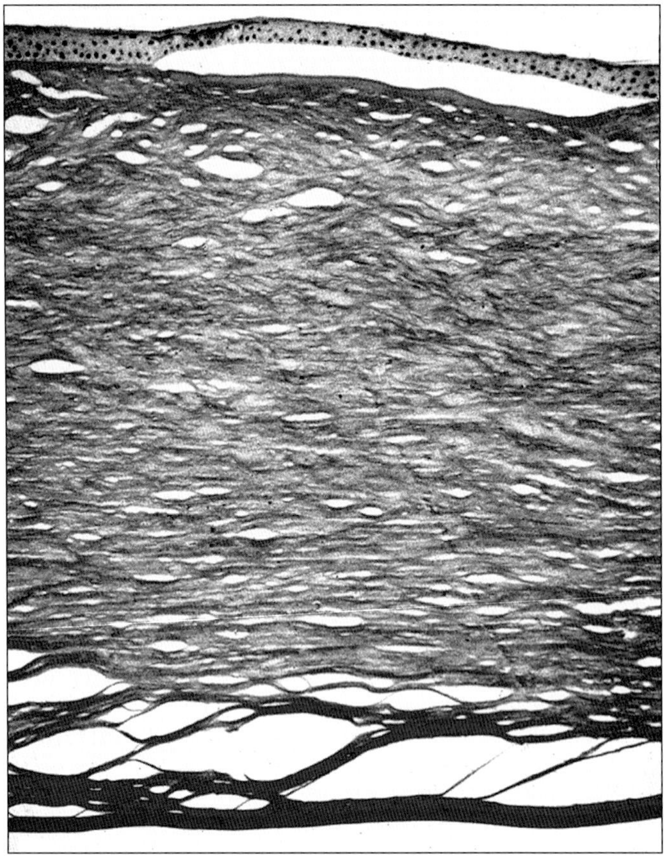

Fig. 73.28 Histology of CHED showing an absence of endothelial cells, a thickened Descemet's membrane, corneal edema, and an epithelial bulla. (Courtesy A Sugar, MD.)

speculated that a loss of regulation of endothelial cell synthesis and secretion produces the abnormal posterior portion of Descemet's membrane.

X-Linked Endothelial Corneal Dystrophy (XECD)

MIM None

Schmid et al. described a large family with a sex-linked endothelial corneal dystrophy mapped to the genetic locus Xq25.[24] The gene has not been identified. As such, it is considered category 2 in the IC3D classification with a genetic locus mapped without a specific genetic mutation identified.

Males are more severely affected than females. Two male probands presented with congenital corneal clouding described as a milky, ground-glass appearance. Seven other males had abnormalities of the endothelium resembling moon craters as well as visually debilitating subepithelial band keratopathy requiring corneal transplantation. Female probands were asymptomatic and presented with moon crater-like appearance of the posterior cornea and a peau d'orange texture including the mothers of the two males with congenital corneal clouding.

Corneal transplantation was performed in 10 eyes of six males. Light microscopy revealed irregular thinning of the epithelium and Bowman's layer. Descemet's membrane was thickened with atypical multilayered endothelial cells present in some areas and absent in others. Transmission electron microscopy showed subepithelial amorphous deposits of granular material consistent with band keratopathy. There was a thickened Descemet's membrane with an abnormal anterior banded zone, evidence that the onset of the dystrophy began prior to birth.

References

1. Koeppe L. Klinische beobachtungen mit der nerstspaltlampe und der hornhautmikroskop. *Graefe's Arch Clin Exp Ophthalmol.* 1916;91: 375–379.
2. Cibis GW, et al. The clinical spectrum of posterior polymorphous dystrophy. *Arch Ophthalmol.* 1977;95:1529–1537.
3. Waring GO, Rodrigues MM, Laibson PR. Corneal dystrophies. II. Endothelial dystrophies. *Surv Ophthalmol.* 1978;23:147–168.
4. Laganowski HC, Sherrard ES, Kerr Muir MG. The posterior corneal surface in posterior polymorphous dystrophy: a specular microscopical study. *Cornea.* 1991;10:224–232.
5. Krachmer JH. Posterior polymorphous corneal dystrophy: a disease characterized by epithelial-like endothelial cells which influence management and prognosis. *Trans Am Ophthalmol Soc.* 1985;83:413–475.
6. Weisenthal RW, Krachmer JH. Posterior polymorphous corneal dystrophy: ten years of progress. In: Cavanagh HD, ed. *The cornea: transactions of the World Congress on the Cornea III.* New York: Raven; 1988.
7. Hirst LW, Waring GO. Clinical specular microscopy of the posterior polymorphous endothelial dystrophy. *Am J Ophthalmol.* 1983; 95:143–155.
8. Laganowski HC, et al. Distinguishing features of iridocorneal endothelial syndrome and posterior polymorphous dystrophy: value of endothelial specular microscopy. *Br J Ophthalmol.* 1991;75:212–216.
9. Cibis GW, Tripathi RC. The differential diagnosis of Descemet's tears (Haab's striae) and posterior polymorphous dystrophy bands: a clinicopathological study. *Ophthalmology.* 1982;89:614–620.
10. Rodrigues MM, et al. Glaucoma due to endothelialization of the anterior chamber angle: a comparison of posterior polymorphous dystrophy of the cornea and Chandler's syndrome. *Arch Ophthalmol.* 1980;98: 688–696.
11. Bourgeois J, Shields MB, Thresher R. Open angle glaucoma associated with posterior polymorphous dystrophy. *Ophthalmology.* 1984;91: 420–423.
12. Bechara SJ, et al. Keratoconus associated with posterior polymorphous dystrophy. *Am J Ophthalmol.* 1991;112:729–731.
13. Cremona FA, Ghosheh FR, Rapuano CR, et al. Keratoconus associated with other corneal dystrophies. *Cornea.* 2009;28:127–135.
14. Shields MB, Campbell DG, Simmons RJ. The essential iris atrophies. *Am J Ophthalmol.* 1978;85:749–759.
15. Hemady RK, et al. Bilateral iridocorneal endothelial syndrome: case report and review of the literature. *Cornea.* 1994;13:368–372.
16. Blair SD, et al. Bilateral progressive essential iris atrophy and keratoconus with coincident features of posterior polymorphous dystrophy: a case report and proposed pathogenesis. *Cornea.* 1992;11:255–261.
17. Hirst LW. Bilateral iridocorneal endothelial syndrome. *Cornea.* 1995;14:331.
18. Sherrard ES, Frangoulis MA, Kerr Muir MG. On the morphology of cells of posterior cornea in the iridocorneal endothelial syndrome. *Cornea.* 1991;10:233–243.
19. Hirst LW. Differential diagnosis of iridocorneal endothelial syndrome and posterior polymorphous endothelial dystrophy. *Br J Ophthalmol.* 1993;77:610.
20. Pardos GJ, Krachmer JH, Mannis MJ. Posterior corneal vesicles. *Arch Ophthalmol.* 1981;99:1573–1577.
21. Harada T, et al. Specular microscopic observation of posterior corneal vesicles. *Ophthalmologica.* 1990;201:122–127.
22. Sekundo W, et al. An ultrastructural investigation of an early manifestation of posterior polymorphous dystrophy of the cornea. *Ophthalmology.* 1994;101:1422–1431.
23. Levy SG, et al. Early onset posterior polymorphous dystrophy. *Arch Ophthalmol.* 1996;114:1265–1268.
24. Schmid E, Lisch W, et al. A new X-linked endothelial corneal dystrophy. *Am J Ophthalmol.* 2006;141:478–487.
25. Boruchoff SA, Weiner MJ, Albert DM. Recurrence of posterior polymorphous dystrophy after penetrating keratoplasty. *Am J Ophthalmol.* 1990;109:323–328.
26. Sekundo W, et al. Multirecurrence of corneal posterior polymorphous dystrophy. An ultrastructural study. *Cornea.* 1994;13:509–515.
27. Boruchoff SA, Kuwabara T. Electron microscopy of posterior polymorphous degeneration. *Am J Ophthalmol.* 1971;72:879–887.
28. Rodrigues MM, et al. Endothelial alterations in congenital corneal dystrophies. *Am J Ophthalmol.* 1975;80:678–698.
29. Polack FM, et al. Scanning electron microscopy of posterior polymorphous corneal dystrophy. *Am J Ophthalmol.* 1980;89:575–584.
30. Henriquez AS, et al. Morphologic characteristics of posterior polymorphous dystrophy. A study of nine corneas and review of the literature. *Surv Ophthalmol.* 1984;29:139–147.
31. Richardson WP, Hettinger ME. Endothelial and epithelial-like cell formations in a case of posterior polymorphous dystrophy. *Arch Ophthalmol.* 1985;103:1520–1524.
32. Johnson BL, Brown SI. Posterior polymorphous dystrophy: a light and electron microscopic study. *Br J Ophthalmol.* 1978;62:89–96.
33. Waring GO, Laibson PR, Rodrigues M. Clinical and pathologic alteration of Descemet's membrane with emphasis on endothelial metaplasia. *Surv Ophthalmol.* 1974;18:325–368.
34. Rodrigues MM, et al. Epithelialization of the corneal endothelium in posterior polymorphous dystrophy. *Invest Ophthalmol Vis Sci.* 1980;19:832–835.
35. Rodrigues MM, et al. Posterior polymorphous dystrophy of the cornea: cell culture studies. *Exp Eye Res.* 1981;33:535–544.
36. Cockerham GC, et al. An immunohistochemical analysis and comparison of posterior polymorphous dystrophy with congenital hereditary endothelial dystrophy. *Cornea.* 2002;21:787–791.
37. Levy SG, et al. The composition of wide-spaced collagen in normal and diseased Descemet's membrane. *Curr Eye Res.* 1996;15:45–52.
38. Murphy C, Alvarado J, Juster R. Prenatal and postnatal growth of the human Descemet's membrane. *Invest Ophthalmol Vis Sci.* 1984;25: 1402–1415.
39. McCartney ACE, Kirkness CM. Comparison between posterior polymorphous dystrophy and congenital hereditary endothelial dystrophy of the cornea. *Eye.* 1988;2:63–70.
40. Weiss JS , Moller HU, Lisch WL, et al. The IC3D classification of the corneal dystrophies. *Cornea.* 2008;27(Suppl 2):S1–S42.
41. Heon E, et al. Linkage of posterior polymorphous corneal dystrophy to 20q11. *Hum Mol Genet.* 1995;4:485–488.
42. Heon E, et al. VSX1: a gene for posterior polymorphous dystrophy and keratoconus. *Hum Mol Genet.* 2002;11:1029–1036.
43. Aldave AJ, et al. Candidate gene screening for posterior polymorphous dystrophy. *Cornea.* 2005;24:151–155.
44. Krafchak CM, et al. Mutations in TCF8 cause posterior polymorphous corneal dystrophy and ectopic expression of COL4A3 by corneal endothelial cells. *Am J Hum Genet.* 2005;77:694–708.
45. Gwilliam R, et al. Posterior polymorphous dystrophy in Czech families maps to chromosome 20 and excludes the VSX1 gene. *Invest Ophthalmol Vis Sci.* 2006;46:4480–4484.
46. Biswas S, et al. Missense mutations in COL8A2, the gene encoding the alpha 2 chain of type VIII collagen, cause two forms of corneal endothelial dystrophy. *Hum Mol Genet.* 2001;10:2415–2423.
47. Yellore VS, et al. No pathogenic mutations identified in the COL8A2 gene or four positional candidate genes in patients with posterior polymorphous corneal dystrophy. *Invest Ophthalmol Vis Sci.* 2005;46: 1599–1603.
48. Morio SE, et al. Clinicopathological correlation and genetic analysis in a case of posterior polymorphous dystrophy. *Am J Ophthalmol.* 2003;135:461–470.
49. Shimizu S, et al. A locus for posterior polymorphous corneal dystrophy (PPCD 3) maps to chromosome 10. *Am J Med Genet A.* 2004;130(4): 372–377.
50. Grooteclaes MI, et al. Evidence for a function of CtBP in epithelial gene regulation and anoikis. *Oncogene.* 2000;19:3823–3828.
51. Liskova P, et al. Novel mutations in the ZEB1 gene identified in Czech and British patients with posterior polymorphous dystrophy corneal dystrophy. *Hum Mutat* 2007;28:638.
52. Aldave AJ, et al. Posterior polymorphous corneal dystrophy is associated with TCF8 gene mutations and abdominal hernia. *Am J Med Genet Part A.* 2007;143A:2549–2556.
53. Aldave AJ, Sonmez B. Elucidating the molecular genetic basis of the corneal dystrophies. *Arch Ophthalmol.* 2007;125:177–186.

54. Teekhasaenee C, et al. Posterior polymorphous dystrophy and Alport syndrome. *Ophthalmology.* 1991;98:1207–1215.
55. Antignac C. Molecular genetics of basement membrane: the paradigm of Alport's syndrome. *Kidney Int.* 1995;47:529–533.
56. Fuchs E. Dystrophia epithelialis corneae. *Graefe's Arch Clin Exp Ophthalmol.* 1910;76:478–508.
57. Krachmer JH, et al. A study of sixty-four families with corneal endothelial dystrophy. *Arch Ophthalmol.* 1978;96:2035–2039.
58. Cross HE, Maumenee AE, Cantolino SJ. Inheritance of Fuchs's endothelial dystrophy. *Arch Ophthalmol.* 1971;85:268–272.
59. Magovern M, et al. Inheritance of Fuchs' combined dystrophy. *Ophthalmology.* 1979;86:1897–1920.
60. Rosenblum P, et al. Hereditary Fuchs' dystrophy. *Am J Ophthalmol.* 1980;90:455–462.
61. Adamis AP, et al. Fuchs' endothelial dystrophy of the cornea. *Surv Ophthalmol.* 1993;38:149–168.
62. Gottsch JD, et al. Inheritance of a Novel COL8A2 mutation defines a distinct early-onset subtype of Fuchs corneal dystrophy. *Invest Ophthalmol Vis Sci.* 2005;46:1934–1939.
63. Hogan MJ, Wood I, Fine M. Fuchs' endothelial dystrophy of the cornea. *Am J Ophthalmol.* 1974;78:363–383.
64. Kaufman SC, et al. Diagnosis of advanced Fuchs' dystrophy with the confocal microscope. *Am J Ophthalmol.* 1993;116: 652–653.
65. Abbott RL, et al. Specular microscopic and histologic observations in nonguttate corneal endothelial degeneration. *Ophthalmology.* 1981;88:788–800.
66. Waring GO, et al. Alterations of Descemet's membrane in interstitial keratitis. *Am J Ophthalmol.* 1976;81:773–785.
67. Krachmer JH, Schnitzer JI, Fratkin J. Corneal pseudoguttata: a clinical and histopathological description of endothelial cell edema. *Arch Ophthalmol.* 1981;99:1377–1381.
68. Eye Banking Statistical Report 2007 EBAA www.restoresight.org
69. Dawson DG, et al. Cornea and sclera. In: *Adler's physiology of the eye.* 11 ed. Elsevier 2009. in press.
70. Geroski DH, et al. Pump functions of the human corneal endothelium. Effects of the age and cornea guttatae. *Opthalmology.* 1985;92:759–763.
71. Edelhauser HF. The resiliency of the corneal endothelium to refractive and intraocular sugery. *Cornea.* 2000;19:263–273.
72. Basic Clinical and Science Course Section 8, External Disease and Cornea. American Academy of Ophthalmology, p. 325.
73. Seitzman GD, Gottsch JD, Stark WJ, et al. Cataract surgery in patients with Fuchs corneal dystrophy. Expanding recommendations for cataract surgery without simualtaneous keratoplasty. *Opthalmlology.* 2005;112:441–446.
74. Price FW, Whitson WE, Marks RG. Graft survival in four common groups of patients undergoing penetrating keratoplasty. *Ophthalmology.* 1991;98:322–328.
75. Johnson DH, Bourne WM, Campbell RJ. The ultrastructure of Descemet's membrane I. *Arch Ophthalmol.* 1982;100:1942–1947.
76. Bourne WM, Johnson DH, Campbell RJ. The ultrastructure of Descemet's membrane. III. Fuchs' dystrophy. *Arch Ophthalmol.* 1982;100: 1952–1955.
77. Sawada H, Konomi H, Hirosawa, K. Characterization of the collagen in the hexagonal lattice of Descemet's membrane: its relation to type VIII collagen. *J Cell Biol.* 1990;110:219–227.
78. Iwamoto T, DeVoe AG. Electron microscopic studies on Fuchs' combined dystrophy. I. Posterior portion of the cornea. *Invest Ophthalmol Vis Sci.* 1971;10:9–28.
79. Alexander RA, Grierson I, Garner A. Oxytalan fibers in Fuchs' endothelial dystrophy. *Arch Ophthalmol.* 1981;99:1622–1627.
80. Gottsch JD, et al. Fuchs corneal dystrophy: abberant collagen distribution in an L450W mutant of the COL8A2 gene. *Invest Ophthalmol Vis Sci.* 2005;46:4504–4511.
81. Zhang C, et al. Immunohistochemistry and electron microscopy of early onset Fuchs corneal dystrophy in three cases with the same L450W COL8A2 mutation. *Trans Am Ophthalmol Soc.* 2006;104:85–97.
82. Sundin OH, et al. Linkage of late onset Fuchs corneal dystrophy to a novel locus at 13pTel-13q.12.13. *Invest Ophthalmol Vis Sci.* 2006;47:140–145.
83. Sundin OH, et al. A common locus for late onset Fuchs corneal dystrophy maps to 18q21.2-q21.32. *Invest Ophthalmol Vis Sci.* 2006; 47:3919–3926.
84. Vithana EN, et al. SLC4A11 mutations in Fuchs endothelial corneal dystrophy. *Hum Mol Genet.* 2008;17:656–666.
85. Kobayashi A, et al. Analysis of the COL8A2 gene mutation in Japanese patients with Fuchs endothelial dystophy and posterior polymorphous dystrophy. *Jpn J Ophthalmol.* 2004;48:195–198.
86. Aldave AJ, et al. No pathogenic mutations identified in the COL8A1 and COL8A2 genes in familial Fuchs corneal dystrophy. *Invest Ophthalmol Vis Sci.* 2006;47:3787–3790.
87. Mehta JS, et al. Analysis of the posterior polymorphous corneal dystrophy 3 gene, TCF8, in late onset Fuchs endothelial corneal dystrophy. *Invest Ophthalmol Vis Sci.* 2008;49:184–188.
88. Al Faran MF, Tabbara KF. Corneal dystrophies among patients undergoing keratoplasty in Saudi Arabia. *Cornea.* 1991;10:13–16.
89. Pandrowala H, et al. Frequency, distribution and outcome of keratoplasty for corneal dystrophies at a tertiary eye care center in South India. *Cornea.* 2004;23;541–546.
90. Laurence GZ. Corneitis interstitialis in utero. *Klin Monat Augenheilkunde.* 1893;1:351.
91. Maumenee AE. Congenital hereditary corneal dystrophy. *Am J Ophthalmol.* 1960;50:1114–1124.
92. Kenyon KR, Maumenee AE. The histological and ultrastructural pathology of congenital hereditary corneal dystrophy. A case report. *Invest Ophthalmol.* 1968;7:475–500.
93. Pearce WG, Tripathi RC, Morgan G. Congenital endothelial corneal dystrophy: clinical, pathological and genetic study. *Br J Ophthalmol.* 1969;53:577–591.
94. Kenyon KR, Maumenee AE. Further studies of congenital hereditary endothelial dystrophy of the cornea. *Am J Ophthalmol.* 1973;76: 419.
95. Toma NMG, et al. Linkage of congenital hereditary endothelial dystrophy to chromosome 20. *Hum Mol Gen.* 1995;4:2395–2398.
96. Vithana EN, et al. Mutations in sodium-borate cotransporter SLC4A11 cause recessive congenital hereditary endothelial dystrophy (CHED2). *Nat Genet.* 2006;38;755–757.
97. Jiao X, Sultana P, et al. Autosomal recessive corneal endothelial dystrophy (CHED2) is associated with mutations in SLC4A11. *J Med Genet.* 2007;44;64–68.
98. Kumar A, et al. Genetic analysis of two Indian families affected with congenital hereditary endothelial dystrophy: two novel mutations in SLC4A11. *Mol Vis.* 2007;13:39–46.
99. Sultana A, et al. Mutational spectrum of the SLC4A11 gene in autosomal recessive congenital hereditary endothelial dystrophy. *Mol Vis.* 2007;13:1327–1332.
100. Aldave A, Yellore VS, et al. Autosomal recessive CHED associated with novel compound heteryzgous mutations in SLC4A11. *Cornea.* 2007;26:896–900.
101. Desir J, Moya G, et al. Borate transporter SLC4A11 mutations cause both Harboyan syndrome and non-syndromic corneal endothelial dystrophy. *J Med Genet.* 2007;44;322–326.
102. Judisch GF, Maumenee IH. Clinical differentiation of recessive congenital hereditary endothelial dystrophy and dominant hereditary endothelial dystrophy. *Am J Ophthalmol.* 1978;85:606–612.
103. Kirkness CM. The corneal endothelial dystrophies. *Ann Acad Med.* 1989;18:158–164.
104. Kirkness CM, et al. Congenital hereditary corneal oedema of Maumenee: its clinical features, management and pathology. *Br J Ophthalmol.* 1987;71:130–144.
105. Al-Rajhi AA, Wagoner MD. Penetrating keratoplasty in congenital hereditary endothelial dystrophy. *Ophthalmology.* 1997;104:956–961.
106. Witschel H, et al. Congenital hereditary stromal dystrophy of the cornea. *Arch Ophthalmol.* 1978;96:1043–1051.
107. Schaumberg DA, et al. Corneal transplantation in young children with congenital hereditary endothelial dystrophy. *Am J Ophthalmol.* 1999;127:373–378.
108. Sajjadi H, et al. Results of penetrating keratoplasty in CHED (congenital hereditary endothelial dystrophy). *Cornea.* 1995;14:18–25.
109. Antine B. Histology of congenital hereditary corneal dystrophy. *Am J Ophthalmol.* 1970;69:964–969.
110. Kenyon KR, Antine B. The pathogenesis of congenital hereditary endothelial dystrophy of the cornea. *Am J Ophthalmol.* 1971;72:787–795.

Chapter 74

Noninflammatory Ectatic Disorders

Robert S. Feder, Theresa J. Gan

The noninflammatory ectatic diseases of the cornea discussed in this chapter are keratoconus, pellucid marginal degeneration, keratoglobus, and posterior keratoconus. Beside the similarities in name, these conditions, to varying degrees, are similar in clinical presentation (Table 74.1). The first three disorders may actually represent variations in the phenotypic expression of the same pathogenetic mechanism.

Corneal thinning is a hallmark of these ectatic diseases. The area of maximal thinning, relative to the location of maximal corneal protrusion, is helpful in differentiating these conditions. Distortion of the anterior corneal curvature occurs in keratoconus, pellucid marginal degeneration, and keratoglobus (Fig. 74.1). The resultant reduction in visual function can vary from mild to severe.

Computer-assisted topographical and pachymetric analyses have dramatically improved the sensitivity of detection of these ectatic disorders, particularly in the case of keratoconus. This has prompted debate on appropriate terminology for the patient with topographical evidence of inferior steepening, eccentric elevation or thinning, but without clinical signs of keratoconus. Keratoconus suspect or subclinical keratoconus are commonly used terms.

This type of analysis has been of great value in refining study populations for genetic studies and is an integral part of the screening examination of the prospective keratorefractive surgery patient.

Keratoconus, pellucid marginal degeneration, and keratoglobus share a basic treatment algorithm. Visual correction begins with glasses, followed by contact lens fitting. Failing these modalities, a surgical approach, designed to restore a more normal corneal contour, is planned.

Posterior keratoconus differs from the other noninflammatory thinning disorders in many respects. To reduce the confusion caused by the similarity in name, it is included in the discussion that follows.

Keratoconus

Definition

Keratoconus is a clinical term used to describe a condition in which the cornea assumes a conical shape because of thinning and protrusion. The process is noninflammatory. Cellular infiltration and vascularization do not occur. It is usually bilateral and, although it involves the central two-thirds of the cornea, the apex of the cone is usually centered just below the visual axis. This disease process results in mild to marked impairment of visual function.

Prevalence, distribution, and course

Reported estimates of the prevalence of keratoconus vary widely, because of the variation in diagnostic criteria. Most estimates fall between 50 and 230 per 100 000.[1] Keratoconus occurs in people of all races. There is no significant gender predominance.

Keratoconus usually occurs bilaterally. Unilateral cases occur. However, it has been convincingly shown[2–4] that when diagnostic criteria and computer-assisted topographical analysis allow the detection of very early keratoconus in the fellow eye the incidence of unilateral involvement is probably in the range of 2–4%.

The onset of keratoconus occurs at about the age of puberty. The cornea begins to thin and protrude, resulting in irregular astigmatism with what is usually a steep curvature. Typically, over a period of 10 to 20 years the process continues until the progression gradually stops. If a faint, broad iron ring is present, it becomes a thinner, more discrete ring. The rate of progression is variable. The severity of the disorder at the time progression stops can range from very mild irregular astigmatism to severe thinning, protrusion, and scarring requiring keratoplasty.

Associated disease

Systemic disease

Over the past half century much has been written linking keratoconus to atopic disease.[5–7] The largest controlled study[8,9] found a positive history of atopic disease in 35% of 182 keratoconus patients as compared to 12% of 100 normal control patients.

The thorough evaluation of the keratoconus patient should include a complete history of atopic disease. Appropriate referrals can be made if significant atopic disease is newly revealed. Allergic lid and conjunctival disease can affect contact lens tolerance adversely. As a result, surgical intervention may be required earlier in the course of the disease to achieve visual rehabilitation. Cataract related

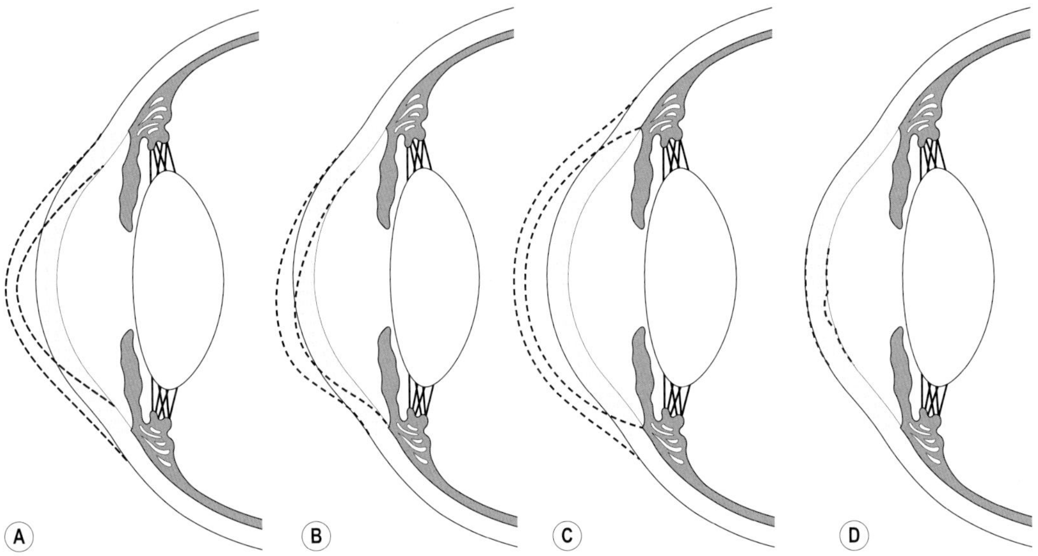

Fig. 74.1 The presence of corneal thinning and the type of contour abnormality can be helpful in recognizing the type of ectatic disorder. (**A**) Keratoconus; (**B**) pellucid marginal degeneration; (**C**) keratoglobus; and (**D**) posterior keratoconus.

Table 74.1 Noninflammatory ectatic disorders – clinical presentation and appearance compared and contrasted

	Keratoconus	Pellucid marginal degeneration	Keratoglobus	Posterior keratoconus
Frequency	Most common	Less common	Rare	Least common
Laterality	Usually bilateral	Bilateral	Bilateral	Usually unilateral
Age at onset	Puberty	Age 20 to 40 years	Usually at birth	Birth
Thinning	Inferior paracentral	Inferior band 1 to 2 mm wide	Greatest in periphery	Paracentral posterior excavation
Protrusion	Thinnest at apex	Superior to band of thinning	Generalized	Usually none
Iron line	Fleischer ring	Sometimes	None	Sometimes
Scarring	Common	Only after hydrops	Mild	Common
Striae	Common	Sometimes	Sometimes	None

either to atopy or to the use of steroid medication may complicate the management of the atopic keratoconus patient.

Rados[10] was the first to report an association between Down's syndrome and keratoconus. Most series report the incidence between 5.5% and 15%.[11–13] Keratoconus also occurs with increased frequency among developmentally delayed individuals without Down's syndrome, and the incidence of unilateral disease may be substantially higher in this group compared with the general population.[14]

Two plausible explanations for this association with keratoconus are that genetic abnormalities induce structural or biochemical changes resulting in the well-recognized phenotype or that eye rubbing causes the condition. Corneal hydrops occurs with increased frequency in patients with Down's syndrome or other forms of intellectual impairment and this may also result from habitual ocular massage.

Keratoconus has long been known to occur in patients with noninflammatory connective tissue disorders.[15,16] Most notable among these are Ehlers-Danlos syndrome and osteogenesis imperfecta. Robertson found the prevalence of hypermobility of the joints to be 50% in 44 consecutive keratoconus patients.[17] Joint hypermobility in keratoconus has subsequently been confirmed,[18,19] especially for the metacarpophalangeal and wrist joints.

An increased prevalence (38%[20] to 58%[21]) of mitral valve prolapse has been found in keratoconus patients. The prevalence appears to increase with severity of the corneal disease.

Lichter et al.[22] studied a group of mitral valve prolapse patients and found an increased prevalence of keratoconus. In contrast, Street et al.[23] were unable to confirm the association of keratoconus, mitral valve prolapse, and joint hypermobility in a well-controlled study of 95 keratoconus patients. While the association with floppy eyelid syndrome had been documented in case reports,[24,25] Lee and colleagues found a prevalence of 17% (3/18) in a group of patients with floppy eyelid syndrome.[26] Keratoconus has been associated with other disorders of connective tissue, such as congenital hip dysplasia,[27] oculodentodigital syndrome, Rieger's syndrome,[28] anetoderma,[29] and focal dermal hypoplasia.[30] It has also been reported in nail-patella syndrome,[28] Apert's syndrome,[31] craniofacial dysostosis (Crouzon's syndrome),[32,33] and Marfan's syndrome.[34] Turner's syndrome, which is sometimes associated with disorders in tissues of mesodermal origin, has also been found in association with keratoconus.[35,36]

In a large case-controlled study, comparing keratoconus and normal patients, the incidence of manifest diabetes was significantly lower in the keratoconus group. Seiler and colleagues[37] theorized that diabetes offered a protective effect regarding keratoconus.

Keratoconus patients are said to exhibit characteristic personality traits. Studies have sought to determine if these so-called traits actually exist, if they are related to the chronic progressive visual disability, or if they are specific for keratoconus. While no specific personality disorder has ever been identified in keratoconus patients, certain tendencies have been detected. Mannis et al.[38] found patients with keratoconus and other chronic eye diseases to be less conforming and more passive-aggressive, paranoid, and hypomanic than normal control individuals. In a small study, Swartz et al.[39] found that the incidence of abnormalities in psychologic testing was less in keratoconus patients after penetrating keratoplasty than before surgery.

Ocular disease

Keratoconus may appear in the presence of isolated ocular pathology. A classic example is retinitis pigmentosa. Many authors over the past 50 years have reported this association.[1] Infantile tapetoretinal degeneration (Leber's congenital amaurosis) is frequently complicated by keratoconus and cataract. In a classic, large study by Alstrom and Olson,[40] more than one-third of those patients over age 45 years old had keratoconus. Keratoconus occurring with advancing age was more recently confirmed.[41] Moschos et al.[42] studied a large group of keratoconus patients and found 2.6% (6/233) with electroretinogram abnormalities and 3.9% (9/233) with abnormal visual evoked response, confirming the presence of diffuse or central tapetoretinal degeneration. Elder found a much higher incidence of keratoconus among children with Leber's congenital amaurosis compared with a group of blind children from other causes. As a result of this study, a genetic basis, rather than an environmental cause such as eye rubbing, was suspected to explain this association.[43]

Conical cornea has also been reported with retinopathy of prematurity,[44] progressive cone dystrophy,[45] aniridia,[46] iridoschisis,[47] and essential iris atrophy.[48] In addition, associations between keratoconus and Fuchs' dystrophy,[49,50] posterior polymorphous dystrophy,[48,51–53] and granular[54–56] and lattice dystrophies[57,58] have been described.

Finally, the relationship between vernal conjunctivitis and keratoconus has been widely reported.[1,59] Totan and his associates[60] evaluated 82 vernal patients with videokeratography and found evidence of keratoconus in 26.8%. Only 8.5% were diagnosed using biomicroscopy. Tuft et al.[61] found keratoconus to be an important cause of vision loss in a study of 37 patients with atopic keratoconjunctivitis.

Etiology

The various associations with systemic and ocular diseases have led to the development of many theories regarding the etiology of keratoconus. Nevertheless, the cause of this corneal disorder remains an enigma. Keratoconus may represent a general phenotype, the cause of which may vary considerably depending on the clinical setting, e.g. long-term contact lens wear, atopy, or identical twins with conical cornea. It has been suggested that investigations into the etiology of the condition focus on keratoconus found in similar clinical settings in order to isolate a specific cause.

Results from biochemical, histopathological, and molecular genetic studies have provided new insights into the cause of keratoconus. The discussion of the etiology of keratoconus in this chapter is begun here, but continues in the subsequent sections on biochemistry, heredity, and pathology.

Early theories attempted to link the systemic and ocular diseases associated with keratoconus. For example, if keratoconus was primarily an ectodermal disease, then associations with atopic disease and tapetoretinal degenerations (neuroectodermal origin) seem logical. Several reports have implicated eye rubbing as an important etiologic factor in the development of keratoconus.[6,9,62] The reported prevalence among keratoconus patients ranges from 66% to 73%.[1] The microtrauma associated with eye rubbing may be the etiologic link between conical cornea and associated systemic and ocular diseases. Itching, ocular irritation, and eye rubbing are common features of vernal keratoconjunctivitis and atopic disease. Vigorous eye rubbing has frequently been observed in patients with Down's syndrome and may explain the high incidence of associated corneal hydrops. Finally, eye rubbing is commonly seen in poorly sighted patients with Leber's tapetoretinal degeneration and retinopathy of prematurity, both of which are associated with keratoconus.

Contact lens wear is another form of corneal microtrauma that seems to be associated with keratoconus. Retrospective studies have found a history of contact lens wear before the diagnosis of keratoconus in 17.5%[63] to 26.5%[64] of cases. Macsai et al.,[65] in a retrospective review, identified a subgroup of keratoconus patients who were not felt to have had the condition before beginning contact lens wear. This group of long-term contact lens wearers was older and tended to have central cones with a flatter corneal curvature than keratoconus patients with no history of contact lens wear before the diagnosis. While a cause and effect relationship may be impossible to prove, this study provides suggestive evidence.

Biochemistry

Over the past two decades, biochemistry has provided an important line of research into the etiology of keratoconus. Since much of the work has been done on host corneas following penetrating keratoplasty, it is important to keep in mind that the results of many of these studies relate more to advanced keratoconus rather than early disease.

The total amount of protein has been shown to be decreased in keratoconus.[66] Theoretically, an up-regulation of degradative enzymes and the down-regulation of proteinase inhibitors could result in a degradation of the extracellular matrix of the stroma. The level of degradative lysosomal enzymes, such as acid esterase and acid phosphatase, cathepsins B and G, and some matrix metalloproteinases, has been shown to be elevated in keratoconus corneas.[67,68]

If keratoconus were simply caused by an increase in proteolytic enzymes and decrease proteinase inhibitors in the corneal epithelium, one might expect a significant recurrence rate following a corneal graft after the graft epithelium was replaced by the epithelium of the host. In fact, the recurrence rate following penetrating keratoplasty is low. One must assume that the pathogenesis of keratoconus is more complex than the preceding theory would suggest.

Keratocytes from keratoconus corneas have been found to have four times the interleukin-1 binding sites, when compared to nonkeratoconus corneas.[69,70] This may result in an increased sensitivity of the keratocytes in keratoconus to the effects of interleukin-1. Interleukin-1 has also been shown to induce apoptosis or controlled cell death of stromal keratocytes in vitro. Apoptosis has been found in the stromal keratocytes of keratoconus corneas, but not in normal controls.[71] Wilson et al.[72] postulated that the corneal epithelium might release interleukin-1 in response to microtrauma occurring after eye rubbing or contact lens wear. This in turn would be more likely to trigger apoptosis of stromal keratocytes in patients with a heightened sensitivity to interleukin-1, such as occurs in keratoconus.

Heredity

The most compelling evidence for a genetic origin in some forms of keratoconus is the degree of concordance between monozygotic twins. There are reports of at least 18 sets of monozygotic twins[73] that identify one or both siblings in the pair with evidence of keratoconus. Seven of the 13 pairs, evaluated without corneal topography, were concordant for keratoconus. Edwards et al.[73] point out that the evidence of discordance cannot be considered conclusive in the absence of corneal topography. In addition, evaluations may have been performed in younger patients, prior to the development of keratoconus. At least six concordant pairs have been reported since the advent of corneal topography.[74–76]

McMahon et al.[77] described two pairs of discordant monozygotic twins in which one of each pair had keratoconus and the other had normal corneal topography in both eyes. It was suggested that an environmental trigger might be necessary in addition to a genetic predisposition or that genetic differences between the individuals may exist, even in monozygotic twins.

The frequency of inheritance has been estimated to be 6%.[78] Computer-assisted topography has been used to examine family members of keratoconus patients.[79–81] Corneal contour abnormalities were uncovered in some clinically unaffected relatives. Whether these patients would progress to clinically significant disease is unknown. This evidence has supported an autosomal dominant inheritance pattern with incomplete penetrance. The information gathered using corneal topography may help create more accurate pedigrees in families with keratoconus, which could be used in future genetic study.

The results of earlier attempts to correlate certain HLA types with keratoconus[7,63] were inconclusive. HLA-A26, B40, and DR9, frequently found in the elderly Japanese population, have recently been found to be associated with keratoconus in younger individuals.[82]

Molecular genetic techniques are being used to study candidate genes for proteins that may be involved in the development of keratoconus such as the interleukin-1 system, proteases, and protease inhibitors.[6,73,81] Phenotypic and genetic heterogeneity make this investigation particularly challenging. Rabinowitz et al.[16,81] have studied various collagen genes, excluding several such as *COL6A1*, the gene encoding the alpha 1 chain of type VI collagen.[81]

Aldave et al. reported that mutations in genes encoding alpha 1 and alpha 2 chains of type VIII collagen, *COL8A1* and *COL8A2*, were not present in keratoconus or keratoglobus patients.[83]

Hameed and his colleagues[84] have applied linkage analysis in a two-generation consanguineous family with autosomal recessive Leber's congenital amaurosis and keratoconus. It is suggested that the combined phenotype is due to a gene within the 17p13 chromosomal region. Damji et al. described families with Leber's congenital amaurosis and keratoconus in which a Trp278X mutation in the *AIPL1* gene on 17p was found.[85]

Keratoconus has been found in association with chromosomal abnormalities other than Down's syndrome. It has been associated with a chromosome 7,11 translocation[86] and with a chromosome 13 ring abnormality.[87]

Patients commonly ask if keratoconus is inherited and if their children will develop the disorder. Using clinical evaluation and three keratographic indices, Wang et al.[88] found the keratoconus prevalence of first-degree relatives to be 3.34%, which is up to 68 times that found in the general population. It seems reasonable to tell them the chance that a first-degree relative would be found to have symptoms of the disease, while significantly greater than the general population, is still less than 1 in 20.

The phenotypic appearance commonly recognized as keratoconus may be the result of multiple genotypes. Keratoconus study populations that have associated ocular or systemic diseases in common or topographical characteristics in common may be more likely to share a common genotype. Identifying such specific study groups is essential in the genetic study of keratoconus.[89] While it may be that the development of some forms of keratoconus are under direct genetic control, it is also possible that the genetic influence is more subtle, requiring the effects of environmental stimuli to produce the phenotype characteristic of keratoconus.

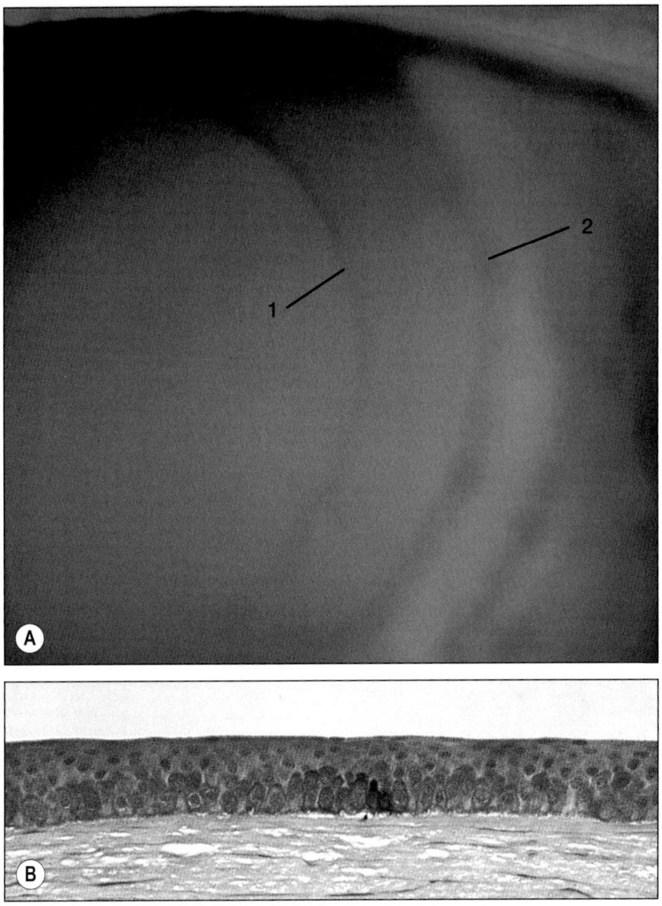

Fig. 74.2 The Fleischer ring in keratoconus. (**A**) The Fleischer ring (*1*) is a landmark indicating the location of the base of the cone; (*2*) pupil margin. (**B**) The ring results from hemosiderin pigment deposited in the basal epithelium. (Prussian blue stain ×200.)

Pathology

Every layer and tissue of the cornea can potentially be involved in the pathologic process of keratoconus. Central epithelial thinning has been found with variable frequency.[90] Specular microscopy of the corneal epithelium has revealed enlargement of the superficial cells and prominence of elongated cells, findings not seen in long-term hard contact lens wearers.[91] Early degeneration of the basal epithelial cells can be followed by disruption of the epithelial basement membrane. Breaks in the epithelial layer can be associated with epithelium growing posteriorly into Bowman's layer and collagen growing anteriorly into the epithelium, forming Z-shaped interruptions at the level of Bowman's layer.[92] These Z-shaped areas are typical of keratoconus. Fragmentation of the Bowman's layer seen with scanning electron microscopy has been described as specific to keratoconus and possibly an early change leading to the disease.[93]

A hallmark of keratoconus is the Fleischer ring found at the base of the cone (Fig. 74.2A). The brown iron ring can be seen histopathologically (Fig. 74.2B). Light and electron microscopy reveal that ferritin particles accumulate within and between the epithelial cells, particularly in the basal epithelium.[94]

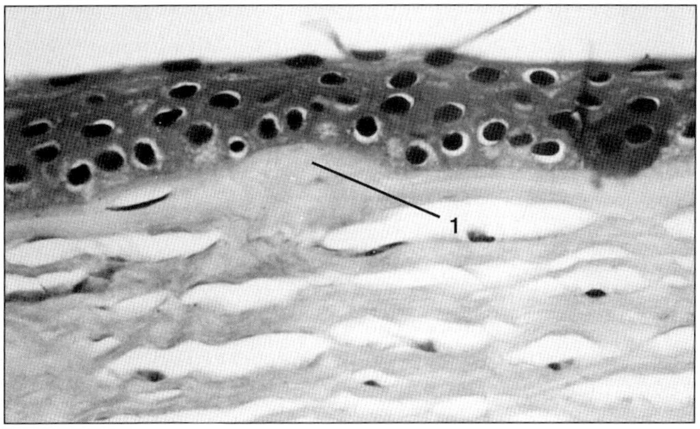

Fig. 74.3 A break in Bowman's layer (*1*) is filled with collagenous scar tissue (hematoxylin and eosin stain, ×400.) Breaks such as those seen here are felt to be related to the subepithelial and anterior stromal scarring typically seen in keratoconus.

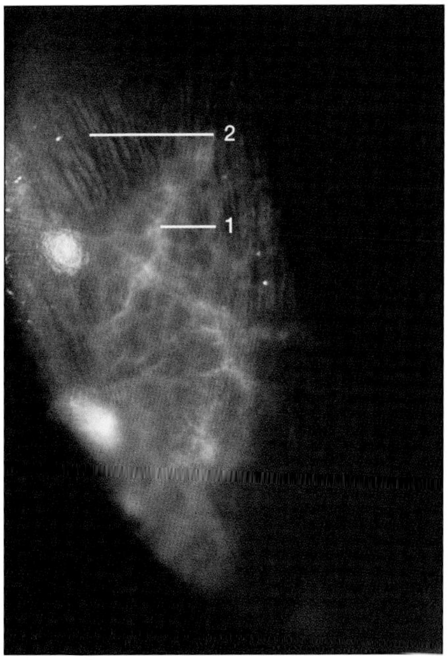

Fig. 74.4 Reticular, subepithelial, and anterior stromal scars (*1*) develop within the cone and result from breaks in Bowman's layer. The typical appearance is seen in this slit lamp photograph. Also present are Vogt's striae (*2*).

Shapiro et al.[95] correlated anterior clear spaces detected clinically within the thinned stroma of the cone with interruptions of Bowman's layer. They postulated that these breaks in Bowman's layer may later fill with scar tissue (Fig. 74.3). Consolidation of these fine scars may result in the reticular branching opacities often seen at this level (Fig. 74.4). Perry et al. found that breaks in Bowman's layer occurred with increased frequency in oval, sagging cones compared with round cones.[96]

Kaas-Hansen suggested that the breaklines in Bowman's layer were a secondary phenomenon, occurring later in the disease, and not fundamental in the pathogenesis of keratoconus, because similar short breaks were found in normal corneas.[97] Scarring of Bowman's layer and the anterior stroma are common and correlate histopathologically with collagen fragmentation, fibrillation, and fibroblastic activity.

The pathology of collagen fibrils in keratoconus has been well studied. Pouliquen et al.[98] have found normal-sized collagen fibers; however, the number of collagen lamellae was abnormally low. The number found within the cone was less than half (41%) the number outside of the cone. Fullwood et al.[99] used synchrotron X-ray diffraction to study keratoconus corneas and found no significant difference in interfibrillar spacing between keratoconus and control corneas. They concluded that the stromal thinning was not the result of closer packing of the stromal collagen fibrils.

It has been suggested that collagen lamellae are released from their interlamellar attachments or from their attachments to Bowman's layer and become free to slide. This results in thinning without collagenolysis.[100] Smolek has found the interlamellar strength profile in the normal cornea to be significantly weaker inferiorly and centrally.[101] Significant alteration of the normal orthogonal arrangement of the collagen fibrils found in keratoconus may be related to this biomechanical instability of the stromal tissue.[102] The most common location for the apex of the cone, in the central or inferior cornea, may be related to this inherent corneal weakness. This may also explain the association of eye rubbing with keratoconus.[103]

Endothelial cell pleomorphism and polymegathism occur in keratoconus. The degree of polymegathism does not differ significantly from normal controls with a similar contact lens history, suggesting that these changes may be related to long-term contact lens wear rather than keratoconus.[104] Patterns of endothelial damage vary from isolated cell membranolysis to denudement of Descemet's membrane. More damage occurs at the base of the cone than at the apex and correlates with the severity and duration of the disease.[105]

Diagnosis

The diagnosis of keratoconus depends first on the suspicion of the condition and then on careful evaluation employing various available diagnostic tools including biomicroscopy, keratometry, keratoscopy, pachymetry, and computer-assisted topography.

Typically, an affected patient in the teens or twenties seeks consultation for symptoms of progressive visual blurring and/or distortion. Photophobia, glare, monocular diplopia, and ocular irritation are also presenting symptoms. Early in the course of the disease, visual acuity may be normal even in symptomatic patients. Contrast sensitivity measurement may, however, uncover visual dysfunction before Snellen visual acuity loss can be measured.[106] High, irregular myopic astigmatism with a scissoring reflex on retinoscopy is typical in established keratoconus. In advanced keratoconus the corneal protrusion may cause angulation of the lower lid on downgaze. This nonspecific finding has been referred to as Munson's sign (Fig. 74.5). Usually the diagnosis of the disease is made long before Munson's sign is evident.

Slit lamp examination reveals characteristic findings. An eccentrically located ectatic protrusion of the cornea is noted (Fig. 74.6). While the apex is usually inferior to an imaginary horizontal line drawn through the pupillary axis, it can be located in the central cornea. Superior keratoconus also can occur.[107–109] Computer-assisted corneal topography has revealed that superior flattening is associated with inferior steepening in keratoconus.[110] Smolek and Klyce used computer-generated surface area measurements to determine that the total corneal surface area tended to be conserved in mild to moderate forms of the disease.[111] They theorize that keratoconus at these stages may not be a true ectasia.

Corneal thinning from one-half to one-fifth of normal thickness is observed at the apex of the protrusion (Fig. 74.7). Two types of cones have been described.[96] The round

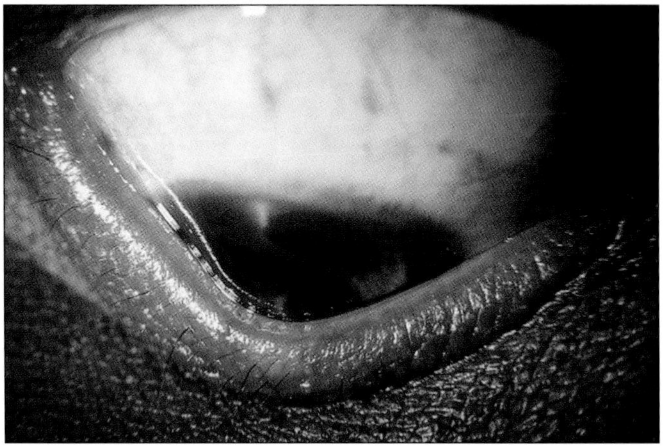

Fig. 74.5 Angulation of the lower lid in downgaze known as Munson's sign, which is a nonspecific sign of advanced keratoconus.

Fig. 74.6 The apex of the cone is usually in the inferior paracentral cornea.

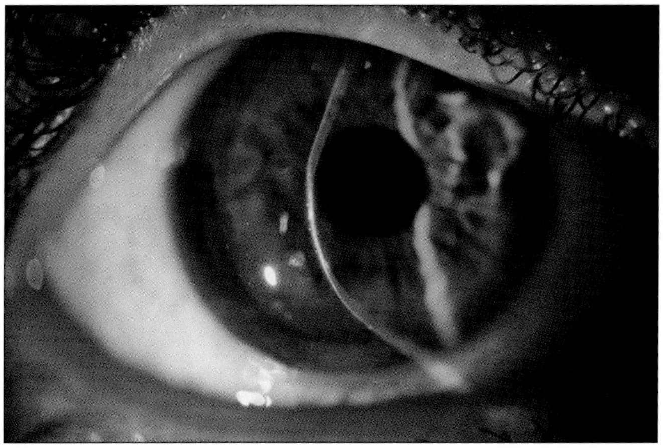

Fig. 74.7 A hallmark of keratoconus is corneal thinning, which occurs at the cone apex, the point of maximal protrusion. Scarring may induce flattening at the apex of the cone. Corneal flattening can sometimes be seen superior and peripheral to the cone.

or nipple-shaped cone is smaller in diameter, while the larger oval or sagging cone may extend to the limbus and is more prone to contact lens fitting problems. Computer-assisted corneal mapping has further characterized these two groups.[110]

Keratoconus is in the differential diagnosis of prominent corneal nerves and when observed it is usually mild and localized.[112] Striae occur in the posterior stroma, just anterior to Descemet's membrane. When the intraocular pressure is transiently raised, by applying external pressure to the globe, the folds disappear (Fig. 74.8). These fine parallel striae described are to be distinguished from the superficial linear scars seen at the corneal apex (see Fig. 74.4). These result from ruptures in Bowman's layer. Subtle anterior clear spaces were identified at the slit lamp in 38% of 69 consecutive keratoconus cases.[95] Light and electron microscopy revealed breaks in Bowman's layer in two corneal buttons of patients with this clinical finding.

The Collaborative Longitudinal Evaluation of Keratoconus (CLEK) study has found that corneal scarring in keratoconus is associated with reduced high- and low-contrast visual acuity and increased symptoms of glare.[113] Factors predictive of incident corneal scarring include corneal curvature greater than 52 diopters (D), contact lens wear, corneal staining, and age less than 20 years.[114] Scarring was more than three times as likely to be found in association with a flat-fitting contact lens.[115] To date, there are no controlled studies on the effect of apical clearance versus flatter-fitting lenses on corneal scarring. Adjusting contact lens fit may reduce the incidence of corneal scarring. However, steeper corneas are more likely to scar even without contact lens wear.[114]

In more advanced cases, deeper opacities can be seen at the apex of the cone resulting from ruptures in Descemet's membrane. Acute keratoconus or corneal hydrops results from stromal imbibition of aqueous through these defects (Fig. 74.9A). The edema may persist for weeks or months, usually diminishing gradually. Eventually, it is replaced by scarring (Fig. 74.9B), which in some cases may result in flattening of the conical contour.

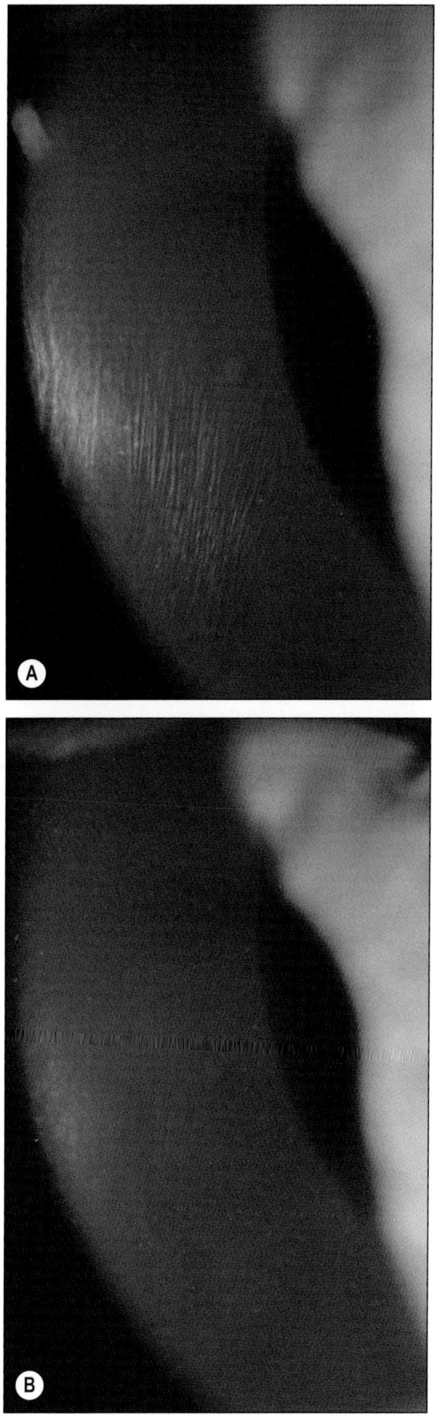

Fig. 74.8 Striae in keratoconus. (**A**) Fine posterior stromal folds known as Vogt's striae are commonly found on slit lamp examination in and near the apex of the cone. (**B**) The striae disappear when external pressure is applied to the globe, as shown here.

Corneal pseudocysts or intrastromal clefts have been described in association with hydrops in keratoconus (Fig. 74.9C).[116,117] Single or multiple clefts can occur, and bilateral involvement is possible. Clefts usually close within 6 months, but stromal neovascularization is common and can affect future graft survival. The presence of large intrastromal clefts

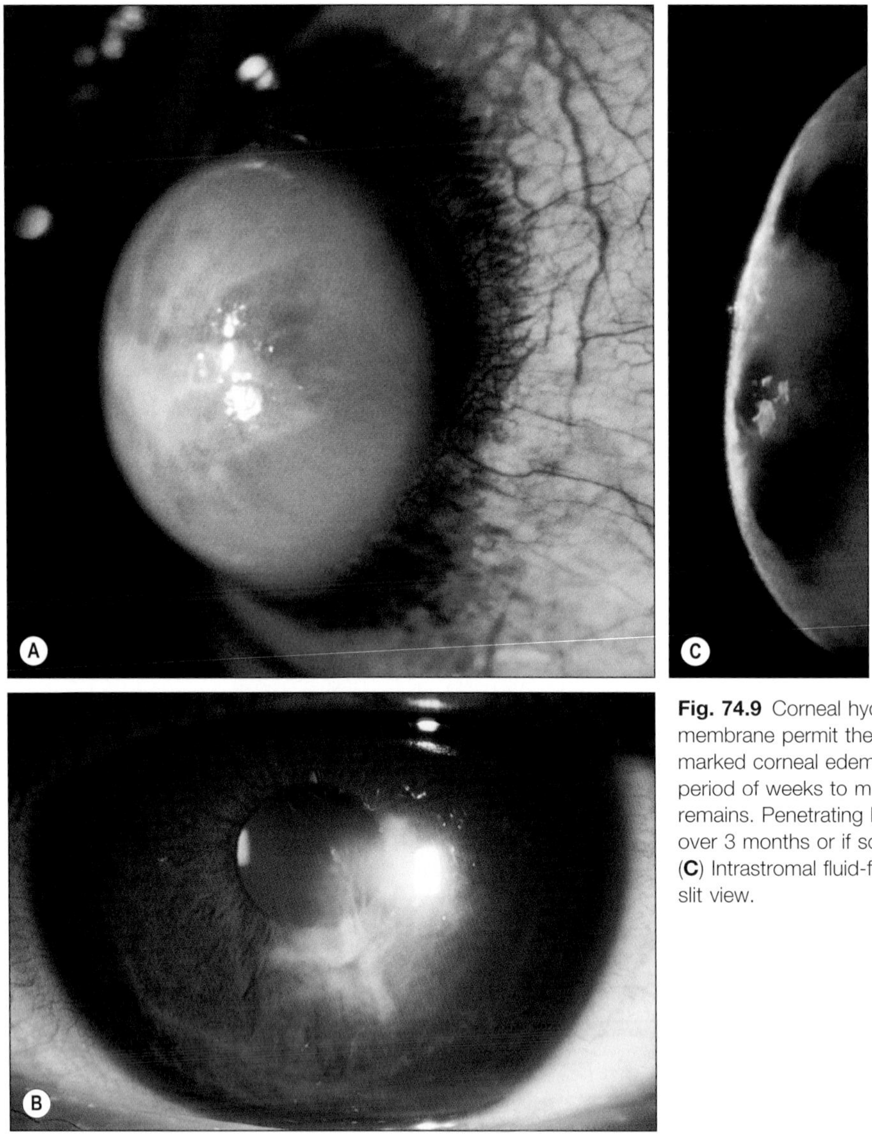

Fig. 74.9 Corneal hydrops in keratoconus. (**A**) Ruptures in Descemet's membrane permit the stromal imbibition of aqueous and result in the marked corneal edema seen in this slit lamp photograph. (**B**) Over a period of weeks to months, the defect closes and deep stromal scarring remains. Penetrating keratoplasty is usually necessary if edema persists over 3 months or if scarring is extensive or is in the central cornea. (**C**) Intrastromal fluid-filled clefts can sometimes occur, as seen in this slit view.

may explain how corneal perforation can occur after minor trauma in cases of keratoconus with hydrops.

The Fleischer ring is a partial or complete annular line commonly seen at the base of the cone. When identified, it provides a landmark for the peripheral edge of the cone. As the ectasia progresses, the ring tends to become more densely pigmented and narrower, and it may completely encircle the cone at its base. Cobalt blue illumination in the widest possible slit beam can be used in early cases to enhance the appearance of a subtle iron ring (see Fig. 74.2A).

The keratometer is an invaluable, widely available tool for measuring corneal curvature. Inability to superimpose the central keratometric rings suggests irregular corneal astigmatism, a hallmark of keratoconus. There is no keratometric value beyond which the diagnosis of keratoconus is definite. There are patients with steep corneas and high astigmatic errors who do not have keratoconus and, conversely, patients with keratoconus who have central corneas of normal steepness. Inferior corneal steepening is also an early sign of keratoconus. By performing central keratometry, followed by keratometry with the patient in upward gaze, steepening in the inferior cornea can be identified and documented.

Keratoscopy or videokeratography, based on the Placido disk, can provide qualitative contour information. In early keratoconus, a focal area of increased corneal curvature appears as an isolated area of smaller ring spacing and distortion. As the condition progresses, the ring spacing decreases overall and becomes increasingly irregular (Fig. 74.10C).

Computer-assisted corneal topography devices have become indispensable for diagnosing subclinical keratoconus and for tracking the progression of the disease (Fig. 74.10A,B,D).[118–120] Placido systems (e.g. TMS, EyeSys, Humphrey), slit-scan systems (Orbscan, Bausch & Lomb), scanning slit combined with a Placido system (Orbscan II, Bausch & Lomb), and rasterstereography (PAR) have all been used for these measurements.[121] Scheimpflug photography is the latest technology to be applied to the analysis of corneal topography and keratoconus detection. Advances in technology have led to changes in the way corneal topography is used to analyze corneal contour. At its inception, corneal

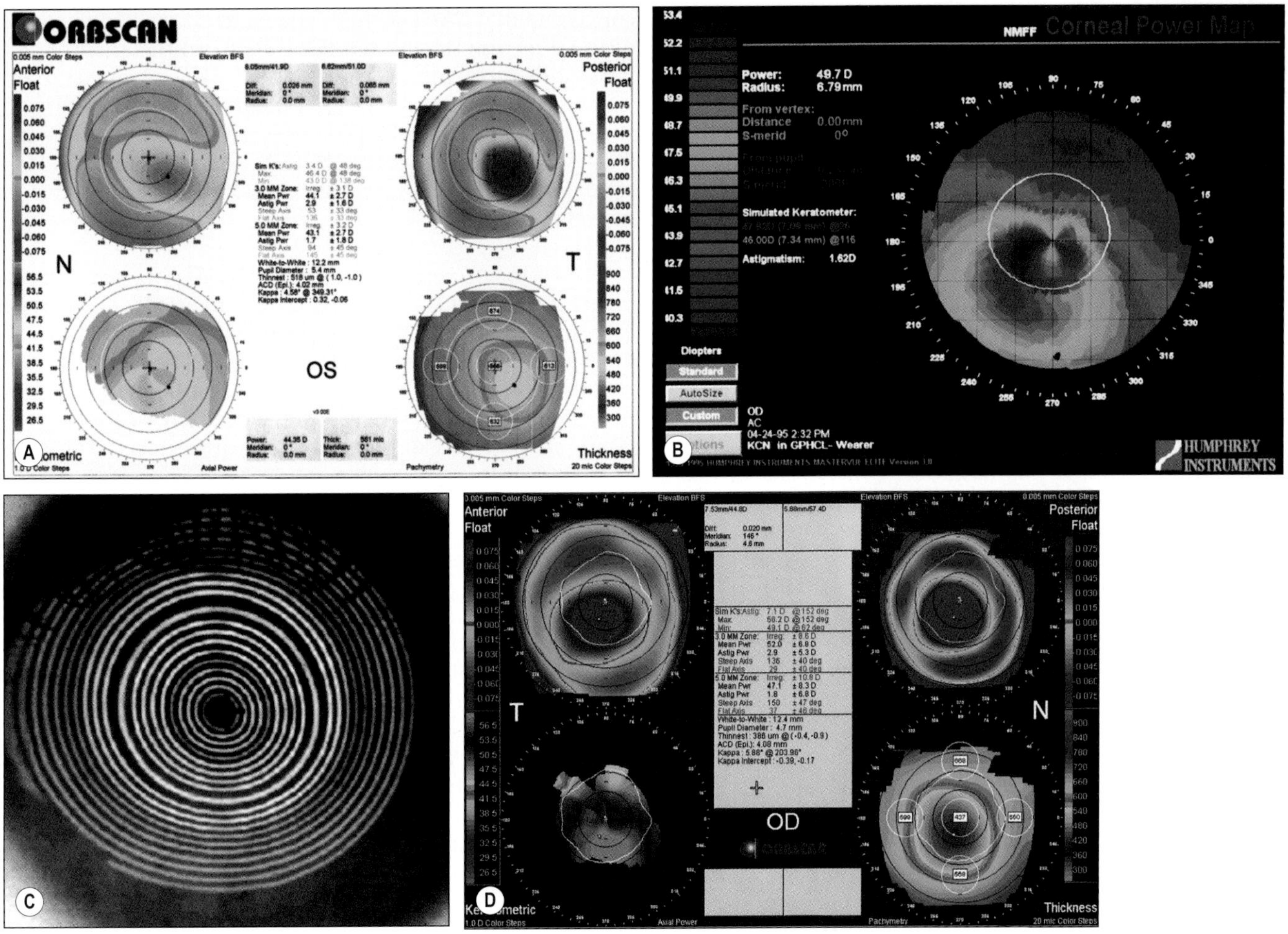

Fig. 74.10 Computer-assisted topography maps and photokeratoscopy are useful in detecting keratoconus at various stages of development. Representative stages of disease are demonstrated. (**A**) Subclinical keratoconus. Orbscan (Bausch & Lomb) (1) anterior elevation map (*upper left*) shows an eccentric area of elevation, (2) posterior float (*upper right*) shows prominent elevation coincident with the anterior elevation, (3) power map (*lower left*) shows asymmetric dumbbell with some skewing of radial axes and superior flattening, (4) pachymetry map (*lower right*) shows point of maximal thinning eccentric and coincident with elevation on anterior and posterior float maps. Even the thinnest part of the cornea could be considered within the normal range. (**B** and **C**) Early keratoconus. (**B**) Power map in early keratoconus demonstrates steep central corneal power inferior steepening, superior flattening, asymmetric dumbbell with skewed radial axes >21 degrees, Sim K astigmatism >1.5 diopters, all findings seen in keratoconus power maps. (**C**) Keratograph in early keratoconus shows decreased ring spacing inferiorly. (**D**) Moderate keratoconus. Orbscan II (Bausch & Lomb): (1) prominent inferior paracentral elevation, (2) marked elevation in posterior float, (3) marked steepening in power map with point of maximal steepening coincident with maximal elevation, (4) pachymetric map illustrates abnormally thin cornea with thinnest part of the cornea at the point of maximal elevation and steepening.

topography referred primarily to the use of a Placido disk-generated power map. The slit-scan device and rasterstereography enabled the computer to provide more accurate anterior elevation data. The Scheimpflug technology in the Pentacam (Oculus, Lynnwood, WA) provides reliable measurement of anterior and posterior corneal elevation and accurate measurement of corneal thickness. Thus, early keratoconus detection has become less dependent on review of a power map and more an evaluation of power, elevation, and pachymetry.

It is unclear whether the keratoconus suspect patient will ultimately develop clinical manifestations of keratoconus, but it is important to detect this condition when refractive surgery is being considered. Of the patients presenting for keratorefractive surgery, 2–6% were suspected to have keratoconus.[122–124] The outcome of refractive surgery in this setting may be unpredictable and may lead to progressive keratectasia.[125] Although investigators have reported successful photorefractive surgery in keratoconus suspects,[126,127] caution is recommended until this issue has been more thoroughly studied.

Rabinowitz has suggested four quantitative videokeratographic indices as an aid for screening patients for keratoconus.[128] These indices include central corneal power value greater than 47.2 D, inferior–superior dioptric asymmetry (I-S value) over 1.2, Sim-K astigmatism greater than 1.5 D, and skewed radial axes (SRAX) greater than 21 degrees. These indices were used to distinguish keratoconus from normal corneas and were most effective when astigmatism was greater than 1.5 D. Maeda et al.[129,130] developed an expert system classifier using eight topographic indices. It was found to be significantly better than keratometry for identifying keratoconus and had greater specificity than either keratometry or the Rabinowitz-McDonnell test, which is based on central corneal power and I-S value. Evolution in keratoconus detection has resulted in continued refinement of the neural network approach by Smolek and Klyce[131] and the KISA% index described by Rabinowitz and Rasheed.[132] Both systems purport an ability to detect keratoconus suspects and grade the severity of keratoconus.

Poor patient fixation,[133] misalignment of the videokeratograph,[134,135] dry spots on the cornea, inferior eyeball compression,[16] and contact lens-related corneal warpage[136] can all result in a pseudokeratoconus appearance on a power map. Suspicion should be raised if the map is grossly inconsistent with other aspects of the examination.

The scanning-slit topography device (Orbscan, Bausch & Lomb), provides the clinician with an anterior elevation map (anterior float) based on a best-fit sphere, a mathematically derived posterior elevation map (posterior float), a power map, and a topographical pachymetry map (see Fig. 74.10A). The point of maximal elevation on the posterior float should be less than 40 microns (μm) greater than the best-fit sphere. Values greater than 50 microns (μm) are suggestive of keratoconus. The posterior float is the least reliable of the four maps. Wilson has discussed the uncertainties regarding the derived posterior curvature.[137] The pachymetry map gives a relative overview of corneal thickness, but the values should not be considered equivalent to pachymetric readings measured by ultrasound.

Scheimpflug photography can be used to provide a more accurate means of measuring corneal thickness and elevation. The Pentacam has a computer program that plots the change in corneal thickness from the thinnest spot moving outward toward the periphery and analyzes the rate of thickness change compared to normative data. A virgin cornea with an isolated island of anterior elevation greater than 11 microns (μm) as detected by the Pentacam, and posterior elevation greater than 20 microns (μm) is suspicious for an ectatic corneal contour.

The ophthalmologist should make use of all available modalities to evaluate the contour and thickness of the paracentral as well as the central cornea. Since keratoconus progresses, measurements of contour and thickness taken over time can help to confirm the diagnosis.

Corneal ectasia following keratorefractive surgery

One of the challenges in evaluating patients for keratorefractive surgery is determining which patient is at risk to develop postoperative corneal ectasia. This condition resembles keratoconus, with typical clinical and topographic findings of progressive thinning and protrusion and resultant loss of visual function. Ectasia can present years after refractive surgery and can occur in some patients in the absence of any apparent risk factors.[138,139]

An understanding of cornea stromal ultrastructure and biomechanics can help explain how ectasia can develop in some cases. Dawson et al. have shown that the anterior and peripheral stroma is more rigid with greater cohesive tensile strength than the posterior two-thirds of the stroma. They concluded that this is perhaps related to observed differences in the direction of collagen fibrils between the anterior and posterior stroma and/or the degree of collagen lamellar interweaving in Bowman's layer.[140] LASIK surgery resulting in stromal ablation into the posterior stroma would potentially create a postsurgical cornea with less rigidity and cohesive tensile strength. This situation would arise if the degree of myopia is high, the cornea is thin, or the flap is unintentionally thick.

Some patients are predisposed to developing ectasia even in the absence of surgery. The onset of keratoconus is typically in puberty, but it may develop later. The onset of pellucid marginal degeneration occurs later. Patients with an abortive form of ectasia, the so-called forme fruste disease, may remain in the subclinical state if left untouched. A young patient may develop manifest disease in the absence of surgery if followed over time. It is imperative to successfully identify these patients and counsel them against LASIK surgery.

Inferior steepening, asymmetric dumbbell, skewed radial axes, crab-claw configuration, high astigmatism, and I/S ratios determined from power maps have long been helpful findings used to diagnose the at-risk patient. With the advent of newer technologies, more accurate elevation maps have become useful tools for detecting forme fruste disease. An area of off-center elevation either anteriorly or posteriorly when compared with a best-fit sphere is a helpful indicator. Programs have been developed which modify the classic best-fit sphere to alter the sensitivity of keratoconus detection. Finally, more accurate pachymetry maps created using Scheimpflug technology can help identify significant differences between the two eyes or areas of off-center thinning in an eye. Proper preoperative evaluation requires the refractive surgeon to use multiple maps and analyses before concluding that the risk of ectasia is minimal.

Randleman et al. studied patients with post-LASIK ectasia and identified five main risk factors for this complication. Young age at the time of surgery, abnormal preoperative topography, reduced residual stromal bed thickness, decreased preoperative cornea thickness, and high myopia were significant factors in patients who developed ectasia after LASIK surgery.[141] These variables were incorporated into a scoring algorithm to quantitatively assess the risk of ectasia. The scoring method provides a model for systematically screening high-risk patients.

Treatment

The management of keratoconus begins with spectacle correction. Once glasses fail to provide adequate visual function, contact lens fitting is required. Contact lens wear improves visual function by creating a new anterior refractive surface (Fig. 74.11). Contact lenses do not prevent progression of corneal ectasia. While they seem to be associated with the development of keratoconus in some cases, this important mode of therapy should never be withheld for fear of causing progressive disease.

Contact lenses must be tailored to the individual's visual needs and comfort tolerance. Given ample time and motivation, fitting expertise, and access to all available contact lens modalities, many keratoconus patients can be successfully

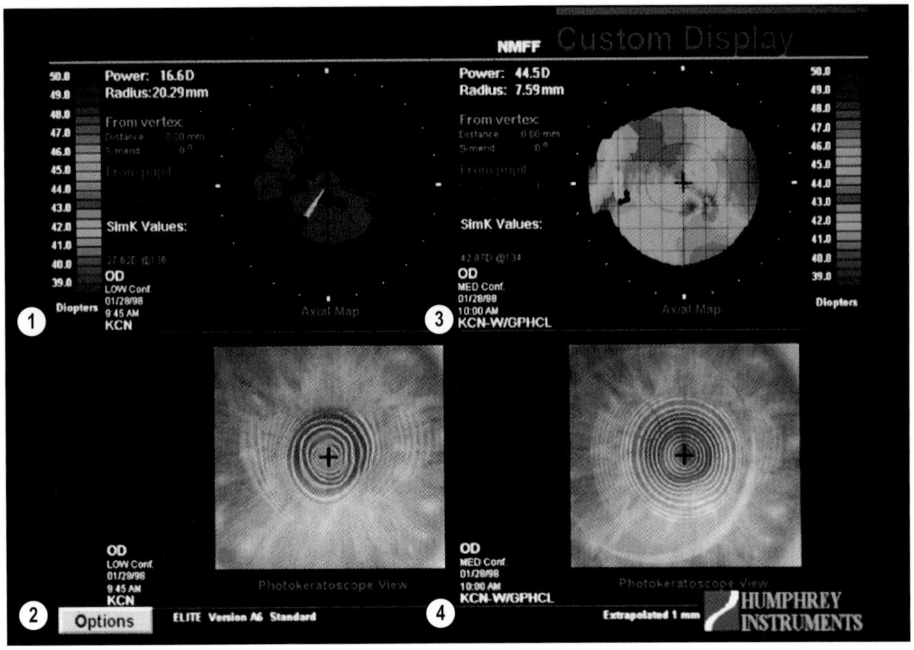

Fig. 74.11 The effect of hard contact lens wear on the anterior refractive surface in a case of advanced keratoconus. (*1*) Without the contact lens a scarred, markedly flat cone apex is seen. (*2*) This correlates with the widely spaced and irregular keratograph. (*3*) With a hard contact lens on the same cornea the power map has an appearance approaching normal. (*4*) This is verified in the keratograph on the lower left in which the edge of the contact lens can be seen.

refitted, achieving good visual function with a stable, well-tolerated lens.

Relatively flat-fitting, rigid gas-permeable (RGP), hard contact lenses with light apical corneal touch, the so-called three-point touch technique, remain the mainstay of contact lens treatment for keratoconus.[142,143] An apical clearance fitting technique is also commonly used. Other options include soft toric lenses, standard bicurved hard lenses, custom-back toric lenses, piggyback systems, hybrid lenses made of combined hard lens with a soft skirt, scleral lenses, and mini scleral lenses.[144,145]

Hybrid lenses, such as the SoftPerm lens (CIBA Vision Corp., Duluth, GA) and the newer SynergEyes KC lens (SynergEyes, Inc., Carlsbad, CA) may be more comfortable for patients who cannot tolerate an RGP alone. The SoftPerm lens has an optic zone diameter of 7.0 mm and a permeability of 14.0×10^{-11} (cm^2/s) (mL O_2/mL × mmHg).[146] The newer SynergEyes KC has a rigid optic of 7.8 mm made of highly oxygen permeable material Paragon HDS 100 (*paflufocon* D) bonded to a soft outer skirt composed of PolyHEMA (hemiberfilcon A). SynergEyes offers a significantly higher Dk of 100×10^{-11} (cm^2/s) (mL O_2/mL × mmHg) which may improve patient comfort. Lenses are available in base curve radii as steep as 5.7 mm.[147]

Mini-scleral lenses have a diameter of 14–17 mm compared to scleral lenses with a diameter of 20–24 mm. Mini-scleral lenses are designed to offer the benefits of scleral lenses such as vaulting the cornea to limit cornea touch, providing a tear fluid reservoir, correcting astigmatism, and improving vision, in addition to offering practitioners and patients greater ease in fitting and handling.[148,149]

One form of contact lens intolerance may result from epithelial breakdown overlying a subepithelial fibrotic scar occurring at the apex of the cone. Using a self-retaining wire speculum and topical anesthesia, this can easily be debrided at the slit lamp. After the cornea has healed, the patient may resume contact lens wear, obviating the need for more invasive surgery. Phototherapeutic keratectomy (PTK) has also been used in this setting as well as in cases of advanced keratoconus to reduce contact lens intolerance.[150,151] While it may be helpful in some cases, PTK may cause keratolysis,[152] increased scarring, and ectasia, and thereby hasten the need for penetrating keratoplasty.

Contact lens-intolerant keratoconus patients without central scarring, who have mild or moderate disease, may be candidates for intrastromal ring segment insertion. The ideal candidates also have low spherical equivalents and average keratometry readings of less than 53 D. The procedure improves visual acuity by flattening the central cornea, reducing astigmatism and centering the cone.[153–156] The goal of the procedure is to improve contact lens fit and comfort. It may also improve best-spectacle-corrected visual acuity (BSCVA). It is important to set proper patient expectations prior to surgery and inform the patient that glasses and/or contact lenses will still be needed after surgery.

Ferrara rings (Ferrara Ophthalmics, Belo Horizonte, Brazil) and Intacs (Addition Technology Inc, Des Plaines, IL, USA), commonly used ring segments, are made of rigid polymethyl methacrylate. Ferrara rings have a fixed inner diameter of 5.0 mm and a triangular anterior contour.[156] Intacs have an inner diameter of 6.8 mm, a flat anterior surface, and are available in thicknesses of 0.25–0.45 mm, in 0.05 mm increments.[155] The thickest segments are not currently available in the USA. Enhanced effect is generally achieved with the thicker segments.

To achieve the desired effect, the ring segments must be inserted at approximately two-thirds depth; therefore, the cornea should be at least 450 μm thick (Fig. 74.12). Stromal channels have traditionally been prepared with a specially designed keratome. Some femtosecond lasers can now be

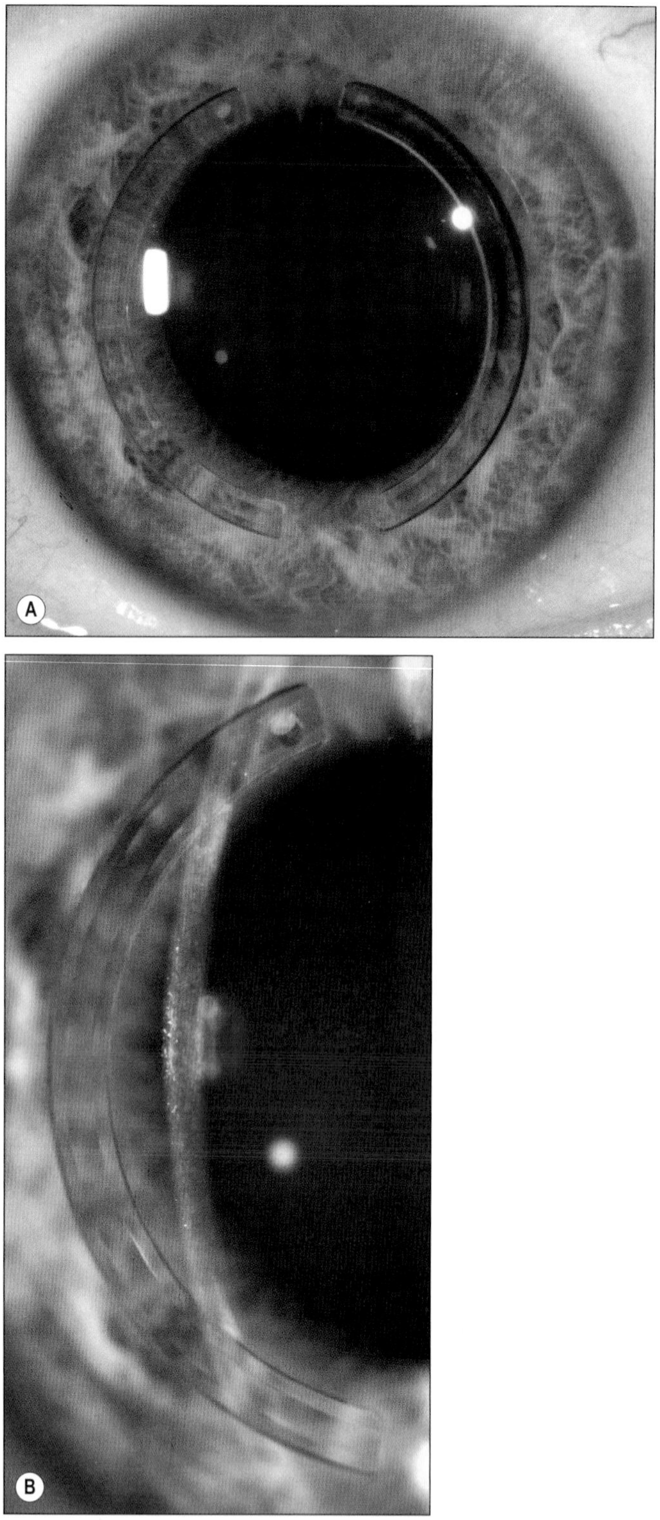

Fig. 74.12 Intracorneal ring segments (**A**) Diffuse illumination reveals two ring segments in a keratoconus cornea. (**B**) Slit view demonstrates the appropriate depth for ring segment placement.

programmed to create stromal channels of the appropriate width and depth.[157] While wide channels make insertion easy, the desired effect can only be obtained with a snug fit.

Colin and Malet reported that contact lens wear was restored in over 80% of cases. The 2-year best-corrected visual acuity (BCVA) improved in 68.3% of eyes ($p < 0.001$), and the manifest refraction spherical equivalent improved from a mean of −6.93 D ± 3.91 (SD) preoperatively to −3.80 ± 2.73 D at 2 years ($p < 0.001$). Measurements of mean keratometry decreased from 50.1 ± 5.6 D to 46.8 ± 4.9 D at 2 years ($p < 0.001$).[155]

While the ring segments are removable, the procedure should not be considered completely reversible. The ring segments do not prevent progression of the underlying disease. If keratoplasty later becomes necessary, the surgery should occur at least 1 month following ring removal.

Collagen cross-linking (CXL or C3-R) is the most recent addition to the surgical armamentarium and may slow or halt the progression of keratoconus by using a photo-oxidative treatment to increase the rigidity of the corneal stroma (Fig. 74.13A).[158–160] At the time of this writing, CXL is not FDA approved for use in the USA, but a prospective, multicenter study is under way.

The procedure begins with the removal of the central epithelium to enhance stromal saturation with the topically applied riboflavin (vitamin B_2). The cornea is then irradiated with ultraviolet A (UVA) light at 370 nm for 30 minutes using a special UVA generating device (Fig. 74.13B). The irradiation of the riboflavin results in chemical reactions that create covalent bonds, which bridge amino groups of the stromal collagen fibrils.[161]

The principal effects of cross-linking are localized to the anterior 300 μm of the stroma.[162] The biomechanical effect in human corneas has been shown to be a 328.9% increase in corneal rigidity.[163] Morphologically, the formation of cross-links increases intermolecular spacing as the collagen polypeptide chains are pushed apart.[161] Increased resistance to enzymatic degradation shown in porcine eyes following cross-linking may also contribute to biomechanical stability.[164]

The improvement in visual acuity after CXL is the result of decreasing both corneal curvature and astigmatism. Raiskup-Wolf et al. reported a 2.68 D reduction in corneal power at 1 year postoperatively.[158] Three years after the treatment, the BCVA improved one line in 58% of 33 eyes and remained stable in 29% of eyes ($p < 0.01$). The astigmatism had diminished by a mean of 1.45 D in 54% of eyes. These topographical changes have the potential to improve contact lens fit. CXL appears to be most beneficial for patients with mild progressive keratoconus. It is less effective in patients with advanced keratoconus and may be less effective in patients with ectasia following LASIK surgery.

CXL poses a risk of dose-dependent keratocyte apoptosis affecting the anterior 300 μm of the cornea (Fig. 74.13C). UVA irradiance of 0.36 mW/cm^2 has been found to be cytotoxic to the rabbit corneal endothelium, which corresponded to a human corneal stromal thickness of less than 400 μm.[165,166] Therefore, pachymetry should be performed preoperatively to confirm that the corneal stroma is greater than 400 μm thick. Preliminary studies have shown that the lens and retina are not adversely affected.[167]

When a stable, comfortable contact lens fit cannot be obtained or fails to provide adequate vision, more invasive surgery such as keratoplasty is recommended. The type of keratoplasty surgery depends greatly on the individual patient's needs and the surgeon's preferred technique. While

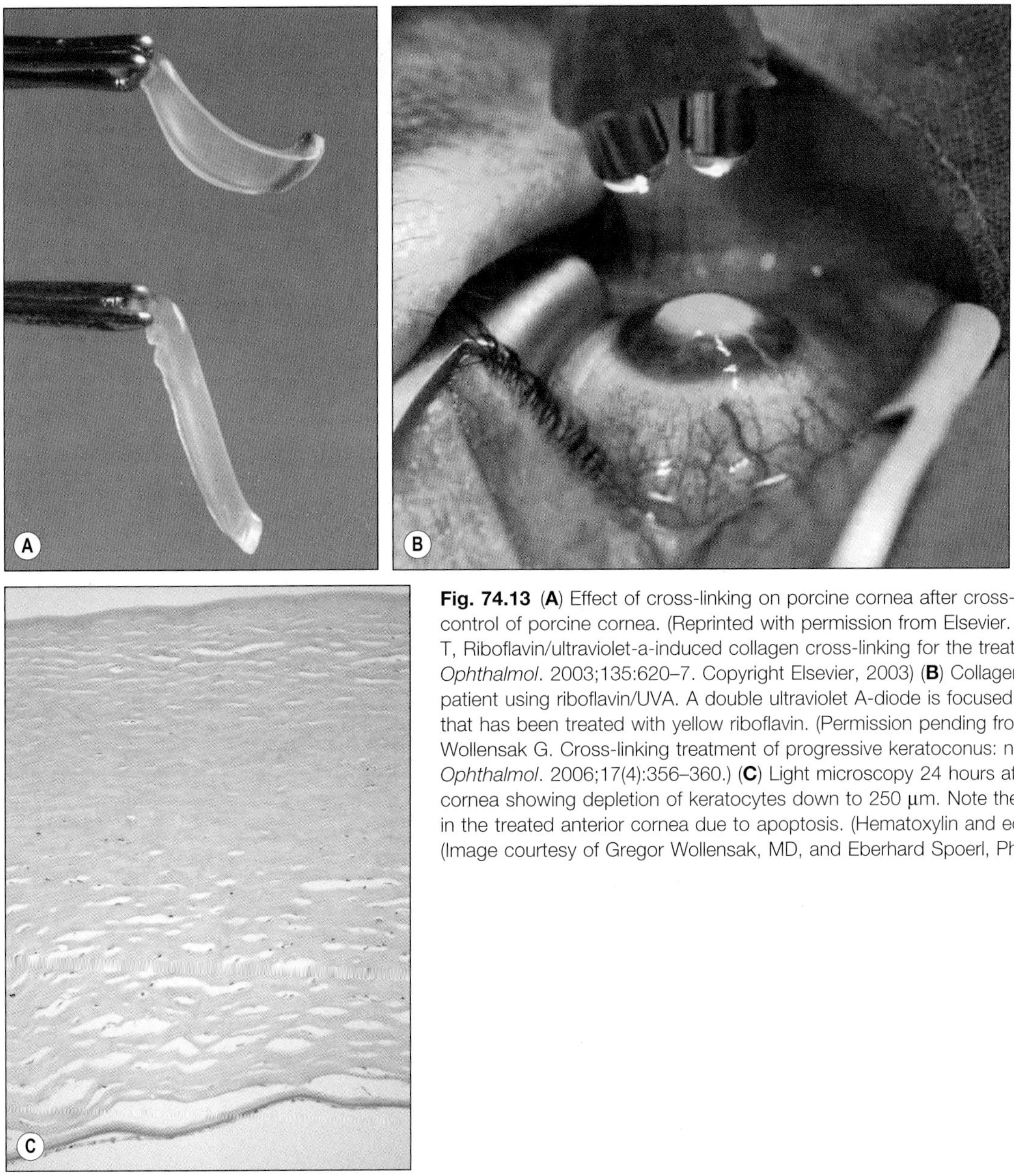

Fig. 74.13 (**A**) Effect of cross-linking on porcine cornea after cross-linking. *Below*: Untreated control of porcine cornea. (Reprinted with permission from Elsevier. Wollensak G, Spoerl E, Seiler T, Riboflavin/ultraviolet-a-induced collagen cross-linking for the treatment of keratoconus. *Am J Ophthalmol*. 2003;135:620–7. Copyright Elsevier, 2003) (**B**) Collagen cross-linking treatment on a patient using riboflavin/UVA. A double ultraviolet A-diode is focused 1 cm from the abraded cornea that has been treated with yellow riboflavin. (Permission pending from Lippincott Williams & Wilkins. Wollensak G. Cross-linking treatment of progressive keratoconus: new hope. *Curr Opin Ophthalmol*. 2006;17(4):356–360.) (**C**) Light microscopy 24 hours after cross-linking in human cornea showing depletion of keratocytes down to 250 μm. Note the absence of inflammatory cells in the treated anterior cornea due to apoptosis. (Hematoxylin and eosin stain, magnification ×200.) (Image courtesy of Gregor Wollensak, MD, and Eberhard Spoerl, PhD.)

penetrating keratoplasty has traditionally been the surgery of choice, lamellar surgery is becoming more popular for patients with mild to moderate disease. Recurrent keratoconus in the donor following cornea transplant has been reported;[168,169] however, recurrent keratoconus is far more likely to be related to incomplete excision of the cone. The iron ring, found at the base of the cone, should be used as a reference when planning graft size. Permanent mydriasis after penetrating keratoplasty described by Urrets-Zavalia[170] rarely occurs with modern microsurgical techniques.

Postkeratoplasty myopia can be reduced by using the same-sized donor and host corneal buttons.[171–174] Some have even suggested undersizing the donor to further flatten the postoperative corneal contour.[175] Axial length can be an important factor in the refractive error outcome following keratoplasty.[176] Ultrasound axial length measured from the anterior lens capsule to retina reveals a broad range in length from 18.77 to 25.65 mm.[177] Reducing donor size, in a relatively short eye, could result in significant postoperative hyperopia. The flattened corneal contour could complicate contact lens fitting in the anisometropic patient. Same-size donor and host corneal buttons should not be used when the anterior lens-to-retina length is less than 20.19 mm, the mean length for nonkeratoconic individuals with emmetropia.

Deep anterior lamellar keratoplasty (DALK) is a recently developed alternative to traditional lamellar keratoplasty as well as penetrating keratoplasty (PK). One advantage of the procedure is that the host endothelium is preserved, thus reducing the risk of rejection. The risk of endophthalmitis is theoretically less because this is largely an extraocular procedure. Intact host Descemet's membrane may afford greater wound stability than occurs in penetrating keratoplasty. In addition, the reduced need for topical steroid may help the DALK patient to heal faster than the PK patient. Visual outcomes are comparable to PK.[178–180] The main drawbacks are that DALK is technically more challenging and time consuming.

The procedure involves a staged dissection of stroma down to the level of Descemet's membrane and transplantation of donor tissue that has had Descemet's membrane removed. Anwar and Teichmann introduced the big bubble technique in which air is injected into the deep stroma after an initial stromal dissection. This acts to safely separate the posterior stroma from Descemet's membrane, resulting in a shorter and safer surgery.[181] Viscoelastic has also been used to separate the host Descemet's membrane. Reducing the intraocular pressure (IOP) with a paracentesis also helps to prevent perforation. Melles et al. has described using intracameral air as a reference to help judge the depth of the host stromal dissection.[182]

The treatment of keratoconus is rarely an emergency. The exception is corneal hydrops, resulting from a rupture in Descemet's membrane (see Fig. 74.9). This may be a finding at presentation in the patient with developmental delay, such as in Down's syndrome. A dramatic reduction in vision occurs as a result of stromal edema. This may be accompanied by redness, discomfort, and photophobia. Proper management includes patching or bandage contact lens, cycloplegia, hypertonic sodium chloride ointment and/or drops, and reassurance. Topical steroids are rarely needed, and their use has been implicated in rare cases of hydrops with perforation.

Intracameral air has been used in the management of corneal hydrops. The air acts as a mechanical barrier, reducing aqueous flow into the stroma through the rupture in Descemet's membrane. Because the air is absorbed over a few days, the intracameral gases sulfur hexafluoride (SF_6) and perfluoropropane (C_3F_8), in isoexpansile concentrations, have been used.[183,184] Perfluoropropane in 14% dilution persists in the anterior chamber for about 6 weeks. A concentration of 20% SF_6 gas is nontoxic to the endothelium and lasts about 2 weeks before reabsorption. Panda et al. reported the safety and efficacy of SF_6 in expediting resolution of corneal edema compared to conventional medical management.[183] Hydrops that does not clear by 3 to 4 months is best treated by penetrating keratoplasty.

Pellucid Marginal Degeneration

Pellucid marginal degeneration (PMD) is a bilateral, peripheral corneal ectatic disorder characterized by a band of thinning 1–2 mm in width, typically in the inferior cornea, extending from the 4 to the 8 o'clock position. The area of thinning is usually found 1–2 mm central to the inferior limbus. Atypical cases of PMD with thinning extending beyond the inferior 4 clock hours occur,[185] as do cases in which the thinning is confined to a superior location.[186,187] Unilateral cases have also been reported.[188,189]

In contrast to keratoconus, maximal corneal protrusion typically occurs just superior to, rather than within, the area of thinning (Fig. 74.14). The result is a corneal contour which is reminiscent of a 'beer belly.' The protruding cornea

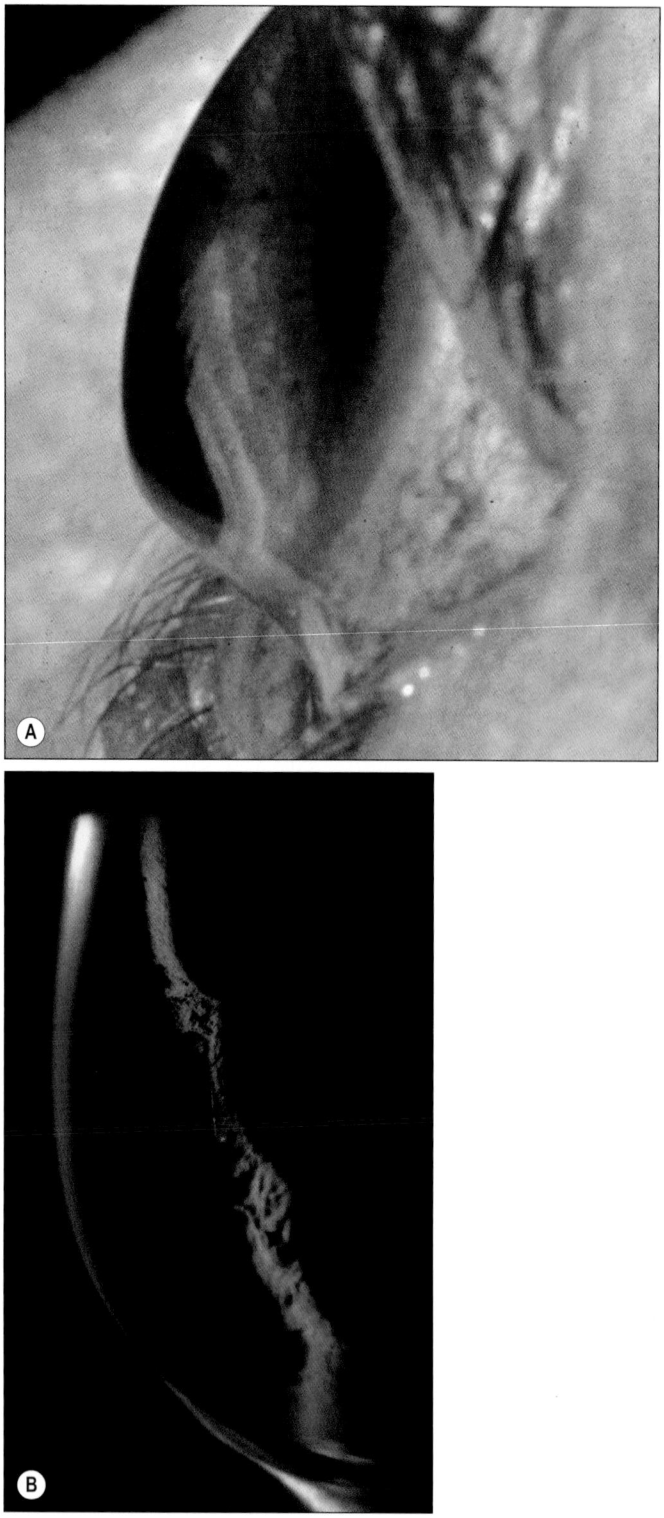

Fig. 74.14 Pellucid marginal degeneration appearance. (**A**) The profile of a cornea with pellucid marginal degeneration shows protrusion and sagging of the inferior cornea. (**B**) This slit lamp photograph demonstrates corneal protrusion superior to the point of maximal thinning.

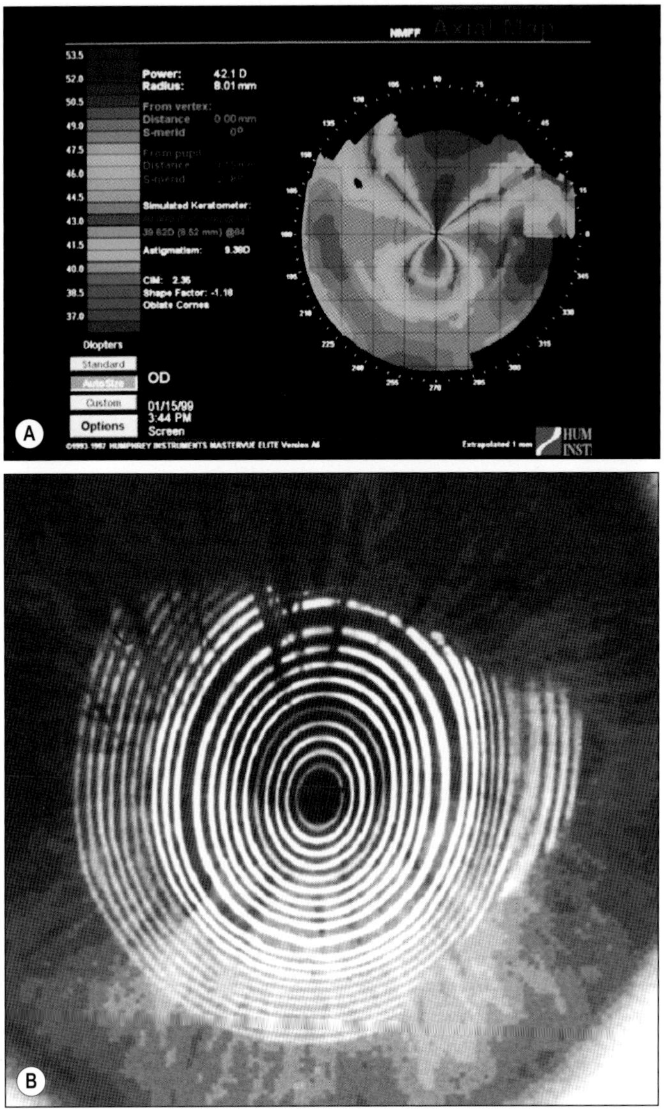

Fig. 74.15 Pellucid marginal degeneration topography. (**A**) The power map shows the classic crab-claw configuration often seen in pellucid marginal degeneration. (**B**) The videokeratograph confirms the presence of superior flattening with against-the-rule astigmatism superiorly and with-the-rule astigmatism inferiorly.

is of normal thickness. The abnormal corneal contour induces a shift in the axis of astigmatism from against-the-rule, superiorly, to with-the-rule, near the point of maximal protrusion. PMD and keratoconus can occur in the same eye.[190] The two diseases can also be seen in the same family.

Maguire et al.[191] have described the corneal contour in PMD using computer-generated power maps. The typical crab-claw (Fig. 74.15) illustrates the shift in astigmatism from the superior to the inferior cornea. The crab-claw appearance on a power map can also occur in patients with inferior keratoconus. Computer-assisted topography may reveal corneal contour abnormalities in asymptomatic family members of a PMD patient even when the slit lamp examination is normal.[192]

Patients with PMD are poor candidates for refractive surgery because of the potential for an undesirable outcome and the risk that the surgical procedure might stimulate progressive ectasia. Ambrosio and Wilson have emphasized the need to screen refractive surgery candidates with corneal topography and regional pachymetry to rule out PMD, even when the best-corrected acuity is 20/20 and the biomicroscopic examination is normal.[193] Review of accurate pachymetric maps can help identify the patient with inferior thinning.

Patients with this condition usually present for treatment between the second and fifth decades of life with complaints of blurred vision resulting from irregular astigmatism. There is no racial or gender predisposition.

Schlaeppi[194] appropriately chose the name *pellucid*, meaning clear, to describe this thinning disorder. These corneas are generally clear and avascular, with no iron ring, infiltrate, or lipid deposition. Stromal scars have been described at the level of Descemet's membrane extending into the mid stroma, located at the superior aspect of the thinned area. Cameron reported such scars in 39% of PMD patients.[195] Subtle Descemet's folds, which are occasionally seen concentric to the inferior limbus, may disappear with external pressure. While the cornea can become quite thin, rupture rarely occurs.[196–198] Acute hydrops can occur and the result is edema, scarring, and vascularization of the inferior cornea.

Pellucid marginal degeneration can be distinguished from other peripheral thinning disorders found in the differential diagnosis (Table 74.2). The findings typical of keratoconus, specifically, protrusion within the area of corneal thinning, striae, and Fleischer's ring, are not seen in PMD. Terrien's marginal degeneration can cause high astigmatism in a similar age group. However, in contrast to pellucid degeneration, this disorder has a male predilection. It commonly affects the cornea, superiorly as well as inferiorly, with vascularization and lipid deposition. When corneal protrusion occurs in Terrien's degeneration, it is usually within the area of thinning. Mooren's ulcer is usually unilateral and is associated with marked inflammation and pain, an epithelial defect in the area of ulceration, undermining of the central edge of the ulcer, and vascularization up to the peripheral edge. Corneal changes in Mooren's ulcer are not confined to the inferior or superior cornea. Finally, idiopathic furrow degeneration, while bilateral and noninflammatory, occurs in the elderly within a corneal arcus.

In PMD the epithelium, Descemet's membrane, and the endothelium are normal. Rodrigues et al. found normal or focal disruption of Bowman's layer.[199] Within the area of corneal thinning, electron microscopy showed electron-dense areas of fibrous long-spacing (FLS) collagen with a periodicity of 100–110 nm, in contrast to a periodicity of 60–64 nm found in normal collagen. Similar FLS collagen has been seen in other conditions, including advanced keratoconus, but is not seen in normal corneal stroma. Weakening in the area of FLS collagen in the corneal stroma could result in the thinning observed in PMD. Since PMD and keratoconus can both occur in the same eye, this finding may also be important in the pathogenesis of keratoconus. As in keratoconus, there is a statistically significant reduction of highly sulfated keratan sulfate epitopes in PMD.[200]

Spectacles usually fail to adequately correct the high irregular astigmatism associated with typical cases of PMD. Large-

Table 74.2 The differential diagnosis of pellucid marginal degeneration – clinical presentation and appearance of other peripheral thinning disorders compared and contrasted

	Pellucid marginal degeneration	Terrien's marginal degeneration	Mooren's ulcer	Furrow degeneration
Age at onset	Second to fifth decade	Usually middle-aged to elderly	Adult to elderly	Elderly
Laterality	Bilateral	Bilateral	Unilateral and bilateral types	Bilateral
Gender	Male = female	Males predominate	Males more common	Male = female
Astigmatism	Common	Common	Sometimes	None
Thinning	Inferior band 1–2 mm wide	Usually starts superiorly	Starts within lid fissure	Occurs within arcus
Inflammation	None	Occasionally	Typical; worse in bilateral type	None
Epithelial defect	None	Usually none	Typical	None
Vascularization	None	Crosses area of thinning	Peripheral edge of thinning	None
Lipid deposition	None	Common; central to thinning	Not acutely	Corneal arcus
Perforation	Hydrops more common	Unusual	Common in bilateral type	Never

diameter, rigid gas-permeable contact lenses can be tried. However, because of the contour abnormality, a stable long-term fit can be difficult to achieve. The hybrid lenses, such as the SoftPerm lens, have been used successfully in PMD.[201] The newer generation of scleral lenses made from gas-permeable plastic may also be of benefit.[202,203]

A surgical approach is often required for visual rehabilitation. Large-diameter or eccentric penetrating keratoplasty may be necessary to encompass the area of peripheral thinning. Placing the graft wound in proximity to the limbal vasculature increases the risk of endothelial rejection. Success with large-diameter keratoplasty in the absence of corneal neovascularization has been reported.[204,205] Varley et al.[205] reported a rejection rate of 64%, but none of the 12 large, eccentric grafts failed because of rejection over a mean follow-up period of 3 years. Kremer et al. described a two-stage procedure in which a large-diameter lamellar keratoplasty is followed by a smaller central penetrating keratoplasty.[206] Rasheed and Rabinowitz have suggested performing these two procedures simultaneously.[207]

Alternative surgical procedures include thermokeratoplasty, crescentic lamellar keratoplasty, and crescentic or wedge excision.[208,209] Long-term astigmatism drift may be a problem following resection procedures.

Keratoglobus

Keratoglobus is a bilateral ectatic disorder that is usually nonprogressive or minimally progressive. The typical globular protrusion of the cornea results from generalized thinning, most marked in the periphery (Fig. 74.16). Associated scleral thinning has also been described.[210] Minimal, if any, corneal scarring may be seen, but an iron ring is not observed. The cornea is of normal or slightly increased diameter. Acute hydrops occurs less frequently than in keratoconus;[211] however, the opposite is true about corneal perforation and rupture. Keratoglobus patients are prone to corneal rupture after minimal trauma, even when there is no history of trauma.

In addition to keratoconus and pellucid marginal degeneration, the differential diagnosis of keratoglobus includes congenital glaucoma and megalocornea (Table 74.3). In contrast to congenital glaucoma, keratoglobus is a thinning disorder without corneal edema or Haab's striae, and the IOP, optic disks, and overall globe size are normal. In congenital megalocornea the horizontal corneal diameter is greater than 12 mm. The thickness and contour of the enlarged cornea are normal.

The computer-assisted corneal topography in patients with keratoglobus has not been well documented. Based on the biomicroscopic findings one would expect to see central and paracentral elevation and steepening with generalized thinning. This is demonstrated in the power map (Fig. 74.17). Keratoglobus can occur in the fellow eye of a patient with PMD and has been reported to develop in a PMD patient after cataract surgery through a limbal approach.[212] Cameron observed the development of keratoglobus after the resolution of hydrops in a keratoconus patient.[213] Pouliquen et al.[214] has also described unilateral keratoglobus occurring in a patient with pre-existing keratoconus.

Unlike keratoconus, keratoglobus is not associated with atopy, tapetoretinal degeneration, or hard contact lens wear. Keratoglobus has been reported in association with inflammatory orbital pseudotumor, chronic marginal blepharitis, chronic eye rubbing, and in glaucoma following penetrating keratoplasty.[213] Acquired keratoglobus has also been described in association with vernal keratoconjunctivitis[213] and hyperthyroidism.[215]

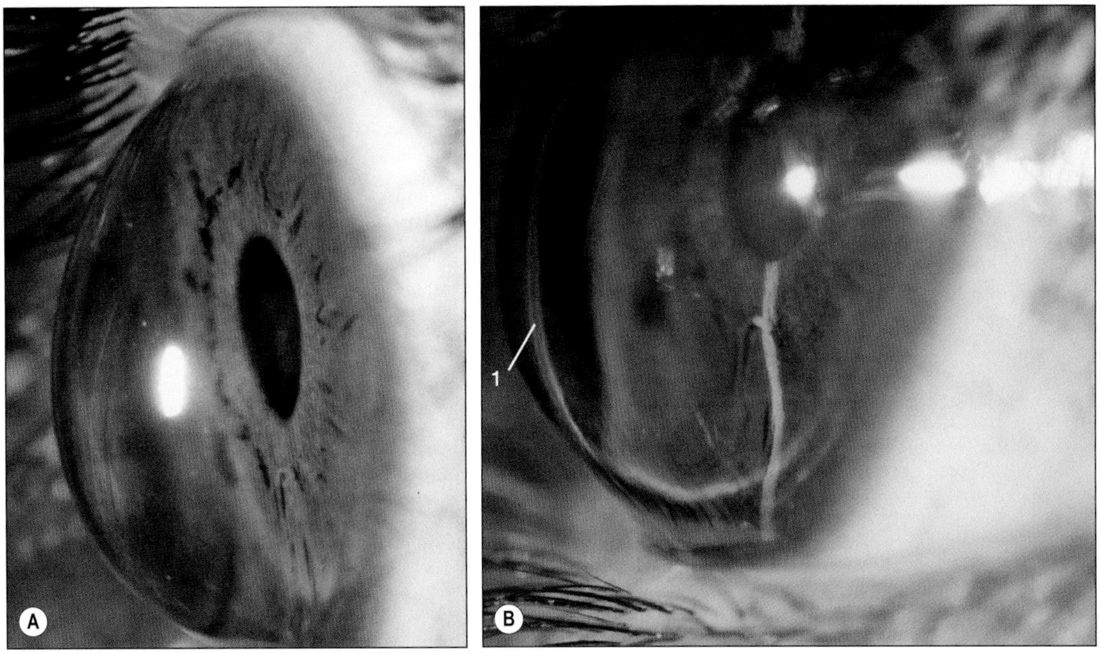

Fig. 74.16 Keratoglobus appearance. (**A**) The typical globular contour of the keratoglobus can be seen in this cornea photographed in profile. (**B**) Generalized thinning is common (*1*), with the greatest thinning found in the periphery.

Table 74.3 The differential diagnosis of keratoglobus – clinical presentation and appearance of commonly confused conditions are compared and contrasted

	Keratoglobus	Megalocornea	Congenital glaucoma
Corneal diameter	Normal or slightly increased	Greater than 12.5 mm	Greater than 12.5 mm
Thickness	Diffuse thinning; greatest in periphery	Normal	Edematous
Protrusion	Marked	None	Moderate
Astigmatism	Moderate to marked	Minimal	Minimal
Hydrops	Rupture more common	None	Common
Scarring	Possible	None	Haab's striae
Intraocular pressure	Normal to low	Normal	Elevated
Disk	Normal	Normal	Cupping
Posterior segment axial length	Normal	Normal	Increased

While there is no association with Down's syndrome, keratoglobus has been reported in association with Rubinstein-Taybi syndrome, in which intellectual impairment occurs.[216] As in keratoconus, there is evidence to suggest an association with abnormalities of connective tissue. Many reports link keratoglobus and blue sclera to other findings, such as hyperextensible joints, abnormalities in teeth and hearing, a high incidence of fractures, and consanguinity.[210,211,217,218]

Hyams et al.[217] considered keratoglobus to be an inherited syndrome involving connective tissue, while Greenfield et al.[28] concluded that this disorder represented a probable abnormality in collagen synthesis and postulated autosomal recessive inheritance. Keratoglobus associated with other disorders of connective tissue bears some resemblance to the ocular form of Ehlers-Danlos syndrome, but these patients do not demonstrate skin hyperelasticity, marked joint laxity, microcornea, or reduced skin collagen hydroxylysine.[210]

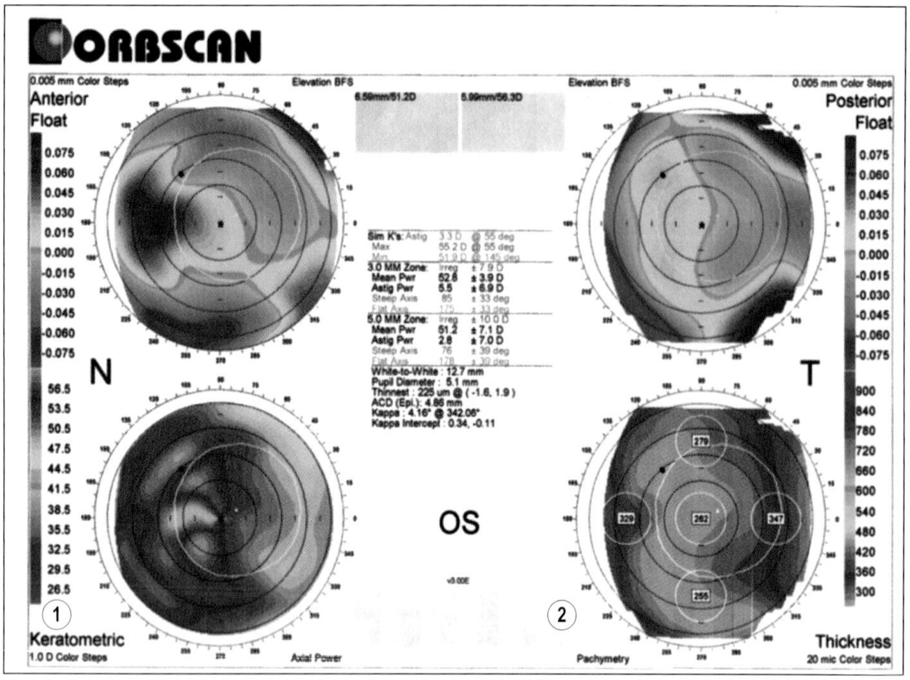

Fig. 74.17 Keratoglobus topography. (*1*) Orbscan (Bausch & Lomb) power map reveals diffuse steepening with the flattest Sim K reading 51.9 diopters, (*2*) Pachymetric map shows diffuse thinning, with the inferior part of the cornea being thinnest.

No definitive inheritance pattern has been demonstrated in keratoglobus. There may, however, be a genetic relationship between keratoglobus and keratoconus. Keratoglobus and keratoconus can be found in different members of the same family.

Spectacle correction is the first step in the management of keratoglobus. Functional vision can sometimes be obtained with glasses. Spectacles also afford the patient some protection from corneal rupture associated with trauma. A stable contact lens fit is difficult to achieve due to the abnormal corneal contour. There may be a role for a rigid gas-permeable scleral lens. One must weigh the advantages of contact lens wear and a nonsurgical approach, against the increased the risk of trauma associated with manipulation during insertion and removal.

Surgical intervention should be considered when functional vision cannot otherwise be obtained. A lamellar graft or epikeratoplasty[219] has the advantage of being an extraocular procedure with no risk of failure resulting from endothelial rejection. Prominent folds can result from compression of the markedly ectatic cornea. The use of partial-thickness corneoscleroplasty to preserve the anterior chamber angle, followed at a later time by a smaller-diameter penetrating keratoplasty has also been recommended.[220,221] Kanellopoulos and Pe describe an alternative, nonpenetrating procedure of suturing a corneoscleral ring graft around the cornea.[222]

As in pellucid marginal degeneration, a large-diameter penetrating keratoplasty would be required to encompass the markedly thin peripheral pathology. Grafts of this size are at greater risk of endothelial rejection. There is also a greater propensity to develop glaucoma caused by outflow channel compromise. In general, surgical intervention should be delayed, when possible.

Posterior Keratoconus

In posterior keratoconus, thinning results from an increase in the curvature of the posterior cornea. Corneal involvement can be diffuse or localized. In keratoconus posticus generalis the entire posterior corneal surface has an increased curvature and the cornea typically remains clear. In the localized form, keratoconus posticus circumscriptus, there may be one, or occasionally more, central or paracentral areas of posterior excavation associated with variable amounts of stromal scarring (Fig. 74.18). Corneal guttae are often seen within the area of involvement, and pigment is sometimes found at the peripheral edge of this posterior lesion.

While corneal astigmatism can occur, it is generally not the high irregular astigmatism seen in keratoconus (anterior keratoconus).[223] This relative lack of involvement of the anterior refractive surface explains why posterior keratoconus results in only mild to moderate reduction in visual function. Vision decrease, when it occurs, is usually caused by stromal scarring, associated ocular disease, or amblyopia. Computer-assisted topographical analysis on a posterior keratoconus patient has demonstrated a central steepening in the area of posterior excavation as well as surrounding flattening. Rao and Padmanabhan[224] have confirmed the presence of steepening when the area of involvement is central or paracentral, but found flattening over the area of peripheral involvement.

Posterior keratoconus is developmental, usually nonprogressive, noninflammatory, and unilateral.[1] Bilateral involvement, however, is not uncommon.[225] Acquired cases occur and are usually associated with trauma.[226,227] The condition has also been reported in a patient with interstitial keratitis after spontaneous intrastromal hemorrhage.[228]

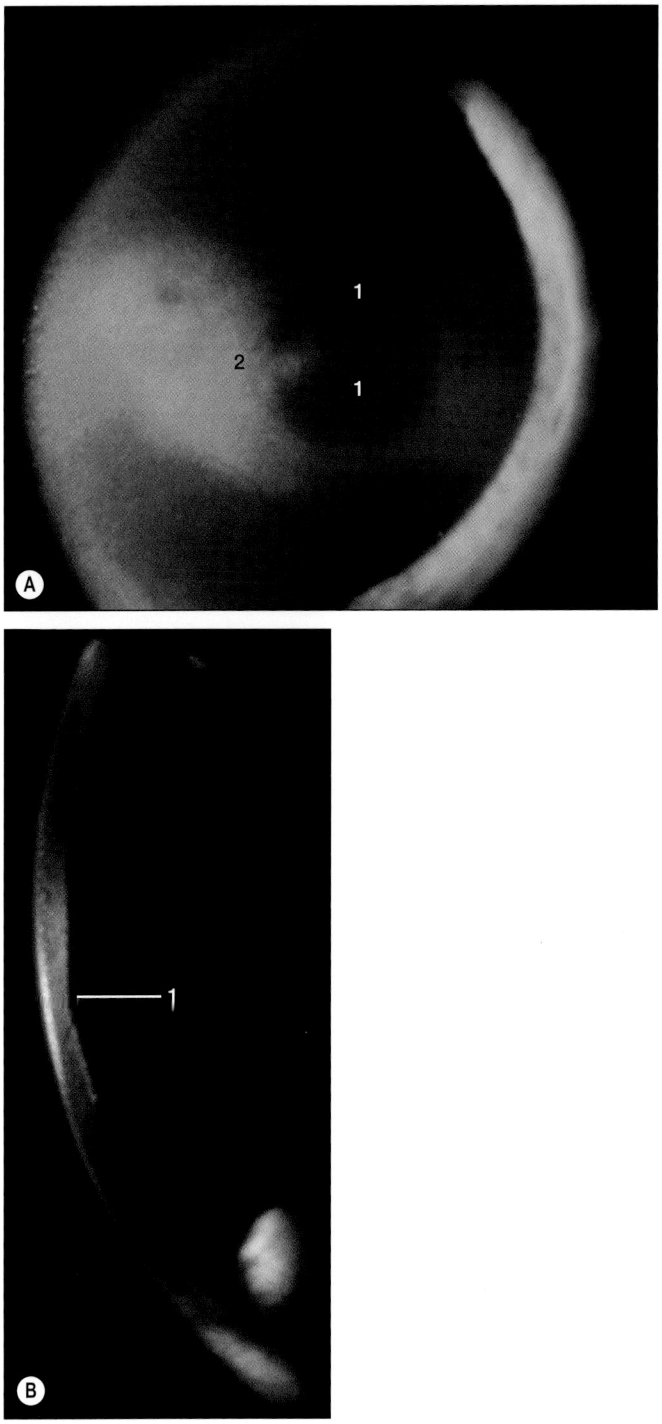

Fig. 74.18 Posterior keratoconus. (**A**) In the localized form an area of relative lucency (*1*), which corresponds to the site of posterior excavation, is surrounded by stromal scarring (*2*). (**B**) This slit view demonstrates thinning (*1*), which results from steepening in the posterior corneal contour. The anterior corneal contour is relatively unaffected.

The histopathologic findings in posterior keratoconus have been described.[223,229,230] Irregular epithelium with focal disruption of the epithelial basement membrane is seen, and Bowman's layer is replaced with fibroblastic proliferation. The stroma is thin, with lamellar disorganization also noted. The central portion of Descemet's membrane is not thin but may show marked disorganization. A ring of thickened Descemet's membrane at the edge of the cone may be associated with pigmented excrescences, although this finding was not confirmed by al-Hazzaa et al.[230] Guttae may be seen within the cone and adjacent to it. The endothelium is intact but is attenuated in the area of guttae. Electron microscopy reveals an abnormal anterior banded layer. This abnormality in Descemet's membrane suggests that the developmental changes, which result in posterior keratoconus, occur before the formation of the anterior banded layer, between 6 and 8 months of gestation.[1,231]

Clinically, there are similarities between posterior keratoconus and Peters' anomaly. However, a difference is observed histopathologically. In Peters' anomaly the corneal endothelium and Descemet's membrane are either absent or markedly thinned,[232] which is not the case in posterior keratoconus.

Keratoconus and posterior keratoconus are similar in name, but the two disorders are distinctly different and except for an isolated report[233] are not associated (see Table 74.1). Posterior keratoconus does not develop into keratoconus, despite the fact that anterior steepening can occur in a central or paracentral affected area.

Many ocular abnormalities have been found in association with posterior keratoconus. Changes consistent with mesodermal dysgenesis, as well as associated aniridia, ectropion uvea, iris atrophy, glaucoma, anterior lenticonus, ectopia lentis, and anterior lens opacities have been described,[234] as have choroidal and retinal sclerosis. Abnormalities other than in the eye have also been reported.[229] These include hypertelorism, a flattened nasal bridge, lateral canthal displacement, cleft lip and palate, webbed neck, brachydactyly, genitourinary anomalies, short stature, and abnormal gait.

The pathogenesis of this disorder is unknown. Its association with other developmental abnormalities of the anterior segment has led Waring et al.[235] to conclude that posterior keratoconus may be a variant of the anomalies of mesodermal dysgenesis.

Posterior keratoconus usually requires no treatment, particularly when the abnormality is outside of the visual axis. Glasses can correct associated refractive error. Visual rehabilitation with a contact lens seems reasonable if a focal area of paracentral steepening or irregular astigmatism is demonstrated. Glasses and contact lenses do little to correct vision loss caused by mid and posterior stromal scarring. Penetrating keratoplasty can be considered in patients with poor vision, although amblyopia may compromise the final visual result. Preoperative potential acuity testing may help identify those patients who would not benefit from surgery.

References

1. Krachmer JH, Feder RS, Belin MW. Keratoconus and related noninflammatory corneal thinning disorders. *Surv Ophthalmol.* 1984;28:293–322.
2. Rabinowitz YS, Nesburn AB, McDonnell PJ. Videokeratography of the fellow eye in unilateral keratoconus. *Ophthalmology.* 1993;100: 181–186.
3. Holland DR, Maeda N, Hannush SB, et al. Unilateral keratoconus. Incidence and quantitative topographic analysis. *Ophthalmology.* 1997;104: 1409–1413.
4. Lee LR, Hirst LW, Readshaw G. Clinical detection of unilateral keratoconus. *Aust N Z J Ophthalmol.* 1995;23:129–133.

5. Copeman PW. Eczema and keratoconus. *Br Med J.* 1965;5468:977–979.
6. Gasset AR, Hinson WA, Frias JL. Keratoconus and atopic diseases. *Ann Ophthalmol.* 1978;10:991–994.
7. Wachtmeister L, Ingemansson SO, Moller E. Atopy and HLA antigens in patients with keratoconus. *Acta Ophthalmol (Copenh).* 1982;60:113–122.
8. Davies PD, Lobascher D, Menon JA, et al. Immunological studies in keratoconus. *Trans Ophthalmol Soc UK.* 1976;96:173–178.
9. Rahi A, Davies P, Ruben M, et al. Keratoconus and coexisting atopic disease. *Br J Ophthalmol.* 1977;61:761–764.
10. Rados A. Conical cornea and mongolism. *Arch Ophtalmol.* 1948;40:454–478.
11. Cullen JF, Butler HG. Mongolism (Down's syndrome) and keratoconus. *Br J Ophthalmol.* 1963;47:321–330.
12. Pierce K, Eustace P. Acute keratoconus in mongols. *Br J Ophthalmol.* 1971;55:50–54.
13. Shapiro M, France TD. The ocular features of Down's syndrome. *Am J Ophthalmol.* 1985;99.
14. Haugen OH. Keratoconus in the mentally retarded. *Acta Ophthalmol (Copenh).* 1992;70:111–114.
15. McKusick VA. *Heritable disorders of connective tissue.* 3rd ed. St. Louis: Mosby; 1966.
16. Rabinowitz YS. Keratoconus. *Surv Ophthalmol.* 1998;42:297–319.
17. Robertson I. Keratoconus and the Ehlers-Danlos syndrome. A new aspect of keratoconus. *Med J Aust.* 1975;1:571–573.
18. Ihalainen A. Clinical and epidemiological features of keratoconus. Genetic and external factors in the pathogenesis of the disease. *Acta Ophthalmol (Copenh).* 1986;64(Suppl.):178.
19. Woodward EG, Morris MT. Joint hypermobility in keratoconus. *Ophthalmic Physiol Opt.* 1990;10:360–362.
20. Beardsley TL, Foulks GN. An association of keratoconus and mitral valve prolapse. *Ophthalmology.* 1982;89:35–37.
21. Sharif KW, Casey TA, Coltart J. Prevalence of mitral valve prolapse in keratoconus patients. *J R Soc Med.* 1992;85:446–448.
22. Lichter H, Loya N, Sagie A, et al. Keratoconus and mitral valve prolapse. *Am J Ophthalmol.* 2000;129:667–668.
23. Street DA, Vinokur ET, Waring GO 3rd, et al. Lack of association between keratoconus, mitral valve prolapse, and joint hypermobility. *Ophthalmology.* 1991;98:170–176.
24. Donnenfeld ED, Perry HD, Gibralter RP, et al. Keratoconus associated with floppy eyelid syndrome. *Ophthalmology.* 1991;98:1674–1678.
25. Negris R. Floppy eyelid syndrome associated with keratoconus. *J Am Optom Assoc.* 1992;63:316–319.
26. Lee WJ, Kim JC, Shyn KH. Clinical evaluation of corneal diseases associated with floppy eyelid syndrome. *Korean J Ophthalmol.* 1996;10:116–121.
27. Nucci P, Brancato R. Keratoconus and congenital hip dysplasia. *Am J Ophthalmol.* 1991;111:775–776.
28. Greenfield G, Stein R, Romano A, Goodman RM. Blue sclerae and keratoconus: key features of a distinct heritable disorder of connective tissue. *Clin Genet.* 1973;4:8–16.
29. Brenner S, Nemet P, Legum C. Jadassohn-type anetoderma in association with keratoconus and cataract. *Ophthalmologica.* 1977;174:181–184.
30. Zala L, Ettlin C, Krebs A. [Focal dermal hypoplasia with keratoconus, papillomatosis of esophagus and hidrocystomas (author's transl)]. *Dermatologica.* 1975;150:176–185.
31. Geerarts WJ. *Ocular syndromes.* 2nd ed. Philadelphia: Lea and Febiger; 1969.
32. Wolter FR. Bilateral keratoconus in Crouzon's syndrome with unilateral acute hydrops. *J Pediatr Ophthalmol.* 1977;14:141–143.
33. Perlman JM, Zaidman GW. Bilateral keratoconus in Crouzon's syndrome. *Cornea.* 1994;13:80–81.
34. Austin MG, Schaefer RF. Marfan's syndrome, with unusual blood vessel manifestations. *Arch Pathol.* 1957;64:205–209.
35. Nucci P, Trabucchi G, Brancato R. Keratoconus and Turner's syndrome: a case report. *Optom Vis Sci.* 1991;68:407–408.
36. Macsai M, Maguen E, Nucci P. Keratoconus and Turner's syndrome. *Cornea.* 1997;16:534–536.
37. Seiler T, Huhle S, Spoerl E, Kunath H. Manifest diabetes and keratoconus: a retrospective case-control study. *Graefe's Arch Clin Exp Ophthalmol.* 2000;238:822–825.
38. Mannis MJ, Morrison TL, Zadnik K, et al. Personality trends in keratoconus. An analysis. *Arch Ophthalmol.* 1987;105:798–800.
39. Swartz NG, Cohen EJ, Scott DG, et al. Personality and keratoconus. *CLAO J.* 1990;16:62–64.
40. Alstrom CH, Olson O. Heredo-retinopathia congenitalis. Monohybride recessiva autosomalis. *Hereditas Genetiskt Arkiv.* 1957;43:1–177.
41. Heher KS, Traboulsi EI, Maumenee IH. The natural history of Leber's congenital amaurosis. *Ophthalmology.* 1992;99:241–245.
42. Moschos M, Droutsas D, Panagakis E, et al. Keratoconus and tapetoretinal degeneration. *Cornea.* 1996;15:473–476.
43. Elder MJ. Leber congenital amaurosis and its association with keratoconus and keratoglobus. *J Pediatr Ophthalmol Strabismus.* 1994;31:38–40.
44. Lorfel RS, Sugar HS. Keratoconus associated with retrolental fibroplasia. *Ann Ophthalmol.* 1976;8:449–450.
45. Wilhelmus KR. Keratoconus and progressive cone dystrophy. *Ophthalmologica.* 1995;209:278–279.
46. Klintworth GK. *Degenerations, depositions, and miscellaneous reactions of the ocular anterior segment.* 2nd ed. New York: Marcel Dekker; 1994; 743–794.
47. Eiferman RA, Law M, Lane L. Iridoschisis and keratoconus. *Cornea.* 1994;13:78–79.
48. Blair SD, Seabrooks D, Shields WJ, et al. Bilateral progressive essential iris atrophy and keratoconus with coincident features of posterior polymorphous dystrophy: a case report and proposed pathogenesis. *Cornea.* 1992;11:255–261.
49. Lipman RM, Rubenstein JB, Torczynski E. Keratoconus and Fuchs' corneal endothelial dystrophy in a patient and her family. *Arch Ophthalmol.* 1990;108:993–994.
50. Lipman RM, Rubenstein JB, Torczynski E. Keratoconus and Fuchs' endothelial dystrophy. *Cornea.* 1991;10:368.
51. Weissman BA, Ehrlich M, Levenson JE, Pettit TH. Four cases of keratoconus and posterior polymorphous corneal dystrophy. *Optom Vis Sci.* 1989;66:243–246.
52. Driver PJ, Reed JW, Davis RM. Familial cases of keratoconus associated with posterior polymorphous dystrophy. *Am J Ophthalmol.* 1994;118:256–257.
53. Bechara SJ, Grossniklaus HE, Waring GO, 3rd, Wells JA, 3rd. Keratoconus associated with posterior polymorphous dystrophy. *Am J Ophthalmol.* 1991;112:729–731.
54. Vajpayee RB, Snibson GR, Taylor HR. Association of keratoconus with granular corneal dystrophy. *Aust N Z J Ophthalmol.* 1996;24:369–371.
55. Wollensak G, Green WR, Temprano J. Keratoconus associated with corneal granular dystrophy in a patient of Italian origin. *Cornea.* 2002;21:121–122.
56. Mitsui M, Sakimoto T, Sawa M, Katami M. Familial case of keratoconus with corneal granular dystrophy. *Jpn J Ophthalmol.* 1998;42:385–388.
57. Sassani JW, Smith SG, Rabinowitz YS. Keratoconus and bilateral lattice-granular corneal dystrophies. *Cornea.* 1992;11:343–350.
58. Smith SG, Rabinowitz YS, Sassani JW, Smith RE. Keratoconus and lattice and granular corneal dystrophies in the same eye. *Am J Ophthalmol.* 1989;108:608–610.
59. Klintworth GK, Damms T. Corneal dystrophies and keratoconus. *Curr Opin Ophthalmol.* 1995;6:44–56.
60. Totan Y, Hepsen IF, Cekic O, et al. Incidence of keratoconus in subjects with vernal keratoconjunctivitis: a videokeratographic study. *Ophthalmology.* 2001;108:824–827.
61. Tuft SJ, Kemeny DM, Dart JK, Buckley RJ. Clinical features of atopic keratoconjunctivitis. *Ophthalmology.* 1991;98:150–158.
62. Karseras AG, Ruben M. Aetiology of keratoconus. *Br J Ophthalmol.* 1976;60:522–525.
63. Karantinos EAD, ed. *Histocompatibility antigens (HLA) in keratoconus.* Vol. 40. London: The Royal Society of Medicine and Academic Press; 1981.
64. Gasset AR, Houde WL, Garcia-Bengochea M. Hard contact lens wear as an environmental risk in keratoconus. *Am J Ophthalmol.* 1978;85:339–341.
65. Macsai MS, Varley GA, Krachmer JH. Development of keratoconus after contact lens wear. Patient characteristics. *Arch Ophthalmol.* 1990;108:534–538.
66. Critchfield JW, Calandra AJ, Nesburn AB, Kenney MC, Keratoconus I. Biochemical studies of normal and keratoconus corneas. *Exp Eye Res.* 1988;46:953–963.
67. Sawaguchi S, Yue BY, Sugar J, Gilboy JE. Lysosomal enzyme abnormalities in keratoconus. *Arch Ophthalmol.* 1989;107:1507–1510.
68. Zhou L, Sawaguchi S, Twining SS, et al. Expression of degradative enzymes and protease inhibitors in corneas with keratoconus. *Invest Ophthalmol Vis Sci.* 1998;39:1117–1124.
69. Fabre EJ, Bureau J, Pouliquen Y, Lorans G. Binding sites for human interleukin 1 alpha, gamma interferon and tumor necrosis factor on cultured fibroblasts of normal cornea and keratoconus. *Curr Eye Res.* 1991;10:585–592.
70. Bureau J, Fabre EJ, Hecquet C, et al. Modification of prostaglandin E2 and collagen synthesis in keratoconus fibroblasts, associated with an

increase of interleukin 1 alpha receptor number. *C R Acad Sci III.* 1993;316:425–430.
71. Kim W, Rabinowitz Y, Meisler D, Wilson S. Keratocyte apoptosis associated with keratoconus. *Exp Eye Res.* 1999;69:475–481.
72. Wilson SE HY, Weng J, Li Q, et al. Epithelial injury induces keratocyte apoptosis: hypothesized role for the interleukin-1 system in the modulation of corneal tissue organization and wound healing. *Exp Eye Res.* 1996;62:325–327.
73. Edwards M, McGhee CN, Dean S. The genetics of keratoconus. *Clin Exp Ophthalmol.* 2001;29:345–351.
74. Bechara SJ, Waring GO, 3rd, Insler MS. Keratoconus in two pairs of identical twins. *Cornea.* 1996;15:90–93.
75. Parker J, Ko WW, Pavlopoulos G, et al. Videokeratography of keratoconus in monozygotic twins. *J Refract Surg.* 1996;12:180–183.
76. Watters HOAG. Keratoconus in monozygotic twins in New Zealand. *Clin Exp Optometry.* 1995;78:125–129.
77. McMahon TT, Shin JA, Newlin A, et al. Discordance for keratoconus in two pairs of monozygotic twins. *Cornea.* 1999;18:444–451.
78. Kennedy RH, Bourne WM, Dyer JA. A 48-year clinical and epidemiologic study of keratoconus. *Am J Ophthalmol.* 1986;101:267–273.
79. Gonzalez V, McDonnell PJ. Computer-assisted corneal topography in parents of patients with keratoconus. *Arch Ophthalmol.* 1992;110: 1413–1414.
80. Rabinowitz YS, Garbus J, McDonnell PJ. Computer-assisted corneal topography in family members of patients with keratoconus. *Arch Ophthalmol.* 1990;108:365–371.
81. Rabinowitz YS, Maumenee IH, Lundergan MK, et al. Molecular genetic analysis in autosomal dominant keratoconus. *Cornea.* 1992;11:302–308.
82. Adachi W, Mitsuishi Y, Terai K, et al. The association of HLA with young-onset keratoconus in Japan. *Am J Ophthalmol.* 2002;133:557–559.
83. Aldave A, Bourla N, Yellore V, et al. Keratoconus is not associated with mutations in *COL8A1* and *COL8A2*. *Cornea.* 2007;26:963–965.
84. Hameed A, Khaliq S, Ismail M, et al. A novel locus for Leber congenital amaurosis (LCA4) with anterior keratoconus mapping to chromosome 17p13. *Invest Ophthalmol Vis Sci.* 2000;41:629–633.
85. Damji KF, Sohocki MM, Khan R, et al. Leber's congenital amaurosis with anterior keratoconus in Pakistani families is caused by the Trp278X mutation in the *AIPL1* gene on 17p. *Can J Ophthalmol.* 2001;36: 252–259.
86. Morrison DA, Rosser EM, Claoue C. Keratoconus associated with a chromosome 7,11 translocation. *Eye.* 2001;15:556–557.
87. Heaven CJ, Lalloo F, McHale E. Keratoconus associated with chromosome 13 ring abnormality. *Br J Ophthalmol.* 2000;84:1079.
88. Wang Y, Rabinowitz YS, Rotter JI, Yang H. Genetic epidemiological study of keratoconus: evidence for major gene determination. *Am J Med Genet.* 2000;93:403–409.
89. Jacobs DS, Dohlman CH. Is keratoconus genetic? *Int Ophthalmol Clin.* 1993;33:249–260.
90. Scroggs MW, Proia AD. Histopathological variation in keratoconus. *Cornea.* 1992;11:553–559.
91. Tsubota K, Mashima Y, Murata H, et al. Corneal epithelium in keratoconus. *Cornea.* 1995;14:77–83.
92. Kanai A. [Electron microscopic studies of keratoconus]. *Nippon Ganka Gakkai Zasshi.* 1968;72:902–918.
93. Sawaguchi S, Fukuchi T, Abe H, et al. Three-dimensional scanning electron microscopic study of keratoconus corneas. *Arch Ophthalmol.* 1998;116:62–68.
94. Iwamoto T, DeVoe AG. Electron microscopical study of the Fleisher ring. *Arch Ophthalmol.* 1976;94:1579–1584.
95. Shapiro MB, Rodrigues MM, Mandel MR, Krachmer JH. Anterior clear spaces in keratoconus. *Ophthalmology.* 1986;93:1316–1319.
96. Perry HD, Buxton JN, Fine BS. Round and oval cones in keratoconus. *Ophthalmology.* 1980;87:905–909.
97. Kaas-Hansen M. The histopathological changes of keratoconus. *Acta Ophthalmol (Copenh).* 1993;71:411–414.
98. Pouliquen Y, Graf B, de Kozak Y, et al. [Morphological study of keratoconus]. *Arch Ophtalmol Rev Gen Ophtalmol.* 1970;30:497–532.
99. Fullwood NJ, Tuft SJ, Malik NS, et al. Synchrotron x-ray diffraction studies of keratoconus corneal stroma. *Invest Ophthalmol Vis Sci.* 1992;33:1734–1741.
100. Polack FM. Contributions of electron microscopy to the study of corneal pathology. *Surv Ophthalmol.* 1976;20:375–414.
101. Smolek M. Interlamellar cohesive strength in the vertical meridian of human eyebank corneas. *Invest Ophthalmol Vis Sci.* 1993;34: 2962–2969.
102. Daxer A, Fratzl P. Collagen fibril orientation in the human corneal stroma and its implication in keratoconus. *Invest Ophthalmol Vis Sci.* 1997;38:121–129.
103. Smolek MK, Beekhuis WH. Collagen fibril orientation in the human corneal stroma and its implications in keratoconus. *Invest Ophthalmol Vis Sci.* 1997;38:1289–1290.
104. Halabis JA. Analysis of the corneal endothelium in keratoconus. *Am J Optom Physiol Opt.* 1987;64:51–53.
105. Sturbaum CW, Peiffer RL Jr. Pathology of corneal endothelium in keratoconus. *Ophthalmologica.* 1993;206:192–208.
106. Zadnik K, Mannis MJ, Johnson CA, Rich D. Rapid contrast sensitivity assessment in keratoconus. *Am J Optom Physiol Opt.* 1987;64:693–697.
107. Eiferman RA, Lane L, Law M, Fields Y. Superior keratoconus. *Refract Corneal Surg.* 1993;394–395.
108. Prisant O, Legeais JM, Renard G. Superior keratoconus. *Cornea.* 1997;6:693–694.
109. Kim T, Khosla-Gupta B, Debacker C. Blepharoptosis-induced superior keratoconus. *Am J Ophthalmol.* 2000;30:232–234.
110. McMahon TT, Robin JB, Scarpulla KM, Putz JL. The spectrum of topography found in keratoconus. *CLAO J.* 1991;7:198–204.
111. Smolek MK, Klyce SD. Is keratoconus a true ectasia? An evaluation of corneal surface area. *Arch Ophthalmol.* 2000;18:1179–1186.
112. Kinoshita S, Tanaka F, Ohashi Y, Ikeda M, Takai S. Incidence of prominent corneal nerves in multiple endocrine neoplasia type 2A. *Am J Ophthalmol.* 1991;11:307–311.
113. Wagner H, Barr J, Zadnik K. Collaborative Longitudinal Evaluation of Keratoconus (CLEK) Study: methods and findings to date. *Cont Lens Anterior Eye.* 2007;30:223–232.
114. Barr J, Wilson B, Gordon M, et al. Estimation of the incidence and factors predictive of corneal scarring in the Collaborative Longitudinal Evaluation of Keratoconus (CLEK) Study. *Cornea.* 2006;25:16–25.
115. Korb DR, Finnemor, BM, Herman JP. Apical changes and scarring in kerartoconus as related to contact lens fitting techniques. *Am J Optom Assoc.* 1982;53:199–205.
116. Margo CE, Mosteller MW. Corneal pseudocyst following acute hydrops. *Br J Ophthalmol.* 1987;71:359–360.
117. Feder RS, Wilhelmus KR, Vold SD, O'Grady RB. Intrastromal clefts in keratoconus patients with hydrops. *Am J Ophthalmol.* 1998;126:9–16.
118. Maguire LJ, Bourne WM. Corneal topography of early keratoconus. *Am J Ophthalmol.* 1989;108:107–112.
119. Maguire LJ, Lowry JC. Identifying progression of subclinical keratoconus by serial topography analysis. *Am J Ophthalmol.* 1991;112: 41–45.
120. Wilson SE, Klyce SD. Advances in the analysis of corneal topography. *Surv Ophthalmol.* 1991;35:269–277.
121. Guarnieri FA, Guarnieri JC. Comparison of Placido-based, rasterstereography, and slit-scan corneal topography systems. *J Refract Surg.* 2002;18: 169–176.
122. Nesburn AB, Bahri S, Salz J, et al. Keratoconus detected by videokeratography in candidates for photorefractive keratectomy. *J Refract Surg.* 1995;11:194–201.
123. Saragoussi JJ, Pouliquen YJ. Does the progressive increasing effect of radial keratotomy (hyperopic shift) correlate with undetected early keratoconus? *J Refract Corneal Surg.* 1994;10:45–48.
124. Wilson SE, Klyce SD. Screening for corneal topographic abnormalities before refractive surgery. *Ophthalmology.* 1994;101:147–152.
125. Hori-Komai Y, Toda I, Asano-Kato N, Tsubota K. Reasons for not performing refractive surgery. *J Cataract Refract Surg.* 2002;28:795–797.
126. Bilgihan K, Ozdek SC, Konuk O, et al. Results of photorefractive keratectomy in keratoconus suspects at 4 years. *J Refract Surg.* 2000; 16:438–443.
127. Sun R, Gimbel HV, Kaye GB. Photorefractive keratectomy in keratoconus suspects. *J Cataract Refract Surg.* 1999;25:1461–1466.
128. Rabinowitz YS. Videokeratographic indices to aid in screening for keratoconus. *J Refract Surg.* 1995;11:371–379.
129. Maeda N, Klyce SD, Smolek MK. Comparison of methods for detecting keratoconus using videokeratography. *Arch Ophthalmol.* 1995;113: 870–874.
130. Maeda N, Klyce SD, Smolek MK, Thompson HW. Automated keratoconus screening with corneal topography analysis. *Invest Ophthalmol Vis Sci.* 1994;35:2749–2757.
131. Smolek MK, Klyce SD. Current keratoconus detection methods compared with a neural network approach. *Invest Ophthalmol Vis Sci.* 1997;38:2290–2299.
132. Rabinowitz YS, Rasheed K. KISA% index: a quantitative videokeratography algorithm embodying minimal topographic criteria for diagnosing keratoconus. *J Cataract Refract Surg.* 1999;25:1327–1335.

133. Hubbe RE, Foulks GN. The effect of poor fixation on computer-assisted topographic corneal analysis. Pseudokeratoconus. *Ophthalmology.* 1994;101:1745–1748.
134. Mandell RB, Chiang CS, Yee L. Asymmetric corneal toricity and pseudokeratoconus in videokeratography. *J Am Optom Assoc.* 1996;67: 540–547.
135. Silverman CM. Misalignment of videokeratoscope produces pseudokeratoconus suspect. *J Refract Corneal Surg.* 1994;10:468.
136. Endl MJ, Klyce SD. *Six pearls for surgical planning with videokeratography.* Thorofare, NJ: Slack, Inc.; 2001.
137. Wilson SE. Cautions regarding measurements of the posterior corneal curvature. *Ophthalmology.* 2000;107:1223.
138. Tabbara K, Kotb A. Risk factors for corneal ectasia after LASIK. *Ophthalmology.* 2006;113:1618–1622.
139. Binder P, Lindstrom R, Stulting R, et al. Keratoconus and corneal ectasia after LASIK. *J Refract Surg.* 2005;21:749–752.
140. Dawson D, Grossniklaus H, McCarey B, Edelhauser H. Biomechanical and wound healing characteristics of corneas after excimer laser keratorefractive surgery: is there a difference between advanced surface ablation and sub-Bowman's keratomileusis? *J Refract Surg.* 2008;24: 90–96.
141. Randleman J, Russell B, Ward M, et al. Risk factors and prognosis for corneal ectasia after LASIK. *Ophthalmology.* 2003;110:267–275.
142. Szczotka LB, Barr JT, Zadnik K. A summary of the findings from the Collaborative Longitudinal Evaluation of Keratoconus (CLEK) Study. CLEK Study Group. *Optometry.* 2001;72:574–584.
143. Edrington TB, Szczotka LB, Barr JT, et al. Rigid contact lens fitting relationships in keratoconus. Collaborative Longitudinal Evaluation of Keratoconus (CLEK) Study Group. *Optom Vis Sci.* 1999;76:692–699.
144. Lim N, Vogt U. Characteristics and functional outcomes of 130 patients with keratoconus attending a specialist contact lens clinic. *Eye.* 2002;16:54–59.
145. Maguen E, Martinez M, Rosner IR, et al. The use of Saturn II lenses in keratoconus. *CLAO J.* 1991;17:41–43.
146. Ozkurt Y, Oral Y, Karaman A, et al. A retrospective case series: use of SoftPerm contact lenses in patients with keratoconus. *Eye Contact Lens.* 2007;33:103–105.
147. Pilskalns B, Fink B, Hill R. Oxygen demands with hybrid contact lenses. *Optom Vis Sci.* 2007;84:334–342.
148. Rosenthal P, Croteau A. Fluid-ventilated, gas-permeable scleral contact lens is an effective option for managing severe ocular surface disease and many corneal disorders that would otherwise require penetrating keratoplasty. *Eye Contact Lens.* 2005;31:130–134.
149. Ye P, Sun A, Weissman B. Role of mini-scleral gas-permeable lenses in the treatment of corneal disorders. *Eye Contact Lens.* 2007;33:80–83.
150. Cochener B, Le Floch G, Volant A, Colin J. [Is there a role for Excimer laser in the treatment of keratoconus?]. *J Fr Ophtalmol.* 1997;20: 758–766.
151. Rapuano CJ. Excimer laser phototherapeutic keratectomy: long-term results and practical considerations. *Cornea.* 1997;16:151–157.
152. Lahners WJ, Russell B, Grossniklaus HE, Stulting RD. Keratolysis following excimer laser phototherapeutic keratectomy in a patient with keratoconus. *J Refract Surg.* 2001;17:555–558.
153. Alio J, Shabayek M, Belda J, et al. Analysis of results related to good and bad outcomes of Intacs implantation for keratoconus correction. *J Cataract Refract Surg.* 2006;32:756–761.
154. Boxer Wachler B, Christie J, Chandra N, et al. Intacs for keratoconus. *Ophthalmology.* 2003;110:1475.
155. Colin J, Malet F. Intacs for the correction of keratoconus: two-year follow-up. *J Cataract Refract Surg.* 2007;33:69–74.
156. Siganos D, Ferrara P, Chatzinikolas K, et al. Ferrara intrastromal corneal rings for the correction of keratoconus. *J Cataract Refract Surg.* 2002;28:1947–1951.
157. Rabinowitz Y, Li X, Ignacio T, Maguen E. INTACS inserts using the femtosecond laser compared to the mechanical spreader in the treatment of keratoconus. *J Refract Surg.* 2006;22:764–771.
158. Raiskup-Wolf F, Hoyer A, Spoerl E, Pillunat L. Collagen crosslinking with riboflavin and ultraviolet-A light in keratoconus: long-term results. *J Cataract Refract Surg.* 2008;34:796–801.
159. Wittig-Silva C, Whiting M, Lamoureux E, et al. A randomized controlled trial of corneal collagen cross-linking in progressive keratoconus: preliminary results. *J Refract Surg.* 2008;24:S720–S725.
160. Wollensak G, Spoerl E, Seiler. Riboflavin/ultraviolet-a-induced collagen crosslinking for the treatment of keratoconus. *Am J Ophthalmol.* 2003;135:620–627.
161. Wollensak G. Crosslinking treatment of progressive keratoconus: new hope. *Curr Opin Ophthalmol.* 2006;17:356–360.
162. Kohlhaas M, Spoerl E, Schilde T, et al. Biomechanical evidence of the distribution of cross-links in corneas treated with riboflavin and ultraviolet A light. *J Cataract Refract Surg.* 2006;32:279–283.
163. Wollensak G, Spoerl E, Seiler T. Stress-strain measurements of human and porcine corneas after riboflavin-ultraviolet-A-induced cross-linking. *J Cataract Refract Surg.* 2003;29:1780–1785.
164. Spoerl E, Wollensak G, Seiler T. Increased resistance of crosslinked cornea against enzymatic digestion. *Curr Eye Res.* 2004;29:35–40.
165. Wollensak G, Spoerl E, Wilsch M, Seiler T. Endothelial cell damage after riboflavin-ultraviolet-A treatment in the rabbit. *J Cataract Refract Surg.* 2003;29:1786–1790.
166. Wollensak G, Spoerl E, Wilsch M, Seiler T. Keratocyte apoptosis after corneal collagen cross-linking using riboflavin/UVA treatment. *Cornea.* 2004;23:43–49.
167. Spoerl E, Mrochen M, Sliney D, et al. Safety of UVA-riboflavin cross-linking of the cornea. *Cornea.* 2007;26:385–389.
168. Kremer I, Eagle RC, Rapuano CJ, Laibson PR. Histologic evidence of recurrent keratoconus seven years after keratoplasty. *Am J Ophthalmol.* 1995;119:511–512.
169. Belmont SC, Muller JW, Draga A, et al. Keratoconus in a donor cornea. *J Refract Corneal Surg.* 1994;10:658.
170. Urrets-Zavalia AJ. Fixed dilated pupil, iris atrophy, and secondary glaucoma. A distinct clinical entity following penetrating keratoplasty in keratoconus. *Am J Ophthalmol.* 1963;56:257–265.
171. Wilson SE, Bourne WM. Effect of recipient–donor trephine size disparity on refractive error in keratoconus. *Ophthalmology.* 1989;96:299–305.
172. Perry HD, Foulks GN. Oversize donor buttons in corneal transplantation surgery for keratoconus. *Ophthalmic Surg.* 1987;18:751–752.
173. Spadea L, Bianco G, Mastrofini MC, Balestrazzi E. Penetrating keratoplasty with donor and recipient corneas of the same diameter. *Ophthalmic Surg Lasers.* 1996;27:425–430.
174. Goble RR, Hardman Lea SJ, Falcon MG. The use of the same size host and donor trephine in penetrating keratoplasty for keratoconus. *Eye.* 1994;8(Pt 3):311–314.
175. Girard LJ, Eguez I, Esnaola N, et al. Effect of penetrating keratoplasty using grafts of various sizes on keratoconic myopia and astigmatism. *J Cataract Refract Surg.* 1988;14:541–547.
176. Lanier JD, Bullington RH, Jr, Prager TC. Axial length in keratoconus. *Cornea.* 1992;11:250–254.
177. Lewyckyj M. Axial length in eyes with keratoconus. *Invest Ophthalmol.* 1991;32:778.
178. Shimazaki J, Shimmura S, Ishioka M, Tsubota K. Randomized clinical trial of deep lamellar keratoplasty vs penetrating keratoplasty. *Am J Ophthalmol.* 2002;134:159–165.
179. Terry M, Ousley P. Deep lamellar endothelial keratoplasty visual acuity, astigmatism, and endothelial survival in a large prospective series. *Ophthalmology.* 2005;112:1541–1548.
180. Watson S, Ramsay A, Dart J, et al. Comparison of deep lamellar keratoplasty and penetrating keratoplasty in patients with keratoconus. *Ophthalmology.* 2004;111:1676–1682.
181. Anwar M, Teichmann K. Big-bubble technique to bare Descemet's membrane in anterior lamellar keratoplasty. *J Cataract Refract Surg.* 2002; 28:398–403.
182. Melles G, Lander F, Rietveld F, et al. A new surgical technique for deep stromal, anterior lamellar keratoplasty. *Br J Ophthalmol.* 1999;83: 327–333.
183. Panda A, Aggarwal A, Madhavi P, et al. Management of acute corneal hydrops secondary to keratoconus with intracameral injection of sulfur hexafluoride (SF_6). *Cornea.* 2007;26:1067–1069.
184. Shah S, Sridhar M, Sangwan V. Acute corneal hydrops treated by intracameral injection of perfluoropropane (C_3F_8) gas. *Am J Ophthalmol.* 2005;139:368–370.
185. Rao SK, Fogla R, Padmanabhan P, Sitalakshmi G. Corneal topography in atypical pellucid marginal degeneration. *Cornea.* 1999;18:265–272.
186. Bower KS, Dhaliwal DK, Barnhorst DA, Jr, Warnicke J. Pellucid marginal degeneration with superior corneal thinning. *Cornea.* 1997;16:483–485.
187. Cameron JA, Mahmood MA. Superior corneal thinning with pellucid marginal corneal degeneration. *Am J Ophthalmol.* 1990;109:486–487.
188. Basak SK, Hazra TK, Bhattacharya D, Sinha TK. Unilateral pellucid marginal degeneration. *Indian J Ophthalmol.* 2000;48:233–234.
189. Wagenhorst BB. Unilateral pellucid marginal degeneration in an elderly patient. *Br J Ophthalmol.* 1996;80:927–928.
190. Kayazawa F, Nishimura K, Kodama Y, et al. Keratoconus with pellucid marginal corneal degeneration. *Arch Ophthalmol.* 1984;102:895–896.
191. Maguire LJ, Klyce SD, McDonald MB, Kaufman HE. Corneal topography of pellucid marginal degeneration. *Ophthalmology.* 1987;94:519–524.

192. Santo RM, Bechara SJ, Kara-Jose N. Corneal topography in asymptomatic family members of a patient with pellucid marginal degeneration. *Am J Ophthalmol.* 1999;127:205–207.
193. Ambrosio R, Jr, Wilson SE. Early pellucid marginal corneal degeneration: case reports of two refractive surgery candidates. *Cornea.* 2002;21:114–117.
194. Schlaeppi V. La dystrophie marginale infericure pellucide de la cornee. *Probl Actuels Ophthalmol.* 1957;1:672–677.
195. Cameron JA. Deep corneal scarring in pellucid marginal corneal degeneration. *Cornea.* 1992;11:309–310.
196. Akpek EK, Altan-Yaycioglu R, Gottsch JD, Stark WJ. Spontaneous corneal perforation in a patient with unusual unilateral pellucid marginal degeneration. *J Cataract Refract Surg.* 2001;27:1698–1700.
197. Lucarelli MJ, Gendelman DS, Talamo JH. Hydrops and spontaneous perforation in pellucid marginal corneal degeneration. *Cornea.* 1997;16:232–234.
198. Orlin SE, Sulewski ME. Spontaneous corneal perforation in pellucid marginal degeneration. *CLAO J.* 1998;24:186–187.
199. Rodrigues MM, Newsome DA, Krachmer JH, Eiferman RA. Pellucid marginal corneal degeneration: a clinicopathologic study of two cases. *Exp Eye Res.* 1981;33:277–288.
200. Funderburgh JL, Funderburgh ML, Rodrigues MM, et al. Altered antigenicity of keratan sulfate proteoglycan in selected corneal diseases. *Invest Ophthalmol Vis Sci.* 1990;31:419–428.
201. Astin CL. The long-term use of the SoftPerm lens on pellucid marginal corneal degeneration. *CLAO J.* 1994;20:258–260.
202. Pullum KW, Buckley RJ. A study of 530 patients referred for rigid gas permeable scleral contact lens assessment. *Cornea.* 1997;16:612–622.
203. Biswas S, Brahma A, Tromans C, Ridgway A. Management of pellucid marginal corneal degeneration. *Eye.* 2000;14(Pt 4):629–634.
204. Speaker MG, Arentsen JJ, Laibson PR. Long-term survival of large diameter penetrating keratoplasties for keratoconus and pellucid marginal degeneration. *Acta Ophthalmol Suppl.* 1989;192:17–19.
205. Varley GA, Macsai MS, Krachmer JH. The results of penetrating keratoplasty for pellucid marginal corneal degeneration. *Am J Ophthalmol.* 1990;10:149–152.
206. Kremer I, Sperber LT, Laibson PR. Pellucid marginal degeneration treated by lamellar and penetrating keratoplasty. *Arch Ophthalmol.* 1993;111:169–170.
207. Rasheed K, Rabinowitz YS. Surgical treatment of advanced pellucid marginal degeneration. *Ophthalmology.* 2000;107:1836–1840.
208. Duran JA, Rodriguez-Ares MT, Torres D. Crescentic resection for the treatment of pellucid corneal marginal degeneration. *Ophthalmic Surg.* 1991;22:153–156.
209. MacLean H, Robinson LP, Wechsler AW. Long-term results of corneal wedge excision for pellucid marginal degeneration. *Eye.* 1997;11(Pt 5):610–617.
210. Biglan AW, Brown SI, Johnson BL. Keratoglobus and blue sclera. *Am J Ophthalmol.* 1977;83:225–233.
211. Gupta VP, Jain RK, Angra SK. Acute hydrops in keratoglobus with vernal keratoconjunctivitis. *Indian J Ophthalmol.* 1985;33:121–123.
212. Rumelt S, Rehany U. Surgically induced keratoglobus in pellucid marginal degeneration. *Eye.* 1998;12(Pt 1):156–158.
213. Cameron JA. Keratoglobus. *Cornea.* 1993;12:124–130.
214. Pouliquen Y, Dhermy P, Espinasse MA, Savoldelli M. [Keratoglobus]. *J Fr Ophtalmol.* 1985;8:43–54.
215. Jacobs DS, Green WR, Maumenee AE. Acquired keratoglobus. *Am J Ophthalmol.* 1974;77:393–399.
216. Nelson ME, Talbot JF. Keratoglobus in the Rubinstein-Taybi syndrome. *Br J Ophthalmol.* 1989;73:385–387.
217. Hyams SW, Kar H, Neumann E. Blue sclerae and keratoglobus. Ocular signs of a systemic connective tissue disorder. *Br J Ophthalmol.* 1969;53:53–58.
218. Reddy SC. Keratoglobus and complicated microphthalmos. *Indian J Ophthalmol.* 1978;26:23–26.
219. Cameron JA, Cotter JB, Risco JM, Alvarez H. Epikeratoplasty for keratoglobus associated with blue sclera. *Ophthalmology.* 1991;98:446–452.
220. Macsai MS, Lemley HL, Schwartz T. Management of oculus fragilis in Ehlers-Danlos type VI. *Cornea.* 2000;19:104–107.
221. Jones DH, Kirkness CM. A new surgical technique for keratoglobus-tectonic lamellar keratoplasty followed by secondary penetrating keratoplasty. *Cornea.* 2001;20:885–887.
222. Kanellopoulos A, Pe L. An alternative surgical procedure for the management of keratoglobus. *Cornea.* 2005:24:1024–1026.
223. Krachmer JH, Rodrigues MM. Posterior keratoconus. *Arch Ophthalmol.* 1978;96:1867–1873.
224. Rao SK, Padmanabhan P. Posterior keratoconus. An expanded classification scheme based on corneal topography. *Ophthalmology.* 1998;105: 1206–1212.
225. Chan DQ. Bilateral circumscribed posterior keratoconus. *J Am Optom Assoc.* 1999;70:581–586.
226. Bareja U, Vajpayee RB. Posterior keratoconus due to iron nail injury – a case report. *Indian J Ophthalmol.* 1991;39:30.
227. Williams R. Acquired posterior keratoconus. *Br J Ophthalmol.* 1987;71:16–17.
228. Cote MA, Gaster RN. Keratohematoma leading to acquired posterior keratoconus. *Cornea.* 1994;13:534–538.
229. Streeten BW, Karpik AG, Spitzer KH. Posterior keratoconus associated with systemic abnormalities. *Arch Ophthalmol.* 1983;101:616–622.
230. al-Hazzaa SA, Specht CS, McLean IW, Harris DJ, Jr. Posterior keratoconus. Case report with scanning electron microscopy. *Cornea.* 1995;14:316–320.
231. Wulle KG. Electron microscopy of the fetal development of the corneal endothelium and Descemet's membrane of the human eye. *Invest Ophthalmol.* 1972;11:897–904.
232. Kuper C, Kuwabara T, Stark WJ. The histopathology of Peters' anomaly. *Am J Ophthalmol.* 1975;80:653–660.
233. Vajpayee RB, Sharma N. Association between anterior and posterior keratoconus. *Aust N Z J Ophthalmol.* 1998;26:181–183.
234. Grayson M. *Diseases of the cornea.* St. Louis: Mosby; 1979.
235. Waring GO, 3rd, Rodrigues MM, Laibson PR. Anterior chamber cleavage syndrome. A stepladder classification. *Surv Ophthalmol.* 1975;20:3–27.

Chapter 75

Iridocorneal Endothelial Syndrome

Emmett F. Carpel

History and Background

In the early part of the twentieth century, several case reports described a curious disorder in which the iris underwent progressive atrophy.[1–6] Patients presented with complaints of blurred vision or changes in the shape of the pupil, although occasionally the iris changes were first noted during a routine examination. In this unilateral condition in young adults, the iris underwent a change from mild eccentricity of the pupil and stromal atrophy to marked corectopia and complete iris hole formation. The pupil remained intact, but was displaced toward the periphery where extensive peripheral anterior synechiae (PAS) were noted.[6] The condition was called essential or progressive iris atrophy to denote the absence of an identifiable cause and its progressive nature.[2,4,5] Glaucoma was a frequent finding in this disorder, and was poorly controlled with medical treatment, although successful filtering operations were described.[3] Later, the description of an abnormal corneal endothelium and the formation of iris nodules were added to the manifestations of essential (progressive) iris atrophy.[7–11]

Chandler[10,12] reported a group of patients with abnormal corneal endothelium, described as a 'hammered silver appearance,' and corneal edema that occurred at a normal or slightly increased intraocular pressure. Iris nodules and PAS were also described, with glaucoma as an associated finding. This unilateral, nonfamilial disorder came to be known as Chandler's syndrome.

Cogan and Reese[13] later described patients with many features in common with those described here. Most often, patients presented with blurred vision or reported noticing spots on the iris. Iris nodules and PAS were clinically the most noticeable part of this disorder. Glaucoma was invariably present. This condition was also nonfamilial and unilateral and came to be termed the Cogan-Reese syndrome.

Scheie and Yanoff[14] reported a series of patients with unilateral glaucoma and iris changes that included heterochromia, ectropion uveae, PAS, and fine iris nodules. Corneal edema occurred at normal or slightly elevated intraocular pressure. Iris nevus cells diffusely infiltrated the anterior iris, which showed a blunted or effaced surface because of abnormal Descemet's membrane extending across the chamber angle onto the anterior iris surface. This nonfamilial condition became known as the iris nevus syndrome.

Common threads running through all these conditions included a unilateral, progressive, nonfamilial ocular disorder of young adulthood with abnormal corneal endothelium and peripheral anterior synechiae. Glaucoma, iris atrophy, and nodules were associated findings. Through the accumulated clinical and histopathologic reports, Campbell et al.[11] concluded that an abnormality of the corneal endothelium with production of abnormal basement membrane was the common etiologic basis and unified these disorders. Because corneal endothelial and iris abnormalities were found in all entities, it was termed the iridocorneal endothelial syndrome (ICE syndrome).[8,15–17] This unifying hypothesis has been reviewed extensively and supported.[18–21] Coincidentally, the acronym ICE also signifies commonly used names of these conditions – *I*ris nevus syndrome, *C*handler's syndrome, and *E*ssential (progressive) iris atrophy.

The diagnosis of the ICE syndrome is considered when two of the three main clinical features are present unilaterally: typical iris changes, abnormal corneal endothelium, and PAS.[9,22–25] Because the common etiology and features of these disorders are accepted, as long as a patient is correctly diagnosed with ICE syndrome, labeling of the particular subtype is not necessary. It is still useful for descriptive purposes, however, to categorize the entities separately, since the presentation and clinical course may vary markedly among them (Table 75.1).

Clinical Features

Essential iris atrophy

Essential (progressive) iris atrophy, although described in childhood,[26] first presents typically in young adults, unilaterally, and in women more than men. The presenting symptoms are blurred vision or a noticeable change in the iris substance or pupil. It is also occasionally first observed during a routine eye examination.[9,20,27] Rarely, pain is reported, but usually only in advanced cases with high intraocular pressure and corneal edema.[9,28]

The signs of the disorder are usually unmistakable, but vary from a spectrum of bare eccentricity of the pupil to severe corectopia. Iris atrophy and partial-thickness holes in the iris stroma appear on the side opposite the pupillary eccentricity, and, with continued stretch, full-thickness iris holes develop (Fig. 75.1). Atrophic iris holes also develop in

Table 75.1 Iridocorneal endothelial syndrome: clinical variations

	Progressive (essential) iris atrophy	Chandler's syndrome	Cogan-Reese syndrome	Iris nevus syndrome
Main clinical feature	Marked iris atrophy; holes and corectopia	Corneal edema at normal or slightly elevated intraocular pressure	Pedunculated, pigmented iris nodules	Diffuse nevus or heterochromia of iris
Corneal endothelium abnormal (slit lamp or specular microscopy)	Yes, may be subclinical	Yes	Yes (not originally reported)	Yes
Corneal edema	Variable – late	Present – early	Present	Present
Peripheral anterior synechiae beyond Schwalbe's line	Present	Present	Present	Present
Iris surface change	Present	Present	Present	Present
Iris atrophy	Marked	Minimal	Variable	Variable
Iris nodules	Present – late	Present – late	Present – early	Variable
Ectropion uveae	Present	Infrequent	Present	Present
Glaucoma	Present	Present	Present	Present
Pathogenesis	Abnormal endothelium and basement membrane proliferation	Abnormal endothelium and basement membrane proliferation	Abnormal endothelium and basement membrane proliferation	Abnormal endothelium and basement membrane proliferation
Heterochromia	Absent	Absent	Absent	Present

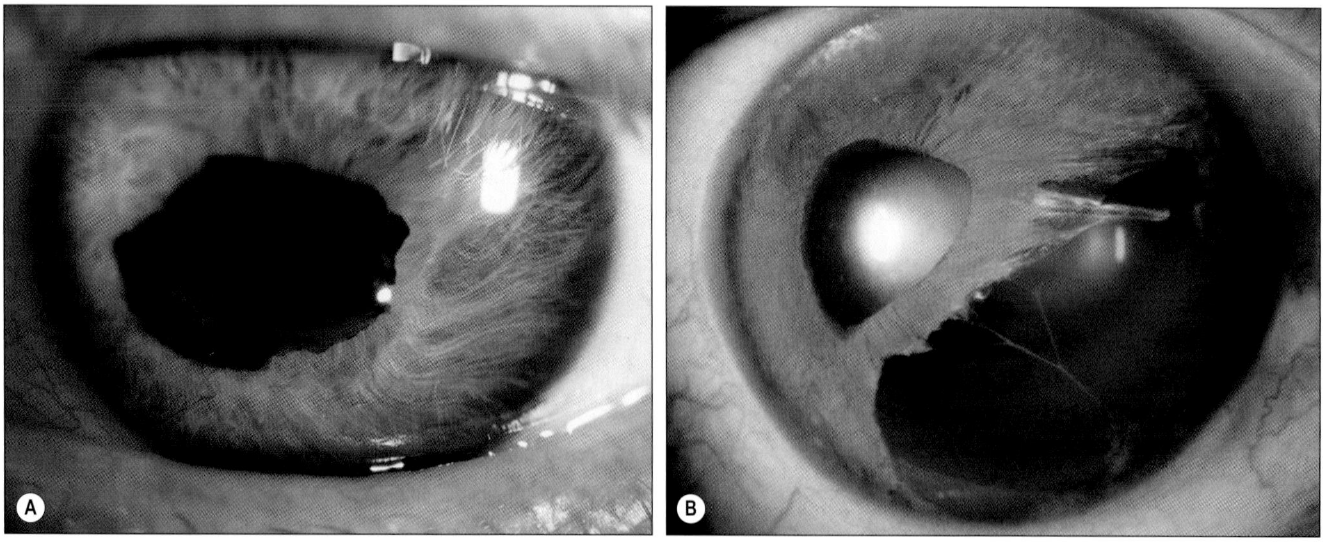

Fig. 75.1 (**A, B**) ICE syndrome. Essential (progressive) iris atrophy. Typical advanced iris changes of corectopia, thinning of iris, and stretch holes. (Courtesy of Jonathan E. Pederson, MD.)

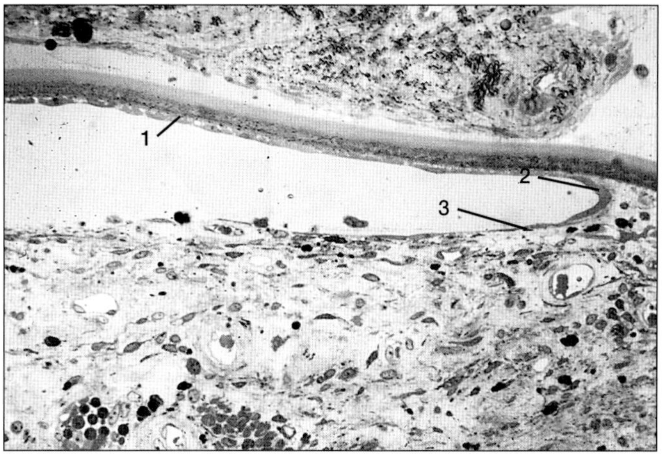

Fig. 75.2 Toluidine blue stain of corneal, anterior angle, and iris tissue in Chandler's syndrome; light microscopy. Degenerating endothelial cells and pathologic basement membrane material on the posterior cornea (*1*), causing peripheral anterior synechiae (*2*), and on the iris surface (*3*).

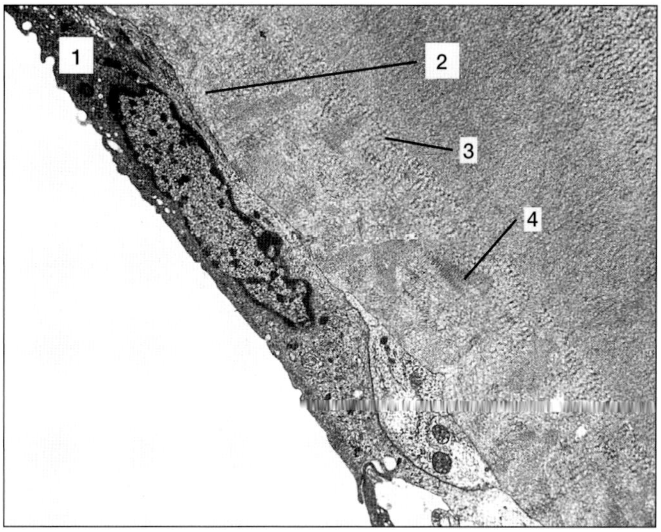

Fig. 75.3 Transmission electron micrograph of Chandler's syndrome cornea. Degenerating endothelial cell (*1*) on pathologic basement membrane material (*2*) containing posterior banding (*3*) and extracollagenous material (*4*).

areas not affected by stretching and are attributed to ischemia.[9,11,29] The underlying pathophysiologic event is an abnormal corneal endothelium, which produces abnormal basement membrane that extends beyond Schwalbe's line, covering the anterior chamber angle and anterior iris surface (Fig. 75.2).[11,30,31] The abnormal basement membrane is referred to by various names in the literature: cuticular membrane, glass membrane, cellular membrane, hyaline membrane, and ectopic Descemet's membrane.[7,14,32–35] Multilayered collagenous tissue posterior to Descemet's membrane associated with abnormal endothelium has been demonstrated by electron microscopy (Fig. 75.3). Contraction of this membrane draws the iris toward that side, resulting in corectopia and stretching atrophy in the opposite iris quadrant.[11] Progressive peripheral anterior synechiae develop, which are usually seen anterior to Schwalbe's line, resulting in progressive angle closure.[25] Even in the absence of PAS, the angle may be functionally closed because of the presence of a clinically invisible membrane overlying the trabecular meshwork.[20,36,37] Thus, there may be no correlation between the degree of PAS and the level of intraocular pressure.

The differences in growth and contracture of this endothelially derived membrane lead to a variable clinical presentation. If there is a 360-degree angle coverage and equal contraction, little corectopia and iris atrophy may be present, but loss of normal iris architecture is generally seen. Later in the clinical course, buds of normal iris stroma, seen as iris nodules, protrude through the membrane-lined iris surface.[8,30,38] The nodules begin as fine, yellow, raised areas and progress from light to dark brown pedunculated forms.[9] The normal architecture of the adjacent iris is lost, giving a flat, effaced surface.

Glaucoma, iris atrophy, or nodules may be seen relatively early or late, depending on the degree of endothelial proliferation and membrane formation in the anterior chamber angle. Corneal edema occurs, usually associated with elevated intraocular pressure, but it may occur early with widespread endothelial dysfunction. On slit lamp examination, the fine, hammered silver appearance of the endothelium described in Chandler's syndrome[10] is not always seen.[24] A total endothelial abnormality may exist, detected only by specular microscopy.[25]

Specular microscopy is an invaluable tool for early or confirmatory diagnosis.[39–41] Although endothelial cell pleomorphism and a decrease in the percentage of hexagonal cells of the contralateral eye have been described,[42,43] typical morphologic specular microscopic changes (ICE cells)[44] are unilateral. The following changes are usually seen in Chandler's syndrome, but may be seen in any of the ICE syndrome patients. The endothelial mosaic may contain a typical ICE cell in which the hexagonal borders are lost, a light or dark area is seen within, and reversal of the usual normal light/dark pattern occurs.[42,44–49] Oval dark and light bodies within cell boundaries and smaller round structures with either a bright or dark appearance near cell centers are thought to be endothelial cell nuclei and blebs of the apical cell membrane.[50] Epithelialization of the endothelial cells are thought to be the histological correlate of the ICE cell seen on specular microscopy.[44]

It must be emphasized, however, that the typical ICE cell is not necessary for the diagnosis in the presence of suspicious clinical findings (i.e. a solitary PAS or unilateral glaucoma in an otherwise normal eye[27,41]), as many unilateral abnormal patterns on specular microscopy also may be seen.[51,52] Partial endothelial involvement and regression of the abnormal endothelium has been reported.[47,48,53] Total cellular disorganization with no identifiable cells may be seen, even with a clinically clear and thin cornea (Fig. 75.4). Patchy areas of diffuse endothelial disorganization or typical ICE cells abruptly adjacent to normal endothelium may occur[18,47] Areas with increased cell density of smaller than normal endothelial cells[18,46] may represent the result of compaction or replication.[18,47] There appears to be no relation between duration of the disease and degree of endothelial abnormality,[42] nor is there a correlation of the ICE cells and endothelial density with corneal edema.[54] Single vesicular

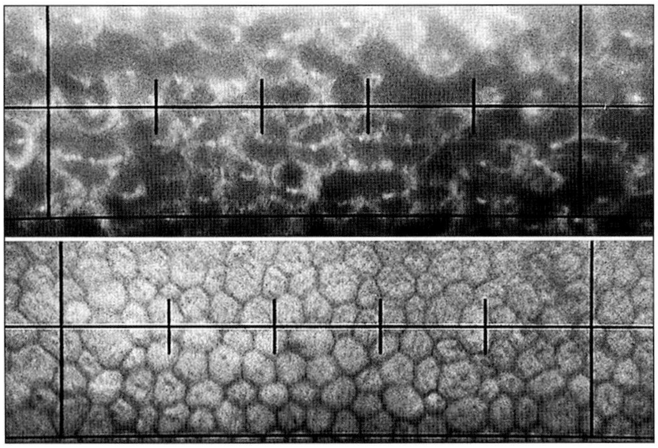

Fig. 75.4 Top, Specular microscopic appearance of patient with ICE syndrome, showing total abnormality of endothelium. ICE cells are seen with dark/light reversal. The patient was asymptomatic, and the pachymetry was normal. **Bottom**, Contralateral normal eye of same patient.

lesions, round doughnut-like elevations, and bands or ridges typical of posterior polymorphous dystrophy (PPD) are not seen.[47,49,54–56] Specular microscopy is very useful in general in distinguishing between ICE syndrome and PPD,[49] but may not always differentiate between progressive PPD and ICE syndrome which may share a final common pathological progression.[57]

Other diagnostic tools of great value in the diagnosis of ICE syndrome are ultrasound biomicroscopy (UBM) and in vivo confocal microscopy. They are especially helpful when corneal edema prevents gonioscopic view of the angles or specular microscopy. UBM has revealed peripheral anterior synechiae, iris atrophy, arborized shape of the iridocorneal angle, and closed angles.[58]

Confocal microscopy has been of great use as an early diagnostic tool, and invaluable in cases with corneal edema.[59–63] Consistent findings are irregular or indistinct endothelial cell borders with bright hyperreflective nuclei, and prominent corneal nerves. There may be small cells or larger epithelioid-like cells detected.[60] A transition between uniform cells with dark nuclei seen with confocal microscopy is consistent with patterns previously described with specular microscopy.

Aside from the unilateral presentation in the ICE syndrome, confocal microscopy also may not always be able to distinguish between ICE syndrome and PPD. Epithelialization of the endothelium characteristic of PPD has been reported in ICE syndrome,[64–67] but endothelial cells retain their typical characteristics and lineage.[31,44,50,68–70]

Chandler's syndrome

The first symptoms of Chandler's syndrome are usually blurred vision or seeing colored halos around lights.[10,27] These symptoms occur unilaterally in young adults as a result of corneal edema and are at first most evident in the morning. Corneal edema was first described as occurring at a normal or slightly elevated intraocular pressure and, because of the abnormal endothelium, is the dominating clinical characteristic of this subtype of ICE syndrome.[10,12] The abnormal corneal endothelium, best seen with specular reflection, has a fine hammered silver appearance (Fig. 75.5), which is finer in appearance than the guttata of Fuchs' endothelial dystrophy.[10,47] Iris changes may occur but are usually minimal and confined to the stroma with no hole formation, although nodules are seen.

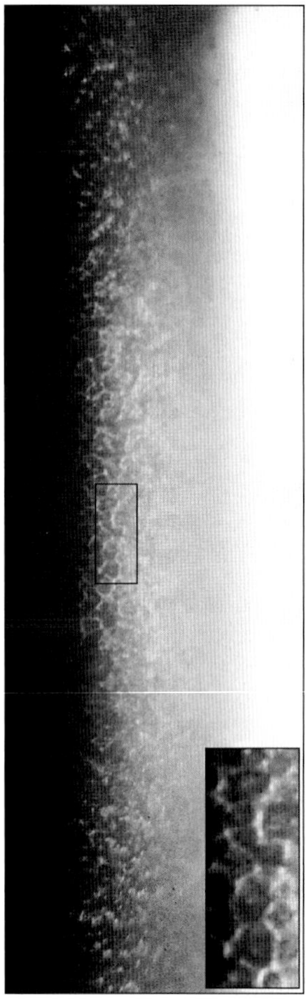

Fig. 75.5 Slit lamp view of patient with early ICE syndrome (Chandler's syndrome). Note fine hammered appearance of endothelium (*inset*) and reversal of cell borders (white instead of normal black).

Considerable endothelial abnormality may exist before extensive PAS are seen,[42] but gonioscopy will usually reveal a membrane or PAS in the angle. Glaucoma eventually occurs, but the syndrome and signs of Chandler's syndrome may be rather advanced before damage from glaucoma develops. Chandler suggested that if intraocular pressure could be normalized, corneal edema might be avoided.[10] Because of the progressive nature of this disorder, one expects corneal decompensation to occur eventually, even with good intraocular pressure control.

Specular microscopy may show all or any of the findings previously described with essential iris atrophy, but often a total diffuse abnormality is seen.[19,45] In extreme cases of corneal edema, specular microscopy may not be possible. Confocal microscopy may be of value in these cases;[60–63,71] however, clinical characteristics and gonioscopy are often adequate to make the diagnosis.

Cogan-Reese syndrome

Cogan-Reese syndrome[13] is the least common of the major variants of ICE syndrome in Caucasians.[40] One series in the Chinese literature found it the most common,[72] as did a more recent report on Thai patients.[73] As originally described, the disorder presented in two patients with unilateral glaucoma and pedunculated iris nodules. A hyaline membrane ('ectopic Descemet's membrane')[13] extending from the posterior surface of the cornea, around the anterior chamber angle, onto the anterior iris surface, and resulting in peripheral anterior synechiae was described. Mild iris atrophy, ectropion uvea, and numerous lightly pigmented pedunculated nodules were also seen. Histopathologic examinations of the nodules revealed a core of normal iris stroma and cells consistent with nevus cells covered by an ectopic Descemet's membrane and endothelium. Klien[74] and Wood[7] had described similar cases. Endothelial changes were not described, nor were holes in the iris or marked distortion of the pupil, and all reported cases occurred in women.

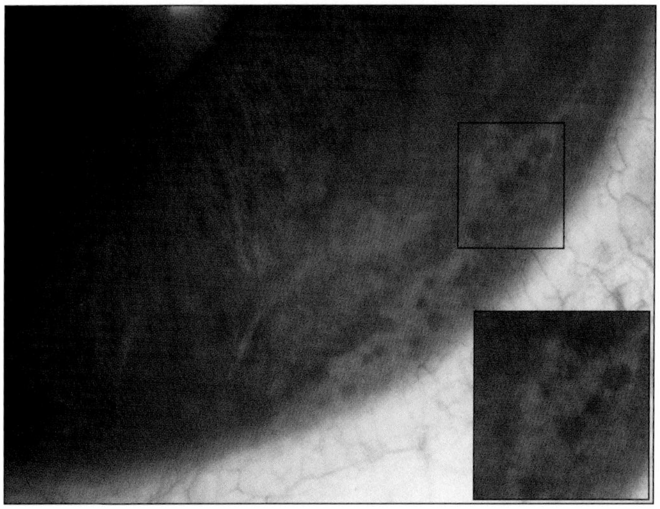

Fig. 75.6 Slit lamp photograph of patient with ICE syndrome (Cogan-Reese). Inferotemporal iris has dark nodules, surrounded by effaced iris architecture. The dark nodules are normal stroma (*inset*).

Iris nevus syndrome

Scheie and Yanoff[14] reported 14 patients with a unilateral diffuse nevus of the iris and several other signs including loss of surface architecture of the iris resulting in a matted appearance, ectropion uvea, heterochromia, PAS, corneal edema, and unilateral glaucoma. Fine iris nodules and mild iris atrophy were also described. This report emphasized the difficulty in distinguishing these patterns from diffuse malignant melanoma on the one hand and essential iris atrophy on the other. The nodules were hypopigmented and clustered; PAS and iris atrophy for the most part did not occur. Heterochromia and blunting of the normal iris architecture were the distinguishing iris features rather than the atrophy and hole formation seen in essential iris atrophy.

Although the Cogan-Reese syndrome and iris nevus syndrome are thought to be part of the ICE syndrome, there is some confusion about whether these are two distinct subtypes,[75] and they are often lumped together and the terms are often used interchangeably.[34,37,47,72,75] This confusion was fostered, in part, by the title of the Scheie and Yanoff report 'Iris nevus (Cogan-Reese) syndrome.'[14] A primary clinical sign in the Cogan-Reese report, iris nodules, is now known to be buds of normal stroma surrounded by an effaced iris covered with endothelium-derived abnormal basement membrane (Figs 75.6, 75.7).[32,33,37,38,76] The clinically striking feature of the iris nevus syndrome was heterochromia or a diffuse iris nevus, although fine nodules and a matted iris architecture were present.[15,34] Referring to the Cogan-Reese entity as the iris nodule syndrome may lessen the confusion. Unilateral endothelial proliferation with excess basement membrane, PAS, iris surface effacement, and glaucoma in young adults places these within the ICE spectrum, whether or not they are a single subtype or two.[9]

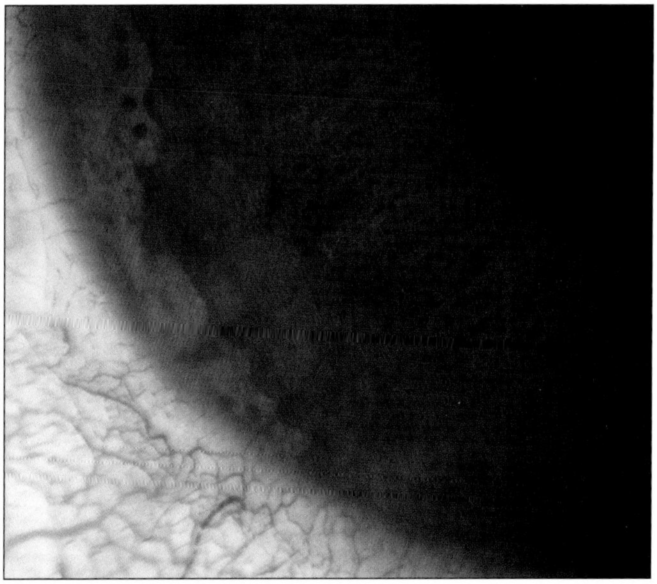

Fig. 75.7 Same patient as in Figure 75.6. View of inferonasal iris.

Etiology

Ischemic,[4,77] toxic,[5] and inflammatory[5,78] etiologies have been reviewed[5,20] and dismissed. The etiology at this time is still unknown. A viral origin has been proposed and supported with laboratory data.[79] Using the polymerase chain reaction, herpes simplex virus (HSV) DNA was reported to be present within the endothelium of a large percentage of ICE syndrome patients.[80,81] This finding is specific for HSV DNA but is not invariably present, and the observation has not been corroborated. Antibodies to Epstein-Barr virus (EBV) were noted in a high percentage of patients with ICE syndrome, but no direct role for EBV as a cause of the ICE syndrome was established.[82] What is certain is that some event, as yet unknown, causes the endothelium and basement membrane to extend beyond the peripheral cornea, leading to the clinical characteristics described (Fig. 75.8).[11,14,15,31,34,45,83] This endothelial cell-derived overgrowth

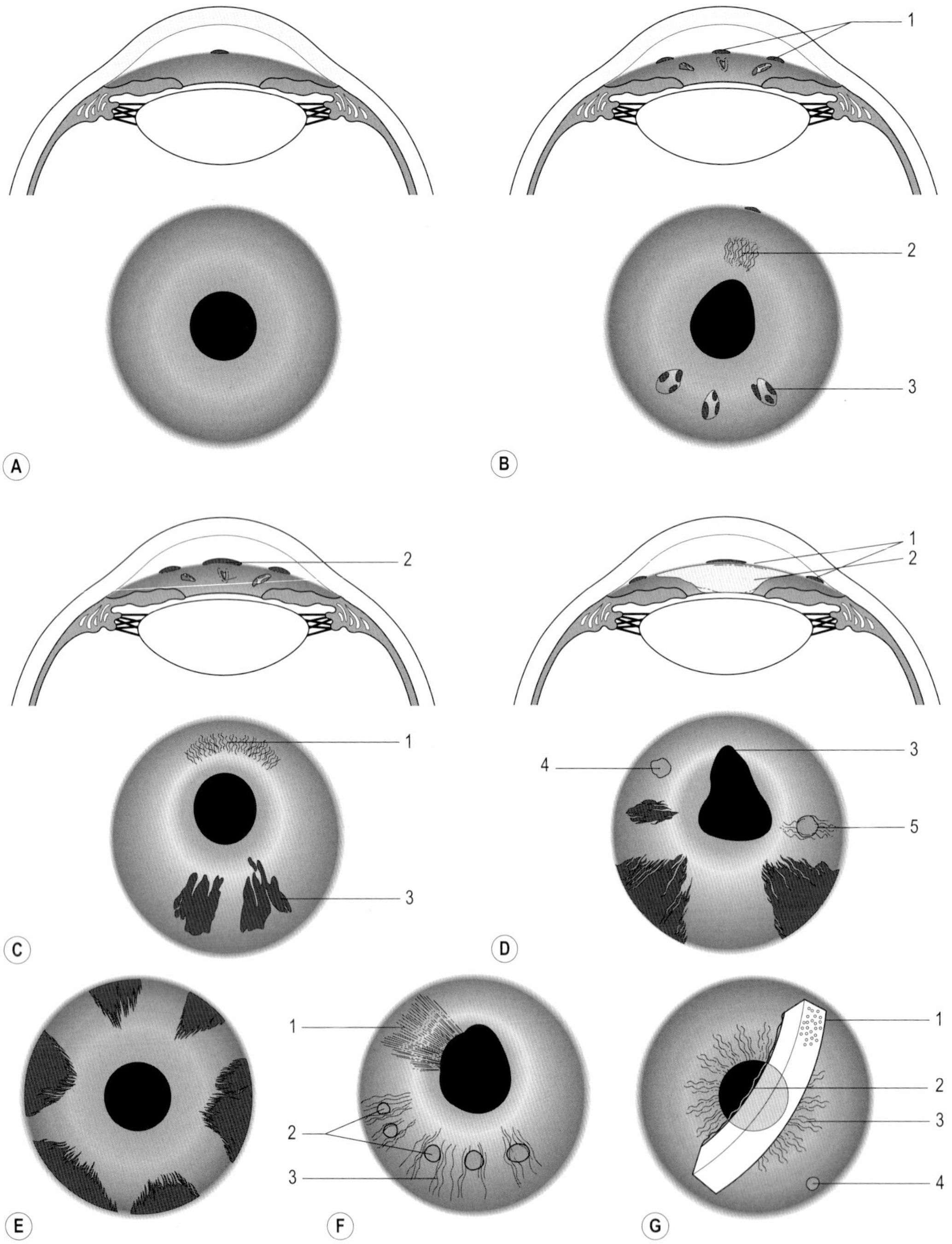

Fig. 75.8 Development and variation of ICE syndrome (after the membrane theory of Campbell). (**A**) Earliest stage of iris and anterior chamber angle involvement. Solitary peripheral anterior synechiae (PAS), but no pupil and iris abnormality. (**B**) Growth and extension of abnormal membrane from posterior corneal surface over the anterior chamber angle onto the surface of the iris. Multiple PAS (*1*), contraction of membrane on iris surface (*2*), and early stretch-induced iris stromal atrophy in the quadrant opposite the membrane (*3*). The pupil is mildly eccentric. (**C**) Diffuse anterior chamber angle and iris involvement with abnormal membrane growth. Matting of iris surface caused by growth and contraction of membrane (*1*), broader PAS, and wider iris and pupil involvement as membrane grows and contracts (*2*), and increase in iris stromal atrophy from increased membrane contraction and PAS 180 degrees opposite (*3*). Pigment epithelium of iris is visible through atrophic holes in iris stroma. (**D**) Progressive (essential) iris atrophy at an advanced stage. Clinically visible membrane covers trabecular meshwork and anterior chamber angle, functionally closing angle between PAS (*1*). Increase in effacement of iris (*2*). Ectropion uveae (*3*). Nonstretch 'melting' hole (*4*), possibly caused by ischemia. Iris 'nodule' (*5*), which is a bud of normal iris protruding through membrane-covered, flattened iris. (**E**) ICE variation: progressive (essential) iris atrophy with 360 degrees of anterior chamber angle involvement. Multiple iris holes but no corectopia because of relatively symmetric 360-degree membrane contraction and PAS. (**F**) ICE variation: iris nevus syndrome (Cogan-Reese syndrome). Diffuse iris lesion–iris nevus (*1*) and multiple iris 'nodules' (*2*), which are really buds of normal iris surrounded by effaced iris architecture. Iris atrophy (*3*) is usually mild, but is variable. (**G**) ICE variation: Chandler's syndrome. Microcystic corneal edema (*1*) and hammered silver appearance of corneal endothelium (*2*). Mild stromal iris atrophy (*3*) and an iris 'nodule' (*4*).

has led to some confusion as these endothelial cells have exhibited epithelial characteristics by electron microscopic (EM) and immunohistochemistry studies.[44,70] Epithelialization of the endothelium was previously thought to be characteristic of PPD. A study of an early case of ICE syndrome reported the appearance of a dual cell population, suggesting a transformation from normal hexagonal endothelial cells to ICE cells.[84] Dual populations of epithelial-like cells and normal endothelial cells were reported in cases of 'subtotal ICE' syndrome.[53] Epithelial characteristics of endothelial cells may be a final common cytologic transformation in these two, as well as other, disorders of the corneal endothelium.[85] Theories put forth to explain this phenomenon include a primordial nest of neural crest-derived pluripotential cells that under the right stimulus proliferate and, more likely, metaplasia of the neuroectoderm-derived endothelial cells.[70,72,85–87] The stimulus for metaplastic transformation is unknown, but a viral cause is considered a good possibility. This also would be consistent with the two-hit hypothesis proposed.[43]

Although there are isolated case reports of familial or bilateral involvement,[20,29,77,88–92] strong evidence indicates that ICE syndrome is nonfamilial[23,47,49] and is unilateral.[23,31,47,51,93,94]

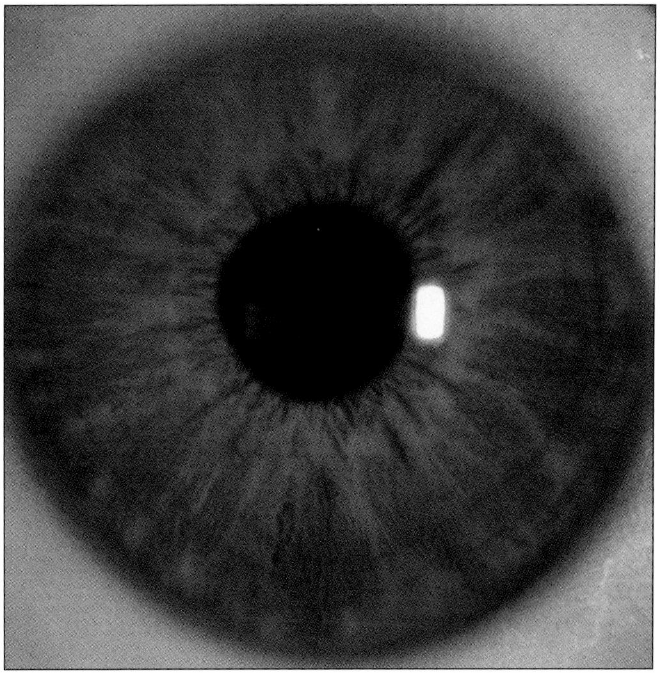

Fig. 75.9 Early ICE syndrome. Subtle eccentricity of pupil in superior quadrant.

Clinical Course

The iridocorneal endothelial syndrome is a progressive disorder,[5,9,10,18,19,48,69] but the subtypes may progress slowly (over decades)[18] or relatively quickly.[10,68] Glaucoma may be an early (before PAS)[11,30,83] or late[5] finding, depending on the degree of trabecular meshwork covered by the endothelial-derived membrane or the number of peripheral anterior synechiae. Scanning electron microscopy of a single surgical specimen revealed a monolayer of corneal endothelium-like cells with a thick basement membrane-like material. Neovascularization was observed in the corneal-scleral trabeculum, posing yet another mechanism of elevation of intraocular pressure in ICE patients.[95] It is important to establish the diagnosis early so that the patients may have realistic expectations and to monitor the progress of the disease, especially if glaucoma is not present and gross corneal changes have not occurred. Careful slit lamp examination and gonioscopy at regular intervals are valuable to assess progression (Figs 75.9, 75.10).[96]

Differential Diagnosis

A variety of different clinical entities must be distinguished from components of the ICE syndrome: (1) Fuchs' endothelial dystrophy;[10,42] (2) iris abnormalities including ischemic atrophy, aniridia, iridoschisis,[20] and PAS from prior trauma or uveitis;[97] (3) angle abnormalities from neovascular glaucoma[97] and trauma;[98] and (4) iris nodules from malignant melanoma and neurofibromatosis.[8,13,14,20] However, careful evaluation of the constellation of symptoms and signs associated with ICE syndrome limits consideration to only two conditions: posterior polymorphous dystrophy (PPD) and Axenfeld-Rieger syndrome (Table 75.2).

Posterior polymorphous dystrophy is an endothelial dystrophy that may have protean manifestations including diffuse corneal edema, corectopia, glass membrane formation, iridocorneal adhesions, and glaucoma.[68,99–102] Generally, the corneal changes are discrete, focal, bilateral, and asymptomatic. Round or oval vesicular changes, irregularly shaped gray opacities and parallel lines or ridges befitting the term polymorphous are observed in Descemet's membrane.[99] The bilateral changes may be rather asymmetric with only a single vesicle or group of vesicles as evidence of involvement.[100] Specular microscopy reveals dark rings, rounded hills or ovals, parallel ridges, and lesions corresponding to the clinical features.[49,55] Epithelialization of the endothelium is thought to be the characteristic endothelial change,[76,101,103–105] although fibroblastic metaplasia has been reported.[106] Epithelial characteristics of endothelial cells include myriad microvilli, keratofibrils, desmosomal attachments, and scant mitochondria in contrast to rich micro-organelles, apical tight junctions, and flat apical surfaces characteristic of endothelium.[68,106] These endothelial cells stain positive for cytokeratins using immunohistochemical techniques.[102]

PPD is inherited, usually in an autosomal dominant mode,[99–101,103] and examination of asymptomatic affected family members reveals characteristic lesions at Descemet's membrane. Although iris atrophy has been described rarely, nodules are not encountered. Glaucoma tends to be associated with significant corneal changes, but may not parallel the presence of PAS.[100] The corneal endothelium in PPD produces an abnormal Descemet's membrane-like material that may extend from the posterior cornea onto the iris, resulting in PAS and corectopia.[99,100] Descemet's membrane appears thickened.[103] A common pathogenesis for PPD

Table 75.2 General characteristics of ICE, posterior polymorphous dystrophy, and Axenfeld-Rieger syndrome

	ICE	PPD	A-RS
Age of onset	Young adult	Congenital	Congenital
Laterality	Unilateral*	Bilateral*	Bilateral*
Sex predilection	F > M	F = M	F = M*
Posterior embryotoxin	No*	No	Yes
Cornea abnormal (slit lamp)	Yes (fine, guttae-like changes, 'hammered silver')	Yes (vesicles, plaques at Descemet's membrane)	No
Specular microscopy	Diffuse changes, ICE cell	Focal change*	Normal
Basic defect	Abnormal proliferation of endothelium	Epithelialization of endothelium	Retention of primordial endothelial layer
Glaucoma	80–100%	25%	50%
Glaucoma mechanism	Membrane or PAS occluding angle	Unknown, membrane or PAS occluding angle	Incomplete or maldevelopment of trabecular meshwork and Schlemm's canal
Iris atrophy	Mild to severe	Minimal	Mild to severe
Iris nodules	Yes	No	No*
Progression	Yes – may be relentless	Minimal	No*
Inheritance	No	Autosomal dominant*	Autosomal dominant

PPD, posterior polymorphous dystrophy; A-RS, Axenfeld-Rieger syndrome; F, female; M, male.
** Denotes rare exceptions.*

Fig. 75.10 Goniophotograph of same patient as in Figure 75.9. View of superior angle showing early PAS, corresponding to pupil eccentricity.

and the iridocorneal endothelial syndrome has been postulated.[30,107]

The difference between ICE syndrome and Axenfeld-Rieger syndrome has been reviewed extensively.[25,108] Axenfeld-Rieger syndrome is a congenital condition that may have dramatic iris atrophy, iris hole formation, and corectopia. Glaucoma is a frequent component of this disorder. Gonioscopy reveals a prominent Schwalbe's line in all cases, with strands of tissue stretching from the iris periphery to Schwalbe's line. In addition to enlargement, Schwalbe's line is often anteriorly displaced, but much variation exists.[25] The corneal endothelium is normal, but specular microscopy may reveal some pleomorphism and intracellular dark spots.[25] It has been postulated that the ocular signs are due to a developmental arrest in gestation of tissues derived from neural crest cells.[25] The bilateral involvement may be asymmetric,[20] and iris nodules are not usually seen. Axenfeld-Rieger syndrome has autosomal dominant inheritance and frequently has associated developmental anomalies.[20,108] Molecular genetic techniques have linked chromosomal loci and phenotypic expression.[109]

Management

Treatment is geared to the dominant clinical type. Because there is no prevention or cure, early endothelial or iris changes are observed only. Until a specific viral origin is firmly established, antiviral therapy cannot be recommended.[81] Medical treatment is generally ineffective,[14,41,96] but when glaucoma develops it may be managed initially with aqueous suppressants. Pilocarpine and other miotics have no place in the management of the glaucoma because the problem is one of access to the trabecular meshwork, not an intrinsic defect in the meshwork itself. Intraocular pressure control with aqueous suppressants is usually short-lived because further angle closure develops (Fig. 75.11). Ultimately, glaucoma filtering surgery is required.[41] Some reports have suggested a bleak prognosis,[9,32,72] but there are many reports of success. In addition to the usual causes of bleb failure, other sources of failure in the ICE syndrome are

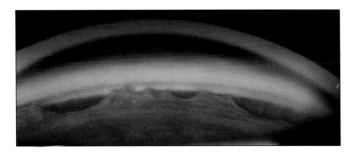

aggressive subconjunctival fibrosis and endothelialization of the bleb.[15,21,31,32,34,72,110] Antifibrotic agents,[111] mini aqueous shunts,[112] and glaucoma drainage implants (GDIs) have been evaluated and used with variable success.[110,112–114] One would generally first use trabeculectomy with mitomycin-C, and then proceed with GDIs if failure occurred. No matter which technique is employed, the success rate often diminishes markedly with time and multiple procedures may be required.[110,113–115]

Early in the clinical course, corneal edema may respond to lowering intraocular pressure.[10,20,24,36] Hypertonic saline solutions and soft contact lenses may be helpful. As the endothelial dysfunction progresses, however, corneal edema may be present even with excellent control of intraocular pressure. Persistent corneal edema may occur at any time because of progressive endothelial degeneration, elevated intraocular pressure, trauma of prior intraocular surgery, or some combination of these. When corneal clarity can no longer be maintained with good intraocular pressure control, and if advanced glaucomatous changes are not present, penetrating keratoplasty and endothelial keratoplasty, both deep lamellar endothelial keratoplasty (DLEK) and Descemet stripping endothelial keratoplasty (DSEK), are therapeutic options.[20,24,111–119] Many successes are reported with Chandler's variation of ICE syndrome,[22,23,28] but penetrating keratoplasty in the progressive iris atrophy variant of ICE syndrome may have a poorer prognosis because of continued inflammation.[120] Heavy use of antiinflammatory medications may improve the outcome in these cases, but multiple grafts may be needed. Control of glaucoma is the key factor in the ultimate visual success of keratoplasty in any of the subtypes of the ICE syndrome.

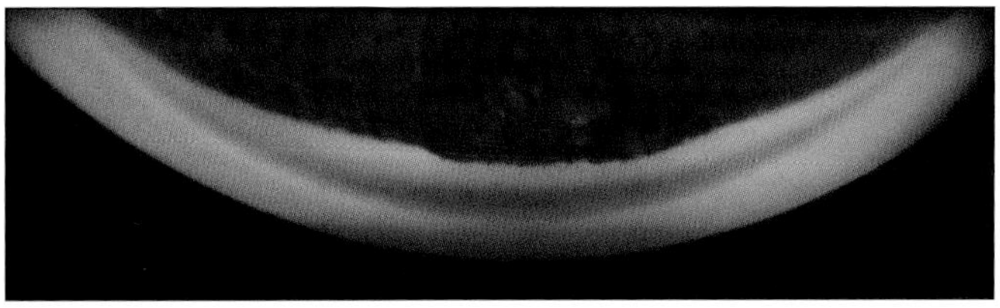

Fig. 75.11 Goniophotograph of inferior angle; patient with ICE syndrome. Note broad PAS extending beyond trabecular meshwork and Schwalbe's line. No normal angle structures are seen.

Cataracts may develop de novo or subsequent to glaucoma or corneal surgery. As part of surgical rehabilitation in patients with iris deficiencies when the iris is not amenable to suturing techniques, iris diaphragm intraocular lenses or iris prostheses have been used.[121–123] In ICE patients, cataract extraction with implantation of an intraocular lens and a multipiece endocapsular iris prosthesis through a small incision can achieve visual rehabilitation while sparing conjunctiva should future glaucoma surgeries be needed (Fig. 75.12).[123] The prosthetic iris helps to minimize postsurgical glare and photophobia.

Summary

The ICE syndrome is a unilateral, acquired corneal endothelial disorder, usually first seen in young adulthood. This abnormal proliferating endothelium produces a basement membrane that extends across the chamber angle onto the anterior iris surface and causes the characteristic clinical picture. Glaucoma may occur early or very late during the development of the clinically characteristic signs, and ICE syndrome should be strongly considered in any case of unilateral glaucoma without other obvious causes.[27,41]

Corneal edema at normal or slightly elevated intraocular pressure and any unilateral change in the iris surface or irregularity of the pupil, in the absence of a history of trauma or inflammation, should raise suspicion for the ICE syndrome. Gonioscopy, when possible, should always be performed. A single PAS,[31] or irregular appearance in the angle, also should suggest the diagnosis of ICE syndrome. Specular microscopy and confocal microscopy are invaluable tools for early diagnosis of ICE syndrome, and any of the previously described unilateral changes will confirm the diagnosis. Bilateral involvement and ocular involvement in family members almost always negate the diagnosis of ICE syndrome, and other causes should be sought. Later in the

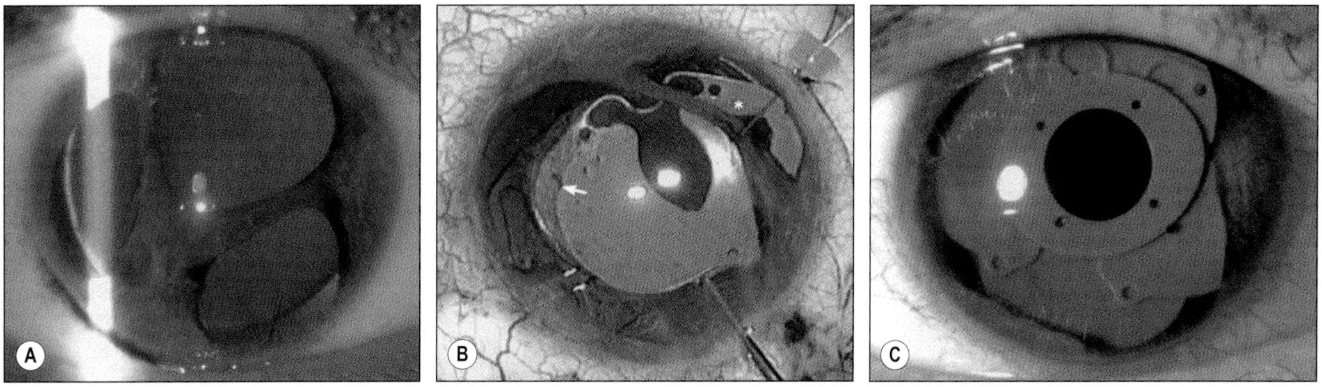

Fig. 75.12 (**A**) Preoperative photograph showing extensive iris abnormalities in ICE syndrome. The lens is cataractous. (**B**) Insertion of iris device into the capsular bag through a small incision. (**C**) Postoperative appearance showing the iris elements aligned and locked. (From Khng C, Snyder ME. Iris reconstruction with a multipiece endocapsular prosthesis in iridocorneal endothelial syndrome. J Cataract Refract Surg 2005;31(11):2051–4. Copyright Elsevier 2005.)

clinical course, progressive unilateral endothelial changes, iris holes, and nodules confirm the diagnosis of ICE syndrome. Treatment ranges from observation to medical management of the glaucoma, to surgical management of the glaucoma, and keratoplasty.

References

1. Harms C. Einseitige spontone Lückenbildung der Iris durch Atrophiè ohne mechanische Zerrung. *Klin Monatsbl Augenheilkd.* 1903;41: 522–528.
2. Waite JH. Essential progressive atrophy of the iris. *Am J Ophthalmol.* 1928;11:187–189.
3. Gifford S. Essential atrophy of iris associated with glaucoma. *Am J Ophthalmol.* 1926;9:548.
4. Zentmayer W. Essential atrophy of the iris. *Am J Ophthalmol.* 1918;1:510.
5. DeSchweinitz GE. Essential progressive atrophy of the iris: a second communication. *Arch Ophthalmol.* 1927;56:10–27.
6. Rochat GF, Mulder W. On progressive atrophy of the iris with formation of holes and glaucoma. *Br J Ophthalmol.* 1924;8:362–366.
7. Wood J. Melanosis of the iris and new formation of a hyaline membrane on its surface. *Br J Ophthalmol.* 1928;12:140–146.
8. Shields MB, et al. Iris nodules in essential iris atrophy. *Arch Ophthalmol.* 1976;94:406–410.
9. Shields MB, Campbell DG, Simmons RJ. The essential iris atrophies. *Am J Ophthalmol.* 1978;85:749–759.
10. Chandler PA. Atrophy of the stroma of the iris. *Am J Ophthalmol.* 1956;41:607–615.
11. Campbell DG, Shields MB, Smith TR. The corneal endothelium and the spectrum of essential iris atrophy. *Am J Ophthalmol.* 1978;86:317–324.
12. Chandler PA. Atrophy of the stroma of the iris, endothelial dystrophy, corneal edema, and glaucoma. *Trans Am Ophthalmol Soc.* 1955; 53:75–93.
13. Cogan DG, Reese AB. A syndrome of the iris nodules, ectopic Descemet's membrane, and unilateral glaucoma. *Doc Ophthalmol.* 1969;26: 425–433.
14. Scheie HG, Yanoff M. Iris nevus (Cogan-Reese) syndrome. *Arch Ophthalmol.* 1975;93:963–970.
15. Eagle RC, et al. Proliferative endotheliopathy with iris abnormalities: the iridocorneal endothelial syndrome. *Arch Ophthalmol.* 1979;97: 2104–2111.
16. Yanoff M. Discussion of presentation by Dr. M Bruce Shields et al. *Trans Am Acad Ophthalmol.* 1979;86:1549–1550.
17. Yanoff M. Iridocorneal endothelial syndrome: unification of a disease spectrum. *Surv Ophthalmol.* 1979;24:1–2.
18. Neubauer L, Lund O, Leibowitz HM. Specular microscopic appearance of the corneal endothelium in iridocorneal endothelial syndrome. *Arch Ophthalmol.* 1983;101:916–918.
19. Hetherington J. The spectrum of Chandler's syndrome. *Ophthalmology.* 1978;85:240–244.
20. Shields MB. Progressive essential iris atrophy, Chandler's syndrome, and the iris nevus (Cogan-Reese) syndrome: a spectrum of disease. *Surv Ophthalmol.* 1979;24:3–20.
21. Daicker B, Sturrock G, Guggenheim R. Zur kenntnis des Cogan-Reese-Syndroms. *Klin Monatsbl Augenheilkd.* 1982;180:531–538.
22. Chang PCT, et al. Prognosis for penetrating keratoplasty in iridocorneal endothelial syndrome. *Refract Corneal Surg.* 1993;9:129–132.
23. Crawford GJ, et al. Penetrating keratoplasty in the management of iridocorneal endothelial syndrome. *Cornea.* 1989;8:34–40.
24. Shields MB, et al. Corneal edema in essential iris atrophy. *Trans Am Acad Ophthalmol.* 1979;86:1533–1548.
25. Sheilds MB. Axenfeld-Rieger syndrome: a theory of mechanism and distinctions from the iridocorneal endothelial syndrome. *Trans Am Ophthalmol Soc.* 1983;81:736–784.
26. Salim S, Shields MB, Walton D. Iridocorneal endothelial syndrome in a child. *J Pediatr Ophthalmol Strabismus.* 2006;43(5):308–310.
27. Lichter PR. The spectrum of Chandler's syndrome: an often overlooked cause of unilateral glaucoma. *Ophthalmology.* 1978;85:245–251.
28. Buxton JN, Lash RS. Results of penetrating keratoplasty in the iridocorneal endothelial syndrome. *Am J Ophthalmol.* 1984;98:297–301.
29. Brancato R, Bandello F, Lattanzio R. Iris fluorescein angiography in clinical practice. *Surv Ophthalmol.* 1997;42:41–70.
30. Kupfer C, et al. The contralateral eye in the iridocorneal endothelial (ICE) syndrome. *Ophthalmology.* 1983;90:1343–1350.
31. Eagle RC, Shields JA. Iridocorneal endothelial syndrome with contralateral guttate endothelial dystrophy. *Ophthalmology.* 1987;94:862–870.
32. Reese AB. Deep-chamber glaucoma due to the formation of a cuticular product in the filtration angle. *Am J Ophthalmol.* 1944;27:1193–1205.
33. Radius RL, Hershcler J. Histopathology in the iris-nevus (Cogan-Reese) syndrome. *Am J Ophthalmol.* 1980;89:780–786.
34. Eagle RC, et al. The iris naevus (Cogan-Reese) syndrome: light and electron microscopic observations. *Br J Ophthalmol.* 1980;64:446–452.
35. Waring GO, Laibson PR, Rodrigues M. Clinical and pathologic alterations of Descemet's membrane: with emphasis on endothelial metaplasia. *Surv Ophthalmol.* 1974;18:325–368.
36. Rodrigues MM, Streeten BW, Spaeth GL. Chandler's syndrome as a variant of essential iris atrophy. *Arch Ophthalmol.* 1978;96:643–652.
37. Weber PA, Gibb G. Iridocorneal endothelial syndrome: glaucoma without peripheral anterior synechias. *Glaucoma.* 1984;6:128–134.
38. Tester RA, et al. Cogan-Reese syndrome. Progressive growth of endothelium over iris. *Arch Ophthalmol.* 1998;116:1126.
39. Kerr-Muir MG, Laganowski HC, Buckley RJ. Differential diagnosis of iridocorneal endothelial syndrome and posterior polymorphous endothelial dystrophy (letter). *Br J Ophthalmol.* 1993;77:610.
40. Laganowski HC, et al. Distinguishing features of the iridocorneal endothelial syndrome and posterior polymorphous dystrophy: value of endothelial specular microscopy. *Br J Ophthalmol.* 1991;75:212–216.
41. Laganowski HC, Kerr-Muir MG, Hitchings RA. Glaucoma and the iridocorneal endothelial syndrome. *Arch Ophthalmol.* 1992;110:346–350.
42. Hirst LW, et al. Specular microscopy of iridocorneal endothelial syndrome. *Am J Ophthalmol.* 1980;89:11–21.
43. Lucas-Glass TC, et al. The contralateral corneal endothelium in the iridocorneal endothelial syndrome. *Arch Ophthalmology.* 1997;115: 40–44.
44. Levy SG, et al. The histopathology of the iridocorneal-endothelial syndrome. *Cornea.* 1996;15:46–54.
45. Patel A, et al. Clinicopathologic features of Chandler's syndrome. *Surv Ophthalmol.* 1983;27:327–344.
46. Sherrard ES, et al. The posterior surface of the cornea in the irido-corneal endothelial syndrome: a specular microscopical study. *Trans Ophthalmol Soc UK.* 1985;104:766–774.
47. Bourne WM. Partial corneal involvement in the iridocorneal endothelial syndrome. *Am J Ophthalmol.* 1982;94:774–871.
48. Bourne WM, Brubaker RF. Progression and regression of partial corneal involvement in the iridocorneal endothelial syndrome. *Trans Am Ophthalmol Soc.* 1992;90:200–219.
49. Laganowski HC, et al. Distinguishing features of the iridocorneal endothelial syndrome and posterior polymorphous dystrophy: value of endothelial specular microscopy. *Br J Ophthalmol.* 1991;75:212–216.
50. Alvarado JA, et al. Pathogenesis of Chandler's syndrome, essential iris atrophy and the Cogan-Reese syndrome. *Invest Ophthalmol Vis Sci.* 1986;27:853–872.
51. Sherrard ES, Frangoulis MA, Kerr-Muir MG. On the morphology of cells of posterior cornea in the iridocorneal endothelial syndrome. *Cornea.* 1991;10:233–243.
52. Setälä K, Vannas A. Corneal endothelial cells in essential iris atrophy. *Acta Ophthalmol (Copenh).* 1979;57:1020–1029.
53. Levy SG, et al. On the pathology of the iridocorneal endothelial syndrome: the ultrastructural appearance of 'subtotal-ICE.' *Eye.* 1995;9:318–323.
54. Liu Y-K, et al. Clinical and specular microscopic manifestations of iridocorneal endothelial syndrome. *Jpn J Ophthalmol.* 2001;45:281–287.
55. Laganowski HC, Sherrard ES, Kerr-Muir MG. The posterior corneal surface in posterior polymorphous dystrophy: a specular microscopical study. *Cornea.* 1991;10:224–232.
56. Brooks AMV, et al. Differentiation of posterior polymorphous dystrophy from other posterior corneal opacities by specular microscopy. *Ophthalmology.* 1989;96:1639–1645.
57. Hirst LW. Differential diagnosis of iridocorneal endothelial syndrome and posterior polymorphous endothelial dystrophy. *Br J Ophthalmol.* 1993;77:610.
58. Zhang M, Chen J, Lang L, et al. Ultrasound biomicroscopy of Chinese eyes with iridocorneal syndrome. *Br J Ophthalmol.* 2006;90(1):64–69.
59. Chiou AGY, et al. Confocal microscopy in the iridocorneal endothelial syndrome. *Br J Ophthalmol.* 1999;83:697–702.
60. Grupcheva CN, McGhee CN, Dean S, Craig JP. In vivo confocal microscopic characteristics of iridocorneal endothelial syndrome. *Clin Experiment Ophthalmol.* 2004;32(3):275–283.
61. Garibaldi DC, Schein OD, Jun A. Features of the iridocorneal endothelial syndrome on confocal microscopy. *Cornea.* 2005;24(3):349–351.
62. Sheppard JD Jr, Lattanzio FA Jr, Williams PB, Mitrev PB, Allen RC. Confocal microscopy used as the definitive, early diagnostic method in Chandler syndrome. *Cornea.* 2005;24(2):227–229.
63. Le QH, Sun XH, Xu JJ. In-vivo confocal microscopy of iridocorneal endothelial syndrome. *Int Ophthalmol.* 2009;29:11–18.

64. Hirst LW, et al. Epithelial characteristics of the endothelium in Chandler's syndrome. *Invest Ophthalmol Vis Sci.* 1983;24:603–611.
65. Portis JM, et al. The corneal endothelium and Descemet's membrane in the iridocorneal endothelial syndrome. *Trans Am Ophthalmol Soc.* 1985;83:316–327.
66. Kramer TR, et al. Cytokeratin expression in corneal endothelium in the iridocorneal endothelial syndrome. *Invest Ophthalmol Vis Sci.* 1992;33:3581–3585.
67. Quigley HA, Forster RF. Histopathology of cornea and iris in Chandler's syndrome. *Arch Ophthalmol.* 1978;96:1878–1882.
68. Rodrigues MM, et al. Glaucoma due to endothelialization of the anterior chamber angle. *Arch Ophthalmol.* 1980;98:688–696.
69. Rodrigues MM, Stulting RD, Waring GO. Clinical, electron microscopic, and immunohistochemical study of the corneal endothelium and Descemet's membrane in the iridocorneal endothelial syndrome. *Am J Ophthalmol.* 1986;101:16–27.
70. Hirst LW, et al. Immunohistochemical pathology of the corneal endothelium in iridocorneal endothelial syndrome. *Invest Ophthalmol Vis Sci.* 1995;36:820–827.
71. Mocan MC, Bozkurt B, Orhan M, Irkec M. Chandler syndrome manifesting as ectropion uvea following laser in situ keratomileusis. *J Cataract Refract Surg.* 2008;34(5):871–873.
72. Ye T, Pang Y, Liu Y. Iris nevus syndrome (report of 9 cases). *Eye Sci.* 1991;7:34–39.
73. Teekhasaenee C, Ritch R. Iridocorneal endothelial syndrome in Thai patients. *Arch Ophthalmology.* 2000;118:187–192.
74. Klien BA. Pseudomelanomas of the iris. *Am J Ophthalmol.* 1941;24:133–138.
75. Sugar HS. The iris nevus and Cogan-Reese syndromes: separate entities? *Ann Ophthalmol.* 1981;13:405–407.
76. Waring GO 3rd, et al. The corneal endothelium. Normal and pathologic structure and function. *Ophthalmology.* 1982;89:531–590.
77. Jampol LM, Rosser MJ, Sears ML. Unusual aspects of progressive essential iris atrophy. *Am J Ophthalmol.* 1974;77:353–357.
78. Inomata H, et al. Iris nevus (Cogan-Reese) syndrome: clinicopathological correlations. *Nippon Ganka Gakkai Zasshi.* 1990;94:80–88.
79. Alvarado JA, et al. Pathogenesis of Chandler's syndrome, essential iris atrophy and Cogan-Reese syndrome. *Invest Ophthalmol Vis Sci.* 1986;27:873–882.
80. Alvarado JA, et al. Further studies to substantiate a viral etiology for the ICE syndrome. *Invest Ophthalmol Vis Sci.* 1993;34(Suppl):994, (abstract).
81. Alvarado JA, et al. Detection of herpes simplex viral DNA in the iridocorneal endothelial syndrome. *Arch Ophthalmol.* 1994;112:1601–1609.
82. Tsai CS, et al. Antibodies to Epstein-Barr virus in iridocorneal endothelial syndrome. *Arch Ophthalmol.* 1990;108:1572–1576.
83. Benedikt O, Roll P. Open-angle glaucoma through endothelialization of the anterior chamber angle. *Glaucoma.* 1980;2:368–380.
84. Lee WR, Marshall GE, Kirkness CM. Corneal endothelial cell abnormalities in an early stage of the iridocorneal endothelial syndrome. *Br J Ophthalmol.* 1994;78:624–631.
85. Howell DN, et al. Endothelial metaplasia in the iridocorneal endothelial syndrome. *Invest Ophthalmol Vis Sci.* 1997;38:1896–1901.
86. Bahn CF, et al. Classification of corneal endothelial disorders based on neural crest origin. *Ophthalmology.* 1984;91:558–563.
87. Levy SG, et al. Pathology of the iridocorneal endothelial syndrome. The ICE cell. *Invest Ophthalmol Vis Sci.* 1995;36:2592–2601.
88. Blum JV, Allen JH, Holland MG. Familial bilateral essential iris atrophy (group 2). *Trans Am Acad Ophthalmol Otolaryngol.* 1962;66:493–500.
89. Kaiser-Kupfer M, Kuwabara T, Kupfer C. Progressive bilateral essential iris atrophy. *Am J Ophthalmol.* 1977;83:340–346.
90. Gedda L, Bérard-Magistretti S. Atrofia ereditaria progressiva dell'iride. *Acta Genet Med Gemellol (Roma).* 1959;8:39–64.
91. Hemady RK, Patel A, Blum S, Nirankari VS. Bilateral iridocorneal endothelial syndrome; case report and review of the literature. *Cornea.* 1994;13:368–372.
92. Des Marchais B, et al. Bilateral Chandler syndrome. *J Glaucoma.* 1999;8:276–277.
93. Bourne WM. Letters to the editor. *Ophthalmology.* 1984;91:884–885.
94. Hirst LW. Bilateral iridocorneal endothelial syndrome. *Cornea.* 1995;14:331.
95. Awai M, Futa R, Hamanaka T, Hirata A, et al. A case of Chandler's syndrome revealed by ultrastructural studies of the trabecular meshwork. *Acta Ophthalmol Scand.* 2005;83(1):113–114.
96. Gazala JR. Progressive essential iris atrophy. *Am J Ophthalmol.* 1960;49:713–723.
97. Gartner S, Taffet S, Friedman AH. The association of rubeosis iridis with endothelialisation of the anterior chamber: report of a clinical case with histopathological review of 16 additional cases. *Br J Ophthalmol.* 1977;61:267–271.
98. Colosi NJ, Yanoff M. Reactive corneal endothelialization. *Am J Ophthalmol.* 1977;83:219–224.
99. Cibis GW, et al. Iridocorneal adhesions in posterior polymorphous dystrophy. *Trans Am Acad Ophthalmol Otolaryngol.* 1976;81:770–777.
100. Cibis GW, et al. The clinical spectrum of posterior polymorphous dystrophy. *Arch Ophthalmol.* 1977;95:1529–1537.
101. Krachmer JH. Posterior polymorphous corneal dystrophy: a disease characterized by epithelial-like endothelial cells which influence management and prognosis. *Trans Am Ophthalmol Soc.* 1985;83:413–475.
102. Anderson NJ, et al. Posterior polymorphous membranous dystrophy with overlapping features of iridocorneal endothelial syndrome. *Arch Ophthalmol.* 2001;119:624–625.
103. Tripathi RC, Casey TA, Wise G. Hereditary posterior polymorphous dystrophy: an ultrastructural and clinical report. *Trans Ophthalmol Soc UK.* 1974;94:211–225.
104. Rodrigues MM, et al. Epithelialization of the corneal endothelium in posterior polymorphous dystrophy. *Invest Ophthalmol Vis Sci.* 1980;19:832–835.
105. Boruchoff SA, Kuwabara T. Electron microscopy of posterior polymorphous degeneration. *Am J Ophthalmol.* 1971;72:879–887.
106. Johnson BL, Brown SI. Posterior polymorphous dystrophy: a light and electron microscopic study. *Br J Ophthalmol.* 1978;62:89–96.
107. Blair SD, et al. Bilateral progressive essential iris atrophy and keratoconus with coincident features of posterior polymorphous dystrophy: a case report and proposed pathogenesis. *Cornea.* 1992;11:255–261.
108. Shields MB. Axenfeld-Rieger and iridocorneal endothelial syndromes: two spectra of disease with striking similarities and differences. *J Glaucoma.* 2001;10(Suppl 1):S36-S38.
109. Alward WLM. Axenfeld-Rieger syndrome in the age of molecular genetics. *Am J Ophthalmol.* 2000;130:107–115.
110. Wright MM, et al. 5-Fluorouracil after trabeculectomy and the iridocorneal endothelial syndrome. *Ophthalmology.* 1991;98:314–316.
111. Yonker JM, Juzych MS. Iridocorneal endothelial syndrome. *Glaucoma Today.* 2007:31.
112. Alvim PT, Cohen EJ, Rapuano CJ, et al. Penetrating keratoplasty in iridocorneal endothelial syndrome. *Cornea.* 2001;20(2):134–140.
113. Doe EA, et al. Long-term surgical outcomes of patients with glaucoma secondary to the iridocorneal endothelial syndrome. *Ophthalmology.* 2001;108:1789–1795.
114. Lanzl IM, et al. Outcome of trabeculectomy with mitomycin-C in the iridocorneal endothelial syndrome. *Ophthalmology.* 2000;107:295–297.
115. Kim DK, et al. Long-term outcome of aqueous shunt surgery in ten patients with iridocorneal endothelial syndrome. *Ophthalmology.* 1999;106:1030–1034.
116. Price MO, Price FW Jr. Descemet stripping with endothelial keratoplasty for treatment of iridocorneal endothelial syndrome. *Cornea.* 2007;26(4):493–497.
117. Bahar I, Kaiserman I, Buys Y, Rootman D. Descemet's stripping with endothelial keratoplasty in iridocorneal endothelial syndrome. *Ophthalmic Surg Lasers Imaging.* 2008;39(1):54–56.
118. Huang T, Yujuan W, Jianping J, et al. Deep lamellar endothelial keratoplasty for iridocorneal endothelial syndrome in phakic eyes. *Arch Ophthalmol.* 2009;127(1):33–36.
119. Bahar I, Kaiserman I, McAllum P, et al. Comparison of posterior lamellar keratoplasty techniques to penetrating keratoplasty. *Ophthalmology.* 2008;115(9):1525–1533.
120. DeBroff BM, Thoft RA. Surgical results of penetrating keratoplasty in essential iris atrophy. *J Refract Corneal Surg.* 1994;10:428–432.
121. Rosenthal KJ. Sutureless phacotrabeculectomy and insertion of an iris diaphragm ring in a patient with the Axenfeld-Reiger syndrome: first reported case. *Video Cataract Refract Surg.* 1997;13(2).
122. Burk SE, DaMata AP, Snyder ME, et al. Prosthetic iris implantation for congenital, traumatic, or functional iris deficiencies. *J Cataract Refract Surg.* 2001;27:1732–1740.
123. King C, Snyder ME. Iris reconstruction with a multipiece endocapsular prosthesis in iridocorneal endothelial syndrome. *J Cataract Refract Surg.* 2005;31(11):2051–2054.

Chapter 76

Corneal and Conjunctival Degenerations

Richard I. Chang, Steven Ching

Degeneration of a tissue is defined as a deterioration and decrease in function. Degenerations have classically been contrasted to the dystrophies. Dystrophies are generally bilateral and symmetric. They are hereditary and usually appear early in life. The dystrophies are avascular and located centrally. Progression occurs slowly and no systemic diseases are associated with the disease.

Conversely, degenerations may be unilateral or bilateral and are often asymmetric. Inheritance patterns are usually not found. Many degenerations occur later in life and are considered aging changes. Degenerations are often eccentric or peripheral and correspond with vascularity. Progression is variable and may be rapid. Local and systemic diseases are commonly associated.

Previous classifications of the degenerations have involved: anterior/posterior, involutional/noninvolutional, aging changes/depositions, and central/marginal degenerations.[1–6] The aforementioned general guidelines have helped us to classify various diseases. This chapter discusses both corneal and conjunctival degenerations. Where appropriate, the treatment modalities are also discussed. Surgical treatments are discussed elsewhere in this text and are only mentioned briefly. The ectatic degenerations are discussed elsewhere.

Corneal Degenerations

The cornea changes with age, and various age-related degenerative changes cannot be classified under any specific disease heading. Flattening in the vertical meridian, inducing increased astigmatism, occurs with age. Additional aging changes include decreasing corneal thickness, increasing thickness of Descemet's membrane, and endothelial cell loss. Corneal luster also diminishes with age.[3]

Arcus senilis

Corneal arcus – also known as arcus senilis (Fig. 76.1) or gerontoxon in the aged and arcus juvenilis or anterior embryotoxon in the young population – is a degenerative change involving lipid deposition in the peripheral cornea. Lipid deposition starts clinically as a gray to yellow arc, first in the inferior cornea then the superior cornea.[7,8] As the deposition progresses, the arcs meet, forming a complete ring.

The arcus has a sharp peripheral border ending at the edge of Bowman's layer with a lucent zone (lucid interval of Vogt) to the limbus. The central edge is more diffuse. Fine dots with interweaving lines can be seen at the slit lamp. Lipid is first deposited at Descemet's membrane and subsequently at Bowman's layer. Histopathologically, the arcus has an hourglass appearance as the opacity extends into the corneal stroma from these two layers.

Histochemically, the opacity is made up of cholesterol, cholesterol esters, phospholipids, and neutral glycerides.[9,10] Pathologically, the lipid is predominantly extracellular cholesteryl ester-rich lipid particles. These corneal lipid particles are similar to a type found in human atherosclerotic lesions but accumulate in the absence of foam cells, unlike atherosclerotic lesions.[11] Deposition is first seen in the anterior layers of Descemet's membrane as a double lamina.[10] Deposition then occurs in Bowman's layer, ending abruptly with the termination of this structure. In advanced stages deposition is seen between the stromal lamellae, sparing the limbus. Similar deposition of lipid can be seen in the perilimbal sclera overlying the ciliary body.

Experiments have shown the lipids to be of vascular origin. Lipids in the form of low-density lipoprotein (LDL) cross the capillary wall.[12] This is independent of arterial blood pressure, unlike the situation in the aorta. The limbal vasculature is part of a low-pressure perfusion system. The endothelium of these blood vessels act as tight junctions but in the presence of elevated circulating LDL may become dysfunctional. Although the lipid in the peripheral cornea likely originates from LDL, it is modified LDL and apo B sparse.[13] Corneal arcus is usually bilaterally symmetric and progresses slowly over years. Hyperemia of the limbal vasculature has been associated with a more rapid rate of arcus formation. Corneal arcus may be deflected by the presence of corneal vascularization. A lucid interval is seen between the vascularization and the arcus, which may be due to the vessel's ability to reabsorb the lipid in this area before it precipitates. Unilateral arcus may be seen with carotid artery occlusion on the side without the arcus.[14]

The prevalence of corneal arcus has been shown to increase with age.[15] The degeneration affects men more than women. The prevalence in women increases significantly in the postmenopausal period. Approximately two-thirds of all men are affected in the 40–60-year-old range. Virtually 100% of the population is affected after age 80.[8,15] Certain ethnic

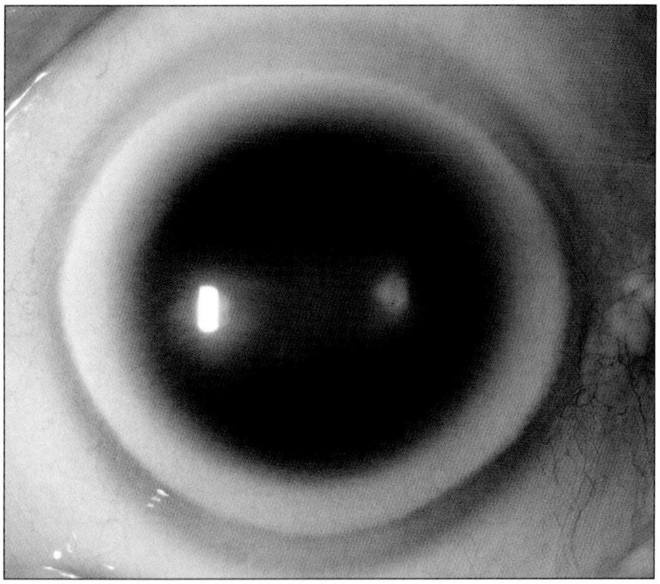

Fig 76.1 Arcus senilis.

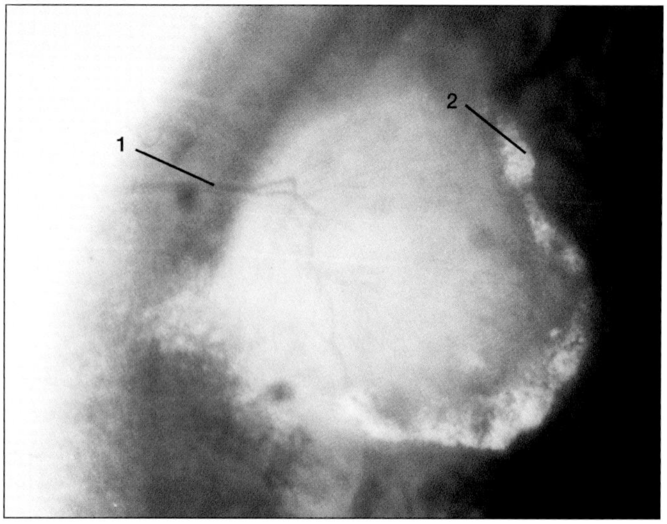

Fig 76.2 Herpes zoster keratitis with neovascularization (*1*). At the leading edge of the scar, secondary lipid degeneration is visible (*2*). These perilimbal lesions are typical in zoster keratitis.

populations are affected less frequently. Black males have the highest incidence, followed by black females, then white males followed by white females.[13] Blacks are affected at a younger age than whites.[15] The opacity remains peripheral but may occasionally extend centrally. Some consider this to represent a lipid keratopathy rather than an arcus senilis.

Corneal arcus has no visual significance, and thus no necessary treatment. However, it can be clinically significant. Patients under the age of 40 with corneal arcus have an increased risk of coronary artery disease and should be evaluated for hyperlipoproteinemia. Hyperlipoproteinemia types IIa and IIb are associated with premature corneal arcus formation, the most commonly observed being type IIa hyperlipoproteinemia.[16] These diseases may be primary or secondary and involve increased levels of β-lipoproteins rich in cholesterol. Primary disease is an autosomal dominant disorder with incomplete penetrance.[8] In addition to corneal arcus, these patients have xanthelasma elsewhere including tendons and the vasculature. Diseases causing a rise in β-lipoproteins include nephrotic syndrome, hypothyroidism, increased cholesterol intake, obstructive jaundice, and diabetic ketoacidosis.

Rare genetic disorders of high-density lipoprotein (HDL) metabolism causing corneal deposits include lecithin cholesterol acyltransferase (LCAT) deficiency, which has an autosomal recessive mode of inheritance with strong penetrance, fish eye disease, whose exact mode of inheritance is unknown, and Tangier disease, which occurs in homozygotically affected individuals with an autosomal recessive mutation. All of these diseases may produce a generalized corneal clouding that may affect visual acuity and manifest at an early age. An arcus may also be observed in LCAT deficiency.[8,13]

Lipid degeneration

Lipid degeneration has a primary and secondary form. Primary lipid degeneration is rare and is described in case reports. Secondary forms are more common and occur in vascularized corneas (Fig. 76.2). Associations of secondary lipid degeneration include interstitial keratitis, trauma, corneal hydrops, corneal ulceration, and mustard gas injuries due to its thrombosing properties.[13]

To classify a patient as having primary lipid degeneration, there should be no prior history of the following: trauma, family history of similar conditions, corneal vascularization, and no known disorders of lipid metabolism. Serum lipids are in the normal range. Lipid deposition is either central or peripheral. Peripheral deposition is usually seen as an extension from an arcus senilis.

Fatty acids in primary degeneration consist of cholesterol, triglycerides, and phospholipids. Extracellular deposition of fats has been demonstrated.[1,2] These components are similar to those found in arcus senilis. It has been suggested that primary degeneration is related to arcus if not an advanced stage of arcus. The cause of the disorder is uncertain but may be due to increased vascular permeability of the limbal vessels. Alternatively, the etiology may be an altered metabolic activity of the keratocytes and release of this fatty material into the stroma from dying cells. Histopathologic studies have shown a decrease in the cellularity of the stroma in areas of lipid degeneration.[17] As in corneal arcus, the fats are usually found in the posterior stroma and Descemet's membrane, in contrast to hereditary crystalline dystrophy of Schnyder in which the deposits are usually found more anteriorly.

Lipid keratopathy is more common in women than men, with a ratio of 70:30. Women have a higher level of HDL, which may play a role since lipid keratopathy invariably develops prior to menopause.[16]

Clinical significance of the disease other than its cosmetic appearance is decreased vision. Penetrating keratoplasty has been used to treat primary lipid degeneration. There is one case report of recurrence in the graft.[18]

Secondary lipid degeneration is associated with corneal neovascularization. These vessels become more permeable and have decreased ability to remove lipid. Local regression is associated with normolipoproteinemia and local progression is associated with hyperlipoproteinemia.[16] The corneal infiltrate is gray to yellow-white. Onset is sudden and may cause a rapid decrease in vision.

The degeneration may be sea fan-shaped with feathery edges or as a dense discoid lesion. The discoid lesion occurs in areas of active inflammation, whereas the sea fan appears in areas of postinflammatory inactive neovascularization. Crystals, representing cholesterol, may be seen at the edges of the lesion. The fats are similar to those found in primary degeneration. Regression of the lesion occurs more often when it is related to active inflammation. Penetrating keratoplasty may be required for improvement in visual function.

Several rare disorders deposit lipid in the cornea. These diseases are autosomally inherited and include familial LCAT deficiency, apolipoprotein A-1 deficiency, Tangier disease, and fish eye disease.[8] Because these disorders are inherited, they are not classified as degenerative corneal diseases. In general the deposition is diffuse and occurs in the first few decades of life.

As in primary lipid keratopathy, keratoplasty may be a therapeutic modality. Photodynamic therapy and verteporfin has been used successfully in animal models and human trials for corneal lipid degeneration associated with neovascularization.[19]

Spheroidal degeneration (climatic droplet keratopathy)

Spheroidal degeneration is known by many different names in the literature, including Bietti's nodular corneal degeneration, Labrador keratopathy, climatic droplet keratopathy, degeneratio corneae sphaerularis elaioides, corneal elastosis, fisherman's keratitis, keratinoid corneal degeneration, and chronic actinic keratopathy.[18,20,21] Spheroidal degeneration and climatic droplet keratopathy are the most commonly used terms. Because this entity can affect both the cornea and conjunctiva, we refer to it here as spheroidal degeneration.

Spheroidal degeneration is classified into three basic types. Type 1 occurs bilaterally in the cornea without evidence of other ocular pathology (Fig. 76.3A) Type 2, or secondary spheroidal degeneration, occurs in the cornea in association with other ocular pathology (Fig. 76.3B). Type 3 is the conjunctival form of the degeneration and may occur with types 1 or 2 (Fig. 76.3C). A grading system ranging from trace to grade 4 is also used. Trace implies small numbers of deposits in either one or both eyes with one end of the interpalpebral space affected. The grading is a continuum to grade 4 in which deposits form elevated nodules and reduce vision.

Clinically, clear to yellow-gold spherules are seen in the subepithelium, within Bowman's, or in the superficial

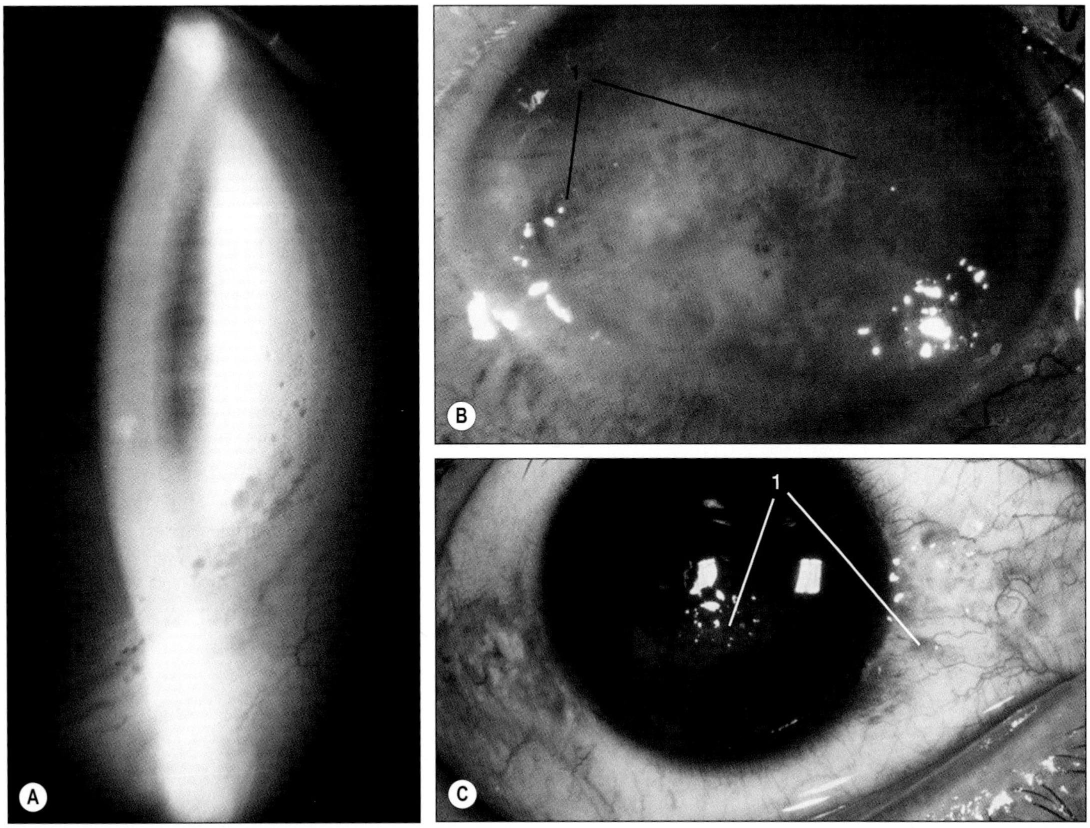

Fig 76.3 (**A**) Spheroidal degeneration, type 1. The degeneration is best seen at the limbus at 8 o'clock in retroillumination. The droplet-like lesions can appear clear or have a yellow tint. (**B**) Spheroidal degeneration (*1*) in a cornea with scarring due to leutic keratitis (type 2). (**C**) Spheroidal degeneration, type 3, demonstrating both corneal and conjunctival elastoid degeneration (*1*).

corneal stroma. They measure from 0.1 to 0.4 mm. In the early stages of type 1, they appear at the limbus in the interpalpebral zone at 3 and 9 o'clock. In type 2 the spherules may be diffuse or begin centrally. The conjunctival form also occurs interpalpebrally in the 3 and 9 o'clock positions. The spherules are generally smaller and less numerous. They sometimes overlay a rectus muscle. Typically they are found in association with pinguecula.[22–24] The spherules may be autofluorescent, and darken with age, progressing from a lighter yellow to a brownish-yellow color.

Etiologies for the primary and conjunctival forms are the same as those for pterygium and pinguecula – ultraviolet radiation and microtrauma including sand, dust, wind, and drying. Studies show a direct correlation between ultraviolet exposure and disease prevalence and severity.[25–27] Primary and conjunctival forms are usually found bilaterally, although unilateral and asymmetric cases have been reported due to exposure differences from such things as unilateral ptosis. These cases have given further credence to ultraviolet radiation as the etiologic factor. Population studies show increased prevalence with advanced age. There is a higher incidence in men, probably because of occupational exposure differences between men and women in these studies.

Secondary degeneration is caused by multiple disease entities. It is associated with corneal neovascularization. A clear interval is observed between the spherules and the neovascularization. Spherules also have been noted in association with herpes keratopathy, glaucoma, and lattice degeneration.[23]

Histopathologically, deposits of hyaline-like material are found in the corneal stroma, Bowman's layer, and subepithelium. Bowman's layer is disrupted, and in advanced cases the epithelium is elevated and thinned. They have a histochemical staining characteristic similar to degenerative connective tissue, such as in pingueculae, but fail to stain for other components found in elastotic material from pingueculae.[28] With continued climatic exposure, corneal deposits coalesce and enlarge, involving the anterior one-third of the stroma and spread across the cornea in a band-shaped distribution.[29] Histochemical analysis demonstrates extracellular deposition of a complex of proteins including tryptophan, cystine, cysteine, and tyrosine. The deposits stain positively for fibrin. Electron microscopy demonstrates abnormal collagen fibers adjacent to the spherules, reminiscent of the elastotic degeneration found in pterygia and pinguecula.

The source of the degenerative material is controversial. It is suggested that the material originates from corneal stroma where it is associated with abnormal collagen. Hanna and Fraunfelder[24] believed the material to be secreted by corneal and conjunctival fibroblasts. The degenerative material is also postulated to be of plasma origin. Experiments have suggested that plasma proteins diffuse into the cornea. These proteins are then precipitated within the superficial cornea after alteration, presumably due to ultraviolet radiation.[24] This may explain the lucent area between the deposits and the limbus or neovascularization. The vasculature may reabsorb the material within this zone faster than it can precipitate.

Another possible pathogenesis of spheroidal degeneration is the deposition of advanced glycation end products (AGEs). AGEs are the end reaction products of sugars and proteins which are closely related to ultraviolet irradiation and the aging process, inducing oxidative stress and molecular damage. There is a similar finding of AGEs in pinguecula, cataracts, and drusen in the retina.[30]

Spheroidal degeneration may be progressive as long as a patient remains exposed to the causative factors. Patients are asymptomatic unless the disease is advanced to the point of decreased vision. Advanced lesions may be nodular and break through the epithelium, causing irritation or foreign body sensation. There is an inherent instability of advanced stage 3 degeneration which may take a relentless downhill course. Cessation of climatic exposure at this stage may have little or no effect. Rapid forming, focal, sterile ulceration may lead to a descemetocele or perforation. The lesions are often hypoesthetic or anesthetic. These areas may also become infected. During the infection, deposits tend to show dissolution in the presence of marked corneal inflammation. End-stage corneal cicatrix with extensive neovascularization and leukoma are not uncommon.[29] Spheroidal degeneration is a major cause of blindness in certain areas of the world including the Dahlak Islands.[18] Treatment is instituted for the symptomatic stage. Dahan et al.[21] have shown regression of the degeneration in patients who have had cataract extraction. The reason for this is unclear; Dahan et al. suggest it is from the aphakic photophobia induced by the surgery.

Conjunctival lesions are directly excised. Lamellar or penetrating keratoplasty is used to treat the corneal form to restore vision. Excimer laser phototherapeutic keratectomy may also be beneficial for treating mild forms of climatic droplet degeneration.[31] The degeneration may recur, as has been seen in conjunctival excision.[32] There is no formal data on recurrence after penetrating keratoplasty.

Climatic proteoglycan stromal keratopathy

Insults from climatic factors such as solar radiation, heat, drying, and microtrauma from snow or sand can produce specific types of corneal degenerations. The most well known is spheroidal climatic keratopathy, which was mentioned previously. In 1995, climatic proteoglycan keratopathy was described. This disorder occurs in the Middle East, predominantly in men (82.7%) with an average age of 64 years. It occurs bilaterally but sometimes asymmetrically. There was no familial pattern discerned. Essential criterion for diagnosis is the clinical presence of a gray, oval or round, ground glass-appearing, stromal corneal opacity that occurs larger anteriorly than posteriorly, and occupies most of the thickness of the corneal stroma. A subset of patients demonstrated prominent discrete white dots at the level of Descemet's membrane. Also, refractile dots or lines were found at any level of the stroma in some patients, which resembled lattice or amyloid degeneration. There may be the presence of other corneal degenerative disorders such as spheroidal keratopathy, band keratopathy, traumatic, and/or postinfectious scars.[33]

Light microscopy demonstrated excess deposits of proteoglycans both intracellularly and extracellularly. Some specimens stained for amyloid. Central corneal thinning and flattening may also be present due to changes in proteoglycan chemistry with resultant changes in corneal hydration.[33]

Amyloid degeneration

The term amyloid applies to a group of proteins that were originally discovered because of starchlike staining characteristics. These serum proteins are found in various body tissues including the eye. Amyloidosis may be local or systemic, and each form may be primary or secondary (Table 76.1). There are familial and nonfamilial forms of primary amyloidosis. Secondary amyloidosis occurs in association with trauma or prolonged inflammatory conditions and is the most common cause of amyloidosis of the cornea.

Histopathologically, amyloid is an amorphous extracellular substance that stains with Congo red and thioflavin T. Congo red-stained amyloid exhibits birefringence in polarized light and dichromism when green light is added. Thioflavin T sections show yellow-green fluorescence of the amyloid deposits.[34] Electron microscopy shows a β-pleated sheet configuration of the protein, which is organized into fibrils.

Systemic amyloidosis rarely has ocular manifestations. Primary amyloidosis of the nonfamilial type typically affects organs such as heart and tongue. This form may be responsible for polyneuropathies and may cause ophthalmoplegia or ptosis.[34] The familial form has been associated with vitreoretinal veils and glaucoma.[5,34] Secondary systemic amyloidosis is the most commonly encountered form. It occurs secondary to chronic diseases including tuberculosis, osteomyelitis, rheumatoid arthritis, syphilis, and leprosy. This form of amyloidosis rarely involves the eye. Amyloid in the form of immunoglobulin can be seen in the cornea and conjunctiva in association with multiple myeloma and paraproteinemia.[35,36]

Eye involvement is most commonly seen in localized amyloidosis. Corneal amyloidosis can occur secondary to local eye disease. Corneal amyloid was thought to be rare until a study by McPherson and Kiffney[37] in 1966 revealed a 3.5% incidence in a review of 200 pathologic specimens. Amyloid has been associated with trauma, retinopathy of prematurity, trachoma, and phlyctenular disease.[37–39] It has been found histologically in a subepithelial nodule or pannus, in deep corneal stroma, or in association with corneal neovascularization.[37]

A primary localized degenerative form of amyloid deposition also affects the cornea. Polymorphic amyloid degeneration (PAD) is seen in patients after age 50.[40,41] This degeneration is characterized by polymorphic punctate or filamentous opacities in the central cornea. Opacities are located throughout the stroma but are typically posterior.[40–43] The lesions appear gray on direct illumination and should not be confused with cornea farinata or the pre-Descemet's dystrophies. When retroilluminated, the lesions appear clear and may look crystalline (Fig. 76.4). Deposits are usually found bilaterally and are asymptomatic. PAD is not associated with any other disease, and no heritability has been demonstrated.[40] In contrast, the lattice dystrophies are typically found in the anterior stroma, may be large and filamentous, cause decreased vision and recurrent erosions, and are inherited and begin early in life. Amyloid degeneration also occurs in association with spheroidal degeneration.[42] These amyloid deposits occur in elderly people without a family history of lattice degeneration. The origin of the corneal deposits is controversial. Fibroblast production, cellular degeneration,[44] or the lack of a serum inhibitory factor[42] may be the source.

Primary localized amyloidosis also may involve the conjunctiva. Conjunctival amyloidosis is a yellow or pinkish mass located in the eyelids or conjunctival fornix. It rarely occurs on the bulbar conjunctiva.[35] Secondary causes should

Table 76.1 Amyloidosis

Type	Protein types	Etiologies	Ocular findings	Systemic findings
Primary localized	AP, AF	None	Lattice dystrophy (I–III) gelatinous drop dystrophy, polymorphic amyloid degeneration, conjunctival amyloid deposits	None, with the exception of type II lattice (Meretoja's syndrome); part of a primary systemic form known as Finnish hereditary amyloidosis, which manifests as facial nerve palsies and peripheral neuropathies
Primary systemic	AP, AF, AL	Familial Nonfamilial	Ophthalmoplegia (orbital and muscle infiltrates), ptosis (nerve infiltrate), vitreous veils, dry eye (lacrimal involvement), pupil abnormalities (neuropathy or direct muscle infiltrate)	Cardiomyopathy, gastrointestinal disease, skin involvement, peripheral neuropathies
Secondary localized	AP	Trauma, retinopathy of prematurity, trachoma, phlyctenulosis	Deposition in cornea, conjunctiva, eyelids	None
Secondary systemic	AP	Chronic inflammation, chronic infection, neoplasms (e.g. rheumatoid arthritis, ulcerative colitis, tuberculosis, syphilis, multiple myeloma, Hodgkin's)	Rare eye involvement usually in the form of immunoglobulin deposits in cornea and conjunctiva	Deposits found in spleen, kidney, liver

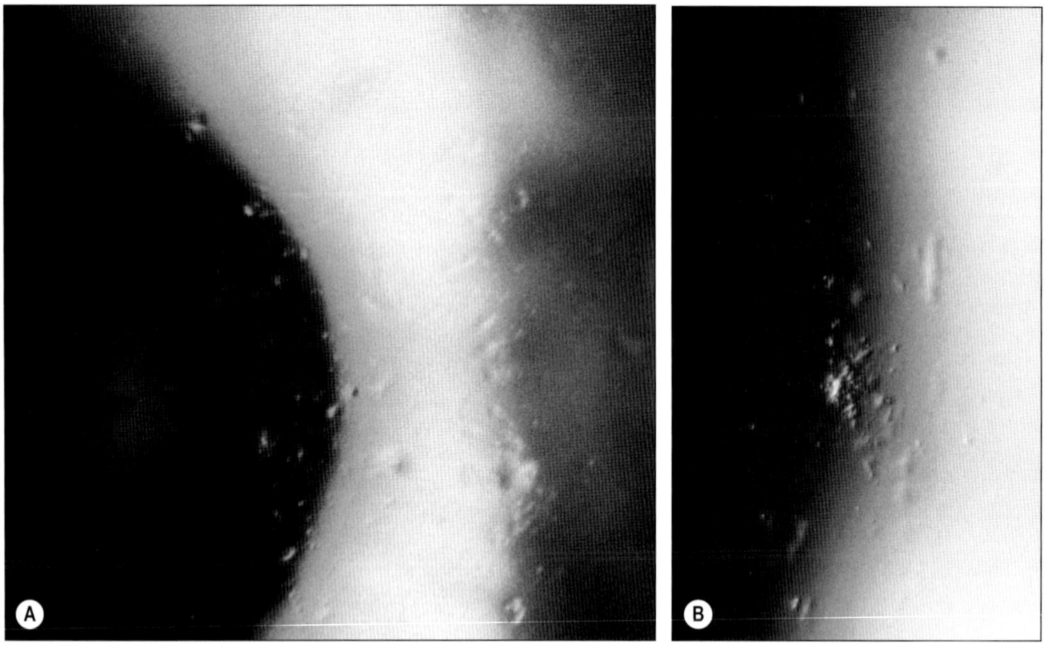

Fig 76.4 (**A**) Polymorphic amyloid degeneration, high magnification. Note that the lesions are best seen with retroillumination off the iris. Lesions are typically deep and central. (**B**) Polymorphic amyloid degeneration, high magnification. The shape of the lesions is typical of amyloid. They often have knoblike excrescenses as well as stellate appendages.

be sought when conjunctival amyloidosis is observed to evaluate for potentially life-threatening illness.

Salzmann's nodular degeneration

Salzmann's nodular degeneration was originally described as a dystrophy in 1925. It has since been defined as a degenerative process that follows episodes of keratitis. It was most commonly associated with a history of phlyctenular disease but was also observed after vernal keratoconjunctivitis, trachoma, measles, scarlet fever, or interstitial keratitis. It is rarely associated with noninflammatory conditions including epithelial basement membrane dystrophy and postoperative corneal surgery.[45,46] The most common setting now seems to be idiopathic or in association with practically any significant corneal inflammatory disease, especially meibomian gland dysfunction (including ocular rosacea) (Fig. 76.5). Some case series show a possible association with contact lens wear, especially in females.[47] Clinically, degenerative lesions appear as yellowish-white to blue elevated nodular lesions. They may be found as single or multiple lesions. Nodules are often annular in location and in the mid periphery. Nodules are often seen adjacent to corneal scarring or a corneal pannus. An iron line may be seen at the edge of the nodules.[48] These lesions are found more often in women than in men[49] and may be either unilateral or bilateral.[49,50] Progression of the lesions is slow. Vascularization may be seen adjacent to, but not as a primary portion of, the lesion.

Histopathologically, dense collagen plaques with hyalinization are located between epithelium and Bowman's layer. Frequently, there is an excessive secretion of basement membrane-like material, Bowman's layer is absent under the lesion, and the overlying epithelium may be atrophic or absent.[45,46]

Salzmann's degeneration is generally asymptomatic. Epithelial erosions may overlie the lesion causing symptoms of lacrimation, photophobia, or irritation. A nodule may also involve the visual axis causing decreased vision. Either of these symptomatic lesions may require treatment. Lubrication can be tried for mildly symptomatic lesions. Superficial keratectomy, by manual dissection or with phototherapeutic keratoablation, may be used for lesions near the visual axis.[51] For lesions extending to the mid stroma, lamellar or penetrating keratoplasty may be necessary. Recurrence is possible after keratoplasty.[49,50] The recurrent lesions are often not clinically similar to the original lesion but are indistinguishable histologically.

Corneal keloids

Keloids of the cornea are rare and may be clinically similar to Salzmann's nodular degeneration. Keloids may occur after trauma or in association with chronic ocular surface inflammation. Corneal keloids have been found in association with Lowe's syndrome[52] and congenitally in Rubinstein-Taybi syndrome.[53] Keloids are rarely found without antecedent ocular disease.[54] Keloids are usually seen in a younger age group than Salzmann's degeneration and occur more frequently in men.[55]

Nodules are white and superficial but may extend deep into the stroma. They may cause irritation or decreased vision. Clinically, they do not retract with time but outgrow their initial boundaries.[56] Treatment should be limited to symptomatic patients. Treatment with superficial keratectomy or penetrating or lamellar keratoplasty may be performed for visually significant lesions. Studies on the incidence of recurrence have not been performed to our knowledge. Topical corticosteroids also have a beneficial effect in terms of limiting progression, but this treatment must be studied further.

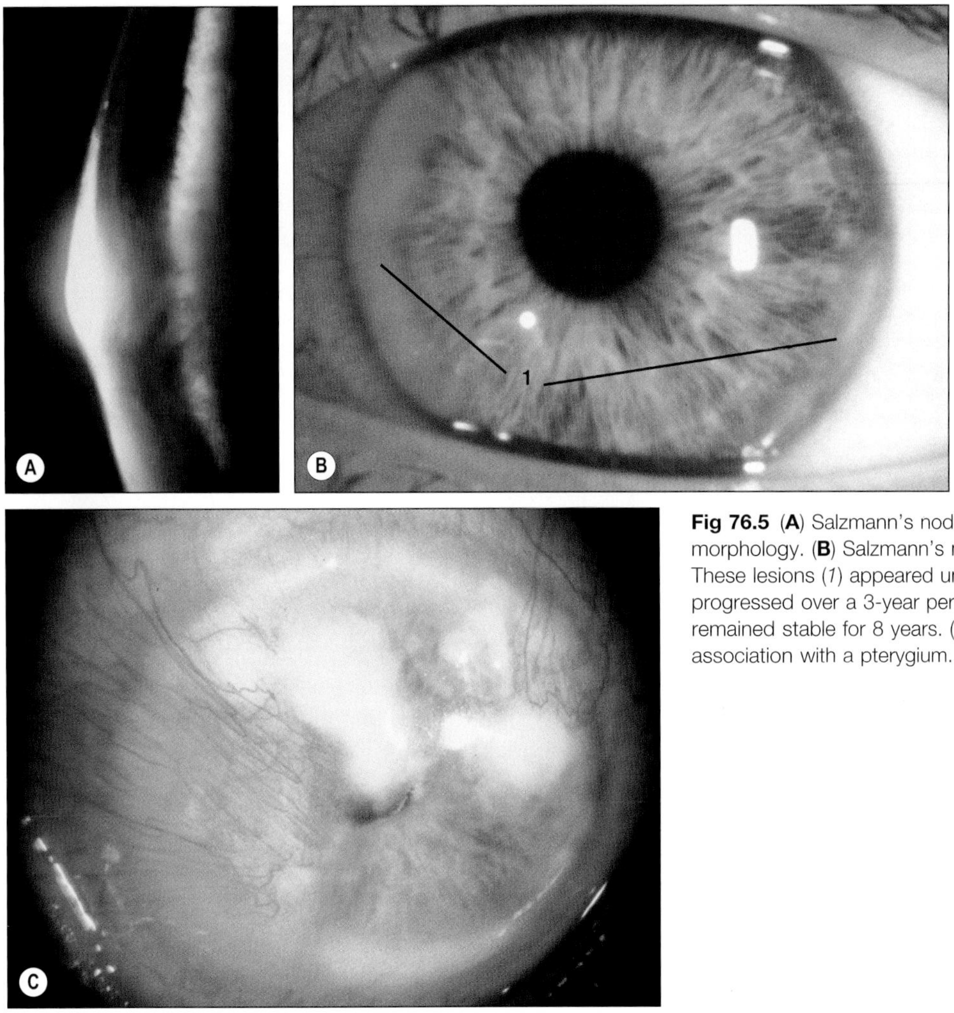

Fig 76.5 (**A**) Salzmann's nodular degeneration, demonstrating its nodular morphology. (**B**) Salzmann's nodular degeneration versus corneal keloid. These lesions (*1*) appeared unilaterally in a 30-year-old woman. They progressed over a 3-year period to the extent pictured here and have remained stable for 8 years. (**C**) Salzmann's nodular degeneration in association with a pterygium.

Histopathologic examination demonstrates fibroblastic proliferation intermixed with hyalinized collagen bundles. Fibroblasts demonstrate myofibroblastic characteristics. Bowman's layer may be fragmented or absent. Histopathologic findings vary according to the stage of the keloid. In the early stages, there is an abundance of type III collagen, myofibroblasts, and new vessel formation. In the late stages, there is haphazardly arranged collagen type I fascicles with little myofibroblasts and involution of blood vessels.[57]

Terrien's marginal corneal degeneration

Terrien's marginal degeneration is a peripheral inflammatory condition often included in the degenerative category. It is a rare disorder of unknown etiology. The condition can be seen at any age[58] but is most common in those between 20 and 40 years of age. Men are affected more than women in a 3:1 ratio.[58] Typically, the disease is bilateral and symmetric, but may be asymmetric, with disease occurring in the second eye decades after the first.[59]

The lesion usually begins superonasally with fine punctate opacities in the anterior stroma with a lucent area to the limbus. Fine superficial vascularization from the limbal arcades leading to the lesion differentiates it from arcus. A gutter similar to marginal furrow degeneration then forms between the opacity and limbus. The stroma progressively thins, usually over many years. The peripheral edge of the gutter gently slopes, whereas the central edge is often steeper. Overlying epithelium remains intact. The gutter becomes more vascularized and wider over time. The lesion may eventually extend circumferentially or centrally.[60] A yellow-white zone of lipid can be seen central to the advancing edge of the gutter (Fig. 76.6).

Two types of Terrien's degeneration have been classified. The more common quiescent type is seen in older patients. These patients may be asymptomatic for a long time because the lesion produces no pain. Inflammatory Terrien's degeneration usually occurs in the younger age groups. These patients may have recurrent episodes of inflammation, episcleritis, or scleritis.[61] This is treated with steroids.

Astigmatism may be produced from the marginal thinning. Typically, the lesion is superior, inducing against-the-rule astigmatism, which may be the presenting symptom. Astigmatism may be treated with glasses or contact lenses.

Histopathologic examination demonstrates fibrillar degeneration of collagen. Epithelium may be normal, thick,

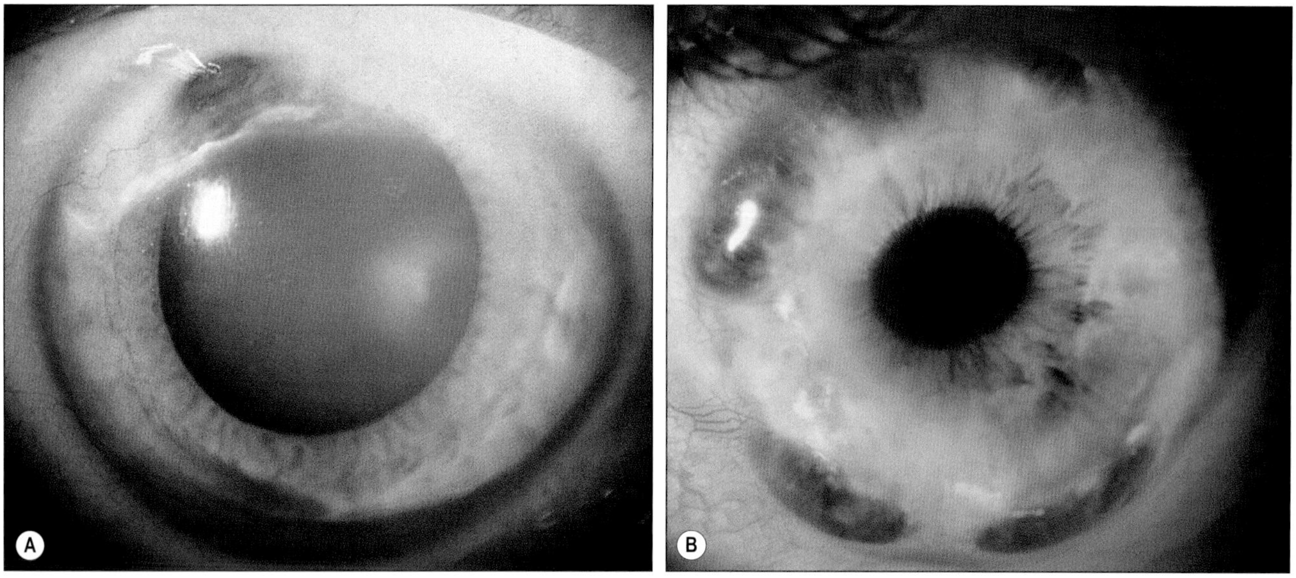

Fig 76.6 (**A**) Terrien's marginal degeneration showing vascularization, lipid deposit centrally, and superior corneal location. (**B**) Terrien's marginal degeneration showing circumferential extension.

or thinned; Bowman's layer is fragmented or absent. Breaks in Descemet's membrane may be seen in thinned areas. When thinning occurs, aqueous pockets occasionally can be seen clinically. Aqueous pockets may even connect to the subepithelial space, causing a filtering bleb and hypotony.[62] Fibrous tissue can be seen repairing Descemet's membrane. Lipid deposition consists of cholesterol crystals. Histiocytes filled with products of collagen phagocytosis also can be seen. Inflammatory cells are sparse, without definite infiltrate. One study has reported a lymphocyte and plasma cell infiltrate, suggesting a relationship between Terrien's degeneration and Mooren's ulcer.[63] Lopez et al.[64] demonstrated a difference in the proportion of B cells, with 5% in Terrien's and 25% in Mooren's. This may represent the difference in the rapidity, activity, and pathogenesis of these two diseases.

A case report has shown Terrien's marginal degeneration with associated posterior polymorphous dystrophy.[65] Another case report has shown an association with a dermatologic disease, erythema elevatum diutinum.[66]

Although there is no treatment to prevent the disease from advancing, progression is slow. Perforation may occur spontaneously or secondary to apparently minor trauma in approximately 15% of patients. Patients may be treated with lamellar or eccentric penetrating grafts in cases of large astigmatism, impending perforation, or perforation.

Limbal girdle (of Vogt)

Vogt described two types of limbal girdle. The girdle is a crescentic yellow-to-white band found in the interpalpebral limbus. It is usually symmetric, occurring in the nasal limbus more frequently than in the temporal.[67] With exposure, the inferior limbus may be involved as well.

Type 1 appears as a white band that may contain holes (Fig. 76.7A). The central border is relatively sharp with no extensions. It is separated from the limbus by a narrow lucent area. Type 1 is generally thought to represent early calcific band keratopathy. Type 2, however, is thought to be a true limbal girdle (Fig. 76.7B). This chalky band has no holes or clear interval to the limbus. Centrally, there are irregular linear extensions.

The incidence of Vogt's limbal girdle increases with age. It has not been found before age 20. The incidence rises to approximately 55% in the 40–60-year age group and 100% in those over 80.[67] Limbal girdle may be seen with direct illumination, but is best seen with a combination of retroillumination and scleral scatter.

Histopathologically, the lesion is subepithelial and may have overlying epithelial atrophy. Destruction and calcification of Bowman's layer have been observed in type 1. Although calcium also has been identified at the level of Bowman's in type 2, the lesion is thought to be in the limbal area peripheral to Bowman's layer. Elastotic degeneration similar to that seen in pinguecula has been found and is discussed later in this chapter. This degeneration is an incidental finding and is asymptomatic. No treatment is required.

Band keratopathy

Band-shaped keratopathy occurs in calcific and noncalcific forms such as in advanced spheroidal degeneration or urate keratopathy. The noncalcific forms are discussed elsewhere. Typically, the term band keratopathy refers to the calcific form of keratopathy.

Calcific band keratopathy, classified as a corneal degeneration, is a deposition across the cornea at the level of Bowman's layer. Band keratopathy is caused by many entities, most commonly with chronic uveitis such as in juvenile rheumatoid arthritis (Fig. 76.8) or in hypercalcemic states such as chronic renal failure (Boxes 76.1 and 76.2).

Clinically, band keratopathy begins at the corneal periphery in the 3 and 9 o'clock positions (Fig. 76.8A). The band may start centrally in cases of chronic ocular inflammation.

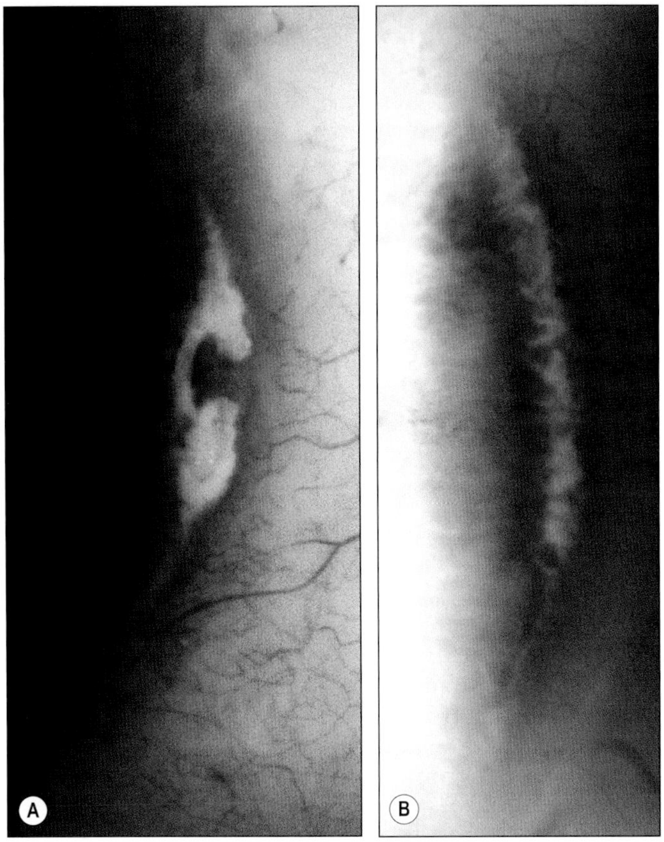

Fig 76.7 (A) Limbal girdle of Vogt, type 1. Note the calcific nature, including clear spaces. (B) Limbal girdle of Vogt, type 2. Note the chalky nature.

The peripheral form has a sharply demarcated peripheral edge separated from the limbus by a lucent zone. This zone is due either to the lack of Bowman's layer at the periphery or from the buffering capacity of the limbal vessels, which prevent precipitation of calcium. The central edge is nondescript and fades into normal cornea. Early, the opacity is gray and later becomes white and chalky. Lucent holes are scattered throughout the opacity and represent penetrating corneal nerves. The lesion is subepithelial but may break through the epithelium in advanced stages. A complete band from limbus to limbus may form in later stages.

Histopathologically, fine basophilic granules are first seen at the level of Bowman's layer. The granules later coalesce.[68] These fragment Bowman's layer and replace the superficial stroma. Hyaline-like material is deposited in subepithelial tissue around the calcific depositions, giving the appearance of reduplication of Bowman's layer. A fibrous pannus, associated with the calcification, also separates epithelium and Bowman's layer. The overlying epithelium may be atrophic.

Box 76.1 General causes of band keratopathy

- Hypercalcemic states
- Chronic ocular disease
- Chemicals (eye drops and irritants)
- Inherited diseases
- Systemic diseases
- Idiopathic

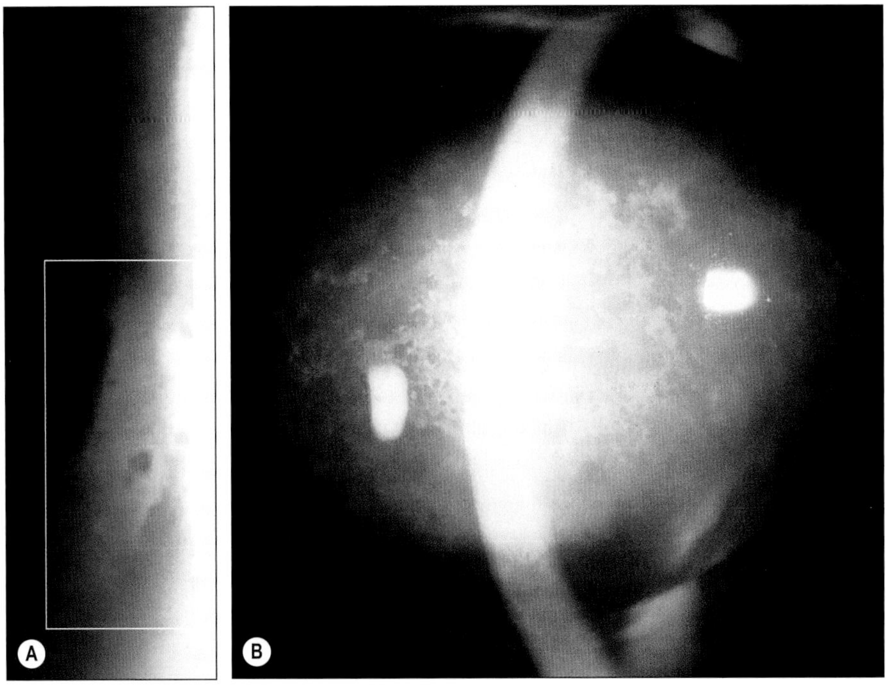

Fig 76.8 (**A**) Calcific band keratopathy (*box*) in a patient with juvenile rheumatoid arthritis. (**B**) Calcific degeneration in an eye with long-standing leutic interstitial keratitis

Box 76.2 Diseases associated with band keratopathy

Congenital hereditary endothelial dystrophy[117]	Nephropathic cystinosis[118]
Chronic uveitis	Norrie's disease
Discoid lupus	Paget's disease
Dry eye syndromes	Phthisis
Fanconi's disease	Prolonged corneal edema
Hyperparathyroid states	Prolonged glaucoma
Hyperphosphatasia	Proteus syndrome[119]
Hypophosphatasia	Sarcoidosis
Ichthyosis	Spheroid degeneration
Interstitial keratitis	Still's disease
Intraocular silicone oil	Thiazides
Lithium	Trachoma
Mercury	Tuberous sclerosis
Metastatic carcinoma to bone	Tumoral calcinosis[120]
Milk-alkali syndrome (Albright-Burnett)	Uremia
Multiple myeloma	Viscoelastics
	Vitamin D toxicity

Calcium deposits are intracellular when associated with hypercalcemia and can be found both intranuclearly and intracytoplasmically on histologic examination.[68,69] The deposits may be found extracellularly when they occur with local disease or renal failure. Conjunctival deposits of calcium may also be found when associated with hypercalcemia. Calcium is deposited in the form of hydroxyapatite, a phosphate salt.

Physiologically, the cause of calcium salt precipitation is speculative. Theories include an alteration of corneal metabolism that causes increased tissue pH and precipitation of calcium, evaporation of the tears because of exposure of the interpalpebral zone, which causes calcium precipitation, or carbon dioxide release and subsequent rise in pH.

Experimentally, Doughman et al.[70] found that band keratopathy did not occur in laboratory animals with induced ocular inflammation and vitamin D overdose unless the lids were kept open. In other case reports band keratopathy occurred in one eye of a patient with chronic renal failure, uveitis, and hypercalcemia, but not in the other eye wearing an aphakic contact lens. It has been proposed that the lack of evaporation in the eye with the contact lens prevented the precipitation of calcium.[71]

These lesions progress slowly over months to years. In patients with dry eye, however, the calcium deposition has been reported to occur over weeks.[72] In most cases, the associated disease causing the band keratopathy is known (Fig. 76.8B). In those patients who present with band keratopathy of unknown etiology, possible systemic causes should be investigated. After obtaining a history and ocular examination, a medical work-up should include serum calcium, phosphorus, uric acid, and renal function measurements. If hyperparathyroidism or sarcoid is suspected, parathyroid hormone (PTH) and angiotensin-converting enzyme (ACE) levels also can be obtained. Patients should be questioned about their supplemental vitamin and calcium intake. In patients who have band keratopathy secondary to hypercalcemia, incomplete regression has been observed when the calcium levels are normalized.[73]

Early stages of band keratopathy are asymptomatic. Later stages can be symptomatic with decreasing vision, foreign body sensation, tearing, or photophobia. When the patient becomes symptomatic, the mainstay of treatment is the application of ethylenediaminetetraacetic acid (EDTA).[74,75] Epithelium is removed after instillation of topical anesthetic since EDTA will not penetrate the epithelium. EDTA is then applied to the calcific areas, in 0.05 molar concentration on saturated cellulose sponges. A diamond burr or No. 15 blade is used to remove any residual calcium and to produce a smooth corneal surface.[74,75] Band keratopathy has been treated successfully using excimer laser phototherapeutic keratectomy.[76–79] The excimer laser has been used to clear the visual axis and improve vision. Laser therapy may be performed directly on smooth band keratopathy. Rough surface keratopathy requires scalpel removal of large plaques and a masking fluid to ablate tissue and leave a smooth surface.[76–79] Amniotic membrane has been used after the primary surgical removal of band keratopathy to quickly restore a stable ocular surface.[80]

Calcareous degeneration

Calcareous degeneration of the cornea is a second type of calcific degeneration. Like band keratopathy, this degeneration occurs in diseased eyes. Unlike band keratopathy, calcareous degeneration involves the posterior stroma. Calcium deposition may be full corneal thickness or may spare Bowman's layer and corneal epithelium. This degeneration is seen in phthisis bulbi, necrotic intraocular neoplasm, multiple ocular surgeries, extensive trauma, and other conditions in which bone is formed in the eye. In eyes with persistent epithelial defects and inflamed stroma, this form of calcification may form rapidly.[81] It also has been reported in a failed corneal graft.[82]

Reticular degeneration of Koby

This is a very rare degenerative disorder whose existence can be disputed. Koby's degeneration consists of a fine white reticulum at the level of Bowman's layer. Overlying epithelium may have a brownish discoloration. This degeneration is most commonly reported in patients with chronic inflammation.

Perry and Scheie[83] and Perry et al.[84] have demonstrated the white reticulum consisting of calcium. The brown reticulated epithelial pattern stained positively for iron. They concluded that this degeneration is an atypical form of band keratopathy. It is usually painless but may lead to decreased vision. They reported a patient who responded well to treatment with EDTA.

Iron lines

Iron, seen as a faint yellow to dark-brown discoloration in the corneal epithelium, is found in many corneal condi-

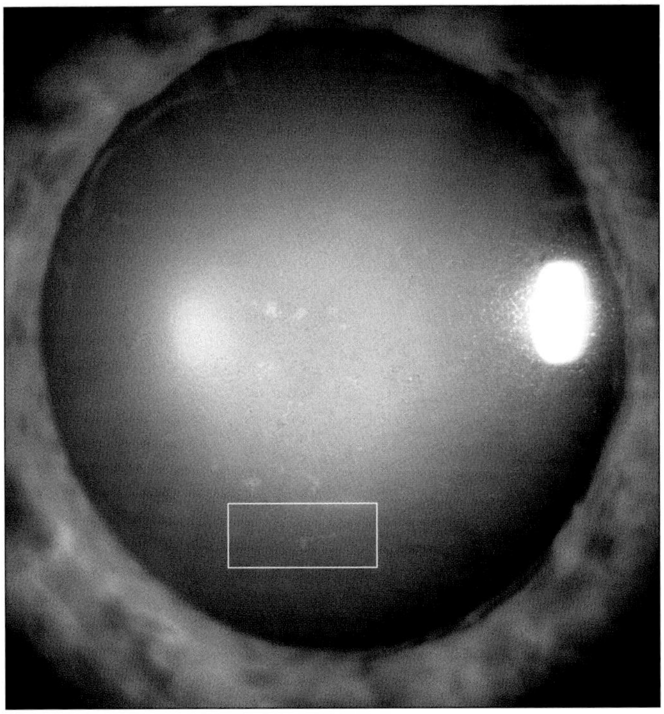

Fig 76.9 Hudson-Stähli line (*box*).

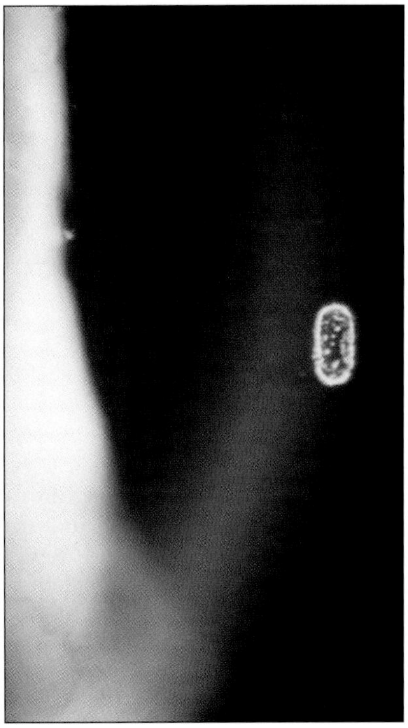

Fig 76.10 Coats' white ring.

tions. Eponyms have been given to some specific iron lines. The most common iron line is the Hudson-Stähli line, which is located in the lower third of the cornea (Fig. 76.9) The line usually runs horizontally, higher nasally and lower temporally. The line may be distinct or may be broad (1–2 mm) and faint, giving rise to a Hudson-Stähli zone, as termed by Rose and Lavin.[85] The end of the line may be split into multiple small dots or lines. Hudson-Stähli lines may be altered by various factors including corneal scars and contact lens wear. The line may be displaced and broadened by either of these factors.[86,87] Hudson-Stähli lines increase in length and density with time. Typically, it is bilateral and symmetric. Studies have shown a unilateral incidence from 4% to 30%. However, faint asymmetric lines may have been missed. Hudson-Stähli lines are seen in individuals as young as 2 years of age.[88] The incidence increases with age up to 70 years. After the age of 70, the incidence decreases for reasons that are unclear. Norn found the overall incidence to be lower in 1988 than 1968 for uncertain reasons.[89]

Iron deposition associated with a filtering bleb after glaucoma surgery was described by Ferry in 1968.[90] It appears on the cornea just anterior to the filtering bleb. He related its incidence to the size of the filtering bleb. Iron may be seen at the advancing edge of a pterygium (Stocker's line) and at the base of the cone in keratoconus (Fleischer ring).

Iron lines have been described after a wide range of refractive corneal procedures, including epikeratophakia, penetrating keratoplasty, keratophakia, keratomileusis, radial keratotomy, excimer photorefractive keratectomy, placement of intrastromal corneal rings, and LASIK.[91] There are also case reports of iron lines forming after orthokeratology.[92] The iron line is found adjacent to the corneal irregularity. Thus, a stellate pattern has been described in relation to radial keratotomy[93] and a semicircular or complete ring of pigmentation associated with penetrating keratoplasty, epikeratophakia, and keratomileusis.[94,95] Irregular iron deposition has been noted with corneal scars.[88]

Histologically, iron, predominantly ferritin, is found intracellularly and extracellularly in the basal epithelial layer of the cornea, regardless of the type of iron line. The source and etiology of the iron have been very controversial. The source has been attributed to the tears, aqueous humor, cellular breakdown, blood breakdown, or blood plasma. Iron is most often deposited in relation to some corneal irregularity, such as a pterygium, filtering bleb, scar, or postsurgical change in the corneal contour. This distribution has led to the various etiologic theories to explain both the source of the iron and why it is only deposited in the basal epithelial layer. The most common theory attributes the deposition to localized trauma at the site of contour change or to a pooling of tears at this site.[88,90,94,95] Another theory relates to epithelial migration and attrition.[87] Convincing arguments have been given for each theory, but the precise etiology remains unclear.

Clinically, iron lines can be seen with direct illumination with a broad white light on slit lamp examination. Fainter lines may be difficult to see and may be made visible with the use of the cobalt blue light on the slit lamp. Iron lines are visually insignificant but may be important surgical landmarks as in keratoconus. No treatment is necessary.

Coats' white ring

Coats first described white rings of the cornea that are usually 1 mm or less in diameter. The rings are located in the inferior portion of the cornea. The ring may be oval and incomplete. Discrete white dots may be seen with areas of coalescence (Fig. 76.10). Lesions are seen at the level of

Bowman's layer or superficial stroma. Epithelium remains intact.

Coats originally thought the lesions were congenital. Histopathologic study has supported their traumatic origin.[96] Histochemical analysis has revealed iron within the lesion, which likely represents an old metallic foreign body. Miller also presented a series of cases in limestone workers, suggesting that injuries with calcium carbonate were the source of the rings.[97] A history of trauma may be difficult to elicit. These lesions represent an incidental finding and are asymptomatic.

Hassall-Henle bodies

Hassall-Henle bodies or Descemet's warts are excrescences of Descemet's membrane found in the peripheral cornea. They are one of the most common aging changes. Descemet's membrane thickens progressively throughout life. Nodular areas of thickening in the periphery extend into the anterior chamber. Excrescences are best seen on specular reflection and appear as dark, round holes in the specular reflection. Histopathologically, they are identical to guttae in the central cornea that are associated with Fuchs' dystrophy.[98]

Crocodile shagreen

A corneal mosaic pattern resembling cobblestone or crocodile skin is seen in the anterior or posterior cornea. Crocodile shagreen is usually bilateral. Both anterior and posterior forms appear clinically as polygonal gray to white 'cracked ice' opacities with central lucent zones (Fig. 76.11).

Histopathologically, the stroma is thrown into folds, either at Bowman's layer in the anterior form or around Descemet's membrane in the posterior form. The sawtooth pattern of irregularly arranged collagen corresponds with the grayish opacity. Calcium may be deposited at the peaks of the sawtooth in anterior shagreen. Fibrous plaques have been seen around Bowman's layer, releasing tension. This pattern is thought to be due to this relaxation of tension. The collagen is thrown into sawtooth folds in the posterior form as well.[99]

The anterior form of this degeneration may be seen as a senile change. The anterior mosaic also has been described in keratoconus patients with hard contact lenses.[100] It also has been associated with trauma, band keratopathy, hypotony, and juvenile X-linked megalocornea. A similar pattern is seen with instillation of fluorescein after pressure is applied to the cornea through the lids.

The posterior form has been described solely as an age-related degeneration. Clinically, it appears similar to central cloudy dystrophy of François, which has an autosomal dominant inheritance pattern.[99,101] The shagreen is most often found to be bilateral and central. A similar age-related change can be found occasionally in the peripheral cornea, resembling corneal arcus. Generally, the opacity is visually insignificant and requires no treatment.

Senile furrow

This rare degeneration is seen in elderly patients. Peripheral thinning is seen in the avascular zone between arcus senilis and the limbal vascular arcades. The thinning may be an illusion caused by the arcus senilis. True thinning also can occur (Fig. 76.12). The thinning is usually shallow and of no visual significance. These lesions are not known to vascularize or perforate. As they are asymptomatic, no treatment is required.

Cornea farinata

Cornea farinata is an asymptomatic degenerative condition characterized by tiny opacities, found bilaterally in the pos-

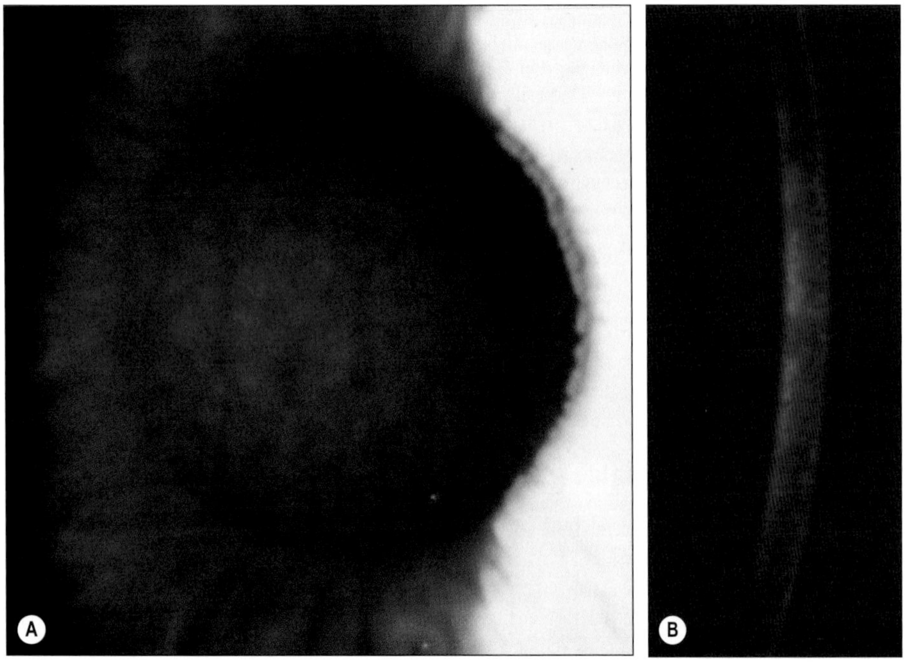

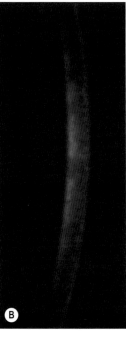

Fig 76.11 (**A**) Posterior crocodile shagreen showing polygonal morphology and central location. (**B**) Posterior crocodile shagreen showing posterior location.

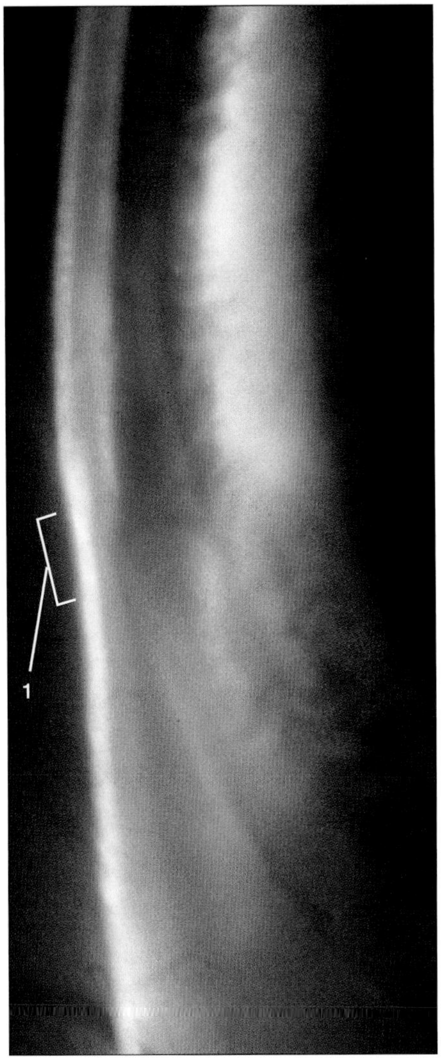

Fig 76.12 Furrow degeneration shows peripheral thinning (*1*).

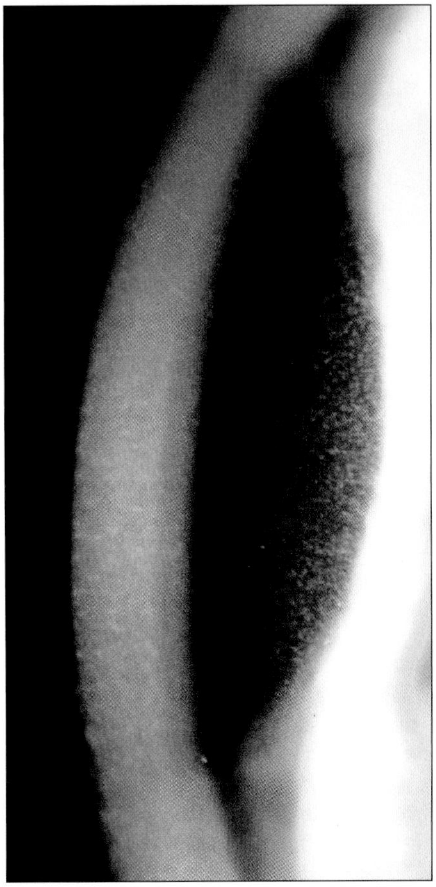

Fig 76.13 Cornea farinata, best seen by indirect illumination. The lesions are pre-Descemet's and are similar to those of pre-Descemet's dystrophy and X-linked ichthyosis.

terior stroma near Descemet's membrane. These opacities are best seen on retroillumination and are gray-brown to white; hence it has been called a 'flour dust' appearance (Fig. 76.13). They do not interfere with vision. The condition may be inherited.[102,103] In general, the opacities associated with the pre-Descemet's dystropy are larger and more pleomorphic than in cornea farinata. Pre-Descemet's opacities may also occur with X-linked ichthyosis, keratoconus, and in PAD. Histopathologically, vacuoles filled with a lipofuscin-like substance have been found in the posterior stromal keratocytes.

Dellen

Dellen or Fuchs' dimples may occur as an age-related change or secondary to other ocular abnormalities. Dellen may last only 24 to 48 hours and are found most commonly in the temporal peripheral cornea, usually adjacent to a paralimbal elevation.

Clinically, dellen are saucer-like depressions in the corneal surface. Although they may be idiopathic, they are more commonly adjacent to elevated areas. Dellen may be found after cataract extraction near areas of conjunctival chemosis or after strabismus or glaucoma filtering surgery. They also may occur adjacent to areas of conjunctival swelling from episcleritis, conjunctivitis, pingueculae, or pterygia. Anesthetics, specifically cocaine use, may cause dellen. They also may be associated with lagophthalmos.

Histopathologically, thinning of the corneal epithelium, Bowman's layer, and anterior stroma is seen. Treatment with ocular lubricants or pressure patching will accelerate the healing process.

Conjunctival Degenerations

The conjunctiva becomes thinner and more fragile with age. Varicosities or microaneurysms of the conjunctival blood vessels may be observed. These degenerative findings are not typically classified and are frequently overlooked, as they are not clinically significant.

Pingueculae

Pingueculae are elevated masses on the conjunctiva, gray-white to yellow in color (Fig. 76.14). They are found in the interpalpebral zone, paralimbal, in the 3 and 9 o'clock posi-

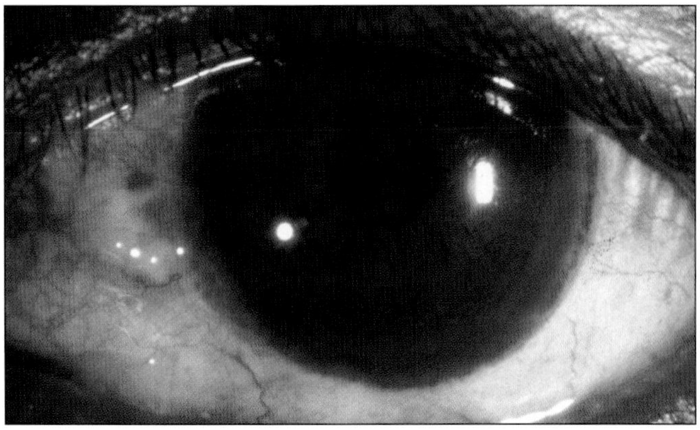

Fig 76.14 Pinguecula, seen in the typical limbal palpebral fissure location.

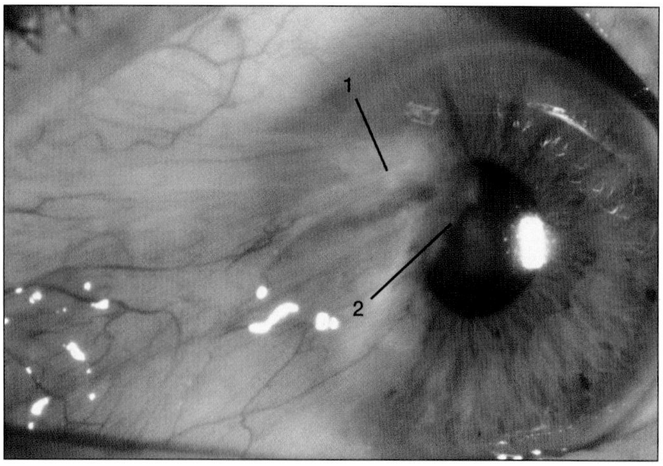

Fig 76.15 Pterygium. Note the fibrovascular component (*1*) and avascular fibrotic leading edge (*2*). This lesion is inactive.

tions. Pingueculae are usually bilateral and are more often found nasally than temporally.[104]

Histopathologically, they may have normal, atrophic, or hyperkeratotic conjunctival epithelium. The substantia propria shows basophilic degeneration on hematoxylin and eosin staining. This material stains for elastin but is not broken down by elastase. Thus it is termed elastotic degeneration.

The cause of a pinguecula is believed to be actinic in origin, similar to skin damage, specifically damage from ultraviolet radiation. There may be a relationship with advanced glycation end products, as mentioned previously under spheroidal degeneration, which is found in UV irradiation and age-related processes.[105] The reason for the nasal predominance is unclear. One theory suggests that more actinic damage occurs in this area because of reflection from the side of the nose.[106] Other possible causes of pingueculae include trauma, wind, sand, or drying that do not account for the nasal predominance.

The masses typically encroach on the corneal limbus. Once they cross the limbus, the term *pterygium* is applied. There is controversy, however, as to their relationship and the actual progression of a pinguecula to a pterygium.

The prevalence of pingueculae increases with age because they are found in virtually all persons in their 80s. These lesions are usually clinically insignificant. They rarely become inflamed and cause irritation. If symptomatic, pingueculitis can be treated with lubricants, topical corticosteroids, or topical NSAIDs.[107] Pingueculae also may be treated by excision, although this is rarely necessary and is usually for cosmetic reasons.

Gaucher's disease can be associated with a pinguecula that is brownish in color. Dyskeratosis or even tumors of the overlying epithelium may occur. These should be differentiated on examination by the epithelial location of the tumors from the subepithelial location of pinguecula.

Pterygium

A pterygium is a winglike mass of fibrovascular tissue extending from the conjunctiva to the cornea. This lesion is highly vascular, as opposed to pingueculae. Pterygia may arise from pingueculae and are histologically similar. The masses are located in the interpalpebral fissure in the horizontal meridian (Fig. 76.15).

Histopathologically, pterygia show changes similar to those of pingueculae. Epithelium may be normal, acanthotic, hyperkeratotic, or even dysplastic. Impression cytology of surface cells directly overlying pterygium is abnormal, demonstrating increased goblet cell density with squamous metaplasia. There was also shown to be abnormal surface cytology of other areas of the bulbar conjunctiva in areas without clinical evidence of pterygium.[108] The substantia propria shows elastotic degeneration of collagen as defined by Austin et al.[109] as elastodysplasia and elastodystrophy. Collagen being produced undergoes abnormal maturation and degeneration. The source of the fibers is thought to be from damaged fibroblasts. Pterygia have three distinct parts. The cap or leading edge is a flat, gray zone on the cornea consisting mainly of fibroblasts. This area invades and destroys Bowman's layer. An iron line (Stocker's line) may be seen anterior to the cap. There also may be areas of corneal drying or even a dellen anterior to the cap. Immediately behind the cap is a whitish, thickened vascular area firmly attached to the cornea, referred to as the head. The body or tail is the fleshy, mobile, vascular area of bulbar conjunctiva, which has distinct edges. This body becomes an important landmark for surgical correction.

Studies have shown an increased prevalence of pterygium as one approaches the equator. They are found more commonly in men than women and in people who work outdoors. The prevalence also increases with age. The incidence of pterygia is greatest in the 20–40 age group.[96,110] One study revealed the highest incidence in people 15 to 25 years of age, in equal male:female ratios, in the Virgin Islands.[96] The Barbados Eye Study recently revealed one-quarter of the black participants had a pterygium, a frequency 2.5 times higher than the white participants. It also showed that pterygium was twice as frequent in people who worked outdoors but was only one-fifth as likely in people who always wore sunglasses.[111]

Pterygium is found more commonly nasally than temporally. There has been much debate about its etiology. It is thought that ultraviolet irradiation is the primary factor. Population studies of pterygium, pinguecula, and spheroidal degeneration have shown a positive relationship between increased ultraviolet exposure and increased prevalence of pinguecula and spheroidal degeneration. These studies, however, did not show a direct relationship to pterygia. There have been theories of microtrauma induced by sand, dust, wind, or drying. Most likely, its occurrence is multifactorial and may include hereditary susceptibility. The cause of the nasal predominance is unclear but has been ascribed to increased ultraviolet damage in this area. One theory suggests reflection of the ultraviolet light off the side of the nose. Coroneo[112] postulates that the cornea itself acts like a side-on lens to focus ultraviolet light into this area. A newer theory postulates that pterygia have some tumor-like features. These characteristics include recurrence following resection, ultraviolet radiation exposure as an etiology, and common treatment modalities (radiation, antimetabolites). The *p53* gene, which is a marker for neoplasia and is known to control cell differentiation, cell cycle, and apoptosis, has been found in the epithelium of pterygium. This raises the possibility that pterygium may be a growth disorder due to uncontrolled cell proliferation rather than a degenerative disorder.[113]

A true pterygium grows across the limbus and destroys Bowman's layer. A recent study demonstrated immunohistochemically the presence of six different matrix metalloproteinases in the pterygium cells invading the cornea. These are probably responsible for the dissolution of Bowman's layer.[114]

A true pterygium must be differentiated from a pseudopterygium, which may occur after trauma. Pseudopterygium has been reported secondary to inflammatory corneal disease. A probe may be passed at the limbus under a pseudopterygium. Further distinction can be made, since pseudopterygia may be found anywhere on the cornea and are usually found obliquely, whereas true pterygia are horizontal in the 3 or 9 o'clock positions.

Pterygium can be seen in various forms on a continuum. Pterygia can be quiescent with little vascularity and no observed growth. They can be active with hyperemia and fairly rapid growth. Patients may be asymptomatic. Most often, the patient presents for evaluation, either worried about the cosmetic appearance or symptomatic with redness, irritation, or visual change. Symptoms may include irritation, foreign body sensation, or photophobia. Decreased vision can occur as the pterygium crosses the visual axis or creates increased astigmatism. A tethering effect may be created by large lesions causing diplopia, most commonly in lateral gaze. This effect will occur more often in recurrent lesions with scar tissue formation.

Many forms of treatment have been advocated for pterygium. The various methods are mentioned here, but the surgical details are discussed elsewhere. In general, primary pterygia are treated more conservatively. A small atrophic pterygium may be observed periodically. Lubricating solutions may be used for irritation. Active pterygia may be treated initially with vasoconstrictors, nonsteroidal antiinflammatory agents, or steroid drops. These may be used alone or before surgical excision. (The surgical management of pterygium is discussed in detail in Chapter 144.)

Concretions

Concretions are white to yellow spots found on the palpebral conjunctiva occasionally encased in clear cysts. They may be found in elderly persons or secondary to inflammation. Most commonly this degeneration is seen in later stages of trachoma. Studies have shown the concurrence of Herbert's pits and conjunctival concretions of the superior tarsus in trachoma.[115]

These concretions contain an amorphous material composed of mucopolysaccharide and mucin. Degenerated organelles and epithelial cell nuclei also have been identified. It is hypothesized that chronic inflammation causes hyperplasia and invagination of the conjunctival epithelium. This new pseudogland may become clogged. If it ruptures into the substantia propria, an inflammatory reaction may ensue.[116]

The degenerated material (concretion) may be found on routine examination. They may come to the surface and cause a foreign body sensation. They may be easily removed for patient comfort.

References

1. Deluise VP. Peripheral corneal degenerations and tumors. *Int Ophthalmol Clin*. 1988;26:49–62.
2. Donaldson DD. Corneal degeneration. *Ann Ophthalmol*. 1973;5:561–565.
3. Duke-Elder S, Leigh AG. System of ophthalmology. In: *Diseases of the outer eye*. Vol 8. St Louis: Mosby; 1965.
4. Friedlaender MH, Smolin G. Corneal degenerations. *Ann Ophthalmol*. 1979;11:1485–1495.
5. Sugar A. Corneal and conjunctival degenerations. In: Kaufman HE, et al, eds. *The cornea*. New York: Churchill Livingstone; 1988.
6. Townsend WM. Pterygium. In: Kaufman HE, et al, eds. *The cornea*. New York: Churchill Livingstone; 1988.
7. François J, Feher J. Arcus senilis. *Docu Ophthalmol*. 1973;34:165–182.
8. Rifkind BM. Corneal arcus and hyperlipoproteinemia. *Surv Ophthalmol*. 1972;16:295–304.
9. Andrews JS. The lipids of arcus senilis. *Arch Ophthalmol*. 1962;68:264.
10. Cogan DG, Kuwabara T. Arcus senilis: its pathology and histochemistry. *Arch Ophthalmol*. 1959;61:553–560.
11. Gaynor PM, Zhang W, Salehizadeh B, et al. Cholesterol accumulation in human cornea: evidence that extracellular cholesterol ester-rich lipid particles deposit independently of foam cells. *J Lipid Res*. 1996;37:1849–1861.
12. Walton KW. Studies on the pathogenesis of corneal arcus formation: the human corneal arcus and its relation to atherosclerosis as studied by immunofluorescence. *J Pathol*. 1973;111:263–274.
13. Barchiesi BJ, Eckel RH, Ellis PP. The cornea and disorders of lipid metabolism. *Surv Ophthalmol*. 1991;36:1–22.
14. Smith JL, Susac JO. Unilateral arcus senilis: sign of occlusive disease of the carotid artery. *JAMA*. 1973;225:676.
15. Cooke NT. Significance of arcus senilis in Caucasians. *J R Soc Med*. 1981;74:201–204.
16. Crispin S. Ocular lipid deposition and hyperlipoproteinaemia. *Prog Retin Eye Res*. 2002;21:169–224.
17. Savino DF, Fine BS, Alldredge Jr OC. Primary lipidic degeneration of the cornea. *Cornea*. 1986;5:191–198.
18. Rodgers FC. Clinical findings, course, and progress of Bietti's corneal degeneration in the Dahlak Islands. *Br J Ophthalmol*. 1973;57:657–664.
19. Brooks BJ, Ambati BK, Marcus DM, et al. Photodynamic therapy for corneal neovascularization and lipid degeneration. *Br J Ophthalmol*. 2004;88(6):840.
20. Young JD, Finlay RD. Primary spheroidal degeneration of the cornea in Labrador and northern Newfoundland. *Am J Ophthalmol*. 1975;79:129–134.
21. Dahan E, Judellson J, Welsh NH. Regression of Labrador keratopathy following cataract extraction. *Br J Ophthalmol*. 1986;70:737–741.

22. Sullivan WR. Bilateral central lipid infiltrates of the cornea. *Am J Ophthalmol.* 1977;84:781–787.
23. Fraunfelder FT, Hanna C, Parker JM. Spheroid degeneration of the cornea and conjunctiva. *Am J Ophthalmol.* 1972;74:821–828.
24. Hanna C, Fraunfelder FT. Spheroid degeneration of the cornea and conjunctiva. *Am J Ophthalmol.* 1972;74:829–839.
25. Norn M, Franck C. Long-term changes in the outer part of the eye in welders. Prevalence of spheroid degeneration, pinguecula, pterygium, and corneal cicatrices. *Acta Ophthalmol (Copenh).* 1991;69:382–386.
26. Norn M. Spheroid degeneration, keratopathy, pinguecula, and pterygium in Japan (Kyoto). *Acta Ophthalmol (Copenh).* 1984;62:54–60.
27. Norn MS. Spheroid degeneration, pinguecula, and pterygium among Arabs in the Red Sea territory, Jordan. *Acta Ophthalmol (Copenh).* 1982;60(6):949–954.
28. Gray RH, Johnson GJ, Freedman A. Climatic droplet keratopathy. *Surv Ophthalmol.* 1992;36(4):241–253.
29. Ormerod LD, Dahan E, Hagele JE, et al. Serious occurrences in the natural history of advanced climatic keratopathy. *Ophthalmology.* 1994;101(3):448–453.
30. Kaji Y, Nagai R, Amano S, et al. Advanced glycation end product deposits in climatic droplet keratopathy. *Br J Ophthalmol.* 2007;91:85–88.
31. Ayres BD, Rapuano CJ. Excimer laser phototherapeutic keratectomy. *Ocul Surf.* 2006;4(4):196–206.
32. Norn MS. Conjunctival spheroid degeneration. *Acta Ophthalmol (Copenh).* 1982;60:434–438.
33. Waring GO, Malaty A, Grossniklaus H, et al. Climatic proteoglycan stromal keratopathy: a new corneal degeneration. *Am J Ophthalmology.* 1995;120:330–341.
34. Blodi FC, Apple DJ. Localized conjunctival amyloidosis. *Am J Ophthalmol.* 1979;88:346–350.
35. Gorevic PD, et al. Lack of evidence for protein AA reactivity in amyloid deposits of lattice corneal dystrophy and amyloid corneal degeneration. *Am J Ophthalmol.* 1984;98:216–224.
36. D'Amico DJ, Kenyon KR, Ruskin JN. Amiodarone keratopathy: drug-induced lipid storage disease. *Arch Ophthalmol.* 1981;99:257–261.
37. McPherson SD, Kiffney GT. Corneal amyloidosis. *Am J Ophthalmol.* 1966;62:1025–1033.
38. Collyer RT. Amyloidosis of the cornea. *Can J Ophthalmol.* 1968; 3:35–38.
39. Garner A. Amyloidosis of the cornea. *Br J Ophthalmol.* 1969;53:73–81.
40. Mannis MJ, Krachmer JH, Rodrigues MM, Pardos GJ. Polymorphic amyloid degeneration of the cornea: a histopathologic study. *Arch Ophthalmol.* 1981;99:1217–1223.
41. Nirankari V, Rodrigues MM, Rajagopalan S, Brown D. Polymorphic amyloid degeneration. *Arch Ophthalmol.* 1989;107:598.
42. Matta CS, et al. Climatic droplet keratopathy with corneal amyloidosis. *Ophthalmology.* 1991;98:192–195.
43. Krachmer JH, Dubord PJ, Rodrigues MM, Mannis MJ. Corneal posterior crocodile shagreen and polymorphic amyloid degeneration. *Arch Ophthalmol.* 1983;101:54–59.
44. Takahashi T, Kondo T, Isobe T, Okada S. A case of corneal amyloidosis. *Acta Ophthalmol (Copenh).* 1983;61:150–156.
45. Wood TO. Salzmann's nodular degeneration. *Cornea.* 1990;9:17–22.
46. Werner LP, Issis K, Werner LP, et al. Salzmann's corneal degeneration associated with epithelial basement membrane dystrophy. *Cornea.* 2000;19(1):121–123.
47. Farjo AA, Halperin GI, Syed N, et al. Salzmann's nodular corneal degeneration clinical characteristics and surgical outcomes. *Cornea.* 2006;25(1):11–15.
48. Farjo AA, Halperin GI, Syed N, et al. Salzmann's nodular corneal degeneration clinical characteristics and surgical outcomes. *Cornea.* 2006;25(1):11–15.
49. Severin M, Kirchhof B. Recurrent Salzmann's corneal degeneration. *Graefe's Arch Clin Exp Ophthalmol.* 1990;228:101–104.
50. Vannas A, Hogan MJ, Wood I. Saltzmann's nodular degeneration of the cornea. *Am J Ophthalmol.* 1975;79:211–219.
51. Das S, Link B, Seitz B. Salzmann's nodular degeneration of the cornea. *Cornea.* 2005;24:772–777.
52. Cibis GW, Tripathi RC, Tripathi BJ, Harris DJ. Corneal keloid in Lowe's syndrome. *Arch Ophthalmol.* 1982;100(11):1795–1799.
53. Rao SK, Fan DSP, Pang CP, et al. Bilateral congenital corneal keloids and anterior segment mesenchymal dysgenesis in a case of Rubinstein-Taybi syndrome. *Cornea.* 2002;21(1):126–130.
54. Holbach LM, Font RL, Shivitz IA, Jones DB. Bilateral keloid-like myofibroblastic proliferations of the cornea in children. *Ophthalmology.* 1990;97:1188–1193.
55. Mullaney PB, Teichmann K, Huaman A, et al. Corneal keloid from unusual penetrating trauma. *J Pediatr Ophthalmol Strabismus.* 1995; 32:331–334.
56. Mejia LF, Acosta C, Santamaria JP. Clinical, surgical, and histopathologic characteristics of corneal keloid. *Cornea.* 2001;20(4):421–424.
57. Risco JM, Huaman A, Antonios SR. A case of corneal keloid: clinical, surgical, pathological and ultrastructural characteristics. *Br J Ophthalmol.* 1994;78:568–571.
58. Beauchamp GR. Terrien's marginal corneal degeneration. *J Pediatr Ophthalmol Strabismus.* 1982;19:97–99.
59. Goldman KN, Kaufman HE. Atypical pterygium: a clinical feature of Terrien's marginal degeneration. *Arch Ophthalmol.* 1978;96: 1027–1029.
60. Nirankari V, Kelman S, Richards R. Central involvement in Terrien's degeneration. *Ophthalmic Surg.* 1983;14:245–247.
61. Austin P, Brown SI. Inflammatory Terrien's marginal corneal disease. *Am J Ophthalmol.* 1981;92:189–192.
62. Romanschuk KG, Hamilton WK, Braig RF. Terrien's marginal degeneration with corneal cyst. *Cornea.* 1990;9:86–87.
63. Binder PS, Zavala EY, Stainer GA. Noninfectious peripheral corneal ulceration: Mooren's ulcer or Terrien's marginal degeneration? *Ann Ophthalmol.* 1982;14:425–435.
64. Lopez JS, et al. Immunohistochemistry of Terrien's and Mooren's corneal degeneration. *Arch Ophthalmol.* 1991;109:988–992.
65. Wagoner MD, Teichmann KD. Terrien's marginal degeneration associated with posterior polymorphous dystrophy. *Cornea.* 1999;18(5): 612–615.
66. Shimazaki J, Yang H, Shimmura S, et al. Terrien's marginal degeneration associated with erythema elevatum diutinum. *Cornea.* 1998;17(3): 342–344.
67. Sugar HS, Kobernick S. The white limbus girdle of Vogt. *Am J Ophthalmol.* 1960;50:101–107.
68. Cursino JW, Fine BS. A histologic study of calcific and noncalcific band keratopathies. *Am J Ophthalmol.* 1976;82:395–404.
69. Berkow JW, Fine BS, Zimmerman LE. Unusual ocular calcification in hyperparathyroidism. *Am J Ophthalmol.* 1968;66:812–824.
70. Doughman DJ, Olson GA, Nolan S, Hajny RG. Experimental band keratopathy. *Arch Ophthalmol.* 1969;81:264.
71. Feist RM, Tessler H, Chandler JW. Transient calcific band-shaped keratopathy associated with increased serum calcium. *Am J Ophthalmol.* 1992;113:459–461.
72. Lemp MA, Ralph RA. Rapid development of band keratopathy in dry eyes. *Am J Ophthalmol.* 1977;83:657–659.
73. Porter R, Crombie AL. Corneal calcification as a presenting and diagnostic sign in hyperparathyroidism. *Br J Ophthalmol.* 1973;57:655–658.
74. Bokosky JE, Meyer RF, Sugar A. Surgical treatment of calcified band keratopathy. *Ophthalmic Res.* 1985;16:645–647.
75. Wood TO, Walker GG. Treatment of band keratopathy. *Am J Ophthalmol.* 1975;80:553.
76. O'Brart DPS, et al. Treatment of band keratopathy by excimer laser phototherapeutic keratectomy: surgical techniques and long term follow up. *Br J Ophthalmol.* 1993;77:702–708.
77. Amano S, Oshika T, Tazawa Y, et al. Long-term follow-up of excimer laser phototherapeutic keratectomy. *Jpn J Ophthalmol.* 1999;43: 513–516.
78. Dogru M, Katakami C, Miyashita M, et al. Ocular surface changes after excimer laser phototherapeutic keratectomy. *Ophthalmology.* 2000;107: 1144–1152.
79. Rapuano CJ. Excimer laser phototherapeutic keratectomy: long-term results and practical considerations. *Cornea.* 1997;16(2):151–157.
80. Anderson DF, Prabhasawat P, Alfonso E, et al. Amniotic membrane transplantation after the primary surgical management of band keratopathy. *Cornea.* 2001;20(4):354–361.
81. Lavid FJ, Herreras JM, Calonge M, et al. Calcareous corneal degeneration: report of two cases. *Cornea.* 1995;14(1):97–102.
82. Duffey RJ, LoCascio JA. Calcium deposition in a corneal graft. *Cornea.* 1987;6:212–215.
83. Perry HD, Scheie HG. Superficial reticular degeneration of Koby. *Br J Ophthalmol.* 1980;64:841–844.
84. Perry HD, Leonard ER, Yourish NB. Superficial reticular degeneration of Koby. *Ophthalmology.* 1985;92:1570–1573.
85. Rose GE, Lavin MJ. The Hudson-Stahli line. I: An epidemiological study. *Eye.* 1987;1:466–470.
86. Rose GE, Lavin MJ. The Hudson-Stahli line. II: A comparison of properties in eyes with and without long-term contact lens wear. *Eye.* 1987;1:471–474.
87. Rose GE, Lavin MJ. The Hudson-Stahli line. III: Observations on morphology, a critical review of aetiology and a unified theory for the formation of iron lines of the corneal epithelium. *Eye.* 1987;1: 475–479.
88. Barraquer-Somers E, Chan CC, Green WR. Corneal epithelial iron deposition. *Ophthalmology.* 1983;90:729–734.

89. Norn M. Hudson-Stahli's iron line in the cornea. *Acta Ophthalmol (Copenh)*. 1990;68:339–340.
90. Ferry AP. A 'new' iron line of the superficial cornea. *Arch Ophthalmol*. 1968;79:142–145.
91. Vongthongsri A, Chuck RS, Pepose JS. Corneal iron deposits after laser in situ keratomileusis. *Am J Ophthalmol*. 1999;127:85–86.
92. Hiraoka T, Furuya A, Okamoto F, et al. Corneal iron ring formation associated with overnight orthokeratology. *Cornea*. 2004;23(8 suppl):S78–S81.
93. Steinberg EB, et al. Stellate iron lines in the corneal epithelium after radial keratotomy. *Am J Ophthalmol*. 1984;98:416–421.
94. Koenig SB, et al. Corneal iron lines after refractive keratoplasty. *Arch Ophthalmol*. 1983;101:1862–1865.
95. Mannis MJ. Iron deposition in the corneal graft. *Arch Ophthalmol*. 1983;101:1858–1861.
96. Anduze AL, Merritt JC. Pterygium: clinical classification and management in Virgin Islands. *Ann Ophthalmol*. 1985;17:92–95.
97. Miller EM. Genesis of white rings of the cornea. *Am J Ophthalmol*. 1966;61:904–907.
98. Yanoff M, Fine BS. *Ocular pathology*. 5th ed. St. Louis: Mosby; 2002.
99. Meyer JC, Quantock AJ, Kincaid MC, et al. Characterization of a central corneal cloudiness sharing features of posterior crocodile shagreen and central cloudy dystrophy of François. *Cornea*. 1996;15(4):347–354.
100. Dangel ME, Krachmer GP, Stark WJ. Anterior corneal mosaic in eyes with keratoconus wearing hard contact lenses. *Arch Ophthalmol*. 1984;102:888–890.
101. Bramsen T, Ehlers N, Braggesen LH. Central cloudy corneal dystrophy of François. *Acta Ophthalmol (Copenh)*. 1976;54:221–226.
102. Curran RE, Kenyon KR, Green WR. Pre-Descemet's membrane corneal dystrophy. *Am J Ophthalmol*. 1974;77:711–716.
103. Grayson M, Wilbrandt H. Pre-Descemet dystrophy. *Am J Ophthalmol*. 1967;64:276–282.
104. Taylor HR, et al. Corneal changes associated with chronic UV irradiation. *Arch Ophthalmol*. 1989;107:1481–1484.
105. Kaji Y, Oshika T, Amano S, et al. Immunohistocheical localization of advanced glycation end products in pinguecula. *Graefe's Arch Clin Exp Ophthalmol*. 2006;244(1):104–108.
106. Perkins ES. The association between pinguecula, sunlight, and cataract. *Ophthalmic Res*. 1985;17:325–330.
107. Frucht-Pery J, Siganos CS, Solomon A, et al. Topical indomethacin solution versus dexamethasone solution for treatment of inflamed pterygium and pinguecula: a prospective randomized clinical study. *Am J Ophthalmol*. 1999;127:148–152.
108. Chan CML, Liu YP, Tan DTH. Ocular surface changes in pterygium. *Cornea*. 2002;21(1):38–42.
109. Austin P, Jakobiec A, Iwamoto T. Elastodysplasia and elastodystrophy as the pathologic bases of ocular pterygia and pinguecula. *Ophthalmology*. 1983;90:96–109.
110. Hill JC, Maske R. Pathogenesis of pterygium. *Eye*. 1989;3:218–226.
111. Luthra R, Nemesure BB, Wu S, et al. Frequency and risk factors for pterygium in the Barbados Eye Study. *Arch Ophthalmol*. 2001;119:1827–1832.
112. Coroneo MT. Pterygium as an early indicator of ultraviolet insolation: a hypothesis. *Br J Ophthalmol*. 1993;77:734–739.
113. Weinstein O, Rosenthal G, Zirkin H, et al. Overexpression of p53 tumor suppressor gene in pterygia. *Eye*. 2002;16:619–621.
114. Dushku N, John MK, Schultz GS, et al. Pterygia pathogenesis: corneal invasion by matrix metalloproteinase expressing altered limbal epithelial basal cells. *Arch Ophthalmol*. 2001;119:695–706.
115. Chumbley LC. Herbert's pits and lid secretions: an important association. *Eye*. 1988;2:476–477.
116. Chang S, Hou P, Chen M. Conjunctival secretions. *Arch Ophthalmol*. 1990;108:405–407.
117. Akhtar S, Bron AJ, Meek KM, Bennett L. Congenital hereditary endothelial dystrophy and band keratopathy in an infant with corpus callosum agenesis. *Cornea*. 2001;20(5):547–552.
118. Tsilou ET, Rubin BI, Reed GT, et al. Age-related prevalence of anterior segment complications in patients with infantile cystinosis. *Cornea*. 2002;21(2):173–176.
119. Sheard RM, Pope FM, Snead MP. A novel ophthalmic presentation of proteus syndrome. *Ophthalmology*. 2002;109:1192–1195.
120. Ghanchi R, Ramsay A, Coupland S, et al. Ocular tumoral calcinosis. *Arch Ophthalmol*. 1996;114:341–345.

Chapter 77

Bacterial Keratitis

Sean L. Edelstein, Pongmas Wichiensin, Andrew J.W. Huang

Introduction

Microbial keratitis or infectious corneal ulcer is due to the proliferation of microorganisms (including bacteria, fungi, viruses, and parasites) and associated inflammation and tissue destruction within the corneal tissue. It is a potentially sight-threatening condition and frequently presents as an ocular emergency. However, it is often challenging to distinguish microbial keratitis from other noninfectious or inflammatory corneal conditions resulting from trauma or immune-mediated reactions. Bacterial keratitis is the most common cause of suppurative corneal ulceration, which rarely occurs in the normal eye because of the human cornea's natural resistance to infection. However, predisposing factors including contact lens wear, trauma, corneal surgery, ocular surface disease, systemic diseases,[1] and immunosuppression may alter the defense mechanisms of the ocular surface and permit bacteria to invade the cornea. There are no specific clinical signs to help confirm a definite bacterial cause in microbial keratitis, but clinicians should identify the risk factors for ocular infection and assess the distinctive corneal findings to determine potential etiologies. When there is strong suspicion for a possible infectious keratitis, laboratory investigations should be considered in order to identify and confirm the causal organisms. Based on the clinical and laboratory findings, a therapeutic plan can then be initiated.[2] It is sometimes necessary to modify the therapeutic plan based on clinical response and tolerance of the antimicrobial agents. The goals for treating bacterial keratitis are to treat the corneal infection and associated inflammation, and to restore corneal integrity and visual function. Medical therapy with appropriate antibiotics is the mainstay of treatment. The outcome usually depends on the preceding pathology and the extent of ulceration at the time of presentation.[3] Surgery may be considered if medical therapy fails to eradicate the pathogens or if the vision is markedly threatened by the infection or resultant scar.

Epidemiology

The accurate incidence of bacterial keratitis is not known. It is estimated that 30 000 cases of microbial keratitis occur in the USA annually.[4] An estimated 10 to 30 individuals per 100 000 contact lens wearers develop microbial keratitis annually in the USA,[5,6] with estimated costs of US$50 million in annual expenditures for medical care of this condition. A recent large prospective, population-based surveillance study from Australia similarly reported microbial keratitis affecting 4.2 per 10 000 contact lens wearers per year.[7] Similar estimates for Great Britain show approximately 1500 annual cases of microbial keratitis from all causes.[8]

Complete epidemiological information for developing countries is lacking. Bacterial keratitis is a leading cause of corneal blindness in developing nations, usually caused by ocular trauma.[9] The changing patterns of risk factors (such as HIV and AIDS) and causal microorganisms are likely to affect the global statistics of bacterial keratitis.

Occasionally, severe or refractory bacterial keratitis requires surgery. Statistics from the Eye Bank Association of America demonstrate that approximately 1% of all corneal transplants are performed as a result of microbial keratitis. Based upon the annual incidence of bacterial keratitis, we estimate that approximately 0.5–1% of infectious keratitis cases require surgical intervention in the USA.

Host Defense and Risk Factors

Defense of the ocular surface

Bacterial keratitis usually occurs in patients with predisposing factors, which can compromise normal ocular surface defenses.[10] These natural defenses include the eyelid, tear film, corneal epithelium, and normal ocular flora. The eyelids and adnexae provide a physical barrier to the ocular surface against noxious external irritations and exogenous microorganisms. Normal blinking also provides a good distribution of tear film to wash away such organisms. Eyelid trauma or any abnormality of the lid closure can compromise this defense mechanism. Older individuals and debilitated or unconscious patients lacking adequate Bell reflexes or with poor blinking and corneal exposure are at particular risk for bacterial keratitis. The rinsing action of the tear film and its constituents provide additional protective effects.[11] Abnormalities of tear components, tear volume, or tear drainage system are the principal causes of a compromised ocular surface. Many proteins in the tear film, such as secretory immunoglobulins, complement components, and various enzymes including lysozyme, lactoferrin, betalysins, orosomucoid, and ceruloplasmin have antibacterial effects.[12] Chronic colonization and infection of the eyelid margin or lacrimal outflow system can predispose cornea to bacterial infection when minor trauma occurs. Chronic epiphora due to nasolacrimal duct obstruction can lead to reduced concentrations of certain antibacterial substances in the tear film.[13] More frequently, a dry eye with aqueous deficiency and poor corneal wetting from rheumatologic diseases, HIV infection, and conjunctival scarring predisposes the cornea to bacterial invasion.[14] Deficiency of the mucin or lipid layers in the tear film can also facilitate corneal infection.[15]

An intact corneal epithelium is an important defense factor. Only a few bacteria, such as *Neisseria gonorrhoeae, Corynebacterium diphtheriae, Haemophilus aegyptius*, and *Listeria monocytogenes* can penetrate an intact corneal epithelium, while most cannot. Compromised corneal epithelial integrity caused by contact lens wear, corneal trauma, or corneal surgery is the important predisposing factor to bacterial ulcers. Furthermore, corneal epithelial cells are capable of phagocytosis and intercellular transport of ingested particles, potentially providing additional defenses to eradicate the invading microorganisms. Normal conjunctival flora includes both planktonic bacteria suspended in the tears and sessile bacteria adherent to the ocular surface, which help to prevent overgrowth of exogenous organisms. Inappropriate use of topical antibiotics could eliminate the natural protection by normal flora and predispose the cornea to development of opportunistic infections, particularly when combined with corneal disease or trauma. The biofilm, a slimy layer composed of organic polymers produced by embedded bacteria on contact lenses, can protect adherent bacteria from antibacterial substances and provides a nidus for infection.[16,17] The conjunctiva contains subepithelial mucosal-associated lymphoid tissue (MALT), which is a collection of lymphoid cells, and can provide specific immune-mediated defenses to the ocular surface.

Other local corneal conditions that predispose to corneal infection include bullous corneal edema from corneal injury or surgery, absence of corneal sensation from herpetic corneal infection or topical anesthetic abuse, and local immunosuppression from prolonged use of topical corticosteroids.

External risk factors

Trauma, including chemical and thermal injuries, foreign bodies, and local irradiation can predispose to bacterial keratitis. This is more likely in cases of corneal trauma associated with an agricultural rather than an industrial setting,[18] and is more likely to be caused by unusual organisms such as *Nocardia*. Exposure to contaminated water or other solutions following corneal trauma can lead to bacterial keratitis. Prior contamination of ophthalmic solutions, such as nonpreserved fluorescein eye drops,[19] led to the adoption of guidelines for the preparation of sterile topical solutions[20] and preservatives are now routinely added to multiuse topical ophthalmic medications. Nonetheless, corneal infection continues to occur from contamination of topical solutions and the tips or caps of eye dropper bottles.[21]

Chronic abuse of topical anesthetics can disrupt the corneal epithelium and render it at risk for microbial infection (Fig. 77.1).[22] Crack cocaine smoking has also been associated with corneal infection, probably caused by disrupting corneal epithelium via associated cellular and neuronal toxicity.[23] Nosocomial corneal infections have occurred in unconscious patients during general anesthesia or coma[24] as a result of lagophthalmos and corneal exposure. Inadvertent contamination of the eyes or skin can occur by the tubings or solutions used for aspirating the airways.[25,26] Geographic and climatic factors can also influence the prevalence of bacterial keratitis. The variation of habitats and microorganism exposure, such as living in rural versus urban areas, can lead to differences in infectious keratitis profile.

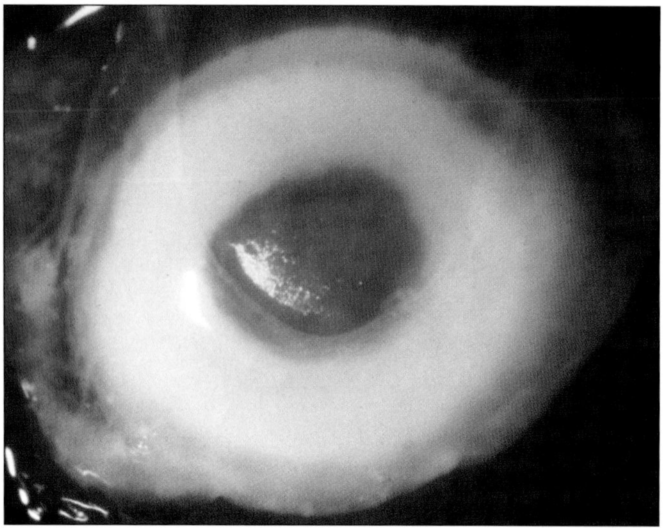

Fig. 77.1 *Bacillus* keratitis associated with trauma and topical anesthetic abuse. Aggressive peripheral stromal necrosis with a ring ulcer.

Contact lens use

Contact lens wear has been identified as the most common risk factor for bacterial keratitis in developed countries.[27] Recent studies suggest there are as many as 36 million contact lens wearers in the USA.[28] All types of contact lenses, including hard, gas-permeable, soft, disposable, and cosmetic lenses, have been implicated in microbial keratitis.[29–31] On average, contact lens users have a 1.5% chance of developing infectious keratitis during a lifetime of contact lens wear. The incidence has been estimated at 2.7 to 4.1 per 10000 wearers per year for daily-wear soft contact lens use and at 9.3 to 20.9 per 10000 wearers per year for extended wear contact lens use.[6,29,30] The incidence is lowest for rigid gas-permeable lenses, estimated to be 0.4 to 4 per 10000. The risk of microbial keratitis has not been significantly reduced in daily disposable contact lens users,[31,32] even though it eliminated lens storage and hygiene steps. Continuous lens wear increases the risk of infectious keratitis by approximately tenfold[33,34] and the risk of infection is enhanced incrementally with each consecutive night of lens wear. Although there is less corneal hypoxia associated with the use of silicone hydrogel lenses, the risk for microbial keratitis has been reported to be comparable between extended wear of silicone hydrogel lenses and overnight wear of hydrogel lenses.[35] Orthokeratology, which involves the programmed overnight application of a rigid contact lens for the transient reduction of myopia, has been associated with increased risk for infectious keratitis in several case reports.[36,37]

Three groups of patients have an increased risk of contact lens-related infectious keratitis, with the incidence reported at between 1% and 5%: aphakes,[38] patients with a corneal transplant, and patients wearing a bandage lens for chronic keratopathy. Pre-existing keratopathy also predisposes therapeutic contact lens wearers to infection by less common microbes.[39]

Contamination of contact lenses by *Pseudomonas* spp. or fungi was occasionally encountered in the early years of contact lens manufacturing. Better industrial manufacturing standards with improved packaging have ensured the sterility of new lenses. However, contamination from improper subsequent lens handling frequently occurs.[40] Many patients with contact lens-associated bacterial keratitis often fail to practice recommended lens care regimens,[41] and the same organisms can sometimes be isolated from corneal scrapings and the contact lens case or solutions.[42] *Pseudomonas* spp. is the most common isolate of bacterial keratitis associated with contact lens wear (Fig. 77.2).[43,44] *Pseudomonas aeruginosa* and other microorganisms have been frequently recovered from tap and bottled water used to prepare contact lens saline solutions. Bacteria can adhere to a contact lens regardless of lens materials[45] and microbes can survive in the moist chamber of a contact lens case (Fig. 77.3).[46] Worn contact lenses with surface protein and mucin deposits or irregularities are more susceptible to bacterial adhesion.[47,48] The polysaccharide layer of encapsulated bacteria can facilitate colonization of the contact lens surface. A biofilm can protect bacteria from antibacterial agents. Extended wear contact lenses augment the risks of infection by accumulating coatings or debris under the lens[49] and by enhancing bacterial colonization on the cornea.[50] A seasonal variation in the incidence of contact lens-associated bacterial keratitis might be due to activities such as swimming in the summer.[51] Contact lens wear does not necessarily affect normal conjunctival flora,[52] but some lens disinfectants may influence microbial flora.[53] Although healthcare workers wearing contact lenses do not necessarily have altered conjunctival flora,[54] they are prone to develop bacterial keratitis caused by antibiotic-resistant strains.

Contact lens use can adversely affect the healthy cornea[55] by causing hypoxia and altering epithelial hemostasis. Corneal hypoxia and related endothelial dysfunction can result in acute epithelial edema and compromised epithelial integrity. A tight lens syndrome can be precipitated by poor lens hydration, inadequate oxygen permeability of the lens, and repeated overnight hypoxic stress. Contact lens wear slows corneal epithelial hemostasis by suppressing cell proliferation,[56] impairing cell migration,[57] and reducing the rate of cell exfoliation.[58] Corneal abrasion may occur during lens insertion or removal.

Ocular surface pathologies

Ocular surface diseases such as cicatricial pemphigoid, Stevens-Johnson syndrome, atopic keratoconjunctivitis, radiation and chemical injury, and vitamin A deficiency can lead to squamous metaplasia of the ocular surface epithelia and cause an unstable tear film.[59] Disruption of the epithelial glycocalyx leads to ocular surface breakdown that encourages bacterial adherence and subsequent keratitis.[60] Bacterial keratitis can complicate corneal epithelial erosions associated with corneal epithelial basement membrane dystrophy,[61] lattice corneal dystrophy, and vernal or atopic keratoconjunctivitis.[62]

Bacterial keratitis after corneal transplantation can occur at any time postoperatively[63] and retrospective reviews have reported an incidence of approximately 2–5%.[64–66] Post-keratoplasty use of extended wear soft contact lenses has been a major risk factor.[67,68] Other predisposing factors include chronic epithelial defects, frequent application of topical corticosteroids and other agents, and concurrent dry eye syndrome.[69–71] Loose, broken, or exposed sutures can

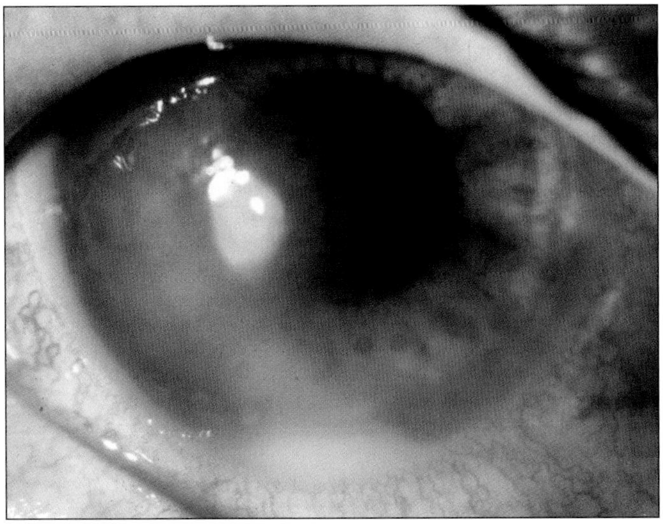

Fig. 77.2 *Pseudomonas* keratitis associated with extended wear soft contact lens. A paracentral corneal infiltrate with surrounding corneal edema and hypopyon.

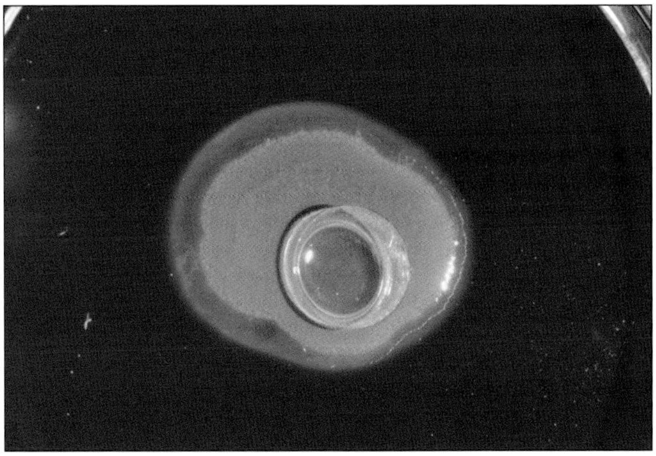

Fig. 77.3 Culture of the contact lens from a patient with *Pseudomonas* keratitis. Confluent growth of *Pseudomonas* around the contact lens on a blood agar plate.

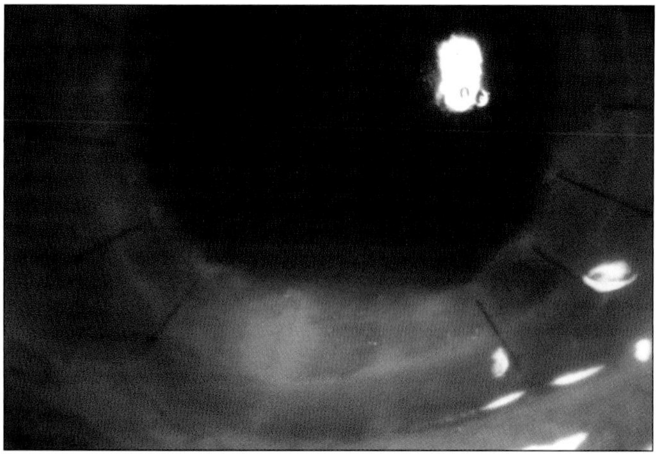

Fig. 77.4 A stromal infiltrate from coagulase-negative *Staphylococcus* in the deep stroma around the suture track of a corneal graft. The condition developed after suture removal.

harbor ocular flora and permit an entry site for microbes, and suture removal can drag surface microorganisms into the corneal stroma (Fig. 77.4).[72] Chronic inflammation associated with infectious keratitis tends to progress into the graft–host junction or along a lamellar wound interface such as infectious crystalline keratopathy.

Bacterial keratitis has been reported after refractive surgeries such as radial keratotomy and LASIK.[73–77] Corneal infection may occur shortly after surgery or several years later.[78] Bacterial keratitis has been reported to occur with less frequency in other types of keratorefractive procedures such as postkeratoplasty relaxing incisions, and excimer laser phototherapeutic[79] or photorefractive keratectomy.[80,81] In addition to the common organisms associated with refractive surgeries,[82] unusual microbes such as *Mycobacterium* have been encountered in LASIK with higher frequency (Fig. 77.5).[75,76] Similar to refractive keratotomy procedures, contaminated surgical instruments have been implicated in many cases of post-LASIK keratitis.[83]

Systemic conditions such as malnutrition, diabetes, collagen vascular diseases, or chronic alcoholism may also compromise the ocular surface and increase the risk of microbial keratitis caused by unusual organisms such as *Moraxella* (Fig. 77.6).[84] In patients with acquired immunodeficiency syndrome (AIDS), microbial keratitis does not appear to be more prevalent than in the normal population. However, the keratitis tends to be more severe and more resistant to therapy in these patients.[85,86]

Pathogenesis

Bacterial keratitis can be caused by multiple microorganisms (Table 77.1). *Staphylococci* and *Pseudomonas* are the most common organisms in the USA.[87] In contrast, streptococci, particularly *Streptococcus pneumoniae*, are a predominant cause of bacterial keratitis in many developing nations.[88,89] The smallest inoculum that can produce infection in the human cornea remains undetermined. A single viable organism can theoretically initiate corneal infection. Animal models of bacterial keratitis show that only about 50 *P. aeruginosa* or 100 *Staphylococcus aureus* are needed to initiate corneal infection.[90,91]

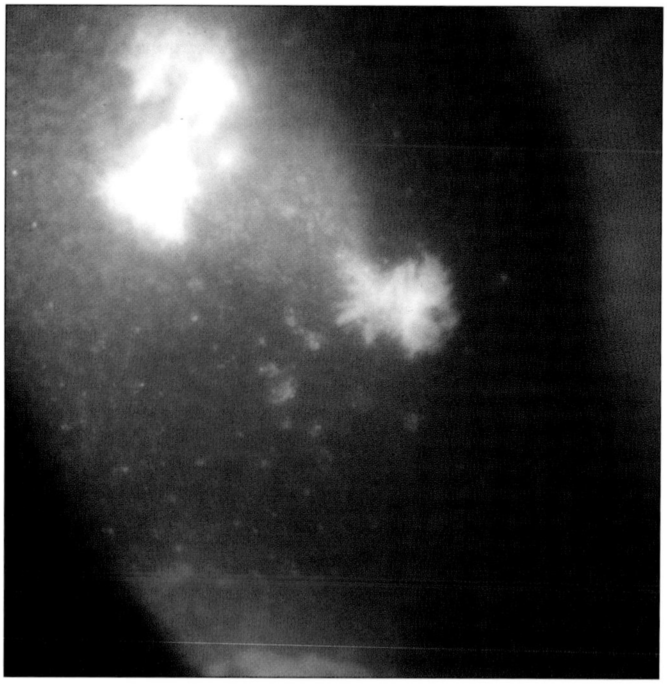

Fig. 77.5 An indolent nontuberculous *Mycobacterium* keratitis with several intralamellar infiltrates with feathery edge and mild surrounding stromal inflammation after LASIK surgery.

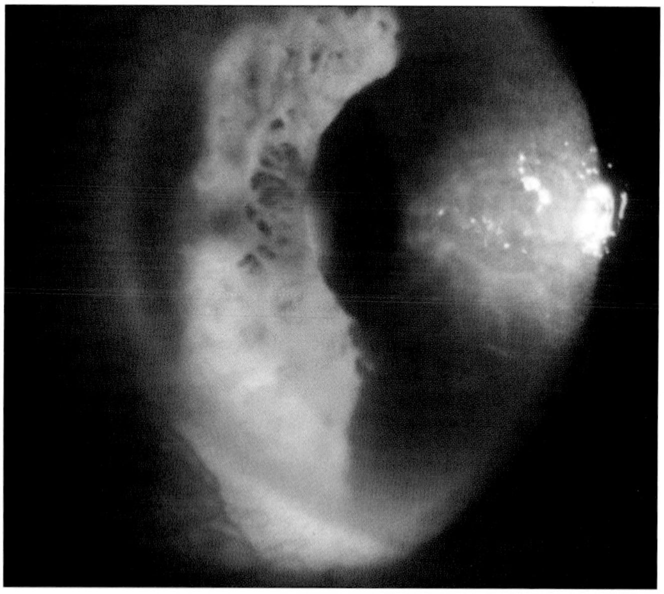

Fig. 77.6 A superficial indolent corneal ulcer with moderate corneal edema and mild infiltrates in a diabetic patient with *Moraxella* keratitis.

Bacterial adherence

Bacterial keratitis occurs when microorganisms overcome host defenses. The pathogen adheres to the wounded corneal surface and avoids the clearance mechanisms of the tear film

Table 77.1 Common etiologic agents of bacterial keratitis in the USA

Class/organism	Common isolates*	Cases (%)
Gram-positive isolates		**29–53**
Gram-positive cocci	*Staphylococcus aureus*	4–19
	Coagulase-negative staphylococci	1–45.5
	Streptococcus pneumoniae	0–3
	Streptococcus viridans group	1–6
Gram-positive bacilli	*Propionibacterium* species	4–7
	Mycobacterium species	3
Gram-negative isolates		**47–50**
Gram-negative bacilli	*Pseudomonas aeruginosa*	3–33
	Serratia marcescens	3–13.5
	Proteus mirabilis	4
	Enteric Gram-negative bacilli, other	1–10
Gram-negative	*Haemophilus influenzae*, other *Haemophilus* species	2.5
Coccobacillary organisms	*Moraxella* species and related species	1
Gram-negative cocci	*Neisseria* species	1

*Regional differences may affect the order and percentage of pathogens.
Data from Preferred practice pattern: bacterial keratitis. *American Academy of Ophthalmology, 2008.*[234]

and lid blinking. Shortly after injury, viable bacteria adhere to the damaged edges of corneal epithelial cells[92] and to the basement membrane or the bare stroma near the wound edge.[93] The glycocalyx of injured epithelium is particularly susceptible to attachment by microorganisms.

Microbial attachment is initiated by the interaction of bacterial adhesins with glycoprotein receptors of the ocular surface.[94,95] The ability of certain bacteria to adhere to an epithelial defect may account for the frequent occurrence of *S. aureus*, *S. pneumoniae*, and *P. aeruginosa* infection.[96] Biofilm production enhances bacterial aggregation, protects adherent microorganisms, and helps growth during these early stages of infection.[97] Pili (fimbriae) are thin (4–10 nm in diameter) protein filaments located on the surfaces of many bacteria. Pili facilitate adherence of *P. aeruginosa* and *Neisseria* spp. to epithelium.

Bacterial invasion

The bacterial capsule and other surface components are important in corneal invasion. For example, some bacteria avoid activation of the alternate complement pathway because of their capsular polysaccharide. Lipopolysaccharides, the subcapsular constituents of bacteria, are the major mediators of corneal inflammation. Intrastromal inoculation of endotoxin induces an inflammatory response.[98] Bacterial invasion into surface epithelial cells is partially mediated by the interactions between the bacterial cell-surface proteins, integrins, epithelial cell-surface proteins, and the release of proteases by bacteria. Organisms such as *N. gonorrhoeae*,[99] *N. meningitidis*,[100] *Corynebacterium diphtheriae*, *Haemophilus aegyptius*, and *Listeria monocytogenes* can penetrate the intact corneal epithelial surface via these types of mechanisms.

Colonization of the corneal surface sometimes precedes stromal invasion. Without antibiotics or other intervening factors, bacteria continue to invade and replicate in the corneal stroma. Keratocytes are also capable of phagocytosis,[101] but the exposed, avascular stroma provides little protection to the cornea. Microorganisms in the anterior stromal lamellae produce proteolytic enzymes[102,103] that destroy stromal matrices and collagen fibrils. Bacterial invasion begins within hours after exogenous contamination of a corneal wound[97] or after the application of a heavily contaminated contact lens.[104] The largest increase in a bacterial population occurs within the first 2 days of stromal infection.[90]

After inoculation, bacteria infiltrate the surrounding epithelium and into the deeper stroma around the initial site of infection. Viable bacteria tend to be found at the peripheral margins of the infiltrate or deep within a central ulcer crater. Unchecked bacterial multiplication in the corneal stroma results in progressive enlargement or extension of infectious foci into the surrounding cornea.

Corneal inflammation and tissue damage

Various soluble mediators and inflammatory cells can be induced by bacterial invasion and cause corneal inflammation with eventual tissue destruction. Soluble mediators of inflammation include the kinin-forming system, the clotting and fibrinolytic systems, immunoglobulins, complement components, vasoactive amines, eicosanoids, neuropeptides, and cytokines. The complement cascade can be triggered to kill bacteria but complement-dependent chemotaxins[105] can initiate focal inflammation.

The production of cytokines such as tumor necrosis factor (TNF)-alpha and interleukin-1[106] results in the adherence and extravasation of neutrophils in limbal blood vessels. This process is mediated by cell adhesion glycoproteins such as integrins and selectins and members of the immunoglobulin superfamily such as intercellular adhesion molecules (ICAMs) on vascular endothelial cells and on leukocytes.

Vascular dilation of the conjunctival and limbal blood vessels is associated with increased permeability, resulting in an inflammatory exudate into the tear film and peripheral cornea. Polymorphonuclear neutrophils (PMNs) can enter the injured cornea anteriorly via tear film through an epithelial defect, but most migrate from the limbus.[107]

Recruitment of acute inflammatory cells occurs within a few hours after bacterial inoculation. As neutrophils accumulate at the infected site, more cytokines such as leukotrienes and complement components are presumably released to attract additional leukocytes. Macrophages subsequently begin to migrate to the cornea to ingest invading bacteria and degenerating neutrophils. Extensive stromal inflammation eventually leads to proteolytic stromal degradation and liquefactive tissue necrosis.

Natural History

While some bacteria (e.g. *Gonococcus*) can invade an intact corneal epithelium, most cases of bacterial keratitis develop at the site of an epithelial abnormality or defect in the corneal surface. The rate of disease progression is dependent on the virulence of the infecting organism and on host factors. For example, highly virulent organisms such as *Pseudomonas, Streptococcus pneumoniae*, or *Gonococcus* cause rapid tissue destruction, while other organisms such as nontuberculous *Mycobacterium* and *Streptococcus viridans* are usually associated with a more indolent keratitis. Some bacteria that are considered to be normal conjunctival flora (e.g. *Corynebacterium*) may become opportunistic pathogens in the compromised eye.

Bacterial keratitis can occur in any part of the cornea, but infections involving the central cornea have a worse prognosis. Scarring in this location is likely to cause visual loss, even if the causal organism is successfully eradicated. Untreated or severe bacterial keratitis may result in corneal perforation and has the potential to develop into endophthalmitis and result in loss of the eye.[87] Because the destruction of corneal tissues can take place rapidly (within 24 hours by a virulent organism), optimal management requires rapid recognition, timely institution of therapy, and appropriate follow-up.

Presentation

The clinical signs and symptoms of microbial keratitis are variable and they depend on the virulence of the organism, duration of infection, pre-existing corneal conditions, immune status of the host, and previous use of antibiotics or corticosteroids. Severe bacterial keratitis usually has a history of rapid onset of pain, photophobia, decreased vision, conjunctival injection, anterior chamber reaction, and/or hypopyon. However, keratitis caused by nontuberculous *Mycobacterium* may present with an insidious onset or indolent course. The clinical findings usually cannot readily distinguish the causing organism. Nonetheless, clinical diagnosis is possible when a pertinent history is available or the organisms present with characteristic features, such as a rapidly progressive stromal necrosis with mucopurulent discharge in *Pseudomonas aeruginosa* keratitis in a young patient with extended contact lens wear. However, many microorganisms such as fungi or *Acanthamoeba* can cause masquerading syndromes mimicking bacterial keratitis.

Differential Diagnosis

The differential diagnosis includes infectious and noninfectious causes of infiltrates. Nonbacterial corneal pathogens include fungi (both yeast and mold), parasites (including protozoa such as *Acanthamoeba*), nematodes (such as *Onchocerca*), and viral infection. Viruses including herpes simplex virus (HSV), varicella-zoster virus (VZV), and Epstein-Barr virus (EBV) produce immunologically mediated corneal infiltrates that may resemble a bacterial, fungal, or *Acanthamoeba* keratitis. Eyes with viral keratitis are also prone to microbial superinfection. Viruses can also cause a true suppurative keratitis, as in necrotizing stromal disease. Noninfectious stromal infiltration may be associated with contact lens wear or antigens from local and systemic bacterial infections. Systemic diseases, such as collagen vascular disorders (e.g. rheumatoid arthritis, systemic lupus erythematosus), vasculitic disorders (e.g. polyarteritis nodosa, Wegener's granulomatosis), and other inflammatory disorders such as sarcoidosis may produce infiltrative keratitis. Other causes include dermatologic disorders (e.g. severe ocular rosacea) and allergic conditions (e.g. vernal and atopic keratoconjunctivitis). Corneal trauma, including chemical and thermal injury, and corneal foreign bodies, including exposed or loose sutures, may also lead to infiltrative keratitis, which may be infectious or noninfectious in nature.

Clinical Examination

The purpose of clinical evaluation of bacterial keratitis is to evaluate predisposing or aggravating factors in order to construct a differential diagnosis, to assess the severity of the disease and the associated complications, and to initiate appropriate management in a timely manner. Obtaining a detailed history is important and should include ocular symptoms (e.g. degree of pain, redness, discharge, blurred vision, photophobia, duration of symptoms, circumstances surrounding the onset of symptoms) and review of prior ocular history (including previous infectious keratitis, ocular surgery, contact lens wear,[33,34,108] trauma, and dry eye).[109]

In many cases, patient discomfort, tearing, and inflammation will compromise visual acuity. It is useful, however, to document baseline visual acuity and to ascertain that it is consistent with the anterior segment examination. An external examination should be performed with particular attention to the followings: general appearance of the patient, including skin conditions, facial examination, eyelids and lid closure, conjunctiva, nasolacrimal apparatus, and corneal sensation (assess prior to instillation of topical anesthetic).

Detailed slit lamp biomicroscopy should include evaluation of the following: eyelid margins (meibomian gland dysfunction, ulceration, eyelash abnormalities including trichiasis, irregularities, nasolacrimal obstructions or punctal anomalies), tear film (dry eye or debris), conjunctiva (discharge, erythema, follicles, papillae, cicatrization, keratinization, membrane, pseudomembrane, ulceration, scars, foreign bodies), sclera (inflammation, ulceration, nodules or ischemia), and cornea (epithelial defects, punctate keratopathy, edema, stromal infiltrates, thinning, or perforation). The location (central, peripheral, perineural, or adjacent surgical or traumatic wound), density, size, shape (ring [Figs 77.7, 77.8], or satellite lesions), depth, character of infiltrate margin (suppurative, necrotic, feathery, soft, crystalline), and color of the corneal ulcer should be carefully evaluated and documented. The endothelium and

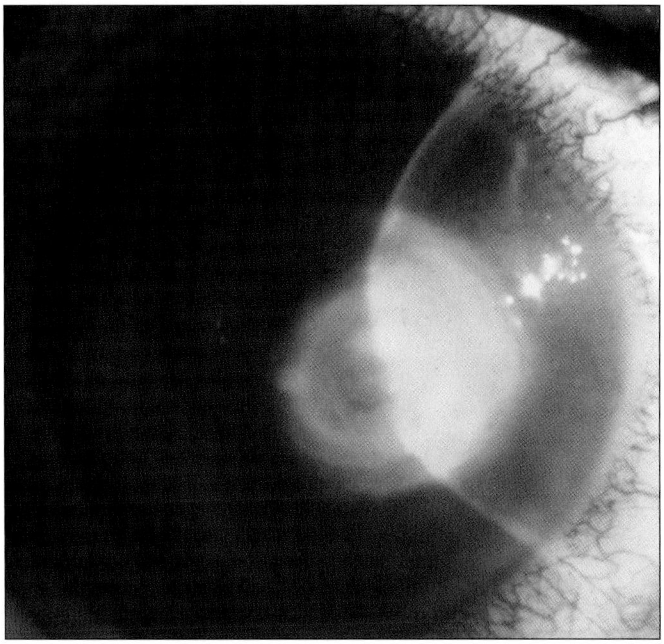

Fig. 77.7 Nontuberculous *Mycobacterium* keratitis with a ring infiltrate with stromal necrosis and central thinning, mimicking *Acanthamoeba* keratitis.

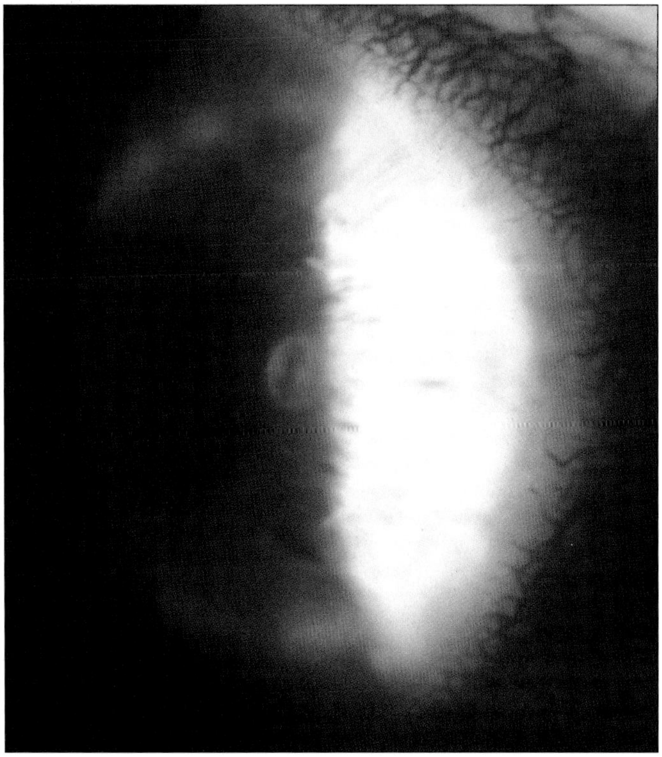

Fig. 77.8 A small superficial *Staphylococcus aureus* keratitis with a large, noninfectious immune ring.

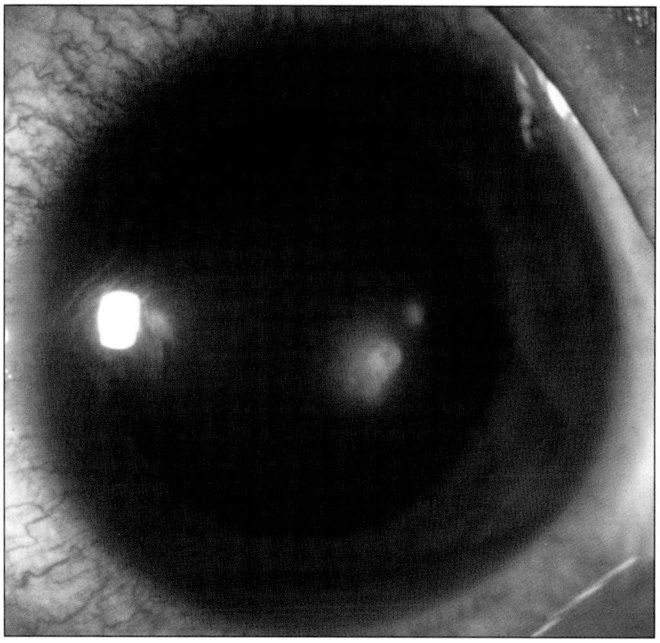

Fig. 77.9 A small and dense localized infiltrate with a small satellite lesion in a *Serratia* keratitis.

associated anterior chamber inflammation (cell, flare, hypopyon, or fibrin) should not be overlooked. Other findings such as foreign bodies, exposed or broken sutures, signs of corneal dystrophies (e.g. epithelial basement membrane dystrophy), previous corneal inflammation (thinning, scarring, or neovascularization), and signs of previous corneal or refractive surgery are also important. Fluorescein or rose Bengal staining may provide additional information, such as the presence of dendrites, pseudodendrites, loose or exposed sutures, and epithelial defects. Intraocular extension of infection or infectious endophthalmitis, though rarely directly caused by the microbial keratitis without corneal perforation, should be ruled out by inspecting the anterior chamber and vitreous cavity with regard to inflammation and clarity. Attention should also be directed to the contralateral eye for clues to etiology as well as possible similar pathology.

Clinical features suggestive of bacterial keratitis include suppurative stromal infiltrate (particularly those greater than 1 mm in size) with indistinct edges, edema, and white cell infiltration in surrounding stroma. An epithelial defect is typically present. An anterior chamber reaction is often seen. The corneal ulcer is considered to be severe if the lesion progresses rapidly, has an infiltration dimension larger than 6 mm, involves deeper than one-third of the corneal thickness, presents with impending or overt perforation, or has scleral involvement.[110] The microbial organisms that usually produce these severe and rapidly progressive corneal ulcers include *S. aureus*, *S. pneumoniae*, β-hemolytic *streptococcus*, and *P. aeruginosa*. On the other hand, less severe or slowly progressive corneal ulcers usually are caused by organisms such as coagulase-negative *staphylococcus*, *S. viridans*, *Actinomyces*, *Nocardia*, *Moraxella*, and *Serratia* (Fig. 77.9).

Specific Bacterial Ulcers

The most common pathogenic organisms identified in bacterial keratitis include *staphylococci* and Gram-negative rods (*Pseudomonas* species). In bacterial keratitis associated with the use of cosmetic contact lenses, *Pseudomonas* is the most commonly identified etiologic agent, accounting for up to two-thirds of cases.[111–113] However, a review from Florida found that *Serratia marcescens* was isolated as frequently as *Pseudomonas aeruginosa* in contact lens-associated keratitis[114] and a review from Melbourne, Australia, found that *Pseudomonas* was isolated in only 7% of contact lens-associated keratitis.[115] *Pseudomonas* is also a common pathogen in bacterial keratitis that occurs in hospitalized infants and in adults who are respirator dependent.[116] A review of 30 years of cultures for suspected infectious keratitis in south Florida showed that Gram-positive isolates remained relatively stable whereas Gram-negative isolates declined.[117] A review of 5 years of bacterial isolates from bacterial keratitis in Pittsburgh showed Gram-positive isolates decreasing while Gram-negative isolates remained relatively stable.[118] In comparison, a review of 15 years of bacterial isolates from cases of keratitis in Great Britain showed that the *Pseudomonas* species increased in proportion to organisms identified, but there was no overall increase in the proportion of Gram-negative isolates.[119]

Not only are there no specific signs or symptoms that are pathognomonic to distinguish the bacteria responsible for bacterial keratitis but also there are many factors that may alter the clinical presentation, such as previous use of topical antibiotics or corticosteroids or underlying systemic diseases. Nonetheless, some characteristic features of the infiltrative ulcer may provide clues to the causal microorganisms.

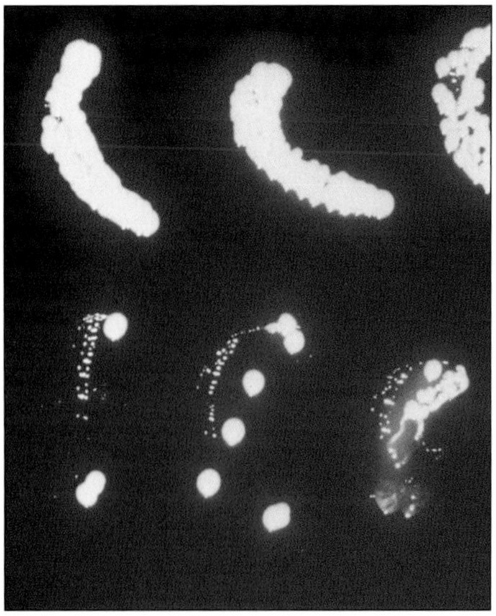

Fig. 77.10 Pearly-white colonies of *Staphylococcus aureus* in C streaks on a blood agar plate from a corneal ulcer. Diminishing numbers of colonies are noted in the consecutive C streaks, indicating the organisms are from bona fide infection rather than contamination of the plate.

Staphylococci

Staphylococcus, the most common Gram-positive organism, is usually present in normal ocular flora. The bacteria grow easily on routine culture media as pearly white colonies (Fig. 77.10). *Staphylococcus* keratitis occurs more frequently in compromised cornea cases such as bullous keratopathy, chronic herpetic keratitis, keratoconjunctivitis sicca, ocular rosacea, or atopic keratoconjunctivitis.

S. aureus tends to produce a rapidly progressive corneal infiltration and moderate anterior chamber reactions with endothelial plaques or hypopyon. The corneal lesions usually are round or oval with dense infiltration and a distinct border (Fig. 77.11), but occasionally a stromal microabscess with an ill-defined border may develop. Methicillin-resistant *Staphylococcus aureus* (MRSA) has been isolated with increasing frequency from patients with bacterial keratitis[120] and has been reported following keratorefractive surgery.[121]

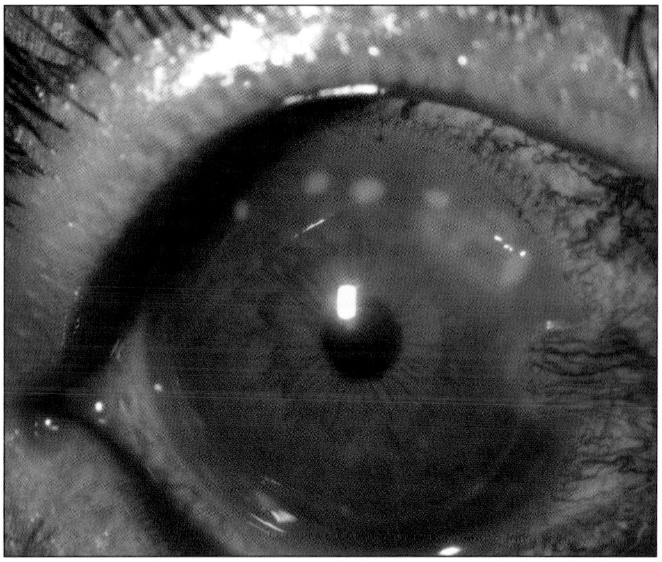

Fig. 77.11 A large peripheral corneal ulcer of *Staphylococcus aureus* with several smaller infiltrates in a patient with marked blepharitis.

Coagulase-negative *staphylococci* usually cause opportunistic infection in the compromised cornea. More than 85% of eyelid cultures from the normal population are positive for nonaureus *staphylococcus*,[122] and this is the most frequently isolated organism from bacterial keratitis.[123] The infection tends to progress slowly and the infiltrates are usually superficial, localized with the surrounding cornea clear. However, severe ulcers with dense infiltrates can occur if untreated.

Streptococci

Streptococcus pneumoniae keratitis usually occurs after corneal trauma, dacryocystitis, or filtering bleb infection. The ulcer tends to be acute, purulent, and rapidly progressive with a deep stromal abscess (Fig. 77.12). The anterior chamber reaction is usually severe with marked hypopyon and retrocorneal fibrin coagulation. A culture appears nonhemolytic on a blood or chocolate agar plate (Fig. 77.13). Perforation secondary to ulcer is common. A distinct, indolent crystalline keratopathy has also been reported.[124]

Nocardia

Nocardia asteroides grow slowly as small white colonies on the culture plate (Fig. 77.14), and is a variably acid-fast and Gram-positive bacillus in branching filaments (Fig. 77.15).

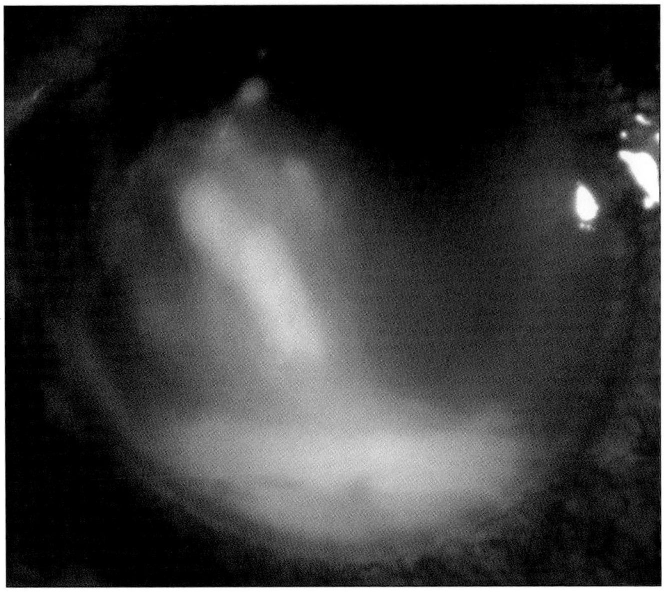

Fig. 77.12 A *Streptococcus pneumoniae* corneal ulcer in an immunocompromised patient with deep stromal infiltrates and dense hypopyon.

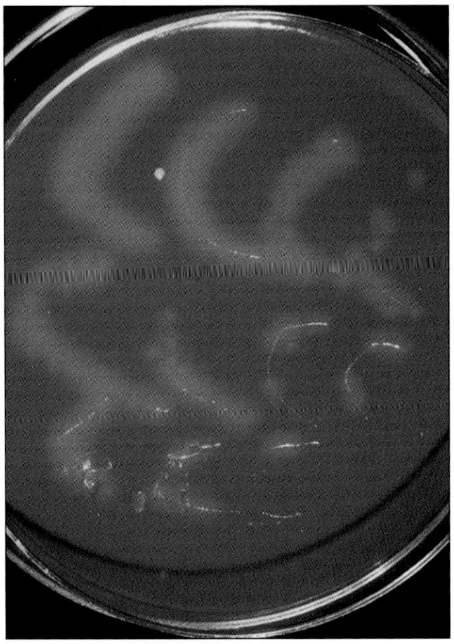

Fig. 77.13 Heavy growth of nonhemolytic *Streptococcus pneumoniae* on a chocolate agar plate.

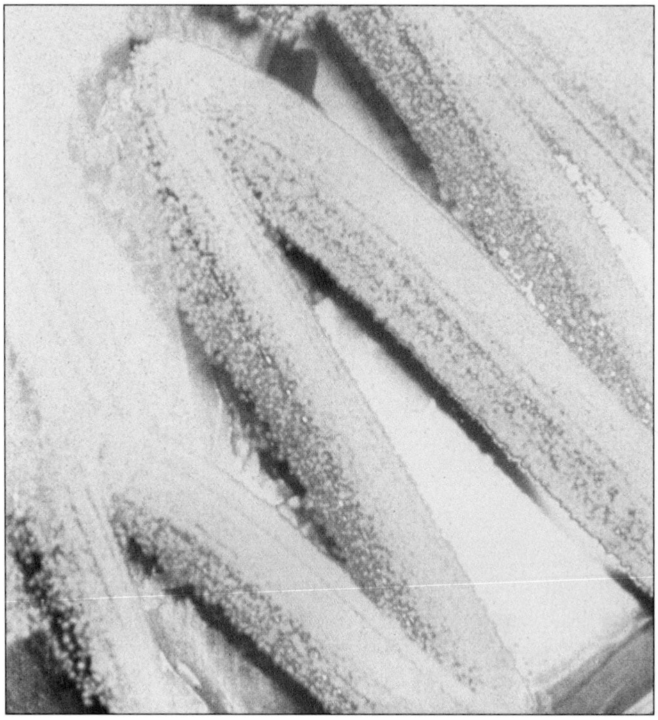

Fig. 77.14 Confluent growth of small white colonies of *Nocardia asteroides*.

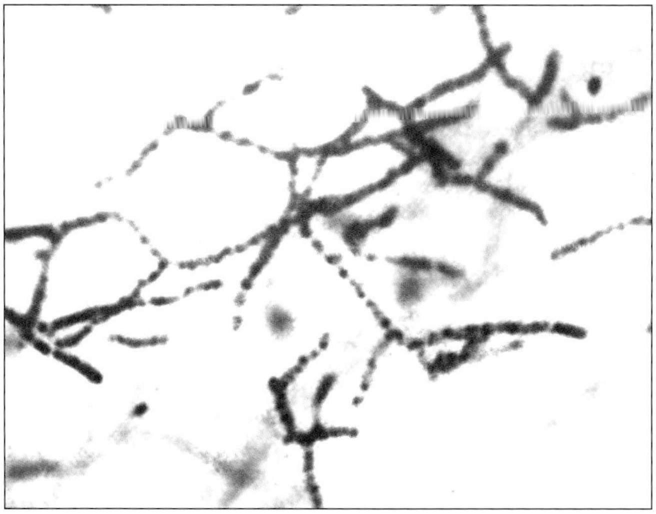

Fig. 77.15 Branching Gram-positive and variably acid-fast *Nocardia* arranged as pseudohyphae from a corneal scraping.

It tends to produce indolent ulcer after minor trauma, particularly with exposure to contaminated soil.[125] The keratitis usually waxes and wanes. *Nocardia* can survive within neutrophils and macrophages associated with production of superoxide dismutase. The characteristic features of *Nocardia* keratitis include raised, superficial pinhead-like infiltrates in a wreathlike configuration (Fig. 77.16), brush fire border, cracked windshield appearance, and multifocal or satellite lesions. The keratitis may simulate mycotic infection.

Nontuberculous mycobacteria

This is a class of rapidy growing and acid-fast mycobacteria, previously known as atypical mycobacteria. The most common pathogens are *Mycobacterium fortuitum* and *M. chelonei*, which may be found in soil and water. These organisms tend to cause a slowly progressive keratitis, and usually occur after a corneal foreign body, corneal trauma (Fig. 77.17) or following corneal surgery, particularly after LASIK

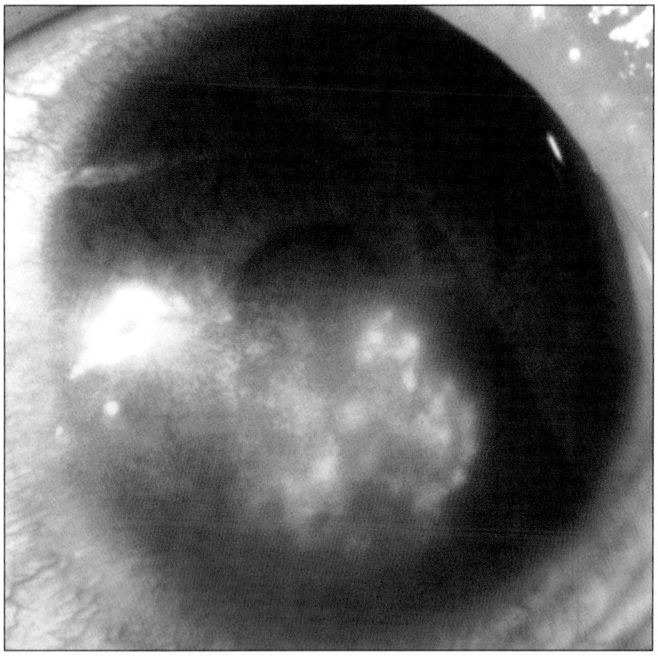

Fig. 77.16 Trauma-related *Nocardia* keratitis with multifocal chalky white infiltrates in a wreathlike configuration on the leading edge.

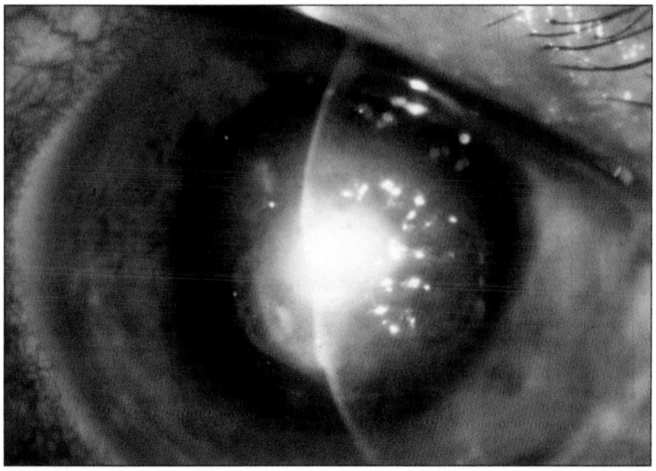

Fig. 77.17 Nontuberculous *Mycobacterium* keratitis with a central stromal infiltrate with surrounding corneal edema and minimum associated inflammation.

(see Fig. 77.5).[75,76,126,127] Keratitis from nontuberculous mycobacteria is often associated with delayed onset of symptoms, and severe ocular pain can develop from 2 to 8 weeks after exposure to the organism. Infiltrates are typically nonsuppurative and can be solitary or multifocal, with variable anterior chamber reactions. Delay in diagnosis is common due to the protracted clinical course and difficulty of isolating the organism from culture. The diagnosis may be confirmed with acid-fast stain or culture on Lowenstein-Jensen medium. (Fig. 77.18). Lack of response to conventional antibiotic therapy is usually a clue to the diagnosis of this unusual keratitis.

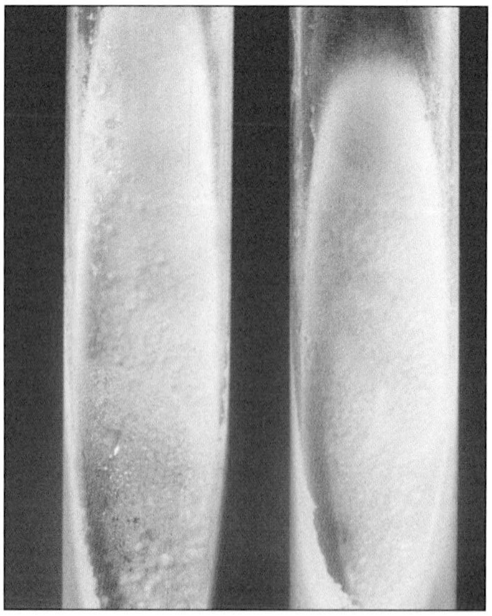

Fig. 77.18 Confluent growth of small colonies of nontuberculous *Mycobacterium* on Lowenstein-Jensen medium.

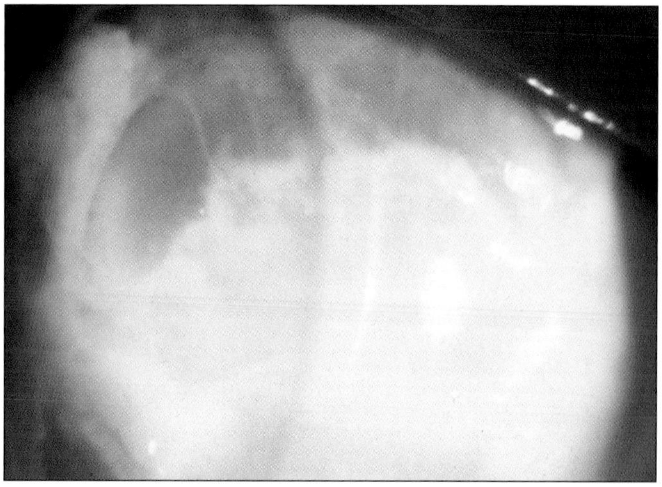

Fig. 77.19 Extensive stromal necrosis with mucopurulent discharge in a *Pseudomonas* keratitis.

Pseudomonas

Pseuodmonas aeruginosa is the most common Gram-negative pathogen isolated from severe keratitis. The increasing prevalence of *Pseudomonas* keratitis in otherwise healthy individuals has been largely associated with the use of soft contact lenses. Rapid progression, dense stromal infiltrate, marked suppuration, liquefactive necrosis, and descemetocele formation or corneal perforation are the characteristics of this pathogen (Fig. 77.19). The remaining uninvolved cornea usually has a ground-glass appearance and diffuse graying of epithelium. Despite appropriate treatment, the keratitis may progress rapidly into a deep stromal abscess and stromal keratolysis with perforation may occur. A corneal ring infiltrate, which is a dense accumulation and aggregation of polymorphonuclear leukocytes, can also be

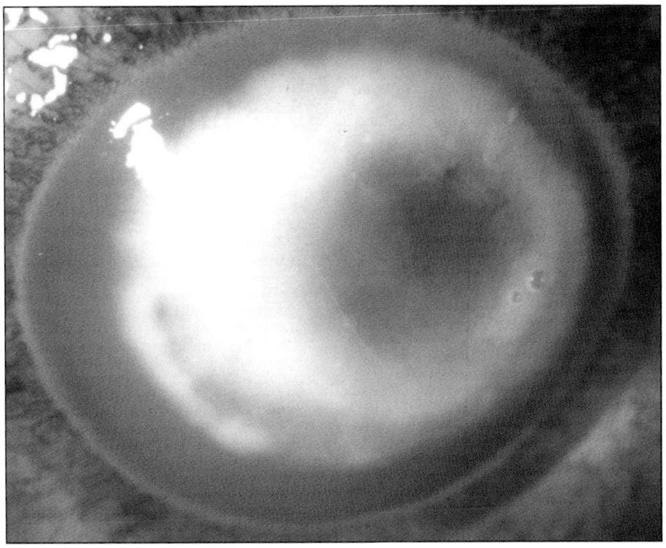

Fig. 77.20 A ring of necrotic stromal infiltrate in a *Pseudomonas* keratitis, simulating *Acanthamoeba* keratitis.

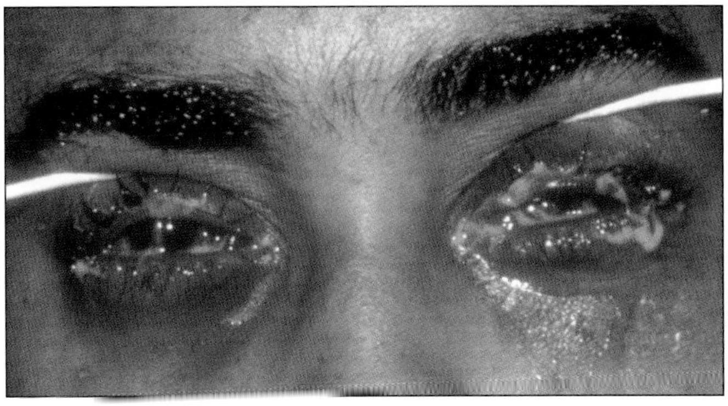

Fig. 77.21 Acute mucopurulent discharge in a patient with *Neisseria gonorrhoeae* keratoconjunctivitis.

present (Fig. 77.20). The other less common clinical presentation of *Pseudomonas* keratitis associated with contact lens use is multiple elevated granular opacities caused by less virulent species with a more indolent course.[128,129]

Neisseria

Keratitis caused by *N. gonorrhoeae* or *N. meningitides* is usually presented with rapidly progressive, hyperpurulent conjunctivitis and chemosis (Fig. 77.21).[130] These organisms are obligate intracellular Gram-negative cocci. These ulcers can lead to rapid corneal perforation. Conjunctivitis and keratitis caused by *N. gonorrhoeae* needs to be treated aggressively with systemic ceftriaxone because of its destructive nature and ability to penetrate intact corneal epithelium.[131]

Bacillus

Bacillus cereus, a Gram-positive bacillus, can cause a rapid and devastating keratitis following trauma or wound contamination. *B. cereus* keratitis is characterized by a distinctive stromal ring infiltrate (see Fig. 77.1) remote from the site of injury, with rapid progression to stromal abscess, corneal perforation, and intraocular extension with destruction mediated by specific exotoxins.[132,133]

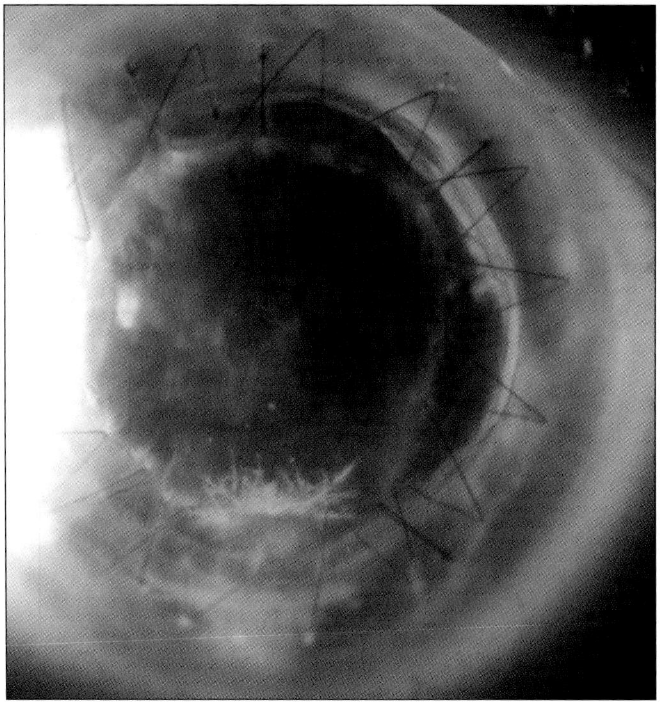

Fig. 77.22 Infectious crystalline keratitis from *Streptococcus viridans* in a corneal graft with chronic corticosteroid use.

Infectious crystalline keratopathy

The condition is characterized by minimal stromal inflammation with fine needle-like extensions in the corneal stroma, resembling a snowflake (Fig. 77.22). The most common causative organism is alpha-hemolytic *streptococci*.[134] Other organisms include *Streptococcus pneumoniae*,[124] *Staphylococcus epidermidis*,[135] *Peptostreptococcus*, *Haemophilus aphrophilus*,[136] *Pseudomonas*,[137] *Acinetobacter*, *Citrobacter*, *Enterobacter*, and *Stenotrophomonas*.[138] *Mycobacterium fortuitum*,[137] *Candida albicans*,[139] and other fungi[140] have also been isolated. Organisms with low virulence invade the cornea and replicate, but incite little host response. Colonies of bacteria grow into the cornea through interlamellar spaces, so the keratitis can be seen as linear, crystal-like structures in the stroma. Unlike other bacterial corneal ulcers, infectious crystalline keratopathy usually has an intact epithelium and is not associated with severe stromal inflammation. Risk factors include prior surgery, particularly after penetrating keratoplasty, wearing a therapeutic contact lens, chronic use of topical corticosteroids, and topical anesthetic abuse. Definitive diagnosis requires isolation of the causative organisms. To obtain an adequate corneal specimen for diagnosis of this type of keratitis, use of a 25-gauge needle or corneal biopsy to get crystalline lesions in deep stroma may be considered.

Laboratory Investigations

Cultures and smears

Laboratory investigations of microbial keratitis include corneal scraping to obtain specimens for microbiological stainings and cultures to isolate the causative organism[141] and determine sensitivity to antibiotics.[142] The majority of community-acquired cases of bacterial keratitis resolve with empirical therapy and are managed without smears or cultures.[143,144] Prior to initiating antimicrobial therapy, smears and cultures are indicated in cases where the corneal infiltrate is central, large, deep, is chronic in nature, or has atypical clinical features suggestive of fungal, amoebic, or mycobacterial keratitis. In addition, cultures are helpful to guide modification of therapy in patients with a poor clinical response to empirical treatment[145] and to decrease toxicity by eliminating unnecessary drugs. The hypopyon that occurs in eyes with bacterial keratitis is usually sterile (see Fig. 77.12) and aqueous or vitreous taps should not be performed in order to avoid intraocular inoculation of the microorganisms, unless there is a high suspicion of microbial endophthalmitis.

Culture

Obtaining corneal materials for microbial culture is most easily performed with slit lamp magnification under topical anesthesia. Proparacaine hydrochloride 0.5% is the preferred anesthetic agent because of its minimal inhibitory effects on organism recovery. Use of other topical anesthetics, such as tetracaine, may significantly reduce organism recovery due to their bacteriostatic effects. Culture yield may be improved by avoiding anesthetics with preservatives.[146] Corneal material is obtained by scraping corneal tissues from the advancing borders of the infected area using either a wet Dacron/calcium alginate or sterile cotton swab,[147] a heat-sterilized platinum (Kimura) spatula, a No. 15 Bard-Parker blade,[147] a jeweler's forceps, a large-gauge disposable needle, or a Minitip Culturette.[148] A small trephine may be necessary to obtain an adequate corneal biopsy specimen for ulcers with primary deep stromal involvement. Multiple samples from the advancing borders of representative areas of the ulcer are often required to achieve maximal yield of organisms.[142] Obtaining only purulent material usually results in inadequate yield. Corneal specimens obtained from corneal scrapings are usually small in quantity and should be inoculated directly onto appropriate culture media in order to maximize culture yield (Table 77.2).[149] If this is not feasible, specimens should be placed into a broth culture medium (Fig. 77.23) prior to transportation. This has been reported to generate satisfactory yields of causative organisms.[150] Cultures of contact lenses, lens case, and contact lens solution may provide additional information to guide therapy.

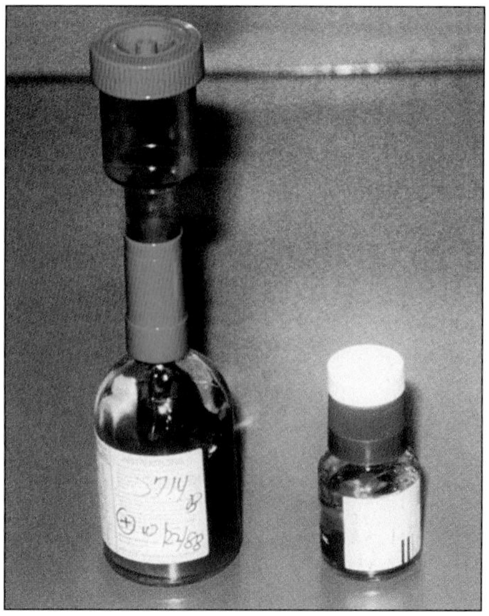

Fig. 77.23 Broth medium can be used to transport culture materials.

Table 77.2 Culture media for bacterial keratitis

Standard media	Common isolates
Blood agar	Aerobic and facultative, anaerobic bacteria, including *P. aeruginosa*, *S. aureus*, *S. epidermidis*, *S. pneumoniae*
Chocolate agar	Aerobic and facultative, anaerobic bacteria, including *H. influenzae*, *N. gonorrhoeae*, and *Bartonella* species
Thioglycollate broth	Aerobic and facultative, anaerobic bacteria
Supplemental media	
Anaerobic blood agar (CDC, Schaediler, Brucella)	*P. acnes*, *Peptostreptococcus*
Lowenstein-Jensen medium	*Mycobacterium* species, *Nocardia* species
Middlebrook agar	*Mycobacterium* species
Thayer-Martin agar	Pathogenic *Neisseria* species

Note: Fungi and Acanthamoeba *can be recovered on blood agar. However, more specific media are available (for fungi: Sabouraud's dextrose agar, brain-heart infusion; for* Acanthamoeba*: buffered charcoal yeast extract, blood agar with* E. coli *overlay).*
Data from Preferred practice pattern: bacterial keratitis. *American Academy of Ophthalmology, 2008.*[234]

The commonly used culture media for bacterial keratitis are listed in Table 77.2. Blood agar is a standard medium for isolation of aerobic bacteria at 35°C (see Fig. 77.10). It also supports the growth of saprophytic fungi and *Nocardia* at room temperature. The agar is derived from seaweed with the addition of 5–10% red blood cells to provide nutrients as well as an index of hemolysis. Chocolate agar is incubated at 35°C with 10% carbon dioxide to isolate facultative organisms. It is prepared by heat denaturation of blood to provide hemin and diphosphopyridine nucleotide for the growth of *Neisseria*, *Moraxella*, and *Haemophilus* (Fig. 77.24). Thioglycolate broth is a liquid medium and is incubated at 35°C for aerobic and anaerobic bacteria. Sabouraud agar is incubated at room temperature for fungi and *Nocardia* (see

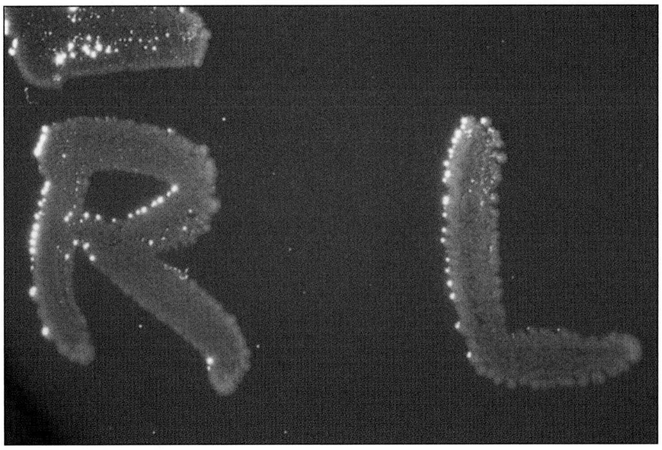

Fig. 77.24 Confluent growth of *Haemophilus influenzae* from eyelid culture on a chocolate agar plate.

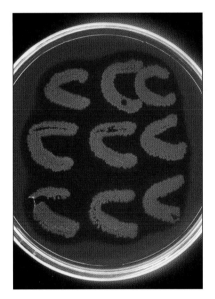

Fig. 77.25 Growth of *Pseudomonas aeruginosa* in C streaks on a blood agar plate.

Fig. 77.14). Lowenstein-Jensen medium incubated at 35°C is used specifically to isolate mycobacteria (see Fig. 77.18). The Thayer-Martin medium is a selective, chemically enriched, chocolate agar that allows the isolation of *Neisseria gonorrhoeae* by suppressing the growth of other inhibitory bacteria and fungi. Brain-heart infusion (BHI) broth, is used to enhance the recovery of filamentous fungi and yeasts.

While plating the culture medium, the specimen should be inoculated in C streaks to distinguish valid bacterial growth from plating contamination (Fig. 77.25).[151] If the quantity of specimen is limited, a single inoculation into chocolate agar or thioglycolate broth can be considered.[149] For aerobic and anaerobic cultures of ocular specimens, the cornea should be held for 7 days and 7 to 14 days, respectively, before being reported as no-growth. Mycobacterial and fungal cultures should be held for 4 to 6 weeks before being reported as no-growth.

Indications for reculture

Lack of a favorable clinical response, particularly in the setting of negative cultures results, suggest the need for reculture and/or corneal biopsy. Toxicity from medications or corticosteroid withdrawal may be confused with antibiotic failure, and medicamentosa may be a potential cause of an apparent lack of clinical improvement. Discontinuation of antibiotics for 12 to 24 hours prior to reculture may increase culture yield, as may avoidance of preserved solutions, such as anesthetics or cycloplegic agents.

Stains

Microbial pathogens may be categorized by examining stained smears of corneal scrapings.[143,152] The material for smear is applied to a clean glass microscope slide in an even, thin layer for microbial staining (Table 77.3 for specific diagnostic stains). Immersion of the slide in methanol 95% or cold acetone in a Coplin jar for 5 to 10 minutes is preferable to heat fixation because this preserves a better morphology of cells and microorganisms.

Gram stain is used routinely to stain the corneal specimens. This stain can confirm the presence of a microorganism with a sensitivity of 55–79%.[143,153] It can also distinguish bacteria from fungi. Gram-positive bacteria retain the gentian violet–iodine complex and appear bluish-purple. Gram-negative bacteria lose the gentian violet–iodine complex by decolorization with acid alcohol and appear pink when counterstained with safranin.

Giemsa stain is primarily used to distinguish the types of inflammatory cells and intracytoplasmic inclusions, and can distinguish bacteria from fungi. Bacteria appear dark blue and fungi appear purple or blue. *Acanthamoeba* and *Chlamydia* inclusion bodies may be identified with Giemsa stains (Fig. 77.26). Acridine orange stain is also a useful screening test. It is a fluorochromatic dye that binds to ribonucleic acid. Microorganisms fluoresce orange whereas epithelial cells and polymorphonuclear leukocytes fluoresce green. An epifluorescence microscope is needed to visualize organisms and cells. The organisms that can be visualized by acridine orange include bacteria, fungi, *Acanthamoeba*, and *Mycobacterium* (weakly staining). The acridine orange stain accurately predicts culture results in 71–84% of the cases and has been reported to be more sensitive than Gram stain.[154] Calcofluor white, another fluorochromatic dye, binds to chitin and cellulose in the cell wall of fungi and *Acanthamoeba* cysts. These organisms stain bright green under epifluorescence microscopy.

Carbol fuchsin or Ziehl-Neelsen acid-fast stains are for identification of suspected *Mycobacterium*, *Actinomyces*, or *Nocardia*. Some of these organisms contain a specific lipid wax fraction that is resistant to decolorization by strong mineral acids after being stained by basic carbol fuchsin. Mycobacteria are acid-fast. *Nocardia* is variably stained (see Fig. 77.15), while *Actinomyces* is not acid-fast.

Antimicrobial susceptibility testing

Organisms that are often considered as nonpathogenic in a general laboratory can still be corneal pathogens. The anti-

Table 77.3 Diagnostic stains for bacterial keratitis

Type of stain	Organisms visualized	Comments
Gram stain*	Best for bacteria; can also visualize fungi,† *Acanthamoeba*	Distinguishes Gram-positive from Gram-negative organisms; widely available; rapid (5 minutes)
Giemsa stain*	Bacteria, fungi,† *Chlamydia*, *Acanthamoeba*‡	Basis for Aema-color and Diff-Quik tests; widely available; rapid (2 minutes)
Acid fast	*Mycobacterium*, *Nocardia*	Widely available; takes 1 hour; reliable stain for *Mycobacterium*
Acridine orange*	Bacteria, fungi,† *Acanthamoeba*‡	Requires use of epifluorescence microscope; rapid (2 minutes)
Calcofluor white	Fungi,† *Acanthamoeba*‡	Requires use of epifluorescence microscope; rapid (2 minutes)

**Most useful stains for screening purposes.*
†PAS (periodic acid-Schiff) and GMS (Gomori methenamine silver) also can be used to identify fungi.
‡H&E (hematoxylin and eosin) and PAS also can be used to identify Acanthamoeba.
Data from Preferred practice pattern: bacterial keratitis. *American Academy of Ophthalmology, 2008.*[234]

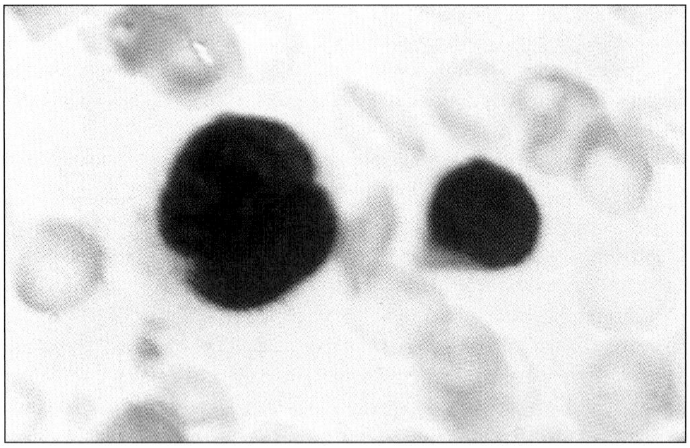

Fig. 77.26 Inclusion bodies of *Chlamydia* by Giemsa stain.

biotics chosen for sensitivity testing should be appropriate and include agents readily available for topical ophthalmic preparations.[155] Standard disk diffusion or microdilution techniques are the preferred laboratory methods for antimicrobial susceptibility testing of bacterial ocular isolates. However, the results of disk diffusion relate to levels of drug in serum rather than the high concentration achievable in ocular tissues. Minimal inhibitory concentration (MIC) may provide more useful information, however, for microbial keratitis. It approximates drug levels at the site of infection based on experimental data. The precise resistance breakpoints for ocular isolates have not been well determined because of lack of data on actual drug concentrations in ocular tissues when affected by bacterial keratitis.[156]

Other Diagnostic Tools

Corneal biopsy

Corneal biopsy may be indicated if there has been a lack of response to treatment[157–159] or if cultures have been negative on more than one occasion and the clinical picture continues to suggest strongly an infectious process. It may also be indicated if the infiltrate is located in the mid or deep stroma with overlying uninvolved tissue that yield little material with scraping.[157,158] In a cooperative patient, corneal biopsy may be performed while at the slit lamp or operating microscope. Using topical anesthesia, a 2–3-mm circular trephine can be used to outline the area to be biopsied. The stromal tissue specimen should be large enough to allow bisection so that one portion can be sent for culture and the other for histopathology. Biopsy should be planned in consultation with microbiologists and pathologists to ensure proper specimen handling and tissue fixation.[160] The biopsy specimen should be delivered to the laboratory in a timely fashion. The biopsy may also help ulcer healing by debulking or debridement of necrotic tissue. Biopsy from below a lamellar flap can be considered for a midstromal lesion such as infectious crystalline keratopathy, or a deep stromal lesion such as fungal keratitis. An option for a deep corneal abscess may be to use a suture that can be passed through the abscess without disturbing the overlying intact corneal epithelium and stroma. A 7-0 or 8-0 Vicryl or silk suture can be passed through the abscess. The pathogen may attach to the fibers of the suture, and the suture can then be cultured.

Impression cytology

Impression cytology has been used as a simple biopsy technique for diagnosing a variety of ocular surface diseases.[161] A millipore filter is pressed on the cornea or conjunctiva to effectively remove cells from the surface of the epithelium. Many investigators have used this technique to acquire cells for cytologic analysis of dry eye conditions and ocular surface neoplasia.[162–167] Impression cytology also has been used to debride dendritic epithelial keratitis by herpes simplex virus.[168,169] It can also isolate *Acanthamoeba* from superficial *Acanthamoeba* keratitis.[170,171] It can also facilitate organism identification by collecting microbial nucleic acids for molecular microbiology or collecting microbial antigens for immunocytochemistry.

Polymerase chain reaction (PCR) and immunodiagnostic techniques may be useful,[172,173] but they are not widely available in microbiology laboratories. Confocal microscopy is a noninvasive in vivo diagnostic method for microbial keratitis.[174] The tandem scanning slit lamp of the confocal microscope permits real-time viewing of structures in the living cornea at the cellular level in four dimensions (*x*, *y*, *z*, and time). It has been successfully used to distinguish some unusual pathogens such as *Acanthamoeba* cysts or fungal hyphae. However, the current resolution of the commercially available confocal microscopes limits their use as a diagnostic tool for bacterial keratitis.[175]

Specific Therapeutic Agents

Cephalosporins

Like penicillins, cephalosporins contain a β-lactam ring that is necessary for bactericidal activity. The nucleus of cephalosporins is 7-aminocephalosporanic acid, which is resistant to the action of penicillinases produced by staphylococci.

Cefazolin, with an excellent activity against Gram-positive pathogens and minimal toxicity after topical administration, has been the most commonly used first-generation cephalosporin for bacterial keratitis. It is most frequently used in combination with other agents against Gram-negative bacteria to provide a broad spectrum of coverage for polymicrobial keratitis, or if the causative organisms are unknown.

Ceftazidime is a third-generation cephalosporin with antipseudomonal activity. It is used in *Pseudomonas* keratitis with resistance to aminoglycosides or fluoroquinolones. Ceftazidime also has some activity against Gram-positive organisms.

Topical β-lactam antibiotics have never been available commercially because they are somewhat unstable in solution and tend to break down in days or weeks. A fresh preparation must be provided every 4–5 days.

Glycopeptides

Vancomycin is a glycopeptide antibiotic with activity against penicillin-resistant staphylococci. Its bactericidal effect is related to the inhibition of biosynthesis of peptidoglycan polymers during bacterial cell wall formation. It is primarily active against Gram-positive bacteria and remains one of the most potent antibiotics against methicillin-resistant *S. aureus* and coagulase-negative *staphylococci*. Vancomycin should be reserved for cephalosporin-resistant *staphylococci*. *Streptococci* (including penicillin-resistant strains) are also highly susceptible to vancomycin. Vancomycin has excellent activity against a variety of other Gram-positive bacilli including *Clostridium*, *Corynebacterium*, *Bacillus*, *L. monocytogenes*, *Actinomyces*, and *Lactobacillus*.

Aminoglycosides

Aminoglycosides have a selective affinity to the bacterial 30-S and 50-S ribosomal subunits to produce a nonfunctional 70-S initiation complex that, in turn, facilitates the inhibition of bacterial protein synthesis. Aminoglycosides have a bactericidal effect against aerobic and facultative Gram-negative bacilli. However, there is emergence of *Pseudomonas* resistance to gentamicin,[118] tobramycin, and to a lesser extent, amikacin. For severe *Pseudomonas* keratitis, aminoglycosides may be combined with an antipseudomonal cephalosporin. For *Nocardia* keratitis, amikacin has also been reported to be effective[176] and remains the drug of choice.[125] Although commercially prepared aminoglycosides are adequate for mild to moderate keratoconjunctivitis, many ophthalmologists prefer to use more concentrated preparations for severe bacterial keratitis (Table 77.4 and Box 77.1).

Macrolides

Macrolides such as erythromycin contain a macrocyclic lactone ring for sugar attachment. They inhibit bacterial protein synthesis by reversibly binding to the 50-S ribosomal subunit, thereby preventing elongation of the peptide chain in susceptible bacteria. Erythromycin has a relatively broad spectrum of activity, especially against most Gram-positive and some Gram-negative bacteria. Erythromycin may be either bacteriostatic or bactericidal, depending on the concentration of drug, organism susceptibility, growth rate, and size of the inoculum. *S. pneumoniae* and *S. pyogenes* are both highly susceptible to erythromycin with occasional resistant strains. Erythromycin also has generally good activity against most *S. viridans* and anaerobic *streptococci*. It has variable activity against *Enterococcus*, *Actinomyces*, *Nocardia*, *Chlamydia*, and certain nontuberculous *mycobacteria*.[177] Many *S. aureus* and coagulase-negative *staphylococci* are susceptible, although there may be increasing resistance.[177] Most strains of *N. gonorrhoeae* and *N. meningitides* are susceptible to erythromycin. Many strains of *H. influenzae* are only moderately susceptible. Erythromycin is rarely, if ever, indicated in infection caused by Gram-negative bacteria due to their resistance to the antibiotic. The cell walls of most Gram-negative bacilli prevent the passive diffusion of erythromycin into the cell.

Erythromycin ointment is one of the best-tolerated and least toxic topical ophthalmic antibiotics, commonly used for blepharitis. However, its penetration into the cornea is suboptimal secondary to its relative lack of solubility and bioavailability.

Newer macrolides including azithromycin, clarithromycin, and roxithromycin have higher tissue levels and are more favorable for treating intracellular pathogens, including *C. trachomatis* and nontuberculous *mycobacteria*. Topical suspensions of clarithromycin[178–180] and azithromycin[179] have been used to treat of nontuberculous *mycobacterial* infections. Because of their poor solubility and limited corneal penetration, topical preparations of these newer macrolides may have a limited role for bacterial keratitis.

Fluoroquinolones

The newest family of antibacterial agents to receive US Food and Drug Administration approval for bacterial keratitis is that of the fluoroquinolone compounds. The bactericidal action is due to inhibition of bacterial DNA gyrase and topoisomerase IV, which are enzymes essential for bacterial DNA synthesis. The second and third generation of fluoroquinolones, such as ciprofloxacin, ofloxacin, and levofloxacin, are commercially available for ophthalmic use and

Table 77.4 Antibiotic therapy of bacterial keratitis

Organism	Antibiotic	Topical concentration	Subconjunctival dose
No organism identified or multiple types of organisms	Cefazolin with Tobramycin or gentamicin or Fluoroquinolones*	50 mg/mL 9–14 mg/mL Various†	100 mg in 0.5 mL 20 mg in 0.5 mL
Gram-positive cocci	Cefazolin Vancomycin‡ Bacitracin‡ Fluoroquinolones*	50 mg/mL 15–50 mg/mL 10 000 IU Various†	100 mg in 0.5 mL 25 mg in 0.5 mL
Gram-negative rods	Tobramycin or gentamicin Ceftazidime Fluoroquinolones	9–14 mg/mL 50 mg/mL Various†	20 mg in 0.5 mL 100 mg in 0.5 mL
Gram-negative cocci§	Ceftriaxone Ceftazidime Fluoroquinolones	50 mg/mL 50 mg/mL Various†	100 mg in 0.5 mL 100 mg in 0.5 mL
Nontuberculous mycobacteria	Amikacin Clarithromycin Azithromycin Fluoroquinolones	20–40 mg/mL 10 mg/mL 10 mg/mL Various†	20 mg in 0.5 mL
Nocardia	Sulfacetamide Amikacin Trimethoprim/sulfamethoxazole: Trimethoprim Sulfamethoxazole	100 mg/mL 20–40 mg/mL 16 mg/mL 80 mg/mL	20 mg in 0.5 mL

**Fewer Gram-positive cocci are resistant to gatifloxacin and moxifloxacin than other fluoroquinolones.*
†Ciprofloxacin 3 mg/mL; gatifloxacin 3 mg/mL; levofloxacin 15 mg/mL; moxifloxacin 5 mg/mL; ofloxacin 3 mg/mL, all commercially available at these concentrations.
‡For resistant Enterococcus *and* Staphylococcus *species and penicillin allergy. Vancomycin and bacitracin have no Gram-negative activity and should not be used as a single agent in empirically treating bacterial keratitis.*
§Systemic therapy is necessary for suspected gonococcal infection.
Data from Basic Clinical and Science Course 2008–2009, Section 8; External Disease and Cornea. *Table 7-7. American Academy of Ophthalmology.*

have similar antimicrobial spectra, including most Gram-negative and some Gram-positive bacteria.[181] The first two agents have been tested by double-masked clinical trials to compare their efficacy with conventional fortified antibiotics.[182] No difference in efficacy was noted for the treatment of common ocular pathogens.[183–186] Among those pathogens tested, *Streptococcus pneumoniae* was noted to respond less to fluoroquinolone than to conventional fortified cefazolin. Other organisms that responded less favorably to fluoroquinolone monotherapy include *S. viridans*, anaerobic *Streptococcus* in crystalline keratopathy,[187] methicillin-resistant *Staphylococcus aureus*,[188,189] non-aeruginosa *Pseudomonas*, and anaerobes.

The wide use of fluoroquinolone monotherapy has imposed a risk of emergence of resistant strains of microorganisms.[118,190–193] Increasing resistance of *Pseudomonas aeruginosa*[194,195] and Gram-positive organisms such as *Staphylococcus aureus* and streptococcus species[118] to fluoroquinolones has been reported. There is also growing evidence for resistance of *Staphylococcus aureus* to third-generation fluoroquinolones, from 5.8% in 1993 to 35% in 1997.[190]

The latest fourth-generation fluoroquinolones such as gatifloxacin and moxifloxacin have been developed with an expanded antimicrobial spectrum to combat these resistant strains.[196] In randomized, controlled trials, both moxifloxacin and gatifloxacin performed at least as well as standard therapy, fortified cefazolin/tobramycin combination therapy, and potentially better than an earlier-generation fluoroquinolone, ciprofloxacin.[197,198] The fourth-generation fluoroquinolones have been reported to have better coverage of Gram-positive pathogens as compared to earlier-generation fluoroquinolones in head-to-head in vitro studies.[199]

Side effects of fluoroquinolone are minimal. The incidence of ocular discomfort for patients receiving topical fluoroquinolone is significantly less when compared with patients receiving fortified antibiotics (5.7% vs 13.4%).[184] Crystalline corneal deposits after use of ciprofloxacin[200] (Fig. 77.27), norfloxacin,[201] and ofloxacin[202] have been reported. These deposits occur with higher frequency in ciprofloxacin-treated eyes, consistent with the pH solubility profile of fluoroquinolone compounds in that ciprofloxacin is less soluble at physiological pH.[203] However, these deposits are precipitates of the antibiotics and do not appear to diminish the antimicrobial effect.[204] Although there have been some concerns of increased risk of corneal perforation with fluoroquinolones in the treatment of severe bacterial keratitis compared with traditional fortified topical antibiotics (cefazolin and tobramycin),[205] these reports are retrospective, not from randomized, controlled trials, and will need confirmation in

Box 77.1 Preparation of fortified topical antibiotics

Cefazolin 50 mg/mL or ceftazidime 50 mg/mL
1. Add 9.2 mL of artificial tears to a vial of cefazolin, 1 g (powder for injection)
2. Dissolve. Take 5 mL of this solution and add it to 5 mL of artificial tears
3. Refrigerate and shake well before instillation

Tobramycin 14 mg/mL or gentamicin 14 mg/mL
1. Withdraw 2 mL from an injectable vial of intravenous tobramycin or gentamicin (40 mg/mL)
2. Add the withdrawn 2 mL to 5 mL of commercial tobramycin or gentamicin ophthalmic solution (3 mg/mL) to give a 14 mg/mL solution

Vancomycin 15 mg/mL, vancomycin 25 mg/mL, or vancomycin 50 mg/mL
1. To a 500-mg vial of vancomycin:
   a. Add 33 mL of 0.9% sodium chloride for injection USP (no preservatives) or artificial tears to produce a solution of 15 mg/mL
   b. Add 20 mL of 0.9% sodium chloride for injection USP (no preservatives) or artificial tears to produce a solution of 25 mg/mL
   c. Add 10 mL of 0.9% sodium chloride for injection USP (no preservatives) or artificial tears to produce a solution of 50 mg/mL
2. Refrigerate and shake well before instillation

Amikacin
Intravenous formulation can be used (80 mg/2 cc ampules)

Trimethoprim/sulfamethoxazole
16 mg/mL and 80 mg/mL commercial preparation can be used

Adapted from Basic Clinical and Science Course 2008–2009, Section 8; External Disease and Cornea. *Table 7-7. American Academy of Ophthalmology.*

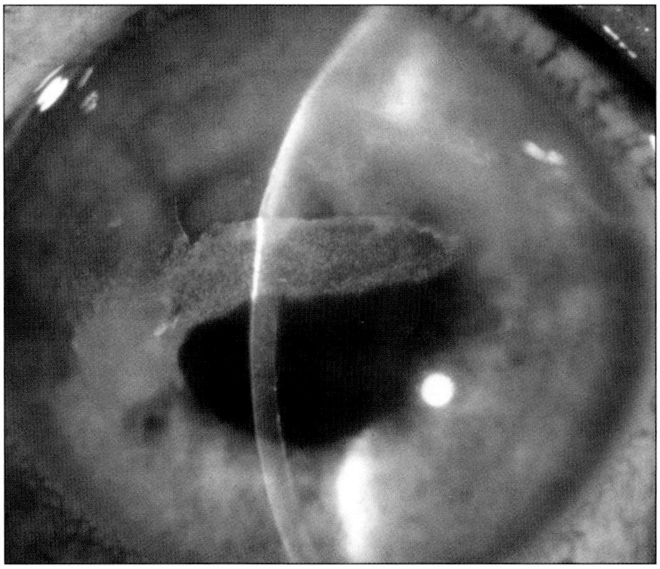

Fig. 77.27 Crystalline deposits of ciprofloxacin in a partially resolved bacterial keratitis with mild stromal thinning.

future studies. Alteration of corneal collagens or keratocyte functions has been attributed to fluoroquinolones.[205]

The greater potency and resistance-thwarting capabilities of the fourth-generation fluoroquinolones is due to strategic modifications to the molecule that have allowed it to overcome several bacterial defenses effectively. The third-generation fluoroquinolones only target DNA gyrase for Gram-negative organisms and topoisomerase IV for Gram-positive organisms. In contrast, the methoxy group (OCH_3) substitution at the eighth carbon on the basic ring of the fourth-generation quinolones enhances their antibacterial potency. The C8-methoxy group can tightly bind to both the bacterial enzymes DNA gyrase and topoisomerase IV. All bacteria contain at least one and usually both of these enzymes, which allows bacterial DNA to supercoil during replication. The C8-methoxy fluoroquinolones block the bacteria's ability to supercoil and cause DNA gyrase to nick bacterial DNA. With two killing mechanisms (i.e. activity against both topoisomerase IV and DNA gyrase), resistance to a C8-methoxy fluoroquinolone requires a bacterial strain to alter two target sites rather than one, and two simultaneous mutations are far less probable than a single-step mutation.[196] The result of this dual mechanism of action in fourth-generation fluoroquinolones is heightened efficacy against Gram-positive species with less propensity for bacteria to develop mutations and drug resistance. The C8-methoxy fluoroquinolones may also be effective against nontuberculosis *mycobacteria* and *Nocardia*.

Sulfonamide and trimethoprim

Sulfonamides have a structure similar to that of para-aminobenzoic acid (PABA). The mechanism of action is to competitively inhibit the bacterial synthesis of folic acid. The sulfonamides are primarily bacteriostatic at therapeutic concentrations.

Sulfonamides are active against Gram-positive and Gram-negative bacteria, although susceptibilities often are variable, even among susceptible pathogens. Many bacteria become highly resistant to sulfonamides during therapy because of chromosomal or plasmid-mediated transference. Topical sulfonamides are not first-line medications for most bacterial keratitis. However, they are conventionally used for *Nocardia* keratitis,[206] although a combination of trimethoprim and sulfamethoxazole (Bactrim) is proven to be more effective against *Nocardia*.[207]

Trimethoprim is a 2,4-diamino-pyrimidine that also inhibits bacterial folic acid synthesis. Trimethoprim is often combined with a sulfonamide to produce a synergistic antibacterial effect. Trimethoprim may be bacteriostatic or bactericidal, depending on the clinical situation. Trimethoprim is active against many Gram-positive cocci in vitro, although increasing resistance is observed among *staphylococci*. Trimethoprim has only minimal activity against *enterococci*. *P. aeruginosa* and most anaerobes are resistant to it.

Strategies for Initial Management

Topical antibiotic eye drops are capable of achieving high levels of tissue concentration and are the preferred method of treatment in most cases. Ointments may be useful adjunctive therapy and for use at bedtime in less severe cases, but may impair the penetration of concomitant topical eye drops.[153] Subconjunctival antibiotics may be helpful where there is imminent scleral spread or perforation or in cases where compliance with the treatment regimen is questionable. Systemic antibiotics may be considered in severe cases with scleral or intraocular extension of infection. Systemic therapy is necessary in cases of gonococcal keratitis due to its fulminant nature and systemic involvement.[131,208] Collagen shields[209,210] or soft contact lenses soaked in antibiotics are sometimes used and may enhance drug delivery. They may also be useful in cases where there is an anticipated delay in initiating appropriate therapy, but these modalities have not been fully evaluated in terms of the potential risk for inducing drug toxicity.[210,211] In addition, they can become displaced or lost, leading to unrecognized interruption of drug delivery. In selected cases, the choice of initial treatment may be guided by the results obtained from smears that are diagnostic.[153,212]

Topical broad-spectrum antibiotics are used initially in the empirical treatment of bacterial keratitis (see Table 77.4).[117,213,214] For central or severe keratitis, a loading dose every 5 to 15 minutes for the first hour, followed by applications every 15 minutes to 1 hour around the clock to achieve a sustained therapeutic level, is recommended.[215] For less severe keratitis, a regimen with less frequent dosing is appropriate. Cycloplegic agents may be used to decrease synechia formation and to decrease pain and ciliary spasm in more severe cases. Single-drug therapy using a fluoroquinolone (e.g. third or fourth generation) has been shown to be as effective as combination therapy utilizing antibiotics that are fortified by increasing their concentrations over those of commercially available topical antibiotics.[182,184] Some pathogens (e.g. *streptococci*, anaerobes) reportedly have variable susceptibility to fluoroquinolones,[216,217] and the prevalence of resistance to the fluoroquinolones appears to be increasing.[114,118,194,216] Combination fortified antibiotic therapy is an alternative to consider for severe infection and for eyes unresponsive to treatment.[191] Fluoroquinolones are poorly effective against methicillin-resistant *Staphylococcus aureus* (MRSA) ocular isolates,[218] which generally are sensitive to vancomycin. Due to the global emergence of MRSA, vancomycin should not be used routinely for Gram-positive cocci and should be reserved for severe or refractory infections. Treatment with more than one agent may be necessary for nontuberculous mycobacteria, which has been reported in association with LASIK.[75,76] Treatment options for nontuberculous mycobacteria include oral and topical clarithromycin, moxifloxacin, and gatifloxacin.[126,127] Amikacin, previously the only treatment option, has been largely replaced by these new treatment options.

Table 77.4 summarizes current recommendations by the American Academy of Ophthalmology in using antibiotic therapy for bacterial keratitis and Box 77.1 describes instructions for the preparation of fortified topical ophthalmic antibiotics. Frequency of reevaluation of the patient with bacterial keratitis depends on the extent of disease, but severe cases (e.g. deep stromal involvement or larger than 2 mm with extensive suppuration) initially should be followed at least daily until clinical improvement is documented. Several strategies for initial management of keratitis have been employed by ophthalmologists.[151,215,219–221]

Culture-guided approach

In this traditional approach, corneal scrapings for staining and microbiological culture are performed in all cases of microbial keratitis[222] before treatment is started. In partially treated patients, suspending the treatment for 12 to 24 hours before obtaining corneal specimens for culture may be necessary to improve the yield and decrease false-negative culture results. The initial therapy is based on the clinical and epidemiological information and may be modified according to microbiological results. These patients are more likely to have severe corneal ulcers or infections caused by atypical pathogens. This approach is also beneficial to monitor infectious trends through epidemiological surveys.

The major disadvantage of this approach is the inconvenience and cost. Cultures from routine corneal scrapings are positive in only 60% of patients.[145] In addition, antibiotic sensitivity is usually extrapolated from therapeutic antibiotic concentrations in serum, rather than from local ocular concentrations. Discrepancy between in vitro sensitivity and clinical response is often encountered.[153] It has been suggested that, if a cornea-specific sensitivity method could be routinely employed, the clinical choice of antibiotics would be greatly facilitated.[223]

Empirical approach

This approach is based on the pre-existing culture and sensitivity data without specifically obtaining corneal specimens from the patients. Clinicians use broad-spectrum antibiotics to cover potential causative organisms. Fortified antibiotics such as cefazolin or vancomycin for Gram-positive organisms and tobramycin or ceftazidime for Gram-negative organisms are used (see Table 77.4). However, prolonged and nonelective use of these fortified antibiotics may cause ocular discomfort and epithelial toxicity.

The important breakthrough in this empirical approach is the introduction of fluoroquinolone antibiotics, which have been shown by clinical trials to have an efficacy for common ocular pathogens equivalent to that of the fortified antibiotics.[183] However, there are potential gaps in the antibacterial spectrum of fluoroquinolone monotherapy. Therapy with cephalosporin or vancomycin is preferable in cases with suspected streptococcal infection in trauma-related keratitis. In the past, monotherapy with fluoroquinolone was generally recommended for contact lens-related *Pseudomonas* keratitis; however, increasing emergence of ciprofloxacin-resistant *P. aeruginosa* has been reported, and this treatment strategy should be exercised with caution.[194,195]

The advantages of this approach are convenience and cost-effectiveness. It is a preferred option for clinical practices outside academic centers.[224] A community survey demonstrated that in the USA approximately 50% of patients with microbial keratitis were treated without microbiologic work-ups. Only 6.3% of these patients failed to respond to treatment and required further subspecialty care.[145] This study also demonstrated that the cultures obtained after ineffective topical antibiotic therapy were usually positive for bacteria and the cultures were helpful in guiding subsequent appropriate therapy. One important drawback of this approach is that epidemiological data can no longer be collected for future reference and for monitoring of the potential emergence of resistant organisms.

Case-based approach

In this option, clinicians obtain corneal specimens before initial treatment only in selective cases with ulceration involving visual axis or with large, deep ulcers.[219] Microbiologic testing is also performed in keratitis associated with trauma, or contamination by vegetation materials or unsanitized water.

For small and peripheral ulcers, it is generally acceptable to initiate treatment without performing corneal cultures. Broad-spectrum antibiotics, either fortified or commercial preparations, are chosen based on the pre-existing community data. For central, large, and deep ulcers, the antibiotic should be chosen based on the microbiological information (Fig. 77.28).

This approach is practical, because a central corneal ulcer has a tendency to be more severe and sight-threatening than a peripheral ulcer. Clinicians can continue to obtain corneal specimens from keratitis suspected of atypical organisms and it is therefore possible to record these for epidemiological surveillance.

Modification of Therapy

The clinical response to treatment is multifactorial, taking into account the severity of the initial clinical picture, the virulence of the pathogen, and the presence of systemic or ocular immunocompromise.[225] The clinical response is best assessed after 48 hours of treatment, as earlier evaluation is usually inconclusive and not helpful in assessing the efficacy of antibiotic treatment. Keratitis due to *Pseudomonas* and other Gram-negative organisms may exhibit increased inflammation during the first 24 to 48 hours despite appropriate therapy.[151,153] In general, the initial therapeutic regimen should be modified when the eye shows a lack of improvement or stabilization within 48 hours. Several clinical features suggestive of a positive response to antibiotic therapy[226] include reduction in pain, reduced amount of discharge, less eyelid edema or conjunctival injection, consolidation and sharper demarcation of the perimeter of the stromal infiltrate, decreased density of the stromal infiltrate, reduced stromal edema and endothelial inflammatory plaque, reduced anterior chamber inflammation, and reepithelialization. The culture/sensitivity data should only be used as a guide to modify therapy for patients with definite worsening of the clinical findings (Fig. 77.29).

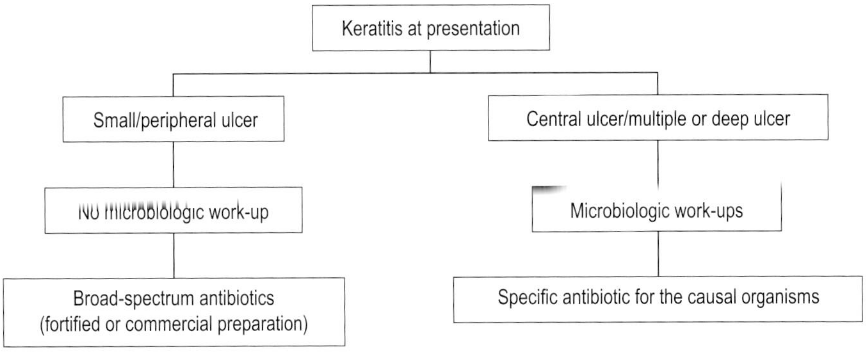

Fig. 77.28 Initial evaluation of microbial keratitis.

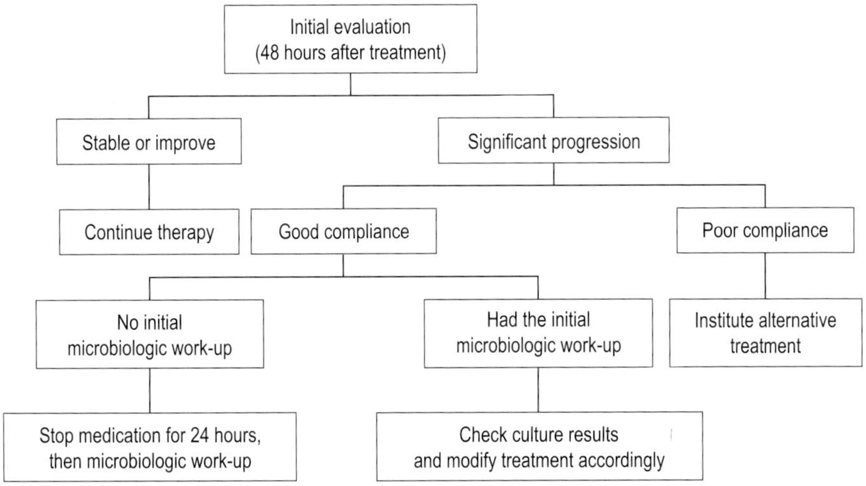

Fig. 77.29 Initial management of microbial keratitis.

Progression after 48 hours of treatment implies that organisms are not sensitive to selected agents or the patient is not compliant. For nonresponsive cases, one should consider stopping the antibiotics for at least 24 hours (prior to corneal scraping) to increase the yield for microbiology cultures. Topical therapy is tapered according to clinical response, taking into account the severity of the initial clinical picture and the virulence of the pathogen. More prolonged therapy may be mandated by the presence of virulent or indolent organisms or ocular immunocompromise.

Review after 1 week

After 1 week of specific treatment, the clinical findings and response to antibiotics should be reviewed (Fig. 77.30). If complete resolution is noted, the medication can be discontinued. In this nonurgent phase, if the ulcer is still progressing and the previous culture remains negative, the medication should be stopped for at least 24 hours prior to repeating the microbiological work-up. Special staining/culture media or corneal biopsy may be required. Noninfectious causes or atypical organisms such as nontuberculous *mycobacteria*, *Nocardia*, or *Acanthamoeba* should be suspected. The antibiotic should be modified accordingly.

In progressive ulcer with a prior positive culture and proper therapy, the existence of a resistant strain should be suspected. Polymicrobial infection, which has been observed in 6–56% of the overall cases, should also be considered.[227] The antibiotic sensitivity should be reevaluated and the therapy modified if necessary. For an unresponsive keratitis on seemingly appropriate treatment, one should consider possible drug toxicity or underlying ocular surface problems. Promotion of epithelial healing is the mainstay for a nonhealing sterile ulcer. The indolent, nonhealing ulcer sometimes can be improved by debridement of necrotic corneal stroma, frequent lubrication, and/or temporary tarsorrhaphy.

Corticosteroid Therapy

Topical corticosteroid therapy may have a beneficial role in treating some cases of bacterial keratitis; however, its use remains controversial, as there is no conclusive scientific evidence that corticosteroids alter clinical outcome. The potential advantage of corticosteroids is the possible suppression of inflammation, which may reduce subsequent corneal scarring and associated visual loss. Potential disadvantages include recrudescence of infection, local immunosuppression, inhibition of collagen synthesis predisposing to corneal melting, and increased intraocular pressure or cataract formation. Topical corticosteroids, used without antibiotics, worsen experimental *Pseudomonas* keratitis and may promote recurrence of apparently healed *Pseudomonas* keratitis after discontinuing antibiotics. In contrast, in *pneumococcal* keratitis, administration of topical corticosteroids in the absence of topical antibiotics does not worsen the disease.[228,229] In prospective studies, no difference was found between the patients with microbial keratitis treated with or without corticosteroids in terms of time to cure, final visual acuity,[184] and complications.[230] In other studies, patients who received corticosteroids before being diagnosed with microbial keratitis had a significantly greater chance of antibiotic treatment failure and related complications.[231,232] Despite the risks involved, many experts believe that the judicious use of topical corticosteroids in the treatment of bacterial keratitis can reduce morbidity.[222,233] Patients being treated with topical corticosteroids at the time of presentation with suspected bacterial keratitis should have their topical steroids reduced or eliminated until the infection has been controlled. Inflammation may temporarily worsen as the corticosteroid is reduced.

The objective in topical corticosteroid therapy is to use the minimum amount of corticosteroid required to achieve control of inflammation. Successful treatment requires optimal timing, careful dose regulation, use of adequate concomitant antibacterial medication, and close follow-up. Corticosteroids should not be part of initial treatment of presumed bacterial ulcers, and ideally they should not be used until the organism has been determined by cultures. The use of corticosteroids in the initial treatment of corneal ulcers has been determined to be a risk factor for requiring a penetrating keratoplasty.[231]

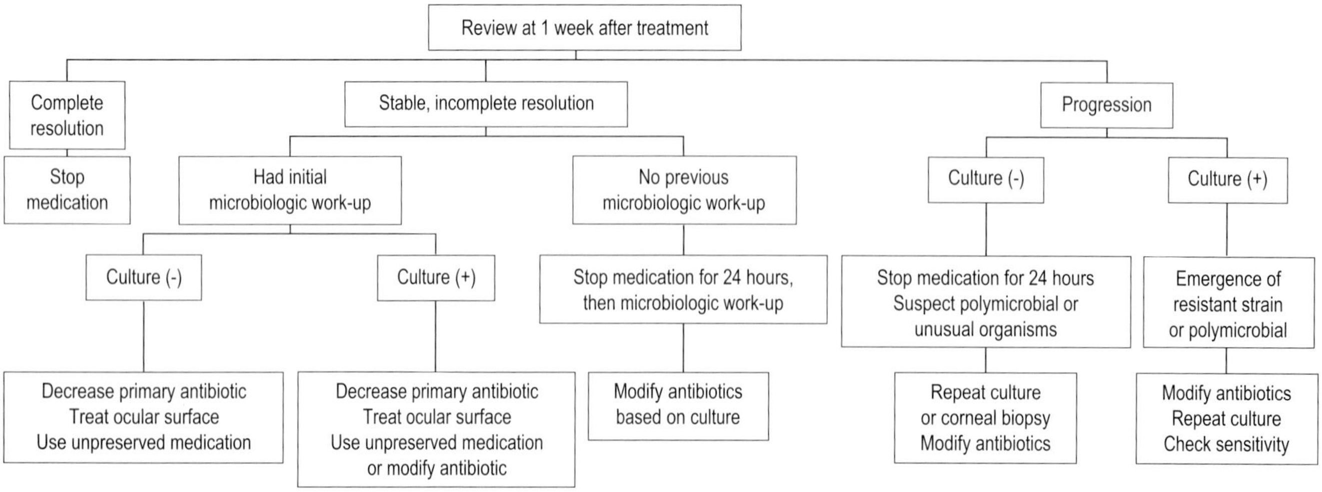

Fig. 77.30 Reevaluation after 1 week of antimicrobial therapy.

In cases where the corneal infiltrate compromises the visual axis, topical corticosteroid therapy may be added to the regimen following at least 2 to 3 days of progressive improvement with topical antibiotic treatment.[234] Topical antibiotics, which are generally administered more frequently than corticosteroids during treatment of active infection, are continued at high levels with gradual tapering. Patient compliance is essential, and the intraocular pressure must be monitored frequently. The patient should be reexamined within 1 to 2 days after initiation of topical corticosteroid therapy. Corticosteroids should not be used in eyes with significant corneal thinning or impending perforation due to their adverse effects of activating collagenolytic enzymes and suppressing collagen synthesis.

Therapy for Complicated Cases

Coexisting risk factors, such as eyelid abnormalities, should be corrected for optimal results. Additional treatment is necessary in cases where the integrity of the eye is compromised, such as when there is an extremely thin cornea, impending or frank perforation, progressive or unresponsive disease, or endophthalmitis.[235] Application of tissue adhesive, therapeutic contact lens, penetrating keratoplasty, and, rarely, lamellar keratectomy are among the treatment options.

Cyanoacrylate tissue adhesives

Cyanoacrylate tissue adhesive (*N*-butyl-2-cyanoacrylate) is approved for dermatologic use but not for ophthalmic use. It has been used to treat progressive corneal thinning, descemetocele, and corneal perforation with satisfactory results.[236,237] In addition to its tectonic support and bacteriostatic effects, the tissue glue can arrest keratolysis by blocking leukocytic proteases from the corneal wound. Perforations up to 2–3 mm in diameter can be sealed by the tissue adhesive. Necrotic tissue and debris should be removed from the ulcer bed prior to application of the glue. Due to potential corneal toxicity, only the minimum amount of glue required to cover the defect should be used. A bandage contact lens is then placed to ensure patient comfort and proper placement of the glue. The adhesive is usually left in place until it dislodges spontaneously or a keratoplasty is performed.

Therapeutic soft contact lenses

After eradication of the causative bacteria, therapeutic contact lenses may be applied to facilitate epithelial healing.[238] Antibiotic administration should continue over the therapeutic soft contact lens. Caution should be exercised, as recurrent infection may occasionally complicate the use of a therapeutic contact lens. A therapeutic lens may also provide some tectonic support for impending or microscopic corneal perforation.

Surgical Management

Conjunctival flap

Conjunctival flap has been used to treat recalcitrant microbial keratitis.[239] The flap can bring blood vessels to the infected area, promote healing, and provides a stable surface covering. A conjunctival flap should not be placed over a necrotic area with active infection because the flap can become infected and necrotic. A conjunctival flap is particularly useful in cases of nonhealing peripheral corneal ulcer, where the flap can be placed without compromising vision.

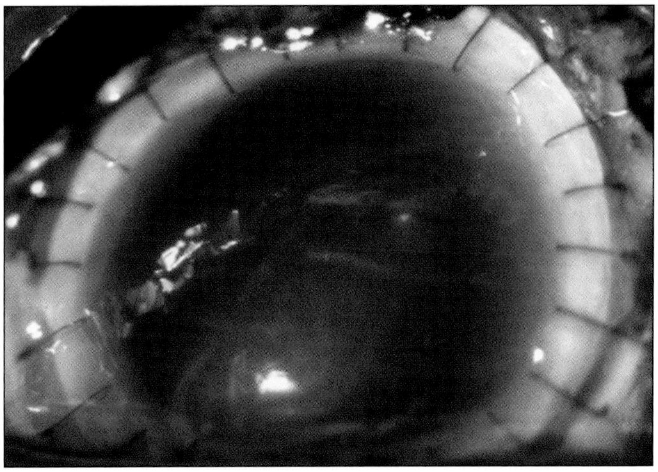

Fig. 77.31 A large therapeutic penetrating keratoplasty performed on the patient with severe *Pseudomonas* keratitis in Figure 77.19.

Penetrating keratoplasty

Major factors that can necessitate penetrating keratoplasty for patients with bacterial keratitis include older age, delay in referral, injudicious steroid treatment, past ocular surgery, large size of ulcer, and central location of the ulcer.[231,240,241] A therapeutic penetrating keratoplasty performed at the acute stage of microbial keratitis is difficult[242–244] and is associated with a higher complication rate and lower graft survival, as compared to perfoming an optical keratoplasty for corneal scarring. The indications for emergency therapeutic penetrating keratoplasty are uncontrolled progression of the infiltrates (Fig. 77.31), limbal involvement with impending scleritis, or corneal perforation. Intensive antibiotics should be administered for 48 hours before surgery to minimize the risks of recurrent infection or development of endophthalmitis. It is preferable to defer penetrating keratoplasty at an acute stage of bacterial keratitis to avoid potentially incomplete excision of infected tissues or intraocular extension of the infection. After complete resolution of the corneal infection, optical penetrating keratoplasty can be used to remove corneal scarring and to rehabilitate vision.

Prevention and Early Detection

Early detection and appropriate treatment are imperative in order to prevent permanent visual loss from bacterial keratitis.[215] The risk may be reduced by avoiding or correcting predisposing factors. For example, screening patients for predisposing factors and educating them about the risks of extended-wear lenses[245] and the importance of adherence to techniques that promote contact lens hygiene[6] may reduce the incidence of bacterial keratitis in contact lens users. Most ocular trauma can be avoided by using protective eyewear for sports and other high-risk activities.[246,247]

Patients should be acquainted with the signs and symptoms of infection, and be informed that they should consult an ophthalmologist promptly if they experience these. Ocular surface disease such as corneal epithelial defects, severe tear deficiency, or lagophthalmos should be treated. Prophylactic antibiotics can be considered for patients with chronic epithelial defects; however, the routine use of prophylactic topical antibiotics in this setting is controversial, because their efficacy has not been established and chronic use may promote growth of resistant organisms.

Counseling and Referral

The diagnosis and management of patients with bacterial keratitis require the clinical training and experience of an ophthalmologist, because the disease has the potential to cause visual loss or blindness. Severe cases, or those that fail to respond to treatment, may be best managed by an ophthalmologist who has expertise and experience in the management of bacterial keratitis. The majority of patients can be treated on an outpatient basis. Hospitalization may be necessary if the keratitis is severe or vision-threatening, if compliance is poor, if pain is severe, or if surgical intervention is necessary.[224] Compliance may be difficult to achieve due to the requirement for frequent instillation of eye drops, the patient's inability to instill the eye drops because of age, mental or physical disability, or the lack of an adequate support system at home. Patients and care providers should be educated about the destructive nature of bacterial keratitis and the need for strict adherence to the therapeutic regimen. The possibility of permanent visual loss and need for future visual rehabilitation should be discussed. Patients with significant visual impairment should be referred for vision rehabilitation if they are not candidates for surgical visual rehabilitation. A social service referral may be also appropriate in cases of severe visual impairment.

References

1. Wilhelmus KR. Review of clinical experience with microbial keratitis associated with contact lenses. *CLAO J.* 1987;13:211–214.
2. Tuft SJ. Suppurative keratitis. *Br J Ophthalmol.* 2003;87:127.
3. Coster DJ, Badenoch PR. Host, microbial, and pharmacological factors affecting the outcome of suppurative keratitis. *Br J Ophthalmol.* 1987; 71:96–101.
4. Pepose JS, Wilhelmus KR. Divergent approaches to the management of corneal ulcers. *Am J Ophthalmol.* 1992;114:630–632.
5. MacRae S, Herman C, Stulting RD, et al. Corneal ulcer and adverse reaction rates in pre-market contact lens studies. *Am J Ophthalmol.* 1991; 111:457–465.
6. Poggio EC, Glynn RJ, Schein OD, et al. The incidence of ulcerative keratitis among users of daily-wear and extended-wear soft contact lenses. *N Engl J Med.* 1989;321:779–783.
7. Stapleton F, Keay L, Edwards K, et al. The incidence of contact-lens related microbial keratitis in Australia. *Ophthalmology.* 2008;115: 1655–1662.
8. Dart JKG. Disease and risks associated with contact lenses. *Br J Ophthalmol.* 1993;77:49–53.
9. Upadhyay MP, Karmacharya PCD, Koirala S, et al. Epidemiologic characteristics, predisposing factors, and etiologic diagnosis of corneal ulceration in Nepal. *Am J Ophthalmol.* 1991;111:92–99.
10. Bourcier T, Thomas F, Borderie V, et al. Bacterial keratitis: predisposing factors, clinical and microbiological review of 300 cases. *Br J Ophthalmol.* 2003;87:834–838.
11. Smolin G. The role of tears in the prevention of infections. *Int Ophthalmol Clin.* 1987;27:25–26.
12. Selinger DS, Selinger RC, Reed WP. Resistance to infection of the external eye: the role of tears. *Surv Ophthalmol.* 1979/1980;24:33–38.
13. Jensen OL, Gluud BS. Bacterial growth in the conjunctival sac and the local defense of the outer eye. *Acta Ophthalmol.* 1985;63(Suppl 173): 80–82.
14. Lemp MA. Is the dry eye contact lens wearer at risk? Yes. *Cornea.* 1990;9(Suppl I):S48–S50.
15. Sommer A. Effects of vitamin A deficiency on the ocular surface. *Ophthalmology.* 1983;90:592–600.
16. Characklis WG, Marshall KC. *Biofilms.* New York: Wiley Interscience; 1990.
17. Zegans ME, Becker HI, Budzik J, O'Toole G. The role of bacterial biofilms in ocular infections. *DNA Cell Biol.* 2002;21:415–420.
18. Upadhyay MP, Rai NC, Brandt F, et al. Corneal ulcers in Nepal. *Graefe's Arch Clin Exp Ophthalmol.* 1982;219:55–59.
19. Vaughan DG Jr. The contamination of fluorescein solutions: with special reference to *Pseudomonas aeruginosa* (bacillus pyocyanene). *Am J Ophthalmol.* 1955;39:55–61.
20. Theodore FH, Feinstein R. Preparation and maintenance of sterile ophthalmic solutions. *JAMA.* 1953;152:1631–1633.
21. Schein OD, Wasson PI, Boruchoff SA, Kenyon KR. Microbial keratitis associated with contaminated ocular medications. *Am J Ophthalmol.* 1988;105:361–365.
22. Rosenwasser GOD, Holland S, Pflugfelder SC, et al. Topical anesthetic abuse. *Ophthalmology.* 1990;97:967–972.
23. Sachs R, Zagelbaum BM, Hersh PS. Corneal complications associated with the use of crack cocaine. *Ophthalmology.* 1993;100:187–191.
24. Dua HS. Bacterial keratitis in the critically ill and comatose patient. *Lancet.* 1998;351:381–388.
25. Hilton E, Adams AA, Uliss A, et al. Nosocomial bacterial eye infections in intensive-care units. *Lancet.* 1983;1:1318–1320.
26. Kirwan JF, Potamitis T, el-Kasaby H, et al. Microbial keratitis in intensive care. *Br Med J.* 1997;314:433–434.
27. Liesegang TJ. Contact lens-related microbial keratitis: Part I: Epidemiology. *Cornea.* 1997;16:125–131.
28. Saviola JF. Contact lens safety and the FDA: 1976 to the present. *Eye Contact Lens.* 2007;33:404–409.
29. Cheng KH, Leung SL, Hoekman HW, et al. Incidence of contact lens-associated microbial keratitis and its related morbidity. *Lancet.* 1999; 354:181–185.
30. Cohen EJ, Fulton JC, Hoffman CJ, et al. Trends in contact lens-associated corneal ulcers. *Cornea.* 1996;15:566–570.
31. Keay L, Edwards K, Stapleton F, et al. Perspective on 15 years of research: reduced risk of microbial keratitis in frequent-replacement contact lenses with wider use. *Eye Contact Lens.* 2007;33:167–168.
32. Dart JK, Radford CF, Minassian D, et al. Risk factors for microbial keratitis with contemporary contact lenses. *Ophthalmology.* 2008;115:1647–1654.
33. Buehler PO, Schein OD, Stamler JF, et al. The increased risk of ulcerative keratitis among disposable soft contact lens users. *Arch Ophthalmol.* 1992;110:1555–1558.
34. Matthews TD, Frazer DG, Minassian DC, et al. Risks of keratitis and patterns of use with disposable contact lenses. *Arch Ophthalmol.* 1992; 110:1559–1562.
35. Schein O, McNally J, Katz J, et al. The incidence of microbial keratitis among wearers of a 30-day silicone hydrogel extended wear contact lens. *Ophthalmology.* 2005;112:2172–2179.
36. Hsiao CH, Lin HC, Chen YF, et al. Infectious keratitis related to overnight orthokeratology. *Cornea.* 2005;24:783–788.
37. Tseng CH, Fong CF, Chen WL, et al. Overnight orthokeratology-associated microbial keratitis. *Cornea.* 2005;24:778–782.
38. Glynn RJ, Schein CD, Seddon IM, et al. The incidence of ulcerative keratitis among aphakic contact lens wearers in New England. *Arch Ophthalmol.* 1991;109:104–107.
39. Kent HD, Cohen EJ, Laibson PR, Arentsen JJ. Microbial keratitis and cortical ulceration associated with therapeutic soft contact lenses. *CLAO J.* 1990;16:49–52.
40. Aswad MI, Baum J, Barza M. The effect of cleaning and disinfection of soft contact lenses on corneal infectivity in an animal model. *Am J Ophthalmol.* 1995;119:738–743.
41. Bowden III FW, Cohen EJ, Arentsen JJ, Laibson PR. Patterns of lens care practices and lens product contamination in contact lens associated microbial keratitis, *CLAO J.* 1989;15:49–54.
42. Martins EN, Farah ME, Alvarenga LS, et al. Infectious keratitis: correlation between corneal and contact lens cultures. *CLAO J.* 2002;28:146–148.
43. Koidou-Tsiligianni A, Alfonso E, Forster RK. Ulcerative keratitis associated with contact lens wear. *Am J Ophthalmol.* 1989;108:64–67.

44. Schein OD, Ormerod LD, Barraquer E, et al. Microbiology of contact lens-related keratitis. *Cornea*. 1989;8:281–285.
45. Ren DH, Yamamoto K, Ladage PM, et al. Adaptive effects of 30-night wear of hyper-O_2 transmissible contact lenses on bacterial binding and corneal epithelium: a 1-year clinical trial. *Ophthalmology*. 2002;109: 27–40.
46. Lawin-Brussel CA, Refojo MF, Leong FL, Kenyon KR. *Pseudomonas* attachment to low-water and high-water, ionic and nonionic new and rabbit-worn soft contact lenses. *Invest Ophthalmol Vis Sci*. 1991;32: 657–662.
47. Butrus SI, Klotz SA. Contact lens surface deposits increase the adhesion of *Pseudomonas aeruginosa*. *Curr Eye Res*. 1990;9:717–724.
48. Stern GA, Zam AS. The pathogenesis of contact lens-associated *Pseudomonas aeruginosa* corneal ulceration. I. The effect of contact lens coatings on adherence of *Pseudomonas aeruginosa* to soft contact lenses. *Cornea*. 1986;5:41–45.
49. Aswad MI, John T, Barza M, et al. Bacterial adherence to extended-wear soft contact lenses. *Ophthalmology*. 1990;97:296–302.
50. Fleiszig SMJ, Efron N, Pier GB. Extended contact lens wear enhances *Pseudomonas aeruginosa* adherence to human corneal epithelium. *Invest Ophthalmol Vis Sci*. 1992;33:2908–2916.
51. Rabinovitch J, Cohen EJ, Genvert GI, et al. Seasonal variation in contact lens-associated conical ulcers. *Can J Ophthalmol*. 1987;22: 155–156.
52. Elander TR, Goldberg MA, Salinger CL, et al. Microbial changes in the ocular environment with contact lens wear. *CLAO J*. 1992;18:53–55.
53. Fleiszig SMJ, Efron N. Microbial flora in eyes of current and former contact lens wearers. *J Clin Microbiol*. 1992;30:1156–1161.
54. Chambers WA, Belin MW, Parenti DM, Simon GL. Corneal ulcers in house staff: are risk factors identifiable? *Ann Ophthalmol*. 1988;20: 172–175.
55. Cavanagh HD, Ladage PM, Li SL, et al. Effects of daily and overnight wear of a novel hyper oxygen-transmissible soft contact lens on bacterial binding and corneal epithelium: a 13-month clinical trial. *Ophthalmology*. 2002;109:1957–1969.
56. Ladage PM, Ren DH, Petroll WM, et al. Effects of eyelid closure and disposable and silicone hydrogel extended contact lens wear on rabbit corneal epithelial proliferation. *Invest Ophthalmol Vis Sci*. 2003;44: 1843–1849.
57. Ladage PM, Jester JV, Petroll WM, et al. Vertical movement of epithelial basal cells towards the corneal surface during use of extended-wear contact lenses. *Invest Ophthalmol Vis Sci*. 2003;44:1056–1063.
58. Ladage PM, Yamamoto K, Ren DH, et al. Effects of rigid and soft contact lens daily wear on corneal epithelium, tear lactate dehydrogenase, and bacterial binding to exfoliated epithelial cells. *Ophthalmology*. 2001;108:1279–1288.
59. DeCarlo ID, Van Horn DL, Hyndiuk RA, Davis SD. Increased susceptibility to infection in experimental xerophthalmia. *Arch Ophthalmol*. 1981;99:1614–1617.
60. Klotz SA, Au YK, Misra RP. A partial-thickness epithelial defect increases the adherence of *Pseudomonas aeruginosa* to the cornea. *Invest Ophthalmol Vis Sci*. 1989,30.1069–1074.
61. Luchs JI, d'Aversa G, Udell IJ. Ulcerative keratitis associated with spontaneous corneal erosions. *Invest Ophthalmol Vis Sci*. 1995;36:540.
62. Kerr N, Stern GA. Bacterial keratitis associated with vernal keratoconjunctivitis. *Cornea*. 1992;11:355–359.
63. Lomholt JA, Ehlers N. Graft survival and risk factors of penetrating keratoplasty for microbial keratitis. *Acta Ophthalmol Scand*. 1997;75: 418–422.
64. Tseng SH, Ling KC. Late microbial keratitis after corneal transplantation. *Cornea*. 1995;14:591–594.
65. Tuberville AW, Wood TO. Corneal ulcers in corneal transplants. *Curr Eye Res*. 1981;1:479–485.
66. Akova YA, Onat M, Koc F, et al. Microbial keratitis following penetrating keratoplasty. *Ophthalmic Surg Lasers*. 1999;30:449–455.
67. Saini JS, Rao GN, Aquavella JV. Post-keratoplasty corneal ulcers and bandage lenses. *Acta Ophthalmol*. 1988;66:99–103.
68. Smith SG, Lindstrom RL, Nelson JD, et al. Corneal ulcer-infiltrate associated with soft contact lens use following penetrating keratoplasty. *Cornea*. 1984;3:131–134.
69. Al'Hazzaa SAF, Tabbara KF. Bacterial keratitis after penetrating keratoplasty. *Ophthalmology*. 1988;95:1504–1508.
70. Bates AK, Kirkness CM, Ficker LA, et al. Microbial keratitis after penetrating keratoplasty. *Eye*. 1990;4:74–78.
71. Fong LP, Ormerod LD, Kenyon KR, Foster CS. Microbial keratitis complicating penetrating keratoplasty. *Ophthalmology*. 1988;95:1269–1275.
72. Leahey AB, Avery RL, Gottsch JD, et al. Suture abscesses after penetrating keratoplasty. *Cornea*. 1993;12:489–492.
73. Gussler JR, Miller D, Jaffe M, Alfonso EC. Infection after radial keratotomy. *Am J Ophthalmol*. 1995;119:798–799.
74. Heidemann DG, Dunn SP, Chow CY. Early- versus late-onset infectious keratitis after radial and astigmatic keratotomy: clinical spectrum in a referral practice. *J Cataract Refract Surg*. 1999;25:1615–1619.
75. Solomon A, Karp CL, Miller D, et al. *Mycobacterium* interface keratitis after laser in situ keratomileusis. *Ophthalmology*. 2001;108:2201–2208.
76. Karp CL, Tuli SS, Yoo SH, et al. Infectious keratitis after LASIK. *Ophthalmology*. 2003;110:503–510.
77. Quiros PA, Chuck RS, Smith RE, et al. Infectious ulcerative keratitis after laser in situ keratomileusis. *Arch Ophthalmol*. 1999;117:1423–1427.
78. Mandelbaum S, Waring III GO, Forster RK, et al. Late development of ulcerative keratitis in radial keratotomy scars. *Arch Ophthalmol*. 1986; 104:1156–1160.
79. al-Rajhi AA, Wagoner MD, Badr IA, et al. Bacterial keratitis following phototherapeutic keratectomy. *J Refract Surg*. 1996;12:123–127.
80. Amayem A, Ali AT, Waring III GO, Ibrahim O. Bacterial keratitis after photorefractive keratectomy. *J Refract Surg*. 1996;12:642–644.
81. Donnenfeld ED, O'Brien TP, Solomon R, et al. Infectious keratitis after photorefractive keratectomy. *Ophthalmology*. 2003;110:743–747.
82. Dantas PE, Nishiwaki-Dantas MC, Ojeda VH, et al. Microbiological study of disposable soft contact lenses after photorefractive keratectomy. *CLAO J*. 2000;26:26–29.
83. Melki SA, Azar DT. LASIK complications: etiology, management, and prevention. *Surv Ophthalmol*. 2001;46:95–116.
84. Garg P, Mathur U, Athmanathan S, Rao GN. Treatment outcome of *Moraxella* keratitis: our experience with 18 cases – a retrospective review. *Cornea*. 1999;18:176–181.
85. Nanda M, Pflugfelder SC. Fulminant pseudomonal keratitis and scleritis in human immunodeficiency virus-infected patients. *Arch Ophthalmol*. 1991;109:503–505.
86. Hemady RK. Microbial keratitis in patients infected with the human immunodeficiency virus. *Ophthalmology*. 1995;102:1026–1030.
87. Scott IU, Flynn Jr HW, Feuer W, et al. Endophthalmitis associated with microbial keratitis. *Ophthalmology*. 1996;103:1864–1870.
88. Carmichael TR, Wolpert M, Koornhof HI. Corneal ulceration at an urban African hospital. *Br J Ophthalmol*. 1985;69:920–926.
89. Williams G, Billson F, Husain R, et al. Microbiological diagnosis of suppurative keratitis in Bangladesh. *Br J Ophthalmol*. 1987;71:315–321.
90. Kupferman A, Leibowitz HM. Quantitation of bacterial infection and antibiotic effect in the cornea. *Arch Ophthalmol*. 1976;94:1981–1984.
91. Kupferman A, Leibowitz HM. Topical antibiotic therapy of *Pseudomonas aeruginosa* keratitis. *Arch Ophthalmol*. 1979;97:1699–1702.
92. Stern GA, Lubniewski A, Allen C. The interaction between *Pseudomonas aeruginosa* and the corneal epithelium: an electron microscopic study. *Arch Ophthalmol*. 1985;103:1221–1225.
93. Spurr-Michaud SJ, Barza M, Gipson IK. An organ culture system for study of adherence of *Pseudomonas aeruginosa* to normal and wounded corneas. *Invest Ophthalmol Vis Sci*. 1988;29:379–386.
94. Panjwani N, Zaidi TS, Gigstad JE, et al. Binding of *Pseudomonas aeruginosa* to neutral glycosphingolipids of rabbit conical epithelium. *Infect Immun*. 1990;58:114–118.
95. Singh A, Hazlett L, Berk RS. Characterization of pseudomonal adherence to unwounded cornea. *Invest Ophthalmol Vis Sci*. 1991;32:2096–2104.
96. Reichert R, Stern GA. Quantitative adherence of bacteria to human corneal epithelial cells. *Arch Ophthalmol*. 1984;102:1394.
97. Hyndiuk RA. Experimental *Pseudomonas* keratitis. I. Sequential electron microscopy. II. Comparative therapy trials. *Trans Am Ophthalmol Soc*. 1981;79:541–624.
98. Trinkaus-Randall V, Leibowitz HM, Ryan WI, Kupferman A. Quantification of stroma destruction in the inflamed cornea. *Invest Ophthalmol Vis Sci*. 1991;32:603–609.
99. Tjia KF, van Putten JP, Pels E, Zanen HC. The interaction between *Neisseria gonorrhoeae* and the human cornea in organ culture: an electron microscopic study. *Graefe's Arch Clin Exp Ophthalmol*. 1988;226:341–345.
100. Barquet N, Gasser I, Domingo P, et al. Primary meningococcal conjunctivitis: report of 21 patients and review. *Rev Infect Dis*. 1990;12:838–847.
101. Lande MA, Birk DE, Nagpal ML, Rader RL. Phagocytic properties of human keratocyte cultures. *Invest Ophthalmol Vis Sci*. 1981;20:481–489.
102. Alionte LG, Cannon BM, White CD, et al. *Pseudomonas aeruginosa* LasA protease and corneal infections. *Curr Eye Res*. 2001;22:266–271.
103. Kernacki KA, Hobden JA, Hazlett LD, et al. In vivo bacterial protease production during *Pseudomonas aeruginosa* corneal infection. *Invest Ophthalmol Vis Sci*. 1995;36:1371–1378. Erratum in: *Invest Ophthalmol Vis Sci*. 1995;36:1947.

104. Lawin-Brussel CA, Refojo MF, Leong FL, et al. Time course of experimental *Pseudomonas aeruginosa* keratitis in contact lens overwear. *Arch Ophthalmol*. 1990;108:1012–1019.
105. Mondino BI, Sumner HI. Generation of complement-derived anaphylatoxins in normal human donor corneas. *Invest Ophthalmol Vis Sci*. 1990;31:1945–1949.
106. Shams NB, Sigel MM, Davis RM. Interferon-gamma, *Staphylococcus aureus*, and lipopolysaccharide/silica enhance interleukin-1 beta production by human corneal cells. *Reg Immunol*. 1989;2:136–148.
107. Chusid MJ, Davis SD. Polymorphonuclear leukocyte kinetics in experimentally induced keratitis. *Arch Ophthalmol*. 1985;103:270–274.
108. Schein OD, Buehler PO, Stamier JF, et al. The impact of overnight wear on the risk of contact lens-associated ulcerative keratitis. *Arch Ophthalmol*. 1994;112:186–190.
109. Ormerod LD, Fong LP, Foster CS. Corneal infection in mucosal scarring disorders and Sjögren's syndrome. *Am J Ophthalmol*. 1988;105:512–518.
110. Jones DB. Decision making in the management of microbial keratitis. *Ophthalmology*. 1981;88:814–820.
111. Alfonso E, Mandelbaum S, Fox MJ, Forster BK. Ulcerative keratitis associated with contact lens wear. *Am J Ophthalmol*. 1986;101:429–433.
112. Cohen EJ, Laibson PR, Arentsen JJ, Clemons CS. Corneal ulcers associated with cosmetic extended-wear soft contact lenses. *Ophthalmology*. 1987;94:109–114.
113. Mah-Sadorra JH, Yavuz SG, Najjar DM, et al. Trends in contact lens-related corneal ulcers. *Cornea*. 2005;24:51–58.
114. Alexandrakis G, Alfonso EC, Miller D. Shifting trends in bacterial keratitis in South Florida and emerging resistance to fluoroquinolones. *Ophthalmology*. 2000;107:1497–1502.
115. Keay L, Edwards K, Naduvilath T, et al. Microbial keratitis predisposing factors and morbidity. *Ophthalmology*. 2006;113:109–116.
116. Burns RP, Rhodes Jr DH. *Pseudomonas* eye infection as a cause of death in premature infants. *Arch Ophthalmol*. 1961;65:517–525.
117. Forster RK. The management of infectious keratitis as we approach the 21st century. *CLAO J*. 1998;24:175–180.
118. Goldstein MH, Kowalski RP, Gordon YJ. Emerging fluoroquinolone resistance in bacterial keratitis: a 5-year review. *Ophthalmology*. 1999;106:1313–1318.
119. Tuft SJ, Matheson M. In vitro antibiotic resistance in bacterial keratitis in London. *Br J Ophthalmol*. 2000;84:687–691.
120. Marangon FB, Miller D, Muallem MS, et al. Ciprofloxacin and levofloxacin resistance among methicillin-sensitive *Staphylococcus aureus* isolates from keratitis and conjunctivitis. *Am J Ophthalmol*. 2004;137:453–458.
121. Solomon R, Donnenfeld ED, Perry HD, et al. Methicillin-resistant *Staphylococcus aureus* infectious keratitis following refractive surgery. *Am J Ophthalmol*. 2007;143:629–634.
122. McCulley JP, Dougherty JM. Blepharitis associated with acne rosacea and seborrheic dermatitis. *Int Ophthalmol Clin*. 1985;25:159–172.
123. Pinna A, Zanetti S, Sotgiu M, et al. Identification and antibiotic susceptibility of coagulase negative staphylococci isolated in corneal/external infections. *Br J Ophthalmol*. 1999;83:771–773.
124. Matoba AY, O'Brien TP, Wilhelmus KR, Jones DB. Infectious crystalline keratopathy due to *Streptococcus pneumoniae*: possible association with serotype. *Ophthalmology*. 1994;101:1000–1004.
125. Sridhar MS, Sharma S, Garg P, et al. Treatment and outcome of *Nocardia* keratitis. *Cornea*. 2001;20:458–462.
126. Daines BS, Vroman DT, Sandoval HP, et al. Rapid diagnosis and treatment of mycobacterial keratitis after laser in situ keratomileusis. *J Cataract Refract Surg*. 2003;29:1014–1018.
127. John T, Velotta E. Nontuberculous (atypical) mycobacterial keratitis after LASIK: current status and clinical implications. *Cornea*. 2005;24:245–255.
128. McLeod SD, Goei SL, Taglia DP, McMahon TT. Nonulcerating bacterial keratitis associated with soft and rigid contact lens wear. *Ophthalmology*. 1998;105:517–521.
129. Rosenfeld SI, Mandelbaum S, Corrent GF, et al. Granular epithelial keratopathy as an unusual manifestation of *Pseudomonas* keratitis associated with extended-wear soft contact lenses. *Am J Ophthalmol*. 1990;109:17–22.
130. Lee JS, Choi HY, Lee JE, et al. Gonococcal keratoconjunctivitis in adults. *Eye*. 2002;16:646–649.
131. Ullman S, Roussel TJ, Forster RK. Gonococcal keratoconjunctivitis. *Surv Ophthalmol*. 32(3):199–208. 1987.
132. O'Day DM, Smith RS, Gregg CR, et al. The problem of *Bacillus* species infection with special emphasis on the virulence of *Bacillus cereus*. *Ophthalmology*. 1981;88:833–838.
133. Choudhuri KK, Sharma S, Garg P, Rao GN. Clinical and microbiological profile of *Bacillus* keratitis. *Cornea*. 2000;19:301–306.
134. Meisler DM, Langston RH, Naab TJ, et al. Infectious crystalline keratopathy. *Am J Ophthalmol*. 1984;97:337–343.
135. Lubniewski AJ, Houchin KW, Holland EJ, et al. Posterior infectious crystalline keratopathy with *Staphylococcus epidermidis*. *Ophthalmology*. 1990;97:1454–1459.
136. Groden LR, Pascucci SE, Brinser JH. *Haemophilus aphrophilus* as a cause of crystalline keratopathy. *Am J Ophthalmol*. 1987;104:89–90.
137. Hu FR. Infectious crystalline keratopathy caused by *Mycobacterium fortuitum* and *Pseudomonas aeruginosa*. *Am J Ophthalmol*. 1990;109:738–739.
138. Khater TT, Jones DB, Wilhelmus KR. Infectious crystalline keratopathy caused by Gram-negative bacteria. *Am J Ophthalmol*. 1997;124:19–23.
139. Wilhelmus KR, Robinson NM. Infectious crystalline keratopathy caused by *Candida albicans*. *Am J Ophthalmol*. 1991;112:322–325.
140. Weisenthal RW, Krachmer JH, Folberg R. Postkeratoplasty crystalline deposits mimicking bacterial infectious crystalline keratopathy. *Am J Ophthalmol*. 1998;105:70–74.
141. Allan BD, Morlet N, Dart JK. Microbiologic investigation of suspected microbial keratitis. *Ophthalmology*. 1996;103:1165–1166.
142. Levey SB, Katz HR, Abrams DA, et al. The role of cultures in the management of ulcerative keratitis. *Cornea*. 1997;16:383–386.
143. McLeod SD, Kolahdouz-Isfahani A, Rostamian K, et al. The role of smears, cultures, and antibiotic sensitivity testing in the management of suspected infectious keratitis. *Ophthalmology*. 1996;103:23–28.
144. Rodman RC, Spisak S, Sugar A, et al. The utility of culturing corneal ulcers in a tertiary referral center versus a general ophthalmology clinic. *Ophthalmology*. 1997;104:1897–1901.
145. McDonnell PJ, Nobe J, Gauderman WJ, et al. Community care of corneal ulcer. *Am J Ophthalmol*. 1992;114:531–538.
146. Labetoulle M, Frau E, Offret H, et al. Non-preserved 1% lidocaine solution has less antibacterial properties than currently available anaesthetic eye-drops. *Curr Eye Res*. 2002;25:91–97.
147. Jacob P, Gopinathan U, Sharma S, Rao GN. Calcium alginate swab versus Parker blade in the diagnosis of microbial keratitis. *Cornea*. 1995;14:360–364.
148. Epley KD, Katz HR, Herling I, Lasky JB. Platinum spatula versus mini-tip culturette in culturing bacterial keratitis. *Cornea*. 1998;17:74–78.
149. Waxman E, Checheinitsky M, Mannis MJ, Schwab IR. Single culture media in infectious keratitis. *Cornea*. 1999;18:257–261.
150. Schonheyder HC, Pederson JK, Naesar K. Experience with a broth culture technique for diagnosis of bacterial keratitis. *Acta Ophthalmol Scand*. 1997;75:592–594.
151. Allan BDS, Dart JKC. Strategies for the management of microbial keratitis. *Br J Ophthalmol*. 1995;79:777–786.
152. Sharma S, Kunimoto DY, Gopinathan U, et al. Evaluation of corneal scraping smear examination methods in the diagnosis of bacterial and fungal keratitis: a survey of eight years of laboratory experience. *Cornea*. 2002;21:643–647.
153. Jones DB. Initial therapy of suspected microbial corneal ulcers. II. Specific antibiotic therapy based on corneal smears. *Surv Ophthalmol*. 1979;24:105–116.
154. Groden LR, Rodnite J, Brinser JH, Genvert GI. Acridine orange and Gram stain in infectious keratitis. *Cornea*. 1990;9:122.
155. Kowal VO, Levey SB, Laibson PR, et al. Use of routine antibiotic sensitivity testing for the management of corneal ulcers. *Arch Ophthalmol*. 1997;115:462–465.
156. Morlet N, Dart J. Routine antibiotic sensitivity testing for corneal ulcers. *Arch Ophthalmol*. 1998;116:1262–1263.
157. Newton C, Moore MB, Kaufman HE. Corneal biopsy in chronic keratitis. *Arch Ophthalmol*. 1987;105:577–578.
158. Alexandrakis G, Haimovici R, Miller D, Alfonso EC. Corneal biopsy in the management of progressive microbial keratitis. *Am J Ophthalmol*. 2000;129:571–576.
159. Garg P, Sharma S. Corneal biopsy in the management of progressive microbial keratitis. *Am J Ophthalmol*. 2002;133:291–292.
160. Lee P, Green R. Corneal biopsy: indications, techniques, and a report of a series of 87 cases. *Ophthalmology*. 1990;97:718–721.
161. Egbert PR, Lauber S, Maurice DM. A simple conjunctival biopsy. *Am J Ophthalmol*. 1977;84:798–801.
162. Nelson JD. Ocular surface impressions using cellulose acetate filter material. Ocular pemphigoid. *Surv Ophthalmol*. 1982;27:67.
163. Nelson JD, Havener VR, Cameron JD. Cellulose acetate impressions of ocular surface. Dry eye states. *Arch Ophthalmol*. 1983;101:1869–1872.
164. Tseng SC. Staging of conjunctival squamous metaplasia by impression cytology. *Ophthalmology*. 1985;92(6):728–733.
165. Wittpenn JR, Tseng SCG, Sommer A. Detection of early xerophthalmia by impression cytology. *Arch Ophthalmol*. 1986;104(2):237–239.

166. Natadisastra G, Wittpenn JR, West Jr KP, et al. Impression cytology for detection of vitamin-A deficiency. *Arch Ophthalmol*. 1987;105: 1224–1228.
167. Sawada Y, Fischer JL, Verm AM, et al. Detection by impression cytology of conjunctival intraepithelial invasion from eyelid sebaceous cell carcinoma. *Ophthalmology*. 2003;110:2045–2050.
168. Wittpenn JR, Pepose JS. Impression debridement of herpes simplex dendritic keratitis. *Cornea*. 1987;5:245–248.
169. Nakagawa H, Uchida Y, Takamura E, et al. Diagnostic impression cytology for herpes simplex keratitis. *Jpn J Ophthalmol*. 1993;37: 505–513.
170. Sawada Y, Yuan C, Huang AJW. Impression cytology in the diagnosis of *Acanthamoeba* keratitis with surface involvement. *Am J Ophthalmol*. 2004;137:323–328.
171. Florakis GJ, Folberg R, Krachmer JH, et al. Elevated corneal epithelial lines in *Acanthamoeba* keratitis. *Arch Ophthalmol*. 1988;106:1202–1206.
172. Rudolph T, Welinder-Olsson C, Lind-Brandberg L, Stenevi U. 16S rDNA PCR analysis of infectious keratitis: a case series. *Acta Ophthalmol Scand*. 2004;82:463–467.
173. Butler TK, Spencer NA, Chan CC, et al. Infective keratitis in older patients: a 4 year review, 1998–2002. *Br J Ophthalmol*. 2005;89:591–596.
174. Petroll WM, Cavanagh HD, Jester JV. Clinical confocal microscopy. *Curr Opin Ophthalmol*. 1998;9:59–65.
175. Irvine JA, Ariyasu R. Limitations in tandem scanning confocal microscopy as a diagnostic tool for microbial keratitis. *Scanning*. 1994;16: 307–311.
176. Denk PO, Thanas S, Thiel HJ. Amikin may be a drug of choice of *Nocardia* keratitis. *Br J Ophthalmol*. 1996;80:928.
177. Washington JA II, Wilson WR. Erythromycin: microbial and clinical prospective after thirty years of clinical use. Parts I and II. *Mayo Clin Proc*. 1985;60:189–271.
178. Field AJ, Backhoff IK, Dick JD, O'Brien TP. Comparative topical treatment of *Mycobacterium fortuitum* keratitis in rabbits. *Invest Ophthalmol Vis Sci*. 1993;34:737.
179. Husain SE, Matoba AY, Husain N, Jones DB. Antimicrobial efficacy of clarithromycin and azithromycin against *Mycobacterium chelonae* and *Mycobacterium abscessus*. *Invest Ophthalmol Vis Sci*. 1993;34:729.
180. Ford J, Huang AJW, Pflugfelder SCP, et al. Nontuberculous mycobacterial keratitis in south Florida. *Ophthalmology*. 1998;105:1652–1658.
181. Diamond JP, White L, Leeming JP, et al. Topical 0.3% ciprofloxacin, norfloxacin, and ofloxacin in treatment of bacterial keratitis: a new method for comparative evaluation of ocular drug penetration. *Br J Ophthalmol*. 1995;79:606–609.
182. The Ofloxacin Study Group. Ofloxacin monotherapy for the primary treatment of microbial keratitis: a double-masked, randomized, controlled trial with conventional dual therapy. *Ophthalmology*. 1997;104: 1902–1909.
183. O'Brien T, and the Bacterial Keratitis Study Research Group. Efficacy of ofloxacin vs cefazolin and tobramycin in the therapy for bacterial keratitis. *Arch Ophthalmol*. 1995;113:1257–1265.
184. Hyndiuk RA, Eiferman RA, Calwell DR, et al. Comparison of ciprofloxacin ophthalmic solution 0.3% to fortified tobramycin-cefazolin in treating bacterial corneal ulcers. *Ophthalmology*. 1996;103:1854–1863.
185. Baker RS, Flowers Jr CW, Casey R, et al. Efficacy of ofloxacin versus cefazolin and tobramycin in the therapy for bacterial keratitis. *Arch Ophthalmol*. 1996;114:632–633.
186. Gangopadhyay N, Daniell M, Weih L, Taylor HR. Fluoroquinolone and fortified antibiotics for treating bacterial corneal ulcers. *Br J Ophthalmol*. 2000;84:378–384.
187. Ormerod LD, Ruoff KL, Meisler DM, et al. Infectious crystalline keratopathy. Role of nutritionally variant streptococci and other bacterial factors. *Ophthalmology*. 1991;98:159–169.
188. Maffett M, O'Day DM. Ciprofloxacin-resistant bacterial keratitis. *Am J Ophthalmol*. 1993;115:545.
189. Wilhelmus KR, Abshire RL, Schlech BA. Influence of fluoroquinolone susceptibility on the therapeutic response of fluoroquinolone-treated bacterial keratitis. *Arch Ophthalmol*. 2003;121:1229–1233.
190. Snyder ME, Katz HR. Ciprofloxacin-resistant bacterial keratitis. *Am J Ophthalmol*. 1992;114:336–338.
191. Bower KS, Kowalski RP, Gordon YJ. Fluoroquinolones in the treatment of bacterial keratitis. *Am J Ophthalmol*. 1996;121:712–715.
192. Honig MA, Cohen EJ, Rapuano CJ, Laibson PR. Corneal ulcers and the use of topical fluoroquinolones. *CLAO J*. 1999;25:200–203.
193. Kunimoto DY, Sharma S, Garg P, Rao GN. In vitro susceptibility of bacterial keratitis pathogens to ciprofloxacin. Emerging resistance. *Ophthalmology*. 1999;106:80–85.
194. Garg P, Shama S, Rao GN. Ciprofloxacin-resistant *Pseudomonas* keratitis. *Ophthamology*. 1999;106:1319–1323.
195. Chaudhry NA, Flynn HW, Murray TG, et al. Emerging ciprofloxacin-resistant *Pseudomonas aeruginosa*. *Am J Ophthalmol*. 1999;128:509.
196. Mather R, Karenchak LM, Romanowski EG, Kowalski RP. Fourth generation fluoroquinolones: new weapons in the arsenal of ophthalmic antibiotics. *Am J Ophthalmol*. 2002;133:463–466.
197. Constantinou M, Daniell M, Snibson GR, et al. Clinical efficacy of moxifloxacin in the treatment of bacterial keratitis: a randomized clinical trial. *Ophthalmology*. 2007;114:1622–1629.
198. Parmar P, Salman A, Kalavathy CM, et al. Comparison of topical gatifloxacin 0.3% and ciprofloxacin 0.3% for the treatment of bacterial keratitis. *Am J Ophthalmol*. 2006;141:282–286.
199. Kowalski RP, Dhaliwal DK, Karenchak LM, et al. Gatifloxacin and moxifloxacin: an in vitro susceptibility comparison to levofloxacin, ciprofloxacin, and ofloxacin using bacterial keratitis isolates. *Am J Ophthalmol*. 2003;136:500–505.
200. Madhavan HN, Rao SK. Ciprofloxacin precipitates in the corneal epithelium. *J Cataract Refract Surg*. 2002;28:909.
201. Castillo A, Castillo JMBD, Toledano N, et al. Deposition of topical norfloxacin in the treatment of bacterial keratitis. *Cornea*. 1997;16:420–423.
202. Mitra A, Tsesmetzoglou E, McElvanney A. Corneal deposits and topical ofloxacin – the effect of polypharmacy in the management of microbial keratitis. *Eye*. 2007;21:410–412.
203. Essepian JP, Rajpal R, O'Brien TP. Tandem scanning confocal microscopic analysis of ciprofloxacin corneal deposit in vivo. *Cornea*. 1995;14:402.
204. Wihelmus KR, Abshire RL. Corneal ciprofloxacin precipitation during bacterial keratitis. *Am J Ophthalmol*. 2003;136:1032–1037.
205. Mallari PL, McCarty DJ, Daniell M, et al. Increased incidence of corneal perforation after topical fluoroquinolone treatment for microbial keratitis. *Am J Ophthalmol*. 2001;131:131–133.
206. Sridhar MS, Sharma S, Reddy MK, et al. Clinicomicrobiological review of *Nocardia* keratitis. *Cornea*. 1998;17:17–22.
207. Lee LH, Zaidman GW, Van Horn K. Topical bactrim versus trimethoprim and sulfonamide against *Nocardia* keratitis. *Cornea*. 2001;20: 179–182.
208. Centers for Disease Control (CDC). 1998 Guidelines for treatment of sexually transmitted diseases. *MMWR*, vol. 47. Atlanta: US DHHS, PHS Publ No. RR-1; January 23, 1998.
209. Willoughby CE, Batterbury M, Kaye SB. Collagen corneal shields. *Surv Ophthalmol*. 2002;47:174–182.
210. Mondino BJ. Collagen shields. *Am J Ophthalmol*. 1991;112:587–589.
211. Lee BL, Matoba AY, Osato MS, Robinson NM. The solubility of antibiotic and corticosteroid combinations. *Am J Ophthalmol*. 1992;114:212–215.
212. Daniell M. Overview: initial antimicrobial therapy for microbial keratitis. *Br J Ophthalmol*. 2003;87:1172–1174.
213. Baum JL. Initial therapy of suspected microbial corneal ulcers. I. Broad antibiotic therapy based on prevalence of organisms. *Surv Ophthalmol*. 1979;24:97–105.
214. Cokingtin CD, Hyndiuk RA. Insights from experimental data on ciprofloxacin in the treatment of bacterial keratitis and ocular infections. *Am J Ophthaimol*. 1991;112(Suppl):25S-28S.
215. Mcleod SD, Labree LD, Tayyanipour R, et al. The importance of initial management in treatment of severe infectious corneal ulcers. *Ophthalmology*. 1995;102:1943–1948.
216. Knauf HP, Silvany R, Southern Jr PM, et al. Susceptibility of corneal and conjunctival pathogens to ciprofloxacin. *Cornea*. 1996;15:66–71.
217. Osato MS, Jensen HG, Trousdale MD, et al. The comparative in vitro activity of ofloxacin and selected ophthalmic antimicrobial agents against ocular bacterial isolates. *Am J Ophthalmol*. 1989;108:380–386.
218. Asbell PA, Colby KA, Deng S, et al. Ocular TRUST: nationwide antimicrobial susceptibility patterns in ocular isolates. *Am J Ophthalmol*. 2008;145:951–958.
219. Mcdonnell PJ. Empirical or culture-guided therapy for microbial keratitis. *Arch Ophthalmol*. 1996;114:84–87.
220. Baum J. Diagnosing and treating bacterial corneal ulcers. *Ophthalmology*. 1996;103:1332–1333.
221. Daniell M, Mills R, Morlet N. Microbial keratitis: what's the preferred initial therapy? *Br J Ophthalmol*. 2003;87:1167.
222. Wilhelmus KR. Indecision about corticosteroids for bacterial keratitis: an evidence-based update. *Ophthalmology*. 2002;109:835–842.
223. Kowalski RP, Karenchak LM. Comparison of ciprofloxacin and ofloxacin using human corneal susceptibility levels. *Cornea*. 1998;17:282–287.
224. McLeod SD, DeBacker CM, Viana MA. Differential care of corneal ulcer in the community based on apparent severity. *Ophthalmology*. 1996;103: 479–484.
225. Kim RY, Cooper KL, Kelly LD. Predictive factors for response to medical therapy in bacterial ulcerative keratitis. *Graefe's Arch Clin Exp Ophthalmol*. 1996;234:731–738.

226. American Academy of Ophthalmology Basic and Clinical Science Course Subcommittee. Basic and Clinical Science Course. *External Disease and Cornea: Section 8, 2008–2009*. San Francisco, CA: American Academy of Ophthalmology; 2008:183.
227. Benson WH, Lanier JD. Comparison of techniques for culturing corneal ulcers. *Ophthalmology*. 1992;99:800–804.
228. Stern G, Buttross M. Use of corticosteroids in combination with antimicrobial drugs in the treatment of infectious corneal disease. *Ophthalmology*. 1991;98:847–853.
229. Gritz DC, Lee TY, Kwitko S, McDonnell PJ. Topical anti-inflammatory agents in an animal model of microbial keratitis. *Arch Ophthalmol*. 1990;108:1001–1005.
230. Carmichael TR, Gelfand Y, Welsh NH. Topical steroids in the management of central and paracentral corneal ulcers. *Br J Ophthalmol*. 1990; 74:528–531.
231. Miedziak AL, Miller MR, Rapuano CJ. Risk factors in microbial keratitis leading to penetrating keratoplasty. *Ophthalmology*. 1999;106:1166–1170.
232. Morlet N, Minassian D, Butcher J. Risk factors for treatment outcome of suspected microbial keratitis. Ofloxacin Study Group. *Br J Ophthalmol*. 1999;83:1027–1031.
233. Liebowitz HM, Kupferman A. Topically administered corticosteroids: effect on antibiotic-treated bacterial keratitis. *Arch Ophthalmol*. 1980; 98:1287–1290.
234. American Academy of Ophthalmology. *Preferred practice pattern: bacterial keratitis*. San Francisco: American Academy of Ophthalmology; 2008.
235. Pineda II R, Dohlman CH. Adjunctive therapy and surgical considerations in the management of bacterial ulcerative keratitis. *Int Ophthalmol Clin*. 1996;36:37–48.
236. Leahy AB, Gottsch JD, Stark WK. Clinical experience with N-butyl cyanoacrylate tissue adhesive. *Ophthalmology*. 1993;100:173–180.
237. Weiss JL, William P, Linstrom RL. The use of tissue adhesive in corneal perforations. *Ophthalmology*. 1983;90:610–615.
238. Lois N, Cohen EJ, Rapuano CJ, Laibson PR. Contact lens use after contact lens-associated infectious ulcers. *CLAO J*. 1997;23:192–195.
239. Buxton JN, Fox ML. Conjunctival flaps in the treatment of refractory *Pseudomonas* corneal abscess. *Ann Ophthalmol*. 1986;18:315–318.
240. Diamant JI, Abbott RL. Surgical management of infectious and noninfectious keratitis. *Int Ophthalmol Clin*. 1998;38:197–217.
241. Miedziak AI, Miller MR, Rapuano CJ, et al. Risk factors in microbial keratitis leading to penetrating keratoplasty. *Ophthalmology*. 1999;106:1166–1171.
242. Killingsworth DW, Stern GA, Driebe WT, et al. Results of therapeutic penetrating keratoplasty. *Ophthalmology*. 1993;100:534–541.
243. Hill JC. Use of penetrating keratoplasty in acute bacterial keratitis. *Br J Ophthalmol*. 1986;70:502–506.
244. Cristol SM, Alfonso EC, Guildford JH, et al. Results of large penetrating keratoplasty in microbial keratitis. *Cornea*. 1996;15:571–576.
245. Dart JK. Extended-wear contact lenses, microbial keratitis, and public health. *Lancet*. 1999;354(9174):174–175.
246. American Academy of Ophthalmology. *Protective eyewear for young athletes, policy statement*. San Francisco: American Academy of Ophthalmology; 2003. ⟨http://www.aao.org/aao/member/policy/sports.cfm⟩
247. American Academy of Ophthalmology. *Preventive eye care, information statement*. San Francisco: American Academy of Ophthalmology; 1993.

Chapter 78

Nontuberculous Mycobacteria Keratitis

Joseph M. Biber, Joung Y. Kim

Overview

Nontuberculous or 'atypical' mycobacteria keratitis continues to be a diagnostic and therapeutic challenge. In 1965, Turner and Stinson reported the first case of keratitis secondary to *Mycobacterium fortuitum* following the removal of a corneal foreign body.[1] Since their initial report, numerous individual case reports and small case series have been published. Nontuberculous mycobacteria (NTM) have emerged as major pathogens causing severe postoperative microbial keratitis following laser in situ keratomileusis (LASIK).

NTM keratitis is characterized by a delayed onset of symptoms of 1–14 weeks following corneal trauma or surgery followed by an even further delay in diagnosis. Medical treatment can be quite difficult and often requires prolonged and intensive topical and systemic therapy. Surgical intervention including lamellar keratectomy, penetrating keratoplasty (PKP), and in LASIK-associated cases, flap removal, is frequently needed.

Classification

Nontuberculous mycobacteria are composed of all species of the family Mycobacteriaceae apart from *Mycobacterium tuberculosis* and *Mycobacterium leprae*. They are aerobic, nonmotile, nonspore-forming bacilli. NTM were classified by Runyon into four groups based on growth rate and pigment production.[2] Groups I–III are slow growers requiring 2–3 weeks to form colonies in culture at room temperature and are differentiated by pigment production. Group IV are rapid growers forming nonpigmented colonies in culture in 3–5 days. The group classification of NTM identified in keratitis cases is shown in Table 78.1.

The great majority of reported cases of NTM keratitis have been caused by the group IV organisms *M. chelonae*[3–9] and *M. fortuitum*,[3,4,9] with the former being the primary species identified in post-LASIK cases. Other species isolated in reported keratitis cases include *M. marinum*,[10] *M. flavescens*,[5] *M. gordonae*,[11,12] *M. szulgai*,[13] *M. avium-intracellulare*,[3] *M. asiaticum*, *M. nonchromogenicum*,[3] *M. triviale*,[3] *M. abscessus*,[8,14] and *M. mucogenicum*.[14]

Risk Factors

Nontuberculous mycobacteria keratitis is considered uncommon, representing 1.1% (24/2134) of all cases of microbial keratitis over 15 years at one institution.[3] NTM are ubiquitous in soil and water[15] and have been found as normal flora of skin, sputum, and gastric contents.[16] They are resistant to chlorine, 2% formaldehyde and glutaraldehyde, and other commonly used disinfectants.[17] Nosocomial outbreaks of systemic NTM disease have been associated with contaminated tap water,[18] saline and disinfecting solutions,[19] and hemodialyzers.[20]

NTM are opportunistic pathogens requiring some alteration in the normal ocular environment to produce infection. In nearly all reports, a previous history of minor ocular trauma, particularly superficial foreign bodies, or previous ocular surgery is present. In one report, 91% of cases of NTM keratitis had an antecedent history of trauma or ocular surgery.[4] Of the two nontraumatic cases, one had ocular cicatricial pemphigoid and the other had neurotrophic keratopathy.[4] Other associations include contact lens wear,[3] radial keratotomy,[3,21] photorefractive keratectomy,[22] cataract surgery,[5,23] and PKP.[23]

Recently, LASIK has been the most identified risk factor. While the overall rate of microbial keratitis after LASIK is low, NTM have been responsible for a high proportion of reported cases.[14,24–34] In a review of all reported cases of bacterial keratitis after LASIK, NTM keratitis accounted for 64% (50/78) of cases.[35] Of these cases, *M. chelonae* was the most commonly identified subtype (66%, 33/50).[35] The source of the infection in isolated cases is usually unknown. Nearly every case describes infiltrates within the interface, implicating introduction of the organism at the time of the procedure. However, postoperative environmental exposure cannot always be excluded. Infections have occurred following primary procedures, enhancements,[14] and flap lifting to treat epithelial ingrowth.[25] Several factors may contribute to the development of microbial keratitis following LASIK. LASIK is often performed utilizing aseptic, but nonsterile techniques. The motor compartment of the microkeratome cannot be heat sterilized, which brings a nonsterile instrument in close proximity to the surgical field. However, a

Table 78.1 Classification of nontuberculous *Mycobacterium*

Runyon group	Pigment formation	Species
I	Photochromogens	*M. marinum*
II	Scotochromogens	*M. flavescens* *M. gordonae* *M. szulgai*
III	Nonchromogens	*M. avium-intracellulare* *M. asiaticum* *M. nonchromogenicum* *M. triviale*
IV	Rapid growers	*M. chelonae* *M. fortuitum* *M. abscessus* *M. mucogenicum*

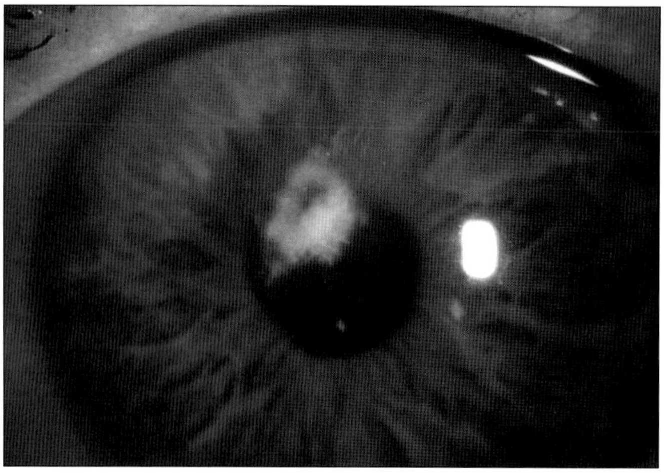

Fig. 78.1 Nontuberculous mycobacterial infection. Note the feathery, indistinct margins and satellite lesions. (Courtesy Edward J. Holland, MD.)

recent case reported infection of *M. abscessus* after LASIK using a femtosecond laser.[36] During the procedure, there is direct exposure of the corneal stroma, which allows these usually low-virulence organisms to bypass the normal ocular surface and epithelial defense mechanisms. Postoperatively, the presence of the flap may provide protection from antibiotic treatment and allow the infection to spread along the interface. Additional risk factors include excessive surgical manipulation of the flap,[14,25,27] epithelial defects, and prior radial keratotomy.[25]

Three single-center outbreaks of NTM keratitis following LASIK have been reported. In one outbreak involving *M. chelonae*, the environmental source of the organism was not isolated; however, a soft contact lens was used as a masking agent during each case. A second outbreak identified *M. szulgai* from a hospital ice machine. The ice was used in a bath to cool a syringe of balanced salt solution used for intraoperative irrigation.[32,37] In a third outbreak involving *M. chelonae*, the suspected source was water from the portable steamer used to clean the microkeratome.[33] These outbreaks emphasize that NTM keratitis can occur in epidemic fashion following LASIK and should be thoroughly evaluated.

Another consistent feature in reported cases is the use of topical corticosteroids either prior to the onset of the infection (e.g. postkeratoplasty, post-LASIK) or during the course of the active infection. In an animal model of *M. fortuitum* keratitis, Paschal and colleagues showed that inoculation of *M. fortuitum* alone in rabbit corneas resulted in a self-limited keratitis of short duration. Early histopathology showed intrastromal granulomatous inflammation or mixed acute and chronic inflammation. By 3–4 weeks postinoculation, there was no evidence of active inflammation or organisms. In contrast, rabbit eyes that were given a single subconjunctival injection of methylprednisolone at the time of inoculation developed indolent corneal ulcerations and satellite lesions that slowly enlarged. Histopathologic examination showed acute inflammation and microorganisms over the 4-week study period. Granulomatous inflammation was not seen until week four.[38] Similar findings were reported in a clinical series. Histologic specimens from patients not treated with corticosteroids showed dense inflammatory infiltrates with few organisms compared to sections from patients who had been treated with corticosteroids, which showed minimal inflammatory cellular reaction and a large number of organisms.[3] Corticosteroid therapy suppresses granulomatous inflammation,[39] which is thought to be necessary to limit the spread of mycobacteria. Through this suppression, corticosteroids may potentiate mycobacterial disease and facilitate the establishment of a chronic infection.[40]

Clinical Features

The typical clinical picture of NTM keratitis not associated with LASIK is a chronic, indolent ulcer that develops several days to several weeks following minor ocular trauma or surgery and is recalcitrant to conventional antibiotic treatment. Patients may complain of moderate pain and photophobia. The lesion is characterized by an irregular infiltrate with indistinct or feathery margins (Fig. 78.1). Overlying epithelial defects are commonly seen. Satellite lesions, a feature characteristic of fungal keratitis, have been reported in NTM infections.[4,41] A partial or complete ring infiltrate can also be seen.[4,11] A crystalline or 'cracked windshield' stromal lesion, which is considered by some authors to be diagnostic of NTM keratitis,[42] is not commonly seen. An anterior chamber reaction is often seen along with a hypopyon. Enlargement with necrosis of the overlying tissue can occur (Fig. 78.2).

NTM keratitis following LASIK is typically associated with mild to moderate pain, photophobia, and varying degrees of visual loss. However, some patients may be entirely asymptomatic.[28,32] Despite the frequent occurrence of bilateral surgery, most reported cases have been unilateral (86%).[35] Symptoms occasionally develop within the first week following surgery; however, in most reported cases there is a delay of 2–14 weeks following the procedure to the development of keratitis. In a review article, the average time of onset for group IV organisms (*M. chelonae*, *M. abscessus*, etc.) was 3.4

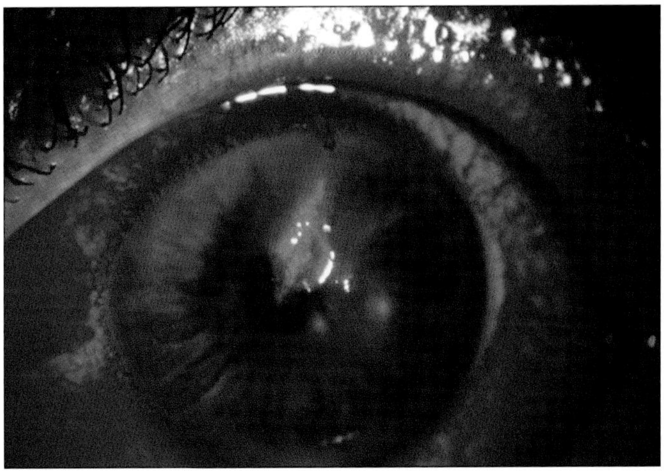

Fig. 78.2 Same patient as in Figure 78.1. Progression of the lesion with necrosis of the overlying stroma and enlargement of the satellite lesions is seen. (Courtesy Edward J. Holland, MD.)

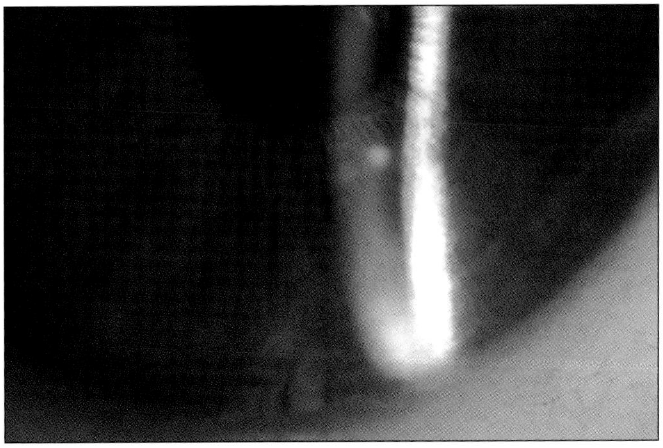

Fig. 78.3 *M. chelonae* keratitis, post-LASIK. A single nummular infiltrate in the flap–stroma interface with minimal surrounding edema. The epithelium was intact and the patient was asymptomatic. (Courtesy Naveen S. Chandra, MD.)

weeks compared to 10 weeks for group II species (*M. szulgai*).[35] There is frequently a further delay from the onset of infection to accurate diagnosis, as patients are often treated empirically without obtaining microbiologic specimens or may be treated for other conditions such as diffuse lamellar keratitis.[28] Solomon reported a mean of 20 days (range, 11–42 days) between the last refractive procedure and the onset of symptoms in four patients. This was followed by an additional period of time (average 4.5 weeks; range, 12–56 days) from the initial onset of symptoms until the patients were correctly diagnosed.[14]

The typical finding is a single or multifocal infiltrate within the interface (Fig. 78.3). Due to its location under the flap, an epithelial defect may be absent. While many patients present with associated nonspecific findings of conjunctival injection and anterior chamber inflammation, this may be absent, particularly in the setting of chronic topical corticosteroid use. The lesion may evolve into a larger infiltrate

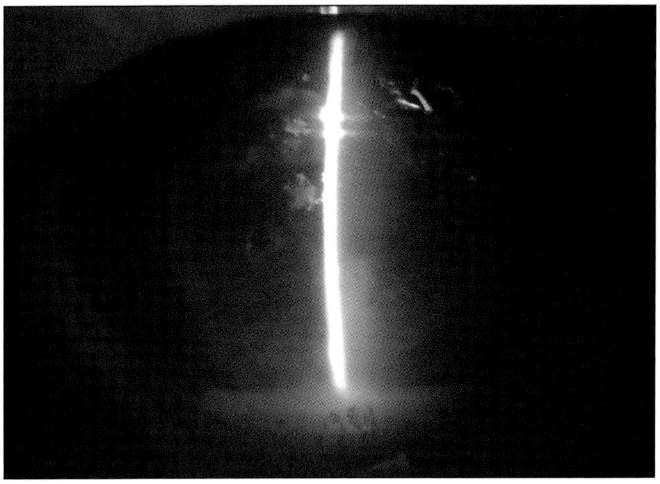

Fig. 78.4 Advanced *M. chelonae* keratitis, post-LASIK. Focal areas of necrosis of the overlying flap with diffuse edema and hypopyon. (Courtesy Naveen S. Chandra, MD.)

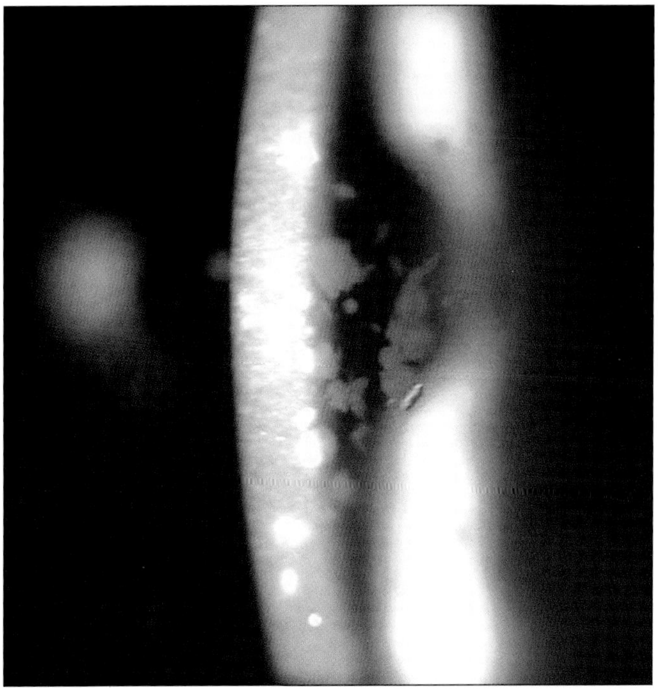

Fig. 78.5 *M. chelonae* keratitis, post-LASIK. Multifocal, crystalline keratopathy developed 2 weeks after LASIK. (Courtesy Naveen S. Chandra, MD.)

with satellite lesions, and necrosis of the overlying flap may occur as the disease progresses (Fig. 78.4).[25] A crystalline or 'cracked windshield' appearance has also been described in LASIK-associated infections as well[31,33] (Fig. 78.5) which may aid in the diagnosis. However, the majority of infiltrates have a nonspecific appearance, and bacterial, fungal, viral, or protozoan etiologies cannot be ruled out on the basis of clinical appearance alone.

The differential diagnosis often includes diffuse lamellar keratitis (DLK), fungal keratitis, and infectious crystalline keratopathy. Differentiation between DLK and NTM keratitis can be difficult but is very important as steroids are critical for treatment of DLK, but may potentiate worsening of NTM keratitis. The infiltrates in DLK are almost always confined to the interface, whereas spread into the anterior or posterior stroma is frequently seen with NTM keratitis. The onset of clinical findings may be helpful also as DLK typically presents earlier than NTM keratitis.

Laboratory Diagnosis

The key to diagnosing NTM keratitis is maintaining a high index of suspicion as the optimal stain and culture media are not obtained in the 'routine' microbial keratitis work-up. A corneal biopsy may be required for infections involving the deeper stroma, and in post-LASIK cases lifting of the flap to access the infiltrate is usually required. A positive culture from a contact lens of an infected patient[3] has been reported and may be an additional source of culture material in these patients. If a biopsy or therapeutic PKP is performed, it is important to submit the specimen for histopathologic (Fig. 78.6) and microbiological examination.

The nontuberculous mycobacteria are acid-fast aerobic bacilli. They do not stain well with Gram stain, although they are considered Gram positive. Microscopically, NTM have been misidentified as *Nocardia*[27,31] or *Corynebacterium*.[6] Ziehl-Neelson acid-fast stain is the primary method used to detect acid-fast organisms. The fluorochrome (auramine and/or auramine-rhodamine) method may also be used with equal or greater sensitivity results.[43] The bacilli appear as bright red thin rods with Ziehl-Neelson acid-fast stain (Fig. 78.7). However, these small organisms can be easily overlooked or not seen at all when adequate samples are not obtained. In Huang's series, only 50% of patients had a positive acid-fast smear.[4]

While NTM will often grow on standard media, inspissated egg media (Löwenstein-Jensen media) and broth media (Middlebrook 7H9 and 7H12) provide more optimal and specific growth conditions. The group IV organisms will typically grow in 3–5 days; however, occasionally, growth is not recorded for over 7 days for the 'rapid growers' and for several weeks for the other species.[13] The microbiology lab needs to be instructed to maintain these plates for extended time periods. Identification of nontuberculous mycobacteria using genetic methods such as polymerase chain reaction (PCR) restriction enzyme analysis[44] or 16S rDNA sequence analysis[45] can provide a more rapid diagnosis of NTM infections; however, these methods are not widely available. In the setting of a LASIK-related outbreak, the Centers for Disease Control and Prevention may process all positive cultures for PCR analysis.

Medical Treatment

The treatment of NTM keratitis is difficult and both the patient and treating physician should be prepared for a protracted disease course. Due to this difficulty and increasing concerns of resistance, a multidrug regimen is often employed. Antibiotics commonly used in the treatment of NTM keratitis are listed in Table 78.2. Nontuberculous mycobacteria are generally resistant to the usual antituberculous antibiotics including isoniazid, ethambutol, and rifampin.[46]

The aminoglycoside amikacin has historically been the antibiotic of choice to treat ocular NTM. Amikacin and tobramycin are bactericidal and inhibit protein synthesis by selectively binding to bacterial 30S and 50S ribosomal subunits.[47] Amikacin at concentrations of 8 mg/mL (0.8%) to 50 mg/mL (5%) has been commonly used; however, treatment failures have been reported even when used at concentrations up to 100 mg/mL.[40] It has been shown to have poor penetration through intact corneal epithelium[48] and can be associated with significant ocular surface toxicity.[49] Despite documented sensitivity, treatment with amikacin alone was successful in only 30% of cases in one series[4] and 40% in another.[50]

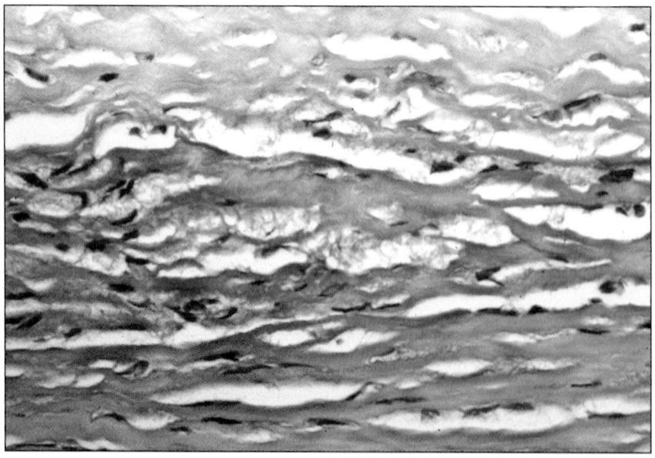

Fig. 78.6 Corneal button from patient with *M. gordonae* keratitis (hematoxylin-eosin stain). Infiltrates of fibrillar material in the stroma with only scattered mononuclear inflammatory cells. The patient had been on chronic topical corticosteroids. (Courtesy Hans E. Grossniklaus, MD.)

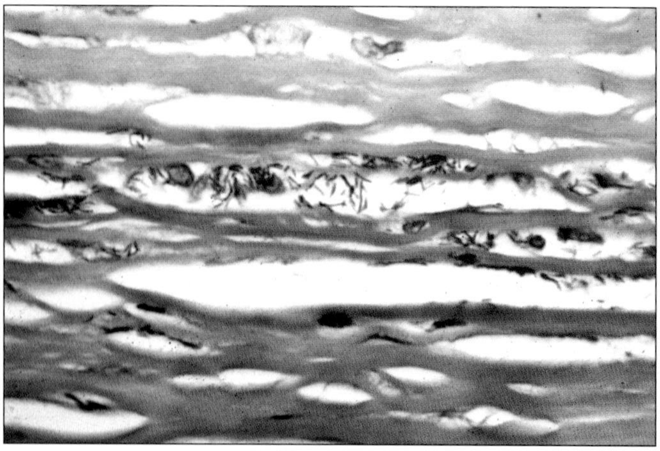

Fig. 78.7 Same specimen as in Figure 78.6. Numerous acid-fast bacilli are seen within the fibrillar material in the stroma. (Ziehl-Neelson acid-fast stain) (Courtesy Hans E. Grossniklaus, MD.)

Table 78.2 Antibiotics that may be effective against NTM

Aminoglycosides	Amikacin Tobramycin
Macrolides	Clarithromycin Azithromycin
Fluoroquinolones	Ciprofloxacin Ofloxacin Moxifloxacin Gatifloxacin
Others	Imipenem Doxycycline Trimethoprim/sulfamethoxazole

Clarithromycin is a macrolide antibiotic that has been found to be effective in treating both ocular and systemic NTM infections. It is bacteriostatic, but may be bactericidal depending on the concentration, the organism involved, and the size of the inoculum.[51] It has been used both topically and orally in the treatment of NTM keratitis. A topical formulation is not commercially available, but may be formulated from granules used for the oral suspension.[52] In a rabbit model, 1–4% solutions of clarithromycin achieved therapeutic corneal concentrations against many NTM after topical application every 2 hours for 12 hours, even in corneas with intact epithelium.[53] The topical solution may be poorly tolerated, leading to the discontinuation by the patient.[3,18,28] Clarithromycin concentrates in tissues following oral administration at levels 2–20 times serum levels[54] and systemic administration may be an alternative for patients who cannot tolerate it topically.[55] Another oral medication that has shown variable effectivity is doxycycline (100 mg Po bid).[35] Azithromycin is a second macrolide antibiotic. A topical preparation of azithromycin 1% is now comercially available, but its use in the treatment on NTM keratitis has not been documented. A topical formulation of 2 mg/mL of azithromycin, made from the powder used for intravenous injection, was used with topical amikacin, topical ciprofloxacin, and oral clarithromycin to successfully treat multiple cases of *M. chelonae* keratitis following LASIK.[28] It was better tolerated than clarithromycin, but, as it was not used as monotherapy, its efficacy could not be established conclusively. Topical clarithromycin has been shown to be more effective than azithromycin in vitro,[55] particularly against *M. chelonae*.

Fluoroquinolones are the only commercially available topical antibiotics that have been shown to have good activity against mycobacteria.[56] However, in vitro sensitivities of NTM keratitis isolates to fluoroquinolones have been variable. In some studies, the newer fourth-generation fluoroquinolones gatifloxacin and moxifloxacin have demonstrated significantly better in vitro activity than ciprofloxacin against rapidly growing NTM.[57,58] Abshire et al. reported effective MIC_{90} (minimium concentration at which 90% of isolates were inhibited) of the fourth-generation fluoroquinolones against *M. fortuitum* and *M. chelonae*.[59] However, Hofling-Lima identified 17 isolates of *M. chelonae* and *M. abscessus* that were not susceptible to all of the fluoroquinolones.[60] Hu et al. reported good activity of ciprofloxacin against 15 isolates of *M. chelonae*. But two other fluoroquinolones, norfloxacin and ofloxacin, showed moderate activity only.[61] Topical ciprofloxacin has been used successfully as single-agent therapy.[7,9] However, ciprofloxacin has been shown to be more effective against *M. fortuitum* than *M. chelonae* in vitro[56,62] and clinically[9]. A rabbit model of *M. chelonae* keratitis demonstrated better activity with a fourth-generation fluoroquinolone, gatifloxacin, compared to ciprofloxacin.[63]

As stated above, corticosteroids appear to contribute to the onset and prolong the course of NTM keratitis. Ford et al. showed a trend for patients treated with topical corticosteroids after diagnosis to be more likely to fail medical therapy than those not so treated.[3] Other authors have reported recurrence of disease with the initiation of topical corticosteroids even after the infection was thought to be under control.[14,26] The use of topical corticosteroids in the management of active mycobacterial infections is not recommended[3,14] and they should be used cautiously when the keratitis appears to be resolving.

The length of medical treatment is typically prolonged and no specific guidelines regarding the duration of treatment have been determined. Active organisms have been recovered after 2 weeks of topical treatment in animal models of NTM keratitis.[64] Viable organisms have been seen in histological sections of an amputated LASIK flap even after 9 weeks of intensive antibiotic therapy,[14] and progression or recurrence of infection after 2 months of treatment have been reported.[30] For patients who were successfully cured with medical therapy alone, the average duration of treatment was 40 days in one study.[50] In post-LASIK cases, treatment duration has ranged from 4 weeks[14] to 9 months,[33] with most resolving after 6–8 weeks of treatment.

Many studies have not shown improved efficacy of multi-agent therapy over single-agent therapy in vitro[61] and in animal models[52,64] for susceptible organisms. However, due to the variable drug sensitivities, multi-agent therapy should be considered until drug sensitivities are available. A triple-drug therapy was required in 49% of cases of NTM keratitis after LASIK, with an additional 21% requiring four agents.[35] In one report, most strains of *M. chelonae* were sensitive to amikacin; however, all isolates of *M. chelonae* were found to be resistant to ciprofloxacin. Clarithromycin was the only drug effective against all isolates of *M. chelonae* and *M. fortuitum* (Table 78.3).[3] It has also shown excellent activity against other strains of NTM, including *M. szulgai*.[32] Multi-agent therapy may also decrease the risk of developing antibiotic resistance during the course of treatment. There have been reports of fourth-generation fluoroquinolone-resistant mycobacterial keratitis.[65] The rapid development of resistance to ciprofloxacin and clarithromycin when used as monotherapy in systemic infections has been described.[56,66]

A starting regimen including fortified amikacin, clarithromycin, and a fourth-generation fluoroquinolone has been

Table 78.3 In vitro sensitivities for NTM isolates (% sensitive [No.])

Drug	*M. chelonae*	*M. fortuitum*
Amikacin	70 (9/13)	100 (2/2)
Clarithromycin	100 (9/9)	100 (2/2)
Ciprofloxacin	0 (0/12)	50 (1/2)
Cefoxitin	22 (2/9)	0 (0/3)
Doxycycline	0 (0/3)	0 (0/2)
Imipenem	50 (4/8)	0 (0/1)
Trimethoprim/sulfamethaxozole	0 (0/5)	100 (1/1)
Tobramycin	73 (8/11)	50 (1/2)

From Ford JG, et al: Nontuberculous mycobacterial keratitis in south Florida, Ophthalmology *105(9):1652–1658, 1998.*

advocated.[67] This regimen may be adjusted when antibiotic sensitivities are obtained. It is important to recognize that the in vivo response to treatment often does not correlate with in vitro drug sensitivities. Factors responsible for this discrepancy may include the frequent delay in diagnosis, inadequate drug penetration, and the slow growth rate of the organism, in addition to the emergence of a resistant strain.[23]

Surgical Treatment

Due to the frequent unresponsiveness of NTM keratitis cases to medical therapy, early surgical intervention should be considered for any patient who does not improve with appropriate antibiotic treatment or has unacceptable toxicity from antibiotic therapy. One study in 2004 found 85% of NTM keratitis cases ultimately required surgical intervention to control the infection.[68]

Therapeutic lamellar keratectomy has been advocated by several authors to surgically manage NTM keratitis.[4,23,50] Hu performed extensive lamellar keratectomies on nine patients who failed to respond to medical therapy and had infiltrates of less than 80% of corneal thickness. The infection was eradicated in seven patients while two patients required a second keratectomy to control the infection. Visual acuity improved in seven patients and remained the same in two.[23] This procedure provides a tissue source for culture and histology, decreases the organism load, facilitates antibiotic penetration, and removes necrotic tissue to allow reepithelialization. It may allow the eye to stabilize before undergoing PKP and, in some cases, may obviate the need for PKP.[4] Topical antibiotic therapy is continued, but often at a lower concentration and frequency, and a shorter duration.

Surgical intervention may be even more essential in post-LASIK infections. Immediate lifting of the flap to obtain adequate specimens for culture and smears and to irrigate with appropriate antibiotics is recommended.[14] Flap removal may play an important role in the resolution of post-LASIK NTM keratitis. Early flap amputation is indicated in cases when the flap is melting, is densely infiltrated, or when there is no significant clinical improvement.[14] The benefit of increased antibiotic access outweighs the probable scarring of the cornea. In one review, 54% of cases required flap amputation and 10% required therapeutic PKP. In 54% of cases, patients ultimately achieved best-corrected visual acuity (BCVA) of 20/40 or better, while 14% were worse than 20/200.[35]

Therapuetic keratoplasty should be considered in cases medically unresponsive, extensive or full-thickness, and/or nearing perforation. Recently, deep anterior lamellar keratoplasty (DALK) has been suggessted as an alternative to therapeutic PKP in some cases of infectious keratitis.[69] A primary advantage of DALK in this settting is the reduction of organism entry into the anterior chamber.[70] The area of trephination should encompass 1–1.5 mm of clinically uninvolved cornea and the specimen should be submitted to pathology and microbiology for evaluation. Topical antibiotic therapy should be continued initially. Corticosteroids should be used judiciously postoperatively with the primary goal of surgery being eradication of infection. Careful postoperative evaluation is required as multiple recurrences in the graft have been described.[3,12,33,71]

Summary

While once considered a rare disease, the incidence of NTM keratitis has been increasing with the increase in popularity of LASIK. The diagnosis should be considered in any chronic ulcer that does not respond to conventional treatments. Acid-fast staining and mycobacteria-specific culture media should be obtained in addition to the routine microbial keratitis work-up. Corticosteroids should be discontinued during the active phase of the infection and used judiciously in the later phases of treatment. Further investigation into the most ideal antibiotic regimen is needed to improve the rate of medical cures. The clinician should be prepared to intervene surgically in cases unresponsive to appropriate medical treatment.

References

1. Turner L, Stinson I. *Mycobacterium fortuitum* as a cause of corneal ulcer. *Am J Ophthamlol.* 1965;60:329–331.
2. Runyon EH. Anonymous mycobacteria in pulmonary disease. *Med Clin N Am.* 1959;43:273–289.
3. Ford JG, Huang AJ, Pflugfelder SC, et al. Nontuberculous mycobacterial keratitis in south Florida. *Ophthalmology.* 1998;105(9):1652–1658.
4. Huang SC, Soong HK, Chang JS, et al. Non-tuberculous mycobacterial keratitis: a study of 22 cases. *Br J Ophthalmol.* 1996;80(11):962–968.
5. Bullington RH Jr, Lanier JD, Font RL. Nontuberculous mycobacterial keratitis. Report of two cases and review of the literature. *Arch Ophthalmol.* 1992;110(4):519–524.
6. Garg P, Athmanathan S, Rao GN. *Mycobacterium chelonae* masquerading as *Corynebacterium* in a case of infectious keratitis: a diagnostic dilemma. *Cornea.* 1998;17(2):230–232.
7. Hwang DG, Biswell R. Ciprofloxacin therapy of *Mycobacterium chelonae* keratitis. *Am J Ophthalmol.* 1993;115(1):114–115.
8. Labalette P, Maurage CA, Jourdel D, et al. Nontuberculous mycobacterial keratitis: report of two cases causing infectious crystalline keratopathy. *J Fr Ophtalmol.* 2003;26(2):175–181.

9. Hu FR, Luh KT. Topical ciprofloxacin for treating nontuberculous mycobacterial keratitis. *Ophthalmology.* 1998;105(2):269–722.
10. David DB, Hirst LW, McMillen J, Whitby M. *Mycobacterium marinum* keratitis: pigmentation a clue to diagnosis. *Eye.* 1999;13(Pt 3a):377–379.
11. Moore MB, Newton C, Kaufman HE. Chronic keratitis caused by *Mycobacterium gordonae. Am J Ophthalmol.* 1986;102(4):516–521.
12. Telahun A, Waring GO, Grossniklaus HE. *Mycobacterium gordonae* keratitis. *Cornea.* 1992;11(1):77–82.
13. Frueh BE, Dubuis O, Imesch P, et al. *Mycobacterium szulgai* keratitis. *Arch Ophthalmol.* 2000;118(8):1123–1124.
14. Solomon A, Karp CL, Miller D, et al. *Mycobacterium* interface keratitis after laser in situ keratomileusis. *Ophthalmology.* 2001;108(12):2201–2208.
15. Wallace RJ Jr, Swenson JM, Silcox VA, et al. Spectrum of disease due to rapidly growing mycobacteria. *Rev Infect Dis.* 1983;5:657–679.
16. Kiewiet AA, Thompson JE. Isolation of 'atypical' mycobacteria from healthy individuals in tropical Australia. *Tubercle.* 1970;51:296–299.
17. Panwalker AP, Fuhse E. Nosocomial *Mycobacterium gordonae* pseudoinfection from contaminated ice machines. *Infect Control.* 1986;7(2):67–70.
18. Chadha R, Grover M, Sharma A, et al. An outbreak of post-surgical wound infections due to *Mycobacterium abscessus. Pediatr Surg Int.* 1998;13(5–6):406–410.
19. Tiwari TS, Ray B, Jost KC Jr, et al. Forty years of disinfectant failure: outbreak of postinjection *Mycobacterium abscessus* infection caused by contamination of benzalkonium chloride. *Clin Infect Dis.* 2003;36(8):954–962.
20. Bolan G, Reingold AL, Carson LA, et al. Infections with *Mycobacterium chelonae* in patients receiving dialysis and using processed hemodialyzers. *J Infect Dis.* 1985;152(5):1013–1019.
21. Robin JB, Beatty RF, Dunn S, et al. *Mycobacterium chelonae* keratitis after radial keratotomy. *Am J Ophthalmol.* 1986;102(1):72–79.
22. Brancato R, Carones F, Venturi E, et al. *Mycobacterium chelonae* keratitis after excimer laser photorefractive keratectomy. *Arch Ophthalmol.* 1997;115(10):1316–1318.
23. Hu FR. Extensive lamellar keratectomy for treatment of nontuberculous mycobacterial keratitis. *Am J Ophthalmol.* 1995;120(1):47–54.
24. Reviglio V, Rodriguez ML, Picotti GS, et al. *Mycobacterium chelonae* keratitis following laser in situ keratomileusis. *J Refract Surg.* 1998;14(3):357–360.
25. Gelender H, Carter HL, Bowman B, et al. *Mycobacterium* keratitis after laser in situ keratomileusis. *J Refract Surg.* 2000;16(2):191–195.
26. Garg P, Bansal AK, Sharma S, Vemuganti GK. Bilateral infectious keratitis after laser in situ keratomileusis: a case report and review of the literature. *Ophthalmology.* 2001;108(1):121–125.
27. Kouyoumdjian GA, Forstot SL, Durairaj VD, et al. Infectious keratitis after laser refractive surgery. *Ophthalmology.* 2001;108(7):1266–1268.
28. Chandra NS, Torres MF, Winthrop KL, et al. Cluster of *Mycobacterium chelonae* keratitis cases following laser in-situ keratomileusis. *Am J Ophthalmol.* 2001;132(6):819–830.
29. Becero F, Maestre JR, Buezas V, et al. [Keratitis due to *Mycobacterium chelonae* after refractive surgery with LASIK (letter)]. *Enferm Infecc Microbiol Clin.* 2002;20(1):44–45.
30. Seo KY, Lee JB, Lee K, et al. Non-tuberculous mycobacterial keratitis at the interface after laser in situ keratomileusis. *J Refract Surg.* 2002;18(1):81–85.
31. Alvarenga L, Freitas D, Hofling-Lima AL, et al. Infectious post-LASIK crystalline keratopathy caused by nontuberculous mycobacteria. *Cornea.* 2002;21(4):426–429.
32. Fulcher SF, Fader RC, Rosa Jr RH, et al. Delayed-onset mycobacterial keratitis after LASIK. *Cornea.* 2002;21(6):546–554.
33. Freitas D, Alvarenga L, Sampaio J, et al. An outbreak of *Mycobacterium chelonae* infection after LASIK. *Ophthalmology.* 2003;110(2):276–285.
34. Daines BS, Vroman DT, Sandoval HP, et al. Rapid diagnosis and treatment of mycobacterial keratitis after laser in situ keratomileusis. *J Cataract Refract Surg.* 2003;29(5):1014–1018.
35. John T, Velotta E. Nontuberculous (atypical) mycobacterial keratitis after LASIK. *Cornea.* 2005;24(3):245–255.
36. Chung SH, Roh MI, Park MS, et al. *Mycobacterium abscessus* keratitis after LASIK with IntraLase femtosecond laser. *Ophthalmologica.* 2006;220(4):277–280.
37. Holmes GP, Bond GB, Fader RC, et al. A cluster of cases of *Mycobacterium szulgai* keratitis that occurred after laser-assisted in situ keratomileusis. *Clin Infect Dis.* 2002;34(8):1039–1046.
38. Paschal JF, Holland GN, Sison RF, et al. *Mycobacterium fortuitum* keratitis. Clinicopathologic correlates and corticosteroid effects in an animal model. *Cornea.* 1992;11(6):493–499.
39. Polansky JR, Weinreb RN. Anti-inflammatory agents: steroids as anti-inflammatory agents. In: Sears ML, ed. *Pharmacology of the eye.* Berlin: Springer-Verlag; 1984:459–538.
40. Dugel PU, Holland GN, Brown HH, et al. *Mycobacterium fortuitum* keratitis. *Am J Ophthalmol.* 1988;105(6):661–669.
41. Hu FR, Huang WJ, Huang SF. Clinicopathologic study of satellite lesions in nontuberculous mycobacterial keratitis. *Jpn J Ophthalmol.* 1998;42(2):115–118.
42. Lazar M, Nemet P, Bracha R, et al. *Mycobacterium fortuitum* keratitis. *Am J Ophthalmol.* 1974;78(3):530–532.
43. Somoskovi A, Hotaling JE, Fitzgerald M, et al. Lessons from a proficiency testing event for acid-fast microscopy. *Chest.* 2001;120(1):250–257.
44. Chen KH, Sheu MM, Lin SR. Rapid identification of mycobacteria to the species level by polymerase chain reaction and restriction enzyme analysis – a case report of corneal ulcer. *Kaohsiung J Med Sci.* 1997;13(9):583–588.
45. Brown-Elliott BA, Griffith DE, Wallace RJ Jr. Diagnosis of nontuberculous mycobacterial infections. *Clin Lab Med.* 2002;22(4):911–925.
46. Sanders WE Jr, Hartwig EC, Schneider NJ, et al. Susceptibility of organisms in the *Mycobacterium fortuitum* complex to antituberculous and other antimicrobial agents. *Antimicrob Agents Chemother.* 1977;12(2):295–297.
47. Tanaka N. Mechanism of action of aminoglycoside antibiotics. In: Umezawa H, Hooper IR, eds. *Handbook of experimental pharmacology.* Vol 62. New York: Springer-Verlag; 1982.
48. Eiferman RA, Stagner JI. Intraocular penetration of amikacin. Iris binding and bioavailability. *Arch Ophthalmol.* 1982;100(11):1817–1819.
49. Davison CR, Tuft SJ, Dart JK. Conjunctival necrosis after administration of topical fortified aminoglycosides. *Am J Ophthalmol.* 1991;111(6):690–693.
50. Tseng SH, Hsiao WC. Therapeutic lamellar keratectomy in the management of nontuberculous *Mycobacterium keratitis* refractory to medical treatments. *Cornea.* 1995;14(2):161–166.
51. Bahal N, Nahata MC. The new macrolide antibiotics: azithromycin, clarithromycin, dirithromycin, and roxithromycin. *Ann Pharmacother.* 1992;26(1):46–55.
52. Helm CJ, Holland GN, Lin R, et al. Comparison of topical antibiotics for treating *Mycobacterium fortuitum* keratitis in an animal model. *Am J Ophthalmol.* 1993;116(6):700–707.
53. Gross RH, Holland GN, Elias SJ, et al. Corneal pharmacokinetics of topical clarithromycin. *Invest Ophthalmol Vis Sci.* 1995;36(5):965–968.
54. Whitman MS, Tunkel AR. Azithromycin and clarithromycin: overview and comparison with erythromycin. *Infect Control Hosp Epidemiol.* 1992;13(6):357–368.
55. Brown BA, Wallace RJ Jr, Onyi GO, et al. Activities of four macrolides, including clarithromycin, against *Mycobacterium fortuitum, Mycobacterium chelonae,* and *M. chelonae*-like organisms. *Antimicrob Agents Chemother.* 1992;36(1):180–184.
56. Wallace RJ Jr, Bedsole G, Sumter G, et al. Activities of ciprofloxacin and ofloxacin against rapidly growing mycobacteria with demonstration of acquired resistance following single-drug therapy. *Antimicrob Agents Chemother.* 1990;34(1):65–70.
57. Brown-Elliott BA, Wallace RJ Jr, Crist CJ, et al. Comparison of in vitro activities of gatifloxacin and ciprofloxacin against four taxa of rapidly growing mycobacteria. *Antimicrob Agents Chemother.* 2002;46(10):3283–3285.
58. Gillespie SH, Billington O. Activity of moxifloxacin against mycobacteria. *J Antimicrob Chemother.* 1999;44: 393–395.
59. Abshire R, Cockrum P, Crider J, et al. Topical antibacterial therapy for mycobacterial keratitis: potential for surgical prophylaxis and treatment. *Clin Ther.* 2004;26:191–196.
60. Hofling-Lima AI, de Freitas D, Sampaio JL, et al. In vitro activity of fluoroquinolones against *Mycobacterium abscessus* and *Mycobacterium chelonae* causing infectious keratitis after LASIK in Brazil. *Cornea.* 2005;24(6):730–734.
61. Hu FR, Chang SC, Luh KT, et al. The antimicrobial susceptibility of *Mycobacterium chelonae* isolated from corneal ulcer. *Curr Eye Res.* 1997;16(10):1056–1060.
62. Lin R, Holland GN, Helm CJ, et al. Comparative efficacy of topical ciprofloxacin for treating *Mycobacterium fortuitum* and *Mycobacterium chelonae* keratitis in an animal model. *Am J Ophthalmol.* 1994;117(5):657–662.
63. Sarayba MA, Shamie N, Reiser BJ, et al. Fluoroquinolone therapy in *Mycobacterium chelonae* keraitis after lamellar keratectomy. *J Cataract Refract Surg.* 2005;31(7):1396–1402.
64. Hu FR, Wang IJ. Comparison of topical antibiotics for treating *Mycobacterium chelonae* keratitis in a rabbit model. *Curr Eye Res.* 1998;17(5):478–482.

65. Moshifar M, Meyer JJ, Espandar L. Fourth-generation fluoroquinolone-resistant mycobacterial keratitis after laser in situ keratomileusis. *J Cataract Refract Surg*. 2007;33(11):1978–1981.
66. Tebas P, Sultan F, Wallace RJ Jr, et al. Rapid development of resistance to clarithromycin following monotherapy for disseminated *Mycobacterium chelonae* infection in a heart transplant patient. *Clin Infect Dis*. 1995;20:443–444.
67. Hamam RN, Noureddin B, Salti HI, et al. Recalcitrant post-LASIK *Mycobacterium chelonae* keratitis eradicated after the use of fourth-generation fluoroquinolone. *Ophthalmology*. 2006;113(6):950–954.
68. Fong CF, Tseng CH, Hu FR, et al. Clinical characteristics of microbial keratitis in a university hospital in Tiawan. *Am J Ophthalmol*. 2004;137(2):329–336.
69. Ti S-E, Scott JA, Janardhanan P, Tan DTH. Therapeutic keratoplasty for advanced suppurative keratitis. *Am J Ophthalmol*. 2007;143:755–762.
70. Susiyanti M, Mehta JS, Tan DT. Bilateral deep anterior lamellar keratoplasty for the management of bilateral post-LASIK mycobacterial keratitis. *J Cataract Refract Surg*. 2007;33(9):1641–1643.
71. Sossi N, Feldman RM, Feldman ST, et al. *Mycobacterium gordonae* keratitis after penetrating keratoplasty. *Arch Ophthalmol*. 1991;109(8):1064–1065.

Chapter 79

Herpes Simplex Keratitis

Edward J. Holland, Gary S. Schwartz, Kristiana D. Neff

The herpes simplex viruses (HSV) are ubiquitous human pathogens capable of causing both asymptomatic infection and active disease in a wide variety of end organs. Virus-specific antigens differentiate HSV into two types: type 1 (HSV-1) and type 2 (HSV-2). Although HSV-1 usually involves the oropharynx and HSV-2 usually involves the genital area, both types can infect either location as has been demonstrated by polymerase chain reaction (PCR) and in situ hybridization.[1] Typically, ocular disease is caused by type 1 rather than type 2, with the exception of herpetic keratitis in neonates in which 75% is caused by HSV-2.[2] Primary infection can be either asymptomatic or active and is followed by a latent state of nonreplication characteristic of herpesviruses.[3] HSV is capable of causing severe primary disease in children and neonates and has been known to cause a variety of ocular diseases in addition to oral-facial infections, encephalitis, meningitis, myelitis, erythema multiforme, hepatitis, and disseminated infection resulting in death.[3] More common infections include recurrent herpes labialis caused by HSV-1, which occurs in 20–45% of the world population, and herpes genitalis caused by HSV-2, which causes an estimated 100 000 new cases each year in the United States, with an increasing seroprevalence, estimated at 21.9% in the last NHANES (National Health and Nutrition Evaluation Survey).[4–8] A longitudinal study by Liesegang et al.[9] extrapolated data to an estimated 20 000 new cases of ocular HSV in the United States per year and more than 48 000 episodes annually. Although research has resulted in a better understanding of the molecular biology and pathogenesis of HSV, HSV infection remains a serious public health problem associated with significant morbidity and mortality.

Viral Structure and Classification

Both HSV-1 and HSV-2 are similar morphologically to other herpesviruses including varicella-zoster, Epstein-Barr, and cytomegalovirus. An icosahedral-shaped capsid surrounds the core, which contains the double-stranded deoxyribonucleic acid (DNA) and associated phosphoproteins of the viral chromatin. The capsid is surrounded by an envelope of glycoproteins, carbohydrates, and lipids. The glycoproteins arise from de novo synthesis via virus specification or from modification to host cell proteins.[10] HSV-1 and HSV-2 share about 50% homology of their DNA, but the sequence variability is enough to allow for different cleavage patterns with restriction endonucleases.[3]

Digestion by restriction endonucleases allows for DNA mapping and subsequent differentiation of viral strains. A viral strain is thought of as a single viral isolate that may be propagated from person to person. Therefore, DNA mapping and subsequent identification of a viral strain can be useful in epidemiologic studies of viral transmission. Different viral strains may produce different patterns of ocular disease, as was shown by Wander et al.[11] Viral DNA sequencing of HSV-1 isolates has identified three distinct genotypes, arbitrarily called A, B, and C, based on the sequencing of the unique short region of the genome.[12]

Receptor specificity and host cell factors determine the ability of a particular virus to infect a cell type. It is thought that HSV binds to one or more cellular receptors, heparin sulfate probably being one of them.[13] The virus fuses with the cell membrane and, after entering the cell, it is brought to the nucleus where transcription of viral DNA occurs with subsequent synthesis of more than 70 proteins. Two virion proteins act on the infected cell before transcription. The first stops the synthesis of host cell macromolecules, and the second interacts with the nucleus to initiate transcription of HSV RNA.[3] HSV DNA alone is considered infectious. Viral DNA begins replication 3 to 4 hours after infection, with complete virions being secreted when infected cells lyse.

Epidemiology

Humans are the only natural reservoir of HSV despite experimental models using other hosts. Close personal contact is thought to be necessary for the spread of HSV because of the physical instability of the virus and the fact that the major portals of entry are the mucous membranes and external skin. Primary exposure and infection may be asymptomatic and are seen earlier and more frequently among lower socioeconomic classes.[4] There is no documentation of viral spread through aerosolization, fomites, or swimming pools. As mentioned earlier, initial end-organ infection can be asymptomatic and unrecognized and is followed by latency in sensory ganglia. In fact, primary infection manifests clinically in only 1–6% of people infected with the virus. The oral route can provide access to the trigeminal ganglion and subsequently the eye.[6,14] Because many patients with HSV infection do not have definitive contact with a source, it has been suggested that asymptomatic shedding of virus is an important source of transmission.[4] In addition, clinical appearance of an infection may represent earlier primary infection at a different end organ. Therefore, what appears to be a primary ocular infection may indeed be an attack in a new end organ within a previously infected host. The time between contact and disease is typically between 3 and 9 days.

Exposure to HSV-1 usually occurs during childhood through contact with oral lesions and secretions. Except in populations where sexual activity includes frequent oral-genital contact, few cases of orolabial infections are caused by HSV-2. On the other hand, HSV-1 is increasingly associated with genital infection, as more adolescents escape orofacial HSV-1 infection in childhood in the developed world and are then, without immunity, involved in orogenital practices. Passive transfer of maternal antibody accounts for the high incidence of antibodies to HSV-1 in children less than 6 months of age. This incidence is about 20% from 6 to 12 months of age and then rises to about 60% between 15 and 25 years.[15,16]

Liesegang et al.[9] were the first to study extensively the epidemiology of ocular involvement with HSV. In 1956, Thygeson et al.[17] reviewed a series of 200 cases of herpetic keratitis, which included only passing mention of epidemiology. Reference to an association between herpes labialis in the parents of children with herpetic keratitis was made, as well as observations of an occupational relationship between herpes keratitis and the practice of dentistry. Other studies have evaluated the epidemiology more carefully and are presented here. In a 5-year study of 152 patients with herpetic keratitis, Wilhelmus et al.[18] found that 64.5% of their group were male and 35.5% female. Nineteen (12%) had concurrent herpes labialis, and 91 (60%) had a previous episode of cutaneous herpes. Forty percent experienced at least one recurrence of corneal ulceration during the study. In addition, 53% of patients presenting with a history of previous ulceration and 28% of those with a primary ulceration experienced a recurrence during the study period. More men (50%) than women (22%) experienced recurrent ulceration.

Bell et al.[19] reviewed 141 records of patients with acute epithelial HSV keratitis and found a high male:female ratio (1.67:1) in patients more than 40 years of age. In younger patients, no difference was observed. A majority of patients (55%) had at least one previous episode of epithelial ulceration. Of the 65 patients with more than one episode, 22 (34%) had an average annual recurrence of one or more episodes, and 44 (68%) had an average of one or more every 2 years. They found no statistical difference in recurrence rate in terms of age at entry into the study, age at occurrence of the first episode, gender, or race. It was also found that recurrent episodes of HSV keratitis were more likely to happen from November through February. Because of the higher incidence of viral upper respiratory infections (URIs) during this time of the year, an association was suggested between URI and the triggering of recurrent HSV keratitis.

The presentation of ocular HSV as conjunctivitis in adults was emphasized for the first time in 1978;[20] 21% of all acute conjunctivitis was thought to be of herpetic origin in a later report.[21] It was again Darougar et al.[22] who studied 108 patients with primary HSV ocular infection. A predominant number (64%) were 15 years of age or older, with only 7% less than 5 years. Moderate and severe conjunctivitis and blepharitis were observed in 84% and 38% of patients, respectively. Eight patients (7%) presented with an acute follicular conjunctivitis without eyelid or corneal lesions. Sixteen patients (15%) developed a chronic blepharoconjunctivitis. Dendritic ulcers represented 15% of the group and, interestingly, 2% presented with 'disciform keratitis.' In a later study by the same authors, 35 (32%) patients experienced one or more recurrent attacks when followed for 2 to 15 years.[23] This incidence was higher in patients less than 20, and no gender predilection was observed. They also found that the more severe the conjunctivitis and eyelid lesions during primary disease, the higher the incidence of recurrent infection. This relationship was not found with corneal lesions.

In another longitudinal, 5-year follow-up of patients with infectious epithelial HSV keratitis, a recurrence rate of epithelial disease of 40% was calculated, with multiple recurrences in half of cases; a 25% rate of stromal keratitis and 6% rate of ocular hypertension was estimated with these recurrences.[24]

Liesegang et al.[9,25] evaluated 122 patients presenting with a first episode of HSV ocular infection over a 33-year period and followed the natural history. The mean age at onset was 37.4 years. Males and females were affected equally after adjustment for age. An age- and sex-adjusted incidence of 8.4 new cases/100 000 person-years was found. Initial episodes involved the eyelid or conjunctiva (54%), superficial cornea (63%), deeper cornea including stroma (6%), and uvea (4%). Although no seasonal trends in incidence were observed, the incidence rate did increase with time. The prevalence of a history of ocular herpes simplex infection was 149/100 000 population. Further evaluation of natural history[25] revealed a recurrence rate after the first episode of 9.6% at 1 year, 22.9% at 2 years, and 63.2% at 20 years. These rates did rise with subsequent repeated episodes, while the interval between episodes shortened. In fact, 70–80% of patients can have a recurrent episode within 10 years of their second attack. Bilateral disease at the same time or at different times occurred in 11.9% of patients. Other studies have reported bilateral disease in 1–10% of cases.[17,26] The eyelid, conjunctiva, and superficial cornea were the most commonly affected sites of recurrent disease. However, the incidence of stromal disease and uveitis did rise with recurrent disease. Another study found recurrence of ocular HSV to be 24% at 1 and 33% at 2 years.[27] In the HEDS study, a recurrence rate of 18% was estimated for both epithelial and stromal HSV keratitis.[28] While a history of previous epithelial keratitis did not alter the likelihood of subsequent episodes, prior stromal keratitis episodes did increase the risk 10-fold in the case of stromal keratitis.

The epidemiology of herpetic eye disease has been studied with greater attention and detail in recent years. Advances in this area will allow the clinician to better understand the disease and improve diagnostic acumen. A comprehensive understanding of clinical presentations and epidemiology in both primary and recurrent disease will not only improve clinical sensitivity but also allow for accurate counseling of patients.

Pathogenesis

Latency and reactivation

The spectrum of ocular disease caused by HSV is broad and is underscored by the ability of HSV to infect a host and establish an indefinite and latent presence in ganglionic neurons. Latency allows for spontaneous and recurrent reactivation of the disease and provides a viral reservoir within the population.[29] The clinical sequelae of HSV infection are largely a result of recurrent disease and the immunologic response associated with each episode. This section describes the mechanisms of latency and reactivation and reviews the available information in this developing area.

After peripheral entry into the host and primary infection with viral replication within an end organ, HSV travels in a retrograde fashion to various ganglia including the trigeminal, cervical, and sympathetic gangliae, and possibly the brain stem.[30–32] Here it resides during the lifespan of the host. This process usually begins within 1 to 2 days of the primary infection and may take several weeks to complete.[33–39] Despite an early immune response by the host, ganglionic infection occurs rapidly and does not require virus replication.[4] Once ganglionic presence has been established, active replication in neurons and surrounding cells leads to cell death.[4] It has been suggested that virus replication within the trigeminal ganglion is of paramount importance for viral spread to sites other than the inoculation site; no periocular virus activity was seen in mice whose corneas were inoculated with a virus mutant defective in its replication in nerve tissue.[40] Regardless, latency can be established and is thought to represent the presence of the viral genome within the neuronal cells.[4,41,42] Using a variety of molecular biologic techniques, HSV DNA has been detected in the culture-negative ganglia of latently infected hosts.[39,43–48] The cornea itself has also been found to host latent HSV virus, with potential for reactivation.

Latently infected neurons have not been found to produce infectious virus. However, a region of the viral genome that is retained within the host cell nucleus during latency is responsible for RNA transcripts termed latency-associated transcripts (LATS).[4] This region of the viral genome also contains part of the gene encoding an important early transcriptional protein of HSV termed IEO. These LATS are made from the opposite (complementary) DNA strand that is responsible for the normal IEO message. The role of LATS is unknown. They are thought to be produced in large amounts during reactivation from latency and ultimately act as a type of regulator in the production of viral proteins and infectious virions. Reactivation of HSV results in virus shedding with or without clinical signs.

Although the cornea itself can be a source of virus in recurrent disease,[49,50] the trigeminal ganglion is the most common source of recurrent HSV infection. Recurrent infection can occur in a different end organ than the primary site. A primary oral or facial infection may subsequently reactivate by traveling via the ophthalmic division of the fifth cranial nerve to the eye instead of recurring at the site of primary infection. The presence of pre-existing antigen-specific T cells and humoral antibodies from primary infection can result in a less severe infection during recurrence; moreover, first-time ocular involvement after infection in another end organ resembles recurrent ocular disease.

Systemic antibodies have no known role in the development of recurrent disease despite their role in the host response to active primary and recurrent infection. It has been demonstrated that antibody titers remain unchanged during and between episodes of recurrent HSV. These titers may even increase without evidence of active infection.[15,51–56]

The study of HSV, particularly the differences in strains, has been a frequently updated area of investigation. Some strains have been reported to cause predominantly epithelial disease and even specific patterns of dendritic ulcers. Other strains have a tendency to produce more severe stromal disease, and some are more likely to cause recurrences.[12,57–59] In one study by Centifanto et al.,[57] DNA analysis revealed that differences in disease patterns may be determined genetically by a specific site on the genome of a virus substrain. A clinical isolate may be composed of several substrains and therefore be competent to produce a spectrum of disease.[60] It also has been demonstrated that some strains cause an epithelial keratitis that is made worse by corticosteroids.[58] There is no clear explanation of this effect, which is further confounded by the observation that the same effect can be seen in vitro where no host-mediated immune system is present.[61]

It has been proposed that the first viral strain to infect the host and establish latency can prevent subsequent infections by a different strain of HSV.[62] This effect was thought to be due to a blocking mechanism whereby other strains could infect the end organ, but could not superinfect the associated ganglion. Evidence to the contrary developed when more than one strain of HSV was found in the same trigeminal ganglion of several animals.[63,64] Previous inoculation with a less virulent strain of virus did provide protection from a more virulent strain, including a decrease in the severity of keratitis and a decrease in the frequency of recovery of latent virions. This protection is incomplete, however, and is demonstrated by the recovery of multiple strains of HSV from the same host. In another study, superinfection with a different viral strain, as opposed to recurrence of the original strain, was seen in one-third of cases of recrudescent herpetic keratitis.[65] The implications of such findings would make the development of vaccinations for HSV difficult to perfect because of both the large number of strains and the possibility of several substrains of HSV existing in a single human host.

Many factors have been implicated in the activation of recurrent HSV ocular disease. The mechanisms that control HSV latency are key to viral shedding and reactivation of disease. Intuitively, the immune system should be the core of regulation in infections, and this has been demonstrated to be a factor in reactivation of latent infection. Recent studies of CD8+ T-cell inhibition of HSV-1 reactivation show viral inactivation via the use of lytic granules degrading precursors to viral gene expression.[66] These CD8+ T cells maintain latency without causing neuronal apoptosis. Sunlight, trauma (including surgery), heat, abnormal body temperature, menstruation, other infectious diseases, and emotional stress have all been implicated in the activation of herpetic disease in human beings.[37,67–70] Prostaglandin F2 alpha analog and prostamide glaucoma medications latanoprost and bimatoprost have also been implicated in ocular or even periocular HSV reactivation.[71–76] Although some type of immunoregulation may exist in all of these circumstances, it has not been clearly demonstrated. Reactivation of disease has been achieved in experimental animals with immunosuppression.[77] However, this is generally not well demonstrated in human beings. The incidence of bilateral disease is, nonetheless, higher in immunocompromised patients.[78,79] Psychological stress, systemic infection, sunlight exposure, menstrual period, contact lens wear, and eye injury were studied as potential triggers of ocular HSV recurrences; 308 immunocompetent adults were observed for 18 months, weekly logs were kept on those five factors and were considered only if completed before the onset of symptoms. With 33 valid recurrences, none of these factors was associated with a recurrence of ocular HSV. When the 26 recurrences excluded for being reported late were examined, high stress and systemic infection were found to have been reported significantly more frequently than in the 33 valid responses. This was a very characteristic example of recall bias in a prospective cohort study.[80]

Overall, the severity and frequency of disease are multifactorial and may depend not only on emotional, physical, and immunologic stress but also on the viral genome and its virulence.

Immune defense mechanisms

Both humoral and cellular responses are part of the host response to HSV infection and may indeed be responsible for limiting spread of disease and for the pathologic sequelae in the local tissue. In ocular infection, viral replication and immunologic response from infection are responsible for destructive changes associated with necrotizing stromal keratitis, immune stromal keratitis, and endotheliitis.[70,81,82] The pathogenesis associated with these manifestations of HSV infection are not clearly understood and have been the focus of many investigations.

Stromal inflammation from HSV keratitis is thought to be due to either replicating virus or the alteration of antigenicity of the stromal cells, allowing for recurrent immune-mediated cycles of inflammation. Details of this process were made more clear by Easty,[83] who summarized his studies of HSV stromal keratitis. He showed that HSV may enter stromal keratocytes where it can be eliminated or escape the immune response and persist within this layer. The virus also can exist within the stroma as a whole virion shed into the stroma from neurons to incite an inflammatory response, or as a slowly proliferating intracellular virus while altering the antigenicity of the cell wall and eliciting an immune response. Latent existence, during which the cell remains antigenically unchanged and there is no active clinical disease, also may occur. In this case, a reactivation would result in disease. In some patients, the disease process is caused by an alteration in cell antigenicity that can lead to an autoimmune-mediated response. Because intact HSV is rarely found in human corneal transplant specimens of patients with a history of HSV keratitis,[84] it has been proposed that residual viral antigens, along with the viral immune alteration of cell membranes in the corneal stroma, can produce an inflammatory response. This response involves lymphocytes, bystander activation of CD4+ T cells,[85] antiviral antibodies, serum complement, polymorphonuclear leukocytes (PMNs), and macrophages.[53,67,86,87]

Molecular mimicry mechanisms have also been proposed for autoimmune disease after HSV infection: viral determinants, such as coat proteins, mimic host antigens, to trigger self-reactive T cells and destroy host tissue.[88]

The endotheliitis seen with HSV and described in a later section also has been studied. Sundmacher et al.[89] proposed that endothelial cells become infected with HSV and therefore elicit a cellular and humoral response. In this theory, cell lysis is thought to be a product of the immune response, with release of infectious virus into the aqueous. Microscopic examination of endothelium in such cases, however, has failed to show viral particles. A delayed-type hypersensitivity response to herpes antigens within the stroma or endothelium also has been proposed as a mechanism responsible for endotheliitis and overlying stromal edema.[83] Furthermore, the delayed-type hypersensitivity reaction not only plays a protective role but also has been implicated in the cause of corneal opacification following HSV infection.[90–94]

Secretion of glycoproteins by HSV also has been implicated in the immune response. Strains of HSV capable of causing stromal disease release greater amounts of glycoprotein than those that cause primarily epithelial disease.[60,95] The exact types of glycoprotein and their roles may be unclear; however, the antigenicity of this protein is thought to be one factor in stimulating the host immune response.

One other puzzling and clinically pivotal aspect of stromal inflammation is neovascularization. In contrast with human herpesvirus 8, responsible for Kaposi's sarcoma,[96] HSV-1 and HSV-2 are not thought to produce proteins that are directly angiogenic. Vascular endothelial growth factor (VEGF), a group of proteins that are the most important thus far studied specific mediators of angiogenesis, have been detected in various inflammatory corneal conditions.[97] VEGF is expressed rapidly, within 24 hours of HSV-1 virus inoculation in mice, by cells other than those directly infected;[98] severity of stromal inflammation was reduced with a VEGF inhibitor in that same experiment and with an endothelial cell inhibitor in another study by the same investigators.[99] Similarly, matrix metalloproteinase-9, up-regulated by HSV infection and produced by neutrophils, induces angiogenesis in mice, and its inhibition appeared to diminish the rate of neovascularization.[100] The role of and the potential for inhibition of angiogenesis in the pathogenesis of stromal keratitis unravels a fascinating area of research, as previously done with retinal neovascularization.

Although the immune defense mechanisms of HSV infection require further investigation, it is clear that there are both beneficial and harmful effects. We know that host defense is mandatory in eliminating virions and thus in preventing the direct toxicity associated with infection. The detrimental effects of this response include local tissue destruction, scarring, and recurrent inflammation. Although this phenomenon may occur in many organs and with many infections, ophthalmologists have the capability of monitoring these secondary effects under microscopic view. Unfortunately, the detrimental effects of the immune response associated with HSV keratitis can result in devastating visual results. Therefore, we are challenged to distinguish the dual role of immunity; to do so allows for the most timely and appropriate medical management.

Clinical Manifestations

Congenital and neonatal ocular herpes

Fortunately, congenital ocular herpetic disease is rare. When all cases of HSV ocular disease are considered, HSV-1 accounts for most cases. Because most congenital cases are acquired in conjunction with genital herpes in the mother and during parturition, HSV-2 accounts for 80% of cases.[101] In general, HSV infects between 1500 and 2000 neonates each year in the United States:[102] 4% are acquired congenitally, 86% natally, and 10% postnatally.[103] In most cases, infection of the mother is a primary genital infection occurring during early to mid gestation,[104] with 60–80% being asymptomatic or unrecognized at the time of delivery.[105] It is important to recognize that other routes of acquisition are also possible and include oral lesions, maternal breast lesions, and nosocomial transmission.[106–108] In addition, infection localized to the skin, eye, or mouth will progress to disseminated disease and/or central nervous system involvement in 75% of cases if not treated.[105]

Ocular manifestations include periocular skin lesions, conjunctivitis, epithelial keratitis, stromal keratitis, and cataracts.[109,110] Posterior ocular findings are discussed elsewhere. Although maternal IgG to HSV may cross the placenta, it does not appear to be sufficient to prevent ocular disease completely. Maternal IgG, however, may quell the clinical course in both systemic and ocular infection. The use of antibody titers for diagnosis is not useful because of preexisting maternal antibody and the delayed production of IgM.[102] The clinical course of congenital and neonatal ocular herpes is similar to primary disease and is discussed later.

Because of the potentially serious complications of congenital and neonatal ocular HSV disease, prompt medical treatment is mandated in conjunction with amblyopia therapy. Moreover, skin vesicles, mouth ulcers, conjunctivitis, or other ocular manifestations suggestive of HSV are all indications for empiric treatment with acyclovir, which should be started in conjunction with a pediatric infectious disease consultation.[102]

Primary ocular herpes

The passage of maternal anti-HSV IgG allows for partial immunity for 6 months. At this point, the passive immunity has diminished to levels that allow for a primary infection of HSV. By the age of 5 years, nearly 60% of the population has been infected with HSV.[3] Latent infection is the usual course and a viral carrier state is established. Only 6% of those infected actually develop clinical manifestations, which typically affect the perioral region rather than the eye.

The presentation of primary ocular HSV is varied and may include acute follicular conjunctivitis, keratoconjunctivitis, preauricular adenopathy, and periocular and eyelid skin vesicles (Fig. 79.1). Adenoviral infections can mimic these findings except where typical vesicular skin lesions are present. Pseudomembranes also may be present and can further confuse the diagnosis in some cases.

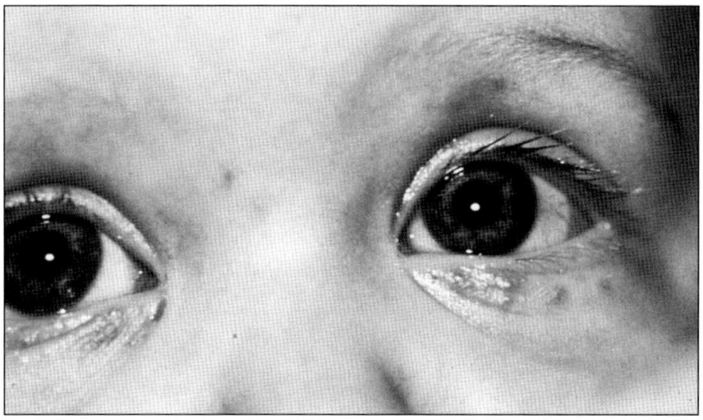

Fig. 79.1 Primary HSV presenting as bilateral blepharitis.

Although rarely a cause, primary HSV should be considered in all cases of keratitis. Early involvement of the cornea may present as a diffuse punctate keratopathy as well as corneal vesicles. During the early stages of infection, epithelial cysts may form and stain negatively with fluorescein. These findings are best appreciated with broad slit lamp illumination. It is thought that this stage of HSV keratitis is similar to the early vesicular lesions of the skin. Eventually these microcysts evolve to erode the overlying epithelium to form microdendritic lesions. Although primary disease is thought to be confined to the epithelium because of a lack of previous immunologic stimulus, it also may be the reason why a large and diffuse involvement of this layer is not uncommon.

Recurrent ocular herpes

In Liesegang's review of the epidemiology of the clinical manifestations of ocular HSV, recurrence rates were 36% at 5 years and 63% at 20 years after a primary episode. After a second episode, 70–80% of patients had another recurrence within 10 years.[25] Schuster et al.[111] reported a 33% recurrence within 2 years in patients with two prior infectious epithelial keratitis episodes. The HEDS study reported an 18% recurrence rate for epithelial keratitis and for stromal keratitis within 18 months in 346 patients with history of ocular HSV within the previous year.[28]

Blepharitis

Herpetic blepharitis can result from a primary infection or recrudescence. The clinical appearance is a vesicular lesion involving a focal area of the eyelid with surrounding erythema similar to that seen at the mucocutaneous junction of the mouth or nose (Fig. 79.2). The typical lesion progresses to ulceration and crusting and heals without a scar unless secondarily infected. Many patients with herpes blepharitis experience recurrences of their lid disease only. Some patients, however, may develop subsequent keratitis after any episode of HSV blepharitis; therefore, this lesion should

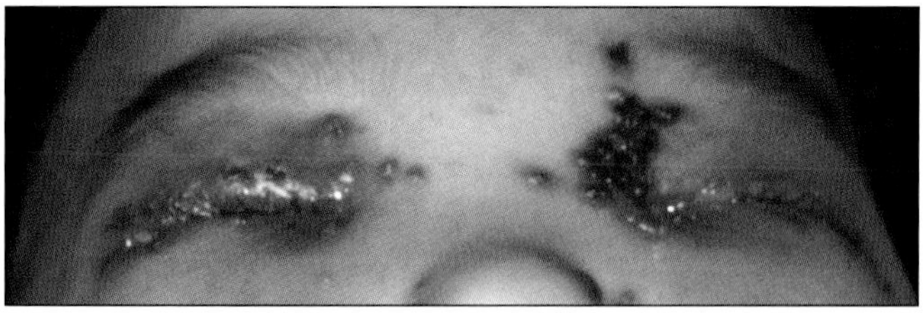

Fig. 79.2 HSV blepharitis presenting as a vesicular lesion with surrounding erythema.

be recognized and properly treated. Because this lesion is relatively uncommon, it is often misdiagnosed. However, it can be separated from more common causes of blepharitis, such as staphylococci, seborrhea, or meibomian gland disease, which tend to involve the entire lid and do not cause vesicles. Diagnosis of HSV blepharitis can be made on the typical clinical appearance and course of a recurrent, focal, vesicular lesion, and through viral culture.

Conjunctivitis

Primary infection with HSV can present as a follicular conjunctivitis. In many patients, this conjunctivitis is self-limiting, but in some it may lead to a subsequent keratitis. One manifestation of HSV is recurrent follicular conjunctivitis. Wishart et al.[23] reported that conjunctivitis with lid lesions was the most common form of recurrence of HSV and accounted for 83% of recurrences. In addition, acute follicular conjunctivitis without lid lesions was seen in 17% of recurrences, and infectious epithelial keratitis was seen in 9%. Other studies have indicated that HSV may constitute up to 23% of cases of acute conjunctivitis presenting to an outpatient ophthalmology clinic and may frequently present without corneal or lid lesions.[112,113]

Some patients with recurrent HSV conjunctivitis may develop a conjunctival dendritic ulcer, which can be best seen with fluorescein. A dendritic ulcer is not always seen, however, and HSV conjunctivitis must be considered in the differential diagnosis of recurrent follicular conjunctivitis. This diagnosis is important because if left unrecognized and treated with topical corticosteroids, the infection has the potential to cause significant ocular damage.

Keratitis

From a diagnostic and therapeutic perspective, HSV keratitis is one of the most challenging entities confronting the clinician. A variety of clinical manifestations of not only infectious keratitis but also immunologic disease can affect all levels of the cornea. Corneal disease includes infectious epithelial keratitis, neurotrophic keratopathy, immune stromal (interstitial) keratitis, necrotizing stromal keratitis, and endotheliitis (Box 79.1; Table 79.1). Recurrent HSV keratitis is typically a unilateral disease. Bilateral herpetic keratitis occurs in approximately 3% of patients with ocular HSV.[114] About 40% of patients with bilateral disease have a history of atopy. In addition, bilateral involvement is more common in younger patients.[26] A sound understanding of the clinical manifestations of HSV keratitis is imperative to treat this disease properly.

Box 79.1 Classification of HSV keratitis

I. Infectious epithelial keratitis
   A. Cornea vesicles
   B. Dendritic ulcer
   C. Geographic ulcer
   D. Marginal ulcer
II. Neurotrophic keratopathy
III. Stromal keratitis
   A. Necrotizing stromal keratitis
   B. Immune stromal (interstitial) keratitis
IV. Endotheliitis
   A. Disciform
   B. Diffuse
   C. Linear

Table 79.1 Common terminology in HSV keratitis

Recommended nomenclature	Alternate terms
Infectious epithelial keratitis (cornea vesicles, dendritic ulcer, geographic ulcer, marginal ulcer)	Dendrite Herpetic epithelial keratitis Infectious epithelial herpes Limbal keratoconjunctivitis
Neurotrophic keratopathy (punctate epithelial erosions, neurotrophic ulcer)	Trophic ulcer Neurotrophic ulcer Metaherpetic ulcer Indolent ulcer
Necrotizing stromal keratitis	Viral necrotizing keratitis Ulcerating interstitial keratitis
Immune stromal keratitis	Interstitial keratitis Disciform keratitis Herpetic disciform keratitis Herpetic stromal keratitis Stromal keratitis Non-necrotizing stromal keratitis Immune ring Wessely ring Limbal vasculitis
Endotheliitis (disciform, diffuse, linear)	Disciform keratitis Disciform edema Disciform disease with endotheliitis Central disciform endotheliitis Central endotheliitis Peripheral endotheliitis Keratouveitis

Infectious epithelial keratitis

All types of recurrent infectious epithelial keratitis are caused by reactivation of live virus. The most commonly recognized clinical manifestations of infectious epithelial keratitis are the dendritic and geographic ulcers. Corneal vesicles and marginal keratitis are less common and may go unrecognized as active infections. Most patients with infectious epithelial keratitis complain of photophobia, pain, and a thin,

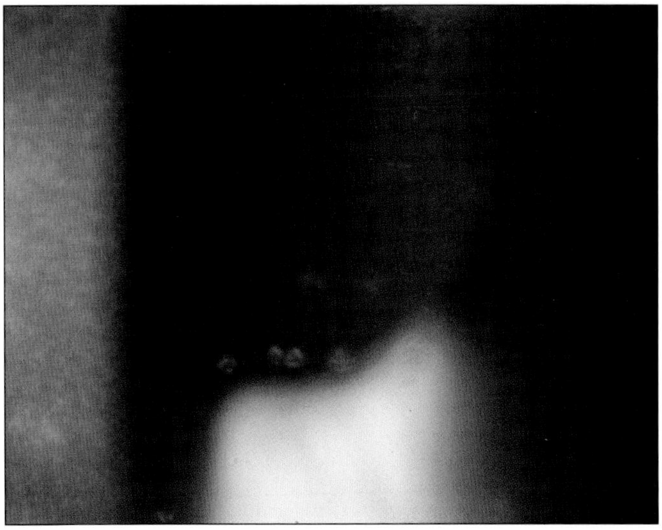

Fig. 79.3 HSV corneal vesicles in an immunocompetent host. These lesions are minute, raised, clear vesicles that stain negatively with fluorescein.

watery discharge; those with central lesions also may present with decreased vision.

The earliest epithelial lesions of reactivated HSV are small vesicles in the epithelium, which in past reports have been described as punctate epithelial keratopathy (PEK).[10,115] In fact, careful examination of these lesions demonstrates minute, raised, clear vesicles that correspond to the vesicular eruptions seen in the skin or mucous membranes elsewhere in the body (Fig. 79.3). These lesions are important to recognize. Many patients with recurrent infectious epithelial keratitis have these vesicles in the early stages of a recurrence, usually before examination by a clinician. Within 24 hours, the vesicles coalesce to form the typical dendritic and geographic ulcers. In some patients, especially those who are immunocompromised, the infectious keratitis is arrested at the vesicle stage. The vesicles may coalesce to form a raised, dendritic lesion (Fig. 79.4), which displaces fluorescein (negative staining). This raised lesion, which is clinically the precursor to the dendritic ulcer in the immunocompetent host, may not progress to a dendritic ulcer in the immunocompromised host and therefore may not be recognized as infectious epithelial keratitis (Fig. 79.5). All patients with HSV corneal vesicles should be recognized as having infectious keratitis and treated promptly.

The most common presentation of HSV keratitis is the dendritic ulcer, a derivative of *dendron*, the Greek word for tree. The features of a dendritic ulcer include a branching, linear lesion with terminal bulbs and swollen epithelial borders that contain live virus. This lesion represents a true ulcer in that it extends through the basement membrane. This clinical feature is important to recognize because it aids in differentiating a true dendritic ulcer from the many other branching lesions of the corneal epithelium. Recently healed epithelial defects and varicella-zoster pseudodendrites are often misdiagnosed as HSV dendritic ulcers. They can be differentiated from HSV because they are raised, rather than ulcerated, and do not stain with fluorescein.

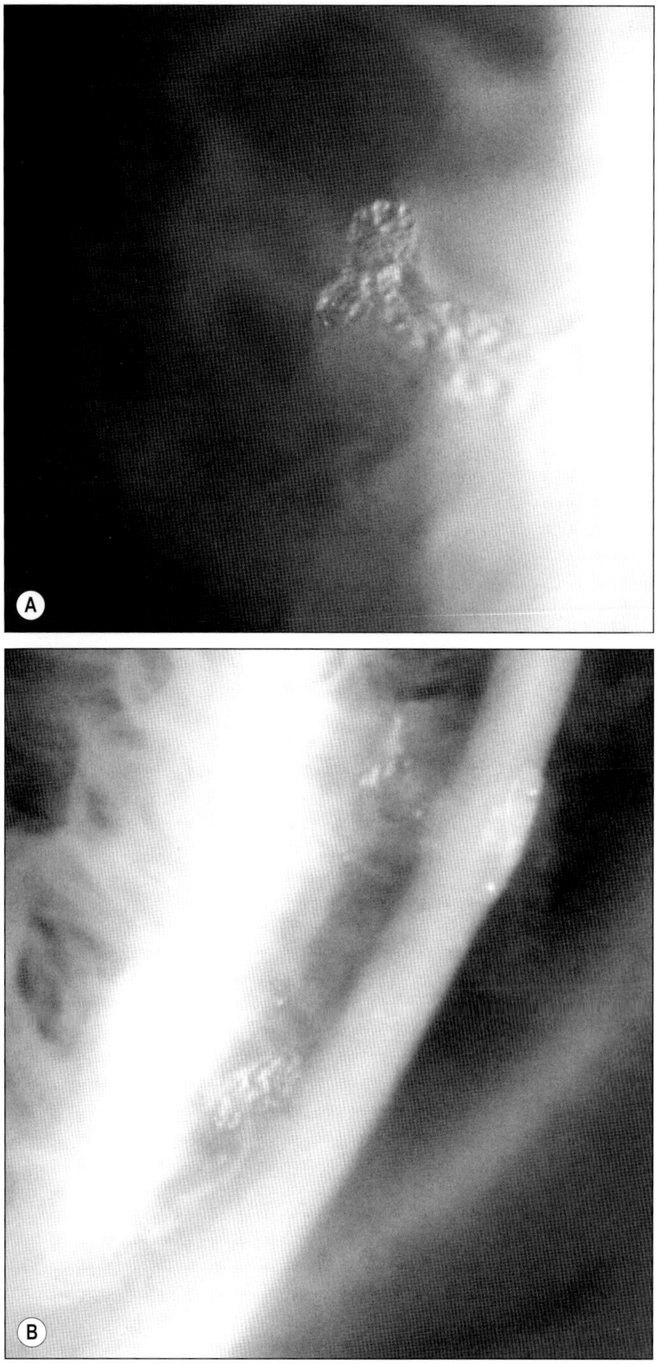

Fig. 79.4 HSV corneal vesicles in an immunocompetent host. (**A**) The cornea vesicles have coalesced. Note the raised appearance indicating that ulceration has not yet occurred. (**B**) The slit beam shows the area of coalesced vesicles to be raised rather than ulcerated.

Classic dendritic ulcers have staining properties that assist the clinician in making the correct diagnosis. Because it is a true ulcer, the dendritic ulcer in HSV stains positively for fluorescein along the length of the lesion (see Fig. 79.5). However, the swollen epithelial borders are actually raised, when compared to the neighboring epithelium, and stain negatively with fluorescein. Rose Bengal, which stains devitalized cells, is typically taken up by the swollen epithelial

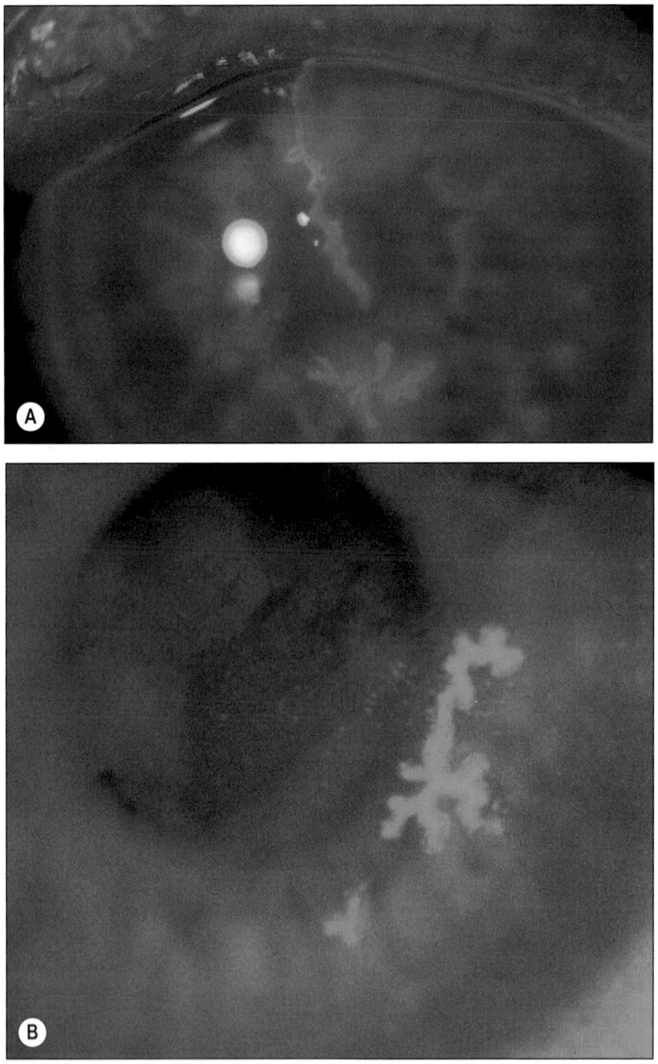

Fig. 79.5 HSV corneal vesicles. (**A**) Branching vesicular lesion of HSV in an immunocompetent patient. (**B**) HSV dendritic ulcer in another immunocompetent patient. Note confluent fluorescein staining centrally, indicating ulceration and late staining peripherally of swollen epithelial borders.

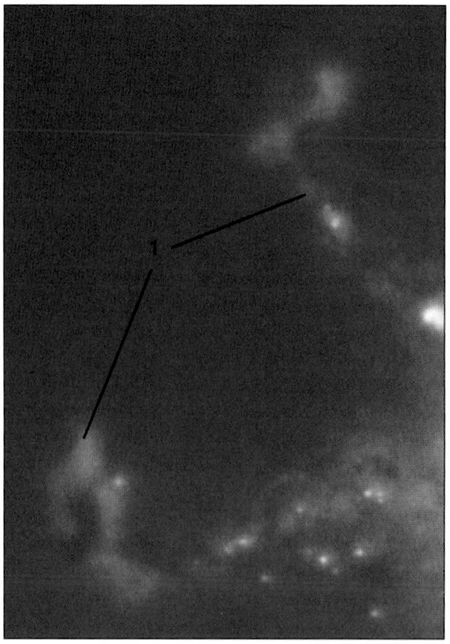

Fig. 79.6 HSV dendritic epitheliopathy. This lesion represents healing epithelium after a dendritic ulcer. Although the epithelium is intact, this branching lesion (*1*) is often misdiagnosed as persistence of the dendritic ulcer.

cells at the ulcer's border. If viral cultures are to be undertaken, rose Bengal staining should not be performed before culturing because rose Bengal is toxic to HSV and will decrease the yield of the culture.[116]

The clinician should realize that the HSV dendritic ulcer may result in an abnormal-appearing epithelium for several weeks after the ulcer heals. We refer to this condition as HSV dendritic epitheliopathy (Fig. 79.6). This lesion is dendritic in shape; however, it is not ulcerated and simply represents healing epithelium after the infection. The toxic effect of antiviral medications on the healing epithelium also may contribute to the formation of this epitheliopathy. Fluorescein staining reveals negative staining along the length of the dendritic lesion and can confuse the clinician into believing the initial dendritic ulcer is persisting and therefore is resistant to current medical therapy.

An enlarged dendritic ulcer that is no longer linear is referred to as a geographic ulcer. This lesion can be thought of as a widened dendritic ulcer. Like a dendritic ulcer, it is a true ulcer in that it is an epithelial lesion that extends through the basement membrane. Also like a dendritic ulcer, it has swollen epithelial borders that contain live virus. The scalloped or geographic borders of the HSV geographic ulcer are important to recognize to differentiate this lesion from healing abrasions and neurotrophic keratopathy, which tend to have smooth borders (Fig. 79.7).

In an epidemiologic study by Wilhelmus et al.,[18] geographic ulcers accounted for 22% of all cases of initial infectious epithelial keratitis and were associated with longer duration of symptoms and time to healing than dendritic ulcers. In addition, geographic ulcers were associated with the previous use of topical corticosteroids. Liesegang,[25] on the other hand, reported that geographic ulcers accounted for only 4% of initial presentations of infectious epithelial keratitis and were not associated with the use of topical corticosteroids.

Another manifestation of HSV infectious epithelial keratitis is the marginal ulcer.[117] This lesion results from active viral disease like that of the dendritic ulcer. However, the proximity of this lesion to the limbus, with its accompanying blood vessels, accounts for the unique clinical features. The epithelial lesion is quickly infiltrated with white blood cells from the nearby limbal blood vessels. The resultant lesion typically seen on presentation has an anterior stromal infiltrate underlying the ulcer and adjacent limbal injection (Fig. 79.8). Careful inspection may show a dendritic ulcer overlying the stromal infiltrate, but in some patients the ulcer may lack the typical dendritic shape (Fig. 79.9).

Patients with HSV marginal ulcers are typically more symptomatic than those with central dendritic ulcers because of the intense inflammation associated with the marginal

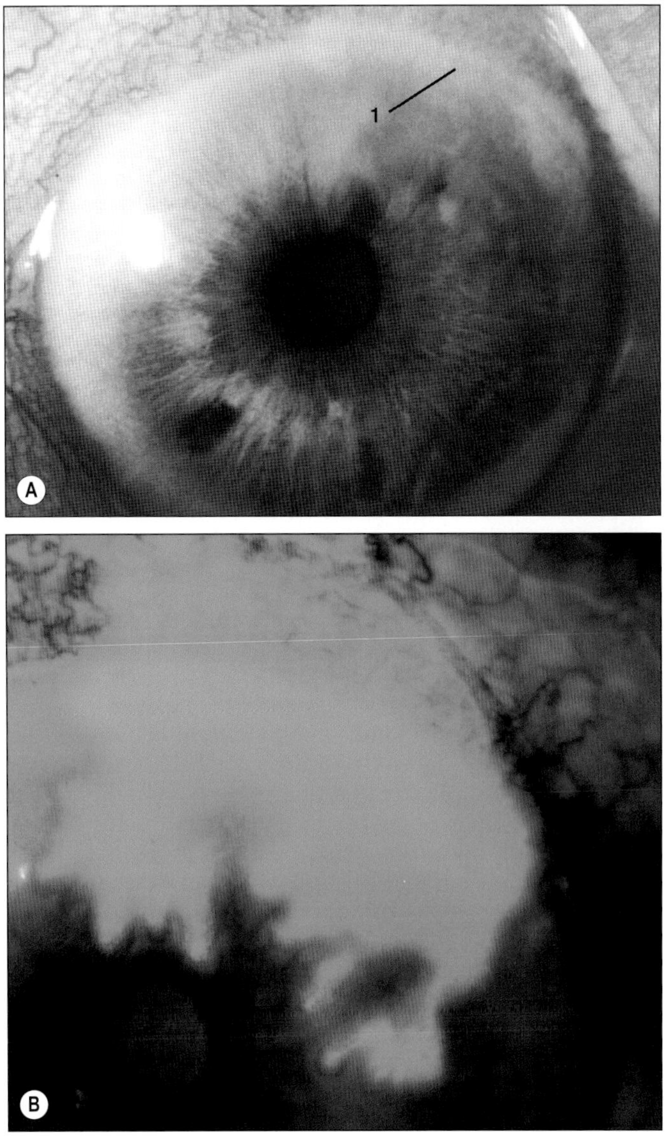

Fig. 79.7 Geographic ulcer. (**A**) Geographic ulcer (*1*) of the cornea and conjunctiva displaying scalloped borders of swollen epithelial cells. (**B**) Fluorescein staining reveals true ulceration of cornea and conjunctiva.

lesion. Authors have stated that this lesion is more difficult to treat than a central dendritic ulcer.[10,115] The infectious aspect of the lesion responds quite well to antiviral treatment; it is the immune response that gives the appearance of more intense and longer-lasting disease. Some patients require topical corticosteroids after initiation of topical antivirals to suppress this immune reaction.

HSV marginal ulcer is uncommon and is most often confused with staphylococcal marginal (catarrhal) disease. If improperly treated with topical antibiotics, and especially with topical corticosteroids without antivirals, this lesion progresses centrally with ulceration and subepithelial infiltration. This central progression more typically has the dendritic presentation and can help in making the proper diagnosis. HSV marginal ulcer can be differentiated from staphylococcal marginal disease based on several clinical

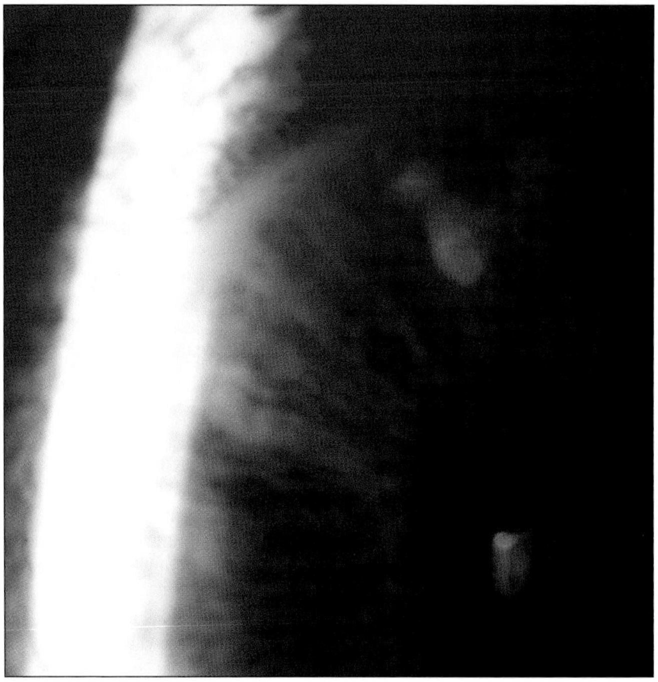

Fig. 79.8 HSV marginal ulcer. This patient had a previous history of a central dendritic ulcer and presented with limbal injection and epithelial defect overlying anterior stromal infiltrate. Culture was positive for HSV.

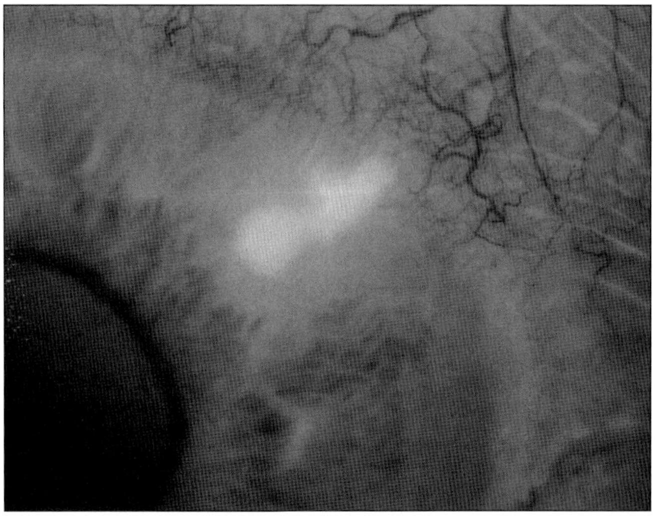

Fig. 79.9 HSV marginal ulcer. Fluorescein staining reveals ulceration, but note that the ulceration is not dendritic in shape. This lesion cultured positive for HSV.

findings (Table 79.2). First, the HSV marginal ulcer starts as an ulcer and is followed by the infiltrate, although both are usually seen at time of presentation. Staphylococcal marginal infiltrate presents as an infiltrate with intact epithelium, but prolonged inflammation can eventually lead to subsequent ulceration. Second, the HSV marginal ulcer is accompanied by limbal injection that often results in early neovascularization of the infiltration. With staphylococcal marginal infiltrates, there is a lucid interval between the limbus and the infiltrate. Third, if untreated, the HSV

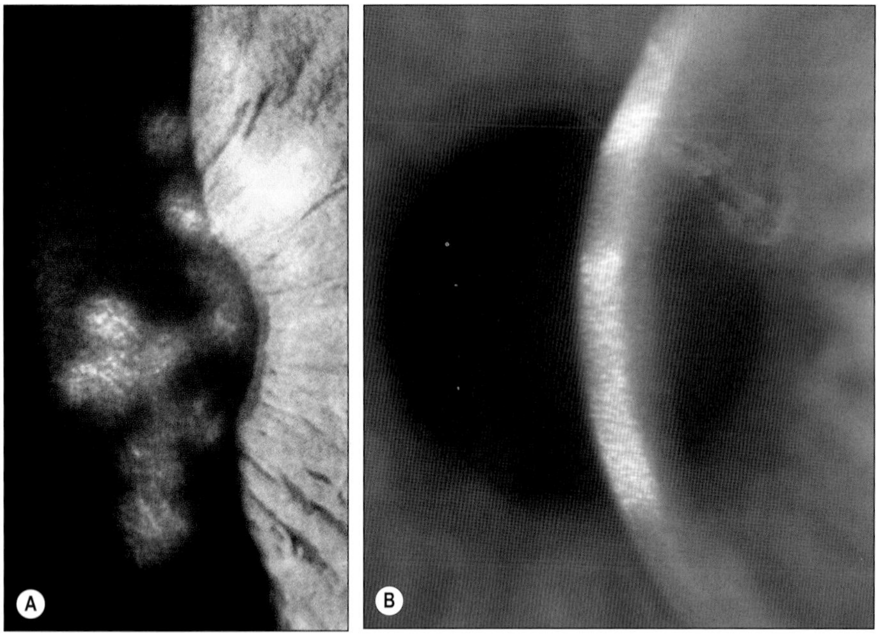

Fig. 79.10 HSV subepithelial scarring. (**A**) The branching pattern of subepithelial scarring referred to as 'ghost figures' or 'footprints' of HSV. (**B**) Slit beam showing the subepithelial location of the scarring.

Table 79.2 Features of herpes simplex marginal ulcer compared to those of staphylococcal marginal infiltrate

Features	HSV marginal ulcer	Staphylococcal marginal infiltrate
Etiology	Active HSV	Immunologic response to staphylococcal antigen
Epithelial defect	Always	Absent (if present, late)
Neovascularization	Often	Never
Progression	Centrally	Circumferentially
Blepharitis	Unrelated	Usually
Location	Any meridian	Typically 2, 4, 8, 10 o'clock meridians

marginal ulcer progresses centrally, as opposed to the staphylococcal marginal infiltrate, which may spread circumferentially but not centrally. Fourth, HSV marginal ulcer is usually not associated with blepharitis, whereas staphylococcal marginal infiltrate is almost always accompanied by blepharitis. Finally, HSV marginal ulcers may occur in any meridian, but staphylococcal marginal infiltrates are most typically seen at the 2, 4, 8, and 10 o'clock meridians, where the lids are in apposition to the cornea.

Sequelae of infectious epithelial keratitis

There are four recognized sequelae of infectious epithelial keratitis. In some patients with a dendritic or geographic ulcer, there can be complete resolution of the infectious lesion without residual evidence of prior infection.

As stated previously, some patients with infectious epithelial keratitis may develop dendritic epitheliopathy. It is important to reemphasize that this lesion does not represent active infection and should not be treated as such.

A potentially sight-threatening sequela of infectious epithelial keratitis is stromal scarring. Scars can range from the faint, gray-white, subepithelial opacities commonly referred to as the 'ghost figures' or 'footprints' of HSV (Fig. 79.10) to dense stromal scarring (Fig. 79.11) accompanied by thinning and decreased vision. The ghost figure of HSV is important to recognize because it is an important clue for making the correct diagnosis in future episodes. This scarring is best seen on slit lamp examination using diffuse or broad, oblique illumination. The patient with recurrent unilateral keratoconjunctivitis should be evaluated carefully for ghost figures. The duration of inflammation and number of episodes appear to correlate with severity of scarring. The immune response, however, varies among patients. Some patients scar severely with one episode, and others may have many repeated episodes with no to minimal scarring.

The last sequela of infectious epithelial keratitis is stromal disease. In a prospective study of patients with infectious epithelial keratitis, Wilhelmus et al.[18] found that 25% of patients develop subsequent stromal inflammation. The stromal disease may be either infectious or immune. Necrotizing keratitis represents true viral infection of the stroma, whereas immune stromal keratitis is mediated by antibody–complement reactions to viral antigen.

Neurotrophic keratopathy

Patients who have had infectious epithelial keratitis are at risk to develop neurotrophic keratopathy. This clinical entity is unique because it is neither immune nor infectious. Rather, it arises from impaired corneal innervation in combination with decreased tear secretion. The keratopathy may

Table 79.3 Features of infectious epithelial keratitis compared to neurotrophic ulcer

Features	Infectious epithelial keratitis	Neurotrophic keratopathy
Staining	Positive fluorescein staining with dendritic or geographic ulcer Rarely negative staining if detected at vesicle stage	Negative staining with intact epithelium Positive staining with epithelial defect
Morphology	Dendritic ulcer: branching shape, terminal bulbs, swollen epithelium at borders Geographic ulcer: scallop shaped, swollen epithelium at borders	PEK and boggy epithelium; may have dendritic shape Neurotrophic ulcer: smooth, typically round or oval with heaped-up epithelium at border
Location	No specific predilection	Most often interpalpebral cornea
Etiology	Active viral infection	Impaired corneal innervation, damaged epithelial BM, stromal inflammation, toxicity from topical medications
Treatment	Topical antivirals, debridement	Lubrication, elimination of toxic topical medications, tape or surgical tarsorrhaphy
Course	Usually resolves within 2 weeks	Chronic, may occur after infectious epithelial keratitis, suspect if infectious epithelial keratitis lasts more than 14 days

PEK, punctate epithelial keratopathy; BM, basement membrane.

Fig. 79.11 HSV stromal scarring. Anterior and midstromal scarring with thinning occurring after infectious epithelial keratitis.

be exacerbated by chronic use of topical medications, especially antivirals.

The early findings of neurotrophic keratopathy include irregularity of the corneal surface and lack of the normal corneal luster. Punctate epithelial erosions may then develop and may progress to a persistent epithelial defect. The epithelial defect in neurotrophic keratopathy is oval in shape with smooth borders, in direct contrast to the geographic ulcer, which is irregular in shape with scalloped borders (Table 79.3). Persistence of the epithelial defect in neurotrophic keratopathy eventually leads to stromal ulceration. The lesion at this stage also can be referred to as a neurotrophic ulcer (Fig. 79.12). The neurotrophic ulcer maintains the same round shape with smooth borders as the epithelial defect, and the stroma at the ulcer bed typically develops a gray-white opacification. The neurotrophic ulcer has a thickened border formed by heaped-up epithelium. Complications of neurotrophic keratopathy include stromal scarring, neovascularization, necrosis, perforation, and secondary bacterial infection.

Stromal disease

Although stromal disease accounts for approximately 2% of initial episodes of ocular HSV disease,[22,25] it accounts for 20–48% of recurrent ocular HSV disease.[25,26,118,119] Stromal involvement in HSV disease is commonly confused and poorly categorized. Unfortunately, many clinicians lump all stromal involvement under the heading of 'stromal keratitis.' This broad categorization neglects the specific etiologies of the different forms of stromal involvement with this disease and can lead to improper treatment.

The corneal stroma may be affected in HSV disease through a variety of mechanisms, either primarily or secondarily (Table 79.4). Secondary involvement may occur as a sequela to infectious epithelial keratitis, neurotrophic keratopathy, or endotheliitis. As previously stated, epithelial disease such as infectious epithelial keratitis may lead to secondary stromal scarring. Neurotrophic keratopathy can also lead to secondary stromal scarring and thinning. Endotheliitis, which results from an inflammatory reaction of the endothelium, leads to secondary stromal edema and, if chronic, can result in scarring. When stromal involvement occurs secondarily to infectious epithelial keratitis, neurotrophic keratopathy, or endotheliitis, the source of inflammation is in the epithelium or endothelium, and treatment must be focused toward the proper origin of inflammation if stromal injury is to be minimized. The stromal involvement from endotheliitis is described in more detail later.

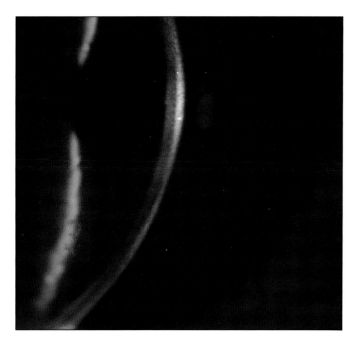

Table 79.4 Causes of stromal disease in herpes simplex keratitis

Clinical manifestation	Associated stromal disease	Other corneal involvement	Mechanism
Infectious epithelial keratitis	Secondary scarring in response to epithelial disease	Dendritic, geographic, or marginal ulcer	Live virus in epithelium; immune response in stroma
Neurotrophic keratopathy	Ulceration and scarring	Epitheliopathy leads to persistent epithelial defect	Impaired corneal innervation, damaged epithelial BM, stromal inflammation, toxicity from topical medications
Necrotizing stromal keratitis	Necrosis and ulceration with dense infiltration	Epithelial defect	Direct viral invasion of stroma with severe immune reaction
Immune stromal keratitis	Infiltrate, neovascularization, immune ring, scarring and thinning	May have antecedent, concurrent or subsequent infectious epithelial keratitis	Ag-Ab complement mediated. Possible role of live virus
Endotheliitis	Secondary stromal edema due to endothelial reaction; chronic edema may lead to scarring	KP in disciform, linear, or diffuse distribution	Immune reaction involving the endothelium Possible role of live virus

BM, basement membrane; KP, keratic precipitates.

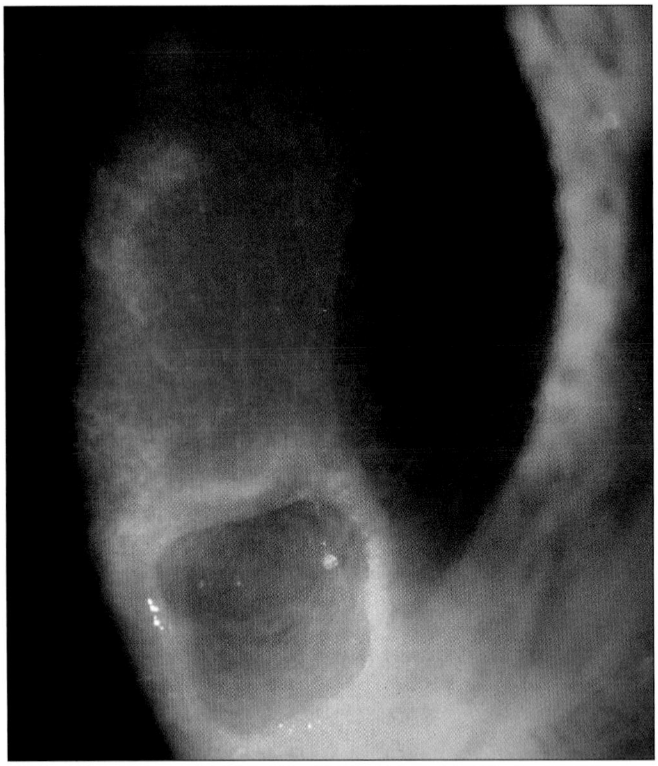

Fig. 79.12 Neurotrophic ulcer. This lesion has a round or oval shape with smooth borders.

Two manifestations of stromal disease from HSV involve the stroma primarily. Necrotizing stromal keratitis occurs from direct viral invasion of the stroma, whereas immune stromal keratitis is the result of an immune reaction within the stroma.

Necrotizing stromal keratitis

Necrotizing stromal keratitis is a rare manifestation of HSV that is thought to result from direct viral invasion of the corneal stroma.[117] The clinical findings are necrosis, ulceration, and dense infiltration of the stroma with an overlying epithelial defect. The combination of replicating virus and severe host inflammatory response leads to destructive intrastromal inflammation that is often refractory to treatment with high-dose antiinflammatory and antiviral medications. The severe inflammation may lead to thinning and perforation within a short period of time (Fig. 79.13). The clinical findings of necrotizing stromal keratitis may resemble those of infectious keratitis secondary to microbial invasion. Therefore, bacterial and fungal pathogens must be considered when treating for necrotizing stromal keratitis. The use of topical corticosteroids without antiviral coverage has been implicated as a possible risk factor.[120,121] Intact virions have been detected in stromal keratocytes and lamellae on electron microscopic examination of pathologic tissue from patients with necrotizing stromal keratitis.[122]

Immune stromal (interstitial) keratitis

We believe that the term immune stromal keratitis is synonymous with interstitial keratitis. Review of this subject is confusing because some authors use interstitial keratitis to refer to stromal neovascularization with inflammation. Others reserve the term for posterior neovascularization only. Still others limit this term for the description of syphilitic keratitis. We recommend that the term interstitial keratitis be used to refer to any inflammatory condition of the stroma that has an immunologic etiology and should not be restricted by the presence or absence of neovascularization, the depth of stromal inflammation, or the etiology of the inflammation. Although either immune stromal keratitis or interstitial keratitis can be used to describe the immune stromal inflammation seen in HSV, we choose to use the term immune stromal keratitis because it is more descriptive of the pathology involved.

Immune stromal keratitis is a common chronic recurrent manifestation of HSV, occurring in 20% of patients with ocular HSV.[18,25] Additional studies have reported the

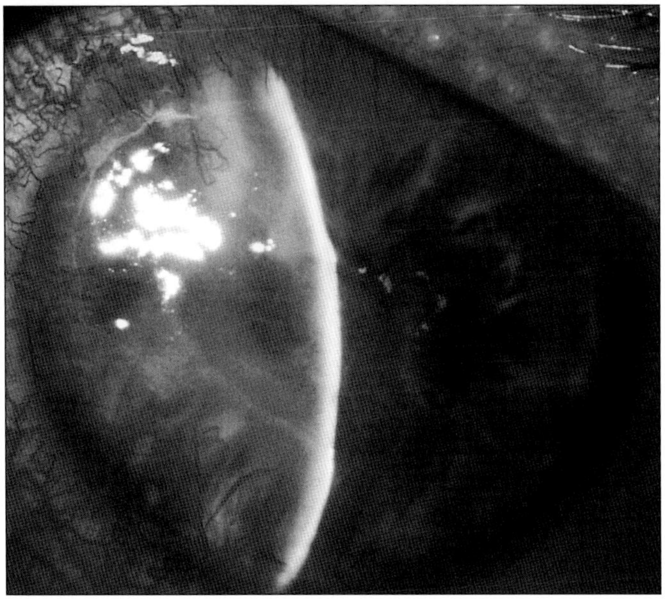

Fig. 79.13 Necrotizing stromal keratitis. Note the necrotic ulceration with dense stromal infiltration.

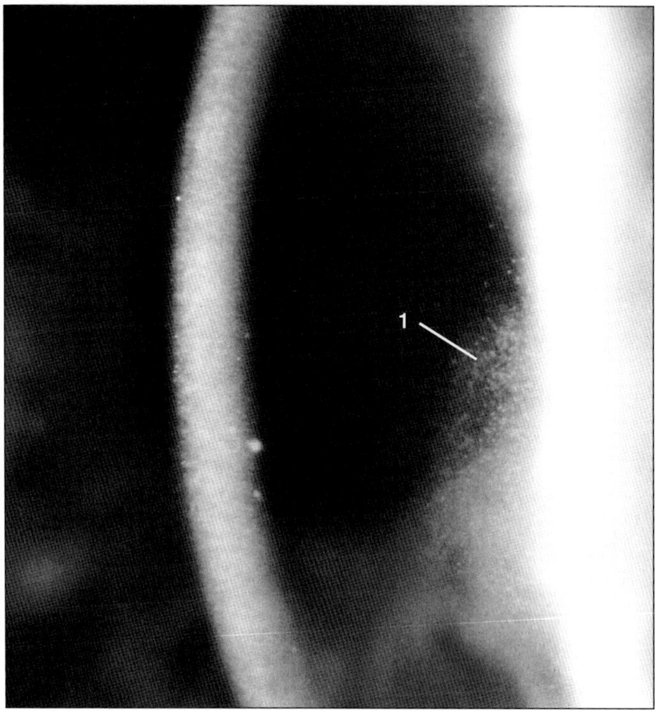

Fig. 79.14 Immune stromal keratitis. Note the fine punctate opacities (*1*) of the mid stroma, which represent AAC immune complexes.

incidences of stromal disease of 21%[123] within 2 years and 26%[124] to 48%[125] within 7 years of infectious epithelial keratitis. The inflammation is thought to be due to retained viral antigen within the stroma. This antigen triggers an antigen-antibody-complement (AAC) cascade that results in intrastromal inflammation. The role of retained viral antigen as a stimulus for chronic inflammation has been implicated because of the finding of viral particles in the stroma of pathology specimens from patients with immune stromal keratitis.[86] Molecular mimicry has been linked with activation of T-cell-mediated autoimmune responses in murine models.[88] The role of live virus in the pathogenesis of immune stromal keratitis has not been elucidated fully.

The unifying characteristic of all presentations of immune stromal keratitis is stromal inflammation. The overlying epithelium is almost always intact except in the situation of combined infectious epithelial keratitis and immune stromal keratitis. The inflammation of immune stromal keratitis can take one or a combination of forms. A common stromal opacity in HSV keratitis is the subepithelial haze and scarring seen after a dendritic ulcer. As stated earlier, when these lesions are permanent, they are referred to as 'ghost scarring' or 'footprints' of HSV keratitis. The degree of anterior stromal scarring may depend on the strain of virus and the severity of the host immune response. When it occurs, ghost scarring is always evident within a few weeks of the episode of infectious epithelial keratitis.

Stromal infiltration is the most common finding in recurrent immune stromal keratitis and can present as punctate stromal opacities that most likely represent AAC immune complexes (Fig. 79.14). In the acute phase, these opacities may be accompanied by haze that is indicative of inflammatory cellular infiltrate of the stroma. The haze and punctate lesions may become permanent opacities. The pattern of stromal inflammation may be focal, multifocal, or diffuse.[126] Stromal infiltration is often accompanied by anterior chamber inflammation, ciliary flush, and significant discomfort. Stromal edema also can accompany this reaction. The edema most likely results from the consequences of stromal inflammation rather than endothelial dysfunction. Severe inflammation can lead to dense infiltration with subsequent scarring and profound visual loss. Vision loss from HSV immune stromal keratitis is the main reason that 3% of all penetrating keratoplasties have been performed in the United States in recent years.[127–129]

A specific form of stromal infiltration secondary to HSV is the immune ring. This ring is also thought to be an AAC precipitate similar to a Wessely ring. It can form an incomplete or complete ring and can be singular or multiple (Fig. 79.15). It is most commonly found in the mid stroma of the central or paracentral cornea.

Another finding of immune stromal keratitis is stromal neovascularization, the pathogenesis and clinical significance of which were discussed in the section of this chapter on immune defense mechanisms. Neovascularization may occur at any level of the cornea. In some cases of severe inflammation, there can be rapid neovascularization with multiple fronds of new vessels associated with intense infiltration, a response similar to the classic descriptions of syphilitic interstitial keratitis (Fig. 79.16). This rapid neovascularization can range from sectoral, with a single frond of vessels, to complete, involving all quadrants of the cornea (Fig. 79.17). Neovascularization also can progress in a subacute or chronic fashion in response to persistent, low-grade stromal inflammation. The neovascularization in these less acute cases tends to be sectoral rather than circumferential. Aggressive treatment of inflammation can result in complete resolution of the blood vessels. Ghost vessels, which

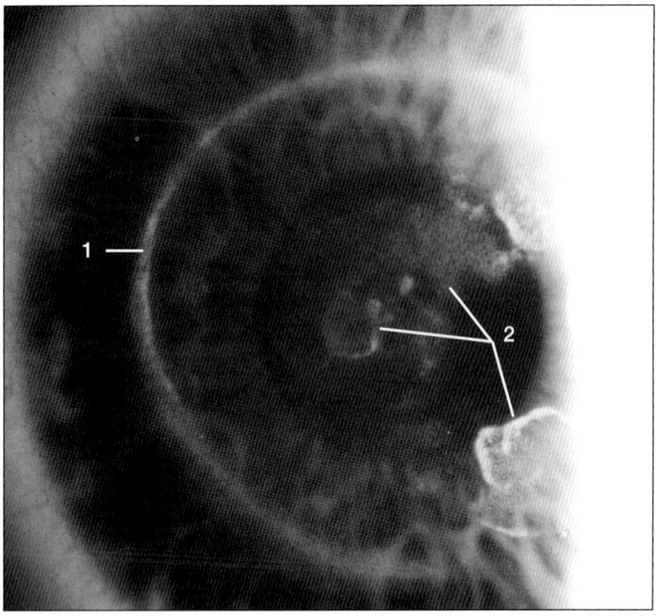

Fig. 79.15 Immune stromal keratitis. Sclerotic scatter reveals a stromal immune ring (*1*) and anterior stromal scarring (*2*) from previous HSV disease.

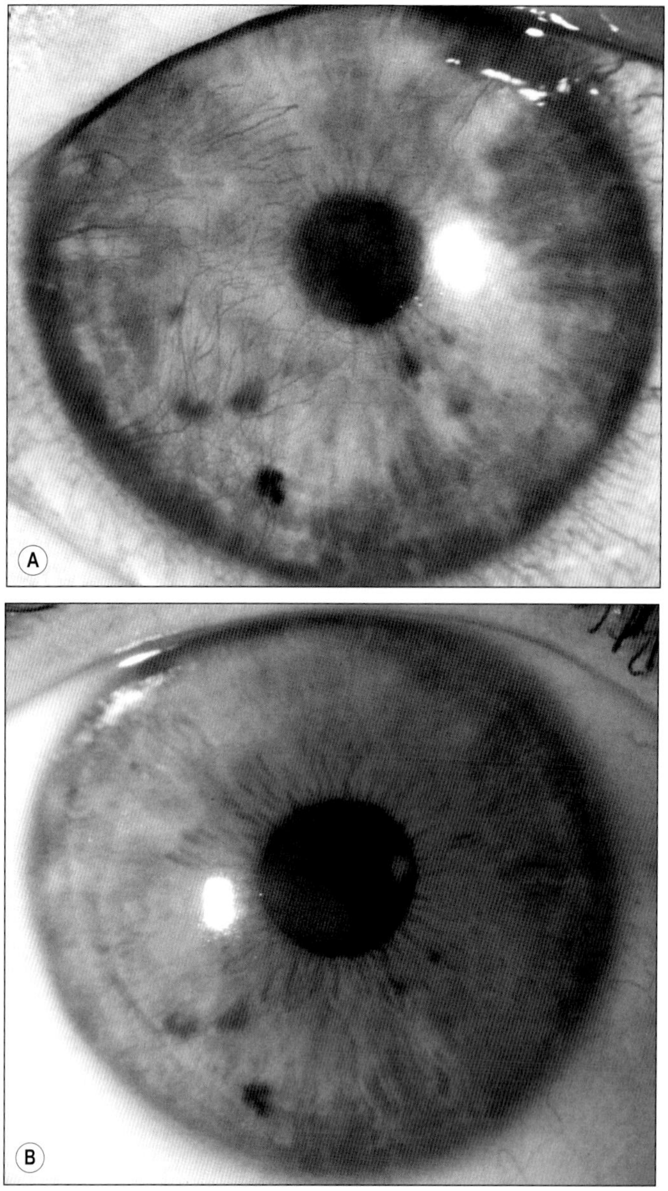

Fig. 79.16 Immune stromal keratitis. (**A**) Acute stromal inflammation presenting with rapid stromal neovascularization in a patient with a history of a dendritic ulcer. (**B**) Treatment with topical corticosteroids resulted in a decrease of the stromal haze and resolution of the neovascularization.

represent empty vessel channels within the stroma, can occur if the inflammation and neovascularization is longstanding before it is quieted. Ghost vessels, in and of themselves, do not cause decreased vision or increased risk of penetrating keratoplasty rejection. If ghost vessels are present, however, there is almost always significant accompanying stromal scarring and thinning because of the chronicity of the inflammation.

Lipid keratopathy can follow stromal neovascularization and can lead to further scarring and loss of vision (Fig. 79.18). A more serious sequela of stromal neovascularization is permanent neovascularization of the cornea, which will decrease the success rate of penetrating keratoplasty because of increased risk of rejection (Fig. 79.19).

Immune stromal keratitis may present days to years after an episode of infectious epithelial keratitis. In some cases, there may be no history of a dendritic ulcer; in other cases, the first documented ulcer may actually occur after an episode of immune stromal keratitis. In cases where there is no antecedent dendritic ulcer, the diagnosis of HSV immune stromal keratitis usually is made presumptively. The astute clinician, when examining a patient with immune stromal keratitis without a known history of herpes simplex disease, should carefully interview the patient to uncover a history of a recurrent unilateral red eye and should examine the cornea for areas of ghost scarring and/or decreased sensation (Fig. 79.20).

The clinical course of immune stromal keratitis is chronic, recurrent inflammation that can persist for years. Patients may experience constant low-grade inflammation with mild fluctuations in severity. Other patients may have periods of complete resolution of inflammation with intermittent flare-ups of severe inflammation. Long-term topical corticosteroids may be required to suppress the inflammatory reaction of immune stromal keratitis. Some patients are exquisitely sensitive to mild reductions in topical corticosteroid. Untreated or undertreated inflammation can lead to stromal scarring, thinning, persistent neovascularization, lipid deposition, and severe loss of vision.

Many clinicians use the terms disciform keratitis or disciform edema as a category of stromal keratitis. We feel these terms are confusing and misleading for two specific reasons. First, the word disciform, meaning round, simply describes the shape of a lesion. Because numerous round lesions of the cornea are seen in HSV keratitis, including a round infiltrate, a ring infiltrate (immune ring), a round scar, or a round area of edema (so-called disciform edema), it carries little meaning

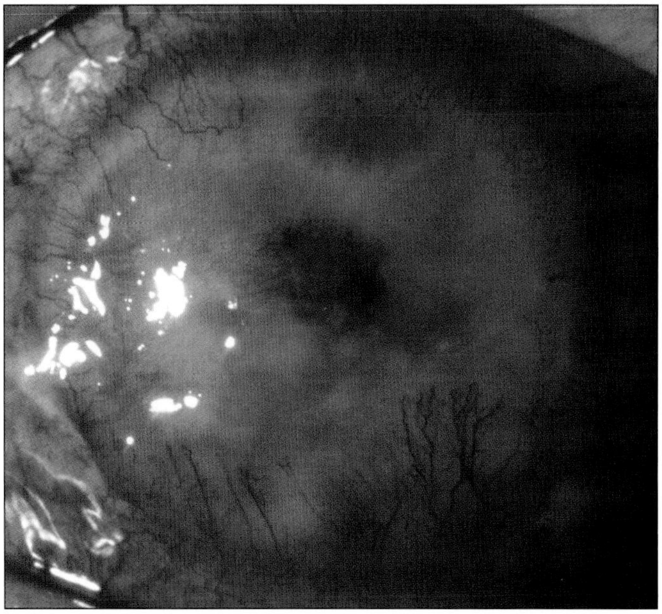

Fig. 79.17 Immune stromal keratitis. Acute, severe stromal inflammation and neovascularization in a patient with a history of previous HSV epithelial keratitis.

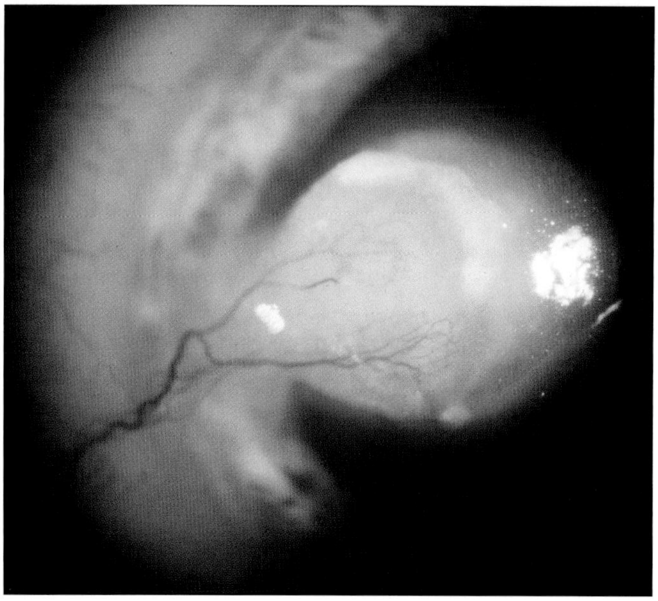

Fig. 79.19 Immune stromal keratitis. Residual scarring, neovascularization, and heavy lipid deposition in a patient with HSV keratitis.

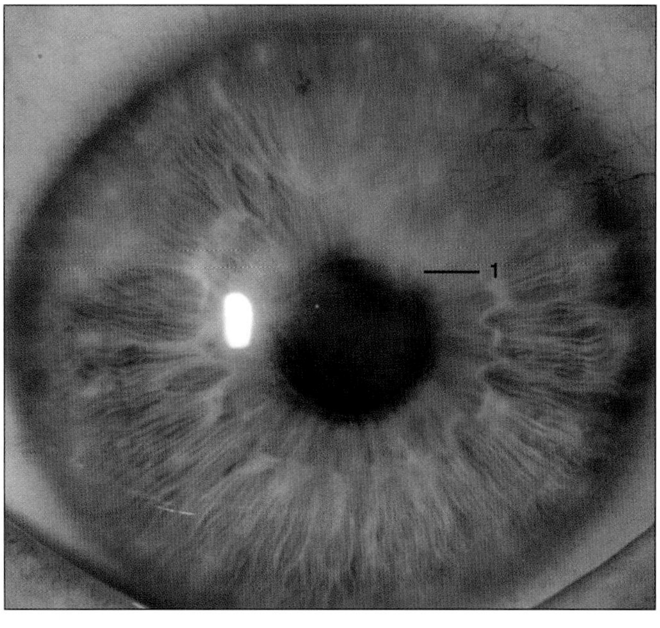

Fig. 79.18 Immune stromal keratitis. A patient with a history of HSV infectious epithelial keratitis has decreased vision secondary to chronic stromal inflammation, neovascularization, and lipid deposition (*1*).

in terms of the pathophysiology. Unfortunately, many clinicians apply the term disciform keratitis to any round lesion of the cornea. Second, this disciform edema or disciform keratitis reaction is not a reaction of the stroma and should not be classified or treated as a stromal keratitis. Careful observation of the patient with disciform edema reveals that this process is an inflammatory reaction of the endothelium, with only secondary stromal and epithelial edema. This distinction between stromal and endothelial inflammation is important because the prognosis and clinical course are different, and visual outcome depends on proper recognition and treatment of the endothelium as the primary site of inflammation. Therefore, we classify this reaction as an endotheliitis rather than a stromal keratitis and discuss it more fully in the next section.

Endotheliitis

Many patients with HSV disease develop corneal stromal edema without stromal infiltrate. These patients all share the following findings: keratic precipitates (KP), overlying stromal and epithelial edema, and iritis. In some patients, the edema is so extensive that the KP cannot be seen on the initial examination. With resolution of the edema, the KP can be visualized as they tend to resolve after the resolution of the stromal edema. We believe this clinical entity is an inflammatory reaction at the level of the endothelium and therefore recommend classifying it as an endotheliitis rather than a stromal keratitis. Certain observations support the argument that the target of inflammation is endothelium. First, the fact that there are KP suggests that the inflammation is at the level of the endothelium. That the KP are always present under the areas of edema and absent under the areas of the nonedematous cornea lends support to the notion that the inflammation is closely related to local endothelial decompensation. An additional argument that the endothelium, and not the stroma, is the primary site of inflammation is the fact that the only stromal finding is edema. Stromal infiltrate and neovascularization, which are signs of stromal inflammation, are notably absent. If untreated, or if severe, however, stromal edema may persist and lead to secondary neovascularization and scarring in a clinical picture that looks similar to immune stromal

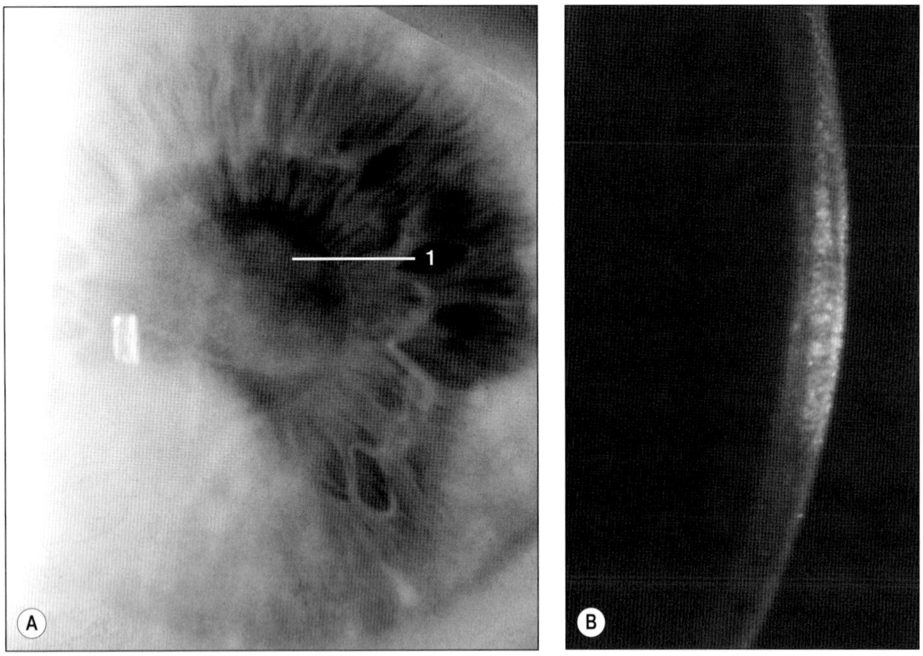

Fig. 79.20 Immune stromal keratitis. (**A**) A patient with a history of a recurrent, irritated, red left eye presents with a sectoral area of immune stromal keratitis characterized by stromal infiltration and neovascularization. Careful examination reveals subepithelial scarring (*1*) of the central cornea consistent with 'ghost scarring' of HSV. (**B**) Slit beam better delineates subepithelial ghost scarring.

keratitis. A consequence of chronic endotheliitis may be the permanent loss of endothelial cells with subsequent intractable corneal edema.[130]

The exact pathogenesis of endotheliitis in HSV is unknown. It certainly appears that reaction at the level of the endothelium is immunologic because of the clinical findings of KP and iritis. That resolution usually can be obtained with topical corticosteroids further supports the immunologic nature of this condition. The role of live virus also has been speculated as contributing to this clinical entity,[131–137] and one immunohistologic study of tissue from patients with previous disciform endotheliitis confirmed the presence of HSV-1 antigen in corneal endothelial cells.[87]

HSV endotheliitis can be classified based on the distribution of the KP and the configuration of the overlying stromal and epithelial edema. The three forms of HSV endotheliitis are disciform, diffuse, and linear (Table 79.5).

Disciform endotheliitis

Disciform endotheliitis is far and away the most common presentation of endotheliitis. As previously stated, the term disciform is commonly applied to the clinical picture of any round lesion of the cornea. For the clinical entity of a round area of stromal edema overlying KP, the most common terms used are disciform edema and disciform keratitis, neither of which is specific as to the etiology of the specific disease entity. Although disciform is a term that, in and of itself, carries little meaning and might best be eliminated, we have chosen to retain it because of its extensive use in the literature and hope that the newly proposed term, disciform endotheliitis, will direct clinicians to a better understanding of this entity.

Patients with disciform endotheliitis present with photophobia and mild to moderate ocular discomfort. Limbal injection is usually seen, as these patients have an accompanying iritis. Visual acuity may range from normal to severely reduced, depending on the location and severity of the stromal edema.

The most striking finding of disciform endotheliitis on slit lamp examination is a round or disc-shaped area of stromal edema. This edema may be in central or paracentral cornea. The edema usually spans the entire stromal thickness, resulting in the usual ground-glass appearance seen with corneal edema from other entities of endothelial decompensation. Typically, in disciform endotheliitis, the edema is within a strikingly focal pattern with a definite demarcation between involved and uninvolved cornea. In the acute setting, the stroma is void of infiltrate and neovascularization (Fig. 79.21).

The epithelium shows microcystic edema overlying the areas of stromal edema. If the stromal edema is mild, however, the epithelium may appear normal. In the most severe cases, epithelial bullae may form.

In all cases of disciform endotheliitis, KP are present. The KP underlie the distribution of stromal edema and are not found in the nonedematous areas. It is sometimes difficult to see the KP because of the severity of the stromal edema. In these cases, it is useful to view the endothelium obliquely to detect the KP. Often, as the stromal edema resolves, the hidden KP become visible because the KP tend to resolve at a slower rate than the edema.

A mild to moderate iritis almost always accompanies disciform endotheliitis. The etiology of the iritis is unclear, but it is apparent that the immune reaction is directed at the corneal endothelium. The accompanying edema from endothelial decompensation seen with disciform endotheliitis is in marked contrast to the lack of corneal edema seen in other causes of acute anterior uveitis. Although most cases of acute anterior uveitis are associated with KP,

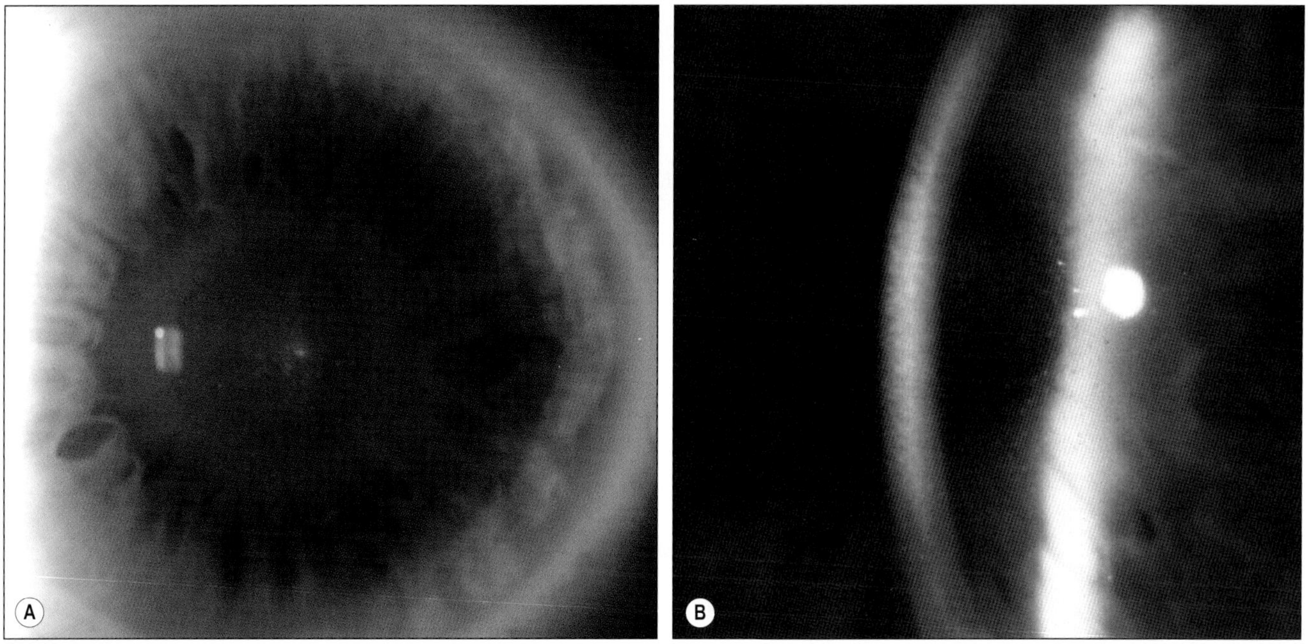

Fig. 79.21 Disciform endotheliitis. (**A**) A patient presented with a central round area of stromal haze caused by edema of the stroma. The edema results from an immune response at the level of the endothelium as evidenced by the keratic precipitates. (**B**) Slit beam shows that the stroma is free of infiltrate. KP can be seen underlying the area of edema.

Table 79.5 Classification of HSV endotheliitis

	Disciform	Diffuse	Linear
Keratitic precipitates	Disc-shaped distribution in central or paracentral cornea	Scattered KP spread over the entire endothelium	Line of KP progressing from the limbus May be sectoral or circumferential
Stroma	Disc-shaped area of edema corresponding to distribution of KP	Stromal edema involving the entire cornea	Edema present peripheral to the line of KP, extending to the limbus
Epithelium	Microcystic edema corresponds to severe stromal edema	Microcystic edema corresponds to severe stromal edema	Microcystic edema corresponds to severe stromal edema
Clinical course	Usually responsive to topical corticosteroids	Treatment with topical and systemic corticosteroids and possibly antivirals will lead to resolution	Requires aggressive treatment with topical and systemic antivirals and corticosteroids Corneal decompensation common

KP, keratic precipitates.
Graft survival rates have been found to be roughly similar between grafts for herpetic keratitis and grafts for other indications, though more rejection episodes are experienced with the former.[224]
Endotheliitis with sensorineural hearing loss due to HSV has been described.[225]

corneal edema is not present with them because these inflammatory cells merely come to rest on the endothelium and do not result from an immune response targeting the endothelium.

The iritis accompanying disciform endotheliitis can be difficult to detect through the edematous cornea. In addition, elevated intraocular pressure, which may be severe, is often present. The increased pressure may be due either to inflammatory cells blocking aqueous outflow or to a primary trabeculitis.

As with the cases of immune stromal keratitis, an episode of disciform endotheliitis may occur months to years after a documented episode of infectious epithelial keratitis. Often, there will not be a documented history of HSV disease, and a careful examination looking for footprints of HSV is helpful in making the proper diagnosis. Occasionally, the first documented dendritic ulcer occurs after an episode of disciform endotheliitis.[138] Although HSV is probably the most common cause of the idiopathic cases of disciform endotheliitis, other causes such as varicella-zoster virus (VZV) can produce an identical clinical picture.

Disciform endotheliitis is normally exquisitely sensitive to topical corticosteroids, and early intervention usually leads to complete resolution of the edema and KP without

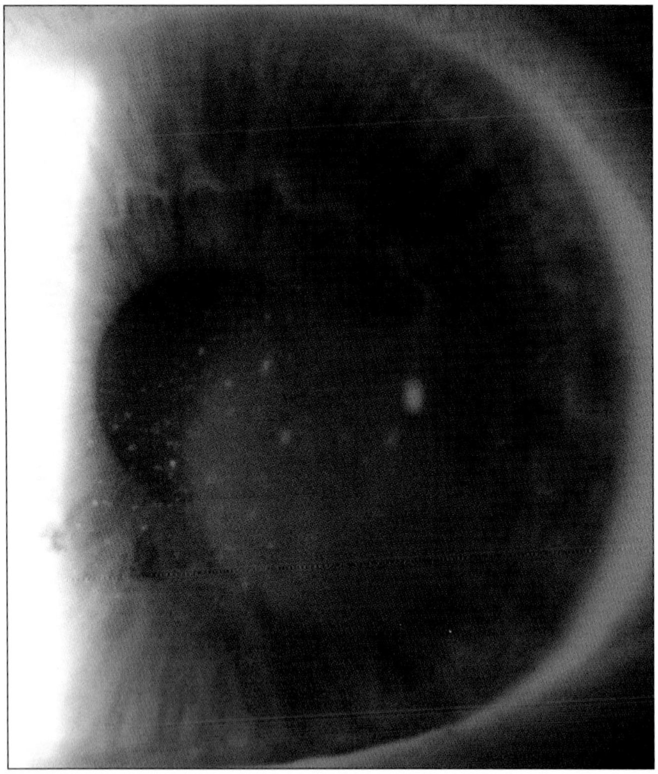

Fig. 79.22 Disciform endotheliitis. Chronic stromal and epithelial edema caused by severe disciform endotheliitis.

stromal scarring or loss of vision. Many cases of disciform endotheliitis are self-limited and completely resolve even if left untreated. Severe cases, however, can lead to permanent edema, scarring, and neovascularization if untreated (Fig. 79.22). For specific recommendations for the treatment of this disorder, see the section on Management.

Diffuse endotheliitis

A rare presentation of HSV keratitis is diffuse endotheliitis. Like patients with disciform endotheliitis, these patients also experience pain, photophobia, injection, and decreased vision. Patients with diffuse endotheliitis typically have scattered KP over the entire cornea with overlying diffuse stromal edema. A mild to moderate iritis is usually present, although it may be difficult to detect because of the corneal edema. Epithelial edema is present in cases of significant stromal edema. It is our clinical impression that the KP may either present in a scattered configuration or spread from a focus of previous disciform endotheliitis. In severe cases, a dense, retrocorneal plaque of inflammatory cells accompanied by hypopyon may be seen (Fig. 79.23).

As in the case of disciform endotheliitis, diffuse endotheliitis represents an immune reaction targeted against the corneal endothelium. This reaction against the endothelium is evident because of the marked stromal edema accompanying the KP.

The clinical course of diffuse endotheliitis is similar to disciform endotheliitis. This similarity is evident because of its exquisite sensitivity to topical corticosteroids and relatively good prognosis. Aggressive treatment with topical corticosteroids typically results in complete resolution of the inflammation and edema. Failure to control the inflammation leads to scarring, neovascularization, persistent edema, and loss of vision.

Linear endotheliitis

Symptoms of linear endotheliitis are similar to those seen with disciform and diffuse endotheliitis where the major complaints are pain, photophobia, and injection. Linear endotheliitis appears clinically as a line of KP on the corneal endothelium that progresses centrally from the limbus. It is accompanied by peripheral stromal and epithelial edema between the KP and the limbus (Fig. 79.24). The line of KP can be sectoral or, in some cases, circumferential (Fig. 79.25). It may have a distinct linear pattern as it moves centrally, but in some cases it may have a more serpiginous appearance. There is usually a well-demarcated line between the area of edematous and nonedematous cornea, with the KP located at the leading edge of the edema.

Sixteen eyes of 12 patients with a clinical appearance consistent with linear endotheliitis have been described in the literature.[139–143] A variety of names have been given to this clinical entity including keratitis linearis migrans, presumed autoimmune corneal endotheliopathy, progressive herpetic corneal endotheliitis, and idiopathic corneal endotheliopathy. Hakin et al.[143] used the term linear endotheliitis in a classification of idiopathic primary endotheliitis, but did not report any cases of linear endotheliitis.

A review of the published cases with findings consistent with linear endotheliitis reveals an association with HSV in only two cases. One patient had a typical HSV dendritic ulcer,[144] and another patient had an anterior chamber paracentesis that disclosed a positive antibody to HSV-1 antigen.[141] Four unilateral cases occurred at the surgical wound after an otherwise uneventful cataract extraction. All patients were primarily treated with topical corticosteroids, two were also treated with topical antiviral medications, and one was treated with oral acyclovir. Of the 16 eyes, five progressed to total corneal edema, and 10 had varying amounts of residual edema. Insufficient data were given on the final case.

We subsequently reported six eyes of five patients with linear endotheliitis.[132] One eye had a dendritic ulcer that was culture-proven for HSV-1, and two eyes had uncomplicated cataract extraction before developing linear endotheliitis at the cataract wound. All cases were treated aggressively with a combination of corticosteroids and topical antivirals, and in four of the patients oral acyclovir was needed to control the inflammation. All patients responded favorably, with complete resolution of the edema and inflammation.

Several observations suggest that linear endotheliitis may be immunologically mediated. First, linear endotheliitis is similar in appearance to the endothelial line seen with allograft rejection after a corneal transplant. Second, several reported cases have been bilateral; approximately half of the cases that do not follow cataract extraction are bilateral. Third, progression of the line occurs from the corneoscleral limbus centrally. Finally, corticosteroids are essential to successful treatment.

Although a definitive association with HSV has been seen in only three of 17 published cases (22 eyes), we believe that

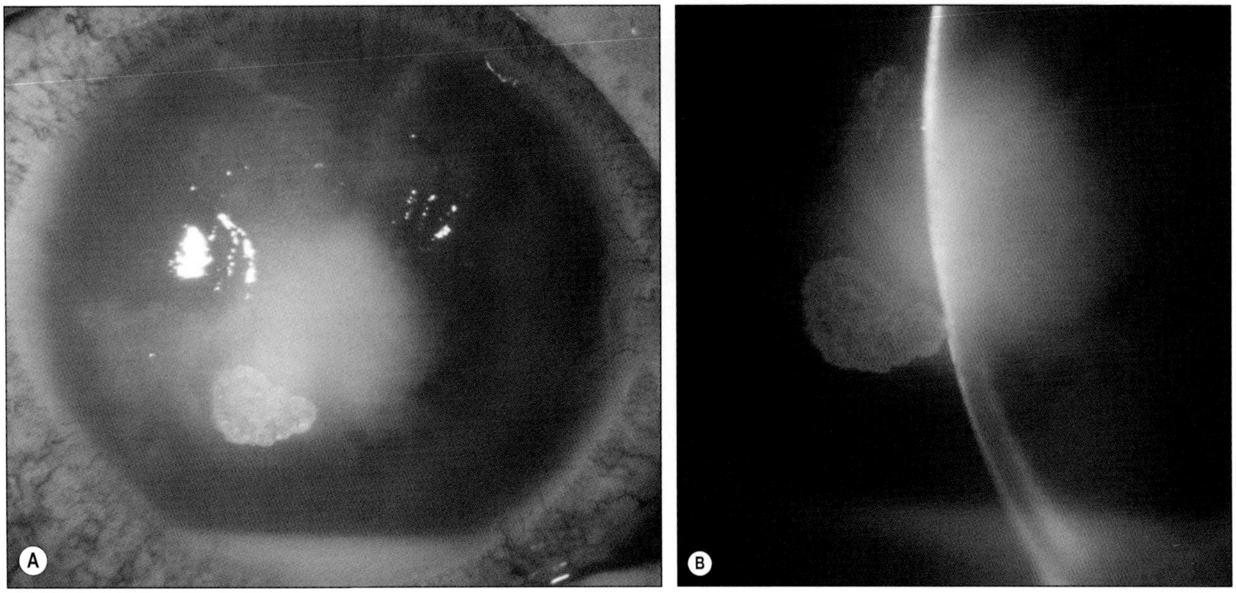

Fig. 79.23 Diffuse endotheliitis. (**A**) Dense retrocorneal plaque in a patient with severe diffuse endotheliitis and a previous history of HSV dendritic ulcer. (**B**) Careful examination with a slit beam reveals that the white lesion is retrocorneal and does not represent stromal inflammation.

many of the idiopathic cases are also due to HSV. The fact that patients treated with oral acyclovir respond favorably is compelling evidence for the role of HSV in this disease entity. Also of interest is the association of linear endotheliitis with a cataract incision. Presumably, a cataract wound causes trauma to corneal nerves that can lead to recrudescence of latent virus in the adjacent tissue.

Unlike disciform and diffuse endotheliitis, linear endotheliitis is quite difficult to treat. Failure to recognize and properly treat this condition leads to corneal decompensation. We believe that linear endotheliitis should be treated aggressively with both corticosteroids and antiviral agents. Oral acyclovir may have a beneficial role and should be considered in all cases.

Iridocyclitis

Patients with HSV keratitis may develop a concomitant or subsequent iridocyclitis. In addition, this iridocyclitis can occur without prior history of a keratitis. Patients present with signs and symptoms typical of iridocyclitis including photophobia, pain, and ciliary flush. Slit lamp examination reveals fine KP and an anterior chamber cellular reaction that can range from mild to severe. Segmental iris atrophy, similar to that seen with VZV iridocyclitis, is not uncommon and results from ischemic necrosis of the iris stroma. These areas of atrophy are seen as transillumination defects when performing a slit lamp examination (Fig. 79.26). Posterior synechiae may develop. Iris masses, hemorrhages, or hyphema, although unusual, also may occur (Fig. 79.27). The iridocyclitis in HSV most commonly accompanies immune stromal keratitis or endotheliitis, but, as previously stated, it may occur as the only inflammatory finding.

Clinical entities such as iridocorneal endothelial syndrome,[145] Fuchs' heterochromic iridocyclitis,[146] and Posner-Schlossman syndrome[147] have been approached in a different light recently in an attempt to link their pathogenesis with HSV. HSV viral DNA has been reported in the aqueous humor of three patients in the acute phase of Posner-Schlossman syndrome and one patient with Fuchs' heterochromic iridocyclitis, opening new possible interpretations for those disorders.

A trabeculitis may occur, which usually results in acute severe elevation of intraocular pressure. The pressure rise in these cases typically responds quickly to topical corticosteroids. Chronic inflammation often leads to secondary glaucoma from inflammatory cells blocking aqueous outflow. Glaucoma from chronic causes is much more difficult to manage.

Although the mechanism of HSV iridocyclitis is not fully understood, live virus appears to have a role in its development. Witmer and Iwamoto[148] described electron microscopic evidence of iris cell invasion by HSV particles. In several reports, viral organisms have been isolated from the anterior chambers of patients with HSV iridocyclitis.[131,149–153]

HSV should be suspected in patients with iridocyclitis who have corneal ghost scarring indicative of a previous infectious epithelial keratitis. We also suspect HSV in a group of patients without prior history or evidence of HSV keratitis who possess the following findings: chronic iridocyclitis that is refractory to topical corticosteroids, segmental iris atrophy, and anterior chamber pigment dispersion. We have had success in resolving inflammation with oral acyclovir in these selected cases.

Diagnosis

Although the diagnosis of primary and recurrent ocular HSV infection relies on a thorough ophthalmic examination, viral culture can help make a definitive diagnosis. This

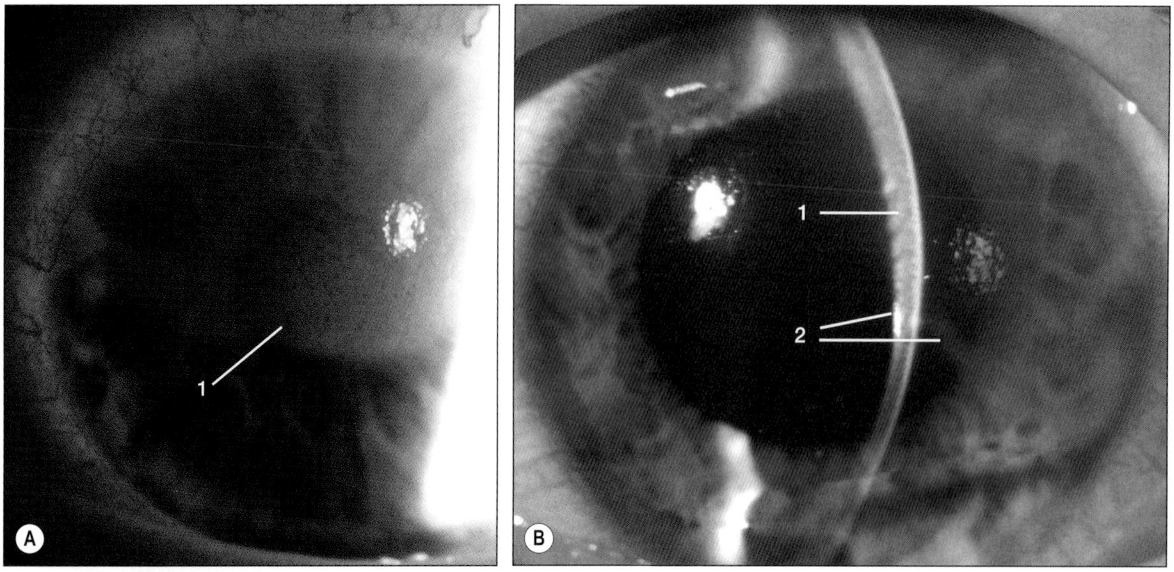

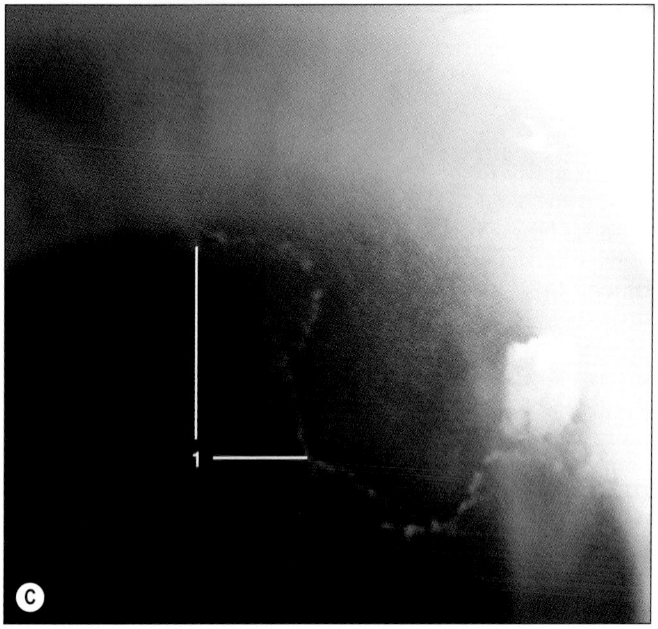

Fig. 79.24 Linear endotheliitis. (**A**) Advancing stromal and epithelial edema (*1*) progressing centrally from the superior limbus. (**B**) Slit beam reveals stroma to be edematous (*1*) but free of infiltrate peripheral to the line (*2*) of KP. (**C**) In another case of linear endotheliitis, linear KP (*1*) are more evident.

requires early culturing (usually within several days of the onset) and may require up to 1 week of incubation. Cell culture systems that require less time would be desirable; 24-hour enzyme-linked or shell vial culture assays have recently been developed with reportedly similar sensitivity and specificity as the traditional culture.[154–157] Viral isolates may then be typed as HSV-1 or HSV-2.[70,157] Typically, skin vesicles contain high viral titers, which can be detected in 90% of cultures,[3] and 70–80% of ulcerations (skin or cornea) are culture positive.[115] If previous antiviral therapy has been used, the yield is much lower.

Cytologic examination of specimens stained with Giemsa or Wright stains may provide rapid clues to diagnosis. Multinucleated giant cells may be seen, but this finding is nonspecific and may be caused by VZV or HSV. These staining techniques also may reveal intranuclear inclusions typical of infection by herpesviruses.[3] These more rapid techniques are not as sensitive as cultures, and negative results do not exclude HSV infection.

Cell culture may reveal characteristic cytopathic effects in cell lines from most species including early granular changes of the cytoplasm followed by cell rounding, enlargement, and finally detachment resulting in plaques; these effects are usually evident within 18 to 72 hours but may require 5 to 10 days.[3] Because this modality is technically demanding and may significantly delay the diagnosis, other more rapid tests are preferred.

Immunologic tests for the detection of ocular HSV have become commercially available. The Herpchek™, Virogen-latex agglutination, enzyme immunofiltration, and the 1-hour enzyme-linked immunoassay can detect HSV antigen in cell culture and direct specimens within 5 hours.[158]

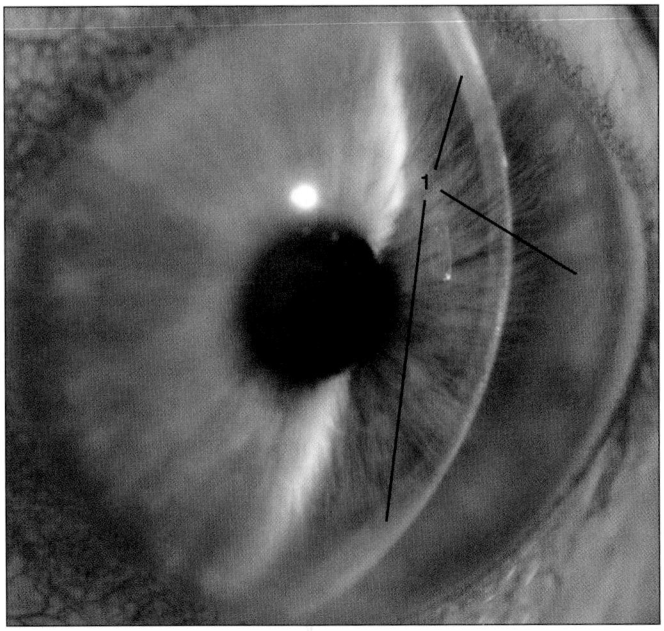

Fig. 79.25 Linear endotheliitis: 360 degrees of peripheral stromal and epithelial edema (*1*) associated with a ring of keratic precipitates in a patient with a history of HSV keratitis. An anterior stromal scar, indicating prior HSV disease, is also evident.

Kowalski and Gordon[158] reviewed these tests in 37 conjunctival or corneal specimens from patients with HSV infection as proven by culture and found that clinical examination alone was just as sensitive as any immunologic test and that the combination of clinical examination with Herpchek™ immunologic testing did not provide any greater cumulative sensititivity.[158] It was suggested that a positive Herpchek™ test would provide a quicker diagnosis than culture isolation and that immunologic testing may be useful when there is a diagnostic dilemma.

Polymerase chain reaction (PCR) in the diagnosis of HSV has been developed and used and is claimed to be equally specific and possibly more sensitive than cell cultures.[159] It targets viral DNA polymerase and, for confirmation, viral thymidine kinase. PCR is still not widely used, however, because it requires a skilled technician, and special equipment not accessible to most clinicians, at a much higher cost.

Other diagnostic tools have been described including electron microscopy to directly view herpes virions and DNA hybridization techniques using HSV nucleic acid probes. Although the latter are highly specific and sensitive, the technical difficulties associated with them preclude widespread clinical use.

Serum antibody titers can be used to differentiate primary herpetic infection from first ocular occurrence of recurrent disease. As discussed in the section on pathogenesis, antibody titers can fluctuate independently from clinical recurrences and therefore are only useful in the diagnosis of primary infection. IgM antibodies are found and can be detected in early primary infection. It is also found in some recurrences, however. Seroconversion with IgG usually occurs within 2 to 4 weeks of primary infection, and any

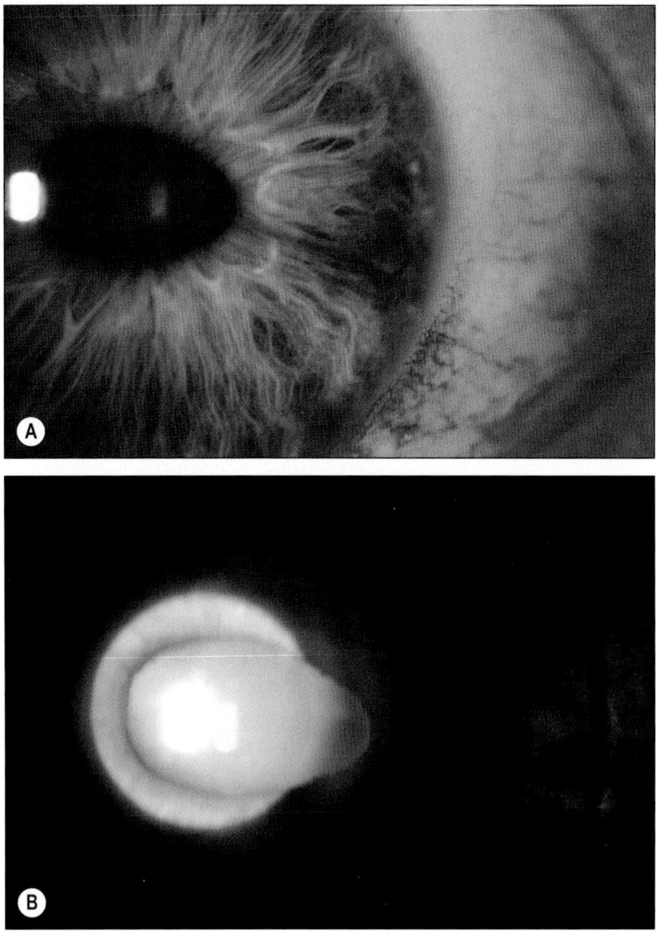

Fig. 79.26 HSV iridocyclitis. (**A**) Diffuse illumination reveals an irregularly shaped pupil in a patient with a history of HSV iridocyclitis. (**B**) When viewed with retroillumination, central areas of iris atrophy are apparent.

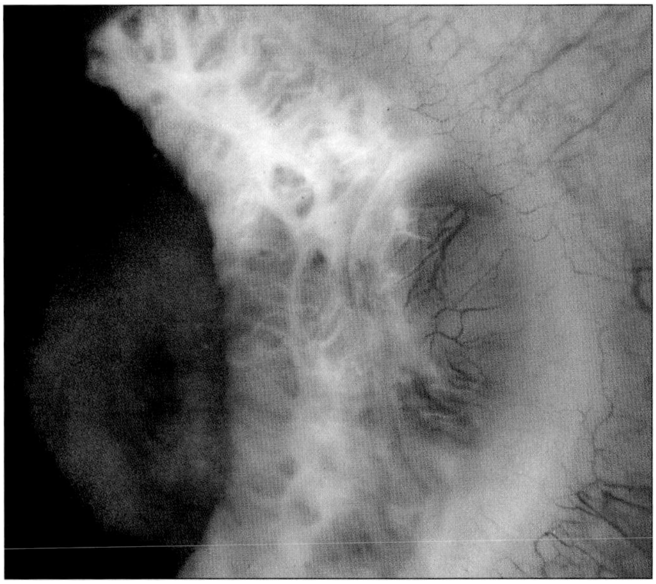

Fig. 79.27 HSV iridocyclitis. A basal iris mass lesion with hemorrhage is seen in a patient with chronic HSV iridocyclitis. Also note subepithelial scarring from previous HSV infectious epithelial keratitis. The mass resolved rapidly with oral acyclovir and prednisone therapy.

serologic evaluation should include paired samples with IgM + IgG in mind. Although serologic testing is seldom used clinically, antibodies to type-specific antigens (glycoprotein gG of HSV-2) may be detected using immunoblotting and enzyme-linked immunosorbent assay methods.[3] These methods would allow for the diagnosis of past HSV-2 infection.

Management

Herpetic Eye Disease Study

A set of multicenter, randomized, placebo-controlled trials under the name Herpetic Eye Disease Study (HEDS) sponsored by the National Eye Institute was designed to address the following HSV-associated clinical questions:

1. Topical corticosteroids in treating stromal keratitis already on a topical antiviral[160]
2. Oral acyclovir in treating stromal keratitis already on a topical steroid and antiviral[161]
3. Oral acyclovir in treating iridocyclitis already on topical steroid[162]
4. Oral acyclovir in preventing recurrence of epithelial and stromal keratitis[163,164]
5. Demographic and disease-specific predictors of recurrent HSV keratitis[28]
6. Risk factors for recurrence of ocular HSV.[80]

The trial of corticosteroids for herpetic stromal keratitis involved 106 patients. All patients in the treatment group received the same schedule of steroid eyedrop taper, regardless of clinical course. After 4 weeks, prednisolone phosphate 1% was reduced to once daily, after 7 weeks a 0.125% concentration eyedrop was reduced to once daily, for a total of 10 weeks. Failure was defined as new focal stromal inflammation, or increase in the area of inflamed cornea, or of the anterior chamber reaction beyond a certain proportion. Time to failure comparison was highly in favor of the treatment group at 10 weeks (26% vs 73%); half the benefit, however, was lost by 6 weeks after the treatment schedule was completed (49% vs 76%). The 95% confidence interval for time to failure in the treatment group was entirely beyond the 10-week treatment period (81–120 weeks). This finding is very suggestive of the treatment and prophylactic effect of corticosteroids in herpetic stromal keratitis. As a commentary on this trial, we believe that the benefit would very likely have been greater had individualized dosage been used; the cohort of treatment failures right after the 10 weeks of treatment were finished could potentially have been avoided if tapering had been tailored to each patient's inflammation. These limitations of the study design were acknowledged and accounted for by the authors; we also recommend a very cautious, gradual, and individualized taper of corticosteroid eyedrops in patients with HSV-ISK.

The efficacy of oral acyclovir in the treatment of HSV-ISK already on topical steroid and antiviral treatment was the object of another HEDS study. One hundred and four patients with HSV-ISK who had used topical steroid and were not eligible for the aforementioned topical steroid for stromal keratitis HEDS trial were randomized to oral acyclovir, 400 mg five times daily, or placebo. Treatment was continued for 10 weeks with an additional 6-week period of observation and a 6-month evaluation. Time to failure was again the principal studied outcome; rate of failure or resolution at 16 weeks, as well as best vision at 6 months were also compared. Time to treatment failure was not delayed significantly in the treatment group. The only positive finding of this trial was an apparent marginally significant treatment benefit on vision at 6 months, which was derived mainly from patients with initial visual acuity worse than 20/200; the crude nature of quantitating count-finger vision, as well as the fact that treatment after 16 weeks was left to the discretion of the ophthalmologist, both limit the validity of any inferences on this finding.

A similar 10-week treatment design and 6-month follow-up period were implemented in the trial of oral acyclovir for iridocyclitis, while on topical steroid and antiviral medications. The goal of 104 patients was hardly reached in this trial; with only 50 patients recruited in 4 years, the decision was made to end the study and release the results. A persistence or increase in the severity of either iridocyclitis or stromal keratitis, as well as a drop in vision or persistent rise in intraocular pressure, were determined to be treatment failures. The rate ratio for the protective effect of acyclovir on time to failure bordered on the significant when intention to treat was studied and was significant with a p value of 0.04 when voluntary or toxicity-related withdrawals were excluded. The protective effect appeared with a 3-week delay after initiation of treatment, presumably due to the more powerful treatment effect of intense topical steroid treatment in these first weeks. We need to comment on the nature of herpetic disease recruited in this study; including stromal keratitis with iridocyclitis could have diluted the findings of the trial. It appears that stromal keratitis and iridocyclitis are two different entities and active virus may be associated with iridocyclitis, while stromal keratitis, an immune reaction, is often accompanied by reactive anterior chamber inflammation. Oral acyclovir had not produced any benefit when added to topical antiviral and corticosteroid in herpetic stromal keratitis, again as part of the HEDS trials. Had the study involved only patients with primary iridocyclitis and not stromal keratitis, the results may have been different, possibly more supportive of a protective effect of the antiviral.

A prophylactic dosage regimen for acyclovir at 400 mg twice daily was used in the treatment group when 703 immunocompetent patients with a history of ocular HSV within the previous year were recruited and randomized to acyclovir or placebo. Treatment carried on for 12 months with an additional 6-month-long observation period. The two groups were similar in baseline characteristics and in reasons for early withdrawal. Acyclovir prophylaxis reduced recurrence of ocular HSV from 32% to 19%, and this protective effect was consistent in a subsequent subgroup analysis. This effect applied both to epithelial and stromal keratitis; it was, however, greatest for stromal keratitis patients with at least one prior episode. Orofacial HSV recurrences were also reduced. Follow-up of the placebo group also provided valuable information, in that it demonstrated that, unlike with stromal keratitis, a history of epithelial keratitis was not a risk factor for recurrent epithelial keratitis; on the other hand, the more the prior episodes of stromal keratitis, the higher the likelihood of recurrence.

Of plausible risk factors for ocular HSV recurrence, stress, systemic infection, sunlight exposure, menstruation, contact lens wear, and eye injury were not deemed significant, when the weekly log was completed prior to recurrence symptoms, to prevent recall bias.

The HEDS studies have provided us with valuable insight in dealing with treatment and prognostic dilemmas in patients with herpetic keratitis. In brief:

1. Oral antiviral prophylaxis reduces recurrences of epithelial and of stromal keratitis.
2. Use of topical corticosteroids is of benefit in stromal keratitis.
3. Use of oral acyclovir may be of help in iridocyclitis.
4. Prophylactic oral acyclovir helps prevent recurrences of herpetic keratitis, particularly stromal with a history of recurrence.

Medical management

Antiviral agents

Current topical antiviral agents used in the treatment of human HSV ocular disease include idoxuridine (IDU), vidarabine or Ara-A, trifluridine (F3T), acyclovir, ganciclovir, and bromovinyldeoxyuridine (BVDU). The first agent developed, IDU, was employed as an anticancer agent in the early 1950s.[10] IDU is a thymidine analog that incorporates into RNA, which then codes for abnormal proteins that impair viral replication and/or effectively inhibits DNA polymerization by binding to the responsible enzyme. It also incorporates into normal host cells, which accounts for the toxicity seen with both topical and systemic treatment. Solubility of the drug is low and, therefore, it is only available in low concentrations. Although IDU is effective in inhibiting viral replication, newer antivirals are considered more potent.

Vidarabine was the second agent developed for human use. It also inhibits viral DNA polymerase, but acts as a DNA chain terminator and is incorporated into both viral and host DNA to a small extent. It is regarded as a safe drug with little toxicity, especially when used systemically, and is used topically in ocular infections as well as systemically when acyclovir resistance is suspected. Vidarabine is highly insoluble and is only available as an ointment. Except in cases of viral strain resistance to other antiviral drugs, vidarabine is considered less potent than other available agents.

Trifluridine was developed as an anticancer agent and later became known as an effective antiviral agent.[165,166] It is now considered the drug of choice in the treatment of infectious epithelial keratitis caused by HSV. Trifluridine works by a similar mechanism of action to IDU and, therefore, can result in significant toxicity including superficial punctate keratitis, lacrimal punctal occlusion, follicular conjunctivitis, and localized contact dermatitis. Studies have indicated that this agent is superior to IDU and Ara-A with a 90–95% efficacy in eliminating dendritic ulcers.[167–173] It appears that F3T is more effective than IDU or vidarabine in antagonizing the stimulus for viral replication caused by the use of corticosteroids. This agent is rapidly degraded in the bloodstream and is not effective systemically.

The three remaining agents, acyclovir, ganciclovir, and BVDU, are considered more specific and therefore less toxic. Although all of these antiviral agents require phosphorylation to be effective, the thymidine kinase required to accomplish phosphorylation is located in both host and viral cells. After the initial phosphorylation, two additional phosphates are attached to form an active triphosphate form. The toxicity to host cells appears to occur because of this phenomenon and has been the basis for the development of selective antiviral agents. Selective antiviral agents are not activated by phosphorylation in host cells but only by virus-infected cells containing viral thymidine kinase. Acyclovir, ganciclovir, and BVDU act in this way and are considered selective agents. Acyclovir can preferentially inhibit HSV DNA by binding to DNA polymerase and acting as a chain terminator. Host cells are affected to a lesser degree. Studies have shown the efficacy of acyclovir ointment in the treatment of ocular herpes infection when compared to vidarabine or IDU with less toxicity.[169,170,174,175]

The issue of toxicity has been debated, with evidence showing that topical administration of these thymidine kinase-selective agents does not provide much benefit.[176] BVDU is not available in the United States, but has been used in Europe; BVDU has the potential for liver toxicity.[68] In a study comparing 0.15% ganciclovir gel and 3% acyclovir ointment, similar therapeutic effacacy shown as epithelial healing rates was noted between each group.[177] Ganciclovir was also noted to be significantly better tolerated by patients and was recently released in the United States as a 0.15% ophthalmic gel. Low solubility and systemic side effects of therapeutic corneal concentrations had limited its use in the past.[178,179]

A recent meta-analysis of therapeutic interventions for herpes simplex virus epithelial keratitis (including dendritic and geographic keratitis) assessed the relative effects of the above antiviral agents and physical interventions including physical debridement and chemical cauterization.[180] Ninety-nine trials published between 1963 and 2007 were included from the worldwide literature. The review found the commercially available and investigational antiviral agents effective versus placebo. Trifluridine, acyclovir, vidarabine, and ganciclovir showed significantly better epithelial healing by 1 week than IDU at the time points of 7 and 14 days. Of those four agents, no treatment emerged as significantly better than the rest. The most commonly used antivirals, trifluridine and acyclovir, appeared equivalent in effect at all timepoints. Interestingly, the combination of interferon or physicochemical treatment with an antiviral agent was significantly better than a single antiviral agent at 7 days but not 14 days.

Resistance to therapy is a known problem in the treatment of HSV. Widespread use of acyclovir has led to the emergence of HSV strains resistant to acyclovir, especially in severely immunocompromised patients. Until recently, few antedotal case reports existed demonstrating resistance in herpetic keratitis.[181] A recent study of 173 immunocompetent patients with herpetic keratitis showed 6.4% of viral isolates to be acyclovir resistant.[182,183] The majority of mutations causing acyclovir resistance occur in the thymidine kinase gene, causing loss or alteration in activity or substrate specificity.[184] Mutant viral cells deficient in thymidine kinase continue to replicate. They can take advantage of the presence of host thymidine kinase and, therefore, may be unaffected by the antiviral agents, especially those that are specific. Other known mutations include alterations in DNA polymerase activity. Although virulent strains are not necessarily magnified with mutation and resistance, several reports have been published on the virulence of mutated virions after treatment.[185–187] Acyclovir has been the mainstay of systemic treatment for HSV for several decades. Gertrude Elion and George Hitchins received the 1988 Nobel prize for the development of acyclovir, among other drugs. Acyclovir acts by competing for viral thymidine kinase and, after phosphorylation, by inhibiting and also acting as a substrate for DNA polymerase. At a dose of 400 mg five times daily, therapeutic aqueous humor levels can be achieved.[188]

Newer oral antivirals have been made available which simplify the dosing regimen of acyclovir. Valacyclovir, a prodrug, converts to acyclovir and has a higher bioavailability than acyclovir. Famciclovir is a prodrug for penciclovir. Both these medications act through inhibition of viral DNA polymerase, like acyclovir. Even though their effectiveness in ocular HSV has not been formally assessed in humans, convenient twice-a-day dosage (once, for prophylaxis) explains their widespread use, despite higher cost. Of note, long-term acyclovir prophylaxis in a formal cost-effectiveness analysis was not deemed to be cost efficient.[189] In clinical practice, however, the results of preventing corneal scarring and penetrating keratoplasties warrant long-term prophylaxis in at least selected cases.

Corticosteroids

Corticosteroids suppress inflammation by interfering with the normal immunologic response to various stimuli. Interference with lymphocyte function, migration, and the release of cellular digestive enzymes are all part of the mechanism of action seen clinically. The use of these agents in the setting of HSV ocular disease presents a challenge requiring both knowledge and experience. The use of antivirals is essential in the elimination of virions in the setting of active infection. However, the benefit of these agents when the disease has an immunologic component is controversial.

Corticosteroids have been found to suppress the local antibody-forming B lymphocytes of the cornea and uveal tract. This effect lasts only as long as the treatment, with a competent immune response once treatment is withdrawn.[190] Inhibition of corneal mucopolysaccharides and collagen also has been reported, as well as the potential for enhancing corneal thinning by stimulating collagenolytic enzymes. However, Lass et al.[191] treated herpetic keratitis with medroxyprogesterone acetate, which resulted in suppression of collagenase. A significant reduction in the infiltration of PMNs was also observed, as well as a reduction of stromal neovascularization. In addition, they found that epithelial disease was exacerbated with this agent, but that it could be eliminated with concurrent use of antiviral therapy.

The use of corticosteroids, both topically and systemically, can predispose the host to severe HSV disease of the eye. It has been suggested, however, that these agents do not increase the incidence of recurrence but only the severity of disease if it were to occur.[192] Advantages of steroid use in ocular disease include inhibition of cellular infiltration and, therefore, opacification and scarring, inhibition of the release of toxic enzymes, and inhibition of neovascularization. Disadvantages include exacerbation and spread of active viral infection by suppression of the normal host immune response and stimulation of viral replication, enhancement of collagenolytic enzyme production with subsequent corneal thinning, creation of a steroid-dependent ocular tissue by allowing for the build-up of viral antigens, the increased risk of opportunistic superinfections, and, finally, steroid-induced glaucoma and cataracts.

Recommendations for clinical manifestations

To treat HSV keratitis successfully, the clinician must recognize the infectious as well as immune components of the keratitis being treated. One can then modulate treatment with antiviral and antiinflammatory medications to eradicate the live virus, decrease the chance for future recurrence, and minimize scarring from inflammation (Box 79.2).

Infectious epithelial keratitis

The goal of treatment of infectious epithelial keratitis is to rid the cornea of live virus in a timely manner. Physical debridement of the ulcer with a sterile cotton-tipped applicator is the first step to undertake. If viral cultures are to be performed, tissue for culture should be obtained before debridement. After debridement, the patient should be placed on topical antiviral medications. The recommended medical regimen is ganciclovir gel 0.15% every 3 hours while awake or trifluridine 1% drops every 2 hours while awake. Vidarabine 3% ointment five times a day may be used as an alternative and is particularly useful in pediatric cases because of the difficulty of administering topical medications in eyedrop form to young children. Topical cycloplegics may be beneficial in patients with significant photophobia or ciliary spasm. Prophylaxis with a broad-spectrum antibiotic may be prudent when treating large geographic ulcers that may take many days to heal. Even though not substantiated in the literature, we and several other clinicians also use oral antiviral medications in the treatment of infectious epithelial keratitis, particularly with the newer agents and their more convenient dosing schedule, but also with acyclovir, when cost is a consideration. Although infectious epithelial keratitis is usually a self-limited disease, benefits exist for timely diagnosis and treatment. These benefits include reduction in patient morbidity, subepithelial scarring, and the potential risk of immune-mediated diseases of the cornea.

Topical antiviral therapy should be continued for 10 to 14 days. After 5 to 7 days, ganciclovir is usually tapered to 3 times a day for the duration of the treatment period, and trifluridine is usually tapered to five times a day for the rest of the treatment period. Vidarabine ointment, similarly, can be tapered to three times a day after 5 to 7 days.

If infectious epithelial keratitis has not healed after 2 weeks of treatment, careful inspection of the lesion should be undertaken to be certain that the lesion being treated is,

Box 79.2 Indications for corticosteroids and antivirals in the treatment of different forms of HSV keratitis

No corticosteroids
- HSV conjunctivitis
- Infectious epithelial keratitis
- Mild immune stromal keratitis without prior corticosteroid use
- Mild disciform endotheliitis without prior corticosteroid use
- Mild diffuse endotheliitis without prior corticosteroid use
- Noninflamed neurotrophic keratopathy

Topical corticosteroids
- Marginal keratitis
- Moderate immune stromal keratitis
- Moderate disciform endotheliitis
- Moderate diffuse endotheliitis
- Inflamed neurotrophic keratopathy
- Moderate iridocyclitis/trabeculitis

Oral corticosteroids (used in conjunction with topical corticosteroids)
- Severe immune stromal keratitis
- Severe disciform endotheliitis
- Severe diffuse endotheliitis
- All cases of linear endotheliitis
- Severe iridocyclitis/trabeculitis

Topical antivirals
- HSV blepharitis
- HSV conjunctivitis
- Infectious epithelial keratitis
- Prophylaxis for corticosteroid treatment of immune stromal keratitis (drop for drop with topical corticosteroid)

Oral antivirals
- Primary HSV infection
- Selected cases of severe diffuse endotheliitis
- Selected cases of severe iridocyclitis/trabeculitis
- Linear endotheliitis
- Immunocompromised patients
- Pediatric patients refractory to topical medications
- Prophylaxis against recurrent infectious epithelial keratitis
- Prophylaxis for post-PK patients with history of HSV keratitis

in fact, an ulcer. Often, the epithelium at the site of the healing ulcer appears abnormal for several weeks. This epitheliopathy takes a dendritic shape but is not ulcerated and represents healing epithelium after the infection. We refer to this abnormal epithelium as HSV dendritic epitheliopathy. The misdiagnosis of this lesion as active virus typically leads to the continued use of topical antivirals, often with the addition of a second or third agent, and propagation of the abnormal epitheliopathy and development of a secondary follicular conjunctivitis. In fact, in the immunocompetent patient, it is extremely rare for treatment of an HSV dendritic ulcer to require more than 14 days of antiviral medication. If antiviral medications are to be given for more than 2 weeks, careful evaluation of the remaining lesion must be undertaken to be certain that it is a dendritic ulcer rather than merely dendritic epitheliopathy.

If a true ulceration persists after 14 days of treatment, one must distinguish between a neurotrophic ulcer and persistent infectious epithelial keratitis. A neurotrophic ulcer has smooth borders and lacks the scalloped edges of infectious epithelial keratitis. If the lesion is persistent infectious epithelial keratitis, resistance to the antiviral medication must be considered, and an alternative medication can be initiated. It must be borne in mind that both trifluridine and acyclovir rely on the enzyme thymidine kinase for activation; therefore, a strain of HSV resistant to one medication often will also be resistant to the other. Vidarabine, on the other hand, is activated by cellular enzymes and is often effective against strains of HSV that are resistant to trifluridine and acyclovir. A true, persistent, infectious epithelial keratitis caused by resistance is exceedingly rare; however, resistant strains of HSV are becoming more common, especially in the immunocompromised patient. Fortunately, ulcers from resistant strains of HSV usually resolve within a few weeks even if left untreated. Overtreatment of infectious epithelial keratitis with topical antivirals is much more common than undertreatment.

Topical corticosteroid medications are not recommended for the treatment of infectious epithelial keratitis unless severe immune stromal inflammation is also present.

Neurotrophic keratopathy

Neurotrophic keratopathy results from impaired corneal innervation and decreased tear secretion. Chronic use of topical medications often contributes to this disease entity. Therapy must be aimed at decreasing exposure of the cornea to toxic substances while increasing lubrication. When a lesion is recognized as neurotrophic keratopathy, the first step in treatment is discontinuation of all unnecessary topical medications, especially topical antivirals. Frequent use of nonpreserved artificial tears promotes epithelial healing. In cases of significant ulceration, prophylactic treatment with a broad-spectrum antibiotic may be considered.

In severe cases of neurotrophic keratopathy, the above treatment regimen may be inadequate. Some patients have boggy, rolled epithelium at the borders of the ulcer. This abnormal epithelium may act as a mechanical barrier to new epithelial migration. These patients may benefit from gentle debridement of this abnormal epithelium at the ulcer edge.

Other patients may have persistent ulceration secondary to chronic low-grade inflammation at the base of the ulcer. These patients usually benefit from the administration of mild topical corticosteroid.

An additional treatment option for the nonhealing neurotrophic ulcer is a therapeutic soft contact lens. When a soft contact lens is used for this purpose, it should be accompanied by a broad-spectrum topical antibiotic once a day. This method only should be used for a short time because of the risk of infectious bacterial keratitis with prolonged contact lens wear.

Tape tarsorrhaphy also may be useful in the treatment of neurotrophic keratopathy. This solution usually works only for the short term because of patient inconvenience. A temporary tarsorrhaphy that lasts up to 3 months may be performed by injecting botulinum toxin into the levator muscle in a technique that was described by Wuebolt and Drummond.[193] In our experience, surgical tarsorrhaphy is the most effective treatment for severe neurotrophic keratopathy. This procedure can easily be accomplished in most office settings; however, it is underused in the management of this disorder. Although the tarsorrhaphy does not need to be so extensive as to cover the entire area of keratopathy, it should result in complete lid coverage of the area of ulceration. Neurotrophic ulcers that have persisted for months often resolve in just a few days after surgical tarsorrhaphy.

Historically, a conjunctival flap has been an important and effective treatment option for neurotrophic keratopathy. This procedure should still be considered, although it requires taking the patient to the operating room. Surgical tarsorrhaphy appears to be equally as effective as conjunctival flap and can be performed in the office setting.

Immunologic disease

Topical corticosteroids are valuable therapeutic agents in the management of HSV keratitis. The Herpetic Eye Disease Study (HEDS)[194] evaluated the efficacy of topical corticosteroids used in conjunction with topical antiviral coverage in the treatment of HSV immune stromal keratitis. The results showed that the topical corticosteroid regimen used resulted in a significant reduction of stromal inflammation and decrease in the duration of immune stromal keratitis.

The clinician must weigh the benefits against the risks of corticosteroid use when initiating therapy. Significant advantages of topical corticosteroids are the rapid and effective response of inflammation of the cornea and other parts of the anterior segment, the reduction of corneal scarring and neovascularization, and the reduction of intraocular sequelae of HSV such as secondary glaucoma and posterior synechiae. In addition to the development of cataract and glaucoma, specific potential complications of topical corticosteroids in the treatment of HSV include the facilitation of viral penetration into the cornea[195] and viral invasion of individual keratocytes.[196] The potential increased risk of viral invasion may contribute to prolonged stromal inflammation. Additional complications associated with topical corticosteroids are stromal necrosis and perforation and secondary microbial infection.

Topical corticosteroids may be beneficial in the treatment of a variety of HSV presentations, including marginal keratitis, immune stromal keratitis, endotheliitis, iridocyclitis, and trabeculitis. The following guidelines may be useful in treating patients with ocular inflammation from HSV. In patients with mild inflammation, such as early immune stromal keratitis or mild disciform endotheliitis, and no history of prior corticosteroid use, the clinician may elect not to initiate corticosteroid therapy. In some of these patients, the inflammation will resolve on its own without the patient being committed to a course of corticosteroids. However, if the inflammation is moderate to severe, there is a significant decrease in visual acuity from stromal inflammation or edema, or the patient is symptomatic with photophobia and discomfort, topical steroids may be indicated. If the decision is made to use topical corticosteroids, a significant strength and frequency should be used to suppress the inflammation.

There is some controversy regarding the starting dose of corticosteroids when treating patients with immune stromal keratitis. One option is to start the corticosteroids at a low dose and slowly increase until the minimal necessary dose to control inflammation is achieved.[197] Another option calls for a high initial corticosteroid dose to control inflammation rapidly, followed by a slow tapering course.[198] A final option, and one with which we agree, is to customize the initial corticosteroid dose according to the level of inflammation.[123] It is important to avoid rapid tapering or abrupt discontinuation of topical corticosteroids to prevent rebound inflammation.

The frequency and duration of treatment for immune stromal keratitis are also controversial. It is interesting to note that in the HEDS at 6 months, no clinically significant difference in visual acuity was seen between the corticosteroid-treated group and control subjects.[194] One criticism of the HEDS is that all patients were treated using the same protocol. Fifty percent of patients treated with corticosteroids who 'failed' treatment did so during the 6 weeks of observation just after the 10-week treatment period had ended. One conclusion that can be drawn from this observation is that each patient treated for HSV immune stromal keratitis must have an individualized treatment regimen, and treatment with corticosteroids often must continue for longer than 10 weeks.

When treating HSV patients with topical corticosteroids, it is important for the clinician to understand the concept of flare dose, which was not evaluated in the HEDS. Inflammation often flares when topical corticosteroids are tapered below a certain level. This level is called the flare dose, and the clinician should not attempt to taper the topical medications below it until the inflammation is quiet for several months. Vanishingly low-dose topical corticosteroids, such as prednisolone acetate $\frac{1}{8}$% or even $\frac{1}{16}$% once a day or every other day, may be necessary to prevent recurrence of inflammation in some patients.

Oral corticosteroids are also useful in selected patients with HSV keratitis. In patients with severe immune stromal keratitis, disciform endotheliitis, diffuse endotheliitis and iritis, and all cases of linear endotheliitis, oral corticosteroids are indicated. Oral corticosteroids also may prove more beneficial than topical corticosteroids in patients with persistent epithelial defects and significant immune response.

A common situation in management of HSV disease is the underusage of corticosteroids for the immunologic components. Many patients may require long-term, low-dose, topical corticosteroids to suppress inflammation and prevent the sequelae of scarring, neovascularization, and loss of vision. Many clinicians repeatedly attempt to discontinue corticosteroids in patients with persistent inflammation because of the fear of the development of corticosteroid-related side effects such as cataracts, increased intraocular pressure, and secondary microbial keratitis. The prevention of cataract and steroid-response increased intraocular pressure in an eye that goes on to develop an opaque cornea from chronic inflammation from HSV should be considered a treatment failure. Less morbidity occurs in treating a patient for cataract or increased intraocular pressure and a clear cornea than treating a patient with no cataract or glaucoma and a cornea that is opaque from chronic inflammation. The risk of microbial keratitis is very low, and this entity can be treated with antibiotics.

Topical corticosteroids should not be used in a cavalier manner. Except under unusual circumstances, topical corticosteroids should be avoided when treating infectious epithelial keratitis or neurotrophic keratopathy. Some investigators believe that the use of topical corticosteroids for immune HSV disease enhances viral replication and therefore makes the patient more susceptible to future episodes of infectious keratitis.[199]

Most clinicians recommend topical antiviral coverage for patients receiving topical corticosteroids in the treatment of immunologic HSV disease. The most common recommendation is to use topical antivirals and corticosteroids with equal frequency ('drop for drop') until the corticosteroids are reduced to a dose equivalent to prednisolone phosphate 0.1% once a day. Because lower doses of topical corticosteroid appear to carry a lesser risk of recurrent infectious epithelial keratitis,[200] the antiviral can be discontinued at this point. This regimen was developed to reduce the risk of developing infectious HSV disease in patients treated with corticosteroids.[197,201] Few studies have looked at the long-term effects of topical antiviral prophylaxis. Long-term (several months) use of topical antivirals, including trifluridine, results in significant complications such as toxic keratoconjunctivitis, allergic conjunctivitis, or punctal stenosis. Therefore, we rarely use topical antivirals for longer than a few weeks, and we prefer the use of oral acyclovir for long-term prophylaxis.

In those patients with recurrent infectious epithelial keratitis and chronic immunologic disease, we treat each infectious episode with a 10–14-day course of topical antivirals and discontinuation or reduction of corticosteroids. Many chronic immunologic patients have rapid recurrence of the inflammatory reaction when topical corticosteroids are stopped. To prevent this rebound inflammation, either topical corticosteroids may be resumed after 3 to 4 days of antiviral treatment, or a short course of oral corticosteroids may be used. In patients who require chronic prophylactic coverage, oral acyclovir, 400 mg twice a day, can be used. This medication is more effective against viral recurrences than topical antivirals and eliminates the problems associated with the toxicity of the topical medications.

Iridocyclitis/trabeculitis

The primary cause of inflammation from HSV iridocyclitis is immune, and therefore corticosteroids are indicated in its treatment. Frequent topical drops accompanied by ointment at night may be needed to suppress the inflammatory reaction. In the most severe cases, oral corticosteroids may be of benefit.

Some patients with chronic iridocyclitis, with or without history of HSV keratitis, do not respond to large-dose topical corticosteroids. These patients may show resolution of their inflammation when oral acyclovir, 400 mg five times a day, is used in addition to topical corticosteroids. This response to oral acyclovir may be clinical evidence for the role of active virus in the etiology of HSV iridocyclitis.

A trabeculitis often accompanies episodes of HSV iridocyclitis. This trabeculitis manifests as an acute and severe elevation of intraocular pressure. Antiglaucoma medications are useful in the acute phase to decrease the intraocular pressure. However, because the etiology of the increased pressure is an immune reaction at the level of the trabecular meshwork, it is necessary to use topical corticosteroids to treat this disorder properly and return the intraocular pressure to normal.

Indications for oral acyclovir

The indications for oral acyclovir can be divided into treatment of active viral disease and prophylaxis against recurrence. In some patients, topical antiviral therapy may not be effective in treating active infections. These patients include those with primary HSV infection, immunocompromised patients, infants, and other patients with iridocyclitis not responsive to topical corticosteroids.

The patient with a significant primary HSV infection may benefit from oral acyclovir. In selected cases, use of acyclovir may shorten the course of the disease, reduce the chance of corneal involvement, and decrease patient morbidity and the likelihood of recurrence.

Immunocompromised patients may be either medically immunosuppressed from organ transplantation or cancer chemotherapy, or immunodeficient from a systemic disease such as AIDS. These patients lack the normal immunologic response that is important in controlling active virus and may not respond to topical antiviral therapy alone. Immunocompromised patients with active viral disease often require systemic administration of acyclovir to resolve the infection. For the moderately immunocompromised patients, oral acyclovir is probably adequate. For the severely immunocompromised patient, however, intravenous acyclovir may be necessary to achieve predictably high levels of medication to treat the infection effectively.[202]

Oral acyclovir is effective in treating infectious epithelial keratitis in adults.[203–205] In our experience, oral acyclovir is quite useful for treating infants and children with infectious epithelial keratitis. We have treated several patients in whom standard topical therapy with antiviral drops and ointments has failed. Oral acyclovir may have certain advantages over topical antiviral agents in treating this patient population. First, it is difficult to administer topical medications to patients in this age group. Second, it may be difficult to examine these patients appropriately in the office setting. Third, infants and children tend to express a severe immune reaction associated with their epithelial disease not typically seen in adults. For these reasons, infectious epithelial keratitis in these patients inadequately treated with a regimen of topical antiviral medications may resolve much more quickly on oral acyclovir, offering the benefit of fast visual rehabilitation and protection from amblyogenesis. We have reported on seven patients between the ages of 6 weeks and 5 years whom we treated with systemic acyclovir, with no adverse effects, for epithelial keratitis, which resolved in all cases.[206]

Iridocyclitis patients, as mentioned earlier, may have active virus as part of the etiology of their disease. In these patients, topical antiviral medications do not penetrate into the anterior chamber at a high enough concentration to control the infection.[207] Oral acyclovir results in therapeutic levels of medication in the tear film[203,208] and aqueous humor,[209] and when used with corticosteroids, has been effective in treating selected patients with HSV iridocyclitis, as supported by the HEDS study.

There are two specific populations of patients who may benefit from long-term oral acyclovir as a prophylactic agent. Included in this group are patients with frequently recurrent infectious epithelial keratitis and postpenetrating keratoplasty patients with history of HSV keratitis. Patients who experience two or more episodes of infectious epithelial keratitis per year may be candidates for prophylactic treatment with oral acyclovir, 400 mg twice a day. Patients with frequently recurrent infectious epithelial keratitis will benefit from prophylaxis because frequent recurrent disease not only causes pain but also increases the risk of corneal scarring and loss of vision. Prophylaxis with oral acyclovir has two specific advantages over prophylaxis with topical antivirals. First, prophylactic use of topical antiviral agents does not prevent the recurrence of infectious epithelial keratitis. Second, chronic usage of topical antiviral medications leads to toxic keratopathy and conjunctival scarring. There have been limited studies on the use of oral acyclovir in this setting. We and others[3] found that oral acyclovir is effective prophylaxis in the patient with frequent recurrent infectious epithelial keratitis. Studies on the efficacy of oral acyclovir on recurrent genital HSV indicate a significant reduction in frequency and severity of episodes.[4] However, discontinuation of prophylactic therapy leads to an increase in the recurrence rate similar to that seen before prophylactic treatment.

Patients who undergo penetrating keratoplasty (PK) for the treatment of visual loss associated with HSV keratitis are at significant risk for recurrence of active infection in the graft. In addition, HSV endotheliitis in the post-PK patient may be indistinguishable from allograft rejection and thus may confuse the clinician. We advocate the use of long-term prophylaxis with oral acyclovir, 400 mg twice a day, in our post-PK patients. A recent study has shown the efficacy of this treatment regimen in preventing recurrence of HSV in the graft.[210,211]

Several attempts have been made at developing HSV vaccines, which have mainly focused on controlling genital herpes.[212] Recently, HSV-1 immunization against murine herpetic stromal keratitis has been demonstrated with a vaccine based on the envelope glycoprotein D. As shown in this study, the new area of DNA vaccines may have future impact against HSV-1.[213]

Surgical

Occasionally, adjuvant therapy is indicated in the treatment of HSV ocular disease. These approaches include the use of therapeutic contact lenses, collagenase inhibitors, tarsorrhaphy, conjunctival flap, cyanoacrylate gluing, and lamellar or penetrating keratoplasty.

In cases of persistent epithelial defects and ulceration, a therapeutic contact lens may be considered. However, we do not recommend this practice in all cases because of the increased likelihood of opportunistic infections. Tarsorrhaphy would be preferred in these cases and should be the first modality of treatment before the use of a contact lens.

The use of the conjunctival flap was described by Gundersen,[214] in 1958, but its need is diminishing with the advancement of medical therapy. Nevertheless, it may still be useful in those patients with chronic ulcers failing conventional therapy and who have functional vision in the fellow eye and a contraindication to immediate PK, especially if the visual potential is limited or when a delay in more definitive surgery (i.e. keratoplasty) is necessary. Performing a PK in the setting of severe inflammation carries a much higher incidence of failure and will certainly present a difficult and unrewarding postoperative course for both physician and patient.

If corneal perforation were to occur from HSV disease, corneal gluing could be considered if the perforation were small (see Ch. 139). Lamellar keratoplasy may also be considered in these situations but should not be considered in lieu of penetrating keratoplasty because of low success rates in achieving good visual results and a risk of reactivation of the diseases in the interface.[122,215,216]

Penetrating keratoplasty should be considered when there is corneal perforation that cannot be treated with other modalities, or when there is a central stromal scar that precludes adequate vision. Foster and Duncan[217] also have suggested this option to eliminate the antigenic material responsible for repeated episodes of immune-mediated keratitis. In two reports, HSV-1 has also been implicated in the causation of primary graft failure.[218,219] In the setting of perforation, active HSV is likely with significant ocular inflammation. Therefore standard postoperative care must be modified to improve the likelihood of graft survival. In addition to standard postoperative topical medications, we recommend the use of perioperative topical antivirals, oral acyclovir, and, in selected cases, systemic corticosteroids, if not contraindicated. When PK is performed for corneal scarring, the risk of recurrent HSV disease is 12–19%,[220–223] and perioperative therapy should again be tailored. We recommend the additional use of oral acyclovir for at least 1 year postoperatively.

References

1. Obara Y, et al. Distribution of herpes simplex virus types 1 and 2 genomes in human spinal ganglia studied by PCR and in situ hybridization. *J Med Virol.* 1997;52(2):136–142.
2. Waggoner-Fountain LA, Grossman LB. Herpes simplex virus. *Pediatr Rev.* 2004;25:86–93.
3. Goodman JL. Infections caused by herpes simplex viruses. In: Hoeprich PD, Jordan C, Ronald AR, eds. *Infectious diseases.* 5th ed. Philadelphia: JB Lippincott; 1994.
4. Kaplowitz L, et al. Prolonged continuous acyclovir treatment of normal adults with frequently recurring genital herpes simplex virus infection. *JAMA.* 1991;265:747.
5. Lehner T, Wilton J, Shilltoe E. Immunological basis for latency, recurrences and putative oncogenicity of herpes simplex virus. *Lancet.* 1975;2:60.
6. Workshop on the treatment and prevention of herpes simplex virus infection. *J Infect Dis.* 1973;127:117.
7. Fleming DT, et al. Herpes simplex virus type 2 in the United States, 1976 to 1994. *N Engl J Med.* 1997;337(16):1105–1111.
8. Armstrong GL, et al. Incidence of herpes simplex virus type 2 infection in the United States. *Am J Epidemiol.* 2001;153(9):912–920.
9. Liesegang TJ, Melton J III, Daly PJ, Ilstrup DM. Epidemiology of ocular herpes simplex. *Arch Ophthalmol.* 1989;107:1155–1159.
10. Kaufman HE, Rayfield MA. Viral conjunctivitis and keratitis: herpes simplex virus. In: Kaufman H, et al, eds. *The cornea.* New York: Churchill Livingstone; 1988.
11. Wander AH, Centifanto YM, Kaufmam HE. Strain specificity of clinical isolates of herpes simplex virus. *Arch Ophthalmol.* 1980;98:1458–1461.
12. Norberg P, et al. Phylogenetic analysis of clinical herpes simplex virus type 1 isolates identified three genetic groups and recombinant viruses. *J Virol.* 2004;78(19):10755–10764.

13. Kinchington PR. Viral keratitis and conjunctivitis: virology. In: Smolin G, Thoft RA, eds. *The cornea.* 3rd ed. Boston: Little, Brown; 1994.
14. Spence J, Miller F, Court D. *Thousand family survey.* London: Oxford University Press; 1954.
15. Buddingh G, et al. Studies on the natural history of herpes simplex infections. *Pediatrics.* 1953;11:595.
16. Scott T. Epidemiology of herpetic infection. *Am J Ophthalmol.* 1957; 43:134.
17. Thygeson P, Kimura SJ, Hogan MJ. Observations on herpetic keratitis and keratoconjunctivitis. *Arch Ophthalmol.* 1956;56:375–388.
18. Wilhelmus KR, et al. Prognostic indicators of herpetic keratitis: analysis of a five-year observation period after corneal ulceration. *Arch Ophthalmol.* 1981;99:1578–1582.
19. Bell DM, Holman RC, Pavan-Langston D. Herpes simplex keratitis: epidemiological aspects. *Ann Ophthalmol.* 1982;14:421–424.
20. Darougar S, et al. Acute follicular conjunctivitis and keratoconjunctivitis due to herpes simplex virus in London. *Br J Ophthalmol.* 1978;62(12): 843–849.
21. Wishart PK, et al. Prevalence of acute conjunctivitis caused by chlamydia, adenovirus, and herpes simplex virus in an ophthalmic casualty department. *Br J Ophthalmol.* 1984;68(9):653–655.
22. Darougar S, Wishart MS, Viswalingam ND. Epidemiological and clinical features of primary herpes simplex virus ocular infection. *Br J Ophthalmol.* 1985;69:2–6.
23. Wishart MS, Darougar S, Viswalingam ND. Recurrent herpes simplex virus ocular infection: epidemiological and clinical features. *Br J Ophthalmol.* 1987;71:669–672.
24. Wilhelmus KR, et al. Prognosis indicators of herpetic keratitis. Analysis of a five-year observation period after corneal ulceration. *Arch Ophthalmol.* 1984;99(9):1578–1582.
25. Liesegang TJ. Epidemiology of ocular herpes simplex. *Arch Ophthalmol.* 1989;107:1160–1165.
26. Norn MS. Dendritic (herpetic) keratitis, I: incidence-seasonal variations-recurrence rates-visual impairment-therapy. *Acta Ophthalmol (Copenh).* 1970;48:91–107.
27. Shuster JJ, Kaufman HE, Nesburn AB. Statistical analysis of the rate of recurrence of herpesvirus ocular epithelial disease. *Am J Ophthalmol.* 1981;91(3):328–331.
28. Herpetic Eye Disease Study Group. Predictors of recurrent herpes simplex virus keratitis. *Cornea.* 2001;20(2):123–128.
29. Wechsler SL, Nesburn AB. Recent advances in the molecular biology of herpes simplex latency: a short review. In: Cavanagh HD, ed. *The cornea: transactions of the World Congress on the Cornea III.* New York: Raven Press; 1988.
30. Stevens JG, Nesburn AB, Cook ML. Latent herpes simplex virus from trigeminal ganglia of rabbits with recurrent eye infection. *Nature.* 1972;235:216.
31. Stevens JG, Cook ML. Latent herpes simplex virus in spinal ganglia of mice. *Science.* 1971;173:843.
32. Fraser N, et al. Herpes simplex type 1 DNA in human brain tissue. *Proc Natl Acad Sci USA.* 1981;78:843.
33. Balfour H. Resistance of herpes simplex to acyclovir. *Ann Intern Med.* 1983;98:404.
34. Baringer J. The virology of herpes simplex virus infection in humans. *Surv Ophthalmol.* 1976;21:171.
35. Baringer J, Swoveland P. Recovery of herpes simplex virus from human trigeminal ganglions. *N Engl J Med.* 1973;288:648.
36. Bastian F, et al. Herpes hominus: isolation from human trigeminal ganglion. *Science.* 1972;178:306.
37. Klein R. Pathogenic mechanisms of recurrent herpes simplex virus infections. *Arch Virol.* 1976;51:1.
38. Roizman B, Sears A. Herpes simplex viruses and their replication. In: Fields B, Knipe D, eds. *Virology.* vol. 2. 2nd ed. New York: Raven Press; 1990.
39. Strauss S. Clinical and biological differences between recurrent herpes simplex virus and varicella-zoster virus infections. *JAMA.* 1989;262:3455.
40. Summers BC, Margolis TP, Leib DA. Herpes simplex virus type 1 corneal infection results in periocular disease by zosteriform spread. *J Virol.* 2001;75(11):5069–5075.
41. Chang TW. Recurrent viral infection. *N Engl J Med.* 1971;284:765–771.
42. Meyers RL, Petit TH. The pathogenesis of cornea inflammation due to herpes simplex virus. *J Immunol.* 1973;111:1031–1042.
43. Dunkel E, et al. Molecular biology of ocular viral infections. In: *Molecular biology of the eye.* New York: Alan Liss; 1988.
44. Liesegang T. Biology and molecular aspects of herpes simplex and varicella-zoster virus infections. *Ophthalmology.* 1992;99:781.
45. Pavan-Langston D, Rong B, Dunkel E. Extraneuronal herpetic latency: animal and human corneal studies. *Acta Ophthalmol Suppl (Copenh).* 1989;192:135.
46. Puga A, et al. Herpes simplex virus DNA and mRNA sequences in acutely and chronically infected trigeminal ganglia of mice. *Virology.* 1978; 89:102.
47. Rong BL, et al. Detection of HSV thymidine kinase and latency-associated transcript gene expression in human herpetic corneas by polymerase chain reaction. *Invest Ophthalmol Vis Sci.* 1991;32:1808.
48. Sabbaga E, et al. Detection of HSV nucleic acid sequences in the cornea during acute and latent ocular disease. *Exp Eye Res.* 1988;47:545.
49. Kaye SB, et al. Evidence for herpes simplex viral latency in the human cornea. *Br J Ophthalmol.* 1991;75:195–200.
50. Cook SD, Hill JH. Herpes simplex virus: molecular biology and the possibility of corneal latency. *Surv Ophthalmol.* 1991;36:140–148.
51. Centifanto Y, Little J, Kaufman H. Relationship between virus chemotherapy secretory antibody formation and recurrent herpetic disease. *Ann NY Acad Sci.* 1973;173:649.
52. Hammer H, Dobozy A. Cell-mediated immunity to herpes virus type 1 in patients with recurrent corneal herpes simplex. *Acta Ophthalmol (Copenh).* 1980;58:161–166.
53. Meyers R. Immunology of herpes simplex virus infection. *Int Ophthalmol Clin.* 1975;15:37.
54. Meyers R, Chitjian P. Immunology of herpesvirus infections: immunity to herpes simplex virus in eye infections. *Surv Ophthalmol.* 1976;21:194.
55. Meyers-Elliott R, Pettit T, Maxwell W. Viral antigens in the immune rings of herpes simplex stromal keratitis. *Arch Ophthalmol.* 1980;98:897.
56. Meyers-Elliott R, et al. HLA antigens in herpes stromal keratitis. *Am J Ophthalmol.* 1980;89:54.
57. Centifanto YM, et al. Ocular disease pattern induced by herpes simplex virus is genetically determined by a specific region of viral DNA. *J Exp Med.* 1982;155:475.
58. Kaufman H, et al. Effect of the herpes simplex virus genome on the response of infection to corticosteroids. *Am J Ophthalmol.* 1985;100:114.
59. Spear P. Glycoproteins specified by herpes simplex viruses. In: Roizman B, ed. *The herpesviruses.* vol. 3. New York: Plenum Press; 1985.
60. Hubbard A, Centifanto-Fitzgerald Y. Variability among HSV-1 strains Herpesvirus Workshop and its importance in disease. In: *Proceedings of the Ninth International.* Seattle; 1984.
61. Nishiyama Y, Rapp F. Regulation of persistent infection with herpes simplex virus in vitro by hydrocortisone. *J Virol.* 1979;31:841.
62. Centifanto-Fitzgerald Y, Varnell E, Kaufman H. Initial HSV-1 injection prevents ganglionic superinfection by other strains. *Infect Immun.* 1982;35:1125.
63. Gordon Y, Araullo-Cruz T. Herpesvirus inoculation of cornea. *Am J Ophthalmol.* 1984;97:482.
64. Varnell E, Centifanto-Fitzgerald Y, Kaufman HE. Herpesvirus infection and its effect on virulent superinfections, ganglionic colonization and shedding. Presented to the Association for Research in Vision and Ophthalmology. Florida: Sarasota; April 1981.
65. Remeijer L, et al. Corneal herpes simplex virus type 1 superinfection in patients with recrudescent herpetic keratitis. *Invest Ophthalmol Vis Sci.* 2002;43(2):358–363.
66. Knickelbein JE, et al. Noncytotoxic lytic granule-mediated CD8+ T cell inhibition of HSV-1 reactiviation from neuronal latency. *Science.* 2008;322(5899):268–271.
67. Liesegang T. Ocular herpes simplex infection: pathogenesis and current therapy. *Mayo Clin Proc.* 1988;63:1092.
68. Liesegang T. Diagnosis and therapy of herpes zoster ophthalmicus. *Ophthalmology.* 1991;98:1216.
69. Pavan-Langston D. Major ocular viral infections. In: Galasso G, Whitley R, Merigan T, eds. *Antivral agents and viral diseases of man.* 3rd ed. New York: Raven Press; 1990.
70. Pavan-Langston D. Viral disease of the cornea and external eye. In: Albert D, Jakobiec F, eds. *System of ophthalmology.* Philadelphia: WB Saunders; 1994.
71. Kroll DM, Schuman JS. Reactivation of herpes simplex virus keratitis after initiating bimatoprost treatment for glaucoma. *Am J Ophthalmol.* 2002;133(3):401–403.
72. Morales J, et al. Herpes simplex virus dermatitis in patients using latanoprost. *Am J Ophthalmol.* 2001;132(1):114–116.
73. Kaufman HE, et al. Effects of topical unoprostone and latanoprost on acute and recurrent herpetic keratitis in the rabbit. *Am J Ophthalmol.* 2001;131(5):643–646.
74. Camras CB. Latanoprost increases the severity and recurrence of herpetic keratitis in the rabbit; latanoprost and herpes simplex keratitis. *Am J Ophthalmol.* 2000;129(2):271–272; author reply 2000:272–273.
75. Wand M, Gilbert CM, Liesegang TJ. Latanoprost and herpes simplex keratitis. *Am J Ophthalmol.* 1999;127(5):602–604.
76. Kaufman HE, Varnell ED, Thompson HW. Latanoprost increases the severity and recurrence of herpetic keratitis in the rabbit. *Am J Ophthalmol.* 1999;127(5):531–536.

77. Openshaw H, et al. Acute and latent infection of sensory ganglia with herpes simplex virus. immune control and virus reactivation. *J Gen Virol.* 1979;44:205.
78. Garrity J, Liesegang T. Ocular complications of atopic dermatitis. *Can J Ophthalmol.* 1984;19:21.
79. Margolis T, Ostler HB. Treatment of ocular disease in eczema herpeticum. *Am J Ophthalmol.* 1990;110:274.
80. Herpetic Eye Disease Study Group. Psychological stress and other potential triggers for recurrences of herpes simplex virus eye infections. *Arch Ophthalmol.* 2000;118(12):1617–1625.
81. Jones B, et al. Symposium on herpes simplex eye disease. Objectives of therapy of herpetic eye disease. *Trans Ophthalmol Soc UK.* 1977;97: 305.
82. Levy D, Banerjee A, Glenny H. Cimetidine in the treatment of herpes zoster. *J R Coll Physicians Lond.* 1985;19:96.
83. Easty DL. Pathogenesis of herpes simplex stromal keratitis: role of replicating virus. In: Cavanagh HD, ed. *The cornea: transactions of the World Congress on the Cornea III.* New York: Raven Press; 1988.
84. Pepose JS. Herpes simplex keratitis. role of viral infection versus immune response. *Surv Ophthalmol.* 1991;35:345–352.
85. Gangappa S, Deshpande SP, Rouse BT. Bystander activation of CD4+ T cells accounts for herpetic ocular lesions. *Invest Ophthalmol Vis Sci.* 2000;41(2):453–459.
86. Dawson C, Togni B, Moore R. Structural changes in chronic herpetic keratitis. *Arch Ophthalmol.* 1968;79:740.
87. Holbach L, Font R, Naumann G. Herpes simplex stromal and endothelial keratitis. *Ophthalmology.* 1990;97:722.
88. Zhao ZS, et al. Molecular mimicry by herpes simplex virus-type 1: autoimmune disease after viral infection. *Science.* 1998;279(5355): 1344–1347.
89. Sundmacher R, Neumann-Haefelin D. Herpes simplex virus isolierung aus dem Kammerwasser bei fokaler iritis, endotheliitis und langdauernder keratitis disciformis mit sekundarglaukom. *Klin Monatsbl Augenheilkd.* 1979;175:488.
90. Meyers-Elliott RH, Chitjian PA, Dethlefs BA. Experimental herpesvirus keratitis in the rabbit. topical versus intrastromal infection routes. *Ophthalmic Res.* 1983;15:240–256.
91. Kimura T, Murata K, Okumura K, Nakajima A. Immunopathological analysis of corneal inflammation caused by HSV type-1 infection. In: Cavanagh HD, ed. *The cornea: transactions of the World Congress on the Cornea III.* New York: Raven Press; 1988.
92. Peeler J, Niederkorn J, Matoba A. Corneal allografts induce cytotoxic T cell but not delayed hypersensitivity responses in mice. *Invest Ophthalmol Vis Sci.* 1985;26:1516–1523.
93. Lausch RN, et al. Resolution of HSV corneal infection in the absence of delayed-type hypersensitivity. *Invest Ophthalmol Vis Sci.* 1985;26: 1509–1515.
94. Larsen HS, Russell RG, Rouse BT. Recovery from lethal herpes simplex virus type 1 infection is mediated by cytotoxic T lymphocytes. *Infect Immun.* 1983;41:197–204.
95. Smeraglias R, et al. The role of herpes simplex virus secreted glycoproteins in herpetic keratitis. *Exp Eye Res.* 1982;35:443–459.
96. Boshoff C. Kaposi's sarcoma. Coupling herpesvirus to angiogenesis. *Nature.* 1998;391(6662):24–25.
97. Philipp W, Speicher L, Humpel C. Expression of vascular endothelial growth factor and its receptors in inflamed and vascularized human corneas. *Invest Ophthalmol Vis Sci.* 2000;41(9):2514–2522.
98. Zheng M, et al. Contribution of vascular endothelial growth factor in the neovascularization process during the pathogenesis of herpetic stromal keratitis. *J Virol.* 2001;75(20):9828–9835.
99. Zheng M, et al. Control of stromal keratitis by inhibition of neovascularization. *Am J Pathol.* 2001;159(3):1021–1029.
100. Lee S, et al. Role of matrix metalloproteinase-9 in angiogenesis caused by ocular infection with herpes simplex virus. *J Clin Invest.* 2002;110(8):1105–1111.
101. Nahmias A, Alford C, Korones S. Infection of the newborn with herpesvirus hominis. *Adv Pediatr.* 1970;17:185.
102. Overall JC. Herpes simplex virus infection of the fetus and newborn. *Pediatr Ann.* 1994;23:131–136.
103. Whitley R, et al. Predictors of morbidity and mortality in neonates with herpes simplex virus infections. *N Engl J Med.* 1991;324:45–54.
104. Hutto C, et al. Intrauterine herpes simplex virus infections. *J Pediatr.* 1987;110:97–101.
105. Whitley RJ. Herpes simplex virus infections. In: Remington JS, Klein JO, eds. *Infectious diseases of the fetus and newborn infant.* 3rd ed. Philadelphia: WB Saunders; 1990.
106. Douglas JM, Schmidt O, Corey L. Acquisition of neonatal HSV-1 infection from a paternal source contact. *J Pediatr.* 1983;103:908–910.
107. Light IJ. Postnatal acquisition of herpes simplex by the newborn infant: a review of the literature. *Pediatrics.* 1979;63:480–482.
108. Yeager AS, Arvin AM. Reasons for the absence of a history of recurrent genital infections in mothers of neonatal herpes simplex virus infections. *Pediatrics.* 1984;73:188–193.
109. Hagler W, Walters P, Nahmias A. Ocular involvement in neonatal herpes simplex virus infection. *Arch Ophthalmol.* 1969;82:169.
110. Cibis A, Bunde R. Herpes simplex virus induced congenital cataracts. *Arch Ophthalmol.* 1971;85:220.
111. Shuster JJ, Kaufman HE, Nesburn AB. Statistical analysis of the rate of recurrence of herpesvirus ocular epithelial disease. *Am J Ophthalmol.* 1981;91:328–331.
112. Wishart PK, et al. Prevalence of acute conjunctivitis caused by chlamydia, adenovirus and herpes simplex virus in an ophthalmic casualty department. *Br J Ophthalmol.* 1984;68:653–655.
113. Darougar S, et al. Acute follicular conjunctivitis and keratoconjunctivitis due to herpes simplex virus in London. *Br J Ophthalmol.* 1978;62: 843–849.
114. Wilhelmus KR, Falcon MG, Jones BR. Bilateral herpetic keratitis. *Br J Ophthalmol.* 1981;65:385–387.
115. Pavan-Langston D. Herpetic infections. In: Smolin G, Throft RA, eds. *The cornea.* Boston: Little, Brown; 1994.
116. Roat ME, et al. The antiviral effects of rose bengal and fluorescein. *Arch Ophthalmol.* 1987;105:1415–1417.
117. Thygeson P. Marginal herpes simplex keratitis simulating catarrhal ulcer. *Invest Ophthalmol Vis Sci.* 1971;10:1006.
118. McGill J, et al. Reassessment of idoxuridine therapy of herpetic keratitis. *Eye.* 1974;94:542–552.
119. Whitcher JP, et al. Herpes simplex keratitis in a developing country. *Arch Ophthalmol.* 1976;94:587–592.
120. Shimeld C, et al. Isolation of herpes simplex virus from the cornea in chronic stromal keratitis. *Br J Ophthalmol.* 1982;66:643.
121. Sanitato JJ, et al. Acyclovir in the treatment of herpetic stromal disease. *Am J Ophthalmol.* 1984;98:537.
122. Brik D, Dunkel E, Pavan-Langston D. Persistent herpes simplex virus in the corneal stroma despite topical and systemic antiviral therapy. *Arch Ophthalmol.* 1993;111:522.
123. Williams HP, Falcon MG, Jones BR. Corticosteroids in the management of herpetic eye disease. *Trans Ophthalmol Soc UK.* 1977;97:341–344.
124. McGill J, et al. Reassessment of idoxuridine therapy of herpetic keratitis. *Trans Ophthalmol Soc UK.* 1974;94:542–552.
125. Kobayashi S, Shogi K, Ishizu M. Electron microscopic demonstration of viral particles in keratitis. *Jpn J Ophthalmol.* 1972;16:247–250.
126. Wilhelmus KR. Diagnosis and management of herpes simplex stromal keratitis. *Cornea.* 1987;6:286–291.
127. Brady SE, et al. Clinical indications for and procedures associated with penetrating keratoplasty, 1983–1988. *Am J Ophthalmol.* 1989;108: 118–122.
128. Mohamedi P, et al. Changing indications for penetrating keratoplasty, 1984–1988 (letter). *Am J Ophthalmol.* 1989;107:550–552.
129. Mamalis N, et al. Changing trends in the indications for penetrating keratoplasty. *Arch Ophthalmol.* 1992;110:1409–1411.
130. Vannas A, Ahonen R, Makitie J. Corneal endothelium in herpetic keratouveitis. *Arch Ophthalmol.* 1983;101:913–915.
131. Kaufman HE, Kanai A, Ellison ED. Herpetic iritis: demonstration of virus in the anterior chamber by fluorescent antibody techniques and electron microscopy. *Am J Ophthalmol.* 1971;71:465.
132. Olsen TW, et al. Linear endotheliitis. *Am J Ophthalmol.* 1994;117: 468–474.
133. Vannas A, Ahonen R. Herpetic endothelial keratitis. *Acta Ophthalmol (Copenh).* 1981;59:296.
134. Robin JB, et al. Progressive herpetic corneal endotheliitis. *Am J Ophthalmol.* 1985;100:336.
135. Oh JO. Endothelial lesions of rabbit cornea produced by herpes simplex virus. *Invest Ophthalmol Vis Sci.* 1970;9:196.
136. Reijo A, Antti V, Jukka M. Endothelial cell loss in herpes zoster keratouveitis. *Br J Ophthalmol.* 1983;67:751.
137. Sundmacher R, et al. Connatal monosymptomatic corneal endotheliitis by cytomegalovirus. In: Sundmacher R, ed. *Herpetic eye diseases.* Munich: JF Bergmann Verlag; 1981.
138. Sutcliffe E, Baum J. Acute idiopathic corneal endotheliitis. *Ophthalmology.* 1984;91:1161.
139. Fuchs A. Keratitis linearis migrans. *Z Augenheilkd.* 1926;58:315.
140. Khodadoust AA, Attarzadeh A. Presumed autoimmune corneal endotheliopathy. *Am J Ophthalmol.* 1982;93:718.
141. Robin JB, Steigner JB, Kaufman HE. Progressive herpetic corneal endotheliitis. *Am J Ophthalmol.* 1985;100:336.
142. Ohashi Y, et al. Idiopathic corneal endotheliopathy. *Arch Ophthalmol.* 1985;103:1666.

143. Hakin KN, Dart JK, Sherrard E. Sporadic diffuse corneal endotheliitis. *Am J Ophthalmol.* 1989;108:509.
144. Sugar A, Smith T. Presumed autoimmune corneal endotheliopathy. *Am J Ophthalmol.* 1982;94:689.
145. Alvarado JA, et al. Detection of herpes simplex viral DNA in the iridocorneal endothelial syndrome. *Arch Ophthalmol.* 1994;112(12): 1601–1609.
146. Barequet IS, et al. Herpes simplex virus DNA identification from aqueous fluid in Fuchs' heterochromic iridocyclitis. *Am J Ophthalmol.* 2000;129(5):672–673.
147. Yamamoto S, et al. Possible role of herpes simplex virus in the origin of Posner-Schlossman syndrome. *Am J Ophthalmol.* 1995;119(6): 796–798.
148. Witmer R, Iwamoto T. Electron microscope observation of herpes-like particles in the iris. *Arch Ophthalmol.* 1968;79:331.
149. Sundmacher R. A clinico-virologic classification of herpetic anterior segment disease with special reference to intraocular herpes. In: Sundmacher R, ed. *Herpetic eye diseases.* Munich: JF Bergmann Verlag; 1981.
150. Ahonen R, Vannas A. Clinical comparison between herpes simplex and herpes zoster ocular infections. In: Maudgal PC, Missotten L, eds. *Herpetic eye diseases.* The Netherlands: Dr W Junk Publishers; 1985.
151. Collin B, Abelson M. Herpes simplex virus in human cornea, retrocorneal fibrous membrane, and vitreous. *Arch Ophthalmol.* 1976;94:1726.
152. Pavan-Langston D, Brockhurst R. Herpes simplex panuveitis. *Arch Ophthalmol.* 1969;81:783.
153. Sundmacher R, Neumann-Haefelin D. Herpes simplex virus isolations from the aqueous of patients suffering from focal iritis, endotheliitis, and prolonged disciform keratitis with glaucoma. *Surv Ophthalmol.* 1981;27:342.
154. Kowalski RP, et al. ELVIS: a new 24-hour culture test for detecting herpes simplex virus from ocular samples. *Arch Ophthalmol.* 2002;120(7): 960–962.
155. Athmanathan S, Bandlapally S, Rao GN. Comparison of the sensitivity of a 24 h-shell vial assay, and conventional tube culture, in the isolation of herpes simplex virus-1 from corneal scrapings. *Clin Pathol.* 2002;2(1):1.
156. Athmanathan S, Bandlapally S, Rao GN. Collection of corneal impression cytology directly on a sterile glass slide for the detection of viral antigen. An inexpensive and simple technique for the diagnosis of HSV epithelial keratitis – a pilot study. *Ophthalmology.* 2001;1(1):3.
157. Hyndiuk R, Glasser D. Herpes simplex keratitis. In: Tabbara KF, Hyndiuk RA, eds. *Infections of the eye.* Boston: Little, Brown; 1986.
158. Kowalski RP, Gordon YJ. Evaluation of immunologic tests for the detection of ocular herpes simplex virus. *Ophthalmology.* 1989;9:1583–1586.
159. Espy MJ, et al. Evaluation of LightCycler PCR for implementation of laboratory diagnosis of herpes simplex virus infections. *J Clin Microbiol.* 2000;38(8):3116–3118.
160. Wilhelmus KR, et al. Herpetic Eye Disease Study. A controlled trial of topical corticosteroids for herpes simplex stromal keratitis. *Ophthalmology.* 1994;101(12):1883–1895; discussion 1994:1895–1896.
161. Barron BA, et al. Herpetic Eye Disease Study. A controlled trial of oral acyclovir for herpes simplex stromal keratitis. *Ophthalmology.* 1994; 101(12):1871–1882.
162. The Herpetic Eye Disease Study Group. A controlled trial of oral acyclovir for iridocyclitis caused by herpes simplex virus. *Arch Ophthalmol.* 1996;114(9):1065–1072.
163. The Herpetic Eye Disease Study Group. Oral acyclovir for herpes simplex virus eye disease: effect on prevention of epithelial keratitis and stromal keratitis. *Arch Ophthalmol.* 2000;118(8):1030–1036.
164. The Herpetic Eye Disease Study Group. Acyclovir for the prevention of recurrent herpes simplex virus eye disease. *N Engl J Med.* 1998; 339(5):300–306.
165. Heidelberger C, Parsons DG, Remy DC. Syntheses of 5-trifluoromethyluracil and 5-trifluoromethyl-2′-deoxyuridine. *J Med Chem.* 1964;7:1.
166. Kaufman HE, Heidelberger C. Therapeutic antiviral action of 5-trifluoromethyl-2′-deoxyuridine. *Science.* 1964;145:585.
167. Wellings PC, et al. Clinical evaluation of trifluorothymidine in the treatment of herpes simplex corneal ulcers. *Am J Ophthalmol.* 1972; 73:932.
168. Heidelberger C, King DH. Trifluorothymidine. *Pharmacol Ther.* 1979;6: 427.
169. Collum L, Benedict-Smith A, Hillary I. Randomized double-blind trial of acyclovir and idoxuridine in dendritic corneal ulceration. *Br J Ophthalmol.* 1980;64:766.
170. Coster D, et al. Clinical evaluation of adenine arabinoside and trifluorothymidine in the treatment of corneal ulcers caused by herpes simplex virus. *J Infect Dis.* 1976;133(suppl):A173.
171. Pavan-Langston D. Clinical evaluation of adenine arabinoside and idoxuridine in treatment of ocular herpes simplex. *Am J Ophthalmol.* 1975;80:495.
172. Pavan-Langston D, Buchannan R. Vidarabine therapy of simple and IDU-complicated herpetic keratitis. *Trans Am Acad Ophthalmol Otolaryngol.* 1976;74:81.
173. Pavan-Langston D, Foster CS. Trifluorothymidine and idoxuridine therapy of ocular herpes. *Am J Ophthalmol.* 1977;84:818.
174. Coster D, et al. A comparison of acyclovir and idoxuridine as treatment for ulcerative herpetic keratitis. *Br J Ophthalmol.* 1980;64:763.
175. Pavan-Langston D, et al. Acyclovir and vidarabine in therapy of ulcerative herpes simplex keratitis – a comparative masked clinical trial. *Am J Ophthalmol.* 1981;92:829.
176. McCulley JP, et al. A double-blind, multicenter clinical trial of acyclovir vs idoxuridine for treatment of epithelial herpes simplex keratitis. *Ophthalmology.* 1982;89:1195.
177. Colin J, et al. Ganciclovir ophthalmic gel (Virgan; 0.15%) in the treatment of herpes simplex keratitis. *Cornea.* 1997;16(4):393–399.
178. Hoh, HB, et al. Randomized trial of ganciclovir and acyclovir in the treatment of herpes simplex dendritic keratitis: a multicenter study. *Br J Ophthalmol.* 1996;80:140–143.
179. Majumdar SS, et al. Dipeptide monoester ganciclovir prodrugs for treating HSV-1-induced corneal epithelial and stromal keratitis: in vitro and in vivo evaluations. *J Ocul Pharmacol Ther.* 2005;21(6):463–474.
180. Wilhelmus KR. Therapeutic interventions for herpes simplex virus epithelial keratitis. *Cochrane Database of Systematic Reviews.* 2008;1: CD002898.
181. Zhang W, et al. Dendritic keratitis caused by an acyclovir-resistant herpes simplex virus with frameshift mutation. *Cornea.* 2007;26(1): 105–106.
182. Duan R, et al. Acyclovir-resistant corneal HSV-1 isolates from patients with herpetic keratitis. *J Infect Dis.* 2008;198:659–663.
183. Sarisky RT, et al. Biochemical characterization of a virus isolate, recovered from a patient with herpes keratitis, that was clinically resistant to acyclovir. *Clin Infect Dis.* 2001. 33:2034–2039.
184. Morfin F, Thouvenot D. Herpes simplex virus resistance to antiviral drugs. *J Clin Virol.* 2003;26:29–37.
185. Crumpacker CS, et al. Resistance to antiviral drugs of herpes simplex virus isolated from a patient treated with acyclovir. *N Engl J Med.* 1982;306:343.
186. Burns WH, et al. Isolation and characterization of resistant herpes simplex virus after acyclovir therapy. *Lancet.* 1982;1:421.
187. Sibrack CD, et al. Pathogenecity of acyclovir-resistant herpes simplex virus type 1 from an immunodeficient child. *J Infect Dis.* 1982;146:673.
188. Hung SO, et al. Oral acyclovir in the management of dendritic herpetic corneal ulceration. *Br J Ophthalmol.* 1984;68(6):398–400.
189. Lairson DR, et al. Prevention of herpes simplex virus eye disease. a cost-effectiveness analysis. *Arch Ophthalmol.* 2003;121(1):108–112.
190. Meyers R, et al. Effect of local corticosteroids on antibody-forming cells in the eye and draining lymph nodes. *Invest Ophthalmol.* 1975;14:138.
191. Lass J, Pavan-Langston D, Berman M. Treatment of experimental herpetic interstitial keratitis with medroxyprogesterone. *Arch Ophthalmol.* 1980;98:520.
192. Kilbrick S, et al. Local corticosteroid therapy and reactivation of herpetic keratitis. *Arch Ophthalmol.* 1971;86:694.
193. Wuebolt GE, Drummond G. Temporary tarsorrhaphy induced with type A botulinum toxin. *Can J Ophthalmol.* 1991;26:383–385.
194. Wilhelmus KR, et al. Herpetic Eye Disease Study: a controlled trial of topical corticosteroids for herpes simplex stromal keratitis. *Ophthalmology.* 1994;101:1883–1896.
195. Robbins RM, Galin MA. A model of steroid effects in herpes keratitis. *Arch Ophthalmol.* 1975;93:828–830.
196. Dawson C, et al. Herpes virus infection of human mesodermal tissue (cornea) detected by electron microscopy. *Nature.* 1968;217:460.
197. Patterson A, Jones BR. The management of ocular herpes. *Trans Ophthalmol Soc UK.* 1967;87:59–84.
198. Aronson SB, Moore TE. Corticosteroid therapy in central stromal keratitis. *Am J Ophthalmol.* 1969;67:873–896.
199. Easterbrook M, et al. The effect of topical corticosteroid on the susceptibility of immune animals to reinoculation with herpes complex. *Invest Ophthalmol Vis Sci.* 1973;2:181–184.
200. Mukherjee G, Mohan M, Angra SK. Topical corticosteroid in herpetic keratitis. *East Arch Ophthalmol.* 1979;7:34–40.
201. Sundmacher R. Trifluorthymidineprophylaxe bei der steroidtherapie herpetischer keratouveitiden. *Klin Monatsbl Augenheilkd.* 1978;173: 516–519.
202. Young T, et al. Herpes simplex keratitis in patients with acquired immune deficiency syndrome. *Ophthalmology.* 1989;96:1476.
203. Collum LMT, Akhtar J, McGettrick P. Oral acyclovir in herpetic keratitis. *Trans Ophthalmol Soc UK.* 1985;104:629–632.
204. Schwab IR. Oral acyclovir in the management of herpes simplex ocular infections. *Ophthalmology.* 1988;95:423–430.

205. Hung SO, et al. Oral acyclovir in the management of dendritic herpetic corneal ulceration. *Br J Ophthalmol.* 1984;68:398–400.
206. Schwartz GS, Holland EJ. Oral acyclovir for the management of herpes simplex virus keratitis in children. *Ophthalmology.* 2000;107(2): 278–282.
207. Poirier RH, et al. Intraocular antiviral penetration. *Arch Ophthalmol.* 1982;100:1964–1967.
208. Collum LMT, et al. Oral acyclovir (Zovirax) in herpes simplex dendritic corneal ulceration. *Br J Ophthalmol.* 1986;70:435–438.
209. Hung SO, Patterson A, Rees PJ. Pharmacokinetics of oral acyclovir (Zovirax) in the eye. *Br J Ophthalmol.* 1984;68:192–195.
210. Barney NP, Foster CS. A prospective randomized trial of oral acyclovir after penetrating keratoplasty for herpes simplex keratitis. *Cornea.* 1994;13:232–236.
211. Barron BA, et al. Herpetic Eye Disease Study: a controlled trial of oral acyclovir for herpes simplex stromal keratitis. *Ophthalmology.* 1994;101: 1871–1882.
212. Stanberry LR. Herpes vaccines for HSV. *Dermatol Clin.* 1998;16(4): 811–816.
213. Inoue T, et al. Effect of herpes simplex virus-1 gD or gD-IL-2 DNA vaccine on herpetic keratitis. *Cornea.* 2002;21(Suppl 2):79–85.
214. Gundersen T. Conjunctival flaps in treatment of corneal diseases. *Arch Ophthalmol.* 1958;6:880.
215. Fine M. Lamellar corneal transplant. In: *Symp. Cornea Transactions of the New Orleans Academy of Ophthalmology.* St Louis: Mosby; 1972.
216. Tullo AB, et al. Isolation of herpes simplex virus from corneal discs of patients with chronic stromal keratitis. In: Maugdal PC, Missotten L, eds. *Herpetic eye diseases.* Dordrecht, Netherlands: Junk Publishers; 1984.
217. Foster CS, Duncan J. Penetrating keratoplasty for herpes simplex keratitis. *Am J Ophthalmol.* 1981;92:336.
218. Cockerham GC, Krafft AE, McLean IW. Herpes simplex virus in primary graft failure. *Arch Ophthalmol.* 1997;115(5):586–589.
219. De Kesel RJ, et al. Primary graft failure caused by herpes simplex virus type 1. *Cornea.* 2001;20(2):187–190.
220. Langston R, Pavan-Langston D, Dohlman CH. Penetrating keratoplasty for herpetic keratitis. *Trans Am Acad Ophthalmol Otolaryngol.* 1975;79: 577.
221. Cohen E, Laibson P, Arensten J. Corneal transplantation for herpes simplex keratitis. *Am J Ophthalmol.* 1983;95:645.
222. Fine M, Cignetti F. Penetrating keratoplasty in herpes simplex keratitis. *Arch Ophthalmol.* 1977;95:613.
223. Ficker L, et al. Changing management and improved prognosis for corneal grafting and herpes simplex keratitis. *Ophthalmology.* 1989; 96:1587.
224. Halberstadt M, et al. The outcome of corneal grafting in patients with stromal keratitis of herpetic and non-herpetic origin. *Br J Ophthalmol.* 2002;86(6):646–652.
225. Mimura T, et al. Corneal endotheliitis and idiopathic sudden sensorineural hearing loss. *Am J Ophthalmol.* 2002;133(5):699–700.

Chapter 80

Herpes Zoster Keratitis

W. Barry Lee, Thomas J. Liesegang

Varicella-zoster virus (VZV), also referred to as human herpesvirus type 3, is a ubiquitous virus that causes two distinct clinical conditions, varicella (chickenpox) and herpes zoster (shingles).[1] Varicella represents a primary infection with VZV, and herpes zoster results from a reactivation of the latent VZV within the sensory spinal or cerebral ganglia. Steiner[2] first demonstrated varicella to represent an infectious disease in 1875 after inoculation of participants from an infected individual reproduced the disease. While the relationship between varicella and herpes zoster was first noted in 1888,[3] laboratory research only later confirmed VZV as the etiology of both disorders by direct isolation and later by restriction endonuclease patterns.[4,5]

Epidemiology

Serological evidence of prior VZV infection is present in 95% of the population within the United States.[6] Varicella represents a primary infection after exposure of a susceptible or seronegative individual to VZV. Prior to the introduction of varicella vaccination in 1995, approximately 4 million cases (15–16 cases/1000 person-years) of VZV infection occurred annually within the USA, with the peak age of varicella occurrence at 5 to 9 years of age, and over 90% of children infected by the age of 15.[7,8] Prior to vaccination introduction, approximately 12000 to 13000 patients were hospitalized annually in the USA with 100 to 150 annual deaths from varicella complications. After the implementation of the varicella vaccine in 1995, the incidence of varicella in the USA has declined by 57–90% with a similar decrease in hospitalizations by 75–88%, deaths by >74%, and direct inpatient and outpatient medical expenditures by 74%.[9,10]

The second clinical entity of VZV, herpes zoster, derives its name from the Greek words *herpein*, meaning 'to spread' or 'to creep,' and *zoster*, meaning 'girdle' or 'zone.' The lifetime risk of herpes zoster is estimated to be 10–30%.[11] The reported incidence of herpes zoster prior to vaccination ranged from 1.2 to 6.5 cases/1000 person-years, with approximately 500000 cases annually in the United States.[12] With the advent of varicella vaccination, it remains to be seen how herpes zoster incidence will be affected as the population ages. A number of studies have reported on herpes zoster incidence in the post-vaccination era in comparison to the pre-vaccination era.[12–14] The data remain inconclusive, as some studies have found a small increase in incidence of herpes zoster while others have found no change in herpes zoster in the post-vaccination era.

Increasing age represents a significant risk factor for the development of herpes zoster, and the likelihood of infection increases directly in proportion to age. The incidence in persons older than 75 years of age exceeds 10/1000 cases annually.[15] In addition, an 85-year-old individual has a 50% probability of developing herpes zoster once and a 1% chance of herpes zoster appearing twice.[15] Herpes zoster makes no distinction between gender, race, or seasonal preference.[15] Another important risk factor for the development of herpes zoster is altered cell-mediated immunity. Patients with neoplastic diseases, those taking immunosuppressive drugs, and organ transplant recipients are particularly at risk for herpes zoster. Other predisposing factors include syphilis, tuberculosis, malaria, and emotional and physical trauma. Patients who are seropositive for human immunodeficiency virus (HIV) also develop herpes zoster with a higher frequency than the normal population. A longitudinal study confirmed an incidence of 29.4/1000 cases annually in HIV-seropositive patients compared to 2.0/1000 cases annually in HIV-seronegative controls.[16] The likelihood of infection with zoster is inversely proportional to the host's immune response.

Herpes zoster in children represents an uncommon finding with potentially devastating sequelae. The incidence of herpes zoster in children is estimated at 0.2/1000 cases per year in those less than 5 years of age, but increases to 0.6/1000 cases per year at age 15 to 19 years. The incidence of childhood zoster is 122 times higher in children with a childhood malignancy.[17] Other risk factors for childhood zoster include maternal infection with varicella during pregnancy and varicella in the first year of life. Varicella vaccination can also be a risk factor for development of infection because current vaccines are made from live attenuated viruses.[18] Children who develop varicella before 1 year of age have a relative risk between 2.8 and 20.9 of developing herpes zoster in childhood.[17] In children and young adults, serum antibody directed against VZV represents a good surrogate marker for cell-mediated immunity (i.e. antibody correlates with T-cell reactivity to VZV). In elderly persons, the presence of antibody does not always indicate T-cell reactivity to VZV. Contrary to earlier information, zoster is rarely a primary marker for increased risk of subsequent cancer in either adults or children.[17,19]

Viral structure and pathogenesis

Humans are the only known natural host of VZV. VZV is a heat-labile virus, which spreads from cell to cell by direct contact. VZV is among the smallest of the viral genomes within the herpesvirus family. Its viral structure includes a core of double-stranded DNA surrounded by an icosahedral nucleocapsid, with an outer cell membrane containing glycoproteins, carbohydrates, and lipids. The outer viral envelope aids in attachment and penetration of the virus into human cells. The virus attaches to host cells by binding to heparan sulfate proteoglycans and mannose-6-phosphate receptors.[20] After attachment, the glycoproteins within the viral envelope fuse with the host cell membrane, leading to viral entry into the host cell, at which time the virus uncoats and travels to the nucleus where it initiates transcription of viral genomes.

After primary infection, VZV is transported from the varicella vesicular lesions along sensory axons or via hematogenous spread to the various dorsal roots or trigeminal ganglia and neural cell bodies. VZV can travel to ganglions at multiple levels of the neuraxis.[21] VZV then enters a state of latency in either the ganglion satellite cells or within the neurons as it incorporates into the host genome.[22] Little is known about the mechanism of how VZV establishes latency in the central nervous system or the specific pathways responsible for viral reactivation from the latency stage. However, it is known that during latency there is a continual active transcription of selected VZV genes.[6,22]

Disturbance of the symbiosis of the virus and host initiates reactivation of VZV. Once reactivated, the virus replicates within cells of the dorsal root ganglion and virions travel to the skin or mucous membrane via axonal transport. Virion transport produces associated abnormal skin sensations, pain, and tenderness followed by the characteristic unilateral dermatomal eruption of herpes zoster. The dermatomes most frequently involved in the infection are those in the lower thoracic to upper lumbar distribution, which accounts for about 50% of cases. Cranial nerve involvement occurs in 13–20% of cases, with the trigeminal nerve seen most frequently.[15] Reactivation involves an alteration of the immune system in association with age, trauma, and neural degeneration. Impairment of the host's cellular immunity plays an important role in initiating reactivation from latency. There is a direct correlation between increasing age, zoster recurrence, and a decline in cell-mediated immunity as measured by in vitro lymphocyte response to VZV antigen or skin testing.[23–25] Immunologic study of VZV latency in humans suggests that frequent dynamic reactivations of VZV occur, but the reactivations are confined by the host defenses; only when cell-mediated immunity drops below a certain critical level does the virus manifest with the clinical syndrome of herpes zoster.[26,27]

Clinical Disorders

Varicella

Clinical findings

Varicella is the clinical entity caused by primary infection from transmission of VZV through respiratory secretions or from direct contact with cutaneous lesions. The virus enters the conjunctiva or respiratory tract mucosa during primary infection. After an incubation period of 10–21 days, it replicates in the regional lymphatic tissues and disseminates via a primary viremia.[28] Clinical manifestations include prodomal symptoms of fever, malaise, myalgias, and anorexia, along with the classic pruritic vesicular exanthem. The characteristic rash initially appears as small red papules and progresses to generalized vesicular lesions. The diffuse exanthem is usually more numerous on the face and trunk with rare occurrence on mucosal surfaces.

Although varicella is generally a mild disease, it is more severe in neonates, adults, and immunosuppressed individuals. A variety of systemic and neurologic complications can contribute to increased morbidity and mortality with varicella infection (Box 80.1). Pneumonia is the most common complication of adult varicella and can range from no symptoms to a fatal illness in susceptible adults and neonates.[29] Varicella can also be a fatal disorder in infants and adults who are immunocompromised with potential involvement of the viscera, vascular system, or central nervous system. Central nervous system manifestations include cerebellar ataxia, diffuse meningoencephalitis, meningitis, myelitis,

Box 80.1 Varicella

Systemic manifestations
- Superinfection and septicemia
- Varicella pneumonia
- Myocarditis
- Glomerulonephritis
- Pancreatitis
- Hepatitis
- Vasculitis
- Athritis
- Orchitis

Neurologic manifestations
- Acute cerebellar ataxia
- Diffuse meningoencephalitis
- Meningitis
- Myelitis
- Guillain-Barré syndrome (polyneuritis)
- Reye syndrome
- Delayed cerebral vasculitis
- Optic neuritis
- Internal ophthalmoplegia
- Tonic pupil
- Cranial nerve paresis
- Facial nerve palsy

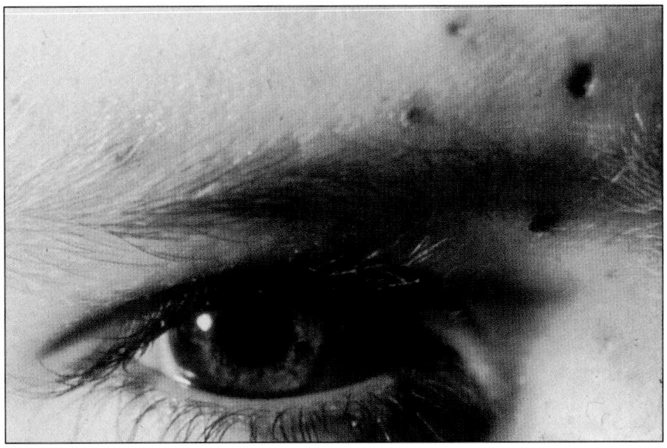

Fig. 80.1 Primary varicella. A vesicular eruption from varicella infection on the periocular skin and eyelids in this 8-year-old child. This is a common finding of primary varicella infection.

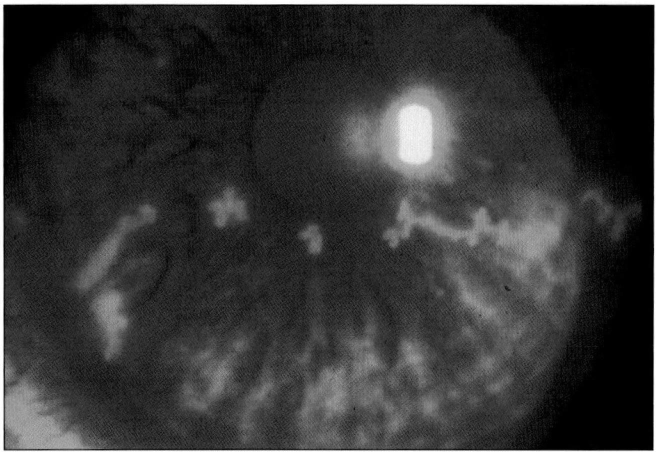

Fig. 80.2 Varicella dendritic keratitis. Numerous dendrites are seen in this slit lamp photograph with fluorescein staining of the dendritic lesions from active viral growth in the corneal epithelium.

Guillain-Barré syndrome, delayed cerebral vasculitis, and optic neuritis.[30]

Congenital varicella syndrome (CVS) is a severe consequence of VZV in neonates after transplacental infection of VZV in a newly infected pregnant female. While 5% of pregnant women in the United States are susceptible to VZV, most do not develop CVS, with the risk of transplacental infection following maternal infection at 25%. The risk of CVS in the offspring of mothers infected in the first half of pregnancy is 2–5%, while development of CVS in the latter half of pregnancy is extremely rare.[29] The most frequent findings of CVS include cutaneous scars, cardiac anomalies, skeletal anomalies, ocular anomalies, deafness, and neurological manifestations such as microcephaly and cortical atrophy.

Ophthalmic manifestations

The ocular manifestations of varicella can occur on the periocular skin, eyelids, conjunctiva, and cornea, with rare intraocular involvement. A vesicular eruption on the periocular skin and eyelids is a common finding in varicella infection (Fig. 80.1). Vesicles can cause scarring if there is secondary bacterial infection or deep dermal involvement. The vesicles (or 'pocks') can also involve the conjunctiva or cornea and may lead to scarring and vascularization. Nonspecific papillary conjunctivitis is another common finding of varicella infection. Less commonly, a punctate or dendritic keratitis from active viral growth in the corneal epithelium can occur in varicella,[31] or a delayed disciform keratitis from presumed immunologic stromal reaction (with or without uveitis) can occur (Fig. 80.2).[32] The keratitis can progress to mucous plaque or neurotrophic keratopathy. Rare ocular complications of varicella include gangrene of the eyelids, corneal melting, interstitial keratitis, chronic uveitis, cataract, extraocular muscle palsies, internal ophthalmoplegia, retinopathy, and optic neuritis. Most of these manifestations are presumably immunologic.

Ocular findings in neonates with CVS include microphthalmia, chorioretinitis, cataracts, optic nerve atrophy and hypoplasia, and Horner's syndrome.[33]

Herpes zoster ophthalmicus

Clinical findings

Herpes zoster is the clinical entity caused by reactivation of the latent VZV from sensory ganglia. Acute herpes zoster includes 1–4 days of prodromal symptoms including fever, malaise, headaches, and hypoesthesias, with pain, burning, itching, erythema, and edema in the affected dermatome. Viral release from the sensory nerve endings results in a macular rash, which becomes papular and then vesicular within 24 hours. The grouped vesicles usually involve one dermatome, but can include up to three adjacent dermatomes. New vesicles continue to develop for about 4 days and may continue for weeks in immunosuppressed patients. The vesicles become pustular and may eventually rupture or hemorrhage. Hemorrhagic necrosis of the deeper dermal tissues may occur, with a propensity for permanent pigmentation and residual scarring. Occasionally an attack will occur without the cutaneous skin eruption (zoster sine herpete).[34] Hematogenous spread of virus is possible and results in the appearance of remote grouped vesicles in a site distant from the involved dermatome. Visceral dissemination is a more severe complication of herpes zoster, with the lungs and gastrointestinal system most commonly involved.[30] After 2 to 3 weeks, the acute phase subsides and the rash crusts over and dissipates, yet the pain may persist in the dermatome affected, resulting in a condition known as postherpetic neuralgia.

While any sensory ganglia may be involved with herpes zoster, herpes zoster ophthalmicus (HZO) is used to describe reactivation from the trigeminal ganglia with ocular involvement. Hutchinson was the first to describe the signs and symptoms of herpes zoster ophthalmicus in 1865.[35] Of the three divisions of the trigeminal nerve (ophthalmic, maxillary, and mandibular), the ophthalmic division is most commonly affected in herpes zoster in 8–56% of cases (Fig. 80.3).[15,36–38] The ophthalmic division further divides into the nasociliary, frontal, and lacrimal branches, of which the frontal nerve is most commonly involved and the lacrimal

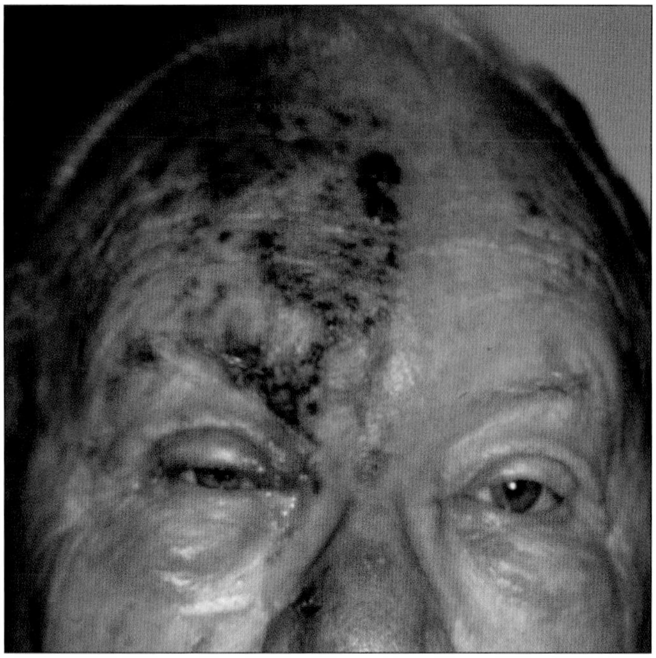

Fig. 80.3 Herpes zoster involving the ophthalmic nerve distribution of the trigeminal nerve. An elderly man with eschars of the forehead, brow, periocular, and nasal skin.

branch is least commonly involved in HZO.[39] The nasociliary nerve innervates the anterior and posterior ethmoidal sinuses, the skin of both eyelids, and the tip of the nose, conjunctiva, sclera, cornea, iris, and the choroid. Because of the extensive innervations of the nasociliary nerve, its involvement in HZO is associated with a 50–76% chance of ocular complications, which lowers to 34% in cases of HZO without nasociliary involvement.[40–42] Vesicles at the side of the tip of the nose are known as Hutchinson's sign and are indicators of potential ocular disease.

Ophthalmic manifestations

Approximately 10–20% of herpes zoster cases involve the ophthalmic nerve division, with 20–70% developing ocular findings.[43–45] The presence of Hutchinson's sign is a poor prognostic indicator because of the increased risk of ocular sequelae secondary to its extensive intraocular innervations. Ocular involvement is not correlated with age, sex, or severity of the skin rash.[43] The diffuse and multiple ocular complications of HZO are related to different mechanisms of disease, including antigenic viral components, immune reaction, vasculitis, neural involvement, and scarring. The disease may manifest with acute, chronic, or relapsing phases, depending on the mechanisms involved. Chronic disease can be present in 20–30% of HZO cases.[42–45] While the visual outcome in HZO is extremely variable, the visual prognosis in African-Americans with a high prevalence of human immunodeficiency virus (HIV) infection carries a much worse prognosis.[46]

Periocular skin and eyelids

Lid edema is usually the first sign of HZO, accompanied with pruritus, hypoesthesia, or pain. A maculopapular rash follows the initial findings and progresses to a vesicular skin eruption. VZV can be cultured from the skin vesicles for up to 5 to 7 days. Depending on the depth of dermal involvement and the presence of a secondary bacterial infection (usually *Streptococcus* species or *Staphylococcus aureus*), there can be variable sloughing of the skin with resultant cicatricial contracture or gangrene. In most patients, the vesicles heal within 2 to 3 weeks, leaving some residual pitting or pigmentation change. Other lid changes include trichiasis, ectropion, entropion, madarosis, or poliosis. A hemorrhagic vesicular eruption in the skin may be indicative of anticoagulant use, a hematologic disease, or a severe vasculitis; this eruption heralds severe dermal scarring and postherpetic neuralgia.[47] Cicatricial contraction of the eyelids may lead to chronic corneal exposure and may require plastic surgical repair to protect the integrity of the globe. Other chronic changes include excavated scars, pigment changes, lid margin notching, ptosis, and sloughing of the skin.

Conjunctiva

The conjunctival changes in HZO can include a papillary or follicular reaction, chronic hyperemia, and/or pseudomembrane formation. A vesicular eruption may occur within the conjunctiva, leading to vesicle rupture with possible hemorrhagic changes. With severe conjunctival changes, extensive conjunctival scarring and symblepharon formation may ensue. Extension of the conjunctival changes to the lacrimal puncta may result in punctal scarring, punctal occlusion, and epiphora. The conjunctival cytology consists of mononuclear cells and lymphocytes.

Episclera, sclera

Herpes zoster ophthalmicus can cause an episcleritis, anterior scleritis, or posterior scleritis. Both episclera and sclera can become affected during the acute stages of HZO or months later after the disappearance of vesicles. While episcleritis is typically found early in the course of HZO, it may persist up to and beyond 3 months in a significant number of patients.[40] Scleritis is usually diffuse anterior or nodular in nature and has a tendency to progress toward the perilimbal area, resulting in a peripheral limbal vasculitis.[48] Scleral thinning and staphyloma formation can occur as a result of chronic scleritis.[49] Posterior scleritis is less common and typically results from an infiltrative process involving the perivascular and perineural tissue.

Cornea

The cornea has multiple manifestations probably related to different mechanisms of disease. Corneal manifestations occur in about two-thirds of patients with ocular disease in acute HZO. It appears chronologically as punctate epithelial keratitis, early pseudodendrites, anterior stromal infiltrates, sclerokeratitis, keratouveitis/endotheliitis, serpiginous ulceration, neurotrophic keratopathy, and exposure keratopathy (Table 80.1).[47,50–52]

Punctate epithelial keratitis. The initial corneal manifestation is a coarse punctate epithelial keratitis with blotchy, swollen epithelial cells. They are usually peripheral, multiple, raised, small, and focal, and they stain with rose Bengal. A conjunctivitis usually accompanies the lesions. VZV has been cultured from these lesions.[53]

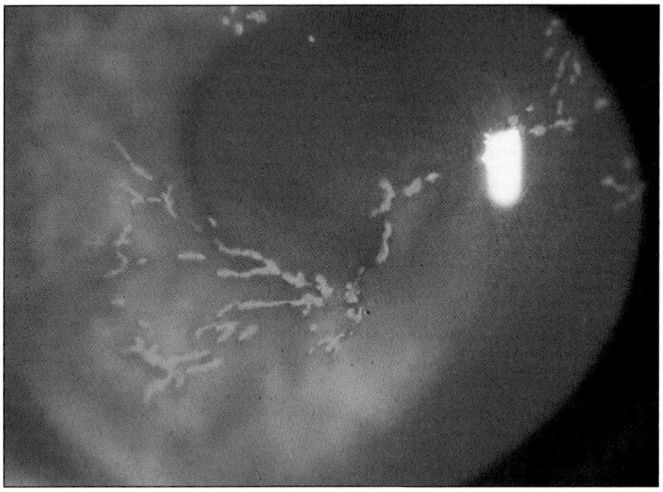

Fig. 80.4 Pseudodendrites in HZO. Numerous pseudodendrites can be seen along the cornea in an immunosuppressed individual with AIDS.

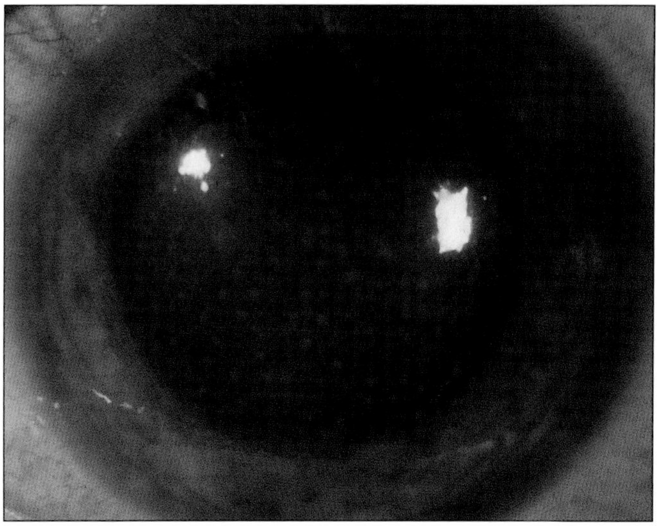

Fig. 80.5 HZ keratouveitis. This photograph depicts mild corneal edema with diffusely scattered granulomatous keratic precipitates, anterior chamber reaction, and mild injection of the episclera after onset of HZO.

Table 80.1 Corneal changes in HZO

Morphology/pathogenesis	Frequency (%)	Usual onset
Punctate epithelial keratitis	50	2 days
Pseudodendritic keratitis	50	4–6 days
Anterior stromal keratitis	40	10 days
Keratouveitis/endotheliitis	34	7 days
Serpiginous ulceration	7	1 month
Sclerokeratitis	1	1 month
Corneal mucous plaques	13	2–3 months
Disciform keratitis	10	3–4 months
Neurotrophic keratopathy	25	2 months
Exposure keratopathy	11	2–3 months
Interstitial keratitis/lipid keratopathy	15	1–2 years
Permanent corneal edema	5	1–2 years

Pseudodendrites. Multiple dendritic or stellate lesions of edematous, raised epithelial cells occur within a few days. They are typically found in the corneal periphery and probably represent a coalescence of previous punctate epithelial keratitis (Fig. 80.4). They differ from herpes simplex viral dendrites in that they are more superficial, have blunt ends, lack central ulceration, and stain minimally with fluorescein and rose Bengal. VZV has been cultured from these lesions,[51,53] and corneal cytology shows multinucleated giant cells and intranuclear inclusion bodies.[54]

Anterior stromal infiltrates. Isolated or multiple patches of a hazy, granular, dry infiltrate just under Bowman's layer occur at about 10 days. They frequently underlie the previous epithelial lesions and probably represent either stromal reaction to soluble viral antigen diffusing into the anterior stroma or direct viral cytotoxicity. These stromal infiltrations may be missed in the presence of stromal edema. The residual nummular scars are a marker of previous herpes zoster corneal inflammation.

Keratouveitis/endotheliitis. A sudden onset of Descemet's folds and subsequent stromal and epithelial edema may occur about 1 week into the disease course. The folds may be diffuse or localized and can have underlying keratic precipitates and associated uveitis (Fig. 80.5). This manifestation may represent direct viral invasion of the endothelium with an immune reaction varying from mild disciform keratitis to a severe granulomatous inflammatory reaction. A secondary glaucoma can also occur in association with the inflammation in which a hypopyon or hyphema may be found. The etiology of the glaucoma may result from extension of VZV to the trabecular meshwork or a severe ischemic vasculitis of the pars plicata.

Serpiginous ulceration. Peripheral crescentic corneal thinning with a gray-white base may occur with associated vascularization or with progression to perforation (Fig. 80.6). This thinning may be initiated by a limbal vasculitis or an immune mechanism.[53]

Sclerokeratitis. An extension of scleritis onto the cornea may occur approximately 1 month after the onset of HZO, creating a limbal vascular keratitis (Fig. 80.7). It may manifest with scleralization, vascularization, stromal thinning, or peripheral faceting of the cornea. The underlying etiology is probably a vasculitis or immune complex deposition.[47]

Corneal mucous plaques. This corneal finding typically occurs several months after HZO in a quiescent eye or in an eye with minimal smoldering keratitis. These plaques occur suddenly as elevated coarse gray-white branching lesions on

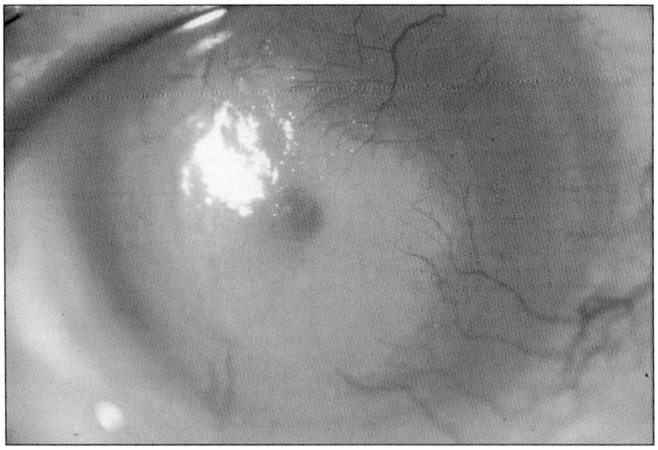

Fig. 80.6 Healed corneal melt from HZV serpiginous ulceration, 3 months after cyanoacrylate glue and therapeutic bandage lens placement with subsequent removal. The photograph demonstrates diffuse corneal scarring, vascularization, and halted ulceration and thinning after treatment.

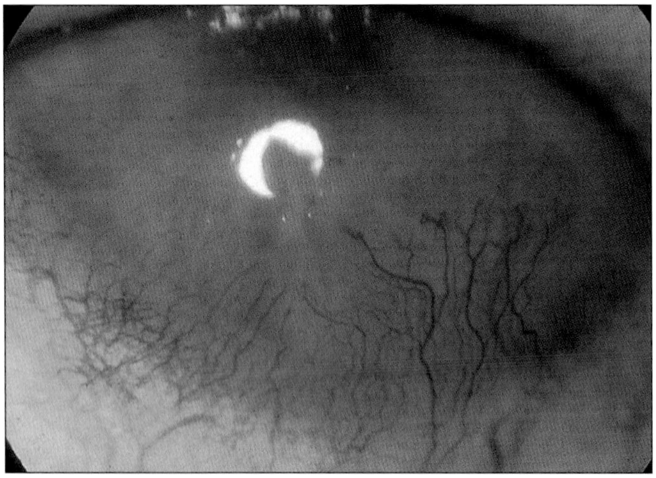

Fig. 80.7 Sclerokeratitis. A patient with sclerokeratitis 1 month out from HZO infection. Note the scleralization, vascularization, and mild thinning of the peripheral area of involved cornea.

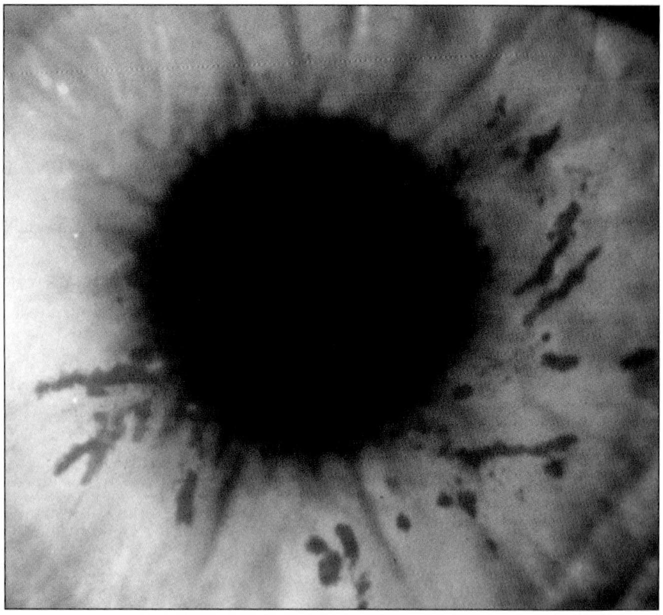

Fig. 80.8 HZ mucous plaque keratopathy. Mucous plaques on the cornea 2 months after HZO in a relatively quiescent eye. These can be wiped from the cornea but tend to be transient and variable in location.

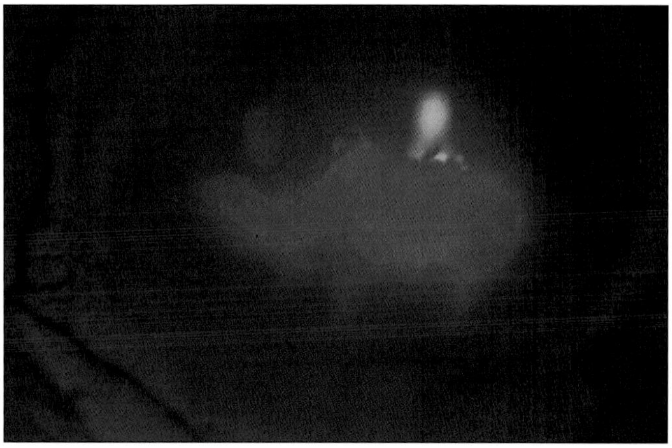

Fig. 80.9 HZ neurotrophic keratopathy. Note the neurotrophic ulceration in the inferior paracentral cornea surrounded by diffuse punctate epithelial keratopathy 7 months after HZO.

the surface of edematous epithelial cells (Fig. 80.8). They have sharp margins and lack terminal branches seen in true dendrites.[51,55] In addition, these plaques stain with rose Bengal but sparingly with fluorescein. The mucous plaques are variable in size, migratory in nature, and transitory around the cornea. The etiology of these lesions is unclear but may represent either an immune origin or mechanical causes such as neurotrophic changes or an abnormal epithelial receptor site, similar to a large filament.[47,51] Pavan-Langston and colleagues postulate a possible infectious etiology as indicated by polymerase chain reaction (PCR) detection of VZV viral DNA within the lesions and response to certain antiviral regimens.[54] The lesions were previously mistaken for superimposed herpes simplex virus. They can be removed from the surface of the cornea, leaving an abnormal but intact epithelium.

Disciform keratitis. Several weeks or months after acute HZO, a deep central or peripheral disc-shaped area of stromal edema may develop with minimal infiltrate and an intact epithelium. The cornea can show multiple areas of corneal edema in a relatively quiescent eye. The etiology of the disciform keratitis is most likely analogous to herpes simplex disciform keratitis and may represent either a VZV viral infection of the endothelium or an immune reaction to soluble antigen or viral particles in the corneal stroma.[56] Immune rings can also be associated with disciform keratitis in HZO and are most commonly seen in the central or paracentral cornea. This form of stromal inflammation is similar to the antigen-antibody complex seen in a Wessely ring.

Neurotrophic keratopathy. Neurotrophic keratopathy represents a diminution of corneal sensation with loss of epithelial integrity and subsequent epithelial breakdown. It usually occurs in the first few months of infection, but can develop

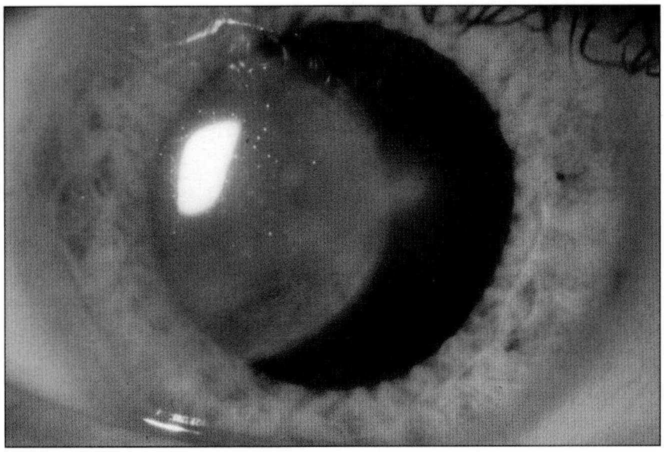

Fig. 80.10 HZ interstitial keratitis. The photograph depicts central corneal scarring with diffuse corneal haze and peripheral corneal neovascularization with early lipid deposition.

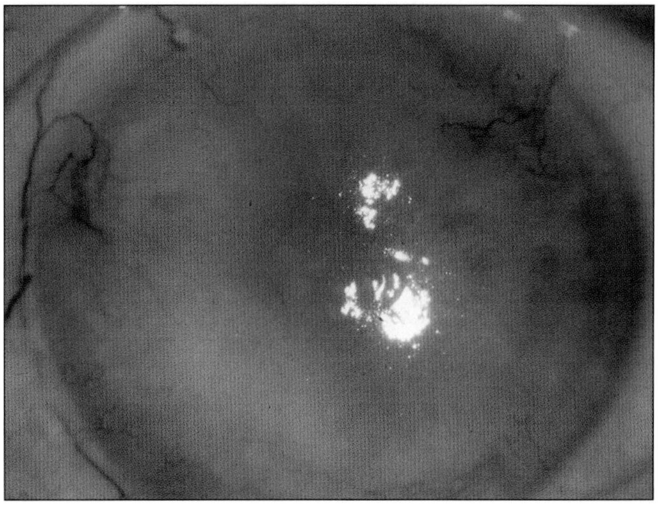

Fig. 80.11 HZ stromal scarring. Persistent stromal inflammation leading to corneal stromal vascularization with early lipid deposition towards the apex of the scarring.

months after the acute infection. While hyperesthesia of the cornea has been reported following HZO,[57] the majority of patients with corneal findings associated with HZO have depressed corneal sensation. The altered corneal sensation resolves in most patients, but some patients never regain normal sensation, while others have progressively diminished sensation. An estimated 20% of patients with HZO will have some degree of decreased corneal sensitivity after 1 year.[40,51] The initial signs of a neurotrophic cornea may be subtle: a lack of corneal luster, an irregular corneal surface, or mild coarse punctate epithelial erosions. Over time, a gray haze or edema of the epithelium develops with fine intraepithelial vesicles visualized. Horizontal, oval epithelial defects with boggy stromal ulcers finally develop in the lower aspect of the cornea (Fig. 80.9). Ominous complications such as superinfection, corneal thinning, corneal perforation, and fibrovascular scarring may ensue. The etiology of this disorder is complex and includes neurotransmitter reduction, delayed epithelial turnover, lower blink frequency, diminished corneal lubrication, meibomian gland dysfunction, and tear dysfunction.[51,58]

Exposure keratopathy. Exposure keratopathy is caused by cicatricial eyelid changes resulting from HZO. Several factors contribute to corneal desiccation in the setting of these eyelid changes including a frozen or poorly mobile upper lid from dermal contracture, associated lid thickening and irregularity, ectropion, meibomian gland dysfunction, and aberrant lashes.[51,59]

Interstitial keratitis/lipid keratopathy. The extensive corneal inflammation created by HZO results in significant corneal scarring with vascularization and lipid deposition (Fig. 80.10). This interstitial keratitis characteristically is paracentral or peripheral with a vascular leash and lipid deposits in the horizontal corneal meridian. The interstitial keratitis may progress to cause a complete corneal opacification (Fig. 80.11). Laser closure of the inciting blood vessels may be helpful in selected circumstances.[60] Persistence of the virus in a latent form or persistent reactivation of the virus may be an underlying mechanism creating this appearance, as VZV DNA has been detected years after an attack.[61]

Corneal edema. HZO can create temporary or permanent corneal edema. Permanent corneal endothelial decompensation may result even in the absence of scarring and vascularization. The probable mechanism is likely either endothelial destruction by VZV, a vasculitis, or an immune reaction.[62] Specular microscopy following HZO has shown spotty loss of endothelial cells along with bleb formation.[62,63] Anterior segment ischemia from ciliary body necrosis is another potential contributory cause.[64] Corneal perforation can accompany an associated neurotrophic keratopathy.[51,60,65] Peripheral corneal ulcers may occasionally heal spontaneously, whereas a central perforation has a grave prognosis.[46]

Uveal tract

Uveitis tends to accompany most forms of keratitis, but it is especially prevalent and difficult to manage in herpes zoster keratouveitis. Up to 40% of patients with HZO may develop anterior uveitis.[41] The inflammation can be granulomatous or nongranulomatous and is typically associated with extensive keratic precipitates, corneal edema, and posterior synechiae. Less frequently, the uveitis occurs independent of the corneal disease or may be delayed by several months. In either circumstance, there is usually intense photophobia, ciliary injection, corneal edema, hyperemia of the iris, and anterior chamber reaction. An associated anterior chamber fibrin reaction can occur with a hypopyon or a hyphema and elevated intraocular pressure. Endothelial decompensation can occur with chronic infection leading to persistent corneal edema. Zoster iritis may result from an ischemic occlusive vasculitis with ciliary body inflammation and segmental iris distortion and sectoral iris atrophy (Fig. 80.12). Hypotony, cyclitic membrane formation, and phthisis bulbi may develop. Fluorescein angiography demonstrates occlusion of iris vasculature with sectoral iris atrophy and iris pigment epithelial loss.[66] A retrospective study on uveitis in HZO found that secondary glaucoma occurred in 56% of the patient population.[67] The inflammatory glaucoma

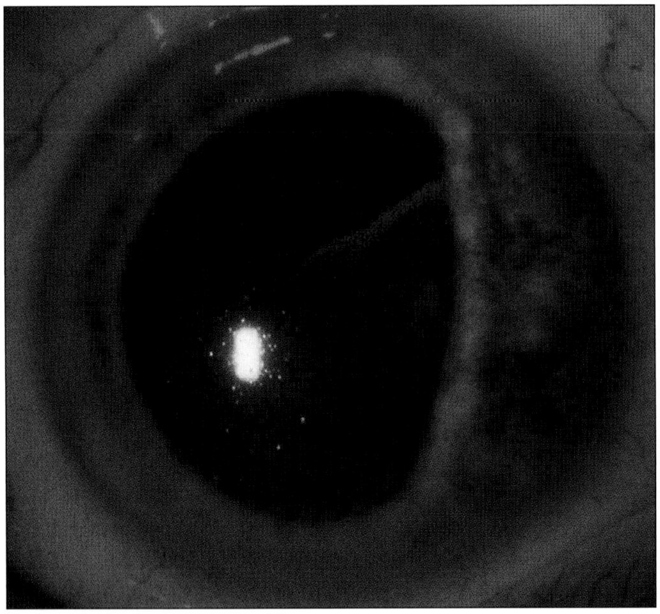

Fig. 80.12 Sectoral iris atrophy. Infection with VZV in HZO can lead to sectoral iris atrophy and segmental iris distortion from an ischemic occlusive vasculitis with ciliary body inflammation. Note the iris distortion and atrophy contributing to the inability of dilation in the involved sector upon cylcoplegia.

Box 80.2 Herpes zoster ophthalmicus

Systemic manifestations
- Cutaneous dissemination
- Visceral dissemination
  - Varicella pneumonia
  - Hepatitis

Neurologic manifestations
- Acute neuralgia
- Segmental motor weakness
- Cranial neuropathies
- Encephalitis, myelitis, and encephalomyelitis
- Guillain-Barré syndrome
- Delayed cerebral vasculitis
- Multifocal leukoencephalitis
- Postherpetic neuralgia

accompanying HZO uveitis may have several underlying mechanisms: (1) trabecular meshwork blockage by cellular debris, iris pigment, or blood; (2) peripheral anterior synechiae; (3) pupillary block glaucoma from posterior synechiae; or (4) structural changes through the trabecular meshwork. Less frequently, hypotony may result from the necrosis in the area of the pars plicata.[48] Posterior subcapsular cataract formation develops from prolonged chronic uveitis or chronic steroid administration for uveitis treatment.

Neurologic manifestations

Acute neuralgia is one of the most common debilitating findings during the initial reactivation in herpes zoster and occurs in approximately 93% of cases.[41] The pain is localized along the affected dermatome and corresponds to the severity of the rash. The acute neuralgia is described as aching, itching, or burning in association with a superimposed lancinating pain. The pain may be associated with sympathetic hyperactivity such as tachypnea, tachycardia, diaphoresis, mydriasis, and anxiety. Although the acute pain tends to remit in the majority of patients as the disease course progresses, an estimated 10–30% of patients have unremitting pain lasting months to years after the acute infection has resolved, a phenomenon known as postherpetic neuralgia (PHN).[9–11,15,45]

PHN is the most common complication of herpes zoster, occurring in 9.3–17% of patients with increased incidence and severity in the sixth to eight decades of life.[45,68] PHN is defined as pain persisting beyond 1 month after rash onset or rash resolution.[45,68–70] A correlation exists between PHN and the severity of the rash, the presence of ocular involvement, the decline in corneal sensation, and the presence of early neuralgia.[50] While PHN resolves in most patients within 1 year,[43] it is still the primary cause of intractable debilitating pain in elderly patients and is the leading cause of suicide in patients older than 70 years of age with chronic pain.[69,70] It does appear to be more severe, more widespread, and more recalcitrant as age increases in the elderly. The pain has variable manifestations from allodynia (superficial hypersensitive burning pain) to deep aching pain, to sharp intermittent lancinating pain. Some cases include the entire gamut of pain levels.

The pathogenic mechanisms of PHN are multifactorial and not completely understood. Changes in both peripheral and central nervous system (CNS) afferent pathways may contribute to the pain of PHN. Convincing evidence points to CNS disease as a potential cause in regards to peripheral C-fiber degeneration resulting in abnormal CNS processing of pain signals. Further postulation of a CNS role stems from persistent pain despite sectioning of peripheral nerves and presence of stimulus-evoked pain in large areas of skin surrounding the infected dermatome, suggesting abnormal CNS sensory processing.[70,71] Another theory relates to a preferential loss of normal descending inhibitory inputs with a subsequent hyperexcitable state of the ascending nociceptive fibers. The presence of acute pain in HZO may also contribute to PHN in that it initiates spinal cord hyperreflexia and produces axonal damage, creating ectopically discharging nociceptors. Other research suggests susceptibility genes to PHN may exist within the human histocompatibility leukocyte antigen region.[72] Regardless of whether these internal factors contribute to PHN alone or in combination, external factors such as advanced age, organ transplantation, malignancy with chemotherapy, HIV infection, and long-term corticosteroid use likely have a role in PHN as well.[73,74] A multivariate analyses of 1178 patients with herpes zoster found that a severe rash is a significant risk factor for the development of PHN; thus, patients with more severe pain and older age are more likely to develop severe rash and subsequent PHN.[75]

Additional neurological findings include cerebral infarction and acute inflammatory neurologic disorders such as aseptic meningitis, encephalitis, myelitis, cranial polyneuropathy, or acute polyneuritis (Guillain-Barré syndrome) (Box 80.2).[76,77] These disorders represent a central spread of VZV from the dorsal root ganglion and occur with increased risk in immunodeficiency and cutaneous dissemination. Abnormal mentation, fever, headache, nuchal rigidity, ataxia, and cranial palsies are clinical signs of encephalitis while ipsilateral leg weakness, sensory loss, and ultimate paraparesis and paraplegia represent findings of myelitis. Ramsay Hunt syndrome occurs when herpes zoster involves the seventh cranial nerve (geniculate ganglion). This syndrome consists of facial muscle weakness with additional loss of taste over the anterior two-thirds of the tongue, ear pain, and vesicles in the external auditory canal or pinna.[78] Additionally, an affective disorder with anorexia, lassitude, mood changes, antisocial behavior, severe depression, and insomnia may accompany herpes zoster. Neurological findings may occur in the absence of cutaneous lesions, representing a forme fruste of zoster sine herpete.[76,79]

Immunosuppression in herpes zoster

With the exception of advanced age, decreased cellular immunity remains one of the main risk factors for herpes zoster. Conditions with depressed cellular immunity include any form of cancer, especially leukemia and lymphoma, radiation, chemotherapy, organ trasnplantation, HIV infection, and systemic immunosuppression to treat autoimmune or hematologic disorders.[15,80–82] In the immunosuppressed patient, zoster causes more severe involvement within the dermatome, with an increased risk of progression to both cutaneous and visceral dissemination. Dissemination is highest in patients with lymphoproliferative malignancies (approximately 25% without antiviral therapy).[82] About 10–50% of patients with cutaneous dissemination will also develop visceral dissemination (pneumonia, meningoencephalitis, hepatitis) with a more ominous prognosis.[15,81] Even with antiviral therapy, the mortality for herpes zoster with visceral disease is 5–15%, mostly attributable to pneumonitis.[81]

The appearance of herpes zoster in HIV-seropositive individuals indicates declining immune function in this patient subset and has predicted the onset of AIDS in patients in the United States and other countries.[82–85] The development of zoster in healthy young adults should raise suspicion of HIV seropositivity as a possible underlying disorder. Kestelyn and colleagues described a series of 19 patients with an average age of 28 of whom nearly 80% were healthy, but found to be seropositive for HIV.[86] The majority of cases of zoster in HIV-seropositive patients are clinically similar to zoster in other immunosuppressed hosts except that recurrences are more frequent and cutaneous lesions can appear atypical.[87] Skin lesions associated with VZV in HIV-seropositive individuals occasionally are larger (10–20 mm), multiple, punched-out, and ulcerated with a central black eschar and a peripheral rim of vesiculation yielding a positive VZV culture. Alternatively, multiple hyperkeratotic ulcerated erythematous-based lesions with no dermatomal distribution have been described.[82]

Histopathology of VZV

Tissue damage from HZV infection occurs as a result of a combination of factors including chronic inflammation, vasculitis, and necrosis in response to direct viral invasion within host tissues. Reactivation of VZV in the ganglion causes a chronic inflammatory reaction with associated hemorrhagic necrosis in the dorsal root ganglion and the adjacent perineural tissues.[88] The associated cellular infiltrate in the acute infectious process is primarily mononuclear cells along with typical eosinophilic intranuclear inclusions found in the neurons and glial cells. The amount of inflammation correlates with the clinical picture. The virus can then spread peripherally and centrally. CNS vasculitis is attributed to viral spread directly from the trigeminal ganglion to adjacent blood vessels in the CNS. Viral particles have been demonstrated by electron microscopy in the blood vessels of patients with disseminated herpes zoster and in patients with CNS angiitis.[89] With peripheral viral spread, VZV travels down the sensory axons toward the skin, producing demyelination, cellular infiltration, and subsequent scarring with fibrosis of the peripheral nerves. A granulomatous inflammatory reaction is also seen within the peripheral nerves. Fluorescent antibody and electron microscopy studies have detected VZV and its associated antigen in neuronal and satellite cells as well as their corresponding sensory nerves before the onset of the characteristic zoster skin rash.[90]

Once VZV reaches the skin after retrograde travel from the ganglia, the host reaction results in a mononuclear and multinucleated giant cell infiltration within the subepithelial and dermal tissues. With continued VZV replication, the epithelial cells undergo degenerative changes characterized by ballooning and cell fusion, thus creating multinucleated giant cells. Eosinophilic intranuclear inclusions labeled Lipschutz bodies (Cowdry type A intranuclear inclusions) also develop within the tissues, indicating active VZV replication. These histopathologic findings can be associated with an angiitis with subsequent creation of ischemia, necrosis, and hemorrhage within the dermis. Although depressed cellular immunity is an important factor for stimulating the onset of herpes zoster, the presence and localization of antibody related to the immune response may be an important factor in causing certain sequelae (i.e. granulomatous vasculitis, ischemic optic neuropathy, orbital vasculitis).

A combination of factors results in the variety of ocular sequelae of HZO including direct viral invasion and the host inflammatory, immune, and vascular reactions. In the early stages of HZO a nongranulomatous (lymphocytes and plasma cells) infiltration is initiated within the iris, trabecular meshwork, ciliary body, retinal vasculature, and optic nerve.[64] The lymphocytic and plasma cell infiltration of the posterior ciliary artery and nerves in the retrobulbar region appears to be unique to HZO.[48] This early inflammatory reaction is reversible, but with more severe inflammation the ciliary body and choroid can develop necrosis with the onset of granulomatous infiltration of epithelioid and giant cells.[64] Late findings include chronic inflammation and vasculitis of the iris and ciliary body, granulomatous choroiditis, perivascular inflammation of retinal vessels, lymphocytic infiltration of the posterior ciliary nerves and vessels, and perineuritis and perivasculitis of the ocular muscles.

The corneal changes in HZO stem from a combination of host inflammatory responses and immune-mediated reactions secondary to viral invasion and replication. Disciform keratitis may occur as a result of lymphocyte-mediated responses to viral antigen in the stroma or to direct viral invasion of the endothelium.[56] The focal ischemic necrosis that can occur within the iris and retina may be related to immune complexes with antigen in the nerve fiber bundle and antibody in the adjacent blood vessels. Necrotizing retinitis, as seen in acute retinal necrosis, is likely a result of direct viral invasion of the retina.[91] Damage to the optic nerve may be related to a vasculitis with resultant ischemia and chronic inflammation. While viral replication has not been demonstrated in the eye, viral DNA has been found postmortem in corneal tissues and ocular neurovascular bundles.[50]

Diagnosis of herpes zoster ophthalmicus

The diagnosis of HZO is most often a clinical diagnosis based on the characteristic signs and symptoms of the infection, frequently negating the need for laboratory testing. However, zoster can mimic other diseases on occasion, such as herpes simplex virus or impetigo, necessitating laboratory testing to make a rapid diagnosis and aid in prompt management. Laboratory testing for VZV includes morphologic and immunomorphologic tests, viral isolation, serologic tests, and cellular immunity tests.[92]

Morphologic tests can identify the herpes virus, but they cannot differentiate between the specific types of herpes viruses. The simplest morphologic test for identification of herpes virus is the Tzanck smear. Several stains can be used to confirm multinucleated giant cells and the characteristic acidophilic intranuclear inclusions in material scraped from the cornea or the base of a vesicle. The giant cells are due to epithelial cell fusion that is mediated by viral glycoproteins. A variety of stains can be used to evaluate these findings, such as hematoxylin and eosin, Giemsa, Papanicolaou, Wright, and toluidine blue. In addition, light microscopy or electron microscopy can confirm a herpetic infection from a skin biopsy.

Immunologic tests, while requiring greater expertise, can help detect herpetic viral antigen or nucleic acid from vesicular fluid. Immunofluorescent and immunoenzyme stains (immunoperoxidase or enzyme-linked immunosorbent assay) are more sensitive than culture and can detect relatively few viral particles late in the disease course.[93] The polymerase chain reaction technique can also detect viral particles from skin vesicles in a timely manner with extreme sensitivity, but it is difficult to determine whether one is detecting active disease, inactive viral particles, or recrudescent disease.[94,95] The definitive technique of identification is direct isolation of VZV from a culture of vesicular fluid. Material from the base of a skin vesicle can be cultured on monolayers from a variety of cells with specific recognizable cytopathic effects. Unfortunately, the virus is very heat-labile and growth is slow.

Serologic tests can also aid in identification of VZV exposure when acute and convalescent sera are available for comparison. A number of assays can be used to measure anti-VZV antibodies for indication of prior or recurrent infection. Some of these assays include complement fixation, immune adherence hemagglutination, passive hemagglutination, radioimmunoassay, immunoblot, latex agglutination, fluorescent-antibody-to-membrane antigen test (FAMA), immunofluorescence, and enzyme-linked immunosorbent assay (ELISA).[81] The FAMA is the most reliable for VZV-specific antibodies.[81,96] A fourfold or greater rise in IgM antibody titer provides laboratory evidence of recent infection. The serologic diagnosis of reactivated herpes zoster is somewhat more complicated than identifying acute infection, because it involves an amnestic response, and exogenous reexposure, asymptomatic reactivations of latent VZV, and symptomatic herpes zoster can all induce VZV-specific IgM. Regardless, a single serum sample with a high titer of antibody against VZV suggests a recent exposure to VZV.

Another important laboratory test involves detection of cell-mediated immunity status of an individual since zoster develops only in patients with depressed VZV cell-mediated immunity. Measurements of in vitro proliferative responses of peripheral lymphocytes to VZV antigen can distinguish immune individuals from those susceptible to VZV. This test remains a cumbersome task at the present time. An additional test of the skin can confirm a defect in cell-mediated immunity, but its significance is unclear.[92]

Therapy of VZV infection

Medical treatment

Treatment of varicella is supportive and directed at treating the various symptoms of infection. Therapy includes maintenance of hydration with adequate fluid intake, nonaspirin antipyretics, cool baths, and careful hygiene to prevent secondary bacterial infection from pruritic skin lesions. High-risk children can receive benefit with the use of leukocyte interferon, vidarabine, or acyclovir.[97–99] Some cases of varicella in immunocompromised individuals require intravenous acyclovir. Oral acyclovir shortens the duration of illness by accelerating cutaneous healing and decreasing new lesion formation; however, it is unclear whether the medication cost justifies use in otherwise healthy children.[100–102] Zoster immune globulin is not effective once the disease is contracted, but it can induce passive immunity within 96 hours of exposure in susceptible individuals at risk for severe infection, such as premature infants, neonates, the immunocompromised, and adults.[103]

Treatment of the vesicular eruption in zoster with topical acyclovir shows only minimal benefit. Most dermatologists prefer open wet dressing with an antiseptic such as Burow's solution or emulsion or a dressing soaked in acetic acid, zinc sulfate, copper sulfate, or permanganate. After drying of the lesions, a topical antibiotic ointment can be applied to soften the lesions and prevent secondary bacterial infection.

Treatment of herpes zoster is aimed at accelerating healing, limiting severity and duration of pain, reducing complications, and avoiding disseminated disease. Three drugs (acyclovir, valacyclovir, and famciclovir) are currently FDA-approved for treatment of herpes zoster in the United

States. These antiviral agents are guanosine analogs and act to interfere with viral thymidine kinase and DNA polymerase, resulting in viral DNA chain termination. In particular, acyclovir has an excellent safety profile, but limitations include only modest activity against VZV in vitro and low bioavailability after oral administration.[42] Valacyclovir is a prodrug of acyclovir and produces serum acyclovir levels three to five times as high as those achieved with oral acyclovir.[87] Famciclovir is a prodrug of penciclovir and acts in a similar fashion to the above antivirals. Both valacyclovir and famciclovir were therapeutically equivalent to acyclovir in treatment of herpes zoster in immunocompetent patients in regards to the rate of cutaneous healing and pain resolution.[104] All three drugs are exceptionally well tolerated with minimal contraindications, although dose adjustments must be made in renal insufficiency. Valacyclovir and famciclovir show superior pharmacokinetics and simpler dosing regimens compared with acyclovir, but they are more expensive. Other antiherpetic medications include foscarnet, cidofovir, sorivudine, and brivudin (Table 80.2). The latter two drugs inhibit viral DNA polymerase by acting as pyrimidine nucleoside analogs, and they are more active against VZV in vitro in comparison to acyclovir.[105,106] Foscarnet and cidofovir may provide benefit in acyclovir-resistant VZV isolates because they do not act on viral thymidine kinase for their antiviral activity.[107]

Controversy exists regarding the use of oral acyclovir for localized zoster in the normal host. In some placebo-controlled trials, acyclovir at a dose of 800 mg five times daily shortened viral shedding duration, hastened the cessation of new lesion formation, accelerated the rate of healing, and reduced the severity of acute pain.[108–110] Other studies indicate that acyclovir use in HZO leads to a reduced incidence of dendritic keratopathy, episcleritis, iritis, and stromal keratitis.[43,111,112] Cobo and colleagues found a reduced incidence of pseudodendritic keratopathy, stromal keratitis, and iritis, but no effect of oral acyclovir on episcleritis, corneal hypoesthesias, neurotrophic keratitis, or PHN.[113] A large, prospective, double-blind, controlled study comparing acyclovir with placebo treatment found that late ocular inflammatory complications occurred in 29% of treated patients versus 50–71% of untreated patients.[114] Without antiviral therapy in HZO, an estimated 50% of patients develop ocular complications, some of which are potentially vision threatening.[40] In contrast, a retrospective, paired, controlled study failed to confirm a beneficial effect of acyclovir on prevention of corneal complications.[115] In addition, the cost-to-benefit ratio for treatment of individuals in developing countries indicates that acyclovir may not be cost effective.[116] Therefore, although systemic antivirals may lessen some of the complications of ocular zoster, these cases are usually less severe. There does not appear to be convincing or consistent evidence of the benefit of the systemic antivirals in preventing or treating the most severe complications of HZO, including intraocular involvement, optic nerve disease, or retinal diseases. Anecdotal reports of improvement are reported but these major eye complications still occur in many individuals given the recommended doses of systemic antivirals. Ocular VZV disease has not gone away in this era of potent antivirals. This is probably related to the multifaceted pathophysiology of VZV disease.

Intravenous acyclovir is the treatment of choice for severely immunosuppressed individuals (organ transplantation, acquired immune deficiency syndrome, leukopenia) at a dose of 15–20 mg/kg per day in adults and up to 30 mg/kg per day in patients with disseminated zoster. Treatment with intravenous acyclovir is effective at avoiding the complication of disseminated infection. Immunocompromised individuals with uncomplicated and localized herpes zoster can receive treatment with oral acyclovir, valacyclovir or famciclovir, but careful monitoring is essential for signs of disseminated disease in order to switch to intravenous acyclovir therapy.[117] Long-term oral acyclovir prophylaxis has been advocated for certain immunocompromised patients such as organ transplant recipients, as some studies have confirmed delayed VZV reactivation and lowered morbidity with treatment.[117] Immunocompetent patients with HZO should receive high-dose oral acyclovir (800 mg five times a day for 7 to 10 days) beginning within 72 hours of rash onset. Patients must be instructed that the benefits of therapy are modest and a risk of significant ocular complications and PHN still remains.

Therapy for selected complications of HZO requires individual considerations. Corneal complications relate to multiple mechanisms of disease including host inflammatory response, immune mechanisms, and a vasculitis. The early punctate epithelial keratitis and pseudodendrites are probably related to epithelial viral infection. Topical ophthalmic acyclovir (not available in the USA) and ganciclovir gel (soon to be available in the USA) may be effective in treatment. Systemic acyclovir may be beneficial but no studies have verified its effectiveness. Topical corticosteroids are beneficial in decreasing the vasculitis, inflammation, and immune

Table 80.2 Antiviral treatment of acute herpes zoster

Drug	Dose	Duration of therapy
IV acyclovir	Immunocompetent: • 3 months to 12 years (30 mg/kg/day div q8h) • >12 years (use oral or 30 mg/kg/day div q8h) Immunocompromised: • 3 months to 12 years (60 mg/kg/day div q8h) • >12 years (30 mg/kg/day div q8h)	 7–10 days 7–10 days 7–10 days 7–10 days
Oral acyclovir	Adults: 800 mg five times daily	7–10 days
Oral famciclovir	Adults: 250 mg three times daily	7 days
Oral valacyclovir	Adults: 1000 mg three times daily	7 days
Brivudin	<12 years: 15 mg/kg/day div q 8h >12 years: 125 mg four times daily	5 days; 7–10 days in severe disease

reactions in some of the corneal and uveal manifestations, such as keratouveitis, disciform keratitis, sclerokeratitis, interstitial keratitis, episcleritis, and trabeculitis. Conversely, topical corticosteroids should be used with caution because they predispose to prolonged treatment and recurrences. The addition of a nonsteroidal antiinflammatory drug is indicated (and steroid-sparing) for some inflammatory conditions such as scleritis, sclerokeratitis, and episcleritis with deeper inflammation. Many forms of inflammation (i.e. interstitial keratitis) may progress despite all treatment and lead to vascularization and lipid keratopathy. Systemic corticosteroids in conjunction with antivirals are indicated for vitritis, retinitis, optic neuritis, and acute retinal necrosis. Severe inflammatory glaucoma is treated with topical corticosteroids and antiglaucoma medications.

Therapy for neurotrophic keratopathy from HZO remains largely a surgical treatment, but some medical therapies can stabilize the ocular surface until a tarsorraphy or other surgical modality is performed. Frequent preservative-free artificial tears or liquid gels along with lubricant ointments can provide increased tear volume. Topical antibiotic ointments may also be used to prevent secondary bacterial infections. Topical ciclosporin can be a useful treatment adjunct by increasing tear volume and goblet cell density; however, its use should be carefully monitored as it is an immunosupressant with a potential for increased risk of secondary infection. A variety of compounded growth factors have shown benefit with epithelial healing in neurotrophic keratopathy when applied topically such as autologous serum, substance-P-derived peptide (FGLM), and insulin-like growth factor I.[118,119]

Systemic corticosteroids in herpes zoster

Controlled clinical trials have evaluated the role of corticosteroids in combination with acyclovir for the treatment of herpes zoster. These studies indicate that patients receiving corticosteroids and antivirals have a moderate but statistically significant acceleration in cutaneous healing rates and alleviation of acute pain compared to antivirals alone.[120,121] This combination therapy resulted in a better quality of life, decreased use of analgesics, a decrease in the time to uninterrupted sleep, and a decrease in time to resumption of normal activities of daily living.[121] Corticosteroid use did not demonstrate a beneficial effect on reduction of incidence or duration of PHN. The use of corticosteroids for herpes zoster without concomitant antiviral therapy is not recommended and can cause detrimental ophthalmologic complications. In addition, corticosteroids are contraindicated in some specific forms of keratopathy from HZO and in patients at risk for corticosteroid-induced toxicity such as diabetes mellitus or gastritis. Indications for systemic corticosteroids in the treatment of some form of HZO complications include large hemorrhagic skin bullae, progressive proptosis with ophthalmoplegia (orbital apex syndrome), optic neuritis, and cerebral angiitis.

Surgical treatment

Surgical management of herpes zoster may become necessary to control certain corneal complications of HZO including nonhealing corneal epithelial defects, corneal scarring, melting, and perforation. Punctal occlusion, whether with plugs or cautery, may provide an increase in tear volume. A partial or total conjunctival flap or amniotic membrane transplantation may facilitate coverage of nonhealing corneal epithelial defects. In less severe cases of exposure keratopathy, a reconstructive eyelid surgery or botulinum-induced ptosis may be helpful. Tarsorrhaphy remains the gold standard for treatment of a nonhealing epithelial defect, neurotrophic keratopathy, and early keratolysis. While a tarsorrhaphy can be performed with adhesive glue, tape, or Breathe Right® strips, sutures remain the most permanent and definitive method of treatment. In cases of small perforations, treatment alternatives may include glue adhesives and a bandage contact lens with a future corneal patch graft or therapeutic keratoplasty as needed. Deep anterior lamellar keratoplasty (DALK), penetrating keratoplasty (PK), and prosthokeratoplasty may be utilized in cases of severe corneal scarring with subsequent lateral tarsorrhaphy placement. Large corneal perforations require urgent therapeutic PK and tarsorrhaphy.

Although PK in HZO has demonstrated poor results in previous reports,[122–124] some studies suggest effective visual rehabilitation can be achieved in patients with corneal lesions secondary to VZV using frequent lubrication and lateral tarsorrhaphy.[125–127] Reed and colleagues retrospectively reviewed 12 patients undergoing penetrating keratoplasty for complications related to HZO. Ten of 12 grafts remained clear after an average follow-up of 3 years, with nine patients having a visual acuity of 20/80 or better.[125] Tanure and colleagues retrospectively reviewed patients undergoing penetrating keratoplasty for complications of HZO and found that 87% of grafts remained clear at an average follow-up of 50 months with 53% of grafts seeing 20/100 or better.[126] Conversely, many ophthalmologists recommend a graft be performed only for tectonic reasons in HZO complications because of the high risk of failure. When considering penetrating keratoplasty, higher success rates may be achieved by waiting as long as possible after active inflammation subsides before performing the graft.[127] While more studies are needed documenting outcomes of prosthokeratoplasty for the surgical treatment of herpes zoster keratitis, the Boston keratoprosthesis has successfully salvaged and restored vision in a high-risk herpes zoster eye in which standard keratoplasty would almost certainly have failed, restoring vision from light perception to 20/60 Snellen acuity.[128]

Therapy of neuralgia

Acute neuralgia in HZO usually responds moderately to mild analgesics. Although topical dermatologic acyclovir is generally not effective in controlling the acute pain, 40% idoxuridine in dimethyl sulfoxide has been reported to help in nonophthalmic zoster.[129] Burow's solution and cool compresses can help the dermatologic rash and alleviate pain, but drying of the lesions must be avoided to prevent cicatrization. Oral and intravenous acyclovir in controlled trials has been effective, with acute neuralgia pain relief. Systemic corticosteroids have also been reported to alleviate acute pain, and are additive to acyclovir in the initial weeks of the disease. Some anesthesiologists advocate repetitive stellate

Table 80.3 Stepwise therapy of postherpetic neuralgia

Mild analgesics	
Cimetidine	300 mg orally three times daily
Capsaicin cream	0.025–0.075% three to four times daily
Lidocaine/prilocaine	three times/day
Lidocaine patch	5% patch; up to three patches at a maximum of 12 hours
Tricyclic antidepressants	10–25 mg orally qhs initially; total dose (75–100 mg daily as tolerated)
Gabapentin	300 mg orally daily; increase to 600 mg 2–6 times a day (3600 mg daily; maximum dose)
Pregabalin	300 mg orally daily (600 mg daily; maximum dose)
Hydroxyzine	25 mg three times daily (postherpetic itch)
Opioids	oxycodone (5 mg orally every 6 hours)
Stellate ganglion block	Daily
Physiotherapy Transcutaneous electric nerve stimulation Shortwave diathermy Ultrasound	

ganglion blocks of the sympathetic nervous system, although no large controlled studies document benefit.[130,131]

PHN is best prevented by prophylactic vaccination with the herpes zoster vaccine. For those with herpes zoster, oral valacyclovir or famciclovir within 72 hours of rash onset, showed statistical superiority over acyclovir in reducing the incidence, severity, and duration of PHN.[132,133] For persistent cases, management in conjunction with a pain expert is recommended. A variety of pharmacologic therapies exist for those who are not helped by mild analgesia (Table 80.3). Systemic cimetidine may alter endomorphins, modulate pain receptors in the brain, or cause blockade of H_2-receptors in the peripheral and CNS as well as T lymphocytes.[134,135] Topical therapeutic agents include aspirin dissolved in chloroform, lidocaine/prilocaine cream, lidocaine 5% ointment or patch, and capsaicin cream 0.025%. Capsaicin is an extract of hot chili peppers that depletes the pain neurotransmitter, substance P, while lidocaine blocks sodium channels to prevent conduction of nerve impulses.[136–140] Tricyclic antidepressants (TCAs) have shown effectiveness in treating PHN by blocking reuptake of serotonin and norepinephrine, leading to inhibition of conscious pain perception and blockage of chronic neuropathic pain. Amitriptyline in particular was highly effective in two placebo-controlled trials and it was effective in counteracting the depression that frequently accompanies herpes zoster.[45,141,142] Because little difference in pain control efficacy exists among various TCAs, drug selection may depend on side effects, as tertiary amines such as amitriptyline, imipramine, and doxepin have more anticholinergic, cardiac, and CNS effects compared to demethylated secondary amines nortriptyline and desipramine. Anticonvulsants have also traditionally been used to manage chronic neuropathic pain. Randomized, double-blind, placebo-controlled trials have shown effectiveness of gabapentin and pregabalin in PHN with equal effectiveness in management of neuropathic pain compared to TCAs.[143–146] Opioid drugs such as morphine, oxycodone, and methadone can also provide analgesic benefit in PHN alone or in combination with other drug classes listed.[45] Various forms of physiotherapy with transcutaneous electric nerve stimulators, diathermy, or ultrasound have been effective in anecdotal reports as have repetitive stellate ganglion blocks.[147–149] Intrathecal injection of methylprednisolone acetate once weekly for 4 weeks resulted in significant pain relief of intractable PHN in one study.[150] Despite all the different therapies, patients should understand that not all patients benefit from treatment of PHN.[151]

Varicella and herpes zoster vaccination

A live attenuated vaccine for varicella was approved by the US FDA and incorporated into the recommended immunization schedule for children starting in 1995.[152,153] The vaccine, known as the Oka/Merck VZV vaccine (Varivax, Merck & Co., NJ, US), was recommended for any infants, children, adolescents, and adults in the United States without previous chickenpox and without concurrent pregnancy. A mass vaccination program was begun for children aged 12–18 months in the USA beginning in 1996. The vaccine has prevented disease in 80–85% receiving one dose with >95% effectiveness at preventing severe varicella since its introduction. While the decline in disease was greatest among preschool children, every age group including infants and adults showed a significant decline.[17] A decade of the vaccination program has shown disease incidence reduced by 57–90%, accompanied by hospitalizations reduced by 75–88%, and deaths from severe varicella reduced by >74%, yet a plateau in disease reduction was achieved between 2003 and 2006.[9,10,17] While a reported 2–3% of healthy childhood vaccinees and 30–40% of adult vaccinees develop breakthrough infection, this form of varicella is much less severe than primary varicella.[17] In fact, outbreaks of varicella in highly vaccinated school populations have developed, albeit small in number and less than in the prevaccine era. These breakthrough infections led the Advisory Committee on Immunization Practices to recommend a two-dose childhood varicella vaccination program beginning in 2006, with the second vaccination given at 4–6 years of age. A second booster dose has been recommended for children who received only one dose under the previous recommendations. The second dose is felt to reduce varicella disease an additional 79%.[10]

Although the varicella vaccine has created a decline in varicella disease, controversy still surrounds the continued use of the vaccine. The main concerns regarding infant varicella vaccination include the continued costs of vaccination, given the new two-dose vaccination program, the long-term efficacy of vaccination, whether the vaccine could lead to an increase in adult disease, and whether it could lead to an increase in the incidence of herpes zoster.[154] Brisson et al[155] have modeled changes in herpes zoster epidemiology and predict that the more effective vaccination is at preventing varicella, the larger the increase in zoster incidence. They predict an increase in the incidence of zoster over the next 5 to 40 years, but state that the increase will exist temporarily because the risk of reactivation of the vaccine virus is much lower than the risk of the wild virus. Eventually the vaccine virus will replace all wild-type virus and the risk of herpes zoster will decline progressively.[156] Studies comparing herpes zoster incidence before and after the vaccination program remain inconclusive thus far.[157] A double-blind, placebo-controlled vaccine trial is currently underway to assess whether varicella immunization of children affects the incidence of herpes zoster later in life. While several questions regarding the vaccine remain unanswered, reports since its administration in 1995 seem very encouraging for a potential to eradicate VZV.

In 2006, the US FDA approved the use of a high-potency live attentuated Oka/Merck VZV vaccine (Zostavax, Merck & Co., NJ, USA) for the prevention of herpes zoster in immunocompetent individuals 60 years of age and older. A randomized, double-blind, placebo-controlled, multicenter trial, The Shingles Prevention Study, found that the vaccine reduced the overall incidence of herpes zoster by 51%, the burden of illness by 61%, and the incidence of PHN by 66%.[158] Vaccine implementation remains in its infancy; however, it is felt that 250 000 cases of herpes zoster in the USA will be prevented each year by the vaccine.[159] The zoster vaccine has not been demonstrated in clinical studies to prevent repeated episodes of herpes zoster in patients with prior disease and studies are underway to assess whether the vaccine can be used in immunocompromised individuals. In addition, the duration of the vaccine's protective effect and whether a booster vaccination will be necessary to maintain its efficacy have not been determined.

References

1. Corey L. Herpesviruses. In: Sherris JC, ed. *Medical microbiology.* New York: Elsevier; 1984:411–426.
2. Steiner P. Zur inoculation der varicellen. *Wein Med Wochenschr.* 1875;25:306.
3. Von Bokay J. Das auftreten der schafblattern unter besonderen umstanden. *Unger Arch Med.* 1892;1:159.
4. Weller TH, Stoddard MB. Intranuclear inclusion bodies in cultures of human tissue inoculated with varicella vesicle fluid. *J Immunol.* 1952;68:311–319.
5. Straus SE, Reinhold, Smith HA, et al. Endonuclease analysis of viral DNA from varicella and subsequent zoster infections in the same patient. *N Engl J Med.* 1984;311:1362–1364.
6. Straus SE. Overview: the biology of varicella-zoster virus infection. *Ann Neurol.* 1994;35:S4–S8.
7. Nguyen HQ, Jumaan AO, Seward JF. Decline in mortality due to varicella after implementation of varicella vaccination in the United States. *N Engl J Med.* 2005;352:450–458.
8. Marin M, Guris D, Chaves SS, et al. Prevention of varicella. Recommendations of the Advisory Committee on Immunization Practices (ACIP). *MMWR Recomm Rep.* 2007;56:1–40.
9. Zhou F, Harpaz R, Jumaan AO, et al. Impact of varicella vaccination on health care utilization. *JAMA.* 2005;294:797–802.
10. Marin M, Meissner HC, Seward JF. Varicella prevention in the United States: a review of successes and challenges. *Pediatrics.* 2008;122: 744–751.
11. Liesegang TJ. The varicella-zoster virus disease. *Contemp Ophthalmol.* 2006;5:1–7.
12. Jumaan AO, Yu O, Jackson LA, et al. Incidence of herpes zoster, before and after varicella-vaccination-associated decreased in the incidence of varicella, 1992–2002. *J Infect Dis.* 2005;191:2000–2007.
13. Yih WK, Brooks DR, Lett SM, et al. The incidence of varicella and herpes zoster in Massachusetts as measured by the Behavioral Risk Factor Surveillance System (BRFSS) during a period of increasing varicella vaccine coverage, 1998–2003. *BMC Public Health.* 2005;5:68.
14. Mullooly JP, Riedlinger K, Chun C, et al. Incidence of herpes zoster, 1997–2002. *Epidemiol Infect.* 2005;133:245–253.
15. Liesegang TJ. Herpes zoster ophthalmicus. natural history, risk factors, clinical presentation, and morbidity. *Ophthalmology.* 2008;115:S3–S12.
16. Buchbinder SP, Katz MH, Hessol NA, et al. Herpes zoster and human immunodeficiency virus infection. *J Infect Dis.* 1992;166:1153–1156.
17. Guess HA, Broughton DD, Melton LJ 3rd, Kurland LT. Epidemiology of herpes zoster in children and adolescents. a population-based study. *Pediatrics.* 1985;76:512–517.
18. Breuer J. Live attenuated vaccine for the prevention of varicella-zoster virus infection. Does it work, is it safe and do we really need it in the UK? *J Med Microbiol.* 2003;52:1–3.
19. Ragozzino MW, Melton LJ 3rd, Kurland LT, et al. Risk of cancer after herpes zoster. A population-based study. *N Engl J Med.* 1982;307: 393–397.
20. Zhu Z, Gershon MD, Ambron R, et al. Infection of cells by varicella zoster virus. inhibition of viral entry by mannose 6-phosphate and heparin. *Proc Natl Acad Sci USA.* 1995;92:3546–3550.
21. Mahalingam R, Wellish M, Wolf W, et al. Latent varicella zoster viral DNA in human trigeminal and thoracic ganglia. *N Engl J Med.* 1990;323:627–631.
22. Gilden DH, Mahalingam R, Dueland AN, Cohrs R. Herpes zoster: pathogenesis and latency. *Prog Med Virol.* 1992;39:19–75.
23. Cooper M. The epidemiology of herpes zoster. *Eye.* 1987;1:413–421.
24. Miller AE. Selective decline in cellular immune response to varicella-zoster in the elderly. *Neurology.* 1980;30:582–5871.
25. Burke BL, Steele RW, Beard OW, et al. Immune responses to varicella-zoster in the aged. *Arch Intern Med.* 1982;142:291–293.
26. Weigle KA, Grose C. Molecular dissection of the humoral immune response to individual VZV proteins during chickenpox, quiescence, reinfection and reactivation. *J Infect Dis.* 1984;149:741–749.
27. Ljungman P, Lonnqvist B, Gahrton G, et al. Clinical and subclinical reactivations of varicella-zoster virus in immunocompromised patients. *J Infect Dis.* 1986;153:840–847.
28. Cherry JD. Chickenpox transmission. *JAMA.* 1983;250:2060.
29. Wiesenfeld HC, Sweet RL. Perinatal infections. In: Scott JR, Disaia PJ, Hammond CB, Spellacy WN, eds. *Danforth's obstetrics and gyncecology.* 7th ed. Philadelphia: JB Lippincott; 1994:480–481.
30. Rockley PF, Tyring SK. Pathophysiology and clinical manifestations of varicella zoster virus infections. *Int J Dermatol.* 1994;33:227–232.
31. Nesburn AB, Borit A, Pentelei-Molnar J, Lazaro R. Varicella dendritic keratitis. *Invest Ophthalmol.* 1974;13:764–770.
32. Wilhelmus KR, Hamill MB, Jones DB. Varicella disciform stromal keratitis. *Am J Ophthalmol.* 1991;111:575–580.
33. Lambert SR, Taylor D, Kriss A, et al. Ocular manifestations of the congenital varicella syndrome. *Arch Ophthalmol.* 1989;107:52–56.
34. Lewis GW. Zoster sine herpete. *Br Med J.* 1958;2:418–421.
35. Hutchinson J. A clinical report on herpes zoster frontalis ophthalmicus (shingles affecting the forehead and nose). *R London Ophthalmol Hosp Rep.* 1865;5:191.
36. Hope-Simpson RE. The nature of herpes zoster. a long-term study and a new hypothesis. *Proc R Soc Med.* 1965;58:9–20.
37. Scott TFM. Epidemiology of herpetic infections. *Am J Ophthalmol.* 1957;43:134–147.
38. Weller TH. Varicella and herpes zoster, changing concepts of natural history, control and importance of a not-so-benign virus, Part II. *N Engl J Med.* 1983;309:1434–1440.
39. Edgerton AE. Herpes zoster ophthalmicus. Report of cases and review of literature. *Arch Ophthalmol.* 1945;34:40–62, 114–153.
40. Cobo M, Foulks GN, Liesegang T, et al. Observations on the natural history of herpes zoster ophthalmicus. *Curr Eye Res.* 1987;6:195–199.
41. Womack LW, Liesegang TJ. Complications of herpes zoster ophthalmicus. *Arch Ophthalmol.* 1983;101:42–45.
42. Harding SP, Lipton JR, Wells JCD. Management of ophthalmic zoster. *J Med Virol.* 1993;1:S97–101.
43. Harding SP, Lipton JR, Wells JCD. Natural history of herpes zoster ophthalmicus. predictors of postherpetic neuralgia and ocular involvement. *Br J Ophthalmol.* 1987;1:353–358.
44. Liesegang TJ. Herpes zoster virus infection. *Curr Opin Ophthalmol.* 2004;15:531–536.
45. Pavan-Langston D. Herpes zoster. antivirals and pain management. *Ophthalmology.* 2008;115:S13–S20.

46. Lewallen S. Herpes zoster ophthalmicus in Malawi. *Ophthalmology.* 1994;101:1801–1804.
47. Marsh RJ. Herpes zoster keratitis. *Trans Ophthalmol Soc UK.* 1973;93: 181–192.
48. Naumann G, Gass JDM, Font RL. Histopathology of herpes zoster ophthalmicus. *Am J Ophthalmol.* 1968;65:533–541.
49. Penman GG. Scleritis as a sequel of herpes ophthalmicus. *Br J Ophthalmol.* 1931;15:585–588.
50. Marsh RJ, Cooper M. Ophthalmic herpes zoster. *Eye.* 1993;7:350–370.
51. Liesegang TJ. Corneal complications from herpes zoster ophthalmicus. *Ophthalmology.* 1985;92:316–324.
52. Cobo LM. Corneal complications of herpes zoster ophthalmicus. *Cornea.* 1988;7:50–56.
53. Pavan-Langston D, McCulley JP. Herpes zoster dendritic keratitis. *Arch Ophthalmol.* 1973;89:25–29.
54. Pavan-Langston D, Yamamoto S, Dunkel EC. Delayed herpes zoster pseudodendrites. *Arch Ophthalmol.* 1995;113:1381–1835.
55. Marsh RJ, Cooper M. Ophthalmic zoster: mucous plaque keratitis. *Br J Ophthalmol.* 1987;71:725–728.
56. Yu DD, Lemp MA, Mathers WD, et al. Detection of varicella-zoster virus DNA in disciform keratitis using polymerase chain reaction. *Arch Ophthalmol.* 1993;111:167–168.
57. Tullo AB, et al. Corneal hyperesthesia after herpes zoster ophthalmicus. *Cornea.* 1983;2:115–117.
58. Mackie IA. Role of the corneal nerves in destructive disease of the cornea. *Trans Ophthamlol Soc UK.* 1978;98:343–347.
59. Waring GO, Ekins MB. Corneal perforation in herpes zoster ophthalmicus caused by eyelid scarring with exposure keratitis. In: Sundmacher R, ed. *Herpetische augenkrankungen; Herpetic Eye Diseases.* Munchen: JF Bergmann; 1981.
60. Marsh RJ. Argon laser treatment of lipid keratopathy. *Br J Ophthalmol.* 1988;72:900–904.
61. Wenkel H, Rummelt C, Rummelt V, et al. Detection of varicella zoster virus DNA and viral antigen in human cornea after herpes zoster ophthalmicus. *Cornea.* 1993;12:131–137.
62. Reijo A, Anti V, Jukka M. Endothelial cell loss in herpes zoster keratouveitis. *Br J Ophthalmol.* 1983;67:751–754.
63. Sundmacher R, Miller O. The corneal endothelium in ophthalmic zoster. *Klin Monatsbl Augenheilkd.* 1982;180:271–274.
64. Hedges TR III, Albert DM. The progression of the ocular abnormalities of herpes zoster: histopathologic observations of nine cases. *Ophthalmology.* 1982;89:165–177.
65. Mondino BJ, Brown SI, Mondzelewski JP. Peripheral corneal ulcers with herpes zoster ophthalmicus. *Am J Ophthalmol.* 1978;86:611–614.
66. Marsh RJ, Easty DL, Jone BR. Iritis and iris atrophy in herpes zoster ophthalmicus. *Am J Ophthalmol.* 1974;78:255–261.
67. Thean JH, Hall AJ, Stawell RJ. Uveitis in herpes zoster ophthalmicus. *Clin Exp Ophthalmol.* 2001;29:406–410.
68. [illegible] JH. Prognostic factors of postherpetic neuralgia. *J Korean Med Sci.* 2002;17:655–659.
69. Hess TM, Lutz LJ, Nauss LA, Lamer TJ. Treatment of acute herpetic neuralgia: a case report and review of the literature. *Minn Med.* 1990;73:37–40.
70. Rowbotham MC, Fields HL. Post-herpetic neuralgia: the relation of pain complaint, sensory disturbance, and skin temperature. *Pain.* 1989; 39:129–144.
71. Watson CPN, Deck JH. The neuropathology of herpes zoster with particular reference to postherpetic neuralgia and its pathogenesis. In: Watson CPN, ed. *Herpes zoster and postherpetic neuralgia: pain research and clinical management*, vol. 8. Amsterdam: Elsevier; 1993: 139–157.
72. Sato M, Ohashi J, Tsuchiya N, et al. Association of HLA-A 3303-B-4403-DRB1-1302 haplotype, but not of TNFA promoter and NKp30 polymorphism, with PHN in the Japanese population. *Genes Immun.* 2002;3:477–481.
73. Choo PW, Galil K, Donahue JG, et al. Risk factors for postherpetic neuralgia. *Arch Intern Med.* 1997;157:1217–1224.
74. Meister W, Neiss A, Gross G, et al. A prognostic score for postherpetic neuralgia in ambulatory patients. *Infection.* 1998;26:359–363.
75. Nagasako EM, Johnson RW, Griffin DRJ, et al. Rash severity in herpes zoster: correlates and relationship to postherpetic neuralgia. *J Am Acad Dermatol.* 2002;46:834–839.
76. Hirschmann JV. Herpes zoster. *Semin Neurol.* 1992;12:322–328.
77. Elliott KJ. Other neurological complications of herpes zoster and their management. *Ann Neurol.* 1994;35:S57–S61.
78. Devriese PP, Moesker WH. The natural history of facial paralysis in herpes zoster. *Clin Otolaryngol.* 1988;13:289–298.
79. Mayo DR, Boos J. Varicella zoster-associated neurologic disease without skin lesions. *Arch Neurol.* 1989;46:313–315.
80. Hirsch M. Herpes group in the immunocompromised host. In: Rubin R, Young L, eds. *Clinical approach to infection in the compromised host.* New York: Plenum; 1988:347–365.
81. Liesegang TJ. Varicella-zoster virus eye disease. *Cornea.* 1999;18: 511–531.
82. Weksler ME. Immune senescence. *Ann Neurol.* 1994;35:S35–S37.
83. Panda S, Sarkar S, Mandal BK, et al. Epidemic of herpes zoster following HIV epidemic in Manipur. *India J Infect.* 1994;28:167–173.
84. van Griesven GJ. Risk factor for progression of human immunodeficiency virus (HIV) infection among seroconverted and seropositive homosexual men. *Am J Epidemiol.* 1990;132:203–210.
85. van de Perre P, Bakkers E, Batungwanayo J. Herpes zoster in African patients: an early manifestation of HIV infection. *Scand J Infect Dis.* 1988;20:277–282.
86. Kestelyn P, Stevens AM, Bakkers E, et al. Severe herpes zoster ophthalmicus in young African adults: a marker for HTLV-III seropositivity. *Br J Ophthalmol.* 1987;71:806–809.
87. Gnann JW, Whitley RJ. Herpes zoster. *N Engl J Med.* 2002;347: 340–346.
88. Ghatak NR, Zimmerman HM. Spinal ganglion in herpes zoster. *Arch Pathol.* 1973;95:411–415.
89. Karbassi M, Raizman MB, Schuman JS. Herpes zoster ophthalmicus. *Surv Ophthalmol.* 1992;36:395–410.
90. Esiri MM, Tomlinson AH. Herpes zoster. Demonstration of virus in trigeminal nerve and ganglion by immunofluorescence and electron microscopy. *J Neurol Sci.* 1972;15:35–38.
91. Schwartz JN, Cashwell F, Hawkins HK. Necrotizing retinopathy with herpes zoster ophthalmicus: a light and electron microscopical study. *Arch Pathol Lab Med.* 1976;100:386–391.
92. Liesegang TJ. Diagnosis and therapy of herpes zoster ophthalmicus. *Ophthalmology.* 1991;98:1216–1229.
93. Dahl H, Marcoccia J, Linde A. Antigen detection: the method of choice in comparison with virus isolation and serology for laboratory diagnosis of herpes zoster in human immunodeficiency virus-infected patients. *J Clin Microbiol.* 1997;35:347–349.
94. Dlugosch D, Eis-Hubinger AM, Kleim JP, et al. Diagnosis of acute and latent varicella-zoster virus infections using the polymerase chain reaction. *J Med Virol.* 1991;35:136–141.
95. Nahass GT, Goldstein BA, Zhu WY, et al. Comparison of Tzanck smear, viral culture, and DNA diagnostic methods in detection of herpes simplex and varicella-zoster infection. *JAMA.* 1992;268:2541–2544.
96. Cohen PR. Tests for detecting herpes simplex virus and varicella-zoster virus infections. *Dermatol Clin.* 1994;12:51–68.
97. Arvin AM, Kushner JH, Feldman S, et al. Human leukocyte interferon for treatment of varicella in children with cancer. *N Engl J Med.* 1982;306:761–765.
98. Whitley RJ, Soong SJ, Dolin R, et al. Early vidarabine therapy to control the complications of herpes zoster in immunosuppressed patients. *N Engl J Med.* 1982;307:971–975.
99. Prober CG, Kirk LE, Keeney RE. Acyclovir therapy of chickenpox in immunosuppressed children – a collaborative study. *J Pediatr.* 1982;101:622–625.
100. Balfour HH Jr, Kelly JM, Suarez CS, et al. Acyclovir treatment of varicella in otherwise healthy children. *J Pediatr.* 1990;116:633–639.
101. Balfour HH. Clinical aspects of chickenpox and herpes zoster. *J Int Med Res.* 1994;22S:3A–12A.
102. Rothe MJ, Feder HM, Grant-Kels JM. Oral acyclovir therapy for varicella and zoster infections in pediatric and pregnant patients: a brief review. *Pediatr Dermatol.* 1991;8:236–242.
103. Prince A. Infectious diseases. In Behrman RE, Kliegman, RM, eds. *Essentials of pediatrics.* 2nd ed. Philadelphia: WB Saunders; 1994:297–394.
104. Tyring SK, Beutner KR, Tucker BA, et al. Antiviral therapy for herpes zoster: randomized, controlled clinical trial of valacyclovir and famciclovir therapy in immunocompetent patients 50 years and older. *Arch Fam Med.* 2000;9:863–869.
105. Snoeck R, Andrei G, De Clercq E. Chemotherapy of varicella zoster virus infections. *Int J Antimicrob Agents.* 1994;4:211–226.
106. Wutzler P. Antiviral therapy of herpes simplex and varicella-zoster virus infections. *Intervirology.* 1997;40:343–356.
107. Smith KJ, Kahlter DC, Davis C, et al. Acyclovir-resistant zoster responsiveness to foscarnet. *Arch Dermatol.* 1991;127:1069–1071.
108. Huff JC, Bean B, Balfour HH, et al. Therapy of herpes zoster with oral acyclovir. *Am J Med.* 1988;85:S84–S88.
109. Morton P, Thomson AN. Oral acyclovir in the treatment of herpes zoster in general practice. *N Z Med J.* 1989;102:93–95.

110. McKendrick MW, McGill JI, White JE, Wood MJ. Oral acyclovir in acute herpes zoster. *Br Med J*. 1986;293:1529–1532.
111. Herbort CP, Buechi ER, Piguet B, et al. High-dose oral acyclovir in acute herpes zoster ophthalmicus: the end of the corticosteroid era. *Curr Eye Res*. 1991;10:171–175.
112. Harding SP, Porter SM. Oral acyclovir in herpes zoster ophthalmicus. *Curr Eye Res*. 1991;10:177–182.
113. Cobo LM, Foulks GN, Liesegang T, et al. Oral acyclovir in the therapy of acute herpes zoster ophthalmicus. An interim report. *Ophthalmology*. 1985;92:1574–1583.
114. Hoang-Xuan T, Buchi ER, Herbort CP, et al. Oral acyclovir for herpes zoster ophthalmicus. *Ophthalmology*. 1992;99:1062–1071.
115. Aylward GW, Claoue CM, Marsh RJ, Yasseem N. Influence of oral acyclovir on ocular compilations of herpes zoster ophthalmicus. *Eye*. 1994;8:70–74.
116. Kubeyinje EP. Cost-benefit of oral acyclovir in the treatment of herpes zoster. *Int J Dermatol*. 1997;36:457–459.
117. Nikkels AF, Pierard GE. Oral antivirals revisited in the treatment of herpes zoster. *Am J Clin Dermatol*. 2002;3:591–598.
118. Chikama T, Fukuda K, Morishige N, Nishida T. Treatment of neurotrophic keratopathy with substance-P-derived peptide (FGLM) and insulin-like growth factor I. *Lancet*. 1998;351:1783–1784.
119. Matsumoto Y, Dogru M, Goto E, et al. Autolgous serum application in the treatment of neurotrophic keratopathy. *Ophthalmology*. 2004;111:1115–1120.
120. Wood MJ, Johnson RW, McKendrick MW, et al. A randomized trial of acyclovir for 7 days and 21 days with and without prednisolone for treatment of acute herpes zoster. *N Engl J Med*. 1994;330:896–900.
121. Whitley RJ, Weiss H, Gnann JW, et al. Acyclovir with and without prednisone for the treatment of herpes zoster: a randomized, placebo-controlled trial. *Ann Intern Med*. 1996;125:376–383.
122. Pavan-Langston D. Viral diseases. Herpetic diseases. In: Smolin G, Thoft RA, eds. *The cornea. Scientific foundations and clinical practice*. Boston: Litlle, Brown; 1987:261.
123. Raber I, Laibson P. Herpes zoster ophthalmicus. In: Leibowitz HM, ed. *Corneal disorders. Clinical diagnosis and management*. Philadelphia: WB Saunders; 1984:418.
124. Marsh RJ. Herpes zoster. In: Fraundfelder FT, Roy RH, eds. *Current ocular therapy 2*. Philadelphia: WB Saunders; 1985:54.
125. Reed JW, Joyner SJ, Knauer WJ III. Penetrating keratoplasty for herpes zoster keratopathy. *Am J Ophthalmol* . 1989;107:257–261.
126. Tanure MAG, Cohen EJ, Grewal S, et al. Penetrating keratoplasty for varicella-zoster virus keratopathy. *Cornea*. 2000;19:135–139.
127. Soong HK, Schwartz AE, Meyer RF, Sugar A. Penetrating keratoplasty for corneal scarring due to herpes zoster ophthalmicus. *Br J Ophthalmol*. 1989;73:19–21.
128. Pavan-Langston D, Dohman CH. Boston keratoprosthesis treatment of herpes zoster neutrophic keratopathy. *Ophthalmology*. 2008;115:S21–S23.
129. Aliaga A, Armijo M, Camacho F, et al. A topical solution of 40% idoxuridine in dimethyl sulfoxide compared to oral acyclovir in the treatment of herpes zoster. A double-blind multicenter clinical trial. *Med Clin (Barc)*. 1992;92:245–249.
130. Colding A. The effect of sympathetic blocks on herpes zoster. *Acta Anaesthesiol Scand*. 1964;13:133–141.
131. Harding SP, Lipton JR, Wells JC, Campbell JA. Relief of acute pain in herpes zoster ophthalmicus by stellate ganglion block. *Br Med J*. 1986;292:1428.
132. McKendrick MW, McGill JI, Wood MJ. Lack of effect of acyclovir on postherpetic neuralgia. *Br Med J*. 1989;298:431.
133. Vander SM, Carrasco D, Lee P, Tyring SK. Reduction of postherpetic neuralgia in herpes zoster. *J Cutan Med Surg*. 2001;5:409–416.
134. Magligit GM, Talpaz M. Cimetidine for herpes zoster. *N Engl J Med*. 1984;310:318–319.
135. Levy DW, Banerjee AK, Glenny HP. Cimetidine in treatment of herpes zoster. *J Roy Coll Physicians Lond*. 1985;19:96–98.
136. Bernstein JE, Korman NJ, Bickers DR, et al. Topical capsaicin treatment of chronic postherpetic neuralgia. *J Am Acad Dermatol*. 1989; 21:265–270.
137. Peikert A, Hentrich M, Ochs G. Topical 0.025% capsaicin in chronic post-herpetic neuralgia: efficacy, predictors of response and long-term course. *J Neurol*. 1991;238:452–456.
138. King RB. Topical aspirin in chloroform and the relief of pain due to herpes zoster and postherpetic neuralgia. *Arch Neurol*. 1993;50: 1046–1053.
139. Stow PJ, Glynn CJ, Minor B. EMLA cream in the treatment of post-herpetic neuralgia. Efficacy and pharmacokinetic profile. *Pain*. 1989; 39:301–305.
140. Rowbotham MC, Davies PS, Verkempinck C, et al. Lidocaine patch: double-blind controlled study of a new treatment method for post-herpetic neuralgia. *Pain*. 1996;65:39–44.
141. Watson CP, Evans RJ, Reed K, et al. Amitriptyline versus placebo in postherpetic neuralgia. *Neurology*. 1982;32:671–673.
142. Max MB. Treatment of post-herpetic neuralgia: antidepressants. *Ann Neurol*. 1994;35:S50–S53.
143. Dworkin RH, Corbin AE, Young JP Jr, et al. Pregabalin for the treatment of postherpetic neuralgia: a randomized, placebo-controlled trial. *Neurology*. 2003;60:1274–1283.
144. Rowbotham M, Harden N, Stacey B, et al. Gabapentin for the treatment of postherpetic neuralgia. *JAMA*. 1998;280:1837–1842.
145. Rice ASC, Maton S, Postherpetic Study Group. Gabapentin in postherpetic neuralgia: a randomised, double blind, placebo controlled study. *Pain*. 2001;94:215–224.
146. Dallocchio C, Buffa C, Mazzarello P, et al. Gabapentin vs. amitriptyline in painful diabetic neuropathy: an open-label pilot study. *J Pain Symptom Manage*. 2000;20:280–285.
147. Loeser JD, Black RG, Christman A. Relief of pain by transcutaneous electrical stimulation. *J Neurosurg*. 1975;42:308–314.
148. Long DM. External electrical stimulation as a treatment of chronic pain. *Minn Med*. 1973;57:195–198.
149. Currey TA, Dalsania J. Treatment for herpes zoster ophthalmicus: stellate ganglion block as a treatment for acute pain and prevention of postherpetic neuralgia. *Ann Ophthalmol*. 1991;23:188–189.
150. Kotani N, Kushikata T, Hashimoto H. Intrathecal methylprednisolone for intractable postherpetic neuralgia. *N Engl J Med*. 2000;343: 1514–1519.
151. Hempenstall K, Nurmikko TJ, Johnson RW, et al. Analgesic therapy in postherpetic neuralgia: a quantitative systematic review. *PLoS Med*. 2005;2:e164.
152. Halloran ME, Cochi SL, Lieu TA, et al. Theoretical epidemiologic and morbidity effects of routine varicella immunization of preschool children in the United States. *Am J Epidemiol*. 1994;140:81–104.
153. Lieu TA, Cochi SL, Black SB, et al. Cost-effectiveness of a routine varicella vaccination program for US children. *JAMA*. 1994;271:375–381.
154. Edmunds WJ, Brisson M. The effect of vaccination on the epidemiology of varicella zoster virus. *J Infect*. 2002;44:211–219.
155. Brisson M, Edmunds WJ, Gay NJ, et al. Modelling the impact of immunization on the epidemiology of varicella zoster virus. *Epidemiol Infect*. 2000;125:651–659.
156. Quirk M. Varicella vaccination reduces risk of herpes zoster. *Lancet*. 2002;2:454.
157. Seward JF. Update on varicella and varicella vaccine, US. 41st Interscience Conference on Antimicrobial Agents and Chemotherapy, 2001.
158. Oxman MN, Levin MJ, Johnson GR, et al. A vaccine to prevent herpes zoster and postherpetic neuralgia in older adults. *N Engl J Med*. 2005;352:2271–2284.
159. Betts RF. Vaccination strategies for the prevention of herpes zoster and postherpetic neuralgia. *J Am Acad Dermatol*. 2007;57:S143–S147.

Chapter 81

Less Common Viral Corneal Infections

Kenneth C. Chern, David M. Meisler

This chapter addresses the anterior segment manifestations of the less common viral infections (summarized in Table 81.1). Clues from systemic manifestations may help identify the specific causative virus. This chapter describes DNA viruses from the Poxviridae, Herpesviridae (excluding herpes simplex and herpes zoster), and Papovaviridae families. The RNA viruses affecting the eye are members of the Picornaviridae, Togaviridae, Paramyxoviridae, and Orthomyxoviridae families. The Flaviviridae and Bunyaviridae families have only isolated cases of ocular involvement.[1,2]

DNA Viruses

Poxviridae

Poxviridae are large, encapsulated, double-stranded DNA viruses that most commonly affect the skin. Variola, and its counterpart, vaccinia, and molluscum contagiosum have been reported to affect the eye and ocular adnexa. A handful of reports describe ocular involvement by cowpox or orf.[3,4]

Variola (smallpox)

Variola, the causative agent for smallpox, was declared eradicated by the World Health Organization in May 1980 after worldwide mass vaccination programs.[5] Resurgence of this infection has been a concern since this virus has been implicated as a possible pathogen in bioterrorism.[6] Smallpox is transmitted by the inhalation of airborne secretions and is highly contagious. The virus multiplies in regional lymphoid tissues and, after a 2–3-day viremic phase, localizes in mucous membranes, skin, and internal organs. The maculopapular rash develops into vesicles and then into pustules. Healing of the pustules leaves depigmented scars and pits. Secondary infection of pustules may lead to life-threatening complications.

Involvement of the lids with vesicles causes severe edema with closure of the lids. Cicatrization of pustules occurring at the ciliary border may result in entropion, madarosis, trichiasis, and punctual stenosis. In severe cases, there is a catarrhal or purulent conjunctivitis. In less than 1% of cases, exquisitely painful pustules form on the conjunctiva and rapidly progress to membrane formation and tissue necrosis. Inflammation extending onto the limbus and cornea can become secondarily infected, producing ulceration, interstitial or disciform keratitis, and perforation of the globe.[7]

No specific treatment is available. Routine vaccination of the general public, the primary means of prophylaxis, has been discontinued after global eradication of the virus.

Vaccinia

Vaccinia has been encountered infrequently since the discontinuation of vaccinia inoculation as a prophylaxis for smallpox. Vaccinia infection is usually mild, conferring immunity against variola (smallpox), cowpox, and monkeypox. Cell-mediated immunity is critical in containing and eliminating vaccinia infection. Pregnant women, immunocompromised individuals, and atopic persons with eczema or chronic dermatitis may develop disseminated vaccinia.

Ocular involvement is thought to be by autoinoculation from the vaccination site by hand-to-eye contact.[8] Primary vaccinees are at a higher risk for ocular involvement. Vaccinial vesicles on the eyelid coalesce on an erythematous base accompanied by severe edema that may mimic orbital cellulitis.[9] Vesicular lesions of the eyelid margin may scar, leading to loss of eyelashes, distortion of the eyelid, and epiphora. Vesicles may spread to the conjunctiva and involve the cornea as a marginal infiltrate or stromal keratitis. The inflammatory keratitis may result in permanent corneal scarring.

Treatments for ocular vaccinia include intramuscular hyperimmune vaccinia immunoglobulin,[10–12] topical vidarabine,[13] trifluorothymidine,[14] and idoxuridine.[15,16]

Molluscum contagiosum

The molluscum contagiosum virus produces raised umbilicated nodules on the face, abdomen, and the genital region.[17] In children, transmission occurs by direct contact; in adults, by sexual contact. Atypical and disseminated infection may occur in immunodeficient conditions such as acquired immunodeficiency syndrome (AIDS),[18,19] immunosuppression by corticosteroids or chemotherapeutic drugs,[20,21] and atopic dermatitis.[22]

Eyelid margin involvement of the warty growths (Fig. 81.1A) produces a chronic follicular conjunctivitis (Fig. 81.1B) that has been associated with the shedding of viral particles into the tear film. Punctate keratopathy, subepithelial infiltrates, and a corneal pannus resembling trachoma

Table 81.1 Anterior segment and systemic manifestations of less common viral infections

Virus	Anterior segment findings	Nonocular findings
DNA viruses		
Poxviridae		
Variola virus	Cicatrizing pustules, catarrhal conjunctivitis, stromal keratitis	Maculopapular rash, vesicles, and pustules; pitting scars and skin depigmentation; fever
Vaccinia virus	Superficial punctate keratopathy, stromal keratitis and scarring, extensive lid edema	Disseminated vaccinia
Molluscum contagiosum virus	Chronic follicular conjunctivitis; rare punctate keratitis; raised, umbilicated lid margin lesions	Molluscum nodules on face and genital region
Herpesviridae		
Cytomegalovirus	Catarrhal conjunctivitis, dendritic keratitis, stromal keratitis, iridocyclitis	Mononucleosis-like infection, chorioretinitis, congenital anomalies
Epstein-Barr virus	Follicular conjunctivitis, stromal keratitis, nummular keratitis	Infectious mononucleosis
Papovaviridae		
Human papillomavirus	Lid margin and conjunctival papillomas, squamous cell cancer	Papillomas and cancer of the cervical, anogenital region, respiratory tract, and skin
RNA viruses		
Picornaviridae		
Enterovirus and coxsackievirus	Acute hemorrhagic conjunctivitis, rare epithelial keratopathy	Lymphadenopathy, fever, malaise, upper respiratory infection
Togaviridae		
Rubella (German measles) virus		
Acquired	Mild epithelial keratitis, follicular conjunctivitis	Thrombocytopenia, encephalitis
Congenital	Microphthalmos, congenital cataracts	Cardiac malformations, deafness, dental anomalies, intellectual impairment
Flaviviridae and Bunyaviridae	Ocular irritation	Dengue, yellow fever, West Nile fever, sandfly fever, Rift Valley fever
Paramyxoviridae		
Rubeola (measles) virus	Acute follicular conjunctivitis, superficial punctate keratopathy, conjunctival Koplik's spots	Morbilliform rash, fever, cough, coryza
Mumps virus	Follicular keratitis, rare stromal keratitis	Parotitis, orchitis, meningitis
Newcastle disease virus	Follicular conjunctivitis, rare punctate keratitis or subepithelial infiltrates	Encephalitis, gastroenteritis
Orthomyxoviridae		
Influenzavirus	Mild catarrhal conjunctivitis	Fever, chills, myalgias, malaise

also may be present.[23] Limbal or corneal molluscum lesions[24] and palpebral conjunctival lesions[25] are exceedingly rare.

The diagnosis can be made by expressing and smearing the core of a molluscum lesion on a slide. Under light microscopy, epidermal cells with large intracytoplasmic inclusions (molluscum bodies) rupture, releasing the material into the central cavity of the lesion.[17]

Molluscum contagiosum is usually a self-limited disease that resolves over 2 to 3 months. Surgical treatments include excision, curettage, and cryotherapy. Chemical cauterization of skin lesions with trichloroacetic acid, phenol, iodine, tretinoin, and other compounds has been used in the past with variable success.[26] More recently, immunomodulatory therapy with imiquimod and related medications,[27,28]

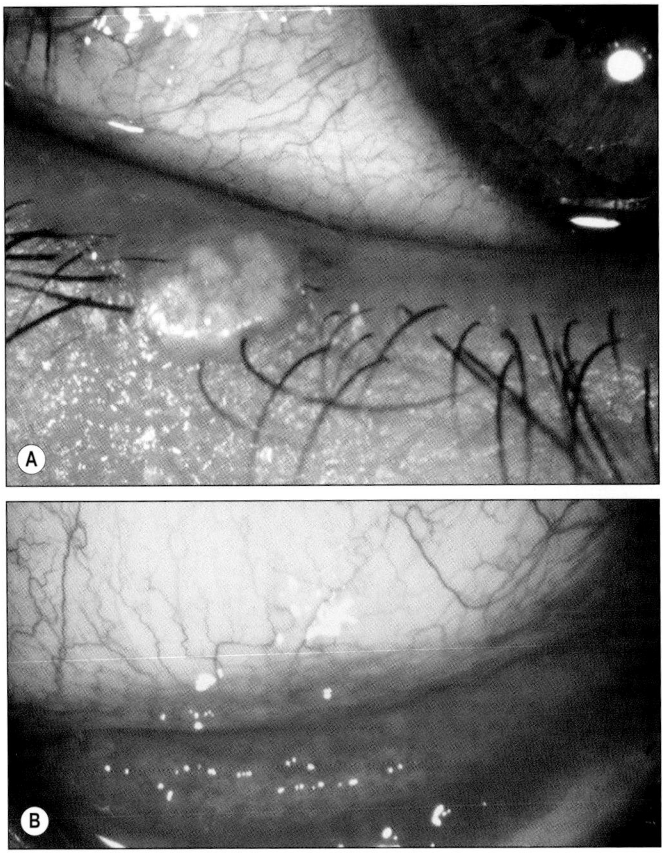

Fig. 81.1 Molluscum contagiosum. (**A**) Molluscum contagiosum lesion of the lower eyelid. (**B**) Follicular conjunctivitis secondary to virus shedding from the eyelid lesion.

photodynamic therapy,[29] and pulsed dye laser treatments[30] have been shown to eliminate molluscum skin lesions. The follicular conjunctivitis resolves slowly after treatment of the eyelid margin lesions.[23] In patients with AIDS, the lesions may persist, be difficult to eradicate, and recur frequently.[31]

Herpesviridae

The herpes viruses are enveloped, icosahedral, double-stranded DNA viruses that cause a wide variety of ocular infections. Herpes simplex and herpes zoster infections are discussed elsewhere (see Chs 80 and 81). Cytomegalovirus and Epstein-Barr virus less frequently involve the anterior segment.

Cytomegalovirus

Cytomegalovirus (CMV) is a ubiquitous herpesvirus, with seropositivity in humans exceeding 50% of the population. CMV infection can range from subclinical and asymptomatic infection to an infectious mononucleosis-like illness in young adults to severe pneumonia, hepatitis, and colitis in immunocompromised individuals. Transplacental CMV infection can be severe, with jaundice, hepatosplenomegaly, thrombocytopenia, anemia, pneumonia, microcephaly, seizures, and cerebral calcification.[32,33] Primary ocular disease manifests as chorioretinitis and is seen in more than 20% of infected infants. Optic nerve hypoplasia and coloboma, optic nerve atrophy, cataracts, Peters' anomaly, microphthalmia, and anophthalmia have been reported in association with congenital CMV infection.[33]

In patients with AIDS, CMV causes a devastating necrotizing retinochoroiditis indicative of a severely weakened immune system.[34,35] With the development of highly active antiretroviral therapy (HAART), the incidence of CMV retinitis is much lower and the presentation of this infection has changed.[36,37]

Anterior segment manifestations of CMV are very rare. CMV has been cultured from tears of patients with acute catarrhal conjunctivitis and CMV mononucleosis,[38] as well as from the tears of eight children immunosuppressed with acute lymphocytic lymphoma with CMV present in the urine or saliva.[39] In a patient with AIDS, CMV was cultured from corneal scrapings of an epithelial lesion. These slightly elevated, branching, nonulcerative dendrites recurred after debridement and were associated with an underlying stromal keratitis and iritis. This epithelial keratitis was unresponsive to oral and topical antiviral therapy.[40] Histologic evidence of CMV has been demonstrated in a conjunctival specimen[41] and a caruncle lesion[42] from AIDS patients with CMV. CMV transmission through infected tears may also be possible. The risk of CMV transmission from penetrating keratoplasty is as yet unproven.[43,44]

Epstein-Barr virus

The Epstein-Barr virus (EBV) is a widespread virus transmitted through oral secretions. EBV has been implicated in infectious mononucleosis, nasopharyngeal carcinoma, Sjögren's syndrome, oral hairy leukoplakia, and Burkitt's lymphoma.[45,46]

Infectious mononucleosis, a disease commonly affecting adolescents, is a self-limited infection characterized by fever, lymphadenopathy, pharyngitis, and splenomegaly.[45] Diagnosis is confirmed with the heterophil antibody test and by elevation of antibody titers against the viral capsid, nuclear, and envelope antigens. The most common ocular manifestation is a transient, monocular follicular conjunctivitis. Two distinct types of stromal keratitis have been described: (1) discrete, sharply demarcated, multifocal, pleomorphic, ring-shaped granular anterior stromal opacities and (2) soft, blotchy, pleomorphic, multifocal infiltrates predominantly involving the peripheral cornea.[47–49] Subepithelial infiltrates resembling those found in adenoviral keratitis,[50] stellate microdendrites,[51] and nummular keratitis[52] also may be observed. Other manifestations that occur less frequently include conjunctival nodules (Fig. 81.2),[53] periorbital edema, episcleritis, and uveitis.[48,54]

EBV has been postulated as the pathogenetic factor in the irido-corneal-endothelial syndrome[55] and Parinaud's oculoglandular syndrome.[56]

Papovaviridae

Human papillomavirus

The human papillomavirus (HPV) has a predilection for infecting epithelium. HPV has been implicated in causing a

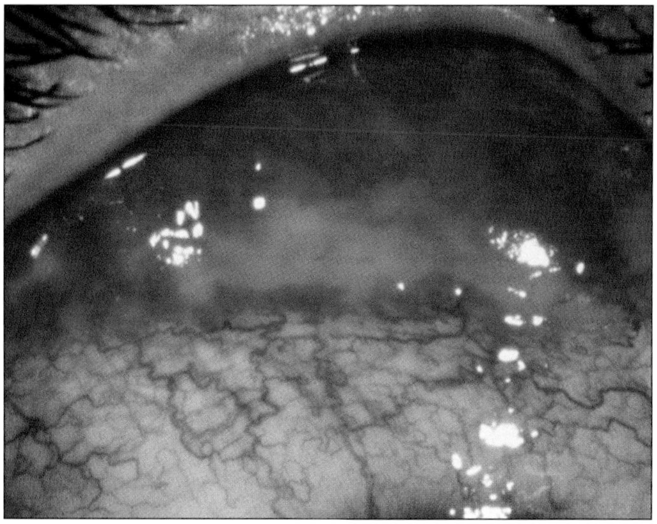

Fig. 81.2 Epstein-Barr virus associated conjunctival nodule.

wide variety of benign and malignant epithelial neoplasms involving the cervix, anogenital region, respiratory tract, and skin.[57]

The relationship between HPV and conjunctival papillomas (Fig. 81.3A), dysplasia, and carcinoma is unclear. HPV viral capsid antigen has been detected in 46% of conjunctival papillomas and 8.2% of conjunctival dysplasia or carcinoma.[58] HPV types 6 and 11 have been linked to benign epithelial proliferations such as conjunctival papillomas.[59] In particular, HPV type 6/11 DNA probes hybridize to conjunctival papilloma samples, but not to conjunctival dysplasia or to negative conjunctival controls (Fig. 81.3B).[60]

In contrast, HPV types 16 and 18 have been strongly linked to carcinomas of the cervix and anogenital region. Recently, DNA of HPV types 16 and 18 has been identified in conjunctival epithelial dysplasia and carcinoma using polymerase chain reaction amplification.[61,62] HPV type 16 also has been recovered from conjunctival swabs of asymptomatic patients with known cervical HPV infection. It is unclear whether these patients are at a higher risk of developing ocular papillomas and neoplasia.[63]

Surgical resection, carbon dioxide laser cauterization,[64–66] and cryotherapy[67] have been tried; however, there may be recurrence of the lesions. Immunotherapy with systemic interferon-α in patients after surgical resection of conjunctival papillomas reduced the rate of recurrence; however, after discontinuation of the therapy, the papillomas may reappear.[68] Dinitrochlorobenzene, when applied topically, has successfully eradicated conjunctival papilloma recalcitrant to other therapy.[69]

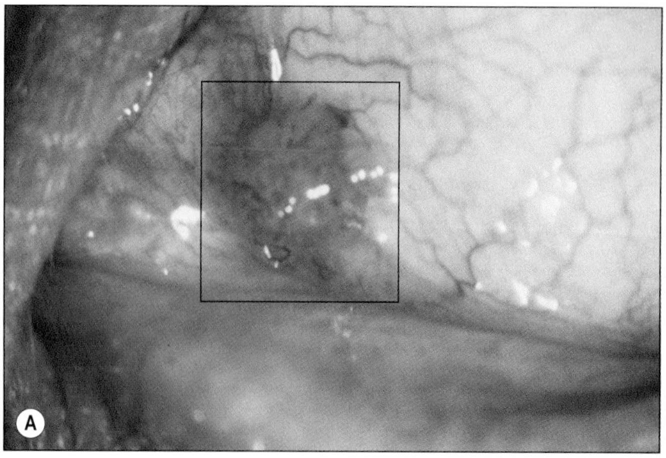

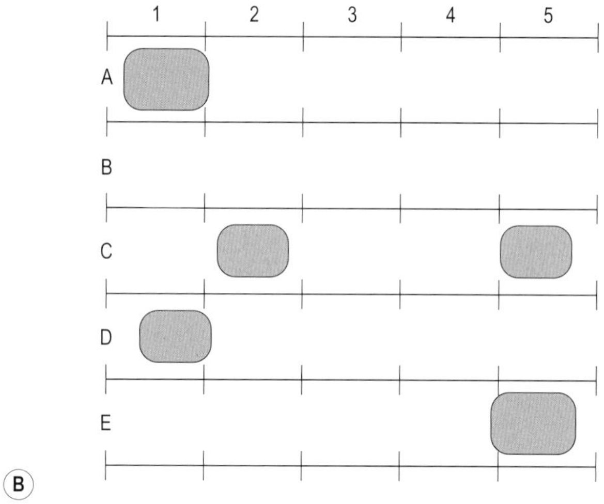

Fig. 81.3 Human papillomavirus. (A) Conjunctival papilloma (*box*). (B) Blot of hybridization of a probe complementary to HPV 6/11 DNA. The strong signal in position A1 corresponds to a positive HPV 6/11 control. Position D1 containing DNA from the conjunctival lesion is also positive.

RNA Viruses

Picornaviridae

Acute hemorrhagic conjunctivitis

Acute hemorrhagic conjunctivitis (AHC) is a highly contagious disease first described in the epidemic outbreak in Ghana in 1969, when almost 9000 people were infected.[70] AHC has been called 'Apollo 11 disease' because of its coincidental occurrence with the Apollo 11 moon landing. Hand-to-eye contact is the most probable means of transmission. Crowding and poor hygiene in tropical, developing countries have led to severe outbreaks.[71] This disease has swept across Africa,[72] southeast Asia,[73,74] and Japan.[75,76] In the western hemisphere, outbreaks have occurred in southern Florida,[77] Central and South America,[78,79] and the Caribbean.[80,81]

The most common viruses isolated are picornavirus subtypes enterovirus 70[78,81] and coxsackie A24.[82,83] Confirmatory diagnosis is through isolation of the virus from conjunctival swabs as serum antibody titers may be low or undetectable.[84] An immunofluorescence test has been used for more rapid diagnosis of enterovirus 70 in one outbreak.[85]

Within 24 hours of inoculation, infected patients have a sudden unilateral conjunctivitis, with the fellow eye involved soon thereafter. Severe pain, foreign body sensation, photophobia, and watery discharge develop within hours after infection. The most characteristic findings are bulbar subconjunctival hemorrhages ranging in size from pinpoint petechiae to large, flat hemorrhages.[70] In rare instances, superficial punctate keratopathy or subepithelial infiltrates may be present predominantly in the inferior half of the cornea.[82,84] Patients also may have lymphadenopathy, fever, malaise, and symptoms of an upper respiratory infection.[84]

The disease usually remits in 7 to 10 days without treatment and with no residua. There are rare reports of neurologic sequelae including radiculomyelitis,[85A,85B] muscle dysfunction,[86] and Bell's palsy.[77]

Togaviridae

Rubella (German measles) virus

Rubella is less commonly seen since the licensure of a vaccine in 1969. Nevertheless, outbreaks continue to occur, predominantly affecting children and young adults in which unvaccinated persons congregate in close proximity. Immigrants from foreign countries that do not routinely immunize against rubella also pose a risk for rubella exposure and transmission in the United States. In 1993, 190 cases of postnatally acquired rubella and no cases of congenital rubella syndrome were reported to the National Notifiable Disease Surveillance System.[87] Acquired rubella is usually mild and self-limiting, whereas congenital rubella infection disrupts fetal development and maturation.

Acquired rubella

Infected individuals may have a mild catarrhal or follicular conjunctivitis. A small proportion of patients develop bilateral, fine, punctate, epithelial keratopathy, concentrated centrally and appearing a week after the skin rash.[88,89] The keratitis and conjunctivitis resolve within 7 days with no sequelae.[89]

Congenital rubella

Maternal–fetal transmission of the rubella virus occurs during the viremic stage 10 to 12 days after maternal infection. In the mother, rubella may produce a fever, malaise, and lymphadenopathy, and may or may not be accompanied by a morbilliform rash.

Gestational age is an important factor in assessing the degree of fetal involvement. Infection during the first or second trimester is more serious, with the virus disrupting organogenesis and differentiation. Many fetal tissues are susceptible to infection, leading to the abnormalities found in the congenital rubella syndrome: congenital deafness, cardiac malformations, bony and dental abnormalities, ocular malformations, and intellectual impairment.[90]

Retinopathy, described as a 'salt and pepper' appearance of the retinal pigment epithelium, is the most common ocular disorder, occurring in 24% of congenital cases. Other ocular manifestations of congenital rubella include microphthalmos, strabismus, congenital cataracts, transient corneal leucoma, iris atrophy and hypoplasia, and glaucoma.[90] Keratoconus and hydrops have been reported in patients with congenital rubella, with a history of intellectual impairment and eye rubbing.[91]

Paramyxoviridae

Rubeola (measles)

Rubeola continues to be a cause of epidemics in children and young adults despite the availability of a vaccine since 1963.[92,93] Transmission is via inhalation of aerosolized respiratory secretions from infected individuals. After an 11-day incubation period, patients develop cough, coryza, Koplik's spots, fever, and a morbilliform rash. The ocular manifestations are limited predominantly to the epithelium of the conjunctiva and cornea. The conjunctivitis is mild and watery with no prominent follicular or papillary reaction, or pseudomembrane formation. Koplik's spots similar in appearance to those found on other mucous membranes have been reported to occur on the semilunar fold or the caruncle.[94,95] Subconjunctival hemorrhages, sometimes bilateral, have been found coincident with the conjunctivitis.[96]

Fine, superficial punctate epithelial erosions and subepithelial infiltrates may be found on the conjunctiva and cornea. Larger stellate lesions of the cornea also have been described. The central cornea and interpalpebral fissure are most commonly involved with the keratitis. Patients complain of tearing, photophobia, decreased vision, and foreign body sensation. Treatment is symptomatic and ocular findings usually resolve within a few weeks of onset without permanent sequelae; however, the keratitis may persist for as long as 4 months.[92,97]

In developing countries, malnutrition, vitamin A deficiency, herpes simplex infection, and traditional medical therapy lead to a high incidence of corneal ulceration and bacterial superinfection concomitant with measles infection.[98–101]

No specific treatment or cure is available. Immunization with attenuated measles virus is effective prophylaxis.

Mumps

The mumps virus is transmitted by inhalation of airborne secretions. The classic presentation is a child with bilateral, swollen, tender parotid and other salivary glands. Systemic viremia may produce meningitis, orchitis, and pancreatitis.[102]

Dacryoadenitis is the most common ocular manifestation.[103] Bilateral involvement of the lacrimal glands occurs coincident with or preceding the swelling of the parotids. Painful swelling, proptosis of the orbit, and conjunctival chemosis or injection may herald viral infiltration. Resolution occurs without treatment within several days, without residua in many instances.

Mumps produces a mild follicular conjunctivitis, mild hyperemia and edema of the conjunctiva and lids, and occasionally chemosis.[103,104] Bonnet[105] proposed that the mumps virus causes an adenitis of the accessory lacrimal glands. Treatment is symptomatic and resolution occurs spontaneously in 4 to 6 days.

Corneal involvement is rare.[106] The keratitis associated with mumps typically occurs 5 to 11 days after the onset of the parotitis. There is rapid, unilateral, relatively painless visual loss, in some cases to the level of light perception, accompanied by tearing and photophobia. Full-thickness stromal infiltration with white, interlacing fimbriae and white dotlike opacities in the anterior stroma have been described.[103] A region of lucent stroma may remain near the limbus.[105] In 1 to 5 weeks, the stromal process resolves without vascularization, leaving a fine nebula, and a return to normal vision. The epithelium is usually unaffected, but ulceration and punctate keratitis have been described.[103]

Other manifestations include extraocular muscle palsies, tenonitis, iritis, scleritis, and secondary infections.[103] Topical corticosteroids may hasten the resolution of the keratitis, iritis, and scleritis.[107]

Live attenuated mumps vaccine is effective prophylaxis and is often given in combination with measles and rubella vaccines.

Newcastle disease

The Newcastle disease virus (NDV) predominantly infects poultry and other avian species, causing diarrhea, intestinal hemorrhage, respiratory distress, and nasal and ocular discharge.[108,109] The virus is highly contagious and may be spread through contact with infected secretions, eggs, and feces, as well as through inhalation of viral particles.[108,109] In humans, NDV has been linked to encephalitis[110] and gastroenteritis.[111]

Isolated cases of ocular involvement with NDV in humans were first reported in 1949.[112–114] The first identified epidemic occurred among workers at a Utah turkey processing plant in 1965.[115] Sporadic reports today have been associated with poultry workers, veterinarians, and laboratory technicians. The virus produces a self-limiting infection characterized by marked preauricular adenopathy and a follicular conjunctivitis. Corneal involvement is rare, but may present as superficial punctate keratitis or subepithelial infiltrates.[116]

Treatment is symptomatic and the infection usually clears without sequelae within 2 weeks. Subepithelial infiltrates may resolve more slowly over 18 months.[116]

Orthomyxoviridae

Influenza

Influenza infection produces acute, usually self-limiting febrile illnesses with outbreaks every winter. Antigenic variation of influenza strains A, B, and C makes lifelong immunity impossible. Infection is transmitted by contact with infected secretions or inhalation of droplets aerosolized by coughing or sneezing. Affected patients have a sudden onset of fever, chills, myalgia, anorexia, malaise, and headache. Significant mortality occurs from viral pneumonia, secondary bacterial pneumonia, and exacerbation of chronic bronchitis.[117]

In most cases, influenza virus causes a mild catarrhal conjunctivitis. No treatment is required. Keratitis, uveitis, retinal hemorrhages, and optic neuritis are exceedingly rare.

References

1. Peters CJ, Johnson KM. California encephalitis viruses, Hantaviruses, and other Bunyaviridae. In: Mandell GL, Bennett JC, Dolin R, eds. *Principles and practice of infectious disease*. 4th ed. New York: Churchill Livingstone; 1995.
2. Monath TP. Flaviviruses (yellow fever, dengue, dengue hemorrhagic fever, Japanese encephalitis, St Louis encephalitis, tick-borne encephalitis). In: Mandell GL, Bennett JC, Dolin R, eds. *Principles and practice of infectious disease*. 4th ed. New York: Churchill Livingstone; 1995.
3. Hall CJ, Stevens JD. Ocular cowpox. *Lancet*. 1987;1:111.
4. Duke-Elder S, MacFaul PA. *System of ophthalmology*. vol XIII. St Louis: Mosby; 1965.
5. World Health Organization. *Wkly Epidemiol Rec*. 1980;55:148.
6. Drazen JM. Smallpox and bioterrorism. *N Engl J Med*. 2002;346:1262–1263.
7. Duke-Elder S, MacFaul PA. *System of ophthalmology*. vol. XV. St Louis: Mosby; 1965.
8. Lane JM, Ruben FL, Neff JM, Millar JD. Complications of smallpox vaccination, 1968. *N Engl J Med*. 1969;281:1201–1208.
9. Duke-Elder S, MacFaul PA. *System of ophthalmology*. vol XIII. St Louis: Mosby; 1965.
10. Ellis PP, Winograd LA. Ocular vaccinia. *Arch Ophthalmol*. 1962;68:600–609.
11. Ruben FL, Lane JM. Ocular vaccinia. *Arch Ophthalmol*. 1970;84:45–48.
12. Rydberg M, Pandolfi M. Treatment of vaccinia keratitis with post-vaccinial gamma globulin. *Acta Ophthalmol (Copenh)*. 1963;41:713–718.
13. Hyndiuk RA, et al. Treatment of vaccinial keratitis with vidarabine. *Arch Ophthalmol*. 1976;94:1363–1364.
14. Hyndiuk RA, Seideman S, Leibsohn JM. Treatment of vaccinial keratitis with trifluorothymidine. *Arch Ophthalmol*. 1976;94:1785–1786.
15. Jack MK, Sorenson RW. Vaccinal keratitis treated with IDU. *Arch Ophthalmol*. 1962;69:730–732.
16. Fulginiti VA, Winograd LA, Jackson M, Ellis P. Therapy of experimental vaccinal keratitis. *Arch Ophthalmol*. 1965;74:539–544.
17. Jordan MC. Molluscum contagiosum. In: Hoeprich PD, Jordan MC, Ronald AR, eds. *Infectious diseases: a treatise of infectious processes*. 5th ed. Philadelphia: JB Lippincott; 1994.
18. Kohn SR. Molluscum contagiosum in patients with acquired immunodeficiency syndrome. *Arch Ophthalmol*. 1987;105:458.
19. Lombardo PC. Molluscum contagiosum and the acquired immunodeficiency syndrome. *Arch Dermatol*. 1985;121:834–835.
20. Cotton DW, Cooper C, Barret DF, Leppard BJ. Severe atypical molluscum contagiosum infection in an immunocompromised host. *Br J Dermatol*. 1987;116:871–876.
21. Rosenberg EW, Yusk JW. Molluscum contagiosum: eruption following treatment with prednisone and methotrexate. *Arch Dermatol*. 1970;101:439–441.
22. Pauly CR, Artis WM, Jones HE. Atopic dermatitis, impaired cellular immunity, and molluscum contagiosum. *Arch Dermatol*. 1978;114:391–393.
23. Curtin BJ, Theodore FH. Ocular molluscum contagiosum. *Am J Ophthalmol*. 1955;39:302–307.
24. Charles NC, Friedberg DN. Epibulbar molluscum contagiosum in acquired immune deficiency syndrome. *Ophthalmology*. 1992;99:1123–1126.
25. Hindaal CH, van Bijsterveld OP. Molluscom contagiosum of the palpebral conjunctiva. Report of a case. *Ophthalmologica*. 1979;178:137–141.
26. Williams LR, Webster G. Warts and molluscum contagiosum. *Clin Dermatol*. 1991;9:87–93.
27. Arican O. Topical treatment of molluscom contagiosum with imiquimod 5% cream in Turkish children. *Pediatr Int*. 2006;48:403–405.
28. Hourihane J, et al. Interferon alpha treatment of molluscum contagiosum in immunodeficiency. *Arch Dise Child*. 1999;80:77–79.
29. Gold MH, Moiin A. Treatment of verrucae vulgaris and molluscum contagiosum with photodynamic therapy. *Dermatolo Clin*. 2007;25:75–80.
30. Chatproedprai S, et al. Efficacy of pulsed dye laser (585 nm) in the treatment of molluscum contagiosum subtype 1. *Southeast Asian J Trop Med Public Health*. 2007;38:849–854.
31. Robinson MR, et al. Molluscum contagiosum of the eyelids in patients with acquired immune deficiency syndrome. *Ophthalmology*. 1992;99:1745–1747.
32. Matoba A. Ocular viral infections. *Pediatr Infect Dis*. 1984;3:358–368.
33. McCarthy RW, Frenkel LD, Kollarits CR, Keys MP. Clinical anophthalmia associated with congenital cytomegalovirus infection. *Am J Ophthalmol*. 1980;90:558–561.
34. Holland GN, Gottleib MS, Yee RD, et al. Ocular disorders associated with a new severe acquired cellular immunodeficiency syndrome. *Am J Ophthalmol*. 1982;93:393–402.

35. Holland GN, Pepose JS, Pettit TH, et al. Acquired immune deficiency syndrome: ocular manifestations. *Ophthalmology.* 1983;90:859–873.
36. Zegans ME, Walton RC, Holland GN, et al. Transient vitreous inflammatory reactions associated with combination antiretroviral therapy in patients with AIDS and cytomegalovirus retinitis. *Am J Ophthalmol.* 1998;125:292–300.
37. Jacobson MA, Zegans M, Pavan PR, et al. Cytomegalovirus retinitis after initiation of highly active antiretroviral therapy. *Lancet.* 1997;349:1443–1445.
38. Garau J, et al. Spontaneous cytomegalovirus mononucleosis with conjunctivitis. *Arch Intern Med.* 1977;137:1631–1632.
39. Cox F, Meyer D, Hughes WT. Cytomegalovirus in tears from patients with normal eyes and with acute cytomegalovirus chorioretinitis. *Am J Ophthalmol.* 1975;80:817–824.
40. Wilhelmhus KR, Font RL, Lehmann RP, Cernoch PL. Cytomegalovirus keratitis in acquired immunodeficiency syndrome. *Arch Ophthalmol.* 1996;114:869–872.
41. Brown HH, Glasgow BJ, Holland GN, Foos RY. Cytomegalovirus infection of the conjunctiva in AIDS. *Am J Ophthalmol.* 1988;106:102–104.
42. Espana-Gregori E, et al. Cytomegalovirus infection of the caruncle in the acquired immunodeficiency syndrome. *Am J Ophthalmol.* 1994;117:406–407.
43. Holland EJ, et al. The risk of cytomegalovirus transmission by penetrating keratoplasty. *Am J Ophthalmol.* 1988;105:357–360.
44. Pepose JS. The risk of cytomegalovirus transmission by penetrating keratoplasty. *Am J Ophthalmol.* 1988;106:238–240.
45. Niederman JC. Infectious mononucleosis. In: Hoeprich PD, Jordan MC, Ronald AR, eds. *Infectious diseases: a treatise of infectious processes.* 5th ed. Philadelphia: JB Lippincott; 1994.
46. Chodosh J. Epstein-Barr virus stromal keratitis. *Ophthalmol Clin North Am.* 1994;7:549–556.
47. Matoba AY, Wilhelmus KR, Jones DB. Epstein-Barr viral stromal keratitis. *Ophthalmology.* 1986;93:746–751.
48. Wong KW, et al. Ocular involvement associated with chronic Epstein-Barr virus disease. *Arch Ophthalmol.* 1987;105:788–792.
49. Palay DA, Litoff D, Krachmer JH. Stromal keratitis associated with Epstein-Barr virus infection in a young child. *Arch Ophthalmol.* 1993; 111:1323–1324.
50. Matoba AY, Jones DB. Corneal subepithelial infiltrates associated with Epstein-Barr viral infection. *Ophthalmology.* 1987;94:1669–1671.
51. Wilhelmus KR. Ocular involvement in infectious mononucleosis. *Am J Ophthalmol.* 1981;91:117–118.
52. Pinnolis M, McCulley JP, Urman JD. Nummular keratitis associated with infectious mononucleosis. *Am J Ophthalmol.* 1980;89:791–794.
53. Gardner BP, Margolis TP, Mondino BJ. Conjunctival lymphocytic nodule associated with the Epstein-Barr virus. *Am J Ophthalmol.* 1991;112:567–571.
54. Tanner OR. Ocular manifestations of infectious mononucleosis. *Arch Ophthalmol.* 1954;51:229–241.
55. Tsai CS, et al. Antibodies to Epstein-Barr virus in iridocorneal endothelial syndrome. *Arch Ophthalmol.* 1990;108:1572–1576.
56. Meisler DM, Bosworth DE, Krachmer JH. Ocular infectious mononucleosis manifested as Parinaud's oculoglandular syndrome. *Am J Ophthalmol.* 1981;92:722–726.
57. Fife KH. Papillomaviruses and human warts. In: Hoeprich PD, Jordan MC, Ronald AR, eds. *Infectious diseases: a treatise of infectious processes.* 5th ed. Philadelphia: JB Lippincott; 1994.
58. McDonnell JM, et al. Demonstration of papillomavirus capsid antigen in human conjunctival neoplasia. *Arch Ophthalmol.* 1986;104:1801–1805.
59. Lass JH, Jenson AB, Papale JJ, Albert DM. Papillomavirus in human conjunctival papillomas. *Am J Ophthalmol.* 1983;95:364–368.
60. McDonnell PJ, et al. Detection of human papillomavirus type 6/11 DNA in conjunctival papillomas by in situ hybridization with radioactive probes. *Hum Pathol.* 1987;18:1115–1119.
61. McDonnell JM, McDonnell PJ, Sun YY. Human papillomavirus DNA in tissues and ocular surface swabs of patients with conjunctival epithelial neoplasia. *Invest Ophthalmol Vis Sci.* 1992;33:184–189.
62. Odrich MG, et al. A spectrum of bilateral squamous conjunctival tumors associated with human papillomavirus type 16. *Ophthalmology.* 1991;98:628–635.
63. McDonnell JM, et al. Human papillomavirus type 16 DNA in ocular and cervical swabs of women with genital tract condylomata. *Am J Ophthalmol.* 1991;112:61–66.
64. Bosniak SL, Novick NL, Sachs ME. Treatment of recurrent squamous papillomata of the conjunctiva by carbon dioxide laser vaporization. *Ophthalmology.* 1986;93:1078–1082.
65. Jackson WB, Beraja R, Codere F. Laser therapy of conjunctival papillomas. *Can J Ophthalmol.* 1987;22:45–47.
66. Schachat A, Iliff WJ, Kashima HK. Carbon dioxide laser therapy of recurrent squamous papilloma of the conjunctiva. *Ophthalmic Surg.* 1982;13:916–918.
67. Omohundro JM, Elliott JH. Cryotherapy of conjunctival papillomas. *Arch Ophthalmol.* 1970;84:609–610.
68. Lass JH, et al. Interferon-alpha therapy of recurrent conjunctival papillomas. *Am J Ophthalmol.* 1987;103:294–301.
69. Petrelli R, Cotlier E, Robins S, Stoessel K. Dinitrochlorobenzene immunotherapy of recurrent squamous papilloma of the conjunctiva. *Ophthalmology.* 1981;88:1221–1225.
70. Chatterjee S, Quarcoopome CO, Apenteng A. Unusual type of epidemic conjunctivitis in Ghana. *Br J Ophthalmol.* 1970;54:628–631.
71. Reeves WC, et al. Acute hemorrhagic conjunctivitis epidemic in Colon, Republic of Panama. *Am J Epidemiol.* 1986;123:325–335.
72. Quarcoopome CO. Epidemic haemorrhagic conjunctivitis in Ghana. *Br J Ophthalmol.* 1973;57:692–693.
73. Yin-Murphy M, Baharuddin-Ishak, Phoon MC, Chow VTK. A recent epidemic of coxsackie virus type A24 acute haemorrhagic conjunctivitis in Singapore. *Br J Ophthalmol.* 1986;70:869–873.
74. Chou M-Y, Malison MD. Outbreak of acute hemorrhagic conjunctivitis due to coxsackie A24 variant-Taiwan. *Am J Epidemiol.* 1988; 127:795–800.
75. Kono R. Apollo 11 disease or acute hemorrhagic conjunctivitis: a pandemic of a new enterovirus infection of the eye. *Am J Epidemiol.* 1975;101:33–390.
76. Kono R, et al. Pandemic of new type of conjunctivitis. *Lancet.* 1972;1:1191–1194.
77. Sklar VEF, et al. Clinical findings and results of treatment in an outbreak of acute hemorrhagic conjunctivitis in southern Florida. *Am J Ophthalmol.* 1983;95:45–54.
78. Asbell PA, et al. Acute hemorrhagic conjunctivitis in Central America: first enterovirus epidemic in the western hemisphere. *Ann Ophthalmol.* 1985;17:205–210.
79. Centers for Disease Control. Acute hemorrhagic conjunctivitis – Mexico. *MMWR.* 1989;38:327–330.
80. Centers for Disease Control. Acute hemorrhagic conjunctivitis caused by coxsackievirus A24 – Caribbean. *MMWR.* 1987;36:245–251.
81. Onorato IM, et al. Acute hemorrhagic conjunctivitis caused by enterovirus type 70: an epidemic in American Samoa. *Am J Trop Med Hyg.* 1985;34:984–991.
82. Wolken SH. Acute hemorrhagic conjunctivitis. *Surv Ophthalmol.* 1974;19:71–84.
83. Lin K-H, et al. Molecular epidemiology of a variant of coxsackievirus A24 in Taiwan: two epidemics caused by phylogenetically distinct viruses from 1985 to 1989. *J Clin Microbiol.* 1993;31:1160–1166.
84. Christopher S, et al. An epidemic of acute hemorrhagic conjunctivitis due to coxsackievirus A24. *J Infect Dis.* 1982;146:16–19.
85. Pal SR, et al. Rapid immunofluorescence diagnosis of acute hemorrhagic conjunctivitis caused by enterovirus 70. *Intervirology.* 1983;20: 19–22.
85A. Wright PW, Strauss GH, Langford MP. Acute hemorrhagic conjunctivitis. *Am Fam Physician.* 1992;45:173–178.
85B. Kono R, et al. Neurologic complications associated with acute hemorrhagic conjunctivitis virus infection and its serologic confirmation. *J Infect Dis.* 1974;129:590–593.
86. Chopra JS, et al. Neurological complications of acute haemorrhagic conjunctivitis. *J Neurol Sci.* 1986;73:177–191.
87. Centers for Disease Control. Rubella and congenital rubella syndrome – United States, January 1, 1991–May 7, 1994. *MMWR.* 1994; 43:391–401.
88. Hara J, et al. Ocular manifestations of the 1976 rubella epidemic in Japan. *Am J Ophthalmol.* 1979;87:642–945.
89. Smolin G. Report of a case of rubella keratitis. *Am J Ophthalmol.* 1972;74:436–647.
90. Wolff SM. The ocular manifestations of congenital rubella. *J Pediatr Ophthalmol.* 1973;10:101–141.
91. Boger WP 3rd, Petersen RA, Robb RM. Keratoconus and acute hydrops in mentally retarded patients with congenital rubella syndrome. *Am J Ophthalmol.* 1981;91:231–233.
92. Deckard PS, Bergstrom TJ. Rubeola keratitis. *Ophthalmology.* 1981;88:810–813.
93. Smoak BL, Novakoski WL, Mason CJ, Erickson RL. Evidence for a recent decrease in measles susceptibility among young American adults. *J Infect Dis.* 1994;170:216–219.
94. Bonamour G. La participation de la cornée à l'éruption cutanée de la face au cours des maladies infectieuses éruptives de l'enfance: rougeole et scarlatine. *Bull Soc Ophtalmol.* 1953;82:95–97.
95. Gaud F. Les complications oculaires des maladies infectieuses éruptives de l'enfance. *Arch Ophthalmol (Paris).* 1958;18:25–26.

96. Kayikcioglu O, Kir E, Soyler M, et al. Ocular findings in a measles epidemic among young adults. *Ocul Immunol Inflamm.* 2000;8:59–62.
97. Florman AL, Agaston HJ. Keratoconjunctivitis as a diagnostic aid in measles. *JAMA.* 1962;179:568–570.
98. Sandford-Smith JH, Whittle HC. Corneal ulceration following measles in Nigerian children. *Br J Ophthalmol.* 1979;63:720–724.
99. Foster A, Sommer A. Corneal ulceration, measles, and childhood blindness in Tanzania. *Br J Ophthalmol.* 1987;71:331–343.
100. Frederique G, Howard RO, Boniuk V. Corneal ulcers in rubeola. *Am J Ophthalmol.* 1970;68:996–1003.
101. Foster A, Sommer A. Childhood blindness from corneal ulceration in Africa: causes, prevention, and treatment. *Bull World Health Organ.* 1986;74:619–623.
102. Pomeroy C, Jordan MC. Mumps. In: Hoeprich PD, Jordan MC, Ronald AR, eds. *Infectious diseases: a treatise of infectious processes.* 5th ed. Philadelphia: JB Lippincott; 1994.
103. Riffenburgh RS. Ocular manifestations of mumps. *Arch Ophthalmol.* 1961;66:739–743.
104. Meyer RF, Sullivan JH, Oh JO. Mumps conjunctivitis. *Am J Ophthalmol.* 1974;78:1022–1024.
105. Bonnet P. Les complications oculaires des oreillons: manifestations oculaires de l'infection ourlienne. *J Med Lyon.* 1938;19:171–182.
106. Fields J. Ocular manifestations of mumps. *Am J Ophthalmol.* 1947;30:591–595.
107. Sutphin JE. Mumps keratitis. *Ophthalmol Clin North Am.* 1994;7:557–566.
108. Pringle CR, Heath RB. Paramyxoviridae. In: Parker MT, Collier LH, eds. *Topley and Wilson's principles of bacteriology, virology, and immunity.* 8th ed. Philadelphia: BC Decker; 1990.
109. Keeney AH, Hunter MC. Human infection with the Newcastle virus of fowls. *Arch Ophthalmol.* 1950;44:573–580.
110. Howitt BF, Bishop LK, Kissling RE. Presence of neutralizing antibodies to Newcastle disease virus in human sera. *Am J Public Health.* 1948;38:1263–1272.
111. McGough TF. Outbreak of Newcastle disease in Ohio. *Ohio State Med J.* 1949;45:25.
112. Freymann MW, Bang FB. Human conjunctivitis due to Newcastle virus. *Bull Johns Hopkins Hosp.* 1949;84:409–413.
113. Ingalls WL, Mahoney A. Isolation of Newcastle virus from humans. *Am J Public Health.* 1949;39:737–740.
114. Shimkin NI. Conjunctival hemorrhage due to an infection of Newcastle virus of fowls in man. *Br J Ophthalmol.* 1946;30:260–264.
115. Trott DG, Pilsworth R. Outbreaks of conjunctivitis due to Newcastle disease virus in chicken broiler factory workers. *Br Med J.* 1965;2:1514–1517.
116. Hales RH, Ostler HB. Newcastle disease conjunctivitis with subepithelial infiltrates. *Br J Ophthalmol.* 1973;57:694–697.
117. Betts RF. Influenza virus. In: Mandell GL, Bennett JC, Dolin R, eds. *Principles and practice of infectious disease.* 4th ed. New York: Churchill Livingstone; 1995.

Chapter 82

Fungal Keratitis

Eduardo C. Alfonso, Anat Galor, Darlene Miller

Fungal keratitis represents one of the most difficult forms of microbial keratitis for the ophthalmologist to diagnose and treat successfully. Difficulties arise in making the correct diagnosis, establishing the clinical characteristics of fungal keratitis, and obtaining confirmation from the microbiology laboratory. Other problems relate to treatment. It is difficult to obtain topical antifungal preparations, they do not work as effectively as antibiotics for bacterial infections, and the infection is often more advanced because of delays in making the correct diagnosis. Medical or surgical success, therefore, may be limited.

There has been an increase in the number of reported cases of fungal keratitis.[1–4] The increasing use of broad-spectrum topical antibiotics may provide a noncompetitive environment for fungi to grow. In addition, the use of topical corticosteroid enhances the growth of fungi while suppressing host immune response. There has also been an increase in fungal keratitis related to the use of soft contact lenses.[4–7] The increasing laboratory capability for recovery of fungi from infected corneas has increased our awareness of fungal keratitis. The treatment of fungal keratitis can be quite challenging, often requiring prolonged and intensive topical and systemic antifungal therapy, with surgical intervention in the form of penetrating keratoplasty, conjunctival flap, or cryotherapy required when medical treatment fails.

Pathogenesis

Fungi are eukaryotic and heterotrophic organisms. That is, they have a membrane-bound nucleus within which the genome of the cell is stored as chromosomes of DNA, and they require organic compounds for growth and reproduction. They are nonphotosynthetic and typically form reproductive spores. Many fungi exhibit both sexual and asexual forms of reproduction. Some fungi are unicellular, but most form filaments of vegetative cells known as mycelia. The mycelia usually exhibit branching and are typically surrounded by cell walls containing chitin or cellulose.[8]

Fungi are ubiquitous, saprophytic, and/or pathogenic organisms. Saprophytic fungi obtain their nutrients from decaying organic matter, whereas pathogenic fungi feed on living cells. Pathogenic fungi are actually saprobes, which are known to cause disease in humans. Many of the fungi associated with ocular infections are saprophytic and have been reported as causes of infection only in the ophthalmic literature. A convenient method of classifying fungal isolates has been reported in the ophthalmic literature. It includes four diagnostic/laboratory groups: yeasts which include *Candida* spp.; filamentous septated fungi, which include both nonpigmented hyphae (*Fusarium* spp. and *Aspergillus* spp.) and pigmented hyphae (*Alternaria* spp. and *Curvularia* spp.); filamentous nonseptated fungi, which include *Mucor* spp.; and other fungi (Box 82.1).[9–12]

Fungi gain access into the corneal stroma through a defect in the epithelial barrier. This defect may be due to external trauma, including epithelial trauma caused by wearing contact lenses, a compromised ocular surface, or previous surgery. Once in the stroma, they multiply and can cause tissue necrosis and a host inflammatory reaction. Organisms can penetrate deep into the stroma and through an intact Descemet's membrane. It is thought that once organisms gain access into the anterior chamber or to the iris and lens, eradication of the organism becomes extremely difficult. Likewise, organisms that extend from the cornea into the sclera become difficult to control. Blood-borne, growth-inhibiting factors may not reach the avascular tissues of the eye such as the cornea, anterior chamber, and sclera, which may explain why fungi continue to grow and persist despite treatment. It also may be the reason why a conjunctival flap helps control fungal growth (i.e. by bringing to avascular tissue blood-borne, growth-inhibiting factors).

Epidemiology

Fungi may be part of the normal external ocular flora. They have been isolated from the conjunctival sac in 3–28% of healthy eyes in various series.[11–15] They can be recovered from diseased eyes with even greater frequency (17–37%).[11,12] The organisms most commonly found in healthy eyes include *Aspergillus* spp., *Rhodotorula* spp., *Candida* spp., *Penicillium* spp., *Cladosporium* spp., and *Alternaria* spp. In southern Florida, *Candida parapsilosis* was the most frequently isolated fungal organism from the normal eye.[15] Overall, the incidence of fungal keratitis is low (6–20%) when compared to bacterial keratitis in various series of microbial corneal ulcers, with more numerous reports of fungal keratitis from the southern United States.[1–3] It continues to be a disease most commonly encountered in patients who come from a rural setting. *Aspergillus* spp. is the most common organism responsible for fungal keratitis worldwide.[9] In the United

Box 82.1 Fungi causing human keratitis

Yeast
- *Candida* species
  - *albicans, parapsilosis, krusei, tropicalis, guillermondii*
- *Trichosporon beigelii*
- *Pichia ohmeria*
- *Cryptococcus uniguttulans*
- *Malassezia restricta*
- *Blastoschizomyces capitatus*

Filamentous septated
- Nonpigmented hyphae (hyaline)
- *Fusarium* species
  - *solani, oxysporum, moniliforme, episphaesia*
- *Aspergillus* species
  - *fumigatus, flavus, terreus, glaucus, niger*
- *Acremonium* species
- *Cylindocarpon* species
- *Paecilomyces* species
- *Scedosporium apiosperum (Pseudoallescheria boydii)*
- *Trichophyton mentagrophytes*
- *Arthrographis kalrae*
- *Beauveria bassiana*
- Pigmented hyphae (dematiaceous)
- *Alternaria* species
- *Curvularia* species
  - *senegelensis, verruculosa*
- *Cladosporium* species
- *Colleotricum* species
  - *dematium, gloeosporoides*
- *Exopilia philophora*
- *Histoplasma capsulatum*
- *Lasiodiplodia threobromae*
- *Scytalidium* species

Filamentous nonseptated
- *Mucor* species
- *Rhizopus* species

Box 82.2 Most common risk factors for the development of fungal keratitis

Trauma (including contact lenses)

Topical medications (corticosteroids and others)

Corneal surgery (penetrating keratoplasty, LASIK, radial keratotomy)

Chronic keratitis (herpes simplex, herpes zoster, vernal/allergic conjunctivitis)

States, *Candida* spp. and *Aspergillus* spp. are most frequently isolated in fungal keratitis, whereas *Fusarium* spp. predominates in the southern United States.[9,16–18] In two series of fungal keratitis from southern Florida, *Fusarium solani* was the most commonly isolated organism.[3,19] In a more recent study by Rosa et al.,[20] *Fusarium oxysporum* was the most common species (37%), followed by *Fusarium solani* (24%) using the McGinnis classification scheme.[21] In the same study, *Candida* spp., *Curvularia* spp., and *Aspergillis* spp. were the next most common fungal isolates in order of decreasing frequency. *Fusarium* spp. has been reported as an isolate in fungal keratitis in many regions of the world, including the Americas, Europe, Africa, India, China, and Japan.[22–27] The largest series of fungal keratitis outside of southern Florida are reported from India, with the most common fungal isolates being *Aspergillus* spp. (27–64%), followed by *Penicillium* spp. (2–29%), *Fusarium* spp. (6–32%), and a number of other rare organisms.[24,28–33] With newer methods for DNA molecular identification, such as polymerase chain reaction (PCR), the classification of fungi known to be ocular pathogens will likely change.[34–36] Numerous case reports of less usual organisms have been reported as a cause of fungal keratitis. Proper identification is important for future exposure prevention and determining the best treatment modalities.[37–43]

Risk Factors

For the onset of fungal keratitis, trauma is the most frequent risk factor (Box 82.2), and in a study from Miami, trauma was the major risk factor in 44% of patients.[21] Trauma most often occurs outdoors and involves plant matter. Gardeners using motorized lawn mowers and trimmers are specially predisposed.[21,44,45] Fungi also may be responsible for some cases of microbial keratitis associated with contact lens wear.[2,3,5,21,45–48] Starting in 2005, an increase in fungal keratitis caused by *Fusarium* spp. was observed in contact lens wearers and was linked to the contact lens solution ReNu with MoistureLoc.[4,7] Several studies reported on patients affected by this worldwide outbreak.[4,6,7,49] An epidemiological investigation of *Fusarium* keratitis identified 164 cases in 33 states and 1 US territory. The median age of affected patients was 41 years; 94% wore soft contact lenses. One-third of eyes required corneal transplantation. A case-control study of 45 cases and 78 controls found that cases were significantly more likely to report using ReNu with MoistureLoc as a solution to clean and store soft contact (odds ratio, 13.3; 95% confidence interval, 3.1–119.5). No fungal contamination of the MoistureLoc product was found as *Fusarium* was not recovered from the factory, warehouse, solution filtrate, or unopened solution bottles.[4] A potential explanation for the increased risk seen with MoistureLoc is its loss of in vitro fungistatic activity after prolonged temperature elevation.[50] Since MoistureLoc was permanently withdrawn from the market in May 2006, fungal keratitis levels have returned to pre-outbreak levels. Although *Fusarium* was the predominant fungi found in association with soft contact lens wear, other fungi such as *Acremonium*, *Alternaria*, *Aspergillus*, *Candida*, *Collectotrichum*, and *Curvularia* species were also found. Fungi have been shown to grow within the matrix of soft contact lenses.[51,52] Wilhemus et al.[53] and Wilhemus[54] reported fungal infection in 4 of 90 (4%) cosmetic (phakic and aphakic) contact lens wearers and in 4 of 15 (27%) therapeutic lens users. Filamentous fungi are more commonly associated with cosmetic lens wear, and yeasts with therapeutic lens use.[55] In spite of these findings, bacterial infections are still more common than fungal ones in the setting of contact lens-associated keratitis.

The use of topical corticosteroids has been associated with the development and worsening of fungal keratitis.[56–59] They appear to activate and increase the virulence of fungi.[60,61] Systemic use of corticosteroids may predispose the patient to fungal keratitis by rendering the patient immunosuppressed. Topical anesthetic abuse has also been associated as a risk factor.[62] More recently, topical moxifloxacin was found to be a risk factor for fungal keratitis in a retrospective case-control study comparing patients with fungal (n = 29) and bacterial keratitis (n = 82).[63] Furthermore, 13 of 32 moxifloxacin bottles grew fungus on culture. Other less common risk factors for fungal keratitis include vernal or allergic keratoconjunctivitis, incisional refractive surgery, neurotrophic ulcers secondary to varicella-zoster or herpes simplex viruses, keratoplasty, and amniotic membrane transplantation.[64–68] Predisposing factors for the development of fungal keratitis in patients after keratoplasty include suture problems, topical steroid use, antibiotic use, contact lens wear, graft failure, and persistent epithelial defects.[69–73] The contamination of donor corneas is of special concern because no antifungal is routinely used in the preparation of the donor globe or in the solution used to preserve the tissue before transplantation.[74,75] Routine culture of donor rims and media may aid in the identification of the organism and prompt initiation of antifungal treatment.[76] Fungal keratitis has been recently reported associated to refractive surgery.[77,78] It can occur in the immediate postoperative period or later. The early form may be associated with the direct surgical contamination of the cornea. The late form is usually associated with trauma.[79] In one case it was associated with contamination from a pet.[80] Trauma has not been clearly identified in these cases, and they represent the ability of organisms to penetrate through diseased epithelium directly into the stroma, avoiding Bowman's layer.[67,81,82] Delayed diagnosis also plays a role in the outcome of fungal keratitis after refractive surgery.[83–85] It has also been reported after enhancement procedures.[86]

Some systemic diseases may increase the risk for the development of fungal keratitis, especially diseases associated with immunosuppression. One series reported a 12% incidence of diabetes mellitus in a group of patients with fungal keratitis; the incidence of diabetes mellitus in the United States is estimated to be only 1% of the population.[21,87] Patients chronically ill and hospitalized in intensive care units also may be predisposed to the development of fungal keratitis, usually with *Candida* spp. In a series from Africa, HIV-positive patients were more likely to develop fungal keratitis compared to non-HIV patients.[88] In patients with leprosy, fungal ulcers may be more common.[89]

Fungal keratitis in children is rare and is seen when trauma with organic matter has taken place. In one series, fungal keratitis composed 18% of all cases of keratitis cultured in children.[81] In most cases, it is impossible to establish the initial event because history is unavailable. All children with a suspected keratitis should be cultured for fungi, as discussed in the section on laboratory diagnosis.[90]

Clinical Features

The symptoms of fungal keratitis may not present as acutely as with other forms of microbial keratitis, especially bacterial. Patients may report the initial symptom of a foreign body sensation for several days with a slow onset of increasing pain. The most frequently encountered external and slit lamp signs of fungal keratitis are commonly seen in other forms of microbial keratitis and include suppuration, conjunctival injection, epithelial defect, stromal infiltration, and anterior chamber reaction or hypopyon (Box 82.3). Some findings such as elevated areas, hypate (branching) ulcers, irregular feathery margins, a dry rough texture, and satellite lesions (Figs 82.1-82.5),[91] can be helpful in suggesting the diagnosis keratitis caused by filamentous fungi. The appearance of macroscopic brown pigmentation in fungal keratitis may be due to the presence of a dematiaceous fungus (*Curvularia lunata*) (Fig. 82.6).[92] The presence of an intact epithelium with a deep stromal infiltrate may also be found in fungal keratitis (Fig. 82.7). Despite these descriptive findings, studies to assess the clinical manifestations of suppurative (bacterial) versus fungal keratitis have demonstrated that it was not possible to differentiate clinically between

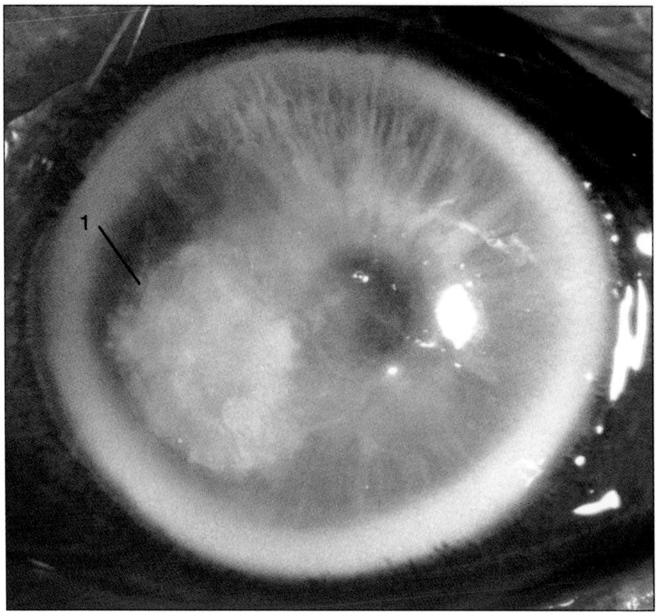

Fig. 82.1 Stromal infiltrate in fungal keratitis. Note feathering margins (*1*).

Box 82.3 Presenting clinical features of fungal keratitis

Nonspecific
- Conjunctival injection
- Epithelial defect
- Anterior chamber reaction

Specific
- Infiltrate:
- Feathery margins
- Gray/brown pigmentation
- Elevated edges
- Rough texture
- Satellite lesions

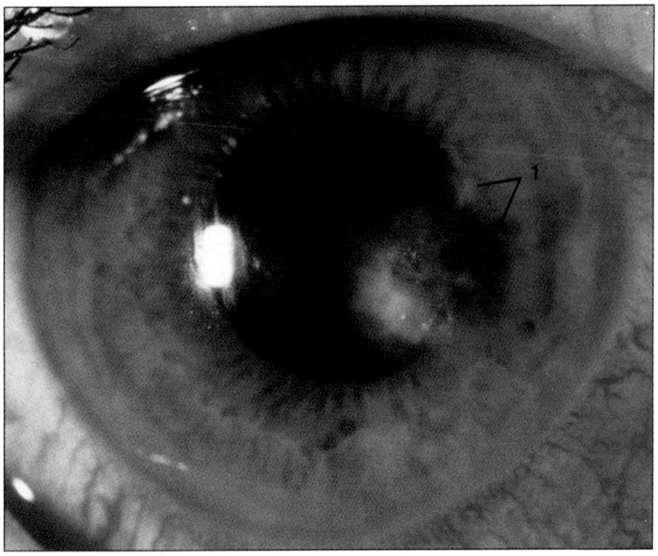

Fig. 82.2 Fungal keratitis with satellite lesions (*1*).

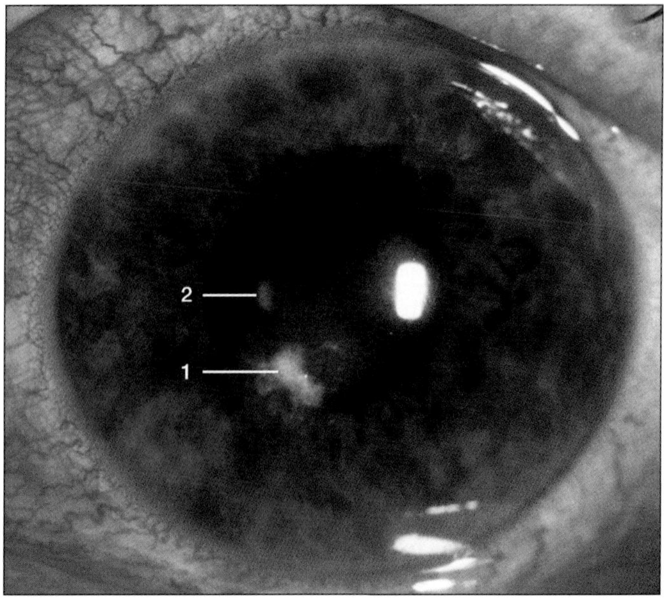

Fig. 82.4 Dry rough texture (*1*), satellite lesions (*2*).

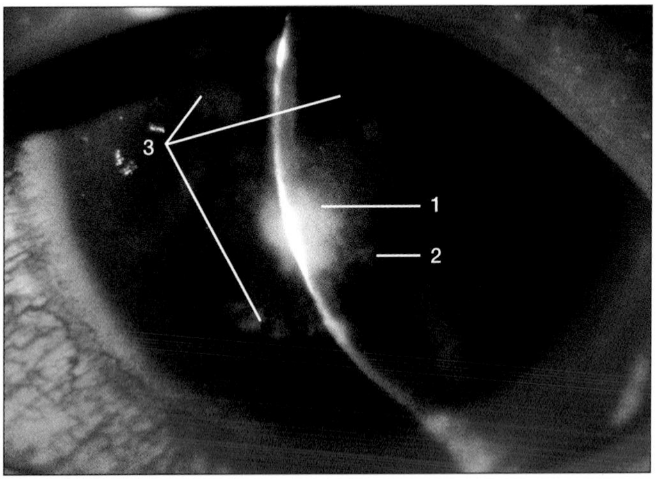

Fig. 82.3 Fungal keratitis with nummular midstromal infiltrate (*1*) with irregular feathery margins (*2*) and satellite lesions (*3*).

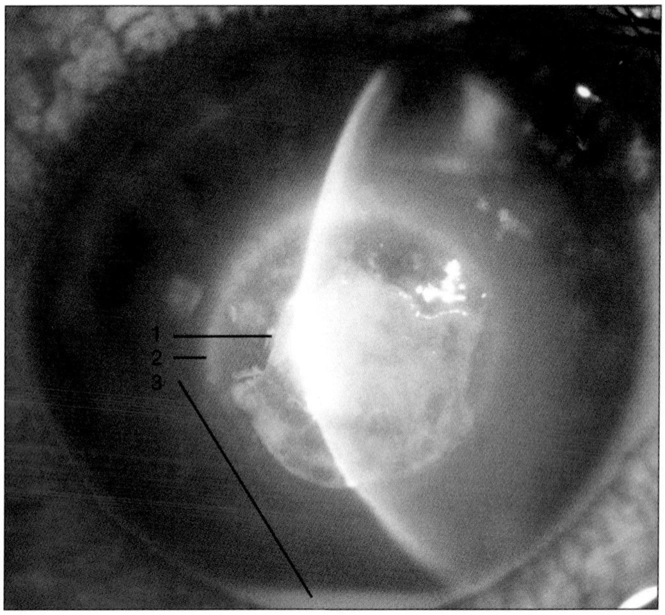

Fig. 82.5 Elevated corneal lesion (*1*), gray/dirty white surface, a ring infiltrate (*2*), and a hypopyon (*3*).

bacterial and fungal keratitis, especially in cases where yeasts are the infecting fungi.[93]

The confocal microscope is a useful clinical tool for the diagnosis of fungal keratitis. Its use is currently limited, even though the instrument is commercially available. The limitations to its current use are the cost of the instrument and the lack of clinical experience with its use. With increasing availability, these two barriers may be overcome.[94–97]

Laboratory Diagnosis

Because it is difficult to clinically establish a diagnosis of fungal keratitis, the use of smears and cultures is of extreme importance. The Gram and Giemsa stains are the most common initial stains used for the rapid identification of fungi. Initial studies reported the detection of hyphal fragments of filamentous fungi, blastopores, or pseudohyphae of yeasts in 78% of smears of fungal keratitis.[98] More recent studies suggest that the percentages of positive smears revealing fungal elements are less than previously reported (27–33% versus 43–66%, respectively).[3,19,21,98] Other methods of examining smears in patients with suspected fungal keratitis are potassium hydroxide (10–20%) wet mounts,[99] acridine orange staining, Grocott's methenaminesilver technique,[100] lectins,[101] and calcofluor white preparations.[102–106]

Culture media for suspected fungal keratitis should include the same culture media used for a general infectious keratitis work-up. These include sheep blood agar, chocolate agar, Sabouraud's dextrose agar, and thioglycollate broth.

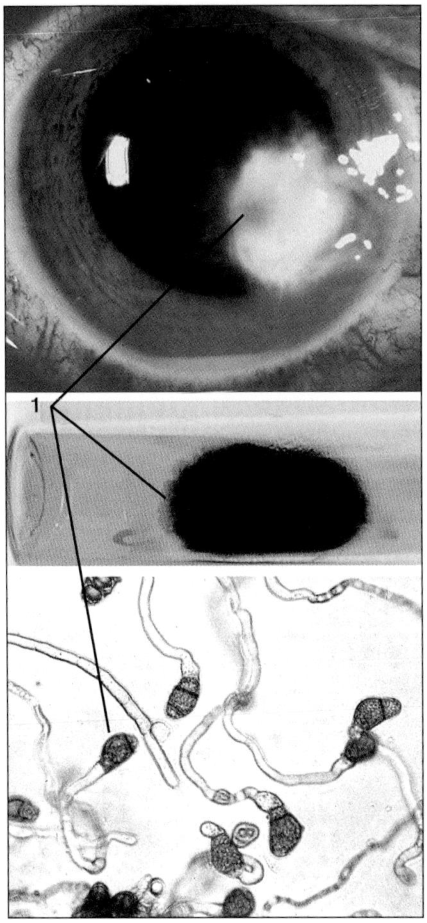

Fig. 82.6 *Curvularia* keratitis showing brown pigmentation (*1*) in the corneal infiltrate (*top*), culture (*middle*), and slide preparation (*bottom*). (Courtesy Mario Brunzini, MD.)

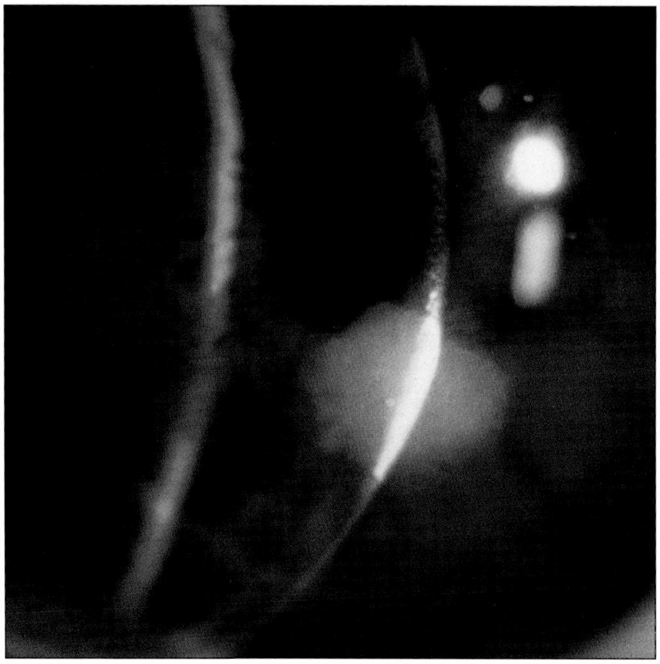

Fig. 82.7 *Candida* keratitis with overlying intact epithelium.

Positive cultures should be expected in 90% of cases. Initial growth occurs within 72 hours in 83% of cultures and within 1 week in 97% of cultures.[21] Because both yeast and hyphae readily grow in sheep blood agar and Sabouraud's dextrose agar at room temperature, other media such as brain-heart infusion need not be used initially, unless the clinical suspicion for fungal keratitis is high.[95] Excellent recovery rates of fungal isolates with brain-heart infusion broth or solid media have been obtained, especially when constant agitation of the liquid medium is used.[98,105,107] Increasing the humidity of the medium by placing the inoculated agar plates in plastic bags has also been recommended for enhancement of fungal growth.[108] Other less widely used methods for the identification of fungi include immunofluorescence staining, electron microscopy, and polymerase chain reaction (PCR).[34,109–113] These newer methods will provide a more sensitive and specific identification as well as providing immediate information on pathogenesis and treatment.

Along with assisting in a diagnosis, scraping also provides for initial debridement of organisms and of epithelium, which can improve penetration of the antifungal medication. We have also used a diamond-tipped motorized burr to obtain the scrapings. If corneal scrapings for smears and cultures are negative, a diagnostic superficial keratectomy or corneal biopsy may prove necessary. The biopsy can be performed in the minor operating room or at the slit lamp after topical anesthesia using tetracaine, proparacaine, or lidocaine. In some cases, eyelid and retrobulbar anesthesia may be required. Under the microscope, a round 2–3-mm sterile disposable dermatologic trephine is advanced into the anterior corneal stroma to incorporate both clinically infected and adjacent clear cornea. Care is taken to avoid the visual axis if possible. The base is then undermined with a surgical blade to complete the lamellar keratectomy.[114,115] The femtosecond laser has also been used to obtain biopsy specimens.[116,117] The main advantages of the laser include the uniformity and size of the corneal button created and the potential for less induced astigmatism. Its main disadvantages are the cost and availability of the laser. The corneal biopsy specimen should be submitted for smears, cultures, and histopathologic examination. In some cases of deep keratitis with an intact overlying epithelium and stroma, a 27-gauge hypodermic needle or a 6-0 silk suture can be introduced into the infiltrate to obtain a specimen for culture. Corneal biopsy is superior to scraping for recovering fungi. In animal experiments, corneal scrapings found 3 of 10 specimens positive for *C. albicans*, 5 of 10 for *F. solani*, and 6 of 10 for *A. fumigatus*; corneal biopsy specimens demonstrated fungal elements in all inoculated eyes.[118] Furthermore, comparing the value of direct examination and culture of biopsy specimens, cultures found 7 of 10 specimens positive for *C. albicans* and 8 of 10 for *F. solani* and *A. fumigatus*; direct examination demonstrated culture-positive fungal elements in all specimens.[119] Alexandrakis et al.[114] also demonstrated an increased recovery rate of organisms from corneal biopsy specimens from recalcitrant culture-negative cases. In a series of fungal keratitis, Rosa et al.[20] reported a 78% culture-positive rate from corneal biopsies performed in initial cases of keratitis. Cultures of the biopsied specimens in two patients with suspected recurrent fungal keratitis were negative, resulting in cessation of antifungal therapy and resolution.

An anterior chamber tap may be useful in the isolation of fungal organisms that may have penetrated through an intact Descemet's membrane. Under aseptic conditions, the hypopyon and/or endothelial plaque can be aspirated and submitted for laboratory examination.[120]

It is important to submit surgical specimens from cases of microbial keratitis for histopathologic examination, especially if the microbiologic diagnosis is not known. Histopathologic examination of corneal buttons can reveal the presence of fungal elements in 75% of patients.[20] It has been shown that 59% of corneas infected by fungi are still culture-positive at the time of keratoplasty, with 90% of eyes exhibiting hyphal elements on pathologic examination.[121] Fungal hyphae usually lie parallel to the corneal surface and lamellae.[122–124] A vertical or perpendicular arrangement of fungal hyphae in the corneal stroma has been associated with increased virulence and in patients on topical corticosteroid therapy.[123,124] Descemet's membrane may function as a barrier for invasion of microorganisms; however, fungi have been shown to penetrate through an intact Descemet's membrane.[122,123]

Fungi also have been removed from topically applied medications, cosmetics, contact lenses, and their storage and cleaning solutions in patients with fungal keratitis. These items should be obtained from the patient at the initial visit. Cultures and smears can be obtained to increase the chances of identifying the causative organism.[125–128]

With the advent of molecular diagnostic techniques, the manner by which fungal keratitis is detected may change. The superiority of molecular diagnostics over currently used techniques has been demonstrated in several studies.[34,129,130] Polymerase chain reaction was compared to microbial culture in 108 consecutive corneal ulcers.[130] A positive PCR for fungi was obtained in 29 of 31 culture-positive samples, with good concordance between the culture and PCR results. A positive PCR result was also obtained in 46 of 52 culture-negative samples, of which 28 were fungal products.[130] Oechsler et al. evaluated molecular sequence analysis of nuclear ribosomal RNA internal transcribed spacer regions for the detection and differentiation of *Fusarium* spp.[34] They were able to identify *Fusarium* as the causative pathogen in 15 of 58 ocular specimens, 75% of which were *F. solani* and 16% of which were *F. oxysporum*. Furthermore, they demonstrated that molecular sequence analysis correctly identified subspecies with more accuracy than morphologic classifications. So far, these comparisons have been performed in research or academic centers. Lack of commercial detection kits, expense of equipment, and shortage of skilled personnel will make the transition to routine microbiology laboratories more difficult but necessary to improve the speed of identification, sensitivity, and specificity and to reduce the morbidity associated with the current delayed identification.

Medical Therapy

It is often difficult for a clinician faced with the possibility of a fungal keratitis to decide both which antifungal to use and the route of administration. O'Day has pointed out that current selection of antifungals is based on animal experiments, clinical experience, and published sensitivity data (Table 82.1).[108] In vitro sensitivity testing of a particular isolate is rarely indicated.[131] The data obtained from individual testing are difficult to interpret, and the tests are expensive to set up. In addition, by the time results are obtained, the clinical appearance of the keratitis will determine whether it is responding to medical treatment or whether surgery is indicated. Recent studies suggest that careful clinical monitoring of the infiltrate and antifungal testing may play a role in the outcome of the treatment.[132]

Many chemicals have been tried for the treatment of fungal keratitis.[133] These have ranged from antiseptics to antibiotics. Four groups of compounds have become the principal drugs for the treatment of fungal disease (Table 82.2). These are the polyenes, the azoles (imidazoles and triazoles), the pyrimidines, and the echinocandins. Among the polyenes, the most commonly used compounds have been amphotericin B and natamycin. The only commercially available topical antifungal in the United States is natamycin 5%. Most other topical antifungals must be prepared extemporaneously.[134] In a study from southern Florida, natamycin was the initial topical antifungal agent used in 91% (107/118) of patients.[19] Jones et al.[135] reported 18 consecutive cases of *F. solani* keratitis treated successfully with natamycin.[134] In cases of *Candida* spp., amphotericin B may be the drug of choice (see Table 82.1).[108,133,136,137] A 0.15% concentration of topical amphotericin B is usually sufficient to treat fungal keratitis and to avoid ocular toxicity from higher concentrations.[138]

Among the azoles, the most commonly used compounds have been topical voriconazole and oral ketoconazole and itraconazole. Vemulakonda et al. analyzed the aqueous and vitreous penetration of topically administered voriconazole 1% (1 drop every 2 hours for 1 day) in noninflamed human eyes undergoing planned vitrecomy.[139] The aqueous and vitreous levels exceeded or met the MIC_{90} for most pathogens, demonstrating that voriconazole can be suitable as an ophthalmic drop. Several clinical case reports have reported on the successful use of voriconazole on fungal keratitis which failed to respond to conventional agents.[140] Most patients were treated with a combination of topical, oral, and intravenous voriconazole. However, there is ongoing debate on whether voriconazole's in vivo effect is as good as predicted by in vitro studies. Marangon et al. reported that while voriconazole had good in vitro susceptibility, it was not effective as a topical 1% solution in two patients with keratitis, one with *Fusarium* species and the other with *Colletotrichum*.[141] Voriconazole (50 μg/0.1 mL) has also been used successfully as an intrastromal injection in three patients with deep fungal keratitis recalcitrant to topical therapy alone.[142] Data on the use of posaconazole in the treatment of fungal keratitis is limited; a few case reports described rapid resolution of infection after oral posaconazole was used as salvage therapy.[140,143,144] Miconazole is the drug of choice for *Paecilomyces* spp.[133]

The echinocandins (caspofungin and micafungin) have also been used in the treatment of fungal keratitis. Topical caspofungin 0.5% in conjunction with intrastromal voriconazole successfully treated a patient with *Alternaria* keratitis.[145] Likewise, micafungin 0.1%, used as a single

Table 82.1 Antimicrobial activity of antifungal agents based on published reports

Antifungal agent	*Alternaria*	*Aspergillus*	*Candida*	*Cephalosporium*	*Cladosporium*	*Curvularia*	*Fusarium*	*Paecilomyces*	*Penicillium*
Polyenes									
Amphotericin	S	S	S		S	S	S	R	S
Nystatin		S	S						S
Natamycin		S	S	S	S		S	R	
Imidazoles									
Clotrimazole	S	S	S		S	S	I	S	
Miconazole		S	S		S		I	I	
Econazole		S	I		S		S	I	
Ketoconazole		I	S		S		S		S
Fluconazole		S	S						
Itraconazole		I	I			I	R	R	
Voriconazole		S	S			S	I	S	
Posaconazole		S	S				I		
Pyrimidines									
5-Fluorocytosine	R	S		S		R	R	I	

Modified from Benson WH, Lanier JD. Ophthalmology 99:800–804, 1992.
S, susceptible; I, variable susceptibility; R, resistant.

agent, successfully treated three patients with *Candida* keratitis.[146]

Several topical antifungal medications may act synergistically against a particular fungal organism.[147–150] Amphotericin B 0.15% and subconjunctival rifampin were more effective than amphotericin alone.[151] Amphotericin B and flucytosine (5-flurocytosine) have synergistic effects.[152] Natamycin and ketoconazole have been used effectively in an animal model of *Aspergillus* keratitis.[148] Likewise, experimental models have demonstrated the potential antagonism between antifungals such as amphotericin B and the imidazoles. Antagonism also has been described when amphotericin B and the imidazoles have been used systemically.[153] Clinically, it is difficult to interpret these studies because they are performed in vitro or in animals.[135] Resistance to an antifungal is rare except in the case of flucytosine, in which resistance has been documented when used for systemic mycoses and could potentially occur if used alone for the topical treatment of yeast keratitis.[154] Competition for volume in the precorneal tear film and washout may be of more concern when using two topical antifungals. In clinical series, more than one concurrent topical antifungal has been needed 5% of the time.[19]

Clinically, commercially available natamycin 5% suspension is the initial drug of choice for fungal keratitis. If worsening of the keratitis is observed on topical natamycin, topical amphotericin B 0.15% can be substituted in cases of *Candida* spp. keratitis and *Apergillus* keratitis. An oral or topical azole can be substituted or added in cases *Fusarium* spp. keratitis. The length of time required for topical treatment has not been firmly established clinically or experimentally. Guidelines have been derived from retrospective clinical reviews. Jones et al.[135] reported an average of 30 days of treatment for *Fusarium* keratitis with natamycin.[115] The average length of treatment with topical treatment was 39 days.[19] In general, the length of treatment is longer than that for cases of bacterial keratitis. The clinician must determine the length of treatment for each individual based on clinical response. Problems that can arise from prolonged treatment are due to toxicity. The inflammatory response from this toxicity can be confused with persistent infection. If toxicity is suspected and if adequate treatment has been given for at least 4 to 6 weeks, treatment should be discontinued and the patient carefully observed for evidence of recurrence.

Subconjunctival injections of antifungal agents are not routinely used in the treatment of fungal keratitis because of toxicity and the intense pain induced. Miconazole is perhaps the least toxic and best-tolerated antifungal agent (5–10 mg of 10 mg/mL suspension).[107,136,155] Subconjunctival injections should be reserved for cases of severe keratitis,

Table 82.2 Classification and doses of antifungals

Antifungal	Eyedrop	Intracameral	Intravitreal	Oral	Intravenous
Polyenes					
Amphotericin B	0.15–0.20%	0.8–1.0 mg	5 μg/0.1 mL		0.5–0.7 mg/kg
Natamycin	5%				
Azoles					
Econazole	2%				
Miconazole	1%	5 mg /0.5 mL	25–50 μg/0.1 mL		
Ketoconazole				200–400 mg daily	
Fluconazole	0.2%			100–400 mg daily	200–400 mg daily
Itraconazole	1%		5 μg/0.05 mL	200–400 mg daily	200 mg daily
Voriconazole	1%		50–200 μg/0.1 mL	200 mg twice daily	3–6 mg/kg twice daily
Posaconazole	4%			200 mg three times daily	
Pyrimidines					
5-Fluorocytosine				25–37.5 mg/kg/day four times daily	
Allylamines					
Terbinafine				250 mg daily	
Echinocandins					
Caspofungin	0.5%				50 mg daily
Micafungin	0.1%				

scleritis, and endophthalmitis.[156] Corneal intrastromal injections of agents such as voriconazole are used when the infiltrate is recalcitrant to topical treatment or due to its depth into the cornea. Likewise, intraocular injections into the anterior chamber are now more commonly used. The use of systemic antifungal agents is generally not indicated in the management of fungal keratitis, but can be considered for deep lesions that do not respond adequately to topical therapy. Several clinical and experimental studies have reported favorable results in the treatment of fungal keratitis with systemic ketoconazole, itraconazole, miconazole, fluconazole, voriconazole, and posaconazole.[140,157–162] A commonly used first choice for an oral antifungal agent is voriconazole as it has a favorable side-effect profile. Treatment with a systemic antifungal agent is recommended in cases of severe deep keratitis, scleritis, and endophthalmitis. Systemic antifungals also may be used as prophylactic treatment after penetrating keratoplasty for fungal keratitis.

The corneal epithelium serves as a barrier to the penetration of most topical antifungal agents. Debridement of the corneal epithelium is an essential component of the medical management of fungal keratitis, especially early in the course of treatment. O'Day et al. have demonstrated experimentally that corneal debridement significantly increases the antifungal effect of topical antifungals.[163,164]

Antibiotics have also been evaluated as potential fungicidal agents in vitro.[165] Chloramphenicol had some activity against both *Fusarium* and *Aspergillus*, and moxifloxacin and tobramycin had activity against *Fusarium*. In the recent epidemic of soft contact lens related *Fusarium* keratis, several cases had clinical resolution with the use of topical fluoroquinolones.[166] However, these effects were modest compared to the MIC_{90} of antifungal agents. Antiseptics have received a mixed review in the literature as to their effectiveness in the treatment of fungal keratitis. Povidone-iodine, polyhexamethylene biguanide and others have been used in animal models.[167,168] Chlorhexidine has been suggested as a potential treatment for fungal keratitis.[169]

Other potential antifungal treatments have been evaluated in animal models. Collagen shields have been soaked in amphotericin to increase the concentration of the drug in the initial treatment periods (in *Aspergillus* keratomycosis).[170] The excimer laser has been used in rabbits to ablate surface infection of fungal organisms.[171] Garg et al.[172] showed the potential fungistatic capabilities of tissue glue. Collagen cross-linking has been suggested as a potential adjunct to medical therapy. Future treatment modalities will hopefully be based on better understanding of the pathophysiology of fungal keratitis. As we gain more knowledge at the molecular level, better medical treatments will become available.[173] Future medical therapy will also be directed at control of the damage caused by fungal mycotoxins. Mycotoxins exhibit varying degrees of toxicity in human and animal cell lines and most likely have a role in the pathogenesis and tissue destruction associated with mycotic keratitis infections.[174]

The use of topical corticosteroids in the treatment of fungal keratitis must be approached cautiously. O'Day et al. reported that the efficacy of amphotericin B appeared unaffected when used in conjunction with topical 1% prednisolone acetate in a rabbit model of *Candida* spp. keratitis.[175,176] However, the topical corticosteroid worsened the disease when given alone and adversely influenced the efficacy of natamycin, flucytosine, and miconazole when given in combination. In another series, 15% (19/125) of patients received topical corticosteroids (for an average of 24 days) to decrease corneal inflammation and scarring after the diagnosis of fungal keratitis had been established and after an average of 2 weeks of antifungal therapy had been completed. Two patients worsened after starting topical corticosteroids within 1 to 3 days of beginning topical antifungal therapy. Previous to this study, Stern and Buttross had concluded that topical corticosteroids were contraindicated in the treatment of fungal keratitis.[177] An animal study model of *Candida* keratitis suggests that topical steroids started after the infectious keratitis has been controlled may be beneficial.[178] Our current regimen is to not consider topical steroids until after at least 2 weeks of antifungal treatment and clear clinical evidence of control of the infection. Careful follow-up is required to ensure that improvement is taking place. The steroid drop is used in conjunction with the topical antifungal and never without. Usually, steroid treatment is carried on for 2 to 3 weeks.

Surgical Therapy

Fungal keratitis is a surgical disease in most parts of the world because of the delay in initiating medical treatment or the inability to obtain antifungal medications. Daily debridement with a spatula or blade is the simplest form of surgical intervention and is usually performed at the slit lamp under topical anesthesia. Debridement is performed every 24 to 48 hours and works by debulking organisms and necrotic material and by enhancing the penetration of the topical antifungal. A biopsy may be used not only for diagnosis but also as a therapeutic intervention.[179] Approximately one-third of fungal infections result in either medical treatment failures or corneal perforations.[121]

The majority of surgical procedures reported are therapeutic penetrating keratoplasty, and a small percentage have been treated with a conjunctival flap (Fig. 82.8). A series of

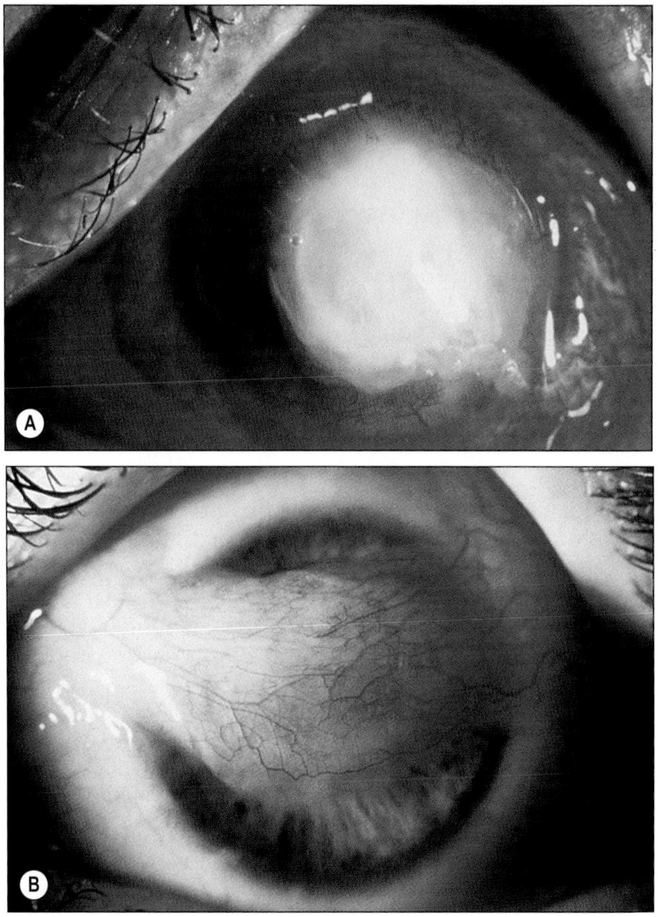

Fig. 82.8 *Fusarium* keratitis treated with conjunctival flap. (**A**) Preoperative photograph. (**B**) Postoperative photograph. (Courtesy Mario Brunzini, MD.)

patients that responded to lamellar keratoplasty have been reported in the literature.[180,181] The main goals are to control the infection and maintain the integrity of the globe. An optical keratoplasty can then be performed at a later time.[19,182] The timing of the therapeutic keratoplasty is important. Most retrospective series indicate that keratoplasty was performed within 4 weeks of presentation, primarily because of medical treatment failure; in some cases it may be required because of recurrence of infection.[20] When progression of the keratitis is noted, penetrating keratoplasty should be performed. If the infectious process is allowed to progress until it involves the limbus or sclera, unfavorable outcomes secondary to scleritis, endophthalmitis, and recurrences are more common.[180,181,183,184] Tissue adhesive can be used to delay or prevent the need for corneal transplant in patients with severe thinning or perforation. The use of N-butyl cyanoacrylate tissue adhesive and bandage contact lens was evaluated in 73 patients with fungal keratitis.[172] Outcome measures included resolution of the infiltrate and preservation of the integrity of the globe. The infiltrate resolved in 42 of 66 eyes and structural integrity was maintained in eight additional patients as a bridge to penetrating keratoplasty.

The technique of the keratoplasty is similar to that performed for other forms of microbial keratitis.[185] The size of the trephination should leave a 1–1.5 mm clear zone of clinically uninvolved cornea to reduce the possibility of residual fungal organisms peripheral to the trephination.[9,119] Interrupted sutures with slightly longer bites should be used to avoid cheese-wiring of the suture if the edge of the recipient becomes involved with a persistent organism.[119] Irrigation of the anterior segment should be performed to eliminate any organisms. Affected intraocular structures including the iris, lens, and vitreous should be excised. The specimens removed should be submitted to both the microbiology and pathology laboratories for culture and fixed-section examination. Once the infected tissue is removed, surgical instrumentation should be changed to sterile ones to avoid recontamination of the donor tissue. If involvement of intraocular structures or endophthalmitis is suspected, an antifungal agent should be injected intraocularly at the time of keratoplasty. Recommended intraocular antifungal agents include amphotericin B.

After penetrating keratoplasty, topical antifungal agents should be continued to prevent recurrence of infection (Fig. 82.9). Postoperatively, systemic antifungals such as ketoconazole, fluconazole, or voriconazole may be used in addition to topical antifungal agents.[186] If the pathology laboratory reports that no organisms were seen at the edge of the corneal specimen, antifungals could be stopped after 2 weeks and the patient followed carefully for recurrences. A report from the microbiology laboratory regarding growth of organisms from the corneal or intraocular tissues should indicate the need for more prolonged topical and systemic antifungal therapy, possibly for 6 to 8 weeks.

The use of topical corticosteroids in the postoperative management of fungal keratitis is controversial. At the time of keratoplasty, if the infection has been controlled clinically, topical corticosteroids may be used. If it is not known whether the infection is controlled, corticosteroids should be avoided during the early postoperative period.[16] Although the main goal of penetrating keratoplasty in fungal keratitis is to eliminate the infecting organism, a secondary goal is the maintenance of a clear corneal transplant for optical reasons. Even if graft failure or rejection occurs, the patient can undergo a second optical keratoplasty once the rejection is controlled.[187] The effects of other immunosuppressive medications such as ciclosporin A have been shown in the laboratory and clinically to be of help in postkeratoplasty patients. Ciclosporin A is an antifungal that can also help prevent the immune response. This dual action makes it ideal for use in this clinical condition.[188,189]

The success of therapeutic penetrating keratoplasty has been reported as better than medical therapy by several authors.[181,190] Xie et al. reported on 108 cases where penetrating keratoplasty was performed as a treatment for severe fungal keratitis that could not be cured by antifungal medication. Corneal grafts in 86 eyes remained clear during follow-up. Complications included recurrent fungal infection in eight eyes and corneal graft rejection in 32 eyes.[181] Other possible surgical modalities include conjunctival flap, flap plus keratectomy, flap plus penetrating graft, and lamellar graft.[191] Several authors have recommended excisional keratectomy and inlay conjunctival flap as the procedure of choice in fungal keratitis, especially in peripheral ulcers refractory to medical therapy.[91,192,193] This procedure and the other procedures described earlier may be particularly useful in situations in which access to topical antifungal agents and the availability of donor corneal tissue are limited. A lamellar keratoplasty is generally contraindicated in the treatment of active fungal keratitis unless it is possible to remove all the infected tissue. Otherwise, the fungal organisms can be trapped in the intralamellar space, keeping them isolated from the antifungal therapy and the host immune response, thereby leading to the potential for persistence or recurrence of the infection.[16,91,121,191]

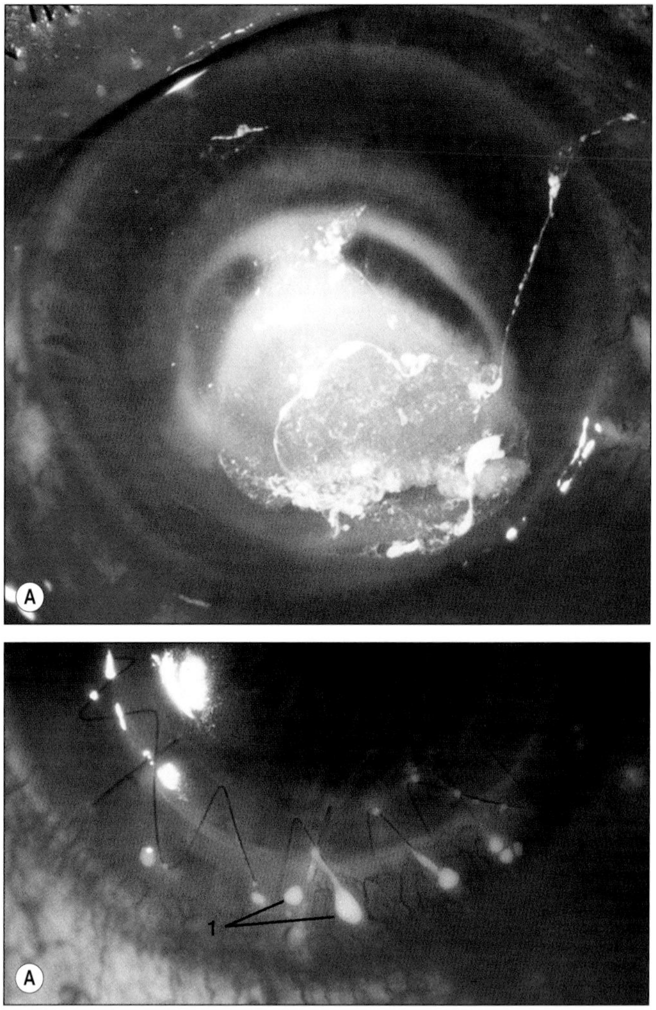

Fig. 82.9 Penetrating keratoplasty for *Candida* keratitis. (**A**) Preoperative photograph. (**B**) Postoperative photograph showing recurrence (*1*) of *Candida* in the graft.

Cryotherapy may be used in conjunction with topical antifungal agents and/or a corneoscleral graft in cases of fungal scleritis and keratoscleritis.[194] Retrobulbar anesthesia is usually required, and a conjunctival recession is performed to expose the infected sclera. Using a retinal cryoprobe, two freeze–thaw cycles of several seconds are applied primarily to the borders of the infection where the organisms are presumably replicating and invading. The area is left exposed and subconjunctival antifungals injected.[195] These patients are usually continued on both topical and systemic antifungal agents.

Considering visual rehabilitation after a treated fungal infection, a stepwise approach should be implemented beginning with spectacle correction and hard contact lenses. If these modalities fail to improve vision sufficiently, surgical procedures should be considered. In a patient with healed infection, a lamellar procedure can be considered. However, a deep anterior lamellar procedure (e.g Anwar's big bubble technique) may be preferable as it removes all the stromal tissue, decreasing the risk for residual organisms. A rotational graft can be considered for patients with off-center scars. Finally, traditional penetrating keratoplasty in patients with inactive fungal keratitis can yield successful results.

Prognosis

The prognosis of fungal keratitis varies depending on the depth and size of the lesion and the causative organism. In general, small superficial infections respond well to topical therapy. Deep stromal infections and infections with concomitant scleral or intraocular involvement are much more difficult to eradicate. One prospective, interventional study of 115 consecutive patients with fungal keratitis assessed treatment outcomes after 1 month of topical natamycin use.[196] Of 115 patients included in the study, 52 were considered treatment successes, 27 had slow-healing ulcers, and 36 were considered treatment failures. Multivariate analysis demonstrated that the three factors significantly associated with treatment failure were large ulcer size (greater than 14 mm^2), the presence of a hypopyon, and *Aspergillus* as the causative organism. Surgical therapy can prove successful when medical treatment fails,[181] or as a secondary measure to visually rehabilitate the eye.

Conclusion

In summary, the diagnosis and treatment of fungal keratitis can be quite challenging. Information derived from the microbiology laboratory is required to make a correct diagnosis. Molecular diagnosis may improve detection rates and earlier clinical diagnosis. Prolonged medical treatment and prompt timing of surgical intervention are required to increase the chances of a cure.

References

1. Koidou-Tsiligianni A, Alfonso E, Forster RK. Ulcerative keratitis associated with contact lens wear. *Am J Ophthalmol.* 1989;108(1):64–67.
2. Alfonso E, Mandelbaum S, Fox MJ, Forster RK. Ulcerative keratitis associated with contact lens wear. *Am J Ophthalmol.* 1986;101(4):429–433.
3. Liesegang TJ, Forster RK. Spectrum of microbial keratitis in south Florida. *Am J Ophthalmol.* 1980;90(1):38–47.
4. Chang DC, Grant GB, O'Donnell K, et al. Multistate outbreak of *Fusarium* keratitis associated with use of a contact lens solution. *JAMA.* 2006;296(8):953–963.
5. Alfonso EC, Cantu-Dibildox J, Munir WM, et al. Insurgence of *Fusarium* keratitis associated with contact lens wear. *Arch Ophthalmol.* 2006;124(7):941–947.
6. Gaujoux T, Chatel MA, Chaumeil C, et al. Outbreak of contact lens-related *Fusarium* keratitis in France. *Cornea.* 2008;27(9):1018–1021.
7. Ma SK, So K, Chung PH, et al. A multi-country outbreak of fungal keratitis associated with a brand of contact lens solution: the Hong Kong experience. *Int J Infect Dis.* 2008.
8. Atlas R. *Basic and practical microbiology.* New York: Macmillan; 1986.
9. Foster CS. Fungal keratitis. *Infect Dis Clin North Am.* 1992;6(4):851–857.
10. Forster RK, Rebell G. The diagnosis and management of keratomycoses. I. Cause and diagnosis. *Arch Ophthalmol.* 1975;93(10):975–978.
11. Ainley R, Smith B. Fungal flora of the conjunctival sac in healthy and diseased eyes. *Br J Ophthalmol.* 1965;49(10):505–515.
12. Ando N, Takatori K. Fungal flora of the conjunctival sac. *Am J Ophthalmol.* 1982;94(1):67–74.
13. Hammeke JC, Ellis PP. Mycotic flora of the conjunctiva. *Am J Ophthalmol.* 1960;49:1174–1178.
14. Williamson J, Gordon AM, Wood R, et al. Fungal flora of the conjunctival sac in health and disease. Influence of topical and systemic steroids. *Br J Ophthalmol.* 1968;52(2):127–137.
15. Wilson LA, Ahearn DG, Jones DB, Sexton RR. Fungi from the normal outer eye. *Am J Ophthalmol.* 1969;67(1):52–56.
16. Jones D. Diagnosis and management of fungal keratitis. In: Tasman W, Jaeger EA, eds. *Duane's clinical ophthalmology.* Vol. 4. Philadelphia: JB Lippincott; 1993.
17. Chin GN, Hyndiuk RA, Kwasny GP, Schultz RO. Keratomycosis in Wisconsin. *Am J Ophthalmol.* 1975;79(1):121–125.
18. Doughman DJ, Leavenworth NM, Campbell RC, Lindstrom RL. Fungal keratitis at the University of Minnesota: 1971–1981. *Trans Am Ophthalmol Soc.* 1982;80:235–247.
19. Jones DB, Sexton R, Rebell G. Mycotic keratitis in south Florida: a review of thirty-nine cases. *Trans Ophthalmol Soc UK.* 1970;89:781–797.
20. Rosa RH Jr, Miller D, Alfonso EC. The changing spectrum of fungal keratitis in south Florida. *Ophthalmology.* 1994;101(6):1005–1013.
21. McGinnis M. *Laboratory handbook of medical mycology.* New York: Academic Press; 1980.
22. Gugnani HC, Talwar RS, Njoku-Obi AN, Kodilinye HC. Mycotic keratitis in Nigeria. A study of 21 cases. *Br J Ophthalmol.* 1976;60(9):607–613.
23. Khairallah SH, Byrne KA, Tabbara KF. Fungal keratitis in Saudi Arabia. *Doc Ophthalmol.* 1992;79(3):269–276.
24. Srinivasan R, Kanungo R, Goyal JL. Spectrum of oculomycosis in South India. *Acta Ophthalmol (Copenh).* 1991;69(6):744–749.
25. Cuero RG. Ecological distribution of *Fusarium solani* and its opportunistic action related to mycotic keratitis in Cali, Colombia. *J Clin Microbiol.* 1980;12(3):455–461.
26. Hemo I, Pe'er J, Polacheck I. *Fusarium oxysporum* keratitis. *Ophthalmologica.* 1989;198(1):3–7.
27. Zapater RC, Arrechea A. Mycotic keratitis by *Fusarium*. A review and report of two cases. *Ophthalmologica.* 1975;170(1):1–12.
28. Gopinathan U, Garg P, Fernandes M, et al. The epidemiological features and laboratory results of fungal keratitis: a 10-year review at a referral eye care center in South India. *Cornea.* 2002;21(6):555–559.
29. Leck AK, Thomas PA, Hagan M, et al. Aetiology of suppurative corneal ulcers in Ghana and south India, and epidemiology of fungal keratitis. *Br J Ophthalmol.* 2002;86(11):1211–1215.
30. Poria VC, Bharad VR, Dongre DS, Kulkarni MV. Study of mycotic keratitis. *Indian J Ophthalmol.* 1985;33(4):229–231.
31. Reddy PS, Satyendran OM, Satapathy M, et al. Mycotic keratitis. *Indian J Ophthalmol.* 1972;20(3):101–108.
32. Grover S, Jagtap P, Sharma KD. Mycotic keratitis. *Indian J Ophthalmol.* 1975;23(2):7–10.
33. Sundaram BM, Badrinath S, Subramanian S. Studies on mycotic keratitis. *Mycoses.* 1989;32(11):568–572.
34. Oechsler RA, Feilmeier MR, Ledee D, et al. Utility of molecular sequence analysis of the ITS rRNA region for identification of *Fusarium* spp. from ocular sources. *Invest Ophthalmol Vis Sci.* 2009;50:2230–2236.
35. Alfonso EC. Genotypic identification of *Fusarium* species from ocular sources: comparison to morphologic classification and antifungal sensitivity testing (an AOS thesis). *Trans Am Ophthalmol Soc.* 2008;106:227–239.
36. Bagyalakshmi R, Therese KL, Prasanna S, Madhavan HN. Newer emerging pathogens of ocular non-sporulating molds (NSM) identified by polymerase chain reaction (PCR)-based DNA sequencing technique targeting internal transcribed spacer (ITS) region. *Curr Eye Res.* 2008;33(2):139–147.
37. Wilhelmus KR, Jones DB. *Curvularia* keratitis. *Trans Am Ophthalmol Soc.* 2001;99:111–130; discussion 30–32.
38. Rishi K, Font RL. Keratitis caused by an unusual fungus, *Phoma* species. *Cornea.* 2003;22(2):166–168.
39. Guarro J, Hofling-Lima AL, Gene J, et al. Corneal ulcer caused by the new fungal species *Sarcopodium oculorum.* *J Clin Microbiol.* 2002;40(8):3071–3075.
40. Wu Z, Ying H, Yiu S, et al. Fungal keratitis caused by *Scedosporium apiospermum*: report of two cases and review of treatment. *Cornea.* 2002;21(5):519–523.

41. Shin JY, Kim HM, Hong JW. Keratitis caused by *Verticillium* species. *Cornea.* 2002;21(2):240–242.
42. Yamamoto N, Matsumoto T, Ishibashi Y. Fungal keratitis caused by *Colletotrichum gloeosporioides*. *Cornea.* 2001;20(8):902–903.
43. Jani BR, Rinaldi MG, Reinhart WJ. An unusual case of fungal keratitis: *Metarrhizium anisopliae*. *Cornea.* 2001;20(7):765–768.
44. Clinch TE, Robinson MJ, Barron BA, et al. Fungal keratitis from nylon line lawn trimmers. *Am J Ophthalmol.* 1992;114(4):437–440.
45. Strelow SA, Kent HD, Eagle RC Jr, Cohen EJ. A case of contact lens related *Fusarium solani* keratitis. *CLAO J.* 1992;18(2):125–127.
46. Alfonso EC, Miller D, Cantu-Dibildox J, et al. Fungal keratitis associated with non-therapeutic soft contact lenses. *Am J Ophthalmol.* 2006;142(1):154–155.
47. Kremer I, Goldenfeld M, Shmueli D. Fungal keratitis associated with contact lens wear after penetrating keratoplasty. *Ann Ophthalmol.* 1991;23(9):342–345.
48. Yamamoto GK, Pavan-Langston D, Stowe GC 3rd, Albert DM. Fungal invasion of a therapeutic soft contact lens and cornea. *Ann Ophthalmol.* 1979;11(11):1731–1735.
49. Rao SK, Lam PT, Li EY, et al. A case series of contact lens-associated *Fusarium* keratitis in Hong Kong. *Cornea.* 2007;26(10):1205–1209.
50. Bullock JD, Warwar RE, Elder BL, Northern WI. Temperature instability of ReNu with MoistureLoc: a new theory to explain the worldwide *Fusarium* keratitis epidemic of 2004–2006. *Arch Ophthalmol.* 2008;126(11):1493–1498.
51. Churner R, Cunningham RD. Fungal-contaminated soft contact lenses. *Ann Ophthalmol.* 1983;15(8):724–727.
52. Berger RO, Streeten BW. Fungal growth in aphakic soft contact lenses. *Am J Ophthalmol.* 1981;91(5):630–633.
53. Wilhelmus KR, Robinson NM, Font RA, et al. Fungal keratitis in contact lens wearers. *Am J Ophthalmol.* 1988;106(6):708–714.
54. Wilhelmus KR. Review of clinical experience with microbial keratitis associated with contact lenses. *CLAO J.* 1987;13(4):211–214.
55. Hoflin-Lima AL, Roizenblatt R. Therapeutic contact lens-related bilateral fungal keratitis. *CLAO J.* 2002;28(3):149–150.
56. Hogan MJ, Thygeson P, Kimura S. Uses and abuses of adrenal steroids and corticotropin. *Trans Am Ophthalmol Soc.* 1954;52:145–171.
57. Jones BR. Principles in the management of oculomycosis. XXXI Edward Jackson Memorial Lecture. *Am J Ophthalmol.* 1975;79(5):719–751.
58. Berson EL, Kobayashi GS, Becker B, Rosenbaum L. Topical corticosteroids and fungal keratitis. *Invest Ophthalmol.* 1967;6(5):512–517.
59. Mitsui Y, Hanabusa J. Corneal infections after cortisone therapy. *Br J Ophthalmol.* 1955;39(4):244–250.
60. Agarwal LP, Malik SR, Mohan M, Khosla PK. Mycotic corneal ulcers. *Br J Ophthalmol.* 1963;47:109–115.
61. Forster RK, Rebell G. Animal model of *Fusarium solani* keratitis. *Am J Ophthalmol.* 1975;79(3):510–515.
62. Chern KC, Meisler DM, Wilhelmus KR, et al. Corneal anesthetic abuse and *Candida* keratitis. *Ophthalmology.* 1996;103(1):37–40.
63. Mack RJ, Shott S, Schatz S, Farley SJ. Association between moxifloxacin ophthalmic solution and fungal infection in patients with corneal ulcers and microbial keratitis. *J Ocul Pharmacol Ther.* 2009;25:279–284.
64. Sridhar MS, Gopinathan U, Rao GN. Fungal keratitis associated with vernal keratoconjunctivitis. *Cornea.* 2003;22(1):80–81.
65. Verma S, Tuft SJ. *Fusarium solani* keratitis following LASIK for myopia. *Br J Ophthalmol.* 2002;86(10):1190–1191.
66. Vajpayee RB, Gupta SK, Bareja U, Kishore K. Ocular atopy and mycotic keratitis. *Ann Ophthalmol.* 1990;22(10):369–372.
67. Maskin SL, Alfonso E. Fungal keratitis after radial keratotomy. *Am J Ophthalmol.* 1992;114(3):369–370.
68. Das S, Ramamurthy B, Sangwan VS. Fungal keratitis following amniotic membrane transplantation. *Int Ophthalmol.* 2009;29(1):49–51.
69. Fong LP, Ormerod LD, Kenyon KR, Foster CS. Microbial keratitis complicating penetrating keratoplasty. *Ophthalmology.* 1988;95(9):1269–1275.
70. Das S, Constantinou M, Ong T, Taylor HR. Microbial keratitis following corneal transplantation. *Clin Experiment Ophthalmol.* 2007;35(5):427–431.
71. Harris DJ Jr, Stulting RD, Waring GO 3rd, Wilson LA. Late bacterial and fungal keratitis after corneal transplantation. Spectrum of pathogens, graft survival, and visual prognosis. *Ophthalmology.* 1988;95(10):1450–1457.
72. Wright TM, Afshari NA. Microbial keratitis following corneal transplantation. *Am J Ophthalmol.* 2006;142(6):1061–1062.
73. Tseng SH, Ling KC. Late microbial keratitis after corneal transplantation. *Cornea.* 1995;14(6):591–594.
74. Kloess PM, Stulting RD, Waring GO 3rd, Wilson LA. Bacterial and fungal endophthalmitis after penetrating keratoplasty. *Am J Ophthalmol.* 1993;115(3):309–316.
75. Tappeiner C, Goldblum D, Zimmerli S, et al. Donor-to-host transmission of *Candida glabrata* to both recipients of corneal transplants from the same donor. *Cornea.* 2009;28(2):228–230.
76. Sutphin JE, Pfaller MA, Hollis RJ, Wagoner MD. Donor-to-host transmission of *Candida albicans* after corneal transplantation. *Am J Ophthalmol.* 2002;134(1):120–121.
77. Panda A, Das GK, Vanathi M, Kumar A. Corneal infection after radial keratotomy. *J Cataract Refract Surg.* 1998;24(3):331–334.
78. Chen WL, Tsai YY, Lin JM, Chiang CC. Unilateral *Candida parapsilosis* interface keratitis after laser in situ keratomileusis: case report and review of the literature. *Cornea.* 2009;28(1):105–107.
79. Karp CL, Tuli SS, Yoo SH, et al. Infectious keratitis after LASIK. *Ophthalmology.* 2003;110(3):503–510.
80. Tuli SS, Yoo SH. *Curvularia* keratitis after laser in situ keratomileusis from a feline source. *J Cataract Refract Surg.* 2003;29(5):1019–1021.
81. Cruz OA, Sabir SM, Capo H, Alfonso EC. Microbial keratitis in childhood. *Ophthalmology.* 1993;100(2):192–196.
82. Gussler JR, Miller D, Jaffe M, Alfonso EC. Infection after radial keratotomy. *Am J Ophthalmol.* 1995;119(6):798–799.
83. Periman LM, Harrison DA, Kim J. Fungal keratitis after photorefractive keratectomy: delayed diagnosis and treatment in a co-managed setting. *J Refract Surg.* 2003;19(3):364–366.
84. Pushker N, Dada T, Sony P, et al. Microbial keratitis after laser in situ keratomileusis. *J Refract Surg.* 2002;18(3):280–286.
85. Kouyoumdjian GA, Forstot SL, Durairaj VD, Damiano RE. Infectious keratitis after laser refractive surgery. *Ophthalmology.* 2001;108(7):1266–1268.
86. Kuo IC, Margolis TP, Cevallos V, Hwang DG. *Aspergillus fumigatus* keratitis after laser in situ keratomileusis. *Cornea.* 2001;20(3):342–344.
87. Braunwald E. *Harrison's principles of internal medicine.* 11 ed. New York: McGraw-Hill Books; 1987.
88. Mselle J. Fungal keratitis as an indicator of HIV infection in Africa. *Trop Doct.* 1999;29(3):133–135.
89. John D, Daniel E. Infectious keratitis in leprosy. *Br J Ophthalmol.* 1999;83(2):173–176.
90. Panda A, Sharma N, Das G, et al. Mycotic keratitis in children: epidemiologic and microbiologic evaluation. *Cornea.* 1997;16(3):295–299.
91. Kaufman HE, Wood RM. Mycotic keratitis. *Am J Ophthalmol.* 1965;59:993–1000.
92. Berger ST, Katsev DA, Mondino BJ, Pettit TH. Macroscopic pigmentation in a dematiaceous fungal keratitis. *Cornea.* 1991;10(3):272–276.
93. Sevel D, Kassar B. Suppurative keratitis and fungal keratitis. *Trans Ophthalmol Soc N Z.* 1973;25:228–232.
94. Chew SJ, Beuerman RW, Assouline M, et al. Early diagnosis of infectious keratitis with in vivo real time confocal microscopy. *CLAO J.* 1992;18(3):197–201.
95. Irvine JA, Ariyasu R. Limitations in tandem scanning confocal microscopy as a diagnostic tool for microbial keratitis. *Scanning.* 1994;16(5):307–311.
96. Winchester K, Mathers WD, Sutphin JE. Diagnosis of *Aspergillus* keratitis in vivo with confocal microscopy. *Cornea.* 1997;16(1):27–31.
97. Avunduk AM, Beuerman RW, Varnell ED, Kaufman HE. Confocal microscopy of *Aspergillus fumigatus* keratitis. *Br J Ophthalmol.* 2003;87(4):409–410.
98. Jones DB, Wilson L, Sexton R, Rebell G. Early diagnosis of mycotic keratitis. *Trans Ophthalmol Soc UK.* 1970;89:805–813.
99. Sharma S, Silverberg M, Mehta P, et al. Early diagnosis of mycotic keratitis: predictive value of potassium hydroxide preparation. *Indian J Ophthalmol.* 1998;46(1):31–35.
100. Vemuganti GK, Naidu C, Gopinathan U. Rapid detection of fungal filaments in corneal scrapings by microwave heating-assisted Grocott's methenamine silver staining. *Indian J Ophthalmol.* 2002;50(4):326–328.
101. Garcia ML, Herreras JM, Dios E, et al. Evaluation of lectin staining in the diagnosis of fungal keratitis in an experimental rabbit model. *Mol Vis.* 2002;8:10–16.
102. Sharma S, Kunimoto DY, Gopinathan U, et al. Evaluation of corneal scraping smear examination methods in the diagnosis of bacterial and fungal keratitis: a survey of eight years of laboratory experience. *Cornea.* 2002;21(7):643–647.
103. Forster RK, Wirta MG, Solis M, Rebell G. Methenamine-silver-stained corneal scrapings in keratomycosis. *Am J Ophthalmol.* 1976;82(2):261–265.

104. Kanungo R, Srinivasan R, Rao RS. Acridine orange staining in early diagnosis of mycotic keratitis. *Acta Ophthalmol (Copenh).* 1991;69(6):750–753.
105. Wilson LA, Sexton RR. Laboratory diagnosis in fungal keratitis. *Am J Ophthalmol.* 1968;66(4):646–653.
106. Thomas PA. Mycotic keratitis – an underestimated mycosis. *J Med Vet Mycol.* 1994;32(4):235–256.
107. O'Day DM, Akrabawi PL, Head WS, Ratner HB. Laboratory isolation techniques in human and experimental fungal infections. *Am J Ophthalmol.* 1979;87(5):688–693.
108. O'Day DM. Selection of appropriate antifungal therapy. *Cornea.* 1987;6(4):238–245.
109. Bock M, Maiwald M, Kappe R, et al. Polymerase chain reaction-based detection of dermatophyte DNA with a fungus-specific primer system. *Mycoses.* 1994;37(3–4):79–84.
110. Makimura K, Murayama SY, Yamaguchi H. Specific detection of *Aspergillus* and *Penicillium* species from respiratory specimens by polymerase chain reaction (PCR). *Jpn J Med Sci Biol.* 1994;47(3):141–156.
111. Gaudio PA, Gopinathan U, Sangwan V, Hughes TE. Polymerase chain reaction based detection of fungi in infected corneas. *Br J Ophthalmol.* 2002;86(7):755–760.
112. Ferrer C, Munoz G, Alio JL, et al. Polymerase chain reaction diagnosis in fungal keratitis caused by *Alternaria alternata. Am J Ophthalmol.* 2002;133(3):398–399.
113. Ferrer C, Colom F, Frases S, et al. Detection and identification of fungal pathogens by PCR and by ITS2 and 5.8S ribosomal DNA typing in ocular infections. *J Clin Microbiol.* 2001;39(8):2873–2879.
114. Alexandrakis G, Haimovici R, Miller D, Alfonso EC. Corneal biopsy in the management of progressive microbial keratitis. *Am J Ophthalmol.* 2000;129(5):571–576.
115. Rosa R, Alfonso E. Infectious keratitis: fungal keratitis. In: Stenson S, ed. *Surgical management in external diseases of the eye.* New York: Igaku-Shoin; 1995.
116. Kim JH, Yum JH, Lee D, Oh SH. Novel technique of corneal biopsy by using a femtosecond laser in infectious ulcers. *Cornea.* 2008;27(3):363–365.
117. Yoo SH, Kymionis GD, O'Brien TP, et al. Femtosecond-assisted diagnostic corneal biopsy (FAB) in keratitis. *Graefe's Arch Clin Exp Ophthalmol.* 2008;246(5):759–762.
118. Ishibashi Y, Kaufman HE. Corneal biopsy in the diagnosis of keratomycosis. *Am J Ophthalmol.* 1986;101(3):288–293.
119. Ishibashi Y, Hommura S, Matsumoto Y. Direct examination vs culture of biopsy specimens for the diagnosis of keratomycosis. *Am J Ophthalmol.* 1987;103(5):636–640.
120. Sridhar MS, Sharma S, Gopinathan U, Rao GN. Anterior chamber tap: diagnostic and therapeutic indications in the management of ocular infections. *Cornea.* 2002;21(7):718–722.
121. Forster R. The role of excisional keratoplasty in microbial keratitis. In: Cavanagh H, ed. *The cornea: transactions of the World Congress of the Cornea III.* New York: Raven Press; 1988.
122. Ishida N, Brown AC, Rao GN, et al. Recurrent *Fusarium* keratomycosis: a light and electron microscopic study. *Ann Ophthalmol.* 1984;16(4):354–356, 8–60, 62–66.
123. Zimmerman LE. Mycotic keratitis. *Lab Invest.* 1962;11:1151–1160.
124. Panda A, Mohan M, Mukherjee G. Mycotic keratitis in Indian patients (a histopathological study of corneal buttons). *Indian J Ophthalmol.* 1984;32(5):311–315.
125. Feghhi M, Mahmoudabadi AZ, Mehdinejad M. Evaluation of fungal and bacterial contaminations of patient-used ocular drops. *Med Mycol.* 2008;46(1):17–21.
126. Schein OD, Hibberd PL, Starck T, et al. Microbial contamination of in-use ocular medications. *Arch Ophthalmol.* 1992;110(1):82–85.
127. Schein OD, Wasson PJ, Boruchoff SA, Kenyon KR. Microbial keratitis associated with contaminated ocular medications. *Am J Ophthalmol.* 1988;105(4):361–365.
128. Martins EN, Farah ME, Alvarenga LS, et al. Infectious keratitis: correlation between corneal and contact lens cultures. *CLAO J.* 2002;28(3):146–148.
129. Vengayil S, Panda A, Satpathy G, et al. Polymerase chain reaction-guided diagnosis of mycotic keratitis: a prospective evaluation of its efficacy and limitations. *Invest Ophthalmol Vis Sci.* 2009;50(1):152–156.
130. Kim E, Chidambaram JD, Srinivasan M, et al. Prospective comparison of microbial culture and polymerase chain reaction in the diagnosis of corneal ulcer. *Am J Ophthalmol.* 2008;146(5):714–723, 23 e1.
131. O'Day DM, Ray WA, Robinson RD, et al. In vitro and in vivo susceptibility of *Candida* keratitis to topical polyenes. *Invest Ophthalmol Vis Sci.* 1987;28(5):874–880.
132. Vemuganti GK, Garg P, Gopinathan U, et al. Evaluation of agent and host factors in progression of mycotic keratitis: a histologic and microbiologic study of 167 corneal buttons. *Ophthalmology.* 2002;109(8):1538–1546.
133. Alfonso E. Antifungal agents. In: Albert D, Jakobiec F, eds. *Principles and practice of ophthalmology – basic sciences.* Philadelphia: WB Saunders; 1994.
134. Reynolds L, Closson R. *Extemporaneous ophthalmic preparations.* Vancouver; 1993.
135. Jones DB, Forster FK, Rebell G. *Fusarium solani* keratitis treated with natamycin (pimaricin): eighteen consecutive cases. *Arch Ophthalmol.* 1972;88(2):147–154.
136. Johns KJ, O'Day DM. Pharmacologic management of keratomycoses. *Surv Ophthalmol.* 1988;33(3):178–188.
137. Jones DB. Decision-making in the management of microbial keratitis. *Ophthalmology.* 1981;88(8):814–820.
138. Wood TO, Williford W. Treatment of keratomycosis with amphotericin B 0.15%. *Am J Ophthalmol.* 1976;81(6):847–849.
139. Vemulakonda GA, Hariprasad SM, Mieler WF, et al. Aqueous and vitreous concentrations following topical administration of 1% voriconazole in humans. *Arch Ophthalmol.* 2008;126(1):18–22.
140. Hariprasad SM, Mieler WF, Lin TK, et al. Voriconazole in the treatment of fungal eye infections: a review of current literature. *Br J Ophthalmol.* 2008;92(7):871–878.
141. Marangon FB, Miller D, Giaconi JA, Alfonso EC. In vitro investigation of voriconazole susceptibility for keratitis and endophthalmitis fungal pathogens. *Am J Ophthalmol.* 2004;137(5):820–825.
142. Prakash G, Sharma N, Goel M, et al. Evaluation of intrastromal injection of voriconazole as a therapeutic adjunctive for the management of deep recalcitrant fungal keratitis. *Am J Ophthalmol.* 2008;146(1):56–59.
143. Tu EY, McCartney DL, Beatty RF, et al. Successful treatment of resistant ocular fusariosis with posaconazole (SCH-56592). *Am J Ophthalmol.* 2007;143(2):222–227.
144. Tu EY, Park AJ. Recalcitrant *Beauveria bassiana* keratitis: confocal microscopy findings and treatment with posaconazole (Noxafil). *Cornea.* 2007;26(8):1008–1010.
145. Tu EY. *Alternaria* keratitis: clinical presentation and resolution with topical fluconazole or intrastromal voriconazole and topical caspofungin. *Cornea.* 2009;28(1):116–119.
146. Matsumoto Y, Dogru M, Goto E, et al. Successful topical application of a new antifungal agent, micafungin, in the treatment of refractory fungal corneal ulcers: report of three cases and literature review. *Cornea.* 2005;24(6):748–753.
147. Searl SS, Udell IJ, Sadun A, et al. *Aspergillus* keratitis with intraocular invasion. *Ophthalmology.* 1981;88(12):1244–1250.
148. Komadina TG, Wilkes TD, Shock JP, et al. Treatment of *Aspergillus fumigatus* keratitis in rabbits with oral and topical ketoconazole. *Am J Ophthalmol.* 1985;99(4):476–479.
149. Fitzsimons R, Peters AL. Miconazole and ketoconazole as a satisfactory first-line treatment for keratomycosis. *Am J Ophthalmol.* 1986;101(5):605–608.
150. Minogue MJ, Francis IC, Quatermass P, et al. Successful treatment of fungal keratitis caused by *Paecilomyces lilacinus. Am J Ophthalmol.* 1984;98(5):626–627.
151. Stern GA, Okumoto M, Smolin G. Combined amphotericin B and rifampin treatment of experimental *Candida albicans* keratitis. *Arch Ophthalmol.* 1979;97(4):721–722.
152. Beggs WH. Mechanisms of synergistic interactions between amphotericin B and flucytosine. *J Antimicrob Chemother.* 1986;17(4):402–404.
153. Brajtburg J, Kobayashi D, Medoff G, Kobayashi GS. Antifungal action of amphotericin B in combination with other polyene or imidazole antibiotics. *J Infect Dis.* 1982;146(2):138–146.
154. Hoeprich PD, Ingraham JL, Kleker E, Winship MJ. Development of resistance to 5-fluorocytosine in *Candida parapsilosis* during therapy. *J Infect Dis.* 1974;130(2):112–118.
155. Foster CS. Miconazole therapy for keratomycosis. *Am J Ophthalmol.* 1981;91(5):622–629.
156. Scott IU, Flynn HW Jr, Feuer W, et al. Endophthalmitis associated with microbial keratitis. *Ophthalmology.* 1996;103(11):1864–1870.
157. Ishibashi Y, Matsumoto Y, Takei K. The effects of intravenous miconazole on fungal keratitis. *Am J Ophthalmol.* 1984;98(4):433–437.
158. Hemady RK, Chu W, Foster CS. Intraocular penetration of ketoconazole in rabbits. *Cornea.* 1992;11(4):329–333.
159. Ishibashi Y. Oral ketoconazole therapy for keratomycosis. *Am J Ophthalmol.* 1983;95(3):342–345.
160. Singh SM, Sharma S, Chatterjee PK. Clinical and experimental mycotic keratitis caused by *Aspergillus terreus* and the effect of subconjunctival

oxiconazole treatment in the animal model. *Mycopathologia*. 1990; 112(3):127–137.
161 Torres MA, Mohamed J, Cavazos-Adame H, Martinez LA. Topical ketoconazole for fungal keratitis. *Am J Ophthalmol*. 1985;100(2): 293–298.
162. O'Day DM. Orally administered antifungal therapy for experimental keratomycosis. *Trans Am Ophthalmol Soc*. 1990;88:685–725.
163. O'Day DM, Head WS, Robinson RD, Clanton JA. Corneal penetration of topical amphotericin B and natamycin. *Curr Eye Res*. 1986;5(11): 877–882.
164. O'Day DM, Ray WA, Head WS, Robinson RD. Influence of the corneal epithelium on the efficacy of topical antifungal agents. *Invest Ophthalmol Vis Sci*. 1984;25(7):855–859.
165. Day S, Lalitha P, Haug S, et al. Activity of antibiotics against *Fusarium* and *Aspergillus*. *Br J Ophthalmol*. 2009;93(1):116–119.
166. Munir WM, Rosenfeld SI, Udell I, et al. Clinical response of contact lens-associated fungal keratitis to topical fluoroquinolone therapy. *Cornea*. 2007;26(5):621–624.
167. Panda A, Ahuja R, Biswas NR, et al. Role of 0.02% polyhexamethylene biguanide and 1% povidone iodine in experimental *Aspergillus* keratitis. *Cornea*. 2003;22(2):138–141.
168. Fiscella RG, Moshifar M, Messick CR, et al. Polyhexamethylene biguanide (PHMB) in the treatment of experimental *Fusarium* keratomycosis. *Cornea*. 1997;16(4):447–449.
169. Rahman MR, Johnson GJ, Husain R, et al. Randomised trial of 0.2% chlorhexidine gluconate and 2.5% natamycin for fungal keratitis in Bangladesh. *Br J Ophthalmol*. 1998;82(8):919–925.
170. Schwartz SD, Harrison SA, Engstrom RE Jr, et al. Collagen shield delivery of amphotericin B. *Am J Ophthalmol*. 1990;109(6):701–704.
171. Frucht-Pery J, Mor M, Evron R, et al. The effect of the ArF excimer laser on *Candida albicans* in vitro. *Graefe's Arch Clin Exp Ophthalmol*. 1993;231(7):413–415.
172. Garg P, Gopinathan U, Nutheti R, Rao GN. Clinical experience with N-butyl cyanoacrylate tissue adhesive in fungal keratitis. *Cornea*. 2003;22(5):405–408.
173. Gopinathan U, Ramakrishna T, Willcox M, et al. Enzymatic, clinical and histologic evaluation of corneal tissues in experimental fungal keratitis in rabbits. *Exp Eye Res*. 2001;72(4):433–442.
174. Naiker S, Odhav B. Mycotic keratitis: profile of *Fusarium* species and their mycotoxins. *Mycoses*. 2004;47(1–2):50–56.
175. O'Day DM, Ray WA, Robinson R, Head WS. Efficacy of antifungal agents in the cornea. II. Influence of corticosteroids. *Invest Ophthalmol Vis Sci*. 1984;25(3):331–335.
176. O'Day DM, Robinson R, Head WS. Efficacy of antifungal agents in the cornea. I. A comparative study. *Invest Ophthalmol Vis Sci*. 1983;24(8): 1098–1102.
177. Stern GA, Buttross M. Use of corticosteroids in combination with antimicrobial drugs in the treatment of infectious corneal disease. *Ophthalmology*. 1991;98(6):847–853.
178. Schreiber W, Olbrisch A, Vorwerk CK, et al. Combined topical fluconazole and corticosteroid treatment for experimental *Candida albicans* keratomycosis. *Invest Ophthalmol Vis Sci*. 2003;44(6):2634–2643.
179. Kompa S, Langefeld S, Kirchhof B, Schrage N. Corneal biopsy in keratitis performed with the microtrephine. *Graefe's Arch Clin Exp Ophthalmol*. 1999;237(11):915–919.
180. Xie L, Zhai H, Shi W. Penetrating keratoplasty for corneal perforations in fungal keratitis. *Cornea*. 2007;26(2):158–162.
181. Xie L, Dong X, Shi W. Treatment of fungal keratitis by penetrating keratoplasty. *Br J Ophthalmol*. 2001;85(9):1070–1074.
182. Forster RK, Rebell G. The diagnosis and management of keratomycoses. II. Medical and surgical management. *Arch Ophthalmol*. 1975;93(11): 1134–1136.
183. Dursun D, Fernandez V, Miller D, Alfonso EC. Advanced *Fusarium* keratitis progressing to endophthalmitis. *Cornea*. 2003;22(4):300–303.
184. Wang MX, Shen DJ, Liu JC, et al. Recurrent fungal keratitis and endophthalmitis. *Cornea*. 2000;19(4):558–560.
185. Sony P, Sharma N, Vajpayee RB, Ray M. Therapeutic keratoplasty for infectious keratitis: a review of the literature. *CLAO J*. 2002;28(3): 111–118.
186. Avunduk AM, Beuerman RW, Warnel ED, et al. Comparison of efficacy of topical and oral fluconazole treatment in experimental *Aspergillus* keratitis. *Curr Eye Res*. 2003;26(2):113–117.
187. Cristol SM, Alfonso EC, Guildford JH, et al. Results of large penetrating keratoplasty in microbial keratitis. *Cornea*. 1996;15(6):571–576.
188. Bell NP, Karp CL, Alfonso EC, et al. Effects of methylprednisolone and cyclosporine A on fungal growth in vitro. *Cornea*. 1999;18(3): 306–313.
189. Perry HD, Doshi SJ, Donnenfeld ED, Bai GS. Topical cyclosporin A in the management of therapeutic keratoplasty for mycotic keratitis. *Cornea*. 2002;21(2):161–163.
190. Killingsworth DW, Stern GA, Driebe WT, et al. Results of therapeutic penetrating keratoplasty. *Ophthalmology*. 1993;100(4):534–541.
191. Polack FM, Kaufman HE, Newmark E. Keratomycosis. Medical and surgical treatment. *Arch Ophthalmol*. 1971;85(4):410–416.
192. DeVoe AG. Keratomycosis. *Am J Ophthalmol*. 1971;71(1 Part 2):406–414.
193. Sanitato JJ, Kelley CG, Kaufman HE. Surgical management of peripheral fungal keratitis (keratomycosis). *Arch Ophthalmol*. 1984;102(10): 1506–1509.
194. Reynolds MG, Alfonso E. Treatment of infectious scleritis and keratoscleritis. *Am J Ophthalmol*. 1991;112(5):543–547.
195. Alfonso E. Surgical management of ocular infections. In: Bialasciewicz A, ed. *Infectious disease of the eye*. New York: Springer Verlag; 1993.
196. Lalitha P, Prajna NV, Kabra A, et al. Risk factors for treatment outcome in fungal keratitis. *Ophthalmology*. 2006;113(4):526–530.

Chapter 83

Acanthamoeba and Other Parasitic Corneal Infections

Elmer Y. Tu

Introduction

Acanthamoeba keratitis is a chronic, primarily contact lens-related, infection caused by a free-living amoeba found ubiquitously in water and soil. Although classically presenting with radial keratoneuritis, a corneal ring infiltrate and/or disproportionate, incapacitating pain, most patients will initially present with less characteristic signs and symptoms frequently contributing to diagnostic delay (Fig. 83.1). Commonly mistaken for noninfectious as well as bacterial, fungal, or viral causes of chronic keratitis, the amoebic infection is resistant to commonly utilized ophthalmic antimicrobial agents, but may become transiently asymptomatic with the use of corticosteroids. Excellent outcomes are probable when the infection is diagnosed and treatment initiated before deep infiltration.[1] Medical cure requires the specific use of biguanides alone or in combination with a diamidine for weeks to months or longer.[2,3] Clinical resistance does occur and may require more aggressive medical or surgical therapy.

Incidence

Since its first description in 1973,[4] *Acanthamoeba* keratitis has been recognized as a generally rare infection characterized by periodic outbreaks.[5–12] Incidence is expressed relative to the overall number of contact lens wearers, the group at far greatest risk of infection, but limited knowledge of baseline rates is available since most estimates are based on outbreak analyses. An analysis of the only comprehensive effort to identify cases in the USA encompassing an outbreak of *Acanthamoeba* keratitis estimated an incidence of 1.49–2.01 cases per million contact lens users per year.[5,11,12] With the exception of a regional outbreak in Iowa,[8] a consistently greater incidence, as high as 1 in 30 000 contact lens users per year or higher, had been found in the United Kingdom (UK) during the 1990s.[9,10] However, since 2003, another US outbreak has been recognized and, while no comprehensive US data has been collected, regional incidence estimates for the Chicago area now approach the rates reported in the UK.[6,7,13,14] *Acanthamoeba* keratitis remains less common than other forms of contact lens-related and unrelated microbial keratitis. Contact lens-related microbial keratitis occurs in 1–25 cases per 10 000 wearers per year, primarily dependent on wear regimen.[15,16] In India, *Acanthamoeba* was identified in 1% of all patients cultured for possible infectious keratitis regardless of etiology.[17]

Risk Factors

Contact lens wear in otherwise healthy individuals of any age is the primary risk factor for the development of *Acanthamoeba* keratitis, with greater than 90% of cases associated with any contact lens use.[5,12,18–20] Initially described in contaminated or agricultural corneal injuries, few cases were reported in the following decade until the early to mid-1980s contemporaneous to a dramatic increase in the popularity of soft contact lenses.[12] Although greater than 90% of contact lens wearers who suffer *Acanthamoeba* keratitis wear soft contact lenses, the remainder are rigid lens wearers, their total only slightly below their statistical share of overall lens wearers. The significantly lower risk of bacterial keratitis in rigid lens wear does not extend to amoebic keratitis, albeit occurring at a lower rate than in soft contact lens wear. Recently, the reemergence of rigid lens use for orthokeratology has highlighted this increased risk of *Acanthamoeba* keratitis where epithelial thinning, inadequate hygiene, and routine tap water exposure during care may be contributing factors.[21]

In both soft and rigid lens wearers, trauma, swimming in lenses, and noncompliance with contact lens disinfection systems are associated with an increased risk of *Acanthamoeba* keratitis.[10] Other hygiene-related variables include contact lens wear during hot tub use as well as rinsing lenses or cases in nonsterile water.[7,9,10,19,20] A case-control study of the national US outbreak of the mid-1980s found the main association was the use of homemade saline utilizing salt tablets and nonsterile water (odds ratio [OR], infinity) with a smaller association with swimming in lenses (OR, 6.2) and less frequent disinfection (OR, 5.8).[20] Overall, compliance with contact lens wear and care regimens has been and continues to be universally poor. Despite numerous changes in contact lens materials and disinfection systems to improve this, little change has been seen in the rates of other forms of contact lens-related microbial keratitis in the last two decades, further suggesting that periodic outbreaks of *Acanthamoeba* keratitis may be due to other factors.[16,22]

While no specific soft lens type has yet been associated with *Acanthamoeba* keratitis, specific contact lens care

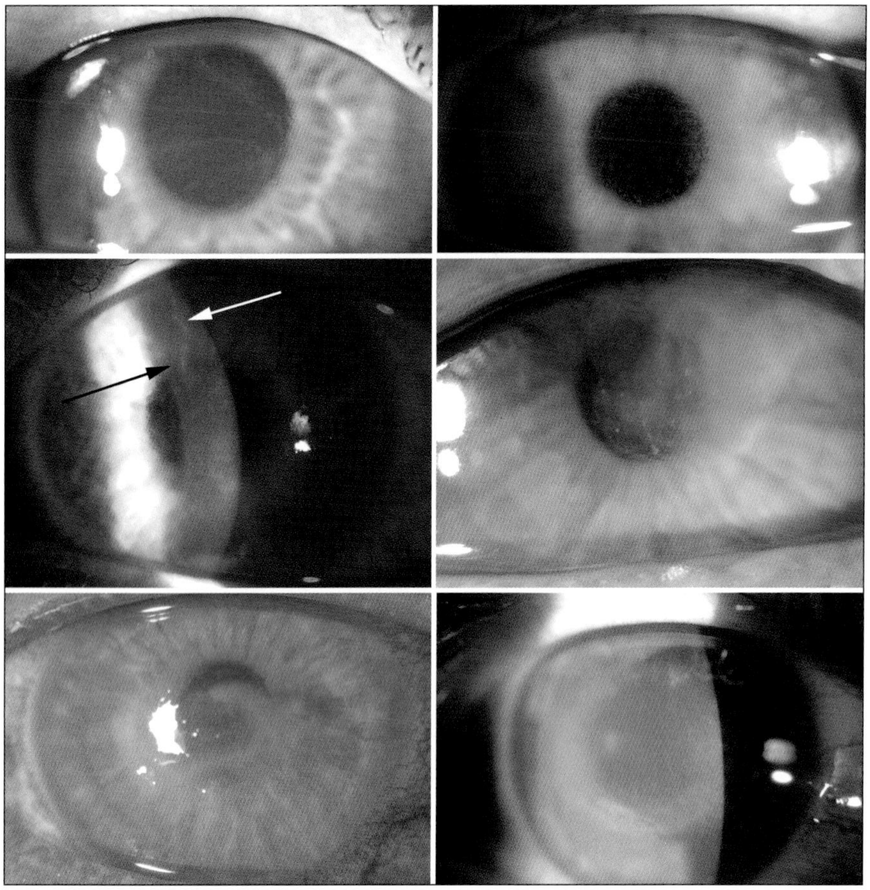

Fig. 83.1 Slit lamp photographs of *Acanthamoeba* keratitis. *Top right* & *top left* Isolated epitheliitis. Two patients with an isolated epithelial presentation of *Acanthamoeba* keratitis. Note the granular, cystic-appearing epithelium with little or no stromal inflammation. *Middle left* Epitheliitis with radial neuritis. A patient with very irregular-appearing epithelium and an inflamed, nodular corneal nerve superiorly. *Middle right* Anterior stromal disease. A patient with anterior stromal involvement with clear surrounding cornea and without associated deep inflammation. *Bottom left* Deep stromal keratitis. Note the diffuse central infiltrate with generalized central haze without a clear lateral or deep border. *Bottom right* Ring infiltrate. An early ring infiltrate demonstrating an area of central corneal haze with a relative paracentral demarcation ring characteristic of an immune *Acanthamoeba* ring. (From Tu EY, Joslin CE, Sugar J, Shoff ME, Booton GC. Prognostic factors affecting visual outcome in *Acanthamoeba* keratitis. *Ophthalmology*. 2008;115(11): 1998–2003.)

systems have been associated with greater risk. The systems most effective against both forms of the amoeba are heat and hydrogen peroxide disinfection, specifically the two-step type which ensures extended disinfectant exposure time prior to neutralization. Cysts are highly resistant to chlorine and most current multipurpose solutions (MPS).[19,23,24] Consequently, the use of one-step hydrogen peroxide systems,[10] chlorine-based disinfection,[19] and, most recently, AMO Complete MoisturePlus, an MPS, have been associated with an increased risk of *Acanthamoeba* keratitis.[7,13] Despite this specific association, it should be noted that nearly 50% of patients in the recent US outbreak were using other disinfectants, mostly other MPSs, suggesting that these systems may also present additional risk.[7] Similarly, no wearing schedule, e.g. overnight wear or frequent replacement, has yet been associated with *Acanthamoeba* keratitis, but daily replacement lenses may be protective since solutions and repeated handling are not involved in their care.[10] Other lens care practices such as solution reuse ('topping off'), not rubbing or rinsing lenses, and domestic water exposure during lens care or wear have also been suggested as risk factors.[7,10] A moderate decline in cases of *Acanthamoeba* keratitis in the UK was thought to be, in part, due to education and modification of these factors.[10]

Regardless, the geographical variation found in larger outbreaks remains unexplained. It has been suggested that variations in the level of contamination of the domestic water supply may play a role.[6,8,10] Previous surveys have demonstrated a significant geographic variation in *Acanthamoeba* household water contamination.[25,26] Further, the risk in counties most affected by severe regional flooding was significantly higher (OR, 10.83) while those with private wells rather than municipal water were protected (OR, 0.12) during an outbreak in Iowa.[27] The hardness of domestic water (relative risk [RR], 3.37) and the use of rooftop cisterns have also been identified as risk factors with microbiologic studies confirming the presence of genotypically identical organisms from keratitis patients and their cold water taps.[10,26] The nonrandom distribution of cases in the Chicago area also suggests a geographic risk factor which has been hypothesized to be due to changing domestic water disinfection standards combined with an extended water distribution system,[6] and is consistent with the common use of MPS systems more reliant on environmental control of *Acanthamoeba* rather than direct sterilization efficacy.[6,7]

Pathogenesis

Acanthamoebae are free-living organisms commonly found in water and soil which prey on other microorganisms. They exist as a more vulnerable, freely mobile trophozoite and as a characteristic double-walled cyst (Fig. 83.2) extremely resistant to extremes of temperature, desiccation, irradiation, antimicrobial agents, and other changes in environment.[28] Further, when challenged, trophozoites can encyst rapidly, within hours, preserving the ability to produce viable trophozoites decades later. Its primary manifestation is keratitis, but it is, in immunocompromised hosts, associated with the rare conditions granulomatous amoebic encephalitis (GAE), disseminated cutaneous amoebiasis, as well as visceral forms.[29] *A. castellanii* is the most common species associated with keratitis with *A. polyphaga* and *A. hatchetti* also commonly identified in larger series. *A. culbertsoni, A. rhysodes, A. lugdunesis, A. quina*, and *A. griffini* have also been described. Although 18S ribosomal DNA typing does not correlate well with earlier nomenclature, it permits consistent genotypic classification, with most keratitis isolates grouped as T4, with T3 second in frequency.[30] Other genotype groups have constituted a small minority of reported keratitis isolates.

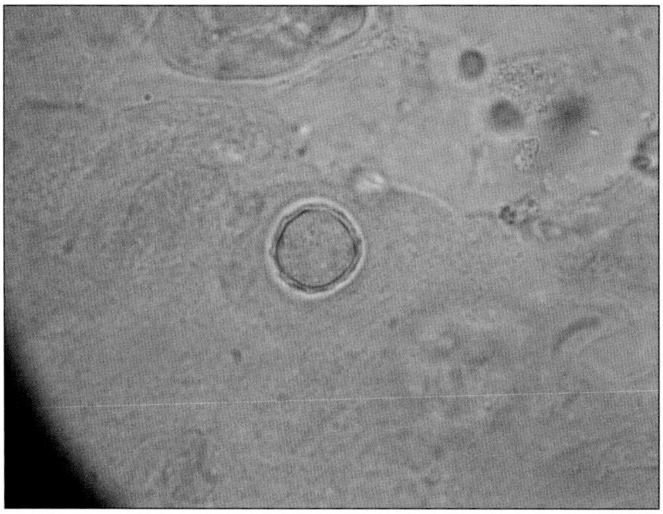

Fig. 83.2 *Acanthamoeba* cyst from a superficial corneal scraping. (Diff-Quik stain, original magnification 100×)

The mechanism and progression of human infection has been inferred from animal models of *Acanthamoeba* keratitis (Fig. 83.3). Initial attachment of the amoeba is facilitated by its expression of a mannose-binding protein which binds to corneal epithelial cell-expressed mannosylated glycoprotein.[31] Corneal injury such as contact lens wear may increase its expression as well as measured cytopathic effects.[31,32] Once bound, acanthamoebae then express proteases such as MIP-133 which degrade both corneal epithelium and corneal stroma, promoting invasion and ulceration. In the corneal stroma, the organism can proliferate, subsisting on bacterial prey or, possibly, resident keratocytes.[32]

In animal models, *Acanthamoeba* keratitis does not induce systemic IgG production. Human studies indicate that a majority of subjects express serum anti-*Acanthamoeba* IgG, probably from other exposures.[33] Once acanthamoebae are established in the stroma, however, both clinically in

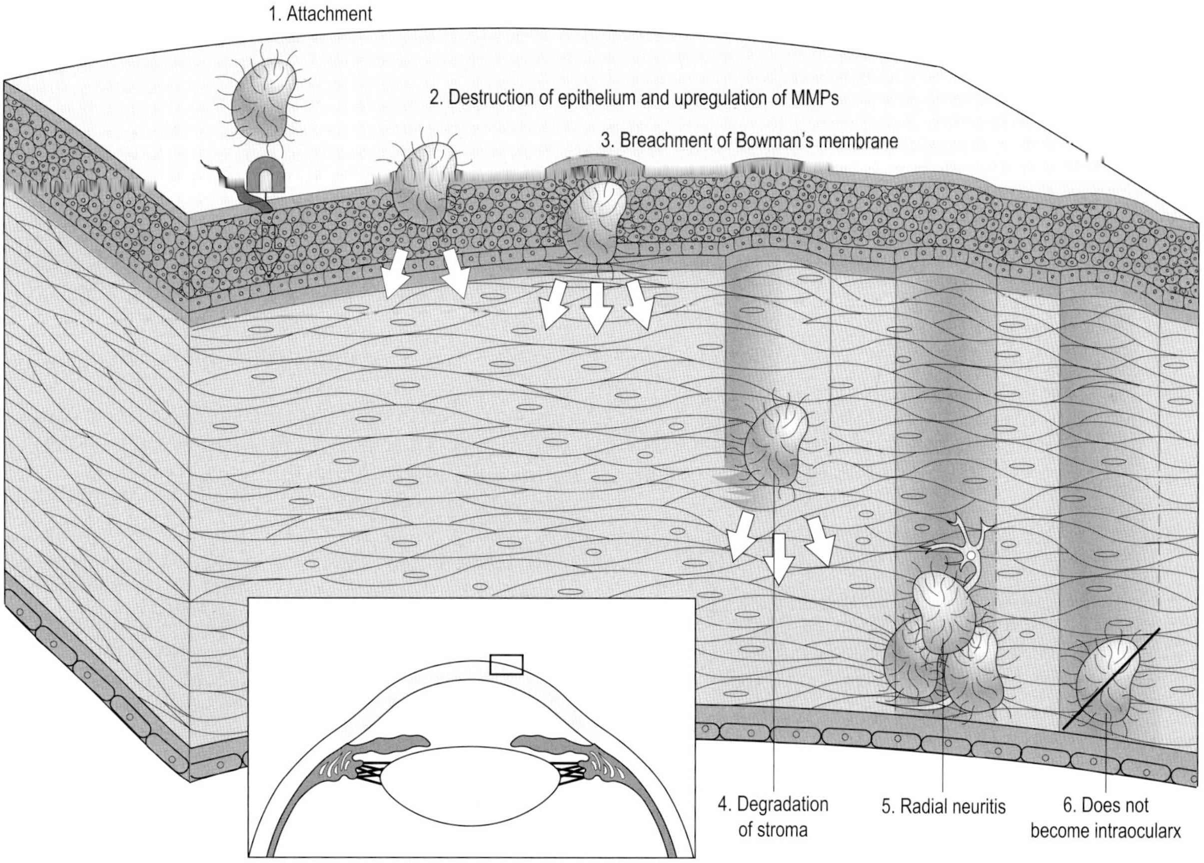

Fig. 83.3 Proposed pathogenesis of acanthamoebal corneal infection. (From Clarke DW, Niederkorn JY. The pathophysiology of *Acanthamoeba* keratitis. *Trends Parasitol*. 2006;22(4):175–180.)

humans and in animal models, this systemic immune sensitization appears ineffectual at clearing infection.[34] However, experimental studies have demonstrated that inducement of IgA through oral immunization can be effective at preventing or mitigating infection in animals, presumably by preventing initial attachment or, alternatively, by neutralizing the amoeba's proteases to impair further penetration.[35] In fact, human studies have found tear IgA levels to be lower in *Acanthamoeba* keratitis patients versus controls, suggesting that susceptibility may play a role in some patients.[34]

While the precise mechanism of contact lens-induced risk for *Acanthamoeba* infection is unclear, it is known that they cause a significant immunedeviation of the ocular surface, permit binding of microorganisms, and promote biofilm formation on the lens and lens paraphernalia.[36] This provides a stable microorganism-rich food supply to encourage proliferation and extend contact time of the amoeba with corneal epithelium, increasing chances of successful binding. Numerous studies have shown increased pathogenicity of *Acanthamoeba* when co-cultured with organisms commonly associated with human disease and also when incorporated inside the amoeba as endosymbionts.[37] It appears that the pathogenesis of *Acanthamoeba* keratitis is more complex in humans, as evidenced by its nonlinear corneal progression, chronicity of infection, and variations in corneal pathogenicity clinically encountered.

Clinical Features

Acanthamoeba keratitis is often recognized at first presentation only when accompanied by a high index of clinical suspicion. Any age may be affected[38] and no sex predilection has been noted, although a larger number of contact lens wearers are female. *Acanthamoeba* keratitis is bilateral in 7–11% of patients.[1,39] The distribution of other clinical features described in most large series is likely biased toward advanced stages of disease, as would be expected from tertiary care facilities. The spectrum of signs and symptoms, therefore, represents various stages in its chronic, indolent course rather than distinct manifestations of disease. A strong suspicion for *Acanthamoeba* infection should, therefore, include any patient with the risk factors outlined above, primarily contact lens wear with or without significant noncompliance, significant water exposure or contaminated trauma combined with the clinical features of any known presentation of disease. Other commonly reported characteristics, including a history of chronicity, multiple physician referrals, culture-negative scrapings, resistance to antimicrobial agents (bacterial, fungal, and viral), and previous corticosteroid use, are related to the indolent nature of the disease and misdiagnosis or delayed diagnosis rather than being an integral feature of the disease. Accordingly, initial presentation may be virtually asymptomatic or manifest as a nonspecific foreign body sensation, photophobia, sometimes escalating to severe, intractable pain with visual acuity similarly unpredictable in the early stages.

Anatomic classification of clinical signs is consistent with proposed animal models of pathogenesis, correlates loosely with reported duration of disease, and is clinically useful.[1] Epitheliitis represents a predominantly epithelial infestation which may present with a mild foreign body sensation ranging to moderate pain and mild loss of visual acuity. Its flat, diffuse microcystic form exhibits relative perilimbal sparing and may be confused with dry eye or contact lens-associated surface toxicity (see Fig. 83.1).[40] Epithelial ridges, whorls, and pseudodendrites may be commonly confused with epithelial herpetic keratitis as evidenced by the high proportion of antiviral use in patients ultimately diagnosed with *Acanthamoeba* keratitis.[1] Corneal sensation in these early stages may be paradoxically decreased, further mimicking herpetic disease.[41] The disease may remain restricted to the epithelium, sometimes indefinitely. Simple debridement without other medical intervention has been rarely reported to be curative at this stage.[42] Stromal invasion may take the form of anterior stromal disease which is characterized by shallow stromal excavation and/or localized stromal infiltration, with or without an overlying epithelial defect, involving the anterior third of the stroma. These patients may also have moderate to more significant pain, but usually exhibit less global inflammation than more advanced stages of disease (see Fig. 83.1). Visual acuity is dependent on the location of the stromal lesion and inflammatory response.

The most characteristic signs and symptoms include severe, incapacitating pain, the presence of a ring infiltrate, and radial keratoneuritis (see Fig. 83.1).[40] Radial keratoneuritis, representing amoebic migration along the corneal nerves and the host immune response, occurs in mid or deep stroma, beginning centrally or paracentrally and extending toward the limbus. It may accompany any stage of the disease. Although largely pathognomonic for *Acanthamoeba* keratitis, it has also been described in *Pseudomonas* keratitis.[43] The often disproportionate pain, usually more severe than fungal keratitis, in advanced disease invariably includes extreme photophobia related possibly to its neurotrophic nature, its ability to synthesize certain prostaglandins, and the host's reactive immune response. The visible ring infiltrate represents an immune hypersensitivity response which may be related or unrelated to the viability of the organisms.[44] Prior to the formation of a defined ring, herpetic disciform keratitis, other forms of interstitial keratitis, and anesthetic abuse may also mimic this appearance. Accurate diagnosis with these signs of infection is probable, but, with the exception of radial keratoneuritis, represents advanced disease which has been shown to carry with it a poorer prognosis for both medical cure and visual recovery.[1]

Extracorneal manifestations of *Acanthamoeba* include limbitis, scleritis, uveitis (Fig. 83.4) as well as eyelid abnormalities including edema and dacryoadenitis.[45,46] Most of these are thought to be inflammatory rather than infectious, without evident organisms in the region of inflammation, but choroidal and intraocular recovery of organisms has been rarely reported.[47] Similarly, sudden blindness without pathologic evidence of intraocular spread has also been described.[48] Historically, a significant proportion of *Acanthamoeba* keratitis patients have been found to have co-infections involving a second bacterial, fungal, or viral agent. Acanthamoebae are also known to commonly harbor bacterial endosymbionts. Both exogenous and endogenous co-infectious pathogens have been shown to increase virulence, as seen with *Acanthamoeba*-associated infectious

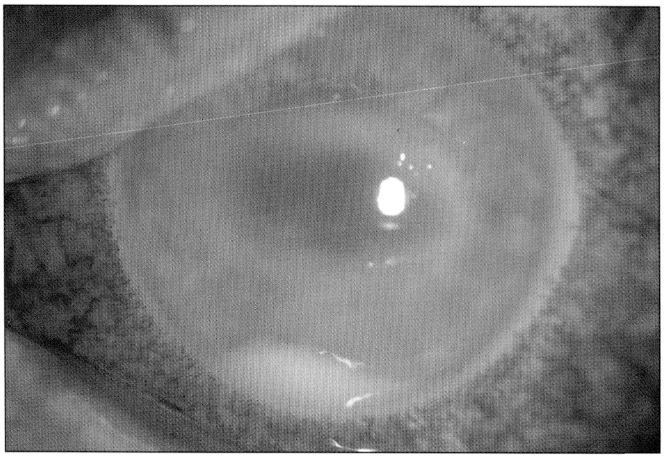

Fig. 83.4 Slit lamp photo of *Acanthamoeba* keratitis with the extracorneal manifestation of anterior uveitis.

crystalline keratopathy, triggering significant deviation from both established clinical presentations and expected treatment response.[48A]

Diagnosis

Culture and isolation of a responsible pathogen is the microbiologic standard for definitive diagnosis of an infectious disease. Unfortunately, the rates of positive culture in patients with a clinical diagnosis of *Acanthamoeba* keratitis range only between 0% and 53%.[8–10,14,40] The diagnosis of many cases of *Acanthamoeba* keratitis patients are then based primarily on clinical features, which are most reliable in advanced disease when prognosis is poorer.[1,14] Individual laboratories vary significantly in their culture success. *Acanthamoeba*, isolated infrequently utilizing common methods used for keratitis,[14] are identified best when provided a bacterial food source, e.g. *E. coli* or, preferably, *E. cloacae*, plated on a non-nutrient agar revealing characteristic 'snail tracks' left by the grazing amoebae.[49] Although previous studies have suggested that superficial scrapings were useful only in earlier disease, a recent study supports its use for any presentation of disease.[40,50] Corneal biopsy for both histology and culture is indicated if less invasive methods are nondiagnostic. Owing to the *Acanthamoeba's* hardy nature, corneal scrapings or deeper tissue samples placed in transport media such as Page's saline require minimal storage and handling. The propensity for co-infection should direct other routine and other indicated cultures based on clinical presentation.[40]

Corneal smears and traditional histopathology have a significantly higher yield than culture and also contribute significant evidence of infection. Various histopathologic methods may be utilized, including KOH, Diff-Quik/ Giemsa (see Fig. 83.2), Gram, acridine orange, impression cytology, and calcafluor white stains with yields reportedly as high as 92%.[17,51] The use of polymerase chain reaction (PCR) has also been described,[52] but has limitations in confirming the presence of viable organisms. Traditional histopathology with epithelial or stromal biopsies may result in even higher yields.[8]

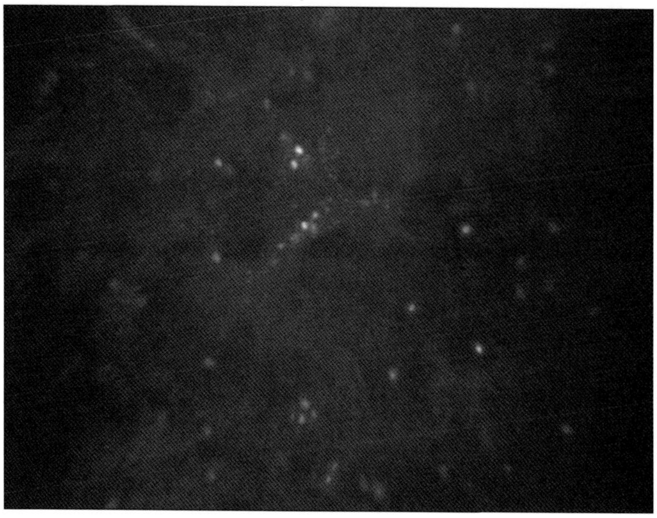

Fig. 83.5 Confocal microscopy of *Acanthamoeba* keratitis. Note the multiple bright white opacities distributed in clusters throughout the scan, The central grouping demonstrates a bright white center surrounded by a halo representing the cyst wall.

Confocal microscopy provides in vivo high-magnification sectioning of the cornea by timing transmission and reception of reflected light to a narrow plane, reducing scatter, to improve optical resolution (Fig. 83.5). Its successful use for *Acanthamoeba* keratitis was first described in 1992.[53] Since that time, a significant divergence between US studies, relying primarily on confocal microscopy but with low rates of culture confirmation, and UK studies, relying primarily on microbiologic and clinic characteristics for diagnosis, has emerged.[8,9,19,54,55] Our center's analysis of the relationship between culture, histology, and confocal microscopy found that the sensitivity of confocal microscopy exceeded 90% in all groups and specificity ranged between 77% and 100% when employing the different diagnostic criteria utilized in previous studies.[50] However, image acquisition and accurate interpretation are critical and the potential for misinterpretation exists. Ultimately, clinical diagnosis is made through a composite of clinical features and supportive evidence gained through both invasive and noninvasive methods.[50] Because of the specific and extended nature of therapy and the negative prognostic impact of misdiagnosis, every effort should be made to obtain any supportive or diagnostic evidence of disease.

Treatment

Early recognition of *Acanthamoeba* keratitis has so far proven to be the strongest predictor of a good visual outcome.[1,55] Previous studies have suggested that disease duration of greater than 3 or 4 weeks prior to diagnosis carries a poorer prognosis.[55,56] While our recent experience supports a correlation of untreated disease duration with clinical staging, there was no independent correlation with visual outcome.[1] Rather, clinical depth of corneal involvement at presentation was strongly predictive of visual outcome, suggesting that the rate of corneal invasion is highly variable among individual cases. Therefore, outcome is poorer in deeper disease where inflammation promotes irreversible corneal scarring and extracorneal sequelae unrelated to disease duration. Most patients have very good visual outcomes with a standard regimen of one- or two-drug therapy.[57] Accordingly, two-thirds of overall patients achieved 20/25 or better vision, but deep stromal disease or an immune ring at initial presentation was strongly associated (OR, 10.27; 95% confidence interval [CI], 2.91–36.17) with a poorer visual outcome.[1] Identifiable at presentation, these patients may benefit from more aggressive observation and medical and surgical therapy.[1] Regardless, standard medical treatment is continued for weeks to years and requires medications to achieve cure.

Medical

Early medical therapy was unsuccessful and, despite penetrating keratoplasty, eventual blindness or loss of the eye was common.[4] The first medical cure was reported a decade later, utilizing the combination of topical propamidine isetionate (Brolene) with previously less effective agents such as neomycin.[58] Along with hexamidine (Desmodine), the diamidines are lethal to the trophozoite form and retard encystment, but are less effective against mature cysts, suggesting that their peak efficacy may be early in the treatment phase when trophozoites are more numerous.[59] Cysts predominate later, often requiring the concomitant and continued use of a cysticidal agent. The drug is normally dosed hourly for the first 3–5 days and tapered over the first 2–6 weeks, depending on clinical response. Toxicity manifests as a painful erosive inferior conjunctivitis that responds to reduction or elimination of the topical diamidine. Both drugs are commercially available outside of the USA, with in vitro efficacy marginally favoring hexamidine.[59] Recently, intravenous pentamidine, another diamidine, given over several days, has been described for recalcitrant disease.

The mainstays of current therapy are the biguanides PHMB (Bacquacil) 0.02% and chlorhexidine 0.02%, which exhibit antitrophozoite activity but are also lethal to the cyst form.[2,3] These agents are not commercially available and each has been shown to be effective as single agents with comparable efficacy.[57] Recommended dosing frequency varies, but they are initially used hourly for the first several days and tapered slowly over the first 4–6 weeks to q.i.d. dosing. This maintenance therapy is tapered more slowly to ensure cyst killing, typically lasting 3–6 months, but occasionally continuing for a year or more. Superficial disease may require significantly less time, with treatment regimens tailored to individual response. All patients require close observation for several months after treatment withdrawal for signs of recrudescence. Their introduction and widespread use in the 1990s led to a dramatic improvement in rates of medical cure and, correspondingly, visual outcomes. Severe intraocular complications characterized by a white cataract and permanent wide mydriasis may occur in some cases of *Acanthamoeba* keratitis after initiation of either PHMB or chlorhexidine treatment.[60] Although thought to be a toxic response to these medications, it may also represent an idiosyncratic response or be related primarily to the disease, since much higher concentrations of chlorhexidine have been safely used.[61]

The majority of patients will achieve successful cure with these agents, but clinical resistance may occur. These cases may respond to increased concentrations of 0.04–0.06% chlorhexidine.[61] In recalcitrant disease, intracameral extension or choroidal invasion, which have been rarely reported, the addition of antifungal agents such as clotrimazole and itraconazole as well as newer antifungals which exhibit better anti-acanthamoebal activity should be considered.[62] Their precise clinical role has not yet been determined. Miltefosine has significant anti-acanthamoebal activity in vitro, but with limited published clinical experience.[62]

Surgical

Our treatment algorithm includes wide mechanical debridement accompanying initial treatment to remove accessible organisms and to improve drug penetration.[1,42] Conversely, persistent epithelial defects related to either a neurotrophic cornea or medication toxicity may complicate treatment. Partial tarsorrhaphy or amniotic membrane grafting is helpful in patients who do not respond to adjustment of their topical medications.[14] Corneal biopsy may be indicated in patients without other sufficient evidence of disease. Cryotherapy may have a role in further reducing the number of organisms and has been previously successfully combined with transplantation. Conjunctival flaps are of uncertain benefit in a disease with a limited response to cell-mediated host immunity.

The most controversial aspect of surgical management in *Acanthamoeba* keratitis is the role of corneal transplantation. A surgical margin clear of infection may be difficult to discern clinically and may be further masked by corticosteroid therapy. As expected, the results of penetrating keratoplasty were universally poor prior to the introduction of effective medical therapy.[4] Recurrence was common since remaining organisms could not be adequately suppressed. Greater awareness and the introduction of more effective drugs have significantly reduced therapeutic transplantation.[40] Patients undergoing keratoplasty once free of infection, defined as 3 months after discontinuation of anti-acanthamoebal medications, have the best outcomes,[63] but a small subset of patients will still experience extended, intractable infection and inflammation unresponsive to medical therapy. Severe extracorneal manifestations, e.g. limbitis, scleritis, and intraocular sequelae (e.g. cataract formation, permanent mydriasis, uveitis, and severe glaucoma as well as debilitating psychological effects), are not uncommon in this setting. A recent report on penetrating keratoplasty in patients receiving effective medical therapy has identified lower recurrence rates, but with a high rate of poor anatomic and visual outcomes related to these secondary sequelae of chronic disease.[64] The appropriate timing for therapeutic keratoplasty may be before these secondary ocular derangements become the greater risk factor for poor outcome.[64]

Role of corticosteroids

The role of corticosteroids in the management of *Acanthamoeba* keratitis remains unclear. In a Chinese hamster model, corticosteroid use induces chronic *Acanthamoeba* keratitis and increases the severity of deep stromal keratitis.[65] However, cell-mediated immunity may be ineffective in moderating disease, potentially damaging tissues without beneficial effect.[34] While the use of corticosteroids in other infectious keratitis is generally contraindicated, especially in untreated disease, none of the human studies, limited in power by the widespread use of corticosteroids prior to diagnosis, to date has identified its use as a risk factor for poor outcome.[1,66] Topical and systemic corticosteroid therapy has been commonly utilized for treatment of the sterile extracorneal manifestations of *Acanthamoeba* keratitis, e.g. limbitis and scleritis, but with vigilance for signs of extracorneal infection.[67] Sterile keratitis may also occur rarely, but persistent inflammation of the cornea should be considered infectious unless proven otherwise.[44] Regardless, corticosteroid use should be discontinued or limited to the lowest effective dose when possible, but has value and necessity in selected patients. In all *Acanthamoeba* keratitis patients, increasing inflammation is a useful guide to *Acanthamoeba* location and activity.

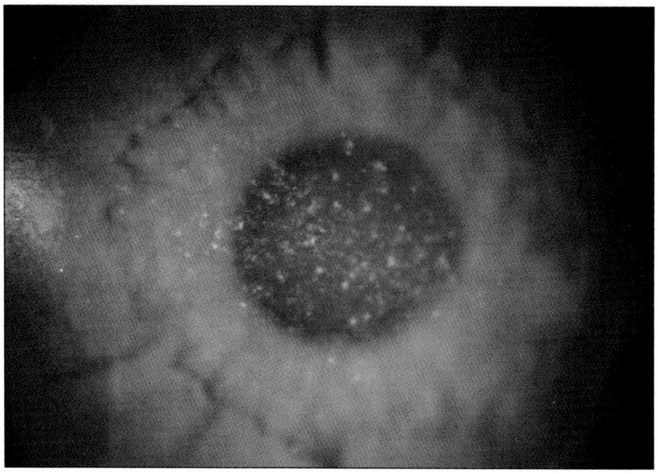

Fig. 83.6 Superficial microsporidial keratoconjunctivitis. An AIDS patient exhibits classic superficial microsporidial keratitis with relatively minimal inflammation.

Other Parasitic Corneal Infections

Non-*Acanthamoeba* amoebic keratitis

A number of other ubiquitous, cosmopolitan, free-living amoebae have been associated with human disease, but only a few have been suspected pathogens in exogenous amoebic keratitis. Most of these cases exhibited signs and symptoms similar to those seen in *Acanthamoeba* keratitis, mostly in contact lens wearers. Of the cases reported in the literature, *Vahlkampfia*, *Hartmannella vermiformis*, and *Naegleria* have been identified individually while most report a mixed population of *Vahlkampfia*, *Paravahlkampfia*, and *Hartmannella* sometimes with *Acanthaomeba*.[68–70] The incidence of infections with these other amoeba is likely higher since identification is even more difficult than in *Acanthamoeba* and is based primarily on morphology or very specific microbiologic methods. Furthermore, they respond well to empiric anti-acanthamoebal regimens, creating a potential source of misclassification, but, in limited published experience, do not commonly require therapeutic surgical intervention.

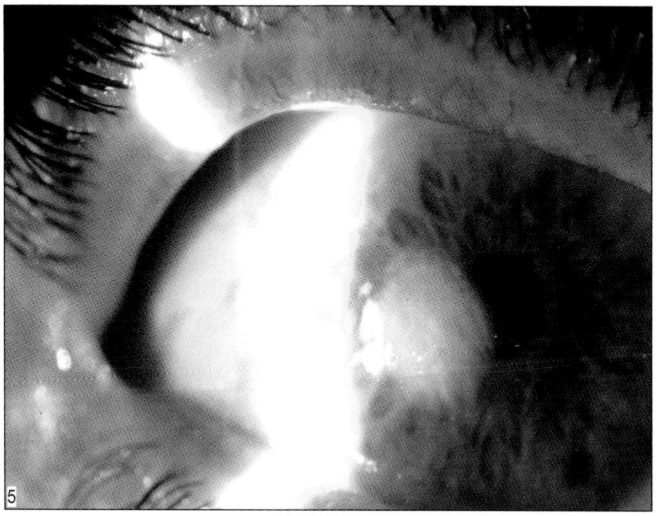

Fig. 83.7 Stromal microsporidial keratitis. Immunocompetent patient with disciform-like microsporidial keratitis. (Courtesy Terry O'Brien, Bascom Palmer Eye Institute, Miami, Florida).

Microsporidia

Microsporidia is a group of obligate intracellular parasites transmitted through air or water by highly efficient spores which utilize an integrated filament to pierce and attach to a target cell's wall. Once bridged by this tubule, the infective sporoplasm enters the host cell's cytoplasm, replicating either freely in the cytoplasm or within a cytoplasmic vacuole, bursting the host once the new spores reach maturity. Originally thought to be protozoan, genetic studies indicate that it is a highly refined fungal organism stripped of morphologic attributes unnecessary for its survival.[71]

Keratitis risk factors for microsporidia are not well defined, but a history of trauma or exposure to contaminated water is most commonly noted. Unlike *Acanthamoeba* keratitis, two largely separate, distinct forms are recognized: a superficial keratoconjunctivitis and a deep stromal keratitis.[72] Microsporidial keratoconjunctivitis was commonly associated with immunocompromised patients and presents with a superficial, multifocal, raised punctuate keratopathy associated with a mild to moderate conjunctivitis (Fig. 83.6).[72,73] Patients complain of redness, pain, photophobia and variably decreased vision. This form is most commonly associated with *Encephalitozoon* spp., but other members of *Microsporidium* have been reported. Microsporidial keratoconjunctivitis is increasingly reported in healthy, noncontact lens wearers mimicking epidemic keratoconjunctivitis or other causes of superficial punctuate keratitis.[74,75] Stromal microsporidiosis is found more commonly in immunocompetent patients as a chronic, progressive keratitis resembling a herpetic disciform disease with pain and, more significantly, decreased vision (Fig. 83.7).[72] Patients may develop uveitis as well as corneal neovascularization, necrosis, and perforation.

Diagnosis is most easily made by identifying the characteristic small oval or oblong spores on a calcafluor white or modified acid fast stain.[76] Culture diagnosis is challenging because specialized cell culture media is required for the growth of this obligate intracellular organism. Electron microscopy is very useful for definitive identification, but other antigen detection or PCR methods remain in development.[77] Corticosteroids appear to be ineffective and may worsen disease in both forms. The use of a number of drugs including albendazole, fumagillin, itraconazole, and propamidine isetionate has been associated with resolution of microsporidial keratoconjunctivitis, but has been less effective in stromal keratitis, where corneal transplantation is often required.[72,75] Although most immunodeficient patients appear unable to clear the pathogen, many cases of superficial keratitis in immunocompetent patients have been reported to resolve without specific treatment. This suggests both that the disease is more likely persistent and, consequently, diagnosed in immunocompromised patients, but that the incidence is significantly higher in immunocompetent patients than previously recognized.[74]

Parasitic Keratitis of Primarily Endogenous Origin

The following parasites produce a keratitis not from direct corneal inoculation, as those noted above, but which are usually the result of a systemic infection. These organisms all utilize an insect vector to penetrate systemic defenses. Once established, spread occurs hematologenously to the limbal end vessels, most commonly resulting in invasion of the corneal stroma to produce a centripetal interstitial keratitis.

Onchocerciasis

Onchocerciasis (river blindness) is caused by the filarial parasite *Onchocerca volvulus* introduced to the host by the bite of a *Simulium* black fly and is a major cause of Third World blindness.[78] Once mature, the adult worm releases microfilariae, which spread hematologenously to the eye and adnexal structures, invading the corneal stroma from the limbus. The microfilariae attract minimal inflammation as they migrate centrally, but create a centripetal sclerosing keratitis as they die, exacerbated by the exposure of their inflammatory endosymbiotic bacteria, *Wolbachia* spp.[78] The diagnosis is confirmed by direct observation of the microfilariae in the cornea or anterior chamber. To minimize scarring, combined treatment of the parasite with ivermectin (single dose, 150 ug/kg) and the endosymbiont with doxycycline is recommended.[79]

Leishmaniasis

Leishmaniasis is caused by protozoa from the genus *Leishmania* transmitted by a sandfly vector and takes two distinct systemic forms, cutaneous and visceral.[80] Corneal involvement occurs in a subset of the cutaneous form, American (mucocutaneous) leishmaniasis, initially manifesting as a sectoral or diffuse interstitial keratitis followed by aggressive neovascularization. Surface inoculation through contact with an eyelid lesion, interestingly, resembles an exogenous parasitic keratitis with suppurative corneal ulceration. Primary therapeutic agents are the pentavalent antimony compounds, sodium stibogluconate and meglumine antimoniate, which, if effective, will treat both the systemic infection and the keratitis.[81] Second-line agents include amphotericin B, pentamidine, and paromycin.[81]

Trypanosomiasis

Trypanosomiasis is caused by protozoa from the genus *Trypanosoma*. Keratitis is a feature of African sleeping sickness (*T. brucei*) transmitted by the tsetse fly. Once introduced, lymph nodes, liver, and spleen are initially affected, spreading hematologenously to the central nervous system (CNS), resulting in characteristic neurologic deficits and somnolence. These patients may exhibit frank corneal ulceration or progressive corneal infiltration and neovascularization, leading to an interstitial keratitis. Early treatment consists of pentamidine or suramin, but requires melarsoprol or eflornithine with or without nifurtimox once it has involved the CNS.[81] American Chagas' disease (*T. cruzi*) through direct inoculation produces a conjunctivitis or periocular infection without keratitis and is responsive to benznidazole and nifurtimox.[80]

References

1. Tu EY, Joslin CE, Sugar J, et al. Prognostic factors affecting visual outcome in *Acanthamoeba* keratitis. *Ophthalmology.* 2008;115(11):1998–2003.
2. Duguid IG, Dart JK, Morlet N, et al. Outcome of *Acanthamoeba* keratitis treated with polyhexamethyl biguanide and propamidine. *Ophthalmology.* 1997;104(10):1587–1592.
3. Seal D, Hay J, Kirkness C, et al. Successful medical therapy of *Acanthamoeba* keratitis with topical chlorhexidine and propamidine. *Eye.* 1996;10(Pt 4):413–421.
4. Jones BR, McGill JI, Steele AD. Recurrent suppurative kerato-uveitis with loss of eye due to infection by *Acanthamoeba castellani. Trans Ophthalmol Soc UK.* 1975;95(2):210–213.
5. *Acanthamoeba* keratitis associated with contact lenses – United States. *MMWR Morb Mortal Wkly Rep.* 1986;35(25):405–408.
6. Joslin CE, Tu EY, McMahon TT, et al. Epidemiological characteristics of a Chicago-area *Acanthamoeba* keratitis outbreak. *Am J Ophthalmol.* 2006;142(2):212–217.
7. Joslin CE, Tu EY, Shoff ME, et al. The association of contact lens solution use and *Acanthamoeba* keratitis. *Am J Ophthalmol.* 2007;144(2):169–180.
8. Mathers WD, Sutphin JE, Folberg R, et al. Outbreak of keratitis presumed to be caused by *Acanthamoeba*. *Am J Ophthalmol.* 1996;121(2):129–142.
9. Radford CF, Lehmann OJ, Dart JK. *Acanthamoeba* keratitis: multicentre survey in England 1992–6. National Acanthamoeba Keratitis Study Group. *Br J Ophthalmol.* 1998;82(12):1387–1392.
10. Radford CF, Minassian DC, Dart JK. *Acanthamoeba* keratitis in England and Wales: incidence, outcome, and risk factors. *Br J Ophthalmol.* 2002;86(5):536–542.
11. Schaumberg DA, Snow KK, Dana MR. The epidemic of *Acanthamoeba* keratitis: where do we stand? *Cornea.* 1998;17(1):3–10.
12. Stehr-Green JK, Bailey TM, Visvesvara GS. The epidemiology of *Acanthamoeba* keratitis in the United States. *Am J Ophthalmol.* 1989; 107(4):331–336.
13. *Acanthamoeba* keratitis multiple states, 2005–2007. *MMWR Morb Mortal Wkly Rep.* 2007;56(21):532–534.
14. Thebpatiphat N, Hammersmith KM, Rocha FN, et al. *Acanthamoeba* keratitis: a parasite on the rise. *Cornea.* 2007;26(6):701–706.
15. Dart JK, Radford CF, Minassian D, et al. Risk factors for microbial keratitis with contemporary contact lenses: a case-control study. *Ophthalmology.* 2008;115(10):1647–1654.
16. Stapleton F, Keay L, Edwards K, et al. The incidence of contact lens-related microbial keratitis in Australia. *Ophthalmology.* 2008;115(10): 1655–1662.

17. Bharathi MJ, Ramakrishnan R, Meenakshi R, et al. Microbiological diagnosis of infective keratitis: comparative evaluation of direct microscopy and culture results. *Br J Ophthalmol.* 2006;90(10):1271–1276.
18. *Acanthamoeba* keratitis in soft-contact-lens wearers. *MMWR Morb Mortal Wkly Rep.* 1987;36(25):397–398, 403–394.
19. Radford CF, Bacon AS, Dart JK, et al. Risk factors for *Acanthamoeba* keratitis in contact lens users: a case-control study. *BMJ.* 1995;310(6994): 1567–1570.
20. Stehr-Green JK, Bailey TM, Brandt FH, et al. *Acanthamoeba* keratitis in soft contact lens wearers. A case-control study. *JAMA.* 1987;258(1):57–60.
21. Van Meter WS, Musch DC, Jacobs DS, et al. Safety of overnight orthokeratology for myopia: a report by the American Academy of Ophthalmology. *Ophthalmology.* 2008;115(12):2301–2313 e2301.
22. Poggio EC, Glynn RJ, Schein OD, et al. The incidence of ulcerative keratitis among users of daily-wear and extended-wear soft contact lenses. *N Engl J Med.* 1989;321(12):779–783.
23. Hiti K, Walochnik J, Haller-Schober EM, et al. Viability of *Acanthamoeba* after exposure to a multipurpose disinfecting contact lens solution and two hydrogen peroxide systems. *Br J Ophthalmol.* 2002;86(2):144–146.
24. Shoff ME, Joslin CE, Tu EY, et al. Efficacy of contact lens systems against recent clinical and tap water *Acanthamoeba* isolates. *Cornea.* 2008; 27(6):713–719.
25. Shoff ME, Rogerson A, Kessler K, et al. Prevalence of *Acanthamoeba* and other naked amoebae in South Florida domestic water. *J Water Health.* 2008;6(1):99–104.
26. Kilvington S, Gray T, Dart J, et al. *Acanthamoeba* keratitis: the role of domestic tap water contamination in the United Kingdom. *Invest Ophthalmol Vis Sci.* 2004;45(1):165–169.
27. Meier PA, Mathers WD, Sutphin JE, et al. An epidemic of presumed *Acanthamoeba* keratitis that followed regional flooding. Results of a case-control investigation. *Arch Ophthalmol.* 1998;116(8):1090–1094.
28. Aksozek A, McClellan K, Howard K, et al. Resistance of *Acanthamoeba castellanii* cysts to physical, chemical, and radiological conditions. *J Parasitol.* 2002;88(3):621–623.
29. Schuster FL, Visvesvara GS. Free-living amoebae as opportunistic and non-opportunistic pathogens of humans and animals. *Int J Parasitol.* 2004;34(9):1001–1027.
30. Booton GC, Kelly DJ, Chu YW, et al. 18S ribosomal DNA typing and tracking of *Acanthamoeba* species isolates from corneal scrape specimens, contact lenses, lens cases, and home water supplies of *Acanthamoeba* keratitis patients in Hong Kong. *J Clin Microbiol.* 2002;40(5):1621–1625.
31. Garate M, Marchant J, Cubillos I, et al. In vitro pathogenicity of *Acanthamoeba* is associated with the expression of the mannose-binding protein. *Invest Ophthalmol Vis Sci.* 2006;47(3):1056–1062.
32. Clarke DW, Niederkorn JY. The pathophysiology of *Acanthamoeba* keratitis. *Trends Parasitol.* 2006;22(4):175–180.
33. Cerva L. *Acanthamoeba culbertsoni* and *Naegleria fowleri*: occurrence of antibodies in man. *J Hyg Epidemiol Microbiol Immunol.* 1989;33(1). 99–103.
34. Clarke DW, Niederkorn JY. The immunobiology of *Acanthamoeba* keratitis. *Microbes Infect.* 2006;8(5):1400–1405.
35. Garate M, Alizadeh H, Neelam S, et al. Oral immunization with *Acanthamoeba castellanii* mannose-binding protein ameliorates amoebic keratitis. *Infect Immun.* 2006;74(12):7032–7034.
36. Gray TB, Cursons RT, Sherwan JF, et al. *Acanthamoeba*, bacterial, and fungal contamination of contact lens storage cases. *Br J Ophthalmol.* 1995;79(6):601–605.
37. Fritsche TR, Sobek D, Gautom RK. Enhancement of in vitro cytopathogenicity by *Acanthamoeba* spp. following acquisition of bacterial endosymbionts. *FEMS Microbiol Lett.* 1998;166(2):231–236.
38. Tseng CH, Fong CF, Chen WL, et al. Overnight orthokeratology-associated microbial keratitis. *Cornea.* 2005;24(7):778–782.
39. Wilhelmus KR, Jones DB, Matoba AY, et al. Bilateral *Acanthamoeba* keratitis. *Am J Ophthalmol.* 2008;145(2):193–197.
40. Bacon AS, Frazer DG, Dart JK, et al. A review of 72 consecutive cases of *Acanthamoeba* keratitis, 1984–1992. *Eye.* 1993;7(Pt 6):719–725.
41. Perry HD, Donnenfeld ED, Foulks GN, et al. Decreased corneal sensation as an initial feature of *Acanthamoeba* keratitis. *Ophthalmology.* 1995; 102(10):1565–1568.
42. Holland GN, Donzis PB. Rapid resolution of early *Acanthamoeba* keratitis after epithelial debridement. *Am J Ophthalmol.* 1987;104(1):87–89.
43. Feist RM, Sugar J, Tessler H. Radial keratoneuritis in *Pseudomonas* keratitis. *Arch Ophthalmol.* 1991;109(6):774–775.
44. Yang YF, Matheson M, Dart JK, et al. Persistence of *Acanthamoeba* antigen following *Acanthamoeba* keratitis. *Br J Ophthalmol.* 2001;85(3):277–280.
45. Tomita M, Shimmura S, Tsubota K, et al. Dacryoadenitis associated with *Acanthamoeba* keratitis. *Arch Ophthalmol.* 2006;124(9):1239–1242.
46. Mannis MJ, Tamaru R, Roth AM, et al. *Acanthamoeba* sclerokeratitis. Determining diagnostic criteria. *Arch Ophthalmol.* 1986;104(9):1313–1317.
47. Moshari A, McLean IW, Dodds MT, et al. Chorioretinitis after keratitis caused by *Acanthamoeba*: case report and review of the literature. *Ophthalmology.* 2001;108(12):2232–2236.
48. Awwad ST, Heilman M, Hogan RN, et al. Severe reactive ischemic posterior segment inflammation in *Acanthamoeba* keratitis: a new potentially blinding syndrome. *Ophthalmology.* 2007;114(2):313–320.
48A. Tu EY, Joslin CE, Nijm LM, et al. Polymicrobial Keratitis: *Acanthamoeba* and Infectious Crystalline Keratopathy. *Am J Ophthalmol.* 2009;148(1):13–19.e2. Epub 2009 Mar 27.
49. Penland RL, Wilhelmus KR. Laboratory diagnosis of *Acanthamoeba* keratitis using buffered charcoal-yeast extract agar. *Am J Ophthalmol.* 1998;126(4):590–592.
50. Tu EY, Joslin CE, Sugar J, et al. The relative value of confocal microscopy and superficial corneal scrapings in the diagnosis of *Acanthamoeba* keratitis. *Cornea.* 2008;27(7):764–772.
51. Sawada Y, Yuan C, Huang AJ. Impression cytology in the diagnosis of *Acanthamoeba* keratitis with surface involvement. *Am J Ophthalmol.* 2004;137(2):323–328.
52. Mathers WD, Nelson SE, Lane JL, et al. Confirmation of confocal microscopy diagnosis of *Acanthamoeba* keratitis using polymerase chain reaction analysis. *Arch Ophthalmol.* 2000;118(2):178–183.
53. Chew SJ, Beuerman RW, Assouline M, et al. Early diagnosis of infectious keratitis with in vivo real time confocal microscopy. *CLAO J.* 1992;18(3):197–201.
54. Parmar DN, Awwad ST, Petroll WM, et al. Tandem scanning confocal corneal microscopy in the diagnosis of suspected *Acanthamoeba* keratitis. *Ophthalmology.* 2006;113(4):538–547.
55. Bacon AS, Dart JK, Ficker LA, et al. *Acanthamoeba* keratitis. The value of early diagnosis. *Ophthalmology.* 1993;100(8):1238–1243.
56. Claerhout I, Goegebuer A, Van Den Broecke C, et al. Delay in diagnosis and outcome of *Acanthamoeba* keratitis. *Graefe's Arch Clin Exp Ophthalmol.* 2004;242(8):648–653.
57. Lim N, Goh D, Bunce C, et al. Comparison of polyhexamethylene biguanide and chlorhexidine as monotherapy agents in the treatment of *Acanthamoeba* keratitis. *Am J Ophthalmol.* 2008;145(1):130–135.
58. Moore MB, McCulley JP, Luckenbach M, et al. *Acanthamoeba* keratitis associated with soft contact lenses. *Am J Ophthalmol.* 1985;100(3): 396–403.
59. Perrine D, Chenu JP, Georges P, et al. Amoebicidal efficiencies of various diamidines against two strains of *Acanthamoeba* polyphaga. *Antimicrob Agents Chemother.* 1995;39(2):339–342.
60. Herz NL, Matoba AY, Wilhelmus KR. Rapidly progressive cataract and iris atrophy during treatment of *Acanthamoeba* keratitis. *Ophthalmology.* 2008;115(5):866–869.
61. Mathers W. Use of higher medication concentrations in the treatment of *Acanthamoeba* keratitis. *Arch Ophthalmol.* 2006;124(6):923.
62. Schuster FL, Guglielmo BJ, Visvesvara GS. In-vitro activity of miltefosine and voriconazole on clinical isolates of free-living amebas: *Balamuthia mandrillaris, Acanthamoeba* spp., and *Naegleria fowleri. J Eukaryot Microbiol.* 2006;53(2):121–126.
63. Awwad ST, Parmar DN, Heilman M, et al. Results of penetrating keratoplasty for visual rehabilitation after *Acanthamoeba* keratitis. *Am J Ophthalmol.* 2005;140(6):1080–1084.
64. Kashiwabuchi RT, de Freitas D, Alvarenga LS, et al. Corneal graft survival after therapeutic keratoplasty for *Acanthamoeba* keratitis. *Acta Ophthalmol.* 2008;86(6):666–669.
65. McClellan K, Howard K, Niederkorn JY, et al. Effect of steroids on *Acanthamoeba* cysts and trophozoites. *Invest Ophthalmol Vis Sci.* 2001; 42(12):2885–2893.
66. Park DH, Palay DA, Daya SM, et al. The role of topical corticosteroids in the management of *Acanthamoeba* keratitis. *Cornea.* 1997;16(3):277–283.
67. Lee GA, Gray TB, Dart JK, et al. *Acanthamoeba* sclerokeratitis: treatment with systemic immunosuppression. *Ophthalmology.* 2002;109(6):1178–1182.
68. Aitken D, Hay J, Kinnear FB, et al. Amebic keratitis in a wearer of disposable contact lenses due to a mixed *Vahlkampfia* and *Hartmannella* infection. *Ophthalmology.* 1996;103(3):485–494.
69. Lorenzo-Morales J, Martinez-Carretero E, Batista N, et al. Early diagnosis of amoebic keratitis due to a mixed infection with *Acanthamoeba* and *Hartmannella*. *Parasitol Res.* 2007;102(1):167–169.
70. Ozkoc S, Tuncay S, Delibas SB, et al. Identification of *Acanthamoeba* genotype T4 and *Paravahlkampfia* sp. from two clinical samples. *J Med Microbiol.* 2008;57(Pt 3):392–396.
71. Thomarat F, Vivares CP, Gouy M. Phylogenetic analysis of the complete genome sequence of *Encephalitozoon cuniculi* supports the fungal origin of microsporidia and reveals a high frequency of fast-evolving genes. *J Mol Evol.* 2004;59(6):780–791.
72. Joseph J, Vemuganti GK, Sharma S. Microsporidia: emerging ocular pathogens. *Indian J Med Microbiol.* 2005;23(2):80–91.

73. Friedberg DN, Stenson SM, Orenstein JM, et al. Microsporidial keratoconjunctivitis in acquired immunodeficiency syndrome. *Arch Ophthalmol.* 1990;108(4):504–508.
74. Das S, Sharma S, Sahu SK, et al. New microbial spectrum of epidemic keratoconjunctivitis: clinical and laboratory aspects of an outbreak. *Br J Ophthalmol.* 2008;92(6):861–862.
75. Chan CM, Theng JT, Li L, et al. Microsporidial keratoconjunctivitis in healthy individuals: a case series. *Ophthalmology.* 2003;110(7):1420–1425.
76. Joseph J, Sridhar MS, Murthy S, et al. Clinical and microbiological profile of microsporidial keratoconjunctivitis in southern India. *Ophthalmology.* 2006;113(4):531–537.
77. Conners MS, Gibler TS, Van Gelder RN. Diagnosis of microsporidia keratitis by polymerase chain reaction. *Arch Ophthalmol.* 2004;122(2):283–284.
78. Pearlman E, Gillette-Ferguson I. *Onchocerca volvulus, Wolbachia* and river blindness. *Chem Immunol Allergy.* 2007;92:254–265.
79. Hoerauf A, Specht S, Buttner M, et al. *Wolbachia* endobacteria depletion by doxycycline as antifilarial therapy has macrofilaricidal activity in onchocerciasis: a randomized placebo-controlled study. *Med Microbiol Immunol.* 2008;197(3):295–311.
80. Lam S. Keratitis caused by leishmaniasis and trypanosomiasis. *Ophthalmol Clin N Am.* 1994;7(4):635–639.
81. Croft SL, Barrett MP, Urbina JA. Chemotherapy of trypanosomiases and leishmaniasis. *Trends Parasitol.* 2005;21(11):508–512.

Chapter 84

Corneal Diseases in the Developing World

Pravin K. Vaddavalli, Prashant Garg, Gullapalli N. Rao

The World Health Organization defines health as 'a state of complete physical, mental, and social well-being and not merely the absence of disease or infirmity.' More recently, this concept has been extended to include health-related quality of life and applies to vision too. Impairment, disability, and handicap are all related directly to the concept of health and visual function. Impairment concerns the physical aspects of health; disability has to do with the loss of functional capacity resulting from an impaired organ; handicap is a measure of the social and cultural consequences of an impairment or disability; and health-related quality of life means health as assessed by the individual concerned.

Worldwide, more than 161 million people are visually impaired; among them, 124 million have low vision and 37 million are blind. Another 153 million people live with visual impairment due to uncorrected refractive errors (nearsightedness, far-sightedness or astigmatism). More than 90% of the world's visually impaired people live in low- and middle-income countries. Except in the most developed countries, cataract remains the leading cause of blindness. The good news is that up to 75% of all blindness in adults is avoidable through prevention or treatment. Worldwide, corneal scarring is the single most important cause of avoidable blindness, followed by cataract and retinopathy of prematurity (ROP).

Diseases affecting the cornea are a major cause of blindness worldwide, second only to cataract in overall importance. The epidemiology of corneal blindness is complicated and encompasses a wide variety of infectious and inflammatory eye diseases that cause corneal scarring, which ultimately leads to functional blindness. In addition, the prevalence of corneal disease varies from country to country and even from one population to another.[1]

Corneal disease ranges from nonsignificant diseases such as simple climactic droplet keratopathy to blinding diseases such as keratitis. The impact that the blinding diseases have on the individual and on society is much larger than nonblinding ones.

The prevalence of these disorders and the effects they have on visual disability in developing countries assumes great significance for two reasons. Firstly, the epidemiology of corneal diseases varies widely based on geography and local environmental conditions as compared to more developed nations. More importantly, the impact these disorders have on the visual outcome is to a large extent magnified by the inadequate levels of eye care available in most developing nations. Medical and surgical interventions for visual disability caused by corneal disease are usually inadequate and are accessible only to a small minority of patients needing them.

Corneal Blindness

While cataract is responsible for nearly 20 million of the 45 million blind people in the world, the next major cause is trachoma, which blinds 4.9 million individuals, mainly as a result of corneal scarring and vascularization. Ocular trauma and corneal ulceration are significant causes of corneal blindness that are often underreported but may be responsible for 1.5–2.0 million new cases of monocular blindness every year. Causes of childhood blindness (about 1.5 million worldwide with 5 million visually disabled) include xerophthalmia (350 000 cases annually), ophthalmia neonatorum, and less frequently seen ocular diseases such as herpes simplex virus infections and vernal keratoconjunctivitis.[1]

The global distribution of blindness by economic regions as published by WHO in 1995 is shown in Table 84.1.[2] To provide an easy means of comparison, the authors described what is known as a regional burden of blindness (RBB) (Table 84.2).[2] The data clearly show that 75% of world blindness currently occurs in Asia and Africa.

Approximately 50% of all blindness is due to cataract, 15% due to trachoma, up to 10% due to uncorrected refractive error, 4% due to childhood blindness, and 1% due to onchocerciasis. These five diseases are responsible for up to 80% of the world's blindness.[3] Other causes of blindness include glaucoma, diabetic retinopathy, trauma, and age-related macular degeneration. The relative importance of diseases causing blindness varies greatly by region.[4] Table 84.3 shows regional estimates of the major causes of blindness. The Eye Diseases Prevalence Research Group estimated that the leading cause of blindness among white persons older than 40 years is age-related macular degeneration, accounting for 54% of all blindness, compared to 8.7% by cataract. However, cataract and glaucoma accounted for over 60% of blindness among black persons in the same age group.[5] Data from Europe and Australia show that

Table 84.1 Global magnitude of blindness by economic regions

World Bank regions	Prevalence of blindness (%)	Number blind (millions)	Major causes
Established market economies (EME)	0.3	2.4	Cataract
Former socialist economies of Europe	0.3	1.1	Retinal diseases
Latin America & Caribbean	0.5	2.3	Cataract
Middle Eastern crescent	0.7	3.6	Cataract
China	0.6	6.7	Cataract
India	10	8.9	Cataract
Rest of Asia	0.8	5.8	Refractive errors
Sub-Saharan Africa	1.4	7.1	Cataract

From Thylefors B, Negrel AD, Pararajasegaram R, Dadzie KY. Global data on blindness. Bull World Health Organ. 1995;73:115–2.

Table 84.2 Regional burden of blindness (RBB)

World Bank regions	Percent of global population	Percent of global blindness	Regional burden of blindness (RBB)
Established market economies (EME)	15.1	6.3	0.41
Former socialist economies of Europe	6.6	2.9	0.44
Latin America & Caribbean	8.4	61	0.72
Middle Eastern crescent	9.6	9.5	0.99
China	21.4	17.6	0.82
India	16.1	23.5	1.46
Rest of Asia	13	15.3	1.18
Sub-Saharan Africa	9.7	18.8	1.93

From Thylefors B, Negrel AD, Pararajasegaram R, Dadzie KY. Global data on blindness. Bull World Health Organ. 1995;73:115–2.

Table 84.3 Regional variations in the causes of blindness (%)

	EME	FSE	Latin America & Caribbean	Middle Eastern crescent	China	India	OAI	SSA
Cataract	3.5	8.3	57.6	45.2	32.4	51.2	39.8	43.6
Corneal scar			6.8	25.7	17.6	9.7	23.6	19.4
Glaucoma	7.5	6.8	8.0	5.7	2.7	12.8	16.7	12.0
Others	89.0	84.9	27.5	23.4	27.3	26.3	19.9	25.0

EME, established market economies; FSE, former socialist economies of Europe; OAI, other Asia and Islands; SSA, sub-Saharan Africa.
From Thylefors B, Negrel AD, Pararajasegaram R, Dadzie KY. Global data on blindness. Bull World Health Organ. 1995;73:115–2.

age-related macular degeneration and uncorrected refractive errors are leading causes of blindness.[6–8] In India, important causes of blindness in various epidemiological surveys are cataract (44–77.5%), uncorrected refractive error (16.3%), retinal diseases (2–10.9%), glaucoma (7.9–10.2%), and corneal diseases (2–7.1%).[9–11] Other less-developed countries, too, have a similar distribution of blindness.[12–15] In the Eastern Mediterranean countries, common causes of blindness are cataract (45.2%), trachoma and nontrachomatous corneal scar (25.7%), and glaucoma (5.7%).[12] The data clearly show that corneal diseases are important as a cause of blindness in nations with less-developed economies which are already burdened by a higher prevalence of blindness.

There is a strong correlation between aging and blindness; approximately 58% of all blind persons are aged more than 60 years and only 3.8% of the global total are between 0 and 14 years.[16] However, this prevalence of blindness in children is an underestimate of the magnitude of the problem, because the mortality among blind children, particularly in the developing world, is higher than their sighted counterparts and the prevalence takes into account only children who survive.[17] In addition, childhood blindness must be considered a priority because blind children have many years of blindness ahead of them and the visual loss affects all aspects of their development. Current estimates suggest that globally there are 1.4 million blind children.[16] The prevalence of blindness in children also varies according to socioeconomic status and under-5 mortality rates. In low-income countries with high under-5 mortality, the prevalence may be as high as 1.5 per 1000 children compared to 0.3 per 1000 children in high-income countries.[18] Nearly 22.9% of blind children live in sub-Saharan Africa and approximately three-quarters of the world's blind children live in the African and Asian continents (Table 84.4).[17]

Of the 1.4 million blind children worldwide, an estimated 25% are blind from retinal diseases, 20% from corneal

Table 84.4 Estimates of prevalence of childhood blindness by World Bank regions

World Bank regions	Estimated regional prevalence	Estimated No. of blind children	Percent of global childhood blindness
Established market economies (EME)	0.3	50000	3.57
Former socialist economies of Europe	0.51	40000	2.85
Latin America & Caribbean	0.6	100000	7.14
Middle Eastern crescent	0.8	190000	13.5
China	0.5	210000	15
India	0.8	270000	19.3
Rest of Asia	0.83	220000	15.7
Sub-Saharan Africa	1.24	320000	22.9

From Gilbert CE, Anderton L, Dandona L, et al. Prevalence of blindness and visual impairment in children – a review of available data. Ophthalmic Epidemiol 1999;6:73–81.

pathology, 13% due to cataract, 6% from glaucoma, and 17% due to anomalies affecting the whole globe.[19] The causes of childhood blindness are also different in developed countries and countries with less-developed economies. In poor countries of the world, corneal scarring due to vitamin A deficiency, measles, ophthalmia neonatorum, and the effects of harmful traditional eye remedies predominate,[20–25] while at the other end of the socioeconomic spectrum, retinal diseases, and optic nerve affections due to genetic or perinatal causes, are important causes of blindness.[16,17] Corneal disease is responsible for less than 2% of blindness in children in industrialized countries, while in the poorest areas of Africa and Asia corneal scarring accounts for 25–50% of childhood blindness.[19] Thus, corneal disease is an important cause of blindness among children living in developing nations, which already carry a major burden of blindness.

These studies in adults and children clearly show that corneal diseases are important causes of blindness in both adults and children and that the major burden of these diseases is in developing countries with less-developed economies.

Causes of Corneal Blindness

The epidemiology of corneal diseases resulting in blindness is varied and largely depends on the ocular diseases that are endemic in each geographical area. Traditionally, important diseases responsible for corneal blindness include xerophthalmia, trachoma, onchocerciasis, leprosy, and ophthalmia neonatorum.[26,27]

Xerophthalmia

Xerophthalmia, caused by vitamin A deficiency, is still the leading cause of childhood blindness. Of approximately 1.5 million children blind, and 5 million visually disabled worldwide, 350000 are blinded every year as a result of vitamin A deficiency. The subsequent high mortality in these children, initially documented by Sommer et al.,[28] explains the relatively low prevalence of xerophthalmia in developing countries in spite of its high incidence. In other words, the majority of children who have vitamin A deficiency severe enough to cause the bilateral corneal melting, perforation, and blindness associated with xerophthalmia die within the first year. An even more tragic aspect of xerophthalmia is its close association with measles epidemics. Malnourished children who are on the edge of developing xerophthalmia frequently do so after contracting measles from a sibling or a classmate.[29]

Clinical features

Xerophthalmia is a term that describes the ocular changes resulting from vitamin A deficiency. Xerosis implies drying of the conjunctival or corneal epithelium. While conjunctival xerosis may signal mild disease, corneal xerosis indicates more severe deficiency. Other clinical findings in the spectrum include Bitot's spots on the conjunctiva, fundus changes, and nyctalopia (night blindness). Keratomalacia is the most severe ocular form of vitamin A deficiency, resulting in rapid sterile melt of the cornea, leading to corneal perforation and secondary infection often resulting in permanent blindness. Children with vitamin A deficiency are also likely to suffer from systemic illnesses such as diarrhea, respiratory illnesses, and measles. The presence of keratomalacia indicates a poor prognosis for health and life, with more than 50% percent of children with xerophthalmia dying due to associated poor nutritional status and susceptibility to disease.

Management

Xerophthalmia should not be considered an isolated ocular disease because it generally occurs with generalized malnutrition and is an ocular and a medical emergency.

Xerophthalmia treatment schedules for children between 1 and 6 years of age are:[27,28]

- immediately on diagnosis: 200 000 IU of vitamin A orally
- following day: 200 000 IU of vitamin A orally
- 4 weeks later: 200 000 IU of vitamin A orally.

Vitamin A deficiency is not an isolated entity and is dependent on many dietary, social, and economic factors. Community interventions and education therefore play equally, if not more important, roles in the prevention and management of this disease. Other preventive strategies include increasing awareness about breast-feeding, dietary fortification, and improvement of general nutrition. Measles also contributes significantly to the morbidity and mortality of vitamin A deficiency syndromes by precipitating acute deficiency and unmasking borderline malnutrition. Immunization of children against measles is also an important health strategy in the prevention of vitamin A deficiency states.[27,30]

Trachoma

Trachoma is a chronic keratoconjunctivitis caused by the bacterium *Chlamydia trachomatis* and primarily affects the superior and inferior tarsal conjunctiva and the cornea.

Currently, trachoma is the world's leading infectious cause of blindness and the leading cause of ocular morbidity. Regions and countries where trachoma remains a major cause of external ocular disease and blindness include:

- Africa: western, eastern and southern Africa and Sudan
- Mediterranean and Middle East: Morocco, Tunisia, Libya, Egypt, Djibouti, Saudi Arabia, the Gulf States, Iran, Afghanistan, Pakistan
- Asia: India, Nepal, Myanmar, China
- Southeast Asia: Laos, Vietnam, Philippines, Australia, some Pacific islands
- Americas: Mexico, Guatemala, Brazil, Bolivia, Peru.

Trachoma is a disease of overcrowded and unclean living environments and is spread by poor hygiene, contaminated water, and houseflies. Patients most severely affected by trachoma are usually infected early in childhood and remain infected most of their lives.[31]

Clinical diagnosis

Trachoma is nearly always bilateral. The infection begins in the upper tarsal conjunctiva but also involves the lower fornix. Initial response to infection includes a widespread papillary reaction and a diffuse follicular response, which indicates active infection. Follicles also appear at the limbus and, when healed, leave characteristic scars known as Herbert's pits. It often results in corneal scarring with dense vascularization, ocular surface problems, and invariable presence of entropion and trichiasis. Corneal changes during the acute stage include development of a superior pannus; punctuate keratitis eventually resulting in various grades of cornea scarring. Chronic disease results in conjunctival scarring, which results in entropion and trichiasis, chiefly of the upper lid, with further damage to the cornea. Trachoma often leads to an increased susceptibility to microbial keratitis and dacryocystitis. A detailed grading system and description of the clinical manifestations are beyond the scope of this chapter and may be referred to in other chapters of this book.

Management

Tetracyclines form the mainstay of the medical management of trachoma. Topical tetracycline 1% ointment or suspension three times a day for a minimum of 6 weeks is the current recommended treatment for active disease by the WHO.[27]

Oral azithromycin is a new antibiotic that has shown great promise in treating trachoma as a single 1 g dose.[32]

Surgical management of the complications of trachoma is equally important in dealing with the late sequelae of the disease. Surgical strategies may range from simple procedures such as epilation of trichiatic eyelashes to electrolysis and cryoablation of the lash follicles. More complex procedures to correct associated entropion depend on the degree of disability and severity of scarring on the tarsal plate.[27]

Public health strategies

An important cog in the wheel of preventing trachoma is tackling it at the community level. Improving the standard of living in the community along with better sanitation best controls trachoma. A simple strategy for promotion of hygiene, blindness prevention, and community support is the SAFE strategy, which is an acronym for:

S – Surgery for trachoma
A – Antibiotics to treat inflammatory disease
F – Face washing, especially in children
E – Environmental changes, including provision of clean water and improvement of sanitation.[32]

In 1996, an alliance for the global elimination of trachoma was formed under the aegis of the Vision 2020 program with a goal to eradicate trachoma by the year 2020.[32]

It is estimated by WHO that at present there are about 4.9 million people blind from trachomatous corneal scarring and 10 million suffering from trichiasis and thus at risk of corneal blindness.[26]

Onchocerciasis

Onchocerciasis (river blindness) is a chronic parasitic infection that can lead to corneal and retinal scarring and intraocular damage from uveitis. Onchocerciasis results in severe blinding keratitis due to an inflammatory response to dead and degenerating microfilaria in the corneal stroma. The end result is severe corneal scarring and vascularization. Approximately 18 million people are infected with the disease in 30 African and six Latin American countries, but the great majority of the 270 000 people blind from onchocerciasis are from Africa.

Clinical features

Common clinical signs of systemic onchocerciasis are skin nodules and patchy loss of skin pigment along with skin rashes and itching. In patients with severe infection, dead microfilariae may be seen in the cornea as straight transparent needle-like structures, while living microfilariae are coiled up and are usually seen in the peripheral cornea, particularly at the 3 and 9 o'clock positions. Punctate keratitis with snowflake-like stromal opacities may occur with deep stromal scarring resembling sclerosing keratitis. Other causes of blindness are chronic uveitis, chorioretinitis, and optic atrophy from microfilarial invasion.

Management

Systemic treatment of onchocerciasis can control generalized infection and, though it cannot reverse permanent visual disability, it can halt further progression of the disease. In the past, diethlycarbamazine citrate (DEC) and suramin sodium were used but have now been replaced by ivermectin, a broad-spectrum antiparasitic agent, a much safer drug for human use. Although uveitis and chorioretinitis can be managed with topical and systemic therapy, visual disability resulting from corneal scarring has a poor prognosis due to the associated vascularity.[1,27] Until 15 years ago the outlook for eradicating onchocerciasis was dismal. Public health projects that focused on reducing the habitat of the vector of the parasite, a small black fly that breeds in freshwater streams and rivers, were frustratingly ineffective and destructive to the environment. The development of ivermectin in the 1980s and its widespread distribution since 1987 have led to a remarkable decrease in the number of new cases of onchocerciasis in endemic areas. With the administration of one tablet of ivermectin twice a year to all individuals in endemic areas, it is estimated that there will be no new cases of onchocerciasis by the year 2020.[1] The African Program for Onchocerciasis Control (APOC) in Africa and the Onchocerciasis Elimination Program of the Americas (OEPA), both managed by the WHO with support from the World Bank and Merck & Co Inc., are community health initiatives to halt the spread of onchocerciasis.[27]

Current data from West Africa show that blindness rates due to onchocerciasis are below 1% in communities that had up to 10% blindness rates at the onset of the onchocerciasis control program. The incidence of the onchocerciasis-related blindness in West Africa is now zero.[32]

Leprosy

Leprosy is a chronic, slowly progressive debilitating disease that primarily affects skin, peripheral nerves, and extremities. Leprosy affects 10–12 million people, the majority of whom are in Africa and the southern portion of the Indian subcontinent. There are approximately 250 000 blind from the disease.[33] Regions where leprosy is primarily concentrated include sub-Saharan Africa, the Middle East, the Indian subcontinent, Indochina, and islands in the western Pacific.

Clinical features

Corneal involvement in leprosy may be due to direct invasion by *Mycobacterium leprae* resulting in loss of corneal sensation and corneal opacities. These corneal lesions are further complicated by the frequent presence of lagophthalmos resulting from paralysis of the seventh cranial (facial) nerve that leads to exposure keratitis, repeated corneal ulcers, and eventually corneal scarring and vascularization. Interstitial keratitis may also occur as a result of direct corneal infiltration by *M. leprae*. Other pathways of blindness in leprosy include chronic uveitis, secondary glaucoma, and cataract formation.

Management

Medical treatment of leprosy is primary oral multidrug therapy (MDT) with rifampicin, clofazimine, and dapsone. Surgical correction of lid deformities including simple tarsorraphy forms the mainstay in preventing and managing corneal complications along with topical palliative therapy. Visual rehabilitation by corneal transplantation has limited success due to the corneal vascularity, recurrent uveitis, and frequently anesthetic corneas.

A comprehensive national leprosy program is necessary for control of the disease. In India, the National Leprosy Control Program (NLCP) and in Africa, the All Africa Leprosy Rehabilitation and Training (ALERT) center in Addis Ababa, Ethiopia, are such successful programs. Today, the prevalence of leprosy is rapidly declining in most countries around the world as a direct result of widespread public health efforts, especially the administration of multidrug therapy. The introduction of MDT by the World Health Organization in 1982 for the treatment of multibacillary leprosy has led to a shortened treatment time of 2 years and a high degree of bacterial eradication (99.9%).[1,27,33]

Ophthalmia Neonatorum

Ophthalmia neonatorum, or conjunctivitis of the newborn, refers to any conjunctivitis with discharge that occurs in the first 28 days of life.[34] The risk of blindness is high in infections caused by *Neisseria gonorrhoeae*, especially since ocular gonorrhea in the newborn is frequently bilateral. If the infection is caused by *Chlamydia trachomatis* or other less virulent pathogens, the risk of blindness is low. In the past century there has been a significant change in the spectrum of organisms causing ophthalmia neonatorum as the incidence of chlamydial infections has risen dramatically in relation to gonorrheal infections, especially in industrialized countries.[35] In developing countries the prevalence of chlamydial infection in pregnant women ranges from 7% to 29%. One-third of infants exposed at birth develop a chlamydial infection. Similar studies of gonorrheal infection in Africa indicate a maternal infection prevalence of 3–22%, with gonorrheal ophthalmia developing in 30–50% of exposed neonates.[36]

Although the worldwide incidence of ophthalmia neonatorum is not known, it represents a significant cause of childhood corneal blindness, especially in developing countries. Prevention of sexually transmitted diseases in adults, antenatal screening of pregnant women, ocular prophylaxis at birth, and early diagnosis and treatment of ocular infections in neonates are important strategies in reducing the incidence of ophthalmia neonatorum. Studies have shown that a 2.5% solution of aqueous povidone-iodine applied to the eyes of neonates is just as effective and is cheaper than erythromycin ointment or 1% silver nitrate (Crede's prophylaxis) in preventing the majority of cases of chlamydial and gonorrheal ophthalmia neonatorum.[37] Tetracycline ointment may also be used. If prophylaxis fails, a single intramuscular injection of cefotaxime (100 mg/kg) is effective against gonorrhea in the newborn, and a 2-week course of erythromycin orally (50 mg/kg daily in four divided doses) is recommended for the treatment of chlamydia.[1]

Although these diseases still remain important causes of blindness, the recent success of public health programs in controlling onchocerciasis and leprosy as well as a gradual worldwide decline in the number of cases of trachoma has generated new interest in other causes of corneal blindness. These include corneal trauma, corneal ulceration, and complications from the use of traditional eye medicines.

Corneal Trauma

In 1992, Thylefors and Négrel drew attention to the fact that trauma is often the most important cause of unilateral loss of vision in developing countries.[38,39] They estimated that approximately 1.6 million people are blind from injuries, 2.3 million had bilateral low vision, and 19 million are unilateral blind or had low vision.[39] Though corneal trauma can range from innocuous corneal abrasions to sight-threatening penetrating ocular injuries, even minor corneal trauma that breaches the epithelium has potential to result in microbial keratitis and its associated complications.

Even though ocular trauma is a global problem, the burden of blindness from eye injuries falls most heavily on developing countries, especially those where war and civil unrest have left a legacy of eye trauma from weapons such as land mines.[40] A country-wide, population-based survey in Nepal reported that trauma was responsible for 7.7% of all monocular blindness.[41] A more recent population-based prospective study in Bhaktapur District in Kathmandu Valley, Nepal, revealed that the annual incidence of ocular injury is 1788 per 100000 people, with 789 of the injuries due to corneal abrasions.[42] In other words, 1.8% of the residents of Bhaktapur District experience some form of ocular injury every year. In Nepal and other developing countries, injuries are usually associated with agricultural work, but a much higher rate of ocular trauma can occur in specialized situations, such as foundries. Data from the Andhra Pradesh Eye Disease Study (APEDS), which sampled 11786 people of all ages from 94 clusters representative of the population of the Indian state of Andhra Pradesh, revealed corneal trauma accounted for 28.6% of all corneal blindness, second only to corneal scars secondary to keratitis in childhood, which accounted for 36.7%.[43]

Chemical injuries from both acids and alkalis are common causes of corneal injury due to the easy availability and lax regulations regarding their use. A commonly used edible calcium hydroxide paste (chuna) in India and injuries with cement in construction sites cause a significant number of corneal injuries every year.[44] Though epidemiological data on the magnitude of chemical injuries causing corneal involvement and leading to blindness are largely unavailable, a study on the etiology of corneal perforations from Shandung province in China revealed that primary corneal perforations were caused by ocular trauma in 715 eyes (66.8%) and thermal burns and chemical injury accounted for 34 eyes (4.8%), and 29 eyes (4.1%), respectively.[45]

Infectious Keratitis

Corneal ulceration has been recognized as a silent epidemic in developing countries. Gonzales et al. reported that the annual incidence of corneal ulceration in Madurai District in South India was 113 per 100000 people,[46] approximately 10 times the annual incidence of 11 per 100000 reported from developed countries.[47] By applying the 1993 corneal ulcer incidence rate in Madurai District to all of India, there are an estimated 840000 people a year in the country who develop an ulcer. This figure is 30 times the number of corneal ulcers seen in the United States.[47] Extrapolating the Indian estimates further to the rest of Africa and Asia, the number of corneal ulcers occurring annually in the developing world is approximately 1.5–2 million, and the actual number is probably greater. Invariably, corneal blindness is the end result in the majority of these infections, or the outcomes may be even more disastrous, such as corneal perforation, endophthalmitis, or phthisis. In a prospective population-based study by Upadhyay et al. in Bhaktapur District, Nepal, the annual incidence of corneal ulceration was found to be 799 per 100000 people.[42] This extraordinarily high rate is seven times the incidence reported in South India and 70 times the rate in the United States. These reports suggest that corneal ulceration may be much more common in developing countries than previously recognized. The Andhra Pradesh Eye Disease Study (APEDS) conducted at LV Prasad Eye Institute, Hyderabad, estimated that the prevalence of corneal blindness in at least one eye was 0.66% (95% CI, 0.49–0.86). The most frequent causes of corneal blindness included keratitis in childhood (36.7%), trauma (28.6%), and keratitis during adulthood (17.7%).[43]

In addition to these high incidence rates, antibiotic and antifungal treatment for microbial keratitis is relatively costly and the visual outcome is almost invariably poor. In many developing countries antifungal medications are not available at any price. With such a dismal prospect for both medical and surgical treatment for corneal ulcers, the public health solution for this enormous problem is logically a strategy for prevention. Upadhyay et al. recently proved the efficacy of such a program.[42] Since the majority of corneal ulcers follow the occurrence of trivial corneal abrasions, post-traumatic corneal ulceration can be prevented by timely application of antibiotic ointment to eyes with corneal abrasions, but prophylaxis must be started within 18 hours after injury for maximum benefit to be obtained.[42] A similar study to examine the prophylactic effect of a combination of 1% chloramphenicol eye ointment and 1% clotrimazole eye ointment seemed promising in preventing bacterial and fungal keratitis following corneal abrasions in South India.[42,48]

Traditional Eye Medicines

In addition, the use of traditional eye medicines is a public health problem in many developing nations and an important risk factor for corneal blindness. These products are often contaminated and provide the vehicle for the spread of the pathogens. In Tanzania, 25% of corneal ulcers were associated with traditional eye medicine use.[49]

The etiology of microbial keratitis also varies widely between developed countries and the developing world. While bacteria account for the majority of the cases of microbial keratitis in the developed countries, fungi are the causative organisms in over 40% of microbial keratitis in literature from India, Nepal, Ghana, and Bangladesh. Amongst fungi, the filamentous fungi are the causative organisms in the overwhelming majority of fungal keratitis.[50]

Keratoconus

Keratoconus, a noninflammatory ectatic disorder of the cornea, is believed to be more prevalent in the Asian countries than in the West. Though large epidemiological studies do not exist, the prevalence of keratoconus in Saudi Arabia has been estimated to be about 20 per 100 000 population. The disease has also been reported to have an earlier age of onset (17.7 ± 3.6 years) and present with more severe forms in developing countries. The high association with atopic ocular disease in these patients may partially explain the high incidence rates but genetics are believed to play a role too.[51] This stems from the fact that studies investigating the role of ethnic origin in the incidence of keratoconus reveal that incidence of keratoconus of 25 per 100 000 (1 in 4000) per year for Asians, compared with 3.3 per 100 000 (1 in 30 000) per year for white people ($p < 0.001$). Asians presented significantly younger than white patients. The incidence of atopic disease was found to be significantly higher in white compared to Asian keratoconic patients.[52,53]

Corneal Dystrophy

Though lower in the order of importance from the point of view of relative prevalence compared to other, more potentially morbid cornea conditions, some corneal dystrophies appear to be seen more commonly in developing countries compared to the West, probably due to socioeconomic factors such as consanguinity. Among indications for keratoplasty, dystrophies account for 9.6% of all corneal grafts in India, 6.47% in Iran, and 4% in Northern China.[54–56] In a retrospective analysis done at LV Prasad Eye Institute, India, corneal dystrophies accounted for 8.1% of all corneal transplantations done in the study period, with a history of consanguinity present in 26% of these patients. The commonest dystrophy was congenital hereditary endothelial dystrophy (34.8%), followed by macular dystrophy (29.3%), Fuchs' endothelial dystrophy (16.6%), and lattice dystrophy (15%); the remaining 11% included granular dystrophy, gelatinous drop-like keratopathy, Reis-Bücklers dystrophy, and posterior polymorphous dystrophy. Outcomes of keratoplasty in this group of patients was relatively good, with a graft survival for all dystrophies at the end of 1 year being 94.3 ± 1.7%, and at the end of 5 years being 74.4 ± 4.5%.[57] Among patients undergoing keratoplasty for corneal dystrophies in Saudi Arabia, 62% patients had macular dystrophy, followed by congenital hereditary endothelial dystrophy, Fuchs' corneal dystrophy, lattice corneal dystrophy, and granular dystrophy, in reducing order of prevalence. A high prevalence of consanguinity was also identified amongst these patients.[58]

Keratoplasty

An alternative way of analyzing corneal diseases prevalent in a community is to look at the indications for keratoplasty. Table 84.5 provides information on important indications for keratoplasty in different geographical locations.[59] As the table shows, the important causes of corneal blindness (based on indications of keratoplasty) in established economies are pseudophakic bullous keratopathy (PBK), keratoconus, failed grafts, and corneal dystrophy. In contrast, in less-developed economies corneal scar and active keratitis are the most common indications for penetrating keratoplasty. Keratoconus and other dystrophies occur less often in these countries (4% vs 15%).

Table 84.5 Indications of keratoplasty based on different geographical locations

Indication	USA	Canada	UK	France	India	Nepal	Taiwan	Brazil
PBK	27.2	28.5	7.6	9.9	10.6	6.0	17.6	14.7
Fuchs' dystrophy	15.2	7.7	9.3	9.4	1.2		4.5	
Keratoconus	15.4	10	15	28.8	6.0	4.0	2.5	13.1
Corneal dystrophy	1.3		3.6		7.2		1.6	
Corneal scar	.8	2.9	5.9	7.7	28.1	37.0	27.9	6.6
Keratitis	2.9	8.5	8.3	10.9	12.2	9.0	17.9	17.9
Failed graft	18.1	22.3	40.9	9.9	17.1	13.3	21	12.8
Others		20.2	21.5	23.4	17.7		6.9	16

From Garg P, Krishna PV, Stratis AK, et al. The value of corneal transplantation in reducing corneal blindness. Eye. 2005;19(10):1106–14.

The data on repeat keratoplasty, an important indication of the procedure both in developed and developing countries, also show similar trends.[60] Even among the pediatric age group, indications for keratoplasty differ in developing and developed nations. While congenital opacities are the most common indications for penetrating keratoplasty in developed countries, acquired nontraumatic scars are the most common indications in developing nations.[61]

From these data on the indications for keratoplasty in developing countries, it is obvious that the most frequent indications would probably result in poor graft survival as compared to graft survival outcomes in developed countries where the most common indications are, by default, the ones that have the best outcome. In the state of Andhra Pradesh in Southern India, Dandona and associates analyzed 1-, 2-, and 5-year survival rates of 1725 corneal transplants performed at a tertiary eye care center in India.[56] The survival rates were 79.6% (95% CI, 77.3–81.9%), 68.7% (CI, 65.7–71.7%), and 46.5% (CI, 41.7–51.3%), respectively. Preoperative diagnosis was the most significant variable affecting transplant survival in the multivariate Cox regression model. Keratoconus had the highest 1- and 5-year survival rate of 96.4% (CI, 93–99.8%) and 95.1% (CI, 84.8–100%), respectively. Five-year survival for other indications in that study were 56% (CI, 45.2–66.8%) for corneal dystrophies; 52.2% (CI, 43.9–60.5%) for corneal scar other than adherent leukoma, 44.1% (CI, 28.8–59.4%) for PBK; 31.5% (CI, 16.1–46.8%) for adherent leukoma, 21.5% (CI, 8.5–34.5%) for aphakic bullous keratopathy, and 21.2% (CI, 13.8–26.6%) for repeat transplants after failure of the first transplant. Other factors that affected graft survival in the study were socioeconomic status, age at surgery, vascularization of host cornea, and quality of donor cornea. The odds of the eye being blind after transplantation were high for indications such as adherent leukoma, failed graft, and aphakic bullous keratopathy, presence of deep vascularization, lower socioeconomic status, and age less than 10 years.[56]

Table 84.6 shows the outcome of keratoplasty based on published reports from both established and less-developed economies.[59] Overall survival of corneal grafts is much better in developed countries (64.5–91% 5-year survival) than reported by Dandona et al. (46.5%). One of the factors responsible for better outcome in some of these series is that the principal indications for keratoplasty (55–68%), namely PBK, keratoconus, and corneal dystrophies, carry a much better prognosis than vascularized corneal scar, adherent leukoma, and active keratitis, which are the most common indications of keratoplasty (40.3%) in developed countries.

Keratoplasty is considered a high-risk procedure in the pediatric age group. In a multicenter study by Dana et al. the overall survival rate was 80.2% (CI, 72.9–87.4%) at 1 year and 67.4% (CI, 58.3–76.4%) at 2 years.[62] In a study published from LV Prasad Eye Institute in India 66.2% eyes had clear graft at the last follow-up (mean follow-up 1.3 years).[63]

Extrapolation of the data from these studies clearly indicates that the outcome of corneal transplantation is likely to be poor in situations where corneal blindness is caused mainly by vascularized corneal scar and adherent leukoma, or where the socioeconomic status is poor, and where this form of blindness is in children.

Other factors that are critical for the success of corneal transplants are quality and efficiency of eye banking, availability of trained corneal surgeons, quality of clinical facilities for surgery, and availability of potent corticosteroids and other immunomodulatory agents at affordable cost. Follow-up care for corneal transplants is a lifelong commitment and access to care by ophthalmologists who have been exposed to the care of corneal transplants is also a major determinant of success.

In India, with a population close to one billion, only 20 514 donor corneas were procured in the year 2003.[64] Of these, only 8426 could be utilized for transplantation. The requirement for donor corneas per year in India is estimated to be 20 times the current procurement. This clearly shows that there is a huge gap between demand and supply of donor corneal tissues in India, and probably in other countries where corneal blindness is most prevalent. Thus, there is lack of quality corneal tissues in these countries. This may not only affect the number of transplants that can be performed but also graft outcome.

Table 84.6 Outcomes of keratoplasty in various indications

Series	1-yr outcome	2-yr outcome	5-yr outcome	10-yr outcome	Keratoconus	PBK	Dystrophy	Scar	Regraft
Dandona et al.[56]	79.6	68.7	46.5		95.1	44.1	56	31.5	21.2
Price et al. 1993	97	95	91		98	91	98		70
Thompson et al. 2003				82	92	74	90		41
Inoue et al. 2000				72.2	98.8	51.1	76.9		61.8
Sit et al. 2001		78.8	64.5		95.9	50	85.2	73.5	
Williams et al. 2003	90.8	84.1	72.2	59	97.5	57.8	75.8	56.5	413
Ing et al. 1998				78	96	76	81	46	

From Garg P, Krishna PV, Stratis AK, et al. The value of corneal transplantation in reducing corneal blindness. Eye. 2005;19(10):1106–14.

Conclusion

The spectrum of corneal diseases seen in developing countries seems to vary greatly from that seen in more developed countries. The magnitude of importance these diseases assume is also higher in these countries due to the potential blinding nature of many of them and the fact that a majority of them are preventable. While the majority of these differences could be explained by socioeconomic factors alone, geographical location, environmental influences, genetic trends, and cultural variations are confounding factors. It is important for all cornea specialists to recognize these trends and contribute towards better understanding of these diseases and join the battle against the scourge of preventable corneal blindness. In the last few decades since corneal blindness has been recognized as a significant contributor to the global pool of blindness, a number of changes have helped reduce the scourge. Paradigm shifts in the management of diseases, with more emphasis on community-based treatment rather than individual treatment and improvements directed against socioeconomic conditions, have helped ease the burden of corneal disease and consequently blindness. Numerous organizations such as the WHO, ORBIS, various nongovernmental organizations, and IAPB, have played, and continue to play, stellar roles in these areas but there is still a long way to go before corneal diseases in the developing world, especially the preventable ones, are reduced significantly and no longer contribute significantly to blindness.

References

1. Whitcher JP, Srinivasan M, Upadhyay MP. Corneal blindness: a global perspective. *Bull World Health Organ.* 2001;79:214–221.
2. Thylefors B, Négrel AD, Pararajasegaram R, Dadzie KY. Global data on blindness. *Bull World Health Organ.* 1995;73:115–121.
3. Foster A. Vision 2020 – the right to sight (editorial). *Trop Doct.* 2003;33:193–194.
4. Pascolini D, Mariotti SP, Pokharel GP, et al. 2002 global update of available data on visual impairment: a compilation of population-based prevalence studies. *Ophthalmic Epidemiol.* 2004;11:67–115.
5. Congdon N, O'Colmain B, Klaver CC, et al. Causes and prevalence of visual impairment among adults in the United States. *Arch Ophthalmol.* 2004;122:477–485.
6. Klaver CC, Wolfs RC, Vingerling JR, Hofman A, de Jong PT. Age-specific prevalence and causes of blindness and visual impairment in an older population: the Rotterdam Study. *Arch Ophthalmol.* 1998;116: 653–658.
7. VanNewkirk MR, Weih L, McCarty CA, Taylor HR. Cause-specific prevalence of bilateral visual impairment in Victoria, Australia: the Visual Impairment Project. *Ophthalmology.* 2001;108: 960–967.
8. Attebo K, Mitchell P, Smith W. Visual acuity and the causes of visual loss in Australia: the Blue Mountain Eye Study. *Ophthalmology.* 1996;103: 357–364.
9. Thulasiraj RD, Nirmalan PK, Ramakrishnan R, et al. Blindness and vision impairment in a rural south Indian population: the Aravind Comprehensive Eye Survey. *Ophthalmology.* 2003;110:1491–1498.
10. Dandona L, Dandona R, Srinivas M, et al. Blindness in the Indian state of Andhra Pradesh. *Invest Ophthalmol Vis Sci.* 2001;42:908–916.
11. National programme for control of blindness, Directorate General of Health Services, Ministry of Health and Family Welfare Government of India. National survey on blindness and visual outcome after cataract surgery. New Delhi 2002.
12. Tabbara KF. Blindness in the eastern Mediterranean countries. *Br J Ophthalmol.* 2001;85:771–775.
13. Fotouhi A, Hashemi H, Mohammad K, Jalali KH, Tehran Eye Study. The prevalence and causes of visual impairment in Tehran: the Tehran Eye Study. *Br J Ophthalmol.* 2004;88:740–745.
14. Farber MD. National Registry for the Blind in Israel: estimation of prevalence and incidence rates and causes of blindness. *Ophthalmic Epidemiol.* 2003;10:267–277.
15. Saw SM, Husain R, Gazzard GM, et al. Causes of low vision and blindness in rural Indonesia. *Br J Ophthalmol.* 2003;87:1075–1078.
16. Gilbert C, Foster A. Childhood blindness in the context of VISION 2020 – the right to sight. *Bull World Health Organ.* 2001;79:227–232.
17. Gilbert CE, Anderton L, Dandona L, et al. Prevalence of blindness and visual impairment in children – a review of available data. *Ophthalmic Epidemiol.* 1999;6:73–81.
18. Gilbert CE, Foster A. Blindness in children: control priorities and research opportunities. *Br J Ophthalmol.* 2001;85:1025–1027.
19. Dandona R, Dandona L. Childhood blindness in India: a population based perspective. *Br J Ophthalmol.* 2003;87:263–265.
20. Rahi JS, Sripathi S, Gilbert CE, Foster A. Childhood blindness in India: causes in 1318 blind school students in nine states. *Eye.* 1995;9:545–550.
21. Lewallen S, Courtright P. Blindness in Africa: present situation and future needs. *Br J Ophthalmol.* 2001;85:897–903.
22. Ezegwui IR, Umeh RE, Ezepue UF. Causes of childhood blindness: results from schools for the blind in southeastern Nigeria. *Br J Ophthalmol.* 2003;87:20–23.
23. Wedner SH, Ross DA, Balira R, Kaji L, Foster A. Prevalence of eye diseases in primary school children in a rural area of Tanzania. *Br J Ophthalmol.* 2000;84:1291–1297.
24. Hornby SJ, Gilbert CE, Foster A, et al. Causes of childhood blindness in the People's Republic of China: results from 1131 blind school students in 18 provinces. *Br J Ophthalmol.* 1999;83:929–932.
25. Whitcher JP, Srinivasan M, Upadhyay MP. Corneal blindness: a global perspective. *Bull World Health Organ.* 2001;79:214–221.
26. World Health Organization. *Global initiative for the elimination of avoidable blindness.* Geneva: World Health Organization; 1997 (unpublished document WHO/PBL/97.61/Rev1).
27. Schwab L. *Eye care in developing nations.* 4th ed. Manson Publishing, London. UK. 2007:117–126.
28. Sommer A, et al. Impact of vitamin A supplementation on childhood mortality. *Lancet.* 1986,1:1169–1173.
29. Schwab L, Kagame K. Blindness in Africa: Zimbabwe schools for the blind survey. *Br J Ophthalmol.* 1993,77:410–412.
30. Semba RD, Bloem MW. Measles blindness. *Surv Ophthalmol.* 2004 Mar-Apr;49(2):243–255.
31. Mabey DC, Solomon AW, Foster A. Trachoma. *Lancet.* 2003; 362(9379):223–229.
32. Boatin BA. The current state of the onchocerciasis control program in West Africa. *Trop Doct.* 2003;33:210–214.
33. John D, Daniel E. Infectious keratitis in leprosy. *Br J Ophthalmol.* 1999;83:173–176.
34. Foster A, Volker K. Ophthalmia neonatorum in developing countries [editorial]. *N Engl J Med.* 1995;332:600–601.
35. Whitcher JP. Neonatal ophthalmia: have we advanced in the last 20 years? *International Ophthalmology Clinics.* 1990,30:39–41.
36. Laga M, et al. Epidermiology and control of gonococcal ophthalmia neonatorum. *Bull World Health Organ.* 1989;64:471–477.
37. Isenberg SJ, et al. A controlled trial of povidone-iodine as prophylaxis against ophthalmia neonatorum. *N Engl J Med.* 1995;332:562–566.
38. Thylefors B. Present challenges in the global prevention of blindness. *Aust NZ J Ophthalmol.* 1992;20:89–94.
39. Négrel AD, Thylefors B. The global impact of eye injuries. *Ophthalmic Epidemiol.* 1998;5:143–167.
40. Jackson H. Bilateral blindness due to trauma in Cambodia. *Eye.* 1996;10:517–520.
41. Brilliant LB, et al. Epidemiology of blindness in Nepal. *Bull World Health Organ.* 1985;63:375–386.
42. Upadhyay MP, Karmacharya PC, Koirala S, et al. The Bhaktapur Eye Study: ocular trauma and antibiotic prophylaxis for the prevention of corneal ulceration in Nepal. *Br J Ophthalmol.* 2001;85(4):388–392.
43. Dandona R, Dandona L. Corneal blindness in a southern Indian population: need for health promotion strategies. *Br J Ophthalmol.* 2003; 87(2):133–141.
44. Agarwal T, Vajpayee RB, Sharma N, Tandon R. Severe ocular injury resulting from chuna packets. *Ophthalmology.* 2006;113(6):961.
45. Xie L, Zhai H, Dong X, Shi W. Primary diseases of corneal perforation in Shandong Province, China: a 10-year retrospective study. *Am J Ophthalmol.* 2008;145(4):662–666.
46. Gonzales CA, et al. Incidence of corneal ulceration in Madurai District, South India. *Ophthalmic Epidemiol.* 1996;3:159–166.
47. Erie JC, et al. Incidence of ulcerative keratitis in a defined population from 1950 through 1988. *Arch Ophthalmol.* 1993;111:1665–1671.

48. Srinivasan M, Upadhyay MP, Priyadarsini B, Mahalakshmi R, Whitcher JP. Corneal ulceration in south-east Asia III: prevention of fungal keratitis at the village level in south India using topical antibiotics. *Br J Ophthalmol.* 2006;90(12):1472–1475.
49. Yorston D, Foster A. Traditional eye medicines and corneal ulceration in Tanzania. *J Trop Med Hyg.* 1994;97:211–214.
50. Gopinathan U, Garg P, Fernandes M, et al. The epidemiological features and laboratory results of fungal keratitis: a 10-year review at a referral eye care center in South India. *Cornea.* 2002;21(6):555–559.
51. Assiri AA, Yousuf BI, Quantock AJ, Murphy PJ. Incidence and severity of keratoconus in Asir province, Saudi Arabia. *Br J Ophthalmol.* 2006; 90(8):1071.
52. Georgiou T, Funnell CL, Cassels-Brown A, O'Conor R. Influence of ethnic origin on the incidence of keratoconus and associated atopic disease in Asians and white patients. *Eye.* 2004;18(4):379–383.
53. Pearson AR, Soneji B, Sarvananthan N, Sandford-Smith JH. Does ethnic origin influence the incidence or severity of keratoconus? *Eye.* 2000;14 (Pt 4):625–628.
54. Kanavi MR, Javadi MA, Sanagoo M. Indications for penetrating keratoplasty in Iran. *Cornea.* 2007;26(5):561–563.
55. Xie L, Song Z, Zhao J, Shi W, Wang F. Indications for penetrating keratoplasty in north China. *Cornea.* 2007;26(9):1070–1073.
56. Dandona L, Naduvilath TJ, Janarthanan M, Ragu K, Rao GN. Survival analysis and visual outcome in a large series of corneal transplants in India. *Br J Ophthalmol.* 1997;81:726–731.
57. Pandrowala H, Bansal A, Vemuganti GK, Rao GN. Frequency, distribution, and outcome of keratoplasty for corneal dystrophies at a tertiary eye care center in South India. *Cornea.* 2004;23(6):541–546.
58. al Faran MF, Tabbara KF Corneal dystrophies among patients undergoing keratoplasty in Saudi Arabia. *Cornea.* 1991;10(1):13–16.
59. Garg P, Krishna PV, Stratis AK, Gopinathan U. The value of corneal transplantation in reducing corneal blindness. *Eye.* 2005;19(10):1106–1114.
60. Tabin GC, Gurung R, Paudyal G, et al. Penetrating keratoplasty in Nepal. *Cornea.* 2004;23:589–596.
61. Dada T, Sharma N, Vajpayee RB. Indications for pediatric keratoplasty in India. *Cornea.* 1999;18:296–298.
62. Dana MR, Moyes AL, Gomes JA, et al. The indications for and outcome in pediatric keratoplasty. A multicenter study. *Ophthalmology.* 1995;102: 1129–1138.
63. Aasuri MK, Garg P, Gokhale N, Gupta S. Penetrating keratoplasty in Children. *Cornea.* 2000;19:140–144.
64. The Eye Bank Association of India. About us. ⟨http:www.ebai.org⟩.

Chapter 85

Syphilitic Stromal Keratitis

Kirk R. Wilhelmus

Historical Background

The great pox

Syphilis emerged in the late 15th century. As this malign infection spread across Europe and Asia, some developed blepharoconjunctivitis, others uveitis.[1] Syphilis affected infants,[2,3] who were sometimes born with inflamed eyes.[4,5] Syphilologists, though, overlooked corneal complications of sexually transmitted disease.[6–8] Even when keratitis was acknowledged to arise during *lues venerea* or to afflict children of syphilitic parents,[9] many commingled ocular syphilis and gonorrheal conjunctivitis.[10,11] *Strumous ophthalmia* was largely attributed to tuberculosis and called scrofulous corneitis.[12,13] Then, a Victorian polymath deduced that stromal keratitis during adolescence was often consequent on late congenital syphilis.[14,15]

Hutchinson's revelation

Jonathan Hutchinson (1828–1913)[16–25] recognized his first case of keratitis associated with congenital syphilis in 1849 and collated his articles dating from 1858 into a monograph in 1863 (Box. 85.1).[14,26,27] Hutchinson described syphilitic keratitis (Fig. 85.1) 'as a diffuse haziness near the centre of the cornea of one eye' that became 'densely opaque by the spreading and confluence of these interstitial opacities.' He noticed that 'after from one to two months, the other cornea is attacked and goes through the same stages, but rather faster than the first.'[27] Almost all had a distinctive physiognomy, with 'old fissures at the angles of the mouth, a sunken bridge to the nose, and a set of permanent teeth peculiar for their smallness, bad colour, and the vertically notched edges of the central upper incisors.'[27] Fifteen percent were deaf. The combination of stromal keratitis, notched teeth, and deafness was dubbed Hutchinson's triad.[28]

Discovery and description

The groundbreaking idea linking childhood corneal inflammation to prenatal infection was not immediately accepted,[22,23,29] but opinion duly changed as an average of one report per year endorsed Hutchinson's discovery.[30–32] By 1900, congenital syphilis was diagnosed in 50–75% of patients with nonulcerative stromal keratitis (Fig. 85.2).[33] Hutchinson originally thought that keratitis did not occur during acquired syphilis,[27] but when others did[34–37] he conceded its rare occurrence.[38] Despite persistent skeptics,[39] conventional wisdom eventually accepted the concept of acquired syphilitic keratitis.[40]

Treponema pallidum was discovered in 1905, and the following year a complement-fixation test was developed, soon used for diagnosing syphilitic eye disease.[41] Seroscreening confirmed that syphilis was an important cause of corneal blindness during the early 20th century.[42] Clinical research extended Hutchinson's observations,[43–45] and texts[46–49] set forth the gamut of syphilitic keratitis (Table 85.1).

Origins of medical therapy

Hot baths and heat cabinets were early treatments for syphilis and syphilitic keratitis.[50] Thermal spas at Aachen and other sulfur springs attracted thousands. Therapeutic hyperthermia was also induced by iatrogenic malaria[51] and by injecting milk or typhoid vaccine. Some syphilitics benefited from 'artificial fever,' perhaps because *T. pallidum* cannot mount a heat-shock response and is susceptible to increased temperature.

Some eyes were irradiated with ultraviolet light or X-rays, and others were subjected to conjunctival peritomy, corneal puncture or trephination, and subconjunctival injections.[52] Blood-letting by incision or leeches became popular. Traceable to Arabic physicians' use of mercury, quicksilver[46] was often prescribed, though sometimes by a quacksalver.

In 1909, systematic research yielded arsenical compounds. Arsphenamine and its soluble derivative neoarsphenamine could palliate syphilis and control experimental primary syphilitic keratitis,[53] but proved disappointing for stromal keratitis.[54–56] Systemic treatment did not prevent syphilitic keratitis,[57,58] had no consistently beneficial effect on its course,[59–61] and did not avert recurrent keratitis or involvement of the second eye.

Penicillin was a breakthrough, first shown in the 1940s to cure early syphilis. Treating syphilitic mothers obviated neonatal transmission,[62] and the incidence of stromal keratitis due to congenital syphilis declined dramatically. Yet, irrespective of conflicting reports,[63] penicillin proved ineffective for syphilitic keratitis.[64,65] Corneal disease still occurred after systemic treatment of syphilitic toddlers, and the clinical course of stromal keratitis was usually not influenced by penicillin.[66]

Antiinflammatory therapy came about during the 1950s.[67–70] Within a year of the initial ophthalmic use of a corticosteroid, syphilitic keratitis could at last be quelled.[71] A topical corticosteroid effectively suppressed stromal keratitis,[50,72] and its dosage was soon refined.[73–76]

Box 85.1 Events in the history of syphilitic stromal keratitis

1858	First report in the ophthalmic literature of stromal keratitis during late congenital syphilis
1863	Hutchinson publishes book on syphilitic keratitis
1873	First report by Fournier of stromal keratitis during acquired syphilis
1881	First experiments on keratitis of primary ocular syphilis
1897	First clinicopathologic correlation of syphilitic keratitis
1908	Treponemes found in stromal keratitis of early congenital syphilis
1910	Serologic testing first used in diagnosis of syphilitic keratitis
1914	Arsenicals and mercurials found usually ineffective for treating keratitis; first penetrating keratoplasty for syphilitic keratitis
1925	Treponemes not found in stromal keratitis of late congenital syphilis
1931	First experiments on keratitis of secondary syphilis
1944	Rate of syphilitic keratitis declines due to improved prenatal care and maternal treatment
1945	Corneal donor serologic testing for syphilis begun by eye banks
1947	Penicillin found usually ineffective for treating syphilitic keratitis
1950	Topical corticosteroid first used for syphilitic keratitis
1990	Corneal donor serologic testing for syphilis required by Eye Bank Association of America
1997	Corneal donor serologic testing for syphilis not required by Eye Bank Association of America
2002	Recipient syphilitic keratitis removed from list of keratoplasty indications by the Eye Bank Association of America
2005	Corneal donor serologic testing for syphilis required by the US Food and Drug Administration

Evolution of corneal surgery

In the late 19th century syphilitic keratopathy was an occasional indication for anterior lamellar keratoplasty, but graft failure was common.[77] After the first penetrating corneal transplant for syphilitic keratopathy in 1914,[78] corneal surgeons realized that transplantation should be delayed until well after the ocular inflammation had resolved. Syphilitic keratopathy remained a reason for keratoplasty during the first half of the 20th century,[79–81] accounting for about 15% of corneal transplants. Half of corneal grafts, whether small and round[82] or square,[83] succeeded, but postoperative uveitis and other complications were common.[84] With the introduction of topical cortisone, corneal grafts stayed clear in 75% of recipients.[85] After 1950 syphilitic keratopathy dwindled as a surgical indication.[86,87]

Epidemiology

Before penicillin

During the 19th and early 20th centuries, one in 10 young adults acquired syphilis, but less than 5% of syphilitic keratitis was associated with acquired disease.[48,88,89] In contrast, about one in every 100 babies was born with congenital syphilis,[90] and 10–50% of children with late congenital syphilis developed stromal keratitis.[91–94] Hutchinson's observation was sound: stromal keratitis was largely due to congenital syphilis rather than acquired syphilis.

Before penicillin, stromal keratitis comprised 5–15% of ocular syphilitic manifestations[46,95,96] and 0.5% of all eye disturbances.[88,97–99] Approximately 3% of blindness was linked to syphilitic keratitis,[42,100,101] mostly from congenital syphilis.[102] Extrapolating prevalence data,[103] by the middle of the 20th century approximately one million people worldwide had had syphilitic keratitis. Although they were bled, injected, or given arsenicals, some nevertheless recovered.

The antibiotic era

Antibiotics curbed the syphilis epidemic. Maternal therapy before the second trimester or early treatment of the infant often prevented ocular involvement caused by congenital syphilis and reduced the prevalence of syphilitic corneal disease.[104,105] The chance that a parent who had had

Table 85.1 Syphilis and the cornea

Stage	Onset	Laterality	Prevalence
Early congenital syphilis	Birth	Usually bilateral	Rare
Late congenital syphilis	5–20 years of age	Usually bilateral	Occasional
Early acquired syphilis	6 weeks to 6 months after primary chancre	Usually unilateral	Rare
Late acquired syphilis	1–20 years after primary chancre	Usually unilateral	Uncommon

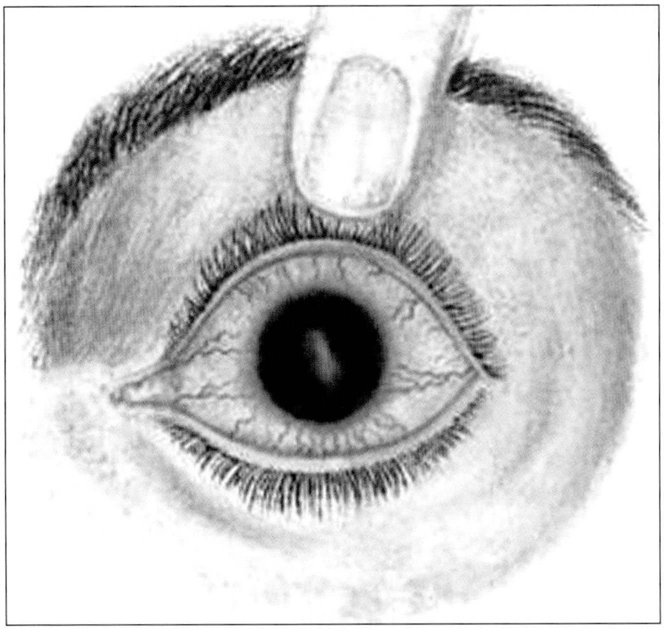

Fig. 85.1 Early stage of syphilitic keratitis. Acute stromal keratitis with 'cherry-red' limbal congestion in a malnourished 12-year-old girl treated by Hutchinson in 1859. (From Hutchinson J. *A clinical memoir on certain diseases of the eye and ear, consequent on inherited syphilis.* London: John Churchill, 1863, facing page 66.)

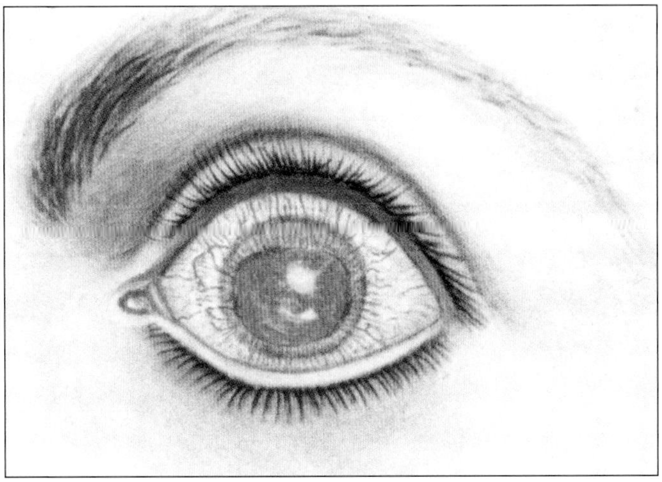

Fig. 85.2 Early 20th century drawing of stromal keratitis caused by congenital syphilis, showing central corneal inflammation with edema and peripheral corneal neovascularization. (From Hazen HH. *Syphilis, a treatise on etiology, pathology, diagnosis, prognosis, prophylaxis, and treatment.* St. Louis: Mosby, 1919: 450.)

syphilitic keratitis would give birth to their own syphilitic infant, once a feared prospect,[106,107] became practically unheard of.[108,109]

Syphilis brings about a wide range of eye diseases,[110,111] but stromal keratitis and keratopathy currently constitute less than 5% of all forms of ocular syphilis. Over 10 million cases of syphilis occur globally each year, with perhaps 10000 annual cases of syphilitic stromal keratitis. Residual corneal scarring exists in about 10% of those with late con-

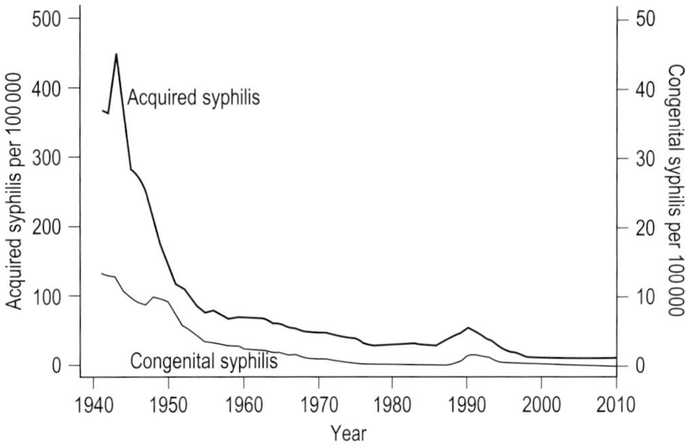

Fig. 85.3 Syphilis statistics in the United States showing annual rates of acquired syphilis and congenital syphilis per 100 000 population. Comparable statistics are available for the United Kingdom (www.hpa.org.uk) and other countries (www.who.int). (Data from the Centers for Disease Control and Prevention. Copyright American Medical Association. All rights reserved.)

genital syphilis.[112–116] Worldwide, an estimated 50000–200000 people have sight-limiting corneal opacification due to syphilis.

Global burden of syphilitic keratitis

The annual rate of acquired syphilis in North America and Europe is about 5 per 100000 persons, and the annual rate of congenital syphilis is 8 per 100000 live births (Fig. 85.3). At the beginning of the 21st century, public health officials in industrialized nations optimistically talked of eliminating syphilis.[117]

Syphilis accounts for less than 0.5% of new patients in a referral eye-care practice[110] and 0.05% of general ophthalmic outpatients.[118,119] Less than 1% of active stromal keratitis is attributed to syphilis.[120,121] Ophthalmologists more often see postinflammatory scarring and vessels than syphilitic keratitis.[122]

Meanwhile, syphilis surged in developing countries. In sub-Saharan villages, where 10% of pregnant women have syphilis, the infant mortality rate is 50% among seropositive newborns. In some regions 2% of African children are born with congenital syphilis,[123] and 10% of survivors later develop keratitis. The reprovable tragedy of congenital syphilis is that it inflicts preventable suffering and blindness among the poor.[124]

Stromal Keratitis in Congenital Syphilis

Onset

Stromal keratitis is the most common, and sometimes the only, sign of late congenital syphilis.[94,125–127] Rare before age 2,[128] keratitis typically begins between 5 and 15 years of age (Fig. 85.4),[88,103,129,130] and hardly ever after age 30.[131] Nearly twice as many girls are affected as boys, but among young adults this gender imbalance disappears. Onset in females clusters between 7 and 13 years of age,[56] suggesting a possible hormonal influence.[132,133]

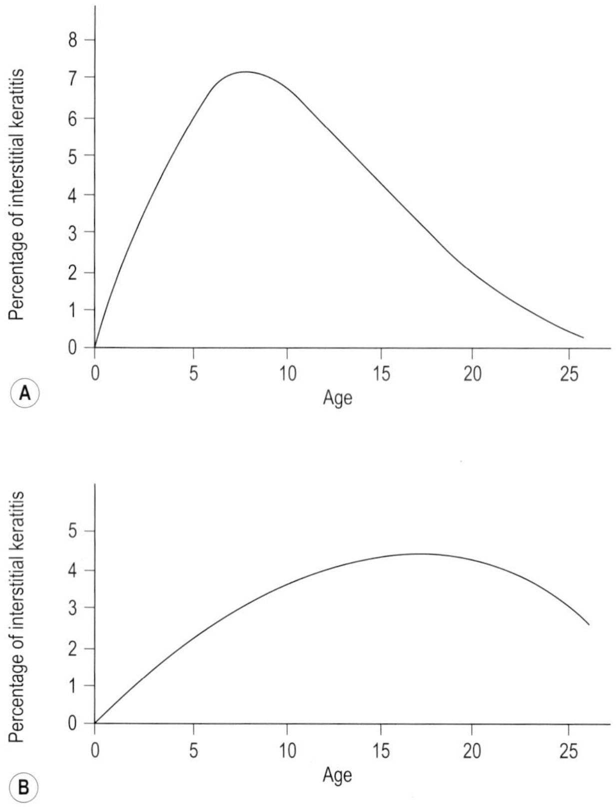

Fig. 85.4 Age distribution at onset of stromal keratitis among 1010 patients with untreated late congenital syphilis at five centers in the USA. (**A**) Age-specific prevalence of stromal keratitis among all patients developing syphilitic keratitis. (**B**) Age-specific incidence of stromal keratitis, showing relatively linear risk of syphilitic keratitis until 25 years of age assuming patients with late congenital syphilis remain at constant risk of developing corneal involvement. (From Cole HN, et al. *Arch Dermatol Syph* 1937; 35: 563–579.)

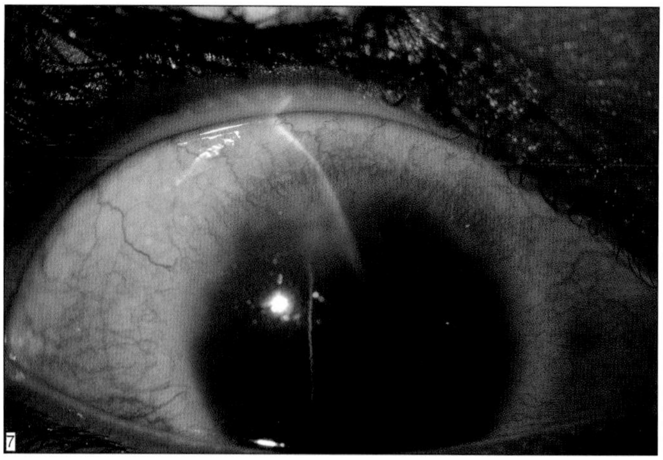

Fig. 85.5 Acute stromal keratitis with active corneal neovascularization. A thirteen-year-old boy was treated during infancy for congenital syphilis but developed bilateral hearing loss at age 12 years. One month later multifocal stromal keratitis with peripheral neovascularization affected the left eye. Six months later, as shown, peripheral stromal keratitis of the right eye occurred.

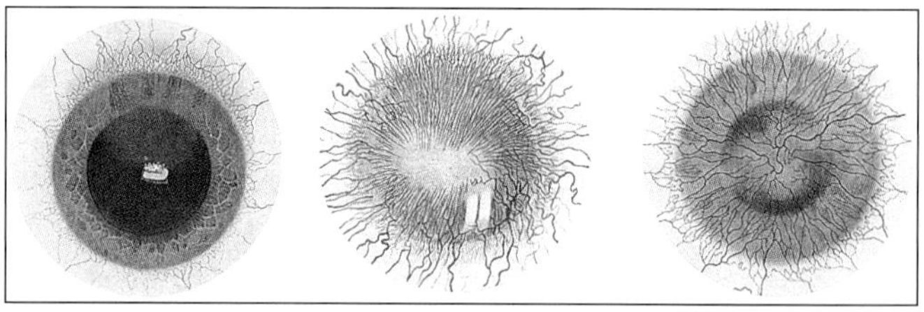

Fig. 85.6 Progression of syphilitic stromal keratitis. *Left*, Acute stromal inflammatory edema with neovascularization. *Middle*, Corneal inflammation with dense superficial and deep neovascularization. *Right*, Partial clearing with regression of vascularization. (Adapted from Theil R. *Atlas der Augenkrankheiten; Sammlung typischer krankheitshilder mit kurzen diagnostschen und therapeutischen Hinweisen.* Vol. 1. Leipzig: Thieme, 1936: 192–193.)

Trauma is thought to provoke its development.[134,135] Up to 5–10% of cases follow ocular injury,[136] an association that in the past set a legal precedent of occupational liability.[137,138] Surgery for congenital cataract or secondary glaucoma may induce keratitis.[139,140] Fever, the common cold, menarche, pregnancy, and even antisyphilitic treatment[141,142] have rarely preceded its inception. A reputed link with psychological stress[143] is likely explained by recall bias.[144]

Corneal inflammation

Stromal keratitis usually begins as an inflammatory infiltration that has a slight preference for the superior cornea and deeper stroma (Fig. 85.5). A faint stromal haze and swollen endothelial cells may appear before symptoms are noticeable. Without corticosteroid therapy, corneal inflammation may remain mild and localized, but often blooms into diffuse stromal keratouveitis and inflammatory edema (Fig. 85.6), resembling a *ground-glass cornea.*

Stromal keratitis due to syphilis was formerly called *interstitial keratitis* or *parenchymatous keratitis* (*keratitis parenchymatosa*). Clinicians still use 'IK' as a metonym to encompass the spectrum of inflammatory and postinflammatory corneal changes. *Luetic keratitis* (from *lues venerea)* is an occasional epithet.

Syphilitic corneal corruption takes myriad forms. The epithelium stays intact but can temporarily erode over superficial opacities.[145] Nascent punctate infiltrates clump together or align parallel to the limbus before coalescing.[146] Multiple stromal infiltrates may arise at varying levels in the cornea.[147] Curvilinear inflammation in the deep stroma is an odd phenomenon called *keratitis linearis migrans* or *keratitis parenchymatosa annularis* that starts with one or more spindly infiltrates that lengthen, extend posteriorly, and then advance.[148–151]

Atypically, an eruption of necrotizing or granulomatous inflammation soaks the deep cornea, known formerly as *keratitis profunda* or *keratitis pustuliformis profunda.*[152–154] This milky reaction may stay focal but can expand circumferentially and suffuse toward the opposite limbus, rarely breaking through Descemet's membrane[155] or draining

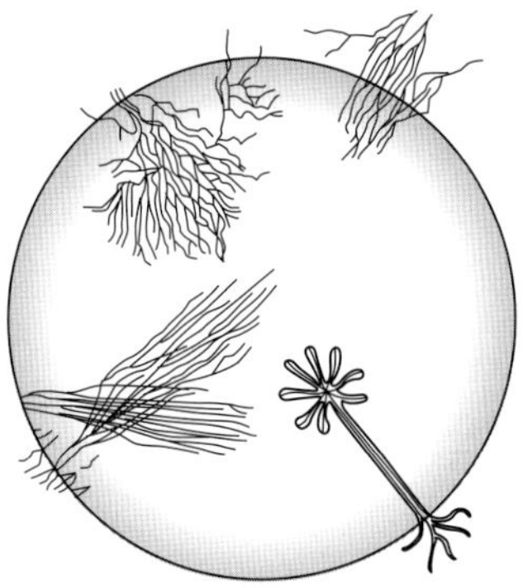

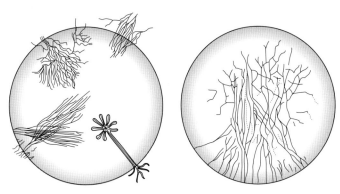

Fig. 85.7 Corneal neovascularization associated with syphilitic stromal keratitis. The left drawing shows various forms of superficial stromal vessels that form terminal loops and arborescent or brush forms. The right-hand figure depicts radiating vessels of the deep stroma. Holmes Spicer WT. *Br J Ophthalmol* 1924;8(Suppl 1):1–63.

externally.[156] Exceptionally, keratoscleritis produces a peripheral ring infiltrate.[157] A discus of stromal infiltration may leave a band in the deep stroma, like a high-water mark from an inflammatory wave.[158]

Corneal endothelial pseudoguttae accompany stromal keratouveitis.[159] Microcystic epithelial edema is common, and bullae may form. The stroma can thicken to 600 μm or more.[160,161] Wrinkling of the deep stroma and Descemet's membrane creates stellate, striate, circinate, or crisscross folds. Frosty corneal edema with blunted sensation can resemble disciform endotheliitis.[162]

Corneal neovascularization

New blood and lymphatic vessels often – but not always[102] – invade the cornea during syphilitic keratitis. Superficial capillaries bud from venules of the limbal arcades. Deeper vessels arise as terminal branches of the anterior ciliary vessels. Vascular tufts insinuate between stromal lamellae to head for the inflamed zone. Stromal vessels may conform to a fascicular pattern in one sector, or invade radially from various directions (Fig. 85.7). A rosy pannus of intertwining vessels on a wan stromal backdrop produces a *salmon-colored patch*. Limbal inflammation might resemble a fleshy tumor of the peripheral cornea.[163]

As capillaries sprout into the cornea some peripheral clearing begins, making it appear that ingrowing vessels push inflammation ahead as they sweep through the clear periphery towards the turbid zone. Anfractuous arterioles brush the central cornea and exude a perivascular haze, at times bleeding into the stroma. The cornea becomes a dirty red, blending into the surrounding ciliary flush and episcleritis. Serried deep vessels empurple stromal inflammation to create a *plum-colored eye*.

The extent of neovascularization depends on the severity of inflammation and the use of antiinflammatory drugs. Without corticosteroid treatment, a neovascular fretwork forms over several weeks. Ultimately a florid stage is reached at the peak of the inflammatory reaction. Once the cornea is vascularized, the inflammatory process subsides.

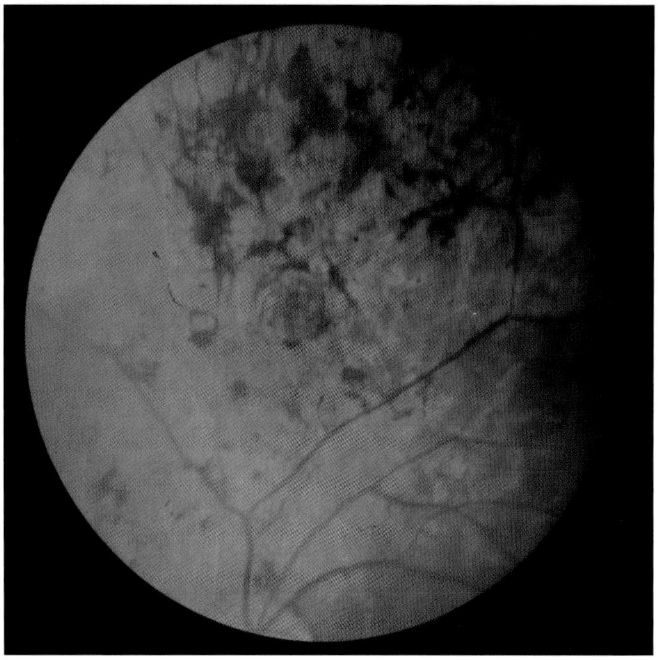

Fig. 85.8 Chorioretinal atrophy after subclinical chorioretinitis caused by congenital syphilis. Characteristics include patchy intraretinal and perivascular pigmentation, narrowed blood vessels, and mild optic atrophy.

Uveitis

Anterior uveitis

Iridocyclitis commonly attends stromal keratitis,[88,103] and iritis can precede the onset of syphilitic keratitis.[illegible] Keratic precipitates are usually small, but can sometimes be confluent and retiform or large and granulomatous.[166] The number of cells and amount of flare range from minimal to marked, although a hypopyon is unusual. Either increased intraocular pressure or hypotony can be a transient feature. Iris blood vessels become engorged, and a small hyphema can rarely occur. If synechiae form, the pupil may bind down.

Posterior uveitis

Intermediate uveitis, posterior uveitis,[141,167,168] or retinal vasculitis[169,170] seldom occur during active stromal keratitis. On the other hand, because stromal keratitis presents during late congenital syphilis, the sequelae of prior chorioretinitis that occurred during early congenital syphilis may be present when corneal inflammation begins.[43] Subclinical, multifocal inflammation of the choriocapillaris leads to scattered chorioretinal atrophy, patchy proliferation of the retinal pigment epithelium (sometimes called 'bone spicules'), and narrowed retinal blood vessels.[171] Pigmentary chorioretinopathy (graphically described as a *salt-and-pepper fundus*) can be focal or diffuse (Fig. 85.8) and shows window defects on fluorescein angiography. Between 10% and 50% of children with syphilitic keratitis have chorioretinal pigmentation, perivascular fibrotic sheathing, or optic atrophy.[56,172]

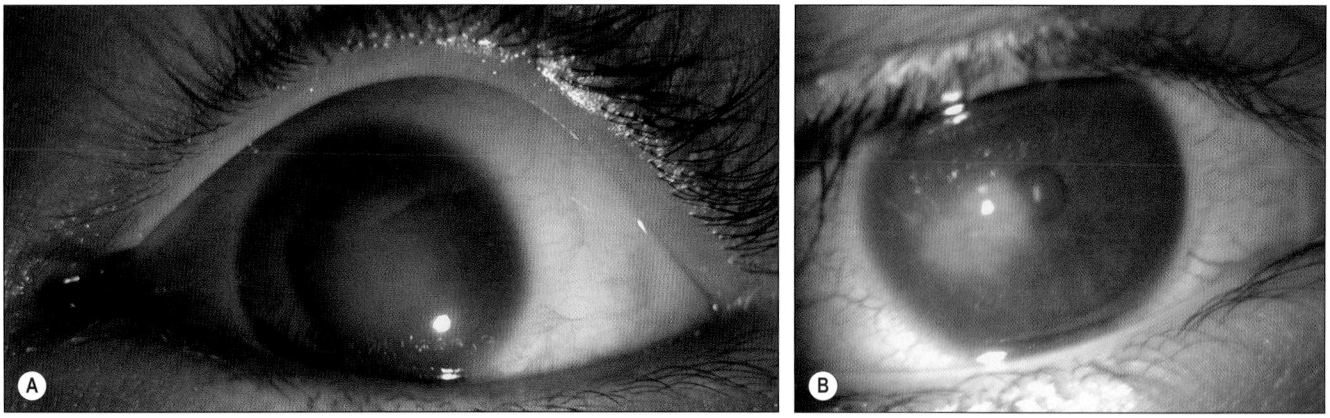

Fig. 85.9 Bilateral, recurrent syphilitic keratitis. (**A**) An eight-year-old boy developed stromal keratouveitis of his left eye during late congenital syphilis (reactive TP-PA, 1:1024 RPR, nonreactive CSF VDRL, and negative herpes simplex virus antibodies). (**B**) Despite intravenous penicillin and treatment with topical prednisolone, stromal keratouveitis occurred 3 months later in his right eye, then recurred twice later in the left eye.

Bilateral keratitis

Unilateral stromal keratitis due to late congenital syphilis is not a typical pattern.[173,174] In 80% of patients with stromal keratitis caused by congenital syphilis the contralateral cornea becomes inflamed.[94] Bilateral involvement may happen simultaneously. More often, inflammation of the other cornea begins a few weeks later (Fig. 85.9) – within 3 months in 75% of cases.[56] The interval does not correlate with severity. With time, the opposite eye becomes less likely to be affected: only 2% develop keratitis of the second eye more than 5 years later, although delays over 15 years are recorded.

Recurrent ocular inflammation

Approximately 5–15% of patients have another episode in the same eye.[88,103,175] Recrudescence is rebound inflammation when corticosteroid therapy is stopped prematurely.[176] Recurrence is a separate relapse months or years after resolution of the preceding episode with subsequent quietude.[168] Ocular trauma can reopen existing ghost vessels and trigger repeat inflammation in a vulnerable cornea. A recurrence is usually unilateral and tends to be milder than the first episode,[94,177] although multiple recurrences can ensue. Focal stromal keratitis may occur at the site of previous disease or elsewhere in the cornea.[177] Syphilitic keratitis was once thought to be able to recur in a corneal graft, but this post-operative complication now seems implausible. Recurrences may be episodes of iridocyclitis rather than stromal keratitis.[178] Episcleritis, scleritis, and posterior uveitis have arisen after resolution of syphilitic keratitis.[179]

Physical findings of early congenital syphilis

Skin

Stigmata of early congenital syphilis[113,126,180] are found in about 50% of untreated patients with syphilitic stromal keratitis or keratopathy (Table 85.2). A cutaneous rash during infancy leads to dry, wrinkled skin. Rhagades are perioral radiating fissures at the labial commissures, producing a withered mouth in 10% of people with congenital syphilitic keratitis. Premature crow's feet may occur at the outer canthi, and periorbital cicatrices contribute to ectropion in later life.[181]

Skull

Anomalies of the facial bones create a distinctive, often asymmetric physiognomy.[182] Cranial malformations include frontal bossing, supraorbital thickening, a sloping cranium with enlarged forehead (*leontiasis ossea*), short maxillae, a high-arched or perforated palate, and a prominent mandible (Fig. 85.10). Prior inflammation of the nasal cartilage or bones can lead to a flattened nasal bridge with depression of the nasal dorsum and over-rotation of the nasal tip. This saddle-nose deformity, occurring in 5% of patients with syphilitic keratitis,[56] predisposes to dacryocystitis.

Bones

Skeletal aberrations arise as bones grow. Sternoclavicular thickening and a flared scapula may develop during childhood. A sabre shin on one or both legs is the most common bony abnormality, affecting 15% of patients with syphilitic keratitis,[56] but may be hard to recognize without palpation or X-rays. Radiographic anomalies of long bones occur in one-fifth of seropositive children.

Teeth

Malformed incisors (Hutchinson's teeth) are hallmarks of congenital syphilis.[183–185] Erosion produces notched upper central incisors of the second dentition (Fig. 85.11). When dental serration is not conspicuous, a flaw in the enamel can be seen with transillumination by holding a light behind the front teeth. The incisors resemble screwdrivers, thickened in anteroposterior diameter but narrowed and rounded at their incisal margin. Other teeth tend to be small and widely spaced, with dental hypoplasia found in about a half of patients with syphilitic stromal keratitis.[56,136,186] Caries is common, and teeth are often capped or removed at an early

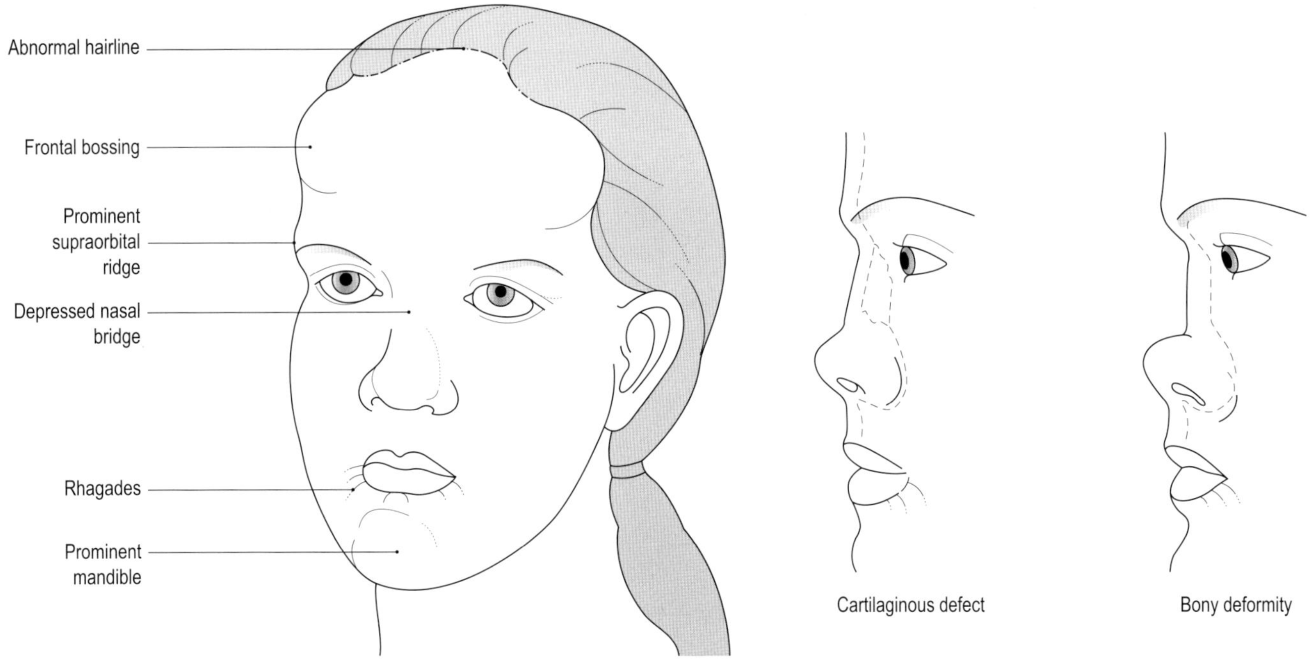

Fig. 85.10 Facial and cranial features of congenital syphilis. Side views depict how a saddle-nose deformity may be produced either by destruction of the nasal cartilage or by collapse of the bony septum. Stepwise hearing loss, beginning with attenuation of high tones, can be characterized by audiometry (From Jerger S, Jerger J: *Auditory Disorders: a manual for clinical evaluation*. Boston: Little Brown, 1981).

Table 85.2 Permanent changes of the teeth and bones caused by congenital syphilis

Structure	Sign	Appearance
Upper central incisors	Hutchinson's teeth	Widely spaced, peg-shaped, stunted central incisors, notched at the cutting edge
First lower molars	Moon's molars	Dome-shaped molars; narrower at the cutting edge; maldevelopment of the usual four cusps produces a mulberry-shaped, bulging crown prone to caries
Frontal and parietal bones	Parrot's nodes	Frontal bossing with rounded bony prominences separated by a groove; exostosis of the supraorbital area produces an 'Olympian brow'
Nasal bones	Saddle-nose deformity	Depressed bridge, often with flattened lower nose and a retroussé tip
Maxillary bones	Short maxillae	Maxillary underdevelopment with midfacial concavity and a high palatal arch
Tibia	Fournier's tibia	Sabre shin with thickening of the forward portion and anterior bowing of the middle tibia

age. Lower incisors, canines, and molars may have defective enamel. Mulberry molars characteristically show many small cusps on the first molars and are narrower at the grinding surface than at the gum. Ectodermal dysplasia and other genodermatoses may simulate congenital syphilis if corneal and dental abnormalities are present.[187]

Physical findings of late congenital syphilis

Hearing loss

Children with congenital syphilis have normal audiological tests before the onset of stromal keratitis or sensorineural deafness.[188] Reduced hearing sometimes occurs around the time of corneal inflammation, but more commonly starts a few years later. Most who lose hearing from congenital syphilis will have had stromal keratitis. Hearing loss afflicts 10–15% of individuals with late congenital syphilis who have had stromal keratitis,[56,186] perhaps more often in those with severe ocular inflammation. Stromal keratitis, deafness, and abnormal teeth form Hutchinson's triad.[189] Females are more often affected, and onset might be related to menarche. Rarely does otosyphilis start in adulthood, although Menière's triad of tinnitus, perceptive hypoacusis, and disequilibrium can be a late manifestation.[190] Stromal keratitis with deafness can also occur with Cogan's syndrome, Wegener's granulomatosis, sarcoidosis, and, rarely, herpes simplex virus infection.[191]

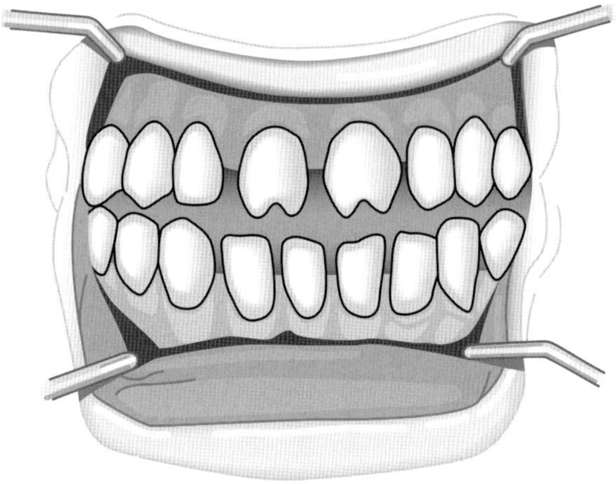

Fig. 85.11 Hutchinson's notched incisors and widely spaced teeth.

The cochlea and vestibule are the principal sites of syphilitic dysfunction.[192] Associated middle ear complications include endolymphatic hydrops, atrophy of the organ of Corti, and osteitis of the otic capsule. The eighth nerve and central auditory pathway can be harmed by basal meningitis during neurosyphilis.

Arthritis

Joint symptoms, typically synovitis of the knees, but also of the ankles, elbows, or shoulders, are a manifestation of late congenital syphilis.[193] Bilateral knee effusion (Clutton's joints)[194–196] formerly occurred in 10% or more of patients with stromal keratitis.[56,197] This now-rare condition begins around puberty, between the ages of 10 and 15 years, in equal numbers of girls and boys. Arthritis may accompany ocular inflammation but more often immediately precedes stromal keratitis.

Neurosyphilis

Neurosyphilis can precede[198] or follow[199] syphilitic corneal disease. Abnormal cerebrospinal fluid can be found in 5–10% of patients with syphilitic keratitis.[100] However, asymptomatic neurosyphilis is no more likely in patients with stromal keratitis than among others with untreated latent syphilis.[56] Neurosyphilis, usually asymptomatic, develops in a quarter to a half of children with untreated congenital syphilis[200] but in less than 5% who receive antibiotics.[209] Juvenile paresis is recognized around puberty as a change in behavior or intellect or as seizures.[198] Juvenile tabes begins at about 20 years of age and may be associated with optic atrophy. Among many neuroophthalmic manifestations are optic neuritis, cranial nerve palsy, and pupillary light–near dissociation.[201–203]

Stromal Keratitis in Acquired Syphilis

Onset

Keratitis is very uncommon in acquired syphilis.[38] Exceptional during early mucocutaneous syphilis[204] and secondary syphilis,[205] stromal keratitis is typically a feature of late syphilis.[206–208] Onset generally starts 2–15 years after acquiring syphilis,[88,209] but has rarely been delayed more than 20 years. Many patients do not recall a primary chancre or previous symptoms of secondary syphilis and usually have few other signs. Keratitis may be more likely if syphilis was acquired at a young age. Corneal trauma can be a precipitating factor.[210] Syphilitic stromal keratitis has not occurred during HIV/AIDS.

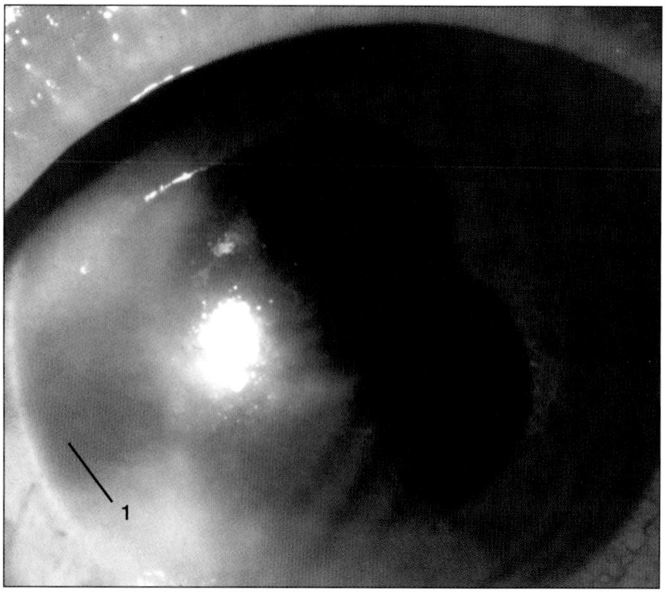

Fig. 85.12 Stromal keratouveitis manifested by extensive stromal edema and deep neovascularization (*1*) in acquired syphilis.

Corneal inflammation

Stromal keratitis associated with acquired syphilis resembles that of congenital syphilis but is usually unilateral and less severe. Stromal inflammation begins with lymphocytes infiltrating the peripheral or central cornea, with a modest predilection for the superior cornea.[211] A limpid haze may resolve and be subclinical, but can evolve to deep stromal keratitis. Corneal inflammation evokes stromal blood vessels (Fig. 85.12), but neovascularization is scarcer and scantier in acquired syphilis than in congenital syphilis.[35] Mild iridocyclitis may be present[212] but is seldom intense.[213]

Keratitis usually remains localized rather than becoming diffuse.[214] Protean variations include multifocal infiltrates[215,216] and marginal ulcerative keratitis.[217] Necrotizing inflammation of the posterior cornea[218] may effloresce centrally or peripherally[219,220] and simulate an abscess.[221–224] A limbal gumma[224–226] is a raised fleshy lesion.

Less than a third of patients develop keratitis of the other eye. When bilateral, the inflammatory reaction in the second eye is usually a milder version of the first. Recrudescent stromal keratitis can follow abrupt discontinuation of topical corticosteroid therapy. Recurrent stromal keratitis (Fig. 85.13), uveitis, and scleritis can occur months to years later.[227] Systemic antisyphilitic treatment does not prevent bilateral keratitis or recurrent ocular inflammation.

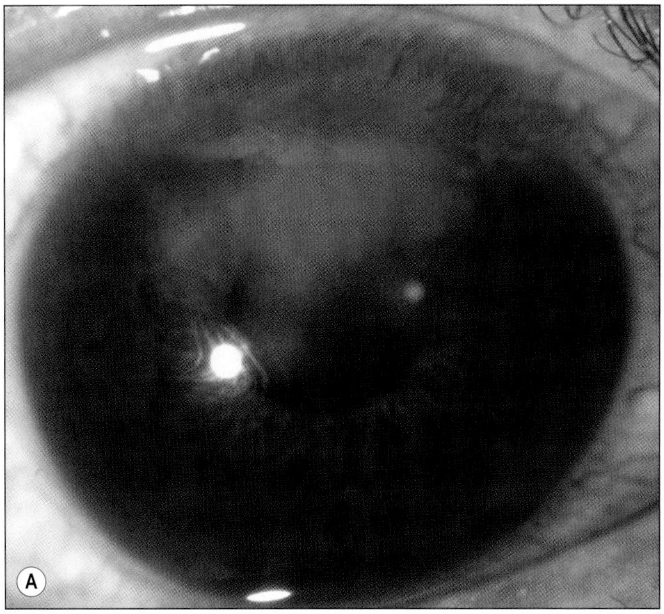

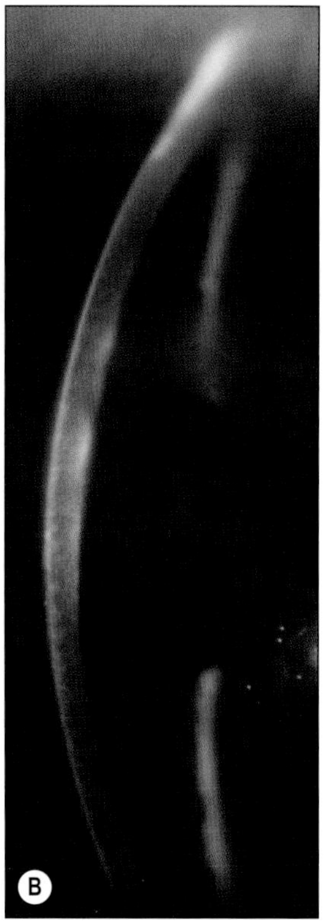

Fig. 85.13 Syphilitic stromal keratitis. (**A**) Inflammatory stromal edema of the superior cornea. (**B**) Recurrent stromal keratitis of the deep central cornea 5 months later. (Adapted from Wilhelmus KR, Jones DB. *Am J Ophthalmol* 2006; 141: 319, published with permission from the *American Journal of Ophthalmology*. Original copyright by the Ophthalmic Publishing Company.)

Physical findings of acquired syphilis

Signs of secondary acquired syphilis are enlarged lymph nodes and a maculopapular rash over the trunk, palms, and soles.[228] Mucous patches are infectious, painless erosions of the mouth and, rarely, the conjunctiva.[229] Sudden hearing loss and acute arthritis[230] rarely occur. Long-lasting stigmata of prior secondary syphilis may be subtle, such as hypo- or hyperpigmented spots on the skin and patchy alopecia of scalp hair, eyebrows, or eyelashes. People with late acquired syphilis who develop stromal keratitis are usually otherwise asymptomatic but can later have cardiovascular complications, gummas, and neurosyphilis. Neurological examination should seek to uncover signs of meningovascular or parenchymatous neurosyphilis, especially in adults with a high titer (≥1:32) of a nontreponemal serologic test.[231,232]

Syphilitic Stromal Keratopathy

Recovery from stromal keratitis

Untreated, stromal inflammation gradually abates over weeks to months. Topical corticosteroid treatment dramatically speeds regression.[74] Resolution usually starts peripherally, often at the place where inflammation began. Lymphatic vessels shrivel,[233] and blood vessels slowly shrink and fade into marcescent remnants that become all but invisible. With corticosteroid treatment, a child's cornea can clear completely.

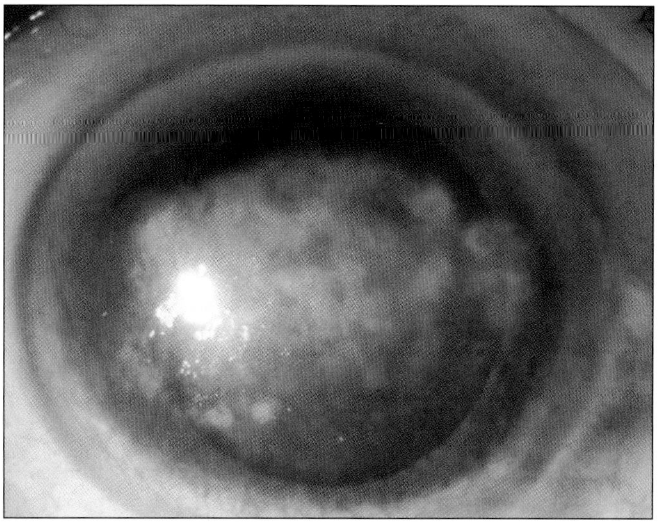

Fig. 85.14 Anterior stromal opacification of an adult who had bilateral keratitis during childhood. A dense corneal arcus blends into the limbus.

Corneal opacity

Corneal opacification is the most visible aftermath of stromal keratitis. Stromal fibrosis produces a diffuse or patchy central corneal haze reminiscent of dried lymph. Peripheral scarring (Fig. 85.14), a vascularized pannus, and a premature arcus

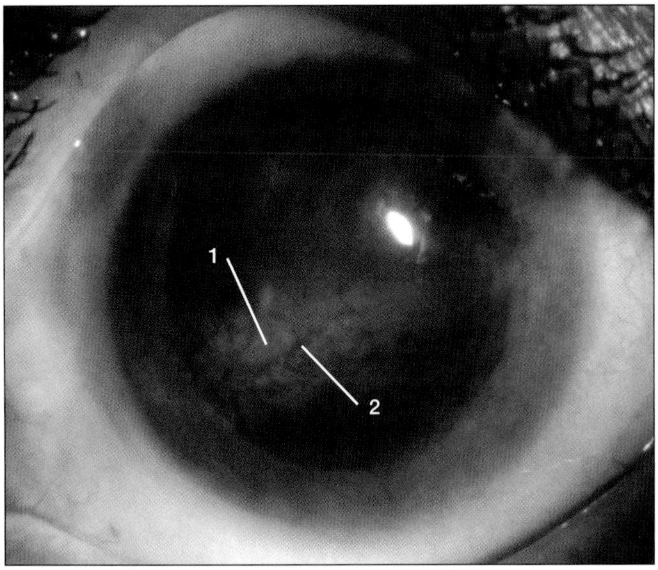

Fig. 85.15 Deep stromal scarring (*1*) canalized by ghost vessels (*2*) in an adult who had bilateral keratitis during childhood.

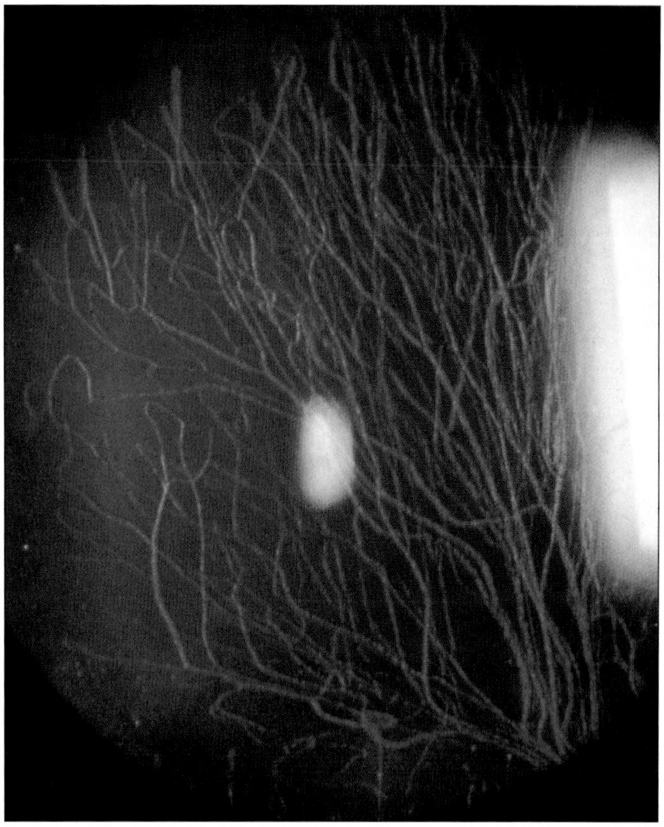

Fig. 85.16 Corneal ghost vessels visualized by retroillumination. (From Lee ME, Lindquist TD. J Am Med Assoc. 1989; 262: 2921. Copyright 1989, American Medical Association. All right reserved.)

can make the cornea appear oval[234] or small.[235] Deep stromal scarring may resemble posterior crocodile shagreen (Fig. 85.15).

Some corneas are thickened by chronic edema or a vascularized, fibromatous mass. Others, ravaged by inflammation, are left thinned, with irregular astigmatism. Anterior inflammation tends to flatten, whereas deep keratitis steepens the cornea's conformation. A weakened cornea can become ectatic and take on a conical contour. Keratectasia can also indicate secondary glaucoma.

Spheroidal degeneration, Salzmann's nodular degeneration, corneal keloid, secondary amyloid degeneration,[236,237] lipid keratopathy, and calcific band keratopathy[238] are possible sequelae. Corneal sensation is typically normal, although hypesthesia[211] and neurotrophic keratopathy[239] have been reported. Bacterial superinfection,[240] perforation,[241] and phthisis bulbi[242] have rarely occurred.

Ghost vessels

A tracery of intertwined phantom vessels may form a threadlike network weaving through a stromal haze,[243] sometimes creating zigzag patterns against a background of chalky white scarring and lipid. A pearly corona may surround a leaky vessel, and deposits can fan out like a palm frond.[244] Vascular channels are visualized by indirect illumination, retroillumination (Fig. 85.16),[245] specular reflection, and confocal microscopy.[246] Though termed *ghost vessels*, corneal angiography shows that many are patent and convey plasma (Fig. 85.17). Some lumina may remain just large enough to carry the occasional red blood cells. Rupture due to sudden increased blood pressure or blunt ocular trauma can bring about an intracorneal hemorrhage,[247] even temporary corneal blood staining.[248]

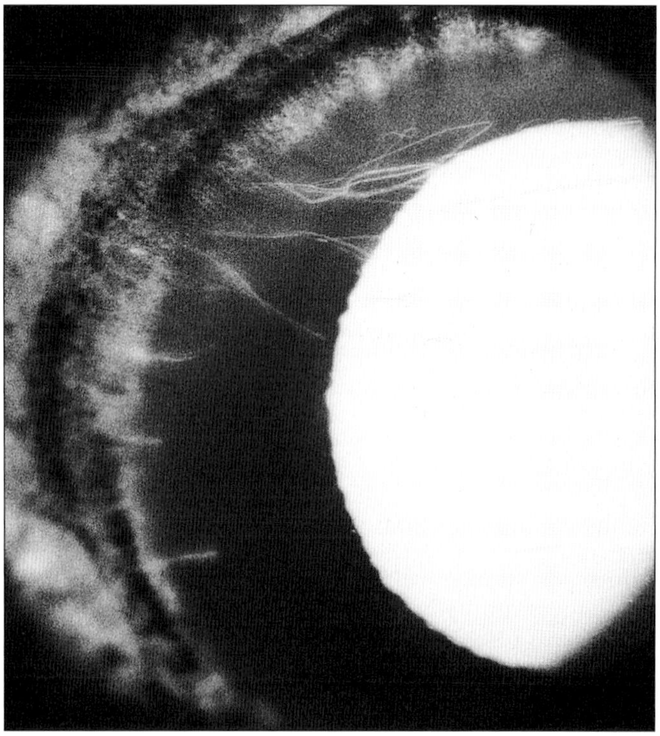

Fig. 85.17 Corneal angiogram showing intrastromal blood vessels in an adult who had syphilitic keratitis during childhood.

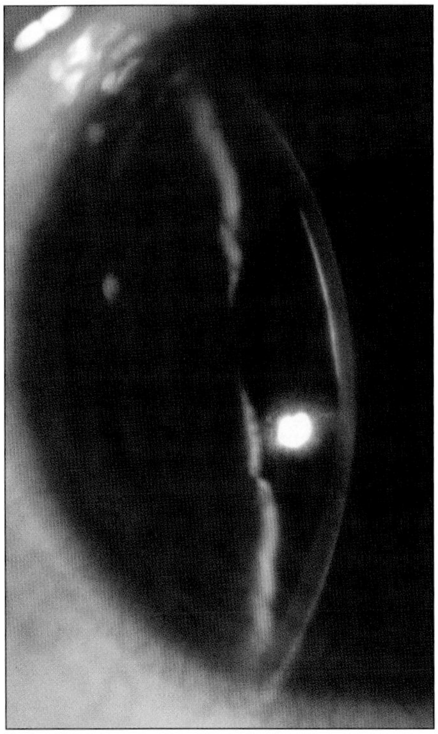

Fig. 85.18 Posterior collagenous layer, seen with a thin slit beam as a white, irregular plaque of the posterior cornea.

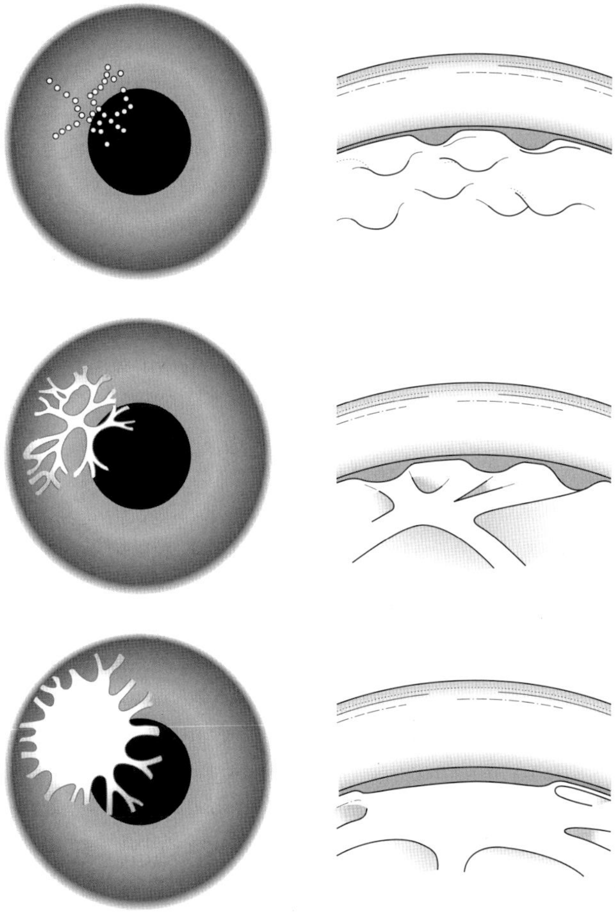

Fig. 85.19 The spectrum of posterior corneal changes following syphilitic keratitis occurring at a young age. Altered edothelial cells produce abnormal collagenous material that may resemble grouped guttae (*top*), a retrocorneal ridge (*center*), and focal plaques (*bottom*) of Descemet's membrane. (Redrawn from Waring GO, et al. *Am J Ophthalmol* 1976; 81: 773–785. Published with permission from the *American Journal of Ophthalmology*. Original copyright by The Ophthalmic Publishing Company.)

Alterations to Descemet's membrane and endothelium

Posterior collagenous layer

Corneal endothelial damage varies from mild pleomorphism to marked cell loss. Injured cells undergo a regenerative response that produces a dove-gray subendothelial film (Fig. 85.18). The term *posterior collagenous layer* was coined to describe the accretion resulting from endothelial mesenchymal transformation.[249] This alteration may be localized to one area or spread across the deeper cornea,[50,250] like a sheet of beaten metal (Fig. 85.19). Endothelial metaplasia also produces knobbles on Descemet's membrane[251] that are scattered, zonally confluent, or aligned. Postinflammatory endothelial dysfunction predisposes to corneal edema later in life and after intraocular surgery (Fig. 85.20).

Retrocorneal scrolls

Before the use of corticosteroids, approximately 2–15% of eyes with syphilitic keratitis developed ridges or bands on Descemet's membrane.[252,253] These multilaminar refractile scrolls look like glass rods (*Glasleisten*) or a delicate lattice.[250–255] A retrocorneal filigree might be mistaken for corneal striae or ghost vessels. Strands of hyaline material can extend into the anterior chamber or fuse into a web of interconnecting fibers (Fig. 85.21). Splits in Descemet's membrane heal as opaline tracks, crescents, or rings, and form linear guttata. Postuveitic fibrin deposits can also leave retrocorneal lines or filaments,[256] and old keratic precipitates persist as deposits and plaques on the endothelium.

Uveal alterations

Iris atrophy can follow syphilitic keratoiritis. Iridoschisis is focal or sectoral anterior stromal atrophy in which radial fibers and iris stroma are preserved, so the iris does not transilluminate.[257–259] Peripheral anterior synechiae persist in a third of eyes following syphilitic keratouveitis.[260] Posterior synechiae may produce pupillary distortion and corectopia. Pigmentary chorioretinopathy and optic atrophy are visible in up to half of patients with syphilitic keratopathy.[203,261] A few have vitreous opacities.[262]

Secondary glaucoma

Ocular hypertension and glaucoma (Table 85.3) are potential sequelae of syphilitic stromal keratouveitis.[203] Up to a fifth

Table 85.3 Glaucoma after syphilitic stromal keratitis

Gonioscopy	Mechanism
Open angle	Trabecular sclerosis Angle endothelialization
Narrow angle	Peripheral anterior synechiae Iridoschisis

of patients with congenital syphilitic keratopathy and a half of those with iridoschisis develop glaucoma,[203,263] typically 15–30 years later in the fifth decade of life. Postuveitic open-angle glaucoma results from reduced outflow[264] due to trabecular meshwork sclerosis or endothelialization of the anterior chamber angle.[263–270] Approximately one-quarter of patients with glaucoma following syphilitic stromal keratitis have a normal angle by gonioscopy. Narrow-angle glaucoma and angle closure may arise from circumferential peripheral anterior synechiae, iris cysts, a dislocated lens, or

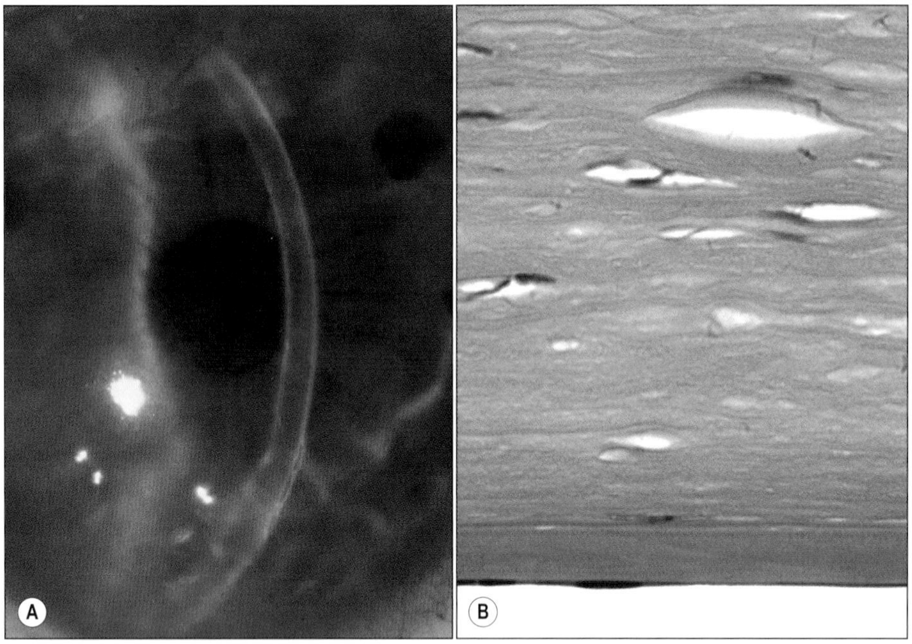

Fig. 85.20 Corneal edema in a 60-year-old woman that followed bilateral stromal keratitis at 6 years of age associated with congenital syphilis. (**A**) Central corneal thickness of 0.69 mm. (**B**) Thickened (16 mm) Descemet's membrane (PAS, ×40). Other sections show deep stromal blood vessels.

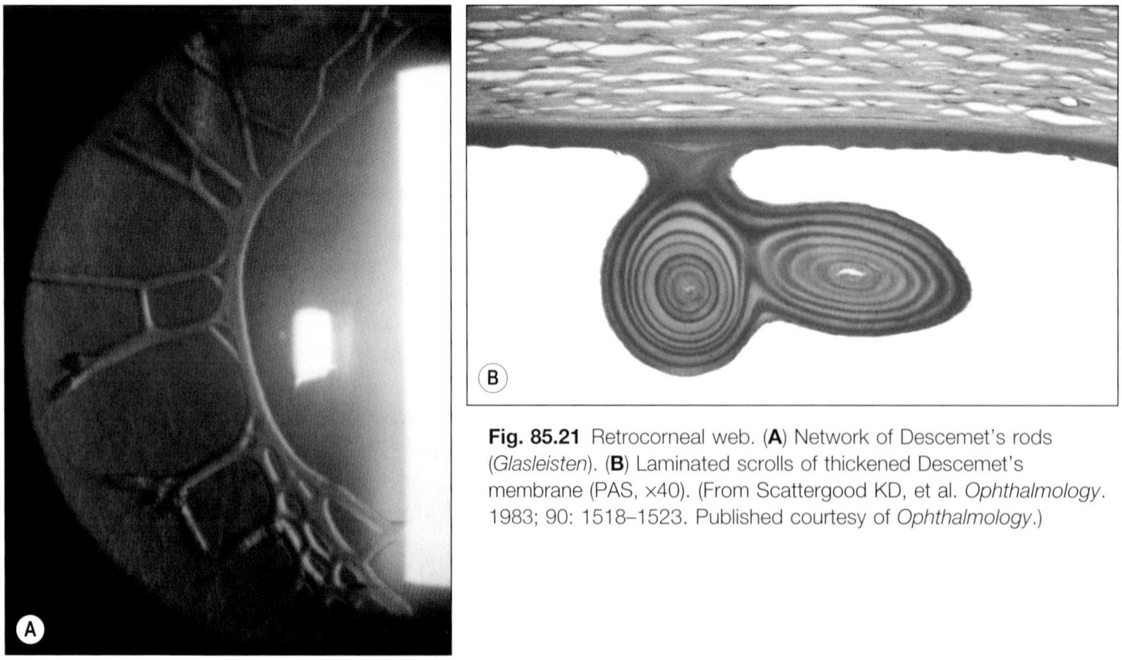

Fig. 85.21 Retrocorneal web. (**A**) Network of Descemet's rods (*Glasleisten*). (**B**) Laminated scrolls of thickened Descemet's membrane (PAS, ×40). (From Scattergood KD, et al. *Ophthalmology*. 1983; 90: 1518–1523. Published courtesy of *Ophthalmology*.)

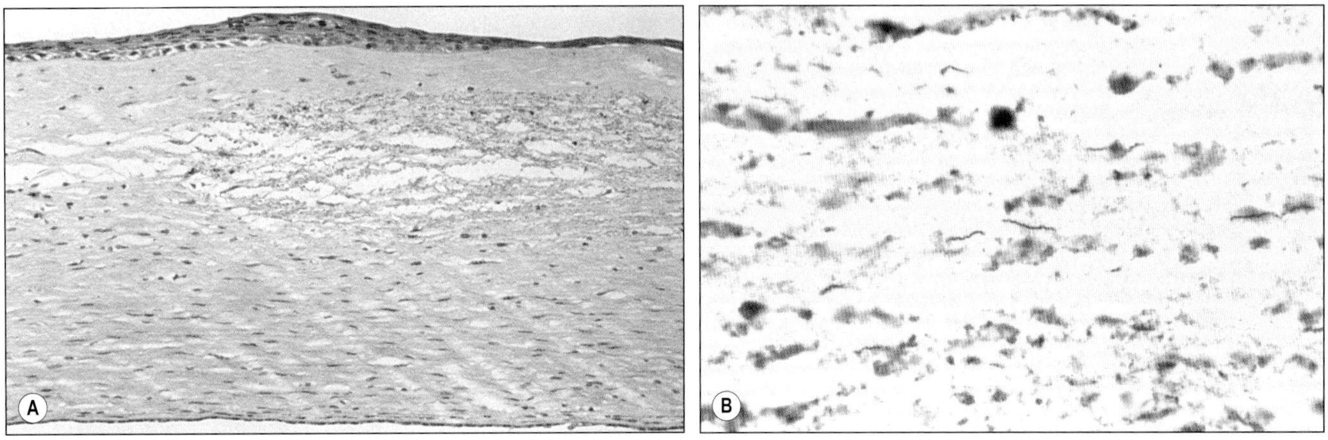

Fig. 85.22 Histopathological section of necrotizing keratitis during early congenital syphilis (PAS, ×40). (**A**) Necrosis of stroma. (**B**) Spirochetes between the stromal lamellae (Warthin Starry, ×400). (From Luckenbach MW. Presented at the Theobald Society meeting, 1985.)

Table 85.4 Intrauterine infections affecting the cornea during infancy and childhood

Structure	Congenital syphilis	Herpes simplex virus	Rubella	Cytomegalovirus
Cornea	Stromal keratitis	Epithelial and stromal keratitis	Congenital corneal edema	Congenital corneal opacity
Retina	Chorioretinopathy	Chorioretinopathy	Chorioretinopathy	Chorioretinopathy
Ears	Hearing loss	Normal	Hearing loss	Hearing loss
Skull	Maldeveloped	Normal	Microcephaly	Microcephaly
Teeth	Maldeveloped	Normal	Maldeveloped	Maldeveloped

a developmentally narrow angle secondary to juvenile ocular inflammation.[111,271,272]

Cataract

Secondary cataract, often cortical,[273] occurs in 5% of patients following severe or prolonged iridocyclitis.[186] Eyes with resolved syphilitic keratouveitis have intact zonules and are probably not at increased risk of lens subluxation.

Pathology

Stromal keratitis of early syphilis

Stillborns with congenital syphilis have treponemes disseminated throughout the body, including the cornea.[274] Their eyes may be clinically normal or extensively inflamed.[275] Microphthalmia or buphthalmos may occur. Syphilitic stromal keratitis in a surviving neonate, albeit rare,[276,277] has treponemes in the midst of an intense inflammatory reaction (Fig. 85.22). Other prenatal infections produce overlapping findings (Table 85.4). A primary conjunctival chancre, as well as conjunctivitis during secondary acquired syphilis, also contains *T. pallidum*.[278] Suppurative or necrotizing corneal infiltrates in secondary syphilis are also presumed but not proven to be infective.

Stromal keratitis of late syphilis

Treponemes are very difficult to find in the eye[279–282] and are not present in the cornea during late congenital or late acquired syphilis. Corneal histopathology shows patches of infiltrates composed of lymphocytes,[283] mainly T cells. The inflammatory process tends towards the deeper layers,[284–287] where macrophages cluster around necrotic keratocytes. A granulomatous reaction can creep along Descemet's membrane and crumple the posterior cornea.[288] Corneal neovascularization gravitates toward the deeper stroma. Ingrowing vessels, stimulated by unsequestered vascular endothelial growth factor, generally stay in the same lamellar plane along their direction of growth unless stromal necrosis and disorganization deflect their path. Inflammatory cells cuff newly formed vessels.[289] The endothelium is often fretted by mononuclear inflammatory cells coming from the deep stroma or anterior chamber (Fig. 85.23).

Anterior uveitis frequently coexists with stromal keratitis. Lymphocytic infiltration of the iris and ciliary body can be severe, sometimes extending toward the anterior choroid or into the sclera. Giant cells are occasionally present in the uveal tract, and leukocytes permeate the trabecular meshwork and surround Schlemm's canal. Iris synechiae and pigment dispersion may alter the anterior chamber angle.

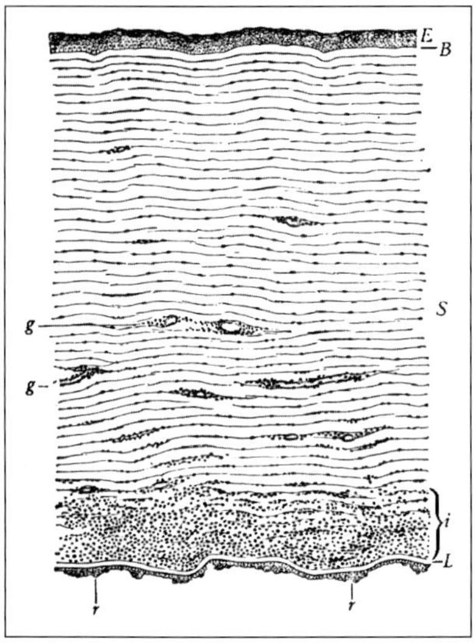

Fig. 85.23 Lymphocytic infiltration of the deep stroma (i) and corneal endothelium (r) with stromal blood vesssels (g) during syphilitic keratitis. (From Fuchs E. *Lehrbuch der Augenheilkunde*. Leipzig: Franz Deuticke, 1889: 178.)

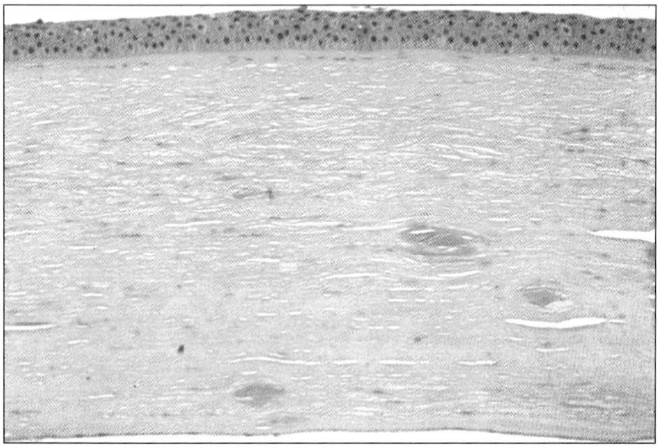

Fig. 85.24 Histopathologic section of syphilitic keratopathy showing localized amyloid deposition around stromal blood vessels (Congo red, ×40). Polarized microscopy demonstrated birefringence and dichromism of these fusiform and linear deposits. (From Dutt S, et al. *Ophthalmology* 1992; 99: 817–823. Published courtesy of *Ophthalmology*.)

Residual stromal keratopathy

The corneal epithelium can vary in thickness. Its basement membrane may be irregularly thickened,[290] and a fibrous pannus may disrupt Bowman's layer. Activated keratocytes lay down collagen in damaged cornea, resulting in stromal scarring.[291] Calcific and lipid deposits are sometimes seen. Small blood vessels remain in various stromal layers, whereas others regress by apoptosis.[292] Fusiform deposits of amyloid are detectable (Fig. 85.24), particularly around ghost vessels.[237] Clumps or rows of guttate excrescences are sometimes present, mingled beneath deep stromal vessels.[293] The endothelial cell density may be reduced, and endothelial cells can be abnormally enlarged and polyploid.[294] Fibrosis replaces keratic precipitates and plaques.

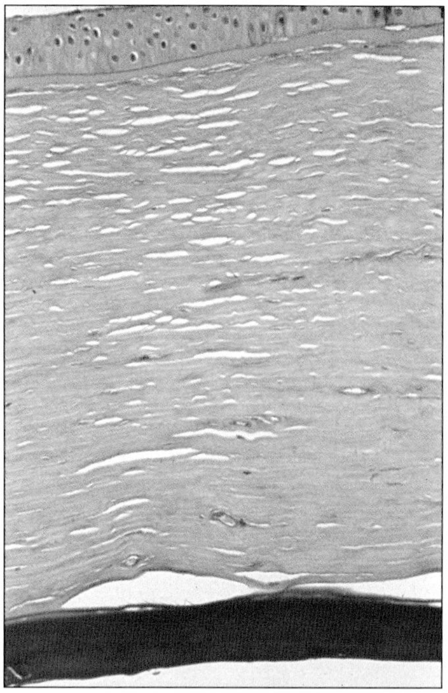

Fig. 85.25 Histopathologic section of syphilitic keratopathy showing thickened Descemet's membrane and stromal blood vessels.

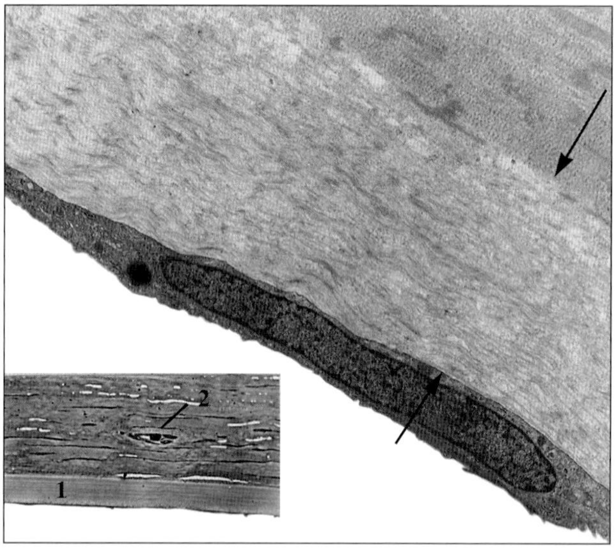

Fig. 85.26 Posterior collagenous layer (between arrows) on electron micrograph (×8000). At lower power (inset), Descemet's membrane is thickened and laminated (*1*) and a deep stromal blood vessel is patent (*2*). (From Scattergood KD, et al. *Ophthalmology* 1983; 90: 1518–1523. Published courtesy of *Ophthalmology*.)

Secondary alterations of Descemet's membrane are accentuated if the inflammatory reaction occurred during childhood and progressed unchecked (Fig. 85.25). Descemet's membrane thickens, frequently more than 15 μm (Fig. 85.26). Formerly said to be reduplicated,[295–298] a posterior collagenous layer occurs when Descemet's membrane has an anterior layer of type IV collagen and slowly accretes a posterior layer of disordered extracellular matrix (Fig. 85.27).[249,299]

Types I, III, IV, and VIII collagens are laid down through posttranslational upregulation of collagen assembly by transformed endothelium,[251,300] stimulated by transforming growth factor-beta and fibroblast growth factor from leukocytes.[301] A cleavage plane at the junction of Descemet's membrane and the posterior collagenous layer may lead to a crinkled split and result in strands or scrolls. Concentric layers of abnormal Descemet's membrane contain long- and short-fiber collagens, fibronectin, laminin, and decorin.[251,302] Ridges,[297,303] scrolls,[304] networks,[256,305] and filaments[306] that extend into the anterior chamber occasionally form an iridocorneal adhesion,[307] retrocorneal fibrous membrane,[287] or intracameral web. Changes in Descemet's membrane remain permanently, as a record of pathological events in the biography of the corneal endothelium.

Pathogenesis

Corneal immunology

Infection is a prerequisite for syphilitic keratitis,[308] but *T. pallidum* lacks virulence factors among its 1039 protein-encoding genes. Immunity has the key role.[309,310] Syphilitic keratitis is characterized by mononuclear cell infiltration,[311–314] indicative of an immune-mediated reaction.[315–317] Historic experiments in ocular immunology showed that corneal[318] or intravenous[319] challenge induced stromal keratitis in a previously exposed eye. Hypersensitivity,[320] stimulated by bacterial proteins[321,322] or autogenous antigens,[285,315,323] spurs corneal inflammation and angiogenesis.[324] Deciphering these inflammatory pathways will answer long-standing questions about syphilitic keratitis and its poor response to antimicrobials.[97]

Keratitis in other spirochetal infections

Stromal keratitis rarely occurs with spirochetoses other than syphilis (Table 85.5). Nonvenereal human treponematoses such as bejel, yaws, and pinta are not transmitted transplacentally and do not cause stromal keratitis, except for a very few cases of yaws.[325,326] Lyme disease is caused by a spirochete, *Borrelia burgdorferi*, that may lead to stromal keratitis[327] and sometimes deafness. Relapsing fever is a tropical disease due to *Borrelia recurrentis* that has rarely caused stromal keratitis.[328] Leptospirosis, caused by *Leptospira interrogans*, is an exceptional reason for stromal keratitis.[329,330]

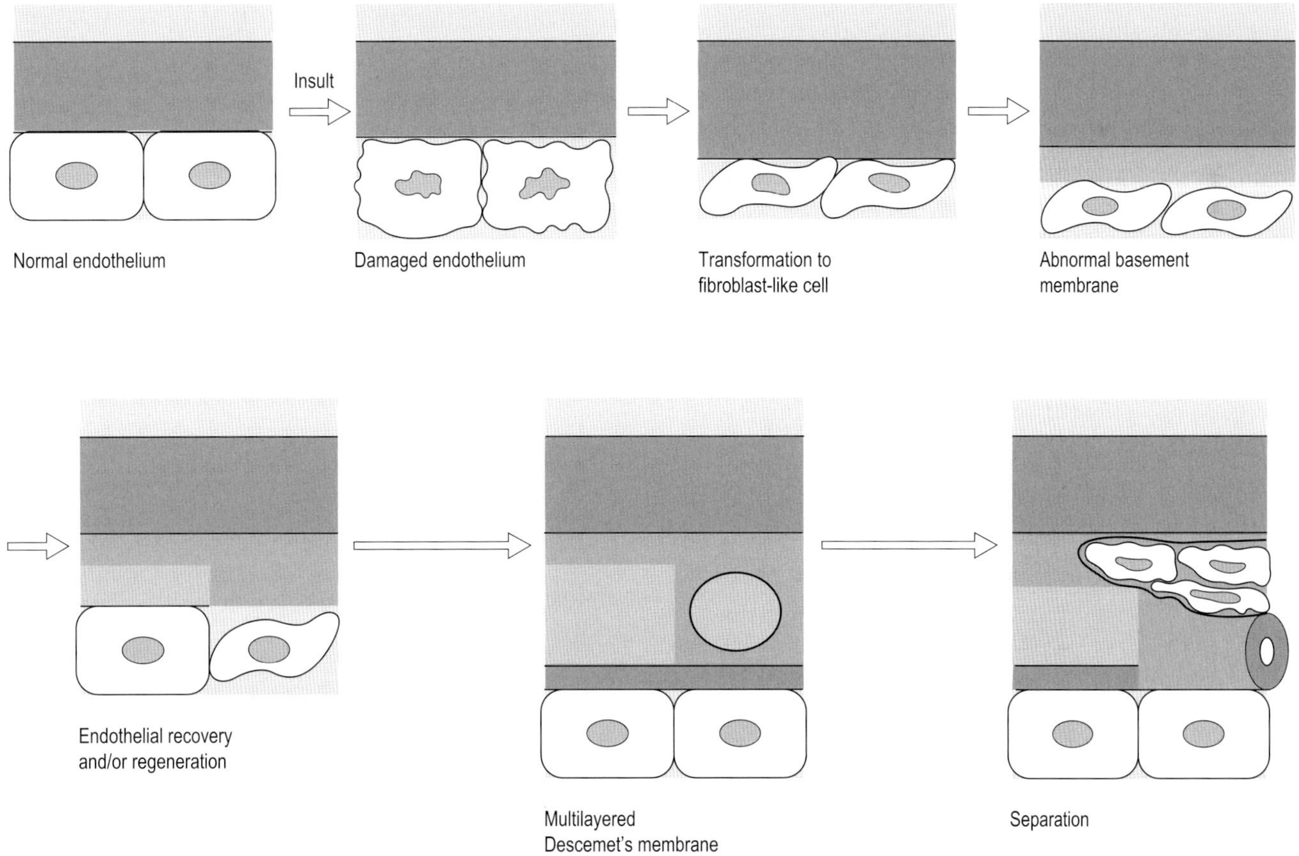

Fig. 85.27 Pathogenesis of altered Descemet's membrane during syphilitic corneal disease. (From Waring GO, et al. *Am J Ophthalmol* 1976; 81: 773–785. Published with permission from the *American Journal of Ophthalmology*. Copyright by the Ophthalmic Publishing Company.)

Table 85.5 Stromal keratitis during human spirochetoses

Disease	Pathogen	Stromal keratitis	Serologic test for syphilis
Congenital syphilis	*T. pallidum* subsp. *pallidum*	Common	Reactive
Acquired syphilis	*T. pallidum* subsp. *pallidum*	Rare	Reactive
Bejel	*T. pallidum* subsp. *endemicum*	None	Reactive
Yaws	*T. pallidum* subsp. *pertenue*	Rare	Reactive
Pinta	*Treponema carateum*	None	Reactive
Lyme disease	*Borrelia burgdorferi*	Rare	Occasionally reactive
Relapsing fever	*Borrelia recurrentis*	Rare	Occasionally reactive
Leptospirosis	*Leptospira interrogans*	Rare	Rarely reactive

Infection *versus* immunity

T. pallidum prefers body sites with a lower temperature and can wriggle into the anterior segment during both early congenital and secondary acquired syphilis.[274,331,332] Although cathelicidins and other antimicrobial peptides at the corneal surface hinder treponemal infection, treponemes are capable of attaching to epithelial cells and fibroblasts, as well as components of the extracellular matrix such as fibronectin, type I collagen, and laminin. *T. pallidum* eludes host clearance mechanisms, and its immunoevasiveness allows stealthy treponemes to circumvent phagocytosis and to persist in extracellular niches.[333] Outer membrane lipoproteins and glycolipids of latent treponemes, exposed by some insult,[321] might enkindle innate inflammation[334,335] via CD14, toll-like receptors, and lymphocyte-attracting chemokines. Waning control over sequestered antigens[336] could also be an impetus to enhanced immunoreactivity.[333] Yet, despite these observations, dissemination to the cornea and subsequent immune recognition of intrastromal *T. pallidum* is unlikely.[226]

Previous reports[44,129] of visualizing treponemes in the inflamed cornea mistook artifacts and nonpathogenic contaminants.[337,338] The cornea of active, untreated interstitial keratitis does not contain treponemes when examined by dark-field microscopy, special stains, or infectivity testing.[129,315] Notwithstanding provocative descriptions of intracameral spiral forms,[166,282,283,288,289,339] treponemes are also not present in the aqueous humor during stromal keratouveitis.[340] Furthermore, transmission by donor eye tissue obtained from donors with syphilis has not been reported.

Stromal keratitis in late syphilis is not a localized treponemal infection.[315] The possibility was once considered that it was a coincidental disease caused by a herpesvirus in a person with syphilis,[341] but viral genes are not present in a cornea affected by syphilitic keratitis.[333,342] Immunity, rather than infection, explains the nature of syphilitic corneal inflammation.[343]

Box 85.2 Serologic tests for syphilis

Treponemal tests
Fluorescent treponemal antibody absorption (FTA-ABS)
T. pallidum immobilization (TPI, Nelson-Mayer test)
Hemagglutination treponemal test for syphilis (HATTS)
Microhemagglutination assay for *T. pallidum* (MHA-TP)
T. pallidum hemagglutination assay (TPHA)
T. pallidum latex agglutination (TPLA)
T. pallidum particle agglutination (TP-PA)
Enzyme immunoassay (EIA) for treponemal antibodies
Nontreponemal tests
Venereal Disease Research Laboratory (VDRL) test
Rapid plasma reagin (RPR) test
Automated reagin test (ART)

Autoimmune hypothesis

Molecular similarities between microbial components and corneal constituents may instigate inflammation.[344] Release of hidden antigens, immunogenic alteration of autoantigens, or mimicry between self-antigens and microbial components are reasons for stromal keratitis in systemic diseases such as Cogan's syndrome,[345] Lyme disease, and leptospirosis.[329,346–351] Corneal inflammation during late syphilis may likewise be due to dysregulated reactions by usurped hypersensitivity. Antibodies against phospholipid epitopes of the treponemal outer membrane might cross-react with corneal lipids such as phosphatidylglycerol and phosphatidylcholine.[352,353] Finding other autoantibodies such as antinuclear and anti-smooth muscle antibodies during chronic syphilitic keratitis also suggests an infection-induced autoimmune process.[354] In a hierogamy of microorganism and lymphocyte, treponemal mimotopes could underlie the pathogenesis of stromal keratitis during late syphilis.

Laboratory Investigation

Serologic tests

Treponemal tests

Treponemal serologic tests (Box 85.2) detect immunoglobulins to *T. pallidum* polypeptides by indirect immunofluorescence (FTA-ABS), hemagglutination (MHA-TP, TPHA, and HATTS), particulate agglutination (TP-PA and TPLA), and enzyme immunoassay (EIA and ELISA). A reactive test confirms prior exposure, whether adequately treated or not, although 10% of children with congenital syphilis are seronegative. A treponemal antibody test remains reactive for life in two-thirds of patients with congenital syphilis and in approximately 80% of adults treated for acquired syphilis.

Nontreponemal tests

The Venereal Disease Research Laboratory (VDRL) and rapid plasma reagin (RPR) tests detect immunoglobulins to treponemal phospholipids. Over time, quantitative VDRL and RPR titers gradually decrease, ultimately becoming undetectable in about a quarter of untreated individuals. Adequate treatment usually induces an ensuing decline, but the antibody titer may fall more slowly in patients who sustain stromal keratitis. Although almost half of treated patients become nonreactive, some retain a 'serofast reaction' with an enduring low titer. A persistently high (≥1 : 32) or increasing titer suggests treatment failure or reinfection.

Diagnostic decision-making

Serodiagnosis of stromal keratitis

The diagnosis and management of a patient with syphilitic corneal disease depends on serologic testing, neurological status, and prior antisyphilitic therapy (Fig. 85.28). Nonulcerative stromal keratitis, especially when unilateral, is associated with several infectious and immune-mediated diseases.[120] Serologic testing for syphilis is considered for patients who have first-episode deep stromal keratitis without a known cause, bilateral stromal keratitis or keratouveitis without another predisposing disease, stromal keratitis during childhood, stromal keratitis associated with pigmentary chorioretinopathy or other developmental consequences of congenital syphilis, necrotizing stromal keratitis during a maculopapular skin rash, stromal keratitis associated with optic atrophy or other neurological signs, and recurrent stromal keratitis or uveitis following previous antisyphilis treatment. For diagnosis a treponemal test such as the MHA-TP or FTA-ABS is preferred to the VDRL or RPR,[211] but a nontreponemal test is usually obtained to judge the effectiveness of systemic treatment. Serologic testing is unlikely to be cost-effective for routine evaluation of unilateral stromal keratitis, but is an option for patients whose initial episode of idiopathic stromal keratitis is not preceded or accompanied by signs of another disorder, such as herpes simplex virus eye disease. Deciding whether seropositive stromal keratitis in an adult is caused by acquired rather than congenital syphilis can be difficult.[355]

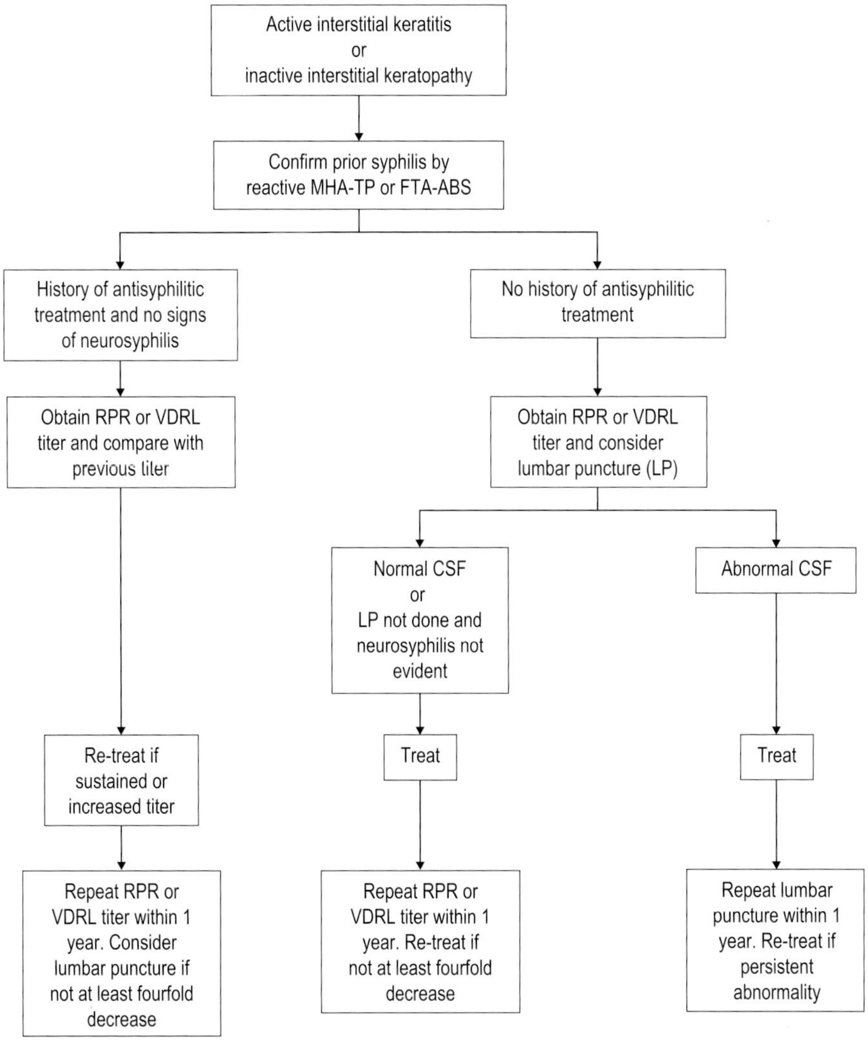

Fig. 85.28 Diagnostic and therapeutic algorithm of syphilitic corneal disease.

Serologic testing of stromal keratopathy

Vascularized corneal opacification is a sign of prior stromal keratitis. Syphilis accounts for up to a third of cases of bilateral postinflammatory stromal opacification but is a very infrequent reason for a unilateral corneal opacity.[120] A patient with residual keratopathy, especially if bilateral, could be suspected to have had congenital syphilis if prolonged ocular inflammation occurred during childhood, if the patient or parents were treated for a sexually transmitted disease, or if stigmata of congenital syphilis are present.[122] Parental testing, though rarely done for ocular syphilis, may help to differentiate congenital and acquired syphilis.[40] A positive serologic test is the only finding in over half of all cases of corneal scarring due to syphilis.

Cerebrospinal fluid testing

Patients with residual syphilitic keratopathy can have asymptomatic neurosyphilis,[271] but the risk–benefit ratio of lumbar puncture[356] is not favorable and so it is often deferred unless there is optic atrophy, pupillary light–near dissociation, or hearing loss. Laboratory-based indications for examining the cerebrospinal fluid (CSF) are a high (≥1 : 32) or increasing (≥fourfold) nontreponemal serum titer and HIV coinfection. The most common CSF abnormalities of neurosyphilis are leukocytosis (≥5 mononuclear cells/mm^3) and elevated protein (>40 mg/dL). A reactive CSF nontreponemal serologic test is specific but not sensitive, having a positive predictive value of 60% for neurosyphilis. A treponemal serologic test of the CSF can yield misleading results because serum antibodies can cross the blood–brain barrier but, when negative, excludes neurosyphilis. Full evaluation of the CSF, which is usually unfeasible, includes IgM immunoblotting, nucleic acid testing, and infectivity assay.[357]

Detection of *T. pallidum*

Dark-field microscopy is insensitive and limited to infective mucocutaneous lesions. The polymerase chain reaction reveals the genomic presence of treponemes in blood, tissue, and body fluids during congenital and acquired syphilis. Nucleic acid testing of aqueous and vitreous samples can verify the diagnosis of syphilitic uveitis. Whether genomic detection of *T. pallidum* from the eye is applicable to syphilitic stromal keratouveitis is doubtful.

Treatment

Antibacterial therapy

Syphilis is treated with penicillin, but stromal keratitis in late congenital syphilis responds slowly, if at all.[358] Penicillin neither reduces the severity of corneal inflammation nor prevents subsequent involvement of the other eye.[65,133,359] Patients with syphilitic keratitis or keratopathy should receive antibacterial dosages used for late syphilis (Table 85.6), not to remedy syphilitic keratitis, sensorineural deafness, or perisynovitis but to control systemic infection and neurosyphilis.[65]

Some treat persons having syphilitic corneal disease with the regimen for asymptomatic neurosyphilis.[360] Others prescribe the dosage for late syphilis if intraocular or neurological signs are not present.[271] With posterior uveitis, deafness, or other signs of neurosyphilis, higher penicillin doses are used.[361]

Table 85.6 Systemic treatment of syphilis

Status	Treatment
Infant with early congenital syphilis	Aqueous penicillin G 50 000 units/kg intravenously every 8–12 hours for 10–14 days
Child (<12 years old) with late congenital syphilis	Aqueous penicillin G 50 000 units/kg intravenously every 8–12 hours for 10–14 days
Adolescent (>12 years old) or adult with late congenital or acquired syphilis but without neurosyphilis	Benzathine penicillin G 2.4 million units (or 50 000 units/kg) intramuscularly once weekly for 3 consecutive weeks
Adolescent or adult with neurosyphilis	Aqueous penicillin G 3–4 million units intravenously every 4 hours for 10–14 days

Adapted from treatment guidelines at cdc.gov.

A lingering quandary is what to do for a patient with residual keratopathy who has no other signs of syphilis and whose history of previous treatment is vague.[199] Young adults with latent syphilis should be tested and treated. For the elderly, the need for testing and the benefit of antisyphilitic treatment are uncertain. Previously, a quarter of patients with syphilitic keratopathy were unaware of their diagnosis.[362] One option is to test and, if seropositive, to treat, then to reexamine and retest later.

Follow-up

The Jarisch–Herxheimer reaction, occurring shortly after beginning penicillin, is caused by the release of proinflammatory treponemal lipoproteins that trigger the production of tumor necrosis factor-α. Acute exacerbation of stromal keratitis and episcleritis, formerly termed 'therapeutic shock,' is very rarely encountered.[65,141] A paradoxical worsening of an ocular gumma can occur during late syphilis as a result of treatment-induced necrosis.[141,363]

Posttreatment serologic testing helps to gauge efficacy of antibiotic therapy. Adequate treatment produces a fourfold or greater reduction in titer of the same nontreponemal test by 3 months after therapy. Treatment failure is suspected if the nontreponemal test persists at a high titer, or if the CSF remains abnormal. Whether recurrent keratitis is an indication for antibacterial re-treatment is unclear.

Antiinflammatory therapy

Topical corticosteroids

Before the introduction of topical corticosteroids, 5–10% of patients were left with an obvious opacity, about one-third

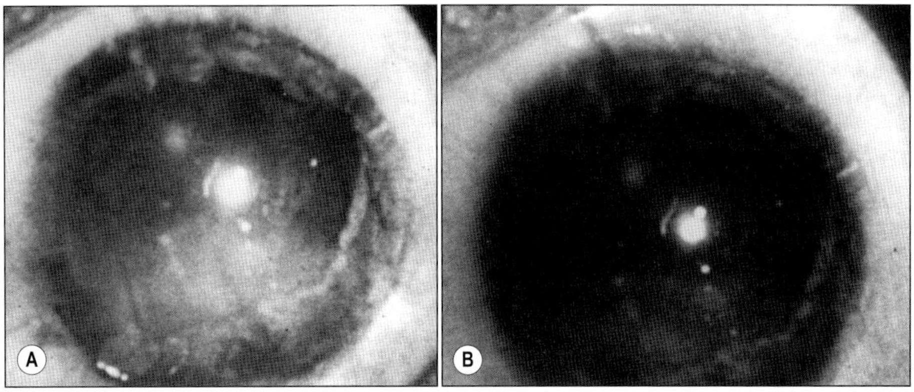

Fig. 85.29 Immediate effect of topical corticosteroid. (**A**) Recurrent stromal keratitis due to congenital syphilis. (**B**) Resolving corneal inflammation 2 days after beginning topical cortisone, followed by complete improvement within 2 weeks. (From Gordon DM. *The clinical use of corticotropin, cortisone and hydrocortisone in eye disease*. Springfield, IL: Charles C Thomas, 1954: 24.)

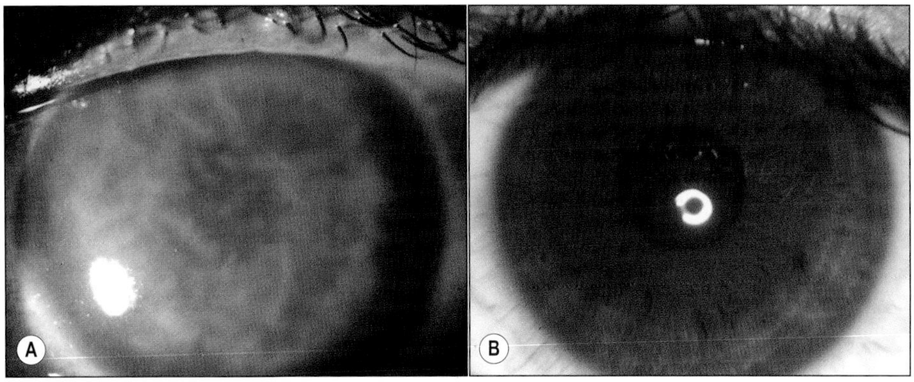

Fig. 85.30 Sustained effect of topical corticosteroid. (**A**) Acute inflammatory corneal edema due to syphilis, possibly acquired. (**B**) Complete resolution 6 months later. (From Dinas da Gama R, Cidade M. *N Engl J Med* 2002; 346: 1799. Copyright by the Massachusetts Medical Society.)

developed a faint haze, and the rest cleared.[364] Without corticosteroids, 25–50% improved to at least 20/30,[56,98,365] whereas 5–10% stayed worse than 20/200,[65,234,253] and up to 5% were bilaterally blinded.[366,367] Untreated syphilitic keratitis in a neonate or young child could induce amblyopia.[368]

A topical corticosteroid shortens the course of active syphilitic keratitis (Fig. 85.29), reduces permanent opacification (Fig. 85.30), and improves vision.[71,73–76,369,370] With a topical corticosteroid the cornea can clear completely.[371] Approximately 90% recover 20/30 vision or better.[372]

Corticosteroid dosage is chosen according to the severity of anterior segment inflammation.[373] The equivalent of prednisolone 1% or dexamethasone 0.1% is usually given four to eight times daily. A mydriatic–cycloplegic agent can be added for concomitant iridocyclitis.[75] Improvement generally occurs within a few days. The frequency of administration is tapered to prevent rebound inflammation. Prolonged topical corticosteroids may be needed to annul the corrosive effect of smoldering inflammation and to avert recrudescence.

Adjunctive antiinflammatory agents

Systemic antiinflammatory treatment is not usually indicated for acute syphilitic keratitis. An oral corticosteroid is reserved to suppress vasculitic and other immune-mediated complications of late syphilis, such as scleritis, sensorineural hearing loss, and synovitis. Topical or oral ciclosporin can be considered for persistent or recurrent stromal keratitis failing topical corticosteroid treatment.[354,374]

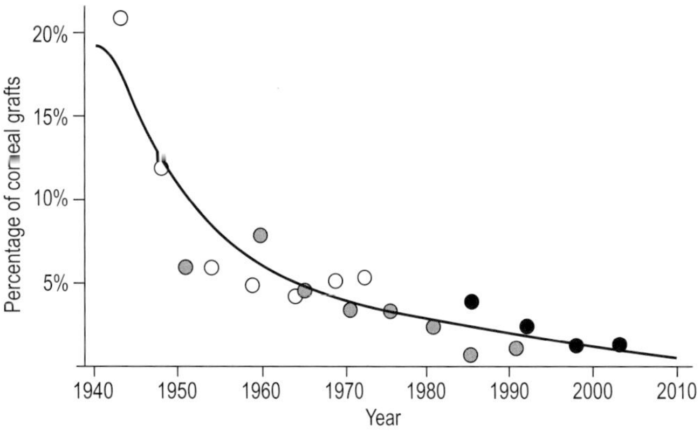

Fig. 85.31 Diminishing prevalence of syphilitic keratopathy as an indication for corneal transplantation in the United States during the 20th century, with an epidemiologic transition at the start of the antibiotic era. White dots, Baltimore; grey dots, Los Angeles; black dots, Philadelphia. (Compiled from references in text).

Surgical management

Preoperative indications

Syphilitic eye disease as a reason for corneal transplantation has declined in the era of antibiotics (Fig. 85.31).[375–379a] At one center, the proportion of grafts performed for syphilitic keratopathy fell fivefold during the late 20th century.[380] Few corneal grafts are now performed for interstitial keratitis or

Table 85.7 Prevention strategies for syphilitic keratitis

Prevention level	General clinical use	High-risk individual
Primary prevention	Provide prenatal screening and prevention practices for sexually transmitted diseases	Treat expectant mothers with syphilis and provide accessible treatment for people with early syphilis
Secondary prevention	Correctly diagnose ocular syphilis by selective serologic testing	Prevent visual loss by early recognition and appropriate treatment of stromal keratitis
Tertiary prevention	Use adequate therapy to reduce sight-threatening complications	Correct permanent visual disability by keratoplasty

keratopathy in the United States (1%),[381,382] Australia (<1%),[383] Canada (1–3%),[383–385] France (3%),[386] Germany (<1%),[387] England (1%),[380] Northern Ireland (7%),[388] and Ireland (<1%).[389] In 2002, the Eye Bank Association of America dropped syphilitic keratitis/keratopathy as a separate indication for keratoplasty.[390]

Corneal surgery is appropriate for patients with visual loss caused by irreversible opacification or edema. Just as stromal keratitis occurs more often in girls than in boys with congenital syphilis, keratoplasty for syphilitic keratopathy is performed nearly twice as often in females as in males.[384] Because both eyes are often affected, sequential, bilateral corneal transplants may be considered.[391] The chance of vision improvement is better if the patient does not have amblyopia, maculopathy, or optic atrophy.

Operative techniques

Penetrating keratoplasty is the preferred surgical procedure for treating residual corneal opacification caused by syphilis.[392,393] A triple procedure of corneal transplantation, cataract extraction, and intraocular lens implantation is an option for syphilitic keratopathy with cataract.[394,395] Care is taken during trephination, as Descemet's membrane can split and be left behind in the anterior chamber.[396] Anterior lamellar keratoplasty might be contemplated for a stromal scar,[397] but penetrating keratoplasty is needed when Descemet's membrane and the endothelium are also altered.

Postoperative complications

Iritis, glaucoma, and rejection jeopardize a successful outcome.[392,398] The presence of corneal blood vessels increases the risk of allograft reaction. Laser photocoagulation, diathermy, photodynamic therapy, and inhibitors of vascular endothelial growth factor have been tried preoperatively. Postoperatively, corticosteroids are important for maintaining a clear graft. Corneal transplantation for syphilitic corneal disease has a reasonably good prognosis: the 10-year graft survival rate is 50–80%.[383,392,399,400] If the transplant fails, regrafting can be carried out.[401]

Prevention

Prenatal care

Congenital syphilis is a lint screen for an unfair health system that leaves poor women and children behind.[402] One in four deliveries of syphilitic mothers results in an infected infant.[403] Serologic testing for syphilis should be offered to couples planning to conceive, and to women during early pregnancy, depending on the population's risk of syphilis.[404,405] Penicillin treatment of an expectant mother with syphilis can prevent stromal keratitis from occurring later in her child.[406,407] Waiting to treat ocular syphilis is unwise.[408–410] Antibacterial treatment of a seropositive child after infancy has no consistently preventive or therapeutic benefit on late syphilitic corneal disease.[411]

Public health ophthalmology

Encountering a patient with ocular syphilis is an opportunity to practice epidemiology.[412–414] Each case has a potentially infected family member or friend. For a child with congenital syphilis, parents and siblings should be tested. For an adult with acquired syphilis, serologic testing should be available to sexual partners and offspring. Newly diagnosed syphilis is reportable to the public health department.

Prevention strategies target communities and individuals.[415] From a community perspective, primary prevention thwarts exposure; secondary prevention reduces complications; and tertiary prevention minimizes vision-limiting sequelae. For individuals, the goal of primary prevention is to preclude ocular disease in infected patients, and secondary and tertiary prevention tactics curtail inflammatory and postinflammatory consequences. Preventive ophthalmology takes both approaches (Table 85.7).

Syphilitic keratitis is a sentinel event signaling a missed opportunity: deterrence is more important than preemption.[90,361] Improved surveillance and health promotion are key strategies to interrupting spread, avoiding complications, and ultimately eliminating syphilis.

References

1. Wilhelmus KR. The history of ocular syphilis. In: Bialasiewicz AA, Schaal KP, eds. *Infectious diseases of the eye*. Buren, The Netherlands: Aeolus; 1994:494–499.
2. Diday P. *Traité de la syphilis des nouveau-nés et des enfants à la mamelle*. Paris: G Masson; 1854:57–96.
3. Quétal C. *History of syphilis*. Baltimore: Johns Hopkins University; 1990:165–170.
4. Bertin RJH. *Traité de la maladie vénérienne chez les enfants nouveau-nés, les femmes enceintes et les nourrices*. Paris: Gabon; 1810.
5. Galligo I. *Trattato teorico-pratico sulle malattie venerea*. Firenze: Cecchi; 1849:449.

6. Lawrence W. *A treatise on the venereal diseases of the eye*. London: John Wilson; 1830:144–145.
7. Wardrop J. *Essays on the morbid anatomy of the human eye*. Edinburgh: George Ramsay; 1808:14–21.
8. Crissey JT, Parish LC. *The dermatology and syphilology of the nineteenth century*. New York: Praeger; 1981:80–94, 352–366.
9. von Plenck JJ. *Doctrina de morbis oculorum*. Vienna: R. Graeffer; 1777:77–85.
10. Scarpa A. *Saggio di osservazioni e d'esperienze sulle principale malattie degli occhi*. Pavia: Baldassare Comino; 1801:179–201.
11. Swediaur F. *Traité complet sur les symptomes, les effets, la nature et le traitement des maladies syphilitiques*. vol. I. Paris: self-published; 1805: 138–148.
12. Mackenzie W. *A practical treatise on the diseases of the eye*. London: Longman, Reese, Orme, Brown & Green; 1833:347–350.
13. Schindler HB. *Die Entzündungsformen der menschlichen Hornhaut*. Leipzig: Weidmann; 1838. p. 267.
14. Kelly EC. Sir Jonathan Hutchinson. Biography and bibliography. *Med Classics*. 1940;5:107–245.
15. McKusik VA. The clinical observations of Jonathan Hutchinson. *Am J Syph Gonorrhea Vener Dis*. 1952;36:101–126.
16. Obituary, Sir Jonathan Hutchinson. *Br Med J*. 1913;1:1398–1401.
17. Hutchinson H. *Jonathan Hutchinson: life and letters*. London: W Heinemann; 1946.
18. Kampmeier RH. Prenatal syphilis and Sir Jonathan Hutchinson. *Sex Transm Dis*. 1977;4:167–169.
19. Greaves D. Sir Jonathan Hutchinson. *Trans Ophthalmol Soc UK*. 1978; 98:176–177.
20. Henkind P. Jonathan Hutchinson – 1823–1913. *Am J Ophthalmol*. 1978; 85:265–266.
21. Jackson R. Jonathan Hutchinson on syphilis. *Sex Transm Dis*. 1980;7:90–96.
22. Hirschberg J, (Blodi FC, transl). *The history of ophthalmology*. vol. 8. Bonn: Wayenborgh; 1987:273–277.
23. Oriel JD. Eminent venereologists 4: Jonathan Hutchinson. *Genitourin Med*. 1990;66:401–406.
24. Ellis H. Jonathan Hutchinson (1828–1913). *J Med Biogr*. 1993;1:11–16.
25. Ferry AP. Ophthalmology and Vanity Fair. *Ophthalmology*. 1993;100: 429–437.
26. Hutchinson J. On the means of recognising the subjects of inherited syphilis in adult life. *Br Med J*. 1858;1:822–823.
27. Hutchinson J. *A clinical memoir on certain diseases of the eye and ear, consequent on inherited syphilis*. London: John Churchill; 1863.
28. Fournier A. *La syphilis héréditaire tardive: Leçons professées*. Paris: G Masson; 1886:63–65, 187–219.
29. Bull CS. A contribution to the study of inherited syphilis of the eye. *Am J Med Sci*. 1877;74:66–74.
30. Lees DB, Barlow T. On lesions of the cranial bones in congenital syphilis. *Trans Pathol Soc Lond*. 1879;30:350–355.
31. Parinaud H. Kératite interstitielle et la syphilis héréditaire. *Arch Gén Méd*. 1883;11:521–524.
32. Evans TC. The ocular manifestations of hereditary syphilis revised. Presented at the Western Ophthalmological, Otological, Laryngological and Rhinological Association, Kansas City, MO, 1896.
33. Marshall CD. On interstitial keratitis and its complications. *Ann Ophthalmol*. 1897;6:479–490.
34. Morton AS. A peculiar form of interstitial keratitis in secondary syphilis. *Roy Lond Ophthalmic Hosp Rep*. 1876;9:50–53.
35. Wilder WH. Corneal lesions in acquired syphilis. *JAMA*. 1901;37: 1669–1671.
36. Stephenson S. The corneal lesions of acquired syphilis. *Ophthalmoscope*. 1903;1:169–173.
37. Carpenter JT. Diffuse interstitial keratitis in acquired syphilis. *Ann Ophthalmol*. 1908;17:617–628.
38. Hutchinson J. *Syphilis*. 2nd ed. London: Cassell; 1913:237–238.
39. Dennie CC. *A history of syphilis*. Springfield, IL: Charles C Thomas; 1962:76.
40. Pariser H. Acquired syphilitic interstitial keratitis: with a report of two cases. *Am J Syph Gonorrhea Vener Dis*. 1939;23:214–219.
41. Leber A. Serodiagnostische Untersuchungen bei Syphilis und Tuberkulose des Auges. *Albrecht von Graefe's Arch Ophthalmol*. 1910;73:1–69.
42. Marshall J, Seiler HE. A statistical analysis of 3,219 persons certified blind at the Regional Clinic for the Certification of the Blind, Glasgow and south-west Scotland, during the period 1929–1935. *Br J Ophthalmol*. 1942;26:339–466.
43. Sidler-Huguenin E. Über die hereditär-syphilitischen Augenhintergrundsveränderungen, nebst einigen allemeinen Bemerkungen über Augenerkrankungen bei angeborener Lues. *Zeitschr Augenheilkd*. 1904; 51:1–256.
44. Igersheimer J. Die Keratitis parenchymatosa eine echtluetische Erkrankung. *Dtsch Med Wochenschr*. 1910;36:938–939.
45. Merté H-J. Die Auffassung von der Pathogenese der Keratitis parenchymatosa im wandel der zeiten. *Hist Ophthalmol Int*. 1979;1:31–47.
46. Alexander L. *Neue Erfahrungen über luetische Augenerkrankungen*. Wiesbaden: JF Bergmann; 1895.
47. Terrien F. *Syphilis de l'oeil et de ses annexes*. Paris: G Steinheil; 1905.
48. Igersheimer J. *Syphilis und Auge*. Berlin: Julius Springer; 1918:183–270.
49. Rosica A. *La cheratiti parenchimatose*. Chieti: Rizzi; 1923.
50. Schofield CB. My choice: Cortisone in the treatment of syphilitic eye disease. *Sex Transm Infect*. 2000;76(Suppl 1):S13–S14.
51. Anderson CR, Wilson WA. Active interstitial keratitis of late prenatal syphilis: its treatment. *Calif West Med*. 1939;50:196–199.
52. Duke-Elder S, Leigh AG. Diseases of the outer eye. In: Duke-Elder S, ed. *System of ophthalmology*. vol. 8, part 2. London: Henry Kimpton; 1965:815–832.
53. Ehrlich P, Hata S. *Die experimentelle Chemotherapie der Spirillosen*. Berlin: Julius Springer; 1910:58–81.
54. Clapp CA. Interstitial keratitis. A review of some of the ideas advanced in the past decade. *Arch Ophthalmol*. 1929;2:580–587.
55. Cole HN, Usilton LF, Moore JE. Late prenatal syphilis, with special reference to interstitial keratitis: its prevention and treatment. *Arch Dermatol Syph*. 1937;35:563–579.
56. Klauder JV, VanDoren E. Interstitial keratitis: analysis of five hundred and thirty-two cases with particular reference to standardization of treatment. *Arch Ophthalmol*. 1941;26:408–429.
57. vom Hofe K. Verhindert die Behandlung einer kongenitalen Lues den Ausbruch einer Keratitis parenchymatosa? Zugleich ein Beitrag zur Frage Keratitis parenchymatosa und Trauma. *Klin Monatsbl Augenheilkd*. 1933;90:492–494.
58. Weber G, Falk U. Katamnese einer mit Ehrlich 606 behandelten Lues connata tarda. *Hautarzt*. 1971;22:521–523.
59. Lawford JB. Discussion on the treatment of syphilitic eye affections by the newer methods. *Trans Ophthalmol Soc UK*. 1916;36:10–62.
60. Weve H. Zur Therapie der Keratitis parenchymatosa luetica. *Arch Augenheilkd*. 1929;100–101:833–852.
61. Klauder JV, Robertson HF. The treatment for interstitial keratitis. *Arch Ophthalmol*. 1931;6:134–135.
62. Oriel JD. *The scars of Venus. A history of venereology*. London: Springer-Verlag; 1994:59–70.
63. Atkinson WS. Interstitial keratitis treated with subconjunctival injections of penicillin. *Arch Ophthalmol*. 1945;34:233.
64. Yampolsky J, Heyman A. Penicillin in the treatment of syphilis in children. *JAMA*. 1946;132:368–371.
65. Klauder JV. Treatment of interstitial keratitis. With particular reference to results of penicillin therapy. *Am J Syph Gonorrhea Vener Dis*. 1947; 31:576–599.
66. Rasmussen DH. The treatment of syphilis. *Surv Ophthalmol*. 1969;14: 184–197.
67. Geddes AK, McCall MF. Interstitial keratitis treated with cortisone. *Can Med Assoc J*. 1950;63:601.
68. Steffensen EH, Olson JA, Margulis RR, et al. The experimental use of cortisone in inflammatory eye disease. *Am J Ophthalmol*. 1950;33:1033–1040.
69. Horne GO. Topical cortisone in treatment of syphilitic ocular disease. *Br Med J*. 1951;1:1289–1291.
70. Simpson WG, Rosenblum BF, Wood CE, et al. Local cortisone acetate therapy in congenital syphilitic interstitial keratitis. A preliminary report. *J Vener Dis Inform*. 1951;32:116–119.
71. Duke-Elder S. A series of cases treated locally by cortisone. A preliminary report to the Medical Research Council by the Panel on Ophthalmological Applications of Cortisone and ACTH. *Br J Ophthalmol*. 1951;35: 672–694.
72. North DP. The treatment of interstitial keratitis. *Br Med J*. 1954;2:7–9.
73. Crane GW Jr, McPherson SD Jr. The effect of local cortisone in the treatment of syphilitic interstitial keratitis. *Am J Syph Gonorrhea Vener Dis*. 1951;35:525–531.
74. Drews LC, Barton GD, Mikkelsen WM. The treatment of acute interstitial keratitis with topical cortisone. *Am J Ophthalmol*. 1953;36:90–103.
75. Oksala A. Interstitial keratitis: its treatment by mydriatics and its recurrence. *Am J Ophthalmol*. 1957;44:217–221.
76. Sédan J. La récidive dans la kératite interstitielle considerée dans ses rapports avec la cortisonothérapie; d'après 146 observations recueillies de 1926 à 1950 et 24 observations recueillies de 1950 à 1956. *Bull Mém Soc Fr Ophtalmol*. 1957;70:138–153.
77. Lohlein W. *Zeitfrogen der Augenhelikunde*. Stuttgart: Enke; 1938:405.
78. Ascher KW. Zur Keratoplastikfrage. Bericht über 49 in den Jahren 1908 bis 1917 ausgeführte Hornhautpfropfungen. *Albrecht von Graefe's Arch Ophthalmol*. 1919;99:339–369.

79. Sourdille GP. Kératites de Hutchinson et kératoplasties: greffes perforantes ou greffes lamellaires? *Ann Oculist*. 1950;183:495–499.
80. Paton RT. *Keratoplasty*. New York: McGraw-Hill; 1955:77–78, 229, 250–254.
81. Ainslie D. A survey of one hundred penetrating corneal grafts. *Trans Ophthalmol Soc UK*. 1959;79:209–220.
82. Elschnig A. Keratoplasty. *Arch Ophthalmol*. 1930;4:165–173.
83. Stansbury FC. Corneal transplantation. I. Visual and cosmetic results. *Arch Ophthalmol*. 1949;42:813–844.
84. Venca L, Rosso L. L'évolution post-opérative des greffes de la cornée dans les kératites parenchymateuses syphilitiques. *Ann Oculist*. 1948;181: 199–212.
85. Owens WC, Frank JJ, Leahey B. Results. *Am J Ophthalmol*. 1948;31: 1394–1399.
86. Brooks AMV, Weiner JM. Indications for penetrating keratoplasty: a clinicopathologic review of 511 corneal specimens. *Aust NZ J Ophthalmol*. 1987;15:277–281.
87. Léger F, Vital C, Négrier M-LM, et al. Histologic findings in a series of 1,540 corneal allografts. *Ann Pathol*. 2001;21:6–14.
88. Spicer WTH. Parenchymatous keratitis: interstitial keratitis: uveitis anterior. *Br J Ophthalmol*. 1924;8(Suppl):1–63.
89. Adamantiadis B. Kératite pustuliforme profonde et les diverses formes de la kératite parenchymateuse syphilitique acquise. *Ann Oculist*. 1935;172:304–311.
90. Parran T. *Shadow on the land: syphilis*. New York: Reynal & Hitchcock; 1937.
91. Fournier A. *Traité de la syphilis*. Paris: Rueff; 1899.
92. Green J Jr. The eye in hereditary syphilis. *Am J Dis Child*. 1920;20: 29–54.
93. Lemoine AN. Ocular manifestations of congenital syphilis and treatment by induced hyperpyrexia. *Trans Am Ophthalmol Soc*. 1934;32: 522–554.
94. Dunlop EMC, Zwink FB. Incidence of corneal changes in congenital syphilis. *Br J Vener Dis*. 1954;30:201–209.
95. Alexander L. *Syphilis und Auge: nach eigenen Beobachtungen*. Wiesbaden: JF Bergmann; 1889:38–47, 207–226.
96. de Schweinitz GE. Ophthalmology in the United States. In: Ireland MW, ed. *The Medical Department of the United States Army in the World War*. vol. 11. part 2. Washington, DC: US Government Printing Office; 1924:555–561.
97. Derby GS, Walker CB. Interstitial keratitis of luetic origin. *Trans Am Ophthalmol Soc*. 1913;13:317–339.
98. Carvill M, Derby GS. Interstitial keratitis. *Boston Med Surg J*. 1925; 193:403–412.
99. Guy WH. Interstitial keratitis in congenital syphilis. Clinical notes on incidence and treatment. *JAMA*. 1926;87:1551–1555.
100. Harman BN. Causes and prevention of blindness. *Am J Ophthalmol*. 1921;4:824–834.
101. Savvaitov AS. [Blindness in the Union of Soviet Socialist Republics]. *Vestn Oftalmol*. 1932;1:291–303.
102. Palich-Szántó O. Über die avaskuläre Form der Keratitis parenchymatosa. *Klin Monatsbl Augenheilkd*. 1959;135:719–724.
103. Oksala A. Studies on interstitial keratitis associated with congenital syphilis occurring in Finland. *Acta Ophthalmol*. 1952;30:1–30.
104. Graham TN, Romaine HH, Rulison RH. Syphilitic interstitial keratitis. Report of 103 cases. *NY State J Med*. 1948;48:1916–1919.
105. Klauder JV. Appreciation of Wassermann in relation to ocular syphilis. *Arch Dermatol Syph*. 1956;73:464–468.
106. Collins ET. On the children of patients who have had interstitial keratitis. *R Lond Ophthalmic Hosp Rep*. 1903;15:206–214.
107. Haldimann C. Über Keratitis parenchymatosa bei Lues congenita der zweiten Generation. *Zeitschr Augenheilkd*. 1937;91:183.
108. Bonugli FS. Third-generation syphilis and bilateral interstitial keratitis occurring in all surviving members of 2 generations. *Br J Vener Dis*. 1954;30:24–27.
109. Rutherford HW. Two cases of third generation syphilis. *Br J Vener Dis*. 1965;41:142–146.
110. Tamesis RR, Foster CS. Ocular syphilis. *Ophthalmology*. 1990;97:1281–1287.
111. Wilhelmus KR, Lukehart SA. Syphilis. In: Pepose JS, Holland GN, Wilhelmus KR, eds. *Ocular infection and immunity*. St Louis: Mosby; 1996:1437–1466.
112. Robinson HM. Interstitial keratitis in late congenital syphilis. *South Med J*. 1932;25:956–960.
113. Robinson RCV. Congenital syphilis. *Arch Dermatol*. 1969;99:599–610.
114. Fiumara NJ, Lessell S. Manifestations of late congenital syphilis. An analysis of 271 patients. *Arch Dermatol*. 1970;102:78–83.
115. Peterson JC. Congenital syphilis: a review of its present status and significance in pediatrics. *South Med J*. 1973;66:78–83.
116. Fiumara NJ, Lessell S. The stigmata of late congenital syphilis: an analysis of 100 patients. *Sex Transm Dis*. 1983;10:126–129.
117. Schmid GP, Stoner BP, Hawkes S. The need and plan for global elimination of congenital syphilis. *Sex Transm Dis*. 2007;34(Suppl):S5–S10.
118. Harden AF, Wright DJM. Clinical aspects of treponemal eye disease. A report of 21 cases. *Proc Roy Soc Med*. 1975;67:817–819.
119. Wilhelmus KR. Prospective evaluation of ocular syphilis in a general ophthalmology clinic. *Invest Ophthalmol Vis Sci*. 1989;30(Suppl):449.
120. Schwartz GS, Harrison AR, Holland EJ. Etiology of immune stromal (interstitial) keratitis. *Cornea*. 1998;17:278–281.
121. Matoba AY, Wilhelmus KR, Jones DB. Etiology of nonsuppurative stromal keratitis. Presented at the American Academy of Ophthalmology, Atlanta, GA, 2008.
122. Hariprasad SM, Moon SJ, Allen RC, et al. Keratopathy from congenital syphilis. *Cornea*. 2002;21:608–609.
123. Shafii T, Radolf JD, Sánchez PJ, et al. Congenital syphilis. In: Holmes KK, Sparling PF, Stamm WE, et al. eds. *Sexually transmitted diseases*. 4th ed. New York: McGraw-Hill; 2008:1577–1612.
124. Saloojee H, Velaphi S, Goga Y, et al. The prevention and management of congenital syphilis: an overview and recommendations. *Bull WHO*. 2004;82:424–430.
125. Ravin LC. Interstitial keratitis as a sign of congenital syphilis: report of two cases. *Ohio State Med J*. 1942;38:760–762.
126. Nabarro D. *Congenital syphilis*. London: Edward Arnold; 1954:329–348.
127. Rossochowitz W. Vorkommen und klinisches Bild der Keratitis parenchymatosa e lue congenita im Wandel der letzen 50 Jahre. *Klin Monatsbl Augenheilkd*. 1964;48:611–619.
128. Devlin PJ. A case of interstitial keratitis at an early age. *Br J Ophthalmol*. 1945;29:155–156.
129. Clausen W. Ätiologische, experimentelle und therapeutische Beiträge zur Kenntnis der Keratitis interstitialis. *Albrecht von Graefe's Arch Ophthalmol*. 1912;83:399–504.
130. Herzau W, Hossman E. Ueber Keratitis parenchymatosa. *Klin Monatsbl Augenheilkd*. 1932;88:467–477.
131. Sherman ES. Interstitial keratitis. *J Med Soc NJ*. 1947;30:591–595.
132. Power H. Relation of ophthalmic disease to certain normal and pathological conditions of the sexual organs. *Trans Ophthalmol Soc UK*. 1888;8:1–39.
133. Klauder JV. Blindness due to syphilis. *J Vener Dis Inform*. 1951;32: 183–192.
134. Mohr T. Beobachtungen über Keratitis parenchymatosa nach Trauma. *Klin Monatsbl Augenheilkd*. 1910;48:611–619.
135. Voisin J, Pouliquen Y. Kératite interstitielle hérédo-syphilitique et traumatisme. *Bull Soc Ophtalmol Fr*. 1957;57:415–418.
136. Barkan H. Luetic interstitial keratitis of traumatic origin. *Trans Am Ophthalmol Soc*. 1926;24:363–384.
137. De Courcy TL. Interstitial keratitis and the Workman's Compensation Act. *Trans Ophthalmol Soc UK*. 1930;50:556–564.
138. Klauder JV. Ocular syphilis: interstitial keratitis and trauma; clinical experimental and medicolegal aspects. *Arch Ophthalmol*. 1933;10: 302–328.
139. Schulman F. Seltene Zwischenfälle nach Elliots Trepanation, zugleich Beitrag zur Frage Keratitis parenchymatosa und Trauma. *Klin Monatsbl Augenheilkd*. 1934;92:522–530.
140. Larsen V. Kératite syphilitique déclanchée par opération. *Acta Ophthalmol*. 1947;25:195–199.
141. Bonamour G. Kératite interstitielle hérédo-spécifique apparue au cours d'une réaction d'Herxheimer déclenchée par un traitement pénicilliné. *Bull Soc Ophtalmol Fr*. 1952;52:99–100.
142. Braley AE. Ocular allergies. *Trans Am Acad Ophthalmol Otolaryngol*. 1958;62:826–834.
143. Inman WS. Emotional factors in diseases of the cornea. *Br J Med Psychol*. 1965;38:277–287.
144. Kip KE, Cohen F, Cole SR, et al. Recall bias in a prospective cohort study of acute time-varying exposures: example from the Herpetic Eye Disease Study. *J Clin Epidemiol*. 2001;54:482–487.
145. Papastathopoulos J. Syphilitic corneal gumma. *Bull Hellen Soc Ophthalmol*. 1960;28:95–97.
146. Rice NSC, Jones BR, Wilkinson AE. Study of late ocular syphilis. Demonstration of treponemes in aqueous humour and cerebrospinal fluid. I. Ocular findings. *Trans Ophthalmol Soc UK*. 1968;88:257–273.
147. Schöninger L. Ueber einen Fall von Keratitis interstitialis punctata bei Lues acquisita und Idiosynkrasie gegen Neosalvarsan. *Klin Monatsbl Augenheilkd*. 1924;73:467–470.
148. Vossius A. Zur Begründung der Keratitis parenchymatosa annularis. *Albrecht von Graefe's Arch Ophthalmol*. 1905;60:116–117.
149. Fuchs A. Über einige seltene luetische Erkrangkungen des Auges. I. Keratitis linearis migrans. *Zeitschr Augenheilkd*. 1926;58:315–321.

150. Wright MH. Keratitis linearis migrans. *Br J Ophthalmol.* 1963;47:504–507.
151. Coop DH. Interstitial linear keratitis. *Br J Ophthalmol.* 1968;52:910–911.
152. Ehlers H. On the formation of precipitates in profound keratitis. *Acta Ophthalmol.* 1927;4:226–236.
153. Woillez M, Dalmas G, Doise O. La gomme de la cornée, forme rare de kératite interstitielle. *Bull Soc Ophtalmol Fr.* 1954;54:636–638.
154. Offret G, Campinchi R. Un aspect classique mais un peu oublié de kératite syphilitique: la kératite pustuliforme postérieure. *Bull Soc Ophtalmol Fr.* 1959;59:51–55.
155. von Hippel E. Über Keratitis parenchymatosa und Ulcus internum corneae. *Albrecht von Graefe's Arch Ophthalmol.* 1908;68:354–380.
156. Terson A. Gummatie of the cornea. *Ann Ophthalmol.* 1906;15:424–427.
157. Suganuma S. Ueber die Pathogenese der Sklero-perikeratitis progressiva. *Klin Monatsbl Augenheilkd.* 1940;105:702–707.
158. Gilbert W. Zur Klinik und Pathologie der angeborenen Augensyphilis. *Arch Augenheilkd.* 1920;87:59–74.
159. Schnyder WF. Untersuchungen des normalen und pathologischen Endothels der Hornhaut mittels der Nernstspaltlampe. *Klin Monatsbl Augenheilkd.* 1920;65:783–812.
160. von Hippel E. Ueber Keratitis parenchymatosa. *Albrecht von Graefe's Arch Ophthalmol.* 1893;39:204–228.
161. Cook C, Langham M. Corneal thickness in interstitial keratitis. *Br J Ophthalmol.* 1953;37:301–304.
162. Granström KO. Die Keratitis parenchymatosa in Späterem alter. *Acta Ophthalmol.* 1934;12:122–136.
163. Stephenson S. A note upon the pseudo-neoplastic form of interstitial keratitis. *Br J Ophthalmol.* 1917;1:754–756.
164. Davidescu G. Hereditary syphilitic parenchymatous keratitis with an unusual beginning. *Spitalul.* 1947;60:1–2.
165. Bonnet P, Bonnet I. Kératite interstitielle à manifestations abnormales. *Bull Soc Ophtalmol Fr.* 1953;53:376–379.
166. Bryn A. Ein Beitrag zur Kenntnis der keratitis punctata syphilitica. *Klin Monatsbl Augenheilkd.* 1927;78:89–92.
167. Ling WP. Interstitial keratitis with unusually marked chorioretinitis. Pathologic–anatomic examination of a case. *Arch Ophthalmol.* 1929;1:207–218.
168. Oksala A. Interstitial keratitis and chorioretinitis. *Acta Ophthalmol.* 1952;30:427–441.
169. Bonnet P, Moreau PG. Kératite interstitielle hérédo-syphilitique et périphlébite de la rétine. *Bull Soc Ophtalmol Fr.* 1951;51:651–652.
170. Campinchi R. Ré post-opératoire de kératite interstitielle avec apparition de périphlébite rétinienne. *Bull Soc Ophtalmol Fr.* 1965;65:183–185.
171. Friedenwald J. Ocular lesions in fetal syphilis. *Trans Am Ophthalmol Soc.* 1929;27:203–218.
172. Schmidt-Rimpler H. *Augenheilkunde und Ophthalmoskopie, für Aerzte und Studirende.* 7th ed. Leipzig: Hirzel; 1901:413.
173. Juhasz-Schäffer A. Ueber einen Fall von Keratitis parenchymatosa avasculosa des einen Auges auf Grundlage einer kongenitalen Lues. *Klin Monatsbl Augenheilkd.* 1938;101:576–579.
174. Remler O. Zur Frage der Einseitigkeit der Keratitis parenchymatosa. *Klin Monatsbl Augenheilkd.* 1952;121:602–609.
175. Kakisu Y. Statistical and epidemiological studies of ocular syphilis. *Acta Soc Ophthalmol Jpn.* 1958;62:2481–2519.
176. Collier M. Récidive unilatérale atypique d'une kératite interstitielle hérédo-syphilitique avasculaire à hypopion. Papillite bilatérale subaiguë choroïdite périphérique cicatricielle. *Bull Soc Ophtalmol Fr.* 1959;4:289–294.
177. Sédan J. Sur la récidive des kératites interstitielles. *Bull Soc Ophtalmol Fr.* 1966;66:432–435.
178. Dalsgaard-Nielsen E. On 'recurrence' of syphilitic interstitial keratitis. *Acta Ophthalmol.* 1939;17:38–42.
179. MacFarlane WV. Progressive blindness due to posterior uveitis following antisyphilitic treatment for interstitial keratitis. *Br J Vener Dis.* 1957;33:165–167.
180. Lazarescu D. Faits résultant de 349 observations de kératite héré. *Arch Ophtalmol.* 1936;53:756–762.
181. Delcourt B, De Laey JP, Dernouchamps JP, et al. Un cas de séquelles oculaires et orbito-faciales de syphilis congénitale. *Bull Soc Belge Ophtalmol.* 1979;184:99–107.
182. Zákoutská H. Syfilis v naši době: démonzace pohlavních nemocí přispívá k jejich šíření. *Vesmír.* 1998;77:506–509.
183. Bradlaw LV. The dental stigmata of prenatal syphilis. *Oral Surg Oral Med Oral Pathol.* 1953;6:147–158.
184. Lawson BJ. Hutchinson's teeth. *Oral Surg Oral Med Oral Pathol.* 1967;24:635–636.
185. Herschfeld JJ. Classics in dental history: Sir Jonathan Hutchinson, the universal specialist: his studies of syphilitic changes in the mouth. *Bull Hist Dent.* 1988;36:34–38.
186. Dalsgaard-Nielsen E. Correlation between syphilitic interstitial keratitis and deafness. *Acta Ophthalmol.* 1938;16:635–647.
187. Takechi K, Sekiguchi K, Goto S. A case of keratitis, ichthyosis, and deafness syndrome with Hutchinson's triad-like symptoms. *Nippon Ganka Gakkai Zasshi.* 1999;103:322–326.
188. Gleich LL, Urbina M, Pincus RL. Asymptomatic congenital syphilis and auditory brainstem response. *Int J Pediatr Otorhinolaryngol.* 1994;30:11–13.
189. Keyes EL. *Syphilis: a treatise for practitioners.* New York: D Appleton; 1908:533.
190. Indesteege F, Verstraete WL. Menière's disease as a late manifestation of congenital syphilis. *Acta Otorhinolaryngol Belg.* 1989;43:327–333.
191. Mimura T, Amano S, Nagahara M, et al. Corneal endotheliitis and idiopathic sudden sensorineural hearing loss. *Am J Ophthalmol.* 2002;133:699–700.
192. Rodger TR. Aural syphilis. *Br J Vener Dis.* 1945;21:115–123.
193. Clutton HH: Symmetrical synovitis of the knee in hereditary syphilis. *Lancet.* 1886;1:391–393. (Reprinted in *Clin Orthop Relat Res* 1968; 57:5–8).
194. Klauder JV, Robertson HF. Symmetrical serous synovitis (Clutton's joints): congenital syphilis and keratitis. *JAMA.* 1934;103:236–240.
195. Thompson RG, Berry CZ. Symmetrical serous synovitis. *US Armed Forces Med J.* 1951;2:1723–1727.
196. Borella L, Goobar JE, Clark GM. Synovitis of the knee joints in late congenital syphilis. Clutton's joints. *JAMA.* 1962;180:190–192.
197. Prech A. De la valeur de l'examen oculaire pour le diagnostic de certaines manifestations de l'hérédo-syphilis. *Bull Mem Soc Fr Ophtalmol.* 1901;21:389–391.
198. Kopp I, Solomon HC. Interstitial keratitis in patients with neurosyphilis of congenital origin, with a discussion of fever as a precipitating factor of keratitis in the paretic variety. *Am J Syph Gonorrhea Vener Dis.* 1939;23:751–758.
199. Probst LE, Wilkinson J, Nichols BD. Diagnosis of congenital syphilis in adults presenting with interstitial keratitis. *Can J Ophthalmol.* 1994;29:77–80.
200. Platou RV. Treatment of congenital syphilis with penicillin. *Adv Pediatr.* 1949;4:39–86.
201. Lesser RL. Spirochetal diseases. In: Miller NR, Newman NJ, eds. *Walsh and Hoyt's clinical neuro-ophthalmology.* 6th ed. vol. 3. Baltimore: Williams & Wilkins; 2005:3077–3114.
202. Luhr AF. Oculomotor palsy with parenchymatous keratitis. *Am J Ophthalmol.* 1924;7:293.
203. Smith JL. Testing for congenital syphilis in interstitial keratitis. *Am J Ophthalmol.* 1971;72:816–820.
204. Lister A. Interstitial keratitis with associated syphilitic penile lesions. *Trans Ophthalmol Soc UK.* 1948;68:288–290.
205. Trematore M. La cheratite parenchimatosa nella silfilide acquisita. *Ross Ital Ottalmol.* 1938;7:520–534.
206. Collins ET. Primary chancre of the conjunctiva and interstitial keratitis. *Roy Lond Ophthalmic Hosp Rep.* 1904;16:16–19.
207. Bonnet J-L. Kératite interstitielle de la syphilis acquise. *Bull Soc Ophtalmol Fr.* 1950;50:499–500.
208. Desbordes P, Biot J. Un cas de syphilis acquise revelée par une kératite unilatérale. *Med Trop.* 1968;28:230–232.
209. Lawford JB. Interstitial keratitis in acquired syphilis. *Trans Ophthalmol Soc UK* 1900;20:67–73.
210. Audéoud-Naville A. Un cas de kératite pustuliforme profunde. *Acta Ophthalmol.* 1935;52:289–300.
211. Wilhelmus KR, Jones DB. Adult-onset syphilitic stromal keratitis. *Am J Ophthalmol.* 2006;141:319–321.
212. Moore JE. Syphilitic iritis. A study of 249 patients. *Am J Ophthalmol.* 1931;14:110–126.
213. Enroth E. Ein Fall von Luetischer Hypopyonkeratitis. *Acta Ophthalmol.* 1927;4:271–273.
214. Shimanovich AN, Platnitskala VS, Khazina BN, et al. [Parenchymatous keratitis in acquired syphilils]. *Vestn Dermatol Venerol.* 1962;36:67–68.
215. Baumert OH. Zur Kenntnis der Keratitis punctata profunda Mauthner. *Klin Monatsbl Augenheilkd.* 1927;79:782–785.
216. Weill G. La kératite ponctuée syphilitique. *Bull Soc Ophtalmol Paris.* 1927;27:332–335.
217. Martinez JA, Sutphin JE. Syphilitic interstitial keratitis masquerading as staphylococcal marginal keratitis. *Am J Ophthalmol.* 1989;107:431–433.
218. Klien BA. Acute metastatic syphilitic corneal abscess. A clinical and histopathologic study. *Arch Ophthalmol.* 1935;14:612–617.
219. Schneider R. Zur Keratitis pustuliformis profunda. *Klin Monatsbl Augenheilkd.* 1922;69:238–241.

220. Bryn A. Ein Beitrag zur Kenntnis des akuten metastatisch syphilitischen Hornhautabszesses. *Klin Monatsbl Augenheilkd.* 1924;73:680–689.
221. Bielschowsky A. Über eine ungewohnliche Form von syphilitscher Hornhautaffektion. *Ber Dtsch Ophthalmol Ges Heidelberg.* 1908;35: 323–325.
222. Granström KO. A case of keratitis pustuliformis profunda. *Acta Ophthalmol.* 1929;7:330–336.
223. Schaefer F. Über einen Fall von Keratitis pustuliformis profunda mit Blutung in die Vorderkammer im Anschluss an eine Neosalvarsaninjektion im Sinne der Jarisch-Herxheimerschen Reaktion. *Arch Augenheilkd.* 1932;106:559–566.
224. Bonnet P, Paufique L, Bonamour G. Gomme syphilitique de la cornée avec hypopyon. *Bull Soc Ophtalmol Paris.* 1933;33:690–693.
225. Uhthoff W. Ein Fall van grosser syphilitischer (gummöser) Ulceration der Cornea, Conjunktiva und Sklera. *Ber Dtsch Ophthalmol Ges Heidelberg.* 1907;34:266–269.
226. Kraupa E. Das spätsyphilitische Hornhautinfiltrat. *Ophthalmologica.* 1950;119:225–226.
227. Wilhelmus KR, Yokoyama CM. Syphilitic episcleritis and scleritis. *Am J Ophthalmol.* 1987;104:595–597.
228. Baughn RE, Musher DM. Secondary syphilitic lesions. *Clin Microbiol Rev.* 2005;18:205–216.
229. Duke-Elder S. Diseases of the outer eye. In: Duke-Elder S, ed. *System of ophthalmology.* vol. 8. part 1. London: Henry Kimpton; 1965:236–243.
230. LeGuillas L, Couloma P, vanVarseveld F. Kératite interstitielle et phénomènes arthropériostiques au cours de la syphilis acquise secondaire. *Arch Ophtalmol.* 1939;3:231–235.
231. Swartz MN, Healy BP, Musher DM. Late syphilis. In: Holmes KK, Sparling PF, Mårdh P-A, et al. eds. *Sexually transmitted diseases.* 3rd ed. New York: McGraw-Hill; 1999:487–509.
232. Sparling PF, Swartz MN, Musher DM, et al. Clinical manifestations of syphilis. In: Holmes KK, Sparling PF, Stamm WE, et al. eds. *Sexually transmitted diseases.* 4th ed. New York: McGraw-Hill; 2008: 661–684.
233. Cursiefen C, Maruyama K, Jackson DG, et al. Time course of angiogenesis and lymphangiogenesis after brief corneal inflammation. *Cornea.* 2006;25:443–447.
234. Hoehne H. Ueber Keratitis parenchymatosa. *Klin Monatsbl Augenheilkd.* 1940;105:656–693.
235. Luyckx-Bacus J, Delmarcelle Y. Recherches biométriques sur des yeux présentant une microcornée ou une megalocornée. *Bull Soc Belge Ophtalmol.* 1968;149:433–437.
236. Hill JC, Maske R, Bowen RM. Secondary localized amyloidosis of the cornea associated with tertiary syphilis. *Cornea.* 1990;9:98–101.
237. Dutt S, Elner VM, Soong HK, et al. Secondary localized amyloidosis in interstitial keratitis. Clinicopathologic findings. *Ophthalmology.* 1992; 99:817–823.
238. Mihara E, Miyata H, Inoue Y, et al. Application of energy-dispersive X-ray microanalysis on the diagnosis of atypical calcific band keratopathy. *Okajimas Folia Anat Jpn.* 2005;82:19–24.
239. Alexander L. *Über die neuroparalytische Hornhaut-Entzündung (bie Syphilis),* Wiesbaden: JF Bergmann; 1880.
240. Kim RY, Cosper KL, Kelly LD. Predictive factors for response to medical therapy in bacterial ulcerative keratitis. *Albrecht von Graefe's Arch Ophthalmol.* 1996;234:731–738.
241. Terson A. Kératite syphilitique ulcérée. *Presse Méd.* 1928;36:1179–1180.
242. Uchiyama K, Tsuchihara K, Horimoto T, et al. Phthisis bulbi caused by late congenital syphilis untreated until adulthood. *Am J Ophthalmol.* 2005;139:545–547.
243. Lee ME, Lindquist TD. Syphilitic interstitial keratitis. *JAMA.* 1989;262:2921.
244. Bonnet P. Les opacités cornéennes 'en feurille de palmier' reliquots de la kératite interstitielle (type annulaire de Vossier). *Arch Ophtalmol.* 1935;52:625–655.
245. Klauder JV, Cowan A. Corneal examination and slit lamp microscopy in diagnosis of late congenital syphilis, especially in adults. *JAMA.* 1939;113:1624–1627.
246. Brooks AMV, Grant G, Gillies WE. Differentiation of posterior polymorphous dystrophy from other posterior corneal opacities by specular microscopy. *Ophthalmology.* 1989;96:1639–1645.
247. Côté MA, Gaster RN. Keratohematoma leading to acquired posterior keratoconus. *Cornea.* 1994;13:534–538.
248. Giessler S, Gross M, Struck HG. Spontane Hämatocornea nach Keratitis verschiedener Genese. *Klin Monatsbl Augenheilkd.* 1997;211:65–67.
249. Waring GO III. Posterior collagenous layer of the cornea. Ultrastructural classification of abnormal collagenous tissue posterior to Descemet's membrane in 30 cases. *Arch Ophthalmol.* 1982;100:122–134.
250. Stähli J. Ueber persistente retrokorneale Glashautleisten in ehedem parenchymatosakranken Augen. *Klin Monatsbl Augenheilkd.* 1919;63: 336–349.
251. Kawaguchi R, Saika S, Wakayama M, et al. Extracellular matrix components in a case of retrocorneal membrane associated with syphilitic interstitial keratitis. *Cornea.* 2001;20:100–103.
252. Lehmann H. Beitrage zur Kenntnis der Glasleistenbildung an der Hornhauthinleifläche bei abfelaufener Keratitis parenchymatosa. *Zeitschr Augenheilkd.* 1927;62:230–245.
253. Dalsgaard-Nielsen E. On the acuity of vision and the causes of impairment of vision in patients with past syphilitic interstitial keratitis. *Acta Ophthalmol.* 1939;17:43–58.
254. Weill G, Jost A. Sur un räseau de trabecules retrocornäens consäcutif à une kératite parenchymateuse hérédospécifique. *Ann Oculist.* 1926; 163:100–114.
255. Balavoine C. Les formations hyalines rétro-cornéennes acquises. *Ann Oculist.* 1953;186:111–140.
256. Swartz J. Retrocorneal hyaline bands in interstitial keratitis. *Br J Ophthalmol.* 1953;37:374–375.
257. Pearson PA, Amrien JM, Baldwin LB, et al. Iridoschisis associated with syphilitic interstitial keratitis. *Am J Ophthalmol.* 1989;107:88–90.
258. Foss AJE, Hykin PG, Benjamin L. Interstitial keratitis and iridoschisis in congenital syphilis. *J Clin Neuroophthalmol.* 1992;12:167–170.
259. Salvador F, Linares F, Merita I, et al. Unilateral iridoschisis associated with syphilitic interstitial keratitis and glaucoma. *Ann Ophthalmol.* 1993;25:328–329.
260. Ruusuvaara P, Setala K, Kivela T. Syphilitic interstitial keratitis with bilateral funnel-shaped iridocorneal adhesions. A case report. *Eur J Ophthalmol.* 1996;61:6–10.
261. Tamotsu H, Tada T, Hara A. [A case of syphilitic keratitis and retinopathy]. *Nippon Ika Daigaku Zasshi.* 1994;61:503–505.
262. Rosa D. Le alterazioni del vitreo nella cheratite parenchimatosa. *Arch Ottalmol.* 1950;54:42–56.
263. Knox DL. Glaucoma following syphilitic interstitial keratitis. *Arch Ophthalmol.* 1961;66:18–25.
264. Britten MJA, Palmer CAL. Glaucoma and inactive syphilitic interstitial keratitis. *Br J Ophthalmol.* 1964;48:181–190.
265. Kraupa E. Das Spätglaukom nach Keratitis parenchymatosa. *Zeitschr Augenheilkd.* 1934;84:43–51.
266. Oksala A. The chamber angle in interstitial keratitis. *Am J Ophthalmol.* 1957;43:719–723.
267. Sugar HS. Late glaucoma associated with inactive syphilitic interstitial keratitis. *Am J Ophthalmol.* 1962;53:602–605.
268. Lichter PR, Schaffer RN. Interstitial keratitis and glaucoma. *Am J Ophthalmol.* 1969;68:241–248.
269. Grant WM. Late glaucoma after interstitial keratitis. *Am J Ophthalmol.* 1975;79:87–91.
270. Tsukahara S. Secondary glaucoma due to inactive congenital syphilitic interstitial keratitis. *Ophthalmologica.* 1977;174:188–194.
271. Brooks AMV, Weiner JM, Robertson IF. Interstitial keratitis in untreated latent (late) syphilis. *Aust NZ J Ophthalmol.* 1986:14:127–132.
272. Akabane N, Hamanaka T, Yamaguchi T, et al. Peripheral anterior synechia of congenital syphilis. *Invest Ophthalmol Vis Sci.* 1995;36(4): S84.
273. Rosen E. Embryonal cataract associated with interstitial keratitis and syphilitic choroiditis. *Arch Ophthalmol.* 1949;42:749–754.
274. Hardy JB, Hardy PH, Oppenheimer EH, et al. Failure of penicillin in a newborn with congenital syphilis. *JAMA.* 1970;212:1345–1349.
275. Contreras F, Pedera J. Congenital syphilis of the eye with lens involvement. *Arch Ophthalmol.* 1978;96:1052–1053.
276. Schlimpert H. Pathologisch-anatomische befunde an den augen bie zwei fällen von lues congenita. *Dtsch Med Wochenschr.* 1906;32:1942–1945.
277. Thiel H-J, Harms D. Pathologisch-anatomische Augenbefunde bei fötaler Lues. *Klin Monatsbl Augenheilkd.* 1969;154:712–716.
278. Spektor FE, Eagle RC Jr, Nichols CW. Granulomatous conjunctivitis secondary to *Treponema pallidum. Ophthalmology.* 1981;88:863–865.
279. Schneider R. Zur Keratitis pustuliformis profunda. *Wien Klin Wochenschr.* 1952;64:949.
280. Goldman JN, Girard KF. Intraocular treponemes in treated congenital syphilis. *Arch Ophthalmol.* 1967;78:47–50.
281. Christman EH, Hamilton RW, Heaton CL, et al. Intraocular treponemes. *Arch Ophthalmol.* 1968;80:303–307.
282. Rios-Montenegro EN, Israel CW, Nicol WG, et al. Histopathologic demonstration of spirochetes in the human eye. *Am J Ophthalmol.* 1969; 67:335–346.
283. Weskamp C. Histopathology of interstitial keratitis due to congenital syphilis. *Am J Ophthalmol.* 1949;32:793–806.
284. Elschnig A. Ueber Keratitis parenchymatosa. *Klin Monatsbl Augenheilkd.* 1905;43:168–170.

285. Elschnig A. Über Keratitis parenchymatosa. *Albrecht von Graefe's Arch Ophthalmol.* 1906;62:481–546.
286. Watanabe B. Pathologisch-anatomischer Befund bei Keratitis parenchymatosa syphilitica congenita mit besonderer Berückfläche der Hornhaut. *Klin Monatsbl Augenheilkd.* 1914;52:408–416.
287. Kunze FE. Anatomische Untersuchung eines Falles von Keratitis parenchymatosa e lue hereditaria. *Albrecht von Graefe's Arch Ophthalmol.* 1920;102:205–228.
288. Igersheimer J. Anatomischer Befund einer Keratitis pustuliformus profunda (Fuchs). *Albrecht von Graefe's Arch Ophthalmol.* 1930;123:468–475.
289. Löwenstein A. Tierversuche zur Frage der Entstehung der Keratitis parenchymatosa. *Klin Monatsbl Augenheilkd.* 1927;78:73–89.
290. Edmonds C, Iwamoto T. Electron microscopy of late interstitial keratitis. *Ann Ophthalmol.* 1972;4:693–696.
291. Braley AE. Pathology of the discs removed for corneal transplantation. *Trans Pa Acad Ophthalmol Otolaryngol.* 1962;15:61–74.
292. Ozaki N, Ishizaki M, Ghazizadeh M, et al. Apoptosis mediates decrease in cellularity during the regression of Arthus reaction in cornea. *Br J Ophthalmol.* 2001;85:613–618.
293. Wolter JR. Secondary cornea guttata. A late change in luetic interstitial keratopathy. *Am J Ophthalmol.* 1960;50:17–25.
294. Ikebe H, Takamatsu T, Itoi M, et al. Changes in nuclear DNA content and cell size of injured human corneal endothelium. *Exp Eye Res.* 1988;47:205–215.
295. Redslob E. Rédoublement et développement de la membrane de Descemet. *Bull Mém Soc Fr Ophtalmol.* 1933;46:216–229.
296. Günther JC. Ein Fall von ungewöhnlicher Verdickung der Descemetschen Membran. *Klin Monatsbl Augenheilkd.* 1962;141:740–743.
297. Nakamura A, Takahashi T, Inoue M, et al. Histopathological study of the retrocorneal hyaline network. *Folia Ophthalmol Jpn.* 1981;32:1603–1606.
298. Renard G, Dhermy P, Pouliquen Y. Dystrophies endothélio-descémétiques secondaires. Etude histologique et ultrastructurale. *J Fr Ophtalmol.* 1981;4:721–739.
299. Waring GO III, Font RL, Rodrigues MM, et al. Alterations of Descemet's membrane in interstitial keratitis. *Am J Ophthalmol.* 1976;81:773–785.
300. Ko MK, Kay EP. Differential interaction of molecular chaperones with procollagen I and type IV collagen in corneal endothelial cells. *Mol Vis.* 2002;8:1–9.
301. Lee JG, Kay EP. FGF-2-mediated signal transduction during endothelial mesenchymal transformation in corneal endothelial cells. *Exp Eye Res.* 2006;83:1309–1316.
302. Dogru M, Kato N, Matsumoto Y, et al. Immunohistochemistry and electron microscopy of retrocorneal scrolls in syphilitic interstitial keratitis. *Curr Eye Res.* 2007;32:863–870.
303. Kanai A, Kaufman HE. The retrocorneal ridge in syphilitic and herpetic interstitial keratitis: an electron-microscopic study. *Ann Ophthalmol.* 1982;14:120–124.
304. Kestenbaum A. Sagenannte Glasleisten nach Keratitis parenchymatosa. *Zeitschr Augenheilkd.* 1924;53:113–115.
305. Scattergood KD, Green WR, Hirst LW. Scrolls of Descemet's membrane in healed syphilitic interstitial keratitis. *Ophthalmology.* 1983;90:1518–1523.
306. Balavoine C. Un noveau cas de réseau hyalin retrocornéen. *Ophthalmologica.* 1951;121:76–79.
307. Stanculéano G. Steltener Befund an der Hinterfläche der Kornea bei einer klinisch diagnostizierten Keratitis parenchymatosa. *Klin Monatsbl Augenheilkd.* 1904;42:456–467.
308. McDannald CE. Twin child with interstitial keratitis. *Arch Ophthalmol.* 1919;48:523.
309. Igersheimer J. Zur Entstehung der luetischen Keratitis parenchymatosa. *Albrecht von Graefe's Arch Ophthalmol.* 1913;85:361–379.
310. Merté H-J. Experimentelle Untersuchungen über einige Probleme der Hornhautanaphylaxie. Ein Beitrag zur Klärung der Pathogenese der Keratitis parenchymatosa und zu deren Therapie. *Albrecht von Graefe's Arch Ophthalmol.* 1960;161:420–465.
311. Reis W. Beiträge zur Histopathologie der parenchymatösen Erkrankungen der Cornea. *Albrecht von Graefe's Arch Ophthalmol.* 1907;66:201–262.
312. Gilbert W. Keratitis parenchymatosa annularis. *Klin Monatsbl Augenheilkd.* 1910;48:460–468.
313. Jaeger E. Ein histologisch untersuchter Fall von Keratitis parenchymatosa. *Klin Monatsbl Augenheilkd.* 1925;74:488–497.
314. Manlinin I, Sharkovski I. [The clinical history and pathologic anatomy of parenchymatous keratitis]. *Vestn Oftalmol.* 1934;4:606–610.
315. Klauder JV. Clinical and experimental study of interstitial keratitis. *J Invest Dermatol.* 1939;2:157–173.
316. Friedman R. *A history of dermatology in Philadelphia.* Fort Pierce Beach: Froben; 1955:542–552.
317. Beerman H. Memoir of Joseph Victor Klauder (1888–1962). *Trans Stud Coll Phys Phila.* 1963;31:77–78.
318. Wessely K. Über anaphylaktische Erscheinungen an der Hornhaut (Experimentelle Erzeugung einer parenchymatösen Keratitis durch arfremdes Serum). *München Med Wschr.* 1911;58:1427.
319. von Szily A. Ueber die Bedeutung der Anaphylaxie in der Augenheilkunde. *Klin Monatsbl Augenheilkd.* 1913;51:164–181.
320. Sugahara M, Iwasaki Y, Inada N, et al. [Immunohistochemical study of interstitial keratitis in an animal model]. *Nippon Ganka Gakkai Zasshi.* 2000;104:779–785.
321. Schieck F. Das Problem der Genese der interstitiellen Keratitis. *Dtsch Med Wochenschr.* 1914;40:890–892.
322. Riehm W. Anaphylaxie und Keratitis parenchymatosa. *Klin Monatsbl Augenheilkd.* 1929;82:648–656.
323. Löwenstein A. Ueber das klinische Bild der ophthalmia anaphylactica nebst Bemerkungen zur Pathogenese der Keratitis parenchymatosa. *Klin Monatsbl Augenheilkd.* 1929;82:64–71.
324. Wessely K. Das Problem der Keratitis parenchymatosa. *München Med Wochenschr.* 1933;80:1673–1676.
325. Hackett CJ. Interstitial keratitis, boomerang legs and yaws in European boy from New Hebrides. *Med J Austr.* 1935;2:213–216.
326. Smith JL, David NJ, Indgin S, et al. Neuro-ophthalmological study of late yaws and pinta II. The Caracas Projects. *Br J Vener Dis.* 1971;47:226–251.
327. Zaidman GW, Wormser GP. Lyme keratitis. *Ophthalmol Clin North Am.* 1994;7:597–604.
328. Nataf R. Les complications oculaires de la fièvre récurrente. *Bull Mém Soc Fr Ophtalmol.* 1946;59:287–291.
329. Mancel E, Merien F, Pesenti L, et al. Clinical aspects of ocular leptospirosis in New Caledonia (South Pacific). *Aust N Z J Ophthalmol.* 1999;27:380–386.
330. Gupta A, Gulnar DP, Srinivasan R, et al. Bilateral acute keratouveitis in leptospirosis: a new entity. *Indian J Ophthalmol.* 2007;55:399.
331. Axenfeld KTPP. *Die Bakteriologie in der Augenheilkunde.* Jena: Gustav Fischer; 1907:357–359.
332. Nicol WG, Rios-Montenegro EN, Smith JL. Congenital ocular syphilis. *Am J Ophthalmol.* 68:467–471, 1969.
333. Radolf JD, Hazlett KRO, Lukehart SA. Pathogenesis of syphilis. In: Radolf JD, Lukehart SA, eds. *Pathogenic Trepenoma: molecular and cellular biology.* Norfolk: Caister Academic Press; 2006:197–236.
334. Schieck F. Kann die Keratitis parenchymatosa auf anaphylaktischen Zuständen beruhen? *Zeitschr Augenheilkd.* 1914;32:95–100.
335. Riehm W. Die Pathogenese der Keratitis parenchymatosa im lichte der Allergieforschung. *Klin Monatsbl Augenheilkd.* 1952;120:50–60.
336. Woods AC, Chesney AM. Relation of the eye to immunity in syphilis, with special reference to the pathogenesis of interstitial keratitis. *Am J Ophthalmol.* 1946;29:389–401.
337. Rios-Montenegro EN, Nicol WG, Smith JL. Treponemalike forms and artifacts. *Am J Ophthalmol.* 1969;68:196–205.
338. Ryan SJ, Nell EE, Hardy PH. A study of aqueous humor for the presence of spirochetes. *Am J Ophthalmol.* 1972;73:250–257.
339. Smith JL. *Spirochetes in late seronegative syphilis, penicillin notwithstanding.* Springfield, IL: Charles C Thomas; 1969:252–260.
340. Sowmini CN. Clinical progression of ocular syphilis and neurosyphilis despite treatment with massive doses of penicillin. Failure to demonstrate treponemes in affected tissues. *Br J Vener Dis.* 1971;47:348–355.
341. Grüter W. Eperimentelle und klinische Beiträge zum Problem der parenchymatösen Keratitis. *Ber Dtsch Ophthalmol Ges Heidelberg.* 1949;55:48–59.
342. Alvarado JA, Underwood J, Green WR, et al. Detection of herpes simplex viral DNA in the iridocorneal endothelial syndrome. *Arch Ophthalmol.* 1994;112:1601–1609.
343. Wicher V, Wicher K. Pathogenesis of maternal-fetal syphilis revisited. *Clin Infect Dis.* 2001;33:354–363.
344. Baughn RE, Jiang A, Abraham R, et al. Molecular mimicry between an immunodominant amino acid motif on the 47-kDa lipoprotein of *Treponema pallidum* (Tpp47) and multiple repeats of analogous sequences in fibronectin. *J Immunol.* 1996;157:720–731.
345. Lunardi C, Bason C, Leandri M, et al. Autoantibodies to inner ear and endothelial antigens in Cogan's syndrome. *Lancet.* 2002;360:915–921.
346. Parma AE, Santisteban CG, Villalba JS, et al. Experimental demonstration of an antigenic relationship between *Leptospira* and equine cornea. *Vet Immunol Immunopathol.* 1985;10:215–224.
347. Parma AE, Fernandez AS, Santisteban CG, et al. Tears and aqueous humor from horses inoculated with *Leptospira* contain antibodies which bind to cornea. *Vet Immunol Immunopathol.* 1987;14:181–185.

348. Parma AE, Sanz ME, Lucchesi PM, et al. Detection of an antigenic protein of *Leptospira interrogans* which shares epitopes with the equine cornea and lens. *Vet J.* 1997;153:75–79.
349. Lucchesi PM, Parma AE. A DNA fragment of *Leptospira interrogans* encodes a protein which shares epitopes with equine cornea. *Vet Immunol Immunopathol.* 1999;71:173–179.
350. Lucchesi PM, Parma AE, Arroyo GH. Serovar distribution of a DNA sequence involved in the antigenic relationship between *Leptospira* and equine cornea. *BMC Microbiol.* 2002;2:3–7.
351. Wada S, Yoshinari M, Katayama Y, et al. Nonulcerative keratouveitis as a manifestation of leptospiral infection in a horse. *Vet Ophthalmol.* 2003;6:191–195.
352. Merchant TE, Lass JH, Roat MI, et al. P-31 NMR analysis of phospholipids from cultured human corneal epithelial, fibroblast and endothelial cells. *Curr Eye Res.* 1990;9:1167–1176.
353. Sachedina S, Greiner JV, Glonek T. Membrane phospholipids of the ocular tunica fibrosa. *Invest Ophthalmol Vis Sci.* 1991;32:625–632.
354. Orsoni JG, Zavota L, Manzotti F, et al. Syphilitic interstitial keratitis: treatment with immunosuppressive drug combination therapy. *Cornea.* 2004;23:530–532.
355. Mendel F. Ueber einen Fall von Keratitis diffusa e lue acquisita. *Centralbl Prakt Augenheilkd.* 1901;25:10–13.
356. Wiesel J, Rose DN, Silver AL, et al. Lumbar puncture in asymptomatic late syphilis. An analysis of the benefits and risks. *Arch Intern Med.* 1985;145:465–468.
357. Michelow IC, Wendel GD Jr, Norgard MV, et al. Central nervous system infection in congenital syphilis. *N Engl J Med.* 2002;346:1792–1798.
358. Benton CD Jr, Heyman A. Treatment of ocular syphilis with penicillin. *Arch Ophthalmol.* 1948;40:302–310.
359. Moore JE. *Penicillin in syphilis.* Springfield, IL: Charles C Thomas; 1946:196–202.
360. Dunlop EMC. Survival of treponemes after treatment: comments, clinical conclusions, and recommendations. *Genitourin Med.* 1985;61:293–301.
361. Workowski KA, Berman SM. Sexually transmitted diseases treatment guidelines, 2006. *MMWR Recomm Rep.* 2006;55:1–94.
362. Dalsgaard-Nielsen E. On disablement and social conditions of patients with past syphilitic interstitial keratitis. *Br J Ophthalmol.* 1939; 23:544–556.
363. Leonhardt V-A. Jarisch-Herxheimersche oder allergische Reaktion am Auge nach Penicillinverabreichung. *Klin Monatsbl Augenheilkd.* 1952; 121:292–297.
364. Assinder EW. Syphilis in ophthalmology. *Br J Ophthalmol.* 1942;26: 1–23.
365. Carvill M. Interstitial keratitis. Further report. *JAMA.* 1931;96:1936–1938.
366. Freeman JDJ. A case of bilateral interstitial keratitis leading to blindness. *Br J Ophthalmol.* 1943;27:104–106.
367. Woods AC. Syphilis of the eye. *Am J Syph Gonorrhea Vener Dis.* 1943;27:133–186.
368. LeMond RF. Syphilitic amblyopia. *Am J Ophthalmol.* 1897;2:301–336.
369. Ashworth AN. Results of local cortisone therapy in syphilitic interstitial keratitis. *Br J Vener Dis.* 1958;34:83–90.
370. Woods AC. Cortisone in interstitial keratitis. *Am J Syph Gonorrhea Vener Dis.* 1958;35:517–524.
371. Dinis da Gama R, Cidade M. Interstitial keratitis as the initial expression of syphilitic reactivation. *N Engl J Med.* 2002;346:1799.
372. Horne GO. Topical cortisone in syphilitic interstitial keratitis. *Br J Vener Dis.* 1955;31:9–24.
373. Gordon DM. *The clinical use of corticotropin, cortisone and hydrocortisone in eye disease.* Springfield, IL: Charles C Thomas; 1954:25.
374. Miserocchi E, Modorati G, Rama P. Effective treatment with topical cyclosporine of a child with steroid-dependent interstitial keratitis. *Eur J Ophthalmol.* 2008;18:816–818.
375. Arentsen JJ, Morgan B, Green WR. Changing indications for keratoplasty. *Am J Ophthalmol.* 1976;81:313–318.
376. Smith RE, McDonald HR, Nesburn AB, et al. Penetrating keratoplasty: changing indications, 1947 to 1978. *Arch Ophthalmol.* 1980;98:1226–1229.
377. Robin JB, Gindi JJ, Koh K, et al. An update of the indications for penetrating keratoplasty: 1979 through 1983. *Arch Ophthalmol.* 1986; 104:87–89.
378. Mohamadi P, McDonnell JM, Irvine JA, et al. Changing indications for penetrating keratoplasty, 1984–1988. *Am J Ophthalmol.* 1989;107:550–552.
379. Flowers CW, Chang KY, McLeod SD, et al. Changing indications for penetrating keratoplasty, 1989–1993. *Cornea.* 1995;14:583–588.
379a. Ghosheh FR, Cremona FR, Rapuano CJ, et al. Trends in penetrating keratoplasty in the United States 1980–2005. *Int Ophthalmol.* 2008;28: 147–153.
380. Al-Yousuf N, Mavrikakis I, Mavrikakis E, et al. Penetrating keratoplasty: indications over a 10 year period. *Br J Ophthalmol.* 2004;88:998–1001.
381. Mannis MJ, Holland EJ, Beck RW, et al. Clinical profile and early surgical complications in the Cornea Donor Study. *Cornea.* 2006;25:164–170.
382. Eye Bank Association of America. *Eye banking statistical report.* Washington, DC: EBAA; 2002:13.
383. Williams KA, Hornsby NB, Bartlett CM, et al. *Australian Corneal Graft Registry 2000 Report.* Adelaide: Snap Printing; 2001:81, 100.
384. Maeno A, Naor J, Lee HM, et al. Three decades of corneal transplantation: indications and patient characteristics. *Cornea.* 2000;19:7–11.
385. Dorrepaal SJ, Cao KY, Slomovic AR. Indications for penetrating keratoplasty in a tertiary referral centre in Canada, 1996–2004. *Can J Ophthalmol.* 2007;42:244–250.
386. Legeais J-M, Parc C, d'Hermies F, et al. Nineteen years of penetrating keratoplasty in the Hotel-Dieu Hospital in Paris. *Cornea.* 2001;20: 603–606.
387. Lang GK, Wilk CM, Nauman GOH. Wandlungen in der Indikationsstellung zur Keratoplastik (Erlangen, 1964–1986). *Fortschr Ophthalmol.* 1988;85:255–258.
388. Kervick GN, Shepherd WFI. Changing indications for penetrating keratoplasty. *Ophthalmic Surg.* 1990;21:227.
389. Collum LMT, Mullaney J, McDermott MA, et al. A comparative analysis over a decade of the changing indications for penetrating keratoplasty in Ireland. *Ir J Med Sci.* 1987;156:262–264.
390. *Medical Advisory Board Minutes.* Washington, DC: Eye Bank Association of America; 2002.
391. Sampaio R, Held E, Cohen EJ, et al. Binocular vision recovery in bilateral keratoplasty. *Cornea.* 2001;20:471–474.
392. Rabb MF, Fine M. Penetrating keratoplasty in interstitial keratitis. *Am J Ophthalmol.* 1969;67:907–917.
393. Lagoutte F, Dupuy P. L'association kératite interstitielle/cataracte sénile. Ses particularités cliniques et chirugicales. A propos de 10 cas. *Bull Soc Ophtalmol Fr.* 1982;82:723–724.
394. Meyer RF, Musch DC. Assessment of success and complications of triple procedure surgery. *Am J Ophthalmol.* 1987;104:233–240.
395. Pedersen OO. Combined corneal transplantation, extracapsular cataract extraction, and artificial lens implantation (triple procedure). *Acta Ophthalmol.* 1987;65(Suppl 182):83–86.
396. Kurz GH, D'Amico RA. Retained Descemet's membrane after keratoplasty for old interstitial keratitis. *Am J Ophthalmol.* 1973;16:51–53.
397. Barraquer J, Rutlán J. *Microsurgery of the cornea: an atlas and textbook.* Barcelona: Ediciones Scriba; 1984:68–69.
398. Goldman JN, Kenneth MD, Girard F. Causes de l'opacité après greffe de cornée dans la kératite interstitielle. *Bull Mém Soc Fr Ophtalmol.* 1967; 80:126–131.
399. Goegebuer A, Ajay L, Claerhout I, et al. Results of penetrating keratoplasty in syphilitic interstitial keratitis. *Bull Soc Belge Ophtalmol.* 2003;35–39.
400. Claerhout I, Kestelyn P. Résultats obtenus par kératoplastie transfixiante dans le cas d'une kératite syphilitique interstitielle. *Rev Belge Med Dent.* 2004;59:34–42.
401. Rapuano CJ, Cohen EJ, Brady SE, et al. Indications for and outcomes of repeat penetrating keratoplasty. *Am J Ophthalmol.* 1990;109:689–695.
402. Southwick KL, Guidry HM, Weldon MM, et al. An epidemic of congenital syphilis in Jefferson County, Texas, 1994–1995: inadequate prenatal syphilis testing after an outbreak in adults. *Am J Publ Health.* 1999;89:557–560.
403. Mobley JA, McKeown RE, Jackson KL, et al. Risk factors for congenital syphilis in infants of women with syphilis in South Carolina. *Am J Publ Health.* 1998;88:597–602.
404. Hollier LM, Hill J, Sheffield JS, et al. State laws regarding prenatal syphilis screening in the United States. *Am J Obstet Gynecol.* 2003;189: 1178–1183.
405. Terris-Prestholt F, Watson-Jones D, Mugeye K, et al. Is antenatal syphilis screening still cost effective in sub-Saharan Africa. *Sex Transm Infect.* 2003;79:375–381.
406. Putkonen T. Does early treatment prevent dental changes in congenital syphilis? *Acta Dermatol Venereol.* 1963;43:240–249.
407. Bernfeld WK. Hutchinson's teeth and early treatment of congenital syphilis. *Br J Vener Dis.* 1971;47:54–56.
408. Ingraham NR Jr. The value of penicillin alone in the prevention and treatment of congenital syphilis. *Acta Dermatol Venereol.* 1951;31(Suppl 24):60–88.

409. Robinson RCV. Syphilitic keratitis after 5 years of seronegativity (following penicillin therapy). *Am J Syphil Gonorrhea Vener Dis*. 1952;36: 92–83.
410. Azimi PH. Interstitial keratitis in a five-year-old. *Pediatr Infect Dis J*. 1999;18:299–311.
411. Oksala A. Interstitial keratitis after adequate penicillin therapy: a case report. *Br J Vener Dis*. 1957;33:113–114.
412. Ullmo A. Kératite parenchymateuse à répétition chez une syphilis congénitale de 2e génération. *Bull Soc Fr Dermatol Syphilig*. 1968;75: 645–656.
413. Arens C. Ein Fall von Keratitis parenchymatosa e Lue connata. *Klin Monatsbl Augenheilkd*. 1981;178:375–376.
414. Ignat F, Davidescu L. Cheratita parenchimatosa sifilitica. *Oftalmologia*. 1997;41:209–212.
415. Rompalo AM. Can syphilis be eradicated from the world? *Curr Opin Infect Dis*. 2001;14:41–44.

Chapter 86

Nonsyphilitic Interstitial Keratitis

Roxana Ursea, Matthew T. Feng, Janine A. Smith

Interstitial keratitis (IK) is a nonsuppurative inflammation characterized by cellular infiltration and vascularization of the corneal stroma with minimal primary involvement of the corneal epithelium or endothelium. Congenital syphilis is classically associated with IK. However, the disorder has a multitude of causes. The disease process can be caused by direct invasion of microorganisms or by an immune response against exogenous or endogenous antigens within the corneal stroma. IK is a clinical manifestation of both infectious and noninfectious diseases; the most common disorders associated with IK are listed in Box 86.1. Syphilitic IK is discussed in Chapter 85. This chapter will discuss nonsyphilitic causes of IK, focusing on Cogan's syndrome.

Cogan's Syndrome

Background

Mogan and Baumgartner first described a patient with Menière's syndrome and IK in 1931.[1] David G. Cogan reported four patients with IK with vestibuloauditory symptoms in 1945 and was the first to differentiate this syndrome from congenital syphilis.[2] He reported an additional four patients with nonsyphilitic IK and vestibuloauditory symptoms in 1949.[3] Since that time, over 200 cases of nonsyphilitic IK and vestibuloauditory dysfunction, now termed Cogan's syndrome, have been reported in the literature.[4–21] Nevertheless, the disease is rare and large case series are rarely reported. One notable exception is a series of 60 patients seen at the Mayo clinic beginning in 1940.[22]

Typical Cogan's syndrome is strictly defined as nonsyphilitic, noninfectious IK associated with vestibuloauditory disease manifested by a sudden, usually bilateral onset of tinnitus, sensorineural hearing loss, vertigo, nausea, and vomiting similar to Menière's disease. However, it is unlikely that Cogan's syndrome represents a single disease. Cases of atypical Cogan's syndrome, where ocular inflammatory disease other than IK is associated with vestibuloauditory disease, have been described.[7] In addition, Cogan's syndrome has been associated with a number of underlying systemic vasculitides such as polyarteritis nodosa,[9,13,23–34] Wegener's granulomatosis,[11,23,35] and rheumatoid arthritis.[36–38] Cogan's syndrome, in its classic description, probably represents the clinical manifestations of an immune response against antigens present in both the corneal stroma and inner ear. This disease process can involve ocular structures in addition to the cornea, such as the choroid (atypical Cogan's syndrome), or cause a systemic vasculitic disease such as polyarteritis nodosa. We prefer a broad definition of Cogan's syndrome to include any presumed immune disorder leading to IK and vestibuloauditory disease, since a common pathophysiology and need for immunosuppressive therapy is shared by all these disorders.

Epidemiology

There are no estimates of prevalence or incidence for this rare syndrome. To date, three-quarters of patients are distributed between ages 14 and 47, with the average age of onset being approximately 30 years.[4] The full range, however, encompasses both pediatric and geriatric populations.[4,39–41] While reported mostly in whites, clear evidence of racial predilection is lacking. Females slightly outnumber males.[4] Cogan's syndrome is not believed to have hereditary transmission.

Clinical manifestations

Approximately half of patients with Cogan's syndrome present with typical and/or atypical ocular symptoms, one-third with vestibuloauditory symptoms, and the remainder with both.[15,42] Patients may also describe a history of fever, headache, bloody diarrhea, anthralgia, myalgia, or preceding upper respiratory infection. Untreated, 75% will experience combined ocular and vestibuloauditory symptoms by 5 months. The subsequent natural history of disease includes vision loss secondary to corneal scarring and permanent hearing loss in 60–80% of patients.

A nonsyphilitic IK is the predominant ocular feature of typical Cogan's syndrome, often accompanied by iritis or subconjunctival hemorrhage. The IK usually has a sudden onset and a more gradual resolution with frequent recurrence over the course of the disease. The IK can be unilateral or bilateral and is often associated with decreased vision, severe eye pain or irritation, lacrimation, and photophobia. Acute signs consist of a patchy infiltration of the midstroma (Fig. 86.1). Corneal neovascularization (Fig. 86.2) from the limbus is common and produces salmon patches, but occurs later in the course of the disease. Late findings include

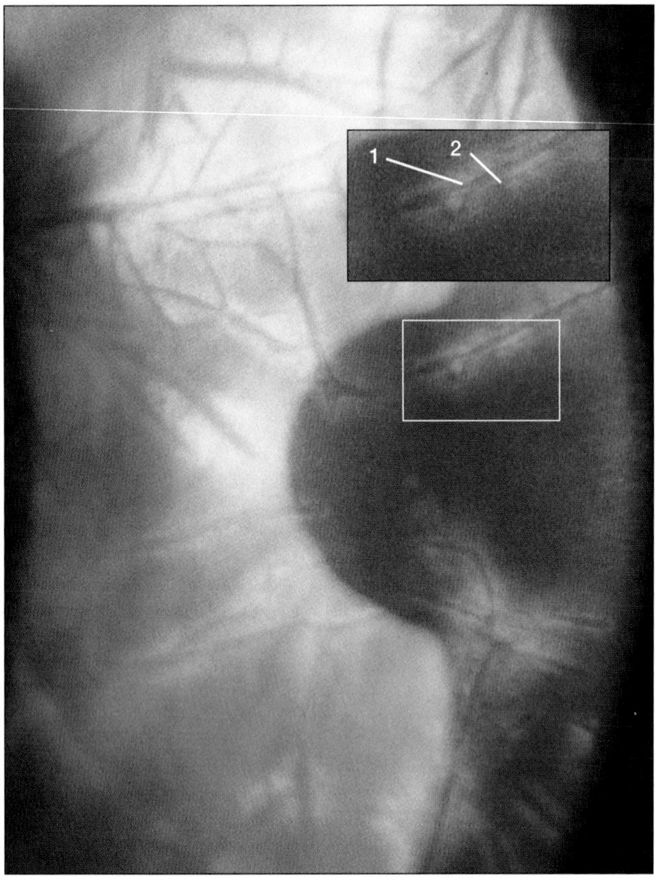

Fig. 86.1 Slit lamp photograph of the cornea with broad oblique illumination shows interstitial keratitis in a patient with Cogan's syndrome. Stromal scarring (*1*) with ghost vessels (*2*) outlined in relief can be seen in the inset. (Courtesy of Muriel I. Kaiser-Kupfer, MD, National Eye Institute.)

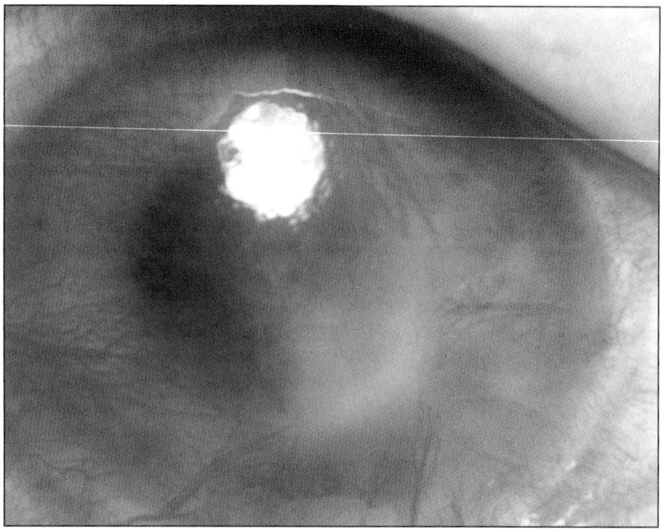

Fig. 86.2 Slit lamp photograph of the cornea in a patient with a long history of Cogan's syndrome shows extensive corneal inflammation with extensive neovascularization and cellular infiltration of the stroma. (Courtesy of David G. Cogan, MD, National Eye Institute.)

Box 86.1 Causes of interstitial keratitis

Bacterial infection	**Parasitic infection**
Syphilis	Leishmaniasis
Tuberculosis	Onchocerciasis
Leprosy	Trypanosomiasis
Lyme disease	*Acanthamoeba* keratitis
Brucellosis	Microsporidiosis
Trachoma	
Viral infection	**Systemic disease**
Herpes simplex virus	Cogan's syndrome
Herpes zoster virus	Sarcoidosis
Epstein-Barr virus	Lymphoma
Mumps	
Rubeola	
HTLV-1	

stromal scarring and ghost vessels. Earlier in the course of the disease, the IK may involve the anterior stroma of the cornea and may be misdiagnosed as a viral keratitis.[43]

Vestibuloauditory dysfunction is also characteristic of typical Cogan's syndrome. Patients complain of nausea and vomiting associated with acute tinnitus, vertigo, and a progressive bilateral loss of hearing. These symptoms may precede the eye disease in some patients, but usually occur no later than 1 to 6 months after the onset of ocular symptoms.[15] The hearing loss was present in almost all the reported cases of Cogan's syndrome and can progress to total deafness within 3 months in untreated patients.

Patients with vestibuloauditory dysfunction and ocular inflammatory disease other than IK and iritis are categorized as atypical Cogan's syndrome. Atypical forms of Cogan's syndrome comprise about 30% of reported cases.[44] Ocular findings in atypical Cogan's syndrome include conjunctivitis, other keratitis, scleritis, episcleritis, posterior uveitis, vitritis, papillitis, disk edema, retinal hemorrhage, retinal artery occlusion, tenonitis, orbital inflammation, and exophthalmos.[4]

As many as 50% of patients with atypical Cogan's syndrome have systemic findings of underlying rheumatologic diseases. Findings of Cogan's syndrome have been associated with a number of rheumatologic diseases, including polyarteritis nodosa, Wegener's granulomatosis, rheumatoid arthritis, Crohn's disease, and relapsing polychondritis.[15,23,37,45,46] Findings of atypical Cogan's syndrome can also be seen in patients with sarcoidosis and Vogt-Koyanagi-Harada's disease.[47] Systemic vasculitis is also associated with 15–20% of Cogan's syndrome, chiefly involving medium and large-sized vessels, most seriously aortitis.[4] Norton and Cogan described a patient with rheumatic fever and aortic insufficiency who later developed typical Cogan's syndrome.[48] Aortic insufficiency has subsequently been noted in patients with both typical and atypical Cogan's syndrome.[14,19,49–52] Gilbert and Talbot described a patient with

Cogan's syndrome with signs of periarteritis nodosa cerebral sinus thrombosis.[13] In fact, some authors have classified Cogan's syndrome among the vasculitides.[4,53] The recognition of underlying systemic vasculitis is important, since these patients require systemic immunosuppressive therapy.[44] Recently, there have also been isolated reports of association with pregnancy,[54] HIV,[55] and mastocytosis.[56]

Etiology and pathogenesis

The exact etiology of Cogan's syndrome remains unknown. Clinical and histologic findings currently favor an autoimmune mechanism against a common antigen in the cornea and inner ear. Majoor et al.[16] detected corneal antibodies in two Cogan's syndrome patients whose titers fell following high-dose corticosteroids. Helmchen et al.[57] analyzed the serum of five Cogan's syndrome patients for antibodies against corneal and inner ear tissue. Three patients demonstrated IgM, but not IgG, antibody against cornea. The serum of four patients intermittently contained low-titer IgG antibodies against inner ear labyrinthine tissue, but without clear correlation to disease activity. Lunardi et al.[58] subsequently analyzed the serum of eight Cogan's syndrome patients and identified IgG antibodies against CD148, a cell-surface marker on the sensory epithelia of the inner ear and on endothelial cells. Although CD148 is not found in the cornea, anti-CD148 IgG cross-reacted with connexin 26. Connexins 43 and 50, corneal gap junction proteins, show homology to connexin 26. In animal models, these antibodies induced hearing loss, corneal involvement, and pathology-proven vasculitis. Cogan's syndrome is often associated with systemic vasculitis, suggesting that the immune-mediated disease is widespread. Immune autoreactivity against widespread cell-surface markers such as CD148 is a plausible mechanism.

The trigger for this presumed immune response is also unknown. Because Cogan's syndrome is often preceded by an upper respiratory prodrome,[1] it is thought that infectious antigens may sensitize the patient's immune system through molecular mimicry against autoantigens found in the cornea, inner ear, and vasculature.[15] Anti-CD148 antibody targets a 12-residue peptide (SGRDTSIQILWI) with homology to reovirus type III core protein,[58] where reovirus causes mild rhinitis and pharyngitis. Additional homology to viral proteins has been reported,[59] including large tegument proteins, which have been separately implicated in mechanistic models of herpes virus IK via cross-reactivity of exogenous viral antigens with corneal autoantigens.[60] The behavior of IK in the context of viremia and immune recovery disease[61] supports this theory. Deposition of immune complexes and cryoglobulinemia have also been reported to play some role in the pathophysiology of the disorder.[15,62]

Histologic studies of the corneas of patients with Cogan's syndrome have demonstrated infiltration of the deep layers of the stroma with lymphocytes and plasma cells (Fig. 86.3),[47,63] supporting a cell-mediated reaction.[64,65] A similar inflammatory infiltrate was found in the conjunctiva of a patient with Cogan's syndrome.[15] Varying degrees of corneal neovascularization were also noted. Neovascularization may result partly via reduced expression of soluble fms-like tyrosine kinase, a VEGF binder in healthy human corneas, that has been reported in two IK corneas.[66] Pathologic studies

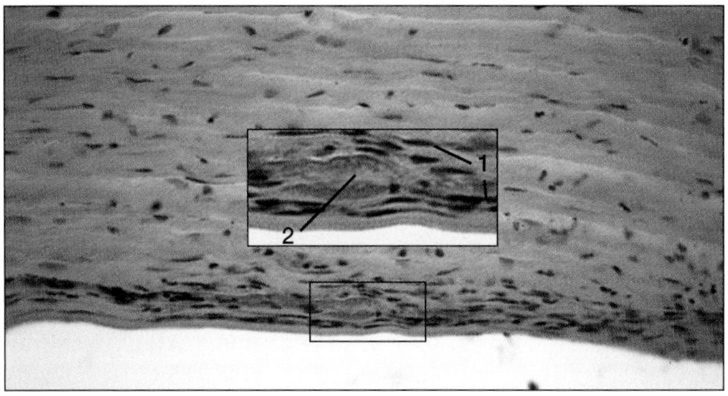

Fig. 86.3 Inset of histologic section of the cornea from a patient with Cogan's syndrome shows interstitial keratitis with infiltration of chronic inflammatory cells (*1*) into the deep stroma and an area of neovascularization (*2*) adjacent to Descemet's membrane. (Hematoxylin and eosin, original magnification ×400.) (Courtesy of David G. Cogan, MD, National Eye Institute.)

have also shown infiltration of the cochlea with plasma cells and lymphocytes in a patient with atypical Cogan's syndrome.[63] These reports suggest that the pathologic findings in Cogan's syndrome are caused by an underlying immune response and not by direct invasion by an infectious agent.

Differential diagnosis

Cogan's syndrome is diagnosed by clinical suspicion and exclusion. As such, key assessments include vestibular function and appropriate imaging and serologic testing. CBC with differential, ESR, CRP, creatinine, urinalysis, FTA-Abs or MHA-TP with RPR, EBV titer, Lyme panel, C3 and C4 levels, p-ANCA, c-ANCA, RF, ANA, and PPD with anergy panel should be considered, based on history and examination findings.[4] Congenital syphilis is the disease that can mimic Cogan's syndrome. Furthermore, it is the most important disease to diagnose correctly, since specific antibiotic therapy is often warranted. A number of factors differentiate congenital syphilis from Cogan's syndrome. IK in congenital syphilis has an insidious onset, a limbal distribution, and frequently causes corneal scarring. The IK of Cogan's syndrome develops suddenly, has a patchy distribution, and rarely causes progressive scarring, probably because of earlier diagnosis and treatment. Although both diseases lead to hearing loss, vestibulatory system dysfunction with vertigo, nausea, and vomiting are rarely found in congenital syphilis. Importantly, patients with congenital syphilis will have positive serologic tests for syphilis and systemic signs of the disease, such as skeletal and dental abnormalities.

A number of other infections are associated with the combination of IK and hearing loss. Chlamydial infection can cause inclusion conjunctivitis, IK, and hearing loss.[67–69] Tuberculosis is another infectious disease that can produce IK and hearing loss. But, like chlamydial infection, tuberculosis does not cause a Menière's-like syndrome of vestibular dysfunction. A number of viral infections, including rubeola, herpes zoster, and mumps, can lead to IK and hearing loss, but again, vestibulatory dysfunction is rare.[15,70,71] Finally, a host of rheumatologic disorders have been associated with IK and vestibulatory dysfunction. Whether these diseases should be considered as other diseases in the differential diagnosis of Cogan's syndrome or causes of the syndrome is debatable. The important point is always to evaluate patients with findings of Cogan's syndrome for an underlying rheumatologic disease that may warrant prompt immunosuppressive therapy.

Laboratory findings

Leukocytosis and a mild eosinophilia have been described in some patients with Cogan's syndrome.[15] Many have an elevated erythrocyte sedimentation rate (ESR), especially those with an active underlying systemic vasculitis. Most patients have normal complement levels and negative antinuclear antibodies. Char, Cogan, and Sullivan suggested a positive association of human leukocyte antigen (HLA) B17 and Cogan's syndrome,[72] which was later confirmed in a report by Del Carpio and colleagues.[73] However, others were unable to establish an association between HLA antigens and Cogan's syndrome.[74,75]

Treatment

In general, initial therapy for Cogan's syndrome consists of low-dose topical steroids for IK and high-dose systemic corticosteroids for inner ear disease. Prednisolone acetate 1% one drop per affected eye may be administered hourly to q.i.d. in tapering doses and is usually effective for both typical and atypical ocular inflammation. Deep ocular inflammation is an exception and, like vestibuloauditory symptoms, requires prompt systemic corticosteroids. Combination immunosuppression may be necessary for steroid-refractory or relapsing disease as described below. Concurrent treatment of systemic associations appears to facilitate the remission of Cogan's syndrome. If medical treatment fails, corneal transplant and cochlear impant can be considered for permanent corneal opacity and permanent deafness, respectively.

In a literature review, Haynes et al. noted that 77 of 81 untreated patients had moderate, severe, or profound hearing loss at 5 years.[15] In contrast, 10 of 18 patients treated with corticosteroids within 2 weeks of onset of hearing loss reported improvement in hearing acuity. Six of six patients demonstrated improved hearing thresholds for pure tones and suprathreshold speech discrimination results within 2 weeks after starting corticosteroid therapy.[76] At mean follow-up of 2.5 years, patients had only mild hearing impairment in the mid- and low-frequency ranges. No patient had severe hearing loss. Three patients were tapered off corticosteroids without further hearing loss. Patients are usually started on 1–2 mg/kg per day of prednisone for the first week and then slowly tapered, depending on the therapeutic response and development of adverse effects. Treatment courses of 2 to 6 months are common. Ocular symptoms of IK and iritis tend to be relatively mild and treated with topical corticosteroids and cycloplegic agents, and most patients maintain good visual acuity. Ocular and vestibuloauditory symptoms may respond to therapy incongruously, with the prognosis for IK usually better than for hearing.[16,77,78] In the only published case of Cogan's syndrome complicating pregnancy, IK resolved after 3 weeks on topical steroids alone.[54]

Prompt and prolonged immunosuppressive therapy is warranted for patients with Cogan's syndrome with an underlying active rheumatologic disease, especially if systemic vasculitis is present. In patients unresponsive to corticosteroids alone, other immunosuppressive agents such as ciclosporin A or cyclophosphamide have been used.[79,80] Recently, successful treatment of Cogan's syndrome with FK 506[81] or methotrexate[82] have been reported, including low-dose methotrexate safely in a child.[83] The efficacy of cytotoxic agents agrees with the view of Cogan's syndrome as a cell-mediated autoimmune disorder. Unfortunately, some cases associated with an underlying systemic vasculitis progress despite immunosuppressive therapy and lead to significant morbidity.[84]

Over the past decade, a number of more specific immunotherapies have become available. Antibodies against proinflammatory cytokines such as tumor necrosis factor-alpha (TNF-α) have been successfully used for the treatment of rheumatologic conditions. Etanercept, an antibody against TNF, was shown to be safe when combined with conventional treatment in Wegener's granulomatosis and a randomized trial of etanercept for this disease is in progress. Infliximab is another anti-TNF-α which can neutralize TNF-α in extracellular and transmembrane forms, like etanercept, as well as the receptor-bound form. Two cases of Cogan's syndrome refractory to combination steroid and cyclophosphamide therapy achieved remission on infliximab at 2 and 3 years.[77] Infliximab dosing was 300 mg every 1 to 3 months and permitted eventual discontinuation of corticosteroids. An antibody against the interleukin-2 receptor was useful in treating patients with uveitis secondary to a number of systemic conditions.[85] These new immunotherapies may be useful in treating immune-mediated ocular inflammatory diseases including Cogan's syndrome. However, clinical trials are needed to define the role of these new medications for this disease, since potentially serious side effects and exacerbation of vasculitis have been reported with the use of these agents.[86]

Nonsyphilitic Bacterial Infection

Mycobacterial infection

Although IK was first coined by Hutchinson in 1858 to describe a pattern of corneal inflammation characteristic of congenital syphilis, several other microorganisms can invade the cornea and elicit an identical response. IK is a well-recognized ocular manifestation of systemic acid-fast mycobacterial infection by tuberculosis (Fig. 86.4) or leprosy. Tuberculosis remains a significant infectious disease problem around the world and has recently reemerged as a public health concern in the United States. *Mycobacterium tuberculosis* enters the body primarily via inhalation. Macrophages deliver the bacilli to the lymphatic system, where they gain access to the bloodstream. Hematogenous spread to the eye can result in uveitis, particularly choroiditis; retinal vasculitis; conjunctivitis; scleritis; and keratitis.[87]

IK is usually associated with systemic tuberculosis, since primary ocular tuberculosis is exceedingly rare.[88] Nevertheless, IK is a rare finding even in patients with active pulmonary disease. Among 12 500 patients in three

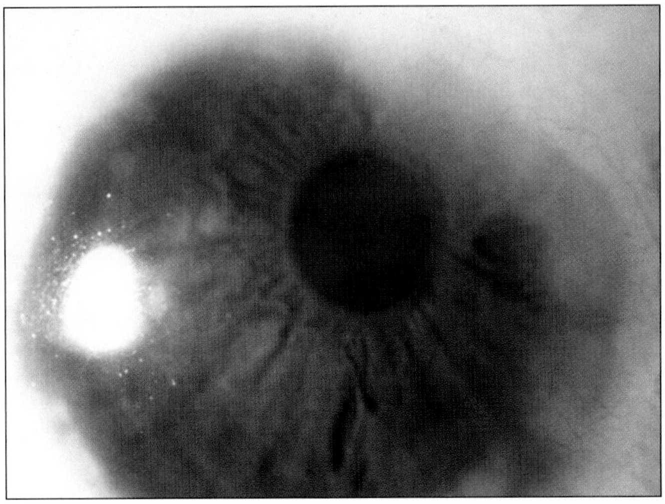

Fig. 86.4 Corneal photograph of a patient with interstitial keratitis associated with tuberculosis. Note characteristic sectoral, peripheral corneal involvement with stromal vascularization. (Courtesy of R. Christopher Walton, MD, Hamilton Eye Institute.)

pulmonary tuberculosis series, IK was found in 0.12%.[89–91] When it occurs, tuberculous IK is generally unilateral. Inflammation may involve either the anterior or posterior stroma, cellular infiltration is often peripheral or quadrantic and is followed by localized edema, and later stromal vascularization may occur with or without development of significant scarring or corneal thinning.[87] The natural course lasts weeks to months. Topical corticosteroids can hasten the resolution of active disease, supporting the theory that the IK results from a localized immune response to tuberculin antigens. Associated uveitis may be treated with topical cycloplegic agents. Treatment for the underlying tuberculosis is required: for example, with the initial regimen of isoniazid, rifampin, pyrazinamide, and streptomycin or ethambutol. These medications can have serious ocular and systemic side effects, so the risk-to-benefit ratio should be carefully considered when treating patients with ocular manifestations of tuberculosis infection, especially if there is no evidence of active systemic disease.[92] A single case report of unexpected improvement of bilateral tuberculous IK in a 21-year-old man on acitretin, a synthetic aromatic retinoid for psoriasis, may prompt further study of vitamin A derivatives for the treatment of corneal diseases.[93]

Mycobacterium leprae characteristically infects skin and peripheral nerves as an obligate intracellular organism, resulting in a spectrum of clinical disease. Lepromatous leprosy occurs secondary to defective cell-mediated immunity against the organism and is characterized by widespread dermal and neural disease and predominanat CD8+ lymphocyte involvement. In contrast, tuberculous leprosy is manifest primarily with nerve involvement and minimal skin disease. CD4+ lymphocytes are observed in typical granuloma formations. These mycobacteria accumulate in cooler tissues such as the cornea, typically in the lepromatous or multibacillary form of disease. In 61 patients with Hansen's disease, ocular findings included punctate epithelial keratopathy (28%), corneal hypoesthesia (16%), corneal pannus (10%), corneal nerve involvement (7%), focal avascular keratitis (5%), and IK (3%).[94] There was no association between these findings and disease stage or classification. In contrast to tuberculous IK, corneal involvement in leprosy is generally bilateral, and the presence of bacilli throughout the stroma supports an infectious rather than an immunologic etiology. The superior cornea is often involved primarily with deep infiltration of lymphocytes, macrophages, and *M. leprae* organisms accompanied by stromal edema, which may progress to involve the central cornea. Vascularization may occur as a late sequela of disease, and corneal opacification is permanent, should it occur. The comorbidity of corneal nerve involvement may contribute to the poorer prognosis of these cases.[95] The World Health Organization advocates a multidrug therapeutic regimen of daily dapsone and clofazimine and monthly rifampin and clofazimine for multibacillary disease. Topical corticosteroids for IK and cycloplegics for uveitis can be employed with careful monitoring of the corneal epithelium for neurotrophic and neuroparalytic disease as well as toxic reactions.

Lyme disease

Lyme disease is caused by infection with the spirochete *Borrelia burgdorferi* via the *Ixodes scapularis* deer tick. The clinical signs of disease have been separated into three stages, with a flulike illness and the pathognomonic skin lesion, erythema migrans, as features of stage 1. Ocular signs manifest during stages 2 and 3, although a follicular conjunctivitis can be seen in stage 1. During stage 2, hematogenous dissemination of the spirochetes results in neurologic, cardiac, and rheumatologic signs. Facial nerve palsy has been reported as a common neurologic manifestation of disease. Ocular inflammatory signs occur in stage 3 disease and include episcleritis, keratitis, uveitis, vasculitis, exudative retinal detachment, and endophthalmitis.

Although keratitis is not a common feature of Lyme disease, the inflammatory pattern is interstitial. Involvement is usually bilateral, although it may present in one eye. This IK is characterized by multiple poorly defined or nebular stromal opacities.[96] These infiltrates have indistinct borders, can be present throughout the corneal stroma, and do not profoundly affect visual acuity.[97] Unlike other forms of IK, stromal edema is not a common feature. Late vascularization and keratic precipitates with uveitis have been reported.[98] Most reported cases of keratitis were empirically treated with topical corticosteroids while one in three untreated patients developed edema, vascularization, and corneal haze. Late administration of corticosteroid drops remained effective.[99] Administration of topical corticosteroids appears to prevent the progression of inflammation to vascularization and scarring; however, appropriate systemic antibiotic treatment with ceftriaxone or tetracycline must be given.

Parasitic Infection

Acanthamoeba keratitis

A history of contact lens wear and the use of homemade saline solutions were found to be linked to this 'new' infection, which was described in 1975.[100,101] Infection with this free-living amoeba (see Ch. 83) is especially difficult to

Table 86.1 Features of parasitic interstitial keratitis (IK) by etiology

Disease	Synonym	Agent (vector)	Endemic areas	Pertinent history	Characteristic corneal findings
Acanthamoeba keratitis	None	*Acanthamoeba*	Worldwide	Contact lens wear/abuse, freshwater exposure	Pain out of proportion to findings. Radial keratoneuritis, early superficial epitheliopathy, stromal infiltration and edema without early stromal neovascularization, late ring infiltrate
Onchocerciasis	River blindness	*Onchocerca volvulus* (black fly)	West and Central Africa, Latin America, Yemen	Travel to endemic areas	Live microfilariae, peripheral stromal edema, centripetal full-thickness stromal vascularization, complete opacification, absence of thinning
Leishmaniasis	Baghdad boils, sandfly disease	*Leishmania* spp. (sandfly)	Asia, Africa, Latin America, Mediterranean	Travel to endemic areas	Focal or diffuse IK with deep neovascularization, late thinning, histologic findings of organisms and granulomatous inflammation
African trypanosomiasis	African sleeping sickness	*Trypanosoma brucei* (tsetse fly)	Africa	Travel to endemic areas	Diffuse neovascularization, severe scarring and thinning, potential perforation
Microsporidiosis	None	Microsporidia	Worldwide	Immunocompromised status	Anterior to midstromal infiltration

eradicate because the trophozoite form can encyst and elude the immune system and pharmacologic agents. Although a superficial epitheliopathy is an early feature, stromal involvement ensues with infiltration accompanied by edema, which is easily mistaken for herpetic stromal disease. At this stage of interstitial inflammation the diagnostic possibilities are myriad and, if the patient does not have a history of contact lens wear or fresh water exposure (Table 86.1), the diagnosis may not be obvious. Careful examination of the corneal epithelium for a band of intra- and intercellular edema and instability with poor adhesion to the underlying basement membrane should give the clinician adequate indication for diagnostic scrapings and culture using specific media to rule out *Acanthamoeba* infection. The infiltrates progress and often coalesce into frank abscesses in a circumferential pattern characteristic of this disease. Stromal neovascularization is typically not an early finding.

Onchocerciasis

Onchocerciasis (see Ch. 84) is the second leading cause of infectious blindness worldwide. The *Simulium* black fly vector of the filarial nematode *Onchocerca volvulus* requires rapidly flowing bodies of water for reproduction, hence the common name 'river blindness.' *Onchocerca* larvae mature, forming nodules in subcutaneous tissue of affected individuals. The microfilariae offspring of the adult female can migrate to the ocular tissues in the thousands. When they die and release parasite antigens, a vigorous helper T-cell type 2 inflammatory response is initiated primarily involving interleukin (IL)-4 and resultant B-cell antibody production, and IL-5 with eosinophil activation. The development of interstitial corneal disease includes a cellular immune response demonstrating increased disease in guinea pigs sensitized to *Onchocerca* antigens before intracorneal injection of bovine *Onchocerca lienalis* microfilariae.[102] Other animal models of *Onchocerca volvulus* infestation confirmed the T-cell dependence of the keratitis, and IL-4 and IL-5 have been found in human pathologic specimens.[103,104] Proteins from both eosinophilic and neutrophilic degranulation can cause direct damage to the corneal stroma resulting in scarring. Chemokines including RANTES and eotaxin, as well as increased vascular cell adhesion molecule-1 expression, are now known to be involved in the inflammatory process. The corneal manifestations of onchocerciasis include the presence of live microfilariae, punctate epitheliopathy, subepithelial infiltration, stromal edema, scarring, and neovascularization. A particular pattern of sclerosing keratitis is frequently encountered among middle-aged people living in savannah regions of West Africa. Taylor et al. have published numerous reports detailing onchocerciasis in Africa, describing a typical pattern of peripheral edema followed by progressive vascularization of all levels of the stroma spreading in a centripetal pattern.[105] Complete opacification of the cornea can result. Corneal thinning is not a feature of long-standing disease. Ivermectin, a microfilariacidal agent, is the mainstay of treatment for onchocerciasis in the absence of vaccines or pharmaceuticals effective against adult and larval forms.

Leishmaniasis

Leishmaniasis is the result of cutaneous or visceral infection with species of the flagellate protozoal genus *Leishmania* transmitted by sandflies found in Asia, Africa, Latin America, and the Mediterranean region. Cutaneous leishmaniasis secondary to *Leishmania braziliensis* is characterized by mucous membrane, nasal, and facial involvement.[106] The eyelids and the cornea can be affected in the facial cutaneous form of leishmaniasis. Ulcerative keratitis may progress to frank abscess formation, corneal necrosis, and perforation. An alternate presentation is IK with focal or diffuse stromal infiltration and characteristic deep vascularization. With resolution, after many years, the cornea may become scarred and thinned. Histopathologic examination shows *Leishmania* organisms and granulomatous inflammation.[107,108] In the visceral form of leishmaniasis, the peripheral cornea is rarely affected with sectoral scarring adjacent to limbal nodules.[109] The treatment of ocular disease is systemic therapy with stibogluconate sodium and meglumine antimonate, which has been used topically for keratitis.[110] Alternative therapy with amphotericin B, ketoconazole, or paromycin may be effective.

Trypanosomiasis

Trypanosomiasis results from infection with the protozoans *Trypanosoma cruzi* and *brucei*, causing the American form, known as Chagas' disease, and the African form, termed sleeping sickness, respectively. The corresponding vectors are the reduviid bug and the tsetse fly. The ocular manifestations of Chagas' disease include conjunctivitis, periorbital edema and discoloration, and dacryocystitis, the full constellation of which is termed Romana's sign. In sleeping sickness, a severe form of IK characterized by diffuse vascularization, scarring, and the potential for corneal perforation can be seen.[111] Anterior segment inflammation can be seen in addition to optic nerve involvement.[109] Treatment requires the use of potent systemic antiprotozoal agents such as nifurtimox and suramin.[110]

Microsporidiosis

Microsporidial keratitis is a rare cause of IK. These minute, obligately intracellular protozoans gained more attention when they were isolated from patients with acquired immunodeficiency syndrome (AIDS) who had superficial keratoconjunctivitis. There have been few reports in the literature documenting stromal keratitis secondary to *Microsporidium* or *Nosema* species occurring in immunocompetent individuals. Presentation has ranged from anterior to midstromal infiltration to anterior uveitis with gross corneal necrosis and perforation.[112–115] Treatment of these few cases has ranged from penetrating keratoplasty to systemic antiprotozoal agents such as itraconazole with mixed results.[116]

Viral Infection

Herpes simplex virus infection

Corneal manifestations of viral infection are myriad, from classic dendritic epithelial disease to fulminant necrotizing stromal keratitis leading to corneal perforation. Interestingly, various forms of stromal keratitis can be caused by several distinct types of viruses. Herpes simplex virus (see Ch. 79) is a principal cause of corneal blindness and, despite years of investigation, remains a formidable opponent for the ophthalmologist and affected patient. Herpetic stromal disease can manifest as IK, nummular keratitis, and ulcerative necrotizing stromal keratitis. The IK hallmarks of edema, new vessel formation, and cellular infiltration may be present to varying degrees and may be accompanied by scleritis and uveitis, which further complicate this serious condition. The pattern of stromal infiltration may be central or peripheral, focal or multifocal, superficial or full thickness. Wessely-type immune rings, if present, support the diagnosis.[117] The pathophysiology of herpetic stromal disease is likely immune mediated with T lymphocytes and macrophages implicated.[118] The Herpetic Eye Disease Study found that patients with a history of stromal keratitis treated with oral acyclovir 400 mg twice daily had a significant decrease in occurrence of recurrent stromal keratitis. Although acyclovir did not reduce established herpetic stromal inflammation, topical corticosteroids with antivirals was found to be superior to placebo with antivirals in hastening resolution of herpetic stromal disease.[119]

Varicella-zoster virus infection

Herpes zoster (see Ch. 80) is another common cause of IK. One of the many ocular manifestations of zoster is stromal infiltration. A careful history and accompanying signs of herpes zoster ophthalmicus will often clarify the diagnosis. While the most common ocular finding in varicella is a vesicular eruption on the periocular skin and eyelids, IK is a rare ocular complication. Reported cases of primary varicella IK tend to lag 1 to 2 months after cutaneous eruption, suggesting an immunologic mechanism.[120,121] A similar lag between cutaneous and ocular manifestations of varicella uveitis coincides closely with the delayed appearance of circulating antibodies.[122] Resolution of varicella IK can be on the order of months.[120]

Other viral infections

Epstein-Barr virus (EBV; see Ch. 81) is another herpes virus that can cause corneal disease. Unilateral, multifocal, discrete anterior stromal infiltrates, as well as bilateral, full-thickness, peripheral infiltrates, have been reported in patients with and without a history of infectious mononucleosis.[123] Ringlike opacities have been reported by multiple authors and a particular pattern of subepithelial infiltrates reminiscent of adenoviral infection has been noted as well.[124] Vascularization is a variable feature. EBV has not been isolated from corneal tissue with documented stromal keratitis, and the mechanism of inflammation remains unclear. There are reports of successful treatment using topical corticosteroids.[125]

Although mumps infection is uncommon in the United States, it remains a significant pediatric public health concern worldwide. Ophthalmic manifestations are uncommon. Conjunctival or lacrimal gland inflammations are most likely to occur. However, corneal involvement may range from punctate epithelial disease to multifocal nummular keratitis. Several authors report 'striate keratitis,' described as lacy, linear opacities.[126] Epithelial edema may be present over stromal infiltrates. Associated uveitis and even optic neuritis have been reported.[127]

Measles is an important cause of childhood blindness in developing countries. Superficial epithelial keratitis is commonly seen near the onset of the rash and usually resolves without sequelae. In some cases, factors such as concomitant vitamin A deficiency, malnutrition, exposure, and the use of traditional medicines combine to result in stromal infiltration and even corneal perforation.[128] The World Health Organization has recommended the use of topical ointments and the administration of systemic vitamin A for all children with measles.

Human T-lymphotrophic virus type 1 (HTLV-1) is one of six distinct retroviruses known to infect human lymphocytes and one of four actively spreading in epidemics (HIV-1, HIV-2, and HTLV-2 being the others). HTLV-1 results in adult T-cell leukemia and is endemic to South and Central Africa, Japan, and Melanesia. The estimated seroprevalence in the United States is less than 0.04% with the highest rates among immigrants, sex workers, and injection drug users. In addition to uveitis, HTLV-1 has been reported to cause a bilateral, peripheral, anterior stromal IK that is chronic and steroid-unresponsive.[129,130]

References

1. Mogan RF, Baumgartner CJ. Meniere's disease complicated by recurrent interstitial keratitis: excellent result following cervical ganglionectomy. *West J Surg.* 1934;42:628.
2. Cogan DG. Syndrome of nonsyphilitic interstitial keratitis and vestibuloauditory symptoms. *Arch Ophthalmol.* 1945;33:144–149.
3. Cogan DG. Nonsyphilitic interstitial keratitis with vestibuloauditory symptoms: report of 4 additional cases. *Arch Ophthalmol.* 1949;42: 42–49.
4. Mazlumzadeh M, Matteson EL. Cogan's syndrome: an audiovestibular, ocular, and systemic autoimmune disease. *Rheum Dis Clin North Am.* 2007;33:855–874, vii–viii.
5. Bernhardt O, et al. Cogan syndrome bei angiitis von hirnnerven, aortitis, endokarditis und glomerulonephritis. *Dtsch Med Wochenschr.* 1976;101:373.
6. Boyd GG. Cogan's syndrome. *Arch Otolaryngol.* 1957;65:24.
7. Cody DTR, Williams HL. Cogan's syndrome. *Laryngoscope.* 1960;70:447.
8. Cody DTR, Williams HL. Cogan's syndrome. *Mayo Clin Proc.* 1962;37:372.
9. Crawford WJ. Cogan's syndrome associated with polyarteritis nodosa: a report of three cases. *Pa Med J.* 1957;60:835.
10. Cote DN, et al. Cogan's syndrome manifesting as sudden bilateral deafness: diagnosis and management. *South Med J.* 1993;86:1056–1060.
11. Fauci AS, Wolff SM. Wegener's granulomatosis: studies in eighteen patients and a review of the literature. *Medicine.* 1973;52:535.
12. Gerber M. Cogan's syndrome, a case report. *Q Bull Northwest Med Sch.* 1958;32:15.
13. Gilbert WS, Talbot FJ. Cogan's syndrome: signs of periarteritis nodosa and cerebral venous sinus thrombosis. *Arch Ophthalmol.* 1969;82:633.
14. Hammer M, et al. Complicated Cogan's syndrome with aortic insufficiency and coronary stenosis. *J Rheumatol.* 1994;21:552–555.
15. Haynes BF, et al. Cogan's syndrome: studies in 13 patients, long-term follow-up and review of the literature. *Medicine (Baltimore).* 1980; 59:426–441.
16. Majoor MH, et al. Corneal autoimmunity in Cogan's syndrome? Report of two cases. *Ann Otol Rhinol Laryngol.* 1992;101:679–684.
17. Ochonisky S, et al. Cogan's syndrome. An unusual etiology of urticarial vasculitis. *Dermatologica.* 1991;183:218–220.
18. Quinn FB, Falls HF. Cogan's syndrome: case report and a review of etiologic concepts. *Trans Am Acad Ophthalmol Otol.* 1958;62:716.
19. Pinals RS. Cogan's syndrome with arthritis and aortic insufficiency. *J Rheumatol.* 1978;5:3.
20. Suzuki Y, et al. Cogan's syndrome, report of a case. *J Otorhinolaryngol Soc (Japan).* 1965;68:54.
21. Wilder-Smith E, Roelcke U. [Cogan syndrome. Case report, review of the literature, therapy]. *Laryngorhinootologie.* 1991;70:90–92.
22. Gluth MB, et al. Cogan syndrome: a retrospective review of 60 patients throughout a half century. *Mayo Clin Proc.* 2006;81:483–488.
23. Cogan DG. Corneoscleral lesions in periarteritis nodosa and Wegener's granulomatosis. *Trans Am Ophthalmol Soc.* 1955;53:321.
24. Lake-Bakaar G. Polyarteritis nodosa presenting with bilateral nerve deafness. *J R Soc Med.* 1978;7:144–146.
25. Weaver M. Profound sensorineural hearing loss associated with collagen disease. *Trans Pac Coast Otol Soc.* 1972;53:83.
26. Frohnert PP, Sheps SG. Long-term follow-up study of periarteritis nodosa. *Am J Med.* 1967;43:8.
27. Gussen R. Polyarteritis nodosa and deafness. A human temporal bone study. *Arch Otorhinolaryngol.* 1977;217:263.
28. Harbart F, McPherson SD. Scleral necrosis in periarteritis nodosa: a case report. *Am J Ophthalmol.* 1947;30:727.
29. Ingalls RG. Bilateral uveitis and keratitis accompanying periarteritis nodosa. *Trans Am Acad Ophthalmol.* 1951;56:630.
30. McNiel NF, et al. Polyarteritis nodosa causing deafness in an adult. Report of a case with special reference to concepts about the disease. *Ann Intern Med.* 1952;37:1253.
31. Oliner L, et al. Nonsyphilitic interstitial keratitis and bilateral deafness (Cogan's syndrome). Associated with essential polyangitis (periarteritis nodosa). *N Engl J Med.* 1953;248:1001.
32. Peitersen E, Carlsen BH. Hearing impairment as the initial sign of polyarteritis nodosa. *Acta Otolaryngol.* 1966;61:189.
33. Rich AR. The role of hypersensitivity in periarteritis nodosa. *Bull Johns Hopkins Hosp.* 1942;71:123.
34. Rose GA, Spencer H. Polyarteritis nodosa. *Q J Med.* 1957;26:43.
35. Haynes BF, et al. The ocular manifestations of Wegener's granulomatosis: fifteen years experience and review of the literature. *Am J Med.* 1977;63:131.
36. Arnold GE, Ohsaki K. Two cases of sudden deafness. *Ann Otol Rhinol Laryngol.* 1963;72:605.
37. Bennett FM. Bilateral recurrent episcleritis associated with posterior corneal changes, vestibulo-auditory symptoms and rheumatoid arthritis. *Am J Ophthalmol.* 1963;55:815.
38. Smith JL. Cogan's syndrome. *Laryngoscope.* 1970;80:121.
39. Kundell SP, Ochs HD. Cogan's syndrome in childhood. *J Pediatr.* 1980;97:96–98.
40. Ndiaye IC, Rassi SJ, Wiener-Vacher SR. Cochleovestibular impairment in pediatric Cogan's syndrome. *Pediatrics.* 2002;109:E38.
41. Martinez-Osorio H, Fuentes-Paez G, Calonge M. Severe keratopathy in paediatric Cogan's syndrome. *Rheumatology (Oxford).* 2006;45:1576–1577.
42. Vollertsen RS, et al. Cogan's syndrome: 18 cases and a review of the literature. *Mayo Clin Proc.* 1986;61:344–361.
43. Cobo LM, Haynes BF. Early corneal findings in Cogan's syndrome. *Ophthalmology.* 1984;91:903.
44. Cobo LM. Cogan's syndrome. In Gold DH, Weingeist TA, eds. *The eye in systemic disease.* Philadelphia: Lippincott; 1990.
45. Froehlich F, et al. Association of Crohn's disease and Cogan's syndrome. *Dig Dis Sci.* 1994;39:1134–1137.
46. McAdam LP, et al. Relapsing polychondritis: prospective study of 23 patients and a review of the literature. *Medicine.* 1976;55:193.
47. Wolff D, et al. The pathology of Cogan's syndrome causing profound deafness. *Ann Otol Rhinol Laryngol.* 1965;74:507.
48. Norton EWD, Cogan DG. Syndrome of nonsyphilitic interstitial keratitis and vestibuloauditory symptoms. *Arch Ophthalmol.* 1959;61:695.
49. Cochrane AD, Tatoulis J. Cogan's syndrome with aortitis, aortic regurgitation, and aortic arch vessel stenoses. *Ann Thorac Surg.* 1991;52: 1166–1167.
50. Gelfand ML, Kantor T, Gorstein F. Cogan's syndrome with cardiovascular involvement: aortic insufficiency. *Bull NY Acad Sci.* 1972;48:647.
51. Paolini G, et al. Aortic valve replacement in Cogan's syndrome. *Eur J Cardiothorac Surg.* 1991;5:549–551.
52. Stewart SR, Robbins DL, Castles JJ. Acute fulminant aortic and mitral insufficiency in ankylosing spondylitis. *N Engl J Med.* 1978;1299:1448.
53. Cheson BD, Bluming AZ, Alroy J. Cogan's syndrome: a systemic vasculitis. *Am J Med.* 1976;60:549.
54. Deliveliotou A, et al. Successful full-term pregnancy in a woman with Cogan's syndrome: a case report. *Clin Rheumatol.* 2007;26:2181–2183.
55. Sheikh SI, et al. Reversible Cogan's syndrome in a patient with human immunodeficiency virus (HIV) infection. *J Clin Neurosci.* 2009; 16:154–156.
56. Magone MT, Maric I, Hwang DG. Peripheral interstitial keratitis: a novel manifestation of ocular mastocytosis. *Cornea.* 2006;25:364–367.
57. Helmchen C, et al. Cogan's syndrome: clinical significance of antibodies against the inner ear and cornea. *Acta Otolaryngol.* 1999;119:528.
58. Lunardi C, et al. Autoantibodies to inner ear and endothelial antigens in Cogan's syndrome. *Lancet.* 2002;360:915–921.
59. Benvenga S, Trimarchi F, Facchiano A. Cogan's syndrome as an autoimmune disease. *Lancet.* 2003;361:530–531.
60. Koelle DM, et al. Tegument-specific, virus-reactive CD4 T cells localize to the cornea in herpes simplex virus interstitial keratitis in humans. *J Virol.* 2000;74:10930–10938.
61. Ioannidis AS, et al. Immune recovery disease: a case of interstitial keratitis and tonic pupil following bone marrow transplantation. *Br J Ophthalmol.* 2004;88:1601–1602.

62. Ryan LM, Kozin F, Eiferman R. Immune complex uveitis: a case. *Ann Intern Med.* 1978;88:62.
63. Fisher ER, Hellstrom HR. Cogan's syndrome and systemic vascular disease. *Arch Pathol.* 1961;72:572.
64. Cogan DG, Sullivan Jr WR. Immunologic study of nonsyphilitic interstitial keratitis with vestibuloauditory symptoms. *Am J Ophthalmol.* 1975;80:491–494.
65. Hughes GB, et al. Autoimmune reactivity in Cogan's syndrome: a preliminary report. *Otolaryngol Head Neck Surg.* 1983;91:24–32.
66. Ambati BK, et al. Soluble vascular endothelial growth factor receptor-1 contributes to the corneal antiangiogenic barrier. *Br J Ophthalmol.* 2007;91:505–508.
67. Gow JA, Ostler HB, Schachter J. Inclusion conjunctivitis with hearing loss. *JAMA.* 1974;229:519.
68. Darougar S, et al. Isolation of *Chlamydia psittaci* from a patient with interstitial keratitis and uveitis associated with otological and cardiovascular lesions. *Br J Ophthalmol.* 1978;62:709.
69. Dawson CR, et al. Experimental inclusion conjunctivitis in man. III. Keratitis and other complications. *Arch Ophthalmol.* 1967;78:341.
70. Pau H. *Differential diagnosis of eye diseases.* Philadelphia: Saunders; 1978.
71. Marcy SM, Kibrick S. Mumps. In Hoeprich P, ed. *Infectious diseases: a modern treatise of infectious processes.* Hagerstown, MD: Harper & Row; 1977.
72. Char DH, Cogan DG, Sullivan WR. Immunologic study of nonsyphilitic interstitial keratitis with vestibuloauditory symptoms. *Am J Ophthalmol.* 1975;80:491.
73. Del Carpio J, Espinoza LR, Osterland CK. Cogan's syndrome and HLA BW17. *N Engl J Med.* 1976;295:1276.
74. Cheson BD, Garevoy MR. Cogan's syndrome and BW17 revisited. *N Engl J Med.* 1977;297:62.
75. Kaiser-Kupfer MI, et al. The HLA antigens in Cogan's syndrome. *Am J Ophthalmol.* 1978;86:314.
76. Haynes BF, et al. Successful treatment of sudden hearing loss in Cogan's syndrome with corticosteroids. *Arthritis Rheum.* 1981;24:501–503.
77. Fricker M, et al. A novel therapeutic option in Cogan diseases? TNF-alpha blockers. *Rheumatol Int.* 2007;27:493–495.
78. Cundiff J, et al. Cogan's syndrome: a cause of progressive hearing deafness. *Am J Otolaryngol.* 2006;27:68–70.
79. Fauci AS, et al. Cyclophosphamide therapy of severe systemic necrotizing vasculitis. *N Engl J Med.* 1979;301:235–238.
80. Pevetti-Pezzi P, et al. Immunosuppressive therapy for Cogan's syndrome. In Nussenblatt RB et al, eds. *Advances in ocular immunology.* Amsterdam: Elsevier; 1994.
81. Roat MI, et al. Treatment of Cogan's syndrome with FK 506: a case report. *Transplant Proc* 23:3347, 1991.
82. Matteson EL, et al. Open trial of methotrexate as treatment for autoimmune hearing loss. *Arthritis Rheum.* 2001;45:146–150.
83. Inoue Y, et al. Low-dose oral methotrexate for the management of childhood Cogan's syndrome: a case report. *Clin Rheumatol.* 2007; 26:2201–2203.
84. Vaiopoulos G, et al. Lack of response to corticosteroids and pulse cyclophosphamide therapy in Cogan's syndrome. *Clin Rheumatol.* 1994;13: 110–112.
85. Nussenblatt RB, et al. Treatment of noninfectious intermediate and posterior uveitis with the humanized anti-Tac mAb: a phase I/II clinical trial. *Proc Natl Acad Sci USA.* 1999;96:7462.
86. Cunnane G, et al. Accelerated nodulosis and vasculitis following etanercept therapy for rheumatoid arthritis. *Arthritis Rheum.* 2002;47:445.
87. Duke-Elder S. Tuberculous interstitial keratitis. In: *System of ophthalmology. Diseases of the outer eye.* vol VIII, part 2. London: Klimpton; 1965.
88. Anhalt EF, et al. Conjunctival tuberculosis. *Am J Ophthalmol.* 1960; 50:265–269.
89. Glover LP. Some eye observations in tuberculosis patients at the state sanitorium, Cresson, PA. *Am J Ophthalmol.* 1930;13:411–412.
90. Goldenburg M, Fabricant ND. The eye in the tuberculous patient. *Trans Sect Ophthalmol Am Med Assn.* 1930;135–165.
91. Donahue HC. Ophthalmologic experience in tuberculosis sanitorium. *Am J Ophthalmol.* 1967;64:742–748.
92. Helen CJ, Holand GN. Ocular tuberculosis. *Surv Ophthalmol.* 1993;38:229.
93. Labouteoulle M, et al. Rapid improvement of chronic interstitial keratitis with acitretin. *Br J Opthalmol.* 2002;86:1445–1446.
94. Dana MR, et al. Ocular manifestations of leprosy in a noninstitutionalized community in the United States. *Arch Ophthalmol.* 1991;15: 289–293.
95. Ffytche TJ. Ocular leprosy: the continuing challenge. *Int Ophthalmol.* 1991;15:289–293.
96. Miyashiro MJ, et al. Lyme disease associated with unilateral interstitial keratitis. *Cornea.* 1999;18:115–116.
97. Baum J, et al. Bilateral keratitis as a manifestation of Lyme disease. *Am J Ophthalmol.* 1988;105:75–77.
98. Zaidman GW. The ocular manifestations of Lyme disease. *Int Ophthalmol Clin.* 1993;3:9.
99. Rommehl EW, et al. Bilateral keratitis in Lyme disease. *Ophthalmology.* 1989;96:1194–1197.
100. Jones BR, McGill JI, Steele ADM. Recurrent suppurative keratouveitis with loss of eye due to infection by *Acanthamoeba castellani. Trans Ophthal Soc UK.* 1975;95:210–213.
101. Jones DB, Visvesvara GS, Robinson NM. *Acanthamoeba* polyphage keratitis and *Acanthomoeba* uveitis with fatal meningoencephalitis. *Trans Ophthal Soc UK.* 1975;95:221–232.
102. Donnelly JJ, Rockey JH, Bianco AE, et al. Ocular immunopathologic findings of experimental onchocerciasis. *Arch Ophthalmol.* 1984; 102:628–634.
103. Pealmen E, et al. Sclerosing keratitis induced by *Onchocerca volvulus* correlates with production of Th-2 associated cytokines. *Invest Ophthalmol Vis Sci ARVO.* 1993;34:3329.
104. Limaye AP, et al. IL-2 and past history of eosinophilia in patients with onchocerciasis. *J Clin Invest.* 1991;88:1418–1421.
105. Taylor HR, et al. Ivermectin treatment of patients with severe ocular onchocerciasis. *Am J Trop Med Hyg.* 1989;40:494.
106. Cairns JE. Cutaneous leishmaniasis (oriental sore): a case with corneal involvement. *Br J Ophthalmol.* 1968;52:481–483.
107. Duke-Elder S. Disease of the outer eye. In: *System of ophthalmology.* vol VIII, part 21. London: Klimpton; 1965.
108. Roizenblatt J. Interstitial keratitis caused by American (mucocutaneous) leishmaniasis. *Am J Ophthalmol.* 1979;87:175–179.
109. Rodger FC. Ophthalmology in the tropics. In Manson-Bahr PEC, Apted FIC, eds. *Manson's tropical disease.* 18th ed. London: Baillière Tindall; 1982.
110. Webster LT. Chemotherapy of parasitic infections. In Gilman AG et al, *eds. The pharmacologic basis of therapeutics.* 8th ed. New York: Pergamon; 1990.
111. Duke-Elder S, Leigh AG. Diseases of the outer eye. In: *System of ophthalmology.* vol VIII, part 2. London: Klimpton; 1965.
112. Ashton W, Wirasinha PA. Encephalitozoonosis (nosematosis) of the cornea. *Br J Ophthalmol.* 1973;57:669.
113. Pinolis M, et al. Nosematosis of the cornea. Case report, including electron microscopic studies. *Arch Ophthalmol.* 1981;99:1044–1047.
114. Davis RM, et al. Corneal microsporidiosis. A case report including ultrastructural observations. *Ophthalmology.* 1990;97:953–957.
115. Cali A, et al. Corneal microsporidiosis. Characterization and identification. *J Protozool.* 1991;39:215.
116. Yee RW, et al. Resolution of microsporidial epithelial keratopathy in a patient with AIDS. *Ophthalmology.* 1991;98:196.
117. Meyers R. Immunology of herpes simplex virus infection. *Int Ophthalmol Clin.* 1975;15:37.
118. Pepose JS. Herpes simplex keratitis. Role of viral infection vs. immune response. *Surv Ophthalmol.* 1991;35:345.
119. Herpetic Eye Disease Study Group. Oral acyclovir for herpes simplex virus disease: effect on prevention of epithelial keratitis and stromal keratitis. *Arch Ophthalmol.* 2000;118:1030–1036.
120. Fernandez de Castro LE, et al. Ocular manifestations after primary varicella infection. *Cornea.* 2006;25:866–867.
121. Ostler HB, Thygeson P. The ocular manifestations of herpes zoster, varicella, infectious mononucleosis, and cytomegalovirus disease. *Surv Ophthalmol.* 1976;21:148–159.
122. Appel I, et al. Uveitis and ophthalmoplegia complicating chickenpox. *J Pediatr Ophthalmol.* 1977;14:346–348.
123. Matoba AY, Wilhelmus KR, Jones DB. Epstein-Barr viral stromal keratitis. *Ophthalmology.* 1986;93:746.
124. Pflugfelser SC, Huang A, Crouse C. Epstein-Barr viral keratitis after a chemical facial peel. *Am J Ophthalmol.* 1990;110:571.
125. Matoba AY. Ocular disease associated with Epstein-Barr virus infection. *Surv Ophthalmol.* 1990;35:145.
126. Nectoux R. Keratitie ourlienne. *Ann Ocul* 1946;179:597–599.
127. Onal S, Toker E. A rare ocular complication of mumps: kerato-uveitis. *Ocul Immunol Inflamm.* 2005;13:395–397.
128. Dekkers NW, Treskes M. Measles keratitis. *Ophthalmol Clin North Am.* 1994;74:574.
129. Merle H, et al. A description of human T-lymphotropic virus type 1-related chronic interstitial keratitis in 20 patients. *Am J Ophthalmol.* 2001;131:305–308.
130. Merle H, et al. Ocular lesions in 200 patients infected by the human T-lymphotropic virus type 1 in Martinique (French West Indies). *Am J Ophthalmol.* 2002;134:190–195.

Chapter 87

Corneal Micropuncture in Recurrent Erosion Syndromes

Roy Scott Rubinfeld

Commonly encountered in ophthalmic practice, recurrent erosion syndrome is a painful, often frightening, and sometimes incapacitating condition for many patients worldwide. In this syndrome, as implied by its name, corneal epithelial cells erode, resulting in denuded areas on the corneal surface. These areas then reepithelialize, and the process recurs when the epithelial cells slough again at a later time. Erosions are characteristically episodic in nature, with many patients free of symptoms other than perhaps a mild ocular foreign body sensation or vague 'awareness' of the affected eye between erosions. This sensation of awareness can be most noticeable in dry, cold or windy environments. Most erosions occur during the evening or early morning hours and are described as an abrupt 'ripping' or 'tearing' sensation generally followed immediately by sharp pain, a marked foreign body sensation, epiphora, photophobia, visual disturbances, and often lid swelling.

These attacks may vary greatly in pattern and intensity. Some patients have mild symptoms every few months or years, and some experience severe, incapacitating, frequent erosions causing pain and other symptoms lasting for hours or days at a time. In some patients with recurrent erosion, the epithelial defects never fully close, and loose sheets of epithelium slide over the surface of the eye with each blink. These patients experience constant pain and can be some of the most distraught individuals encountered in clinical practice.

The unpredictable nature of recurrent erosions often heightens patient anxiety. For active people, the knowledge that, on any given day, they may suddenly experience acute pain and be unable to work or participate in normal activities for hours or days at a time can be extremely disturbing. It is not uncommon for patients with severe erosions to begin displaying signs of depression and anxiety disorders. Since most erosions occur during sleep or on awakening, some patients come to fear falling asleep and experience varying degrees of insomnia. The resulting disruption in normal sleep patterns may exacerbate the patient's psychologic stress as well as their experience of the symptoms. Anxiety may even make erosions more frequent by causing patients to open their eyes more quickly on awakening and by inducing more rapid eye movements as well as interfering with normal blinking and tear production.

Pathophysiology

The pathophysiology of recurrent erosion syndrome is only partially understood. Normal adhesion of the corneal epithelium depends primarily on structures known as attachment complexes, which are composed of elements from the basal epithelial cell, basement membrane, Bowman's layer, and corneal stroma. Through electron microscopic and immunohistochemical staining methods, these elements are thought to include hemidesmosomes, basal lamina, lamina densa, lamina lucida, anchoring fibrils, laminin, fibronectin, and types IV and VII collagen.

Abnormalities of epithelial adhesion resulting in recurrent erosion can be associated with previous traumatic abrasions or with corneal dystrophies. In the case of erosions associated with previous trauma, superficial injury to the cornea may damage the basement membrane. Some corneas appear unable to re-form normal attachment complexes, resulting in recurrent erosions occurring up to many years after the original injury.

Many ophthalmic or systemic diseases are associated with an increased incidence of recurrent erosions. A partial list of these includes lattice, Reis-Bücklers', macular, granular, and Meesmann's dystrophies; diabetes mellitus; and bullous keratopathy. Anterior basement (Cogan's or map-dot) corneal dystrophy is the dystrophy most commonly responsible for recurrent corneal erosion. Basement membrane abnormalities, including reduplication of basement membrane within the epithelium (maps) and cystic degeneration of cells (microcysts), have been reported present in between 6% and 42% of the general population.[1,2]

Diagnosis

For clinicians familiar with the common features of recurrent erosion syndrome, a patient with a history of previous trauma to the involved eye, episodes of pain on awakening, and a ragged, grayish-staining area of epithelium (Fig. 87.1) constitutes little or no diagnostic challenge. The diagnosis of recurrent erosion syndrome in more subtle cases, however, can be quite difficult.

The clinician should carefully inquire about trauma to the involved eye. Often, the patient will describe previous milder

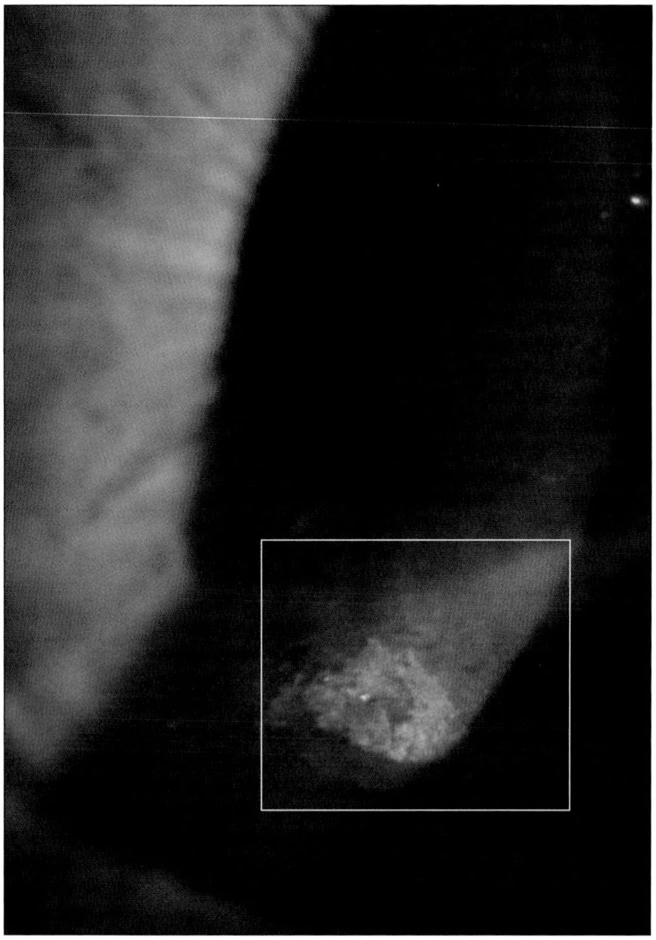

Fig. 87.1 Slit lamp appearance of active recurrent erosion showing ragged, edematous, disrupted gray epithelium (*box*). Note that the area of erosion is surrounded by apparently intact but also edematous grayish epithelium. (Courtesy of Peter R Laibson, MD; from Rubinfeld RS: Recurrent corneal erosion. In Roy FH, editor: *Master techniques in ophthalmic surgery*, Baltimore, 1995, Williams & Wilkins.)

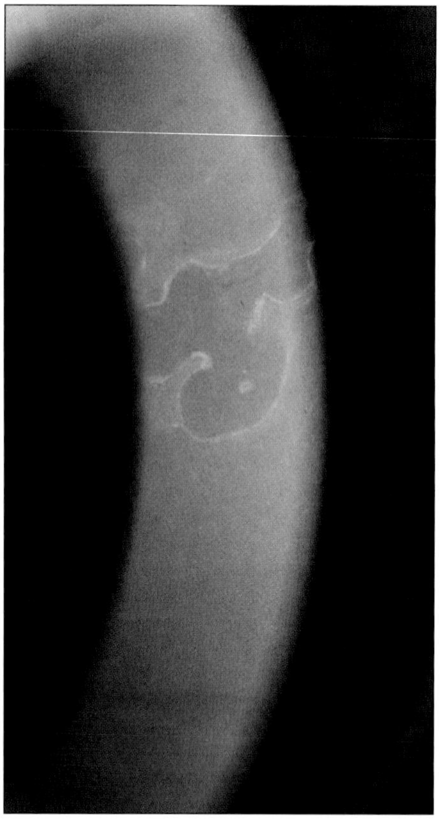

Fig. 87.2 Broad-beam slit lamp appearance of anterior basement membrane lines present in recurrent erosion patient. This pathology was much less obvious using standard narrow slit beam illumination.

episodes of erosion, which helps support the diagnosis. Keen slit lamp examination is often required to find subtle signs of erosion. Several different examination techniques can be helpful in this situation. Broad, angled slit beam examination of both eyes before and after instillation of fluorescein (Figs 87.2, 87.3) should be performed as well as a retroillumination examination of the cornea with dilation of the pupil to discern signs of basement membrane dystrophy or sites of previous erosion. This careful examination may not only confirm the diagnosis but may also indicate which areas will need to be treated. Gentle pressure applied to the cornea through the eyelid may demonstrate wrinkling of loosely adherent epithelium. A fine slit beam examination may reveal subtle, residual brown granularity of the stroma (brawny edema), which persists briefly after restoration of epithelial integrity.

Sometimes even the best observer will discern no visible corneal abnormalities on slit lamp examination because the epithelial defect has resolved in the time between the occurrence of the erosion and the examination of the patient. In this situation the clinician should be especially careful not to label the distraught patient with complaints of eye pain and no visible signs of disease as 'functional' or 'psychoneurotic.' Clinicians should remember that recurrent erosion patients often display signs of anxiety and depression, as previously described. In these situations when the diagnosis is in question, the patient should be instructed to return for examination immediately after the next episode of pain without allowing time for the epithelium to heal and cover the erosion. Usually this approach will not only confirm the diagnosis but also will help in choosing the correct treatment as well as the areas to be treated.

Medical Treatment

For decades, recurrent erosion syndrome remained one of the more frustrating ophthalmologic problems encountered in clinical practice because of its occasional resistance to available treatments and prolonged course. Today, new therapies and a rational stepwise approach to management of erosions provide opportunities to convert distraught individuals suffering from persistent recurrent erosion into some of the most grateful patients in a clinician's practice.

Topical agents

A mainstay of medical treatment that remains effective to this day for the vast majority of patients with corneal erosions involves the long-term nightly use of hyperosmotic

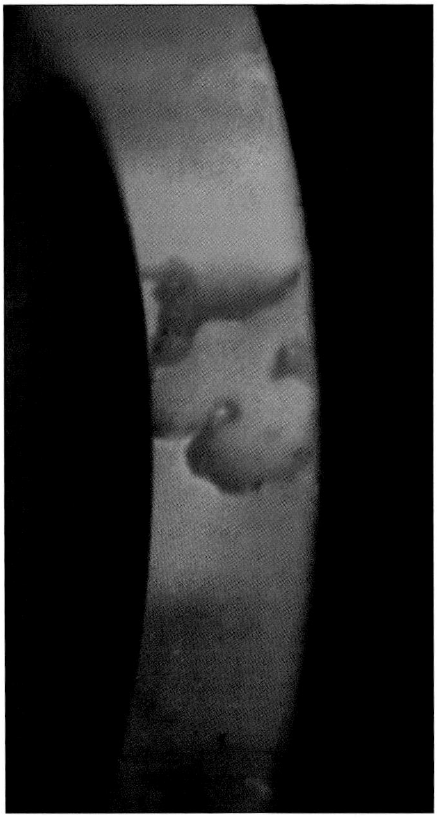

Fig. 87.3 Slit lamp appearance of the same patient's eye as in Figure 87.2 in which visualization of the basement membrane lines is enhanced with a tear film thickly stained with fluorescein.

lubricating ointments. The rationale for this treatment derives from the concept of nocturnal relative hypotonicity of the preocular tear film. At night, with the eyes closed, tear evaporation is reduced. The resultant lowered concentration of dissolved salts in the tears is postulated to shift the osmotic gradients, resulting in a relative increase in corneal epithelial edema and consequent reduction in epithelial adhesion. The vehicle (e.g. petrolatum) serves also to prevent erosions by keeping the eye lubricated during rapid eye movements or while opening the eyes in the morning. Hyperosmotic eyedrops during the daytime are sometimes added to this approach in an effort to minimize epithelial edema during waking hours as well, thus allowing re-formation of more normal attachment complexes. These agents must be used consistently for at least 6 to 12 months after the patient's last erosion, since it often takes this much time for re-formation of normal attachment complexes. Unfortunately, patients frequently decide to stop the use of these topical agents soon after the erosions resolve, only to have a recurrence, which may prolong the time required for the attachment complexes to re-form. It is essential to query and educate patients in this regard. Some clinicians use only bland lubricants without a hyperosmotic component, but this approach may be less effective. Currently available hyperosmotic ointments include sodium chloride 5% (Muro-128, Bausch and Lomb), and sulfacetamide 10% (Bleph-10, AK-Sulf).

In addition to the hyperosmotic agents that are now available, other topical preparations may be of value in treating some patients with recurrent erosions. Some promising results have been reported in early studies using topical osmotic colloidal solutions[3] and clinical trials are now under way to further evaluate these preparations. Topical autologous serum eyedrops[4] as well as numerous investigational trophic growth factors may be demonstrated to be effective in treating some erosion patients, especially in patients with more severe types of epitheliopathy, such as those associated with long-term diabetes or neurotrophic keratitis.

Some investigators[5] have suggested that topical corticosteroids combined with oral doxycycline may help treat recurrent erosions by inhibition of matrix metalloproteinase-9. The use of topical steroids in the treatment of recurrent erosion must, however, be weighed against the potential risks of infection, cataract, and intraocular pressure elevation.

Patching and bandage lenses

Patching during acute erosions in conjunction with lubricant/antibiotic agents is another effective treatment that helps to resolve the acute erosion in the vast majority of patients. Bandage contact lenses may be helpful in the case of acute erosions, but there appears to be an increased risk of microbial keratitis associated with their use.[6,7] In addition, they are often not effective in preventing further erosions except in cases where abnormalities in lid anatomy play a significant causative role in the erosions. Patching acute erosions and the consistent long-term nightly use of hyperosmotic ointments effectively resolve recurrent erosion syndrome for the vast majority of patients.

In addition to lid abnormalities or corneal inflammation, patients with recurrent erosions may be found, on careful examination, to have other concomitant ophthalmic diseases. Conditions such as dry eye syndrome or meibomian gland dysfunction blepharitis should be treated aggressively with frequent nonpreserved tear supplements or systemic tetracycline (such as doxycycline 50 or 100 mg orally each day), respectively.

Surgical Treatment

For patients in whom consistent, aggressive medical management fails to resolve the erosions, there exist several effective surgical options. The indication for surgical intervention is any situation in which aggressive medical management does not improve the symptoms and signs of erosions, and when the patient's continued pain and epithelial defects interfere with normal activities. The presence of recurring epithelial defects may result in infectious keratitis. This risk of infection, in conjunction with the prospect of continued patient disability and pain, generally overshadows the limited risks of appropriate surgical treatment of recalcitrant recurrent erosions. The choice of surgical approach is determined by the frequency and severity of erosions, the presence of concomitant dystrophies or other diseases, the etiology and location of the erosions, and the patient's needs and desires (Table 87.1).

Table 87.1 Surgical therapies for recurrent erosion syndromes

Procedure	ASP (ER)	Epithelial keratectomy	Debridement	Excimer PTK/PRK	YAG procedures
Optimum candidate	Localized erosions with or without mild to moderate ABM dystrophy	Erosions in multiple areas, moderate to severe ABM, with decreased VA; loose sheet of floppy epithelium	Single area of erosion with localized loose sheets of epithelium, localized areas of abnormal epithelium affecting best corrected vision	Erosions in multiple areas, moderate to severe ABM, with decreased VA, loose sheets of epithelium with myopia	Unclear
Availability	Worldwide	May require operating microscope and diamond burr apparatus	Worldwide	Limited	Moderately limited
Cost	Very inexpensive	Moderate	Very inexpensive	Extremely expensive	Moderately expensive
Debridement required	–	+	+	+	Debridement required only with older technique
Efficacy	Excellent	Excellent	Mixed	Good?	Some early reports encouraging

ASP, anterior stromal puncture; ER, epithelial reinforcement; PTK, phototherapeutic keratectomy; PRK, photorefractive keratectomy; ABM, anterior basement membrane; VA, visual acuity; YAG, yttrium–aluminum–garnet.

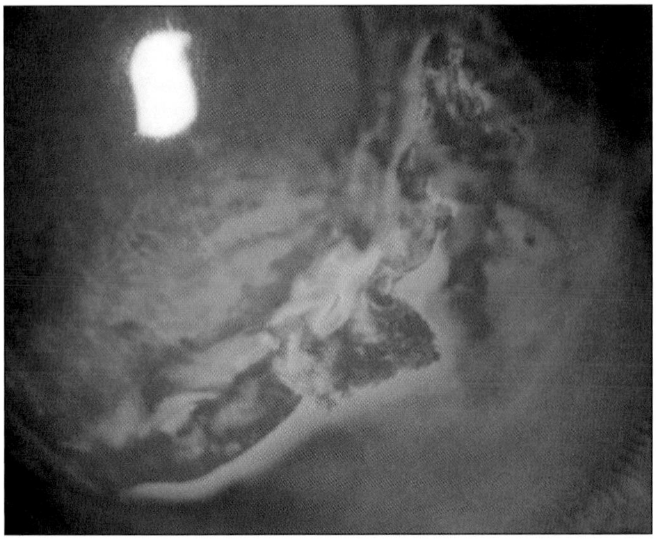

Fig. 87.4 Slit lamp appearance of loosely adherent sheet of floppy epithelium in a recurrent erosion patient. This sheet slid back and forth across the cornea with each blink. Note that fluorescein staining of the tear film helps make the loose epithelium more visible.

Debridement and superficial keratectomy

Historically, debridement[8,9] and then superficial keratectomy[10] were the first surgical approaches to the treatment of recurrent corneal erosions, and these procedures remain in use today.[11] Debridement may be useful for removing a localized area of very loosely adherent 'floppy' sheet of epithelium in a limited number of erosion patients (Fig. 87.4). This technique requires only a cotton swab or blunt instrument and can be performed at the slit lamp with topical anesthesia. The suboptimal efficacy and limitations of this procedure derive from the fact that no significant modifications to enhance epithelial adhesion are made in Bowman's layer or other deeper corneal structures. A more aggressive approach, generally requiring the use of an operating microscope, is that of a large superficial epithelial keratectomy. This technique is much more likely to benefit recurrent erosion patients. The optimum candidate for this procedure has spontaneous multiple erosions in different areas of the cornea, no history of trauma, and severe basement membrane dystrophy, resulting in poor vision and large areas of loosely adherent irregular epithelium. After subconjunctival, peribulbar, or retrobulbar injections of a local anesthetic agent (or, in some highly cooperative patients, the use of topical anesthetic agents) a lid speculum is inserted to hold the eye open. A superficial plane of dissection using a steel or jewel blade is established in the perilimbal area. Leaving approximately 1 mm of intact perilimbal epithelium, the rest of the epithelium and its basement membrane, if possible, are lifted and dissected free. An attempt should be made to peel and dissect away the epithelium in a continuous sheet. Persistent epithelial fragments may be visualized by instilling fluorescein. Bowman's layer should not be incised but should be scraped with a blade oriented perpendicular to the surface of the cornea, taking care not to produce linear scars in Bowman's layer. Alternatively, a diamond burr may be used to gently polish Bowman's layer to enhance epithelial adhesion.[11] Preoperatively, the instillation of several drops of topical nonsteroidal antiinflammatory agents such as bromfenac (Xibrom), ketorolac tromethamine (Acular) or diclofenac (Voltaren) generally helps greatly with pain management in patients undergoing debridement or superficial epithelial keratectomy procedures. Postoperatively, the use of these drops, 2 to 3 times daily as needed for pain, in conjunction with a well-fitted bandage contact lens for up to 3 to 5 days, usually improves patient comfort during the early postoperative period. More recently, a technique known as alcohol delamination of the corneal epithelium[12] has been proposed to improve the efficacy of debridement in the treatment of recurrent erosions. Debridement and removal of abnormal or reduplicated epithelium is most effective in cases where localized areas of such epithelium interfere with visual acuity by inducing refractive changes (Figs 87.5–87.9).

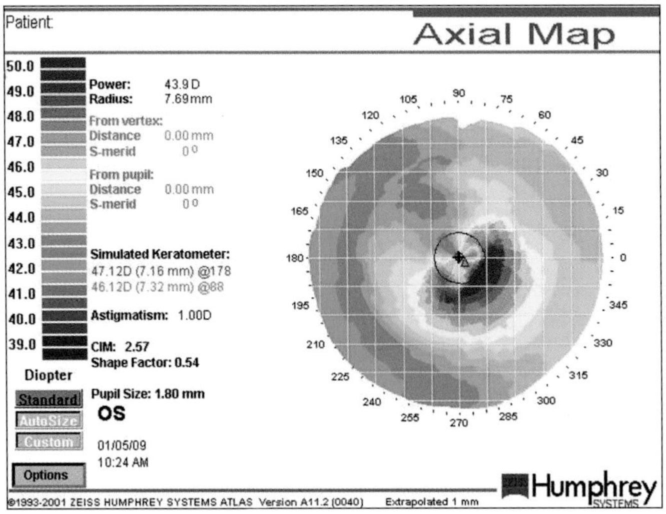

Fig. 87.5 Placido disk topographic map of a patient who complained of poor quality of vision and foreign body sensation following cataract surgery with an intraoperative corneal abrasion. In spite of excellent lens implant position, the best corrected vision was a poor quality 20/25. This appearance is suggestive of pericentral keratoconus.

Anterior stromal puncture (epithelial reinforcement, corneal micropuncture)

In 1986 McLean et al.[13] described a significant innovation in the surgical management of resistant corneal erosions, which they termed 'anterior stromal puncture.' This highly effective office technique involved the use of a straight 20-gauge needle to make multiple shallow penetrations through the epithelium into anterior corneal stroma to improve epithelial adhesion, apparently by forming tiny scarring attachments similar to the metalworking technique of spot welding. Laibson[14] and others expressed concerns about the possibility of corneal perforation with a straight needle, and several perforations have been reported using a 20-gauge needle.[15] Despite a high level of surgeon's skill, these perforations may occur because of the natural tendency for many patients undergoing stromal puncture to slowly back away from the slit lamp during the procedure and then jerk forward unpredictably once they realize their head position is wrong.

Concerns regarding this possibility of perforation, as well as questions regarding depth of penetration, the possibility of excessive scarring, and the reproducibility of results with stromal puncture, prompted the design of a disposable, inexpensive, specialized instrument for use in corneal micropuncture.[16] In histopathologic studies of cadavers and in clinical trials, this instrument has been shown to produce consistent, shallow penetrations (Figs 87.10, 87.11), minimal scarring (Figs 87.12, 87.13), and has virtually eliminated the possibility of perforation while retaining the high success rate of anterior stromal puncture with a straight needle.[15,16]

Anterior stromal puncture or micropuncture is an office procedure performed conveniently at the slit lamp under

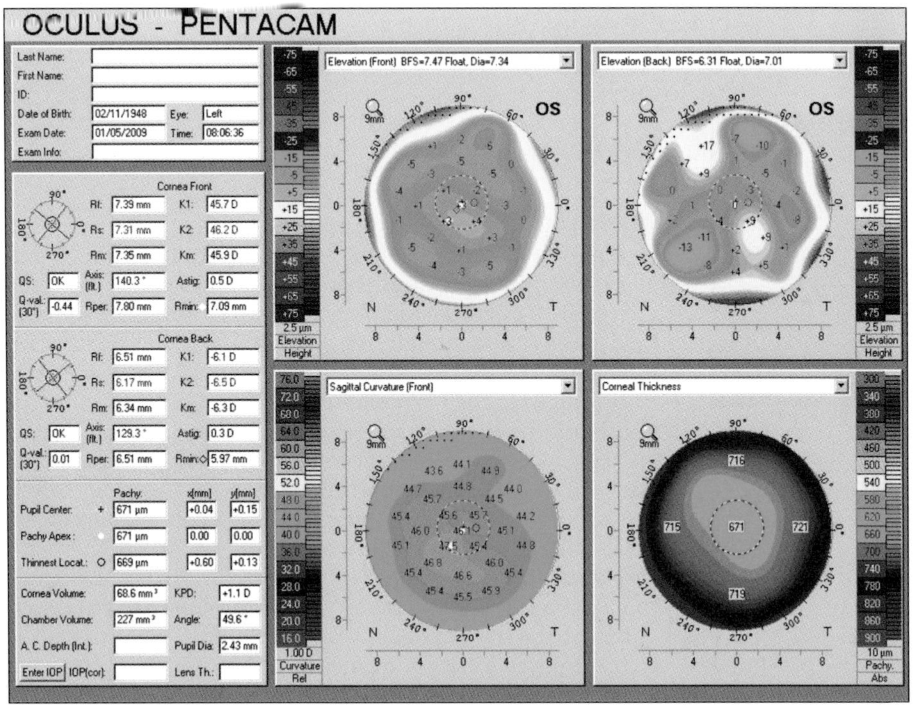

Fig. 87.6 Pentacam advanced imaging scan of the same eye demonstrating no signs of keratoconus.

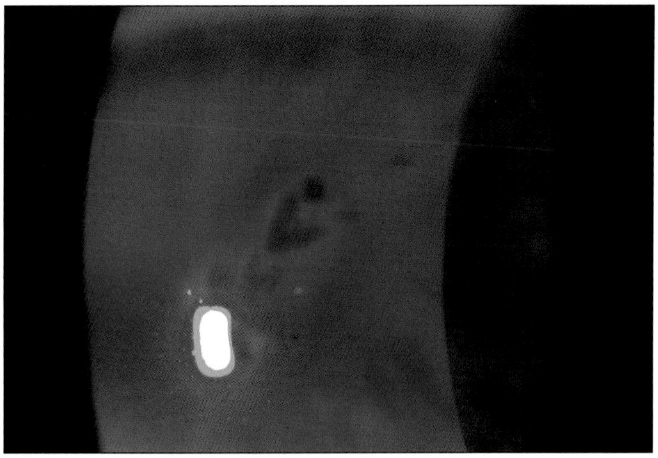

Fig. 87.7 Slit lamp appearance with thick fluorescein layer of localized area of abnormal, reduplicated epithelium in the same eye. Localized debridement improved the patient's vision and comfort.

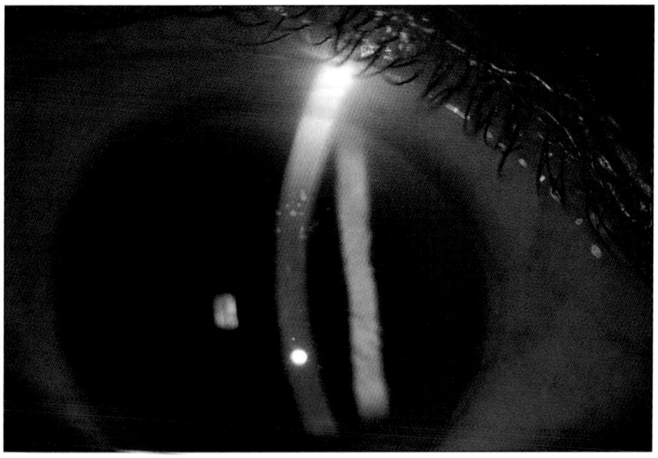

Fig. 87.8 Slit lamp appearance of a patient with unexpected, increased astigmatism after LASIK with a corneal abrasion.

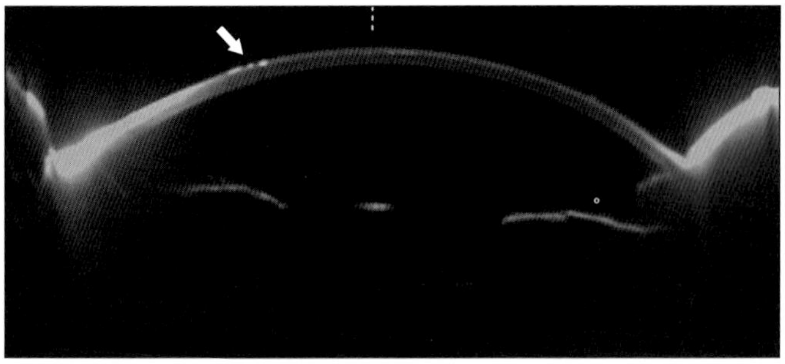

Fig. 87.9 Pentacam image of the reduplicated abnormal epithelium causing the astigmatism in the same eye as Figure 87.8. Debridement of this epithelium improved the astigmatism, vision, and comfort.

topical anesthetic. When discussing this procedure with patients, the term epithelial reinforcement may be substituted for stromal puncture to allay patient anxiety.[17] In my experience, for most patients the use of the word 'puncture' is the most frightening aspect of this technique. Before the

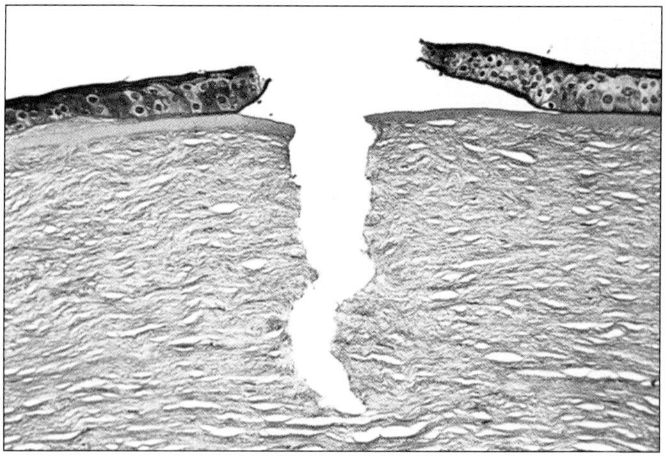

Fig. 87.10 Hematoxylin and eosin-stained human cadaver eye after stromal puncture with conventional straight needle. The mean penetration depth with this technique was 208 μm. (Original magnification ×50) (From Rubinfeld RS et al: Successful treatment of recurrent corneal erosion with Nd:YAG anterior stromal pressure. *Am J Ophthalmol* 111:252–254, 1991.)

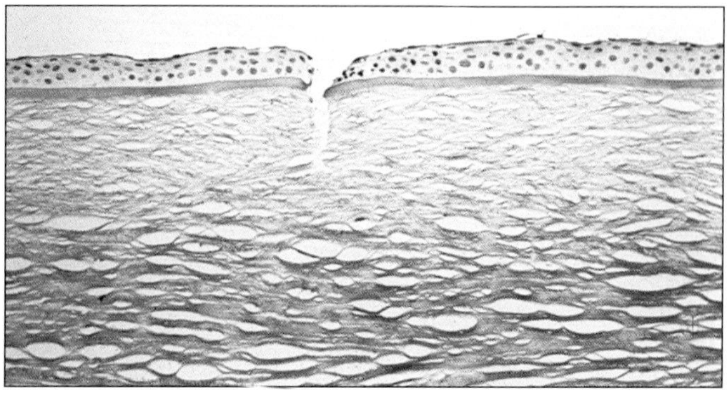

Fig. 87.11 Hematoxylin and eosin-stained histopathology slide of human cadaver eye after stromal puncture with a standardized specially designed needle. Mean penetration with this needle was 108 μm. (Original magnification ×50.) (From Rubinfeld RS et al: Successful treatment of recurrent corneal erosion with Nd:YAG anterior stromal pressure. *Am J Ophthalmol* 111:252–254, 1991.)

procedure (CPT Code 65600), the chart should be reviewed and drawings of previous erosions studied to determine the area to be treated. A careful preoperative slit lamp examination should also include retroillumination. Epithelial reinforcement may be performed either between erosive episodes or through loose, irregular epithelium during an active erosion without the need for debridement. Topical nonsteroidal drops such as ketorolac or diclofenac should be instilled every 10 to 15 minutes, starting 30 minutes to 1 hour before the procedure to aid in postoperative pain management. Also, several drops of a fluoroquinolone, or other broad-spectrum antibiotic, may be used preoperatively to reduce the likelihood of infection by decreasing the bacterial population of the external eye. Fortunately, however, infections after epithelial reinforcement (stromal puncture) are extremely rare.

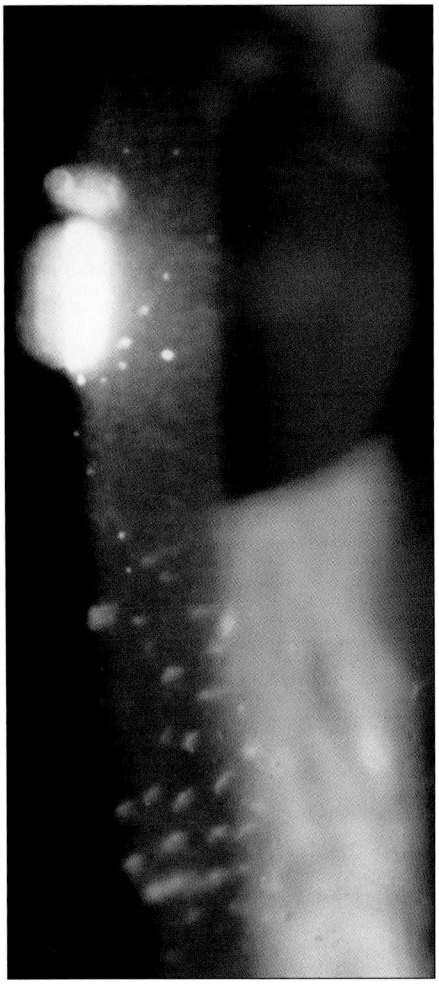

Fig. 87.12 Slit lamp photograph showing corneal scarring 3 months after anterior stromal puncture with a 25-gauge straight needle. This scarring faded slowly, becoming nearly invisible by 2 years after surgery. (From Rubinfeld RS et al: *Ophthalmic Surg* 21:318–326, 1990, by kind permission of Slack, Inc.)

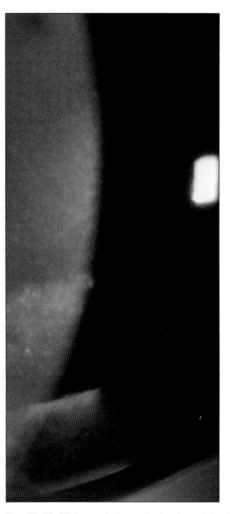

Fig. 87.13 Slit lamp photograph showing minimal corneal scarring only 2 weeks after anterior stromal puncture with a standardized, specially designed needle. This haze resolved completely by 2 months after surgery and was no longer visible by slit lamp examination. (From Rubinfeld RS et al: *Ophthalmic Surg* 21:318–326, 1990, by kind permission of SLACK, Inc.)

Fluorescein, along with several drops of topical anesthetic, should be applied to help visualize the puncture marks. The patient is admonished not to move or blink without warning the surgeon and is assured that the procedure itself is completely painless because of the use of the topical anesthetic. A drop of anesthetic in the nonoperative eye may help to control the urge to blink during the procedure. The standardized disposable stromal puncture needle* is mounted on a tuberculin syringe. The angled tip of the needle is kept perpendicular to the surface of the cornea and a few punctures are made. It is helpful to pause at this point to confirm for the patient that the procedure is truly painless. Patient anxiety will thereby be lessened and cooperation enhanced. Generally, the design of the needle prohibits the patient from even visualizing the device during the procedure, which also helps allay patient anxiety (Fig. 87.14).

Closely placed, generally nonconfluent punctures should cover the entire erosive area and should also include 1–2 mm of apparently normal margins outside the visible limits of the erosive area. Treatment of these apparently normal margins is necessary because the loose epithelium usually extends beyond the visible limits of the erosion, as can sometimes be demonstrated by retroillumination (Fig. 87.15). Treatment within the pupillary space should be minimized if possible, although in our experience subjective and objective glare testing has revealed no problems in patients who have been treated with the standardized needle in the pupillary space.[16] A topical antibiotic drop or ointment such as tobramycin ointment or fluoroquinolone drops, a cycloplegic agent such as scopolamine 0.25%, and more topical nonsteroidal drops are instilled postoperatively. A hydrophilic bandage lens can be applied and left in place for 1 or 2 days, but this may increase the risks of postoperative infection and, in the author's experience, this has not

* Available from Sharpoint Surgical Specialties Corporation, Reading, PA (order number 3800) 1.800.523.3332 www.surgicalspecialties.com (or www.angiotech.com) or Bausch and Lomb/Storz, Rochester, NY (Stromal Puncture Cannula) 1.800.338.2020 (order number E7185) www.storz.com.

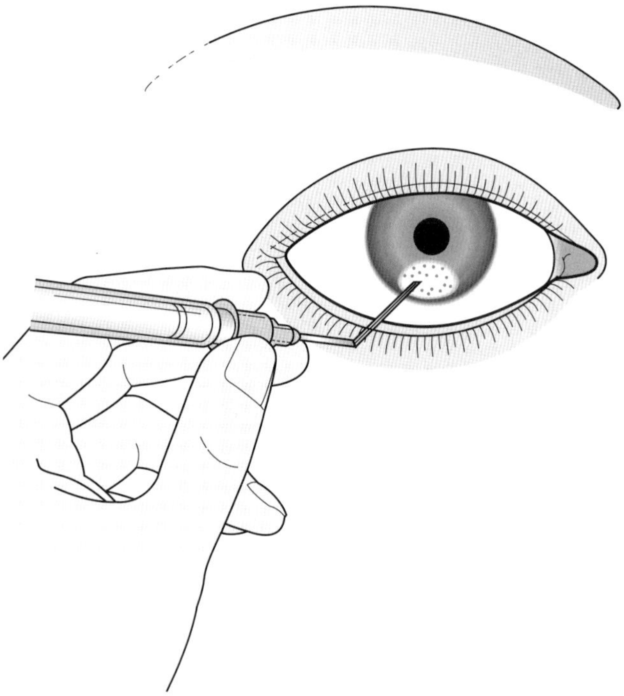

Fig. 87.14 Epithelial reinforcement technique (stromal puncture). The two preset bends in the standardized needle prevent the patient from visualizing the needle tip and shaft, thereby reducing patient anxiety. (From Rubinfeld RS: Recurrent corneal erosion. In Roy FH, editor: *Master techniques in ophthalmic surgery*, Baltimore, 1995, Williams & Wilkins.)

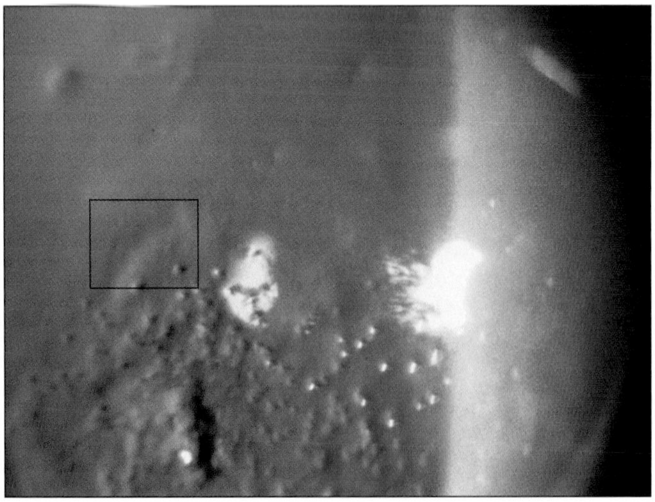

Fig. 87.15 Retroillumination slit lamp photograph taken immediately after anterior stromal puncture. Note that the area of anterior basement membrane abnormality (*box*) extends beyond the limits of the treated fluorescein-stained erosive epithelium. (Reproduced from Rubinfeld RS et al: Anterior stromal puncture for recurrent erosion: further experience and new instrumentation, *Ophthalmic Surg* 21:318–326, 1990, by kind permission of Slack Inc.)

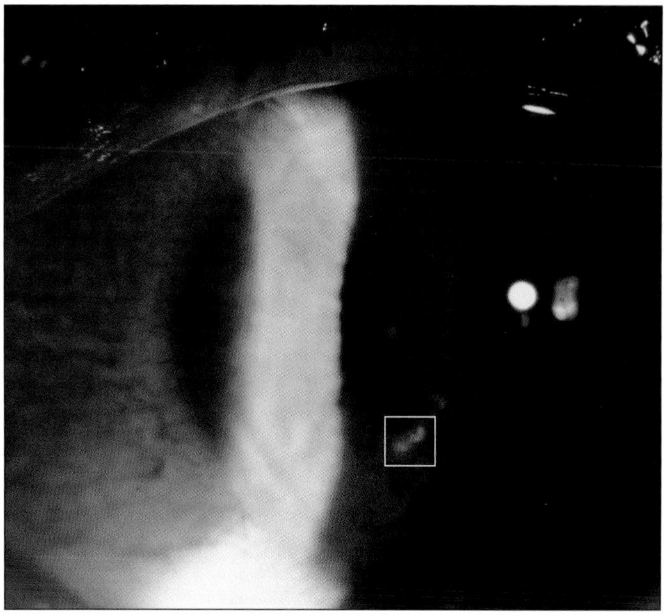

Fig. 87.16 Slit lamp photograph of small erosion (*box*) that occurred 4 days after stromal puncture in an untreated area adjacent to the original erosion. This is the same patient as shown in Figure 87.15. (Reproduced from Rubinfeld RS et al: Anterior stromal puncture for recurrent erosion: further experience and new instrumentation, *Ophthalmic Surg* 21:318–326, 1990, by kind permission of Slack Inc.)

improved postoperative comfort significantly. Patients may use the topical nonsteroidal agent up to three times daily as needed for pain over the next 2 to 3 days. Alternatively, the eye may be patched without a bandage lens after the nonsteroidal and antibiotic drops or ointments are instilled. Oral oxycodone or codeine–acetaminophen tablets or a systemic nonsteroidal agent should be prescribed. Once reepithelialization has occurred, hyperosmotic ointments are used three or four times daily to lubricate and protect the delicate healing epithelial tissue for several weeks postoperatively. Hyperosmotic ointments should then consistently be used at bedtime for 6 to 12 months (and occasionally longer) after stromal puncture while attachment complexes and other ultrastructural components are re-forming to achieve maximal epithelial adhesion.

Postoperatively, following micropuncture it is not uncommon for patients to experience a foreign body sensation and occasionally some subtle discomfort on awakening in the morning or at other times when the eye is poorly lubricated. Also, patients often experience an 'awareness' of the eye for many months or more after their erosions resolve. As with most erosion patients, this is particularly noticeable on exposure to wind or dry air currents. In our experience with several years' follow-up, a single anterior stromal puncture (epithelial reinforcement) procedure is effective approximately 80% of the time in selected recurrent erosion patients.[18,19] Treatment failure generally tends to occur when the surgeon treats too small an area, and erosions then develop outside of the treated area (Fig. 87.16). A second, larger treatment can often resolve the erosions in patients in whom the initial epithelial

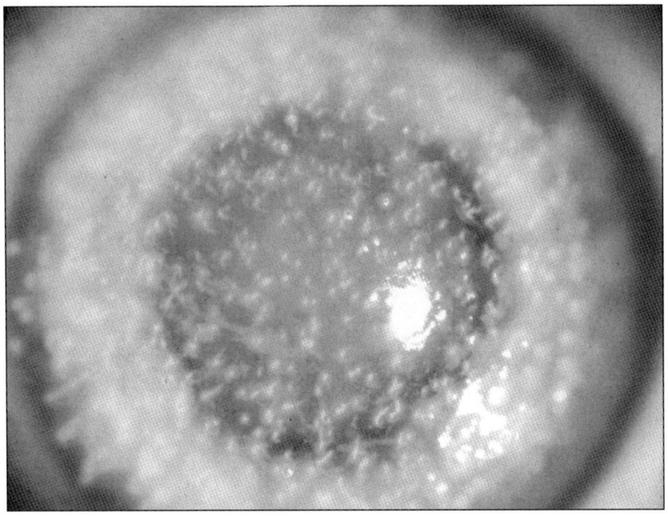

Fig. 87.17 Slit lamp photograph taken immediately after epithelial reinforcement in a patient with moderate degrees of diffuse basement membrane dystrophy and multiple recurrent corneal erosions. This technique has been dubbed 'pancorneal puncture.'

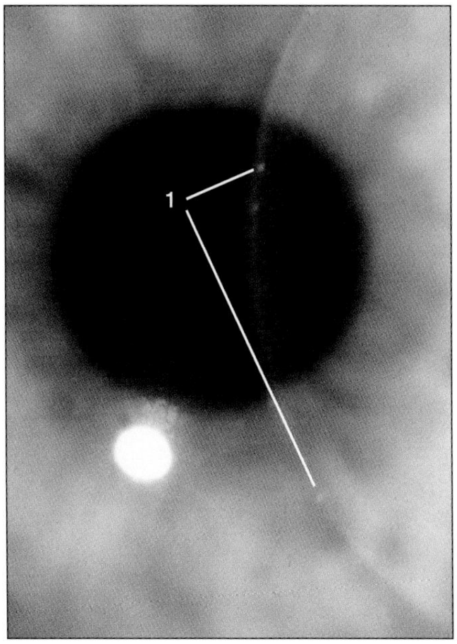

Fig. 87.18 Slit lamp photograph of the same patient as in Figure 87.17 taken 2 months after pancorneal puncture treatment. The patient is completely free of erosions at this point and remains so throughout 2 years of follow-up. Note that almost no scarring (*1*) is visible.

reinforcement procedure was unsuccessful. The optimum candidate for anterior stromal puncture or epithelial reinforcement is the patient with a single persistent area of erosion associated with previous trauma or minimal anterior basement membrane dystrophy.

A technique dubbed pancorneal puncture by MacRae, in which large areas of the cornea are treated in patients with moderate amounts of basement membrane dystrophy, can be quite effective (Figs 87.17, 87.18). Patients with severe basement membrane dystrophy, however, with consequent loss of visual acuity and numerous spontaneous, multifocal erosions are better candidates for superficial keratectomy than anterior stromal puncture.

Although the efficacy of anterior stromal puncture has been established, the mechanism of action of this technique has not been fully elucidated. It has been postulated that multiple plugs of epithelium fill the puncture sites and function as a series of 'spot welds,' focally binding the loosened sheets of corneal epithelium to the underlying edematous stroma until more normal ultrastructural architecture and attachment complexes can form.[15,20] Katsev et al.[21] described a case of stromal puncture in which punctures of 0.1 mm depth caused a fibrotic reaction and new basement membrane formed as well. Hsu et al.[22] performed electron microscopic and immunohistochemical studies of stromal puncture in human corneas with bullous keratopathy. Fibronectin, type IV collagen, and laminin were found within the puncture sites and in the reactive subepithelial pannus adjacent to the puncture site. They postulated that stimulation of production of these extracellular matrix proteins may be important in the attachment of epithelial cells to the underlying connective tissue. Epithelial–stromal reactions in the development of subepithelial fibrosis may also play a role in reestablishing epithelial attachment.

Encouraged by the success of anterior stromal puncture in recurrent erosion patients without corneal dystrophies and in those with basement membrane dystrophy, some surgeons have used this technique on patients whose corneal erosions are associated with bullous keratopathy. Although corneal stromal edema is generally well tolerated, rupture of epithelial bullae and the resulting corneal erosions in these patients can be very painful. For some of these bullous keratopathy patients with erosions who are poor candidates for penetrating keratoplasty because of poor visual potential or medical contraindications, stromal puncture has been shown to be a useful treatment.[15,18,22,23] Epithelial reinforcement can also be used to control painful erosions in patients with bullous keratopathy who are awaiting corneal transplantation. The optimum candidates for this type of treatment are those whose bullae are localized[22,23] and not diffusely distributed throughout the cornea (Figs 87.19, 87.20).

YAG laser procedures

Several investigators have suggested the use of YAG laser treatments for resistant corneal erosions. Geggel[24] initially proposed a technique in which epithelial debridement was performed and then photodisruption of the anterior corneal stroma was induced with the YAG laser. Katz et al.[25] reported modifying the procedure so that debridement was not necessary. They renamed this technique Nd:YAG laser photo-induced adhesion. Extensive experience and long-term follow-up are not available with these techniques, and they involve more expensive technology than stromal puncture.[16] However, these approaches, especially the technique that eliminates the need for debridement, may have some role in the treatment of patients with resistant corneal erosions.

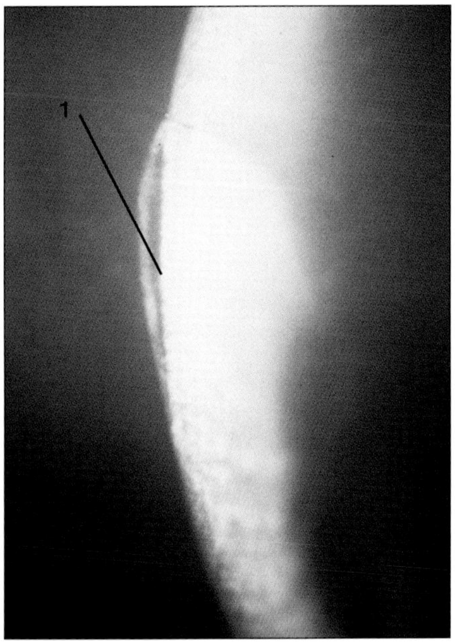

Fig. 87.19 Slit lamp photograph of patient with bullous keratopathy and secondary painful corneal erosions. Note bullous elevation of the corneal epithelium (*1*). (Reproduced from Hsu JKW et al: Anterior stromal puncture. Immunohistochemical studies in human corneas. *Arch Ophthalmol* 111:1057–1063, 1993. © 1993 American Medical Association. All rights reserved.)

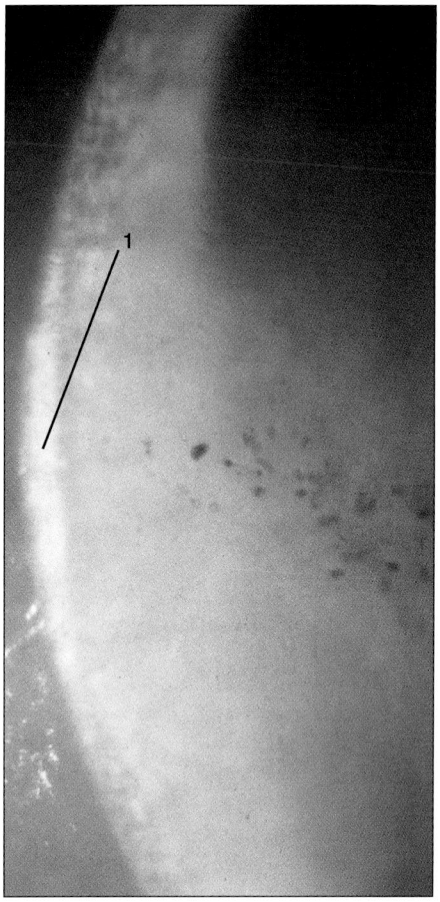

Fig. 87.20 Slit lamp photograph of the same patient as in Figure 87.19, 8 months after anterior stromal puncture treatment. This patient remained free of any further painful corneal erosions for over 4 years of follow-up. Note the resolution of the subepithelial bullae and the formation of subepithelial fibrosis/pannus (*1*). (Reproduced from Hsu JKW et al: Anterior stromal puncture. Immunohistochemical studies in human corneas. *Arch Ophthalmol* 111:1057–1063, 1993. © 1993 American Medical Association. All rights reserved.)

Excimer phototherapeutic keratectomy

The ArFl excimer laser has been used to treat patients with recurrent corneal erosions.[26–28] This application of the excimer laser is covered more extensively elsewhere in Chapter 89. However, a limited discussion of this approach is appropriate here. Phototherapeutic keratectomy (PTK) using the excimer laser involves treating Bowman's layer or anterior stroma, resulting in an ultramicroscopically modified, roughened surface to anchor the corneal epithelium.[29] This approach involves extremely expensive technology, and clinical experience, and long-term follow-up data are limited. Also, surgical technique and success rates vary widely with individual surgeons, patient characteristics, and laser techniques. One group of investigators has, in fact, reported that symptoms of recurrent erosion were more common and more pronounced in patients who had PRK than in patients who had LASIK for the correction of myopia.[30]

The patient's epithelium is usually removed mechanically by scraping with a spatula or blade, since using the laser to ablate the epithelium in patients with severe basement membrane dystrophy can induce irregularities in the deeper corneal tissues. Development of better coupling or masking agents may eliminate this problem in the future. Once the epithelium is removed, the laser is used to treat or 'dust' Bowman's layer.

Excimer PTK usually results in a postoperative refractive shift toward hyperopia. In patients with myopia and corneal erosions associated with marked basement membrane dystrophy the excimer laser can be used to perform a combined PTK and photorefractive keratectomy (PRK) procedure. In this case, the PRK parameters and techniques are determined in part by the patient's preoperative refractive status. Combining PTK and PRK can reduce or eliminate ametropia, improve the best corrected vision by reducing the surface irregularity of the dystrophic epithelium, and resolve the recurrent corneal erosions. Postoperatively, bandage contact lenses along with topical nonsteroidal agents and antibiotics are generally used.

Despite questions regarding cost, refractive shift, long-term success rates, and wide variation in technique, excimer PTK may be an important treatment for recurrent erosions, especially in patients whose corneal erosions are associated with marked basement membrane dystrophy and ametropia. In addition, patients with corneal erosions caused by other corneal dystrophies, such as superficial variant of granular dystrophy, Reis-Bücklers' dystrophy, and other similar conditions involving the anterior cornea, may be excellent candidates for excimer PTK.

Disclaimer

The author has no proprietary interest in any of the devices or techniques described herein.

References

1. Trobe JD, Laibson PR. Dystrophic changes in the anterior cornea. *Arch Ophthalmol.* 1972;87:378–382.
2. Werblin TP, et al. Prevalence of map-dot-fingerprint changes in the cornea. *Br J Ophthalmol.* 1981;65:401–409.
3. Foulks GN. Treatment of recurrent corneal erosion and corneal edema with topical osmotic colloidal solution. *Ophthalmology.* 1981;88:801–803.
4. Benitez del Castillo JM, et al. Treatment of recurrent corneal erosions using autologous serum. *Cornea.* 2002;21:781–783.
5. Dursun D, Kim MC, Solomon A. Treatment of recalcitrant recurrent erosions with inhibitors of matrix metalloproteinase-9, doxycycline, and corticosteroids. *Am J Ophthalmol.* 2001;132:781–783.
6. Thoft RA, Mobilia EF. Complications with therapeutic extended-wear soft contact lenses. *Int Ophthalmol Clin.* 1981;21:197–208.
7. Williams R, Buckley RJ. Pathogenesis and treatment of recurrent erosion. *Br J Ophthalmol.* 1985;69:435–437.
8. Trobe JD, Laibson PR. Dystrophic changes in the anterior cornea. *Arch Ophthalmol.* 1972;87:378–382.
9. Galbavy EJ, Mobilia EF, Kenyon KR. Recurrent corneal erosions. *Int Ophthalmol Clin.* 1984;24:107–131.
10. Buxton JN, Constad WH. Superficial epithelial keratectomy in the treatment of epithelial basement membrane dystrophy. *Ann Ophthalmol.* 1987;19:92–96.
11. Forstot SL, et al. Diamond burr keratectomy for the treatment of recurrent erosion syndrome. *Ophthalmology.* Sept 1994;(Suppl): poster.
12. Dua HS, et al. Alcohol delamination of the corneal epithelium: an alternative in the management of recurrent corneal erosions. *Ophthalmology.* 2006;113:404–411.
13. McLean EN, MacRae SM, Rich LF. Recurrent erosion: treatment by anterior stromal puncture. *Ophthalmology.* 1986;93:784–788.
14. Laibson PR. Recurrent erosion: treatment by anterior stromal puncture; discussion. *Ophthalmology.* 1986;93:787–788.
15. Rubinfeld RS, et al. Anterior stromal puncture for recurrent erosion: further experience and new instrumentation. *Ophthalmic Surg.* 1990; 21:318–326.
16. Rubinfeld RS, MacRae SM, Laibson PR. Correspondence regarding successful treatment of recurrent corneal erosion with Nd:YAG anterior stromal puncture. *Am J Ophthalmol.* 1991;111:252–254, (letter).
17. Lindstrom RL. Personal communication, June 23, 1994.
18. Rubinfeld RS. Recurrent corneal erosion. In: Roy FH, ed. *Master techniques in ophthalmic surgery.* Baltimore: Williams & Wilkins; 1995.
19. Laibson PR. *Personal communication.* Oct 1991.
20. Judge D, et al. Anterior stromal micropuncture electron microscopic changes in the rabbit cornea. *Cornea.* 1991;10:418–423.
21. Katsev DA, et al. Recurrent corneal erosion: pathology of corneal puncture. *Cornea.* 1990;9:152–160.
22. Hsu JKW, et al. Anterior stromal puncture. Immunohistochemical studies in human corneas. *Arch Ophthalmol.* 1993;111:1057–1063.
23. Cormier G, et al. Anterior stromal punctures for bullous keratopathy. *Arch Ophthalmol.* 1996;114:654–658.
24. Geggel HS. Successful treatment of recurrent corneal erosion with Nd-YAG anterior stromal puncture. *Am J Ophthalmol.* 1990;110: 404–407.
25. Katz HR, et al. Nd:YAG laser photo-induced adhesion of the corneal epithelium. *Am J Ophthalmol.* 1994;118:612–622.
26. Campos M, et al. Clinical follow-up of phototherapeutic keratectomy for treatment of corneal opacities. *Am J Ophthalmol.* 1993;115:433–440.
27. Rapuano CJ, Laibson PR. Excimer laser phototherapeutic keratectomy. *CLAO J.* 1993;19:235–240.
28. Jain S, Austin DJ. Phototherapeutic keratectomy for treatment of recurrent corneal erosion. *J Cataract Refract Surg.* 1999;25:1610–1614.
29. Stein RM. Unpublished data.
30. Hovanesian JA, Sujal SS, Maloney RK. Symptoms of dry eye and recurrent erosion syndrome after refractive surgery. *J Cataract Refract Surg.* 2001;27:577–584.

Chapter 88

Filamentary Keratitis

Richard S. Davidson, Mark J. Mannis

Filamentary keratitis may present a therapeutic challenge for the treating ophthalmologist. Filamentary keratitis describes a condition in which filaments – adherent complexes of mucus and corneal epithelium – are present on the corneal surface. Although generally uncommon, filamentary keratitis is associated with a number of conditions in which the ocular surface is abnormal, and patients that are affected are highly symptomatic. There has been debate in the literature over the cause and pathophysiology of corneal filaments. Most agree, however, that filaments consist of a variable combination of degenerated epithelial cells and mucus that are firmly attached to the corneal surface at one end.[1–5] Filaments appear as small, gelatinous strands on the anterior surface of the cornea and may differ in size (as small as 0.5 mm and as long as 10 mm), shape, composition, and distribution.[6] Long-term treatment of filamentary keratitis is often challenging, and recurrences are common.

Background

Filamentary keratitis may occur whenever there is a disruption in the tear film or the corneal surface. The corneal epithelial surface consists of nonkeratinized, squamous epithelium five to seven cells thick. The basal cells comprise the innermost layer of the epithelium. As the surface is approached, cells undergo modification to wing cells and then to flattened squamous superficial epithelial cells. The basal epithelium is attached to the underlying cornea by basement membrane, hemidesmosomes, and anchoring fibrils. The superficial corneal epithelial cells are characterized by numerous microvilli that interdigitate with the mucus layer of the tear film.

Definition

There is some inconsistency in the literature regarding the exact definition of filaments. In all cases, filaments are attached to the corneal surface at their base. Consisting of degenerated epithelial cells surrounding a mucus core,[7] filaments may be broad and short or long and stringy. They may also take the form of broad-based plaques, variably covered with epithelium. The clinical variants observed are not cause specific, and most respond similarly to treatment.

Pathophysiology

Work by Zaidman et al.,[5] along with studies by Lohman et al.[1] and Maudgal et al.,[2] support the theory that abnormalities of the corneal surface are responsible for the origin of filaments. Microscopic analysis performed on postmortem eyes demonstrated scattered groups of inflammatory cells and fibroblasts just below the basement membrane of the corneal epithelium. These cells violated the epithelial basement membrane and infiltrated Bowman's membrane.[5] Vacuoles and fibrillar material replaced the epithelial basement membrane in segments. On the basis of these histologic findings, the authors hypothesized that an underlying process damages the basal epithelium, which leads to focal areas of basement membrane detachment. The raised epithelium then acts as a receptor site for mucus and degenerated cells (Fig. 88.1).[5] Tabery recently confirmed these findings with an in vivo photomicrographic study of the human cornea. Her study revealed that the in vivo morphology of filamentary keratitis is consistent with aggregations of mucus and cell debris adhering to the corneal surface.[8]

Filamentary keratitis is associated with a variety of disease processes (Box 88.1). The most frequently associated disorder is keratoconjunctivitis sicca with or without Sjögren's syndrome. However, filamentary keratitis has also been associated with recurrent erosion syndrome and epithelial keratitis of any cause.[6] There is evidence that a change in the ratio of mucus to aqueous may predispose to the formation of filaments.[9] A lack of tear production may result in the increased production of mucus by conjunctival goblet cells. Since mucus serves as a disposal system for exfoliated epithelial cells, the requisite elements for filament formation may be present in dry eye states.[10] An increase in the amount or viscosity of the lipid layer may fracture the mucus layer into strands and damage the epithelial layer. Changes in the chemical composition of the tear film may result in a shift in the glycoproteins produced. In certain pathologic corneal states, there is a shift toward sulfomucin, which is more viscous than the normally predominant sialomucin.[8–14] Furthermore, a change in the composition of the mucus layer may alter the polarity at the surface, which can lead to the adherence of mucus to the epithelium.[15] The epithelial surface of the cornea may be pathologic in some systemic disease states, offering the substrates and attachment sites for filaments. Finally, mechanical damage to the ocular

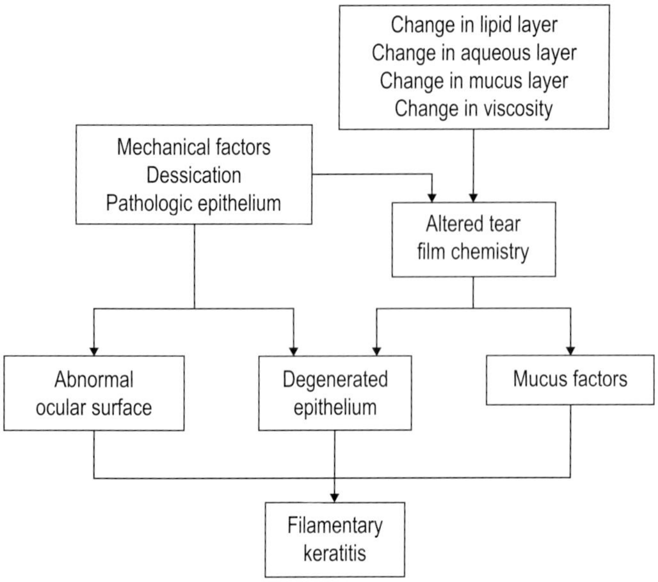

Fig. 88.1 Pathophysiology of filament formation. Filaments arise when there is an alteration of the composition of the tear film and an abnormal ocular surface.

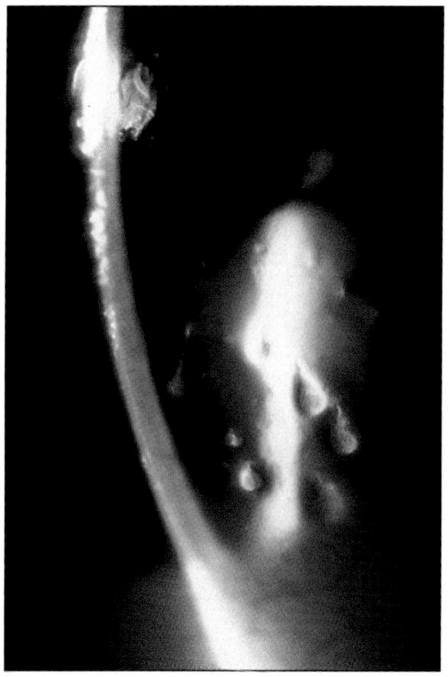

Fig. 88.2 Typical clinical appearance of filamentary keratitis.

Box 88.1 Associations with filamentary keratitis

Ocular trauma/surgery
- Abrasion/erosion
- Contact lens overwear
- Cataract extraction
- Penetrating keratoplasty

Ophthalmic disorders
- Keratoconjunctivitis sicca
- Superior limbic keratitis
- Neurotrophic keratopathy
- Prolonged patching
- Ptosis
- Aniridia
- Ocular albinism

Systemic disorders
- Sarcoid
- Diabetes mellitus
- Hereditary hemorrhagic telangiectasia
- Ectodermal dysplasia
- Psoriasis
- Atopic dermatitis
- Brain stem injury

Medication
- Diphenhydramine hydrochloride

surface can result in attachment sites for filaments. These variables of abnormal ocular surface, altered mucus or tear chemistry, and degenerated epithelium seem to comprise the final common pathway for filament formation.

Keratoconjunctivitis sicca is associated with a number of tear film abnormalities that predispose the corneal surface to filament formation. The aqueous tear deficiency both diminishes lubrication and also alters the viscosity of the mucus layer, leading to frequent epithelial defects. Moreoever, many patients have concurrent blepharitis and secrete an abnormally viscous, lipid layer that can attenuate the tear break-up time, fractionate the mucus layer, and desiccate the epithelial layer. The increased blink rate present in keratoconjunctivitis sicca may further injure a tenuous corneal surface.

Other clinical situations leading to desiccation of the ocular surface may lead to filament formation. These include the use of systemic anticholinergic drugs, seventh cranial nerve palsy, and severe intracranial or systemic disease with an altered mental status, resulting in decreased blink.[16] Seedor et al. reported a case of corneal filaments after the administration of diphenhydramine hydrochloride, perhaps secondary to its anticholinergic effect of decreased tear production.[17] Any trauma to the ocular surface may predispose to filament formation. Corneal abrasions or erosions may be accompanied by the development of filamentary keratitis. Contact lens overwear, likewise, has been implicated in filamentary keratitis, with corneal edema leading to an erosion, forming a site for filament formation.[18] Prolonged occlusion from ptosis, therapeutic patching, or severe strabismus may both damage and dry the surface.[19] Aniridia and ocular albinism have been associated with filaments, perhaps secondary to photophobia and blepharospasm, which may interfere with the competency of the epithelial barrier.[20] Tight apposition of the lids to the globe has been postulated as the cause of filament formation in superior limbic keratoconjunctivitis.

Surgical conditions have also been associated with filament formation. Dodds and Laibson reported several cases of filamentary keratitis after extracapsular cataract extraction.[20] They noted that filaments in these cases only occurred early in the postoperative course and only in the operated eye.[20] Filaments are commonly seen after penetrating keratoplasty (Fig. 88.2). Rotkis et al. reported a series of 114 patients who had had penetrating keratoplasty; 27% developed filaments.[21] Patients having penetrating keratoplasty for keratoconus were found to have the highest incidence of filament formation.[21] In addition, Mannis et al. showed that recipient age is of key importance in the development of surface disease, including filamentary keratitis following penetrating keratoplasty.[22] As donor epithelium is replaced with recipient epithelium in the corneal transplant bed, disruption of the ocular surface may foster filament formation. An interruption in corneal sensation in the postoperative period may also be a contributing factor. Fifth cranial nerve paralysis, ectodermal dysplasia, and herpetic infectious keratopathy may also contribute to neurotrophic keratitis and filament formation.

Miscellaneous clinical conditions have also been associated with corneal filaments. Wolper and Laibson reported a case of filamentary keratitis with hereditary hemorrhagic telangiectasia.[23] The authors postulated that conjunctival vascular abnormalities absorb constituents from the lipid or mucoid layer, altering the constituents of the tear film. Diabetes mellitus appears to cause a basic alteration in the epithelium and its attachment to the stroma.[15] In the case of irritant disorders, such as psoriasis or atopic diseases, goblet cells are triggered to increase mucus secretions in the setting of an already compromised surface.[19] Although the causes of filamentary keratitis are numerous, Hamilton and Wood described a case in which no cause could be identified; they called this essential filamentary keratitis.[24] Brain stem injury has also been associated with filamentary keratitis.[6]

The location of the filaments may provide a clue as to the cause. Filaments associated with keratoconjunctivitis sicca, pharmacologic dry eye, or exposure keratopathy are often found in the interpalpebral space. Filaments found on the superior cornea are associated with superior limbic keratoconjunctivitis, ptosis, or other causes of prolonged lid closure. Filaments after corneal transplantation are usually found on the graft in direct association with a suture or at the graft–host interface. After cataract extraction, filaments are usually found superiorly.

Clinical Manifestations

Symptoms of filamentary keratitis may vary from mild to severe foreign body sensation with photophobia, blepharospasm, and epiphora. The blepharospasm results from the pain caused by the filaments.[6] Symptoms are often most prominent with blinking, and patients may be less symptomatic with eyes closed.

Filaments generally vary in size from 0.5 mm to several millimeters in length (Fig. 88.3). There may be a small gray subepithelial opacity beneath the filament.[13] The filaments are generally firmly adherent to the cornea, although sometimes the force generated by blinking may break this attachment. This results in an epithelial defect that can perpetuate further filament formation.

Filaments stain with rose Bengal and less brightly with fluorescein. The underlying epithelial defect will stain prominently with fluorescein. The elevated filament appears as a dark spot in the fluorescein pool, producing negative fluorescein staining.

Treatment

The treatment of filamentary keratitis can be challenging. In rare circumstances, there is spontaneous resolution. In general, however, the treatment of filamentary keratitis is chronic and can be frustrating for both patient and ophthalmologist. Any underlying cause of filament formation, such as keratoconjunctivitis sicca, contact lens overwear, medication toxicity, or prolonged occlusion, should be identified and treated. Recently Kakizaki et al. showed improvement in filamentary keratitis by performing blepharoptosis surgery on two patients in whom they felt blepharoptosis was the underlying cause for the filamentary keratitis.[25]

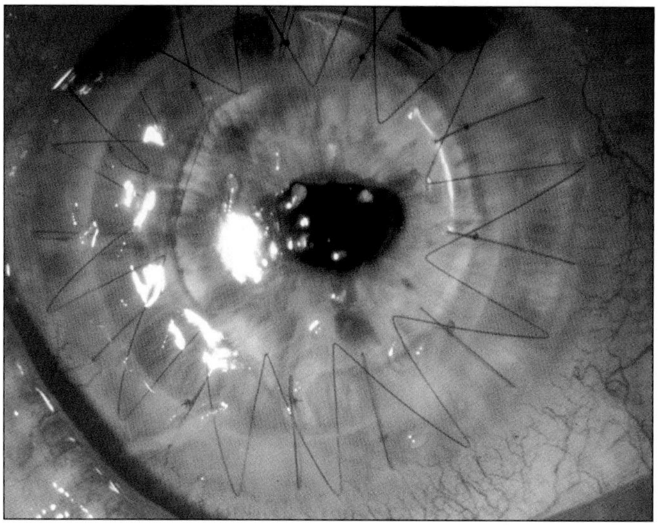

Fig. 88.3 Filamentary keratitis following penetrating keratoplasty.

Mechanical debridement of the filaments may be helpful as a temporizing measure but is rarely permanently successful. The filaments may be removed with a jeweler's or tying forceps. Care should be taken not to disrupt the epithelium at the base of the filament, since this may provide receptor sites for new filaments.

Topical tear substitutes administered throughout the day in conjunction with ointments at bedtime may provide some symptomatic relief. Some patients benefit from more viscous tear substitute products. One should remember that ointments and viscous tear substitutes may also act to alter the composition of the tear film and further compound the problem. Care should be taken to use tear substitutes that do not contain preservatives that may be toxic to the epithelium. Newer, oil-based tear substitutes may provide additional relief by stabilizing the lipid layer of the tear film and preventing desiccation. Finally, punctal occlusion may be helpful in dry eye states.

Hamilton and Wood reported a 95% success rate with the use of 5% sodium chloride ophthalmic solution, administered topically three to four times daily.[24] The ointment form may be used at night. This regimen appears to work directly at the level of the corneal epithelium by reducing edema and promoting better adhesion. Another hypothesis is that conjunctival interstitial fluid is drawn osmotically to the corneal surface, reversing the dry eye state.[26] Hypotonic preparations that provide a fluid gradient to increase surface lubrication have also been used.

N-acetylcysteine (10%) has been used successfully to treat filamentary keratitis.[26] Acetylcysteine is a sulfhydryl compound that serves as a mucolytic agent by decreasing the viscosity of mucus. The ocular solution is a respiratory preparation without preservative but can be stored safely in the refrigerator for 3 to 4 weeks.

Bloomfield et al. have advocated the use of a bandage soft contact lens.[27] They reported 100% success in treating a series of 20 patients. The soft contact lenses were removed within 24 hours of the disappearance of filaments. Patients were treated with topical corticosteroids and artificial tears to decrease inflammation and increase lubrication. The contact lens appears to protect against the shearing forces of the lids.[27] The contact lens should have a high oxygen permeability and should be well lubricated with frequent topical artificial tears. The ideal contact lens for this purpose is a thin, low water content, hydrogel soft contact lens. Bloomfield et al. noted that none of their patients had recurrences of filamentary keratitis. However, these patients must be monitored closely due to the risk of complications from prolonged contact lens wear.

Recently, Hadassah et al. evaluated the functionality of using a succinylated collagen bandage lens (SCBL) in the treatment of filamentary keratitis. While this study did show that the use of these lenses was well-tolerated and maintained good transparency, it did not comment on the effectiveness of the lens in treating the filamentary keratitis.[28]

Grinbaum et al. have shown success in the treatment of filamentary keratitis with the use of 0.1% diclofenac sodium either as a sole treatment or in conjunction with other modalities.[29] Avisar et al. demonstrated diclofenac sodium 0.1% to be as effective as sodium chloride 5% drops in the treatment of filamentary keratitis. In their study of 32 patients, the 16 patients that received diclofenac sodium 1% had a significantly more rapid improvement of the clinical symptoms as compared with those receiving topical sodium chloride 5%.[30] Additional treatments without proven value include pharmacologically active peptides such as eledoisin,[31] beta irradiation,[32] topical heparin, topical dextran, and systemic mucolytics.

Summary

Filamentary keratitis is a clinical entity encountered in various corneal conditions. These conditions have in common a disruption of the ocular surface and the precorneal tear film. There is a wide range of clinical anatomic variants, and it can be a frustrating ocular condition because of the severity of symptoms and the chronicity of the problem.

References

1. Lohman LE, Rao GN, Aquavella JV. In vivo microscopic observations of human corneal epithelial abnormalities. *Am J Ophthalmol.* 1982;93:210–217.
2. Maudgal PC, Missotten L, Van Deuren H. Study of filamentary keratitis by replica technique. *Graefe's Arch Ophthalmol.* 1979;211:11–21.
3. Theodore FH. Filamentary keratitis. *Contact Lens J.* 1982;8:137–146.
4. Thygeson P. Filamentary keratitis. *Trans Am Acad Ophthalmol Otolaryngol 112th Meeting.* 1963.
5. Zaidman GW, et al. The histopathology of filamentary keratitis. *Arch Ophthalmol.* 1985;103:1178–1181.
6. Tuberville AW, Wood TO. Filamentary keratitis. In: Fraunfelder FT, Roy FH, eds. *Current Ocular Therapy 2.* Philadelphia: WB Saunders; 1985.
7. Lamberts DW. Dry eye syndromes. In: Foster CS, ed. *Corneal and external disease.* Chicago: Year Book; 1985.
8. Tabery, HM. Filamentary keratopathy: a non-contact photomicrographic in vivo study in the human cornea. *Eur J Ophthalmol* 2003;13(7):599–605.
9. Wright P. Filamentary keratitis. *Trans Ophthalmol Soc UK.* 1975;95(2):260–266.
10. Adams AD. The morphology of human conjunctival mucus. *Arch Ophthalmol.* 1979;97(4):730–734.
11. Theodore FH. Corneal filaments. *Eye Ear Nose Throat Monthly.* 1966;45(9):104.
12. Weskamp C. Parenchymatous origin of filamentary keratitis; new histopathologic concepts. *Am J Ophthalmol.* 1956;42:115–120.
13. Jones B, Coop H. The management of keratoconjunctivitis sicca. *Trans Ophthalmol Soc UK.* 1965;42:115–120.
14. Wright P, Mackie IA. Mucus in the healthy and diseased eye. *Trans Ophthalmol Soc UK.* 1978;98(3):335–338.
15. Holly FJ. Biophysical aspects of epithelial adhesion to stroma. *Invest Ophthalmol Vis Sci.* 1978;17(6):552–557.
16. Davis W, Drewry R, Wood T. Filamentary keratitis and stromal neovascularization associated with brain stem injury. *Am J Ophthalmol.* 1980;90:489–491.
17. Seedor JA, et al. Filamentary keratitis associated with diphenhydramine hydrochloride. *Am J Ophthalmol.* 1986;101(3):376–377.
18. Dada V, Zisman Z. Contact lens induced filamentary keratitis. *Am J Optom Physiol Optics.* 1975;52:545–546.
19. Good WV, Whitcher JP. Filamentary keratitis caused by corneal occlusion. *Ophthalmic Surg.* 1992;23(1):66.
20. Dodds H, Laibson P. Filamentary keratitis following cataract extraction. *Arch Ophthalmol.* 1972;88:609–612.
21. Rotkis W, Chandler J, Forstot S. Filamentary keratitis following penetrating keratoplasty. *Ophthalmology.* 1982;89:946–949.
22. Mannis MJ, et al. Preoperative risk factors for surface disease after penetrating keratoplasty. *Cornea.* 1997;16(1):7–11.
23. Wolper JW, Laibson PR. Hereditary hemorrhagic telangiectasis (Rendu-Osler-Weber disease) with filamentary keratitis. *Arch Ophthalmol.* 1969;81:272–277.
24. Hamilton W, Wood TO. Filamentary keratitis. *Am J Ophthalmol.* 1982;93:466–469.
25. Kakizaki H, et al. Filamentary keratitis improved by blepharoptosis surgery: two cases. *Acta Ophthalmol Scand.* 2003;81(6):669–671.
26. Marsh P, Pflugfelder SC. Topical nonpreserved methylprednisolone therapy for keratoconjunctivitis sicca in Sjögren syndrome. *Ophthalmology.* 1999;106(4):811–816.
27. Bloomfield SE, et al. Treatment of filamentary keratitis. *Am J Ophthalmol.* 1973;76(6):978–980.
28. Hadassah J, et al. Clinical evaluation of succinylated collagen bandage lenses for ophthalmic applications. *Ophthalmic Res.* 2008; 40:257–266
29. Grinbaum A, et al. The beneficial effect of diclofenac sodium in the treatment of filamentary keratitis. *Arch Ophthalmol.* 2001;119(6):926–927.
30. Avisar, R, et al. Diclofenac sodium, 0.1% (Voltaren Ophtha), versus sodium chloride, 5%, in the treatment of filamentary keratitis. *Cornea.* 2000;19(2):145–147.
31. Jaeger W, Gotz M, Kaercher T. Eledoisin. A successful therapeutic concept for filamentary keratitis. *Trans Ophthalmol Soc UK.* 1985;104:496.
32. Winters DM, Asbury T. Filamentary keratitis. Response to beta radiation. *Am J Ophthalmol.* 1961;51:1292.

Chapter 89

Thygeson's Superficial Punctate Keratitis

Ivan R. Schwab, Ana Carolina Vieira

The superficial punctate keratitis of Thygeson is an uncommon epithelial keratopathy of unknown cause. It has no known association with other ocular or systemic disease. It is characterized by a coarse punctate epithelial keratitis with little or no hyperemia of the bulbar or palpebral conjunctiva. This condition is paradoxical, as it is often considered to be infectious in origin (but not so proven) and yet is successfully treated with corticosteroids. It appears to be an active keratitis but incites no neovascularization. This disorder is an enigmatic disease that is often misdiagnosed.

History

In 1889, Ernst Fuchs[1] first defined the term keratitis punctata superficialis or superficial punctate keratitis (SPK). He used the term to describe an epidemic keratoconjunctivitis that affected patients in the Third Clinic in Vienna. Although the condition was usually bilateral, it began unilaterally and was worse in the first eye to be affected. These patients had an associated follicular conjunctivitis and punctate keratitis. We now believe these patients had epidemic keratoconjunctivitis (EKC), and that this epidemic was probably caused by a strain of adenovirus. Subsequently, the term EKC was employed to describe such epidemics, and the term SPK was no longer used.

In 1950, Phillips Thygeson first reported 26 cases of what has become known as superficial punctate keratitis of Thygeson (SPKT). Some of these patients had been followed in his office for as long as 24 years.[2] In this initial publication, Thygeson discussed the individual lesions in detail. He described individual evanescent opacities that would change position over time. He noted that each opacity comprised a group of smaller intraepithelial opacities. There was little edema and no cellular infiltration. He noted mild conjunctival inflammation accompanying the lesions, with a mild papillary response on the palpebral surface of the upper lid. In this initial publication, Thygeson discussed the term superficial punctate keratitis (SPK). Despite Thygeson's description of SPKT, the term superficial punctate keratitis has been, and continues to be, used incorrectly to describe many different forms of superficial keratitis.[3]

In 1961, Thygeson added 29 cases and described the five diagnostic features that differentiate SPKT from other epithelial keratopathies: (1) a chronic, bilateral, punctate epithelial keratitis; (2) long duration with remissions and exacerbations; (3) eventual healing without scars; (4) lack of response to systemic or topical antibiotics or sulfonamides or to the removal of the corneal epithelium; and (5) a striking symptomatic response to topical corticosteroids.[3]

In 1963, Jones[4] reported 27 cases of SPKT and added additional features to the physical findings. He reported a faint opacification of the superficial stroma underlying the epithelial opacity. He believed this stromal change had the gray appearance of lamellar separation caused by edema, rather than the hard or dotlike appearance of cellular infiltration. Additionally, in retroillumination this stromal change was transparent or translucent, suggesting edema. Jones also emphasized that the disease should be called SPKT and that SPK should not be used to describe other forms of keratitis.[5]

In 1966, Thygeson[6] described another 27 previously unreported cases and distinguished superior limbic keratoconjunctivitis from SPKT. Thygeson thought that a viral cause of SPKT was strongly suggested by: (1) the absence of bacteria or other microorganisms; (2) the resistance of the disease to antibacterial agents; (3) the scanty mononuclear cell exudate on conjunctival scrapings; and (4) the viral appearance of the epithelial lesions.[6]

In 1968, Quere et al.[7] described three stages in SPKT: (1) the onset, lasting 1–2 weeks, characterized by catarrhal inflammation, photophobia, and tearing; (2) a developmental stage of up to 8 months in which the signs of conjunctival inflammation disappeared, leaving the epithelial lesions; and (3) a stage of regression of several months to 3 years, during which the lesions became fewer in number and smaller until they finally vanished. Quere et al. also suggested that this disease was chronic.[7] The total duration of the disease in these patients, many of whom had been treated with steroids, ranged from 4 months to 30 years, with an average of 7.5 years and a median of 4 years. The longest reported case of SPKT was 40 years, reported by Tanzer and Smith in 1999.[8]

In 1971, Wakui et al.[9] described the ultrastructural characteristics of the disease. Their electron microscopic findings of the corneal epithelium from patients with SPKT failed to reveal viral particles but did show cell destruction confined to one discrete area, which contrasted with the cell-to-cell spread of herpes simplex keratitis.

In 1974, Lemp et al.[10] isolated varicella-zoster from a patient with SPKT, but this may have been a laboratory accident or even spontaneous shedding. Current investigators do not believe varicella-zoster virus to be a likely cause.

In 1981, Darrell[11] reviewed the disease and described 36 patients with SPKT in whom there was a significant incidence of the histocompatibility antigen HLA-DR3.

In 1981, Tabbara et al.[12] reported 45 cases. These authors believed that corticosteroids prolonged the course of the disease, based on the natural history of many of these patients compared to the reported natural history of the disease described by Thygeson before the introduction of corticosteroids.

In 2003, Watson et al.[13] performed confocal microscopy on six patients with SPKT and found changes not only in the corneal epithelium: irregular nerve fibers and haze in the subepithelial nerve plexus were also found. Generalized haze and areas of high reflectivity, microdots and reflective bodies in the anterior stroma, and keratocytes with reflective nuclei and cell bodies of irregular size and shape were also reported. The images suggested that wound healing and cell death were occurring in the anterior stroma. These findings were related to the duration of SPKT, were not seen in normal fellow eyes and were also present diffusely in areas without lesions.[13]

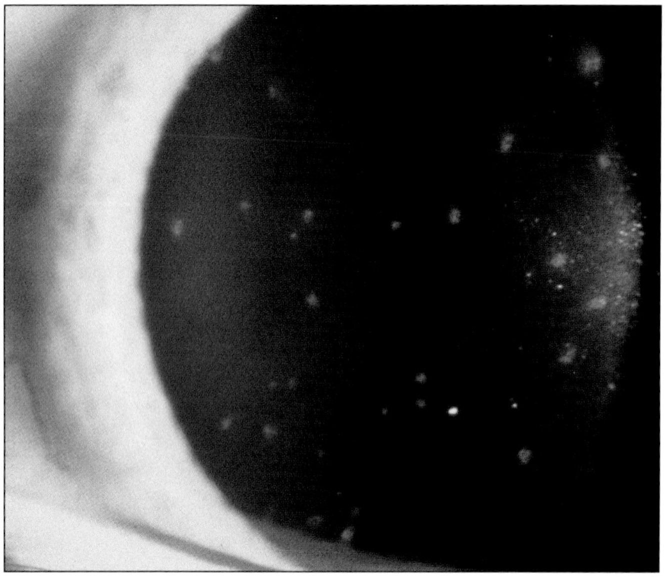

Fig. 89.1 Superficial punctate keratitis of Thygeson. Coarse epithelial keratitis with discrete round to oval lesions scattered diffusely across the cornea, although usually the lesions are concentrated in the central to paracentral cornea. The lesions are entirely intraepithelial, although there may be associated subepithelial haze or mild edema.

Epidemiology

Most authors report no sex predilection, although Darrell[11] did find a mild female preponderance (25 women and seven men). Van Bijsterveld et al.,[14] in a large series (54 cases) of SPKT, found significantly more women affected than men. These investigators also suggested that the median age of onset was younger for women than for men. Conversely, Tabbara et al.,[12] in his series of 45 patients, had 28 men and 17 women. Without gender-specific population rates or properly performed prevalence studies, however, these numbers mean very little. Patients have been reported ranging from as young as 2.5 years of age to over 70, with a mean age of 29.[15] The onset of the disease is frequently documented during the second and third decades.

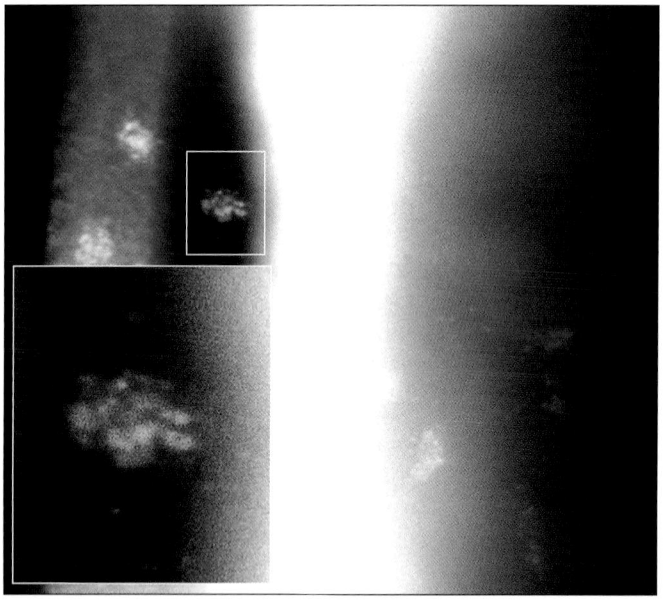

Fig. 89.2 Superficial punctate keratitis of Thygeson. A closer view of the individual lesions (box). Each discrete lesion is composed of many smaller grains, making a round to vertically oval translucent to opaque deposit.

Disease Course and Clinical Manifestations

Patients usually have a long history of exacerbations and spontaneous remissions of foreign body sensation. Other symptoms include photophobia, burning, tearing, and occasional blurring of vision.

The conjunctiva may be mildly injected or completely quiet. Classic clinical signs include oval or round, grouped punctate intraepithelial deposits composed of numerous discrete, fine, granular, white to gray, dotlike opacities (Figs 89.1 and 89.2). These three-dimensional opacities often have a raised center that breaks through the epithelial surface and may show tiny hairlike filaments that are almost certainly mucus. The corneal lesions may have a ragged edge or a stellate appearance that has, on occasion, led to an incorrect diagnosis of herpes simplex keratitis. Mild epithelial and subepithelial edema, without infiltration, is occasionally seen associated with the opacities. The opacities are evanescent and migratory, but favor the central cornea and visual axis. On average, there are 15–20 corneal lesions, but the range is between 1 and 50.[3,6,12] If the classic grouped intraepithelial deposits are not found on first examination, SPKT can still be considered based on atypical epithelial findings and a history of recurrent keratitis, absence of other corneal disease, and response to topical corticosteroids.[11] Salzmann's nodular degeneration has been reported in association with prolonged SPKT.[16]

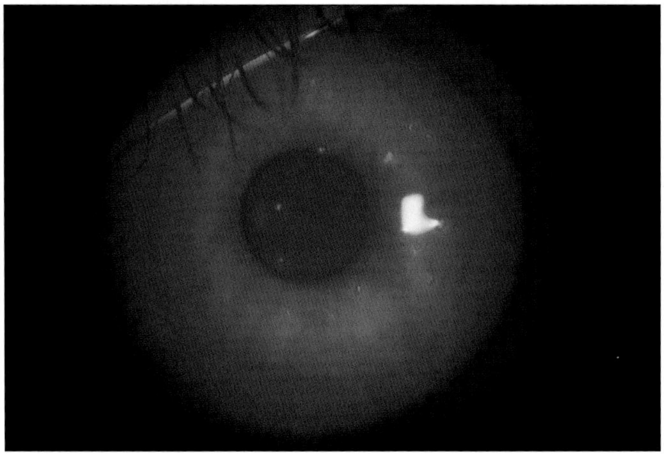

Fig. 89.3 Superficial punctate keratitis of Thygeson. During exacerbations, the focal opacities are elevated above the superficial epithelium and stain with fluorescein.

Untreated individual attacks usually last 1–2 months and then resolve, only to recur 6–8 weeks later. However, the time course is quite variable. During exacerbations these focal opacities are elevated above the superficial epithelium and stain with fluorescein (Fig. 89.3) and rose Bengal. During remissions, lesions may disappear completely unless subepithelial scarring has left a 'footprint.'[6] These inactive lesions appear to be flat, intraepithelial, gray dots and do not stain with fluorescein or rose Bengal. There may be periods of months to years with no visible lesions and no clinical symptoms.

Corneal sensation is not generally affected, although occasional patients have mild corneal hypesthesia.

This disease is almost exclusively bilateral, with only one in 20 patients having unilateral disease. There might, however, be marked asymmetry on presentation.[17]

Although the course is chronic and may last more than two decades, signs and symptoms often resolve spontaneously. Visual prognosis in patients with SPKT is generally excellent. Nagra et al.[17] found visual acuities of 20/30 or better during active disease in 80% of their patients, and improvement with treatment in patients whose initial visual acuities were between 20/40 and 20/50. A prolonged course may sometimes be complicated by topical treatment with steroids.

Differential Diagnosis

The differential diagnosis should not be difficult, as the disease is so distinctive. Thygeson suggested several possible diagnoses that might confuse the ophthalmologist, including the epithelial keratitis of staphylococcal blepharitis, pneumococcal conjunctivitis, seborrheic blepharitis, keratoconjunctivitis sicca, neurotrophic and exposure keratopathy, vernal keratitis, molluscum contagiosum, verruca, and occupational and traumatic keratopathy. Other observers have included herpes zoster and herpes simplex, recurrent erosion syndrome, rosacea, Reiter's syndrome, leprosy, and keratitis medicamentosa. It is most important to rule out herpes simplex keratitis as this is aggravated by topical corticosteroids, whereas SPKT benefits from their use.

Treatment

Low-dose topical corticosteroids are commonly used during acute exacerbations of SPKT. However, response to corticosteroids varies[18] and some believe the average course of the disease to be prolonged by corticosteroid therapy.[6,12] Corticosteroids should be used sparingly and in very low pulsed doses. Medrysone 1% has been used by the authors with success. Theoretically, because it has less antiinflammatory potency than dexamethasone 0.1%, there is less potential for corticosteroid-induced complications.

Therapeutic soft contact lenses offer an alternative treatment to be used during exacerbations.[18,19] These lenses offer immediate symptomatic relief and, usually, rapid resolution of the epithelial lesions, but may expose the patient to the complications of lens wear, including bacterial keratitis.[17,20]

Studies have reported good outcomes with the use of ciclosporin A.[21,22] Reinhard and Sundmacher[22] treated 31 eyes of 17 patients with SPKT using 2% topical ciclosporin A with a slow taper. Of the 31 eyes treated, 68% had complete suppression of SPKT after 4 weeks of therapy. The only reported side effect of ciclosporin was a burning sensation noted by all patients. Another immunosuppressant, FK506, has also been used to treat a patient with SPKT.[23]

Other topical agents have been tried with little or no success. Idoxuridine (IDU), specifically, may produce subepithelial scarring and is contraindicated.[5,12] Nesburn et al.[24] treated six eyes in four patients with SPKT with topical trifluridine 1% and reported improvement in five of them. However, the authors noted that the signs and symptoms disappeared more slowly than when treated with corticosteroids. Nesburn et al. concluded that trifluridine is an effective and safe alternative to corticosteroids, noting only mild irritation and transient limbal follicle formation as side effects.

Epithelial debridement has no effect on the course of the diasease. Chemical cauterization (previously done with iodine) of the active lesions does not improve symptoms and may produce scarring and even ulceration.[12]

Goldstein et al.[25] reported a case of SPKT that was successfully treated with combined PRK–PTK procedures. A case of recurrent SPKT in a patient submitted to PRK in one eye and LASIK in the fellow eye was reported and it was suggested that PRK may be a better option than LASIK in patients with this condition.[26]

Pathogenesis

The pathogenesis of SPKT is yet not understood. Conjunctival scrapings show scant mononuclear cells and corneal scrapings show slightly abnormal epithelial cells with vacuolated cytoplasm, occasional neutrophils, mononuclear cells, degenerating epithelial cells and mucus.[6] Bacterial cultures have shown normal conjunctival flora.[2] The epithelial basement membrane and its hemidesmosomal attachments are intact.[12]

In 1971, Wakui et al.[9] described the clinical and electron microscopy (EM) of SPKT. EM did not reveal virus particles and showed cell destruction confined to a single, discrete area, in contrast to the cell-to-cell spread of destruction observed in herpes simplex keratitis. Other investigators in more recent studies have also not detected viruses by electron microscopy.[12,18] Although in the past viruses have been isolated from corneas of patients with SPKT,[10,27] viral cultures performed by several different investigators have been negative.[3,6,7,11,12,15,18,28] Curiously, the lesions of SPKT do resemble viral lesions and the tendency to recur over years suggests a viral cause. Also, SPKT has several features in common with known viral infections of the cornea. These include intraepithelial lesions, the long duration, exacerbations and remissions, and a mononuclear cell response, all suggesting a latent virus or defective virion as the causative agent. Adenovirus and measles can have similar characteristics to SPKT. Human papillomavirus (HPV) has been mentioned as a possible source, as it causes minimal inflammation. We have examined corneal scrapings from two patients with SPKT using polymerase chain reaction to evaluate HPV as the infective agent, but both patients were negative with our testing. HPV remains an interesting possibility, however. Ostler[29] has suggested that a slow virus may be responsible.

In 1968 and 1973, Quere et al.[7,15] suggested an allergic cause, because some of their patients had eczema, urticaria, or asthma, and also because the lesions responded to corticosteroids. The lack of eosinophils in smears and the lack of other signs or symptoms of ocular allergy make this possibility less likely. Physical examination and clinical history have failed to reveal any consistent associated systemic disease. Van Bijsterveld evaluated plasma cortisol levels in patients with SPKT and found them to be within normal limits for both sexes, but significantly higher in females. In these same patients, the serum protein and protein fraction concentrations were normal.

HLA-DR3 antigens have been associated with SPKT.[11] An increased frequency of HLA-Dw3 and HLA-DR3 antigens is associated with several autoimmune diseases, including gluten-sensitive enteropathy, dermatitis herpetiformis, chronic hepatitis, Addison's disease, Sjögren's syndrome, Graves' disease, insulin-dependent diabetes mellitus, and systemic lupus erythematosus. For this reason, it is likely that an immune mechanism also plays a role in SPKT. Conceivably, SPKT may be caused by a common virus whose clinical effect on the corneal epithelium and stroma is determined by the presence of HLA-DR3. However, this is represented by a single study, and there has been no independent confirmation from other investigators. Indeed, certain features of SPKT imply an immune process. The lymphocytes in corneal epithelium, the marked effect of corticosteroids on the corneal lesions, and the chronic course of SPKT with remissions and exacerbations all suggest an immune mechanism.

Fite et al.[30] reported a case in which a patient with SPKT underwent photorefractive keratectomy for myopia. Seventeen months after surgery, symptomatic SPKT lesions occurred in the periphery but not in the treated central cornea. This suggests that an inflammatory signal from the limbus or anterior stroma may contribute to the pathogenesis of SPKT.

A study using corneal noncontact photomicrography suggested that the morphology of the epithelial changes is compatible with an immunologically mediated injury.[31]

References

1. Fuchs E. Keratitis punctate superficialis. *Klin Wochenschr.* 1889;2:837–839.
2. Thygeson P. Superficial punctate keratitis. *JAMA.* 1950;144:1544–1549.
3. Thygeson P. Further observations on superficial punctate keratitis. *Arch Ophthalmol.* 1961;66:34–38.
4. Jones BR. Thygeson's superficial punctate keratitis. *Trans Ophthalmol Soc UK.* 1963;83:245–253.
5. Jones BR. The differential diagnosis of punctate keratitis. *Trans Ophthalmol Soc UK.* 1960;80:665–675.
6. Thygeson P. Clinical and laboratory observations on superficial punctate keratitis. *Am J Ophthalmol.* 1966;61:1344–1349.
7. Quere MA, Diallo J, Rogez JP. La kératite de Thygeson (à propos de 16 cas de kératite ponctuée superficielle). *Bull Soc Ophtalmol Fr.* 1968;68:276–280.
8. Tanzer DJ, Smith RE. Superficial punctate keratitis of Thygeson: the longest course on record? *Cornea.* 1999;18(6):729–730.
9. Wakui K, Komoriya S, Hayashi E, et al. Corneal and epithelial dystrophies. *Rinsho Ganka.* 1971;25:1103–1123.
10. Lemp MA, Chambers RW Jr, Lundy J. Viral isolate in superficial punctate keratitis. *Arch Ophthalmol.* 1974;91:8–10.
11. Darrell RW. Thygeson's superficial punctate keratitis: natural history and association with HLA-DR3. *Trans Am Ophthalmol Soc.* 1981;74:486–516.
12. Tabbara KF, Ostler HB, Dawson C, et al. Thygeson's superficial punctate keratitis. *Ophthalmology.* 1981;88:75–77.
13. Watson SL, Hollingsworth J, Tullo AB. Confocal microscopy of Thygeson's superficial punctate keratopathy. *Cornea.* 2003;22(4):294–299.
14. van Bijsterveld OP, Mansour KH, Dubois FJ. Thygeson's superficial punctate keratitis. *Ann Ophthalmol.* 1985;17(2):150–153.
15. Quere MA, Delplace MP, Rossazza C, et al. Frequence et etiopathogenie de la keratitie de Thygeson. *Bull Soc Ophtalmol Fr.* 1973;73:629–631.
16. Abbott RL, Forster RK. Superficial punctate keratitis of Thygeson associated with scarring and Salzmann's nodular degeneration. *Am J Ophthalmol.* 1977;87:296–298.
17. Nagra PK, Rapuano CJ, Cohen EJ, et al. Thygeson's superficial punstate keratitis. Ten years' experience. *Ophthalmol.* 2004;111:34–37.
18. Sundmacher R, Press M, Neumann-Haefelin D, et al. Keratitis superficialis punctata Thygeson. *Klin Monatsbl Augenheilkd.* 1977;170:908–916.
19. Goldberg DB, Schanzlin DJ, Brown SI. Management of Thygeson's superficial punctate keratitis. *Am J Ophthalmol.* 1980;89:22–24.
20. Forstot SL, Binder PS. Treatment of Thygeson's superficial punctate keratopathy with soft contact lenses. *Am J Ophthalmol.* 1979;88:186–189.
21. Del Castillo JM, Del Castillo JB, Garcia-Sanchez J. Effect of topical cyclosporin A on Thygeson's superficial punctate keratitis. *Doc Ophthalmol.* 1996–1997;93(3):193–198.
22. Reinhard T, Sundmacher R. Topical cyclosporin A in Thygeson's superficial punctate keratitis. *Graefes Arch Clin Exp Ophthalmol.* 1999;237(2):109–112.
23. Reinhard T, Reis A, Mayweg S, et al. Topical Fk506 in inflammatory corneal and conjunctival diseases. *Klin Monatsbl Augenheilkd.* 2002;219(3):125–131.
24. Nesburn AB, Lowe III GH, Lepoff NJ, et al. Effect of topical trifluridine on Thygeson's superficial punctate keratitis. *Ophthalmology.* 1984;91:1188–1192.
25. Goldstein MH, Feistmann JA, Bhatti MT. PRK-pTK as a treatment for a patient with Thygeson's superficial punctate keratitopathy. *CLAO J.* 2002;28(4):172–173.
26. Netto MV, Chalita MR, Krueger RR. Thygeson's superficial punctate keratitis recurrence after laser in situ keratomileusis. *Am J Ophthalmol.* 2004;138:507–508.
27. Braley AE, Alexander RC. Superficial punctate keratitis: isolation of a virus. *Arch Ophthalmol.* 1953;50:147–154.
28. Reinhard T, Roggendorf M, Fengler I, et al. PCR for varicella zoster virus genome negative in corneal epithelial cells of patients with Thygeson's punctate keratitis. *Eye.* 2004;18:304–305.
29. Ostler HB. Suspected infectious etiology. In: Smolin G, Thoft RA, eds. *The cornea: scientific foundations and clinical practice.* Boston: Little Brown;1983.
30. Fite SW, Chodosh J. Photorefractive keratectomy for myopia in the setting of Thygeson's superficial punctate keratitis. *Cornea.* 2001;20(4):425–426.
31. Tabery HM. Corneal surface changes in Thygeson's superficial punctate keratitis: a clinical and non-contact photomicrographic in vivo study in the human cornea. *Eur J Ophthalmol.* 2004;14(2):85–93.

Chapter 90

Neurotrophic Keratitis

Bernard H. Chang, Erich B. Groos, Jr.

Neurotrophic keratitis is a degenerative disease of corneal epithelium characterized by impaired healing. Absence of corneal sensitivity is the hallmark of the condition, which may end in corneal stromal melting and perforation.[1] The causes of decreased corneal sensation are myriad and may affect sensory nerve supply from the trigeminal nucleus to the corneal nerve endings.[2] Reduced corneal sensation renders the corneal surface prone to occult injury and decreases reflex tearing; it also appears to decrease healing rates of corneal epithelial injuries. Vulnerability and poor healing secondary to corneal sensory denervation favor the formation of nonhealing epithelial defects that tend to ulcerate and ultimately perforate if not appropriately treated in a timely fashion.

The initial clinical appearance of an anesthetic cornea pairs loss of the usual corneal epithelial sheen with mild disruptions in the tear surface.[1] Even in the absence of injury, the condition may progress to punctate keratitis, epithelial loss, and finally stromal ulceration. Evaluation of a patient found to have impaired or absent corneal sensation should include careful review of previous surgical procedures, concomitant systemic diseases, and topical and systemic medications. A careful and complete ocular examination should follow to elucidate clues to local disease processes causing corneal anesthesia and to identify defects in other external ocular structures that may contribute to poor corneal epithelial healing. Management should emphasize the prevention of epithelial defects because of profoundly impaired healing of the epithelium. An epithelial defect in the setting of corneal anesthesia is a serious ocular condition requiring prompt and aggressive therapy to prevent ulceration and possible perforation.

Clinical Causes

Both local ocular and distant neurologic conditions may impair corneal sensation. The most common causes for corneal anesthesia are herpes simplex and herpes zoster virus infections of the ocular surface.[1–5] Next in frequency are tumors and surgical procedures that damage the ophthalmic branch of the trigeminal nerve. Other causes include congenital syndromes, corneal dystrophies, local trauma to the corneal nerves, infections such as leprosy, systemic disease, topical medications, and exposure to toxins. Also, chronic corneal epithelial injury or severe stromal inflammation may cause corneal hypoesthesia (Box 90.1). Although any cornea afflicted with decreased sensation may develop neurotrophic keratitis, conditions that result in more profound corneal anesthesia are more likely to develop neurotrophic changes.[6]

Herpes simplex and herpes zoster infections of the cornea have characteristic clinical appearances that are described in detail in other chapters. The extent of corneal anesthesia in both entities is well known, with herpes zoster causing more segmental hypoesthesia than herpes simplex.[6] Although the lack of corneal sensation plays a central role in the development of persistent epithelial defects and corneal ulceration in herpes simplex corneal disease, herpes zoster keratitis promotes more classic neurotrophic lesions, which often occur without viral epithelial infection. Twenty-one percent of patients with herpes zoster ophthalmicus will demonstrate decreased central corneal sensitivity.[6] Forty-nine percent will develop corneal hypoesthesia to some degree within 1 year, and one-third of that total will have persistent decreased sensation beyond 1 year.[6] Despite improving methods for treatment, both conditions can lead to ulceration and perforation of the cornea, significantly affecting vision.

Pure neuroparalytic keratitis secondary to fifth nerve palsy is second to herpetic infection in terms of the incidence of persistent corneal epithelial defects and subsequent perforations. The condition may occur secondary to intentional or inadvertent damage to the trigeminal nucleus, root, ganglion, or any segment of the ophthalmic branch of this cranial nerve.[2] Most frequently, the nerve is damaged during attempted ablative procedures for trigeminal neuralgia.[3] Surgical procedures to repair maxillary fractures may also damage the fifth cranial nerves, resulting in neurotrophic keratitis.[14] A fertile setting for neurotrophic keratitis occurs after resection of an acoustic neuroma, particularly when both the fifth and seventh cranial nerves are affected.[2] With concomitant facial nerve paralysis the anesthetic cornea suffers chronic exposure, a combination that, despite aggressive therapy, favors recurrent or persistent epithelial defects, stromal lysis, and ultimately perforation.

Another cause of corneal anesthesia that may predispose to neurotrophic keratitis is diabetes mellitus.[28,29] Diabetics have decreased corneal sensation that increases in severity and prevalence in proportion to the duration of their diabetes. Corneal sensory loss is another manifestation of

Box 90.1 Causes of corneal hypoesthesia

Infection
- Herpes simplex[4,7]
- Herpes zoster[6,8]
- Leprosy[9]

Fifth nerve palsy
- Surgery (as for trigeminal neuralgia)[3,10,11]
- Neoplasia (such as acoustic neuroma)[12,13]
- Aneurysms[2]
- Facial trauma[14]
- Congenital[15,16]
- Familial dysautonomia (Riley-Day syndrome)[17]
- Goldenhar-Gorlin syndrome[18]
- Möbius syndrome[16]
- Familial corneal hypesthesia[19]
- Congenital insensitivity to pain with anhidrosis[20]

Topical medications
- Anesthetics[21–23]
- Timolol[24,25]
- Betaxolol[24]
- Sulfacetamide 30%[26]
- Diclofenac sodium[27]

Corneal dystrophies
- Lattice
- Granular (rare)

Systemic disease
- Diabetes mellitus[28–30]
- Vitamin A deficiency[2]

Iatrogenic
- Contact lens wear[32]
- Trauma to ciliary nerves by laser and surgery (primarily for retinal conditions)[30,31]
- Corneal incisions[33]
- LASIK[34]

Toxic
- Chemical burns
- Carbon disulfide exposure[2,19]
- Hydrogen sulfide exposure[2,19]

Miscellaneous
- Increasing age[2]
- Dark eye color[2]
- Adie's syndrome[35]
- Any condition causing chronic corneal epithelial injury or inflammation

the generalized peripheral neuropathy often found with long-standing diabetes. Peripheral panretinal photocoagulation for neovascular retinal disease often deepens the hypoesthesia already present.[30] Because these patients are at risk for developing proliferative vitreoretinopathy and vitreous hemorrhage requiring surgical intervention, they are also at risk for developing persistent nonhealing corneal epithelial defects in the immediate postoperative period. Some diabetics, however, may develop neurotrophic keratitis without previous surgical injury.[29]

Chronic use of various topical medications will cause corneal sensory loss. These medications include timolol, betaxolol, 30% sulfacetamide, and diclofenac sodium. When used after keratorefractive surgery, this effect of diclofenac sodium aids pain control but may aggravate epithelial integrity in an environment of temporary corneal hypoesthesia seen with LASIK and photorefractive keratectomy (PRK).[27] Moreover, the illicit use of topical anesthetics produces a profound and predictable course of corneal ulceration (Fig. 90.1).[21–23] The most frequent cases appear in the setting of cocaine abuse or the use of a diagnostic topical anesthetic, usually by a healthcare professional, as an analgesic for the relief of eye pain after an ocular injury. In the latter situation, topical anesthetics are used more frequently and with increasingly inadequate results until the cornea is severely damaged. The epithelium will not heal with continued use of the topical anesthetic, promoting frequent infectious keratitis and occasional corneal perforation in these patients.

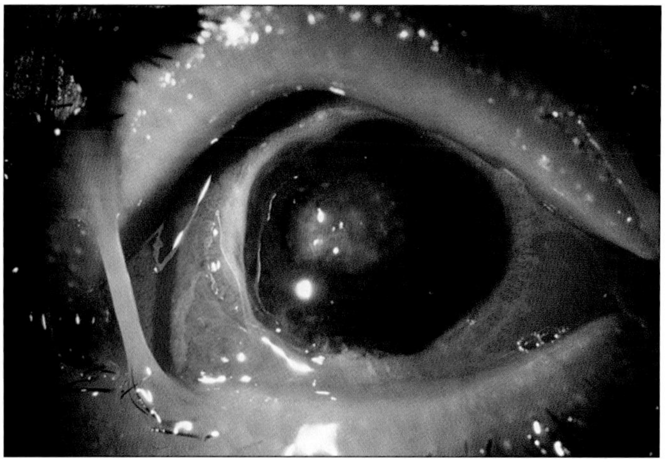

Fig. 90.1 Complete corneal necrosis secondary to topical anesthetic abuse. (Courtesy Mark J. Mannis, MD.)

Biochemical Basis

The search for the molecular basis of neurotrophic keratitis began when a 1954 animal study showed that sectioning the trigeminal nerve results in characteristic corneal findings of neurotrophic keratitis despite tarsorrhaphy.[36] Before this finding, dry eye was cited as the cause for the progressive corneal epithelial changes seen in denervated corneas.[37] Cavanagh and colleagues theorized that corneal epithelial proliferation is regulated bidirectionally by controls linked to the sensory and sympathetic nerves and their neurotransmitters.[5,37] A recent study supported this theory by demonstrating corneal limbal stem cell deficiency in eyes with neurotrophic keratitis.[38] There is evidence as well to suggest that sensory neurons directly affect the development of corneal epithelial cell characteristics that are critical to the maintenance of good epithelial layer integrity.[39] A decrease in epithelial cell mitosis eventually leads to a deficit in corneal epithelial cells even in the absence of a pre-existing defect or accelerated cell death.[40,41] The subsequent defect occurs centrally because the corneal epithelium is persistently regenerated centripetally from the periphery and sheds old cells at its apex, as described by Thoft in his *X, Y, Z Hypothesis*.[41]

Epithelial mitosis in both the cornea and skin is reduced by rising levels of intracellular cyclic adenosine monophosphate (cAMP) and increased by rising intranuclear levels of cyclic guanosine monophosphate (cGMP).[37] Adrenergic neurotransmitters and prostaglandins raise intracellular cAMP levels, thereby reducing epithelial mitosis, whereas acetylcholine (ACh) derived from sensory neurons increases intranuclear cGMP levels and epithelial growth. In the setting of sensory denervation of the cornea, severe depletion of ACh in otherwise ACh-rich tissue occurs and causes a decrease in epithelial growth. The effects of prostaglandins help explain the delay in corneal wound healing found in the presence of significant inflammation. Adrenergic stimulation in turn has been shown to reverse partially the effects of sensory denervation created by ipsilateral sympathetic denervation.[42–44] In animal studies in which corneal anesthesia is obtained either chemically or surgically, corneal epithelial effects are mitigated by cervical sympathetic denervation.[44] These findings support Cavanagh's proposed dual and antagonistic control system of corneal epithelial regeneration.[37,42]

Substance P is a neuropeptide present in the cornea and is depleted with sensory denervation, specifically with capsaicin.[45] Animal models involving the use of capsaicin show classic changes of neurotrophic keratitis, lending credence to the role of substance P as a direct trophic molecule on corneal epithelial growth.[45] Substance P alone has also been found to stimulate DNA synthesis and corneal epithelial cell growth.[46] In the same study, calcitonin gene-related peptide (CGRP), which is present in nearly all substance P-containing neurons in the cornea, showed synergism with substance P but no trophic effect on its own. More recent research challenges the role of substance P as a trophic influence and supports its indirect effects on epithelial cell adhesion.[47] Research continues along several avenues to develop specific medical therapy for neurotrophic keratitis.

Clinical Findings

Corneal anesthesia triggers a cascade of ocular surface abnormalities that promote the development of ulceration.[1,3,48] Reflex tearing decreases secondary to the lack of the afferent limb of the reflex.[2] Blink rates are decreased for the same reason.[2] Tear mucus secretions increase and become more viscous in character.[49] The resulting tear surface abnormalities, aggravated by progressive abnormalities of the corneal epithelial microvilli, impair ocular surface lubrication to the extent that the cornea is vulnerable to injury and poorly capable of repairing itself once an injury occurs.[1,3,48]

The earliest sign of sensory denervation is rose Bengal staining of the inferior palpebral conjunctival surface.[1,3] The tear surface is disrupted several seconds after each blink, forming geographic dry spots on the corneal epithelium, a finding seen readily with the aid of topical fluorescein. Increased viscosity of tear mucus contributes to this abnormal surface wetting.[49] At this point, punctate fluorescein staining of the corneal epithelium may be present, but only after several minutes of fluorescein exposure.[1,3] Some anesthetic corneas may even show gray punctate superficial lesions that stain readily.[1,3] Small facets of drying epithelium, also known as Gaule spots, may be seen in retroillumination.[1] These have been compared to dellen that may appear at the limbus in early neurotrophic keratitis. The preceding findings constitute the extent of Mackie's stage I of neurotrophic keratitis (Box 90.2).[1,3] This stage may become chronic, resulting in superficial vascularization, stromal scarring, and epithelial hyperplasia and irregularity. Rarely, a hyperplastic precorneal membrane will grow centrally from the limbus to cover intact corneal epithelium.[50]

Box 90.2 Clinical stages of neurotrophic keratitis[1,3]

Stage 1
- Rose Bengal staining of the palpebral conjunctivae
- Decreased tear break-up time
- Increased viscosity of tear mucus
- Punctate epithelial staining with fluorescein
- Scattered small facets of dried epithelium (Gaule spots)

Stage 2
- Acute loss of epithelium, usually under the upper lid
- Surrounding rim of loose epithelium
- Stromal edema
- Aqueous cell and flare
- Edges of the defect become smooth and rolled with time

Stage 3
- Stromal lysis, sometimes resulting in corneal perforation

Adapted from Mackie IA: Neuroparalytic (neurotrophic) keratitis. In Symposium on contact lenses: transactions of the New Orleans Academy of Ophthalmology, *St Louis, 1973, Mosby; Mackie IA:* Trans Ophthalmol Soc UK *93:343, 1978.*

Stage 2 involves the acute loss of epithelium, often in an area covered by the upper lid.[1,3] The mechanism of loss is similar to that for recurrent erosions and is encouraged by the milieu of poor tear wetting of a rough and abnormal corneal epithelium. The area of epithelial loss is usually surrounded by a large area of loose epithelium. Folds develop in Descemet's membrane as the stroma begins to swell. Often, aqueous cell and flare are present. Rarely, a sterile hypopyon will form (Fig. 90.2). This stage is an indication for urgent and appropriate treatment. As this stage persists, the surrounding epithelial cells become hazy, edematous, and poorly adherent to Bowman's membrane. The edges of the defect become smooth and rolled as the defect ages without appreciable epithelial growth.[1,3–5] The punched-out horizontal, oval, or circular shape of these chronic defects is characteristic of neurotrophic keratitis (Figs 90.3, 90.4).

Stage 3 often ensues in the absence of adequate treatment of stages 1 and 2, and sometimes despite appropriate treatment. Stromal lysis is the hallmark of this stage, and sometimes perforation ensues (Fig. 90.5).[1,3–5] Inflammation, secondary infection, and the imprudent use of topical corticosteroids promote stromal lysis and increase the risk for perforation.[4]

Histopathologic Findings

Histopathologic changes of the corneal epithelium are consistent with the resulting clinical pathology. The epithelial thickness is decreased in the setting of chronic anesthesia

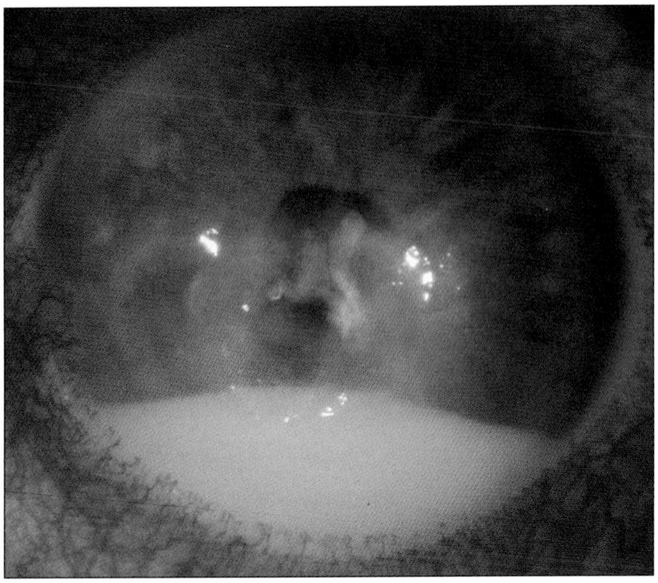

Fig. 90.2 Neurotrophic ulceration with hypopyon. (Courtesy Mark J. Mannis, MD.)

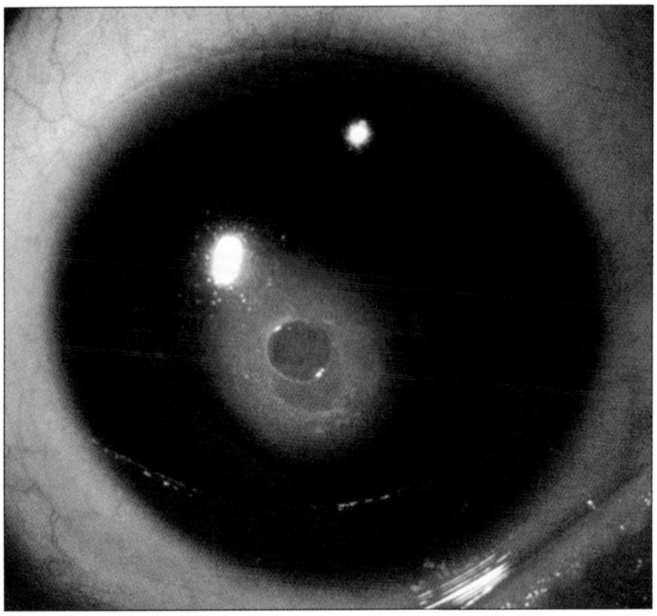

Fig. 90.3 Central, circular, punched-out epithelial defect secondary to and classic for neurotrophic keratitis. (Courtesy Ivan R. Schwab, MD.)

with complete loss of the normal surface desquamating layer.[50] Epithelial cell glycogen is decreased as well.[48] The surface cells lose all microvilli, leading to impaired adherence of the tear film.[3] The remaining surface epithelial cells show intracellular swelling. Abnormal synthesis of basal lamina as well as complete loss of the same in other areas helps to explain defective epithelial adhesion.[3]

Conjunctival changes include decreased goblet cell density and an increase in the length of surface microvilli.[48,51] Impression cytology reveals loss of goblet cells as well as their migration onto the corneal surface.[38] Most of these

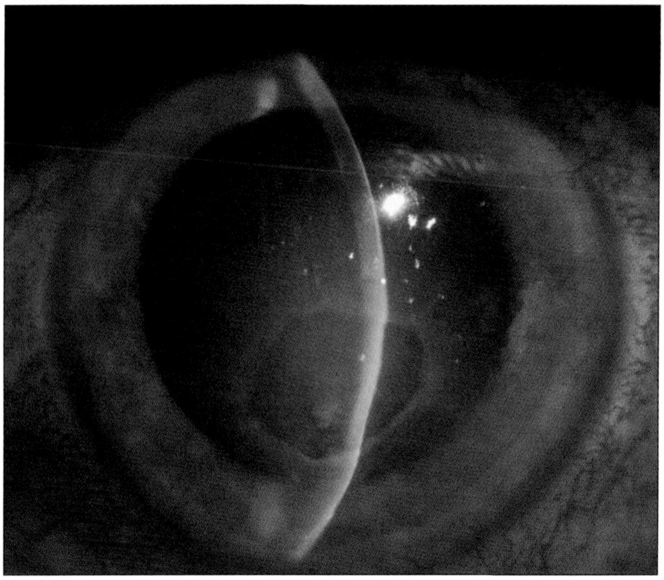

Fig. 90.4 A border of hazy epithelium surrounds a large inferior epithelial defect, which demonstrates impaired healing secondary to corneal anesthesia. (Courtesy Mark J. Mannis, MD.)

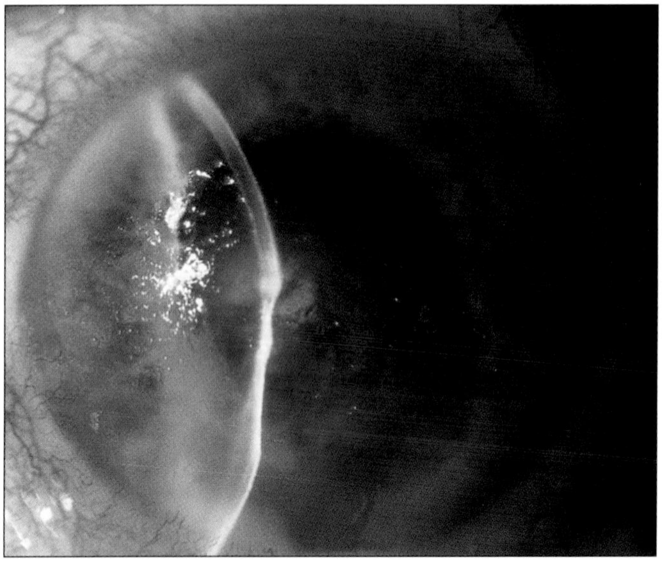

Fig. 90.5 Stromal lysis with thinning in a cornea that suffers decreased sensation. (Courtesy Mark J. Mannis, MD.)

corneal and conjunctival epithelial changes are found in keratitis sicca as well, but not to the degree that they are found in neurotrophic keratitis.[48]

Clinical Evaluation

The causes of corneal hypoesthesia are legion and include a broad spectrum of ocular and systemic conditions. A careful ocular examination supplemented by thorough medical and surgical history taking should enable one to determine the cause for any loss of sensation.[2] Medical and surgical history reveals previous surgical or traumatic injury to the trigeminal nerve, diabetes mellitus, the use of various topical medications known to decrease corneal sensation, previous ocular laser or surgical procedures, and the use of contact lenses. Direct ocular exposure to caustic chemicals or chronic exposure to carbon disulfide and hydrogen sulfide must be identified, if present, during the initial interview. The absence of any identifiable cause for corneal anesthesia, particularly in the setting of severely damaged corneas with advanced stomal lysis, should trigger suspicion of topical anesthetic abuse, especially with the history of a recent corneal erosion.[21]

The presence of other neurologic deficits may help to localize neoplasms, injuries, or vascular accidents, which include the fifth cranial nerve or its brainstem nucleus, among other local structures.[2] Of particular interest is seventh and eighth nerve function, especially with respect to acoustic neuromas and subsequent surgery to remove them. Corneal hypoesthesia is the second most common finding (after decreased hearing) in acoustic neuromas.[2] Ocular motility may reveal associated dysfunction of cranial nerves III, IV, and VI that may localize an aneurysm or cavernous sinus pathology. Pupillary abnormalities auger the status of cranial nerve II as well as defects in the sympathetic innervation of the iris. The presence of an afferent papillary defect in association with corneal hypoesthesia would localize the lesion to the intraconal orbit. Pupil reactions consistent with Adie's pupil have also been associated with alterations in corneal sensation.[35] Any associated neurologic deficit found in association with corneal sensory loss should be investigated thoroughly under the direction of an internist or neurologist.

Normal eyelid function is critical to the prognosis of neurotrophic keratitis. The presence of eyelid defects or the absence of normal lid closure promotes corneal epithelial exposure and drying and hastens the progression to stage 3 keratopathy. The lids may be scarred secondary to removal of periocular infiltrative tumors or chemical or thermal burns. Thyroid ophthalmopathy may present with proptosis and upper eyelid retraction, both of which favor exposure keratopathy. Poor lid closure from cranial nerve VII palsy is sometimes seen in association with severe corneal hypoesthesia, particularly after resection of an acoustic neuroma, and favors corneal ulceration.[2]

Ocular surface examination should include careful analysis of qualitative and quantitative tear function. Absence of the nasal-lacrimal tearing reflex along with ipsilateral loss of sensation in the nasal mucosa presents a high risk for subsequent neurotrophic corneal ulceration.[52] The corneal examination begins with assessment of the pattern and degree of corneal sensory deficit. The most useful instrument for this is the esthesiometer of Cochet-Bonnet, which measures corneal sensitivity by the length of nylon line (between 0 and 6 cm in length) required to elicit a lid blink or patient response.[2] Patchy hypoesthesia may indicate a local ocular condition such as previous herpes zoster keratitis.[6] Measuring the depth of corneal anesthesia is important, since lower levels of sensation tend toward more severe corneal epithelial disease. In one series using the Cochet-Bonnet device to measure the depth of corneal sensation loss in herpes zoster keratitis, only corneas with readings of 2 cm or less underwent epithelial sloughing and stromal ulceration.[6]

Direct biomicroscopic examination of the cornea is essential to identify local corneal conditions that may predispose to corneal sensory deficits. Signs of epithelial disease, particularly of a dendritic nature, identify herpetic disease as the probable underlying cause. One must be careful to distinguish the dendritic patterns of herpes simplex and herpes zoster. Sometimes, only culture identification or direct immunofluorescence staining of infected cells can differentiate the two. Characteristics of these lesions are discussed at length in Chapters 79 and 80. In some instances, a healing epithelial defect may assume a dendritic shape but be distinguished from herpetic keratitis by the absence of branching. The presence of stromal scarring may indicate previous infection. Prominence and beading of the corneal nerves may be subtle signs of lepromatous anterior segment involvement.[9] Corneal hypoesthesia also occurs in advanced stromal dystrophies such as lattice and granular, which have characteristic clinical appearances described in detail in Chapter 72.

Attention to the condition of the corneal epithelium is important once the degree of sensory dysfunction has been measured. The presence of significant epithelial fluorescein staining or of a frank epithelial defect calls for immediate and aggressive treatment. Dense anterior stromal infiltrate indicates infectious keratitis. In this situation, cultures should be taken before instituting the appropriate broad-spectrum topical antibiotic therapy. The presence of stromal lysis and thinning requires even more aggressive therapy to maintain structural integrity of the cornea.

Other ocular findings may aid the search for underlying causes of a corneal sensory deficit. Iris atrophy with or without associated anterior chamber inflammation is often seen with herpes zoster and simplex keratouveitis and may also be seen with leprosy.[8,9] Mild anterior chamber cell and flare may be seen with neurogenic causes of corneal anesthesia.[51] Poor accommodation may also signal herpes zoster as the cause for corneal sensory loss since the virus may damage ciliary ganglion motor nerve fibers. Dilated fundus examination may reveal optic nerve pallor or swelling on the affected side. These findings may localize the lesion to the orbit or retro-orbital region. The presence of background diabetic retinopathy or laser scars from treatment of retinopathy may also shed light on the cause of corneal sensory loss.

Management

Management of a hypoesthetic cornea depends on the condition of the epithelium at initial presentation and the degree to which the sensation is impaired. Stage 1 findings require simple topical lubrication, preferably with preservative-free solutions or ointments, to prevent preservative-induced epithelial toxicity. The use of a therapeutic soft contact lens at this stage may be effective but increases the risk for infectious keratitis.[19,53] Eyelid dysfunction must be carefully assessed and remedied to prevent exposure keratopathy and progression to stage 2 disease. Although many hypoesthetic corneas never progress to more severe clinical stages, the presence of sensory loss places the cornea at risk for the duration of the loss. In general, the more severe the sensory deficit, the more likely it is that the cornea will develop epithelial ulceration as a result.[6,52] In some cases in which there is severe or total loss of corneal sensation, a lateral tarsorrhaphy often prevents epithelial defects.[3,54] The use of a palpebral spring or botulinum A toxin injection of the levator has been reported as possible substitutes for lateral tarsorrhaphy.[55,56] With any of these options the advantages of access for medications and improved oxygen supply to the ocular surface exist when compared to serial patching. The key to successful management of an anesthetic cornea is fastidious care of the corneal epithelial surface to prevent progression to more advanced stages of neurotrophic keratitis.

Because deficits in corneal sensory innervation impair corneal epithelial growth, the presence of an epithelial defect on an anesthetic cornea requires immediate and appropriate therapy. A marginally anesthetic cornea may respond well to lubricants and topical prophylactic antibiotics, whereas the presence of severe or complete loss of sensation requires a more aggressive approach. Silicone plugs of the lower puncta alone or in combination with the upper puncta can greatly improve tear function.[57] There is some evidence that topical tetracycline speeds healing of epithelial defects. Oral doxycycline or minocycline serves to remedy qualitative tear dysfunction through its action in the meibomian glands and may even aid in preventing corneal stromal lysis. Even in the absence of eyelid defects or dysfunction, a tarsorrhaphy that covers most, if not all, of the defect will often effect closure of an epithelial defect.[54]

Until recently, adjunctive medical therapy to promote epithelial growth had proved elusive. Recent studies in humans have shown that substance P and insulin-like growth factor 1 (IGF-1) together and nerve growth factor alone accelerate epithelial healing in neurotrophic corneas.[58–60] The expense of formulation and short shelf-lives of these peptides has led to trials of naturally occurring substances to promote growth. Published studies have shown a role for both umbilical cord serum and platelet-rich autologous serum eyedrops for the treatment of neurotrophic ulcers.[61,62] Autologous serum tear preparations were first described in 1984 to have beneficial effects in patients with keratoconjunctivitis sicca.[63] This therapeutic effect is believed to be secondary to the growth factors, fibronectin, vitamins, and immunoglobulins found in serum.[64] Several recent reports describe enhanced epithelial healing in recalcitrant corneal ulcers.[64] Over the past four years, our clinical experience with autologous serum (20%) has been positive, making it an integral part of the aggressive management of stages 1 and 2 neurotrophic keratitis.

The presence of inflammation in conjunction with a neurotrophic corneal ulceration renders treatment even more complicated. The inflammatory response inhibits corneal epithelial growth in concert with the absence of sensory innervation.[4,5,37] Although the use of topical corticosteroids is indicated in rare cases in which inflammation is the driving cause of the persistent defect, particularly in chemical burns, one should follow patients using corticosteroids in these cases very carefully because of the risk of precipitous stromal lysis and perforation. Although theoretically the use of topical nonsteroidal agents would block the influence of prostaglandins locally on corneal epithelial growth, their use clinically has not had dramatic trophic effects on wound healing.[65] In difficult cases, one should consider the use of preservative-free solutions of steroid in combination with a broad-spectrum antibiotic such as cefazolin. Diclofenac sodium in particular should be avoided because of its tendency to cause corneal hypoesthesia with topical use.[27]

Stage 3 neurotrophic keratitis involves stromal ulceration and lysis with thinning of the cornea. Corneas showing progressive thinning despite lubrication, autologous serum, aggressive treatment of stromal inflammation, and tarsorrhaphy require immediate attention to arrest stromal lysis and subsequent progression to corneal perforation. Cyanoacrylate glue, tectonic lamellar keratoplasty, conjunctival flaps, and, more recently, multilayer amniotic membrane transplantation may all serve to halt progression of stromal lysis to perforation.[54,66–72] Use of amniotic membrane shows additional promise not only for arresting progressive melting but also for eliminating the surrounding stromal infiltrate.[68–71] When an eye is initially seen at this stage, preserving the structural integrity of the globe takes precedence over visual rehabilitation. Application of cyanoacrylate glue followed by a bandage soft contact lens is a noninvasive and very effective approach to address impending perforation.[72] In the case of perforation, glue may be applied if the opening is smaller than 2 mm.[54,73,74] The overall results for treating perforated eyes have improved since the use of glue became a common approach.[54,73] Larger defects require lamellar or penetrating keratoplasty.[54,73] The lamellar graft, because of its lower rejection rate and more rapid healing, is the procedure of choice for small to intermediate-sized holes and will preserve most of the endothelium. Recently, good results have been reported with lamellar grafting using multilayer amniotic membrane.[71,75] Conjunctival flaps, despite their effectiveness at arresting stromal lysis and creating a new epithelial barrier, have assumed a diminished role in the approach to these ulcerations and perforations because of the poor cosmetic and visual result.[54,67,73]

The issue of performing penetrating keratoplasty on anesthetic corneas for visual rehabilitation has not been addressed by any large series in the literature. Stromal neovascularization, which often attends scarring from severe neurotrophic ulceration, and the persistence of poor epithelial sensation combine to add significant risk against graft survival (Fig. 90.6). Careful maintenance of the ocular surface and partial tarsorrhaphy are vital to success in these cases.[76] In one series of patients with corneal scarring secondary to herpes zoster keratitis, a favorable success rate was reported with corneal transplantation protected by lateral tarsorrhaphy.[76] Preliminary experience in our clinic using perioperative nonpreserved steroids and antibiotics along with long-term maintenance using autologous serum has shown promise in maintaining the grafts in these challenging cases. Further study is necessary to delineate protocols and long-term complications of such an aggressive approach. In any eye that has suffered ulceration, neurotrophic or otherwise, a 6-month period of clinical stability is recommended before considering penetrating keratoplasty.

Summary

A corneal surface lacking adequate sensory innervation is at risk to develop progressive epitheliopathy resulting in

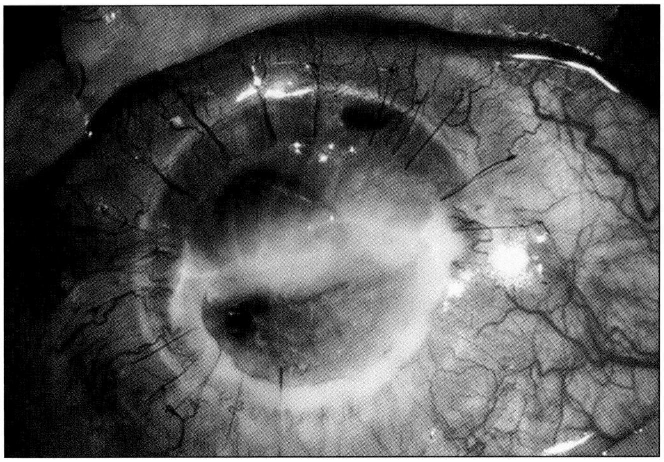

Fig. 90.6 Stromal lysis and thinning with perforation in a corneal graft performed on a patient with previous herpes zoster keratitis. (Courtesy Ivan R. Schwab, MD.)

epithelial sloughing, stromal lysis, and subsequent corneal perforation in the absence of timely and appropriate therapy. The causes of corneal hypoesthesia are numerous, but herpetic infections and damage to the ophthalmic division of the trigeminal nerve are most likely to result in clinical corneal disease. The trophic effect of cholinergic sensory nerve fibers on corneal epithelial cells is lost in any condition that impairs corneal sensation. The resultant decrease in epithelial growth rate slows wound healing and may cause epithelial defects even in the absence of frank trauma. Initial evaluation should identify the underlying cause of the corneal sensory loss, with particular attention to potential pathology of the central nervous system along the path of the trigeminal nerve. In the absence of an obvious cause, topical anesthetic abuse should be considered. Treatment should be directed toward preventing epithelial defects and promoting epithelial cell regeneration. Preservative-free lubricants, autologous serum, and tarsorrhaphy are the mainstays of this approach. Autologous serum provides growth factors that research may eventually provide in pharmacologic form. Corneal perforation should be addressed with cyanoacrylate glue for impending and small perforations and with lamellar or penetrating keratoplasty for larger defects. Prompt identification of corneal anesthesia in the setting of an epithelial defect will allow appropriate and aggressive therapy directed toward avoidance of severe stage 3 neurotrophic keratitis.

References

1. Mackie IA. Neuroparalytic (neurotrophic) keratitis. In: *Symposium on contact lenses: transactions of the New Orleans Academy of Ophthalmology.* St Louis: Mosby; 1973.
2. Miller NR. *Walsh and Hoyt's clinical neuro-ophthalmology.* Baltimore: Williams & Wilkins; 1985.
3. Mackie IA. Role of the corneal nerves in destructive disease of the cornea. *Trans Ophthalmol Soc UK.* 1978;93:373.
4. Cavanagh HD, et al. The pathogenesis and treatment of persistent epithelial defects. *Trans Am Acad Ophthalmol Otol.* 1976;81:754.
5. Cavanagh HD, Colley AM, Pihlaja DJ. Persistent corneal epithelial defects. *Int Ophthalmol Clin.* 1979;19:197.
6. Cobo ML. Corneal complications of herpes zoster ophthalmicus: prevention and treatment. *Cornea.* 1988;7:50.
7. Liesegang TJ. Ocular herpes simplex infection: pathogenesis and current therapy. *Mayo Clin Proc.* 1988;63:1092.
8. Liesegang TJ. Corneal complications from herpes zoster ophthalmicus. *Ophthalmology.* 1985;92:316.
9. Karaçorlu MA, Çakiner T, Saylan T. Corneal sensitivity and correlations between decreased sensitivity and anterior segment pathology in ocular leprosy. *Br J Ophthalmol.* 1991;75:117.
10. Onofrio BM. Radiofrequency percutaneous Gasserian ganglion lesions. Results in 140 patients with trigeminal pain. *J Neurosurg.* 1975;42:132.
11. Davies MS. Corneal anaesthesia after alcohol injection of the trigeminal sensory root: examination of 100 anaesthetic corneae. *Br J Ophthalmol.* 1970;54:577.
12. Sterkers JM, et al. Preservation of facial, cochlear, and other nerve functions in acoustic neuroma treatment. *Otolaryngol Head Neck Surg.* 1994;110:146.
13. Tos M, Drozdziewicz D, Thomsen J. Medial acoustic neuromas. A new clinical entity. *Arch Otorhinolaryng Head Neck Surg.* 1992;118:127.
14. Lanigan DT, Romanchuk K, Olson CK. Ophthalmic complications associated with orthognathic surgery. *J Oral Maxillofac Surg.* 1993;51:480.
15. Rosenberg ML. Congenital trigeminal anaesthesia: a review and classification. *Brain.* 1984;107:1073.
16. Donaghy M, et al. Hereditary sensory neuropathy with neurotrophic keratitis. Description of an autosomal recessive disorder with a selective reduction of small myelinated nerve fibres and a discussion of the classification of the hereditary sensory neuropathies. *Brain.* 1987;110:563.
17. Goldberg MF, Payne JW, Brunt PW. Ophthalmologic studies of familial dysautonomia. *Arch Ophthalmol.* 1968;80:733.
18. Baum JL, Feingold M. Ocular aspects of Goldenhar's syndrome. *Am J Ophthalmol.* 1973;75:253.
19. Purcell JJ, Krachmer JH, Thompson HS. Corneal sensation in Adie's syndrome. *Am J Ophthalmol.* 1977;84:496.
20. Yagev R, Levy J, Shorer Z, et al. Congenital insensitivity to pain with anhidrosis: ocular and systemic manifestations. *Ophthalmology.* 1999; 127(3):322–326.
21. Rosenwasser GOD. Complications of topical anesthetics. *Int Ophthalmol Clin.* 1989;30(3):153.
22. Rosenwasser GOD, et al. Topical anesthetic abuse. *Ophthalmology.* 1990;97:967.
23. Willis WE, Laibson PR. Corneal complications of topical anesthetic abuse. *Can J Ophthalmol.* 1970;5:239.
24. Weissman SS, Asbell PA. Effects of topical timolol (0.5%) and betaxolol (0.5%) on corneal sensitivity. *Br J Ophthalmol.* 1990;74:409.
25. Van Buskirk EM. Corneal anesthesia after timolol maleate therapy. *Am J Ophthalmol.* 1979;88:739.
26. Chung FW, Reinhart J, Fraser NM. Effect of 30% sulfacetamide on corneal sensitivity. *Am J Optom Physiol Opt.* 1984;61:318.
27. Szerenyi K, et al. Decrease in normal human corneal sensitivity with topical diclofenac sodium. *Am J Ophthalmol.* 1994;118:312.
28. Schwartz DE. Corneal sensitivity in diabetics. *Arch Ophthalmol.* 1974; 91:175.
29. Lockwood A, Hope-Ross M, Chell P. Neurotrophic keratopathy and diabetes mellitus. *Eye.* 2006;20(7):837–839.
30. Menchini U, et al. Argon versus krypton panretinal photocoagulation side effects on the anterior segment. *Ophthalmologica.* 1990;201:66.
31. Johnson SM. Neurotrophic corneal defects after diode laser cycloablation. *Am J Ophthalmol.* 1998;126(5):725–727.
32. Velasco MJ, et al. Variations in corneal sensitivity with hydrogel contact lenses. *Acta Ophthalmol.* 1994;72:53.
33. Campos M, et al. Corneal sensitivity after photorefractive keratectomy. *Am J Ophthalmol.* 1992;114:51.
34. Breil P, Frisch L, Dick HB. Diagnostik und Therapie der LASIK-induzierten neurotrophen Epitheliopathie. *Ophthalmologe.* 2002;99(1):53–57.
35. Purcell JJ, Krachmer JH. Familial corneal hypesthesia. *Arch Ophthalmol.* 1979;97:872.
36. Sigelman S, Friedenwald JS. Mitotic and wound-healing activities of the corneal epithelium: effect of sensory denervation. *Arch Ophthalmol.* 1954;52:46.
37. Cavanagh HD, Colley AM. The molecular basis of neurotrophic keratitis. *Acta Ophthalmol Suppl.* 1989;192:115.
38. Puangsricharern V, Tseng SC. Cytologic evidence of corneal diseases with limbal stem cell deficiency. *Ophthalmology.* 1995;102(10): 1476–1485.
39. Baker KS, et al. Trigeminal ganglion neurons affect corneal epithelial phenotype. *Invest Ophthalmol Vis Sci.* 1993;34:137.
40. Lemp MA, Mathers WD. Corneal epithelial cell movement in humans. *Eye.* 1989;3:438.
41. Thoft RA. The X, Y, Z hypothesis of corneal epithelial maintenance. *Invest Ophthalmol Vis Sci.* 1983;24(10):1441.

42. Abelli L, Geppetti P, Maggi CA. Relative contribution of sympathetic and sensory nerves to thermal nociception and tissue trophism in rats. *Neuroscience.* 1993;57:739.
43. Perez E, et al. Effects of chronic sympathetic stimulation on corneal wound healing. *Invest Ophthalmol Vis Sci.* 1987;28:221.
44. Shimizu T, et al. Capsaicin-induced corneal lesions in mice and the effects of chemical sympathectomy. *J Pharmacol Exp Ther.* 1986;243: 690.
45. Fujita S, et al. Capsaicin-induced neuroparalytic keratitis-like corneal changes in the mouse. *Exp Eye Res.* 1984;38:165.
46. Reid TW, et al. Stimulation of epithelial cell growth by the neuropeptide substance P. *J Cell Biochem.* 1993;52:476.
47. Araki-Sasaki K, Aizawa S, Hiramoto M, et al. Substance P-induced cadherin expression and its signal transduction in a cloned human corneal epithelial cell line. *J Cell Physiol.* 2000;182(2):189–195.
48. Gilbard JP, Rossi SR. Tear film and ocular surface changes in a rabbit model of neurotrophic keratitis. *Ophthalmology.* 1990;97:308.
49. Wright P, Mackie IA. Mucus in the healthy and diseased eye. *Trans Ophthalmol Soc UK.* 1977;97:1.
50. Zabel RW, Mintsioulis G. Hyperplastic precorneal membranes. Extending the spectrum of neurotropic keratitis. *Cornea.* 1988;7:50.
51. Alper MG. The anesthetic eye: an investigation of changes in the anterior ocular segment of the monkey caused by interrupting the trigeminal nerve at various levels along its course. *Trans Am Ophthalmol Soc.* 1975;73:323.
52. Heigle TJ, Pflugfelder SC. Aqueous tear production in patients with neurotrophic keratitis. *Cornea.* 1996;15(2):135–138.
53. Kent HD, et al. Microbial keratitis and corneal ulceration associated with therapeutic soft contact lenses. *CLAO J.* 1990;16:49.
54. Donzis PB, Mondino BJ. Management of noninfectious corneal ulcers. *Surv Ophthalmol.* 1987;32:94.
55. McNeill JI, Oh YH. An improved palpebral spring for the management of paralytic lagophthalmos. *Ophthalmology.* 1991;98:715.
56. Kandarakis AS, Page C, Kaufman HE. The effect of epidermal growth factor on epithelial healing after penetrating keratoplasty in human eyes. *Am J Ophthalmol.* 1984;98:411.
57. Tai MC, Cosar CB, Cohen EJ, et al. The clinical efficacy of silicone punctal plug therapy. *Cornea.* 2002;21(2):135–139.
58. Nishida T, Chikama T, Morishige N, et al. Persistent epithelial defects due to neurotrophic keratopathy treated with a substance P-derived peptide and insulin-like growth factor 1. *Jpn J Ophthalmol.* 2007;51(6): 442–447.
59. Tan MH, Bryars J, Moore J. Use of nerve growth factor to treat congenital neurotrophic corneal ulceration. *Cornea.* 2006;25(3):352–355.
60. Bonini S, Lambiase A, Rama P, et al. Topical treatment with nerve growth factor for neurotrophic keratitis. *Ophthalmology.* 2000;107(7):1347–1351.
61. Yoon KC, You IC, Im SK, Jeong TS, Park YG, Choi J. Application of umbilical cord serum eyedrops for the treatment of neurotrophic keratitis. *Ophthalmology.* 2007;114(9):1637–1642.
62. Alio JL, Abad M, Artola A, et al. Use of autologous platelet-rich plasma in the treatment of dormant corneal ulcers. *Ophthalmology.* 2007;114(7): 1286–1293.
63. Fox RI, Chan R, Michelson JB, et al. Beneficial effect of artificial tears made with autologous serum in patients with keratoconjunctivitis sicca. *Arthritis Rheum.* 1984;27:459–461.
64. Poon AC, Geerling G, Dart JK, et al. Autologous serum eyedrops and epithelial defects: clinical and in vitro toxicity studies. *Br J Ophthalmol.* 2001;85:1188–1197.
65. Hersh PS, et al. Topical nonsteroidal agents and corneal wound healing. *Arch Ophthalmol.* 1990;108:577.
66. Alino AM, Perry HD, Kanellopoulos AJ, et al. Conjunctival flaps [see comments]. *Ophthalmology.* 1998;105(6):1120–1123.
67. Lugo M, Arentsen JJ. Treatment of neurotrophic ulcers with conjunctival flaps. *Am J Ophthalmol.* 1987;103:711.
68. Chen HJ, Pires RT, Tseng SC. Amniotic membrane transplantation for severe neurotrophic corneal ulcers. *Br J Ophthalmol.* 2000;84(8): 826–833.
69. Kruse FE, Rohrschneider K, Volcker HE. Multilayer amniotic membrane transplantation for reconstruction of deep corneal ulcers. *Ophthalmology.* 1999;106(8):1504–1510.
70. Khokhar S, Natung T, Sony P, et al. Amniotic membrane transplantation in refractory neurotrophic corneal ulcers: a randomized, controlled clinical trial. *Cornea.* 2005;24(6):654–660.
71. Hick S, Demers PE, Brunette I, et al. Amniotic membrane transplantation and fibrin glue in the management of corneal ulcers and perforations: a review of 33 cases. *Cornea.* 2005;24(4):369–377.
72. Fogle JA, Kenyon KR, Foster CS. Tissue adhesive arrests stromal melting in the human cornea. *Am J Ophthalmol.* 1980;89:795.
73. Hirst LW, Smiddy WE, Stark WJ. Corneal perforations: changing methods of treatment, 1960–1980. *Ophthalmology.* 1982;89:630.
74. Webster RG, et al. The use of adhesive for the closure of corneal perforations. *Arch Ophthalmol.* 1968;80:705.
75. Rodríguez-Ares MT, Touriño R, López-Valladares MJ, Gude F. Multilayer amniotic membrane transplantation in the treatment of corneal perforations. *Cornea.* 2004;23(6):577–583.
76. Reed JW, Joyner SJ, Knauer WJ. Penetrating keratoplasty for herpes zoster keratopathy. *Am J Ophthalmol.* 1989;107:257.

Chapter **91**

Factitious Keratoconjunctivitis

Lisa M. Nijm, Matthew R. Parsons

One of the most difficult diagnoses to make in the field of medicine is that of self-inflicted injury. Factitious keratoconjunctivitis is no exception. By virtue of our own training, we seek to discover the etiology underlying every ocular disease, but the thought that it may be self-inflicted often eludes even the most trained ophthalmologist. Voutilainen and Tuppurainen[1] felt that self-injuring patients were expressing a strong cry for help but at the same time were incapable of describing what kind of help they needed. Factitious behavior may be difficult to comprehend at times, but it must be exposed. Failure to diagnose such disease may result in delay of appropriate therapy to prevent permanent damage as well as enormous unnecessary costs to the medical system.[2] This chapter will discuss the diagnosis and treatment of factitious keratoconjunctivitis and the related, but distinct disorders of ocular Munchausen, malingering, and other self-induced causes of ocular trauma.

Factitious Disorders Defined

The term factitious disorders, when used correctly, describes only disorders where symptoms or physical findings are intentionally produced by the patient in order to assume the sick role.[3] Unfortunately, outside the psychiatric literature, the term factitious is used more broadly to describe any self-induced injury. Factitious disorders must be distinguished from malingering and somatoform disorders. While malingering also results in intentionally produced symptoms or physical findings, in contrast, there is always evidence of external incentive. Secondary gain provides the motivation for malingering and is often easily understood if the entire situation is known. Malingering can be adaptive in certain situations (e.g. with prisoners of war) and does not necessarily imply psychopathology. Somatoform disorders include hysteria, conversion disorder, and hypochondriasis. These disorders also produce physical or mental findings that are not fully explained. However, in contrast to factitious disorders and malingering, these symptoms are not voluntarily produced and are not under conscious control. Somatoform disorders rarely, if ever, result in corneal or conjunctival disease and will not be discussed further.

Factitious disorders, by definition, imply psychopathology.[3] The patient possesses a pathologic need to assume the sick role and be involved in the medical system. This drive is so strong that all sorts of self-induced injury, in any degree, may result. Achieving the sick role is the sole motivation for the behavior. External incentives, such as financial gain or avoiding responsibility, are characteristically absent. Patients repeatedly victimize themselves, often with disastrous results, while masking the true nature of their illness.[3] The true source of the pathology is often overlooked for several reasons. First, the patients often emphatically deny any trauma – self-induced or accidental. Second, the motivation for the self-destructive behavior is deeply seated in the patient's psyche and is difficult for the physician to understand. Third, the physician is often reluctant to consider the possibility of self-induced disease because of an inherent desire to trust the patient's history as factual or because of a long-standing relationship with the patient. Manifestations of factitious disorders are wide and varied. Some examples in the literature are recurrent skin ulceration by auto-injection of bacteria,[4,5] subcutaneous emphysema,[6] simulated herpes zoster,[7] hematuria,[8,9] feigned sickle cell crisis,[10] iron deficiency anemia,[11,12] epilepsy,[13] acquired immunodeficiency syndrome (AIDS),[14] arthritis,[15] purpura,[16] hypercalcemia,[17] cancer,[18,19] septicemia,[20] fatal asthma,[21] fatal water intoxication,[22] fatal hypoglycemia,[23,24] and a whole host of other manifestations.[25–31] Understanding that fatalities often result from factitious disease puts in perspective some of the bizarre ophthalmic injuries that result from this disorder.

Factitious keratoconjunctivitis

In 1990, a classic case of bilateral factitious crystalline keratopathy was reported.[32] An 18-year-old male presented with bilateral corneal ulcers involving the deep stroma associated with bilateral hypopyon (Fig. 91.1). Peculiar blue, refractile, crystalline stromal deposits surrounding both ulcers were noted. The patient emphatically denied any exposure to contact lenses or any traumatic injury. After extensive diagnostic and therapeutic intervention, no etiology could be discovered. After the parents discovered a powdered eye shadow product along with one of his father's insulin syringes and a liquid mixture of the eye shadow, self-induced trauma was suspected. On confrontation with the eye shadow, the patient admitted injecting his corneas with the mixture on several occasions.

In 1982, Jay et al. reported six cases of self-inflicted eye injury.[33] All six cases showed evidence of mechanical injury

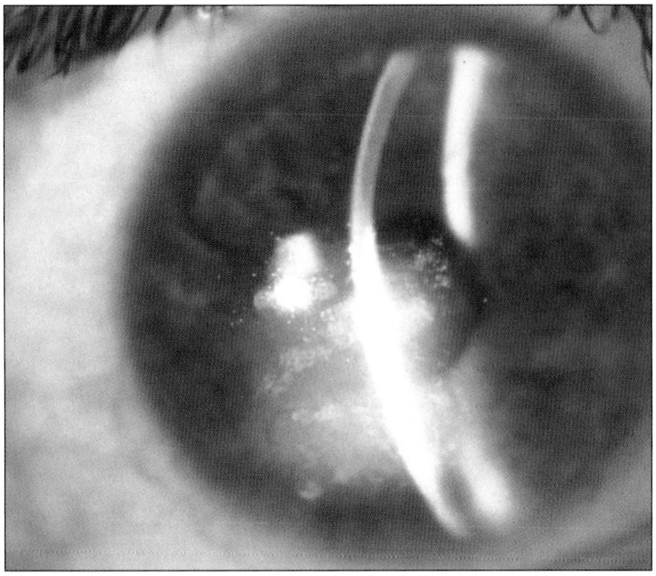

Fig. 91.1 An 18-year-old with bilateral self-induced corneal ulcers produced by injecting each cornea with a solution mixed from eye shadow. Peculiar blue refractile crystals were visible in the corneal stroma. (Reproduced with permission from Lembach RG, Ringel DM: *Cornea* 9(3):246–248, 1990.)

to the inferior and nasal quadrants of the cornea and conjunctiva. The areas of involvement showed sharply delineated borders – linear or square. Three of the six patients either had medical training or worked in a medical office. Five of the six were between 18 and 32 years old. Characteristically, they showed an attitude of serene indifference. Pathologic examination of detached conjunctival epithelium showed no evidence of inflammation. Many had associated self-induced injury elsewhere on the body and all patients had associated psychopathology.

In 1963, Segal et al. reported 22 cases of self-inflicted corneal and conjunctival injuries among prisoners in whom malingering was not involved.[34] A total of 166 injuries to 43 eyes were described. Of these, 148 were chemical injuries (crystal violet, lime, and Lysol), 29 were mechanical (ground glass, metal, wood slivers, and pencils), and 3 were thermal (a lighted cigarette applied to the cornea). Of the 22 patients, 10 eyes suffered complete blindness. Six patients had a best visual acuity of less than 0.1 (20/200) in the best eye. A lack of interest in seeking medical care was characteristic and contributed significantly to a poor outcome.

In 1989, Errico et al.[35] reported a case of factitious hypermineralocorticoidism by chronic use of 9-alpha-fluoroprednisolone. In 1990, Karnik et al. reported a case of an 18-year-old female who was discovered to be injecting air in the face, chest, and around the eye, resulting in subcutaneous, orbital, and subconjunctival emphysema.[36]

In 1995, Heinz et al. reported a one-eyed diabetic male with therapy-resistant superficial punctate keratopathy.[37] This healed promptly with ocular occlusion. Anterior scleritis and cicatricial conjunctivitis have also been reported as factitious disorders.[38,39]

A peculiar type of factitious keratoconjunctivitis was reported by Fells and Bors in 1970.[40,41] A 25-year-old man undertook a deliberate, systematic effort to eliminate vitamin A and beta-carotene from all aspects of his diet for 5.5 years. Rouland et al. reported a second case in 1989.[42,43] Predictably, corneal xerosis, a crocodile pattern to the conjunctiva, poor wetting, and corneal perforation occurred. Yellow retinal spots and nonrecordable electroretinogram (ERG) and electro-oculogram (EOG) tracings were found. Interestingly, in the absence of generalized poor nutrition, Bitot's spots were not found. The patient continually refused to receive vitamin A therapy.

Munchausen syndrome (chronic factitious disorder)

Munchausen syndrome is a chronic form of factitious disease characterized by frequent hospitalizations, self-inflicted injuries, dramatic medical histories, and multiple unnecessary invasive procedures resulting in massive, often unpaid, medical bills.[20] The patient's entire life may consist of trying to gain admission to hospitals.[3]

Ocular Munchausen syndrome was best described by Rosenberg et al. in 1986.[44] Rosenberg et al. described a case series of ocular Munchausen involving four female patients, ranging from 21 to 27 years, three of whom worked in the medical field. The cases ranged from one patient who suffered recurrent, bilateral corneal ulcerations resulting from self-inflicted trauma that eventually led to two corneal transplants and subsequent enucleation of one eye, to self-induced alkali burns, which eventually resulted in uveoblepharon (attachment of the iris to the eyelid) and blindness. Voutilainen and Tuppurainen reported a case in 1989 of an 18-year-old woman who repeatedly inflicted damage to both eyes over a period of several years by applying various chemicals and perforating the corneas with a safety pin.[1] Winans et al. described a 23-year-old woman in 1983 who repeatedly injected air into her right orbit and periocular tissues.[45] Eventual enucleation was required, after which she resumed the behavior on the opposite side. In 2000, Tahir et al.[46] reported a case of a 30-year-old woman who had injected a mixture of saliva and tap water into both eyes, resulting in endophthalmitis. Further questioning revealed previous admissions for extensive burns, chronic urinary tract infections, chronic anemia, numerous endoscopic procedures, osteomyelitis, pneumonia, and multiple surgical procedures, all felt to be factitious in nature.

Of note, Munchausen syndrome by proxy occurs when a parent is unable to distinguish the child's needs from his or her own and submits the child to multiple unnecessary procedures and dangerous treatments while feigning laboratory results and concocting medical history to perpetuate the deception.[47] Though no cases of ocular Munchausen syndrome by proxy have been reported to date, it is an important syndrome that all ophthalmologists should be aware of in perplexing cases of childhood ocular trauma.

Diagnosis of factitious keratoconjunctivitis

The diagnosis of factitious keratoconjunctivitis should be included in the differential diagnosis of any case in which the trauma sustained arises under suspicious or poorly explained circumstances. In the context of corneal disease, bilateral presentation of suspicious corneal lesions should always be suspect. Any patient exhibiting poor healing or recurrent breakdown in which the clinical context does not support such occurrences should also be suspect. As illustrated above, patients with factitious injuries often have associated psychologic stresses or other internal conflicts occurring simultaneously that may increase the risk of self-destructive behavior.[33]

In general, factitious disease most commonly presents in patients in the second or third decade of life and more often among medical or health allied professionals, possibly due to greater accessibility to medical devices and medication.[33] Frequently, these patients will display less concern for the presenting problem than would normally be appropriate. Serene indifference is of cardinal importance in suggesting the diagnosis. Finally, the location of the trauma may also serve as an identifying factor in diagnosis. Factitious ocular disease is nearly always found in the inferior or nasal quadrants,[33] very rarely in the superior quadrant.

Patients with chronic factitious disease typically either emphatically deny any history of trauma or have an explanation that incompletely explains the severity or true nature of the injury. A history of multiple recurrent episodes of poorly explained disease is typical. The patients often improve dramatically when placed on a 24-hour watch. Devastating consequences are common. Patients often refuse psychiatric care and seem inappropriately willing to accept the devastating consequences of their abusive behavior. Often, it is difficult and frustrating for the physician to understand the motivation behind the behavior.

Treatment of factitious disease

Several authors suggest using a treatment approach known as sympathetic authority once the diagnosis of factitious disease has been made.[33,48,49] Using this technique, a diagnosis of unexplained injury is made. The physician then presents the patient with the conflicting evidence in a non-threatening manner, which, in some cases, may result in an admission of involvement. If the patient's confidence can be maintained, the patient's need to depend on the physician may be met while, at the same time, gradually decreasing the frequency and length of visits. Some patients only participate in factitious behavior just prior to a visit to the physician. Most patients, however, remain resistant to treatment and refuse to cooperate with efforts to decrease the incidence of injury.[50] A complete discussion of the treatment of these patients is beyond the scope of this text.[51,52] Psychiatric referral should be considered in all cases, since various psychosocial stresses and internal conflicts are often involved. Despite appropriate therapy, a large percentage of patients are destined for prolonged physical and psychologic morbidity.

Treatment of Munchausen syndrome is much less hopeful than that of isolated factitious disease. At various times, hypnosis, insulin coma, electroshock, lobotomy, and psychotherapy have been employed, then abandoned because of poor results.[44] Psychiatrists generally agree that treatment of Munchausen syndrome is seldom successful.[53]

Miscellaneous Types of Self-Induced Trauma

Malingering

Malingering differs from factitious disease in that there is a definite (although usually hidden) motive for the claimed pathology. Most commonly, the patient claims visual loss or other feigned symptoms and carefully avoids inflicting any injury. However, under various circumstances, the patient does produce self-inflicted injury.[54,55] For instance, malingering is quite common among prison inmates in order to escape the rigors of detention.[56] Therefore, malingering cannot be ruled out even if the traumatic injury is severe.

Mucus fishing syndrome

In 1985, McCulley et al.[57] report a case series of twenty-five patients who had a well-circumscribed pattern of rose Bengal staining on the nasal and inferior bulbar conjunctiva. All patients had a history of increased mucus production as a non-specific response to ocular surface damage. The inciting event was typically keratoconjunctivitis sicca. However, allergic conjunctivitis, atopic keratoconjunctivitis, corneal foreign body, and conjunctival squamous cell carcinoma were also found. The patients admitted to mechanical removal of the mucus strands (mucus fishing) and, on demonstrating their method of removal, the source of the persistent ocular surface irritation became apparent. The epithelial injury created by mucus fishing propagates the ocular surface irritation, resulting in further mucus production, creating a vicious cycle. The nasal and inferior bulbar conjunctiva are the most frequently involved, as these seem to be the most accessible areas.

Treatment consists of eliminating the digital manipulation (if possible), mechanically removing the mucus plaques and strands, treating the underlying condition (such as dry eye), and using mucolytic agents, such as acetylcysteine 10% topically, in order to reduce mucus production.

Congenital corneal anesthesia

Corneal ulceration has long been recognized as a complication of congenital corneal anesthesia. However, repeated self-induced trauma is not typically involved. In 1985, Trope et al. reported four boys under 2.5 years of age in whom severe corneal ulceration developed as a result of self-inflicted injury.[58] Eye scratching was observed, and healing occurred with arm splinting. Congenital corneal anesthesia was diagnosed in each case. Corneal ulceration recurred after removal of the elbow splints. Two of the four boys had clinical evidence of mild brainstem or cerebellar maldevelopment. However, these cases essentially represented an isolated congenital corneal anesthesia. None of the patients had familial dysautonomia (Riley-Day syndrome). Since 1985, three similar cases have been reported.[59–61] In 1999, Yagev et al.[62] reported 15 Bedouin children afflicted with congenital insensitivity to pain and commented that all of the children had self-inflicted injuries, both ocular and nonocular. Self-induced trauma should be suspected in any infant in whom corneal ulceration fails to heal with standard therapy, and the possibility of congenital corneal anesthesia should be explored.

Inadvertent or unintentionally self-induced trauma

At times, patients are aware that they have caused the physical signs for which they are presenting but are unwilling to admit it to the physician for reasons of embarrassment or unwillingness to accept responsibility. This is to be distinguished from malingering, since the actual trauma was produced in an inadvertent, rather than a purposeful, manner. For example, a patient who experiences ultraviolet light-induced keratitis from inadequately protected eyes in a tanning booth may be embarrassed and therefore attempt to conceal the true history behind the injury. A common cause of unintentional trauma is medicamentosa, either iatrogenic or unintentionally self-induced. For various reasons, the patient may be slow to report the use of non-prescribed medications. Many over-the-counter medications contain preservatives that interfere with epithelial cell membrane physiology. Patients may obtain eyedrops such as gentamicin, trifluridine, and even proparacaine from a friend or family member. In some countries, topical anesthetics are available over the counter. Patients with pre-existing ocular surface disease may switch from nonpreserved tears to preserved tears in an effort to save money without informing their physician – not realizing the potential toxicity. Schwab and Abbott reported 19 patients in 1989 who developed a much more serious toxic ulcerative keratopathy from this type of chemically induced trauma.[63]

Neurologic disorders

Gilles de la Tourette syndrome is a rare neurologic disorder in which there are motor and behavioral abnormalities.[64] The onset is normally in childhood. Waxing and waning ticlike muscle movements are the initial symptom. As progression occurs, grunting, echolalia, coprolalia, and self-mutilation occur. Self-injury occurs in 43% of cases.[65]

Self-mutilation of the oral and facial region is a major symptom in Lesch-Nyhan syndrome.[65] This is a sex-linked recessive inborn error of purine metabolism. Injuries can be severe and do not appear to be under voluntary control.[66] Patients with Cornelia de Lange syndrome also may show self-mutilating behavior.[67] Auto-aggression syndrome has been associated with self-induced blepharoconjunctivitis.[68] While eye injuries are not the focus in these syndromes, they can occur as part of the general tendency toward self-mutilation.

Self-inflicted injuries in children

Ocular injuries from self-mutilation are not uncommon in severely mentally challenged children. Noel and Clarke reported four cases of self-inflicted ocular injuries in children in 1982.[69] Corneal laceration, iris prolapse, and corneal and conjunctival abrasions were found. Additionally, vitreous hemorrhage and retinal detachments were described from repeated striking of the eyes. A careful, complete ophthalmic examination is indicated in any child exhibiting self-mutilating behavior because potentially blinding injuries may otherwise go unnoticed.

Eye poking, by contrast, is a distinct clinical entity found in severely disabled children.[70] Profound intellectual impairment is always present. Eye poking is to be distinguished from eye rubbing, which may be found normally in children, and also from eye pressing, which is a steady, prolonged, nonpainful pressure exerted on one or both globes in an attempt to stimulate phosphenes in children with profound noncortical visual loss.

Eye poking may be found in children with impaired (71%) or normal (29%) vision. Eye poking is diagnosed when children episodically exert intense pressure with the tips of their fingers on the side of one or both globes. This causes intense pain and is one of the most disturbing behaviors to watch in these children. Eye poking, also in contrast to eye pressing, usually results in tissue damage, which may be severe. Jan et al.[70] reported corneal scarring, infectious keratitis, retinal detachments, and cataracts. In one case, the trauma was severe enough to require enucleation. Behavioral modification and other forms of treatment have been largely unsuccessful.

Topical Anesthetic Abuse

By far, topical anesthetic abuse represents one of the most common and destructive forms of self-induced ocular injury. Anesthetic abuse may be factitious in nature, most often as a means to gain access to the medical system. On the other hand, it may also be iatrogenic, with the agents occasionally being supplied by primary care physicians, optometrists, emergency room physicians, and even ophthalmologists.[71,72] Inadvertent abuse may be found if the patient obtains eyedrops from an acquaintance and is unfamiliar with its destructive effects. Unfortunately, topical anesthetic agents are still available over the counter in many countries.[73–75] Often, the patient may demonstrate abuse as a manifestation of addictive behavior. These patients may remove bottles of anesthetic from the office during a visit without the physician's knowledge. Many of the patients are medical personnel with easy access to the drug.[76] In addition, abusers of street drugs may apply cocaine powder directly to the eyes.[77]

Local effects on the corneal surface

While the molecular and cellular mechanisms of local anesthetic toxicity have not yet been satisfactorily clarified, much has been learned in recent years about the mechanisms of corneal damage. It is generally well accepted that anesthetic agents inhibit the ability of the epithelium to migrate and divide, yet the ultrastructural alterations corresponding to this are just beginning to be elucidated.

In 1994, Boljka et al. explored the effects of 0.5% tetracaine on the surface of freshly enucleated human corneas.[78] Half of each cornea was treated with three drops of tetracaine at 2-minute intervals. The other half was treated with 0.9% normal saline and served as a control. The cytotoxicity of tetracaine was demonstrated according to the morphologic changes of the epithelial cells as seen by scanning electron microscopy. Treated cells showed loss of microvilli (Fig. 91.2). Tetracaine deposits were present on

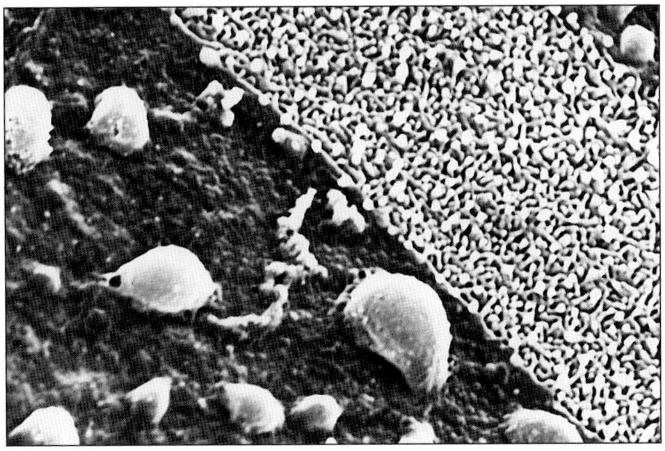

Fig. 91.2 Epithelial surface of a freshly enucleated human cornea treated with three drops of 0.5% tetracaine. Multiple tetracaine deposits can be seen on the epithelial surface. Note that the cell on the left is completely devoid of microvilli. (Scanning electron micrograph ×7500.) (Reproduced from Boljka M et al.: Toxic side effects of local anaesthetics on the human cornea. *Br J Ophthalmol* 78:386–389, 1994, with permission from BMJ Publishing Group.)

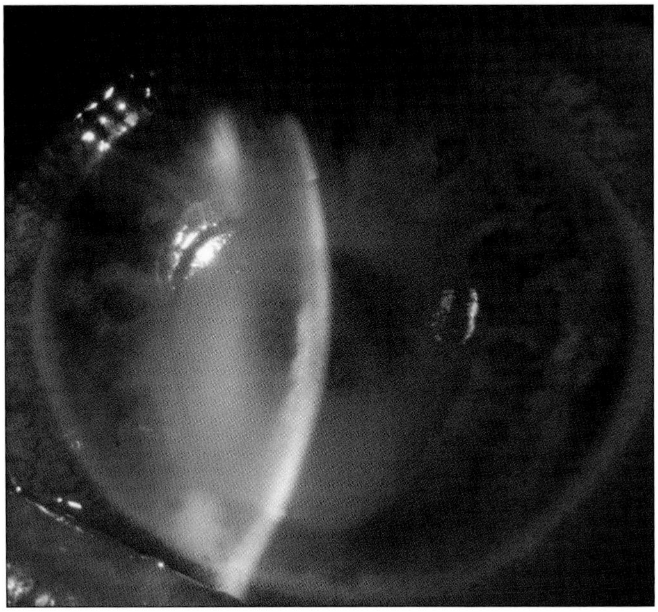

Fig. 91.3 Corneal surface subjected to topical anesthetic abuse. Note the small hypopyon, the stromal opacification, and the trophic-like edge to the epithelial defect. (Courtesy Edward J. Holland, MD.)

microvilli or on cell membranes (if no microvilli were present) in the treated cells. Treated cells showed increased desquamation on scanning electron microscopy. The loss of microvilli and other intercellular contacts may lead to increased desquamation. Animal studies have shown a reduced number of desmosomes and an increased tendency for cellular membrane rupture in eyes treated with anesthetic agents.[79] Corneal epithelium has been shown to increase in thickness after several drops of proparacaine.[80]

Local anesthetics are also known to inhibit epithelial sliding.[81] Actin filaments are known to be increased in density at the leading edges of migrating corneal epithelial cells.[82] These are felt to be part of the cytoplasmic machinery responsible for cellular motility. Local anesthetics also act directly at the level of the plasma membrane to alter osmotic fragility and inhibit cellular movement. They also interact with acidic phospholipids and are able to displace calcium ions from the cell membrane. Swelling of mitochondria and lysosomes has also been described.[83]

In addition to the effect on epithelial cells, Risco and Millar described similar changes in the endothelium of a cornea replaced by an allograft because of anesthetic abuse.[84] The endothelial cells were varied in size and shape, and the normal mosaic was absent. The edges of the cells were rounded up with a prominent intercellular gap. Many cells were devoid of microvilli. Intercellular junctions were markedly abnormal.

Clinical presentation

The clinical features of anesthetic abuse abound in the ophthalmic literature.[71,72,75–77,83–89] The earliest feature of anesthetic abuse is the failure of the presenting problem (corneal abrasion, contact lens overwear, infectious keratitis, etc.) to respond to appropriate therapy. Initially, a punctate keratitis is seen. As the patient continues to administer the anesthetic, the eye becomes more injected and epithelial defects appear or transform to a neurotrophic-like appearance. The resultant pain increases and causes the patient to administer the drops with increasing frequency, thus compounding the situation. It is not uncommon for patients to put drops in their eye every 5 to 15 minutes – at the same time concealing this information from the physician.

As the process progresses, the eye becomes increasingly inflamed. It is common to see keratic precipitates and hypopyon at the initial examination (Fig. 91.3). The epithelial defect enlarges and becomes increasingly trophic. Eventually, only a thin rim of epithelium may be present inside the limbus. Visual acuity markedly declines. The corneal clarity in and around the epithelial defect begins to decrease. Diffuse stromal edema, full-thickness stromal infiltration, and a ring infiltrate are common presenting signs. Stromal vascularization will occur with chronic ulceration. If the cause of the insult is not discovered, stromal thinning and perforation may occur. Infectious crystalline keratopathy has been reported in two cases where topical anesthetic abuse was the only known risk factor.[89] Four cases of *Candida albicans* keratitis superinfection with known topical anesthetic abuse were also reported in 1996 by Chern et al.[90]

Diagnosis

A high index of suspicion is crucial in cases of suspected anesthetic abuse, as often the patient has a well thought out, complete history. In particular, suspicion should be heightened if the patient is associated with the medical field in any way (e.g. veterinary nurse or medical technician). Because of the presence of corneal infiltrates and anterior segment inflammation, infectious keratitis must be ruled out with corneal scrapings, culture, and antibiotic therapy. Differential diagnosis includes bacterial, fungal, herpetic, and amoebic keratitis. Suspicion should be maintained in the face of negative cultures in any patient who is not responding to appropriate therapy. If pain seems out of proportion to the physical findings, this may be a clue to suspect anesthetic abuse. At some point the patient should be confronted, and 24-hour observation may be necessary. Many times, the diagnosis is only made when the patient is discovered concealing the anesthetic drops.

Treatment

Even after diagnosis, it is sometimes impossible to outwit a determined anesthetic abuser. Once the diagnosis is made and secondary infectious keratitis is ruled out, corneal healing usually occurs if all exposure to anesthetics is removed. Oral analgesics or narcotics are indicated to break the vicious cycle of topical anesthetic abuse. Topical cycloplegics may help to decrease inflammation and diminish pain. Topical corticosteroids are rarely necessary and may potentiate corneal thinning. A mild topical antibiotic may help prevent secondary infection, but epithelially toxic antibiotics (such as aminoglycosides) should be avoided. In advanced cases, or where abuse cannot be terminated, permanent corneal scarring or corneal perforation may occur, necessitating corneal transplantation. Occasionally, anesthetic abuse continues after surgery, resulting in loss of the graft. Psychiatric consultation is occasionally helpful.[72]

Conclusion

Because of the potentially serious and permanent damage that may result from anesthetic agents, all ophthalmologists should be extremely cautious with these drugs and carefully guard against theft from their office, by either office personnel or by patients. These medications should routinely be kept under monitored conditions and out of reach of unsupervised patients. The actual dispensing of these drops for patient self-administration constitutes negligence on the part of the practitioner, even if the patient is instructed to discontinue the drops in a few days. Even today, education of primary care providers, optometrists, and pharmacists concerning the toxicity of these drops and the potential for abuse is of paramount importance.

References

1. Voutilainen R, Tuppurainen K. Ocular Munchausen syndrome induced by incest. *Acta Ophthalmol.* 1989;67:319–321.
2. Sutherland AJ, Rodin GM. Factitious disorders in a general hospital setting: clinical features and a review of the literature. *Psychosomatics.* 1990;31(4):392–399.
3. American Psychiatric Association. Factitious disorders. In: *Diagnostic and statistical manual of mental disorders (DSM IV).* 4th ed. Washington, DC: American Psychiatric Association; 1994.
4. Martinez Salazar F, et al. Bacteremia and multiple and recurrent skin ulcers due to *Brucella melitensis. Med Clin.* 1993;100(11):417–419.
5. Garcia-Blazquez R, Puras A. Bacteremia and multiple and recurrent skin ulcers due to *Brucella melitensis.* A new modality of self-induced infection. *Med Clin.* 1993;100(11):417–419.
6. Mackersie RC. Self-induced subcutaneous air mimicking a gas-forming infection. *Ann Emerg Med.* 1986;15(11):1357–1359.
7. Levitz SM, Tan OT. Factitious dermatosis masquerading as recurrent herpes zoster. *Am J Med.* 1988;84(4):781–783.
8. Abrol RP, et al. Self-induced hematuria. *J Natl Med Assoc.* 1990; 82(2):127–128.
9. Gordon GH, Chrys R. Factitious hematuria and self-induced *Candida albicans* fungemia. *West J Med.* 1985;143(2):246–249.
10. Ballas SK. Munchausen sickle cell painful crisis. *Ann Clin Lab Sci.* 1992;22(4):226–228.
11. Nishimura S, et al. Munchausen syndrome with severe iron deficiency anemia. *Jpn J Clin Hematol.* 1992;33(4):478–482.
12. McIntyre AS, Kamm MA. A case of factitious colonic bleeding. *J R Soc Med.* 1990;83(7):465–466.
13. Christensen RC, Szlabowicz JW. Factitious status epilepticus as a particular form of Munchausen's syndrome. *Neurology.* 1991;41(12): 2009–2010.
14. Sno HN, Storosum JG, Wortel CH. Psychogenic HIV infection. *Intern J Psychiatry Med.* 1991;21(1):93–98.
15. Samaniah N, et al. An unusual case of factitious arthritis. *J Rheumatol.* 1991;18(9):1424–1426.
16. Yates VM. Factitious purpura. *Clin Exp Dermatol.* 1992;17(4):238–239.
17. Darras C, et al. Factitious acute hypercalcemia biological interference between calcium and lipids. *Intensive Care Med.* 1992;18(2):131–132.
18. Bruns AD, et al. Munchausen's syndrome and cancer. *J Surg Oncol.* 1994;56(2):136–138.
19. Baile WF, Kuehn CV, Straker D. Factitious cancer. *Psychosomatics.* 1992;33(1):100–105.
20. Castor B, et al. Infected wounds and repeated septicemia in a case of factitious illness. *Scand J Infect Dis.* 1990;22(2):227–232.
21. Bernstein JA, et al. Potentially fatal asthma and syncope. A new variant of Munchausen's syndrome in sports medicine. *Chest.* 1991;99(3): 763–765.
22. Vieweg WV, et al. Death from self-induced water intoxication among patients with schizophrenic disorders. *J Nerv Ment Dis.* 1985;173(3): 161–165.
23. Given BD, et al. Hypoglycemia due to surreptitious injection of insulin. *Diabetes Care.* 1991;14(7):544–547.
24. Patel F. Fatal self-induced hyperinsulinemia: a delayed post-mortem analytical detection. *Med Sci Law.* 1992;32(2):151–159.
25. McDaniel JS, et al. Factitious disorder resulting in bilateral mastectomies. *Gen Hosp Psychiatry.* 1992;14(5):355–356.
26. Bouillon R, et al. The measurement of fecal thyroxine in the diagnosis of thyrotoxicosis factitia. *Thyroid.* 1993;3(2):101–103.
27. Alarcon GS, et al. Hip osteonecrosis secondary to the administration of corticosteroids for feigned bronchial asthma. *Arth Rheum.* 1994; 37(1):139–141.
28. Topazian M, Binder HJ. Brief report: factitious diarrhea detected by measurement of stool osmolality. *N Engl J Med.* 1994;330(20):1418–1419.
29. Okimoto N, Soejima R. Factitious hemoptysis and anemia. *Chest.* 1994;105(5):1629.
30. Apfelbaum JD, Williams HJ. Factitious simulation of systemic lupus erythematosus. *West J Med.* 1994;160(3):259–261.
31. Solyom C, Solyom L. A treatment program for functional parpaplegia/ Munchausen syndrome. *J Behav Ther Exp Psychiatry.* 1990;21(3): 225–230.
32. Lembach RG, Ringel DM. Factitious bilateral crystalline keratopathy. *Cornea.* 1990;9(3):246–248.
33. Jay JL, Grant S, Murray SB. Keratoconjunctivitis artefacta. *Br J Ophthalmol.* 1982;66:781–785.
34. Segal P, et al. Self-inflicted eye injuries. *Am J Ophthalmol.* 1963;55: 349–362.
35. Errico M, Freda M, Zingrillo M, Grilli M. Factitious hypermineralcorticoidism by chronic use of 9-alpha-fluoroprednisolone containing collyrium. *J Endocrinol Invest.* 1989;12(4):277–278.
36. Karnik AM, et al. A unique case of Munchausen's syndrome. *Br J Clin Pract.* 1990;44(12):699–701.
37. Heinz P, Bodanowitz S, Hesse L. Keratitis punctata superficialis caused by self-injury. *Klin Monatsbl Augenheilkd.* 1995;207(2):130–132.
38. Zamir E, Read RW, Rao NA. Self-inflicted anterior scleritis. *Ophthalmology.* 2001;108(1):192–195.
39. Chapman FM, Dickinson AJ. Self-induced cicatricial conjunctivitis. *Eye.* 1999;13(Pt 5):674–676.
40. Fells P, Bors F. Ocular complications of self-induced vitamin A deficiency. *Trans Ophthalmol Soc UK.* 1970;89:221–228.
41. Bors F, Fells P. Reversal of the complications of self-induced vitamin A deficiency. *Br J Ophthalmol.* 1971;55:210–214.
42. Rouland JF, et al. Xerophthalmia caused by self-induced deficiency disease. *J Fr Ophtalmol.* 1989;12(4):273–277.
43. Rouland JF, Amzallag T, Bale F. Xerophthalmia caused by self-induced deficiency. *Bull Soc Ophtalmol France.* 1989;89(12):1425–1427.
44. Rosenberg PN, et al. Ocular Munchausen's syndrome. *Ophthalmology.* 1986;93(8):1120–1123.
45. Winans JM, House LR, Robinson JE. Self-induced orbital emphysema as a presenting sign of Munchausen's syndrome. *Laryngoscope.* 1983;93: 1209–1211.

46. Tahir RM, Singh AD, Hazariwala K. Ocular factitious disorder presenting as endophthalmitis. *Can J Ophthalmol.* 2000;35(5):247–248.
47. Eminson DM, Postlethwaite RJ. Factitious illness: recognition and management. *Arch Dis Child.* 1992;67(12):1510–1516.
48. Parker G, Barrett E. Factitious patients with fictitious disorders: a note on Munchausen's syndrome. *Med J Aust.* 1991;155:772–775.
49. Drews RC. Organic functional ophthalmic problems. *Int Opthalmol Clin.* 1967;7:665–696.
50. Taylor S, Hyler SE. Update on factitious disorders. *Int J Psychiatry Med.* 1993;23(1):81–94.
51. Spivak H, Rodin G, Sutherland A. The psychology of factitious disorders. A reconsideration. *Psychosomatics.* 1994;35(1):25–34.
52. Schoen M. Resistance to health: when the mind interferes with the desire to become well. *Am J Clin Hypn.* 1993;36(1):47–54.
53. Bursten B. On Munchausen's syndrome. *Arch Gen Psychiatry.* 1965; 13:261–268.
54. Braude L. Chronic unilateral inferior membranous conjunctivitis (factitious conjunctivitis). *Arch Ophthalmol.* 1994;112:1488–1489.
55. Boni BM, Schmidt N. Self-induced epidemic keratoconjunctivitis. *JAMA.* 1977;238(5):396–397.
56. Lozzi O. Notes on some self-induced diseases in prison communities. *Quad Criminol Clin.* 1978;20(1):87–98.
57. McCulley JP, Moore MB, Matoba A. Mucus fishing syndrome. *Ophthalmology.* 1985;92(9):1262–1265.
58. Trope GE, et al. Self-inflicted corneal injuries in children with congenital corneal anaesthesia. *Br J Ophthalmol.* 1985;69:551–554.
59. Gaonker CH, Mukherjee AK, Gawns SY. Self-inflicted corneal injuries in a child with congenital sensory neuropathy. *Indian J Ophthalmol.* 1991;39(2):68–69.
60 Shorey P, Lobo G. Congenital corneal anesthesia: problems in diagnosis. *J Ped Ophthalmol Strabismus.* 1990;27(3):143–147.
61. Momtchilova M, Pelosse B, Mathieu S, et al. Congenital corneal anesthesia in children: diagnostic and therapeutic problems. *J Fr Ophtalmol.* 2000;23(3):245–248.
62. Yagev R, Levy J, Shorer Z, Lifshitz T. Congenital insensitivity to pain with anhidrosis: ocular and systemic manifestations. *Am J Ophthalmol.* 1999; 127(3):322–326.
63. Schwab IR, Abbott RL. Toxic ulcerative keratopathy: an unrecognized problem. *Ophthalmology.* 1989;96(8):1187–1193.
64. Steingard R, Dillon-Stout D. Tourette's syndrome and obsessive compulsive disorder – clinical aspects. *Psych Clin North Am.* 1992;15(4): 849–860.
65. Van Woert MH, Yip LC, Balis ME. Purine phosphoribosyltransferase in Gilles de la Tourette syndrome. *N Engl J Med.* 1977;296(4):210–212.
66. Evans J, Sirikumara M, Gregory M. Lesch-Nyhan syndrome and the lower lip guard. *Oral Surg Oral Med Oral Pathol.* 1993;76(4):437–440.
67. Shear CS, et al. Self-mutilative behavior as a feature of the de Lange syndrome. *J Pediatr.* 1971;78:506.
68. Assadoullina A, Bialasiewicz AA, Richard G. Therapy refractory unilateral chronic blepharokeratoconjunctivitis as the chief manifestation of autoaggression syndrome. *Ophthalmologe.* 1999;96(5):319–324.
69. Noel LP, Clarke WN. Self-inflicted ocular injuries in children. *Am J Ophthalmol.* 1982;94:630–633.
70. Jan JE, et al. Eye-poking. *Dev Med Child Neurol.* 1994;36(4):321–325.
71. Epstein DL, Paton D. Keratitis from misuse of corneal anesthetics. *N Engl J Med.* 1968;279(8):396–399.
72. Rosenwasser GO, et al. Topical anesthetic abuse. *Ophthalmology.* 1990;97(8):967–972.
73. Perry HD, Kasper WS, Donnenfeld ED. Colirio oculos antiseptico sedante. *Cornea.* 1990;9(4):362–364.
74. Moreira H, Kureski ML, Fasano AP. Topical anesthetic abuse in Brazil. *Ophthalmology.* 1991;98(9):1322.
75. Penna EP, Tabbara KF. Oxybuprocaine keratopathy: a preventable disease. *Br J Ophthalmol.* 1986;70:202–204.
76. Rapuano CJ. Topical anesthetic abuse: a case report of bilateral corneal ring infiltrates. *J Ophthalmol Nurs Technol.* 1990;9(3):94–95.
77. Zagelbaum BM, et al. Corneal ulcer caused by combined intravenous and anesthetic abuse of cocaine. *Am J Ophthalmol.* 1993;116(2):241–242.
78. Boljka M, Kolar G, Vidensek J. Toxic side effects of local anaesthetics on the human cornea. *Br J Ophthalmol.* 1994;78:386–389.
79. Leuenberger P. Die stereo-ultrastrukture der kornealoberfläche bei der ratte. *Graefe's Arch Klin Exp Ophthalmol.* 1970;180:182–192.
80. Herse P, Siu A. Short-term effects of proparacaine on human corneal thickness. *Acta Ophthalmol.* 1992;70(6):740–744.
81. Marr WG, et al. Effect of topical anesthetics. *Am J Ophthalmol.* 1957;43:606–610.
82. Gipson IK, Anderson RA. Actin filaments in normal and migrating corneal epithelial cells. *Invest Ophthalmol Vis Sci.* 1977;16:161–166.
83. Zagelbaum BM, et al. Topical lidocaine and proparacaine abuse. *Am J Emerg Med.* 1994;12(1):96–97.
84. Risco JM, Millar LC. Ultrastructural alterations in the endothelium in a patient with topical anesthetic abuse keratopathy. *Ophthalmology.* 1992;99(4):629–633.
85. Duffin RM, Olson RJ. Tetracaine toxicity. *Ann Ophthalmol.* 1984; 16(9):836–838.
86. Reiser HJ, Laibson PR. Anesthetic abuse of the cornea (letter). *Ophthalmic Surg.* 1989;20(1):72–73.
87. Arffa RC. *Grayson's diseases of the cornea.* 3rd ed. St. Louis: Mosby; 1991.
88. Willis WE, Laibson PR. Corneal complications of topical anesthetic abuse. *Can J Ophthalmol.* 1970;5(3):239–243.
89. Kintner JC, et al. Infectious crystalline keratopathy associated with topical anesthetic abuse. *Cornea.* 1990;9(1):77–80.
90. Chern KC, Meisler DM, Wilhelmus KR, et al. Corneal anesthetic abuse and *Candida* keratitis. *Ophthalmology.* 1996;103(1):37–40.

Chapter 92

Corneal Disease in Rheumatoid Arthritis

Vanee V. Virasch, Richard D. Brasington, Anthony J. Lubniewski

Introduction

Rheumatoid arthritis (RA) is the prototype of the systemic, autoimmune disease. It is a chronic inflammatory disease of unknown etiology, affecting primarily synovial joints, and less frequently extra-articular tissues, such as the eye, pleura, pericardium, and nerve. The incidence of RA is about 1%, affecting women approximately three times as often as men. Although disease occurs at any age, the incidence increases with advancing age. Onset is most common in women between the fourth and sixth decades. RA most commonly presents as a symmetrical polyarthritis, involving the small joints of the hands and feet, as well as larger joints such as the wrists, elbows, shoulders, knees, and ankles.[1]

The diagnosis of RA is currently based on a set of seven criteria put forth by the American Rheumatism Association. These criteria include the presence, for greater than 6 weeks, of either morning stiffness, polyarthritis, arthritis involving hand joints, or symmetric arthritis, in addition to rheumatoid nodules, positive serum rheumatoid factor, or characteristic radiographic changes of the joints. Satisfying four of these seven criteria allows for high sensitivity and specificity in diagnosing RA.[2]

It is now recognized that, unless treated aggressively, RA is a chronic, progressive disease, resulting in substantial disability and increased mortality.[3] Studies from the last two decades have clearly demonstrated that inadequately treated patients with RA have mortality of about 40–50% at 5 years.[4] The patients who present with ophthalmic disease tend to be patients with severe, long-standing RA and high titers of rheumatoid factor.[5] Fortunately, extra-articular disease is now less common than before, due to the current approach of treating RA aggressively early in the course of the disease.

Pathogenesis

The etiopathogenesis of RA is unknown. The current model holds that the disease develops in the genetically predisposed host upon exposure to an as yet unknown stimulus or antigen in the environment. We know, for example, that many patients with RA have in common a highly conserved region in the antigen-binding region of the third hypervariable region of the HLA class II beta chain molecule between amino acids 67 and 74, the so-called 'shared epitope.'[6] The hypothesis is that an interaction between host and foreign antigen (such as an unidentified infectious agent) sets off an immunological reaction to self which is inappropriately perpetuated, resulting in damage to articular structures. While we do not understand all the fine details of this immunological response, we do know that the inflammatory cytokines tumor necrosis factor alpha (TNF-α) and interleukin-1 (IL-1) appear to be largely responsible for driving the inflammatory cascade which leads to inflammation of synovial joints and the damage to the articular structures.[7,8] Moreover, the recognition of the imbalance between these proinflammatory mediators, and their naturally occurring inhibitors (soluble TNF receptor and IL-1 receptor antagonist), has led to remarkably effective treatments.

Rheumatoid factors are antibodies, most commonly IgM, with affinity for the Fc region of human IgG. Serum rheumatoid factors can be detected in 70–90% of RA patients as compared to 1–5% of the general population. In patients with an established diagnosis of RA, high titers of rheumatoid factor are associated with a higher incidence of extra-articular manifestations, more severe joint destruction, and worse prognosis. Additionally, the presence of rheumatoid factor and increasing titers of the antibody are predictive for the development of RA in patients without active disease.[9]

The advent of detection of antibody to cyclic citrullinated proteins has been a major advance in the diagnosis of early RA. Citrullination (conversion of peptidyl-arginine to peptidyl-citrulline) is a post-translational modification of proteins which is thought to be important in the initiation of the autoimmune response which leads to the development of RA. Antibodies to CCP (anti-CCP) are highly specific for RA, and can be detected very early in disease.[10] The combination of a positive anti-CCP with a positive RF further increases the specificity for RA.[11] A Swedish study of blood bank samples showed that each of these tests had about a 70% sensitivity for detecting the individuals who ultimately developed RA, and the combination of these two tests resulted in 99% specificity.[12] Thus, seropositivity for either of these tests, in a patient with symmetrical polyarthritis in the hands and feet, makes the diagnosis of RA quite likely.

Clinical Manifestations

Articular manifestations

The initial clinical presentation of RA can be quite variable, although typically the patient displays swelling in the small joints of the hands and feet, morning stiffness, and fatigue. Most commonly, the onset is insidious, but occasionally may be abrupt, with a transition from wellness to disease occurring overnight. RA almost always involves the small joints of the hands and feet; in fact, the absence of involvement of the proximal interphalangeal joints (PIP), metacarpal–phalangeal joints (MCP), wrists, and forefeet casts doubt on the validity of the diagnosis of RA.

Symmetry in joint involvement is a hallmark of the disease. As a practical matter, a patient with symmetrical swelling of the small joints of the hands, morning stiffness lasting more than 1 hour, and a positive rheumatoid factor most likely has RA.

Extra-articular manifestations

There are a variety of extra-articular manifestations of RA. Rheumatoid nodules affect about 30% of all RA patients and are present in about 50% of patients with RA and scleritis.[13] Episcleral, scleral, choroidal, and orbital nodules have been described but are rare.[14–18] The classic histologic features of the rheumatoid nodule include a zone of central necrosis surrounded by a densely cellular corona of pallisading fibroblasts, and collagen fibers, in turn surrounded by an outer more vascular capsular zone less densely infiltrated with lymphocytes, plasma cells, mast cells, perivascular histiocytes, and macrophages.[15,19]

Vasculitis of variable-sized vessels, particularly smaller vessels including vasa nervorum and digital vessels, is another recognized RA-associated phenomenon.[20] The activity of the vasculitis in these patients seems to correlate well with serum rheumatoid factor levels.[21] Immunoglobulin and complement deposition within blood vessel walls, infiltration with lymphocytes, and in some instances neutrophils, and focal areas of vessel wall necrosis have been demonstrated in rheumatoid vasculitis.[22,23] Rheumatoid vasculitis may first manifest itself in the eye with the presence of peripheral ulcerative keratitis or necrotizing scleritis.[24] Other nonocular extra-articular manifestations of RA may involve the lungs, heart, skin, muscles, bones, central and peripheral nervous system, and hematopoietic and lymphoreticular systems.[25–30] Of these extra-articular manifestations, necrotizing scleritis, peripheral ulcerative keratitis, cryoglobulinemia, neuropathy, skin ulceration, and vasculitic rash are the best identifiers of patients with poor life prognosis.[31,32]

Ocular manifestations

Keratoconjunctivitis sicca

There are a variety of ocular manifestations of rheumatoid arthritis. The most common associated disorder is keratoconjunctivitis sicca (KCS), or secondary Sjögren's syndrome (SS), which is clinically evident in 15–25% of RA patients.[33,34]

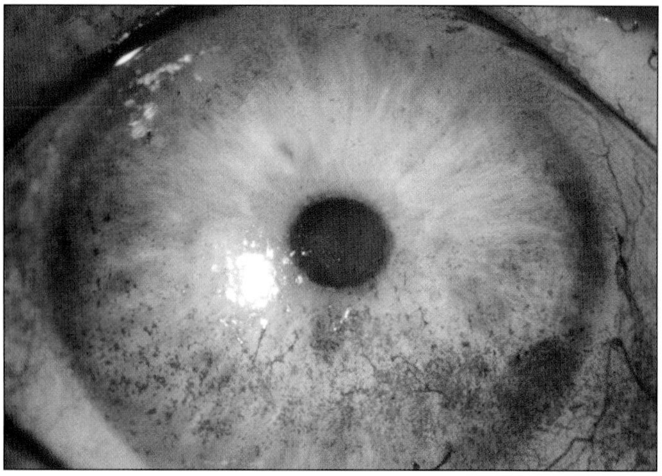

Fig. 92.1 Slit lamp photograph of severe keratoconjunctivitis sicca in a patient with RA. Note intense rose Bengal staining of superficial punctate keratopathy on the inferior cornea and interpalpebral conjunctiva as well as uptake by corneal filaments.

It remains a matter of debate whether 'secondary Sjögren's syndrome' represents a separate coexisting entity from a rheumatic disease or is a clinical manifestation as part of a rheumatic disorder. A recent study suggests that the etiology of dry eye may be different in RA patients with secondary SS and patients without secondary SS.[35] The symptoms, nevertheless, are similar to primary Sjögren's syndrome. Ocular sicca usually develops in the setting of long-standing rheumatoid disease, although it may be an early or presenting manifestation of RA. Patients may complain of gritty or sandy foreign body sensation, burning, irritation, mucus discharge, and photophobia. On examination, patients have a diminished tear meniscus, and Schirmer testing reveals decreased tear production. Punctate epithelial keratopathy, mucus stranding, and filamentary keratitis may be found on examination. Corneal and conjunctival findings are most easily seen with fluorescein, rose Bengal, or lissamine green stains (Fig. 92.1). Staining of the nasal and temporal interpalpebral conjunctiva is typical early in the disease, with diffuse confluent corneal staining occurring subsequently with progression of disease. Determination of tear lysozyme or lactoferrin concentration may be a useful diagnostic adjunct.[36,37] A severity scale for dry eye was recently introduced based on a Delphi panel that provides a useful clinical schema to aid in assessing severity of disease and can help guide treatment of the dry eye patient.[38]

The pathogenesis of keratoconjunctivitis sicca in secondary Sjögren's syndrome is lacrimal gland hyposecretion and conjunctival changes leading to tear hyperosmolarity and tear film instability. Hyposecretion is amplified by a neurosecretory block due to the effects of inflammatory cytokines, such as IL-1β, IL-6, and TNF-α, or to the presence of circulating antibodies directed against muscarinic receptors within the glands.[39–41] Inflammatory mediators are present in the tears and within the conjunctiva, although it is not clear whether they originate from the lacrimal gland or the conjunctiva itself.[39]

Histopathologic examination of lacrimal and salivary glands in Sjögren's syndrome reveals infiltration and

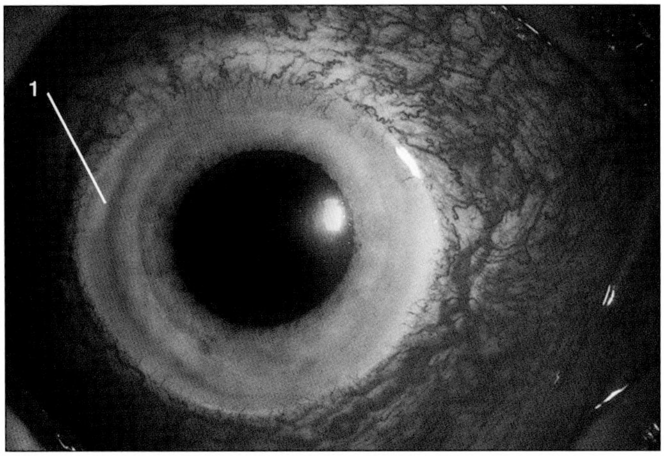

Fig. 92.2 Slit lamp photograph of a 65-year-old patient with RA demonstrating diffuse anterior scleritis associated with marginal infiltrates (*1*) and posterior scleritis. (Courtesy of Edward J. Holland, MD, Cincinnati, OH.)

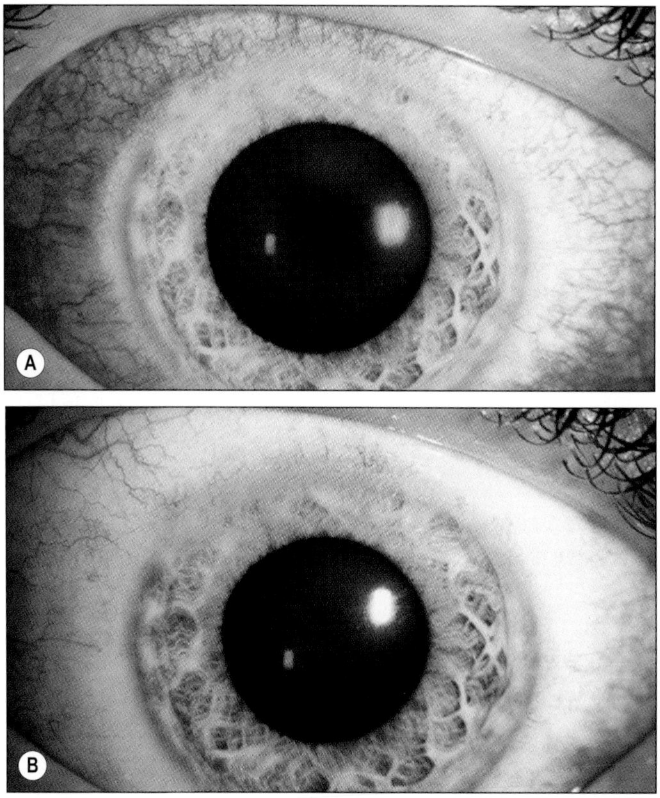

Fig. 92.3 Scleritis. (**A**) Slit lamp photograph of a patient with diffuse episcleritis before instillation of neosynephrine. (**B**) Same patient minutes after instillation of one drop of 2.5% neosynephrine ophthalmic solution. Note blanching of the superficial vessels. (Courtesy of D. Doughman, MD, Minneapolis, MN.)

replacement of normal lacrimal and salivary glandular structures by both T and B lymphocytes. The central portion of affected gland lobules is often densely infiltrated, with relative sparing of the lobule periphery.[42] Plasma cells, macrophages, and histiocytes may also be present. The extent of histopathologic change found in the lacrimal gland has been shown to correlate with the duration of KCS.[43] Histopathologic findings are not limited to the lacrimal gland, as conjunctival impression cytology specimens in patients with primary Sjögren's syndrome demonstrated squamous metaplasia, goblet cell loss, and lymphocytic infiltration more frequently than in non-Sjögren's dry eye patients.[44]

Scleritis

After KCS, scleritis is the most common ocular manifestation of RA, occurring in up to 20% of RA patients with isolated episcleritis in up to 11%.[13,45–48] Scleritis usually occurs in patients with well-established RA who have other extra-articular manifestations of the disease. The occurrence of scleritis or episcleritis is often a harbinger of worsening systemic disease and warrants reevaluation of the existing medical therapy in these patients.[49] In contrast to patients with episcleritis, who complain of only mild to moderate pain or irritation, patients with scleritis often complain of severe boring ocular pain and photophobia. However, the finding of episcleritis should not be taken lightly as up to 36% of patients may have a systemic disease association, with 14% having a systemic vasculitic-autoimmune condition.[47] Disease activity in the setting of RA or other autoimmune diseases is often more severe than in idiopathic scleritis cases.[46] All types of anterior scleritis, including diffuse, nodular, necrotizing scleritis with inflammation and necrotizing scleritis without inflammation (scleromalacia perforans), as well as posterior scleritis, have been documented in patients with RA.[45]

Diffuse anterior scleritis is the most common and the most benign scleritis variant (Fig. 92.2). Sectoral or widespread inflammation of the ocular surface may be encountered with scleral and episcleral edema and chemosis, as well as distortion and engorgement of the superficial radial and deep interwoven episcleral vessels. These vessels do not typically blanch with topical application of neosynephrine as they do in episcleritis (Fig. 92.3).[48,50]

In nodular scleritis, single or multiple, firm, tender nodules anchored to underlying stroma can be seen (Fig. 92.4). Nodular scleritis tends to be intermediate in severity between diffuse anterior scleritis and necrotizing scleritis with respect to signs and symptoms of disease and final visual outcome.[45,50]

Patients with necrotizing scleritis with inflammation exhibit zones of intense scleral inflammation, edema, and necrosis with overlying epithelial defects (Fig. 92.5). Patients most often have severe pain. Some patients, however, can exhibit large areas of necrosis and thinning and be relatively pain free.[51] During active episodes of necrotizing scleritis, overlying epithelial integrity needs to be carefully assessed. Change in the size of epithelial defects, extent of stromal necrosis, depth of underlying stromal loss, and presence of adjacent keratitis all need to be followed closely during an acute episode.[48,49] Secondary bacterial and fungal infections can occur and must be considered in the diagnosis and management.

Patients with necrotizing scleritis without inflammation, also referred to as scleromalacia perforans, have usually had severe RA for many years.[52] Severe scleral thinning may be

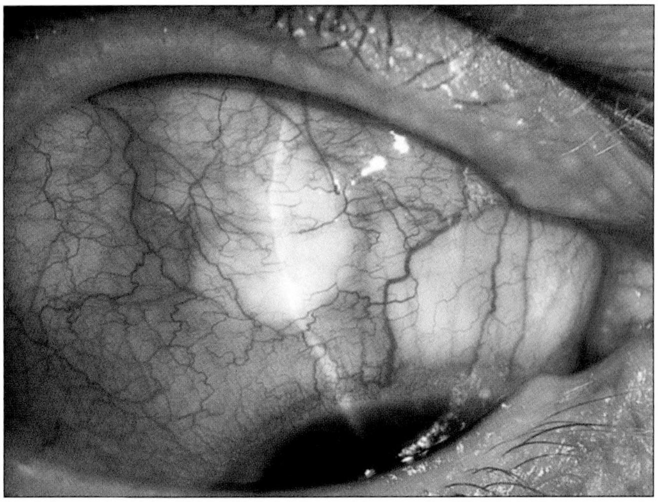

Fig. 92.4 Slit lamp photograph demonstrating a thickened scleral nodule in a 53-year-old patient with RA and diffuse nodular scleritis.

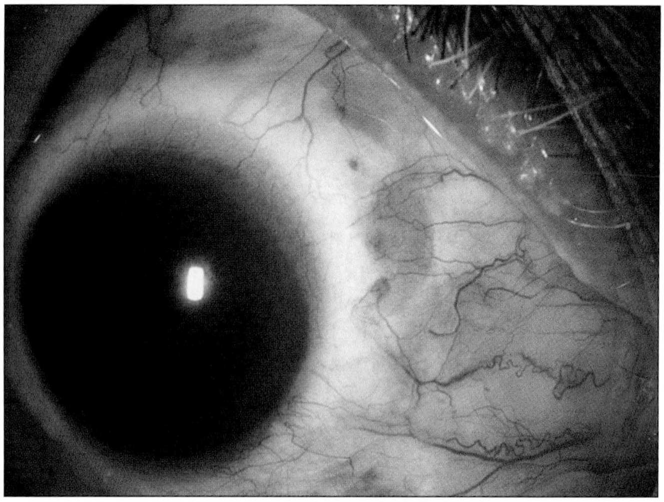

Fig. 92.6 Slit lamp photograph of diffuse scleromalacia perforans in a 70-year-old patient with long-standing RA.

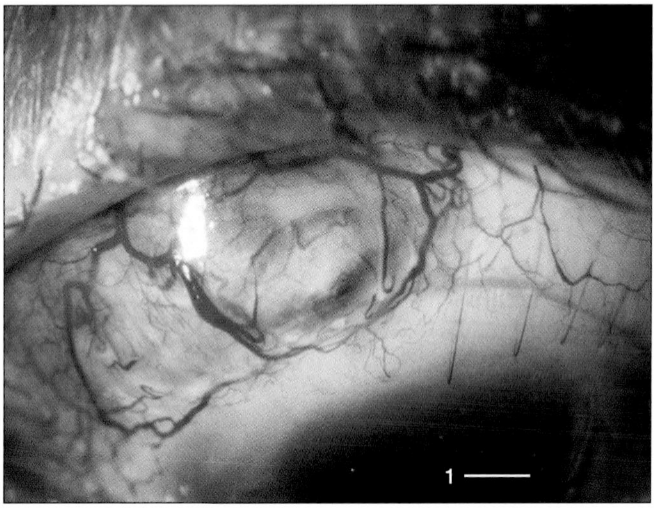

Fig. 92.5 Slit lamp photograph demonstrating necrotizing scleritis overlying the nasal aspect of a cataract incision 3 months after extracapsular cataract extraction with intraocular lens implant. Also note the filamentary keratitis (*1*).

present and manifest as blue-gray areas of sclera on slit lamp examination. An exaggerated eye wall convexity or brown discoloration indicates areas of extreme scleral thinning where uvea may be covered only by conjunctiva and episclera (Fig. 92.6). These eyes are at increased risk for rupture secondary to minor trauma.

Posterior scleritis is also seen in patients with RA. Its signs and symptoms may include a concurrent anterior scleritis, proptosis, ocular pain worsening with eye movement, and exudative retinal detachment (Fig. 92.7A,B).[45,50] Evidence of posterior scleral edema and inflammation can often be demonstrated on ultrasonography.[53] Orbital imaging studies using magnetic resonance imaging (MRI) or computed tomography (CT) scanning, with and without contrast, can help distinguish posterior scleritis from other disease processes such as orbital pseudotumor or orbital cellulites (Fig. 92.7C).

Histopathologic evaluation of scleritis in RA patients suggests contributions of both type III (immune complex) and type IV (cell-mediated) hypersensitivity reactions in the pathogenesis of scleritis. The histopathologic changes seen in scleritis include a zonal granulomatous inflammation with central necrosis surrounded by neutrophils, histiocytes, and giant cells, in turn surrounded by lymphocytes and plasma cells, with unravelling of scleral fibers adjacent to the areas of necrosis and inflammatory cell infiltration.[51] Additionally, vasculitis with vessel wall immune complex deposition, inflammatory cell infiltration, fibrinoid necrosis, and resultant vessel thrombosis has been described.[50,54] Histopathologic examination of rheumatoid scleritis also reveals a distinct lack of lymphoid follicles and often a lack of evidence of accumulation of granulation tissue in the areas of scleral destruction, suggesting an aberrant wound healing response in this setting.[51] Based on histopathologic changes, immune-mediated scleritis can be differentiated from idiopathic or infectious scleritis; however, the changes seen in rheumatoid scleritis are not specific enough to differentiate this entity from other immune-mediated causes.[55]

Keratitis

Keratitis in RA occurs most often contiguous with adjacent scleritis, but it may occur as an isolated finding.[48,56] It may also occur following previous episodes of scleritis, even in the setting of previous successful scleritis treatment with immunosuppressive agents. The corneal findings associated with scleritis, including sclerosing keratitis, acute stromal keratitis, limbal guttering, peripheral ulcerative keratitis, and keratolysis, have been well described and occur in up to 50% of patients with scleritis.[24,45]

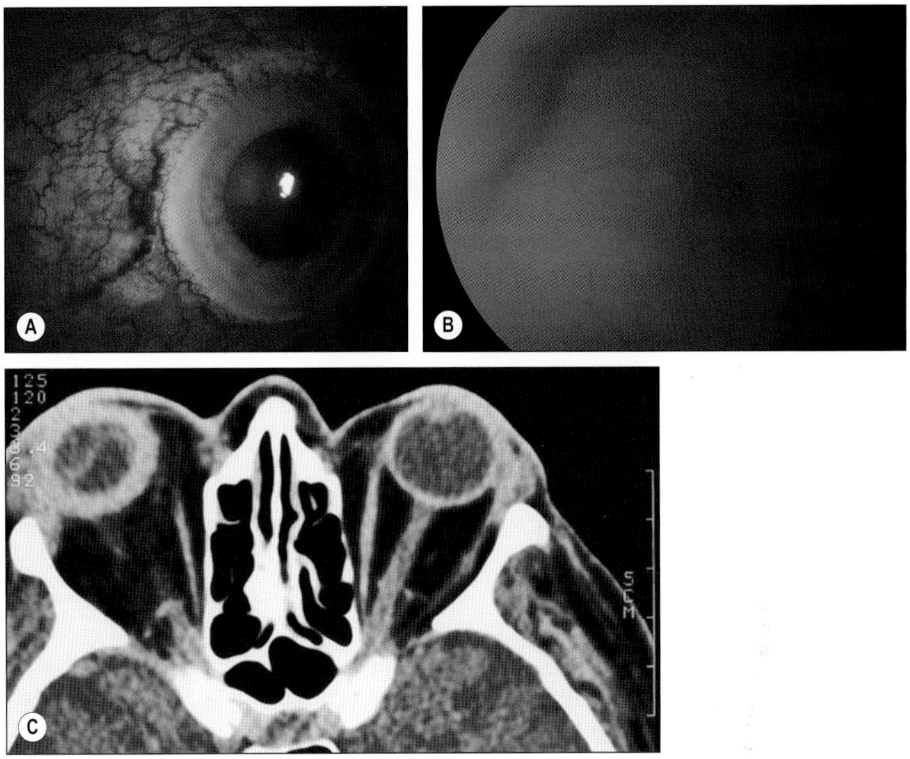

Fig. 92.7 Scleritis. (**A**) Slit lamp photograph of diffuse anterior and posterior scleritis in a 67-year-old patient with RA. (**B**) Fundus photograph of an exudative retinal detachment in the same patient. (**C**) Axial noncontrast CT image of same patient demonstrating diffuse anterior and posterior scleral thickening.

Sclerosing keratitis occurs most frequently adjacent to an area of active scleritis.[13] In sclerosing keratitis, the peripheral cornea becomes thickened and opacified and may become secondarily vascularized. These changes may extend centripetally over time and may leave the cornea completely opacified, particularly when the patient is untreated or when severe circumferential disease is manifest.[32]

Acute stromal keratitis can manifest as stromal opacities at any level of the cornea with accompanying stromal edema (Fig. 92.8). The opacities may coalesce if left untreated. Overlying epithelium may break down with the development of peripheral ulcerative keratitis (PUK) (Fig. 92.9).[57] Vascularization and thinning of the cornea may occur as well. Many of these findings may resolve, however, with appropriate treatment and resolution of the accompanying scleritis.[58]

Limbal guttering has also been reported both adjacent to an area of active scleritis and as an isolated finding (Fig. 92.10). In limbal guttering, the corneal epithelium generally remains intact and the extent of peripheral thinning may be variable. In severe cases, limbal guttering may progress to perforation with or without trauma.

Peripheral ulcerative keratitis is often associated with necrotizing scleritis and may carry the same guarded prognosis. The current proposed scheme for the pathogenesis of PUK is immune complex deposition in the limbal vessels leading to immune-mediated vasculitis that results in leakage of inflammatory cells and proteins. This subsequently activates the complement system and increases cytokine production, recruiting neutrophils and macrophages that release collagenases and other proteases that in turn cause corneal tissue destruction.[24,56,59] Studies have shown that increased cytokines may also stimulate an increase in matrix

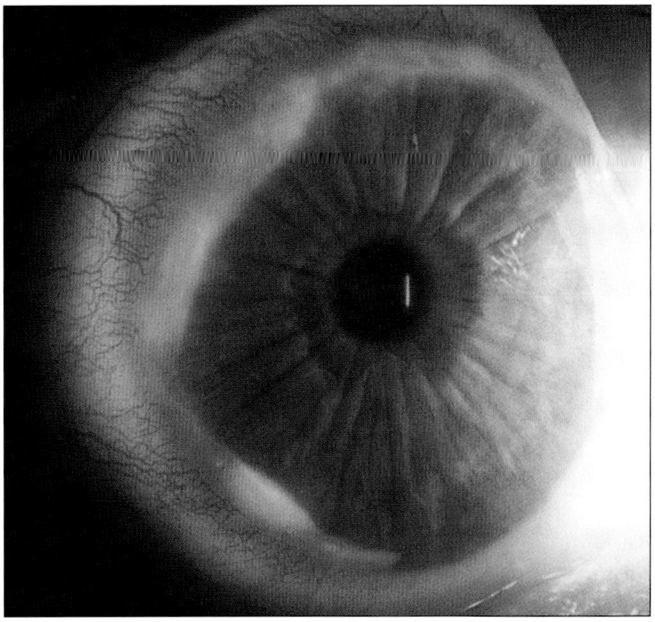

Fig. 92.8 Slit lamp photograph of the right eye of a 50-year-old patient with RA and acute marginal stromal infiltrates.

metalloproteinase production by keratocytes themselves, contributing further to the rapid corneal destruction seen in PUK.[60] Occlusion of adjacent limbal vessels, antibodies to corneal antigens, limbal conjunctival collagenase production, and decreased local expression of collagenase

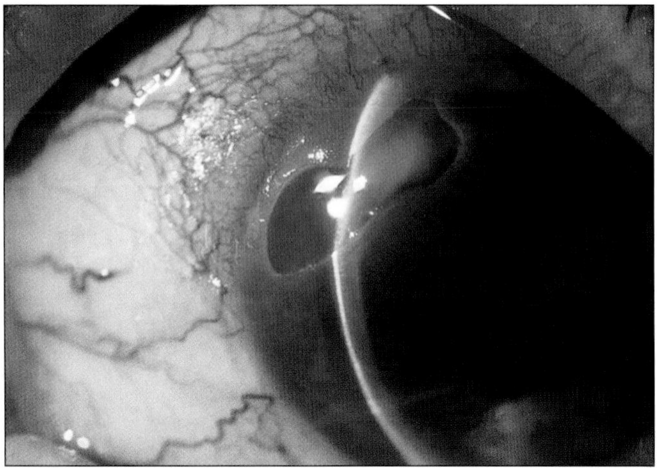

Fig. 92.9 Slit lamp photograph of a patient with peripheral ulcerative keratitis (PUK). Note the sectoral location with associated scleritis, corneal infiltrate, and overlying epithelial defect.

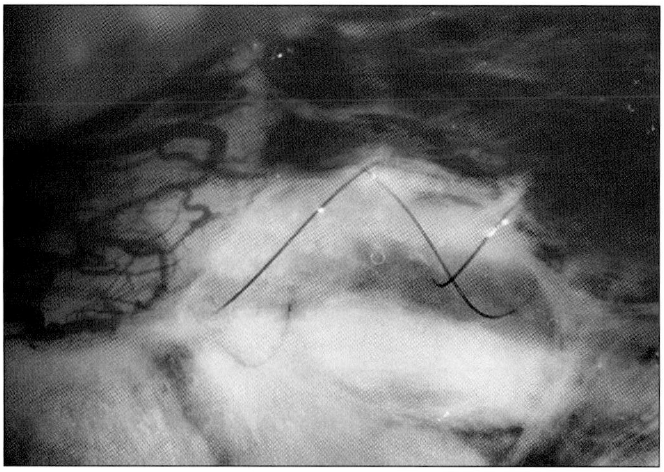

Fig. 92.11 Slit lamp photograph of necrotizing scleritis 1 week after phacoemulsification with intraocular lens implantation. Note eroded running suture and prolapsed uveal tissue. (Courtesy of Edward J. Holland, MD, Cincinnati, OH.)

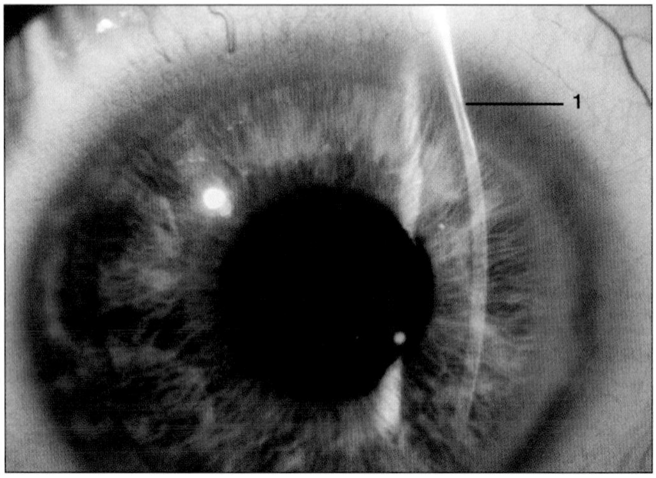

Fig. 92.10 Slit lamp photograph of a patient with limbal guttering (*1*). Note the absence of stromal infiltrate.

inhibitors have all been described and are thought to be important pathogenetically in PUK.[61–65] Patients can also have secondary infectious keratitis or scleritis associated with rheumatoid marginal keratitis, PUK, or necrotizing scleritis.[66,67] A high index of suspicion along with frequent reassessment will assist in early diagnosis and subsequent treatment of these secondary complications.

Keratolysis may occur associated with necrotizing scleritis in inflamed or noninflamed eyes. Loss of stroma occurs in regions of clear cornea and may progress to descemetocele formation.[68] Corneal and scleral stromal lysis with wound dehiscence has also been described after cataract, strabismus, and other intraocular surgeries in patients with RA, often in patients with preoperative KCS (Fig. 92.11).[69–71] Postoperative scleral or corneal necrosis may, in fact, be the first manifestation of a systemic vasculitic process, and such patients should receive an appropriate autoimmune work-up with a consulting rheumatologist to rule out RA or other autoimmune disorders.[72]

Additional ocular disease

There are several ocular manifestations of RA in addition to the corneal and scleral manifestations, including orbital myositis,[73] Brown's syndrome,[74,75] cranial nerve palsies,[76] scleritis-associated nongranulomatous anterior uveitis,[77] rubeosis,[78] cataracts and glaucoma,[45,46,49] complications secondary to posterior scleritis including optic neuritis, choroidal masses, chorioretinal scarring, choroidal and retinal detachment,[53,79] retinal microangiopathy with cottonwool spots,[80,81] and posterior segment vasculitis.[82,83]

Treatment

Systemic disease

The treatment of RA is controversial, since the disease varies with respect to clinical course and outcome. The primary goals of treatment are to slow or reduce the inflammatory process in the hope of minimizing joint and muscle damage as well to relieve pain in order to maintain functional status. It is now understood that damage may progress in patients with persistent synovial proliferation, even if their symptoms are well controlled, leading to progressive disability. This recognition, as well as the understanding that the mortality of individuals with severe RA is increased, has resulted in the contemporary view that rheumatoid arthritis should be treated aggressively as soon as the disease is diagnosed.[84,85] Three major classes of therapeutics are used: nonsteroidal antiinflammatory drugs (NSAIDs), corticosteroids, and disease-modifying antirheumatic drugs (DMARDs).

Nonsteroidal antiinflammatory drugs (NSAIDs) improve the quality of life for patients with RA by reducing pain and inflammation, and should be part of the medical regimen for most patients.[84] However, NSAIDs do nothing to prevent joint damage and disability. Systemic corticosteroids, especially prednisone, also provide dramatic relief of symptoms,[86,87] although they are not as effective as the so-called disease-modifying antirheumatic drugs (DMARDs). Clinical evidence demonstrates that DMARDs prevent bone and cartilage damage and improve signs, symptoms, and quality of life for patients with RA.[88] Thus, initial therapy for a patient with RA will almost always include a NSAID, a DMARD, and sometimes oral prednisone.

The choice of an initial DMARD depends very much upon the training and experience of the individual rheumatologist, but it would be fair to say that most rheumatologists begin with methotrexate.[84] Methotrexate is well known as an antagonist of tetrahydrofolic acid, but its mechanism of action in the treatment of RA may also entail its effects on adenosine metabolism and purine synthesis. The oral route of administration is most common, in doses of 7.5–20 mg once a week. The most common untoward effects of methotrexate administration are aphthous stomatitis, nausea, diarrhea, elevation of hepatic transaminases, and cytopenias. Co-administration of folic acid, 1–2 mg daily, can prevent or reduce such problems. Periodic laboratory monitoring of complete blood count (CBC) and chemistry profile including albumin, aspartate aminotransferase (AST), alanine aminotransferase (ALT), and creatinine is essential.

Sulfasalazine is preferred as the initial DMARD by some.[89] Its mechanism of action is not fully understood. It is administered orally on a daily basis in two or three divided doses. Patients are generally started on 500 mg b.i.d. and the dose increased to a total of 2–3 g daily. Gastrointestinal tolerability is better with an enteric-coated preparation. Periodic laboratory monitoring is also necessary with sulfasalazine.

Leflunomide (Arava) is the newest orally administered small-molecule DMARD. Leflunomide's active metabolite inhibits the enzyme dihydroorotate dehydrogenase, thereby blocking the synthesis of de novo pyrimidines in activated lymphocytes. The dose of leflunomide is either 10 or 20 mg daily. Diarrhea, rash, and hair loss are the common symptomatic toxicities, and monitoring of AST and ALT is critical, since serious hepatic toxicity has been observed. Direct comparison trials have shown that leflunomide is comparable to methotrexate, and probably superior to sulfasalazine, in terms of symptom relief and prevention of radiographic progression.[90]

Other DMARD agents occasionally used for systemic rheumatoid arthritis include ciclosporin,[91,92] penicillamine,[93] antimalarials (hydroxychloroquine),[94] and oral and injectable gold.[94] Ciclosporin has been used effectively to treat ocular manifestations of rheumatoid vasculitis[95] at a dose of 2–4 mg/kg in two divided doses. Close monitoring of renal function is critical; dose reduction or cessation of treatment is indicated if the serum creatinine rises more than 30% above baseline. Rigorous control of blood pressure is also essential. Permanent renal impairment can result if the above guidelines are not followed closely.[95,96] Despite their decreased use, the above-mentioned DMARDs have a history of proven efficacy and continue to be used worldwide.[97]

The availability of agents that effectively block TNF has revolutionized the treatment of RA. The first agent to obtain FDA approval (1998) was etanercept (Enbrel), which exploits the naturally occurring inhibitor of TNF, soluble TNF receptor (sTNFR). This agent is given as a twice-weekly subcutaneous dose of 25 mg. Etanercept has been shown to have efficacy comparable to methotrexate, but works more rapidly, with onset of improvement often occurring within 1–2 weeks.[98] Etanercept may be given as a single agent, or in combination with methotrexate.[99]

Infliximab (Remicade) is a monoclonal antibody to TNF created by immunization of mice with purified human TNF. Genetic manipulation converts the constant portion of this immunoglobulin molecule to human sequences, resulting in a 'chimeric' monoclonal antibody. Infliximab therapy is more effective when co-administered with methotrexate, perhaps because the immunosuppressive effect of the methotrexate may suppress the patient's formation of human antichimeric antibodies, which might neutralize the infliximab. Infliximab is given intravenously at a starting dose of 3 mg/kg, followed by similar doses 2 and 6 weeks later, then every 8 weeks. Patients with a suboptimal response to this regimen are often treated with a higher dose of infliximab, or a shorter interval of 4 weeks between infusions.[100]

The most recently available TNF blocker is adalimumab (Humira). Unlike infliximab, it is derived entirely from human immunoglobulin sequences, and is a genetically engineered anti-TNF antibody. Because its half-life is 10–20 days, it can be administered subcutaneously every other week. Efficacy and prevention of radiographic progression seems to be comparable to that seen with etanercept and infliximab. Clinical trial data support its use both with and without methotrexate.[101]

IL-1 is the other proinflammatory cytokine that drives the rheumatoid inflammatory process. Modern therapeutics takes advantage of the fact that a natural inhibitor, IL-1 receptor antagonist (IL-1ra), blocks the activity of IL-1 by binding to its receptor without generating a transmembrane signal. Recombinant genetic technology has produced anakinra (Kineret), which is administered as a daily dose of 100 mg.[102] Although this agent does not produce dramatic relief of symptoms in as large a percentage of patients as the TNF blockers, for some patients it is very effective.

In 2007, two additional biologic DMARDS were FDA approved for the treatment of RA. In general, these agents are considered after unsuccessful treatment with one or more of the TNF antagonists. Two biologics should never be used in combination; all the evidence to date for such combinations shows no increase in efficacy and a definite increase in infectious toxicity.

Abatacept is a fusion protein joining the T-cell surface protein CTLA4 (cytotoxic lymphocyte-associated antigen 4) to the Fc fragment of the IgG_1 molecule. Intravenous administration of CTLA4-Ig (abatacept) retards the excessive T-cell activation that is believed to be pathologic in some patients with RA. Abatacept is FDA approved for the treatment of RA which does not respond adequately to methotrexate, although it is most commonly prescribed for RA unresponsive to TNF antagonists.

Rituximab is a chimeric monoclonal antibody to a unique B-lymphocytes surface antigen CD20, which has been FDA approved since 1997 for the treatment of lymphoma. Administration results in rapid and complete depletion of peripheral blood B cells in RA patients. About one-quarter of patients treated in phase III clinical trials achieved at least 50% improvement, and the mean duration of response is 7 months. Repeated courses of this agent can be given.

At this writing, additional TNF antagonists are awaiting FDA approval. Golimumab is a monoclonal anti-TNF antibody administered once monthly. Certolizumab pegol is a unique fusion protein combining the Fab′ fragment of an anti-TNF monoclonal antibody fused to a polyethylene glycol base, also parenterally administered. Finally, tocilizumab is a monoclonal antibody to the interleukin-6 receptor. All three of these agents have shown efficacy in treating RA.

Extra-articular manifestations of RA are generally regarded as less common in the current era, perhaps because of the current aggressive approach to the treatment of RA. Nonetheless, occasionally patients with severe, seropositive, nodular, destructive RA will experience nonarticular complications such as interstitial lung disease, cutaneous and systemic vasculitis, pericarditis, and ocular inflammatory disease. There are no prospective, controlled, double-masked, randomized, placebo-controlled trials evaluating the above agents in the treatment of these extra-articular manifestations. Yet, clinical experience and case reports suggest that some of the above agents may be of benefit in treating ocular inflammatory disease.[103–106]

Potent immunosuppressive drugs such as azathioprine and cyclophosphamide are used for the treatment of rheumatoid vasculitis and other severe systemic extra-articular problems.[95] The dose for each agent is 1–2 mg/kg/day in a single oral dose. Close monitoring of the CBC is critical, since profound cytopenias can result, leading to bleeding and/or opportunistic infections. The metabolites of cyclophosphamide can damage the bladder mucosa, resulting in hemorrhagic cystitis and bladder cancer. Therefore, morning dosing and vigorous oral hydration with maintenance of high urine output is important during the administration of cyclosphosphamide. The agent can also be given in an intravenous bolus every 1–3 months.[95]

Ocular disease

Therapy for patients with ocular manifestations of RA is also tailored to individual patients' symptoms and findings. KCS and mild to moderate anterior scleritis can often be successfully managed with topical agents by the ophthalmologist. More severe disease may involve the addition of systemic steroids. Treating necrotizing scleritis and peripheral ulcerative keratitis with the addition of systemic immunosuppressives (DMARDs) often requires close teamwork between the ophthalmologist and consulting rheumatologist.

Keratoconjunctivitis sicca (KCS)

The principles of treatment of secondary Sjögren's syndrome in patients with RA are the same as for KCS from other causes. Stepwise progressive therapy is directed at maintenance of the ocular surface while providing relief from symptoms. Underlying systemic diseases, blepharitis, allergic conditions, environmental triggers, concurrent systemic and topical medications, and abnormalities of eyelid position or function must be identified and addressed when possible. More recently, the control of ocular surface inflammation with resultant improvement in KCS signs and symptoms has revolutionized dry eye therapy.[107]

The initial treatment of KCS remains ocular surface lubrication with artificial tear substitutes, fornicial lubricating inserts, and lubricating ointments. In eyes that are not responsive to topical lubrication alone, additional medical interventions can be considered. A trial of moderate doses of topical steroids can be beneficial in treating the underlying inflammatory component often associated with dry eye.[108] Topical application of 20–50% autologous serum prepared sterile in saline has also shown efficacy in ocular surface disease. The replacement of biologically active tear components to help rehabilitate the ocular surface is the premise behind this therapy. However, issues regarding preparation, storage, and prevention of contamination remain.[109–111] Pharmacological stimulation of natural tear production by oral pilocarpine has been objectively shown to increase tear production and flow and to improve symptoms of dry eye and mouth in Sjögren's patients.[112] However, tolerance to the side effects including nausea, gastrointestinal cramping, palpitations, and sweating remains problematic. Newer parasympathomimetics, such as cevimeline, have been shown to be equally effective with a much lower side-effect profile.[113] Topical secretagogues, such as diquafosol, rebamipide, and ecabet sodium, are currently under development and have been shown to stimulate aqueous secretion, mucin secretion, or both.[39] A large, randomized study has shown diquafosol, a P2Y2 receptor agonist, to be well tolerated and superior to placebo in reducing corneal staining and symptoms in dry eye patients.[114] Other agents including acetylcysteine, sex hormones (androgens), and topical vitamin A have given variable results.[107]

Randomized clinical trials using topical ciclosporin A drops twice daily for management of dry eye have demonstrated significant improvement in the objective and subjective measurements of moderate and severe dry eye as well as symptoms with no significant topical or systemic adverse events.[115–117] A more recent study has also shown efficacy in patients with mild dry eye disease.[118] Conjunctival biopsies of patients with Sjögren's and non-Sjögren's-related KCS showed decreased levels of interleukin-6, decreased levels of lymphocyte activation markers CD11a and HLA-DR, and elevated goblet cell density following treatment with topical ciclosporin A when compared to baseline.[119–121]

Use of oral tetracycline derivatives has shown a significant beneficial effect on the treatment of eyelid margin disease as well as ocular surface inflammation.[122–124] Although their exact mechanisms of action remain poorly understood, proposed therapeutic actions include lowering the melting point of meibomian secretions, inhibition of cytokine production, protease and lipase inhibition, and antimicrobial activity.[122,123,125–129] Further, the use of tetracyclines has been shown to be effective in improving the symptoms of rheumatoid arthritis, perhaps providing a dual benefit in these patients.[130–132]

The use of nutritional supplementation such as omega-3, omega-6, linoleic acid, linolenic acid, and other essential fatty acids has been shown to improve quality of life and decrease systemic symptoms in rheumatoid patients, again providing a potential dual benefit.[133–136]

Additional medical and surgical interventions may be necessary for advanced disease secondary to KCS with persistent epithelial defects, sterile corneal ulceration, and significant exposure keratoconjunctivitis. Environmental modulators such as moisture chambers or commercially available goggles and a room humidifier may be beneficial. If nocturnal lagophthalmos is present, the use of a lubricating ointment in addition to the above measures or further surgical manipulation of the eyelids may be necessary.[137,138] Punctal occlusion is a very common technique used to maintain and prevent tear drainage from the ocular surface.[139] Punctal occlusion may worsen symptoms in the face of significant ocular surface inflammation, moderate eyelid margin disease, or allergic conjunctivitis, as delayed tear clearance may exacerbate irritation of the ocular surface secondary to an increase in the concentration of inflammatory mediators with delayed clearance from the tear film.[140,141]

For more severe disease, medial canthoplasty and/or lateral tarsorrhaphy can be performed and are generally underused. These techniques are particularly helpful for patients with persistent epithelial defects and sterile corneal ulcers, either from sicca syndrome or as an adjunct in keratolysis secondary to rheumatologic disease.[142] Either suture or chemical tarsorrhaphy, with botulinum type A, can be used on a temporary basis to promote healing of an acute exacerbation of severe keratitis.[139]

Keratitis

Oral corticosteroid and topical ciclosporin A play a major role in the treatment of RA-associated keratitis, particularly nonulcerative keratitis, keratolysis, and peripheral ulcerative keratitis (PUK) (Fig. 92.12).[68,143,144] Topical steroids should be used only with great caution in rheumatoid marginal furrowing with epithelial defects and sterile keratolysis, since they may lead to hastened thinning and perforation.[145–148] As described above, suture or chemical tarsorrhaphy can be a useful adjunct to help promote healing of persistent epithelial defects. Contact lens therapy with low water content lenses has been utilized as well; however, frequent assessment is necessary in order to prevent mechanical, hypoxic, and infectious complications.[149–152] Since protease activity has been documented in both PUK and paracentral keratolysis,[64,153–155] the use of inhibitors of these enzymes has been studied, with some success in delaying the progression of ulceration and promoting healing of epithelial defects.[155–157] Cytokine activity has also been documented in rheumatoid corneal ulcerations;[64] however, the use of inhibitors of these mediators has yet to be tested. The immunosuppressive treatment of patients with peripheral ulcerative keratitis, or severe recalcitrant keratitis or keratolysis, is similar to treatment of patients with necrotizing scleritis and is addressed below.

Scleritis

Non-necrotizing scleritis

Systemic medical therapy for RA-associated non-necrotizing scleritis and keratitis is successful in most cases.[48] As in the treatment of systemic RA, a stepwise approach to treatment is commonly applied. Initial treatment for mild to moderate non-necrotizing scleritis may include oral NSAIDs. Indometacin (25 mg) or ibuprofen (600 mg) three times a day or naproxen (500 mg) twice a day can be effective in rapidly relieving ocular pain and inflammation, often within the first few days of therapy.[45,48] Gastrointestinal side effects remain a significant problem with the use of oral NSAIDs. The use of more selective NSAIDs may hopefully reduce these side effects while maintaining efficacy, but these agents have yet to be formally studied in scleritis.[158,159] Topical steroid drops and ointments can be used initially in combination with oral NSAIDs or can be added to this initial NSAID therapy if there is no symptomatic relief or improvement in the clinical picture within the first weeks of NSAID therapy alone. Topical steroids alone are not as efficacious in the treatment of anterior scleritis.[160] However, in the management of noninfectious, non-necrotizing anterior scleritis, subconjunctival corticosteroid injections have shown significant benefit without adverse side effects.[161–163] Topical NSAIDs may play a role in early stages as well. These agents are less well tolerated, and patients often complain of burning with instillation, but they avoid the problems of glaucoma and cataract formation sometimes seen with

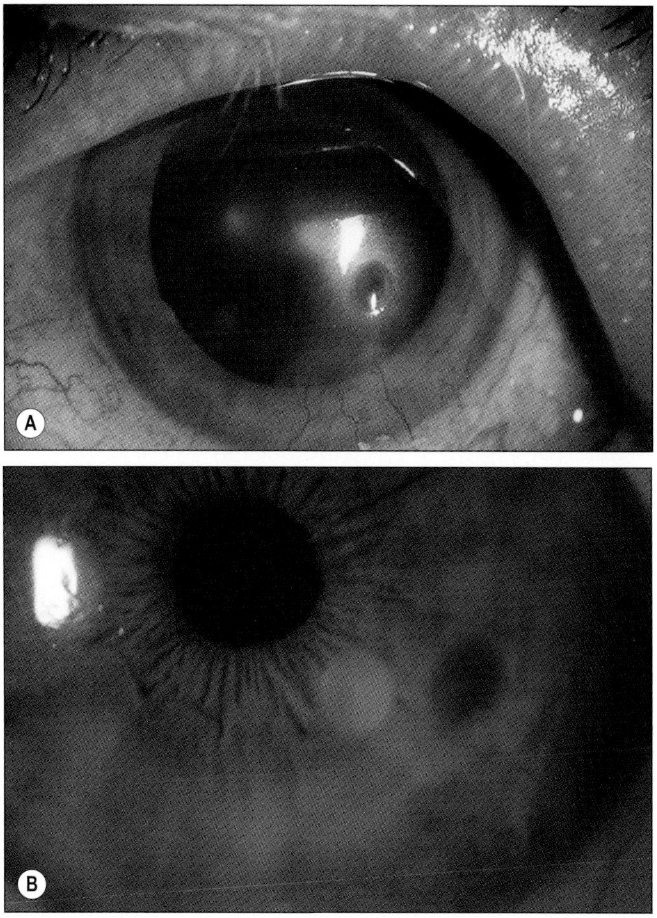

Fig. 92.12 Keratitis. (**A**) Slit lamp photograph of paracentral keratolysis in a patient with RA. (**B**) Subsequent healing with minimal scar formation with the use of topical ciclosporin 0.5% in nonpreserved artificial tears.

topical steroid use. Problems with corneal complications such as keratitis and frank melting have been reported and are presumably secondary to stimulation of protease activity, potentially limiting their use for these conditions.[164,165]

Regarding necrotizing scleritis without inflammation, scleromalacia perforans, treatment is generally observation, eye protection, and therapeutic modulation of systemic disease. In the absence of trauma, this condition tends to be slowly progressive and does not require aggressive management.[166] However, with trauma, perforation may occur, necessitating tectonic reconstruction.

Necrotizing scleritis and peripheral ulcerative keratitis (PUK)

Necrotizing scleritis with inflammation is the ocular manifestation of a systemic vasculitic process and is a particularly ominous finding. It should be addressed with ophthalmic and medical urgency. Ocular morbidity is high, and, more importantly, without appropriate systemic immunosuppression, more than half of these patients may die within 5 years of onset of their disease.[13,32,167] Internal medicine or rheumatologic consultation is imperative for the diagnosis and management of associated systemic findings. Therapy initiated for other systemic findings may, in fact, have beneficial effects on the ocular manifestations.

The etiology of necrotizing scleritis or PUK must be addressed, as the differential diagnosis is broad.[57] Infectious etiologies must be initially ruled out, as treatment with immunosuppression could lead to exacerbation.[168–170] Such patients need to undergo corneal scrapings for Gram and KOH stains, and for bacterial and fungal culture. Appropriate intensive, broad-spectrum, fortified, topical antimicrobial therapy must be started immediately in such cases.

The goal of medical treatment in patients with necrotizing scleritis and PUK is to reduce inflammation, promote epithelial healing, and minimize stromal loss. Preservative-free lubricating agents are helpful in managing the ocular surface. Initiation of topical therapy with immunomodulators such as ciclosporin A may be considered after secondary fungal and bacterial ulceration have been ruled out or treated. Unlike with noninfectious, non-necrotizing scleritis, subconjunctival steroid injection in necrotizing scleritis is thought to be contraindicated despite an unclear history to support the proposed tendency to induce corneal and scleral stromal lyses.[78,161,163,171] These agents, though effective topically, do not treat the underlying vasculitis and this must be taken into consideration with the addition of systemic immunosuppression in order to influence the mortality rate.[32,172] As described above, increased protease activity has been documented in eyes with PUK and scleritis;[154,173] therefore, the use of protease inhibitors such as tetracycline derivatives may provide additional benefit in preventing further stromal loss. Adjunctive surgical procedures for tectonic support are sometimes required in severe cases.

In the setting of acute inflammation associated with severe scleritis or keratitis, oral prednisone at an initial dose of 1 mg/kg/day may be initiated in an attempt to reduce inflammation rapidly. If the desired clinical response is achieved, prednisone may be tapered rapidly to a 20 mg/day dosage over the second week, with a subsequent slower tapering of drug over subsequent weeks. Patients not responsive to oral prednisone may benefit from high-dose intravenous pulse methylprednisolone at initial doses as high as 1 g per day for 3 consecutive days followed by oral therapy.[95] It must be stressed, however, that despite a profound effect on ocular and systemic symptoms, systemic steroids fail to influence the high mortality rate of patients with rheumatoid vasculitis.[32] Therefore, the addition of cytotoxic chemotherapy is necessary to successfully treat these patients.[172]

Immunosuppressive drugs are the next line of therapy and, as previously stated, are truly mandatory in order to delay or prevent mortality secondary to rheumatoid vasculitis. They are used in recalcitrant cases of scleritis or keratitis, including necrotizing scleritis, PUK, and keratolysis.[24,48,95,172] Patients who have responded to oral steroids but who cannot be tapered off steroids without return of active disease may also be considered as candidates for immunosuppressive therapy. In this subset of patients, the initiation of immunosuppressive drugs may avoid complications of long-term systemic corticosteroids such as osteoporosis, worsening of hypertension and diabetes, electrolyte imbalances, and gastrointestinal bleeding.[95]

Immunosuppressive therapy in ocular inflammation

The therapeutic agents to be described have been found to be effective in cases poorly responsive to corticosteroids and other antiinflammatory agents. An excellent review of immunosuppressive therapy by Jabs and colleagues[95] and several subsequent studies have documented guidelines regarding the recommended choice, dosing, and application of the most utilized therapies and provides the basis for the following recommendations as well.[174,175] Immunomodulators available for use in ocular inflammatory diseases comprise antimetabolites, alkylating agents, T-cell inhibitors, and biologic agents.

Antimetabolites include methotrexate, azathioprine, mycophenolate mofetil, and leflunomide. Oral methotrexate in doses ranging from 7.5 to 25 mg/week has been shown to be effective in cases of scleritis unresponsive to oral corticosteroid.[95,176] Azathioprine (1–2.5 mg/kg/day) has also been used in the setting of severe or recalcitrant rheumatoid scleritis and peripheral ulcerative keratitis with varying degrees of success.[32,45,177] Recent studies have shown favorable results for mycophenolate motefil (1 g twice daily) as a monotherapy and adjunctive therapy for scleritis and also suggested better inflammatory control when compared with methotrexate, with fewer side effects than azathioprine.[178–180] Leflunomide is the newest of this class and at this writing, animal studies and a few clinical reports suggest there may be some efficacy in treatment of ocular inflammation.[181,182]

Alkylating agents consist of cyclophosphamide and chlorambucil. Cyclophosphamide can be effective in the setting of severe progressive scleritis and PUK, or when methotrexate or other immunosuppressive therapy has proven ineffective. It may be given at oral doses of 1–2 mg/kg/day, or as pulsed intravenous therapy every 3–4 weeks under rheumatologic or internal medicine guidance.[32,95,183,184] Messmer and Foster reported a retrospective case series of 25 eyes in 16 RA patients with PUK and/or necrotizing scleritis unresponsive to conventional topical and systemic steroids who were managed with cytotoxic immunosuppressive agents and aggressive early surgical intervention.[172] Such intervention preserved the integrity of the globe in 23 of 25 eyes, but final visual outcomes were disappointing. Cyclophosphamide (Cytoxan) appeared to be the most effective agent in this series. Methotrexate was also very effective, and with less potential for toxicity may be preferable as an initial agent. Development of PUK and/or necrotizing scleritis was associated with prior cataract surgery in 31% of the study population, suggesting that high-risk RA patients with high serum levels of rheumatoid factor may benefit from systemic immunosuppression prior to elective cataract surgery.[172] Chlorambucil (0.1–0.2 mg/kg/day) is used when other cytotoxic agents have failed in severe disease, and has shown considerable efficacy.[95,185] Both these medications, however, are limited by their potential for serious toxicity.

The T-cell inhibitor ciclosporin A has also been used in the setting of recalcitrant disease at doses of 2–5 mg/kg/day with frequent monitoring of blood pressure and renal function.[95] One case series of six patients with RA and necrotizing scleritis or keratolysis unresponsive to treatment with steroids and other immunosuppressive agents reported improvement in the ocular as well as systemic manifestations of the underlying disease with the initiation of oral ciclosporin A. Dosing was introduced at 2.5 mg/kg/day and adjusted to maintain trough levels of whole blood ciclosporin in the 150–200 ng/mL range.[186] Tacrolimus, working by a mechanism similar to ciclosporin A, may actually be more efficacious and has shown promise in immune-mediated ocular surface inflammation, both systemically and topically.[95,187–192] Combination therapy, as used in rheumatic diseases, may also prove to be more effective than monotherapy and perhaps limit the side-effect profile.[95]

The newest class of DMARDs, the biological response modifiers, are currently being assessed for efficacy towards ocular inflammation. Despite showing significant efficacy in treating rheumatoid arthritis, mixed results including increased ocular surface inflammation have been documented.[95,103–106] Several reports have documented successful treatment of refractory PUK with infliximab, a TNF blocker.[193,194]

There are multiple potentially severe adverse side effects associated with immunosuppressive therapy, as mentioned above.[95] In addition, patients starting therapy with any of the immunosuppressive agents must be warned of increased susceptibility to infection as well as the possible carcinogenicity of these drugs, in particular the potential increased risk of developing hematopoietic malignancies, though this concept is still debated.[95,195]

Surgical management

In cases in which scleral necrosis and thinning have progressed to impending perforation, tectonic procedures may be necessary to maintain the integrity of the globe. Cyanoacrylate glue application with oversized bandage contact lens placement may be effective as a temporizing measure in this setting (Fig. 92.13).[196–199] However, scleral grafting with donor sclera often becomes a necessary intervention.[52,172,200–202] Attempts should be made during scleral grafting to preserve as much healthy conjunctiva surrounding a necrotic scleral bed as possible. This will reduce the size of the postoperative epithelial defect overlying the scleral graft and speed epithelial healing. Other tissues used for tectonic support have been studied due to difficulties with homogeneous sclera, including limited vascularization, necrosis, and sloughing.[203–209]

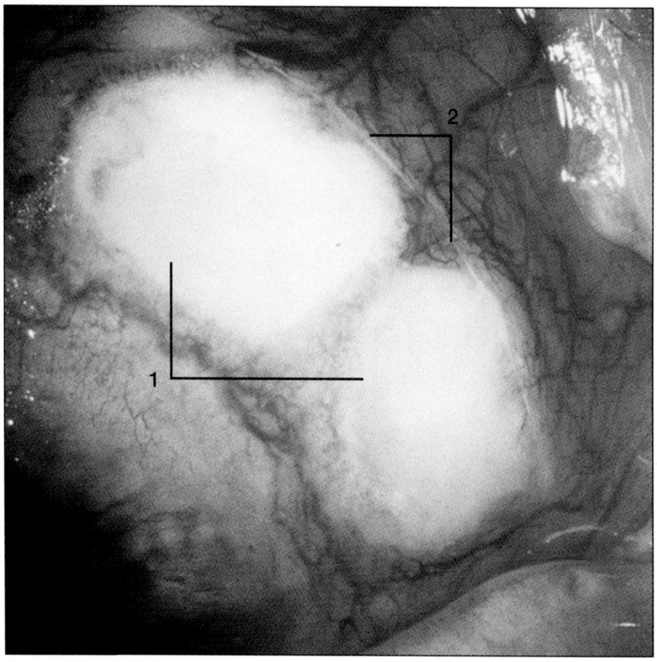

Fig. 92.13 Slit lamp photograph of a 67-year-old patient with severe necrotizing scleritis. Note the two large areas of scleral thinning and associated necrotizing scleritis, which have been covered with *N*-butylacrylate tissue glue (*1*) and an oversized bandage contact lens (*2*).

Peripheral ulcerative keratitis unresponsive to medical therapy may respond to conjunctival resection,[210–212] or application of tissue adhesive,[172,213–215] but may require conjunctival flaps,[216–219] or annular lamellar corneoscleral patch grafting if there is impending perforation.[24,172,220–222] Once stabilized and appropriately immunosuppressed, penetrating keratoplasty may be performed for visual rehabilitation (Fig. 92.14).

In the setting of severe keratolysis, cyanoacrylate glue application,[197,213–215,223] lamellar or penetrating keratoplasty may be effective therapy, although visual prognosis in these cases is guarded.[172,221,222,224–226]

More recently, amniotic membrane transplantation (AMT) has been attempted in the management of deep corneal ulceration, corneal perforation, and scleral ulceration from a variety of causes with relative success.[227,228] One retrospective case series of 34 eyes with nontraumatic corneal perforation or descemetocele treated with AMT reported a successful outcome (defined as cessation of aqueous leak, presence of a deep anterior chamber, complete epithelialization over the amniotic membrane, and formation of visible stromal thickness) in 28 of 34 eyes. Success in patients with RA was less promising, as 3 of the 6 patients in this series with rheumatoid ulceration failed AMT and required additional tectonic procedures.[229] However, in the management of scleromalacia, AMT is useful in providing tectonic support when used with scleral grafting.[230]

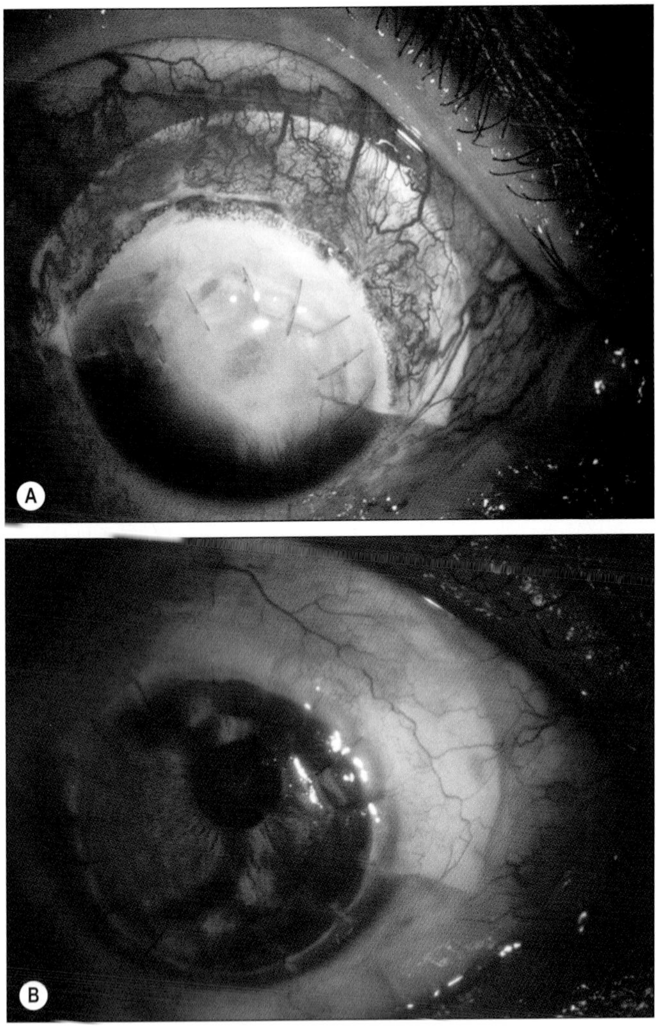

Fig. 92.14 Penetrating keratoplasty. (**A**) Slit lamp photograph of an annular lamellar keratoplasty performed for PUK with impending perforation. (**B**) Slit lamp photograph of same patient 9 months after stabilization with penetrating keratoplasty and clear corneal graft.

For severe disease requiring rehabilitation of vision, prosthetic corneas have been developed; however, their success with associated corneal melting syndromes has been limited, requiring additional treatments to help stabilize the ocular surface.[231–233] Research in this area continues and may provide benefit to patients in underserved areas where transplant tissue may be limited.

As described earlier, the addition of aggressive lubrication and tarsorrhaphy may enhance surgical success. However, it is important to realize that surgical treatment, though often necessary to maintain tectonic support for the eye, will not prevent further progression of disease and potential mortality without the concomitant use of immunosuppressive therapy.

References

1. Goronzy JJ, Weyand CM. Rheumatoid arthritis. Epidemiology, pathology, and pathogenesis in rheumatoid arthritis. In: Klippel JH, ed. In: *Primer on the rheumatic diseases*. 12th ed. Atlanta: Arthritis Foundation; 2001.
2. Arnett FC, Edworthy SM, Bloch DA, et al. The American Rheumatism Association 1987 revised criteria for the classification of rheumatoid arthritis. *Arthritis Rheum*. 1988;31:315–324.
3. Sharp JT, Wolfe F, Mitchell DM, et al. The progression of erosion and joint space narrowing scores in rheumatoid arthritis during the first twenty-five years of disease. *Arthritis Rheum*. 1991;34:660–668.
4. Pincus T, Callahan LF. Early mortality in RA predicted by poor clinical status. *Bull Rheum Dis*. 1992;41:1–4.
5. O'Day D, Horn JF. The eye and rheumatic disease. In: Ruddy S, Harris ED, and Sledge CM, eds. *Kelley's textbook of rheumatology*. 6th ed. Philadelphia: Saunders; 2001.
6. Gregersen PK, Silver J, Winchester RJ. The shared epitope hypothesis. An approach to understanding the molecular genetics of susceptibility to rheumatoid arthritis. *Arthritis Rheum*. 1987;30:1205–1213.
7. Brennan FM, Maini RN, Feldmann M. Role of pro-inflammatory cytokines in rheumatoid arthritis. *Springer Semin Immunopathol*. 1998;20:133–147.
8. Choy EH, Panayi GS. Cytokine pathways and joint inflammation in rheumatoid arthritis. *N Engl J Med*. 2001;344:907–916.
9. Anderson RJ. Rheumatoid arthritis. Clinical and laboratory features. In: Klippel JH, ed. *Primer on the rheumatic diseases*. 12th ed. Atlanta: Arthritis Foundation; 2001.
10. Visser H, le Cessie S, Vos K, et al. How to diagnose rheumatoid arthritis early: a prediction model for persistent (erosive) arthritis. *Arthritis Rheum*. 2002;46:357–365.
11. Schellekens GA, Visser H, de Jong BA, et al. The diagnostic properties of rheumatoid arthritis antibodies recognizing a cyclic citrullinated peptide. *Arthritis Rheum*. 2000;43:155–163.
12. Rantapaa-Dahlqvist S, de Jong BA, Berglin E, et al. Antibodies against cyclic citrullinated peptide and IgA rheumatoid factor predict the development of rheumatoid arthritis. *Arthritis Rheum*. 2003;48:2741–2749.
13. McGavin DD, Williamson J, Forrester JV, et al. Episcleritis and scleritis. A study of their clinical manifestations and association with rheumatoid arthritis. *Br J Ophthalmol*. 1976;60:192–226.
14. Sevel D. Rheumatoid nodule of the sclera. (a type of necrogranulomatous scleritis). *Trans Ophthalmol Soc UK*. 1965;85:357–367.
15. Ferry AP. The histopathology of rheumatoid episcleral nodules. An extra-articular manifestation of rheumatoid arthritis. *Arch Ophthalmol*. 1969;82:77–78.
16. Hurd ER, Snyder WB, Ziff M. Choroidal nodules and retinal detachments in rheumatoid arthritis. Improvement with fall in immunoglobulin levels following prednisolone and cyclophosphamide therapy. *Am J Med*. 1970;48:273–278.
17. Rao NA, Font RL. Pseudorheumatoid nodules of the ocular adnexa. *Am J Ophthalmol*. 1975;79:471–478.
18. Lebowitz MA, Jakobiec FA, Donnenfeld ED, et al. Bilateral epibulbar rheumatoid nodulosis. A new ocular entity. *Ophthalmology*. 1988;95:1256–1259.
19. Cochrane W, Davies DV, Dorling J, et al. Ultramicroscopic structure of the rheumatoid nodule. *Ann Rheum Dis*. 1964;23:345–363.
20. Scott DG, Bacon PA, Tribe CR. Systemic rheumatoid vasculitis: a clinical and laboratory study of 50 cases. *Medicine (Baltimore)*. 1981;60:288–297.
21. Voskuyl AE, Zwinderman AH, Westedt ML, et al. Factors associated with the development of vasculitis in rheumatoid arthritis: results of a case-control study. *Ann Rheum Dis*. 1996;55:190–192.
22. Conn DL, McDuffie FC, Dyck PJ. Immunopathologic study of sural nerves in rheumatoid arthritis. *Arthritis Rheum*. 1972;15:135–143.
23. Schmid FR, Cooper NS, Ziff M, et al. Arteritis in rheumatoid arthritis. *Am J Med*. 1961;30:56–83.
24. Messmer EM, Foster CS. Vasculitic peripheral ulcerative keratitis. *Surv Ophthalmol*. 1999;43:379–396.
25. Hunder GG, McDuffie FC. Hypocomplementemia in rheumatoid arthritis. *Am J Med*. 1973;54:461–472.
26. Husby G. Amyloidosis in rheumatoid arthritis. *Ann Clin Res*. 1975;7:154–167.
27. Reimer KA, Rodgers RF, Oyasu R. Rheumatoid arthritis with rheumatoid heart disease and granulomatous aortitis. *JAMA*. 1976;235:2510–2512.
28. Voyles WF, Searles RP, Bankhurst AD. Myocardial infarction caused by rheumatoid vasculitis. *Arthritis Rheum*. 1980;23:860–863.
29. Hyland RH, Gordon DA, Broder I, et al. A systematic controlled study of pulmonary abnormalities in rheumatoid arthritis. *J Rheumatol*. 1983;10:395–405.
30. Hara KS, Ballard DJ, Ilstrup DM, et al. Rheumatoid pericarditis: clinical features and survival. *Medicine (Baltimore)*. 1990;69:81–91.
31. Erhardt CC, Mumford PA, Venables PJ, et al. Factors predicting a poor life prognosis in rheumatoid arthritis: an eight year prospective study. *Ann Rheum Dis*. 1989;48:7–13.

32. Foster CS, Forstot SL, Wilson LA. Mortality rate in rheumatoid arthritis patients developing necrotizing scleritis or peripheral ulcerative keratitis. Effects of systemic immunosuppression. *Ophthalmology.* 1984;91:1253–1263.
33. Mody GM, Hill JC, Meyers OL. Keratoconjunctivitis sicca in rheumatoid arthritis. *Clin Rheumatol.* 1988;7:237–241.
34. Matsuo T, Kono R, Matsuo N, et al. Incidence of ocular complications in rheumatoid arthritis and the relation of keratoconjunctivitis sicca with its systemic activity. *Scand J Rheumatol.* 1997;26:113–116.
35. Fujita M, Igarashi T, Kurai T, et al. Correlation between dry eye and rheumatoid arthritis activity. *Am J Ophthalmol.* 2005;140:808–813.
36. Danjo Y, Lee M, Horimoto K, et al. Ocular surface damage and tear lactoferrin in dry eye syndrome. *Acta Ophthalmol (Copenh).* 1994;72:433–437.
37. Pflugfelder SC, Solomon A, Stern ME. The diagnosis and management of dry eye: a twenty-five-year review. *Cornea.* 2000;19:644–649.
38. Behrens A, Doyle JJ, Stern L, et al. Dysfunctional tear syndrome: a Delphi approach to treatment recommendations. *Cornea.* 2006;25: 900–907.
39. Lemp MA, Baudoin C, Baum J, et al. The definition and classification of dry eye disease: report of the Definition and Classification Subcommittee of the International Dry Eye Workshop (2007). *Ocul Surf.* 2007; 5:75–92.
40. Yoon KC, Jeong IY, Park YG, et al. Interleukin-6 and tumor necrosis factor-alpha levels in tears of patients with dry eye syndrome. *Cornea.* 2007;26:431–437.
41. Zoukhri D. Effect of inflammation on lacrimal gland function. *Exp Eye Res.* 2006;82:885–898.
42. Fox RI, Kang HI. Pathogenesis of Sjögren's syndrome. *Rheum Dis Clin North Am.* 1992;18:517–538.
43. Williamson J, Gibson AA, Wilson T, et al. Histology of the lacrimal gland in keratoconjunctivitis sicca. *Br J Ophthalmol.* 1973;57:852–858.
44. Pflugfelder SC, Huang AJ, Feuer W, et al. Conjunctival cytologic features of primary Sjögren's syndrome. *Ophthalmology.* 1990;97:985–991.
45. Tuft SJ, Watson PG. Progression of scleral disease. *Ophthalmology.* 1991;98:467–471.
46. Sainz de la Maza M, Foster CS, Jabbur NS. Scleritis associated with rheumatoid arthritis and with other systemic immune-mediated diseases. *Ophthalmology.* 1994;101:1281–1286; discussion 7–8.
47. Akpek EK, Uy HS, Christen W, et al. Severity of episcleritis and systemic disease association. *Ophthalmology.* 1999;106:729–731.
48. Jabs DA, Mudun A, Dunn JP, et al. Episcleritis and scleritis: clinical features and treatment results. *Am J Ophthalmol.* 2000;130:469–476.
49. Sainz de la Maza M, Jabbur NS, Foster CS. Severity of scleritis and episcleritis. *Ophthalmology.* 1994;101:389–396
50. Watson PG, Young RD. Scleral structure, organisation and disease. A review. *Exp Eye Res.* 2004;78:609–623.
51. Rao NA, Marak GE, Hidayat AA. Necrotizing scleritis. A clinico-pathologic study of 41 cases. *Ophthalmology.* 1985;92:1542–1549.
52. Rosenthal JW, Williams GT. Scleromalacia perforans as a complication of rheumatoid arthritis. *Am J Ophthalmol.* 1962;54:862–864.
53. McCluskey PJ, Watson PG, Lightman S, et al. Posterior scleritis: clinical features, systemic associations, and outcome in a large series of patients. *Ophthalmology.* 1999;106:2380–2386.
54. Fong LP, Sainz de la Maza M, Rice BA, et al. Immunopathology of scleritis. *Ophthalmology.* 1991;98:472–479.
55. Riono WP, Hidayat AA, Rao NA. Scleritis: a clinicopathologic study of 55 cases. *Ophthalmology.* 1999;106:1328–1333.
56. Shiuey Y, Foster CS. Peripheral ulcerative keratitis and collagen vascular disease. *Int Ophthalmol Clin.* 1998;38:21–32.
57. Dana MR, Qian Y, Hamrah P. Twenty-five-year panorama of corneal immunology: emerging concepts in the immunopathogenesis of microbial keratitis, peripheral ulcerative keratitis, and corneal transplant rejection. *Cornea.* 2000;19:625–643.
58. Tauber J, Sainz de la Maza M, Hoang-Xuan T, et al. An analysis of therapeutic decision making regarding immunosuppressive chemotherapy for peripheral ulcerative keratitis. *Cornea.* 1990;9:66–73.
59. Mondino BJ. Inflammatory diseases of the peripheral cornea. *Ophthalmology.* 1988;95:463–472.
60. Squirrell DM, Winfield J, Amos RS. Peripheral ulcerative keratitis 'corneal melt' and rheumatoid arthritis: a case series. *Rheumatology (Oxford).* 1999;38:1245–1248.
61. Berman M, Dohlman CH, Gnadinger M, et al. Characterization of collagenolytic activity in the ulcerating cornea. *Exp Eye Res.* 1971;11:255–257.
62. Watson PG. Vascular changes in peripheral corneal destructive disease. *Eye.* 1990;4(Pt 1):65–73.
63. John SL, Morgan K, Tullo AB, et al. Corneal autoimmunity in patients with peripheral ulcerative keratitis (PUK) in association with rheumatoid arthritis and Wegener's granulomatosis. *Eye.* 1992;6(Pt6):630–636.
64. Riley GP, Harrall RL, Watson PG, et al. Collagenase (MMP-1) and TIMP-1 in destructive corneal disease associated with rheumatoid arthritis. *Eye.* 1995;9(Pt 6):703–718.
65. Prada J, Noelle B, Baatz H, et al. Tumour necrosis factor alpha and interleukin 6 gene expression in keratocytes from patients with rheumatoid corneal ulcerations. *Br J Ophthalmol.* 2003;87:548–550.
66. Ormerod LD, Fong LP, Foster CS. Corneal infection in mucosal scarring disorders and Sjögren's syndrome. *Am J Ophthalmol.* 1988;105:512–518.
67. Hamideh F, Prete PE. Ophthalmologic manifestations of rheumatic diseases. *Semin Arthritis Rheum.* 2001;30:217–241.
68. Kervick GN, Pflugfelder SC, Haimovici R, et al. Paracentral rheumatoid corneal ulceration. Clinical features and cyclosporine therapy. *Ophthalmology.* 1992;99:80–88.
69. Insler MS, Boutros G, Boulware DW. Corneal ulceration following cataract surgery in patients with rheumatoid arthritis. *J Am Intraocul Implant Soc.* 1985;11:594–597.
70. Mamalis N, Johnson MD, Haines JM, et al. Corneal-scleral melt in association with cataract surgery and intraocular lenses: a report of four cases. *J Cataract Refract Surg.* 1990;16:108–115.
71. Glasser DB, Bellor J. Necrotizing scleritis of scleral flaps after transscleral suture fixation of an intraocular lens. *Am J Ophthalmol.* 1992; 113:529–532.
72. Sainz de la Maza M, Foster CS. Necrotizing scleritis after ocular surgery. A clinicopathologic study. *Ophthalmology.* 1991;98:1720–1726.
73. Nabili S, McCarey DW, Browne B, et al. A case of orbital myositis associated with rheumatoid arthritis. *Ann Rheum Dis.* 2002;61:938–939.
74. Killian PJ, McClain B, Lawless OJ. Brown's syndrome. An unusual manifestation of rheumatoid arthritis. *Arthritis Rheum.* 1977;20:1080–1084.
75. Beck M, Hickling P. Treatment of bilateral superior oblique tendon sheath syndrome complicating rheumatoid arthritis. *Br J Ophthalmol.* 1980;64:358–361.
76. Sigal LH. The neurologic presentation of vasculitic and rheumatologic syndromes. A review. *Medicine (Baltimore).* 1987;66:157–180.
77. Sainz de la Maza M, Foster CS, Jabbur NS. Scleritis-associated uveitis. *Ophthalmology* 1997;104:58–63.
78. Fraunfelder FT, Watson PG. Evaluation of eyes enucleated for scleritis. *Br J Ophthalmol.* 1976;60:227–230.
79. Gupta A, Bansal RK, Bambery P. Posterior scleritis related fundal mass in a patient with rheumatoid arthritis. *Scand J Rheumatol.* 1992;21: 254–256
80. Meyer E, Schart J, Miller B, et al. Fundus lesions in rheumatoid arthritis. *Ann Ophthalmol.* 1978;10:1583–1584.
81. Rezai KA, Patel SC, Eliott D, et al. Rheumatoid hyperviscosity syndrome: reversibility of microvascular abnormalities after treatment. *Am J Ophthalmol.* 2002;134:130–132.
82. Matsuo T, Koyama T, Morimoto N, et al. Retinal vasculitis as a complication of rheumatoid arthritis. *Ophthalmologica.* 1990;201:196–200.
83. Matsuo T, Masuda I, Matsuo N. Geographic choroiditis and retinal vasculitis in rheumatoid arthritis. *Jpn J Ophthalmol.* 1998;42:51–55.
84. American College of Rheumatology Subcommittee on Rheumatoid Arthritis Guidelines. Guidelines for the management of rheumatoid arthritis: 2002 update. *Arthritis Rheum.* 2002;46:328–346.
85. Mottonen T, Hannonen P, Korpela M, et al. Delay to institution of therapy and induction of remission using single-drug or combination-disease-modifying antirheumatic drug therapy in early rheumatoid arthritis. *Arthritis Rheum.* 2002;46:894–898.
86. Kirwan JR. The effect of glucocorticoids on joint destruction in rheumatoid arthritis. The Arthritis and Rheumatism Council Low-Dose Glucocorticoid Study Group. *N Engl J Med.* 1995;333:142–146.
87. Moreland LW, O'Dell JR. Glucocorticoids and rheumatoid arthritis: back to the future? *Arthritis Rheum.* 2002;46:2553–2563.
88. Jones G, Halbert J, Crotty M, et al. The effect of treatment on radiological progression in rheumatoid arthritis: a systematic review of randomized placebo-controlled trials. *Rheumatology (Oxford).* 2003;42:6–13.
89. Smolen JS, Kalden JR, Scott DL, et al. Efficacy and safety of leflunomide compared with placebo and sulphasalazine in active rheumatoid arthritis: a double-blind, randomised, multicentre trial. European Leflunomide Study Group. *Lancet.* 1999;353:259–266.
90. Sharp JT, Strand V, Leung H, et al. Treatment with leflunomide slows radiographic progression of rheumatoid arthritis: results from three randomized controlled trials of leflunomide in patients with active rheumatoid arthritis. Leflunomide Rheumatoid Arthritis Investigators Group. *Arthritis Rheum.* 2000;43:495–505.

91. Yocum DE, Klippel JH, Wilder RL, et al. Cyclosporin a in severe, treatment-refractory rheumatoid arthritis. A randomized study. *Ann Intern Med.* 1988;109:863–869.
92. Tugwell P, Bombardier C, Gent M, et al. Low-dose cyclosporin versus placebo in patients with rheumatoid arthritis. *Lancet.* 1990;335: 1051–1055.
93. Suarez-Almazor ME, Spooner C, Belseck E. Penicillamine for treating rheumatoid arthritis. *Cochrane Database Syst Rev.* 2000;CD001460.
94. Sanders M. A review of controlled clinical trials examining the effects of antimalarial compounds and gold compounds on radiographic progression in rheumatoid arthritis. *J Rheumatol.* 2000;27:523–529.
95. Jabs DA, Rosenbaum JT, Foster CS, et al. Guidelines for the use of immunosuppressive drugs in patients with ocular inflammatory disorders: recommendations of an expert panel. *Am J Ophthalmol.* 2000;130:492–513.
96. Faulds D, Goa KL, Benfield P. Cyclosporin. A review of its pharmacodynamic and pharmacokinetic properties, and therapeutic use in immunoregulatory disorders. *Drugs.* 1993;45:953–1040.
97. Jessop JD, O'Sullivan MM, Lewis PA, et al. A long-term five-year randomized controlled trial of hydroxychloroquine, sodium aurothiomalate, auranofin and penicillamine in the treatment of patients with rheumatoid arthritis. *Br J Rheumatol.* 1998;37:992–1002.
98. Moreland LW, Baumgartner SW, Schiff MH, et al. Treatment of rheumatoid arthritis with a recombinant human tumor necrosis factor receptor (p75)-fc fusion protein. *N Engl J Med.* 1997;337:141–147.
99. Bathon JM, Martin RW, Fleischmann RM, et al. A comparison of etanercept and methotrexate in patients with early rheumatoid arthritis. *N Engl J Med.* 2000;343:1586–1593.
100. Lipsky PE, van der Heijde DM, St Clair EW, et al. Infliximab and methotrexate in the treatment of rheumatoid arthritis. Anti-Tumor Necrosis Factor Trial in Rheumatoid Arthritis with Concomitant Therapy Study Group. *N Engl J Med.* 2000;343:1594–1602.
101. Weinblatt ME, Keystone EC, Furst DE, et al. Adalimumab, a fully human anti-tumor necrosis factor alpha monoclonal antibody, for the treatment of rheumatoid arthritis in patients taking concomitant methotrexate: the Armada Trial. *Arthritis Rheum.* 2003;48:35–45.
102. Cohen S, Hurd E, Cush J, et al. Treatment of rheumatoid arthritis with anakinra, a recombinant human interleukin-1 receptor antagonist, in combination with methotrexate: results of a twenty-four-week, multicenter, randomized, double-blind, placebo-controlled trial. *Arthritis Rheum.* 2002;46:614–624.
103. Smith JR, Levinson RD, Holland GN, et al. Differential efficacy of tumor necrosis factor inhibition in the management of inflammatory eye disease and associated rheumatic disease. *Arthritis Rheum.* 2001;45:252–257.
104. Aeberli D, Oertle S, Mauron H, et al. Inhibition of the TNF-pathway: use of infliximab and etanercept as remission-inducing agents in cases of therapy-resistant chronic inflammatory disorders. *Swiss Med Wkly.* 2002;132:414–422.
105. Sfikakis PP. Behçet's disease: a new target for anti-tumour necrosis factor treatment. *Ann Rheum Dis.* 2002;61(Suppl 2):ii51–ii53.
106. Papaliodis GN, Chu D, Foster CS. Treatment of ocular inflammatory disorders with daclizumab. *Ophthalmology.* 2003;110:786–789.
107. Calonge M. The treatment of dry eye. *Surv Ophthalmol.* 2001;45(Suppl 2):S227–S239.
108. Marsh P, Pflugfelder SC. Topical nonpreserved methylprednisolone therapy for keratoconjunctivitis sicca in Sjögren syndrome. *Ophthalmology.* 1999;106:811–816.
109. Tsubota K, Goto E, Fujita H, et al. Treatment of dry eye by autologous serum application in Sjögren's syndrome. *Br J Ophthalmol.* 1999; 83:390–395.
110. Tananuvat N, Daniell M, Sullivan LJ, et al. Controlled study of the use of autologous serum in dry eye patients. *Cornea.* 2001;20:802–806.
111. Noble BA, Loh RS, MacLennan S, et al. Comparison of autologous serum eye drops with conventional therapy in a randomised controlled crossover trial for ocular surface disease. *Br J Ophthalmol.* 2004;88:647–652.
112. Vivino FB, Al-Hashimi I, Khan Z, et al. Pilocarpine tablets for the treatment of dry mouth and dry eye symptoms in patients with Sjögren syndrome: a randomized, placebo-controlled, fixed-dose, multicenter trial. P92-01 Study Group. *Arch Intern Med.* 1999;159:174–181.
113. Ono M, Takamura E, Shinozaki K, et al. Therapeutic effect of cevimeline on dry eye in patients with Sjögren's syndrome: a randomized, double-blind clinical study. *Am J Ophthalmol.* 2004;138:6–17.
114. Tauber J, Davitt WF, Bokosky JE, et al. Double-masked, placebo-controlled safety and efficacy trial of diquafosol tetrasodium (INS365) ophthalmic solution for the treatment of dry eye. *Cornea.* 2004;23:784–792.
115. Stevenson D, Tauber J, Reis BL. Efficacy and safety of cyclosporin a ophthalmic emulsion in the treatment of moderate-to-severe dry eye disease: A dose-ranging, randomized trial. The Cyclosporin A Phase 2 Study Group. *Ophthalmology.* 2000;107:967–974.
116. Sall K, Stevenson OD, Mundorf TK, et al. Two multicenter, randomized studies of the efficacy and safety of cyclosporine ophthalmic emulsion in moderate to severe dry eye disease. CsA Phase 3 Study Group. *Ophthalmology.* 2000;107:631–639.
117. Small DS, Acheampong A, Reis B, et al. Blood concentrations of cyclosporin a during long-term treatment with cyclosporin A ophthalmic emulsions in patients with moderate to severe dry eye disease. *J Ocul Pharmacol Ther.* 2002;18:411–418.
118. Perry HD, Solomon R, Donnenfeld ED, et al. Evaluation of topical cyclosporine for the treatment of dry eye disease. *Arch Ophthalmol.* 2008;126:1046–1050.
119. Turner K, Pflugfelder SC, Ji Z, et al. Interleukin-6 levels in the conjunctival epithelium of patients with dry eye disease treated with cyclosporine ophthalmic emulsion. *Cornea.* 2000;19:492–496.
120. Kunert KS, Tisdale AS, Stern ME, et al. Analysis of topical cyclosporine treatment of patients with dry eye syndrome: effect on conjunctival lymphocytes. *Arch Ophthalmol.* 2000;118:1489–1496.
121. Kunert KS, Tisdale AS, Gipson IK. Goblet cell numbers and epithelial proliferation in the conjunctiva of patients with dry eye syndrome treated with cyclosporine. *Arch Ophthalmol.* 2002;120:330–337.
122. Dougherty JM, McCulley JP, Silvany RE, et al. The role of tetracycline in chronic blepharitis. Inhibition of lipase production in staphylococci. *Invest Ophthalmol Vis Sci.* 1991;32:2970–2975.
123. Beardsley RM, De Paiva CS, Power DF, et al. Desiccating stress decreases apical corneal epithelial cell size – modulation by the metalloproteinase inhibitor doxycycline. *Cornea.* 2008;27:935–940.
124. Stone DU, Chodosh J. Oral tetracyclines for ocular rosacea: an evidence-based review of the literature. *Cornea.* 2004;23:106–109.
125. Paemen L, Martens E, Norga K, et al. The gelatinase inhibitory activity of tetracyclines and chemically modified tetracycline analogues as measured by a novel microtiter assay for inhibitors. *Biochem Pharmacol.* 1996;52:105–111.
126. Quarterman MJ, Johnson DW, Abele DC, et al. Ocular rosacea. Signs, symptoms, and tear studies before and after treatment with doxycycline. *Arch Dermatol.* 1997;133:49–54.
127. Solomon A, Rosenblatt M, Li D, et al. Doxycycline inhibition of interleukin-1 in the corneal epithelium. *Am J Ophthalmol.* 2000;130: 688.
128. Shine WE, McCulley JP, Pandya AG. Minocycline effect on meibomian gland lipids in meibomianitis patients. *Exp Eye Res.* 2003;76:417–420.
129. De Paiva CS, Corrales RM, Villarreal AL, et al. Corticosteroid and doxycycline suppress MMP-9 and inflammatory cytokine expression, MAPK activation in the corneal epithelium in experimental dry eye. *Exp Eye Res.* 2006;83:526–535.
130. Nordstrom D, Lindy O, Lauhio A, et al. Anti-collagenolytic mechanism of action of doxycycline treatment in rheumatoid arthritis. *Rheumatol Int.* 1998;17:175–180.
131. O'Dell JR, Paulsen G, Haire CE, et al. Treatment of early seropositive rheumatoid arthritis with minocycline: four-year followup of a double-blind, placebo-controlled trial. *Arthritis Rheum.* 1999;42:1691–1695.
132. Alarcon GS. Tetracyclines for the treatment of rheumatoid arthritis. *Expert Opin Investig Drugs.* 2000;9:1491–1498.
133. Brown NA, Bron AJ, Harding JJ, et al. Nutrition supplements and the eye. *Eye.* 1998;12 (Pt 1):127–133.
134. Barabino S, Rolando M, Camicione P, et al. Systemic linoleic and gamma-linolenic acid therapy in dry eye syndrome with an inflammatory component. *Cornea.* 2003;22:97–101.
135. Zurier RB, Rossetti RG, Jacobson EW, et al. Gamma-linolenic acid treatment of rheumatoid arthritis. A randomized, placebo-controlled trial. *Arthritis Rheum.* 1996;39:1808–1817.
136. Volker D, Fitzgerald P, Major G, et al. Efficacy of fish oil concentrate in the treatment of rheumatoid arthritis. *J Rheumatol.* 2000;27: 2343–2346.
137. Lemp MA. Management of dry eye disease. *Am J Manag Care.* 2008;14:S88–101.
138. Tsubota K. New approaches to dry-eye therapy. *Int Ophthalmol Clin.* 1994;34:115–128.
139. Murube J, Murube E. Treatment of dry eye by blocking the lacrimal canaliculi. *Surv Ophthalmol.* 1996;40:463–480.
140. Pflugfelder SC, Jones D, Ji Z, et al. Altered cytokine balance in the tear fluid and conjunctiva of patients with Sjögren's syndrome keratoconjunctivitis sicca. *Curr Eye Res.* 1999;19:201–211.
141. Yen MT, Pflugfelder SC, Feuer WJ. The effect of punctal occlusion on tear production, tear clearance, and ocular surface sensation in normal subjects. *Am J Ophthalmol.* 2001;131:314–323.
142. Welch C, Baum J. Tarsorrhaphy for corneal disease in patients with rheumatoid arthritis. *Ophthalmic Surg.* 1988;19:31–32.

143. Liegner JT, Yee RW, Wild JH. Topical cyclosporine therapy for ulcerative keratitis associated with rheumatoid arthritis. *Am J Ophthalmol.* 1990;109:610–612.
144. Holland EJ, Olsen TW, Ketcham JM, et al. Topical cyclosporin A in the treatment of anterior segment inflammatory disease. *Cornea.* 1993;12:413–419.
145. Brown SI, Grayson M. Marginal furrows. A characteristic corneal lesion of rheumatoid arthritis. *Arch Ophthalmol.* 1968;79:563–567.
146. Krachmer JH, Laibson PR. Corneal thinning and perforation in Sjögren's syndrome. *Am J Ophthalmol.* 1974;78:917–920.
147. Pfister RR, Murphy GE. Corneal ulceration and perforation associated with Sjögren's syndrome. *Arch Ophthalmol.* 1980;98:89–94.
148. Kenyon KR. Decision-making in the therapy of external eye disease: noninfected corneal ulcers. *Ophthalmology.* 1982;89:44–51.
149. Bruce AS, Brennan NA. Corneal pathophysiology with contact lens wear. *Surv Ophthalmol.* 1990;35:25–58.
150. Romero-Rangel T, Stavrou P, Cotter J, et al. Gas-permeable scleral contact lens therapy in ocular surface disease. *Am J Ophthalmol.* 2000;130:25–32.
151. Montero J, Sparholt J, Mely R. Retrospective case series of therapeutic applications of a lotrafilcon a silicone hydrogel soft contact lens. *Eye Contact Lens.* 2003;29:S54–S56; discussion S7–9, S192–4.
152. Shah C, Raj CV, Foulks GN. The evolution in therapeutic contact lenses. *Ophthalmol Clin North Am.* 2003;16:95–101, vii.
153. Geerling G, Joussen AM, Daniels JT, et al. Matrix metalloproteinases in sterile corneal melts. *Ann NY Acad Sci.* 1999;878:571–574.
154. Smith VA, Hoh HB, Easty DL. Role of ocular matrix metalloproteinases in peripheral ulcerative keratitis. *Br J Ophthalmol.* 1999;83:1376–1383.
155. Perry HD, Golub LM. Systemic tetracyclines in the treatment of noninfected corneal ulcers: a case report and proposed new mechanism of action. *Ann Ophthalmol.* 1985;17:742–744.
156. Golub LM, Ramamurthy NS, McNamara TF, et al. Tetracyclines inhibit connective tissue breakdown: new therapeutic implications for an old family of drugs. *Crit Rev Oral Biol Med.* 1991;2:297–321.
157. Ralph RA. Tetracyclines and the treatment of corneal stromal ulceration: a review. *Cornea.* 2000;19:274–277.
158. Lipsky PE, Isakson PC. Outcome of specific COX-2 inhibition in rheumatoid arthritis. *J Rheumatol Suppl.* 1997;49:9–14.
159. Davies NM, Teng XW, Skjodt NM. Pharmacokinetics of rofecoxib: a specific cyclo-oxygenase-2 inhibitor. *Clin Pharmacokinet.* 2003;42:545–556.
160. McMullen M, Kovarik G, Hodge WG. Use of topical steroid therapy in the management of nonnecrotizing anterior scleritis. *Can J Ophthalmol.* 1999;34:217–221.
161. Tu EY, Culbertson WW, Pflugfelder SC, et al. Therapy of nonnecrotizing anterior scleritis with subconjunctival corticosteroid injection. *Ophthalmology.* 1995;102:718–724.
162. Croasdale CR, Brightbill FS. Subconjunctival corticosteroid injections for nonnecrotizing anterior scleritis. *Arch Ophthalmol.* 1999;117:966–968.
163. Zamir E, Read RW, Smith RE, et al. A prospective evaluation of subconjunctival injection of triamcinolone acetonide for resistant anterior scleritis. *Ophthalmology.* 2002;109:798–805; discussion 807.
164. Guidera AC, Luchs JI, Udell IJ. Keratitis, ulceration, and perforation associated with topical nonsteroidal antiinflammatory drugs. *Ophthalmology.* 2001;108:936–944.
165. Reviglio VE, Rana TS, Li QJ, et al. Effects of topical nonsteroidal antiinflammatory drugs on the expression of matrix metalloproteinases in the cornea. *J Cataract Refract Surg.* 2003;29:989–997.
166. Harper SL, Foster CS. The ocular manifestations of rheumatoid disease. *Int Ophthalmol Clin.* 1998;38:1–19.
167. Watson PG. The diagnosis and management of scleritis. *Ophthalmology.* 1980;87:716–720.
168. Hemady R, Sainz de la Maza M, Raizman MB, et al. Six cases of scleritis associated with systemic infection. *Am J Ophthalmol.* 1992;114:55–62.
169. Sykes SO, Riemann C, Santos CI, et al. *Haemophilus influenzae* associated scleritis. *Br J Ophthalmol.* 1999;83:410–413.
170. Hwang YS, Chen YF, Lai CC, et al. Infectious scleritis after use of immunomodulators. *Arch Ophthalmol.* 2002;120:1093–1094.
171. Sainz de la Maza M, Jabbur NS, Foster CS. An analysis of therapeutic decision for scleritis. *Ophthalmology.* 1993;100:1372–1376.
172. Messmer EM, Foster CS. Destructive corneal and scleral disease associated with rheumatoid arthritis. Medical and surgical management. *Cornea.* 1995;14:408–417.
173. Di Girolamo N, Lloyd A, McCluskey P, et al. Increased expression of matrix metalloproteinases in vivo in scleritis tissue and in vitro in cultured human scleral fibroblasts. *Am J Pathol.* 1997;150:653–666.
174. Kim EC, Foster CS. Immunomodulatory therapy for the treatment of ocular inflammatory disease: evidence-based medicine recommendations for use. *Int Ophthalmol Clin.* 2006;46:141–164.
175. Lim L, Suhler EB, Smith JR. Biologic therapies for inflammatory eye disease. *Clin Exp Ophthalmol.* 2006;34:365–374.
176. Shah SS, Lowder CY, Schmitt MA, et al. Low-dose methotrexate therapy for ocular inflammatory disease. *Ophthalmology.* 1992;99:1419–1423.
177. Jifi-Bahlool H, Saadeh C, O'Connor J. Peripheral ulcerative keratitis in the setting of rheumatoid arthritis: treatment with immunosuppressive therapy. *Semin Arthritis Rheum.* 1995;25:67–73.
178. Galor A, Jabs DA, Leder HA, et al. Comparison of antimetabolite drugs as corticosteroid-sparing therapy for noninfectious ocular inflammation. *Ophthalmology.* 2008;115:1826–1832.
179. Thorne JE, Jabs DA, Qazi FA, et al. Mycophenolate mofetil therapy for inflammatory eye disease. *Ophthalmology.* 2005;112:1472–1477.
180. Sobrin L, Christen W, Foster CS. Mycophenolate mofetil after methotrexate failure or intolerance in the treatment of scleritis and uveitis. *Ophthalmology.* 2008;115:1416–1421, 21 e1.
181. Niederkorn JY, Lang LS, Ross J, et al. Promotion of corneal allograft survival with leflunomide. *Invest Ophthalmol Vis Sci.* 1994;35:3783–3785.
182. Robertson SM, Lang LS. Leflunomide: inhibition of S-antigen induced autoimmune uveitis in Lewis rats. *Agents Actions.* 1994;42:167–172.
183. Jampol LM, West C, Goldberg MF. Therapy of scleritis with cytotoxic agents. *Am J Ophthalmol.* 1978;86:266–271.
184. Hemady R, Tauber J, Foster CS. Immunosuppressive drugs in immune and inflammatory ocular disease. *Surv Ophthalmol.* 1991;35:369–385.
185. Goldstein DA, Fontanilla FA, Kaul S, et al. Long-term follow-up of patients treated with short-term high-dose chlorambucil for sight-threatening ocular inflammation. *Ophthalmology.* 2002;109:370–377.
186. McCarthy JM, Dubord PJ, Chalmers A, et al. Cyclosporine A for the treatment of necrotizing scleritis and corneal melting in patients with rheumatoid arthritis. *J Rheumatol.* 1992;19:1358–1361.
187. Kilmartin DJ, Forrester JV, Dick AD. Tacrolimus (FK506) in failed cyclosporin A therapy in endogenous posterior uveitis. *Ocul Immunol Inflamm.* 1998;6:101–109.
188. Reis A, Reinhard T, Sundmacher R, et al. A comparative investigation of FK506 and cyclosporin A in murine corneal transplantation. *Graefe's Arch Clin Exp Ophthalmol.* 1998;236:785–789.
189. Sloper CM, Powell RJ, Dua HS. Tacrolimus (FK506) in the management of high-risk corneal and limbal grafts. *Ophthalmology.* 2001;108:1838–1844.
190. Ahmad SM, Stegman Z, Fructhman S, et al. Successful treatment of acute ocular graft-versus-host disease with tacrolimus (FK506). *Cornea.* 2002;21:432–433.
191. Reinhard T, Reis A, Mayweg S, et al. [Topical FK506 in inflammatory corneal and conjunctival diseases. A pilot study] *Klin Monatsbl Augenheilkd.* 2002;219:125–131.
192. Miyazaki D, Tominaga T, Kakimaru-Hasegawa A, et al. Therapeutic effects of tacrolimus ointment for refractory ocular surface inflammatory diseases. *Ophthalmology.* 2008;115:988–992 e5.
193. Thomas JW, Pflugfelder SC. Therapy of progressive rheumatoid arthritis-associated corneal ulceration with infliximab. *Cornea.* 2005;24:742–744.
194. Atchia II, Kidd CE, Bell RW. Rheumatoid arthritis-associated necrotizing scleritis and peripheral ulcerative keratitis treated successfully with infliximab. *J Clin Rheumatol.* 2006;12:291–293.
195. Lane L, Tamesis R, Rodriguez A, et al. Systemic immunosuppressive therapy and the occurrence of malignancy in patients with ocular inflammatory disease. *Ophthalmology.* 1995;102:1530–1535.
196. Ohrstrom A, Stenkula S, Berglin L, et al. Scleral reinforcement by a teflon graft and a tissue adhesive. *Acta Ophthalmol (Copenh).* 1988;66:643–646.
197. Leahey AB, Gottsch JD, Stark WJ. Clinical experience with *N*-butyl cyanoacrylate (Nexacryl) tissue adhesive. *Ophthalmology.* 1993;100:173–180.
198. Lin CP, Tsai MC, Wu YH, et al. Repair of a giant scleral ulcer with preserved sclera and tissue adhesive. *Ophthalmic Surg Lasers.* 1996;27:995–999.
199. Sharma A, Pandey S, Sharma R, et al. Cyanoacrylate tissue adhesive augmented tenoplasty: a new surgical procedure for bilateral severe chemical eye burns. *Cornea.* 1999;18:366–369.
200. Obear MF, Winter FC. Technique of overlay scleral homograft. *Arch Ophthalmol.* 1964;71:837–838.
201. Sevel D, Abramson A. Necrogranulomatous scleritis treated by an onlay scleral graft. *Br J Ophthalmol.* 1972;56:791–799.
202. Sainz de la Maza M, Tauber J, Foster CS. Scleral grafting for necrotizing scleritis. *Ophthalmology.* 1989;96:306–310.
203. Taffet S, Carter GZ. The use of a fascia lata graft in the treatment of scleromalacia perforans. *Am J Ophthalmol.* 1961;52:693–696.
204. Blum FG Jr, Salamoun SG. Scleromalacia perforans. A useful surgical modification in fascia lata or scleral grafting. *Arch Ophthalmol.* 1963;69:287–289.

205. Torchia RT, Dunn RE, Pease PJ. Fascia lata grafting in scleromalacia perforans with lamellar corneal-scleral dissection. *Am J Ophthalmol.* 1968;66:705–709.
206. Breslin CW, Katz JI, Kaufman HE. Surgical management of necrotizing scleritis. *Arch Ophthalmol.* 1977;95:2038–2040.
207. Koenig SB, Sanitato JJ, Kaufman HE. Long-term follow-up study of scleroplasty using autogenous periosteum. *Cornea.* 1990;9:139–143.
208. Mauriello JA Jr, Pokorny K. Use of split-thickness dermal grafts to repair corneal and scleral defects – a study of 10 patients. *Br J Ophthalmol.* 1993;77:327–331.
209. Nguyen QD, Foster CS. Scleral patch graft in the management of necrotizing scleritis. *Int Ophthalmol Clin.* 1999;39:109–131.
210. Eiferman RA, Carothers DJ, Yankeelov JA Jr. Peripheral rheumatoid ulceration and evidence for conjunctival collagenase production. *Am J Ophthalmol.* 1979;87:703–709.
211. Wilson FM 2nd, Grayson M, Ellis FD. Treatment of peripheral corneal ulcers by limlial conjunctivectomy. *Br J Ophthalmol.* 1976;60:713–719.
212. Feder RS, Krachmer JH. Conjunctival resection for the treatment of the rheumatoid corneal ulceration. *Ophthalmology.* 1984;91:111–115.
213. Fogle JA, Kenyon KR, Foster CS. Tissue adhesive arrests stromal melting in the human cornea. *Am J Ophthalmol.* 1980;89:795–802.
214. Weiss JL, Williams P, Lindstrom RL, et al. The use of tissue adhesive in corneal perforations. *Ophthalmology.* 1983;90:610–615.
215. Bernauer W, Ficker LA, Watson PG, et al. The management of corneal perforations associated with rheumatoid arthritis. An analysis of 32 eyes. *Ophthalmology.* 1995;102:1325–1337.
216. Gundersen T. Conjunctival flaps in the treatment of corneal disease with reference to a new technique of application. *AMA Arch Ophthalmol.* 1958;60:880–888.
217. Insler MS, Pechous B. Conjunctival flaps revisited. *Ophthalmic Surg.* 1987;18:455–458.
218. Maguire LJ, Shearer DR. A simple method of conjunctival dissection for Gunderson flaps. *Arch Ophthalmol.* 1991;109:1168–1169.
219. Alino AM, Perry HD, Kanellopoulos AJ, et al. Conjunctival flaps. *Ophthalmology.* 1998;105:1120–1123.
220. Pettit TH. Corneoscleral freehand lamellar keratoplasty in Terrien's marginal degeneration of the cornea – long-term results. *Refract Corneal Surg.* 1991;7:28–32.
221. Bessant DA, Dart JK. Lamellar keratoplasty in the management of inflammatory corneal ulceration and perforation. *Eye.* 1994;8(Pt 1):22–28.
222. Soong HK, Farjo AA, Katz D, et al. Lamellar corneal patch grafts in the management of corneal melting. *Cornea.* 2000;19:126–134.
223. Hirst LW, Stark WJ, Jensen AD. Tissue adhesives: new perspectives in corneal perforations. *Ophthalmic Surg.* 1979;10:58–64.
224. Portnoy SL, Insler MS, Kaufman HE. Surgical management of corneal ulceration and perforation. *Surv Ophthalmol.* 1989;34:47–58.
225. Palay DA, Stulting RD, Waring GO 3rd, et al. Penetrating keratoplasty in patients with rheumatoid arthritis. *Ophthalmology.* 1992;99:622–627.
226. Pleyer U, Bertelmann E, Rieck P, et al. Outcome of penetrating keratoplasty in rheumatoid arthritis. *Ophthalmologica.* 2002;216:249–255.
227. Lee SH, Tseng SC. Amniotic membrane transplantation for persistent epithelial defects with ulceration. *Am J Ophthalmol.* 1997;123:303–312.
228. Hanada K, Shimazaki J, Shimmura S, et al. Multilayered amniotic membrane transplantation for severe ulceration of the cornea and sclera. *Am J Ophthalmol.* 2001;131:324–331.
229. Solomon A, Meller D, Prabhasawat P, et al. Amniotic membrane grafts for nontraumatic corneal perforations, descemetoceles, and deep ulcers. *Ophthalmology.* 2002;109:694–703.
230. Oh JH, Kim JC. Repair of scleromalacia using preserved scleral graft with amniotic membrane transplantation. *Cornea.* 2003;22:288–293.
231. Khan B, Dudenhoefer EJ, Dohlman CH. Keratoprosthesis: an update. *Curr Opin Ophthalmol.* 2001;12:282–287.
232. Dohlman CH, Dudenhoefer EJ, Khan BF, et al. Protection of the ocular surface after keratoprosthesis surgery: the role of soft contact lenses. *CLAO J.* 2002;28:72–74.
233. Hicks CR, Crawford GJ, Lou X, et al. Corneal replacement using a synthetic hydrogel cornea, AlphaCor: device, preliminary outcomes and complications. *Eye.* 2003;17:385–392.

Chapter 93

Corneal Disease Associated with Nonrheumatoid Collagen-Vascular Disease

Joel Sugar, M. Soledad Cortina

The immune-mediated systemic disorders cover a broad spectrum. These so-called collagen-vascular diseases include the rheumatoid arthropathies, the collagenoses, and the vasculitides. While these groupings are not clear-cut, they allow for a structure for discussion of these disorders. The arthritides (rheumatoid arthritis, juvenile rheumatoid arthritis, etc.) are discussed elsewhere (see Ch. 92), as are the other inflammatory disorders with associated arthropathy such as ankylosing spondylitis (see Ch. 107) and inflammatory bowel disease (see Ch. 61). The collagen-vascular diseases have often been thought of as autoimmune disorders. In most instances the etiology is uncertain, although immune mechanisms play a definite role.

The Collagenoses

The collagenoses refer to a group of disorders in which connective tissues are involved in destructive and inflammatory processes. Vasculitis may occur, and the distinction between the collagenoses and the vasculitides is somewhat arbitrary.

Systemic lupus erythematosus

Systemic lupus erythematosus (SLE) is the prototypical collagenosis. It is a disorder of unknown etiology, markedly more frequent in women than in men (9:1), with higher mortality observed in black females.[1] It has a definite genetic predisposition, and HLA class II antigens DR2 and DR3 and class III C4AQ0 are highly associated.[2] T- and B-cell hyperreactivity lead to production of autoantibodies and immune complex deposition leading to chronic inflammation and organ damage.

Clinical manifestations are multisystemic. The American College of Rheumatology 1982 criteria for the diagnosis include any four of the 11 findings listed in Box 93.1.[3] Clinical disease is widespread, and patients often have arthralgias and myalgias (95%), cutaneous rashes and photosensitivity (80%), glomerulonephritis (50%), neurologic symptoms (60%), pleuritis (60%), and other symptoms. Almost all patients experience fatigue, fever, anorexia, and weight loss.

The diagnosis is made on the basis of clinical findings in addition to the presence of autoantibodies on serologic testing. Antinuclear antibodies (ANAs) are present in 95% of patients and anti-DNAs are common (70%), with anti-double-stranded DNA being relatively specific to lupus. Numerous other autoantibodies are found as well, including anti-Ro (SSA) and anti-La (SSB) as well as anticardiolipin (lupus anticoagulant). Complement levels are decreased with active disease. Complete blood count and urinalysis are also appropriate in the work-up.

Ocular manifestations are seen in a minority of patients but any portion of the eye can be affected. The most frequent finding is cotton-wool spots in the retina, which are independent of hypertension and central nervous system involvement.[4] A severe occlusive retinal vasculitis associated with central nervous system involvement has also been described.[5] Neuro-ophthalmic complications include cranial nerve palsies, visual field loss, cortical blindness, gaze palsies, etc.[6] Local involvement of the small vessels of the optic nerve can lead to optic neuropathy.[7] Choroidopathy with uveal effusion and serous detachments may occasionally occur.[8]

Eyelid involvement with lid erythema, scaling plaques, and loss of lashes has been described in the discoid or localized cutaneous form of lupus, which may present as a chronic blepharitis.[9] Anterior segment abnormalities in lupus are infrequent, with the exception of those related to secondary Sjögren's syndrome which develops in one out of five patients with SLE.[10] Conjunctival involvement is infrequent. Conjunctival scarring and even symblepharon formation have also been reported, especially in discoid lupus. Interestingly, linear deposits of immunoreactants have been found in the basement membrane zones of the bulbar conjunctiva in a high proportion of patients with systemic and cutaneous lupus.[11] Conjunctival chemosis has been reported as a presenting finding in SLE,[12] although this is uncommon, as are periorbital edema[13] and orbital inflammation.[14]

Recurrent episcleritis may be seen and in one series was found in 28% of patients.[11] Scleritis is less common, although it can occur. Typically, the scleritis is nodular.[15] Uveitis is infrequently seen.[16] An elevated conjunctival mass with chronic blepharoconjunctivitis has been reported in discoid lupus.[17]

Box 93.1 Criteria for the classification of SLE

Malar rash
Discoid rash
Photosensitivity
Oral ulcers
Nonerosive arthritis
Serositis – pleuritis or pericarditis
Renal disorder – proteinuria or casts
Neurologic disorder – seizures or psychosis
Hematologic disorder – hemolytic anemia, leukopenia, lymphopenia, or thrombocytopenia
Immunologic disorder – positive lupus erythematosus preparation, anti-double-stranded DNA, anti-smooth muscle, or false-positive venereal disease research laboratory test for syphilis
Antinuclear antibodies

From Hahn BH. Systemic Lupus erythematosus. In: Isselbacher KJ et al. (eds) Harrison's principles of internal medicine, New York, 1994 McGraw-Hill.

Corneal involvement in systemic and cutaneous lupus is uncommon. Corneal staining, usually in a nonspecific pattern, has been reported in 6.5%[3] to as high as 88% of patients.[18] While in some patients this may result from tear insufficiency, in others, without dry eyes, superficial keratopathy has nonetheless been reported.[19] Asymptomatic dry eye with abnormal Schirmer testing is also commonly found.[20] A case of bilateral deep stromal haze consistent with deep stromal keratitis[21] and another case of deep 'band-shaped' stromal infiltration with uveitis have been reported,[22] but the incidence of corneal stromal involvement in systemic lupus is exceedingly low. Peripheral ulcerative keratitis responsive to the control of the systemic disease has been reported.[23]

Corneal endotheliitis with bilateral corneal edema responsive to corticosteroids has also been reported in systemic lupus.[24] In discoid lupus, epithelial keratopathy has been reported.[25] Sterile corneal ulceration after cataract extraction in lupus patients because of tear insufficiency, or possibly an immune mechanism, has also been seen.[26] Significant late corneal scarring has been reported in a patient 1 year after photorefractive keratectomy for myopia.[27]

Treatment of systemic lupus is with systemic corticosteroids for acute disease. Hydroxychloroquine (Plaquenil) may be effective for chronic disease, while lower doses of corticosteroids may be necessary as well. Cytotoxic agents such as azathioprine, chlorambucil, and cyclophosphamide may also be useful. Ocular disease treatment depends primarily on the treatment of the systemic disease. The dry eye is treated with lubricants. Rituximab has been shown to induce remissions in refractory patients, usually given in combination with cyclophosphamide and methylprednisolone.[28]

The ophthalmologist is often involved in the evaluation of patients with lupus who are being treated with hydroxychloroquine. Hydroxychloroquine can cause a 'bull's-eye' maculopathy with paracentral scotoma.[29] The American Academy of Ophthalmology has published recommendations on screening for chloroquine and hydroxychloroquine (Plaquenil) retinopathy. They consider patients who use less than 6.5 mg/kg of hydroxychloroquine or 3 mg/kg of chloroquine daily, who are lean or average in body fat, have used the drug for less than 5 years, are under age 60, and have no retinal or renal/liver disease to be at low risk. These patients need comprehensive eye evaluation once between ages 20 and 29, twice from ages 30 to 39, every 2 to 4 years between 40 and 64, and every 1 to 2 years at 65 and older. High-risk patients need annual screening. The screening should consist of complete eye examination with visual acuity and dilated fundus examination, visual field testing with Amsler grid or Humphrey 10-2 fields, and optional color vision testing, baseline fundus photography, and, in the case of underlying maculopathy, fluorescein angiography or multifocal electroretinogram (ERG).[30] Evidence is showing that multifocal ERG is able to detect decreased retinal function in patients with an otherwise normal examination. This test may be indicated in patients considered high risk for developing toxicity and, if abnormal, it may dictate need for closer monitoring.[31]

Systemic sclerosis

Like lupus, systemic sclerosis is a multisystem disorder. Synonyms include scleroderma and progressive systemic sclerosis. Fibrosis of the skin and viscera is the hallmark. Overproduction of collagen in the skin and viscera and vascular damage with endothelial injury, intimal thickening, and vascular occlusion are seen.[32] The vast majority of patients are women. Clinical manifestations vary with the disease type but include skin thickening diffusely or in the limited form on the face and distal extremities. The epidermis is thin, skin appendages are lost, and fibrosis extends from the dermis to below the epidermis, leading to skin tightening. Visceral involvement includes fibrosis in the gastrointestinal tract with dysphagia, esophagitis, and poor motility; interstitial fibrosis in the lungs with dyspnea and cough; myocardial fibrosis with heart failure, arrhythmia, and pericarditis; and renal vascular involvement with renal failure and severe hypertension. In the limited form, visceral involvement is less common, but often features of the CREST syndrome are present, with calcinosis, Raynaud's phenomenon, esophageal dysmotility, sclerodactyly, and telangiectasia. Raynaud's phenomenon occurs in 95% of patients with systemic sclerosis, and is caused by vasoconstriction in the arteries and arterioles of the digits, typically brought on by cold, with pallor and numbness followed by redness and pain in the affected digits.

Localized forms of scleroderma occur as well. One is linear scleroderma, which typically occurs in children or young adults beginning as an erythematous band of skin that becomes thickened and adherent to the underlying tissues. The underlying tissues become atrophied, and an entire extremity may become involved. Facial involvement (scleroderma en coup de sabre) in children may lead to hemifacial atrophy. Disease activity may abate after 2 to 3 years. Morphea is an even more localized form of scleroderma, characterized by patches of scleroderma-like skin change that evolve over months to years and spontaneously improve.[33]

The etiology of scleroderma is unknown. Laboratory findings may include an elevated sedimentation rate and elevated serum globulin levels. Rheumatoid factor is positive in 25% of patients. ANA tests are positive in up to 90% of patients. Antibodies to the nucleolus are most specific for scleroderma, as are antibodies to Scl-70, a nuclear enzyme topoisomerase-1.[34] Varying subsets of systemic sclerosis have different ANAs, with anticentromere antibodies being seen in the CREST group.[35]

Ocular manifestations of systemic sclerosis are common. Eyelid tightening with blepharophimosis and lid telangiectases is frequent, with 65% of patients having eyelid tightening and 17% lid telangiectasia.[36,37] Corneal exposure may be seen but is infrequent. Conjunctival vascular changes with sludging and telangiectasia are frequent. Shallow conjunctival fornices caused by subconjunctival fibrosis may occur. Conjunctival biopsy shows dense subconjunctival fibrosis around capillaries with minimal lymphocytic infiltrate, but high numbers of mast cells are present and attenuation in capillary walls occurs in some cases with endothelial cell disruption and vessel occlusion.[38]

Keratoconjunctivitis sicca is very common (37–76%).[37,38] Whether to consider this a form of secondary Sjögren's syndrome is uncertain. A minority of scleroderma patients show the lymphocytic infiltrate characteristic of Sjögren's syndrome on salivary gland biopsy, and glandular fibrosis is more frequent.[39,40] Conjunctival biopsies from Sjögren's patients show lymphocytic infiltrate with the absence of fibrosis and the absence of the numerous mast cells seen in scleroderma.[38]

Orbital findings are rare in systemic sclerosis. Enophthalmos from orbital fat atrophy may be seen in both the systemic and localized forms.[41] Scleritis is very uncommon. Myositis may occur. Neuro-ophthalmic complications of intracranial aneurysms secondary to the vascular involvement of scleroderma have been reported infrequently.[42] Retinal changes are typically those of the hypertension associated with the renal involvement. Central retinal vein occlusion has been reported.[43] Retinal pigment epithelial defects were shown on fluorescein angiography in 26% of a series of patients and postulated to be caused by microvascular involvement of the choroid.[44] A case of choroidal sclerosis in localized scleroderma has also been reported.[45]

Corneal involvement is predominantly secondary to the eyelid changes and tear insufficiency. Corneal inflammatory disease is extremely unusual. A case was reported of bilateral peripheral corneal melting with perforation thought to be caused by T-cell-mediated inflammation in a patient with systemic sclerosis.[46] Corneal superficial infiltrates were reported in a case of localized scleroderma.[47]

In the past, options for treating systemic sclerosis were few and not very successful in altering the course of the disease.[33] However, recent studies have shown clinical benefit in patients treated with high immunosuppressive doses of cyclophosphamide.[48] Corticosteroids may be beneficial for associated myositis and myalgias and arthralgias. Future clinical trials for treatment of systemic sclerosis are planned which include autologous hematopoietic stem cell transplantation, and other immunomodulators such as interferon gamma, mycophenolate, and antibodies directed to several cytokines.[49] D-Penicillamine, which interferes with collagen cross-linking, has been used for decades to treat the skin fibrosis; a multicenter, controlled trial showed no difference between high- and low-dose treatments.[49,50] Alternative treatments for fibrosis include ultraviolet A therapy, minocyline, methotrexate, and mycophenolate. Ophthalmic treatment is symptomatic, with management of the eyelids and dry eyes.

Mixed connective tissue disease

A number of overlap syndromes with the features of various collagenoses have been described. Mixed connective tissue disease (MCTD) is such a syndrome, with features of systemic lupus, systemic sclerosis, and polymyositis. High ANA titers are present. Autoantibodies to an extractable nuclear antigen (U_1RNP) are common.[51] Clinical features include hand edema, synovitis, myositis, Raynaud's phenomenon, and sclerosis of the digits (acrosclerosis).[52]

Ophthalmic findings are few.

Polymyositis and dermatomyositis

Polymyositis and dermatomyositis are inflammatory myopathies of unknown cause characterized by the presence of lymphocytic inflammation in skeletal muscles leading to muscle weakness. In dermatomyositis, skin lesions are present as well. Symmetrical muscle weakness, elevated serum muscle enzyme levels, especially creatine phosphokinase (CK), SGOT, SGPT, and LDH, as well as elevated ANA levels are seen. Electromyography shows characteristic changes. The most frequent antibody is to Jo-1, a cytoplasmic transfer RNA synthetase. Skin findings include a heliotrope discoloration of the eyelids and a scaly erythematous dermatitis involving especially the skin over the joints of the fingers (Gottron's sign), elbows, and knees (Fig. 93.1), as well as the face, neck, and torso. Pulmonary fibrosis may occur, as may myocardial inflammation and cardiac failure.[53] There is a well-known association between dermatomyositis and underlying malignancy in patients over 40 years of age.

Ocular findings are few. The myositis does not commonly involve the extraocular muscles. Retinopathy is infrequent,[54] but proliferative vascular retinopathy has been observed in an overlap syndrome with scleroderma.[55]

Anterior segment findings include the classic heliotrope or lilac discoloration of the eyelids (Fig. 93.2) and conjunc-

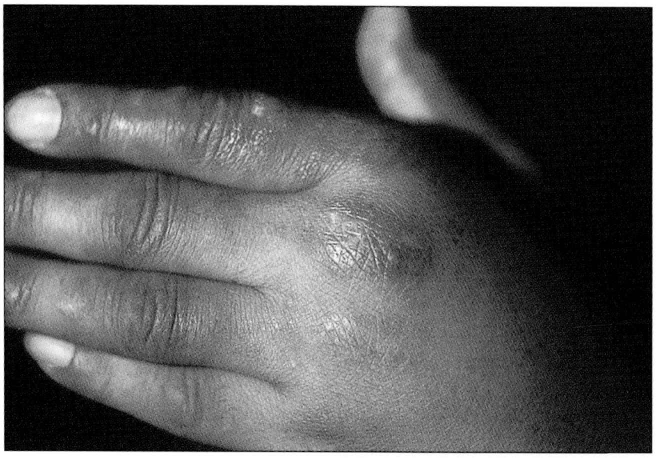

Fig. 93.1 Changes over the joints of the hand in dermatomyositis (Gottron's papules).

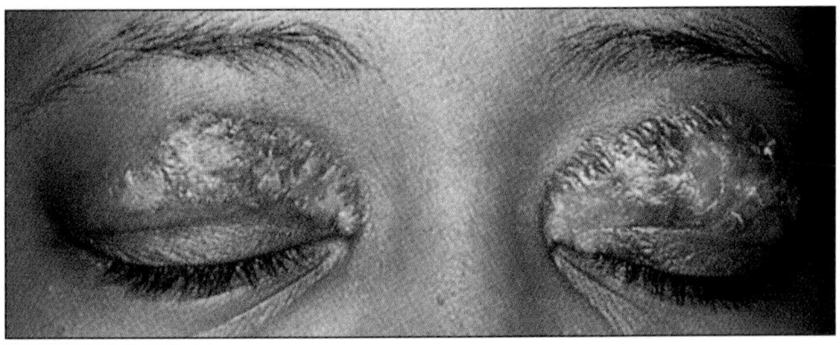

Fig. 93.2 Lid edema and discoloration in dermatomyositis.

tival chemosis. Conjunctival and episcleral vascular tortuosity have been reported with juvenile dermatomyositis but these findings were of low sensitivity and specificity.[56] Periorbital edema is common and may occur in acute presentations of the disease.[57] Avascular patches on the bulbar conjunctiva have been reported, presumably as a result of vasculitis.[58] Corneal changes have been only rarely reported, but Sjögren's syndrome with dry eye occurs.[59]

Treatment of polymyositis and dermatomyositis is with systemic corticosteroids. Unfortunately, not all patients respond to steroid therapy and combination with azathioprine is most commonly used in these cases.[60] Intravenous immunoglobulins are used in resistant patients and other stronger immunosuppressants may be considered as well such as ciclosporin, mycophenolate, and methotrexate.[60]

Relapsing polychondritis

Relapsing polychondritis is a disorder in which three or more of the following are present: recurrent chondritis of both auricles, nonerosive inflammatory polyarthritis, chondritis of the nasal cartilages, ocular inflammation, chondritis of the respiratory tract involving laryngeal and/or tracheal cartilage, and cochlear and/or vestibular damage manifested by hearing loss, tinnitus, and/or vertigo. This is the McAdam classification.[61] These criteria have been modified to include patients with one or more of McAdam's criteria plus histologic confirmation, or patients with chondritis involving two or more anatomic sites, which responds to steroids and/or dapsone treatment.[62] Men and women are affected with equal frequency, and occurrence is usually in midlife. The frequency of the findings varies, but auricular chondritis occurs in 85% (Fig. 93.3), arteritis in 52%, and respiratory disease in 48%.[63] Skin disease, renal disease, and cardiovascular disease – especially aortic root – occur, but much less frequently. Survival is 74% at 5 years and 55% at 10 years, with death being secondary to systemic vasculitis, infection, and malignancy.[64]

No specific laboratory test exists to confirm the diagnosis, which is usually made on clinical grounds. The etiology is unknown but certainly involves autoimmune phenomena. Antibodies to cartilage are frequent, and antibodies to type II collagen may be found as well.[65]

Ocular manifestations are a significant aspect of relapsing polychondritis with, in one large series, 51% of patients having ophthalmologic disease.[63] Lid edema and tarsal as well as orbital inflammation may occur.[66] Extraocular muscle palsy may occur from vasculitis involving the muscles or the

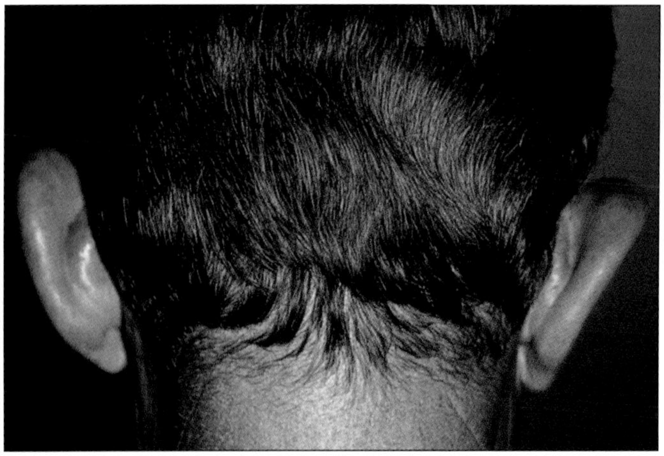

Fig. 93.3 Auricular swelling and erythema in relapsing polychondritis.

cranial nerves.[63] Conjunctival nonspecific edema may occur, as can keratoconjunctivitis sicca, although this was seen in only about 10% of patients.[63] Scleritis and episcleritis are the most common findings. Diffuse, nodular, and necrotizing scleritis can occur and may be unilateral or bilateral. Both may correlate with occult systemic inflammation; it is believed that scleritis is a marker of severity of the underlying disease that warrants aggressive immunomodulatory treatment.[63,67] Conjunctival and scleral biopsies show perivasculitis, vasculitis, and infiltration with mast cells, plasma cells, and lymphocytes.[67] A case of chronic conjunctivitis with obliterative microangiopathy observed in the conjunctival biopsy has been reported.[68] Uveitis is usually seen in association with scleritis or keratitis. Severe nongranulomatous anterior segment or diffuse inflammation may occur.[69]

Retinal involvement has included chorioretinal infiltrates, exudative retinal detachment, hemorrhage, exudates, cotton-wool spots, and vein occlusion. Optic neuritis and ischemic optic neuropathy have been reported as well.[63]

Corneal findings include peripheral stromal and epithelial infiltrates with edema,[69] peripheral corneal thinning with crystalline deposits and pannus formation,[63] and peripheral ulcerative keratitis with at times spontaneous perforation.[70] The keratitis may occur in the absence of scleritis[71] or may be part of a sclerokeratitis.[72]

Treatment of relapsing polychondritis varies with the severity of the manifestations. Topical steroids are not effective in controlling the inflammation. Nonsteroidal antiinflammatory agents may be of benefit for mild symptoms. Dapsone, which may act by inhibiting lysosomal enzyme release, is beneficial and moderately successful in some patients. Systemic corticosteroids are helpful for acute exacerbations. Cytotoxic agents and ciclosporin A can also be considered.

The Vasculitides

The vasculitides are a heterogeneous group of disorders that have in common inflammation of vessels and probably immune complex deposition. The type of vessels involved, the distribution of involvement, and the type of inflammation varies among the different vasculitic syndromes. While ophthalmic involvement varies from syndrome to syndrome, the ophthalmologist may play a very important role in raising suspicion of the diagnosis as a vasculitis. This is perhaps most true in Wegener's granulomatosis.

Wegener's granulomatosis

Wegener's granulomatosis is a systemic vasculitis characterized by necrotizing and granulomatous inflammation of the vessels of the upper and lower respiratory tract, glomerulonephritis, and other organ involvement with small vessel inflammation. The etiology is unknown. A 'limited form' of Wegener's granulomatosis without renal involvement has been described, although this may represent early cases. The American College of Rheumatology (ACR) has established criteria for the diagnosis of Wegener's granulomatosis, with the presence of at least two of the four criteria making the diagnosis with a sensitivity of 88% and a specificity of 92%. Hemoptysis can serve as a surrogate criterion in the absence of biopsy data. Box 93.2 lists the ACR criteria.[73] Wegener's granulomatosis typically has its onset in the mid-40s and involves males twice as frequently as females. However, it can present in children, with ocular involvement as the initial manifestation.[74] Presentation may include, as in the other collagen-vascular diseases, nonspecific complaints of fever, malaise, joint and muscle pain, and weight loss. Upper airway symptoms of sinusitis are common (67%), with discharge, rhinorrhea, epistaxis, and otitis. Pulmonary infiltrates are seen on chest roentgenogram (71%), and hemoptysis may be a presenting finding (18%). Renal failure is less common as a presenting occurrence (11%). Ocular inflammation is a presenting finding in 16%.[75]

Laboratory findings include a normocytic normochromic anemia, elevated sedimentation rate, and often a positive rheumatoid factor. Circulating immune complexes may be found during disease activity. ANAs are not found.[75] The antineutrophil cytoplasmic antibody (ANCA) appears to be the most sensitive and specific test outside of biopsy for the diagnosis of Wegener's granulomatosis. ANCA tests for antibodies to a neutrophil serine proteinase, proteinase 3, in the classic diffuse cytoplasmic staining pattern (C-ANCA) or to myeloperoxidase or other lysosomal enzymes in the perinuclear staining pattern (P-ANCA).[76] The C-ANCA appears to be highly specific for Wegener's, while the P-ANCA is less specific and is seen in microscopic polyarteritis as well.[77] Sensitivity and specifiity of the ANCA test are high (93% and 97%, respectively),[78] but depend on extent and activity of the disease. Titers tend to decrease during remission and increase prior to clinical relapse.[78,79] In an evaluation of scleritis patients, ANCA testing appeared to be both extremely sensitive and specific, with all of seven Wegener's scleritis patients having positive C- or P-ANCA and none of 54 patients with other sources of ocular inflammation being positive.[76] A high prevalence of circulating autoantibodies to two corneal epithelial antigens has been demonstrated in this disorder.[80] Cytokeratin 3 appears to be an autoantigen in patients with peripheral ulcerative keratitis in Wegener's.[81]

Box 93.2 Criteria for the classification of Wegener's granulomatosis

Nasal or oral inflammation

Abnormal chest radiograph

Urinary sediment – microhematuria or red blood cell casts

Granulomatous inflammation on biopsy

From Reynolds I, Tullo AB, John SL et al. Corneal epithelial-specific cytokeratin 3 is an autoantigen in Wegener's granulomatosis-associated peripheral ulcerative keratitis. Invest Ophthalmol Vis Sci 1999;40:2147.

Histopathology of Wegener's granulomatosis shows necrotizing granulomas as well as necrotizing or granulomatous vasculitis.[82]

Ocular involvement is common, in one series occurring in 58% of patients,[75] and may be present in the absence of obvious systemic manifestations.[83] Proptosis with orbital pseudotumor or orbital inflammation is not infrequent, being reported in 22% of Wegener's patients in one series[84] and 45% of patients with ocular involvement in another series.[85] Orbital biopsy showed classic granulomatous inflammation, tissue necrosis, and vasculitis in just over 50% of such patients.[86] Extension of nasopharyngeal disease may lead to nasolacrimal duct obstruction.[87] Retinal vasculitis and vasculitis involving the vessels of the optic nerve causing ischemic optic neuropathy occur, as may retinal artery or vein occlusion. Cotton-wool spots may also be present.[85,88]

Anterior segment findings of Wegener's granulomatosis include conjunctivitis, episcleritis, scleritis, keratitis, and uveitis. Secondary Sjögren's syndrome with dry eye is frequent, occurring in 55% of patients in one series.[88] Conjunctivitis and episcleritis are relatively common, although granulomatous conjunctival nodules are rare.[89] Conjunctival ulceration may occur.[90] Tarsal conjunctival disease with areas of necrosis and fibrovascular changes may be observed more frequently in the palpebral side leading to entropion and trichiasis.[91] Association of conjunctival fibrosis, nasolacrimal duct obstruction, and subglottis stenosis has been reported and ENT referral should be considered in patients with tarsal-conjunctival disease.[91] Scleritis and keratitis are often the presenting findings of Wegener's granulomatosis to the corneal specialist (Fig. 93.4). The incidence appears to be about 12–13% of Wegener's patients.[84,88] Scleritis may be an anterior sectorial scleritis without scleral necrosis. Peripheral corneal subepithelial infiltrates (Fig. 93.5) may be associated and may develop into grainy anterior stromal opacities (Fig. 93.6). More severe scleritis with scleral necrosis can occur with yellow sequestrae of necrotic sclera, often with loss of overlying conjunctiva (Fig. 93.7). Peripheral corneal changes may be the same as with non-necrotizing disease, or deep stromal infiltration may occur and extend centrally (Fig. 93.8). In areas of contiguous scleral necrosis, corneal guttering may occur and may extend both centrally and circumferentially.[92] Corneal ulceration may lead to perforation.

Treatment of Wegener's granulomatosis is essential, as the diffuse form of the disease is life-threatening. Before treatment was available, the mean survival was only 5 months.[93] Treatment focuses on the systemic disorder, although

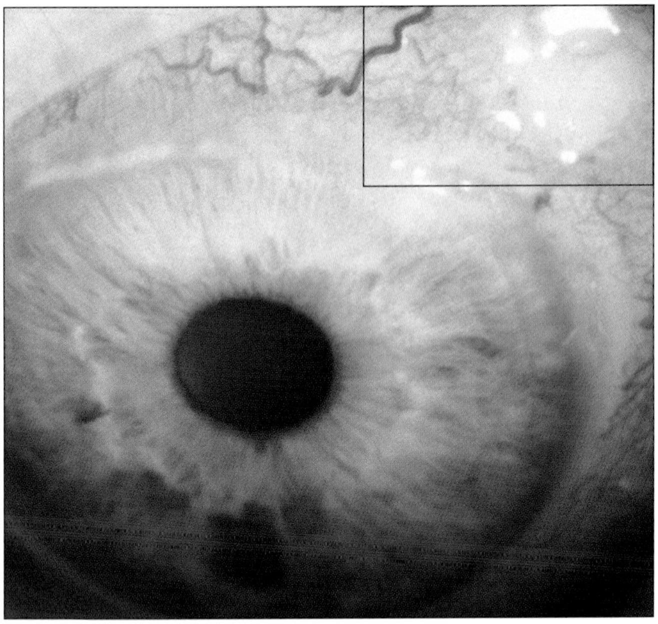

Fig. 93.4 Focal necrotizing scleritis with peripheral keratitis (*box*) in Wegener's granulomatosis.

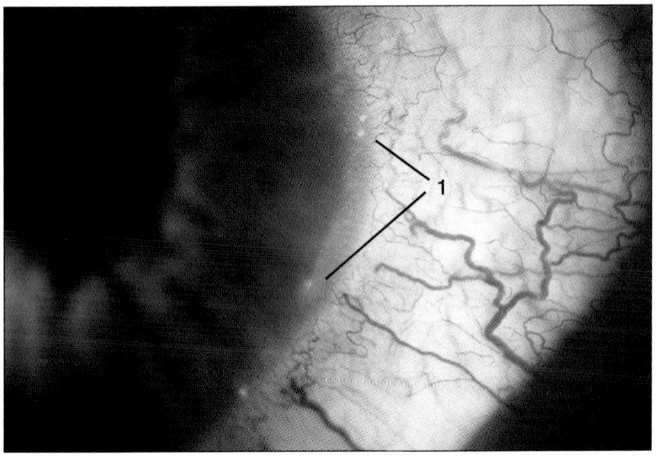

Fig. 93.5 Peripheral anterior stromal and subepithelial infiltrates (*1*) in Wegener's granulomatosis.

artificial tears for dry eyes and topical corticosteroids for mild conjunctivitis and episcleritis are beneficial. The mainstay of treatment is the use of a combination of systemic corticosteroids and cytotoxic agents. Typically, oral prednisone (1 mg/kg) and cyclophosphamide (2 mg/kg) orally are used for initial therapy, with the prednisone tapered after 2 to 4 weeks but continued over many months while the cyclophosphamide is continued for at least 1 year. The goal is to keep the leukocyte count in the 3000 to 4000 cells/mm^3 range.[75] Alternatively, 'pulsed' intravenous methylprednisolone (500 mg to 1 g) and cyclophosphamide (500 mg or more) may be used.[94] The side effects of systemic corticosteroids are well known. Cyclophosphamide can cause bone marrow suppression, hemorrhagic cystitis, alopecia, ovarian failure and azoospermia, pulmonary fibrosis, and malignancy. Complete blood count is essential frequently at the

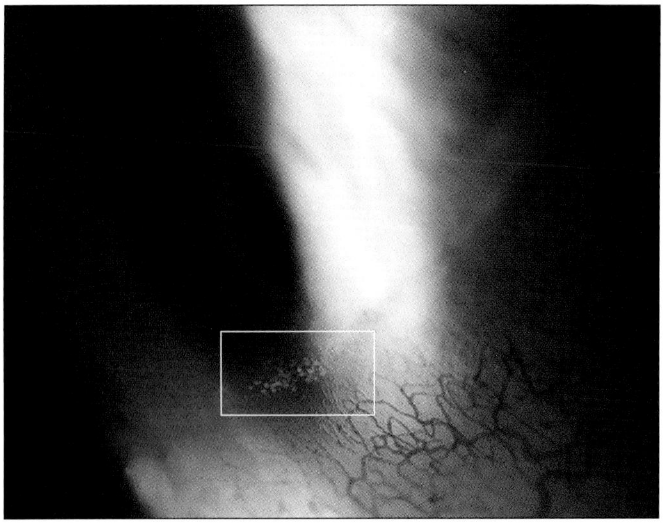

Fig. 93.6 Residual grainy anterior stromal opacities (*box*) in Wegener's granulomatosis.

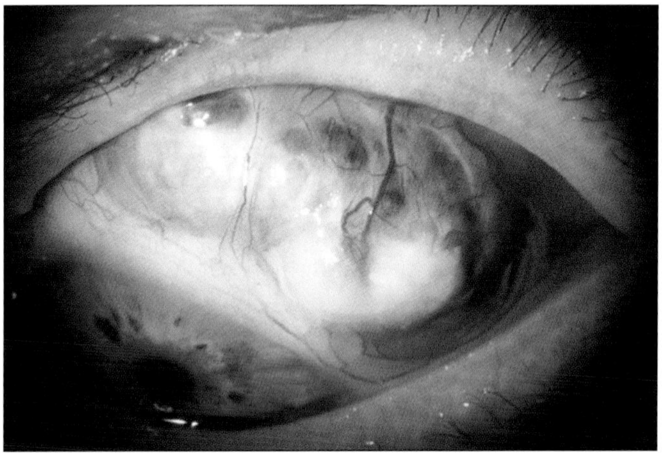

Fig. 93.7 Sequelae of necrotizing scleritis in Wegener's granulomatosis.

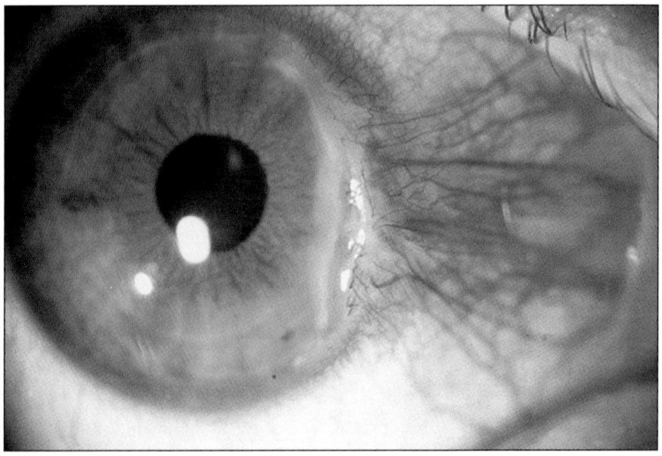

Fig. 93.8 Peripheral ulcerative keratitis in a patient with polyarteritis nodosa. (Courtesy of Paul J. Dubord, MD.)

initiation of therapy, with monitoring at least monthly once the treatment is stabilized. Approximately 50% of patients experience a relapse after discontinuation of therapy. Therefore, treatment planning needs to incorporate less toxic agents that are able to maintain remissions. The most commonly used agents for this purpose are trimethoprim-sulfamethoxazole and methotrexate.[95] Treatment effectiveness can be monitored by serial ANCA levels as well as by clinical response. This has been debated, however,[96,97] and current guidelines state that serial ANCA levels alone are insufficient to monitor disease activity or predict relapse and should not guide treatment but may be helpful in selected patients.[98] Antitumor necrosis factor and tumor necrosis factor receptor agents such as infliximab and etanercept appear beneficial. Intravenous immunoglobulin, which has been helpful in the systemic disease manifestations, has been reported to worsen ocular symptoms, and in one patient induced a retinal vasculitis.[99]

Polyarteritis nodosa

Polyarteritis nodosa, also called periarteritis nodosa, is a vasculitis of small and medium-sized arteries leading to multiple organ system disease. Occurrence is usually in middle age, and males are more frequently affected than females. The American College of Rheumatology criteria for the diagnosis include the presence of at least three of the following 10 findings: weight loss greater than or equal to 4 kg; livedo reticularis – mottling of the skin over the torso or extremities; testicular pain or tenderness; myalgias, weakness, or leg tenderness; mononeuropathy or polyneuropathy; systemic hypertension with diastolic greater than 90 mmHg; elevated blood urea nitrogen or creatinine level; presence of hepatitis B surface antigen or antibody in serum; arteriographic evidence of aneurysms or occlusions (nonarteriosclerotic); polymorphonuclear leukocytes or polymorphonuclear and mononuclear cells present in artery walls on biopsy of small or medium-sized arteries.[100] The etiology is unknown, although in some patients it may be related to hepatitis B antigen-associated immune complex disease or other immune complexes.

The systemic findings can be assumed from the preceding diagnostic criteria, with renal disease (70%), visceral infarctions, peripheral neuropathy (50–70%), and arthritis and arthralgias (50%). No specific laboratory finding makes the diagnosis. Hepatitis B surface antigens have been found in as many as half of all patients with polyarteritis nodosa.[101] Biopsy showing small and medium arterial vasculitis and angiography showing aneurysms and vascular narrowing confirm the diagnosis.[102] P-ANCA testing is positive in the microscopic form.

Ocular findings occur in a minority of patients (10–20%),[103] most commonly involving the retinal vessels. This may occur secondary to the hypertension or there may be vasculitis involving retinal vessels.[104] Central nervous system involvement or direct nerve involvement may lead to extraocular muscle palsies and optic nerve infarction. Orbital involvement with a pseudotumor-like lesion has been reported.[105] Conjunctival nodules caused by edema and necrosis of conjunctival vessels as well as uveitis have also been reported.[106]

Anterior segment findings are infrequent but include scleritis, sclerokeratitis, and peripheral ulcerative keratitis (see Fig. 93.8). The scleritis may be diffuse and associated with peripheral keratitis and ulceration,[107] or more focal with peripheral corneal Mooren's-like ulceration.[108] Bilateral peripheral ulceration with perforation in a patient with microscopic polyarteritis has also been reported.[109]

Treatment focuses on the systemic disease and involves the use of corticosteroids and, more importantly, cytotoxic agents, which have markedly improved the outcome.[109]

Churg-Strauss syndrome

Churg-Strauss syndrome or allergic granulomatosis and angiitis is a vasculitic syndrome similar to Wegener's granulomatosis and polyarteritis nodosa but with allergy, asthma, and inflammation of small arteries and veins with eosinophils. The ACR 1990 criteria for the diagnosis include at least four of the following six: asthma; eosinophilia greater than 10% on white blood cell differential count; mononeuropathy or polyneuropathy; pulmonary infiltrates that are transitory on chest X-ray films; paranasal sinus pain, tenderness, or opacification on X-ray films; and extravascular eosinophils on tissue biopsy, which includes artery, arteriole, or venule.[110] Patients have allergic symptoms, including asthma, often for many years, followed by eosinophilia in blood and tissues, followed by vasculitis. The disorder is most common in males, with onset around 40 years of age. The cause is unknown. Histopathology shows necrotizing vasculitis of small arteries and venules, and granulomas with an eosinophilic core and a dominant eosinophilic cellular infiltrate near the vessels.[102]

Ophthalmic manifestations of this uncommon disorder have been infrequently reported. Branch retinal artery occlusion was reported in two cases,[111] and extraocular muscle palsy and ischemic optic neuropathy have been described.[112] Conjunctival waxy yellow nodules[113] and diffuse nodular conjunctival thickening have been observed.[114] Episcleritis and severe uveitis, scleritis, and disk edema have also been reported.[115]

Corneal involvement appears to be exceedingly rare, with a single case of peripheral corneal ulceration being reported.[23]

Treatment of Churg-Strauss syndrome is with systemic corticosteroids. Use of antimetabolites has been less well demonstrated to be effective.[102]

Cogan syndrome

Cogan syndrome of interstitial keratitis and deafness may be considered among the vasculitides. It is reviewed in Chapter 86.

Behçet's disease

Behçet's disease involves vasculitis and uveitis. Scleritis and keratitis occur. This disorder is discussed in Chapter 109.

Giant cell arteritis

Giant cell arteritis (GCA) or temporal arteritis is a systemic vasculitis of medium to large vessels. The ACR criteria for

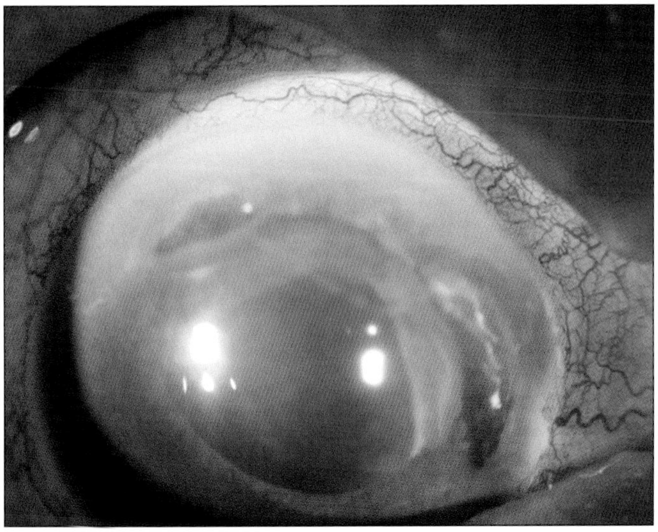

Fig. 93.9 Peripheral ulcerative keratitis in a patient with giant cell arteritis.

the diagnosis include age over 50, new-onset headache, temporal artery tenderness or decreased pulsation, elevated sedimentation rate (50 mm or greater by the Westergren method), and positive temporal artery biopsy. The presence of three or more of these five criteria has a sensitivity of 93.5% and specificity of 91.2%.[116] In addition to these criteria, patients often have arthralgias and myalgias, fever, weight loss, anorexia, malaise, jaw claudication, leg claudication, and symptoms of polymyalgia rheumatica. Affected individuals have a median age in the 70s, with increasing prevalence with advancing age. The etiology is unknown. Laboratory findings usually include a markedly elevated sedimentation rate and C-reactive protein, elevated fibrinogen levels, anemia, elevated platelet count, and abnormal liver function. Temporal artery biopsy shows vessel occlusion and granulomatous inflammation in vessel walls and is generally considered the gold standard for diagnosis.

Ocular manifestations include ischemic optic neuropathy, amaurosis fugax, diplopia and ophthalmoplegia, and retinal vessel occlusion. Formed visual hallucinations have also been reported.[117] Anterior segment findings are infrequent. Scleritis has been reported.[118] Anterior segment ischemia with diffuse corneal edema, hypotony, and keratic precipitates has been reported, presumably secondary to inflammation involving the long posterior ciliary arteries.[119] Bilateral peripheral corneal ulceration without infiltration has been reported in a single case of temporal arteritis,[120] and we have recently treated a patient with biopsy-proven CGA that developed peripheral corneal ulceration while being tapered off oral prednisone (Fig. 93.9).

Treatment of giant cell arteritis is prompt initiation of systemic corticosteroids. Initial intravenous steroid therapy has been suggested to decrease the total dose needed.[121] Temporal artery biopsy can be carried out subsequently. Steroid sparing agents such as methotrexate, infliximab, and etanercept have been used in an attempt to reduce the required steroid dosage with some success, but further studies are needed to demonstrate their efficacy.[122] Methotrexate has been most extensively studied and is likely to be beneficial as an adjunctive therapy with steroid sparing effect.[123] Aspirin may help prevent stroke and vision loss.[123]

Conclusion

The collagenoses and vasculitides have many similar findings, especially in the eye. Patients with scleritis, sclerokeratitis, and peripheral keratitis require a systemic evaluation and appropriate laboratory studies to establish specific diagnoses in these potentially life-threatening disorders. Familiarity with these disorders and appropriate collaboration with internists and rheumatologists is essential.

References

1. Kotzin BL, West SG. Systemic lupus erythematosus. In: Rich RR, Fleisher TA, Shearer WT, Kotzin BL, Schroeder HW, eds. *Clinical immunology and practice*. 2nd ed. London: Mosby; 2001:60.1–60.24.
2. Hahn BH. Systemic lupus erythematosus. In: Isselbacher KJ, et al, eds. *Harrison's principles of internal medicine*. New York: McGraw-Hill; 1994.
3. Tan EM, et al. The 1982 revised criteria for the classification of systemic lupus erythematosus. *Arthritis Rheum*. 1982;25:1271.
4. Gold DH, Morris DA, Henkind P. Ocular findings in systemic lupus erythematosus. *Br J Ophthalmol*. 1972;56:800.
5. Jabs DA, et al. Severe retinal vaso-occlusive disease in systemic lupus erythematosus. *Arch Ophthalmol*. 1986;104:558.
6. Borruat F-X, et al. Complications neuro-ophthalmologiques du lupus erythemateux dissemine. *Klin Monatsbl Augenheilkd*. 1994;204:403.
7. Jabs DA, et al. Optic neuropathy in systemic lupus erythematosus. *Arch Ophthalmol*. 1986;104:564.
8. Davies JB, Rao PK. Ocular manifesstations of systemic lupus erythematosus. *Curr Opin Opthalmol*. 2008;19:512–518.
9. Huey C, et al. Discoid lupus erythematosus of the eyelids. *Ophthalmology*. 1983;90:1389.
10 Hochberg MC, et al. Systemic lupus erythematosus: a review of clinicolaboratory features and immunogenetic markers in 150 patients with emphasis on demographic subsets. *Medicine*. 1985;64:285.
11. Frith P, et al. External ocular findings in lupus erythematosus: a clinical and immunopathological study. *Br J Ophthalmol*. 1990;74:163.
12. Leahy AB, Connor TB, Gottsch JD. Chemosis as a presenting sign of systemic lupus erythematosus. *Arch Ophthalmol*. 1992;110:609.
13. Norden D, et al. Bilateral periorbital edema in systemic lupus erythematosus. *J Rheumatol*. 1993;20:2158.
14. Feinfeld RE, Hesse RJ, Rosenberg SA. Orbital inflammatory disease associated with systemic lupus erythematosus. *South Med J*. 1991;84: 98.
15. Foster CS. Immunosuppressive therapy for external ocular inflammatory disease. *Ophthalmology*. 1980;87:140.
16. Williamson J. Incidence of eye disease in cases of connective tissue disease. *Trans Ophthalmol Soc UK*. 1974;94:742.
17. Uy HS, Pineda R, Shore JW, et al. Hypertrophic discoid lupus erythematosus of the conjunctiva. *Am J Ophthalmol*. 1999;127:604.
18. Heiligenhaus A, Dutt JE, Foster CS. Histology and immunopathology of systemic lupus erythematosus affecting the conjunctiva. *Eye*. 1996;10:425.
19. Spaeth GL. Corneal staining in systemic lupus erythematosus. *N Engl J Med*. 1967;276:1168.
20. Soo MP, Chow SK, Tan CT, et al. The spectrum of ocular involvement in patients with systemic lupus erythematosus without ocular symptoms. *Lupus*. 2000;9:555.
21. Reeves JA. Keratopathy associated with systemic lupus erythematosus. *Arch Ophthalmol*. 1965;74:159.
22. Halmay O, Ludwig K. Bilateral band-shaped deep keratitis and iridocyclitis in systemic lupus erythematosus. *Br J Ophthalmol*. 1964;48: 558.
23. Messmer EM, Foster CS. Vasculitic peripheral ulcerative keratitis. *Surv Ophthalmol*. 1999;43:379.
24. Varga JH, Wolf TC. Bilateral transient keratoendotheliitis associated with systemic lupus erythematosus. *Ann Ophthalmol*. 1993;25:222.
25. ten Doesschate J. Corneal complications in lupus erythematosus discoides. *Ophthalmologica*. 1956;132:153.
26. Maffett MJ, et al. Sterile corneal ulceration after cataract extraction in patients with collagen vascular disease. *Cornea*. 1990;9:279.

27. Cua IY, Pepose JS. Late corneal scarring after photorefractive keratectomy concurrent with development of systemic lupus erythematosus. *J Refract Surg.* 2002;18:750.
28. Camous L, Melander C, Vallet M, et al. Complete remission of lupus nephritis with rituximab and steroids for induction and rituximab alone for maintenance therapy. *Am J Kidney Dis.* 2008;52:346–352.
29. Weiner A, et al. Hydroxychloroquine retinopathy. *Am J Ophthalmol.* 1991;112:528.
30. Marmor MF, Carr RF, Easterbrook M, Farjo A, Mieler WF. Recommendations on screening for chloroquine and hydroxychloroquine retinopathy. *Ophthalmology.* 2002;109:1377.
31. Chang WH, Katz BJ, Warner JE, et al. A novel method for screening the multifocal electroretinogram in patients using hydroxychloroquine. *Retina.* 2008;28:1478–1486.
32. Gilliland BC. Systemic sclerosis (scleroderma). In: Isselbacher KJ, et al, eds. *Harrison's principles of internal medicine.* New York: McGraw-Hill; 1994.
33. Seibold JR. Scleroderma. In: Kelley WN, et al, eds. *Textbook of rheumatology.* Philadelphia: Saunders; 1993.
34. Sturgess A. Recently characterised autoantibodies and their clinical significance. *Aust NZ J Med.* 1992;22:279.
35. Fritzler MJ, Kinsella TD, Garbutt E. The CREST syndrome: a distinct serologic entity with anticentromere antibodies. *Am J Med.* 1980;69:520.
36. Schwab IR, DiBartolomeo A, Farber M. Ocular changes in scleroderma. *Invest Ophthalmol Vis Sci.* 1986;27(Suppl):97.
37. West RH, Barnett AJ. Ocular involvement in scleroderma. *Br J Ophthalmol.* 1979;63:845.
38. Mancel E, et al. Conjunctival biopsy in scleroderma and primary Sjögren's syndrome. *Am J Ophthalmol.* 1993;115:792.
39. Osial TA, et al. Clinical and serologic study of Sjögren's syndrome in patients with progressive systemic sclerosis. *Arthritis Rheum.* 1983;26:500.
40. Janin A, et al. Histological criteria of Sjögren's syndrome in scleroderma. *Clin Exp Rheumatol.* 1989;7:167.
41. Kirkali PA, Kansu T, Sanac AS. Unilateral enophthalmos in systemic scleroderma. *J Clin Neuro-Ophthalmol.* 1991;11:43.
42. Ortiz JR, Newman NJ, Barrow DL. CREST-associated multiple intracranial aneurysms and bilateral optic neuropathies. *J Clin Neuro-Ophthalmol.* 1991;11:233.
43. Saari KM, Rudenberg HA, Laitinen O. Bilateral central retinal vein occlusion in a patient with scleroderma. *Ophthalmologica.* 1981;182:7.
44. Kraus A, et al. Defects of the retinal pigment epithelium in scleroderma. *Br J Rheumatol.* 1991;30:112.
45. Milenkovic S, Petrovic L, Risimic D, et al. Choroidal sclerosis in localized scleroderma (morphea en Plaque). *Ophthalmic Res.* 2008;40:101–104.
46. Horie K, et al. A case of peripheral corneal ulcer accompanied by progressive systemic sclerosis. *Acta Ophthalmol Soc Jpn.* 1992;96:922.
47. Coyle EF. Scleroderma of the cornea. *Br J Ophthalmol.* 1956;40:239.
48. Nannini C, West CP, Erwin PJ, Matteson EL. Effects of cyclophosphamide on pulmonary function in patients with scleroderma and interstitial lung disease: a systematic revew and meta-analysis of randomized controlled trials and observational prospective cohort studies. *Arthritis Res Ther.* 2008;10(5):R124.
49. Varga J. Systemic sclerosis: an update. *Bull NYU Hosp Jt Dis.* 2008;66:198–202.
50. De Clerck LS, et al. D-Penicillamine therapy and interstitial lung disease in scleroderma: a long-term follow-up study. *Arthritis Rheum.* 1987;30:643.
51. Bennett RM. Mixed connective tissue disease and other overlap syndromes. In: Kelley WN, et al, eds. *Textbook of rheumatology.* Philadelphia: Saunders; 1993.
52. Alarcon-Segovia D, Cardial MH. Comparison between three diagnostic criteria for mixed connective tissue disease: study of 593 patients. *J Rheumatol.* 1989;16:328.
53. Wortmann RL. Inflammatory diseases of muscle. In: Kelley WN, et al, eds. *Textbook of rheumatology.* Philadelphia: Saunders; 1993.
54. Liebman S, Cook C. Retinopathy in dermatomyositis. *Arch Ophthalmol.* 1965;74:704.
55. Venkatesh P, Bhaskar VM, Keshavamurthy R, Garg S. Proliferative vascular retinopathy in polymyositis and dermatomyositis with scleroderma (overlap syndrome). *Ocul Immunol Inflamm.* 2007;15:45–49.
56. Young TA, Al-Mayouf S, Feldman BM, Levin AV. Clinical assessment of conjunctival and episcleral vessel tortuousity in juvenile dermatomyositis. *J AAPOS.* 2002;6:238.
57. Dicken CH. Periorbital edema: an important physical finding in dermatomyositis. *Cutis.* 1991;48:116.
58. van Nouhuys CE, Sengers RCA. Bilateral avascular zones of the conjunctiva in a patient with juvenile dermatomyositis. *Am J Ophthalmol.* 1987;104:440.
59. Ringel SP, et al. Sjögren's syndrome and polymyositis or dermatomyositis. *Arch Neurol.* 1982;39:157.
60. Wiendl H. Idiopathic inflamatory myopathies: current and future therapeutic options. *Neurotherapeutics.* 2008;5:548–557.
61. McAdam LP, et al. Relapsing polychondritis: prospective study of 23 patients and review of the literature. *Medicine.* 1976;55:193.
62. Damiani JM, Levine HL. Relapsing polychondritis – report of ten cases. *Laryngoscope.* 1979;89:929.
63. Isaak BL, Liesegang TJ, Michet CJ. Ocular and systemic findings in relapsing polychondritis. *Ophthalmology.* 1986;93:681.
64. Michet CJ, et al. Relapsing polychondritis: survival and predictive role of early disease manifestations. *Ann Intern Med.* 1986;104:74.
65. Ebringer R, et al. Autoantibodies to cartilage and type II collagen in relapsing polychondritis and other rheumatic diseases. *Ann Rheum Dis.* 1981;40:473.
66. Tucker SM, Linberg JV, Doshi HM. Relapsing polychondritis, another cause for a 'salmon patch.' *Ann Ophthalmol.* 1993;25:389.
67. Hoang-Xuan T, Foster CS, Rice BA. Scleritis in relapsing polychondritis: response to therapy. *Ophthalmology.* 1990;97:892.
68. Yu EN, Jurkunas U, Rubin PAD, Baltatzis S, Foster CS. Obliterative micorangiopathy presenting as chronic conjunctivitis in a patient with relapsing polychondritis. *Cornea.* 2006;25:621–622.
69. Matas BR. Iridocyclitis associated with relapsing polychondritis. *Arch Ophthalmol.* 1970;84:474.
70. Matoba A, et al. Keratitis in relapsing polychondritis. *Ann Ophthalmol.* 1984;16:367.
71. Barth WF, Berson EL. Relapsing polychondritis, rheumatoid arthritis and blindness. *Am J Ophthalmol.* 1968;66:890.
72. Michelson JB, et al. Melting corneas with collapsing nose. *Surv Ophthalmol.* 1984;29:148.
73. Leavitt RY, et al. The American College of Rheumatology 1990 criteria for the classification of Wegener's granulomatosis. *Arthritis Rheum.* 1990;33:1101.
74. Levi M, Kodsi SR, Rubin SE, et al. Ocular involvement as the initial manifestation of Wegener's granumomatosis in children. *J AAPOS.* 2008;12:94–96.
75. Fauci AS, et al. Wegener's granulomatosis: prospective clinical and therapeutic experience with 85 patients for 21 years. *Ann Intern Med.* 1983;98:76.
76. Soukiasian SH, et al. Diagnostic value of antineutrophil cytoplasmic antibodies in scleritis associated with Wegener's granulomatosis. *Ophthalmology.* 1992;99:125.
77. Ramirez G, Khamashta MA, Hughes GRV. The ANCA test: its clinical relevance. *Ann Rheum Dis.* 1990;45:741.
78. Cohen Tervaert JW, et al. Association between active Wegener's granulomatosis and anticytoplasmic antibodies. *Arch Intern Med.* 1989;149:2461.
79. Specks U, et al. Anticytoplasmic autoantibodies in the diagnosis and follow-up of Wegener's granulomatosis. *Mayo Clin Proc.* 1989;64:28.
80. Reynolds I, John SL, Tullo AB, et al. Characterization of two corneal epithelium-derived antigens associated with vasculitis. *Invest Ophthalmol Vis Sci.* 1998;39:2594.
81. Reynolds I, Tullo AB, John SL, et al. Corneal epithelial-specific cytokeratin 3 is an autoantigen in Wegener's granulomatosis-associated peripheral ulcerative keratitis. *Invest Ophthalmol Vis Sci.* 1999;40:2147.
82. Lie JT. Illustrated histopathologic classification criteria for selected vasculitis syndromes. *Arthritis Rheum.* 1990;33:1074.
83. Harper SL, Letko E, Samson CM, et al. Wegener's granulomatosis: the relationship between ocular and systemic disease. *J Rheumatol.* 2001;28:1025.
84. Haynes BF, et al. The ocular manifestations of Wegener's granulomatosis: fifteen years experience and review of the literature. *Am J Med.* 1977;63:131.
85. Bullen CL, et al. Ocular complications of Wegener's granulomatosis. *Ophthalmology.* 1983;90:279.
86. Kalina PH, et al. Diagnostic value and limitations of orbital biopsy in Wegener's granulomatosis. *Ophthalmology.* 1992;99:120.
87. Hardwig PW, Bartley GW, Garrity JA. Surgical management of nasolacrimal duct obstruction in patients with Wegener's granulomatosis. *Ophthalmology.* 1992;99:133.
88. Stavrou P, et al. Ocular manifestations of classical and limited Wegener's granulomatosis. *Q J Med.* 1993;86:719.
89. Jordan DR, Addison DJ. Wegener's granulomatosis: eyelid and conjunctival manifestations as the presenting feature in two individuals. *Ophthalmology.* 1994;101:602.
90. Fortney AC, Chodosh J. Conjunctival ulceration in recurrent Wegener granulomatosis. *Cornea.* 2002;21:623.

91. Pakrou N, Selva D, Leibovitch I. Wegener's Granulomatosis: ophthalmic manifestations and management. *Semin Arthritis Rheum.* 2006;35:284–292.
92. Charles SJ, Meyer PAR, Watson PG. Diagnosis and management of systemic Wegener's granulomatosis presenting with anterior ocular inflammatory disease. *Br J Ophthalmol.* 1991;75:201.
93. Walton EW. Giant-cell granuloma of the respiratory tract (Wegener's granulomatosis). *Br Med J.* 1958;2:265.
94. Meyer PA, et al. 'Pulsed' immunosuppressive therapy in the treatment of immunologically induced corneal and scleral disease. *Eye.* 1987;1:487.
95. White ES, Lynch III JP. Pharmacological therapy for Wegener's granulomatosis. *Drugs.* 2006;66:1209–1228.
96. Kerr GS, et al. Limited prognostic value of changes in antineutrophil cytoplasmic antibody titer in patients with Wegener's granulomatosis. *Arthritis Rheum.* 1993;36:365.
97. Power WJ, et al. Disease response in patients with ocular manifestations of Wegener's granulomatosis. *Ophthalmology.* 1995;102:154.
98. Luxton G, Langham R, Caring for Australians with renal impairment. *Nephrology.* 2008;13:S17–S23.
99. Blum M, Andrassy K, Adler D, et al. Early experience with intravenous immunoglobulin treatment in Wegener's granulomatosis with ocular involovement. *Graefe's Arch Clin Exp Ophthalmol.* 1997;235:599.
100. Lightfoot RW, et al. The American College of Rheumatology 1990 criteria for the classification of polyarteritis nodosa. *Arthritis Rheum.* 1990;33:1088.
101. Trepo CG, et al. The role of circulating hepatitis B antigen/antibody immune complexes in the pathogenesis of vascular and hepatic manifestations in polyarteritis nodosa. *J Clin Pathol.* 1974;27:863.
102. Conn DL, Hunder GG, O'Duffy JD. Vasculitis and related disorders. In: Kelley WN, et al, eds. *Textbook of rheumatology.* Philadelphia: Saunders; 1993.
103. Wise GN. Ocular periarteritis nodosa. *Arch Ophthalmol.* 1952;48:1.
104. Morgan CM, et al. Retinal vasculitis in polyarteritis nodosa. *Retina.* 1986;6:205.
105. van Wien S, Merz EH. Exophthalmos secondary to periarteritis nodosa. *Am J Ophthalmol.* 1963;56:204.
106. Purcell JJ, Birkenkamp R, Tsai CC. Conjunctival lesions in periarteritis nodosa: a clinical and immunopathologic study. *Arch Ophthalmol.* 1984;102:736.
107. Moore JG, Sevel D. Corneo-scleral ulceration in periarteritis nodosa. *Br J Ophthalmol.* 1966;50:651.
108. Cogan DG. Corneoscleral lesions in periarteritis nodosa and Wegener's granulomatosis. *Trans Am Ophthalmol Soc.* 1955;53:321.
109. Akova YA, Jabbur NS, Foster CS. Ocular presentation of polyarteritis nodosa: clinical course and management with steroid and cytotoxic therapy. *Ophthalmology.* 1993;100:1775.
110. Masi A, et al. The American College of Rheumatology 1990 criteria for the classification of Churg-Strauss syndrome (allergic granulomatosis and angiitis). *Arthritis Rheum.* 1990;33:1094.
111. Dagi LR, Currie J. Branch retinal artery occlusion in the Churg-Strauss syndrome. *J Clin Neuro-Ophthalmol.* 1985;5:229.
112. Weinstein JM, et al. Churg-Strauss syndrome (allergic granulomatous angiitis): neuro-ophthalmic manifestations. *Arch Ophthalmol.* 1983;101:1217.
113. Meisler DM, et al. Conjunctival inflammation and amyloidosis in allergic granulomatosis and angiitis (Churg-Strauss syndrome). *Am J Ophthalmol.* 1981;91:216.
114. Shields CL, Shields JA, Rozanski TI. Conjunctival involvement in Churg-Strauss syndrome. *Am J Ophthalmol.* 1986;102:601.
115. Cury D, Breakey AS, Payne BF. Allergic granulomatous angiitis associated with uveoscleritis and papilledema. *Arch Ophthalmol.* 1956;55:261.
116. Hunder GG, et al. The American College of Rheumatology 1990 criteria for the classification of giant cell arteritis. *Arthritis Rheum.* 1990;33:1122.
117. Cullen JF, Coleiro JA. Ophthalmic complications of giant cell arteritis. *Surv Ophthalmol.* 1976;20:247.
118. Long RG, Friedmann AI, James DG. Scleritis and temporal arteritis. *Postgrad Med J.* 1976;52:689.
119. Zion VM, Goodside V. Anterior segment ischemia with ischemic optic neuropathy. *Surv Ophthalmol.* 1974;19:19.
120. Gerstle CC, Friedman AH. Marginal corneal ulceration (limbal guttering) as a presenting sign of temporal arteritis. *Ophthalmology.* 1980;87:1173.
121. Mazlumzadeh M, Hunder GG, Easley KA, etal. Treatment of giant cell arteritis using induction therapy with high-dose glucocorticoids: a double-blind, placebo-controlled, randomized prospective clinical trial. *Arthritis Rheum.* 2006;54:3310–3318.
122. Hall JK. Giant-cell arteritis. *Curr Opin Ophthalmol.* 2008;19:454–460.
123. Mahr AD, Jover JA, Spiera RF, et al. Adjunctive methotrexate for treatment of giant cell arteritis: an individual patient data meta-analysis. *Arthritis Rheum.* 2007;56:2789–2797.

Chapter 94

Phlyctenular Keratoconjunctivitis and Marginal Staphylococcal Keratitis

Gary Chung

Phlyctenular keratoconjunctivitis (PKC) and marginal staphylococcal keratitis are noninfectious inflammatory processes of the ocular surface. Although clinically distinct entities, these two conditions share a common pathophysiologic mechanism: an immune reaction to a microbial antigen. This immune reaction can lead to corneal and conjunctival nodules (PKC) or peripheral corneal infiltrates (marginal staphylococcal keratitis). Both conditions are usually self-limiting. However, diagnostic dilemmas can occur, and clinicians must be able to differentiate these entities from acute infections to avoid inappropriate treatment.

Phlyctenular Keratoconjunctivitis

Background and history

Phlyctenular keratoconjunctivitis, or phlyctenulosis, is thought to represent a bacterial allergy to a number of antigens, the most common being tuberculoprotein and staphylococcal antigen. The term phlyctenule is derived from the Greek word *phlyctena*, which means 'blister.' This was likely a reference to the appearance of a conjunctival or corneal nodule after undergoing necrosis and ulceration. The earliest description of phlyctenulosis is found in a textbook written by C. de St. Yves in 1722, according to Duke-Elder.[1]

Phlyctenular keratoconjunctivitis was classically described as a disease of sickly children in areas of endemic tuberculosis.[2] In the 1940s, Sorsby was the first to confirm the strong correlation when he reported that 85% of patients with PKC tested positive to the tuberculin skin test versus 15% in a control group in the same hospital.[3] Fritz et al.[4] and Philip et al.[5] later made similar observations in studies of impoverished Alaskan villages with high rates of tuberculosis, noting that the prevalence of PKC correlated directly with tuberculin skin sensitivity. There was also increased morbidity in children with PKC, who had greater odds of developing clinical tuberculosis.[5,5a]

Etiology and epidemiology

Following the eradication of tuberculosis in developed countries, the overall incidence of PKC has declined dramatically. Even among patients who have active tuberculosis, PKC is now rare. In a recent study of 1005 patients with active systemic tuberculosis, there was only one case of phlyctenulosis.[6] *Staphylococcus* has emerged as the most common pathogen associated with this disorder. The association of PKC and *Staphylococcus* was actually reported as early as the 1950s by Thygeson[7] and then characterized further by Ostler and Lanier[8] who reported five patients with PKC and positive skin tests to *Staphylococcus* antigens. Other antigens have been implicated as well such as *Chlamydia*,[7,9] *Coccidioides*,[7] *Candida*,[7] herpes simplex virus,[10] and parasites.[11–13]

In early studies when tuberculosis was endemic,[3,5] PKC was described as a condition that occurred most often in the first two decades of life, with a peak incidence in the midteens, and rarely occurred before 5 years of age. A higher incidence in females was consistently reported. A peak incidence in the spring and summer has been reported.[3] A review of the more recent reports on PKC in the United States[8,9,14,15] still shows this to be a disease most commonly presenting in the teenage years with a preference towards females.

Pathogenesis

Phlyctenular keratoconjunctivitis is considered a hypersensitivity reaction to a specific antigen and thus requires (1) sensitization of the cornea or conjunctiva to a microbial antigen and (2) repeated exposure to that microbial antigen. Mondino and Kowalski[16] demonstrated this in an experimental model in which rabbits were immunized intradermally with staphylococcal cell wall antigens. After a topical ocular challenge with viable *S. aureus*, phlyctenules and catarrhal infiltrates developed in the immunized rabbits, but not in the nonimmunized rabbits.

In tuberculoprotein-induced PKC, the host becomes sensitized presumably from a bacteremia associated with a past pulmonary infection. An attack of PKC is then precipitated when tuberculous antigens are presented to the eye either from an endogenous source (via the bloodstream) or an exogenous source (external inoculation of the conjunctival sac).[17]

Several clinical observations support the concept of an *exogenous source* for tuberculous antigens. First, PKC seemed to be prevalent only in crowded communities with a high rate of tuberculosis, while it was rarely observed among infected persons who lived in areas with low tuberculosis infection rates. This led Philip et al.[5] to postulate that a 'highly contaminated environment' was necessary to provide the external inoculums needed to trigger attacks of PKC. Next, Thygeson routinely questioned all patients with PKC about family medical history and agreed that 'phlyctenulosis in a child is usually an indication that an active case of tuberculosis is present in his environment.'[7] Environments with heavy tuberculous contamination like those described above are infrequent today, which may explain the remarkably low rate of PKC among patients with active tuberculosis, as mentioned before.[6]

In staphylococcal-induced PKC, sensitization of the eye could occur via many routes since staphylococcal colonization of the skin and mucous membranes is common. Mondino et al.[18] showed that rabbits could be immunized with just topical application of viable *S. aureus* to the conjunctival sac. Therefore, it is conceivable that chronic staphylococcal colonization of the eyelids offers enough antigen for the host tissues to be sensitized. In this case, the same bacterial antigens will be lingering locally to trigger a hypersensitivity attack once the ocular tissue becomes adequately sensitized. These antigens are allowed to pass the corneal epithelial barrier, likely with the help of exotoxins that cause epithelial breakdown.[19]

Immunologically, the pathogenesis of PKC is presumed to be a cell-mediated type IV hypersensitivity reaction to microbial antigens. The histological findings in phlyctenule biopsies included a predominance of monocyte-derived cells (macrophages and dendritic Langerhans cells) with a moderate amount of T lymphocytes.[20] These findings are comparable to what is seen in the human skin tuberculin reaction, which is considered to be a classic example of delayed-type hypersensitivity. The inflammatory infiltrate is found just beneath the epithelium and also includes neutrophils which may be a response to necrosis that has occurred in these lesions. Aberrant HLA-DR4 antigen expression was present in the basal epithelium of the phlyctenule, and similar aberrant expression has been seen by keratinocytes in the tuberculin reaction.[20] No microorganisms have been found in phlyctenule samples.

Clinical features

Classic descriptions of children with phlyctenules by Duke-Elder are of a child who 'hides away in a dark corner, burying his face in his hands.'[1] Beauchamp et al.[14] reported two cases in which the children were suspected of having psychiatric disorders presumably due to the social awkwardness that a chronically photophobic child exudes. Recognizing and appropriately handling these cases when they do occur can have a significant impact on the lives of such children and their families.

In general, the severity of the symptoms depends on the location of the phlyctenule. In a conjunctival lesion, the symptoms are mild. Tearing, foreign body sensation, and some itching are common. Corneal lesions cause the same symptoms but with more intensity and are also characterized by significant photophobia. Staphylococcal-related

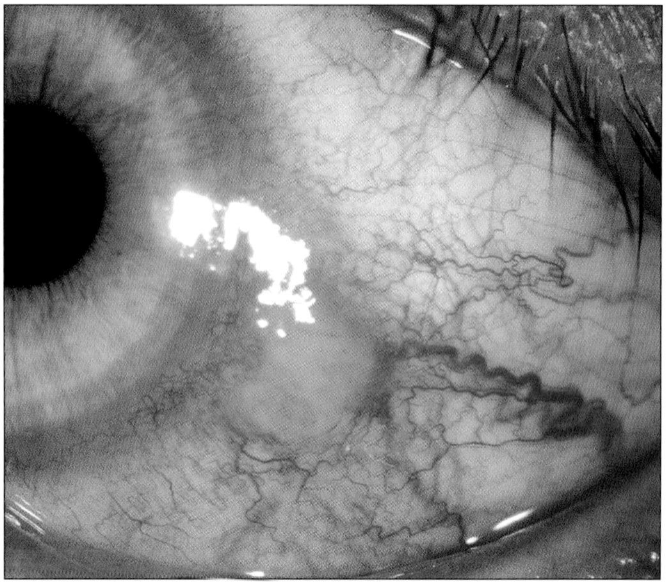

Fig. 94.1 Conjunctival phlyctenule. Phlyctenulosis is a type IV hypersensitivity reaction associated with a response to some antigen. It has been shown to occur in the presence of many organisms. The lesions start as elevated areas of conjunctiva and can ulcerate and eventually heal over 2 weeks.

phlyctenules may cause less photophobia than the classic descriptions of tuberculous phlyctenules.[8]

Conjunctival phlyctenules occur most commonly near the limbus, but can occur anywhere on the bulbar conjunctiva. Lesions rarely occur on the palpebral conjunctiva. Classically, conjunctival phlyctenules occur at the limbus and appear as a pink fleshy nodule standing out in the background of surrounding conjunctival injection (Fig. 94.1). They are usually 1–2 mm in diameter, but can vary in size from a pinpoint lesion to several millimeters in diameter. After a few days, the central, superficial portion usually turns yellow or gray and becomes soft. This central portion sloughs off, creating an ulcer, which then reepithelializes. This cycle of infiltration, ulceration, and resolution usually takes 1 to 2 weeks to complete. Some phlyctenules resolve prior to ulcerating. After resolution, no conjunctival scarring is seen.

Corneal phlyctenules typically appear at the limbus as a small white nodule with adjacent intense conjunctival injection (Fig. 94.2). These phlyctenules often undergo necrosis, forming a marginal ulcer. The ulcer resolves, resulting in anterior stromal scarring, typically triangular in shape with the base of the triangle at the limbus. Superficial corneal neovascularization (pannus) can also develop. The pannus formation can be fascicular or broader, as seen in trachoma. Unlike trachoma, a broad pannus in PKC typically is inferiorly located and has an irregular border.[4,14] Subsequent corneal phlyctenules can arise at the central edge of a pannus from prior attacks. This can happen multiple times such that the phlyctenule can appear to 'wander' across the cornea (Fig. 94.3).

There are other less common corneal manifestations of PKC. Multiple small phlyctenular lesions may be distributed diffusely over the entire corneal surface (i.e. miliary

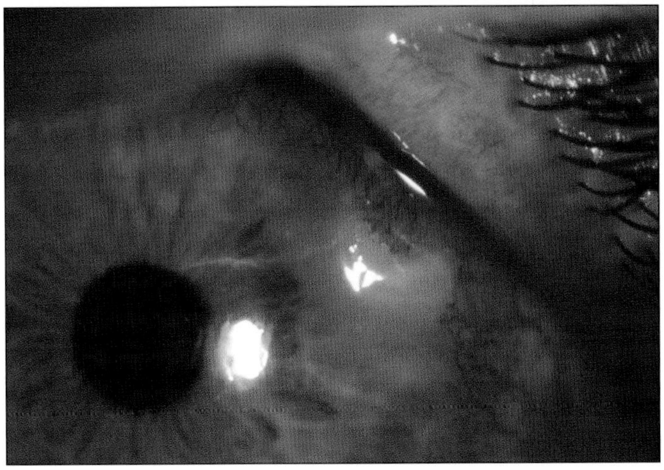

Fig. 94.2 Corneal phlyctenule. More severe symptoms are associated with corneal disease, and sequelae such as scarring are more common. It is important to differentiate this lesion from an infectious process.

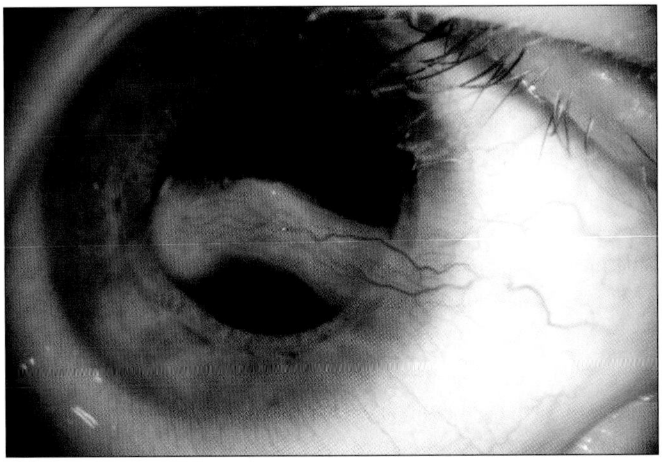

Fig. 94.3 Corneal phlyctenule. These lesions can spread across the cornea, bringing a band of vascularization and scarring.

phlyctenulosis).[4] Corneal perforation secondary to phlyctenulosis is uncommon but can occur.[8,9,14]

Differential diagnosis

During the nodular stage, the phlyctenular lesions may resemble Salzmann's corneal nodules, limbal papillae in vernal keratoconjunctivitis, inflamed pinguecula, and nodular episcleritis. Unlike phlyctenular patients, Salzmann's corneal nodules are typically not inflamed and are not as rapidly progressive. In vernal keratoconjunctivitis, the findings are usually bilateral and distinguishing features include marked itching, thick ropy mucoid discharge, more diffuse limbal hypertrophy, and cobblestone-like conjunctival papillae. Inflamed pinguecula do not ulcerate or migrate quickly onto the cornea, and they are characteristically located at the 3 or 9 o'clock position. Lesions in nodular episcleritis can be differentiated from phlyctenulosis, since the former do not migrate or ulcerate.

During the ulcerative stages, corneal phlyctenular lesions may resemble infectious corneal ulcers, herpes simplex virus (HSV) keratitis, catarrhal ulcers, and ulcers associated with collagen vascular diseases. Catarrhal ulcers have a clear intervening space between the lesion and the limbus. Further, the long axis of the marginal infiltrate is parallel to the circumference of the cornea, whereas the long axis of ulcerated phlyctenule is frequently perpendicular to it.[17] The other lesions will be discussed in the differential diagnosis of marginal staphylococcal keratitis.

In the healing stages, phlyctenulosis can resemble trachoma, luetic keratitis, and rosacea. Trachoma is characterized by Herbert's pits, tarsal conjunctival scarring (Arlt's line), and a superior pannus with a uniform leading edge. PKC can also present as a broad pannus but it is often inferiorly located with an irregular border.[4,14] The differentiation from trachoma is complicated by the fact that *Chlamydia* infection has been associated with PKC.[7,9] Luetic keratitis involves the deeper cornea with ghost vessels and there may be evidence of past iritis (i.e. synechiae). Differentiating PKC from corneal findings in acne rosacea may be challenging. In acne rosacea, inferior diffuse superficial vascularization with punctate epithelial erosions or infiltrates may resemble PKC. Further, facial pustules and telangiectasias have been reported in children with PKC.[9,15] However, rosacea is a disease that affects adults (typically 30–40 years old) and prolonged remission after oral antibiotics does not occur, as can be seen in PKC.[9,15]

Careful evaluation during treatment also confirms the diagnosis. Phlyctenular ulcers usually resolve rapidly with topical corticosteroid therapy alone, whereas topical steroid therapy may worsen the course of infectious corneal ulcers.

Diagnostic evaluation

A deliberate history and examination should be performed, bearing in mind the known organisms implicated in PKC (see previous section). Diagnostic testing should be considered if there is suspicion of a past or present microbial infection. A history of travel to endemic areas for tuberculosis or unexplained pulmonary symptoms should warrant skin testing and a chest radiograph. If positive, household members should be tested for tuberculosis as well. Testing for *Chlamydia* may be indicated in young adults with a history of sexual risk factors or with suspicious examination findings. Culbertson et al. actually had a 50% (5 of 10 patients) positivity rate for *Chlamydia* testing in his series of patients with PKC.[9] In cases where an infectious ulcer is suspected, corneal scrapings and cultures should be obtained.

Treatment

The short-term treatment goal for phlyctenular keratoconjunctivitis is to reduce the active inflammatory response with topical corticosteroids. Prednisolone acetate 1% given six times daily can be used as a starting dose. Tapering may begin within the first week and should be based on the clinical response. Nontuberculosis-related phlyctenules have been noted to be less responsive to topical corticosteroids and may have a more protracted course.[3,8] A topical antibiotic is recommended before corticosteroid use if a corneal lesion has an overlying epithelial defect, whereas conjunctival lesions can be treated right away with corticosteroids. A cycloplegic agent and dark sunglasses may be helpful in photophobic patients.

The long-term treatment goal for PKC is to eliminate recurrences by reducing the antigenic load to the ocular surface. In the rare case of tuberculoprotein-induced PKC, treatment of the primary infection should occur to prevent future clinical tuberculosis and to reduce potential sources of endogenous antigen. Treating household members who are tuberculin positive will eliminate potential sources of exogenous antigen. In most cases, PKC will be triggered by staphylococcal bacterial antigens in sensitized individuals. Minimizing staphylococcal colonization of the lid margins involves removal of bacteria with lid scrubs and the use of topical antibiotic ointments.

Oral tetracycline has been shown to be an effective adjunctive treatment in difficult cases of PKC. Studies by Zaidman and Brown[15] and Culbertson et al.[9] showed rapid relief and halting of the disease progression with oral tetracycline in cases of recurrent or resistant nontuberculous PKC. Based on the positive and sometimes lasting results achieved in patients, oral tetracycline can be taken for refractory cases at a dose of 250 mg three times a day until 3 weeks after the patient is completely asymptomatic. The dosage is then decreased by 250 mg a day every 3 to 4 weeks until the patient is using tetracycline once a day.[15]

Tetracycline may deposit in developing teeth, causing discoloration, and therefore is contraindicated for patients under the age of 8, pregnant women, or nursing mothers. Erythromycin is an alternative in these cases.

In patients with significant scarring, penetrating keratoplasty has been performed with good results.[21]

Staphylococcal Marginal Keratitis

Background

Staphylococcal marginal keratitis, also referred to as catarrhal infiltrates or ulcers, is a peripheral corneal disorder characterized by inflammatory infiltration that may lead to ulceration. It is likely the most common disorder of the peripheral cornea. Thygeson[22] first reported the frequent association of catarrhal infiltrates with chronic conjunctivitis due to *Staphylococcus*. These peripheral ulcers differed from central ulcers in their relatively benign course and the lack of bacteria found in corneal scrapings. Accordingly, these lesions are thought to represent an antibody response to toxins rather than direct bacterial invasion.

Pathogenesis

Similar to phlyctenulosis, bacterial antigens from chronic staphylococcal colonization of the eyelids are thought to trigger an immune response in a sensitized cornea. The immune response is most likely a type III hypersensitivity reaction resulting in immune complex deposition in the peripheral cornea.[23] These complexes activate the complement pathway, attracting neutrophils to the site forming an opacity (catarrhal infiltrate). In support of this theory, immunoglobins and C3 complement have been demonstrated in marginal infiltrates.[17] Further, Gram and Giemsa staining of corneal scrapings show neutrophils but no organisms.

The size of immune complexes is dependent upon the ratio of antigen to antibodies present locally. The circular zone of the cornea that is 2 mm from the limbus may have an antigen-to-antibody ratio that is conducive to the larger, more inflammagenic immune complexes (a zone of optimal proportions).[23] Further, antibody and antigen complexes would activate the classic complement pathway most vigorously in the peripheral cornea, since there is much more complement component C1 in the peripheral cornea versus the central cornea.[17]

Catarrhal infiltrates are associated with staphylococcal blepharoconjunctivitis in an overwhelming majority of cases. Colonization is common, as positive lid cultures for *S. aureus* have been seen in up to 90% of normal patients,[24] with high colonization rates usually occurring in warmer climates.[19] Other associations such as acute β-hemolytic streptococcal conjunctivitis and chronic dacryocystitis have been reported.[25] Other bacteria that have been isolated in patients with catarrhal infiltrates include *Moraxella*, *Haemophilus*, and other streptococcal species.[22]

Clinical features

Patients with staphylococcal marginal keratitis usually present with pain, photophobia, foreign body sensation, and conjunctival injection. The symptoms are typically mild to moderate and are not specific.

Staphylococcal marginal keratitis begins with one or more localized peripheral stromal infiltrates, which tend to occur in locations where the lid margin crosses the limbus (i.e. 2, 4, 8, 10 o'clock positions). Classically, these lesions are parallel to the limbus and separated from the limbus by 1–2 mm of clear cornea (Fig. 94.4A). The infiltrates are usually round but can coalesce into broader lesions (Fig 94.4B). With prolonged inflammation, the corneal epithelium overlying the stromal infiltrates can break down, leading to ulceration (Fig. 94.5). Blood vessels may bridge this area once necrosis occurs. The natural course of the disease is spontaneous resolution in 2 to 3 weeks with few long-term sequelae. Recurrences are common, especially if an associated blepharitis is left untreated.

Staphylococcal blepharitis has distinctive features which include hard, brittle, fibrinous scales (squamous type) and matted crusts on the lid margin that can leave an ulcer when removed (ulcerative type). Other signs include dilated blood vessels on the lid margins, white lashes, lash loss, trichiasis, and collarettes.[26]

Differential diagnosis

Staphylococcal marginal keratitis begins with an infiltrate that has an intact epithelium but may ulcerate with prolonged inflammation. In cases with ulceration, staphylococcal marginal keratitis may resemble infectious corneal ulcers. Infectious ulcers are usually more painful, more central in location, and have a modest anterior chamber reaction.

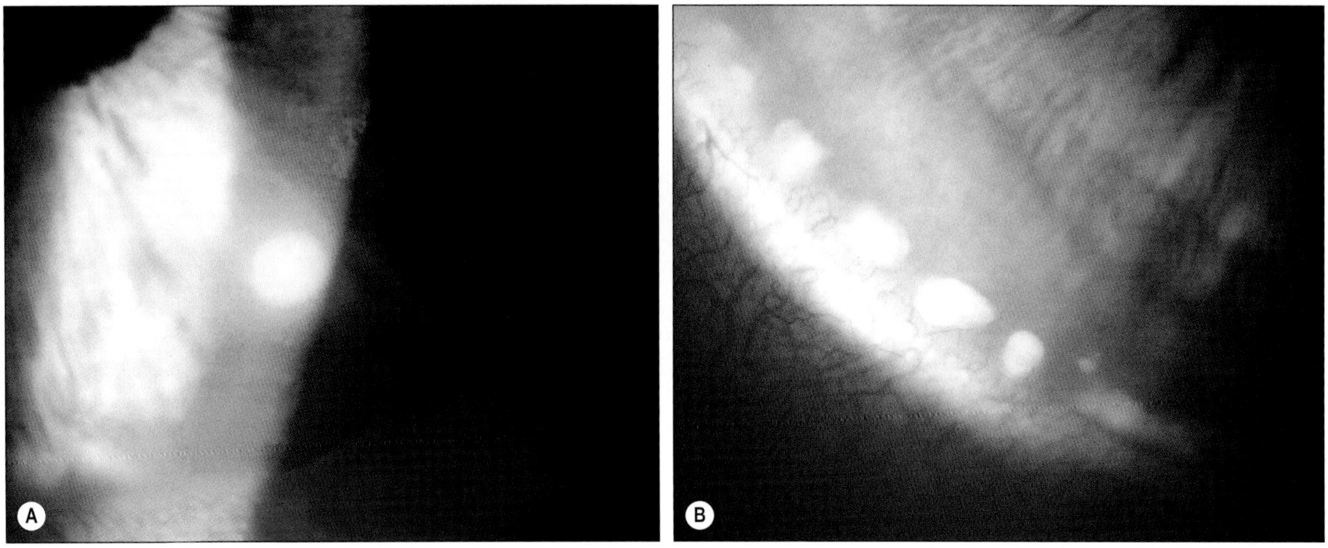

Fig. 94.4 Staphylococcal marginal keratitis. (**A**) These infiltrates are hypersensitivity reactions to staphylococcal antigen usually associated with blepharitis. There is a clear 'lucid' interval between the infiltrate and the limbus. These lesions respond well to topical corticosteroids. (**B**) Multiple marginal infiltrates near the limbus. Some of these may coalesce into broader lesions.

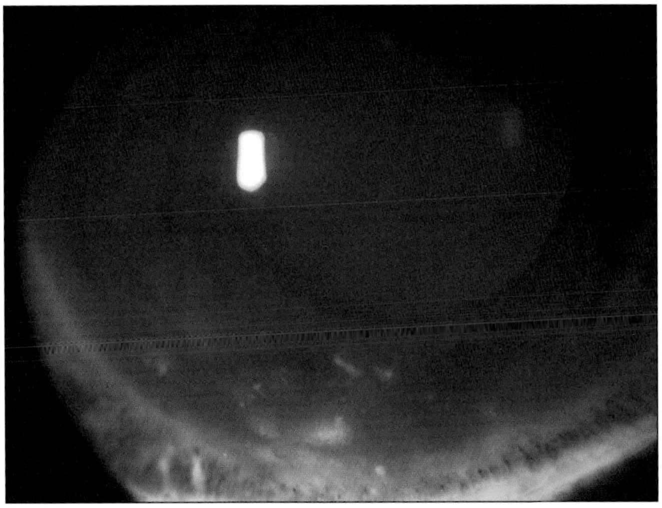

Fig. 94.5 Staphylococcal marginal keratitis. Fluorescein examination reveals overlying epithelial defects. These lesions can be confused with infectious keratitis, and microbial evaluation may be indicated.

Herpes simplex virus keratitis with both epithelial and stromal involvement can be difficult to distinguish from marginal staphylococcal keratitis. One important difference is the evolution of the lesions: HSV infection begins with an epithelial defect followed by an infiltrate, which is the reverse order in staphylococcal marginal keratitis. Dendritic or geographic epithelial lesions and profound corneal hypoesthesia are other distinguishing features of herpes simplex keratitis.

An ulcerated staphylococcal marginal infiltrate may be difficult to distinguish from peripheral ulcerative keratitis caused by collagen vascular diseases (e.g. rheumatoid arthritis). If there is suspicion for the latter, the natural progression and/or response to treatment may ultimately reveal the diagnosis. If observed, staphylococcal marginal keratitis tends to have a benign course, whereas the course of collagen vascular-associated ulcers tends to be more severe and progressive. If treated, staphylococcal marginal keratitis responds rapidly to topical corticosteroids, whereas patients with peripheral corneal ulcers related to collagen-vascular disease often need systemic immunosuppression to control inflammation and may worsen on topical corticosteroids.

Diagnostic evaluation

The diagnosis of staphylococcal marginal keratitis is usually made based on clinical findings. In cases where there is an overlying epithelial defect, exclusion of infectious processes is important. If the clinical diagnosis of staphylococcal marginal keratitis is equivocal, we recommend corneal scrapings for culture, particularly in situations with an associated epithelial defect and a significant anterior chamber reaction. Microbial evaluation is also recommended if clinical improvement is not observed or if the infiltrates progress despite therapy.

Treatment

Similar to the treatment paradigm of phlyctenulosis, the treatment of staphylococcal marginal keratitis involves suppressing the acute immune response and reducing the stimulus for future attacks (bacterial antigens). Topical corticosteroids (i.e. fluorometholone, loteprednol, and prednisolone acetate) are the mainstay in the treatment of acute marginal staphylococcal infiltrates. In cases of corneal stromal infiltrates without epithelial breakdown, topical corticosteroids may be used immediately. In cases with epithelial breakdown and stromal ulceration, a broad-spectrum topical antibiotic should be used briefly prior to starting topical corticosteroids.

Eyelid hygiene is used to remove bacteria from the lashes and lid margins, while antibiotic ointments are used to limit bacterial colonization. Systemic antibiotics (i.e. tetracycline, doxycycline, erythromycin) may be indicated when the disease is recurrent or if there is significant meibomian gland disease. Recently, a topical form of azithromycin has become commercially available that is applied to the eyelid and may provide broad-spectrum antibioisis with once-daily dosing.

Acknowledgments

The author and editors would like to recognize the work of Reza M. Mozayeni and Sheridan Lam for their contributions from the original chapter.

References

1. Duke-Elder S. *System of ophthalmology*. St Louis: Mosby; 1965.
2. Gibson SW. The etiology of phlyctenular conjunctivitis. *Am J Dis Child.* 1917;15(2):81–115.
3. Sorsby A. The etiology of phlyctenular ophthalmia. *Br J Ophthalmol.* 1942;159:189.
4. Fritz MN, Thygeson P, Durham DG. Phlyctenular keratoconjunctivitis among Alaska natives. *Am J Ophthalmol* 1951;34:177–184.
5. Philip RN, Comstock GW, Shelton JH. Phlyctenular keratoconjunctivitis among Eskimos in southwestern Alaska. *Am Rev Respir Dis.* 1965;91(2): 171–187.
5a. Thygeson P. The etiology and treatment of phlyctenular keratoconjunctivitis. *Am J Ophthalmol.* 1951;34(9):1217–1236.
6. Biswas J, Badrinath SS. Ocular morbidity in patients with active systemic tuberculosis. *Int Ophthalmol.* 1995–1996;19(5):293–298.
7. Thygeson P. Observations on nontuberculous phlyctenular keratoconjunctivitis. *Trans Am Acad Ophthalmol Otolaryngol.* 1954;58:128–132.
8. Ostler HB, Lanier JD. Phlyctenular keratoconjunctivitis with special reference to the staphylococcal type. *Trans Pac Coast Oto-Ophthalmol Soc Annu Meet.* 1974;55:237–252.
9. Culbertson WW, et al. Effective treatment of phlyctenular keratoconjunctivitis with oral tetracycline. *Ophthalmology.* 1993;100:1358–1366.
10. Holland EJ, et al. Ocular involvement in an outbreak of herpes gladiatorum. *Am J Ophthalmol.* 1992;114:680–684.
11. Jeffery MP. Ocular diseases caused by nematodes. *Am J Ophthalmol.* 1955;40:41.
12. Hussein AA, Nasr ME. The role of parasitic infection in the etiology of phlyctenular eye disease. *J Egypt Soc Parasitol.* 1991;21:865–868.
13. Ghosh JB. Phlyctenular conjunctivitis in kala-azar (letter). *Indian Pediatr.* 1991;28:1531.
14. Beauchamp GR, Gillette TE, Friendly DS. Phlyctenular keratoconjunctivitis. *J Pediatr Ophthalmol Strabismus.* 1981;18:22–28.
15. Zaidman GW, Brown SI. Orally administered tetracycline for phlyctenular keratoconjunctivitis. *Am J Ophthalmol.* 1981;92:178–182.
16. Mondino BJ, Kowalski RP. Phlyctenulae and catarrhal infiltrates. Occurrence in rabbits immunized with staphylococcal cell walls. *Arch Ophthalmol.* 1982;100:1968–1971.
17. Mondino BJ. Inflammatory disease of the peripheral cornea. *Ophthalmology.* 1988;95:463–472.
18. Mondino BJ, Brawman-Mintzer O, Adamu SA. Corneal antibody levels to ribitol teichoic acid in rabbits immunized with staphylococcal antigens using various routes. *Invest Ophthalmol Vis Sci.* 1987;28: 1533–1558.
19. Smolin G, Okumoto M. Staphylococcal blepharitis. *Arch Ophthalmol.* 1977;95(5):812–816.
20. Abu el-Asrar AM, et al. Phenotypic characteristics of inflammatory cells in phlyctenular eye disease. *Doc Ophthalmol.* 1989;70:353–362.
21. Smith RE, Dippe DW, Miller SD. Phlyctenular keratoconjunctivitis: results of penetrating keratoplasty in Alaskan native. *Ophthalmic Surg.* 1975;6:62–66.
22. Thygeson P. Marginal corneal infiltrates and ulcers. *Trans Am Acad Ophthalmol Otolaryngol.* 1946;51:198–209.
23. Smolin G. Hypersensitivity reactions. In: Smolin G, ed. *Ocular immunology*. 2nd ed. Boston: Little, Brown; 1986.
24. Tomar VPS, Sharma OP, Joski K. Bacterial and fungal flora of normal conjunctiva. *Ann Ophthalmol.* 1971;3:669.
25. Cohn H, et al. Marginal corneal ulcers with acute beta streptococcal conjunctivitis and chronic dacryocystitis. *Am J Ophthalmol.* 1979;87: 541–543.
26. McCulley JP, Dougherty JM, Deneau DG. Classification of chronic blepharitis. *Ophthalmology.* 1982;89:1173.
27. Abelson MB, et al. Clinical cure of bacterial conjunctivitis with azithromycin 1%: vehicle-controlled, double-masked clinical trial. *Am J Ophthalmol.* 2008;145:959–965.

Chapter **95**

Mooren's Ulcer

Prashant Garg, Virender S. Sangwan

Introduction

Mooren's ulcer is a painful, progressive, chronic ulcerative keratitis that begins peripherally and progresses circumferentially and centrally. It is an idiopathic disease occurring in complete absence of any diagnosable systemic disorder that could be responsible for the progressive destruction of the cornea. The disease is strictly a peripheral ulcerative keratitis (PUK), with no associated scleritis. Bowman published the first report of Mooren's ulcer in 1849. Later, in 1854, McKenzie described it as 'chronic serpiginous ulcer of the cornea or *ulcus roden*.'[1] The disorder was named as Mooren's ulcer after Dr Mooren, who was the first to clearly describe this insidious corneal problem and define it as a clinical entity in 1863 and 1867.[2] In 1902, Nettleship et al. published a review of 67 previously published cases and 11 new cases from their experience.[3] Subsequently, a large number of reports have been published describing the etiology, pathogenesis, clinical presentations, and treatment outcome.

Epidemiology

Wood and Kaufman described two clinical types of Mooren's ulcer.[4] The first, limited type, is usually unilateral, with mild to moderate symptoms, and generally responds well to medical and surgical treatment. This type is believed to occur in older patients and is known as typical or benign Mooren's ulcer. The second type is bilateral although both eyes may not be affected simultaneously, with relatively more pain and generally a poor response to therapy. The bilateral variety primarily occurs in younger patients and is known as atypical or malignant Mooren's ulcer. This variety of the ulcer progresses relentlessly and is more likely to result in corneal perforation. It is also believed that the atypical Mooren's ulcer has a predilection for young black males.[5] However, in 1990, Lewallen and Courtright, in their review of the published series of Mooren's ulcer, found that 43% of older patients had bilateral disease, whereas bilateral disease was present in only one-third of patients younger than 35 years.[6] Also, more whites were affected with bilateral disease than blacks. They concluded that the current understanding of the epidemiology of Mooren's ulcer might be flawed because of inconsistent definition of the disease, poor documentation and follow-up, and problems inherent in non-population-based data collection.

Watson, based on clinical presentation and anterior segment fluorescein angiographic findings, divided Mooren's ulcer into three distinct varieties.[7] *Unilateral Mooren's ulceration* is a painful progressive corneal ulceration in elderly patients and is associated with nonperfusion of the superficial vascular plexus of the anterior segment. *Bilateral aggressive Mooren's ulceration*, which occurs in young patients, progresses circumferentially, then centrally in the cornea. There is vascular leakage and new vessel formation, extending into the base of the ulcer. *Bilateral indolent Mooren's ulceration* usually occurs in middle-aged patients presenting with progressive peripheral corneal guttering in both eyes, with little inflammatory response. There is no change from normal vascular architecture except an extension of new vessels into the ulcer.

Mooren's ulcer can occur in all age groups, but the vast majority of them present between 40 and 70 years. The disease can occur in either sex, but men outnumber women. Unilateral involvement is more common overall, and the majority of affected eyes have partial peripheral corneal ulceration. The interpalpabral limbus is involved most often, followed by the inferior and then the superior limbus.[8,9]

Etiology

Mooren's ulcer has been associated with different entities, often leading to the conjecture that there may be a causal relationship. Multiple studies including collaborative studies have reported association between Mooren's ulcer and hepatitis C infection.[10–12] Many of these patients responded to interferon therapy.[13,14] Infectious associations have been reported with hookworm infestation.[15–18] These authors proposed that molecular mimicry might be involved, with the infecting agent stimulating an autoimmune response to corneal antigens through cross-reacting epitopes. Alternatively, they also proposed that deposition of immune complexes in limbal or peripheral corneal tissues led to an immune response and release of proteolytic enzymes.

Pathogenesis

The pathogenesis of Mooren's ulcer remains uncertain. Mooren's ulcer has the characteristics of an autoimmune process, and various authors have documented autoimmune phenomena, both in the eye and systemically, in patients suffering from this disorder.

The cellular population found in the conjunctiva adjacent to the ulcer and in the peripheral edge of the ulcer is primarily plasma cells, lymphocytes, and macrophages.[19–21] In addition, there are neutrophils, eosinophils, and mast cells. There is increased binding of IgG, IgM, and C3 to the epithelium of conjunctiva adjacent to the ulcer.[19] Kafkala et al., in a recent publication, demonstrated upregulation of various adhesion and co-stimulatory molecules in epithelial cells in the conjunctiva of Mooren's ulcer patients.[22] In this study, the ratio of CD4/CD8 cells and B7-2/antigen-presenting cells were significantly higher in Mooren's ulcer specimen. Systemically, Mooren's ulcer patients have a decrease in number of suppressor T cells relative to number of helper T cells, elevated IgA levels, and circulating IgG antibodies and immune complexes to human corneal and conjunctival epithelium.[19,23] Gottsch and colleagues demonstrated antibodies to an autoantigen that exists in corneal stroma.[24] The antigen, known as 'cornea-associated antigen', has an amino acid sequence identical to that of calgranulin C of neutrophils. The human leukocyte antigen (HLA) system is a critical component for immune recognition and various studies have identified association between HLA-DR17 and the occurrence of Mooren's ulcer.[25,26] All this evidence supports an autoimmune basis for the disease.

Mooren's ulcer may represent a final common pathway to a variety of insults to the cornea in susceptible patients. Trauma or infection may alter normal corneal antigens, which may lead to an autoimmune response. Altered antigen is taken up by macrophages that move through the conjunctival vessels to the peripheral lymph nodes, eventually resulting in T-cell activation, differentiation, and proliferation. The lymphocytes return to the conjunctival vessels and cause ocular inflammation. The corneal edema from inflammation allows easier diffusion of immune components into pericentral and central cornea from the limbal vessels, which may explain why Mooren's ulcers typically begin in the periphery. The cornea is thus damaged, liberating more altered corneal antigens that aggravate and perpetuate the process until the corneal stroma is completely destroyed.

Clinical Features

Symptoms

Patients with Mooren's ulcer usually complain of redness, tearing, and photophobia, but pain is typically the outstanding feature. The pain often is incapacitating and may well be out of proportion to the inflammation. There may also be a complaint of decreased visual acuity, which may be secondary to associated iritis, central corneal involvement, or irregular astigmatism due to peripheral corneal thinning.

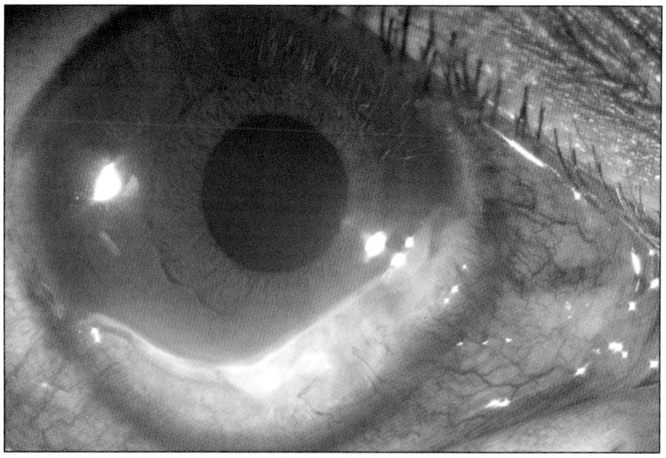

Fig. 95.1 An early Mooren's ulcer characterized by a crescent-shaped peripheral ulcer concentric to limbus; the leading edges are undermined and infiltrated.

Signs

Typically, Mooren's ulcer begins as a crescent-shaped gray-white infiltrate in the peripheral cornea. Epithelial breakdown and stromal melting follow this. Eventually it develops into a characteristic chronic crescent-shaped peripheral ulcer. The ulcer is concentric to limbus; the leading edges are undermined, infiltrated, and deepithelialized. The ulcer progresses circumferentially and centrally. As it progresses, it creates an overhanging edge at its central border (Fig. 95.1). Though the ulcer may begin as a shallow furrow in the peripheral cornea, over time it may involve the limbus. The adjacent conjunctiva and sclera are usually inflamed and hyperemic.

As the disease progresses, the ulcer spreads in three directions: peripherally, centrally, and rarely into sclera. Behind the advancing edge of the ulcer, healing may take place. This healing is in the form of corneal epithelialization and vascularization. Associated with this is scarring and thinning. The healed area remains clouded. In an advanced case of Mooren's ulcer most of the cornea is lost, leaving behind a central island surrounded by area of grossly thinned, scarred, and vascularized tissue (Fig. 95.2). Although the disease is characterized by progressive thinning, corneal perforation is uncommon and is more common in eyes with peripheral as compared to total ulceration.[8,9] Iritis sometimes is associated with Mooren's ulcer. Hypopyon is rare unless secondary infection is present. Glaucoma and cataract may complicate the process.

Differential Diagnosis

Although Mooren's ulcer has a characteristic clinical picture, several other diseases can present with peripheral keratitis and ulceration. The differential diagnosis of Mooren's ulcer includes other inflammatory and noninflammatory causes of peripheral thinning and ulceration (Table 95.1).

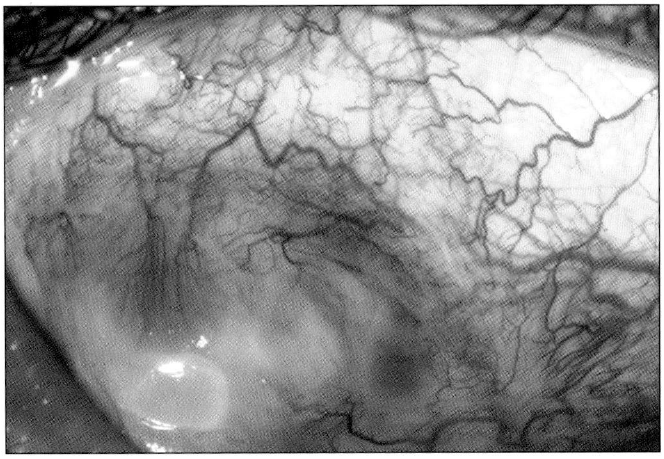

Fig. 95.2 Advanced Mooren's ulcer characterized by gross destruction of cornea, leaving behind a central island of tissue.

Table 95.1 Differential diagnosis of Mooren's ulcer

Ocular
Terrien's marginal degeneration
Pellucid marginal degeneration
Idiopathic furrow degeneration
Staphylococcal marginal keratitis
Rosacea keratitis
Exposure keratitis
Systemic
Tuberculosis
Syphilis
Varicella-zoster
Sarcoidosis
Collagen vascular diseases
Rheumatoid arthritis
Wegener's granulomatosis
Polyarteritis nodosa
Systemic lupus erythematosus
Relapsing polychondritis

Diagnosis

As previously stated, Mooren's ulcer is idiopathic, and the characteristic features must occur in the absence of any systemic process that may cause PUK. Thus, it is a diagnosis of exclusion. To make the distinction between all the diseases, all patients presenting with peripheral keratitis and ulceration must undergo a detailed history with specific attention to history of systemic illness, and a complete ocular and systemic examination. A careful review of systems can often narrow the differential to a limited number of entities. The laboratory studies should include complete and differential blood cell counts, platelet counts, erythrocyte sedimentation rate, rheumatoid factor, antinuclear antibody, antineutrophil cytoplasmic antibodies, chest X-ray examination, liver enzymes, and fluorescent treponemal antibody absorption test. Additional testing is done as indicated by the review of systems and physical examination. Infectious etiologies should be excluded by appropriate cultures, because microbial keratitis can rapidly progress and is usually amenable to antibiotic therapy.

Treatment

The goals of treatment in Mooren's ulcer are to stop the ulcerative process and allow reepithelialization of the cornea. A wide variety of medical and surgical approaches have been advocated over the years, ranging from systemic immunosuppression through excision of the limbal conjunctiva adjacent to the ulcer, conjunctival flaps over the ulcer, beta-irradiation, lamellar keratoplasty, antihelminthics, and cauterization. Four strategies underlie most of these treatments: (1) local immunosuppression, (2) systemic immunosuppression, (3) removal of local stimulatory antigens, and (4) removal of distant stimulatory antigens.

The following stepwise approach to management is recommended: (1) topical corticosteroids, (2) conjunctival resection, (3) systemic immunosuppression, and (4) additional surgery.[27]

Topical corticosteroids: These are used aggressively on an hourly basis, along with topical prophylactic antibiotics and cycloplegic medications. When the cornea shows signs of reepithelialization the steroid therapy is tapered gradually over months. It is important to monitor for cataracts and an increase in intraocular pressure.

Conjunctival resection: This removes involved conjunctiva and blocks collagenase and the immune response to corneal antigen by providing a biological barrier. In this procedure, conjunctiva adjacent to the corneal ulcer is resected up to 2 clock hours on either side to bare sclera and extends 3–4 mm from the limbus. Postoperatively, topical corticosteroids and antibiotics are continued.

Systemic immunosuppression

Those cases of bilateral or progressive Mooren's ulcer that fail therapeutic steroids and conjunctival resection will require systemic cytotoxic chemotherapy to bring a halt to the progressive corneal destruction. It is better to start this treatment sooner rather than later, before the corneal destruction has become too extensive for surgery.

Systemic corticosteroids can be given to suppress inflammation and arrest progressive corneal thinning. The recommended dosage for oral prednisolone is 1–1.5 mg/kg body weight/day. The dosage is adjusted according to the severity of the disease and is tapered slowly when improvement occurs. Alternatively, to avoid side effects associated with long-term corticosteroid therapy, patients can be given intravenous pulse therapy of methylprednisolone.

Other systemic immunosuppressants used in the management of Mooren's ulcer are: cyclophosphamide (2 mg/kg/day), methotrexate (7.5–15 mg once weekly), and azathioprine (2 mg/kg/day). The degree of fall in white blood cell count is considered as the most reliable indicator of immunosuppression produced by cyclophosphamide.

Oral ciclosporin A (3–4 mg/kg/day) has been successfully used to treat a case of bilateral Mooren's ulcer unresponsive to local therapy as well as systemic immunosuppression.[28] Ciclosporin A works by suppression of the helper T-cell population and stimulation of the depressed population of suppressor and cytotoxic T cells present in these patients.

Although immunosuppression is effective, close follow-up is necessary to ensure that the white blood cell count does not reach a dangerously low level. The administering physician must be vigilant about adverse effects of these cytotoxic and immunosuppressive medications.

Other agents

Topical ciclosporin: Recently, topical ciclosporin 0.5% ophthalmic solution 4 to 6 times daily has been successfully used to treat Mooren's ulcer without the potential side effects of oral immunosuppressants.[29] Topical ciclosporin penetrates corneal epithelium to reach the stroma and cause local suppression of ocular immune reactions in the cornea and conjunctiva.

Interferon alpha-2b: Treating chronic hepatitis C patients with subconjunctival injections of interferon alpha-2b over a 6-month period has been shown to improve healing of Mooren's ulcer after other more conventional forms of treatment for the ulcer have failed.[11,12]

Additional Surgery

Additional surgical procedures can be performed to control the ulcerative disease, repair corneal perforation, or improve vision after final healing of the ulcer. Various surgical procedures used are:

- *Keratoepithelioplasty*: In this procedure the ulcerated corneal tissue and adjacent conjunctiva are removed and donor corneal lenticules with intact epithelium are sutured onto bare sclera.[30] There are two theories to explain success with this procedure. According to one theory, intact corneal epithelium has antiangiogenic properties and the Bowman's layer is quite resistant to cell invasion. Another theory is that the transplanted lenticules mask the biological signal of surgical damage to corneoscleral tissue. In a series published by Kinoshita et al., all nine eyes that were not cured by conjunctival resection alone demonstrated good results with keratoepithelioplasty.[30]
- *Lamellar keratectomy*: In this procedure four-fifths of the corneal thickness is excised. The procedure controls the inflammatory process by removal of the corneal antigenic stimulus. A lamellar keratoplasty is required for visual rehabilitation. This procedure should be used after more conservative treatments have failed.
- *Lamellar keratoplasty* (LKP): LKP is widely used at present for the treatment of Mooren's ulcer. The procedure removes antigenic targets of the cornea, prevents immunological reactions, reconstructs the anatomy and prevents it from perforating, and improves vision. The surgical procedure involves removal of necrotic ulcerative cornea and reconstruction of anatomical structure using lamellar donor lenticule. The surgical plan depends on the shape of the ulcer and infiltration of the cornea. If the ulcer is smaller than a half circle of the limbus and the central cornea is not involved, a crescent-shaped lamellar graft is used. If the ulcer is larger than two-thirds of a circle of the limbus and the central cornea is intact, then a doughnut-shaped lamellar graft is used. If the central cornea is involved, a full lamellar graft is used to maintain visual acuity. For perforation of peripheral cornea, double lamellar grafts comprising a thin inner graft with endothelium for repair of perforation and another lamellar graft on the surface whose shape depends on the shape of the ulcer is used. Chen at al. reported a cure rate of 73.7% after the first procedure of LKP plus 1% ciclosporin A eyedrops and a final cure rate of 95.6%.[9]
- *Tissue adhesive and bandage contact lens*: In cases of perforation or impending perforation, tissue adhesive with bandage contact lens may be used to seal small perforations.
- *Tectonic grafts (patch graft or penetrating keratoplasty)*: Large perforations cannot be managed by tissue adhesive and require tectonic grafts such as a patch graft or penetrating keratoplasty. Since Mooren's ulcer is an autoimmune reaction, a Mooren-type melt might develop in the donor graft and, as with any corneal graft procedure, adjunctive immunosuppression is advisable to decrease the chances of graft failure.

At the L V Prasad Eye Institute, a stepwise approach to treatment of Mooren's ulcer is used. Treatment proceeds from topical corticosteroids to conjunctival excision with or without lamellar keratectomy and, finally, to systemic immunosuppression. However, if a patient presents with bilateral simultaneous ulcer or advanced disease or progresses rapidly, little time is spent waiting for a therapeutic response to topical therapy, and treatment consisting of conjunctival excision with systemic immunosuppression is undertaken.

Prognosis

The clinical course, response to therapy, and eventual prognosis of Mooren's ulcer are related to disease presentation. The disease can present as a unilateral disorder, a bilateral nonsimultaneous disorder, or a bilateral simultaneous disorder. Patients with unilateral disease usually respond best to therapy and have the best prognosis. Patients with simultaneous bilateral disease usually do the worst. Patients with nonsimultaneous bilateral disease fall in between.

Summary

Mooren's ulcer is an uncommon, painful ulceration of the peripheral cornea. The etiology has yet to be determined; however, histologic and serologic evidence suggest an autoimmune mechanism. The diagnosis is one of exclusion. Therefore, Mooren's ulcer is diagnosed based on the presence of classical clinical features after all other causes of peripheral corneal ulcer are excluded, using detailed clinical assessment and appropriate laboratory tests. The goals of treatment are control of inflammation and tissue destruction, and promotion of corneal epithelialization. Classically, a stepwise approach is used in the treatment of this disorder; however, in a patient with rapidly progressive and bilateral disease, a more aggressive approach must be adopted.

References

1. Duke-Elder S, Leigh AG. Diseases of the outer eye, part 2. In: Duke Elder S, ed. *System of ophthalmology*. Vol. VIII, London: Henry Kimpton; 1977:916.
2. Mooren A. Ulcus Rodens. *Ophthalmiatrische Beobachtungen*. Berlin: A. Hirschwald; 1867:107–110.
3. Nettleship A, Brkic S, Vackonic S. Chronic serpiginous ulcer of the cornea (Mooren's ulcer). *Trans Ophthalmol Soc UK*. 1902;22:103–144.
4. Wood T, Kaufman H. Mooren's ulcer. *Am J Ophthalmol*. 1971;71: 417–422.
5. Keitzman B. Mooren's ulcer in Nigeria. *Am J Ophthalmol*. 1968;65: 679–685.
6. Lewallen S, Courtright P. Problems with current concepts of the epidemiology of Mooren's corneal ulcer. *Ann Ophthalmol*. 1990;22:52–55.
7. Watson PG. Management of Mooren's ulceration. *Eye*. 1997;11: 349–356.
8. Srinivasan M, Zegans ME, Zelefsky JR, et al. Clinical characteristics of Mooren's ulcer in South India. *Br J Ophthalmol*. 2007;91:570–575.
9. Chen J, Xie H, Wang Z, et al. Mooren's ulcer in China: a study of clinical characteristics and treatment. *Br J Ophthalmol*. 2000;84:1244–1249.
10. Wilson SE, Lee WM, Murakami C, Weng J, Moninger GA. Mooren's corneal ulcers and hepatitis C virus infection. *N Engl J Med*. 1993;329: 62.
11. Baratz KH, Fulcher S, Bourne WM. Hepatitis C associated keratitis. *Arch Ophthalmol*. 1998;116:529–530.
12. Pluznik D, Butrus SI. Hepatitis C associated peripheral corneal ulceration: rapid response to intravenous steroids. *Cornea*. 2001;20:888–889.
13. Moazami G, Auran JD, Florakis GJ, Wilson SE, Srinivasan DB. Interferon treatment of Mooren's ulcers associated with hepatitis C. *Am J Ophthalmol*. 1995;119:365–366.
14. Erdem U, Kerimoglu H, Gundogan FC, Dagli S. Treatment of Mooren's ulcer with topical administration of interferon alfa-2a. *Ophthalmology*. 2007;114:446–449.
15. Kuriakose ET. Mooren's ulcer: etiology and treatment. *Am J Ophthalmol*. 1963;55:1064–1069.
16. Majekodunmi AA. Ecology of Mooren's ulcer in Nigeria. *Doc Ophthalmol*. 1980;49:211–219.
17. van der Gaag R, Abdillahi H, Stilma JS, Vetter JC. Circulating antibodies against corneal epithelium and hookworm in patients with Mooren's ulcer from Sierra Leone. *Br J Ophthalmol*. 1983;67:623–628.
18. Zelefsky JR, Srinivasan M, Kundu A, et al. Hookworm infestation as a risk factor for Mooren's ulcer in South India. *Ophthalmology*. 2007;114:450–453.
19. Brown S, Mondino B, Rabin B. Autoimmune phenomenon in Mooren's ulcer. *Am J Ophthlamol*. 1976;82:835–840.
20. Foster CS, Kenyon K, Greiner G, Greineder D. The immunopathology of Mooren's ulcer. *Am J Ophthalmol*. 1979;88:149–159.
21. Murray P, Rahi A. Pathogenesis of Mooren's ulcer: some new concepts. *Br J Ophthalmol*. 1984;68:182–186,.
22. Kafkala C, Choi J, Zafirakis P, et al. Mooren ulcer: an immunopathologic study. *Cornea*. 2006;25:667–673.
23. Schapp OL, Feltkemp TE, Breebart AC. Circulating antibodies to corneal tissue in a patient suffering from Mooren's ulcer (ulcus rodens cornea). *Clin Exp Immunol*. 1969;5:365–370.
24. Gottsch J, Liu S, Minkovitz JB, et al. Autoimmunity to a cornea-associated stromal antigen in patients with Mooren's ulcer. *Invest Ophthalmol Vis Sci*. 1995;36:1541–1547.
25. Zelefsky JR, Taylor CJ, Srinivasan M, et al. HLS-DR17 and Mooren's ulcer in South India. *Br J Ophthalmol*. 2008;92:179–181.
26. Liang CK, Chen KH, Hsu WM, Chen KH. Association of HLA type and Mooren's ulcer in Chinese in Taiwan. *Br J Ophthalmol*. 2003;87: 797–798.
27. Sangwan VS, Zafirakis P, Foster CS. Mooren's ulcer: current concepts in management. *Indian J Ophthalmol*. 1997;45:7–17.
28. Hill J, Potter P. Treatment of Mooren's ulcer with cyclosporine A: report of three cases. *Br J Ophthalmol*. 1987;71:11–15.
29. Zhao JC, Jin XY. Immunological analysis and treatment of Mooren's ulcer with cyclosporin A applied topically. *Cornea*. 1993;12:481–488.
30. Kinoshita S, Ohashi Y, Ohji M, Manabe R. Long-term results of keratoepithelioplasty in Mooren's ulcer. *Ophthalmology*. 1991;98:438–445.

Chapter 96

Corneal Complications of Intraocular Surgery

Shahzad I. Mian, Alan Sugar

Corneal complications after intraocular surgery are common, but can range from small epithelial defects to persistent edema from endothelial decompensation (Table 96.1). With recent advances in technology and improvement in surgical technique, the rate of complications secondary to intraocular surgery has decreased. However, the number of intraocular surgeries, especially cataract extraction, is increasing due to the rapidly increasing prevalence of patients with functionally significant cataracts. The number of cataract surgeries performed in the United States has grown to over 2.3 million per year.[1] The Collaborative Eye Disease Prevalence Study predicts a 50% increase in the rate of cataract surgery over the next two decades from 6.7 million patients post cataract surgery in 2000 to 10 million patients in 2020.[2] Therefore, a low rate of complications can still affect large numbers of patients.[3] The course and treatment of these complications can incur considerable human and financial cost. Recognition of corneal complications associated with surgery is essential to early recognition, management, and prevention of these complications.

Epithelial Complications

Epithelial defects are a common complication which can occur from surgical trauma or toxicity of medications and antiseptics. Excessive dryness can occur with use of topical anesthetics with prolonged preoperative application. Patients with dry eye syndromes, exposure keratopathy, anterior basement membrane dystrophy, diabetes mellitus, and undergoing vitrectomy are at increased risk for developing epithelial defects, especially with minor trauma to the corneal surface.

Epithelial edema may also develop intraoperatively with a history of dry eyes, surgical trauma, elevated intraocular pressure, prolonged surgical times, and endothelial injury. Epithelial edema can result in an irregular light reflex and decreased clarity of intraocular structures, requiring central corneal epithelial debridement. Filamentary keratitis may also develop postoperatively in patients with ptosis or dry eyes.

Management involves frequent lubrication with artificial tears, and use of gels or ointments. Some patients may benefit from therapeutic soft contact lens use. A tarsorrhaphy and/or amniotic membrane graft may be necessary to treat chronic \ epithelial defects. Use of autologous serum may decrease time to reepithelialization by 40%.[3] Patients at risk may benefit from preoperative use of lubricants and topical ciclosporin 0.05% and intraoperative use of viscoadhesives on the corneal surface. Most epithelial defects resolve promptly but may result in infectious keratitis, corneal scarring, and neovascularization with loss of vision, especially after retinal surgery.

Thermal Burns

Thermal burns to the cornea can occur with use of cautery and phacoemulsification ultrasonic handpieces. Coagulation of corneal tissue results in collagen shrinkage with focal opacification, scar tissue formation, and induction of astigmatism. Central corneal injury has more significant sequelae as compared to peripheral burns. The phacoemulsification handpiece generates significant heat due to friction between the vibrating needle and silicone sleeve with use of ultrasound energy which must be adequately cooled down with flow of irrigation fluid.[4] Constriction of the silicone sleeve, disruption of this irrigation, and prolonged phacoemulsification times can result in sudden thermal burn to the incisional corneal tissue, resulting in corneal contraction, wound gape, and leaky incisions (Fig. 96.1). Thermal burns during phacoemulsification can occur due to hydration of an incision during surgery resulting in a tight entrance wound, during lens fragment removal, and with dense nucleus removal requiring high degrees of ultrasound energy.[5]

Prevention and early recognition of thermal injury is essential to minimizing morbidity associated with thermal burns. Phacoemulsification must be discontinued with loss of irrigation flow or tight incisions. Improvements in phacoemulsification technology and cataract extraction techniques have significantly reduced thermal wound injuries with cataract extraction.[6] Hyperpulse and microburst settings as well as torsional phacoemulsification handpieces generate less heat when compared to longitudinal handpieces, which can reduce the risk of thermal burns during surgery.[7]

Descemet's Membrane Tear/Detachment

Small tears in Descemet's membrane occur frequently, especially adjacent to corneal incisions; however, they remain localized and do not result in vision loss. Small Descemet's tears can enlarge during surgery to become detachments

Table 96.1 Corneal complications of intraocular surgery

Epithelial	Abrasion
	Edema
	Filaments
	Toxic keratopathy
Thermal burns	Cautery
	Phacoemulsification probe
Infection	Bacterial
	Fungal
	Herpes simplex keratitis
Descemet's membrane	Tear
	Detachment
Endothelial injury	Aphakic bullous keratopathy
	Pseudophakic bullous keratopathy
	Brown-McLean syndrome
	Phakic bullous keratopathy
	TASS

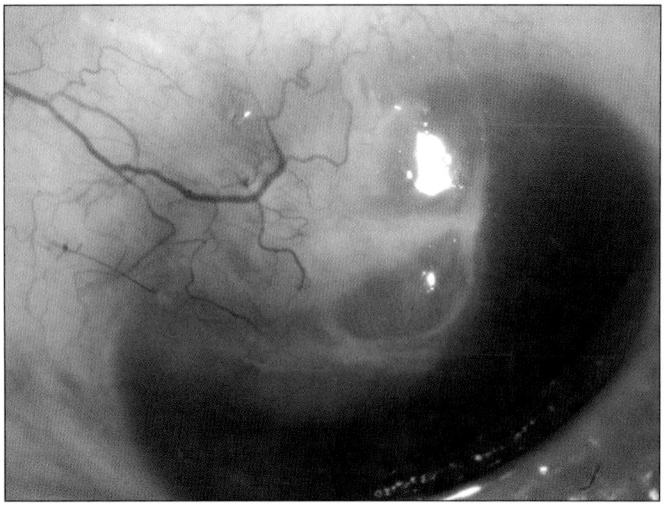

Fig. 96.1 Corneal scar and neovascularization after phacoemulsification burn at the clear corneal incision.

associated with corneal edema and vision loss. Descemet's membrane detachment has been reported with cataract extraction, iridectomy, trabeculectomy, penetrating keratoplasty, pars plana vitrectomy, deep sclerectomy, and viscocanalostomy.[8–30] Risk factors for Descemet's membrane detachment include blunt knife entry, oblique insertion of instruments, entry of instruments or viscoelastics into a false plane above Descemet's membrane, or history of ocular conditions disrupting Descemet's membrane such as congenital glaucoma, birth forceps injury, keratoconus, and Terrien's marginal degeneration (Fig. 96.2). Clear corneal phacoemulsification incisions have an increased association with Descemet's tears when compared to scleral tunnel incisions with extracapsular cataract extraction due to repeat insertion and removal of the phacoemulsification probe with high-flow irrigation and a tight incision which can strip the Descemet's membrane.[31] The detachment can be noted in the immediate postoperative period or weeks later.

Descemet's membrane detachments can spontaneously reattach with medical treatment alone, with a mean resolution time of 10 weeks.[31] Detachments with planar separations between the stroma and Descemet's membrane are more likely to reattach spontaneously. With large detachments or slow resolution, descemetopexy with air, sulfur hexafluoride (SF_6), perfluoropropane 14% (C_3F_8) gas injections, sodium hyaluronate or through-and-through

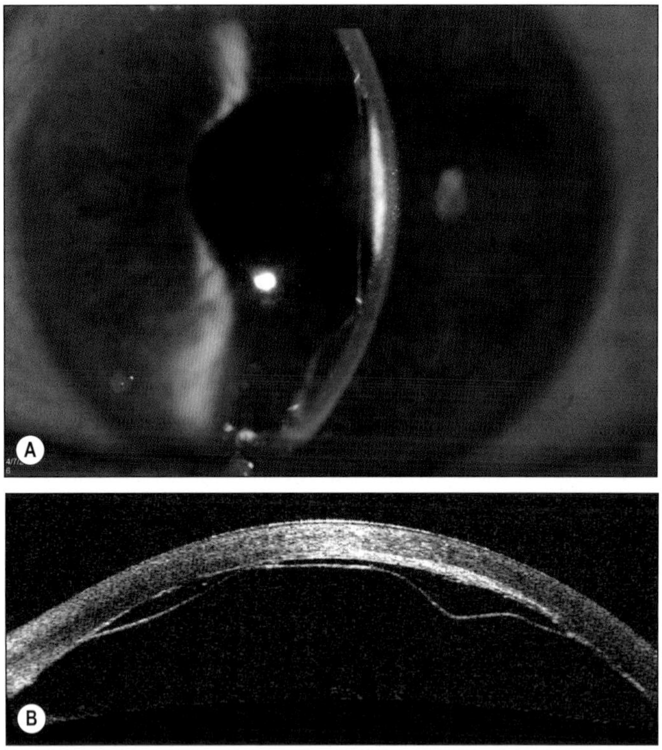

Fig. 96.2 Descemet's membrane detachment: (**A**) slit lamp photo, (**B**) anterior segment OCT.

corneal mattress sutures may help and can be repeated.[32–35] Bullous keratopathy or corneal scarring may occur, requiring endothelial or penetrating keratoplasty in 7–8% of cases.[11,19,21,23–25,36,37]

Infectious Keratitis

Infectious keratitis with permanent corneal scarring can occur with clear corneal surgery, with bacterial keratitis presenting more commonly in the early and fungal keratitis in the late postoperative period. Infectious keratitis is more commonly seen adjacent to the corneal incision site, with use of sutures, and in association with endophthalmitis. Herpes simplex keratitis can flare in patients with previous history of disease. Early recognition of infectious keratitis can allow for better resolution. Corneal cultures can help guide treatment of the keratitis and possible associated endophthalmitis. Prophylaxis with povidone-iodine, intracameral cephalosporins, and postoperative antibiotics may reduce risk of endophthalmitis and keratitis. Patients with history of herpes simplex keratitis may need oral antiviral prophylaxis to reduce risk of flare-ups.

Endothelial Injury

Injury to the endothelium during intraocular surgery can result in corneal edema, which can result in formation of bullae and is commonly known as bullous keratopathy. Corneal edema secondary to endothelial injury is a major cause of poor visual outcomes after intraocular surgery and a leading indication for keratoplasty.[38] Bullous keratopathy may present gradually in the setting of aphakia, and pseudophakia or with an acute onset with an inflammatory reaction known as toxic anterior segment syndrome (TASS). Our progressive understanding of the causes of bullous keratopathy has helped both to reduce the rate of their occurrence and to direct improvements in surgical techniques, and instrument design and manufacture.

Incidence

Aphakic bullous keratopathy (ABK) has been known for over 100 years as a leading cause of secondary corneal degeneration,[39] although it was described as 'corneal dystrophy' or 'bullous keratitis' in much of the earlier literature.[40] The relationship of edema to corneal endothelial degeneration has been widely recognized only since the 1960s.[41] It is difficult to determine the incidence of bullous keratopathy in aphakic eyes from the pre-intraocular lens (pre-IOL) era, but before the successful application of keratoplasty in aphakic eyes in the 1960s it was considered a hopeless complication of cataract extraction.[42]

When IOLs were first enthusiastically used in large numbers of cataract patients, their acceptance, particularly in the United States, was significantly delayed by rates of permanent corneal edema as high as 50% over 5 years. Barraquer inserted almost 500 anterior chamber lenses in the late 1950s, but corneal edema and chronic inflammation led him to remove half of them by 1970.[43] These complications were not recognized until several years after surgery. With improvements in IOL design and surgical techniques the incidence of this complication is decreasing, but it is unlikely to disappear. Past rates of ABK (Fig. 96.3) are difficult to determine. Comparative series in the period of early IOL use give rates of 0–0.8% with intracapsular extraction and no IOL.[44–46] Rates in eyes with vitreous loss during intracapsular cataract extraction ranged from 0.9% to 11.3% before the availability of vitrectomy techniques.[47]

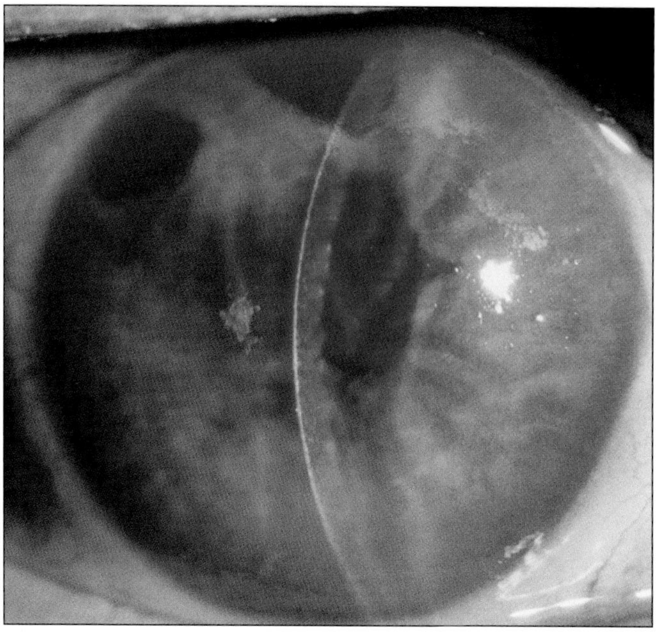

Fig. 96.3 Aphakic bullous keratopathy.

While much more information is available on corneal complications with the use of IOLs, it is possible to attribute the development of edema to the IOL itself only in limited circumstances, as the underlying rate without IOL use in controlled comparisons is usually not available. The rate has dropped with improved techniques,[38] but has been quite high in some early series and with some relatively disastrous lens designs. Binkhorst noted over 9% corneal decompensation in an early series of 694 iris clip lens patients. The edema occurred 3 years after cataract surgery, on average, and caused loss of useful vision in 5.5% of patients.[48] Pseudophakic bullous keratopathy (PBK) occurred in 9% of 354 patients in a later series with iris clip lens insertion and intracapsular cataract extraction.[48] Pearce found a 2.7% incidence of PBK in a 4-year follow-up of eyes with Binkhorst-type lenses.[49] In early American studies of iris-plane Copeland lenses, the first lens widely used in the United States, 6% developed PBK with 5-year follow-up.[50] Drews combined several series to derive a $3.2 \pm 4.35\%$ incidence of permanent corneal edema in 8515 cataract and IOL eyes operated on in the 1960s and early 1970s.[51] In most of these patients, intracapsular cataract extraction was combined with iris-supported or anterior chamber IOL insertion. Tennant, however, reported a 15% PBK incidence in the same era using extracapsular extraction and anterior chamber IOLs.[52]

With the widespread acceptance of IOL use in the United States by the early 1980s, data became available on large numbers of patients. The requirement of premarket approval by the US Food and Drug Administration (FDA) mandated the collection of data on patients having investigational IOLs inserted after 1978. The initial report from the FDA, on 409 000 lenses inserted between 1978 and 1982, found only 0.06% corneal endothelial decompensation at 1 year for the newly popular posterior chamber IOLs, 1.2% for anterior chamber IOLs, and 1.5% for iris-fixated lenses.[53] There was

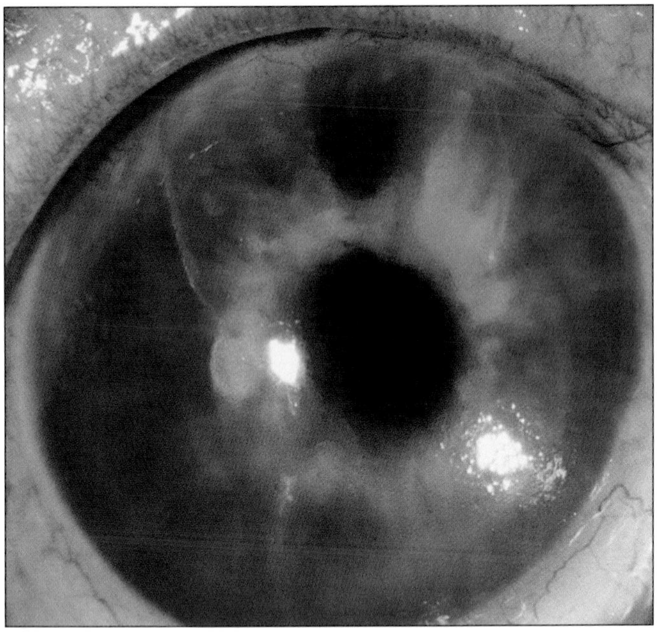

Fig. 96.4 PBK in an eye with an Azar 91Z closed-loop anterior chamber IOL.

concern that the rate of significant complications was underreported in these series.[54]

In the mid-1980s, when patient and surgeon acceptance of IOLs made them the standard of care for cataract surgery in adults, several new IOL designs were tried and enthusiastically promoted. Some of these lenses were of the 'closed-loop' anterior chamber type. The first IOL design recognized to be associated with a high incidence of bullous keratopathy was the Azar 91Z lens, reported to have the 'highest postoperative complication rate of any implant of contemporary design and manufacture' (Fig. 96.4).[55] A rate at 1 year of 5.1% PBK led to withdrawal of this lens from the market in 1983.[56] Similar problems occurred with the Leiske (Surgidev style 10) lens and the ORC stableflex lens, which caused greater than 5% PBK,[56–58] and these were withdrawn from use in 1986 and 1987, respectively.[54] Other styles, such as the Hessburg lens, were initially reported to do well[59] and only much later reported to cause bullous keratopathy.[60] Other anterior chamber lens styles have also been found to cause corneal decompensation. The Dubroff lens, reported to cause PBK at an average of 4 years after insertion, has small loops in the angle[61] and may act similarly to open-loop posterior chamber IOLs placed in the anterior chamber, which also cause endothelial damage.[62] The denominators for these series, necessary to give incidence rates, are not available, but the prevalence of complications suggests very high rates of corneal damage. Estimates comparing the proportion of closed-loop anterior chamber lenses removed to the total number inserted confirm a high relative risk of corneal and other complications compared to posterior chamber or open-loop semiflexible anterior chamber lenses.[63]

The rate of corneal decompensation with currently used posterior chamber IOLs is felt to be low. In Switzerland, a rate of 0.1–0.3% was reported with extracapsular cataract extraction.[64] Estimates from extensive Medicare data on patients having cataract surgery in 1984 gave a 0.47% rate for phacoemulsification or extracapsular cataract extraction with posterior chamber IOL insertion.[65] Waring estimated in 1989 that a contemporary rate of 0.1% would lead to a tapering off of the PBK 'epidemic.'[38]

Another approach to estimating the relative size of the aphakic and pseudophakic corneal edema problem is to examine the rates of keratoplasty for these indications. The rate of success for keratoplasty in aphakic eyes was low until the mid-1960s, so earlier data on keratoplasty rates may underestimate the incidence.[42,66] Similarly, very few keratoplasties were done for PBK before the mid-1970s. In a series of keratoplasty buttons examined from 1948 to 1978, no keratoplasties were performed for ABK from 1947 to 1961.[67] From 1974 to 1978, ABK was the leading indication, accounting for 30% of the cases. No cases of PBK were seen through 1973, but by 1978 two-thirds of bullous keratopathy cases were in eyes with intraocular lenses.[67] An update 5 years later showed PBK alone as the leading indication for keratoplasty (17.5%), and ABK (10.9%) declining.[68] Although the total number of penetrating keratoplasties has been declining, PBK continues to be the leading indication. In one series, the rate of PBK has increased from 22.9% (1983–1988) to 27.2% (1996–2000).[69,70] A similar trend was also seen in Canada, where PBK emerged as the leading indication for penetrating keratoplasty in the early 1980s, and has been rapidly increasing.[71] At our institution, PBK accounted for 2% of keratoplasties in 1976 and had increased to 26% by 1984 and had remained at this level through the early 1990s.[72,73] Similar trends have also been described in other large series.[64,73–76] However, there is evidence to suggest a decline in incidence of PBK in the 1990s after a peak in the late 1980s, including a decreased rate of IOL explantations.[38,77–83] In addition, when comparing the last 100 cases requiring penetrating keratoplasty over three decades, there was a trend towards a decrease in the number of keratoplasties performed due to PBK and ABK.[83] The most recent Eye Bank Association of America statistical report shows that corneal edema after cataract surgery still accounts for 15.7% of the 40000 corneal transplants performed in the United States.[84]

Histopathology of ABK and PBK

The corneal histopathology of ABK and PBK has been generally nonspecific. The prime feature is attenuation and loss of corneal endothelial cells with associated epithelial bullae and stromal edema, resulting in pain and loss of vision.[85] There is thickening of the posterior collagenous layer of Descemet's membrane and a decrease in stromal keratocytes.[86] Subepithelial and retrocorneal fibrous proliferation occurs due to structural and compositional changes in glycosaminoglycans and extracellular matrix proteins.[87] The epithelial basement membrane has decreased amounts of fibronectin, laminin, and collagen type IV, which function as adhesive proteins for normal epithelium. The lack of these adhesive proteins and accumulation of antiadhesive proteins, such as tenascin-C and thrombospondin-1, leads to loss of contact of epithelial cells with each other and with underlying subepithelial tissue, resulting in subepithelial bullae and fibrosis.[88–92] There are increased levels of insulin-like growth factor-I, bone morphogenetic protein, interleukin-8 and interleukin-1, which lead to abnormal accumulation of basement membrane and extracellular matrix proteins, including fibronectin, laminin, type IV collagen, TGFBI, and fibrillin, resulting in subepithelial fibrosis and thickening of the posterior collagenous layer.[93–98] The changes in the basement membrane and extracellular matrix are noted only in ABK and PBK and not in routine postcataract surgery corneas.

Inflammatory cells and macrophages are seen in the deep corneal stroma and deposited as keratic precipitates on the endothelium.[99] Many studies have documented the deposits of inflammatory cells on the intraocular lens and inflammation at the site of haptic to angle or ciliary body touch.[86] The complex range of histopathologic changes in pseudophakic eyes with various types of intraocular lenses are thoroughly described by Apple et al.[100] Endothelial degeneration and posterior proliferation of collagen was previously described in aphakic eyes without IOLs.[101] Histopathologic evidence of underlying corneal endothelial dystrophy as a pre-existing risk factor for postcataract endothelial degeneration has been seen in both aphakic and pseudophakic corneas having keratoplasty for corneal edema.[101,102]

Pathogenesis

The final process in development of aphakic and pseudophakic corneal edema is loss of adequate endothelial pumping function secondary to many potential causes. The study of the response of the corneal endothelium to cataract surgery and its modern modifications was greatly enhanced by the development of clinical specular microscopy. Specular microscopy (see Ch. 14) was first applied to eyes having cataract surgery by Bourne and Kaufman in 1976.[103] Their finding of a 12% reduction of the central corneal endothelial cell density in eyes having intracapsular cataract extraction, and 62% in eyes with IOLs, led to intense study of the effects of variations in surgical technique and IOL type on the endothelium.[104] Initial studies examined short-term endothelial loss and suggest stabilization of the initial effects of surgery over a 3-month period.[105–107] Cell loss after intracapsular cataract extraction without IOLs ranged from 4% to 21%, averaging about 12%.[104–111] Significant differences were not seen when comparing intracapsular and extracapsular extraction (17% and 14%).[112] In early studies, phacoemulsification was associated with 16% to 67% endothelial cell loss, correlating with the degree of trauma at surgery.[113] Short-term studies of various IOL types have also been reported.

Of greater importance for understanding the development of PBK is the long-term course of endothelial cell damage after cataract extraction. Liesegang et al.[114] followed patients having intracapsular cataract extraction with or without an iris-support IOL and extracapsular extraction with or without a posterior chamber lens with specular microscopy over a 2-year period. The cell loss at 2 years ranged from 7.6% for extracapsular extraction without IOL to 24.5% for intracapsular extraction with IOL.[114] The most important finding, however, was that cell loss, which had ranged from 11% to 16% at 2 months in all groups, continued to progress over the period of follow-up in all groups. A randomized trial assigned patients to receive intracapsular cataract extraction with contact lens fitting, intracapsular extraction with iris-support IOL, or extracapsular extraction with iridocapsular IOL.[115] There was greater cell loss in the implant groups, and cell loss appeared to slow after 3 years. Martin et al.[116] confirmed continued cell loss for up to 5 years after intracapsular extraction with or without an iris clip IOL.

Rates of cell loss with the most recent forms of cataract extraction are relatively low compared to studies using early cataract extraction techniques and IOL types. Werblin found 9% central endothelial cell loss at 1 year after phacoemulsification and posterior chamber lens insertion, with 11.5% loss at 3 years, followed by only 0.3% per year greater loss than in control eyes.[117] Others have found 2.71% to 16.7% loss at 3 months with phacoemulsification and posterior chamber IOLs.[118–129] Continuous improvement in phacoemulsification techniques offers possible increased safety, although microincision methods still yield about 8% loss.[130]

Bates et al.[131] proposed a model of cell loss after cataract extraction that was exponential, with different reduction rates for complicated and uncomplicated cases. This model predicts decompensation of the cornea at 542 cells/mm^2 and a time to decompensation of almost 40 years for uncomplicated cases. Liesegang et al.[132] and Bourne et al.[133] prospectively followed patients having various types of cataract surgery with or without IOLs. They found a 2.5% per year cell loss in all groups over 10 years, predicting 60 years to reach 500 cells/mm^2 in eyes with 2200 cells/mm^2 at 1 year postoperatively.

The density of endothelial cells required to maintain corneal deturgescence is unknown, but has been reported to be 515 cells/mm^2 at the time of onset of bullous keratopathy in one prospective study and may be even lower in some cases.[134,135] Localized corneal edema can develop, however, and may be related to regional loss of endothelial cells. Hoffer and Phillippi noted that cell loss was greatest near the site of superior cataract wounds and decreased with distance from the wound.[136] Olsen noted a similar vertical disparity, which was greatest in older patients, presumably because of the decreased ability to redistribute the endothelial cell population.[137]

Brown-McLean Syndrome

An interesting and unusual form of peripheral corneal edema occurring long after cataract surgery was described by Brown and McLean in 1969 and is now referred to as the Brown-McLean syndrome.[138,139] Peripheral corneal edema develops many years after cataract extraction in these patients, with the diagnosis made almost 16 years after surgery on average and as long as 34 years later.[140,141] The edema extends 2–3 mm centrally from the limbus and up to 360 degrees, although the superior limbus may remain clear, particularly if there is a superior sector iridectomy (Fig. 96.5). Fine brown or orange pigment is deposited on or in the endothelium in the involved areas in most cases. The central corneal endothelium may have decreased cell density but rarely becomes edematous, even after prolonged follow-up.[140–144] Histopathology is similar to other forms of bullous keratopathy.[142] The etiology is unknown, but altered aqueous

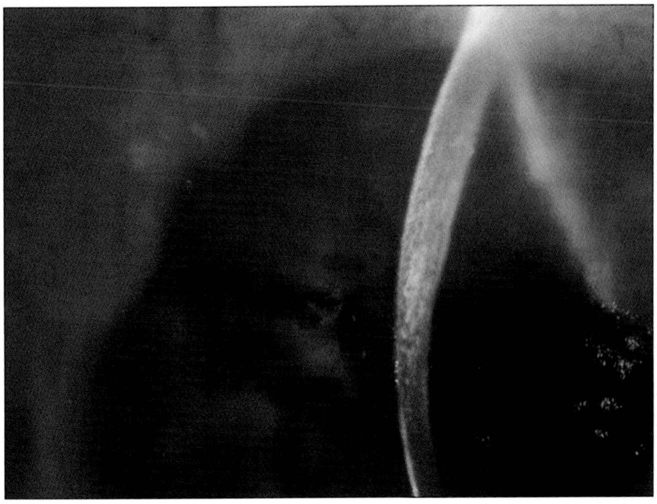

Fig. 96.5 Peripheral corneal edema in an eye with Brown-McLean syndrome.

dynamics and iridodonesis or movement of other tissues or an IOL have been proposed as etiologies. The frequent bilaterality and a report of involved siblings have been considered by some to suggest a possible hereditary factor.[138,140] This syndrome has been reported to occur more often in patients with anterior chamber than posterior chamber lenses, but may appear in more posterior chamber IOL eyes with longer follow-up. Peripheral stromal and epithelial edema, with pigmentation of the endothelium, consistent with Brown-McLean syndrome, has also been observed in a corneal graft 9 years after keratoplasty.[145] Brown-McLean syndrome has been reported after angle-closure glaucoma in phakic eyes, with spontaneous lens absorption and iridodonesis, and in association with myotonic dystrophy, suggesting that nonsurgical endothelial trauma may also result in this syndrome.[140,143] While keratoplasty has been reportedly used for control of pain, peripheral conjunctival flaps have also been successful.[142] Most patients require no therapy.

Toxic Anterior Segment Syndrome

Toxic anterior segment syndrome (TASS) is a sterile postoperative inflammatory reaction most likely caused by a noninfectious agent that gains entry into the anterior segment at the time of surgery and results in toxic damage to intraocular lenses. This typically presents 12 to 48 hours after anterior segment surgery, including cataract and penetrating keratoplasty.[146,147] The hallmark of this inflammation, which distinguishes it from infectious endophthalmitis is Gram stain and culture negativity. Possible causes of TASS include intraocular solutions with inappropriate chemical composition, concentration, pH, osmolality; denatured ophthalmic viscosurgical devices; enzymatic detergents; bacterial endotoxin; oxidized metal deposits; and factors related to intraocular lenses such as residues from polishing or sterilizing compounds. An outbreak of TASS in 2005 involved 112 patients at seven centers. Patients present with blurred vision (60%), anterior segment inflammation (49%), classically with limbus-to-limbus diffuse corneal edema and cell deposition. In this outbreak, 89% of the patients had been exposed to a single brand of balanced salt solution manufactured by Cytosol Laboratories and distributed by Advanced Medical Optics as AMO Endosol.[148] TASS associated with mild antigenic load resolves rapidly with clearing of corneal edema but more severe TASS can result in permanent endothelial cell loss and associated bullous keratopathy.

Table 96.2 Causes of ABK and PBK

Pre-existing endothelial disease
Fuchs' dystrophy, cornea guttata
Pseudoexfoliation
Trauma
Angle-closure glaucoma
Intraoperative factors
IOL-to-cornea touch
Irrigating solutions
Instrumentation
Sterilization technique
Ultrasound damage
Vitreous loss, nuclear loss
Drug toxicity
Intracameral anesthesia
Descemet's membrane detachment
Postoperative factors
Long-term cell loss
Vitreous-to-endothelial touch
IOL dislocation – touch
Flat anterior chamber
Peripheral anterior synechiae
Pseudophakodonesis
Inflammation
Toxic materials

Specific Etiologic Factors in ABK and PBK

Preoperative factors: pre-existing disease

One of the potential factors in the development of postcataract corneal edema is a pre-existing abnormality of the endothelium leading to decompensation of the cornea after the superimposed trauma of cataract surgery (Table 96.2). Waltman noted that the unoperated eyes of 25% of patients presenting with pseudophakic bullous keratopathy in one eye had abnormally low cell counts, with 17% below 1000 cells/mm^2, and 8% between 1000 and 1500 cells/mm^2, suggesting a predisposition on the basis of a reduced endothelial reserve.[149] Rao et al.[150] prospectively examined patients having intracapsular cataract extraction and iris-support IOL insertion. While 10% of patients developed PBK requiring penetrating keratoplasty, there was no difference in preoperative cell counts between eyes with and without bullous keratopathy. These authors did, however, find a significant correlation between variation in cell size, polymegathism, and development of corneal edema.[150] The coefficient of variation of cell area, a measure of variability in cell size, was 40.7 in those developing edema and 27.4 in those without edema. The same group had earlier correlated polymegathism with increased corneal thickness after cataract surgery, independent of cell loss.[151] Cheng et al., however, in their prospective randomized IOL study, correlated postoperative corneal thickness with cell loss rather than preoperative cell morphology.[152] They were unable to find any predictive value of measurement of endothelial cell size or shape variability.[153] Bourne et al.,[133] in their 10-year follow-up of cataract patients, were unable to correlate preoperative cell density or coefficient of variation of cell area with postoperative cell loss.

Several groups have found that the presence of corneal guttae is associated with the development of PBK. Bourne et al. found greater long-term cell loss in patients with cornea guttata. Taylor et al.[46] had found guttae to be a risk factor for ABK. Koenig and Schultz found that 15 of 17 contralateral eyes of patients having keratoplasty for PBK had cornea guttata or frank Fuchs' dystrophy.[154] Histopathologic study of corneas removed at keratoplasty for PBK with posterior chamber IOLs found evidence of endothelial dystrophy in 67%.[102] In contrast, only 12% of corneal buttons from PBK patients with anterior chamber IOLs had similar findings, suggesting that endothelial dystrophy is a major cause of PBK in patients having contemporary cataract surgery, whereas the IOL used may have been more etiologic with older lens types. Current techniques allow performance of phacoemulsification in eyes with Fuchs' dystrophy and mild edema (thickness <640 microns (μm)) without frank decompensation in most cases.[155]

Pseudoexfoliation syndrome can predispose to higher risk of ABK and PBK, not only due to higher rate of vitreous loss during cataract extraction but also due to a clinically and histopathologically distinct keratopathy. Naumann and Schlotzer-Schrehardt reviewed 22 patients with clinically diagnosed pseudoexfoliation syndrome undergoing penetrating keratoplasty.[156] Clinically, the patients showed diffuse corneal edema, with pleomorphic and reduced endothelial cells, including retrocorneal flakes of pseudoexfoliation in three patients. Histopathologically, there was diffuse, irregular thickening of Descemet's membrane and focal accumulation of locally produced pseudoexfoliation material. There was absence of guttae, presence of a higher degree of fibroblastic transformation and melanin phagocytosis of endothelial cells, and more pronounced cell loss when compared to Fuchs' dystrophy. A reduced preoperative endothelial cell count of 10.5–11.1% has also been demonstrated in patients with pseudoexfoliation syndrome undergoing cataract extraction.[123,126]

Other risk factors for poor endothelial reserve before cataract surgery have also been reported. Ishikawa, in a retrospective review of patients who had cataract surgery, noted preoperative endothelial cell density to be less than 2000 cells/mm^2 in patients with previous history of corneal diseases, angle-closure glaucoma, pseudoexfoliation, and a history of trauma.[157] Advanced nuclear cataract and chronic pulmonary disease were also significant risk factors. Recognition of these factors preoperatively may help predict postoperative corneal decompensation.

From the foregoing considerations, it is apparent that clinical specular microscopy of the corneal endothelium is of value in research studies of cataract surgery.[158] It is not reasonable to recommend its routine clinical use because corneal guttae are detectable on slit lamp examination and the clinical plan is unlikely to be altered by specular microscopic findings. However, preoperative risk factors for endothelial cell loss should be considered in surgical planning. Similarly, it has been shown that with current cataract and IOL techniques the risk of developing bullous keratopathy is low, even when preoperative endothelial cell counts are very low.[159]

Intraoperative factors

While many aspects of the surgical procedure have potential to damage the corneal endothelium and lead to bullous keratopathy, most have not been well studied or well quantified. Most of the clinical information available is from retrospective studies. Limbal or corneal incisions alone, without lens extraction, cause some endothelial cell loss centrally in animal models, which correlates with incision length.[160] It would be expected that large incisions for intracapsular or planned extracapsular surgery would cause more cell loss when compared to small incisions (<3 mm) used for phacoemulsification. Reduced cell loss with current techniques appears to confirm this trend.[124,159–161] With corneal incisions entering central to the limbus, a greater central cell loss might be anticipated with superior incisions compared to the more peripheral temporal incisions.[162]

Although increased instrumentation with current techniques may be expected to increase endothelial damage, there is no clinical evidence to support this hypothesis. While current cataract techniques require more intraocular manipulation and time than older techniques, they are done with maintenance of the corneal dome and cause less endothelial damage than the older techniques. Earlier studies of phacoemulsification showed central endothelial loss as high as 34%, twice as much as when compared with intracapsular cataract extraction.[113] Moving phacoemulsification from the anterior to the posterior chamber significantly decreases cell loss,[117,122,163] and endocapsular emulsification, including quick-chop and soft-shell, techniques have improved this further.[119,128,130,161]

Ophthalmic instrument sterilization techniques have been reported to cause toxic endothelial cell destruction syndrome. AbTox Plazlyte, a sterilization technique that can degrade brass to copper and zinc on cannulated surgical instruments, resulted in irreversible endothelial cell destruction.[164] In another epidemic, instruments sterilized with a new plasma gas protocol led to corneal decompensation in ten patients, with six requiring penetrating keratoplasty.[165] Use of 2% glutaraldehyde for sterilization of small lumen instruments has also been linked to an epidemic of corneal decompensation after cataract extraction.[166]

Intraocular irrigating solutions have the potential for endothelial toxicity, as shown by Edelhauser et al. in a series of laboratory studies.[167–169] They showed that physiologic saline solution caused corneal swelling and endothelial damage. Ringer's solution did so to a lesser degree, and balanced salt solution (BSS) maintained endothelial structure and function from several hours to indefinitely when bicarbonate, adenosine, and reduced glutathione were included.[167] The osmotic and pH values of solutions must be kept within a relative physiologic range.[168,169] Laboratory and clinical studies in human corneas have confirmed the tendency of solutions not specifically designed for intraocular use to cause corneal edema.[170,171] Balanced salt solution enriched with bicarbonate, dextrose, and glutathione (BSS Plus) has been shown in the laboratory to protect the endothelium better than BSS alone,[172] but clinical trials have not shown an apparent long-term difference.[173] Although these solutions have theoretical and possibly clinical advantages, they require that an additive vial be injected into the larger solution container just before use. There is a risk of toxicity to the endothelium with unsupplemented irrigant.

Topical and intracameral anesthesia have become popular options for pain control in cataract surgery. Topical anesthesia is safe and effective when compared to retrobulbar and peribulbar anesthesia.[174,175] Intracameral use of preservative-free lidocaine 1% from 0.1 mL to 0.5 mL has shown no change in endothelial cell counts up to 3 months after surgery.[176,177] However, lidocaine 5% and 10% causes significant corneal endothelial loss.[178] In addition, intracameral undiluted bupivacaine HCl 0.5%, bupivacaine HCl 0.75%, and proparacaine HCl 0.5% produce endothelial toxicity with significant corneal thickening and opacification.[179]

Medications introduced into the anterior chamber during cataract extraction have the potential for endothelial toxicity as well. Epinephrine is often added to irrigating solutions to maximize pupillary dilation. Reports of corneal edema after intraocular epinephrine use have been attributed to pH and to toxicity of sodium bisulfite preservatives.[180] Preservative-free epinephrine solutions irrigated directly into the anterior chamber assist in pupil dilation and decrease the severity of floppy iris syndrome related to alpha antagonists used systemically to treat urinary obstruction.[181] Benzalkonium chloride-preserved viscoelastic during cataract surgery can lead to immediate postoperative striate keratopathy. Eleftheriadis et al.[182] reported decreased vision and corneal edema with decreased endothelial cell count and density 14 to 16 months after cataract surgery, with two patients requiring penetrating keratoplasty. Intraocular miotics have also been shown to have endothelial toxicity potential. Acetylcholine 1% (Miochol) in vitro alters endothelial function and structure.[183] In a similar test system, carbachol 0.01% (Miostat) is well tolerated by the endothelium.[184] In vivo, both solutions appear to be well tolerated.[185] Immediate corneal edema has followed irrigation of improperly prepared acetylcholine when distilled water, the diluent alone, was instilled.[186] Vancomycin in the irrigating solution has been used as a prophylaxis for postoperative endophthalmitis; however, concentrations greater than 1.0 mg/mL can lead to corneal endothelial toxicity and decompensation.[187] Povidone-iodine is routinely used as an antiseptic solution in preparing eyes for surgery and is also used as an alternative to postoperative topical antibiotics. Povidone-iodine in both 5% and 10% concentrations can lead to severe endothelial toxicity with one drop placed directly in the anterior chamber.[188] Intraoperative leakage of povidone-iodine into the anterior chamber must be prevented.

Trauma directly caused by the IOL is a major concern. Touch of the surface of polymethyl methacrylate (PMMA) intraocular lenses to the endothelium causes adherence of endothelial cells to the IOL surface, with removal or lysis as the implant is moved away.[189] This lens touch is probably a major cause of the decline in endothelial density noted in the early specular microscopic studies.[190] However, the South Asian Cataract Management Study reported endothelial cell loss after intracapsular cataract extraction with anterior chamber IOL implantation to be greater only 6 weeks after surgery and no different at 2 years when compared to no IOL implantation.[191] To prevent IOL contact, air bubbles were used initially to keep the IOL back from the cornea.[192] Air has, however, been shown to damage the endothelium.[193] When compared with other endothelial protective agents in a controlled trial, air caused severe cell loss.[194] Viscoelastics were introduced to prevent endothelial damage in cataract surgery in the late 1970s. Sodium hyaluronate has been shown to prevent the endothelial damage caused by direct IOL-to-cornea touch.[195] In the first clinical studies, sodium hyaluronate decreased cell loss from intracapsular cataract extraction from 17% to 7%.[196] With intracapsular extraction and an iris-supported IOL, cell loss was dramatically reduced from 47% to 17%.[197] There was little benefit with early study of the effect of viscoelastics on posterior chamber lens insertion with phacoemulsification.[198] However, more recent studies stress that the benefit of these agents is great.[194,199] Chondroitin sulfate–sodium hyaluronate combination viscoelastics (Viscoat) have been claimed to adhere to the endothelium better than sodium hyaluronate alone and provide better protection during phacoemulsification and posterior chamber IOL insertion.[200] It appeared that this effect was related to prolonged retention of Viscoat and of hydroxypropyl methylcellulose-based viscoelastics (OcuCoat). Viscoat has also been shown to be effective in reducing postoperative corneal edema compared to Healon GV (sodium hyaluronate 1.4%) when used during phacoemulsification.[201] Healon 5, a high molecular weight viscoelastic agent, showed decreased endothelial cell loss compared to Viscoat and Healon GV.[128] The value of the more adherent and retained material appears to be greatest when emulsification is performed anterior to the lens capsule.[119] Cell loss did not differ between these agents in other studies.[202] These agents are also useful when cataract extraction or IOL insertion is unusually complicated or traumatic.[200]

Complicated cataract surgery has been associated with both increased cell loss and increased bullous keratopathy. Vitreous loss led to an increased incidence of ABK before the availability of vitrectomy.[47] It appears that careful anterior vitrectomy followed by posterior or anterior chamber IOL insertion gives a rate of corneal edema development of 1–2%, which does not contraindicate the use of the IOL after vitrectomy.[203] In the study of 1984 Medicare patients, there was a threefold increase in the rate of corneal edema development when an anterior vitrectomy was performed at cataract extraction (2.4% vs 0.9%).[65] Loss of lens nuclear fragments into the vitreous, usually occurring with vitreous loss and later requiring retinal evaluation, was associated with corneal edema after vitrectomy in 9–34% of patients,[204,205] whereas corneal edema was present in almost half before vitrectomy.[205] Retained lens capsular and nuclear fragments in the anterior chamber can also lead to corneal decompensation and vision loss requiring surgical intervention.[206] Minimizing trauma from attempting to retrieve the nuclear fragment from an anterior approach during the initial cataract surgery may decrease corneal complications.

Postoperative causes of corneal edema

The endothelial cell loss associated with initial surgery and superimposed long-term loss related to aging and to IOL presence may lead to corneal edema, as discussed earlier. Prevention of corneal edema by medical treatment in the postoperative period has been disputed. Treatment with oral nonsteroidal agents to decrease inflammation was associated with decreased endothelial cell loss in one trial.[207] Use of subconjunctival injection of depot steroids, however, was felt to cause greater long-term cell loss by altering endothelial repair.[208]

Vitreous touch to the corneal endothelium was considered to be a major cause of bullous keratopathy before the use of intraocular lenses, which tend to hold the vitreous back.[209] It is said that corneal decompensation is more likely if the vitreous face is intact than if it is broken. Several medical treatments to induce vitreous retraction were proposed in the past, with questionable effect.[210] Pars plana vitrectomy has been used with early endothelial decompensation.[211] In a series of 17 such eyes, decreased corneal edema occurred in nine. Early vitrectomy, good preoperative visual acuity, and a broken vitreous face were associated with a good outcome.[212] Vitreous adherent to the cataract wound may be associated with localized edema of the cornea. It may cause continued endothelial damage directly or by causing chronic anterior segment inflammation.

IOL touch to the cornea after cataract surgery may occur in several settings. A flat anterior chamber can occur immediately with wound leakage or may be delayed with pupillary block. These conditions require urgent treatment when pupil-supported lenses are present so that corneal damage can be limited. In one series, a flat anterior chamber with IOL-to-cornea touch after glaucoma filtering surgery related to overfiltration or choroidal hemorrhage led to corneal edema in two of eight cases, although only one of eight was pseudophakic. Two eyes required cataract extraction after re-formation of the chamber and developed PBK.[213] Dislocated or subluxed IOLs can directly touch the endothelium. This was a problem with anterior loop dislocation of pupil-supported IOLs.[214] It also occurs with anterior chamber lenses when a lens haptic slips into a peripheral iridectomy, tilting the opposite haptic forward against the cornea. This problem can be prevented by using midperipheral rather than peripheral iridectomies when anterior chamber IOLs are inserted. Even with posterior chamber lenses, haptic or optic subluxation may rarely lead to endothelial touch and localized or diffuse edema (Fig. 96.6).

Iris adhesions to the cornea may contribute to corneal damage by allowing endothelial cells to migrate off Descemet's membrane[215] or by tearing them away when synechiae are broken. They also may be associated with chronic inflammation damaging to the cornea. Synechiae have been a problem with anterior chamber lenses of all types. Particularly, they have been associated with closed-loop anterior chamber lenses. Synechiae, along with chronic inflammation, may be related to the high rate of PBK with these lenses.

Chronic uveitis has long been considered a factor in corneal damage. The causes of inflammation after cataract surgery are many and complex. They have been extensively

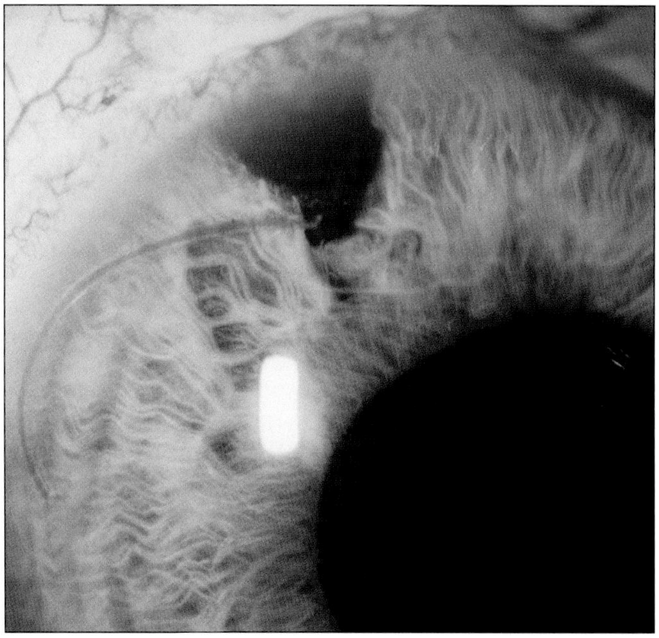

Fig. 96.6 The loop of a sulcus-placed posterior chamber IOL touching the endothelium after slipping anteriorly through a peripheral iridectomy.

examined by Apple et al.[100] and include mechanical, toxic, biocompatibility, infectious, and immune problems. Review of these factors is beyond the scope of this chapter. The mechanisms by which chronic inflammation damages the cornea are complex also, and not well understood.[215] Release of inflammatory mediators and their diffusion to the endothelium may cause direct damage or initiate a cytotoxic cellular response. Induction of oxidative damage by release of oxygen free radicals may play a final toxic role.[216,217] Substances derived from intraocular lenses that are directly toxic to the corneal endothelium may be produced from polymerization of IOL materials.[218] This is unlikely to be a clinically significant factor because of the low levels of such substances and their rapid clearance from the aqueous humor.

Epithelial downgrowth after cataract surgery is a rare cause of corneal edema.[219] Epithelial cells grow through the cataract wound, usually when there has been delayed wound healing or a fistula, and cover the endothelium as well as other intraocular surfaces.[220] Surgical treatment is difficult, and results are variable.[221,222] There is an undocumented perception that current cataract techniques have greatly decreased the rate of this complication.

Corneal Edema with Intraocular Lenses in Phakic Eyes

Intraocular lenses have been inserted in phakic eyes for the treatment of high myopia in limited trials beginning in the 1950s. The acceptable tolerance for corneal damage must be very low if the risk-to-benefit ratio in refractive surgery is fairly considered. There are three types of intraocular lenses being evaluated in phakic eyes for treatment of myopia, hyperopia, and astigmatism: angle-fixated anterior chamber

IOLs, iris-fixated anterior chamber IOLs, and phakic posterior chamber IOLs.

The initial anterior chamber lenses were abandoned because of poor design and manufacture causing uveitis and corneal edema. The myopic anterior chamber lenses of Baikoff, as originally designed, caused excessive corneal damage because of peripheral lens-to-cornea touch.[223] In 1991, the lens was modified to have a convex-concave shape, less angulation, and thinner optic edge to increase the lens–cornea spacing by 0.6 mm.[224] The endothelial cell loss with the modified Baikoff lens was reported to be between 20% and 28% at 2 years.[225] Further modifications have decreased the endothelial cell loss to 5.6–6.8% at 2 years and 5.5–7.5% at 3 years.[226] The third-generation Baikoff lens is the Nuvita lens, which is being evaluated by Bausch & Lomb Surgical (Irvine, CA). This lens has a larger optic diameter, and improved vaulting to minimize further potential contact between the footplate and the iris. However, initial studies demonstrate endothelial loss.[227] The Vivarte lens distributed by Ciba Vision and the Alcon angle-fixated anterior chamber lenses are both foldable, have acrylic optic and footplates, and have been investigated in the past.[228,229]

The iris-claw anterior chamber lens has also been used for myopia for many years, being marketed as the Artisan/Verisyse lens (Ophtec USA, Boca Raton, FL) with endothelial cell loss ranging from 0.7% to 10.9% at 3 years and 14.05% at 5 years and a suggestion of continuing significant cell loss.[230,231] The foldable Artiflex phakic intraocular lens for correction of myopia shows no loss of endothelial cells at 2 years.[232] The criteria for inclusion for most phakic anterior chamber lenses include endothelial cell count greater than 2300 cells/mm^2 and an anterior chamber depth greater than 3.2 mm measured by ultrasonography.

Phakic posterior chamber IOLs have undergone many modifications in design to minimize the rate of complications; however, the risk of corneal decompensation is low due to the location of these lenses.[229] The mean endothelial cell loss at 10 years is 4.7% with posterior chamber IOLs. The Visian ICL (STAAR Surgical Co., Monrovia, CA) is a collagen /HEMA copolymer posterior chamber lens aproved by the FDA in 2005 for use in the USA.

Treatment

Treatment of ABK and PBK is largely covered elsewhere in this book. Medical treatment of corneal edema is discussed in Chapter 21. Anterior stromal puncture may help reduce tearing and pain, and improve vision through regression of epithelial bullae and epithelial edema in patients with early corneal edema and those awaiting penetrating keratoplasty.[233] Annular keratotomy has also been reported with good success for patients with pain and poor visual potential.[234] The ultimate treatment for ABK and PBK is keratoplasty when visual loss and discomfort become medically untreatable. Corneal opacification in ABK and PBK may not allow full evaluation of anterior synechiae, posterior synechiae, iridectomies, intraocular lens haptic and optic positioning, and residual capsular support. The preoperative planning and prognosis can be aided with the use of ultrasound biomicroscopy.[235] The issues involved relate primarily to handling of the intraocular lens in PBK, or insertion of a secondary intraocular lens in ABK. Treatments short of keratoplasty play a limited role but are sufficient in many cases. Endokeratoplasty has become the treatment of choice over conventional penetrating keratoplasty for patients with diseased endothelium.[236]

A few treatments are specific to pseudophakic corneal edema. IOL subluxation or dislocation, causing localized or diffuse corneal edema, is treated by either repositioning or exchange of the IOL. The suturing techniques described by McCannel for stabilizing iris-support lenses are useful in various situations and should be familiar to anterior segment surgeons.[237] These techniques have been useful in repositioning posterior chamber lenses as well.[238] IOL removal has been advocated for the treatment of early corneal decompensation in the past, especially for defective IOL types such as the closed-loop anterior chamber lenses.[239] More recently, the trend has been to exchange defective lens types for posterior chamber lenses, sutured to the iris or sclera if necessary, when early edema occurs.[240] It is often difficult to determine when this approach should be used, as opposed to temporizing with topical hyperosmotic agents until vision decreases enough to warrant keratoplasty. Coli et al.[241] replaced 102 anterior chamber lenses with posterior chamber lenses, in most cases sutured to the iris, in eyes with early corneal edema. With a mean of 18 months of follow-up, vision was stabilized in about 75%. A little less than one-quarter (23.5%) had progression to frank endothelial decompensation. Of those corneas decompensating, 75% had preoperative cell counts of 500 cells/mm^2 or less.

Future Considerations

The emphasis on corneal complications of intraocular surgery has shifted over the past two decades from recognition to management and to prevention. Through this process, surgical techniques and IOL design, materials, and manufacture have greatly improved. Continued awareness of the relationship between intraocular surgery and corneal structure and function will be necessary to minimize this problem in the future. Specifically, the effects of new instrumentation, IOL materials, and direct corneal incisions should be studied carefully in prospective long-term investigations.

References

1. Hall MJ, Lawrence L. *Ambulatory surgery in the United States, 1996, advance data from vital and health statistics; no. 300.* Hyattsville, Maryland: National Center for Health Statistics, 1998.
2. Congdon N, Friedman D, Kempen J, O'Colmain J. The prevalence of clinically significant cataract, cataract surgery and related disabilities in the United States. *Invest Ophthalmol Vis Sci.* 2002;43:E-Abstract 937.
3. Schulze SD, Sekundo W, Kroll P. Autologous serum for the treatment of corneal epithelial abrasions in diabetic patients undergoing vitrectomy. *Am J Ophthalmol.* 2006;142:207–211.
4. Ernest P, Rhem M, McDermott M, Lavery K, Sensoli A. Phacoemulsification conditions resulting in thermal wound injury. *J Cataract Refract Surg.* 2001;27:1829–1839.
5. Bradley MJ, Olson, RJ. A survey about phacoemulsification incision thermal contraction incidence and causal relationships. *Am J Ophthalmol.* 2006;141:222–224.
6. Sippel KC, Pineda R. Phacoemulsification and thermal wound injury. *Semin Ophthalmol.* 2002;17:102–109.

7. Braga-Mele R. Thermal effect of microburst and hyperpulse settings during sleeveless bimanual phacoemulsification with advanced power modulations. *J Cataract Refract Surg*. 2006;32:639–642.
8. Liu DT, Lai JS, Lam DS. Descemet membrane detachment after sequential argon-neodymium:YAG laser peripheral iridotomy. *Am J Ophthalmol*. 2002;134:621.
9. Ocakoglu O, Ustundag C, Devranoglu K, et al. Repair of Descemet's membrane detachment after viscocanalostomy. *J Cataract Refract Surg*. 2002;28:1703.
10. Kozlova T, Zagorski ZF, Rakowska E. A simplified technique for non-penetrating deep sclerectomy. *Eur J Ophthalmol*. 2002;12:188.
11. Sugar HS. Prognosis in stripping of Descemet's membrane. *Am J Ophthalmol*. 1967;63:140–143.
12. Sparks GM. Descemetopexy. Surgical reattachment of stripped Descemet's membrane. *Arch Ophthalmol*. 1967;78:31–34.
13. Wyatt H, Ghosh J. Reposition of Descemet's membrane after cataract extraction. A case report. *Br J Ophthalmol*. 1959;53:267–269.
14. Greenhut J, Sargent R, Pilkerton R. Descemetopexy. A report of two cases. *Ann Ophthalmol*. 1971;3:1244–1246 passim.
15. Mackool RJ, Holtz SJ. Descemet membrane detachment. *Arch Ophthalmol*. 1977;95:459–463.
16. Makley TA, Keates RH. Detachment of Descemet's membrane (an early complication of cataract surgery). *Ophthalmic Surg*. 1980;11:189–191.
17. Dowlut SM, Brunet M. Décollement de la membrane de Descemet dans la chirurgie de la cataracte. *Can J Ophthalmol*. 1980;15:122–124.
18. Merrick C. Descemet's membrane detachment treated by penetrating keratoplasty. *Ophthalmic Surg*. 1991;22:753–755.
19. Hagan III JC. Treatment of progressive Descemet's membrane detachment [letter]. *Ophthalmic Surg*. 1992;23:641–642.
20. Anderson CJ. Gonioscopy in no-stitch cataract incisions. *J Cataract Refract Surg*. 1993;19:620–621.
21. Minkovitz JB, Schrenk LC, Pepose JS. Spontaneous resolution of an extensive detachment of Descemet's membrane following phacoemulsification. *Arch Ophthalmol*. 1994;112:551–552.
22. Ellis DR, Cohen KL. Sulfur hexafluoride gas in the repair of Descemet's membrane detachment. *Cornea*. 1995;14:436–437.
23. Walland MJ, Stevens JD, Steele ADM. Repair of Descemet's membrane detachment after intraocular surgery. *J Cataract Refract Surg*. 1995;21: 250–253.
24. Assia EI, Levkovich-Verbin H, Blumenthal M. Management of Descemet's membrane detachment. *J Cataract Refract Surg*. 1995 21:714–717.
25. Gault JA, Raber IM. Repair of Descemet's membrane detachment with intracameral injection of 20% sulfur hexafluoride gas. *Cornea*. 1996;15: 483–489.
26. Kremer I, Stiebel H, Yassur Y, Weinberger D. Sulfur hexafluoride injection for Descemet's membrane detachment in cataract surgery. *J Cataract Refract Surg*. 1997;23:1449–1453.
27. Macsai MS, Gainer KM, Chisholm L. Repair of Descemet's membrane detachment with perfluoropropane (C_3F_8). *Cornea*. 1998;17:129–134.
28. Mahmood MA, Teichmann KD, Tomey KF, Al-Rashed D. Detachment of Descemet's membrane. *J Cataract Refract Surg*. 1998;24:827–833.
29. Kansal S, Sugar J. Consecutive Descemet membrane detachment after successive phacoemulsification. *Cornea*. 2001;20:670–671.
30. Donzis PB, Karcioglu ZA, Insler MS. Sodium hyaluronate (Healon®) in the surgical repair of Descemet's membrane detachment. *Ophthalmic Surg*. 1986;17:735–737.
31. Marcon AS, Rapuano CJ, Jones MR, et al. Descemet's membrane detachment after cataract surgery: management and outcome. *Ophthalmology*. 2002;109:2325.
32. Vastine DW, et al. Stripping of Descemet's membrane associated with intraocular lens implantation. *Arch Ophthalmol*. 1983;101:1042.
33. Zeiter HJ, Zeiter JT. Descemet's membrane separation during five hundred forty-four intraocular lens implantations; 1975 through 1982. *Am Intraocular Implant Soc J*. 1983;9:36.
34. Kremer I, Stiebel H, Yassur Y, et al. Sulfur hexafluoride injection for Descemet's membrane detachment in cataract surgery. *J Cataract Refract Surg*. 1997;23:1449.
35. Macsai MS, Gainer KM, Chisholm L. Repair of Descemet's membrane detachment with perfluoropropane (C_3F_8). *Cornea*. 1998;17:129.
36. Morrison LK, Talley TW, Waltman SR. Spontaneous detachment of Descemet's membrane. Case report and literature review. *Cornea*. 1989;8:303–305.
37. Bergsma DR, McCaa CS. Extensive detachment of Descemet membrane after holmium laser sclerostomy. *Ophthalmology*. 1996;103:678–680.
38. Waring GO. The 50-year epidemic of pseudophakic corneal edema. *Arch Ophthalmol*. 1989;107:657.
39. Hess C. Klinische und experimintelle studie uber die entstehung der streifenformigen hornhauttraubung nach starextraktion. *Graefe's Arch Clin Exp Ophthalmol*. 1892;38:1.
40. Cogan DG. Experimental production of so-called bullous keratitis. *Arch Ophthalmol*. 1940;23:918.
41. Stocker FW. *The endothelium of the cornea and its clinical implications*. Springfield, IL: Charles C Thomas; 1971.
42. Fine M. Penetrating keratoplasty in aphakia. *Arch Ophthalmol*. 1964;72:50.
43. Nordlohne ME. *The intraocular implant lens: development and results with special reference to the Binkhorst lens*. Baltimore: Williams & Wilkins; 1975.
44. Oxford Cataract Treatment and Evaluation Team (OCTET). I. Cataract surgery: interim results and complications of a randomized controlled trial. *Br J Ophthalmol*. 1986;70:402.
45. Jaffe NS, et al. A comparison of 500 Binkhorst implants with 500 routine intracapsular cataract extractions. *Am J Ophthalmol*. 1978;85:24.
46. Taylor DM, et al. Pseudophakic bullous keratopathy. *Ophthalmology*. 1983;90:19.
47. Vail D. After-results of vitreous loss. *Am J Ophthalmol*. 1965;59:573.
48. Binkhorst CD. The iridocapsular (two-loop) lens and the iris-clip (4-loop) lens in pseudophakia. *Trans Am Acad Ophthalmol Otolaryngol*. 1973;77:589.
49. Pearce JL. Long-term results of the Binkhorst iris-clip lens in senile cataract. *Br J Ophthalmol*. 1972;56:319.
50. Jaffe NS, Duffner LR. The iris-plane (Copeland) pseudophakos. *Arch Ophthalmol*. 1976;94:420.
51. Drews RC. Inflammatory response, endophthalmitis, corneal dystrophy, glaucoma, retinal detachment, dislocation, refractive error, lens removal and enucleation. *Trans Am Acad Ophthalmol Otolaryngol*. 1978;85:164.
52. Tennant JL. Results of primary and secondary implants using Choyce mark VIII lens. *Ophthalmic Surg*. 1977;8:54.
53. Stark WJ, et al. The FDA report on intraocular lenses. *Ophthalmology*. 1983;90:311.
54. Stark WJ, et al. Closed-loop anterior chamber lenses. *Arch Ophthalmol*. 1987;105:20.
55. Hagan JC. A clinical review of the IOLAB Azar model 91Z flexible anterior chamber intraocular lens. *Ophthalmic Surg*. 1987;18:258.
56. Apple DJ, Olson RJ. Closed-loop anterior chamber lenses. *Arch Ophthalmol*. 1987;105:19.
57. Smith PW, et al. Complications of semi-flexible, closed-loop anterior chamber intraocular lenses. *Arch Ophthalmol*. 1987;105:52.
58. Beehler CC. Follow-up of the Stableflex lens. *J Cataract Refract Surg*. 1987;13:84.
59. Stokes HR. The Hessburg flexible anterior chamber intraocular lens. *Ophthalmic Surg*. 1984;15:985.
60. Sugar J, Wiet SP, Meisler DM. Pseudophakic bullous keratopathy with Intermedics model 024 (Hessburg) anterior chamber intraocular lens. *Arch Ophthalmol*. 1988;106:1575.
61. Lee DA, Price FW, Whitson WE. Intraocular complications associated with the Dubroff anterior chamber lens. *J Cataract Refract Surg*. 1994;20:421.
62. Liu JF, Koch DD, Emery JM. Complications of implanting three-piece C-loop posterior chamber lenses in the anterior chamber. *Ophthalmic Surg*. 1988;19:802.
63. Lim ES, et al. An analysis of flexible anterior chamber lenses with special reference to the normalized rate of lens explantation. *Ophthalmology*. 1991;98:243.
64. Bigar F. Pseudophakic bullous keratopathy in Switzerland. *Dev Ophthalmol*. 1989;18:154.
65. Canner JK, Javitt JC, McBean AM. National outcomes of cataract extraction. III. Corneal edema and transplant following inpatient surgery. *Arch Ophthalmol*. 1992;110:1137.
66. Sanders N. Penetrating keratoplasty for aphakic bullous keratopathy. *South Med J*. 1968;61:869.
67. Smith RE, et al. Penetrating keratoplasty, changing indications, 1947 to 1978. *Arch Ophthalmol*. 1980;98:1226.
68. Robin JB, et al. An update of the indications for penetrating keratoplasty. 1979 through 1983. *Arch Ophthalmol*. 1986;104:87.
69. Brady SE, Rapuano CJ, Arentsen JJ, et al. Clinical indications for and procedures associated with penetrating keratoplasty. 1983–1988. *Am J Ophthalmol*. 1989;108:118.
70. Cosar CB, Sridhar MS, Cohen E, et al. Indications for penetrating keratoplasty and associated procedures, 1996–2000. *Cornea*. 2002;21:148.
71. Maeno A, Naor J, Lee HM, et al. Three decades of corneal transplantation: indications and patient characteristics. *Cornea*. 2000;19:7.
72. Sugar A, et al. Specular microscopic follow-up of corneal grafts for pseudophakic bullous keratopathy. *Ophthalmology*. 1985;92:325.
73. Haamann P, Jensen DM, Schmidt P. Changing indications for penetrating keratoplasty. *Acta Ophthalmol*. 1994;72:443.
74. Lindquist TD, McGlothan JS, Rotkis WM, et al. Indications for penetrating keratoplasty: 1980–1988. *Cornea*. 1991;10:210.

75. Sharif KW, Casey TA. Changing indications for penetrating keratoplasty. 1971 through 1990. *Eye*. 1993;7:485.
76. Edwards M, Clover GM, Brookes N, et al. Indications for corneal transplantation in New Zealand: 1991–1999. *Cornea*. 2002;21:152.
77. Chan CM, Wong TY, Yeong SM, et al. Penetrating keratoplasty in the Singapore National Eye Centre and donor cornea acquisition in the Singapore Eye Bank. *Ann Acad Med Singapore*. 1997;26:395.
78. Cursiefen C, Küchle M, Naumann G. Changing indications for penetrating keratoplasty: histopathology of 1,250 corneal buttons. *Cornea*. 1998;17:468.
79. Chen WL, Hu FR, Wang IJ. Changing indications for penetrating keratoplasty in Taiwan from 1987 to 1999. *Cornea*. 2001;20:141.
80. Dobbins K, Price F, Whitson W. Trends in the indications for penetrating keratoplasty in the midwestern United States. *Cornea*. 2000;19:813.
81. Mamalis N, Anderson CW, Kreisler KR, et al. Changing trends in the indications for penetrating keratoplasty. *Arch Ophthalmol*. 1992;110:1409.
82. Solomon KD, et al. Complications of intraocular lenses with special reference to an analysis of 2,500 explanted intraocular lenses (IOLs). *Eur J Implant Refract Surg*. 1991;3:195.
83. Sugar A, Sugar J. Techniques in penetrating keratoplasty. *Cornea*. 2000;19:603.
84. Eye Bank Association of America. *2007 Eye Banking Statistical Report*. Washington, DC: 11–12.
85. Liu G, et al. Histopathological study of pseudophakic bullous keratopathy developing after anterior chamber or iris-supported intraocular lens implantation. *Jpn J Ophthalmol*. 1993;37:414,.
86. Champion R, Green WR. Intraocular lenses. A histopathologic study of eyes, ocular tissues, and intraocular lenses obtained surgically. *Ophthalmology*. 1985;92:1628.
87. Ljubimov AV, Burgeson RE, Butkowski RJ, et al. Extracellular matrix alterations in human corneas with bullous keratopathy. *Invest Ophthalmol Vis Sci*. 1996;37:997.
88. Maseruka H, Ataullah SM, Zardi L, et al. Tenascin-cytotactin (TN-C) variants in pseudophakic/aphakic bullous keratopathy corneas. *Eye*. 1998;12:729.
89. Quantock AJ, Meek KM, Brittain P, et al. Alteration of stromal architecture and depletion of keratan sulphate proteoglycans in oedematous human corneas: histological, immunochemical and X-ray diffraction evidence. *Tissue Cell*. 1991;23:593.
90. Hsu JK, Rubinfeld RS, Barry P, et al. Anterior stromal puncture: immunohistochemical studies in human corneas. *Arch Ophthalmol*. 1993;111:1057.
91. Ljubimov AV, Saghizadeh M, Spirin KS, et al. Expression of tenascin-C splice variants in normal and bullous keratopathy human corneas. *Invest Ophthalmol Vis Sci*. 1998;39:1135.
92. Saghizadeh M, Khin HL, Bourdon MA, et al. Novel splice variants of human tenascin-C mRNA identified in normal and bullous keratopathy corneas. *Cornea*. 1998;17:326.
93. Rosenbaum JT, Planck ST, Huang XN, et al. Detection of mRNA for the cytokines, interleukin-1 alpha and interleukin-8, in corneas from patients with pseudophakic bullous keratopathy. *Invest Ophthalmol Vis Sci*. 1995;36:2151.
94. Ljubimov AV, Saghizadeh M, Pytela R, et al. Increased expression of tenascin-C binding epithelial integrins in human bullous keratopathy corneas. *J Histochem Cytochem*. 2001;49:1341.
95. Ljubimov AV, Saghizadeh M, Spirin KS, et al. Increased expression of fibrillin-1 in human corneas with bullous keratopathy. *Cornea*. 1998;17:309.
96. Akhtar S, Bron AJ, Hawksworth NR, et al. Ultrastructural morphology and expression of proteoglycans, Big-h3, tenascin-C, fibrillin-1, and fibronectin in bullous keratopathy. *Br J Ophthalmol*. 2001;85:720.
97. Saghizadeh M, Chwa M, Aoki A, et al. Altered expression of growth factors and cytokines in keratoconus, bullous keratopathy and diabetic human corneas. *Exp Eye Res*. 2001;73:179.
98. Spirin KS, Ljubimov AV, Castellon R, et al. Analysis of gene expression in human bullous keratopathy corneas containing limiting amounts of RNA. *Invest Ophthalmol Vis Sci*. 1999;40:3108.
99. Wolter JR. Pathologie des hornahautendothels bei pseudophaker keratopathie. *Fortschr Ophthalmol*. 1987;84:109.
100. Apple DJ, et al. *Intraocular lenses: evolution, designs, complications and pathology*. Baltimore: Williams & Wilkins; 1989.
101. Kenyon KR, VanHorn DL, Edelhauser HF. Endothelial degeneration and posterior collagenous proliferation in aphakic bullous keratopathy. *Am J Ophthalmol*. 1978;85:329.
102. Lugo M, et al. The incidence of preoperative endothelial dystrophy in pseudophakic bullous keratopathy. *Ophthalmic Surg*. 1988;19:16.
103. Bourne WM, Kaufman HE. Cataract extraction and the corneal endothelium. *Am J Ophthalmol*. 1976;82:44.
104. Bourne WM, Kaufman HE. Endothelial damage associated with intraocular lenses. *Am J Ophthalmol*. 1976;81:482.
105. Sugar A, et al. Endothelial cell loss from intraocular lens insertion. *Ophthalmology*. 1978;85:394.
106. Galin M, et al. Time analysis of corneal endothelial cell density after cataract extraction. *Am J Ophthalmol*. 1979;88:93.
107. Schultz RO, et al. Response of the corneal endothelium to cataract surgery. *Arch Ophthalmol*. 1986;104:1164.
108. Drews RC, Waltman SR. Endothelial cell loss and intraocular lens placement. *Am Intraocular Implant Soc J*. 1978;4:14.
109. Forstot SL, et al. The effect of intraocular lens implantation on the corneal endothelium. *Trans Am Acad Ophthalmol Otolaryngol*. 1977;83:195.
110. Hirst LW, et al. Quantitative corneal endothelial evaluation in intraocular lens implantation and cataract surgery. *Am J Ophthalmol*. 1977;84:775.
111. Cheng H, et al. Endothelial cell loss and corneal thickness after intracapsular extraction and iris clip lens implantation: a randomized controlled trial. *Br J Ophthalmol*. 1977;61:785.
112. Bourne WM, et al. Corneal trauma in intracapsular and extracapsular cataract extraction with lens implantation. *Arch Ophthalmol*. 1981;99:1375.
113. Sugar J, Mitchelson J, Kraff M. The effect of phacoemulsification on corneal endothelial cell density. *Arch Ophthalmol*. 1978;96:446.
114. Liesegang TJ, Bourne WM, Ilstrup DM. Short- and long-term endothelial cell loss associated with cataract extraction and intraocular lens implantation. *Am J Ophthalmol*. 1984;97:32.
115. Oxford Cataract Treatment and Evaluation Team (OCTET). Long-term corneal endothelial cell loss after cataract surgery. *Arch Ophthalmol*. 1986;104:1170.
116. Martin NF, Stark WJ, Maumenee AE. Continuing corneal endothelial loss in intracapsular surgery with and without Binkhorst four-loop lenses: a long-term specular microscopy study. *Ophthalmic Surg*. 1987;18:867.
117. Werblin TP. Long-term endothelial cell loss following phacoemulsification: model for evaluating endothelial damage after intraocular surgery. *Refract Corneal Surg*. 1993;9:29.
118. Levy JH, Pisacano AM. Endothelial cell loss in four types of intraocular lens implant procedures. *J Am Intraocul Implant Soc*. 1985;11:465.
119. Rafuse PE, Nichols BD. Effects of Healon vs. Viscoat on endothelial cell count and morphology after phacoemulsification and posterior chamber lens implantation. *Can J Ophthalmol*. 1992;27:125.
120. Koch DD, et al. A comparison of corneal endothelial change after use of Healon or Viscoat during phacoemulsification. *Am J Ophthalmol*. 1993;115:188.
121. Hayasaki K, Nakao F, Hayashi F. Corneal endothelial cell loss after phacoemulsification using nuclear cracking technique. *J Cataract Refract Surg*. 1994;20:44.
122. Zetterstrom C, Laurell CG. Comparison of endothelial cell loss and phacoemulsification energy during endocapsular phacoemulsification surgery. *J Cataract & Refract Surg*. 1995;21:55.
123. Wirbelauer C, Anders N, Pham DT, et al. Early postoperative endothelial cell loss after corneoscleral tunnel incision and phacoemulsification in pseudoexfoliation syndrome. *Ophthalmologe*. 1997;94:332.
124. Ravalico G, Tognetto D, Palomba MA, et al. Corneal endothelial function after extracapsular cataract extraction and phacoemulsification. *J Cataract Refract Surg*. 1997;23:1000.
125. Lee JH, Oh SY. Corneal endothelial cell loss from suture fixation of a posterior chamber intraocular lens. *J Cataract Refract Surg*. 1997;23:1020.
126. Wirbelauer C, Anders N, Pham DT, et al. Corneal endothelial cell changes in pseudoexfoliation syndrome after cataract surgery. *Arch Ophthalmol*. 1998;116:145.
127. Ventura AC, Walti R, Bohnke M. Corneal thickness and endothelial density before and after cataract surgery. *Br J Ophthalmol*. 2001;85:18.
128. Holzer MP, Tetz MR, Auffarth GU, et al. Effect of Healon 5 and 4 other viscoelastic substances on intraocular pressure and endothelium after cataract surgery. *J Cataract Refract Surg*. 2001;27:213.
129. Miyata K, Maruoka S, Nakahara M, et al. Corneal endothelial cell protection during phacoemulsification: low- versus high-molecular-weight sodium hyaluronate. *J Cataract Refract Surg*. 2002;28:1557.
130. Mathys KC, Cohen KL, Armstrong BD. Determining factors for corneal endothelial cell loss by using bimanual microincision phacoemulsification and power modulation. *Cornea*. 2007;26:1049.
131. Bates AK, Hiorns RW, Cheng H. Modelling of changes in the corneal endothelium after cataract surgery and penetrating keratoplasty. *Br J Ophthalmol*. 1992;76:32.
132. Liesegang TJ, Bourne WM, Ilstrup DM. Prospective 5-year postoperative study of cataract extraction and lens implantation. *Trans Am Ophthalmol Soc*. 1989;87:57.

133. Bourne WM, Nelson LR, Hodge DO. Continued endothelial cell loss ten years after lens implantation. *Ophthalmology*. 1994;101:1014.
134. Bates AK, Cheng H, Hiorns RW. Pseudophakic bullous keratopathy: relationship with endothelial cell density and use of a predictive cell loss model. *Curr Eye Res*. 1986;5:363.
135. Hoffer KJ. Corneal decompensation after corneal endothelium cell count. *Am J Ophthalmol*. 1979;87:252.
136. Hoffer KJ, Phillippi G. Vertical endothelial cell disparity. *Am J Ophthalmol*. 1979;87:344.
137. Olsen T. Corneal thickness and endothelial damage after intracapsular cataract extraction. *Acta Ophthalmol*. 1980;58:424.
138. Brown SI, McLean JM. Peripheral corneal edema after cataract extraction, a new clinical entity. *Trans Am Acad Ophthalmol Otolaryngol*. 1969;73:465,.
139. Brown SI. Peripheral corneal edema after cataract extraction. *Am J Ophthalmol*. 1970;70:326.
140. Gothard TW, et al. Clinical findings in Brown-McLean syndrome. *Am J Ophthalmol*. 1993;115:729.
141. Lim JI, Lam S, Sugar J. Brown-McLean syndrome. *Arch Ophthalmol*. 1991;109:22.
142. Reed JW, Cain LR, Weaver RG, et al. Clinical and pathologic findings of aphakic peripheral corneal edema: Brown-McLean syndrome. *Cornea*. 1992;11:577.
143. Charlin R. Peripheral corneal edema after cataract extraction. *Am J Ophthalmol*. 1985;99:298.
144. Tuft SJ, Kerr MM, Sherrard ES, et al. Peripheral corneal oedema following cataract extraction (Brown-McLean syndrome). *Eye*. 1992;6:502.
145. Sugar A. Brown-McLean syndrome occurring in a corneal graft. *Cornea*. 1997;16:493.
146. Mamalis N, Edelhauser HF, Dawson DG, et al. Toxic anterior segment syndrome. *J Cataract Refract Surg*. 2006;32:324–333.
147. Maier P, Birnbaum F, Böhringer D, Reinhard T. Toxic anterior segment syndrome following penetrating keratoplasty. *Arch Ophthalmol*. 2008;126:1677–1681.
148. Kutty PK, Forster TS, Wood-Koob C, et al. Multistate outbreak of toxic anterior segment syndrome, 2005. *J Cataract Refract Surg*. 2008;34:585–590.
149. Waltman SR. Penetrating keratoplasty for pseudophakic bullous keratopathy. *Arch Ophthalmol*. 1981;99:415,.
150. Rao GN, et al. Pseudophakic bullous keratopathy. Relationship to preoperative corneal endothelial status. *Ophthalmology*. 1984;91:1135.
151. Rao GN, et al. Endothelial cell morphology and corneal deturgescence. *Ann Ophthalmol*. 1979;11:885.
152. Cheng H, et al. Positive correlation of corneal thickness and endothelial cell loss. Serial measurements after cataract surgery. *Arch Ophthalmol*. 1988;106:920.
153. Bates AK, Cheng H. Bullous keratopathy: a study of endothelial cell morphology in patients undergoing cataract surgery. *Br J Ophthalmol*. 1988;72:409.
154. Koenig SB, Schultz RO. Penetrating keratoplasty for pseudophakic bullous keratopathy after extracapsular cataract extraction. *Am J Ophthalmol*. 1988;105:348.
155. Seitzman GD, Gottsch JD, Stark WJ. Cataract surgery in patients with Fuchs' corneal dystrophy: expanding recommendations for cataract surgery without simultaneous keratoplasty. *Ophthalmology*. 2005;112:441.
156. Naumann GO, Schlotzer-Schrehardt U. Keratopathy in pseudoexfoliation syndrome as a cause of corneal endothelial decompensation: a clinico-pathologic study. *Ophthalmology*. 2000;107:1111.
157. Ishikawa A. Risk factors for reduced corneal endothelial cell density before cataract surgery. *J Cataract Refract Surg*. 2002;28:1982.
158. American Academy of Ophthalmology. Ophthalmic procedures assessment, corneal endothelial photography. *Ophthalmology*. 1991;98:1464.
159. Kiessling LA, Ernest PH, Lavery KT. Scleral tunnel incision with internal corneal lip in patients with low preoperative endothelial cell counts. *J Cataract Refract Surg*. 1993;19:610.
160. Galin MA, et al. Experimental cataract surgery. *Ophthalmology*. 1979;86:213.
161. Amon M, et al. Endothelial cell density and corneal pachymetry after no-stitch, small incision cataract surgery. *Doc Ophthalmol*. 1992;81:301.
162. Hoffer KJ. Cell loss with superior and temporal incisions. *J Cataract Refract Surg*. 1994;20:368.
163. Kraff MC, Sanders DR, Lieberman HL. Monitoring for continuing endothelial cell loss with cataract extraction and intraocular lens implantation. *Ophthalmology*. 1982;89:30.
164. Duffy RE, Brown SE, Caldwell KL, et al. An epidemic of corneal destruction caused by plasma gas sterilization. The Toxic Cell Destruction Syndrome Investigative Team. *Arch Ophthalmol*. 2000;118:1167.
165. Smith CA, Khoury JM, Shields SM, et al. Unexpected corneal endothelial cell decompensation after intraocular surgery with instruments sterilized by plasma gas. *Ophthalmology*. 2000;107:1561.
166. Courtright P, Lewallen S, Holland SP, et al. Corneal decompensation after cataract surgery. An outbreak investigation in Asia. *Ophthalmology*. 1995;102:1461.
167. Edelhauser HF, et al. Intraocular irrigating solutions: their effect on the corneal endothelium. *Arch Ophthalmol*. 1975;93:648.
168. Edelhauser HF, et al. Osmotic tolerance of rabbit and human corneal endothelium. *Arch Ophthalmol*. 1981;99:1281.
169. Gonnering R, et al. The pH tolerance of rabbit and human corneal endothelium. *Invest Ophthalmol Vis Sci*. 1979;18:373.
170. Edelhauser HF, Gonnering R, VanHorn DL. Intraocular irrigating solutions: a comparative study of BSS Plus and lactated Ringer's solution. *Arch Ophthalmol*. 1978;96:516.
171. Claoue C, et al. A prospective randomized double-masked clinical comparison of Hartman's solution and balanced salt solution in phacoemulsification. *Eur J Implant Ref Surg*. 1994;6:54.
172. Li J, et al. Effects of BSS and BSS+ irrigation solutions on rabbit corneal transendothelial electrical potential differences. *Cornea*. 1993;12:199.
173. Benson WE, Diamond JG, Tasman W. Intraocular irrigating solutions for pars plana vitrectomy. *Arch Ophthalmol*. 1981;99:1013.
174. Patel BCK, Byrnes TA, Crandall A, et al. A comparison of topical and retrobulbar anesthesia for cataract surgery. *Ophthalmology*. 1996;103:1196.
175. Karp CL, Cox TA, Wagoner MD, et al. Intracameral anesthesia. *Ophthalmology*. 2001;108:1704.
176. Martin RG, Miller JD, Cox CC 3rd, et al. Safety and efficacy of intracameral injections of unpreserved lidocaine to reduce intraocular sensation. *J Cataract Refract Surg*. 1998;24:961.
177. Elvira JC, Hueso JR, Martinez-Toldos J, et al. Induced endothelial cell loss in phacoemulsification using topical anesthesia plus intracameral lidocaine. *J Cataract Refract Surg*. 1999;25:640.
178. Eggeling P, Pleyer U, Hartmann C, et al. Corneal endothelial toxicity of different lidocaine concentrations. *J Cataract Refract Surg*. 2000;26:1403.
179. Judge AJ, Najafi K, Lee DA, Miller KM. Corneal endothelial toxicity of topical anesthesia. *Ophthalmology*. 1997;104:1373–1379.
180. Edelhauser HF, et al. Corneal edema and the intraocular use of epinephrine. *Am J Ophthalmol*. 1982;93:327.
181. Myers WG, Shugar JK. Optimizing the intracameral dilation regimen for cataract surgery. *J Cataract Refract Surg*. 2009;35:273.
182. Eleftheriadis H, Cheong M, Sandeman S, et al. Corneal toxicity secondary to inadvertent use of benzalkonium chloride preserved viscoelastic material in cataract surgery. *Br J Ophthalmol*. 2002;86:299.
183. Yee RW, Edelhauser HF. Comparison of intraocular acetylcholine and carbachol. *J Cataract Refract Surg*. 1986;12:18.
184. Birmbaum DB, et al. Effect of carbachol on rabbit corneal endothelium. *Arch Ophthalmol*. 1987;105:253.
185. Olson RJ, et al. Commonly used intraocular medications and the corneal endothelium. *Arch Ophthalmol*. 1980;98:2224.
186. Grimmett MR, et al. Corneal edema after Miochol. *Am J Ophthalmol*. 1993;116:236.
187. Sandboe FD, Medin W, Bjerknes R. Toxicity of vancomycin on corneal endothelium in rabbits. *Acta Ophthalmologica Scand*. 1998;76:675.
188. Alp BN, Elibol O, Sargon MF, et al. The effect of povidone iodine on the corneal endothelium. *Cornea*. 2000;19:546.
189. Kaufman HE, Katz JC. Endothelial damage from intraocular lens insertion. *Invest Ophthalmol*. 1976;15:996.
190. Sugar J, Mitchelson J, Kraff M. Endothelial trauma and cell loss from intraocular lens insertion. *Arch Ophthalmol*. 1978;96:449.
191. Snellingen T, Shrestha JK, Huq F, et al. The South Asian Cataract Management Study: complications, vision outcomes, and corneal endothelial cell loss in a randomized multicenter clinical trial comparing intracapsular cataract extraction with and without anterior chamber intraocular lens implantation. *Ophthalmology*. 2000;107:231.
192. Bourne WM, Brubaker RF, O'Fallon WM. Use of air to decrease endothelial cell loss during intraocular lens implantation. *Arch Ophthalmol*. 1979;97:1473.
193. Eiferman RA, Wilkins EL. The effect of air on human corneal endothelium. *Am J Ophthalmol*. 1981;92:328.
194. Kerr Muir MG, et al. Air, methylcellulose, sodium hyaluronate and the corneal endothelium. *Eye*. 1987;1:480.
195. Katz J, et al. Process of endothelial damage from intraocular lens insertion. *Trans Am Acad Ophthalmol Otolaryngol*. 1977;83:204.

196. Pape LG, Balazs E. The use of sodium hyaluronate (Healon) in human anterior segment surgery. *Ophthalmology*. 1980;87:699.
197. Miller D, Stegman R. Use of Na-hyaluronate in anterior segment surgery. *Am Intraocular Implant Soc J*. 1980;6:13.
198. Hoffer AJ. Effects of extracapsular implant techniques on endothelial density. *Arch Ophthalmol*. 1982;100:791.
199. Pedersen OO. Comparison of the protective effects of methylcellulose and sodium hyaluronate on corneal swelling following phacoemulsification of senile cataracts. *J Cataract Refract Surg*. 1990;16:594.
200. Glasser DB, et al. Endothelial protection and viscoelastic retention during phacoemulsi?cation and intraocular lens implantation. *Arch Ophthalmol*. 1991;109:1438.
201. Behndig A, Lundberg B. Transient corneal edema after phacoemulsification: comparison of 3 viscoelastic regimens. *J Cataract Refract Surg*. 2002;28:1551.
202. Probst LE, Nichols BD. Corneal endothelial and intraocular pressure changes after phacoemulsification with Amvisc plus and Viscoat. *J Cataract Refract Surg*. 1993;19:725.
203. Balent A, Civerchia LL, Mohamadi P. Visual outcomes of cataract extraction and lens implantation complicated by vitreous loss. *J Cataract Refract Surg*. 1988;14:158.
204. Blodi BA, et al. Retained nuclei after cataract extraction. *Ophthalmology*. 1992;99:41.
205. Gilliland GD, Hutton WL, Fuller DG. Retained intravitreal lens fragments after cataract surgery. *Ophthalmology*. 1992;99:1263.
206. Bohigian GM, Wexler SA. Complications of retained nuclear fragments in the anterior chamber after phacoemulsification with posterior chamber lens implant. *Am J Ophthalmol*. 1997;123:546.
207. Nielsen CB. The effect of prostaglandin-inhibitor naproxen on the endothelial cell loss after cataract extraction. *Acta Ophthalmol*. 1983;61:102.
208. Evans K, O'Brien C, Patterson A. Corneal endothelial response to corticosteroid in cataract surgery. *Eur J Implant Refract Surg*. 1994;6:74.
209. Leahey BD. Bullous keratitis from vitreous contact: edema of cornea secondary to vitreous contact. *Arch Ophthalmol*. 1951;46:22.
210. Sears ML, McLean EB, Bellows AR. Drug-induced retraction of the vitreous face after cataract extraction. *Trans Am Acad Ophthalmol Otolaryngol*. 1972;76:498.
211. Homer PI, Peyman GA, Sugar J. Automated vitrectomy in eyes with vitreocorneal touch associated with corneal dysfunction. *Am J Ophthalmol*. 1980;89:500.
212. Fourman S. Management of cornea-lens touch after filtering surgery for glaucoma. *Ophthalmology*. 1990;97:424.
213. Richards BW, et al. The effects of nonfixated lower lens haptics of Binkhorst lens on corneal endothelial cell density. *Ophthalmic Surg*. 1986;17:286.
214. Jacobs PM, Cheng H, Price NC. Pseudophakodonesis and corneal endothelial contact: direct observations by high-speed cinematography. *Br J Ophthalmol*. 1983;67:650.
215. Obstbaum SA, Galin MA. Cystoid macular oedema and ocular inflammation; the corneo-retinal inflammatory syndrome. *Trans Ophthalmol Soc UK*. 1979;99:187.
216. Hull DS, et al. Hydrogen peroxide-mediated corneal endothelial damage; induction by oxygen free radical. *Invest Ophthalmol Vis Sci*. 1984;25:1246.
217. Rao NA, et al. Modulation of lens-induced uveitis by superoxide dismutase. *Ophthalmic Res*. 1986;18:41.
218. Holyk PR, Eifrig DE. Effects of monomeric methylmethacrylate on ocular tissues. *Am J Ophthalmol*. 1979;88:385.
219. Weiner MJ, et al. Epithelial downgrowth: a 30-year clinicopathologic review. *Br J Ophthalmol*. 1989;73:6.
220. Maumenee AE. Treatment of epithelial downgrowth and intraocular fistula following cataract extraction. *Trans Am Ophthalmol Soc*. 1964;62:153.
221. Stark WJ, et al. Surgical management of epithelial ingrowth. *Am J Ophthalmol*. 1978;85:772.
222. Naumann GOH, Rummelt V. Block excision of cystic and diffuse epithelial ingrowth of the anterior chamber. *Arch Ophthalmol*. 1992;110:223.
223. Mimouni F, et al. Damage to the corneal endothelium from anterior chamber intraocular lenses in phakic myopic eyes. *Refract Corneal Surg*. 1991;7:277.
224. Waring GO. Phakic intraocular lenses for high myopia: where do we go from here? *Refract Corneal Surg*. 1991;7:275.
225. Baikoff G. Phakic anterior chamber intraocular lenses. *Int Ophthalmol Clin*. 1991;31:75.
226. Baikoff G, Arne J, Bokobza Y, et al. Angle-fixated anterior chamber phakic intraocular lens for myopia of –7 to –19 diopters. *J Refract Surg*. 1998;14:282.
227. Alió JL, de la Hoz F, Pérez S, et al. Phakic anterior chamber lenses for the correction of myopia: a 7-year cumulative analysis of complications in 263 cases. *Ophthalmology*. 1999;106:458.
228. Kohnen T, Baumeister M, Magdowski G. Scanning electron microscopic characteristics of phakic intraocular lenses. *Ophthalmology*. 2000;107:934.
229. Guell JL, Velasco F. Phakic intraocular lens implantation. *Int Ophthalmol Clin*. 2002;42:119.
230. Saxena R, Boekhoorn SS, Mulder PG, et al. Long-term follow-up of endothelial cell change after Artisan phakic intraocular lens implantation. *Ophthalmology*. 2008;115:608.
231. Silva RA, Jain A, Manche EE. Prospective long-term evaluation of the efficacy, safety, and stability of the phakic intraocular lens for high myopia. *Arch Ophthalmol*. 2008;126:775–781.
232. Dick HB, Budo C, Malecaze F, et al. Foldable Artiflex phakic intraocular lens for the correction of myopia: two-year follow-up results of a prospective European multicenter study. *Ophthalmology*. 2009;116:671–677.
233. Sridhar MS, Vemuganti GK, Bansal AK, et al. Anterior stromal puncture in bullous keratopathy: a clinicopathologic study. *Cornea*. 2001;20:573.
234. Koenig SB. Annular keratotomy for the treatment of painful bullous keratopathy. *Am J Ophthalmol*. 1996;121:93.
235. Madhavan C, Basti S, Naduvilath TH, et al. Use of ultrasound biomicroscopic evaluation in preoperative planning of penetrating keratoplasty. *Cornea*. 2000;19:17.
236. Busin M, Arffa RC, Sebastiani A. Endokeratoplasty as an alternative to penetrating keratoplasty for the surgical treatment of diseased endothelium. *Ophthalmology*. 2000;107:2077.
237. McCannel MA. A retrievable suture idea for anterior uveal problems. *Ophthalmic Surg*. 1976;7:98.
238. Panton RW, et al. Surgical management of subluxated posterior-chamber intraocular lenses. *Arch Ophthalmol*. 1993;111:919.
239. Alpar JJ. Removal of intraocular lenses: explantation and/or lens exchange. *Ann Ophthalmol*. 1987;19:194.
240. Pande M, Noble BA. The role of intraocular lens exchange in the management of major implant-related complications. *Eye*. 1993;7:34.
241. Coli AF, Price FW, Whitson WE. Intraocular lens exchange for anterior chamber intraocular lens-induced corneal endothelial damage. *Ophthalmology*. 1993;100:384.

Chapter 97

Mechanical Injury

M. Bowes Hamill

The cornea, as the most anterior structure of the eye, is exposed to various hazards ranging from airborne debris to blunt trauma of sufficient force to disrupt the globe itself. As a result, corneal injury may assume multiple forms and clinical presentations. Because the cornea is also the major refracting surface of the eye, even minor changes in its contour result in significant visual problems. This chapter deals with the diagnosis and management of different types of nonpenetrating corneal trauma.

Approach to the Patient with a Corneal Injury

History

A careful history is important in the setting of trauma. The data gathered in this process direct the subsequent physical examination and provide the examiner with the information needed to begin assessing risks for occult injuries and emergent conditions. The history also contributes greatly to the determination of the need for and the selection of ancillary testing.

The history should begin with a complete description of the traumatic event. This description will allow the examiner to estimate the risk for various types of ocular involvement such as foreign body penetration or occult rupture of the globe. Different situations dictate specific lines of inquiry. For example, when dealing with injuries involving foreign bodies, attention should be directed at identifying the foreign body source material, since some materials are relatively inert (glass, plastic), while others are highly inflammatory (certain metals, vegetable materials, or insect parts). The risk of microbial contamination should also be assessed. When injuries result from blunt or contusive trauma, the patient should be questioned as to the physical characteristics of the injuring object and an estimate made as to the amount of energy transferred. In situations in which radiant or ionizing energy sources have resulted in corneal damage, the examiner should question the patient about the wavelength, the power of the source, and the duration of exposure. Each injury setting is unique, and the examiner must obtain an accurate and detailed history specific to the individual case.

Examination

The examination should begin with a general inspection of the patient for the presence of life-threatening or emergent conditions. Inspection of the cornea and surrounding skin with a penlight may reveal the presence of foreign particles or chemical residues, which would indicate that a search for corneal foreign bodies or examination for chemical injury should be made. A general inspection may also reveal lacerations or abrasions of the lids, which should signal to the examiner that similar injuries may have occurred to the underlying or adjacent cornea. A detailed examination of the cornea requires magnification. Ideally, the patient should be evaluated at the slit lamp. Unfortunately, in the emergency setting, this equipment is often not available. While a portable slit lamp or loupes with good illumination are helpful, every attempt should be made to examine the patient at the slit lamp at the soonest appropriate time.

One of the most important caveats for the examiner is the need to perform a complete examination and not to become distracted by the injury itself. In the treatment of injury, errors are rarely made by commission; rather, errors of omission are the rule. For this reason the slit lamp evaluation of the cornea should follow a logical, orderly sequence similar to that used in the nontrauma patient. This approach will ensure that all corneal and surrounding tissues are carefully inspected. Special efforts should be made to detect occult damage, and an initial inspection of the cornea using the illumination technique of sclerotic scatter is helpful to identify subtle changes in corneal transparency which may indicate injury. The entire cornea should be inspected at both medium and high magnification using all illumination techniques. Diagnostic dyes, such as fluorescein or rose Bengal, can also be of benefit in the detection of corneal injury. It is recommended that instillation of these dyes follows rather than precedes a complete corneal examination in order to avoid masking or hiding subtle corneal findings.

Abrading Injuries

Epithelial abrasions

Etiology

Corneal abrasions (removal of part or all of the corneal epithelium) are one of the most common ophthalmic injuries. In one English series, corneal abrasions were the cause of 10% of new patient visits to the ophthalmic emergency room.[1] In a study of corneal abrasions in Bhaktapur, Nepal, evaluating sequential corneal ulceration, the annual incidence of corneal abrasion was estimated at 789 per 100 000.[2] These injuries result from various causes, although tangential impact from a foreign body is one of the most frequent etiologies. The common causative agents include fingernails, paper, mascara brushes, and plants. Important noncontact sources of epithelial injury include chemicals, radiation, and heat.

The attachment structures of the corneal epithelium to the stroma are complex. The basal cells of the epithelium rest on a basement membrane and are anchored to the stroma by hemidesmosomes. The lamina lucida, lying just beneath the basal cell membrane, contains a variety of specialized components including bullous pemphigoid antigen and laminin. Immediately below the lamina lucida is the lamina densa, composed of type IV collagen.[3] When tangential force is applied, the epithelial cells separate from their underlying attachments at the junction between the bullous pemphigoid antigen and the laminin layer.[4] If Bowman's membrane has not been disturbed, the surface will heal without scarring. If Bowman's membrane is removed, or the corneal stroma is involved, corneal scarring of some degree will result.

Clinical signs and findings

The patient with a corneal abrasion can generally tell the examiner the exact time of the injury and is usually quite symptomatic, often out of proportion to the degree of visible injury. The exception to this rule is found in patients with ultraviolet keratitis (welder's 'burn') or contact lens overwear. In these situations, symptoms may be delayed up to 8 hours after exposure to the welding arc or contact lens.

The most common symptoms of corneal abrasion are pain, photophobia, foreign body sensation, and tearing. The pain and photophobia can be so intense that even visual acuity testing is not possible. For this reason a drop of topical anesthetic, such as proparacaine 0.5%, can greatly facilitate the examination. Within seconds of instillation of the anesthetic the patient generally experiences almost complete relief, allowing a thorough evaluation of the eye. In addition to pain and photophobia, visual acuity may be decreased because of the irregularity of the denuded ocular surface. The decreased visual acuity can be overcome somewhat with a pinhole, although, commonly, the visual acuity is not completely normal. Examination of the abraded cornea with a penlight frequently reveals a roughening of the normal corneal light reflex in the area of epithelial loss, and occasionally a loose flap of epithelium can be seen. The edges of the epithelial defect can be appreciated with the slit lamp either by direct or sclerotic scatter illumination. The presence of an abrasion can be confirmed with the application of fluorescein dye that, when illuminated with a light source through a cobalt blue filter, will stain the defect apple green. In most circumstances, it is not absolutely necessary to use a blue light to visualize the area of denuded epithelium, since the fluorescein staining is visible in white light, although not as distinctly as with blue illumination.

The slit lamp evaluation should be directed at determining the extent of the abrasion, the extent of underlying stromal involvement, and the presence of any other associated injuries. When examining a patient with a corneal abrasion, as in all trauma, the examiner should be alert to the possibility of unsuspected, occult injury, such as globe perforation. It is not uncommon for a high-velocity, sharp-edged foreign body to pass completely through the cornea, leaving virtually no evidence save for a small epithelial disturbance (Fig. 97.1).

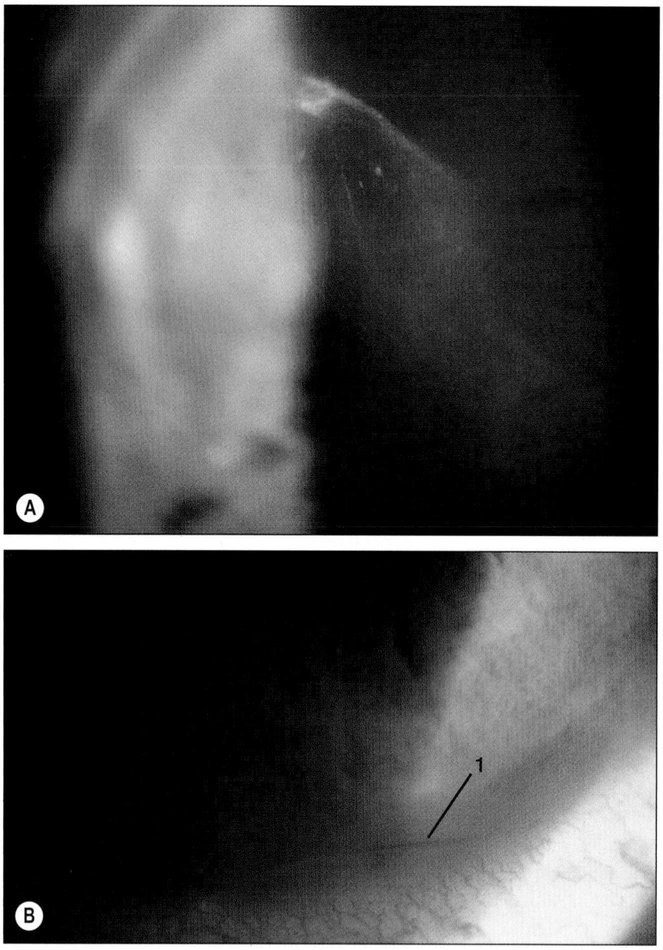

Fig. 97.1 This patient was the victim of aggravated assault during which his spectacles were broken by impact from a blunt object. High-magnification cornea photography demonstrates very little stromal damage, (**A**) The only visible wound at the time of initial injury was a small epithelial defect. (**B**) A large glass fragment (*1*) has passed completely through the cornea stroma and is lying in the inferior angle. This case illustrates how little corneal trauma can accompany a high-velocity sharp foreign body as it penetrates the cornea.

If the patient is examined soon after the injury, the corneal stroma underlying the abrasion is usually clear. If the injury has been present for 12 to 24 hours, some white blood cell recruitment may occur, resulting in a mild granular anterior stromal infiltrate underlying the defect. This is frequently accompanied by anterior chamber cell and flare reaction. Because the corneal epithelium represents a major line of defense against external pathogens, the treating physician must carefully evaluate the presence and progression of any corneal infiltrate in the abraded cornea for the development of microbial keratitis.

Treatment

Treatment of corneal abrasion is directed toward alleviating the patient's symptoms, preventing complications, and protecting the healing epithelium. The three modalities usually employed are the instillation of a cycloplegic agent, topical antibiotics, and application of a tight patch. While most authors accept cycloplegia as a mainstay of therapy, recent data have suggested that there may be better alternatives than tight patching and topical antibiotics in some patients.

Cycloplegic agents paralyze the ciliary body, decreasing ciliary body spasm, thereby significantly reducing the deep pain and photophobia associated with abrading injuries of the cornea. The choice of the agent used should be dictated by the size and clinical setting of the abrasion. Very small abrasions may not require any cycloplegia. Short-acting agents, such as cyclopentolate hydrochloride 0.5% or 1%, are appropriate for small to moderately sized abrasions, which can be expected to heal within 12 to 24 hours. Longer-acting cycloplegics, such as homatropine hydrobromide 5% or scopolamine hydrobromide 0.25%, may be more appropriate for larger defects or those patients who will require longer to heal.

Tight patching, either of the injured eye only or of both eyes, has been used for many years as the definitive treatment of corneal abrasion. The application of the tight patch in itself reduces patient discomfort and, theoretically, by eliminating blinking of the involved eye, aids the epithelial healing process. Patching, however, increases corneal temperature, which may facilitate replication of microorganisms in the tear film and thus, potentially, increase the risk of secondary microbial keratitis after abrasion.[5] In addition, the presence of the patch may also reduce available oxygen to the healing epithelium, thus slowing reepithelialization. In one study, corneal abrasion patients treated with antibiotic and cycloplegic agents alone healed faster than those treated with antibiotics, cycloplegics, and a patch.[6] This has led some authors to recommend not patching routine corneal abrasions.[7] A review of relevant published literature performed by Mackway-Jones at the Manchester Royal Infirmary found no benefit from treatment with a patch and a positive benefit from no patch in the treatment of corneal abrasions.[8] A similar outcome was reported in a study of children with corneal abrasions.[9] In a review of the available literature on the subject, Turner and Rabiu performed a meta-analysis of eleven studies involving 1014 patients for the Cochrane Collaboration.[10] The results of this analysis revealed that for smaller injury (less than 10 mm^2) the groups treated without a patch healed significantly faster on day one without any difference in pain scores compared to the groups treated by patching. The conclusion was that it was 'reasonable to conclude that patching the eye is not useful for the treatment of simple traumatic corneal abrasions.' In a national survey of corneal abrasion treatment, Sabri et al.[11] reported that topical antibiotic alone with a cycloplegic agent is currently the most commonly employed immediate treatment in the United Kingdom.

Bandage soft contact lenses for the treatment of corneal abrasion have several theoretical advantages over a tight patch and may offer an attractive therapeutic alternative in abrasion therapy. Like a patch, the lens covers and protects the epithelium, allowing healing and reducing patient discomfort. Unlike the opaque eye pad, however, the lens permits vision during the healing process. This may be very important in allowing patients to continue to work and perform their daily activities. The bandage lens is also much more cosmetically acceptable and rarely results in discomfort when compared to a tight patch. In one reported series, 40% of patients patched for corneal abrasions removed their patch because of discomfort.[6] Bandage contact lenses are not without potential problems. In a study of epithelial wound healing in the rabbit model, Ali and Insler found that a high water content lens (Softcon, 55% water content) resulted in a slower healing rate than treatment with tarsorrhaphy or topical medications alone.[12] Epithelial adhesion may also be affected by the use of an extended-wear contact lens. In a study investigating epithelial adherence in cats, Madigan et al.[13] noted decreased epithelial adherence in those eyes that had been wearing a high water content lens (71% water) for 1 year before epithelial removal. These theoretical issues notwithstanding, bandage contact lenses can be employed for several days without complications in the treatment of routine corneal abrasions in patients requiring binocular vision during the healing process. Vandorselaer et al. reported the successful use of therapeutic soft contact lenses in a prospective series of 176 consecutive patients. The authors noted that 80% of patients were able to return to work immediately and that no serious complications were noted during treatment.[14]

The third arm of therapy is topical antibiotics. One of the concerns in the treatment of corneal abrasion is the development of subsequent microbial keratitis. With any break in normal host defenses, in this case the corneal epithelium, there is a risk of subsequent microbial infection. It is generally agreed that most cases of microbial keratitis begin with a defect in the corneal epithelium that allows the microorganisms resident in the preocular tear film access to the underlying tissue where replication and keratitis ensues. Experimental studies investigating adherence of *Pseudomonas aeruginosa* to the corneas of rabbits, cattle, and sheep have demonstrated increased adherence to both partial- as well as full-thickness epithelial abrasions.[15] In the case of partial-thickness epithelial defects, adherence was increased 20 times over that in the uninjured rabbit eye. For these reasons, most authors recommend instillation of a broad-spectrum topical antibiotic as a prophylactic measure in addition to a cycloplegic agent when treating all but the most minor abrasions.

Various agents have been proposed, but, practically speaking, any of the broad-spectrum agents is probably acceptable from an antimicrobial standpoint. In the Bhaktapur eye study in Nepal, 96% of traumatic epithelial defects (551 total abrasion cases), healed without infection and none of the patients treated with a topical antibiotic (1% chloramphenicol ophthalmic ointment) within 18 hours following injury developed an infection. Of those patients treated between 18 and 48 hours following abrasion, 11% (18 of 158) developed a corneal ulcer. It should be noted that Bhaktapur is a community in the Katmandu valley whose corneal ulcer rate is 70 times higher than in the USA.[2] It is important to appreciate, also, that almost all drugs retard epithelial healing to some degree.[16] The need for antimicrobial prophylaxis, therefore, must be balanced against the toxic effects of the drug itself. In a study of the effect of topical antibiotics on corneal epithelial wound healing rates, gentamicin sulfate 0.3%, tobramycin 0.3%, and chloramphenicol 0.5% were all associated with delayed healing rates.[17] Interestingly, in the same study, healing rates were better with fortified gentamicin. This difference was thought to result from the decreased concentration of the preservative benzalkonium chloride in the fortified preparation.[17] In a similar study of rabbit corneal abrasions, topical chloramphenicol 0.5% without preservatives was found to result in healing rates identical to that in the untreated control eye.[12] Given the relative rarity of microbial keratitis in corneal abrasion patients and the potential for delaying epithelial healing, each clinician must decide on a case-by-case basis as to whether antibiotic prophylaxis is indicated.

Because pain is a major complaint in patients with corneal abrasions, pain control is a significant issue. Although the patient frequently requests it, under no circumstances should the patient be prescribed a topical anesthetic for self-administration. With prolonged use of these agents, corneal sensation and immune function are compromised and severe sight-threatening complications may result. Good results, however, have been achieved utilizing nonsteroidal antiinflammatory agents (NSAIDs) for pain control in abrasion patients. In a recent article, Weaver and Terrell reviewed five randomized, placebo-controlled, blinded trials of nonsteroidal antiinflammatory agents (diclofenac, ketorolac, indometacin) for both effectiveness in reducing pain and evidence of healing delay in patients with corneal abrasions.[18] These investigators found that the use of NSAIDs did not result in a delay in healing in the studies reviewed and that these agents were also effective in pain control.

Healing

Healing of a corneal epithelial defect occurs in several stages. The first is the latent phase, lasting approximately 1 hour. During the latent phase the surrounding basal cells undergo a series of biochemical and ultrastructural changes, resulting in the production of actin filaments in the leading edges of the basal cells and increased desquamation of epithelial surface cells.[19,20] This stage is followed by a period of epithelial cell migration of the now thinned leading edge of the epithelium across the defect. This migration appears to proceed by a 'front wheel drive' mechanism involving the production of focal adhesion plaques containing vinculin (a 130-kDa protein) at the leading edges of the migrating cell connected to actin stress fibers within the cell body.[21] While epithelial migration seems to begin along the entire circumference of the defect, with time the migrating epithelial cells tend to form sheets of advancing epithelium derived from separate regions of the defect perimeter. These sheets appear as convex fronts of thin epithelium moving toward the defect center.[22] The clinical appearance of this phenomenon is quite typical. As the epithelial sheets come into contact with one another, an epithelial healing line is formed that has the appearance of one or more 'Y's joined at the base. These healing lines can be mistaken for an atypical herpetic epithelial dendrite if a history of trauma is not appreciated. Immediately after closure of the defect, the epithelium in the area of and surrounding the defect has a peculiar pebbled appearance that remains for 1 or 2 days following fluorescein instillation. With thickening of the epithelium and smoothing of the surface, this surface change disappears.

After the denuded area has been covered by epithelium sliding in from the periphery, the replicative phase begins. This phase of healing is characterized by the proliferation of epithelial cells within and adjacent to the defect areas until the new epithelium achieves normal thickness. With the closure of the defect and the proliferation of the new epithelial layer, the basal epithelial cells reestablish their hemidesmosomal attachments to the basement membrane. This process requires up to 6 weeks after the abrasion for completion. In some cases of corneal abrasion, especially abrasions after trauma with a fingernail, paper, or vegetable matter, the basement membrane attachments are abnormal and the new epithelium spontaneously sloughs from the surface of the cornea. This condition is termed recurrent corneal erosion and has been reported to occur after 7.7% of traumatic abrasions.[23] Recurrent corneal erosions can cause significant difficulties for the patient. The treatment of recurrent erosion is discussed in detail in Chapter 87.

Complications

Most corneal abrasions heal spontaneously without difficulty in 24 to 48 hours and without scarring if Bowman's membrane is uninvolved.

Stromal abrasions

Etiology

While abrading injuries of the corneal epithelium are common, abrasions extending into the stroma are quite unusual. These injuries generally occur in the setting of a tangential blow with an abrasive or sharp object. The most common circumstance involves sports (especially basketball) with a fingernail as the causative agent. In the majority of these situations, a partial-thickness corneal flap is created that may be of varying thickness and can remain attached (Fig. 97.2) or be completely avulsed, leaving a bed of bare stroma. Rarely, stromal abrasions can be seen as part of a larger facial injury, such as are associated with motorcycle accidents, involving substantial abrading trauma to the lids, brow, and orbital rim.

Clinical signs and findings

As in injuries involving the epithelium, the stromal abrasion appears as an area of cornea that has lost its normal luster and light reflex. The surface appears quite rough, and, if it has been present for more than a short time, local edema underlying the area of involvement may be present. Determination of the depth and degree of corneal involvement, especially in the setting of a corneal flap, usually requires the use of a slit lamp. As in all corneal injuries, it is incumbent on the examiner to rule out a perforating injury.

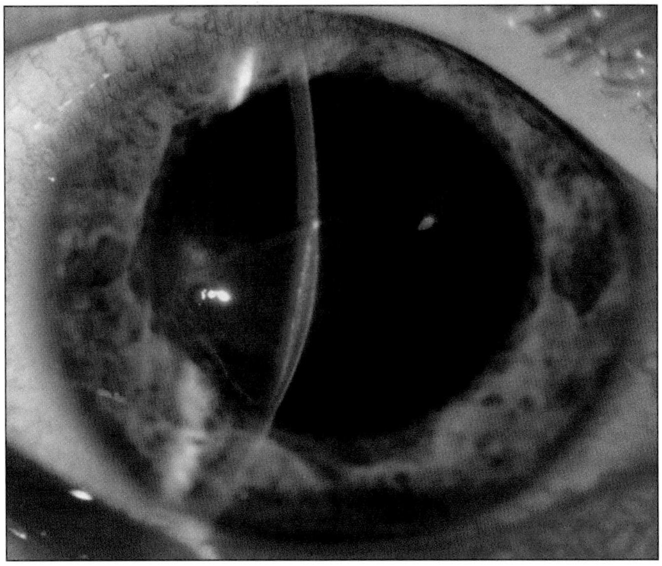

Fig. 97.2 This patient was playing basketball when he was hit in the right cornea by an opponent's thumbnail, resulting in a corneal flap. This flap is 60–70% deep at its deepest point. Treatment was limited to the application of a bandage contact lens. This injury healed well without significant corneal opacification or topographic sequelae.

Treatment

In the event of an abrasion without a flap, the therapeutic options depend on the amount of tissue remaining. If the abraded area is relatively thick, treatment can proceed as with an epithelial abrasion with the application of a bandage contact lens to allow the epithelium to heal over the bare stroma. Decisions regarding the keratorefractive effect and management (e.g. hard contact lens or penetrating keratoplasty) can be deferred until epithelial healing is complete. If the remaining stroma is thin, consideration of a primary penetrating or lamellar keratoplasty may be appropriate, although, if at all possible, the epithelium should be allowed to heal and inflammation resolve before reconstructive efforts are undertaken.

If a corneal flap is present, the therapeutic goal becomes stabilization of the remaining tissue in its proper anatomic location. For patients with little distortion of the flap, a bandage contact lens may be sufficient for this purpose. After epithelialization, the flap becomes stable and stromal healing proceeds. If the flap is distorted or there has been significant delay in seeking treatment so that exposure or edema of the flap or bed is present, sutures may be necessary to reapproximate the avulsed tissue and allow healing.

Complications

Complications of stromal abrasions and partial-thickness corneal lacerations are similar to those of corneal epithelial abrasions, although with involvement of the deeper layers the risk of complications, such as infection, is increased over cases with epithelial involvement alone. Unlike epithelial abrasions, however, injury to the stroma will result in scar formation. One of the major complications seen in these patients is keratorefractive alteration, which can be difficult to correct.

Blunt Trauma

Blunt trauma refers to injuries that result from an impact with a noncutting instrument, in which the tissue damage is the result of a rapid transfer of compressive force. Injuries of this type involving the face and head (and incidentally the eye) are relatively common. Blunt trauma can be further broken down into two types: contusive and concussive. Contusion injuries result from direct impact and may involve tissue bruising and fractures. Concussion injuries, on the other hand, arise from the rapid acceleration, deceleration, or oscillation of tissues as a result of the impact and energy transfer to the surrounding tissues. As an example, explosion injuries can result in ocular contusion after impact with flying debris. Explosions can also cause concussive injuries from the hydrostatic shockwaves in the tissues generated by the atmospheric high and low pressure waves caused by the blast. Shockwaves can also be generated by the impact of foreign material onto the ocular surface.

Contusion injuries

With the application of force to the cornea, the surface is compressed and displaced posteriorly. The degree and type of injury that result from the blunt impact depend in large measure on the amount and vector of the force, the area over which it is applied, and the rate at which the force loading occurs. For example, tangentially applied forces frequently result in abrasions. Forces applied over a large area will result in less energy transfer per area of tissue and therefore a less severe injury than the same force applied to a small area. Finally, increasing rates of energy transfer are associated with increased severity of injuries, both to the surface and to the deep tissues, because of a greater likelihood of transmitted hydrostatic shockwaves.

Clinical signs and findings

The historical inquiry in the patient with blunt trauma should be directed at estimating the factors just discussed above so as to allow the examiner to make risk assessments concerning the degree and nature of the tissue injury. Several aspects of the injury setting should be addressed specifically in the history. The object causing the injury should be described in terms of both its physical characteristics (sharp edges, weight, size) and its velocity at the time of impact. This information should be coupled with a description of the circumstances of the injury, including how the blow was struck, and where an assailant was standing. This provides the examiner with the necessary data to evaluate the relative risks of various possible sequelae.

Diffuse endotheliopathy

One of the most frequently injured corneal tissues in blunt trauma, after the epithelium, is the endothelium. Rapid energy transfer to the cornea produces a posterior displacement and infolding of the cornea as well as a hydrostatic

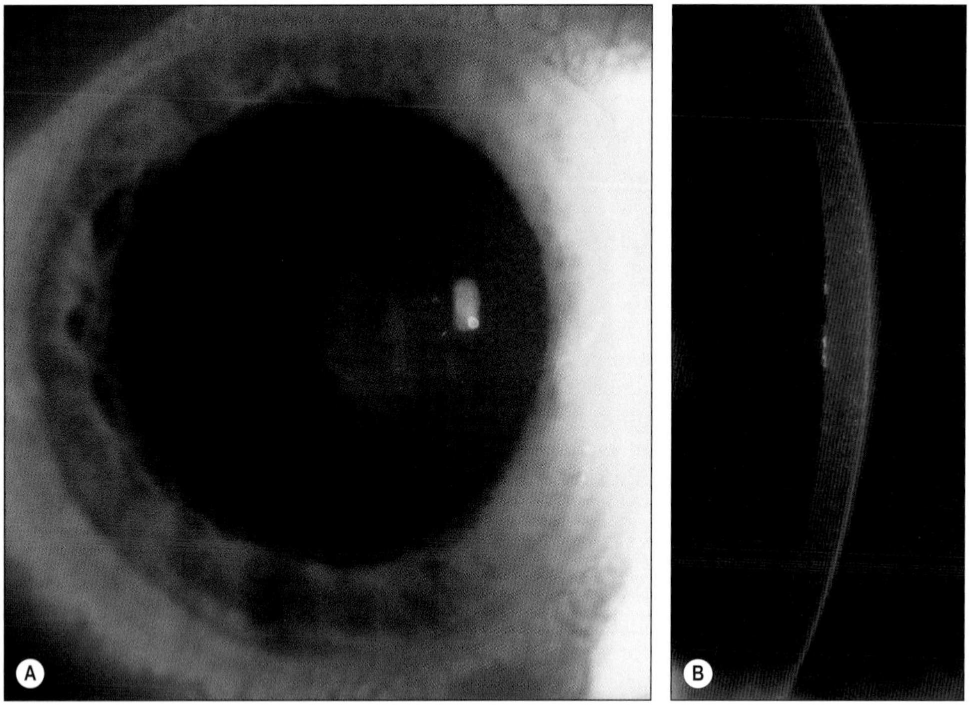

Fig. 97.3 This patient is a 27-year-old oil rig worker who was hit in the central cornea with a jet of high-pressure air (7500 psi). (**A**) Sclerotic scatter demonstrates an area of stromal edema in the area of the impact. (**B**) A thin slit lamp examination in direct focal illumination shows keratic precipitates and a thickened cornea. This clinical appearance can also be seen after nonpenetrating impacts by blunt objects such as BB pellets.

shockwave that propagates posteriorly. The degree of endothelial compromise depends on the amount and speed of energy transfer. In some cases the cornea is physically pushed posteriorly to impact the lens. In this situation there may be contusion of the endothelium from lens impact as well as lens injury from the same mechanism. These injuries generally result in widespread corneal edema with diffuse striate keratopathy. More frequently, the corneal endothelium is injured without apparent impact with other structures. Classically, these injuries result from high-speed impacts such as those generated from elastic 'bungee' cords and nonpenetrating BB gun projectiles. The clinical picture is one of localized or zonal corneal edema underlying the area of impact (Fig. 97.3). There is frequently an inflammatory (cell and flare) response in the anterior chamber and associated injuries to other anterior segment structures, such as angle recession, iris sphincter tears, and hyphema. Even though the cornea recovers clarity in the majority of these patients, studies have shown that after corneal injury there is permanent endothelial cell loss.[24,25] In a study of endothelial cell loss after blunt trauma, Slingsby and Forstot found that, while there was a large variability in the percentage of cells lost, blunt trauma did result in a significant reduction in endothelial cell density.[24] In this study, eyes with angle recession had a 12% decrease in endothelial cell density compared to the fellow uninjured eye. When eyes were stratified to greater than or less than 180 degrees of angle recession, eyes with greater than 180 degrees of recession had a 21.2% decrease compared to their fellow eyes.

Treatment of concussive/contusive endothelial injury is expectant and directed at controlling inflammation and ensuring that other injuries are managed appropriately. In most patients, the edema generally subsides as the damaged endothelial cells recover or are replaced by enlargement of the surrounding cells, and the cornea recovers its preinjury clarity.

Endothelial rings

An interesting subtype of traumatic endotheliopathy can be seen associated with small high-speed nonpenetrating foreign bodies.[26–28] These small ring-shaped endothelial lesions were probably first described by Pichler in 1916 in patients after explosion injuries.[29] In an experimental study, Cibis et al. were able to produce these lesions in monkeys and rabbits when graphite particles were shot from an air rifle.[30] Importantly, the authors noted that the force required to produce the rings was relatively specific; too little force produced no changes, while too much force resulted in perforating injuries or deep penetration by the foreign bodies, both of which produced sheets of endothelial destruction rather than discrete rings. Examination of these lesions by light and scanning electron microscopy (SEM) revealed that the rings consisted of swollen or disrupted endothelial cells with adherent fibrin and leukocytes. The cells in the center of the rings were normal. No alterations in the structure of the stroma or Descemet's membrane were found.[30] Maloney et al. examined two patients with this condition by specular microscopy and serial slit lamp photography.[31] In these patients, specular microscopy revealed that during the acute phase the involved endothelium was swollen and had lost its usual well-defined architecture. With time (4.5 months after trauma), no endothelial abnormality was noted in areas of previous rings despite careful searching with the specular microscope.[31]

The precise etiology of this phenomenon is unclear, but it probably results from the transmission of a hydrostatic shockwave from the impacting foreign body to the endothelium.[30,31] The role, if any, of actual corneal stretch or displacement is unknown. With time, these lesions fade, first to partial C-shaped rings, next to areas of punctate endothelial change, and finally to normal-appearing endothelium.

Stromal injuries and fractures

When substantial force is applied to the cornea, the corneal tissues may be sufficiently posteriorly displaced so as to result in fractures of the stroma.[32] The fracture may involve Bowman's membrane or, in some cases, be associated with an intact Bowman's and epithelium. If Descemet's membrane is involved, these fractures may be obscured in the early phases by overlying corneal edema.

Over the past 15 years, the rapid acceptance of radial keratotomy (RK) and laser in situ keratomileusis (LASIK) in the United States has resulted in a large number of patients who have had this procedure on one or both eyes. The effect of RK incisions on the cornea's ability to withstand impact is unknown in any individual patient. Despite several published case reports of corneas with radial keratotomy incisions surviving trauma,[33,34] the impression among most ophthalmologists is that corneas that have undergone RK are at an increased risk of rupture following impact, and several reports have been published detailing accounts of patients who have had corneal ruptures of the incision sites after injury.[35–39] It is interesting to note that many of these cases have occurred months to years after the procedure, indicating that corneal wound healing in this procedure is quite prolonged. For these reasons, RK patients who have had significant blunt trauma should be examined carefully for wound dehiscence and possible globe rupture. Patients who have had lamellar refractive procedures are also at risk for late sequelae from blunt trauma. Although following the procedure the corneal flap adheres well to the underlying surface, the junction never achieves the strength of the surrounding tissue. With blunt tangential force, as is seen with air bag injuries, the flap may become dislodged.[40]

Obstetric injuries

One subtype of blunt corneal injury is that caused at delivery either as a result of the birth process per se or secondary to the application of instruments to assist with the delivery, such as obstetric forceps or vacuum extraction devices. Injuries to the eye resulting from delivery have been reported as relatively common. Duke-Elder estimated that injury to the eye or adnexa may occur in as many as 20–25% of normal births, and, with prolonged or instrumented labor and delivery, the incidence may increase to as much as 40–50%.[41] In general, most of these injuries are minimal and resolve without sequelae. In a review of all babies born in the Nehru Hospital in Chandigarh, India, Jain et al. found 243 ocular injuries in 2016 infants.[42] Of these, 238 (98%) were retinal hemorrhages, subconjunctival hemorrhages, or lid ecchymoses.

Corneal birth injuries are relatively infrequent, however, and only one case of corneal edema was reported in Jain's series. This infant had a forceps-assisted delivery.[42] Although rare, corneal birth injuries have been recognized since the end of the nineteenth century. De Wecker, in a report published in 1896, and Truc, in a paper in 1898, both described cases of a unilateral linear corneal opacity after forceps-assisted delivery.[43,44] In the case described by de Wecker, dense corneal edema with a visible forceps mark across the brow was present at birth. The edema resolved over the first month of life, although a hazy linear opacity remained. Truc's patient was 4 years old at the time of examination, presenting with strabismus. Examination of the cornea revealed a dense linear opacity in the oblique meridian (1 to 7 o'clock). Two additional cases of corneal birth injury were published at about the same time by Noyes and Dujardin.[45,46] These accounts described infants with total corneal edema that resolved rapidly with minimal sequelae. In an excellent review of ocular birth injuries published in 1903, Thomson and Buchanan concluded that injury to the cornea occurred in three patterns: a diffuse opacity that is temporary, a diffuse opacity that is permanent, and a linear opacity that is permanent.[47] They postulated that the first form is caused by edema without inflammation, the second by diffuse edema associated with inflammation, with or without diffuse stripping of Descemet's membrane, and the third by linear breaks in Descemet's membrane. Since that time, several other clinical signs have been reported, including the presence of 'glass' membranes derived from the stripped Descemet's membrane, cyst formation in the region of Descemet's membrane ruptures, and transient parallel lines of blood in the cornea, oriented in the oblique axis, which resolved shortly after birth.[48] The source for the blood was felt by the authors to be the peripheral cornea.

Pathogenesis

Corneal birth injuries arise from the compression of the globe against the roof of the orbit during delivery. The resultant force causes a horizontal expansion of the cornea, leading to vertically oriented splits or tears in Descemet's membrane. Subsequently, the overlying cornea becomes edematous. While the majority of these injuries are felt to result from application of obstetric forceps, identical injuries can be the result of the birth process itself, specifically fetal passage through a deformed pelvis with compression from a prominent sacral promontory.[49]

Clinical signs

Although these injuries are present at birth, they may go unrecognized for several days because of the accompanyng lid edema.[48] As previously discussed, the injured cornea may initially be totally or regionally opaque. Over the succeeding weeks with reformation of Descemet's membrane, the edema generally resolves, and subsequent examinations reveal single or multiple breaks in Descemet's membrane, which may appear as linear or crescentic lines or opacities, generally oriented in the vertical oblique meridian. Stromal scarring over the breaks may be present in some cases. The edges of the breaks are rolled at the margins and may form free strands of Descemet's membrane in the aqueous attached only at the ends.[41] Microscopic examination reveals that Descemet's membrane is of variable thickness at the edges of the rupture with a folded or scrolled appearance. One case of epithelial transformation of the endothelium in the area of rupture has been reported in a corneal button removed for keratoplasty.[50] Injury may not be limited to the cornea, however. Reports have been published documenting cases involving adults with visible contralateral occipital depression and ipsilateral periorbital depressions associated with the typical corneal changes as a result of forceps trauma at birth.[51]

The differential diagnosis for this condition includes congenital glaucoma, congenital hereditary endothelial dystrophy (CHED), von Hippel's internal ulcer, and Peters' anomaly. With resolution of the edema, the appearance of the stromal breaks is relatively typical, however.

Although in most cases the corneal edema clears within days to weeks, the refractive consequences of breaks in Descemet's membrane may be profound. Large astigmatic errors with the keratometric steep axes parallel to the breaks are the rule. It has been postulated that breaks in Descemet's membrane allow expansion of the cornea in a direction perpendicular to the long axis of the break. This expansion results in flattening in that meridian and compensatory steepening at 90 degrees.[52] The degree of induced astigmatism can be severe, as seen in a series of patients reported by Angell et al.[53] in which the mean cylinder in the involved eyes was 6.9 diopter (D) (3.0–10.50 D) compared to 0.36 D (0.0–1.50D) in the noninvolved eyes. This degree of induced astigmatism may account for reports of amblyopia seemingly out of proportion to local corneal changes.[49] In addition to astigmatic changes, the involved eyes also demonstrate significant myopia as compared to their fellow eyes. In the series of Angell et al. the average increase in myopia was 7.8 D more myopia in affected than unaffected eyes. This myopic shift is felt to be axial in most cases, and these authors suggested that the process of axial lengthening in birth injuries may be similar to that seen in experimental studies in young animals after corneal opacification or lid fusion.[53]

The long-term sequelae of this injury are not limited to keratorefractive changes. With injury to Descemet's membrane also comes damage to the endothelium. McDonald and Burgess, in a review of four patients suspected to have had forceps injury to the cornea, noted that in the three cases in which specular microscopy was performed, the injured eyes showed decreases in endothelial cell density.[51] This relative lack of endothelial cells caused by the injury may explain the tendency of these corneas to develop spontaneous, visually significant corneal edema later in life.

Management

In most cases, since the edema present at birth resolves over the first few weeks of life, no acute treatment is required. Efforts, rather, should be directed at recognition and treatment of subsequent refractive errors by frequent cycloplegic refractions and prescription of spectacles or contact lenses as necessary. The benefits of corneal transplantation for persistent central corneal opacification in childhood must be considered on a case-by-case basis, although vigorous prevention of amblyopia may significantly increase the visual success of corneal transplantation later in life, should corneal edema develop.

Injuries Caused by Radiant Energy

Ultraviolet radiation

The electromagnetic spectrum encompasses a vast spread of radiant energy wavelengths from the very short (10^{-16}: cosmic and gamma rays) to the very long (10^{8}: sound waves). Near the middle of the spectrum are located the visible wavelengths. Immediately 'below' the visible spectrum is the ultraviolet (UV). For convenience, and based on biologic effects, the ultraviolet spectrum has been further subdivided into UVC (200–290 nm), UVB (290–320 nm), and UVA (320–400 nm). While the cornea transmits the majority of visible light, greater and greater amounts of ultraviolet light are absorbed by the cornea as the wavelength decreases (Fig. 97.4).[54] The wavelengths between 200 and 300 nm are strongly absorbed by the cellular elements in the cornea, whereas the wavelengths from 300 to 400 nm are transmitted by the cornea and absorbed by the lens. The energy per photon increases with decreasing wavelength, and, at short wavelengths, each photon has sufficient energy to cause photochemical reactions in nucleic acids and proteins within the cell. Because of the relatively high energy of photons in the far ultraviolet, fewer 'hits' are required to result in cellular damage.[55] The action spectrum (threshold of exposure) for corneal damage has been estimated to begin at about 210 nm and extend to 360 nm.[54] Because of absorption and energy considerations, however, the exposure necessary for clinical effect varies considerably over this range, as illustrated in Figure 97.5. As can be seen, the cornea is maximally sensitive to UV radiation (UVR) in the wavelengths between 260 and 280 nm because these wavelengths represent the first absorption bands of the common bases of nucleic acids and aromatic amino acids. Because of the photochemical nature of the injury, repeated exposures should be expected to result in cumulative damage over time. This has been investigated by Zuchlich, who found that, while repeated exposure did result in cumulative damage, the additive effect leveled off, indicating that a repair mechanism is present for UV-induced damage in the cornea.[54] Antioxidant defense mechanisms may play an important role in corneal healing following UV exposure. In a study of glucose-6-phosphate dehydrogenase (G6PDH) levels, the rate-limiting enzyme in the pentose phosphate pathway and important in the production of reduced glutathione, an antioxidant enzyme, corneal exposure to small doses of UVA and UVC enhanced G6PDH activity in porcine corneas. With larger doses of UVC, however, the pathway was damaged.[56]

Corneal effects of UV irradiation

The corneal epithelium is the first tissue layer exposed to incoming light and consequently shows the most absorption and tissue damage from UVR. With moderate exposure

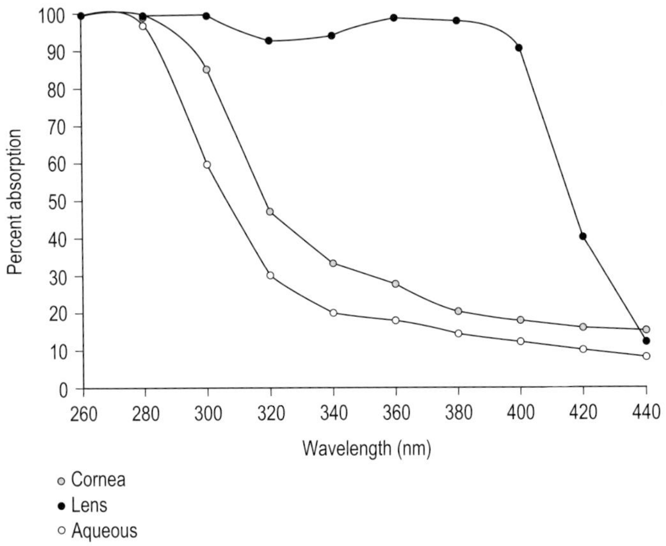

Fig. 97.4 Shown above is a chart of the absorption spectra of the cornea, the lens, and the aqueous in the primate eye. The cornea absorbs almost all wavelengths below 290 nm and becomes reasonably transparent as the wavelength increases. The lens absorbs significantly more in the longer wavelengths. (Adapted from Zuchlich JA: *Health Physics* 56(3):671–682, 1989.)

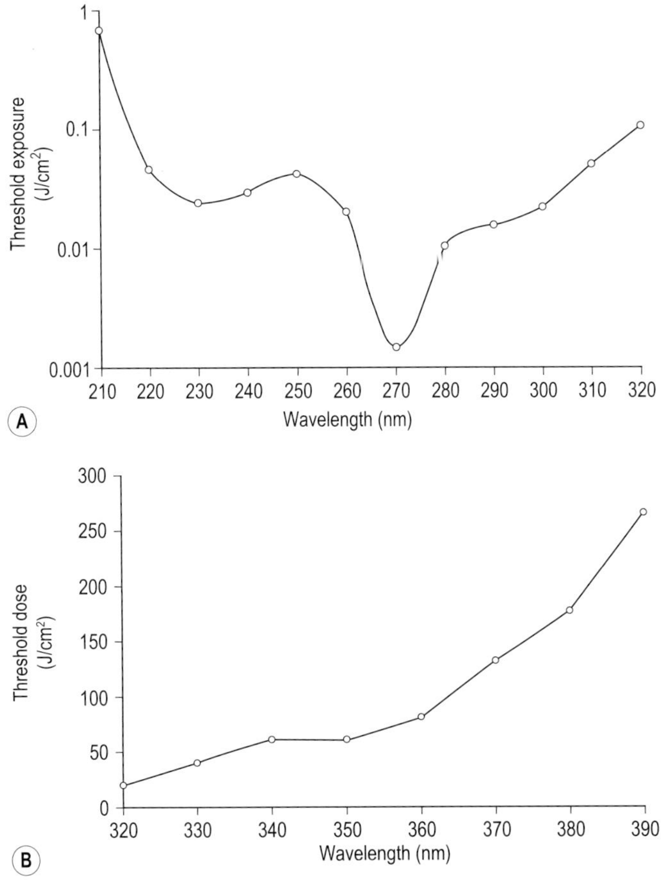

Fig. 97.5 These curves illustrate the action spectrum for both far (**A**) and near (**B**) UV-induced corneal damage. In the far UV, the corneal action spectrum peaks at approximately 270 nm. (Adapted from Zuchlich JA: *Health Physics* 56(3):671–682, 1989.)

(0.08 J/cm^2 at 300 nm) in primates, Bergmanson noted areas of full-thickness epithelial changes with separation of superficial epithelial cells, and nuclear and cytoplasmic damage in the remaining attached cells.[57] There was selective sparing of basal and wing cells. With increased exposure (0.225 J/cm^2 at 300 nm) the entire epithelial layer sloughed, leaving an intact basement membrane. In a similar study in pigmented rabbits, Clarke et al. irradiated the entire corneal surface with 300 nm UVR (0.05 J/cm^2).[58] Within 24 hours the corneas in experimental animals showed a decreased corneal light reflex with granularity of the epithelium visible by retroillumination. By 48 hours, electron microscopy revealed severely damaged central corneal epithelial cells with exfoliation of superficial cells into the tear film and edema of the remaining cells. The authors postulated that this clinical picture resulted from UVR-induced damage to the cellular components, causing increased membrane permeability. The epithelial cells became edematous, with decreased numbers of microplicae, and eventually sloughed into the tear film.[58] This reaction developed over time, with 50% of epithelial cells showing damage in 24 hours and 100% involvement at 48 hours. In this study, even though the entire cornea was radiated, the majority of the damage was noted in the central cornea because of the effects of corneal curvature on collimated irradiation. As an example of the effect of wavelength on corneal damage, Zuchlich required 90 J/cm^2 at 350 nm to achieve epithelial cell sloughing and epithelial thinning in the rhesus monkey.[54]

These epithelial toxic effects of UVB radiation seem to be ameliorated somewhat by the presence of macrophage migration inhibitory factor (MIF) . In a mouse study utilizing MIF-overexpressed transgenic, wild type (WT), and MIF knock out (KO) mice, Kitaichi and colleagues noted that both WT and KO mice showed much more acute damage from UVB exposure than MIF overexpressing mice. Additionally, MIF overexpressing mice had significantly fewer TUNEL positive nuclei than the other groups.[59] Although it was initially thought that keratocytes were resistant to the effects of UVR, since early studies with high exposures (1 J/cm^2) failed to produce stromal changes, these studies used short wavelengths (280–290 nm), which are absorbed by epithelium.[60] Using longer 300 nm UVR, after moderate exposures (0.08 J/cm^2), Bergmanson noted spaces around keratocytes. As the exposure increased to 0.225 J/cm^2, keratocytes throughout the stroma were described as 'severely traumatized.'[57] Pitts et al., in a similar study also using primates, noted increasing keratocyte damage with increasing exposure to 300 nm UVR.[60] Initially, keratocytes were seen to develop intracellular vacuoles followed by fragmentation of cellular processes, and finally nuclear disintegration. The authors interpreted the spaces around the keratocytes and within the lamellae as edema and felt that this indicated endothelial dysfunction in addition to stromal damage. UVR can affect corneal nerves as well as keratocytes, although the degree of exposure at 300 nm necessary to cause changes is much higher than for the epithelium. With exposures of 0.225 J/cm^2, some axonal swelling in the subepithelial zones has been noted, along with an absence of epithelial terminals.[57]

The endothelium also absorbs UVR with resultant damage. In a study by Riley et al.,[61] rabbit corneas exhibited edema after UVR, which spontaneously resolved after 4 days. The degree of edema and the duration of the swelling depended on the duration of exposure to 300 nm UVR. In this study, exposures ranged from 0.1 to 0.2 J/cm^2. Changes in the cellular architecture ranging from irregularity in the posterior endothelial contour to extensive intracellular edema have also been noted by other investigators after exposure to 300 nm UVR in exposure ranges from 0.08 to 0.225 J/cm^2.[57,61–63] In addition to light and electron microscopy, specular microscopy has also revealed UVR-induced endothelial changes. Ringvold et al., after exposing albino rabbits to a commercially available sun lamp for 5 to 20 minutes, noted specular microscopic changes that persisted from 1 week to 8 months after exposure.[62] These changes were characterized by endothelial pleomorphism and rosette formation.

Clinical signs and findings

The most common types of human UVR injury are welder's keratitis, snow blindness, and keratitis after exposure to tanning sun lamps. Similar to findings in animal studies, the acute effects of UVR in humans are generally delayed for 8 to 12 hours after exposure. Early symptoms include generalized ocular surface discomfort, followed by pain, photophobia, and a foreign body sensation. Individuals suffering from this condition report intense discomfort. Millodot and Earlam reported that corneal sensitivity was reduced immediately after corneal UVR but recovered rapidly.[63] The decrease in corneal sensitivity peaked at 1.75 hours, and corneal sensation returned to baseline in all subjects by 4 hours. Interestingly, in five of the seven subjects the cornea became more sensitive than baseline by 4 hours after exposure.[63] Although Bergmanson noted relative resistance to damage by UVR in corneal nerves, this intense discomfort after UV injury may result from a direct effect of UVR on the corneal nerve or its relationship with the overlying epithelium.[57]

Slit lamp examination of human corneas after welding arc exposure reveals a loss of the normal corneal luster and light reflex. Depending on the wavelength encountered and the duration of the exposure, the epithelium may show a roughened surface with epithelial erosions or, occasionally, frank epithelial defects that stain with fluorescein. The cornea may also be slightly edematous. In general, there is minimal anterior cell inflammatory reaction, although some cell and flare may be present. Treatment is similar to that for corneal abrasion and includes cycloplegia and oral analgesics. The pain and discomfort subside and resolve over the next 24 to 48 hours, and full recovery is the rule.

The corneal sequelae of chronic exposure to UVR are not well understood but may include such conditions as pterygium, climatic droplet keratopathy (CDK), and permanent endothelial morphologic changes.[64–67] Because of the possible significant deleterious effects of both acute and chronic UVR to the cornea and other ocular structures, there is increasing interest in measures to protect the eye from exposure to that portion of the spectrum. Several contact lenses have been manufactured that contain UV chromophores; examples include the Sofscreen U4 series lens and Vistakon UV-BLOC(Rx) (now discontinued). Both lenses showed significant absorption of UVR below 350 nm, although the Vistakon lens blocked transmittance up to 400 nm and seemed to decrease overall UV transmittance to lower levels than the Sofscreen U4. Both lenses were effective in reducing the clinical effects of UVR in rabbit studies.[68,69] Using a different approach, Oldenburg et al. evaluated the efficacy of UV chromophores applied topically to the preocular tear film in rabbits.[70] Their studies did not reveal any apparent toxicity and demonstrated a significant protective effect to exposure from a 308-nm UVR source. This protective effect persisted even if exposure to UVR was delayed for up to 60 minutes after instillation.[70]

Infrared radiation

The infrared portion of the spectrum lies just above the visible spectrum, with wavelengths of approximately 10^{-4} m. Fortunately, corneal injuries from infrared (heat) radiation are relatively rare because of the blink reflex and head turn avoidance behavior that accompany exposure of the face and eyes to intense heat. Duke-Elder and MacFaul summarized the results of several investigations into the effects of infrared radiation on the cornea.[71] They reported that with exposure to radiant heat the epithelium is destroyed and the underlying stroma becomes opacified because of the coagulation of the stromal proteins. There is a tendency for the stroma to be more easily damaged than the epithelium as a result of the localized cooling influences of the tear film and the air–epithelium interface. Although corneal changes are noted early—that is, within 20 minutes after exposure—the full clinical picture generally progresses over 24 hours. At that time, significant stromal edema develops and the corneal lamellae lose their architecture. The transition between affected and normal tissue tends to be sharply demarcated.[71]

Although injuries caused by infrared radiation are unusual, a case of corneal edema after xenon arc photocoagulation has been reported.[72] In this case, the authors postulated that the thermal energy of the xenon arc was absorbed by the iris, with secondary heating of the aqueous and damage to the corneal endothelium. This hypothesis is supported by the prolonged and significant iritis that followed the procedure, requiring oral prednisone for control, as well as the presence of iris transillumination defects 11 months postoperatively. The authors also suggested that the development of corneal edema during the procedure may have resulted in further scattering of light and increased absorption by the iris. It would also seem possible, however, that the development of corneal edema with resultant loss of corneal transparency would result in decreased transmission and increased absorption of the incoming light by the cornea, per se, with resultant local heating. In the reported case, almost complete corneal clearing occurred within 6 months.

Thermal Burns

In addition to infrared radiation, thermal injury (burn injuries) can occur by contact. Multiple studies have been performed to investigate the effect of the direct application of heat to the cornea.[73–75] In early studies using cautery applied to rabbit corneas, Shahan and Lamb noted that the initial result was a loss of epithelium and localized edema, followed by the development of an opaque corneal scar.[73] If the injury was located near the limbus, a triangular pannus of vessels developed. In a similar series of experiments, Campbell and Michaelson found that if the thermal insult occurred 4.2 mm or more from the limbus, no vascularization took place.[74] Angiogenesis after localized thermal injury probably results from release of an angiogenic factor(s) by the injured tissue, producing a proliferation of vessels from the limbus. The vascular response after this type of trauma seems to follow a typical pattern, with DNA synthesis beginning first in the endothelial cells of the venules and capillaries, peaking 40 hours after injury, and then increased DNA synthetic activity in the lymphatic endothelium over the next 2 to 3 days.[76]

In an effort to determine the heat tolerance of the cornea, Goldblatt et al. sewed an etched conductive heating element to rabbit corneas and applied controlled heat over time.[77] Their studies indicated that the rabbit cornea could tolerate heating to 45°C for 15 minutes without visible damage by light microscopy. With heating to 52°C for 5 minutes, the corneas appeared normal to inspection initially, but stromal edema developed over the subsequent 24 hours and resolved over the following week. After heating to 59°C for 5 minutes the corneas were grossly clouded, with pathologic findings of stromal edema, vacuole formation, nuclear destruction, and stromal disorganization. This damage was noted 1 week after injury, although the authors also found some indication of repair. When a temperature of 59°C was maintained for 15 minutes, the result was total cellular dropout and massive stromal edema.

Duke-Elder subdivides burn injuries into two groups: flame burns and contact burns. Flame burns, as the name implies, are those caused by fire, whereas contact burns result from contact with hot objects or liquids. Flame burns involving the face and lids are relatively common, although corneal involvement is rare because of the rapidity of lid closure and the insulating quality of the lids. With significant burns involving the face, involvement of the eyes has been reported to be as high as 20% in some series.[78] In a review of 400 consecutive patients admitted to a regional burn center, Guy et al. found that 47% of patients had facial involvement, 27% had involvement of the eyes or lids, and 11% of patients had ocular injuries sufficient to warrant an ophthalmic evaluation.[79] In their series, 31% of the eye injuries were corneal burns or abrasions, of which only 7% resulted in permanent corneal scarring. When the cornea is involved in a flame burn, it is generally the result of a devastating injury causing loss of the lids and destruction of the anterior segment. An example of a typical flame burn of the face and lids is illustrated in Figure 97.6. This individual attempted suicide by dousing herself with gasoline and setting herself on fire. Despite significant involvement of the face, the anterior segment is relatively untouched.

Contact burns are a more frequent cause of corneal injury than flame burns, although they are also uncommon. Contact burns occur when a hot object or fluid comes into direct contact with the corneal surface. The most frequent causes of this type of burn in the industrial setting include hot metal fragments and solder. In the home, these injuries are more commonly caused by hot grease or oil. In a series of 59 contact burns of the cornea reported from India in 1991, Vajpayee et al. noted that boiling fluid and hot oil resulted in 42% and 32% of cases, respectively, followed by fireworks and match heads (18% and 17%).[80] An increasingly frequent cause of corneal contact burns in the United States is the curling iron (Fig. 97.7).[81–83]

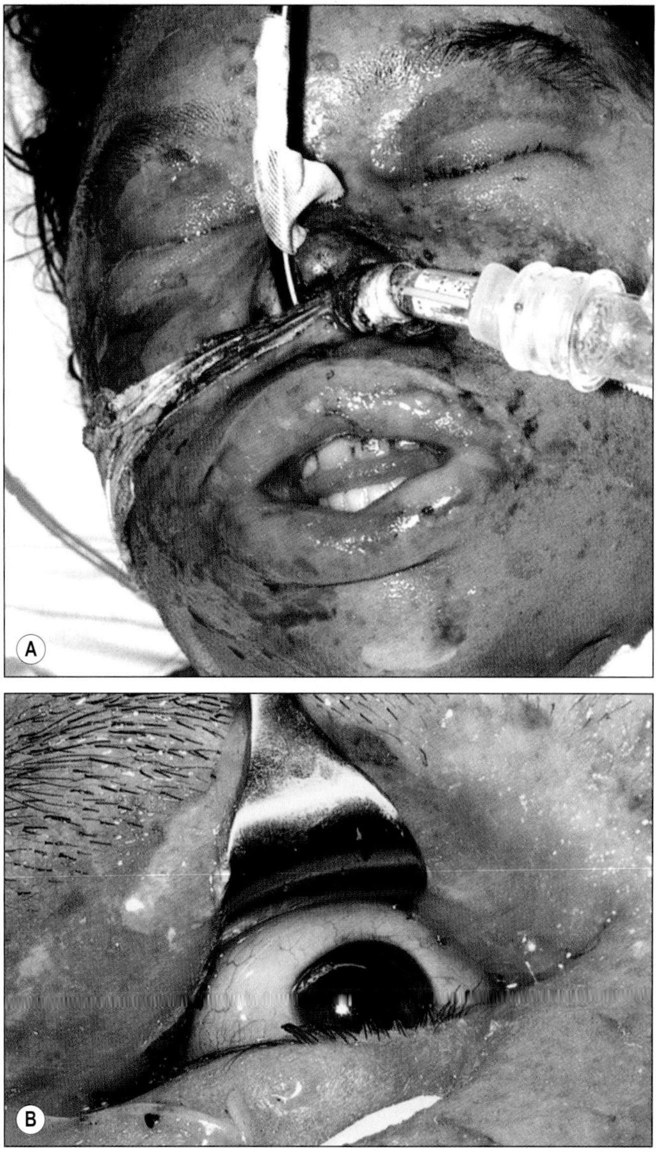

Fig. 97.6 This young girl attempted suicide by dousing herself with gasoline and setting herself on fire. (**A**) As can be seen, she has suffered extensive burns of the face with loss of parts of the brow and eyelashes. (**B**) The globe was well protected by both the blink reflex and the thermal insulating quality of the lids. This is fairly typical of most facial thermal burns unless they are extremely severe.

Clinical signs and findings

The clinical result of a contact burn to the cornea depends on four factors: the temperature of the agent, the heat-retaining capacity of the material, the duration of contact, and the area over which the heat is applied. As can be seen

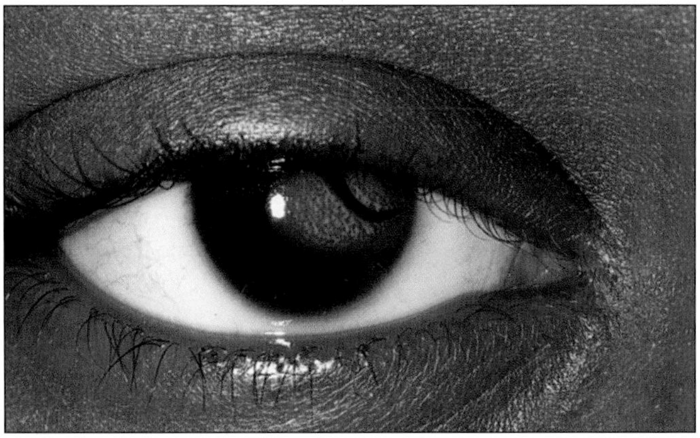

Fig. 97.7 This patient inadvertently struck her cornea with a curling iron. The cornea shows the typical appearance of white epithelium, which subsequently sloughed to reveal clear underlying stroma. This injury healed without visible sequelae, although the patient had significant local corneal flattening that persisted for several months after the injury.

from Goldblatt's work, even moderate heat applied to the cornea for a prolonged time can result in significant tissue damage.[77] Most traumatic events, however, involve heat sources of higher temperatures applied for much shorter times.

In clinical practice, two different types of tissue reaction are generally produced, depending on the temperature of the heat source. If the source is hot (>1000°C) with significant heat retention capacity, such as molten metal or glass, the result may be a severe burn with involvement of the deeper layers of the cornea. The involved tissue becomes opaque, with what has been described as a porcelain or ground-glass appearance. This eschar eventually sloughs, leaving thinned tissue behind that may later become ectatic or staphylomatous.[71] An interesting phenomenon occurs with contact burns caused by low-melting-temperature metals. In these cases, the cooling effect of the tear film may be sufficient to protect the cornea, so that the corneal tissue is unaffected, and a cast of the anterior surface of the eye may be produced.[71]

Management

Management of minor contact burns is similar to that of corneal epithelial abrasions. In most cases the damage is limited to the epithelial layers only and heals within 24 to 48 hours without sequelae. The corneal flattening resulting from the stromal heating may persist for several weeks. With more severe burns, efforts must be directed at the control of inflammation and prevention of infection. Surgery may be needed later in the course to manage corneal thinning and corneal symblepharon if they occur. In the most severe injuries, necrosis of the entire cornea may result in subsequent sloughing of the cornea, extrusion of intraocular contents, and loss of the globe.[71] In general, however, burns with stromal involvement heal with a permanent scar, the density and size of which depend on the initial injury. Although these scars tend to fade with time, a case report of squamous cell carcinoma arising in a contact thermal burn of the cornea and limbus occurring 15 years after the injury has been published.[84]

Foreign Body Injuries

Second to corneal abrasions, corneal foreign bodies are the most common form of ophthalmic trauma. In a recent study in northern Sweden, the incidence of eye injuries was estimated to be 8.1 per 1000 population, with corneal and conjunctival foreign bodies comprising 40% of these.[85] Banerjee, in a similar study, found that of 25 000 new patients seen in an emergency room in England over a 6-month period, 472 (1.8%) were patients who had ocular foreign bodies that occurred at work.[86] He made the further point that only 60% of patients were wearing eye protection at the time of injury, even though the activities at the time of injury were ones that would be considered 'high risk' for foreign body generation (grinding, drilling, hammering, and welding). The issue of protective eye wear is an important one, as most authorities feel that the use of well-fitting, proper eye protection could prevent most commonly encountered corneal foreign body injuries. Unfortunately, compliance with the use of safety eye wear is less than optimal. During the 1991 Gulf War, ocular injuries accounted for 14% of injuries seen at a one army field hospital. Of these, 17% were corneal foreign bodies.[87] Only 3% of injured soldiers were injured while wearing protective eye wear, although most US Army troops were issued goggles on deployment.

Fortunately, most corneal foreign body injuries are not severe and do not result in prolonged morbidity. In a study of 504 corneal foreign body injuries at the Southampton Eye Hospital, most patients took no time off from work as a result of their injury and only 37 (7.3%) lost more than 12 hours.[88] In this group of patients the median time lost to work was 4 hours. Some corneal foreign bodies can, however, result in significant ocular problems.

Clinical signs and findings

When a foreign body injury is suspected, the examiner must positively rule out the presence of intraocular foreign material. A variety of diagnostic choices is available for this purpose, ranging from inspection of the intraocular contents by gonioscopy and indirect ophthalmoscopy to computed tomography (CT) scanning. Most corneal foreign bodies are visible by careful slit lamp examination, although the findings may be subtle. This is fortunate, as the patient's ability to localize his or her own corneal foreign body is less than absolute. In one series, while patients were able to localize the foreign body as either to the side (medial, central, or lateral anterior ocular surface) or to the level (upper, middle, or lower cornea) 78% of the time, they were correct only 28% of the time in predicting both the side and the level.[89]

The slit lamp evaluation in the setting of foreign body injury should be thorough and meticulous. A standard routine should be followed, avoiding examination of the most obvious injury first because multiple foreign bodies are not uncommon and care should be taken to eliminate this possibility. Use of various illumination techniques is helpful. Sclerotic scatter may highlight transparent intrastromal foreign material, whereas retroillumination from the iris or fundus will help delineate discontinuities in the stroma. The application of fluorescein to the tear film may also be of assistance with small foreign bodies by staining surrounding epithelial defects and pooling in and around irregularities in the epithelial contour. Care should be taken to determine the depth of the material in the stroma using high magnification and narrow slit width, since this will assist with the decision for and technique of subsequent removal (Fig. 97.8).

Foreign bodies located on the surface can be removed using various approaches. If the material is superficial, gentle application of a cotton swab may be sufficient. For more adherent material, a sharp instrument may be required. Various instruments have been proposed to assist with this procedure, including the use of an electromagnet for magnetic foreign bodies.[90–93] In most cases of superficial foreign bodies, a tuberculin syringe with an attached 27- or 30-gauge needle is an effective instrument for removal. The needle is small enough to delicately remove even minute particles, while the barrel of the syringe provides a comfortable grip for easy maneuverability.

Ferrous foreign bodies pose a special problem when embedded in the cornea, since they rust on contact with the tear film, forming rust rings (Fig. 97.9). Rusting begins almost immediately after the object is embedded, and a ring may begin to form as early as 3 hours after injury.[94] The presence of the rust in the tissue not only interferes with vision but also may retard healing.[95] Rust rings can be removed either by scraping with a small needle or by the application of a rotating burr to the involved area. While both methods are effective, in a study of rust rings in a rabbit model, scraping with a needle tended to result in slightly larger epithelial defects and slower epithelial healing compared to the rotating burr.[96]

After removal of the foreign body, the eye should be treated as with a corneal abrasion, with the application of a broad-spectrum antibiotic and a cycloplegic agent, if necessary. As in studies of small abrasions, investigations into the use of eye patching after small foreign body removal showed increased patient comfort when patching was not employed.[97] Almost all epithelial defects from small inert foreign bodies heal without sequelae within 24 to 48 hours.

Plant and insect corneal foreign bodies deserve special mention, since these types of materials may result in injuries with long-term corneal and ocular sequelae. Foreign material of plant origin has a high incidence of microbial contamination. For this reason, any patient with a plant-derived foreign body should be followed closely for the development of a subsequent infection, and, in the event infection develops, appropriate laboratory studies must be performed, with special attention to fungal cultures. In addition to the risk of microbial contamination, some vegetable materials are highly antigenic, and corneal implantation results in significant corneal inflammation.[98] On the other hand, cases of plant-derived stromal foreign bodies retained for many years have been reported.[99] Insect and arachnid parts can also result in significant foreign body reactions within the cornea. One of the classic examples results from exposure to tarantulas. New World tarantulas have a dense covering of hairs on their dorsal abdomens, and, when threatened, these spiders vibrate their hind legs across their abdomens, releasing these hairs into the air. Tarantula hairs have been classified into four types by Cooke et al; one of these (type III) is described as long and thin (0.3–1.2 mm) with sharp points and multiple sturdy barbs capable of penetrating the skin.[100] One of the more popular tarantulas imported from Mexico as a pet is the red knee tarantula (*Brachypelma smithi*), whose

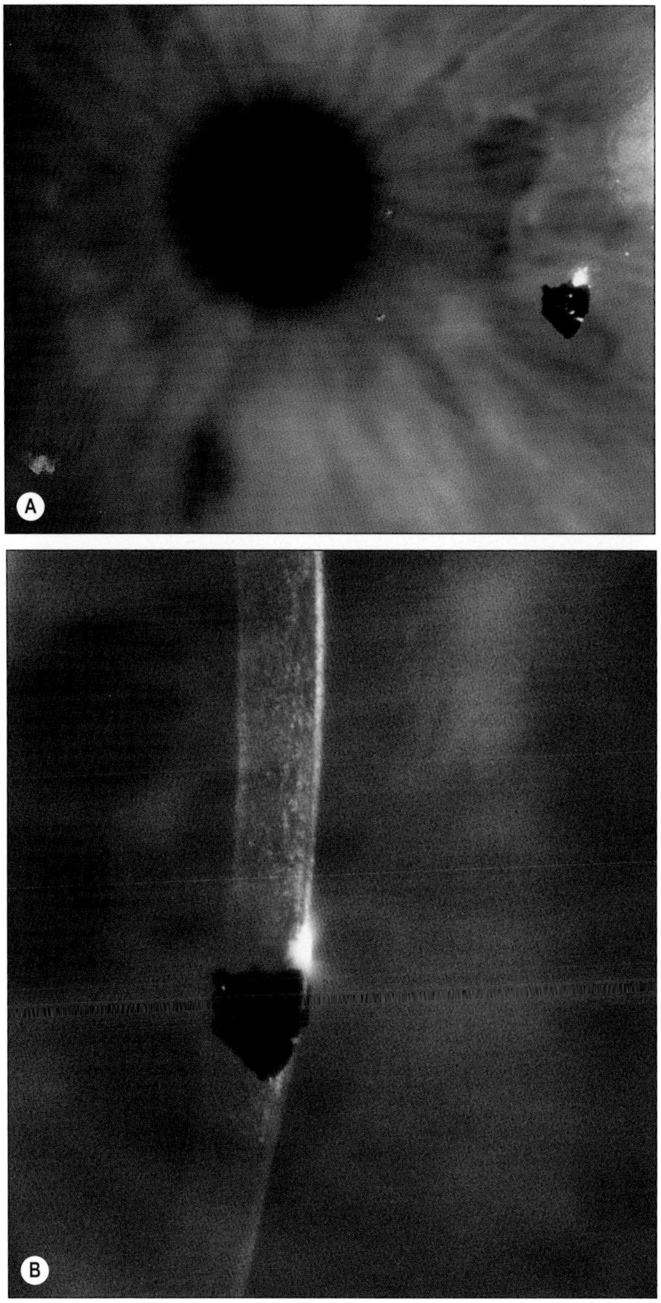

Fig. 97.8 This patient was struck in the eye while performing yard work. Careful examination using diffuse light (**A**) and a thin slit lamp (**B**) revealed that this foreign material was adherent to the epithelium and consequently could be removed by simple washing. Care should be taken when examining patients with corneal foreign bodies to determine the depth of the material so that appropriate removal measures can be undertaken.

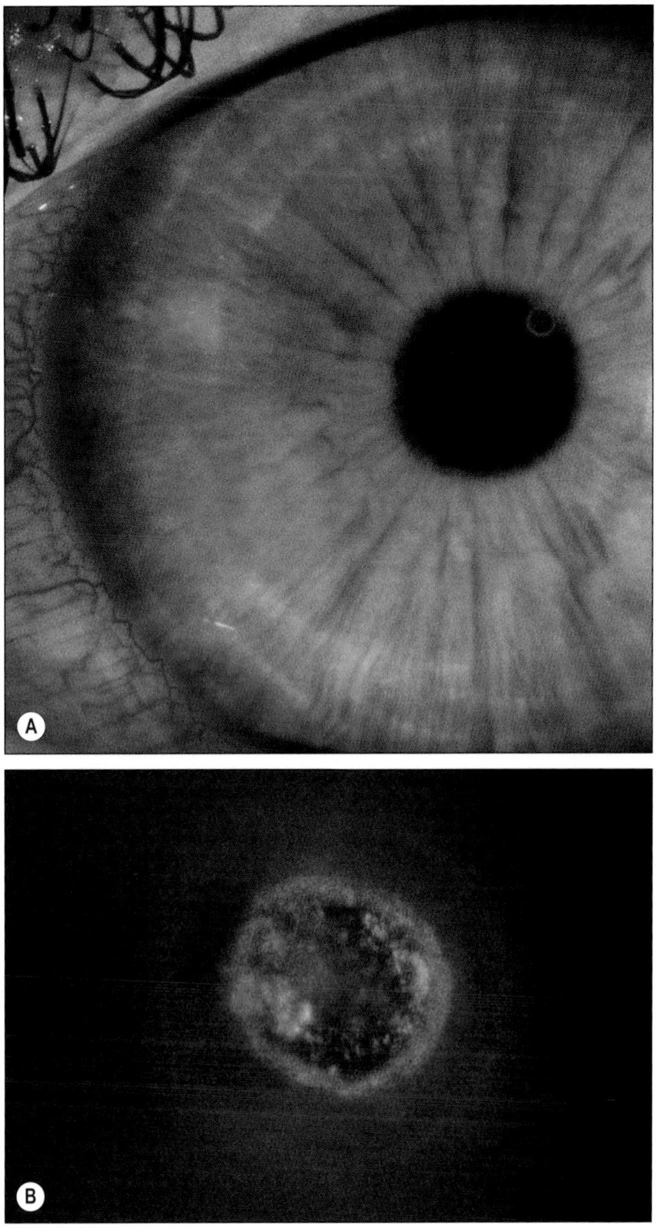

Fig. 97.9 Corneal foreign bodies derived from ferrous materials can rust. As can be seen in this patient, under low (**A**) and high (**B**) magnification, these rust marks are brownish-red in color and slightly irregular. If the material has been present for some time, the iron foreign body can completely degrade, leaving a pastelike material adherent to the corneal surface.

abdomen is well supplied with type III hairs. Once released into the air or carried to the ocular surface by the fingers after contact with the spider or its enclosure, the hairs can become embedded in the cornea, where they cause irritation and itching. With time, they can migrate into the deep stroma and even into the anterior chamber.[101,102] Therapy should be directed at controlling inflammation and removal of hairs that protrude from the epithelial surface, if possible. With time and corticosteroid therapy, hairs remaining in the cornea are reported to resorb.[101] A similar reaction occurs with exposure to caterpillar hairs (setae).[103–106]

Stings

In addition to other types of trauma, the cornea can be injured as a result of stings. These events are relatively rare, but when they occur can result in significant pain and vision loss. The two most frequent types of sting encountered are those resulting from bees and wasps and those from jellyfish.

Bee and wasp stings

Both bees and wasps are members of the order Hymenoptera. This order contains over 100 000 species, of which bees comprise about 20 000 species and wasps 30 000. Other members of the family include ants and sawflies. While some members of both bee and wasp families are nonstinging (such as the wasp suborder Symphyta), many species have the ability to inflict a painful sting if disturbed. Although the majority of case reports of Hymenoptera stings result from bees and wasps, the fire ant (*Solenopsis invicta*) represents a growing problem, especially in the southwestern United States, and has been responsible for corneal sting injuries.[107]

The stinger of both bees and wasps is a modified ovipositor and thus is present only in females. In bees, the stinger is composed of three sections: a single dorsal section, which is hollow, and two thin, straight, barbed darts located in grooves in the ventral surface of the dorsal section. These three pieces fit together as a tube connected to the poison sac at the apex of the insect's abdomen. In the honeybee, as opposed to most bees, the stinger and attached poison sacs are left embedded in the victim. After the sting, the musculature surrounding the sac continues to pump venom. For this reason, when removing an embedded honeybee stinger, care should be taken to avoid pressure on the poison sac.

Bee and wasp venoms are similar, although not identical. In bee venom there are several biogenic amines, polypeptide toxins, and enzymes. The amines (histamine and dopamine) result in immediate pain and discomfort, whereas the polypeptides are the main toxic agents. These polypeptides include melittin, apamin, mast cell degranulating polypeptide, and minimine. The enzymatic components, phospholipase A and B, along with hyaluronidase, are the major antigenic moieties, of which phospholipase A is the most antigenic.[108,109] Wasp venom differs from bee venom in that it contains acetylcysteine, which may account for the increased pain noted in wasp stings.[110] Because of the multiple compounds in the venom of these insects, the local and systemic reaction to envenomization is both toxic and allergic.

Multiple case reports of corneal bee and wasp stings have been published, and these injuries tend to produce a characteristic clinical picture.[110–117] The presentation is generally one of immediate and occasionally severe pain, tearing, and decreased vision. In some cases the lids have been swollen and in others the lids remain normal. The bulbar conjunctiva is generally injected and chemotic. The cornea shows an infiltrate of varying density at the site of the sting, with edema either confined to the epithelium and anterior stroma or full thickness, involving up to one half of the cornea (Fig. 97.10). There may be an epithelial defect at the site of the

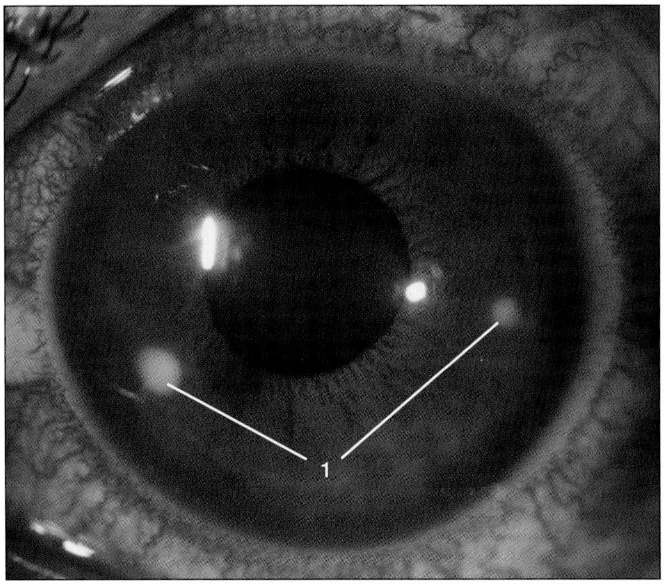

Fig. 97.10 This patient was working in the garden when he was stung twice in the cornea by a bee. The clinical picture of his injured cornea reveals two areas of localized infiltrate (*1*) and corneal opacity with pinpoint epithelial defects overlying the center of each area of cornea infiltrate. These stromal changes resolved over the next 2 to 3 weeks with topical corticosteroid therapy.

stinger entry. Within several days, some patients have developed a fine network of epithelial wrinkles or ridges associated with striate keratopathy. Many authors report an active iritis with keratic precipitates, and one patient has been reported who developed a hyphema.[108] The lens is also frequently involved, with many patients developing anterior subcapsular opacities. Interestingly, the same patient who developed a hyphema also developed spontaneous subluxation of the lens in the area of the sting.[108] The injection of venom into the cornea may also affect the iris, and there are several reports of patients whose pupils were either mid-dilated and fixed or segmentally dilated in the area of the sting. The iris may become atrophic in the area of the envenomation. Most reported cases of bee and wasp stings to the cornea did not have posterior segment involvement, although in a recently reported case of wasp sting to the cornea, where the patient was known to be allergic to wasp venom, a nonrecordable electroretinogram (ERG) occurred 3 days after the incident.[111]

The previous case notwithstanding, most patients with this type of injury respond well to topical corticosteroids and cycloplegic agents, with good recovery of function, although some corneal vascularization may develop in the area of the sting. After the acute event, the retained stinger may be well tolerated in the cornea for many years, indicating that the cause of the reaction is probably the venom rather than a toxic or antigenic property of the stinger.[110,115]

Jellyfish stings

Corneal jellyfish stings are another unusual injury caused by toxin injection into the cornea. While generally rare, in some areas of the USA, notably the Chesapeake Bay, they may be relatively common. Rapoza et al. reported that of the 110 Chesapeake Bay watermen examined as part of a study of cataractogenesis, 90 (82%) gave a history of having sustained ocular jellyfish stings at some time.[118] This regional frequency of jellyfish injuries was supported by the report of Glasser et al., also from the Chesapeake Bay, detailing five cases over 3 years.[119]

Like bee and wasp stings, jellyfish stings result in a relatively typical clinical picture.[118–121] Initially, the patient complains of severe burning pain, tearing, and photophobia. These symptoms may be so severe as to be incapacitating. Rapoza et al. reported that many watermen on the Chesapeake Bay routinely carry proparacaine on their boats to allow them to continue to function after these injuries.[118] On examination, the cornea demonstrates punctate epithelial keratitis with epithelial and stromal edema. Nematocysts of the jellyfish may be adherent to the epithelium. In some cases the anterior chamber shows a significant inflammatory reaction, while in others there is relatively little cell and flare response. Glasser et al. reported that four out of five patients in their series developed dilated and sluggish pupils on the side of the injury, with decreased amplitudes of accommodation in some of those patients.[119] All five patients in their series developed elevations of intraocular pressure, which persisted for up to 4 years in one patient.[119]

Treatment is generally supportive with topical corticosteroids, cycloplegia, and antiocular hypertensives as necessary. In most cases, the injury resolves without sequelae in 24 hours to several weeks. In some cases, however, abnormalities such as pupillary dilation, increased intraocular pressure, and decreased accommodative amplitudes may persist for months.[121] A similar type of injury may also result from the nematocysts of certain corals, such as the red coral (phylum Cnidaria).[122]

References

1. Chiapella AP, Rosenthal AR. One year in an eye casualty. *Br J Ophthalmol.* 1985;69:865–870.
2. Upadhyay MP, Karmacharya PC, Koirala S, et al. The Bhaktapur eye study: ocular trauma and antibiotic prophylaxis for the prevention of corneal ulceration in Nepal. *Br J Ophthalmol.* 2001;85:388–392.
3. Fujikawa LS, et al. Basement membrane components in healing rabbit corneal epithelial wounds: immunofluorescence and ultrastructural studies. *J Cell Biol.* 1984;98:128–138.
4. Parrish CM, Chandler JW. Corneal trauma. In: Kaufman HE, et al, eds. *The cornea.* New York: Churchill Livingstone; 1988.
5. Parrish CM, Chandler JW. Non-perforating mechanical injuries. In: Kaufman HE. et al, eds. *The cornea.* New York: Churchill Livingstone; 1988.
6. Kirkpatrick JNP, Hoh HB, Cook SD. No eye pad for corneal abrasion. *Eye.* 1993;7:468–471.
7. Easty DL. Is an eye pad needed in cases of corneal abrasion? *Br Med J.* 1993;307:1022.
8. Mackway-Jones K. Towards evidence based emergency medicine: best BETS from the Manchester Royal Infirmary. *J Accid Emerg Med.* 1999;16:136–141.
9. Michael JG, Hug D, Dowd MD. Management of corneal abrasion in children: a randomized clinical trial. *Ann Emerg Med.* 2002;40:67–72.
10. Turner A, Rabiu M, Patching for corneal abrasions, The Cochrane Collaboration. *The Cochrane Library Issue.* 2009;1:1–32.
11. Sabri K, et al. National survey of corneal abrasion treatment. *Eye.* 1998;12:278–281.
12. Ali Z, Insler MS. A comparison of therapeutic bandage lenses, tarsorrhaphy, and antibiotic and hypertonic saline on corneal wound healing. *Ann Ophthalmol.* 1986;18:22–24.

13. Madigan MC, Holden BA, Kwok LS. Extended wear of contact lenses can compromise corneal epithelial adhesion. *Curr Eye Res.* 1987;6(10): 1257–1260.
14. Vandorselaer T, Youssfi H, Caspers-Valu LE, Dumont P, Vauthier L. Treatment of traumatic corneal abrasion with contact lens associated with topical nonsteroid anti-inflammatory agent (NSAID) and antibiotic: a safe and effective and comfortable solution. *J Fr Ophtalmol.* 2001;24(10) 1025–1033.
15. Klotz SA, Yue-Kong A, Raghunath PM. A partial-thickness epithelial defect increases the adherence of *Pseudomonas aeruginosa* to the cornea. *Invest Ophthalmol Vis Sci.* 1989;30(6):1069–1074.
16. Pfister RR, Burnstein NL. The effects of ophthalmic drugs, vehicles, and preservatives on corneal epithelium: a scanning electron microscope study. *Invest Ophthalmol Vis Sci.* 1976;15:246–259.
17. Stern GA, et al. Effect of topical antibiotic solutions on corneal epithelial wound healing. *Arch Ophthalmol.* 1993;101:644–647, 1983;3(7):468–471.
18. Weaver CS, Terrell KM. Evidence-based emergency medicine. Update. Do ophthalmic non-steroidal inflammatory drugs reduce the pain associated with simple corneal abrasion without delaying healing? *Ann Emerg Med.* 2003;41(1):134–140.
19. Gipson IK, Keezer L. Effects of cytochalasins and colchicine on the ultrastructure of migrating corneal epithelium. *Invest Ophthalmol Vis Sci.* 1982;22:643–650.
20. McDonnell PJ, Green WR, Schanzlin DJ. Corneal trauma. In: Spoor TC, Nisi FA, eds. *Management of ocular, orbital, and adnexal trauma.* New York: Raven Press; 1988.
21. Soong HK. Vinculin in focal cell-to-substrate attachments of spreading corneal epithelial cells. *Arch Ophthalmol.* 1987;105:1129–1132.
22. Dua HS, Forrester JV. Clinical patterns of corneal epithelial wound healing. *Am J Ophthalmol.* 1987;104:481–489.
23. Weene LE. Recurrent corneal erosion after trauma: a statistical study. *Ann Ophthalmol.* 1985;17:521–524.
24. Slingsby JG, Forstot SL. Effect of blunt trauma on the corneal endothelium. *Arch Ophthalmol.* 1981;99:1041–1043.
25. Roper-Hall MJ, Wilson RS, Thompson SM. Changes in endothelial cell density following accidental trauma. *Br J Ophthalmol.* 1982;66: 518–519.
26. Löwenstein A. Überlegungen zu einem fall von traumatischer hornhautquellung nebst bemerkungen über die bedeutung des hornhautendothels, *Albrecht von Graefe's Arch Klin Ophthalmol.* 1931;127:598–605.
27. Payrau P, Raynaud G. Lésions de la cornée par souffle: corps étrangers perforants microscopiques; anneaux veloutés postérieurs. *Ann Oculist.* 1965;198:1057–1074.
28. Forstot SL, Gasset AR. Transient traumatic posterior annular keratopathy of Payrau. *Arch Ophthalmol.* 1974;92:527–528.
29. Pichler A. Die Casparsche ringtrübung der Hornhaut. *Z Augenheilkd.* 1916;35:311–313.
30. Cibis GW, Weingeist TA, Krachmer JH. Traumatic corneal endothelial rings. *Arch Ophthalmol.* 1978;96:485–488.
31. Maloney WF, et al. Specular microscopy of traumatic posterior annular keratopathy. *Arch Ophthalmol.* 1979;97:1647–1650.
32. Duke-Elder S, MacFaul PA. Lacerations of the cornea. In: Duke-Elder S, ed. *System of ophthalmology.* vol. XIV, part 1. St Louis: Mosby; 1972.
33. John ME, Schmitt TE. Traumatic hyphema after radial keratotomy. *Ann Ophthalmol.* 1988;15:930–932.
34. Spivack LE. Case report: radial keratotomy incisions remain intact despite facial trauma from plane crash. *J Refract Surg.* 1987;4:59–60.
35. Forstot SL, Damiano RE. Trauma after radial keratotomy. *Ophthalmology.* 1988;95:833–835.
36. Simons KB, Linsalata RP, Zaragosa AM. Ruptured globe secondary to blunt trauma following radial keratotomy. *J Refract Surg.* 1988;4: 132–135.
37. Pearlstein ES, et al. Ruptured globe after radial keratotomy. *Am J Ophthalmol.* 1988;106:755–756.
38. Binder P, et al. Histopathology of traumatic corneal rupture after radial keratotomy. *Arch Ophthalmol.* 1988;106:1584–1590.
39. Bloom HR, Sands J, Schneider D. Corneal rupture from blunt trauma 22 months after radial keratotomy. *Refract Corneal Surg.* 1990;6:197–199.
40. Norden RA, et al. Air bag-induced corneal flap folds after in situ keratomileusis. *Am J Ophthalmol.* 2000;130(2):234–235.
41. Duke-Elder S, MacFaul PA. Birth injuries. In: Duke-Elder S, ed. *System of ophthalmology.* vol. XIV, part 2. St Louis: Mosby; 1972.
42. Jain IS, et al. Ocular hazards during birth. *J Pediatr Ophthalmol Strabis.* 1980;17(1):14–16.
43. De Wecker L. Les lésions oculaires obstétricales. *Ann d'Ocul.* 1896; 116:140–145.
44. Truc H. Lésions obstétricales de l'oeil et de ses annexes. *Ann d'Ocul.* 1898;119(3):161.
45. Noyes H. Traumatic keratitis caused by forceps delivery of an infant. *Trans Am Ophthalmol.* 1896;Soc 7(session 1895):454.
46. Dujardin. Keratite obstétricale. *J Sci Med de Lille.* 1896;48:521–526.
47. Thomson WE, Buchanan L. A clinical and pathological account of some of the injuries to the eye of the child during labour. *Trans Ophthalmol Soc UK.* 1903;23:296–319.
48. Sugar HS, Airala MA. Birth injuries of the cornea. *J Pediatr Ophthalmol.* 1971;8(1):26–28.
49. Lloyd RI. Birth injuries of the cornea and allied conditions. *Am J Ophthalmol.* 1938;21(4):359–365.
50. Tetsumoto K, et al. Epithelial transformation of the corneal endothelium in forceps birth-injury-associated keratopathy. *Cornea.* 1993;12(1):65–71.
51. McDonald MB, Burgess SK. Contralateral occipital depression related to obstetric forceps injury to the eye. *Am J Ophthalmol.* 1992;114(3): 318–321.
52. Hofmann RF, Paul TO, Penteli-Molnar J. The management of corneal birth trauma. *J Pediatr Ophthalmol Strabis.* 1981;18(1):45–47.
53. Angell LK, Robb RM, Berson FG. Visual prognosis in patients with ruptures in Descemet's membrane due to forceps injuries. *Arch Ophthalmol.* 1981;99:2137–2139.
54. Zuchlich JA. Ultraviolet-induced photochemical damage in ocular tissues. *Health Physics.* 1989;56(3):671–682.
55. Tsubai T, Matsuo M. Ultraviolet light induced changes in the glucose-6-phosphate dehydrogenase activity of porcine corneas. *Cornea.* 2002;21(5):495–500.
56. Lattimore MR. Effects of ultraviolet radiation on the oxygen uptake rate of the rabbit cornea. *Optom Vis Sci.* 1989;66(2):117–122.
57. Bergmanson JPG. Corneal damage in photokeratitis – why is it so painful? *Optom Vis Sci.* 1990;67(6):407–413.
58. Clarke SM, Doughty MJ, Cullen AP. Acute effects of ultraviolet-B irradiation on the corneal surface of the pigmented rabbit studied by scanning electron microscopy. *Acta Ophthalmol.* 1990;68:639–650.
59. Kitaichi N, Shimizu T, Yoshida K, et al. Macrophage migration inhibitory factor ameliorates UV-induced photokeratitis in mice. *Exp Eye Res.* 2008;86, 929–935.
60. Pitts DG, Bergmanson JPG, Chu LW. Ultrastructural analysis of corneal exposure to UV radiation. *Acta Ophthalmol.* 1987;65:263–273.
61. Riley MV, et al. The effects of UV-B irradiation on the corneal endothelium. *Curr Eye Res.* 1987;6(8):1021–1033.
62. Ringvold A, Davanger M, Olsen EG. Changes of the cornea endothelium after ultraviolet irradiation. *Acta Ophthalmol.* 1982;60:41–53.
63. Millodot M, Earlam RA. Sensitivity of the cornea after exposure to ultraviolet light. *Ophthal Res.* 1984;16:325–328.
64. Taylor HR, et al. The long-term effects of visible light on the eye. *Arch Ophthalmol.* 1992;110:99–104.
65. Hill JC, Maske R. Pathogenesis of pterygium. *Eye.* 1989;3:218–226.
66. Karai I, et al. Morphological change in corneal endothelium due to ultraviolet radiation in welders. *Br J Ophthalmol.* 1984;68:544–548.
67. Olsen EG, Ringvold A. Human cornea endothelium and ultraviolet radiation. *Acta Ophthalmol.* 1982;60:54–56.
68. Cullen AP, Dumbleton KA, Chou BR. Contact lenses and acute exposure to ultraviolet radiation. *Optom Vis Sci.* 1989;66(6):407–411.
69. Bergmanson JPG, Pitts DG, Chu LW. The efficacy of a UV-blocking soft contact lens in protecting cornea against UV radiation. *Acta Ophthalmol.* 1987;65:278–286.
70. Oldenburg JB, Gritz DC, McDonnell PJ. Topical ultraviolet light-absorbing chromophore protects against experimental photokeratitis. *Arch Ophthalmol.* 1990;108:1142–1144.
71. Duke-Elder S, MacFaul PA. Radiation injuries. In: Duke-Elder S, ed. *System of ophthalmology.* vol. XIV, part 2. St Louis: Mosby; 1972.
72. Pfister RR, et al. Photocoagulation keratopathy. *Ophthalmology.* 1971;86:94–96.
73. Shahan WE, Lamb HD. Histologic effect of heat on the eye. *Am J Ophthalmol.* 1916;33(8):225.
74. Campbell FW, Michaelson IC. Blood-vessel formation in the cornea. *Br J Ophthalmol.* 1949;33:238–255.
75. Lister A, Greaves DP. Effect of cortisone upon the vascularization which follows corneal burns. *Br J Ophthalmol.* 1951;35:725–729.
76. Junghans BM, Collin HB. Limbal lymphangiogenesis after corneal injury: an autoradiographic study. *Curr Eye Res.* 1989;8(1):91–100.
77. Goldblatt WS, et al. Hyperthermic treatment of rabbit corneas. *Invest Ophthalmol Vis Sci.* 1989;30(8):1778–1783.
78. Linhart RW. Burns of the eyes and eyelids. *Ann Ophthalmol.* 1978;10:999–1000.
79. Guy RJ, et al. Three-years experience in a regional burn center with burns of the eyes and eyelids. *Ophthalmic Surg.* 1982;13(5):383–386.

80. Vajpayee RB, et al. Contact thermal burns of the cornea. *Can J Ophthalmol.* 1991;26(4):215–218.
81. Mannis MJ, Miller RB, Krachmer JH. Contact thermal burns of the cornea from electric curling irons. *Am J Ophthalmol.* 1984;98:336–339.
82. Bloom SM, Gittinger JW, Kazarian EL. Management of corneal contact thermal burns. *Am J Ophthalmol.* 1986;100:536.
83. Awan KJ. Contact thermal burns of the cornea from electric curling irons (letter). *Am J Ophthalmol.* 1985;99(1):90–91.
84. Margo CE, Groden LR. Squamous cell carcinoma of the cornea and conjunctiva following a thermal burn of the eye. *Cornea.* 1986;5(3): 185–188.
85. Mönestam E, Björnstig: Eye injuries in northern Sweden. *Acta Ophthalmol.* 1991;69:1–5.
86. Banerjee A. Effectiveness of eye protection in the metal working industry. *Br Med J.* 1990;301:645–646.
87. Heiner JS, et al. Ocular injuries and diseases at a combat supported hospital in support of operations Desert Shield and Desert Storm. *Arch Ophthalmol.* 1993;111:795–798.
88. Alexamder MM, et al. More than meets the eye: a study of time lost from work by patients who incurred injuries from corneal foreign bodies. *Br J Ophthalmol.* 1991;75:740–742.
89. Kaye-Wilson LG. Localization of corneal foreign bodies. *Br Med J.* 1992;76:741–742.
90. Weaver JH. A needle for corneal foreign body removal. *Trans Am Acad Ophthalmol Otolaryngol.* 1971;75(3):660–661.
91. Huismans H. Kombinierte fremdkörper-und parazentesenadel mit auswechselbarem aufsatz. *Klin Monatsbl Augenheilkd.* 1990;197:441.
92. Arnold RW, Erie JC. Magnetized forceps for metallic corneal foreign bodies (letter). *Arch Ophthalmol.* 1988;106:1502.
93. Weiss JS, Kachadoorian H. Removal of corneal foreign bodies with ocular magnet (letter). *Ophthalmic Surg.* 1989;20(5):378–379.
94. Zuckerman B, Lieberman TW. Corneal rust ring. *Arch Ophthalmol.* 1960;63:254–264.
95. Jayamanne DGR, Bell RW. Non-penetrating corneal foreign body injuries: factors affecting delay in rehabilitation of patients. *J Accident Emerg Med.* 1994;11:195–197.
96. Liston RL, Olson RJ, Mamalis N. A comparison of rust-ring removal methods in a rabbit model: small-gauge hypodermic needle versus electric drill. *Ann Ophthalmol.* 1991;23:24–27.
97. Hulbert MFG. Efficacy of eyepad in corneal healing after corneal foreign body removal. *Lancet.* 1991;337:643.
98. Steahly LP, Almquist HT. Corneal foreign bodies of coconut origin. *Ann Ophthalmol.* 1977;9(8):1017–1021.
99. Dahlan F, Milam DF, Bunt-Milam AH. Long-term corneal retention of a plant foreign body. *Cornea.* 1989;8(1);72–74
100. Cooke JAL, et al. Urticaria caused by tarantula hairs. *Am J Trop Med Hyg.* 1973;22:130–133.
101. Chang PCT, Soong HK, Barnett JM. Corneal penetration by tarantula hairs (letter). *Br J Ophthalmol.* 1991;75(4):253–254.
102. Hered RW, et al. Ophthalmia nodosa caused by tarantula hairs. *Ophthalmology.* 1988;95(2):166–169.
103. Teske SAH, et al. Caterpillar-induced keratitis. *Cornea.* 1991;10(4): 317–321.
104. Haluska FG, et al. Experimental gypsy moth (*Lymantria dispar*) ophthalmia nodosa. *Arch Ophthalmol.* 1983;101:799–801.
105. Conrath J, et al. Caterpillar setae-induced acute anterior uveitis: a case report. *Am J Ophthalmol.* 2000;130(6):841–843.
106. Horng C, Chou P, Liang J. Caterpillar setae in the deep cornea and anterior chamber. *Am J Ophthalmol.* 2000;129(3):384–385.
107. Amador M, Busse FK. Corneal injury caused by imported fire ants in a child with neurological compromise. *J Pediatr Ophthalmol Strabis.* 1998;34:55–57.
108. Chen CJ, Richardson CD. Bee sting-induced ocular changes. *Ann Ophthalmol.* 1986;18:285–286.
109. Sobotka AK, et al. Allergy to insect stings. *J Allergy Clin Immunol.* 1976;57(1):29–40.
110. Gilboa M, Gdal-on M, Zonis S. Bee and wasp stings of the eye. Retained intralenticular wasp sting: a case report. *Br J Ophthalmol.* 1977;61: 662–664.
111. Kitagawa K, Hayasaka S, Setogawa T. Wasp sting-induced retinal damage. *Ann Ophthalmol.* 1993;25:157–158.
112. Smolin G, Wong I. Bee sting of the cornea: case reports. *Ann Ophthalmol.* 1982;14(4):342–343.
113. Young CA. Bee sting of the cornea with case report. *Am J Ophthalmol.* 1931;14:208–216.
114. Singh G. Bee sting of the cornea. *Ann Ophthalmol.* 1984;16(4): 320–322.
115. Tuft SJ, Crompton DO, Coster DJ. Insect sting in a cornea (letter). *Am J Ophthalmol.* 1985;99(6):727–728.
116. Smith DG, Roberge RJ. Corneal bee sting with retained stinger. *J Emerg Med.* 2001;20(2):125–128.
117. Yildirim N, Erol N. Bee sting of the cornea: a case report. *Cornea.* 1998;17(3):333–334.
118. Rapoza PA, et al. Ocular jellyfish stings in Chesapeake Bay watermen (letter). *Am J Ophthalmol.* 1986;102(4):536–537.
119. Glasser DB, et al. Ocular jellyfish stings. *Ophthalmology.* 1992;99(9): 1414–1418.
120. Wong SK, Matoba AY. Jellyfish sting of the cornea. *Am J Ophthalmol.* 1985;100(5):739–740.
121. Hercus J. An unusual eye condition. *Med J Aust.* 1944;1:98–99.
122. Keamy J, Umlas J, Lee Y. Red coral keratitis. *Cornea.* 2000;19(6): 859–860.

Chapter 98

Acid Injuries of the Eye

Daryl A. Pfister, Roswell R. Pfister

Introduction

Ocular chemical and thermal injuries represent between 8% and 18% of ocular trauma.[1] Acid injuries to the eye are not uncommon due to the fact that strong acids are encountered throughout our society. In our homes, acids are components in rust removal products, pool cleaners, and car batteries. Depending upon the source quoted, between 49% and 76.5% of ocular chemical injuries occur in the workplace[2,3] where acids are used as reagents in the manufacture of dyes, PVC pipe, fertilizer, explosives, and many other applications. Mustard gas, which was used as recently as in the Iran–Iraq war, forms hydrochloric acid upon hydrolysis, and it could also be used as a terrorist weapon.[4,5]

Occasionally, acids are used as a means of assault, where the injuries sustained are frequently bilateral and are often more severe than accidental exposures.[1] Traditionally, acid injuries have been considered less destructive to the eye than alkali injuries. However, strong acids can cause devastating ocular injuries mimicking alkali exposure, and knowledge about the interaction of acid with the eye and treatment modalities is important to all healthcare providers (Fig. 98.1).

The Chemistry of Acids

There are many classification systems of acids. The simplest scheme refers to a pH range below 7.0 denoting acids and above 7.0 for bases or alkaline substances. Under this scheme, physiologic pH is usually slightly basic at about 7.4. In terms of injury prediction, a more useful concept might be strong versus weak acids. A strong acid or base can be thought of as being more or almost completely dissociated into cations (+) and anions (–) in solution. The more fully an acid or base is dissociated, the stronger it is. In the case of acids, strong ones form more free hydrogen ions (H^+) in solution and, by definition, have a lower pH. Obviously, the anion of an acid determines the amount of dissociation, and therefore its strength. Examples of strong acids include hydrochloric, nitric, and sulfuric acids. Strong acids are often additionally referred to as inorganic or mineral. In contrast, organic acids are usually weak, such as acetic and carbonic acids. Weak acids are not completely dissociated in solution and have higher pH readings. The interaction of strong and weak acids with tissues is somewhat different, as discussed in the next section.

The Biochemistry of Acids

An injury resulting from any chemical introduced into a biologic system relates to the volume, concentration, and toxicity, as well as its penetration, and duration of exposure.[6] Breaking down this statement, it is easy to see how volume and concentration directly affect the degree of injury. Because all acids in solution form hydrogen ions, toxicity from an acid is proportionally related to the identity of the acid's anion. Some anions, such as the fluoride ion in hydrofluoric acid, are particularly noxious, resulting in more damage at similar volume and concentration than others. Several acids that cause relatively distinctive ocular injuries are listed in Table 98.1.

Acids and alkalis interact with tissues in fundamentally differently ways. In biologic systems, alkaline agents saponify the lipids of cell membranes, causing both rapid and deep penetration.[7] Acids, on the other hand, precipitate and denature proteins somewhat limiting further penetration. Alkalis penetrate lipid layers more readily and rapidly; however, acids bind proteins, limiting penetration but potentially increasing the local duration of exposure to the anion. Acid anions with higher binding potentials can cause damage at higher pH than anions with lower binding potentials.

An important topic to address when discussing acids and alkalis in biologic systems is buffers. Buffering capacity refers to the amount of acid or base that can be absorbed before rapid pH swings occur. If there were no buffering capacity available, most cellular reactions halt. The cornea does have some buffering capacity,[8,9] and its pH begins to neutralize within 15 minutes after exposure to weak acids and is probably normalized by 1 hour.[10] Since biologic systems are meant to neutralize only small amounts of weak acids and bases, these systems are quickly overwhelmed during exposure to strong acids or bases.

An amphoteric substance is loosely related to buffers in that it is capable of acting like either an acid or a base, and as such, it can neutralize both acids and bases. Two products have been introduced taking advantage of this phenomenon: Diphoterine, and Hexafluorine, both developed by Prevor Laboratories in France. Diphoterine is an amphoteric, hypertonic, polyvalent compound for use in ocular and skin decontaminations of about 600 chemicals, including acids, alkalis, reducers, oxidizers, alkylating agents, and radionucleotides. Additionally, the binding reaction is not exothermic.[11,12] Hexafluorine is its counterpart for ocular and dermal exposures to hydrofluoric acid as well as fluorides in acidic environments.[13] While the science behind these compounds sounds promising, the experimental studies and clinical observations with these compounds in both the dermal and ocular literature do not always agree as to their effectiveness. In fact, the experimental dermatological literature (rat model) suggests that Hexafluorine treatment outcomes are worse than standard treatment with water and calcium gluconate.[14,15] The clinical literature seems to suggest otherwise; however, there are shortcomings. Most of the clinical literature suggests that both compounds lessen the effects of chemical injury on the eye and skin in splash injuries in the workplace.[13,16] Substantial limitations in these studies include the lack of both controls and grading of the injuries. One clinical study using controls and grading shows that diphoterine does significantly improve reepithelialization in human alkali injuries for grade I and II injuries; however, there were insignificant numbers to draw conclusions for higher-grade injuries.[17] Perhaps the discrepancy in the experimental and clinical literature lies with the lack of grading, and for milder chemical injuries these new agents may be effective. Further rigorous experimental and clinical studies are needed to determine ultimate effectiveness of these new compounds.

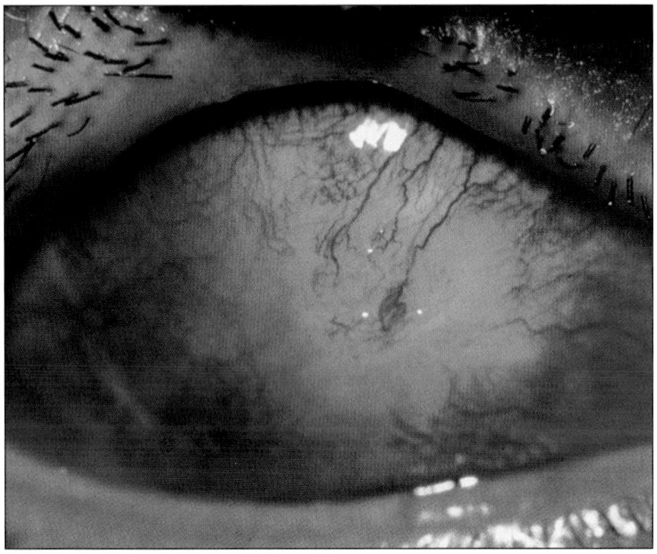

Fig. 98.1 External photograph showing a very severe acid injury, indistinguishable from very severe alkali injury.

Ocular Effects of Acid

A cascade of events occurs upon exposure of the eye to acid beyond the denaturation and precipitation of proteins. Collagen shrinkage immediately raises the intraocular pressure, and the effect persists for at least 3 hours through the elaboration of prostaglandins, possibly from the presence of H^+ ions in the aqueous.[18,19] Additionally, the stroma liberates ascorbic acid (vitamin C). In severe acid injuries, ascorbate levels in the aqueous plummet after 24 hours, probably due to either breakdown of the blood–aqueous barrier or damage to the active transport mechanism of the ciliary body.[10,20] Ascorbate is an essential element in the elaboration of collagen, and its loss can lead to stromal ulceration.[21,22]

During the first week after injury, mucopolysaccharides, which are initially unharmed by acid, are either liberated from damaged tissue or destroyed, contributing to decreased tear breakup time, punctate staining (PEE), or slow-healing epithelial defects.[23,24] Even mild injuries may exhibit these changes. Epithelial breakdown can result in stromal edema, especially in the first 24–36 hours; however, as long as the endothelium is undamaged, stromal hydration largely normalizes upon reepithelialization. Energy production through glycolysis tumbles in the first 3 or 4 days after injury, becoming supernormal at a week.[10] Glycolysis levels may correspond to either increases for repairing injured tissue or from the influx of polymorphonuclear neutrophils (PMNs) leading to tissue breakdown and ulceration. Depending upon which process succeeds, the result can vary from complete repair to scar formation with neovascularization to perforation.

Table 98.1 Special-mention acids

Acid	Strength	Use	Distinctive ocular effects
Sulfuric (H_2SO_4)	Strong	Car batteries, fertilizer, making other acids, explosives, dyes, refining petroleum	Car battery explosions causing acid injury and concussive damage
Nitric (HNO_3)	Strong	Fertilizers, explosives, rocket propellant, production of nylon	Yellowish epithelial opacity
Chromic (H_2CrO_4)	Strong	An intermediate in electroplating, ceramic glazes, wood preservation	Brown discoloration of conjunctiva, chronic conjunctivitis
Hydrofluoric (HF)	Weak, but most reactive anion	Etching glass, semiconductor production, rust remover	Acts like alkali to saponify lipids, causing deep, rapid penetration, extensive ischemia, and calcific plaques in corneal stroma

Table 98.2 Classification* and prognosis in acid injuries of the eye

Grade	Epithelial opacity, defect	Stromal edema, opacity	Conjunctival involvement	Limbal ischemia	Recovery	1 Vision impairment, 2 scarring, 3 vessels
(I) Mild	Opacified white†	None to minimal, none	Erythema, opacification, chemosis	None	Rapid	1, 2, 3 none to little
(II) Moderate	Opacified white,† common at 24–36 hours	Mild to moderate, none	Opacification, chemosis, petechia or subconjunctival hemorrhage	None to minimal	Epithelial healing likely within 10 days	1 mild, 2 faint anterior scar possible, 3 little tendency
(III) Severe	Entire epithelium opacified white†	Moderate to severe, mild opacity obscures iris details	Opacification, hemorrhages, necrosis	≤1/3	Epithelial healing possible in weeks to months, ulcers/ perforation possible	1 moderate to severe, 2 moderate anterior scar, 3 peripheral usual
(IV) Very severe	Opacified white† (if present) and sloughs rapidly	Marked, severe	Necrosis may be extensive	>1/3	Protracted (months–years), sloughing of stroma possible with ulceration/perforation	1, 2, 3 extensive, like severe alkali injuries

* Accurate determination of grade may have to be delayed by 24 to 48 hours.
† With chromic or nitric acid, the epithelium may be brown or yellow.

Classification and Prognosis of Acid Injuries

This classification scheme for acid injury is a modification of the one used for alkali injuries and represents a further adaptation of the 1–4 grading system first proposed by Hughes (Table 98.2).[9] Classes of injury for acids are differentiated based upon the extent of epithelial damage, stromal edema denoting degree of penetration,[25] and limbal ischemia (whitening), as in alkali injuries. While using the classification system, a delay of 24 to 48 hours may be indicated, for the initial clinical impression may be better or worse than the actual injury (Fig. 98.2). The classification system is meant only as a general guide to help determine prognosis and treatment. Fortunately, most acid injuries are moderate (grade II or less) and carry relatively good prognoses.

Treatment

Immediate

Chemical injuries have mostly been treated similarly, with copious and continuous irrigation of clean water or other nontoxic irrigant as quickly as possible after exposure (see also Ch. 99 for alkali injuries). In this manner, dilution is the solution, as it helps remove and decrease the potency of the noxious agent. Of note, never use a base to neutralize an acid because it can magnify the injury.

Relatively recently, some debate on the osmotic component of irrigation solutions has evolved. Some experimental literature suggests that low osmolarity may be better by increasing stromal hydration, and this theory is supported by pH measurements in the anterior chamber of rabbits,[26,27] by diluting the agent in the stroma and flushing it out. Other literature suggests that hyposmotic rinsing may cause deeper penetration due to stromal swelling;[28] however, no experimental documentation is offered with this hypothesis. Several experimental articles suggest that isosmotic solutions such as physiologic saline and Ringer's lactate may be disadvantageous by both lacking buffer capacity and inducing less stromal edema.[26,29] An interesting work studying all the major solutions in an experimental rabbit alkali injury model found that while none of the solutions normalized pH in the anterior chamber, both diphoterine and Cederroth Eye Wash Solution (including borate buffer) (Cederroth Industrial Products, Upplands Väasby, Sweden) were the best, tap water was intermediate, and physiologic saline and phosphate buffer were not effective.[30] Current recommendations might be summed up by suggesting that either low osmotic washes such as tap water or high buffer capacity agents such as diphoterine or Cederroth Eye Wash Solution should be considered for use as initial rinsing agents.[27] Clearly, more work needs to be done to answer the question about the best solution to use with chemical injuries.

Acute care

While irrigation continues, transfer to an emergency facility should be arranged, and if possible, irrigation should continue during transport. An irrigating contact lens (Morgan therapeutic lens or Mor-FLEX® Lens (MT2000), Mor-Tan Inc., PO Box 8719, Missoula, MT 59807) is preferable to simple irrigation, and the lens can be used with or without a drop of topical anesthetic. Note that the irrigating lens should be inserted into the fornices while the solution is flowing.

In the emergency department, irrigation should continue after checking the fornices for particulate matter by double

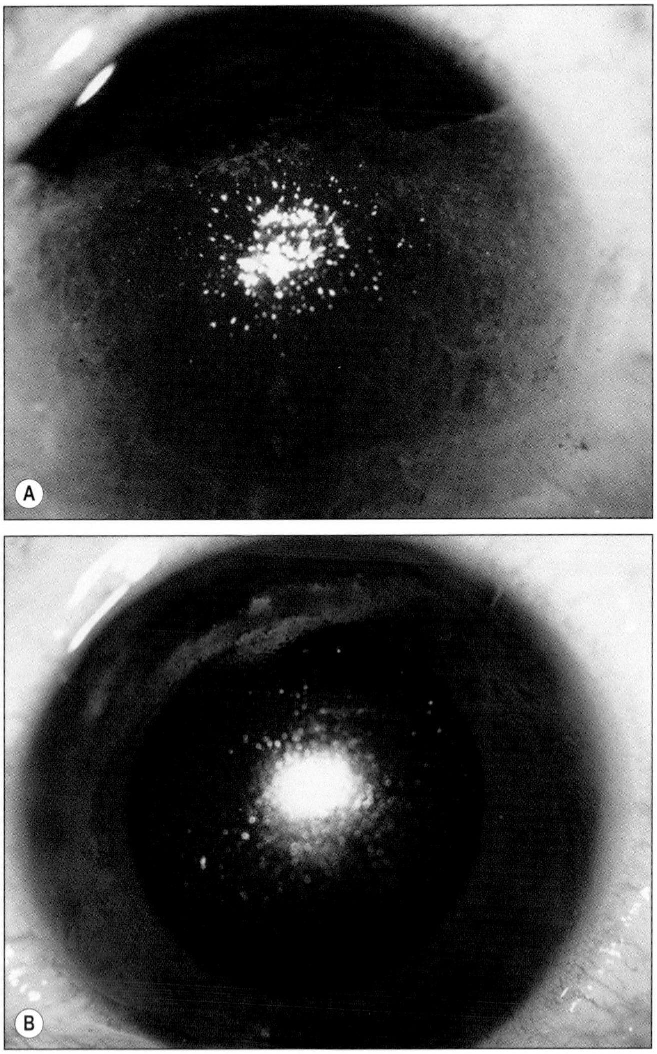

Fig. 98.2 External photograph showing (A) a mild acid injury (grade I) on presentation with white opacified epithelium partially protected above by the superior lid. (B) The same eye 24 hours later: after sloughing, the epithelium reveals minimal stromal involvement.

inversion of the lids and sweeping them with moist, sterile cotton swabs. If the injury included an explosion, as occurs frequently with a car battery, ocular integrity should be verified prior to manipulation.[31] Irrigation is paramount, with 1 to 2 liters over 1 to 2 hours being associated with shorter overall treatment courses and better outcomes.[32] Indeed, there may be merit to irrigating longer, such as 2 to 4 hours.[33] As an end point, a pH check of the tears 5 to 10 minutes following irrigation might be useful, and if the pH is less than 7, irrigation should continue.

Following irrigation, a more thorough ophthalmologic examination should ensue, including vision, external and slit lamp examinations, epithelial and limbal involvement, stromal edema, and intraocular pressure. Initial evaluation of the stroma may prove difficult if epithelial opacity exists, but limbal involvement should be apparent in higher-grade injuries. A delay in the assessment of stromal edema by 24 to 48 hours may be needed due to epithelial opacity or false impressions of corneal hydration from irrigation.

Subacute and intermediate care

Following rinsing and initial assessment, treatment includes coverage with a broad-spectrum topical antibiotic to guard against infection in the face of an epithelial defect. With moderate or large epithelial defects, consideration can be given to prescribing antibiotic ointment such as ciprofloxacin (Ciloxan® ointment, Alcon Laboratories, Inc., 6201 S. Freeway, Ft. Worth, TX 76134). Moderately long-acting cycloplegic agents can decrease painful ciliary spasm. If glaucoma is present, topical or oral agents can be used. Recalcitrant cases might require periodic paracentesis, which may be therapeutic, by allowing rapid normalization of the anterior chamber pH, especially if balanced salt solution is used to re-form it. Topical nonsteroidal antiinflammatory drugs should be used cautiously due to the possibility of corneal melting in conjunction with epithelial defects.[34,35] Patients without pain may have severe injuries due to anesthesia from nerve damage. Injuries with significant inflammation and/or secondary iritis may benefit from cautious use of topical steroids in the first 7 to 10 days; however, the use of steroids beyond this time may increase corneal ulcerations or perforations.[36] It is difficult to know whether topical steroids diminish corneal scarring. Damage to the eye or/and eyelids can create abnormal blinking and lagophthalmos. Ointments, nonpreserved artificial tears, or gels can help, but taping or patching the lids closed, partial tarsorrhaphy, or early skin grafting may be required.

Systemic ascorbic acid (vitamin C) has been shown in an animal study to reduce the rate of corneal ulceration in acid injuries.[37] Moderate or higher-grade acid injuries may benefit from the addition of oral vitamin C and/or citrate, but without further human studies we are unable to definitively conclude that these supplements are favorable (see Ch. 99).

Newer strategies involving human amniotic membrane transplantation (AMT) are being utilized in both acute and chronic chemical injuries. AMT may help decrease a number of potential sequelae, including speeding reepithelialization of both the corneal and conjunctival surfaces, reducing ocular surface inflammation and symblepharon formation, and reducing pain. In acute cases, a literature review suggests that AMT be performed within 2–3 weeks of injury;[38–41] however, one paper studied temporary sutured AMT patching,[42] and another utilized a sutureless temporary amniotic membrane patch (ProKera; Bio-Tissue, Inc, Miami, FL), with reapplication if needed.[43] A prospective, randomized clinical trial studying AMT with adjunctive therapy versus medical therapy alone in grade II to IV chemical injuries found that for moderate cases, the AMT-treated group had less subjective discomfort and faster reepithelialization; however, grade IV injuries showed no statistical difference. Additionally, between the treatment group and controls, there was no difference in final vision, corneal neovascularization, symblepharon formation, or tear function.[38] AMT can be useful in chemical injury cases, but there are unanswered questions requiring more research.

Limbal stem cell[44] deficiency (LSCD) occurs most frequently in high-grade chemical injuries with extensive perilimbal ischemia. LSCD causes persistent epithelial defects, and healing occurs by conjunctival epithelial and vascular ingrowth with persistent stromal inflammation. Sources for limbal stem cell transplants range from conjunctival limbal autografts (CLAU), living related and cadaveric donors, to ex vivo culture expanded limbal epithelium.[45] Limbal stem cell transplants can be combined with AMT. Although the surgery can be long and tedious, in some cases this is the only hope to salvage a chemically injured eye. Additionally, one drawback of utilizing allogeneic material is the need for long-term systemic immune suppression.[46,47] Some success has been reported combining deep anterior lamellar keratoplasty (DALK) with limbal stem cell transplantation with or without AMT.[48] In severe cases with both extensive or total LSCD and large ulcers or perforations, limbus-to-limbus penetrating grafts may be attempted to provide both a healthy cornea and stem cell mass.[49] Glaucoma and graft rejection are problematic following large grafts, however.

Long term

The long-term treatment of acid injuries involves the maximization of function and restoration of vision. The process of visual rehabilitation is often delayed for 1 to 2 years to allow a quiet, stable eye. Before contemplating keratoplasty, lid abnormalities and secondary glaucoma should be addressed. Seton valves are frequently required due to extensive conjunctival scarring. LSCD must be addressed with or without amniotic membrane transplantation to provide a stable ocular surface prior to keratoplasty. These procedures can be performed separately or in conjunction with keratoplasty. Symblephara can be freed from their anterior attachments and can then be used to re-form the palpebral conjunctiva by reflection posteriorly and suturing in place.[50] Fresh donor material with intact epithelium is essential along with efforts to protect the epithelium during the procedure, including frequent application of viscoelastic and balanced salt solution to the graft's surface. Oversizing the donor button and placing interrupted nylon sutures tied relatively tightly may be used in vascularized corneas to allow for wound contraction. In cases in which lid function is imperfect, surgical correction should be sought prior to undertaking visual rehabilitation. In cases where dry eye is a factor, punctal occlusion should be considered preoperatively and partial tarsorrhaphy should be considered intraoperatively or immediately postoperatively. As with alkali injuries, a keratoprosthesis can be considered for those bilateral cases in which vision cannot be restored otherwise or in bilateral cases that have undergone multiple previous failed grafts.

References

1. Merle H, Gérard M, Schrage N. [Ocular burns]. *J Fr Ophtalmol.* 2008;31(7):723–734. [French].
2. Adepoju FG, Adeboye A, Adigun IA. Chemical eye injuries: presentation and management difficulties. *Ann Afr Med.* 2007;6(1):7–11.
3. Midelfart A, Hagen YC, Myhre GB. [Chemical burns to the eye]. *Tidsskr Nor Laegeforen.* 2004;124(1):49–51. [Norwegian].
4. Solberg Y, Alcalay M, Belkin M. Ocular injury by mustard gas. *Surv Ophthalmol.* 1997;41(6):461–466.
5. Kehe K, Balszuweit F, Emmler J, et al. Sulfur mustard research-strategies for the development of improved medical therapy. *Eplasty.* 2008;8: e32.
6. Hughes WF Jr. Alkali injuries of the eye. I. Review of the literature and summary of present knowledge. *Arch Ophthalmol.* 1946;35:423–449.
7. Pfister RR. Chemical injuries of the eye. *Ophthalmology.* 1983;90: 1246–1253.
8. Schultz G, Henkind P, Gross E. Acid injuries of the eye. *Am J Ophthalmol.* 1968;66:654–657.
9. Friedenwald JS, Hughes WF Jr, Herrmann H. Acid–base tolerance of the cornea. *Arch Ophthalmol.* 1944;31:279–283.
10. Guidry MA, Allen JH, Kelly JB. Some biochemical characteristics of acid injury of the cornea. I. Ascorbic acid studies. *Am J Ophthalmol.* 1955;40:111–119.
11. Hall AH, Blomet J, Mathieu L. Diphoterine for emergent eye/skin chemical splash decontamination: a review. *Vet Hum Toxicol.* 2002;44(4): 228–231.
12. Langefeld S, Press UP, Frentz M, et al. [Use of lavage fluid containing diphoterine for irrigation of eyes in first aid emergency treatment]. *Ophthalmologe.* 2003;100(9):727–731, [German].
13. Soderberg K, Kuusinen P, Mathieu L, Hall AH. An improved method for emergent decontamination of ocular and dermal hydrofluoric acid splashes. *Vet Hum Toxicol.* 2003;46(4):216–218.
14. Höjer J, Personne M, Hultén P, Ludwigs U. Topical treatments for hydrofluoric acid burns: a blind controlled experimental study. *J Toxicol Clin Toxicl.* 2002;40(7):861–866.
15. Hultén P, Höjer J, Ludwigs U, Janson A. Hexafluorine vs. standard decontamination to reduce systemic toxicity after dermal exposure to hydrofluoric acid. *J Toxicol Clin Toxicol.* 2004;42(4):355–361.
16. Mathieu L, Nehles J, Blomet J, Hall AH. Efficacy of hexafluorine for emergent decontamination of hydrofluoric acid eye and skin splashes. *Vet Hum Toxicol.* 2001;43(5):263–265.
17. Merle H, Donnio A, Ayeboua L, et al. Alkali ocular burns in Martinique (French West Indies). Evaluation of the use of an amphoteric solution as the rinsing product. *Burns.* 2005;31(2):205–211.
18. Chiang TS, Moorman LR, Thomas RP. Ocular hypertensive response following acid and alkali injuries in rabbits. *Invest Ophthalmol.* 1971;10: 270–273.
19. Paterson CA, et al. The ocular hypertensive response following experimental acid injuries in the rabbit eye. *Invest Ophthalmol Vis Sci.* 1979; 18:67–74.
20. Friedenwald JS. Discussion. *Am J Ophthalmol.* 1955;40:119–120.
21. Musselmann K, Kane B, Alexandrou B, Hassell JR. Stimulation of collagen synthesis by insulin and proteoglycan accumulation by ascorbate in bovine keratocytes in vitro. *Invest Ophthalmol Vis Sci.* 2006;47(12): 5260–5266.
22. Pfister RR, Paterson CA. Ascorbic acid in the treatment of alkali burns of the eye. *Ophthalmology.* 1980;87(10):1050–1057.
23. Friedenwald JS, Hughes WF Jr, Herrmann H. Acid injuries of the eye. *Arch Ophthalmol.* 1946;35:98–108.
24. Schultz G, Henkind P, Gross E. Acid injuries of the eye. *Am J Ophthalmol.* 1968;66:654–657.
25. McCulley JP, et al. Hydrofluoric acid injuries of the eye. *J Occup Med.* 1983;25:447–450.
26. Kompa S, Redbrake C, Hilgers C, et al. Effect of different irrigating solutions on aqueous humour pH changes, intraocular pressure and histological findings after induced alkali burns. *Acta Ophthalmol Scand.* 2005; 83(4):467–470.
27. Kompa S, Schareck B, Tympner J, et al. Comparison of emergency eyewash products in burned porcine eyes. *Graefe's Arch Clin Exp Ophthalmol.* 2002;240(4):308–313.
28. Kuckelkorn R, Schrage N, Keller G, Redbrake C. Emergency treatment of chemical and thermal eye burns. *Acta Ophthalmol Scand.* 2002;80(1): 4–10.
29. Rihawi S, Frentz M, Reim M, Schrage NF. Rinsing with isotonic saline solution for eye burns should be avoided. *Burns.* 2008;34(7):1027–1032.
30. Rihawi S, Frentz M, Schrage NF. Emergency treatment of eye burns: which rinsing solution should we choose? *Graefe's Arch Clin Exp Ophthalmol.* 2006;244(7):845–854.
31. Moore AT, Cheng H, Boase DL. Eye injuries from car battery explosions. *Br J Ophthalmol.* 1982;66(2):141–144.
32. Saari KM, Leinonen J, Aine E. Management of chemical eye injuries with prolonged irrigation. *Acta Ophthalmol.* 1984;(Suppl 161):52–59.
33. Pfister RR. Chemical corneal injuries. *Int Ophthalmol Clin.* 1984;24: 157–168.
34. Di Pascuale MA, Whitson JT, Mootha VV. Corneal melting after use of nepafenac in a patient with chronic cystoid macular edema after cataract surgery. *Eye Contact Lens.* 2008;34(2):129–130.

35. Asai T, Nakagami T, Mochizuki M, et al. Three cases of corneal melting after instillation of a new nonsteroidal anti-inflammatory drug. *Cornea.* 2006;25(2):224–227.
36. Donshik PC, et al. Effect of topical corticosteroids on ulceration in alkali-burned corneas. *Arch Ophthalmol.* 1978;96:2117–2120.
37. Wishard P, Paterson CA. The effect of ascorbic acid on experimental acid injuries of the rabbit cornea. *Invest Ophthalmol Vis Sci.* 1980;19:564–566.
38. Tamhane A, Vajpayee RB, Biswas NR, et al. Evaluation of amniotic membrane transplantation as an adjunct to medical therapy as compared with medical therapy alone in acute ocular burns. *Ophthalmology.* 2005;112(11):1963–1969.
39. Meller D, Pires RT, Mack RJ, et al. Amniotic membrane transplantation for acute chemical or thermal burns. *Ophthalmology.* 2000;107(5):980–989; discussion 990.
40. Arora R, Mehta D, Jain V. Amniotic membrane transplantation in acute chemical burns. *Eye.* 2005;19(3):273–278.
41. Tejwani S, Kolari RS, Sangwan VS, Rao GN. Role of amniotic membrane graft for ocular chemical and thermal injuries. *Cornea.* 2007;26(1):21–26.
42. Kobayashi A, Shirao Y, Yoshita T, et al. Temporary amniotic membrane patching for acute chemical burns. *Eye.* 2003;17(2):149–158.
43. Kheirkhah A, Johnson DA, Paranjpe DR, et al. Temporary sutureless amniotic membrane patch for acute alkaline burns. *Arch Ophthalmol.* 2008;126(8):1059–1066.
44. Pfister RR. Corneal stem cell disease: concepts, categorization, and treatment by auto- and homotransplantation of limbal stem cells. *CLAO J.* 1994;20:64–72.
45. Djalilian AR, Wadia HP, Balali S, et al. Epithelial transplantation for the management of severe ocular surface disease. In: Brightbill FS, ed. *Corneal surgery: theory, technique, and tissue.* 4th ed. St. Louis: Elsevier; 2009.
46. Sangwan VS, Matalia HP, Vemuganti GK, et al. Early results of penetrating keratoplasty after cultivated limbal epithelium transplantation. *Arch Ophthalmol.* 2005;123(3):334–340.
47. Solomon A, Ellies P, Anderson DF, et al. Long-term outcome of keratolimbal allograft with or without penetrating keratoplasty for total limbal stem cell deficiency. *Ophthalmology.* 2002;109(6):1159–1166.
48. Fogla R, Padmanabhan P. Deep anterior lamellar keratoplasty combined with autologous limbal stem cell transplantation in unilateral severe chemical injury. *Cornea.* 2005;24(4):421–425.
49. Wagoner MD. Chemical injuries of the eye: current concepts in pathophysiology and therapy. *Surv Ophthalmol.* 1997;41(4):275–313.
50. Pfister DR, Holland EJ. Keratoepithelioplasty in the management of severe ocular surface disease. *Invest Ophthalmol Vis Sci.* 1995;(Suppl 36):195.

Chapter 99

Alkali Injuries of the Eye

Roswell R. Pfister, Daryl R. Pfister

The entire anterior segment of the eye is seriously jeopardized by exposure to alkali. Nonperforating ocular injuries of this type result in destruction of cellular components, denaturation and degradation of collagenous tissues, and release of inflammatory mediators by alkaline hydrolysis of a broad range of intracellular and extracellular proteins, invading cells, and basal epithelial cells. The extraordinary inflammatory reaction that supervenes is the pivot around which most complications revolve. In the absence of treatment, the best attainable result is an eye with a scarred, vascularized cornea that has not ulcerated or developed glaucoma and is amenable to visual rehabilitation by conjunctival and/or corneal surgery.

Epidemiology

There are profound psychologic, social, and economic repercussions that occur after alkali injury. Injury of one eye often results in costly medical care dependency, loss of job, interpersonal conflicts, and isolation for the period of time necessary to stabilize the injured eye. Blindness resulting from bilateral injury usually adds restriction of job and economic opportunities with a further burden placed on the social system for subsistence as well as loss of taxable income.

The type of alkali causing eye injury can be ammonia, lye, potassium hydroxide, magnesium hydroxide, or lime.[1] Table 99.1 summarizes the possible source and relevant comments pertaining to each type of chemical injury. In addition, a comprehensive review of chemical injuries is presented by Wagoner.[2] Data gathered from a large urban hospital show that young black men are at greatest risk of a severe alkali injury assault, usually in a domestic setting, where there is low-income, high-density housing, and a record of alcoholism and prior assaults.[3] In the industrial sector, approximately 10% of 52 142 cases of ocular trauma reported from 16 states were chemical burns (1.6% acid and 0.6% alkali). Safety monitors have reduced the incidence of job-related eye injuries, but despite such programs the storage and use of powerful alkalis, under extreme pressure and high temperature, continue to pose serious threats, even to the properly attired worker wearing protective clothing and goggles.

Of 221 chemical injuries reported in 180 patients at the Croydon Eye Unit, United Kingdom, almost half were caused by alkali in males (75.6%) between the ages of 16 and 25.[4] Accidental injuries accounted for 89.4%; the remainder were assaults. Work-related accidents numbered 63%, 33% occurred at home, and 3% at school.

Two large series of chemical injuries were reported by Kuckelkorn et al.[5,6] in Aachen, Germany, in 1990–91. In the first report,[5] 236 injuries occurred in 171 patients, of which 70% were males. Industrial accidents numbered 61%, 37% were household, and 2% unknown. Most injuries were classified as mild (88%). In the second series, 42 patients had sustained severe alkali injuries occurring over a 7-year period.[6] The industrial sector contributed 73.8% while the rest were sustained at home.

Farmers using liquid ammonia as fertilizer and homeowners using powerful cleansing agents, without eye protection, continue to be at special risk.

Last, the deployment of automobile airbags, occasionally releasing sodium hydroxide as part of the chemically driven, rapid inflation process, can cause corneal abrasions and mild alkali injuries. Although these cases make up 21.6% of eye injury cases, in most cases they constitute less severe injuries and tend to heal readily.[7]

Pathophysiology and Natural Clinical History

The pain, lacrimation, and blepharospasm following an ocular alkali injury result from direct injury of free nerve endings located in the epithelium of the cornea, conjunctiva, and eyelids. Ammonia penetrates the eye almost instantaneously but a delay of 3 to 5 minutes occurs after sodium hydroxide.[8] Depending on the severity of the injury, a wave of hydroxyl ions rapidly penetrates the eye, causing saponification of cellular membranes with massive cell death and partial hydrolysis of corneal glycosaminoglycans and collagen.

With severe alkali injuries of cornea and sclera, there is a sudden, spiking rise in the intraocular pressure, lasting about 10 minutes, caused primarily by shrinkage of the collagenous envelope of the eye. A more prolonged rise in pressure quickly follows, secondary to prostaglandin release.[9] Strong alkali rapidly penetrates into the eye, overcoming the poor buffering capacity of anterior segment tissues and aqueous humor. Within 1 minute, the severe rise in aqueous humor pH causes lysis of corneal cells as well as those lining and

Table 99.1 Chemical injuries

Class	Compound	Common source/uses	Comments
Alkali	Ammonia [NH_3]	Fertilizers Refrigerants Cleaning agents (7% solution)	Combines with water to form NH_4OH fumes Very rapid penetration
	Lye [NaOH]	Drain cleaners	Penetrates almost as rapidly as ammonia
	Potassium hydroxide [KOH]	Caustic potash	Severity similar to that of lye
	Magnesium hydroxide [$Mg(OH)_2$]	Sparklers	Produces combined thermal and alkali injury
	Lime [$Ca(OH)_2$]	Plaster Mortar Cement Whitewash	Most common cause of chemical injury in workplace Poor penetration Toxicity increased by retained particulate matter

From Wagoner M, Kenyon K: Chemical injuries of the eye. In: Albert D, Jakobiac F, eds. Principles and Practice of Ophthalmology: Clinical Practice, vol. 1, Philadelphia, 1994, W.B. Saunders. pp. 234–245.

adjacent to the anterior chamber, compromising the blood–aqueous barrier and releasing necrotic debris into the aqueous humor. This leads to a severe fibrinous inflammatory reaction in the entire anterior segment of the eye.

Glaucoma may ensue from inflammatory products accumulating in the aqueous humor and chamber angle, promoting closure by anterior synechiae, especially inferiorly. The trabecula and ciliary body may be injured directly by penetration of alkali through the sclera or by contact with alkalotic aqueous humor percolating through the meshwork. Ocular hypertension, hypotension, or both may occur at different time periods, depending on the predominance of one or more factors. Chemical injury to iris, crystalline lens, and ciliary body may produce mydriasis, cataract, and even phthisis bulbi, respectively. Externally, this inflammatory reaction may be so profound as to lead to extensive symblephara and even ankyloblepharon from the apposition of raw conjunctival surfaces.

Repair

Repair of the eye after an alkali injury is a complex process that involves each cellular and extracellular tissue layer, including the eyelids, corneal and conjunctival epithelium, fibroblasts and collagen, endothelium, and all other tissues contiguous to the anterior chamber.

Epithelium

Destruction of the corneal epithelium alone in a mild injury might lead, at most, to a recurrent corneal erosion, resulting from injury to basal lamina and anterior corneal stroma. When a portion of the limbal stem cells is destroyed, the remaining stem cell population heals first by the propagation of pluripotential epithelial stem cells around the corneal periphery and then by centripetal growth of cells phenotypic for cornea. If the injury destroys the entire limbal palisades of Vogt, then the phenotypic source of corneal epithelium is lost. To resurface the cornea, the remaining conjunctival epithelial cells must first spread over collagenous tissues of the episclera and then continue over corneal stroma. On the cornea, this rate of epithelial motility is initially similar to epithelial recovery occurring after a simple abrasion but then breaks down, creating a persistent epithelial defect.[10,11] Unfortunately, when conjunctival epithelium grows over the cornea, fibrous tissue and neovasculatization advance behind the growing epithelial edge to create a pannus covering some or all of the cornea.

When injury to the cornea is very severe, but the corneal epithelial stem cell population is left intact, then initial epithelial healing still proceeds at a rate similar to that when the stem cell population has been destroyed.[10] An experimental severe alkali injury of 12 mm, which does not destroy the limbal stem cells, later showed substantial epithelial adhesion problems leading to persistent epithelial defects. At 84 hours, epithelial movement usually stops when the leading edge loses its adherence and then subsequently peels back from the stroma as a sheet (96 hours), thereafter maintaining a persistent epithelial defect. It has been suggested that this loss of epithelial adhesion might result from accelerated degradation of fibrinogen by plasminogen activator, a substance probably secreted in excessive amounts by the basal epithelial cells in the alkali-injured eye.[12] From these experiments it can therefore be concluded that in the severely alkali-injured cornea, the presence of a normal corneal stem cell population does not necessarily imply that epithelial healing is assured. In fact, persistent epithelial defects might also result from the consequences of a denatured framework of the stroma. Clearly, epithelial–stromal interaction plays an important role in the adhesion of epithelium to stroma.

Stroma

Healing of the corneal stroma in a timely manner is the key to avoidance of ulceration and perforation of the globe. Two events proceed simultaneously in the repair process: (1) degradation and removal of necrotic debris, and (2) replacement of portions of the fixed cells, collagenous matrix, and glycosaminoglycans. Concentrated alkali exposure strips the cornea of its vital cells and glycosaminoglycans, leaving behind the skeletal framework of the collagen in a partially denatured form. Extensive high-pressure liquid chromatography studies have revealed that direct alkaline hydrolysis of cellular and extracellular proteins yields inflammatory mediators, which are chemotactic to neutrophils.[13] At high concentrations, these simple tripeptides, consisting of acetylated or methylated proline-glycine-proline, constitute powerful attractive agents that diffuse to the limbal vasculature where they initiate and promote neutrophilic invasion into the cornea within hours of the injury. These chemoattractants might also play a role as one of the signals from the wound inducing the secretion of adhesion molecules from the vascular endothelium (E-selectin) and the intravascular leukocytes (L-selectin) to incite leukocyte rolling and adhesion to the vascular endothelium.

Once neutrophils accumulate, their release of leukotrienes, and the presence of interleukin-1 alpha and interleukin-6 serve to recruit successive waves of inflammatory cells.[14] These inflammatory components serve to perpetuate stromal inflammation, with continued release of a variety of degradative enzymes including *N*-acetylglucosaminidase and cathepsin-D into the tissues and tear film. The positive side of neutrophil presence is the finding that they seem to stimulate epithelial proliferation when examined by its proliferative cellular nuclear expression.[15] In this study, neutrophils appear to act as the initiating messenger promoting the process of corneal vascularization.

Alkali injury of collagen also releases a second inflammatory mediator that metabolically stimulates the neutrophils to undergo a respiratory burst. Prodigious oxygen utilization by the stimulated neutrophils results in the by-product superoxide radicals, an unstable form of oxygen that is highly destructive of tissues. When the mediator is present in excess there is extreme stimulation, causing neutrophil lysis with the release of granules containing a wide variety of enzymes. The release and activation of degrader enzymes from the specific and azurophilic granules of neutrophils act to destroy tissue by cleaving proteins and other molecular species. These responses serve to promote dissolution of the remaining corneal stroma, tipping the scales toward corneal ulceration and perforation.

Interleukin (IL)-1 and IL-6 production appears to have dual roles after alkali injury to the cornea.[16] Up-regulation of inflammatory cytokines after alkali injury is thought to play an important role in corneal healing but also in inflammatory cell infiltration and tissue destruction as a consequence of matrix metalloproteinase (MMP) production. Furthermore, topical application of a synthetic MMP inhibitor to alkali-injured mouse cornea reduced the expression of inflammatory cytokines and MMP expression. It is hypothesized that a vicious cycle may be initiated after the alkali injury to the cornea, with second injury occurring as a consequence of inflammatory cytokine release.

Fibroblasts invading the cornea after severe alkali injuries are immature, with their polysomal systems in disarray. The proline in collagen produced from these cells is underhydroxylated, preventing it from winding into the triple helical structure of normal collagen. These individual strands of amino acids are as vulnerable to enzymatic lysis as the alkali-denatured collagen. These histologic features of corneal tissues are the sine qua non of tissue scorbutus.[17] Corneal tissue scorbutus results when alkali damage to the nonpigmented ciliary epithelium compromises its ability to concentrate ascorbate in the aqueous humor, denying this important reducing substance from hydroxylating proline as collagen is being produced in the endoplasmic reticulum of fibroblasts. As a result of this ascorbate deficiency, the repair process is faulty, with the destruction–repair equation shifted in the direction of tissue disappearance, and hence corneal ulceration. In very severe injuries, fibroblasts invade the cornea slowly, or not at all, resulting in rapid conversion of stroma to a necrotic sequestrum.

Endothelium

In mild injuries, penetration of alkali is minimal and the endothelium is undamaged. Moderate injuries probably cause some endothelial cell death but mostly interfere with the pump mechanism, leading to a variable degree of reversible corneal edema. Severe injuries will destroy endothelium, which leads to severe corneal thickening. Alternately, the simultaneous loss of glycosaminoglycans, which bind water in the cornea, might result in no significant net gain or loss of thickness during the early stages, only an opaque cornea.

Classification of Alkali Injuries: Clinical Technique

Understanding and documenting the salient findings in an alkali injury of the eye permits proper classification so that appropriate immediate treatment can be initiated and accurate prognostication adduced. Documentation of the following physical data is recommended in the form of a labeled drawing:

1. Epithelial defect: Instill fluorescein and measure the size and draw the shape of the defect. Include any conjunctival epithelial defects, especially as it relates to the perilimbal conjunctiva (stem cells).
2. Stromal opacity: Gradations are made on the basis of a penlight examination. Grade 0 – clear cornea; grade 1 – mild corneal haze; grade 2 – mild to moderate opacity; grade 3 – moderate opacity; grade 4 – moderate to severe opacity, details of iris trabeculae cannot be seen but pupil visible; grade 5 – severe corneal opacity, pupil not visible with penlight.
3. Perilimbal ischemia: Document the clock hours where the conjunctiva is whitened. In these areas the conjunctiva

and episclera are devoid of blood vessels. This whitening is not to be confused with less severe injury where there is chemosis and thrombosed blood vessels but some of the conjunctiva is still viable. Although not originally planned, perilimbal whitening has proved to be a useful parameter by which to judge the extent of corneal stem cell damage and, indirectly, injury of the underlying ciliary body and trabecular meshwork. Documentation of these findings allows for a later, and more accurate, determination of the necessity for corneal stem cell transplantation.

4. Adnexa: The blinking pattern, exposure and/or lagophthalmos should be measured and documented.

These measurements and findings can then be applied to the classification of alkali injuries as described by Hughes and modified by Pfister and Koski.[18] This classification, with accompanying drawings, represents the span of damage encountered after alkali injury (Fig. 99.1). The accuracy of early assessment becomes very important in subsequent evaluation and treatment plans.

Regarding terminology, the literature is replete with allusions to alkali 'burns,' potentially confusing the alkali injury terminology with a thermal component that might not exist. Herein, we recommend the designation of alkali injury or acid injury of the eye to distinguish chemical injuries from true thermal burns. When both injuries occur simultaneously, then alkali-thermal injury or thermal-alkali injury might be used, with what is thought to be the most prominent injurious agent stated first. Acid injuries should be referred to in a similar way.

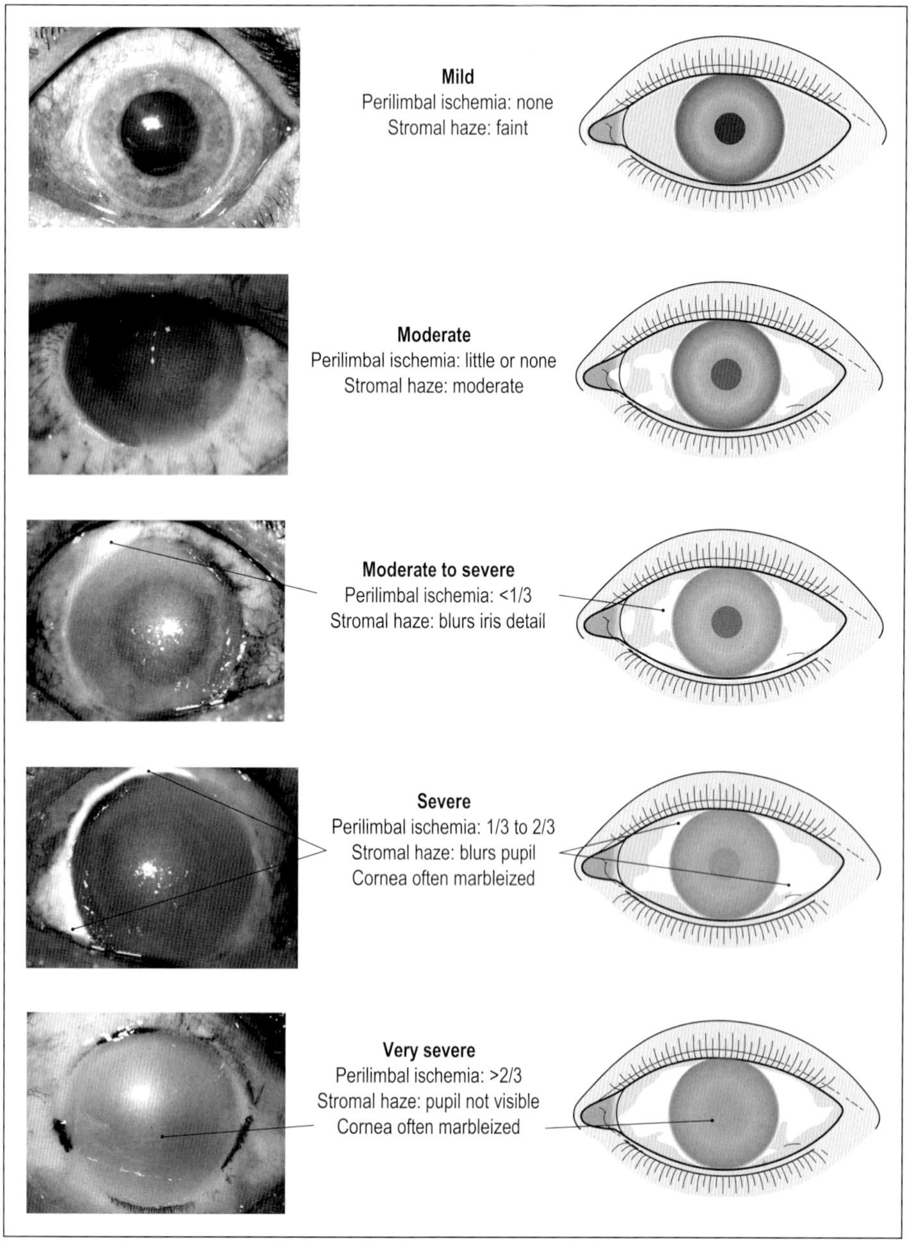

Fig. 99.1 Classification of alkali-burned eyes.
Mild: Corneal epithelial erosion, faint anterior stromal haziness, no ischemic necrosis of perilimbal conjunctiva and sclera. Prognosis: healing with little or no corneal scarring; visual loss usually no greater than one to two lines.
Moderate: Moderate corneal opacity, little or no significant ischemic necrosis of perilimbal conjunctiva. Prognosis: slow healing of epithelium with moderate scarring, peripheral corneal vascularization, and visual loss of two to seven lines.
Moderate to severe: Corneal opacity blurring iris details, ischemic necrosis of conjunctiva limited to less than one-third of perilimbal conjunctiva. Prognosis: prolonged corneal healing with significant corneal vascularization and scarring; vision usually limited to 20/200 or less.
Severe: Blurring of pupillary outline, ischemia of approximately one-third to two-thirds of perilimbal conjunctiva, cornea often marbleized. Prognosis: very prolonged corneal healing with inflammation and high incidence of corneal ulceration and perforation. In the best cases, severe corneal vascularization and scarring with counting-fingers vision.
Very severe: Pupil not visible, greater than two-thirds ischemia of perilimbal conjunctiva, cornea often marbleized. Prognosis: very prolonged corneal healing with inflammation and high incidence of corneal ulceration and perforation. In the best cases, severe corneal vascularization and scarring with counting-fingers vision.

Emergency Treatment

The harm caused by alkali injury is predicated on the concentration of the cation, the duration of exposure, the pH of the solution, and both the extent and specific areas of ocular tissue exposure. Remove the source of the caustic agent from the external eye by immediate irrigation at the scene of the accident with clear water and subsequently the emergency room for 1 to 2 hours with isotonic buffered saline. Using this technique alone to reduce the alkali concentration in the corneal stroma and aqueous humor after a severe alkali injury is open to question. Studies on the effect of 90 minutes of external irrigation on intraocular pH in an animal model have shown only a 1.5 pH unit reduction of the elevated pH.[8] It is necessary to lavage the external eye, but relatively little immediate progress can be made to end the intraocular cauterization by alkali using this technique alone. Removal of the aqueous by paracentesis lowered the pH by 1.5 pH units. Reformation of the aqueous humor with buffered phosphate solution lowered the pH by an additional 1.5 pH units. It is premature to suggest that all severe alkali injuries should undergo paracentesis. However, in the absence of strict scientific information in human eyes, it is reasonable to suggest in severe injuries, occurring 1 to 2 hours previously, that paracentesis and removal of an aliquot of aqueous humor be performed. This can be accomplished at the slit lamp or in the minor operating room suite. Under topical anesthesia, a supersharp 15-degree blade can create a partial-thickness, self-sealing tunnel at the limbus down which a 25-gauge needle is inserted, finally penetrating into the anterior chamber. If available, it is preferable to replace the aqueous humor with a buffered phosphate solution or balanced salt solution to reduce the intraocular pH to near-normal levels.

Diphoterine (Prevor) is a proprietary amphoteric compound which has been much heralded as a universal emergency irrigant for eyes injured with acidic or alkaline compounds. There are numerous individual accounts of success with this agent but relatively little scientific evidence for its efficacy in a controlled study. While many workplaces have embraced Diphoterine as a first-response irrigant, the final decision regarding its efficacy must await scrupulous scientific investigation.

There are several chemical injuries that require special treatment. For example, the pultaceous character of lime used in cement compounds clings to the conjunctiva. The bulk of material can be removed with a cotton-tipped applicator but the sticky paste in contact with the conjunctiva can be loosened and removed with greater ease by irrigation with a solution of ethylene diaminetetraacetic acid (EDTA 0.01 M).

The intraocular pressure rise after alkali injury can usually be treated by topical alpha- or beta-blockers and topical and/or systemically administered carbonic anhydrase inhibitors. If the pressure fails to respond, temporary control of an acute pressure rise can be achieved by a beveled paracentesis incision at the limbus, under topical anesthesia, followed by periodic release of aqueous humor at the slit lamp or in the minor surgical suite.

The presence of necrotic tissue in the eye gives rise to inflammatory mediators that attract polymorphonuclear neutrophils (PMNs) into the damaged cornea and stimulate the full range of PMN enzyme and metabolic products destructive to even the remaining normal tissues. To avert some of these devastating consequences, careful excision of superficial necrotic tissues might be carried out to reduce the mediator load encouraging this process.[13]

The degree of eyelid dysfunction after alkali injury is usually dependent on the severity of orbital and periorbital skin and conjunctival injury. Immediately after injury and for several days, eyelid edema makes eye observations difficult. The eyelid position and periodic blinking required to resurface the exposed cornea and conjunctiva with tears are usually disturbed, at least temporarily, even in the mildest injuries. More often, the intense blepharospasm and photophobia induced by a more severe injury persist until the inflammatory or ulcerative process has subsided, sometimes for years. Some injuries can render the skin white or charred, the latter signaling third-degree dermal injury with eventual sloughing of eyelid tissue.

Alkali destruction of conjunctival epithelium, in combination with the inflammatory reaction, causes fibrinous adhesions that must be opened periodically under topical anesthesia. When extensive damage of conjunctiva has occurred, fibrous proliferation in the subconjunctival tissues shrinks the linear surface of conjunctiva and promotes the formation of symblephara, particularly by contact between the raw surfaces of naturally apposed conjunctiva. In the most severe cases the eyelids become scarred to the globe (ankyloblepharon), causing the exposed cornea to dry with resultant epithelial defects, leading to PMN infiltration, ulceration, infection, and, potentially, perforation.

Prophylactic approaches to maintain eyelid mobility and limit conjunctival and forniceal contracture can be tried but are of unproven value. These consist of lining the palpebral conjunctiva with a thin plastic wrap, which is secured by sutures passing through the upper and lower fornices. A more physiologic and anatomic approach is to line the conjunctival tissues with amniotic membrane shortly after the injury or later when lid mobility has already been compromised by scarring. Recreated tissue planes can seldom be covered by rearrangement of existing conjunctiva. Alternatively, amniotic membrane sutured to the raw, exposed surfaces offers not only an opportunity to cover denuded tissues but also provides innate antiinflammatory agents to these healing tissues. In the more severe injuries of natural conjunctiva, coverage of these raw areas with mucous membrane obtained from the mouth might have a better chance of remaining open. Unfortunately, the phenotype of buccal mucosal epithelium is not conducive to any subsequent efforts to rehabilitate the eye by corneal transplantation. When ankyloblepharon is present, any known effort to reconstitute a semblance of the natural conjunctival environment, for the purpose of preparation for corneal transplantation, has been unsuccessful.

Pain management during this stage of the disease is not complicated. The pain at the time of injury is excruciating, but usually short-lived. Pain receptors are destroyed by the alkali; hence they do not continue to transmit a pain response. When necessary, pain control might be required for several days – rarely greater than 1 week. Photophobia can be extreme, creating a painful environment that can be improved only with UV protective, dark wraparound sunglasses with which to carry on daily activities.

Transitional-Stage Medical Treatment

The transitional-stage treatment of the alkali-injured eye begins as early as 1 to 2 weeks in milder injuries and as late as 1 to 2 months in more severe cases. Problems such as epithelial defects, inflammation and ulceration, glaucoma, symblephara, and eyelid dysfunction might appear and/or continue from the acute stage through the subacute to the chronic stage imperceptibly and without interruption.

Epithelium

The healing of a corneal epithelial defect after alkali injury is largely predicated upon the severity of the injury and the extent of perilimbal injury. Part of the significance of perilimbal injury is the finding that the stem cell phenotype for corneal epithelial cells resides deep within a narrow band of cells located on, and partially straddling, the limbus. Loss of some portion of the stem cells requires that corneal epithelium be repopulated from the geographically distant remaining stem cells around the limbal circumference. If all corneal stem cells have been destroyed, then corneal reepithelialization proceeds from the viable edge of the conjunctival epithelium with cells phenotypic for conjunctiva. If the conjunctival stem cells, located in the fornices, are also destroyed, then the deepithelialized and inflamed conjunctival surfaces are likely to result in extensive symblephara or ankyloblepharon. The formulation and frequency of applied medications used during this period can be toxic to fresh epithelium covering the alkali-injured cornea. Preservatives, such as benzalkonium chloride, and ointments, especially those containing lanolin, can perpetuate or create epithelial defects. It is wise to avoid topical treatment with multiple medications in the hope of preventing corneal ulceration when there is no clear-cut indication to do so. At most, initial treatment with an antibiotic (q.i.d.) and dilator (b.i.d.) is indicated. If the patient is participating in a clinical trial or new therapies prove efficacious, topical applications would begin immediately after injury.

Inflammation and corneal ulceration

Alkali injury of the cornea has been shown to trigger the release of inflammatory mediators, which are believed to be responsible for chemoattraction and subsequent activation of neutrophils (PMNs) within the corneal stroma. The density of the PMN infiltrate appears to be directly related to the severity of the injury and to the likelihood of subsequent ulceration. Although all cells of the cornea have been shown to be capable of releasing a broad spectrum of enzymes destructive of collagen and glycosaminoglycans, the presence of enormous numbers of PMNs and the absence of any other cells in significant numbers suggest that PMNs and their products are the major cellular elements associated with ulceration.

Historically, treatment of ulcers resulting from alkali injuries has been directed at the inhibition of type I collagenase, produced by keratocytes, and capable of cleavage of the collagen molecule into one-quarter and three-quarter fragments. Newer data have identified the collagenases as a family of enzymes, referred to as metalloproteinases (MMPs) and consisting of collagenase type I (MMP-1 degrades type I, II, and III collagen), stromelysin (MMP-3 degrades casein, proteoglycan, and fibronectin and to a limited extent laminin, elastin, gelatin, and type IV collagen), and gelatinase (MMP-9, which degrades gelatin, type IV, V, and VI collagen, and fibronectin).[19] When activated, this full array of enzymes is available to degrade both the residual normal cornea as well as denatured corneal matrix.

Although controversy still exists, acetylcysteine, L-cysteine, and EDTA have all been reported to inhibit mammalian collagenase in vitro and significantly reduce the incidence of ulceration in animal corneas after alkali injuries. In contrast, one study in extreme alkali-injured animal eyes showed no favorable effect of acetylcysteine when compared to control eyes (81% vs 75%).[20] In an open clinical study, L-cysteine (0.2 M solution) was begun on the seventh day after a 'total' alkali injury in 33 human eyes, and only one eye perforated.[21] An alkali-injury study including 28 human eyes substantiated the favorable effect of L-cysteine in the acute stage, in the presence of an ulcer, and before or after corneal transplantation. In 35 patients with corneal ulceration (diseases unspecified) treated with 0.2 M EDTA, 86% healed or remained unchanged compared to 46% of the 26 control eyes.[22] Cysteine and acetylcysteine are both effective inhibitors of collagenase, but the latter has the advantage of greater stability and ready availability in the marketplace. Although it is suspected that acetylcysteine has a favorable effect in some human alkali-injured corneas, this has not yet been proven by clinical trial. If desired, acetylcysteine (Mucomyst 10% or 20%) or L-cysteine drops should commence 7 days after the injury.

The use of topical steroids after chemical injury is controversial. If used for the first 7 days after injury, they are believed to decrease the inflammatory reaction of the entire anterior segment, possibly reducing some of the late side effects, such as glaucoma.[23] This paper reported that if used for longer than 10 days, topical steroids might interfere with the repair process and therefore enhance the opportunity for corneal ulceration and perforation. Subsequent research in human eyes by Davis et al.[24] has confirmed that simultaneous use of 10% ascorbate topically hourly and 1 g of ascorbate orally per day prevents ulceration if used up to the time of corneal reepithelization.

A surgical emergency arises when a leaking descemetocele or frank perforation supervenes. If the perforation is smaller than 1.0 mm in diameter (the ulcer itself is usually much larger) and relatively free of blood vessels, then adhesive closure with cyanoacrylate is the least invasive and the most effective way of reestablishing the integrity of the eye.[25] A soft contact lens diminishes the discomfort of the adhesive. The adhesive remains in place for 2 to 10 weeks, after which it falls off or is loosened enough to be picked off with a jeweler's forceps. Large corneal ulcerations and perforations require a corneal patch graft to replace tissue lost from ulceration. The ulcer bed and edges are cleaned of epithelium and inflammatory debris. Necrotic tissue is excised from the edges and base to create a viable bed of stroma into which the transplanted tissue is positioned. The donor patch graft is cut larger than the recipient bed, cut to fit the contours of the ulceration, and fastened to the edges of the ulcer with interrupted sutures of 10-0 nylon with their knots buried into the stroma.[26]

Glaucoma

Any caustic agent might damage the trabecular meshwork directly, and/or necrotic and inflammatory debris can clog the outflow channels. Organization of this inflammatory sediment results in fibroproliferation, scar contraction, and the formation of extensive anterior synechiae, further embarrassing outflow facility.

Treatment of this type of glaucoma initially consists of oral carbonic anhydrase inhibitors, topical beta-blockers, and alpha-blockers to control pressure. Severe scarring of the perilimbal conjunctiva and bulbar conjunctiva, combined with foreshortening of the fornices, makes conventional filtration surgery much less successful. Cautious use of wound-modifying agents such as mitomycin-C can improve success significantly. Cyclocryothermy is a viable option but the destructive nature of this treatment of the ciliary body in an already damaged eye limits its utility. Depending on the conjunctival condition, the use of translimbal intraocular setons, linked to equatorial filtration plates, might offer the only effective way to siphon aqueous from a severely glaucomatous eye.

Transitional-Stage Surgical Treatment

Tenon-plasty

Very severely alkali-injured eyes and anterior segment necrosis share some properties, in particular, vascular insufficiency. To improve vascular support of the anterior segment in alkali-injured eyes, Reim has popularized excision of necrotic conjunctiva and advancement of Tenon's capsule over the cornea, employing careful dissection to preserve the vascular supply of the capsule located posteriorly.[27] The procedure, referred to as tenon-plasty, prevented or arrested corneal ulceration in 24 eyes of 21 patients sustaining severe alkali injuries of the eyes.

Persistent corneal epithelial defects

For inflammation to subside, and the anterior surface to stabilize, it is necessary for the epithelium to be intact, with a normal complement of five layers and with a stable tear film. One or more of these requirements are commonly deficient in alkali injuries, generically referred to as ocular surface disease, resulting in an abnormal epithelial surface which can lead to persistant corneal epithelial defects. Eyelid incongruities, incomplete blinking, toxicity of preservatives in eyedrops, tear film deficiencies, or other factors influencing the vitality of the corneal epithelium must be discovered and removed or corrected medically or surgically.

Soft contact lenses have been employed to protect the epithelium from a variety of surface problems. Mixed results are cited in individual accounts and in sparse literature. Although soft contact lenses, fit with high water content, are useful to attempt to gain epithelial stability, they must not be relied on to solve stem cell or other more deep-seated problems alone. The primary problem must be uncovered and addressed.

Autologous serum eyedrops have been rediscovered as a method of establishing epithelial integrity by growth and migration in a variety of diseases. There are no FDA or other specified guidelines to make serum drops. The authors' own approach is to draw two tubes of citrated blood from the patient, centrifuge, and decant the serum into separate tubes. Under sterile conditions, the top of a tear substitute bottle is removed and the serum drawn up into a 3-cc syringe and injected directly into the bottle, creating a 20–40% solution. Any bottles not being used are kept frozen. Serum drops are used every 2 to 3 hours initially, reducing to 4 times a day and only stopping weeks after the defect has disappeared. Patients are cautioned to keep the bottles in the refrigerator even though a preservative is present in the original bottle. Salutory results are common in 1 to 2 weeks but failure suggests that a stem cell deficiency or other factors are operative.

Corneal stem cell replacement

Replacement of the corneal stem cells lost from disease or injury is now established as required when complete loss of limbal stem cells has occurred.[28–30] If the injury is monocular, then autotransplantation of the limbal stem cells from the uninjured eye offers the best opportunity to replenish the stem cell supply. The use of lenticular grafts, pioneered by Thoft,[28] led the way to a variety of surgical approaches to replenish the corneal stem cell population from related or unrelated donors. Research by Pfister indicated that, when the injury is bilateral, allografted limbal tissue was capable of restoring the stem cell population from an unrelated donor.[30] Replacement of the entire cornea and adjacent stem cells by a very large penetrating keratoplasty has been performed successfully and reported in two different series.[31,32] Kukelkorn et al. replaced the entire cornea in sterile, ulcerating, alkali-injured eyes, preserving an intact epithelium and absence of ulceration over a 1-year period.[31] Redbrake et al. reported nine eyes operated on in this way, preserving the epithelium but only maintaining clarity in two.[32] Nevertheless, under the circumstances, these results should be considered a successful outcome. One potential danger might be that such large transplants might interfere with the episcleral aqueous outflow channels and hence increase the likelihood of glaucoma. The use of a 12- or 13-mm lamellar corneal transplant, including the limbal epithelial stem cell population, managed to restore the epithelial integrity, without complications, in an average of 5.2 days.[33] The latter approach, performed an average of 29.5 months after injury, might gain all the advantages of replacement of the cornea and associated stem cells but reduce the risk of consequent glaucoma. When there is deep corneal ulceration, descemetocele, or frank corneal perforation, suturing a piece of cornea into the ulcerated bed reestablishes integrity of the globe. The optimal medical and surgical conditions necessary to promote allografted corneal stem cell growth and to protect them from the immune process are currently in discovery. It is clear, however, that immunosuppression is required to sustain the vitality of these allografted tissues.

Amniotic Membrane Transplantation

Following a chemical injury, placement of amniotic membrane over the cornea and adjacent conjunctiva helps in ocular surface reconstruction, promotes rapid epithelial healing, and may help to partially restore limbal stem cell function. Amniotic membrane was surgically placed over 72 eyes of 69 patients of which 24 were acute cases and 48 were chronic cases. The main clinical findings were symblephara (52.8%), corneal vascularization (51.3%), conjunctivalization (45.8%), limbal ischemia (45.8%), limbal stem cell deficiency (55.5%), and epithelial defect (48.6%). Eighteen cases were due to acid injuries (5 acute, 13 chronic), 52 were due to alkali (18 acute and 34 chronic), and 2 cases were due to thermal burns (1 each acute and chronic). Overall success rate was 87.5% in acute cases and 72.9% in chronic cases. Indication-wise, success rates were 94.3% for epithelial defect healing, 88.2% for symptomatic relief, 59.7% for ocular surface reconstruction, and 55% for improving limbal stem cell function. Success was not achieved in any outcome measure in 1/24 (4.2%) in the acute group and 6/48 (12.5%) in the chronic group. Success rates in acute and chronic cases are comparable.[34]

As an adjunct, amniotic membrane stretched over the alkali-injured cornea has proved to be useful when transplanting corneal stem cells by replacing the abnormal surface of the cornea with a new surface, tending to quiet the inflammatory process.[34,35] The amniotic membrane is first sutured over the entire cornea and perilimbal tissues, followed by the corneal stem cells layered on top and sutured at the limbus. Amniotic membrane alone does not substitute for corneal stem cells in a severe alkali injury where there is a stem cell deficiency or complete loss. The advent of in vitro techniques to culture and expand corneal stem cells might soon provide a new and immunologically more suitable source of corneal stem cells.[36]

Visual Rehabilitation

The prospects for restoration of vision after alkali injury have been substantially improved over the past decade. To achieve success, it is imperative that the intraocular and extraocular milieu be favorable to support the special conditions required for the corneal transplant. Success in any type of restorative surgery will be governed by (1) lid–globe congruity with normal blinking and the absence of corneal exposure, (2) sufficient resurfacing of a near-normal tear film layer to which a transplanted cornea can adapt, (3) the presence of epithelial stem cells phenotypic for cornea, (4) the absence of any current ulceration, inflammation, and/or uncontrolled glaucoma, (5) flawless surgical technique, and (6) fresh corneal transplant tissue.

Preparatory procedures to lyse symblephara, expand cul-de-sacs, and eliminate lagophthalmos are often required to reestablish normal lid physiology and anatomy. Secondary glaucoma must also be controlled with medications, cyclocryothermy, or filtration surgery of some type. Laser of large feeder vessels at the limbus might be done to reduce the vascular supply and control bleeding at the time of surgery.

If corneal surgery is delayed for 18 months to 2 years after a chemical injury, it increases the chances of success, especially without pre-existing ulceration, perforation, or glaucoma.[37] Corneal surgery is indicated for the worst eye in bilateral burns when serviceable vision is not available. In some patients with severe monocular injuries, if a definite need for binocularity does not exist, the option of corneal transplantation must be balanced against the expectation of the higher incidence of complications.

If corneal transplantation is indicated, it is important to pay meticulous attention to the rigorous protocol of fine corneal surgery. A few points of importance will be mentioned. Trephination with a vacuum cutter and vertical section of remaining attachments with scissors improves the quality of the wound architecture. It is often necessary to oversize the donor corneal button by 0.5 mm or even 0.75 mm to compensate for retraction of the scarred and vascularized recipient bed. If suction cannot be achieved due to surface irregularity, layering a ring of viscoelastic on the peripheral cornea usually assists vacuum adherence. Absorb fresh blood from the wound edges with cellulose sponges, applying pressure to active bleeders by squeezing with fine-toothed forceps until bleeding stops or until suture placement closes the vessel. Light applications of wetfield cautery are not recommended, but if used, should be used sparingly.

The donor cornea should be fresh, with intact epithelium, cut 0.50–0.75 mm larger than the recipient bed. Donor tissue is age-matched but HLA or blood typing is not usually done for the first transplant. After placement of four cardinal interrupted sutures, a single continuous 10-0 nylon suture provides optimal wound closure. The cardinal sutures are then removed and the continuous knot buried. This leaves the corneal surface smooth and uninterrupted postoperatively. This is especially true for more extensively vascularized corneas. The interrupted knots must be buried to avoid epithelial defects and limit portals for infection. If the recipient corneal tissue is thin and of poor qjuality to hold sutures then it is generally safer to use 18 to 24 interrupted sutures, depending on corneal tissue quality. It is rarely necessary to thicken the recipient bed by a lamellar graft in preparation for penetrating keratoplasty 3 to 6 months later.

An attractive alternative approach, utilizing a large-diameter lamellar keratoplasty, including corneal stem cells in the periphery, restored vision in nine eyes an average of 29 months after injury. Six eyes obtained significant visual improvement, while none developed corneal vascularization or signs of rejection after 7.4 months. One persistent epithelial defect healed under a soft contact lens.[33]

When cataract is present, it is usually wisest to remove it at the time of penetrating keratoplasty. Cataract surgery should follow modern techniques with special emphasis on the approach to the open eye. If preoperative pressure devices reduce the vitreous volume such that the crystalline lens has no tendency to prolapse forward, then a curvilinear capsulorrhexis (CCR) can be performed. Efforts to create a CCR, in the presence of positive vitreous pressure, can result in a radial tear across the equator, zonular dehiscence, and possible vitreous loss. To avert this, if positive vitreous pressure is noted, a 'can opener' technique should be employed while placing mild pressure on the anterior lens capsule with a surgical sponge. In either case, hydrodissection of the lens usually prolapses the lens nucleus for easy removal. Cortical cleanup with an irrigation and aspiration handpiece followed by intracapsular placement of an intraocular lens can then be accomplished. Choice of the intraocular lens should be dictated mostly by haptic design, in particular, torsional strength, easy collapsibility, and null anteroposterior movement as the haptic is collapsed. These criteria are met with the Bausch & Lomb model 122 lens, which has the strength to support the posterior capsule while the cornea is sutured in place.

In the immediate postoperative period, a topical steroid and antibiotic is used four times a day. Frequent examinations are necessary to determine if ocular surface disease supervenes, in particular, epithelial irregularities and frank epithelial defects. These events might signal tear deficiency problems, previously determined, or corneal stem cell failure. Later, if epithelial defects are noted, a soft contact lens, fitted for continuous wear, or a one- or two-pillar tarsorrhaphy might solve the problem. Ultimately, if stem cell replacement has not already been performed, then it might be considered at that time. It is critical to remove interrupted sutures that become loose and/or break through the epithelium as soon as this occurs.

In the most severe cases, implantation of a keratoprosthesis might afford the only means by which vision can be restored.[38] Corneas exhibiting exuberant vascularity, repeated failures of fresh transplanted corneal tissue, and the inability to restore normal lid anatomy are potential indications for this procedure. The operation is advisable only in those with severe bilateral injuries where serviceable vision is not present in either eye. All currently available devices are investigational and are difficult to implant. A surprising degree of success has been achieved, but this must be balanced against the sometimes serious and untreatable complications that can occur.

New Research Initiatives

Our concept of the basic biochemical, physiologic, and anatomic changes in the anterior segment of the eye after alkali injury has matured substantially in recent years. This better understanding has been driven by the evolution of the disciplines of molecular biology and biochemistry as applied to ocular disease. As a result, we are now able to employ orthomolecular approaches to supplement our traditional treatment.

Experimental treatment modalities

The aqueous humor ascorbic acid level is depressed to one-third of normal in an animal model of severe alkali injury to the eye. Topically or subcutaneously administered ascorbate (10%) significantly decreases the incidence of corneal ulcerations and perforations when the aqueous humor ascorbate level is elevated above 15 mg/dL.[16] Light and electron microscopy and radioactive tracer experiments show that the mechanism of action is replenishment of ascorbic acid to the scorbutic fibroblasts of the cornea. Ascorbic acid is a powerful reducing agent required by fibroblasts to hydroxylate proline while the collagen strand is being synthesized in the ribosomes. Synthesis of collagen thereby promotes healing of damaged corneal tissues.

Citrate has been shown to be extremely effective in decreasing the incidence of corneal ulceration after alkali injury by acting as a chelator of extracellular calcium.[19] Calcium, located in the plasma membrane of the neutrophil, is necessary for all physiologic activities of the cell by acting as calcium calmodulin, an important intracellular second messenger. Inhibition of the neutrophils through calcium depletion may be caused by interference with calcium–calmodulin microfilament or microtubule interfaces in the plasma membrane.[39] Hence, topical treatment with citrate can entirely halt virtually all neutrophilic activities.

Citrate also inhibits the efferent limb of the inflammatory response by interfering with the adherence of neutrophils to perilimbal vascular endothelium. This effect decreases the migration of neutrophils into the damaged cornea, thus diminishing the number of neutrophils discharging hydrolytic enzymes into the corneal stroma.

Ascorbate and citrate reduce the incidence of corneal ulceration in alkali-injured eyes by different mechanisms, which accounts for the substantial further reduction in corneal ulceration in alkali-injured animals when these compounds are used together. Corneal ulcers decreased from an untreated incidence of 80% to a transitory 4.6% when citrate and ascorbate eyedrops were alternated hourly throughout the day.[40]

Using the Roper-Hall modification of Hughes's classification of alkali injuries, Brodovsky et al.[41] showed that grade III injuries treated with a combination of ascorbate, citrate, and fluorometholone attained vision of 20/40 or better in the treated group including 27 of 29 eyes (93%) compared to 3 of 6 eyes (50%) in the control group. There was also a trend toward shorter hospital stays in the treatment group. Specific topical treatment consisted of 10% ascorbate, 10% citrate, and fluorometholone every 2 hours, day and night, 1% atropine t.i.d. and chloramphenicol q.i.d. To this was added 500 mg ascorbate q.i.d. and 4 g of a proprietary urinary alkalinizer containing 720 mg of citric acid anhydrous and 620 mg of sodium citrate anhydrous t.i.d. In groups graded as I, II, and IV, there was no statistical difference between the treated and control groups.

Other putative treatments to prevent corneal ulceration in severe alkali injury, such as oral tetracycline, subconjunctival progesterone, intramuscular nortestosterone, and thiol dipeptides, have all shown favorable effects in limited animal studies of alkali injuries. However, a clinical trial will be needed before any of these approaches can be considered for routine human use.

Other possible chemical therapies

Fibronectin has been implicated as a key element in wound healing for its involvement in cell-to-cell and cell-to-matrix adhesion and cell spreading. Eye trauma causes exudation of large proteins such as fibrinogen from conjunctival blood vessels, reaching the bare basement membrane where polymerization and deposition take place. Epithelial defects occurring in herpetic keratitis, trophic corneal ulcers, and after cataract surgery have responded to fibronectin drops when used in an open-labeled study. However, albumin eyedrops were as effective as fibronectin in the treatment of persistent epithelial defects after alkali injuries in rabbits.[42] This suggests a nonspecific response. The determination of the value of fibronectin in persistent epithelial defects again can be gleaned only from a prospective, randomized clinical trial.

Epidermal growth factor (EGF) enhances the rate of healing and induces hyperplasia in corneal epithelium.[43] EGF stimulated complete epithelial healing after alkali injury in two studies, but in each instance recurrent erosions re-established the defect.[44,45] Epithelial proliferation is clearly stimulated by EGF, but its utility in corneal diseases is unknown. Its use may be limited to certain types of persistent epithelial defects where adhesion problems are least significant. Growth factors might find a more favored place in the acceleration of wound strength by enhancement of macromolecular synthesis.

The devastating nature of alkali injuries of the eye that result in severe personal, social, and economic loss attracts the attention of researchers, ophthalmologists, occupational medicine, and employers. The impact of these medical and surgical solutions found for the problems of alkali-injured patients might well find uses in other broad areas of inflammation in the body.

References

1. Wagoner M, Kenyon K. Chemical injuries of the eye. In: Albert D, Jakobiac F, eds. *Principles and practice of ophthalmology: clinical practice.* vol. 1. Philadelphia: WB Saunders; 1994:234–245.
2. Wagoner M. Chemical injuries of the eye: current concepts in pathophysiology and therapy. *Surv Ophthalmol.* 1997;41:275–313.
3. Klein R, Lobes LA. Ocular alkali burns in a large urban area. *Ann Ophthalmol.* 1976;8:1185–1189.
4. Morgan S. Chemical burns of the eye: causes and management. *Br J Ophthalmol.* 1987;71:854–857.
5. Kuckelkorn R, Luft I, Kottek A, et al. Chemical and thermal eye burns in the residential area of RWTH Aachen. Analysis of accidents in 1 year using a new automated documentation of findings. *Klin Monatsbl Augenheikd.* 1993;203:34–42.
6. Kuckelkorn M, Makropoulos W, Kotteck A, Reim M. Retrospective study of severe alkali burns of the eyes. *Klin Monatsbl Augenheikd.* 1993;203: 397–402.
7. Pearlman J, Au Eong K, Kuhn F. Airbags and eye injuries: epidemiology, spectrum of injury, and analysis of risk factors. *Surv Ophthalmol.* 2001; 46:234–243.
8. Paterson CA, Pfister RR, Levinson RA. Aqueous humor pH changes after experimental alkali burns. *Am J Ophthalmol.* 1975;79:414–419.
9. Paterson CA, Pfister RR. Intraocular pressure changes after alkali burns. *Arch Ophthalmol.* 1974;91:211–218.
10. Pfister R, Burstein N. The alkali-burned cornea. I. Epithelial and stromal repair. *Exp Eye Res.* 1976;23:519–535.
11. Dua HS, Forrester JV. The corneoscleral limbus in human corneal epithelial wound healing. *Am J Ophthalmol.* 1990;110:646–656.
12. Berman M, Leary R, Gage G. Evidence for a role of the plasminogen activator-plasmin system in corneal ulceration. *Invest Ophthalmol Vis Sci.* 1980;19:1201–1221.
13. Pfister RR, et al. Identification and synthesis of chemotactic tripeptides from alkali-degraded whole cornea: a study of N-acetyl-Proline-Glycine-Proline and N-methyl-Proline-Glycine-Proline. *Invest Ophthalmol Vis Sci.* 1995;36:1306–1316.
14. Sotozono C, He J, Matsumoto Y, et al. Cytokine expression in the alkali-burned cornea. *Curr Eye Res.* 1997;16:670–676.
15. Gan L, Fagerholm P, Kim H-J. Effect of leukocytes on corneal cellular proliferation and wound healing. *Invest Ophthalmol Vis Sci.* 1999;40: 575–581.
16 Sotozono C. Second injury of the cornea: the role of inflammatory cytokines in corneal damage and repair. *Cornea.* 2000;19:S155–S159.
17. Pfister RR, Paterson C. Additional clinical and morphological observations on the favorable effect of ascorbate in experimental ocular burns. *Invest Ophthmalmol Vis Sci.* 1977;16:478–487.
18. Pfister RR, Koski J. The pathophysiology and treatment of the alkali burned eye. *South Med J.* 1982;75:417–422.
19. Werb Z, Aggeler J. Proteases induce secretion of collagenase and plasminogen activator by fibroblasts. *Proc Natl Acad Aci USA.* 1978;75: 1839–1843.
20. Pfister RR, Nicolaro ML, Paterson CA. Sodium citrate reduces the incidence of corneal ulcerations and perforations in extreme alkali-burned eyes – acetylcysteine and ascorbate have no favorable effect. *Invest Ophthalmol Vis Sci.* 1981;21:486–490.
21. Brown S, Akiya S, Weller CA. Prevention of the ulcers of the alkali-burned cornea: preliminary studies with collagenase inhibitors. *Arch Ophthalmol.* 1969;82:95–97.
22. Slansky HH, Dohlman CH, Berman MB. Prevention of corneal ulcers. *Trans Am Acad Ophthalmol Otolarygol.* 1971;75:1208–1211.
23. Donshik PC, Berman MB, Donlman CH, et al. Effect of topical corticosteroids on corneal ulceration in alkali-burned corneas. *Arch Ophthalmol.* 1978;96:2117–2120.
24. Davis A, Ali Q, Aclimandos W. Topical steroid use in the treatment of ocular alkali burns. *Br J Ophthalmol.* 1997;81:732–734.
25. Fogle J, Kenyon K, Foster C. Tissue adhesive arrests stromal melting in the human cornea. *Am J Ophthalmol.* 1980;89:795–802.
26. Abel R, Binder P, Polack F, Kaufman J. The results of penetrating keratoplasty after chemical burns. *Trans Am Acad Ophthalmol Otolarygol.* 1975;79:584–595.
27. Reim M, Overkamping B, Kuckelkorn R. 2 years experience with tenonplasty. *Ophthalmologe.* 1992;89:524–530.
28. Thoft R. Indications for conjunctival transplantation. *Ophthalmology.* 1982;89:335–339.
29. Kenyon KR. Conjunctival autograft transplantation for advanced and recurrent pterygium. *Ophthalmology.* 1985;92:1461–1470.
30. Pfister RR. Stem cell disease. *CLAO J.* 1993;20:64–72.
31. Kukelkorn R, Redbrake C, Schrage N, Reim M. Keratoplasty with 11–12 mm diameter for management of severely chemically burned eyes. *Ophthalmologe.* 1993;90:683–687.
32. Redbrake C, Buchal V, Reim M. Keratoplasty with a scleral rim after most severe eye burns. *Klin Monatsbl Augenheilkd.* 1996;208:145–151.
33. Vajpayee R, Thomas S, Sharma N, et al. Large-diameter lamellar keratoplasty in severe ocular alkali burns. *Ophthalmology.* 2000;107: 1765–1768.
34. Tsai R, Tseng S. Human allograft limbal transplantation for corneal surface reconstruction. *Cornea.* 1994;13:389–400.
35. Meller D, et al. Amniotic membrane transplantation for acute chemical or thermal burns. *Invest Ophthalmol Vis Sci.* 2000;107:980–990.
36. Grueterich M, Espana E, Touhami A, et al. Phenotypic study of a case with successful transplantation of ex vivo expanded human limbal epithelium for unilateral total limbal stem cell deficiency. *Ophthalmology.* 2002;109:1547–1552.
37. Kramer S. Late numerical grading of alkali burns to determine keratoplasty prognosis. *Trans Am Ophthalmol Soc.* 1983;81:97–106.
38. Dohlman C, Doane M. Keratoprosthesis in end stage dry eye. *Adv Exp Med Biol.* 1994;350:561–564.
39. Pfister R, Haddox J, Dodson B. Polymorphonuclear leukocytic inhibition by citrate, other metal chelators and trifluoperazine: evidence to support calcium binding protein involvement. *Invest Ophthalmol Vis Sci.* 1984;25:955–970.
40. Pfister R, Haddox J, Barr D. The combined effect of citrate/ascorbate treatment in alkali-injured rabbit eyes. *Cornea.* 1991;10:100B–104B.
41. Brodovsky S, McCarty C, Snibson G. Management of alkali burns: an 11-year retrospective review. *Ophthalmology.* 2000;107(10):1829–1835.
42. Boisjoly H, et al. The effect of fibronectin compared to albumin on rabbit epithelial wound healing. *Invest Ophthalmol Vis Sci (Suppl).* 1987; 28:52.
43. Ho P, et al. Kinetics of corneal epithelial regeneration and epidermal growth factor. *Invest Ophthalmol Vis Sci.* 1974;13:804.
44. Eiferman R, Schultz G. Treatment of alkali burns in rabbits with epidermal growth factor. *Invest Ophthalmol Vis Sci.* 1987;28:52.
45. Singh G, Foster CS. Epidermal growth factor in alkali-burned corneal epithelial wound healing. *Am J Ophthalmol.* 1987;103:802–807.

Chapter 100

External Eye Manifestations of Biological and Chemical Warfare

Craig A. Skolnick

The spectrum of biological and chemical agents that can be used in warfare is frightening. Healthcare providers must be alert to patterns of illness and the constellation of clinical findings associated with an outbreak of biological or chemical warfare. The intentional release of an unusual infectious agent can be difficult to recognize since many of the commonly used organisms are rarely seen in their natural form. When used as weapons, there is potential for an immense number of casualties due to ease of dispersal, rapid onset of effect, and lack of preparation for containment and defense. Timely recognition of symptoms and early treatment are key to victim survival.

Background

The deliberate use of microorganisms and toxins as weapons dates back to the middle ages. During the fourteenth-century siege of Kaffa (now Feodossia, Ukraine), the attacking Tatars catapulted plague infested cadavers into the city in order to initiate an epidemic.[1] South American aboriginals are well known for using curare and amphibian-derived toxins as arrow poisons, and British forces used smallpox against native North Americans during the French and Indian War of the mid-eighteenth century. The advent of modern microbiology and Koch's postulates during the nineteenthth century afforded the opportunity to isolate and produce stockpiles of specific pathogens. There is evidence that Germany developed an aggressive biological warfare program during World War I, including operations to infect livestock and contaminate animal feed of the Allied forces using *Bacillus anthracis* and *Burkholderia* (*Pseudomonas*) *mallei*, the etiologic agents of anthrax and glanders.

The first widespread use of chemical weapons occurred during World War I, when more than 1 million casualties resulted from the use of sulfur, mustard, and chlorine gases. These horrors led to the first international diplomatic efforts to limit weapons of mass destruction. The 1925 Geneva Protocol for the Prohibition of the Use in War of Asphyxiating, Poisonous, or Other Gases, and of Bacteriological Methods of Warfare was enacted to prohibit the use of biological weapons.[2] Unfortunately, there were no provisions for inspection, and many countries that ratified the treaty still began research programs to develop biological weapons.

During World War II, Japan conducted experiments in which prisoners were infected with various bacterial pathogens, which led to at least 10000 deaths.[3] Many Chinese cities were attacked by contaminating water supplies and food items with pure cultures of *B. anthracis*, *Vibrio cholerae*, *Shigella* spp., *Salmonella* spp., and *Yersinia pestis*. International concern heightened during the late 1960s, which led to the signing of the 1972 Biological and Toxin Weapons Convention. The treaty prohibited the development, possession, and stockpiling of pathogens or toxins in 'quantities that have no justification for prophylactic, protective or other peaceful purposes.'[4] Transferring technology or expertise between countries was also prohibited. In 1979, the ineffectiveness of the convention was demonstrated by an accidental airborne release of anthrax spores by a Soviet military microbiology facility in Sverdlovsk (now Ekaterinburg, Russia), which led to numerous deaths.[5] Non-state-sponsored biological terrorism began to surface in the 1980s, which culminated with the 1995 sarin gas attack of the Tokyo, Japan, subway system by the Aum Shinrikyo cult.

Mechanism of Attack

A biological weapon is more than a microorganism or toxin. It is a system composed of four major components: payload (the biological agent), munition (a container that keeps the payload intact and virulent during delivery), delivery system (missile, artillery shell, aircraft, etc.), and dispersal mechanism (an explosive force or spray device to dispense the agent to the target population).[6] Certain agents are attractive because of low visibility, small volume, high potency, and easy delivery. Aerosolization would be the predominant method of dissemination because advanced delivery systems are not required, and small quantities make transportation and concealment quite easy. In 1970, the World Health Organization predicted the effect of an aerosol release of 50 kg of biological weapon over a city of 500000 people (Table 100.1).[7,8] Highly contagious organisms with delayed onset of symptoms make ideal weapons for a covert attack. In an overt attack, chemical agents are likely to be deployed,

Table 100.1 Estimated casualties for a hypothetical biological warfare attack on a city of 500000*

Agent	Downwind reach (km)	No. dead	No. incapacitated
Rift Valley fever	1	400	35000
Tick-borne encephalitis	1	9500	35000
Typhus	5	19000	85000
Brucellosis	10	500	100000
Q fever	>20	150	125000
Tularemia	>20	30000	125000
Anthrax	>20	950000	125000

* This model assumes that 50 kg of agent is deployed from an aircraft along a 2 km line upwind from the city.
From McGovern TW, Christopher GW, Eitzen EM: Cutaneous manifestations of biological warfare and related threat agents, Arch Dermatol 135:311–322, 1999. Copyright © (1999) American Medical Association. All rights reserved.

Box 100.1 Biological diseases

Anthrax (*Bacillus anthracis*)

Botulism (*Clostridium botulinum* toxin)

Plague (*Yersinia pestis*)

Smallpox (Variola major and minor)

Tularemia (*Francisella tularensis*)

Viral hemorrhagic fevers

Filoviruses – Ebola, Marburg

Arenaviruses – Lassa, Machupo

From Centers for Disease Control and Prevention: Biological Diseases/ Agents List. Available at http://www.bt.cdc.gov/agent/agentlist-category. asp, accessed 02/28/09.

causing rapid onset of symptoms and an overwhelming demand for emergency medical services. Both biological and chemical weapons can incapacitate an entire city and impede the mobilization of military personnel.

Warning Signs

In order to recognize a bioterror attack, one must be familiar with the various clinical presentations of these agents. The American College of Physicians and the American Society of Internal Medicine have suggested that the following epidemiological clues be considered:[9]

1. Unusual temporal or geographic clustering of illness.
2. Unusual age distribution of common disease (i.e. an illness that appears to be chickenpox in adults but is really smallpox).
3. Large epidemic, with greater case loads than expected, especially in a discrete population.
4. More severe disease than expected.
5. Unusual route of exposure.
6. A disease that is outside its normal transmission season, or is impossible to transmit naturally in the absence of its normal vector.
7. Multiple simultaneous epidemics of different diseases.
8. A disease outbreak with health consequences to humans and animals.
9. Unusual strains or variants of organisms or antimicrobial resistance patterns.

The Centers for Disease Control and Prevention (CDC) of the United States has listed the high-priority biological diseases (Box 100.1)[10] that pose significant risk to national security based on the following: can be easily disseminated and/or transmitted from person to person; result in high mortality rates and have the potential for major public health impact; might cause public panic and social disruption; and require special action for public health preparedness.[11] Most of these agents have significant ophthalmic manifestations that may aid in diagnosis or complicate management.

Biological Diseases

Anthrax

Bacillus anthracis is the ideal biologic weapon because of its stability in spore form, its ease to grow in culture, the lack of natural immunity in many industrialized nations, and the severity of infection.

Microbiology/epidemiology

Bacillus anthracis is an encapsulated, aerobic, Gram-positive, spore-forming, rod-shaped bacterium. Spores form when environmental nutrients are depleted, such as occurs with dry soil, the natural reservoir. Spores can survive for decades in contaminated soils or workplaces and can resist temperatures of over 10°C for prolonged periods.[12,13] Inhalation (wool-sorter's disease) can occur from animal products, such as wool fibers or bone meal, leading to outbreaks in slaughterhouses, textile industries, and tanneries.[14] Herbivores such as cattle, goats, and sheep ingest spores and serve as the natural transmitters of infection. Humans become infected through direct contact with contaminated carcasses or from eating infected meat. Animal husbandmen, butchers, and veterinarians are most susceptible.[12]

Clinical manifestations

Three principal forms of anthrax occur in humans: cutaneous, inhalational, and gastrointestinal. The majority of naturally occurring disease is cutaneous, comprising more than 95% of cases.[12] Spores sent in mailed letters or packages can lead to either cutaneous or inhalational anthrax. The differential diagnosis of cutaneous anthrax includes cowpox, spider bite, ecthyma gangrenosum, ulceroglandular tularemia, plague, scrub typhus, rickettsial spotted fever, rat bite fever, staphylococcal or streptococcal cellulitis, and herpes simplex virus.[15,16]

Cutaneous anthrax

Cutaneous disease begins as a small, painless, pruritic, red macule that progresses to a papule which vesiculates, ruptures, and ulcerates. It then forms a classic 1–5 cm brown or coal-black eschar surrounded by significant nonpitting edema.[8] The term anthrax is derived from the Greek *anthrakos* meaning 'coal.' It appears at the site of inoculation (spores or bacilli) within 3 to 10 days. The edema can spread, and translucent epidermal bullae vesicles often surround the lesion – the so-called 'pearly wreath.'[13] After 2 to 4 weeks the eschar sloughs away, leaving an exposed area of granulation tissue. Although fatalities due to cutaneous disease are rare, 10–20% of untreated patients develop malignant edema, septicemia, shock, renal failure, and death.[8]

Ophthalmic manifestations

Ocular findings in cutaneous anthrax relate to eyelid involvement.[13,17–20] The main complication is cicatricial ectropion due to late eyelid scarring (Fig. 100.1).[21] Lid malposition causes exposure keratopathy which can lead to epithelial breakdown and secondary infectious keratitis. Corneal scarring is more likely to occur in patients who present late without treatment during the acute stage. It appears that upper eyelid involvement is more likely to result in ectropion. Severely affected patients have undergone release of contractures and full-thickness postauricular skin grafts with satisfactory resolution of ectropion.[13] Temporal artery inflammation has been reported as a complication of overlying cutaneous anthrax.[22]

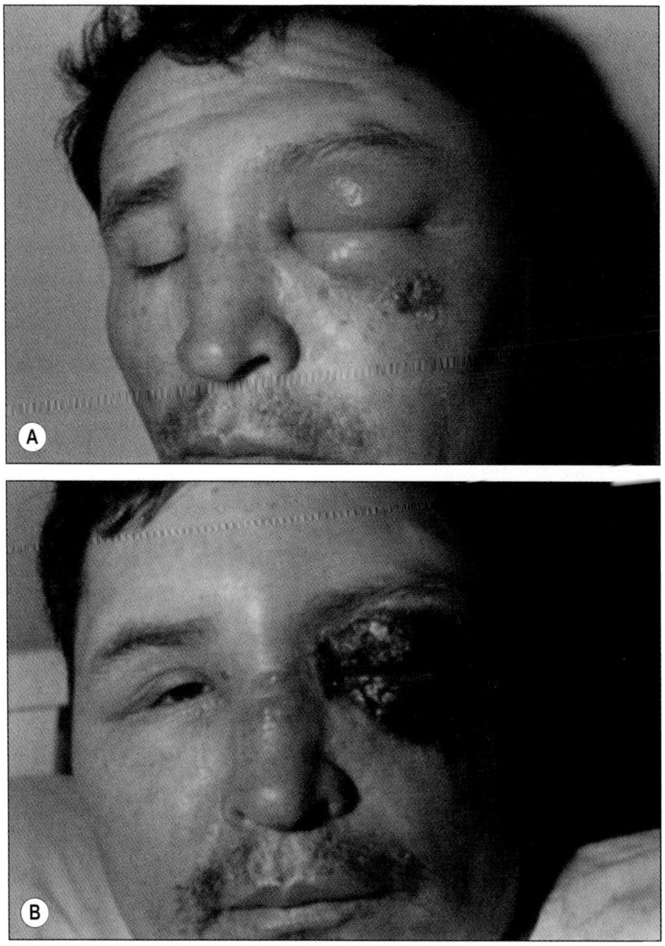

Fig. 100.1 Cutaneous anthrax. (**A**) Swelling and erythema in the early phase. (**B**) Central ulceration with black, necrotic tissue in the latter phase. (From Noeller TP: Biological and chemical terrorism: recognition and management, *Cleve Clin J Med* 68(12):1001–1016, 2001.)

Diagnosis

Anthrax bacilli can be visualized by Wright or Gram stain of peripheral blood or isolated by blood culture. Diagnostic testing for cutaneous disease includes Gram stain and culture of vesicular fluid, tissue biopsy, specific enzyme-linked immunosorbent assays (ELISAs) to measure antibody titers, immunomagnetic-electrochemiluminescence (ECL) assays for antigen detection, and polymerase chain reaction (PCR) for nucleic acid detection.[14] Spores have a diameter of 2–6 mm, which is ideal for entrapment in the lower respiratory tract. The time for infection is variable because spores must germinate into bacilli after phagocytosis by tissue macrophages. The dose of anthrax in an exposure is inversely correlated with incubation time. Cases in the accidental release in Sverdlovsk developed 2 to 43 days after exposure.[14] Thus it may be hard to trace the onset of an attack, making response and containment more difficult.

Treatment

Treatment of inhalational and gastrointestinal anthrax should begin with intravenous ciprofloxacin 400 mg every 12 hours (Table 100.2).[21] Doxycycline 100 mg every 12 hours can be used, but has poorer central nervous system penetration. One or two of the following additional antibiotics should be added until susceptibility testing is performed: rifampin, vancomycin, penicillin, ampicillin, chloramphenicol, imipenem, clindamycin, and clarithromycin. Cutaneous disease can be treated with either oral ciprofloxacin or doxycycline alone. Treatment should be continued for 60 days because of the possibility of delayed germination of spores.[16] Direct contact with wound or wound drainage should be avoided when caring for a patient with cutaneous anthrax.

Despite aggressive supportive therapy and antibiotics, fatality is very high. In the twentieth-century series of 18 patients in the United States, the mortality rate of occupationally acquired inhalational anthrax was 89%, but the majority of these cases occurred before the development of critical care units and antibiotics.[23] After the September 2001 terrorist attacks on the United States, anthrax spores were sent to various locations via the postal service, resulting in 11 cases of inhalational anthrax with five deaths.[16]

Prevention

Since there are no data to support person-to-person transmission of anthrax, patient contacts do not need immunization or prophylactic treatment unless they were exposed to the aerosol or surface contamination at the time of attack. A vaccine derived from an attenuated strain of anthrax is available, and studies in rhesus monkeys indicate that it is

Table 100.2 CDC recommendations for antimicrobial therapy against anthrax

Indication	Adults	Children
Postexposure prophylaxis	Ciprofloxacin 500 mg by mouth twice a day OR Doxycycline 100 mg by mouth twice a day	Ciprofloxacin 10–15 mg/kg by mouth every 12 hrs* OR Doxycycline: >8 yrs and >45 kg 100 mg by mouth every 12 hrs >8 yrs and ≤45 kg 2.2 mg/kg by mouth every 12 hrs ≤8 yrs: 2.2 mg/kg by mouth every 12 hrs
Cutaneous anthrax	Ciprofloxacin 500 mg by mouth twice a day OR Doxycycline 100 mg by mouth twice a day	Ciprofloxacin 10–15 mg/kg by mouth every 12 hrs* OR Doxycycline: >8 yrs and >45 kg: 100 mg by mouth every 12 hrs >8 yrs and ≤45 kg: 2.2 mg/kg by mouth every 12 hrs ≤8 yrs: 2.2 mg/kg by mouth every 12 hrs
Inhalational anthrax	Ciprofloxacin 400 mg intravenously every 12 hrs OR Doxycycline 100 mg intravenously every 12 hrs PLUS (for either drug) One or two additional antibiotics (e.g. rifampin, vancomycin, penicillin, ampicillin, chloramphenicol, imipenem, clindamycin, clarithromycin)	Ciprofloxacin 10–15 mg/kg intravenously every 12 hrs* OR Doxycycline: >8 yrs and >45 kg: 100 mg intravenously every 12 hrs >8 yrs and ≤45 kg: 2.2 mg/kg intravenously every 12 hrs ≤8 yrs: 2.2 mg/kg intravenously every 12 hrs PLUS (for either drug) One or two additional antibiotics

* *Ciprofloxacin dose in children not to exceed 1 g/day.*
From Noeller TP: Biological and chemical terrorism: recognition and management, Cleve Clin J Med *68(12):1001–1016, 2001.*

protective for inhalational anthrax.[24] Should an attack occur, those exposed must be vaccinated and receive chemoprophylaxis with either ciprofloxacin or doxycycline orally until at least three doses of vaccine have been administered.[25] The safety of the vaccine was studied in military personnel, and 1% of inoculations were associated with one or more systemic events (i.e. headache, malaise, blurred vision, nausea). Isolated cases of optic neuritis have been reported after anthrax booster vaccination,[26] but a matched case-controlled study among US military personnel from 1998 through 2003 showed no statistically significant association.[27] One case of unilateral optic neuropathy, bilateral anterior uveitis, bilateral posterior scleritis, bilateral sensorineural hearing loss, and focal segmental glomerulosclerosis has been reported,[28] as well as a patient who developed central serous chorioretinopathy after vaccination.[29]

Botulism

Botulism is a serious paralytic illness caused by a nerve toxin produced by the bacterium *Clostridium botulinum*. Three forms of naturally occurring botulism exist: food-borne, wound, and intestinal. The oldest and most common form observed on a worldwide basis is food-borne, which typically occurs after ingestion of improperly prepared home-canned food that contains preformed neurotoxin.[30] It poses a major bioweapons threat because of its extreme potency and lethality, its ease of production, transportation, and misuse, and the need for prolonged intensive care among affected persons.[31]

Microbiology

Clostridium botulinum is a rod-shaped, spore-forming, obligate anaerobe commonly found in soil. There are seven types of toxin designated A through G, which are defined by their absence of cross-neutralization (i.e. anti-A antitoxin does not neutralize toxin types B–G).[31] Types A, B, and E account for greater than 99% of human botulism.[30] Type A toxin is the most potent poison known to humans, 100000 times more toxic than sarin nerve gas.[25] Once absorbed, the toxin is carried via the blood to peripheral cholinergic synapses. It irreversibly binds to the presynaptic neuromuscular junction, where it is internalized and blocks acetylcholine release, causing paralysis. Interestingly, a vial of therapeutic Botox® (Allergan, Irvine, CA, USA) contains only about 0.3% of the estimated human lethal inhalational dose and 0.005% of the estimated lethal oral dose.[30]

Clinical manifestations

During an attack, botulinum toxin would likely be used as an inhalational agent or to deliberately contaminate food, since it does not penetrate intact skin and is not transmitted from person to person.[31] Symptoms generally begin 12 to 72 hours after ingestion. The time of onset after an inhalational exposure is not known, but experimentally is similar to food-borne exposure.[25]

Botulism classically presents as an acute, afebrile, symmetric, descending flaccid paralysis that always begins in the bulbar musculature (Box 100.2).[31,30] Patients have a clear sensorium because the toxin does not penetrate the brain tissue. The prominent bulbar palsies (the 4Ds) include diplopia, dysarthria, dysphonia, and dysphagia. If the origin is food-borne, the neurologic signs may be preceded by abdominal cramps, nausea, vomiting, or diarrhea.[32] Sensory changes are not present. As the disease progresses, weakness extends below the neck with loss of deep tendon reflexes, constipation, and unsteady gait. Severe cases lead to respiratory collapse from diaphragm and intercostal muscle involvement and airway obstruction from pharyngeal muscle paralysis.[31] Autonomic nervous system involvement can lead to cardiovascular lability.

Ophthalmic manifestations

Visual symptoms of diplopia, photophobia, and blurred vision are present early (Table 100.3).[30] Accommodative paresis and mydriasis account for the blurred vision and photophobia, respectively. Blepharoptosis, gaze paralysis, pupillary dilation, and nystagmus are common ophthalmic signs. Dry eye and dry mouth from parasympathetic cholinergic blockade can also be prominent.

Box 100.2 Signs and symptoms of food-borne and wound botulism

Signs
- Ventilatory (respiratory) problems
- Extraocular muscle paresis or paralysis (including eyelids)
- Muscle paresis or paralysis
- Dry mucous membranes in mouth, throat
- Dilated, fixed pupils
- Ataxia
- Somnolence
- Hypotension (including postural)
- Nystagmus
- Decreased to absent deep tendon reflexes
- Fever (more common for wound botulism)
- Sensory deficits (very rare)

Symptoms
- Visual disturbances (blurred vision, diplopia, photophobia)
- Dysphagia
- Dry mouth
- Generalized weakness (usually bilateral)
- Nausea or vomiting
- Dizziness or vertigo
- Abdominal pain, cramps, discomfort
- Diarrhea
- Urinary retention or incontinence
- Sore throat
- Constipation
- Parasthesias

Adapted from Caya JG: Clostridium botulinum *and the ophthalmologist: a review of botulism, including biological warfare ramifications of botulinum toxin,* Surv Ophthalmol *46:25–34, 2001.*

Table 100.3 Ophthalmic signs and symptoms of botulism

Signs and symptoms	Frequency
Blurred vision	89%
Ptosis	80%
Diplopia	59%
Abnormal pupil reaction to light	59%
Impaired accommodation	59%
Nystagmus	56%
Mydriasis	52%
Extraocular muscle dysfunction on examination	36%

Adapted from Caya JG: Clostridium botulinum *and the ophthalmologist: a review of botulism, including biological warfare ramifications of botulinum toxin,* Surv Ophthalmol *46:25–34, 2001.*

Uncommon neuro-ophthalmic manifestations include complete bilateral internal ophthalmoplegia[33] which can include both permanent and transient tonic pupils. A dilated and poorly reactive pupil with loss of accommodation are typical findings. Light-near dissociation, sectoral iris contractions, and supersensitivity of the iris sphincter muscle to weak miotics (pilocarpine 0.1%) are also hallmark findings of a tonic pupil.

Diagnosis

Early diagnosis of botulism is made by the history and physical examination. The differential diagnosis includes Guillain-Barré and the Miller-Fisher variant, myasthenia gravis, Lambert-Eaton syndrome, tick paralysis, stroke, and various central nervous system disorders.[21,31] Botulism differs from other causes of flaccid paralyses in that there is the presence of symmetry, absence of sensory nerve damage, and disproportionate involvement of cranial nerves compared to muscles below the neck.[31] An electromyogram can be diagnostic. Demonstration of toxin by mouse bioassay is diagnostic in samples of serum, stool, gastric aspirate, and suspect food.[31] Studies suggest that aerosolized toxin is usually not identifiable in serum or stool, but may be present on nasal mucous membranes and detected by ELISA for up to 24 hours after exposure.[25] Fecal, wound, and gastric specimens can be cultured anaerobically if a food-borne or wound source of *C. botulinum* is suspected.

Treatment

Management is primarily supportive, with ventilatory assistance essential in advanced cases. Early administration with equine-derived trivalent (types A, B, E) antitoxin can minimize subsequent nerve damage and severity of disease, but will not reverse existing paralysis, which can last from weeks to months.[34] In a large outbreak of botulism, the need for mechanical ventilators, critical care beds, and skilled personnel might quickly exceed capacity. Research directed at recombinant vaccines and human antibody may eventually minimize the threat of botulinum toxin as a weapon of mass destruction.

Smallpox

Smallpox is one of the most dreaded diseases in the history of humankind. It raged in epidemic and endemic forms for more than 3000 years, killing hundreds of millions of people. In 1966, the World Health Organization established a vaccination program with extensive educational and surveillance programs for global eradication. Smallpox was successfully eradicated in 1977, with the last case documented in Somalia.[35]

Microbiology

Variola is a large, double-stranded DNA virus and member of the genus orthopoxvirus. The viruses are complex, and the virion is brick-shaped with a diameter of about 200 nm.[14] Three other members of this genus (monkeypox, vaccinia, and cowpox) can infect humans but are not highly contagious.[36]

Epidemiology

There are two clinical forms of smallpox, variola major and a much milder form, variola minor. Typical variola major epidemics resulted in mortality rates of greater than 30%

among unvaccinated persons.[36] Smallpox spreads from person to person primarily in droplet form or aerosols expelled from the oropharynx of infected persons. Contaminated bedding and clothing can also spread the virus via direct contact.[37] Smallpox would likely be used in aerosol form during a biological assault, given both its small infectious dose and significant stability.

Clinical manifestations

After an incubation period of about 12 days, patients become febrile and often develop severe constitutional symptoms.[38] Headache, backache, vomiting, abdominal pain, and malaise are common. The clinical presentation of smallpox is heralded by a diffuse maculopapular rash beginning 2 to 3 days after this prodromal phase.[39] Lesions first appear on the mucous membranes of the oropharynx. Skin lesions appear mostly on the head, torso, and extremities in a centrifugal pattern, evolving from a flat rash to a papule, a vesicle, and then a pustule which becomes crusted and scabbed. This leads to permanent scarring, usually most extensive on the face. Classically, the lesions are at one stage of development at a given point and can affect the palms and soles. Chickenpox (varicella), the disease most frequently confused with smallpox, differs in that lesions are in various stages of development at a given point. Varicella lesions are more superficial, rarely found on the palms and soles, and the distribution is centripetal, with the trunk affected more than the face and extremities.[37]

Nearly one-third of patients with smallpox will die, usually during the second week of illness. This most likely results from the toxemia and cardiovascular collapse associated with circulating immune complexes and soluble variola antigens.[36] Pneumonia, encephalitis, osteomyelitis, orchitis, sepsis, and overwhelming hemorrhage into the skin and mucous membranes can complicate smallpox infection.[40] Variola minor, the less severe form of smallpox, results in milder symptoms with only a sparse rash and less than 1% mortality.[36] Patients are most infectious during the first week of the illness; however, some risk of transmission is present until all scabs have fallen off.[37] It is thought that smallpox cannot be transmitted until the onset of the rash,[25,37] so diagnosis during the prodromal stage with subsequent quarantine would be essential to limit additional exposure.

Ophthalmic manifestations

Smallpox led to blindness in 2–5% of students in blind schools of developing countries in Africa.[41] Typically, a mild conjunctivitis appears around the fifth day of illness with subconjunctival hemorrhage in some cases. Actual pustules which resemble phlyctenules may form on the bulbar or tarsal conjunctiva and even involve the limbus.[42] These lesions are very inflamed and painful and can lead to infiltration and ulceration of the cornea. Less frequently, an interstitial or disciform keratitis evolves (Fig. 100.2). Lid alopecia and punctal stenosis may result when pustules involve the cilia and puncta, respectively. Ankyloblepharon has also been reported due to severe eyelid adhesions between the upper and lower canthi.[43] Secondary infectious keratitis can occur late and lead to significant morbidity; therefore, antibiotic prophylaxis is warranted. Dense corneal scarring can leave patients phthisical and blind.

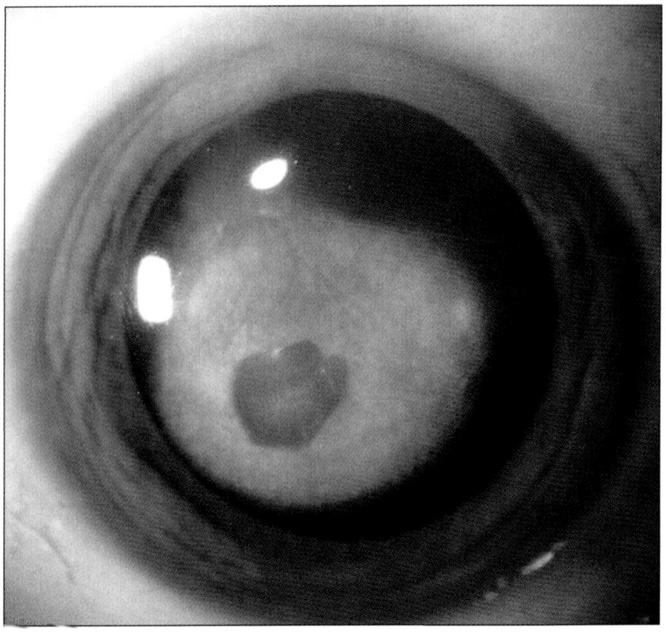

Fig. 100.2 Variola (smallpox). This patient demonstrates a central corneal scar from a smallpox or variola infection.

Diagnosis

Laboratory diagnosis of smallpox can be confirmed with electron microscopy of vesicular or pustular fluid, or characteristic Guarnieri bodies can be visualized under light microscopy.[25] Virus culture of skin lesions, oropharynx, conjunctiva, and urine is definitive. PCR techniques can discriminate between strains and offer a more rapid result.[37]

Treatment and vaccination

There is no specific systemic or ocular treatment for smallpox, although cidofovir has in vitro and in vivo activity against Poxviridae.[25] In 1796, Edward Jenner demonstrated that an infection caused by cowpox protected against smallpox, which led to the worldwide practice of vaccination.[44] Currently, smallpox vaccine is prepared from live vaccinia virus using cell culture techniques.[14]

The interval between an aerosol release of variola and diagnosis of the first cases is as much as 2 weeks.[37] Fortunately, the virus is inactivated after 2 days, eliminating further exposure. Individuals in whom infection is suspected should be vaccinated within 4 days of exposure and placed under surveillance. Vaccination programs ended in 1972 in the United States, and it is presumed that few people who were vaccinated have lasting protective levels of immunity.

Complications of vaccination

Vaccination is not without risk. Life-threatening encephalitis occurs at a rate of 1 case per 300000.[45] Progressive

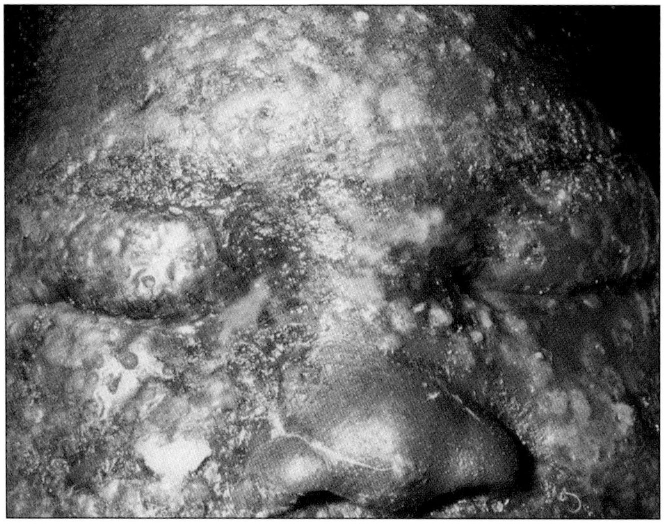

Fig. 100.3 Eczema vaccinatum. Vaccinial skin lesions extending over the area currently afflicted with eczema. (Courtesy of Richard K. Forster, MD.)

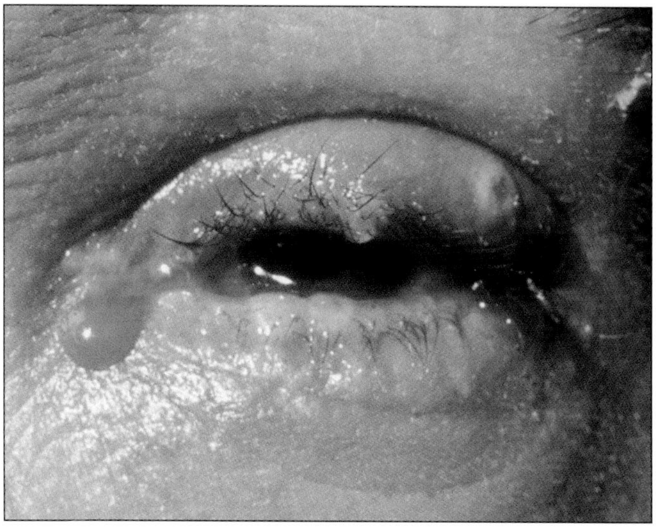

Fig. 100.4 Ocular vaccinia blepharoconjunctivitis with typical umbilicated pustules. (Courtesy of Richard K. Forster, MD.)

vaccinia or vaccinia gangrenosum results from necrosis of the skin at the vaccination site, with advanced cases involving underlying bone and viscera.[37] Patients with a history of eczema are at risk of developing extensive vaccinial lesions (eczema vaccinatum) over affected sites (Fig. 100.3). In some vaccine recipients, blood-borne dissemination of virus leads to a self-limiting generalized vaccinial rash. Transmission of vaccinia from the site of vaccination to close contacts, or autoinoculation to sites such as face, mouth, eyelid, and genitalia, can take place. Vaccinia immune globulin is used to treat these complications with variable success.

Vaccinia ophthalmic manifestations

Inadvertent autoinoculation of vaccinia from the deltoid site accounts for the ophthalmic complications of vaccination, which has an incidence of 3.6 per 100 000 inoculations.[46] The majority of patients have vaccinia of the eyelids or conjunctiva, but a smaller percentage have corneal involvement. Typically, patients present 4 to 7 days after vaccination with advanced blepharoconjunctivitis and pustules commonly affecting both lids (Fig. 100.4). The conjunctivitis is usually purulent and ulceration can occur with adherent membrane formation and preauricular lymphadenopathy.[42] Severe cases present with periorbital edema mimicking orbital cellulitis.[47]

Vaccinial keratitis is the most feared ophthalmic complication. Corneal involvement develops in 20–37% of cases of ocular vaccinia.[48] When virus infects the corneal epithelium it produces a grayish, fine granular opacity with mild epithelial edema.[47] Diseased cells stain with rose Bengal, and dendritic lesions are occasionally present. Subepithelial infiltrates may form and lead to peripheral neovascularization and ulceration. Some patients develop a disciform or necrotizing stromal keratitis with possible perforation.[42,47] The diseased epithelium is less opaque and swollen than that in herpes simplex and a conjunctival follicular reaction is usually absent. The ulceration is more rapid, extensive, and irregular than in herpes.[47] Permanent sequelae include corneal scarring, punctal stenosis, eyelid scarring, and loss of lashes.

Treatment

Topical steroids are effective for stromal opacities, neovascularization, and uveitis; however, treatment of the acute infection requires viral inactivation and steroids are contraindicated. Topical and parenteral vaccinia immune globulin is effective for ocular vaccinia,[49,50] especially with orbital inflammation.[47] Idoxuridine, an antiviral used for herpes simplex, can be used to treat early vaccinial keratitis.[51] It is likely that newer antivirals (trifluridine) would be at least as effective as idoxuridine, as both inhibit viral DNA synthesis by thymidine kinase phosphorylation. Most of the cases that occurred in the Department of Defense Smallpox Vaccination Program (2002–03) were treated successfully with trifluridine 1%.[46]

Tularemia

Microbiology and epidemiology

The causative bacterial agent of tularemia, *Francisella tularensis*, is a highly infectious, aerobic, Gram-negative coccobacillus found in widely diverse animal hosts and habitats throughout the world. Tularemia has epidemic potential, but typically occurs in isolated cases in rural areas. The natural reservoirs for infection are various small animals including rabbits, squirrels, voles, mice, and water rats that become infected through bites from ticks, flies, and mosquitoes, and through contact with contaminated soil, water, and vegetation.[52] Humans become infected by various modes, including bites by arthropods, handling infectious animal tissues or fluids, direct contact with or ingestion of contaminated water, food, or soil, and inhalation of infective aerosols.

Clinical manifestations

The clinical forms of tularemia depend on the virulence of the bacteria as well as the site of inoculation. Disease presentations include ulceroglandular, glandular, oculoglandular, oropharyngeal, pneumonic, typhoidal, and septic forms.[8,52,53] After an incubation of 2 to 10 days, there is rapid onset of fever, chills, rigors, headache, myalgias, coryza, and sore throat. Frequently, there is a dry or slightly productive cough with substernal pain.[52] Nausea, vomiting, and diarrhea can occur and nearly half of patients demonstrate a pulse–temperature dissociation.[54]

Intentional aerosol release of *F. tularensis* would lead to the generalized illness with a significant number of patients developing pleuropneumonitis. Hematogenous spread may occur, with death resulting from sepsis, disseminated intravascular coagulation, adult respiratory distress syndrome, and multiple organ failure.[53,55] The largest recorded airborne outbreak of tularemia occurred in a farming community in Sweden in 1966–67. The strain was a less virulent form, but still led to 140 serologically confirmed cases. Pulmonary symptoms were present in 10%, conjunctivitis in 26%, skin ulceration in 12%, pharyngitis in 31%, oral ulcers in 9%, and 32% had various exanthemas, such as erythema multiforme and erythema nodosum.[48] Person-to-person transmission is not known to occur.[52]

Ophthalmic manifestations

Tularemia is one of the causes of Parinaud's oculoglandular syndrome.[56] Direct contamination of the eye leads to conjunctival ulceration, chemosis, and tender lymphadenopathy of the preauricular, submandibular, and cervical regions.[53] The conjunctivitis is unilateral (90%) and granulomatous, typically with multiple yellow nodules involving the tarsal or bulbar surface.[57] Rare ocular effects include corneal ulceration,[56,57] dacryocystitis,[58] acute glaucoma,[59] endogenous retinitis,[60] and optic neuritis.[58] The differential diagnosis includes bacterial conjunctivitis, adenoviral, syphilis, cat-scratch disease, herpes simplex infection, and other rare causes of Parinaud's oculoglandular syndrome.[53,58]

Diagnosis

F. tularensis can be identified by examination of secretions or biopsy specimens using direct fluorescent antibody or immunohistochemical stains.[52] Cultures are definitive, but must be performed with cysteine-enriched media.[52,53] Serological testing can be diagnostic; however, it can take longer than 10 days after the onset of illness for a significant change in titers, proving less useful in an outbreak.[52] Several PCR assays have been developed that would give faster results.[14]

Treatment

Treatment is with streptomycin 1 g IM b.i.d. for 10 days, with gentamicin (5 mg/kg IM or IV) as an alternative. Fluoroquinolones are probably as effective.[52,59] In a mass exposure situation or for postexposure prophylaxis, oral doxycycline 100 mg b.i.d. or ciprofloxacin 500 mg b.i.d. can be used for 14 days.[52] Treatment for ocular disease should include frequent topical gentamicin.[57,58]

Viral hemorrhagic fever

Microbiology and epidemiology

Viral hemorrhagic fever is a clinical illness associated with fever and bleeding diathesis caused by a virus belonging to one of four families: Filoviridae, Arenaviridae, Bunyaviridae, and Flaviviridae (Table 100.4).[61] All are RNA viruses that in nature reside in animal hosts or arthropod vectors. Humans are infected by the bite of an infected arthropod, via aerosol (the mechanism in a biological attack) generated from infected rodent excreta, or by direct contact with infected animal carcasses. Some viruses can lead to human-to-human transmission via direct contact with blood, secretions (oral and conjunctival), or tissues of infected patients or needlestick injuries.[61]

Clinical manifestations

The vascular system is primarily targeted by these viruses. Microvascular damage with changes in vascular permeability lead to a coagulopathy and signs of bleeding which include conjunctival hemorrhage, mild hypotension, flushing, and petechiae.[61] Symptoms of fatigue, dizziness, and myalgias are present during the first week of illness. Nausea and nonbloody diarrhea may accompany the high fevers after an incubation period that ranges from 2 to 21 days.[61] Disseminated intravascular coagulation with hematuria, hematemesis, and melena occurs as a late ominous sign. In severe cases, shock and generalized mucous membrane hemorrhage results with end-organ damage and death within 1 to 2 weeks.

Some viral hemorrhagic fevers present with suggestive clinical features.[61] Ebola and Marburg (Filoviridae family) are especially virulent and can cause necrosis of visceral organs (liver, spleen, kidneys). Adult respiratory distress syndrome is a sequela of one species of Hantavirus. Nephropathia epidemica is caused by Puumala virus, and leads to an acute hemorrhagic tubular and interstitial nephritis.

Ophthalmic manifestations

Filoviridae

Due to high mortality rates, Ebola and Marburg hemorrhagic fever are two of the most feared illnesses. Eye involvement presents with symptoms of pain, photophobia, tearing, and blurred vision.[62] Conjunctival injection is seen in at least one-half of patients during the acute phase, and may present with subconjunctival hemorrhage. Fifteen percent (3/20) of patients who survived the 1995 Ebola outbreak in the Democratic Republic of Congo developed acute anterior uveitis with vitreous opacities in one patient.[62] The onset of uveitis was 1 to 2 months after initial infection. Treatment with topical cycloplegics and steroids was effective in all patients. A case of recurrent anterior uveitis with elevated intraocular pressure occurred after a small outbreak of Marburg virus in Johannesburg, South Africa, in 1975. Virus was cultured from the anterior chamber aspirate at presentation, 80 days after initial infection.[63]

Table 100.4 Hemorrhagic fever viruses*

Family	Genus	Virus	Disease	Vector in nature	Geographic distribution
Filoviridae	Filovirus	**Ebola**†	Ebola hemorrhagic fever	Unknown	Africa
		Marburg	Marburg hemorrhagic fever	Unknown	Africa
Arenaviridae	Arenavirus	**Lassa**	Lassa fever	Rodent	West Africa
		New World Arenaviridae‡	New World hemorrhagic fever	Rodent	Americas
Bunyaviridae	Nairovirus	Crimean-Congo hemorrhagic fever	Crimean-Congo hemorrhagic fever	Tick	Africa, central Asia, Eastern Europe, Middle East
	Phlebovirus	**Rift Valley fever**	Rift Valley fever	Mosquito	Africa, Saudi Arabia, Yemen
	Hantavirus	Agents of hemorrhagic fever with renal syndrome	Hemorrhagic fever with renal syndrome	Rodent	Asia, Balkans, Europe, Eurasia§
Flaviviridae	Flavivirus	Dengue	Dengue fever, Dengue hemorrhagic fever, and Dengue shock syndrome	Mosquito	Asia, Africa, Pacific, Americas
		Yellow fever	Yellow fever	Mosquito	Africa, tropical Americas
		Omsk hemorrhagic fever	Omsk hemorrhagic fever	Tick	Central Asia
		Kyasanur Forest disease	Kyasanur Forest disease	Tick	India

** Bold indicates hemorrhagic fever viruses that pose serious risk as biological weapons.*
† There are four subtypes of Ebola: Zaire, Sudan, Ivory Coast, and Reston.
‡ The New World Arenaviridae include Muchupo, the cause of Bolivian hemorrhagic fever; Junin, the cause of Argentine hemorrhagic fever; Guanarito, the cause of Venezuelan hemorrhagic fever; and Sabia, the cause of Brazilian hemorrhagic fever. An additional arenavirus has been isolated following three fatal cases of hemorrhagic fever in California, 1999–2000.
§ Additionally, the agents of Hantavirus pulmonary syndrome have been isolated in North America.
From Borio L, Inglesby T, Peters CJ et al: Hemorrhagic fever virus as biological weapons: medical and public health management, JAMA 287(18):2391–2405, 2002.

Nephropathia epidemica

Some of the other less virulent causes of viral hemorrhagic fever also have ophthalmic signs. Patients affected with nephropathia epidemica can present with eye pain, blurred vision, and photophobia. The most prominent eye finding is transient myopia due to forward movement of the anterior diaphragm and thickening of the crystalline lens.[64] Usually, the intraocular pressure is slightly lowered;[65] however, acute glaucoma has been observed.[66] Other findings include conjunctival injection and hemorrhage, iritis, and retinal edema with hemorrhage.[67] Neuro-ophthalmic findings include tonic pupils[68] and isolated abducens palsy.[69]

Rift Valley fever

Rift Valley fever presents predominantly with retinal findings, although conjunctival injection with photophobia and retroorbital pain is present initially. Fundus examination typically reveals cotton-wool exudates and hemorrhage in the macula and paramacular area, vascular occlusions and sheathing, macular edema, and optic pallor.[70] Vitreous hemorrhage, retinal detachment, and epiretinal membranes may also develop. Uveitis with occasional anterior chamber reaction occurs in less than one-third of patients.

Diagnosis

Travel history and clinical presentation can aid in the diagnosis and help determine the type of hemorrhagic fever virus. Occasionally, thrombocytopenia or leukopenia may be present. Viral cultures, rapid enzyme immunoassays (ELISA, reverse transcription-PCR), and electron microscopy can identify the specific subtype of virus.[25]

Treatment

Treatment is supportive, but ribavirin may be beneficial in Arenaviruses or Bunyaviruses.[61] With the exception of yellow fever and Argentine hemorrhagic fever, there is no licensed vaccine for any of the viral hemorrhagic fevers.

Others

The CDC has listed additional biological agents that pose significant but lower risk to public health than the agents already described. The known ophthalmic associations of these are listed in Box 100.3.[10,71–94]

Chemical Agents

Chemical attacks can easily overwhelm medical resources, especially in urban areas. Materials to manufacture chemical weapons are inexpensive and easy to obtain. The categories and types used by the CDC are listed in Box 100.4.[95] They can be found as solids, liquids, gases, vapors, and aerosols.[96] The state of an agent is chosen depending on its intended use and desired duration of exposure or persistence. Liquids and solids persist the longest, with variables that include temperature, wind conditions, agent–surface interactions, and the agent's volatility.

The efficacy of a chemical agent is determined by its degree of absorption and its toxicity. Chemicals penetrate epidermal surfaces due to their lipophilic nature and are often mixed with additional substances to enhance diffusion through protective clothing and other barriers.[96] Toxicity is determined by the dose or concentration (gas or vapor) and

Box 100.3 Biological agents of second-highest priority and ophthalmic manifestations

Brucellosis (*Brucella* spp.) – uveitis[71,72] with iridocyclitis (acute or chronic, granulomatous or nongranulomatous) and multifocal choroiditis (nodular or geographic[73]), nummular keratitis,[74] recurrent episcleritis,[75] optic neuritis,[76] dacryoadenitis,[77] endogenous endophthalmitis[78]

Epsilon toxin of *Clostridium perfringens* – corneal ulcer,[79] endogenous endophthalmitis[80]

Salmonella spp. – Reiter's syndrome,[81] peripheral ulcerative keratitis,[82] stellate maculopathy and chorioretinitis,[83] endogenous endophthalmitis[84]

Escherichia coli O157:H7 – keratitis,[85] endogenous endophthalmitis[86]

Shigella spp. – Reiter's syndrome, keratitis[87], orbital inflammation[88]

Glanders (*Burkholderia mallei*) – none

Melioidosis (*Burkholderia pseudomallei*) – anophthalmic socket infection,[89] keratitis with endophthalmitis[90]

Psittacosis (*Chlamydia psittaci*) – conjunctivitis, uveitis,[91] interstitial keratitis[92]

Q fever (*Coxiella burnetii*) – choroidal neovascularization,[93] optic neuritis[94]

Ricin toxin from *Ricinus communis* (castor beans) – none

Staphylococcal enterotoxin B – none

Trichothecene mycotoxins – none

Typhus fever (*Rickettsia prowazekii*) – none

Vibrio cholerae – none, keratitis in other *Vibrio* species

Viral encephalitis (alphaviruses, i.e. Venezuelan equine encephalitis, eastern equine encephalitis, western equine encephalitis) – none

List from Medline search for ophthalmic involvement, Centers for Disease Control and Prevention: Biological Diseases/Agents List. Available at http://www.bt.cdc.gov/agent/agentlist-category.asp, accessed 02/28/09.

length of exposure. Most chemical agents produce at least mild eye irritation, but nerve agents and vesicants have particular interest to ophthalmologists.

Nerve agents

Nerve agents are potent organophosphate compounds that inhibit acetylcholinesterase, leading to excessive acetylcholine neurotransmitter at its postsynaptic receptor sites. Both muscarinic and nicotinic receptors are affected, causing cholinergic crisis (Box 100.5).[96] Muscarinic effects involve the smooth muscles (bronchoconstriction, increased gastric motility, miosis), the glands (lacrimation, rhinorrhea, salivation, increased secretion – gastrointestinal and airway), and the heart (bradycardia). Nicotinic effects include fasciculations, twitching, fatigue, tachycardia, hypertension, and paralysis. Nerve agents cross the blood–brain barrier and can lead to confusion, altered consciousness, seizures, apnea, coma, and death. Small exposures are associated with transient effects such as poor concentration, and disturbances of vision, sleep, and emotions.

Ophthalmic manifestations

On March 20, 1995, the Aum Shinrikyo cult released sarin (isopropyl methylphosphonofluoridate) gas at several points in the Tokyo, Japan, subway system.[97] A similar incident occurred on June 27, 1994, in Matsumoto, Japan.[98] Pure sarin is colorless and odorless, and when vaporized is absorbed through the respiratory tract and conjunctiva. Within minutes of exposure victims noted a sensation of darkness related to miosis. Many had conjunctival injection, with pain and impaired accommodation related to ciliary spasm. In nearly one-third of patients, there was an approximate 3 mmHg lowering of intraocular pressure. Ocular signs and symptoms resolved within several days to several weeks after treatment with topical cycloplegics.

Treatment

Management includes basic life resuscitation, decontamination, drug therapy, and supportive care. Removal of clothing and jewelry, and forceful soap and water washing of the skin is recommended. Hypochlorite (0.5% solution) can be used instead of water as it inactivates nerve agents.[99] Despite decontamination, the effects may worsen with time because these agents can accumulate in fat and release slowly.[96] Atropine is a competitive inhibitor of acetylcholine at muscarinic receptors, and thus reverses the hypersecretory, bronchoconstrictive, bradycardic, and gastrointestinal effects of nerve agents.[100] Pralidoxime (Protopam, 2-PAM) can counteract nicotinic (primarily muscle weakness) effects by binding to the nerve agent and reactivating acetylcholinesterase.

Vesicants

Vesicants are oily liquids that become aerosolized when dispersed by an explosive blast from a bomb or when released under high ambient temperatures. Sulfur mustard is the most common vesicant used in chemical weapons. It is lipophilic and readily penetrates skin, most textiles, and rubber.[100] Skin penetration occurs in less than 2 minutes, but there is a delay of minutes to hours in the onset of a burning sensation. In contrast, lewisite causes almost immediate burning. Once absorbed, it alkylates and denatures DNA, RNA, and proteins, leading to cell death.

Clinical manifestations

Clinical effects usually appear within 4 to 8 hours after exposure to mustard. Dermal exposure produces superficial (erythema, pain) to partial-thickness (bullae) burns with uncommon full-thickness (deep bullae, ulcer) involvement.[100] Inhalation of mustard vapor can cause bronchospasm, mucosal sloughing, and hemorrhagic pulmonary edema in severe cases. Large exposure can lead to bone marrow suppression and gastrointestinal effects which may lead to secondary infection, sepsis, and death.

Ophthalmic manifestations

Ocular effects range from a mild conjunctivitis to corneal burns. The eye is very susceptible to damage due to the enhanced absorption by the aqueous–mucous surface and the tendency for concentration in the oily layer of the tear

Box 100.4 Chemical agents

Biotoxins

Poisons that come from plants or animals
- Abrin
- Brevetoxin
- Colchicine
- Digitalis
- Nicotine
- Ricin
- Saxitoxin
- Strychnine
- Tetrodotoxin
- Trichothecene

Blister agents/vesicants

Chemicals that severely blister the eyes, respiratory tract, and skin on contact
- Mustards
  - Distilled mustard (HD)
  - Mustard gas (H) (sulfur mustard)
  - Mustard/lewisite (HL)
  - Mustard/T
  - Nitrogen mustard (HN-1, HN-2, HN-3)
  - Sesqui mustard
  - Sulfur mustard (H) (mustard gas)
- Lewisites/chloroarsine agents
  - Lewisite (L, L-1, L-2, L-3)
  - Mustard/lewisite (HL)
- Phosgene oxime (CX)

Blood agents

Poisons that affect the body by being absorbed into the blood
- Arsine (SA)
- Carbon monoxide
- Cyanide
  - Cyanogen chloride (CK)
  - Hydrogen cyanide (AC)
  - Potassium cyanide (KCN)
  - Sodium cyanide (NaCN)
- Sodium monofluoroacetate (compound 1080)

Caustics (acids)

Chemicals that burn or corrode people's skin, eyes, and mucous membranes (lining of the nose, mouth, throat, and lungs) on contact
- Hydrofluoric acid (hydrogen fluoride)

Choking/lung/pulmonary agents

Chemicals that cause severe irritation or swelling of the respiratory tract (lining of the nose, throat, and lungs)
- Ammonia
- Bromine (CA)
- Chlorine (CL)
- Hydrogen chloride
- Methyl bromide
- Methyl isocyanate
- Osmium tetroxide
- Phosgene
  - Diphosgene (DP)
  - Phosgene (CG)
- Phosphine
- Phosphorus, elemental, white or yellow
- Sulfuryl fluoride

Incapacitating agents

Drugs that make people unable to think clearly or that cause an altered state of consciousness (possibly unconsciousness)
- BZ
- Fentanyls & other opioids

Long-acting anticoagulants

Poisons that prevent blood from clotting properly, which can lead to uncontrolled bleeding
- Super warfarin

Metals

Agents that consist of metallic poisons
- Arsenic
- Barium
- Mercury
- Thallium

Nerve agents

Highly poisonous chemicals that work by preventing the nervous system from working properly
- G agents
  - Sarin (GB)
  - Soman (GD)
  - Tabun (GA)
- V agents
  - VX

Organic solvents

Agents that damage the tissues of living things by dissolving fats and oils
- Benzene

Riot control agents/tear gas

Highly irritating agents normally used by law enforcement for crowd control or by individuals for protection (for example, mace)
- Bromobenzylcyanide (CA)
- Chloroacetophenone (CN)
- Chlorobenzylidenemalononitrile (CS)
- Chloropicrin (PS)
- Dibenzoxazepine (CR)

Toxic alcohols

Poisonous alcohols that can damage the heart, kidneys, and nervous system
- Ethylene glycol

Vomiting agents

Chemicals that cause nausea and vomiting
- Adamsite (DM)

From Centers for Disease Control and Prevention: Chemical Agents List and Information. Available at http://emergency.cdc.gov/agent/agentlistchem-category.asp, last updated 04/01/08.

Box 100.5 Nerve agent signs

Muscarinic
- Smooth muscle
- Bronchoconstriction
- Increased gastric motility
- Miosis
- Glands
- Lacrimation
- Rhinorrhea
- Salivation
- Increased gastrointestinal secretions
- Bronchorrhea
- Diaphoresis
- Other
  - Bradycardia
  - Heart block
  - Hypotension
  - Urinary incontinence

Nicotinic
- Muscle
- Fasciculations
- Twitching
- Fatigue
- Flaccid paralysis
- Other
  - Tachycardia
  - Hypertension

Central nervous system
- Headaches
- Vertigo
- Agitation
- Anxiety
- Slurred speech
- Delirium
- Coma
- Seizures
- Central respiratory depression

Adapted from American College of Physicians-American Society of Internal Medicine: Bioterrorism Summaries from Annual Session 2002. Available at http://www.acponline.org/bioterro/as_sum1.htm, last accessed 11/05/02.

film due to mustard's lipophilic quality.[101] The cornea is thus exposed for a prolonged period of time, leading to pain from loosening of the epithelial layer, which exposes the free unmyelinated nerve endings.

Symptoms begin with eye pain, photophobia, lacrimation, and blurred vision. A mild conjunctivitis is commonly seen within an hour of exposure and is one of the earliest clinical signs.[101] Mild injury causes blepharospasm, eyelid erythema, and lacrimation. Moderate injury leads to periorbital edema, corneal epithelial edema, and punctate corneal erosions. Vesication of the cornea can lead to complete sloughing of the epithelium. Microscopically, there is loss of conjunctival mucus with occlusion of blood vessels due to goblet and endothelial cell injury, respectively.[102] Recovery typically occurs without significant adverse sequelae; however, about 90% of mildly affected patients are visually disabled for approximately 10 days.[103]

Severe injury (about 10% of patients) can result in conjunctival chemosis and blanching due to destruction of conjunctival and limbal blood vessels. There is corneal stromal edema with diminished or absent sensation, which can lead to ulceration, secondary microbial keratitis, and perforation. Deeper penetration may result in anterior uveitis, the formation of posterior synechiae, a transient elevation of intraocular pressure, and lens opacification. Corneal pannus formation begins within a few weeks due to persistent inflammation and limbal stem cell deficiency. Corneal scarring and conjunctivalization lead to impaired vision in the months that follow the acute injury. Conjunctival scrape cytology in soldiers with chronic eye problems after exposure to mustard gas during the Iraq–Iran war has shown dysplasia in 41% (9 of 22) studied, but none with squamous cell carcinoma.[104] Chronic angle closure glaucoma and phthisis can lead to blindness.

An unusual delayed type of keratopathy develops in 0.5% of patients up to 40 years after severe exposure to mustard gas.[101] After an inactive period, the patient experiences a recurrent attack of stromal keratitis starting near the limbus and advancing centrally. There is a pathognomonic porcelain-white episcleral area adjacent to the peripheral corneal ulceration.[105] Areas of stromal calcification with overlying epithelial breakdown are characteristically located in the lower and central cornea.[106] Aneurysmatic dilatations and tortuosity of conjunctival and corneal vessels exists with intracorneal hemorrhage. Advanced cases lead to corneal opacification with crystal and cholesterol deposits. The pathogenesis is unknown, but may involve degenerative processes that accompany the deposition of cholesterol, as well as immunological reaction to corneal proteins that were structurally modified by the mustard.[101]

Treatment

Management of acute exposure should include removal of contaminated clothes and flushing of the skin with soap and water. Absorbent powders, such as calcium chloride and magnesium oxide, are also effective if available.[107] The eyes of both symptomatic and asymptomatic patients should be irrigated with tap water as soon as possible. Topical antibiotics and cycloplegics should be prescribed, but the use of topical steroids is controversial. Steroid use within 7 to 10 days can limit polymorphonuclear cell migration, inhibit collagenolysis and quell chemical anterior uveitis. The disadvantage is impaired epithelial wound healing with the possibility of subsequent corneal ulceration and perforation. Vitamin C (ascorbate), citrate, and N-acetylcysteine (Mucomyst) may be beneficial adjunctive therapies. Frequent lubrication, bandage contact lenses, and tarsorrhaphy aid in management. Ocular surface reconstruction with amniotic membrane and/or limbal stem cell transplantation along with penetrating keratoplasty may be required for full visual rehabilitation.

References

1. Christopher GW, Cieslak TJ, Pavlin JA, et al. Biological warfare: a historical perspective. *JAMA*. 1997;258(5):412–417.
2. Geissler E. *Biological and toxin weapons today*. New York: Oxford University Press; 1986.

3. Harris S. Japanese biological warfare research on humans: a case study of microbiology and ethics. *Ann NY Acad Sci.* 1992;666:21–52.
4. Sims NA. *The diplomacy of biological disarmament.* New York: Plenum Press; 1983.
5. Meselson M, Guillemin J, Hugh-Jones M, et al. The Sverdlovsk anthrax outbreak of 1979. *Science.* 1994;266:1202–1208.
6. Zilinskas RA. Iraq's biological weapons: the past as future. *JAMA.* 1997; 278(5):418–424.
7. WHO Group of Consultants. *Health aspects of chemical and biological weapons.* Geneva, Switzerland: World Health Organization; 1970:72–99.
8. McGovern TW, Christopher GW, Eitzen EM. Cutaneous manifestations of biological warfare and related threat agents. *Arch Dermatol.* 1999;135: 311–322.
9. American College of Physicians–American Society of Internal Medicine: ACP–ASIM Guide to Bioterrorism Identification, 2002.
10. Centers for Disease Control and Prevention. Biological Diseases/Agents List. Available at http://www.bt.cdc.gov/agent/agentlist-category.asp, accessed 02/28/09.
11. Centers for Disease Control and Prevention. Chemical Agents List and Information. Available at http://www.bt.cdc.gov/agent/agentlistchem.asp, accessed 02/28/09.
12. Klotz SA. Anthrax. In: Gorbach S, Bartlett J, Blacklow N, eds. *Infectious diseases.* Philadelphia, PA: WB Saunders; 1992:1291–1293.
13. Yorston D, Foster A. Cutaneous anthrax leading to corneal scarring from cicatricial ectropion. *Br J Ophthalmol.* 1989;73:809–811.
14. Broussard LA. Biological agents: weapons of warfare and bioterrorism. *Mol Diagn.* 2001;6(4):323–333.
15. Centers for Disease Control and Prevention. Anthrax, Lab and Health Professionals, Training Material. Available at http://www.bt.cdc.gov/Agent/anthrax/SlideSetAnthrax.pdf, 10/31/2001.
16. Inglesby TV, O'Toole T, Henderson DA, et al. Anthrax as a biological weapon, 2002: updated recommendations for management. *JAMA.* 2002;287(17):2236–2252.
17. Celebi S, Aykan U, Alagoz G, et al. Palpebral anthrax. *Eur J Ophthalmol.* 2001;11(2):171–174.
18. Soysal HG, Kiratli H, Recep OF. Anthrax as the cause of preseptal cellulitis and cicatricial ectropion. *Acta Ophthalmol Scand.* 2001;79(2): 208–209.
19. Aslan G, Terzioglu A. Surgical management of cutaneous anthrax. *Ann Plast Surg.* 1998;41(5):468–470.
20. Chovet M, Ducam M, Negrel AD, et al. [Late aspects of palpebral anthrax (author's transl.)]. *Med Trop.* 1979;39(1):91–96.
21. Noeller TP. Biological and chemical terrorism: recognition and management. *Cleve Clin J Med.* 2001;68(12):1001–1016.
22. Doganay M, Aygen B, Inan M, et al. Temporal artery inflammation as a complication of anthrax. *J Infect.* 1994;28(3):311–314.
23. Brachman P, Friedlander A. Inhalation anthrax. *Ann NY Acad Sci.* 1980;353:83–93.
24. Friedlander AM, Welkos SL, Pitt ML. Postexposure prophylaxis against experimental inhalation anthrax. *J Infect Dis.* 1993;167:1239–1242.
25. Franz DR, Jahrling PB, Friedlander AM, et al. Clinical recognition and management of patients exposed to biological warfare agents. *JAMA.* 1997;278(5):399–411.
26. Kerrison JB, Lounsbury D, Thirkill CE, et al. Optic neuritis after anthrax vaccination. *Ophthalmology.* 2002;109:99–104.
27. Payne DC, Rose CE Jr, Kerrison J, et al. Anthrax vaccination and risk of optic neuritis in the United States military, 1998–2003. *Arch Neurol.* 2006;63(6):871–875.
28. Syed NA, Glazer-Hockstein C, Kolasinski SL. *Bilateral anterior uveitis, posterior scleritis and optic neuropathy following anthrax vaccination.* Orlando, Florida: American Academy of Ophthalmology scientific poster; 2002.
29. Foster BS, Agahigian DD. Central serous chorioretinopathy associated with anthrax vaccination. *Retina.* 2004;24(4):624–625.
30. Caya JG. *Clostridium botulinum* and the ophthalmologist: a review of botulism, including biological warfare ramifications of botulinum toxin. *Surv Ophthalmol.* 2001;46:25–34.
31. Arnon SS, Schecter R, Inglesby TV, et al. Botulinum toxin as a biological weapon: medical and public health management. *JAMA.* 2001;285(8): 1059–1070.
32. Hughes JM, Blumenthal JR, Merson MH, et al. Clinical features of types A and B food-borne botulism. *Ann Intern Med.* 1981;95:442–445.
33. Ehrenreich H, Garner CG, Witt TN. Complete bilateral internal ophthalmoplegia as sole clinical sign of botulism: confirmation of diagnosis by single fibre electromyography. *J Neurol.* 1989;236:243–245.
34. Tacket CO, Shandera WX, Mann JM, et al. Equine antitoxin use and other factors that predict outcome in type A foodborne botulism. *Am J Med.* 1984;76:794–798.
35. World Health Organization. *The global elimination of smallpox: final report of the global commission for the certification of smallpox eradication.* Geneva, Switzerland: World Health Organization; 1980.
36. Fenner F, Henderson DA, Arita I, et al. *Smallpox and its eradication.* Geneva, Switzerland: World Health Organization; 1988; 1460.
37. Henderson DA, Inglesby TV, Bartlett JG, et al. Smallpox as a biological weapon: medical and public health management. *JAMA.* 1999;281(22): 2127–2137.
38. Noble J. Smallpox. In: Gorbach S, Bartlett J, Blacklow N, eds. *Infectious diseases.* Philadelphia, PA: WB Saunders; 1992:1112–1113.
39. World Health Organization. Available at http://www.who.int/emc/diseases/smallpox/slideset/pages/spox_015.htm, accessed 02/28/09.
40. American College of Physicians–American Society of Internal Medicine. Bioterrorism. Quick Facts about Smallpox. Available at http://www.acponline.org/bioterro/smallpox_facts.htm, last accessed 02/28/09.
41. Olurin O. Etiology of blindness in Nigerian children. *Am J Ophthalmol.* 1970;70(4):533–540.
42. Duke-Elder S. *Diseases of the outer eye, viral kerato-conjunctivitis.* London: Henry Kingston; 1965;359–360.
43. Saxena RC, Garg KC, Ramchand S. Ankyloblepharon following smallpox. *Am J Ophthalmol.* 1966;61:169–171.
44. Sutcliffe J, Duin N. *A history of medicine.* London: Morgan Samuel Editions; 1992:40.
45. Lane JM, Ruben FL, Neff JM, et al. Complications of smallpox vaccination, 1968: national surveillance in the United States. *N Engl J Med.* 1969;281:1201–1208.
46. Fillmore GL, Ward TP, Bower KS, et al. Ocular complications in the Department of Defense Smallpox Vaccination Program. *Ophthalmology.* 2004;111(11):2086–2093.
47. Jones BR, Al-Hussaini MK. Therapeutic considerations in ocular vaccinia. *Trans Ophthalmol Soc UK.* 1963;83:613–631.
48. Dahlstrand S, Ringertz O, Zetterberg B. Airborne tularemia in Sweden. *Scand J Infect Dis.* 1971;3(1):7–16.
49. Ellis PP, Winograd LA. Ocular vaccinia: a specific treatment. *Arch Ophthalmol.* 1962;68:600–609.
50. Rydberg M, Pandolfi M. Treatment of vaccinia keratitis with post-vaccinial gamma globulin. *Acta Ophthalmol.* 1963;41:713–718.
51. Jack MK, Sorenson RW. Vaccinial keratitis treated with IDU. *Arch Ophthalmol.* 1963;69:730–732.
52. Dennis DT, Inglesby TV, Henderson DA, et al. Tularemia as a biological weapon: medical and public health management. *JAMA.* 2001;285(21): 2763–2773.
53. Cross JT, Penn RL. *Francisella tularensis* (tularemia). In: Mandell GL, Bennett JE, Dolin R, eds. *Principles and practice of infectious diseases.* 5th ed. Philadelphia, PA: Churchill Livingstone; 2000:2393–2402.
54. Evans ME, Gregory DW, Schaffner W, et al. Tularemia: a 30-year experience with 88 cases. *Medicine.* 1985;64:251–269.
55. American College of Physicians – American Society of Internal Medicine. Bioterrorism, Quick Facts about Tularemia. Available at http://www.acponline.org/bioterro/tularemia.htm, last accessed 02/28/09.
56. Francis E. Oculoglandular tularemia. *Arch Ophthalmol.* 1942;28:711.
57. Steinemann TL, Sheikholeslami MR, Brown HH, et al. Oculoglandular tularemia. *Arch Ophthalmol.* 1999;117:132–133.
58. Chin GN. Parinaud's oculoglandular conjunctivitis. In: Tasman W, Jaeger EA, Schwab IR, eds. *Duane's clinical ophthalmology.* vol. 4. Philadelphia, PA: Lippincott-Raven; 1996.
59. Pärssinen O, Rummukainen M. Acute glaucoma and acute corneal oedema in association with tularemia. *Acta Ophthalmol Scand.* 1997;75: 732–734.
60. Marcus DM, Frederick AR Jr, Hodges T, et al. Typhoidal tularemia. *Arch Ophthalmol.* 1990;108:118–119.
61. Borio L, Inglesby T, Peters CJ, et al. Hemorrhagic fever virus as biological weapons: medical and public health management. *JAMA.* 2002;287(18): 2391–2405.
62. Kibadi K, Mupapa K, Kuvula K, et al. Late ophthalmologic manifestations in survivors of the 1995 Ebola virus epidemic in Kikwit, Democratic Republic of the Congo. *J Infect Dis.* 1999;179(Suppl 1):S13-S14.
63. Kuming BS, Kokoris N. Uveal involvement in Marburg virus disease. *Br J Ophthalmol.* 1977;61:265–266.
64. Kontkanen M, Puustjärvi T, Kauppi P. Ocular characteristics in nephropathia epidemica or puumula virus infection. *Acta Ophthalmol Scand.* 1996;74:621–625.
65. Kontkanen MI, Puustjärvi TJ, Lähdevirta JK. Intraocular pressure changes in nephropathia epidemica: a prospective study of 37 patients with acute systemic puumula virus infection. *Ophthalmology.* 1995; 102:1813–1817.
66. Saari KM. Acute glaucoma in hemorrhagic fever with renal syndrome (nephropathia epidemica). *Am J Ophthalmol.* 1976;81(4):455–461.

67. Saari KM, Luoto S. Ophthalmological findings in nephropathia epidemica in Lapland. *Acta Ophthalmol.* 1984;62:235–243.
68. Pärssinen O, Kuronen J. Tonic pupillary reaction after epidemic nephropathy and transient myopia. *Am J Ophthalmol.* 1989;108(2):201–202.
69. Lee EY, Choi SO, Choi GB, et al. Isolated abducens nerve palsy as a complication of haemorrhagic fever with renal syndrome. *Nephrol Dial Transplant.* 1998;13:2113–2114.
70. Yoser SL, Forster DJ, Rao NA. Systemic viral infections and their retinal and choroidal manifestations. *Surv Ophthalmol.* 1993;37(5):313–352.
71. Al-Kaff AS. Ocular brucellosis. *Int Ophthalmol Clin.* 1995;35(3):139–145.
72. Walker J, Sharma OP, Rao NA. Brucellosis and uveitis. *Am J Ophthalmol.* 1992;114(3):374–375.
73. Tabbara KF, Al-Kassimi H. Ocular brucellosis. *Br J Ophthalmol.* 1990; 74(4):249–250.
74. Woods AC. Nummular keratitis and ocular brucellosis. *Arch Ophthalmol.* 1946;35:490.
75. Güngör K, Bekir NA, Namiduru M. Recurrent episcleritis associated with brucellosis. *Acta Ophthalmol Scand.* 2001;79:76–78.
76. Puig Solanes M, Heatley J, Arenas F, et al. Ocular complications in brucellosis. *Am J Ophthalmol.* 1953;36:675–689.
77. Bekir NA, Güngör K. Bilateral dacryoadenitis associated with brucellosis. *Acta Ophthalmol Scand.* 1999;77(3):357–358.
78. al Faran MF. *Brucella melitensis* endogenous endophthalmitis. *Ophthalmologica.* 1990;201(1):19–22.
79. Stern GA, Hodes BL, Stock EL. *Costridium perfringens* corneal ulcer. *Arch Ophthalmol.* 1979;97(4):661–663.
80. Nangia V, Hutchinson C. Metastatic endophthalmitis caused by *Clostridium perfringens. Br J Ophthalmol.* 1992;76(4):252–253.
81. Saari KM, Vilppula A, Lassus A, et al. Ocular inflammation in Reiter's disease after *Salmonella* enteritis. *Am J Ophthalmol.* 1980;90(1):63–68.
82. Yang J, Baltatzis S, Foster CS. Peripheral ulcerative keratitis after *Salmonella* gastroenteritis. *Cornea.* 1998;17(6):672–674.
83. Fusco R, Magli A, Guacci P. Stellate maculopathy due to *Salmonella typhi.* A case report. *Ophthalmologica.* 1986;192(3):154–158.
84. Senft SH, Awad A, Batholomew L. *Salmonella* endophthalmitis in an infant with presumed retinopathy of prematurity. *Eye.* 1993;7(Pt 1): 190–191.
85. Leahey AB, Avery RL, Gottsch JD, et al. Suture abscesses after penetrating keratoplasty. *Cornea.* 1993;12(6):489–492.
86. Tseng CY, Liu PY, Shi ZY, et al. Endogenous endophthalmitis due to *Escherichia coli*: a case report and review. *Clin Infect Dis.* 1996;22(6): 1107–1108.
87. Kelinske M, Poirer R. Corneal ulceration due to *Shigella flexneri. J Pediatr Ophthalmol Strabismus.* 1980;17(1):48–51.
88. Ronen S, Rozenmann Y, Zylbermann R, et al. Orbital inflammation: an unusual extraintestinal complication of shigellosis. Report of a case. *Ophthalmologica.* 1980;180(1):46–50.
89. Nussbaum JJ, Hull DS, Carter MJ. *Pseudomonas pseudomallei* in an anophthalmic orbit. *Arch Ophthalmol.* 1980;98(7):1224–1225.
90. Srimuang S, Roongruangchai K, Lawtiantong T, et al. Immunobiological diagnosis of tropical ocular diseases: *Toxocara, Pythium insidiosum, Pseudomonas (Burkholderia) pseudomallei, Mycobacterium chelonei* and *Toxoplasma gondii. Int J Tissue React.* 1996;18(1):23–25.
91. Adachi K, Hosokawa T, Watanabe Y, et al. [A case of psittacosis meningitis with uveitis]. *Rinsho Shinkeigaku.* 1989;29(1):122–124.
92. Darougar S, John AC, Viswalingam M, et al. Isolation of *Chlamydia psittaci* from a patient with interstitial keratitis and uveitis associated with otological and cardiovascular lesions. *Br J Ophthalmol.* 1978;62(10): 709–714.
93. Ruiz-Moreno JM. Choroidal neovascularization in the course of Q fever. *Retina.* 1997;17(6):553–555.
94. Schuil J, Richardus JH, Baarsma GS, et al. Q fever as a possible cause of bilateral optic neuritis. *Br J Ophthalmol.* 1985;69(8):580–583.
95. Centers for Disease Control and Prevention. Chemical Agents List and Information. Available at http://emergency.cdc.gov/agent/agentlistchem-category.asp, last updated 04/01/08.
96. American College of Physicians–American Society of Internal Medicine. Bioterrorism Summaries from Annual Session 2002. Available at http://www.acponline.org/bioterro/as_sum1.htm, accessed 11/05/02.
97. Kato T, Hamanaka T. Ocular signs and symptoms caused by exposure to sarin gas. *Am J Ophthalmol.* 1996;121(2):209–210.
98. Nohara M, Segawa K. Ocular symptoms due to organophosphorus gas (sarin) poisoning in Matsumoto. *Br J Ophthalmol.* 1996;80:1023.
99. Macintyre AG, Christopher GW, Eitzen E. Weapons of mass destruction events with contaminated casualties: effective planning for health care facilities. *JAMA.* 2000;283(2):242–249.
100. Prevention and treatment of injury from chemical warfare agents. *The Medical Letter.* January 7, 2002;44(1121):1–4.
101. Solberg Y, Alcalay M, Belkin M. Ocular injury by mustard gas. *Surv Ophthalmol.* 1997;41(6):461–466.
102. Maumenee AE, Scholtz RO. The histopathology of ocular lesions produced by sulfur and nitrogen mustards. *Bull Johns Hopkins Hosp.* 1948;82:121–147.
103. Safarinejad MR, Moosavi SA, Montazeri B. Ocular injuries caused by mustard gas: diagnosis, treatment, and medical defense. *Mil Med.* 2001;166(1):67–70.
104. Safaei A, Saluti R, Kumar PV. Conjunctival dysplasia in soldiers exposed to mustard gas during the Iraq–Iran war: scrape cytology. *Acta Cytol.* 2001;45(6):909–913.
105. Pleyer U, Sherif Z, Baatz H, et al. Delayed mustard gas keratopathy: clinical findings and confocal microscopy. *Am J Ophthalmol.* 1999;128:506–507.
106. Blodi FC. Mustard gas keratopathy. *Int Ophthalmol Clin.* 1971;2(3): 1–13.
107. Aasted A, Darre E, Wulf HC. Mustard gas: clinical, toxicological and mutagenic aspects based on modern experience. *Ann Plast Surg.* 1987; 19:330–333.

Chapter 101

Contact Lens Applications in Corneal Disease

Danielle Robertson, H. Dwight Cavanagh

Since the early 1900s contact lenses have evolved from non-oxygen-permeable rigid lenses made of glass or polymethylmethacrylate to the comfort of modern lenses composed of soft silicone hydrogel materials. With the introduction of the first commercially available soft lens by Otto Wichterle in 1971,[1] low-cost contact lenses became widely available for patients who were unable to tolerate wear of the hard, oxygen-impermeable materials. As the popularity of these lenses grew, so did the apparent need for improvement in physiological performance. The continued advances in designs over several decades led to the development of newer lenses that are physiologically superior to their original soft lens counterparts, in that their constituent polymers allow more oxygen to reach the surface of the eye, thereby reducing the incidence of lens-related complications. While these new hyper-oxygen-transmissible lenses have been widely accepted into routine clinical practice for the correction of refractive error, they also offer significant advantages in the visual rehabilitation of patients with abnormal corneas who demonstrate an increased demand for oxygen, and for therapeutic use in wound healing and ocular surface disease.

In the nonpathological cornea, contact lenses are routinely used as the primary mode of vision correction by approximately 125 million wearers worldwide.[2] Many patients opt for contact lenses in lieu of spectacles primarily for cosmetic reasons, including the use of tinted lenses for a change of eye color. In addition to cosmesis, contact lenses can be used to eliminate the magnification or minification effect seen in patients with high myopic or hyperopic refractive errors due to the increased vertex distance of the lens in the spectacle plane; they have a well-centered optical zone that moves in the direction of gaze, thereby improving peripheral vision by eliminating prismatic effects and distortion, and they enhance binocularity in patients with significant degrees of anisometropia by eliminating the large differences in retinal image size produced by spectacles. For patients with uncorrected regular and irregular astigmatism, both soft and rigid lenses can also provide visual benefit, with rigid lenses often providing superior visual acuity through the formation of an aqueous 'lens' in the postlens tear film which optically neutralizes any residual refractive error. Regardless of the underlying reason for lens wear, there is an increasing range of choices available to meet each individual patient's specific needs.

Contact Lens Materials and Complications

The applications of contact lenses for diseased and altered corneas requires careful consideration of appropriate lens materials to meet individual needs, whether it be a hard, RGP lens without flexure to provide optimal visual acuity in an advanced cone, or high oxygen transmissibility in a soft lens to enhance corneal physiology during wound healing, particularly during long periods of extended wear. To meet the increased demand for newer lens designs aimed at optimizing wear for these patients, along with the ongoing quest for safer lens wear and increased ocular surface biocompatibility, contact lens materials have evolved continuously over the past several decades. Traditional hard, inflexible contact lenses, commonly prescribed until the early 1980s, were made of polymethylmethacrylate (PMMA), an oxygen-impermeable rigid material. In addition to the lack of comfort these lenses produced, complications driven by the diminished supply of oxygen to the central cornea included corneal warpage, vascularization, central corneal clouding or edema, and endothelial cell polymegathism. To increase comfort and oxygen supply to the cornea, soft hydrogel lenses were introduced. These conventional soft, flexible lenses are composed of a HEMA (2-hydroxyethylmethacrylate) core polymer, a hydrophilic monomer which functions to absorb water. Alone, HEMA-based lenses contain 38% water and are considered low-water lenses. The addition of co-monomers such as *N*-vinyl-pyrrolidone (NVP) and methacrylic acid (MAA) increases the overall water content of the lens material from 38% to as high as 70%.

Water content is especially important in understanding oxygen transmissibility in conventional soft lenses. The increased proportion of absorbed water in a specific lens material will result in a corresponding exponential increase in oxygen permeability, defined as Dk, where D is the diffusion coefficient of the material and k is the solubility constant. The oxygen transmissibility of a specific lens is a measure of oxygen permeability as a function of lens thickness, Dk/t.[3] As a general rule, lenses with a higher percentage of water transmit higher levels of oxygen to the cornea; however, as seen above, lens thickness must also be taken into account. An increased amount of water within the lens does not come without inherent disadvantages, as high-water lenses tend to be more fragile and require thicker

Table 101.1 FDA classification of hydrogel lenses

Group	Water	Ionicity
1	Low (<50%)	Nonionic
2	High (>50%)	Nonionic
3	Low (<50%)	Ionic
4	High (>50%)	Ionic

designs, which in turn reduces oxygen transmission; they have higher evaporation rates, leading to lens dehydration on the eye; and they attract a higher amount of adherent lipoprotein surface deposits. In theory, although high-water lenses should provide better comfort and be ideally suited for patients experiencing difficulty with lens wear, such as those suffering from dry eye, thinner, low-water designs with the same Dk/t are paradoxically often better tolerated for longer-wearing regimens.

Lens hydration or water content is also one of two factors used by the US Food and Drug Administration to classify hydrogel lens materials into four different groups to enable prediction of their performance with different contact lens care solutions.[4] The second factor in the classification guidelines is the electrostatic charge or ionic property of the lens material. Ionic lenses are composed of materials that carry a negative electrical charge, which can react with positively charged tear film components and solutions. These lenses tend to have a higher rate of surface deposits. Nonionic lenses are considered electrically neutral and possess an intrinsic resistance to surface deposits. A familiarity with lenses belonging to each class is important when fitting patients experiencing issues with lens dryness and/or surface deposits. The FDA lens material classification guidelines are shown in Table 101.1.

In the early 1980s, traditional hard lens materials were revamped and newer rigid gas-permeable (RGP) designs emerged. These lenses offered significant oxygen benefit to the cornea and had improved comfort over PMMA lenses. The advantages of these RGP lenses over soft HEMA lenses included an enhancement in visual acuity, due to the innate ability of the RGP to mask both regular and irregular astigmatism, a decrease in the frequency of ocular sequelae from chemically preserved contact lens care solutions, as RGP lenses do not bind solution components as soft lenses do, and increased durability. Further, due to corneal complications such as neovascularization, which is seen with low oxygen-transmissible soft lens wear, particularly following extended wear, high-oxygen RGP lenses that do not cover the entire corneal surface provided a more physiological alternative for patients wishing to continue lens wear.

Currently, despite the improved safety profile seen with RGP lenses, a majority of the contact lens market is still dominated by soft lenses.[5] Specifically, recent studies have shown that soft lens wear carries an increased risk of infection compared to RGP lenses, regardless of the modality of

Table 101.2 Currently available silicone hydrogel soft lenses

Manufacturer	Trade name	Lens material	Dk/t*
Bausch & Lomb	Purevision	Balafilcon A	110
Ciba Vision	O2 Optix	Lotrafilcon B	138
Ciba Vision	O2 Optix Custom	Sifilcon A	117
Ciba Vision	Air Optix Aqua	Lotrafilcon B	138
Ciba Vision**	Air Optix Night and Day Aqua	Lotrafilcon A	175
Cooper Vision	Biofinity	Comfilcon A	160
CooperVision	Avaira	Enfilcon A	125
Menicon	PremiO	Asmofilcon A	161
Vistakon	Acuvue Advance	Galyfilcon A	86
Vistakon	Acuvue Oasys	Senofilcon A	147

* *Dk/t: 10^{-9} (cm × mL O_2) (sec × mL × mm Hg).*
** *Air Optix Night and Day Aqua has replaced Focus Night and Day. Focus Night and Day is no longer available.*

wear.[6] Benchmark studies on the incidence of microbial infection associated with soft lens wear have reported rates of 4.1 cases per 10 000 persons per year for daily wear (DW), and 20.9 per 10 000 persons per year for extended wear (EW).[7,8] The primary causative agent in contact lens-related microbial infections of the cornea over three decades remains the pathogenic Gram-negative bacterium *Pseudomonas aeruginosa*.[9–11] In an effort to reduce the incidence of lens-related infections, a flurry of studies over the past two decades have focused on the pathophysiological response of the ocular surface to contact lens wear and have sought to increase lens–cornea biocompatibility. As a result of these studies, oxygen was established as a key mediator of lens-induced complications and a new generation of hypertransmissible lens materials was born.[12]

Silicone hydrogel lenses, which are comprised of a mix of hydrophobic silicone and hydrophilic hydrogel monomers, offer the advantage of hyper-oxygen transmissibility. Owing to the silicone component, these lenses require surface modifications to enhance wettability. First-generation lenses used plasma surface treatments and coatings, whereas newer designs incorporate wetting agents into the polymer matrix. Unlike conventional hydrogel lenses, silicone hydrogel lenses are low water, despite their increased oxygen transmission, classifying them as group I or group III lenses. Table 101.2 lists all currently available silicone hydrogel lenses. The increased oxygen supply to the corneal surface has reduced the number of hypoxia-related complications, including bulbar and limbal redness, neovascularization, corneal edema, epithelial microcysts, stromal striae, folds and thinning, and endothelial cell changes in density, shape and size.[13] Although these effects emphasize the importance of increased oxygen supply to the cornea, it is important to note that silicone hydrogel lenses have not reduced the overall incidence of contact lens-related inflammatory events or microbial infection.[14] Silicone materials have also been used in the manufacturing of RGP lenses. At present, there are several RGP lens materials available with exceedingly high Dk values, among the highest of which are the Boston XO_2 lens with a Dk of 141 (Bausch & Lomb, Rochester, NY), the Fluoroperm 151 lens with a Dk of 151 (Paragon Vision Sciences, Mesa, AZ), and the Menicon Z lens, which has a Dk of 175 (Menicon, Nagoya, Japan), and is the only hyper-Dk RGP approved for overnight wear by the FDA. When fitted in an alignment lens–cornea relationship, the Z material has been shown to have the lowest risk of infection compared to silicone hydrogel soft lenses, even when worn on a 30-day extended-wear basis.[6]

Contact Lenses in Corneal Disease and Surface Abnormalities

In patients with corneal disease and surface irregularities, management of contact lens wear can be challenging. In these patients the cornea often has increased oxygen demands as well as abnormal topographies that prohibit the use of standard lens designs. Common indications for contact lenses includes their therapeutic use as a bandage to support and protect the cornea, manage pain, and aid in epithelial healing following abrasions or recurrent corneal erosions; and in situations where there is a dramatic alteration in corneal shape, as seen following refractive surgery, corneal grafting, and keratectasia. Bandage lenses, which are primarily worn on an extended-wear basis in patients with pre-existing epithelial defects, require the patient to be monitored for a host of complications arising from overnight wear, including hypoxia and risk of microbial infection. In postoperative corneas and cases of keratectasia, the severe abnormal shape changes can lead to substantial increases in irregular astigmatism and anisometropia, rendering spectacle correction inadequate. Moreover, the altered corneal topography can make the ideal lens–cornea relationship obsolete, requiring skill and expertise from the contact lens practitioner to minimize complications such as epithelial damage, scarring and graft rejection.

Therapeutic Uses for Contact Lenses

Contact lenses are commonly used as bandages to provide relief for a wide range of ocular surface disorders, including trauma. Bandage lenses function to protect the epithelium during blinking, encourage epithelial regeneration, maintain corneal hydration, aid in pain control, preserve fornices by inhibiting symblepharon formation, and enhance drug delivery.[15,16] Unlike most forms of contact lens wear, an improvement in visual acuity is not the primary aim. Indications for the use of bandage lenses include trauma such as corneal abrasions and chemical burns, persistent or recurrent epithelial abnormalities, lid irregularities, bullous keratopathy, severe ocular surface disease such as keratoconjunctivitis sicca, ocular cicatricial pemphigoid, Stevens–Johnson syndrome, and postoperatively.[17] A detailed summary of therapeutic indications for contact lens wear is given in Table 101.3.

Table 101.3 Indications for therapeutic bandage lens wear

Bullous keratopathy
Lid abnormalities
Ocular surface disease
Keratoconjunctivitis sicca
Ocular cicatricial pemphigoid
Stephens–Johnson syndrome
Neurotrophic keratitis
Persistent/recurrent epithelial abnormalities
Filamentary keratitis
Persistent epithelial defects
Recurrent corneal erosions
Postinfectious ulcers (herpes, bacteria, fungi)
Trichiasis
Postoperative
PRK/LASEK
Delayed epithelial healing
Poor wound apposition after PKP
Trauma
Chemical burn
Corneal abrasion
Corneal perforation

The most common lenses used for therapeutic measures are conventional hydrogel and silicone hydrogel, limbal, and more recently, scleral RGPs, and collagen shields. Hydrogel and silicone hydrogel lenses are the mainstay for bandage use. With the increasing popularity of silicone hydrogels and the benefits of improved corneal physiology, however, silicone hydrogel lenses have become the preferred form. Recent studies evaluating the use of silicone hydrogels for pain relief and epithelial wound closure have confirmed these benefits.[18–20] In a retrospective study examining the efficacy of silicone hydrogel lenses worn in a therapeutic modality, 91.6% of patients achieved pain relief and 83.78% demonstrated complete corneal recovery without complications.[21] With any soft lens, the initial fit is dependent on the indication for use. In the presence of an epithelial defect, a tighter lens is typically more effective by reducing lens movement over the indicated region. After re-epithelialization is complete, a flatter-fitting lens with improved movement may be beneficial. If the cornea is perforated, a bandage lens combined with cyanoacrylate tissue adhesive glue may be indicated.

When sufficient corneal protection from a rigid lens is required, intralimbal or large-diameter RGP lenses are an excellent alternative. These lenses have an overall diameter of 10.0–11.5 mm, extending across the entire corneal surface just inside the limbus. Fitting strategies are aimed at optimizing the lens–cornea relationship to optimize movement and enhance tear flow. One primary therapeutic indication for large-diameter RGP lenses is dry eye arising from underlying etiologies such as rheumatoid arthritis or ocular cicatricial pemphigoid.[16] RGP lenses offer the added benefit of improved visual acuity and ease of handling, which is often advantageous over larger, scleral designs. Proprietary intralimbal designs such as the Dyna-Intralimbal lens (Lens Dynamics,

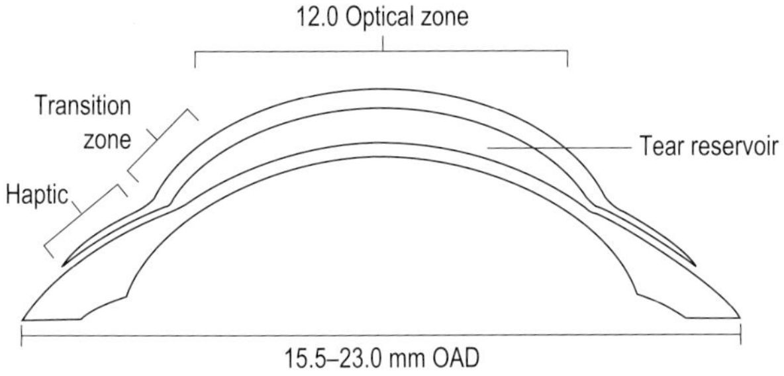

Fig. 101.1 Schematic of the Boston scleral lens. The peripheral haptic rests on the sclera, allowing the lens to vault over the abnormal or diseased cornea, creating a tear reservoir which can bathe the damaged epithelium to facilitate healing or to create a new refractive surface for optimal visual acuity.

Golden, CO) are available. These lenses are available with a plasma-treated surface coating to enhance wettability and comfort and reduce deposits. Most lenses, however, are custom and can be manufactured in high-Dk material to reap the benefits of increased oxygen.

The use of scleral lenses to treat advanced ocular surface disease was previously limited by the low oxygen transmissibility of the available lens materials and difficulty in manufacturing on a large scale. The recent reintroduction of these lenses using newer hyper-oxygen-transmitting materials and lathe-cut designs based upon optical spline functions has had encouraging reports.[22,23] The advantage of using scleral lenses in severe ocular surface disease derives from the fact that the lenses rest on the sclera and vault over the cornea and limbus, forming an aqueous reservoir that continuously bathes the damaged epithelium (Fig. 101.1). This aqueous buffer protects the eye from the mechanical friction of the eyelid during blinking, and maintains the eye in a well-hydrated environment. One example of a currently available scleral lens is the Boston lens, made of a fluorosilicone/acrylate polymer, which has a Dk value of 127.[24] Compared to a standard RGP lens, the overall diameter of the lens is significantly larger, with a total diameter ranging from 15.0 to 24.0 mm. Outside the large 12.0–14.0 mm optical zone there is a 2.0 mm transition zone. The center thickness for these lenses varies, ranging from 0.25 to 0.39 mm. Lenses are fitted using a diagnostic set. Care should be made when fitting to ensure there is no blanching of underlying scleral blood vessels. Lens suction is reduced by the incorporation of fluid-ventilated channels to allow for adequate tear exchange.[23] Success with this device has been reported in end-stage ocular cicatricial pemphigoid, Stevens–Johnson syndrome, graft-versus-host disease, and end-stage dry eye.[25–27]

Collagen shields are composed of a collagen protein matrix, either porcine or bovine in nature, which will dissolve when placed on the eye.[28] Typical dissolution times for most range from 12 to 72 hours. Shaped like a contact lens, collagen shields have an overall diameter similar in size to a soft lens (14.5–16.0 mm) and a 9 mm base curve. The initial center thickness of the shield ranges from 0.15 to 0.19 mm with a Dk/t of 27.[28] With dissolution of the lens, Dk/t rapidly increases as the center thickness is reduced. Compared to a conventional soft lens, 24 hours of lens wear with the collagen shield resulted in a 3% increase in corneal thickness, compared to a 4% increase as seen with a 70% water soft lens.[29] Collagen shields have been used clinically to promote epithelial wound healing and in drug delivery systems, as will be described below.[28] Collagen shields have also been reported to be used as a carrier for transplantation of amniotic epithelial cells to the corneal surface for the treatment of persistent epithelial defects.[30] These lenses are fitted solely for therapeutic applications and do not correct or improve visual acuity. As with any lens type, patients with active infections or ocular surface disease must be closely monitored during treatment.

Contact Lenses for Drug Delivery

Because of the reduced costs and its efficacy of use, topical therapy remains the mainstay in the management of ocular disease and postoperative procedures. Drawbacks to traditional eye drops, however, include the minimal amount of drug that ultimately arrives at the target tissue, and systemic uptake. Disposable contact lenses and collagen shields have been suggested as a potential vehicle for ophthalmic drug delivery to increase contact time, reduce systemic absorption, and increase bioavailability. Studies evaluating specific drug–lens combinations have investigated pilocarpine and beta-blockers for glaucoma,[31,32] fluoroquinolones for microbial keratitis,[33,34] ciclosporin for dry eye,[35] and various antiallergy and antiinflammatory agents.[36] These studies have shown that lenses soaked in these respective compounds can deliver an increased amount of drug to the ocular surface. Intrinsic problems associated with lens soaking include cost, the limited uptake of the drug into the lens polymer, and the inability of the lens to maintain a sustained-release effect. More recent lens designs are evaluating the use of surfactants and matrices that will produce a time-release effect and increase the duration the lens can be used.[35,37,38] Although these innovative designs have yet to be tested extensively in vivo, as lens materials continue to improve, the future is promising provided costs for the devices can be made comparable to the use of simple topical drops alone.

Irregular Cornea and Ectasia

Noninflammatory corneal ectasias consist of a group of diseases including keratoconus, pellucid marginal degeneration (PMD), Terrien's marginal degeneration, and keratoglobus. Of these, the most common indication for contact lenses in the visual rehabilitation of a patient with ectasia is keratoconus. Keratoconus is a progressive disease characterized by thinning of the central or inferior cornea, producing defined areas of corneal steepening. The disease typically presents during the second decade of life and is bilateral, but often asymmetric. This asymmetry creates variable amounts of spherical and astigmatic anisometropia, which can be extreme when associated with advanced disease. Pellucid marginal degeneration is a second cause of irregular cornea that can mimic keratoconus. It is a relatively uncommon disease characterized by a flattened cornea centrally and severe inferior ectasia running from 4 o'clock to 8 o'clock. Unlike keratoconus, PMD has a characteristic topographical pattern seen as 'kissing pigeons.' The disease is bilateral, occurring in patients aged 20–40, in both males and females. The severe ectasia seen in PMD creates significant against-the-rule astigmatism and is often harder to fit than keratoconus, owing to problems with lens dislocation secondary to excessive edge lift.[39]

It falls to the skilled lens practitioner to determine the appropriate optical correction to optimize visual acuity and patient comfort until a decline in best-corrected visual acuity, coupled with extensive corneal scarring, necessitates surgical intervention. Whereas RGP lenses represent the gold standard for many of these patients, in the early stages of the disease spectacles or soft contact lenses may provide adequate refractive correction. For early cones, soft lenses are also advantageous as patients often experience a marked increase in corneal hypersensitivity. This is thought to be due to the stretching of nerve fibers within the steepened region of the cornea, and may render some patients intolerant to RGP lens wear.

Unlike RGP lenses, hydrogel contact lenses offer the patient the advantage of comfort, but because of the low modulus of elasticity of the lens material, they tend to drape over the cornea. This draping phenomenon is responsible for the inability of the soft lens to mask corneal surface abnormalities and subsequent correction of any irregular astigmatism induced from the ectatic regions. Silicone hydrogel lenses offer the advantage of a higher modulus of elasticity, which eliminates some of the drape seen with traditional hydrogel lenses and can conceal mild surface abnormalities. Custom soft lenses for keratoconus are also readily available. Examples of these include the Eni-Eye Soft lens (Acculens, Denver, CO), the Flexlens Harrison Keratoconus and Tricurve Keratoconus designs (X-cell Contacts, Duluth, GA), and the Super Nova Hydrokone (Innovations in Sight, Front Royal, VA). These lenses are thicker centrally than conventional soft lenses, eliminating drape and resulting in the formation of a true aqueous tear lake beneath the lens which enhances the ability to correct for irregular astigmatism. Lenses are available in both spherical tricurve and aspheric designs, with a large range of parameters.

In more advanced cones the cornea tends to develop a hyposensitivity, also known as Axenfeld's sign, which often facilitates RGP lens wear. Further, as the cone progresses, the substantial increase in irregular astigmatism limits the effectiveness of soft lenses to provide acceptable levels of vision correction. Owing to the ability of RGP lenses to mask corneal topographical irregularities, essentially providing a new refractive surface, RGP lenses, either alone or in a combination system, are typically indicated for patients with intermediate to advanced disease. When fitting RGP lenses, it is important to remember that there is no standard fitting algorithm for every cone. Therefore, it is imperative to have a variety of lens designs within the fitting arsenal to address individual cases.

The first step in fitting any irregular cornea is to obtain an accurate assessment of corneal shape and curvature. Whereas keratometry readings are heavily utilized when fitting standard alignment fit RGP lenses, when obtaining keratometry measurements on a keratoconic patient, mires may appear distorted or irregular. Depending on the overall shape of the cornea, keratometry measurements that describe the central corneal curvature may not be suitable for use in contact lens fitting. Corneal topography, which gives a complete description of the total surface of the cornea, is ideal in identifying the type of cone and proper lens selection. If topography is not available, then photodiagnosis of the cone based on the fundus reflex is suggested.

Whereas early cones may only show small regions or islands of corneal steepening, more advanced ones can be classified into one of three shapes: nipple, oval, or globus. For all cones, the more advanced the disease, the more one sees larger cones with greater degrees of apex decentration. Nipple cones are small cones characterized by the presence of a 5 mm steepened region surrounded by normal peripheral cornea. The apex of a nipple cone is typically located centrally or decentered inferonasally. Oval cones, which are the most common, are larger than nipple cones. They are characterized by an inferior area of steepening with a displaced apex inferotemporally. In early stages of the disease the remainder of the cornea in the superior meridian is relatively normal. As the oval cone progresses, it proceeds in a radial fashion, with ectasia spreading into the temporal cornea, and in later stages it encompasses the superior cornea as well. Often a small island of normal cornea will persist in the superior nasal quadrant. Unlike nipple cones, oval cones show greater destruction of the underlying corneal layers. In contrast, globus cones are the largest and generally involve at least 75% of the corneal surface. Corneas with globus cones are usually positive for Munson's sign.

Lenses for keratoconus are fitted through careful diagnostic lens selection and fluorescein pattern assessment. Keep in mind that multiple lenses are typically required to achieve the desired lens–cornea relationship. It is also important when fitting keratoconic patients to administer an anesthetic prior to the diagnostic assessment to eliminate excess tearing, which could disturb normal lens centration and complicate the fluorescein pattern assessment. The most common lens–cornea relationship used in keratoconus is the three-point touch. This is defined by a central 'feathery' touch with bearing in the mid-periphery, and is used to distribute the weight of the lens evenly across the corneal surface. In general, too much bearing at any one point can lead to epithelial compromise, as seen in a flat- or steep-fitting lens. Flat-fitting lenses, which may provide the best visual acuity, have excess apical bearing which can damage the epithelium and lead to corneal scarring as well as lens intolerance, whereas a smaller steep-fitting lens will show excess pooling centrally with air bubbles underneath, leading to epithelial damage and edema along with a reduction in vision.

Because patients with keratoconus are dependent solely on their contact lenses, necessitating extensive wearing schedules, the selection of lens materials should be directed at polymers with relatively high oxygen transmissibility. Increased oxygen to the epithelial surface will result in improved physiology as well as a reduced risk of corneal hypoxia and erosions. Additional complications with RGP lenses in keratoconus arise from poor lens–cornea relationships, and can range from mild to more serious. For flat-fitting lenses, epithelial erosions are common over the central area of the cone. When treating erosions, refitting the lens so that it vaults the area of the defect is usually necessary. Scarring induced by flat-fitting lenses can significantly reduce visual acuity in addition to making the patient contact lens intolerant. For patients with nipple cones, RGP lenses may erode the nodule over time, necessitating a soft lens or a combination hybrid or 'piggyback' system. Assessment of lenses after fitting and after longer periods of wear with fluorescein staining is essential for both RGPs and soft lenses to rule out lens tightening on the eye.

For early to moderate cones, multicurve RGP lenses with flat peripheral curves provide the best fitting relationship.[40] The primary advantage of these lenses is that individual parameters can be easily modified as needed. The overall diameter of these lenses will vary depending on their centration and movement. With a central cone, a smaller overall diameter will facilitate a well-centered lens; in contrast, a peripheral cone requires a larger-diameter lens with a larger optical zone. As lenses will decenter toward the apex of the cone, it becomes more difficult to align the optic zone over the pupil area. Aspheric RGP lens designs are also useful in managing early to moderate cones due to improved cornea–lens alignment; however, power changes throughout the lens resulting from the aspheric design can reduce visual acuity if the lens is not adequately centered.

For more advanced cones, specialized RGP designs are available. Of these, the newly popular Rose K lens (Menicon USA, Clovis, CA) is most the common and has shown the greatest success for centrally placed cones.[41] The Rose K lens is designed with steeper than normal base curves designed to fit the central cone while aligning the lens in the otherwise normal periphery (Fig. 101.2). The lens is available in overall

(A)

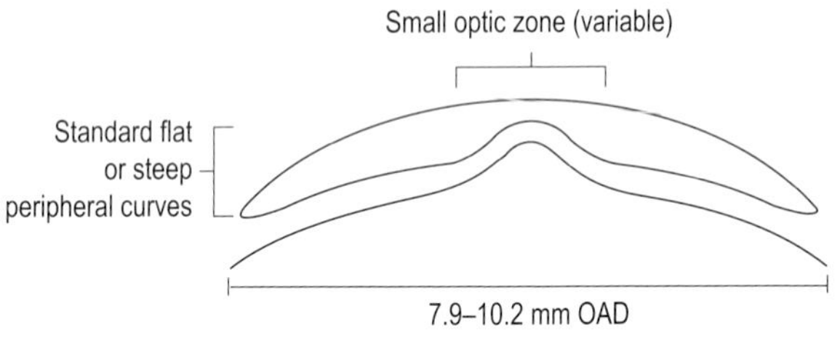

(B)

	Rose K	Soper	McGuire
OAD (mm)	7.9–10.2	7.5–9.5	8.6–9.6
OZ (mm)	OZD decreases with steeper BC	6.0–8.0	Dependent on cone type
BC (mm)	4.75–8.00	Steepens as OAD increases	5.60–7.35
PC design	Std/flat/steep	Bicurve	4 PC

Fig. 101.2 Specialized RGP lens designs for keratoconus. (**A**) The Rose K lens, with its small optical zone (OZ) and peripheral curve (PC) design, fits directly over the cone while minimizing peripheral tear pooling. (**B**) Comparison of the most commonly used RGP proprietary lens designs for keratoconus. OAD, overall diameter; OZD, optical zone diameter; BC, base curve.

diameters of 7.9–10.2 mm, with base curves ranging from 4.75 to 8 mm and flat, steep, or standard peripheral curves for attaining the recommended edge lift of 0.8 mm. A new version of the Rose K lens, the Rose K2, is now available, incorporating an aspheric design into the posterior optical zone. Other proprietary lens designs commonly used in keratoconus include the Soper Cone and the McGuire lens. The Soper Cone is a bicurve lens that is available in three different fitting sets depending on the stage of the disease. For mild cones, smaller lenses with smaller optical zones are sufficient. For more advanced cones, larger-diameter lenses with larger optical zones are required to enhance centration. Lens fit is adjusted by varying the diameter, thereby steepening the fit, with base curve and peripheral curves held constant. This allows for vaulting over the corneal surface and eliminates any harsh bearing over the cone apex. The McGuire lens, whose design was based upon a modification of the Soper Cone, employs four peripheral curves to maximize an alignment three-point touch fit. Three fitting sets are available depending on the shape of the cone, with the larger lenses for more advanced oval and globus cones.

Some clinicians report success when using ultralarge diameter and intralimbal designs in fitting cones.[42] Intralimbal lenses offer several of the advantages of a scleral lens, such as a large overall diameter, ranging from 10.4 to 12.0 mm, and a correspondingly larger optical zone (9.4 mm) that allows for good centration of the pupil in line with the optics of the lens, but is smaller and therefore fits within the limbal margin, which can be easier to handle and ideal for patients intimidated by scleral lenses. Good candidates for these lenses have ectasia at either 4 or 8 o'clock or in the far periphery, as seen with inferior cones or in PMD and patients with globus cones. Intralimbal lenses are best fitted using corneal topography. The temporal 4.0 mm point from the topography is used for base curve selection. Keratometry can be used in place of a topographer, with the starting base curve fit slightly flatter than the mean values. An excessively flat-fitting lens will have unacceptable inferior edge lift requiring a steeper lens fit; if air bubbles are present or the patient reports lens sensation superiorly, a flatter lens is necessary. The primary drawback to these larger lenses is that they may be hard to handle for new wearers.

With advanced cones or eyes with significant amounts of irregular astigmatism, semiscleral and scleral lenses may be the optimum choice for best vision.[27,43] Scleral lenses, as their name implies, are designed to rest on the scleral surface, thereby vaulting the entire cornea and limbus. Semiscleral lenses, such as the Macrolens (C&H Contact Lenses, Dallas, TX) and the Epicon (Specialty Ultravision, Campbell, CA), are slightly smaller than scleral lenses but offer many of the same advantages. Semiscleral and full scleral designs are ideal for cones where the clinician is unable to achieve adequate lens centration and stability with other RGP designs. These lenses offer the additional advantage of comfort by eliminating edge effects on the eyelids. Scleral lenses are currently available in spherical and toric designs, including front- and back-surface torics as well as bitorics. Fitting is either through diagnostic lens assessment using trial lenses or by molding.

For patients requiring the visual correction associated with an RGP lens but who are intolerant of these designs,

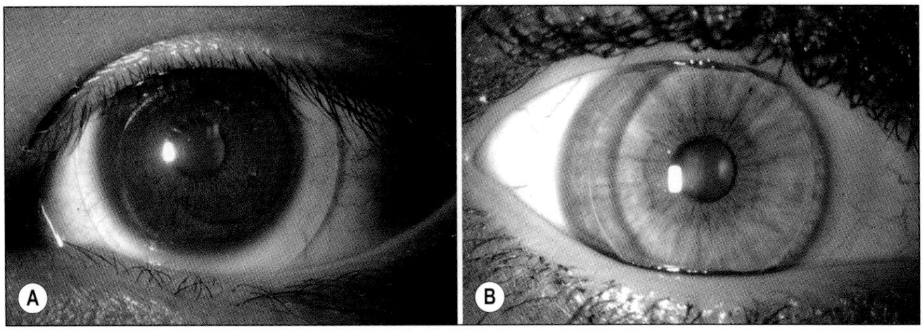

Fig. 101.3 Combination lens systems allow for the comfort of a soft lens while providing the visual acuity of an RGP. (**A**) SoftPerm lens (Ciba Vision) is composed of an RGP center surrounded by a soft hema skirt. (**B**) Piggyback design consisting of a 9.0 mm diameter RGP lens fitted over a silicone hydrogel soft lens.

hybrid lenses can often be a promising alternative (Fig. 101.3).[44] There are two hybrid lenses currently available: the SoftPerm from Ciba (Ciba Vision, Duluth, GA) and the SynergEyes KC (SynergEyes, Carlsbad, CA). SoftPerm lenses are composed of an RGP center made of Pentasilcon P and a soft hema skirt from synergicon A material, which gives the advantage of vision obtained with an RGP and the comfort of a soft lens. Studies evaluating the efficacy of SoftPerms in RGP-intolerant cases have reported an increase in visual acuity in 83.3% of all patients examined.[45] There are several drawbacks to the SoftPerm lens, however, including care of the lens, tearing of the lens between the soft and the RGP junction, and cost. SoftPerms also have a very low Dk (Dk/t of 14 at center; skirt is low water), contributing to an increased risk for neovascularization in an already diseased cornea, which may contribute to graft rejection if PKP is later required. Additionally, these lenses are available in a limited range of parameters and are not always well tolerated by the patient. More recently, the SynergEyes KC has been introduced which is composed of high-Dk materials, paflufocon D – hem-iberfilcon A, making it the lens of choice when selecting a hybrid lens system.[46] This lens has an 8.4 mm aspheric RGP center (Dk 100) surrounded by a flatter-fitting soft skirt with a total overall diameter of 14.5 mm. Because of the HEMA component, these lenses are fitted using high molecular weight fluorescein. When assessing the fit, the central fluorescein pattern should show an area of apical clearance. Adequate movement will show 0.5 mm on excursion. The SynergEyes also uses an advanced bonding system at the rigid–soft lens interface to eliminate frequent tearing or separation of the two lens components. Although the SynergEyes eliminates many of the complications of SoftPerms arising from hypoxia, such as corneal edema and neovascularization, care should be made to fit the lens to prevent tightening, abrasions, or corneal staining. Giant papillary conjunctivitis has also been reported with this form of lens.[47]

Piggyback systems are another alternative for the RGP-intolerant patient (Fig. 101.3).[48] This combination lens fit is accomplished by first fitting a low plus-power lens. Silicone hydrogel lenses are best to optimize oxygen transmissibility.[49] Corneal topography or keratometry of the new surface formed from the soft lens is then performed to facilitate a flat-fitting large-diameter RGP lens (9.0–9.5 mm OAD). The ideal fluorescein pattern will demonstrate pooling centrally, as apical bearing could lead to lens instability and peripheral touch at 3 and 9 o'clock. The increased center thickness in

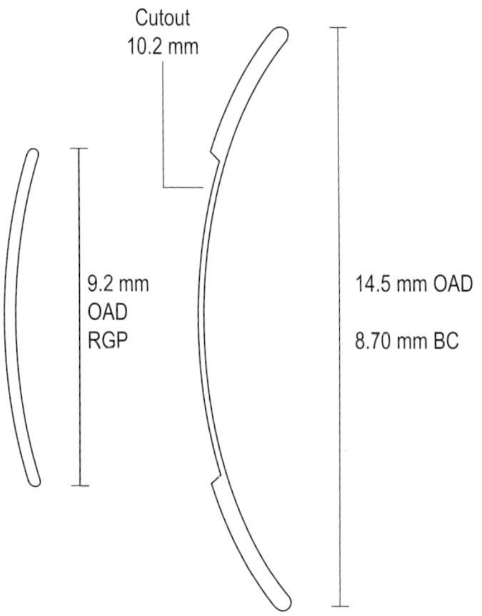

Fig. 101.4 The Flexlens Piggyback Lens. The RGP cutout maintains adequate centration of the RGP lens over the visual axis.

the plus-power lens design helps to center the RGP. Custom soft lens designs are available that possess a cutout or depression to hold the RGP lens and maintain optimal centration (Fig. 101.4; X-Cel Laboratories, Duluth, GA). Adequate RGP lens movement during blinking is essential to facilitate effective tear exchange under the lens. PMMA lenses, which have been used previously, are contraindicated as they create an anoxic post-lens environment. One of the drawbacks to fitting piggyback systems is patient compliance. The use of both soft and RGP lenses requires dual cleaning systems. Replacing a conventional hydrogel with a disposable soft lens that eliminates a cleaning step is advantageous. A summary of lens designs used in the treatment of keratoconus is given in Table 101.4.

Intacs

Patients with advanced disease and intolerant of RGP lenses often require full-thickness corneal grafts. In a subset of these patients, Intacs (Addition Technology, Fremont, CA) have been used to restore tolerance and postpone the need for surgery. Intacs are intrastromal implants which were originally developed to treat low to mild levels of myopia. For use in the visual rehabilitation of patients with

Table 101.4 Available contact lens designs for keratoconus

Conventional hydrogels	Early cones with little astigmatism, will drape cornea
Silicone hydrogels	Early cones, less drape due to higher modulus
Torics	Early cones with regular astigmatism
Soft keratoconic designs	Early to moderate cones, thicker centrally to mask irregular astigmatism
RGP multicurve	Early to moderate cones, individual parameters can all be modified to enhance fit
Aspheric RGP	Early to moderate cones, decentration can cause problems with vision
RGP keratoconic designs	Moderate to advanced cones, can add toric surfaces
Semisclerals and sclerals	Advanced cones, vaults apex, can add toric surfaces
Hybrids and piggybacks	Moderate to advanced cones, comfort of soft lens, vision of RGP, use higher Dk materials
Intacs	Used to restore contact lens tolerance

keratoconus, Intacs have now gained FDA approval as a surgical alternative to reduce irregular astigmatism, thereby improving visual acuity and facilitating contact lens fitting in advanced cones. The advantage of these intrastromal rings is that they offer a fully reversible means of correction and may delay the need for penetrating keratoplasty; however, their effects on disease progression are still unknown. Studies on the reestablishment of contact lens tolerance following Intacs use demonstrate that this procedure reduces the corneal steepening seen in advanced disease and results in a corresponding increase in visual acuity.[50] Successful contact lens fitting using reverse geometry RGP lens designs, as well as hydrogel torics, scleral lenses, and piggy systems have all been reported in the literature [51–53], but long-term success rates and tolerance of the disease have yet to be established.

Wavefront Customized Contact Lens Designs

The primary aim of contact lens wear for patients with abnormal corneal surfaces is visual rehabilitation and the achievement of optimal visual acuity. In many of these conditions, rapid changes in corneal steepening throughout the once prolate cornea result in an increase in aberrations and further visual compromise. Although RGP lenses can correct for the irregular astigmatism seen in many of these conditions, they are unable to fully correct for all of the unwanted aberrations and restore the altered corneal surface back to normal, baseline levels. With the continued advancement in wavefront technology, it is now possible to map out the aberration profile for these abnormal corneas and theoretically design a contact lens in either a soft or an RGP material to neutralize existing aberrations.[54,55] Current studies in keratoconic patients are evaluating the use of wavefront-guided custom soft lenses for this reason.[56] In these studies, soft lenses were designed with both the spherical correction for the habitual refraction and calculated aberration correction on the anterior surface coupled with a toric posterior curve based on the patient's corneal topography. Lenses were stabilized using a prism ballast design. Regardless of the small sample size evaluated, prototype early lenses have shown improvements in visual acuity, with results comparable to those of RGP lenses. Additional studies are needed to examine a host of interactive factors, such as corneal changes over time and the effect of pupil size under various light conditions. As lens designs continue to progress, the ability to significantly enhance visual outcome using soft hydrogel lenses may eliminate some of the corneal complications arising from RGP lens wear in keratoconic patients, and may offer alternatives to those who currently require RGP lenses for visual correction but are intolerant of lens wear.

Postoperative Corneas: Contact Lens Fitting after PKP

There is a wide range of indications for penetrating keratoplasty, including corneal ectasia, corneal dystrophies, and scarring secondary to trauma or disease. Patients who have undergone PKP experience dramatic alterations in corneal shape which render spectacles largely ineffective for visual correction. Binocularity is typically affected by significant amounts of spherical and astigmatic anisometropia, which can result in symptoms of asthenopia, including eye strain, headaches, diplopia, and ocular fatigue. As many as 20% of PKP patients have significant amounts of corneal astigmatism postoperatively, requiring contact lenses for improvement of visual acuity; of these, more than 90% report satisfactory visual acuity with contact lenses, defined as 20/40 or better, compared to those electing to wear spectacles.[57–59] When fitting contact lenses on a postoperative cornea, the primary goal is to reduce additional stress or mechanical trauma to the graft which could lead to rejection. High-Dk RGP lenses are the lenses of choice, as they offer substantial oxygen benefits which are necessary for graft survival, correct for any irregular astigmatism and surface irregularities, providing optimal visual correction, and carry the lowest risk of infection compared to soft lenses.[57]

The greatest challenge in fitting contact lenses after PKP is the resulting shape of the donor graft. Approximately one-third of grafts are prolate or proud, another one-third can be described as oblate or plateau, and a smaller proportion demonstrate a mixed prolate/oblate shape (18%), asymmetric astigmatism (9%), or a steep to flat pattern (13%).[60] Sutures can play a large role in the outcome of the postoperative corneal topography: the number and type of sutures, and the timing of their removal. Prior to lens fitting, it is also important to assess the sutures for epithelialization and healing at the host–graft interface. Provided the condition necessitating grafting has not damaged or depleted the host's limbal stem cell compartment, epithelialization of the stromal graft is accomplished through the host's stem cells. Reepithelialization of corneal epithelium usually occurs by postoperative day 4, but the graft is not completely healed for 18–24 months.

Contact lenses can be fitted as early as 3 months postoperatively, depending on the overall condition of the eye; however, this will require more frequent lens changes as lenses will need to be modified as sutures are removed. Greater stability is seen when fitting lenses between 6 and 12 months. In general, when fitting lenses on a post-graft cornea, it is important to vault the graft and the graft–host interface by resting the lens on the host tissue, as a lens bearing on the grafted tissue can induce neovascularization. Lens bearing over the wound margin can also lead to corneal chafing. The mean size of the corneal graft will range from 7.5 to 8.5 mm in diameter. Therefore, larger overall diameters ranging from 10.0 to 11.0 mm, with fairly large optical zones (9.0 mm), are required. Several proprietary designs are available, including the Rose K Post-Graft Lens and the 10.4 diameter post-graft lens (Lens Dynamics, Golden, CO). These lenses offer the additional benefit of improved centration, which can be quite challenging in the post-graft cornea, particularly with tilted grafts. Smaller optical zones that do not exceed the size of the donor graft can lead to visual complaints of glare. Scleral lenses, with their large optical zone, have also been reported with great success for these patients.[43] In extreme cases in which the patient is resistant to RGP lens wear, toric or reverse geometry hydrogel lenses may be used.[61]

It is imperative that patients wearing contact lenses for visual rehabilitation following PKP are monitored closely for complications, which range from minor to severe, and include superficial punctuate keratitis and ulceration, problems of allergic etiology such as giant papillary conjunctivitis, broken or loose sutures, development of subepithelial haze, graft thickening, corneal chafing, neurotrophic keratitis, dry eye, discomfort, neovascularization, infection and immune-mediated graft failure, as listed in Table 101.5. Proper patient education is also essential, as redness, pain, or visual changes could signify changes in graft stability necessitating intervention. For selected cases, either LASIK or PRK can be used to reduce post-PKP refractive errors so that successful contact lens wear can be achieved.

Table 101.5 Complications of postoperative lens wear

Penetrating keratoplasty	Refractive surgery
Broken/loose sutures	Discomfort
Discomfort	Epithelial sloughing
Dry eye	Flap disruption if RGP fit too early
Graft failure	Hypoxia from overnight wear
Graft thickening	Infection
	Neovascularization of incisions
Infection	(RK)
Neurotrophic keratitis	
Supepithelial haze	
Giant papillary conjunctivitis	
Corneal ulceration	
Conjunctivitis	
Superficial punctate keratitis	
Corneal chafing at wound margin	
Neovascularization	

Postoperative Corneas: Contact Lenses after Refractive Surgery

Despite the increasing number of patients electing to undergo refractive surgery as their primary form of vision correction, there remains a continuous influx of patients who require postoperative visual correction. Poor surgical outcomes following these procedures can result in a large number of visual disturbances, including haloes and ghosting, monocular diplopia, residual ametropia, and irregular astigmatism. Dry eye, which leads to contact lens intolerance preoperatively, is a common complication of the procedure that may or may not resolve over time. As seen following keratoplasty, the abnormal topography after refractive surgery complicates lens fitting, as the cornea has changed from a natural prolate to a more flattened, oblate shape. Lens fitting is further confounded by the patient's desire to not have to wear glasses or contacts, which was likely their main motivation for surgery. This alone represents the largest challenge in contact lens fitting, as patients who have just undergone keratorefractive surgery are usually not pleased to return to contact lens wear.

Radial Keratotomy (RK)

Radial keratotomy was the first incisional corneal refractive procedure, where a series of deep, radial stromal incisions are made throughout the mid-peripheral cornea. Incisions serve to weaken this region structurally, thereby allowing for the alteration or flattening of the central cornea by aqueous forces within the anterior chamber pushing outward in the mid-periphery, reducing axial length and correcting myopia. Although RK is no longer the refractive procedure of choice owing to secondary hyperopia, there is a subpopulation of RK patients who still must cope with the visual complications of this procedure. When fitting these patients, several options exist for both soft and RGP lens designs. If a soft lens is chosen, the use of a lens with high oxygen transmissibility, such as a silicone hydrogel, is a must. This reduces the unwanted complication of neovascularization of the incisions, which is seen in more than 50% of post-RK patients fitted with traditional soft lenses.[62] For patients with substantial amounts of regular astigmatism, toric lenses are now available in this material. Because of the altered corneal shape, a careful trial assessment is required, as these lenses often may not rotate appropriately or may be rotationally unstable.

For patients who are unable to achieve acceptable visual acuity with soft lenses due to astigmatism or monocular polyopia arising from corneal surface irregularities, RGP lenses are required. Despite the many designs available, reverse geometry RGP lenses typically provide the best centration and visual acuity (Fig. 101.5).[63] Several proprietary designs are available which have been successfully used in RK patients. Examples include the Menicon Plateau lens (Menicon, Nagoya, Japan), the OK lens (Contex, Sherman Oaks, CA), and the RK Bridge lens (Conforma, Norfolk, VA). Diagnostic lenses are selected to fit more steeply than the flattest postoperative keratometry value. If using topography, the measurement of the corneal curvature at a point

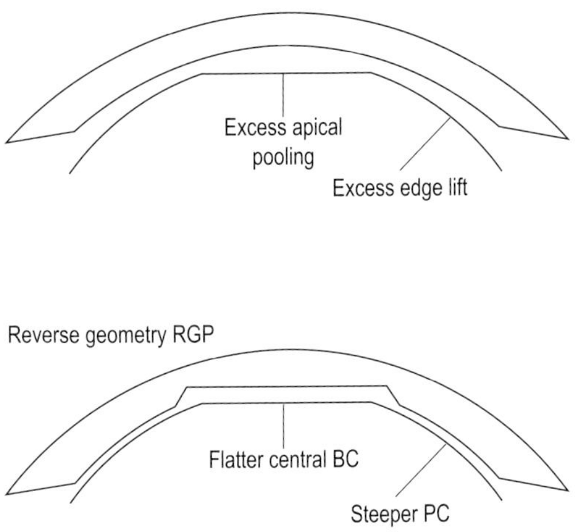

Fig. 101.5 Following refractive surgery, the new oblate corneal shape often precludes successful fitting of a traditional RGP design. Reverse geometry lenses, which are flatter centrally than peripherally, eliminate many of the fitting complications associated with postoperative RGP lens wear.

3.5 mm superior to the visual axis is used for initial base curve selection. The optimal fit for these patients is an alignment fit in the mid-periphery; however, the goal is to achieve the best fit that will not further compromise the already damaged cornea. As with any oblate cornea, it is common to have problems with lens decentration, which is normally overcome by using a larger lens. For patients intolerant of RGP lenses, combination systems such as a hybrid lens or piggyback may be used in high-Dk materials.

Photorefractive Keratectomy (PRK)

PRK is a refractive procedure in which the epithelium is removed and the anterior stroma ablated until the desired effect is achieved. As a result of the longer recovery time, the increased pain associated with the procedure, and the potential for haze, PRK is not the procedure of choice for patients seeking to undergo refractive surgery. However, it remains a viable option for patients who do not meet the required criteria for LASIK. These include patients who have a thin cornea preoperatively, creating a potential risk for keratectasia, and patients with occupations where flap stability is critical, such as the military, or in certain sports where there is a risk of trauma that could dislocate the flap.

The removal of the epithelium in PRK is associated with a significant increase in pain compared to LASIK. For this reason, bandage lenses are commonly worn on an extended basis for up to 3–5 days postoperatively, to alleviate pain and provide protection to the wounded corneal surface. Bandage lenses are also used to facilitate reepithelialization of the cornea, with an average healing time of 3–4 days. Laser-assisted subepithelial keratectomy (LASEK) is a variant of PRK in which the epithelium is removed following dilute alcohol exposure and then replaced following laser ablation. Similar to PRK, a bandage lens is required postoperatively to facilitate adhesion of the epithelial flap and control pain. Complications of bandage lens wear after PRK and LASEK include the increased risk of infection seen with extended wear of soft contact lenses, as well as signs of corneal hypoxia, including overnight swelling and epithelial sloughing during the healing process.

The use of silicone hydrogel lenses as a bandage has been heavily investigated in recent years as an alternative to traditional hydrogel lenses. Studies comparing the effectiveness of these materials suggest that there is an increase in the rate of reepithelialization with silicone hydrogel lenses: some studies report epithelialization a full day sooner than with low-Dk lenses.[64,65] This phenomenon is attributed to increased bioavailability of oxygen to the corneal surface, leading to substantial improvements in corneal epithelial physiology. These higher-Dk lenses may also provide better control over initial postoperative pain levels. In terms of visual outcome, higher-Dk lenses may offer the additional benefits of improved visual acuity at earlier time points and potentially facilitate a reduced incidence of stromal haze.[66] The drawback to the use of silicone hydrogel materials for bandage lenses is the potential for an increased number of corneal infiltrative events. Corneal infiltrates have been reported to occur more frequently in patients wearing silicone hydrogel lenses, presumably due to a combination of factors, including mechanical irritation and increased lens deposition.[67]

Following healing, in some patients contact lenses are indicated for visual correction. As with all refractive surgery, patient motivation to eliminate the need for spectacles and contact lenses is often a complicating factor in fitting contact lenses after surgery. For some, soft lenses are a viable option, and success rates up to 36% for soft contact lens wear in post-PRK patients have been reported.[68] Soft lenses will drape the cornea, and in many instances will have improved centration and movement over RGP designs. When fitting soft lenses, the final lens power is similar to the postoperative manifest refraction. If irregular astigmatism is present, RGP lenses are necessary for optimal visual acuity. Unlike soft lenses, RGP lenses are fitted with apical clearance over the ablation zone, mid-peripheral touch, and adequate edge lift. Apical clearance results in a vaulting of the flattened corneal surface. The resulting lens power is then similar to the preoperative refraction due to the plus-powered tear lens under the vault. As the lens has an alignment fit in the mid-peripheral cornea outside the ablation zone, base curves for the initial diagnostic lens are chosen based on preoperative keratometry values. The overall diameter for these lenses is typically fairly small, with a range of 9.2–9.6 mm. Lens over-refraction is imperative for the determination of final lens power. Problems with lens decentration have been reported and may lead to discomfort and subsequently shortened duration of wear.

Laser in situ Keratomileusis (LASIK)

LASIK is a refractive surgery procedure which differs from PRK by creating an anterior stromal flap to expose the underlying stroma. Following laser ablation of the exposed tissue, the flap is then replaced with the epithelium intact, allowing for a rapid recovery in visual acuity and minimal pain.

Owing to the stability of the procedure and the absence of corneal haze as seen in PRK, LASIK is the refractive procedure of choice and is used to treat higher degrees of refractive error. Despite the significant advantages associated with this procedure, complications such as decentered optical zones, flap loss, irregular astigmatism, and iatrogenic keratectasia may all require additional forms of vision correction. In these cases, contact lenses are usually indicated.[69] For treatment of higher degrees of refractive error, the corresponding increase in the rate of change between the flatter central cornea and the steeper periphery for myopic procedures can make contact lens fitting challenging.[70] This dramatic increase can lead to problems with lens instability, excessive apical clearance, and bubbles beneath the lens. In contrast, hyperopic LASIK removes tissue mid-peripherally, resulting in a steeper than normal central cornea. Hyperopic ablation zones also tend to be larger than myopic zones. Together these changes can create additional difficulties with lens centration.

Unlike PRK, bandage lenses are typically not required following LASIK. In re-treatment cases a bandage lens may be indicated. Bandage lenses are also frequently required to treat recurrent corneal erosions after LASIK. When fitting contact lenses for therapeutic management of these conditions, microbial infection, swelling and discomfort are all complications to watch for. When contact lenses are indicated for visual correction, it is imperative that healing is achieved prior to lens fitting to avoid mechanical disruption of the flap. For soft lenses, fitting can be initiated between 4 and 12 weeks, after stable visual acuity has been achieved.[71] Higher myopes or patients who have had multiple repeat procedures may take longer. Individual consideration for the elastic modulus of the lens is important and may adversely affect lens fit. Lenses with a higher modulus will be stiffer and may result in edge fluting, whereas lenses with a lower modulus will drape the cornea. A general rule of thumb for soft lenses is to select a base curve that is flatter than the flattest postoperative keratometry reading by 0.3 mm. This should allow for good lens movement and prevention of tightening. Lens centration and movement should be adequate, with 0.5–1.5 mm movement on excursion. Importantly, lens over-refraction and visual acuity need to be stable. Owing to their oblate corneal shape, toric lenses do not rotate the same as when fitted on a prolate cornea. For low levels of astigmatism these lenses may suffice; however, for higher levels or irregular astigmatism, RGP lenses are required.

RGP lenses can usually be fitted 2–3 months after surgery, but some recommend waiting as long as 6 months to ensure flap integrity.[69,71] Fitting RGP lenses earlier than this can lead to flap disruption as a result of mechanical irritation from the lens. Aspheric lenses often work well. Selection of the trial lens is based on the postoperative keratometry reading. It is recommended to fit 1.00–1.50 D steeper than the flattest keratometry value. As in RK and PRK, with a steeper-fitting lens a positive lacrimal lens is formed from apical pooling. This is corrected by the minus power of the lens; thus, the final lens power is often significantly higher in power than the postoperative manifest refraction. The optimal fluorescein pattern will show apical and peripheral clearance with little fluorescein over the ablation zone. Bearing should occur in the mid-periphery, approximately 3–4 mm from the center. Selection of lens material is also an important parameter. Higher-Dk lenses may be more prone to flexure. In these cases, stiffer low-Dk materials may be required. It is best to fit standard RGP lenses with larger overall diameters to allow for vaulting and enhanced centration and stability. This is particularly important for patients who have had larger amounts of ametropia corrected. For standard tricurve designs, diameters range from 9.2 to 10 mm. As with most lens designs, pupil size is a consideration. Larger optical zones are required for larger pupils; this becomes particularly important if any decentration issues are present. When fitting reverse geometry lenses, trial lens selection should be based upon the secondary or reverse curve. It is recommended that the reverse curve be fitted 1.0–5.0 D steeper than the base curve. Similar to standard RGP designs, lenses with larger overall diameters tend to have improved centration and better stability. Typical overall diameters for reverse geometry lenses range from 9.5 to 11.5 mm, with an optical zone from 6.0 to 8.0 mm. For selected patients scleral lenses or combination designs may be needed.

Iatrogenic keratectasia following LASIK is defined as corneal thinning resulting in a continuous, progressive loss of visual acuity that is not correctable with spectacles or soft lenses. The etiology of iatrogenic keratectasia is unknown. It can occur months after surgery and is most commonly seen in patients with high preoperative myopic refractive errors and *forme fruste* keratoconus.[72] Although not as common, it has been reported after low myopic LASIK.[73] Diagnostic criteria for iatrogenic keratectasia include myopic regression, an abnormal pupillary scissor reflex, a progressive decline in visual acuity, and a change in corneal topography. Treatment options include contact lenses or penetrating keratoplasty. When fitting traditional RGP lens designs, the same problems arise as with any refractive surgical patient due to corneal shape and topography; however, there may also be pain associated with lens wear, which may lead to intolerance. The best RGP lens options for iatrogenic keratectasia are similar to those for keratoconus. This includes multicurve lens designs and aspherics.[74] The Rose K lens, designed for patients with keratoconus, is advantageous if the area of ectasia is central. If there are ectatic changes in the periphery of the ablation zone, a reverse geometry lens will provide better centration. The lens is fitted using the mid-peripheral curve and the fluorescein pattern should look similar to that of the three-point touch pattern seen in keratoconus.

Contact lenses are also recommended for the treatment of irregular astigmatism following LASIK.[75] Irregular astigmatism can be caused by flap displacement, the formation of an epithelial ingrowth, scarring secondary to infection, diffuse lamellar keratitis, a decentered ablation, or the formation of central islands leading to monocular diplopia or polyopia, glare, haloes, and distortion. For the majority of these complications, the size of the pupil is critical to the type of symptoms the patient will experience. Larger pupils (6–7 mm) often result in increased visual complaints. In these cases, larger-diameter RGP lenses with larger optical zones are required, designed to not overlap the pupil margin. Decentered ablations can also result in visual complaints arising from residual ametropia created by the edge of the ablation zone crossing the visual axis and the formation of a multifocal cornea, defined by the presence of monocular diplopia and haloes. Lens fitting is further complicated by difficulties with centration. In addition to larger optical zones, reverse geometry designs may be needed.

Prosthetic Contact Lenses

Prosthetic lenses are primarily used for cosmetic purposes when a patient presents with significant corneal scarring, or for iris problems to create a new aperture to control light entering the eye, thereby improving vision.[76–78] Managing realistic patient expectations is imperative for successful lens fitting. Depending on the underlying diagnosis, the lens material, base curve, diameter, and movement of the lens are all key considerations. Prism ballasted lens designs are used for stabilization to achieve the optimal cosmetic effect. The pupil can be either clear or opaque. In the case of corneal scarring in which maximizing visual acuity is not a factor, opaque pupils are used and the optimal pupil size for cosmesis will be determined. For patients requiring visual correction, typically a 4.0 mm clear pupil is used to achieve best corrected visual acuity. Smaller pupils can be used but may blur images. Iris size is also critical to enhance the final outcome, as is color selection to ensure that the lens matches the corresponding eye as closely as possible. There are numerous companies that will custom manufacture prosthetic contact lenses.[79] Some of these fabricate their own lenses; others simply add the color to the lens surface after the ideal lens fit is achieved. Color may fade over time. Complications associated with prosthetic contact lenses are the same as those with conventional lenses; however, it has been reported that prosthetic lens wearers have a higher incidence of complications.[80] This is probably due to the lenses being fitted on an already compromised cornea and further emphasizes the importance of patient selection and monitoring.

Summary

Contact lenses play a pivotal role in the management of refractive errors, particularly in the abnormal cornea. Although advances in lens materials have led to substantial improvements in corneal physiology, for even the most skilled practitioner extreme irregularities in the corneal surface arising from pathological and postoperative conditions can pose a significant challenge in lens fitting and maintenance of a healthy lens–cornea relationship. A thorough understanding of lens materials and designs, as well as fitting strategies and complications, is imperative to maximize success and minimize risk associated with lens wear.

References

1. Wichterle O, Lim D. Hydrophilic gels for biological use. *Nature.* 1960;185:117–118.
2. Key JE. Development of contact lenses and their worldwide use. *Eye Contact Lens.* 2007;33(6 Pt. 2):343–345.
3. Nicolson PC, Vogt J. Soft contact lens polymers: an evolution. *Biomaterials.* 2001;22:3273–3283.
4. Dillehay SM, Henry VA. *Material selection.* 2nd ed. Philadelphia: Lippincott Williams & Wilkins; 2000.
5. Morgan PB, Efron N. A decade of contact lens prescribing trends in the United Kingdom (1996–2005). *Contact Lens Anterior Eye.* 2006;29:59–68.
6. Ren DH, Yamamoto K, Ladage PM, et al. Adaptive effects of 30-night wear of hyper-O2 transmissible contact lenses on bacterial binding and corneal epithelium. *Ophthalmology.* 2002;109(1):27–39.
7. Schein OD, Glynn RJ, Poggio EC, Seddon JM, Kenyon KR. The relative risk of ulcerative keratitis among users of daily-wear and extended-wear soft contact lenses. A case–control study. Microbial Keratitis Study Group. *N Engl J Med.* 1989;321(12):773–778.
8. Poggio EC, Glynn RJ, Schein OD, et al. The incidence of ulcerative keratitis among users of daily-wear and extended-wear soft contact lenses. *N Engl J Med.* 1989;321(12):779–783.
9. Ormerod LD, Smith RE. Contact lens-associated microbial keratitis. *Arch Ophthalmol.* 1986;104:79–83.
10. Pachigolla G, Blomquist P, Cavanagh HD. Microbial keratitis pathogens and antibiotic susceptibilities: a 5-year review of cases at an urban county hospital in North Texas. *Eye Contact Lens.* 2007;33:45–49.
11. Mondino BJ, Weissman BA, Farb MD, Pettit TH. Corneal ulcers associated with daily-wear and extended-wear contact lenses. *Am J Ophthalmol.* 1986;102(1):58–65.
12. Holden BA, Mertz GW. Critical oxygen levels to avoid corneal edema for daily and extended wear contact lenses. *Invest Ophthalmol Vis Sci.* 1984;25:1161–1167.
13. Stapleton F, Stretton S, Papas E, Skotnitsky C, Sweeney DF. Silicone hydrogel contact lenses and the ocular surface. *Ocul Surf.* 2006;4(1):24–43.
14. Dumbleton K. Adverse events with silicone hydrogel continuous wear. *Contact Lens Anterior Eye.* 2002;25(3):137–146.
15. Lattimore MR, Schallhorn SS, Lewis RB, Kaupp S. Bandage soft contact lens barrier function: a clinical research note. *Contact Lens Anterior Eye.* 2000;23:124–127.
16. Rubinstein MP. Applications of contact lens devices in the management of corneal disease. *Eye.* 2003;17:872–876.
17. Karlgard CCS, Jones LW, Moresoli C. Survey of bandage lens use in North America, October–December 2002. *Eye Contact Lens.* 2004;30(1):25–30.
18. Arora R, Jain S, Monga S, Narayanan R, Raina UK, Mehta DK. Efficacy of continuous wear PureVision contact lenses for therapeutic use. *Contact Lens Anterior Eye.* 2004;27:39–43.
19. Montero J, Sparholt J, Mely R. Retrospective case series of therapeutic applications of a Lotrafilcon A silicone hydrogel soft contact lens. *Eye Contact Lens.* 2003;29(1S):S54-S56.
20. Kanpolat A, Ucakhan OO. Therapeutic use of Focus Night & Day contact lenses. *Cornea.* 2003;22(8):726–734.
21. Ozkurt Y, Rodop O, Oral Y, Comez A, Kandemir B, Dogan OK. Therapeutic applications of Lotrafilcon A silicone hydrogel soft contact lenses. *Eye Contact Lens.* 2005;31(6):268–269.
22. Romero-Rangel T, Stavrou P, Cotter J, Rosenthal P, Baltatzis S, Foster CS. Gas-permeable scleral contact lens therapy in ocular surface disease. *Am J Ophthalmol.* 2000;130:25–32.
23. Rosenthal P, Croteau A. Fluid-ventilated, gas-permeable scleral contact lens is an effective option for managing severe ocular surface disease and many corneal disorders that would otherwise require penetrating keratoplasty. *Eye Contact Lens.* 2005;31(3):130–134.
24. Rosenthal P, Cotter J. The Boston Scleral Lens in the management of severe ocular surface disease. *Ophthalmol Clin North Am.* 2003;16(1):89–93.
25. Schornack MM, Baratz KH, Patel SV, Maguire LJ. Jupiter scleral lenses in the management of chronic graft versus host disease. *Eye Contact Lens.* 2008;34(6):302–305.
26. Segal O, Barkana Y, Hourovitz D, et al. Scleral contact lenses may help where other modalities fail. *Cornea.* 2003;22(4):308–310.
27. Pullum KW, Whiting MA, Buckley RJ. Scleral contact lenses: the expanding role. *Cornea.* 2005;24(3):269–277.
28. Willoughby CE, Batterbury M, Kaye SB. Collagen corneal shields. *Surv Ophthalmol.* 2002;47:174–182.
29. Ros FE, Tijl JW, Faber JAJ. Bandage lenses: collagen shield vs. hydrogel lens. *CLAO J.* 1991;17:187–189.
30. Parmar DN, Alizadeh H, Awwad ST, et al. Ocular surface restoration using non-surgical transplantation of tissue-cultured human amniotic epithelial cells. *Am J Ophthalmol.* 2006;141(2):299–307.
31. Hillman JS. Management of acute glaucoma with pilocarpine-soaked hydrophilic lens. *Br J Ophthalmol.* 1974;58(7):674–679.
32. Alvarez-Lorenzo C, Hiratani H, Gomez-Amoza JL, Martinez-Pacheco R, Souto C, Concheiro A. Soft contact lenses capable of sustained delivery of timolol. *J Pharm Sci.* 2002;91(10):2182–2192.
33. Tian X, Iwatsu M, Sado K, Kanai A. Studies on the uptake and release of fluoroquinolones by disposable contact lenses. *CLAO J.* 2001;27:216–220.

34. Hui A, Boone A, Jones L. Uptake and release of ciprofloxacin-HCl from conventional and silicone hydrogel contact lens materials. *Eye Contact Lens.* 2008;34(5):266–271.
35. Kapoor Y, Chauhan A. Ophthalmic delivery of cyclosporine A from Brij-97 microemulsion and surfactant-laden p-HEMA hydrogels. *Int J Pharm.* 2008;361:222–229.
36. Karlgard CC, Wong NS, Jones LW, Moresoli C. In vitro uptake and release studies of ocular pharmaceutical agents by silicon-containing and p-HEMA hydrogel contact lens materials. *Int J Pharm.* 2003;257: 141–151.
37. Kapoor Y, Thomas JC, Tan G, John VT, Chauhan A. Surfactant-laden soft contact lenses for extended delivery of ophthalmic drugs. *Biomaterials.* 2009;30:867–878.
38. Rosa dos Santos J-F, Alvarez-Lorenzo C, Silva M, et al. Soft contact lenses functionalized with pendant cyclodextrins for controlled drug delivery. *Biomaterials.* 2009; in press.
39. Kompella VB, Aasuri MK, Rao G. Management of pellucid marginal corneal degeneration with rigid gas permeable contact lenses. *CLAO J.* 2002;28(3):140–145.
40. Lee J-L, Kim M-K. Clinical performance and fitting characteristics with a multicurve lens for keratoconus. *Eye Contact Lens.* 2004;30(1):20–24.
41. Ozkurt YB, Sengor T, Kurna S, et al. Rose K contact lens fitting for keratoconus. *Int Ophthalmol.* 2008;28:395–398.
42. Ozbek Z, Cohen EJ. Use of intralimbal rigid gas-permeable lenses for pellucid marginal degeneration, keratoconus, and after penetrating keratoplasty. *Eye Contact Lens.* 2006;32(1):33–36.
43. Visser E-S, Visser R, van Lier HJJ, Otten HM. Modern scleral lenses Part I: clinical features. *Eye Contact Lens.* 2007;33(1):13–20.
44. Rubinstein MP, Sud S. The use of hybrid lenses in management of the irregular cornea. *Contact Lens Anterior Eye.* 1999;22(3):87–90.
45. Ozkurt Y, Oral Y, Karaman A, Ozgur O, Dogan OK. A retrospective case series: use of SoftPerm contact lenses in patients with keratoconus. *Eye Contact Lens.* 2007;33(2):103–105.
46. Nau AC. A comparison of SynergEyes versus traditional rigid gas permeable lens designs for patients with irregular corneas. *Eye Contact Lens.* 2008;2008(34):4.
47. Chung CW, Santim R, Heng WJ, Cohen EJ. Use of SoftPerm contact lenses when rigid gas permeable lenses fail. *CLAO J.* 2001;27(4): 202–208.
48. O'Donnell C, Maldonado-Codina C. A hyper-Dk piggyback contact lens system for keratoconus. *Eye Contact Lens.* 2004;30(1):44–48.
49. Lopez-Alemany A, Gonzalez-Meijome JM, Almeida JB, Parafita MA, Refojo MF. Oxygen transmissibility of piggyback systems with conventional soft and silicone hydrogel contact lenses. *Cornea.* 2006;25(2):214–219.
50. Colin J, Cochener B, Savary G, Malet F, Holmes-Higgin D. INTACS inserts for treating keratoconus. *Ophthalmology.* 2001;108(8):1409–1414.
51. Nepomuceno RL, Boxer Wachler BS, Weissman BA. Feasibility of contact lens fitting on keratoconus patients with INTACS inserts. *Contact Lens Anterior Eye.* 2003;26:175–180.
52. Smith KA, Carrell JD. High-Dk piggyback contact lenses over Intacs for keratoconus: a case report. *Eye Contact Lens.* 2008;34(4):238–241.
53. Ucakhan OO, Kanpolat A, Ozdemir O. Contact lens fitting for keratoconus after intacts placement. *Eye Contact Lens.* 2006;32(2):75–77.
54. Marsack JD, Parker KE, Pesudovs K, Donnelly WJ, Applegate RA. Uncorrected wavefront error and visual performance during RGP wear in keratoconus. *Optom Vis Sci.* 2007;84(6):463–470.
55. Marsack JD, Parker KE, Niu Y, Pesudovs K, Applegate RA. On-eye performance of custom wavefront-guided soft contact lenses in a habitual soft lens-wearing keratoconic patient. *J Refract Surg.* 2007;23:960–964.
56. Marsack JD, Parker KE, Applegate RA. Performance of wavefront-guided soft lenses in three keratoconus subjects. *Optom Vis Sci.* 2008;85(12): 1172–1178.
57. Wietharn BE, Driebe WT. Fitting contact lenses for visual rehabilitation after penetrating keratoplasty. *Eye Contact Lens.* 2004;30(1):31–33.
58. Genvert GI, Cohen EJ, Arentsen JJ, Laibson PR. Fitting gas-permeable contact lenses after penetrating keratoplasty. *Am J Ophthalmol.* 1985;1985(99):5.
59. Szczotka-Flynn L, Lindsay RG. Contact lens fitting following corneal graft surgery. *Clin Exp Optom.* 2003;86:244–249.
60. Waring G, Hannush S, Bogan S, Maloney R. *Classification of corneal topography with videokeratography.* New York: Springer; 1992.
61. Costas K, Nick V, Lefteris K, Theodore M. Fitting the post-keratoplasty cornea with hydrogel lenses. *Contact Lens Anterior Eye.* 2009;32(1):22–26.
62. Yeung KK, Olson MD, Weissman BA. Complexity of contact lens fitting after refractive surgery. *Am J Ophthalmol.* 2002;133:607–612.
63. Mathur A, Jones L, Sorbara L. Use of reverse geometry rigid gas permeable contact lenses in the management of the postradial keratotomy patient: review and case report. *Int Contact Lens Clin.* 2001;26(5):121–127.
64. Engle AT, Laurent JM, Schallhorn SC, et al. Masked comparison of silicone hydrogel lotrafilcon A and etafilcon A extended-wear bandage contact lenses after photorefractive keratectomy. *J Cataract Refract Surg.* 2005;31:681–686.
65. Szaflik JP, Ambroziak AM, Szaflik J. Therapeutic use of a Lotrafilcon A silicone hydrogel soft contact lens as a bandage after LASEK surgery. *Eye Contact Lens.* 2004;30(1):59–62.
66. Edwards JD, Bower KS, Sediq DA, et al. Effects of lotrafilcon A and omafilcon A bandage contact lenses on visual outcomes after photorefractive keratectomy. *J Cataract Refract Surg.* 2008;34:1288–1294.
67. Szczotka-Flynn L, Diaz M. Risk of corneal inflammatory events with silicone hydrogel and low dk hydrogel extended contact lens wear: a meta-analysis. *Optom Vis Sci.* 2007;84(4):247–256.
68. Lim L, Siow K-L, Chong JSC, Tan DTH. Contact lens wear after photorefractive keratectomy: comparison between rigid gas permeable and soft contact lenses. *CLAO J.* 1999;25(4):222–227.
69. Steele C, Davidson J. Contact lens fitting post-laser-in situ keratomileusis (LASIK). *Contact Lens Anterior Eye.* 2007;30:84–93.
70. Bufidis T, Konstas AGP, Pallikaris IG, Siganos DS, Georgiadis N. Contact lens fitting difficulties following refractive surgery for high myopia. *CLAO J.* 2000;26(2):106–110.
71. Zadnik K. Contact lens management of patients who have had unsuccessful refractive surgery. *Curr Opin Ophthalmol.* 1999;10:260–263.
72. Randleman JB, Russell B, Ward MA, Thompson KP, Stulting RD. Risk factors and prognosis for corneal ectasia after LASIK. *Ophthalmology.* 2003;110(2):267–275.
73. Amoils SP, Deist MB, Gous P, Amoils PM. Iatrogenic keratectasia after laser in situ keratomileusis for less than -4.0 to -7.0 diopters of myopia. *J Cataract Refract Surg.* 2000;26:967–977.
74. Choi H-J, Kim M-K, Lee J-L. Optimization of contact lens fitting in keratectasia patients after laser in situ keratomileusis. *J Cataract Refract Surg.* 2004;30:1057–1066.
75. Alio JL, Belda JI, Artola A, Garcia-Lledo M, Osman A. Contact lens fitting to correct irregular astigmatism after corneal refractive surgery. *J Cataract Refract Surg.* 2002;28:1750–1757.
76. Olali C, Mohammed M, Ahmed S, Gupta M. Contact lens for failed pupilloplasty. *J Cataract Refract Surg.* 2008;34:1995–1996.
77. Cole CJ, Vogt U. Medical uses of cosmetic colored contact lenses. *Eye Contact Lens.* 2006;32(4):230–206.
78. Yildirim N, Basmak H, Sahin A. Prosthetic contact lenses: adventure or miracle. *Eye Contact Lens.* 2006;32(2):102–103.
79. Bator KK, Salituro SM. Prosthetic soft contact lenses and you. *Eye Contact Lens.* 2005;31(5):215–218.
80. Kanemoto M, Toshida H, Takahiro I, Murakami A. Prosthetic soft contact lenses in Japan. *Eye Contact Lens.* 2007;33(6):300–303.

Chapter 102

Complications of Contact Lens Wear

Elisabeth J. Cohen

As of 2006, 33 million people in the USA and 125 million people worldwide were estimated to wear contact lenses, and the numbers are increasing.[1,2] Given the enormous number of contact lens wearers, even when the rate is very low, complications will occur in large numbers of people and be frequently seen in practice. Whether or not ophthalmologists fit contact lenses, it is necessary that they are able to diagnosis contact lens-related complications. In addition, every eye examination of a patient wearing contacts is an opportunity to educate the patient with regard to proper lens hygiene, including regular disinfection and avoidance of exposure of contact lenses and cases to water.

Contact lens complications vary greatly in severity and frequency. Infections can result not only in loss of vision but also in loss of the eye. Prevention, early diagnosis, and appropriate treatment of contact lens-related infections are of critical importance. Infiltrates and abrasions in contact lens patients have the risk of being or becoming infections. Contact lens keratopathy, due to reactions to preservatives in lens care solutions, remains a problem which needs to be recognized so that, after resolution, contact lens use can be resumed successfully. Problems related to allergies and hypoxia have decreased in recent years with the evolution toward use of daily wear, frequent replacement lenses, and the development of more oxygen-permeable contact lens materials. Dry eyes in contact lens wearers remain a frequent problem that can reduce contact lens tolerance if not treated adequately. Corneal warpage is less frequent now that polymethyl methacrylate (PMMA) hard lenses are rarely used, but still occurs and needs to be resolved before lens refitting or refractive surgery.

The first step, as always in patient care, is to obtain a careful and complete history. It is necessary to ask every patient if they have a history of contact lens use. Most symptomatic patients have discontinued wearing contacts and may not offer this information unless asked. In older patients, especially, past use of contact lenses may be overlooked. The ocular history of pain and discomfort is very helpful in making an accurate diagnosis. Pain that continues to increase after lens removal suggests an infection. More specifically, acute pain for hours to days favors a bacterial infection, and subacute pain lasting weeks and often unresponsive to initial treatment suggests infection by an unusual organism, such as *Acanthamoeba* or fungus. Pain or discomfort that subsides following lens removal favors a sterile problem. If the symptoms recur with the resumption of contact lens use, contact lenses are the likely cause of the problem. Itching is associated with allergies, which are frequently aggravated and sometimes caused by contact lens use. Burning on insertion of contacts points to a problem with the disinfecting system used. Burning or dryness later in the day after several hours of lens use is consistent with dry eyes and/or tight lenses.

In addition to the ocular history, a careful contact lens history is important. This can be deferred in patients with severe, acute pain caused by an infection until after necessary treatment is begun, but should be documented in the medical record. It is important to obtain as much specific information as possible regarding contact lenses and lens care regimens used. In 2008, 90% of lenses worn in the USA were soft and 10% were rigid gas-permeable (RGP).[2] Soft contact lenses (SCL) should be correctly described as frequent replacement (replaced after 2 weeks to 3 months), disposable (single use), or conventional. It should be noted if they are used for daily wear, extended wear, or both. The brand and specific name of the lens is important to determine so that one knows if it was approved for extended wear or is a silicone hydrogel lens. Use of special lenses such as cosmetic/costume, orthokeratology, therapeutic, and aphakic lenses should be recorded. In addition, the lens care regimen should be determined, including the names of the products used, trying to be as specific as possible, and the level of compliance with recommended lens care regimens. Recent changes in types of lenses and brands of solutions used prior to the onset of symptoms are also frequently important in order to determine the correct diagnosis and treatment. It is helpful to ask the patient to bring in packages of contact lenses and bottles of the solutions, as it is difficult to get an accurate history.

Infiltrates

Contact lens-related infiltrates are common and discussed in detail elsewhere (see Ch. 23). The critical issue is to distinguish sterile infiltrates from early infections. Sterile infiltrates are typically associated with mild pain that decreases after lens removal, and are not associated with anterior chamber reaction or surrounding corneal edema (Fig. 102.1).[3]

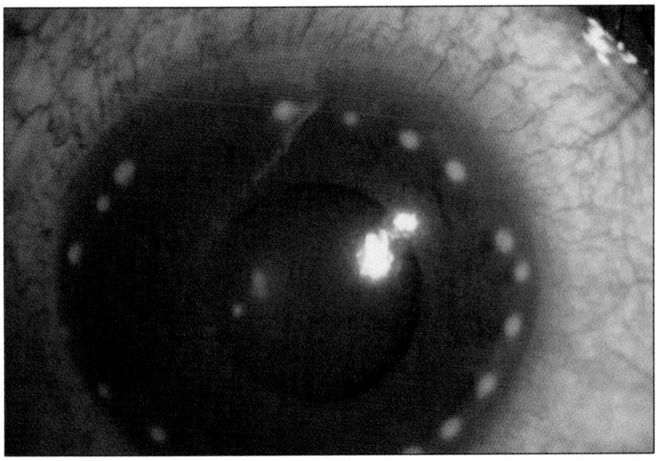

Fig. 102.1 Multiple peripheral, presumed sterile, infiltrates associated with soft contact lens use. This unusual presentation is of uncertain etiology. Treatment with frequent topical antibiotics and close follow-up is recommended. Mid-strength topical steroids can be added at a follow-up visit if inflammation is not resolving and there is no evidence of infection.

In this study, small infiltrates, less than 1 mm, were culture positive in one-third of cases. If in doubt, it is safer to treat as infectious with intensive topical antibiotics and close follow-up. Topical steroids are not indicated acutely and may not be needed, as sterile infiltrates are usually a self-limited problem.

Abrasions

Corneal abrasions in patients who wear contacts are a potentially serious complication. It is important to look for any evidence of a corneal infiltrate and, if present, to treat it as a corneal ulcer. They should never be patched, because they can become serious *Pseudomonas* infections overnight (Fig. 102.2).[4] They should be treated intensively with adequate antibiotic coverage for *Pseudomonas*, such as bacitracin/polymxyin, tobramycin, or ciloxan ointment every 2 hours, and not just erythromycin or bacitracin four times a day. Patients should be advised to return for follow-up in 1 day, and sooner if they are getting worse, as manifest by increased pain, decreased vision, or a change in the appearance of their eye with the development of a white area in the cornea. Cycloplegia and oral pain medications can be prescribed, similar to noncontact lens-related abrasions. Topical steroids should not be used in the initial treatment of contact lens-related abrasions.

Infections

Microbial keratitis is the most serious complication of contact lens use, and contact lenses are a major risk factor for corneal ulcers. Corneal ulcers associated with use of non-therapeutic soft contact lenses are most often caused by bacterial infection, especially *Pseudomonas*, but in recent years there has been an epidemic of fungal keratitis and an ongoing resurgence of *Acanthamoeba* keratitis. Corneal infections are more often associated with the use of soft contact lenses than rigid gas-permeable lenses. However, use of RGP lenses for orthokeratology has been associated with bacterial infections and *Acanthamoeba* keratitis.[5] Understanding of risk factors for various corneal infections can facilitate their prevention and prompt diagnosis. Early diagnosis and appropriate treatment of infections are necessary to reduce loss of vision and, in the most severe cases, loss of the eye. Small ulcers, less than 1 mm, are often treated with intensive hourly topical fourth-generation fluoroquinolones, although this is an off-label use of gatifloxacin and moxifloxacin (Fig. 102.3). Larger ulcers, or those unresponsive to this treatment, are cultured and treated with intensive, every 30 minutes, fortified tobramycin and hourly cefazolin/vancomycin (Fig. 102.4). Topical steroids are avoided in the

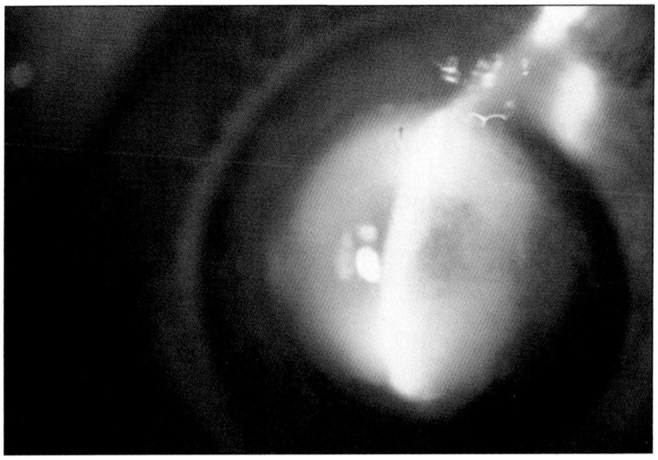

Fig. 102.2 A severe *Pseudomonas* ulcer developed one day after patching an abrasion in a patient who used extended-wear soft lenses. This resulted in severe scarring, and a penetrating keratoplasty was necessary for visual rehabilitation. Patching is contraindicated in contact lens-related abrasions. Treatment should include frequent topical antibiotic ointment or drops with good coverage for *Pseudomonas* and immediate follow-up for increased pain, decreased vision, or a change in the appearance of the eye.

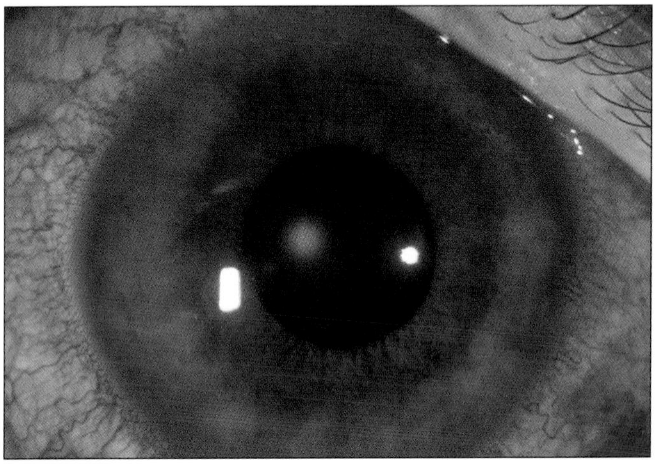

Fig. 102.3 A small central corneal ulcer can be treated with topical intensive fluoroquinolone drops every 30–60 minutes around the clock without performing cultures. If the ulcer worsens after 1 day of treatment, cultures should be performed and fortified antibiotics started.

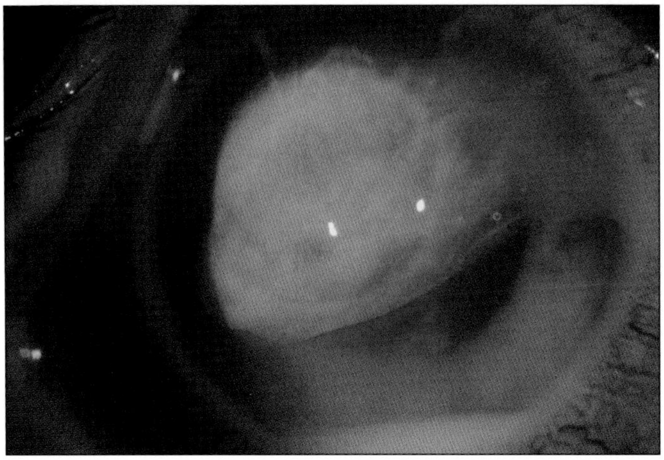

Fig. 102.4 Severe contact lens-related infections require cultures and immediate intensive treatment with fortified antibiotics. Since *Pseudomonas* is the most common cause, initial treatment included fortified tobramycin every 30 minutes around the clock and cefazolin every hour around the clock, after an initial loading dose of 1 drop every 5 minutes 5 times. Ceftazidime can be added every hour around the clock initially or after 1–2 days of treatment if there is not improvement. If cultures grow *Pseudomonas*, then cefazolin can be discontinued.

initial management and, in some cases, added cautiously after the organism is identified and the infection is responding to treatment.

Soft contact lens use has been associated with bacterial keratitis since the 1980s. In landmark articles by Schein and associates and Poggio and coworkers, published in the *New England Journal of Medicine* in 1989, the major risk factor for ulcerative keratitis was determined to be extended, overnight wear of contact lenses.[6,7] Daily disposable lenses became available in 1995 and silicone hydrogel lenses in 1999. Despite advances in contact lens materials and the introduction of frequent-replacement and single-use disposable lenses, recent landmark articles provide evidence that the incidence of and risk factors for contact lens-related microbial keratitis have not changed greatly, with the important exception that single-use, daily-disposable contacts have significantly decreased the number of ulcers associated with vision loss.[8,9]

These studies by Dart and associates Stapleton and coworkers contain very important information. The risk factor study, by Dart and colleagues,[8] reports the result of a well-designed, major case-control study conducted by investigators at Moorfields Eye Hospital in London during 2004 and 2005. The relative risk (RR) of microbial keratitis was compared to the risk associated with daily-wear, planned (frequent)-replacement lenses to facilitate comparison of risk associated with use of various soft contact lenses. The risk associated with RGP lenses was significantly less, 0.16. Although, RGP lenses account for only 5–10% of lenses worn in the USA, they are the safest from the point of view of infection. Although the overall RR of single-use, daily-disposable lenses was higher (1.56) than frequent-replacement lenses, the risk of vision loss was significantly less. No daily-disposable lens wearer lost vision, defined as less than or equal to 20/40 Snellen acuity. This definition of vision loss is notable since microbial keratitis can result in much more severe vision loss. The grading system of disease severity is described and tested in another paper.[10] The decrease in severity of microbial keratitis associated with daily disposables was attributed to avoidance of exposure to pathogens in contact lens cases. Another interesting finding was that different brands of daily-disposable lenses had different relative risks; 1-day Acuvues (Johnson & Johnson, Langhorne, PA) had the lowest risk, similar to planned-replacement lenses, and two other commonly used brands had significantly higher risk. The RR associated with overnight wear was 5.4, and did not differ among different lenses, including silicone hydrogel lenses. The hyper-oxygen transmissible lenses reduce hypoxia associated with overnight wear, but not microbial keratitis. Other significant risk factors observed in this study included occasional overnight wear, increased number of days per week of contact lens wear, with 2 or less days associated with significantly less risk, lenses worn for hyperopia or to change the color of eye, irregular hand washing, younger age (less than or equal to 49 years), and male sex. There appears to be a dose-dependent quality to the risk associated with lens wear, with less use being safer. Other than handwashing, hygiene was not found to be significant.

The companion incidence study by Stapleton and associates had findings consistent with the case-control study and previous reports.[9] It was a 1-year prospective study conducted during 2003–2004 in Australia. The overall incidence of microbial keratitis was similar in frequent-replacement and daily-disposable lenses wearers, 1.9 and 2.2 cases per 10 000 per year, respectively, but the risk of severe infection, defined as vision less than or equal to 20/40, was significantly lower with daily-disposable contacts. The incidence for daily wear of silicone hydrogels was 11.9, with a *P* value of 0.06, suggesting no advantage of silicone hydrogels for daily wear in terms of infection. Overnight wear had a significantly increased incidence of 19.5 for hydrogel soft contacts and 25.4 for silicone hydrogels. The difference between hydrogel soft contacts and silicone hydrogels was not significant, but the numbers do not suggest any advantage of silicone hydrogrels in this regard. Increased risk for occasional overnight wear, defined as less than one time per week, was observed. In addition to overnight wear, other significant risk factors included poor contact lens case hygiene, smoking, internet purchase of contacts, less than 6 months of extended wear of contact lenses, and higher socioeconomic class. Other than care of the case, lens hygiene was not significant. Further studies regarding the role of internet purchase, duration of extended wear, and socioeconomic status are necessary, as these have not been previously reported. The case-control study by Schein and associates in 1989 reported a four times increased risk for smokers, that was not statistically significant.[6] The data suggest that risk of contact lens-related infection is one more reason to encourage patients to stop smoking. Daily-disposable lenses have significantly decreased the severity of microbial keratitis, but the increased incidence associated with even occasional overnight wear persists despite the use of silicone hydrogel lenses.

These researchers in Australia have done other important studies on contact lens-related microbial keratitis. In a study on factors affecting morbidity, they reported that 14.3% lost two or more lines of vision, and that the causative organism was the major determinant of severity, although delay in treatment beyond 12 hours was also significant.[11] In another study on climate, disease severity, and organism, they found that severe infections were significantly more common in warmer and more humid locations.[12] *Pseudomonas* was the most common isolate and accounted for most of the cases with vision loss. This is in keeping with our clinical impression that severe *Pseudomonas* infections are most common during the warm summer months in the northeastern USA. Other researchers in Australia studied the correlation between cultures of corneal scrapings and contact lens cases and found that contact lenses were culture positive twice as often (70% vs 34%) and that the same organism was found in a majority (13/17) of eyes with positive corneal cultures from the contact lens cultures. In this series, the Gram-negative rod *Serratia marcescens* was the most common isolate. Contact lens cultures may be useful, but are not the same as corneal cultures, which provide definitive information, but are less likely to be positive.

Trends in contact lens-related corneal ulcers on the Cornea Service at Wills Eye Institute have been reported over the past 25 years.[13,14] In the 1990s, there was a decrease in the percentage of contact lens-related ulcers followed by a significant increase beginning in 1999. From 1999 to 2002, at Wills, 30%, of corneal ulcers were contact lens related. This is similar to the report that at a tertiary eye center in Australia, from 2001 to 2003, 33.7% of ulcers were lens related.[15] In 2006 and 2007, the percentage of contact lens-related ulcers has increased to over 50% at Wills, while the total number of ulcers has also gone up (Airiani S. ARVO Symposium 2009). *Pseudomonas* was the most common bacteria isolated. Approximately 75% of contact lens-related infections were presumed or proven bacterial in etiology and 25% caused by *Acanthamoeba* or fungal organisms.

Fungal infections

Fungal infections associated with nontherapeutic soft contact lenses were uncommon until recently. Trauma with vegetable-contaminated matter has been the major risk for fungal keratitis caused by filamentous organisms, including *Fusarium*. There is evidence that the percentage of fungal infections associated with use of contact lenses began to increase, at least in one center in Florida, before the *Fusarium* outbreak in 2005 and 2006.[16] In the same series, beginning in 2005, contact lens use was the most common risk factor for fungal keratitis, accounting for 52% of cases, compared to 29% associated with trauma. In Miami, the percent of fungal keratitis in contact lens-related ulcers in general, and *Fusarium* in particular, doubled from 2004 to 2005, leading to the conclusion that contact lens wear may be a risk factor for fungal keratitis.[17,18]

In 2005 and 2006 there was an international outbreak of contact lens-related *Fusarium* keratitis that was first reported in Hong Kong and Singapore and subsequently in the USA that was associated with the use of ReNu with MoistureLoc (Bausch & Lomb, Rochester, NY) contact lens multipurpose solution.[19–23] The Centers for Disease Control and Prevention (CDC) investigation determined that the outbreak was

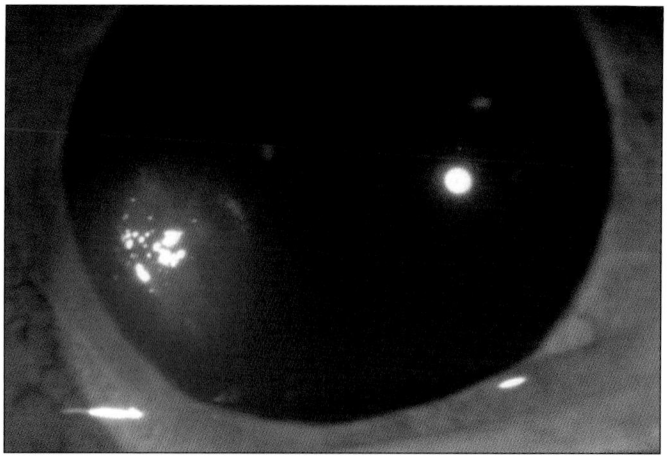

Fig. 102.5 This ulcer was caused by *Fusarium* and occurred during the outbreak. The patient had a smaller infiltrate in the other eye which also grew out *Fusarium*.

associated with the use of ReNu with MoistureLoc, and sales of this product were halted in the USA in April 2006, and it was withdrawn from the market worldwide in May 2006.[19] After the withdrawal of ReNu ML, the number of cases of contact lens-related *Fusarium* infections declined. In view of the genetic diversity and groups of *Fusarium* isolated, the likely source of *Fusarium* was thought to be water in the patients' sinks and showers. ReNu MoistureLoc passed the current stand-alone tests for multipurpose solutions, including biocidal activity against *Fusarium solani*, one of the test organisms. The *Fusarium* outbreak was one factor, the other being the *Acanthamoeba* outbreak discussed below, leading to changes in standards for multipurpose disinfecting solutions currently under consideration at the Food and Drug Administration (FDA).[24]

The *Fusarium* outbreak at Wills Eye Institute was reported in collaboration with the experience at the University of Medicine and Dentistry of New Jersey (Fig. 102.5).[25] The incidence of *Fusarium* keratatis at these centers in northeastern USA increased almost sevenfold during the epidemic, compared to the previous time period. Two-thirds (10/15) of the patients, who all wore soft contacts, used tap water to rinse their cases, a noncompliant behavior. The infections were serious, with 40% requiring therapeutic keratoplasties to control infection. Since this time, the number of contact lens-related *Fusarium* infections decreased in 2007 and 2008, but the overall number of fungal infections has remained elevated, and five contact lens-related fungal infections caused by *Alternaria* and *Paecilomyces* infections have occurred (Yildiz unpublished data).

A raised index of suspicion for contact lens-related fungal infections is indicated, since the occurrence of just three infections in a short period of time may represent an outbreak when these infections have previously been rare.[26] In addition, the possibility of fungal infection makes it appropriate to avoid the use of topical steroids in the treatment of corneal infections of unknown etiology, since steroids enhance fungal infection. Also, the indication for corneal cultures of contact lens-related infections may be lowered to enable the diagnosis and appropriate treatment of fungal infections. In view of the report of the favorable response of some ulcers later proven to be caused by *Fusarium* to initial treatment with topical fluoroquinolones, fungal infections may be more common than realized, and response to topical antibiotics does not rule out a fungal etiology.[27] The development of new standards for contact lens solution efficacy testing is very important, but will take years to be developed and implemented. In the meantime, it is necessary to educate all patients wearing contacts regarding current lens care recommendations, including avoidance of exposure of contact lenses and lens cases to water.

Acanthamoeba

Contact lens-related *Acanthamoeba* infections have increased in recent years and continue to be more frequent than in previous years, despite the withdrawal of one multipurpose solution associated with increased risk. In the 1980s, in a landmark article, risk factors for *Acanthamoeba* keratitis were determined to be use of soft contact lenses, disinfection using homemade saline, infrequent disinfection, and exposure to water by swimming in contacts.[28] In contrast to bacterial infections, overnight wear is not the major risk factor. In the 1990s, *Acanthamoeba* keratitis decreased in frequency in the USA, although there was an outbreak in 1993–1994 in Iowa, thought to be related to flooding and subsequent exposure to contaminated water.[29]

A significant increase in *Acanthamoeba* keratitis has been reported beginning in 2003 in Chicago and 2004 in Philadelphia.[30,31] In the Chicago area, it was determined that there was an increased risk associated with living in the counties surrounding Chicago than in central Cook County. A possible explanation for the geographical distribution was the implementation of US Environmental Protection Agency (EPA) policies to decrease disinfection by-products, such as chlorine, in the water supply in 2002. As a result, it was thought that water users further away from Lake Michigan water treatment would be exposed to water with biofilms containing more microorganisms to support the growth of *Acanthamoeba*. In Philadelphia, it was also observed that many of the *Acanthamoeba* patients lived further away from the city, and that a number used well water.

In another important paper by investigators at the University of Illinois at Chicago, use of Complete MoisturePlus Multi-Purpose Solution (Advanced Medical Optics [AMO], Santa Ana, CA) was determined in a case-control study to be a significant risk factor for *Acanthamoeba* keratitis (odds ratio 16.67), although 38.8% of cases had no history of its use.[32] A positive, but not statistically significant, association of three hygiene variables—solution reuse, lack of rubbing, and showering with lenses—with *Acanthamoeba* keratitis was observed. Reuse is a noncompliant behavior, but no-rub is recommended with many multipurpose solutions, and showering with lenses is not included in standard care directions, but can be assumed to be compliant behavior in lenses approved for extended wear.

The CDC, after being informed of the Illinois outbreak, conducted an investigation and also found an association of *Acanthamoeba* keratitis with use of Complete MoisturePlus. This was reported in *MMWR* on May 26, 2007, and AMO voluntarily recalled the product at this time.[33] The increased number of infections in the Philadelphia area has persisted since recall of the product (unpublished data).

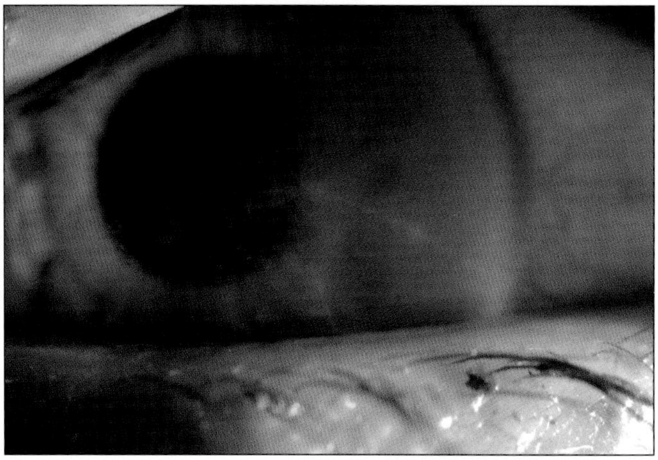

Fig. 102.6 Epithelial keratitis and radial neuritis due to *Acanthamoeba* infection. It is important to consider the diagnosis of *Acanthamoeba* keratitis in patients with epithelial keratitis or atypical herpes simplex viral keratitis. The prognosis is much better when the diagnosis is made in the early stages of disease.

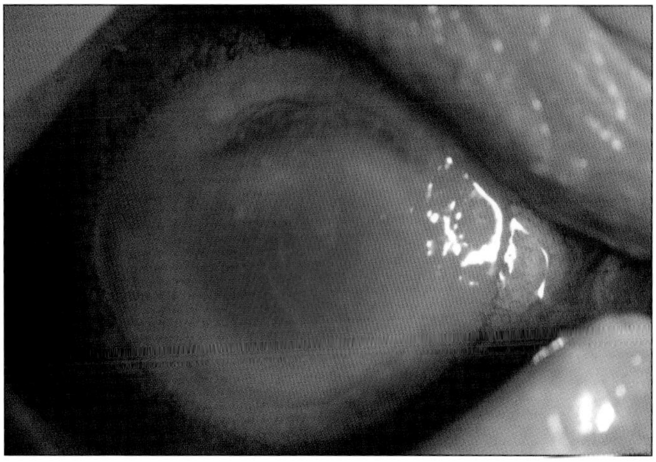

Fig. 102.7 This patient with *Acanthamoeba* keratitis presented with a ring infiltrate. Treatment was complicated by streptococcal superinfection, delayed healing, and refractory glaucoma resulting in NLP vision. The eye was enucleated due to pain. A ring infiltrate is the hallmark of *Acanthamoeba* keratitis, but it is a late sign and associated with a poorer prognosis.

Diagnosis of *Acanthamoeba* keratitis in the early stages of disease, with epithelial keratitis and radial keratoneuritis, is associated with a better outcome than is later diagnosis, with deep stromal keratitis or the classic ring infiltrate (Figs 102.6 and 102.7).[31,34] The differential diagnosis is herpes simplex keratitis due to epitheliopathy, dendritiform keratitis, and non-specific stromal keratitis in *Acanthamoeba* keratitis. It is important to suspect the diagnosis in any patient wearing contacts who presents with epithelial changes, often associated with pain and upper lid swelling, unresponsive to treatment including lubrication, antiviral medication, antibiotics, and steroids. Herpes keratitis is usually responsive to treatment, and *Acanthamoeba* infection must be considered in any patient with atypical dendritic keratitis or who is unresponsive to treatment. *Acanthamoeba* keratitis is usually unilateral, but can be bilateral. *Acanthamoeba* keratitis is most frequently associated with use of soft contact lenses, but can occur in association with rigid gas-permeable lenses, especially for orthokeratology.[35] It is important to ask about a history of using tap water for rinsing contact lenses or cases in all patients wearing contacts, since this will increase the index of suspicion for *Acanthamoeba* keratitis. As soon as the diagnosis is suspected, smears and cultures should be obtained and treatment should be begun immediately, usually including polyhexamethylene biguanide 0.02% (PHMB) or chlorhexidine 0.02% and, often, propamidine isethionate 0.1%.[36]

Due to the frequently devastating nature of *Acanthamoeba* keratitis with a prolonged painful course, guarded prognosis, and potential irreversible loss of vision and the eye, prevention is of the utmost importance. Currently, *Acanthamoeba* is not one of the standard test organisms that contact lens disinfection systems are required to be effective against. Revising current standards is under discussion at the FDA, but changes are complex and will take time to come about.[37] Some solutions for rigid gas-permeable lenses are effective in killing *Acanthamoeba* cysts, but soft lens multipurpose solutions are not.[38] The increased risk associated with Complete MoisturePlus and *Acanthamoeba* keratitis compared to other multipurpose solutions may be due to the presence of propylene glycol in the formulation, which is associated with encystment of *Acanthamoeba*.[39] Hydrogen peroxide systems are more effective than multipurpose solutions, but ones that are currently available in the USA are not entirely effective.[40] Prolonged exposure to hydrogen peroxide prior to neutralization is necessary for efficacy.[41] There is concern that some silicone hydrogel lenses may be more prone to attachment of *Acanthamoeba* trophozoites than other silicone hydrogel lenses or conventional soft lenses.[42]

In the absence of multipurpose solutions effective against *Acanthamoeba*, we recommend the use of single-use, daily-disposable lenses whenever possible. When not, we recommend hydrogen peroxide systems. All patients wearing contacts must be educated at each office visit against exposure of contact lenses and cases to water, including showering or washing one's face while wearing contacts.

Contact Lens-Induced Keratopathy

Contact lens-induced keratopathy is a better term to use than contact lens-superior limbic keratitis (SLK) to describe a keratitis that begins superiorly, but in advanced cases can involve the entire cornea with superficial punctate keratitis, neovascularization, and scarring.[43–45] It is thought to be an allergic and/or toxic response to preservatives, usually thimerosal, used in contact lens solutions, and is unrelated to the etiology of Theodore's SLK.[46] In the past, thimerosal was the preservative in many but not all cases.[47,48] It can take months to resolve after discontinuation of contact lenses, and, if lens use persists, significant permanent visually scarring can develop. Since use of thimerosal was discontinued and the shift from conventional to frequent-replacement lenses, the problem has decreased in frequency.

Reactions to current preservatives in multipurpose solutions can cause a similar keratoconjunctivitis that is often greatest superiorly (Fig. 102.8). It is thought to be a form of localized limbal stem cell deficiency. Resolution after contact lens discontinuation is slow. Treatment consists primarily of lubrication with preservative-free, unit-dose tears. Following resolution, contact lenses can be resumed successfully using single-use, daily-disposable lenses, or, if this is not possible, hydrogen peroxide systems, since these are neutralized to saline, prior to lens reinsertion. Follicular conjunctivitis, peripheral infiltrates, and peripheral scars can occur. The differential diagnosis includes *Chlamydia* keratoconjunctivitis and staphylococcal hypersensitivity keratitis. Contact lens keratopathy is almost always bilateral, and if not, the possibility of *Acanthamoeba* keratitis must be considered in unilateral epitheliopathy and nonspecific keratitis. A history of improvement when contact lenses are discontinued and recurrence when lenses are resumed supports a contact lens solution-related etiology. Often there is a history of changing multipurpose solutions several months prior to the onset of symptoms.

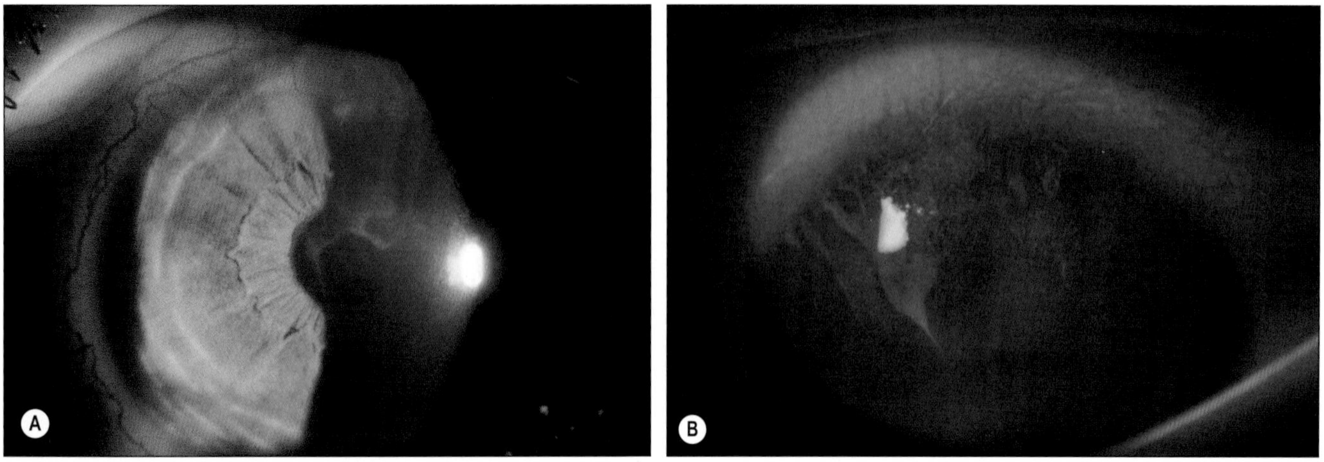

Fig. 102.8 (**A**) Contact lens-induced keratopathy, presumably due to a reaction to preservatives in contact lens solutions, can cause superior superficial corneal scarring and surface irregularity. (**B**) Fluorescein stain reveals changes consistent with limbal stem cell deficiency.

Giant Papillary Conjunctivitis and Other Allergies

Giant papillary conjunctivitis (GPC) has become less common in recent years with the increased use of frequent-replacement lenses. Excellent review articles summarize the current understanding of GPC, or contact lens-induced giant papillary conjunctivitis.[49,50] Coating on contact lenses stimulates an immune response and is thought to also cause conjunctival trauma. The more frequent replacement of contacts, the less the problem of GPC, with the ideal lens, in this regard, being a single-use, daily-disposable contact lens.

GPC was first reported in the 1970s and was described in detail by Allansmith and colleagues.[51] The problem occurs most frequently in patients wearing soft contact lenses, but also occurs in patients wearing RGP lenses, hybrid lenses, ocular prostheses, and sclera lenses.[52,53] With RGP lenses, it takes longer for GPC to develop, and the papillary reaction tends to be more localized on the superior tarsus.[51] A localized GPC can also occur due to exposed sutures after ocular surgery. The variety of foreign bodies associated with a similar reaction supports the etiology as a response to the coating on a foreign body, rather than the specific nature of the foreign body. GPC is usually bilateral, but can be asymmetric, especially in patients who wear different types of lenses and/or replace them at different intervals in their eyes.

GPC refers to symptoms associated with a papillary reaction of the superior tarsus. Eversion of the upper lid is necessary to make the diagnosis and should be a part of the routine examination of patients who wear contacts. Symptoms include decreased lens tolerance, increased mucus, and itching. Papillae on the superior tarsus that are greater than 0.3 mm are considered pathologic, unless they are located along the superior border of the tarsal plate, where they can occur in normal people or be associated with seasonal allergies. Allansmith described four stages of GPC. Stage 1 is preclinical, in which symptoms of mucus and itching precede signs. In stage 2, mild GPC, there are more symptoms and a mild papillary reaction of the tarsus, which can be better seen with fluorescein dye. In stage 3, moderate GPC, there may be excessive lens movement, the papillae are elevated, and the apices of the papillae may be white due to scarring, and stain with fluorescein (Fig. 102.9). In stage 4, severe GPC, patients are unable to wear contacts, papillae are larger (>1 mm) and may appear similar to those in vernal conjunctivitis. Histology of the conjunctiva in GPC is also similar to vernal conjunctivitis.[54] Numerous mediators of inflammation are elevated in the tears of patients with GPC.[50] In severe GPC, ptosis can develop. Instead of this staging system, it is common to rate the papillae 1–4 plus. Symptoms and signs may not correlate, as some patients are very symptomatic with mild findings and others are relatively free of symptoms with more findings. Symptoms are more important than signs, since they determine contact lens tolerance.

Treatment of GPC involves decreasing both the coating on contact lenses and the immune response. Replacing contacts is effective in enabling most patients to resume lens wear, and discontinuing lens wear for 3 to 4 weeks and then

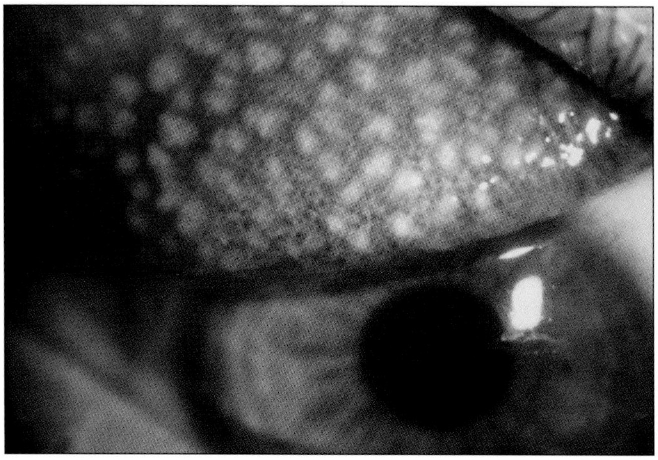

Fig. 102.9 Giant papillary conjunctivitis is associated with a papillary reaction of the body of the superior tarsus. Fibrosis causes whitening of the papillae, obscuring the fibrovascular core.

refitting patients with frequent-replacement or disposable daily-wear lenses is even more effective.[55] If patients are asymptomatic after discontinuing lens use, they can often resume lens wear with new contacts successfully, without staying out of contacts. A single-use, disposable daily-wear contact is the ideal lens for prevention and treatment of GPC. When not available, the next best approach is a frequent-replacement, daily-wear contact that is preferably replaced at least every 2 weeks.[56] Use of hydrogen peroxide solutions for disinfection and weekly enzymatic cleaning of frequent-replacement lenses are recommended.[49]

Standard treatment to reduce the immune response includes the use of mast cell stabilizers.[57] Chronic use of combination mast cell stabilizer and antihistamine drops are helpful to prevent recurrent mucus production and itching. These drops should be instilled before and after contact lens use. It is safest to avoid use of topical steroids, but in severe cases low- or mid-strength steroids can be used to control symptoms when patients discontinue contact lenses, prior to refitting. Necessary treatment depends on the severity of GPC at the time of diagnosis. The goal is to enable patients to wear contact lenses without recurrent symptoms. The papillae often persist, but can decrease slowly over a period of years. With proper management, over 90% of patients with GPC are able to wear contact lenses successfully.

Seasonal and perennial ocular allergies also reduce contact lens tolerance. Approximately 20% of the population has hay fever. Seasonal increase of symptoms associated with contact lens use is significantly higher in patients with than in those without allergies.[58] Environmental antigens are part of the coating on contact lenses, and contact lenses prolong antigenic exposure. Contact lenses have been described as an 'antigen depot.'[59] Contact lenses are inert plastics. The allergic response is to the coating on lenses, and not the lenses themselves. Extended wear of contact lenses is contraindicated in patients with ocular allergy.[59] Single-use dailies improved comfort in 67% of patients, compared to 18% with improvement by replacement of the same contacts.[60] Contact lens use should be discontinued temporarily when allergies are moderate to severe until they improve with treatment and/or there is a change in seasons.

Treatment of ocular allergies can enhance contact lens tolerance in patients with mild to moderate symptoms. Lubrication with tears can help to increase contact lens tolerance. In addition, topical mast cell stabilizer and or antihistamine eyedrops can be used before lens insertion and after lens removal, but not while lenses are being worn, in patients who have mild symptoms. Systemic antihistamine used to control allergic rhinitis can increase dry eyes. If adequate control of allergies is not possible with these measures, the addition of topical 0.05% ciclosporin for treatment of dry eyes and off-label treatment of allergies can be helpful, especially in patients with perennial allergies. Optimal management of ocular allergies is especially important in keratoconus patients who require RGP lenses for visual rehabilitation. Contact lens tolerance can decrease during the allergy season in these patients to the point of developing corneal abrasions. Use of lubricating gels and ointments at bedtime, in addition to the other treatment, can help to prevent this complication. More frequent replacement of RGP lenses, every 4 to 12 months, may also be necessary.

In addition to GPC, there are other contact lens-related causes of ptosis. A retained, lost RGP lens can cause unilateral ptosis with or without inflammation.[61,62] A mass may be present on lid eversion. Patients who wear RGP lenses can develop ptosis with disinsertion of the levator aponeurosis, probably due to pulling and stretching of the lids during lens removal.[63] Unilateral ptosis that is reversible can develop in patients who wear RGP lenses in one eye, such as for the correction of keratoconus, and does not require a neurological work-up for acquired ptosis.

Dry Eyes

Similar to allergies, contact lens use can both aggravate and cause dry eyes. Dry eyes is a frequent complaint in people wearing contacts, occurring in up to 75%, and the most common reason for discontinuing lens use.[64] The International Dry Eye Workshop has defined dry eye as a 'disease of the tears and ocular surface that results in symptoms of discomfort ... and is accompanied by increased osmolality of the tear film and inflammation of the ocular surface.'[65] The major advantage of silicone hydrogel lenses with increased oxygen permeability is for extended wear, but there are reports that people who are refitted with them have significantly fewer dry eye symptoms than with their previous hydrogel soft lenses.[66–68] Dehydration of silicone hydrogel lenses increases their oxygen permeability, in contrast to hydrogel lenses. Contact lens solutions also may affect dry eye symptoms.[64]

There is evidence that dehydration of the lens surface by evaporation is more important than water loss from the contact lens itself.[69] Evaporation of the tear film over a contact lens is higher than without a contact, and is independent of the lens water content or material.[70,71] Wearing contacts in normal humidity produces more tear film evaporation than without a contact lens in low humidity.[72] Evaporation of the tear film leads to a thinner, unstable tear film with decreased break-up time.[65] In addition, evaporation results in increased tear osmolality.[73] In this study, over half of the patients had contact lens-related dry eye by self-report. Significant factors associated with dry eye included female sex and use of high water (over 50%) content lenses, in addition to rapid prelens tear film thinning (evaporation) and increased tear film osmolality. Women have dry eye more often than men in general, so it is to be expected they would also have contact lens-related dry eye more often. High water contact lenses are used more often since the introduction of frequent-replacement and daily-disposable lenses, whereas, in the past, many conventional daily-wear contacts had low water content.

Contact lenses often increase dry eye symptoms. Patients may be asymptomatic without contacts and very symptomatic with them. Symptoms that increase later in the day, with longer duration of contact lens use, suggest the possibility of dry eyes. Worse symptoms in dry environments, including indoor heat in the winter and air conditioning in the summer, as well as activities involving prolonged use of the eyes, such as reading or computer work, also point to dry eyes. Lenses become tighter with increased hours of wear and can cause symptoms of dryness and burning. Difficulty in removing lenses also points to tight lenses. Fitting looser contacts can increase contact lens tolerance in many patients with dry eye symptoms.

Diagnosis and treatment of dry eyes can enhance contact lens tolerance in many patients. Blepharitis and meibomian gland disease cause evaporative dry eye which is aggravated by contact lens use. Treatment with warm compresses, artificial tears, antibiotic ointment at bedtime, topical ciclosporin 0.05% and, if needed, oral doxycycline can be very effective. It is important to recognize that blepharitis is a chronic condition that requires long-term treatment to be controlled. Aqueous deficient dry eye is also common. Treatment includes artificial tears, preferably unit-dose, preservative-free tears if used more than four times daily, topical ciclosporin 0.05% twice daily (before and after lens use), and punctal plugs. Lubricating drops can be used with lenses, and it is more effective to use them regularly in dry eye patients, rather than to wait until symptoms develop. Both lack of effect and benefit have been reported for topical ciclosporin 0.05% treatment of dry eye in contact lens wearers.[74,75] Beneficial effect or oral omega-6 fatty acids for contact lens-associated dry eye has been reported.[76] Many systemic medications can worsen dry eyes, including over-the-counter antihistamines. Oral contraceptives sometimes also can be associated with the development of dry eyes and contact lens intolerance. A careful history may determine if recent changes in systemic medications are factors which could be potentially modified, in collaboration with the patient's other physicians. Patients with mild to moderate dry eye can be successful wearing contact lenses, but contact lenses are contraindicated in patients with severe dry eye.[65]

Hypoxia

Acute hypoxia causes corneal swelling and, in extreme cases, a hypopyon, and chronic hypoxia results in corneal neovascularization and, in severe cases, sterile corneal infiltrates. These manifestations of moderate to severe acute and chronic hypoxia are less common than in the past due to the development of more gas-permeable materials for rigid, soft, and hybrid contact lenses. Acute edema due to contact lens overwear can occur in patients who use daily-wear lenses overnight. They can present with central full-thickness corneal edema, with or without a hypopyon, with an intact corneal epithelium, and without a corneal infiltrate. Acute symptoms of pain begin to diminish follow lens removal. Initial treatment includes cycloplegia and low-dose prophylactic topical antibiotics, and follow-up within 1 to 2 days. If improvement is not evident, and there continues to be no evidence of infection, topical steroids can be added and close follow-up continued. Following resolution, patients can resume use of daily-wear soft contacts only if improved compliance is assured. Chronic hypoxia can occur with overwear of low gas-permeable lenses, even on a daily-wear basis, such as early-generation hybrid lenses and high-powered (plus and minus) daily-wear soft contact lenses. Patients have relatively mild to moderate symptoms of redness and reduced contact lens tolerance. On examination, the findings of superficial and stromal corneal neovascularization, with and without corneal infiltrates and lipid deposits, are often greater than the symptoms. It is necessary to reduce or preferably discontinue wear of the offending contacts and refit the patient with more gas-permeable, looser lenses. The vessels often become inactive, but permanent scarring remains that varies in severity. Close follow-up every 3 to 4 months is necessary to make sure the corneal neovascularization is stable and the patient is compliant with recommended lens use.

Currently, lens materials are available that provide adequate oxygen transmission for daily- and extended-wear of soft and gas-permeable lenses. Although this represents a clinically important advance in contact lens technology, the new silicone hydrogel hyper-oxygen transmissible lenses have not reduced the problem of soft contact lens-associated infections, as was hoped.[8,9] Although these lenses have eliminated lens-induced hypoxia, the mechanical interaction with the cornea and the effects on the tear film are similar to other hydrogel lenses.[77] Studies have shown that both hypoxia and tear stagnation during overnight wear significantly impair the epithelial barrier function and that elimination of lens-induced hypoxia alone does not improve the epithelium.[78] The conclusion was that it is necessary to eliminate both hypoxia and tear stagnation to prevent damage to the corneal epithelium associated with extended wear of contact lenses. Epithelial damage is considered a prerequisite for bacteria (and other organisms) bound to contact lenses to infiltrate the cornea and cause microbial keratitis.[79] Although the advent of silicone hydrogel lenses has not reduced the risk of contact lens-associated corneal infections, there is evidence that they have improved comfort and reduced dryness and redness.[68]

Hypoxia is a major issue for overnight wear of contact lens, but less of an issue for daily wear of contacts. Since elimination of hypoxia has not reduced the risk of corneal infections associated with extended wear, daily wear is preferred, and patients need to be informed regarding the continued increased risk of overnight wear. Increasing the oxygen transmissibility of lens materials sometimes has adverse effects on other properties. For example, RGP wearers may have decreased lens tolerance with high-Dk materials, compared with mid-Dk materials. In 2008 in the USA, silicone hydrogel lenses were fit in over half (54%) of people wearing contacts, lenses were used for daily wear in 65%, and a 2-week replacement schedule in almost half (44%).[2] Advantages of silicone hydrogel lenses for daily wear in people who are asymptomatic in other soft lenses have not been documented.

Corneal Warpage

Corneal warpage refers to contact lens-induced irregular astigmatism. It is reversible over a period of weeks. It causes spectacle blur when glasses are used after contact lens removal. In addition, the manifest refraction changes, and patients may not be correctable to 20/20 visual acuity. On topography, irregular astigmatism is present, often with inferior steepening that can appear similar to keratoconus (Fig. 102.10). There is no corneal thinning or other signs of

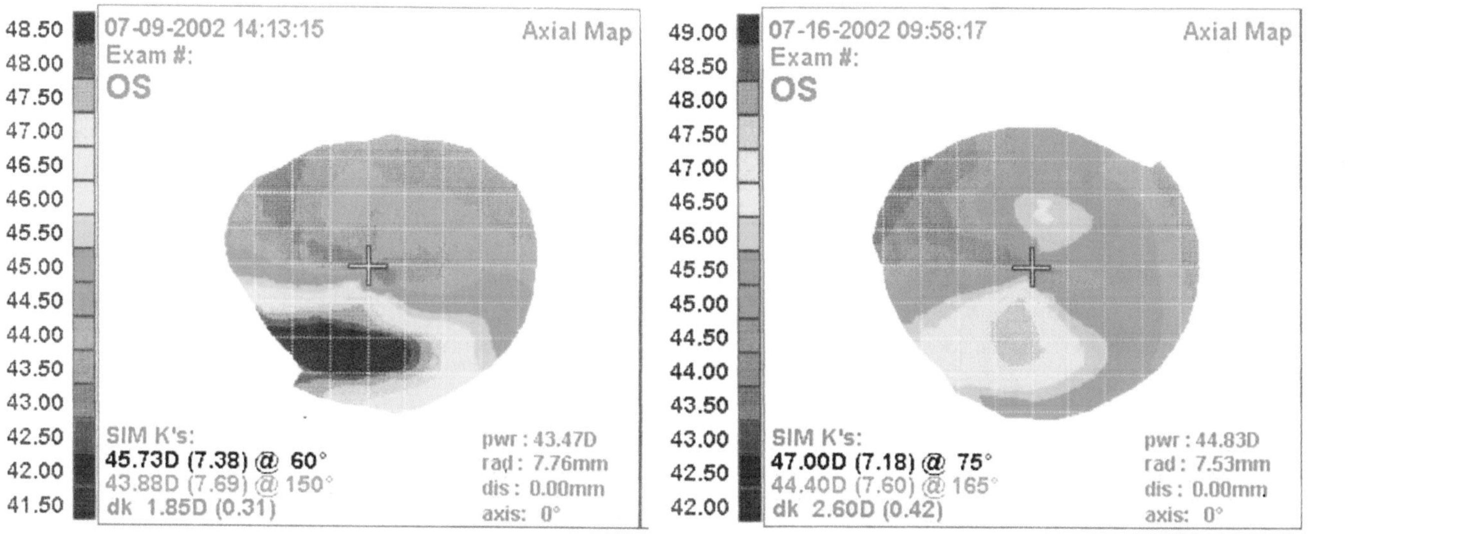

Fig. 102.10 Corneal warpage induced by a bifocal rigid gas-permeable lens resulted in inferior steepening (*left*). One week after discontinuing lens wear in that eye, irregular astigmatism is resolving (*right*).

keratoconus. Corneal warpage was much more common in the past, associated with the use of PMMA lenses, but still occurs in association with gas-permeable and, occasionally, soft contacts. Patients who wear contacts should also have glasses so that they can monitor their vision with glasses, and also so they do not overwear contacts if they develop symptoms.

When corneal warpage is suspected, contact lens wear should be discontinued until the refraction and topography stabilize. This is often difficult to do because patients can't see well with glasses and their manifest refraction is variable. Frequently, it is helpful to discontinue lenses one eye at a time and prescribe temporary glasses. It can take weeks for the cornea to recover, and recovery is slower in patients with a history of rigid gas-permeable lens use than soft contact lens use. After the topography and refraction are stable for consecutive visits, glasses are prescribed, contact lenses can be refitted using a different type of contact, and patients are monitored closely to be sure the problem does not recur. Patients with corneal warpage are not candidates for refractive surgery until the problem resolves and their refractions and topographies are determined to be stable. As mild degrees of corneal warpage are more frequent and less symptomatic, people wearing contacts are routinely asked to discontinue lenses at least 2 (soft contacts) to 3 (RGP contacts) weeks prior to refractive surgery and to have stability of their refraction and topography documented.[80] If patients have slit lamp signs of keratoconus, such as thinning and ectasia, they have keratoconus and not warpage, and should not be advised to discontinue contact lens use.

Conclusions

Contact lenses are worn by millions of people and are generally very safe. There is a wide range of contact lens-related complications that vary greatly in severity. A history regarding contact lens use is important in all patients. Early diagnosis and treatment are necessary to optimize the outcomes of patients with complications and enable many of them to successfully resume contact lens wear. Single-use, daily-disposable lenses have advantages with regard to both serious and nonserious complications. Patients who wear contact lenses are also at risk for ocular problems unrelated to lenses, especially associated with myopia, and should receive comprehensive eye care. Every eye examination is an opportunity for patient education to reduce complications.

References

1. Barr JT. 20 years of contact lenses. *Contact Lens Spectrum.* 2006;21: 28–38.
2. Nichols JJ. Contact lenses 2008. *Contact Lens Spectrum.* 2009;24:24–32.
3. Stein RM, Clinch TE, Cohen EJ, et al. Infected versus sterile corneal infiltrates in contact lens wear. *Am J Ophthalmol.* 1988;105:632–636.
4. Clemons CS, Cohen EJ, Arentsen JJ, Donnenfeld ED, Laibson PR. *Pseudomonas* ulcers following patching of corneal abrasions associated with contact lens wear. *CLAO.* 1987;13:161–164.
5. Van Meter WS, Musch DC, Jacobs DS, et al. Safety of overnight orthokeratology for myopia. A report by the American Academy of Ophthalmology. *Ophthalmology.* 2008;115:2301–2313.
6. Schein OD, Glynn RJ, Poggio EC. The relative risk of ulcerative keratitis among daily-wear and extended-wear soft contact lenses. *N Engl J Med.* 1989;321:773–778.
7. Poggio EC, Gl;ynn RJ, Schein OD. The incidence of ulcerative keratitis among users of daily-wear and extended-wear soft contact lenses. *N Engl J Med.* 1989;321:779–783.
8. Dart JKG, Radford CF, Minassian D, Verma S, Stapleton F. Risk factors for microbial keratitis with contemporary contact lenses. *Ophthalmology.* 2008;115:1647–1654.
9. Stapleton F, Keary L, Edwards K, et al. The incidence of contact lens-related microbial keratitis in Australia. *Ophthalmology.* 2008;115:1655–1162.
10. Keay L, Edwards K, Dart J, Stapleton F. Grading contact lens-related microbial keratitis: relevance to disease burden. *Optom Vis Sci.* 2008;85: 531–537.
11. Keay L, Edwards K, Naduvilath T, Forde K, Stapleton F. Factors affecting the morbidity of contact lens-related microbial keratitis: a population study. *Invest Ophthalmol Vis Sci.* 2006;47:4302–4308.
12. Stapleton F, Keay LJ, Sanfilippo PG, et al. Relationship between climate, disease severity, and causative organism for contact lens-associated microbial keratitis in Australia. *Am J Ophthalmol.* 2007;144:690–698.
13. Rattanatam T, Heng WJ, Rapuano CJ, Laibson PR, Cohen EJ. Trends in contact lens-related corneal ulcers. *Cornea.* 2001;20:290–294.
14. Mah-Sadorra JH, Yavuz SGA, Najjar DM, et al. *Cornea.* 2005;24:51–58.
15. Keay L, Edwards K, Naduvilath T, et al. Microbial keratitis predisposing factors and morbidity. *Ophthalmology.* 2006;113:109–116.
16. Iyer SA, Tuli SS, Wagoner RC. Fungal keratitis: emerging trends and treatment outcomes. *Eye Contact Lens.* 2006;32:267–271.
17. Alfonso EC, Miller D, Cantu-Dibildox J, O'Brien, TP, Schein OD. Fungal keratitis associated with non-therapeutic soft contact lenses. *Am J Ophthalmol.* 2006;142:154–155.
18. Alfonso EC, Cantu-Dibildox J, Munir WM, et al. Insurgence of *Fusarium* keratitis associated with contact lens wear. *Arch Ophthalmol.* 2006;124: 941–947.
19. Chang DC, Grant GB, O'Donnell, et al. Multistate outbreak of *Fusarium* keratitis associated with use of a contact lens solution. *JAMA.* 2006; 296:953–963.
20. Rao SK, Lam PT, Li EY, Yuen HK, Lam DS. A case series of contact lens-associated *Fusarium* keratitis in Hong Kong. *Cornea.* 2007;26:1205–1209.
21. Yu DK, Ng AS, Lau WW, Wong CC, Chan CW. Recent pattern of contact lens-related keratitis in Hong Kong. *Eye Contact Lens.* 2007;33:284–287.
22. Khor WB, Aung T, Saw SM, et al. An outbreak of *Fusarium* keratitis associated with contact lens wear in Singapore. *JAMA.* 2006;295:2867–2873.
23. Saw SM, Ooi PL, Tan DT, et al. Risk factors for contact lens-related *Fusarium* keratitis: a case-control study in Singapore. *Arch Ophthalmol.* 2007;125:611–617.
24. Saviola JF. New directions in contact lens care testing. *Eye Contact Lens.* 2008;300–301.
25. Gorscak JJ, Ayres BD, Bhagat N, et al. An outbreak of *Fusarium* keratitis associated with contact lens use in the northeastern United States. *Cornea.* 2007;26:1187–1194.
26. Bullock JD. Use of the Poisson probability mass function in a retrospective evaluation of the worldwide *Fusarium* keratitis epidemic of 2004–6. *Cornea.* 2008;1013–1017.
27. Munir WM, Rosenfeld SI, Udell I, et al. Clinical response of contact lens-associated fungal keratitis to topical fluoroquinolone therapy. *Cornea.* 2007;26:621–624.
28. Stehr-Green JK, Bailey TM, Brandt FH, et al. *Acanthamoeba* keratitis in soft contact lens wearers; a case-control study. *JAMA.* 1987;258:57–60.
29. Meier PA, Mathers WD, Sutphin JE, et al. An epidemic of presumed *Acnathamoeba* keratitis that followed regional flooding: results of a case-control investigation. *Arch Ophthalmol.* 1998;116:1090–1094.
30. Joslin CE, Tu EY, McMahon TT, et al. Epidemiological characteristics of a Chicago-area *Acanthamoeba* keratitis outbreak. *Am J Ophthalmol.* 2006; 142:212–217.
31. Thebpatiphat N, Hammersmith KM, Rocha FN, et al. *Acanthamoeba* keratitis: a parasite on the rise. *Cornea.* 2007;26:701–706.
32. Joslin CE, Tu EY, Shoff ME, et al. The association of contact lens solution use and *Acanthamoeba* keratitis. *Am J Ophthalmol.* 2007;144:169–180.
33. MMWR *Acanthamoeba* keratitis – multiple states, 2005–2007. May 26, 2007;56;1–3. http://www.cdc.gov/mmwr.
34. Tu ET, Joslin CE, Sugar J, Shoff ME, Booten GC. Prognostic factors affecting visual outcome in *Acanthamoeba* keratitis. *Ophthalmology.* 2008;115: 1998–2003.
35. Sun X, Zhang Y, Li R, et al. *Acanthamoeba* keratitis. *Ophthalmology.* 2006;113:412–416.
36. Lim N, Goh D, Bunce C, et al. Comparison of polyhexamethylene biguanide and chlorhexidine as monotherapy agents in the treatment of *Acanthamoeba* keratitis. *Am J Ophthalmol.* 2008;145:130–135.

37. Anger C, Lally JM. *Acanthamoeba*: a review of its potential to cause keratitis, current lens care solution disinfection standards and methodologies, and strategies to reduce patient risk. *Eye Contact Lens.* 2008;34:247–253.
38. Hiti K, Walochnik J, Haller-Schober EM, Fashinger C, Aspock H. Efficacy of contact lens storage solutions against different *Acanthamoeba* strains. *Cornea.* 2006;25:423–427.
39. Kilvington S, Heaselgrave W, Lally JM, Ambrus K, Powell H. Encystment of *Acanthamoeba* during incubation in multipurpose contact lens disinfectant solutions and experimental formulations. *Eye Contact Lens.* 2008;34:133–139.
40. Shoff ME, Joslin CE, Kubatko L, Fuerst PA. Efficacy of contact lens systems against recent clinical and tap water *Acanthamoeba* isolates. *Cornea.* 2008;27:713–719.
41. Mowrey-McKee M, George M. Contact lens solution efficacy against *Acanthamoeba castellani. Eye Contact Lens.* 2007;33:211–215.
42. Beattie TK, Tomlinson A, McFadyen AK. Attachment of *Acanthamoeba* to first- and second-generation silicone hydrogel contact lenses. *Ophthalmology.* 2006;113:117–125.
43. Miller RA, Brightbill FS, Slama SL. Superior limbic keratoconjunctivitis in soft contact lens wearers. *Cornea.* 1982;1:293.
44. Stenson S. Superior limbic keratitis associated with soft contact lens use. *Arch Ophthalmol.* 1983;101:4-2-404.
45. Bloomfield SE, Jakobiec FA, Theodore FH. Contact lens induced keratopathy: a severe complication extending the spectrum of keratoconjunctivitis in contact lens wearers. *Ophthalmology.* 1984;91:290–294.
46. Mondino BJ, Brawman-Mintzer O, Boothe WA. Immunological complications of soft contact lenses. *J Am Optom Assoc.* 1987;58:832–835.
47. Sendele DD, Kenyon KR, Mobilia EF. Superior limbic keratoconjunctivitis in contact lens wearers. *Ophthalmology.* 1982;90:616–622.
48. Fuerst DJ, Sugar J, Worobec S. Superior limbic keratoconjunctivitis associated with cosmetic soft contact lens wear. *Arch Ophthalmol.* 1983;101:1214–1216.
49. Donshik PC, Ehlers WH, Ballow M. Giant papillary conjunctivitis. *Immunol Allergy Clin N Am.* 2008;28:83–103.
50. Elhers WH, Donshik PC. Giant papillary conjunctivitis. *Curr Opin Allergy Clin Immunol.* 2008;8:445–449.
51. Allansmith MR, Korb, DR, Greiner JV, et al. Giant papillary conjunctivitis in contact lens wearers. *Am J Ophthalmol.* 1977;83:697–698.
52. Chung CW, Santim R, Heng W, et al. Use of SoftPerm contact lenses when rigid gas permeable lenses fail. *CLAO J.* 2001;27:202–208.
53. Ozkurt Y, Karaman OY, Ozgur O, Dogan OK. A retrospective case series: use of SoftPerm contact lenses in patients with keratoconus. *Eye Contact Lens.* 2007;33:103–105.
54. Allansmith MR, Baird RS, Greiner JV. Vernal conjunctivitis and contact lens-associated giant papillary conjunctivitis compared and contrasted. *Am J Ophthalmol.* 1979;87:544–555.
55. Donshik PC. Giant papillary conjunctivitis. *Trans Am Ophthalmol Soc.* 1994;92:687–744.
56. Porazinski AD, Donshik PC. Giant papillary conjunctivitis in frequent replacement contact lens wearers: a retrospective study. *CLAO J.* 1999;25:142–147.
57. Lustine T, Bouchard CS, Cavanagh HD. Continued contact lens wear in patients with giant papillary conjunctivitis. *CLAO J.* 1991;17:104–107.
58. Kumar P, Elston R, Black D, et al. Allergic rhinoconjunctivitis and contact lens intolerance. *CLAO J.* 1991;17:31–34.
59. Lemp MA, Bielory L. Contact lenses and associated anterior segment disorders: dry eye disease, blepharitis, and allergy. *Immunol Allergy Clin N Am.* 2008;28:105–107.
60. Hayes VY, Schnider CM, Veys J. An evaluation of 1-day disposable contact lens wear in a population of allergy sufferers. *Cont Lens Anterior Eye.* 2003;26:85–93.
61. Yassin JG, White RH, Shannon GM. Blepharoptosis as a complication of contact lens migration. *Am J Ophthalmol.* 1971;72:536–537.
62. Zola E, van der Meulen IJ, Lapid-Gortzak R, van Vliet JM, Nieuwendaal CP. A conjunctival mass in the deep fornix after a long retained hard contact lens in a patient with keloids. *Cornea.* 2008;27:1204–1206.
63. van den Bosch WA, Lemij HG. Blepharoptosis induced by prolonged hard contact lens wear. *Ophthalmology.* 1992;99:1759–1765.
64. Sindt CW, Longmuir RA. Contact lens strategies for the patient with dry eye. *Ocul Surf.* 2007;5:294–307.
65. Lemp MA. The definition and classification of dry eye disease: report of the definition and classification subcommittee of the international dry eye workshop. *Ocul Surf.* 2007;5:75–92.
66. Dillehay SM, Miller MB. Performance of Lotrafilcon B silicone hydrogel contact lenses in experienced low-Dk/t daily lens wearers. *Eye Contact Lens.* 2007;33:272–277.
67. Schafer J, Mitchell GL, Chalmers RL, et al. The stability of dryness symptoms after refitting with silicone hydrogel contact lenses over 3 years. *Eye Contact Lens.* 2007;33:247–252.
68. Dillehay SM. Does the level of available oxygen impact comfort in contact lens wear?: review of the literature. *Eye Contact Lens.* 2007;3:148–155.
69. Ketelson HA, Meadows DL, Stone RP. Dynamic wetability properties of a soft contact lens hydrogel. *Colloids Surf B Biointerfaces.* 2005;40:1–9.
70. Holly F. Tear film physiology and contact lens wear II. Contact lens–tear film interaction. *Am J Optom Physiol Opt.* 1981;58:331–341.
71. Thai LC, Tomlinson A, Doane MG. Effect of contact lens materials on tear physiology. *Optom Vis Sci.* 2004;81:194–204.
72. Guillon M, Maissa C. Contact lens wear affects tear film evaporation. *Eye Contact Lens.* 2008;3:326–330.
73. Nichols JJ, Sinnott, LT. Tear film, contact lens, and patient-related factors associated with contact lens-related dry eye. *Invest Ophthalmol Vis Sci.* 2006;47:1319–1328.
74. Willen CM, McGwin G, Liu B, Owsley C, Rosenstiel C. Efficacy of cyclosporine 0.05% ophthalmic emulsion in contact lens wearers with dry eyes. *Eye Contact Lens.* 2008;34:43–45.
75. Hom MM. Use of cyclosporine 0.05% ophthalmic emulsion for contact lens-intolerant patients. *Eye Contact Lens.* 2006;32:109–111.
76. Kokke KH, Morris JA, Lawrenson JG. Oral omega-6 essential fatty acid treatment in contact lens associated dry eye. *Cont Lens Anterior Eye.* 2008;31:141–146.
77. Stapleton F, Stretton, S Papas E, Skotnitsky C, Sweeney DF. Silicone hydrogel contact lenses and the ocular surface. *Ocul Surf.* 2006;4:24–43.
78. Lin MC, Polse KA. Hypoxia, overnight-wear, and tear stagnation effects on the corneal epithelium: data and a proposed model. *Eye Contact Lens.* 2007;33:378–381.
79. McGlinchey SM, McCoy CP, Gorman Sp, Jones DS. Key biological issues in contact lens development. *Expert Rev Med Devices.* 2008;5:581–590.
80. Hashemi H, Firoozabadi MR, Mehravaran S, Gorouhi F. Corneal stability after discontinued soft contact lens wear. *Cont Lens Anterior Eye.* 2008;31:122–125.

PART VIII

THE SCLERA AND ANTERIOR UVEA

Chapter 103

Episcleritis

Eric S. Pearlstein

Episcleritis is a relatively benign, self-limiting condition affecting the outer coat of the eye. There are few if any serious sequelae, and it therefore demands little in terms of evaluation and treatment. Clinically, the condition is categorized as either simple or nodular.[1] Nodular episcleritis has a well-demarcated, elevated area of inflamed episcleral tissue. The simple form demonstrates vascular congestion of the episclera but without a discrete nodule.

Episcleritis should not be thought of as simply a mild version of scleritis. These two diseases should instead be regarded as distinct clinical entities, since the implications of the usually harmless episcleritis differ significantly from the more ominous scleritis.

Anatomy

The episclera is comparable to a synovial membrane, allowing smooth movements of the globe as would the synovial tissue in a ball-and-socket joint.[2] The rheumatologic analogy goes further when one considers the higher incidence of scleral and episcleral inflammatory conditions associated with rheumatologic conditions.

The episclera is a fibroelastic structure consisting of collagen bundles, fibroblasts, melanocytes, proteoglycans, and glycoproteins.[3,4] It has two layers: an outer parietal layer and a deep visceral layer. These two layers are loosely fused by fine connecting fibers.[2] The outer parietal layer, which is the more superficial, is vascularized by the superficial episcleral capillary plexus. This capillary plexus with its uniquely straight and radially oriented vessels helps distinguish this layer from the deep visceral layer (Fig. 103.1). The outer parietal layer fuses with the muscle sheaths. As it approaches the limbus, the outer parietal layer also fuses with conjunctiva and the deep visceral layer of episclera.

The visceral layer, which is closely adherent to the sclera, contains the deep episcleral capillary plexus. The freely anastomosing configuration of this capillary plexus characterizes this layer. Both the superficial and deep plexuses derive their blood supply predominantly from the anterior ciliary arteries. However, the posterior ciliary arteries do provide some episcleral circulation posterior to the muscle insertions.[3]

While the vascular plexus of the conjunctiva is also somewhat interlacing, it is readily distinguished from the two deeper layers by its free mobility over them.

Incidence

Episcleritis is not a very common condition. The true incidence is difficult to determine, however, since patients often do not seek medical advice for self-limiting, asymptomatic conditions. Williamson has suggested that 0.08% of new hospital visits may be attributable to episcleritis.[5]

Several large studies have been conducted that offer significant insight into the characteristics of patients with episcleritis: Watson and Hayreh's[1] reported cases from the Moorfield's Eye Hospital (group I), Sainz de la Maza et al.[6] study from The Massachusetts Eye and Ear Infirmary (group II), Akpek et al.[7] also from The Massachusetts Eye and Ear Infirmary (group III), Jabs et al.[8] from The Wilmer Eye Institute (group IV), and the pediatric study by Read et al.[9] at the University of Washington (group V). Table 103.1 provides an overview of their findings. The adult groups found either no significant sex predilection or a predominance of women affected. The pediatric group demonstrated mostly male involvement. All study groups found the simple variety of episcleritis to be the most common. Sixty-seven percent of simple episcleritis is so-called sectoral, involving only one sector (Fig. 103.2), and 33% have the diffuse variety of simple episcleritis, according to study group I.

Clinical Manifestations

History

Episcleritis generally has an acute onset, particularly in the simple form. A patient is often able to pinpoint the exact time that a painful episode began. Nodular episcleritis may have a somewhat more insidious onset. However, approximately half of the time discomfort may not be the presenting complaint, since the condition may be asymptomatic.[1] An area of episcleral painless injection may be noted incidentally.

When pain is present in episcleritis, it is usually a mild discomfort. The terms hot, prickly, and foreign body-like are most commonly used to describe the sensation. It is possible, although quite rare, to have severe pain in episcleritis. If pain of this degree is present, the diagnosis of episcleritis is in question, and one should suspect scleritis.

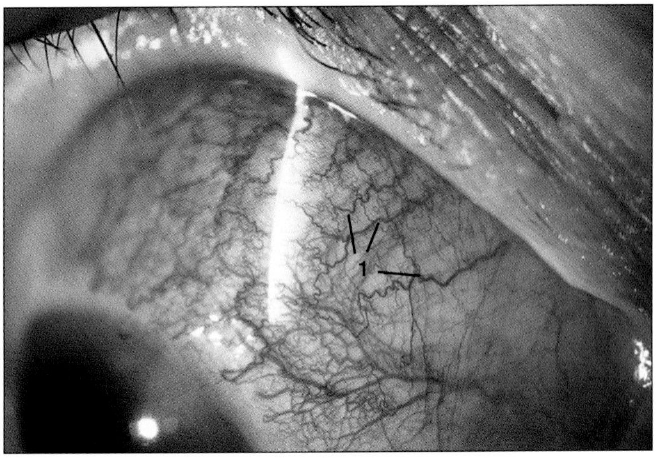

Fig. 103.1 Simple episcleritis. Note the engorgement of the radially oriented superficial episcleral vessels (*1*).

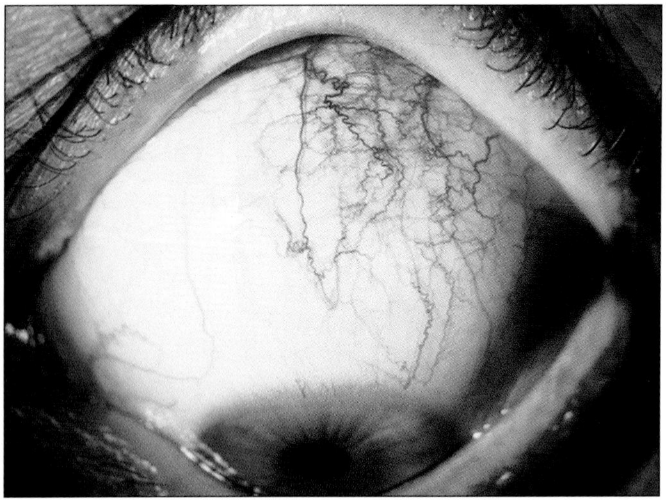

Fig. 103.2 Simple episcleritis. Note the sectoral involvement of vascular dilation. The conjunctival and superficial episcleral vessels are particularly prominent.

Table 103.1 Characteristics of patients with episcleritis

	Group I*	Group II†	Group III#	Group IV+	Group V@
Number of eyes	217	127	132	55	18
Simple/nodular	78%/22%	83%/17%	84%/16%	81%/19%	92%/8%
Sex (% female)	45	74	69	70	17
Average age	Fourth to fifth decade	43 years	43 years	45 years	9 years
Bilaterality	37%	35%	32%	49%	50%
Associated diseases	26%	32%	36%	35%	50%

* *Data from Watson PG, Hayreh SS.* Br J Ophthalmol *60:163, 1976.*
† *Data from Sainz de la Maza M et al.* Ophthalmology *101:389, 1994.*
# *Data from Akpek EK et al.* Ophthalmology *106:729, 1999*
+ *Data from Jabs DA et al.* Am J Ophthalmol *130:469, 2000*
@ *Data from Read RW et al.* Ophthalmology *106:2377, 1999*

Photophobia is present in a small number of patients.[1] Tenderness may also be described and is usually localized to the inflamed area. An important historical point is the exclusion of ocular discharge. While infectious conditions typically cause either a purulent or a mucopurulent discharge, episcleritis causes only a watery discharge.

Physical examination

Visual acuity in episcleritis patients is typically unaffected. Lid edema as well as chemosis may be present in severe cases.[2] Bulbar injection, which may be diffuse or sectoral, is typically fiery or brick red. Natural sunlight and an unmagnified view can be useful in distinguishing the redness of episcleritis from the violaceous hue of scleritis. The injection of episcleritis occurs typically in the interpalpebral area.[10] Although engorged, the radially oriented vessels of the superficial episcleral capillary plexus maintain a normal architecture. The use of the red-free light is quite helpful to delineate clearly the vascular pattern. Should there appear to be any distortion of the normal vascular anatomy, one should suspect deeper inflammation involving the sclera.

A useful technique to aid in visualizing the vascular anatomy involves topical phenylephrine.[11] Phenylephrine at a concentration of 2.5% will blanch only the conjunctival vasculature, thus permitting one to examine clearly the vascular pattern of the deeper layers. This aids, therefore, in the distinction of conjunctivitis from episcleritis. The use of 10% phenylephrine will blanch not only the superficial layer of conjunctiva but also the superficial episcleral capillary plexus. It will not, however, blanch the deep plexus, thus aiding in the distinction between episcleritis and scleritis.

The use of a narrow, bright slit beam is crucial in distinguishing the nodule of episcleritis from scleritis. Noting the relation of the innermost reflection of light, which rests on the sclera and the visceral layer, to the more superficial

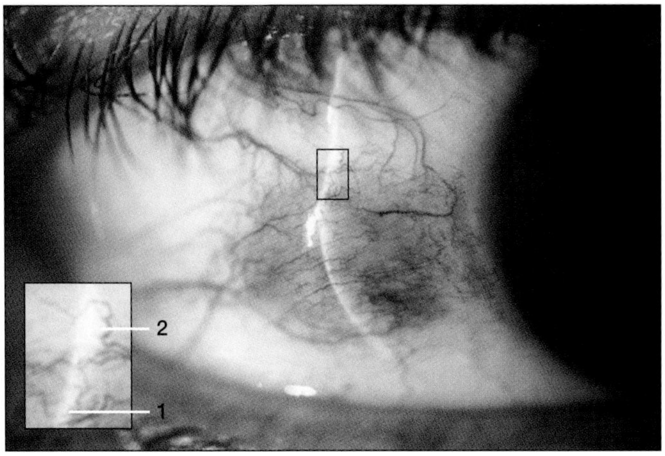

Fig. 103.3 Nodular episcleritis. In the enlarged inset, note that the nodule is displacing the anterior reflection of light (*1*), while the light reflected from the sclera shows no displacement (*2*).

reflection, which arises from the outer parietal layer, is most important. In nodular episcleritis the inner reflection of light will appear undisturbed, whereas the outer reflection will be clearly displaced forward (Fig. 103.3). In nodular scleritis, both beams will be displaced forward.

The cornea in episcleritis is typically unaffected. Although rare, corneal involvement may be cause for excessive lacrimation, photophobia, and temporary diminution of visual acuity. (For a further discussion of corneal complications, see Complications below.)

Course

The natural history of the disease is determined by the variety of episcleritis. Simple episcleritis is bilateral in 40% of cases, whereas nodular episcleritis is bilateral 13% of the time.[6] There are two classic presentations of episcleritis. The first presentation typically peaks 24 hours after the onset of symptoms. A slow improvement develops in 5 to 10 days, with complete resolution usually by 2 to 3 weeks. This form has a tendency to recur either in the same eye, the fellow eye, a different sector, or even interchangeably between simple and nodular episcleritis. Recurrence rates as high as 60% have been noted, with the first recurrence typically within 2 months of the first attack. Recurrences may then continue for 3 to 6 years, with decreasing frequency after 3 to 4 years.[3,12] These patients typically have a moderate or severe attack and usually have no associated systemic disease.

The other presentation of episcleritis is milder, with more prolonged attacks and no regularity to the intervals between attacks. These are typically the patients with associated systemic diseases.[1,3]

The nodular variety is usually more uncomfortable than the simple variety and also has a more protracted course. The firm nodule is freely mobile over the underlying tissues and may either be solitary or appear as multiple lesions. Although the diameter is typically 2–3 mm, nodules as large as 6 mm have been described.[3] The nodule will increase in size for 2 to 3 days and may persist for 2 months, although 4 to 5 weeks would be an average duration. The nodule of episcleritis does not necrose.

Recurrent attacks of episcleritis in the same location may lead to an alteration of the superficial scleral lamellae. These variably sized lamellae, which consist of collagen and elastic tissue, are arranged in a random orientation. The orientation and irregular size of the lamellae account in part for the opaque nature of the sclera.[2] Recurrent episodes may change this random orientation to a more regular one, as one sees in the cornea, and thus increase the scleral translucency. The underlying blue color of the uveal tissue may then be more visible and should not be mistaken for an area of scleral thinning, which may occur in scleritis but not in episcleritis.

Differential Diagnosis

Conjunctivitis must be considered in the differential diagnosis of episcleritis. Viral conjunctivitis, with its classic watery discharge, may be mistaken for episcleritis. However, the presence of palpebral conjunctival injection, conjunctival follicles, and preauricular adenopathy is useful in the diagnosis of conjunctivitis.

Phlyctenular conjunctivitis may be confused with nodular episcleritis. However, the conjunctiva is mobile over an episcleral nodule, whereas a phlyctenule lies within the conjunctiva.[13] In addition, phlyctenules may ulcerate.

Scleritis can be mistakenly diagnosed as episcleritis. The distinguishing clinical features have already been discussed.

An isolated episcleral plasmacytoma has been misdiagnosed as nodular epislceritis.[14]

Pathology

The histopathology reveals a nongranulomatous inflammation with vascular dilation and perivascular infiltration of lymphocytes and plasma cells.[2,3] Extracellular accumulation of proteinaceous fluid is also typically present. Biopsy of episcleral nodules in rheumatoid arthritis patients has shown the histopathology to be similar to that of subcutaneous rheumatoid nodules.[3,4]

Angiography

Angiography is rarely necessary for episcleritis. Investigations using fluorescein and indocyanine green[15] have shown the vascular pattern of the episcleral vessels to maintain a normal configuration while demonstrating an accelerated transit time and increased vascular permeability.[16] Once the inflammatory episode has resolved, no angiographically demonstrable evidence of the attack remains.[8,16]

Complications

Fortunately, complications are uncommon in episcleritis. However, patients with recurrent disease do have a higher rate of complications.[7]

Box 103.1 Diseases associated with episcleritis

A. Collagen-vascular and other inflammatory diseases
  1. Rheumatoid arthritis*
  2. Inflammatory bowel disease
    a. Crohn's disease*
    b. Ulcerative colitis
  3. Psoriatic arthritis
  4. Systemic lupus erythematosus
  5. Reiter's syndrome
  6. Relapsing polychondritis
  7. Ankylosing spondylitis
  8. Pustulotic arthro-osteitis (PAO)[41]

B. Vasculitic diseases
  1. Polyarteritis nodosa
  2. Temporal arteritis
  3. Cogan's syndrome
  4. Churg-Strauss syndrome
  5. Wegener's granulomatosis
  6. Behçet's disease

C. Dermatologic diseases
  1. Rosacea*
  2. Pyoderma gangrenosum
  3. Sweet's syndrome (acute febrile neutrophilic dermatosis)[42]

D. Metabolic diseases
  1. Gout*

E. Atopy*

F. Malignancies
  1. T-cell leukemia
  2. Hodgkin's lymphoma

G. Foreign body
  1. Vegetable matter
  2. Animal matter (insect hairs)
  3. Mineral matter (suture, talc, stones)

H. Chemical injury

I. Infectious
  1. Bacteria
  2. *Mycobacteria*
    a. Atypical mycobacterial disease
    b. Tuberculosis
    c. Hansen's disease
  3. Spirochetes
    a. Syphilis
    b. Lyme disease
  4. *Chlamydia*
  5. *Actinomyces*
    a. Nocardiosis
  6. Fungi
    a. Filamentous
    b. Dimorphic
  7. Viruses
    a. Herpes zoster*
    b. Herpes simplex
    c. Mumps
    d. Chikungunya
  8. Parasites
    a. Protozoa
      i. *Acanthamoeba*
      ii. Toxoplasmosis
    b. Helminths
      i. Toxocariasis

J. Medications
  1. Topiramate
  2. Pamidronate disodium
  3. Erlotinib
  4. Risedronate

** Most common associations.*
Adapted from Foster CS, Sainz de la Maza M. The sclera, *New York, 1994, Springer-Verlag.*

Mild anterior uveitis has been reported to occur in as many as 11% of patients.[1,5,7] Intermediate uveitis (pars planitis) is rarely seen with episcleritis.

Corneal changes are uncommon and mild. Corneal dellen formation may occur adjacent to an episcleral nodule close to the limbus. Infiltrates in the corneal periphery may also develop in an area adjacent to the episcleral inflammation, but these are usually transient and never progress to an ulcerative keratitis.[6] The highest reported rate of decreased vision occurred in 2% of patients followed over 11 years, in study group II. Most reduction in visual acuity associated with episcleritis is secondary to naturally progressing cataractous lens changes. Glaucoma was present in 4% of patients in group II and 8% in group III. Therefore, any lens opacification or glaucoma may be a reflection of natural development or a complication of steroid use rather than a complication of episcleritis.

Etiology

The majority of episcleritis cases in adults are idiopathic in nature. However, a significant number of patients have an associated systemic condition (Box 103.1). From 26% to 36% of adult patients have an associated disorder.[1,6,7] From 5% to 14% have collagen vascular disease or vasculitis, with rheumatoid arthritis as the most common association. Episcleritis has actually been the presenting sign of a vasculitic condition (Wegener's granulomatosis and Cogan's syndrome) in a number of patients.[7] Akpek et al.[7] found 51% of patients to have some concurrent eye disease. These associated eye conditions include ocular rosacea, keratoconjunctivitis sicca, and atopic keratoconjunctivitis. Acne rosacea with its associated lid disease is seen in 2% to 24%.[1,6,7] From 1% to 4% of patients have inflammatory bowel disease (IBD), usually Crohn's disease. In fact, the tendency of IBD patients to have Crohn's disease, rather than ulcerative colitis, is so strong that if a patient with ulcerative colitis is noted to have epislceritis the gastroenterologic diagnosis should be seriously reconsidered.[17] From 1% to 12% of atopic patients, with seasonal as well as perennial allergies, have episcleritis.[1,6,7] Interestingly, the incidence of atopy in episcleritis patients was found to be the same as in the general population.[18] Two to seven percent of episcleritis patients have herpes zoster ophthalmicus with a self-resolving episcleritis that left no sequelae.[1,6] Herpes simplex-induced episcleritis (1%) also usually resolves without sequelae. One percent of patients may have had a chemical injury inducing the episcleritis.[2,6] Foreign materials, whether talc, animal, or vegetable matter, may induce episcleritis. A transcleral suture used to support an intraocular lens has been reported to induce episcleritis.[19] Children between ages 5 and 16 years, who were diagnosed with episcleritis, had an associated systemic disease 67% of the time.[9]

Gout is certainly associated with episcleritis. Eleven percent of episcleritis patients have an elevated serum uric acid level and 7% have clinical gout.[1] Episcleritis has been reported as the initial presentation of patients with Hodgkin's lymphoma[20] and pyoderma gangrenosum.[21] Infectious diseases such as tuberculosis,[1] leprosy,[3] Lyme disease,[22] brucellosis,[23] mumps,[24] *Acanthamoeba* infection,[6] toxoplasmosis,[25] and chikungunya[26] are associated with episcleritis. Syphilis in the primary, secondary, or tertiary form may be associated with episcleritis.[27]

Episcleritis has been described as an adverse ocular event with the following drugs: topiramate,[28] pamidronate disodium,[29] risedronate,[30] and erlotinib.[31] Stress and hormonal changes are often mentioned as a possible precipitating factor for episcleritis, but most of the reports are anecdotal. The physician who developed recurrent episcleritis whenever he had a stressful situation, such as a school examination or oral presentation, certainly lends support to the emotional triggers.[32] Also, the effect of hormonal fluctuations is suspected from reports of women having recurrent bouts of episcleritis associated with particular times in their menstrual cycle.[33]

Any genetic tendencies toward episcleritis are thought to be related to the associated systemic diseases that have a genetic basis.

Laboratory Evaluation

All patients who are diagnosed as having episcleritis should be afforded a complete ophthalmic evaluation. In this way, associated conditions such as acne rosacea, foreign bodies, herpes simplex, or herpes zoster would not go undetected. However, should a patient continue to have persistent or recurrent attacks, and no obvious disease associations, further systemic evaluation may be warranted.

Etiologic investigation is begun by obtaining a thorough review of systems, with particular emphasis on collagen vascular, inflammatory, vasculitic, or atopic diseases. This investigation should be repeated with each subsequent attack or at least annually. A screening evaluation as illustrated in Box 103.2 may be useful for these patients. It must be emphasized, however, that the review of systems and the physical examination should be used to tailor this list. Obtaining all possible tests for all known associations with episcleritis would be impractical, cost prohibitive, and misleading. It may be helpful to enlist the aid of an internist or rheumatologist. It is, however, important to help direct the investigating physician toward the most likely disease entities so that a 'shotgun' approach is avoided.

Box 103.2 Basic laboratory evaluation of episcleritis*

- Rheumatoid factor
- Antinuclear antibody
- Serum uric acid
- Erythrocyte sedimentation rate
- Complete blood count with differential
- VDRL-FTA
- Urinalysis
- PPD
- Chest X-ray film

** For recurrent or persistent disease.*

Treatment

The natural history of simple episcleritis is such that treatment is usually not necessary, especially since the disease is often asymptomatic. While it has been clearly stated in the literature that episcleritis does not progress to scleritis,[1,3] some reports indicate that there may be some exceptions to this rule.[7,8,34,35] To avoid any risk of progression to scleritis, it may be prudent to consider early treatment of severe cases and to follow all cases of episcleritis through to their resolution. Treatment may also be justified if the condition is persistent or recurrent, or if nodular episcleritis is present.

The treatment of episcleritis should be directed initially at any underlying disease process. For example, a patient with acne rosacea may require systemic tetracycline or doxycycline, while a patient with gout may require allopurinol.[3] Any possible allergens or irritants should be eliminated, particularly in the atopic individual. The use of mast cell stabilizers as indicated for underlying diseases is also quite useful. However, since most patients have no underlying disorder or precipitating factors, their treatment should be largely empiric. For those patients who are not bothered by the appearance or discomfort, simple reassurance that there is no serious ophthalmic disorder may be all that is required. If, however, there is significant discomfort or if cosmesis presents a problem, treatment may be justified.

Supportive therapy such as cold compresses and iced artificial tears offer little risk. Their lubricating and vasoconstricting effect, as well as any placebo effect, may go a long way to satisfy the patient.

Since their introduction, topical nonsteroidal antiinflammatory drugs (NSAIDs) in the form of ophthalmic solutions have been discussed as a treatment for episcleritis. Both topical flurbiprofen[34]and topical ketorolac[36] have been shown to be no more effective than placebo in eradicating episcleral inflammation. While oxyphenbutazone has been effective as a topical treatment, it is an ointment, which many patients find undesirable, and it is not commercially available in the United States.[37] A newer, investigational antiinflammatory, 2-(2-hydroxy-4-methylphenyl) aminothiazole hydrochloride 0.1%, which effectively reduces the signs of mild episcleritis, may find some place in the treatment of episcleritis.[35] It is not yet commercially available.

Ocular decongestant eyedrops have long been used for this condition and do offer the advantage of temporary vasoconstriction.

The use of topical corticosteroids presents a dilemma. It is unquestionable that the signs and symptoms of episcleritis are effectively and quickly eradicated with the use of these agents.[18,37] The dilemma is, however, whether it is worth the risk of using a topical steroid for the treatment of a relatively benign disease with a short natural history. Foster and Sainz de la Maza reported anecdotally that the use of any topical steroids should be contraindicated in episcleritis patients.[3] There is concern that the use of these drops will not only increase the risk for recurrent disease but also will create a 'rebound effect' in which a more intense episcleritis develops with each subsequent attack. These authors therefore recommended the use of systemic NSAIDs, should treatment beyond supportive therapy be required.[3] Jabs et al.[8] suggest that the use of topical steroids is justified, although they may first wait to see whether the inflammation resolves spontaneously.[8] They begin with fluorometholone 0.1%, four times per day. Should this be ineffective, then prednisolone acetate 1% is used. Although the risks of topical steroids may be minimized by the use of hourly pulse therapy with rapid tapering of the drops when signs and symptoms have improved, there still is some risk, particularly in recurrent cases.

Should it become necessary to treat a patient who is unresponsive to topical steroids, or if one elects to avoid the use of steroids, then systemic NSAIDs may be used. Indometacin (Indocin SR 75 mg two times per day)[3] or flurbiprofen (100 mg three times daily)[2] is usually effective. Other NSAIDs may also be effective and should probably be administered at a dosage recommended to control the pain of rheumatoid arthritis. Should one NSAID be ineffective, it may be necessary to experiment with others until a good clinical response is obtained. Some feel that NSAIDs may be terminated abruptly once the patient no longer demonstrates signs or symptoms of episcleritis.[2] Others feel that the patient must continue treatment uninterrupted for a period of at least 6 months.[3] A compromise approach may be to reduce the NSAID dosage once an improvement is noted and maintain this lowered dosage until resolution is complete. Rapid tapering may then be done. Another alternative to topical steroids is topical tacrolimus.[38]

The use of more potent systemic medicines is rarely indicated for the treatment of episcleritis that is not associated with a systemic disease. However, some patients with an underlying disease, such as rheumatoid arthritis, may require medicines such as prednisone, hydroxychloroquine (Plaquenil),[39] or even low-dose methotrexate[39] to control their episcleritis. The response to treatment of episcleritis patients was delayed significantly if the patient smoked. Smokers may therefore require more intensive therapy to achieve resolution as quickly as nonsmokers.[40]

References

1. Watson PG, Hayreh SS. Scleritis and episcleritis. *Br J Ophthalmol.* 1976;60:163.
2. Watson PG. Diseases of the sclera and episclera. In: Tasman W, Jaeger EA, eds. *Duane's clinical ophthalmology.* rev edn. Philadelphia: Lippincott; 1992.
3. Foster CS, Sainz de la Maza M. *The sclera.* New York: Springer-Verlag; 1994.
4. Spencer WH. Sclera. In: Spencer WH, ed: *Ophthalmic pathology.* 3rd ed. Philadelphia: Saunders; 1985.
5. Williamson J. Incidence of eye disease in cases of connective tissue disease. *Trans Ophthalmol Soc UK.* 1974;94:742.
6. Sainz de la Maza M, Jabbur NS, Foster CS. Severity of scleritis and episcleritis. *Ophthalmology.* 1994;101:389.
7. Akpek EK, Uy H, Christen W, et al. Severity of episcleritis and systemic disease association. *Ophthalmology.* 1999;106:729.
8. Jabs DA, Mudun A, Dunn JP, Marsh MJ. Episcleritis and scleritis: clinical features and treatment results. *Am J Ophthalmol.* 2000;130:469.
9. Read RW, Weiss AH, Sherry DD. Episcleritis in childhood. *Ophthalmology.* 1999;106:2377.
10. Lyne AJ, Pitkeathley DA. Episcleritis and scleritis. *Arch Ophthalmol.* 1968;80:171.
11. Watson PG, Hazleman BL. *The sclera and systemic disorders.* Philadelphia: Saunders; 1976.
12. Watson PG. Doyne memorial lecture, 1982. The nature and the treatment of scleral inflammation. *Trans Ophthalmol Soc UK.* 1982;102:257.
13. Duke-Elder S, Leigh AG. Diseases of the outer eye. Cornea and sclera. In: Duke-Elder S, ed. *System of ophthalmology.* vol. 8. Part 2. St Louis: Mosby; 1965.
14. Auw-Haedrich C, Schmitt-Graff A, Witschel H. Isolated episcleral plasmacytoma mimicking episcleritis in a patient with benign monoclonal gammopathy. *Br J Ophthalmol.* 2001;85:1264.
15. Aydin P, Akova YA, Kadayifcilar S. Anterior segment indocyanine green angiography in scleral inflammation. *Eye.* 2000;14:211.
16. Watson PG, Bovey E. Anterior segment fluorescein angiography in the diagnosis of scleral inflammation. *Ophthalmology.* 1985;92:1.
17. Knox DL, Schachat AP, Mustonen E. Primary, secondary and coincidental ocular complications of Crohn's disease. *Ophthalmology.* 1984;91:163.
18. Buckley RJ. Atopic disease of the cornea. In: Cavanagh HD, ed. *The cornea: transactions of the World Congress of the Cornea III.* New York: Raven; 1988.
19. Palmer DJ, Leo RL. Episcleritis and secondary glaucoma after transcleral fixation of a posterior chamber intraocular lens. *Arch Ophthalmol.* 1991;109:617.
20. Thakker MM, Perez VL, Moulin A, et al. Multifocal nodular episcleritis and scleritis with undiagnosed Hodgkin's lymphoma. *Ophthalmology.* 2003;110:1057.
21. Miserocchi E, Modorati G, Foster CS, et al. Ocular and extracutaneous involvement in pyoderma gangrenosum. *Ophthalmology.* 2002;109:1941.
22. Flach AJ, Lavoie PE. Episcleritis, conjunctivitis and keratitis as ocular manifestations of Lyme disease. *Ophthalmology.* 1990;97:973.
23. Gungor K, Bekir NA, Namiduru M. Recurrent episcleritis associated with brucellosis. *Acta Ophthalmol Scand.* 2001;79:76.
24. North DP. Ocular complications of mumps. *Br J Ophthalmol.* 1953;37:99.
25. Zimmerman LE. Ocular pathology of toxoplasmosis. *Surv Ophthalmol.* 1961;6:832.
26. Mahendradas P, Ranganna SK, Shetty R, et al. Ocular manifestations associated with chikungunya. *Ophthalmology.* 2008;115:287.
27. Wilhelmus KT, Yokoyama CM. Syphilitic episcleritis and scleritis. *Am J Ophthalmol.* 1987;104:595.
28. Fraunfelder FW, Fraunfelder FT, Keates EU. Topiramate-associated acute, bilateral, secondary angle-closure glaucoma. *Ophthalmology.* 2004;111:109.
29. Fraunfelder FW, Fraunfelder FT, Jensvold B. Scleritis and other ocular side effects associated with pamidronate disodium. *Am J Ophthalmol.* 2003;135:219.
30. Aurich-Barrera B, Wilton L, Harris S, et al. Ophthalmological events in patients receiving risedronate: summary of information gained through follow-up in a prescription-event monitoring study in England. *Drug Saf.* 2006;29:151.
31. Shahrokni A, Matuszczak J, Rajebi MR, et al. Erlotinib-induced episcleritis in a patient with pancreatic cancer. *JOP.* 2008;9:216.
32. Margo CE. Recurrent episcleritis and emotional stress. *Arch Ophthalmol.* 1984;102:821.
33. Moench LM. Gynaecologic foci in relation to scleritis and episcleritis and other ocular infections. *Am J Med Sci.* 1927;174:439.
34. Lyons CJ, Hakin KN, Watson PG. Topical flurbiprofen: an effective treatment for episcleritis? *Eye.* 1990;4:521.
35. Liu CSC, Ramirez-Florez S, Watson PG. A randomised double blind trial comparing the treatment of episcleritis with topical 2-(2-hydroxy-4-methylphenyl) aminothiazole hydrochloride 0.1% (CBS 113A) and placebo. *Eye.* 1991;5:678.
36. Williams CPR, Browning AC, Sleep TJ, et al. A randomised, double-blind trial of topical ketorolac vs artificial tears for the treatment of episcleritis. *Eye.* 2005;19:739.

37. Watson PG, McKay DA, Clemett RS, et al. Treatment of episcleritis. A double blind trial comparing betamethasone 0.1%, oxyphenbutazone 10% and placebo eye ointment. *Br J Ophthalmol.* 1973;57:866.
38. Miyazaki D, Tominaga T, Kakimaru-Hasegawa A, et al. Therapeutic effects of tacrolimus ointment for refractory ocular surface inflammatory diseases. *Ophthalmology.* 2008;115:988.
39. Soukiasian SH, Foster CS, Raizman MB. Treatment strategies for scleritis and uveitis associated with inflammatory bowel disease. *Am J Ophthalmol.* 1994;118:601.
40. Boonman ZFHM, de Keizer RJW, Watson PG. Smoking delays the response to treatment in episcleritis and scleritis. *Eye.* 2005;19:949.
41. Ikegawa S, Urano F, Suzuki S, et al. Three cases of pustulotic arthro-osteitis associated with episcleritis. *J Am Acad Dermatol.* 1999;41:845.
42. Kato T, Kunikata N, Taira H, et al. Acute febrile neutrophilic dermatosis (Sweet's syndrome) with nodular episcleritis and polyneuropathy. *Int J Dermatol.* 2002;41:107.

Chapter 104

Scleritis

Joseph M. Biber, Brian L. Schwam, Michael B. Raizman

Inflammatory diseases of the sclera may present in various ways, from subclinical or self-limiting episodes to rapidly progressive and destructive processes. In general, scleritis can be divided into two major categories based on cause. The first, noninfectious scleritis, is most commonly caused by immune-mediated disorders, including primary vasculitides and vasculitides associated with inflammatory diseases. The systemic autoimmune conditions, especially the vasculitides, tend to underlie the most severe and fulminant processes that may involve the sclera. The second group, infectious scleritis, is most commonly initiated by surgery or local extension from adjacent ocular tissues. While the clinical presentation of infectious scleritis may be similar to, if not indistinguishable from, that associated with systemic immune-mediated diseases, scleritis of infectious etiology occurs more rarely, and their history will usually aid in differentiating the two. The challenge for the clinician is to diagnose and treat promptly any underlying systemic disorder while preventing long-term ocular sequelae and vision loss.

Immune-mediated Scleritis

Epidemiology

Scleritis can occur in patients of any age, but most commonly occurs in the fourth to sixth decades, with the mode in the fifth decade.[1–3] It affects more women than men in a ratio of 1.6 : 1. The condition is bilateral in 52% of patients, with half of these cases occurring in both eyes simultaneously.[1–3] Scleritis occurs in all races without any predilection.[3] Inflammation of the sclera is present in 14% of patients with relapsing polychondritis,[4] 10% of patients with Wegener's granulomatosis (WG),[5,6] 10% of patients with inflammatory bowel disease,[2] and in 6% of those with polyarteritis nodosa[2,7] or rheumatoid arthritis (RA).[8] Patients with scleritis have a 25–50% chance of harboring a systemic disease responsible for the ocular inflammation. Of patients with a systemic disease, 77.6% have a previously diagnosed disease, 14.0% have conditions diagnosed as a result of the initial evaluation, and 8.4% develop a systemic disease during follow-up. Rheumatic disease is more likely to be have been diagnosed at initial presentation than systemic vasculitis.[9] The incidence and prevalence of scleritis in the general population is not known.

Pathogenesis and risk factors

The exact pathogenic mechanisms that incite scleral inflammation are unknown. However, it is generally accepted that a disordered immune response leads to both tissue and blood vessel damage. Genetic factors, such as major histocompatibility complex expression, may predispose to ocular disease as in some systemic vasculitides. In vitro expression of cartilage-associated genes, such as Indian hedgehog, type-X collagen, and matrix metalloproteinase-13, demonstrate the chondrogenic potential of human sclera and may further explain why the sclera and joint cartilage are common targets of inflammatory cells.[10] Preceding viral infection or self-antigens to connective tissue molecules found in the sclera and elsewhere may provoke an autoimmune response, as has been proposed in RA.[11–14] Lack of scleral inflammation in an animal model of experimentally induced autoimmunity to collagen and the finding of normal levels of anticollagen type I antibody in patients with necrotizing scleritis suggest that autoimmunity to collagen may not play a role in the pathogenesis of scleritis.[3]

The interaction of genetically controlled mechanisms with environmental factors or endogenous substances gives rise to an autoimmune process that damages the episcleral and scleral perforating capillary and postcapillary venules, causing inflammatory microangiopathy.[15] Histopathologic studies suggest that immune complex deposition (type III hypersensitivity) in vessels is important in this process, especially in necrotizing and recurrent non-necrotizing scleritis.[16] Complement components already contained in the sclera are activated by immune deposits via the classic pathway. Scleral fibroblasts probably participate by presenting antigen to T-helper cells.[16] An overall increase of inflammatory cells, including T cells of all types, macrophages, and B cells, has been found in the sclera and overlying conjunctiva.[16] T lymphocytes are the predominant infiltrating cells around scleral fibers, while clusters of B lymphocytes have been found in perivascular areas.[17] Although both T-helper/inducer lymphocytes (CD4) and T-suppressor/cytotoxic (CD8) lymphocytes are increased, there is a predominance of the former.[15] Inflammatory mediators such as interleukin-1α, -2, -3, -6, interferon-γ, tumor necrosis factor-α, and matrix metalloproteinases are elevated in patients with scleritis compared to normal individuals and may influence scleral breakdown.[15,18] These findings demonstrate the participation of T-helper 1 lymphocytes in necrotizing scleritis.[15]

Scleritis, especially necrotizing scleritis, is more common in those with an underlying systemic vasculitis. Trauma to the sclera, most commonly after surgery, may further enhance the likelihood of scleral inflammation in those patients with systemic vasculitis. In one study, 96% of patients with surgically-induced scleritis had necrotizing scleritis.[19] Three-quarters of those with scleritis after surgery had two or more antecedent surgical procedures. Although the most common surgical procedure in this group was cataract extraction through a limbal incision, scleritis also developed after glaucoma, strabismus, and retinal detachment surgeries.[19] Numerous other studies in the literature report scleritis after ocular surgery, including cataract surgery,[20] transcleral suture fixation of an intraocular lens,[21] strabismus surgery,[22] glaucoma filtering surgery,[23] pterygium excision,[24,25] penetrating keratoplasty,[26] diode laser transcleral cyclophotocoagulation,[27,28] and ganciclovir implants.[29] Sterile foreign bodies can incite a granulomatous scleritis. Several cases have been attributed to suture material, including polyglactin[30] and polyester.[31] Chemical injuries cause scleral inflammation directly. In most cases of surgically induced scleritis, necrotizing scleritis developed[19–22,25,32] and was associated with an underlying systemic vasculitic disease (63–90% of patients).[19,32] Therefore, patients who develop scleritis after ocular surgery, especially necrotizing scleritis, should be evaluated for a systemic vasculitic disease.

Scleritis has been reported as an adverse side effect of medications, primarily bisphosphonates.[33–35] Although the exact mechanism is unknown, it is believed to be in part due to a cytokine release from T cells that are activated because of the chemical composition of the drug.[36]

Clinical findings

Scleritis may be classified on the basis of clinical appearance. The most accepted classification was proposed by Watson and Hayreh and divides scleritis into anterior and posterior forms (Box 104.1). Anterior scleritis is further divided into diffuse, nodular, necrotizing with inflammation (necrotizing), and necrotizing without inflammation (scleromalacia perforans).[7] Classification can assist in determining the severity of the disease and selecting appropriate therapy. Certain forms of scleritis are more often associated with systemic disease, as will be discussed later.

Diffuse anterior scleritis is the most common clinical presentation and is the least severe type of scleritis. It often has an insidious onset and may resemble diffuse episcleritis, as overlying episcleral injection is present. Examination reveals distortion and tortuosity of both superficial and deep vascular networks with loss of the normal radial pattern. The sclera often takes on a violet, blue, or salmon color (Fig. 104.1). After resolution, the involved areas of the sclera may appear somewhat translucent or bluish-gray because of rearrangement of collagen fibers. Progression to either nodular or, less commonly, necrotizing scleritis is possible, although most cases do not progress.[2] Loss of vision secondary to associated ocular complications is less likely than in necrotizing forms.[3] An associated systemic disease may be found in 25–45% of patients with diffuse anterior scleritis, most commonly RA.[1,3,37]

Nodular anterior scleritis presents with a nodule (or nodules) that is firm, immobile, and tender to palpation. The nodule varies from yellow to deep red, depending on the local vascular congestion and is usually in the interpalpebral zone, close to the limbus (but can occur anywhere) (Fig. 104.2). The underlying sclera may become transparent, but not necrotic. Like diffuse anterior scleritis, permanent visual loss and progression to necrotizing scleritis is uncommon.[2]

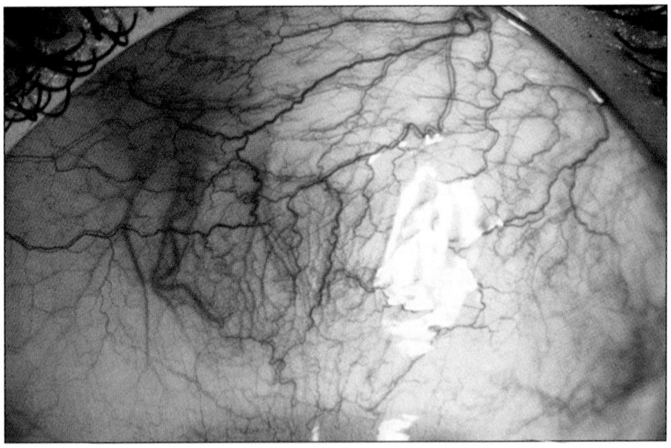

Fig. 104.1 Diffuse anterior scleritis. Note the salmon color of the sclera underlying the inflamed episclera.

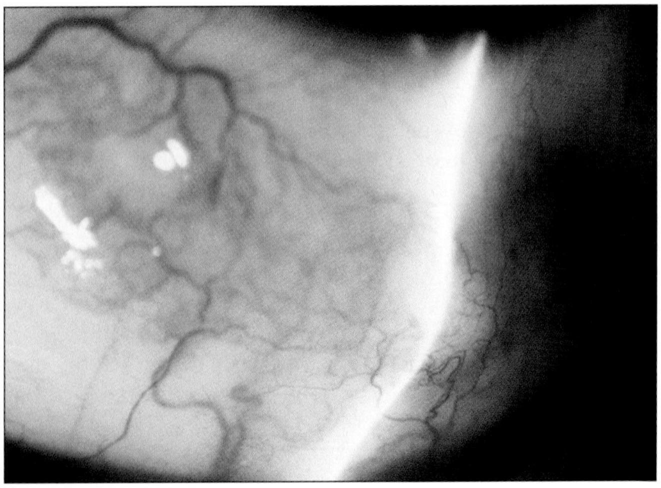

Fig. 104.2 Nodular scleritis in the eye of a patient with inflammatory bowel disease.

Box 104.1 Classification of noninfectious scleritis

- Anterior
  - Diffuse
  - Nodular
  - Necrotizing with inflammation (necrotizing)
  - Necrotizing without inflammation (scleromalacia perforans)
- Posterior

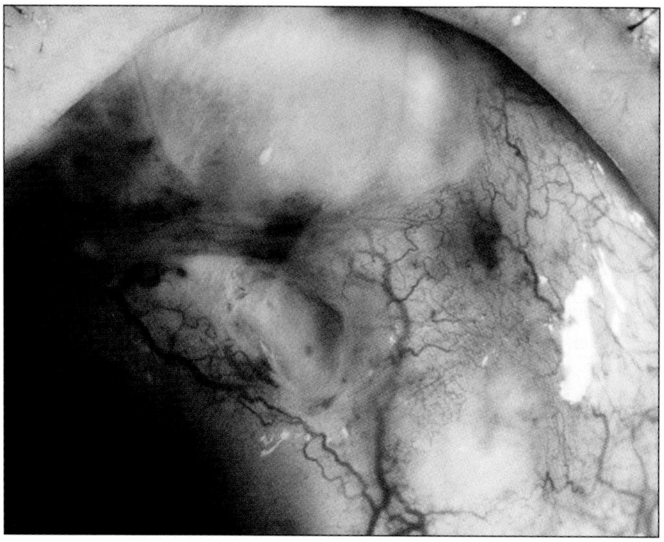

Fig. 104.3 Severe necrotizing scleritis in the eye of a patient with Wegener's granulomatosis.

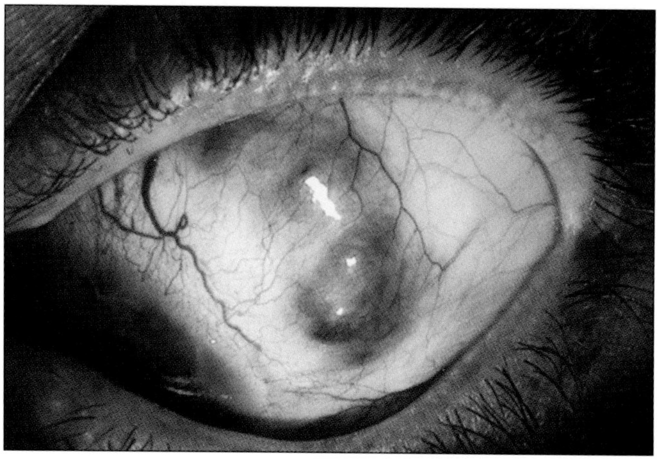

Fig. 104.4 Scleromalacia perforans from rheumatoid arthritis in a blind eye with elevated intraocular pressure.

An associated systemic disease may be found in 44–50% of patients with nodular scleritis, most commonly RA.[1,3]

Of all types of scleritis, necrotizing anterior scleritis with inflammation (necrotizing scleritis) is the most severe and is associated with the greatest potential for visual loss (Fig. 104.3).[1,3,37] Patients often present in extreme discomfort and may be in severe distress. Examination reveals white, avascular areas of sclera and conjunctiva, with surrounding scleral edema and congestion. Uveal tissue may appear as the overlying sclera becomes thin and translucent. Some areas of ciliary body or choroid may remain covered only by conjunctiva. Despite pronounced thinning in some cases, perforation is rare without scleral trauma or a markedly elevated intraocular pressure (IOP). If untreated, areas of inflammation may widen to involve the entire anterior globe and peripheral cornea. Sight-threatening complications include peripheral ulcerative keratitis, uveitis, and glaucoma. Involved sclera can heal remarkably well when inflammation ceases. Rapidly progressive necrotizing scleritis is often bilateral and associated with an acute exacerbation of systemic vasculitis.[37] Visual loss is common in necrotizing scleritis; in one study, 82% of patients lost visual acuity.[3] From 50% to 81% of patients were found to have an underlying connective tissue disease or vasculitis,[1,3] most commonly WG, RA, and relapsing polychondritis.[3]

Necrotizing scleritis without inflammation, also termed scleromalacia perforans, is characterized by an almost total lack of symptoms. Patients may present with blurred vision because of astigmatism or may notice a discoloration of the sclera. Examination shows thinned and avascular areas of episclera and sclera with no surrounding inflammation (Fig. 104.4). These regions develop a porcelain appearance. As in necrotizing scleritis, only conjunctiva may cover prolapsed uvea, but perforation is uncommon without trauma. Unlike necrotizing scleritis, even small areas of extreme thinning or perforation show little healing. Visual loss is uncommon. Necrotizing scleritis without inflammation is most common in elderly women with long-standing RA, and 66% of patients will have some associated systemic disease.[1,3,37]

Posterior scleritis may be difficult to diagnose unless accompanied by anterior scleritis.[38] Posterior scleritis may be confused with other posterior segment or orbital processes, including choroidal melanoma,[39] orbital lymphoma,[40] acute posterior multifocal placoid pigment epitheliopathy,[41] and serpiginous choroiditis.[42] The condition is underdiagnosed and frequently leads to sight-threatening complications. Patients may complain of loss of vision, pain, or diplopia, and findings may include hyperopia, conjunctival chemosis, proptosis, lid edema or retraction, and ophthalmoplegia.[13,14,43] Posterior segment findings include optic nerve edema, optic neuritis, serous and exudative retinal detachment, macular edema, annular ciliochoroidal detachment and choroidal thickening, mass and folds, all commonly associated with visual loss (Fig. 104.5).[3,11,43] Roughly 16–35% of the cases are bilateral.[43,44] Only 29% of patients with posterior scleritis have an associated systemic disease. The systemic associations were similar to those seen in anterior scleritis. Patients with associated systemic disease more frequently had accompanying anterior scleritis.[44] Posterior scleritis may accompany orbital inflammatory pseudotumor; these two conditions may share similar clinical presentation and radiographic findings.[45]

Associated systemic diseases

Approximately half of patients with scleritis have an associated systemic disease, most commonly seen in patients with necrotizing scleritis and scleromalacia perforans, followed by those with diffuse anterior, nodular anterior, and posterior types.[1,3] Patients with scleritis and peripheral keratopathy are especially likely to have an associated systemic disease.[46] The most common associated disease is RA (Fig. 104.6),[1,3,37,47] followed by WG[1,3,37,47] and relapsing polychondritis.[1,3,37] The list of other associated systemic diseases is extensive (Box 104.2). The ocular prognosis of scleritis with systemic vasculitic diseases varies depending on the specific systemic disease. Necrotizing scleritis in WG is a severe disease that can lead to permanent visual loss.[48,49] Scleritis in spondyloarthropathies or in systemic lupus erythematosus is usually a benign and self-limiting condition, whereas scleritis in RA

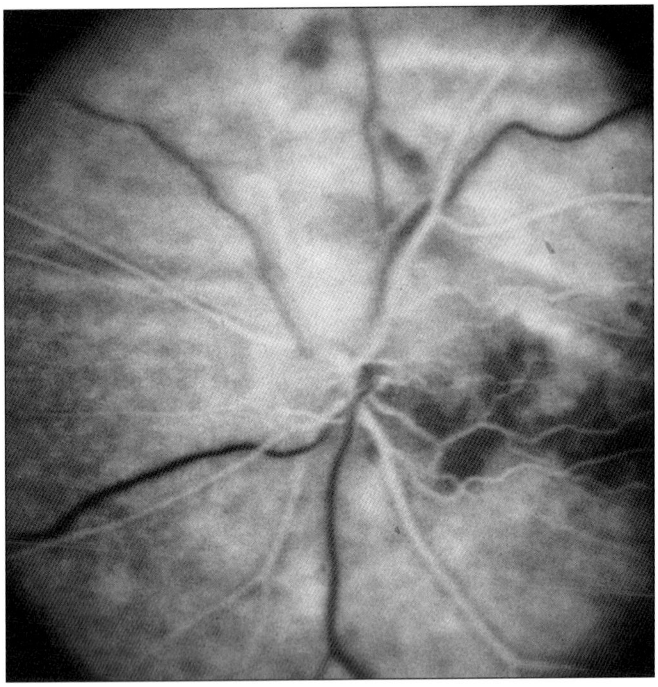

Fig. 104.5 Choroidal folds visible on fluorescein angiography in an eye with posterior scleritis.

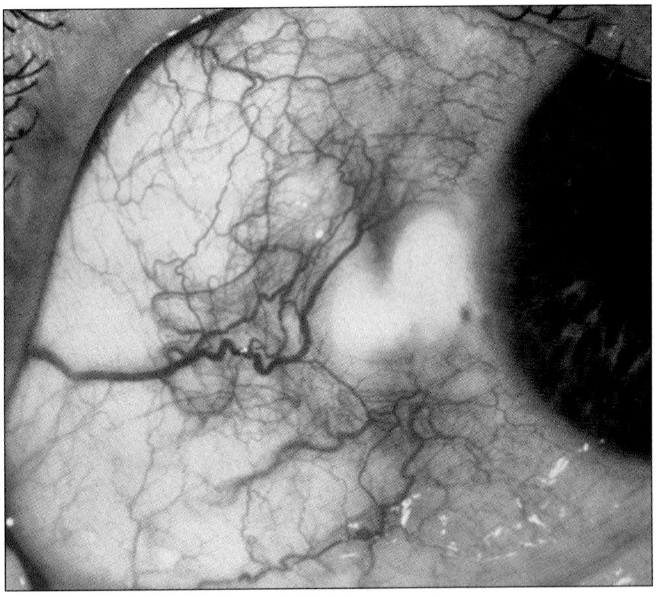

Fig. 104.6 Necrotizing scleritis in the eye of a patient with rheumatoid arthritis. Note the avascular region adjacent to the limbus.

Box 104.2 Associated systemic vasculitic and connective tissue diseases

Rheumatoid arthritis
Wegener's granulomatosis
Relapsing polychondritis
Polyarteritis nodosa
Inflammatory bowel disease
Systemic lupus erythematosus
Ankylosing spondylitis
Reiter's syndrome
Psoriatic arthritis
Giant cell arteritis
Behçet's disease
Churg-Strauss syndrome
Cogan's syndrome
Takayasu's disease
Limited scleroderma
Hypocomplementeric urticarial vasculitis
Other associated systemic diseases:
- Infections
- Sarcoidosis
- Congenital erythropoietic porphyria
- Antiphospholipid syndrome
- Polymyalgia rheumatica
- Pyoderma gangrenosum
- Graft-versus-host disease
- Gout
- Atopy
- Medication induced
- Rosacea
- Rheumatic fever
- Pernicious anemia
- Fibromyalgia
- Sweet's syndrome
- Stevens-Johnson syndrome
- Stiff-person syndrome
- Tubulointerstial nephritis and uveitis syndrome
- Non-Hodgkin's lymphoma
- Multiple myeloma
- Erythema elevatum diutinum

or relapsing polychondritis tends to be a disease of intermediate severity.[48]

At the time of presentation with scleritis, most patients with an associated systemic disease already carry the medical diagnosis. However, 15–59% of patients will present with scleritis as the first manifestation of a systemic vasculitis or connective tissue disease.[3,50] This presentation is especially true for patients with necrotizing anterior scleritis with inflammation.[3] Laboratory testing for antineutrophil cytoplasmic antibodies (ANCA) in the setting of scleritis has facilitated the diagnosis of WG in its limited (ocular) form.[51–53]

Scleritis is an uncommon adverse effect of medications. Reported cases of scleritis have been attributed to bisphosphonates, including pamidronate, alendronic acid, risedronate, and zoledronate, and topiramate.[33–35] Etanercept has been associated with cases of ocular inflammation, including scleritis.[54] The mechanism of medication-induced scleritis is unknown and discontinuation of the medicine is often recommended.

Complications

Complications generally occur late in the disease course and are most commonly seen in necrotizing scleritis. In a retrospective review, nearly 60% of scleritis patients developed an ocular complication.[47] Visual loss may be found in 16–37% of patients and is secondary to uveitis, keratitis, glaucoma, cataract, or fundus abnormalities.[1,47,55] Patients with scleritis associated with uveitis and glaucoma often have severe visual loss, and it is these eyes that most commonly require enucleation.[56,57]

Uveitis develops in more than one-third of patients with scleritis,[1,55,58] arising as a direct extension of scleral inflammation to the adjacent uveal tract. The anterior chamber reaction is usually not severe, although anterior and posterior synechiae may develop. Uveitis is highly associated with complications that lead to visual loss, including peripheral ulcerative keratitis and glaucoma, and may be a poor prognostic sign.[3,58] Anterior uveitis is most often present in necrotizing scleritis, whereas posterior uveitis is more common with posterior scleritis. The presence of scleritis-associated uveitis does not seem to correlate with the presence of systemic diseases.[58]

In general, keratitis associated with scleral inflammation involves the adjacent peripheral cornea and may be present in 14–37% of patients.[1,55] Peripheral corneal thinning, corneal infiltrates, interstitial keratitis, and peripheral ulcerative keratitis are possible complications; they may even precede the scleritis.[59] Peripheral corneal thinning is most often seen in diffuse anterior scleritis, but is not uncommon in patients with long-standing RA.[7] Grayish discoloration may occur in areas of thinning and, later, localized vascularization with subsequent lipid deposition. Thinning can lead to irregular astigmatism and visual loss. Perforation is rare unless the eye is traumatized. Small, superficial, peripheral corneal infiltrates are not unusual and occur adjacent to areas of scleritis.

Interstitial keratitis is characterized by corneal edema, intact epithelium, and one or more gray opacities. It is usually peripheral, but may be central. If not treated, the opacities can progress centrally and coalesce, resulting in a sclerotic appearance. White opacities may develop peripheral to the advancing edge and take on a crystalline appearance. Stromal vessels peripheral to the leading edge may become permanent, with subsequent lipid deposition in the opacities, giving a 'candy floss' appearance.[7] Visual loss occurs with extension into the visual axis.

Peripheral ulcerative keratitis is the most severe form of keratitis associated with scleritis and usually occurs in necrotizing scleritis. Progressive thinning and ulceration with vascularization, white cell infiltration, and loss of stroma occur. Without treatment, spontaneous perforation can occur. Visual loss can result from irregular astigmatism, progression into the visual axis, or perforation. Peripheral ulcerative keratitis is highly associated with visual loss and occult systemic vasculitic disease.[3]

Elevated IOP is present in approximately 13% of patients with scleritis[1,55] and may occur transiently during acute inflammatory episodes. Permanent visual field changes in these patients are less frequent.[1] Scleral edema and increased episcleral venous pressure from vascular congestion are probably important. However, increased IOP in this setting may also be caused by steroid treatment, open-angle glaucoma from uveitis, or angle-closure mechanisms.

Posterior subcapsular cataract formation develops from intraocular inflammation or steroid treatment. Cataract removal, when inflammation has resolved, must be undertaken with caution because of the risk of recurrent scleral inflammation after surgery.[21]

Fundus abnormalities related to scleral inflammation may occur in 6% of patients,[3] most commonly cystoid macular edema, optic nerve edema, retinal detachment, and choroidal folds. Retinal pigment epithelial migration as a result of pars plana inflammation may lead to characteristic peripheral retinal changes.[1] Combined retinal and choroidal detachments can arise.[60] Choroidal folds and exudative retinal detachment may lead to relative hyperopia, which usually resolves spontaneously with appropriate treatment. If any of these fundus changes are long-standing, permanent visual loss can occur. Posterior segment complications are mostly seen in posterior scleritis. Posterior segment inflammation in an eye with anterior scleritis should raise suspicion of concomitant posterior scleral disease.

Signs aiding in differential diagnosis

Prompt diagnosis of scleritis is essential because of its possible association with systemic disease and its potential to cause permanent visual loss. Differentiation from the more benign episcleritis can often be made by history and examination. Patients presenting with scleritis will often complain of pain, which may radiate to the forehead, brow, or jaw, and can be severe enough to awaken the patient at night. History of a red eye, focal or diffuse, accompanied by photophobia, blurred vision, and tenderness to touch will often accompany the ocular pain. The patient with episcleritis describes mild discomfort or foreign body sensation, and photophobia. In scleritis, the sclera in natural light will have a deep violet, blue, or salmon color; in episcleritis, the conjunctiva appears fiery or brick red with only superficial vascular involvement. On examination, scleral edema with overlying superficial and deep episcleral vascular engorgement is common. Avascular areas with blood vessel closure are sure signs of scleritis and do not occur in episcleritis. Such an appearance strongly suggests necrotizing scleritis and possible systemic vasculitis. Additionally, decreased vision and uveitis, which can be seen in scleritis, are rarely present in episcleritis.

Peripheral corneal ulceration can accompany scleritis, typically occurring in a setting of systemic vasculitis. Mooren's ulcer usually lacks scleral inflammation. By definition, Mooren's ulcer is diagnosed in the absence of systemic disease. Reports indicate an association between hepatitis C and Mooren's ulcer.[61,62] It is likely that some forms of scleritis and peripheral ulcerative keratitis are caused by currently unrecognized systemic diseases.

Laboratory investigations

Laboratory investigation should follow, based on a careful history and physical examination. Various blood tests, X-rays, and a urinalysis may be helpful in selected patients (Box 104.3). There is no single correct set of tests for every patient with scleritis. Increased erythrocyte sedimentation rate, anemia, leukocytosis, depletion of complement, and detection of circulating immune complexes may be clues to an underlying systemic connective tissue disease and/or vasculitis, but are nonspecific.

Box 104.3 Common laboratory tests for work-up of associated systemic disease

Antineutrophil cytoplasmic antibodies
Complete blood count
Erythrocyte sedimentation rate
Circulating immune complexes
Complement
Antinuclear antibodies
Rheumatoid factor
HLA typing
Urinalysis
Blood urea nitrogen
Serum creatinine
Chest X-ray
Joint X-rays
Blood cultures and serologies (infectious)

A positive test for serum antineutrophil cytoplasmic autoantibody (ANCA), especially the cytoplasmic staining pattern (C-ANCA), is highly specific for WG. Since scleritis can be a harbinger of a potentially fatal systemic disease, and is often the initial presentation of WG, a case can be made for ordering an ANCA evaluation in every patient with scleritis.[63] One study found that patients with a positive ANCA test are more likely to have severe ocular disease and an undiagnosed primary vasculitis than those with a negative ANCA test.[64] For ANCA testing, laboratories no longer identify neutrophil staining patterns, but assay for antibodies directed against specific proteins. Antibodies to proteinase-3 are associated with the C-ANCA staining pattern and are highly specific for WG. Antibodies to myeloperoxidase are associated with the P-ANCA (perinuclear) staining pattern and are usually associated with idiopathic necrotizing crescentic glomerulonephritis or microscopic polyarteritis (and less commonly with WG).[63] Microscopic polyarteritis has been associated with scleritis and other posterior segment diseases.[65] Serum levels of ANCA may be helpful in monitoring the response to systemic treatment.[51,52] Increased serum blood urea nitrogen and creatinine along with proteinuria and/or hematuria are indicators of associated renal disease. Repeating a previously negative ANCA test should be considered if additional signs of systemic disease, such as glomerulonephritis,[64] or if necrotizing scleritis recurs.

Elevated antinuclear antibody (ANA) and rheumatoid factor levels, although not specific for a particular disease, are suggestive of systemic lupus erythematosus (and related disorders) and RA, respectively. Even though it is unusual for scleritis to be the intial presentation of RA, patients with idiopathic scleritis and a positive rheumatoid factor are more likely to develop RA even without joint complaints.[66] However, obtaining an ANA level in the absence of symptoms or signs of lupus is not likely to be of value because scleritis is rarely the presenting manifestation of lupus. In fact, a positive ANA test can be misleading in the absence of other criteria for the diagnosis of lupus.[67]

Testing for HLA-B27 may be helpful when considering inflammatory bowel disease as a cause of scleritis.[68] Other conditions associated with the B27 antigen, such as Reiter's syndrome and ankylosing spondylitis, are less commonly associated with scleritis.

Chest X-ray films are useful in the diagnosis of WG and less common causes of scleritis such as sarcoidosis and Churg-Strauss syndrome. X-ray films of symptomatic joints may reveal arthritic changes. Computed tomography[43] and magnetic resonance imaging can show scleral thickening in posterior scleritis and reveal associated orbital inflammation.

A-scan and B-scan ultrasonography are most useful in the diagnosis of posterior scleritis when thickening of the posterior sclera is not visible by ophthalmoscopy.[38,43,69] Typical features of posterior scleritis include diffuse choroidal edema, high reflectivity of the inner sclera and low to medium reflectivity of scleral swelling, retrobulbar edema, and appearance of the T sign.[43,70] High-frequency ultrasound biomicroscopy has been used in the diagnosis of scleritis,[71] but may not be useful in the clinical setting since it does not always contribute additional information.[72] Optical coherence tomography may provide additional information in cases of posterior scleritis.[73]

Anterior segment indocyanine green angiography can be used to help differentiate from severe episcleritis and scleritis.[74] Anterior segment indocyanine green angiography can also be used in conjunction with fluorescein angiography to detect areas of vasculitis not clinically seen, and to monitor treatment response.[75]

Scleral biopsy is rarely necessary, but may help define a systemic vasculitis or infection.[3] Histopathologic findings of neutrophilic and lymphocytic infiltration of vessel walls suggest a vasculitic process,[16,76] but may be hard to confirm in the small scleral vessels. Evidence of either granulomatous or nongranulomatous inflammation in scleral tissue can be present, depending on the severity of disease.[16,76] Biopsy is probably not necessary in necrotizing scleritis, where a high correlation with systemic vasculitic disease is already recognized.[3,19] When sclera is biopsied, avoid thin regions that might be prone to uveal prolapse. Inflamed sclera may heal poorly after biopsy and patch grafting could be required.[1]

Therapy

Oral nonsteroidal antiinflammatory drugs (NSAIDs) are usually effective, by reducing pain and inflammation, in non-necrotizing scleritis. In some cases, months or years of therapy are required. There is no conclusive evidence that one NSAID is better than another. A good response to indometacin, naproxen, diflunisal, nabumetone, and others has been reported. If one NSAID is ineffective, another may be tried.[1,3] NSAIDs are not sufficient in the initial management of necrotizing scleritis. Due to concerns for increased renal and cardiovascular events, the selective COX-2 inhibitors rofecoxib[77] and celecoxib are no longer recommended for treatment of non-necrotizing scleritis.

Topical corticosteroids and topical NSAIDs are usually inadequate in scleritis cases. A few reports suggest that topical ciclosporin A may be effective in the treatment of necrotizing scleritis that does not respond to conventional therapy.[78–80] Topical tacrolimus (0.02%) may be helpful in treating refractory sclerokeratitis as an adjunctive immunosuppressant.[81]

Systemic corticosteroids are indicated in some cases of severe non-necrotizing scleritis unresponsive to oral NSAIDs, and in necrotizing scleritis. Oral prednisone at a starting dose of 1 mg/kg per day is appropriate, followed by a slow taper according to response. Potential side effects of systemic steroids need to be monitored.[3,82] Subconjunctival injections of triamcinolone may be a safe and effective treatment for resistant, non-necrotizing anterior scleritis.[83,84] One study found complete resolution of the signs and symptoms of scleritis in 94% of eyes treated, with no scleral necrosis or perforation.[83] Cases of scleral perforation after subconjunctival steroid injections[1] raise concern, but we and others do not believe injections of corticosteroids are contraindicated in non-necrotizing scleritis.[3,82–84] Injections of intraorbital steroids may be helpful in selected cases, especially when contraindications to systemic corticosteroid use exist.[3,82] Deep intramuscular methylprednisolone injections (2.5–3.0 mg/kg) can be used alternatively to ensure compliance with fewer systemic side effects.[85]

Systemic immunosuppressive agents are required in cases of severe necrotizing scleritis, and scleritis of any type in the setting of WG or polyarteritis nodosa. These vasculitides are associated with destructive renal, pulmonary, and other organ disease, and with high mortality.[3] Cyclophosphamide is the drug of choice in WG.[1,3,86,87] A starting dose of 2.5 mg/kg per day is reasonable, but should be adjusted based on clinical response and white blood count. In most cases, a good reduction in ocular inflammation will occur without the white blood cell (WBC) count falling below 3000/μL, but some reduction in the WBC count is usually necessary to achieve a therapeutic response.

Systemic immunosuppressive agents should also be considered in cases of idiopathic scleritis if vision is threatened or pain is intolerable. Systemic NSAID and corticosteroid failure or unacceptably high maintenance doses of steroid are other indications for alternative immunosuppressive therapy. Systemic immunosuppression may be required in over 25% of scleritis cases.[47] Use of methotrexate (up to 20–25 mg/week), azathioprine (starting dose of approximately 2.5 mg/kg/day and ciclosporin (2.5–5.0 mg/kg/day) in the therapy of scleritis is well documented.[1,3,68,86,88–90] Mycophenolate mofetil (2–3 g/day) has been found to be an effective immunosuppressive and steroid-sparing agent for controlling severe anterior and posterior scleritis with minimal side effects.[91,92]

Several new biologic agents are being studied for their safety and efficacy in controlling severe recalcitrant ocular inflammation, including scleritis. These agents include the tumor necrosis factor inhibitors, etanercept and infliximab; the antilymphocyte medications, rituximab and alemtuzumab; the interleukin-2 receptor blocker, daclizumab; and the interleukin-1 receptor antagonist, anakinra. Infliximab (5 mg/kg infusions every 2–8 weeks) has demonstrated efficacy in treating ocular inflammation[93,94] and has been shown to be more effective than etanercept.[95] Etanercept has been implicated in some cases of scleritis.[54] Rituximab, an anti-CD20 monoclonal antibody, may be useful in treating refractory cases of ocular inflammation, including scleritis in WG.[96,97] Further investigation is needed to determine the efficacy of these medications in controlling severe ocular inflammatory diseases. Some patients with relapsing polychondritis have scleritis that is resistant to all immunosuppressive agents, but dapsone can help the scleritis in some cases.[3,98] Corticosteroids may be useful as an adjunct to systemic immunosuppressive agents in scleritis associated with systemic vasculitis.[3] One report suggested that trimethoprim–sulfamethoxazole may help in the treatment of limited WG.[52]

It may be difficult to determine the appropriate point at which to halt immunosuppressive therapy. If scleritis is controlled for 1 year, the medication may be stopped. Any signs of reactivation warrants reinstitution of the previously effective drug. In cases of scleritis associated with ANCA, serum levels of ANCA may correlate with disease activity and help in determining response to therapy and appropriate times to stop and start cyclophosphamide therapy. One study suggests that smoking may delay the response to treatment in patients with scleritis, irrespective of disease type or treatment.[99]

The management of posterior scleritis is controversial. Oral NSAIDs, oral corticosteroids, intraorbital steroids, immunosuppressive agents, and some biologic agents have all been used successfully.

Although rare, surgical management may be necessary in necrotizing scleritis and scleromalacia perforans. Unless an emergent perforation is present, appropriate control of the inflammation with medical therapy should be obtained prior to any surgical procedures, to increase the chance of success and prevent relapses. Tectonic scleral and peripheral corneal patch grafting can be performed with autologous or homologous sclera, fascia lata, dermis, periostium, aortic tissue, and synthetic material (Gore Tex).[100] Two newer surgical techniques advocate using a conjunctiva-Müller muscle pedicle-flap[101] or a tarsoconjunctival pedicle-flap[102] to manage large scleral defects.

Surgically induced scleritis has shown a wide range of responses to a variety of treatments depending on the type of ocular surgery previously performed, the severity of the scleritis, and the association of a systemic disease. Some cases have had a favorable response to a combination therapy with topical corticosteroids and topical ciclosporin A[20] or topical corticosteroids and oral NSAIDs.[23,103] Some required oral corticosteroids[25] or immunosuppressive agents.[104] Surgical treatment to cover the exposed sclera with conjunctiva or lamellar patch grafting has been necessary in some cases associated with cataract surgery[105] and pterygium excision[106] after failure to respond to medical treatment.

Infectious Scleritis

Scleritis is most often immune-mediated. Infections of the sclera are rare, accounting for approximately 4–18% of cases in a tertiary-care setting.[7,76,107] In general, scleral infections may be classified into two groups. The first, exogenous infections, are most common and include post-traumatic and postsurgical infections and extensions from adjacent ocular infections. These exogenous infections tend to be acute, suppurative, and destructive. Less common are those cases

Box 104.4 Infectious agents associated with scleritis

Bacteria
- *Pseudomonas aeruginosa*
- *Pseudomonas fluorescens*
- *Staphylococcus aureus*
- Methicillin-resistant *Staphylococcus aureus*
- *Staphylococcus epidermidis*
- *Streptococcus pneumoniae*
- *Streptococcus equinus*
- *Streptococcus pyogenes*
- *Serratia marcescens*
- *Corynebacterium* spp.
- *Proteus* spp.
- *Moraxella* spp.
- *Nocardia* spp.
- *Escherichia coli*
- *Mycobacterium tuberculosis*
- *Mycobacterium chelonei*
- *Mycobacterium leprae*
- *Treponema pallidum*
- *Borrelia burgdorferi*
- *Haemophilus influenzae*
- *Listeria monocytogenes*
- *Stenotrophomonas maltophilia*

Fungi
- *Aspergillus* spp.
- *Paecilomyces* spp.
- *Sporothrix schenckii*
- *Blastomyces* spp.
- *Acremonium* spp.
- *Scedosporium* spp.
- *Rhizopus*
- *Pseudallescheria boydii*
- *Metarrhizium* spp.

Parasites
- *Acanthamoeba* spp.
- *Toxoplasma gondii*
- *Toxocara canis*
- *Microsporidia*
- *Onchocerca*
- Insect larva

Viruses
- Varicella zoster
- Herpes simplex

of scleritis in the second group, endogenous infections. These cases often resemble noninfectious diffuse, nodular, or necrotizing scleritis. Scleritis associated with systemic infections such as syphilis and tuberculosis fall into this category.

Bacteria, viruses, fungi, and parasites are all able to infect the sclera (Box 104.4). Organisms reach and infect the sclera in various ways (Box 104.5). The most likely source of scleral infection is spread from contiguous ocular structures. Most commonly, the sclera is infected by migration of organisms from the adjacent cornea in cases of keratitis.[108–112] Infections of the conjunctiva or orbital tissues almost never involve the sclera, but rarely scleritis will follow orbital cellulitis, dacryocystitis, sinusitis, or severe conjunctivitis.[113]

Box 104.5 Causes of infectious scleritis

Extension from other structures
- Keratitis
- Choroiditis
- Endophthalmitis
- Conjunctivitis
- Orbital cellulitis
- Dacryocystitis
- Sinusitis

Traumatic, with or without foreign body

Postsurgical
- Scleral buckle
- Pterygium excision, especially with β-irradiation or mitomycin application
- Cataract extraction
- Glaucoma filtration surgery
- Strabismus surgery
- Vitrectomy
- Suture abscess
- Combined penetrating keratoplasty and cataract extraction
- Sub-Tenon's injection of Kenalog

Organisms may reach the sclera via the circulation with deposition of septic emboli in or near the sclera. This is the presumed mechanism of infection in cases without antecedent trauma, surgery, or associated corneal infection. While organisms may directly infect the sclera, it is also possible that scleral inflammation may represent an immune response in the absence of scleral organisms. Scleritis may arise in response to foreign antigen or autoantigen in the sclera in association with infection rather than actual invasion by replicating organisms, but this mechanism remains hypothetical, without solid clinical or experimental support.

Trauma can introduce organisms directly into the sclera in penetrating injuries. Foreign bodies that lodge in or pass through the sclera may harbor organisms.[114,115] Still, infectious scleritis after trauma is quite rare, compared to post-traumatic endophthalmitis. Postsurgical infections of the sclera are also rare, but can develop any time from days to years after surgery.

Systemic immunosuppression is a risk factor for infectious scleritis. Cases associated with acquired immunodeficiency syndrome,[112] chemotherapy,[116] and diabetes mellitus[117] have been reported.

Clinical Findings

Keratoscleritis

Most cases of infectious scleritis result from severe bacterial infections of the cornea, but viral, fungal, and parasitic keratitis may also evolve into a keratoscleritis. Gram-negative bacteria, most commonly *Pseudomonas aeruginosa*, can spread from the cornea to the sclera (Fig. 104.7).[108,110,112,118] *Pseudomonas* scleritis without keratitis has also been reported.[119] *Staphylococcus aureus*,[113,120] *Streptococcus pneumoniae*,[111] *Mycobacterium chelonei*,[111] herpes simplex,[1] herpes zoster,[118,121]

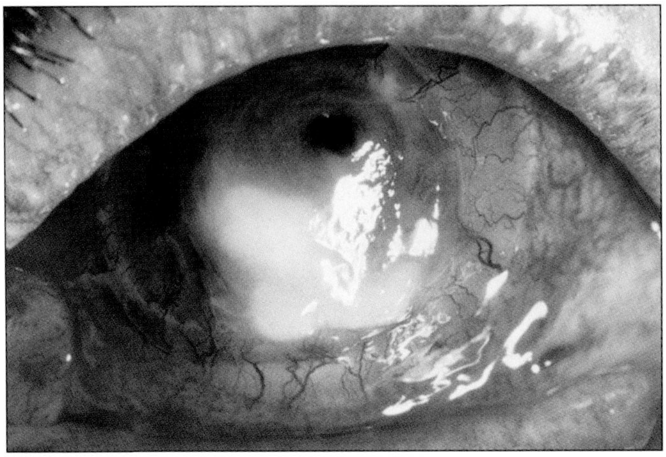

Fig. 104.7 Severe *Pseudomonas* sclerokeratitis.

Aspergillus,[122] *Acremonium*,[111] and *Acanthamoeba*[109,123,124] have also been reported to cause keratoscleritis. Immunosuppressed patients, especially those with acquired immunodeficiency syndrome, can have fulminant keratoscleritis with poor response to therapy.[112]

Infection of the peripheral cornea that spreads to the limbus will first demonstrate limbal erythema, usually with edema and infiltrate. There may be no conjunctival epithelial defect. Pain may increase with infection of the sclera. Scleral involvement in cases of keratitis decreases the prognosis for control of the infection, but can be successfully treated, as outlined below.

Panophthalmitis

Scleritis may result from progression of severe endophthalmitis of any cause. Most cases occur after trauma or surgery. Eyes with endophthalmitis are usually intensely hyperemic, so the first sign of scleral infection may be scleral thinning, uveal prolapse, or scleral perforation. Many of these eyes are hypotonous with poor visual prognosis. Abscesses and necrosis in a scleral tunnel after cataract extraction in two patients were associated with *S. aureus* and *S. equinus* endophthalmitis, respectively.[125]

Less commonly, intraocular infections from endogenous causes may extend into the sclera and present as a scleritis. Such cases of *Toxoplasma*[126] and *Toxocara*-induced scleritis[107,127] have been reported.

Scleritis after scleral buckling surgery[128,129]

Infection associated with a scleral buckle may present in several ways. The patient may experience pain and a foreign body sensation. Signs and symptoms of uveitis may develop. An abscess may be seen in the choroid or retina. The buckle may extrude and be evident on examination. A subconjunctival abscess can be seen in some cases. In others, a purulent discharge is noted. Additional signs may include subconjunctival hemorrhage, conjunctival granuloma, recurrent retinal detachment, proliferative vitreoretinopathy, and scleral perforation. Scleral infection from a buckle may develop immediately after surgery, or years later. Reported causative genera include *Staphylococcus*, *Pseudomonas*, *Proteus*, and fungi.[129–131]

Post-pterygium excision scleritis

Infections after pterygium excision are rare. When infections arise after this common procedure, they are usually associated with the use of mitomycin-C[132,133] or β-irradiation[122,134–136] at the excision site. Reports of infectious scleritis associated with bare sclera closure technique without the use of adjunctive therapy have been described.[137,138] Interestingly, infectious scleritis after pterygium surgery can have a long latency period (1–36 years), which is similar to surgically induced necrotizing scleritis.[139] Patients may have pain, redness, scleral necrosis, and a purulent discharge. *P. aeruginosa* is the most common organism in postsurgical infectious scleritis.[139] Other causes include *S. pneumoniae*[140] and methicillin-resistant *S. aureus*.[138] An analogous streptococcal infection may occur in the setting of chronic scleritis without previous surgery,[141] suggesting that *S. pneumoniae* organisms have a predilection for necrotic tissue.

Other postsurgical infectious scleritis

Scleral inflammation at the site of recent or remote surgery should prompt consideration of an infectious process. Infections of the sclera can occur after cataract surgery,[125,142,143] strabismus surgery,[107] glaucoma filtering surgery,[111,143,144] and vitrectomy.[129,145,146] Two cases of methicillin-resistant *S. aureus* have been reported following vitrectomy.[129,146] Pain, hyperemia, a purulent discharge, and scleral necrosis are typical signs. While bacterial infections are most likely in this setting, fungi and *Nocardia* have been implicated after cataract surgery.[106]

Herpetic scleritis

Although not commonly recognized, scleral involvement in primary varicella zoster can occur and may be associated with stromal keratitis.[121] The severity of symptoms, such as pain and blurry vision, probably reflects the degree of corneal involvement. Ocular signs may include diffuse or focal conjunctival and scleral edema and hyperemia, tenderness to palpation, and concurrent corneal infiltrates.

Similar signs and symptoms can follow herpes zoster ophthalmicus with involvement of the sclera.[1,118,121] Ischemia with occlusion of conjunctival and scleral vessels is typical. In one series of 86 patients with herpes zoster ophthalmicus, three patients developed scleral inflammation.[118] Scleritis in this setting is usually accompanied by keratitis and uveitis. Chronic inflammation can lead to scleral nodules, thinning, and uveal prolapse.

Herpes simplex virus rarely infects the sclera. If epithelial herpetic disease spreads or involves the limbal conjunctiva (primarily), the underlying sclera may become inflamed.

Syphilitic scleritis[147–149]

Syphilis can lead to inflammation in any ocular structure. Syphilitic scleritis is rare (probably less than 5% of cases of scleritis in a referral practice), but has been reported with the secondary, tertiary, and congenital forms of the disease.

Inflammation may be restricted to the episclera or be associated with diffuse inflammation, including uveitis. Evidence of associated interstitial keratitis will be found in cases of congenital syphilis. Patients usually have positive serologic tests for *Treponema pallidum* and usually respond to systemic penicillin or other appropriate antibiotics. However, the role of the spirochete in causing scleritis is uncertain. Rather than direct infection of the sclera, the inflammation may result from vasculitis. The diagnosis may be hard to prove, but response to antibiotic therapy and the absence of connective tissue disorders strongly suggests syphilis as a cause for scleritis in such cases.

Mycobacterium tuberculosis scleritis[107,147–149]

Although the incidence of tuberculosis in the United States is rising, ocular tuberculosis remains rare.[149] Even more rare is scleral involvement.[107] Of 10 524 patients with tuberculosis examined in a sanitarium between 1940 and 1966, only 14 had evidence of scleritis.[147] Rarely are bacilli found on biopsy of the sclera, suggesting a hypersensitivity reaction rather than direct infection of the sclera, making definitive diagnosis difficult. Patients may be asymptomatic or may have pain, redness, and a mucopurulent discharge. Diffuse scleritis, ulceration, or nodules of the sclera may be seen. Uveitis with corneal opacification and vascularization will often accompany tubercular scleritis.

Signs aiding in differential diagnosis

The clinical findings in a case of infectious scleritis, including the presentation, natural history, and disease course, depend on the precipitating cause of the infection. Symptoms are nonspecific and often similar to those in keratitis. The potential clinical signs are myriad (Box 104.6). When present, subconjunctival nodules may be yellow or red in color. The overlying conjunctiva may be intact or ulcerated. The appearance may be identical to noninfectious diffuse, nodular, or necrotizing scleritis.

In most cases of infectious scleritis, the cause is readily apparent, for example with obvious concurrent keratitis, recent trauma, or previous ocular surgery. Infection of the sclera in association with systemic infection is less common and can be more difficult to diagnose, requiring a careful history, review of systems, physical examination, and laboratory investigation. Scleritis associated with systemic infection may appear similar to noninfectious scleritis. These cases require an investigation for noninfectious causes of scleritis, as outlined above.

Box 104.6 Clinical signs of infectious scleritis

- Subconjunctival nodule
- Subconjunctival abscess
- Scleral necrosis
- Nodular or diffuse scleritis
- Conjunctival or episcleral hyperemia
- Mucopurulent discharge
- Subconjunctival hemorrhage
- Uveitis
- Uveal prolapse
- Scleral perforation
- Conjunctival ulceration

Laboratory investigations

Because most cases of infectious scleritis are associated with other ocular infection, the diagnosis will often come by culturing the cornea or vitreous. In cases of scleritis where no obvious infection is present, a careful history is required. Previous surgery, trauma, known systemic diseases, and risk for tuberculosis and syphilis should be determined.

Laboratory and imaging studies may be helpful, especially if systemic disease cannot be ruled out. Cultures of infected tissues should be performed. As with corneal ulcers, Gram and Giemsa stains should be obtained with placement of scrapings on blood, chocolate, and Sabouraud agar. If tuberculosis is a consideration, specimens should be stained for acid-fast bacilli and cultures performed on Lowenstein-Jensen medium. Scleritis with possible *Acanthamoeba* infection requires additional staining with calcofluor white or specific antibodies, and plating on non-nutrient agar overlaid with *Escherichia coli*.

Biopsy of inflamed sclera should be reserved for cases in which a diagnosis is not determined by the preceding steps, and intervention altered based on the results. A number of case reports include rare organisms,[107,117,120,131,150–155] some found only by culture or microscopic evaluation of biopsy material.

Therapy

Effective treatment of infectious scleritis usually requires culture or pathologic evidence of a causative organism. In cases of scleritis suspected to arise from tuberculosis, herpes zoster or simplex, or syphilis, presumptive therapy may be considered. Therapy of mycobacterial tuberculosis scleritis should be with multiple agents and may include isoniazid, rifampin, pyrazinamide, and ethambutol or streptomycin. Herpes zoster scleritis may respond to topical or systemic corticosteroids. Acyclovir appears to be helpful for many forms of ocular inflammation related to zoster infections. Herpes simplex scleritis is usually responsive to topical antiviral agents and can worsen if active infection is treated with corticosteroids. Syphilitic scleritis usually responds to systemic penicillin therapy. Topical and systemic corticosteroids may be helpful, depending on the degree of ocular inflammation. The management of fungal scleritis is usually difficult. Prolonged systemic and topical antifungal therapy such as oral itraconazole and topical amphotericin B should be initiated, but may not eradicate the infection. A combination of voriconazole and caspofungin has been used to treat *Aspergillus flavus* scleritis.[156] Surgical management may improve the outcome.[115,143]

Foreign bodies and foreign material such as sutures or scleral buckling components must be removed if associated with infection. Retinal detachment after the removal of infected elements is unusual, although scleral perforation can occur. Scleral grafts may be required after removal of the buckle.

Medical treatment of scleritis caused by bacteria can be successful. The prognosis is worse with bacterial keratoscleritis. Initial therapy of scleritis follows that for bacterial keratitis, with intensive topical broad-spectrum antibiotics. Topical therapy may be altered based on Gram stain, culture, and sensitivity results. It is common for clinicians to add intravenous antibiotics when infection of the sclera is associated with keratitis. Parenteral therapy is a generally accepted clinical practice, although controlled studies have not been done to clarify the added benefit. Given the poor outcome in most cases of bacterial keratoscleritis treated with drops alone, more aggressive approaches would seem reasonable. Use of a combination of intravenous ceftazidime and an aminoglycoside (tobramycin or gentamicin) in combination with topical fortified antibiotics has been reported to be effective in three patients with *Pseudomonas* scleritis or sclerokeratitis.[157] Topical third- and fourth-generation fluoroquinolones can also be used to treat *Pseudomonas* scleritis or sclerokeratitis. Fortified vancomycin and intravenous vancomycin are recommended to treat cases of methicillin-resistant *S. aureus*.[138] Antibiotic treatment via subpalpebral lavage may provide an alternative route to improve scleral penetration in severe infections.[158]

Several series support surgical intervention in cases of keratoscleritis. Cryotherapy appears to be a useful and safe adjunct to antibiotics, especially in cases of *Pseudomonas* infection.[111] Direct treatment of necrotic sclera with the cryoprobe after conjunctival resection may be effective for several reasons, including organism destruction, altering the host tissue to enhance the elimination of organisms and the healing process, and better antibiotic penetration.

Aggressive surgical debridement of infected tissue with appropiate antibiotic therapy may further improve response.[159] Severe destruction of the cornea or scleral perforation may require lamellar or full-thickness grafting.[159] Penetrating keratoplasty may be indicated in some cases of keratitis threatening scleral invasion. Grafting should probably be reserved for scleritis cases that do not respond to cryotherapy or surgical debridement in combination with topical and parenteral antibiotics, or in those cases where globe perforation has occurred or is imminent. Despite these aggressive treatments, 60% of eyes with infectious scleritis may require evisceration, enucleation, or have no light perception.[110,111]

References

1. Watson P. Diseases of the sclera and episclera. In: Tasman W, Jaeger E, eds. *Duane's clinical ophthalmology*. Vol. 4. Philadelphia: Lippincott; 1987:23.21–23.43.
2. Tuft SJ, Watson PG. Progression of scleral disease. *Ophthalmology.* 1991;98:467.
3. Foster CS, Sainz de la Maza M. *The sclera.* New York: Springer-Verlag; 1994.
4. Isaak BL, Liesegang TJ, Michet CJ Jr. Ocular and systemic findings in relapsing polychondritis. *Ophthalmology.* 1986;681–689.
5. Bullen CL, Liesegang TJ, McDonald TJ, DeRemee RA. Ocular complications of Wegener's granulomatosis. *Ophthalmology.* 1983;90:279–290.
6. Haynes BF, Fishman ML, Fauci AS, Wolff SM. The ocular manifestations of Wegener's granulomatosis. Fifteen years experience and review of the literature. *Am J Med.* 1977;63:131–141.
7. Watson PG, Hayreh SS. Scleritis and episcleritis. *Br J Ophthalmol.* 1976;60:163–191.
8. McGavin DD, Williamson J, Forrester JV, et al. Episcleritis and scleritis: a study of their clinical manifestations and association with rheumatoid arthritis. *Br J Ophthalmol.* 1976;60:192–226.
9. Akpek EK, Thorne JE, Qazi FA, Do DV, Jabs DA. Evaluation of patients with scleritis for systemic disease. *Ophthalmology.* 2004;111:501–506.
10. Seko Y, Azuma N, Takahashi Y, et al. Human sclera maintains common characteristics with cartilage throughout evolution. *Public Libr Sci ONE.* 2008;3:e3709 [E-pub; PMID: 19002264].
11. Phillips PE. Evidence implicating infectious agents in rheumatoid arthritis and juvenile rheumatoid arthritis. *Clin Exp Rheumatol.* 1988; 6:87–94.
12. Gedde SJ, Augsburger JJ. Posterior scleritis as a fundus mass. *Ophthalmic Surg.* 1994;25:119–121.
13. Watson PG, Hazleman BL. *The sclera and systemic disorders.* Philadelphia: Saunders; 1976.
14. Calthorpe CM, Watson PG, McCartney ACE. Posterior scleritis: a clinical and histopathological survey. *Eye.* 1988;2:267–277.
15. Sainz de la Maza M. Scleritis immunopathology and therapy. *Dev Ophthalmol.* 1999;30:84.
16. Fong LP, Sainz de la Maza M, Rice BA, et al. Immunopathology of scleritis. *Ophthalmology.* 1991;98:472–479.
17. Bernauer W, Watson PG, Daicker B, et al. Cells perpetuating the inflammatory response in scleritis. *Br J Ophthalmol.* 1994;78:381–385.
18. Seo KY, Lee HK, Kim EK, et al. Expression of tumor necrosis factor alpha and matrix metalloproteinase-9 in surgically induced necrotizing scleritis. *Ophthalmic Res.* 2006;38:66–70.
19. O'Donoghue E, Lightman S, Tuft S, et al. Surgically-induced necrotising sclerokeratitis (SINS) – precipitating factors and response to treatment. *Br J Ophthalmol.* 1992;76:17–21.
20. Díaz-Valle D, Benítez del Castillo JM, Castillo A, et al. Immunologic and clinical evaluation of postsurgical necrotizing sclerocorneal ulceration. *Cornea.* 1998;17:371–375.
21. Glasser DB, Bellor J. Necrotizing scleritis of scleral flaps after transscleral suture fixation of an intraocular lens. *Am J Ophthalmol.* 1992;113: 529–532.
22. Gross SA, von Noorden GK, Jones DB. Necrotizing scleritis and transient myopia following strabismus surgery. *Ophthalmic Surg.* 1993;24: 839–841.
23. Fourman S. Scleritis after glaucoma filtering surgery with mitomycin C. *Ophthalmology.* 1995;102:1569–1571.
24. Alsagoff Z, Tan DT, Chee SP. Necrotizing scleritis after bare sclera excision of pterygium. *Br J Ophthalmol.* 2000;84:1050–1052.
25. Sridhar MS, Bansal AK, Rao GN. Surgically induced necrotizing scleritis after pterygium excision and conjunctival autograft. *Cornea.* 2002;21:305–307.
26. Lyons CJ, Dart JK, Aclimandos WA, et al. Sclerokeratitis after keratoplasty in atopy. *Ophthalmology.* 1990;97:729–733.
27. Shen SY, Lai JS, Lam DS. Necrotizing scleritis following diode laser transscleral cyclophotocoagulation. *Ophthalmic Surg Lasers Imaging.* 2004; 35:251–253
28. Ganesh SK, Rishi K. Necrotizing scleritis following diode laser trans-scleral cyclophotocoagulation. *Indian J Ophthalmol.* 2006;54:199–200.
29. Srivastava S, Taylor P, Wood LV, et al. Post-surgical scleritis associated with the ganciclovir implant. *Ophthalmic Surg Lasers Imaging.* 2004; 35:254–255.
30. Salamon SM, Mondino BJ, Zaidman GW. Peripheral corneal ulcers, conjunctival ulcers, and scleritis after cataract surgery. *Am J Ophthalmol.* 1982;93:334–337.
31. Stokes J, Wright M, Ramaesh K, et al. Necrotizing scleritis after intraocular surgery associated with the use of polyester nonabsorbable sutures. *J Cataract Refract Surg.* 2003;29:1827–1830.
32. Sainz de la Maza M, Foster CS. Necrotizing scleritis after ocular surgery. A clinicopathologic study. *Ophthalmology.* 1991;98:1720–1726.
33. Fraunfelder FW, Fraunfelder FT, Jensvold B. Scleritis and other ocular side effects associated with pamidronate disodium. *Am J Ophthalmol.* 2003;135:219–222.
34. Fraunfelder FW, Fraunfelder FT, Keates EU. Topiramate-associated acute, bilateral, secondary angle-closure glaucoma. *Ophthalmology.* 2004; 111:109–111.
35. Fraunfelder FW, Fraunfelder FT. Adverse ocular drug reactions recently identified by the National Registry of Drug-Induced Ocular Side Effects. *Ophthalmology.* 2004;111:1275–1279.
36. Macarol V, Fraunfelder FT. Pamidronate disodium and possible ocular adverse drug reactions. *Am J Ophthalmol.* 1994;118:220–224.
37. Hakin KM, Watson PG. Systemic associations of scleritis. *Int Ophthalmol Clin.* 1991;31:111–129.

38. Rosenbaum JT, Robertson JE Jr. Recognition of posterior scleritis and its treatment with indomethacin. *Retina.* 1993;13:17–21.
39. Shukla D, Kim R. Giant nodular posterior scleritis simulating choroidal melanoma. *Indian J Ophthalmol.* 2006;54:120–122.
40. Dorey SE, Clark BJ, Christopoulos VA, et al. Orbital lymphoma misdiagnosed as scleritis. *Ophthalmology.* 2002;109:2347–2350.
41. Laghmari M, Boutimzine N, Karim A, et al. Posterior scleritis simulating acute posterior multifocal placoid pigment epitheliopathy. *J Fr Ophtalmol.* 2004;27:174–178.
42. Narang S, Kochhar S, Srivastava M, et al. Posterior scleritis mimicking macular serpiginous choroiditis. *Indian J Ophthalmol.* 2003;51:351–353.
43. Benson WE. Posterior scleritis. *Surv Ophthalmol.* 1988;32:297–316.
44. McCluskey PJ, Watson PG, Lightman S, et al. Posterior scleritis: clinical features, systemic associations, and outcome in a large series of patients. *Ophthalmology.* 1999;106:2380–2386.
45. Uy HS, Nguyen QD, Arbour J, et al. Sclerosing inflammatory pseudotumor of the eye. *Arch Ophthalmol.* 2001;119:603–607.
46. Sainz de la Maza M, Foster CS, Jabbur NS, et al. Ocular characteristics and disease associations in scleritis-associated peripheral keratopathy. *Arch Ophthalmol.* 2002;120:15–19.
47. Jabs DA, Mudun A, Dunn JP, et al. Episcleritis and scleritis: clinical features and treatment results. *Am J Ophthalmol.* 2000;130:469–476.
48. Sainz de la Maza M, Foster CS, Jabbur NS. Scleritis associated with systemic vasculitic diseases. *Ophthalmology.* 1995;102:687–692.
49. Pakrou N, Selva D, Leibovitch I. Wegener's granulomatosis: ophthalmic manifestations and management. *Semin Arthritis Rheum.* 2006;35:284–292.
50. Carrasco MA, Cohen EJ, Rapuano CJ, et al. Therapeutic decision in anterior scleritis: our experience at a tertiary care eye center. *J Fr Ophtalmol.* 2005;28:1065–1069.
51. Soukiasian SH, Foster CS, Niles JL, et al. Diagnostic value of anti-neutrophil cytoplasmic antibodies in scleritis associated with Wegener's granulomatosis. *Ophthalmology.* 1992;99:125–132.
52. Soukiasian SH, Jakobiec FA, Niles JL, et al. Trimethoprim-sulfamethoxazole for scleritis associated with limited Wegener's granulomatosis: use of histopathology and anti-neutrophil cytoplasmic antibody (ANCA) test. *Cornea.* 1993;12:174–180.
53. Ahmed M, Niffenegger JH, Jakobiec FA, et al. Diagnosis of limited ophthalmic Wegener's granulomatosis: distinctive pathologic features with ANCA test confirmation. *Int Ophthalmol.* 2008;28:35–46.
54. Taban M, Dupps WJ, Mandell B, et al. Etanercept (enbrel)-associated inflammatory eye disease: case report and review of the literature. *Ocul Immunol Inflamm.* 2006;14:145–150.
55. Sainz de la Maza M, Jabbur NS, Foster CS. Severity of scleritis and episcleritis. *Ophthalmology.* 1994;101:389–396.
56. Wilhelmus KR, Grierson I, Watson PG. Histopathologic and clinical associations of scleritis and glaucoma. *Am J Ophthalmol.* 1981;91:697–705.
57. Fraunfelder FT, Watson PG. Evaluation of eyes enucleated for scleritis. *Br J Ophthalmol.* 1976;60:227–230.
58. Sainz de la Maza M, Foster CS, Jabbur NS. Scleritis-associated uveitis. *Ophthalmology.* 1997;104:58–63 [Comments in: *Ophthalmology.* 1997; 1104:1207–1208].
59. Ferry AP, Leopold IH. Marginal (ring) comeal ulcer as a presenting manifestation of Wegener's granulomatosis. *Trans Am Acad Ophthalmol Otolaryngol.* 1970;74:1276–1282.
60. Matthews BN, Stavrou P. Bilateral combined retinal and choroidal detachment in antineutrophil cytoplasmic antibody-positive scleritis. *Acta Ophthalmol Scand.* 2003;81:405–407.
61. Moazami G, Auran JD, Florakis GJ, et al. Interferon treatment of Mooren's ulcers associated with hepatitis C. *Am J Ophthalmol.* 1995; 119:365–366.
62. Wilson SE, Lee WM, Murakami C, et al. Mooren-type hepatitis C virus-associaled corneal ulceration. *Ophthalmology.* 1994;101:736–745.
63. Falk RJ, Jennette JC. Antineutrophil cytoplasmic autoantibodies with specificity for myeloperoxidase in patients with systemic vasculitis and idiopathic necrotizing and crescentic glomerulonephritis. *N Engl J Med.* 1988;318:1651–1657.
64. Hoang LT, Lim LL, Vaillant B, et al. Antineutrophil cytoplasmic antibody-associated active scleritis. *Arch Ophthalmol.* 2008;126:651–655.
65. Matsuo T. Eye manifestations in patients with perinuclear antineutrophil cytoplasmic antibody-associated vasculitis: case series and literature review. *Jpn J Ophthalmol.* 2007;51:131–138.
66. Lin P, Bhullar SS, Tessler HH, et al. Immunologic markers as potential predictors of systemic autoimmune disease in patients with idiopathic scleritis. *Am J Ophthalmol.* 2008;145:463–471 [Erratum in: *Am J Ophthalmol.* 2008;145:111].
67. Rosenbaum JT, Wernick R. The utility of routine screening of patients with uveitis for systemic lupus erythematosus or tuberculosis. A Bayesian analysis. *Arch Ophthalmol.* 1990;108:1291–1293.
68. Soukiasian SH, Foster CS, Raizman MB. Treatment strategies for scleritis and uveitis associated with inflammatory bowel disease. *Am J Ophthalmol.* 1994;118:601–611.
69. Benson WE, Shields JA, Tasman W, et al. Posterior scleritis. A cause of diagnostic confusion. *Arch Ophthalmol.* 1979;97:1482–1486.
70. Perri P, Mazzeo V, De Palma P, et al. Posterior scleritis: ultrasound findings in two cases. *Ophthalmologica.* 1998;212(Suppl 1):110–112.
71. Pavlin CJ, Easterbrook M, Hurwitz JJ, et al. Ultrasound biomicroscopy in the assessment of anterior scleral disease. *Am J Ophthalmol.* 1993;116:628–635.
72. Tran VT, LeHoang P, Herbort CP. Value of high-frequency ultrasound biomicroscopy in uveitis. *Eye.* 2001;15:23–30.
73. Erdol H, Kola M, Turk A. Optical coherence tomography findings in a child with posterior scleritis. *Eur J Ophthalmol.* 2008;18:1007–1010.
74. Guex-Crosier Y, Durig J. Anterior segment indocyanine green angiography in anterior scleritis and episcleritis. *Ophthalmology.* 2003;110: 1756–1763.
75. Nieuwenhuizen J, Watson PG, Emmanouilidis-van der Spek K, et al. The value of combining anterior segment fluorescein angiography with indocyanine green angiography in scleral inflammation. *Ophthalmology.* 2003;110:1653–1666 [Erratum in: *Ophthalmology.* 2004;111:331].
76. Rao NA, Marak GE, Hydayat AA. Necrotizing scleritis: a clinicopathologic study of 41 cases. *Ophthalmology.* 1985;92:1542–1549.
77. Zhang J, Ding EL, Song Y. Adverse effects of cyclooxygenase 2 inhibitors on renal and arrhythmia events: meta-analysis of randomized trials. *JAMA.* 2006;296:1619–1632.
78. Holland EJ, Olsen TW, Ketcham JM, et al. Topical cyclosporine A in the treatment of anterior segment inflammatory disease. *Cornea.* 1993; 12:413–419.
79. Rosenfeld SI, Kronish JW, Schweitzer WA, et al. Topical cyclosporine for treating necrotizing scleritis. *Arch Ophthalmol.* 1995;113:20–21.
80. Shimura M, Yasuda K, Fuse N, et al. Effective treatment with topical cyclosporin A of a patient with Cogan syndrome. *Ophthalmologica.* 2000;214:429–432.
81. Miyazaki D, Tominaga T, Kakimaru-Hasegawa A, et al. Therapeutic effects of tacrolimus ointment for refractory ocular surface inflammatory diseases. *Ophthalmology.* 2008;115:988–992.e985.
82. Hakin KN, Ham J, Lightman SL. Use of orbital floor steroids in the management of patients with uniocular non-necrotising scleritis. *Br J Ophthalmol.* 1991;75:337–339.
83. Albini TA, Zamir E, Read RW, et al. Evaluation of subconjunctival triamcinolone for nonnecrotizing anterior scleritis. *Ophthalmology.* 2005;112:1814–1820.
84. Zamir E, Read RW, Smith RE, et al. A prospective evaluation of subconjunctival injection of triamcinolone acetonide for resistant anterior scleritis. *Ophthalmology.* 2002;109:798–805.
85. Deokule S, Saeed T, Murray PI. Deep intramuscular methylprednisolone treatment of recurrent scleritis. *Ocul Immunol Inflamm.* 2005;67–71.
86. Hemady R, Tauber J, Foster CS. Immunosuppressive drugs in immune and inflammatory ocular disease. *Surv Ophthalmol.* 1991;35:369–385.
87. Charles SJ, Mayer PA, Watson PG. Diagnosis and management of systemic Wegener's granulomatosis presenting with anterior ocular inflammatory disease. *Br J Ophthalmol.* 1991;75:201–207.
88. Hakin KN, Ham J, Lightman SL. Use of cyclosporin in the management of steroid dependent non-necrotising scleritis. *Br J Ophthalmol.* 1991; 75:340–341.
89. Priori R, Paroli MP, Luan FL, et al. Cyclosporin A in the treatment of relapsing polychondritis with severe recurrent eye involvement. *Br J Rheumatol.* 1993;32:352.
90. Jachens AW, Chu DS. Retrospective review of methotrexate therapy in the treatment of chronic, noninfectious, nonnecrotizing scleritis. *Am J Ophthalmol.* 2008;145:487–492.
91. Larkin G, Lightman SL. Mycophenolate mofetil. A useful immunosuppressive in inflammatory eye disease. *Ophthalmology.* 1999;106:370–374.
92. Thorne JE, Jabs DA, Qazi FA, et al. Mycophenolate mofetil therapy for inflammatory eye disease. *Ophthalmology.* 2005;112:1472–1477.
93. Murphy CC, Ayliffe WH, Booth A, et al. Tumor necrosis factor alpha blockade with infliximab for refractory uveitis and scleritis. *Ophthalmology.* 2004;111:352–356.
94. Sobrin L, Christen W, Foster CS. Mycophenolate mofetil after methotrexate failure or intolerance in the treatment of scleritis and uveitis. *Ophthalmology.* 2008;115:1416–1421.
95. Galor A, Perez VL, Hammel JP, et al. Differential effectiveness of etanercept and infliximab in the treatment of ocular inflammation. *Ophthalmology.* 2006;113:2317–2323.

96. Cheung CM, Murray PI, Savage CO. Successful treatment of Wegener's granulomatosis associated scleritis with rituximab. *Br J Ophthalmol.* 2005;89:1542.
97. Onal S, Kazokoglu H, Koc A, et al. Rituximab for remission induction in a patient with relapsing necrotizing scleritis associated with limited Wegener's granulomatosis. *Ocul Immunol Inflamm.* 2008;16:230–232.
98. Hoang-Xuan T, Foster CS, Rice BA. Scleritis in relapsing polychondritis. Response to therapy. *Ophthalmology.* 1990;97:892–898.
99. Boonman ZF, de Keizer RJ, Watson PG. Smoking delays the response to treatment in episcleritis and scleritis. *Eye.* 2005;19:949–955.
100. Nguyen QD, Foster CS. Scleral patch graft in the management of necrotizing scleritis. *Int Ophthalmol Clin.* 1999;39:109–131.
101. Yazici B. Use of conjunctiva-Müller muscle pedicle flap in surgical treatment of necrotizing scleritis. *Ophthal Plast Reconstr Surg.* 2008; 24:19–23.
102. Davidson RS, Erlanger M, Taravella M, et al. Tarsoconjunctival pedicle flap for the management of a severe scleral melt. *Cornea.* 2007;26: 235–237.
103. Sen J, Kamath GG, Clearkin LG. Surgically-induced diffuse scleritis: comparison of incidence in phacoemulsification and conventional extracapsular cataract extraction. *Br J Ophthalmol.* 2002;86:701–707.
104. Karia N, Doran J, Watson SL, et al. Surgically-induced necrotizing scleritis in a patient with ankylosing spondylitis. *J Cataract Refract Surg.* 1999;25:597–600.
105. Mansour AM, Bashshur Z. Surgically-induced scleral necrosis. *Eye.* 1999;13:723–724.
106. Jain V, Garg P, Sharma S. Microbial scleritis—experience from a developing country. *Eye.* 2009;23:255–261.
107. Hemady R, Sainz de la Maza M, Raizman MB, et al. Six cases of scleritis associated with systemic infection. *Am J Ophthalmol.* 1992;114:55–62.
108. Raber IM, Laibson PR, Kurz GH, et al. *Pseudomonas* corneoscleral ulcers. *Am J Ophthalmol.* 1981;92:353–362.
109. Mannis MJ, Tamaru R, Roth AM, et al. *Acanthamoeba* sclerokeratitis. Determining diagnostic criteria. *Arch Ophthalmol.* 1986;104:1313–1317.
110. Alfonso E, Kenyon KR, Ormerod LD, et al. *Pseudomonas* corneoscleritis. *Am J Ophthalmol.* 1987;103:90–98.
111. Reynolds MG, Alfonso E. Treatment of infectious scleritis and keratoscleritis. *Am J Ophthalmol.* 1991;112:543–547.
112. Nanda M, Pflugfelder SC, Holland S. Fulminant pseudomonal keratitis and scleritis in human immunodeficiency virus-infected patients. *Arch Ophthalmol.* 1991;109:503–505.
113. Lebensohn JE. Suppurative conjunctivitis with scleral involvement. *Am J Ophthalmol.* 1974;78:856–857.
114. Cobo M. Inflammation of the sclera. *Int Ophthalmol Clin.* 1983; 23:159–171.
115. Rodriguez-Ares MT, De Rojas Silva MV, Pereiro M, et al. *Aspergillus fumigatus* scleritis. *Acta Ophthalmol Scand.* 1995;73:467–469.
116. Hwang YS, Chen YF, Lai CC, et al. Infectious scleritis after use of immuno modulators. *Arch Ophthalmol.* 2002;120:1093–1094.
117. Maskin SL. Infectious scleritis after a diabetic foot ulcer. *Am J Ophthalmol.* 1993;115:254–255.
118. Womack LW, Liesegang TJ. Complications of herpes zoster ophthalmicus. *Arch Ophthalmol.* 1983;101:42–45.
119. Codere F, Brownstein S, Jackson WB. *Pseudomonas aeruginosa* scleritis. *Am J Ophthalmol.* 1981;91:706–710.
120. Sainz de la Maza M, Hemady RK, Foster CS. Infectious scleritis: report of four cases. *Doc Ophthalmol.* 1993;83:33–41.
121. Threlkeld AB, Eliott D, O'Brien TP. Scleritis associated with varicella zoster disciform stromal keratitis. *Am J Ophthalmol.* 1992;113:721–722.
122. Margo CE, Polack FM, Mood CI. *Aspergillus* panophthalmitis complicating treatment of pterygium. *Cornea.* 1988;7:285–289 [Erratum in: *Cornea.* 1989;1988:1158].
123. Lee GA, Gray TB, Dart JK, et al. *Acanthamoeba* sclerokeratitis: treatment with systemic immunosuppression. *Ophthalmology.* 2002;109:1178–1182.
124. Ebrahimi KB, Green WR, Grebe R, et al. *Acanthamoeba* sclerokeratitis. *Graefe's Arch Clin Exp Ophthalmol.* 2009;247:283–286.
125. Ormerod LD, Puklin JE, McHenry JG, et al. Scleral-flap necrosis and infectious endophthalmitis after cataract surgery with a scleral tunnel incision. *Ophthalmology.* 1993;100:159–163.
126. Schuman JS, Weinberg RS, Ferry AP, et al. Toxoplasmic scleritis. *Ophthalmology.* 1988;95:1399–1403.
127. Shields JA. Ocular toxocariasis. A review. *Surv Ophthalmol.* 1984; 28:361–381.
128. Zinn KM, Ferry AP. Massive scleral necrosis from a *Pseudomonas* infection following scleral buckling and pars plana vitrectomy surgery. *Mt Sinai J Med.* 1980;47:618–621.
129. Rich RM, Smiddy WE, Davis JL. Infectious scleritis after retinal surgery. *Am J Ophthalmol.* 2008;145:695–699.
130. Hagler WS, Jarrett WH 2nd, Smith JA. Infections after retinal detachment surgery. *South Med J.* 1975;68:1564–1569.
131. Bhermi G, Gillespie I, Mathalone B. *Scedosporium* (*Pseudallescheria*) fungal infection of a sponge explant. *Eye.* 2000;14:247–249.
132. Rubinfeld RS, Pfister RR, Stein RM, et al. Serious complications of topical mitomycin-C after pterygium surgery. *Ophthalmology.* 1992;99:1647–1654. [Comments in: *Ophthalmology.* 1992;99:1645–1646; 1993;100: 292–293; 1993;100:976–978].
133. Carrasco MA, Rapuano CJ, Cohen EJ, et al. Scleral ulceration after preoperative injection of mitomycin C in the pterygium head. *Arch Ophthalmol.* 2002;120:1585–1586.
134. Tarr KH, Constable IJ. *Pseudomonas* endophthalmitis associated with scleral necrosis. *Br J Ophthalmol.* 1980;64:676–679.
135. Cameron ME. Preventable complications of pterygium excision with beta-irradiation. *Br J Ophthalmol.* 1972;56:52–56.
136. Hanssens M. A peculiar case of necrotizing sclerokeratitis with *Pseudomonas* infection. *Bull Soc Belge Ophthalmol.* 1995;259:45–52.
137. Huang SC, Lai HC, Lai IC. The treatment of *Pseudomonas* keratoscleritis after pterygium excision. *Cornea.* 1999;18:608–611.
138. Lee JE, Oum BS, Choi HY, et al. Methicillin-resistant *Staphylococcus aureus* sclerokeratitis after pterygium excision. *Cornea.* 2007;26: 744–746.
139. Su CY, Tsai JJ, Chang YC, et al. Immunologic and clinical manifestations of infectious scleritis after pterygium excision. *Cornea.* 2006; 25:663–666.
140. Paula JS, Simão ML, Rocha EM, et al. Atypical pneumococcal scleritis after pterygium excision: case report and literature review. *Cornea.* 2006;25:115–117.
141. Altman AJ, Cohen EJ, Berger ST, et al. Scleritis and *Streptococcus* pneumoniae. *Cornea.* 1991;10:341–345.
142. Berler DK, Alper MG. Scleral abscesses and ectasia caused by *Pseudomonas aeruginosa.* *Ann Ophthalmol.* 1982;14:665–667.
143. Bernauer W, Allan BD, Dart JK. Successful management of *Aspergillus* scleritis by medical and surgical treatment. *Eye.* 1998;12(Pt2):311–316.
144. Orengo-Nania S, Best SJ, Spaeth GL, et al. Early successful treatment of postoperative necrotizing *Pseudomonas* scleritis after trabeculectomy. *J Glaucoma.* 1997;6:433–435.
145. Margo CE, Pavan PR. *Mycobacterium chelonae* conjunctivitis and scleritis following vitrectomy. *Arch Ophthalmol.* 2000;118:1125–1128.
146. Feiz V, Redline DE. Infectious scleritis after pars plana vitrectomy because of methicillin-resistant *Staphylococcus aureus* resistant to fourth-generation fluoroquinolones. *Cornea.* 2007;26:238–240.
147. Donahue HC. Ophthalmologic experience in a tuberculosis sanatorium. *Am J Ophthalmol.* 1967;64:742–748.
148. Nanda M, Pflugfelder SC, Holland S. *Mycobacterium tuberculosis* scleritis. *Am J Ophthalmol.* 1989;108:736–737.
149. Helm CJ, Holland GN. Ocular tuberculosis. *Surv Ophthalmol.* 1993;38:229.
150. Tabbara KF. Other parasitic infections. In: Tabbara K, Hyndiuk R, eds. *Infections of the eye.* Boston: Little Brown; 1986
151. Brooks JG Jr, Mills RA, Coster DJ. Nocardial scleritis. *Am J Ophthalmol.* 1992;114:371–372.
152. Brunette I, Stulting RD. *Sporothrix schenckii* scleritis. *Am J Ophthalmol.* 1992;114:370–371.
153. Taravella MJ, Johnson DW, Petty JG, et al. Infectious posterior scleritis caused by *Pseudallescheria boydii.* Clinicopathologic findings. *Ophthalmology.* 1997;104:1312–1316.
154. Sykes SO, Riemann C, Santos CI, et al. *Haemophilus influenzae*-associated scleritis. *Br J Ophthalmol.* 1999;83:410–413.
155. Mietz H, Franzen C, Hoppe T, et al. Microsporidia-induced sclerouveitis with retinal detachment. *Arch Ophthalmol.* 2002;120:864–865.
156. Howell A, Midturi J, Sierra-Hoffman M, et al. *Aspergillus flavus* scleritis: Successful treatment with voriconazole and caspofungin. *Med Mycol.* 2005;43:651–655.
157. Helm CJ, Holland GN, Webster RGJ, et al. Combination intravenous ceftazidime and aminoglycosides in the treatment of pseudomonal scleritis. *Ophthalmology.* 1997;104:838–843.
158. Meallet MA. Subpalpebral lavage antibiotic treatment for severe infectious scleritis and keratitis. *Cornea.* 2006;25:159–163.
159. Huang FC, Huang SP, Tseng SH. Management of infectious scleritis after pterygium excision. *Cornea.* 2000;19:34–39.

Chapter 105

Classification and Diagnosis of Anterior Uveitis

Andrea D. Birnbaum, Chloe Gottlieb, Robert B. Nussenblatt, Nida Sen

Anterior uveitis is the most common form of uveitis.[1,2] The term anterior uveitis is used to describe inflammation confined to the iris (iritis), ciliary body (cyclitis), or both (iridocyclitis).[3] This chapter describes the methods used for accurate diagnosis, classification, and management of patients with anterior uveitis. Using a systematic approach, a limited differential diagnosis can be established, appropriate diagnostic studies selected, and a final diagnosis made in most patients.

Diagnosis

The Standardization of Uveitis Nomenclature (SUN) Working Group developed criteria for reporting clinical data in uveitis.[3] Disease is classified based on onset, duration, and course. Onset of inflammation is considered either sudden or insidious. Duration is divided into limited (≤3 months) and persistent (>3 months). Disease course can be described as acute, recurrent, or chronic. Acute anterior uveitis refers to an episode of sudden onset and limited duration. Recurrent uveitis describes repeated episodes of uveitis with periods of quiescence off all treatment for more than 3 months. In chronic uveitis, a patient is not free of inflammation for longer than 3 months while off treatment.

Symptoms of Anterior Uveitis

Characteristic symptoms of acute anterior uveitis include pain, redness, photophobia, and occasional tearing. Their severity may vary with the underlying etiology, abruptness of onset, and tolerance of the patient. The pain of anterior ocular inflammation results from congestion and irritation of the anterior ciliary nerves and, if severe, can produce ciliary spasm and photophobia.[4] Pain is often localized to the eye, but also can be referred to the periorbital region, forehead, or temple. Nausea and vomiting may occur if there is accompanying angle closure glaucoma. Blurred vision may be seen in cases of severe inflammation with fibrin or with reactive cystoid macular edema (CME).

Pain is uncommon in chronic anterior uveitis. Instead, blurred vision and dull ache are the more common presenting symptoms; however, many cases will be asymptomatic. Associated redness is typically mild. Decreased vision is more common in chronic anterior uveitis because of extensive posterior synechiae formation, pupillary seclusion, cataract, glaucoma, cyclitic membrane formation, or CME.

History

The chief complaint and history of present illness are important in the diagnosis of uveitis. Pertinent history includes symptoms at onset, duration, laterality, clinical course, prior treatment and response, and history of antecedent illnesses.

Historical information should include details of any similar episodes. Previous diagnoses that can complicate the management of the disorder, such as steroid-induced intraocular pressure changes, glaucoma, and herpes keratitis, also should be documented. Finally, a detailed history of previous ocular surgery, including strabismus and cyclodestructive procedures, or a history of penetrating trauma or foreign body, is crucial when considering a diagnosis of sympathetic ophthalmia or exogenous endophthalmitis. In this situation timing is important, with exogenous endophthalmitis more common after recent trauma or surgery.

Demographic Information

Certain types of uveitis are more common in particular age groups (Table 105.1). These groups are not intended to be mutually exclusive, but instead should serve as general guidelines for establishing a differential diagnosis.

Consideration of gender, race, and ethnicity of the patient also may prove useful when considering several diagnoses. For example, ankylosing spondylitis is more common in males, whereas pauciarticular juvenile idiopathic (rheumatoid) arthritis (JIA) occurs most frequently in females.

Occupation may provide clues to possible infectious etiologies. Slaughterhouse workers, butchers, veterinarians, and farmers may be exposed to tissues or milk products infected with *Brucella*. Medical workers are at risk for a variety of infectious agents, such as tuberculosis, herpes simplex, and human immunodeficiency virus (HIV).

Current and past residences and recent travel provide information on possible exposure to infectious agents. A history of tick bites or traveling in wooded areas, particularly in endemic regions such as Connecticut or Wisconsin,

Table 105.1 Age-based differential diagnosis of anterior uveitis

<5 years	5–15 years	16–35 years	36–64 years	>65 years
Juvenile idiopathic uveitis	Juvenile idiopathic uveitis	HLA-B27 associated*	Idiopathic	Idiopathic
Toxocariasis	Toxocariasis	Herpetic	HLA-B27 associated*	IOL-associated uveitis†
Post-viral	Sarcoidosis	Sarcoidosis	Herpetic	Herpetic
Retinoblastoma	Kawasaki's disease	Toxoplasmosis	Fuchs' heterochromic iridocyclitis	Intraocular lymphoma
JXG	Leukemia	Behçet's	Sarcoidosis	Ocular ischemia
Leukemia	Lyme	Syphilis	Toxoplasmosis	

JXG, juvenile xanthogranuloma; VKH, Vogt–Koyanagi–Harada syndrome; IOL, intraocular lens.
* *Ankylosing spondylitis, reactive arthritis, psoriatic arthritis.*
† *Includes* P. acnes *endophthalmitis and uveitis–glaucoma–hyphema syndrome.*

should raise the possibility of Lyme disease. Individuals residing in the southwestern United States, Mexico, or Central and South America may be exposed to coccidioidomycosis. Leprosy should be considered in immigrants from developing regions. Onchocerciasis, or river blindness, is endemic in Africa and Central America. Fuchs' heterochromic iridocyclitis may be more common in patients from countries without a rubella vaccination program.[5]

Past Medical History and Review of Systems

The past medical history should include specific questions regarding infectious diseases or exposure, including sexually transmitted diseases, as well as other past conditions, such as autoimmune and rheumatologic diseases. Certain medications, such as rifabutin, bisphosphonates, sulfonamide and cidofovir, can cause or exacerbate anterior uveitis.[6] The historical belief that prostaglandin analogs are associated with anterior segment inflammation and cystoid macular edema has been recently disproved.[7]

The review of systems is directed toward specific signs and symptoms suggestive of an underlying etiology for the uveitis (Table 105.2). These findings help provide the basis for the selection of appropriate diagnostic tests.

Social and Family History

Social history should include dietary history, pet exposure, and history of drug abuse. Information regarding the consumption of raw meat (toxoplasmosis), raw fish, or unpasteurized dairy products (brucellosis) may yield further diagnostic clues. Exposure to cats may be associated with toxoplasmosis and bartonellosis, whereas contact with puppies is a risk factor for toxocariasis. Patients with a history of intravenous drug abuse are at increased risk for metastatic endophthalmitis, particularly with fungal organisms. Family history is occasionally useful in the diagnosis of uveitis, especially in the human leukocyte antigen (HLA)-linked disorders. For example, there is a strong genetic influence in HLA-B27-associated anterior uveitis and spondyloarthropathies.[8] Chronic anterior uveitis is more common in patients with a family history of inflammatory bowel disease than in the general population.[9]

Physical Examination

External

The external examination of the patient with uveitis can be invaluable in establishing a differential diagnosis. In most cases of anterior uveitis this would include examination of the skin, joints, oral cavity, and lymphoid organs, as well as a neurologic evaluation as appropriate. Examination of the ocular adnexa should focus on the presence or absence of skin lesions, lacrimal gland swelling, and pigmentary changes of the skin and lashes.

Pupils

In many cases of anterior uveitis the pupils will exhibit decreased reactivity, or they may be nonreactive as a result of posterior synechiae or seclusion of the pupil. In patients with herpetic iritis the pupil may be dilated in the absence of dilating drops or posterior synechiae. Intense inflammation of the iris also can result in a poorly reactive pupil in the absence of synechiae. Testing for an afferent pupillary defect can provide evidence of posterior segment disease.

Sclera and conjunctiva

The inflamed sclera should first be examined in daylight followed by slit lamp evaluation. In scleritis, the episclera and sclera are both inflamed and may assume a violaceous hue. The normal radial configuration of scleral vessels is altered. Avascular areas may be seen in patients with necrotizing scleritis. In the more benign episcleritis, the eye is pink or red in appearance, with congestion of the episcleral vessels, but there is no underlying scleral edema. The application of 2.5% phenylephrine will significantly blanch congested episcleral vessels but will have minimal effect on dilated scleral vessels.

Table 105.2 Systemic associations in anterior uveitis

Sign or symptom	Associated conditions
Head	
Headaches	Sarcoidosis, VKH, Behçet's, intraocular lymphoma, Lyme
Alopecia	VKH, syphilis
Lacrimal swelling	Sarcoidosis
Tinnitus/hearing loss	VKH, sarcoidosis, MS
Vertigo	VKH, MS
Sinusitis	Wegener's
Oral sores/ulcers	Behçet's, HSV
Pharyngitis–tonsillitis	Sarcoidosis, toxoplasmosis
Respiratory	
Cough	TB, sarcoidosis, toxocariasis, coccidioidomycosis
Wheezing	Sarcoidosis, toxocariasis
Hilar adenopathy	Sarcoidosis
Pneumonia	Coccidioidomycosis, sarcoidosis, Wegener's
Cardiovascular	
Pericarditis	Reactive arthritis, Kawasaki's, Lyme, sarcoidosis
Myocarditis	Kawasaki's
Thrombophlebitis	Behçet's
Gastrointestinal	
Diarrhea	IBD, Whipple's, *Giardia*
Hepatomegaly	Sarcoidosis, toxocariasis
Genitourinary	
Urethritis	Reactive arthritis, syphilis
Epididymitis	Reactive arthritis, Behçet's
Genital sores/ulcers	Reactive arthritis, Behçet's, syphilis, HSV
Neurologic	
Meningitis	Sarcoidosis, Behçet's, Lyme, VKH
CSF pleocytosis	VKH, Behçet's, sarcoidosis
Psychosis	VKH, Behçet's, sarcoidosis
Cranial nerve palsies	Sarcoidosis, Lyme, intraocular lymphoma, MS, Whipple's
Weakness/paresthesias	MS
Transient ischemic attacks	Ocular ischemia
Incontinence	MS
Musculoskeletal	
Arthritis/arthralgias	Sarcoidosis, Behçet's, syphilis, AS, IBD, reactive arthritis, psoriasis, Lyme
Sacroiliitis	Ankylosing spondylitis, reactive arthritis, IBD
Fasciitis/tendonitis	Reactive arthritis
Lymphoid	
Lymphadenopathy	Sarcoidosis, toxoplasmosis, Lyme, Kawasaki's
Splenomegaly	Sarcoidosis, Lyme, brucellosis
Skin	
Folliculitis	Behçet's
Vitiligo	VKH
Erythema nodosum	Sarcoidosis, Behçet's, IBD
Nodules	Sarcoidosis, IBD, leprosy
Scaling lesions	Psoriasis, reactive arthritis
Erythema chronicum migrans	Lyme
Macules/papules	Sarcoidosis, syphilis
Superficial thrombophlebitis	Behçet's
Pustules	HZV

MS, multiple sclerosis; IBD, inflammatory bowel disease; AS, ankylosing spondylitis; VKH, Vogt–Koyanagi–Harada syndrome; CSF, cerebrospinal fluid; HSV, herpes simplex virus; HZV, herpes zoster virus.

The palpebral conjunctiva should be examined for the presence of nodules. If present, conjunctival nodules suggest a diagnosis of sarcoidosis or tuberculosis. These lesions may be biopsied prior to the initiation of topical steroids to confirm the clinical suspicion.

Diffuse or circumcorneal injection of the bulbar conjunctiva is common in acute anterior uveitis. Sectoral inflammation of the conjunctival vessels or nodular elevations suggest a more localized process, such as scleritis or episcleritis. Absent or minimal conjunctival injection is frequently seen in chronic anterior uveitis.

Cornea

Simultaneous inflammation of the anterior uvea and corneal stroma may also occur. Disorders that result in a significant keratouveitis include infectious diseases such as herpes simplex, varicella-zoster, syphilis, tuberculosis, and leprosy. Peripheral keratitis also may be associated with anterior uveitis in a variety of systemic vasculitides, such as rheumatoid arthritis, systemic lupus erythematosus, Wegener's granulomatosis, and polyarteritis nodosa. Reduced corneal sensation supports the diagnosis of herpes (both simplex and zoster) and should be evaluated in all cases when herpetic disease is in the differential.

Secondary corneal changes such as keratitis, stromal edema, and bullous keratopathy may occur as a result of long-standing anterior uveitis. Autoimmune endotheliopathy similar in appearance to an endothelial rejection line also has been described in some patients with pars planitis and herpetic uveitis.[10] Band keratopathy results from calcium deposition in Bowman's layer and is a frequent complication in chronic anterior uveitis. It occurs more commonly in younger individuals, such as those with JIA. In many cases, band keratopathy begins in the nasal and temporal peripheral cornea; however, the entire interpalpebral region may eventually be involved.

Keratic precipitates (KPs) are the most common corneal findings in anterior uveitis. They consist of clusters of inflammatory cells that accumulate on the corneal endothelium, frequently in a triangular configuration (Arlt's triangle) with the base down. Two types of KPs have been described clinically: nongranulomatous and granulomatous. Small to medium-sized keratic precipitates are more common in acute nongranulomatous inflammation and are usually composed of lymphocytes. They are typically white or slightly pigmented and round in appearance. These KPs are most commonly found over the middle and lower cornea. On the other hand, in Fuchs' heterochromic iridocyclitis they are often diffusely distributed over the endothelium, and fine filaments may be seen adjacent to the precipitates, giving a stellate appearance (Fig. 105.1). Stellate KPs may also be seen in herpetic uveitis.

Mutton-fat KPs are large collections of macrophages that typically occur in granulomatous inflammation. These deposits are large, with slightly irregular margins, and are characteristically located on the middle and lower cornea (Fig. 105.2). They have a greasy appearance, and unlike the small–medium KPs seen in acute inflammation they may increase in size by coalescence. The presence of mutton-fat KPs and iris nodules is strong evidence of a granulomatous

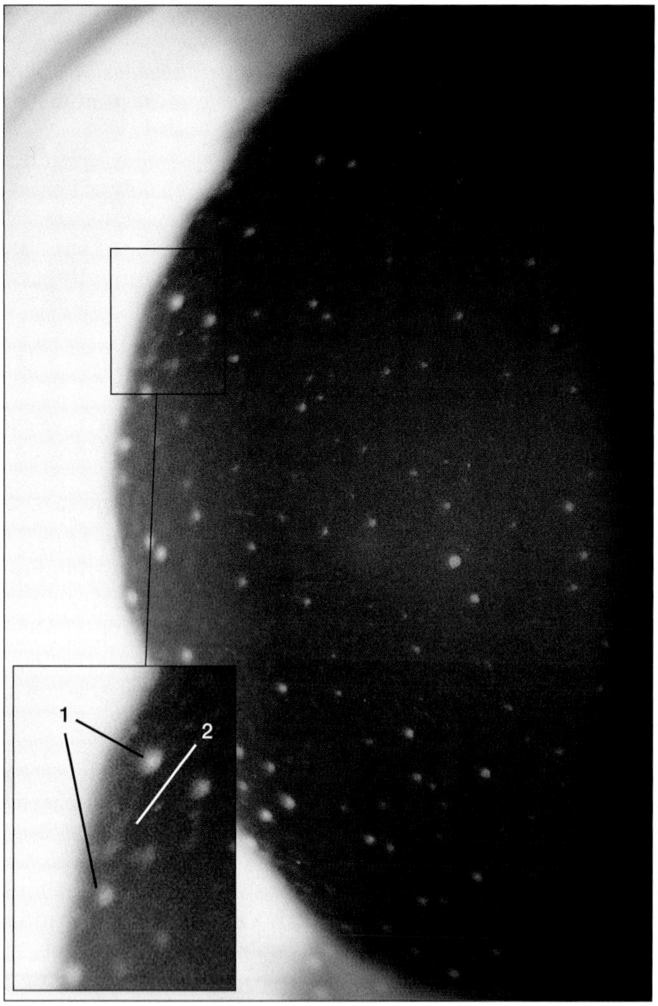

Fig. 105.1 Diffuse small–medium keratic precipitates (1) with adjacent fine filaments (2, inset) in a patient with Fuchs' heterochromic iridocyclitis.

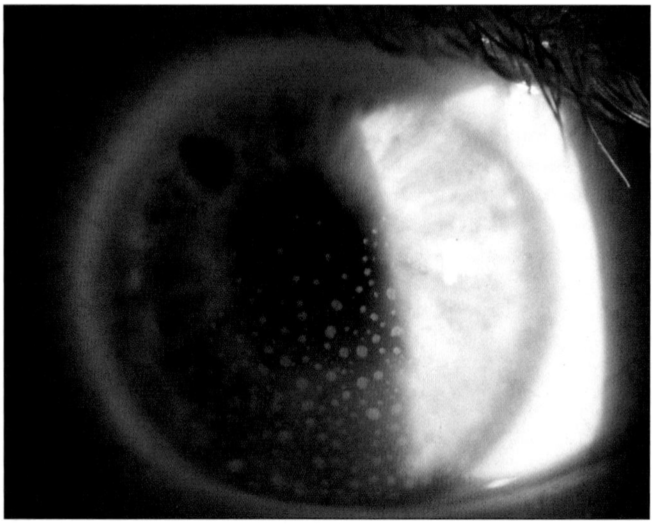

Fig. 105.2 Mutton-fat keratic precipitates in a patient with sarcoidosis.

Table 105.3 Grading of anterior chamber cells and flare (SUN criteria, Modified from Nussenblatt RB, Whitcup SM, Palestine AG: Uveitis. Fundamentals and clinical practice, St Louis, 1996, Mosby.)

Cells		Flare	
Grade	*Cells*	*Grade*	*Flare*
0	0	0	Complete absence
Trace	1–5	1+	Very slight
1+	6–15	2+	Moderate (iris and lens clear)
2+	16–25	3+	Marked (iris and lens hazy)
3+	26–50	4+	Intense (fibrin, plastic aqueous)
4+	>50		

inflammatory response. In the past, small-to-medium KPs have been referred to as 'nongranulomatous.' However, they can also be seen in granulomatous inflammation, especially after treatment or late in the course of the disease.

As inflammation subsides, larger KPs become smaller and translucent or accumulate pigment, whereas smaller KPs decrease in size or disappear completely. Treatment with corticosteroids also may alter the shape and size of the precipitates.

Anterior chamber, anterior chamber angle, and iris

The presence of inflammatory cells and flare in the anterior chamber is the hallmark of anterior uveitis and should be quantified and assigned a grade according to the SUN criteria (Table 105.3).[3] Anterior chamber cells represent a spillover from the actively inflamed iris and/or ciliary body. The grading of anterior chamber cells provides an index of disease activity and is therefore useful in evaluating the response to therapy. If the inflammatory reaction is especially severe, cells may collect in the inferior portion of the anterior chamber to form a hypopyon. In most cases the hypopyon is clearly visible, although in mild reactions or early in the course of the disease the cells may be confined to the anterior chamber angle (Fig. 105.3). The hypopyon can be quantified according to its height in millimeters or the percentage of the anterior chamber involved. HLA-B27, Behçet's disease and infections are the most common causes of hypopyon uveitis. A pseudohypopyon can be seen in several of the masquerade syndromes, including retinoblastoma, leukemia, intraocular lymphoma and choroidal melanoma.[11]

Anterior chamber flare represents an increase in the protein concentration of the anterior chamber. It frequently accompanies anterior chamber cells, but may persist after the cells have disappeared as a result of persistent leakage from the blood–aqueous barrier. Therefore, the presence of flare alone is a less reliable sign of active inflammation. In

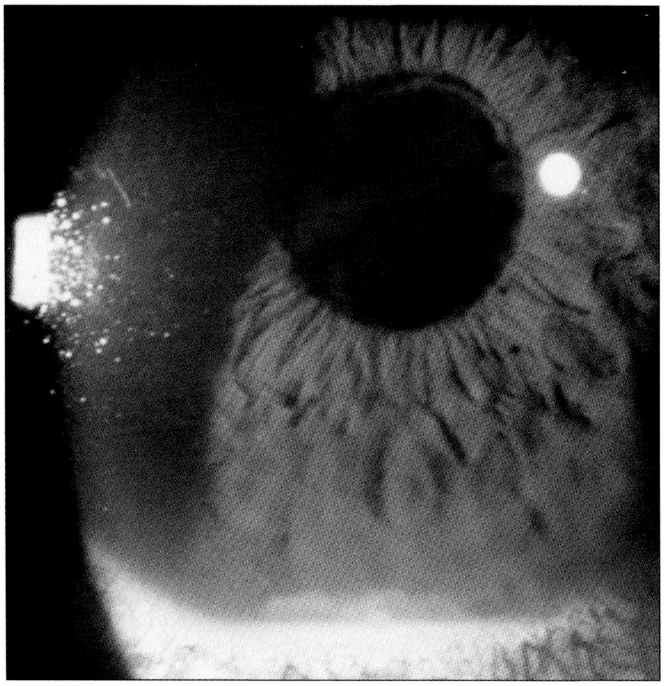

Fig. 105.3 Minimal hypopyon in a patient with Behçet's disease.

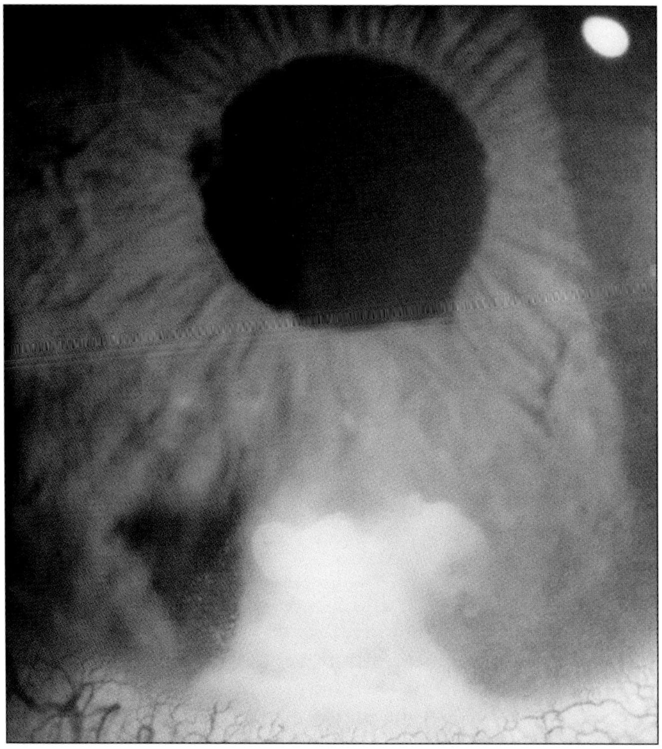

Fig. 105.4 Fibrin coagulum adherent to the corneal endothelium.

cases with an intense fibrin response, a fibrin coagulum may form in the lower portion of the anterior chamber (Fig. 105.4).

Hyphema is an uncommon complication of anterior uveitis. Specific inflammatory diseases associated with a spontaneous hyphema include herpetic uveitis and Fuchs' heterochromic iridocyclitis.[12] Spontaneous bleeding into the

Box 105.1 Etiologies of anterior uveitis

HLA-B27 associated
Ocular disease only (no systemic disease)
Ankylosing spondylitis
Reactive arthritis (formerly Reiter's syndrome)
Psoriatic arthropathy
Inflammatory bowel disease

Juvenile idiopathic (rheumatoid) arthritis

Fuchs' heterochromic iridocyclitis

Herpetic disease

Glaucomatocyclitic crisis
Sarcoidosis*
Syphilis*
Lyme disease*

** Granulomatous inflammation.*

anterior chamber also can be seen in juvenile xanthogranuloma, retinoblastoma, leukemia, and neovascularization of the iris.

Examination of the anterior chamber angle can reveal further information about the severity of the inflammation and mechanism of any secondary glaucoma. Subclinical hypopyon, trabecular precipitates, pigment, and peripheral anterior synechiae may be visible and contribute to trabecular meshwork dysfunction. Abnormal angle vessels can be seen in Fuchs' heterochromic iridocyclitis. Gonioscopy should be performed routinely on patients with uveitis and in cases where the intraocular pressure is elevated.

The iris should be evaluated carefully, searching for the presence of atrophic areas, nodules or granulomas, abnormal vasculature, and posterior synechiae. The pattern of iris atrophy, if present, can suggest either an etiology or the relative duration of the inflammation. Diffuse stromal or pigment epithelial atrophy is characteristic of chronic inflammation, whereas a patchy pattern typically develops after the resolution of iris nodules. Sectoral iris atrophy is most commonly seen in uveitis associated with herpes zoster or simplex.[13] Posterior pigment epithelial atrophy is classically seen in herpetic disease, whereas Fuchs' heterochromic iridocyclitis typically results in atrophy of anterior iris stroma, with loss of the normal pattern of iris crypts.[14]

Iris nodules are focal collections of inflammatory cells located in the iris stroma. They are commonly seen in granulomatous forms of uveitis and can be a useful clinical sign in establishing a limited differential diagnosis (Box 105.1). Koeppe nodules are located on the pupillary margin and can be present in both granulomatous and nongranulomatous uveitis, whereas Busacca nodules are pathognomonic of granulomatous disease and found throughout the remainder of the iris (Fig. 105.5). Iris nodules also may be present during the early stages of Fuchs' heterochromic iridocyclitis, where they are typically small and transparent.[15]

Posterior synechiae represent areas of adhesion between the iris and the anterior lens capsule. The adhesions are typically located along the pupillary zone of the iris, but can occur anywhere along the posterior surface of the iris.

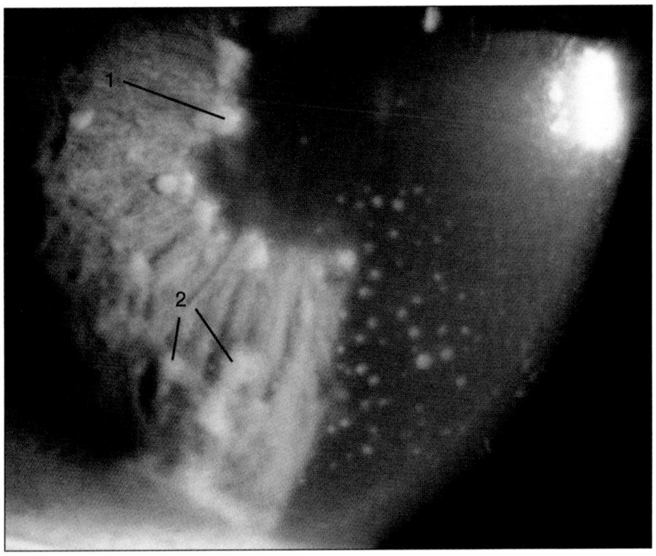

Fig. 105.5 Koeppe (1) and Busacca (2) nodules in a patient with Vogt–Koyanagi–Harada syndrome. (From Nussenblatt RB, Palestine AG: *Uveitis. Fundamentals and clinical practice*, St Louis: Mosby; 1989.)

Synechiae formation is more common in chronic anterior uveitis, but can occur after a single episode of intense inflammation. Extensive posterior synechiae can lead to pupillary seclusion and pupillary block glaucoma. An inflammatory pupillary membrane also may form, leading to pupillary occlusion. The iris may also adhere to the trabecular meshwork (TM), forming peripheral anterior synechiae (PAS). When severe, this can lead to secondary angle-closure glaucoma.

Lens and anterior vitreous

Clumped pigment deposits on the anterior capsule are remnants of posterior synechiae that rarely interfere with visual function. They are common sequelae of chronic anterior uveitis, and may develop after an especially severe episode of acute inflammation.

Posterior subcapsular cataracts are a frequent finding in chronic inflammation. They develop as a result of the inflammatory process, as well as the use of corticosteroids in the treatment of the disease. In long-standing inflammation opacities also may develop in the lens cortex and nucleus.

In pseudophakic patients the position of the intraocular lens (IOL) and haptics should be inspected for the possibility of chronic irritation of the iris or ciliary body (uveitis–glaucoma–hyphema syndrome). In patients with prolonged or chronic postoperative inflammation a thorough search for retained lens fragments as well as plaques on the lens capsule, suggesting chronic endophthalmitis related to *P. acnes*, should be made. Inflammatory deposits, analogous to KP, frequently form on IOLs.

Inflammatory cells in the anterior vitreous are seen in cases of iridocyclitis; therefore slit lamp examination includes assessment of the retrolental space. With severe inflammation, a cyclitic membrane may form along the anterior hyaloid face.

Intraocular pressure

Intraocular pressure is reduced in most cases of severe acute iridocyclitis because of a decrease in aqueous production by the inflamed ciliary body. In severe inflammatory episodes, however, intraocular pressure may increase as a result of altered aqueous outflow, secondary to clogging of the TM with cells and debris. Elevated intraocular pressure in the setting of mild to moderate acute anterior uveitis suggests a diagnosis of Posner–Schlossman syndrome or herpetic uveitis (herpes simplex, varicella-zoster). Elevation in intraocular pressure is frequent in chronic uveitis. It may be the result of angle closure from progressive PAS, iris bombe due to 360° of posterior synechiae, or angle neovascularization. Open-angle glaucoma often occurs due to inflammatory changes to the TM or steroid use.

Retina and optic nerve

A thorough dilated examination of the posterior segment is essential in every patient with anterior uveitis. Significant inflammation in the vitreous suggests concomitant intermediate and/or posterior uveitis. The retina should be examined for any inflammatory lesions, such as toxoplasmosis scars, Dalen–Fuchs nodules, or signs of retinitis. Careful examination of the macula is essential to look for cystoid macular edema. Optic nerve inflammation may occur as part of severe anterior inflammation, or as part of multiple sclerosis, or granulomatous involvement. A posterior examination should also be carried out to rule out conditions such as foreign bodies, tumors, or undiagnosed retinal detachment.

Classification

The classification of a patient with uveitis serves to establish a limited differential diagnosis, guide the selection of diagnostic studies, suggest medical consultation in cases with possible systemic associations, choose appropriate therapy, and provide prognostic information. Following completion of the history and physical examination, the disorder is classified based on the following criteria: onset, severity, duration, pattern, type of inflammatory response, anatomic position, response to therapy, demographic data, and associated conditions.

Response to Therapy

In most cases of isolated anterior uveitis, topical corticosteroids are the mainstay of therapy. Initially, corticosteroids may be administered every 1–2 hours for several days, followed by a slow taper and eventual cessation. Episodes considered responsive to this form of therapy should respond rapidly to treatment and may resolve after several weeks. Inactive disease is defined as zero cells in the anterior chamber. A person is considered to be in remission only after demonstrating inactive disease for 3 or more months while off all therapy.[3] Chronic anterior uveitis may require long-term low-dose therapy to suppress inflammation and prevent recurrence. A few patients will require systemic therapy for treatment of anterior uveitis.

Diagnostic Evaluation

The diagnostic evaluation of patients with anterior uveitis is the final step in establishing a diagnosis. The approach is to select tests that have a high predictive value based on a likely diagnosis or narrow differential diagnosis. Unlike sensitivity and specificity, the positive predictive value of a given test depends on the prevalence of the disease in a given population.

There are no strict guidelines regarding when and how to work-up patients with anterior uveitis. First episodes of acute anterior uveitis, especially if mild, unilateral, non-granulomatous, and responsive to topical corticosteroids probably do not require diagnostic evaluation unless there is evidence for an underlying etiology. We recommend diagnostic testing for first episodes of uveitis when there is a high index of suspicion regarding an underlying cause, the inflammatory response appears granulomatous, or the inflammation fails to respond to therapy within a reasonable time. Diagnostic evaluation is also recommended for all patients with recurrent or chronic inflammation. The work-up should be directed by the results of the history and physical examination. Table 105.4 lists some useful diagnostic studies for the most common etiologies of anterior uveitis. Whenever the uveitis is part of a systemic disorder, consultation with an appropriate specialist may be indicated.

In cases where the history and examination do not suggest any specific diagnoses, we recommend a limited work-up. This may include some or most of the following tests, depending on the clinical spectrum and patient demographics: HLA-B27 for cases that are acute in nature; fluorescent treponemal antibody absorption or other specific treponemal test; antinuclear antibody and rheumatoid factor for children with chronic iritis or iridocyclitis; angiotensin-converting enzyme and lysozyme; and chest X-ray or CT scanning. Testing for tuberculosis (TB) is warranted in cases of granulomatous anterior uveitis, posterior uveitis, and in patients with systemic signs and symptoms of TB or risk factors for TB (recent emigration from an endemic area, history of exposure). An evaluation by an internist or infectious disease specialist can help to clarify a patient's TB status and risk. QuantiFERON TB Gold is a new interferon-gamma release assay used to identify exposure to certain mycobacterial antigens; however, it has not been validated in screening community or hospital-based patients, and has not been investigated in screening patients with ocular inflammation for TB. Of great importance in patients with uveitis is clarifying their TB status before starting immunosuppressive therapy. In endemic areas, we also consider a Lyme titer. It is important to explain to the patient that in nearly half of all cases an underlying condition is never found and the patient is considered to have idiopathic anterior uveitis.

The role of invasive diagnostic testing in anterior uveitis is limited. In patients with suspected sarcoidosis, biopsy of conjunctival nodules or enlarged lacrimal glands may be useful. Iris biopsy occasionally provides diagnostic information, although it is typically not useful in the initial stages of the disease. The biopsy is usually performed at the time of cataract extraction or glaucoma filtering surgery and may be diagnostic in cases of unspecified granulomatous uveitis, as well as juvenile xanthogranuloma.

Anterior chamber paracentesis may be valuable in evaluating a possible infectious uveitis or masquerade syndrome. The use of polymerase chain reaction (PCR) techniques can aid in the diagnosis of conditions such as herpes simplex[13] and zoster, cytomegalovirus, or toxoplasmosis. Quantitative PCR performed on aqueous samples can detect not only the presence of deoxyribonucleic acid (DNA) from the infectious agent, but also provides the number of copies of DNA per volume of sample. In our experience, an aqueous tap obtained through clear cornea gives the best result, and copies of HSV DNA, for example, often number thousands per milliliter of aqueous. Theoretically, this also reduces contamination from infectious agents in the serum. A positive result with PCR should be correlated with levels from aqueous cultures and serologies as well as clinically. Careful cytologic examination of cells obtained by paracentesis can establish a diagnosis in some of the masquerade syndromes, such as intraocular lymphoma and leukemia.

Fluorescein angiography and optical coherence tomography (OCT) may be indicated in patients with suspected posterior disease, or to determine the presence of macular edema secondary to anterior uveitis.

Treatment

Topical corticosteroids are effective for most forms of anterior uveitis. Prednisolone is the most commonly used preparation and is available as an acetate suspension or phosphate solution. The acetate suspension has better corneal penetration, but both preparations appear to be effective when used frequently. Severe inflammatory reactions may require aggressive treatment, with initial dosing every hour followed by a slow taper over 4–6 weeks. Failure to use adequate doses of topical corticosteroids, or tapering the dose too rapidly, are the most common reasons for treatment failure or recurrent inflammation. The risk of complications such as elevated intraocular pressure and cataract formation can be reduced by using the lowest dose and shortest duration to control the inflammation. For maintenance therapy weaker steroids may be considered, such as rimexolone, or loteprednol, a synthetic corticosteroid that becomes deactivated by the esterases in the tissues or aqueous.

Cycloplegics are useful in the control of pain associated with ciliary spasm, as well as limiting or preventing the formation of synechiae. Intermediate duration cycloplegics such as scopolamine 0.25% or homatropine 5% are effective in most situations. Atropine sulfate should be avoided because it causes prolonged iris–cornea contact. Cyclopentolate is also not recommended because of its chemoattractant properties, which may aggravate the inflammation.[16]

Occasionally, when the acute inflammation cannot be controlled adequately with topical steroids, a periocular injection may be considered. We recommend a subconjunctival injection of triamcinolone acetonide or a short-acting preparation such as dexamethasone phosphate when steroid response may be a concern. Alternatively, a short course of systemic steroids may be used to control the inflammation in the acute stage. Patients who require long-term treatment are often started on steroid-sparing agents, such as antimetabolites, ciclosporin, and tumor necrosis

Table 105.4 Diagnostic studies in anterior uveitis

Diagnosis	Diagnostic studies
Ankylosing spondylitis	HLA-B27, sacroiliac X-rays, rheumatology consultation
Reactive arthritis	HLA-B27
Inflammatory bowel disease	Gastroenterology consultation, Promethius IBD Serology 7
Herpes simplex	Clinical appearance, corneal sensation, serology, PCR of aqueous
Varicella-zoster	Clinical appearance, corneal sensation, quantitative PCR of aqueous
Behçet's disease	Established clinical criteria, HLA-B51
Juvenile idiopathic uveitis (formerly JRA)	ANA, pediatric rheumatology consultation
Fuchs' heterochromic iridocyclitis	Clinical appearance
Sarcoidosis	Serum ACE and lysozyme, chest X-ray, consider CT chest, gallium scan, pulmonary function tests, biopsy: conjunctival nodule, lacrimal gland
Toxocariasis	Clinical appearance ELISA
Brucellosis	Serology
Leptospirosis	Serology
Tuberculosis	Tuberculin skin testing, chest X-ray
Syphilis	FTA-ABS with VDRL or RPR
Sympathetic ophthalmia	History and clinical appearance
Lyme disease	ELISA: if positive, confirm with Western blot
Birdshot retinochoroidopathy	HLA-A29
Multiple sclerosis	Neurology consultation, MRI
Intraocular lymphoma	Oncology consultation, lumbar puncture, MRI of the head, vitreous biopsy
Tubulointerstitial nephritis and uveitis	Urinalysis, urine β-2 microglobulin
Lupus	ANA
Wegener's granulomatosis	ANCA

HLA, human leukocyte antigen; JRA, juvenile rheumatoid arthritis; ANA, antinuclear antibody; ACE, angiotensin-converting enzyme; ELISA, enzyme-linked immunosorbent assay; FTA-ABS, fluorescent treponemal antibody absorption; VDRL, Venereal Disease Research Laboratory; MRI, magnetic resonance imaging; PCR, polymerase chain reaction; ANCA, anti-neutrophil cytoplasmic antibody; CT, computed tomography; RPR, rapid plasma reagin.

factor (TNF)-alfa inhibitors to avoid the complications of chronic steroid use.

Ciclosporin A exerts its immunosuppressive effects by interfering with factors involved in T-cell recruitment and activation. One study demonstrated effectiveness in treating methotrexate-resistant inflammation in JIA.[17] Common side effects are nephrotoxicity and hypertension.[18]

The antimetabolites used to treat ocular disease include azathioprine (Imuran), methotrexate (Rheumatrex) and mycophenolate mofetil (MMF, CellCept). Bone marrow suppression and hepatotoxicity are side effects of these drugs; therefore, patients must be monitored with frequent blood tests while on treatment. Women should undergo pregnancy testing before starting on these compounds and should be counseled not to become pregnant while taking them.

TNF-alfa inhibitors have demonstrated efficacy in the systemic management of arthritic conditions such as rheumatoid arthritis and ankylosing spondilitis.[19] They have shown effectiveness in all forms of uveitis, but they are most commonly used for posterior uveitis and should be reserved for cases of sight-threatening uveitis when other agents have failed. Currently there are three forms of TNF-alfa inhibitor available for clinical use: etanercept (Enbrel), infliximab (Remicade) and adalimumab (Humira).

Etanercept is administered by subcutaneous injection to control the joint disease in rheumatoid arthritis and JIA. It was shown to be less effective than placebo in treating ocular inflammation, and is thought by some to be less effective than the other TNF-alfa inhibitors for treatment of ocular disease.[20,21]

Infliximab is approved for rheumatoid arthritis, Crohn's disease, and psoriatic arthritis. In one study it was shown to be effective in reducing inflammation in 80% of patients with recalcitrant uveitis, particularly that secondary to Behçet's disease.[22] It is generally administered intravenously. Infliximab is a chimeric murine–human antibody; co-administration of antimetabolites or T-cell inhibitors may reduce the risk of developing antichimeric antibodies. Several patients stopped using the drug after they suffered infusion-related allergic reactions, presumably after developing antibodies to the mouse component of the antibody.[23]

Adalimumab is a fully humanized antibody, so the theoretical risk of developing antidrug antibodies is much lower than that of infliximab. It is given by subcutaneous injection and has shown success in treatment of childhood uveitis such as JIA. Over 80% of patients in two studies were able to stop other forms of immunosuppression while on adalimumab.[24,25]

Overall, TNF inhibitors are well-tolerated immunosuppressive medications. Reported side effects include tuberculosis (or activation of latent tuberculosis), multiple sclerosis, and a lupus-like reaction. There is an increased risk of malignancy with biologic agents.[26] Further studies are needed to better define the role of TNF inhibitors in the treatment of uveitis.

Summary

Using a systematic approach, most cases of anterior uveitis can be accurately diagnosed, a limited differential diagnosis generated, and appropriate diagnostic studies selected to confirm the likely diagnosis. In most cases topical steroids provide adequate control of the inflammatory disease, although long-term complications such cataracts and glaucoma are common.

References

1. Chan SM, Hudson M, Weis E. Anterior and intermediate uveitis cases referred to a tertiary centre in Alberta. *Can J Ophthalmol.* 2007;42:860–864.
2. Suhler EB, Lloyd MJ, Choi D, et al. Incidence and prevalence of uveitis in Veterans Affairs Medical Centers of the Pacific Northwest. *Am J Ophthalmol.* 2008;146:890–896.
3. Jabs DA, Nussenblatt RB, Rosenbaum JT. Standardization of uveitis nomenclature for reporting clinical data. Results of the first international workshop. *Am J Ophthalmol.* 2005;140:509–516.
4. Hogan MJ, Kimura SJ, Thygeson P. Signs and symptoms of uveitis. I. Anterior uveitis. *Am J Ophthalmol.* 1959;47:155–170.
5. Birnbaum AD, Tessler HH, Schultz KL, et al. Epidemiologic relationship between Fuchs heterochromic iridocyclitis and the United States rubella vaccination program. *Am J Ophthalmol.* 2007;144:424–428.
6. Fraunfelder FW, Rosenbaum JT. Drug-induced uveitis. Incidence, prevention and treatment. *Drug Saf.* 1997;17:197–207.
7. Chang JH, McCluskey P, Missotten T, et al. Use of ocular hypotensive prostaglandin analogues in patients with uveitis: Does their use increase anterior uveitis and cystoid macular oedema? *Br J Ophthalmol.* 2008;92:916–921.
8. Martin TM, Rosenbaum JT. Identifying genes that cause disease: HLA-B27, the paradigm, the promise, the perplexity. *Br J Ophthalmol.* 1998;82:1354–1355.
9. Lin P, Tessler HH, Goldstein DA. Family history of inflammatory bowel disease in patients with idiopathic ocular inflammation. *Am J Ophthalmol.* 2006;141:1097–1104.
10. Khodadoust AA, Karnama Y, Stoessel KM, Puklin JE. Pars planitis and autoimmune endotheliopathy. *Am J Ophthalmol.* 1986;102:633–639.
11. Birnbaum AD, Tessler HH, Goldstein DA. A case of hypopyon uveitis nonresponsive to steroid therapy and a review of anterior segment masquerade syndromes in childhood. *J Pediatr Ophthalmol Strabismus.* 2005;42:372–377.
12. Howard GM. Spontaneous hyphema in infancy and childhood. *Arch Ophthalmol.* 1962;68:615–620.
13. Sugita S, Shimizu N, Watanabe K, et al. Use of multiplex PCR and real-time PCR to detect human herpes virus genome in ocular fluids of patients with uveitis. *Br J Ophthalmol.* 2008;92:928–932.
14. Van der Lelij A, Ooijman FM, Kijlstra A, Rothova A. Anterior uveitis with sectoral iris atrophy in the absence of keratitis: a distinct clinical entity among herpetic eye diseases. *Ophthalmology.* 2000;107:1164–1170.
15. Rothova A, La Hey E, Baarsma GS, Breebaart AC. Iris nodules in Fuchs' heterochromic uveitis. *Am J Ophthalmol.* 1994;118:338–342.
16. Tsai E, Till GO, Marak GE. Effects of mydriatic agents on neutrophil migration. *Ophthalmic Res.* 1988;20:14–19.
17. Tappeiner C, Roesel M, Heinz C, et al. Limited value of cyclosporine A for the treatment of patients with uveitis associated with juvenile idiopathic arthritis, *Eye.* 2009;23:1192–1198.
18. Nussenblatt RP, Palestine AG. Cyclosporin: immunology, pharmacology, and therapeutic uses. *Surv Ophthalmol.* 1986;31:159–169.
19. Smith JR, Levinson RD, Holland GN, et al. Differential efficacy of tumor necrosis factor inhibition in the management of inflammatory eye disease and associated rheumatic disease. *Arthritis Rheum.* 2001;45:252–257.
20. Smith JA, Thompson DJ, Whitcup SM, et al. A randomized, placebo-controlled, double-masked clinical trial of etanercept for the treatment of uveitis associated with juvenile idiopathic arthritis. *Arthritis Rheum.* 2005;53:18–23.
21. Baughman RP, Lower EE, Bradley DA, et al. Etanercept for refractory ocular sarcoidosis: results of a double-blind randomized trial. *Chest.* 2005;128:1062–1067.
22. Niccoli L, Nannini C, Benucci M, et al. Long-term efficacy of infliximab in refractory posterior uveitis of Behçet's disease: a 24-month follow-up study. *Rheumatology.* 2007;46:1161–1164.
23. Imrie FR, Dick AD. Biologics in the treatment of uveitis. *Curr Opin Ophthalmol.* 2007;18:481–486.
24. Biester S, Deuter C, Michels H, et al. Adalimumab in the therapy of uveitis in childhood. *Br J Ophthalmol.* 2007;91:319–324.
25. Vazquez-Cobian LB, Flynn T, Lehman TJ. Adalimumab therapy for childhood uveitis. *J Pediatr.* 2006;149:572–575.
26. Brown SL, Greene MH, Gershon SK, et al. Tumor necrosis factor antagonist therapy and lymphoma development: twenty-six cases reported to the Food and Drug Administration. *Arthritis Rheum.* 2002;46:3151–3158.

Chapter 106

Idiopathic Uveitis

Kevin J. Warrian, William G. Hodge

Idiopathic intraocular inflammation is an extremely undesirable diagnosis. Without a specific etiologic diagnosis, both prognosis and treatment become less precise. Unfortunately, a significant percentage of uveitis cases fall into this category. In two large independent descriptive studies at tertiary referral centers,[1,2] approximately half of anterior uveitis cases were classified as idiopathic; two-thirds of cases of intermediate uveitis were idiopathic.[3,4] In cases of posterior segment inflammation, a cause cannot be found in approximately one-fourth of cases.[1] Finally, in patients with panuveitis, no cause can be found in 5–10% of cases.[2]

Because this is a diagnosis of exclusion, the clinician must use a diagnostic approach. This approach includes classifying the disease process, performing a careful history and physical examination, ordering appropriate laboratory tests, and seeking appropriate consultation. Only after this protocol has been followed should a case be considered idiopathic. It is also important to realize that, not uncommonly, a case will present as idiopathic but in time will declare itself more clearly.

When one is forced to accept this diagnosis, the condition must be treated nonspecifically. Treatment may entail topical, periocular, oral, or intravenous medication. Idiopathic uveitis should be managed in an algorithmic fashion.

Uveitis Classification

One of the most useful steps in the systematic approach to the uveitis patient is to classify the disease based on as many of the following descriptions as possible: anatomic location, onset, severity, pattern, duration, 'clinical pathology,' patient demographics, and associated features (Table 106.1). In essence, one is stepping back from the details of the case and looking at the big picture. For example, an acute, severe nongranulomatous iridocyclitis in a 25-year-old white patient with morning back pain would make a diagnosis of ankylosing spondylitis very likely. Alternatively, an 80-year-old patient who is experiencing an insidious, mild, chronic vitritis for the first time is not likely to have an intraocular autoimmune process, but more likely has a malignancy or low-grade intraocular infection. Even if this approach simply rules out an entity, it can be very useful. For example, a young man with acquired immunodeficiency syndrome (AIDS) and a low CD4 count who presents with an acute painful retinitis and a marked vitreous cellular reaction may have one of many uveitic entities but does not have cytomegalovirus (CMV) retinitis because of the pain and vitreous reaction. Hence, inappropriate anti-CMV therapy, with all its inherent drawbacks and toxicities, can be avoided simply by appropriate classification.

Uveitis History

The most important part of the uveitis evaluation is a careful anamnesis. When a specific diagnosis is made, the history usually leads the way. The most important aspect of the patient history is the description of symptoms. In someone who presents with severe pain, redness, and photophobia, the diagnosis has already been narrowed down to one of the acute iridocyclitis entities. Patients whose main symptoms are black floaters most likely have an intermediate uveitis. Retinitis that involves the macula presents as a painless loss of central vision, usually with metamorphopsia. Choroiditis that does not affect the macula is usually asymptomatic. Virtually any uveitis patient may have cystoid macular edema. In these individuals, blurry vision that fluctuates unpredictably during the day is characteristic. This can be a valuable piece of history when cystoid macular edema (CME) is possible but difficult to diagnose on examination because of a media abnormality. Determining the most important aspects of the uveitic symptoms requires an assessment of the degree of inflammation and a description of the nature of the visual abnormality.

Other useful components of the history include the geographic history, family history, patient demographics, personal history, systemic disease, ocular history, and history of the present illness. A summary of the components of the history that can lead to specific diagnoses is presented in Table 106.2.

Physical Examination

By the time the physical examination is performed, a differential diagnosis may have already been formulated. Both the visual acuity and penlight examination can provide much information. Besides taking corrected visual acuity, pinhole vision can be valuable. If a patient's vision is worse with pinhole, then macular disease is very likely. Because CME is the most common macular disease seen in uveitis

Table 106.1 Classification of uveitis

Anatomic location	Anterior	Intermediate	Posterior	Panuveitis
Onset	Insidious[5]	Sudden[5]		
Severity	Mild	Moderate	Severe	
Pattern	Acute[5]	Recurrent[5]	Chronic[5]	
Duration	Limited (≤3 months)[5]	Persistent (>3 months)[5]		
Clinical pathology	Granulomatous	Nongranulomatous		
Demographics	Age	Sex	Race	
Associated features problems (?)	Joint complaints (?)	Lung complaints (?)	Skin rashes (?)	GI

Table 106.2 Keys from the history in patients with uveitis

Subdivision	Examples	Diseases
Geographic	Ohio, Mississippi, Missouri, St. Lawrence rivers	Ocular histoplasmosis
Age	Childhood Teenage/young adults	JRA Uveitis of young girls Pars planitis Fuchs' malignancy infection
Gender	Male	HLA-B27 uveitis Behçet's
Race	White Black Oriental Mediterranean	HLA-B27 uveitis Sarcoid VKH syndrome Behçet's Behçet's
Other	Pets Sexual history	Toxoplasmosis Toxocara Syphilis Reiter's AIDS

JRA, juvenile rheumatoid arthritis; HLA, human leukocyte antigen; VKH, Vogt-Koyanagi-Harada syndrome; AIDS, acquired immunodeficiency syndrome.

Table 106.3 SUN anterior chamber cell and flare grading systems[5]

Grade	Cells*	Flare*
0	<1	None
0.5+	1–5	
1+	6–15	Faint
2+	16–25	Moderate (iris and lens details clear)
3+	26–50	Marked (iris and lens details hazy)
4+	>50	Intense (fibrin and plastic aqueous)

* *Using a 1 × 1 mm slit.*

patients, someone with decreased vision that worsens with a pinhole examination probably has CME. Penlight examination can reveal an afferent pupillary defect, which may occur from occlusive vasculitis; this is especially common with Behçet's disease. The penlight examination will also be able to spot the ciliary flush and miotic pupil characteristic of acute iridocyclitis.

Slit lamp examination of the lids and conjunctiva may reveal granulomas and nodules. Examination of the cornea, however, is the most important qualitative part of the anterior segment examination. Keratic precipitates (KPs) should be examined in terms of both character and location. Granulomatous KPs are large, greasy, and often confluent. Although not pathognomonic for granulomatous uveitic entities such as sarcoidosis, they are highly suggestive. Old KPs are typically pigmented. In most uveitic entities, KPs are concentrated on the inferior third of the corneal endothelium. When they are found diffusely over the endothelium, they are usually stellate in character, i.e. the KPs have linear extensions radiating from their center. Diffuse stellate KP narrows the differential diagnosis to three entities: CMV retinitis, Fuchs' heterochromatic iridocyclitis, and herpes simplex keratouveitis. Decreased corneal sensation helps in diagnosing the latter.

The most important quantitative aspect of the anterior segment examination is grading the amount of inflammation. Both the flare (protein exudate) and cell can be graded. The latter, however, is more reproducible and valuable. The international Standardization of Uveitis Nomenclature (SUN) Working Group has provided grading systems for both indicators of anterior segment inflammation (Table 106.3).[5] For iridocyclitis, anterior segment inflammation is usually the end point on which treatment is titrated.

Measuring the intraocular pressure can be another important clue to the etiology of the uveitis. Most uveitic entities

Table 106.4 Grading of vitreous opacities

Grade	Description
0	No inflammation
1	Mild blurring of retinal vessels and optic nerve
2	Moderate blurring of optic nerve head
3	Marked blurring of optic nerve head
4	Optic nerve head not visible

From Nussenblatt RB, Palastine AG. Uveitis: Fundamentals and Clinical Practice. St Louis, 1989, Mosby.

cause a decrease in intraocular pressure in the acute phase. However, five entities are more commonly associated with increased intraocular pressure during acute attacks of uveitis: herpes simplex, herpes zoster, glaucomatocyclitic crisis, toxoplasmosis, and occasionally sarcoidosis. Of course, after multiple bouts of uveitis, any disease process can cause increased intraocular pressure from inflammatory or pigment cell blockage of the trabecular meshwork, posterior synechiae and iris bombé, peripheral anterior synechiae, or forward rotation of the ciliary body.

Indirect ophthalmoscopy and fundus contact lenses allow for examination of the vitreous and fundus. Vitreous inflammation has been quantified for both the direct[6] and indirect ophthalmoscopes.[7] Because the latter is much more commonly used, however, it is probably wiser to become familiar with its classification (Table 106.4). Important in the fundus examination is to determine whether the inflammation is primarily a retinitis or choroiditis, whether it is focal or diffuse, and whether or not a vasculitis is present. As already mentioned, one of the most important aspects of the examination is determining the status of the macula, especially to determine if CME is present.

Laboratory Evaluation

It is important to determine when a laboratory work-up is necessary and what tests should be ordered. Most would agree that a case should be evaluated with ancillary tests if it falls into one of the following categories: (1) bilateral; (2) chronic; (3) recurrent; (4) unresponsive to the initial steps of nonspecific therapy; or (5) warranted based on clues from the history and physical examination. These criteria exclude unilateral cases of mild iridocyclitis that quickly respond to topical steroids and never recur.

To describe the details of all possible laboratory testing in all possible uveitic situations would require a complete textbook; the reader is referred to two comprehensive sources.[7,8] However, some generalities can be made. Any uveitic case that warrants work-up could turn out to be one of the imitators in ophthalmology, including syphilis, tuberculosis, sarcoidosis, Lyme disease, and herpes simplex. These diseases may affect any or all anatomic aspects of the eye and may be acute or chronic, mild or severe, granulomatous or nongranulomatous. Furthermore, all are treatable or curable. Syphilis can be evaluated with both nonspecific (Venereal Disease Research Laboratory [VDRL], Rapid Plasma Reagin [RPR]) and specific (fluorescent treponemal antibody absorption, microhemagglutination-*Treponema pallidum*) treponemal tests. A chest radiograph and skin testing are useful in the diagnosis of both tuberculosis and sarcoidosis. Angiotensin-converting enzyme (ACE) also may be useful in the latter; serum calcium and lysozyme are of questionable usefulness because of their low sensitivity. In patients who have lived in endemic areas for Lyme disease (Connecticut, California, Minnesota, Wisconsin), Lyme titers should be obtained. Finally, herpes simplex should always be considered in this group. Unfortunately, serum antibody titers to herpes simplex virus are so prevalent in the population that a positive test is rarely useful. However, a negative test rules out this entity. In time, molecular techniques applied to ocular fluids may provide a test with a high positive predictive value for herpes simplex uveitis.

It is important to point out, however, that whenever the history or physical examination provides enough information to warrant a laboratory test, it should be performed even if it is a first bout of uveitis. A patient with complaints of problems with night vision who has multifocal nonpigmented lesions of the retinal pigment epithelium, along with poor color vision, should have human leukocyte antigen-A29 (HLA-A29) typing performed to support the diagnosis of birdshot choroidopathy.

Consultation

Consultation is the simplest but, perhaps, most poorly understood aspect of the uveitis evaluation. Appropriate consultation is invaluable both as an aid to diagnosis and as an aid to management with complicated medical treatment. It should be undertaken only after the previous steps have been completed. A specific question should be addressed: Does this patient with uveitis and a PPD of 17 mm warrant antituberculous treatment? Does this patient with retinal vasculitis and nonspecific joint pains have a collagen vascular disease? Can you help manage the blood levels of ciclosporin in order to minimize the many side effects of this drug? In general, supplying all the ocular details of the case to the consultant is not useful, because this is the ophthalmologist's area of expertise. Likewise, consulting a nonophthalmologist early in the work-up to ask for the appropriate laboratory tests and diagnosis will usually be of less value. Only an ophthalmologist can classify the uveitis properly and perform the appropriate ocular history and examination to direct focused laboratory testing.

Nonspecific Treatment of Uvetis

When the classification, history, examination, laboratory evaluation, and consultations cannot uncover a cause for the uveitis, the diagnosis of idiopathic uveitis can be made. The need for treatment depends on several factors.

What to treat

In general, it is most important to treat uveitis for its actual or potential sequelae. The most common of these are posterior synechiae and CME. Cell and flare are most useful primarily as indicators of the end point of treatment. Other sequelae are certainly worth treating, including retinal vasculitis, retinal infiltrates, and neovascularization. Vitreous cells, like their anterior chamber counterparts, are not, in themselves, usually worthy of great concern.

Principles of treatment

Several basic principles of management should be mentioned. First, treatment can be divided into acute and chronic types. Acute therapy is the use of medication to treat a sudden, severe attack of uveitis such as acute anterior iridocyclitis. In this case, treatment must be swift, intense, and tapered slowly. Typically, topical prednisolone acetate 1% is used because of its better intraocular penetration. A typical dosage schedule would be hourly instillation for several days with a slow taper of the drops over several weeks. Chronic treatment is used to decrease the long-term incidence and severity of the consequences of intraocular inflammation (usually CME) when persistent low-grade inflammation is present. Usually nonsteroidal antiinflammatory medications are used at a constant dose (three to four times a day). Additional treatment modalities for the delivery of steroids and other medical therapies include sub-Tenon injection, intravitreal administration, and oral therapy. In an effort to limit potential systemic complications, significant research has been dedicated toward the development of localized drug delivery systems. Currently, clinical trials involving intraocular sustained release devices are ongoing and may proivde a more efficacious treatment system that comes with a lower incidence of systemic side effects.[9,10]

Whenever the potential for posterior synechiae exists, a short-acting mydriatic/cycloplegic (such as homatropine 5%, two to three times a day) should be used to keep the pupil moving. If posterior synechiae have already formed, frequent applications of phenylephrine 2.5% to 10% (beware in patients with hypertension or cardiac disease) and atropine 1% can be used. If unsuccessful, a pledget of cotton can be soaked with these agents and left in the superior or inferior cul-de-sacs. Finally, dilating agents can be injected subconjunctivally at the apex of synechiae with the hope of 'unzipping' the adhesions (Fig. 106.1).[8] A typical algorithm of treatment for idiopathic uveitis is presented in Figure 106.2.

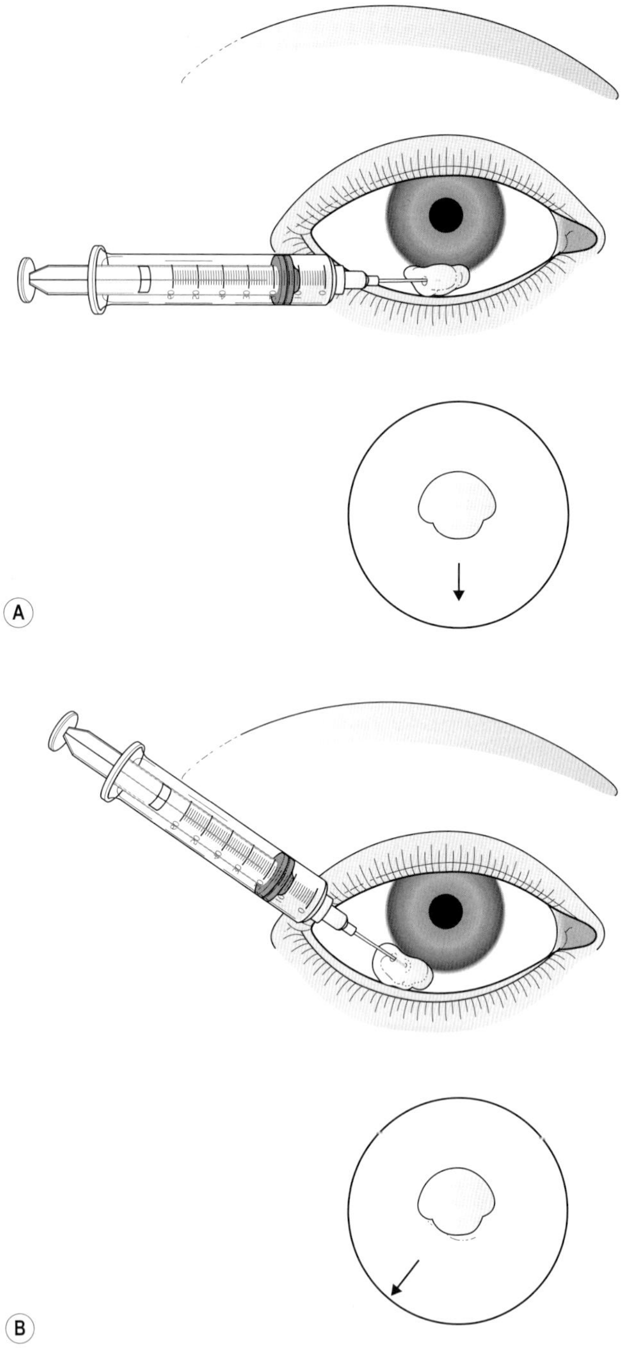

Fig. 106.1 (**A**) Subconjunctival injection of dilating agents performed incorrectly. By placing the injection opposite the midpoint of the synechia, its effectiveness is minimized. (**B**) Subconjunctival injection of dilating agents performed correctly. By placing the injection at the edge of the synechia, its effectiveness has been maximized. (After Smith RE, Nozik RA: *Uveitis: a clinical approach to diagnosis and management*, edn 2, Baltimore, 1989, Williams & Wilkins.)

Nonsteroidal antiinflammatory agents

The principal mechanism of action of nonsteroidal antiinflammatory agents (NSAIDs) is to decrease prostaglandin (PG) synthesis. They have been demonstrated to be useful with angiographic evidence of CME in eyes after cataract surgery.[11,12] As yet, no published studies demonstrate a benefit against CME in eyes with uveitis. Nevertheless, many individuals who treat patients with uveitis believe that these drugs decrease the incidence and severity of CME over the long term. However, they probably do little to treat CME once it is present. They have been shown to be safe and effective in the treatment of acute ocular inflammation after cataract surgery.[13] The principal topical agents in this category include indometacin (Indocid), flurbiprofen (Ocufen), diclofenac (Voltaren), ketorolac (Acular), and nepafenac (Nevanac). When these drugs are used topically, they cause very few side effects except for toxicity from or allergy to the vehicles used to preserve the medications. When given systemically, NSAIDs have potential side effects including

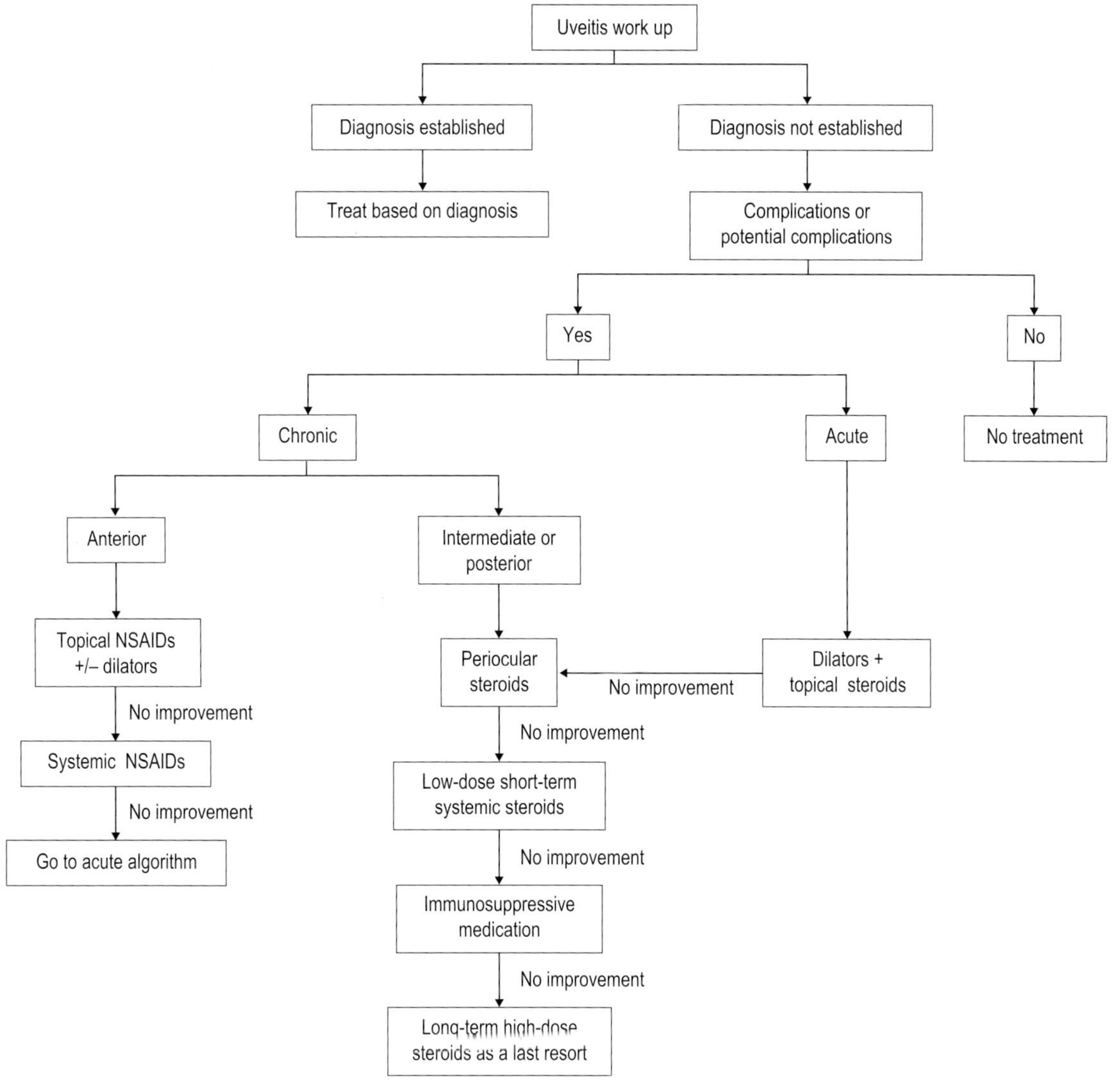

Fig. 106.2 Algorithmic approach to the treatment of idiopathic uveitis.

blood dyscrasias, fluid retention, renal decompensation, liver dysfunction, gastrointestinal upset, and peptic ulceration.

Most side effects of systemic NSAIDs are felt to be due to the nonselective inhibition of two isoforms of the enzyme cyclooxygenase (COX). COX-1 is involved in basal PG production required for normal physiological functions, e.g. gastric cytoprotection. COX-2 is an inducible enzyme which accounts for large amounts of PG production during inflammation. It is felt that COX-2 induction within the eye is responsible for large increases in PGs in various inflammatory conditions and therefore use of COX-2 inhibitors may prove beneficial in the treatment of various forms of uveitis.[14] COX-2 inhibitors currently available worldwide include celecoxib (Celebrex), valdecoxib (Bextra), lumiracoxib (Prexige), and etoricoxib (Arcoxia). Preliminary human studies indicate that COX-2 inhibitors may be useful in treating CME, and animal models have demonstrated the potential for using these agents to treat uveitis.[15,16]

Corticosteroids

Corticosteroids are the mainstay of treatment for idiopathic uveitis. They are powerful, antiinflammatory, and, in high doses, immunosuppressive medications. Their mechanism of action is complex and multifaceted. They are able to decrease the synthesis of arachidonic acid, decrease the release of vasoactive amines from basophils and mast cells, decrease the level of complement, and produce a relative lymphopenia. Although generalizations can be made about the mechanism of action of these agents, there are tremendous practical differences, depending on how they are administered.

Topical corticosteroids are the mainstay of treatment for acute iridocyclitis. Because prednisolone acetate 1% penetrates the anterior chamber well, it is the drug of choice for acute iridocyclitis. Because the acetate form of the drug is a suspension, it is essential that the bottle be shaken multiple times before it is used. In our experience, the most common

Table 106.5 Side effects of systemic steroids

System	Side effects
General	Fever, hypertension
Ocular	Glaucoma, posterior subcapsular cataracts, exophthalmos
Gastrointestinal	Gastric/peptic ulcers
Neuro/CNS	Elevated intracranial pressure, seizures, euphoria, psychosis
Hematologic	Hypercoagulability, leukocytosis
Infectious	Suppression of inflammatory response to infection (especially fungal and viral)
Dermatologic	Delayed tissue healing, hirsutism, acne
Musculoskeletal	Osteoporosis, femur head necrosis
Metabolic	Hyperacidity, diabetes mellitus, hyperosmotic coma

reason for consultation to our uveitis survey unit for anterior segment uveitis is persistent inflammation, which is invariably cured by asking the patient to shake the bottle at least 30 times before use. Phosphate solutions of corticosteroid do not penetrate the anterior chamber well and therefore have less use in the treatment of uveitis. The main side effects of topical corticosteroid preparations occur with long-term use and include increased intraocular pressure (IOP), posterior subcapsular cataracts (PSCC), and temporary pseudoptosis. Rimexolone 1% ophthalmic suspension (Vexol 1%) is a newer, 'site-active,' topical corticosteroid that has significant antiinflammatory activity. One study has shown it to be just as effective as prednisolone 1% in controlling ocular inflammation but it is much less likely to increase IOP.[17]

When anterior uveitis does not respond adequately to topical medication, when the uveitis is predominantly intermediate or posterior, or when CME requires acute treatment, a periocular depot steroid injection is the treatment of choice and most commonly involves a sub-Tenon method (Fig. 106.3). This technique can be repeated monthly if needed. The potential complications include PSCC, increased IOP, conjunctival scarring, ptosis, and rarely intraocular perforation. Retrobulbar hemorrhage, optic nerve injury, and systemic steroid complications are extremely rare with this method.

Although topical and posterior sub-Tenon steroids are common modalities for treating idiopathic uveitis, systemic steroids are rarely justified because they may cause numerous side effects (Table 106.5). In fact, when systemic medication is required, all other things being equal, systemic immunosuppressive therapy should probably be considered before systemic corticosteroids, especially if long-term treatment is likely.

Patients resistant to topical, periocular, and systemic medication can be considered for intraocular steroid treatment. Intravitreal injection of triamcinolone (2–4 mg/0.1 mL) has been shown to induce anatomic resolution of CME and moderate visual improvement in some patients with chronic uveitis.[18] The use of intraocular sustained steroid delivery devices has recently been introduced as another alternative. Further clinical trials with steroid implants are ongoing; however, elevated IOP and cataract formation remain significant side effects with the use of intraocular steroids.

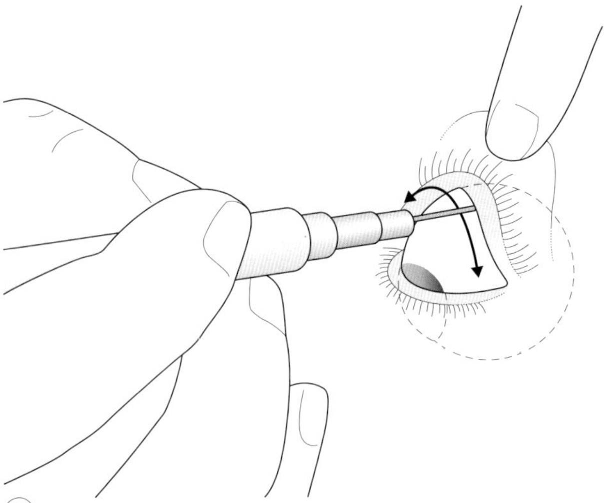
A

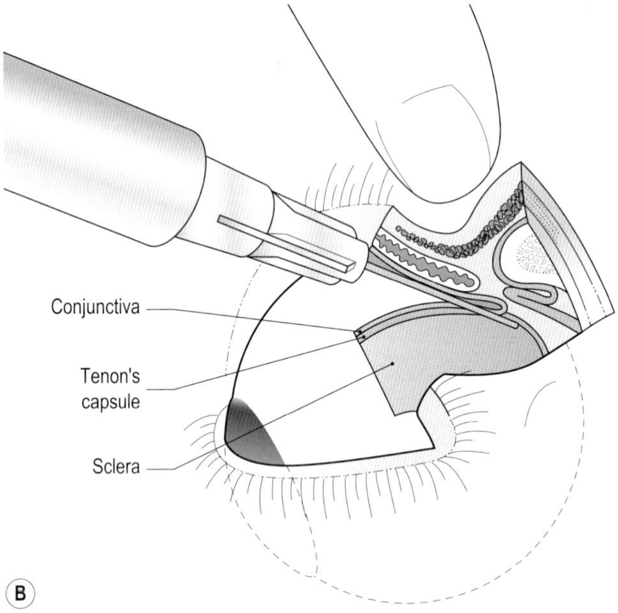

B

Fig. 106.3 (**A**) Posterior sub-Tenon injection. The drawing indicates the correct position of the operator's hands and the needle for posterior sub-Tenon injection. Arrows indicate the direction of the side-to-side circumferential motion. (**B**) Posterior sub-Tenon injection. Drawing indicates the positioning of the tip of the needle in its ideal location between Tenon's capsule and the sclera. (From Smith RE, Nozik RA: *Uveitis: a clinical approach to diagnosis and management*, edn 2, Baltimore, 1989, Williams & Wilkins.)

Immunosuppressive agents

Immunosuppressive agents used in uveitis can be divided into four broad categories: alkylating agents (chlorambucil, cyclophosphamide), antimetabolites (azathioprine, methotrexate), molecules targeting the interleukin-2 (IL-2) pathway (ciclosporin, tacrolimus, sirolimus), and biological response modifiers (BRMs). These immunosuppressive medications often have a narrow therapeutic window and should be used only in severe refractory cases of uveitis. An internist familiar with these drugs should always follow the patient concurrently. An excellent review of the use of immunosuppressive medications in ophthalmology is a valuable reference for anyone using these medications.[19]

The alkylating agents act by transferring an alkyl group to DNA in the N-7 position of guanine during cell division, thus disrupting normal DNA synthesis. Chlorambucil is a more potent agent than cyclophosphamide, but also has more side effects. Antimetabolites are analogs of normal metabolites and are potent immunosuppressive agents. Azathioprine alters purine metabolism, whereas methotrexate is a folate analog. Mycophenolic acid is available as either the prodrug mycophenolate mofetil (MMF/CellCept) or mycophenolate sodium (Myfortic) and has a similar clinical effect as the antimetabolites on lymphocyte proliferation. In its active form, mycophenolic acid inhibits inosine monophosphate dehydrogenase, which is a key enzyme in the purine synthesis pathway that controls the rate of production of guanine monophosphate. Inhibition of this enzymatic step decreases the proliferation of both B- and T-cell lymphocytes and it has proven to be an effective agent in the treatment of chronic uveitis.[20]

Agents employed to either reduce IL-2 production or its action have been used to control ocular inflammation. Ciclosporin is a naturally occurring fungal product that works primarily by decreasing the production of IL-2. In our experience, the beneficial effects of this agent are similar to the previously mentioned immunosuppressives, but the inflammation often rebounds when the drug is tapered. Hence, long-term treatment is often necessary. Tacrolimus, also referred to as FK506 or fujimycin (Prograf/Advagraf/Protopic) has been demonstrated to be as effective as ciclosporin in long-term treatment of uveitis, has a wider theraputic index, and an excellent side-effect profile.[21,22] Unlike either ciclosporin or tacrolimus, which both inhibit the production of IL-2, sirolimus (Rapamune) is a third agent in this class that reduces inflammation by inhibiting the action of IL-2, and preliminary clinical investigation has indicated that it can be used to successfully treat uveitis.[23]

Biological response modifiers (BRMs) include a range of molecules that interrupt the inflammatory cascade at various points in the biochemical sequence. Our ever-increasing understanding of the biochemical mechanisms leading to inflammation has provided a wide range of targets for new medical therapies. The prototypical agent in this class is the monoclonal antibody infliximab (Remicade) which binds to and inactivates tumor necrosis factor-alpha (TNF-α). A more complete listing of availible and investigational BRMs is presented in Table 106.6. To date, preliminary clinical research and case reports have demonstrated a role for infliximab,[24] anakinra,[25] rituximab,[26] abatacept,[27] and daclizumab[28] in treating uveitis.

Table 106.6 Biological response modifiers (BRMs)

Name	Trade name	Target
Adalimumab	Humira	TNF-α
Golimumab	N/A	TNF-α
Certolizumab	Cimiza	TNF-α
Anakinra	Kineret	IL-1
Daclizumab	Zenapax	IL-2
Tocilizumab	Actemra	IL-6
Rituximab	Rituxan	CD20+ B cell
Ocrelizumab	Simponi	CD20+ B cell
Ofatumumab	Arzerra	CD20+ B cell
Abatacept	Orencia	T cell

Summary

The most important lesson in dealing with idiopathic uveitis is to make this a diagnosis of exclusion. When this diagnosis must be considered, a rational treatment approach depends on three principles: (1) treating complications and potential complications of the inflammation instead of the inflammation itself; (2) considering the need to treat both acute and chronic complications; and (3) using the least-toxic medication and the least-invasive delivery system to achieve these goals.

References

1. Wakefield D, Dunlop I, McCluskey PJ, Penny R. Uveitis: aetiology and disease associations in an Australian population. *Aust NZ J Ophthalmol.* 1986;14:181–187.
2. Weiner A, BenEzra D. Clinical patterns and associated conditions in chronic uveitis. *Am J Ophthalmol.* 1991;112:151–158.
3. Boskovich SA, Lowder CY, Meisler DM, Gutman FA. Systemic diseases associated with intermediate uveitis. *Cleve Clin J Med.* 1993;60:460–465.
4. Priem H, Verbraeken H, de Laey JJ. Diagnostic problems in chronic vitreous inflammation. *Graefe's Arch Clin Exp Ophthalmol.* 1993;231: 453–456.
5. Jabs DA, Nussenblatt RB, Rosenbaum JT. Standardization of uveitis nomenclature for reporting clinical data. Results of the First International Workshop. *Am J Ophthalmol.* 2005;140:509–516.
6. Kimura SJ, Thygeson P, Hogan MJ. Signs and symptoms of uveitis. II. Classification of the posterior manifestations of uveitis. *Am J Ophthalmol.* 1959;47:171–176.
7. Nussenblatt RB, Palestine AG. *Uveitis: fundamentals and clinical practice.* St Louis: Mosby; 1989.
8. Smith RE, Nozik RA. *Uveitis: a clinical approach to diagnosis and management.* 2nd ed. Baltimore: Williams & Wilkins; 1989.
9. Jaffe GJ, Martin D, Callanan D, et al. Fluocinolone acetonide implant (Retisert) for noninfectious posterior uveitis: thirty-four-week results of a multicenter randomized clinical study. *Ophthalmology.* 2006;113: 1020–1027.
10. Kane FE, Burdan J, Cutino A, Green KE. Iluvien: a new sustained delivery technology for posterior eye disease. *Expert Opin Drug Deliv.* 2008;5: 1039–1046.
11. Flach AJ, Stegman RC, Graham J, Kruger LP. Prophylaxis of aphakic cystoid macular edema without corticosteroids. A paired-comparison, placebo-controlled double-masked study. *Ophthalmology.* 1990;97: 1253–1258.
12. Flach AJ, Dolan BJ, Irvine AR. Effectiveness of ketorolac tromethamine 0.5% ophthalmic solution for chronic aphakic and pseudophakic cystoid macular edema. *Am J Ophthalmol.* 1987;103:479–486.

13. Solomon KD, Cheetham JK, DeGryse R, Brint SF, Rosenthal A. Topical ketorolac tromethamine 0.5% ophthalmic solution in ocular inflammation after cataract surgery. *Ophthalmology.* 2001;108:331–337.
14. Masferrer JL, Kulkarni PS. Cyclooxygenase-2 inhibitors: a new approach to the therapy of ocular inflammation. *Surv Ophthalmol.* 1997;41(Suppl 2):S35–S40.
15. Reis A, Birnbaum F, Hansen LL, Reinhard T. Successful treatment of cystoid macular edema with valdecoxib. *J Cataract Refract Surg.* 2007; 33:682–685.
16. Bora NS, Sohn JH, Bora PS, Kaplan HJ, Kulkarni P. Anti-inflammatory effects of specific cyclooxygenase 2,5-lipoxygenase, and inducible nitric oxide synthase inhibitors on experimental autoimmune anterior uveitis (EAAU). *Ocul Immunol Inflamm.* 2005;13:183–189.
17. Foster CS, Alter G, DeBarge LR, et al. Efficacy and safety of rimexolone 1% ophthalmic suspension vs 1% prednisolone acetate in the treatment of uveitis. *Am J Ophthalmol.* 1996;122:171–182.
18. Antcliff RJ, Spalton DJ, Stanford MR, et al. Intravitreal triamcinolone for uveitic cystoid macular edema: an optical coherence tomography study. *Ophthalmology.* 2001;108:765–772.
19. Jabs DA, Rosenbaum JT, Foster CS, et al. Guidelines for the use of immunosuppressive drugs in patients with ocular inflammatory disorders: recommendations of an expert panel. *Am J Ophthalmol.* 2000;130:492–513.
20. Teoh SC, Hogan AC, Dick AD, Lee RW. Mycophenolate mofetil for the treatment of uveitis. *Am J Ophthalmol.* 2008;146:752–760.
21. Hogan AC, McAvoy CE, Dick AD, Lee RW. Long-term efficacy and tolerance of tacrolimus for the treatment of uveitis. *Ophthalmology.* 2007; 114:1000–1006.
22. Figueroa MS, Ciancas E, Orte L. Long-term follow-up of tacrolimus treatment in immune posterior uveitis. *Eur J Ophthalmol.* 2007;17:69–74.
23. Shanmuganathan VA, Casely EM, Raj D, et al. The efficacy of sirolimus in the treatment of patients with refractory uveitis. *Br J Ophthalmol.* 2005;89:666–669.
24. Hale S, Lightman S. Anti-TNF therapies in the management of acute and chronic uveitis. *Cytokine.* 2006;33:231–237.
25. Botsios C, Sfriso P, Furlan A, Punzi L, Dinarello CA. Resistant Behçet disease responsive to anakinra. *Ann Intern Med.* 2008;149:284–286.
26. Tappeiner C, Heinz C, Specker C, Heiligenhaus A. Rituximab as a treatment option for refractory endogenous anterior uveitis. *Ophthalmic Res.* 2007;39:184–186.
27. Angeles-Han S, Flynn T, Lehman T. Abatacept for refractory juvenile idiopathic arthritis-associated uveitis – a case report. *J Rheumatol.* 2008;35:1897–1898.
28. Nussenblatt RB, Peterson JS, Foster CS, et al. Initial evaluation of subcutaneous daclizumab treatments for noninfectious uveitis: a multicenter noncomparative interventional case series. *Ophthalmology.* 2005;112: 764–770.

Chapter 107

HLA-B27-Related Uveitis

M. Camille Almond, Jenny V. Ongkosuwito, Marc D. De Smet

Acute anterior uveitis (AAU) is associated with human leukocyte antigen (HLA)-B27 in approximately 50% of cases. This association is more commonly found in males, and, after frequent recurrences, it leads to more long-term complications than in patients with recurrent HLA-B27-negative anterior uveitis.[1,2] Numerous syndromes associated with HLA-B27 have ocular manifestations, most commonly involving the anterior segment.

The association between AAU and HLA-B27 was first reported in 1973.[3] Strong associations were also observed between HLA-B27 and seronegative spondyloarthropathies (SSAs) such as ankylosing spondylitis (AS),[4] psoriatic arthritis (PsA), inflammatory bowel disease (IBD), and reactive arthritis (ReA).[5] The parallel between some of these diseases, uveitis, and HLA-B27 is quite striking. Nearly 100% of AS patients with uveitis are HLA-B27 positive, and uveitis is part of the definition for ReA.[6] Thirty percent of AS patients have AAU, which is much more than the normal prevalence of AAU (1%) among HLA-B27-positive individuals.[3] In parallel with these findings, and as far back as the turn of the twentieth century, a temporal association was noted between these arthropathies and extra-articular infections, particularly those due to enteric organisms.[7,8] As with the SSAs, indirect evidence also linked Gram-negative organisms to AAU,[9–17] the association being strongest after acute symptomatic infections rather than with a chronic carrier state. However, a direct connection has not been demonstrated. Major strides have been made in the last few years in our understanding of the role of HLA-B27 and bacterial antigens on the onset and perpetuation of disease.

HLA-B27 and Pathogenesis of Disease

The HLA system is genetically encoded by the major histocompatibility complex (MHC) located on chromosome 6. The MHC are glycoproteins found on human cell-surface membranes and are divided into three classes.[18] HLA-B27 belongs to the class I antigens, which play an important role both in the development of tolerance to 'self' antigens (by presentation of endogenous proteins) and in the destruction of infected or anomalous cells (by presentation of viral or aberrant peptides) to cytotoxic (CD8) T cells.[19] This occurs by insertion of the cytosol-derived peptide into a groove located on the surface of the class I antigen.[20,21] This complex can then interact with presensitized T cells to incite an inflammatory response.[22–24]

HLA-B27 exists as 24[25] different subtypes, most of which have been associated with either SSAs or AAU; no definite association has been demonstrated for B*2703 in West Africa, B*2706 in Southeast Asia, and B*2709 in Sardinia.[26] The prevalence of HLA-B27 positivity varies greatly among populations, as does its association with inflammatory disease. Four percent to 13% of Caucasians carry the gene, whereas 50% of all Haida Indians are HLA-B27 positive.[24] In Western countries, HLA-B27-associated AAU accounts for 18–32% of anterior uveitis cases, whereas only 6–13% of cases in Asia demonstrate this association.[27] This is due, in part, of course, to the relatively lower frequency of HLA-B27 positivity in Asian countries. The variability among races and ethnicities almost certainly indicates a variable influence of other genetically and environmentally determined factors that have yet to be elucidated.

A link between HLA-B27, enteric bacteria, and inflammatory disease has been demonstrated in transgenic animals. Rats that express both the *HLA-B27* gene and human β_2-microglobulin spontaneously develop an inflammatory illness at about 10 weeks of age that is characterized by diarrhea, arthritis, nail changes, psoriasis-like lesions, and male genital tract lesions. However, these animals do not seem to develop uveitis. Some transgenic lines are prone to disease, whereas others are resistant. Disease susceptibility is related to a high transgene product copy number in lymphoid cells,[28] is T-cell dependent,[29] and can be transferred to irradiated nontransgenic animals.[30] Of particular interest, susceptible transgenic animals maintained in a germ-free state did not develop any joint disease, although they did develop skin changes.[31]

There are many theories as to how infection triggers inflammatory syndromes. One mechanism suggests that the microorganism must be present in the target organ. Using polymerase chain reaction (PCR), chlamydial RNA was found in joints of newly diagnosed ReA patients.[8] Molecular mimicry between bacterial and organ-specific proteins also has been proposed.[22] In this model, bacteria carry sequence motifs that are similar to peptides present in the joint or eye. In the course of the immune response to the infecting microorganism, T cells are redirected against host tissue. HLA-B27 itself also contains peptide sequences that are homologous with S-Ag, a known uveitogenic peptide.[32,33] Breakdown of HLA-B27 during an inflammatory episode could lead to a secondary immune response directed against eye proteins. Earlier, we indicated that the immune response generated by HLA-B27 is directed mainly by CD8 cells, yet it is known that most autoimmune diseases are mediated by CD4 cells. There is recent evidence that HLA-B27 has the unusual ability to form stable heavy chain homodimers, and that these homodimers are capable of presenting antigen to CD4 cells, suggesting that this process may be involved in the pathogenesis of spondyloarthritis.[34,35]

Acute Anterior Uveitis

Acute anterior uveitis is a common form of intraocular inflammation, with an annual incidence of about 8.2 new cases per 100 000 in a white population.[36] This is, by definition, a self-limited disease of less than 3 months' duration that is characterized by recurrent attacks. Fifty percent of patients are HLA-B27 positive, but if one tests patients with recurrent disease, this incidence increases to more than 70%.[37] About half of patients with new-onset AAU have an associated spondyloarthropathy.[1] Eighty percent have AS; the rest are split among ReA, PsA, and other spondyloarthropathies.[1] Patients who are HLA-B27 positive tend to have more recurrent episodes with long disease-free periods. Disease in HLA-B27-negative patients usually occurs later in life (>50 years) and is associated with fewer exacerbations, and a better overall prognosis than in HLA-B27-positive patients with or without systemic manifestations.[38]

AAU in HLA-B27-positive patients presents classically as a nongranulomatous anterior uveitis characterized by an acute onset, mild to severe ocular pain, red eye, photophobia, and a mild decrease in visual acuity.[1,39,40] Men are affected twice as often as women.[1,39] In women, AAU is relatively common in pregnancy, particularly if associated with AS.[41,42] The disease is most often unilateral, but both eyes can be involved if the disease becomes recurrent. Unilateral alternating disease occurs in 38% of patients.[1] On slit lamp examination, small keratic precipitates are seen on the corneal endothelial surface, but mutton-fat precipitates are absent.[39]Fibrin is often present in the anterior chamber,[1] a hypopyon may develop in up to 15% of patients,[43–45] and on rare occasion a hyphema may be seen.[46]

Most AAU episodes resolve with prompt and aggressive topical corticosteroid administration in association with a topical cycloplegic. Therapy should be sustained until there is evidence of quiescence. If, in the initial stages, there is already evidence of a significant fibrin reaction, a subconjunctival steroid injection may help to clear the inflammation. Persistent or very severe inflammation may require the use of sub-Tenon's steroid injection or systemic treatment with immunosuppressive agents. According to Rothova et al.[47] about 32% of cases of AAU require the addition of periocular steroid injections. Resolution generally takes several weeks to occur, on average about 8 weeks in HLA-B27-positive patients, slightly less in HLA-B27-negative individuals.

Complications and Posterior Pole Involvement in HLA-B27-Positive Patients

Chronic inflammation or recurrent attacks of AAU can lead to severe ocular complications. Posterior synechiae can be found in 10% of patients after their first attack, but are present in 40% of patients that have had multiple flare-ups. Cataracts develop in 15% of patients with more than one relapse. Glaucoma, which may require a filtering procedure, is present in only 8–10% of HLA-B27-positive patients, a much lower incidence than in HLA-B27-negative anterior uveitis where the incidence is closer to 40%.[1,42] Glaucoma is more common in HLA-B27-positive patients who have developed posterior pole complications, where it is reported to occur in about one-third of patients.[48] However, these numbers could be confounded by the fact that about 6% of patients are steroid responders.

Posterior pole changes occur more commonly in patients with more prolonged disease (average 4.5 months) and after they have suffered five or more recurrent attacks.[39,45,48,49] They are also more common in patients with associated systemic disease.[50] In the majority of cases (84% in one study), only one eye is affected.[48] Spillover into the anterior vitreous is not uncommon and is related to the severity and duration of anterior segment inflammation, and in particular to the severity of ciliary body involvement.[51] Once present in the vitreous, inflammatory debris can take a considerable time to clear, and with recurrent or prolonged attacks, more debris can accumulate. On careful examination, an anterior vitritis is not uncommon during the acute episode, which is distinguishable from vitreous debris by the presence of discrete cellular elements; it is seen in 30–63% of HLA-B27-positive patients.[40,45,47] Cystoid macular edema (CME), a major cause of permanent visual impairment, is also common in these patients, occurring in up to 30% of patients as compared to 8% of HLA-B27-negative patients.[42,45,47,52] Other posterior pole manifestations include pars plana exudates, papillitis, retinal vasculitis (occasionally severe enough to cause a vascular occlusion), optic disk neovascularization, and epiretinal membrane formation.[4,48,50,53,54]

In patients who develop CME or other posterior changes, more aggressive treatment may be necessary. The majority of patients will need one or more sub-Tenon's injections of depot steroids.[55] Approximately half may require systemic corticosteroids to control the inflammation, which can be administered orally or as pulse intravenous therapy depending on the severity of the inflammation.[48,56,57] About one-third of patients will require more aggressive immunosuppression with methotrexate, cytotoxic agents, or ciclosporin.[48,58] Despite these treatments, progressive vitreous opacification may occur in about 10% of patients with significant posterior pole disease. In these patients, visual improvement can be achieved with a pars plana vitrectomy, often with complete elimination of recurrences.[48,54,59] In patients with recalcitrant disease, some advocate use of intraocular triamcinolone, wherein 4 mg (0.1 mL) of triamcinolone acetonide is injected via the pars plana into the vitreous cavity.[60] In a series of uveitis patients followed by optical coherence tomography (OCT), three HLA-B27-

positive patients with CME who received this injection experienced 6 months of resolution prior to recurrence. This procedure has, however, been associated with cataract and glaucoma when used in other uveitic conditions.[61] Another approach consists of placing a sustained drug delivery system inside the eye.[62] Two hundred and seventy-eight patients with noninfectious posterior uveitis were treated with a fluocinolone implant as part of a multicenter randomized clinical study. Three-year follow-up revealed improved vision, decreased number of recurrences, and decreased need for other adjunctive treatments. However, many patients developed ocular hypertension, 40% of whom required glaucoma filtration surgery. The rate of cataract extraction increased to 93% in implanted phakic eyes (vs 20% in nonimplanted phakic eyes).[63]

Recently, systemically administered anti-TNF antibodies have been investigated for use as steroid-sparing therapy for intraocular inflammation, with mixed results. Although in some cases a single injection has led to a rapid and sustained remission lasting several months, recurrence is common, leading some to question how this effect differs from the natural course of AAU.[25,64] Although anti-TNF agents have been shown to improve arthritis symptoms in SSAs, their utility for AAU is less clear.[65] Success with the use of sulfa antibiotics such as sulfasalazine for the treatment of chronic inflammatory diseases such as IBD has led to their use in recurrent AAU with some promising results. In a prospective study of 10 patients with recurrent AAU, seven of whom were HLA-B27 positive, oral sulfasalazine therapy reduced flare frequency from an average of 3.4 per year to 0.9 per year after 12 months of therapy.[66] Similar results have been demonstrated in another study in patients with both AAU and AS,[67] though this treatment has not yet gained widespread use for uveitis.

A novel therapeutic approach is based on the concept of oral tolerance, where oral administration of an antigen can produce peripheral tolerance to that antigen. Amino acid sequence homology that exists between retinal antigens and certain HLA molecules is thought to contribute to the development of T-cell sensitivity to intraocular antigens in uveitis. Based on this mimicry model, investigators administered HLA-B27 PD protein, found in B-27, -51, and -44, to patients with therapy-refractory uveitis (chronic and acute) and demonstrated decreased intraocular inflammation in all and decreased steroid requirement in most (7/9) of the patients studied.[68] Though still in the early stages of development, this concept is exciting, as it offers the possibility of a targeted systemic treatment for refractory uveitis that does not result in generalized immunosuppression and the inherent risks associated with it.

Other Associated Conditions

Ankylosing spondylitis

Ankylosing spondylitis has a male:female predominance of 3:1. It tends to appear in the third decade of life, often insidiously, with low back pain. The symptoms are worse at rest and improve with exercise. The sacroiliac spine is affected in 100% of patients. As the disease progresses, most patients develop severe axial rigidity, usually starting in the lower spine. Peripheral arthritis is occasionally seen. It affects most commonly the lower extremities and may be the initial presentation in children. AAU is seen in 25% of AS patients. Other rarer manifestations include aortic regurgitation (5%), atrioventricular conductance disturbances, and apical pulmonary fibrosis. Systemic amyloidosis develops in 4% of these patients. Reportedly, 40–80% of patients with AS alone are HLA-B27 positive, whereas positivity reaches 100% in patients with AS and AAU.[27] Patients with AS benefit from an early referral to a rheumatologist. Proper posturing and physical therapy can help to prevent the severe scoliosis associated with this disease.

Psoriatic arthritis

Psoriasis is a chronic inflammatory dermatologic condition that is classically characterized by scattered erythematous plaques with an overlying silvery scale, which can vary from pruritic to painful. As the name implies, PsA is the association of joint involvement with the dermatologic findings of psoriasis, often (in up to 84% of patients) following the development of skin findings by an average of 12 years.[69] The five classic clinical subtypes, based on the 1973 Moll and Wright classification criteria, include polyarticular symmetric, oligoarticular asymmetric, distal interphalangeal (DIP) predominant, spondylitis predominant, and arthritis mutilans. With dactylitis or enthesitis of the digits, patients may develop the 'sausage digit' deformity, and with involvement of the DIP joint, one may also see nailbed pitting, subungual hyperkeratosis, and onycholysis. Rates of PsA in HIV-positive individuals are from 10 to 40 times greater than in the general population.[70]

With a reported prevalence of 7–25%, patients with PsA may also develop AAU, most commonly in those patients who are HLA-B27 positive and exhibit associated sacroiliitis.[71] Rates of HLA-B27 positivity in PsA are reportedly between 40% and 50% in persons of Western European ancestry.[27]

Idiopathic inflammatory bowel disease

Idiopathic inflammatory bowel disease refers to two clinical entities, both included with the spondyloarthropathies: Crohn's disease and ulcerative colitis. Although 10% of these patients have sacroiliitis, and 7% will have AS, eye manifestations are more common in IBD patients who are HLA-B27 negative. Crohn's disease is characterized in the gut by transmural inflammation, with the formation of noncaseating granulomas that affect most commonly the distal ileum and the proximal colon. Ulcerative colitis is primarily a mucosal disease limited to the large intestine and characterized by inflammation and diffuse vascular congestion. In 4–10% of cases, Crohn's disease is associated with a variety of eye lesions (Table 107.1),[72] whereas ulcerative colitis is almost exclusively associated with anterior segment inflammation. The presence of arthritis or active bowel disease, particularly at the level of the large intestine, is associated with more severe ocular inflammation, but the overall incidence of ocular inflammation is not closely related to the presence of active bowel disease.[72,73] Uveitis is the most

Table 107.1 Ocular involvement in inflammatory bowel disease

	Crohn's disease		Ulcerative colitis	
Author	**Hopkins et al.[92]**	**Salmon et al.[72]**	**Korelitz and Coles[93]**	**Wright and Wathinson[94]**
Year	1974	1991	1967	1965
Ocular manifestations		9.1%	1.9%	8.9%
Number of cases				
Crohn's disease		19	4	
Ulcerative colitis		9	24	
Male/Female		5/14	4/9	
Mean age		30.3	27.5	
Uveitis	8	7	13	24
Episcleritis	2	8		
Acute anterior scleritis		4		
Corneal infiltrates	4	2		
Corneal ulcerations				
Arthritis/arthralgia (%)		15 (79%)	11 (85%)	8 (33%)
Erythema nodosum	5	5		

common ocular manifestation seen in Crohn's disease. In children, asymptomatic uveitis (as defined by increased flare or cells) has been detected in 6–12.5% during an active period of systemic disease,[74,75] in contrast to none of the adult patient population.[76] Episcleritis is also very often seen in patients with Crohn's disease. Occasionally, necrotizing scleritis may be seen, but it is a rare manifestation. Large peripheral corneal infiltrates occasionally occur and are sometimes associated with scleritis (Fig. 107.1).[72,77,78] The uveitis seen in this context mainly affects the anterior segment, but rarely a panuveitis or retinal vasculitis may be seen.[72,78] The vasculitis involves both the arterioles and venules and is associated with occlusions. Other rare ocular manifestations associated with Crohn's disease include Sjögren's syndrome, myositis, orbital and eyelid edema, and optic neuritis.

Reactive arthritis

Reactive arthritis (previously known as Reiter's syndrome) is clinically characterized by the triad of arthritis, conjunctivitis, and nongonococcal urethritis occurring simultaneously or sequentially over a short time.[79,80] Ocular manifestations seen in association with ReA are summarized in Table 107.2. The conjunctivitis tends to be papillary, associated with a mucocutaneous discharge but without a preauricular node. Keratitis, when it develops, is best characterized as a punctate epithelial keratitis with pleomorphic infiltrates of the anterior peripheral stroma and micropannus (Fig. 107.2).[81,82] The uveitis is largely limited to the anterior segment, but a spillover into the anterior vitreous is not uncommon.

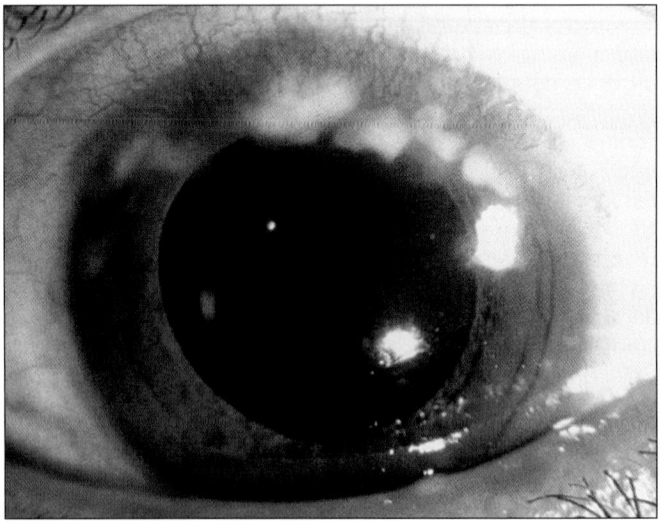

Fig. 107.1 Patient with scleritis and peripheral corneal infiltrates in the setting of Crohn's disease. (From Salmon et al. *Ophthalmology.* 1991;98:480–484. Copyright Elsevier 1991.)

Table 107.2 Ocular involvement in reactive arthritis

	Immunocompetent					Immunodeficiency syndrome
Author	**Csonka**[89]	**Ostler et al.**[95]	**Leirisalo et al.**[83]	**Prakash et al.**[96]	**Lee et al.**[81]	**Winchester et al.**[91]
Year	1958	1970	1982	1983	1986	1987
Number of cases	185	23	160	36	113	13
Male/Female	182/3	22/1	152/8	29/7	102/11	
Mean age	20–40	25	29.6	23.8	28	
HLA-B27			81.3%	83.3%	71.7%	69%
Conjunctivitis	60 (3.3%)	17 (74%)	65 (40.6%)	14 (39%)	66 (58%)	10 (77%)
Uveitis	21 (10.8%)	9 (39%)	6 (3.8%)	7 (19%)	13 (12%)	1 (7%)
Keratitis	5 (2.7%)	8 (35%)	1 (0.6%)		4 (4%)	
Episcleritis					1 (1%)	

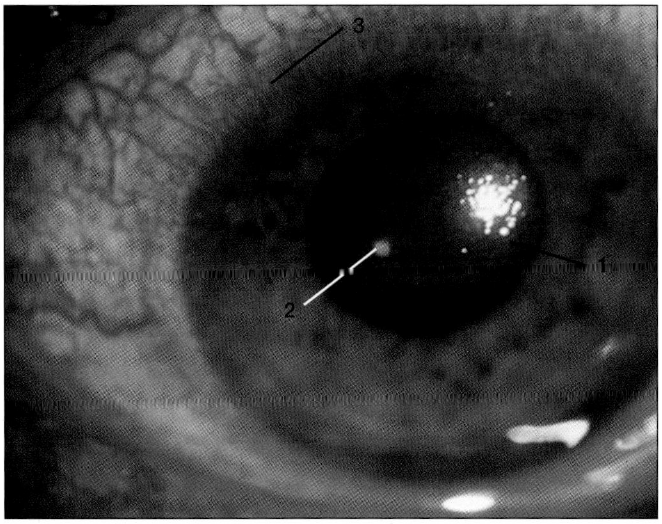

Fig. 107.2 Punctate epithelial keratitis (*1*), anterior stromal infiltrates (*2*), and micropannus (*3*) in the setting of reactive arthritis. (From Lee et al: *Ophthalmology.* 1986;93:350–356. Copyright Elsevier 1986.)

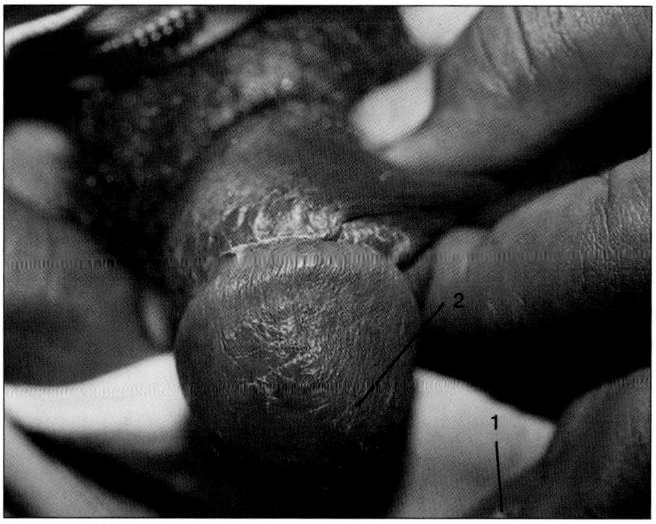

Fig. 107.3 Keratoderma blennorrhagicum lesions on the hand (*1*) and circinate balanitis (*2*) in a patient with reactive arthritis. (Courtesy Thomas Darling, MD, Dermatology Division, National Cancer Institute, National Institutes of Health.)

Joint disease is predominantly seen in the knees, ankles, feet, and wrists in an asymmetric and oligoarticular pattern.[83,84] There are also characteristic skin and nail changes present in 30–40% of patients. Keratoderma blennorrhagicum, which consists of papules, vesicles, or pustules, is usually located on the palms and soles (Fig. 107.3). Nails can develop subungual pustules and hyperkeratosis; however, nail pitting characteristic of psoriasis does not occur. Painless mucous membrane lesions can develop in the oral mucosa or circinate balanitis on the glans penis (Fig. 107.3).[85] Other, less common, systemic manifestations include fever, pericarditis, aortic insufficiency, cardiac conduction defects, systemic amyloidosis, and neurologic problems.

More than 75% of patients with ReA carry the HLA-B27 antigen.[86] In a series of 113 patients, only about half met all major criteria for ReA.[81] Patients with incomplete ReA characteristically had arthritis and a positive HLA-B27, but did not have conjunctivitis or urethritis.[87] Two types of infection may lead to ReA: genitourinary (postvenereal), mainly *Chlamydia*, and gastrointestinal (postdysenteric), Gram-negative organisms including *Yersinia*, *Salmonella*, *Shigella*, and *Campylobacter*.[7,85] Approximately 0.9% of men with non-specific urethritis,[88] and 0.2% of patients following epidemic dysentery will develop ReA.[89] In ReA patients with urethritis, tetracycline or erythromycin seemed to decrease the rate of arthritis to 10% as compared to 37% with penicillin. However, this may be due to an effect of tetracycline on immunocompetent cells rather than on its ability to kill bacteria.[8] ReA is seen in up to 10% of patients who develop acquired immunodeficiency syndrome (AIDS), although these patients do not typically present with the classic triad.[70,90] In 9 of 13 patients described by Winchester et al.,[91] ReA followed or appeared almost simultaneously with clinical evidence of immunodeficiency. The increased incidence of ReA in patients with AIDS (100–200 times that seen in non-AIDS patients) seems to point to the important role of CD8-positive cells in the pathogenesis of this disorder, and by extension the probable role of these cells in other HLA-B27-positive related disease.[70] A simpler explanation may be that these patients develop more frequent acute intestinal infections and are thus more prone to develop ReA.

Individual manifestations in ReA usually evolve over a long period of time, often over 12 to 18 months. Lee et al. found that the complete complex of symptoms took about 2.7 years to develop.[81] A permanent disability, mainly musculoskeletal, occurs in 20% of patients. Nonsteroidal antiinflammatory medication and physical therapy can be helpful in the management of these patients.

Summary

HLA-B27-related uveitis is a common disorder. When a patient presents with a first attack of AAU, a thorough family history is warranted. If other family members are affected by an HLA-B27-related disorder, or if an individual presents with symptoms associated with one of these inflammatory complexes, testing is warranted; otherwise, it is best to wait until the patient has had at least one AAU recurrence. It is probably wise to refer HLA-B27-positive patients to an internist or a rheumatologist for a thorough systemic workup. Proper posturing can avoid some of the late complications of AS, and a judicious antibiotic regimen can prevent some of the manifestations of ReA. Patients should be questioned carefully for a history of conjunctivitis, urethritis, or diarrhea. In many cases of ReA, all signs do not appear concomitantly. Uveitis may follow initial manifestations by 1 or more months. In the presence of ReA, the patient may be an HIV carrier. On slit lamp examination, the presence of conjunctivitis or scleritis should be carefully sought and is indicative of ReA or IBD. HLA-B27 uveitis is not necessarily limited to the anterior segment, as unexplained visual loss may be due to posterior pole involvement, which generally requires more aggressive therapy. In all cases of HLA-B27 uveitis, prompt and assertive therapy is mandatory.

References

1. Rothova A, et al. Clinical features of acute anterior uveitis. *Am J Ophthalmol.* 1987;103:137–145.
2. Rothova A, et al. Acute anterior uveitis (AAU) and HLA-B27. *Br J Rheumatol.* 1983;22:144–145.
3. Brewerton DA, et al. Acute anterior uveitis and HL-A 27. *Lancet.* 1973;2:994–996.
4. Brewerton DA, et al. Ankylosing spondylitis and HL-A 27. *Lancet.* 1973;1:904–907.
5. Calin A. Spondylarthropathy, undifferentiated spondylarthritis, and overlap. In: Maddison BJ, et al, eds. *Oxford textbook of rheumatology*. vol. 2. Oxford: Oxford University Press; 1993:666–674.
6. Derhaag PJ. Genetical factors – other than HLA-B27-associated diseases. *Scand J Rheumatol Suppl.* 1990;87:122–126.
7. Inman RD, et al. Postdysenteric reactive arthritis. *Arthritis Rheum.* 1988;31:1377–1383.
8. Inman RD, Scofield RH. Etiopathogenesis of ankylosing spondylitis and reactive arthritis. *Curr Opin Rheumatol.* 1994;6:360–370.
9. Eastmond CJ, et al. Frequency of faecal *Klebsiella aerogenes* in patients with ankylosing spondylitis and controls with respect to individual features of the disease. *Ann Rheum Dis.* 1980;39:118–123.
10. Holland EJ, et al. Acute anterior uveitis in association with *Klebsiella pneumoniae* and HLA-B27. *Kurume Med J.* 1981;28:181–187.
11. White L, et al. A search for Gram-negative enteric micro-organisms in acute anterior uveitis: association of *Klebsiella* with recent onset of disease, HLA-B27, and B7 CREG. *Br J Ophthalmol.* 1984;68:750–755.
12. Beckingsale AB, et al. *Klebsiella* and acute anterior uveitis. *Br J Ophthalmol.* 1984;68:866–868.
13. Ashaye AO, Perkins ES. Cross reactivity between *Klebsiella pneumoniae* and ocular tissue. *Afr J Med Sci.* 1992;21:73–78.
14. Dequeker J, et al. HLA-B27, arthritis and *Yersinia enterocolitica* infection. *J Rheumatol.* 1980;7:706–710.
15. Ebringer R, et al. *Yersinia enterocolitica* biotype I. Diarrhoea and episodes of HLA B27 related ocular and rheumatic inflammatory disease in South-East England. *Scand J Rheumatol.* 1982;11:171–176.
16. Goh BT, et al. Isolation of *Chlamydia trachomatis* from prostatic fluid in association with inflammatory joint or eye disease. *Br J Vener Dis.* 1983;59:373–375.
17. Wakefield D, Penny R. Cell-mediated immune response to *Chlamydia* in anterior uveitis: role of HLA B27. *Clin Exp Immunol.* 1983;51:191–196.
18. Altman DM, Trowsdale J. Major histocompatibility complex structure and function. *Curr Opin Immunol.* 1990;2:93–98.
19. Murray N, McMichael A. Antigen presentation in virus infection. *Curr Opin Immunol.* 1992;4:401–407.
20. Wakefield D, et al. Acute anterior uveitis and HLA-B27. *Surv Ophthalmol.* 1991;36:223–232.
21. Madden DR, et al. The structure of HLA-B27 reveals nonamer self-peptides bound in an extended conformation. *Nature.* 1991;353: 321–325.
22. Benjamin R, Parham P. HLA-B27 and diseases: a consequence of inadvertent antigen presentation? *Rheum Dis Clin North Am.* 1992;18:11–21.
23. Ivanyi P. Immunogenetics of the spondyloarthropathies. *Curr Opin Rheumatol.* 1993;5:436–445.
24. Kellner H, Yu D. The pathogenetic aspects of spondyloarthropathies from the point of view of HLA-B27. *Rheumatol Int.* 1992;12:121–127.
25. Suhler EB, et al. HLA-B27-associated uveitis: overview and current perspectives. *Curr Opin Ophthalmol.* 2003;14:378–383.
26. Chang JH, et al. Acute anterior uveitis and HLA-B27. *Surv Ophthalmol.* 2005;50:364–388.
27. Khan MA. Update on spondyloarthropathies. *Ann Intern Med.* 2002;136:896–907.
28. Taurog JD, et al. Susceptibility to inflammatory disease in HLA-B27 transgenic rat lines correlates with the level of B27 expression. *J Immunol.* 1993;150:4168–4178.
29. Breban M, et al. T cells but not thymic exposure to B27 are required for the inflammatory disease of HLA-B27 transgenic rats. *Arthritis Rheum.* 1993;36:S73.
30. Breban M, et al. Transfer of the inflammatory disease of HLA-B27 transgenic rats by bone marrow engraftment. *J Exp Med.* 1993;178: 1607–1616.
31. Taurog JD, et al. The germfree state prevents development of gut and joint inflammatory disease in HLA-B27 transgenic rats. *J Exp Med* 1994;180:2359–2364.
32. Wildner G, Thurau SR. Cross-reactivity between an HLA-B27-derived peptide and a retinal autoantigen peptide: a clue to major histocompatibility complex association with autoimmune disease. *Eur J Immunol.* 1994;4:2579–2585.
33. Wildner G, Diedrichs-Mohring M, Thurau SR. Induction of arthritis and uveitis in Lewis rats by antigenic mimicry of peptides from HLA-B27 and cytokeratin. *Eur J Immunol.* 2002;32:299–306.
34. Bowness P. HLA B27 in health and disease: a double-edged sword? *Rheumatology (Oxford).* 2002;41:857–868.
35. Allen RL, O'Callaghan CA, McMichael AJ, Bowness P. Cutting edge: HLA-B27 can form a novel beta 2-microglobulin-free heavy chain homodimer structure. *J Immunol.* 1999;162:5045–5048.
36. Vadot E, et al. Epidemiology of uveitis. Preliminary results of a prospective study in Savoy. In: Saari KM, ed. *Uveitis update*. Amsterdam: Elsevier; 1984:16.

37. Ehlers N, et al. HLA-B27 in acute and chronic uveitis. *Lancet.* 1974;1:99.
38. Power WJ, Rodriguez A, Pedroza-Seres M, et al. Outcomes in anterior uveitis associated with the HLA-B27 haplotype. *Ophthalmology.* 1998; 105:1646–1651.
39. Mapstone R, Woodrow JC. HLA 27 and acute anterior uveitis. *Br J Ophthalmol.* 1975;59:270–275.
40. Zervas J, et al. HLA-B27 frequency in Greek patients with acute anterior uveitis. *Br J Ophthalmol.* 1977;61:699–701.
41. Bennett PH, Burch TA. New York symposium on population studies in the rheumatic diseases: new diagnostic criteria. *Bull Rheum Dis.* 1967;17:453–458.
42. Rosenbaum JT. Characterization of uveitis associated with spondyloarthritis. *J Rheumatol.* 1989;16:792–796.
43. D'Alessandro LP, et al. Anterior uveitis and hypopyon. *Am J Ophthalmol.* 1991;112:317–321.
44. Pearce A, Sugar A. Anterior uveitis and hypopyon. *Am J Ophthalmol.* 1992;113:471–472.
45. Bayen H, et al. Involvement of the posterior eye segment in HLA B27(+) iridocyclitis. Incidence. Value of surgical treatment. *J Fr Ophtalmol.* 1988;11:561–566.
46. Klemperer I, et al. Spontaneous hyphema: an unusual complication of uveitis associated with ankylosing spondylitis. *Ann Ophthalmol.* 1992;24:177–179.
47. Rothova A, et al. HLA B27 associated uveitis. A distinct clinical entity? In: Saari KM, ed. *Uveitis update.* Amsterdam: Elsevier; 1984:91–95.
48. Rodriguez A, et al. Posterior segment ocular manifestations in patients with HLA-B27-associated uveitis. *Ophthalmology.* 1994;101:1267–1274.
49. Saari KM, et al. Ocular inflammation associated with *Yersinia* infection. *Am J Ophthalmol.* 1980;89:84–95.
50. Dodds EM, Lowder CY, Meisler DM. Posterior segment inflammation in HLA-B27+ acute anterior uveitis: clinical characteristics. *Ocular Immunol Inflamm.* 2000;8:73–75.
51. Belmont JB, Michelson JB. Vitrectomy in uveitis associated with ankylosing spondylitis. *Am J Ophthalmol.* 1982;94:300–304.
52. Uy HS, Christen WG, Foster CS. HLA-B27-associated uveitis and cystoid macular edema. *Ocul Immunol Inflamm.* 2001;9:177–183.
53. Pach JM, et al. Disk neovascularization in chronic anterior uveitis. *Am J Ophthalmol.* 1991;111:241–244.
54. Diamond JG, Kaplan HJ. Uveitis: effect of vitrectomy combined with lensectomy. *Ophthalmology.* 1978;86:1320–1329.
55. Smith RE, Nozik RA. *Uveitis. A clinical approach to diagnosis and management.* 2nd ed. Baltimore: William & Wilkins; 1989:63–66.
56. Wakefield D. Methylprednisolone pulse therapy in severe anterior uveitis. *Aust N Z J Ophthalmol.* 1985;13:411–415.
57. Mochizuki M, de Smet MD. Use of immunosuppressive agents in ocular diseases. *Prog Retin Eye Res.* 1994;13:479–506.
58. de Smet MD, Nussenblatt RB. Clinical use of cyclosporine in ocular disease. *Int Ophthalmol Clin.* 1993;33:31–45.
59. Dugel PU, et al. Pars plana vitrectomy for intraocular inflammation-related cystoid macular edema. A preliminary study. *Ophthalmology.* 1992;99:1535–1541
60. Antcliff RJ, Spalton DJ, Stanford MR, et al. Intravitreal triamcinolone for uveitic cystoid macular edema: an optical coherence tomography study. *Ophthalmology.* 2001;108:765–772.
61. Young S, Larkin G, Branley M, Lightman S. Safety and efficacy of intravitreal triamcinolone for cystoid macular oedema in uveitis. *Clin Experiment Ophthalmol.* 2001;29:2–6.
62. Jaffe GJ, Ben-Nun J, Guo H, et al. Fluocinolone acetonide sustained drug delivery device to treat severe uveitis. *Ophthalmology.* 2000;107: 2024–2033.
63. Callanan DG, et al. Treatment of posterior uveitis with a fluocinolone acetonide implant; three-year clinical trial results. *Arch Ophthalmol.* 2008;1226:1191–1201.
64. El-Shabrawi Y, Hermann J. Anti-tumor necrosis factor-alpha therapy with infliximab as an alternative to corticosteroids in the treatment of human leukocyte antigen b27-associated acute anterior uveitis. *Ophthalmology.* 2002;109:2342–2346.
65. Smith JR, et al. Differential efficacy of tumor necrosis factor inhibition in the management of inflammatory eye disease and associated rheumatic disease. *Arthritis Rheum.* 2001;45:252–257.
66. Munoz-Fernandez S, et al. Sulfasalazine reduces the number of flares of acute anterior uveitis over a one-year period. *J Rheumatol.* 2003;30: 1277–1279.
67. Benitez-Del Castillo JM, et al. Sulfasalazine in the prevention of anterior uveitis associated with ankylosing spondylitis. *Eye.* 2000;14:340–343.
68. Thurau SR, Diedrichs-Mohring M, Fricke H, et al. Oral tolerance with an HLA-peptide mimicking retinal autoantigen as a treatment of autoimmune uveitis. *Immunol Lett.* 1999;68:205–212.
69. Gottlieb A, et al. Guidelines of care for the management of psoriasis and psoriatic arthritis Section 2. Psoriatic arthritis: overview and guidelines of care for treatment with an emphasis on the biologics. *J Am Acad Dermatol.* 2008;58:851–864.
70. Tehranzadeh J, et al. Musculoskeletal disorders associated with HIV infection and AIDS. Part II: Non-infectious musculoskeletal conditions. *Skeletal Radiol.* 2004;33:311–320.
71. Durrani K, Foster CS. Psoriatic uveitis: a distinct clinical entity? *Am J Ophthalmol.* 2005;139:106–111.
72. Salmon JF, et al. Ocular inflammation in Crohn's disease. *Ophthalmology.* 1991;98:480–484.
73. Breenstein AJ, et al. The extra-intestinal complications in Crohn's disease and ulcerative colitis. *Medicine.* 1976;55:401–412.
74. Hofley P, Roarty J, McGinnity G, et al. Asymptomatic uveitis in children with chronic inflammatory bowel diseases. *J Pediatr Gastroenterol Nutr.* 1993;17:397–400.
75. Rychwalski PJ, Cruz OA, Alanis-Lambreton G, et al. Asymptomatic uveitis in young people with inflammatory bowel disease. *J AAPOS.* 1997; 1:111–114.
76. Verbraak FD, Schreinemachers MC, Tiller A, et al. Prevalence of subclinical anterior uveitis in adult patients with inflammatory bowel disease. *Br J Ophthalmol.* 2001;85:219–221.
77. Macoul KL. Ocular changes in granulomatous ileocolitis. *Arch Ophthalmol.* 1970;84:95–97.
78. Ruby AJ, Jampol LM. Crohn's disease and retinal vascular disease. *Am J Ophthalmol.* 1990;110:349–353.
79. Reiter H. Ueber eine bisher unerkannte Spirocheteninfektion (Spirochaetosis arthritica). *Dtsch Med Wochenschr.* 1916;42:1535–1536.
80. Sairanen E, et al. Reiter's syndrome: a follow-up study. *Acta Med Scand.* 1969;185:57–63.
81. Lee DA, et al. The clinical diagnosis of Reiter's syndrome. Ophthalmic and nonophthalmic aspects. *Ophthalmology.* 1986;93:350–356.
82. Wiggens RE, et al. Reiter's keratoconjunctivitis. *Arch Ophthalmol.* 1990;108:280–281.
83. Leirisalo M, et al. Follow-up study on patients with Reiter's disease and reactive arthritis, with special reference to HLA-B27. *Arthritis Rheum.* 1982;25:249–259.
84. Fan PT, Yu DTY. Reiter's syndrome. In: Kelley WN, et al, eds. *Textbook of rheumatology.* Philadelphia: WB Saunders; 1993:973.
85. Keat A. Reiter's syndrome and reactive arthritis in perspective. *N Engl J Med.* 1983;309:1606–1613.
86. Brewerton DA, et al. HL-A 27 and arthropathies associated with ulcerative colitis and psoriasis. *Lancet.* 1974;1:956–958.
87. Arnett FC, et al. Incomplete Reiter's syndrome: discriminating features and HL-A W27 in diagnosis. *Ann Intern Med.* 1976;84:8–12.
88. Paronen I. Reiter's disease: A study of 344 cases observed in Finland. *Acta Med Scand Suppl.* 1948;212:1.
89. Csonka GW. The course of Reiter's syndrome. *Br Med J.* 1958;1: 1088–1090.
90. Kaye BR. Rheumatologic manifestations of infection with human immunodeficiency virus (HIV). *Ann Intern Med.* 1989;111:158–167.
91. Winchester R, et al. The co-occurence of Reiter's syndrome and acquired immunodeficiency. *Arch Intern Med.* 1987;106:19–26.
92. Hopkins DJ, et al. Ocular disorders in a series of 332 patients with Crohn's disease. *Br J Ophthalmol.* 1974;58:732–737.
93. Korelitz BI, Coles RS. Uveitis (iritis) associated with ulcerative and granulomatous colitis. *Gastroenterology.* 1967;52:78–82.
94. Wright V, Wathinson G. The arthritis of ulcerative colitis. *Br Med J.* 1965;2:670–675.
95. Ostler BH, et al. Reiter's syndrome. *Am J Ophthalmol.* 1970;71:986–991.
96. Prakash S, et al. Reiter's disease in northern India. A clinical and immunogenetic study. *Rheumatol Int.* 1983;3:101–104.

Chapter 108

Sarcoidosis

Miriam T. Schteingart, Howard H. Tessler

Sarcoidosis is a multisystem chronic inflammatory disorder characterized by the presence of noncaseating granulomas in affected tissues. While the exact cause of the disease is unknown, it is felt to result when genetically susceptible individuals are exposed to particular antigens, triggering an exaggerated cellular immune response.[1] Prolonged antigenic stimulation and/or persistent dysregulation of the immune response could result in chronic disease.[2] Most likely, exposure to a variety of antigens, both infectious and environmental, can trigger the disorder. Mycobacterial DNA and protein antigens have been identified in significant numbers of patients with sarcoidosis.[3,4] Associations with exposure to a variety of organic and inorganic substances have also been described.[5] Certain human leukocyte antigen (HLA) genes, particularly variants of HLA-DRB1, have been associated with differences in disease susceptibility, severity, and clinical course. These genes have the common factor of modifying antigen presentation and elimination as well as the T-cell immune response.[6,7]

The reported incidence of sarcoidosis varies from 10 to 200/100000 depending on the population sampled.[8,9] Sarcoidosis is more common in women than in men and is seen most commonly between the ages of 20 and 40 years. A second peak has been described, primarily in women, with onset between the ages of 45 and 65.[10,11] Sarcoidosis may also present in the pediatric age group. In the United States, the disease is more common in African-Americans than whites, but any ethnic group may be affected.

Sarcoidosis can affect virtually any part of the body and consequently has diverse clinical presentations. Pulmonary involvement is the most frequent form of the disease and usually presents as bilateral hilar adenopathy with or without parenchymal involvement.[9] Ocular involvement is the second most common manifestation, seen in up to 50% of affected patients.[12] Cutaneous involvement is also common, occurring in up to one-third of patients. Involvement of the heart, joints, central nervous system (CNS), liver, and endocrine glands also may be seen.[9]

The eyes may become involved at any time in the course of the disease. Ocular symptoms may be the patient's presenting complaint, or eye involvement may be found incidentally in an asymptomatic patient who is evaluated because of other signs of sarcoidosis. As many as half of patients with ocular involvement have no ocular symptoms, especially early in the course of the disease.[13]

Ocular Manifestations

Eyelids

Small ('millet seed') or large nodules may be seen in the eyelid skin and in the canthal region. The lesions are usually nontender but can rarely ulcerate.[14] Occasionally, the lesions may appear papular or verrucous. More rarely, the eyelid skin may be involved by lupus pernio, a violaceous, nodular, or plaquelike eruption, which frequently results in scarring and fibrosis.[9]

Lacrimal gland

Lacrimal gland involvement occurs in approximately 7% of patients with sarcoidosis and in up to 25% of patients with ocular involvement.[15,16] Involvement is usually bilateral, but may be unilateral.[17] Enlargement of the lacrimal glands may be noted visibly or by palpation. Loss of functioning glandular tissue can result in keratoconjunctivitis sicca. When the salivary glands are also involved, the clinical picture resembles that of typical Sjögren's syndrome.[18] Decreased lacrimal function may improve with resolution of the systemic disease or become permanent, depending on the amount of fibrosis.[19]

Lacrimal drainage system

Involvement of the lacrimal drainage pathway is rare and is usually associated with involvement of the upper respiratory tract.[20] Dacryostenosis may occur secondary to granulomatous inflammation of the nasolacrimal duct, with resulting epiphora and acute or chronic dacryocystitis.[19] Dacryocystitis also may result from granulomatous involvement of the nasolacrimal sac.[20]

Orbit

Aside from the lacrimal gland, orbital involvement is uncommon, occurring in only 1% of patients with ocular sarcoid. Granulomatous inflammation of the orbit may result in unilateral or bilateral proptosis.[17,21] Involvement of the extraocular muscles is rare and may be asymptomatic or present as a painful external ophthalmoplegia. Computed tomography or magnetic resonance imaging may reveal diffuse enlargement of the muscle and its tendon.[22] The differential diagnosis includes thyroid ophthalmopathy, orbital pseudotumor, lymphoma, neoplasm, and trichinosis.

Conjunctiva

Conjunctival involvement has been reported in 4–13% of all patients with sarcoidosis[15,19] and in 17–20% of patients with ocular sarcoidosis.[12,15,16,19] Up to 25% of patients with sarcoid uveitis may have conjunctival changes.[19] The most common conjunctival lesion is the granuloma. Visible granulomas have been reported in as few as 4% and as many as 17% of patients with ocular sarcoidosis.[16,19] Granulomas present as small, round, or oval nodules that are yellow-brown or red in color. There may be surrounding erythema or edema. The nodules vary in size from pinpoint to several millimeters and are most commonly seen in the inferior palpebral conjunctiva and fornix. The nodules are often single and may be unilateral or bilateral.[19] Most patients with conjunctival involvement are asymptomatic. Identification of conjunctival granulomas may be difficult. The nodules are often small and may be easily overlooked by those unfamiliar with their appearance. In addition, distinction from normal conjunctival follicles may be difficult.

Although less common, conjunctival sarcoidosis may also present as a chronic follicular conjunctivitis involving the upper and/or lower palpebral conjunctiva.[23,24] In some cases, cicatricial changes with symblepharon formation can occur.[25,26]

Cornea

The most common corneal manifestation of sarcoidosis is calcific band keratopathy, which is usually associated with elevated serum calcium levels, but is occasionally seen in patients with normal serum calcium.[17,19] Corneal involvement also may take the form of a nummular keratitis (Fig. 108.1) consisting of round, white stromal opacities with indistinct borders and intervening clear areas. Bilateral involvement is common, and multiple opacities may be present in each eye. Although the opacities may be found at any level in the stroma, they tend to occur at the same level in any given patient. Usually, the patient is asymptomatic.[8,27] Nummular keratitis can also be seen in tuberculosis, herpes simplex, herpes zoster, syphilis, and onchocerciasis. Corneal involvement also may present as thickening and opacification of Descemet's membrane and endothelium in the inferior cornea (Fig. 108.2). Deep stromal vessels may be noted in the area of thickening, but the overlying stroma is usually clear.[27] It has been suggested that the opacification results from fibrous metaplasia of the endothelial cells, presumably secondary to the irritating effects of keratic precipitates and chronic inflammation.[27] The presence of inferior corneal opacification in a patient with chronic iridocyclitis should raise the suspicion of sarcoidosis.

Iris

Iris nodules are seen in up to 11% of patients with ocular sarcoidoisis[17] and in approximately 25% of patients with

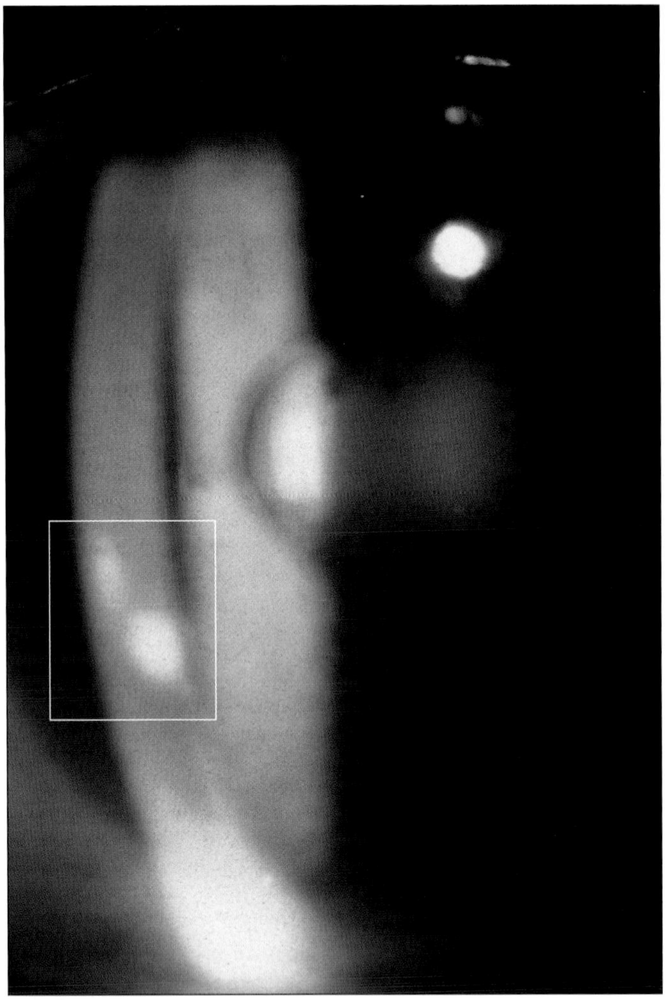

Fig. 108.1 Nummular keratitis. These opacities (*box*) are present at the same level within the corneal stroma.

anterior sarcoid uveitis.[12] Nodules may occur at the pupillary margin (Koeppe nodules) or within the iris stroma (Busacca nodules). The nodules are often yellow-gray or grayish-red in color with overlying dilated vessels. Although nodules are usually small, large nodules may occur and can be mistaken for iris tumors. Large nodules also may result in sector cataract formation.[28] The differential diagnosis of iris nodules includes amelanotic melanoma, metastatic tumors including leukemia and lymphoma, tuberculous granulomas, foreign body granulomas, and juvenile xanthogranulomatosis.

Anterior uveitis

Uveitis is the most common ocular manifestation of sarcoidosis, occurring in up to two-thirds of patients with ocular involvement.[16,29] In addition, sarcoidosis is found in 7% of all patients with uveitis, making it the most commonly associated systemic disease in this group of patients.[30] Sarcoid uveitis may be acute or chronic, granulomatous or nongranulomatous, and unilateral or bilateral. Acute iridocyclitis presents with abrupt onset of pain, redness, photophobia, and blurred vision. Examination reveals cells and

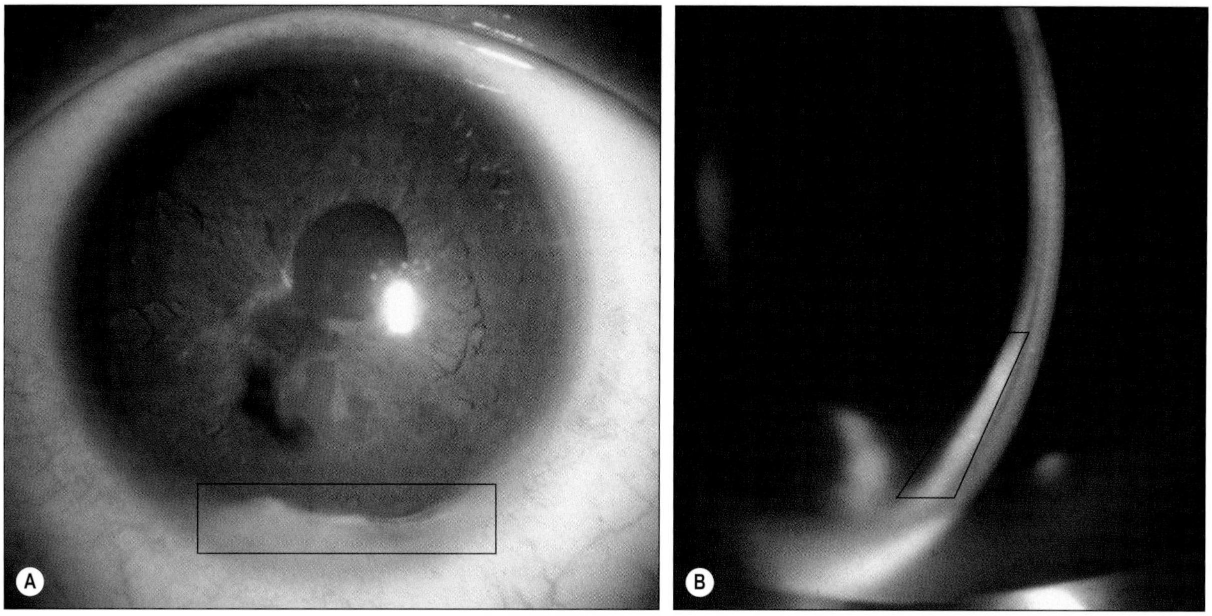

Fig. 108.2 Opacification of corneal endothelium and Descemet's membrane in a patient with sarcoid uveitis (*boxes*). Fine vessels are present within the deep stroma, but are not visualized here.

flare in the anterior chamber and fine keratic precipitates on the corneal endothelium. Acute iridocyclitis is frequently unilateral, is more likely to occur at the onset of the systemic disease, and usually responds well to treatment. Although it usually occurs as a single, isolated episode, recurrent disease may occur.[16] Chronic iridocyclitis is more common than acute iridocyclitis, has a more insidious onset, and tends to be seen in a slightly older age group.[16] Granulomatous inflammation, with mutton-fat keratic precipitates, iris nodules, and synechia formation, is characteristic (Fig. 108.3). Gonioscopy may reveal nodules on the trabecular meshwork and tentlike peripheral anterior synechiae.[29] Chronic iridocyclitis is more difficult to treat and has a higher incidence of complications and a worse prognosis than acute iridocyclitis. The course of the uveitis appears to be somewhat independent of the systemic disease. Uveitis may persist or recur despite resolution of clinical and radiologic evidence of pulmonary disease.[12] Several classic syndromes of sarcoidosis are associated with uveitis. Löfgren's syndrome consists of erythema nodosum, bilateral hilar adenopathy, fever, and acute iridocyclitis. This syndrome often occurs at the onset of the disease and has a very favorable prognosis, tending to resolve within a few weeks.[12] Heerfordt's syndrome (uveoparotid fever) consists of uveitis, parotitis, fever, and facial or other cranial nerve palsies.

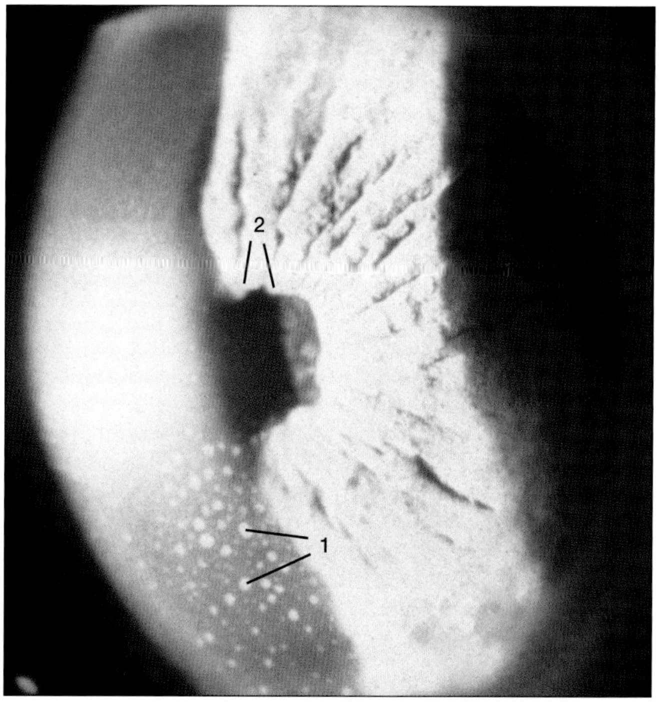

Fig. 108.3 Granulomatous uveitis with muttòn-fat keratic precipitates (*1*) and Koeppe nodules (*2*) along the pupillary border.

Posterior uveitis

Twenty-five percent of patients with ocular sarcoidosis have posterior segment involvement. Although usually seen in association with anterior uveitis, isolated involvement of the posterior segment may occur in up to 20% of patients with sarcoid uveitis.[31] Posterior uveitis is especially common in white patients, especially in elderly females.[32] Vitreous involvement is common. In addition to the presence of vitreous cells, vitreous 'snowballs' (gray-white nodules) are frequently seen in the inferior vitreous, especially in a preretinal location. Periphlebitis is the most common fundus finding (Fig. 108.4).[8] Venous sheathing may be subtle, or

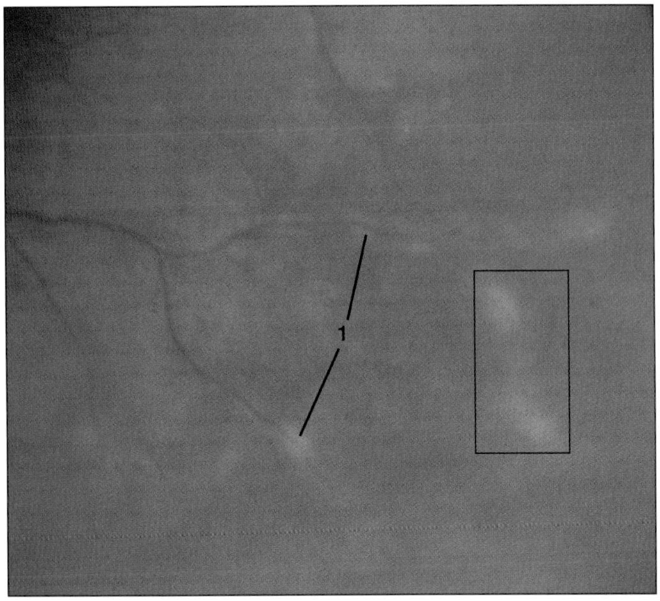

Fig. 108.4 Granulomatous retinal periphlebitis (*1*). This appearance is often referred to as 'candle wax drippings' (*box*).

gray-white exudates may envelop the vein, giving the appearance of 'candle wax drippings.' Increased vascular permeability may result in retinal hemorrhages and retinal or macular edema. Cystoid macular edema (CME) is a relatively frequent finding in any patient with chronic ocular inflammation, but does not appear to be more common in patients with sarcoidosis than in other patients with chronic uveitis.[19] CME should always be suspected as a cause of decreased vision in patients with sarcoid uveitis and is a more frequent cause of visual loss than vitreous haze. Retinal inflammation often leads to disturbance of the underlying retinal pigment epithelium (RPE), with resulting focal areas of RPE mottling and atrophy, particularly at the inferior equator. Peripheral capillary closure may occur with subsequent neovascularization. Choroidal granulomas are seen in 5% of patients with ocular sarcoidosis and appear as yellow-gray or white lesions that may be small (<0.5 disc diameters) or large (>4 disc diameters). They are frequently solitary, but can be multiple.[33] Large granulomas may have an overlying serous detachment of the retina and can be mistaken for choroidal metastases or choroidal melanoma.[34,35] Multifocal choroiditis can be seen and result in round, punched-out lesions, especially in the inferior peripheral retina.[32]

Optic nerve

Optic nerve involvement is uncommon. Four types of optic nerve disease have been described: (1) optic disc swelling secondary to severe intraocular inflammation, (2) papilledema secondary to increased intracranial pressure with CNS involvement, (3) retrobulbar neuritis, and (4) infiltration of the optic nerve by noncaseating granulomas. When the granulomas are present on the optic nerve head, the appearance is that of a yellow mass with surrounding edema.[36] Ultimately, optic atrophy may result. Neuro-ophthalmic involvement in the form of cranial neuropathy, Horner's syndrome, tonic pupil, and involvement of the optic tract with granulomas can also infrequently be seen.[37]

Diagnosis

Sarcoidosis often remains a diagnosis of exclusion, ideally requiring a compatible clinical picture, exclusion of other granulomatous diseases, and histologic evidence of noncaseating granulomas in affected tissues.[38] Ophthalmologists are frequently at a disadvantage when diagnosing sarcoidosis. Often, only the eye appears to be involved, and evidence of systemic disease is lacking. Although purists may insist that the above criteria be met to definitively diagnose sarcoidosis, the ophthalmologist may diagnose presumed or possible sarcoidosis on lesser evidence. Such a diagnosis may not alter the patient's current therapy, but may be helpful if the patient should later develop disease elsewhere in the body.

In a patient with clinical findings suggestive of sarcoidosis, the diagnosis can be supported by a variety of laboratory tests. Elevation of serum angiotensin-converting enzyme (ACE) level occurs in 60–90% of patients with active sarcoidosis.[13] ACE is produced by epithelioid cells within granulomas. The serum ACE level therefore reflects the total body mass of granulomatous tissue. ACE levels have also been found to be elevated in tears and aqueous humor of patients with ocular sarcoidosis, even in the presence of normal serum ACE levels.[39–41] While an elevated ACE level can be helpful in confirming a diagnosis of sarcoidosis, ACE levels may be normal early in the disease when there are few granulomas, or in chronic, relatively quiescent disease.[42] In addition, allelic polymorphisms of the *ACE* gene can affect baseline plasma ACE levels, and may affect the sensitivity of the test.[43] Significant declines in serum ACE levels are seen after treatment with both systemic and local steroids.[13] Lysozyme is also produced by epithelioid cells and serum lysozyme levels may be elevated in patients with active sarcoidosis. Although most patients with elevated serum lysozyme will also have elevated serum ACE levels, occasionally only the lysozyme level is elevated.[13] The combination of elevations of both serum ACE and serum lysozyme levels appears to have a higher predictive value than elevation of either of these values alone.[44] Both ACE and lysozyme are nonspecific, and elevations of these enzymes may be seen in a variety of other disorders, such as leprosy, mycobacterial infection, and histoplasmosis.[45]

A chest radiograph will demonstrate bilateral hilar adenopathy in up to 75% of patients with sarcoidosis.[46] Although the presence of bilateral hilar adenopathy is helpful in confirming the diagnosis, its absence on chest radiograph does not rule out the possibility of sarcoidosis, as ocular disease may precede chest radiographic findings by as much as 9 years[19] or continue years after radiological evidence of systemic disease has resolved.[45] Gallium scanning has also been used to support the diagnosis of sarcoidosis. Typically, increased uptake is noted in the lungs, parotid glands, and lacrimal glands.[47] A positive gallium scan may be seen, even when the chest radiograph is normal. A conventional or high-resolution chest computed tomograph with infusion may also demonstrate mediastinal or hilar adenopathy not seen on chest X-ray.[32,48,49] Newer PET scanning technologies may also be of value in evaluating areas of inflammatory activity.[43,49]

Definitive diagnosis of sarcoidosis requires histologic confirmation. When strong clinical evidence of sarcoidosis exists, however, biopsy may not be necessary. For example, the presence of uveitis and bilateral hilar adenopathy may be considered strong enough evidence of sarcoidosis to obviate the need for tissue biopsy.[46]

If pathologic confirmation is required, any clinically involved tissues may be biopsied. The most common sites for biopsy include the skin, salivary glands, lung, and mediastinal lymph nodes. There is significant debate in the literature regarding the usefulness of conjunctival biopsy. Conjunctival biopsy can be performed easily under local anesthesia with minimal morbidity. The yield from conjunctival biopsies depends heavily on biopsy technique. In general, biopsy of suspicious lesions (conjunctival granulomas) results in a higher percentage of positive biopsies than does blind conjunctival biopsy (20–50% vs 6–30%).[50–52] Bilateral biopsies with examination of multiple tissue sections, however, can increase the yield of blind biopsies, with reports of up to 55% positivity.[53] When clinical involvement of the lacrimal gland is noted, transconjunctival biopsy of the lacrimal gland also may be performed, with positive results in up to 60% of patients. There is a small risk of damage to the lacrimal ducts with resulting dry eye.[13] Rarely, chorioretinal biopsy has been performed to confirm the diagnosis in cases of refractory posterior uveitis.[54]

In summary, a patient suspected of having sarcoidosis based on clinical findings should be further evaluated with ACE and lysozyme levels, as well as a chest radiograph or gallium scan. If the results of these tests are positive, the diagnosis may be confirmed by biopsy of clinically involved and/or readily accessible tissues, including the conjunctiva or lacrimal gland. If biopsy of these sites is negative and the suspicion of sarcoidosis is high, more invasive procedures (e.g. transbronchial lung biopsy) may be considered.[13]

Course and Management

Ocular sarcoidosis may follow an acute, monophasic course associated with a good prognosis, or, more commonly, a chronic or relapsing course, which may last for several years.[55] Patients with chronic uveitis have a higher incidence of complications, including cataract, glaucoma, macular edema, neovascularization, and hypotony. Patients with secondary glaucoma or posterior pole involvement have a particularly poor prognosis.[15,56] The risk of severe visual loss in patients with chronic sarcoid uveitis has been reported as high as 13–20%.[45,57] More aggressive treatment and earlier referral to a uveitis subspecialist for severe cases can reduce the risk of visual loss significantly.[45,58]

The mainstay of treatment for ocular sarcoidosis is corticosteroids in topical, periocular, or systemic form. Long-term treatment is often necessary. Patients who fail to respond adequately to steroid treatment or are intolerant of steroids may require treatment with immunosuppressive agents. Methotrexate has proven effective and relatively safe in the treatment of both systemic[59,60] and ocular[56] disease, allowing for reduction or even discontinuation of systemic steroids in many patients. Azathioprine, chlorambucil, and cyclophosphamide have also been effective in some patients with refractory disease.[59,61] The tumor necrosis factor blocker infliximab has been shown to be very effective in treating sarcoid ocular inflammation,[62] while etanercept has not been shown to be helpful and, in fact, has been associated with onset of sarcoidosis in rare cases.[63,64] Cataract extraction with intraocular lens implantation can be performed successfully in patients whose uveitis has been well controlled for at least 3 months. Exacerbation of inflammation, CME, and posterior capsule opacification are common postoperative complications.[65]

References

1. Newman LS, Rose CS, Maier LA. Sarcoidosis. *N Engl J Med.* 1997;336:1224–1234.
2. Moller DR. Etiology of sarcoidosis. *Clin Chest Med.* 1997;18:695–706.
3. Drake WP, Newman LS. Mycobacterial antigens may be important in sarcoidosis pathogenesis. *Curr Opin Pulm Med.* 2006;12:359–363.
4. Chen ES, Moller DR. Etiology of sarcoidosis. *Clin Chest Med.* 2008;29:365–377.
5. Margolis R, Lowder CY. Sarcoidosis. *Curr Opin Ophthalmol.* 2007;18:470–475.
6. Grunewald J. Genetics of sarcoidosis. *Curr Opin Pulm Med.* 2008;14:434–439.
7. Muller-Quernheim J, Schurmann M, et al. Genetics of sarcoidosis. *Clin Chest Med.* 2008;29:391–414.
8. Mayers M. Ocular sarcoidosis. *Int Ophthalmol Clin.* 1990;30:257–263.
9. Kerdel FA, Moschella SL. Sarcoidosis: an updated review. *J Am Acad Dermatol.* 1984;11:1–19.
10. Hoover DL, Khan JA, Giangiacomo J. Pediatric ocular sarcoidosis. *Surv Ophthalmol.* 1986;30:215–228.
11. Hershey JM, et al. Non-caseating conjunctival granulomas in patients with multifocal choroiditis and panuveitis. *Ophthalmology.* 101:596–601, 1994.
12. Crick RP, Hoyle C, Smellie H. The eyes in sarcoidosis. *Br J Ophthalmol.* 1961;45:461–481.
13. Weinreb RN, Tessler H. Laboratory diagnosis of ophthalmic sarcoidosis. *Surv Ophthalmol.* 1984;28:653–664.
14. Brownstein S, et al. Sarcoidosis of the eyelid skin. *Can J Ophthalmol.* 1990;25:256–259.
15. Jabs DA, Johns CJ. Ocular involvement in chronic sarcoidosis. *Am J Ophthalmol.* 1986;102:297–301.
16. James DG. Ocular sarcoidosis. *Ann N Y Acad Sci.* 1986;465:551.
17. Obenauf CD, et al. Sarcoidosis and its ophthalmic manifestations. *Am J Ophthalmol.* 1978;86:648–655.
18. Melsom RD, et al. Sarcoidosis in a patient presenting with clinical and histological features of primary Sjögren's syndrome. *Ann Rheum Dis.* 1988;47:166–168.
19. Karma A. Ophthalmic changes in sarcoidosis. *Acta Ophthalmol Suppl (Copenh).* 1979;141:1–94.
20. Harris GJ, Williams GA, Clarke GP. Sarcoidosis of the lacrimal sac. *Arch Ophthalmol.* 1981;99:1198–1201.
21. Imes RK, Reifschneider JS, O'Connor LE. Systemic sarcoidosis presenting initially with bilateral orbital and upper lid masses. *Ann Ophthalmol.* 1988;20:466, 467, 469.
22. Cornblath WT, Elner V, Rolfe M. Extraocular muscle involvement in sarcoidosis. *Ophthalmology.* 1993;100:501–505.
23. Bastiaensen LAK, et al. Conjunctival sarcoidosis. *Doc Ophthalmol.* 1985;59:5–9.
24. Dios E, Saornil MA, Herreras JM. Conjunctival biopsy in the diagnosis of ocular sarcoidosis. *Ocular Immunol Inflamm.* 2001;9:59–64.
25. Geggel HS, Mensher JH. Cicatricial conjunctivitis in sarcoidosis: recognition and treatment. *Ann Ophthalmol.* 1989;21:92–94.
26. Flach A. Symblepharon in sarcoidosis. *Am J Ophthalmol.* 1978;85:210–214.
27. Lucchese N, Tessler H. Keratitis associated with chronic iridocyclitis. *Am J Ophthalmol.* 1981;92:717–721.
28. Mader TH, Chismire KJ, Cornell FM. The treatment of an enlarged sarcoid iris nodule with injectable corticosteroids. *Am J Ophthalmol.* 1988;106:365–366.
29. Ohara K, et al. Intraocular manifestations of systemic sarcoidosis. *Jpn J Ophthalmol.* 1992;36:452–457.
30. Rothova A, et al. Uveitis and systemic disease. *Br J Ophthalmol.* 1992;76:137–141.

31. Spalton DJ, Sanders MD. Fundus changes in histologically confirmed sarcoidosis. *Br J Ophthalmol*. 1981;65:348–358.
32. Rothova A. Ocular involvement in sarcoidosis. *Br J Ophthalmol*. 2000;84:110–116.
33. Desai UR, Tawansky KA, Joondeph BC, et al. Choroidal granulomas in systemic sarcoidosis. *Retina*. 2001;21:40–47.
34. Campo RV, Aaberg TM. Choroidal granuloma in sarcoidosis. *Am J Ophthalmol*. 1984;97:419–427.
35. Tingey DP, Gonder JR. Ocular sarcoidosis presenting as a solitary choroidal mass. *Can J Ophthalmol*. 1992;27:25–29.
36. Beardsley TL, et al. Eleven cases of sarcoidosis of the optic nerve. *Am J Ophthalmol*. 1984;97:62–77.
37. Koczman JJ, Rouleau J, et al. Neuro-ophthalmic sarcoidosis: The University of Iowa Experience. *Seminars Ophthalmol*. 2008;23:157–168.
38. Johns CJ, Michele TM. The clinical management of sarcoidosis: a 50 year experience at Johns Hopkins Hospital. *Medicine (Baltimore)*. 1999;78: 65–111.
39. Sharma OP, Vita JB. Determination of angiotensin-converting enzyme activity in tears: a non-invasive test for evaluation of ocular sarcoidosis. *Arch Ophthalmol*. 1983;101:559–561.
40. Immonen I, et al. Concentration of angiotensin-converting enzyme in tears of patients with sarcoidosis. *Acta Ophthalmol (Copenh)*. 1987;65:27–29.
41. Weinreb RN, et al. Angiotensin converting enzyme activity in human aqueous humor. *Arch Ophthalmol*. 1985;103:34–36.
42. Krzystolik M, Power WJ, Foster CS. Diagnostic and therapeutic challenges of sarcoidosis. *Int Ophthalmol Clin*. 1998;38:61–76.
43. Costabel U, Ohshimo S, et al. Diagnosis of sarcoidosis. *Curr Opin Pulm Med*. 2008;14:455–461.
44. Baarsma GS, et al. The predictive value of serum angiotensin converting enzyme and lysozyme levels in the diagnosis of ocular sarcoidosis. *Am J Ophthalmol*. 1987;104:211–217.
45. Stavrou P, Linton S, Young DW, et al. Clinical diagnosis of ocular sarcoidosis. *Eye*. 1997;11:365–370.
46. Winterbauer RH, Belic N, Moores KD. A clinical interpretation of bilateral hilar adenopathy. *Ann Intern Med*. 1973;78:65–71.
47. Karma A, Poukkula AA, Ruokonen AO. Assessment of activity of ocular sarcoidosis by gallium scanning. *Br J Ophthalmol*. 1987;71:361–367.
48. Kaiser PK, Lowder CY, Sullivan P, et al. Chest computerized tomography in the evaluation of uveitis in elderly women. *Am J Ophthalmol*. 2002;133:499–505.
49. Akbar JJ, Meyer CA, et al. Cardiopulmonary imaging in sarcoidosis. *Clin Chest Med*. 2008;29:429–443.
50. Khan F, et al. Conjunctival biopsy in sarcoidosis: a simple, safe, and specific diagnostic procedure. *Ann Ophthalmol*. 1977;9:671–676.
51. Spaide RF, Ward DL. Conjunctival biopsy in the diagnosis of sarcoidosis. *Br J Ophthalmol*. 1990;74:469–471.
52. Elliott JH. Conjunctival biopsy as an aid in the evaluation of the patient with suspected sarcoidosis, discussion. *Ophthalmology*. 1980;87:289–291.
53. Nichols CW, et al. Conjunctival biopsy as an aid in the evaluation of the patient with suspected sarcoidosis. *Ophthalmology*. 1980;87:287–289.
54. Whitcup SM, Chan C. Diagnosis of corticosteroid resistant ocular sarcoidosis by chorioretinal biopsy. *Br J Ophthalmol*. 1999;83:504–505.
55. Karma A, Huhti E, Poukkula A. Course and outcome of ocular sarcoidosis. *Am J Ophthalmol*. 1988;106:467–472.
56. Dev S, McCallum RM, Jaffe GJ. Methotrexate treatment for sarcoid-associated panuveitis. *Ophthalmology*. 1999;106:111–118.
57. Uyama M. Uveitis in sarcoidosis. *Int Ophthalmol Clin*. 42:143–150, 2002.
58. Dana MR, Meray-Lloves J, Schaumberg DA, et al. Prognosticators for visual outcome in sarcoid uveitis. *Ophthalmology*. 1996;103:1846–1853.
59. Baughman RP, Lower EE. Alternatives to corticosteroids in the treatment of sarcoidosis. *Sarcoidosis Vasc Diffuse Lung Dis*. 1997;14:121–130.
60. Lower EE, Baughman RP. Prolonged use of methotrexate for sarcoidosis. *Arch Intern Med*. 1995;155:846–851.
61. Baughman RP, Costabell U, et al. Treatment of sarcoidosis. *Clin Chest Med*. 2008;29:533–548.
62. Baughman RP, Bradley DA, et al. Infliximab in chronic ocular inflammation. *Int J Clin Pharmacol Ther*. 2005;43:7–11.
63. Baughman RP, Lower EE, et al. Etanercept for refractory ocular sarcoidosis. *Chest*. 2005;128:1062–1947.
64. Ishiguro T, Takayanagi N, et al. Development of sarcoidosis during etanercept therapy. *Intern Med*. 2008;47:1021–1025.
65. Akova YA, Foster CS. Cataract surgery in patients with sarcoidosis-associated uveitis. *Ophthalmology*. 1994;101:473–479.

Chapter 109

Behçet's Disease

David C. Herman

Behçet's disease is a systemic vascular disease that affects many organ systems. Although the first description of the disease is attributed to Hippocrates,[1] the modern description of the disease was provided by the Turkish dermatologist Dr. Hulusi Behçet.[2]

The most common criteria employed for the diagnosis of Behçet's disease are those of the International Study Group for Behçet's Disease (Table 109.1).[3] These criteria require oral ulceration recurring at least three times over a 12-month period, and two of the following associated symptoms: recurrent genital ulceration, anterior or posterior uveitis, skins lesions characteristic of Behçet's disease, and a positive pathergy skin test. Other diagnostic criteria are employed, particularly in Japan,[4] but many of the features of the criteria are shared. It has been long recognized that geographic location plays a factor in Behçet's disease. The highest prevalence of the disease occurs along the 'Silk Route,' which extends from the Orient through the Middle East. Even within this geographic region the prevalence is variable. The prevalence of the disease in Japan has been reported to be 8/100000, whereas the prevalence of the disease in Turkey has been reported as high as 80/100000.[5]

Etiology of Behçet's Disease

Although the etiology of Behçet's disease has not been defined, investigations into its pathogenesis have garnered much information and many speculative mechanisms. Herpes simplex virus (HSV) has been speculated to play a role, and investigations employing polymerase chain reaction (PCR) have identified HSV in the tissues of patients with Behçet's disease.[6] Mycobacterial heat shock proteins have been postulated to play a role, but no definitive pathophysiologic connection has been identified.[7]

A genetic predisposition to Behçet's disease probably exists. HLA-B51, and in particular the HLA-B5101 allele, has been associated with Behçet's disease, but the true nature of this association has not been well defined.[8] It is rare to see more than one member of a family with Behçet's disease, even though a large number of family members are HLA-B51 positive, casting the presence of HLA-B51 alone as a minor factor. *TAP* genes, which encode proteins that regulate the transport of antigens, may play a stronger role in the development of Behçet's disease.[9] Factor V Leiden mutation has been identified as an additional risk factor for the development of vasculo-occlusive retinal disease in patients with Behçet's disease.[10]

Although the factor or factors that incite and sustain the inflammation in Behçet's disease are as yet unknown, there is substantial evidence regarding the increase in immune activity in patients with Behçet's disease. Neutrophil phagocytosis and chemotaxis are increased in patients with Behçet's disease when compared to normal controls.[11] Abnormalities in serum and ocular cytokine levels have also been found in patients with Behçet's disease.[12–14]

Clinical Manifestations of Behçet's's Disease

Although the manifestations of Behçet's disease can affect all organ systems either directly or indirectly, the most common symptoms are mucocutaneous, musculoskeletal, ophthalmological, vascular, and neurological in origin.

Mucocutaneous

Oral aphthae are the most common finding, occurring in as many as 96% of patients. These aphthae are most commonly found on the oral, cheek, and lip mucosa. In general, they can be classified as either minor, major, or herpetiform, based on size and location. Minor aphthae are the most common (Fig. 109.1). These lesions are less than 1 cm in diameter, and are usually multiple and found on the lips and oral mucosa. Although painful, and often inhibiting eating, these lesions most often heal within 15 days without scarring. Major oral aphthae are less frequent and more painful. These lesions are more than 1 cm in diameter, with a gray-white base. These lesions can occur deep within the oropharynx, and heal in 2 to 6 weeks, often with scarring that can affect the function of the oropharynx. Herpetiform lesions are the smallest and least common lesions. They occur in crops of multiple lesions and heal in a short period of time without scarring.[15]

The genital ulcers of Behçet's disease occur in men and women. In men, the most common locations are the scrotum and penis, and in women the vulva and labia are most commonly involved. Lesions may occur within the vagina as well. These lesions begin as papules and pustules that quickly ulcerate into more substantial, more painful lesions. Healing occurs in approximately 3 weeks, and is often accompanied by scarring. Although the mucocutaneous findings may

Table 109.1 Diagnostic criteria for the diagnosis of Behçet's disease

Recurrent oral ulceration	Minor aphthous, major aphthous, or herpetiform ulceration observed by physician or patient, which recurred at least 3 times in one 12-month period
Plus 2 of:	
Recurrent genital ulceration	Aphthous ulceration or scarring, observed by physician or patient
Eye lesions	Anterior uveitis, posterior uveitis, or cells in vitreous on slit lamp examination; or retinal vasculitis observed by ophthalmologist
Skin lesions	Erythema nodosum observed by physician or patient, pseudofolliculitis, or papulopustular lesions; or acneiform nodules observed by physician in postadolescent patients not on corticosteroid treatment
Positive pathergy test	Read by physician at 24–48 hours

Findings applicable only in absence of other clinical explanations.
From International Study Group for Behçet's Disease: Criteria for diagnosis of Behçet's disease, Lancet *335:1078–1080, 1990.*

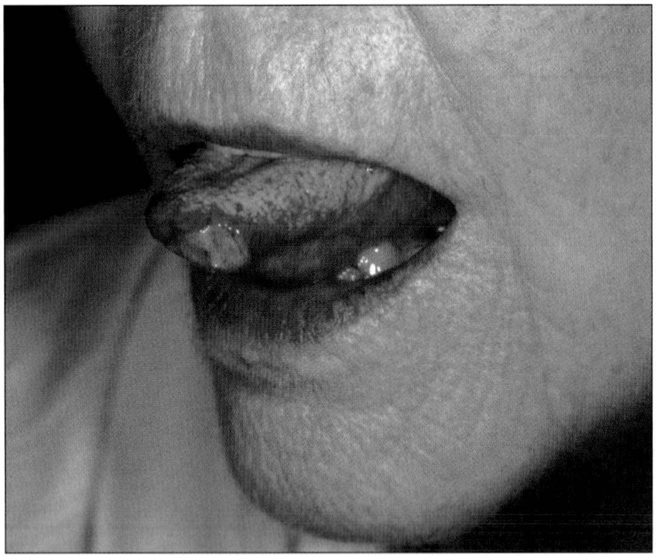

Fig. 109.1 Oral aphthous ulcer on tongue in Behçet's disease.

occur in cycles, with resolution between cycles, one may also encounter lesions in various stages of evolution during the same examination on a patient. A less severe finding than the oral and genital ulcers is a papulopustular skin rash that may occur on multiple areas of the skin at the same time. The back, face, and chest are common areas of occurrence, and the rash can be indistinguishable from acne.

Erythema nodosum, painful, purple-colored nodules usually found on the lower extremities, are another skin finding common in patients with Behçet's disease. These lesions generally occur three to five at a time, although there may be more in some patients with a flare-up of the disease. They are often surrounded by a halo, and resolve as the disease remits, either spontaneously or with treatment.

The pathergy skin reaction is unique to Behçet's disease, and as such has been included in most diagnostic criteria. A positive pathergy skin test is characterized by the appearance of a 1–2-mm cutaneous papule 24 to 48 hours after the skin has been punctured by a needle. There is significant geographic variability in the positivity of this test in patients with Behçet's disease, and regions where the test was often positive have shown a decrease in the incidence of a positive test in patients with Behçet's disease. The decline in positivity of this test has diminished its diagnostic sensitivity for Behçet's disease.[6]

Eye disease

Inflammatory eye disease associated with Behçet's disease affects 60–90% of patients and is the most frequent cause of morbidity and loss of function in these patients. It is most often manifest as a relapsing and remitting panuveitis with destructive features in the anterior and posterior segment of the eye. Ocular inflammation in Behçet's disease is most often bilateral, but can be asymmetric. Retinal vasculitis with vascular occlusions is the direct cause of most visual loss in these patients, and the cumulative destruction of the retina and optic nerve over a span of several years can leave the patient with significant visual disability.[16,17] Although anterior inflammation with hypopyon is considered a hallmark of the disease, limited anterior segment involvement is uncommon, and occurs in only 6–15% of patients. Hypopyon has been reported to occur in 6–30% of patients.

Anterior segment findings include inflammatory cells, keratic precipitates, posterior synechia, peripheral anterior synechia, and cataract. The recurrent nature of the disease, with the accompanying severe bouts of anterior segment inflammation with damage, make glaucoma a common late feature of patients with Behçet's disease. Vascular compromise of the optic nerve from posterior segment inflammation and vasculitis involving the vessels of the optic nerve may make the optic nerve more susceptible to pressure-induced damage, so particular vigilance is warranted in these patients.

An anterior segment finding seen in Behçet's disease is the 'cold hypopyon' (Fig. 109.2), which is characterized by inflammatory cells layered inferiorly in the anterior chamber without the red and painful eye generally associated with hypopyon. The onset of hypopyon may be explosive, and is generally accompanied by posterior segment inflammation. Such explosive exacerbations can significantly decrease visual function within a matter of several hours in some patients.

The posterior aspects of ocular inflammation associated with Behçet's disease are the manifestations most often

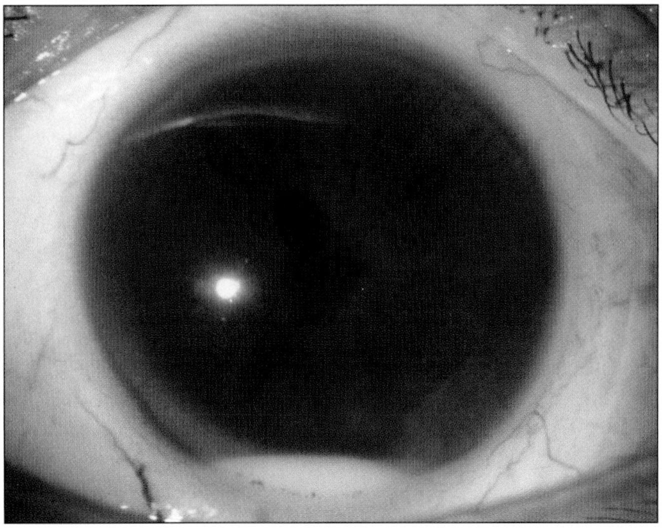

Fig. 109.2 'Cold hypopyon' of Behçet's disease. Note lack of ciliary flush or other signs of inflammation.

associated with loss of visual function. Vitreous cells and haze can appear abruptly and may obscure the view of the retina and choroid. Vasculitis and perivasculitis involving both arteries and veins may cause hemorrhage, and vascular occlusions may lead to infarction of the retina and optic nerve. Optic nerve involvement is not uncommon and may lead to the most rapid and visually devastating loss of vision in patients with Behçet's disease. Inflammation or vascular compromise of the nerve often leads to swelling and a congested appearance of the nerve head on fundus examination (Fig. 109.3). Late findings may show optic nerve atrophy and pallor. Postinflammatory vascular findings include thread-like arterioles and veins, with completely occluded vessels appearing as white lines within atrophic retina. Chronic or relapsing and remitting macular edema may result in pigment hypertrophy with retinal pigment epithelial clumping in the macula. Most studies involving significant numbers of Behçet's disease patients have shown that the ocular inflammatory findings and sequelae are more common in male patients than in females.[18]

The initial presentation of Behçet's disease as an ophthalmic disease can present a differential diagnostic dilemma. Patients presenting with hypopyon can sometimes be distinguished by other factors. The hypopyon associated with idiopathic or HLA-B27-associated anterior uveitis is most often accompanied by pain, severe conjunctival and ciliary injection, and photophobia. Young patients with juvenile rheumatoid arthritis (JRA)-associated anterior uveitis can manifest hypopyon without pain and redness, but the young age of most of these patients makes Behçet's disease unlikely.[19] A detailed history and brief physical examination focused upon the mucocutaneous manifestations of Behçet's disease can often make the diagnosis in an otherwise undifferentiated patient. Ophthalmologists may be uncomfortable asking for manifestations such as genital ulcers, but such information can be invaluable, and allow for the right diagnosis to be made and correct treatment to be rapidly instigated.

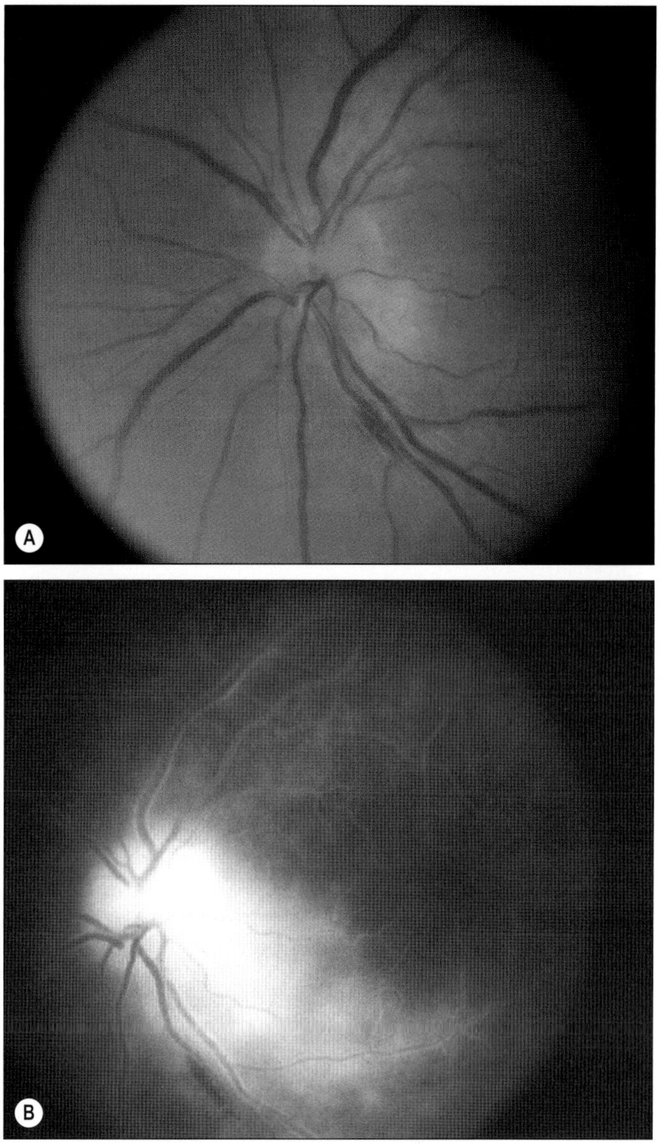

Fig. 109.3 Behçet's disease. (**A**) Fundus photo of retinal and optic nerve inflammation in Behçet's disease. (**B**) Fluorescein angiogram shows diffuse late staining of nerve and surrounding retina, with staining of blood vessel walls.

Posterior segment involvement can present an even greater diagnostic challenge. Detailed examination of the fundus, if the view is allowed through the inflammatory cells in the vitreous, should help determine whether veins, arteries, or both are involved with vasculitic changes. Connective tissue diseases rarely affect both arteries and veins, although this can be seen in systemic lupus erythematosus.[20] Perhaps the most difficult differential diagnosis is that of viral retinitis with acute retinal necrosis. For this, the history is especially important, with focus upon the other manifestations of Behçet's disease, as well as a history of exposure to herpes virus diseases. If acute retinal necrosis is suspected, anterior and posterior chamber taps with PCR for herpes virus should be obtained quickly. Institution of antiviral therapy while waiting for the results of PCR testing has little risk to the patient, and may preserve valuable retina and vision.[21]

Vascular findings

Thrombophlebitis is relatively common in Behçet's disease, and has been reported to occur in more than one-third of patients with the disease. It is most commonly found in the deep veins of the legs, but has been reported in the superior vena cava, the inferior vena cava, dural sinuses, axillary veins, portal vein, and hepatic vein. The risk of embolization is low. The explanation of the low embolic rate has been postulated to be due to the inflammatory nature of the thrombophlebitis, which may increase adhesion of the clot to the vessel wall, making embolism less likely.[22] Patients with Factor V Leiden trait, which is manifest by activated protein C resistance and reduced feedback inhibition of the clotting cascade, have been reported to have higher risk of thrombophlebitis than other patients with Behçet's disease.[23]

Systemic arterial involvement in Behçet's disease is less common than venous, but can be more devastating. Arterial involvement often leads to aneurysm formation and arterial occlusion and may involve the pulmonary arteries, femoral, popliteal, subclavian, and carotid arteries. Behçet's disease is the only known vasculitis that causes pulmonary artery aneurysms. This occurs most commonly in males, and the usual presenting sign is hemoptysis. The risk of mortality is high, particularly if the patient is anticoagulated. For this reason, and because thromboembolism is rare in Behçet's disease, patients with Behçet's disease presenting with hemoptysis should not be anticoagulated and should have bronchoscopy as soon as possible.[24]

Central nervous system

Central nervous system (CNS) manifestations of Behçet's disease are uncommon, occurring in less than 5% of patients in most series,[6] but have been reported in as many as 44% of patients in Saudi Arabia.[25] Computed tomography (CT) and magnetic resonance imaging (MRI) scanning have shown the anatomic findings to be both vascular and parenchymal. Physical findings of CNS disease can be as diverse as the anatomic findings, and include brainstem-related deficits, sphincter problems, and thought disorders. Thought disorders can sometimes occur secondary to high-dose ciclosporin treatment, and distinguishing disease activity from medication side effects can be a challenge in those patients.[26]

Other organ systems can be involved in Behçet's disease. Some patients with Behçet's disease develop a Crohn's-like inflammatory bowel disease that can be difficult to treat. Renal involvement is rare, and shows a nephrotic syndrome picture. Amyloidosis, myositis, and epididymitis can also be present as manifestations of active Behçet's disease.

Treatment of Behçet's Disease

Many medications have been used, with variable effectiveness, to treat Behçet's disease. The types of therapies used have been dependent upon the organ system involved, the severity of the inflammation, and the chronicity of the inflammation. Some medications that have been shown to have short-term efficacy have been found inadequate in controlling the disease long term. The toxicity and low therapeutic index of some medications have limited their long-term use in patients.

Despite the prevalence and morbidity of Behçet's disease, few masked, randomized studies have been performed to evaluate the efficacy of medications used in the treatment of Behçet's disease. There are several factors that explain this. First is the nature of Behçet's disease itself. The relapsing–remitting nature of Behçet's disease makes it difficult to evaluate the response to any particular medication or therapeutic regimen without large numbers of patients over an extended period of time. There also appears to be a regional variability in the response to medications, where some therapies work well in one area of the world, and yet are not adequate in other areas. Indeed, the nature of Behçet's disease itself appears to be changing, with a drift in the primary manifestations of the disease over time.

Azathioprine

Azathioprine, a purine-based antimetabolite, has been shown of significant benefit in the treatment of Behçet's disease in a controlled, randomized study.[27] Patients who received azathioprine 2.5 mg/kg/day showed significantly fewer episodes of inflammation than the control group who received corticosteroids and colchicine only. There was significantly less visual loss in the azathioprine group. This beneficial therapeutic affect also extended to Behçet's disease-related arthritis and genital ulcers. The incidence of thrombophlebitis was also reduced in the azathioprine group. Oral ulcers and papulopustular lesions were not affected. The relatively rare incidence of neurologic disease made it impossible to judge the affect of azathioprine on that particular manifestation of Behçet's disease in this study.

The side effects of azathioprine are primarily hematologic, and close monitoring of these patients is required. Although some patients require a reduction or temporary discontinuation of azathioprine, few patients are required to discontinue the therapy altogether. The long-term side effects of azathioprine, particularly hematologic malignancies, are worrisome although uncommon, and are outweighed by the risks of the disease in patients with life- or sight-threatening Behçet's disease.

Ciclosporin

Ciclosporin (CSA), an interleukin-2 (IL-2) receptor-mediated immunosuppressant, has also been shown to be effective in randomized trials.[17] CSA 5 mg/kg may be the most rapidly acting therapy for an acute attack of uveitis, although antitumor necrosis factor (TNF) medications show promise in this regard. Long-term therapy with CSA has been demonstrated to be more effective in controlling disease than pulsed cyclophosphamide therapy.[28] CSA is often used in conjunction with other immunosuppressives, and the combination may allow each medication to be used below the threshold of its most significant toxicity or adverse side effects.

CSA is nephrotoxic, and renal clearance should be evaluated prior to initiation of therapy. Serum creatinine should be checked at baseline and regularly thereafter to monitor any renal damage. Most acute elevations in serum creatinine are reversible with a decrease in dosage of CSA. Patients should be monitored for hypertension and should be treated aggressively as the renal damage from CSA and hypertension may be synergistic. Nonsteroidal antiinflammatory agents may enhance the nephrotoxic effects of CSA and patients must be warned to avoid these medications while on CSA. The most significant renal damage occurs with doses of CSA at 4 mg/kg/day or higher, and damage may be minimized by using doses less than 3 mg/kg/day.[29]

Corticosteroids

Corticosteroids are useful for acute exacerbations and provide a relatively quick immunosuppressive effect during the sometimes explosive onset of Behçet's uveitis.[17] However, the high doses required and the side effects associated with high-dose corticosteroids make them less useful for long-term therapy. Corticosteroids can be used in conjunction with other immunosuppressive agents, and this is their most beneficial systemic use. Topical corticosteroid therapy for oral or genital ulcers often decreases the discomfort and may hasten the resolution of these ulcers.

Interferon-α

Reported experience has demonstrated a significant reduction in activity of ocular inflammation in nearly 95% of patients treated with interferon-α over a 42-week period. Induction therapy was instituted with 6×10^6 IU three times per week, and then 3×10^6 IU three times per week for maintenance.[30] Side effects limit the usefulness of interferon-α in many patients. Virtually all patients experience aches and fever with administration of the medication, some patients to an intolerable degree. Most disturbingly, the emergence of a Behçet's-like syndrome in patients treated with interferon-α for chronic myeloid leukemia has been reported.[31] Retinopathy has been reported in patients treated with interferon-α for hepatitis as well.[32,33] Lower-dose interferon-α2a has been shown to significantly reduce the relapse rate in patients with Behçet's disease, and appears to be safe and well tolerated over a period of years.[34]

Antitumor necrosis factor medications

Tumor necrosis factor (TNF), an inflammatory cytokine, has been shown to play an active role in the inflammatory cascade of diseases such as rheumatoid arthritis, Crohn's disease, JRA, ankylosing spondylitis, and psoriasis. Anti-TNF medications such as infliximab, a chimeric monoclonal antibody to the TNF receptor, have shown positive results in the treatment of uveitis in several series of Behçet's disease patients.[35–37] Intravenous administration of infliximab has shown a quick and sustained improvement in ocular inflammation in patients who have not responded adequately to conventional therapies.[37] This drug, as well, has its side effects. A lupus-like syndrome develops in some patients, requiring the discontinuation of infliximab.[38] Antibodies to double-stranded DNA have also been noted in some patients.[39] An increased incidence of infection, primarily upper respiratory tract infections, has been observed in patients on anti-TNF medications.[40] Increased incidence of malignancy is always a concern in patients with long-term immunosuppression, but the current short experience with anti-TNF medications precludes a judgment in this area. The development of multiple sclerosis in some patients treated with anti-TNF therapy has raised serious questions regarding its therapeutic index.[41]

Mycophenolate mofetil

Mycophenolate mofetil (MMF) has been used as a standard immunosuppressant after solid organ transplantation, and may be useful in the treatment of ocular inflammation, including that associated with Behçet's disease.[42,43] MMF as an adjunct to CSA or corticosteroids has been shown to decrease ocular inflammation in experimental models and human series.[42,44,45] MMF can be given orally at doses of 1 g b.i.d., and is generally well tolerated. Side effects include gastrointestinal upset and diarrhea, cytomegalovirus (CMV) infection, and *Pneumocystis carinii* pneumonia. Lymphocyte counts must be closely monitored, and patients with combination immunosuppression therapy that includes MMF should be covered for infection with Bactrim SS three times per week or a similar regimen.

Other medications

Colchicine has been used successfully for many years to treat the mucocutaneous manifestations of Behçet's disease. Although colchicine seldom eliminates ulcers, it may reduce them to a more acceptable level, and decrease the severity. There is evidence that colchicine may be more effective in women than in men in reducing the severity of aphthous and genital ulcers, and effective in reducing arthritis and erythema nodosum in both males and females.[46] Evidence for the successful treatment of Behçet's uveitis with colchicine is questionable at best, and it should not be considered an adequate therapy.

Thalidomide may be useful in the treatment of mucocutaneous disease not responsive to colchicine.[47] However, the side effects of this medication severely limit its usefulness. The teratogenic effects of thalidomide are well known, and thus it should not be used in any patient with child-bearing potential. Peripheral neuropathy is common with long-term use. The sedating effect of thalidomide also limits its usefulness, and many patients find that they can tolerate it only when taken at bedtime.

Surgical Therapy in Behçet's Disease

Intraocular surgery in any patient with chronic inflammation requires careful consideration before surgery is attempted. In general, significant visual disability is the most common reason for surgical intervention. Mild visual disability due to cataract or other media opacity is not considered sufficient reason for intervention due to the risks of severe postoperative inflammation and subsequent visual loss from inflammatory sequelae.

Behçet's patients considered for surgery should be treated with systemic therapy to obtain an eye that is free of inflammation before surgery. Increases in medication may be considered before surgery to prevent an explosive increase in inflammation during the immediate postoperative period. Extracapsular cataract extraction or phacoemulsification removal of a cataract has been shown to have similar satisfactory results.[48,49] The same studies have shown that intraocular lens implantation can be safely accomplished in these patients, although vision may be limited by posterior disease, including vascular occlusions and chronic macular edema.[50] Vitreoretinal surgery can also be safely accomplished in these patients, with an increase in visual function without an increase in the frequency or severity of inflammation.[51]

Summary

Behçet's disease is a multisystem disease with significant ocular manifestations that can lead to profound loss of visual function. Proper care of these patients requires knowledge of the disease and a multispecialty approach to medical care. New medications have the potential to change the course and prognosis of a disease that has been recognized for centuries.

References

1. Feigenbaum A. Description of Behçet's syndrome in the Hippocratic third book of endemic diseases. *Br J Ophthalmol.* 1956;40:355–357.
2. Behçet H. Über rezidivierende Aphthose, durch ein Virus verursachte Geshwüre am Munde, am Auge und an den Genitalien. *Dermatol Wochenschr.* 1937;105:1152–1157.
3. International Study Group for Behçet's Disease. Criteria for diagnosis of Behçet's disease. *Lancet.* 1990;335:1078–1080.
4. Behçet's Disease Research Committee of Japan. Behçet's disease: guide to diagnosis of Behçet's disease. *Jpn J Ophthalmol.* 1974;18:291–294.
5. Saylan T, et al. Behçet's disease in the Middle East. *Clin Dermatol.* 1999;17:209–223.
6. Studd M, et al. Detection of HSV-1 DNA in patients with Behçet's syndrome and in patients with recurrent oral ulcers by the polymerase chain reaction. *J Med Microbiol.* 1991;34:39–43.
7. Pervin K, et al. T cell epitope expression of mycobacterial and homologous human 65-kilodalton heat shock protein peptides in short term cell lines from patients with Behçet's disease. *J Immunol.* 1993;151: 2273–2282.
8. Mizuki N, et al. Behçet's disease associated with one of the HLA-B51 subantigens, HLA-B* 5101. *Am J Ophthalmol.* 1993;116:406–409.
9. Gonzalez-Escribano MF, et al. TAP polymorphism in patients with Behçet's disease. *Ann Rheum Dis.* 1995;54:386–388.
10. Verity DH, et al. Factor V Leiden mutation in association with ocular involvement in Behçet's disease. *Am J Ophthalmol.* 1999;128:352–356.
11. Takeno M, et al. Excessive function of peripheral blood neutrophils from patients with Behçet's disease and from HLA-B51 transgenic mice. *Arthritis Rheum.* 1995;38:426–433.
12. BenEzra D, et al. Blood serum interleukin-1 receptor antagonist in pars planitis and ocular Behçet's disease. *Am J Ophthalmol.* 1997;123: 593–598.
13. BenEzra D, et al. Serum levels of interleukin-2 receptor in ocular Behçet's disease. *Am J Ophthalmol.* 1993;115:26–30.
14. Turan B, et al. Systemic levels of the T cell regulatory cytokines IL-10 and IL-12 in Behçet's disease; soluble TNFR-75 as a biological marker of disease activity. *J Rheumatol.* 1997;24:128–132.
15. Main DM, Chamberlain MA. Clinical differentiation of oral ulceration in Behçet's disease. *Br J Rheumatol.* 1992;31:767–770.
16. Nussenblatt RB. Uveitis in Behçet's disease. *Int Rev Immunol.* 1997; 14:67–79.
17. Kaçmaz RO, et al. Ocular inflammation in Beçhet disease: incidence of ocular complications and loss of visual acuity. *Am J Ophthalmol.* 2008;146:828–836.
18. Yazici H, et al. Influence of age of onset and patient's sex on the prevalence and severity of manifestations of Behçet's syndrome. *Ann Rheum Dis.* 1984;43:783–789.
19. Kesen MR, et al. Uveitis associated with pediatric Behçet disease in the American Midwest. *Am J Ophthalmol.* 2008;146:819–827.
20. Jabs DA, et al. Severe retinal vaso-occlusive disease in systemic lupus erythematosus. *Arch Ophthalmol.* 1986;104:558–563.
21. BenEzra D. Clinical aspects and diagnostic guidelines of ocular Behçet's disease. *Dev Ophthalmol.* 1999;31:109–117.
22. Sagdic K, et al. Venous lesions in Behçet's disease. *Eur J Vasc Endovasc Surg.* 1996;11:437–440.
23. Gul A, et al. Coagulation factor V gene mutation increases the risk of venous thrombosis in Behçet's disease. *Br J Rheumatol.* 1996;35: 1178–1180.
24. Pickering MC, Haskard DO. Behçet's syndrome. *J R Coll Phys Lond.* 2000;34:169–177.
25. Stigsby B, et al. Evoked potential findings in Behçet's disease. Brain-stem auditory, visual, and somatosensory evoked potentials in 44 patients. *Electroencephalogr Clin Neurophysiol.* 1994;92:273–281.
26. Kato Y, et al. Central nervous system symptoms in a population of Behçet's disease patients with refractory uveitis treated with cyclosporin A. *Clin Exp Ophthalmol.* 2001;29:335–336.
27. Yazici H, et al. A controlled trial of azathioprine in Behçet's syndrome. *N Engl J Med.* 1990;322:281–285.
28. Ozyazgan Y, et al. Low dose cyclosporin A versus pulsed cyclophosphamide in Behçet's syndrome: a single masked trial. *Br J Ophthalmol.* 1992;76:241–243.
29. Bagnis CI, et al. Long-term renal effects of low dose cyclosporin in uveitis-treated patients: follow-up study. *J Am Soc Nephrol.* 2002;13: 2962–2968.
30. Feron EJ, et al. Interferon-alpha 2b for refractory ocular Behçet's disease. *Lancet.* 1994;343:1428.
31. Budak-Alpdogan T, et al. Skin hyperreactivity of Behçet's patients (pathergy reaction) is also positive in interferon alpha-treated chronic myeloid leukaemia patients, indicating similarly altered neutrophil functions in both disorders. *Br J Rheumatol.* 1998;37:1148–1151.
32. Kawano T, et al. Retinal complications during interferon therapy for chronic hepatitis C. *Am J Gastroenterol.* 1996;91:309–313.
33. Schulman JA, et al. Posterior segment complications in patients with hepatitis C treated with interferon and ribvirin. *Ophthalmology.* 2003; 110:437–442.
34. Gueudry J, et al. Long-term efficacy and safety of low-dose interferon alpha 2a therapy in severe uveitis associated with Behçet disease. *Am J Ophthalmol.* 2008;146:837–844.
35. Sfikakis PP, et al. Effect of infliximab on sight-threatening panuveitis in Behçet's disease. *Lancet.* 2001;358:295–296.
36. Muñoz-Fernandez S, et al. Effect of infliximab on threatening panuveitis in Behçet's disease. *Lancet.* 2001;358:1644–2001.
37. Tabbara KF, et al. Infliximab effects compared to conventional therapy in the management of retinal vasculitis in Behçet disease. *Am J Ophthalmol.* 2008;146:845–850.
38. Feldmann M, et al. Anti-tumor necrosis factor-alpha therapy of rheumatoid arthritis. *Adv Immunol.* 1997;64:283–350.
39. Charles PJ, et al. Assessment of antibodies to double-stranded DNA induced in rheumatoid arthritis patients following treatment with infliximab, a monoclonal antibody to tumor necrosis factor alpha: findings in open-label and randomized placebo-controlled trials. *Arthritis Rheum.* 2000;43:2383–2390.
40. Maini R, et al. Infliximab (chimeric anti-tumour necrosis factor alpha monoclonal antibody) versus placebo in rheumatoid arthritis patients receiving concomitant methotrexate: a randomised phase III trial. ATTRACT Study Group. *Lancet.* 1999;354:1932–1939.
41. Sicotte NL, Voskuhl RR. Onset of multiple sclerosis associated with anti-TNF therapy. *Neurology.* 2001;57:1885–1888.
42. Kilmartin DJ, et al. Rescue therapy with mycophenolate mofetil in refractory uveitis. *Lancet.* 1998;352:35–36.
43. Larkin G, Lightman S. Mycophenolate mofetil. A useful immunosuppressive in inflammatory eye disease. *Ophthalmology.* 1999;106:370–374.
44. Chanaud NP 3rd, et al. Inhibition of experimental autoimmune uveoretinitis by mycophenolate mofetil, an inhibitor of purine metabolism. *Exp Eye Res.* 1995;61:429–434.
45. Teoh SC, et al. Mycophenolate mofetil for the treatment of uveitis. *Am J Ophthalmol.* 2008;146:752–760.
46. Yurdakul S, et al. A double blind study of colchicine in Behçet's syndrome. *Arthritis Rheum.* 1998;41(Suppl):S356.

47. Hamuryudan V, et al. Thalidomide in the treatment of the mucocutaneous lesions of the Behçet's syndrome. A randomized, double-blind, placebo-controlled trial. *Ann Intern Med.* 1998;128:443–450.
48. Kadayifcilar S, et al. Cataract surgery in patients with Behçet's disease. *J Cataract Refract Surg.* 2002;28:316–320.
49. Matsuo T, et al. Ocular attacks after phacoemulsification and intraocular lens implantation in patients with Behçet's disease. *Ophthalmologica.* 2001;215:179–182.
50. Sullu Y, et al. The results of cataract extraction and intraocular lens implantation in patients with Behçet's disease. *Acta Ophthalmol Scand.* 2000;78:680–683.
51. Özertürk Y, et al. Vitreoretinal surgery in Behçet's disease with severe ocular complications. *Acta Ophthalmol Scand.* 2001;79:192–196.

Chapter 110

Fuchs' Heterochromic Iridocyclitis

Debra A. Goldstein, Andrea D. Birnbaum, Howard H. Tessler

Fuchs' heterochromic iridocyclitis (FHI) is a form of chronic iridocyclitis with rather distinctive features. Its characteristic features include (1) unilaterality, (2) characteristic keratic precipitates, (3) iris heterochromia, (4) lack of synechiae, (5) early-onset cataract, (6) vitreous cells and strands, and (7) lack of fundus pathology, although not all findings must be present to make the diagnosis.

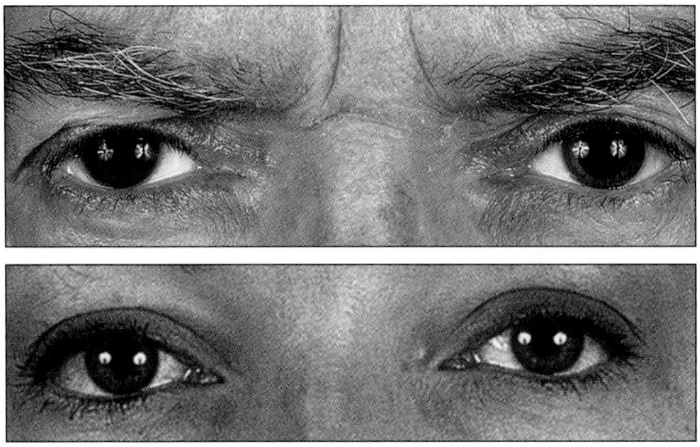

Fig. 110.1 *Top*, Heterochromic iridocyclitis in a brown-eyed patient. The left eye is involved, with lighter iris color. *Bottom*, Heterochromic iridocyclitis in a blue-eyed patient. The right eye is involved, with darker iris color.

Clinical Features

Fuchs' heterochromic iridocyclitis is usually unilateral, although 7–15% of cases are bilateral.[1] It accounts for approximately 2% of uveitis cases.[2] Unlike other forms of iridocyclitis, FHI almost never causes pain, redness, or photophobia. During the early stage, patients with FHI are typically asymptomatic. The diagnosis may be made on routine examination, or when the patient seeks medical attention because of decreased vision due to cataract.

As its name implies, FHI is typically characterized by the color difference between the irides. However, iris heterochromia is not present in all patients. Gross inspection with diffuse white lighting, preferably sunlight, is the most sensitive method of observing subtle heterochromia. On slit lamp examination, subtle iris atrophy may be seen in the involved eye, with loss of anterior stromal details and loss of iris crypts. The amount of iris heterochromia varies considerably and is usually more obvious in Caucasian patients than in African-American or Asian patients. Heterochromia may not be obvious in bilateral cases in which the degree of iris change is similar. Generally speaking, the iris color of the involved eye is darker (more blue) in blue-eyed patients, whereas in brown-eyed patients, the iris color is lighter in the involved eye (Fig. 110.1). In patients with gray eyes, the involved eye may appear more green. The change of iris color in FHI is due to atrophy of the iris stroma.[3] On occasion, rubeosis iridis, inflammatory nodules (Koeppe and Busacca nodules), and iris crystals also may be present.[3–5] Anterior and posterior iris synechiae are rarely seen in FHI.

The most characteristic corneal sign of FHI is the appearance of keratic precipitates (KP), which are white in color and small to medium-sized. The KP tend to be stellate in shape and interconnected by fine fibrin bridges (Fig. 110.2). They are present to a level above the midline of the cornea in almost all cases and are usually evenly scattered over the entire corneal endothelium. This finding is in contradistinc-

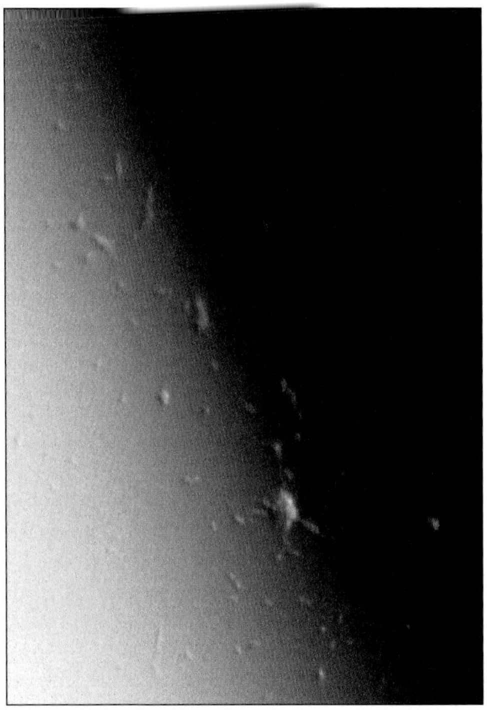

Fig. 110.2 Keratic precipitates in an eye with heterochromic iridocyclitis.

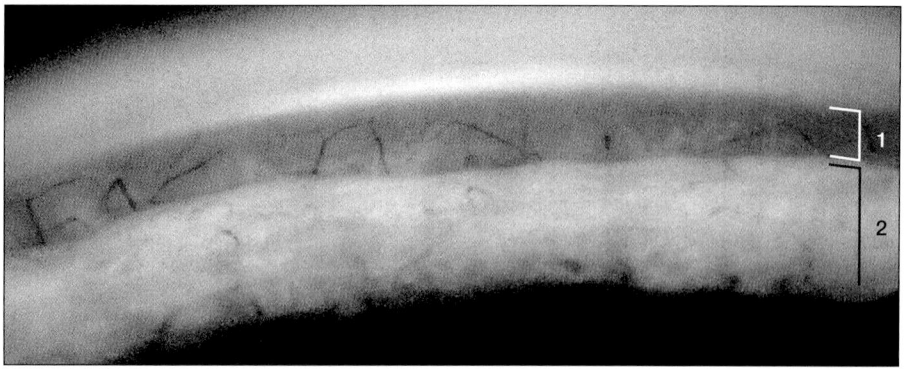

Fig. 110.3 Fine blood vessels course over the trabecular meshwork (*1*) and iris (*2*) in an eye with Fuchs' iridocyclitis. A paracentesis characteristically produces bleeding from these vessels.

tion to most other types of chronic anterior uveitis in which KP concentrate inferiorly.

The anterior chamber usually has a mild to moderate inflammatory reaction, with 1+ to 2+ cells. Fine blood vessels may be seen bridging the angle on gonioscopy (Fig. 110.3). There is a 15–30% incidence of glaucoma and a 75% incidence of posterior subcapsular cataract (Fig. 110.4).[6,7] The glaucoma may be difficult to treat medically, and often requires surgical management.[8]

Anterior vitreous strands or cells (or both) also must be present to make the diagnosis of FHI, which is a form of iridocyclitis, with cells emanating into the vitreous from the ciliary body. Classically, these patients do not develop cystoid macular edema or fundus pathology.

Pathology

The histopathologic features of FHI are similar to those seen in other types of chronic iridocyclitis.[9] Iris stromal atrophy and infiltration of the iris stroma and ciliary body with lymphocytes and plasma cells are the most common features.[10] Russell bodies, which lead to iris crystals clinically, also may be present.[4]

The cause of FHI is unknown, although an association between FHI and infection with the rubella virus has been suggested by several studies. Elevated intraocular titers against rubella virus have been found in patients with FHI, and many FHI patients also have evidence of virus genome in their aqueous fluid.[11,12] Rubella virus-associated uveitis, confirmed by the presence of elevated intraocular antibody production against rubella virus and/or polymerase chain reaction (PCR), presents with many clinical similarities to FHI when compared to idiopathic chronic anterior uveitis.[13] An overall decrease in the incidence of FHI in the United States has been demonstrated in patients targeted by the rubella vaccination program, providing epidemiological support for the rubella association.[14] Additional causes of FHI cannot be excluded, however, and the condition has been associated with other infectious agents, including herpes simples virus and toxoplasmosis. Herpes simplex virus DNA has been identified in the aqueous of a few patients with FHI but not others.[15,16] Focal peripheral chorioretinal scars have been reported in eyes with FHI. In most reports, these lesions are characterized as resembling

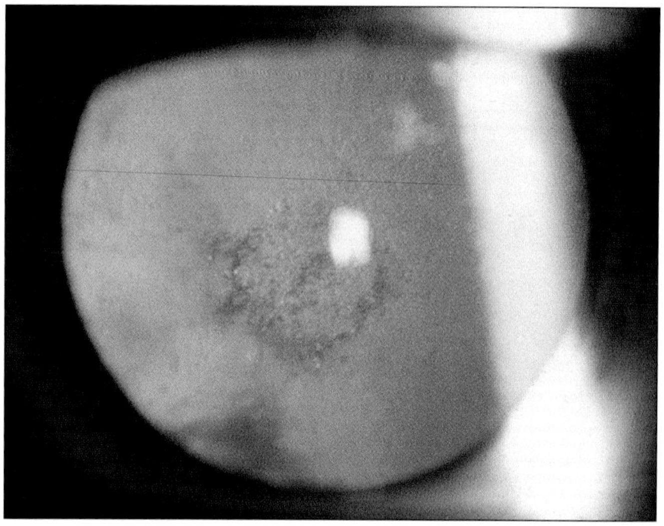

Fig. 110.4 Posterior subcapsular cataract in an eye with heterochromic iridocyclitis as seen in retroillumination.

the fundus lesions seen in ocular toxoplasmosis.[17,18] Interestingly, chorioretinal scars also have been reported in the uninvolved eye in cases of unilateral FHI.[18,19] In some cases, chorioretinal lesions also have resembled those seen in presumed ocular histoplasmosis syndrome.[17] It has been theorized that ocular toxoplasmosis leads to sensitization of the host immune system to retinal antigens (e.g. S-antigen), which later leads to the development of FHI.[20,21] However, autoimmunity to retinal S-antigen has also been reported in patients with FHI without retinal lesions.[20,21] Currently, the exact linkage between ocular toxoplasmosis and FHI is unknown and controversial. FHI may represent a clinical phenotype, with more than one possible etiology.

Differential Diagnosis

Fuchs' heterochromic iridocyclitis is frequently underdiagnosed and overtreated. It may be confused with other forms of chronic iridocyclitis. In both FHI and other forms of chronic iridocyclitis, cells and flare are present in the anterior chamber. In 80–90% of cases of FHI, however, only one eye is involved, whereas other types of chronic iridocyclitis are usually bilateral. As noted previously, the KP in FHI are generally small to medium-sized with stellate outlines and fine interconnecting filaments (i.e. fibrin bridges). In contrast, KP in other forms of chronic iridocyclitis may vary from small to large and usually have rounded contours. In FHI, the distribution of KP is typically throughout the whole cornea, whereas the KP in other types of chronic iridocyclitis are more concentrated inferiorly. One exception to this rule is herpes iritis, where the KP may also be small, stellate, and evenly distributed through the cornea. Herpetic iritis is also often associated with a high intraocular pressure (IOP). Features suggesting the diagnosis of herpes rather than FHI include evidence of corneal stromal disease, ipsilateral pupillary dilation,[22] and iris posterior pigment epithelial atrophy with transillumination defects. Iris transillumination is not characteristic of FHI, since the atrophy tends to involve the anterior stroma.

In the evaluation of heterochromia, causes other than FHI should be considered. In FHI, heterochromia results from stromal atrophy, whereas stromal atrophy is usually not present in other forms of heterochromia. In congenital Horner's syndrome, the involved eye is lighter and the difference usually present from birth, rather than acquired, as in FHI. Meiosis and mild ptosis also may be present. In Waardenburg's syndrome, heterochromia may be present, along with deafness and a white forelock. In Hirschsprung's disease, two distinctive colors (i.e. blue and brown) may be present on the same iris, and the term iris bicolor has been coined to describe this condition.[23] It has been theorized that the variation in iris color in Waardenburg's syndrome and Hirschsprung's disease is due to abnormal migration of neural crest cells. In ocular melanosis, the involved eye is typically darker along with ipsilateral increased pigmentation of the sclera. Darker pigmentation of ipsilateral lids also may be present. Diffuse iris melanoma also may present as heterochromia with the involved eye being darker. Ocular siderosis caused by retained iron foreign body also may darken the iris of the involved eye. In the majority of these conditions, KP and anterior chamber inflammation are absent. However, anterior chamber inflammatory cells may be present in ocular siderosis, and melanoma cells may be present in the anterior chamber of patients with iris melanoma.

Posner-Schlossman syndrome (glaucomatocyclitic crisis) may mimic FHI, as unilateral elevation of intraocular pressure associated with mild anterior chamber reaction may occur in both. The onset of Posner-Schlossman syndrome, however, is acute and symptomatic, whereas the onset of FHI is insidious. Also, the pupil is frequently somewhat dilated during an attack of Posner-Schlossman, whereas in FHI the pupil remains normal. Although a few fine KP may be seen in Posner-Schlossman syndrome, the diffuse stellate KP throughout the cornea of FHI are not seen. In contradistinction to FHI, the eye appears normal between attacks in Posner-Schlossman syndrome, although mild iris stromal hypochromia can occur after multiple attacks. It is important to distinguish these two entities because topical corticosteroids may be effective in lowering intraocular pressure in Posner-Schlossman syndrome, but are ineffective in lowering intraocular pressure in FHI.

Treatment

It is important to separate FHI from other types of chronic iridocyclitis because it is usually unnecessary to treat the inflammation in an eye with FHI. The inflammation of FHI is usually mild and asymptomatic and rarely results in anterior or posterior synechiae or cystoid macular edema. It is actually inadvisable to routinely treat FHI eyes with mild inflammation with topical corticosteroids, as the drops may worsen the glaucoma and hasten the development of cataract.

Since the prevalence of glaucoma in FHI is at least 15%,[10,24] intraocular pressure should be measured at least yearly, and the optic nerve assessed for glaucomatous changes. Approximately 75% of FHI eyes with glaucoma fail maximal medical therapy, and require surgical management with augmented trabeculectomy or tube shunt.[8]

Cataracts in eyes with FHI can be managed successfully with phacoemulsification and implantation of a posterior chamber intraocular lens (IOL). We prefer in the bag to sulcus placement of the IOL. The use of anterior chamber lenses is strongly discouraged in eyes with FHI as in any other eyes with chronic iridocyclitis. In contrast to other types of chronic iridocyclitis, the postoperative course in FHI does not involve severe inflammation, and perioperative oral steroids are usually not required. After cataract surgery, eyes with FHI generally show only mild to moderate anterior chamber reaction that can usually be treated successfully with topical steroids. Postoperative cycloplegia is generally unnecessary because posterior synechiae are rarely encountered in FHI.[25] Hyphema may develop intraoperatively or immediately postoperatively in up to 15–30% of cases. This likely occurs because of the abnormal angle vessels (Amsler sign), and almost always resolves spontaneously.[26,27]

Prognosis

The prognosis of FHI is generally excellent. It is important to make the diagnosis of FHI and avoid unnecessary steroid therapy. Patients should be reassured that the condition is usually unilateral with excellent prognosis for vision. They should also be counseled, however, regarding the need for follow-up because of the high incidence of glaucoma.

References

1. Nussenblatt RB, Palestine AG. *Uveitis: fundamentals and clinical practice.* St Louis: Mosby; 1989.
2. Yaldo MK, Lieberman MF. The management of secondary glaucoma in the uveitis patient. *Ophthalmol Clin North Am.* 1993;6:147–157.
3. Liesegang TJ. Clinical features and prognosis in Fuchs' uveitis syndrome. *Arch Ophthalmol.* 1982;100:1622–1626.
4. Goldstein DA, Edward DP, Tessler HH. Iris crystals in Fuchs' heterochromic iridocyclitis. *Arch Ophthalmol.* 1998;116:1692–1693.
5. Rothova A, La Hey E, Baarsma GS, Breebaart AC. Iris nodules in Fuchs' heterochromic uveitis. *Am J Ophthalmol.* 1994;118:338–342.
6. Tabbut BR, Tessler HH, Williams D. Fuchs' heterochromic iridocyclitis in blacks. *Arch Ophthalmol.* 1988;106:1688–1690.
7. Velilla S, Dios E, Herreras JM, Calonge M. Fuchs' heterochromic iridocyclitis: a review of 26 cases. *Ocul Immunol Inflamm.* 2001;9:169–175.
8. La Hey E, de Vries J, Langerhorst CT, et al. Treatment and prognosis of secondary glaucoma in Fuchs' heterochromic iridocyclitis. *Am J Ophthalmol.* 1993;116:327–340.

9. Goldberg MF, Erozan YS, Duke JR, Frost JK. Cytopathologic and histopathologic aspects of Fuchs' heterochromic iridocyclitis. *Arch Ophthalmol.* 1965;74:604–609.
10. Loewenfeld IE, Thompson HS. Fuchs' heterochromic cyclitis: a critical review of the literature: I. Clinical characteristics of the syndrome. *Surv Ophthalmol.* 1973;17:394–457.
11. Quentin CD, Reiber H. Fuchs heterochromic cyclitis: rubella virus antibodies and genome in aqueous humor. *Am J Ophthalmol.* 2004;138:46–54.
12. De Groot-Mijnes JD, de Visser L, Rothova A, et al. Rubella virus is associated with Fuchs heterochromic iridocyclitis. *Am J Ophthalmol.* 2006;141:212–214.
13. De Visser L, Braakenburg A, Rothova A, de Boer JH. Rubella virus-associated uveitis: clinical manifestations and visual prognosis. *Am J Ophthalmol.* 2008;146:292–297.
14. Birnbaum AD, Tessler HH, Schultz KL, et al. Epidemiologic relationship between Fuchs heterochromic iridocyclitis and the United States rubella vaccination program. *Am J Ophthalmol.* 2007;144:424–428.
15. Mitchel SM, Phylactou L, Fox JD, et al. The detection of herpes viral DNA in aqueous fluid samples from patients with Fuchs' heterochromic cyclitis. *Ocular Immonol Inflamm.* 1996;4:33–38.
16. Barequet IS, Li Q, Wang Y, et al. Herpes simplex virus DNA identification from aqueous fluids in Fuchs' heterochromic iridocyclitis. *Am J Ophthalmol.* 2000;129:672–673.
17. Arffa RC, Schlaegel TF Jr. Chorioretinal scars in Fuchs' heterochromic iridocyclitis. *Arch Ophthalmol.* 1984;102:1153–1155.
18. De Abreu MT, Belfort R Jr, Hirata PS. Fuchs' heterochromic cyclitis and ocular toxoplasmosis. *Am J Ophthalmol.* 1982;93:739–744.
19. Norrsell K, Sjödell L. Fuchs' heterochromic uveitis: a longitudinal clinical study. *Acta Ophthalmol.* 2008;86:58–64.
20. Jones NP. Fuchs' heterochromic uveitis: an update. *Surv Ophthalmol.* 1993;37:253–272.
21. La Hey E, Broersma L, van der Gaag R, et al. Does autoimmunity to S-antigen play a role in Fuchs' heterochromic cyclitis? *Br J Ophthalmol.* 1993;77:436–439.
22. Goldstein DA, Mis AA, Oh FS, Deschenes JG. Persistent pupillary dilation in herpes simplex uveitis. *Can J Ophthalmol.* 2009;44:314–316.
23. Liang JC, Juarez CP, Goldberg MF. Bilateral bicolored irides with Hirschsprung's disease. A neural crest syndrome. *Arch Ophthalmol.* 1983;101:69–73.
24. O'Connor GR. Heterochromic iridocyclitis. *Trans Ophthalmol Soc UK.* 1985;104:219–231.
25. Tejwani S, Murthys, Sangwan VS. Cataract extraction outcomes in patients with Fuchs's heterochromic iridocyclitis. *J Cataract Refract Surg.* 2006;32:1678–1682.
26. Budak K, Akova YA, Yalvac I, et al. Cataract surgery in patients with Fuchs' heterochromic iridocyclitis. *Jap J Ophthalmol.* 1999;43:308–311.
27. Ram J, Kaushik S, Brar GS, et al. Phacoemulsification in patients with Fuchs' heterochromic iridocyclitis. *J Cataract Refract Surg.* 2002;28:1372–1378.

Chapter 111

Juvenile Idiopathic Arthritis

Joseph Tauber

More than 100 illnesses affecting children are associated with arthritis or musculoskeletal complaints.[1] *Juvenile arthritis*, defined as objective synovitis lasting 6 or more weeks before the age of 16, is a generic term for several heterogeneous diseases which fall into two broad groups, differentiated by clinical features, laboratory findings, and long-term course. First are the human leukocyte antigen (HLA)-B27-associated spondyloarthropathies, including juvenile spondylitis, juvenile psoriatic arthritis, juvenile Reiter's syndrome, and juvenile bowel-associated arthritis.[2–5] The second group, which includes any child whose arthritis is of unknown etiology and persists for longer than 3 months, has been traditionally termed *juvenile rheumatoid arthritis* (JRA), and encompasses three subgroups (pauciarticular, polyarticular, and systemic) differentiated by clinical features evident during the first 3 to 6 months after onset.[1,6–9]

Although traditional teaching is that JRA is clinically and genetically unique from adult rheumatoid arthritis, long-term clinical follow up and recent immunogenetic findings have blurred the distinction between some subgroups of JRA and certain adult rheumatic diseases.[10,11] No single clinical finding or laboratory test is diagnostic of JRA, although radiographic findings, HLA associations, and certain laboratory findings (antinuclear antibodies [ANA] and rheumatoid factor [RF]) support suggestive clinical features. Diagnostic criteria for JRA published by the American Rheumatism Association are widely used in the United States (Box 111.1),[12] although European classification systems differ.[13]

Multiple classification schemes for the pediatric arthropathies have been published. Early classification schemes by Brewer et al.[12,14] used the term JRA, while the European League Against Rheumatism (EULAR) popularized the term *juvenile chronic arthritis* (JCA). Both have been superseded by the 2004 ILAR classification,[15] which recommends the term *juvenile idiopathic arthritis* (JIA).

Box 111.1 Diagnostic criteria for the classification of juvenile rheumatoid arthritis

1. Age of onset <16 years
2. Arthritis in one or more joints, defined as swelling or effusion, or by the presence of two or more of the following signs:
   a. Limitation of range of motion
   b. Tenderness or pain on motion
   c. Increased heat
3. Duration of disease of 6 weeks to 3 months
4. Type of onset of disease during the first 4 to 6 months classified as:
   a. Polyarthritis – five joints or more
   b. Oligoarthritis – four joints or less
   c. Systemic disease – intermittent fever, rheumatoid rash, arthritis, visceral disease (hepatosplenomegaly, lymphadenopathy, etc.)
5. Exclusion of other rheumatic diseases

Epidemiology

Five percent of all rheumatic disease in the United States occur during childhood.[4] Estimates of the prevalence of JIA in the United States have ranged from 60000 to 250000 cases, representing 40–50% of all children in the United States with rheumatic conditions.[1,16] Annual disease incidence has been estimated between 0.09 to 1.13 per thousand.[17,18] JIA affects children of all races and ages, females more than males,[1,4,6] but significant demographic differences are seen between subgroups. The peak age at onset of JIA is 2 to 4 years.

Clinical Features

Children with JIA are classified into subgroups based on clinical features noted during the initial 3 to 6 months after the onset of symptoms or the recognition of characteristic signs (Table 111.1). Pauciarticular onset (involving up to four joints) is seen in 40–50% of JIA patients.[1,4–6] Most often, only one or two joints are affected, especially the knee, followed by ankle or elbow.[1,4,19] Subsequent polyarticular involvement is seen in 32–50% of patients ('extending pauciarticular'),[6,10,20] but classification as pauciarticular is based on the initial findings. Pauciarticular JIA patients are usually classified into two types.[1,6–8,10,11,21] Type I is composed mainly of girls, with peak age at onset between 1 and 3 years. This group has mild arthritis and is typically ANA positive and RF negative. Type II patients are mostly older boys (bimodal age peaks at 2 and 9 years) with spondyloarthropathy. More than 50% of type II patients are HLA-B27 positive and ANA and RF negative.[1]

Table 111.1 Juvenile idiopathic arthritis – features of clinical subgroups

	Pauciarticular	Polyarticular	Systemic
Percentage of all JIA	40–50%	40–50%	10–20%
Peak age at onset	<4	Females 1–3, males 2–9	<5
Female : male ratio	3–4 : 1	2–3 : 1	1 : 1
Number of joints involved	Four or less	Five or more	Variable
Systemic features	Up to 12%	Up to 30%	100%
Incidence of uveitis	20–50%	10%	Rare
ANA positivity	75–90%	25–40% (75% of RF+, 10% of RF–)	<10%
RF positivity	<10%	20%	<10%
ELISA RF positivity	71%	85%	60%
Synovitis 10-year remission rate	60%	50%	55%
Severe chronic arthritis	Uncommon	55% seropositive 15% seronegative	25%

ANA, antinuclear antibody; RF, rheumatoid factor; ELISA, enzyme-linked immunosorbent assay.

JIA may be described as a progression from joint inflammation to joint contracture to joint damage and ultimately to alteration or change in overall body growth. Clinical findings include joint pain, swelling, warmth, effusion, and decreased range of motion. Morning 'gelling' and stiffness after periods of inactivity are common. It must be remembered that young children often do not complain of pain even in the presence of severe inflammation.[22,23] Radiographic findings include soft tissue swelling, juxta-articular osteoporosis or erosions, periosteal new bone formation, and expansion of the growth plates.[4,6,24,25] With the exception of ocular involvement, extra-articular findings are unusual in the pauciarticular-onset subgroup.[20] Iridocyclitis occurs in 20–50% of these patients and is often the major source of morbidity.[4,6,20] Laboratory evaluation reveals a positive ANA in 75% or more of pauciarticular JIA patients, especially type I, and RF in 10%, especially type II.[4,19]

A polyarticular onset is seen in 40–50% of patients with JIA, affecting children of all ages, girls twice as often as boys.[1,4,6] Resembling the presentation of adult rheumatoid arthritis, synovitis commonly involves the small joints of the hands and feet, but may involve larger joints including knees, ankles, elbows, wrists, or the cervical spine. Systemic features including fever, lymphadenopathy, hepatosplenomegaly, myositis, pulmonary fibrosis, pericarditis, and vasculitis are reported in 11% of patients.[20] Iridocyclitis occurs in 7–14% of this JIA subgroup.[5] Laboratory findings include elevated sedimentation rate and normochromic, normocytic anemia. Twenty-five percent to 40% of patients will be ANA positive.[1,4] In one study, girls were more than twice as likely as boys to be ANA positive (58% vs 24%).[26] Fifteen percent to 20% of patients will be RF positive, generally boys older than 8 years. These patients have a worse prognosis; 50% of seropositive patients develop destructive arthritis compared with 10–15% of seronegative polyarticular-onset patients.[2] Seropositive, late-onset, polyarticular patients are thought to have childhood-onset rheumatoid arthritis, sharing HLA associations and clinical features with their adult counterparts.[4,10,11]

Systemic onset occurs in approximately 10–20% of cases of JIA affecting boys and girls equally, usually by age 5 years.[1,4,6,10] Resembling Still's disease seen in adults, this presentation may be difficult to differentiate from nonrheumatic systemic disorders, including bacterial or viral infections such as acute rheumatic fever and bacterial septicemia. Synovitis may be absent, pauciarticular, or may evolve into polyarthritis.[1,4,6,10] Other features include weight loss, intermittent fever as high as 104°F, lymphadenopathy, and hepatosplenomegaly. A red to salmon-colored macular rash may appear transiently over the trunk and proximal extremities during febrile episodes. Pericarditis, pleuritis, hepatic, cerebral, and hematologic involvement have been reported.[1,4,6,10] Iridocyclitis is rare in these patients.[4,10,19,20,27] The systemic features are generally self-limited.[6,19] Laboratory findings include elevated sedimentation rate, leukocytosis or leukemoid reaction, and negative screening for antinuclear antibodies (ANA) or IgM rheumatoid factor.[1]

Ocular Clinical Features

Ocular involvement, usually anterior uveitis, is reported in 10–20% of all JIA patients and in 75% of pauciarticular patients.[1,5,20,26,27] Uveitis develops by age 2 years in 53% and by age 7 years in 90%, after the onset of arthritis in 94% of patients, usually within 1 to 2 years, and within 7 years in 90%.[20,25] Though it is generally believed that uveitis rarely presents longer than 7 years following arthritis, onset over a decade later has been reported.[26] Also, uveitis may precede the onset of arthritis in 6–24% of patients.[29] Among patients with JIA uveitis, 88–96% of cases occur in pauciarticular and 7–14% in polyarticular patients. Girls are affected three to four times as often as boys.[5,20,27,29] Uveitis patients are more likely to be ANA positive (71–93%) than patients without uveitis (30%).[5] The level of ANA titer is unrelated to severity of ocular involvement as is the severity of arthritis.[5]

JIA patients usually come for ophthalmic evaluation by referral for screening from the primary care physician or because of a failed school vision examination. Fewer patients are noted to have an injected eye, irregular pupil shape or anisocoria, band keratopathy or leukocoria. Usually asymptomatic,[5,17,19,29] with symptoms reported by only 20–24% of patients,[27] uveitis is bilateral in 70–90% of patients.[5,17,30,31] In unilateral presentations, the second eye is usually involved within several months and rarely after 1 year.[32] Nongranulomatous iridocyclitis is the most common finding, although endothelial glazing, keratic precipitates, and Koeppe nodules may be seen.[5] Twenty percent to 25% of patients have iridocyclitis that is relatively easy to bring under control, 20–25% have chronic, unremitting ocular inflammation, and the remaining 50–60% have a course of recurrent inflammation.[5,17] Posterior segment manifestations are less common, but may include cyclitic membranes, vitritis, macular cysts, holes, edema, and tractional retinal detachments.[33]

Uncontrolled, chronic inflammation leads to ocular complications. Band keratopathy is seen in up to 30% of patients,[27] beginning as paralimbal, calcific deposits at the 3 and 9 o'clock meridians within Bowman's membrane (Fig. 111.1), and later progressing in a bandlike pattern over the visual axis, limiting visualization of intraocular structures.[17] Posterior synechiae are noted at onset in 35% of patients and ultimately are present in 55%.[27] Cataract occurs in 28–46% and glaucoma in 14–27% of patients.[27,32] Glaucoma is often multifactorial, with elements of angle closure by peripheral anterior synechia, trabeculitis, steroid response, and, less often, ciliary effusion or angle neovascularization.[34]

The risk of ocular complications is related most importantly to the severity of involvement at presentation. Patients with severe ocular involvement at first examination (presence of posterior synechiae) are more likely to develop band keratopathy (77% vs 5%), cataract (81% vs 28%), glaucoma (47% vs 17%), phthisis (13% vs 0%) and visual loss (58% vs 35%) than patients with mild ocular involvement.[27] However, one published study showed that 12 of 29 patients with ocular complications had only mild disease at onset.[35] Treatment with systemic corticosteroids also increases the likelihood of ocular complications. In one study that analyzed groups treated with high-dose, low-dose, or no steroids, cataract developed in 100%, 22%, and 13%, respectively, and glaucoma developed in 40% of high-dose and 13% of low-dose patients.[27]

A poor visual outcome (<20/200) occurs in 67% of patients in whom uveitis is diagnosed before arthritis.[27] The presence of glaucoma carries an especially poor prognosis, with 35% of affected eyes losing light perception.[5] The highest risk for poor visual outcome is in young, female, pauciarticular-onset, ANA-positive, RF-negative, patients in whom uveitis is diagnosed before arthritis and who have posterior synechiae at the first ophthalmic examination.[29,36]

Etiology

Despite tremendous advances in our understanding of immunogenetic associations, cellular immune system involvement, and the role of autoantibodies, the pathophysiology of JIA remains speculative. Limited histopathologic studies of ocular tissues in JIA have been published, as only highly diseased eyes with advanced stages of involvement have become available for analysis. Inflammatory infiltrates have been noted in the iris and ciliary body, consisting mainly of plasma cells and scattered giant cells.[38,39] Available information suggests an autoimmune mechanism, but the

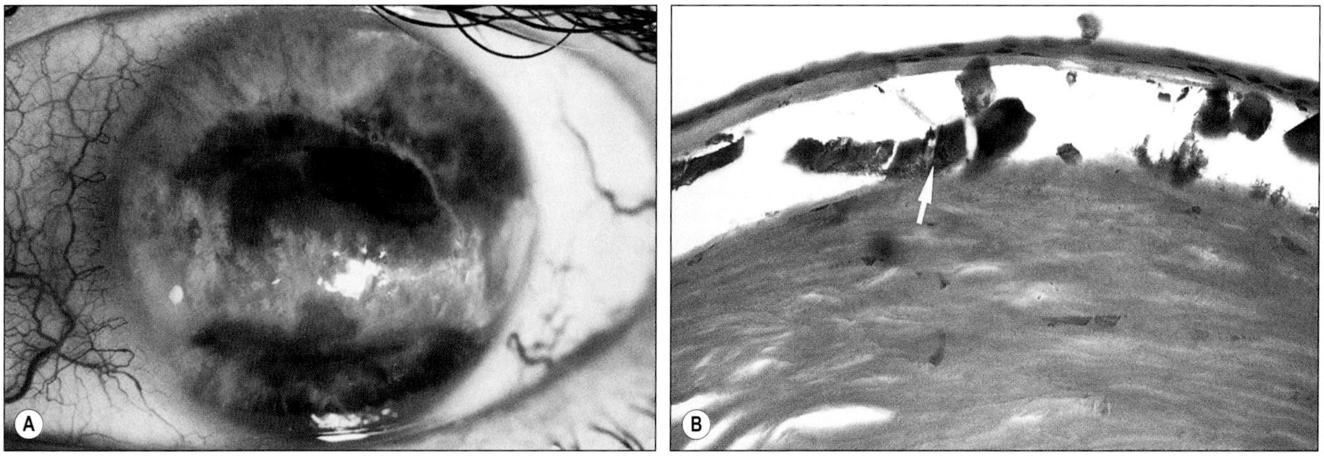

Fig. 111.1 Ocular clinical features. (**A**) Band keratopathy in a young female with advanced JRA uveitis. (**B**) Calcium is deposited within Bowman's membrane.

'trigger' and even the effector mechanism are unknown. Several studies suggest the 'trimolecular complex' (an arthritogenic peptide, HLA molecule, and a T-cell receptor) is central in the pathogenesis of JIA,[2,3] while others point to the macrophage.[40] A full discussion of these concepts is beyond the scope of this chapter.[2,38,41,42,51]

HLA associations differ among JIA subgroups. Alleles from three different regions, HLA-A2, HLA-DR5/DR8, and DPB1*0201, carry independent risk for the development of early-onset, pauciarticular JIA,[2,4,11,37,42–44] and some specific HLA loci carry risk for the development of uveitis.[4,43,45] Polyarticular-onset patients are more likely to have HLA-DR4, especially the Dw4 and Dw14 subtypes.[4] These markers are also present in adult rheumatoid arthritis (RA) patients, supporting the concept that some children with later-onset polyarticular disease, especially those who are seropositive, have childhood-onset RA. HLA-DR5 is associated with uveitis in children with pauciarticular JIA.

Studies of abnormalities in cellular immunity in JIA have been inconsistent.[43,46] Findings of increased activated T cells in JIA synovial fluid but not in serum suggest that 'locally' inappropriate T-cell activity could be pathogenic.[43] A mild increase in numbers of CD5+ B cells, thought to produce autoantibodies, also has been shown in JIA patients.[43,47,48] Numerous autoantibodies have been demonstrated in JIA patients, including antinuclear, antihistone, antiocular, anticardiolipin, anticollagen, anti-T cell, rheumatoid factor, and 'hidden' rheumatoid factors,[49] but their pathogenic significance is unknown. Hidden rheumatoid factors are IgM antibodies directed against IgG molecules, to which they are normally bound in vivo, preventing their detection by usual methods. Enzyme-linked immunosorbent assay (ELISA) methods can detect such antibodies in 85% of polyarticular, 71% of pauciarticular, and 60% of systemic-onset JIA patients.[49,50]

Finally, the potential role of infectious agents such as antigenic triggers for autoimmune processes in JIA has been investigated, especially rubella, parvovirus, and Epstein-Barr virus.[3,10,43,50] Although infection has been reported to precede flare-ups in JIA patients, clear evidence of a causal role for any microorganism is tenuous.

Treatment of Systemic Disease

Detailed reviews of treatment of the rheumatologic aspects of JIA have been published.[6,52–58] Optimal care of the JIA patient (and family) incorporates a multidisciplinary team effort, including the primary care physician (pediatrician or family physician) and the pediatric rheumatologist, the ophthalmologist, physiatrist, orthopedist, nurses, occupational therapists, physical therapists, social workers, and psychologists.

Pharmacologic treatment of JIA has historically followed a stepladder approach,[6,52–59] although there is a definite trend toward earlier institution of immunomodulating drugs.[25,57,60] Initial treatment is usually aspirin administered at 80–120 mg/kg per day, to achieve a serum salicylate level of 20–30 mg/100 mL.[1,6,54,61] If inflammation is not controlled within 4 to 6 months, nonsteroidal antiinflammatory drugs (NSAIDs) will be successful in about 50% of patients[46,53–55,57,68] after 1 or several months. For children younger than 14 years, only tolmetin, naproxen, ibuprofen, and fenoprofen have been approved by the Food and Drug Administration; for older children, any available NSAID may be prescribed.[46,53–55]

Although many JIA patients can be successfully managed with this first level of treatment, inflammation may persist in others. Slow-acting, disease-modifying antirheumatic drugs (DMARDs), which are reported to reduce the rate of bone loss, include hydroxychloroquine, *d*-penicillamine, and sulfasalazine.[63] Although some reports are encouraging, other studies suggest the efficacy of these agents may not be much greater than placebo. Mixed results also have been reported for gold therapy in JIA. Intramuscular administration of gold may be effective in 50–75% of cases,[59,62,68,69] but anecdotal reports suggest oral administration is less effective.[70,71] One multicenter, double-blind study of 231 patients reported improvement in disease indices of 66% with oral gold therapy compared to 56% for placebo.[62] The mechanism by which administration of gold relieves inflammation in JIA is unknown, although some have reported inhibited migration of inflammatory cells and suppression of lysosomal enzymes.[59]

Although corticosteroids are effective in controlling inflammation, their long-term use and tolerability are limited by numerous and serious side effects, including hypertension, diabetes, weight gain, myopathy, and, especially in children, growth retardation and osteoporosis.[52–54,59] Systemic administration of corticosteroids is appropriate during the time required for DMARDs to reach therapeutic levels or in such extreme situations as total failure or intolerance of aspirin and NSAIDs or severe pericarditis.[1,52] Newer corticosteroids such as deflazacort have been shown to retain antiinflammatory efficacy while showing a sparing effect on bone mineralization.[72–75] Rarely, intravenous pulse methylprednisolone may be used for life-threatening complications.[54,76] Intra-articular administration of corticosteroid has become popular as a safe and effective therapeutic modality, especially for pauciarticular disease.[52,77–79]

Immunomodulating and immunosuppressive drugs have been used in JIA for many years, despite limited published controlled studies. Multiple mechanisms of action, both antiinflammatory and immunosuppressive, have been suggested[54] to explain the efficacy of methotrexate in rheumatoid arthritis affecting adults and children,[54,72,81–85] but concerns about toxicity with long-term use have limited its use in children.[54,59,72] Nonetheless, in recent years, a consensus favoring weekly low-dose methotrexate therapy (0.3–0.5 mg/kg/week, typically 7.5–12.5 mg/week for a 25-kg child) for refractory cases is emerging,[80,86,87] influenced at least in part by a large, international, controlled clinical trial.[88] Anecdotal reports suggest substantial toxicity and only limited efficacy for ciclosporin A at doses evaluated.[89] Case reports of the successful use of azathioprine, chlorambucil, and cyclophosphamide in JIA have been published,[54,72] but most agree that the potential toxicity and mutagenicity of these agents are serious enough to limit their use to the rare JIA patient.[3–5,54] Intravenous gammaglobulin administration has also been reported effective in anecdotal cases.[90] The therapeutic role of biologic agents is increasing.[91,92]

Treatment of Ocular Disease

Topical corticosteroids are the mainstay of treatment for uveitis in JIA.[19] It is important to follow the principle of treating anterior chamber cell and not flare, as chronic flare may persist indefinitely. Topical application may be indicated as frequently as every hour or as infrequently as every other day, according to the degree of inflammation present. No prospective, controlled studies have compared specific dosing regimens. However, one review found that 25% of patients had uveitis easily controlled with topical corticosteroids, 50% had a prolonged course, and 25% had a complicated course.[28,29] In one study, 41% of children required 6 months or longer to control uveitis.[93] Although, according to traditional teaching, it is often impossible to totally eliminate anterior chamber cell, recent reports have emphasized the importance of complete eradication of inflammation.[31,94] Oral administration of corticosteroids is rarely successful in cases of inadequate response to topical corticosteroids, but periocular injections of depot preparations such as triamcinolone hexacetonide may be highly effective without the side effects of systemic administration.[93] General anesthesia may be necessary to safely administer these injections in young patients. There is clearly a role for oral NSAIDs as adjunctive treatment facilitating reduction in corticosteroid doses in JIA uveitis.[95] There is also an important place for short-acting mydriatics (1% tropicamide) for the prevention and/or treatment of posterior synechia formation.

Despite the use of corticosteroids and NSAIDs, 20–25% of JIA uveitis patients will have uncontrolled inflammation and ocular complications. The search for steroid-sparing treatment strategies for JIA uveitis has not yielded risk-free alternatives. Anecdotal reports of immunosuppressive treatment in JIA uveitis suggest chlorambucil and methotrexate are valuable in selected cases.[19,27,29,32,96,97] In one study, systemic immunosuppressive therapy was efficacious in six of eight JIA patients with severe, unresponsive ocular inflammation.[32] Although the *potential* side effects of cytotoxic agents must be balanced against the *likely* consequences of systemic corticosteroids, the use of potentially toxic immunosuppressive agents should be limited to persons with experience in their administration, side effects, and appropriate follow-up.

Ocular complications may develop as a result of inadequate control of inflammation or excessive use of corticosteroids as therapy. Band keratopathy is managed with chemical chelation using a 1–2% solution of ethylenediaminetetraacetic acid (EDTA) (0.37 mol) in water or saline, following mechanical removal of the epithelium using a spatula or the edge of a No. 15 blade.

Treatment of glaucoma in JIA includes both medical and surgical approaches.[34] Although miotics should be avoided in patients with uveitis, the use of standard antiglaucoma medications is reported to achieve short-term control of intraocular pressure in 50% and long-term in 30% of patients.[5] Because of the risk of increasing intraocular inflammation, laser trabeculoplasty probably has no significant role. Surgical results are poor, with only 18–50% success rate after trabeculectomy,[5,98] although trabeculodialysis, a variant of a goniotomy procedure, was successful in 18 of 30 (60%) eyes with JIA.[99]

Historically, cataract surgery in uveitis patients has yielded poor results, with only 15–60% of patients reaching 20/40 or better postoperatively. Poor visualization because of band keratopathy or corneal scars; pupillary sclerosis because of synechia formation, iris stromal, and vascular fragility; an increased incidence of glaucoma and sometimes profound postoperative inflammation with glaucoma, pupillary membranes, and hyphema all contribute to intraoperative and postoperative problems in JIA.[94] The results of surgery for cataract in JIA have improved greatly during the last two decades, with postoperative acuity of 20/40 or better achieved in 70–75% of patients.[94,100,101] Reasons include judicious patient selection and proper timing of surgery, an increasing understanding of the importance of complete preoperative control of intraocular inflammation,[5,101] and recognition of the importance of anterior vitrectomy and posterior capsulectomy to remove the scaffold for inflammatory membrane formation postoperatively.[94] Some surgeons advocate phacoemulsification and others pars plana vitrectomy with lensectomy, but intraocular lens implantation is generally contraindicated in JIA.[19,94,102]

Prognosis

Approximately 50% of systemic-onset JIA patients are in remission 5 and 10 years after the onset of disease and 50% have recurrent exacerbations.[10,103] Twenty-five percent of these children develop severe destructive arthritis,[6] the major form of morbidity in this group of patients. Among polyarticular patients, 10–15% of seronegative and 50% of seropositive patients develop severe destructive arthritis, with 10-year remission rates of 60% and 0%, respectively.[6] In pauciarticular patients, early onset is associated with 70% remission and late onset with 55% remission.[103]

According to traditional teaching, 75% of all children with JIA will be inflammation-free as adults,[1] but long-term follow-up data suggest a less optimistic view. A review of multiple studies with follow-up of 10 or more years revealed that persistent arthritis was present in 31–55% of JIA patients and that significant functional limitation affects approximately 31% of patients.[26] Mortality was roughly estimated at 1% for JIA patients, which is increased from 0.08% for normal children between the ages of 1 and 24 years.[25]

In patients with pauciarticular JIA, ocular involvement is typically the major source of morbidity. Twenty percent will have unremitting uveitis,[19] more than 50% will have vision of 20/200 or worse, and 12% will become blind as a result of band keratopathy, cataract, glaucoma, and uveitis.[17,27] One study has shown that although the prevalence of uveitis is lower in ANA-positive patients, the incidence of ocular complications was higher, raising questions about the implications of less frequent screening examinations.[104] Another study demonstrated that, after negative findings on slit lamp examination, in the absence of ocular symptoms, only 1.3% of 76 JIA patients developed uveitis.[105] The serious sequela of ocular involvement has led to numerous recommendations about what is appropriate ophthalmologic screening for JIA patients.[5,44,106] Most recommend annual examinations for systemic-onset patients and biannual examinations for ANA-negative, pauciarticular, or polyarticular children. The highest-risk children – young, ANA-positive, and

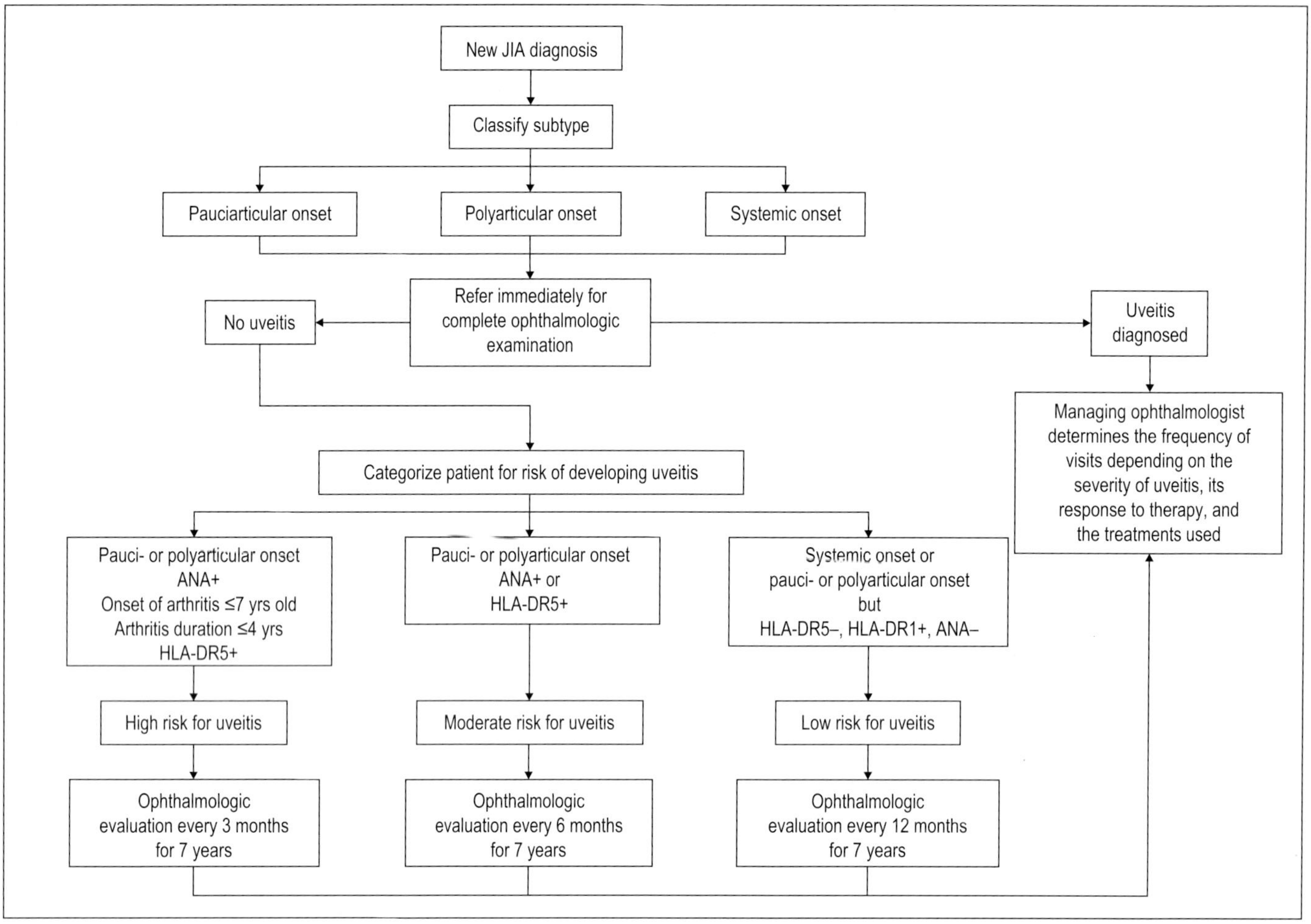

Fig. 111.2 Screening algorithm for JIA patients. Adapted from the Massachusetts Eye and Ear Infirmary website, with permission.

pauciarticular – should be examined every 2 to 3 months. Children diagnosed with JIA who do not develop ocular involvement during the first 7 years may be screened annually, as the risk of uveitis is small.[29] A screening algorithm popularized by the Massachusetts Eye and Ear Infirmary Immunology Service summarizes a useful approach (Fig. 111.2).

Conclusion

Juvenile idiopathic arthritis is among the most devastating of childhood diseases, resulting in lifelong functional disability for many patients. Despite the absence of a diagnostic laboratory test for JIA and a clear understanding of pathogenesis, immunogenetic advances and improved recognition of high-risk patients have allowed for improved outcomes. One encouraging report noted a decreased prevalence of chronic uveitis (45% vs 13%) and a reduced rate of severe visual loss (21% vs 0%) between 1975 and 1989.[107] With 200 000 to 250 000 cases of JIA and 30 000 cases of JIA-associated uveitis in the United States at any given time, this decrease would represent a tremendous reduction of morbidity. More studies are needed to provide a better rationale for choosing between the many available medications for JIA and to understand better the proper place of immunosuppressive therapy in the treatment plan for these children. For now, early recognition of disease and aggressive prevention of ocular complications are primary goals.

References

1. Singsen BH. Pediatric rheumatic diseases. In: Rodnan GP, Schumaker HR, eds. *Primer on the rheumatic diseases*. 9th ed. Atlanta: Arthritis Foundation; 1988:160–164.
2. Weiss JE, Ilowite NT. Juvenile idiopathic arthritis. *Rheum Dis Clin North Am*. 2008;33(3):441–470.
3. Ravelli A, Martini A. Juvenile idiopathic arthritis. *Lancet*. 2007;369(9573):1602.
4. Braun AL, Hoffman RW. Clinical and genetic features of juvenile rheumatoid arthritis. *Mo Med*. 1988;85:799–803.
5. Kanski JJ. Juvenile arthritis and uveitis. *Surv Ophthalmol*. 1990;34:253–267.
6. Borchers AT, Selmi C, Cheema G, et al. Juvenile idiopathic arthritis. *Autoimmune Rev*. 2006;5(4):279–298.
7. Cassidy JT, Petty RE. *Textbook of pediatric rheumatology*. 2nd ed. Philadelphia: WB Saunders; 1990.
8. Jacobs JC. *Pediatric rheumatology for the practitioner*. 2nd ed. New York: Springer Verlag; 1993.
9. Cassiy JT, Petty RE. *Textbook of pediatric rheumatology*. 3rd ed. Philadelphia: WB Saunders; 1994.
10. Allen RC, Ansell BM. Juvenile chronic arthritis – clinical sub-groups with particular relationship to adult patterns of disease. *Postgrad Med J*. 1986;62:821–826.
11. Maksymowych WP, Kerckhove CV, Glass DN. Juvenile rheumatoid arthritis, human leukocyte antigen and other immunoglobulin supergene family polymorphisms. *Am J Med*. 1988;85(Suppl 6A):26–28.
12. Brewer EJ, et al. Current proposed revision of JRA criteria. *Arthritis Rheumatol*. 1977;20:195–199.

13. Prieur AM, et al. Is onset type evaluated during the first 3 months of disease satisfactory for defining the sub-groups of juvenile chronic arthritis? A EULAR cooperative study. *Clin Exp Rheumatol.* 1990;8:321–325.
14. Brewer EJ, et al. Criteria for the classification of juvenile rheumatoid arthritis. *Bull Rheum Dis.* 1973;23:712–719.
15. Duffy CM, et al. Nomenclature and classification in chronic childhood arthritis. *Arthritis Rheum.* 2005;52(2):382–385.
16. Cassidy JT, Nelson AM. The frequency of juvenile arthritis (editorial). *J Rheumatol.* 1988;15:535–536.
17. Rosenberg AM. Uveitis associated with juvenile rheumatoid arthritis. *Semin Arthritis Rheumatol.* 1987;16:158–173.
18. Towner SR, Michet Jr CJ, O'Fallon WM, et al. The epidemiology of juvenile rheumatoid arthritis in Rochester, Minnesota, 1960–1979. *Arthritis Rheum.* 1983;26:1208–1213.
19. OBrien JM, Albert DM. Therapeutic approaches for ophthalmic problems in juvenile rheumatoid arthritis. *Rheum Dis Clin North Am.* 1989;15:413–437.
20. Kanski JJ. Screening for uveitis in juvenile chronic arthritis. *Br J Ophthalmol.* 1989;73:225–228.
21. Ansell BM. Juvenile rheumatoid arthritis, juvenile chronic arthritis and juvenile spondyloarthropathies. *Curr Opin Rheumatol.* 1992;4:706–712.
22. Beales JG, Keen JH, Holt PJL. The child's perception of the disease and the experience of pain in juvenile chronic arthritis. *J Rheumatol.* 1983;10:61–65.
23. Scott PJ, Ansell BM, Huskisson EC. Measurement of pain in juvenile chronic arthritis. *Ann Rheum Dis.* 1977;36:186–187.
24. Reed MH, Wilmot DM. The radiology of juvenile rheumatoid arthritis: a review of the English language literature. *J Rheumatol.* 1991;18(Suppl 31):2–22.
25. Wallace CA, Levinson JE. Juvenile rheumatoid arthritis: outcome and treatment for the 1990s. *Rheum Clin North Am.* 1991;17:891–905.
26. Akduman L, Kaplan HJ, Tychsen L. Prevalence of uveitis in an outpatient juvenile arthritis clinic: onset of uveitis more than a decade after the onset of arthritis. *J Ped Ophthalmol Strabismus.* 1997;34:101–106.
27. Wolf MD, Lichter PR, Ragsdale CG. Prognostic factors in the uveitis of in juvenile rheumatoid arthritis. *Ophthalmology.* 1987;94:1242–1248.
28. Lipton NL, Crawford JS, Greenberg ML. The risk of iridocyclitis in juvenile rheumatoid arthritis. *Can J Ophthalmol.* 1976;11:26–30.
29. Kanski, JJ. Uveitis in juvenile chronic arthritis. *Clin Exp Rheumatol.* 1990;8:499–503.
30. Key SN, Kimura SJ. Iridocyclitis associated with juvenile rheumatoid arthritis. *Am J Ophthalmol.* 1975;80:425–429.
31. Foster CS, Barrett F. Cataract development and cataract surgery in patients with juvenile rheumatoid arthritis-associated iridocyclitis. *Ophthalmology.* 1993;100:809–817.
32. Hemady RK, Baer JC, Foster CS. Immunosuppressive drugs in the management of progressive, corticosteroid-resistant uveitis associated with juvenile rheumatoid arthritis. *Int Ophthalmol Clin.* 1992;32:241–252.
33. Okada AA, Foster CS. Posterior uveitis in the pediatric population. *Int Ophthalmol Clin.* 1992;32:121.
34. Yaldo MK, Lieberman MF. The management of secondary glaucoma in the uveitis patient. *Ophthalmol Clin North Am.* 1993;6:147–157.
35. Edelsten C, Lee V, Bentley CR, et al. An evaluation of baseline risk factors predicting severity in juvenile rheumatoid arthritis associated uveitis and other chronic anterior uveitis in early childhood. *Br J Ophthalmol.* 2002;86:51–56.
36. Dana MR, Merayo Lloves J, Schaumberg DA, et al. Visual outcomes prognosticators in juvenile rheumatoid arthritis associated uveitis. *Ophthalmology.* 1997;104:236–244.
37. Nepom B. The immunogenetics of juvenile rheumatoid arthritis. *Rheum Dis Clin North Am.* 1991;17:825–842.
38. Merriam JC, Chylack LT, Albert DM: Early-onset pauciarticular juvenile rheumatoid arthritis: a histopathologic study. *Arch Ophthalmol.* 1983;101:1085–1092.
39. Sabates R, Smith T, Apple D. Ocular histopathology in juvenile rheumatoid arthritis. *Ann Ophthalmol.* 1979;11:733–737.
40. Behrens EM. Macrophage activation syndrome in rheumatic disease: what is the role of the antigen presenting cell? *Autoimmun Rev.* 2008;7(4):305–308.
41. Bluestone JA, Spencer C, Hirsch R. The T cell receptor in autoimmune disease. *J Rheumatol.* 1992;19:75–77.
42. Maksymowych WP, Glass DN. Population genetics and molecular biology of the childhood chronic arthropathies. *Baillieres Clin Rheumatol.* 1988;2:649–671.
43. Tucker LB. Juvenile rheumatoid arthritis. *Curr Opin Rheumatol.* 1993;5:619–628.
44. Nepom B, Glass D. Juvenile rheumatoid arthritis and HLA: report of the Park City III workshop. *J Rheumatol.* 1992;19:70–74.
45. Prahalad S, Glass DN. A comprehensive review of the genetics of juvenile idiopathic arthritis. *Pediatr Rheumatol Online.* 2008;6:11.
46. Petty RE. Juvenile rheumatoid arthritis and the spondyloarthropathies in children. *Curr Opin Rheumatol.* 1989;1:248–256.
47. Jarvis JN, Kaplan J, Fine N. Increase in CD5+ B cells in juvenile rheumatoid arthritis. *Arthritis Rheum.* 1992;35:204–207.
48. Yoshino K. Immunological aspects of juvenile rheumatoid arthritis. *Acta Paediatr Jpn.* 1993;35:427–438.
49. Lawrence JM, et al. Autoantibody studies in juvenile rheumatoid arthritis. *Semin Arthritis Rheum.* 1993;22:265–274.
50. Moore TL, Dorner RW. Rheumatoid factors. *Clin Biochem.* 1993;26:75–84.
51. Phillips PE. Evidence implicating infectious agents in rheumatoid arthritis and juvenile rheumatoid arthritis. *Clin Exp Rheumatol.* 1988;6:87–94.
52. Prieur AM. The place of corticosteroid therapy in juvenile chronic arthritis in 1992. *J Rheumatol.* 1993;20(Suppl 37):32–34.
53. Silver RM. Nonsteroidal anti-inflammatory drugs in the management of juvenile arthritis. *J Clin Pharmacol.* 1988;28:566–570.
54. Rose CD, Doughty RA. Pharmacological management of juvenile rheumatoid arthritis. *Drugs.* 1992;43:849–863.
55. Hollingsworth P. The use of non-steroidal anti-inflammatory drugs in paediatric rheumatic diseases. *Br J Rheumatol.* 1993;32:73–77.
56. Rooney M. Is there a disease modifying drug for juvenile chronic arthritis? *Br J Rheumatol.* 1992;31:635–641.
57. Levinson J, Wallace C. Dismantling the pyramid. *J Rheumatol.* 1992;19(Suppl 33):6–10.
58. Paulus HE. Antimalarial agents compared with or in combination with other disease-modifying antirheumatic drugs. *Am J Med.* 1988;85(Suppl 4A):45–52.
59. Fink CW. Medical treatment of juvenile arthritis. *Clin Orthop.* 1990;259:60–69.
60. Wilske KR, Healey LA. Challenging the therapeutic pyramid: a new look at treatment strategies for rheumatoid arthritis. *J Rheumatol.* 1990; 17:4–7.
61. Baum J. Aspirin in the treatment of juvenile arthritis. *Am J Med.* 1983;74(6A):10–15.
62. Giannini EH, et al. Auranofin in the treatment of juvenile rheumatoid arthritis. *Arthritis Rheum.* 1990;33:466–476.
63. Brewer EJ, et al. Penicillamine and hydroxychloroquine in the treatment of severe juvenile rheumatoid arthritis. *N Engl J Med.* 1986;314: 1269–1276.
64. Hoyeraal HM. Immunoregulatory drugs in the treatment of juvenile rheumatoid arthritis (JRA). *Scand J Rheumatol.* 1988;76(Suppl): 305–310.
65. Giannini EH, et al. Characteristics of responders and nonresponders to slow-acting antirheumatic drugs in juvenile rheumatoid arthritis. *Arthritis Rheum.* 1989;31:15–20.
66. Van Kerckhove C, Giannini EH, Lovell DJ. Temporal patterns of response to d-penicillamine, hydroxychloroquine and placebo in juvenile rheumatoid arthritis patients. *Arthritis Rheum.* 1988;31: 1252–1258.
67. Kvien TK, Hoyeraal HM, Sandstad B. Slow-acting antirheumatic drugs in patients with juvenile rheumatoid arthritis evaluated in a randomized, parallel 50 week clinical study. *J Rheumatol.* 1985;12: 533–539.
68. Giannini EH, et al. Auranofin therapy for JRA: results of the five year open label extension trial. *J Rheumatol.* 1991;18:1240–1242.
69. Levinson JE, Balz GP, Bondi S. Gold therapy. *Arthritis Rheum.* 1977;20(Suppl):531–535.
70. Marcolongo R, et al. The efficacy and safety of auranofin in the treatment of juvenile rheumatoid arthritis: a long-term open study. *Arthritis Rheum.* 1988;31:979–983.
71. Brewer EJ, Kuzmina N, Giannini EH. Auranofin in juvenile rheumatoid arthritis – results of the USA–USSR double-blind placebo controlled trial (abstract). *Arthritis Rheum.* 1988;31(Suppl):S26.
72. Emery HM. Treatment of juvenile rheumatoid arthritis. *Curr Opin Rheumatol.* 1993;5:629–633.
73. Ferraris J, et al. Effect of therapy with a new glucocorticoid, deflazacort, on linear growth and growth hormone secretion after renal transplantation. *J Pediatr.* 1992;121:809–813.
74. Loftus J, et al. Randomized, double-blind trial of deflazacort versus prednisone in juvenile chronic (or rheumatoid) arthritis: a relative bone-sparing effect of deflazacort. *Pediatrics.* 1991;88:428–436.
75. Vignolo M, et al. Statural growth and skeletal maturation in rheumatic prepubertal children treated with a third generation glucocorticoid (deflazacort) versus prednisone; an interim study. *Clin Exp Rheumatol.* 1991;9:41–45.

76. Bisagni-Faure A, Job-Deslandre C, Menkes C. Intravenous methylprednisolone pulse therapy in Still's disease. *J Rheumatol*. 1992;19:1487–1488.
77. Balogh Z, Ruzsonyi E. Triamcinolone hexacetonide versus betamethasone: a double-blind comparative study of the long-term effects of intra-articular steroids in patients with juvenile rheumatoid arthritis. *Scand J Rheumatol*. 1988;67(Suppl):80–82.
78. Earley A, et al. Triamcinolone into the knee joint in juvenile chronic arthritis. *Clin Exp Rheumatol*. 1988;6:153–155.
79. Sparling M, et al. Radiographic follow-up of joints injected with triamcinolone hexacetonide for the management of childhood arthritis. *Arthritis Rheum*. 1990;33:821–826.
80. Giannini EH, et al. Methotrexate in resistant juvenile rheumatoid arthritis. *N Engl J Med*. 1992;326:1043–1049.
81. Wallace C, et al. Predicting remission in juvenile rheumatoid arthritis with methotrexate treatment. *J Rheumatol*. 1993;20:118–122.
82. Sobrin L, Christen W, Foster CS. Mycophenolate mofetil after methotrexate failure or intolerance in the treatment of scleritis and uveitis. *Ophthalmology*. 2008;115(8):1416–1421.
83. Heiligenhaus A, Mingels A, Heinz C, Ganser G. Methotrexate for uveitis associated with juvenile idiopathic arthritis: value and requirement for additional anti-inflammatory medication. *Eur J Ophthalmol*. 2007;17(5):743–748.
84. Bartoli M, Tara M, Magni-Manzoni S, et al. The magnitude of early response to methotrexate therapy predicts long-term outcome of patients with juvenile idiopathic arthritis. *Ann Rheum Dis*. 2008; 67(3):370–374.
85. Halle F, Prieur AM. Evaluation of methotrexate in the treatment of juvenile chronic arthritis according to the subtype. *Clin Exp Rheumatol*. 1991;9:297–302.
86. Samson CM, Waheed N, Baltatzis S, Foster CS. Methotrexate therapy for chronic non-infectious uveitis; analysis of a case series of 160 patients. *Ophthalmology*. 2001;108:1134–1139.
87. Ramadan A, Nussenblatt R. Cytotoxic agents in ocular inflammation. *Ophthalmol Clin North Am*. 1997;10:377–387.
88. Giannini EH, Brewer EJ Kuzmina N, et al. Methotrexate in resistant juvenile rheumatoid arthritis – results of the USA–USSR double-blind, placebo controlled trial. *N Engl J Med*. 1995;326:1043–1049.
89. Tappeiner C, Roesel M, Heinz C, et al. Limited value of cyclosporine A for the treatment of patients with uveitis associated with juvenile rheumatoid arthritis. *Eye*. 2008;10:1038.
90. Barron K, Sher M, Silverman E. Intravenous immunoglobulin therapy: magic or black magic? *J Rheumatol*. 1992;19:94–97.
91. Furst DE, Breedveld FC, Kalden JR, et al. Updated consensus statement on biological agents for the treatment of rheumatic diseases, 2007. *Ann Rheum Dis*. 2007;66(Suppl 3):iii2–22.
92. Ilowite NT. Update on biologics in juvenile idiopathic arthritis. *Curr Opin Rheumatol*. 2008;20(5):613–618.
93. Chylack LT. The ocular manifestations of juvenile rheumatoid arthritis, *Arthritis Rheum*. 1977;20:217–223.
94. Foster CS, Vitale AT. Cataract surgery in uveitis. *Ophthalmol Clin North Am*. 1993;6:139–146.
95. Olson NY, Lindsley CB, Godfrey WA. Nonsteroidal anti-inflammatory drug therapy in chronic childhood iridocyclitis. *Am J Dis Child*. 1988;142:1289–1292.
96. Godfrey WA, et al. The use of chlorambucil in intractable idiopathic uveitis. *Am J Ophthalmol*. 1974;78:415–428.
97. Miserocchi E, Baltatzis S, Ekong A, et al. Efficacy and safety of chlorambucil in intractable noninfectious uveitis. The Massachusetts Eye and Ear Infirmary experience. *Ophthalmology*. 2002;109:137–142.
98. Beauchamp GR, Parks MM. Filtering surgery in children: barriers to success. *Ophthalmology*. 1979;86:170–180.
99. Kanski J, McAllister JA. Trabeculodialysis for inflammatory glaucoma in children and young adults. *Ophthalmology*. 1985;92:927–929.
100. Flynn HW, Davis JL, Culbertson WW. Pars plana lensectomy and vitrectomy for complicated cataracts in juvenile rheumatoid arthritis. *Ophthalmology*. 1988;95:1114–1119.
101. Smiley WK. The eye in juvenile rheumatoid arthritis. *Trans Ophthalmol Soc UK*. 1974;94:817–829.
102. Hooper PL, Rao NA, Smith RE. Cataract extraction in uveitis patients. *Surv Ophthalmol*. 1990;35:120–144.
103. Ansell BM. Juvenile chronic arthritis. *Scand J Rheumatol*. 1987;66(Suppl):1156.
104. Chalom EC, Goldsmith DP, Koehler MA. Prevalence and outcome of uveitis in a regional cohort of patients with juvenile rheumatoid arthritis. *J Rheumatol*. 1997;24:2031–2034.
105. Oren B, Sehgal A, Simon JW, et al. The prevalence of uveitis in juvenile rheumatoid arthritis. *J AAPOS*. 2001;5:2–4.
106. Section on Rheumatology and Section on Ophthalmology. Guidelines for ophthalmic examinations in children with juvenile rheumatoid arthritis. *Pediatrics*. 1993;92:295–296.
107. Sherry D, Mellins ED, Wedgwood RJ. Decreasing severity of chronic uveitis in children with pauciarticular arthritis. *Am J Dis Child*. 1991;145:1026–1028.

Index

B

D

E

F

G

H

I

J

K

L

M

N

O

P

S

T

U

V

W

X

Y

Z